PRIMARY PEDIATRIC CARE

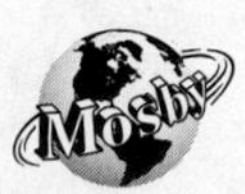

Visit our website at **www.mosby.com**

PRIMARY PEDIATRIC CARE

Editor-in-Chief

ROBERT A. HOEKELMAN, M.D.

Professor and Chairman Emeritus, Department of Pediatrics
University of Rochester, School of Medicine and Dentistry
Rochester, New York

Co-editors

Henry M. Adam, M.D.

Professor of Clinical Pediatrics, Albert Einstein College of Medicine
Director, Pediatric Residency Training Program, Children's Hospital at Montefiore
Bronx, New York

Nicholas M. Nelson, M.D.

Professor Emeritus of Pediatrics
The Pennsylvania State University, The Milton S. Hershey Medical Center
Hershey, Pennsylvania

Michael L. Weitzman, M.D.

Executive Director, American Academy of Pediatrics Center for Child Health Research
Professor and Associate Chairman, Department of Pediatrics
University of Rochester, School of Medicine and Dentistry
Rochester, New York

Modena Hoover Wilson, M.D.

Professor of Pediatrics, The Johns Hopkins University School of Medicine
Baltimore, Maryland
Director, Department of Committees and Sections
American Academy of Pediatrics
Chicago, Illinois

FOURTH EDITION

With 453 illustrations

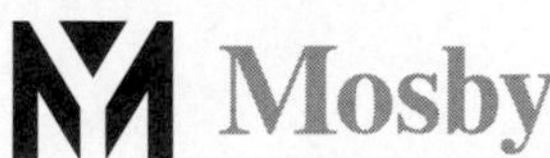

A Harcourt Health Sciences Company

St. Louis London Philadelphia Sydney Toronto

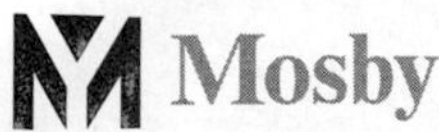

A Harcourt Health Sciences Company

Editor: Elizabeth M. Fathman
Senior Developmental Editor: Ellen Baker Geisel
Project Manager: Patricia Tannian
Project Specialist: Anne Salmo
Book Design Manager: Gail Morey Hudson
Cover Design: Teresa Breckwoldt

FOURTH EDITION

NOTICE

Pharmacology is an ever-changing field. Standard safety precautions must be followed, but as new research and clinical experience broaden our knowledge, changes in treatment and drug therapy may become necessary or appropriate. Readers are advised to check the most current product information provided by the manufacturer of each drug to be administered to verify the recommended dose, the method and duration of administration, and contraindications. It is the responsibility of the licensed prescriber, relying on experience and knowledge of the patient, to determine dosages and the best treatment for each individual patient. Neither the publisher nor the editor assumes any liability for any injury and/or damage to persons or property arising from this publication.

Mosby, Inc.
A Harcourt Health Sciences Company
11830 Westline Industrial Drive
St. Louis, Missouri 63146

Printed in the United States of America

Library of Congress Cataloging in Publication Data

Primary pediatric care / editor-in-chief, Robert A. Hoekelman ; co-editors, Henry M. Adam ... [et al.]. -- 4th ed.
p. ; cm.
Includes bibliographical references and index.
ISBN 0-323-00831-3
1. Pediatrics. I. Hoekelman, Robert A.
[DNLM: 1. Pediatrics. 2. Primary Health Care. WS 100 P9526 2000]
RJ45 .P673 2000
618.92—dc21

00-033917

00 01 02 03 04 GW/MVY 9 8 7 6 5 4 3 2 1

Contributors

ALICE D. ACKERMAN, M.D.
Associate Professor of Pediatrics and Head
Division of Pediatric Critical Care Medicine
University of Maryland School of Medicine
Medical Director, PICU, Pediatrics
Critical Care Transport and Respiratory Care
University of Maryland Hospital for Children
Baltimore, Maryland
29: *Fluid Therapy*

HENRY M. ADAM, M.D.
Professor of Clinical Pediatrics, Albert Einstein College of Medicine
Children's Hospital at Montefiore, Bronx, New York
25: *Management of Fever*

GERALD R. ADAMS, Ph.D.
Professor, Department of Family Relations and Applied Nutrition
University of Guelph, Guelph, Ontario, Canada
109: *Runaway Youth*

ELIZABETH MELLER ALDERMAN, M.D.
Associate Professor of Clinical Pediatrics, Department of Pediatrics
Albert Einstein College of Medicine
Division of Adolescent Medicine
Children's Hospital at Montefiore, Bronx, New York
58: *Child Custody*

CHLOE G. ALEXSON, M.D.
Professor of Pediatrics, University of Rochester School of Medicine
Attending Physician
Children's Hospital at Strong, Rochester, New York
142: *Heart Murmurs*

C. ANDREW ALIGNE, M.D.
Assistant Professor of General Pediatrics, University of Rochester
School of Medicine and Dentistry, Department of Pediatrics
Rochester General Hospital, Rochester, New York
23 (5): *Prevention of Smoking*

JOEL M. ANDRES, M.D.
Chief, Pediatric Gastroenterology
Department of Pediatrics, Arnold Palmer Children's Hospital
Nemours Children's Clinic, Orlando, Florida
152: *Jaundice*

JOHN S. ANDREWS, M.D.
Assistant Professor, Director of Medical Student Education
Johns Hopkins Children's Center, Baltimore, Maryland
245: *Otitis Media and Otitis Externa*
263: *Sinusitis*

TRINA MENDEN ANGLIN, M.D.
Office of Adolescent Health
Maternal and Child Health Bureau, Rockville, Maryland
112: *Violent and Aggressive Behavior*

SUSAN S. ARONSON, M.D.
Clinical Professor of Pediatrics
The Children's Hospital of Philadelphia
University of Pennsylvania, Philadelphia, Pennsylvania
60: *Child Care and Early Education Programs*

BARBARA L. ASSELIN, M.D.
Associate Professor of Pediatrics and Oncology
Department of Pediatrics and The Cancer Center
University of Rochester School of Medicine and Dentistry
Attending Physician, Children's Hospital at Strong
Rochester, New York
232: *Leukemias*

PETER A.M. AULD, M.D.
Director, Pediatrics and Neonatology
Cornell University Medical College
Professor of Pediatrics and Obstetrics
Department of Pediatrics and Neonatology
The New York Presbyterian Hospital, New York, New York
44: *Sequelae to Infertility*

JEFFREY R. AVNER, M.D.
Associate Professor of Pediatrics
Albert Einstein College of Medicine
Director, Pediatric Emergency Service
Department of Pediatrics, Children's Hospital at Montefiore
Bronx, New York
139: *Gastrointestinal Hemorrhage*

JULIE A. BABISH, M.S.W.
Graduate Student, Social Work
Strong Center for Developmental Disabilities
Department of Pediatrics, University of Rochester
School of Medicine and Dentistry, Rochester, New York
11: *Communication with Parents and Patients*

EMILY R. BAKER, M.D.
Assistant Professor
Department of Obstetrics and Gynecology and Radiology
Dartmouth Medical School
Director, Maternal-Fetal Medicine
Department of Obstetrics and Gynecology
Dartmouth-Hitchcock Medical Center, Lebanon, New Hampshire
42: *The Fetus at Risk*

NANCY K. BARNETT, M.D.
Formerly Associate Professor of Pediatrics
The Johns Hopkins University School of Medicine,
Baltimore, Maryland
Associate Clinical Professor
Departments of Pediatrics and Dermatology
University of California, San Francisco, San Francisco, California
Medical Director, Pediatric Dermatology
Valley Children's Hospital, Madera, California
115: *Alopecia and Hair Shaft Anomalies*
149: *Hyperhidrosis*
164: *Pruritus*
166: *Rash*
199: *Contact Dermatitis*
227: *Insect Bites and Infestations*

STEPHEN R. BARONE, M.D.
Assistant Professor of Clinical Pediatrics
New York University School of Medicine, New York, New York
Attending Physician, North Shore University Hospital
Manhasset, New York
226: *Infectious Mononucleosis and Other Epstein-Barr Virus Infections*

TODD F. BARRON, M.D.
Associate Professor of Pediatrics
Section Chief of Pediatric Neurology, Department of Pediatrics
The Pennsylvania State University College of Medicine
The Milton S. Hershey Medical Center, Hershey, Pennsylvania
290: *Increased Intracranial Pressure*

JOHN BAUM, M.D.
Professor Emeritus, Departments of Pediatrics and Medicine
University of Rochester School of Medicine and Dentistry
Attending Physician, Children's Hospital at Strong and the
Strong Memorial Hospital, Rochester, New York
153: *Joint Pain*

WILLIAM R. BEARDSLEE, M.D.
Gardner/Monks Professor of Child Psychiatry
Department of Psychiatry, Harvard Medical School
Psychiatrist-in-Chief, Children's Hospital, Boston, Massachusetts
53: *Mental Health of the Young: An Overview*

PETER F. BELAMARICH, M.D.
Associate Professor of Clinical Pediatrics
Albert Einstein College of Medicine
Children's Hospital at Montefiore, Bronx, New York
113: *Abdominal Distention*
121: *Constipation*

MARK F. BELLINGER, M.D.
Professor of Surgery (Urology), University of Pittsburgh
Chief, Pediatric Urology, Children's Hospital of Pittsburgh
Pittsburgh, Pennsylvania
169: *Scrotal Swelling*
234: *Meatal Ulceration*

ROBERT J. BERKOWITZ, D.D.S.
Professor and Chief, Division of Pediatric Dentistry
Eastman Department of Dentistry
University of Rochester School of Medicine and Dentistry
Clinical Service Chief, Department of Pediatric Dentistry
Children's Hospital at Strong, Rochester, New York
23 (1): *Prevention of Dental Caries*

CHESTON M. BERLIN, Jr., M.D.
University Professor of Pediatrics, Professor of Pharmacology
The Pennsylvania State University College of Medicine
Head, Section of General Pediatrics, Hershey Medical Center
Hershey, Pennsylvania
224: *Iatrogenic Disease*
282: *Drug Overdose*

ROBERT J. BIDWELL, M.D.
Associate Professor of Pediatrics
John A. Burns School of Medicine, University of Hawaii
Director of Adolescent Medicine, Department of Pediatrics
Kapiolani Medical Center for Women and Children
Honolulu, Hawaii
104: *Homosexuality: Challenges of Treating Lesbian and Gay Adolescents*

GLENN H. BOCK, M.D.
Clinical Professor of Pediatrics
Georgetown University School of Medicine, Washington, D.C.
Medical Director
Pediatric Kidney Center
Inova Fairfax Hospital for Children, Falls Church, Virginia
213: *Hemolytic-Uremic Syndrome*
215: *Henoch-Schönlein Purpura*
273: *Urinary Tract Infections*
288: *Hypertensive Emergencies*
295: *Renal Failure*

WILLIAM E. BOYLE, Jr., M.D.
Professor of Pediatrics and Community and Family Medicine
Dartmouth Medical School, Hanover, New Hampshire
Attending Physician, Department of Pediatrics
Dartmouth-Hitchcock Medical Center, Lebanon, New Hampshire
7: *The Pediatric History*

NANCY E. BRAVERMAN, M.D.
Assistant Professor, Institute of Genetic Medicine
Johns Hopkins Medical Center, Baltimore, Maryland
20 (3): *Recognition of Genetic-Metabolic Diseases by Clinical Diagnosis and Screening*

T. BERRY BRAZELTON, M.D.
Professor Emeritus, Department of Pediatrics
Harvard Medical School, Children's Hospital
Boston, Massachusetts
78: *Developmental Approach to Behavioral Problems*

DAVID A. BRENT, M.D.
Academic Chief, Child and Adolescent Psychiatry
Professor of Psychiatry, Pediatrics, and Epidemiology
University of Pittsburgh School of Medicine
Western Psychiatric Institute & Clinic, Pittsburgh, Pennsylvania
107: *Mood Disorders in Children and Adolescents*
108: *Suicide and Suicidal Behavior in Children and Adolescents*

DAVID I. BROMBERG, M.D.
Associate Professor of Pediatrics
University of Maryland Medical System, Baltimore, Maryland
79: *Interviewing Children*
84: *Colic*
292: *Pneumothorax and Pneumomediastinum*

JOHN G. BROOKS, M.D.
Professor and Chairman, Department of Pediatrics
Dartmouth Medical School
Hanover, New Hampshire
269: *Sudden Infant Death Syndrome*

MICHAEL G. BURKE, M.D.
Assistant Professor, Department of Pediatrics
The Johns Hopkins University School of Medicine
Chairman, Department of Pediatrics, St. Agnes Hospital
Baltimore, Maryland
132: *Extremity Pain*

MICHAEL T. BUSCH, M.D.
Director of Sports Medicine
Children's Healthcare of Atlanta at Scottish Rite
Atlanta, Georgia
266: *Sports Injuries*

CAROL J. BUZZARD, M.D.
Clinical Assistant Professor of Pediatrics
Division of Pediatric Cardiology
University of Rochester School of Medicine and Dentistry
Director, Pediatric Cardiology Inpatient Service
Department of Pediatrics, Children's Hospital at Strong
Rochester, New York
146: *High Blood Pressure in Infants, Children, and Adolescents*

ROBERT S. BYRD, M.D., M.P.H.
Assistant Professor of Clinical Pediatrics
University of California-Davis Medical Center, Sacramento, California
72: *School Readiness*

DEBORAH E. CAMPBELL, M.D.
Associate Professor, Department of Pediatrics
Albert Einstein College of Medicine
Director, Division of Neonatology, Department of Pediatrics
Children's Hospital at Montefiore, Bronx, New York
20 (7): *Screening for Drugs*

MARY T. CASERTA, M.D.
Assistant Professor of Pediatrics
Division of Pediatric Infectious Diseases
University of Rochester School of Medicine and Dentistry
Attending Physician, Children's Hospital at Strong
Rochester, New York
291: *Meningococcemia*

ROBERT W. CHAMBERLIN, M.D.
Adjunct Professor, Department of Pediatrics
Dartmouth Medical School, Hanover, New Hampshire
5: *Community-Wide Approaches to Promoting the Health and Development of Families and Children*

NANDITA CHAWLA, M.A.
California School of Professional Psychology
San Diego, California
91: *Peer Relationship Problems*

THOMAS CHERIAN, M.D., D.C.H.
Professor of Pediatrics, Department of Child Health
Christian Medical College Hospital, Vellore, Tamilnadu, India
246: *Parasitic Infections*

PATRICIA CHIVERTON, Ed.D., R.N.
Associate Professor of Clinical Nursing
University of Rochester School of Nursing, Rochester, New York
77: *Nursing Roles in School Health*

CYNTHIA CHRISTY, M.D.
Associate Professor of Pediatrics
University of Rochester School of Medicine and Dentistry
Department of Pediatrics, Rochester General Hospital
Rochester, New York
271: *Tuberculosis*

HARVEY J. COHEN, M.D., Ph.D.
Chairman, Department of Pediatrics, Professor of Pediatrics
Stanford University School of Medicine, Stanford, California
117: *Anemia and Pallor*

MICHAEL W. COHEN, M.D.
Clinical Professor of Pediatrics
University of Arizona College of Medicine, Tucson, Arizona
88: *Enuresis*

WILLIAM L. COLEMAN, M.D.
Associate Professor of Pediatrics
Center for Development and Learning
University of North Carolina
University of North Carolina Medical School
Chapel Hill, North Carolina
22: *Family Systems Approach to the Care of Children*

BLAISE L. CONGENI, M.D.
Professor of Pediatrics, Northeastern Ohio College of Medicine
Director, Division of Infectious Disease, Department of Pediatrics
Children's Hospital Medical Center of Akron, Akron, Ohio
31: *Antimicrobial Therapy*

W. CARL COOLEY, M.D.
Associate Professor of Pediatrics
Dartmouth Medical School, Hanover, New Hampshire
Medical Director, Crotched Mountain Rehabilitation Center
Greenfield, New Hampshire
63: *Family-Centered Care in Pediatric Practice*

SUSAN M. COUPEY, M.D.
Professor of Pediatrics, Albert Einstein College of Medicine
Associate Director, Division of Adolescent Medicine
Department of Pediatrics, Children's Hospital at Montefiore
Bronx, New York
103: *Drug, Alcohol, and Tobacco Abuse*
105: *Interviewing Adolescents*
110: *Adolescent Sexuality*

SHARON S. CUMMINGS, M.P.H.
Research Associate
Center for Health Promotion Research and Development
The University of Texas-Houston Health Science Center
School of Public Health, Houston, Texas
71: *School Health Education*

DAVID R. CUNNINGHAM, Ph.D.
Professor and Director
Division of Communicative Disorders, Department of Surgery
University of Louisville School of Medicine, Louisville, Kentucky
20 (10): *Auditory Screening*

JANE A. CURTIS, M.D.
Associate Professor of Clinical Pediatrics
Department of Pediatrics, Albert Einstein College of Medicine
Children's Hospital at Montefiore, Bronx, New York
125: *Dizziness and Vertigo*

JOSEPH R. CUSTER, M.D.
Director, Pediatric Critical Care Medicine
Associate Professor, Department of Pediatrics
University of Michigan, Ann Arbor, Michigan
296: *Shock*
Appendix B: *Special Procedures*

ROBERT A. DARNALL, M.D.
Associate Professor, Department of Pediatrics and Physiology
Dartmouth Medical School
Attending Neonatologist, Department of Pediatrics
Dartmouth-Hitchcock Medical Center, Lebanon, New Hampshire
269: *Sudden Infant Death Syndrome*

PHILIP W. DAVIDSON, Ph.D.
Professor of Pediatrics and Psychiatry
Director, Strong Center for Developmental Disabilities
University of Rochester School of Medicine and Dentistry
Rochester, New York
11: *Communication with Parents and Patients*
Appendix D: *Common Psychological and Educational Tests*

PAMELA K. DEN BESTEN, D.D.S.
Associate Professor and Chair, Division of Pediatric Dentistry
Department of Growth and Development
University of California at San Francisco, School of Dentistry
San Francisco, California
23 (1): *Prevention of Dental Caries*

JOAN DiMARTINO-NARDI, M.D.
Associate Professor, Department of Pediatric Endocrinology
Albert Einstein College of Medicine
Children's Hospital at Montefiore, Bronx, New York
147: *Hirsutism, Hypertrichosis, and Precocious Sexual Hair Development*

JAY N. DOLITSKY, M.D.
Assistant Professor of Otolaryngology
Department of Otolaryngology, New York Medical College
Director of Medical Student Education
New York Eye and Ear Infirmary, New York, New York
207: *Foreign Bodies of the Ear, Nose, Airway, and Esophagus*

NIENKE P. DOSA, M.D.
Fellow, Division of General Pediatrics, Department of Pediatrics
University of Rochester School of Medicine and Dentistry
Rochester, New York
39: *The Chronically Ill and Disabled Child in School*
297: *Status Asthmaticus*

GEORGE T. DRUGAS, M.D.
Assistant Professor of Surgery
Section of Pediatric Surgery
University of Rochester School of Medicine and Dentistry
Children's Hospital at Strong, Rochester, New York
285: *Esophageal Caustic Injury*

ANA M. DUARTE, M.D.
Clinical Instructor, Department of Dermatology
University of Miami
Director, Department of Dermatology
Miami Children's Hospital, Miami, Florida
189: *Atopic Dermatitis*
259: *Seborrheic Dermatitis*

HOWARD DUBOWITZ, M.D.
Professor of Pediatrics
University of Maryland School of Medicine
Director, Child Protection Program
University of Maryland Medical System, Baltimore, Maryland
57: *Child Abuse and Neglect*

DAVID L. DUDGEON, M.D.
Director and Division Chief, Department of Pediatric Surgery
University Hospitals of Cleveland
Case Western Reserve University
Rainbow Babies & Children's Hospital, Cleveland, Ohio
210: *Gastrointestinal Obstruction*

REGGIE E. DUERST, M.D.
Associate Professor, Department of Pediatrics
University of Rochester, School of Medicine and Dentistry
Rochester, New York
161: *Petechiae and Purpura*

WILLIAM JERRY DURBIN, M.D.
Professor of Pediatrics and Medicine
University of Massachusetts, Director, Pediatric Infectious Diseases
UMass Memorial Health Care, Worcester, Massachusetts
122: *Cough*

LUCIAN A. DURHAM III, M.D., Ph.D.
Assistant Professor of Surgery
Director, Pediatric Cardiovascular Surgery
University of Rochester School of Medicine and Dentistry
Rochester, New York
198: *Congenital Heart Disease*

PAUL H. DWORKIN, M.D.
Professor and Chairman, Department of Pediatrics
University of Connecticut School of Medicine
Farmington, Connecticut
Physician-in-Chief, Connecticut Children's Medical Center
Director and Chairman, Department of Pediatrics
St. Francis Hospital and Medical Center, Hartford, Connecticut
20 (1): *Screening—General Considerations*
76: *School Learning Problems and Developmental Differences*

DAVID R. EDELSTEIN, M.D.
Chairman, Department of Otolaryngology
Head and Neck Surgery, Manhattan Eye, Ear, & Throat Hospital
Clinical Professor, Department of Otorhinolaryngology
Weill Medical College of Cornell University
New York, New York
131: *Epistaxis*

WENDI G. EHRMAN, M.D.
Assistant Professor of Pediatrics, Medical College of Wisconsin
Assistant Professor of Pediatrics, Children's Hospital of Wisconsin
Milwaukee, Wisconsin
239: *Obesity*

MARVIN S. EIGER, M.D.
Associate Clinical Professor, Department of Pediatrics
The Mount Sinai School of Medicine
Attending Physician, Department of Pediatrics
The Beth Israel Medical Center, New York, New York
17 (2): *Feeding of Infants and Children*

ALLEN E. ESKENAZI, M.D.
Associate Professor
Department of Pediatrics
Division of Pediatric Hematology/Oncology
University of Maryland School of Medicine
University of Maryland Medical System
Baltimore, Maryland
170: *Splenomegaly*
225: *Idiopathic Thrombocytopenia*

JEFFREY M. EWIG, M.D.
Clinical Associate Professor, Department of Pediatrics
University of South Florida, Tampa, Florida
Medical Director, Department of Pediatric Pulmonology
All Children's Hospital, St. Petersburg, Florida
36: *Cystic Fibrosis*

MARIANNE E. FELICE, M.D.
Professor and Chair, Department of Pediatrics
University of Massachusetts School of Medicine
Pediatrician-in-Chief, Children's Medical Center
UMass Memorial Health Care, Worcester, Massachusetts
24: *The Ill Child*
294: *Rape*

KATHLEEN LORD FEROLI, R.N., M.S., C.P.N.P.
Instructor, University of Maryland School of Nursing and Medicine
Pediatric Nurse Practitioner
Department of Pediatrics and Adolescent Medicine
Baltimore, Maryland
294: *Rape*

MARTIN A. FINKEL, D.O.
Associate Professor of Pediatrics
Medical Director, Center for Children's Support
University of Medicine & Dentistry of New Jersey
School of Osteopathic Medicine, Stratford, New Jersey
57: *Child Abuse and Neglect*

JOANNE L. FIORAVANTI, R.N., M.S., P.N.P.
Pediatric Nurse Practitioner
Division of Pediatric Cardiology
Children's Hospital at Strong, University of Rochester Medical Center, Rochester, New York
142: *Heart Murmurs*

PHILIP FIREMAN, M.D.
Professor of Pediatrics and Medicine
University of Pittsburgh School of Medicine
Director, Laboratory Service, Section of Allergy and Immunology
Children's Hospital, Pittsburgh, Pennsylvania
188: *Asthma*

JUDITH L. FISHER, M.D.
Resident, Department of Dermatology
Johns Hopkins Medical Institutions, Baltimore, Maryland
166: *Rash*

MARTIN MANDELL FISHER, M.D.
Professor of Clinical Pediatrics
New York University School of Medicine, New York, New York
Chief, Division of Adolescent Medicine, Department of Pediatrics
North Shore University Hospital, Manhasset, New York
102: *Anorexia and Bulimia Nervosa*

MICHAEL FISHER, M.D.
Professor and Head, Division of Dermatology
Department of Medicine, Albert Einstein College of Medicine
Attending Physician, Division of Dermatology
Department of Medicine, Montefiore Medical Center
Jacobi Medical Center, Bronx, New York
166: *Rash*

THOMAS P. FOLEY, Jr., M.D.
Professor of Pediatrics, University of Pittsburgh
Professor of Pediatrics, Children's Hospital of Pittsburgh
Pittsburgh, Pennsylvania
223: *Hypothyroidism*

GILBERT B. FORBES, M.D.
Professor Emeritus of Pediatrics
University of Rochester School of Medicine and Dentistry
Children's Hospital at Strong, Rochester, New York
17 (1): *Nutritional Requirements*

LINDA M. FORSYTHE, M.D.
Staff, Child Psychiatry Service, Massachusetts General Hospital
Instructor in Psychiatry, Harvard Medical School
Boston, Massachusetts
85: *Conduct Disorders*

SHARON L. FOSTER, Ph.D.
Professor of Psychology
California School of Professional Psychology
San Diego, California
91: *Peer Relationship Problems*

HOWARD R. FOYE, Jr., M.D.
Clinical Associate Professor of Pediatrics
University of Rochester School of Medicine and Dentistry
Associate Attending Physician
Children's Hospital at Strong, Rochester, New York
16: *Anticipatory Guidance*

MARY PAT FRANCISCO, M.D.
Department of Pediatrics
University of Florida College of Medicine, Gainesville, Florida
152: *Jaundice*

ELAINE M. FRANK, Ph.D.
Associate Professor and Chair
Department of Communication Sciences and Disorders
University of South Carolina, Columbia, South Carolina
20 (9): *Screening: Language and Speech Assessment*

CARL A. FRANKEL, M.D.
Pediatric Ophthalmologist, Department of Surgery
Division of Ophthalmology, Pinnacle Health Hospitals
Harrisburg, Pennsylvania
168: *Red Eye*
171: *Strabismus*
241: *Ocular Foreign Bodies*
242: *Ocular Trauma*
254: *Preseptal and Orbital Cellulitis*

STANFORD B. FRIEDMAN, M.D.
Professor of Pediatrics, Division of Adolescent Medicine
Albert Einstein College of Medicine
Attending Physician, Division of Adolescent Medicine
Department of Pediatrics, Children's Hospital at Montefiore
Bronx, New York
24: *The Ill Child*
80: *Concepts of Psychosomatic Illness*
83: *Consultation and Referral for Behavioral and Developmental Problems*
100: *Conversion Reactions in Adolescents*
195: *Chronic Fatigue Syndrome*

JOHN P. GEARHART, M.D.
Professor and Director of Pediatric Urology
Department of Urology, Brady Urological Institute
The Johns Hopkins Hospital, Baltimore, Maryland
222: *Hypospadias, Epispadias, and Cryptorchism*

WELTON M. GERSONY, M.D.
Professor of Pediatrics, Department of Cardiology
College of Physicians and Surgeon of Columbia University
Director, Pediatric Cardiology, Presbyterian Hospital
New York, New York
257: *Rheumatic Fever*

HARRY L. GEWANTER, M.D.
Assistant Medical Director, Director of Pediatric Rheumatology
Children's Hospital, Richmond, Virginia
229: *Juvenile Arthritis*

KATHLEEN L. GIFFORD, R.N.
Neonatal Research Nurse, Department of Pediatrics
The Pennsylvania State University College of Medicine
The Milton S. Hershey Medical Center, Hershey, Pennsylvania
45 (4): *Neonatal Adaptations—Adjustment Period*

MAUREEN M. GILMORE, M.D.
Assistant Professor of Pediatrics
The Pennsylvania State University College of Medicine
The Milton S. Hershey Medical Center, Hershey, Pennsylvania
45 (1): *Peripartum Considerations*
45 (2): *Physiological Status of the Healthy Infant*
49: *Critical Neonatal Illnesses*

LAURIE J. GLADER, M.D.
Instructor in Pediatrics, Harvard Medical School
Staff Pediatrician, Boston Children's Hospital
Boston, Massachusetts
35: *Children Assisted by Medical Technology*

JULIUS G. GOEPP, M.D.
Assistant Professor of Emergency Medicine and Pediatrics
Director, Pediatric Emergency Medicine
University of Rochester School of Medicine and Dentistry
Rochester, New York
29: *Fluid Therapy*
268: *Stomatitis*
278: *Dehydration*

MELANIE A. GOLD, D.O.
Assistant Professor of Pediatrics, Section of Adolescent Medicine
University of Pittsburgh School of Medicine
Director of Family Planning, Assistant Professor of Pediatrics
Section of Adolescent Medicine, Children's Hospital of Pittsburgh
Pittsburgh, Pennsylvania
56: *Gay- and Lesbian-Parented Families*

ARCHIE S. GOLDEN, M.D., M.P.H.
Associate Professor, Department of Pediatrics
Johns Hopkins Bayview Medical Center, Baltimore, Maryland
196: *Cleft Lip and Cleft Palate*

DAVID L. GOLDMAN, M.D.
Assistant Professor of Pediatrics, Division of Infectious Diseases
Albert Einstein College of Medicine
Assistant Professor of Pediatrics, Division of Infectious Diseases
Children's Hospital at Montefiore, Bronx, New York
167: *Recurrent Infections*

EDWARD M. GOLDSTEIN, M.D.
Medical Director, Muscular Dystrophy Association Clinic
Department of Neurology
Children's Healthcare of Atlanta at Scottish Rite, Atlanta, Georgia
286: *Head Injuries*

PEARL A. GORDON, Ph.D.
Associate Professor
Department of Audiology and Speech Pathology
University of Tennessee, Knoxville, Knoxville, Tennessee
96: *Stuttering*

ROBERT E. GREENBERG, M.D.
Professor Emeritus of Pediatrics
University of New Mexico School of Medicine
Albuquerque, New Mexico
202: *Diabetes Mellitus*
279: *Diabetic Ketoacidosis*

JOSEPH GREENSHER, M.D.
Professor of Pediatrics
State University of New York School of Medicine
Stony Brook, New York
Medical Director and Associate Chairman
Department of Pediatrics
Winthrop-University Hospital, Mineola, New York
Appendix A: *Pediatric Basic and Advanced Life Support*

MELISSA J. GREGORY, M.D.
Assistant Professor of Pediatrics
University of Rochester School of Medicine and Dentistry
Head of Pediatric Dialysis, Division of Pediatric Nephrology
Children's Hospital at Strong, Rochester, New York
186: *Anuria/Oliguria*
240: *Obstructive Uropathy and Vesicoureteral Reflux*

MICHELLE ANN GRENIER, M.D.
Assistant Professor of Pediatrics, Division of Pediatric Cardiology
University of Rochester School of Medicine and Dentistry
Rochester, New York
20 (4): *Cardiovascular Screening*

LINDSEY K. GROSSMAN, M.D.
Chair, Division of General Pediatrics and Emergency Pediatrics
Department of Pediatrics
Medical College of Virginia Commonwealth University
Richmond, Virginia
123: *Dental Stains*
157: *Malocclusion*
217: *Herpes Infections*

JOHN H. GUNDY, M.D.
Associate Clinical Professor of Pediatrics
Yale University School of Medicine, New Haven, Connecticut
Attending in Pediatrics, Danbury Hospital, Danbury, Connecticut
8: *The Pediatric Physical Examination*

BERNARD GUYER, M.D., M.P.H.
Professor and Chair, Population and Family Health Sciences
Johns Hopkins School of Hygiene and Public Health
Baltimore, Maryland
3: *Morbidity and Mortality Among the Young*

CAROLINE BREESE HALL, M.D.
Professor of Pediatrics and Medicine
Division of Infectious Diseases
University of Rochester School of Medicine and Dentistry
Rochester, New York
156: *Lymphadenopathy*
192: *Bronchiolitis*
277: *Croup (Acute Laryngotracheobronchitis)*
284: *Epiglottitis*

DAVID E. HALL, M.D.
Clinical Associate Professor, Department of Pediatrics
Emory University School of Medicine
Director of Residency Programs
Scottish Pediatric and Adolescent Consultants
Children's Healthcare of Atlanta at Scottish Rite, Atlanta, Georgia
266: *Sports Injuries*
286: *Head Injuries*

WILLIAM J. HALL, M.D.
Professor of Medicine and Pediatrics
University of Rochester School of Medicine and Dentistry
Rochester, New York
192: *Bronchiolitis*
277: *Croup (Acute Laryngotracheobronchitis)*
284: *Epiglottitis*

J. ALEX HALLER, Jr., M.D.
Professor Emeritus, Pediatric Surgery,
Pediatrics, and Emergency Surgery
Department of Surgery, Johns Hopkins University
Pediatric Surgeon (Ret.), Johns Hopkins Hospital
Baltimore, Maryland
247: *Pectus Excavatum and Pectus Carinatum*

JILL S. HALTERMAN, M.D.
Academic Pediatrics Fellow, University of Rochester
School of Medicine and Dentistry, Rochester, New York
13: *Compliance with Pediatric Health Care Recommendations*

ADA HAMOSH, M.D.
Assistant Professor of Pediatrics, Institute of Genetic Medicine
The Johns Hopkins University School of Medicine
Assistant Professor of Pediatrics, Johns Hopkins Hospital
Baltimore, Maryland
20 (3): *Screening: Recognition of Genetic-Metabolic Diseases by Clinical Diagnosis and Screening*

CHRISTOPHER E. HARRIS, M.D.
Assistant Professor, Department of Pediatrics
Division of Pulmonary Medicine
Vanderbilt University School of Medicine
Assistant Professor of Pediatrics
Division of Pediatric Pulmonary Medicine
Vanderbilt University Medical Center, Nashville, Tennessee
252: *Pneumonia*

J. PETER HARRIS, M.D.
Associate Professor of Pediatrics
University of Rochester School of Medicine and Dentistry
Rochester, New York
119: *Cardiac Arrhythmias*

THOMAS A. HAZINSKI, M.D.
Professor and Vice Chairman, Department of Pediatrics
Director, Division of Pediatric Pulmonary Medicine
Department of Pediatrics
Vanderbilt University School of Medicine
Professor and Vice Chairman of Pediatrics
Director, Pediatric Pulmonary Medicine
Vanderbilt University Medical Center, Nashville, Tennessee
182: *Wheezing*
252: *Pneumonia*

HOWARD J. HEINZE, M.D.
Assistant Professor of Pediatrics
University of South Carolina Medical School
Director, Division of Pediatric Endocrinology
Department of Pediatrics
Palmetto Richland Memorial Hospital, Columbia, South Carolina
86: *Cross-Sex Behavior and Gender Identity Disorder*

ALICE B. HEISLER, M.D.
Assistant Professor of Pediatrics
University of Maryland Medical System, Baltimore, Maryland
94: *Self-Stimulating Behaviors*

FRED J. HELDRICH, M.D.
Associate Professor of Pediatrics, Johns Hopkins Medical Institutions
Johns Hopkins Hospital, Baltimore, Maryland
129: *Dysuria*
248: *Pertussis (Whooping Cough)*
258: *Rocky Mountain Spotted Fever*

TERESA M. HERBERT, M.D.
Formerly Department of Pediatrics
University of Rochester School of Medicine and Dentistry
Rochester, New York
293: *Poisoning*

NEIL E. HERENDEEN, M.D.
Clinical Assistant Professor of Pediatrics
Division of General Pediatrics
University of Rochester School of Medicine and Dentistry
Rochester, New York
185: *Animal Bites*
201: *Cystic and Solid Masses of the Face and Neck*

PETER L. HIMBER, M.D.
Assistant Clinical Professor, Department of Pediatrics
The Pennsylvania State University Medical Center
Hershey, Pennsylvania
290: *Increased Intracranial Pressure*

ANDREA S. HINKLE, M.D.
Assistant Professor of Pediatrics
Division of Pediatric Hematology-Oncology
Children's Hospital at Strong
University of Rochester School of Medicine and Dentistry
Rochester, New York
193: *Cancers in Childhood*

JEFF C. HOEHNER, M.D., Ph.D.
Assistant Professor of Surgery, Division of Pediatric Surgery
The Johns Hopkins University School of Medicine
Assistant Professor of Surgery
Division of Pediatric Surgery, Johns Hopkins Medical Institutions
Baltimore, Maryland
255: *Pyloric Stenosis*

ROBERT A. HOEKELMAN, M.D.
Professor and Chairman Emeritus, Department of Pediatrics
University of Rochester School of Medicine and Dentistry
Rochester, New York
4: *Child Health Supervision*
7: *The Pediatric History*
11: *Communication with Parents and Patients*
20 (2): *Screening—The Physical Examination as a Screening Test*
138: *Foot and Leg Problems*
270: *Tonsillectomy and Adenoidectomy*

GEORGE W. HOLCOMB III, M.D.
Katherine B. Richardson Professor of Surgery
University of Missouri at Kansas City; Surgeon-in-Chief
Children's Mercy Hospital, Kansas City, Missouri
32: *Minimally Invasive Surgery*

JOHN T. HORAN, M.D.
Fellow in Pediatric Hematologic Oncology
Department of Pediatrics
University of Rochester School of Medicine and Dentistry
Rochester, New York
280: *Disseminated Intravascular Coagulation*

KYLE D. HOUSER, M.Ed., M.A.
Clinical Instructor in Pediatrics, Department of Pediatrics
University of Rochester School of Medicine and Dentistry
Rochester, New York
Appendix D: *Common Psychological and Educational Tests*

BARBARA J. HOWARD, M.D.
Assistant Professor of Pediatrics
The Johns Hopkins University School of Medicine
Baltimore, Maryland
95: *Sleep Disturbances*
231: *Labial Adhesions*

JULIETTE HUKIN, M.D., F.R.C.P. (C)
Assistant Professor of Pediatrics
British Columbia Children's Hospital
Vancouver, British Columbia, Canada
191: *Brain Tumors*

SHARON G. HUMISTON, M.D., M.P.H.
Medical Epidemiologist, National Immunization Program
Centers for Disease Control and Prevention, Atlanta, Georgia
Clinical Faculty, Department of Emergency Medicine
University of Rochester Medical Center, Rochester, New York
18: *Immunizations*

HOLLY M. HUTA, M.S.
Clinical Audiologist
Bill Wilkerson Center for Otolaryngology and Communication Sciences
Vanderbilt University, Nashville, Tennessee
141: *Hearing Loss*

ROBERT IANNONE, M.D.
Senior Clinical Fellow
Department of Pediatric Hematology and Oncology
The Johns Hopkins University School of Medicine
Baltimore, Maryland
200: *Contagious Exanthematous Diseases*

MICHAEL S. JELLINEK, M.D.
Professor of Psychiatry and of Pediatrics, Harvard Medical School
Chief, Child Psychiatry Service, Massachusetts General Hospital
Boston, Massachusetts
20 (14): *Psychosocial Screening*
85: *Conduct Disorders*

JERRI ANN JENISTA, M.D.
Attending Pediatrician
Departments of Pediatrics and Emergency Medicine
St. Joseph Mercy Hospital, Ann Arbor, Michigan
206: *Enterovirus Infections*
218: *Human Herpesvirus-6 and Human Herpesvirus-7 Infections*

ALAIN JOFFE, M.D., M.P.H.
Associate Professor of Pediatrics, Director, Adolescent Medicine
The Johns Hopkins University School of Medicine
Associate Professor of Pediatrics, Director
of Adolescent Medicine
The Johns Hopkins Hospital, Baltimore, Maryland
116: *Amenorrhea*
126: *Dysmenorrhea*
154: *Limp*
177: *Vaginal Bleeding*
178: *Vaginal Discharge*
262: *Sexually Transmitted Diseases*

DENNIS L. JOHNSON, M.D.
Professor, Department of Surgery and Pediatrics
The Pennsylvania State University School of Medicine
The Milton S. Hershey Medical Center, Hershey, Pennsylvania
220: *Hydrocephalus*

R. JOSEPH JOPLING, M.D.
Associate Clinical Professor
Department of Pediatrics, University of Utah School of Medicine
Salt Lake City, Utah
21: *Counseling Families on Healthy Lifestyles*

NICHOLAS JOSPE, M.D.
Associate Professor of Pediatrics
University of Rochester School of Medicine and Dentistry
Department of Pediatrics, Children's Hospital at Strong
Rochester, New York
221: *Hyperthyroidism*

RUTH K. KAMINER, M.D.
Professor of Pediatrics, Albert Einstein College of Medicine
Associate Director for Medical Services
Children's Evaluation and Rehabilitation Center
Rose F. Kennedy Center, Bronx, New York
19: *Identification of Developmental Delays and the Early Intervention System*

JACK KAMINS, Psy.D.
Assistant Superintendent
Department of Psychological Services and Special Education
Great Neck Union Free School District, Great Neck, New York
74: *School Behavioral Problems*

ROBERT K. KANTER, M.D.
Associate Professor of Pediatrics
Director, Division of Pediatric Critical Care Medicine
State University of New York, Upstate Medical University
Syracuse, New York
297: *Status Asthmaticus*

AUBREY J. KATZ, M.D.
Associate Professor in Pediatrics
Tufts University School of Medicine, Associate Staff in Pediatrics
New England Medical Center, Boston, Massachusetts
209: *Gastrointestinal Allergy*
212: *Gluten-Sensitive Enteropathy (Celiac Sprue)*

ALEX R. KEMPER, M.D., M.P.H.
Primary Care Research Fellow, Department of Pediatrics
University of North Carolina, Chapel Hill, North Carolina
20 (11): *Vision Screening*

KATHI J. KEMPER, M.D.
Associate Professor Pediatrics, Harvard Medical School
Director, Center for Holistic Pediatric Education & Research
Boston, Massachusetts
28: *Complementary and Alternative Medical Therapies*

JOHN H. KENNELL, M.D.
Professor of Pediatrics
Case Western Reserve University School of Medicine
Division of Behavioral Pediatrics
Rainbow Babies and Children's Hospital, Cleveland, Ohio
45 (6): *Neonatal Adaptations—Pediatric Support for Parents*

THOMAS J. KENNY, Ph.D.
Professor (Ret.) of Pediatrics
University of Maryland School of Medicine, Baltimore, Maryland
34: *Mental Retardation*

NISSIM KHABIE, M.D.
Senior Resident, Department of Otolaryngology
Head and Neck Surgery, Manhattan Eye, Ear, and Throat Hospital
New York, New York
131: *Epistaxis*

RITA S. KHANDWALA, M.D.
Assistant Professor
Departments of Anesthesiology, Critical Care, and Pediatrics
The Johns Hopkins University School of Medicine
Baltimore, Maryland
26: *Management of Acute Pain in Children*

MARSHALL H. KLAUS, M.D.
Adjunct Professor of Pediatrics
University of California at San Francisco
San Francisco, California
45 (6): *Pediatric Support for Parents*

DAVID N. KORONES, M.D.
Associate Professor of Pediatrics and Oncology
University of Rochester School of Medicine and Dentistry
Attending Physician
Children's Hospital at Strong, Rochester, New York
117: *Anemia and Pallor*
280: *Disseminated Intravascular Coagulation*

SABINE KOST-BYERLY, M.D.
Instructor
Department of Anesthesiology and Critical Care Medicine
The Johns Hopkins Medical Institutions, Baltimore, Maryland
26: *Management of Acute Pain in Children*

RICHARD E. KREIPE, M.D.
Professor of Pediatrics
Chief, Division of Adolescent Medicine
University of Rochester School of Medicine and Dentistry
Attending Physician, Children's Hospital at Strong
Rochester, New York
99: *Challenges of Health Care Delivery to Adolescents*

LEONARD R. KRILOV, M.D.
Associate Professor of Pediatrics
New York University School of Medicine, New York, New York
Chief, Pediatric Infectious Diseases, Department of Pediatrics
North Shore University Hospital, Manhasset, New York
195: *Chronic Fatigue Syndrome*
226: *Infectious Mononucleosis and Other Epstein-Barr Virus Infections*

ROBERT K. KRITZLER, M.D.
Area Medical Director, Kaiser Permanente
Baltimore, Maryland
165: *Puberty: Normal and Abnormal*

JOHN D. LANTOS, M.D.
Associate Professor of Pediatrics
Section Head, General Pediatrics
Associate Director, MacLean Center for Clinical Medicinal Ethics
Co-Director, Robert Wood Johnson Clinical Scholars Program
University of Chicago, Chicago, Illinois
6: *Ethical and Legal Issues for the Primary Care Pediatrician*

PIETER le ROUX, D. Litt. et Ph.D.
Clinical Associate Professor
Department of Psychiatry and Pediatrics
University of Rochester School of Medicine and Dentistry
Co-Director, Behavioral Sciences Program
Department of Pediatrics, ViaHealth Rochester General Hospital
Rochester, New York
92: *Phobias*

JOHN M. LEVENTHAL, M.D.
Professor of Pediatrics, Yale University School of Medicine
Medical Director of Child Abuse Committee
Department of Pediatrics, Yale-New Haven Children's Hospital
New Haven, Connecticut
68: *Sexual Abuse of Children*

SUSAN E. LEVITZKY, M.D.
Assistant Clinical Professor, Department of Pediatrics
Albert Einstein School of Medicine, Bronx, New York
Attending Pediatrician, Beth Israel Medical Center
New York, New York
148: *Hoarseness*

SAMUEL M. LIBBER, M.D.
Assistant Professor of Pediatrics
The Johns Hopkins University School of Medicine
Johns Hopkins Hospital, Baltimore, Maryland
Anne Arundel Medical Center, Annapolis, Maryland
162: *Polyuria*

STEVEN E. LIPSHULTZ, M.D.
Professor of Pediatrics and Oncology
University of Rochester School of Medicine and Dentistry
Chief of Pediatric Cardiology, Children's Hospital at Strong
Rochester, New York
23 (3): *Preventive Cardiology*
146: *High Blood Pressure in Infants, Children, and Adolescents*
287: *Heart Failure*

GREGORY S. LIPTAK, M.D., M.P.H.
Associate Professor of Pediatrics
University of Rochester School of Medicine and Dentistry
Attending Pediatrician, Children's Hospital at Strong
Rochester, New York
33: *Physical Disability and Chronic Illness*
38: *Cerebral Palsy*
39: *The Chronically Ill and Disabled Child in School*
203: *Diaper Rash*
264: *Spina Bifida*

GEORGE A. LITTLE, M.D.
Professor of Pediatrics, Dartmouth-Hitchcock Medical Center
Children's Hospital at Dartmouth, Lebanon, New Hampshire
42: *The Fetus at Risk*
43 (2): *Perinatal Transport*

DONALD P. LOOKINGBILL, M.D.
Professor, Department of Dermatology
Mayo Medical School, Rochester, Minnesota
Chairman, Department of Dermatology
Mayo Clinic Jacksonville, Jacksonville, Florida
183: *Acne*
190: *Bacterial Skin Infections*
205: *Drug Eruptions*
274: *Verrucae (Warts)*

STEVEN E. LUCKING, M.D.
Associate Professor of Pediatrics
Chief, Division of Pediatric Critical Care
The Pennsylvania State University College of Medicine
The Milton S. Hershey Medical Center, Hershey, Pennsylvania
275: *Airway Obstruction*
281: *Drowning and Near-Drowning*

JAMES A. MANNING, M.D.
Professor of Pediatrics
University of Rochester School of Medicine and Dentistry
Attending Physician, Department of Pediatrics
Children's Hospital at Strong, Rochester, New York
142: *Heart Murmurs*

RONALD V. MARINO, D.O., M.P.H.
Professor of Clinical Pediatrics
State University of New York at Stony Brook
Stony Brook, New York
Director, General Pediatrics, Winthrop Pediatrics Associates
Mineola, New York
75: *School Absenteeism and School Refusal*

ROBERT W. MARION, M.D.
Professor of Pediatrics and Obstetrics & Gynecology
Albert Einstein College of Medicine
Director, Division of Pediatrics, Children's Hospital at Montefiore
Bronx, New York
272: *Umbilical Anomalies*

KEITH H. MARKS, M.B., B.Ch.
Professor of Pediatrics
The Pennsylvania State University College of Medicine
The Milton S. Hershey Medical Center, Hershey, Pennsylvania
49: *Critical Neonatal Illnesses*

JUAN C. MARTINEZ, M.D.
Clinical Assistant Professor of Pediatrics
University of South Florida
Director, Cystic Fibrosis Center
Division of Pediatric Pulmonology
All Children's Hospital, St. Petersburg, Florida
36: *Cystic Fibrosis*

LENI G. MATHEW, M.D., D.C.H.
Lecturer in Pediatrics, Department of Child Health
Christian Medical College Hospital, Vellore, Tamilnadu, India
246: *Parasitic Infections*

REBECCA RIBOVICH MATSAKIS, M.D.
Assistant Professor of Pediatrics
The Johns Hopkins University School of Medicine
Attending Pediatrician, Johns Hopkins Hospital
Baltimore, Maryland
256: *Reye's Syndrome*

LYNNE G. MAXWELL, M.D.
Associate Professor
Department of Anesthesiology, Critical Care, and Pediatrics
The Johns Hopkins University School of Medicine
Baltimore, Maryland
9: *Preoperative Assessment*
26: *Management of Acute Pain in Children*
253: *Postoperative Management of the Pediatric Outpatient: Surgical and Anesthetic Aspects*

JAY H. MAYEFSKY, M.D., M.P.H.
Associate Professor of Pediatrics
Finch University of Health Sciences, The Chicago Medical School
Director, Comprehensive Care Clinic, Department of Pediatrics
Cook County Children's Hospital, Chicago, Illinois
128: *Dyspnea*

ELIZABETH R. McANARNEY, M.D.
Professor and Chair of Pediatrics
University of Rochester School of Medicine and Dentistry
Strong Memorial Hospital, Department of Pediatrics
Rochester, New York
111: *Adolescent Pregnancy and Parenthood*

MARGARET C. McBRIDE, M.D.
Associate Professor of Neurology and Pediatrics
University of Rochester School of Medicine and Dentistry
Rochester, New York
260: *Seizure Disorders*
298: *Status Epilepticus*

CHRISTINA M. McCANN, Ph.D.
Postdoctoral Fellow, Department of Pediatrics
University of Rochester School of Medicine and Dentistry
Rochester General Hospital, Rochester, New York
92: *Phobias*

EDITH A. McCARTHY, M.D.
Neonatology Fellow, Division of Perinatology
New York Presbyterian Hospital–Cornell University
New York, New York
44: *Sequelae to Infertility*

LAURA K. McCORMICK, Dr.P.H.
Assistant Professor
Department of Health Promotion and Behavior
University of Georgia, Athens, Georgia
71: *School Health Education*

HIRAM L. McDADE, Ph.D.
Associate Professor and Graduate Director
Department of Communication Sciences and Disorders
University of South Carolina
Adjunct Associate Professor, Department of Pediatrics
University of South Carolina School of Medicine
Columbia, South Carolina
20 (9): *Screening: Language and Speech Assessment*

DIANE L. McDONALD, M.D.
Clinical Instructor of Pediatrics
University of Virginia, Charlottesville, Virginia
Attending Physician, Department of Emergency Medicine
Fairfax Hospital, Fairfax, Virginia
174: *Syncope*

KATHLEEN McGRATH, R.N., M.S., C.P.N.P.
Clinical Instructor of Nursing
University of Rochester School of Nursing
Advanced Practice Nurse, Department of Pediatrics
Children's Hospital at Strong, Rochester, New York
23 (3): *Preventive Cardiology*

ROBERT H. McLEAN, M.D.
Professor of Pediatrics
Department of Pediatric Nephrology & Hypertension
University of Maryland School of Medicine, Baltimore, Maryland
130: *Edema*

JAMES W. McMANAWAY III, M.D.
Associate Professor of Ophthalmology and Pediatrics
The Pennsylvania State University College of Medicine
The Milton S. Hershey Medical Center, Hershey, Pennsylvania
168: *Red Eye*
171: *Strabismus*
179: *Visual Problems*
241: *Ocular Foreign Bodies*
242: *Ocular Trauma*
254: *Preseptal and Orbital Cellulitis*

BERNADETTE MAZUREK MELNYK, Ph.D., R.N.-C.S., P.N.P.
Associate Professor of Nursing and Pediatrics
Associate Dean for Research
Director, Pediatric Nurse Practitioner Program
University of Rochester School of Nursing
University of Rochester School of Medicine and Dentistry
Rochester, New York
77: *Nursing Roles in School Health*

ALAN M. MENDELSOHN, M.D.
Associate Professor of Pediatrics
University of Rochester School of Medicine and Dentistry
Attending Physician
Children's Hospital at Strong, Rochester, New York
198: *Congenital Heart Disease*

RUTH J. MESSINGER, M.S.W.
Associate in Pediatrics and Social Work Coordinator
University of Rochester School of Medicine and Dentistry
Rochester, New York
11: *Communication with Parents and Patients*

KAREN J. MILLER, M.D.
Clinical Assistant Professor of Pediatrics
University of Rochester School of Medicine and Dentistry
Developmental-Behavioral Pediatrician
The Genesee Hospital, Rochester, New York
73: *Attention Deficit/Hyperactivity Disorder*

MARVIN E. MILLER, M.D.
Professor of Pediatrics and Obstetrics/Gynecology
Wright State University School of Medicine
Director of Medical Genetics and Birth Defects
Department of Pediatrics
Children's Medical Center, Dayton, Ohio
40: *Approaches to Genetic Diseases*
46: *Skin Lesions of the Neonate*
133: *Facial Dysmorphism*

MICHAEL MILOBSKY, M.D.
Department of Pediatrics
University of Maryland Hospital, Baltimore, Maryland
292: *Pneumothorax and Pneumomediastinum*

CYNTHIA S. MINKOVITZ, M.D., M.P.P.
Assistant Professor, Department of Population and Family Health Sciences
The Johns Hopkins University, Baltimore, Maryland
3: *Morbidity and Mortality Among the Young*

WILLIAM MOSS, M.D., M.P.H.
Assistant Scientist
International Health and Molecular Microbiology and Immunology
School of Hygiene and Public Health
The Johns Hopkins University, Baltimore, Maryland
219: *Human Immunodeficiency Virus Infection and Acquired Immunodeficiency Syndrome*

RICHARD T. MOXLEY III, M.D.
Professor of Neurology and Pediatrics
Director, Neuromuscular Disease Center
Associate Chair for Academic Affairs, Department of Neurology
University of Rochester School of Medicine and Dentistry
Rochester, New York
37: *Muscular Dystrophy*

DENNIS J. MUJSCE, M.D.
Associate Professor of Pediatrics
The Pennsylvania State University School of Medicine
The Milton S. Hershey Medical Center, Hershey, Pennsylvania
48: *Common Neonatal Illnesses*
51: *High-Risk Follow-up*

PHILIP R. NADER, M.D.
Professor and Division Chief, Community Pediatrics
University of California, San Diego, San Diego, California
70: *Overview of School Health and School Health Program Goals*

PRAMOD NARULA, M.D.
Associate Professor of Pediatrics
University of New York at Stony Brook, Stony Brook, New York
Director, Pediatric Critical Care, Winthrop-University Hospital
Mineola, New York
Appendix A: *Pediatric Basic and Advanced Life Support*

ROBERT D. NEEDLMAN, M.D.
Assistant Professor of Pediatrics
Case Western Reserve University School of Medicine
Attending Pediatrician, Rainbow Babies & Children's Hospital
University Hospitals of Cleveland, Cleveland, Ohio
66: *Latchkey Children: Children in Self-Care*

NICHOLAS M. NELSON, M.D.
Professor Emeritus of Pediatrics, The Pennsylvania State University
The Milton S. Hershey Medical Center, Hershey, Pennsylvania
10: *Structural and Functional Analysis of Body Systems*
43 (1): *Perinatal Medicine—Overview*
45 (1): *Neonatal Adaptations—Peripartum Considerations*
45 (2): *Neonatal Adaptations—Physiological Status of the Healthy Infant*
45 (3): *Neonatal Adaptations—Recovery Period*
45 (4): *Neonatal Adaptations—Adjustment Period*
45 (5): *Neonatal Adaptations—Establishment of Equilibrium*
51: *High-Risk Follow-up*

PERRY SANTOS NEMECHECK, R.N., M.S., P.N.P.
Pediatric Nurse Practitioner, Department of Pediatric Cardiology
Children's Heart Center, University of Rochester Medical Center
Rochester, New York
20 (4): *Cardiovascular Screening*

C. JEAN OGBORN, M.D.
Assistant Professor of Pediatrics
Division of Pediatric Emergency Medicine
The Johns Hopkins University School of Medicine
Assistant Director of the Pediatric Emergency Department
Johns Hopkins Children's Center, Baltimore, Maryland
151: *Irritability*

KAREN N. OLNESS, M.D.
Professor of Pediatrics, Family Medicine, and International Health
Case Western Reserve University
Director of International Child Health
Rainbow Babies and Children's Hospital, Cleveland, Ohio
12: *Cultural Issues in Primary Pediatric Care*

CRAIG C. ORLOWSKI, M.D.
Assistant Clinical Professor of Pediatrics
University of Rochester School of Medicine and Dentistry
Attending Pediatrician, Children's Hospital at Strong,
Rochester, New York
289: *Hypoglycemia*

ENRIQUE M. OSTREA, Jr., M.D.
Professor of Pediatrics, Wayne State University
Chief, Department of Pediatrics, Hutzel Hospital, Detroit, Michigan
50: *Prenatal Drug Abuse and Neonatal Drug Withdrawal Syndrome*

PHILIP O. OZUAH, M.D.
Associate Professor of Clinical Pediatrics
Albert Einstein College of Medicine
Director, Residency Training Program in Social Pediatrics
Children's Hospital at Montefiore, Bronx, New York
135: *Fatigue and Weakness*
145: *Hepatomegaly*
176: *Torticollis*

CHARLES N. PAIDAS, M.D.
Associate Professor of Surgery, Pediatrics, Oncology, Anesthesia and Critical Care Medicine
The Johns Hopkins University School of Medicine
Johns Hopkins Hospital, Baltimore, Maryland
253: *Postoperative Management of the Pediatric Outpatient: Surgical and Anesthetic Aspects*

JUDITH S. PALFREY, M.D.
T. Berry Brazelton Professor of Pediatrics, Harvard Medical School
Chief, Division of General Pediatrics, Children's Hospital
Boston, Massachusetts
35: *Children Assisted by Medical Technology*

JAMES PALIS, M.D.
Associate Professor of Pediatrics and Oncology
University of Rochester School of Medicine and Dentistry
Attending Physician, Children's Hospital at Strong
Rochester, New York
228: *Iron-Deficiency Anemia*

CHARLES PALMER, M.B., Ch.B., F.C.P.
Professor, Department of Pediatrics
The Pennsylvania State University College of Medicine
The Milton S. Hershey Medical Center, Hershey, Pennsylvania
48: *Common Neonatal Illnesses*

FRANCES C. PAOLINI-MASUCCI, M.S.W.
Co-Director of Social Work Services, Montefiore Medical Center
The University Hospital for the Albert Einstein College of Medicine, Bronx, New York
101: *Counseling Parents of Adolescents*

GUY S. PARCEL, Ph.D.
John P. McGovern Professor of Health Promotion
Director, Center for Health Promotion Research and Development
The University of Texas-Houston Health Science Center
School of Public Health, Houston, Texas
71: *School Health Education*

ASHA PAREKH, M.D.
Clinical Fellow in Psychiatry, Harvard Medical School
Resident in Psychiatry, Massachusetts General Hospital
Boston, Massachusetts
85: *Conduct Disorders*

MARGARETE I. PARRISH, Ph.D., M.S.W.
Assistant Professor of Social Work
University of Maryland School of Social Work
Co-Investigator, Survivors/Perpetrators of Violence
University of Maryland System Shock Trauma Center
Baltimore, Maryland
294: *Rape*

WALTER PEGOLI, Jr., M.D.
Associate Professor of Surgery and Pediatrics
Section Chief, Pediatric Surgery
University of Rochester School of Medicine and Dentistry
Rochester, New York
285: *Esophageal Caustic Injury*

DAVID S. PELLEGRINI, Ph.D.
Private Practice, Washington, D.C.
81: *Prediction of Adult Behavior from Childhood*

ROBERT A. PENDERGRAST, Jr., M.D., M.P.H.
Associate Professor of Pediatrics, Director, Adolescent Medicine
Children's Medical Center, Medical College of Georgia
Augusta, Georgia
118: *Back Pain*

ELLEN C. PERRIN, M.D.
Professor of Pediatrics, University of Massachusetts Medical Center
Worcester, Massachusetts
67: *Teaching Parents About Effective Discipline*

DEBORAH PERSAUD, M.D.
Assistant Professor of Pediatrics
The Johns Hopkins University School of Medicine
Baltimore, Maryland
219: *Human Immunodeficiency Virus Infection and Acquired Immunodeficiency Syndrome*

SHERIDAN PHILLIPS, Ph.D.
Associate Professor of Psychiatry
University of Maryland School of Medicine, Baltimore, Maryland
82: *Options for Psychosocial Intervention with Children and Adolescents*
83: *Consultation and Referral for Behavioral and Developmental Problems*

MICHAEL E. PICHICHERO, M.D.
Professor of Microbiology and Immunology
Professor of Pediatrics and Medicine
University of Rochester School of Medicine and Dentistry
Rochester, New York
230: *Kawasaki Disease*
267: *Staphylococcal Toxic Shock Syndrome*

S. MICHAEL PLAUT, Ph.D.
Associate Professor of Psychiatry
University of Maryland School of Medicine, Baltimore, Maryland
15: *Assessing the Medical Literature*

LESLIE P. PLOTNICK, M.D.
Associate Professor of Pediatrics
Johns Hopkins Hospital, Baltimore, Maryland
162: *Polyuria*
165: *Puberty: Normal and Abnormal*

GREGORY E. PRAZAR, M.D.
Pediatric Practitioner
Exeter Pediatric Associates, Exeter, New Hampshire
90: *Lying and Stealing*
97: *Temper Tantrums and Breath-Holding Spells*
100: *Conversion Reactions in Adolescents*

ANDREW D. RACINE, M.D., Ph.D.
Associate Professor of Pediatrics
Albert Einstein College of Medicine
Director, Division of General Pediatrics
Children's Hospital at Montefiore, Bronx, New York
134: *Failure to Thrive*

EVA G. RADEL, M.D.
Professor of Clinical Pediatrics
Albert Einstein College of Medicine
Director, Division of Pediatric Hematology-Oncology
Department of Pediatrics
Children's Hospital at Montefiore, Bronx, New York
30: *Blood Products and Their Uses*
214: *Hemophilia and Other Hereditary Bleeding Disorders*

IRWIN REDLENER, M.D.
Professor of Pediatrics
Director, Division of Community Pediatrics
Albert Einstein College of Medicine
Children's Hospital at Montefiore, Bronx, New York
65: *Homelessness and the Family*

ROBERT F. REISS, M.D.
Professor of Clinical Pathology and Clinical Medicine
College of Physicians and Surgeons, Columbia University
Vice President, Medical Operations, New York Blood Center
New York, New York
20 (5): *Screening for Anemia*

GEORGE A. REKERS, Ph.D.
Professor of Neuropsychiatry & Behavioral Sciences
University of South Carolina Medical School
Clinical Psychologist and Research Director
Division of Child and Adolescent Psychiatry
Hall Psychiatric Institute, Columbia, South Carolina
86: *Cross-Sex Behavior and Gender Identity Disorder*

JULIUS B. RICHMOND, M.D.
John D. McArthur Professor of Health Policy, Emeritus
Department of Social Medicine, Harvard Medical School
Senior Consultant, Boston Children's Hospital
Boston, Massachusetts
53: *Mental Health of the Young: An Overview*

SARAH M. RODDY, M.D.
Associate Professor of Pediatrics and Neurology
Loma Linda University School of Medicine
Loma Linda, California
159: *Nonconvulsive Periodic Disorders*
260: *Seizure Disorders*
298: *Status Epilepticus*

LANCE E. RODEWALD, M.D.
Director of Immunization Services Division
National Immunization Program
Centers for Disease Control and Prevention, Atlanta, Georgia
13: *Compliance with Pediatric Health Care Recommendations*
18: *Immunizations*

PAUL T. ROGERS, M.D.
Facility Medical Director, Bright Oak Pediatric Center
Medstar Physician Partners, Bel Air, Maryland
Neurodevelopmental Consultant, Department of Pediatrics
Franklin Square Medical Center, Baltimore, Maryland
204: *Down Syndrome: Managing the Child and Family*

LAINIE FRIEDMAN ROSS, M.D., Ph.D.
Assistant Professor of Pediatrics
Assistant Director, MacLean Center for Clinical Medical Ethics
University of Chicago, Chicago, Illinois
6: *Ethical and Legal Issues for the Primary Care Pediatrician*

EDWARD J. RULEY, M.D.
Clinical Professor of Pediatrics
Uniformed Services University of Health Sciences
Bethesda, Maryland
Medical Co-Director, Pediatric Kidney Center
Department of Pediatrics, INOVA Fairfax Hospital for Children
Falls Church, Virginia
143: *Hematuria*
163: *Proteinuria*
237: *Nephritis*

OLLE JANE Z. SAHLER, M.D.
Professor of Pediatrics
Psychiatry, Medical Humanities and Oncology
University of Rochester School of Medicine and Dentistry
Director, Psychosocial Services and Research
Division of Hematology/Oncology, Children's Hospital at Strong
Rochester, New York
52: *Theories and Concepts of Development as They Relate to Pediatric Practice*
Appendix D: *Common Psychological and Educational Tests*

STEVEN D. SALHANICK, M.D.
Assistant Professor of Emergency Medicine
University of Rochester School of Medicine and Dentistry
Strong Memorial Hospital, Rochester, New York
283: *Envenomations*

MORTON E. SALOMON, M.D.
Associate Professor
Department of Emergency Medicine and Pediatrics
Albert Einstein College of Medicine
Vice Chairman and Director of Service
Department of Emergency Medicine
Montefiore Medical Center, Bronx, New York
173: *Stridor*

EDWARD J. SALTZMAN, M.D.
Clinical Professor of Pediatrics
University of Miami School of Medicine, Miami, Florida
1: *The Health Care Delivery System*

MAHER SAQQUR, M.D.
Chief Resident, Department of Neurology
The Pennsylvania State University College of Medicine
Hershey, Pennsylvania
290: *Increased Intracranial Pressure*

JOHN SARGENT, M.D.
Director of Education and Research
Dean, Karl Menninger School of Psychiatry and Mental Health Sciences, The Menninger Clinic, Topeka, Kansas
62: *Family Interactions: Children Who Have Unexplained Physical Symptoms*

RICHARD M. SARLES, M.D.
Professor and Director, Division of Child & Adolescent Psychiatry
University of Maryland School of Medicine, Baltimore, Maryland
83: *Consultation and Referral for Behavioral and Developmental Problems*
94: *Self-Stimulating Behaviors*
158: *Nervousness*

LAWRENCE A. SCHACHNER, M.D.
Professor of Dermatology and Pediatrics, University of Miami
Jackson Memorial Hospital, Miami, Florida
189: *Atopic Dermatitis*
259: *Seborrheic Dermatitis*

ERIC A. SCHAFF, M.D.
Associate Professor of Family Medicine and Obstetrics and Gynecology
University of Rochester School of Medicine and Dentistry
Rochester, New York
41: *Contraception and Abortion*

L.R. SCHERER III, M.D.
Clinical Associate Professor of Pediatric Surgery
Director of Kiwanis-Riley Trauma Life Center
Director, Kiwanis-Riley Regional Pediatric Trauma Center
J.W. Riley Hospital for Children, Indianapolis, Indiana
299: *Thermal Injuries*

STEVEN SCHLOZMAN, M.D.
Child Psychiatry Service
Massachusetts General Hospital, Boston, Massachusetts
20 (14): *Psychosocial Screening*

BARTON D. SCHMITT, M.D.
Professor of Pediatrics
University of Colorado School of Medicine
Medical Director, Encopresis-Enuresis Clinic
Department of Pediatrics, The Children's Hospital
Denver, Colorado
87: *Encopresis*

MARCIE B. SCHNEIDER, M.D.
Director, Adolescent Medicine Program
Greenwich Hospital, Greenwich, Connecticut
Assistant Clinical Professor of Pediatrics
Yale University School of Medicine
New Haven, Connecticut
102: *Anorexia and Bulimia Nervosa*

S. KENNETH SCHONBERG, M.D.
Professor of Pediatrics, Albert Einstein College of Medicine
Director, Division of Adolescent Medicine
Department of Pediatrics, Montefiore Medical Center
Bronx, New York
103: *Drug, Alcohol, and Tobacco Abuse*

SCOTT A. SCHROEDER, M.D.
Assistant Professor of Pediatrics
Albert Einstein College of Medicine
Section Chief, Division of Critical Care
Department of Pediatrics and Pulmonary Medicine
Division of Critical Care and Pulmonary Medicine
Children's Hospital at Montefiore, Bronx, New York
120: *Chest Pain*
144: *Hemoptysis*

CINDY L. SCHWARTZ, M.D.
Associate Professor of Oncology and Pediatrics
Associate Director of Pediatric Oncology for Clinical Programs
The Johns Hopkins University School of Medicine
Baltimore, Maryland
193: *Cancers in Childhood*

GEORGE J. SCHWARTZ, M.D.
Professor of Pediatrics and Medicine
Chief, Division of Pediatric Nephrology
University of Rochester School of Medicine and Dentistry
Attending Physician, Children's Hospital at Strong
Rochester, New York
20 (8): *Use of Urinalysis and the Urine Culture in Screening*

KATHLEEN B. SCHWARZ, M.D.
Associate Professor of Pediatrics
Chief, Division of Pediatric Gastroenterology and Nutrition
The Johns Hopkins University School of Medicine
Johns Hopkins Hospital, Baltimore, Maryland
216: *Hepatitis*

EDWARDS P. SCHWENTKER, M.D.
Professor of Orthopaedics & Rehabilitation and Pediatrics
The Pennsylvania State University College of Medicine
Hershey, Pennsylvania
244: *Osteomyelitis*
261: *Septic Arthritis*

ROBERT D. SEGE, M.D., Ph.D.
Associate Professor of Pediatrics
Tufts University School of Medicine
Associate Chief
Division of General Pediatric and Adolescent Medicine
The Floating Hospital for Children, Boston, Massachusetts
23 (4): *Violence Prevention*

GEORGE B. SEGEL, M.D.
Professor of Pediatrics, Medicine, Genetics and Oncology
Chief, Pediatric Hematology/Oncology and Genetics
Director, Division of Pediatric Genetics
University of Rochester School of Medicine and Dentistry
Rochester, New York
156: *Lymphadenopathy*

HENRY M. SEIDEL, M.D.
Professor Emeritus of Pediatrics
The Johns Hopkins School of Medicine
Johns Hopkins Hospital, Baltimore, Maryland
14: *The Art of Consultation*
64: *Health Needs of Parents*
140: *Headache*

PETER SHERMAN, M.D.
Medical Director, New York Children's Health Project
Division of Community Pediatrics, Department of Pediatrics
Albert Einstein College of Medicine
Children's Hospital at Montefiore, Bronx, New York
61: *Domestic Violence and the Family*
65: *Homelessness and the Family*

WILLIAM A. SHINE, Ed.D.
Superintendent of Schools
Great Neck Union Free School District
Great Neck, New York
74: *School Behavioral Problems*

GEORGE K. SIBERRY, M.D.
Chief Resident, Department of Pediatrics
The Johns Hopkins University School of Medicine
Johns Hopkins Hospital, Baltimore, Maryland
194: *Chickenpox*

ERICA M.S. SIBINGA, M.D.
Senior Clinical Fellow, General Academic Pediatrics
The Johns Hopkins University School of Medicine
Johns Hopkins Hospital, Baltimore, Maryland
154: *Limp*

DAVID M. SIEGEL, M.D., M.P.H.
Associate Professor of Pediatrics and Medicine
Co-Director, Pediatric Rheumatology
University of Rochester School of Medicine and Dentistry
Chief of Pediatrics
Rochester General Hospital, Rochester, New York
153: *Joint Pain*
229: *Juvenile Arthritis*
233: *Lyme Disease*

ARNOLD T. SIGLER, M.D.
Associate Professor of Pediatrics
The Johns Hopkins University School of Medicine
Baltimore, Maryland
135: *Fatigue and Weakness*

EDWARD M. SILLS, M.D.
Associate Professor of Pediatrics
The Johns Hopkins University School of Medicine
Director, Pediatric and Adolescent Rheumatology
Department of Pediatrics, Johns Hopkins Hospital
Baltimore, Maryland
243: *Osteochondroses*
265: *Spinal Deformities*

KATHY SILVERMAN, D.O.
Post-Doctoral Fellow, Division of Adolescent Medicine
Albert Einstein College of Medicine
Children's Hospital at Montefiore, Bronx, New York
20 (7): *Screening for Drugs*

NANCY WEST SIMEONSSON, R.N., M.P.H.
Clinical Assistant Professor, School of Nursing
University of North Carolina, Chapel Hill, North Carolina
20 (13): *Developmental Surveillance and Intervention*

RUNE J. SIMEONSSON, Ph.D., M.S.P.H.
Professor of Education, Research Professor of Psychology
University of North Carolina School of Education
Chapel Hill, North Carolina
20 (13): *Developmental Surveillance and Intervention*

JEAN C. SMITH, M.D.
Clinical Associate Professor of Pediatrics
University of North Carolina School of Medicine
Chapel Hill, North Carolina
Director, Crosby Clinic, Wake County Human Services
Raleigh, North Carolina
114: *Abdominal Pain*

SHIRLEY A. SMOYAK, R.N., Ph.D.
Professor of Public Health
Rutgers, the State University of New Jersey
Adjunct Professor, Department of Family Medicine
Robert Wood Johnson Medical School
New Brunswick, New Jersey
55: *Changing American Families*

DAVID M. SNYDER, M.D.
Associate Clinical Professor of Pediatrics
University of California at San Francisco School of Medicine
San Francisco, California
Medical Director, Developmental and Behavioral Pediatrics
Valley Children's Hospital, Madera, California
78: *Developmental Approach to Behavioral Problems*

ALFRED J. SPIRO, M.D.
Professor of Neurology and Pediatrics
Director, MDA Muscle Disease Clinic
Albert Einstein College of Medicine
Attending Physician, Department of Neurology and Pediatrics
Children's Hospital at Montefiore, Bronx, New York
150: *Hypotonia*

ANTHONY STALLION, M.D.
Assistant Professor of Pediatric Surgery
Case Western Reserve University School of Medicine
Rainbow Babies & Children's Hospital, Cleveland, Ohio
210: *Gastrointestinal Obstruction*

THOMAS J. STARC, M.D., M.P.H.
Professor of Clinical Pediatrics, Columbia University
Associate Attending, Department of Pediatrics
New York Presbyterian Medical Center, New York, New York
23 (3): *Preventive Cardiology*
257: *Rheumatic Fever*

BARBARA STARFIELD, M.D., M.P.H.
University Distinguished Professor
Department of Health Policy and Management and Pediatrics
The Johns Hopkins University, Johns Hopkins Hospital
Baltimore, Maryland
1: *The Health Care Delivery System*

JEFFREY R. STARKE, M.D.
Associate Professor of Pediatrics
Baylor University School of Medicine
Director, Children's Tuberculosis Clinic
Ben Taub General Hospital, Houston, Texas
271: *Tuberculosis*

CAROLE A. STASHWICK, M.D., Ph.D.
Associate Professor of Pediatrics, Director of Adolescent Program
Dartmouth Medical School, Hanover, New Hampshire
Children's Hospital at Dartmouth, Lebanon, New Hampshire
181: *Weight Loss*

DAVID H. STEIN, M.D., M.P.H.
Department of Dermatology
School of Medicine
Department of Health Policy and Management
School of Hygiene and Public Health
The Johns Hopkins University
Johns Hopkins Hospital and Hopkins Bayview Hospital
Baltimore, Maryland
199: *Contact Dermatitis*
227: *Insect Bites and Infestations*

CATHERINE STEVENS-SIMON, M.D.
Associate Professor of Pediatrics
University of Colorado Health Science Center
Children's Hospital/University Hospital, Denver, Colorado
111: *Adolescent Pregnancy and Parenthood*

JEFFREY J. STODDARD, M.D.
Senior Physician Researcher
Center for Studying Health System Change, Washington, D.C.
2: *Pediatrics and Managed Care*

R. SCOTT STRAHLMAN, M.D.
Instructor, Department of Pediatrics
The Johns Hopkins University School of Medicine
Baltimore, Maryland
Chief of Pediatrics, Patuxent Medical Group, Columbia, Maryland
187: *Appendicitis*
208: *Fractures and Dislocations*

VICTOR C. STRASBURGER, M.D.
Professor of Pediatrics
Chief, Division of Adolescent Medicine
University of New Mexico School of Medicine
Albuquerque, New Mexico
69: *Children, Adolescents, and the Media*

DONNA STROBINO, Ph.D.
Professor, Department of Population and Family
Johns Hopkins School of Public Health, Baltimore, Maryland
3: *Morbidity and Mortality Among the Young*

LAURENCE I. SUGARMAN, M.D.
Private Practice in Pediatrics
Clinical Assistant Professor of Pediatrics
University of Rochester School of Medicine and Dentistry
Rochester, New York
27: *Self-Regulation Therapies: Hypnosis and Biofeedback*

DENNIS M. SUPER, M.D., M.P.H.
Associate Professor of Pediatrics, Case Western Reserve University
Vice Chairman, Department of Pediatrics
MetroHealth Medical Center, Cleveland, Ohio
45 (5): *Neonatal Adaptations—Establishment of Equilibrium*
250: *Phimosis*

AMY L. SUSS, M.D.
Assistant Professor of Pediatrics
Director, Division of Adolescent Medicine
SUNY-Health Science Center at Brooklyn
Brooklyn, New York
89: *Fire-Setting*

MOIRA SZILAGYI, M.D., Ph.D.
Clinical Assistant Professor of Pediatrics
Department of Pediatrics
University of Rochester School of Medicine and Dentistry
Strong Memorial Hospital, Rochester, New York
54: *Foster Care and Adoption*

PETER G. SZILAGYI, M.D.
Associate Professor of Pediatrics
University of Rochester School of Medicine and Dentistry
Director of Ambulatory Pediatrics
Director, Division of General Pediatrics
Children's Hospital at Strong, Rochester, New York
13: *Compliance with Pediatric Health Care Recommendations*
18: *Immunizations*
185: *Animal Bites*
201: *Cystic and Solid Masses of the Face and Neck*

MARY ANNE TAN-LAXA, M.D.
Fellow in Neonatal-Perinatal Medicine
Hutzel Hospital/Children's Hospital of Michigan
Wayne State University, Detroit, Michigan
50: *Prenatal Drug Abuse and Neonatal Drug Withdrawal Syndrome*

ANNE MARIE THARPE, Ph.D.
Assistant Professor
Bill Wilkerson Center for Otolaryngology and Communication Sciences, Vanderbilt University Medical Center
Nashville, Tennessee
141: *Hearing Loss*

PHILIP E. THUMA M.D.
Senior Research Fellow and Lecturer
Department of Natural Sciences
Messiah College, Grantham, Pennsylvania
197: *Common Cold*
249: *Pharyngitis and Tonsillitis*

KRISTINE TORJESEN, M.D.
Primary Care Research Fellow, Harvard Medical School
Boston Children's Hospital, Boston, Massachusetts
12: *Cultural Issues in Primary Pediatric Care*

JULIAN J. TREVINO, M.D.
Chief, Department of Dermatology
Wright State University School of Medicine
Staff Physician, Department of Medicine
Children's Medical Center, Dayton, Ohio
46: *Skin Lesions of the Neonate*

MARTIN H. ULSHEN, M.D.
Professor of Pediatrics, Attending Pediatric Gastroenterologist
Duke University Medical Center, Durham, North Carolina
124: *Diarrhea and Steatorrhea*
155: *Loss of Appetite*
180: *Vomiting*

ELISE WILLEM VAN DER JAGT, M.D., M.P.H.
Associate Professor of Pediatrics and Critical Care
University of Rochester School of Medicine and Dentistry
Attending Physician, Children's Hospital at Strong
Rochester, New York
136: *Fever*
137: *Fever of Unknown Origin*

WILLIAM S. VARADE, M.D.
Associate Professor of Pediatrics
University of Rochester School of Medicine and Dentistry
Attending Physician, Children's Hospital at Strong
Rochester, New York
237: *Nephritis*
238: *Nephrotic Syndrome*

ROGER P. VERMILION, M.D.
Associate Professor of Pediatrics
University of Rochester School of Medicine and Dentistry
Attending Physician, Children's Hospital at Strong
Rochester, New York
198: *Congenital Heart Disease*

SUSAN VIG, Ph.D.
Associate Professor of Clinical Pediatrics
Albert Einstein College of Medicine
Senior Psychologist
Children's Evaluation and Rehabilitation Center
Rose F. Kennedy Center, Bronx, New York
19: *Identification of Developmental Delays and the Early Intervention System*

ALLEN R. WALKER, M.D.
Director of Pediatric Emergency Medicine
Assistant Professor of Pediatrics
The Johns Hopkins University School of Medicine
Director, Pediatric Emergency Department
The Johns Hopkins Children's Center, Baltimore, Maryland
276: *Coma*

AUDREY WALKER, M.D.
Assistant Clinical Professor
Department of Psychiatry and Pediatrics
Albert Einstein College of Medicine
Children's Hospital at Montefiore, Bronx, New York
172: *Strange Behavior*

ROBERT F. WARD, M.D.
Assistant Professor of Otolaryngology
Cornell University Medical College
Attending Physician, Department of Otolaryngology
The New York Hospital, Assistant Attending Physician
Manhattan Eye, Ear, and Throat Hospital, New York, New York
207: *Foreign Bodies of the Ear, Nose, Airway, and Esophagus*

RICHARD C. WASSERMAN, M.D., M.P.H.
Professor of Pediatrics, University of Vermont College of Medicine
Attending Pediatrician, Children's Health Care Service
Fletcher Allen Health Care, Burlington, Vermont
20 (11): *Vision Screening*

KRISTI L. WATTERBERG, M.D.
Professor of Pediatrics, The Pennsylvania State University
Department of Pediatrics/Division of Newborn Medicine
The Milton S. Hershey Medical Center, Hershey, Pennsylvania
47: *Signs and Symptoms of Neonatal Illness*

GEOFFREY A. WEINBERG, M.D.
Associate Professor of Pediatrics
University of Rochester School of Medicine and Dentistry
Director, Pediatric HIV Program, Children's Hospital at Strong
Rochester, New York
235: *Meningitis*

IRVING B. WEINER, Ph.D.
Professor of Psychiatry and Behavioral Medicine
University of South Florida, Tampa, Florida
93: *Psychosis*
106: *Juvenile Delinquency*

MICHAEL L. WEITZMAN, M.D.
Executive Director, American Academy of Pediatrics Center for Child Health Research
Professor and Associate Chairman
Department of Pediatrics, University of Rochester
School of Medicine and Dentistry, Rochester, New York
20 (6): *Screening for Lead Poisoning*
39: *The Chronically Ill and Disabled Child in School*
59: *Children of Divorce*
293: *Poisoning*

ESTHER H. WENDER, M.D.
Clinical Professor of Pediatrics
Albert Einstein College of Medicine, Bronx, New York
73: *Attention Deficit/Hyperactivity Disorder*
105: *Interviewing Adolescents*

STEVEN L. WERLIN, M.D.
Professor of Pediatrics, The Medical College of Wisconsin
Children's Hospital of Wisconsin, Milwaukee, Wisconsin
127: *Dysphagia*

JOHN S. WERRY, M.D.
Emeritus Professor of Psychiatry
University of Auckland, Auckland, New Zealand
175: *Tics*

CHARLES F. WHITTEN, M.D.
Associate Dean for Special Programs
Distinguished Professor Emeritus
Wayne State University School of Medicine, Detroit, Michigan
20 (12): *Screening—Sickle Cell Conditions*

JUDITH V. WILLIAMS, M.D.
Eastern Virginia Medical School
Division of Internal Medicine
Norfolk, Virginia
183: *Acne*
190: *Bacterial Skin Infections*
205: *Drug Eruptions*
274: *Verrucae (Warts)*

JENNIFER WILLOUGHBY, Ph.D.
Clinical Fellow, Department of Pediatrics
University of Maryland School of Medicine, Baltimore, Maryland
34: *Mental Retardation*

CRAIG M. WILSON, M.D.
Associate Professor
Departments of Pediatrics, Geographic Medicine, Epidemiology and International Health, and Microbiology
University of Alabama at Birmingham, Birmingham, Alabama
211: *Giardiasis*
251: *Pinworm Infestations*

MODENA HOOVER WILSON, M.D.
Professor of Pediatrics
The Johns Hopkins University School of Medicine
Baltimore, Maryland
Director, Department of Committees and Sections
American Academy of Pediatrics, Chicago, Illinois
23 (2): *Injury Control*
160: *Odor (Unusual Urine and Body)*

BEATRICE L. WOOD, Ph.D.
Associate Professor of Psychiatry and Pediatrics
State University of New York at Buffalo School of Medicine
Associate Director of Pediatric Psychiatry
Children's Hospital at Buffalo, Buffalo, New York
52: *Theories and Concepts of Development as They Relate to Pediatric Practice*

ROBERT A. WOOD, M.D.
Associate Professor of Pediatrics
The Johns Hopkins University School of Medicine
Baltimore, Maryland
184: *Allergic Rhinitis*

KATHLEEN A. WOODIN, M.D.
Division of General Pediatrics
Carolinas Medical Center, Charlotte, North Carolina
Appendix C: *Miscellaneous Values*

JEROME Y. YAGER, M.D., F.R.C.P.(C)
Professor of Pediatrics
University of Saskatchewan, Saskatoon, Saskatchewan, Canada
191: *Brain Tumors*

W. SAM YANCY, M.D.
Clinical Professor of Pediatrics, Duke University Medical Center
Attending Pediatrician, Durham Regional Hospital
Durham, North Carolina
98: *Adolescence*

MYRON YASTER, M.D.
Associate Professor
Departments of Anesthesiology, Critical Care Medicine, and Pediatrics
The Johns Hopkins University School of Medicine
Baltimore, Maryland
9: *Preoperative Assessment*
26: *Management of Acute Pain in Children*
253: *Postoperative Management of the Pediatric Outpatient: Surgical and Anesthetic Aspects*

MICHAEL W. YOGMAN, M.D.
Associate in Medicine, Department of Pediatrics
Boston Children's Hospital, Boston, Massachusetts
78: *Developmental Approach to Behavioral Problems*

GUY YOUNG, M.D.
Assistant Professor of Pediatric Hematology/Oncology
University of Maryland, Baltimore, Maryland
225: *Idiopathic Thrombocytopenia*

RICHARD S.K. YOUNG, M.D., M.P.H.
Associate Clinical Professor of Pediatrics and Neurology
Yale University School of Medicine
Chair, Department of Pediatrics, Hospital of Saint Raphael
New Haven, Connecticut
236: *Meningoencephalitis*

AGLAIA ZELLOS, M.D.
Assistant Professor of Pediatrics
Division of Pediatric Gastroenterology and Nutrition
The Johns Hopkins University School of Medicine
Johns Hopkins Hospital, Baltimore, Maryland
216: *Hepatitis*

Foreword

Primary care has become the recognized term for the field of general medicine practiced largely in the office and community. The term now is highly visible, whereas three decades ago it was scarcely known. Our nation's need for more primary care physicians is the subject of great debate, as is how to accomplish this. In contrast to three decades ago, primary care has achieved academic respectability; both faculty and practitioners are in demand. It is a field whose time in the sun is now. This textbook, *Primary Pediatric Care,* now in its fourth edition, has been one of the major forces leading to acceptance of the field because of its contribution to the knowledge base necessary to educate students, residents, fellows, and practitioners in the field. It recognizes that the care of children is broad and complex and requires the ability to synthesize biological and psychosocial data, to have skills of communication, and to understand, as the editors state, "the determinants and reflections of health and disease."

This text also provides essential information about the health care system, as well as knowledge about promotion of health and prevention of disease, aspects of pediatric practice that account for nearly half of pediatric visits. It deals with complex medical-social issues such as substance abuse, contraception and abortion, adoption, children of gay or lesbian parents, school problems, child abuse, and delinquency—topics difficult to find in traditional pediatric texts—but does not neglect presentation of traditional clinical problems. New to this edition are chapters on screening for behavioral problems, managed care, a family systems approach to the care of children, complementary and alternative medicine therapies, homelessness and the family, sequelae to infertility, domestic violence and the family, and school readiness. Its focus is always on prevention and on diagnosis and treatment of disease presenting in the office or primary care setting rather than in the hospital, although some of these conditions, especially if not diagnosed and treated early, require hospitalization. This ability to deal broadly and comprehensively with child health distinguishes the primary care pediatrician. This text provides the knowledge to allow pediatricians to fulfill this role effectively.

In the past, much of this typical information was gained after starting in practice, if ever. Today there is a research-based knowledge of many of these complex issues. This up-to-date text documents this research base, essential for anyone providing continuing health care for children. Textbooks, similar to all species, have a primary task—survival in a changing world. To have reached a fourth edition, *Primary Pediatric Care* demonstrates survival skills in today's rapidly changing world. It provides the primary care pediatrician, as well as the student, resident, fellow, and other practitioners, with the knowledge to survive and to thrive, and more important, to provide health care of high quality to children—the hope for the future of our human species.

Robert J. Haggerty, M.D.

Professor and Chair Emeritus
Department of Pediatrics
University of Rochester
School of Medicine and Dentistry

Preface

The practice of pediatrics has become increasingly complicated over the years, as knowledge of the etiology, pathophysiology, and management of physical, emotional, behavioral, and social ills has developed more rapidly and fully.

Although the dimensions of pediatrics have grown, the education of the pediatrician has remained, for the most part, disease-oriented and pathophysiological in substance. However, educators have demonstrated awareness of the gap between this disease orientation and the actual practice of primary health care, and they have made major efforts to adjust teaching programs to reflect the actual practice of the majority of pediatricians. This has been done, primarily, by placing medical students and residents in primary care pediatricians' offices and within community health–related facilities for significant portions of their training, while the pathophysiological priority has been maintained in the belief that given a sound disease-oriented experience, the primary care provider can acquire the other, softer, "easier" knowledge of health care—"on the job." It now generally is accepted that much of this practice and community-related knowledge needs to be acquired earlier on.

The purpose of this text is to provide much of the pertinent information concerning the determinants and reflections of health and of disease prenatally and perinatally, and during infancy, childhood, and adolescence. The primary provider of health care to the young should be in command of this information, which constitutes a body of knowledge not now conveniently available to the student and practitioner in one repository. It may seem more subjective than the "harder" pathophysiological knowledge base and, therefore, less scientific. It is not. Indeed, its variables are infinite and its experiments more difficult to control. Although pathophysiological knowledge is treated throughout this text, the book focuses on the *determinants* of health and disease; it attempts to be comprehensive only in regard to this body of knowledge. The reader is referred to other sources when information in greater depth in other areas is required. In Parts Seven, Eight, and Nine, our authors have provided suggestions for *when to refer* and *when to hospitalize*. A chapter on complementary and alternative medical therapies has been added to this edition to fill this need in many situations. Cited references to scientific publications are used, and contributors have identified and clarified controversial issues whenever possible.

The scope of this text, then, is different from that of traditional pediatric texts in that *all* aspects of *health* care are considered. The breadth and depth of the discussion of *illness,* however, are limited to that information which the primary care provider needs to function effectively in his or her role. The rarer diseases and the esoteric points in etiological, pathophysiological, and therapeutic considerations of the more common diseases are not included here. The message is that the physical and emotional health of the child can be adequately maintained by the primary care provider (1) through well-child visits, which focus on prevention and early detection of disease and of psychosocial dysfunction, and (2) through competent management of acute and chronic illness with or without the help of other professionals.

In using this text, our readers are asked to keep in mind the following five questions: (1) What does the primary care provider need to know about the condition or disease being described to recognize it? (2) How should the condition be managed? (3) When should consultation be sought or referral to a specialist be made? (4) What can the primary care provider expect the consultant to do for the patient? and (5) What role should the primary care provider play in the management of care after a referral has been made? Certain general considerations to guide one's thinking include prevention, screening, and emergency management, as well as collaborative care, follow-up care, and costs. Family, community, environmental, and political influences on the presentation and outcome of the condition also must be considered.

We hope that this book will provide all primary health care practitioners with most of the information required to understand and manage the various problems they encounter in caring for the young. It would be extremely difficult, if not impossible, for any one text to provide all the information such practitioners require. We do not pretend to do so but urge the reader (medical student, resident, or practitioner) to seek that information not found herein from references we have provided or from other comprehensive pediatric textbooks that emphasize different elements of health care of the young.

This textbook would not have been published without the help and support of many persons. The names and affiliations of the 322 contributing authors are given in the list of contributors.

Our publication staff provided us with the essentials editors need: opportunity, direction, proficiency, provocation, criticism, and, above all, reassurance and patience. Anne Salmo, Ellen Baker Geisel, and Liz Fathman gave us these and more.

Editorial comment and direction were given by Sydney A. Sutherland, based at the University of Rochester. Her assistance in ensuring the seemingly impossible—the smooth and continual communication among authors, editors, and publishers—is especially appreciated.

We thank all of these good people for their interest, expertise, and understanding.

Robert A. Hoekelman
Henry M. Adam
Nicholas M. Nelson
Michael L. Weitzman
Modena Hoover Wilson

Introduction

Robert A. Hoekelman

There is no doubt that those who are concerned with the delivery of child health care face serious difficulties in finding the resources and mechanisms to ensure that all children in need of preventive, maintenance, and curative services receive them. No matter how the pediatric health care pie is sliced, as it currently exists, all the appetites will not be satisfied. This is true for those who seek these services and even more so for the greater numbers who are in need yet do not recognize that need or do not have the resources to seek the appropriate care.

Any review of health care needs and prospects for meeting them demands an assessment of the services that are required, how these can be organized and delivered effectively and efficiently, who will deliver these services, and how these persons can be prepared to do so.

Traditionally, primary care pediatricians have conducted high-volume practices in solo or partnership arrangements. They have provided preventive services and health maintenance supervision and have managed acute minor illnesses on an ambulatory basis. Only a small part of their efforts, however, has been spent in the diagnosis and treatment of serious illness in the hospital, for which most of their postgraduate training prepared them. These problems have increasingly been referred to subspecialty pediatricians located in large medical centers, either because primary care pediatricians have not had the time to deal with such problems or because their knowledge and skills in the management of severe illness have atrophied from disuse.

Most pediatricians have learned to do what they do through on-the-job experience rather than through formal training, albeit this has changed to some extent in recent years with increasing emphasis being placed on ambulatory care training. To many, the content of private practice comes somewhat as a surprise. Some pediatricians are not satisfied with this role and turn to subspecialty training and practice, but most adjust quickly and find primary care practice extremely rewarding.

There are, however, forces coming to bear on the future of primary pediatric practice over which the individual physician has little or no control. These forces are as follows:

1. The incidence of serious disease in childhood is decreasing because of public and individual preventive health measures: therefore, the number of these illnesses occurring in a single practice is diminishing.
2. The reproductive behavior of the population is changing. The use of contraceptive devices and the liberalization of abortion laws have decreased the birth rate significantly, particularly in the populations served by most pediatricians. Infant mortality, prematurity, and morbidity have diminished as well, and the regionalization of perinatal care has transferred the management of most high-risk newborn infants from the primary care pediatrician to neonatologists in regional centers.
3. The rapid increase in medical knowledge and technology has produced methods of treatment for many childhood diseases that can be provided only in large institutions by specialists who devote most of their efforts to these problems. The primary care physician, therefore, cannot morally or ethically elect to continue to care for these patients.
4. Other professionals have demonstrated their ability to provide competently much of the care currently undertaken by the practicing pediatrician. Family practitioners, pediatric nurse practitioners, and physicians' assistants are capable of providing those services, working with or independent of the pediatrician.
5. Private practice has moved toward consumer control. Demands are being made on the practitioner to institute new organizational and financial arrangements in the provision of primary care. Issues of cost, availability, acceptability, accountability, and efficacy of care provided must be dealt with by each practitioner individually or through managed care organizational arrangements.

These forces need not be viewed negatively; rather, they can be used by pediatric practitioners to improve the health care available to children. Pediatric practice needs to be reorganized to meet the needs of all children, not just those for whom care is sought. Care must also become more continuous and comprehensive and must be coordinated with the health-related needs of children that are met by others. Pediatricians have to relate to the broader issues that affect the health of children within the family structure, within the community, and within the greater environment.

The list of these issues, long neglected, is extensive and includes specific problems within the areas of education (attaining full intellectual potential), communication (understanding and being understood), socialization (behaving appropriately with others), and normalization (functioning within acceptable limits) for both well and ill children. Efforts to deal with these issues effectively need to be directed through the community. The prospect for success in effecting improvement in the health of children probably is greater along this avenue than in the provision of individual health care. It is clear that practicing pediatricians cannot accomplish these goals without working collaboratively with other professionals within and outside the practice setting.

This change in the complexion of primary care practice requires changes in our system of undergraduate and graduate medical education. The curriculum must be altered to include educational objectives commensurate with the activities of primary care physicians and to exclude objectives that are no longer pertinent to practice. Early identification and tracking of students who plan to enter primary care versus those who plan on subspecialty practice within academia or outside is needed, and interdisciplinary education with other professionals who will be working collaboratively with physicians in team-oriented care needs to be instituted. In addition, the milieu in which medical education takes place must be supportive of the broader concept of the practice of primary care.

Primary care has been defined to the satisfaction of almost everyone, and educational programs to prepare physicians to provide such care to children have emerged in response to reason, demand, and dictum. Questions now arise as to who should provide the bulk of that care and how it can best be organized to ensure that the health care needs of all our children are met. The politics of primary pediatric care begin to occupy more of our thoughts and discussion.

Part One of this book, Delivering Pediatric Health Care, presents an analysis of pediatric care in the United States, including how it is delivered and paid for, the morbidity and mortality that occur, the application of child health supervision designed to promote health and reduce morbidity and mortality, the legal and ethical issues that affect the way pediatrics is practiced, and the methods used in promoting the health and development of children and their families community-wide.

Part Two, Evaluation and Communication, addresses the diagnostic process, which begins with construction of a database through the gathering of historical information concerning the patient's illness, the conducting of a complete examination to detect deviations from the normal physical status, and the performing of specific tests to analyze the structure and function of the body systems that may be involved. The process continues with assimilation of the information gathered to reach a provisional or definitive diagnosis, with or without assistance from consulting specialists and the medical literature. It moves to communication of the diagnosis to the patient and parents so that they understand the problem, what can be done to solve it, and their role in its management.

Pediatric patients must be managed with the understanding that to a great extent, they depend on others to ensure their optimum growth and development, their protection from the acquisition of disease, and their recovery from illness. Those largely responsible for these assurances, in turn, depend on health professionals to guide them in the use of the means by which those assurances can best be realized.

Part Two continues with a discussion of how practitioners perceive and respond to the cultural issues that affect how medicine is practiced among selected ethnic populations and how compliance with pediatric health care recommendations can be enhanced in general, both at the primary care level and at the level of consultation with subspecialists. It ends with how physicians communicate with one another through the medical literature.

Part Three, Principles of Patient Care, explores the general principles of prevention and treatment that are applicable to the comprehensive care of the young. It deals with the maintenance of health and prevention of disease in well children through screening for and prevention of illnesses, and with conventional and alternative therapies directed to acutely and chronically ill children, stressing aspects of illness care that are unique to the pediatric patient, including complementary and alternative therapies.

Practitioners of medicine in the United States and other highly developed nations often approach health care of children as though it were separate from that of the rest of the family. Yet common sense tells us that attention to the mother, her pregnancy, the fetus, and the birth process is mandatory for optimal care of the child. These are addressed in Part Four, The Reproductive Process.

Understanding the parents' genetic makeup is essential for the physician who is in the position of giving advice about continuing a pregnancy or undertaking another one. Similarly, an understanding of conception control methods and abortion issues is necessary.

The environment of the developing baby likewise influences the outcome of pregnancy; therefore, knowledge of the transfer of noxious substances across the placenta is valuable, as is familiarity with diagnostic methods such as amniocentesis, ultrasound, and fetoscopy.

As the identification of risk during pregnancy becomes better understood, the developing fetus can be made safe from adverse intrauterine influences. Nutritional requirements of the fetus are now better understood, one consequence being that most physicians no longer starve the mother to keep her weight down during pregnancy.

Personal adaptation (both emotional and physical) of women to pregnancy has been given new emphasis in an attempt to provide caring, individual prenatal services. The involvement of physicians, nurse practitioners, other health workers, and laypersons in educational programs for pregnant women has led to improved services for women and children.

Development of regional facilities and programs for high-risk perinatal patients has promoted successful pregnancies, just as tertiary care obstetrical and newborn services have improved the outcome for newborns and older infants who have serious medical problems.

Part Five, The Newborn, addresses the specifics of the care of the newborn baby from the perspective of the primary care practitioner. Even though much of the technology described is applied by neonatologists, the practitioner must be able to recognize those situations in which neonatologists should be consulted and must be able to apply initial therapeutic measures to stabilize the condition of the sick infant until help can be obtained.

Children are the center of a "universe"; they are surrounded in successive rings by the family and the community. In Part Six, Psychosocial Issues in Child Health Care, we address not only specific diagnoses and problems but also the theories of psychological development and the influences of the family, the school, and society on the psychological and physical well-being of infants, children, and adolescents.

Although the pediatric patient's demographic characteristics (age, sex, race, socioeconomic status), ethical influences, and geographic and seasonal environments direct a practitioner's thoughts to specific diagnoses, the presenting signs and symptoms are more persuasive. They immediately bring to mind many diagnostic possibilities and rule out many others. Differential diagnosis begins with consideration of the potential cause of each sign observed by the examiner and each symptom experienced by the patient. It ends when only one cause remains to explain all of the patient's signs and symptoms; at least this usually is the case.

Seventy signs and symptoms commonly encountered in pediatric practice are discussed in Part Seven, Presenting Signs and Symptoms. Most also are mentioned in other parts of the book in discussions of specific diseases.

Pediatric practice surveys, among other things, catalog the diagnoses made by pediatricians for patients they care for in their offices. The 91 diagnoses discussed in Part Eight, Specific Clinical Problems, along with well-child care, constitute the reasons for most office visits made to pediatricians. Almost all the rest of the visits are related to various psychosocial issues discussed in Part Six. These 91 diagnoses also include most of the reasons for hospitalizing pediatric patients beyond the newborn period. The 24 remaining reasons for hospitalization in this age group (except for those resulting from a small number of rare diseases) are discussed in Part Nine, Critical Situations.

The primary care pediatric practitioner is seldom called on to intervene in critical situations that threaten the life of an infant, child, or adolescent. However, regardless of the practice location and the availability of subspecialists who assist in such crises, each practitioner should be prepared to make appropriate decisions or to take immediate actions that will lead to positive outcomes in such situations. To this end, the methods for management of emergency life-threatening conditions are presented. Appendix A details the methods required for Pediatric Basic and Advanced Life Support. Appendix B, Special Procedures, provides detailed instructions for performing the procedures that may be required in the management of the critical situations described.

Appendix C, Miscellaneous Values, and Appendix D, Common Psychological and Educational Tests, provide the balance of the information pediatric practitioners need to aid themselves in the interpretation of data gathered for the assessment and management of their patients.

Contents

PART SEVEN
PRESENTING SIGNS AND SYMPTOMS

PART EIGHT
SPECIFIC CLINICAL PROBLEMS

PART NINE
CRITICAL SITUATIONS

Appendixes

Primary Pediatric Care

part one

Delivering Pediatric Health Care

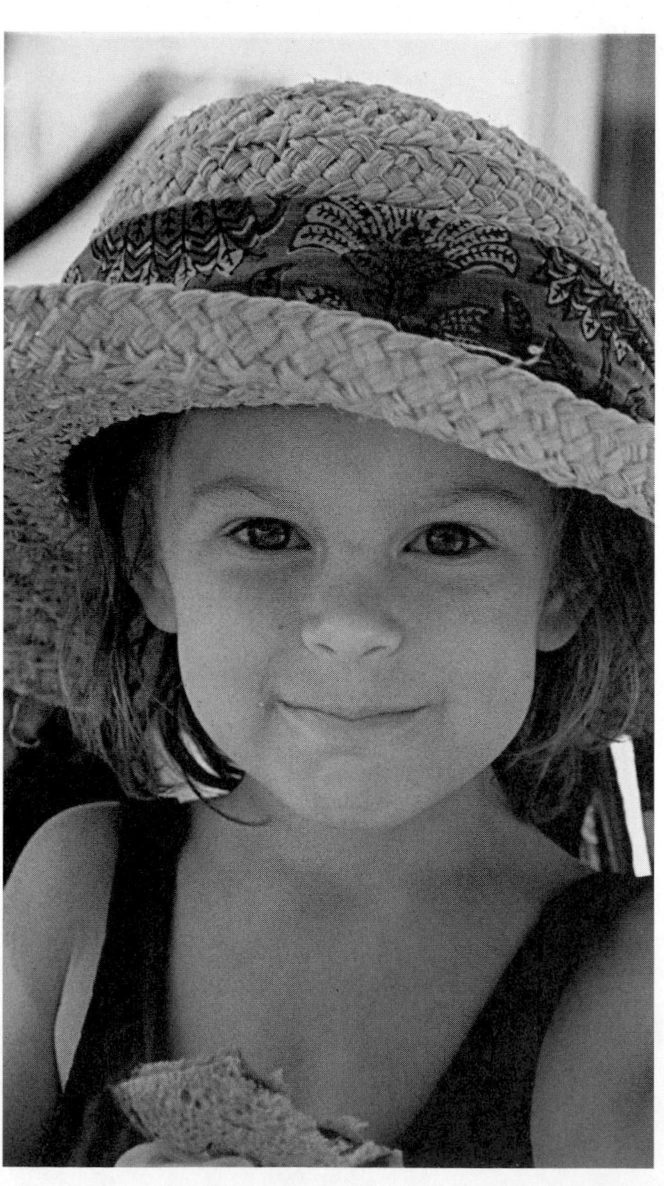

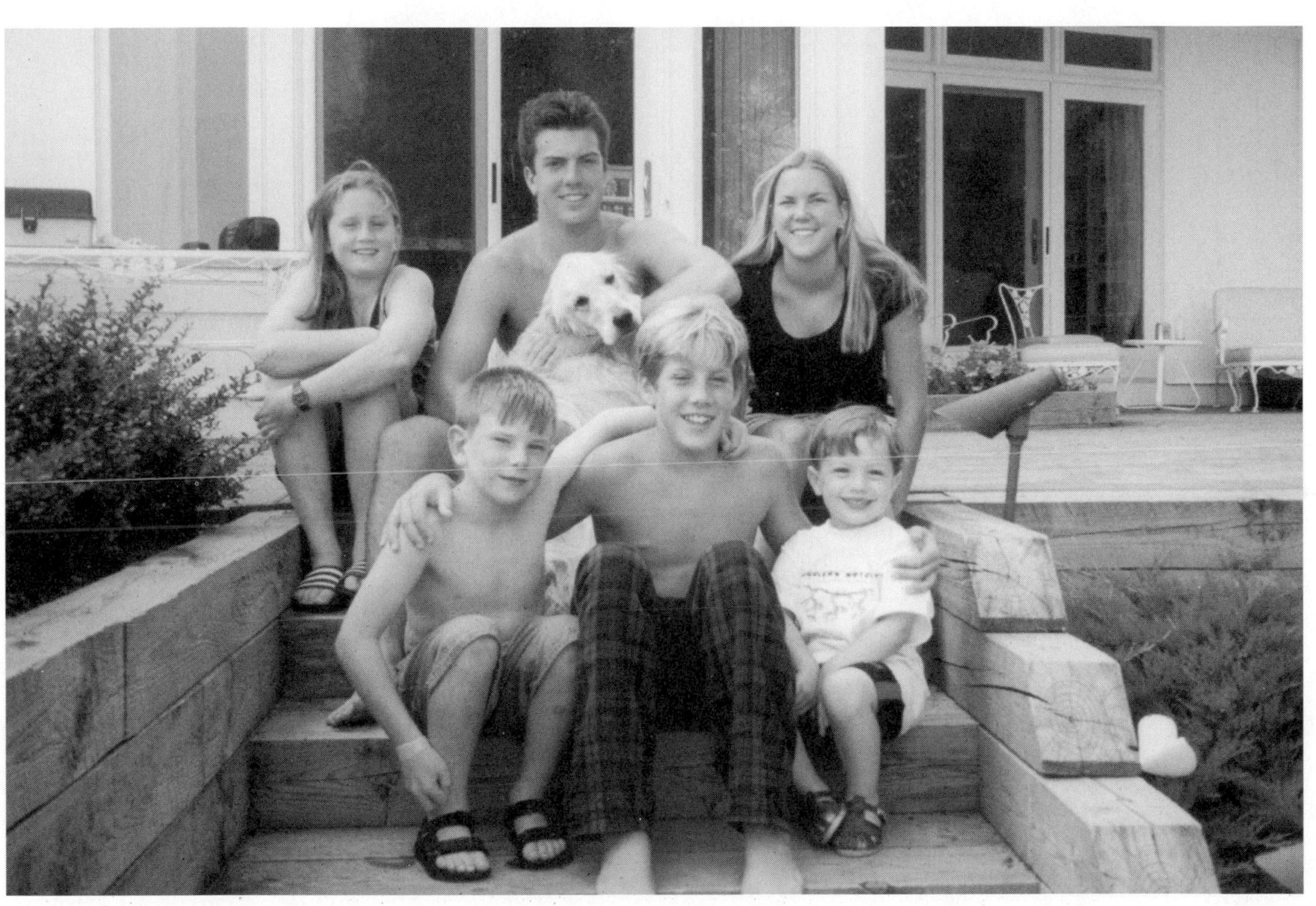

1 The Health Care Delivery System

Edward J. Saltzman • Barbara Starfield

As *the* medical specialty targeted to improving the health of infants, children, adolescents, and young adults, pediatrics plays an important role in the U.S. health care system. Established as a specialty for more than 60 years, it continues to change dramatically in response to vast increases in medical knowledge, preventive health practices, technical advances, and the changing infrastructure of the health care delivery system.

The pediatrician is the major decision maker for care delivered to patients in the above-mentioned age groups.

In 1997, the total number of physicians in the United States was 756,710, with 7.3% (55,240) being self-designated pediatricians—38,988 board certified and 16,252 non-board certified. Women constituted 22% of all physicians and 47% of all U.S. pediatricians were women, a higher percentage than in all other fields of medicine; 64% of 1998 pediatric residents were women. This percentage undoubtedly will increase even further. A large proportion of pediatricians are young; in 1998, only 26% were older than 55 and 58% were younger than age 45, which makes pediatricians, on average, younger than other physicians. Of note is that in 1999, 37% of women physicians had worked part time at some point in their careers, and 21% were currently working part time.

Interest in pediatrics as a career continues to be strong. The National Residency Matching Program (NRMP) results for 1999 showed that 13.3% of U.S. medical school graduates chose pediatric residencies, an increase of 0.4% from 1998. Although more than 50% of U.S. medical school graduates chose primary care specialties, only pediatrics had an increased number of matches. Internal medicine match choices decreased from 34% to 33.2%. Family practice choices decreased from 16% in 1998 to 14.7% in 1999.

Of the new residency positions offered for general pediatrics training in 1998, 82.4% were filled by graduates of U.S. medical schools and 17.4% by international medical graduates. The fill rate of pediatric residency positions was 98.9% in 1998.

In 1999, there were 226 accredited pediatric residency training programs in the United States and 16 in Canada; 9459 pediatricians were enrolled in those programs—7703 in general pediatrics, 1622 in medicine-pediatrics, and 131 in other programs—pediatrics/physical medicine and rehabilitation, pediatrics/emergency medicine, pediatrics/psychiatry/child and adolescent psychiatry. Combined pediatrics/medicine/genetics residency training programs began enrolling residents during the 1998-1999 academic year.

In the 1970s, the American Board of Pediatrics and the American Board of Internal Medicine agreed that individuals who had 2 years of general internal medicine and 2 years of general pediatrics were eligible for board certification in both specialties. In 1998, combined "med-peds" residency programs in the United States offered 456 first-year positions in 106 programs; 89% of the 1622 residents enrolled were graduates of U.S. medical schools. Since 1988, the number of residents entering these positions has increased 135%. The percentage of women enrolled is less than in categorical pediatrics but is increasing annually. Between two thirds and three fourths of "med-peds" residents enter primary care practice; the rest choose subspecialty training. Some 87% of med-peds physicians in community-based general practice care for both adults and children. Med-peds physicians provide 33% to 40% of the care they deliver to families that include children, while family physicians provide between 15% to 27% of the care they deliver to families that include children.

In rural communities or small towns, med-peds physicians may play a role as a consultant in the care of high-risk newborns and children who have a chronic illness or as a hospitalist for children and adults. In more competitive environments, internal medicine and pediatric practices can use the med-peds physician to attract new patients, especially adolescents and families desiring health care for everyone in the same practice.

INTERNATIONAL MEDICAL GRADUATES

By 1998, the number of international medical graduates (IMG) practicing pediatrics in the United States had grown 300% since 1970. In 1997, 9% of the IMG physicians in the United States were pediatricians, comprising 29% of the pediatrician work force. There has been a remarkable decline in the number of IMGs who have started training in the past few years. In 1993, 36.7% of all first-year residency training positions were filled by IMGs. For the 1998-1999 year, this figure was 18%. This change has occurred at a time when overall numbers of categorical pediatricians and medicine/pediatric residents in the first year of training have been relatively constant (3009 in 1993 versus 3063 in 1999).

According to 1998-1999 data collected by the American Board of Pediatrics, approximately 43% of pediatric subspecialty fellows were IMGs, although they constituted only 28% of pediatric residents.

Table 1-1 Number of Board-Certified Pediatric Subspecialists through 1998

	Certified
Adolescent medicine (1994)*	341
Cardiology (1961)	1470
Critical care medicine (1987)	869
Emergency medicine (1992)	949
Endocrinology (1978)	794
Gastroenterology (1990)	587
Hematology-oncology (1974)	1472
Infectious diseases (1994)	670
Medical technology (1994)	20
Neonatology-perinatology (1975)	3382
Nephrology (1974)	529
Pulmonology (1986)	596
Rheumatology (1992)	164
Sports medicine (1993)	46

*Year in parentheses indicates when subspecialty board was established.
Diane Butzin, American Board of Pediatrics: Personal communication, 1999.

Table 1-2 Pediatric Subspecialty Choices of First-Time Takers of the General Pediatrics Certifying Examination: Number of Examinees—1997

	Number
Adolescent medicine	20
Behavioral/developmental	18
Cardiology	82
Critical care medicine	82
Emergency medicine	79
Endocrinology	40
Gastroenterology	48
Hematology-oncology	84
Infectious diseases	49
Neonatal-perinatal medicine	143
Nephrology	26
Pharmacology/toxicology	1
Pulmonology	32
Rheumatology	9
Sports medicine	1

Diane Butzin, American Board of Pediatrics: Personal communication, 1999.

PEDIATRIC SUBSPECIALIZATION

Pediatric training has seen a remarkable growth pattern in recent years. The largest percentage increase among primary care practitioners was in pediatrics (181% from 1970 to 1997); internal medicine grew 135% and family medicine, 72%. In contrast, pediatric subspecialty training growth was 860%. There are 12 areas of pediatric subspecialization certifiable by the American Board of Pediatrics (Table 1-1).

The trend toward pediatric subspecialty training seems to have abated. Data regarding career choice collected from first-time candidates for ABP certifying examinations in 1999 showed that more than 73% chose a career in general pediatrics (57% in 1990), while 25% indicated plans to enter a pediatrics or pediatric-related subspecialty.

The reasons for this downward trend in pediatric subspecialization may indicate a bona fide increased interest in generalist care, accumulated debt that discourages more training, funding limitations for subspecialty training programs, limited future faculty positions, and a concern about the impact of managed care on job availability for pediatric subspecialists.

International medical graduates continue to choose pediatric subspecialty training at higher rates than do American medical graduates. In 1994, 34% of IMGs chose pediatric subspecialty training, while in 1998 approximately 30% did so.

Of those taking the 1997 ABP general pediatric certifying examination who indicated a pediatric subspecialty choice, neonatal-perinatal medicine has remained the most popular. But a relatively new pediatric subspecialty, emergency medicine, is approaching a par with cardiology, critical care medicine, and hematology-oncology as the second most popular choice (Table 1-2).

Only 59% of the certified pediatric subspecialists' time is spent in direct patient care. The remainder is spent in administration, research, and teaching, because 60% practice in academic health centers, compared with fewer than 33% of internal medicine subspecialists who do so. For those not in academia, almost 50% of endocrinologists and gastroenterologists do part-time work in general pediatrics, as do 73% of those entering nephrology. Fourteen percent of those in neonatal-perinatal medicine practice general pediatrics part time.

ALTERNATIVE SOURCES OF CARE FOR CHILDREN

A good deal of pediatric care in the United States is delivered by family practitioners, medicine-pediatric physicians, and internists. It is estimated that 20% of pediatric services are delivered by family practitioners; a smaller percentage is delivered by med-peds physicians and internists. These percentages in rural areas may be slightly higher.

Ancillary clinical personnel—physician extenders—are part of the new staffing and off-hours coverage being used by pediatricians. There is the pressure of the need to increase practice volume, and there is a strong emphasis on office management. The terms *physician extenders* or *mid-level providers* apply to pediatric nurse practitioners (PNPs), physician assistants (PAs), and telephone triage personnel.

PNPs are one category of advanced-practice nurses who are significantly involved in the primary care team. They have, in general, 580 hours of clinical training, are usually prepared at the masters degree level, and also may be certified in a specialty. They conduct physical examinations, track medical histories, make diagnoses, treat minor illnesses and injuries, and provide an array of counseling and educational services. In some states, PNPs prescribe medications, admit patients to hospitals, and make hospital rounds.

PAs are health personnel who typically are trained in 2 or 3 years to render basic health services that also are performed by physicians, mostly under the supervision of pediatricians.

The demand is huge for PNPs (approximately 10,000 in the United States) and for PAs, (approximately 6000 in pediatric activity). It is estimated that 33% of PNPs practice in hospital clinics, 23% in private pediatric practices, 13% in community and public health settings, and 30% in schools and health maintenance organizations. They tend to be less costly than pediatricians, yet patient satisfaction with their services is high. In some underserved and rural areas, they are the only source of primary pediatric care. PNPs and PAs may practice independently in some states. In the late 1990s, 26 states allowed PNPs and PAs to treat patients without physician oversight, and 49 states allow them some type of prescriptive authority.

PATIENT-CALL CENTERS

Traditional pediatric practices have long assumed that answering telephone calls outside of office hours is part of their responsibility. Today, there is an additional need for telephone authorization of care rendered by physicians or at facilities during off hours that requires negotiations on the patients' behalf via telephone.

Because pediatricians' obligations to their patients do not cease when the office closes and because many calls are for nonurgent matters, pediatric call centers have developed in all areas of the United States.

Call centers, or After-Hours Programs (AHP), are staffed by trained personnel on nights, weekends, and holidays. They give advice for symptomatic care and appropriate prescription refills, make referrals to an emergency facility or to an after-hours pediatric office, or advise seeing the patient's own pediatrician during office hours. AHPs operate under professional overview, using protocols provided by pediatricians utilizing their services. Often, health care systems subsidize AHPs on behalf of their network of pediatricians because of the efficiency and cost savings attributed to them.

Before the introduction of AHPs, utilization studies documented that more than 50% of pediatric after-hours visits to emergency rooms were not essential. Data compiled by one AHP showed that 50% of the calls to the center resulted in parents receiving home-care advice, 30% resulted in next-day visits with the child's pediatrician, and only 20% led to after-hours emergency room visits. Thus, the AHP was able to change the utilization of medical resources efficiently and economically, a fact well noticed by third-party payers of health care.

In 1999, call centers served more than 35 million patients in the United States and, at their current rate of growth, could cover 100 million patients by the year 2003.

HOSPITALISTS

The traditional American system of care in which primary care physicians have cared for their hospitalized patients is undergoing a revolutionary change in many urban and suburban areas. A recent alternative allows primary care physicians to relinquish the care of their hospitalized patients voluntarily to a new group of inpatient generalists called *hospitalists*.

Hospitalists are physicians who spend at least 25% of their time serving as the physician of record for hospitalized patients. Patients are referred by their primary care physicians and are referred back to their primary care physician at the time of hospital discharge. Strong emphasis is placed on communication between the two physicians during the patient's hospital stay. Many pediatricians request this type of service from emergency room pediatricians and critical care pediatricians when generalist pediatric hospitalists are not available.

The use of hospitalists allows for increased productivity by the office-based pediatrician. During office hours, it is difficult for a practitioner to leave the office with waiting patients to see a hospitalized patient. Other reported advantages of hospitalist usage include their competency in technical skills—skills easily lost to the physician who visits the hospital only occasionally, shorter patient hospital stays because of constant in-hospital supervision, and the immediate availability of urgent care.

Hospitalist practice is expected to grow, much like other in-hospital specialties such as emergency room pediatricians, critical care pediatricians, and neonatologists.

PRACTICE CHARACTERISTICS

Style and Content

Through much of the early and middle twentieth century, the practicing general pediatrician was the daily expert, always on call in the office for families in need or making frequent house calls and hospital rounds. The practitioner provided care to premature infants, to well and sick newborns, and to well and sick children in and out of the hospital. General pediatricians diagnosed and treated rheumatic fever, glomerulonephritis, all forms of infectious illnesses, and most forms of cardiac, neurological, and allergic diseases. In short, they dealt with all "minor" and most major illnesses. Subspecialists were few and far between, usually found only in academic medical centers. Concepts such as "primary," "secondary," and "tertiary" care were unknown, and pediatric intensivists, neonatologists, and other subspecialists did not exist in community hospitals. There was less time for parental health education because the pediatrician had to provide definitive care in the office, the home, and the hospital for virtually all diseases affecting their patients.

Today, the office-based, primary care pediatrician deals with illnesses that are only potentially serious. The patient almost always is seen in the office, rarely in the hospital, and almost never in the home. The variety of illnesses treated by the primary care pediatrician today does not even remotely resemble those of the past. Upper respiratory tract infections, moderate lower respiratory tract problems, feeding problems, gastrointestinal upsets, and minor trauma account for 75% to 85% of illness care. A large portion of practice time now is spent giving well-child care, dealing with family dynamics, and managing the new morbidities. Most primary care pediatricians devote much of their effort to:

- Providing prenatal counseling
- Providing immunization for all age groups in the practice, with prior educational advice as to the benefit, risk, and alternatives, if any, to immunization
- Preventing injuries by giving advice about seat belts, smoke alarms, water safety, home safety, poison control, and bicycle helmets
- Discussing the child's education with the family and supporting the achievement of educational goals from infancy through adolescence

- Becoming an expert on abuse avoidance, whether it be drug abuse, child abuse, or parental abuse
- Providing advice and support during divorce or other marital crises
- Advising families on lifestyle goals, such as the need for family time and for an understanding of work-related time constraints and stresses, and how the family copes with them
- Promoting good health through advice about a prudent diet and nutrition, exercise, and avoidance of bad health habits, such as smoking
- Encouraging community activism through knowledge and use of common resources and involvement with school boards, religious groups, school athletic programs, and community facilities
- Devoting time to the care of adolescents and young adults, with the twin goals of being able to provide guidance and anticipate problems and to be helpful in solving such problems; areas of special attention include sex education, understanding one's sexuality, avoiding sexually transmitted diseases, preventing drug and alcohol abuse and teenage pregnancy, and advising about education and career goals

The time a pediatrician spends in office practice remains challenging and interesting, although it is channeled differently than in the past.

Because the typical practitioner wants to be (and is becoming) less involved with illnesses that require time-consuming workups or acute care management, either on an outpatient or an inpatient basis, care increasingly is becoming limited to the office. Office-based pediatricians are spending less time in the hospital than in the past; in 1997, practicing pediatricians spent only 15% of their time on hospital rounds, a 9% decrease from 1984.

For example, referrals to hospital-based pediatric generalists and subspecialists have become commonplace for acute care and even normal newborn care and for pediatric representation during cesarean sections and other high-risk deliveries.

Referrals

Referrals are an important, but little understood aspect of practice. Between 2% and 3% of all pediatric visits lead to a referral. Referrals also are made in telephone conversations with parents, which account for about 25% of all referrals. For 75% of referrals, pediatricians anticipate sharing care with, not delegating care entirely to, the specialist; unfortunately, this is not often achieved.

Extended Hours and Satellite Offices

Families in which both parents work and one-parent families now make up the majority of families in the United States. As a result, group or solo practices in which physicians share coverage have been forced to extend their office hours to provide coverage during evenings and on weekends, in addition to on-call coverage at night. This is a radical departure from the office hours that pediatricians traditionally provided.

After-hours coverage is provided in settings that are convenient, such as using the pediatrician's own office or an examination suite at the local community hospital. Many pediatricians join with their colleagues in sharing after-hours or weekend coverage. They take turns covering the telephone and meeting patients' needs, with prompt referral back to the patient's designated doctor. This provides efficient off-hours medical care and affords each practitioner more time for rest, relaxation, and the pursuit of personal interests.

Pediatricians also have embraced the concept of the satellite office as a response to the movement of young families to the suburbs. These offices offer the same complete pediatric care available in the "main" office but are more accessible to suburban dwellers. Satellite offices often outgrow the main office as communities change in character or demographics and establish an identity of their own.

Professional Liability

Pediatricians practice in an environment marked by skyrocketing professional liability claims and, concomitantly, very high malpractice insurance premiums. Some pay annual premiums as high as $25,000, which constitutes a significant percentage of their gross income. In the past, malpractice litigations involved surgeons almost exclusively. During 1997, pediatricians ranked eighth among medical specialists in the number of malpractice claims filed against them (4783) and second in the average payout made ($226,818) (Table 1-3). Common reasons for malpractice lawsuits against pediatricians include failure to diagnose meningitis or sepsis, delay in diagnosing congenital dislocation of the hip or congenital hypothyroidism, and mismanagement of croup and epiglottitis. Because of the variability among states in statutes of limitation for filing malpractice claims on behalf of minors and because of failure to set monetary limits for malpractice awards, pediatricians are at risk not only for high awards but also for settlement many years after the alleged malpractice occurred.

In the 1995 periodic survey by the American Academy of Pediatrics (AAP), it was found that, overall, there had been no change in the frequency or nature of pediatricians' experiences with malpractice suits over the prior 8 years.

The proportion of practicing pediatricians who have ever had a suit brought against them (28%) was similar to that reported in prior years. The proportion of pediatricians who were party to a suit while a resident (10%) also remained constant.

Almost 32% of the pediatric claims closed in 1997 resulted in an indemnity payment to the plaintiff, up from 27% in 1988. This percentage approximated that for all specialty groups (31%). Patients seen when covering another pediatrician's practice and hospitalized patients are most likely to generate malpractice suits.

To avoid malpractice suits, pediatricians should make prudent referrals, test appropriately, maintain good records, spend adequate time with patients, and use other techniques as listed in Box 1-1. However, there is no evidence that either adopting these approaches or attending risk-management educational programs in reducing medical malpractice suits is effective. Defensive medicine has had an economic impact

Table 1-3 1997 Malpractice Claims and Payments by Medical Specialty

	Claims	% Closed with Payout	Average Payout
Neurosurgery	3798	28.74	$235,738
Pediatrics	4783	29.61	226,818
Surgery, Ob/Gyn	22,217	36.43	216,392
Neurology	2194	20.48	215,358
Radiation therapy	1297	22.66	208,879
Pathology (nonsurgical)	1006	30.72	204,955
Cardiology	1978	18.85	182,453
Anesthesiology	5940	36.65	176,544
Surgery, cardiovascular and thoracic	4159	24.01	164,727
Internal medicine	20,319	27.36	153,028
Otorhinolaryngology	2530	32.20	151,282
Surgery, general	16,812	36.06	143,415
Emergency medicine	2217	28.37	140,038
Psychiatry	1557	22.86	136,021
Ophthalmology	4516	30.29	133,252
Surgery, orthopedic	15,729	30.07	130,563
Radiology	8162	29.96	127,466
Gastroenterology	1105	21.88	127,315
Family practitioners/general practitioners	17,372	37.42	122,172
Surgery, urological	3849	30.32	122,087
Gynecology	1812	32.76	109,333
Dermatology (nonsurgical)	1874	32.17	103,285
Surgery, plastic	6105	29.47	83,379

Data based on malpractice claims reported to the Physician Insurers Association of America (Rockville, Maryland) from 1985-1997. Modified from Preston SH: Malpractice danger zones: why primary care is more vulnerable than ever, *Med Econ* 75:106, 1998.

BOX 1-1

WAYS TO AVOID MALPRACTICE SUITS

Standards

- Meet normative standards of health care delivery (i.e., according to expert opinion as found in medical textbooks and articles in scientific journals) and/or empirical standards (i.e., according to local medical practice).

Communication

- Use positive methods in communicating with patients and parents, showing respect, understanding, concern, and compassion.
- Train staff to be sensitive to a patient's needs at all times.
- Train staff to manage patient telephone calls properly and to log all incoming and outgoing telephone calls, including patient problems and instructions given.

Documentation

- Record on the first page of a patient's chart his or her drug allergies and problem list.
- Record for each visit the history, findings on physical examination (including pertinent negative findings), diagnostic tests ordered (including their results), and treatment prescribed in sufficient detail for purposes of recall.
- Record all immunizations given and all screening test results.
- Record all telephone calls during which medical information about the patient was received or advice given; include date and time.
- Place in the patient's chart discharge summaries of hospitalizations and referral letters to and responses from consultants.
- Never alter a chart in response to a claim. If you must change the meaning of your note as a result of newer findings or recollections, write and date a new note referring to the previous note, leaving the original untouched.

Table 1-4 1998 Practice Organization Arrangements by Percentage for Physicians in the United States

	Cardiologists	Family Practitioners	General Practitioners	General Surgeons	Internists	Ob/Gyns	Orthopedic Surgeons	Pediatricians	All Surgical Specialists	All Non-Surgeons
Solo	40.1	53.2	89.4	58.8	52.4	53.7	43.8	42.9	47.9	51.0
Expense-sharers	8.5	8.9	2.9	7.0	8.1	9.7	17.3	3.3	9.4	7.7
Partnerships and groups of 2-3 physicians	13.7	15.7	4.0	14.5	9.5	13.4	9.9	14.6	12.7	11.5
4-9 physicians	17.9	9.9	1.7	11.2	13.0	16.1	18.8	23.8	15.1	14.9
10-24 physicians	11.4	6.2	<1.0	2.4	6.3	3.0	5.8	4.1	7.6	6.7
25-49 physicians	3.2	1.6	<1.0	1.3	3.5	1.3	1.3	3.3	3.1	2.4
50 or more physicians	5.2	4.3	1.7	4.6	7.0	2.7	3.0	8.0	4.1	5.7

Because of rounding, percentages may not total 100.
From Rice B: Flying solo and still flying high, *Med Econ* Pediatric edition, January 1999.

by increasing medical care expenditures. Some of these practice changes may improve medical care; others may be unnecessary or even harmful. Because of a perceived change in physician-patient relationships resulting from the threat of liability, the pleasure of practice has lessened. Changes that are fair and equitable to both the public and the medical profession depend on societal attention to this difficult problem.

Professional Activity

In the mid 1990s, the main professional activity of approximately 93% of pediatricians (both certified and noncertified) was the provision of patient care in the office and hospital. The remainder were engaged primarily in other professional activities such as teaching, research, and administration, or combinations of these.

Most pediatricians who provide patient care do so in group practices because of the overall benefits of merging, the demands of managed care, and the need for off-hours coverage. Still, almost 43% of pediatricians remain in solo practice (Table 1-4).

Pediatricians engaged in direct patient care practice an average of 47.3 weeks a year, a figure that has not changed since 1980. However, pediatricians in group practice spend an average of 2 weeks less per year at work than do those in solo practice.

Practicing pediatricians average 45 hours a week in direct patient contact, 7 hours a week in activities related to patient care (performing and interpreting diagnostic studies, consulting with other physicians, and talking to patients and parents by telephone), and 5 hours a week in administrative, teaching, or research activities. Thus, the average practitioner has a 57-hour work week.

Part-time pediatricians worked 32.3 hours a week in 1998, and the average number of hours did not differ by subspecialty or gender. For both general pediatricians and subspecialty pediatricians, child care responsibility was the primary reason for this "work" preference.

Visits to Pediatricians

In 1996, visits to pediatricians accounted for 96.8 million of the 734.5 million ambulatory care office visits made to primary care physicians in the United States. In 1997, pediatricians averaged 126 total visits per week—99 in the office, 18 as hospital visits, and the remainder in the emergency room and hospital or public health clinics. The greater illness burdens and the "new morbidity" issues among adolescents and young adults in the past decade would be expected to increase the pediatrician's role in the health care of this age group dramatically. Yet, even with this emphasis, adolescent and young adult visits fell from 19.1% of the visits in 1979 to 15.1% in 1994. While this change reflects the changes in the U.S. age-specific population (children younger than 5 years increased by 20.7% and the adolescent population decreased by 7.6% during that span), continued promotion of pediatricians as providers of health care to adolescents and young adults is necessary if pediatricians are to remain important providers of their care.

SCOPE OF PEDIATRIC PRACTICE

Until recently, the types of services provided by the nation's pediatric practitioners were unknown. Because of the rising cost of health care, practitioners increasingly are being required to document services rendered to determine how money is being spent and whether increased costs have resulted in improved health. Although sporadic studies of individual practices have appeared since the 1930s, nothing in the way of national practice data existed until the development of the National Ambulatory Medical Care Survey (NAMCS) by the National Center for Health Statistics in the early 1970s. NAMCS is a periodic survey of office-based practices; in 1992, the survey was expanded to include hospital outpatient departments and emergency rooms. These surveys do not include care provided in tax-supported ambulatory care service programs, although the Bureau of Primary Care with the Department of Health and Human Services conducts similar surveys in community health centers.

Of particular interest are the prescribing practices of the surveyed facilities during 1997-1998, the most recent reported at this writing. Antibiotics are the medications prescribed most frequently; asthma medications rank second; and stimulant medications used to treat ADHD rank third.

ORGANIZATION OF PRACTICE

Only 11% of pediatricians in the United States practice in rural communities to care for the 29% of the childhood population that live therein. By contrast, 37% of the children who live in large metropolitan areas are cared for by almost 59% of practicing pediatricians. The remaining 30% of practicing pediatricians live and practice in suburbia, serving 34% of our children. The 24% growth in child health physicians per 100,000 children younger than 18 years of age during the 1990s has not remedied the geographical disparities in their distribution. Except for pediatricians practicing in sparsely populated areas, which have limited hospital and technical support services and few pediatric specialists, pediatricians generally practice similarly throughout the United States. They, as other specialties, tend to settle in areas that have a high per capita income.

All children are supposed to have a "medical home" that provides continued, integrated care. Even for children who have a regular source of care, this source does not always provide all the required services, nor does it always integrate the services that the child has received elsewhere. Many children who have a physician whom they identify as their regular source of care go to other physicians when they need medical services. Primary care physicians may not be aware of these other visits, even though they may influence the patient's response to subsequent care significantly. Patients often are required to change their primary care provider, when their parents' employer changes its managed health care contract.

This fragmented, uncoordinated care presents a major challenge to our health care goals. If practitioners, health programs, and health institutions continue to function separately, without coordination, and if individuals continue to seek care from several sources, duplication of services will result, with an ever-increasing cost of care without commensurate gains. In fact, effectiveness is likely to diminish because patients often are given conflicting advice and treatment by different practitioners. The extent to which managed care systems alter this fragmentation of care still is unknown.

In most other industrialized nations, health services are regionalized and services are organized according to need. Services required frequently by large portions of the population are provided locally and, thus, are very accessible. These systems constitute primary health care services.

The experience of prepaid group practices, which by definition provide care for a specific population, is useful in determining how many physicians may be needed to ensure accessibility to primary care services. A ratio of 1500 children for every full-time child health physician has proved generally satisfactory, but this ratio varies according to the type and location of pediatric practices.

Physicians providing primary pediatric health care (general pediatricians, family practice physicians, and general internists) should assume responsibility for a broad spectrum of preventive and curative care and for coordinating all the care their patients receive from specialists. When primary care physicians need assistance in diagnosing and managing difficult cases, they should seek appropriate consultation.

REIMBURSEMENT ISSUES

Payment systems are determined largely by third-party insurers. The popular insurance of the past, indemnity insurance (now only 12% to 15% of the insurance sold) generally excludes preventive care. Managed care, with capitation and salary arrangements for physicians, as well as the conventional fee-for-service payments, has changed this. See Chapter 2, Pediatrics and Managed Care, for a complete discussion of managed care in pediatric practice.

In 1992, the Health Care Financing Administration (HCFA) adopted a relative value system of reimbursement to pay physicians for care of the elderly under the Medicare program. This system, called the Resource-Based Relative Value Scale (RBRVS), measures work in four dimensions: (1) time, (2) mental effort and judgment, (3) technical skill and physical effort, and (4) psychological stress. The RBRVS tends to equalize reimbursement by lowering fees for technical procedures and raising fees for "cognitive services." By late 1998, many pediatric RBRVS codes were developed to ensure that pediatricians would be reimbursed according to the same principles as those underlying the HCFA-generated RBRVS fee schedule for Medicare patients.

Impact of Reimbursement on the Scope of Services

Although most Americans are covered by some type of health-benefits package through employer-provided insurance, in 1998 almost 42 million people did not have health insurance; 14 million younger than age 21 years were uninsured. Families insured by managed care plans often discover that their child needs services that either are not covered or are covered only partially. Consequently, even when children are insured privately, they may need additional public sector coverage for needed services.

The two major sources of publicly funded health insurance for financially eligible pediatric patients are Medicaid (Title XIX of the Social Security Act) and the State Children's Health Insurance Program (SCHIP) created in 1997 by Title XXI of the Social Security Act.

Medicaid benefits were "delinked" from welfare benefits in the mid-1980s, leading to an increase in the number of children not covered by health insurance, because of increasing administrative barriers. SCHIP was designed to improve this situation, providing health insurance for children not eligible for Medicaid.

Under both Medicaid and SCHIP, states are required to offer the full spectrum of health benefits to financially eligible children. In some states, Medicaid and SCHIP recipients may have the option to be covered under managed care plans. Uninsured patients should be referred to community social services or health departments for enrollment in Medicaid and SCHIP programs.

Safety net providers. A number of public-sector "safety net" provider systems offer health care services for uninsured and underinsured pediatric patients. These include local public health departments, community and migrant health centers, public hospital systems, and school-based clinic systems. In addition, many not-for-profit organizations assist in meeting the health care needs of uninsured and underinsured children.

Case management and outreach services. The Early and Periodic Screening, Diagnosis and Treatment (EPSDT) component of the Medicaid program requires states to screen Medicaid-eligible children periodically for illnesses and physically disabling conditions and to refer them for definitive treatment. In addition, with EPSDT, there is a federal requirement to provide outreach and case management services for Medicaid-eligible children.

Services for children with special health care needs. The challenge of providing needed services for uninsured and underinsured children with special health care needs (CSHCN) can seem overwhelming for both clinicians and families. In this situation, the two available sources of care are those provided through the federal Title V Maternal and Child Health Block Grant and the Individuals with Disabilities Education Act (IDEA), formerly the Education for all Handicapped Children Act (P.L. 99-457).

In all states, Title V funds may be used for coordination of multidisciplinary health care services and for financing health care not covered by private insurance. Through their education or health systems, states provide early intervention services for infants and toddlers from birth to age 3 years who have special health care needs. Services available through Title V and IDEA are essential for uninsured and underinsured patients. Information on how these services are accessed can be obtained from the local health departments and school systems.

Supplemental Security Income. Supplemental Security Income (SSI) is an entitlement program under which a child who has a documented disability can receive substantially enhanced benefits such as extended eligibility for Medicaid and monthly cash allotments. Disability determination for SSI generally is made by the county social services department and can provide access to a wide array of services and benefits.

Immunization services. The Vaccine for Children (VFC) Program offers routine immunizations, particularly for patients whose health insurance does not provide this service. All county health departments are VFC providers and can provide information about other VFC providers in the community.

Food/nutrition supplementation programs. In most communities, there are several programs that provide food and nutrition supplementation for eligible children and their families. These include Special Supplemental Food Programs for the Women, Infants and Children (WIC), the Community Supplemental Food Program, and the Food Stamps Program. All provide either direct food allotments or coupons redeemable for retail food purchases. Many counties provide nutrition counseling as part of these services. Referral to local social service agencies or health departments should enable eligible families to receive these services.

Subsidized preschool and child care services. While not specifically a health service, preschool and child care services can enhance the development of eligible children and their access to some health services. Federally funded Head Start programs, which serve 3- and 4-year-olds primarily, are available in all communities. Children also receive health screening, immunizations, and meals through these center-based developmental programs.

In addition, many communities support free preschool programs through local school systems. Subsidized child care programs often can be identified by local social services departments. Some provide health screening.

Because, for the foreseeable future, there will be large numbers of uninsured and underinsured children, it is important for pediatricians to be aware of the public-sector health insurance programs, provider systems, and health services available in their communities for their patients.

QUALITY OF CARE

The medical profession has always assumed responsibility for regulating entry into its ranks and for assessing the quality of care provided. Although state boards have the legal authority to dispense licenses to practice, all states delegate this authority to the profession, which nominates candidates, whom the state then licenses. Individuals merely must demonstrate that they graduated from medical school and can achieve a passing grade on a cognitive examination developed by the profession itself, either in the state (state licensing examinations) or nationally (the National Board of Medical Examiners or the Federation of State Licensing Boards, i.e., "Flex" examinations).

The American Board of Pediatrics requires certification renewal every 7 years for pediatricians certified after 1987. This entails successful completion of the Program for Renewal of Certification in Pediatrics (PRCP), which includes a structured home study curriculum and a supervised, open-book written, or computer-based examination. Diplomates certified before 1988 may choose to renew their certification by completing the PRCP voluntarily.

Most health provider organizations use certification and recertification data as one means of ensuring quality of care, requiring their pediatricians to be either board certified (having passed the written examination) or board eligible (having completed 3 years of pediatric residency training in an accredited program) with certification within 5 years of completion of residency training. Whether recertification will be required by these organizations is unclear as yet. There is no requirement that pediatricians demonstrate competence under the conditions of actual practice, either when they enter practice or at any time afterward. However, managed care organizations regularly assess some aspects of quality of care for both adults and children; these efforts may expand in the future.

As of 1997, 73% of the general pediatricians eligible for recertification recertified, and 37% of pediatrician subspecialists recertified in general pediatrics.

Medical School Accreditation

Medical schools are accredited by the Liaison Committee on Medical Education, which is composed of representatives of the American Medical Association and the Association of American Medical Colleges. Medical schools qualify for accreditation by demonstrating to the Liaison Committee that they offer (1) a "sound educational program," which provides students the opportunity to acquire a solid basis of education in medicine and fosters the development of lifelong habits of scholarship and service; (2) scientific research; (3) graduate education through both clinical residency programs and advanced degree programs in the basic medical sciences; and (4) continuing education aimed at maintaining and improving the competence of professionals engaged in caring for patients.

Hospital Accreditation

To be accredited, hospitals must receive approval from the Joint Commission on Accreditation of Health Care Organizations, a council composed of representatives of the American Medical Association, the American Hospital Association, the American College of Surgeons, and the American College of Physicians. Accreditation, both of hospitals and medical schools, is essential to the financial viability of those institutions. Most third-party payers (the government and insurance companies) that reimburse hospitals or contribute to the support of medical schools require them to be accredited as a condition for payment.

Assurance of Quality Care

The passage of federal legislation stimulated the profession to demonstrate its involvement in assuring quality of care. Review of medical activities in hospitals was the first step proposed, largely because hospital costs assume a disproportionate share of the health care dollar. The Professional Standards Review Organization (PSRO) Act, passed in 1972, required that hospital admission of patients covered by government payments be reviewed for justifiability and that hospitals periodically designate individual diagnoses for which all medical records of patients who have those diagnoses would be audited to determine the adequacy of care. However, opposition by the profession, inability to demonstrate unequivocally that costs were reduced as a result of quality assurance activities, and general government policy to reduce government regulation led to severe restrictions in the program and eventually to its demise.

A new program, professional review organizations (PROs), was established by the Tax Equity and Fiscal Responsibility Act (TEFRA) of 1982 as a means of reviewing the completeness, adequacy, and quality of health care, primarily in hospitals. In contrast to the PSROs, which were nonprofit physician organizations, PROs could be for-profit groups and fiscal intermediaries that won the contracts from the federal government for monitoring health care use. Although these PROs currently review diagnostic information and completeness and adequacy of care, as well as appropriateness of admissions, for the elderly (patients covered by Medicare), this type of monitoring may well spread to other groups of patients covered by government and even private insurers.

Studies have shown that the organization in which a physician practices has a greater influence on the quality of practice than the physician's individual characteristics. Team practice, in which nurses and community health workers share responsibility with the physician for certain aspects of care, is likely to result in both greater recognition of patients' problems and the greater probability that they will be addressed by the physician. Prepaid group practices in which several physicians share fiscal accountability also are likely to result in greater consideration of the justifiability of professional actions.

In a health system that allows patients to seek care anywhere they choose, those who fail to obtain relief of their complaints often seek care elsewhere. Thus, physicians may not be in a position to observe the impact of their services. Conversely, no mechanism exists by which patients who are cured can apprise their physician of this. Most physicians are unable to assume responsibility for follow-up care of a patient if the patient does not voluntarily return for care. As the costs of care become an increasing concern of third-party payers (government, insurance companies, and employers), duplication of services, as reflected in visits to different care givers for the same problem, will become evident. As a result, physicians may be encouraged to assume greater responsibility for episodes of illness rather than just for individual visits made by patients; managed care systems will encourage such assumption of responsibility. This is likely to make physicians more aware of deficiencies that may exist in current medical practice.

The historical prerogative by which physicians decide what practices constitute "good quality" is being altered by a movement toward greater public accountability. It appears likely that certain aspects of practice will remain under physicians' control. The first such aspect is the selection of students for entrance into medical school. Ever since the Flexner Report (1910), the upper social classes have been overrepresented in the medical profession compared with their proportion in the general population. The high and continually rising cost of medical education without substantial government subsidy of those who cannot afford it is a powerful deterrent to applications from such students.

The second aspect is practice location. In many countries that have national health insurance programs, physicians are not reimbursed for their services if they locate their practices in areas that already have a sufficient number of physicians. In the United States, there are no deterrents to physicians locating wherever they please.

The third aspect likely to remain in the professional domain is the disciplining of physicians. In some countries, patients' dissatisfaction and complaints can be addressed to government agencies, which consider them and then exonerate the physician or recommend sanctions (usually financial) against him or her. The medical profession in the United States has been impotent in disciplining its members in any meaningful way because there is no way to impose sanctions short of revoking a license, which rarely is done. To date, both professional and legislative bodies have failed to come to grips with this issue.

The fourth aspect likely to remain in the hands of the profession is control over the technical areas of medical care. As new technology is developed, it often is used without adequate prior assessment of its costs and benefits. Although pressure to reduce the rate of growth in medical care costs (which largely are a result of increased use of technology) undoubtedly will lead to attempts to restrain some of physicians' practices, actual control over these practices is likely to be assumed by the organizations that employ or pay physicians. The profession itself, however, may retain development of policies concerning these controls.

Patterns of care in the United States, including the rate of use of tests, procedures, and hospital beds, vary from region to region and from physician to physician by as much as tenfold. What is appropriate usage? Demands are being made for health care outcome data that use various clinical practice guidelines (CPGs) to provide medical management strategies that are thought to be optimal. Once these strategies have been agreed on by the insurer's panel of physician experts, payment for implementing other strategies will be denied, particularly if the other strategies are more costly or less effective than the approved ones. Malpractice liability also has created a need for review of these data in an effort to reduce liability.

An array of initiatives designed to define and improve the quality of health care has been developed during the 1990s. One of these stands out and can be attributed to the writings of W. Edwards Deming, whose work gained wide acceptance in Japanese industries after World War II. Deming and others promoted a specific process for improving quality in manufacturing and other industries. The goal of the process, called continuous quality improvement (CQI), or total quality management (TQM), is to set into motion a permanent method of evaluating production quality by setting standards, improving performance, determining where standards are not being met, changing performance to meet the new standards, and when necessary, redefining the standards based on what was learned throughout the cycle. The goal is a continuous spiral of improved quality in the final product. Some CPGs have been developed by the American Academy of Pediatrics in concert with the American Academy of Family Practice, the federal Agency for Health Care Policy and Research, and other organizations. Many hospitals and managed care organizations already are applying these principles of quality assurance.

Many pediatricians are actively involved in CQI activities; 82% report that their practice staff meets regularly and discusses ways to measure or improve quality. Many are enrolled in voluntary ambulatory quality improvement programs.

The National Committee for Quality Assurance (NCQA), an organization that accredits managed care plans, has developed an overall set of measurements that accredited plans must collect, known as the Health Employer Data and Information Set (HEDIS). HEDIS (regularly updated) measures plans in six areas: effectiveness of care, loss of care, use of services, availability of care, patient satisfaction, and health plan stability. Types of quality-of-care measures for pediatric practice include (1) the percentage of children who have received the standard immunizations and the number of well-child visits recommended at appropriate ages; (2) the number of hospital readmissions within 1 month of hospital discharge for certain diagnoses (e.g., diabetes, asthma); (3) telephone responsiveness of the practice; (4) waiting room experience; and (5) appointment availability. These are all definable and measurable. Many plans encourage data collection and achievement of set goals by financial rewards to those who meet the acceptable criteria or penalties for those who do not.

EFFECTIVENESS OF CARE

Although all practitioners must demonstrate at least a minimal amount of theoretical knowledge as a condition of licensure before they enter practice, the relationship between performance in tests and subsequent quality of practice has never been demonstrated. Even the procedure by which physicians become certified as "specialists" provides dubious assurance of high quality. As previously noted, practice organization (e.g., group practice, teaching hospital practice) is more important as a determinant of quality than are individual physician characteristics. Board certification, apart from its relationship to longer lengths of postgraduate training, appears to have no relationship to practice quality. Continuing education requirements and periodic recertification procedures imposed by professional organizations are unlikely to improve the situation unless the model of quality of care on which the original educational and certification procedures are based is broadened to encompass assessment of the impact of services on health status.

Up to this point, this chapter has examined issues relating to the structure and process of medical care. Manpower, the organization of care, accessibility, and costs reflect the structure, or form, of health services. The process of care has been addressed in the discussion of quality, which involves recognizing patients' problems, further gathering of data to arrive at medical diagnoses, instituting therapy, and reassessing to ensure optimal response to therapy. As has been shown, patients contribute to the process of care by deciding whether to seek it (utilization), accept it, and understand it, and comply with recommendations. The third means by which care may be evaluated is based on the attainment of goals, or outcomes. Outcomes may be divided into four categories: deaths, illness and injury, disability, and others.

Improving Health and Well-Being: Outcomes of Care

The significant declines in mortality over the past century can be attributed more to improvements in public health than to specific technological advances applied to individual patients. The discovery of antibiotics is the only scientific advance applied to individual patients who are ill that has had a major impact in improving length of life; even here, the predominant effect seems to have been to reduce deaths in the elderly from acute infectious complications of chronic illness. The marked improvement in life expectancy over the past century has resulted primarily from lowered infant mortality. Infant mortality began to decline long before specific medical interventions were imposed, and the decline resulted from general improvements in sanitation, maternal nutrition, hygiene, and infant feeding. After infancy, deaths in childhood are so infrequent relatively that they are an insensitive indicator of the value of medical interventions.

Perhaps measuring the value of personal health services delivery in terms of a reduction in mortality is too great an expectation. Rather, some say that the measure of the system should be a reduction in the occurrence of disease and its manifestations—morbidity. But even here, it is unclear that physicians make a critical difference. Certainly the introduction of immunization has been responsible for large declines in the incidence of diphtheria, tetanus, pertussis, poliomyelitis, rubeola, rubella, and *Haemophilus influenzae* type b and hepatitis B infections and for the eradication of smallpox. But once again, it is the public health sector rather than the practice of individual physicians that has been most responsible. Federal funds to support immunizations have been crucial to the effectiveness of these programs; attempts to reduce or eliminate federal support have led to reduced immunization and to disease epidemics among children, particularly the poor.

Illness and injury data are obtainable only for those few conditions for which reporting is mandated by law because of their potential public health impact (contagiousness), such as rubella, rubeola, and hepatitis; however, these causes of morbidity constitute a small proportion of the health problems of children. National health surveys, including household surveys and surveys of practitioners' offices, are an important source of information about the prevalence of other child health conditions.

The ongoing household survey administered by the Department of Health and Human Services' National Center for Health Statistics obtains information about disability from a sample of the population. Disability is ascertained by asking questions about limitations of activity resulting from chronic conditions and about restrictions on usual daily activity.

Increasingly, the impact of medical care is being measured; evidence exists that individuals are more or less comfortable, more or less satisfied with their health, more or less able to achieve their physical and intellectual potential, and more or less able to control physical, emotional, and social threats to their health. The pediatric practitioner of the future will be confronted more with these new concepts of disease

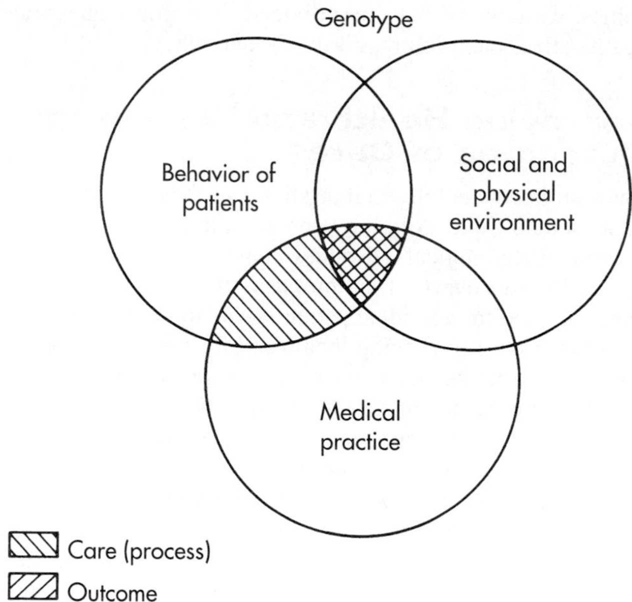

Fig. 1-1 Determinants of health status.

and health than with the acute illnesses that preoccupied the child health practitioner of the past.

The impact that health services can be expected to have, even under the best of circumstances, is limited by the role of other forces. At least four factors determine an individual's state of health (Fig. 1-1). Genetic constitution is the basic determinant. People differ in predisposition to specific illnesses and in response to their treatment largely because of differences in their genotypes. Probably the second most important determinant of an individual's state of health is his or her social and physical environment. Where individuals live, how they work, the food available to them, and the stresses imposed on them by the social system all affect how healthy they are and how well they resist insults to their health. Children particularly are vulnerable to the effects of the physical and social environment, because they are even less able than adults to select their surroundings and exposures. The third most important ingredient is the role that individuals themselves play in their behavior. Although young children are less likely to determine their life patterns than are adults (whose smoking, drinking, eating, and driving behaviors are major underlying causes of death), the patterns set for them by their parents influence not only how ill health is dealt with in childhood but also how well they are taught behavior destined to affect their health in later life. The final and probably least critical determinant of health, except in unusual situations, is the provision of medical services.

Who Defines "Good Care"?

Consumers and providers of health services differ in the priorities they place on the three main elements of care: access, cost, and quality. Costs of and access to medical care are of prime importance to consumers. In contrast, neither access nor cost is an important component of medical school training, which focuses almost exclusively on how to make a diagnosis; how to support this diagnosis with appropriate information from the history, physical examination, and laboratory findings; and how to institute treatment appropriate to the diagnosis. The nature of most educational settings (university-based, research-oriented, with generally a highly specialized faculty) is responsible for the following important limitations in medical training:

1. The educational process focuses largely on the biochemical and biophysical bases of disease processes. In contrast, relatively little attention is devoted to understanding the social, occupational, and environmental causes of ill health, although these are major determinants of disease and dysfunction.
2. The diagnostic process emphasizes assigning single causes for disease and arriving at a single diagnosis. It is more appropriate today to consider multiple causes of a disease. Moreover, one disease often is complicated and modified by the presence of another disease or a genetic, environmental, or psychosocial factor.
3. Insufficient attention is paid to the concept of human variability—to the reasons why some individuals who are predisposed to disease stay well, whereas others succumb, and why some respond to therapy and others do not.
4. Students' exposure to patients' illnesses are short term. Education, composed of blocks of time in various specialties, does not prepare students to assume long-term responsibility for patients, as will be required in the subsequent practice of medicine.
5. Students learn about illnesses either through reading about them or by participating in the care of ill patients. In both instances, their knowledge is derived primarily from experiences with patients at university-affiliated hospitals. Patients appearing for care at such institutions are not representative of the patients whom the students will meet subsequently as practitioners.

In the education of physicians, "quality" of care, characterized by the use of optimal techniques in arriving at diagnostic and therapeutic decisions, is virtually the only dictum emphasized. With this limited concept of "quality," it might be expected that at least diagnosis and therapy would be optimum in clinical practice. Unfortunately, this is not the case, as the following situations indicate.

Many well-accepted diagnostic strategies are of unproved usefulness, and some actually are harmful. For example, studies have shown that patterns of laboratory use may bear little or no relation to patients' needs. The extent of error, both in clinical observations and in laboratory findings, appears largely unrecognized by physicians. Outcome data will help to define these errors.

Many commonly applied therapeutic maneuvers are of unproved usefulness and may be dangerous. For example, several studies demonstrate that surgical rates in the United States are much higher than in other developed countries, without any demonstrable difference in the need for surgery as defined by prevalence of disease or illness. Even within the United States, the number of hospital admissions, the length of stay in the hospital, and the rate of surgical procedures vary markedly from area to area, unrelated to differences in medical need. Outcome data will help determine the usefulness of various therapeutic maneuvers.

Another problem is the misuse of drug therapy. For many physicians, drug manufacturers' representatives and adver-

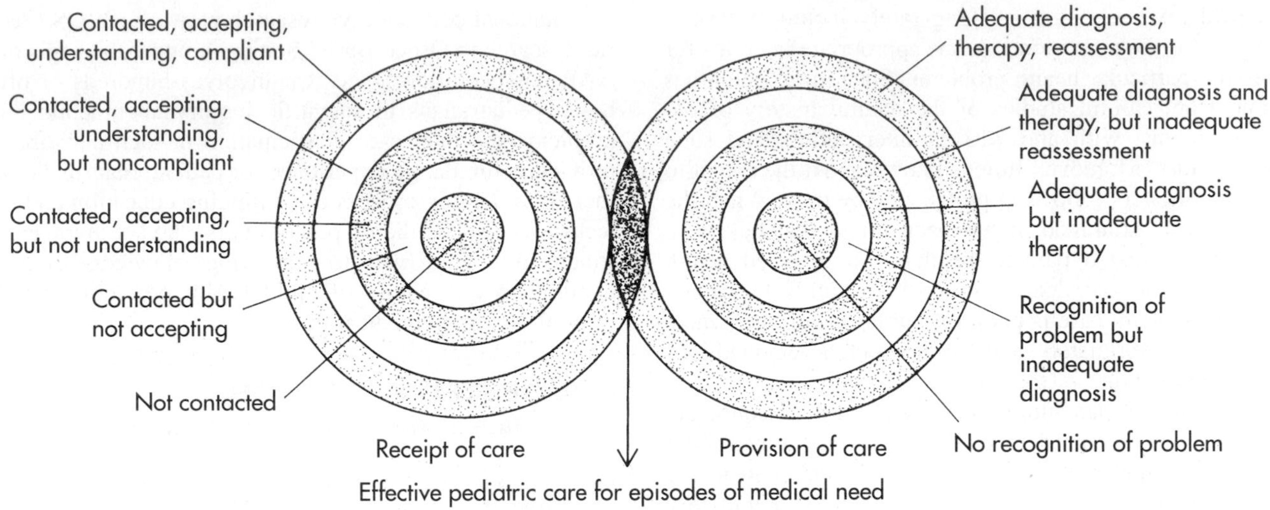

Fig. 1-2 The process of pediatric care.

tisements are the primary sources of information on new drugs. Several surveys have shown a widespread lack of appreciation by physicians of the dangers of many drugs and much unwarranted use of drugs. Outcome data will be helpful in determining the usefulness of drugs by helping physicians prescribe them more appropriately.

Even when diagnostic and therapeutic interventions can be shown to be appropriate and efficacious, applying them does not necessarily produce the desired outcome, because adequate diagnosis and therapy, although necessary for high-quality care, are by themselves insufficient. The treatment of illness and the maintenance of health also require the participation of patients and potential patients and a supportive social and physical environment (see Fig. 1-1). The very best quality of care, defined as efficacious diagnosis and treatment, will fail to achieve its effect if those who require it and can benefit from it do not appear for care, if they fail to understand it, or if they are unwilling to comply with the prescribed therapy (Fig. 1-2).

For these reasons, the traditional definition of quality of care should be broadened from its concentration on diagnostic and therapeutic strategies to include two additional facets of medical practice: problem recognition and follow-up with reassessment.

Problem Recognition

The application of diagnostic or therapeutic strategies requires first that problems, or potential problems, be recognized. Evidence indicates that the existence of many types of health problems often is overlooked.

Physicians are consistently poorer at recognizing the existence of significant behavior problems and social factors related to illness than they are at recognizing problems that have obvious biophysiological or anatomical manifestations. But even organic problems may be neglected. Many children, and adults, too, have health conditions that their physicians fail to follow, even when information about these conditions is available. Failure to recognize the problems that patients bring to physicians is a serious shortcoming in the provision of health services, because it has been shown that this failure is associated both with decreased patient satisfaction and failure to follow medical advice. Without recognizing the full range of patients' problems, no diagnostic strategy or therapeutic intervention can be fully effective.

Problem recognition also extends to prevention of disease. One type of prevention, *primary prevention,* is traditional to pediatricians. It consists of recognizing susceptibility to disease and applying measures to prevent it from occurring. Immunizations are the most obvious example of primary prevention, but prevention goes far beyond this. Sometimes only certain people are at risk of acquiring disease later in life; pediatricians must direct efforts at discovering who these people are, at keeping them under surveillance, and at trying to eliminate the situations that allow the illness to develop. This is known as *secondary prevention.* As social, occupational, environmental, and behavioral factors become recognized as important antecedents of many chronic illnesses, pediatricians will become more involved in activities directed toward preventing them.

Up to now, secondary prevention has not been a common feature of pediatric practice, and when children at risk have been identified, it generally has been at the initiative of government and social agencies. Examples of such efforts include hearing and vision screening in schools, special screening programs for specific disease in special populations (sickle cell anemia, Tay-Sachs disease), and state-mandated neonatal screening for inherited metabolic disorders (e.g., phenylketonuria). A major challenge for pediatricians is recognizing and dealing with occupational hazards that result in parents unknowingly exposing their children to toxic materials invisibly carried home from the workplace. Ultimately, pediatricians must assume responsibility for coordinating all the care of children, including primary and secondary prevention, as well as treating manifest illness.

Follow-up and Reassessment

To ensure that diagnostic procedures and instituted therapy are adequate and that problems are being resolved as expected, patients must be monitored; this is known as *outcomes assessment.*

Medical textbooks and teaching rarely include information that helps the practitioner define appropriate intervals for reassessing particular health problems. Such information has to come from careful studies of the natural history of patients' problems, with and without intervention, and such studies are rare. Moreover, little is known about the extent to which practitioners follow up problems they treat. When the issue has been examined, it has been found that failure to follow up on treated patients results in unresolved health problems. At the very least it produces a highly inefficient health care system: care is paid for, but no benefit is gained. At the most, it ultimately will lead to societal demands for greater accountability of the profession.

It seems likely that future physicians will be encouraged, and perhaps even required, to keep certain types of data about the children in their practices. A data set for hospitals to use for each patient admitted and a similar set for ambulatory care have been accepted by the National Center for Health Statistics and recommended for wide use. These include registration data (patient identification number, name, address, birth date, gender, race, and marital status) and encounter data (facility identification number, provider identification number, patient identification number, source of payment, date of encounter, patient's purpose for visit, physician's diagnosis, diagnostic and management procedures, and disposition). Adoption of this or a similar system for collecting and standardizing information will facilitate the understanding of health and disease processes and the role medical care plays in influencing them.

During the mid 1990s, a movement toward "evidence-based" medicine took hold throughout the world. It is a strategy geared toward using information derived from scientific research to improve practice. Until now, it has been focused largely at major health problems in elderly hospitalized patients. Moreover, its focus largely is on linking interventions with good outcomes rather than on detecting evidence of harm from interventions.

A national collaborative research network, PROS (Pediatric Research in Office-Based Settings), under the aegis of the AAP, has been developed that involves hundreds of office-based pediatricians in scientific inquiry about child health problems and their care. Participation in such networks can provide a stimulating experience for pediatricians and engage them in a lifelong process of continuing education and intellectual renewal. Pediatric practitioners who are involved contribute in a major way to improving knowledge about the distribution and nature of child health problems and their responsiveness to medical therapy.

SUGGESTED READINGS

Albers L: Issues of women in residency and early careers, *Pediatr Ann* 28:171, 1999.

American Association of Physician Assistants: AAPA Census Report, Alexandria, Va, 1998.

American Board of Pediatrics 1999 Annual Report to the American Academy of Pediatrics, Chapel Hill, NC, 1999.

Bellett P, Wachter RM: The hospitalist movement and its implications of the care of hospitalized children, *Pediatrics* 103:473, 1999.

Bocian AB, et al: Size and age-sex distribution of pediatric practice, *Arch Pediatr Adolesc Med* 153:9, 1999.

Broffman G: How can pediatric care be provided in underserved areas? A view of rural pediatric care, *Pediatrics (suppl)* 96:816, 1995.

Brotherton SE, et al: Women in pediatric practice: trends and implications, *Pediatr Ann* 28:177, 1999.

National Ambulatory Medical Care Survey, Series 13:136, Washington, DC, 1998, National Center for Health Statistics.

Onady G: The medicine-pediatrics physician: past, present, and future, *Contemp Pediatr* March 1999, p 129.

Pediatric Workforce Statement, *Pediatrics* 102:2, 1999.

Physician characteristics and distribution in the US, Chicago, 1999, American Medical Association.

Primary care, Washington, DC, 1996, Institute of Medicine, National Academy of Medicine Press.

Stockman J, Tunnessen WW: Pediatric diplomates, Chapel Hill, NC, 1999, American Board of Pediatrics.

Stoddard J, et al: General pediatricians, pediatric subspecialists, and pediatric primary care, *Arch Pediatr Adolesc Med* 152:768, 1998.

2 Pediatrics and Managed Care

Jeffrey J. Stoddard

The U.S. health care system has undergone immense reconfiguration over the past two decades. Skyrocketing health costs resulted in strong, countervailing efforts on the part of the public and private sectors to restrain such costs. Since the defeat in 1994 of sweeping, government-sponsored reform initiatives at the national level, market-based initiatives in health care financing and delivery have emerged as the chief mechanisms used to control health care expenditures. Managed care, which has existed for more than 50 years, has in the past 10 to 15 years become the dominant market mechanism affecting health care costs.

GROWTH IN MANAGED CARE

Although the initial rate of growth of managed care was slow, its rate of growth in the 1980s and 1990s has been astonishing, both with respect to numbers of managed care organizations and the total population enrolled in managed care plans. In 1986, 25.7 million Americans were enrolled in health maintenance organizations (HMOs). By 1995, 59.1 million Americans were enrolled in HMOs, representing a more than doubling in the number of enrollees in less than 10 years. Estimates of managed care enrollment figures for children are variable, due largely to there being no national system for collecting such information longitudinally. The most precise estimates available suggest that approximately 17 million U.S. children (comprising 22% of all children younger than age 20 years) were enrolled in HMOs in 1994. As a group, children have a slightly greater likelihood of being enrolled in HMOs than adults: In 1994, children (<20 years of age) comprised about 33% of total HMO enrollees but only 29% of the U.S. population. Defining managed care more broadly, some 31 million children (46%) were enrolled in managed care in 1996 according to the Medical Expenditure Panel Survey.

The majority of children enrolled in HMOs are privately insured. However, spectacular growth in managed care enrollment also has transpired in public insurance programs, especially Medicaid. From 1982 (when federal regulations pertaining to managed care enrollment for Medicaid beneficiaries were significantly loosened) through 1996, the total number of Medicaid beneficiaries enrolled in HMOs jumped from less than 1 million to more than 8 million. Although separate enrollment estimates for children enrolled in Medicaid managed care plans are not available, it is well known that many state Medicaid programs have selectively targeted child beneficiaries and their families for managed care enrollment.

The dramatic expansion of managed care has generated great controversy. Proponents of the shift argue that managed care organizations provide systematic mechanisms for controlling health care costs while providing families and children with a dedicated and reliable source of health care. Critics maintain that the financial incentives inherent in managed care ultimately will lead to restricted access to needed services and thereby potentially affect quality of care adversely. It must be acknowledged that very little hard evidence can be cited to document such effects. The majority of studies to date that have examined managed care and its effects on quality, outcomes, and satisfaction have focused on adults. Those studies focusing on children primarily analyzed children enrolled in federally sponsored HMO experiments involving Medicaid beneficiaries in the early 1980s. Because so many facets of the health care system have changed in the interim, the applicability of these older studies to the present context is open to question.

WHAT IS MEANT BY MANAGED CARE?

The term *managed care* describes various health care plans and delivery systems that tend to share one or more of the following characteristics: control over payment for medical services, selective contracting with specified providers, case management (often via a primary care gatekeeper), and reliance on utilization review. Integration of health services delivery systems and health care financing mechanisms (insurance functions) represents the *sine qua non* of a fully developed managed care organization.

HOW IS MANAGED CARE AFFECTING PEDIATRICIANS?

Most practicing pediatricians, whether directly involved with managed care, are likely to be significantly affected by it. As managed care has become increasingly common as a mechanism of health care financing and service delivery, it has changed many health care markets in ways that directly or indirectly affect all providers in those markets, including pediatricians. As of the year 2000, few geographical areas remain untouched by managed care. Many pediatricians now work exclusively for managed care organizations; others contract with them. Still others retain independence from managed care organizations but face growing competitive pressures exerted by the marketplace competition that managed care brings with it. For the practicing pediatrician, determining one's level and type of involvement with managed care remains an individual decision. The following general questions have been suggested by the American Academy of Pediatrics' Committee on Child Health Financing as useful in determining whether managed care organizations and strategies are acceptable:[1,2]

1. Will participation in the managed care plan expand or solidify the pediatrician's patient base?
2. Does the plan provide a reasonable level of reimbursement without imposing undue risk?
3. Does the plan provide patients adequate access to pediatric care, including access to pediatric subspecialists?
4. Will involvement with the managed care plan increase or decrease the pediatrician's administrative "hassle factor"?
5. Does the managed care plan compromise the pediatrician's ability to provide high quality medical care?
6. Does the managed care plan contract with hospitals where the pediatrician has (or can receive) clinical privileges?

The pediatrician must consider when analyzing these issues whether the plan will enhance his or her ability to provide medical care to children in the manner in which the pediatrician is comfortable. Practically, the crucial personal consideration for pediatricians in deciding if (or to what degree) to participate in managed care is whether the potential for expansion (or preservation) of one's patient base may be outweighed by lower reimbursement levels, by diminished autonomy, or both.

IMPLICATIONS OF MANAGED CARE FOR PEDIATRICIANS AND THEIR PATIENTS

One positive element of managed care that appeals to many pediatricians is that many managed care organizations emphasize disease prevention and health promotion. This emphasis is manifested by generous (prepaid) health supervision benefits and preventive service coverage. As a principal result of these benefits, many children enrolled in managed care plans make frequent and regular health supervision visits. As a result, pediatricians often are better able to monitor their patients' health. Under the traditional fee-for-service (FFS) system, such services often were not covered by indemnity insurance plans, thus resulting in high out-of-pocket expenses for some families and foregone care or unmet needs for others.

Certain characteristics of managed care plans, however, could negatively affect pediatricians and their patients. Some managed care organizations, for example, prefer to contract with small numbers of large group practices rather than with small groups or multiple solo practitioners. This obviously can result in problems for those independent pediatricians in certain market areas. In many states, "any willing provider" laws protect such physicians. The implications for pediatricians designated as "gatekeepers" within managed care plans also can be profound. Managed care plans that employ gatekeepers who have little or no training or experience in pediatric primary care run the risk of serious compromises in the quality of such care. On the other hand, managed care organizations that employ well-trained pediatricians as gatekeepers could provide these pediatricians with an optimal clinical role. Considerations in this respect relate to the plans' expectations regarding the scope of services to be provided directly by the gatekeepers and the circumstances under which referrals, hospitalizations, and other high-cost services are deemed appropriate. Related to this is the consideration that involves weighing the additional time and effort required to perform gatekeeping functions (i.e., patient care management and coordination services) against the level of additional reimbursement provided for assuming these responsibilities. It is imperative for practicing pediatricians to understand that the financial incentives under managed care are devised such that the pediatrician (as gatekeeper) may be penalized financially for providing costly services and, conversely, financially rewarded for withholding such services. Such a financing arrangement obviously is contrary to traditional fee-for-service medicine in which providers had an economic incentive to do more rather than less on their patients' behalf (without risk to themselves). Financial incentives under managed care now may create tension between pediatricians' interests in serving their patients' needs and their own financial well-being. Under managed care, tremendous pressure is felt by the gatekeepers to practice medicine prudently and cost effectively.

Much debate but few definitive data address concerns such as relative quality of care for children in managed care settings versus traditional settings. This is especially so for at-risk child populations (and the traditional providers of service to such children), including Medicaid beneficiaries and children who have special health care needs. The available data are mixed. For example, Laufenberg found increased physician visits among Medicaid children enrolled in HMOs compared with those in fee-for-service Medicaid plans.[4] On the other hand, Hurley, Freund, and Paul found reductions in physician visits among children enrolled in group and staff model HMOs.[3] But comparisons of managed care with traditional financing systems indicate that timely access to services of high quality for special-needs populations of children remain persistent problems that appear to be exacerbated by some managed care structures. Several localized studies, for example, have shown that vulnerable children tend to experience greater difficulty obtaining specialty services in HMOs regardless of family income.[5] Still, it must be acknowledged that most of these studies are restricted to local areas; thus, it is unclear how generalizable and robust such findings are. Despite the absence of definitive evidence on many questions, large segments of the child population are entering managed care at an astonishing pace.

MANAGED CARE MODELS

It is imperative for pediatricians to be familiar with the various models of managed care.

Staff Model HMO

In a staff model HMO, physicians who provide care to the enrollees of the plan are full-time, salaried employees. Such physician employees generally take care exclusively of the enrollees of the HMO and practice exclusively at the HMO's sites and facilities. Inpatient services may or may not be on-site within the HMO facilities, and certain medical and surgical subspecialists may or may not be represented on the staff. From the standpoint of the pediatrician, the staff model HMO offers these advantages: a predictable, secure salary (with bonus or incentive payments typically contingent upon productivity); a generally well-established patient base; relative freedom from many administrative hassles associated with private practice; consistent schedule and reduced call responsibility; standardized and complete medical records and information systems; and security afforded by a large organizational structure. Disadvantages include: reduced clinical autonomy, which may involve close scrutiny of practice patterns; expectations for provision of a broad scope of service; and cost-effective practice expectations.

Group Model HMO

Under the group model arrangement, the HMO contracts with a multi-specialty medical group to provide medical care to the plan's enrollees. The medical group typically is paid by the HMO on a capitation basis. The medical group may, in turn, compensate its individual physicians by way of a variety of fee-for-service methods or through capitation, salary, or other methods. Advantages offered by the group model HMO include many of those seen with a staff model HMO, including predictable work schedules, freedom from business-related or administrative hassles, an established and self-contained referral network, and availability of comprehensive services on-site. Disadvantages may, again, include diminished physician autonomy in these settings insofar as the group is captive to the HMO for its patient base. Some independent groups, however, may have contracts with multiple HMOs as well as provide care to patients who have other (non-HMO) health insurance coverage.

Network Model HMO

The network model resembles a group model HMO, except that under this model, the HMO contracts with more than one multi-specialty and/or single specialty group practice. Also, as a rule, network model HMOs compensate the medical groups on a capitation basis. In contrast to the closed-panel staff and group models, network models may employ either open-panel or closed-panel plans. Advantages and disadvantages to this sort of arrangement are similar to those associated with the group model HMO arrangement. However, the broader physician participation inherent in some networks may provide a marketing advantage over closed-panel plans, insofar as consumer choice is strengthened.

IPA Model

In an independent practice association (IPA) arrangement, an open-panel organization of independently practicing physicians forms for the purpose of contracting with one or more HMOs. Physicians become members of the IPA, which is a separate legal entity, but continue to practice in their individual offices and also may continue to provide care to non-HMO patients. In some instances, the IPA may have exclusive contracts with one HMO; in others, the IPA may have multiple contracts with several HMOs. In either instance, the IPA typically is paid by the HMO on an all-inclusive capitation basis. Physicians within the IPA are, in turn, generally compensated on a discounted fee-for-service basis and thereby bear some financial risk. This typically translates into some sort of withholding arrangement under which a portion of payment is retained by either the HMO or the IPA and returned at year end if targets are reached. In some IPA arrangements, however, pediatricians (and other primary care physicians) are paid strictly on a capitation basis while specialists are compensated on a fee-for-service basis. IPAs have a broad array of relationships with hospitals, ranging from exclusivity (e.g., hospital-based IPAs) to looser arrangements involving multiple hospitals.

From the perspective of the consumer, IPAs generally provide access to broader pools of physicians than is typical through traditional HMO arrangements, thus yielding a marketing advantage. From the standpoint of the physician, IPAs provide the opportunity for flexibility and more independent practice within a solo or small group setting, while simultaneously providing good access to managed care contracts and the patient populations they bring. This allows physicians relatively greater autonomy compared with the staff, group, or network models. Furthermore, physicians within IPAs can continue to provide care to patients covered by Medicaid, commercial insurance, or indemnity plans and may contract individually (outside the IPA) with other plans, thus allowing considerable flexibility and diversity within the physician's patient panel.

HMO-Controlled Physician Network or Direct Contract Model

This model represents a variation on the IPA model in which the HMO contracts directly with separate and autonomous physicians as opposed to an organized IPA. This type of arrangement has become common in areas where large organized HMOs and IPAs have not yet developed within the local market. Although this type of network is similar in many ways to the IPA arrangement, the absence of the physician organization component poses a potential risk to physicians insofar as no organizational forum for physician decision-making exists to represent physicians' interests.

Preferred Provider Organizations

A preferred provider organization (PPO), unlike an HMO, represents an arrangement that is not an actual organization, but rather a contractual agreement between individual providers and health insurance companies or employers. The critical element of most PPOs is a discounted fee-for-service payment arrangement under which patients are given clear financial incentives to use specified practitioners who are part of the PPO network. PPOs confer maximal flexibility to physicians to continue to provide services in a relatively traditional manner within their own offices, albeit at discounted rates. In addition, PPO arrangements typically provide physicians a relatively risk-free mechanism of entering into managed care (relative to the capitation approach). PPOs often are criticized for being primarily a discounting strategy, with only minimal effort being made to oversee or manage care. Some physicians entering into PPOs question whether the flow of new patients justifies the discounting of fees.

Point of Service Plans

Point of service (POS) plans were developed specifically to provide consumers/enrollees with the joint option of using either the HMO network, or when necessary, non-network providers. Under POS plans, enrollees must select a primary care physician from the HMO network. Care is prepaid as long as enrollees use services from this and other affiliated providers within the network (with cost-sharing kept to a minimum). If, however, the patient chooses to use practitioners outside of the network, varying levels of indemnity insurance coverage exist, but cost-sharing requirements take effect. Financing of care, therefore, is variable depending on the "point of service" where care is provided.

DEVELOPING A MANAGED CARE STRATEGY

Maintaining the viability of one's practice requires an individualized managed care strategy. In so doing, pediatricians should recognize that they have a number of options at their disposal. Strategic planning is essential for all pediatricians and will be shaped largely by the individual pediatrician's personal abilities, aspirations, approaches, preferences, and values, as well as local market forces.

For a few pediatricians, managed care can be ignored altogether or avoided. For others, it may be viewed as a "necessary evil" that must be reluctantly accommodated. For most, managed care will represent a strong (if not dominant) market force that presents a range of opportunities for practice and career development. Thus, decisions relating to involvement in managed care by pediatricians ought to be made on a logical, informed basis by using valid, up-to-date information. General strategies relating to managed care involvement include the following:

1. Seek independent advice from qualified, impartial advisors knowledgeable about the local health care marketplace.
2. Understand the implications of long-term contracts, restrictions, and the fate of agreements if organizational changes ensue.
3. Understand the priorities and needs of organizational administrators, network managers, and other key stakeholders within the organizations.
4. Develop an accurate assessment of the community perception of the quality of care provided by you as an individual physician.
5. Look for special service "carve-out" opportunities that may represent competitive advantages for you or for patients.
6. Examine closely with which pediatric colleagues you wish to affiliate, including such factors as their abilities to deliver high-quality, cost-effective care.

MANAGED CARE EMPLOYMENT/ AFFILIATION ARRANGEMENTS

Full-Time Employment as a Salaried Employee

Many pediatricians, especially younger ones, approach with ease the notion of becoming full-time salaried employees inasmuch as such arrangements might provide them dependable, guaranteed salaries; generous benefits; and immediate access to a well-established panel of patients. More predictable hours, including part-time employment opportunities, often are also feasible in these types of arrangements. The disadvantage to such employment arrangements for the pediatrician is, of course, the loss of autonomy that typically ensues. Whenever a pediatrician embarks on an exclusive employment arrangement with a single managed care organization, that pediatrician must closely scrutinize the employment contract, each and every facet of the health plan, the delivery system, and the structure, function, leadership, market share, and philosophy of the organization.

Exclusivity

Many pediatricians encounter the issue of exclusivity. In many communities and market areas, pediatricians can simultaneously affiliate with multiple managed care organizations or health plans. However, in the more competitive and mature markets (with respect to managed care penetration), physicians, in some instances, are increasingly forced to make decisions in selecting one managed care organization with which to affiliate.

Physician Practice Profiling

Just as physicians scrutinize managed care organizations, so too do managed care organizations increasingly scrutinize physicians—through "profiling." Extensive data are now collected regarding physicians' practice profiles. Information related to quality of care; outcomes; numbers and duration of inpatient admissions; referral rates and patterns; use of laboratory, imaging studies, and ancillary services (comparative resource utilization); and assessment of relative cost-effectiveness of practice patterns is collected on physicians in active practice. Such information is becoming used routinely by some large managed care organizations to monitor providers within their networks. Such data also are reviewed routinely by some prospective employers of physicians. It is essential for individual physicians to know and understand what such practice profiling data reflect about them.

REIMBURSEMENT

Crucial aspects with regard to managed care contracting are the *mechanisms* and the *levels* of reimbursement. There is a continuum of reimbursement methods within managed care. Such reimbursement options that are available in certain markets typically vary according to the extent of managed care penetration and the degree to which financing and service delivery are integrated. In those traditional markets in which fee-for-service payment remains the dominant mode, reimbursement mechanisms based on fee-for-service or modified fee-for-service payment remain largely intact. In those markets in which managed care is beginning to have an influence, discounted fee-for-service and negotiated fee rates are the typical methods of reimbursement. In those markets in which managed care has penetrated to a significant degree, capitation becomes the norm.

Capitation

Capitation is defined as reimbursement to a provider (or group of providers) via the payment of a fixed periodic payment in exchange for delivery of a defined set of health services to a specific patient population. Under capitation, pediatricians are asked to accept a fixed capitation rate (i.e., a dollar amount per member per month) in exchange for providing the full scope of services to that patient. Capitation rates in most instances also entail that the pediatrician will be responsible for serving as the gatekeeper for all specialty and hospital services required by that patient. Capitation amounts are determined actuarially. Because revenues are fixed under capitation, such arrangements frequently are also referred to as *risk contracts*.

Potential advantages of capitation to the pediatrician include ability to control: utilization; stable, regular cash flow; and administrative costs. Potential disadvantages to the pediatrician of capitation include: inability to predict and handle the risks, the burdens of gatekeeper requirements relating to specialty referrals and hospitalization, the requirement for efficient management of the practice, and the administrative costs relating to transition to capitation.

Full-Risk Capitation

Full-risk means that in exchange for a per member, per month payment, the pediatrician agrees to provide the full and comprehensive scope of services without a limit on the number of visits or the total actual cost of providing those services. Managed care organizations prefer this type of capitation because it limits their own risk, shifting it over to the providers.

Shared-Risk Capitation

Shared-risk capitation represents an alternative to full-risk capitation. Under shared-risk plans, physicians are responsible for the delivery of and/or payment for services only if and when certain conditions are met. Such conditions might include a minimum number of enrollees, an income guarantee, a risk pool among a group of physicians or other providers, or stop-loss coverage or reinsurance for particularly high-cost cases. In general, shared-risk is by far the safer choice for those pediatricians who have minimal or modest experience with capitation. Shared-risk arrangements also represent a practical intermediate step for those physicians moving from a fee-for-service or discounted fee-for-service arrangement toward accepting greater risk.

MANAGED CARE CONTRACTING

Before signing a managed care contract, pediatricians need to assess their readiness individually (and the readiness of their practice) for managed care, while also assessing both the strengths and the weaknesses of the managed care plan(s) with which they are considering affiliating. Pediatricians need to review the terms and conditions of the managed care contract carefully. The types of information that pediatricians need to understand include: ownership; market influence and long-range plans (including market share, service area, covered lives, and anticipated change in patient base); administrative issues; participating providers (including physicians, ancillary providers, hospitals, and outpatient facilities); marketing strategy; management; financial data; and external evaluation/accreditation. Specific contract terms and provisions essential for the pediatrician to read carefully and understand fully include: scope of covered services, authorization processes, benefit limitations and exclusions, emergency and after-hours care protocols, formulary issues, eligibility, malpractice insurance, and on-call availability.

Additional specific contract terms and provisions that warrant close attention include automatic renewals, capacity requirements, contract duration, contract assignability, provisions in the event of financial failure of the managed care organization, dispute resolution, final authority, out-of-area coverage, contract changes, termination of agreement with the plan, and gag clauses. Issues relating to selection and ongoing participation, utilization management and cost effectiveness requirements, financial issues (including compensation methods), operational requirements, and relationships within the managed care organization (e.g., exclusivity, hold-harmless clauses) also deserve careful consideration. If provisions within such contracts are not clear or well understood by the pediatrician, expert advice and clarification becomes essential. Although in many cases managed care organizations might be reluctant to alter the terms and conditions within their provider agreements, there typically is some degree of negotiating latitude granted to those physicians who are deemed to be "attractive" providers. Working with professional advisors, pediatricians should attempt to eliminate onerous or burdensome provisions from agreements, including those that might threaten their patients' interests as well as their own. Clearly, careful attention on the part of the pediatrician to managed care organizations' benefit structure, medical management protocols, provider network and delivery system issues, and payment formula from both the pediatrician's and the patient's perspectives are paramount.

RECENT TRENDS

Two major and multifaceted trends that have potentially far-reaching implications have begun to reshape what in the mid-1990s was appearing to be an inexorable drive toward managed care. The first is the rebirth of consumer sovereignty and the second is the organized anti-managed care "backlash."

As consumers increasingly have demanded broad choice among providers, the market has responded. Even as consumers—often at the behest of their employers—have enrolled in ever-increasing numbers into managed care, they have demanded that managed care provide them with broader choices of primary care physicians, specialists, and hospitals. Once thought by managed care theorists to be "transitional" or "vestigial," PPOs and POS plans now are felt to be a permanent part of the health care landscape. Exclusivity often has given way to demand for broad choice, and networks that largely overlap have resulted. One implication of broad and overlapping networks is that the effectiveness of health plan management and support activities will diminish insofar as the importance of any single plan in a physician's practice will be less.

An increasingly visible manifestation of the anti-managed care backlash has been the resurgence of public policy initiatives designed to curb the excesses of market forces. Both consumers and providers have led the push for legislative action to remedy some managed care practices. Consumers pushing for consumer protection and physicians fighting to ensure quality of care have moved the discussion forward through several legislative vehicles (e.g., the "1999 consumer bill of rights"). This activity has engaged lawmakers at both the federal and state levels. States have proceeded more quickly on consumer protection. As of January 2000, more than 40 states had adopted a "Patients' Bill of Rights."

Market forces are moving targets and play out very differently across different communities. Pediatricians cannot afford—either for themselves or for their patients—to be oblivious to the trends affecting the health care market in which they practice.

REFERENCES

1. Committee on Child Health Financing (Berman S, Gross RD, Lewak N, editors): *A pediatrician's guide to managed care,* Elk Grove Village, Ill, 1994, American Academy of Pediatrics.
2. Committee on Child Health Financing: "Strategies for Managed Care" Series, Elk Grove Village, Ill, 1994-1997, American Academy of Pediatrics.
3. Hurley RE, Freund DA, Paul JE: *Managed care in Medicaid: lessons for policy and program design,* Ann Arbor, Mich, 1993, Health Administration Press.
4. Laufenberg HF: Medicaid patients use of HMO services, *WMJ* 88:19, 1989.
5. Rowland D, et al: Medicaid and managed care: lessons from the literature. A report of the Kaiser Commission on the Future of Medicaid, Washington, DC, March 1995.

SUGGESTED READINGS

Kongstvedt PR: *Essentials of managed health care,* Gaithersburg, Md, 1995, Aspen Publishers.

Leatherman S, McCarthy D: Opportunities and challenges for promoting children's health in managed care organizations. In Ruth Stein, editor: *Health care for children: what's right, what's wrong, what's next,* New York, 1997, United Hospital Fund.

Rosenbaum S: Protecting children: defining, measuring, and enforcing quality in managed care. In Ruth Stein, editor: *Health care for children: what's right, what's wrong, what's next,* New York, 1997, United Hospital Fund.

3 Morbidity and Mortality Among the Young

Bernard Guyer • Cynthia S. Minkovitz • Donna Strobino

Over the past few decades, children in the United States have experienced unprecedented improvements in their health status. The infant mortality rate (IMR), for example, one of the most sensitive indicators of the overall health of a population, has declined to 7.1 deaths per 1000 live births in 1997, an all-time low. Life expectancy at birth in the United States reached a new high of 76.5 years in 1997. Age-adjusted death rates declined for almost all diseases and injuries.

These trends toward improvements in child mortality rates, however, do not tell the whole story. Rates of morbidity and disability from some conditions have increased over these decades. Indicators of health care utilization, such as immunization coverage, show that many U.S. children may not be served adequately by the health care system. International comparisons of key indicators, such as IMR, show the United States to be lagging behind other industrialized nations that have better organized primary health care systems and universal health insurance coverage. Finally, disparities in health status among U.S. children continue to persist according to race and socioeconomic status.

Identifying the epidemiological patterns of death and disability among children is an essential component of effective health policy for young Americans. Jameson and Wehr[18] argue that children have medical needs that are different from those of adults because children are dependent on adults, children are on an upward developmental trajectory; and the epidemiology of children's health conditions differs from that of adults. Much of this differential pattern is documented in this chapter.

This chapter also presents the current mortality, morbidity, and demographic profile of U.S. children, highlighting the important trends in health that have occurred over the past 20 years and that may occur in the future. The analysis is restricted to the United States, although in some cases international comparisons are drawn. A more comprehensive, global view of child health mortality and morbidity is beyond the scope of this chapter.

DATA SOURCES AND METHODS

Much of the information used in this chapter is derived from a series of annual publications co-authored by two of the authors of this chapter in collaboration with colleagues from the National Center for Health Statistics.[14] Data on the characteristics of the child population are obtained from the United States Bureau of the Census, the decennial census, and current population surveys conducted in recent years. Finally, data from national health surveys are used to describe chronic conditions and limitations in activity among children in the United States.

Demographic Data from U.S. Census

Data describing the population of children today and in recent decades are derived from U.S. census data and updates of these data between the decennial censuses.[5,8,9] These data, along with data from birth and death certificates and estimates of immigrations, are used by the U.S. Census Bureau to construct population projections reported in this chapter. The approach used to project the population is the cohort component method, in which the three basic demographic components of the population—fertility, life expectancy, and net immigration—are projected over time. A series of projections are estimated by using three assumptions for each population component: a low, middle, and high assumption. The middle series projections are reported here because they represent the most "reasonable" set of assumptions for future population growth.[5,9]

Birth and Death Data from U.S. Vital Statistics

The data presented in this chapter on births and deaths were obtained primarily from two sources—the natality data from certificates of live birth and the mortality data from certificates of death for all residents of the United States. Data for births are final. Data for deaths for 1997 are preliminary and are based on a greater than 85% sample of deaths reported to the National Center for Health Statistics (NCHS).

Natality data are presented for the mother's age, race, Hispanic origin, marital status, use of prenatal care, infant's birth weight, and plurality. Births are tabulated separately by race and Hispanic origin; persons of Hispanic origin may be of any race. Mortality data are presented by age, race, and underlying cause of death. From 1979 to the present, cause of death data in the United States have been classified according to the *9th Revision, International Classification of Diseases.*[37] Population denominators for the calculation of birth, death, and fertility rates are estimates of the United States population as of July 1 of each year, produced by the U.S. Census Bureau.[16]

The data for birthweight-specific infant mortality rates were obtained from linked birth-infant death data.[21] In this data set, death certificates are linked with the corresponding birth certificates for each infant who died in 1996 in the United States. The purpose of this linkage is to use the many additional variables available from the birth certificate to interpret infant mortality patterns better.

Morbidity and Disability Data from National Surveys

National Health Interview Survey (NHIS) data are used to monitor select trends regarding children who have a chronic illness. Information for this population-based survey is gathered through household interviews by the U.S. Census Bureau for the National Center for Health Statistics. Demographic and health data are obtained for each member of the household and are representative of the civilian noninstitutionalized population of the United States. In recent years, the survey has included questions on special health topics relevant to child health, including checklists of childhood health conditions[27] and the presence of childhood disability.[3] Recent supplemental questionnaire components have focused on child health overall (1988) and disability (1994-1995).

DEMOGRAPHIC PROFILE OF U.S. CHILDREN AND POPULATION PROJECTIONS TO THE YEAR 2020

The child population in the United States can be characterized in a number of ways, including its magnitude, percentage of the total population, and racial and ethnic composition. Families that include children also can be characterized by their size, number of parents, and socioeconomic status. These characteristics have important implications for the health and welfare of children.

Current Demographic Profile of U.S. Children

In 1997, more than 69 million children younger than age 18 years were estimated to be in the U.S. population. These children were divided roughly equally between the three age groups: 0 through 5, 6 through 11, and 12 through 17 years. The number of children in the population has fluctuated since the 1950s, primarily because of the high fertility rates during the baby boom years, 1946 to 1964.[30] In 1950, there were an estimated 47,278,000 children younger than age 18 years in the U.S. population. This number increased markedly during the 1950s to more than 64 million in 1960 and exceeded 69 million in 1970, the size of the child population in 1997.[5,8,9]

The percentage of children in the population should be monitored because it provides an overall assessment of the need for investments in future populations. This percentage rose during the 1950s and 1960s from about 31% in 1940 and 1950 to a peak of 36% in 1960. It did not decline much until the late 1970s, when the first half of the baby boom cohorts reached young adult age. Children younger than 18 years constituted 26% of the U.S. population in 1997.[9]

The dependency ratio, a measure of the proportion of persons who are considered dependent, children (<18) and the elderly (≥65 and over), in the population relative to persons eligible to participate in the labor force (18 to 64), is a crude estimate of the extent to which the productive population must provide resources for the dependent population. A youth and an elderly dependency ratio are also computed.[5] The dependency ratio increased dramatically from 64 children and elderly per 100 persons 18 to 64 years old in 1950 to 82 in 1960, due primarily to the rise in the youth dependency ratio. The ratio remained high in 1970, but dropped to 65 in 1980 and has remained slightly below that level since. During this latter period, however, the youth dependency ratio dropped, while the elderly ratio increased from 13.4 in 1950 to 20.3 in 1990.[5,9]

The U.S. child population has become increasingly diverse, racially and ethnically, since 1980 (1980 was the first year for which data on the Hispanic population were available nationally). In 1997, 66% of the child population was non-Hispanic white, 15% was non-Hispanic black, 15% Hispanic, 4% Asian American, and 1% Native American. In contrast, 74% of the child population was non-Hispanic white in 1980 and 9% was Hispanic. The percentage of non-Hispanic black children in the population has remained relatively constant during this time period, while the percentage of Asian American children doubled.[8]

The size of the American family has decreased over the past three decades. The percentage of families having three or more children declined from 21% in 1970 to 10% in 1997. At the same time, the percentage of families having no children younger than age 18 rose from 44% to 51%.[8]

Children increasingly are living in families that have only one parent. In 1996, 68% of children lived in families that had two parents, 24% in families that had a mother only, 4% that had a father only, and 4% that had no parent. In contrast, 88% of children lived in two-parent families in 1960. The decline in two-parent families is due almost entirely to an increase in mother-only families.[7]

The percentage of children living in two-parent families varies markedly by race and ethnicity. Although 75% of white children in 1996 lived in families having two parents, 62% of Hispanic children and only 33% of black children did so. These disparities are due primarily to the greater percentage of black children who live in mother-only families (53%) than white children (18%) or Hispanic children (29%). Children who live in female-headed households have fewer economic resources available to them than do children who live in two-parent families. In 1996, the mean family income for married couple households ($60,854) was 2.8 times greater than the mean for female-headed households ($21,905); these disparities were similar for white, black, and Hispanic families.[7]

The percentage of children living below the U.S. poverty level increased from 15% in 1975 to 22% in 1993, although the percentage dropped to 20% in 1996 (Fig. 3-1). Particularly alarming, however, has been the increase in children living in extremely poor families, below 50% of the poverty level; this percentage rose from 5% in 1975 to 10% in 1993. Although it dropped to 8% in 1996, it still is 1.6 times greater than the percentage in 1975. The percentage of children living in families with incomes below 150% of

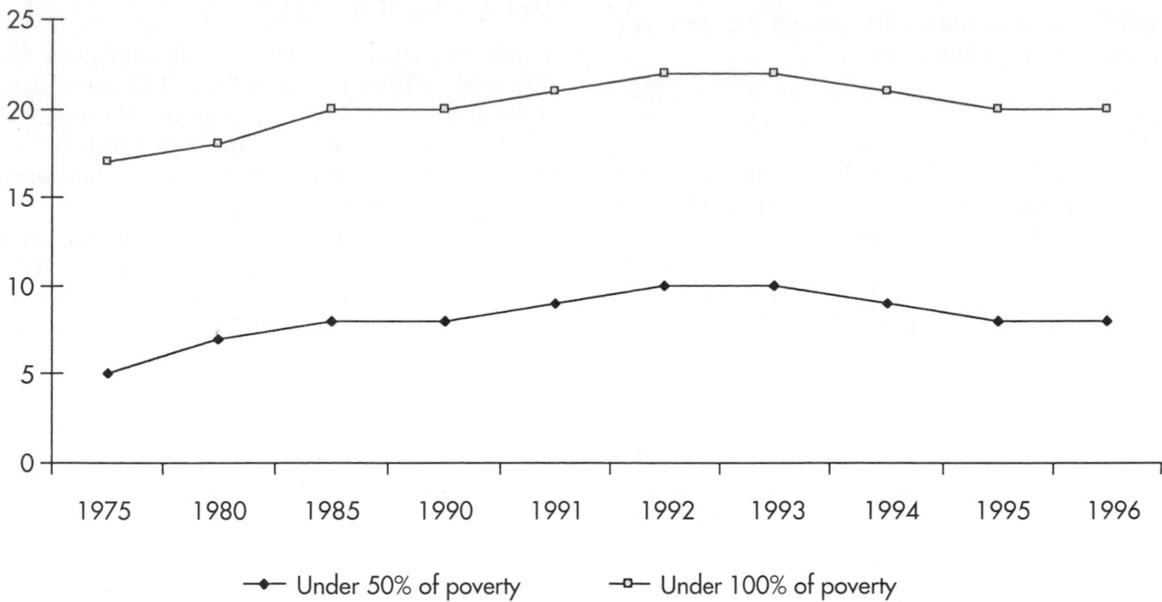

Fig. 3-1 Percentage of children younger than age 18 years living in poverty, 1975 to 1995.

poverty rose only slightly from 30% in 1975 to 33% in 1993 and was followed by a drop to 31% by 1996. The percentage of families living below 200% of poverty remained relatively constant at 43% throughout this period. Although black and Hispanic children are more likely to live in poverty, 32% and 40% respectively in 1989, the secular trends in poverty among children are similar across groups. Native American children are also subject to high rates of poverty; 38% lived in families with incomes below 100% of poverty in 1996.[8]

The majority of children in the United States do not experience poverty while growing up, and most who do have not lived in poverty for more than 5 years. Nevertheless, 14% of children who turned 18 years old between 1988 and 1990 lived in poverty for 6 years or more. Black children are particularly vulnerable to persistent poverty; 47% who turned 18 years old between1988 and 1990 lived in poverty for 6 or more years and 28% for 11 or more years, at least two thirds of their childhood.[7]

Future Population Projections

The population of children in the United States will undergo a number of changes in the next quarter century. To understand these changes, population projections are reported here as estimated by the U.S. Census Bureau.[9]

The number of children in the U.S. population is expected to increase by 10 million by 2020 to about 79 million children. The composition of this population will increasingly include racial and ethnic groups other than non-Hispanic whites. Although black children were the largest minority group in 1996, Hispanic children are expected to surpass them in numbers by 2005, and Asian children are expected to comprise 6% of the U.S. child population by 2020 (Fig. 3-2).[9] This change will occur gradually as new birth cohorts age and as more and more immigrants of Hispanic and Asian heritage are added to the population.[5]

The percentage of children in the total U.S. population is projected to decline slightly over the next quarter century to about 24% of the population; in fact, it is expected never to be as high as it was in the 1960s. The dependency ratio is projected to remain relatively constant through 2010, although a slight decline in the youth ratio and a slight rise in the elderly ratio is suggested. It is expected to rise rapidly, however, between 2010 and 2020, almost entirely because of a rapid increase in the elderly ratio when the first cohorts of the baby boom reach age 65. By 2020, the elderly dependency ratio (27.1) is expected to be about one-third less than the youth dependency ratio (39.9), in contrast to 1990, when the elderly ratio was less than half (20.3) the youth dependency ratio (41.7).[5,9]

These population projections, if correct, have important implications for the health of children, especially relative to the availability and appropriateness of their health services. The changing ethnic and racial diversity of the child population means that those who provide health care to children will need, increasingly, to understand not only the different cultural approaches of their population to health and health care use but also to provide culturally and language-appropriate services and resources to them. Health education, an important component of pediatric care, increasingly will need to address this cultural and language diversity.

The rising elderly dependency ratio means that children will be increasingly less visible in the political world, a world in which they have never been a strong constituent. Debates about allocation of scarce resources will need to achieve a delicate balance between health and the resource needs of our children and those of the elderly, a debate that is likely to become more favorable to the elderly population based on numbers alone. As health care providers and public health professionals, we will continue to need to serve as advocates for our most vulnerable population. The future of our children and subsequent generations depends on our advocacy for them in the ongoing political debate.

BIRTHS

The number of births in 1997 was 3,880,894, the lowest number recorded in the United States since 1987. The birth rate was 14.5 per 1000 total population, the lowest level ever in the nation. The fertility rate, defined as the number of births per 1000 women ages 15 to 44 years, declined slightly to 65.0, reaching the same rate as in 1976 (Table 3-1).

Births to Teenagers

Childbearing among teenagers fell in 1997 to 52.3 births per 1000 females 15 to 19 years of age, 15% lower than the rate for 1991 (Table 3-2). Although teen birth rates have fallen during the 1990s, they still are higher than those reported during the 1980s. The proportion of all births to teen mothers fell slightly to 12.7%.[35]

In 1997, birth rates were higher among non-Hispanic black and Hispanic teenagers than among non-Hispanic white and Asian American teenagers. Since 1991, the largest declines in birth rates—nearly 20%—have been among non-

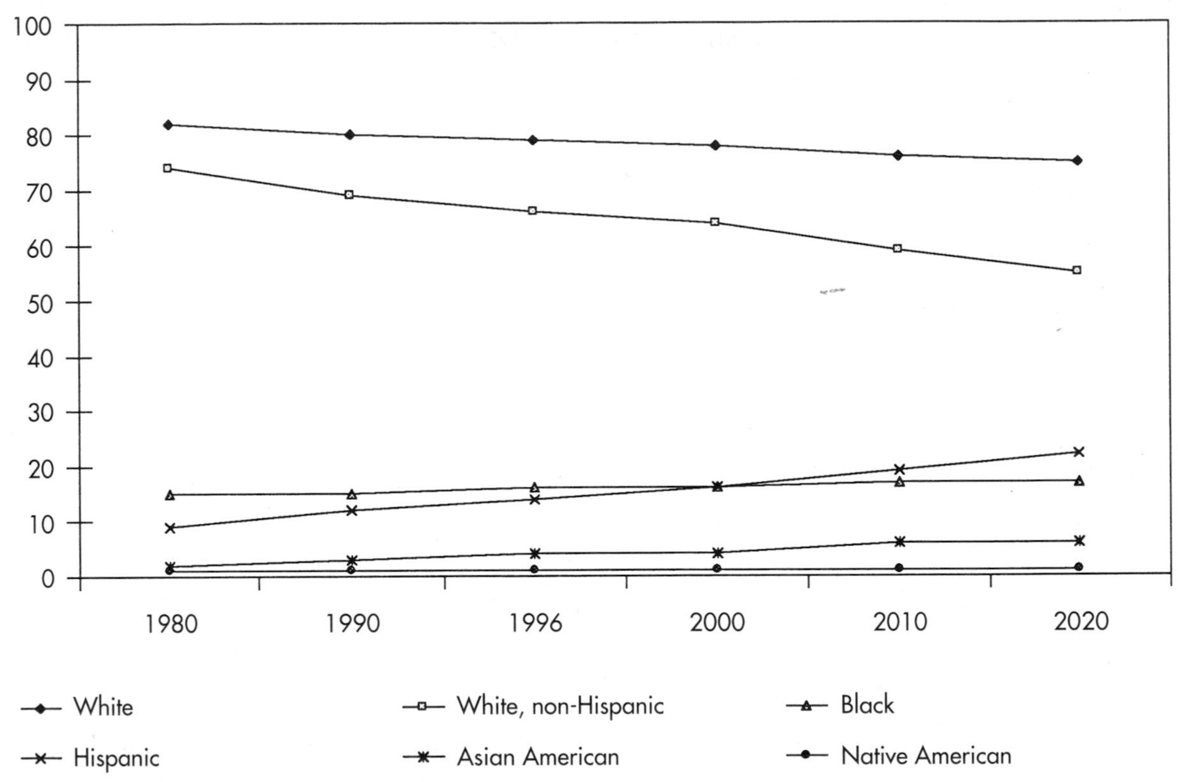

Fig. 3-2 Percentage of children younger than 18 years estimated in U.S. population by race, ethnicity, and year, 1980 to 2020.

Table 3-1 Vital Statistics of the United States, Final 1950-1997 (Selected Years) and Preliminary 1997 Item

	Rate*				
Item	**1997**	**1995**	**1990**	**1980**	**1950**
Birth rate	14.5	14.8	16.7	15.9	24.1
Fertility rate	65.0	65.6	70.9	68.4	106.2
Death rate (crude)†	8.6	8.8	8.6	8.8	9.6
Age-adjusted death rate†	4.8	5.0	5.2	5.9	8.4
Infant mortality	7.1	7.6	9.2	12.6	29.2
Population base (in thousands)	267,636	262,755	248,710	226,546	150,697

From National Center for Health Statistics, National Vital Statistics System and the United States Bureau of the Census. Modified from Guyer B, et al: *Pediatrics* 102:1333, 1998.

*Rates per 1000 population except for fertility, which is per 1000 women ages 15 to 44 years, and infant mortality, which is per 1000 live births.

†Data are preliminary.

Hispanic black teens. The fertility rate for Hispanic teens ages 15 to 19 years dipped below 100 per 1000 in 1997 for the first time since national data became available in 1989.[35]

Births to Women 20 Years of Age and Older

In 1997, birth rates were highest for women ages 20 to 24 years (110.0 births per 1000 women) and for women ages 25 to 29-years (113.8). Rates for women in their twenties declined during the first half of the 1990s but began to rise in 1996, although the rate for women ages 20 to 24 years declined slightly in 1997. Women in their twenties still account for more than 50% of all births. Birth rates for women ages 30 to 34 years (85.3 per 1000), and especially for those ages 35 to 39 years (36.1 per 1000) and 40 to 44 years (7.1 per 1000), have climbed steadily over the past two decades (by 63%, 90%, and 82%, respectively, since the lowest level for each in the late 1970s).[35]

Table 3-2 Birth Rates for Teenagers by Age, Race, and Hispanic Origin: United States, Final 1990-1997

Age, Race, and Hispanic Origin of Mother	Rate 1997	1995	1990	Percent Change, 1990-97
15-19 yr				
All races	52.3	56.8	59.9	−12.7
White, non-Hispanic	36.0	39.3	42.5	−15.3
Black, non-Hispanic	90.8	96.1†	112.8†	−19.5
Hispanic*	97.4	106.7	100.3	−3.0

Modified from Guyer B, et al: *Pediatrics* 102:1333, 1998; and Ventura SJ, et al: Births: final data for 1997. *National Vital Statistics Reports,* vol 47, no 18, Hyattsville, Md, National Center for Health Statistics, 1999.
Note: Rates per 1000 women in specified group.
*Persons of Hispanic origin may be of any race.
†Data for all black women for these years.

Unmarried Mothers

In 1997, 32.4% of all births occurred to unmarried women (Table 3-3). In 1997 the percentage of births to unmarried women was particularly high among mothers younger than 15 years of age (95.7%), mothers ages 15 to 19 years (77.8%), Hispanic women (40.9%), and black women (69.8%). This percentage has increased dramatically over the past three decades, rising from 5% in 1960 to 32% in 1997.[35] The increase in fertility (number of births per 1000 women) for unmarried women since 1980 has occurred in all age groups.[7]

Prenatal Care

The trend toward earlier utilization of prenatal care continued throughout the 1990s, with 82.5% of mothers beginning care in the first trimester of pregnancy in 1997 (see Table 3-3). The percentage of women who had late (beginning in the third trimester) or no care declined 38% since 1989 and was

Table 3-3 Percentage of Births with Selected Characteristics, by Race of Mother: United States, Final 1980-1997

Characteristic	All Races* 1997	1996	1990	1980†	White 1997	1996	1990	1980†	Black 1997	1996	1990	1980†
Mother												
<20 years of age	12.7	12.9	12.8	15.6	11.2	11.3	10.9	13.5	22.2	22.8	23.1	26.5
Unmarried‡	32.4	32.4	28.0	18.4	25.8	25.7	20.4	11.0	69.2	69.8	66.5	55.3
Smoker§	13.2	13.6	18.4	—	14.3	14.7	19.4	—	9.7	10.2	15.9	—
Health Care Utilization												
First-trimester prenatal care‡	82.5	81.9	75.8	76.3	84.7	84.0	79.2	79.2	72.3	71.4	60.6	62.4
Multiple Births, Per 1000												
Live births in twin deliveries (not percent)‡	26.8	25.9	22.6	18.9	28.8	25.8	22.1	18.1	30.0	29.1	26.5	24.0
Live births in higher-order multiple deliveries (not percent)‡	1.7	1.5	0.7	0.4	2.3	1.7	0.8	0.4	0.7	0.7	0.5	0.2
Infant												
Birth weight												
Very low birth weight (VLBW)‖	1.4	1.4	1.3	1.2	1.1	1.1	1.0	0.9	3.0	3.0	2.9	2.5
Low birth weight (LBW)‖	7.5	7.4	7.0	6.8	6.5	6.3	5.7	5.7	13.0	13.0	13.3	12.7

Modified from Guyer B, et al: *Pediatrics* 102:1333, 1998; and Ventura SJ, et al: Births: final data for 1997. *National Vital Statistics Reports,* vol 47, no 18, Hyattsville, Md, National Center for Health Statistics, 1999.
*Includes races other than white and black.
†Data for 1980 based on 100% of births in selected states and on a 50% sample of births in all other states.
‡The 1997 data for multiple births, unmarried mothers, and use of prenatal care are for non-Hispanic whites and non-Hispanic blacks.
§Excludes data for California, Indiana, New York (but includes New York City), and South Dakota, which did not require reporting of tobacco use.
‖Very low birth weight (VLBW) is birth weight of <1500 g (3 lb, 4 oz), and low birth weight (LBW) is birth weight of <2500 g (5 lb, 8 oz).
–, Indicates comparable data not available for this period.

3.9% of births in 1997.[35] The benefits of routine prenatal care are difficult to measure; however, timely, comprehensive prenatal care can promote healthier pregnancies by detecting and managing preexisting maternal medical conditions and providing education about health behaviors.[34]

Since 1989, the percentage of non-Hispanic black mothers who had first-trimester care has risen 21% (from 59.9% to 72.3%); those who had late or no care has declined 39%. Progress in prenatal care utilization has been most pronounced among Hispanic women; first-trimester care climbed 24% since 1989 (from 59.5% to 73.7%), and the percentage of mothers who had late or no care has been halved, dropping from 13.0% to 6.2%.[35]

Multiple Births

The multiple birth rate (defined as the number of births in twin, triplet, and greater deliveries per 1000 live births) was 28.6 per 1000 births in 1997 (see Table 3-3). The vast majority (94%) of multiple births are twins. Since 1980 the number of twin births has risen 52%.[35]

The higher-order multiple birth rate (the number of births in triplet, quadruplet, and greater deliveries per 1000 live births) was 1.74 in 1997, a jump of 14% from the 1996 rate (1.53) following a rise of 20% from 1995 (1.28) to 1996, the largest single year increase in at least 25 years.[14,35] The number and rate of higher-order multiple births has quadrupled since 1980.[22] The dramatic rise in multiple births, and especially of higher-order multiple births, over the past several decades has been attributed to increases in the use of fertility-enhancing therapies and delayed childbearing (the risk of multiple birth increases with maternal age even without the use of fertility enhancing therapies).[19,36]

Non-Hispanic black mothers historically have been, and continue to be, more likely than non-Hispanic white mothers to have a twin birth (30.0 compared with 28.8 per 1000 in 1997), although the racial differential in twin birth rates is narrowing. Non-Hispanic white mothers, however, were more than three times as likely to have a higher-order multiple birth (230.8 compared with 72.7 per 100,000) than non-Hispanic black women in 1997.[35] The greater likelihood of white mothers to seek infertility services likely accounts for much of this difference.[6]

Although multiple births are much more likely than single births to be low-birth-weight or preterm (fewer than 37 completed weeks of gestation), there is evidence that the optimum birth weight and gestational period for multiple births is lower than that of singleton births, and that it continues to decline with increasing plurality.[2] Despite their likely survival advantage over "singletons" at lower birth weights and shorter gestations, however, "multiples" are at greater risk of early death. In 1996, multiple births comprised 16% of all neonatal deaths and were seven times more likely than singletons to die within the first month of life.[21]

Birth Weight

The percentage of low-birth-weight (LBW) infants (<2500 g) was 7.5% in 1997 and has risen by 13% since 1980 (see Table 3-3). When only LBW births among singleton births are analyzed, however, the rate of increase is substantially less—4%. The unprecedented rise in multiple births since the early 1980s has influenced the overall increase in LBW rates.[35]

The percentage of very low–birth-weight (VLBW) infants (<1500 g) was 1.4% in 1997, a rise from 1.2% in 1980 (see Table 3-3).[35] Low birth weight is a major indicator of infant health; despite improvements in survival rates among these smaller infants in recent years, 2 of 100 moderately LBW infants (1500 to 2499 g) and 1 of 4 VLBW infants do not survive the first year of life.[14]

The percentage of LBW infants born to non-Hispanic white mothers has risen 16% since 1989. The VLBW rate for these mothers has increased by more than 20% since the early 1980s. Although much of the increase in LBW and VLBW rates for white births can be attributed to the rise in multiple birth rates,[23] LBW singleton births among non-Hispanic white women have also risen during the 1990s. The percentage of LBW infants among births to non-Hispanic black mothers declined to 13.0% from a high of 13.6% reported for 1991 but remains higher than levels in the early to mid 1980s. In contrast to LBW, however, the percentage of VLBW black births has risen 25% above the VLBW percentages in the 1970s.

The elevated risk of LBW for births to non-Hispanic black women largely can be attributed to their much higher incidence of preterm birth; 17.6% for them compared with 9.8% of births to non-Hispanic white women were shortened gestations in 1997. Infants born preterm are much more likely than those born at longer gestations to weigh less than 2500 g.[35]

DEATHS

Infant Mortality

The preliminary infant mortality rate (IMR) in the United States in 1997 was 7.1 per 1000 live births, the lowest ever recorded in the United States (see Table 3-1). The neonatal mortality rate (NMR; infant deaths under 28 days) declined to 4.7, while the postneonatal mortality rate (PNMR; 28 days through 11 months) fell to 2.4. IMRs were elevated among infants whose mothers were younger than 20 years or 40 years or older, were unmarried, did not complete high school, started prenatal care after the first trimester of pregnancy, or smoked during pregnancy. IMRs were also higher for male infants, multiple births, and infants born preterm or of low birth weight.[21]

Infant mortality in the United States has declined by more than 40% since 1980 (Fig. 3-3). The NMR declined more rapidly during the 1980s, whereas the PNMR has declined more rapidly during the 1990s.

Racial differences in the IMR remain a major national concern. Although all racial groups have experienced declines in IMR, the relative difference in rates between black and white newborns, expressed as the ratio of black to white IMRs, increased from 2.0 in 1980 to 2.4 in 1990. According to preliminary data, the race ratio declined to 2.3 in 1997, the first decline in this ratio since 1973. Although this recent drop is very encouraging, racial disparities in IMR present continued challenges for researchers and health care providers alike.[4,13]

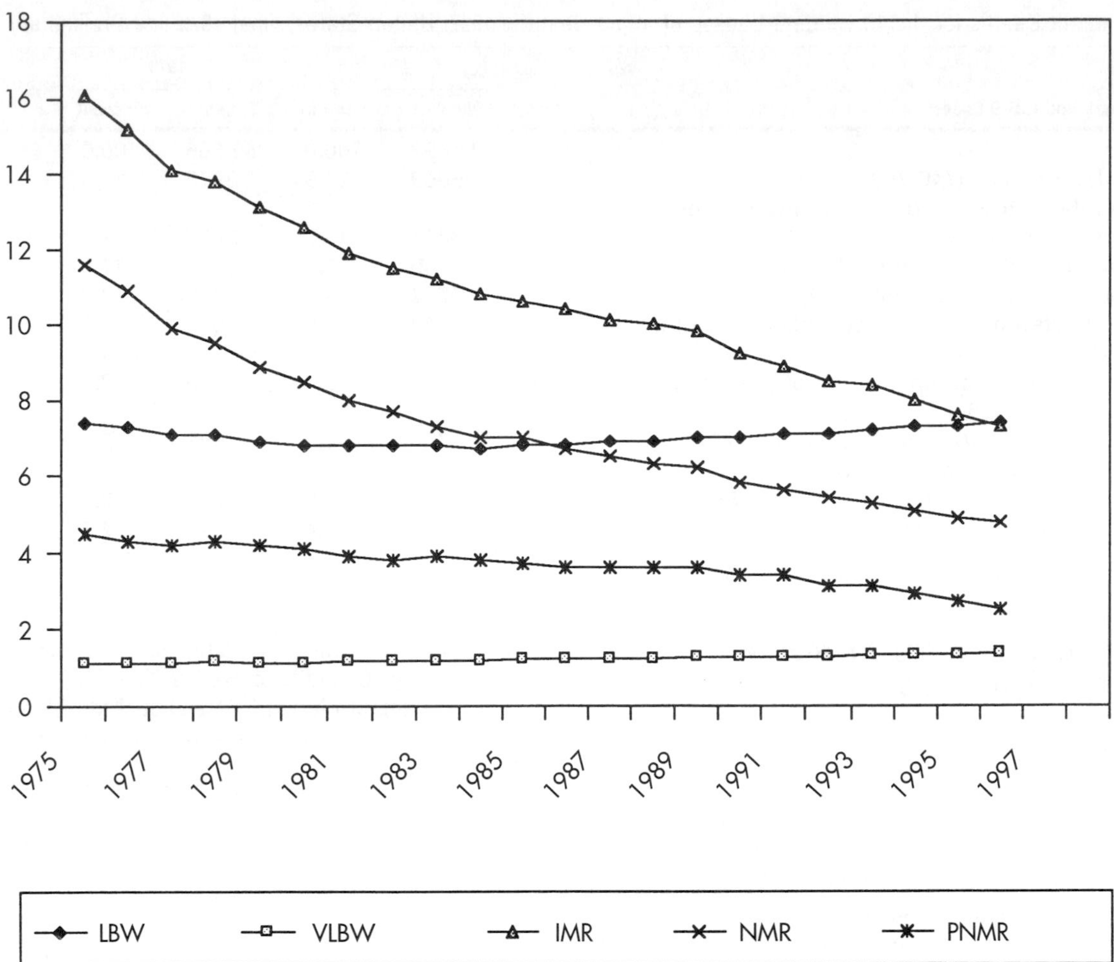

Fig. 3-3 Infant, neonatal, postneonatal mortality, and low- and very low-birth-weight, United States, 1970 to 1994. *IMR,* infant mortality rate; *NMR,* neonatal mortality rate; *PNMR,* postneonatal mortality rate; *LBW,* low birth weight (<2500 g); *VLBW,* very low birth weight (<1500 g).

(With permission of Guyer B, et al: *Pediatrics* 102:1333, 1998.)

Birth Weight–Specific Infant Mortality

Birth weight is one of the most important predictors of infant mortality.[31] The IMR for a given population can be partitioned into two key components: the birth weight distribution and birth weight–specific mortality rates (the death rate for infants at a given weight). The IMR decreases when either the percentage of LBW births decreases or the birth weight–specific mortality rates decrease. All of the decline in the IMR since 1980 (see Fig. 3-3) has been due to declines in birth weight–specific IMRs and not to the prevention of low birth weight.[14] These declines have been attributed primarily to improvements in obstetrical and neonatal care. However, the United States has been unsuccessful in reducing the number of preterm and LBW deliveries, even though preventive efforts have the potential to save many more infant lives and reduce subsequent morbidity.

In 1996, 64% of all infant deaths occurred among the 7.4% of infants who were of low birth weight. Approximately 90% of infants who are of birth weight less than 500 g die within the first year of life and most within the first few days of life. An infant's chances of survival increase rapidly thereafter with increasing birth weight. At birth weights of 1250 to 1499 g, about 95% of babies now survive the first year. IMRs are lowest for infants at birth weights of 4000 to 4499 g, with small increases thereafter among the heaviest infants.[21]

Leading Causes of Infant Death

The 10 leading causes of infant death for 1997 are shown in Table 3-4. Fifty percent of all infant deaths were attributable to four leading causes—congenital anomalies, disorders related to short gestation and unspecified low birth weight, sudden infant death syndrome (SIDS), and respiratory distress syndrome (RDS). IMRs from congenital anomalies declined by 39% from 1979 to 1996, although this decline was less than that for overall infant mortality. SIDS rates have fallen by 42% since 1992, when the American Academy of Pediatrics issued a recommendation to reduce the risk of SIDS by placing infants on their backs or sides to sleep.[1,12] IMRs for RDS have declined by 64% since 1989, when new medical treatments for this condition became widely available.[15,25]

Table 3-4 Infant Deaths for the 10 Leading Causes of Infant Death in 1997: United States, Final 1979 and Preliminary 1997

Cause of Death and ICD-9 Codes	Rank	1997 Number	1997 Percent	1979 Number	1979 Percent	Percent Change 1979-97
All causes	—	27,692	100.0	45,665	100.0	−45.6
Congenital anomalies (740-759)	1	6063	21.9	8923	19.5	−39.0
Disorders related to short gestation and unspecified Low birth weight (765)	2	3727	13.5	3495	7.7	−4.3
Sudden infant death syndrome (798.0)	3	2705	9.8	5279	11.6	−54.1
Respiratory distress syndrome (769)	4	1262	4.6	5458	12.0	−79.3
Newborn affected by maternal complications of pregnancy (761)	5	1242	4.5	1621	3.5	−31.3
Newborn affected by complications of placenta, cord, and membranes (762)	6	927	3.3	970	2.1	−14.4
Infections specific to the perinatal period (771)	7	756	2.7	981	2.1	−31.0
Accidents and adverse effects (E800-E949)	8	753	2.7	1080	2.4	−37.5
Intrauterine hypoxia and birth asphyxia (768)	9	456	1.6	1393	3.1	−70.7
Pneumonia and influenza (480-487)	10	397	1.4	1129	2.5	−68.4

Modified from Guyer B, et al: *Pediatrics* 102:1333, 1998.

International Comparisons of Infant Mortality

Table 3-5 shows infant mortality rates for countries that have at least a population of 2.5 million and for which the IMR was lower than the rate for the United States in 1994, 1995, or 1996.[10] In general, the figures for 1994 and 1995 are based on final reports from each country. Most figures for 1996, apart from the United States, are provisional and may change once final data become available.[14]

The United States' ranking of twenty-third in infant mortality in relation to other developed countries is not enviable, but quick judgments should not be made regarding the reasons for this poor ranking. Reporting of data on live births, especially for the smallest babies with the highest mortality rates, appears to differ across countries, as does the timing of when a live birth must be registered and the reporting of stillbirths.[20] Moreover, the quality of data and coverage of the birth registration systems vary by country, which may affect international comparisons. These differences in reporting, however, do not account for all of the disparity between the IMR in the United States and the other countries. A major reason for the poor ranking of the United States continues to be its persistently high rate of LBW relative to other developed countries.[20]

Table 3-5 Infant Mortality Rates for 1994, 1995, and 1996 for Countries of >2.5 Million Population That Have Infant Mortality Rates Equal to or Less Than the United States Rate for 1994, 1995, or 1996

	Infant Mortality Rate 1996	1995	1994
Singapore	3.8	4.0	4.3
Japan	3.8	4.2	4.3
Finland	4.0	3.9	4.7
Sweden	4.0	3.7	4.4
Norway	4.0	4.0	5.3
Hong Kong	4.0	4.6	4.5
Switzerland	4.7	5.0	5.1
Spain	4.7*	5.5	6.0
France	4.9	4.9	5.9
Germany	5.0	5.3	5.6
Austria	5.1	5.1	6.3
Ireland	5.5	6.4	5.7
Belgium	5.6	6.1	7.6
Canada	5.6	6.1	6.3
Denmark	5.7	5.1	5.5
Netherlands	5.7	5.5	5.6
Australia	5.8	5.7	5.9
Italy	6.0	6.1	6.5
Czech Republic	6.0	7.7	7.9
United Kingdom	6.1	6.2	6.2
New Zealand	†	6.7	7.2
Portugal	6.9	7.5	8.1
United States	7.3	7.6	8.0
Greece	8.1*	7.9	7.9

From United Nations[10] and individual reports by country.
Modified from Guyer B, et al: *Pediatrics* 102:1333, 1998.
*Preliminary data.
†Data not available.

Expectation of Life

The estimated expectation of life at birth for a given year represents the average number of years that a group of infants would be expected to live if, throughout their lifetime, they were to experience the age-specific death rates prevailing during their year of birth. Based on preliminary data for 1997, the expectation of life at birth reached a new record high of 76.5 years. In 1997, life expectancy at birth was 79.8 years for white females, 74.7 years for black females, 74.3 years for white males, and 67.3 years for black males.

Deaths Among Children

In 1997, the death rate for children 1 to 4 years old was 35.6 per 100,000 population, 18.5 per 100,000 population for 5- to 9-year-olds, 23.1 for 10- to 14-year-olds, and 73.3 for 15- to 19-year-olds.[14] Since 1979, death rates have declined by 45% for children 1 to 4 years old, by 41% for children 5 to 9 years old, by 27% for children 10 to 14 years old, and by 26% for teens 15 to 19 years old.

Table 3-6 Death Rate for the Five Leading Causes of Childhood Death in Specified Age Groups in 1997: United States, Final 1979 and Preliminary 1997

Cause of Death and Age	Rank*	1997 Number	1997 Percent	1979 Number	1979 Percent	Percent Change 1979-97
Total: 1-19 yr						
All causes	—	27,489	100.0	40,339	100.0	−35.3
Accidents and adverse effects (E800-E949)	1	11,694	42.5	21,727	53.9	−48.9
Homicide and legal intervention (E960-E978)	2	3228	11.7	2899	7.2	4.8
Suicide (E950-E959)	3	2127	7.7	1940	4.8	3.6
Malignant neoplasms (140-208)	4	2124	7.7	3271	8.1	−38.3
Congenital anomalies (740-759)	5	1216	4.4	1899	4.7	−37.0
1-4 yr						
All causes	—	5471	100.0	8108	100.0	−44.5
Accidents and adverse effects (E800-E949)	1	1958	35.8	3349	41.3	−51.7
Congenital anomalies (740-759)	2	596	10.9	1021	12.6	−51.9
Malignant neoplasms (140-208)	3	458	8.4	578	7.1	−34.8
Homicide and legal intervention (E960-E978)	4	345	6.3	314	3.9	−8.0
Cardiac diseases (390-398, 402, 404-429)	5	195	3.6	265	3.3	−38.1
5-9 yr						
All causes	—	3646	100.0	5278	100.0	−40.5
Accidents and adverse effects (E800-E949)	1	1524	41.8	2707	51.3	−51.9
Malignant neoplasms (140-208)	2	518	14.2	791	15.0	−44.7
Congenital anomalies (740-759)	3	214	5.9	289	5.5	−35.3
Homicide and legal intervention (E960-E978)	4	159	4.4	165	3.1	−20.0
Cardiac diseases (390-398, 402, 404-429)	5	138	3.8	119	2.3	—
10-14 yr						
All causes	—	4398	100.0	5868	100.0	−27.4
Accidents and adverse effects (E800-E949)	1	1805	41.0	2982	50.8	−41.4
Malignant neoplasms (140-208)	2	477	10.9	761	13.0	−39.0
Suicide (E950-E959)	3	308	7.0	151†	2.6	100.0
Homicide and legal intervention (E960-E978)	4	278	6.3	229†	3.9	25.0
Congenital anomalies (740-759)	5	211	4.8	289†	4.9	−31.3
15-19 yr						
All causes	—	13,974	100.0	21,085	100.0	−25.8
Accidents and adverse effects (E800-E949)	1	6407	45.9	12,689	60.2	−43.4
Homicide and legal intervention (E960-E978)	2	2446	17.5	2191	10.4	24.3
Suicide (E950-E959)	3	1814	13.0	1788	8.5	13.1
Malignant neoplasms (140-208)	4	671	4.8	1141	5.4	−34.0
Cardiac diseases (390-398, 402, 404-429)	5	382	2.7	395	1.9	5.3

National Center for Health Statistics, National Vital Statistics System, 1979-97.
Modified from Guyer B, et al: *Pediatrics* 102:1333, 1998.
*Rank based on number of deaths.
†In 1979, congenital anomalies was the third leading cause of death for children 10 to 14 years old, with a total of 289 deaths and a death rate of 1.6; homicide was ranked fourth, suicide sixth, and cardiac diseases fifth.

For children 1 to 4 years old, unintentional injury was the leading cause of death, with congenital anomalies the second and cancer the third leading cause (Table 3-6). Unintentional injuries accounted for 36% of all deaths in this age group, although the rate has declined by 52% since 1979. Death rates for congenital anomalies and cancer have decreased 52% and 35%, respectively, since 1979. Homicide is the fourth leading cause of death in this age group; since 1979, death rates for homicide for this age group have declined by only 8%.

For children 5 to 9 years old (see Table 3-6), unintentional injury, cancer, congenital anomalies, and homicide were the leading causes of death. Unintentional injury accounted for nearly 42% of all deaths in 1997, while cancer accounted for 14% of all deaths in this age group. Since 1979, death rates due to each of the these leading causes of death have declined by at least 20%.

Unintentional injury was the leading cause of death and accounted for 41% of all deaths to children 10 to 14 years old (see Table 3-6). The second leading cause was cancer. The death rate due to unintentional injuries and cancer for this age group declined by 41% and 39%, respectively, since 1979. In contrast, the death rate for suicide doubled during this period. The homicide death rate increased 25% from 1979 to 1996 but declined 17% between 1996 and 1997.

For teens ages 15 to 19 years, unintentional injuries, the leading cause of death, accounted for 46% of all deaths in 1997, although the rate has dropped by 43% since 1979 (see Table 3-6). Homicide, the second leading cause, accounted for 18% of all deaths. The teen homicide rate increased by

24% from 1979 to 1996 but decreased 18% between 1996 and 1997. Suicide was the third leading cause of death for this age group, accounting for 13% of all deaths. Since 1979, suicide rates increased 13% for this age group.

MORBIDITY AND DISABILITY

Identifying epidemiological trends for children who have a chronic illness is important for several reasons. First, although the vast majority of children are healthy, increasing numbers of children, because of advances in medical technology, are growing up with a chronic illness.[24,26,27] Second, children who have a chronic illness receive a disproportionate amount of health care resources, suggesting that these children are particularly vulnerable to insurance policies and health care reforms that limit access to particular services.[17] Third, some children who have a chronic illness have complex medical and other service systems needs that require an array of community resources for optimal functioning. Fourth, children who have a chronic illness have needs distinct from similar adults. Developing policies and allocating resources for health, educational, social service, and other community programs requires knowledge of the characteristics of the target population.

Children with Chronic Conditions

Multiple definitions have been proposed for identifying children who have a chronic illness. These approaches frequently rely on the use of condition lists, functional status and impairments, and the presence of disability or limitation in socially defined roles. However, each of these methods has been noted to have significant limitations. For example, condition lists fail to recognize the variability of an individual's experience with the same chronic condition or similarities across individuals who have different chronic conditions. A new definition for identifying children who have a chronic illness has been proposed by a working group supported by the Federal Maternal and Child Health Bureau's Division of Services for Children with Special Health Care Needs. This definition is as follows:

> "Children with special health care needs are those who have or are at risk for a chronic physical, developmental, behavioral, or emotional condition and who also require health and related services of a type or amount beyond that required by children generally."[24]

This new definition recognizes children who have existing conditions, as well as those at risk, and broadly includes a range of impairments as well as service use.

The historical use of varying definitions of children who have one or more chronic illnesses has contributed to prevalence estimates ranging from 4% to 31%. These differences have dramatic implications for public policy and resource allocation. Applying noncategorical methods and using data from the National Health Interview Survey (NHIS) 1994 Disability Supplement, recent studies have identified overall rates of children younger than 18 years who have chronic conditions to range from 15%[33] to 18%.[28] Differences in prevalence by gender, age, race, and socioeconomic status have been noted across many studies. In general, higher proportions of chronic illness are found among males than females, older than younger children, and black and Hispanic than white children.

The majority of children who have a chronic illness have a single condition rather than multiple conditions, although a small proportion have severe conditions. Using NHIS 1988 data, Newacheck and Taylor[29] reported that among the nearly 20 million children younger than age 18 who had chronic conditions, 70% had one condition; 21% had two conditions; and 9% had three or more conditions. In the same study, the authors found that 65% had mild, 29% moderate, and 6% severe conditions. Children who had multiple conditions and had severe conditions are of interest, because they are at increased risk for developmental, learning, and behavioral problems; having functional limitations; experiencing more bed days and school absences; having poorer overall health status; and using more health care resources.[27]

Limitations in Activity

Data on limitations of activity among children are available from 1984 to 1995 from NHIS data.[11] From 1984 to 1995, the percentage of children ages 0 to 17 who had any limitation in activity resulting from chronic conditions lasting at least 3 months increased slightly from 5% to 6%. Of note, this increase was concentrated in children ages 5 to 17 years (6.1% to 7.4%) rather than younger children ages 0 to 4 years (2.5% to 2.6%). It is possible that children ages 5 to 17 years have higher rates of activity limitation because some limitations are not diagnosed until school entry. Stein and Silver[33] found that 9.5% of all children have functional limitations, 5.1% depend on compensatory mechanisms, and 10.6% have service use or needs above routine care.

There remains a persistent gap in the presence of limitations among children ages 5 to 17 years based on poverty status and race. As shown in Figure 3-4, the percentage of children whose activities are limited is nearly double for children residing in families who have household incomes below the poverty level than for non-poor children. In 1995, 12% of children ages 5 to 17 years living below the poverty level had activity limitation compared with 7% of children in families at or above the poverty level. A similar gap in activity limitation by income is present among younger children, although the overall rates of limitation are lower.[11]

Limitations in activity also vary by gender and race. Among children ages 5 to 17 years, 9% of boys and 6% of girls were limited in activities due to chronic health conditions in 1995. A greater percentage of non-white children report activity limitation. During the same year, rates of limitation by race were 7% for non-Hispanic white, 7.5% for Hispanic, and 9% for non-Hispanic black children ages 5 to 17 years. Similar gaps by gender and race exist for younger children.[11]

Specific Conditions

Respiratory conditions, including hay fever, allergic rhinitis, chronic bronchitis, chronic sinusitis, and asthma account for the chronic conditions most commonly reported in children less than 18 years of age (Table 3-7). Other commonly re-

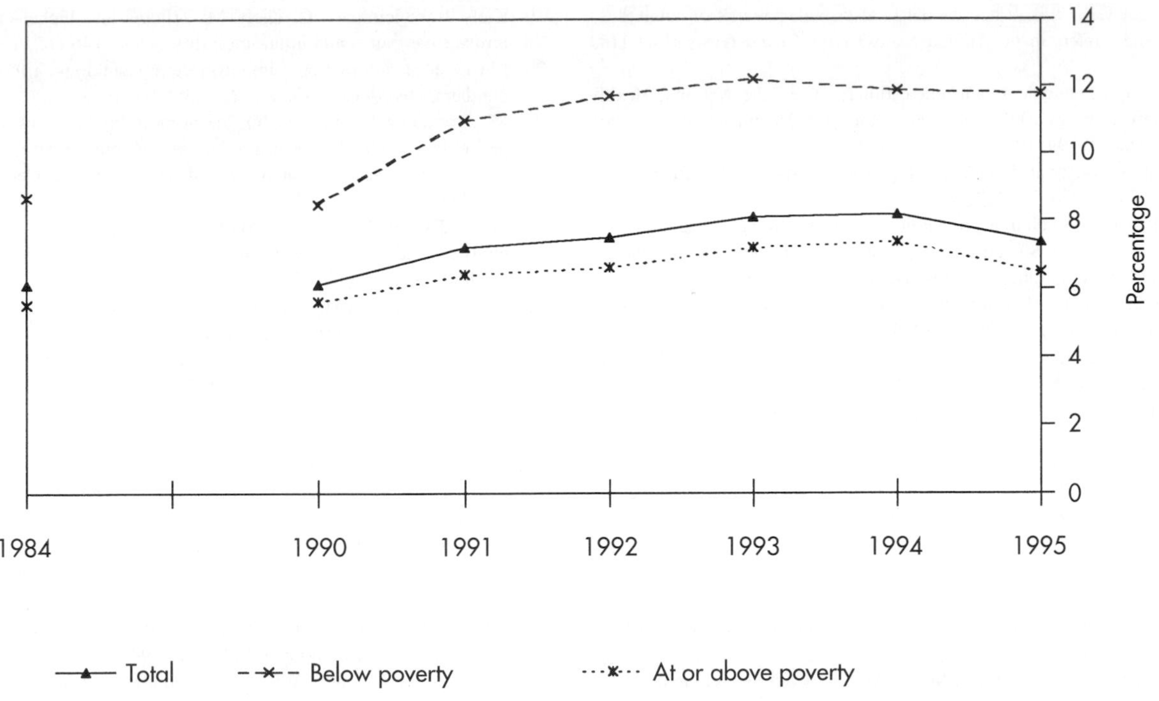

Fig. 3-4 Differences in activity limitation by poverty status for children ages 5 to 17 years.

Table 3-7 Selected Chronic Conditions Per 1000 Persons, Under 18 Years, 1995

Type of Chronic Condition	Number of Chronic Conditions per 1000 Persons
Respiratory Conditions	
Chronic sinusitis	75.6
Asthma	74.9
Hay fever, allergic rhinitis without asthma	66.2
Chronic bronchitis	53.6
Skin Conditions	
Dermatitis	35.2
Serious acne	26.4
Impairments	
Deformity or orthopedic impairment	29.8
Speech impairment	18.1
Hearing impairment	14.9
Visual impairment	7.0
Other Conditions	
Heart disease	18.6
Migraine headache	12.7
Anemia	7.2
Epilepsy	4.0

From Benson V, Marano MA: *Vital Health Stat* 10:199, 1998.

ported conditions tabulated from the 1995 NHIS include skin conditions and impairments. Of note, individual researchers have reanalyzed NHIS data to identify additional conditions of importance for children, including frequent or repeated ear infections and eczema and skin allergies.[27]

CONCLUSION

In general, mortality rates for children in the United States are lower than they have ever been and continue to decline. Yet, differences in health status by socioeconomic status and race persist, as do overall poor health indicators for children in the United States relative to those in other developed countries. These disparities may widen as the numbers and percentages of children in various racial and ethnic groups increase over the next quarter century and as the needs of the elderly place increasing demand on already scarce health care resources for some populations.

Greater investment in the health of our children, including a more effective system of primary care, is needed to address these concerns. Cross-national comparisons demonstrate the association of primary care with greater consumer satisfaction and improved measures of health status such as reduced percentage low-birth-weight, lower death rates from injuries, and higher immunization rates.[32] Ongoing monitoring of the characteristics and health of the child population remains necessary to document the successes and failures of programs and policies designed to improve access to care and the health of children.

Most of the data presented in this chapter are collected routinely through vital records or the census. It would not be possible to make the comparisons noted here or to follow trends over time without careful reporting of these data. It is important that clinicians understand these patterns and remain committed to providing high-quality data through accurate birth and death certificates and medical records.

REFERENCES

1. AAP Task Force on Infant Positioning and SIDS: Positioning and SIDS, *Pediatrics* 87:1120, 1992.

2. Alexander GR, et al: What are the fetal growth patterns of singletons, twins and triplets in the United States? *Clin Obstet Gynecol* 41:115, 1998.
3. Benson V, Marano MA: Current estimates from the National Health Interview Survey, 1995. National Center for Health Statistics, *Vital Health Stat* 10:199, 1998.
4. Blackmore CA, et al: Is race a risk factor or a risk marker for preterm delivery? *Ethn Dis* 3:372, 1993.
5. Campbell PR: Population projections for states, by age, race, and sex: 1993 to 2020, US Bureau of the Census, Current Population Reports, P25-1111, Washington, DC, 1994, US Government Printing Office.
6. Chandra A, Stephen EH: Impaired fecundity in the United States: 1982-95, *Fam Plann Perspect* 30:34, 1998.
7. Child Trends, Inc: *Trends in the well-being of America's children and youth,* 1997 ed. Washington, DC: Office of the Assistant Secretary for Planning and Evaluation, US Department of Health and Human Services, 1997.
8. Child Trends, Inc: *Trends in the well-being of America's children and youth*, 1998 ed. Part 1: Indicators of children's well-being. Washington, DC: Office of the Assistant Secretary for Planning and Evaluation, US Department of Health and Human Services, 1999.
9. Day JC: Population projections of the United States by age, sex, race, and Hispanic origin: 1995 to 2050, US Bureau of the Census, Current Population Reports, P25-1130, US Government Printing Office, Washington, DC, 1996.
10. Department of Economic and Social Affairs: 1996 Demographic Yearbook, New York: United Nations, 1998.
11. Federal Interagency Forum on Child and Family Statistics, America's Children: Key national indicators of well-being, Federal Interagency Forum on Child and Family Statistics, Washington, DC, US Government Printing Office, 1998.
12. Gibson E, et al: Infant sleep position following new AAP guidelines, *Pediatrics* 96:69, 1995.
13. Goldenberg RL, et al: Bacterial colonization of the vagina during pregnancy in four ethnic groups, *Am J Obstet Gynecol* 174:1618, 1996.
14. Guyer B, et al: Annual summary of vital statistics—1997, *Pediatrics* 102:1333, 1998.
15. Hamvas A, et al: The influence of the wider use of surfactant therapy on neonatal mortality among blacks and whites, *N Engl J Med* 334:1635, 1996.
16. Hollmann FW, et al: US population estimates by age, sex, race, and Hispanic origin: 1990 to 1997, Washington, DC, US Bureau of the Census, PPL-91, 1998.
17. Ireys HT, et al: Expenditures for care of children with chronic illnesses enrolled in the Washington State Medicaid Program, fiscal year 1993, *Pediatrics* 100:197, 1997.
18. Jameson EJ, Wehr E: Drafting national health care reform legislation to protect the health interests of children, *Stanford Law Policy Rev* 152-176, Fall 1993.
19. Kiely JL, Kleinman JC, Kiely M: Triplets and higher-order multiple births: time trends and infant mortality, *AJDC* 146:862, 1992.
20. Liu K, et al: International infant mortality rankings: a look behind the numbers, *Health Care Financ Rev* 13:4105, 1992.
21. MacDorman MF, Atkinson JO: Infant mortality statistics from the 1996 period linked birth/infant death data set. Monthly vital statistics report, vol 46, no 12, suppl, Hyattsville, Md, 1998, National Center for Health Statistics.
22. Martin JA, MacDorman MF, Mathews TJ: Triplet and other higher-order multiple births, trends and outcomes, 1971-1994. National Center for Health Statistics, *Vital Health Stat* 55:21, 1997.
23. Martin JA, Taffel SM: Current and future impact of rising multiple birth ratios on low birth weight, *Stat Bull* 76:10, 1995.
24. McPherson M, et al: A new definition of children with special health care needs, *Pediatrics* 102:137, 1998.
25. Modanlou HD, et al: Combined effects of antenatal corticosteroids and surfactant supplementation on the outcome of very low birth weight infants, *J Perinatol* 16:421, 1996.
26. Newacheck PW, Stoddard JJ: Prevalence and impact of multiple childhood chronic illnesses, *J Pediatr* 124:40, 1994.
27. Newacheck PW, Stoddard JJ, McManus M: Ethnocultural variations in the prevalence and impact of childhood chronic conditions, *Pediatrics* 91:1031, 1993.
28. Newacheck PW, et al: An epidemiologic profile of children with special health care needs, *Pediatrics* 102:117, 1998.
29. Newacheck PW, Taylor WR: Childhood chronic illness: prevalence, severity and impact, *Am J Public Health* 82:364, 1992.
30. Philip MS: Characteristic features of modern American fertility, *Popul Dev Rev* 22(S):19, 1996.
31. Shiono PH, Behrman RE: Low birth weight: analysis and recommendations, *Future Child* 5:4, 1995.
32. Starfield B: *Primary care: concept, evaluation, and policy.* New York, 1992, Oxford University Press.
33. Stein REK, Silver EJ: Operationalizing a conceptually based noncategorical definition: a first look at US children with chronic conditions, *Arch Pediatr Adolesc Med* 153:68, 1999.
34. Strobino D, et al: A strategic framework for infant mortality reduction: implementing "Healthy Start." *Milbank Q* 73:507, 1995.
35. Ventura SJ, et al: Births: final data for 1997. National vital statistics reports, vol 47, no 18, Hyattsville, Md, 1999, National Center for Health Statistics.
36. Wilcox LS, et al: Assisted reproductive technologies: estimates of their contribution to multiple births and newborn hospital days in the United States, *Fertil Steril* 65:361, 1996.
37. World Health Organization, Manual of the International Statistical Classification of Diseases, Injuries and the Causes of Death, based on the recommendations of the Ninth Conference: 1975. Geneva, Switzerland, World Health Organization, 1977.

4 Child Health Supervision

Robert A. Hoekelman

We credit George Armstrong as the father of ambulatory pediatrics and the champion of health maintenance and disease prevention in the individual child—this at a time in nineteenth century England when most of his colleagues were concerned only with the treatment of illness. In the United States, child health supervision had its beginnings in the milk stations and child health conferences of our large cities, where babies were brought to be fed, weighed, examined, and immunized against contagious diseases. It was the conviction that child health supervision is vital that provided the fundamental impetus for establishment of the American Academy of Pediatrics (AAP) and that continues to be the principle upon which pediatrics as a special discipline is based. At the American Public Health Association's 1955 conference on health supervision of young children, health was defined as "a state of physical, mental, and social well-being, not merely the absence of disease or infirmity"; the objective of health supervision for children was deemed to be "to keep the well child well and promote the highest possible level of his complete well-being."[6]

It has not been documented how the frequency and content of well-child visits evolved. However, in 1967, the AAP established guidelines (later called *recommendations*) for child health supervision based on observed practices and expert opinion. These were revised twice during the 1970s, three times during the 1980s, again in 1991 and 1995 and, most recently in 2000.[1] These revisions, also based on observations and opinions, in most instances called for an increase in the number of visits and procedures to be conducted during each scheduled visit. Table 4-1 shows the general growth in the number of child health supervision visits recommended by the AAP between 1967 and 1995. The 1995 and 2000 recommendations call for 27 health supervision visits during the first 21 years of life (Fig. 4-1), in addition to a prenatal visit and at least one visit in the hospital after birth. The recommendations are designed for children who receive competent parenting, who have no manifestations of any important health problems, and who are growing and developing satisfactorily. Additional visits may be necessary if circumstances suggest variations from normal.

Over the three decades following the introduction of the first guidelines, many pediatric practitioners and investigators have reexamined the objectives of child health supervision and the methods by which those objectives can be met realistically in terms of needs, costs, and benefits.

OBJECTIVES

The goals of child health supervision have been categorized in several ways. However, there are three basic objectives:

I. Prevention of disease
   A. Immunization
   B. Health education
II. Early detection and treatment of disease
   A. History
   B. Physical examination
   C. Screening
III. Guidance in the psychosocial aspects of child rearing

Prevention of Disease

The first objective is accomplished mostly through immunization against specific communicable diseases and through health education, initially directed to the parents and later to the child when he or she reaches the age of understanding. These educational efforts concern nutrition, dental hygiene, leading healthy lifestyles, and injury prevention. The aim of this approach is to improve individual and public health. These elements of disease prevention are discussed in detail in Chapter 17, Nutrition; Chapter 21, Counseling Families on Healthy Lifestyles; Chapter 23 (One), Prevention of Dental Caries; and Chapter 23 (Two), Injury Control.

Early Detection and Treatment of Disease

The second objective is based on the presumption that early intervention in identified illnesses results in increased cure rates and decreased disability.

Through history-taking and physical assessment of how well or poorly an infant or child is growing and developing compared with suggested norms, invaluable criteria are developed for identifying either wellness or underlying disease. In this sense, these activities are screening tests as much as are the specific tests pediatricians use routinely to detect anemia, tuberculosis, phenylketonuria, sickle cell disease, lead intoxication, and other illnesses in asymptomatic, seemingly normal infants and children.

The principles and techniques of history-taking and the physical examination of infants, young children, and adolescents are detailed in Chapters 7, The Pediatric History, and 8, The Pediatric Physical Examination. The use of the physi-

Table 4-1 American Academy of Pediatrics Recommendations for Child Health Supervision

Number of Visits	Infancy (Birth-1 yr)	Early Childhood (1-4 yr)	Late Childhood (5-12 yr)	Adolescence/ Young Adulthood (13-21 yr)	Total
1967	5	4	3	2	14
1982	6	5	5	4	20
1991	7	5	5	4	21
1995-2000	7	5	6	9	27

cal examination for early detection of disease is discussed in Chapter 20, Screening, as are the specific screening tests used. The methods by which motor, intellectual, social, and emotional development are assessed and monitored in well children are discussed in Chapter 19, Identification of Developmental Delays and the Early Intervention System, and Chapter 78, Developmental Approach to Behavioral Problems.

Guidance in the Psychosocial Aspects of Child Rearing

The psychosocial aspect of child health supervision often is placed under the rubrics of advice, anticipatory guidance, counseling, and reassuring the parents about their concerns and that they are doing a good job. Well-child visits offer an opportunity to identify potential and real problems in psychosocial adjustment, to prevent potential disorders, to treat actual disorders early in their course, and to make referrals for children and their families with gross interpersonal relationship problems that are beyond the therapeutic scope of the primary care practitioner. Anticipatory guidance in these areas is discussed in Chapter 16, Anticipatory Guidance.

Continuity of Care

Some believe that there is a fourth objective of well-child care: continuity of care. This actually can be considered more an outcome of well-child care than an objective, since it speaks to the establishment of a meaningful relationship between the pediatrician and the parents and child. It implies that regular visits produce familiarity, trust, and respect and that these enable the physician to be more effective in managing all aspects of health and illness care.

That continuity of care makes a difference in these respects, however, has not been proven, and although it seems a logical assumption, a physician who demonstrates interest in and concern for the child and family can establish a meaningful relationship instantly without that prior experience of continuity. Conversely, meaningful relationships can dissolve just as quickly if interest and concern are not sustained, regardless of past performance.

Parents, most likely, are not fully cognizant of the objectives for well-child care visits but could be motivated to make visits for other reasons. Included among them are (1) gaining reassurance about their child's health status, (2) obtaining answers to specific questions about child rearing, (3) receiving approval of their parenting skills, (4) doing what is expected of them (if they have been told by their pediatrician), (5) meeting socialization needs (by providing social interactions with nurses, doctors, and other parents immediately and by talking about them afterward with friends, neighbors, and relatives), and (6) establishing a source of care when their child becomes ill. Despite these incentives, most parents do not adhere to the AAP-recommended well-child visits schedule even when the costs of these visits are fully insured.[3]

Some studies have demonstrated that mothers who have the following characteristics are less likely to comply with AAP-recommended well-child care visit schedules: (1) they are employed, (2) they are raising their child alone, (3) they are poor, (4) they are young, (5) they change their residence frequently, (6) they did not utilize prenatal care adequately, (7) they are members of a minority group, and (8) they are poorly educated.[14,15,17] In a study of white, middle-class families with well-educated parents enrolled in a university-affiliated prepaid group practice, Horwitz, Morgenstern, and Berkman[14] found that the highest utilization rates for well-child visits were for younger children and first-born children. Woodward et al[25] confirmed these findings and also found that when a child's physical health status as perceived by the parents was poor, all ambulatory medical care use, including preventive services, increased.

EVALUATION OF THE EFFECTIVENESS OF CHILD HEALTH SUPERVISION

The basis of the effectiveness of child health supervision (and of illness care also) lies in the pediatrician's ability to influence the parents to follow the advice and directions given them. Professional competence is of little use if parental compliance is not obtained. The level of compliance is positively correlated with satisfaction, and satisfaction with effective communication between the parent and the physician, nurse, or other health professional. These interactions are extremely complex and, in part, relate to addressing the parent's concerns and expectations and the need for them to understand the rationale for recommendations made. The degree of satisfaction and compliance achieved depends on the extent to which these needs are acknowledged and met and on the parent's perception of the physician's empathy and view of him or her as a person (reflexive self-concept). These perceptions are formed very rapidly, often in the first moments of communication. The means by which communication and maternal compliance are enhanced are discussed in detail in Chapters 13, Compliance with Pediatric Health Care Recommendations, and 14, The Art of Consultation.

Most of America's children cared for by primary care pediatricians do not receive the AAP's recommended number of well-child visits. In one recent study of urban and subur-

Recommendations for Preventive Pediatric Health Care

Committee on Practice and Ambulatory Medicine

Each child and family is unique; therefore, these **Recommendations for Preventive Pediatric Health Care** are designed for the care of children who are receiving competent parenting, have no manifestations of any important health problems, and are growing and developing in satisfactory fashion. **Additional visits may become necessary** if circumstances suggest variations from normal.

These guidelines represent a consensus by the Committee on Practice and Ambulatory Medicine in consultation with national committees and sections of the American Academy of Pediatrics. The Committee emphasizes the great importance of **continuity of care** in comprehensive health supervision and the need to avoid **fragmentation of care.**

	INFANCY[4]									EARLY CHILDHOOD[4]					MIDDLE CHILDHOOD[4]				ADOLESCENCE[4]										
AGE[5]	PRENATAL[1]	NEWBORN[2]	2-4d[3]	By 1mo	2mo	4mo	6mo	9mo	12mo	15mo	18mo	24mo	3y	4y	5y	6y	8y	10y	11y	12y	13y	14y	15y	16y	17y	18y	19y	20y	21y
HISTORY																													
Initial/Interval	•	•	•	•	•	•	•	•	•	•	•	•	•	•	•	•	•	•	•	•	•	•	•	•	•	•	•	•	•
MEASUREMENTS																													
Height and Weight		•	•	•	•	•	•	•	•	•	•	•	•	•	•	•	•	•	•	•	•	•	•	•	•	•	•	•	•
Head Circumference		•	•	•	•	•	•	•	•	•	•	•																	
Blood Pressure													•	•	•	•	•	•	•	•	•	•	•	•	•	•	•	•	•
SENSORY SCREENING																													
Vision		S	S	S	S	S	S	S	S	S	S	S	O[6]	O	O	O	O	O	S	O	S	S	O	S	S	O	S	S	S
Hearing		O[7]	S	S	S	S	S	S	S	S	S	S	S	O	O	O	O	O	S	O	S	S	O	S	S	O	S	S	S
DEVELOPMENTAL/ BEHAVIORAL ASSESSMENT[8]		•	•	•	•	•	•	•	•	•	•	•	•	•	•	•	•	•	•	•	•	•	•	•	•	•	•	•	•
PHYSICAL EXAMINATION[9]		•	•	•	•	•	•	•	•	•	•	•	•	•	•	•	•	•	•	•	•	•	•	•	•	•	•	•	•
PROCEDURES-GENERAL[10]																													
Hereditary/Metabolic Screening[11]		←	•	→																									
Immunization[12]		•	•	•	•	•	•	•	•	•	•	•	•	•	•	•	•	•	•	•	•	•	•	•	•	•	•	•	•
Hematocrit or Hemoglobin[13]								• →	→	★ →					→				←		•[14]								→
Urinalysis															•				←					•[15]					→
PROCEDURES-PATIENTS AT RISK																													
Lead Screening[16]								★ →	→			★																	
Tuberculin Test[17]									★	★	★	★	★	★	★	★	★	★	★	★	★	★	★	★	★	★	★	★	★
Cholesterol Screening[18]												★	★	★	★	★	★	★	★	★	★	★	★	★	★	★	★	★	★
STD Screening[19]																			★	★	★	★	★	★	★	★	★	★	★
Pelvic Exam[20]																			★	★	★	★	★	★	★	★ ←	★[20]	★	→ ★
ANTICIPATORY GUIDANCE[21]	•	•	•	•	•	•	•	•	•	•	•	•	•	•	•	•	•	•	•	•	•	•	•	•	•	•	•	•	•
Injury Prevention[22]	•	•	•	•	•	•	•	•	•	•	•	•	•	•	•	•	•	•	•	•	•	•	•	•	•	•	•	•	•
Violence Prevention[23]	•	•	•	•	•	•	•	•	•	•	•	•	•	•	•	•	•	•	•	•	•	•	•	•	•	•	•	•	•
Sleep Positioning Counseling[24]	•	•	•	•	•	•	•																						
Nutrition Counseling[25]	•	•	•	•	•	•	•	•	•	•	•	•	•	•	•	•	•	•	•	•	•	•	•	•	•	•	•	•	•
DENTAL REFERRAL[26]									←				•																

1. A prenatal visit is recommended for parents who are at high risk, for first-time parents, and for those who request a conference. The prenatal visit should include anticipatory guidance, pertinent medical history, and a discussion of benefits of breastfeeding and planned method of feeding per AAP statement "The Prenatal Visit" (1996).
2. Every infant should have a newborn evaluation after birth. Breastfeeding should be encouraged and instruction and support offered. Every breastfeeding infant should have an evaluation 48-72 hours after discharge from the hospital to include weight, formal breastfeeding evaluation, encouragement, and instruction as recommended in the AAP statement "Breastfeeding and the Use of Human Milk" (1997).
3. For newborns discharged in less than 48 hours after delivery per AAP statement "Hospital Stay for Healthy Term Newborns" (1995).
4. Developmental, psychosocial, and chronic disease issues for children and adolescents may require frequent counseling and treatment visits separate from preventive care visits.
5. If a child comes under care for the first time at any point on the schedule, or if any items are not accomplished at the suggested age, the schedule should be brought up to date at the earliest possible time.
6. If the patient is uncooperative, rescreen within 6 months.
7. All newborns should be screened per the AAP Task Force on Newborn and Infant Hearing statement, "Newborn and Infant Hearing Loss: Detection and Intervention" (1999).
8. By history and appropriate physical examination: if suspicious, by specific objective developmental testing. Parenting skills should be fostered at every visit.
9. At each visit, a complete physical examination is essential, with infant totally unclothed, older child undressed and suitably draped.
10. These may be modified, depending upon entry point into schedule and individual need.
11. Metabolic screening (eg, thyroid, hemoglobinopathies, PKU, galactosemia) should be done according to state law.
12. Schedule(s) per the Committee on Infectious Diseases, published annually in the January edition of *Pediatrics*. Every visit should be an opportunity to update and complete a child's immunizations.
13. See AAP *Pediatric Nutrition Handbook* (1998) for a discussion of universal and selective screening options. Consider earlier screening for high-risk infants (eg, premature infants and low birth weight infants). See also "Recommendations to Prevent and Control Iron Deficiency in the United States. *MMWR*. 1998;47 (RR-3):1-29.
14. All menstruating adolescents should be screened annually.
15. Conduct dipstick urinalysis for leukocytes annually for sexually active male and female adolescents.
16. For children at risk of lead exposure consult the AAP statement "Screening for Elevated Blood Levels" (1998). Additionally, screening should be done in accordance with state law where applicable.
17. TB testing per recommendations of the Committee on Infectious Diseases, published in the current edition of *Red Book: Report of the Committee on Infectious Diseases*. Testing should be done upon recognition of high-risk factors.
18. Cholesterol screening for high-risk patients per AAP statement "Cholesterol in Childhood" (1998). If family history cannot be ascertained and other risk factors are present, screening should be at the discretion of the physician.
19. All sexually active patients should be screened for sexually transmitted diseases (STDs).
20. All sexually active females should have a pelvic examination. A pelvic examination and routine pap smear should be offered as part of preventive health maintenance between the ages of 18 and 21 years.
21. Age-appropriate discussion and counseling should be an integral part of each visit for care per the AAP *Guidelines for Health Supervision III* (1998).
22. From birth to age 12, refer to the AAP injury prevention program (TIPP®) as described in *A Guide to Safety Counseling in Office Practice* (1994).
23. Violence prevention and management for all patients per AAP Statement "The Role of the Pediatrician in Youth Violence Prevention in Clinical Practice and at the Community Level" (1999).
24. Parents and caregivers should be advised to place healthy infants on their backs when putting them to sleep. Side positioning is a reasonable alternative but carries a slightly higher risk of SIDS. Consult the AAP statement "Positioning and Sudden Infant Death Syndrome (SIDS): Update" (1996).
25. Age-appropriate nutrition counseling should be an integral part of each visit per the AAP *Handbook of Nutrition* (1998).
26. Earlier initial dental examinations may be appropriate for some children. Subsequent examinations as prescribed by dentist.

Key: ● = to be performed; ★ = to be performed for patients at risk; S = subjective, by history; O = objective, by a standard testing method; ←•→ = the range during which a service may be provided, with the dot indicating the preferred age.

NB: Special chemical, immunologic, and endocrine testing is usually carried out upon specific indications. Testing other than newborn (eg, inborn errors of metabolism, sickle disease, etc) is discretionary with the physician.

The recommendations in this statement do not indicate an exclusive course of treatment or standard of medical care. Variations, taking into account individual circumstances, may be appropriate.

American Academy of Pediatrics

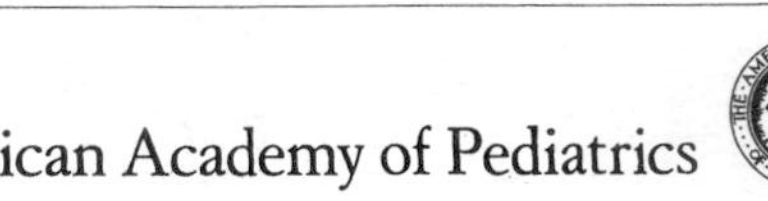

Fig. 4-1 Recommendations for preventive pediatric health care.

ban children younger than 19 years of age who had managed care insurance policies that provided full fees for well-child care visits, only 40% received all of the recommended number of visits, while 25% received no well-child visits at all.[3] These percentages are much lower or higher, respectively, when a portion or all of the visit fee must be borne by the parents.[16,19]

It is difficult to determine why most primary care pediatricians do not do more to ensure that their patients receive the AAP-recommended number of well-child care visits. Mustard et al[15] and Orr, Charney, and Strauss[19] relate the use of health services, including well-child care visits, to the organization and delivery of those services, suggesting that if these elements were improved—made more user friendly—adherence by parents would improve. The amount of effort the AAP has expended in generating its recommendations for preventive pediatric health care should dictate to its members that they do more than they have in adhering to them. However, in a 1992 survey of AAP members, only 59% of respondents reported that they followed the AAP-recommended well-child care visit schedule.[2] Perhaps the experience of those who do not indicates to them that fewer such visits are needed than are recommended, or they understand that the number of recommended visits has not been proven to be of sufficient benefit, given the time and effort they require. Despite such reservations on the part of primary care pediatric practitioners, the number of AAP-recommended well-child care visits has increased steadily.

There are indications that practitioners are not meeting the objectives of well-child care for the vast majority of children whose parents do seek such care for them. Time-motion studies of pediatricians conducting well-child care have shown that very little time is spent on individual well-child visits—12 minutes on average. This has been true for private as well as clinic patients. One must question whether the objectives of well-child care can be reached in such a short time. These studies show that pediatric nurse practitioners working in the same practices spend considerably more time on well-child care (20 to 30 minutes per visit) than do their physician colleagues.

Very few studies have assessed the content of well-child visits in terms of the amount of time pediatricians and parents spend discussing psychosocial issues and concerns. In 1978, Reisinger and Bires[22] demonstrated that anticipatory guidance constituted only about 52 seconds of the 10.3 minutes Pittsburgh pediatricians spent, on average, conducting well-child visits. The practitioners studied spent a high of 97 seconds on anticipatory guidance for visits involving infants 5 months of age or younger and a low of 7 seconds for patients 13 to 18 years of age. Eighteen years later, Goldstein, Dworkin, and Bernstein[10] reported that a sample of Connecticut pediatricians spent on average 17.8 minutes on well-child visits, with 2.4 minutes devoted to anticipatory guidance. Adolescents received 2 to 6 minutes of counseling. Both studies showed that pediatricians trained more recently spent more time overall in anticipatory guidance.

The AAP's guidelines for health supervision are controversial because of concerns that (1) there have been no data to indicate the need for so many visits or the value of what is done during them, save administering immunizations, and (2) there are not nor will there ever be enough health care professionals (pediatricians, family medicine practitioners, nurse practitioners, or physician's assistants) to deliver such care to all or even a significant portion of our children.[5] Others are concerned that adhering to these guidelines ensures that the maldistribution of pediatricians (too many in suburban areas and not enough in inner city, urban, and rural areas) will continue, denying underserved children access to all facets of child health care.[8]

Many investigators have reviewed the overall effectiveness of child health supervision; these reviews were incorporated into a 1988 report by a study group of the Office of Technology Assessment (OTA) of the U.S. Congress. The report was an in-depth study of preventive child health services, including well-child care.[24] The study group's conclusions ranged from strongly negative to strongly positive, based on its opinion regarding intervening or process outcomes the group viewed as bad (high costs, uneven personnel distribution, overdependence of parents on health care providers) or good (parent and provider satisfaction, improved parental compliance with provider instructions, better acute care through establishment of an informed and trusting relationship). However, the study group was unable to base its conclusions on any studies that meet Elinson's accepted criteria for determining the worth of health care intervention.[7] These criteria require that studies be prospective, involve some planned intervention (e.g., child health supervision as recommended by the AAP) designed to achieve specific end points (e.g., improved child health in terms of decreased mortality and morbidity), and include both control and experimental groups. Meeting Elinson's criteria presents some difficulties in evaluating the effectiveness of child health supervision.

In its 1977 report, the AAP's Ad Hoc Committee on the Value of Preventive Child Health Care[13] stated, in applying Elinson's criteria to child health supervision, that preventive child health care is a process applied throughout infancy and childhood and that it would require study over many years if its overall value were to be proven. This creates problems in maintaining sample and investigator continuity, because patient mobility and academic permanency (a condition affecting potential researchers) often is short-lived. Patient mobility could be counteracted by appropriately increasing the size of the initial experimental and control groups to allow for losses. Maintaining investigator continuity would require personal commitment and good health over time; these requisites, particularly that of continuity, are not always assured for academicians, who are most likely to be chosen for principal investigator positions in studies of this type.

The end points chosen could include indices of health and illness, school performance, or psychosocial adjustment. However, new instruments for measuring indices in any of these areas would have to be developed, particularly to maintain uniformity throughout the samples. Large samples would be required, because there would be multiple intervening independent variables, and the differences in the end points most likely would be small. A multicenter study design would be required to overcome geographical, economic, and cultural population variables; this would compound the investigator-continuity problems and create difficulties in standardization.

Any long-range study carries the risk of process and measurement obsolescence. For example, new preventive care procedures could become operative at midpoint and distort planned end point measures; or end points considered significant at the beginning of the study may no longer be significant at the end of the study because of social, political, educational, or medical changes.

The cost of conducting a study of this type would be extremely high, and the prospects for assured, continued funding, even with sanction and direction from the AAP, might not be bright.

Another consideration is the ethical issue of withholding from children in the control group methods of medical management considered valuable. This could be addressed through a passive relationship with the control group and an aggressive promotion of the AAP's preventive care recommendations with the experimental group. A retrospective approach could be used with the control group consisting of children who had received no or few preventive health care services, but this would not meet Elinson's prospective criterion.

The Ad Hoc Committee on the Value of Preventive Child Health Care recognized that the task it recommended is complex and will require considerable time and effort to complete. Nevertheless, it is the only way to determine the overall effectiveness of the child health supervision schedules recommended by the AAP. To date, no such study has been launched.

To these limitations on studying the overall effectiveness of child health supervision, the OTA study group[24] added the observation that: "The health status of children in particular (and the population in general) is far more strongly determined by social and economic factors than by the nature of medical care; hence, the contribution that well-child care can make to health outcomes is likely to be modest, and studies to detect these modest contributions must be based on very large samples. Few available studies of the effectiveness of child health care have had very large samples. None of them directly address the question of the overall effectiveness of well-child care."

The OTA study group's review of the literature evaluating the effectiveness of well-child care as a whole concludes that well-child care as now performed (other than immunization) has no overall effect on childhood mortality or morbidity and exerts little influence on developmental and social functioning outcomes. In 1990, the Canadian Task Force on Periodic Health Examination reached the same conclusion.[4] Despite this, child health supervision remains the basis upon which most pediatric practices are built, because it provides parental and physician satisfaction and reassurance (in some cases, conviction) that well-child visits keep children well and prevent serious illnesses.

ALTERATION OF STANDARDS

If society accepts the premises that large segments of the child population are not receiving what practitioners feel to be optimal health care and that good health care is an inherent right of all citizens and not simply a privilege available to those who can afford it, it becomes obvious that practitioners must compromise their standards of adequate well-child care, the methods of delivering that care, or both.

In regard to changing the standards of child health supervision, practitioners must consider the fact that there is some substantiation that reducing the frequency of visits, at least for infants identified as at low risk, does not alter the outcomes in terms of their physical and developmental status, maternal knowledge of child rearing, maternal anxiety, safety and infant stimulation in the home, and parent-initiated visits as a result of illness.[4,9,12] Thus, the number of visits could be reduced substantially without compromising these aspects of the quality of care. Practitioners must consider that some children may require only minimal health supervision other than completion of immunization schedules and screening tests, whereas others will require much, much more.

Our Canadian colleagues have developed recommendations for the frequency and content of well-baby care during the first 5 years of life, based upon evidence published in scientific journals, and (to a lesser extent) upon opinions of respected authorities or reports of expert committees. Their recommendations are classified as having good, fair, or poor evidence for inclusion or exclusion in a well-child visit. An evidence-based well-baby-care record (the Rourke Baby Record*) incorporates these recommendations to help to simplify and to increase the effectiveness of the preventive care physicians provide for infants and young children.[21]

A method to conserve physician time is to use health care providers other than physicians for child health care. There is good evidence that using nonphysicians, particularly pediatric nurse practitioners, for most elements of well-child care does not reduce the quality of that care. Studies performed in private practices, prepaid group practices, and university hospital clinics have demonstrated that pediatric nurse practitioners are entirely competent to provide well-child care and that the care they render does not result in altered health outcomes, increased utilization, decreased compliance, or decreased parental satisfaction. Equally important, this model is less expensive than that in which the physician provides all elements of well-child care.

Group well-child care (GWCC) visits offer the opportunity to discuss a greater range of issues surrounding child growth and development and to provide anticipatory guidance, leading to greater parental knowledge of child rearing than do individual well-child care (IWCC) visits, using less provider time per patient if the groups are large enough. GWCC visits have been shown to be more fruitful than IWCC visits in these respects among middle-class patients[20] but have not been shown to offer any specific advantages among low-income, high-risk patients.[23]

Consideration of the costs of care must include (1) use of physician time that might be more effectively applied to other health problems, (2) the extent to which taxes should be used to support activities that have so few proven beneficial outcomes, and (3) a family's ability to afford the fees charged, the expenditures for transportation and baby-sitting

*Copies of the Rourke Baby Record can be ordered at no cost from McNeil Consumer Health Care, 890 Woodlawn Road W., Guelph, Ontario, Canada NIK 1A5; 519-836-6500.

services while the parent is away from home, and the loss of income for working parents who must comply with the daytime visit schedules of private practices, clinics, and health centers. Having public health nurses provide all aspects of child health supervision in the homes of underprivileged women and children has proved to be a cost-effective method of delivering such services to a population at high risk that would not receive them otherwise.[18]

DISCUSSION

From the early 1930s through the late 1980s, numerous practice-based studies and those conducted by the National Center for Health Statistics (the National Ambulatory Medical Care Survey) have shown that 30% to 45% of primary care pediatric office visits are for child health supervision and that more than 50% of some primary care pediatricians' office time is spent in this activity. These percentages have risen over time as visits and procedures have been added to the AAP recommendations, and they most surely will rise again with the 1995 increase in recommended visits, from 20 to 27 between birth and age 21.*

In adhering to the AAP's guidelines, pediatricians limit the number of children they can care for who have other health and illness care needs that currently are unmet. It seems that practitioners either must explore further the evidence at hand to determine if they can reduce the frequency of well-child visits or employ others to conduct such visits. Practitioners need to change their perspective on traditional professional roles and methods and focus on the goal of meeting the health supervision and illness care needs of all children.

REFERENCES

1. American Academy of Pediatrics, Committee on Practice and Ambulatory Medicine: Recommendations for preventive pediatric health care, *Pediatrics* 105:645, 2000.
2. Appraising periodicity: *AAP News* 10:6, January 1993.
3. Byrd RS, Hoekelman RA, Auinger P: Adherence to AAP guidelines for well-child care under managed care, *Pediatrics* 104:536, 1999.
4. Canadian Task Force on Periodic Health Examination: Periodic health examination: 1990 update, *Can Med Assoc J* 143:867, 1990.
5. Chamberlin RW, Schiff DW, Rogers KD: Are routine periodic child health visits beneficial? In Smith DH, Hoekelman RA, editors: *Controversies in child health and pediatric practice,* New York, 1981, McGraw-Hill.
6. Committee on Child Health: Health supervision of young children, New York, 1955, American Public Health Association.
7. Elinson J: Effectiveness of social action programs in health and welfare; from Assessing the effectiveness of children's health services, Report of the Fifty-Sixth Ross Conference on Pediatric Research, Columbus, Ohio, 1967, Ross Laboratories.
8. Fossett JW, Peterson JA: Physician supply and Medicaid participation, *Med Care* 27:386, 1989.
9. Gilbert JR et al: How many well-baby visits are necessary in the first 2 years of life? *Can Med Assoc J* 130:857, 1984.
10. Goldstein EN, Dworkin PH, Bernstein B: Time devoted to anticipatory guidance during child health supervision visits: how are we doing? *Amb Child Health* 5:113, 1999.
11. Green M, editor: *Bright futures: guidelines for health supervision of infants, children, and adolescents,* Arlington, Va, 1994, National Center for Education in Maternal and Child Health.
12. Hoekelman RA: What constitutes adequate well-baby care? *Pediatrics* 55:313, 1975.
13. Hoekelman RA, Thompson HC: *Value of preventive child health care,* Evanston, Ill, 1977, American Academy of Pediatrics.
14. Horwitz SM, Morgenstern H, Berkman LF: Factors affecting pediatric preventive care utilization in prepaid group practice, *Pediatrician* 15: 112, 1988.
15. Mustard CA, et al: Continuity of pediatric ambulatory care in a universally insured population, *Pediatrics* 98:1028, 1996.
16. Newacheck PW, Halfon N: Preventive care use by school-age children: differences by socioeconomic status, *Pediatrics* 82:462, 1988.
17. Newacheck PW, Hughes DC, Stoddard JJ: Children's access to primary care: differences by race, income, and insurance status, *Pediatrics* 97: 26, 1996.
18. Olds DL, Kitzman H: Can home visitation improve the health of women and children at environmental risk? *Pediatrics* 86:108, 1990.
19. Orr ST, Charney E, Straus J: Use of health services by black children according to payment mechanisms. *Med Care* 26:939, 1988.
20. Osborn LM, Woolley FR: Use of groups in well-child care, *Pediatrics* 67:701, 1981.
21. Panagiotou L, et al: Evidence-based well-baby care, Parts I & II, *Can Fam Physician* 44:558, 1998.
22. Reisinger KS, Bires JA: Anticipatory guidance in pediatric practice, *Pediatrics* 66:889, 1980.
23. Taylor JA, Kemper KJ: Group well-child care for high-risk families: maternal outcomes, *Arch Pediatr Adolesc Med* 152:579, 1998.
24. US Congress, Office of Technology Assessment: Healthy children: investing in the future, Pub No OTA-H-345, Washington, DC, 1988, US Government Printing Office.
25. Woodward CA, et al: Ontario Child Health Study: Patterns of ambulatory medical care utilization and their correlates, *Pediatrics* 82:425, 1988.

SUGGESTED READING

Canadian Task Force on the Periodic Health Examination: The Canadian Guide to Clinical Preventive Health Care, Ottawa, Canada, 1994, Minister of Supplies and Services Canada.

*This increase was based on the Bright Futures Project, which was sponsored by the U.S. Public Health Service's Maternal and Child Health Bureau and by the Medicaid Bureau of the Health Care Financing Administration. The project's findings were published in 1994[11] and were approved by 16 national medical, nursing, and child advocacy organizations, including the AAP, the American Medical Association (AMA), and the American Nurses Association (ANA). They were officially adopted by the AAP in 1995.

5 Community-Wide Approaches to Promoting the Health and Development of Families and Children

Robert W. Chamberlin

RATIONALE

Many health and developmental problems in children and youth are related to family functioning. These include infant mortality, low birth weight, abuse and neglect, a variety of injuries and illnesses, developmental lags, school failure, delinquency, out-of-wedlock adolescent pregnancy, problems related to substance abuse, and community violence of all kinds.[17] Family well being is, in turn, related to the social environments created by individuals, organizations, local communities, and government policies and actions. Recent reports put out by the U.S. Institute of Medicine on improving health in the community and by the World Health Organization (WHO) on the social determinants of health summarize epidemiological evidence supporting these relationships.[7,19]

Worldwide changes in the economy, family composition, and the role of women have increased the stress on families. At the same time, traditional community support systems have been weakened by families moving away from kinfolk, parents commuting long distances to work, a lack of time for volunteering, and in the United States, cutbacks in government-funded preventive programs.[2] These multiple stresses have overwhelmed the coping capacity of many families, resulting in increased numbers of children displaying the problems noted above (Fig. 5-1).

RESPONSES TO WORLDWIDE CHANGES

Western European countries have responded by building in more support systems for families. Most provide paid pregnancy and child care leave for working mothers and home visitors for new mothers who want them. Most have universal health insurance programs and subsidize high-quality child care for all ages and early-education programs for 3- and 4-year-olds. For older children there are after-school programs, comprehensive health curricula that include sex education and how to use contraceptives, and training to help adolescents cope with stress, to communicate, be assertive, and resist peer pressure to have sex, smoke, and use drugs. All these countries have lower rates of infant mortality, low weight births, child abuse, injuries, community violence of all kinds, and out-of-wedlock adolescent pregnancies and abortions than does the United States.[13,20]

The United States has, until recently, continued to rely on a deficit-oriented system that waits until a family is in crisis and malfunctioning before trying to do anything about it.[1] Although programs for high-risk families are helpful to those they reach, they do nothing to alter the underlying conditions that cause families to falter in the first place.[15] Primary prevention works by preventing families from becoming "high risk." Moreover, demonstration programs in this country also have shown that building community support systems available to all families can reduce these kinds of problems.*

Based on these data, states have been putting together networks of home visiting programs and family resource centers that are open to all community residents regardless of income.[4,12,16] These coordinate services (1) provide opportunities for learning parenting, domestic, and vocational skills; (2) provide safe, developmentally appropriate activities for parents and children; (3) facilitate the formation of support groups for families going through various transitions; and (4) provide transportation to families isolated in rural areas and inner cities. For example, the state of Vermont has at least one parent/child center in each county to coordinate a variety of services for families that have young children. Over the past 10 years they have been able to reduce low weight births, child abuse, adolescent pregnancy, and welfare dependency significantly. Colorado, Kentucky, Maryland, Missouri, Minnesota, Connecticut, and Washington also have statewide family support programs.

In both the United States and Western Europe, community-wide support programs for families that have young children are beginning to merge with more comprehensive approaches to wellness aimed at making cities and communities healthier places to live for all residents. For example, the WHO has been working with Healthy City projects in more than 1000 cities worldwide, including many in the United States and Canada.[8]

The realization that no one agency or provider can cope with all the problems created by the changes affecting families has led individual health care providers and others to work together to create more family-friendly environments at the individual, organizational, community, and governmental levels. Some, like the WHO Healthy Cities projects, start from the top by engaging the political leadership and work their way down to the neighborhood level. Others, such as many family support programs, start locally and work their way up to involve the political establishment. A top-down,

*References 2, 3, 9, 10, 12, 17, 18.

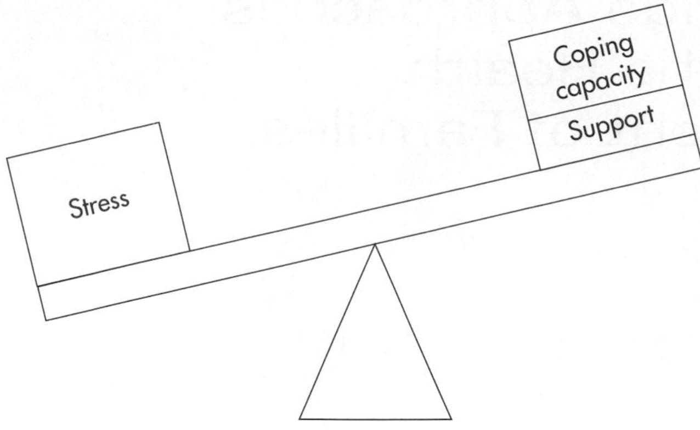

Fig. 5-1 The family balancing act.
(From Chamberlin R: *Pediatr Rev* 13:64, 1992.)

bottom-up combination appears to be the most effective. Without "top support" it is difficult to sustain the needed changes over the many years required before the benefits of these programs show up as improvements in the rates of various health and developmental indicators for the community as a whole. Without "bottom support" what is done often does not meet the most pressing needs of local residents.

IMPLEMENTING COMMUNITY WELLNESS PROGRAMS

Bottom-up efforts to make communities more supportive to families with young children often start with one or two persons concerned about what is happening in their neighborhood or school district. These efforts proceed more or less through the following steps:

1. *Defining a geographical catchment area:* This can be a neighborhood, school district, political ward, small town, clusters of small towns, or even a county. A degree of underlying cohesion that gives residents some common reason for working together is necessary.
2. *Forming a broad-based coalition:* Finding others who share your concerns is the next step. Often this is done by holding a community meeting and having front-line providers such as school teachers, visiting nurses, pediatricians, clergy, local police, and youth workers describe what they are seeing in the community. It also is helpful to invite an outside speaker to provide information about what the community can do to become more supportive.
3. *Developing a community profile:* This involves putting together a database describing the incidence and prevalence of various problems and the resources available in the community.
4. *Identifying short- and long-term action priorities:* The next step is to put the data into some kind of an overall framework that can be used to identify short- and long-term action priorities. The ecological framework used by the Stanford Heart Disease Prevention Programs is a useful example.[11] This approach recognizes the interdependence of the individual, the family, and the community. Data are divided into these three areas. At one end are the health and developmental status indicators for children that one hopes to improve. In the middle are the family and individual behavioral risk and protective factors that will need to be changed to improve the status indicators. At the other end are the changes that need to occur in the way community service providers, organizations, the local media, and local government do business before one can expect much change in individual risk and protective factors. An ecological framework for promoting healthy children and families is shown in Box 5-1. Other models are available.[7,14]
5. *Implementing programs of proven value:* Once short- and long-term priorities are identified, they must be put into action. Promoting programs of proven value, such as preventive health care, home visiting and other family support programs for new parents, quality child care and early-childhood education programs, is important. This requires social marketing skills to convince the community that, in the long run, these programs will benefit everyone.[14]
6. *Monitoring progress and impact:* (See Monitoring and Evaluation section on p. 43.)
7. *Establishing long-term sustainability:* Because it often takes the building of a comprehensive array of preventive programs over a 5- to 10-year period before one reaches

BOX 5-1

ECOLOGICAL FRAMEWORK FOR PROMOTING HEALTHY CHILDREN AND FAMILIES

Environmental Factors

1. Family and peer group: role models and support systems
2. Organizational policies and practices: access to services, family-friendly policies
3. Mass media: education and positive reinforcement
4. Local and state government policies and practices: coordination of services, adequate funding of preventive programs, technical assistance

Individual Factors

1. Knowledge: fetal and child development, reproductive anatomy and physiology, health habits related to pregnancy outcome
2. Feelings, attitudes, and beliefs: self confidence, depression, locus of control, self esteem
3. Behaviors and skills: healthy lifestyle, birthing and parenting skills, domestic and job skills

Status Indicators

1. Birth to age 5 years: low birth weight, immunization status at age 2 years, exposure to abuse or neglect, school readiness
2. Age 6 to 18 years: school achievement, high school graduation rates, post-secondary education, juvenile arrests, out-of-wedlock adolescent pregnancies; sexually transmitted diseases

Modified from Jackson C: A community based approach to preventing heart disease: the Stanford experience. In Chamberlin R, editor: *Beyond individual risk assessment: community-wide approaches to promoting the health and development of families and children,* Washington, DC, 1988, National Center for Education in Maternal and Child Care.

the critical mass needed to demonstrate a positive impact on community base rates, it is necessary to develop a strategy for long-term sustainability. Short-term projects such as developing a community service directory or having an annual family fair are needed to keep momentum going while working on long-term goals such as establishing a home visiting program or family resource center. Once a program is up and running, it is vital to develop an advocacy strategy to head off attempts by short-sighted politicians and agency heads to cut the budgets of preventive programs at the first sign of a budget squeeze.[14]

MONITORING AND EVALUATION ISSUES

These projects are complex, involving many different stakeholders, and they take a number of years to evolve to a level where one can begin to see the effects on community base rates for health and developmental outcomes. Thus, traditional approaches to evaluation are usually not possible or are not very effective.[6,7] Because the energy and, ultimately, the funding to carry out one of these long-term projects must come from the community itself, it is difficult or impossible to pick communities randomly to undergo this kind of long-term commitment. Similarly, it is difficult to find a comparison community that remains sufficiently similar over the long run for one to be able to draw accurate conclusions about whatever differences are or are not found.

An alternative approach is to see if the community is progressing along the lines indicated by ecological theory.[4,11] One, therefore, should expect to see changes in community policies and access to services before one finds significant individual and family changes in wellness behavior. In turn, one would expect to demonstrate individual improvements in birthing and parenting skills in a community sample before finding significant improvements in the health and developmental outcomes of children. With this approach, each community serves as its own control. Although one or more communities could follow this sequence by chance, it is highly unlikely that many communities in different locations would follow the same pattern.

For example, we have considerable data indicating what needs to be done to improve the health and developmental outcomes for young children,[2,9,10,16-18] that is, some combination of access to health information and care, parent education and support with home visitors and/or neighborhood-based family resource centers, and access to quality affordable child care and early-childhood education programs. In addition, safe neighborhoods, adequate housing, good schools, and jobs with family-friendly policies that pay a living wage are needed. Until one sees substantial improvement in access to these kinds of social environments, we cannot expect to see healthier parental behaviors such as earlier onset of prenatal care, decreases in smoking during and after pregnancy, and parenting skills that promote school readiness. Until we see these improvements in parenting behavior, we cannot expect to see decreases in low weight births, children exposed to abuse and neglect, childhood injuries and hospitalizations, and improvements in school readiness and achievement. For some other thoughts about how to approach this complex area, see the recent report of the Institute of Medicine.[7]

CHALLENGES FOR THE FUTURE

We now have considerable knowledge indicating what needs to be done to promote the wellness of families and children. To put this knowledge into practice, however, will require meeting a number of challenges. These include:

- Thinking about health in a context broader than only in terms of the absence of disease
- Overcoming an ideology that says every family should be completely self sufficient and if you get into trouble it's your own fault
- Funding the basic programs that prevent families and children from getting into trouble rather than waiting until the crisis stage to do anything about it
- Supporting community-wide wellness efforts over the long time periods necessary to demonstrate positive results at the community level
- Developing better methods of small-area data analysis to identify neighborhoods, school districts, and small towns that need better access to basic wellness-promoting programs and monitoring the results of efforts to improve the social ecology of these catchment areas
- Bringing together the experience of the WHO Healthy Cities movement for engaging governments and policy makers with the family support movement's experience in developing grass roots neighborhood-based family support programs[5]

ROLE OF THE PEDIATRICIAN

Although few physicians have the time to participate in the many meetings that these coalitions require, pediatricians can facilitate these community efforts in many ways, including the following:

1. *Developing coalitions:* Pediatricians are respected in the community; their endorsement of coalition activity gives it importance and legitimacy.
2. *Building a community profile:* Pediatricians can provide data on what types of child and family problems they are seeing and what resources are present or missing in the community. They also can help coalition members negotiate with the schools, the local hospital, the state health department, the child protection office serving the area, and other organizations that have data needed to develop an accurate baseline community profile.
3. *Establishing short- and long-term priorities:* Attendance at these key meetings is worth the effort.
4. *Implementing programs:* The American Academy of Pediatrics CATCH grants have been used to help develop home visiting programs, family resource centers, and a variety of other programs that promote child and family wellness. Pediatricians also can use their knowledge of growth and development to upgrade area child care by participating in continuing education programs for child care and school health providers.
5. *Advocating:* Testifying at legislative budget hearings about the importance of funding health promotion programs.

Finally, pediatricians can make their own practice more family friendly by developing a "call" hour, a bulletin board to be used by parents to share information and services; support groups for parents undergoing a separation or divorce, or having a child with a disability; or instituting a Reach Out and Read program to encourage positive parent-child interaction and literacy.

IMPLICATIONS FOR TRAINING

Exposing pediatricians in training to community-based programs can be done by having coalitions present "grand rounds" several times during the year. Residents also can "adopt a site" to which to relate over the several years they are in training. This will allow them to see how coalitions function over time, participate in building a community database, and perhaps, act as an advocate at a public hearing. Working in the office of a community-oriented pediatrician will also expose the trainee to a positive role model.

REFERENCES

1. Bronfenbrenner U, Weiss H: Beyond policies without people: an ecologic perspective on child and family policy. In Zigler E, Lynn-Kagan S, Klugman E, editors: *Children, families and government,* New York, 1983, Cambridge University Press.
2. Carnegie Task Force on Meeting the Needs of Young Children: Starting points, New York, 1994, Carnegie Corporation of New York.
3. Chamberlin R: Preventing low birth weight, child abuse, and school failure: the need for comprehensive, community-wide approaches, *Pediatr Rev* 13:64, 1992.
4. Chamberlin R: Primary prevention and the family resource movement. In Singer G, Power L, and Olson A, editors: *Redefining family support: innovations in public-private partnerships,* Baltimore, 1995, Paul Brooks Publishing.
5. Chamberlin R: WHO Healthy Cities and the US family support movements: a marriage made in heaven or estranged bed fellows? *Health Prom Internat* 11:137, 1996.
6. Connell J, et al, editors: *New approaches to evaluating community initiatives,* New York, 1995, Aspen Institute.
7. Durch J, Bailey L, Stoto M, editors: *Improving health in the community,* Washington, DC, 1996, National Academy Press.
8. Flynn B: Healthy cities: toward worldwide health promotion, *Ann Rev Pub Health* 17:299, 1996.
9. Gomby D, et al, editors: *Long-term outcomes of early childhood programs: the future of children,* vol 5, no 3, Los Altos, Calif, 1995, The Center for the Future of Children, The David and Lucile Packard Foundation.
10. Gomby D, Larson C, et al, editors: *Home visiting: the future of children,* vol 3, no 3, Los Altos, Calif, 1993, The Center for the Future of Children. The David and Lucile Packard Foundation.
11. Jackson C: A community based approach to preventing heart disease: the Stanford experience. In Chamberlin R, editor: *Beyond individual risk assessment: community-wide approaches to promoting the health and development of families and children,* Washington, DC, 1988, National Center for Education in Maternal and Child Health.
12. Kagan S, Weissbord B, editors: *Putting families first,* San Francisco, 1994, Jossey-Bass.
13. Miller A: *Maternal health and infant survival,* Arlington, 1987, National Center for Clinical Infant Programs.
14. Minkler M, editor: *Community organizing and community building for health,* New Brunswick, NJ, 1997, Rutgers University Press.
15. Rose G: *The strategy of preventive medicine,* Oxford, 1992, Oxford University Press.
16. Schorr L: *Common purpose: strengthening families and neighborhoods to rebuild America.* New York, 1997, Doubleday.
17. Schorr L: *Within our reach: breaking the cycle of disadvantage,* New York, 1988, Doubleday.
18. Shore R: *Rethinking the brain: new insights into early development,* New York, 1997, Families and Work Institute.
19. Wilkinson R, Marmot M, editors: *Social determinants of health: the solid facts,* Copenhagen, Denmark, 1998, WHO Regional Office for Europe.
20. Williams B, Miller A: *Preventive health care for young children: findings from a 10-country study and directions for United States policy,* Arlington, Va, 1991, National Center for Clinical Infant Programs.

6 Ethical and Legal Issues for the Primary Care Pediatrician

Lainie Friedman Ross • John D. Lantos

The hallmark of clinical ethics in the setting of general internal medicine is its focus on the competent adult patient. Even in cases in which the patient is incompetent, moral reasoning focuses on the prior wishes or values of the patient.[12] The focus also is usually on the doctor-patient dyad. In contrast, the foundation of pediatric clinical ethics is a triad that includes the physician, the child, and his or her parents. Until a few decades ago, all children were presumed to be incompetent, and their opinions were not sought. Instead, parents were legally empowered to make virtually all decisions for their children. Currently there are movements around the world to increase the child's legal power and to give the child, particularly the older child, his or her own voice.[19,34] Some argue that mature children (specifically adolescents) be allowed to make their own decisions without their parents' permission, even without their parents' awareness.[3,5] This is an area of tension and controversy because reasonable people disagree about the degree to which children's values and choices should direct their health care.[31]

Most of the literature of pediatric ethics focuses on the extreme cases: the premature infant who weighs 600 g, the child who has leukemia whose parents refuse chemotherapy, or the child whose sibling needs a kidney transplant. The unique issues that pediatricians in primary care practice face have not received comparable adequate scholarly attention or rigorous analysis. This may be because the ethical issues that arise in the day-to-day practice of pediatrics are usually not concerned with decisions about illnesses that are immediately life-threatening. Nevertheless, pediatricians in primary care practice often face decisions that may have profound effects on a child's physical and mental health and on many emotional, spiritual, and economic elements of family life.

Over the past 30 years, societal standards about difficult moral choices in medicine have evolved through a dialogue among bioethicists, professional societies, and the court system. Legal disputes have been especially important for issues such as do-not-resuscitate (DNR) orders, brain death, and treatment withdrawal. The disputes that arise in primary care are not often the concern of the legal system. When they are, lower courts rather than appeals courts often decide them. Lower-court decisions may not be as carefully reasoned as those of an appeals court, and they do not have broad, direct jurisdiction. As a result, in many cases, neither statutory law nor case law is directly applicable to the issues at hand.

A case-based approach is used in this chapter to examine the ethical issues raised in primary care pediatrics. Every case raises both procedural and substantive issues, that is, how should physicians approach the case (procedural) and what should the final decision be (substantive). In some cases, there are legal constraints on decision making; in others, there is wide consensus or disagreement on the preferable ethical solution.

CASE STUDIES AND ANALYSIS

Case 1

Alan, an 8-year-old boy, presents with multiple plantar warts on his hands. The school is concerned that he is contagious and will not allow him to participate in contact sports until they are treated, or at minimum, are under treatment. You explain to Ms. A, his mother, and to Alan that the two therapeutic options are liquid nitrogen in the office or a salicylate-based therapy that is to be applied nightly. Ms. A requests that you give Alan the in-office treatment. Alan says that he does not want any painful treatment and will apply the ointment nightly. What do you do?

Discussion: On the surface, the case does not appear to involve an ethical issue because Alan, his mother, and the pediatrician all agree that Alan needs treatment. However, there are two very different treatments available. Each has different benefits and burdens. The child prefers one balance of the benefits and burdens, the parent another. Their different values, when brought to play on the therapeutic options, have created a conflict between the parent and child about which the pediatrician may feel indifferent.

The first step in any such conflict is further discussion. It is valuable to understand why Ms. A prefers the liquid nitrogen therapy. Issues to be weighed include efficacy, cost, convenience, attendant risks, and compliance. Ms. A's choice is pragmatic—she sees the liquid nitrogen as being more reliable. Ms. A is afraid, based on experience, that her child will be poorly compliant with the nightly salicylate-based treatment. She does not want to have a nightly battle. Alan has had liquid nitrogen therapy before and finds it quite painful. He promises his mother that he will comply with the nightly ointment applications.

In many such discussions, parents and children will come to consensus, but sometimes their positions are intractable. Who, then, should have the final word? The American Academy of Pediatrics (AAP) Committee on Bioethics published recommendations regarding the roles of parents and children in decision making for children.[5] The committee recommends that the resolution of conflicts between parents and children depend, in part, on the child's decision-making capacity. For children whose decision-making capacity is developed, the committee recommends that the child's decision be final. For the child whose capacity is developing, such as Alan, the committee urges the physician to try to achieve consensus. If the child and parent cannot reach consensus, the AAP supports third-party intervention.[5] Although some may find this reasonable, others might find it hopelessly cumbersome. What third party would be available in a busy pediatric office? Furthermore, there are some parents who would be intolerant of third-party scrutiny. These parents may find even the physician's scrutiny an inappropriate threat to their legitimate parental authority.

What are the pediatrician's options if consensus is not achieved? If she sides with the parent, she will have to give the protesting child a painful treatment. What if the child resists? And what does this tell the child about his right to participate in medical decision making? On the other hand, to side with the child on the grounds of developing maturity places the parent in an awkward position because she now must buy the medicine and apply it to her child's hands nightly. What if the parent resists and says, "OK, doctor, at what time will you come by to place the medicine on Alan's hands?" Her response demonstrates the bind that physicians have in their relationships with their patients. The professionals' challenge, as nonparents, is how to be caring without taking unnecessary control of the life of the child for whom they do not and cannot take full responsibility.[23]

In a case such as this, it appears reasonable that parents have ultimate decision-making authority. For such decisions, where the risks of either treatment are low, as are the burdens of therapy, and where the child is at an age where it is unlikely that he would be capable of taking responsibility for his own medication regimen, parental authority should prevail. Physicians also have the right, and perhaps the obligation, to involve children in the decision-making process and to explain to the child why his wishes and requests are being overridden, even if his parents complain that this threatens their autonomy.

Case 2

Betty, a 15-year-old girl, presents for a yearly physical. Her examination is normal. She attends St. Mary's High School, where she is on the honor roll. She is popular with her friends and tells you that she recently has fallen in love with Bob. She says that she is not sexually active yet, but she asks for birth control pills. She also asks that you not tell her parents because she knows that it is against their moral and religious beliefs and she fears they will prohibit her from seeing Bob.

Case 3

Vicky, a 15-year-old girl, is brought to your office by her mother, Ms. V. Ms. V states that she knows that her daughter is sexually active and she wants her to get long-term contraception to avoid pregnancy. Ms. V is a single mother who became pregnant with Vicky when she was 14, and she wants to protect her daughter from the hardships she faced. Vicky acknowledges that she has a boyfriend and is sexually active. She states that he wants her to get pregnant although she is ambivalent. She does not want contraception because she fears her boyfriend will leave her.

Discussion: By the age of 18, more than 50% of all female adolescents in the United States have had sexual intercourse; even more are sexually active.[4] More than 1 million American adolescents become pregnant every year.[29] Many teens do not seek medical or gynecological care or contraception for months or even years after they initiate sexual activity.[2] Most teens who become pregnant are unmarried, and most of their pregnancies are unplanned.[29] Slightly more than 50% will decide to take the pregnancy to term, and virtually all of these teenagers will take on the responsibilities of parenthood. Pregnant adolescents have a higher incidence of medical complications for themselves and their fetus than do older women.[18] Their children do not fare as well psychosocially as do children of adult mothers.[16] Thus, one can say both that Betty is acting unusually responsible for a 15-year-old and that Ms. V's concerns are well-founded.

Both of their requests should be interpreted as an opportunity for dialogue. Is Bob a classmate or, more typically, an adult male older than 20 years, which may suggest a power differential? Is he willing to take responsibility to avoid pregnancy? What would Betty do if she were to get pregnant, even though she was on the pill? Has she discussed this with Bob? How will Betty's deception affect her relationship with her family? As Vicky's doctor, you may want to address the issue of whether Vicky finds this three-way conversation embarrassing. You might suggest to Ms. V that the best way to protect Vicky from an unwanted pregnancy could be to encourage her to talk with you confidentially. Ms. V and Vicky may be very receptive to this. This does not resolve whether Vicky should receive treatment that her mother requests but Vicky rejects. However, it may give you an opportunity to discuss with Vicky the most likely outcome of adolescent pregnancy: single parenthood and its attendant responsibilities. You may try to encourage her that pregnancy should be a positive decision (i.e., I want to be a parent) and not a passive decision (i.e., it will make my partner happy). You may want to encourage her to get counseling, as it is obvious that her self-esteem is low.

Although parents generally have the legal right and responsibility to make medical decisions for their teenagers, treatment related to reproductive health is an exception under the special consent statutes. These statutes vary in their scope, but all give adolescents the legal autonomy independently to seek and consent to the diagnosis and treatment of drug and alcohol abuse, contraceptive counseling, and/or the procurement of contraceptives.[24] Some states even allow minors to consent to abortions without disclosure or consent from their parents. The statutes were designed to encourage adolescents to seek health care for problems that they might deny or ignore or for which they might delay seeking treatment if they had to get parental permission. Although such statutes *allow* physicians to provide this care, they don't *compel* them to do so. Thus, a pediatrician facing a patient such as Betty has the legal latitude to make a moral decision. The purported purpose of the specialized consent statutes is laudable: to encourage early, responsible sexual health care for adolescents. The pragmatic justification is compelling. Given that adolescents can be and frequently are sexually active even when birth control and other sexual health services are relatively inaccessible, they should be given the opportunity to be responsible for their sexual activity. The pragmatist does not need to concede or refute whether the availability of such services increases the numbers of sexually active adolescents because the number is sufficiently large as to portend a public health crisis, even when such services are unavailable. The pragmatist's position depends on the empirical claim that the statutes will promote better health care for adolescents in the realm of sexual and reproductive services than if parental involvement were required. Nonetheless, empirical data are inconclusive.

It is not clear that the pragmatic arguments are sufficient to justify empowering all adolescents to consent to sexual and reproductive health care. Rather, the pragmatic goal of minimizing adolescent pregnancy may lead one to empower Betty and to disempower Vicky.

The moral argument in support of the specialized consent statutes is based on the claim that if a child is competent to make such decisions, competency should entail autonomy. But this argument implies that these children should have the right to make all health care decisions and not just decisions covered by the special consent statutes. Although some pediatricians lean in this direction, we must ask why health care is exceptional—that is, why don't we allow these same "competent" children to drive, smoke, or make a binding financial contract?

Two moral arguments can be made against the specialized consent statutes. The first is that granting autonomy to adolescents regarding their sexual activity may be autonomy-restricting over a lifetime. As with many decisions that children make, we might justify restricting a child's autonomy now to give her greater lifetime autonomy.[32] The second moral argument against the statutes is that parents have a valid third-party interest in their children's development and activities, even after the children become teenagers and achieve a significant level of competency. To act on those interests and to participate in their child's moral development, they need to have the opportunity to try to inculcate their beliefs through rational discourse.[22,32] They can do this only if they are aware of what their teens are doing—that is, competency is necessary but may not be sufficient to grant an adolescent health care autonomy.

Whether or not one agrees with the specialized consent statutes, they clearly do not apply to Vicky's case. The statutes empower teens to get contraception, but they do not empower them to refuse contraception to which their parents consent on their behalf.[14] Legally, parents can request that physicians provide Depo-Provera to their daughters. However, they cannot demand that a physician do so. Thus, pediatricians must make a personal moral decision about how they will respond.

Case 4

Ms. C calls you the day before she is scheduled to bring her 14-year-old son Charles for his yearly physical examination. She notes that Charles previously was an A-student, but now is getting Cs and Ds. The family is going through turmoil because Mr. C moved out of the house 3 months ago to live with his pregnant girlfriend. Ms. C admits to being depressed and cries easily but has not sought outside help. Charles has been withdrawn and often comes home late and refuses to tell his mother where he has been. She fears that Charles is using drugs and would like you to screen him without telling him what you are doing.

Discussion: Ms. C's request is a call for help. Ms. C and Charles need psychiatric treatment regardless of whether Charles is using drugs. Ideally, both of his parents need to realize how their actions and emotions are affecting their son's behavior. Charles needs parental supervision at a time when both parents are disengaged for different reasons.

The crucial question for Ms. C is, "How will the surreptitious drug testing help?" If it comes back negative, that does not prove that Charles is not using drugs. False-negatives can occur because the half-life of many drugs is less than 24 hours and because urine drug testing tests only for some of the substances more commonly abused. Serum testing is more sensitive but can only be done for specific drugs, so you would need a list of what drugs are suspected. If the screen comes back positive, Ms. C will need to decide how she will approach Charles. Charles presently is not trusting of adults who have betrayed him. Secret testing will increase his distrust.

It would be preferable to ask Ms. C to give you permission to establish a confidential relationship with Charles. You could explain that this is likely to be much better for Charles in the long run. Most parents are willing to do this. If Ms. C gives you such permission, you should arrange to meet with Charles privately and explain the confidential nature of the relationship. You should be honest about when confidentiality would be broken—specifically, in cases in which you believe that Charles is a danger to himself or others.[21]

The opportunity to confide confidentially in his physician may be what Charles needs to help him cope with the turmoil at home.[17] Charles may be willing to discuss whether he is abusing drugs and may be willing to be tested for drugs as well. But there are many other issues that you need to address with Charles that are even more compelling. Is he suicidal? Is he engaging in any other risky behaviors (of which illicit drugs is but one dimension)? Is he depressed? Is he willing to seek psychiatric counseling or begin anti-depressant medication? Are there any adults whom he trusts?

Despite your suggestion, Ms. C may still demand that you test Charles for drugs. There are, in fact, situations in which the grounds for suspecting drug abuse are compelling, and teenagers who are using drugs may not be in a position to assess the risks and benefits of testing or treatment. However, one might also argue that pediatricians should not deceive their patients. Thus, if Charles' mother insists on the testing, the pediatrician should test, but he or she should also insist on informing Charles of the nature of the test. This will help maintain trust and keep the door open for future communication. This approach rests on the moral claim that as a parent, Ms. C has a right and the obligation to care for her son and to determine what medical information she needs to do so. However, this does not give her the right to demand that you lie to him about what you are doing.

The physician also should use this appointment and the discussion about drug testing as an opportunity to encourage Charles and Ms. C to seek counseling and to give Charles anticipatory guidance about any and all risky behaviors in which he is involved.

Case 5

Mr. and Mrs. D are the proud parents of David, a well-appearing 6-week-old boy. During their first well-baby visit, you learn that Mr. D had retinoblastoma as a child and had his left eye removed. You recommend genetic testing to determine if the child is at risk. Mrs. D states that they were offered such testing in utero and that they refused and still refuse genetic testing.

Discussion: Retinoblastoma may be inherited as an autosomal dominant gene or it may develop spontaneously. Given that Mr. D had retinoblastoma, David has a 50% risk for developing retinoblastoma. Before the discovery of the gene for retinoblastoma, children born into families that had a positive history for retinoblastoma underwent ophthalmological surveillance every 3 months. The value of the genetic information is that if David tests negative for the gene, he can avoid frequent eye examinations. If he tests positive, he will need to undergo frequent screening to enhance the likelihood of early detection. If detected early, there is a better prognosis for survival and vision. Testing young children for early-onset conditions encompasses two very different categories of conditions: first, those, such as Duchenne muscular dystrophy and cystic fibrosis, for which early (presymptomatic) diagnosis and treatment do not affect the course of the disease; second, those, such as retinoblastoma, for which early diagnosis and treatment may improve treatment or even save lives.

In the first category of early-onset conditions, the value of presymptomatic diagnosis is to help avoid delay in diagnosis when early symptoms are nonspecific, to target surveillance screening more accurately, to allow parents to prepare for a child who will have special needs, and to give parents information to use in their reproductive planning.[8] On the other hand, early diagnosis may be detrimental in a number of ways. The "vulnerable child" syndrome has been shown to cause morbidity that may be even greater than the morbidity associated with the disease that is diagnosed. Early diagnosis may affect parent-child bonding adversely if the parents hold back on emotional investment because they fear their child will die. In older children, it may adversely affect the child's self image and self-esteem.[8] Finally, in the United States, it may cause difficulties for the parents to obtain appropriate health insurance for the child and even for healthy siblings.[11] Parental expectations for the future also may be limited unnecessarily.[8] Given that early testing has not been shown to improve morbidity or mortality, the risk-benefit balance of presymptomatic testing will depend on the values and needs of each family.[8,30]

The value of presymptomatic testing in the second category is to prevent serious morbidity and mortality. Because it is difficult to come up with a compelling argument why children should not be tested in these circumstances, there is wide consensus that children in families known to carry such genes should be tested.[10] It also is assumed that parents are the child's appropriate decision makers. The question is whether, if parents refuse testing or diagnostic work-ups, physicians should feel compelled to seek state permission to override their refusal.

In such a case, the pediatrician needs to engage Mr. and Mrs. D in dialogue to try to determine why they are refusing testing. They may have refused genetic testing in utero because amniocentesis entails risks of morbidity and mortality and, assuming that a positive test would not have led them to terminate the pregnancy, would not have offered any tangible benefits. However, genetic testing for the gene for retinoblastoma in a 6-week-old child is a simple blood test. Mr. and Mrs. D may continue to refuse testing because of lack of knowledge, fear of stigma or discrimination, or fear that this may interfere with obtaining insurance, particularly if either parent is looking for a new job, which may include a change in insurance.

What should be done if Mr. and Mrs. D continue to refuse testing? Ideally, it would be valuable to know David's genetic status, but as long as Mr. and Mrs. D are compliant with frequent surveillance, their decision is neither abusive nor neglectful. The eye examinations themselves are minimally invasive, although young children may require sedation. Physicians should respect this decision but realize that this adds the additional responsibility that they ensure that David does get appropriate quarterly examinations. If Mr. and Mrs. D refuse or fail to comply with quarterly ophthalmological examinations, this is neglectful and they should be reported to the appropriate child protection authorities.

Case 6

Ms. F delivered Frances, a healthy full-term infant, 24 hours ago. She refused vitamin K and hepatitis B because she did not want to put Frances through any more discomfort than the birth process. You come to draw the screen for phenylketonuria (PKU) and other metabolic conditions before discharge, but she refuses. She agrees to reconsider and will take the card to her private pediatrician, whom she plans to see in 2 days. You suspect that she will again refuse newborn metabolic screening. How should you respond?

Discussion: Each of the conditions screened for is a relatively rare autosomal recessive disease (except for hypothyroidism, which is sporadic.) Thus, there is no way to target "at-risk" couples, and the only way to find affected children is to screen them. The World Health Organization (WHO) has developed criteria for evaluating screening programs First, the disease must represent an important health problem for which there is an accepted treatment that can prevent most or all of the morbidity or mortality associated with the condition. Second, the screening test must be simple and cheap and the follow-up confirmatory testing highly accurate. Third, there must be a system in place to ensure quick communication of results to relevant parties. Lastly, the cost of case finding, diagnosis, and treatment must be economically balanced in relation to expenditures on medial care as a whole.[35]

In the United States, 49 of the 50 states have mandatory universal newborn screening programs Although states have different panels of required tests, the most common tests are those for PKU, hypothyroidism, hemoglobinopathies (including sickle cell disease), congenital adrenal hyperplasia (CAH), and galactosemia.[6] Although screening is thought of as "mandatory," in actual practice, parents can and occasionally do refuse testing. However, they generally are not asked for consent and so, to refuse, they must be informed and proactive. Most parents (and physicians) are unaware of this.

Although it is reasonable to allow parents to refuse screening for rare diseases, mandated medical treatment of any sort overrides important parental rights. Generally, the state should not interfere in the medical decisions that parents make for their children. To do so undermines the family unit. The only exceptions to this are situations in which parental decisions put their children in imminent danger of morbidity or mortality. Thus, parents whose religious beliefs lead them to oppose blood transfusions should not be permitted to refuse blood for their child in a life-threatening situation. Clearly, newborn screening does not present a situation in which children are in immediate danger. Each of these conditions occurs in fewer than 1 in 1000 children, so that a parent who refuses newborn screening is taking a very small, albeit serious risk.

Physicians should educate parents who refuse testing so that they understand why we believe that the benefits greatly outweigh the risks. Most parents agree. In Maryland, where testing is voluntary, fewer than one parent in a thousand refuses testing for their newborns.[15] The risk that these refusals create is much less than the risk of a false-negative test and less than the number of children not tested due to lost and improperly obtained specimens.[26]

Given the experience in Maryland, one might ask whether parental consent should be required for a universal newborn screening program. What are the arguments for seeking parental consent for newborn screening? First, procuring parental consent for newborn screening is a symbol of respect for the family—respect that is well placed, given that families are the primary source of childrearing and given that families, and not the state, will bear the greatest costs if diagnosis is delayed. Second, by requiring consent, parents must be educated about the purpose and limitations of screening, which may give them incentive to follow up on abnormal screening results. Knowledge of negative test results can be reassuring to parents, particularly those who have personal knowledge of any of the conditions for which their infant is being tested.

The major benefit of not requiring consent is to simplify the process of screening. It can be time consuming to obtain parental consent for newborn screening. In this day and age, physicians are more and more pressed for time. In some cases, they may not have time to seek parental consent and newborns may suffer as a result. A related argument is that consent often is perfunctory.[25,33] Neither argument morally justifies circumventing the consent process. Consent is time consuming for all medical conditions, not just newborn tests. In fact, consent ought to be time consuming because parents need information to make well-informed decisions for their children that will promote their children's needs. Pediatricians discuss many issues with parents after the birth of a child. Explaining the screening tests should not add much time to this counseling.

Case 7

Mr. and Ms. G come to the clinic with Gary, their 5-year-old son. Gary was adopted as a newborn. Mr. and Ms. G have told you they plan to tell Gary about his origins, but each time you ask, they give reasons why they have not yet done so. They have kept the adoption secret from all but their immediate family.

Case 8

Mr. and Ms. S bring their 5-year-old child, Sam, for a well-child visit. The family has just moved from California. As you try to take a full past medical history, the parents become visibly uncomfortable. Finally, Mr. S takes Sam out of the room to play in the waiting room, at which time Ms. S explains that they had infertility problems and used donor sperm, so that Mr. S is not Sam's genetic father. They have only sketchy information about the sperm donor, who was a 25-year-old healthy white medical student. They have chosen not to tell Sam about his genetic parentage.

Discussion: Adoption is a legal procedure through which a permanent family is created for a child whose birth parents are unable, are unwilling, or are legally prohibited from caring for their child. Adoption has existed throughout history, although the focus has changed. Historically, "adoption served the needs of adults . . . for the purpose of kinship, religion or the community," in contrast to our current focus on the needs and well-being of the child.[13]

In the United States, formal adoptions peaked in the mid 1960s when there were approximately 240,000 adoptions yearly. Adoptions have decreased because of many social factors, including the decrease in the number of out-of-wedlock pregnancies, the decrease in the stigma of single mothers, and the increased availability of abortion. Nevertheless, 120,000 formal adoptions occur yearly. Despite the large number of children and families who are directly affected by adoption, the medical literature on adoption is scant.

Before World War II, professional adoptions workers advised, if not insisted, that children be told of their adopted status for the pragmatic reason that it was better for the child to learn of adoption from parents in a loving environment than by well-meaning or even malicious neighbors, schoolmates, or relatives. Post-World War II, the professional community, particularly the psychoanalytical community, argued against disclosing. By the mid-1970s, the pendulum returned not only in favor of disclosing adoption but also in openness in all aspects of adoption.[13] Nevertheless, some families do try to keep the adoption a secret.

The new reproductive technologies (NRTs) offer individuals another possible means to achieve parenthood (see Chapter 44, Sequelae to Infertility). The NRTs have offered some new twists. Whereas adoption separated genetic and social parenthood, the NRTs allow individuals to separate genetic, gestational, and social parenthood. For example, through in vitro fertilization, a woman can gestate a fetus who is the product of her husband's sperm and a nongenetically related egg donor whose identity often is unknown. More common are children born by the use of sperm donors such as in the case of Sam. In the early days of donor insemination, the husband's sperm was mixed with the donor's sperm to leave open the possibility that the child was the genetic heir. Now, determination of paternity is widely available and accessible and makes this pretense obsolete. But unlike the adoption literature, very little advice is given to families about disclosure to the child, and the empirical data suggest that most married couples do not disclose this information to the child.[27]

For Gary and Sam, the value of a genetic family history for their pediatrician is to help target medical concerns and to educate families about issues of lifestyle that may exacerbate genetic susceptibilities. As understanding of genetics increases rapidly, genetic family histories become both more and less important. They become more important as we understand that many illnesses have a genetic component. They become less important as we develop the ability to identify particular genes in particular persons without the need to link their genes with family members.

However, there also are the questions of whether children have a right to know their genetic inheritance and whether parents have a right to maintain secrecy. The literature about the psychological risks of disclosure and nondisclosure is small and inconclusive. Nevertheless, most psychologists and psychiatrists support disclosure because of its role in health care screening, diagnosis, and treatment and the importance of genetic identity to one's self-identity. Reasons to respect nondisclosure include that such knowledge may threaten the parent-child relationship and that it might threaten the integrity of the family. Which reasons are stronger depends on how one weighs the advantages and disadvantages.

Although it might be argued that it is better for children to know their biological identity, the physician's right to interfere in interpersonal family dynamics is and ought to be limited to situations of clear-cut abuse or neglect. Nondisclosure of biological relationships does not rise to that level. Pediatricians should encourage disclosure and offer to facilitate or arrange for a facilitator. The physician should encourage disclosure on the grounds that the child otherwise may learn of the genetic discrepancy in a less than ideal setting and that the knowledge will become of greater importance as the child reaches adulthood and begins to make procreative plans. Nevertheless, physicians should not disclose this information to children without the parents' permission.

Case 9

Ms. H brings her 17-year-old son Harold to the clinic for a preparticipation high school basketball sports physical examination. On taking the history, you learn that Harold's father died from a heart condition last year at the age of 40. Harold's uncle died in his late 20s when playing competitive tennis. You are concerned about the possibility of hypertrophic obstructive cardiomyopathy (HOCM, previously known as idiopathic hypertrophic subaortic stenosis [IHSS]). An echocardiogram confirms your diagnosis. You advise against Harold's participation. Harold and his mother are quite angry. Harold already is an all-state player and is being recruited heavily by many universities. The mother plans to take Harold to another physician and demands that you not inform his school or anyone else of your findings. Harold and his mother do not disclose the family history to your colleague, who approves him for interscholastic athletics.

Discussion: HOCM is an autosomal dominant condition that often presents in the late teenage years. It is an idiopathic cause of cardiomyopathy, and the risk of sudden death, particularly during intense athletic activity, increases with age.

Harold has a life-threatening illness that is exacerbated by physical activity. Disclosure of his diagnosis will make him ineligible for sports and will take away his opportunity for a college sports scholarship. Of course, failure to disclose may result in premature death in a high school gymnasium. Competitive sports participation clearly is risky for Harold.

You ask to meet with Harold and his mother. They acknowledge the risks that you mention, but Harold states that basketball is his life and he is willing to risk his life. He and his mother argue that you are no longer his physician and that you no longer are under any obligation to protect him. They are willing to sign papers to release you (and the school) of medical liability.

Harold and Ms. H view the issue as one of autonomy. They understand the risks and benefits of playing, given Harold's cardiac condition, and they believe that it is better for Harold to play basketball despite the risk of sudden death. They also view the issue as one of confidentiality. The physician discovered Harold's cardiac condition within the confidential relationship, and he or she should not disclose without Harold and his mother's explicit consent.

Here is a case in which the parent and child are in consensus but in disagreement with the physician. The family's position for confidentiality and nondisclosure must be weighed against the physician's belief that he or she needs to protect this child from his mother and himself. The physician can and must decide that the harm to patient privacy and confidentiality are outweighed by the life-threatening nature of his cardiac condition. As a moral agent, the physician has an obligation to prevent a serious imminent risk of sudden death to a minor. Harold and his mother cannot waive the physician of this obligation.[28]

The physician also has an obligation to protect the community. Imagine the reaction if Harold were allowed to play and he did die on the basketball court in front of many classmates and their families. Such an event could cause serious psychological trauma to the observers. How would the community respond if they knew that the physician could have prevented this? The physician has an obligation to protect Harold and the community from such unnecessary trauma and should notify the school about Harold's medical condition, and Harold should be prohibited from participating in athletics. Even when Harold turns 18 years old, the school should refuse to let him play basketball or other sports that may lead to his sudden death.[9,28]

Case 10

Mr. K brings Kevin for his prekindergarten examination, during which you notice some linear ecchymoses on his back. You ask Kevin how he got them, and he answers that his father beat him for talking back at dinner last night. Kevin's father confirms this explanation, explaining that he believes that corporal punishment is effective. He admits to using a belt because his hand "did not produce the desired effect." You inform the family that corporal punishment that leaves marks is abusive and that you plan to report your suspicions of child abuse to the department of family services. The father is irate, arguing that discipline is a family matter and that his religious faith supports his convictions of "spare the rod and spoil the child."

Discussion: A recent AAP position statement on guidance for effective discipline begins by noting that "parents often ask pediatricians for advice about the provision of appropriate and effective discipline."[8] The most controversial aspect of this issue is the role, if any, for corporal punishment. Although a recent survey of AAP members found that approximately 85% of respondents generally or completely opposed the use of corporal punishment,[1] more than 90% of American families report having used spanking as a means of discipline at some time.[7]

Kevin's father raises the point that his actions are based on his religious beliefs. Some religious groups take a strong position in support of corporal punishment. Currently, there are religious exemptions to most of the child abuse and neglect statutes, but the exemptions do not apply to corporal punishment, nor should they. The religious exemptions were written to protect those parents who sought prayer-based therapy for their child rather than allopathic medical care; they were not meant to protect a parent from being charged with abuse for beating a child.

To examine the benefits and burdens of corporal punishment, the AAP co-sponsored a consensus conference on this topic in February 1996.[20] The conference concluded with 13 consensus statements that addressed the role of spanking and corporal punishment in parental discipline. Statement No. 6 commented on the lack of data on the effectiveness of spanking in general, and statement No. 8 commented that the data show corporal punishment to be ineffective in older children and adolescents and "is associated with increased risk for dysfunction and aggression later in life."[20] The strongest statement against corporal punishment was Statement No. 12, which stated that the harms of corporal punishment more severe than spanking outweigh any potential benefits.[20]

Despite common usage and acceptance of corporal punishment, the data show that over time, spanking is a less effective strategy than noncorporal methods for reducing undesired behavior. Furthermore, it becomes less effective with continued use.[7] The AAP recommends that parents "be encouraged and assisted in developing methods other than spanking in response to undesired behavior."[7] The AAP statement noted further that many parents go beyond spanking and use an object or other forms of unacceptable corporal punishment: "When punishment fails, parents who rely on it tend to increase the intensity of its use rather than to change strategies." This is no longer discipline but child abuse. The moral objection to corporal punishment is that it teaches the lesson that "might makes right."

Pediatricians should help parents understand the facts about corporal punishment and to realize that any such punishment (beyond an occasional mild spanking) is unacceptable and will be reported.

There is no morally justifiable reason for a parent to inflict physical harm on a child. Although physical manifestations of violence are an imperfect measure of the severity of punishment, they at least define an unacceptable threshold. The marks on Kevin are a sign that his father used more physical force than is morally acceptable. It is appropriate for the physician to work with this family to modify their discipline strategy. If this fails, the parents should be reported to the appropriate authorities. Pediatricians can and should help instill an anti-spanking mindset by enforcing it in their offices or clinics.

CONCLUSION

In the medical care of children, ethical conflicts can develop within the family and between the health care provider and the family, or the health care provider and family may be in conflict with the state. The preceding cases represent different health care scenarios that will be familiar to all who are involved in the primary health care of children. In each, a methodology for resolving conflicts is proposed. The first, and most important, is in-depth discussion among doctors, parents, and children to try to understand why people hold the beliefs that they do. Physicians should be open-minded and willing to compromise, up to a point. The second important consideration is some assessment of the benefits and the burdens of the proposed treatment or action and of the available alternatives. Generally, parents have both the legal responsibility and the moral authority to make medical decisions for their children, but respect for the child's opinion should increase as the child grows older, acquires increased capacity to understand and make decisions, and approaches the age of legal majority. In all of the above situations, pediatricians must balance their own assessments of what is best for the child with an understanding that children benefit from interacting with their families in an environment safe from third-party intrusion. Pediatricians also must remember that their expertise is in deciding what is medically best for a child, whereas parental decisions need to reflect what is best for the child overall, balanced by the parents' right, privilege, and responsibility to preserve their moral values.

REFERENCES

1. AAP survey on corporal punishment reveals divergent views, *AAP News*, September 1998, p 16.
2. Alan Guttmacher Institute: *Sex and America's teenagers,* New York, 1994, The Institute.
3. Alderson P, Montgomery J: *Health care choices: making decisions with children,* London, 1996, Institute for Public Policy Research.
4. American Academy of Pediatrics, Committee on Adolescence: Adolescent pregnancy: current trends and issues: 1998, *Pediatrics* 103:516, 1999.
5. American Academy of Pediatrics, Committee on Bioethics: Informed consent, parental permission, and assent in pediatric practice, *Pediatrics* 95:314, 1995.
6. American Academy of Pediatrics, Committee on Genetics: Newborn screening fact sheets. *Pediatrics* 98:473, 1996.
7. American Academy of Pediatrics, Committee on Psychosocial Aspects of Child and Family Health: Guidance for effective discipline, *Pediatrics* 101:723, 1998.
8. American Society of Human Genetics Board of Directors and American College of Medical Genetics Board of Directors: ASHG/ACMG report. Points to consider: ethical, legal and psychosocial implications of genetic testing in children and adolescents, *Am J Hum Genet* 57:1233, 1995.
9. Anderson V: Court affirms right to disqualify athletes, *Physician Sport Med* 25:19, 1997.
10. Andrews L, et al, editors: *Assessing genetic risks: implications for health and social policy,* Washington, DC, 1994, National Academy Press.
11. Billings P, et al: Discrimination as a consequence of genetic testing. *Am J Hum Genet,* 50:476, 1992.
12. Buchanan A, Brock D: *Deciding for others: the ethics of surrogate decision making,* New York, 1989, Cambridge University Press.
13. Carp EW: *Family matters: secrecy and disclosure in the history of adoption,* Cambridge, Mass, 1998, Harvard University Press.
14. Costello JC: If I can say yes, why can't I say no? Adolescents at risk and the right to give or withhold consent to health care. In Humm SR, et al, editors: *Child, parent and state,* Philadelphia, 1994, Temple University Press.
15. Faden R, et al: A survey To evaluate parental consent as public policy for neonatal screening, *Am Public Health* 72:1347, 1982.
16. Fergusson DM, Woodward LJ: Maternal age and educational and psychosocial outcomes in early adulthood, *J Child Psychol Psychiatry* 40: 479, 1999.
17. Ford CA, et al: Influence of physician confidentiality assurances on

adolescents' willingness to disclose information and seek future health care: a randomized controlled trial. *JAMA* 278:1029, 1997.

18. Fraser AM, Brockert JE, Ward RH: Association of young maternal age with adverse reproductive outcomes, *N Engl J Med* 332:1113, 1995.
19. Freeman M, editor: *Children's rights: a comparative perspective,* Hants, England, 1996, Dartmouth Publishing.
20. Friedman SB, Schonberg SK, editors: The short- and long-term consequences of corporal punishment: proceedings of a conference, *Pediatrics* (suppl 4 Pt 2) 98:i-vi, 803, 1996.
21. Gans GE: *Policy compendium on confidential health services for adolescents,* Chicago, 1993, American Medical Association.
22. Gaylin W: Competence: no longer all or none. In Gaylin W, Macklin R, editors: *Who speaks for the child: the problems of proxy consent,* New York, 1982, Plenum Press.
23. Goldstein J, et al: *In the best interests of the child,* New York, 1986, The Free Press.
24. Holder AR: *Legal issues in pediatrics and adolescent medicine,* ed 2, New Haven, Conn, 1985, Yale University Press.
25. Holtzman NA, et al: Effect of informed parental consent on mothers' knowledge of newborn screening, *Pediatrics* 72:807, 1983.
26. Holtzman NA, Leonard CO, Farfel MR: Issues in antenatal and neonatal screening and surveillance for hereditary and congenital disorders. *Annu Rev Public Health* 2:219, 1981.
27. Lauritzen P: *Pursuing parenthood: ethical issues in assisted reproduction,* Bloomington, Indiana, 1993, Indiana University Press.
28. Mitten MJ: When is disqualification from sports justified? Medical judgment vs patients' rights, *Physician Sports Med* 24:75, 1996.
29. Moore KA: Teen fertility in the United States: 1993 data. Facts at a glance, *Child Trends* January 1996.
30. Report of a Working Party of the Clinical Genetics Society (UK): the genetic testing of children, *J Med Genet* 31:785, 1994.
31. Ross LF: *Children, families, and health care decision-making,* Oxford, UK, 1998, Oxford University Press.
32. Ross LF: Health care decision making by children: is it in their best interest? *Hastings Cent Rep* 27:41, 1997.
33. Statham H, Green J, Snowdon C: Mother's consent to screening newborn babies for disease, *BMJ* 306:858, 1993 (letter).
34. United Nations Convention on the Rights of the Child, 1989.
35. Wilson JMG, Jungner F: Principles and practice of screening for disease. *Public Health Papers* no 34, Geneva, 1968, WHO.

part two

Evaluation and Communication

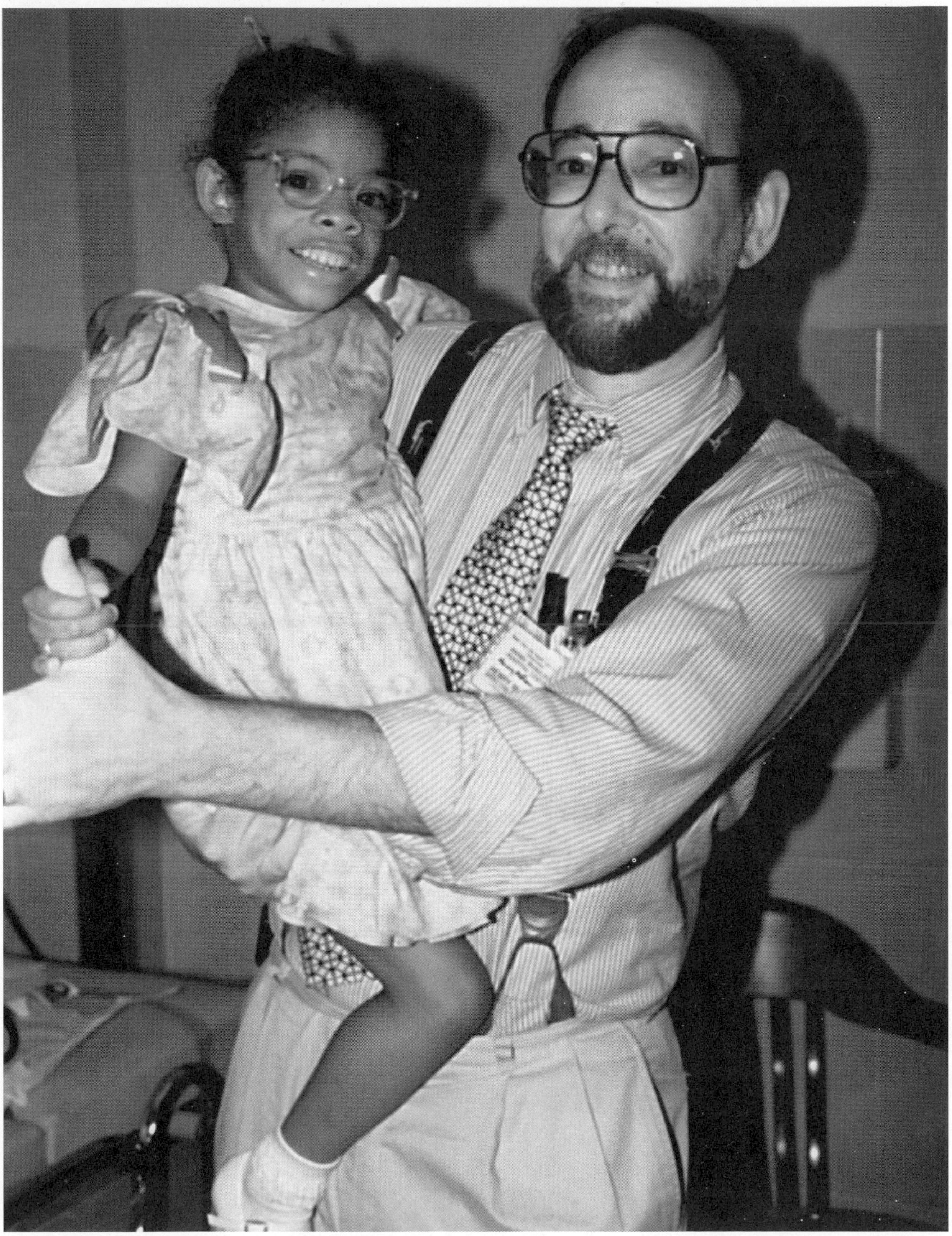

7 The Pediatric History

William E. Boyle, Jr. • Robert A. Hoekelman

"A good history carefully obtained from an intelligent mother . . . puts the physician in possession of a fund of information about the patient which is of greatest value, not only in arriving at a diagnosis in the illness for which he is consulted, but is exceedingly helpful in the future management of the child."

L. EMMETT HOLT, 1908[1]

A history is a narrative related by the patient or his family. It is a unique story in which are embedded the words, phrases, and clues that will direct the physician to the general or specific medical problem of the patient. It requires the physician to pay close attention to this detailed sequence of events, and through careful direct questioning formulate a differential diagnosis. Parents and patients hope the physician will hear their story and interpret it correctly. It in not an easy task.

Perhaps in no other medical field is a history as important as it is in pediatrics. For early detection of problems related to health (including growth, development, and nutrition) and for prevention of future difficulties, the practitioner must have a thorough knowledge of the child and the family, their lifestyle, and their environment. Unlike in most other areas of medicine, the pediatric history usually is given by someone other than the patient. Thus, a certain amount of subjectivity and objectivity is lost. Signs and symptoms are filtered through parental perspectives before emerging as historical data and, therefore, are influenced by parental hopes and fears. A pediatric history is a compilation of information gathered in a variety of ways—through interviews, direct observations, questionnaires, and medical records—that usually provides a concise record of the child and the family.

In the past, training in interviewing and history taking took place for an acute problem in which the concern or complaint was readily stated or easily seen. Today, however, children are treated for an increasing number of psychosocial problems, usually as outpatients. These may include learning difficulties, chronic or disabling conditions, or behavioral or developmental problems—all of which require sensitive, insightful listening. Thus, the pediatrician must have a thorough knowledge of the child's health status, developmental stage, and cognitive level, as well as the family's functional characteristics, belief systems, and socioeconomic circumstances. Much of pediatrics has to do with vague questions or concerns, such as "Why does she cry so much?" "Why is he so thin?" or "Is that cough serious?" These concerns must be answered and expectations dealt with if the encounter is to be fruitful. If the physician and parent or patient have different perceptions of the problem, the physician must attempt to "tease out" and understand the patient's or parent's concerns.

Much transpires during the initial interview between a practitioner and a family other than the gathering of a history. The tone of all future encounters is established, and ideally the family begins to develop a trusting, confident relationship with the practitioner. Just as the practitioner is trying to assess the problem at hand, so, too, are the parents (and child) "sizing up" the clinician and trying to feel comfortable with him or her. A warm, friendly, nonjudgmental, courteous manner certainly facilitates this. History taking requires some degree of decision making on the part of the interviewer as to what is relevant. It is not merely the gathering of a list of all symptoms and pertinent historical "negatives"; it also involves the synthesis of various facts, attitudes, and observations. To do this well requires experience, tact, and some degree of intuition. It is a difficult task. A history is compiled best if, for each visit, the practitioner can obtain the answers to three questions: "Why did you come today?"; "What are you worried about most?"; and "Why does that worry you?" The answers not only direct further inquiry but also provide clues to parent and patient concerns that need to be allayed or dealt with directly during the visit and, perhaps, thereafter. For example, a parent who brings a child to a physician because of swollen cervical lymph nodes may be worried that they represent the first signs of malignancy, because an aunt who died of Hodgkin's disease had the same problem. Parents, older children, and adolescents need to be told what symptoms and signs do *not* represent, as well as what they do represent, especially if the parents and patient are worried that the symptoms and signs indicate a serious or fatal illness.

SETTING AND AMBIANCE

Pediatric histories are taken in a variety of locations, and a comfortable environment should be used to enhance communication. If the practitioner projects courtesy, interest, and a desire to help, a trusting, positive relationship is likely to develop. Patients and parents are acutely aware of what the physician thinks of them or what they perceive the physician's opinion of them to be—the *reflexive self-concept.* ("The doctor thinks I'm a good parent.") If the reflexive self-concept is high, parent (or patient) satisfaction and compliance with recommendations for management are more likely to be high. Some questions to consider are: Does the practitioner imply disinterest in the patient by allowing constant interruptions by others during the history taking? Is privacy ensured? Are children made comfortable? Is there a place for clothing and belongings (other than a lap)? Obviously, seating should be available for all, and the history taker should remain seated for the session. Parents or guardians should be called by their formal names (Mrs. Williams, Mr. Adams), unless a personal relationship has been established that enables the use of first names. "Mother," "Dad," or "Grandma" should never be used. Children should be referred to by their first names—for example, "Chris" or "Jane," rather than "he," "she," or "the baby." Notes can be taken if this does not distract from the continuity or spontaneity of the interview. Most parents find coping with more than one child disruptive and distracting, so seeing more than one child at a time or having others in the room should be discouraged. Toys or books should be available to help quiet infants and toddlers, if necessary.

Clothing and appearance may affect the ease with which a relationship is established. Parents and children view a visit to the pediatrician as a special occasion and frequently dress accordingly. They hope their practitioner will view the visit in the same manner. The practitioner's dress should be appropriate to the population served and consistent with local values. Most pediatricians do not wear a white coat because it may evoke fearful memories for the child, although this has never been substantiated. Whatever the attire, a sense of competence must be conveyed.

TYPES OF INTERVIEWS

The pediatric history is obtained in a variety of settings and for a variety of reasons. The initial history may be taken during an interview with the parents before their baby's birth, in the hospital after the birth, in the physician's office during the first visit for whatever reason, in an emergency room at the time of an acute illness, or in a hospital room after admission for a specific illness or elective surgery. The time devoted to the initial interview and the amount of information gathered depend on the circumstances. Likewise, subsequent history taking will vary in depth and breadth, depending on the reason for the visit and the amount of time that has elapsed since the last visit.

This chapter focuses on the information to be gathered and the techniques used in obtaining the comprehensive pediatric history, which usually is accomplished in a single sitting. Circumstances may preclude completion of this exercise during the initial visit, however, and much of the information will have to be gathered at subsequent visits. For example, the initial history obtained for a child who has acute otitis media and who is "squeezed in" during fully scheduled office hours will be brief and related primarily to the chief complaint. The rest of the history can be obtained during a scheduled follow-up visit when adequate time is allotted for this purpose.

Prenatal Interview

Ideally, the parents should have their first encounter with a pediatrician before their baby is born. To many, the idea of bringing a baby in utero to the pediatrician seems strange, but much information can be gathered at this time, and a strong, understanding relationship between the parents and the pediatrician can be fostered. In addition, problems can be identified and intervention instituted then, rather than waiting until the frantic, unsettled postpartum period. An example is the isolated, deprived, pregnant woman who should be identified before she delivers so that appropriate social and psychological support can be provided. Pregnancy is much more than a period of gestation, growth, and development of a fetus. During this time the mother must adapt to profound psychobiological changes. A life grows within her, distorting her self-image and causing nausea and then fatigue and disequilibrium. She feels obese and uncomfortable. After quickening, she begins to identify this life within her as a separate individual and to fantasize about its gender, size, and soundness. Frequently, she becomes introspective and withdrawn, which may stress her marital relationship. Spousal physical abuse is not uncommon during pregnancy. As her term approaches, the mother wants the discomfort of pregnancy to end, yet she views the work of labor and delivery with some trepidation. All this is hard work for both her body and her psyche. Many women have spent high school or college years preparing for careers, and approaching motherhood frequently means temporarily relinquishing a rewarding position or prestigious job. It means embarking on a new "career" without much training and often without much status. In addition, our society is mobile. There are fewer extended families and, thus, fewer experiences and less advice such families can bring to the task of childrearing. Most young couples live alone and often are far removed from parents and siblings. These couples seldom have a wide range of friends on whom they can rely for help and support. Because of these societal changes, young couples usually find coping with the stresses of parenthood difficult and often turn to professionals for support and assistance.

Ideally, the person who has cared for the woman throughout her pregnancy and delivery and who understands her needs should be the person who will help her understand her new role as a mother. In many communities this is not done. Obstetricians traditionally care for women only throughout pregnancy and the immediate postpartum period. Pediatricians traditionally assume care of the infant at birth. Many women find it difficult to leave someone who has supported them through a difficult psychobiological change and to develop a new relationship while they learn the new role of motherhood. Thus, a prenatal interview can greatly assist in this transition.

Prenatal interviews do not need to be long or detailed; 20 to 30 minutes should suffice. In addition to gathering facts, the pediatrician should set a tone for future encounters. Husband and wife should be interviewed together, if possible, so that parental concerns can be aired and they can be helped to support each other. All parents are anxious about their adequacy and the health of their unborn infant, and a supportive attitude and tacit acknowledgment that these fears are understandable can be most helpful.

Taking a thorough family history is one way of evidencing concern, not just for the child but for the entire family. Parents should understand the physician's interest in them as individuals and not merely as Teddy's or Sarah Jane's mother and father.

During a typical prenatal interview, plans for labor and delivery should be discussed, as well as a program of childbirth education and the type of infant feeding that is contemplated. It is wise at this time to point out certain safety issues to which the parents should attend before their baby comes home, such as obtaining a child safety seat and a smoke detector and setting the hot water heater at a safe temperature (see Chapter 23 [Two], Injury Control). Circumcision should be discussed, unless the couple has learned through tests that their baby is a girl. It also is helpful to point out to the parents that they obviously have imagined a variety of circumstances for their child, which the clinician can understand and help with if they arise. It should be noted whether one or both parents desire a child of a particular gender, which may affect their abilities as parents.

The mother's blood type, medications taken, and rubella status (if known) should be elicited. Genetic information should be gathered about both sets of grandparents. In addition to inherited disorders and birth defects, familial tendencies such as obesity, hypertension, and short stature should be investigated. It also is wise to ask what the couple's own parents were like, because parenting techniques and styles frequently are passed from one generation to the next.

After dealing with the family history, the clinician needs to gather some information about other supportive individuals. Who will help out when the baby comes home? Will the husband have a paternity leave of some sort? Grandparents traditionally visit shortly after delivery, and the pediatrician should point this out and ask if they will be helpful or another burden. He or she also should inquire if transportation and a telephone are readily available. The physician should be alert at all times for evidence of undue stress, isolation, and prior deprivation because these factors are known to be predictors of poor parenting. The parents will want to know when the pediatrician will see the baby in the hospital, what the appointment schedule will be, and how the pediatrician can be reached. Fees for visits also can be discussed at this time.

The parents should be allowed to ask questions about their concerns. It is best to support their instincts rather than to direct and show one's own personal bias. The pediatrician should anticipate certain normal variations such as sleepy babies, the postpartum "blues," and the physiological slump that lasts from 6 to 8 weeks after birth. Parental questions may seem trivial (skin care, type of diapers), but all evolve around the question, "Will we be good parents?" Strong reassurance that their instincts are good serves to reinforce and strengthen the couple's tendencies toward good parenting and leads to a confident beginning as parents.

At the conclusion of the interview the practitioner should have an idea of the parents' lifestyle and coping mechanisms, and they should feel reassured that they have a supportive person who will help them enter parenthood.

As prenatal interviewing has become more widespread, interview requests for second or subsequent pregnancies have become more common. These generally are not quite so formal and can take place during the routine health maintenance visits of an older child. Parental concerns deal not only with the health and soundness of the unborn, but also with coping with another child. "Will I be able to divide myself and still survive?" The mother finds herself torn between her baby in utero and her baby at home, and this issue must be addressed. Inappropriately, she may have her child attempt new developmental tasks such as toilet-training so that in essence she will have only one baby. She also may force a child to "grow up" and relinquish a crib, stroller, or high chair. All these efforts should be discouraged. Separation at the time of delivery can be a problem for a child, who must be told that mommy will leave for a while and then return. This should be done shortly before the expected confinement. The mother's departure can be made easier by having the child help the mother pack for her hospital stay. The separation also will stress the supports the family has developed, and the clinician should review these at this time. It, likewise, is important to recount the previous birth experience, so that conflicts or problems may be identified and, thus, avoided a second time. The mother should be reassured that she will be able to cope and that support will be available.

Comprehensive Pediatric History Interview

Traditionally, history taking has been a stepwise delineation of the events that led to the practitioner-patient encounter. Most clinicians learned this technique while dealing with hospitalized or acutely ill children, where the problem frequently was visible or obvious. Fortunately, a great deal of history taking now takes place in settings other than the hospital and frequently does not involve illness. Therefore, this discussion will focus on the *pediatric interview,* of which historical data are merely a part. The interview should include observation of behavior and family interactions. Essentially, a history is a narrative about an encounter between practitioner and parent and child that includes subjective and objective data and omits some details considered irrelevant.

Box 7-1 is a suggested outline for components of a *comprehensive pediatric history.* In certain settings some of the data already will have been gathered, but a thorough knowledge of each component of the history is essential. Obviously, under certain circumstances it may be necessary to gather other information; the boxed material merely suggests a general format.

Usually the interview begins with the parents stating the concerns that led to the present encounter—the *chief complaint.* The parents should then be allowed, with as little interruption as possible, to relate the history as they recall it. Certain areas may be amplified and clarified, but direct or challenging questions should be avoided. After eliciting the chief complaint, the practitioner should enumerate the events associated with it in an orderly sequence *(present illness).* In addition to facts, parental concerns and feelings about these symptoms should be elicited. The parents should be asked to speculate on what they think is causing the complaint or symptom. This information can be valuable in several respects. First, it demonstrates the level of parental concern, which may influence subsequent care and treatment. Thus, parents who equate nosebleeds with leukemia, for instance, will need more than simple reassurance. Second, parental concerns about causation may "color" the history a great deal; for example, their concern about developmental delay can influence the information they supply about achievement of early milestones. It always is important to discover how the present illness affects the rest of the family. This information will help the physician better understand the family's concerns about and responses to a given symptom or illness and what, if any, secondary gain exists for the child.

BOX 7-1

COMPREHENSIVE PEDIATRIC HISTORY

The following comprehensive pediatric history is exhaustive and obviously not meant to be used in its entirety with all patients. However, depending on the patient's age and gender and the nature of the chief complaint and the present illness, the interviewer will need to explore in depth some or all of the subjects listed. In most instances, common sense must be used in deciding how much information should be gathered.

Date of Interview

Identifying Data

Record the date and place of birth, gender, race, religious preference, nickname (particularly for children 2 to 10 years of age), parents' first names (and last names, if different), and where the parents can be reached during work hours.

Source of and Reason for Referral

Source of the History

This may be the parents, the patient, or sometimes a relative or friend. As a practitioner, you should record your judgment of the validity of the source's reporting. Other possible sources of the history are the patient's medical record or a letter from a referring physician or the school nurse.

Chief Complaints

When possible, quote the parents or the patient. Clarify whether these complaints are the concerns of the parents, the patient, or both. In some instances they are the concerns of a third party, such as a teacher.

Present Illness

This should be a clear, chronological narrative of the problems for which the patient is seeking care. Include the onset of the problem, the setting in which it developed, its manifestations and treatments, its impact on the patient's life, and its meaning to the patient or the parents, or both. Describe the principal symptoms in terms of (1) location, (2) quality, (3) quantity or severity, (4) timing (i.e., onset, duration, and frequency), (5) setting, (6) factors that have aggravated or relieved these symptoms, and (7) associated manifestations. Relevant data from the patient's chart, such as laboratory reports, also belong in the Present Illness section, as do significant negatives (i.e., the absence of certain symptoms that will aid in differential diagnosis). Include how each member of the family responds to the patient's symptoms, their concerns about them, and whether the patient achieves any secondary gains from them.

Past Medical History

General state of health as the parents or patient perceives it

BIRTH HISTORY

This is particularly important during the first 2 years of life and when dealing with neurological and developmental problems. Review the hospital records if preliminary information from the parents indicates significant difficulties before, during, or after delivery.

PRENATAL HISTORY

Determine the mother's health before and during the pregnancy, including nutritional patterns and specific illnesses related to or complicated by the pregnancy; doses and duration of all legal and illegal drugs taken during the pregnancy (including alcohol ingestion and cigarette smoking); weight gain; vaginal bleeding; duration of the pregnancy; and the parents' attitudes toward the pregnancy and parenthood in general and toward this child in particular.

NATAL HISTORY

Determine the nature of the mother's labor and delivery, including degree of difficulty, analgesia used, and complications encountered; birth order, if a multiple birth; and birth weight.

NEONATAL HISTORY

Determine the onset of respirations; resuscitation efforts; Apgar scores and estimation of gestational age; specific problems with feeding, respiratory distress, cyanosis, jaundice, anemia, convulsions, congenital anomalies, or infection; the mother's health after delivery; separation of the mother and infant and the reasons for this; the mother's initial reactions to her baby and the nature of bonding; and patterns of crying and sleeping and of urination and defecation.

Feeding history

This is particularly important during the first 2 years of life and in dealing with problems of undernutrition and overnutrition.

INFANCY

Breast-feeding—frequency and duration of feeds, use of complementary or supplementary artificial (formula) feedings, difficulties encountered, time and method of weaning. *Artificial (formula) feeding*—type, concentration, amount, and frequency of feeds; difficulties encountered (regurgitation, colic, diarrhea); timing and method of weaning. *Vitamin, iron, and fluoride supplements*—type, amount given, frequency, and duration. *Solid foods*—types and amounts of baby foods given; when introduced, and infant's response; introduction of junior and table foods; start of self-foods; start of self-feeding; and the mother's and child's responses to the feeding process.

CHILDHOOD

Eating habits—likes and dislikes, specific types and amounts of food eaten, parents' attitudes toward eating in general and toward this child's undereating or overeating, and parents' response to any feeding problems. With childhood feeding problems, the parents may need to keep a diet diary for 7 to 14 days to allow accurate assessment of the child's food intake.

Modified from Bickley LS, Hoekelman RA: Interviewing and the health history. In Bickley LS, Hoekelman RA, editors: *Bates' guide to physical examination and history taking,* ed 7, Philadelphia, 1999, JB Lippincott.

BOX 7-1

COMPREHENSIVE PEDIATRIC HISTORY—cont'd

Growth and development history

This history is particularly important during infancy and childhood and in dealing with problems such as delayed physical growth, psychomotor and intellectual retardation, and behavioral disturbances.

PHYSICAL GROWTH

Determine the actual (or approximate) weight and height at birth and at 1, 2, 5, and 10 years; record any history of slow or rapid gains or losses; and note the tooth eruption and loss pattern.

DEVELOPMENTAL MILESTONES

Determine the ages at which the patient: held head up while prone; rolled over from front to back and back to front; sat with support and alone; stood with support and alone; walked with support and alone; said first word, combinations of words, and sentences; tied own shoes; and dressed without help.

SOCIAL DEVELOPMENT

Sleep—amount and patterns during the day and at night; bedtime routines; type and location of bed; nightmares, terrors, and somnambulation. *Toileting*—methods of training used; when bladder and bowel control were attained; occurrence of accidents or of enuresis or encopresis; parents' attitudes; terms used in the family for urination and defecation (important to know when a young child is admitted to the hospital). *Speech*—hesitation; stuttering; baby talk; lisping; estimate of the number of words in the child's vocabulary. *Habits*—bed-rocking; head-banging; tics; thumb-sucking; nail-biting; pica; ritualistic behavior; use of tobacco, alcohol, or drugs. *Discipline*—parents' assessment of child's temperament and response to discipline; methods used and their success or failure; negativism; temper tantrums; withdrawal; aggressive behavior. *Schooling*—experience with child care, nursery school, and kindergarten; age and adjustment on entry; current level of parents' and child's satisfaction; academic achievement; school's concerns. *Sexuality*—relationships with members of the opposite gender; inquisitiveness about conception, pregnancy, and girl-boy differences; parents' responses to child's questions, and what they have taught him or her about masturbation, menstruation, nocturnal emissions, the development of secondary sexual characteristics, and sexual urges; dating patterns. *Personality*—degree of independence; relationships with parents, siblings, and peers; group and independent activities and interests; congeniality; special friends (real or imaginary); major assets and skills; self-image.

Childhood illness

Determine the specific illnesses the child has had, as well as any recent exposures to communicable diseases.

Immunizations

Record the specific dates of administration of each vaccine so that a booster program can be maintained throughout childhood and adolescence; also record any untoward reactions to a vaccine. The parents should have their own written record of the child's immunizations.

Screening procedures

Record the dates and results of any screening tests. For all children, these tests should include vision, hearing, urinalysis, and hematocrit, as well as newborn screening for genetic-metabolic disorders. For certain high-risk children, additional tests may include tuberculosis, sickle cell, the human immunodeficiency virus (HIV), blood lead, cholesterol, alpha$_1$-antitrypsin deficiency, and any other screening that may be indicated.

Operations, injuries, and hospitalizations

Elicit the details of these events and the child's and parents' reactions to them. If the child is old enough, ask age-appropriate questions about safety and prevention of injuries.

Allergies

Pay particular attention to the allergic diseases that are more prevalent during infancy and childhood—eczema, urticaria, perennial allergic rhinitis, asthma, food intolerance, and insect venom hypersensitivity.

Current medications

Include home remedies, alternative medicines, nonprescription drugs, and medicines borrowed from family members or friends. If it seems that the patient might be taking one or more medications, survey one 24-hour period in detail: "Take yesterday, for example. Starting from when he woke up, what was the first medicine Thomas took? How much? How often during the day did he take it? What is he taking it for? What other medications . . . ?"

Family history

Record the education attained, job history, emotional health, and family background of each parent or parent substitute; the family's socioeconomic circumstances, including income, type of dwelling, and neighborhood; parents' work schedules; family cohesiveness and interdependence; support available from relatives, friends, and neighbors; ethnic and cultural milieu in which the family lives; parents' expectations of the patient and attitudes toward him or her in relation to siblings. (All or part of this information can be recorded in the Present Illness section, if pertinent to it, or under Psychosocial History.)

Also record the age and health or age and cause of death of each immediate family member, including the parents and siblings (see Fig. 7-1). Ascertain consanguinity of the parents by inquiring if they are "related by blood."

Note the occurrence in the family of any of the following conditions: diabetes, tuberculosis, heart disease, high blood pressure, stroke, kidney disease, cancer, arthritis, anemia, headaches, mental illness, or symptoms resembling those of the patient.

Continued

BOX 7-1

COMPREHENSIVE PEDIATRIC HISTORY—cont'd

Psychosocial history

This is an outline or narrative description that captures the important and relevant information about the patient as a person:

The patient's lifestyle, home situation, and "significant others"

A typical day—how the patient spends his or her time between arising and going to bed

Religious and health beliefs of the family that are relevant to perceptions of wellness, illness, and treatment

The patient's outlook on the future

Review of Systems

General. Usual weight, recent weight change, weakness, fatigue, fever, pallor.

Skin. Rashes, lumps, itching, dryness, color change, changes in hair or nails.

Head. Headache, head injury.

Eyes. Vision, glasses or contact lenses, last eye examination, pain, redness, excessive tearing, double vision.

Ears. Hearing, tinnitus, vertigo, earaches, infection, discharge.

Nose and sinuses. Frequent colds, nasal stuffiness, hay fever, nosebleeds, sinus trouble.

Mouth and throat. Condition of teeth and gums, bleeding gums, last dental examination, frequent sore throats, hoarseness.

Neck. Lumps in the neck, swollen glands, goiter, pain in the neck.

Breasts. Lumps, pain, nipple discharge.

Respiratory. Cough, sputum (color, quantity), hemoptysis, wheezing, asthma, bronchitis, pneumonia, tuberculosis, pleurisy; results of last chest roentgenogram.

Cardiac. High blood pressure, rheumatic fever, heart murmurs; dyspnea, cyanosis, edema; chest pain, palpitations; results of past electrocardiograms or other heart tests.

Gastrointestinal. Trouble swallowing, loss of appetite, nausea, vomiting, hematemesis, indigestion; frequency of bowel movements, change in bowel habits, rectal bleeding or black, tarry stools, constipation, diarrhea; abdominal pain, food intolerance, excessive passing of gas; jaundice, hepatitis.

Urinary. Frequency of urination; polyuria; nocturia; dysuria; hematuria; urgency; hesitancy; incontinence; urinary tract infections.

Genitoreproductive. *Male*—discharge from or sore on penis; history of venereal disease and its treatment; hernias; testicular pain or masses; frequency of intercourse; libido; sexual difficulties; sexual preference.

Female—age at menarche; regularity, frequency, and duration of periods; amount of bleeding, bleeding between periods, last menstrual period; dysmenorrhea; discharge, itching, venereal disease and its treatment; number of pregnancies, number of deliveries, number of abortions (spontaneous and induced); complications of pregnancy; birth control methods; frequency of intercourse; libido; sexual difficulties; sexual preference.

Musculoskeletal. Joint pains or stiffness, arthritis, backache; if these are present, describe location and symptoms (e.g., swelling, redness, pain, stiffness, weakness, limitation of motion or activity); muscle pains or cramps.

Neurological. Fainting, blackouts, seizures, paralysis, local weakness, numbness, tingling, tremors, memory loss.

Psychiatric. Nervousness, tension, moodiness, depression.

Endocrinological. Thyroid trouble, heat or cold intolerance, excessive sweating, diabetes, and excessive thirst, hunger, or urination.

Hematological. Anemia, easy bruising or bleeding, past transfusions and possible reactions to them.

Modified from Bickley LS, Hoekelman RA: Interviewing and the health history. In Bickley LS, Hoekelman RA, editors: *Bates' guide to physical examination and history taking,* ed 7, Philadelphia, 1999, JB Lippincott.

Although the chief complaint must remain the central focus of the interview, it frequently is obvious that it is not the main problem. This especially is true when dealing with very young children. Tired, anxious, or frightened parents often perceive their reactions to an infant as being abnormal in some way; they then project this as something being wrong with the baby. This makes seeking help acceptable. Once the practitioner recognizes this, he or she should try to create an atmosphere that allows the parents to express all their concerns. Questions such as, "Are there any other problems with Kathy you would like to discuss?" or "Is there anything else bothering you about Connor?" might facilitate communication.

After the present illness has been defined and elaborated upon, certain significant events should be enumerated *(past medical history).* Much of this material is factual and can be obtained by using a direct question and answer format. Significant events such as operations, serious injuries, and hospitalizations should be verified by obtaining and reviewing appropriate hospital records.

When obtaining the patient's early history, the practitioner should elicit medically significant facts from conception to the onset of the present illness. All areas delineated in Box 7-1 should be touched on to some degree. The amount of information obtained may vary, but prenatal problems such as bleeding, eclampsia, or infection should be noted, and birth weight, type of delivery, and neonatal problems, if any, must be described. Information about nutrition can reveal a great deal about family dynamics and parental perceptions and expectations. "Tell me how Jennifer eats" frequently

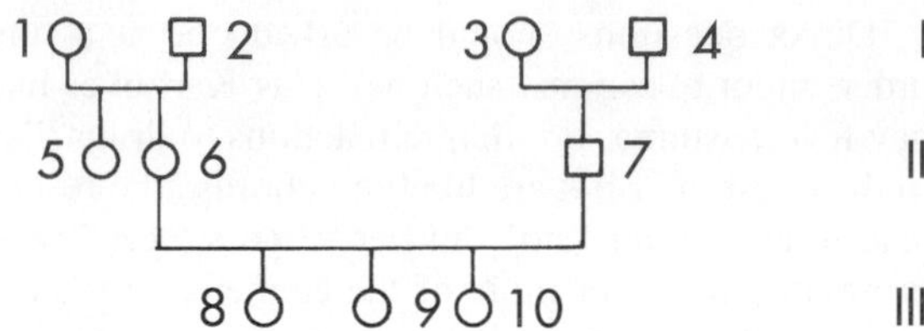

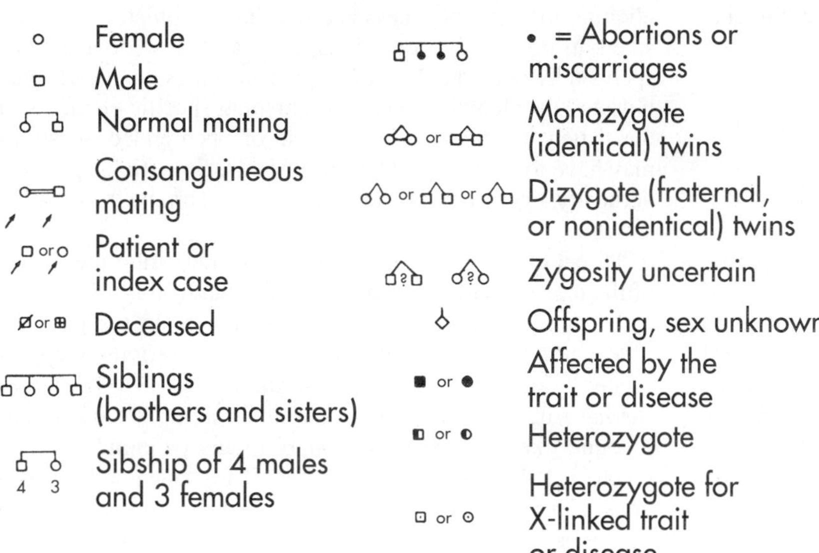

Fig. 7-1 Chart and symbols used to construct a family history, or family pedigree. The Roman numerals indicate generations; the Arabic numerals indicate specific persons.

brings forth a torrent of information, but its value, nutritionally speaking, may be limited. "Good eaters" and "picky eaters" frequently weigh the same, and those who "hardly eat a thing" often are overweight.

In dealing with issues of development, it frequently is best to ask an indirect question, such as "Tell me what Ann did during her first (or second) year." This usually elicits much more information than do direct questions about motor milestones. The clinician should seek information concerning the level of skill rather than the age of achievement; for example, it is more important to know that the child could make simple wants known at age 2 years than the age when the first word was uttered. Some information about social adaptability and temperament should be obtained (see Chapters 79, Interviewing Children, and 105, Interviewing Adolescents).

Previous health care is important, and the child's immunization status is a significant part of the early history. The practitioner should record all immunizations, skin tests, and pertinent screening information on a separate sheet that is readily accessible and retrievable. Filling out a few history forms later for camp or entry into preschool will prove the value of this record.

Allergies and allergic reactions also are an important part of the early history. Specific allergic reactions should be described in as much detail as possible to clarify the reaction. For example, ampicillin can cause a variety of cutaneous and gastrointestinal reactions, but only urticaria and anaphylaxis are true allergic responses to the medication. Idiosyncratic reactions to drugs such as phenothiazides also should be described.

The *family history* contains variable information but often is difficult to construct. An attempt should be made to trace back at least two generations on each side of the family, and any data obtained should be recorded appropriately. Fig. 7-1 shows one method of recording such data. The names, birth dates, and health of the three generations concerned usually are listed below the pedigree (although not shown here), using a number indicating each person. As more data such as births, deaths, and disease become available, they can be added easily.

Consanguinity of parents should be investigated specifically by asking if the parents are related by blood. In addition to seeking known inherited diseases such as diabetes, hemophilia, or neuromuscular disorders, the clinician should note familial tendencies such as obesity, short stature, early heart disease, and hypertension. Sometimes it is appropriate to inquire about the parenting techniques of forebears. It has been shown that abusive parents frequently were deprived or abused as children. It also is important to ask specifically about the health of the parents' brothers or sisters, because they often are overlooked during an interview.

The *psychosocial history* describes the child in his or her present milieu and relationships with family, peers, school, and community. This should include information about the physical setting (e.g., housing), environment, and degree of isolation. Determining how children spend the day, who cares for them, what they like to do, and what their hobbies are is important. Inquiry should be made about the support system within the family; for example, the nature of an extended family, supportive or conflicting roles, the elements of stress that exist for this child, and how the child and family cope with them.

The psychosocial history also should touch on the parents' attitudes toward discipline and expectations about achievement. When appropriate, the practitioner should determine how the parents compare this child to his or her siblings or to other children. It also is appropriate at this time to ask the parents to describe the child's temperament (e.g., "mellow," "feisty," "lazy"), as well as what they see as his or her strengths.

The *review of systems* should be detailed to obtain a baseline evaluation of all systems and their level of function. Children change over time, and various systems may be the target of stress or disease processes. Therefore, the clinician should reassess all organ systems periodically and record their apparent level of function.

INTERVIEWING TECHNIQUES

Although most interviews are direct and straightforward, difficulties occasionally are encountered. Certain pitfalls can be avoided by changing the interview format or adapting particular strategies. Clarification of certain terms always is essential. For example, *diarrhea* and *flu* mean different things to different people, and no true communication can occur until such terms are defined. The temporal nature of complaints also must be assessed carefully. Children who are "always sick" may have recurrent infections that clear in 5 to 7 days, or they may have a perpetually runny nose, which is so in some children who have allergies.

If the patient has been seen before, the clinician should review the child's medical record before the visit to refresh his or her memory on past health and illnesses that may relate to the reason for the current visit. Consultants should review the letter of referral and the reason for and goals of the visit before interviewing the parents and patient.

Many parents see their skills as parents being challenged during the pediatric interview: "After all, if we did things right, we wouldn't need to see the doctor." They become defensive and may answer questions "ideally." At the same time, they want to share fears and worries with a caring, empathetic practitioner. The pediatrician must strive to develop this trusting relationship. By being facilitative, he or she enables the parents to ventilate fears and frustrations and sort out thoughts. Statements such as "That must have worried you" or "I bet that's upsetting" let parents know that the clinician is concerned with much more than the facts in the interview. On the other hand, statements or questions suggesting that the parents have not managed their child's illness properly, such as "You should have brought Gretchen in sooner," or "It would have been better not to have fed Stephanie," or "Why did you do *that?*" always should be avoided.

The techniques used to obtain a complete and accurate history vary with the situation and the person being interviewed.

Types of Questions

In emergencies, the clinician should ask only direct questions (non–open-ended) that quickly elicit the important facts needed to make decisions regarding treatment. In nonemergencies, in which time is not a factor, direct questions should be used to obtain identifying data and information about pregnancy, birth, growth and development, feeding, immunizations, screening tests, previous illnesses, injuries and hospitalizations, family history, and review of systems.

Direct questions should be asked one at a time. Rapid-order direct questions, such as "Has Karl ever had eczema, hay fever, asthma, or allergic reactions to drugs?" are logical to the questioner but are likely to confuse the respondent and lead to an overall "no" answer when a "yes" would be appropriate for one or more of the elements of the question.

Indirect (open-ended) questions are extremely useful in eliciting the present illness and psychosocial history. The answers to open-ended questions, such as "How does Bonnie spend a typical day?", often provide clues to underlying, unstated problems and cues for pursuing specific elements of the patient's illness. However, use of open-ended questions may have to be curtailed because of time limitations, parental verbosity, or the parents' inability to focus on the information sought.

Direct questions also are important in eliciting the details of the present illness and the psychosocial history. For example, if a cough is mentioned as a symptom in the patient's illness, the following sequence of direct questions is appropriate: "How long has Kathy had the cough?"; "When does she have it?"; "Does it wake her up at night?"; "What does it sound like?"; "Does she cough up any phlegm?"; "How much?"; "What does it look like?" Thus, open-ended questions identify the direction for further inquiry, and direct questions help to determine the importance of the symptoms or signs identified.

Leading direct questions—for example, "Does Jane do well in school?"—should be avoided because they are more likely to result in "expected," affirmative answers than are nonleading, direct questions, such as "What kinds of grades does Jane get in school?"

Helping the Parent or Patient Communicate

Throughout the interview the parents or patient should be assisted in several ways to relate all necessary information fully. The practitioner should use medical terminology understood by the parents or patient. Words such as *tinnitus, palpitation,* and *incontinence* may have little meaning to the parents or patient, who often will be too embarrassed to ask for a definition and may simply answer "no" when asked if those signs and symptoms are present.

The interview process is one of interaction between the clinician and the parents or patient. The person providing information should do most of the talking and the practitioner most of the listening. However, the clinician can encourage the parents or patient to communicate their story by using the following seven techniques:

1. *Facilitation.* This is designed to convey interest in what the parent or patient is saying. Maintaining eye contact, leaning forward, nodding in affirmation, and saying "yes," "uh huh," "I see," and the like, all convey interest and encourage the parent or patient to continue. Additional information might be gained by giving an example, such as "In other situations like this, some parents have thought of alternative medicines. Have you thought so, too?"
2. *Reflection.* Repetition of words the parent or patient has said encourages him or her to provide more detail, as is demonstrated in the following example:

Parent: Kara woke up in the middle of the night breathing hard.
Interviewer: Breathing hard?
Parent: Yes, she seemed to be breathing fast and making a wheezing noise.
Interviewer: A wheezing noise?
Parent: Yes, in and out—a musical wheezing sound.

By using reflection, the interviewer was able to elicit the nature of the child's breathing difficulty without influencing its description or diverting the parent's thoughts.

3. *Clarification.* The interviewer often must clarify what the parent or patient has said; for example, "What do you mean by 'Rob wasn't acting right'?"
4. *Empathy.* Recognizing and responding to a parent's or patient's feelings of concern, fear, or embarrassment show understanding and acceptance and encourage continued expression of the emotion. "I can understand why that upset you" or "That must have been difficult to deal with" is an empathetic expression that tells the parent or patient that the clinician appreciates what he or she has been experiencing and is sympathetic. The practitioner also can ask the parent or patient how he or she feels or felt about a particular situation that has been related. This displays an interest in the parent's or patient's feelings as well as in the medical facts.
5. *Confrontation.* This technique is used to clarify what seems to be a contradiction between the parent's or patient's feelings and actions: "You say that Alison loves school but misses a lot because she has an upset stomach most mornings." Although confrontation is used to seek clarification, it also may lead to interpretation of the meaning of the contradiction.
6. *Interpretation.* This technique is used to move beyond clarification to an inference to be made from the circumstances presented. Thus, the above example might lead to the following statement and questions by the practitioner: "Maybe there is some relationship between Alison's upset stomach and her wanting or not wanting to go to school. Do you think that's possible?"
7. *Recapitulation.* This technique is especially useful when a long and complicated or an unusual history is presented. The clinician summarizes to the parent or patient the history as the clinician understands it. This may be done at more than one point during the interview and serves to confirm the validity of the history. It also allows for possible changes.

It sometimes is helpful toward the end of the interview to ask, "Is there anything else you think I should know?" This open-ended inquiry leaves parents with the sense that things were not rushed and that there is still room for discussion.

Hindrances to communication. Although a calm, reserved, interested demeanor is important to enhance communication, the practitioner must guard against appearing casual. Constant eye contact with the parent, interrupted by glances at the child (if present), should be maintained. Evidence of boredom or impatience—looking away from the parents or patient, tapping the fingers or a pencil on a tabletop, or rushing through the interview—must be avoided. Inappropriate smiling or laughter also hinders good communication. The parents or patient always should feel that they have the practitioner's undivided attention. If time is short, the parents or patient should be informed and another appointment made for completing the interview.

Interviewing the Child

A great deal of information can be gained by interviewing the child directly (see Chapter 79, Interviewing Children). Many children interact spontaneously with the pediatrician and answer direct questions readily. Often only the child can reveal the severity of the pain or the extent of the symptoms. Sometimes it is better to approach children indirectly, such as encouraging them to talk about their symptoms, than to seek direct answers. For example, "Tell me about your cold, Gordon" is preferable to "Do you cough?" The pediatrician should always support the child's "own story." It should be taken seriously, and confidences should not be violated except in unusual circumstances.

With chronic problems, such as constipation or enuresis, it is helpful to review with patients their knowledge of the complaint. Patients can be asked what they were told before coming to the physician's office, how they feel about the visit, how their symptoms affect them and alter their lifestyle, and whether they are able to attend school and carry out all their regular activities. It also is important to ask children what they think is causing their symptoms, what they are worried about, and why it worries them.

Interviewing the child provides another opportunity to assess parent-child interaction. Many parents cannot let their child speak without addition, interruption, or correction. A school-age child who clings to a parent and cannot be coaxed to make eye contact with the practitioner or interact in any way probably is overly shy and dependent. As adolescence approaches, parent-child conflicts become more intense. Given the chance, many adolescents will make this obvious. Under these circumstances, separate interviews probably are preferable (see Chapter 105, Interviewing Adolescents).

"Typical day" technique. In many situations, information about a child's typical day can be very helpful and informative, and most parents can relate this information readily. In addition to concrete material (e.g., sleep patterns and feeding activities), much can be learned about areas of stress and harmony within a family. As with other aspects of the history, such information should be obtained as objectively as possible. Parents frequently find it difficult to discuss situations without seeking approval, even if tacit, of their own actions. Mothers who are confused or unsure of themselves frequently may ask advice on a particular aspect of their child's behavior as it is presented in the description of the child's typical day; however, it is best to defer answers until the entire day has been described.

Discussion can begin with an introduction, such as "To find out more about Kim, I am going to ask you to tell me how she spends a typical day." The clinician should then begin by asking what time the patient arises and what happens. Some parents will launch into vivid descriptions and will require little direction, whereas others must be encouraged. Details can be elicited by asking some simple questions, such as "What is her mood on awakening?", "Who takes care of her?", and "What does she usually eat for breakfast?" Discussion can include food likes and dislikes, skill in eating, and conduct at the table. The practitioner also can learn about the child's activities, habits, and television viewing practices. The subject of discipline might come up during this discussion, and the parents' beliefs about prohibitions and punishments can be ascertained.

Lunchtime, afternoon rest periods, and activities are reviewed in much the same way. Descriptions of trips to the market or to other stores can provide information about behavior with others and reactions to new experiences.

The evening meal often is stressful in many families, and how it proceeds can provide many clues to family dynamics. For example, the clinician should find out when the parents arrive home, whether the child eats with the parents, and if so, the types of interactions that occur. Information about the events surrounding preparation for sleep, bedtime rituals, and sleeping patterns also is important.

At the end of such an interview, it should be possible to assess not only the child's style and temperament but also the family's strengths and weaknesses. This information is essential for advising parents of children who are having developmental and maturational problems.

QUESTIONNAIRES

In certain instances, parental questionnaires may be used to supplement the history. Some may be used as part of a general health appraisal; others are more applicable to a specific problem. The Framingham Safety Survey is part of The Injury Prevention Program (TIPP) of the American Academy of Pediatrics. It is the basis of office counseling on injury prevention in child health supervision. Questionnaires are especially helpful for assessing school problems and developmental issues. The Denver Prescreening Developmental Questionnaire-Revised (R-PDQ) and the Achenbach Child Behavior Checklist (CBC) are but two examples (see Appendix D for more information about these questionnaires and others). The wise practitioner will be thoroughly familiar with the questionnaire format and its pitfalls before using it; all such instruments may supply additional information, but all also may be subject to observer bias and should be interpreted accordingly.

RECORDING HISTORICAL INFORMATION

There are two main goals in recording the historical data gained in an interview. First, the patient's symptoms and medical history, which will help in formulating a diagnosis and therapeutic plan, are documented. This serves as a legal record of the practitioner-patient encounter. Second, a reasonable account of the patient's medical status is made available to others who also are involved in the patient's care and to the person who initially gathered the information.

The historical database should contain all the medically significant facts of the child's life. The recorded history is a synthesis of material and observations gained during the interview, compiled in a legible, retrievable form.

The present illness must be recorded clearly and concisely. Consistency is paramount, especially when dealing with events in time. Events must be recorded by using either of these methods: "Dick developed a cough on March 17" or "Dick developed a cough 5 days before our interview on March 23." "Tuesdays" and "Fridays" are difficult to identify 2 weeks after an interview.

Data obtained during an interview can be recorded in a variety of ways, ranging from tape-recording the entire session, a method often used by psychiatrists, to merely noting "Dx—acute otitis media; Rx—amoxicillin × 10 days" on an index card. Records should be legible, and much of the data should be retrievable without having to pore over volumes of paper. This requires some foresight and planning so that different parts of the history can be separated for later use. Ideally, the historical database should be standard and uniform. However, certain problems (hip clicks, birthmarks) change with time and vary by age and gender (menstrual irregularities), by type of population served, and by geographical locale.

A variety of questionnaires have been developed to facilitate development of the database. These are designed to be age appropriate and can be filled out by the parent or by a nurse, physician's assistant, or other office personnel. Such questionnaires can be used to gather a large amount of data quickly, thoroughly, and concisely. However, they also present several drawbacks. First, questions tend to be answered in an idealized way because parents usually have a skewed opinion of their children. Second, all logical sequencing of information gathering is lost, and degrees of concern are not readily expressed. Third, unless the database is updated frequently by subsequent questionnaires, much of the information soon becomes irrelevant.

Gathering and recording a history and communicating compassionately and courteously with patients and their families are difficult tasks. These are not innate skills but rather require work, insight, perseverance, and practice. The work is hard, but the rewards are great.

REFERENCE

1. Holt LE: *The diseases of infancy and childhood,* New York, 1908, Appleton-Century-Crofts.

SUGGESTED READINGS

Bickley LS, Hoekelman RA: Interviewing and the health history. In Bickley LS, Hoekelman, RA, editors: *Bates' guide to physical examination and history taking,* ed 7, Philadelphia, 1999, JB Lippincott.

Cassell EJ: Talking with patients. In *Clinical technique,* vol 2, Cambridge, Mass, 1985, MIT Press.

Feinstein AR: *Clinical judgment,* Baltimore, 1967, Williams & Wilkins.

Klaus MH, Kennell JH: *Parent-infant bonding,* ed 2, St Louis, 1982, Mosby.

Thornton SM, Frankenburg WK, editors: *Child health care communications,* Johnson & Johnson Pediatric Round Table No 8, 1983.

Wessel MA: The prenatal pediatric visit, *Pediatrics* 32:826, 1963.

8 The Pediatric Physical Examination

John H. Gundy

The examination of an infant or child by a physician or nurse practitioner can accomplish several goals simultaneously. With children, as opposed to adults, the physical examination often is the first direct contact between the examiner and the patient, the history having been obtained primarily from a parent. Therefore, one of the crucial outcomes of the examination is the relationship that will be initiated and continued between the physician and the child. The quality and quantity of care plans and the child's future attitude in medical settings will depend in part on this relationship. This chapter emphasizes approaches to examining children of different ages that will enhance the physician-child relationship.

The physician-*parent* relationship, which is initiated when the history is taken, can be enhanced further during the physical examination if the practitioner takes a relaxed, gentle approach toward the child and, no less important, performs a thorough examination appropriate to the setting and the chief complaint. Parents develop trust in physicians in a number of ways, not the least of which is the consideration the practitioner shows for the child's fears and the parents' concern about a particular symptom or sign. For each organ system discussed in this chapter, the common symptoms for which physicians are consulted are linked to a suggested level of "completeness" in performing a physical examination.

The physician must be sensitive to the potential for iatrogenic concerns initiated by his or her comments during the examination and should anticipate the child's wondering, "What's wrong with me?" and the parent's worrying, "What did I do wrong?" Reactions such as these are very common. A thorough grounding in the normal stages of growth and development of the organ systems and the body as a whole allows the examining physician to respond to such questions by emphasizing the normal physical findings, as well as by interpreting abnormal findings in the context of normal developmental patterns. The description of each organ system in this chapter begins with important stages of growth and development, particularly those steps that can be monitored by serial physical examinations. The characteristics of common physical abnormalities will be linked whenever possible to the child's age and stage of growth.

The physical examination has limited value as a screening mechanism for occult disease (see Chapter 20 [Two], The Physical Examination as a Screening Test) and has proved to be much less productive in detecting problems in schoolchildren, for instance, than is a comprehensive history. In general, the physical examination of children confirms abnormalities suggested by the history, as well as normal growth and development. When the child is examined in the presence of one or both parents, the physical examination can provide strong clues about the strength and characteristics of the parent-child relationship.

Each portion of the physical examination is discussed according to the special characteristics of each of five age groups: newborn period, infancy (1 week to 12 months), early childhood (1 through 5 years), late childhood (6 to 12 years), and adolescence (12 to 18 years).

APPROACH TO THE PATIENT

Newborn Period

At least one examination of the newborn infant should be performed in the presence of one or both parents to facilitate both evaluation of the parent-infant relationship and to address the parents' questions about their baby. A newborn infant is examined immediately after birth to assess the adequacy of pulmonary ventilation and the integrity of the cardiovascular system and the central nervous system (CNS). While assessing the need for resuscitation, the examiner should minimize exposure of the wet infant to cool ambient air by drying the infant with a towel and conducting the examination under a warming device.

Recovery from the birth process is measured by using the Apgar scale, with scores of 0, 1, or 2 given for degree of cyanosis, respiratory rate, heart rate, reflex irritability (reaction to a soft catheter introduced into the external nares), and muscle tone (Table 8-1). The infant is rated at 1 and 5 minutes after birth; total scores below 7 or 8 at 1 minute usually indicate some degree of CNS depression, and scores below 3 or 4 indicate severe depression requiring resuscitation. If the Apgar score is 8 or higher at 5 minutes and the baby's airway is clear, the rest of the body is surveyed briefly to identify gross congenital abnormalities and to estimate gestational age (see Figs. 45-8 and 45-9). After the baby is weighed, the weight-gestational age category is determined by using a standard gestational age growth chart (see Fig. 43-4), with certain risks predictable for each group (hypoglycemia and congenital anomalies in babies small for gestational age, hypoglycemia and infant of a diabetic mother in babies large for gestational age). The neuromuscular part of the gestational age determination ideally is postponed until the infant is fully stabilized (12 to 48 hours after birth).

In many hospitals a second, more thorough examination is performed within 12 hours of birth to assess the degree of recovery from the birth process and to determine the presence or absence of signs of respiratory distress and the ability to feed. This examination can serve as a safety check before transferal of the baby from the "transition" nursery to the "routine" nursery. It should take place in a warmed environment with the baby undressed to allow careful observation of the respiratory rate, the degree of respiratory effort, as evidenced by intercostal retractions, the color, and spontaneous activity. Often, quiet babies can arouse themselves with a "startle," or Moro, response that can interfere with the examination. Giving the baby something to suck on (rubber nipple, examiner's finger, or baby's fist) and holding the baby's arms against the sides will help keep the infant as relaxed as possible; performing the examination several hours after a feeding is ideal. Although it is important to assess the intensity and pitch of the cry, as many of the painless parts of the examination as possible should be performed before fully arousing the baby. Therefore, with the baby supine and after making general observations, many examiners begin by listening to the heart and lungs, then palpating the abdomen before examining the remaining systems, leaving the usually uncomfortable abduction of the hips until last.

Examination of the undressed baby with the parents present just before discharge affords the opportunity to point out normal findings, answer questions about perceived imperfections (and sometimes allow both parents a first look at their baby's entire body), discuss care of the circumcision and umbilicus, and observe the quality of the parent-infant attachment while the baby is held or fed. Holding the baby en face (the mother's face is rotated so that her eyes and those of the infant meet fully in the same vertical plane of rotation, as shown in Fig. 8-1), smiling at the baby, responding to signs of hunger or satiation, and talking about the baby positively

Table 8-1 The Apgar Score

Sign	Score 0	Score 1	Score 2
Heart rate	Absent	<100	>100
Respiratory effort	Absent	Weak, irregular	Good, crying
Muscle tone	Flaccid	Some flexion of extremities	Well flexed
Reflex irritability (catheter in nose)	No response	Grimace	Cough or sneeze
Color	Blue, pale	Body pink; extremities blue	Completely pink

From Klaus MH, Fanaroff AA: *Care of the high-risk neonate,* ed 4, Philadelphia, 1993, WB Saunders.

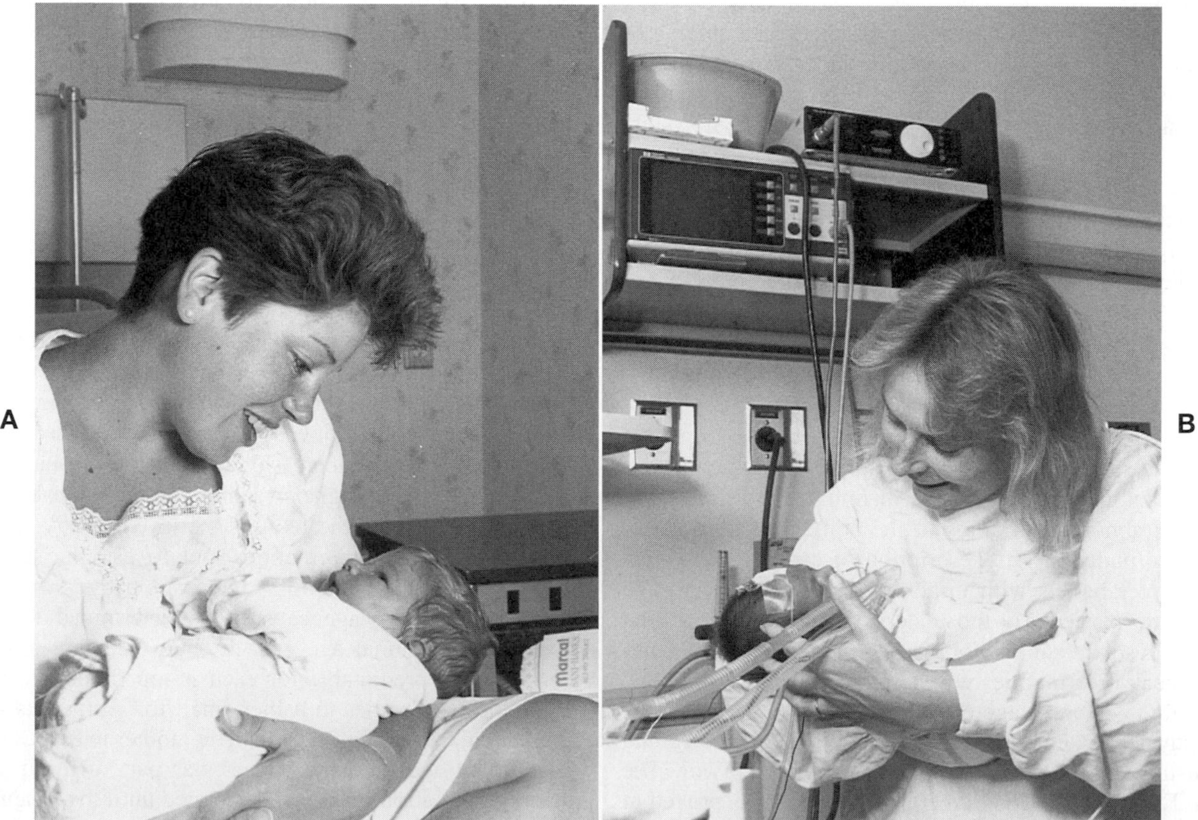

Fig. 8-1 **A,** Full-term 1-day-old infant looking "en face" eye to eye with his mother. **B,** The mother of a 2-day-old, 31-week, 1400-g premature infant on a ventilator positions herself so that she can look eye to eye with her son.

(Courtesy Ruth A. Lawrence, M.D.)

and confidently all are signs that strong parent-infant bonds are being formed and have been enhanced by the hospital experience.

Infancy

Infants between the ages of 1 and 6 months almost always are a pleasure to examine because of their responsiveness to the examiner's face and their increasing interest in environmental objects such as tongue depressors and penlights. At this age infants can be examined successfully on the examination table, with the parent usually standing close beside the table. With the infant unclothed except for the diaper, the practitioner should observe for spontaneous activity, state of alertness, and responsiveness to both the examiner and the parent. The order of the examination varies. If the infant is asleep in the parent's lap or held upright at the breast or shoulder, the heart and respiratory rates can be obtained, and the heart, lungs, and even the abdomen can be examined without waking the baby. Again, the relatively uncomfortable abducting of the hips and speculum examination of the tympanic membranes are best left until last. Prolonged or painful procedures, such as deep palpation of the abdomen or a rectal examination, are best done while the baby is being fed. The infant should be examined as if physically attached to the parent, and the parent's response, especially to painful procedures, should be noted. Sometimes the parent may appropriately thank the examiner for removing an irritable, crying baby to the examining table (or to another room if on a house call), but the physician must never be lulled into thinking that the isolated examination of the infant is a complete examination. With a chronically hospitalized baby, a continuous care nurse may substitute for an absent parent during the examination.

Infants 6 to 12 months of age are increasingly difficult to examine because of their normally developing anxiety about faces other than their parents' and the perceived separation from the parent. Offering interesting objects or allowing infants to sit and reach for objects or to walk or crawl around the office can help distract them. Direct eye contact with the strange face of the examiner can be especially frightening to the baby. Examination at these ages usually is easier if the baby is held in the parent's arms or on the parent's lap. In many clinical situations, direct observation of breast-feeding or bottle-feeding is extremely useful and can help in identifying problems such as improper feeding techniques, weak sucking movements, and dysfunctional swallowing.

Early Childhood

With children 1 to 5 years old, the most effective initial approach is to form a supportive relationship with the parent or an older sibling, who, it is hoped, will become the physician's ally in the examination of the child. This alliance is aided by identifying the parent's emotional state and anxiety level during the history and then "tuning in" nonjudgmentally. For instance, if the parent appears both anxious about the child's symptoms and guilty about having had to bother the physician, the physician might say, "I know it can be frightening to hear a baby cough like that, and I'm glad you brought him in to be examined." A parent who appears angry sometimes can be "defused" by a remark such as, "I know how aggravating it must be to have to bring your child in for so many ear infections." Tired, worn-out parents will work with a physician who is sympathetic, but they can be distracting and even disruptive if they receive nonverbal and verbal messages that they are dressed improperly, somewhat less than adequate as parents, or a general nuisance to those who practice medicine.

In most situations, children in this age group are easiest to examine while being held by the parent, a position that also is comforting to the child when the history is initiated. A few toys and books on a low table, colorful photographs and children's drawings on the walls, and the absence of a white coat on the examiner often lead children to relax and encourage them to leave the parent and explore the office. It can be helpful to offer the child a piece of examining equipment such as a stethoscope or percussion hammer to handle while the history is being taken. The examiner often can alleviate fear by showing the child the otoscope and demonstrating its use before using it on the child. Observing the child's handling of objects and interest and confidence in exploring a new environment, as well as the parent's reaction to the child's curiosity or fear, gives the examiner information important to understanding the child's developmental status and anticipating the parent's ability to cope with any problems the child may have.

In general, older children in this age group are increasingly able to communicate verbally with the examiner. A conversation that starts about the child's cat or siblings can lead to a description of what is about to be done. Continuing to describe what is being done ("I am now listening to your heart beating") can soothe even the child who starts off by screaming and kicking. With a frightened child, the parent may interpret prolonged silence on the examiner's part as disapproval or anger with the child or parent. Also, a continuing conversation with the parent and the child during the examination signals to the child that the examiner is on the parent's side, and this may increase the child's confidence that nothing too drastic will be done.

It is best to have the child remain dressed until just before the examination, some of which can be accomplished by only partly removing pieces of clothing. Even before having the parent undress the child, important general observations about the child can be made, such as the activity level, gross and fine motor coordination, receptive and expressive language function, skin color, respiratory rate, and ability to cope with a foreign environment. Some specific portions of a developmental assessment, such as throwing and catching a ball or drawing a circle, often can break the ice and help the child into a gamelike atmosphere that can be continued throughout the examination.

Again, the order of the examination should be flexible; painful procedures (ears, throat) and frightening ones (anything that requires lying down) should be postponed until last. A steady pace, coupled with gentle but firm anticipatory statements ("Now I'm going to have you lie down so I can listen to your tummy"), enhances a relatively brief encounter, which in turn keeps the parent on the practitioner's side.

It often is necessary to restrain the child, for instance, to accomplish an adequate examination of the tympanic membranes. This can be done in a number of ways, all enhanced by continuing the descriptions and discussions calmly. The parent usually is the best assistant. The child can be restrained by holding the outstretched arms against the child's head or against the child's abdomen while the examiner's body and one elbow immobilize the lower half of the child's body. The parents should be reassured that struggling is a normal response to an examination in this age group, but that it can be aggravated if the parents berate or threaten the child. The examiner's goal should be to evaluate the child's health and illness while maintaining the trust and confidence of both the child and the parent. Achieving this goal requires long hours of practice, the flexibility to ask other professionals for help when the examiner's (or the parent's) patience is about to run out, and, most important, an enjoyment of the diversity, unpredictability, and spontaneity of children.

Late Childhood

Children 6 to 12 years old usually are a pleasure to examine and rarely present any problems. A key ingredient for a successful examination is a relaxed conversation with the child about subjects such as school, hobbies, or favorite friends, interspersed with brief comments about the examination itself. Occasionally a child who had an unpleasant experience with a physician as an infant will need more time for the preparatory description of the examination. School-age children usually prefer to wear a simple drape over their underpants, and they also prefer that siblings of the opposite sex be kept out of the room, particularly when the genitalia are examined. The order of the examination can be the same as for adults (vital signs, then head to foot leaving the genitalia, perineal, and rectal [when required] until last), with care taken to anticipate any painful manipulations or procedures. As with younger children, the examiner can make the following critical observations without the actual "laying on of hands": activity level, ability to follow simple directions, ability to read passages of varying difficulty and to write, clarity of articulation, mood, level of neuromaturational functioning as tested by tasks such as hopping on one foot and rapidly alternating hand movements, and the relationship with the parent.

Adolescence

Most adolescents (12 to 18 years) prefer being examined without their parents in the room. They respect a straightforward, uncondescending approach, and parents respect the examiner who approaches adolescents as though they were adults. Decisions about who will be present *and the issue of confidentiality* should be discussed before the examination. With the parent out of the room, the examiner can review pertinent history or concerns directly with the adolescent. Most pubertal boys and girls have concerns about what is happening to their body, and a physical examination allows the examiner to explain and try to alleviate these concerns. Some special clinics for adolescents use brief, self-administered questionnaires so that the examiner can tune in to the adolescent's present concerns more quickly. While performing the examination, the examiner can reassure the pubertal child about normal developmental stages such as unilateral gynecomastia in boys, rapidly enlarging feet, the beginning of acne, and the interrelationships of the adolescent growth spurt and sexual development. The examiner's ability to approach the child's emerging sexuality factually or nonanxiously will help adolescents view themselves, at least briefly, with objectivity. Instruction in breast and testicular self-examination can help in this regard.

VITAL SIGNS AND EVALUATION OF SOMATIC GROWTH

Just as general observation of a child's behavior can give important clues about the child's general level of functioning, measuring vital signs and the characteristics of somatic growth often provides the basis for decisions about the child's overall health or illness. An abnormal vital sign or physical measurement often is the only outward indication of a problem in a child. Interpretation of vital signs and physical measurements depends on a knowledge of the normal biological changes of the growing infant, child, and adolescent. One principal characteristic of human growth is that different organ systems mature at different rates and times throughout fetal life, infancy, and childhood. Fig. 8-2 compares the longitudinal growth of the body as a whole with three component tissues: lymphoid, neural, and genital.

Temperature

Body temperature usually is measured rectally in infants and in children up to 3 or 4 years of age (because rectal temperatures have been used in clinical studies to determine the significance of temperature levels in infants and young children vis a vis management of potentially life-threatening infectious illnesses) and tympanically in older children. Oral temperatures also can be taken but are less reliable. The axillary temperature sometimes is measured, especially in infants whose bottoms are excoriated or in small premature infants. This reading generally is 2° F lower than the rectal temperature. The rectal temperature usually is measured with the infant or child held prone on the parent's lap (Fig. 8-3). The buttocks are separated, and the lubricated thermometer is inserted through the anal sphincter at an angle of about 20 degrees above the horizontal for a distance of 1½ inches. The thermometer is held in place for approximately 1 minute, either by the examiner or by the parent. Because of the relative thermal instability of newborns, especially prematurely born babies, the ambient temperature often is measured and recorded at the same time and sometimes can explain an abnormally elevated or depressed rectal temperature. Newborns' temperatures normally are higher than those of older children, averaging approximately 99.5° F (37.5° C) during the first 6 months of life. The temperature falls below 99° F (37.2° C) after age 3 and reaches 98° F (36.7° C) by age 11. A circadian rhythm of body temperature is observable by age 2 and is well developed by age 5, with increasingly higher temperatures during the daylight hours and a fall in temperature during the night (Fig. 8-4). In infants and children there often is little relationship between the degree of temperature elevation and the severity of illness. In fact, hypothermia sometimes develops in infants who have profound infection, and children can have rectal temperatures as high as 101° F (38.3° C) after vigorous activity. It is not uncommon for children admitted to the hospital for elective procedures to

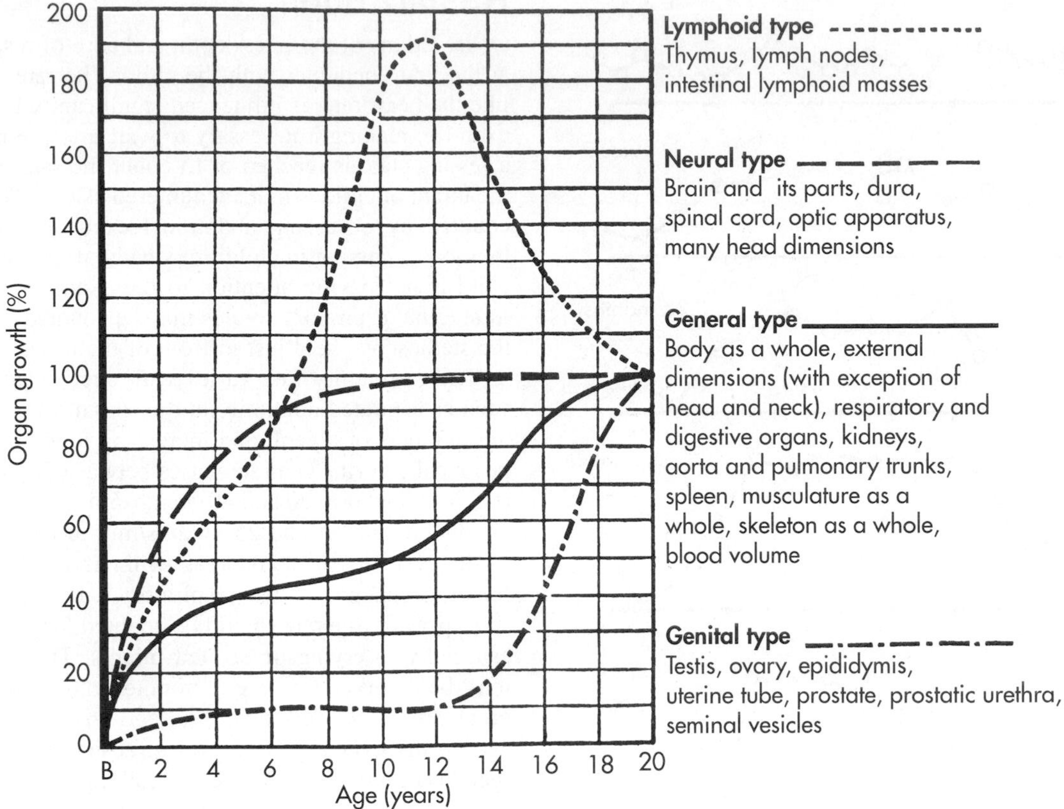

Fig. 8-2 Differential organ growth curves.
(From Harris JA, et al: *The measurement of man,* Minneapolis, 1930, University of Minnesota Press, published in Lowrey GH: *Growth and development of children,* ed 8, Chicago, 1986, Mosby.)

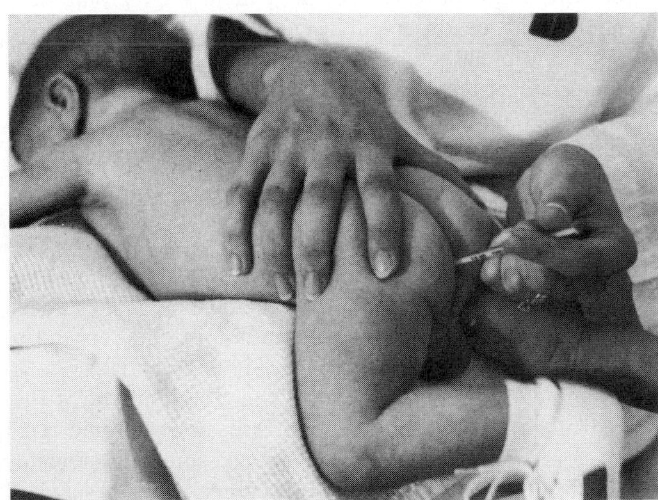

Fig. 8-3 Temperature measurement in infants.
(Photograph by P. Ruben.)

have elevated temperatures initially, probably because of transient anxiety.

Pulse

The heart rate is measured by palpating the peripheral pulse (femoral, radial, or carotid arteries), by observing the pulsating anterior fontanelle, or by palpating or auscultating the heart directly. The pulse can be increased significantly in normal infants and children by anxiety, fever, and exercise before or during the examination, as well as by inflammatory illnesses, shock, and congestive heart failure. Major changes occur in the resting heart rate with increasing age, probably reflecting increasing functional control by the vagus nerve (Table 8-2). A circadian rhythm in the heart rate is observed by age 2, with a fall of 10 to 20 beats/min during sleep; an absence of this rate slowing with sleep can be helpful in diagnosing acute rheumatic fever or thyrotoxicosis.

The examiner also should assess the rhythm of the heartbeat; equal spacing between consecutive beats is recorded as regular sinus rhythm (RSR). The cardiac rhythm more commonly is irregular than regular, especially in early and late childhood, reflecting sinus arrhythmia and increasing vagal control. Extrasystoles, appearing as irregularly spaced beats with or without a compensatory pause, are common in healthy children; usually can be abolished by exercise; and rarely occur as the only physical finding of underlying heart disease. Heart rates above 180 beats/min (especially if rigidly regular) in infants beyond the neonatal period may indicate atrial *tachycardia.* Other arrhythmias in children are rare and occur mostly in those who have underlying heart disease (e.g., congenital heart disease, rheumatic fever, and Kawasaki disease). Tachycardia with shock in infants and children usually is associated with a weak pulse and cold, sweaty extremities. Tachycardia caused by congestive heart failure usually coexists with significant tachypnea, with or without hepatic enlargement. Heart block can occur in children who have Lyme disease with myocardial involvement.

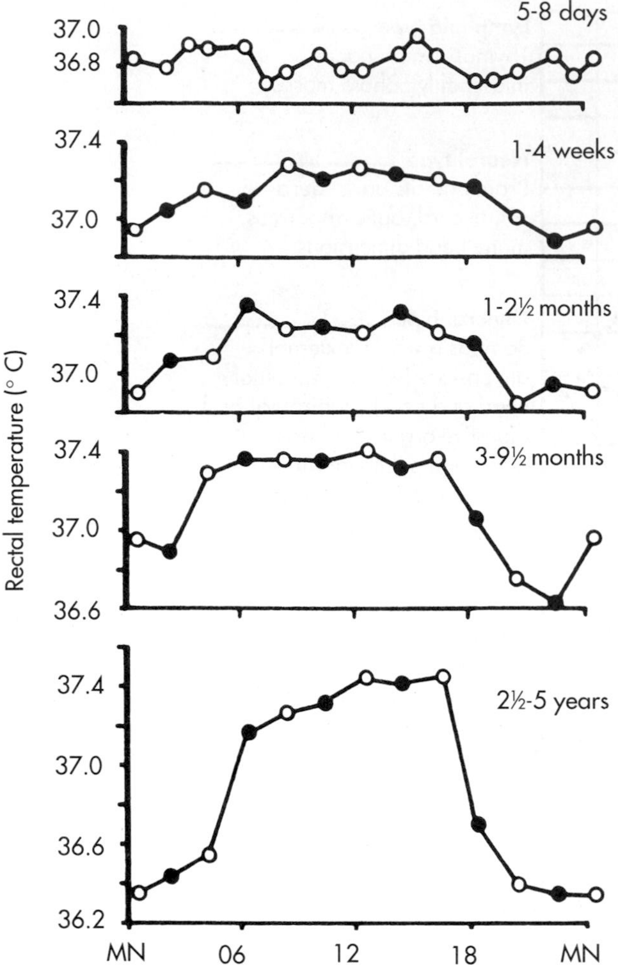

Fig. 8-4 Mean rectal temperature at different hours in groups of infants at different ages. Except in the youngest group, measurements were made every 4 hours. The hollow and solid circles represent different groups of 3 to 18 infants observed over 2 to 11 days. *MN,* Midnight.

(From Davis JA, Dobbing J: *Scientific foundations of pediatrics,* ed 2, Baltimore, 1981, University Park Press.)

Table 8-2 Average Heart Rate for Infants and Children at Rest

Age	Average Rate	Two Standard Deviations
Birth	140	50
First month	130	45
1-6 mo	130	45
6-12 mo	115	40
1-2 yr	110	40
2-4 yr	105	35
6-10 yr	95	30
10-14 yr	85	30
14-18 yr	82	25

From Lowrey GH: *Growth and development of children,* ed 8, Chicago, 1986, Mosby.

Respirations

Observations of the rate, depth, and ease of respiration begin at the first encounter with the child. The rate of respiration, like the heart rate, is influenced significantly by emotion and exercise, making it necessary to wait in some instances until a resting state is reached or to count the rate immediately if the infant or child is first encountered asleep. The rate may be counted by observing abdominal excursion in infants and thoracic excursion in children, ideally at a moment when the child is not paying attention to the examiner. In a sleeping infant, the respiratory sounds may be counted with the bell of the stethoscope held just in front of the nose.

The respiratory rate varies with age, reflecting variables such as aspirated amniotic fluid in the newborn and increasing numbers of alveoli and increasing lung compliance with postnatal growth. The rate varies between 30 and 80 breaths/min in a newborn, 20 and 40 breaths/min in infancy and early childhood, and 15 and 25 breaths/min in late childhood; the adult level of 15 to 20 breaths/min is reached by age 15. Because changes in the respiratory rate are common over short periods, the rate should be counted for at least 1 minute, especially in crying or excited infants. The respiratory rate must be observed for several minutes in newborns, especially premature babies less than 2 kg and 36 weeks of gestational age, to discover apneic episodes (absent respirations for 20 seconds or more) and periodic breathing (apneic periods lasting between 5 and 10 seconds). In early and late childhood, irregular respirations such as Cheyne-Stokes breathing are seen only in severely ill children, such as those who have overwhelming infection or severe head trauma.

Depth of respiration is determined subjectively and compared with norms observed for the patient's age group; deep breathing may be observed in states of metabolic acidosis and shallow breathing in severe obstructive states such as asthma. Ease of respiration is partly a subjective determination, as in estimating the degree of dyspnea, and is discussed in the section of this chapter on the chest and lungs.

Blood Pressure

Because of an interest in the possibility of identifying individuals who have essential hypertension before they reach adulthood, blood pressure is determined in children and in hospitalized infants more regularly. It is essential to measure the blood pressure when evaluating a child who is suspected of having congenital heart disease or chronic renal disease or who is unconscious. Blood pressure measurements in healthy ambulatory patients are compared with standard norms. The auscultatory method of determining blood pressure is useful and is practiced in children over age 5 or 6; between ages 2 and 5, some children are cooperative, but others become agitated and anxious. It is helpful to remember that the blood pressure of hospitalized children, especially those admitted for elective reasons, is higher during the first 1 or 2 days and then tends to plateau at lower levels; the blood pressure of sick, hospitalized children tends to remain constant throughout the hospitalization. Several determinations may be needed to obtain values unaffected by anxiety. Having children "watch the silver column rise" and explaining that the cuff will gently squeeze their arm usually reduces anxiety.

The size of the cuff is important because a cuff that is too small will produce falsely elevated values. The optimal cuff size is one that covers two thirds of the distance between the antecubital fossa and the acromion or between the popliteal fossa and the gluteal fold. The rubber bag inside the cuff should encircle at least 50% of the extremity. Every site where infants and children are examined should have cuffs ranging from 1 to 4 inches in width.

With the auscultation method, the point where the sounds are first heard is recorded as the systolic pressure, and the point where the sounds disappear is recorded as the diastolic pressure. When the pulse sounds cannot be auscultated, a distal artery (radial, popliteal, or dorsalis pedis) can be palpated; the point where the first pulsation is felt is about 10 mm Hg lower than the auscultated systolic pressure. The flush method can be used in infants and young children. The elevated extremity, with the uninflated cuff in place, is stroked and "milked" from the hand to the elbow. The cuff then is inflated to a point above the estimated systolic pressure, and the pressure is slowly released. A sudden flush or reddening of the extremity, compared with the color of the opposite extremity, will occur at a point approximately halfway between the systolic and diastolic pressures. Normally, the systolic pressure is higher in the lower extremities, and the diastolic pressure is the same in the arms and the legs.

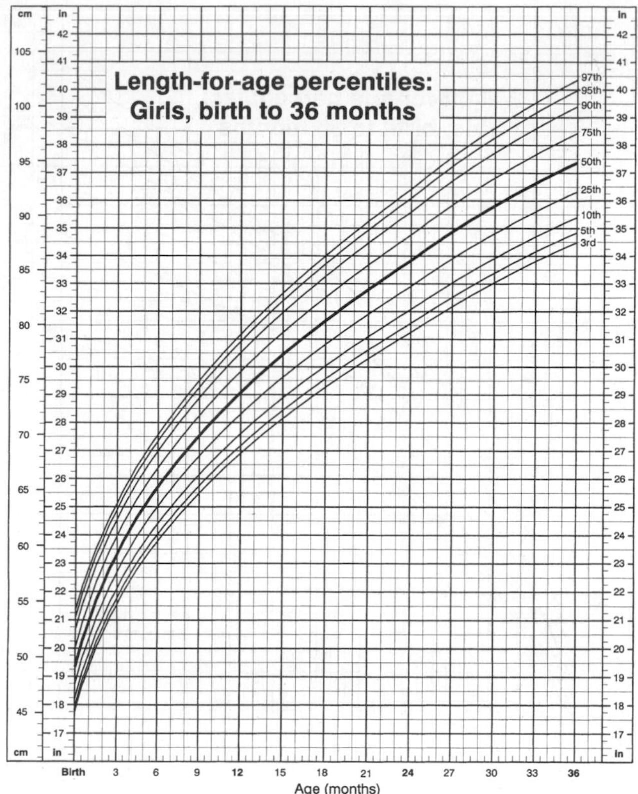

Fig. 8-5 Length-for-age percentiles, girls, birth to 36 months.

(Data from *CDC growth charts: United States,* No 314, US Department of Health and Human Services, Centers for Disease Control and Prevention, National Center for Health Statistics, Hyattsville, Md, 2000.)

Somatic Growth

Assessing somatic growth is crucial in every evaluation of an infant or a child because growth is the central characteristic of normal children and deviations from the child's norm provide an early warning of pathological processes. Several tools are available to aid in this evaluation; the most important, however, are growth charts, constructed either by longitudinal, serial measurements of a single cohort of children or by measurements of large numbers of children of different ages over a brief period. Although physical measurements of a child at a single point in time will give some useful clinical information, serial measurements over months or years provide an accurate record of the infant's or child's overall general pattern of growth, with deviations from the subject's norm indicating some intrinsic defect or environmental insult. The physical measurements used most often in assessing children are height and weight and, in infants and young children, the head circumference, as well. To be clinically useful, all these measurements should be made with care and use of a consistent technique.

Of the different growth charts currently available, the ones used most often are published by the National Center for Health Statistics. These include length for age or stature for age, weight for age, head circumference for age (to 36 months), and weight for length or weight for stature from birth to puberty. Separate charts are available for boys and girls of two age groups: birth to 36 months and 2 to 20 years (Figs. 8-5 to 8-16). The percentile lines on these charts indicate the number of normal children expected to fall above and below the index child's measurement. For instance, a 2-year-old girl whose length is 34 inches is in the 50th percentile for length; 50% of all normal 2-year-old girls will be expected to be taller, and 50% shorter.

Other growth charts indicate the mean and standard deviations from the mean by chronological age. Standard deviations (SD) are defined mathematically; for example, 1 SD above and below the mean includes about 67% of the measurements, and 2 SD above and below the mean includes about 95% of the measurements.

Velocity growth curves (Fig. 8-17) are used to measure differential rates of growth at different ages, especially among adolescents and children suspected of having endocrine disorders. These charts illustrate the two periods of rapid growth—infancy and puberty—and the differences by gender at puberty.

Height. Standing height can be measured fairly accurately in children older than age 2 or 3 years. Some growth charts, such as Stuart's, use standing height measurements beginning at age 6 years; others, such as the National Center for Health Statistics charts, plot standing heights beginning at age 2 years. Stand-up scales with attachments for measuring height generally are inaccurate. Short of buying an expensive wall-mounted apparatus (Stadiometer), accurate measurements can be made by attaching a graduated tape or ruler to a wall and placing a flat surface on top of the head to determine the height (Fig. 8-18). This measurement should be made with the child standing in stockings or bare feet, with his or her heels back and shoulders just touching the wall.

Length of infants. An infant's length is measured most accurately by using flat boards placed across and per-

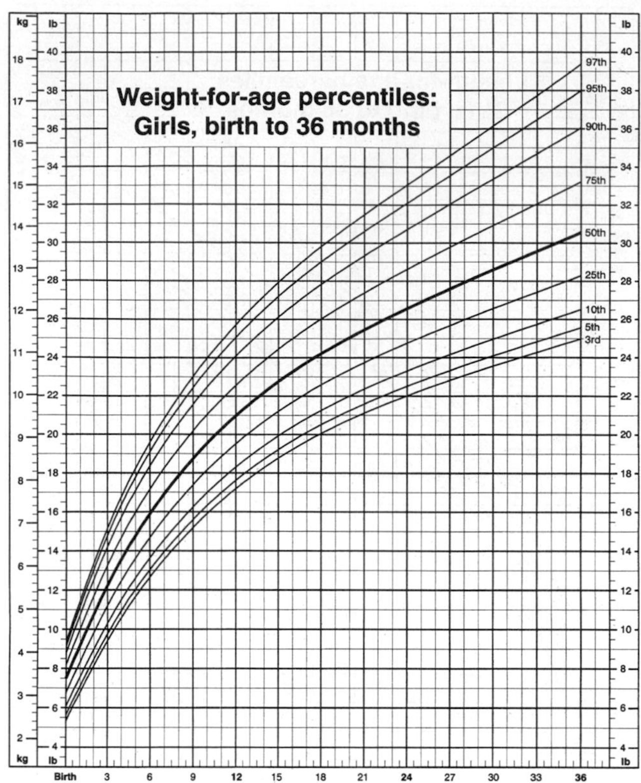

Fig. 8-6 Weight-for-age percentiles, girls, birth to 36 months.

(Data from *CDC growth charts: United States,* No 314, US Department of Health and Human Services, Centers for Disease Control and Prevention, National Center for Health Statistics, Hyattsville, Md, 2000.)

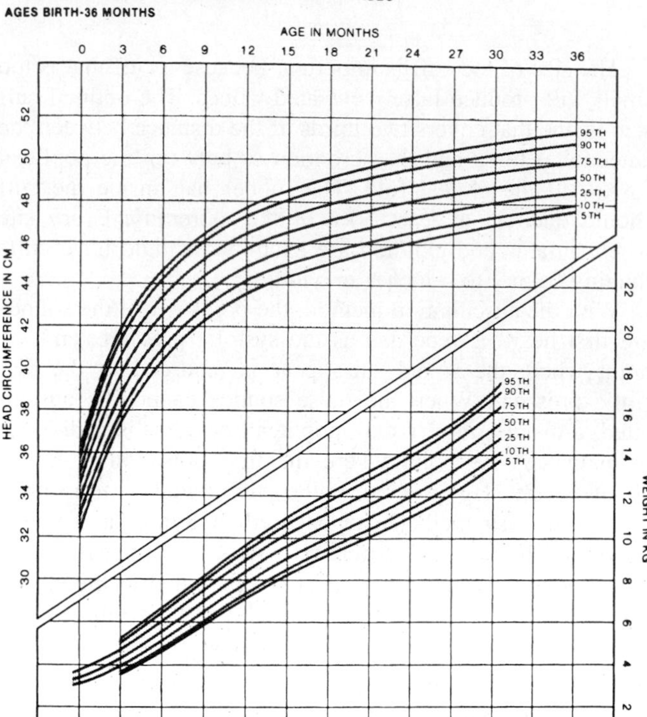

Fig. 8-7 Girls from birth to 36 months: head circumference by age and weight by length.

(Modified from Hamill VV, et al: *Am J Clin Nutr* 32:607, 1979.)

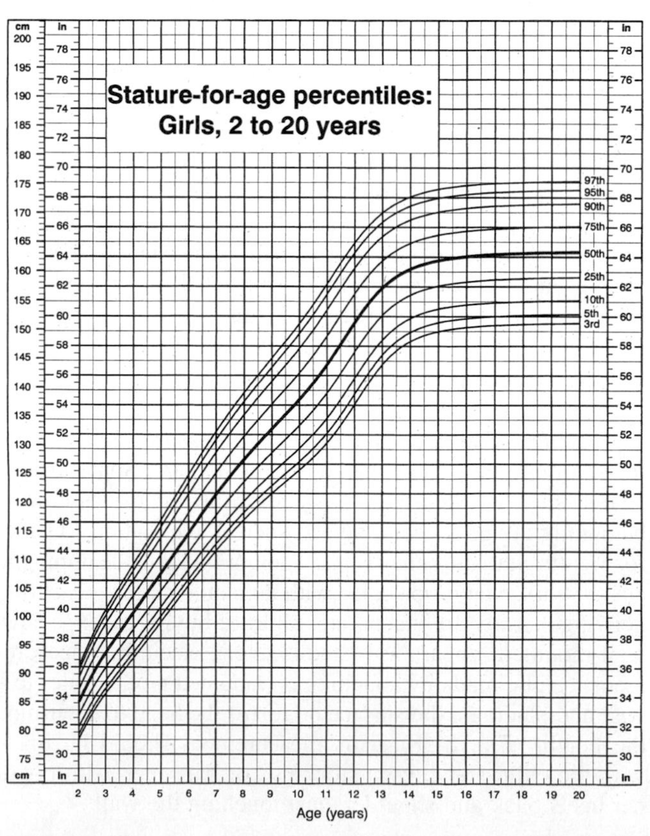

Fig. 8-8 Stature-for-age percentiles, girls, 2 to 20 years.

(Data from *CDC growth charts: United States,* No 314, US Department of Health and Human Services, Centers for Disease Control and Prevention, National Center for Health Statistics, Hyattsville, Md, 2000.)

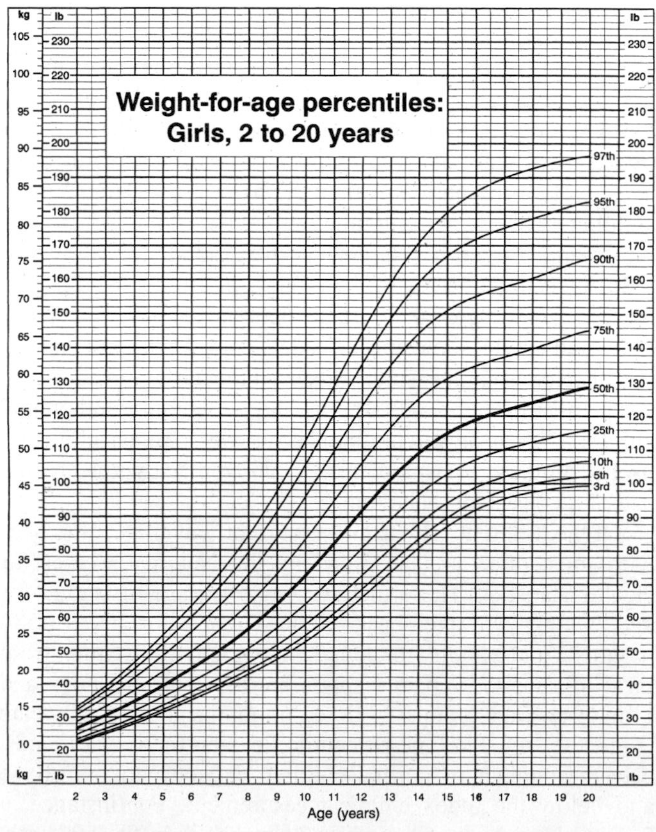

Fig. 8-9 Weight-for-age percentiles, girls, 2 to 20 years.

(Data from *CDC growth charts: United States,* No 314, US Department of Health and Human Services, Centers for Disease Control and Prevention, National Center for Health Statistics, Hyattsville, Md, 2000.)

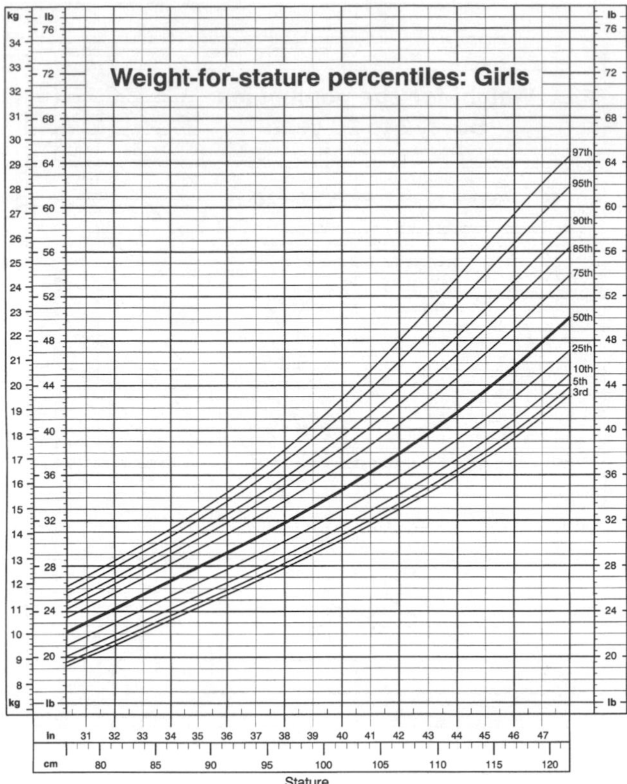

Fig. 8-10 Weight-for-stature percentiles, girls.

(Data from *CDC growth charts: United States,* No 314, US Department of Health and Human Services, Centers for Disease Control and Prevention, National Center for Health Statistics, Hyattsville, Md, 2000.)

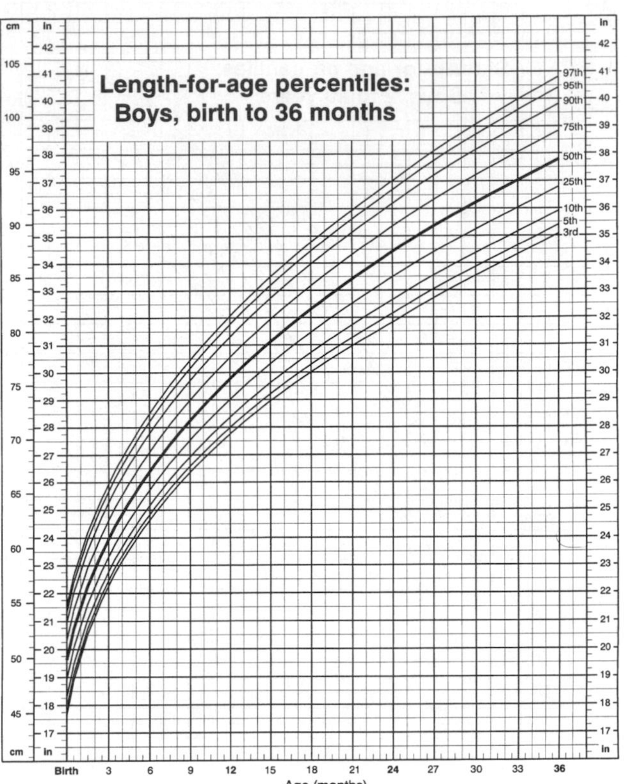

Fig. 8-11 Length-for-age percentiles, boys, birth to 36 months.

(Data from *CDC growth charts: United States,* No 314, US Department of Health and Human Services, Centers for Disease Control and Prevention, National Center for Health Statistics, Hyattsville, Md, 2000.)

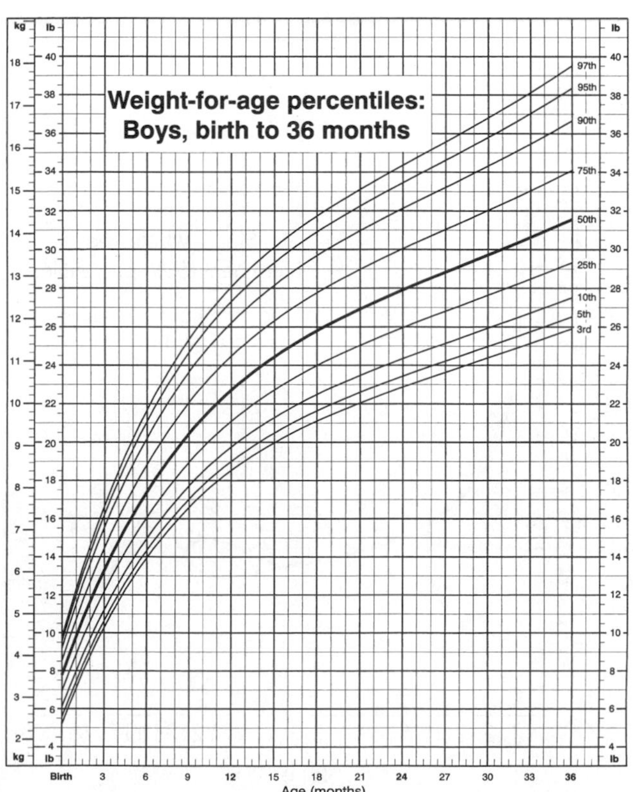

Fig. 8-12 Weight-for-age percentiles, boys, birth to 36 months.

(Data from *CDC growth charts: United States,* No 314, US Department of Health and Human Services, Centers for Disease Control and Prevention, National Center for Health Statistics, Hyattsville, Md, 2000.)

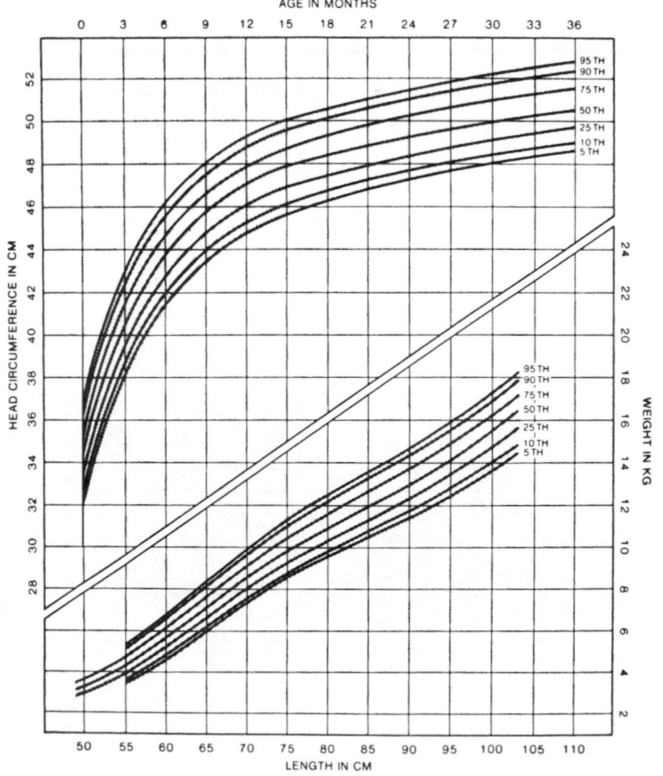

Fig. 8-13 Boys from birth to 36 months: head circumference by age and weight by length.

(Modified from Hamill VV, et al: *Am J Clin Nutr* 32:607, 1979.)

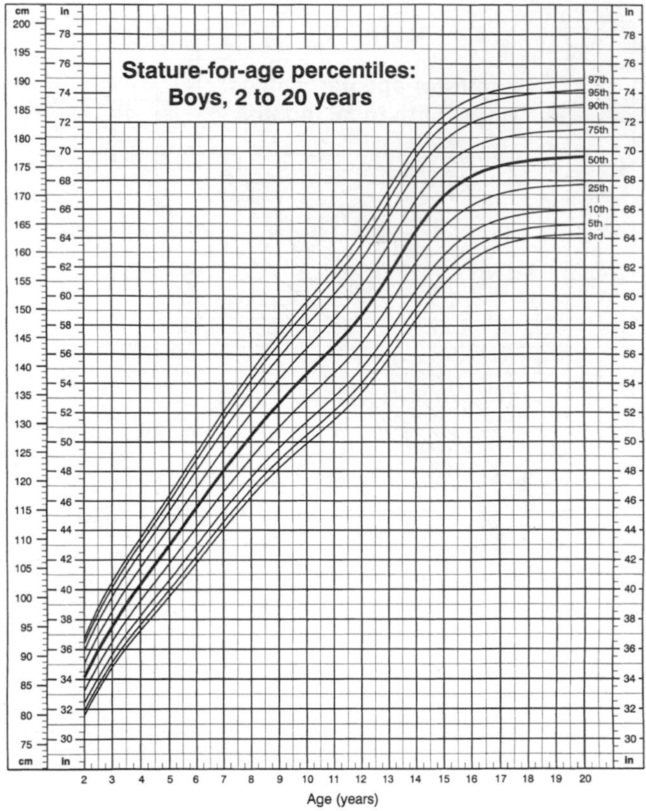

Fig. 8-14 Stature-for-age percentiles, boys, 2 to 20 years.

(Data from *CDC growth charts: United States,* No 314, US Department of Health and Human Services, Centers for Disease Control and Prevention, National Center for Health Statistics, Hyattsville, Md, 2000.)

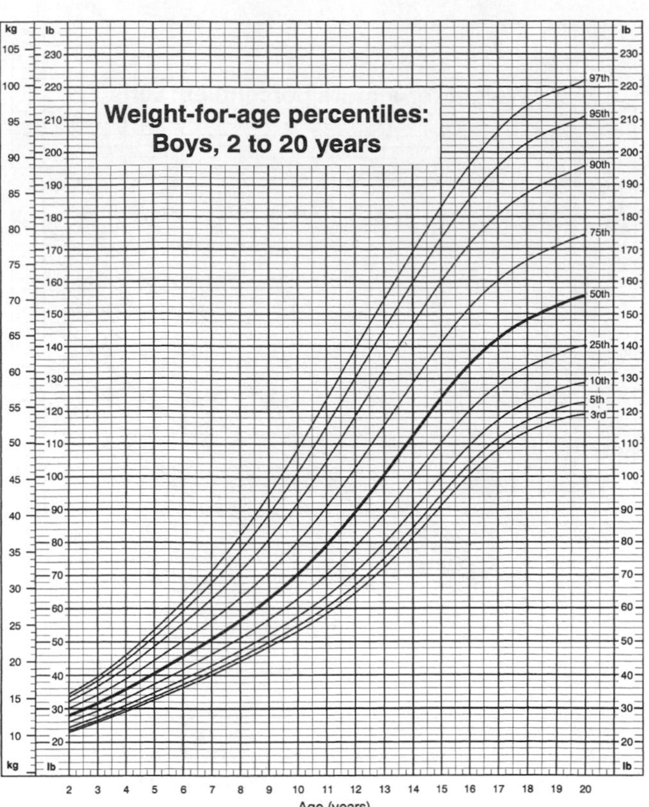

Fig. 8-15 Weight-for-age percentiles, boys, 2 to 20 years.

(Data from *CDC growth charts: United States,* No 314, US Department of Health and Human Services, Centers for Disease Control and Prevention, National Center for Health Statistics, Hyattsville, Md, 2000.)

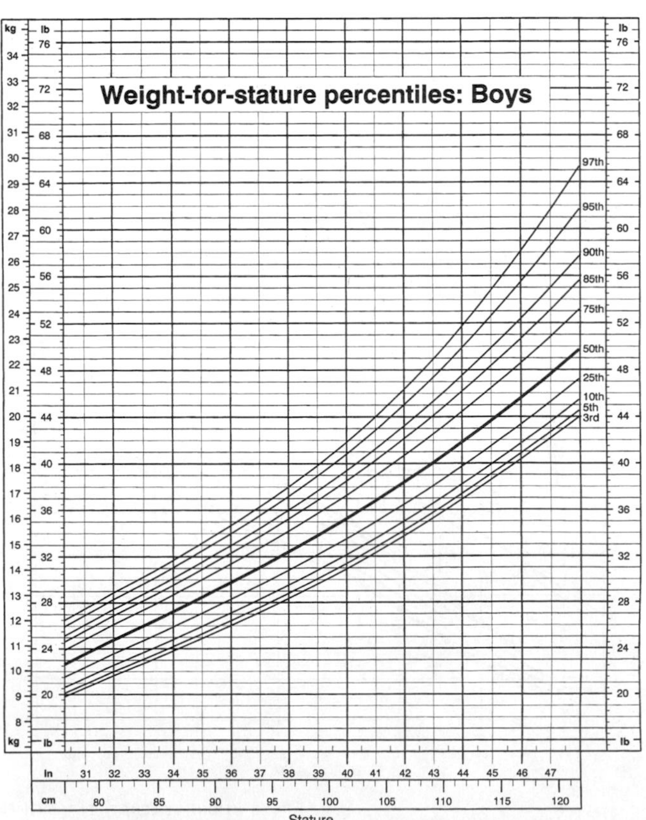

Fig. 8-16 Weight-for-stature percentiles, boys.

(Data from *CDC growth charts: United States,* No 314, US Department of Health and Human Services, Centers for Disease Control and Prevention, National Center for Health Statistics, Hyattsville, Md, 2000.)

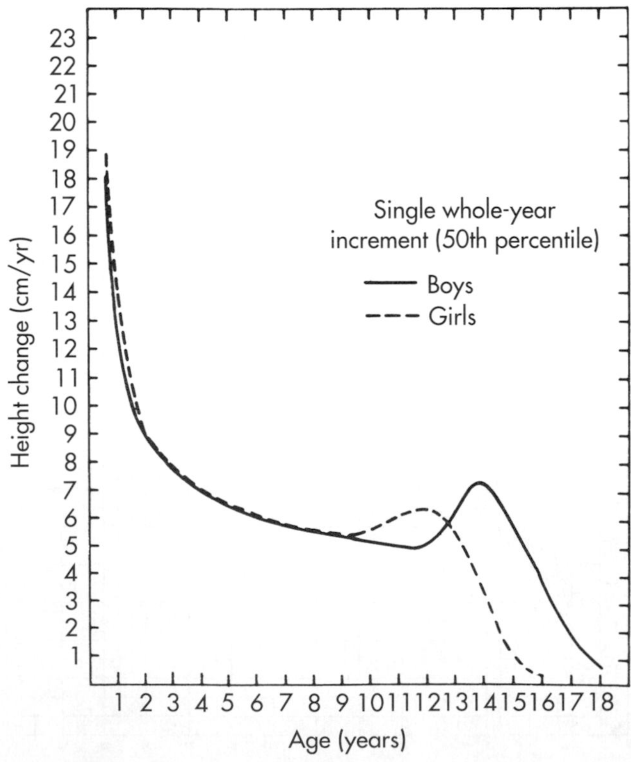

Fig. 8-17 Velocity curves for length and height for boys and girls based on intervals of 1 year.

(From Lowrey GH: *Growth and development of children,* ed 8, Chicago, 1986, Mosby.)

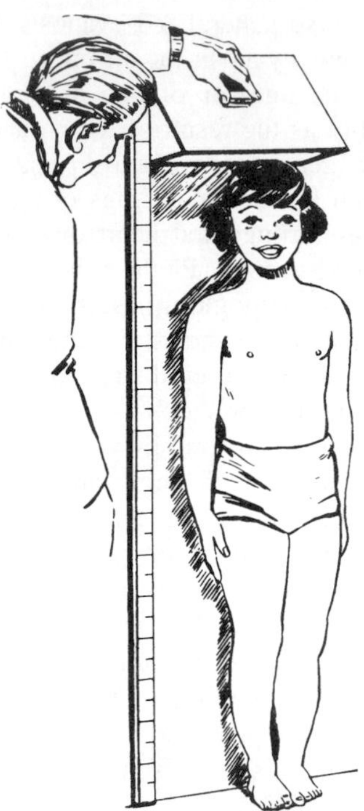

Fig. 8-18 Measurement of height.
(From *Evaluation of body size and physical growth of children,* 1976, Rockville, Md, the Maternal and Child Health Program, US Department of Health, Education, and Welfare.)

pendicular to the examining table in contact with the vertex of the head and the soles of the feet and reading the measurement from a scale attached to the surface of the table (Fig. 8-19); care must be taken, in newborns particularly, to extend the hips and knees fully.

Weight. Infants are weighed on "infant" scales, with the baby clothed only in a diaper. Children old enough to stand are weighed in their underpants on stand-up scales. Stand-up scales, because of their usually wobbly base, may be frightening to children 1 to 3 years old, and sometimes the child must be weighed by subtracting the parent's weight from the combined parent-child weight. Ideally, serial measurements are made using the same scale. In most normally growing children the height and weight measurements, when plotted on growth charts, fall within two standard percentile lines of each other (e.g., the 3rd, 10th, 25th, 50th, 75th, 90th, and 97th percentiles). Children whose measurements are either above the 97th or below the 3rd percentile require further evaluation, as do children whose height and weight differ by more than two percentile lines or categories.

Head circumference. The head circumference is measured and plotted on a standard growth chart during each health maintenance examination from birth to age 2 years, the period of maximum rate of brain growth. With children over age 2 years, head circumference measurements are obtained at the initial examination of any child and when any component of the growth curve has been abnormal.

The measurement is made by placing a cloth tape measure around the maximum occipitofrontal circumference, taking three separate readings and selecting the largest value. When

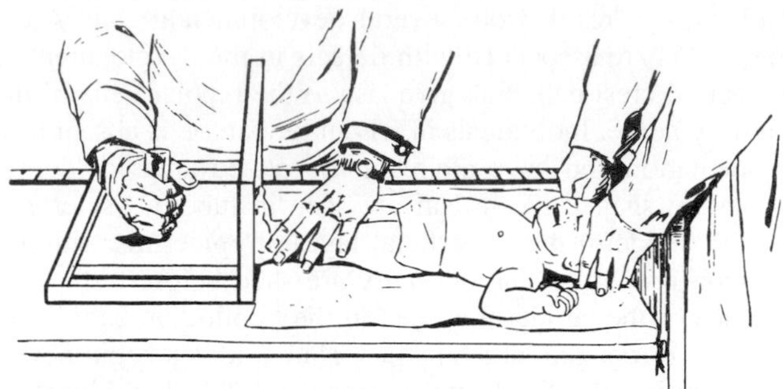

Fig. 8-19 Measurement of length in the infant.
(From *Evaluation of body size and physical growth of children,* 1976, Rockville, Md, the Maternal and Child Health Program, US Department of Health, Education, and Welfare.)

measuring the heads of infants, it usually is necessary to have the infant supine with the arms held firmly against the body by the parent or a nurse; with children, the examiner can improve cooperation by first demonstrating the use of the measuring tape on him- or herself.

Chest and other measurements. In newborns the chest circumference is compared with the head circumference, the head having a larger circumference. The chest circumference normally equals and then exceeds the head circumference during the first year of life. Chest circumference is measured at the level of the nipples midway between expiration and inspiration. Another chest measurement sometimes used in following up children who have chronic pulmonary disease is the thoracic index, obtained by dividing the anteroposterior diameter by the transverse chest diameter. This index normally decreases from 0.85 at birth to 0.74 at age 6 years because of the more rapid growth of the transverse diameter. The transverse (side-to-side) diameter and anteroposterior (sternum-to-vertebrae spinous process) diameter are measured most accurately with special calipers at the level of the nipples. Additional somatic measurements can help in the evaluation of children whose somatic growth is abnormal. The ratio of the upper half of the body to the lower half is obtained by measuring the distance from the crown to the symphysis pubis and then from the symphysis pubis to the floor (or, with an infant, to the heel) while the child is standing. This ratio changes from 1.7:1 in the newborn to 1:1 in the adult. The arm span, normally equal to the standing height, is measured from fingertip to fingertip of the third fingers with the arms outstretched. Norms for these measurements by age and by height are available in pediatric endocrinology textbooks.

ORGAN SYSTEMS

Skin

During the development of the fetus, neural crest cells, or melanoblasts, which have the potential for producing melanin, migrate from the dorsal region of the developing embryo. Under genetic control and mediated by tyrosinase, the melanoblasts produce varying amounts and shades of melanin, which make up the pigment of the skin, hair, and irides. Midline, ventral areas of defective pigmentation, such as piebaldism, can result from several developmental causes and sometimes are associated with defects in the development of the neural crest cells that give rise to the bipolar cells of the auditory nerve. Individuals in whom tyrosinase is absent lack pigmentation and have albinism. Localized areas of depigmentation shaped like a leaf are seen in tuberous sclerosis.

The periderm is a superficial layer of epidermis with absorption properties that normally are shed before birth; persistence of the periderm is seen in the "collodion baby" and in forms of congenital ichthyosis. Hair follicles begin developing during the third fetal month, and skin keratinization first occurs at their openings. Sebaceous glands, whose secretions contribute to the formation of vernix caseosa, are active starting in the latter months of pregnancy; after birth, they are relatively inactive until puberty. Apocrine glands are formed in the fetus but are not developed fully until puberty. Sweat glands, which grow most rapidly between the twenty-second and twenty-fourth fetal weeks, are inactive in the fetus. They become active in the newborn after several weeks and reach a maximal rate of activity by age 2 years. Sweat gland secretion may be under some degree of cortical control, which may explain children's tendency to sweat at all times and adults' tendency to sweat more while asleep.

Adipose tissue begins to develop during fetal life and constitutes 28% of the body weight at term. The number of fat cells increases especially rapidly during the first year of life, with adipose tissue constituting 40% to 70% of the body weight at 4 months of age. Cell numbers increase at a slower rate until puberty, when a second growth spurt occurs. In adults, adipose tissue constitutes 15% to 40% of body weight in men and 25% to 50% in women. The fat content of adipose tissue in a nonobese individual increases from 40% at birth to 80% in the adult.

Examination of the skin often yields important clues to both normal and pathological systemic processes. For instance, the characteristics of the newborn's skin reflect, in part, the length of gestation, and such observations as the opacity of the skin and the distribution of body hair can help determine the gestational age. The onset, distribution, and characteristics of some exanthems are specific for certain infectious diseases of children, and a few lesions are associated with abnormalities of other organ systems, especially the central nervous system (the phakomatoses). The skin, therefore, should be thoroughly examined in each newborn, each acutely ill or febrile child, and each child in whom congenital anomalies are suspected. A thorough examination of the skin involves noting the skin's color, consistency, and turgor; the distribution and type of lesions; and the characteristics of the sweat and sebaceous glands, the body and scalp hair, and the nails.

Newborn period. During the first minutes after birth, the newborn's Apgar score is determined partly by assessment for the presence and distribution of cyanosis. A normal, nonchilled newborn usually progresses from generalized cyanosis to generalized pinkness while normal respirations are established during the first 5 to 10 minutes of extrauterine life. Acrocyanosis, especially on exposure to a cool environment, is common in newborns for several weeks after birth, as is mottling of the skin, a latticelike pattern of pale and dark areas that appear especially on the extremities. Severe cold stress can cause generalized cyanosis. Occasionally, in newborns, transient cyanosis of an entire half of the baby (harlequin color change) or of one or more extremities is noted, presumably as the result of temporary vascular instability. Persistent generalized cyanosis usually is a sign of depression caused by maternal drugs or anesthesia, primary pulmonary disease, congenital heart disease, overwhelming infection, or hypoglycemia. Plethora in newborns may indicate high levels of hemoglobin (seen, for instance, in the twin-to-twin transfusion syndrome), and pallor in newborns may be a sign of anemia or cold stress or, less commonly, of congestive heart failure or shock.

A newborn's skin is covered by varying amounts of white, greasy, vernix caseosa, with larger amounts present in preterm babies. The newborn's skin color is determined partly by the amount of subcutaneous fat present. Premature babies have a smaller amount of subcutaneous fat and generally appear redder than full-term babies; their skin also is more transparent, and therefore subcutaneous blood vessels are more visible. Yellow staining of the vernix by meconium suggests that birth was preceded by acute fetal distress; with more prolonged fetal distress, as in the postmature baby who has placental insufficiency, the yellow (or yellow-green) staining can involve the umbilicus and nails. The skin tends to progress from being smooth to scaly, with varying amounts of desquamation and fissuring as the gestation progresses from preterm to postterm. This latter condition usually changes to normal, smooth skin without specific treatment within 1 to 2 weeks. Nonspecific edema, especially of the hands and feet, is less prominent as the gestational age approaches term. Generalized or localized petechiae, ecchymoses of the scalp or face, lacerations of the external ears, and diffuse or localized scalp edema all can be caused by physical trauma sustained during birth.

Jaundice can be expected to appear in at least 50% of normal term babies and in a higher percentage of preterm babies in the third or fourth day of life, usually indicating the presence of physiological jaundice. However, jaundice appearing at any time during the neonatal period may be an early sign of infection or of metabolic or primary hepatic disease. The early onset of jaundice also raises the question of blood group incompatibility and erythroblastosis. Clinically apparent jaundice usually indicates a serum bilirubin of at least 6 mg/dl, although the lack of subcutaneous fat in premature infants may delay its detection. Because of the variable lighting in many newborn nurseries and maternity units, clinical estimation of the bilirubin level is notoriously inaccurate, although some experienced neonatologists find that jaundice tends to progress from the head to the proximal and then distal extremities with increasing serum concentrations of bilirubin. The most consistent observations can be made by examining the skin in direct daylight. The presence of jaundice is best appreciated after pressure is applied to an area of skin over the forehead or sternum with the flat surface of a glass slide to empty the capillary bed.

The amount of melanin in the skin varies at birth. Babies of black parents may demonstrate very little as neonates. Pigmented areas over the lumbar region and buttocks, known as mongolian spots, commonly are present in black, darker-complexioned white, and Asian babies at birth. They become less prominent and eventually disappear during childhood. A number of other spots can be seen on a healthy newborn's skin, including the common telangiectasias (nevus flammeus) on the eyelids, bridge of the nose, upper lip, and nape of the neck, which usually disappear during infancy; red or purple strawberry hemangiomas or more deep-seated, cavernous hemangiomas; tiny white papules on the nose, cheeks, forehead, and occasionally the trunk caused by plugging of the sebaceous glands (milia); pinpoint vesicles with or without surrounding erythema caused by plugging of the sweat glands (miliaria); erythematous flares with central pinpoint white vesicles or papules, known as erythema toxicum, which may appear and disappear over several hours during the first week of life; and areas of either decreased or increased pigmentation, café-au-lait spots being one example, which may occur in isolation or may be associated with generalized disease, such as neurofibromatosis.

The newborn's skin often is covered with fine lanugo hair, more prominently seen in premature infants, which is lost after several weeks of life. Scalp hair at birth, which varies in amount, commonly is shed and replaced by permanent hair of a different degree of pigmentation. The fingernails may be long in postmature babies, and their color can be influenced by amniotic fluid staining and melanin pigmentation of the nail beds. Incurving of the lateral margins of the toenails is common and can be associated with local inflammation. Examination of the fingerprint and palmar crease patterns in newborns sometimes is useful because of the association of abnormal dermatoglyphics with certain chromosomal abnormalities and intrauterine infections.[4] Magnification is essential in determining the fingerprint pattern on the distal phalanges and the position of the axial triradius of the palm. A single transverse palmar crease (simian line) can occur in normal individuals but more commonly is associated with chromosomal abnormalities such as Down syndrome.

The newborn's skin should be checked carefully for defects and sinus tracts, especially over the entire length of the spine and the midline of the head from the nape of the neck to the bridge of the nose. Sinus tracts sometimes communicate with intracranial and intraspinal spaces or masses, as with dermoid cysts and encephaloceles. Preauricular sinuses may or may not communicate with a persistent brachial cleft space. A more common minor abnormality of the preauricular area is the skin tag, which usually has a cartilaginous core.

Infancy. Careful inspection of a completely undressed infant during health maintenance checks often will reveal minor abnormalities such as cradle cap and diaper dermatitis, the sometimes chronic lesions of infantile acne that first appear at 3 to 4 months of age, and less commonly, scattered ecchymoses of varying ages that can signal child abuse. Palpation of the skin, preferably over the lateral abdominal wall, allows qualitative measurement of subcutaneous adipose tissue during infancy and also observation of skin turgor (the rate of return to resting position after the skin is lifted and released), which is decreased with dehydration.

Early and late childhood. For all children, evaluation of acute or chronic rashes is helped greatly by a careful description of the rash's major characteristics (macular, papular, pustular, vesicular, petechial, ecchymotic, oozing, scaly, exfoliative, abraded, erythematous, or pigmented), location (trunk, face, extremities, or intertriginous or hairy areas), developmental history, and temporal association with other signs and symptoms. In fact, most infectious exanthems of children are diagnosed by certain constellations of these factors. Lyme disease can be diagnosed in its early stages solely by a rash (expanding, red, macular rash with or without a central mark from a tick bite) (see Chapter 227, Insect Bites and Infestations).

Adolescence. Examination of the skin of adolescents allows monitoring of important pubertal changes such as areolar pigmentation, pigmentation of the external genitalia, development of pubic and axillary hair, increased functioning of sweat and apocrine glands, and an increase in subcutaneous fat. The prominent signs of acne vulgaris on the face and trunk can be anticipated in many adolescents.

Head and Face

The rapid rate of brain growth during infancy and childhood explains the increased size of the head relative to body length in newborns and infants compared with that of adults. The facial contours and dimensions change considerably during the first 10 years of life, reflecting the downward and forward growth of the mandible and vertical growth of the maxilla and nasal bones. These changing proportions are best summarized by the proportion of cranium to face volumes at different ages: 8 : 1 at birth, 5 : 1 at age 2, and 2 : 1 by age 18. A thorough examination of the head includes measuring the head circumference and plotting the value on a standard growth chart, observing the shape and symmetry, and palpating the sutures and fontanelles; occasionally, percussion, auscultation, and transillumination are needed. The head should be examined thoroughly in clinical situations involving growth or developmental failure, suspected trauma, a seizure disorder, or fever in an infant and as part of every health maintenance examination from birth to age 2 years.

Newborn period. The newborn's skull is composed of partly calcified, bony plates that interface with each other at predictably located suture lines. The major sutures palpable at birth are the coronal, lambdoid, sagittal, and metopic sutures (Fig. 8-20). Because of overriding of one cranial bone on another after molding of the skull during the descent through the birth canal, the newborn's sutures often feel like ridges. The anterior fontanelle is located at the junction of the sagittal and coronal sutures and varies considerably in size in normal infants; it usually measures about 1 inch at its greatest diameter and is diamond shaped. The posterior fontanelle, found at the junction of the sagittal and lambdoid sutures, only occasionally is palpable at birth. Vascular pulsations, transmitted by the cerebrospinal fluid (CSF), normally can be seen over the anterior fontanelle. With normal CSF pressure and with the infant in an upright position and not crying, the anterior fontanelle is soft and flat on palpation. A bulging fontanelle is a sign of increased intracranial pressure; a depressed fontanelle is a sign of decreased intravascular volume, as in dehydration.

At birth it is common to palpate localized edema over one or more areas of the head. A palpable swelling, particularly

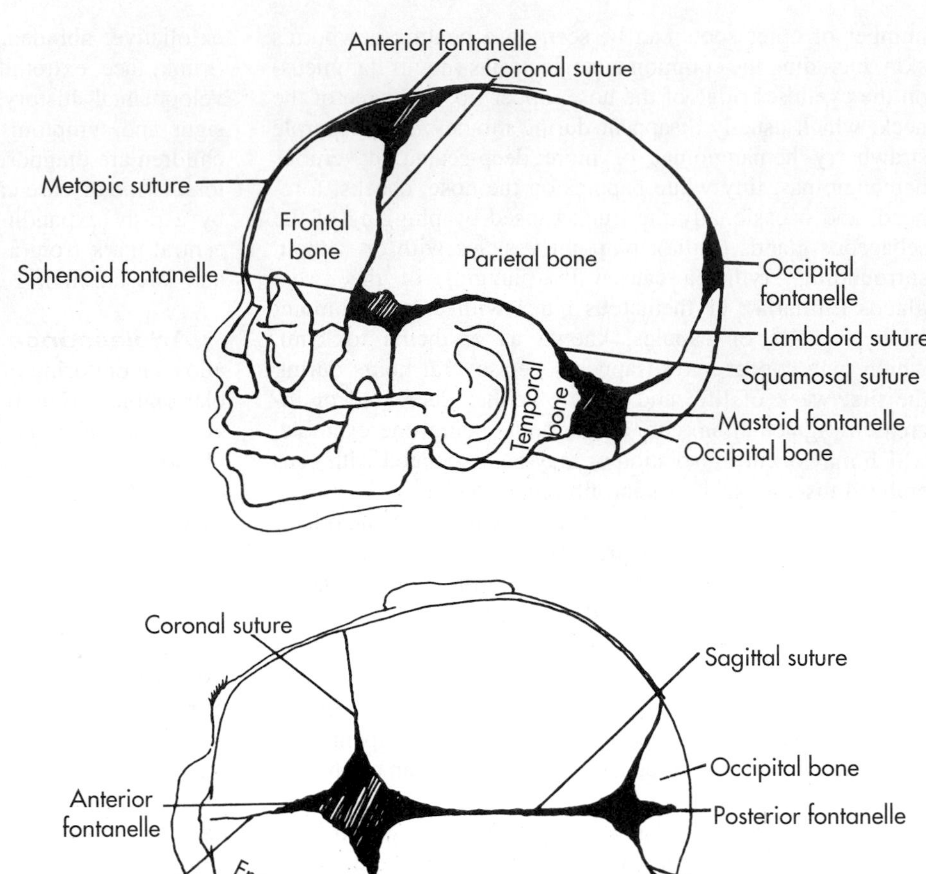

Fig. 8-20 Two views of the neonatal skull, showing clinically important fontanelles and sutures.

(From Scanlon JW, et al: *A system of newborn physical examination,* Baltimore, 1979, University Park Press.)

over the vertex, that recedes after 1 or 2 days represents subcutaneous edema and is called *caput succedaneum.* Swollen areas whose margins are limited to suture lines and that often require weeks to recede represent subperiosteal hemorrhage and are called *cephalhematomas.* These resolve partly by calcification, which initially may feel like a mass with a heaped-up bony rim and a soft center. Other commonly seen effects of the birth process include linear or curved abraded or lacerated areas, especially over the zygomatic arches and preauricular areas, resulting from use of obstetrical forceps. The infant's face may be asymmetrical at birth because of intrauterine positioning with the chin touching one shoulder. Facial palsy, manifested by a drooping corner of the mouth during crying, usually is caused by obstetrical forceps exerting pressure over the facial nerve in the preauricular area.

The cranial bones normally become firmer on palpation with increasing gestational age. One exception occurs when the sutural edges of the cranial bones are pliable and "springy," a condition known as *craniotabes,* which is found in many normal infants and in rare cases is a sign of rickets. A disproportionately large head at birth may indicate hydrocephalus or intrauterine growth retardation (IUGR) in which overall brain growth often is relatively normal.

Transillumination of the newborn and infant head is useful in evaluating asymmetrical or disproportionately large heads, as well as unexplained neurological signs and symptoms. The procedure is accomplished in a completely darkened room by use of a bright light source, such as a three-battery flashlight or a special high-intensity light. If a flashlight is used, it should be fitted with a soft foam rubber collar and held against the head tangentially in such a way as to allow uniform intensity of illumination of the head around the full circumference of the light. Localized bright spots may indicate acquired problems, such as subdural effusions, or congenital defects, such as porencephalic cysts. The entire head will "light up" in the presence of hydranencephaly.

Infancy, childhood, and adolescence. By measuring and plotting serial occipitofrontal head circumferences, the examiner can monitor the normal growth of the brain within the normally yielding cranial bones, which are separated from each other by suture lines that remain open until brain growth is complete. A head circumference that is increasing at an abnormally slow rate may indicate either a slowly growing brain (intrinsic or acquired defect) or cranial sutures that have closed too soon (craniosynostosis). The normally proportioned small head is called *microcephaly,* and a small head associated with premature suture closure is labeled according to the shape distortion caused by the suture involved—scaphocephaly (closure of the sagittal suture, resulting in restricted lateral growth of the head so that it is abnormally long and narrow), plagiocephaly (closure of coronal or lambdoidal suture, resulting in a lopsided appearance to the head so that its maximum length is on a diagonal, rather than along the midline), and acrocephaly (closure of the coronal and sagittal sutures, resulting in an upward growth of the head so that it has a pointed, or conical, shape).

Craniosynostosis, a diagnosis that requires confirmation by roentgenography, often is associated with prominence or ridging of the involved suture line. A head that is growing too rapidly when compared with the rate of height and weight gain always should be evaluated for hydrocephalus and subdural effusions. Sometimes the head is just asymmetrical, with a normally increasing head circumference; this suggests either intrauterine or extrauterine positional effects, such as the flat occiput seen in babies who are left to lie on their backs for long periods and the flattening of one occipital bone and the opposite frontal bone sometimes associated with torticollis (cranioscoliosis). Prominent frontal bone bossing, with or without associated saddle-nose deformity, may be a sign of the developing osteomyelitis associated with congenital syphilis. The anterior fontanelle normally is not palpable after 18 months of age and may disappear as early as 3 months of age.

Percussion of the head by directly tapping with the middle finger normally elicits a flat sound. A "cracked pot" sound may be heard in infants whose fontanelle is open or in infants who have increased intracranial pressure whose fontanelle is closed, as is seen with hydrocephalus. Auscultation of the head for localized bruits, indicating vascular anomalies, is included in the evaluation of children who have seizures or other neurological abnormalities. Up to age 5 years, however, systolic or continuous bruits may be heard over the temporal areas in normal children.

Examination of the face begins with an overall impression, which occasionally yields important diagnostic clues, such as the dull, immobile face associated with hypothyroidism; the open-mouthed expression of the child who has chronic nasopharyngeal obstruction caused by hypertrophied adenoids; the multiply bruised face of the battered child; and the small nose, open mouth, and prominent epicanthal skinfolds of the child who has Down syndrome. Facial puffiness, or edema, especially involving the eyelids, can be an early sign of fluid retention secondary to acute or chronic renal disease or congestive heart failure. The distance between the eyes, usually measured as the interpupillary distance, can be increased as well as decreased in a number of syndromes of chromosomal origin and with other developmental anomalies.

The Chvostek sign, elicited by tapping the cheek just under the zygoma and causing unilateral facial grimacing, sometimes is a sign of hypocalcemia or hyperventilation tetany in older children; it also can be present in normal infants and young children.

Parotid gland swelling often is difficult to distinguish from cervical adenitis. The swollen parotid gland lies mainly anterior to the angle of the mandible and often pushes the ear pinna away from the side of the head, which can be seen when the patient is viewed from behind. Swelling and tenderness below a line drawn from the angle of the mandible to the mastoid process is caused by cervical adenitis. Nonobstructive parotitis usually is viral: when acute, it usually is caused by the mumps virus but can be bacterial; when recurrent or chronic, human immunodeficiency virus (HIV) should be considered (see Chapter 219, Human Immunodeficiency Virus Infection and Acquired Human Immunodeficiency Syndrome).

Eyes

Studies of the process of mother-infant bonding during the neonatal period highlight the functional importance of an intact visual system in babies from the first minutes after birth.[4,5] Although examination of the eye is important in picking up clues to congenital and acquired systemic abnormalities, the overriding goal of examining the eyes of infants and children is to ascertain that normal functioning is taking place and that potentially remediable processes affecting visual acuity are detected early.

At birth the eye is almost full grown compared with the other organs and the body. By this time the retina is completely developed except for the central foveal region, which is fully developed by 4 months of age, as is myelination of the central optic radiations and differentiation of the optic cortex. The cornea increases in diameter from 10 mm at birth to the final adult size of 11.5 mm. The lens doubles in weight between birth and age 20 and then increases another 50% by age 80. The pupillary reflex to light is functioning by 29 to 31 weeks of gestation. At birth the globe tends to be short in relation to the focusing ability of the lens and cornea (hypermetropia), and up to age 12 to 14 years the globe gradually lengthens, with a resulting tendency for visual images to be focused in front of the retina (myopia).[8] At birth, babies can respond to faces, as well as to colored and black and white objects. The fixed focal length of the newborn's eyes (20 cm), along with the aforementioned factors and distracting influences (startle reflex, hunger, temperature changes), limit the newborn's ability to respond visually for more than brief moments.

The ability to accommodate is present by 4 months of age, and the ability to follow a moving light through different planes at various angles from the face is developed fully by 6 months of age.

Examination of the eye is an important part of every examination of an infant or child. The completeness of the examination may vary according to the reason for the visit (health maintenance versus emergency head trauma) and the chief complaint (headaches versus a sprained knee). A thorough examination of the eye includes observation of the lids, including eyelashes, tear ducts, and glands; the conjunctiva; the sclera and cornea; the pupils, including reaction to light and accommodation; and the lens. Globe size and intraocular pressure should be estimated, and the extraocular movements should be tested to note any presence of nystagmus or strabismus. Examination of the fundus includes assessment of the optic disk, macula, retina, and central vessels; this should be done in every child who is examined because of headache, head trauma, or other suspected intracranial lesion. Assessment of visual acuity should be part of every health maintenance examination.

Newborn period. Several attempts may be required to examine a newborn's eyes completely because of transient edema of the eyelids caused by the birth process or by the conjunctivitis induced by antibiotic instillation soon after birth to prevent gonococcal and other bacterial conjunctivitis. The upper eyelid may have a midline notch from incomplete fusion of its embryonic medial and lateral portions. The eyelids normally are fused until the eighth month of gestation. The lids often are slippery with vernix caseosa and conjunctival exudate, which should be removed gently with a dry cloth, allowing separation of the lids with a finger placed on each lid. Occasionally, one or both eyelids will be everted after birth. Episcleral and subconjunctival hemorrhages, either focal or diffuse, commonly are present after birth and can be expected to recede spontaneously. Less commonly, hyphema (blood in the anterior chamber) may be present. Cloudiness of the cornea can be caused by congenital glaucoma and requires ophthalmological consultation. Opaque particles or strands in the lens may be cataracts or remnants of the artery that supplies the lens in its early stages of development (hyaloid artery). This iris often is less pigmented at birth; its final color develops during the first year of life. Although a ring of white specks around the periphery of the iris (Brushfield spots) is present in some normal infants, it is more prominent and common in children who have Down syndrome. Defects in the iris, particularly in the ventral aspect, can be associated with parallel defects in the lens and retina (colobomas) and represent incomplete closure of the embryonic optic fissure.

Careful examination of the newborn's retina is difficult without the use of mydriatics. The appearance of a "red reflex," seen when the ophthalmoscope is held 10 to 12 inches in front of the eye, ascertains that no major obstructions to light and its reflection from the retina are present between the cornea and the retina, such as corneal opacities, cataracts, and retinal tumors. Funduscopic examination of the newborn is indicated in babies in whom the red reflex is absent (leukocoria), in babies who have been given prolonged supplemental oxygen, and in babies in whom CNS trauma or septicemia is suspected. In some newborn nurseries every newborn is given a funduscopic examination. With the ophthalmoscope, the cornea usually can be seen at +20 diopters, the lens at +15 diopters, and the fundus at 0 diopters. The fundus is examined 30 minutes after instillation of a drop of 2.5% phenylephrine (Neo-Synephrine) ophthalmic solution in each eye, optimally with the assistance of another person who can offer the baby a sugar nipple. The physician notes the size and color of the optic disk and macula and any areas of hemorrhage or increased or decreased pigmentation of the retina. In newborns and infants, the optic disk is paler than in older children, the peripheral retina vessels are not well developed, and the foveal light reflection is absent. Papilledema rarely occurs before age 3 because of the ability of the fontanelles and open sutures to absorb increases in intracranial pressure.

Perhaps the most productive method for observing both the structure and function of the newborn's eyes is for the examiner to hold the infant upright, in which position the infant often opens his or her eyes spontaneously. Abnormalities in the size of the eyes should be noted, inasmuch as microphthalmia is a part of several rare congenital defect syndromes. Narrowing of the space between the lids may be an isolated condition, blepharophimosis, or part of Komoto syndrome, which also includes ptosis, epicanthus inversus, and telecanthus; unilateral eyelid droop associated with a constricted pupil indicates Horner's syndrome. Any upward or downward slanting of the axis of the eyelids (palpebral fissures) also should be noted; upward slanting is characteristic of children who have Down syndrome. Although inner epicanthal folds can occur in normal infants, they are common in children who have Down syndrome and in those with other chromosomal abnormalities. The setting-sun sign (a portion of the white sclera is seen between the upper lid margin and the iris) occurs in some normal premature and full-term infants, but persistence suggests the possibility of hydrocephalus.

When the baby is held at arm's length and turned slowly in one direction (Fig. 8-21), the eyes turn toward that direction. When rotation stops, the eyes turn toward the opposite direction after a few quick, unsustained, nystagmoid movements. More sustained nystagmus with this maneuver or at rest may indicate blindness or other CNS problems. When just the head is moved slowly through its full range of motion, the eyes do not move but remain in their original position (doll's eye reflex). This maneuver can demonstrate paresis of the lateral rectus muscle. Strabismus (the condition in which the visual axes of both eyes in fixing a distal point are not parallel) commonly is seen as an intermittent phenomenon in normal newborns and may persist up to 6 months of age (see Chapter 171, Strabismus). The infant should be examined carefully for inward deviation of the eye, or esotropia, and outward deviation, or exotropia—whether alternating, fixed, or transient. Prominent epicanthal folds sometimes can give the erroneous impression of strabismus (pseudostrabismus). Any fixed divergence of the eyes and any transient outward divergence in the newborn require immediate neurological and ophthalmological consultation.

Visual acuity in the newborn is assessed indirectly by means of visual reflexes such as consensual pupillary constriction in response to a bright light; blinking in response to a bright light and to an object moved quickly toward the eyes; and opticokinetic nystagmus, which the normal infant demonstrates when a cylinder that has alternating vertical black and white lines is rotated at specified distances from the eyes.

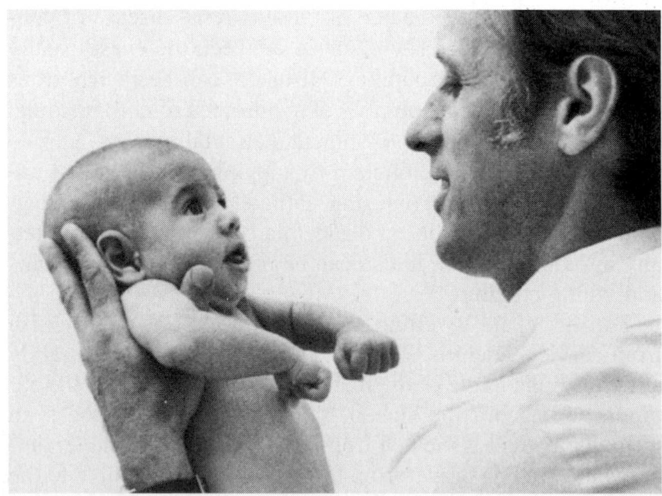

Fig. 8-21 Vestibular function testing in the infant. (Photograph by P. Ruben.)

Infancy. In addition to the findings on the examination described for the newborn, a few common problems particularly affect young infants. Tears often are not present at birth but are produced by 4 months of age. The nasolacrimal duct, however, sometimes is not patent until 1 year of age, leading to a chronically tearing eye with or without purulent discharge. Pressure over the nasolacrimal sac on the medial edge of the lower eyelid will confirm the diagnosis of nasolacrimal duct obstruction by yielding mucoid or purulent fluid. Usually there is minimal or no conjunctival inflammation, and ophthalmological consultation is not indicated unless the tearing and discharge persist beyond 12 months of age.

Although acute conjunctival inflammation with purulent exudate sometimes occurs in neonates in reaction to the routine instillation of antibiotic drops, another cause that must be considered is infection by *Neisseria gonorrhoeae, Staphylococcus aureus,* or *Chlamydia trachomatis. C. trachomatis* can be diagnosed by the presence of cytoplasmic material in the epithelial cells of conjunctival scrapings. An acutely red, tearing eye in infants often is caused by corneal abrasions inflicted by the infant's own fingernails; this diagnosis can be confirmed by placing a damp fluorescein strip in the corner of the eye and observing the green staining of the abraded corneal epithelium.

Unilateral or bilateral ptosis of the lids may be appreciated better after the immediate postbirth period; it may be a familial trait, part of a syndrome of congenital anomalies, or the result of oculomotor nerve palsy. Unilateral exophthalmos, or protrusion of the eye, can result from a retroorbital tumor or abscess.

Childhood and adolescence. After the neonatal period and up to 3 to 5 years of age, visual acuity continues to be determined by the observations of the parents and the examiner. By 4 weeks of age, the infant can fixate on an object; by 6 weeks, coordinated movements in following an object are seen. By 3 months, the infant can follow an object moving across his or her midline, and convergence of the eyes is present. Beginning at 4 to 5 months the infant can reach for and grasp objects. Increasing recognition of familiar objects and faces by 5 to 6 months of age confirms normally developing cortical and visual systems. Between 1 and 3 years of age the infant responds to and uses brightly colored toys and children's books and can circumnavigate the examiner's office. Standardized tests of visual acuity for children under age 3 years have been developed. These tests require the child to "match" a toy or ball with small "test" objects that the examiner holds. These tests, which are not widely known or used, may offer the child health worker a useful screening tool.

Infants and children who fail to perform according to the tests outlined here should be examined further for blindness or mental retardation. Besides instances of blindness that are genetically determined or caused by perinatal insults, amblyopia (or reduced visual acuity) results from suppression of one or two unequal images in the visual cortex. Its importance is that it can be reversed only if diagnosed early enough (by age 6 years at the latest) to allow treatment of the underlying cause. There are two major categories of causes of amblyopia: obstructive amblyopia secondary to a cataract, corneal opacity, or severe ptosis and amblyopia ex anopsia secondary to uniocular squint (strabismus) or refractive (anisometropia) error. Strabismus is detected by using the corneal light reflection (Hirschberg) test and the cover-uncover test. The symmetry of the corneal light reflections is observed while the child focuses on a penlight 12 inches from the eyes; asymmetry indicates esotropia or exotropia. In the cover-uncover test, with the child focusing on the penlight, the visual axis of one eye is interrupted by the examiner's hand; any movement of the uncovered eye indicates strabismus. Similarly, when the examiner's hand is removed, the original uncovered eye moves back to its original position.

Loss of visual acuity in one eye detected during a screening evaluation often is the first indication of amblyopia. Vision is screened by using the Snellen illiterate E chart for children between the ages of 3 and 5 years and the Snellen E chart for children 5 years of age and older (see Chapter 20 [Eleven], Vision Screening).

The most common abnormalities of children's eyes seen in an ambulatory setting are swelling and redness of the eyelids and a red, tearing eye. Swelling and redness of the eyelids occur with obstruction of the nasolacrimal duct, blepharitis, hordeolum, and chalazion. Edema, tenderness, and warmth of the eyelid, usually indicative of periorbital cellulitis, can be caused by infection resulting from local trauma or insect bites, or they can be associated with upper respiratory tract infections and otitis media. Orbital cellulitis is characterized by marked lid edema, proptosis, chemosis, reduced vision, and decreased motility with pain on movement of the globe (see Chapter 254, Preseptal and Orbital Cellulitis). A red, tearing eye can be caused by acute conjunctivitis, subconjunctival hemorrhage, keratitis, acute iridocyclitis, and acute glaucoma. Conjunctivitis characterized by prominence of the conjunctival blood vessels is one of the signs of Kawasaki disease. Evaluation of children who have sustained head trauma or who are suspected of having an overwhelming infection requires careful, repeated testing of the extraocular movements in the six cardinal fields of gaze and of the pupillary light reflex and observation of the conjunctivae and fundi, looking for unilateral abnormalities, hemorrhage, and papilledema. For example, lateral rectus muscle palsy often is the earliest sign of increased intracranial pressure (see Chapter 290, Increased Intracranial Pressure). Retinal hemorrhages can be seen in infants who have the shaken baby syndrome.

Ears

The inner ear develops early in the first trimester of pregnancy, and response to sound can be shown in the twenty-sixth fetal week. At birth the cochlea and vestibule are anatomically mature.

Successful examination of the ears in infants and children, a skill that requires years of practice to develop, is extremely important because of the high incidence of middle ear abnormalities in children. The student should approach the use of the otoscope and the almost universal presence of ceruminous impediments to visualization of the external auditory canal in children with patience and a willingness to ask for confirmation of findings as often as needed. The practitioner should include a thorough examination of the ears in every physical examination, noting the characteristics of the external ear, external canal, and tympanic membrane and assessing hearing acuity.

Newborn period. The external ear is flat and shapeless until 34 weeks of gestation; once folded, it may remain so unless placed back in the flat position. Between 34 and 40 weeks of gestation, an incurving of the periphery of the pinna develops, along with an increasing ability to return spontaneously from the folded to the flat position. Minor anomalies in the shape of the external ear should be noted, including the occasional preauricular skin tags or preauricular sinuses. The position of the upper attachment of the external ears should be noted in relation to a line connecting the inner and outer canthus of the eye. Attachments that fall below this line sometimes are associated with other congenital abnormalities, including renal agenesis. Patency of the external auditory canals can be determined by direct observation after pulling the pinna away from the side of the head. The tympanic membrane is coated with vernix caseosa for several days after birth and usually cannot be visualized.

Auditory screening in neonates begins with identifying those at risk for hearing loss because of a familial hearing disorder; intrauterine viral infection; hyperbilirubinemia, with bilirubin levels above 20 mg/dl; previous treatment with an ototoxic drug (e.g., gentamycin); or defects of the ear, nose, or throat. Neonates with any of these factors should be screened for hearing loss. In some states, all newborns are screened routinely for hearing acuity. Their subsequent language development should be monitored closely, and they should be referred to an audiologist for any signs suggesting hearing loss (see Chapter 20 [Nine] Language and Speech Assessment and Chapter 20 [Ten] Auditory Screening).

Infancy and childhood. Several techniques can help the practitioner visualize the tympanic membrane. The infant's head should be stabilized to prevent painful jamming of the speculum into the ear canal. This sometimes can be accomplished by having the parent or a nurse hold the infant against his or her chest with the infant's head on one and then the opposite shoulder. The head usually is stabilized best by laying the infant supine on the examining table and having the parent or a nurse hold the baby's arms against the body or extended on either side of the head. Providing some type of visual distraction, as well as verbal reassurances, while positioning the infant usually affords the examiner a brief, struggle-free period for performing the otoscopic examination. Varying amounts of resistance are almost universal, however, and a rapid examination is desirable for the infant, the parents, and the examiner. One hand is used to grasp the ear pinna and gently pull it laterally and posteriorly to straighten the lumen of the external canal. In infants, the external canal tends to be perpendicular to the temporal bone, with a slight upward angle (further growth of the skull will give the canal a slightly anterior and downward direction). If the otoscope is held upside down, the infant's head can be stabilized further by the hand holding the ear pinna and the ulnar edge of the hand holding the otoscope (Fig. 8-22).

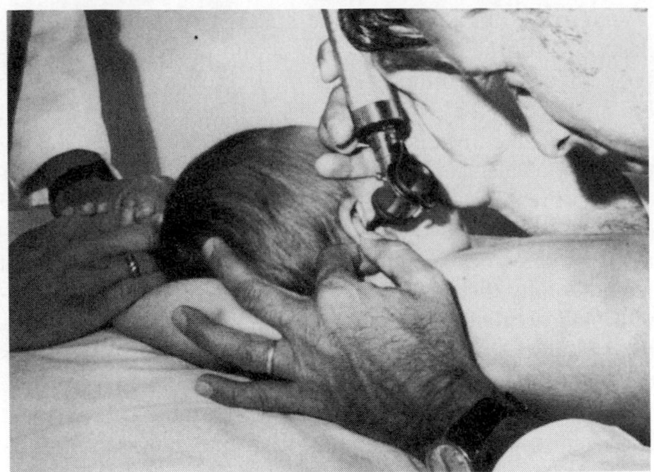

Fig. 8-22 Otoscopic examination of the child. (Photograph by P. Ruben.)

The examiner can further stabilize the infant's body by leaning across the chest and abdomen. The ear speculum then is introduced into the external canal and gently advanced to the point where the bony portion of the canal prevents further entry. Cerumen, which can be soft, firm, or flaky and varies from white to dark brown, may have to be removed. A flexible, wire-loop ear curette can remove small to moderate amounts of soft cerumen and poses less risk of abrading the canal wall or tympanic membrane than does a rigid curette. Curetting is done most safely through the otoscopic head. Larger amounts of hard, inspissated cerumen may require irrigation with warm water and sometimes prior treatment with softening agents such as hydrogen peroxide. An ear canal filled with purulent exudate usually indicates acute otitis media with perforation or otitis externa (the latter is accompanied by pain when the pinna is moved); irrigation usually is unsuccessful and may be dangerous, especially with perforation of the tympanic membrane. Several sizes of specula should be tried to find the largest size that fits into the ear canal, thus allowing visualization of the largest area of tympanic membrane. The otoscope usually must be rotated to view all the important landmarks.

A normal tympanic membrane (Fig. 8-23) is semitransparent, roughly cone shaped, and inclined away from the examiner. The light reflex in the anteroinferior quadrant often is the first landmark seen, with its origin at the central umbo. The examiner, moving the light superiorly from the umbo, can see the long process of the malleus through the membrane, which ends in a bony protuberance that marks the junction of the pars tensa inferiorly and the pars flaccida superiorly. Vague outlines of the incus sometimes can be seen in the posterosuperior quadrant. Air insufflation, by means of a diagnostic otoscopic head fitted with a small bulb, permits direct observation of the eardrum's movement as positive and then negative pressure is applied gently (pneumatoscopy).

As acute otitis media develops, the tympanic membrane becomes increasingly opaque and erythematous, usually progressing superiorly to inferiorly, with progressive outward bulging and eventual loss of the outlines of the malleus and of the light reflex. Air insufflation will demonstrate decreas-

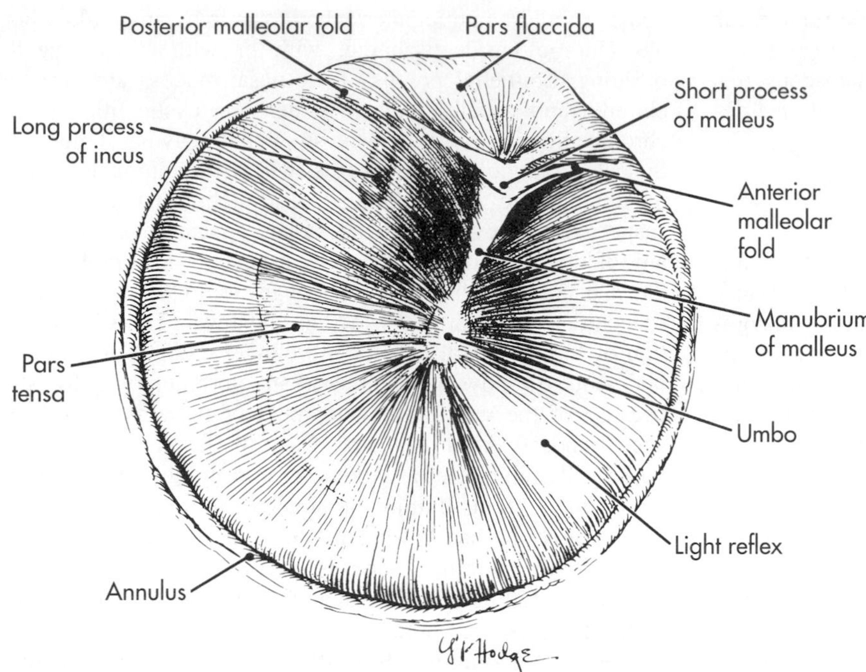

Fig. 8-23 Anatomy of the tympanic membrane.
(From Strome M, editor: *Differential diagnosis in pediatric otolaryngology,* Boston, 1975, Little, Brown.)

ing mobility and sometimes the changing menisci of fluid levels within the middle ear. As the condition heals, these changes resolve inferiorly to superiorly; final resolution of opacity, limited motion, and fluid levels sometimes requires several months.

Bullous myringitis appears as a bubblelike swelling that can almost fill the bony portion of the external ear canal. Blood behind the eardrum, either red or purple, is a sign of basilar skull fracture and should be looked for in children who have suffered head trauma. White plaques on the eardrum are scars from old infections. A white mass in the posterosuperior quadrant may be a cholesteatoma, which is present with chronic obstructive middle ear disease. When examining acutely ill children suspected of having a middle ear infection, the mastoid process should be inspected for overlying swelling and erythema and palpated for tenderness—signs of acute mastoiditis.

In infants, auditory acuity is screened directly and indirectly. The indirect method is based on the effect of normal hearing on language development. Normal infants make cooing sounds (semipurposeful vocalization of vowel sounds) by 6 weeks of age, laugh out loud by 3 months, babble (repetitive sounds, such as "baabaa") by 6 months, echo sounds made in their presence by 9 months, and say their first meaningful word between 12 and 15 months. An infant who fails to progress beyond any of these developmental stages or who regresses should be examined further for hearing loss, as well as for mental retardation.

Hearing can be assessed qualitatively by noting the infant's response to a nearby sound, which is made without visually distracting the infant and without producing vibrations of the air or the surface on which the infant is lying. Responses often are difficult to interpret but include blinking the eyes in a neonate, momentarily ceasing body movements at 1 to 2 months, and turning the eyes or the head toward the sound by 3 to 4 months. The test sounds can be made by snapping the fingers or ringing a bell. With older infants, tongue clucking produces a test sound with the frequencies of normal speech (500 to 2000 Hz). Asking the parents about the infant's responses to sounds may be as reliable as simple office screening.

For children 1 to 5 years of age, normal hearing is necessary for language development beyond the one-word stage. Hearing can be screened by whispering, as softly as possible, a number into the child's ear and asking the child to repeat it or by asking the child if he or she can hear a ticking watch held a few inches from either ear.

Audiometric testing is indicated for any infant or child who fails any of these qualitative tests, and formal testing should be a routine procedure for children before they start school. Because of the high incidence of middle ear infections among infants and preschool children, hearing screening is routine in many offices and well-child clinics, both in following up known infections and as an annual procedure (see Chapter 20 [Ten] Auditory Screening).

Late childhood and adolescence. The tympanic membrane in this age group usually can be examined without resistance, with the child sitting. If the child has ear pain or has had a previous painful examination, the supine position will make head stabilization easier. A qualitative hearing test for children in this age group can be accomplished by using tuning forks, particularly those with frequencies in the human voice range of 500 to 2000 Hz. The examiner's own acuity, presuming that it is normal, can be compared with the child's. Comparing bone and air conduction (Rinne test) and testing for lateralization of bone conduction with the handle of the tuning fork held against the midforehead (Weber test) can distinguish qualitatively between conductive and nerve hearing loss; with conductive loss, air conduction is less than bone conduction, and there is lateralization to the affected ear. Audiometric screening for this age group is routine in many schools. Some children who have chronic middle ear disease have fluctuating hearing loss that can be missed on a single puretone screening. In such cases, pneumatoscopy, impedance audiometry, and tympanometry can provide the definitive diagnosis.

Nose

The relative size and shape of the nose normally are influenced by the downward and forward growth of the maxillary bones and, to a lesser extent, by the increase in the bizygomatic width during childhood. The bony orbits are nearer adult size in the newborn than are the other facial bones, and the palate grows most rapidly during the first year of postnatal life. The paranasal sinuses are represented only by the centrally placed ethmoid sinuses at birth; the maxillary sinuses develop from birth and usually are apparent on roentgenograms by 4 years of age and the sphenoid sinuses by age 6. The frontal sinuses usually have reached the level of the roof of the orbits by age 6 to 7. The nose humidifies incoming air and traps bacteria and noxious materials in its continuous mucous blanket, moving them toward the pharynx by ciliary action. Olfactory function appears to be present at birth and to increase with age.

A thorough examination of the nose involves inspecting the external form, the condition of the external nares, the mucous membranes of the septum, and the turbinates and floor of the nose, as well as noting any exudate present. The nose should be examined in all newborns and in all children who have upper respiratory tract symptoms, noisy breathing, epistaxis, head trauma, headache, and fever.

Newborn period. In examining the newborn's nose, it is important to rule out the presence of unilateral or bilateral choanal atresia, which can produce severe respiratory distress, inasmuch as most newborns are unable to breathe easily through their mouths. This examination is performed by introducing a soft No. 8 feeding tube into each external naris and advancing the catheter to the pharynx. Advancing the feeding tube farther into the stomach rules out esophageal obstructions such as atresia and allows aspiration of the amniotic fluid from the stomach. A simpler technique for testing choanal patency is to close one and then the other nostril while holding the mouth closed. When choanal atresia is present, the infant will struggle for breath when the patent nasal airway is occluded. Obstructed nasal breathing sometimes is seen briefly after birth because of inhaled blood and amniotic debris, which can cause moderate to severe distress, especially in those few infants who have congenitally narrow nasal cavities. A profuse, purulent nasal discharge in the neonatal period could suggest the presence of congenital syphilis.

Infancy, childhood, and adolescence. By elevating the tip of the child's nose and using a nasal speculum, the practitioner can inspect the membranes covering the nasal septum, floor of the nose, and inferior, middle, and superior turbinates in the lateral nasal wall for signs of inflammation and bleeding points. The nasal septum occasionally is deviated to one side, sometimes obstructing breathing on that side. The fairly common occurrence of intranasal foreign bodies should be anticipated when examining any child who has chronic nasal discharge, with or without associated bleeding. Epithelial polyps of the nasal mucosa are rare in children and usually indicate underlying cystic fibrosis or chronic allergic rhinitis. A pale, swollen, boggy nasal mucosa indicates allergic rhinitis, whereas with viral rhinitis the nasal membranes are red and bleed easily. Sinusitis should be suspected whenever purulent exudate appears from beneath any of the three nasal turbinates, especially in a child who has a history of chronic nasal congestion, chronic tracheobronchitis, recurrent otitis media, and fever. Transillumination of the paranasal sinuses in younger children is of limited value to physicians other than otorhinolaryngologists because of the variable development of the sinuses before ages 8 and 10. After 10 years of age the frontal sinuses can be transilluminated in a darkened room by holding a bright light source (transilluminator attachment for an otoscope-ophthalmoscope handle) against the superomedial aspect of the orbit; the maxillary sinuses can be transilluminated by holding the light against the lateral aspects of the hard palate within the closed mouth.

Clear fluid draining from the nose after head trauma should be tested for sugar, which is present with a CSF leak. In a child who has a history of epistaxis, the anteroinferior portion of the septum is a common location of prominent blood vessels (Kiesselbach plexus) that bleed easily, especially when aggravated by local inflammation and self-inflicted abrasions.

Swelling around the bridge of the nose can be caused by a cavernous hemangioma or, less commonly, a nasal encephalocele. Erythematous swelling that involves the lateral portion of the bridge of the nose and adjacent eyelids can be a sign of orbital or periorbital cellulitis, which requires immediate intensive investigation and treatment.

Primary care physicians often are asked to examine a child who has suffered trauma to the nose. Consultation with a subspecialist should be sought immediately if the child has prolonged bleeding from the nose after an injury, there is evidence of a septal hematoma, or there is any question of depression of the base of the nose or of deviation from the nose's normal straight-line vertical axis.

Mouth and Pharynx

The size and shape of the mouth and pharynx change during infancy and childhood, with further growth during the first year of the hard palate and also of the mandible, which expands on all surfaces through the second year, extending downward and forward as a result of mandibular condylar growth. The most useful clinical evidence of growth about the mouth is the eruption, further growth, and shedding of the 20 primary (deciduous) teeth, with subsequent eruption of the 32 secondary (permanent) teeth. Intrauterine tooth growth begins during the second fetal month. The deciduous teeth usually begin to erupt by the sixth month of extrauterine life; roughly one new tooth erupts for each month after 6 months of age, with eruption of all deciduous teeth by 28 to 36 months of age. Table 8-3 summarizes the chronology of eruption and shedding of teeth in the growing human. Shedding of the deciduous teeth and eruption of the permanent teeth normally begins at age 5 in boys and age 5½ in girls and

Table 8-3 Most Common Pattern of Dental Development

Dental Age (yr)	Erupting*		Exfoliating	
0-1	b a	a b		
	b a	a b		
1-2	c	c d		
	d c	c d		
2-3	e	e		
	e	e		
3-4				
4-5				
5-6	6	6		
	6 1	1 6	a	a
6-7	1	1	a	a
	2	2	b	b
7-8	2	2	b	b
8-9				
9-10				
10-11	4	4	d	d
	4 3	3 4	d c	c d
11-12	5 3	3 5	e c	c e
	5	5	e	e
12-13	7	7		
	7	7		
16-24	8	8		
	8	8		

From Barkin RM, Rosen P: *Emergency pediatrics,* ed 4, St Louis, 1994, Mosby.
**a-e,* Primary teeth; *1-8,* secondary teeth.

continues through age 14, with eruption of the permanent teeth completed by age 20.

The pharyngeal tonsils steadily increase in size during childhood and then begin to recede during puberty, a pattern of growth shared with adenoidal lymphoid tissue and peripheral lymph nodes.

The mouth and pharynx should be examined carefully during all health maintenance visits and in all children who have respiratory symptoms, fever of unknown origin, and ear or facial pain. A complete examination involves inspecting and palpating the lips, buccal mucosa, gingiva, hard palate, and mandible, as well as inspecting the teeth, tongue, soft palate, tonsillar pillars, tonsils, and posterior pharyngeal wall.

Newborn period. The newborn's mouth often is examined initially by means of the sucking reflex, with the examiner's finger inside the baby's mouth; this can quiet the baby and expedite other parts of the examination. The relative size of the mandible is noted (small mandibles sometimes are associated with underdevelopment of other facial bones as a result of a generalized or genetic disorder). Clefts of the upper lip may be unilateral, bilateral, or midline and may be associated with palatal clefts. A common normal variant is a prominent mucosal fold connecting the inner midline of the upper lip to the posterior portion of the upper gum, leaving a deep notch in the midline of the gum and spacing of the upper central incisors. The upper and lower gums have finely serrated borders. Occasionally, small white mucus-retention cysts (Bohn nodules), which may be mistaken for teeth, are present. White retention cysts at the midline of the posterior border of the hard palate are known as *Epstein pearls.* Both types of mucus-retention cysts disappear spontaneously within a few months. Filmy, patchy white membranes over the gingiva, inner lips, and buccal mucosa that cannot be removed by scraping and that sometimes overlie an erythematous base can be seen in some healthy newborns; these are characteristics of *Monilia albicans* stomatitis (thrush).

A prominent tongue, which may protrude from the mouth, is seen in congenital hypothyroidism and in Down syndrome. A frenulum attaches to the tongue's inferior surface and may extend almost to its tip. When this is thickened and shortened, protrusion of the tongue is limited. Although a source of concern to parents, this "tongue tie" (ankyloglossia) does not often interfere with speech and rarely requires surgical lysis. Salivation is relatively scanty in a normal newborn; therefore, excessive collection of saliva and mucus in the mouth should prompt investigation for esophageal atresia.

A newborn's pharynx is difficult to visualize except during crying because of the strong gag reflex induced by the tongue blade, which may cause the pharynx to fill with stomach contents. Tonsillar tissue is not visible in newborns.

The quality of the infant's cry should be noted. A strong, lusty cry indicates a healthy baby whose airways and lungs are functioning normally; expiratory grunting is associated with respiratory distress; inspiratory stridor is caused by a number of lesions obstructing upper and lower airways; a high-pitched cry suggests intracranial diseases, either congenital or acquired; a hoarse cry suggests hypocalcemic tetany or cretinism; and absence of a cry suggests severe illness or mental retardation.

Infancy, childhood, and adolescence. Because it usually is difficult to examine the mouth and pharynx of preschool children, these attempts are best saved until the end of the examination. Some manner of restraint usually is required; one of the most effective methods is to have the child seated on the mother's lap with the child's head held stationary by the mother's hand (Fig. 8-24). Some infants and toddlers will permit a brief period of "looking at the teeth," with the tongue depressor used gently to retract the lips and buccal mucosa. A crying infant usually gives the examiner struggle-free glimpses of the mouth and pharynx without the need for manipulation. While adequately restrained, a frightened child with clenched teeth can be examined by slipping the tongue depressor laterally and behind the teeth and onto the tongue. In older children, firm pressure on the anterior half of the tongue, with the tongue not protruded, will allow adequate vision of the whole mouth and pharynx; in infants the gag reflex usually must be induced by slipping the tongue depressor onto the posterior half of the tongue. In general, sick children, including those who have respiratory tract infections, are the most reluctant to have the physician peer into their mouth. Healthy children, on the other hand, sometimes can be persuaded to stick out their tongue and say "aaah" if the practitioner demonstrates how to do so.

Salivation normally increases to full capacity during the third month of life, the age when salivary drooling first is observed because of the infant's limited ability to swallow and the lack of lower front teeth to serve as a dam. Increased salivation associated with respiratory distress and fever usually suggests herpes simplex stomatitis or epiglottitis. Salivation also may increase temporarily with the eruption of new

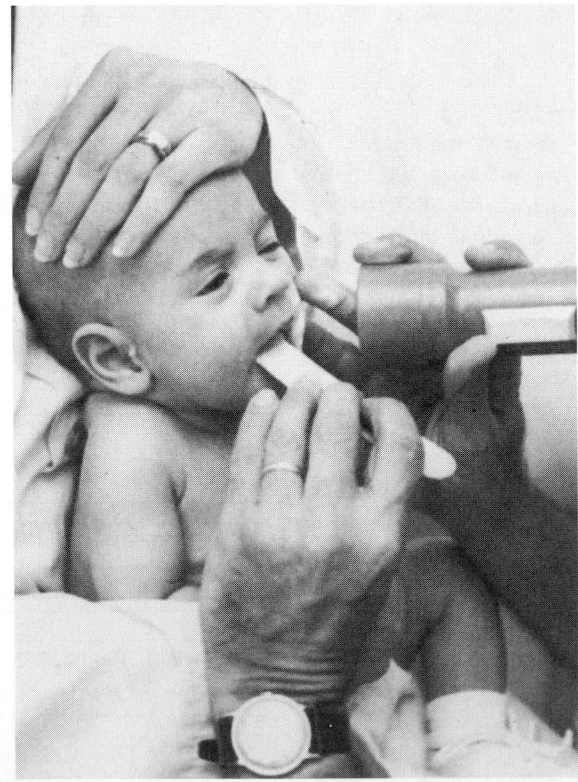

Fig. 8-24 Examination of the pharynx in the infant. (Photograph by P. Ruben.)

teeth. During the winter the lips can be dry and cracked, especially at the corners of the mouth. Deeper fissures at the corners of the mouth, cheilosis, occur in several states of nutritional deficiency and with severe thrush.

The gingivae should be inspected for localized, as well as diffuse, inflammatory lesions. Shallow, white-based ulcers with surrounding erythema can be seen, usually singly, on the gingivae in association with upper respiratory tract infections. Numerous gingival ulcers with concomitant involvement of the tongue and lips associated with increased salivation, fever, and pain usually result from primary herpes simplex infection, which is most common during the first years of life. Recurrent herpes simplex stomatitis, or "cold sores," involving the lips can occur after the primary bout of stomatitis. Localized or diffuse gingival inflammation most often is associated with dental disease, particularly plaque buildup at the gingival borders because of inadequate tooth brushing. Dental abscesses sometimes exhibit an erythematous soft-tissue mass that exudes pus at the dental-gingival border of the involved tooth. Gingivae that bleed easily most often reflect poor mouth hygiene and irritation by bacterial plaque, but the condition can signal, albeit rarely, blood dyscrasia, a clotting deficit, or vitamin C deficiency (scurvy).

The buccal mucosa can be involved with nonspecific ulcerative processes, but occasionally it is the site of important signs of specific infectious diseases. In measles, on the second or third day of the illness, before the onset of the generalized rash, Koplik spots can be seen on the buccal mucosa; these are white pinpoint spots that appear at the level of the lower teeth. In parotitis, usually caused by the mumps virus but occasionally by other organisms, Stensen duct openings, found at the level of the upper molars, are red, swollen, and tender. Scattered white ulcers of varying size can appear on the buccal mucosa in chickenpox. In Kawasaki disease several abnormalities can be seen, including cracked, fissured lips and diffuse redness of the pharynx. Chronic thrush may be an early sign of HIV infection in infants and children.

The teeth are counted with the expectation that the infant will have, on the average, one tooth for each month of age past 6 months up to 28 to 36 months of age, when the full complement of 20 primary teeth will have erupted. Delayed tooth eruption can accompany either serious chronic disease or generalized developmental delay. In infants, the individual teeth are examined for localized or generalized enamel hypoplasia, which can reflect a variety of causes, including hereditary enamel hypoplasia, intrauterine insults such as infections, and prematurity (Fig. 8-25). The infant's teeth may have a permanent yellow, gray, or brown discoloration if the mother took tetracycline during her pregnancy or if the baby was treated with the drug; mottled, pitted teeth with a lusterless, opaque enamel may be the result of an excessive fluoride intake. Oral iron preparations can stain the teeth green, as can an elevated bilirubin level during the neonatal period.

The spacing of the teeth should be observed, giving special attention to teeth that are too close together or too far apart, both of which may cause spacing problems later on. Dental occlusion can be checked by having the child bite down and then observing for maxillary protrusion (overbite) or mandibular protrusion (underbite). Malocclusion has numerous causes, including chronic mouth breathing caused by nasal or nasopharyngeal obstruction, the rare instances of mandibular overgrowth secondary to temporomandibular arthritis in juvenile rheumatoid arthritis, and maxillary overgrowth in untreated hereditary hemolytic anemias, such as Cooley's anemia.

The texture and appearance of the tongue may indicate specific diseases. Dryness, with or without coating, may be seen in chronic mouth breathing or in states of dehydration. Strawberry tongue, a result of the prominence of the papillae, is seen during the course of scarlet fever and in Kawasaki disease. Thrush and herpes simplex, previously described, can involve the tongue. Geographic tongue, in which the surface has the appearance of a relief map, may be nonspecific or may be associated with underlying allergic disease. Deep furrows in the tongue (scrotal tongue) have no significance. Fine and gross tremor of the tongue, including fasciculations and fibrillations, can be seen in both CNS disease (e.g., Sydenham's chorea) and peripheral nerve and neuromuscular junction diseases (Werdnig-Hoffmann disease).

Petechiae sometimes are present on the hard and soft palates in association with pharyngitis, especially streptococcal pharyngitis. The upward motion of the uvula and soft palate should be confirmed during phonation and with the gag reflex to rule out paralysis. A bifid uvula (Fig. 8-26) should be

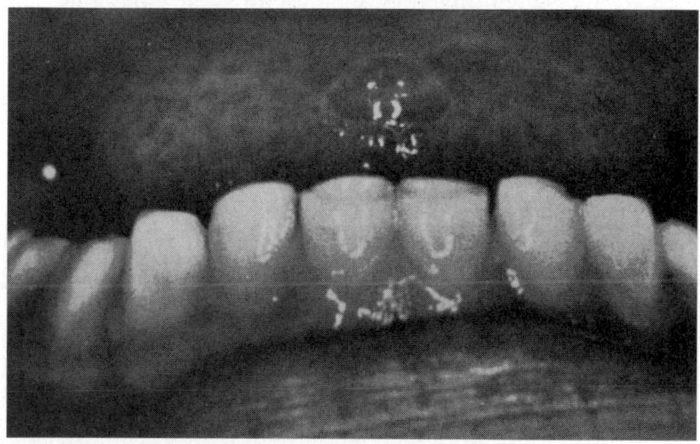

Fig. 8-25 Enamel hypoplasia in a premature child.
(From McDonald RE, Avery DR: *Dentistry for the child and adolescent*, ed 7, St Louis, 2000, Mosby.)

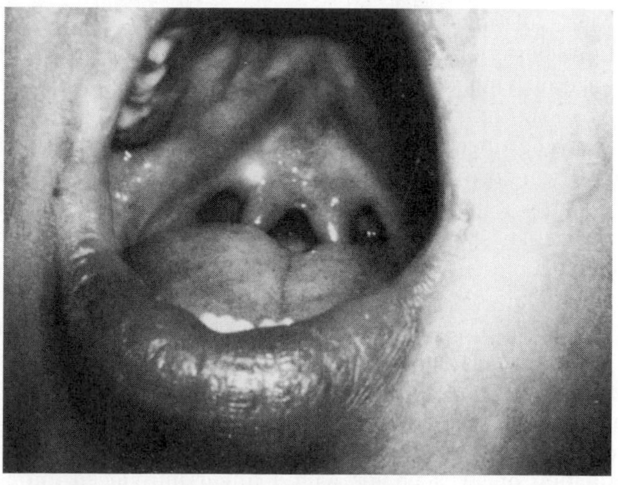

Fig. 8-26 Submucosal cleft palate with bifid uvula.

recognized because it can be associated with a submucous cleft of the soft palate. In this condition the soft palate is relatively short and does not reach the posterior pharyngeal wall. Palatal closure against the posterior pharyngeal wall, essential for normal articulation and voice resonance, can be aided in this condition by the presence of hypertrophied nasopharyngeal lymphoid tissue. Therefore, during the preoperative examination of a child scheduled for adenoidectomy, the practitioner should check for submucous cleft of the palate because it may affect the decision to operate (see Chapter 270, Tonsillectomy and Adenoidectomy).

The anterior and posterior pillars that border the tonsils are difficult to distinguish in most infants. The tonsils (palatal tonsils) are proportionately larger in preschool and school-age children than in adults. Tonsillar size is estimated arbitrarily on a scale of 1 to 4+, 1+ indicating easy visibility and 4+ indicating that the tonsils meet in the midline. The tonsils normally appear more prominent during gagging or crying, and their relative size can be assessed accurately only while the infant or child is at rest. The tonsillar crypts normally contain varying amounts of desquamated cells, which appear as white spots on the surface. However, true tonsillar exudate usually is less localized to the crypts and extends over a greater portion of the surface. Some examiners try to distinguish the color of the exudate—yellow being more common with streptococcal infection, white with viral infections, and gray with diphtheria. A grayish discoloration of the tonsils (rather than an exudate) is sometimes seen with infectious mononucleosis. The only reliable way to determine cause is to obtain a throat culture, especially of the tonsillar exudate in children over 2 to 3 years of age. Tonsillar erythema and edema, which also should be noted, are particularly conspicuous with streptococcal infection.

Shallow, white-based ulcers that have erythematous edges, which may involve the adjacent pillars and posterior pharynx, suggest herpangina, caused by coxsackievirus A, and can be distinguished from the more anterior location of the herpes simplex ulcers. The diphtheritic membrane may be confluent over the tonsils, pharynx, and uvula, and bleeding ensues when the membrane is scraped away with a tongue blade. In infants a diffusely red pharynx and tonsillar area, with or without exudate, most likely has a viral origin. A peritonsillar abscess is suggested by asymmetrical enlargement of the tonsils, often associated with lateral displacement of the uvula toward the unaffected tonsil.

The posterior pharyngeal wall should be inspected for evidence of lymphoid hyperplasia, which has a "cobblestone" appearance and indicates chronic postnasal drainage, as seen in chronic allergic rhinitis or bacterial sinusitis. Postnasal drainage into the pharynx is to be expected in infants and children who have upper respiratory tract infections, and the characteristics of the mucus suggest various causes. Clear mucus is present in allergic rhinitis or in the early stages of acute rhinitis, whereas purulent mucus appears in the late stages of a viral rhinitis or with chronic bacterial sinusitis.

The presence and size of the adenoidal lymphoid tissue can be estimated indirectly by noting the amount of mouth breathing at rest, by observing the ease of breathing through the nostrils, and by noting any nasality to the voice. Direct palpation of the adenoids with a finger introduced through the mouth and around the soft palate is possible only under anesthesia. Using the nasopharyngeal mirror for visualization of the adenoids is most helpful to those who use it every day, such as otolaryngologists.

The epiglottis sometimes is visualized by chance when the throat of a child who has an upper respiratory tract infection is examined. In children who have croupy cough, especially if of sudden onset and associated with high fever, drooling, and signs of upper airway obstruction, the epiglottis must be visualized to rule out acute bacterial epiglottitis, a true emergency in children (see Chapter 284, Epiglottitis). The epiglottis may be swollen several times its usual size and is cherry red. Because of the danger of complete airway obstruction and of cardiac arrest during this examination, endotracheal tubes, a tracheotomy set, and an oxygen source should be at hand. Most primary care physicians choose to rely on a lateral neck roentgenogram initially to evaluate the size of the epiglottis and postpone direct visualization until a surgeon is present.

Neck

The neck is relatively short in infants and lengthens during childhood as a result of vertebral growth. Consequently the epiglottis descends from the level of the first cervical vertebral body at birth to the lower third of the third cervical vertebral body by adulthood. The larynx is one third the adult size at birth. It grows rapidly until age 3, becoming wider and longer, and then grows slowly until puberty, when another rapid increase in all dimensions occurs, especially in boys. The trachea at birth is approximately one third the adult length, and both the anteroposterior and lateral diameters of the trachea increase by nearly 300% from birth to puberty. The thyroid gland increases approximately 10 times in weight from birth through puberty, with most growth occurring during puberty. Cervical lymph nodes, a few of which may be palpable at birth, increase in size, following the growth curve for the body's lymphatic tissues in general; those in most normal children are less than 1 cm in diameter. The neck should be examined thoroughly from time to time in healthy infants and children and always in children who have a respiratory or febrile illness. This examination should include noting the overall neck dimensions; the resistance to passive motion; the size and location of the lymph nodes, thyroid gland, and the trachea; the status of neck vessels; and the presence of masses.

Newborn period. The newborn's relatively short neck should be inspected for position and overall size. Torticollis, a condition in which the head is tilted to one side with the chin rotated toward the opposite shoulder, usually is associated with a palpable hematoma of the involved sternocleidomastoid muscle. It is believed to arise from a birth injury and may require physical therapy. Opisthotonos, in which the neck and back are held in extreme extension, is an ominous sign that indicates either meningeal irritation or, in an infant who has jaundice, kernicterus. In infants, frequent opisthotonic positioning associated with a relative paucity of trunk flexion movements may be an early sign of the spasticity of cerebral palsy. An unusually short neck may indicate cervical spine anomalies (Klippel-Feil syndrome), and a webbed neck is seen in Turner's syndrome. The newborn clavicles should be palpated routinely to rule out clavicular fractures, which usually occur at the junction of the middle and outer thirds of the bone and can occur during birth. Palpable neck masses in the newborn include the midline thyroglossal duct cyst, the supraclavicular cystic hygroma, which transilluminates, and branchial cleft cysts with or without associated skin tags and fistulas along the anterior border of the sternocleidomastoid muscle. Palpable cervical lymph nodes in normal newborns usually are less than 5 mm in diameter. A crackly sensation on palpation in the supraclavicular areas usually indicates pneumomediastinum.

Infancy, childhood, and adolescence. When palpably enlarged lymph nodes are found, the examiner should note their location, size and number, consistency, tenderness, mobility, and attachment to other structures. Anterior cervical lymph nodes commonly enlarge in association with upper respiratory tract infections, dental infections, and stomatitis and less commonly with mycobacterial infection. Enlargement of the posterior cervical nodes is common secondary to insect bites or inflammatory lesions of the scalp. Cervical lymph nodes are enlarged generally with many viral syndromes, especially rubella, measles, and infectious mononucleosis. Lymph nodes enlarged because of an inflammation usually return to normal size days or weeks after the primary infection has subsided. One or more enlarged cervical lymph nodes, combined with other signs, are seen in Kawasaki disease. Lymph nodes that are enlarging without any signs of infection suggest Hodgkin's disease and other lymphomas. Chronically enlarged lymph nodes can be seen throughout the body in HIV infection (see Chapter 219, Human Immunodeficiency Virus Infection and Acquired Immunodeficiency Syndrome).

Every infant and child who has an acute illness should be checked for nuchal rigidity, an important sign of meningeal irritation from meningitis. Ideally the infant or child should be quiet and relaxed, lying supine as the examiner cradles the infant's head with both hands and gently lifts it from the examining table, noting the degree of suppleness and any resistance to flexion. Flexion of the fully extended legs associated with neck flexion (Brudzinsk's sign) and flexion of one fully extended lower extremity while its opposite, flexed 90 degrees at the hip, is fully extended (Kernig's sign) are present less often in infants who have meningitis than in older children and adolescents. A child who has nuchal rigidity is unable to touch the chin to the chest and assumes a tripod position when asked to sit up—that is, rests backward on extended arms while the legs are extended on the examining table.

The thyroid gland normally is difficult to palpate, if palpable at all, before puberty; it should be palpated, as should the trachea, from in front of and from behind the child. An enlarged thyroid can occur in children who have euthyroid, hypothyroid, or hyperthyroid states, and it can be caused by iodine deficiency as well as iodine excess (from cough medicines containing iodine), congenital or familial blockage of thyroxine synthesis, thyroiditis, diffuse or nodular hyperplasia, and, in rare cases, carcinoma. Normally the trachea is slightly deviated to the right; deviation from this norm indicates mediastinal shift, as may occur with foreign body-induced atelectasis and with pneumothorax. Neck venous pulsations and distention, usually difficult to determine in infants because of their relatively short necks, can give clues to heart disease and congestive heart failure in older children.

Children who have painful or limited neck motion should be checked for a full range of flexion, extension, lateral rotation, and lateral flexion. A fairly common cause of limited head motion is wryneck, or torticollis, which can occur after a play injury or sometimes in association with a respiratory tract infection. The head is tilted to one side, with sternocleidomastoid tenderness on the long or stretched side (as distinguished from neonatal torticollis, in which the involved sternocleidomastoid muscle is on the short side); the underlying cause of wryneck is a rotary subluxation of the first two cervical vertebrae.

Chest and Lungs

The chest wall in the fetus and newborn is round; with further growth it gradually flattens, with the lateral diameter exceeding the anteroposterior diameter. The thoracic index (transverse/anteroposterior diameter) is measured serially in some clinics that treat children who have chronic obstructive lung disease, such as cystic fibrosis, as a means of monitoring the degree of formation of a "barrel chest." The infant's chest wall is relatively thin compared with an adult's; therefore, heart and lung sounds are transmitted more clearly. Respirations are predominantly abdominal in infants, reflecting the greater role of the diaphragm in breathing; by age 6 they are predominantly thoracic, reflecting the increased role of the thoracic musculature in normal breathing.

By 16 weeks of gestation the bronchial tree is fully developed, with the adult number of segments and subsegments. Alveoli, in comparison, are just forming by the time of birth, with only 8% of the average adult number present. The number of alveoli increases until age 8, after which they primarily increase in size rather than in number until adulthood. Pulmonary blood vessels develop parallel to the developing bronchial tree and alveoli, and increasing amounts of muscle appear in the walls of the more distal arterioles over time. By 28 weeks of gestation, airway and blood vessel development usually is adequate for gas transfer. By 34 to 36 weeks of gestation, sufficient amounts of a surface-active lipid are present within the alveoli to maintain them in a partly expanded position, rather than remaining collapsed at the end of each expiration. As noted previously, the respiratory rate declines with age, partly because of further postnatal development of the alveoli, with a resulting increase in lung volume.

The breasts of many normal male and female infants are transiently hypertrophied at birth, sometimes producing small amounts of clear or white fluid, called *witch's milk.* This hypertrophy normally disappears by 2 to 3 months of age. Many pubertal boys have transient unilateral or bilateral firm, sometimes painful, subareolar masses that disappear within a year of onset. A girl's pubertal breast development often is asymmetrical and proceeds through several stages, starting with an increase in the areolar diameter between ages 8 and 13, and is completed between ages 12 and 19 (Fig. 8-27).

The chest and lungs should be examined thoroughly in every child who has any respiratory symptoms, fever, abdominal pain, or chest pain. The examiner should note size, symmetry, movement with respirations, localized tenderness

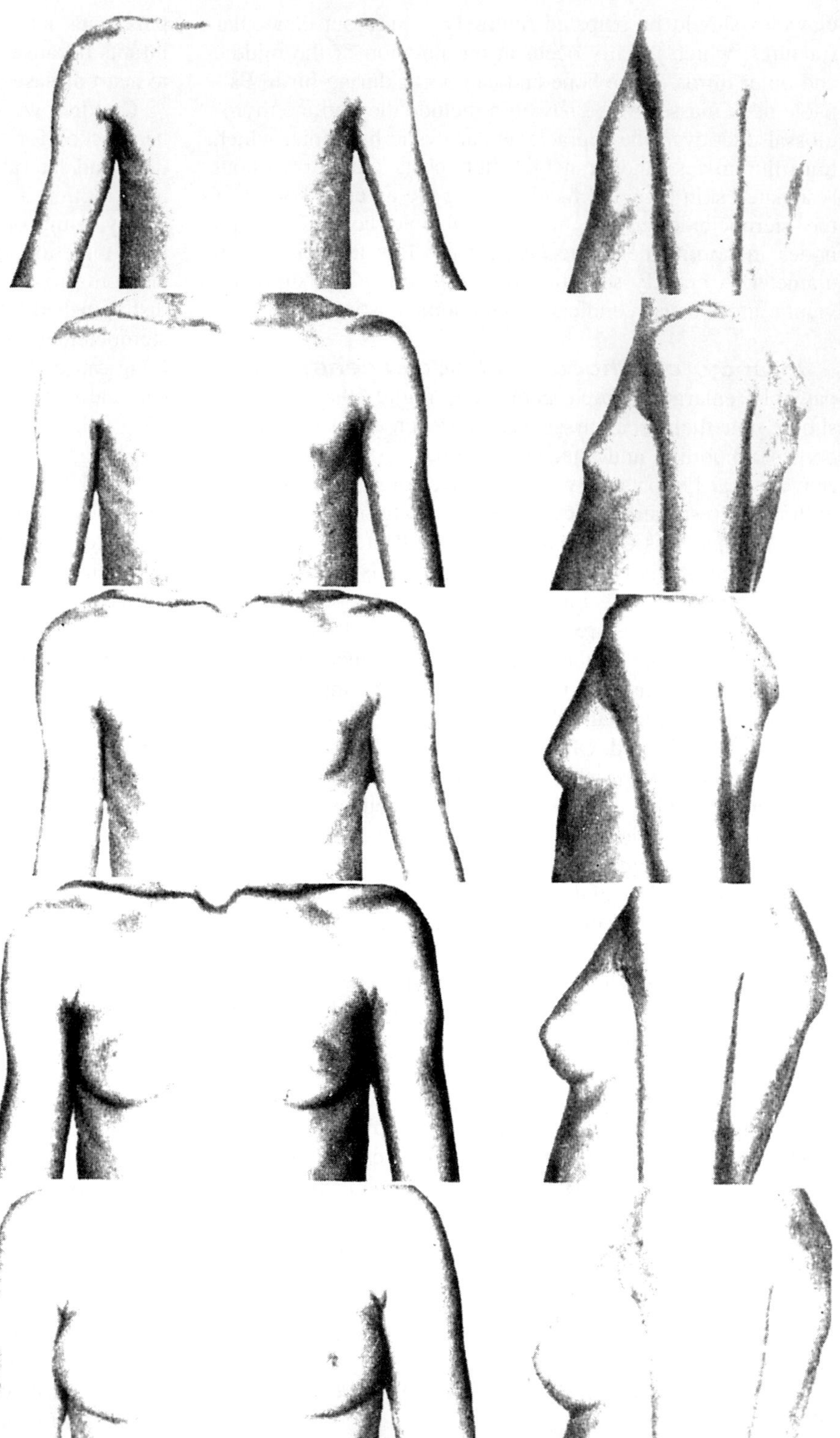

Fig. 8-27 The five stages of development of the female breast.
(From Tanner JM: *Growth at adolescence*, ed 2, Oxford, 1962, Blackwell.)

or masses, and breast characteristics. The three goals of an examination of the lungs using observation, percussion, and auscultation are (1) to determine the nature of respiration, including rate, depth, and ease; (2) to establish the adequacy of gas exchange, as indicated by signs of hypoxia or hypercapnia; and (3) to localize disease. The examiner should use and become familiar with the sound characteristics of one stethoscope. Except when auscultating the chest of a small premature baby, an adult-sized stethoscope with both a bell and a diaphragm generally is effective for examining infants and children of all ages.

Newborn period. During the few moments after birth, the adequacy of the developing lungs for gas exchange (which is influenced by factors such as maternal anesthesia, birth trauma, and the normality of the infant's central nervous and cardiovascular systems) is grossly assessed by the Apgar score (see Table 8-1), which includes observations about the

Table 8-4 Downes Score: A Method for Monitoring Respiratory Distress

Score	0	1	2
Respiratory rate (breaths/min)	60	60-80	>80 or apneic episode
Cyanosis	None	In air	In 40% oxygen
Retractions	None	Mild	Moderate to severe
Grunting	None	Audible with stethoscope	Audible without stethoscope
Air entry (crying)	Clear	Delayed or decreased	Barely audible

From Downes JJ: *Clin Pediatr* 9:326, 1970.

color and initiation of respirations. Once normal respirations have been established, the baby's chest is inspected for deformities, such as a markedly bulging sternum (pectus carinatum) or a markedly concave one (pectus excavatum); asymmetry caused by uneven chest expansion, absence of or deformed ribs, or absence of the pectoral muscle (Poland syndrome); and overall size, inasmuch as small thoracic cages are a feature of several congenital anomalies. The respiratory rate normally falls from as high as 60 breaths/min immediately after birth to 30 to 40 breaths/min by several hours of age. In a normal newborn the auscultated breath sounds are heard easily and have a higher pitch than those in the older child and adult.

A newborn in respiratory distress from any cause exhibits some or all of the following signs: nasal flaring, tachypnea, cyanosis, expiratory grunting, intercostal retractions (subcostal, substernal, and supraclavicular retractions are also possible), and decreased air entry, as measured by decreased breath sounds. If a pulse oximeter is not available, the Downes score (Table 8-4) is a useful clinical tool for serially monitoring the severity of newborn respiratory distress, particularly that caused by hyaline membrane disease. Persistent scores of 5 or higher usually indicate that respiratory assistance is needed. Simple auscultation of a newborn in respiratory distress should aid in the diagnosis of (1) unilateral lesions, such as aspiration pneumonia, congenital diaphragmatic hernia, congenital hypoplastic segments or emphysema, and unilateral pneumothorax and (2) congenital heart disease.

The respiratory rate of newborns, particularly premature newborns, can be quite irregular during the first few days of life and sometimes can slow to the point of apnea. Two patterns should be differentiated in premature infants. *Periodic breathing* is associated with relatively brief periods of apnea lasting 5 to 10 seconds, usually without secondary bradycardia. It occurs more commonly when the baby is awake and is uncommon before 5 days of age. True apneic spells, on the other hand, last longer than 20 seconds, are associated with bradycardia, can be associated with pulmonary disease, and are more common in infants who weigh less than 1250 g.

Infancy, childhood, and adolescence. In these children, auscultation and percussion, along with observation of breathing patterns, are particularly useful techniques for evaluating the chest and lungs. Auscultation often is accomplished most successfully when the infant or child is only minimally aware of being examined—for example, while asleep, being fed, or being held up to the parent's shoulder. When preschool children are asked to "take a deep breath," they often hold their breath. It is easier to start by auscultating while the child breathes at a resting level. If the child is crying, the inspiratory phase can be thoroughly auscultated, but predominantly expiratory adventitious sounds, such as wheezes, can be missed. After the examiner listens to breath sounds at rest or during crying, a useful technique for accentuating adventitious sounds, particularly during the expiratory phase, is inducing forced expiration. The examiner may do this by holding the hands on opposing anterior and posterior sides of the chest, with the stethoscope in one hand held against the chest, and gently squeezing the hands together as expiration is ending.

Breath sounds in infants and children tend to be audible during both inspiration and expiration (i.e., bronchovesicular) and are heard more clearly than in adults. Secretions in any part of the respiratory tree usually are reflected by loudly audible coarse rhonchi heard throughout the chest, and the examiner should repeat his or her observations to rule out transmitted sounds from the nose or pharynx. It is tempting for inexperienced examiners to suspect pneumonia in most children evaluated for acute respiratory illnesses because of the fairly usual occurrence of tracheal and bronchial inflammation with common viral infections. The more or less generalized coarse rhonchi (continuous, low-pitched sounds) from bronchial secretions and the wheezes (higher pitched, predominantly expiratory) from bronchiolar secretions should be distinguished from the much less common, usually localized, crackling rales caused by alveolar fluid or exudate and heard best at the end of inspiration. Pneumonia in infants and young children almost always is accompanied by fever and tachypnea, whereas rales, bronchial breath sounds, dullness to percussion, and a productive cough are less common findings than in adults.

Several objective signs of respiratory distress can be seen in infants and children. Orthopnea occurs in children who have asthma or congestive heart failure. Maximal use of accessory muscles of respiration produces several useful physical signs, including head bobbing, seen especially in infants, with the head bobbing forward in synchrony with each inspiration, and flaring of the nasal alae, resulting from contraction of the anterior and posterior dilator naris muscles. These signs indicate increased work of breathing, or inspiratory efforts shortened by pain, as occurs in pleuritis or thoracic trauma. Intercostal retractions, an exaggerated inspiratory sinking in of intercostal and sometimes supraclavicular soft tissue, indicate increased inspiratory effort and reflect airway obstruction and lung stiffness. Bulging of the intercostal space during expiration occurs with increased expiratory effort, such as in asthma, bronchiolitis, and cystic fibrosis. Subcostal retractions, seen anteriorly at the lower costal margins, reflect flattening of the diaphragm and occur in conditions with diffuse lower airway obstruction. Substernal retractions can be seen in children who have severe upper airway obstruction and in newborns, especially premature infants, who have various pulmonary diseases. Audible wheezes usually indicate obstruction of the larger airways, and grunting can be associated with pneumonia, chest pain, and respiratory distress syndrome in neonates. A "thud" may be heard on inspiration in children who have a tracheal foreign body as the object moves in response to airflow.

The adequacy of gas exchange is judged primarily by seeking signs of hypoxia. Cyanosis, which results when the amount of reduced hemoglobin in the capillaries exceeds 5 g, is either peripheral (as with exposure to a cold environment) or central (seen as blue mucous membranes), the latter being of pulmonary or cardiac origin. Tachycardia, dyspnea on exertion, and CNS depression are additional signs of hypoxia that can be critical in monitoring a child who has marginally adequate gas exchange, as in severe croup. Progressive signs of hypercapnia in acute respiratory illnesses include hot hands, small pupils, engorged fundal veins, muscular twitching, coma, and papilledema.

Localization of intrathoracic lesions in children is aided by palpating for tracheal deviation and observing for unequal respiratory movements of half of the chest, localized areas of dull or flat percussion notes, and the presence of tactile fremitus. Percussion also can be used to delineate the lower boundaries of the lungs in inspiration and expiration.

Heart

The major anatomical characteristics of the heart form long before birth, as do most congenital heart defects. In a normal newborn's heart the right ventricle has a muscle mass equal to that of the left ventricle, reflecting the fetal circulation in which both ventricles pump blood into the systemic circulation, the left through the aorta and the right through the ductus arteriosus. After birth the left ventricle gains weight relative to the right ventricle, reaching the adult weight ratio of approximately 2:1 by age 1, reflecting the major changes in postnatal circulation. At birth, or shortly thereafter, the ductus arteriosus normally closes, and the flap of the foramen ovale is held closed by the rise in pressure in the left atrium. As many as half of all newborns have transient murmurs during the first 24 to 48 hours of life, some of which are caused by a late-closing ductus arteriosus.

Congenital heart defects can be classified according to the embryonic stages of development during which an abnormality arises: position anomalies (dextrocardia with or without situs inversus), anomalous growth of the atrial chambers (atrioventricular canal, ostium primum defect, persistent foramen ovale), anomalous bulboventricular growth and septation (ventricular septal defect, tetralogy of Fallot, double outlet right ventricle, transposition of the great vessels), and maldevelopment of the truncus (truncus arteriosus, patent ductus arteriosus, coarctation of the aorta). See Chapter 198, Congenital Heart Disease.

The significant and normal changes in pulse and blood pressure that occur with age in infants and children have been described earlier in this chapter. It is important to remember that optimal auscultation of the heart requires use of a stethoscope with both a bell and a diaphragm, the bell picking up lower-pitched sounds and the diaphragm picking up higher-pitched ones. Proper use of the bell involves holding it lightly against the chest while the diaphragm is pressed firmly to the chest. Stethoscope tubing should be no more than 10 to 12 inches long. During auscultation, gentle traction on the earpiece end of the stethoscope enhances the audibility of heart sounds by making a tighter seal between the earpiece and the examiner's external auditory canal. Because infants have relatively rapid heart rates, detecting abnormalities in their heart sounds demands that each of the two major heart sounds be listened to in isolation, giving attention to each interval between these sounds. As in adults, the heart is auscultated initially over the four cardinal areas (apex, or *mitral area;* lower left sternal border, or *tricuspid area;* second left intercostal space at the sternal margin, or *pulmonary area;* and second right intercostal space, or *aortic area*). Auscultation then proceeds to the remainder of the precordium and chest, including the infraclavicular and supraclavicular area, the axillae, the back, and the neck.

A thorough examination of the heart should be part of all physical examinations of infants and children; it involves noting the heart rate and rhythm, heart size, and characteristics of the first and second heart sounds, especially in the second left interspace. With murmurs, the following information should be recorded: timing in the cardiac cycle (early, late, or pansystolic; protodiastolic, middiastolic, or presystolic), quality (blowing, harsh, rumbling, musical, or other), grade of maximal intensity (on a scale of I to VI, with V and VI being associated with a palpable thrill), duration, point of maximal intensity, and transmission (see Chapter 142, Heart Murmurs). In all infants and children whose findings suggest congenital heart disease, palpation of peripheral pulses is especially important to determine if the pulses in the lower extremities are diminished and those in the upper extremities increased, as occurs with coarctation of the aorta. Blood pressure is measured as described earlier in this chapter.

Newborn period and infancy. An infant's general appearance can provide clues to underlying heart disease and may mandate a more sophisticated cardiac examination. Examples of conditions frequently associated with congenital heart disease are Down syndrome (endocardial cushion defect), Turner's syndrome (coarctation of the aorta), trisomy 13, trisomy 18, and congenital rubella syndrome (patent ductus arteriosus, pulmonary stenosis). Important clinical signs of significant heart disease include cyanosis, growth failure, and lethargy. The most prominent signs of congestive heart failure in infants are tachypnea, tachycardia, and liver enlargement. Peripheral edema and pulmonary rales are late findings and therefore not as helpful as in adults. Visible chest pulsations can indicate a hyperdynamic state caused by an increased metabolic rate or an inefficient pumping action from valvular or septal incompetency or other defect. Dextrocardia is suggested by a right-sided cardiac impulse and may be associated with abdominal situs inversus (reversal of the position of the liver, spleen, and intestines).

The apical impulse in infants normally is palpated in the fourth left interspace just outside the midclavicular line; after age 7 it is in the adult position of the fifth left interspace in the midclavicular line. The point of maximal impulse of the heart can suggest individual ventricular enlargement. An impulse at the xiphoid process or lower left sternal border suggests right ventricular hypertrophy, whereas an impulse maximal at the apex suggests left ventricular hypertrophy.

Infants' heart sounds often are difficult to differentiate from their breath sounds because the pitches and rates of each can be similar. Watching the abdominal excursions with respiration and palpating a peripheral pulse while auscultating the chest can aid in this differentiation. The examiner should be prepared to spend at least several minutes listening to the precordial area, at which time the heart and respiratory rates and rhythms can be determined. For each heart sound, the intensity, point of maximal intensity, and degrees of splitting should be noted. Normally the second heart sound is louder than the first in the second left interspace and often is split (reflecting the pulmonary valve closing after the aortic valve); the split often widens with inspiration. Examples of abnormalities of the heart sounds are the loud first sound heard at the apex in mitral stenosis; the loud second sound in the pulmonary area, indicating pulmonary hypertension; and the fixed, split second sound in the pulmonary area with atrial septal defect. A third heart sound can be heard at the apex of normal children and should be distinguished from the higher intensity, third-sound gallop that occurs with tachycardia and indicates congestive heart failure.

Heart murmurs are more difficult to localize in infants than in children and adolescents because in infants they often are so well transmitted and heard throughout the chest. Gross anatomical localization can be helpful, however, as illustrated by (1) the prominence over the back of the murmurs of coarctation of the aorta and some cases of patent ductus arteriosus, (2) the precordial systolic murmur of ventricular septal defect growing louder as the examiner descends the left sternal border to the xiphoid, and (3) the murmur or murmurs of peripheral pulmonary artery stenosis becoming louder as the examiner moves the stethoscope laterally from the precordium. On the other hand, the typical to-and-fro continuous murmur of patent ductus arteriosus described in older children may be absent in affected infants and represented only by a precordial systolic murmur.

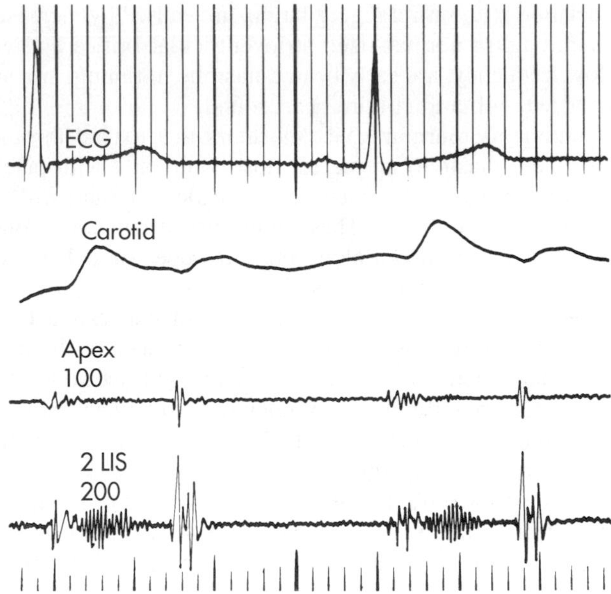

Fig. 8-28 An innocent murmur: phonocardiogram. Note the even harmonic quality of a stringlike murmur. *2 LIS,* Second left intercostal space.

(From Fyler DC: *Nadas' pediatric cardiology,* Chicago, 1992, Mosby.)

Childhood and adolescence. A cardiac examination in children and adolescents follows the outline already given and is different from the examination of infants largely because of the need to distinguish organic murmurs from the "innocent" murmur, which occurs in as many as 50% of normal children. Innocent murmurs are unassociated with any symptomatic, roentgenographic, or electrocardiographic evidence of heart disease, and the three types have several characteristics in common. They usually are low pitched and therefore heard best with the bell. They are musical or vibratory (Fig. 8-28), as distinguished from the more complex range of frequencies of "significant" murmurs. Their intensity usually is no greater than I or II/VI, and both their presence and intensity vary with change in the child's position or respiratory phase. Innocent murmurs are heard most commonly either at the second left interspace or halfway between the lower left sternal border and the apex. At these sites the murmurs are of short duration and occur early in systole. A third common location is above or below either clavicle, where the murmur is called a *venous hum.* This is an impressive sounding murmur, often continuous throughout systole; it is heard best with the child sitting and does not occur in the supine position.

In contrast to innocent murmurs, significant murmurs usually, but not always, are of greater intensity, are less localized, and are more likely to radiate over parts of the chest; they also usually do not change in loudness with a change in the child's position or respiratory phase. Systolic murmurs can be classified as *stenotic, regurgitant,* or *uneven.* Stenotic systolic murmurs are associated with a pressure gradient across the aortic or pulmonary valve and are of high frequency, are diamond shaped, and are transmitted to the neck. Soft systolic murmurs heard in the pulmonary area and associated not with a valvular pressure gradient but with increased flow are present with an atrial septal defect. Atrioventricular valve regurgitant murmurs begin immediately with the first sound, are either decreased or pansystolic, are blowing in character, and are best heard at the lower left sternal border or at the apex, radiating to the axilla and back. The murmur of mitral insufficiency, which is heard at the apex in a large percentage of children who have acute rheumatic fever, can be transient and soft; its discovery can be aided by auscultating over the apex with the child supine and rotated partly onto the left side. The systolic murmur along the left sternal border heard with a ventricular septal defect usually is pansystolic but has a harsher quality than the atrioventricular valve regurgitant murmurs and is transmitted less well to the axilla, neck, and back. An uneven systolic murmur is heard with patent ductus arteriosus along the upper left sternal border. Although pansystolic with or without a diastolic component, the sound of the murmur varies in pitch and intensity from beat to beat.

Most diastolic murmurs are caused by three types of cardiac abnormalities. Protodiastolic murmurs of high pitch with a crescendo-decrescendo pattern are heard with aortic or pulmonary valve regurgitation. Middiastolic murmurs, which are low pitched, rumbling, often crescendo in pattern, preceded by an opening snap and followed by an accentuated first sound, are heard with mitral (and, in rare cases, tricuspid) stenosis. Diastolic flow murmurs, occurring with all large left-to-right shunts and with acute rheumatic fever in association with mitral regurgitation, are caused by increased flow through a normal-sized atrioventricular orifice and are of low frequency, are early or middiastolic in timing, and are associated with a loud third heart sound.

Continuous murmurs (i.e., murmurs that extend through systole into diastole) are heard most commonly with patent ductus arteriosus and sometimes are called "to and fro" or "machinery" murmurs. These murmurs usually are loud, high pitched, and heard along the left upper sternal border, radiating to the neck and back.

The most common presenting signs of congestive heart failure in children, as in infants, are tachypnea, orthopnea, liver enlargement, and sometimes increased sweating. Peripheral edema and pulmonary rales tend to be late findings. In children, the appearance of facial edema more commonly indicates either an allergic reaction or renal disease, such as acute glomerulonephritis. Swelling and redness of the hands and feet are features of Kawasaki disease, as is congestive heart failure (and in a small number, myocardial infarction). Heart failure in children most often occurs with acute or chronic myocarditis (especially acute rheumatic fever), in some children with congenital heart disease, in overwhelming infections, and in hypovolemic states.

Hypertension in children usually is of renal origin, once anxiety has been ruled out. The types of underlying renal disease include acute illnesses such as acute poststreptococcal glomerulonephritis and acute pyelonephritis, end stages of various chronic renal diseases (glomerulonephropathies, chronic obstruction or infection, developmental renal anomalies), kidney tumors such as Wilms' tumor, and renal vessel thrombosis and anomalies. Other causes of hypertension include those related to (1) the central nervous system (poliomyelitis, encephalitis, increasing intracranial pressure of many causes), (2) cardiovascular disease (coarctation of the aorta and aortic run-offs, as with patent ductus arteriosus, anemia, and thyrotoxicosis), (3) endocrine-metabolic disturbances (cortisone therapy, pheochromocytoma, Cushing's disease, congenital adrenal hyperplasia, primary aldosteronism, and porphyria), (4) lead and mercury poisoning, and (5) essential hypertension, in which none of these conditions exists. Increasing experience in the routine measurement of blood pressure in children and adolescents suggests that essential hypertension may be more prevalent among adolescents than was previously believed, especially among those who have a family history of hypertension.

The physical findings of heart disease in infants and children only begin to define the nature of the etiology of the disease. Chest roentgenography and electrocardiography, as well as echocardiography, phonocardiography, and cardiac catheterization, are used to define the diagnosis further. Thus, physical examination of the heart is an important step in cardiac diagnosis but is only the first of many steps that require interpretation by a qualified cardiologist.

Abdomen

The size and shape of the abdomen change with age, reflecting, in part, changes in the intraabdominal and intrathoracic organs. During the neonatal period the abdomen is relatively protuberant because of (1) the intrathoracic expansion of the lungs with downward movement of the diaphragm and (2) the relatively large liver caused by intrauterine extramedullary hematopoiesis. The first meconium stool usually is passed within 24 hours of birth, and intestinal gas is visible by roentgenogram throughout the normal bowel by 48 hours of age. The horizontal position of the stomach within the abdomen in infancy accounts for the increased postprandial protuberance of the epigastric area. The more vertical, adult position of the stomach is developed slowly throughout childhood. The stomach's capacity increases rapidly during the first years of life, from an average of 30 to 90 ml at birth to 210 to 360 ml at age 1 and 500 ml at age 2; it then increases slowly to the adult capacity of 750 to 900 ml. Abdominal protuberance in preschool children is caused by a transient, normal lumbar lordosis. The abdominal musculature is relatively hypotonic at birth, allowing deep palpation. Midline defects include the relatively common and usually transient diastasis recti, the fairly common umbilical hernia, and the rare omphalocele.

The abdomen should be examined thoroughly during all health maintenance examinations and in children who have gastrointestinal symptoms, fever, cough, and any other evidence of acute illness. This examination involves inspection of the abdominal contour and size; palpation for tenderness, an enlarged liver, spleen, or kidneys, and masses; percussion; and auscultation of bowel sounds. Examination of the rectum is indicated in all children who show evidence of an intraabdominal or a pelvic disorder or who have fecal elimination problems or rectal bleeding.

Newborn period and infancy. Absence of the normal prominence of the abdomen in a newborn should lead to further investigation for diaphragmatic hernia or high intestinal atresia. Subcutaneous abdominal wall blood vessels are easily visible in most infants because of their relatively small amount of subcutaneous fat. Abdominal movement is due to the prominent role of the diaphragm in breathing and, in addition, to intestinal peristalsis. Visible peristaltic waves can be observed over any quadrant of the abdomen, especially in premature babies, who have relatively thin abdominal walls. Prominent gastric peristaltic waves moving from left to right across the upper portion of the abdomen are present with congenital pyloric stenosis, which usually manifests by 4 to 6 weeks of age (see Chapter 255, Pyloric Stenosis).

The umbilical stump is inspected at birth for meconium (yellow) staining, a sign associated with chronic fetal distress. The normal umbilicus contains two ventrally placed, thick-walled, smaller arteries and one dorsally placed, thin-walled, larger vein. Infants who have a single umbilical artery may have other congenital malformations, but more often than not it is an isolated anomaly. The umbilical stump, if left uncovered after birth, shrinks to a relatively hard, dark brown eschar, which normally separates from the abdomen by 1 to 2 weeks after birth. The central core area of the umbilicus usually is covered with skin no later than 3 to 4 weeks of age, a process that sometimes is delayed by growth of pink granulation tissue (umbilical granuloma). Transient spotty bleeding of the umbilical area after separation of the umbilical eschar is common and usually lasts no longer than a few days. Chronic drainage of clear fluid from the umbilicus suggests the presence of persistently patent urachus, a urachal cyst, or a communicating Meckel's diverticulum or omphalomesenteric duct. Erythema of the periumbilical skin with or without purulent or foul-smelling discharge suggests omphalitis, a local infection that can spread rapidly to the bloodstream and meninges. Umbilical hernias may be associated with palpable abdominal wall defects that vary from 0.5 to 5 or 6 cm in diameter and that protrude equally as far, especially when the infant is crying or straining.

A light touch of the examining fingers against the infant's abdominal wall usually contacts the liver edge, 1 to 2 cm below the right costal margin. A spleen tip may be palpated in normal infants at the left costal margin. Midline structures such as the enlarged pylorus of infants who have pyloric stenosis sometimes are difficult to palpate because of the contraction of the rectus muscles. Holding the infant's thighs in a flexed position and palpating while the infant is sucking usually will permit deep, midline palpation. The kidneys are accessible to palpation, especially at birth, by the technique of ballottement. One hand is held with the fingers in the costovertebral angle while the other hand presses downward from the anterior costal margin. The posterior hand then "flips" the kidney toward the anterior hand, which usually can "catch" the lower pole of the kidney. It also can be felt as it drops back against the posterior hand. In this manner, symmetry of kidney size can be determined. A unilaterally large kidney occurs with a multicystic kidney, unilateral hydronephrosis, Wilms' tumor, invasive neuroblastoma, or renal vein thrombosis. Other palpable abdominal masses include the dilated bladder secondary to urethral obstruction, the bilateral flank masses of hydronephrosis and polycystic kidney disease, duplications of the bowel, and rare primary hepatic tumors. Palpable masses associated with signs of intestinal obstruction (vomiting, abdominal distention, and failure to pass stool) include the meconium masses associated with imperforate anus, Hirschsprung's disease, meconium plug syndrome, and meconium ileus; midgut volvulus associated with intestinal malrotation; and the sausage-shaped, usually right lower quadrant abdominal mass of intussusception associated with bloody or currant jelly stools. Infants who have signs of intestinal obstruction and no palpable mass require immediate further evaluation for congenital atresia or stenosis of any portion of the bowel, peritonitis, and, in premature infants, necrotizing enterocolitis.

Percussion of an infant's abdomen can be helpful in determining the size of organs or masses and also outlines the relatively large area of the upper portion of the abdomen filled by the stomach. Ascites may accompany peritonitis, liver or kidney disease, and lymphangiomas of the small bowel mesentery. Bowel sounds (peristaltic sounds) are metallic tinkling sounds heard normally every 10 to 30 seconds. They occur more frequently with intestinal obstruction or gastroenteritis and are diminished with ileus, which can accompany almost any infectious process in infants, especially pneumonitis or gastroenteritis.

A rectal examination, performed with the fifth finger, can be useful in differentiating bladder from sacral masses, in palpating the uterus, and in detecting the absence of rectal feces in some infants who have Hirschsprung's disease. Some practitioners prefer to use the index finger for this examination because of its greater length, flexibility, sensitivity, and mobility.

Childhood and adolescence. The shape of the abdomen becomes increasingly scaphoid in school-age children, except for children who have exogenous obesity. Frightened, uncomfortable, or ticklish children can be examined successfully if the thighs are held in partial flexion and the abdomen is approached first with the stethoscope. While listening for bowel sounds, the stethoscope can be pushed gently into the abdomen, and areas of rigidity or tenderness can be noted. The examiner's hands should be warm, and in older children, deep breathing will enhance abdominal palpation. Another useful technique is placing the child's hand between the abdominal wall and the examiner's hand. It can be especially difficult to detect rigidity or tenderness in a crying or nonverbal child. The examiner can watch for facial grimacing and can attempt to "catch" the brief instant of relative relaxation of the abdomen at the end of expiration. The protuberant abdomen of a child whose lungs are hyperexpanded and who experiences forceful abdominal muscle contractions on expiration and sore abdominal muscles (present, for instance, in status asthmaticus) can be especially difficult to examine for intraabdominal abnormalities. Having such a child raise his or her head from the supine position usually lessens intraabdominal pain but increases abdominal muscle soreness.

Abdominal tenderness in children can be localized by the responses to direct palpation, by referred pain on rebound tenderness, by "shake" tenderness in which the child's pelvis is lifted gently off the examining table and gently shaken, by pain accompanying hyperextension of the hips (psoas sign) or external rotation of the hip with the knee held in flexion (obturator sign), and by abdominorectal palpation. Tenderness from an inflamed appendix usually is maximal in the right lower quadrant. Diffuse tenderness can accompany paralytic ileus secondary to extraabdominal or intraabdominal infection, as well as the more serious peritonitis or perforated viscus. Midline tenderness in the lower portion of the abdomen can be elicited by palpating the abdominal aorta or a full bladder.

If the abdomen is soft, the cecum and sigmoid colon often can be rolled between the examining fingers and the adjacent iliac crest. The entire colon sometimes is palpable when filled with feces in association with functional fecal retention. In normal children, the tip of the spleen and the edge of the liver may be palpable, especially on deep inspiration. The spleen commonly enlarges in association with a number of acute infectious diseases and with a number of blood dyscrasias. The liver can enlarge as a result of heart failure, hepatitis, septicemia, a primary or metastatic tumor, blood dyscrasias, and various storage diseases. Upper quadrant direct tenderness and shock tenderness (elicited by gently pounding the lower anterior rib cage), which may be signs of liver or splenic bleeding or rupture, should be investigated in all children who have sustained trauma to the abdomen.

Genitalia

By the end of the third fetal month the undifferentiated fetal gonad has developed into an ovary or, under the influence of the Y chromosome, into a testis. With production of testosterone by the fetal testis (the medulla of the fetal gonad), the wolffian duct system further develops into the epididymis, ductus deferens, and seminal vesicles; development of the müllerian duct system is inhibited by an as yet unidentified factor. The testes descend into the scrotum between the sev-

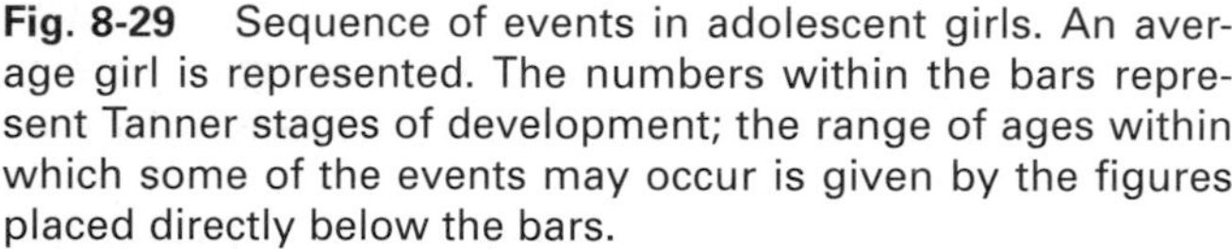

Fig. 8-29 Sequence of events in adolescent girls. An average girl is represented. The numbers within the bars represent Tanner stages of development; the range of ages within which some of the events may occur is given by the figures placed directly below the bars.

(From Marshall WA, Tanner JM: *Arch Dis Child* 45:13, 1970.)

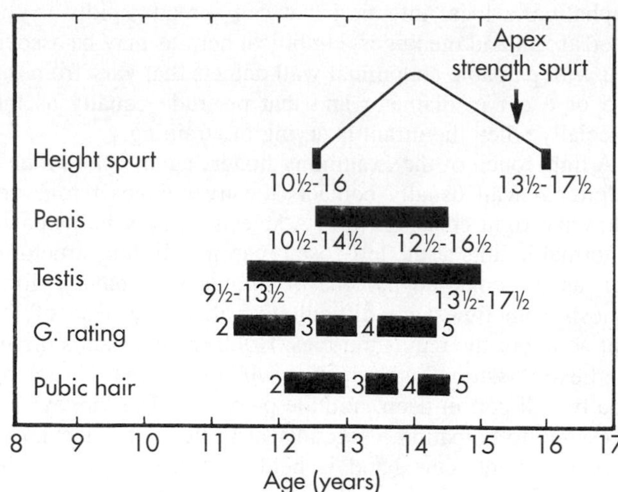

Fig. 8-30 Sequence of events in adolescent boys. An average boy is represented. The numbers within the bars represent Tanner stages of development; the range of ages within which some of the events may occur is given by the figures placed directly below the bars.

(From Marshall WA, Tanner JM: *Arch Dis Child* 45:13, 1970.)

enth and eighth months of gestation, followed by a sleeve of parietal peritoneum, the processus vaginalis, which closes off in most babies by the time of birth. At the time of birth one or more testes are undescended in 3% to 4% of male babies. Most of these descend by 3 months of age, leaving 1% of babies by age 1 year with unilateral or bilateral undescended testes. The processus vaginalis can remain patent and retain its connection with the peritoneal cavity, causing an inguinal hernia that usually is apparent within a few months after birth. A fluid-filled segment of the processus vaginalis within the scrotum, a hydrocele, is present in 10% of male babies and can be associated with an inguinal hernia. Many hydroceles apparent at birth disappear spontaneously within the first few months of life.

In the absence of fetal testosterone and another undetermined factor, the müllerian duct system develops into the fallopian tubes, uterus, and upper vagina. After birth, as a result of withdrawal of maternal estrogen, the uterus decreases in size and then grows slowly back to its birth size by age 5. By age 10 the corpus of the uterus has grown to a size equal to that of the uterine cervix. The cervix grows rapidly again in the premenarcheal years, followed by further growth of the uterine corpus.

The development of secondary sex characteristics during puberty varies considerably as to time of onset, duration, and sequential timing in both boys and girls (Figs. 8-29 and 8-30). In girls, breast development begins between the ages of 8 and 13 and is completed between the ages of 12 and 19. The development of pubic hair roughly parallels breast development. The peak velocity of growth in height occurs, on the average, 1 year after the onset of breast development, whereas menarche occurs approximately 2 years after the onset of breast development. In girls, puberty lasts between 1.5 and 6 years.

In boys, testicular enlargement precedes the development of pubic hair, processes that begin between the ages of 9½ and 13½. An increase in the size of the penis parallels an increase in testicular size, following an initial lag phase. The peak velocity of growth in height occurs later in boys than in girls, commencing at an average age of 14 years. Puberty in boys lasts between 1.8 and 4.7 years.

The stages of development during puberty in boys and girls are illustrated in Figs. 8-31 and 8-32. Sequential recording of a given child's progress can be used both to diagnose abnormal development and to reassure a worried normal adolescent.

Thorough examination of the external genitalia is mandatory immediately after birth to allow rapid evaluation of babies whose genitalia are ambiguous. The external genitalia are examined during all health maintenance examinations and in all children seeking medical attention for abdominal pain. The penis, testes, and external inguinal rings should be examined in boys, and the clitoris, labia majora and minora, vaginal orifice, urethral orifice, and external inguinal rings in girls. Internal inspection of the vagina and cervix and bimanual abdominorectal palpation of the internal genitalia are not part of the routine examination of children; they are, however, performed in the evaluation of problems such as vaginal discharge or bleeding (see the following discussion).

When the primary care physician evaluates an infant, a child, or an adolescent for suspected sexual abuse, the child and parent must be prepared with patience and with attention to their fears and concerns. The child must have some control over the position, draping, and pace of the examination and should not be restrained. The examination is least traumatic to infants and toddlers with the child supine in the mother's lap, although occasionally, other positions are used, such as supine on the examining table in a frog-leg position, in a lateral decubitus position with the knees drawn up to the chest, in a knee-chest supine position, or the knee-chest prone position. The examiner should explain and answer

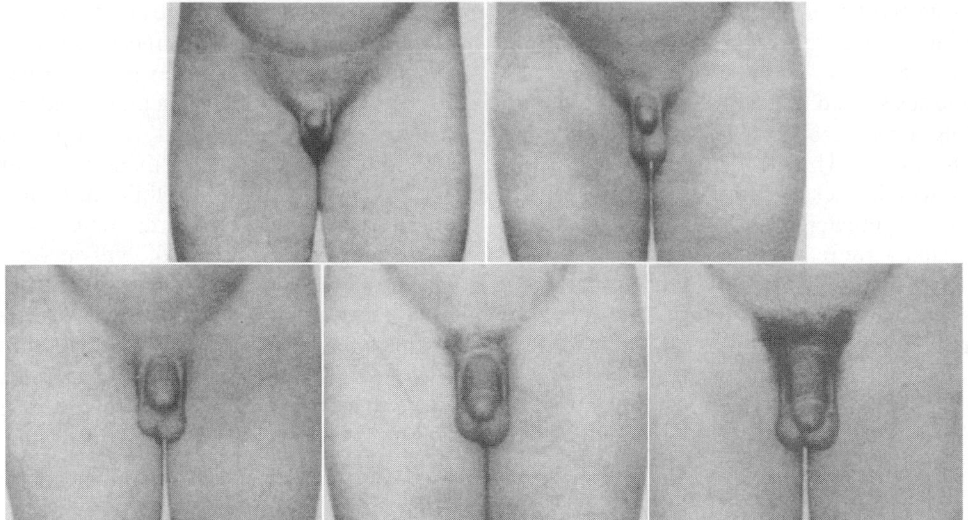

Fig. 8-31 Standards for genitalia maturity ratings in boys. Shown are Tanner stages 1 through 5 of development.

(From Tanner JM: *Growth at adolescence,* ed 2, Oxford, 1962, Blackwell.)

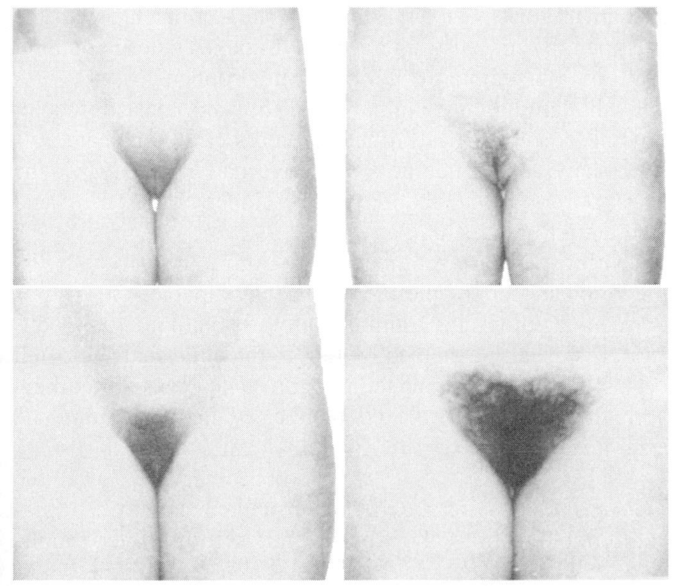

Fig. 8-32 Tanner stages 2 through 5 of development of pubic hair in girls. Stage 1 is not shown, since there is no pubic hair in this stage.

(From Tanner JM: *Growth at adolescence,* ed 2, Oxford, 1962, Blackwell.)

questions both before and during each step. After the body as a whole is inspected for signs of trauma, the external genitalia and anus are observed for old or new abrasions or lacerations (which can be facilitated by prior application of toluidine blue dye), scars, hyperpigmentation, verrucae, and enlarged orifices. The hymen is inspected for shape, stretching, injury, or thickening.[2,3] All findings should be recorded clearly, with diagrams, if necessary, for possible use in future child protective custody hearings. Culture specimens of perineal tissue or exudate, or both, are obtained routinely to detect *Neisseria gonorrhoeae;* if present, and, when otherwise suspected, culture specimens for *Chlamydia trachomatis,* herpes simplex virus, and *Trichomonas* and *Gardnerella* organisms should be obtained. Venereal warts (condyloma acuminatum) can be seen in their earliest stages after application of 3% to 5% acetic acid solution to perineal tissues; their presence suggests sexual molestation.

Newborn period. The appearance of the external genitalia at birth provides information that is useful in assessing gestational age. In boys, the testes are undescended before the thirtieth week of gestation, are high in the inguinal canal between the thirtieth and thirty-sixth weeks, and normally have completely descended into the scrotum by 40 weeks. The scrotal rugae appear, progressing inferiorly to superiorly, between the thirtieth and fortieth weeks. In girls, the labia majora are widely separated and the clitoris is prominent up to the thirty-sixth week; by 40 weeks the labia majora completely cover the labia minora and clitoris.

A white vaginal discharge, occasionally mixed with blood, can be seen for several days after birth, the result of withdrawal from the relatively high levels of maternally derived estrogen. Maternal estrogen also can cause a transient hypertrophy of the labia majora. The urethral and vaginal orifices can be visualized by downward and lateral traction on each side of the perineum (Fig. 8-33). The hymen varies in thickness and size, the central orifice usually measuring up to 4 mm in diameter in infants. Rarely is the hymen imperforate at birth.

The foreskin of the penis usually is nonretractable at birth, a condition that can persist for years. Ordinarily, sufficient retraction is possible to allow visualization of the external urethral meatus at the tip of the glans penis. The ventral surface of the penis should be inspected at birth for hypospadias (an abnormal position of the external urethral meatus located anywhere between the midline scrotum to the tip of the glans), because its presence is a contraindication to circumcision. Hypospadias may be accompanied by chordee, a fixed, downward bowing of the penis. In rare cases the urethral meatus is located on the dorsal surface of the penis, a condition known as *epispadias*. After circumcision the glans penis and the remaining lip of foreskin are swollen and erythematous for several days.

Palpation of the testes should proceed downward from the external inguinal ring to the scrotum to counteract the active cremasteric reflex in infants. This technique is important in diagnosing the undescended testis accurately. Inguinal hernias in infants occur as unilateral or bilateral inguinal and scrotal bulges that usually are reducible and may appear only with crying or straining. Hydroceles are scrotal and sometimes inguinal masses that often are attached to the testes and are nonreducible and nontender and that transilluminate.

In rare cases the appearance of the external genitalia may make it difficult to determine gender. For instance, there may be a midline phallus with apparent scrotal hypospadias and partly fused scrotal-appearing skin with no palpable scrotal masses. In this situation, careful inspection and in some cases probing of the midline of the perineum for a vaginal orifice is an important first step in diagnosing ambiguous external genitalia in a female baby, as is abdominorectal examination to palpate for the presence of a uterus.

Infancy and early childhood. Several minor physical abnormalities are common during the first years of life. In boys, ammoniacal dermatitis involving the perineum (diaper rash) in either a circumcised or an uncircumcised infant can cause balanitis, an acute inflammation of the glans penis, which sometimes is associated with purulent exudate. After an episode of balanitis, the external urethral meatus may become stenotic, causing a narrow urinary stream and prolonged emptying of the bladder. Balanitis in an uncircumcised boy can leave adhesions between the glans penis and the foreskin, preventing retraction of the foreskin.

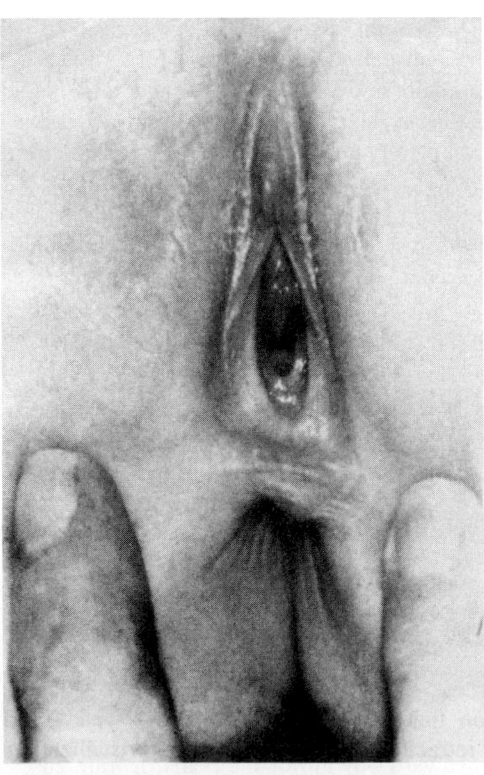

Fig. 8-33 Inspection of the infant vulva.

It is important to diagnose an undescended testis accurately because corrective surgery can protect the functioning of a normal, undescended testis only if performed during the first few years of life. An acutely tender testis may indicate torsion of the testis, orchitis, a complication of mumps that commonly occurs in young men, or epididymitis.

In female infants, paper-thin adhesions between the labia minora are common during the first few years of life, sometimes completely covering the vulvar vestibule, with a small opening through which urine escapes. These labial adhesions sometimes can be parted by applying gentle pressure laterally on the labia majora. They also will disappear if a cream containing estrogen is applied for several weeks.

Vulvovaginal discharge in preschool-age girls most often is caused by vaginal foreign bodies, usually bits of toilet paper; occasionally a specific bacterial organism can be cultured, or pinworms may be discovered. Cultures that are positive for *N. gonorrhoeae* and *C. trachomatis* almost always indicate sexual abuse. Making these diagnoses occasionally requires vaginoscopy with a special instrument, such as the Huffman vaginoscope (Fig. 8-34) or a nasal speculum, although some child abuse experts are against using any instruments when examining for possible sexual abuse. Vaginal specimens for smears and cultures can be obtained with the least pain by first instilling a small amount of sterile nutrient broth into the vagina with a medicine dropper.

Although digital examination of the vagina usually is not possible in prepubertal girls, the uterus can be palpated for size, shape, and tenderness with one hand placed over the lower portion of the abdomen and a finger of the other hand inserted into the rectum.

During a rectal examination in a girl, the cervix is the predominant part of the uterus that is palpable; the ovaries normally are not felt. Examination of the rectum in both boys and girls usually is helped by telling the child that "this will be just like having your temperature taken" and by talking with the child in a relaxed manner while performing the examination.

Late childhood. Children usually begin to have uncomfortable feelings about being undressed in front of adults

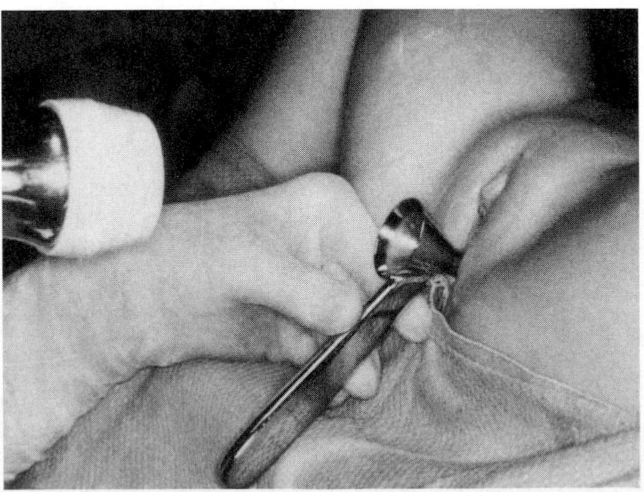

Fig. 8-34 Inspection of the vagina, using a children's vaginoscope and simple illumination with a flashlight.

by the time they reach the age of 5 or 6. Soliciting reassurance from the parent and using drapes or gowns may make the examination of school-age children easier.

Occasionally, secondary sex characteristics begin to develop in children in this age group. Evaluation of such children must distinguish among premature thelarche, premature adrenarche, premature menarche, and precocious puberty, per se.

One method for examining normally retractile testes is to palpate the scrotum with the boy squatting or sitting on the examining table with his legs crossed in the yoga position; the examiner begins to palpate over the inguinal areas and works downward onto the scrotum. This technique is especially helpful when examining boys with exogenous obesity, whose external genitalia may be "engulfed" in excess peripubic and perineal adipose tissue. By age 4 it usually is possible to palpate for an inguinal hernia over the external inguinal ring while the boy coughs, with the examining finger inserted into the scrotal tissue and slid upward into the inguinal canal. Tender, acute swelling of the scrotum can be caused by torsion of the testes, epididymitis, orchitis (often caused by mumps), or an incarcerated inguinal hernia.

Varicoceles are semi-firm masses, sometimes of equal size to the testis, palpable within the spermatic vessels, and are important to find because of their association with infertility unless surgically removed.

Adolescence. Examination of an adolescent's genitalia presents the practitioner with an opportunity to reassure the adolescent about the normal progression of the stages of puberty. The examiner should remember that adolescents have an excellent ability to deny real concerns and worries; therefore, the physician should be especially sensitive to questions that might relate to a concern about venereal disease, pregnancy, or even cancer. Honest, direct answers to the adolescent's questions, coupled with a careful description of the examination before it is performed, will help to establish a trusting relationship.

Bimanual abdominorectal palpation of the uterus, as just described, usually is adequate when examining prepubertal and virginal pubertal girls. A complete pelvic examination is indicated for any adolescent who has vaginal discharge, dysuria, pyuria, lower abdominal pain, irregular vaginal bleeding, or amenorrhea, and for a sexually active adolescent. This examination is aided by proper instruments, including a vaginoscope or small speculum, culture media, glass slides, and a cytology fixative. The physician should be patient and gentle, minimizing painful procedures and embarrassment for the patient. After the external genitalia have been inspected and the internal organs have been examined with a speculum or vaginoscope, the uterus and ovaries are palpated using the bimanual abdominovaginal technique; normally the ovaries are not palpable. Specimens should be obtained periodically in sexually active adolescents to culture for *N. gonorrhoeae* and *C. trachomatis* and to evaluate cervical cytology for herpes virus effects.

Musculoskeletal System

The changes in the musculoskeletal system of infants, children, and adolescents over time give the examiner the most visible evidence of human growth. If a child's sequential measurements of height fall within the norms of a standard growth curve, this is strong evidence not only that bone growth is normal but also that the numerous factors necessary for normal growth are operating appropriately. In addition, because of its visibility, the musculoskeletal system most often is the source of questions from parents concerning possible deviations from normal, including the possible effects of trauma, a leading cause of morbidity and mortality in children.

The outward manifestations of growth of the trunk and extremities reflect primarily growth of bone, muscle, and adipose tissue. Bone grows in the fetus starting with cartilage, then from the primary centers of ossification, primarily in the long bones. Postnatally, new bone formation occurs in secondary centers of ossification at the ends of long bones and the vertebral bodies and in the membranes of the flat bones of the cranium and clavicle. In addition to longitudinal growth of long bones and vertebral bodies, internal remodeling takes place throughout infancy and childhood, resulting in less dense bone, a changing thickness of the bone cortex, and changing amounts of red marrow and fat within the diaphyses of bone. In addition to hormonal factors, bone remodeling is influenced by mechanical forces caused by muscle attachments and gravity. Bone growth is completed with ossification of the growth cartilage and union of the epiphyses and diaphyses of long bones by age 21. The roentgenographic appearance of the onset, size, and shape of secondary ossification centers can be compared with established norms in determining the bone age, a measurement that despite its variability can be helpful in assessing children who are suspected of having abnormal growth.

Growth in stature predominates in the lower extremities before puberty and in the trunk during puberty. The distal extremities reach adult size before the proximal extremities—thus the common complaint of preadolescent children that their feet are too big.

Muscle growth, which results from increases in the number, size, and length of cells, proceeds throughout childhood according to the following increasing proportions of muscle mass to body weight: 1:5 to 1:4 at birth, 1:3 in early adolescence, and 2:5 in early maturity. A spurt in the increase in muscle cell numbers occurs at age 2, and maximal increase occurs between the ages of 10 and 16. Muscle cell size increases faster in girls than in boys between the ages of 3 and 10, but after age 14, boys surpass girls in both the number and size of muscle cells. The number of muscle fibers increases slowly until the fifth decade of life.

A thorough evaluation of the musculoskeletal system should be part of every newborn examination, every child health maintenance examination, and the examination of any child who has an abnormality of growth, stature, or gait. It includes an appraisal of (1) posture, position, and gross deformities, (2) skin color, temperature, and tenderness, (3) bone or joint tenderness, (4) range of joint motion, (5) muscle size, symmetry, and strength, and (6) the configuration and motility of the back.

Newborn period. The position and appearance of the extremities at birth can reflect intrauterine position. The folded position of the lower extremities on the abdomen in the fetus results in the common appearance in newborns of externally rotated, somewhat bowed, lower extremities and inverted feet. A baby born after a breech presentation often has markedly flexed hips and extended knees. Traction on the brachial plexus during delivery can cause what usually is a temporary paresis of the proximal upper extremity muscles (Erb palsy), most often appearing as an asymmetrical Moro reflex (see p. 108). Another common cause of an asymmetrical Moro reflex resulting from a birth injury is a fractured clavicle, which can be confirmed by palpating an area of crepitance, usually over the distal third of the clavicle.

Gross deformities should be recognized at birth, both for early treatment and for possible clues to generalized genetic or metabolic diseases. Relatively common deformities include short or absent extremities, absence of one bone in an extremity, hypertrophy of one bone in an extremity or of an entire half of the body (hemihypertrophy), extra fingers or toes (polydactyly), webbed or fused fingers or toes (syndactyly), and annular constricting bands around a portion of an extremity with or without distal amputation or lack of development. The ratio of extremity length to body length should be noted. In a normal newborn the ratio of the upper segment of the body to the lower segment (above and below the symphysis pubis) is approximately 1.7:1. In various types of dwarfism the extremities alone may be short, as in achondroplasia, or both extremities and trunk may be shortened, as in Morquio's disease. The entire length of the vertebral column should be examined and palpated for bony defects with or without overlying skin defects.

The joints should be tested for range of motion, noting any asymmetry, undue tightness, or contractures, as well as the muscle tone. A floppy or hypotonic baby may have CNS disease, a metabolic disturbance, primary muscle disease, or anterior horn cell disease. Limited unilateral joint motion with or without associated bone or joint tenderness and fever should be investigated extensively as a possible sign of osteomyelitis.

Perhaps the most important part of the examination of a newborn's extremities is the examination of the lower extremities, giving special attention to the hips and feet. The hips are examined particularly to rule out developmental hip dysplasia, a condition that is relatively easy to treat, with good results, *if* treatment is started early. The examiner tests for a dislocated femoral head by abducting one hip at a time and feeling over the greater trochanter for a click or clunk when the femoral head passes back into the acetabulum (Ortolani's sign). This maneuver usually requires 70 to 80 degrees of hip abduction. Downward pressure over the hips transmitted through the flexed knee can be used to attempt to produce posterior dislocation of the femoral head in the Barlow test (Fig. 8-35). The click or clunk of the reducing femoral head should be distinguished from the clicks felt with rotation of the hip and the click felt with simultaneous movement of the knee. After the newborn period, the hip click (Ortolani's sign) heard with congenitally dislocated hips disappears, and other signs become helpful in making this diagnosis. The thigh may appear shorter on the

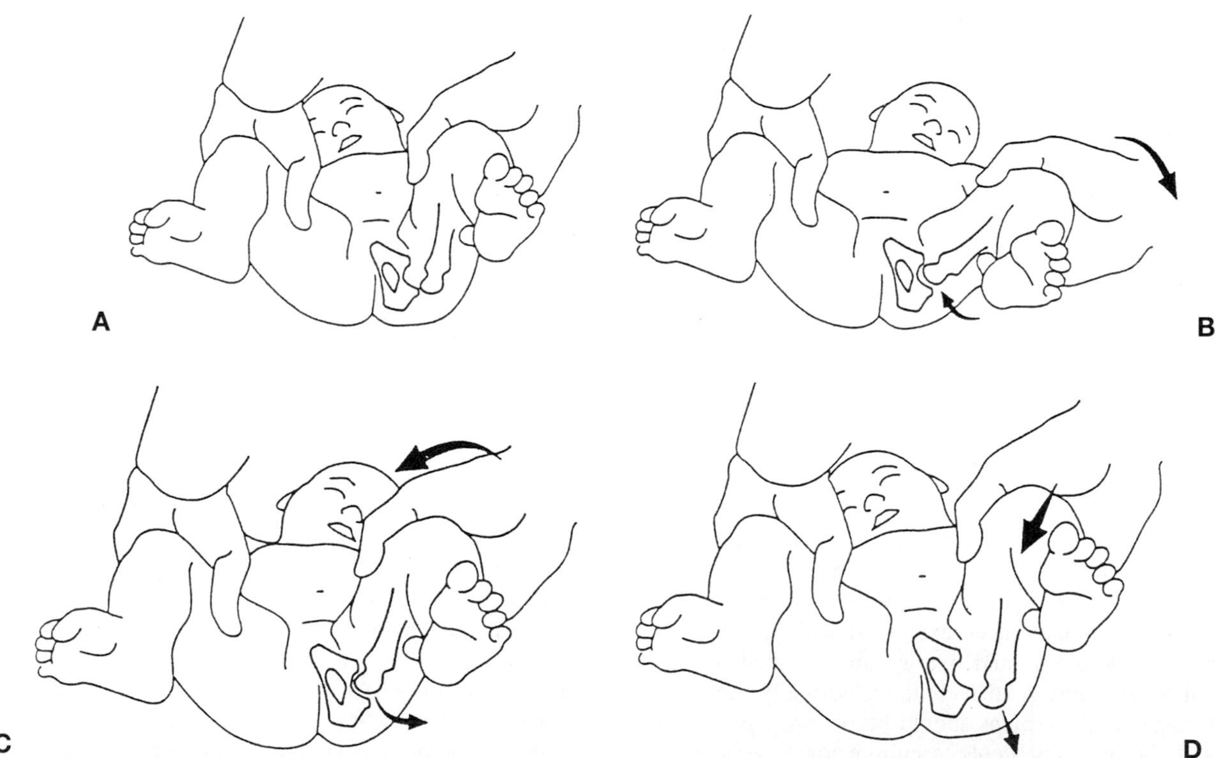

Fig. 8-35 **A** and **B**, The Ortolani maneuver reduces a posteriorly dislocated hip. The affected hip is gently abducted while the femoral head is reduced with an anteriorly directed force provided by the fingers placed over the greater trochanter. **C** and **D**, The Barlow test for dislocation of a located hip. This is done by gently adducting the examined hip, while directing a posterior force across the hip.

(From Pizzutillo PD: *Practical orthopaedics in primary care*, New York, 1977, McGraw-Hill.)

affected side, the thigh skinfolds may be asymmetrical (although this occurs in some normal babies), and the hip will have limited abduction on the affected side. Tight hip abductors in the neonatal period are not a sign of congenital hip dislocation.

A newborn's and an infant's feet often appear flat because of a plantar fat pad that gradually disappears during the first 1 to 2 years of life. The most severe foot deformity at birth is the talipes equinovarus deformity, or clubfoot. True clubfoot deformities cannot be corrected passively, nor do they correct with stroking of the foot's lateral side. This deformity comprises fixed forefoot adduction, fixed inversion especially of the hindfoot, equinus position, internal tibial torsion, and small calf muscles.

Viewing the sole of the resting foot (not spontaneously inverted or everted) allows observation for the normal single anteroposterior plantar axis. In metatarsus varus deformity the forefoot is adducted in relation to the hindfoot, thus describing two anteroposterior axes, and this position is not correctable by stroking the foot's lateral border. In calcaneovalgus deformity the foot is dorsiflexed and everted. See Chapter 138, Foot and Leg Problems, for a complete discussion of developmental orthopedic variations of the lower extremities.

Infancy and early childhood. An infant's lower extremities often remain bowlegged with externally rotated feet for the first 1 to 2 years of life. With ambulation, the feet gradually assume the straight-ahead position, and the knock-knee, or genu valgum, position normally is seen between the ages of 2 and 6 or longer.

Severe bowing of the legs raises the question of rickets or epiphyseal damage from inflammation or trauma (Blount disease). The infant who toes in should be examined for metatarsus varus, internal tibial torsion, or femoral anteversion. Flatfeet, or feet without a longitudinal arch, are common, especially in children who have generalized ligamentous laxity.

A toddler's lower extremities are examined best by first observing the spontaneous gait with the infant undressed. The normal gait usually is wide based and somewhat unstable, with prominent lumbar lordosis. Then, especially if positional deformities are noted, a careful examination of the hips, knees, legs, ankles, and feet with the child in the supine position can confirm the presence of any fixed deformity. A child who has a limp should be examined carefully for signs of trauma; localized bone or joint tenderness from fracture or infection; joint effusions with limited range of motion from trauma, infection, or noninfectious arthritis; peripheral muscle weakness; unilateral or bilateral spasticity, especially manifested by a tight Achilles tendon; and proximal muscle weakness, particularly weakness resulting from unrecognized hip disease such as congenital dislocated hip or coxa vara. Testing for coxa vara can be done by having the child raise one foot while standing. This normally produces an elevation in the contralateral hip. Inability of the hip abductors to elevate the contralateral hip is considered a positive Trendelenburg sign (Fig. 8-36).

Child abuse should be suspected in all cases of trauma if (1) the history of the injury is inconsistent with its severity; (2) there are signs of multiple blunt trauma to the extremities, trunk (especially the buttocks), and face; (3) trauma is recurrent; and (4) significant delay occurs between the episode of injury and the request for medical attention.

The child who has a tender elbow held in pronation, usually after a pulling episode (nursemaid elbow), suffers from

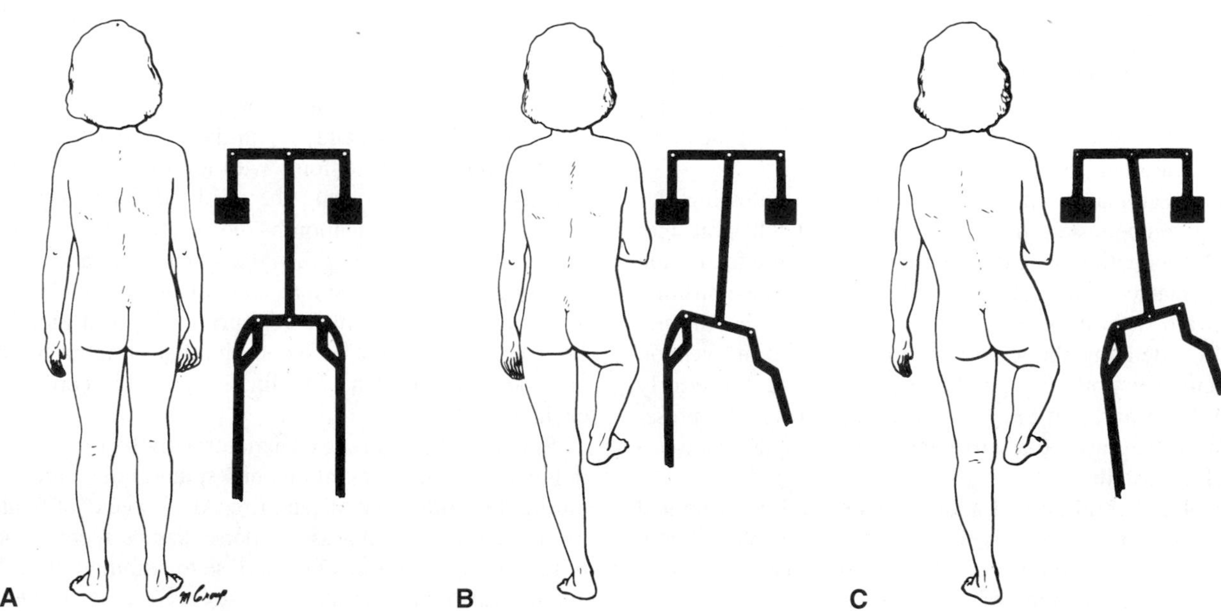

Fig. 8-36 Trendelenburg sign, showing weakness of the gluteus medius muscle. **A,** Normal standing. **B,** Dropping of the pelvis of the contralateral side when standing on the affected leg. **C,** Compensation for weakness when walking by shifting the center of gravity of the trunk to elevate the pelvis on the opposite side.

(From Ferguson AM Jr: *Orthopaedic surgery in infancy and childhood,* ed 5, Baltimore, 1981, Williams & Wilkins.)

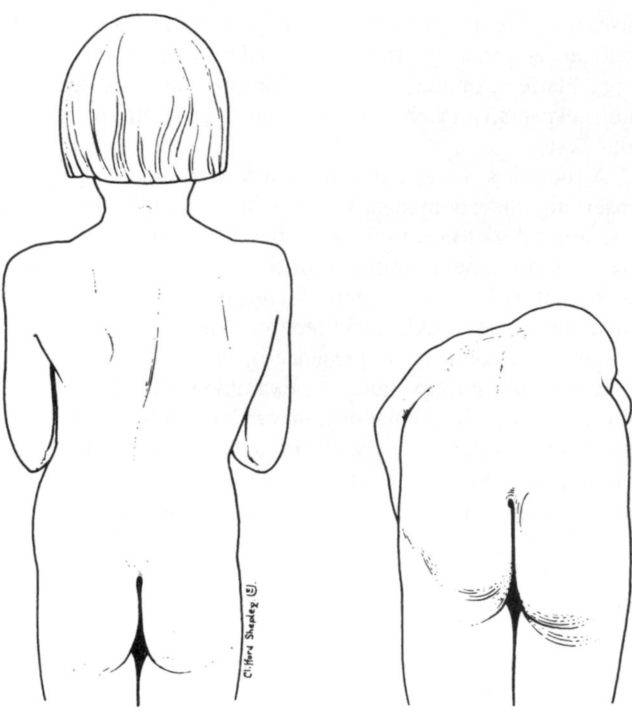

Fig. 8-37 Examination for scoliosis.
(From James JIP: *Scoliosis,* Edinburgh, 1976, E&S Livingstone.)

subluxation of the radial head, which can be reduced easily by supinating the arm while applying pressure to the radial head.

Late childhood and adolescence. A limp in a child between the ages of 4 and 8, especially if accompanied by knee pain, suggests Legg-Calvé-Perthes disease, as well as the conditions previously mentioned. The same symptoms in a child between the ages of 9 and 12 may be caused by a slipped femoral capital epiphysis. Tenderness over the tibial tubercle may be a sign of Osgood-Schlatter disease. Painful heels can be caused by partial evulsion of the Achilles tendon, retrocalcaneal bursitis, or plantar fasciitis.

In the examination of an injured knee, the following elements should be tested: the medial and lateral collateral ligaments, by abducting and adducting the tibia on the femur; the cruciate ligaments, by pulling the tibia forward, then pushing it backward with the knee flexed; the medial and lateral menisci, by extending the knee with the foot held in eversion and then inversion; the patella, by pushing it posteriorly against the femur; and the joint space for effusion, by pressing over the suprapatellar bursa and then attempting ballottement of the patella.

School-age children and adolescents should be examined for scoliosis, or lateral curvature of the vertebral column. Significant spinal curvature can be seen with the child standing erect; lesser degrees of curvature can be observed by having the child bend forward approximately 50 degrees, letting the shoulders droop forward and the arms hang freely. The examiner then looks for a unilateral elevation of the lower thoracic ribs and flank, which accompanies the rotational deformity of scoliosis (Fig. 8-37).

Nervous System

Compared with other organ systems, the manifestations of nervous system growth in infants and children are the most dynamic. Therefore the definitions of normal for any sign that reflects the state of the nervous system or one of its parts are critically age dependent. These norms also demonstrate wide variation among individuals, as well as within a single individual on different days and under variable conditions. The growth and integrity of the growing nervous system can be assessed in two ways. One way is to describe the changes in a child's abilities in various behavioral areas over time, in reference to established norms; this "developmental assessment" is discussed in Chapter 20 (Thirteen), Developmental Surveillance and Intervention. The other method is neurological assessment, in which often-changing physical signs that reflect the state of subsystems of the nervous system are described over time. The developmental stage depends partly on the neurological stage, but it also is influenced greatly by the child's environmental experiences. The major goal of neurological assessment in children is to monitor the maturation of the nervous system, although the methods described for localizing nervous system lesions in adults are useful in evaluating certain problems in children.

The nervous system grows most rapidly during fetal and early postnatal life, reaching approximately one fourth the adult size at birth, half by age 1, four fifths by age 3, and nine tenths by age 7. At the cellular level there are two distinct peaks of growth rate. The first involves neuroblasts, which multiply between 10 and 18 weeks of fetal life; after this time, the number of neuronal cells probably increases very little. The second and more striking spurt of brain growth occurs between midgestation and approximately 18 months of age and reflects multiplication of glial cells, production of myelin by the glial cells, and development of dendrites and synaptic connections. Myelination continues relatively rapidly until age 4, after which it gradually increases to adult levels.

The growth of the spinal cord, after fusion of the neural folds cranially and caudally, initially is most rapid in the lumbar and cervical regions, with the thoracic region developing most rapidly during the third trimester of pregnancy. During the third fetal month, the developing vertebral column grows more rapidly than the spinal cord, and as a result, the cordal end of the spinal cord moves cranially from the level of the fourth lumbar vertebra in the fifth month to the adult level of the first or second lumbar vertebra by the second postnatal month. Myelination of the cord proceeds cephalocaudad.

Spontaneous and reflexive motor activity, reflecting developing muscular innervation and spinal reflex arcs, begins during the tenth week of fetal life. At 12 weeks of fetal age, a primitive rooting and grasp response can be seen; withdrawal of the lower extremities in response to stimulation of the feet and the gastrocnemius stretch reflex are seen at 16 weeks; by 19 weeks, regular respiratory movements are seen in response to hypoxia. Tonic myotactic reflexes, responsible for the recoil of an extended extremity, are well developed in the term infant. The rhythmicity of motor neuron activity, which is responsible for jerky repetitive movements during activity

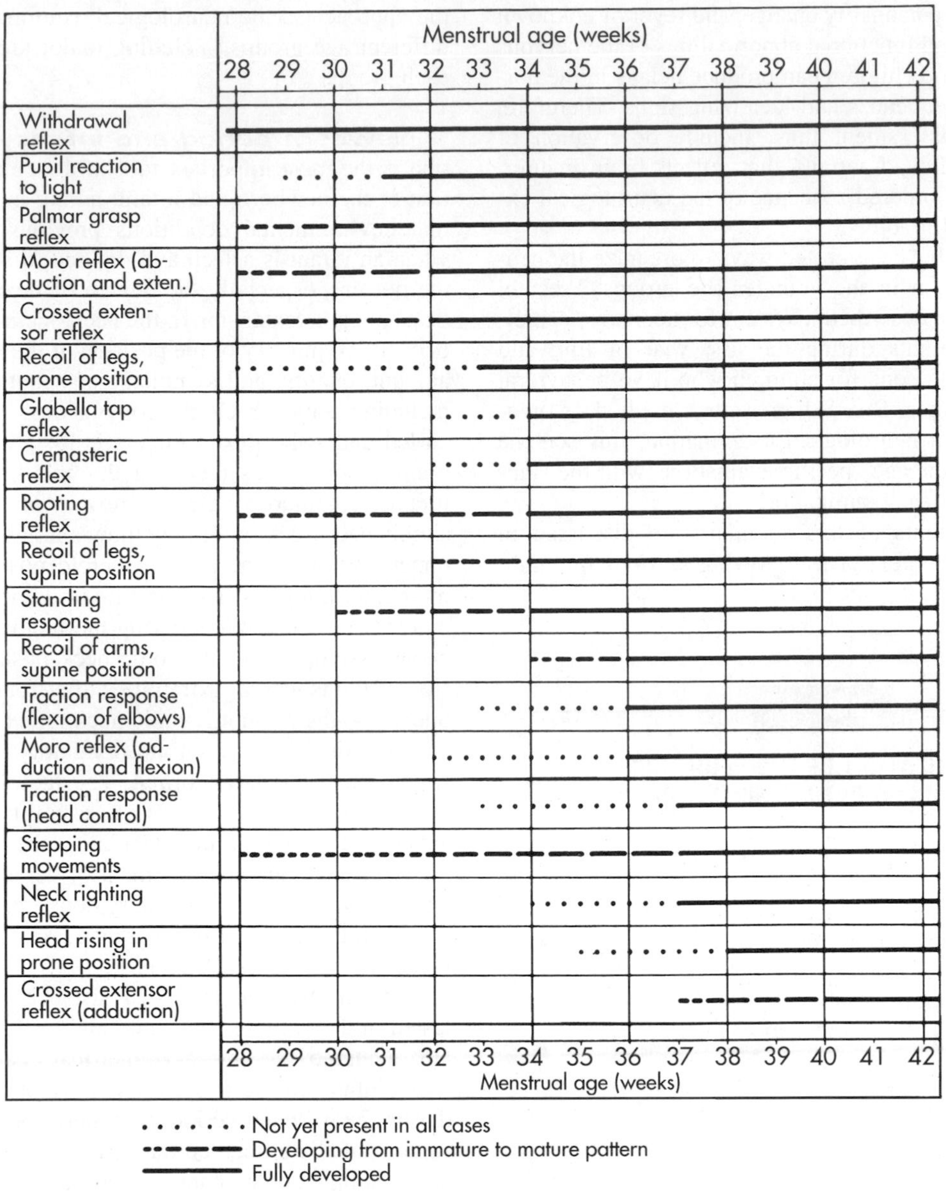

Menstrual age (weeks)
28 29 30 31 32 33 34 35 36 37 38 39 40 41 42

Withdrawal reflex
Pupil reaction to light
Palmar grasp reflex
Moro reflex (abduction and exten.)
Crossed extensor reflex
Recoil of legs, prone position
Glabella tap reflex
Cremasteric reflex
Rooting reflex
Recoil of legs, supine position
Standing response
Recoil of arms, supine position
Traction response (flexion of elbows)
Moro reflex (adduction and flexion)
Traction response (head control)
Stepping movements
Neck righting reflex
Head rising in prone position
Crossed extensor reflex (adduction)

28 29 30 31 32 33 34 35 36 37 38 39 40 41 42
Menstrual age (weeks)

• • • • • • • Not yet present in all cases
- - - - Developing from immature to mature pattern
——— Fully developed

Fig. 8-38 Developmental sequence of various reflexes and motor automatisms.
(From Davis JA, Dobbing J, editors: *Scientific foundations of paediatrics,* ed 2, Baltimore, 1981, University Park Press.)

(e.g., the jerking jaw movements that accompany crying), increases with increasing gestational age. At term, stretch reflexes, such as the knee jerk, are diminished by sleep, whereas exteroceptive reflexes (superficial abdominal and Babinski reflexes) are not.

The normal sequence of changes in an infant's posture, muscle tone, and reflexes that occurs with increasing gestational age from 28 to 40 weeks has been described by several observers and, despite their differences, can be used in assessing a neonate's gestational (menstrual) age (Fig. 8-38). Similarly, the persistence and eventual cessation of certain characteristics of the infant's posture, tone, and reflexes follow a defined pattern with age. Changes in the infant's and child's developmental abilities (see Chapter 20 [Thirteen], Developmental Surveillance and Intervention) also are based on the continuing maturation of the nervous system.

An additional behavioral characteristic of the maturing nervous system is the change in sleep-wake cycles with age. The neonate's sleep-wake cycle usually is quite irregular, but it becomes regular by 15 weeks of age. Rapid eye movement (REM) sleep occurs during a greater proportion of sleeping time in infants than in adults. A small number of neonates are found to have irregular respirations during sleep, sometimes to the point of apnea, a condition that has been discarded as a precursor of sudden infant death syndrome (SIDS; see Chapter 269).

A neurological examination should be performed on every neonate and on infants and preschool children during health maintenance visits. Other indications for a careful neurological assessment include developmental delay, failure in school, abnormal social behavior, headache, head trauma, seizures, sensory disturbances, changes in states of consciousness, abnormal gait, recent personality change, and fever of unknown origin. Structural and functional abnormalities of the nervous system of infants and children can produce delays in the normal maturational sequences and localizing signs. Therefore, the neurological assessment must include observation of spontaneous and elicited activity that reflects brain maturation, as well as the ordered sequence of the neurological examination as used for adults.

Several authors have suggested ways to organize the neurological examination in the younger age groups. Prechtel and Beintema[6] have described a system for neonates; Amiel-Tison,[1] one for infants during the first year of life; and Touwen and Prechtl,[7] one for children who have behavioral or learning disabilities. Box 8-1 presents a method of organizing the data of a neurological examination; this scheme combines parts of the age-specific evaluations with the standard adult neurological examination.

Various components of this summary are discussed in other chapters in this text. The following sections highlight the approach to the neurological examination of children of different age groups, including major areas of emphasis for each group.

BOX 8-1

ORGANIZATION OF THE PEDIATRIC NEUROLOGICAL EXAMINATION

- Conditions under which the examination is conducted
  - Child's behavioral state
  - Environmental conditions
- Mental status
  - State of consciousness
  - Language (receptive and expressive)
  - Cognitive functioning
  - Mood
  - Social and self-awareness
- Station and gait
- Head
  - Skull
  - Cranial nerves I to XII
- Motor
  - Muscle size, symmetry, contractures, tone, and strength
  - Spontaneous activity when prone, supine, sitting, standing, and walking, including fine and gross motor abilities
  - Resistance to passive stretch
  - Coordination
  - Involuntary movements, including fasciculations, tremor, chorea, athetosis, dystonia, and myotonic jerks
- Sensory
- Reflexes
  - Neonatal
  - Deep tendon reflexes, including plantar response
  - Abdominal, cremasteric, and anal reflexes
  - Clonus
- Autonomic nervous system
  - Cardiac and respiratory rate, bladder functioning, temperature control

Newborn period and infancy. Careful observation is the most important tool in the neurological examination of the newborn and infant, taking into account the optimal environmental conditions previously described. Even when an infant is asleep and dressed, the examiner can note the posture, especially the degree of flexion of the extremities; any hyperextension of the neck, including overt opisthotonos; the symmetry of the position of the extremities; and the amount, quality, and symmetry of spontaneous movements, including tonic or clonic convulsions. Holding the thumb curled under the flexed fingers is a sign present with many brain abnormalities (cerebral thumb). In normal premature infants, continuous athetoid movements are common (e.g., simultaneous flexion of the elbow and internal rotation of the upper portion of the arm). Athetoid postures also are common in term infants. Tremor with or without crying is seen in many healthy newborns during the first days of life. Spontaneous assumption of the tonic neck position, that is, extension of the isolateral extremities after rotation of the head to one side—the asymetric tonic neck reflex (ATNR)—may occur in normal infants, but an obligatory ATNR (one that always is present) is abnormal. The face is observed for expression (alert, bland, fussing, crying); symmetry of eye closure after a tap on the glabella (glabella reflex); and symmetry of position and movement of the eyes, including presence of symmetry and pupillary constriction and blinking of the eyelids in response to a hand clap approximately 12 inches from the infant's face.

With the baby undressed, resistance to passive stretch is tested in the extremities, trunk, and neck, noting particularly any symmetrical and asymmetrical increase or decrease. Many infants in whom spasticity develops later are hypotonic during the neonatal period. Symmetry of the biceps, patellar, superficial abdominal, cremasteric, and anal reflexes is noted, and eliciting ankle clonus (recording the number of beats obtained) is attempted. The palmar and plantar grasps are tested (Fig. 8-39) for differences of intensity between the two sides (unilaterally decreased in Erb palsy, for instance) or bilateral absence, as with cord lesions. As shown in Fig. 8-39, it is important to press the infant's palm from the ulnar side, with the infant's head in the midline position. Babinski's reflex (with a flexor response and fanning of the toes), which is expected in normal newborns, is tested for symmetry, as is the withdrawal reflex of the lower extremities.

The rooting response is elicited while the baby's hands are held against the chest (Fig. 8-40). In addition to the response shown, with stimulation of the upper lip, the mouth is opened and the head is retroflexed; with stimulation of the lower lip, the mouth opens and the jaw drops. This reflex is absent in depressed infants; when the examiner's fingers are placed into the depressed infant's mouth, the sucking response is decreased in strength, frequency of sucks, and duration.

In the traction response test (Fig. 8-41), the examiner pulls the supine infant into a sitting position and notes the degree of resistance to extension of the arms at the elbow and the degree to which the head is held upright. In a term infant some degree of flexion of the elbow is maintained, and head

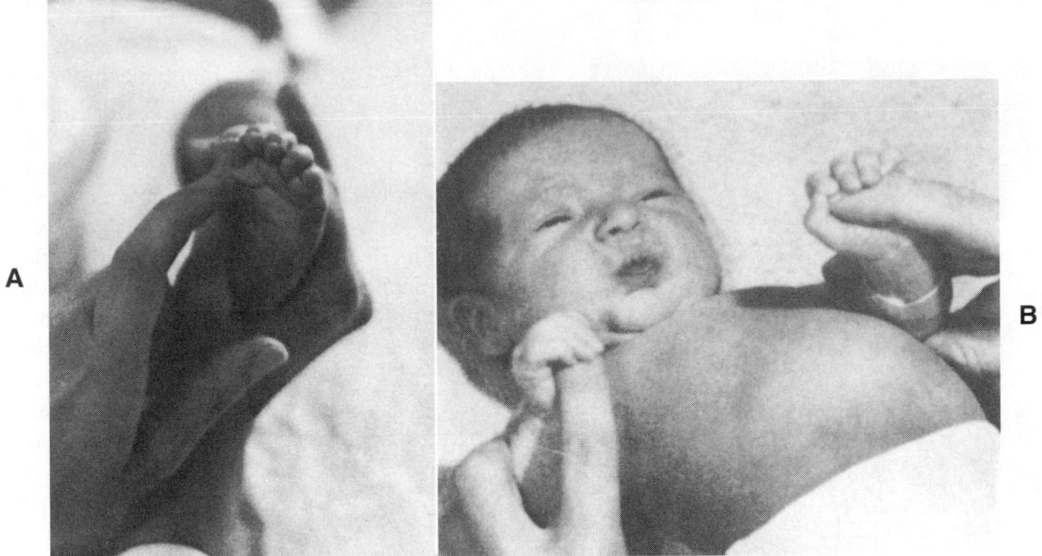

Fig. 8-39 **A,** Plantar grasp. **B,** Palmar grasp.

(**A** from Whaley LF, Wong DL: *Nursing care of infants and children,* ed 4, St Louis, 1991, Mosby; **B** from Prechtl H: *The neurological examination of the full-term newborn infant,* ed 2, London, 1977, Heinemann.)

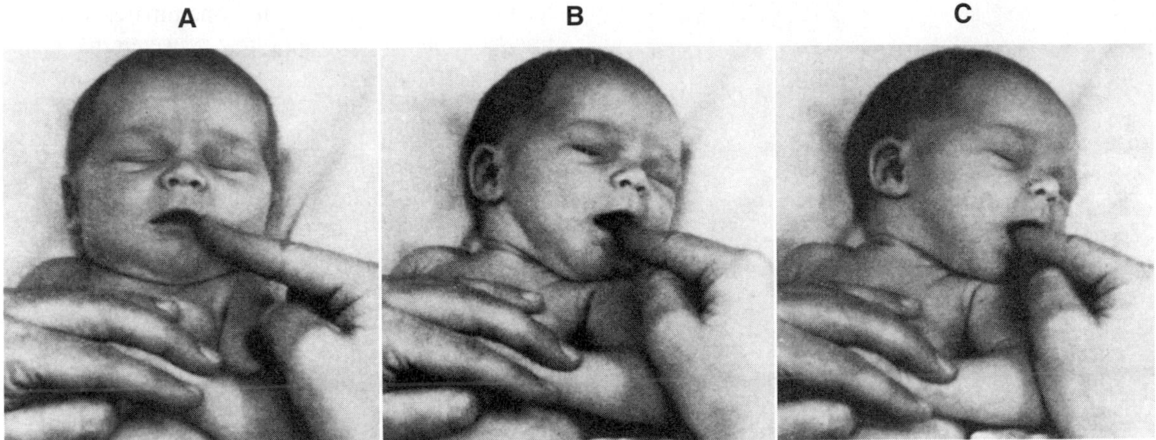

Fig. 8-40 Rooting response. **A,** Stimulation. **B,** Head turning. **C,** Grasping with the mouth.

(From Prechtl H: *The neurological examination of the full-term newborn infant,* ed 2, London, 1977, Heinemann.)

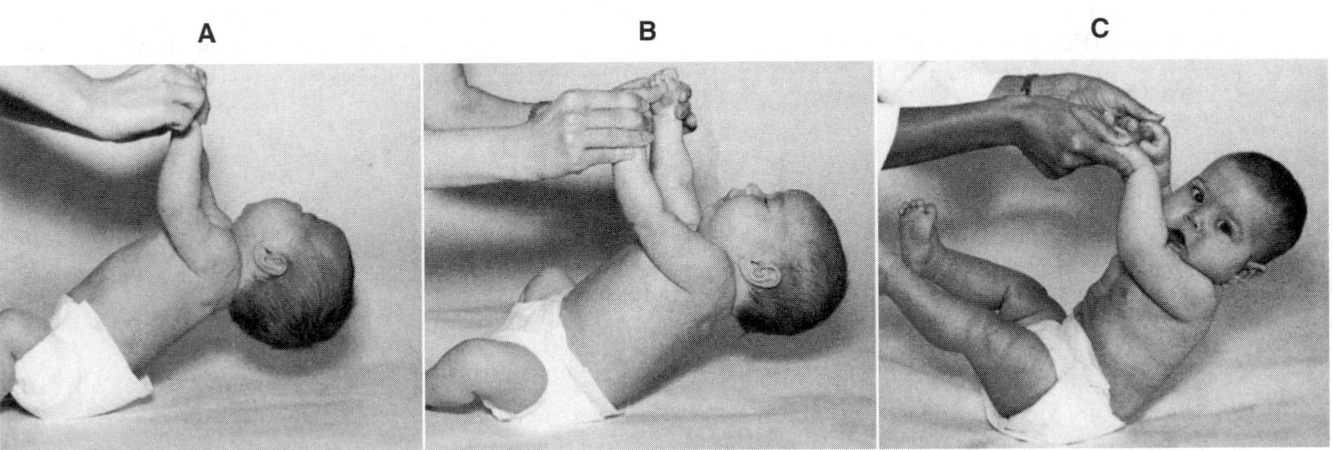

Fig. 8-41 Sitting development. **A,** First 4 weeks or so: complete head lag when being pulled into sitting position. **B,** About 2 months: considerable, but not complete, head lag when being pulled into sitting position. **C,** 4 months: no head lag when being pulled into sitting position.

(From Whaley LF, Wong DL: *Nursing care of infants and children,* ed 4, St Louis, 1991, Mosby.)

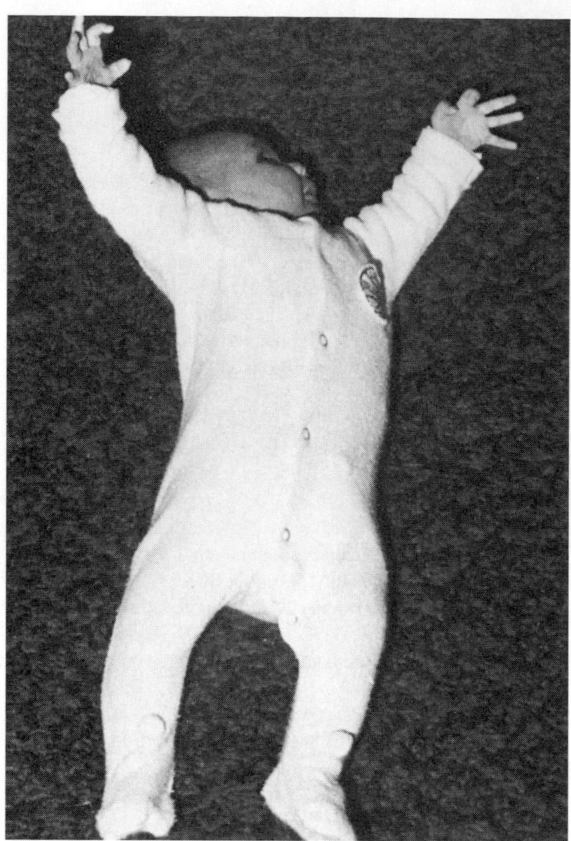

Fig. 8-42 Moro reflex.
(From Whaley LF, Wong DL: *Nursing care of infants and children,* ed 4, St Louis, 1991, Mosby.)

control is relatively weak, with neither head flexors nor extensors predominating.

The Moro reflex is a critically important sign of an intact nervous system, particularly during the neonatal period. It is best elicited by supporting the infant's supine body in one hand, then suddenly allowing the head supported by the other hand to drop a few centimeters during a moment when the head is midline and the neck muscles are relaxed. A complete Moro reflex consists of symmetrical abduction of the arms at the shoulder, extension of the forearm at the elbow, and extension of the fingers (Fig. 8-42), all followed by adduction of the arms at the shoulder and crying. The Moro reflex also can be elicited by holding the supine baby in both arms and then suddenly lowering the entire body about 12 inches *or* by producing a sudden loud noise that startles the baby.

The prone infant is observed for spontaneous head movements (brief lifting or turning from side to side), spontaneous crawling movements, and the incurvation, or Galant, reflex (lateral curvation of the trunk after stimulation with a finger or pin along a paravertebral line from the shoulder to the buttocks about 3 cm from the midline). The infant then is held prone in the air with the examiner's hands around the chest. The normal newborn is somewhat flaccid during this maneuver, but the hypertonic or opisthotonic baby will lift the head and extend the lower extremities to varying degrees. While holding the infant upright with the examiner's hands placed beneath the axillae from behind, the placing and stepping responses are noted. In the placing response, the dorsum of one foot is allowed to brush against the undersurface of a tabletop edge and is followed normally by simultaneous flexion of the knees and hips and placement of the stimulated foot on the table. In the stepping response, the soles of the feet are allowed to touch the surface of the table, which elicits alternating stepping movements with both legs.

Throughout the neurological examination, the practitioner should note the quality and duration of the infant's cry, and he or she should listen for the high-pitched, excessive, or weak cries that can accompany brain lesions. Cranial nerve testing is completed by testing the corneal and jaw jerk reflexes (cranial nerve V); the response during rotation of the upright infant's eyes to turning in the same direction he or she is moved while being held upright facing the examiner with the examiner's hands gripping the baby in the axillae (cranial nerve VIII); the gag reflex, symmetrical elevation of the palate and swallowing movements (cranial nerves IX and X); and by observing for non–injury-related torticollis (cranial nerve XI) and the symmetry of the tongue, including observation for fasciculations (cranial nerve XII).

The results of all these maneuvers occasionally indicate a localized brain lesion, such as hemiparesis secondary to intracranial bleeding. More often, however, the general state of the infant's nervous system is determined to be normal, hyperexcitable, apathetic, or comatose. The physician must then decide what further diagnostic tests are indicated and the frequency of follow-up examinations.

As the infant matures, the neonatal reflexes (automatisms) described above disappear. Persistence of neonatal reflexes beyond age-appropriate norms for their disappearance usually indicates nervous system abnormality. Some of the techniques for examining neonates are continued during the first year to ascertain whether strength and coordination have developed further. For instance, a normal 3-month-old infant no longer demonstrates head lag when pulled to a sitting position; a 5-month-old infant lifts its head from the supine position when about to be pulled up; and he or she sits without support between 5 and 8 months of age. The infant usually walks without support between 12 and 18 months of age.

It is important to monitor the development of hand coordination. A normal infant can reach and grasp objects by 5 months of age, transfer objects from hand to hand by 7 months, and pick up a raisin using a pincer grasp by 10 months (Fig. 8-43). After 8 months of age, a normal infant demonstrates symmetrical parachute and lateral propping reactions. The parachute reflex can be assessed using a flinging motion of the ventrally suspended infant toward the examination table, which should elicit extension of the arms. In the lateral propping reaction, the sitting infant is pushed to one side, and the arms should extend to prevent falling. During these maneuvers the examiner looks for asymmetrical movements.

Early and late childhood. Further growth of the nervous system in infants and children is monitored by observing walking, the development of speech and language abilities, interaction with parents, and the ability to manipulate small objects, use pencils and crayons, climb and run,

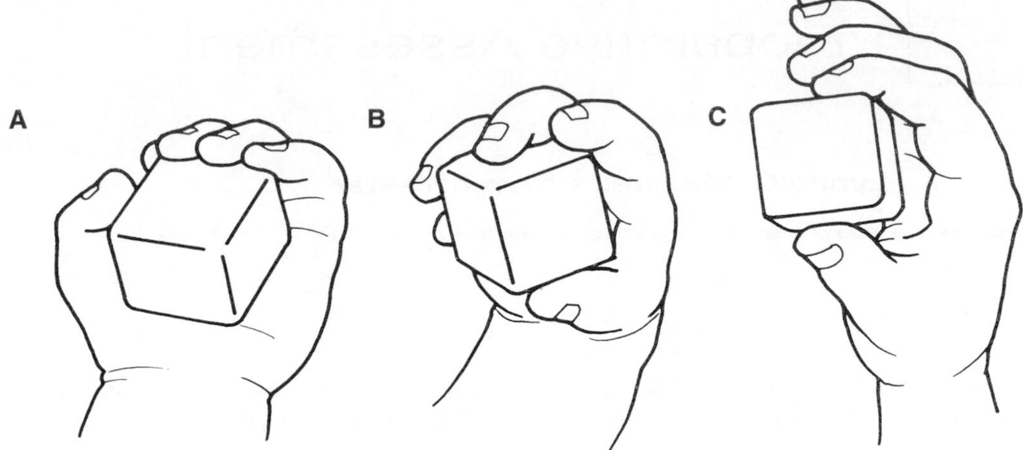

Fig. 8-43 Manipulation. **A,** 6 months: immature palmar grasp of a cube. **B,** 8 months: grasp at the intermediate stage. **C,** 1 year: mature pincer grasp of a cube.

throw and catch a ball, and follow simple directions. Muscle strength in the lower extremities is best tested by observing gait, heel and toe walking, standing and hopping on one leg, and the ability to rise from the floor from a supine position. Coordination can be observed in all these maneuvers, as well as in heel-to-shin, finger-to-nose pointing, and tandem walking. If the child's development is delayed or if the child has a history of school failure, further testing of neurophysiological maturation (described in Chapter 20 [Thirteen], Developmental Surveillance and Intervention) can help define both abilities and areas that need special attention.

As with infants, the neurological examination of school-age children who have nervous system abnormalities usually defines some degree of maturational delay. Localizing neurological signs are less common, occurring in children most often as a result of traumatic intracranial bleeding or brain tumors or after CNS infection.

Adolescence. Although reading ability and comprehension, improved coordination, and increased strength all can be used to monitor further neuromuscular maturation in adolescents, the neurological examination in this age group is similar to the adult examination. When evaluating a young person's mental status, the examiner should remember that many normal adolescents display variable mood swings, confused thinking, and resistance to authority.

REFERENCES

1. Amiel-Tison C: A method for neurological evaluation within the first year of life, *Ciba Found Symb* (59):107, 1978.
2. Berenson AB: A longitudinal study of hymenal morphology, *Pediatrics* 95:490, 1995.
3. Heger A., Emans SJ, editors: *Evaluation of the sexually abused child: a medical textbook and photographic atlas,* New York, 1992, Oxford University Press.
4. Jones Kenneth Lyons: *Smith's recognizable patterns of human malformation,* Philadelphia, 1991, WB Saunders.
5. Klaus MH, Kennell JH: *Bonding: the beginnings of parent-infant attachment,* St Louis, 1983, Mosby.
6. Prechtl H, Beintema D: *The neurological examination of the full term newborn infant,* ed 2, London, 1977, Heinemann.
7. Touwen BCL, Prechtl H: *The neurological examination of the child with minor dysfunction,* London, 1970, Heinemann.
8. Zadnik K, et al: The effect of parental history of myopia in children's eye size, *JAMA* 271:1823, 1994.

SUGGESTED READINGS

American Academy of Pediatrics: Eye examination and vision screening in infants, children and young adults, *Pediatrics* 98:153, 1996.

American Academy of Pediatrics, Task Force on Newborn and Infant Hearing: Newborn and infant hearing loss: detection and intervention, *Pediatrics* 103:527, 1999.

Davis JA, Dobbing J: *Scientific foundations of paediatrics,* ed 2, Baltimore, 1981, University Park Press.

Ferguson AB: *Orthopaedic surgery in infancy and childhood,* ed 5, Baltimore, 1981, Williams & Wilkins.

Fyler DC: *Nadas' pediatric cardiology,* St Louis, 1992, Mosby-Yearbook.

Gammon JA: Visual system screening in infants and young children, *Pediatr Rev* 4:71, 1982.

Hoekelman RA: The pediatric physical examination. In Bickley LS, editor: *Bates' guide to physical examination and history taking,* ed 7, Philadelphia, 1999, JB Lippincott.

James JIP: *Scoliosis,* Edinburgh, 1976, E&S Livingstone.

Lowrey GH: *Growth and development of children,* ed 8, Chicago, 1986, Mosby.

McDowell F, Wolff HG: *Handbook of neurological diagnostic methods,* Baltimore, 1960, Williams & Wilkins.

Monteleone JE: *Recognition of child abuse for the mandated reporter,* ed 2, St Louis, 1996, Mosby.

Pizzutillo D: *Practical orthopaedics in primary practice,* New York, 1997, McGraw-Hill.

Smith TF, O'Day D, Wright PF: Clinical implications of preseptal (periorbital) cellulitis in childhood, *Pediatrics* 62:1006, 1978.

Sperling MA: *Pediatric endocrinology,* Philadelphia, 1996, WB Saunders.

9 Preoperative Assessment

Lynne G. Maxwell • Myron Yaster

Ambulatory or same-day surgery provides significant medical, psychological, and economic benefits to children and their families.[24,27,44] Indeed, it now constitutes more than 50% of all surgery performed in children. Much of the preoperative and postoperative patient care that in the past was provided in the hospital by the surgeon and anesthesiologist now is being performed by the child's pediatrician. Indeed, the pediatrician often is asked "to clear" children for surgery, with little, if any, guidance as to what this means. This chapter reviews the effects of anesthesia on children and highlights those aspects of the child's history and physical examination of particular importance to the anesthesiologist and surgeon.

EFFECTS OF GENERAL ANESTHESIA

General anesthesia abolishes the sensation of pain (analgesia), produces muscle paralysis, amnesia, and a loss of consciousness, and inhibits the adrenal-stress response to pain and surgery. Although the drugs that produce general anesthesia have very narrow therapeutic indices, modern anesthetic practice produces few, if any, perioperative complications. Nevertheless, children and their parents dread the entire experience of surgery. Young children are afraid of separation from their parents, older children fear potential mutilation and death, and teenagers fear all of this plus loss of control.[45] Young children often will struggle, scream, and cry when either separated from their parent(s) or when anesthesia is being induced, particularly if the induction technique is via mask induction of potent volatile vapors such as halothane or sevoflurane. This struggle often leads to a stormy induction of anesthesia and significantly increases the risks of airway compromise (laryngospasm, coughing, breath holding, and so forth), anesthetic overdose (hypotension), and arrhythmias, particularly when halothane is used as the induction agent. Furthermore, memories of this struggle or of the separation from one's parents may be long lasting, indeed, even longer lasting than the experience of surgery itself. Fortunately, the emergence of new drugs for the premedication of pediatric patients such as midazolam (Versed), parental presence during the induction of anesthesia, and improved, faster, and better tolerated volatile anesthetic gases for mask induction (sevoflurane) have lessened the incidence of such terrorizing experiences.

Parents fear for their child's life and safety as well. This sense of terror and foreboding is compounded by a sense of inadequacy and guilt. Rather than protecting their child from pain and suffering, they feel responsible for "causing" it or "allowing" it to happen. Many recent "horror stories" featured on network television "newsmagazines" have added to parental anxiety about their child's safety.

Is this fear and foreboding necessary, and can it be allayed? Ultimately, this depends on how safe anesthesia actually is. Between 1978 and 1982, anesthesia mortality for French children younger than 15 years of age was 1 in 40,000.[39] The incidence of anesthetic complications was 0.7/1000; cardiac arrest occurred in 12 of 40,000 patients but resulted in only one death. The incidence of complications was much higher in infants younger than 1 year (4.3/1000). In a study reviewing the experience in an American hospital from 1969 to 1983, the overall mortality rate was 0.9/10,000 anesthetics, with an incidence of cardiac arrest of 1.7/10,000.[16] In this study, children younger than 12 years of age had a threefold higher incidence of cardiac arrest (4.7/10,000) compared with adult patients (1.4/10,000).[16] Complications leading to cardiac arrest in these studies were due largely to complications of airway management (laryngospasm, difficult intubation, and pulmonary aspiration of gastric contents) or were secondary to halothane overdosage (hypotension, arrhythmia, or both). Infants younger than 1 month of age have the greatest risk of serious intraoperative complications (cardiac arrest) and the highest perioperative death rates because they are more likely to be having major surgery (intrathoracic or intraabdominal) than are older children and are "sicker" (a greater percentage are "ASA physical status 3 to 5") (see below). A recent review of closed anesthesia malpractice claims revealed that complications in pediatric cases were related to respiratory events with a greater frequency than in adult cases (43% versus 30%), and the mortality rate was greater in the affected children (50% versus 35%).[25]

The American Society of Anesthesiologists (ASA) Physical Status classification (Table 9-1) provides a convenient method of summarizing the patient's physical condition and also may provide a means of assessing the relative risk of anesthesia. ASA physical status (PS) 1 patients are healthy and have no underlying disease, whereas ASA PS 4 patients are significantly incapacitated by their underlying disease. Other factors associated with increased preoperative risk are multiple coexistent diseases and the need for emergent surgery. The anesthetic mortality rate in healthy ASA PS 1 children requiring elective surgery is probably less than 1 in 50,000.

Children who are candidates for outpatient surgery generally are in the ASA PS 1 and 2 groups. Therefore, among ASA PS 1 and 2 children who require elective surgery, fac-

Table 9-1 ASA Physical Status Classification for Preoperative Assessment of Patients

PS 1	A normal healthy patient
PS 2	A patient who has mild systemic disease
PS 3	A patient who has severe systemic disease
PS 4	A patient who has a severe systemic disease that is a constant threat to life
PS 5	A moribund patient who is not expected to survive without the operation

American Society of Anesthesiologists, Inc: *ASA relative value guide,* Park Ridge, Ill, 1996.
PS, Physical status.

tors that could impose any additional perioperative risk (e.g., upper respiratory infection, recent meal) are considered unacceptable. Pediatric patients have a higher incidence of respiratory events (laryngospasm and bronchospasm) than do adults. Olsson and Hallen found an incidence of laryngospasm of 17.4:1000 in the 0- to 9-year-old age group, but in patients who had active respiratory infection, the rate increased to 95.8:1000; in patients who had a history of reactive airway disease, the rate rose to 63.9:1000.[26] ASA PS 3 and even 4 patients increasingly are undergoing outpatient surgery because insurance companies are refusing to pay for inpatient care. Unfortunately, whether this is safe or desirable is irrelevant. Because of the increased risk to these children, direct communication between the pediatrician and anesthesiologist is advised well in advance of the planned surgical procedure. Recently, better resources, in addition to this text, have become available to help pediatricians educate themselves and their patients' families about the perioperative experience, from preoperative evaluation to postoperative pain management.[9]

ANESTHETIC RELEVANCE OF THE HISTORY AND PHYSICAL EXAMINATION

The preoperative evaluation is concerned directly with those aspects of the child's history and physical examination that can affect the course of the anesthetic and perioperative management. This evaluation of children for anesthesia depends on an understanding of how anesthesia affects their normal physiology. The areas of primary concern in the history are related to neuromuscular, cardiovascular, respiratory, endocrine, and hematological or oncological diseases. The areas of key interest to the anesthesiologist in the physical examination are related to airway anatomy, the presence of stridor, wheezing, or murmurs, and evidence of preexisting neurological deficit or neuromuscular disease.. Many departments of anesthesiology will provide the pediatrician with a history and physical examination form on which to report the preoperative evaluation (Fig. 9-1).

AIRWAY AND PULMONARY FUNCTION

General anesthesia alters respiratory function significantly at virtually every level. Early effects result from excitation of airway reflexes (laryngospasm, increased secretions, and bronchospasm) during the inhalational induction of general anesthesia before the achievement of a depth of anesthesia appropriate for surgery. The effects of anesthesia include decreased contractility of respiratory muscles, depressed ciliary clearance, depression of the central respiratory response to hypoxia and hypercapnia, decreased lung volume, and increased intrapulmonary shunting. These effects can result in serious and potentially life-threatening consequences, including upper airway obstruction, hypoventilation or apnea, and hypoxemia. The presence of underlying conditions (e.g., prematurity) or respiratory or airway diseases (e.g., asthma or bronchopulmonary dysplasia) compounds the risks of anesthesia greatly for the child. Therefore, detailed information about preexisting respiratory disease should be available for the anesthesiologist.

Upper Respiratory Tract Infections

Children who have acute or recent viral or bacterial upper respiratory infections (URI) are at increased risk for airway and pulmonary complications during anesthesia.[5,23] This risk exists during the acute infection and persists for up to 6 weeks after the infection has run its course.[10] Anesthetic complications that occur commonly in children who have an acute URI or during their convalescence include bronchospasm, laryngospasm, acute subglottic edema with stridor, intraoperative and postoperative hypoxia, atelectasis, and postextubation croup. Endotracheal intubation increases the risk of respiratory complications significantly. Unfortunately, avoiding intubation often is impossible.

Interestingly, several studies have found no significant increase in respiratory complications among children anesthetized because of an acute URI.[31] This has led some to advocate *not* canceling surgery for these children. It is our belief that the physiological, psychological, and financial implications of delays in surgery must be weighed against the risks of increased perioperative complications of anesthetizing a child who has a URI. Patients who have systemic manifestations, such as fever greater than 101.3° F (38.5° C), purulent nasal discharge, and lower respiratory symptoms such as productive cough, crackles, wheezes, or positive chest radiograph findings should have the surgical procedure delayed for 4 to 6 weeks after the resolution of symptoms.[15] Surgery and anesthesia usually can proceed safely in children who have none of these symptoms, particularly if they do not require endotracheal intubation (Fig. 9-2).

Asthma

Asthma is one of the most common and most serious underlying medical conditions that can affect patients undergoing general anesthesia.[14,17] Many procedures performed routinely during anesthetic management, most notably laryngoscopy and intubation, are potent and intense stimuli that produce bronchospasm. Intraoperative bronchospasm can be catastrophic; it may make ventilation difficult, if not impossible, and may result in hypercapnia, acidosis, hypoxia, cardiovascular collapse, and death. Fortunately, this need not and should not happen. Maximal preoperative optimization of a patient's medical management may prevent or, at the very least, limit all of the perioperative complications of

PREOPERATIVE EVALUATION/HISTORY AND PHYSICAL

DATE: ____________ TIME ______ AGE ______ SEX ____ RACE ______

PROCEDURE ____________________

DIAGNOSIS ____________________

MEDICATIONS ____________________

ALLERGIES ____________________

STAMP PATIENT'S IDENTIFICATION OR PRINT CLEARLY

NURSING UNIT / CLINIC

JHH HISTORY NUMBER

PATIENT'S NAME (LAST, FIRST, M.I.)

USE BALLPOINT PEN

PAST MEDICAL HISTORY AND REVIEW OF SYSTEMS

YES	NO	**CARDIOVASCULAR**
□	□	MI
□	□	HYPERTENSION
□	□	ARRHYTHMIA
□	□	ANGINA
□	□	CHF
□	□	VALVULAR DISEASE
□	□	PERIPHERAL VASC. DISEASE
□	□	PAST CARDIAC SURGERY
□	□	OTHER
		PULMONARY
□	□	SMOKING Hx
□	□	ASTHMA
□	□	COPD/EMPHYSEMA/BPD
□	□	OTHER
		RENAL
□	□	RENAL FAILURE
□	□	OTHER

YES	NO	**HEPATIC**
□	□	HEPATITIS
□	□	OTHER
		ENDOCRINE
□	□	DIABETES
□	□	OTHER
		INFECTIOUS
□	□	SEPSIS
□	□	OTHER
		NEUROLOGIC
□	□	SEIZURE
□	□	ELEVATED ICP
□	□	CEREBROVASC. DISEASE
□	□	NEUROMUSCULAR DISORDER
□	□	OTHER
		GASTROINTESTINAL
□	□	G.E. REFLUX/HIATAL HERNIA
□	□	BOWEL OBSTRUCTION
□	□	OTHER

YES	NO	**HEMATOLOGIC**
□	□	SICKLE CELL
□	□	COAGULOPATHY
□	□	PREGNANCY/TRANSFUSION WITHIN LAST 3 MONTHS Y/N
□	□	OTHER
		PEDIATRICS
□	□	PREMATURITY
□	□	CONGENITAL ABN.
□	□	APNEA
□	□	OTHER
		OBSTETRICS
□	□	PREECLAMPSIA/ECLAMPSIA
□	□	PREMATURITY
□	□	PLACENTA PREVIA/ABRUPTIO
□	□	LMP______
□	□	OTHER
		ANESTHETIC DIFFICULTIES
□	□	DIFFICULT INTUBATION
□	□	FAMILY HISTORY
□	□	OTHER
		DRUG USE
□	□	ETOH
□	□	OTHER

□ HISTORY UNKNOWN EXCEPT AS NOTED ABOVE

EXPLANATION OF POSITIVE DATA ____________________

PHYSICAL EXAMINATION BP (RANGE): ____________ P ______ R ______ T ______ WT ______ (lbs.) (Kg.)

LABS:

H&P PERFORMED BY ____________

ECG FINDINGS: ____________

RISK FACTORS:
HEMODYNAMIC COMPROMISE ________ OTHER ________
CRITICAL AIRWAY ________
FULL STOMACH ________ LAST PO ________

IMPRESSION: ASA STATUS | 1 | 2 | 3 | 4 | 5 | E | ____________

REVIEWED BY: ______________ M.D. | DATE ______ TIME ______

CHART COPY

Fig. 9-1 Example of preoperative evaluation/history and physical examination form. (From the Johns Hopkins Hospital, Department of Anesthesiology and Critical Care Medicine, 1988.)

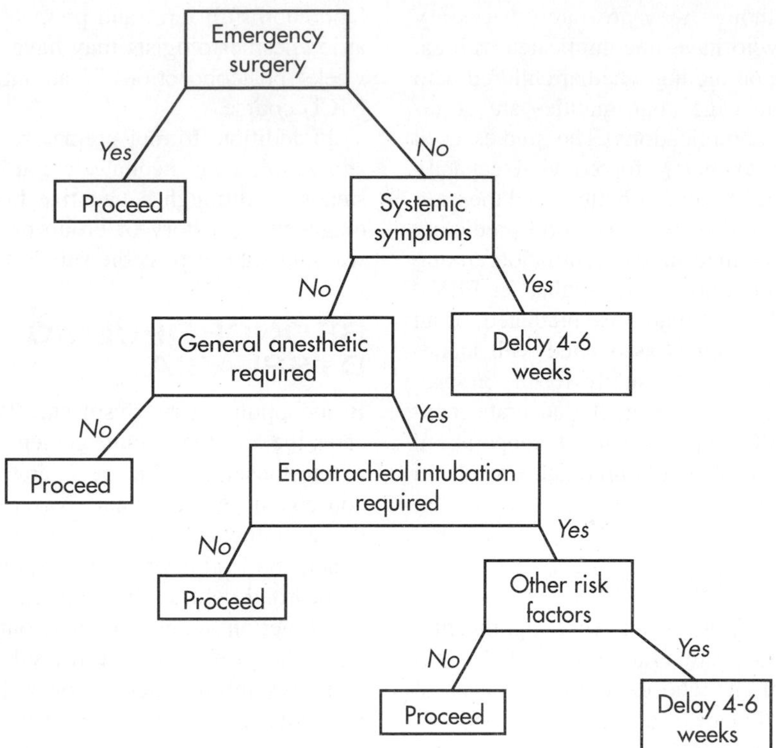

Fig. 9-2 Suggested clinical decision tree for patients who have a recent history of upper respiratory infection being evaluated for surgery.
(From Martin LD: *Pediatr Clin North Am* 41:121, 1994.)

asthma ("the best defense is a good offense"). In general, asthma medical therapy must be escalated preoperatively even in well-controlled or asymptomatic patients to limit or prevent intraoperative bronchospasm. Thus, the child who takes asthma medications only "as needed" ("prn") should begin his or her inhaled beta-agonists or oral medications 3 to 5 days preoperatively.[28,33] The child taking medications on a chronic basis (oral or inhaled) should have steroids added in doses that would be used for an acute exacerbation (prednisone 1 to 2 mg/kg/day, which may be administered as a single morning dose). Finally, the "difficult" asthmatic child who takes bronchodilators and steroids regularly requires either intensification in the frequency of nebulizer treatments, added bronchodilators, increased steroids, or on occasion, all of these.[28]

The child taking theophylline requires special attention. Serum levels (therapeutic range, 10 to 20 μg/ml) should be measured to optimize drug dosing and guide intraoperative bronchodilator therapy. Intraoperatively, the acute administration of intravenous doses of aminophylline is dangerous, even in the setting of low blood levels, because the interaction of high levels of aminophylline and inhalation of general anesthetic agents often produce cardiac dysrhythmias, and wheezing may be treated adequately intraoperatively by the use of beta-agonists, steroids, and intravenous lidocaine (which also suppresses airway reflexes).

Elective surgery should never be performed in children who are wheezing actively or who have had a recent asthma attack. Decreased peak expiratory flow and forced expiratory volume in the first second of expiration (FEV_1) occur in adults and children for up to 6 weeks following an acute asthma attack, and airways are more responsive and prone to bronchospasm in this period (see discussion of upper respiratory tract infections in this chapter). Therefore, a recent asthma exacerbation requiring hospital admission or emergency therapy within 6 weeks of surgery precludes elective surgery. Elective surgery in asthmatic children who have an upper respiratory tract infection should also be delayed 6 weeks, even if they have no wheezing on auscultation, because the incidence of bronchospasm is likely to be increased greatly beyond that seen in nonasthmatic children—an elevenfold increase in respiratory complications when children require endotracheal intubation as part of anesthetic management.

Corticosteroids are extremely effective in preventing perioperative wheezing, even in patients who have severe asthma.[28] Patients should receive 1 mg/kg of prednisone orally once daily for 3 days before surgery and on the morning of surgery. Although the chronic administration of high-dose corticosteroids for the treatment of asthma can be associated with severe systemic side effects, the short-term perioperative administration just described is safe and most effective in decreasing the incidence of perioperative bronchospasm. All oral medications may be taken with small amounts of water on the morning of surgery.

Pulmonary Function Tests

Pulmonary function tests (PFTs) often are used to assess the response to bronchodilator therapy in patients whose bronchospasm is reversible. Although they are rarely necessary preoperatively in patients who have uncomplicated asthma, these tests may be useful in predicting whether children who have pulmonary or thoracic cage abnormalities are at increased risk for anesthetic complications. The studies used most commonly are pulse oximetry, forced vital capacity (FVC), and FEV_1. The absolute values obtained and the ratio of the two measurements (FEV_1/FVC) are useful predictors of the need for postoperative mechanical ventilation among patients at risk (e.g., kyphoscoliosis). In adults, an FEV_1/FVC less than 50%, an FEV_1 less than 35% predicted, or an absolute FVC less than 25 ml/kg is associated with inadequate postoperative ventilation and usually results in prolonged mechanical ventilation. However, the accurate measurement of FEV_1 and FVC requires patient cooperation; therefore, it usually is not possible to obtain reliable results in children younger than 6 years.

PREMATURITY AND APNEA

Infants born prematurely (<37 weeks) have a significantly increased risk of developing postoperative apnea (>15 seconds).[41] Former preterm infants who undergo general anesthesia have an increased incidence of apnea, periodic breathing, and bradycardia for up to 24 hours after surgery compared with full-term infants. Regardless of a patient's age, all general anesthetics, sedatives, hypnotics, and opioids produce dose-dependent and drug-specific alterations in the mechanics and central control of the respiratory system. This places the prematurely born infant at particular risk for developing apnea because the central and peripheral chemoreceptors are immature and limit effective responses to hypoxia and hypercapnia, even without the additional burden of drug-induced depression. Furthermore, the general anesthetics decrease muscle tone in the airways, chest wall, and diaphragm and thereby depress the ventilatory response to hypoxia and hypercapnia further.

Several studies have demonstrated an increased risk for apnea to develop postoperatively in former preterm infants undergoing minor and major surgical procedures.[22] This risk can be minimized by the perioperative administration of caffeine (or theophylline), the use of spinal anesthesia instead of general anesthesia, and the delaying of surgery until the child is older than 48 to 60 postconceptual weeks.[42,43] Welborn et al, in a double-blind study, demonstrated that 10 mg/kg of caffeine base (which is equivalent to 20 mg/kg of caffeine citrate or benzoate) given intravenously after the induction of general anesthesia virtually eliminated postoperative apnea.[42] These same investigators and others also have demonstrated that spinal anesthesia (particularly in inguinal hernia surgery) decreased the risk of postoperative apnea significantly.[43] Nevertheless, it is our belief, albeit conservative, that the risk of postanesthesia apnea has been defined clearly and that the use of caffeine and spinal anesthesia as prophylaxis has been studied only in very small patient populations. Therefore, it is our practice to admit all at-risk patients, regardless of the anesthetic technique used, to monitored, high-surveillance inpatient units for 24 hours after anesthesia and surgery. Galinkin and Kurth have devised a useful algorithm for decision-making on eligibility for day surgery in young infants, both full term and prematurely born,[10] although pediatric anesthesiologists may have more liberal age limits (52 weeks postconception) if an infant had an uncomplicated NICU course.

In addition, former premature infants who were intubated and ventilated as neonates are at increased risk for subglottic stenosis. Although a negative history does not exclude the diagnosis, a history of croup or stridor is a very important warning sign of possible subglottic narrowing.

BRONCHOPULMONARY DYSPLASIA

Bronchopulmonary dysplasia (BPD) significantly complicates the anesthetic management of children. Several effects of anesthesia, together or separately, produce life-threatening consequences. Pulmonary vasoconstriction following anesthetic induction can aggravate ventilation-perfusion mismatch and lead to profound hypoxemia. Anesthetic effects on myocardial contractility can result in impaired right ventricular function, reduced cardiac output, pulmonary hypoperfusion, and profound cardiovascular compromise with hypoxemia resembling acute cor pulmonale. Increased airway reactivity during induction of or emergence from anesthesia can result in a severe exacerbation of BPD, with an increased ventilation-perfusion mismatch. Increased oral and bronchial secretions induced by the anesthetic can compromise airflow and lead to airway or endotracheal tube plugging. Because of diminished respiratory reserves in these patients, such plugging can cause death quickly. These children also may have a degree of increased airway reactivity and tracheomalacia. Intraoperative bronchospasm or airway collapse poses a serious intraoperative risk. Finally, infections of the respiratory tract occur frequently in children who have BPD, and the presence of pneumonia can complicate the perioperative course significantly.

It is essential that the pulmonary status of these children be optimized before anesthesia and surgery. Bronchodilators, antibiotics, diuretics, and corticosteroid therapy all may benefit these children. Respiratory infections or bronchospasm in children who have BPD must be treated thoroughly before elective surgery. For children who have severe BPD and bronchospasm, preoperative treatment with increased inspired oxygen tension may decrease pulmonary vasoreactivity and improve cardiovascular function. The possibility of associated right ventricular dysfunction always should be considered and, where indicated, evaluated with electrocardiogram (ECG) and echocardiography. Because these children are at major risk for perioperative mortality and morbidity, the situation should be explained to parents before surgery. In addition, these children may require continuous postoperative monitoring and ventilation for an extended period (24 to 48 hours). Risks of general anesthesia and intubation in these children sometimes can be avoided with the judicious use of regional anesthesia (caudal or spinal) for operations such as hernia repair in infants younger than 6 months. Parents must be cautioned, however, that regional anesthesia may not be 100% successful and that intubation might still be required.

Some of the most severely affected patients who have

BPD take diuretics such as furosemide or spironolactone, which may result in electrolyte abnormalities. Patients who are on these drugs must have their serum electrolytes assessed preoperatively.

OBSTRUCTIVE SLEEP APNEA

Children who have long-standing obstructive sleep apnea secondary to adenotonsillar hypertrophy, obesity, or other causes also can develop significant pulmonary hypertension and cor pulmonale.[13] Like children who have BPD, these youngsters are at risk for perioperative hypoxemia and acute right heart failure. Patients at greatest risk are those who demonstrate daytime somnolence, complete or frequent obstructive apnea events, cyanosis during sleep, or signs of cardiopulmonary dysfunction.[13] Preoperatively, these children should undergo a hematocrit, chest radiograph, ECG, and echocardiogram. Postoperatively, they should be admitted to the pediatric intensive care unit because the incidence of obstructive events actually may increase during the first 24 hours after surgery.

CARDIOVASCULAR DISEASES

All anesthetic agents can affect the normal cardiovascular system profoundly and adversely. The sinus node, conduction system, and myocardial contractility all can be depressed by general anesthetics. Moreover, general anesthesia alters both preload and afterload by relaxing vascular smooth muscle tone. General anesthetics also attenuate hypoxic pulmonary vasoconstriction and thereby impair ventilation perfusion matching. Finally, halothane, the potent vapor anesthetic, which for many years was used most commonly in pediatric patients, may produce arrhythmias, even in patients who have no underlying conduction defects. Although severe arrhythmias are possible in normal children theoretically, they are more common in those receiving other drugs that are arrhythmogenic, such as epinephrine (often injected by surgeons to cause vasoconstriction and decrease surgical bleeding) or aminophylline. Other patients at increased risk are those who have underlying conduction abnormalities, especially syndromes associated with a prolonged QT interval. More commonly, however, the only manifestations of halothane's effects on the conducting system are occasional PVCs or bigeminy, both of which are seen frequently in association with hypercapnia caused by hypoventilation or with inadequate or "light" anesthesia. These mild dysrhythmias are treated easily by increasing the minute ventilation or the depth of anesthesia.

The newest inhalational anesthetic, sevoflurane, has increasingly replaced halothane for mask induction of anesthesia in children. This is because it is preferable to halothane in having an acceptable odor while having fewer cardiovascular side effects such as bradycardia, hypotension, and ventricular arrhythmias as a result of effects on the myocardial contractility and the conducting system.

Important, common effects of inhalation agents on the cardiovascular system include vasodilation and depression of myocardial contractility. These actions often combine to cause some degree of hypotension, which may be severe in patients who are relatively hypovolemic because of prolonged fasting or extraordinary fluid losses (diarrhea, vomiting, hemorrhage). The presence of underlying heart disease (e.g., congestive heart failure, dysrhythmias, and intracardiac shunts) magnifies the inherent risks of anesthesia. Accordingly, thorough cardiovascular assessment is a critical part of preoperative preparation.

Intracardiac Shunts

Most anesthetic agents decrease vascular tone and thus decrease both pulmonary and systemic vascular resistance. The relative changes in these resistances can alter the dynamics of intracardiac shunts. Thus, during general anesthesia, a left-to-right intracardiac shunt (e.g., ventricular septal defect) may produce pulmonary overcirculation and failure. In contrast, during anesthesia, pulmonary vascular resistance may increase acutely as a consequence of hypoxia, hypercapnia, acidosis, and hypotension. Thus, a predominantly left-to-right shunt can be converted to a right-to-left shunt, which can have catastrophic consequences (e.g., hypoxemia, or acute cor pulmonale). Children who have intracardiac shunts also can have "paradoxical embolism" produced by air or a thrombus traveling from the venous circulation into the systemic circulation (e.g., cerebral arteries). For these reasons, intracardiac shunts must be identified preoperatively.

Murmurs

Cardiac murmurs are common in children (see Chapter 142, Heart Murmurs). Murmurs are either "functional" or pathological. It is imperative that patients who have congenital anomalies of the heart or great vessels be identified before anesthesia is chosen. In general, the child who has a murmur but who has a normal S_1 and S_2, normal exercise tolerance, is acyanotic, and is growing well will tolerate a general anesthetic without complication. However, even asymptomatic patients who have a previously unrecognized pathological murmur should be assessed appropriately and may require antibiotic prophylaxis. Appropriate preoperative evaluation reasonably includes a thorough physical examination and electrocardiogram. If there is any question of a cardiac abnormality, preoperative echocardiography and evaluation by a pediatric cardiologist are necessary.

The presence of an abnormal murmur, cyanosis, decreased exercise tolerance, poor weight gain, sweating, decreased femoral pulses, or a precordial heave necessitates a more complete preoperative evaluation (hematocrit, ECG, chest radiograph, oxygen saturation, and cardiology consultation). If a child who has known congenital heart disease presents for preoperative evaluation, the precise details of any previous surgery, current intracardiac anatomy, cardiac conduction defects, and myocardial function should be documented and the anesthesiologist informed of the findings before surgery. Any anatomical defects should be described and the amount of intracardiac shunting and resting arterial saturation quantified. The pediatrician or cardiologist also should note the cardiac medications the child is taking and any recent changes in the child's status.

Subacute Bacterial Endocarditis Prophylaxis

Antibiotic prophylaxis to prevent bacterial endocarditis is indicated for children who have congenital heart disease and are undergoing any procedure in which the patient is at risk for transient bacteremia (e.g., dental, sinus, airway, genitourinary, gastrointestinal) or when the surgical site, though normally sterile, is contaminated. In addition to patients who have shunts, patients who have hemodynamically insignificant lesions (bicuspid aortic valve, mitral valve prolapse, or a history of infective carditis) also require perioperative prophylaxis. All patients who have undergone palliative or corrective cardiac operations require prophylaxis for the rest of their lives. The only exceptions are those children who have had a patent ductus arteriosus ligated or who have had a primary closure of a secundum atrial septal defect without a prosthetic patch; these two groups of patients require prophylaxis for only the first 6 months postoperatively. Oral endotracheal intubation by itself is not an indication for subacute bacterial endocarditis (SBE) prophylaxis, but nasotracheal intubation does require it. The antibiotic regimen recommended by the American Heart Association[4] should be followed (Box 9-1). It usually is acceptable for the antibiotic to be given when the IV is started after induction of anesthesia because the interval between start of the IV and the incision generally is long enough (5 minutes) to achieve adequate blood levels. Thus, it is unnecessary to start an IV in a child who is awake solely to administer antibiotics for SBE prophylaxis. The necessity for continuing the antibiotic therapy postoperatively should be emphasized to the family because the child may be discharged as soon as 1 to 2 hours after surgery.

NEUROMUSCULAR DISEASES

Anesthetic agents affect the CNS globally in addition to providing anesthesia. Although suppression of awareness and central responses to pain are desirable, anesthetics also inhibit vital central nervous system functions; respiratory depression, inhibition of autonomic tone, and impaired reflex regulation all occur during general anesthesia. Anesthetics also alter cerebrovascular tone, autoregulation, and intracranial fluid dynamics. Thus, anesthetic agents that cause cerebrovascular dilation can alter intracranial space compliance and cerebral perfusion pressure. The potent inhalational agents (halothane, enflurane, isoflurane, desflurane, and sevoflurane) produce sluggish motor reflex responses and impair coordination, effects that may persist for hours after cessation of anesthetic administration. Preexisting neuromuscular weakness may be exacerbated significantly. The normal child may manifest long-tract signs transiently, including hyperextension and hypertonicity associated with extensor plantar reflexes. There may be anisocoria or exacerbation of underlying hemiparesis. Although most general anesthetics are anticonvul-

BOX 9-1

ANTIBIOTIC REGIMENS FOR INFECTIVE ENDOCARDITIS PROPHYLAXIS

Upper Respiratory Tract Surgical Procedures (Including Oral Surgery and Dental Procedures Causing Gingival Bleeding)

1. Standard regimens
   a. Amoxicillin 50 mg/kg (up to 3 g) po 1 hr before the procedure and ½ the initial dose 6 hr later.
   b. For children unable to take oral medications, parenteral ampicillin 50 mg/kg (up to 2 g) 30 min before the procedure and ½ the initial dose 6 hr later.
2. Regimen for those who have intracardiac prosthetic valves or systemic-pulmonary shunts
   Parenteral amipicillin 50 mg/kg (up to 2 g) plus parenteral gentamicin 2.0 mg/kg (up to 80 mg), given 30 min before the procedure. Oral amoxicillin 25 mg/kg (up to 1.5 g) is given 6 hr after the initial antibiotics, or the parenteral regimen can be repeated 8 hr after the first dose. Many authorities recommend one of the above standard regimens for this high-risk group.
3. Regimen for penicillin-allergic patients
   a. Oral: Erythromycin ethylsuccinate or stearate 20 mg/kg (up to 800 mg of erythromycin ethylsuccinate or ≤1 g of erythromycin stearate) 2 hr before the procedure, followed by ½ the initial dose 6 hr later. Alternative regimen: Clindamycin 10 mg/kg (up to 300 mg) po 1 hr before the procedure, followed by ½ the initial dose 6 hr later.
   b. Parenteral: Clindamycin 10 mg/kg IV (up to 300 mg) 30 min before the procedure, followed by ½ the initial dose 6 hr later.
   c. Parenteral for patients who have intracardiac prosthetic material or systemic-pulmonary shunts: Vancomycin 20 mg/kg IV (up to 1 g) given over 1 hr, starting 1 hr before the procedure.

For GI/GU Surgical Procedures

1. Standard regimen: Parenteral ampicillin and gentamicin 30 to 60 min before the procedure and again 8 hr later. Alternatively, oral amoxicillin may be given 6 hr after the initial antibiotics. Dosages are the same as for upper respiratory tract surgery.
2. Oral regimen for minor procedures in a low-risk patient: Amoxicillin 50 mg/kg (up to 3 g) 1 hr before the procedure and ½ the initial dose 6 hr later.
3. Regimen for penicillin-allergic patients: IV vancomycin and gentamicin 1 hr before the procedure, with a repeat dose 8 hr later. Dosages are the same as given for upper respiratory tract surgical procedures.

sants, patients may have seizures after clinically appropriate doses of enflurane and methohexital; thus, these agents usually are avoided in patients who have a known seizure disorder. Finally, chronic or acute preoperative ingestion of CNS stimulants (e.g., methylphenidate, cocaine, and amphetamines) may increase anesthetic requirements significantly.[6]

For these reasons, the presence of central neurological or peripheral neuromuscular abnormalities must be documented preoperatively. Because virtually all anesthetics produce cerebral vasodilation and thereby may increase intracranial pressure, children at risk for intracranial hypertension (e.g., hydrocephalus, brain tumor, and blocked ventriculoperitoneal shunts) must be identified before surgery. Any existing CSF shunt must be evaluated appropriately for patency and proper functioning. In addition, because residual anesthetic effects may impair airway reflexes in the immediate postoperative period, any evidence of brainstem dysfunction (vocal cord paralysis, swallowing dysfunction, and/or aspiration) should be noted in the preoperative evaluation.

Patients who have neuromuscular and degenerative diseases are at increased risk of postoperative weakness. This may require postoperative respiratory care and even prolonged mechanical ventilation. In children who have progressive diseases of nerve or muscle, hyperkalemia or malignant hyperthermia occur more commonly after succinylcholine administration. Indeed, the fear of fatal hyperkalemia following succinylcholine administration in patients who have undiagnosed muscular dystrophy has led the Food and Drug Administration recently to contraindicate the use of succinylcholine in routine intubations in all children. Despite this, because succinylcholine is still the best muscle relaxant for accomplishing rapid intubation, anesthesiologists will still use it for strong indications in children (bowel obstruction, NPO violation). Therefore, communication of signs of possible muscular dystrophy (delayed walking, calf hypertrophy, Gowers' sign) is very appropriate.

Patients receiving anticonvulsant medication should have blood concentrations measured to ensure therapeutic levels perioperatively. These children may require perioperative IV administration of anticonvulsants because postoperative fasting or vomiting may not allow maintenance of therapeutic blood levels with orally administered drugs. However, most anticonvulsants have very long half-lives, and the omission of one dose will not decrease the blood level significantly. Patients who have been seizure-free for 2 years and have had no adjustment of their anticonvulsant dose probably do not require determination of anticonvulsant levels, but the anesthesiologist should be informed to ensure that he or she agrees with this plan.

ENDOCRINOLOGICAL CONSIDERATIONS

Anesthesia and surgery subject the child to significant stresses. Children have greatly increased circulating levels of epinephrine, norepinephrine, and cortisol during surgery. The insulin/glucagon relationship is altered dramatically. Moreover, a stress-related catabolic state persists long after the day of surgery. Therefore, the child undergoing surgery should be in the best nutritional state possible before elective surgery is contemplated.

The stress associated with surgery produces a hyperglycemic response because of increased levels of circulating corticosteroids and catecholamines, even with prolonged preoperative fasting. However, in infants and small children, even mild fasting can be associated with perioperative hypoglycemia, especially in infants younger than 1 year or who have a history of premature birth.

Diabetes Mellitus

The most common endocrinological problem in the perioperative period is diabetes mellitus. Insulin-dependent diabetic children experience significant perioperative difficulties, even when their control is good. Brittle or noncompliant diabetic patients have additional problems, including an increased risk of perioperative hypoglycemia or hyperglycemia, osmotic diuresis, intravascular hypovolemia, and altered mental status. It is essential to document the child's insulin regimen, the degree of compliance, how well the blood glucose concentration is controlled, and whether the child has any adverse effects of a short to moderate fast. A recent growth history also is useful to indicate how well controlled the child's diabetes may be. Various techniques for managing preoperative insulin therapy have been proposed (Table 9-2). It generally is recommended that the child follow routine preoperative fasting guidelines for surgery—namely, not ingesting solid foods or formula (including breast milk) for at least 6 hours before surgery. Patients are allowed to drink clear liquids for up to 2 to 3 hours before surgery.[35,36]

The insulin dose should be decreased to half of the child's usual morning dose on the day of surgery and given as soluble insulin. This seems reasonable because mild to moderate hyperglycemia (without ketosis) usually does not present a

Table 9-2 Protocols for Perioperative Insulin Therapy

Classic regimen (morning of surgery)	Start IV infusion 5% dextrose in 0.45% saline at 1500 ml/m^2/day Administer ½ usual morning insulin dose Check blood glucose before induction and during anesthesia
Continuous insulin infusion (morning of surgery)	Start IV infusion 5% dextrose in 0.45% saline at 1500 ml/m^2/day Add 1-2 units of insulin per ml of 5% dextrose Check blood glucose before induction and during anesthesia
Insulin- and glucose-free regimen (for operative procedures of short duration on the morning of surgery)	Withhold morning insulin dose If indicated for the procedure: glucose-free solution (e.g., lactated Ringer) at maintenance rate Check blood glucose before induction and during anesthesia

serious problem to the child, whereas hypoglycemia has devastating consequences. In the anesthetized child, the usual signs of hypoglycemia (tachycardia, diaphoresis, lethargy progressing to obtunded mental status) are masked, and a significant hypoglycemic insult can occur intraoperatively with little evidence of it until attempts are made to awaken the child. Heavy preoperative sedation also is avoided in diabetic children so that their level of consciousness can be assessed readily during the perioperative period.

Patients on long-term corticosteroid therapy and those who have congenital adrenal insufficiency have suppression of the hypothalamic-pituitary-adrenal axis. Thus, they may be unable to manifest an appropriate stress response and are at risk for severe hemodynamic compromise (Addisonian crisis). Long-term corticosteroid therapy is used commonly for a variety of illnesses. The severity of the underlying disease state and any associated complications must be noted appropriately, as should side effects of steroid therapy, including Cushingoid facies, vascular and bleeding abnormalities, myopathy, and cardiomyopathy. For these reasons, children who are receiving long-term or intermittent corticosteroid therapy should be treated with corticosteroids for 24 hours before surgery. "Stress doses" of steroids are administered commonly to patients on chronic steroid therapy. Although this is of theoretical benefit, the necessity of this regimen has not been substantiated in human studies. In fact, studies in patients undergoing surgery suggest that such stress doses are unnecessary. Even so, until this issue is resolved, a short course of adrenal corticosteroids is relatively harmless. Conservative management would include the administration of 2.5 to 5 mg/m^2 of prednisone orally the night before and 25 to 50 mg/m^2 of hydrocortisone after the IV is started before or after anesthetic induction.

HEMATOLOGICAL CONDITIONS

Hematological conditions that may complicate perioperative management include anemia, sickle cell disease, and the presence of a bleeding diathesis (e.g., factor deficiency syndromes and chronic aspirin therapy). Anemia is associated with a reduction in the oxygen-carrying capacity and a secondary increase in cardiac output. Anemia often is tolerated well; unfortunately, many perioperative events (e.g., blood loss or anesthesia-induced myocardial depression) can subject the child whose cardiac function is intact and compensated to cellular hypoxia and cardiovascular collapse when the stresses of anesthesia and surgery overwhelm the anemic patient's delicate balance of oxygen demand and supply. Furthermore, an anemic child is more likely to need blood transfusions perioperatively if significant bleeding occurs, whereas even in the face of moderate amounts of blood loss, it is common to avoid administrating blood products to children who have normal preoperative hemoglobin levels. Although the hemoglobin value at which individual anesthesiologists choose to transfuse varies greatly, most anesthesiologists allow a normal child's hemoglobin to decline to 7 to 8 g/dl before transfusing blood.

A child who has a previously undiagnosed anemia may have a serious underlying disorder such as sickle cell anemia or a blood dyscrasia that requires additional evaluation before surgery. Thus, the cause of any significant anemia (hemoglobin <9) should be determined preoperatively. Nutritional causes (e.g., iron deficiency) often require relatively brief periods of therapy to improve the child's anemia. The presence of a mild anemia should not delay urgent surgery. For elective surgery, consultation with the anesthesia and surgical team may be required. Because the incidence of previously undetected anemia in children presenting for elective surgery is extremely low, *routine determination of hematocrit and hemoglobin is not necessary* if studies performed previously as part of well-child care have been normal (see discussion of preoperative laboratory testing in this chapter).

Sickle Cell Anemia

Patients who have sickle cell anemia (SSA) have an increased risk of complications from general anesthesia and surgery. Sickling readily occurs with hypoxia, hypercapnia, acidosis, hypothermia, hypovolemia, and hypoperfusion states, all of which can occur perioperatively. Decreased functional residual capacity and altered ventilation-perfusion ratios, which occur commonly during general anesthesia, may give rise to transient hypoxemia, which may precipitate sickling and contribute to postoperative acute chest syndrome. Immobility, vasoconstriction, increased insensible fluid loss, and position on the operating table may produce regional hypoperfusion and stasis. Children who have SSA and who are significantly anemic may benefit from simple red cell transfusions preoperatively to prevent perioperative complications. For minor surgery or surgery not involving the eye or application of a limb tourniquet, simple transfusion to a hemoglobin level of 10 g/dl is associated with an equal incidence of perioperative complications as that seen in patients who received exchange transfusion to a hemoglobin S level of less than 30%.[40] For prolonged or extensive operations, multiple simple or exchange transfusions to achieve hemoglobin S levels less than 30% are recommended.[11] Measures should be taken to ensure adequate perioperative hydration, especially because patients who have SSA and, to a lesser extent, children who have sickle trait have hyposthenuria, and the urine will remain inappropriately dilute, even in the face of significant intravascular volume depletion.

Sickle cell anemia frequently is associated with cardiomyopathy, nephropathy, central and peripheral neuropathy, or chronic respiratory dysfunction—all of which may complicate general anesthesia or the perioperative course. Because of the potential for further impairment during general anesthesia, it is necessary to document the degree of involvement of these organ systems preoperatively. The preoperative assessment also should describe the type of sickle crises the child usually experiences and the date of the most recent crisis. The pediatrician should note the extent of preexisting disease and consult with the anesthesiologist regarding the need for special preoperative preparation, including transfusion therapy. Other forms of hemoglobinopathies such as Cooley's anemia, hemoglobin SC, and thalassemia have important anesthetic implications, and such diagnoses should be communicated to the anesthesiologist.

An underlying bleeding diathesis may create serious problems in the perioperative period because of increased intraoperative and perioperative blood loss and CNS and other organ damage from hemorrhage and hematoma formation. Children who have factor deficiencies are at greatly increased risk for perioperative bleeding unless they receive specific factor replacement before, during, and after surgery. For minor operations the goal is 25% to 40% of normal factor levels preoperatively; for major procedures the target is 50% of normal, with repeat doses administered intraoperatively to maintain that level. Children receiving aspirin or other nonsteroidal antiinflammatory drug (NSAID) therapy may have a higher risk for bleeding because of platelet dysfunction. This usually presents no problems for minor procedures, but such patients may benefit from discontinuation of aspirin therapy 1 week before a major procedure.

Transfusions

Questions frequently are raised by parents regarding transfusion practices. Parents are anxious about the infectious risks of transfusion, and some may have religious objections. Elimination of paid donors, evolution of methods of donor screening, and increasingly sophisticated testing of donated blood have led to a dramatic decrease in the incidence of infection transmitted by transfusion. The biggest remaining threat to safety of the blood supply is donation by someone who is seronegative in the window of time between infection and seroconversion. The incidence of transfusion-associated hepatitis B is 1:63,000.[34] The risk of transfusion-transmitted hepatitis C is 1 in 103,000.[34] Hepatitis A, in which a carrier state is rare, is not usually transmitted by transfusion.

The majority of cases of non-A, non-B, non-C hepatitis are due to an as yet undiscovered viral agent or are of nonviral etiology.[1] Testing for HIV-I antibody was implemented in 1985, in 1992 for HIV-II, and most recently, in 1996 for HIV-I p24 antigen. The risk of transfusion-transmitted HIV is now estimated by at 1:450,000 to 1:600,000.[3,18,34] Cytomegalovirus (CMV) can be transmitted by transfusion, but disease occurs rarely in immunocompetent recipients. Infection can occur and may be devastating in immunocompromised children, such as premature infants, cancer or transplant patients, and those who have congenital immunodeficiency. Testing of donated units for CMV is essential for these immunocompromised patients.

Aside from infectious risks, reactions to transfusion include hemolytic reactions resulting from ABO incompatibility, allergic or anaphylactic reactions, febrile nonhemolytic reactions, and transfusion-associated graft-versus-host disease (TA-GVHD). Proper cross-matching and careful checking of units prior to administration should eliminate most risk of hemolytic reactions, but they still occur in 1:33,000 transfusions, with 1:300,000 to 1:700,000 being fatal (usually due to massive hemolysis and renal failure due to hemoglobinuria).[20,21] Febrile non-hemolytic reactions are immunologically mediated and occur most commonly in patients who have received transfusions previously. TA-GVHD occurs in immunocompromised patients, including those listed above under infectious risks.

Parents should be realistically informed about the risks of excessive blood loss in the operation their child faces. Children as small as 30 kg who have normal hematocrits may donate autologous blood in advance of elective procedures. This should be discussed with the surgeon and arranged through the hospital blood bank. Some blood banks will allow "directed" donation (allogenic or homologous blood), in which a family member who has the same blood type as the patient donates blood for a specific family member, but even if the institution allows this practice, it may take up to a week to prepare such a unit of blood. It must be remembered that some blood banks do not screen directed donor units for HIV or hepatitis and that these units may represent a greater risk of infection than the regular blood supply. Therefore, there may be no actual benefit and a greater risk associated with the administration of directed donor units if those units are not screened.

SPECIAL PROBLEMS

Malignant Hyperthermia

Malignant hyperthermia is a rare (1:15,000 children; 1:40,000 adults), potentially lethal disorder of acute hypermetabolism induced almost exclusively by exposure to volatile anesthetics (halothane, enflurane, and isoflurane) and succinylcholine.[19,37] It is an inherited disorder of intracellular calcium regulation and is due to a widespread membrane defect that exists in many cell types, particularly skeletal muscle. Fortunately, it can be prevented by avoiding triggering agents if the diagnosis is known or suspected. Because of the high risk of mortality, the pediatrician should note any history of anesthetic problems in the patient or family members, especially if high fevers were involved. Preoperative preparation for such children includes consultation with the surgeon and anesthesiologist so that triggering agents can be avoided. Dantrolene sodium, a direct-acting muscle relaxant, has been used with great success in treating the full-blown disease and may be used prophylactically.

Oncology

Children who have received certain chemotherapeutic agents may be at increased risk during the perioperative period. Bleomycin, BCNU, busulfan, cyclophosphamide, and methotrexate all have been associated with pulmonary fibrosis.[2] Exposure to even the modest levels of supplemental oxygen required for all patients who receive general anesthesia may aggravate the underlying lung disease greatly. Myocardial damage has been reported with cyclophosphamide, doxorubicin, adriamycin, m-AMSA, and radiation therapy. Inhalational anesthetics are arrhythmogenic and depress myocardial contractility. Patients who have myocardial damage may develop hypotension, even at low concentrations of inhaled anesthetics. Perioperative stress and hypercapnia can increase the risks of arrhythmia further. Consequently, the preoperative history should include the type and amount of chemotherapy and the extent of any associated complications of its use. In addition to the physical examination, evaluation may include, depending on the history, chest radiographs, arterial blood gas measurements, ECG, and echocardiography to document the extent of cardiorespiratory involvement. A patient who is asymptomatic and whose activity is unrestricted may need no additional laboratory tests. Preoperative communication of this information to the anesthesiologist will help identify children who require further evaluation.

Connective Tissue Disorders

Children who have connective tissue disorders may have multiple organ system involvement. These patients often are treated with aspirin or other NSAIDs, which may complicate their perioperative management further by causing a bleeding diathesis resulting from platelet dysfunction. The effect of aspirin and NSAIDs on platelet function is long-lived, and they should be stopped 1 week preoperatively. If these drugs cannot be stopped, a bleeding time may be performed to evaluate the extent of platelet impairment. Determination of prothrombin and partial thromboplastin times will not reflect this abnormality.

Patients who have connective tissue disorders may have associated dysphagia and esophageal dysmotility, which can predispose patients to pulmonary aspiration of gastric and esophageal contents. Extensive fibrosis of the temporomandibular or cricoarytenoid joint can complicate airway management and endotracheal intubation. Pulmonary infiltration and fibrosis may complicate intraoperative care by causing hypoxemia. Hematological abnormalities, including anemia of chronic disease, may complicate management even further. Again, the history should focus on the extent of disease, the type of treatment, and the child's response to therapy. Laboratory assessment may include an ECG, a chest radiograph, electrolytes, blood urea nitrogen, creatinine, hemoglobin, hematocrit, and platelet levels, as well as evaluation of the peripheral blood smear. A patient who has quiescent disease and who has regular follow-up may need nothing other than his or her hematocrit determined.

MEDICATIONS

Children receive medications regularly for many illnesses. The dosage should be adjusted to ensure adequate therapeutic levels perioperatively. The medications ordinarily are continued at usual doses up to and including the day of surgery. The two current exceptions to this practice are the use of monoamine oxidase (MAO) inhibitors and tricyclic antidepressants (TCA). The MAO inhibitors are encountered infrequently in younger children and adolescents; however, TCAs, such as imipramine and its analogs, are used commonly in the treatment of enuresis. For children receiving MAO inhibitors, the administration of meperidine (Demerol) or pancuronium (Pavulon) can have profound, catastrophic consequences—for example, malignant hypertension and tachycardia.[7] The TCAs can produce significant conduction abnormalities undetected by electrocardiography; moreover, when combined with the volatile anesthetic halothane, TCAs have resulted in life-threatening arrhythmias in the perioperative period. Therefore, it is best to discontinue these agents 2 to 3 weeks before the scheduled operation. If this cannot be done without risk to the patient, preoperative consultation with the anesthesiologist is necessary.

Increasing numbers of children are being treated for behavioral and depressive disorders with selective serotonin reuptake inhibitors (SSRIs) such as fluoxetine (Prozac). Withdrawal can precipitate anxiety, agitation, and diaphoresis; however, most of these drugs have such long elimination half-times that unless prolonged NPO periods are contemplated, withdrawal is unlikely perioperatively. It is important that the anesthesiologist be informed that patients are taking such drugs, because interactions with other drugs administered perioperatively can lead to unexpected side effects. Fluoxetine, like other SSRIs, is a potent inhibitor of the hepatic cytochrome P-450 enzymes and, therefore, may result in elevated blood levels of these other drugs, which depend on these enzymes for metabolism.[38]

In addition, increasing numbers of pediatrics patients, like their parents, are taking herbal or homeopathic medications, which also may lead to unexpected reactions to anesthetic drugs. The use of these substances should be disclosed to the anesthesiologist.

RELEVANT ASPECTS OF THE PHYSICAL EXAMINATION

The physical examination is directed at the general state of health and specifically to discover conditions that could complicate anesthesia. The cardiovascular and respiratory systems demand close attention and documentation. Neurological status should be evaluated, and preexisting deficits specifically documented. Recording of all abnormalities will assist the anesthesiologist in developing an appropriate plan for the anesthesia to be administered.

The pediatrician should note the general body habitus, height, weight (in kg), and percentiles. An obese or Cushingoid child can have significant hypoventilation or airway obstruction in the supine position and under anesthesia and is at increased risk for aspiration pneumonitis. A careful examination of the head and neck is essential. A short neck, large tongue, and a small mandible all constitute sources of airway obstruction and may lead to delay or impossibility in intubating the trachea because of the difficulty in seeing the glottic opening. Midfacial or maxillary hypoplasia may present similar problems. In addition to difficulty with intubation, such patients may have airway obstruction on induction of anesthesia and difficulty with ventilation.

As well as having the aforementioned airway concerns because of large tongues and a relatively hypoplastic midface, patients who have Down syndrome may have atlantoaxial instability. This may manifest only under general anesthesia and neuromuscular blockade and can result in damage to the cervical spinal cord.[29,30] Parents should be questioned about any neurological symptoms such as long-tract signs (hyperreflexia, positive Babinski response, and clonus), hand weakness, or bladder and bowel dysfunction. History of torticollis or neck pain should be elicited. Even in the absence of symptoms, it is recommended that children who have Down syndrome and are 2 years of age or older have lateral flexion and extension radiographs of the cervical spine before anesthesia is given so that patients at risk for subluxation can be identified. Some children older than 5 years of age will have had these films as a requirement for their participation in Special Olympics. If radiographs reveal an atlantodens interval of greater than 5 mm (usually maximal in the flexion view), the child should be referred for orthopedic or neurosurgical consultation before elective surgery.

Some "dwarfing" syndromes can be associated with airway and cardiorespiratory abnormalities that can present significant problems perioperatively. In all children, the presence of loose or fractured teeth must be documented to guard against potential aspiration, because the teeth and oral mucosa may be subject to trauma during airway manipulation.

Preoperative vital signs, including weight in kilograms, temperature, respiratory rate, heart rate, and blood pressure, should be recorded. Accurate weight measurement is essential because anesthetic drug dosing is calculated by weight. Preoperative recognition of any cardiovascular compromise may prevent significant perioperative problems. For example, patients who have significant chest wall or thoracic deformities (e.g., severe scoliosis and dwarfism) can have marked cardiorespiratory compromise manifested as decreased lung volumes and pulmonary function and can have myocardial strain evident on ECG or echocardiogram. Such patients are at risk for intraoperative complications and prolonged postoperative mechanical ventilation. Therefore, they need preoperative pulmonary function studies and their myocardial function evaluated to enable the anesthesiologist to design the optimal anesthetic plan.

LABORATORY EXAMINATION

Laboratory studies are performed to detect significant physiological abnormalities that may prove hazardous to the child perioperatively. In an otherwise healthy child scheduled for outpatient surgery, routine laboratory tests rarely are indicated. Routine preoperative chest radiographs in well children have failed to detect abnormalities of major anesthetic or surgical consequence.[8] Screening tests for hemoglobin and hematocrit values commonly are obtained in the hope of identifying and treating those who have significant anemia. However, recent studies indicate that the incidence of previously undetected anemia in children presenting for elective surgery is extremely low (0.29%).[12,32] Furthermore, outpatient procedures can be performed safely, even in the presence of mild anemia (hematocrit 27% to 35%). Therefore, routine determination of hematocrit and hemoglobin is not advocated if studies performed as part of well-child care have been normal. However, black children who have not had a hemoglobin/hematocrit determination after 6 months of age should have a hemoglobin or hematocrit and a sickle cell screening test. Most surgeons require preoperative determination of coagulation status (prothrombin time [PT], partial thromboplastin time [PTT], and platelet count) in children having procedures with an increased risk of intra- or postoperative bleeding (e.g., tonsillectomy/adenoidectomy, intracranial procedures), even when there is no history of a bleeding disorder in the patient or the patient's family. Electrolyte abnormalities of any consequence are extremely rare in healthy children; preoperative screening for such deviations usually is unhelpful and does not alter the anesthetic management. Even for hospitalized patients who might be expected to have an incidence of laboratory abnormalities higher than that found in "healthy outpatients," routine preoperative testing is not indicated. Screening preoperative urinalysis also has failed to discover serious underlying problems in the vast majority of children studied (99.5% of 1859 patients younger than 19 years of age).[8] Therefore, these tests are not usually performed in healthy children scheduled for elective surgery.

Performing routine preoperative pregnancy tests in adolescent females remains controversial. Because of the high rate of sexual activity among increasingly younger teenagers and because all anesthetic medications increase the incidence of abortion and are potential teratogens at various doses, it is prudent to ask whether the patient is sexually active. The date of the last menstrual period should be documented, and the pediatrician should consider obtaining a screening test for pregnancy and informing the family of potential risks if the test is positive. Some anesthesiologists are reluctant to involve themselves in this aspect of their patient's lives, citing issues of privacy, and are uncomfortable communicating with families about unexpectedly positive results. The pediatrician, having a long-standing relationship with the teenager and family, should be more comfortable dealing with this issue.

Although the healthy child needs almost no preoperative laboratory tests, the situation is entirely different for children who have a history of or the presence of an abnormality. For example, it is helpful to obtain a chest radiograph in a patient who has a history of chronic aspiration or lower airway disease. Knowing the hemoglobin level is important in the child who has sickle cell disease or cardiac disease. A child who has cardiovascular disease and is on digoxin therapy should have his or her serum sodium, potassium, and digoxin levels measured. An ECG is warranted in a child who has obstructive sleep apnea, BPD, congenital heart disease, or severe scoliosis. In these and similar circumstances, preoperative testing is aimed at detecting and quantifying underlying abnormalities associated with known disease that can lead to life-threatening complications during anesthesia.

SUMMARY

Preoperative evaluation and preparation is directed toward minimizing the intrinsic risks of anesthesia and surgery by having the child in the healthiest possible condition before surgery. The pediatrician can contribute to this goal by understanding the effects of general anesthesia on the physiology of children. This allows an appreciation of the anesthesiologist's concerns regarding underlying diseases, which may appear "stable" (and, therefore, of little present concern to the pediatrician) but which may have grave consequences during anesthesia. The preoperative evaluation is designed to ensure that the child's perioperative needs can be met by providing the anesthesiologist both qualitative and quantitative information regarding the child's state of health and disease. The relationship between the child, parents, and pediatrician places the latter in an ideal position to prepare families for their children's surgical experience.

REFERENCES

1. Alter HJ, et al: The incidence of transfusion-associated hepatitis G virus infection and its relation to liver disease, *N Engl J Med* 336:747, 1997.
2. Burrows FA, Hickey PR, Colan S: Perioperative complications in patients with anthracycline chemotherapeutic agents, *Can Anaesth Soc J* 32:149, 1985.
3. Centers for Disease Control and Prevention: US Public Health Service guidelines for testing and counseling blood and plasma donors for human immunodeficiency virus type 1 antigen, *MMWR* 45:1, 1996.
4. Dajani AS, et al: Prevention of bacterial endocarditis: recommendations by the American Heart Association, *JAMA* 264:2919, 1990.
5. DeSoto H, et al: Changes in oxygen saturation following general anesthesia in children with upper respiratory infection signs and symptoms undergoing otolaryngological procedures, *Anesthesiology* 68:276, 1988.
6. Eger EI: MAC. In Eger EI, editor: *Anesthetic uptake and action,* Baltimore, 1974, Williams & Wilkins.

7. Evans-Prosser CD: The use of pethidine and morphine in the presence of monoamine oxidase inhibitors, *Br J Anaesth* 40:279, 1968.
8. Farnsworth PB, et al: The value of routine preoperative chest roentgenograms in infants and children, *JAMA* 244:582, 1980.
9. Ferrari LR, editor: *Anesthesia and pain management for the pediatrician,* Baltimore, 1999, Johns Hopkins.
10. Galinkin JL, Kurth D: Neonatal and pediatric apnea syndromes, *Prob Anesth* 10:444, 1998.
11. Goodwin SR: Perioperative implications of hemoglobinopathies, *Anesth Analg* 86(suppl):39, 1998.
12. Hackmann T, Steward DJ, Sheps SB: Anemia in pediatric day-surgery patients: prevalence and detection, *Anesthesiology* 75:27, 1991.
13. Helfaer MA, Wilson MD: Obstructive sleep apnea, control of ventilation, and anesthesia in children, *Pediatr Clin North Am* 41:131, 1994.
14. Hirshman CA: Airway reactivity in humans: anesthetic implications, *Anesthesiology* 58:170, 1983.
15. Jacoby DB, Hirshman CA: General anesthesia in patients with viral respiratory infections: an unsound sleep? *Anesthesiology* 74:969, 1991.
16. Keenan RL, Boyan CP: Cardiac arrest due to anesthesia: a study of incidence and causes, *JAMA* 253:2373, 1985.
17. Kingston HG, Hirshman CA: Perioperative management of the patient with asthma, *Anesth Analg* 63:844, 1984.
18. Lackritz EM, et al: Estimated risk of transmission of the human immunodeficiency virus by screened blood in the United States, *N Engl J Med* 333:1721, 1996.
19. Larach MG, et al: Prediction of malignant hyperthermia susceptibility by clinical signs, *Anesthesiology* 66:547, 1987.
20. Linden JV, Kaplan HS: Transfusion errors: cause and effects, *Trans Med Rev* 8:169, 1994.
21. Linden JV, Tourault MA, Schribner CL: Decrease in frequency of transfusion fatalities, *Transfusion* 37:243, 1997.
22. Liu LM, et al: Life-threatening apnea in infants recovering from anesthesia, *Anesthesiology* 59:506, 1983.
23. Martin LD: Anesthetic implications of an upper respiratory infection in children, *Pediatr Clin North Am* 41:121, 1994.
24. Maxwell LG, Deshpande JK, Wetzel RC: Preoperative evaluation of children, *Pediatr Clin North Am* 41:93, 1994.
25. Morray JP, et al: A comparison of pediatric and adult anesthesia closed malpractice claims. *Anesthesiology* 78:461, 1993.
26. Olsson GL, Hallen B: Laryngospasm during anesthesia: a computer-aided incidence study of 136,929 patients. *Acta Anaesthesiol Scand* 28: 567, 1984.
27. Pasternak LR: Outpatient anesthesia. In Rogers MC, et al, editors: *Principles and practice of anesthesiology,* St Louis, 1993, Mosby.
28. Pien LC, Grammar LC, Patterson R: Minimal complications in a surgical population with severe asthma receiving prophylactic corticosteroids, *J Allergy Clin Immunol* 82:696, 1988.
29. Pueschel SM: Atlantoaxial instability and Down syndrome, *Pediatrics* 81:879, 1988.
30. Pueschel SM, Scola FH: Atlantoaxial instability in individuals with Down syndrome: epidemiologic, radiographic, and clinical studies, *Pediatrics* 80:555, 1987.
31. Rolf N, Cote CJ: Frequency and severity of desaturation events during general anesthesia in children with and without upper respiratory infections, *J Clin Anesth* 4:200, 1992.
32. Roy WL, Lerman J, McIntyre BG: Is preoperative haemoglobin testing justified in children undergoing minor elective surgery? *Can J Anaesth* 38:700, 1991.
33. Sauder RA, et al: Methylprednisolone increases sensitivity to beta-adrenergic agonists within 48 hours in Basenji greyhounds, *Anesthesiology* 79:1278, 1993.
34. Schreiber GB, et al: The risk of transfusion-transmitted viral infections, *N Engl J Med* 334:1685, 1996.
35. Schreiner MS: Preoperative and postoperative fasting in children, *Pediatr Clin North Am* 41:111, 1994.
36. Schreiner MS, Triebwasser A, Keon TP: Ingestion of liquids compared with preoperative fasting in pediatric outpatients, *Anesthesiology* 72: 593, 1990.
37. Schwartz L, Rockoff MA, Koka BV: Masseter spasm with anesthesia: incidence and implications, *Anesthesiology* 61:772, 1984.
38. Stoelting RJ: *Pharmacology and physiology in anesthetic practice,* ed. 3, Philadelphia, 1999, Lippincott-Raven.
39. Tiret L, et al: Complications related to anaesthesia in infants and children: a prospective survey of 40,240 anaesthetics, *Br J Anaesth* 61:263, 1988.
40. Vichinsky EP, et al.: A comparison of conservative and aggressive transfusion regimens in the perioperative management of sickle cell disease, *N Engl J Med* 333:206, 1995.
41. Welborn LG, Greenspun JC: Anesthesia and apnea: perioperative considerations in the former preterm infant, *Pediatr Clin North Am* 41:181, 1994.
42. Welborn LG, et al: High-dose caffeine suppresses postoperative apnea in former preterm infants, *Anesthesiology* 71:347, 1989.
43. Welborn LG, et al: Postoperative apnea in former preterm infants: prospective comparison of spinal and general anesthesia, *Anesthesiology* 72:838, 1990.
44. Yaster M, et al: The night after surgery: postoperative management of the pediatric outpatient—surgical and anesthetic aspects, *Pediatr Clin North Am* 41:199, 1994.
45. Zuckerberg AL: Perioperative approach to children, *Pediatr Clin North Am* 41:15, 1994.

10 Structural and Functional Analysis of Body Systems

Nicholas M. Nelson

The essential task of the physician, perhaps more than that of the surgeon, is problem delineation. To be sure, the medical practitioner is involved in the solution of problems, once defined, but these solutions tend to emphasize the enhancement of normal and the suppression of abnormal physiological responses, often by pharmacological means, rather than by the surgeon's direct attack on an anatomical structure that has been altered by disease or development.

The symptoms of which the patient complains and the signs that the physician elicits serve to suggest involvement of one or more organ systems, so the patient's history and physical examination together may be viewed as what applied mathematicians and statisticians call exploratory data analysis. In this earliest phase of clinical problem-solving, the physician assembles the differential diagnosis and then orders that list in descending likelihood, based on his or her knowledge of the epidemiology and, particularly, the natural history of the diseases in question.

This chapter is concerned with a succeeding phase of clinical investigation—the "workup," or confirmatory data analysis, wherein the physician's suspicions, intuitions, and knowledge of the location and extent of the patient's condition are confirmed or denied. Of course, many of the problems encountered in primary care are self-evident or otherwise sufficiently familiar as not to require investigation beyond the history or physical examination; yet, no primary care practitioner is likely to see many patients without recourse to the clinical laboratory and radiological or other consultative support of his or her effort to define the patient's problem. During this effort the practitioner must increasingly bear in mind the cost-benefit ratio of the investigations proposed—"cost" to include not only the fiscal but also the morbid and even mortal risks of the procedures under consideration, as constantly displayed against the benefits likely to be returned in the form of useful or definitive diagnostic information. A sequence of investigations should be planned that is pertinent to the organ system indicated by exploratory analysis of the clinical data gathered and that is coordinated with the current differential diagnosis. This list should begin with those procedures that are inexpensive, noninvasive, and of high sensitivity to many diseases ("coarse focus") but of low specificity for any single disease ("fine focus").

GENERAL ASSESSMENT

The quintessence of pediatrics, in contrast to other clinical disciplines, is its constant concern with the changes that accompany the growth and development of its patients. The child seriously involved with disease often announces the intensity of that involvement by primary or secondary disruptions of somatic growth and psychomotor development, almost regardless of precise etiology. These aspects are treated in much greater depth elsewhere in this textbook, but Tables 10-1 and 10-2 set out some of the more important benchmarks against which the pediatrician measures the patient's progress in these areas.

The Lubchenco, Wright, and Babson charts help the neonatologist assess the growth of premature infants, just as the National Center for Health Statistics charts (which largely have displaced the "Harvard" or "Iowa" or "Wetzel grid" standards of an earlier era) serve those who are concerned with the growth of children from term birth through adolescence. The Dubowitz examination inverts the usual approach to developmental assessment by using established age norms of physical and neuromotor characteristics to estimate gestational age; it assumes that the child being assessed is developed normally for his or her gestational age (which is to be estimated), in contrast to the more typical process of referring the assessed stage of growth and development to the child's (known) age.

The available tools for developmental assessment of the young infant necessarily emphasize motor over cognitive phenomena, and many feel that true cognition is estimated best by the adaptive and language components of the various screening instruments. The alleged cultural "loading" of most of the formal psychometric estimators of intelligence (see Table 10-2) has brought them under political and popular critical fire; yet, whatever their "fairness," their position as valid predictors of school performance has not been challenged.

The screening tests noted in Table 10-2 are sufficiently simple and brief to administer, after reasonable practice, to merit consideration for inclusion in a primary care practice, either as a routine assessment or as a preliminary to formal psychometric testing upon symptomatic indication. (See Appendix D, Table D-1 for a description of the tests listed in Table 10-2.)

ORGAN IMAGING

The past two decades have witnessed such rapid and fundamental changes in organ imaging, as scintigraphic, sonographic, magnetic, and computer technologies have intermarried with that of radiation, that some departments of

Table 10-1 Assessment of Growth

Examination	
Basic	**Specialized**
General	
Growth charts	
CROSS SECTIONAL	Cell size (RNA)
Premature infant	Cell number (DNA)
Lubchenco, Usher (weight, length, head)[3,5,9]	
Infant and child	
NCHS (weight, length, head)[4]	
Nellhaus (head)[7]	
LONGITUDINAL	
Premature infant	
Wright (weight)[10]	
Babson, Marks (weight, length, head)[1,6]	
Infant and child	
Tanner (weight, length)[8]	
Chemical	
Alkaline phosphatase	N_2-balance K-balance
Bone Age	
Knee (newborn)	
Hand, wrist (child)	
Body Fat	
Skinfold thickness	Underwater weight
Harpenden calipers	Total body water ^{40}K distribution

radiology have seriously considered changing their names to departments of "medical imaging." In some areas the field also is shifting from one in which the technician occupies the major portion of the patient's experience to one in which the radiologist (imagist?) dominates, especially in the techniques of angiointervention and ultrasound. Throughout the development of the field, the goals of optimum resolution of the tissue of interest and its optimum differentiation from neighboring tissues of noninterest have come into constant conflict with the restraints of cumulative radiation dosage and the desire to minimize invasiveness. Great strides have been made in diminishing risk while increasing definition, but at such an increase in the cost of technology as seriously to question the relative contribution of these techniques toward establishing and maintaining the public health. Before dismissing technological advance in medicine on grounds of cost alone, however, physicians, if not politicians, might well reflect upon the "costs" of the modern computed tomographic or magnetic resonance documentation of a posterior fossa tumor in a 4-year-old (and in *40 minutes*) versus the "lesser costs" of an obsolete evaluation extracted through the pain and risk of a pneumoencephalogram, a ventriculogram, or cerebral angiography (with luck, in *5 days*).

Table 10-3 offers a survey of current imaging techniques and their ability to contribute to our understanding of the patient.

Roentgenography

Still the gold standard against which to measure the resolving power of any imaging technique, classic roentgenography has, nevertheless, rarely been able to differentiate the soft tissues of interest within a body region unless abetted by natural (air) or artificial (barium, iodine, or other radiopaque

Table 10-2 Assessment of Development

	Social Adaptation	Language	Cognition and Intellect	Perception and Motion	Emotion and Projection	Academic Achievement
Screening Tests						
Premature newborn						
Ballard Gestational Aging—expanded				X		
Term newborn						
Brazelton Behavioral Assessment Scale	X					
Infant and child						
Denver Developmental Screening Test	X	X		X		
Developmental Profile II*	X	X	X	X		
Vineland Adaptive Behavior Scales*	X	X		X		
Psychometric Tests						
Bayley Scales of Infant Development II	X	X	X	X		
Developmental Test Visual-Motor Integration				X		
Stanford-Binet Intelligence Scale IV			X			
Test of Language Development		X				
Wechsler Individual Achievement Test						X
Wechsler Intelligence Scale for Children III			X			
Child Behavior Checklist*					X	
Pediatric Behavior Scale*					X	

*Parental observation.

Table 10-3 Imaging Techniques*

Modality	Usefulness for Delineation of: Static Structure	Dynamic Motion	Metabolic Function	Imaging Criterion
Ultrasound	++	+++	0	Acoustic impedance
Magnetic resonance imaging (MRI)				
Hydrogen	++	+	0	Water content
Phosphorus	+	0	++	Energy metabolism
Radionuclide nuclear scintigraphy	+	+	++	Gamma emission
Single photon emission computed tomography (SPECT)	++	++	0	
Positron emission tomography (PET)	+	0	++	Positron emission (metabolic activity)
Roentgenography				
Standard roentgenogram	+++	0	0	Roentgen ray density (enhanced spectrum)
Computed tomography (CT)	++	+	0	
Angiography				
Standard	+++	0	0	
Cine/video	++	+++	0	
Digital subtraction	++	0	0	(reduced background)
Fluoroscopy	++	+++	0	

*In approximate ascending order of energizing radiation sustained by the patient.

compound) increases in contrast. This is because the transmission of roentgen rays through body tissues is a function of their radioabsorption—mineral and bone being the most opaque, water and air being the least. Water, blood, and muscle, unfortunately, are so similar in radiopacity as to render most difficult the precise appreciation of anything more than gross organ dimension within the abdomen, for instance. Angiography, urography, bronchography, and other techniques for instilling contrast agents are very valuable, but all require some level of invasiveness, and many require local or general anesthesia. Moreover, the contrast agents themselves are not benign—for example, they may produce anaphylaxis or hemiplegia after cerebral angiography or myocardial ischemia after coronary angiography. Digital subtraction techniques in venous or arterial angiography can improve differentiation from confusing background structures and even diminish the dose of contrast agent required, but not the necessity for invading the vascular tree.

Radionuclide Imaging

One of the happier aspects of the nuclear age has been the discovery or development of a vast array of radioactive and nonradioactive isotopic tracer elements without which most of modern biochemistry and even archaeology and paleontology could not have proceeded. Nuclear medicine has emphasized the attachment of a radioactive label with requisite physical characteristics to a biologically active carrier molecule, concentrated by natural body processes into the target area or organ, there to emit gamma radiation, which is then recorded, typically by a scintillation camera. This concentration in normal tissues means that diseased areas usually are revealed as areas of altered accumulation of radioactivity.

Because these synthetic radiopharmaceuticals reside and radiate within the body, they must have either a short half-life ($t_{1/2}$) for radiation or be rapidly excreted, or both. On the other hand, the $t_{1/2}$ must be long enough to allow for transport from the site of preparation to that of instillation into the patient. Technetium (Tc) is an element that naturally (without carrier) concentrates especially well in the choroid plexus, the salivary and thyroid glands, and the stomach, but the basic reasons for its prominence as a label in Table 10-4 are its relative ease of preparation, its $t_{1/2}$ of 6 hours, and its gamma emission at energy levels (140 Kv) that prevent absorption by the body (up to 20 Kv), yet are below those levels (above 600 Kv) where radiation scatter becomes so gross as to render organ delineation hopeless. Indeed, wherever the issue has been only that of delineating organ structure, the poor resolving power of most radionuclide techniques has, in many instances, led to their gradual displacement by the equally noninvasive methods of ultrasound, computed tomography (CT), or magnetic resonance imaging (MRI). SPECT (single photon emission computed tomography) scans, in particular, have improved resolution significantly.

The carrier molecules for certain radionuclide techniques are, however, specific examiners of an organ's function (e.g., ^{99m}Tc MAG3 in the assessment of renal tubular function) and, therefore, can challenge nuclear magnetic resonance imaging (MRI) and positron emission tomography (PET) on the grounds of informed functional analysis of certain organs. Few sights, for instance, are more rewarding to the pediatric surgeon, faced with a child who has massive rectal bleeding, than a positive "Meckel diverticulum scan," in which the pertechnetate label has concentrated in the ectopic gastric tissue and thus narrowed the surgeon's otherwise unguided search throughout the intestine for an attackable bleeding site.

Ultrasonography

Ultrasonography has now become the fundamental means for assessment of fetal growth and development, as well as for neonatal and infant intracranial examination, not to mention its contributions in cardiology (echocardiography) and in the examination of the abdominal viscera, the orbit, the hip, and the soft tissues of the neck, the body wall, and the extremities. Although to the untrained eye the current interpretation of ultrasonic scans may seem to approach the mystic, image quality, nonetheless, is vastly superior to that of radionuclide imaging. There is no ionizing radiation, and the sound energy levels used are believed to be far below the threshold for tissue damage.

The critical factor for tissue differentiation is acoustic impedance (analogous to radiodensity), but the range of values displayed by various tissues is much wider than that for radiation. Hence, blood or water in the ultrasonogram (in contrast to the unenhanced roentgenogram) is easily distinguished from connective tissue and muscle; on this fact rests modern echocardiography. Bone and air, however, are nearly opaque to ultrasound, so the cranial and thoracic contents can be examined only through the sonic "windows" offered by the open anterior fontanelle, the subxiphoid region, or the suprasternal notch.

As videorecorded in "real time," examinations by two-dimensional sector or linear array scanning, as well as Doppler scans, form the sonic dynamic equivalents of classic fluoroscopy and cineangiography. By these techniques, the motions of the heart and its valves, the fetus, and the flow of blood can be viewed, reviewed, and analyzed, often by the same analytical formulas developed and substantiated through the more invasive techniques of angiography.

To the advantages of relative safety, high image quality, and the dynamic, as well as static, recording afforded by ultrasonography can be added the highest degree of portability of all the imaging techniques—the equipment is easily brought to the bedside on vehicles substantially smaller and lighter than the usual "portable" roentgenography machine. However, imaging still requires a high degree of patience, experience, and artistry on the part of the examiner wielding the sonic transducer; thus, the interpretability of recordings is much more in direct proportion to the expertise of the physician or sonographer at the bedside than is the case in, say, roentgenography.

Computed Tomography (CT)

Computed tomography is derived from the earlier methods of plain tomography, wherein either the roentgen ray tube or the film cassette (or both) are rotated during exposure so as to blur all tissues except those at the axis of rotation. With CT, a computer enhancement of the digitally analyzed "gray scale" of received roentgen ray transmission vastly widens the scale of appreciable radiodensity differences between tissues beyond that of the "mineral-bone-water-air" scale of classic roentgenography. The body, thus, is viewable as a sequence of axial planar "cuts," reminiscent of the frozen whole-body sections of gross anatomy. These cuts can then be reassembled by the computer for review in ever-larger body segments. Continuous motion of the patient through the scanning gantry ("helical" CT) has reduced the image acquisition time to 1 second per "slice," but iodinated intravenous contrast agents are usually required for suitable enhancement of the image. Moreover, CT is distinctly static, quite expensive, and most cer-

Table 10-4 Radionuclide Scans

Organ	Label	Carrier	Concentration Mechanism
Liver	^{99m}Tc	Sulfur colloid	Phagocytosis (Kuppfer cells)
	^{99m}Tc	HIDA	Active transport (extrahepatic cells)
	^{99m}Tc	PIPIDA	Active transport (biliary cells)
Kidneys	$^{99m}TcO_4$	None	Flow diffusion
	^{99m}Tc	DTPA	Active transport (glomerulus)
	^{125}I	Thalamate	Active transport (glomerulus)
	^{131}I	Hippuran	Active transport (tubule)
Lungs	^{133}Xe	None	Active transport (alveolar gas)
	^{99m}Tc	HSA (macroaggregated)	Capillary blockade
Heart	$^{99m}TcO_4$	None	Flow diffusion
Blood pool	^{99m}Tc	HSA	Compartmentation
	^{99m}Tc	RBC	Compartmentation
Spleen	^{99m}Tc	Sulfur colloid	Phagocytosis (Kuppfer cells)
RE system	^{99m}Tc	RBC	Sequestration
Gut	$^{99m}TcO_4$	None	Active transport (parietal cells)
Abscess, tumor	^{67}Gallium	None	? Transport (inflammatory cells)
			? Diffusion (tumor cells)
Bone	^{99m}Tc	Diphosphonate	Active transport
Thyroid	$^{99m}TcO_4$	None	Flow diffusion
	^{131}I	None	Active transport (thyroid cells)
Adrenal	^{131}I	Cholesterol	Active transport (cortical cells)
	^{125}I		
CSF	^{99m}Tc	HSA	Compartmentation
Brain	$^{99m}TcO_4$	None	Active transport (choroid plexus)

CSF, Cerebrospinal fluid; *DTPA,* diethylenetriamine pentaacetic acid; *HIDA,* hepatoimidodiacetic acid; *HSA,* human serum albumin; *PIPIDA,* paraisopropylimidodiacetic acid; *RBC,* red blood cells; *RE,* reticuloendothelial.

tainly nonportable. Nonetheless, it has revolutionized clinical neurology and has essentially made pneumoencephalography and ventriculography obsolete, while relegating cerebral angiography to the status of a strictly preoperative procedure. The diagnostic acumen and therapeutic capabilities of virtually all the surgical subspecialties have been similarly enhanced by CT cuts through the body part of their interest, from orbit to ankle.

Positron Emission Tomography (PET)

Related to CT scanning in that tomography is used to produce a tissue "slice," PET scans view the positrons emitted by appropriately excited body tissues rather than roentgen rays. If the excitation is produced by isotopes of metabolically active molecules and compounds (e.g., oxygen and glucose), it becomes possible to examine sites of metabolic activity (and blood flow to them). The concept is similar to, but much more rapidly and accurately defined than, radionuclide scans. However, the equipment is expensive, nonportable, and must be close to the cyclotron or other heavy nuclear gear required to produce the short-lived isotopes. PET scanning at most sites, therefore, is much more a research tool than a practical one for clinical evaluation.

Magnetic Resonance Imaging (MRI)

MRI has now assumed a prominent place in the diagnostic imaging armamentarium. It also is noninvasive (and nonportable), but uses no ionizing radiation. It is based on the phenomenon of the magnetic resonance of uniform spin, induced in the atomic particles of all tissues placed in a strong magnetic field and then struck by a radiofrequency pulse delivered at the natural vibrational frequency of the atom in question (e.g., hydrogen). As the imposed radiofrequency pulse subsides, the atomic particles "relax" into their natural random spin orientation and emit a recordable electromagnetic pulse, the density scale of which is a function of the density of that atom in the tissue so bombarded.

If the imposed radiofrequency pulse is "tuned" (like a radio or TV receiver) to resonate in hydrogen nuclei (protons), the emitted electromagnetic pulse reflects the varying water (i.e., hydrogen proton) content of those tissues. If, on the other hand, the pulse is tuned to the phosphorus atom, intimately involved in most of the body's energy-transforming biochemical reactions, the recorded image (as in PET scanning) tends to reflect metabolic activity within the tissues examined. Although the image quality of MRI hydrogen scanning already compares favorably with or exceeds that of CT and PET scanning, it is too early to specify whether the promise of bloodless biochemical biopsy through MRI (phosphorus or other atom) can be realized.

A summary judgment of imaging benefits suggests that MRI is best suited to studies (in nontraumatic clinical settings) of the brain, the spinal cord, and the soft tissues. However, CT is still predominant in the evaluation of head trauma and has not yet been replaced by MRI for the structural examination of the child's chest and abdomen.

SYSTEMIC EVALUATION

The assessment of structure and function of the organ systems within the body involves both biochemical and biophysical means for tracing the effectiveness with which an organ performs its tasks. Disruptions of gross structure need not impair function (e.g., hepatic metastases), and disruptions of function need not impair gross structure (e.g., renal tubular acidosis); thus, evaluation of both is often necessary to rule out disease, especially in those organs that have multiple functions, such as the liver and kidneys.

The functional evaluation of the heart and circulation, the respiratory tract, the neuromotor system, the skin, the eyes, and the ears is accomplished largely by the physician during the physical examination. In contrast, physiological assessment of the hematopoietic, immune, and endocrine systems, the kidneys and the urinary tract, and the liver and intestinal tract depends heavily on laboratory tests. In all, however, a careful medical history designed to test, by system-oriented symptomatic questioning, the presence or absence of normal organ function should direct the exploration of the patient's problem and contribute most to its solution.

Heart and Circulation

Appropriate indicators for investigation of this system (Table 10-5) may range from a presumably innocent cardiac murmur to cyanosis and frank heart failure. The increasing sophistication of echocardiography has relegated formal cardiac catheterization largely to the category of a preoperative and postoperative intervention to be undertaken when accurate measurement of chamber pressures and pulmonary and systemic flow ratios is necessary. Stress (exercise) testing is

Table 10-5 Heart and Circulation

	Examination	
	Basic	**Specialized**
Structure	Chest roentgenogram	Radionuclide scan Echocardiogram Angiography
Function		
Hemodynamics		
Preload	Auscultation	Echocardiogram
Contractility	Sphygmomanometry	Echocardiogram
Afterload	Electrocardiogram	Echocardiogram
Distribution of flow	Oximetry	Radionuclide scan
	Blood gases	Cardiac catheterization Thermodilution Dye dilution Angiography
Microcirculation	Stress exercise testing Maximum O_2 consumption	

Table 10-6 Lungs and Respiratory Tract

	Examination	
	Basic	**Specialized**
Structure		
Overall	Chest roentgenogram Fluoroscopy Sinus roentgenograms, CT scan Barium swallow Sputum Analysis Culture	Nasopharyngoscopy Bronchoscopy (flexible, rigid) Laryngoscopy
Lung volumes	Spirometry Pneumotachometry Tomograms	Gas dilution (N_2, H_2) Body plethysmography Bronchography Angiography Puncture Biopsy
Function		
Ventilation	Spirometry Flow rates	Gas washout (N_2, H_2) Flow-volume loops Occluded breath-mouth pressure Radionuclide scan Body plethysmography
Perfusion		Radionuclide scan Gas absorption (N_2O, acetylene)
Diffusion		Diffusing capacity (CO, O_2)
Gas exchange	Oximetry Transcutaneous blood gases Arterial blood gases	Alveolar-arterial (O_2, CO_2, N_2) gas gradients
Mechanics		Body plethysmography Compliance Resistance
Stress	Exercise Cold air breathing	

used to evaluate the cardiovascular response to the aerobic demands of physical activity.

The hemodynamic stress placed on the heart by excessive venous return (preload) or excessive outflow resistance (afterload) tends to produce dilation or hypertrophy, respectively, of the chamber so loaded. Preload may be estimated clinically by measurement of venous pressure, detection of "flow" murmurs, and roentgenographical assessment of pulmonary vasculature, whereas the more difficult judgment of afterload depends on the site or sites of vascular resistance—at the outflow tract (stenotic semilunar valves), in the great vessels (coarctation), or at the level of the resistance vessels themselves (diastolic hypertension). A sense of chamber wall thickness may be derived from electrocardiography (in the amplitude of QRS deflections), but the echocardiogram has become the modern gold standard for measuring chamber diameters and wall and valve dimensions. Moreover, cardiovascular shunts may be traced during the echocardiogram by simple saline injections or (color) Doppler echocardiography, whereas chamber hemodynamics (ejection fraction, circumferential shortening velocity, and fractional shortening) may be measured accurately and repeatedly as clinical indices of myocardial contractility.

The invasive procedures (cardiac catheterization, angiography, venography) are usually reserved for those situations requiring precise anatomical detail (pulmonary artery) or pressure/flow data, generally in anticipation or documentation of surgical repair or for frank vascular intervention.

Lungs and Respiratory Tract

The patient who has symptoms referable to the respiratory tract (e.g., cough and hyperpnea) may be suffering from more global disease (allergy or diabetic ketoacidosis), but those children who have signs of impending or actual respiratory failure (dyspnea or cyanosis) usually are found to have significant disruption of lung tissue, most often the airways.

The overall aim and usual result of pulmonary function testing (Table 10-6) is the classification of the child's problem as either "obstructive" or "restrictive." Obstructive disease of the airways (asthma or other bronchospastic disease and cystic fibrosis) slows flow rates and alters gaseous outflow curves and flow-volume loops, often producing secondary increases in residual lung volume and functional residual capacity. Restrictive lung disease (pneumonia, respiratory distress syndrome of infancy, neurological disease, or other

Table 10-7 Kidneys and Urinary Tract

	Examination	
	Basic	**Specialized**
Structure	Ultrasound	^{131}I hippuran scan
	Intravenous urography	Angiography
	CT scan	Retrograde cystourethrography
	^{99m}Tc DTPA scan	Cystoscopy
		Biopsy
Function		
Urinary tract	Urinalysis	Voiding cystourethrogram
		Cystometrics
	BUN	Lasix-stimulated diethylene triamine pentaacetic acid (DTPA) scan
	Creatinine	
Glomerulus	Urine flow	^{125}I thalamate scan (captopril-stimulated)
	Creatinine clearance	Inulin clearance
Tubule	Fluid restriction test	Vasopressin test
	Phosphate clearance	Paraamino hippurate (PAH) clearance
	Urine and serum electrolytes	NH_4Cl loading test

conditions that impair the thoracic "bellows") encompasses those processes that restrict or replace alveolar volume and ventilation.

Unfortunately, most of the apparatus and maneuvers developed to assess pulmonary function require a level of understanding and cooperation on the part of the patient that is beyond the capabilities of most children younger than 5 to 7 years of age, unless they are swaddled and satiated (i.e., essentially "thalamic") newborn infants or sedated toddlers. Hence, in practical terms the clinical assessment of pulmonary function is reduced in most cases to simple peak flowmeter studies and estimates of gas exchange (oximetry and transcutaneous or arterial blood gases).

Kidneys and Urinary Tract

Critical disruption of renal function (Table 10-7) can be notoriously subtle and insidious, evoking no detectable symptoms until far advanced. Hence, the cautious physician usually includes a urinalysis, and even in the presence of a normal urinalysis, determinations of blood urea nitrogen (BUN) and creatinine in the evaluation of any child whose growth or general health is at all in question. Manifestation of renal disease in a younger child often is in the form of an abdominal mass (hydronephrosis, Wilms' tumor, or cystic disease), the delineation of which is the special and spectacular province of the ultrasonogram; indeed, these renal lesions can now be detected during careful *fetal* ultrasound examination. Hence, urography now is used only rarely to assess extrarenal retroperitoneal disease, while the function of the lower urinary tract is assessed conveniently by a voiding cystourethrogram, using intravenous radiographic contrast agents or radionuclides.

Intestinal Tract

The modes for investigation of the gastrointestinal tract (endoscopy excepted) have changed less in the last generation, perhaps, than those of any other organ system (Table 10-8); technical improvements have placed nearly the entire alimentary canal under direct scrutiny by endoscopic procedures that, if unpleasant and requiring sedation or anesthesia, nonetheless, are accurate and repeatable. In contrast to the older child and adult, fundamental gastrointestinal disease in the younger child involves malformations nearly as frequently as chronic inflammation (e.g., enteritis and colitis). Nevertheless, acute gastrointestinal intercurrent infectious illnesses are most prominent in any primary pediatric practice.

Liver

Beyond the newborn period, in which hyperbilirubinemia is a daily concern, primary liver disease other than hepatitis is relatively rare among children. However, the liver is frequently yet secondarily involved in multisystemic disease (vascular congestion and obstructions, abscess, storage disease) because of its strategic vascular location and global metabolic activity. The omnipresent, multimembered "liver panels" much beloved by younger house officers often produce information redundant to the usually sufficient items shown in Table 10-9. Bile flow in the jaundiced but acholic young infant can now be assessed accurately by hepatobiliary scintigraphy and confirmed by direct (endoscopic or transhepatic) cholangiography. These measures diminish delay in selecting candidates with biliary atresia for hepatic portoenterostomy (Kasai procedure).

Nervous and Neuromuscular Systems

Perhaps more than in any other organ system, functional assessment of the nervous and neuromuscular systems is accomplished principally during the performance of a careful neurological examination, especially of the older infant and child, for whom communication is not a barrier. The evaluation of no other system, however, has been as revolutionized by the development of ultrasound, CT, and MRI (Table 10-10), which has all but obliterated the need for invasive studies (pneumoencephalography, myelography, ventriculography). Moreover, evoked response testing has placed the

Table 10-8 Intestinal Tract

	Examination	
	Basic	**Specialized**
Structure	Abdominal plain roentgenogram	Computed tomography
	Flat	
	Upright	Radionuclide scan
	Contrast/fluoroscopy	
	Barium esophagogram	
	Upper GI series	Endoscopy
	Barium enema	Esophagoscopy
	Ultrasound scan	Gastroduodenoscopy
		Cholangiopancreatography
		Colonoscopy
		Biopsy
Function		
Peristalsis	Contrast fluoroscopy	Manometry
Secretion	Gastric pH	Duodenal aspiration
		Enzymes
		Bile
Absorption	Fecal analysis	Hydrogen breath test
	Reducing sugar	
	Fat	^{51}CrCl excretion
	Trypsin	
	Alpha$_1$-antitrypsin	Mucosal enzymes (biopsy)
	Loading (tolerance) tests	
	Oral glucose	
	D-xylose	
	Serum carotene	

Table 10-9 Liver

	Examination	
	Basic	**Specialized**
Structure	Ultrasound	Computed tomography
	Radionuclide scan	
	^{131}I rose bengal	
	^{99m}Tc PIPIDA	Endoscopy
		Cholangiopancreatography
		Transhepatic/operative cholangiography
		Biopsy
		Splenoportography
Function		
Protein synthesis	Serum albumin	
	Prothrombin time	
	Gamma globulin	Electrophoresis
Biotransformation	SGOT	5′-Nucleotidase
	SGPT	Gamma-glutamyltransferase
		Leucine aminopeptidase
Conjugation	Bilirubin (direct/total)	
Excretion	Alkaline phosphatase	
Bile flow	Duodenal intubation	^{131}I rose bengal
		Red cell peroxidation
		^{99m}Tc IDA
Special		NH_3
		Alpha$_1$-antitrypsin
		Ceruloplasmin

IDA, Imidodiacetic acid; *PIPIDA,* paraisopropylimidodiacetic acid; *SGOT,* serum glutamic-oxaloacetic transaminase; *SGPT,* serum glutamic-pyruvic transaminase.

Table 10-10 Central and Peripheral Nervous System

	Examination	
	Basic	**Specialized**
Structure	Plain skull roentgenograms Ultrasound	CT MRI Myelography MR angiography Biopsy Muscle Nerve Meninges Brain
Function		
Sensory	Neurological examination	
Vision	Vision testing	VER, ERG, EOG, FPL
Hearing	Audiometry	BAER
Cutaneous		SER
Motor	Neurological examination CPK	EMG, MEP, EOG Nerve conduction study
Integrated	Developmental testing	Psychometric evaluation
Global	CSF EEG	Functional MRI SPECT PET

BAER, Brainstem auditory evoked responses; *CPK,* creatine phosphokinase; *CSF,* cerebrospinal fluid; *CT,* computed tomography; *EEG,* electroencephalogram; *EMG,* electromyogram; *EOG,* electroculogram; *ERG,* electroretinography; *FPL,* forced preferential looking; *MEP,* motor evoked potential; *MR,* magnetic resonance; *MRI,* magnetic resonance imaging; *PET,* positron emission tomography; *SER,* somatosensory evoked responses; *SPECT,* single photon emission computed tomography; *VER,* visual evoked responses.

assessment of the visual and auditory apparatus of the young infant on more secure ground than did the traditional bedside maneuvers. Yet, true vision and hearing require integrated processing of the signals documented (by evoked potentials, say) as being received and sent along the optic and acoustic pathways; so, the possibility of "cortical" blindness or deafness is still investigated best by the behavioral responses of an alert and cooperative patient.

Eye and Ear

The primary care pediatrician's involvement with eyes and ears is properly limited to first aid and functional screening, despite the prominence of conjunctivitis and otitis media and externa in any such practice. His or her role, then, is largely that of prevention and limitation of disease by referral of those patients whose response to relatively straightforward treatment of upper respiratory and ocular problems is unsatisfactory. The development of practical impedance tympanometry has served to sharpen the indications for such referral. Tables 10-11 and 10-12 set out some of those procedures by which the ophthalmologist and otolaryngologist seek to define the finer aspects of structure and function. Both disciplines have developed a number of individuals who confine their practice to children.

Table 10-11 Eye

	Examination	
	Basic	**Specialized**
Structure		
Orbit	CT scan	Ophthalmic ultrasound
Cornea	Fluorescein dye	Slit-lamp biomicroscopy
Media	Fundus red reflex	Slit-lamp biomicroscopy
Retina	Direct ophthalmoscopy	Fluorescein angiography
Function		
Intraocular pressure		Indentation (Schiøtz) tonometry Applanation tonometry
Visual response	Startle reflex Fixation	Optokinetic nystagmus Electroculogram Electroretinogram Visual evoked responses
Ocular alignment	Corneal light reflex (Hirschberg's method) Alternate cover test	
Ocular motility	Conjugate eye movements	Forced duction testing
Visual acuity	Snellen charts Illiterate "E" charts	Refraction Retinoscopy Forced preferential looking
Visual fields	Confrontation Attraction	Perimetry Scotometry
Color vision	Isihara (pseudo-isochromatic) test	Farnsworth-Munsell D-100 color test

Skeleton

Pertinent modalities for assessing the body's bony support are set out in Table 10-13, the radionuclide scans being particularly valuable in the investigation of infectious or metastatic involvement of bone. Radioimmunoassay procedures have brought measurement of the hormones pertinent to bone metabolism (parathyroid hormone, calcitonin, and the vitamin D system) out of the research laboratory and into clinical medicine.

Skin and Appendages

Functional disruptions of cutaneous function are much less frequent causes for presenting complaint than are the itches, rashes, and eruptions that consume much of the pediatrician's day; such disruptions most often reflect general systemic disease, usually of infectious or iatrogenic origin. The hand lens is the technological support used most frequently

Table 10-12 Ear

	Examination	
	Basic	**Specialized**
Structure	Head light and mirror Pneumatic otoscopy	Microscopic otoscopy Computed tomography Magnetic resonance imaging
Function		
Hearing	Visual response Play response Speech response Impedance audiometry Conventional audiometry	BAER* Central auditory processing Cochleography
Vestibular	Bárány chair (or equivalent) Caloric stimulation	Electronystagmography Posturography
Eustachian tube		Pressure-flow study
Sound conduction	Impedance tympanometry	

*Brainstem auditory evoked responses.

Table 10-13 Bone

	Examination	
	Basic	**Specialized**
Structure	Physical examination Plain roentgenograms Ultrasound (joints) CT scan MRI	Radionuclide scan ^{99m}Tc polyphosphate ^{67}Gallium citrate Roentgen-ray absorptiometry Arthrocentesis Bone biopsy
Function	Alkaline phosphatase Ca, P	Parathyroid hormone Calcitonin Vitamin D_3 25-OH-D_3 1,25-$(OH)_2$-D_3

by the inspecting dermatologist, yet exudates, scrapings, and cuttings occasionally require detailed analysis, as indicated in Table 10-14.

Endocrine System

Confirmatory data analysis in this system is almost exclusively functional in nature and dependent on the radioimmunoassay laboratory (Table 10-15), whether the fluid examined be blood or urine, the latter being viewed as an "integrating averager" of hormone secretion (which in blood often displays pulsatile or diurnal rhythms). Roentgenographic, ultrasound, angiographic, MRI, and radionuclide techniques are used to assess endocrine organ size (e.g., pituitary, adrenal cortex, thyroid). Radiology is useful for the detection of some functional tumors of endocrine organs, but hypofunction of these organs, involving picogram quantities of hormones and small clusters of specialized cells often is beyond the powers of even histological techniques for resolution of structure. In most cases in Table 10-15, a "negative feedback axis" is involved that shuts down the hypothalamic activation of the pituitary gland's stimulation of end-organ hormone production. An increased end-organ hormonal level in the blood is the (negative) signal that impedes further trophic hormone release—analogous to the increased heat that shuts off the living room thermostat.

The suspicion of end-organ malfunction and even the measurement of some of the pertinent hormones (especially adrenal and thyroid) are in the province of the primary pediatrician, but detailed assessment of the pituitary and hypothalamic feedback loops by various evocative tests (see Table 10-15) is normally under the proper jurisdiction of the pediatric endocrinologist.

Table 10-14 Skin and Appendages

	Examination	
	Basic	**Specialized**
Structure	Inspection Direct (hand lens) Wood's lamp Exudates (bacteria) Smear Culture Scrapings Direct oil (scabies) KOH (fungi) Tzanck smear (herpes)	Dark field Biopsy Immunofluorescent studies Cuttings (chemical analyses) Hair Nails
Function		
Vasoreactivity		Catechol iontophoresis Skin blood flow
Sweating	Starch-iodine examination Pilocarpine iontophoresis	

Blood

The structural and gross quantitative appraisal of circulating elements in the hematopoietic system is part of any physician's armamentarium, as is an initial "screen" of hemosta-

Table 10-15 Endocrine System

End-organ Hormones	Intermediaries	Releasers
Adrenal cortex	ACTH (corticotropin)	CRH (corticotropin-releasing hormone)
Cortisol		
Aldosterone	Angiotensin II (kidneys)	
Dehydroepiandrosterone		
Adrenal medulla		
Epinephrine		
Norepinephrine		
Dopamine		
Gonads		
Testosterone	FSH (follicle-stimulating hormone)	LH-RH (luteinizing hormone–releasing hormone)
Estradiol	LH (luteinizing hormone)	
Progesterone		
Thyroid		
Triiodothyronine (T_3)	TSH (thyroid-stimulating hormone [thyrotropin])	TRH (thyroid-releasing hormone)
Thyroxine (T_4)		
Parafollicular cells		
Calcitonin		
Parathyroid		
Parathyroid hormone	Vitamin D	
Growth		
Somatomedin action	GH (growth hormone, somatotropin)	GHRH (growth hormone–releasing hormone) Somatostatin (inhibits release)
Lactation		
Direct action	PRL (prolactin)	PRH (prolactin-inhibiting hormone)
Melanocyte	MSH (melanocyte-stimulating hormone)	MRF (melanocyte-releasing factor)
Direct action		
Distal renal tubule		
Direct action	ADH (arginine vasopressin)	
Uterus		
Direct action	Oxytocin	

sis. Central to the assessment of any abnormality is an estimation of the balance between production and destruction of the blood element (or clotting factor) under examination. More specialized tests are the province of the consultant hematologist (Table 10-16). Abnormalities in the hematopoietic system often are the only presenting complaint of patients whose disease is actually of infectious or cancerous origin. But, the pediatrician's most frequent contact with these systems will involve nutritional (primarily iron) deficiencies and ill-defined bleeding tendencies.

Immune System

The body's immunological defenses constitute an elaborate system that has evolved over eons of assault by "nonself" invaders, potential or real. The developmental costs to the species of this system have been the very common occurrence of those atopic individuals who overreact to the antigens in their environment (with eczema, asthma, or rhinitis); the much rarer occurrence of individuals who, by confusing self with nonself, develop "autoimmune" disease (e.g., myasthenia gravis, rheumatic fever, glomerulonephritis, and possibly diabetes); and those whose normal immune defenses have been naturally impaired (through infection with the human immunodeficiency virus [HIV]) or whose immune defenses must be artificially crippled by cancer chemotherapy or to improve the likelihood of successful transplantation of foreign tissues and organs.

The frustrating frequency with which parents and pediatricians deal with infections contracted by the "immunological virgins" who are their children often has led to fruitless attempts to document immunological incompetence. Most often, however, quiet epidemiological reflection will indicate that recurrent infections among otherwise healthy young American children usually are caused by a plethora of microbial invaders (particularly well-concentrated in child care centers) rather than by any paucity of defenses. Relatively simple screening tests of antibody level, as well as of immediate and delayed hypersensitivity, usually can dispel doubt.

The availability of radioallergosorbent tests (RAST) (Table 10-17) for specific antigen-associated IgE has considerably simplified, not to mention humanized, the allergic evaluation of the symptomatic child under consideration for desensitization therapy; however, it should never replace a careful historical review of the onset and offset of those symptoms.

ETIOLOGICAL DELINEATION

It is a sweet irony that a textbook of pediatrics, such as this volume, can now afford a relative neglect of nutritional and infectious disease on the ground that, at least in developed

Table 10-16 Blood and Hematopoietic System

	Examination	
	Basic	**Specialized**
Structure		
Red cells	Hemoglobin Hematocrit Cell volumes (MCV) Smear—morphology (size, shape, inclusions) Reticulocyte count	Bone marrow aspirate Bone marrow biopsy
White cells	Smear—quantitative estimate Smear—morphology (nuclear shape, inclusions)	
Platelets	Smear—quantitative estimate Smear—comparative size (to red cells)	Electron microscopy
Function		
Red cells		
Immune	Coombs test	Antibody panels
Membrane	Osmotic fragility	
Hemoglobin	Electrophoresis	Oxygen dissociation curves Isoelectric focusing electrophoresis
Enzymes	G6PD, PK	Multienzyme panels
White cells		
Chemotaxis		Rebuck skin window Boyden chamber
Phagocytosis		Vital staining (myeloperoxidase)
Bacterial killing	NBT test	
Hemostasis		
Vascular integrity	Tourniquet test	
Platelet function	Bleeding time	Platelet aggregation studies Ristocetin (Willebrand) cofactor
Intrinsic pathway	PTT; Factors VIII, IX, XI, XII	Mixing studies
Extrinsic pathway	PT (prothrombin time)	Factors V, VII, X
Vitamin K	Factors II, VII, IX, X	
Common pathway	Thrombin time Fibrinogen	Heparin titration

G6PD, Glucose 6-phosphate dehydrogenase; *MCV,* mean corpuscular volume; *NBT,* nitroblue tetrazolium test; *PK,* pyruvate kinase, *PTT,* partial thromboplastin time.

Table 10-17 Immune System

	Examination	
	Basic	**Specialized**
Structure		
Lymphocytes		
Overall	Lymphocyte count	Biopsy (node, thymus, spleen, gut)
T cells	Lateral chest roentgenogram Rosette formation (sheep RBC)	Monoclonal markers (helper, suppressor)
B cells	Serum IgG, IgM levels Serum isohemagglutin levels	IgM cell markers
Complement system	Total hemolytic complement level	Specific complement protein levels (C3,C4)
Allergen system	Total IgE (radioimmunoassay)	
Function		
T cell	Skin tests (tuberculin, *Candida*)	Stimulated lymphocyte culture
B cell	Skin tests (Schick test)	Stimulated lymphocyte culture
Allergen	Eosinophils Skin testing Specific radioallergosorbent tests (RAST)	Provocative testing (airways) Prausnitz-Küstner passive transfer Leukocyte histamine release

countries, social, sanitary, economic, and medical advances have diminished the prominence of the serious nutritional and infectious diseases that originally brought pediatrics into being. A concurrent and corollary emphasis on problems of early development (perinatology, neonatology, and congenital anomalies) and behavior (a principal focus of this volume) likely will characterize the pediatrics of the next 100 years. Hence, within the usual etiological classification of disease (Box 10-1), we here will consider only briefly and broadly those of genetic or infectious origin. Discussions of psychogenic disease are found throughout this textbook, whereas the possibility of iatrogenic disease lurks in every contact between child and primary care pediatrician, particularly when the latter is oriented to treatment rather than to thinking and reflecting on the vast majority of his or her sick patients who have self-limited, intercurrent illnesses that usually require only sympathetic support and symptomatic treatment. The pediatrician's therapeutic zeal is better reserved for those few life-threatening emergencies discussed elsewhere in this book.

Genetic Disease

It could be argued that hemolytic disease of the newborn and the prevention of those cases caused by the D-antigen represent a model approach to genetic disease. However, few other, if any, known genetic diseases result in an individual who is phenotypically normal but thrust into the genetically inhospitable environment of a "foreign" amniotic sac (although who now could stipulate that such is not the mechanism for production of some "multifactorial" congenital anomalies?).

A classification of the mechanisms of birth defects is offered in Box 10-2 along with some pertinent examples. Current prenatal diagnostic screening approaches to the prevention of birth defects (actually preventing the birth of defective fetuses) are shown in Box 10-3. Although crude, this scheme can be effective—yet, apart from advanced maternal age (as an index of risk for nondisjunction during meiosis), entry into such a system is, by definition, purchased at the price of a previous genetic disaster. Genetic engineering for gene replacement or alteration of established genetic disease is yet, analogously speaking, somewhere between Isaac Newton's discovery of the law of universal gravitation and human arrival on the surface of the moon—that is, much engineering remains to be done.

BOX 10-1

ETIOLOGICAL CLASSIFICATION OF DISEASE ORIGIN

Genetic and developmental
Nutritional
Infectious
Neoplastic
Traumatic and physical agents
Hypersensitivity
Psychogenic
Unknown or unclassified

The pediatrician, however, is now called on to be aware of and to deal with genetic disease as already established in the patient. He or she must attempt to clarify the clinical presentation, always suspicious of the possibility of an inborn error of metabolism, particularly among those infants who are normal phenotypically, yet give a history of vomiting, dysphagia, and neurological catastrophe (severe alterations in muscle tone, seizures, or coma) after exposure to ingested sugars or protein. A scheme for screening infants with regard to the more common (although all are relatively rare) inborn errors of metabolism is displayed in Table 10-18.

In those infants who are phenotypically abnormal, the pediatrician must strive to identify the dysmorphological pattern presented, often in consultation with an appropriate atlas of known defects or a clinical geneticist. The painstaking work of establishing the family pedigree (often a severe challenge in this nation of mobile immigrants) must be undertaken to provide the essential groundwork for genetic counseling. The genotype must be established, where possible

BOX 10-2

MECHANISMS OF BIRTH DEFECTS

Single Mutant Gene
Autosomal dominant (e.g., achondroplasia, neurofibromatosis, polycystic kidney)
Autosomal recessive (e.g., adrenogenital syndrome, cystic fibrosis, sickle cell disease)
X-linked (e.g., chronic granulomatous disease, glucose 6-phosphate dehydrogenase [G6PD] deficiency, hemophilia A)

Chromosomal Disorders
Aneuploidy
MONOSOMY
XO: Turner's syndrome
TRISOMIES
13: Patau's syndrome
18: Edwards' syndrome
21: Down syndrome
XXY: Klinefelter's syndrome
XYY
XXX

Structural changes
TRANSLOCATIONS (BALANCED, UNBALANCED)
Robertsonian
Reciprocal
DELETIONS
Chromosome 5: cri-du-chat syndrome
BREAKAGE

Multifactorial (gene-environment interaction)
SINGLE CONGENITAL
Cardiac defects
Cleft lip or palate
Meningomyelocele
AGE RELATED
Diabetes
Schizophrenia

BOX 10-3

PRENATAL DIAGNOSTIC SCREENING FOR BIRTH DEFECTS

Indications
Advanced maternal age
Known "carrier"
  Balanced translocation
  X-linked
Previous affected child
  Trisomy
  Neural tube defect

Procedures
Radiography
Ultrasound
Chorionic villus sampling
Amniocentesis
Amniography
Fetoscopy

Amniotic Fluid Analysis
Fluid (secretory products)
  Alpha-fetoprotein
Cultured cells
  Karyotype
  Enzymatic analysis
  Genome (DNA)
    Molecular hybridization
    Restriction endonucleases

Table 10-18 Genetic Screening

Examination: Basic	Examination: Specialized
Newborn (Nonselective Mass Screening)	
Blood bacterial inhibition assay	
(Guthrie test)	
Phenylalanine (phenylketonuria)	
Leucine (maple syrup urine disease)	
Methionine (homocystinuria)	
Tyrosine (tyrosinemia)	
Fluorescent spot test (Beutler)	
Galactose (galactosemia)	
Radioimmunoassay	
Thyroxine (hypothyroidism)	
Infant (Symptomatic)	
Blood	
Ca, Mg, electrolytes	
pH, sugar, ketone, NH_3	
Urine	
Odor	
Sugar	
Ketones	
Amino acids	
Direct reagent spot test	Amino acids
$FeCl_3$	High-pressure liquid chromatography
Dinitrophenylhydrazine	
Ketoacids	Organic acids
Nitrosonaphthol	Gas chromatographic mass spectroscopy
Tyrosine	
Cyanide/nitroprusside	
Cystine	
Homocystine	
Paper or thin-layer chromatography	
Carbohydrates	
Benedict solution	
(Clinitest)	
Reducing sugar	
Glucose oxidase (Labstix)	
Glucose	
Toluidine blue	
Mucopolysaccharides	

(Table 10-19), and biochemical efforts to assay the putative missing enzyme, abnormal substrate (e.g., the glucocerebroside in Gaucher's disease), or deficient protein product (e.g., factor VIII in hemophilia) undertaken to identify the affected biochemical pathway.

Prompt detection of a disease on the growing list of discernible inborn errors of metabolism (e.g., phenylketonuria and maple syrup urine disease) can lead to a rewarding plan for prevention of mental retardation. Some families (those who have a child with trisomy 21 syndrome) will require consistent, sympathetic support over a long period; others (those who have a child with trisomy 13 or 18) may require more intensive support over a shorter period. It is the pediatrician's duty early to decide which type of problem the patient represents and guide the extended family to the appropriate and supportive caregivers.

Infectious Disease

The prior claims to possession of the planet anciently established by the one-celled organisms, the evolution of host defenses by "higher forms" to combat the threat of those microbes, and the genetic ingenuity regularly displayed by such organisms in rapidly developing resistance to human antimicrobials all suggest that infectious diseases will forever remain a fundamental concern for all primary care practitioners, most especially pediatricians. Although most of the great scourges have subsided (for now) in developed countries (e.g., "summer diarrhea," polio, and smallpox), good fortune in genetically driven "antigenic shifts" (e.g., influenza and staphylococcal and streptococcal diseases) has apparently played at least as important a role as have clean water, good housing, antimicrobials, and vaccines. Yet every young child who has intact host defenses can, in any society, be overwhelmed by too large an inoculum in the process of developing immunity firsthand.

The basic diagnostic approaches to the infected child are outlined in Table 10-20, the most powerful tool being the practitioner's constant epidemiological awareness of the endemic or invasive infectious disease currently prevalent in his or her community ("what's going around"). A selected microbial demography of common pediatric infectious diseases is set out in Tables 10-21 to 10-24. Of increasing concern are the many opportunistic infections (Table 10-25) that complicate the course of those patients already suffering from serious primary disease, whose host defenses have been assaulted and diminished by human or natural intervention. The recent development of polymerase chain reaction (PCR) techniques now permits the rapid detection of infectious

Table 10-19 Assessment of Genetic Disease

Examination	
Basic	**Specialized**
Pedigree	Genotype
	Karyotype (cultured)
Proband	Amniotic cells
Phenotype	Leukocytes
Dysmorphological	Bone marrow
Dermatoglyphic	Genome mapping
	Specific protein product
	Enzyme
	Skin fibroblast culture
	Red cells
	Substrate/metabolic product
	Urine
	Blood
	Tissue culture

Table 10-20 Assessment of Infectious Diseases

Examination	
Basic	**Specialized**
Epidemiology	
Body fluids/exudates/tissues	
Direct examination	
Method	
Saline suspension	Special stains
Potassium hydroxide preparation	Dyes
	Fluorescent antibodies
Gram stain	
Tzanck preparation	Electron microscopy
Light microscopy	
Laboratory culture	
Appropriate selective media	
Typing	
Antibiotic sensitivity	Typing
	Phage
Enzymatic screening	Serological
	Specific antibody responses
	Complement fixing
	Neutralizing
	Hemagglutination inhibiting
	Precipitating
	Special serologic assays
	Monospot, Epstein-Barr titer
	Venereal Disease Research Laboratory (VDRL)
	Fluorescent antibodies
	Radioimmunoassay (RIA)
	Enzyme-linked immunosorbent assay (ELISA)

Table 10-21 Perinatal Infections (Relative North American Incidence)

Common	Rare	"Retired"
Viral		
Cytomegalovirus	Varicella	Rubella
Hepatitis B	Coxsackievirus	
Herpes		
Bacterial		
Streptococcus B	*Staphylococcus aureus*	Streptococcus A
Escherichia coli (especially K1)	*Pseudomonas*	Syphilis
Listeria	*Klebsiella-Enterobacter*	Gonorrhea
	Proteus	
	Pneumococcus	
	Pertussis	
	Haemophilus influenzae	
Other		
Chlamydia		
Mycoplasma		
Toxoplasma		

Table 10-22 Respiratory and Pharyngeal Infections (Relative North American Incidence)

Common	Rare	"Retired"
Viral		
Respiratory syncytial virus	Coxsackievirus	Measles
Parainfluenza	Epstein-Barr virus	
Influenza	Herpesvirus	
Rhinovirus	Coronavirus	
Adenovirus		
Bacterial		
Streptococcus A	*Staphylococcus aureus*	Tuberculosis
Pneumococcus	*Legionella*	Diphtheria
Haemophilus influenzae		Pertussis
Other		
Mycoplasma		
Chlamydia		

Table 10-23 Gastrointestinal and Diarrheal Infections (Relative North American Incidence)

Common	Rare	"Retired"
Viral		
Rotavirus	Norwalk virus	Poliovirus
Echovirus		
Coxsackievirus		
Adenovirus		
Bacterial		
Escherichia coli	*Yersinia*	Cholera
Enteropathogenic	*Salmonella*	Typhoid
Enterovirulent	*Shigella*	
Enteroinvasive	*Campylobacter*	
Other		
Giardia	Tapeworm	
	Amebiasis	

Table 10-24 Other Significant Infectious-Disease Agents (Relative North American Incidence)

Common	Rare	"Retired"
Bacteria		
Staphylococcus aureus	*Yersinia*	Tetanus
	Campylobacter	*Haemophilus influenzae* B
	Brucella	
	Meningococcus	
	Clostridium difficile	
	Leptospira	
	Actinomycosis	
	Nocardiosis	
Viruses		
Hepatitis A	Arthropod borne (arbovirus)	Mumps
		Rabies
		Smallpox
		Rubella
		Hepatitis B
		Varicella
Rickettsiae	Spotted fever	Typhus
Fungi/Yeast		
Tinea	Coccidioidomycosis	
Candida	*Cryptococcus*	
	Aspergillosis	
	Histoplasmosis	
Protozoa	Amebiasis	Malaria
	Sporozoea	
	Pneumocystis carinii	
Helminths		
Ascaris	*Toxocara caris*	Hookworm
Enterobius		*Trichinella*

Table 10-25 Opportunistic Infections

Agents
Many
- Low virulence
- Unusual pathogens

Opportunities
Natural

Development
- Anatomical defects of the skin
- Premature infant (small inoculum)
- Term infant (large inoculum)
- Immune defect

Disease
- Cystic fibrosis
- Diabetes
- Malignancy
- Nephrotic syndrome
- Sickle cell disease

Acquired
Acquired immunodeficiency syndrome (AIDS)
Burns
Malnutrition
Trauma

Iatrogenic

Anatomical invasion
- Surgical procedures
- Dental procedures
- Indwelling catheters and shunts
  - Urinary
  - Vascular
  - Peritoneal
  - Ventricular

Ecological disruption
- Antibiotics
- Inhalation therapy

Immune interference
- Suppression
  - Malignancy
  - Transplantation
- Splenectomy

(especially viral) particles in body fluids, obviating the need for time-consuming laboratory culture. Indeed, PCR is becoming the viral equivalent of the bacterial Gram stain and has revolutionized the care of patients with chronic infectious particle loads (e.g., HIV), since it can allow monitoring of treatment in "real time" to assess treatment success or failure months or years in advance of clinical manifestations.

REFERENCES

1. Babson SG: Growth of low-birth-weight infants, *J Pediatr* 77:11, 1970.
2. Ballard JL, et al: New Ballard Score, expanded to include extremely premature infants, *J Pediatr* 119:417, 1991.
3. Battaglia FC, Lubchenco LO: A practical classification of newborn infants by weight and gestational age, *J Pediatr* 71:161, 1967.
4. Hamill PC, et al: Physical growth: National Center for Health Statistics Percentiles, *Am J Clin Nutr* 32:607, 1979.
5. Lubchenco LO, Hansman C, Boyd E: Intrauterine growth in length and head circumference as estimated from live birth at gestational ages from 26 to 42 weeks, *Pediatrics* 37:403, 1966.
6. Marks KH, et al: Head growth in sick premature infants: a longitudinal study, *J Pediatr* 94:282, 1979.
7. Nellhaus G: Head circumference from birth to eighteen years: practical composite international and interracial graphs, *Pediatrics* 41:106, 1968.
8. Tanner JM, Whitehouse RH: Clinical longitudinal standards for height, weight, height velocity, weight velocity, and stages of puberty, *Arch Dis Child* 51:170, 1976.
9. Usher R, McLean F: Intrauterine growth of live-born Caucasian infants at sea level: standards obtained from measurements in 7 dimensions of infants born between 25 and 44 weeks of gestation, *J Pediatr* 74:901, 1969.
10. Wright K, et al: New postnatal growth grids for very low birthweight infants, *Pediatrics* 91:922, 1993.

SUGGESTED READINGS

Frankenburg WK, Camp BW: *Pediatric screening test,* Springfield, Ill, 1975, Charles C Thomas.

Thorpe HS, Werner EE: Developmental screening of preschool children, *Pediatrics* 53:362, 1974.

11 Communication with Parents and Patients

Ruth J. Messinger • Philip W. Davidson
Robert A. Hoekelman • Julie A. Babish

One important goal of any diagnostic procedure is to simplify the choice of treatment and clarify the prognosis. An extremely important component of this goal is conveying pertinent information to the child or to his or her parents or advocates. In most clinical circumstances in which the illness is minor or carries an excellent prognosis, such information is presented straightforwardly by the diagnostician to the patient or the parents. In those cases that involve children who are gravely ill, severely disabled, mentally retarded, learning disabled, or emotionally disturbed, however, the situation becomes far more complex for clinicians, patients, and parents. Parents, years after the fact, vividly remember how and when the "bad news" was told.[7] The interpretive presentation, therefore, must become part of a broader counseling session that deals with feelings and emotions, as well as facts, to ensure understanding of the information being shared.

This chapter focuses on the process of information sharing with parents or patient as an extension of the diagnostic process itself. The goal of interpreting diagnostic findings is more than merely announcing technical information. The real objective in providing that information is to establish a partnership between the provider and parents that will enhance the parents' capacity to respond appropriately to their child's condition, to comply with the recommended treatment, and to become a partner with the rest of the treatment team.

Recent legislative changes that mandate participation by parents in decisions about their children who have special needs and that emphasize family-centered, coordinated, case-managed care make this partnership even more crucial. Part H of the Individuals with Disabilities Education Act (Public Law No. 100-476), for example, specifically mandates parent-driven planning of service provision to their offspring ages 0 to 2 years who have disabilities.

There is no one blueprint for building the very important relationship between clinician and parents; however, interpretation of the physician's findings to parents without unnecessary delay is essential in case management, as is the need to attend to the family's expectations and questions initially and over time. Klein[4] provides an in-depth analysis of how professionals' negative attitudes toward and absence of respect for parents can interfere with constructive communication about a child's diagnosis and treatment. This dialogue may be complicated further when clinicians become frustrated by their inability to cure or "save" the child, when they know that there are no local resources to deal with the child's problem, or when the parents ask questions that the clinician cannot answer.

A professional-parent relationship based on the posture, "I have the information, and I know what's best for your child," represents a basic misinterpretation of the kind of relationship between parent and clinician that is necessary when information about a complex and threatening illness has to be shared. Diagnosis and treatment are biomedical, but psychosocial and educational matters and their presentation to parents are decidedly nonmedical; such presentation is itself a psychosocial process of interpersonal communication. It is inappropriate to assume that simply "having the information" or knowledge about "what's best" for the child is sufficient for communicating diagnostic, therapeutic, and prognostic information to the parents. Parents usually know their child better than anyone else and are central as nurturers, caretakers, and guardians of their children.

To communicate effectively, clinicians must maintain a flow of information between parents and themselves; simply telling parents the facts of an evaluation does not guarantee that they will hear or understand. Lynch and Staloch[6] agree that clinicians must communicate with the parents, and the parents with them, for an understanding to be achieved. Such communication can be described in general terms, but its effective implementation depends on careful individual planning and a reasonable investment of time.

Box 11-1 outlines a method for conducting an "interpretive" conference. The format outlines four major steps, each equally important, that are essential for an effective outcome. It is applicable when the child is evaluated by the clinician (physician, nurse, psychologist, social worker, or educational specialist) alone or when several professionals have been involved as members of an interdisciplinary team in the diagnostic evaluation.

PREPARATION FOR AN INTERPRETIVE CONFERENCE

The interpretive conference must be planned beforehand to ensure that the conference will achieve its purpose. The conference should occur as soon as possible after the examination and testing of the patient. The clinician who conducts the conference is best prepared, both emotionally and cognitively, immediately after the last visit or staffing conference, and parents are anxious to hear about the outcome of the evaluation as soon as possible.

If more than one professional is involved in the conference, the basic aim should be to establish maximum communication between parents and professionals while this exper-

BOX 11-1

INTERPRETIVE CONFERENCE FORMAT OUTLINE

I. Entry pattern
  A. Review of evaluation procedures conducted
  B. Parents' and child's perceptions
  C. Restatement of parental concerns
    1. Main worry
    2. Additional concerns
II. Presentation of findings
  A. Encapsulation: brief overview
  B. Reaction by parents and patient
  C. Detailed findings
    1. Reactions to normal test results
    2. Reactions to abnormal test results
III. Recommendations—only after time has been allowed for reactions
  A. Restatement of concerns with both parents
  B. Recommendations—one at a time
  C. Reactions after each recommendation
  D. Sharing with the child
IV. Summary
  A. Repetition of findings, in varied wording if possible
  B. Restatement by parents or patient
  C. Planning for future contacts

tise is available to ensure that most parental questions can be answered effectively. With certain conditions, such as mental retardation and learning or emotional disorders, the physician may not be included in the conference or may not be the primary spokesperson. In these circumstances the psychologist, special educator, or social work clinician might serve that role.

Sometimes the parents view the physician as the ultimate authority figure. The implication of this perception is that the credibility of a team that does not include the physician may be impaired. On the other hand, the physician need not automatically be cast in the role of leader at an interpretive conference unless the bulk of the information to be discussed is biomedical. In no case should the interpretation of technical material to parents be left in the hands of nonprofessionals or professionals whose lack of expertise could lead to parental misunderstanding. Also, the information should not be revealed by someone who did not participate in the diagnostic workup.

Once the team members have been selected, they should meet long enough to organize the conference, following the outline in Box 11-1. This planning session should allow enough time to ensure that all the team members agree on the major information to be shared with the parents and that all terminology is understood. Team members also should select a leader who will structure the conference. This is of paramount importance because organization of the conference is the key to satisfactory communication. The leader's responsibility is to control the flow of information from professionals to parents and vice versa to ensure two-way communication. *Control* implies not only organization but also a certain empathic sensitivity for the parents' feelings and reactions so that emotional highs and lows can be adequately recognized, permitted, and dealt with respecting families' cultural proscriptions and without the purpose of the conference being disrupted.

The clinician who is to present the information alone also should plan the presentation, following the same procedures recommended for the team. Preparation is especially important for individual presenters because the individual has a more difficult task of control than does a team once the conference has begun. In this circumstance, clinicians must have the chance to listen to other professionals present information and to "pick up" on points that have not been made clear or have not been made at all.

CONDUCTING THE CONFERENCE

Entry Pattern

The beginning of the interview often sets the tone for what follows. It is assumed that planning has included those physical requirements that create an empathic climate, privacy, and freedom from interruption *and that the professional has arranged to arrive on time.*

A review of what has been done diagnostically should be shared with a minimum of technical jargon so that parents will not be intimidated when asked to discuss their "main worry." During such a discussion a "hidden agenda" often surfaces, related either to the cause of the problem or to the problem itself. Therefore, before the information is presented to the parents, the parents' perception of the child and the child's current situation should be sought. For example, the practitioner might ask both parents, "How do you see Mary's problems and strengths today?" Even if both parents have accompanied their child throughout the evaluation, each may have different knowledge about and reactions to what is happening.[1] This also is an appropriate time to ask what others have told them of their child's condition.

Presentation of Findings

Dwelling on technical data that do little to enhance the parents' understanding of their child's disorder accomplishes nothing and may interfere with establishing good professional-parent communication. Such data only serve to confuse, rather than clarify, the parents' concerns. When several different tests have been done in a lengthy, technical evaluation, it is especially helpful for parents to understand that the data presented summarize the results of all those tests.

Some parents need a name for their child's illness or problem. If labels have not already been used by others, they may well be in the future. Most parents want honest appraisals and will resent ambiguous assurances that border on deception. *Honesty with tact is vital.* For example, if an infant has been born having fetal alcohol syndrome, the parents should be told that that is the diagnosis rather than their being given vague or technical terms such as "multiple craniofacial and other anomalies" to explain their child's condition.

The practitioner(s) should focus on the parents' own perceptions of their child when explaining findings, particularly as these may relate to the parent's experiences with other children. Age or grade equivalents rather than ratio scores are useful when it is necessary to convey the presence of developmental delay or immaturity. For example, the clinician might say, "Susan's language development is delayed. You tell me that she, at age 2, babbles but has no words. Babbling is the typical way a 10-month-old communicates." It is clearer to say, "Joey reads and understands written information more like a third grader than a ninth grader" than to say, "Your son's test scores show 'scatter,' and he has a learning disability." It often is said that after the parents hear the bad news, they hear very little else. Krahn, Hallum, and Kime[5] reiterate parents' need to hear something positive in the "informing" interview. For this reason the actual presentation should begin with areas of strength or normality. Abnormal findings, stated honestly but gently, should be restated more than once and by using different words to convey the same findings. Indeed, Kaminer and Cohen[3] emphasize the relationship between empathy and honesty: "The literature documents that communication skills can be taught or at least improved. Acquiring an understanding heart seems to be more difficult." Parents should be encouraged to react to the diagnosis of the problem and to accept their feelings, including the anger that is often directed at the clinician. *Professionals need to learn how to cope with parent anger and not to expect gratitude.* Responses that reflect shock, guilt, bereavement, and inadequacy frequently are seen in various intensities and combinations.[8] *Parents need to be assured of the normalcy of those responses.*[2] Communication at this level also is influenced by any sociocultural and educational differences between the professionals and the parents.

Recommendations

Specific information should be shared at a pace that can be handled emotionally and cognitively. Parents seldom feel comfortable asking for clarification, but if they are asked to restate their "main worry" and other worries, the practitioner's recommendations can become meaningful and relevant. Parents usually find it helpful to receive recommendations that include, among other things, communication with other parents who have a child with a similar problem and referral elsewhere for help.

Recommendations are not complete until the clinician and both parents are able to decide what will be communicated to the child and who will do it. Parents' wishes and the cognitive and emotional development of the child are important considerations in this very important issue.

After recommendations have been shared and before the session is terminated, findings once again should be highlighted. One successful method for obtaining feedback is to ask parents to restate what they heard and what decisions were made. This provides the professional with the parents' perception and understanding of the problem and allows for further clarification, if necessary.

Often, more than one "interpretive" session is indicated. This can be planned by arranging for parents to contact the clinician by telephone (at a specific time) after they have had time to think about and react to the information that was shared or when further questions and concerns arise. The session should be terminated only after the clinician has stated a willingness and an ability to participate in a therapeutic alliance with the parents.

SUMMARY

Discussion of diagnostic findings is a dynamic process that is an initial step in building a therapeutic milieu. The model presented here organizes a typically complex, often unwieldy, process between the professional and the parents that easily can end disastrously and decrease chances for successful therapeutic intervention with the patient. If the clinical findings, diagnosis, and prognosis are presented clearly during the conference, two-way communication will be fostered because both the professional and the parents can identify the limits of the situation and focus on the problems that can be dealt with successfully.[8] This method of imparting information enhances the professional-parent relationship and encourages immediate and future communication and compliance with recommendations.

REFERENCES

1. Bailey D, Blasco P, Simeonsson R: Needs expressed by mothers and fathers of young children with disabilities, *Am J Ment Retard* 97:1, 1992.
2. Girgis A, Sasone-Fisher R: Breaking bad news I: current best advice for clinicians, *Behav Med* 24:2, 1998.
3. Kaminer R, Cohen H: How do you say, "Your child is retarded"? *Contemp Pediatr* 5:36, 1988.
4. Klein S: The challenge of communicating with parents, *Dev Behav Pediatr* 14:3, 1993.
5. Krahn G, Hallum A, Kime C: Are there good ways to give 'bad news'? *Pediatrics* 91:3, 1993.
6. Lynch EG, Staloch NH: Parental perceptions of physicians' communication in the informing process, *Ment Retard* 26:77, 1988.
7. Ptacek JT, Eberhardt TL: Breaking bad news: a review of the literature, *JAMA* 276:496, 1996.
8. Strauss RP et al: Physicians and the communication of bad news: parent experiences of being informed of their child's cleft lip and/or palate, *Pediatrics* 96:1, 1995.

SUGGESTED READINGS

Able-Boone H, Dopecki PR, Smith MS: Parent and health care provider communication and decision making in the intensive care nursery, *Child Health Care* 18:133, 1989.

Briskin H, Liptak G: Helping families with children with developmental disabilities, *Pediatr Ann* 24:5,1995.

Buckman R: *How to break bad news: a guide for health care professionals,* Baltimore, Md, 1992, Johns Hopkins University.

Fletcher AB, Saren AV: Communicating with parents of high-risk infants, *Pediatr Ann* 17:477, 1988.

Myerscough P: *Talking with patients: keys to good communication,* ed 3, New York, 1996, Oxford University Press.

Stone D: A parent speaks: professional perceptions of parental adaptation to a child with special needs, *Child Health Care* 18:174, 1989.

12 Cultural Issues in Primary Pediatric Care

Karen N. Olness • Kristine Torjesen

- You are working in a pediatric emergency room, and you evaluate an 11-month-old child who was born in the Middle East. He has had a fever and cold for a week. On examination you find signs of otitis media and round, ulcerated areas on both wrists. The family explains that they were treating the child with crushed garlic cloves taped onto the child's wrists.
- You are a middle-age pediatrician working in the outpatient department of a large county hospital. A Hmong child is brought in with a cold and fever. You conduct a thorough examination, including otoscopy, and diagnose otitis media. Through the translator you prescribe amoxicillin and arrange for a follow-up appointment. Two days later the child, who is still febrile, returns in the company of 10 adult relatives and the translator. You begin an examination. However, when you reach for the otoscope, the translator says that the family requests that you not use it.
- You are working in a small group practice and have many Mexican-American families as clients. One of the nurse assistants is Mexican-American, and she brings her children to the practice for well-child care. She is well liked by families and colleagues within the practice. One day she mentions that her 4-year-old son is ill, and she asks to leave early. You offer to see him, and she replies that he has *empacho,* a gastrointestinal illness, and that she is taking him to see a healer in the family. She says that empacho cannot be cured by conventional medical treatment.

The above examples represent the types of cross-cultural situations encountered by pediatricians. As they become familiar with the particular belief guiding the use of garlic plasters or the use of an otoscope or the diagnosis of empacho, pediatricians learn how to cope with these situations. More complex cross-cultural issues are those never manifested overtly by clients; they can result in noncompliance, the seeking of another physician, or misinterpretation of the diagnosis and treatment. The goal of cross-cultural medicine, now taught in many medical schools, is not to familiarize physicians with all cultural issues related to medicine but rather to sensitize physicians to different cultural beliefs (Box 12-1). It is hoped that they may take into account different expectations regarding their roles and different explanations for disease that evolve from varying cultural beliefs.

American child health professionals have more cross-cultural issues to consider than do child health professionals in any other country, and they receive little guidance and preparation for these issues. American child health providers encounter cross-cultural issues when diagnosing and treating families who are newcomers to the United States or those whose cultural heritages relate to parents or grandparents who immigrated to the United States. Furthermore, American child health providers are mobile and may themselves work in several different cultural environments during a lifetime. In the future it is likely that the services of American child health experts will be required increasingly in less industrialized countries,[12,32] where 90% of the world's babies are born.

DEFINITIONS

Americans living in urban areas encounter cultural differences every day and may be unaware of them as they work, shop, and play. Culture, cultural norms, and one's perception of social self all play a part in the way reality is defined. *Social self* refers to the way individuals perceive or present themselves to others. It includes the degree of acceptance of the culture or subculture the individuals are in and how they project that acceptance or rejection to those around them. *Culture* is defined as a way of life for a group of people: how they work; how they relax; their values, prejudices, and biases; and the way they interact with one another. This involves *cultural norms,* which are ethical and moral or traditional principles of a given society. Cultural norms usually are unwritten but, nevertheless, are understood as the rules and values by which a culture functions. People are expected to abide by these unwritten rules or norms. When they violate these, they may be criticized or ostracized by others within the culture. Cultural norms include unwritten definitions of health, sickness, and abnormality. Social self, culture, and cultural norms change over generations of families, and it is important to note that persons of the same ethnic group may have very different cultures or cultural norms. Consider, for example, the different cultures of a Chinese farmer living in a rural area of Shanxi province and a fourth-generation American who is ethnically Chinese, has a PhD in economics, and lives in a mostly white suburb of Minneapolis.

It is important to keep in mind that what is typical of a group does not necessarily predict the beliefs of an individual, especially in a multicultural country such as the United States. For this reason, it is preferable to focus on individual families as unique cultural units rather than on the cultural origins or ethnic background of the family.[14] Box 12-1 provides some traditional guidelines to ethnic origins and associated beliefs. During the past generation, the mixing and changing of human societies throughout the world is more

BOX 12-1

HOW TO CULTIVATE CULTURAL SENSITIVITY IN PRIMARY PEDIATRIC CARE

1. Analyze your personal culture and cultural norms.
2. Consider the cultural differences among those working together in a primary pediatric setting.
3. Develop a cultural screening tool for each family.
4. Study specific cultures, especially those represented by your patients.
5. Recognize that ethnic background does not predict the culture of an individual.
6. Be flexible in adapting health care to a family's culture and cultural norms.

rapid than ever before. This is due to rapid information exchange and leads to both positive and negative outcomes. For example, age-old cultural traditions such as caring for one's parents are disappearing. With respect to many areas, including health beliefs, child health professionals must be cautious about making assessments based on ethnic origins alone.

A popular current phrase is "the culture of the workplace." Managers use this phrase often; yet those within a work environment are not provided guidelines for assessing their own cultural norms and how they may fit or conflict with the culture of a workplace. It is possible for a pediatrician to feel comfortable in a children's hospital (i.e., workplace), whether that pediatrician is American or French or Ethiopian, but to feel distinctly out of place in social, recreational, or political aspects of that society. The workplace culture often becomes the principal and most comfortable culture for health professionals, regardless of their own ethnic background, age, gender, or linguistic abilities.

Cross-cultural discomforts in the pediatric workplace may arise from efforts to communicate with families who have different cultural norms.[17] The child health professional may feel uncomfortable despite efforts to be nonjudgmental, because cultural norms are powerful determinants of a person's perceptions. Furthermore, medical training itself is an enculturating process, leading one to hold the same values as one's medical peers.

Explanations of Disease: Cultural Variations

Namboze[21] noted that cultural beliefs about disease causation in Ganda society fall under the following categories: magical, supernatural, infectious, and hereditary. She notes that some of these beliefs are beneficial and can be included in health teaching. Others are harmless and best left alone by child health professionals; some cultural practices, however, are harmful.

Garlic, mentioned in the first vignette, has been part of healing folklore in many cultures. Like many herbal treatments, it may cause multiple adverse effects in addition to local burns.[8]

The National Institutes of Health, responding to congressional demand, developed an Office of Alternative Medicine in 1992 and now a Complementary and Alternative Medicine (CAM) Center in 1999. This center is facilitating research in complementary and alternative medicine and disseminating much information to the public about CAM treatments. There is a new recognition that a majority of Americans use CAM therapies in addition to allopathic medicine.[6,27] (See Chapter 28, Complementary and Alternative Medical Therapies). Some of these therapies are based on cultural traditions and some on recent cultural changes. A great variety of alternative medicine practices are observed among well-educated, middle-class Americans.

An example of CAM therapy based on cultural traditions is found in the treatment of empacho, mentioned in the third vignette, a gastrointestinal disorder attributed to food or saliva getting "stuck." It is believed to be caused by ingesting too much or by eating either the wrong food or at the wrong time. Infants can get empacho by swallowing too much saliva during teething, and adults may get it as a result of anxiety.[24] Folk healers treat empacho with diet change, laxatives, herbal teas, and massage. A study of 67 Puerto Rican parents in Connecticut found that 64% said that at least one of their children had had empacho.[24]

Many ethnic groups within the United States bring their ill children to both pediatricians and traditional healers within the community.[11,14,15,22] Special ceremonies, herbal remedies, chanting, and prayer often are prescribed by the latter. It is unusual for the family to share this information with their pediatricians unless the pediatrician is of the same ethnic group, speaks the same language, or has a long-standing, trusting relationship with the family.

It should be noted that families from many different cultural backgrounds may purchase vitamins, minerals, and food supplements at health food stores or consult chiropractors for their children and also may not inform their pediatricians about all treatments being used.

A recent survey of American adults found that 34% reported using at least one unconventional therapy in the past year. A third of these saw practitioners of unconventional therapy, making an average of 19 visits in 1 year. The type of therapy included relaxation and imagery techniques, chiropractic and spiritual healing, commercial weight-loss programs, megavitamin therapy, homeopathy, acupuncture, and massage.[6]

A Minnesota physician who works at St. Paul-Ramsey Medical Center International Clinic was infertile and decided to consult an herbalist and a shaman while she was visiting a Hmong village in Thailand. Treatment included drinking a mixture of dried bugs, alcohol, and mucus. A year later her daughter was born.[13] She believes that patients should be encouraged to use both their traditional and our medical systems.

CULTURAL ASSESSMENT

Appraising a patient's or parent's cultural beliefs, values, and customs is an essential part of health assessment. A cultural assessment is as important as a physical or psychological assessment. Cultural assessments can be used to understand behavior that otherwise could be interpreted as negative or noncompliant.

The ability to be interculturally sensitive is desirable but difficult. Teufel has noted that ethnocentricity counteracts the ability to be interculturally sensitive and describes six stages of development toward the ideal.[30] Initially the other culture is denied, and cultural differences go unrecognized. The second stage is defensive and a person may either denigrate the other culture or claim one's own to be superior. The third stage is that differences between cultures are trivialized, but such a perspective does not recognize the different social, physical, and spiritual environments in which world views are constructed. In the fourth stage the individual moves toward accepting that a cultural difference exists and that another culture is worthy of understanding. Fifth, the person adapts to the difference and shifts from an ethnocentric world view to one that is ethnorelative. Finally, the ideal is that the difference is integrated. One attains the ability to analyze and evaluate situations from one or more cultural perspectives, and is neither totally a part of nor totally apart from his or her culture but lives on a comfortable boundary.

It is important to remain sensitive to individual differences within the cultural groups while gathering information concerning a particular family; it is important not to make stereotypical assumptions. Problems arise when a negative attitude comes from these erroneous assumptions. For example, although alcoholism is prevalent in many Native American tribes, it would be erroneous to assume that any Native American treated is an alcoholic. There is a tendency to assume that all members of a similar cultural background share commonalties, such as language, religion, and viewpoints. Knowing the differences of the backgrounds within the different cultures is essential to becoming sensitive to variations within a culture. Developing a false sense of cultural knowledge can impede the practitioner from learning specific aspects about a particular culture. An accurate understanding of several cultures would certainly take an anthropologist years of study. The best recommendation is to review the available literature and interview colleagues who are members of a specific cultural group. Observation and interview are two useful tools when assessing cultural background.[28] However, one should be judicious in selecting questions during first visits with a family; it may take years of observation and diplomatic questions to understand the cultural background of a family. Although it may take a relatively short time to gather information about ethnic group affiliation, preferred language, and dietary practices, it may take a long time to know about the values and beliefs, including health beliefs, of a given family.

The American Medical Association distributes a manual on providing culturally competent care to adolescents.[2] This guide lists open-ended questions to facilitate understanding of how an adolescent from another culture perceives his or her health problem; for example, "Apart from me, who do you think can help you get better?"

Ethnic Group Affiliation and Racial Background

Racial background refers to specific physical and structural characteristics. These characteristics are transmitted genetically and distinguish one group from another. Some diseases are more prevalent for genetic reasons in certain racial or ethnic groups, such as sickle cell anemia in blacks and Tay-Sachs disease in families of Ashkenazi Jewish origin.

Within the boundaries of one country, such as Uganda or Laos, there may be scores of different tribes that vary with respect to physical characteristics, genetically transmitted diseases, and health beliefs. On the other hand, some beliefs and lifestyles that affect health are common to ethnic groups that could not have had communication with one another. An example of this is the child-rearing habit that leads to toddler malnutrition. After giving birth, the mother is isolated with the new baby for several weeks. The older toddler, who has been with the mother continually before the sibling's birth, is now rejected. He is depressed, eats poorly, and develops malnutrition. The word *kwashiorkor,* an African tribal word, means "disease of the deposed or separated child."

Health Beliefs and Practices

Viewpoints on health and healing vary from group to group. The basic definition of illness in North America stems from the dominant culture and is based on Western scientific thought, which views illness as a breakdown in a body part because of an infectious organism or injury.[28] Extreme effort is necessary to see illness and healing from a different perspective. The issue of pain is dealt with in Zborowski's classic study.[35] Although the dominant American culture values stoicism and nonemotional expressions of pain, other cultures may express pain through screaming, moaning, and verbal complaining.[31] An understanding of these differences is essential in assessing and treating pain in children.[3] Zatzick and Dimsdale reviewed 13 studies of experiments in which subjects were exposed to various noxious stimuli and pain responses of different cultural groups were compared.[34] None of the studies demonstrated cultural differences in the ability to discriminate painful stimuli. This suggests that differences in expression of pain among cultural groups do not have a neurosensory origin.

Beliefs and perceptions regarding disabilities relate to culture. Many Asian societies are concerned about the spiritual cause of a disability—for example, failure to follow a tradition. A child born with a disability may be the recipient of punishment assigned to a parent or relative.[7] These beliefs are present among Americans from Asian cultures and may affect whether rehabilitation treatment is perceived as important.

Religious Influences or Special Rituals

The dominant culture has separated "church and state" for so many years that it is quite common to separate those entities in health care as well. However, for many cultures, religion still influences beliefs strongly concerning health and illness, death, and treatment. It is important to assess the role of significant religious leaders, especially during times of life-threatening illness. Special religious ceremonies may be comforting to the ill child and to family members. These should be integrated into the treatment. There are recent studies demonstrating the value of prayer in health care.

Language Barriers and Communication Styles

Determining which language is spoken at home is essential in assessing the culture.[28] Although the family and child may speak English, their words and understanding, especially related to abstract concepts, may be limited. It is recommended that a translator accompany the primary caregiver when explaining potentially complex topics. Assessing a family's ability to read and write in English also is important.

Nonverbal communication may have different meanings in different cultures. Many Eastern Asian-Americans nod out of respect, not necessarily out of understanding. Some nonverbal behaviors can lead to alienation and eventually withdrawal; thus, their meanings are essential in keeping communication open. For example, crossing the legs in such a way as to point the sole of the foot toward a person in Southeast Asia is interpreted as an insult. In Bulgaria, one nods the head to mean "no" and moves the head back and forth to denote "yes."

Parenting Styles and Role of Family

Understanding that "parenting is neither good nor bad in any culture, simply different," is the basis of acknowledging differing cultures' attitudes toward the family. It is inaccurate to assume that the dominant American culture has all the answers when it comes to parenting. Although the dominant American culture may value independence in children, another culture may value submissiveness.[28] Attitudes toward family members vary with each culture. Culture will address how different members' advice is regarded and whether those members are involved in decisions. Culture also will affect the values held about children, family structure, and gender.[10] Parental attitudes regarding infant development and sleeping arrangements often reflect cultural values.[19]

Dietary Practices

Diet is an integral part of a person's culture. Dietary practices can include not only preferences and dislikes of particular foods but also food preparation, consumption, frequency, time of eating, and utensils used. When a prescribed diet is part of a patient's treatment, it is essential to assess the cultural influences involved. Consulting a nutritionist, a cultural informant, or colleagues of various ethnic backgrounds can be helpful. In the United States, children from underserved, ethnically diverse population groups are at increased risk for obesity, increased serum lipid levels, and dietary consumption patterns that do not meet the Dietary Guidelines for Americans.[4] However, the overall diet and eating styles in the United States represent a unique culture in the world, generally different from that of the countries of origin, and result in more than 80% of U.S. children consuming more than recommended amounts of total fat and saturated fat. This is a good example of how facets of culture can change dramatically over a few generations.

HOW PEOPLE INTERACT: EXPECTATIONS FOR APPROPRIATE BEHAVIOR

Perhaps in a century, all people of the world will share a common culture with respect to appropriate interactions. The U.S. population has scores of views regarding appropriate interpersonal interactions.[18] More than a common language is required to develop a consensus regarding, for example, eye contact, touching, personal space or territory, appearance, gestures, use of the voice, greetings, partings, and facial expressions. Even responses to pain vary among cultural groups, including subcultures in the United States.[3,35] Most humans tend to use the rules regarding these interactions developed from childhood cultural experiences. Complicating this within the United States is that chaotic living situations for children may not provide models for appropriate interpersonal interactions. Young children who watch television a great deal and who are unable to distinguish what is real from what is not (acting) often imitate unusual or inappropriate interpersonal interactions.

In diplomatic circles there are norms, some of them written, with respect to communication. Diplomats are encouraged to learn about cultural norms within their host country—for example, who can shake hands, how close to another one stands at a reception, and how much eye contact is allowed. Yet diplomats make mistakes and therefore are misinterpreted. American child health professionals who interact with peers from other cultures should study cultural norms before working with foreign colleagues, whether in this country or their own. Visitors from East Africa and Southeast Asia often complain that they find American friendliness superficial. The immediate pleasant friendliness of Americans would represent a more advanced stage of personal intimacy and friendship in their cultures, and they are offended when they discover that it does not necessarily reflect depth. They also find it difficult to accept gifts from Americans because, in many cultures, gifts are only in exchange for something or to acquire an advantage. Direct expression of feelings is inappropriate and considered bizarre in many cultures. In Thailand, for example, one turns anger toward another object, either animate or inanimate, called *prachot.* This is done consciously to alert the person (who is the object of one's displeasure and annoyance) to how the injured party feels. In Southeast Asia, avoiding confrontation is considered positive, and expressing anger, hatred, and annoyance overtly is considered negative.

There are a number of training programs to increase sensitivity among people toward varying cultural norms and values. Pediatricians who plan to work in other cultures may benefit from a game *(Bafa'-bafa')* in which participants are divided into two groups and provided with values, expectations, and customs of a new culture.[26]

PERCEPTUAL DIFFERENCES AMONG CULTURES

Perceptual differences among various groups of humans relate not only to group beliefs, customs, and experiences but also to differences in sensory systems that may have evolved in response to the need for individual survival or to society's needs. These are well-documented differences in auditory, visual, musical, and tactile skills and may relate to differences in eye-hand coordination, information processing, and language and spatial perceptions.

Some of the differences may be genetic, but others reflect the emphasis, focus, and practice of a skill within a culture. For example, an infant's perceptual abilities are modified by listening to a particular language. Syllables, words, and sentences used in all human languages are formed from a set of speech sounds called *phones*. Only part of the phones are used in any particular language. Young infants can discriminate nearly every phonetic contrast, but this broad-based sensitivity declines by 1 year of age.[33] Adults have difficulty discriminating phones that do not connote meaning in their own native language and thus are handicapped when learning a new language. English-speaking natives have difficulty in perceiving the difference between two "k" phonemes (sounds) used in Thai. Japanese-speaking adults have difficulty distinguishing between the English */ra/* and */la/*. Adults who learn another language early but who do not practice the language as they mature may lose their ability to differentiate among its sounds.

Learning the language of another culture is essential to understanding that culture. Dependency on bilingual translators is fraught with the likelihood of misunderstanding, especially in medicine. In some cultures, the status of the translator affects what information is provided by the patient and how it is prepared for the ears of the foreign health professional. If the patient is of "higher" status than the translator, an awkward situation can result for the translator. If the translator has little specific knowledge about health and medical matters, translation is less than ideal. Furthermore, abstract concepts may not translate well from English to other languages. For example, it is much more difficult to express abstract concepts in Norwegian or in Russian than in English. Many words from Western languages do not exist in Asian languages; therefore, the concepts do not exist. Similarly, some Asian concepts cannot be expressed in English. The Lao language, for example, is richer in terms of words related to family relationships than is the English language.

Many studies have demonstrated that information processing differs among cultures. For example, a study of university students from four cultures demonstrated culturally dependent differences in processing information that affected choices of color dominance.[25] Numerous studies have demonstrated cultural differences in children's preferences for colors and shapes. For example, one study demonstrated that African children clearly prefer color to form into their adolescence.[29] Euro-American children, however, selected form over color from kindergarten age into adulthood. Language structure may determine perceptual preference with respect to form or color. For example, Navajo children demonstrate form preferences, and the Navajo language uses different labels for the same objects in different tenses. How often do child health professionals consider how information processing or preferences by a child or his or her parent may depend on the original language or cultural background? Morley[20] has noted that information processing styles, preferences for forms and colors, and educational background must be considered in preparing health education materials for use in developing countries. This also should be an important consideration in planning health education in the United States.

ETHICAL ISSUES IN CROSS-CULTURAL MEDICINE

Many ethical issues operate in making transcultural diagnostic and treatment decisions. These relate to communication barriers, varying explanations for disease, and different expectations regarding what is honest or valuable.

Can an American pediatrician truly explain a surgical consent form to newly arrived parents of a Southeast Asian baby? When newly arrived refugees fear that they will be returned and therefore sign anything or do anything to gain favor, is it ethical to ask them to sign a consent form to have blood drawn for clinical research?

Mental illness is defined very differently among cultures.[16] Is it ethical to use psychotherapy when therapist and patient are unmatched culturally?

Oppenheim and Sprung recently have reviewed cross-cultural differences in ethical decisions related to critical care.[23] They compare Chinese and Israeli cultures with respect to informed consent in intensive care units. For Chinese it is considered callous and inconsiderate to give all information regarding grave decisions directly and openly to the patient or to the parent of the patient. Therefore, informed consent as a Western physician understands it may not be reached. It is important in considering ethical decisions in the intensive care unit to recognize that physicians' attitudes may differ from those of the patient, even when the physician and patient are from the same ethnic group.

REVERSE CULTURE SHOCK

Child health professionals who spend substantial time working in different cultures may find the culture shock when returning to the United States to be as noticeable as the shock when arriving in the new culture. In fact, a benefit of cross-cultural travel (if it goes beyond Western hotels and into indigenous communities) is that one becomes sensitized to cultural norms. We may recognize idiosyncrasies of our own cultures, such as loud voices, frenetic days, instant breakfasts, direct expression of feelings, pampered pets, or written invitations to social events. We may be uncomfortable in our forays to department stores that provide too many choices.

NEED FOR EDUCATION OF HEALTH CARE PROFESSIONALS

Haggerty has noted that megatrends, such as increasing flows of refugees and immigrants, will make all pediatric practices more multicultural and multiethnic.[9] The American Academy of Pediatrics (AAP) recently issued a policy statement defining culturally effective health care and its importance for pediatrics.[1] This statement notes that by the year 2020, approximately 40% of school-age Americans will be minority group children. *Culturally effective pediatric health care* is defined as the delivery of care within the context of appropriate physician knowledge, understanding, and appreciation of cultural distinctions. Such understanding should take into account the beliefs, values, actions, customs, and unique health care needs of distinct population groups. The AAP believes that such knowledge and skills can be taught and acquired through educational courses. It recommends that the pediatric community develop and evaluate curricular programs in medical schools and residency programs to enhance the provision of culturally effective health care and to develop continuing medical education materials for pediatricians and nonpediatricians, with the goal of increasing culturally effective health care. In 1999, the Society for Developmental and Behavioral Pediatrics approved curricular guidelines for residency training in developmental-behavioral pediatrics.[5] These emphasize the need for pediatric residents to develop skills in working with diversity in cultural beliefs. For example, the curriculum suggests that residents, as a routine, identify the relevant racial, cultural, religious, and educational backgrounds of the patient during case presentations.

SUMMARY

Cross-cultural issues in pediatrics affect communication, expectations, and medical explanations. Pediatricians, although enculturated by their specialty training, also have individual ethnic cultural norms that affect their beliefs and values. It, therefore, is helpful for child health professionals to learn about beliefs of their colleagues and patients. Wherever there may be a strong belief in a folk explanation for the cause of an illness, pediatricians are likely to be most successful if they acknowledge the belief and attempt to work with it. When simultaneous use of a traditional and Western medical regimen is possible and will do no harm, it is likely to enhance long-term, trusting relationships. Awareness of cultural evolution, perceptual differences related to cultural background, and implications for decision making with respect to children is essential for child health professionals throughout the world.

REFERENCES

1. American Academy of Pediatrics: Culturally effective pediatric care: education and training issues, *Pediatrics* 103:167, 1999.
2. American Medical Association: *Culturally competent health care for adolescents: a guide for primary care providers,* Chicago, 1994, Department of Adolescent Health, AMA.
3. Bernstein B, Pachter LM: Cultural considerations in children's pain. In Schecter NL, Berde C, Yaster M, editors: *Pain in infants, children, and adolescents,* Baltimore, 1993, Williams & Wilkins.
4. Bronner YL: Nutritional status outcomes for children: ethnic, cultural, and environmental contexts, *J Am Diet Assoc* 96:891, 1996.
5. Coury DL, et al: Curricular guidelines for residency training in developmental-behavioral pediatrics, *J Dev Behav Pediatr* 20:S34, 1999.
6. Eisenberg D, et al: Trends in alternative medicine use in the United States, *JAMA* 280:1569, 1998.
7. Fitzgerald M, Armstrong J: Culture and disability in the Pacific, *International Exchange of Experts and Information in Rehabilitation Newsletter,* Jan 1993.
8. Garty BZ: Garlic burns, *Pediatrics* 91:658, 1993.
9. Haggerty RJ: Child Health 2000: New pediatrics in the changing environment of children's needs in the 21st century, *Pediatrics* 96:805, 1995.
10. Harwood RLK: The influence of culturally derived values on Anglo and Puerto Rican mothers' perception of attachment behavior, *Child Dev* 63:822, 1992.
11. Hufford DJ: Folk medicine and health culture in contemporary society, *Prim Care* 24:723, 1997.
12. Jelliffe DB, Bennett FJ: Indigenous medical systems and child health, *J Pediatr* 57:248, 1960.
13. Kelly M: Healing the transcultural medicine gap, *Health Sciences,* University of Minnesota, Fall 1993.
14. Kinsman SB, Sally M, Fox K: Multicultural issues in pediatric practice, *Pediatr Rev* 17:349, 1996.
15. Krajewski J: Folk-healing among Mexican American families as a consideration in the delivery of child welfare and child health care services, *Child Welfare* 70:157, 1991.
16. Krener PG, Sabin C: Indochinese immigrant children problems in psychiatric diagnosis, *J Am Acad Child Psychiatry* 24:453, 1985.
17. Lynch EW, Hanson MJ, editors: *Developing cross-cultural competence: a guide for working with young children and their families,* Baltimore, 1992, Paul H Brooks.
18. Marsh P: *Eye to eye: how people interact,* Topsfield, Mass, 1988, Salem House.
19. Morelli GA, et al: Cultural variation in infants' sleeping arrangements: questions of independence, *Dev Psychol* 28:604, 1992.
20. Morley D: Beliefs and attitudes to child-rearing and disease. In Morley D, editor: *Paediatric priorities in the developing world,* London, 1973, Butterworth.
21. Namboze JM: Health and culture in an African society, *Soc Sci Med* 17:2041, 1983.
22. Olness KN: Cultural aspects in working with Lao refugees, *Minn Med* 62:871, 1979.
23. Oppenheim A, Sprung CL: Cross-cultural ethical decision-making in critical care, *Crit Care Med* 26:423, 1998.
24. Pachter LM, Bernstein B, Osorio A: Clinical implications of a folk illness: empacho in mainland Puerto Ricans, *Med Anthropol* 13:285, 1992.
25. Schkade LL, Ramani S, Masakazu J: Human information processing and environmental complexity: an experiment in four cultures, *ASCI J Management* 8:56, 1978.
26. Shirts RG: *Bafa'Bafa':* a cross-cultural simulation, Del Mar, Calif, 1977, Simile.
27. Spigelblatt L, et al: The use of alternative medicine by children, *Pediatrics* 94:811, 1994.
28. Stulc DM: The family as a bearer of culture. In Cookfair JM, editor: *Nursing process and practice in the community*, St Louis, 1991, Mosby.
29. Suchman RG: Cultural differences in children's color and form preferences, *J Soc Psychol* 70:3, 1966.
30. Teufel KW: A call for dialogue: health communication interventions in the context of culture, thesis, Antioch College, March 1999.
31. Todd KH: Pain assessment and ethnicity, *Ann Emerg Med* 27:422, 1996.
32. UNICEF: *The state of the world's children,* New York, 1998, UNICEF.
33. Werker JF: Becoming a native listener, *Am Scientist* 77:54, 1989.
34. Zatzick DF, Dimsdale JR: Cultural variations in response to painful stimuli, *Psychosom Med* 52:544,1990.
35. Zborowski M: Cultural components in response to pain, *J Soc Issues* 8:16, 1952.

13 Compliance with Pediatric Health Care Recommendations

Jill S. Halterman • Peter G. Szilagyi • Lance E. Rodewald

Compliance, often referred to as *adherence,* is defined as the extent to which a person's health-related behaviors coincide with medical and health advice given.[31] Difficulties with compliance have been described since the time of Hippocrates. Noncompliance with drug therapy may reflect the failure to fill prescribed medications, delayed or forgotten doses, incorrect amounts of medication or improper dosing intervals, and failure to complete full courses of therapy. For children, the problems surrounding drug compliance are unique because the compliance of the parent as well as the child must be considered. This chapter focuses on compliance with medication use to illustrate the extent and consequences of noncompliance in pediatrics, determinants of noncompliance, and strategies to improve compliance within a pediatric population.

EXTENT OF THE PROBLEM

Many studies describe strikingly low rates of compliance with therapeutic regimens. Because the determined rate of compliance depends on the method of assessment of compliance as well as the particular regimen and setting, published rates vary widely. Some studies estimate that approximately 50% of patients do not comply with a physician's advice on medical therapy.[8,19] When recommendations require the sustained alteration of existing behavior patterns, as in chronic illnesses, the rates of compliance may be even lower.

Many studies document compliance problems for pediatric patients. For example, 40% to 80% of children do not receive a complete 10-day course of treatment prescribed for otitis media or streptococcal pharyngitis.[4,11,13,14,16] Further, for chronic conditions that require a long duration of daily therapy, lack of compliance is cited frequently as a significant problem. In one study, the use of bronchodilators among low-income children who had moderate to severe asthma (estimated from inhalant canister weights at follow-up appointments) was found to be 44%.[10] Further, adherence to penicillin prophylaxis for children who have sickle cell anemia has been determined to be only 43.1% as measured by urine assay.[33] Similar problems have been described among children who have other chronic conditions, including diabetes mellitus, end-stage renal disease, cancer, rheumatic fever, and tuberculosis, where compliance has been as low as 40%.[33] Because patients have been shown to overreport medication use dramatically, compliance rates are likely lower than most health care providers are led to believe.[3]

CONSEQUENCES OF NONCOMPLIANCE

Poor compliance or noncompliance can compromise the efficacy of a medical regimen, leading to adverse patient outcomes. For example, certain children who have diabetes mellitus are hospitalized repeatedly for ketoacidosis and demonstrate highly elevated hemoglobin A_{1c} levels related to noncompliance with the prescribed regimen for insulin therapy. Further, noncompliance can adversely affect medical decisions, leading to inappropriate increases in dosage, changes in the scheduling regimen, or additional medical tests or procedures. For infectious diseases, problems with noncompliance may cause relapses of infections or the emergence of resistant microbial strains. Finally, noncompliance interferes with the physician-parent relationship and prevents accurate evaluations of a treatment's efficacy.

DETERMINANTS OF NONCOMPLIANCE

Physicians tend to overestimate the compliance of their patients and are unable to predict compliance by considering socio-demographic characteristics. Therefore, it is useful to consider factors that may influence compliance among pediatric patients. Such factors include the patient or family's knowledge and recall of the treatment plan, the family's belief system, interactions between the clinician and patient, and characteristics of the treatment regimen (Fig. 13-1).

Patient/Family Knowledge

For a patient to comply with a therapeutic regimen, he or she must comprehend the instructions that are given. However, parents frequently do not possess all the information they need to follow a particular regimen. Confusion about the appropriate use of asthma medications has been shown to be associated with medication noncompliance, with many patients mistaking maintenance medications, which should be administered daily, for symptomatic medications used intermittently (e.g., bronchodilators).[3,6] Further, medical terms that are commonly used during physician/patient encounters are frequently understood poorly by families.[22] A recent study illustrated difficulties with instructions involving dosing of medications, with fewer than 40% of parents correctly identifying a teaspoon from other measuring spoons after liquid medication was prescribed for their child.[1]

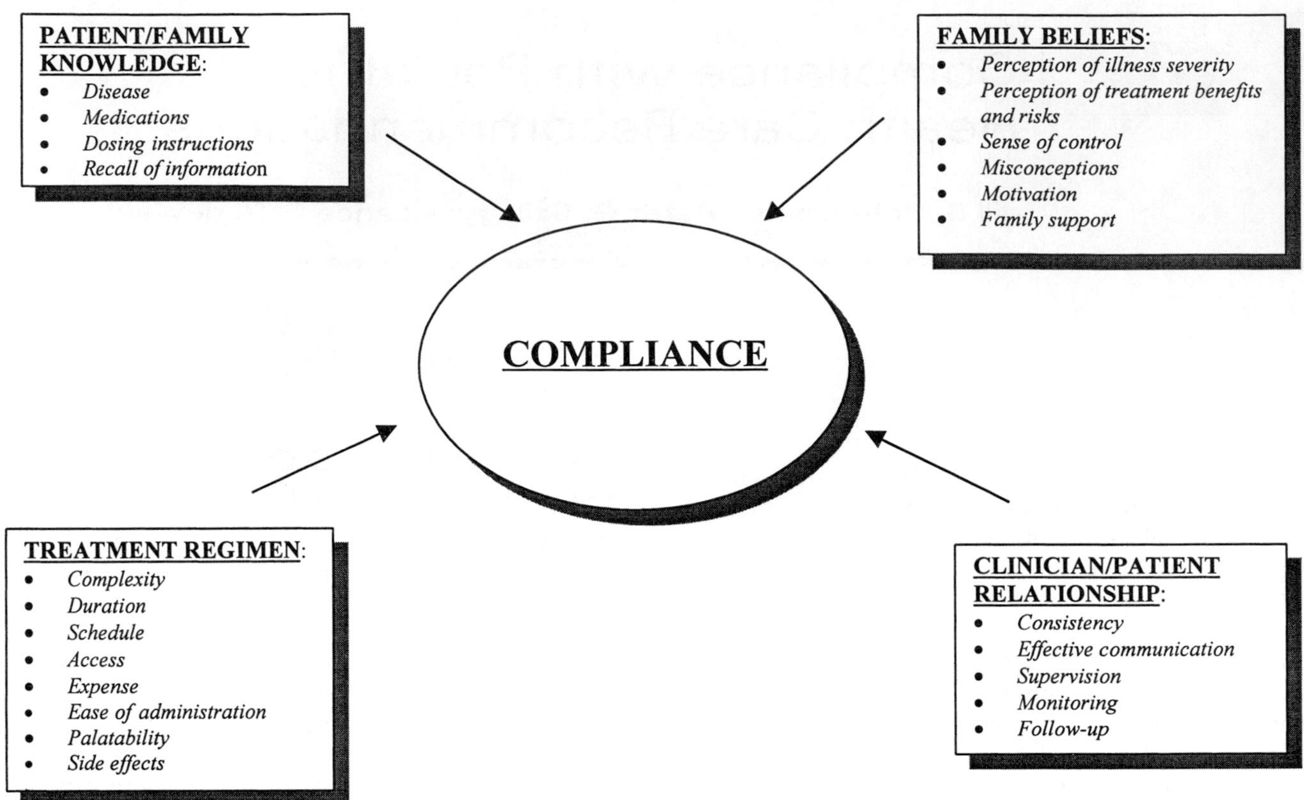

Fig. 13-1 Determinants of compliance among pediatric patients.

Patients also must be able to recall necessary information throughout the duration of therapy to comply with the recommendations. However, patients are known to forget much of what a physician tells them, and the more a patient is told, the greater the proportion he or she will forget.[9] Studies also have shown that patient recall declines rapidly with time. Approximately 50% of the information given to patients is forgotten within 15 minutes following a physician visit.[25,26] Patients tend to remember best what they are told in the first third of a visit.

Family Beliefs

The family's perception of the illness and treatment, as well as their sense of control over the illness, influence their compliance to a therapeutic regimen. Among parents of children who have asthma, fears and misconceptions about preventive medications are common and likely affect patient compliance negatively.[6] Health belief models suggest that an individual's compliance depends on his or her degree of motivation about health-related issues, perception of susceptibility to the illness, perception of disease severity, and feelings about treatment benefits and cost.[21] Mothers who show concern about their child's illness, perceive the illness as a threat, and believe in the accuracy of the diagnosis and the benefits of treatment are more likely to comply with a therapeutic regimen.[2]

Clinician/Patient Relationship

Effective clinician-patient communication enhances patient compliance significantly.[5,17,32] Patients tend to be more compliant when they are treated by the same practitioner consistently.[15,27] Practitioner knowledge of compliance-enhancing techniques also influences patient compliance positively.[28] Patient supervision, monitoring, and consistent follow-up improve compliance, particularly with chronic regimens.[18,30] Studies of asthma have stressed the importance of the development of a long-term partnership for continued care.[23] There also is support for written practitioner-patient contracts to improve compliance.[24]

Treatment Regimen

Lastly, details of the treatment regimen itself can affect patient compliance. Lower rates of compliance are associated with treatments that require long-term medications, multiple medications, complicated or inconvenient schedules, and frequent medication administration.[15,20,29,34] Other important issues include expense and access to appropriate therapies. Further, for pediatric patients, ease of administration, volume of medication, and palatability also must be considered.

STRATEGIES FOR IMPROVING COMPLIANCE

Strategies for improving patient compliance begin with recognizing this widespread problem and considering the aforementioned components and how they may relate to individual patients and families (Table 13-1). Physicians can help improve a patient's understanding of disease and treatment by providing individualized, written information in conjunction with oral instruction. Such information should contain clear, simple, understandable terms and should be relayed

Table 13-1 Strategies for Improving Compliance

Problem	Potential Solution
Patient/family knowledge	Provide individualized, written information
	Give clear, simple instructions
	Address important features early in discussion
	Provide measuring devices, calendars
Family beliefs	Address fears and misconceptions
	• Enlist support from other family members
	Provide families with sense of control over illness
Clinician/patient relationship	Increase continuity of care
	Set treatment goals in collaboration with family
	Consider written contracts
	Provide routine supervision and monitoring
	Utilize a health team approach
Treatment regimen	Use simplified, short regimens
	Tailor dosage intervals to the patient's daily routine
	Consider palatability, volume of medication
	Consider facilitated drug delivery systems

back from patient to physician to ensure understanding. Although important details should be emphasized, an overload of information should be avoided. Further, the most important details should be presented early in the discussion. Providing measuring devices and calendars may also be helpful for patients who have limited resources.

Another means by which physicians can help improve compliance is to address beliefs, fears, and potential misconceptions that the family may hold. Potential solutions may involve encouraging families to disclose worries and concerns, providing accurate information, offering other sources of information, and enlisting support from other family members. Modification of beliefs may be necessary for certain families to increase compliance. Further, patients should be provided with a sense of control over their illness via accurate information in a supportive environment.

Patient-physician interactions can be improved by increasing continuity of care and increasing practitioner awareness of family concerns. Treatment goals should be set in collaboration with the child and his or her family to allow for a therapeutic framework in which the patient and provider can work together. A written contract may be helpful in some cases, particularly when long-term therapy is needed. Further, routine supervision with compliance monitoring may be necessary to ensure continuation of therapies for chronic disease. This may involve follow-up appointments, phone calls, home visits, blood level monitoring, or counting of unused pills. Other members of the health care team, including nurses and social workers, can help provide support for families to improve compliance as well as assist with contracts, monitoring, and education. Information and counseling from pharmacists also have been shown to be helpful.[7]

Finally, a treatment should be as simple as possible to maximize the likelihood of patient compliance. Medications should be prescribed by using the shortest regimen that is reasonable, and dosing should be tailored to the patient's daily routine. When possible, single agents should be prescribed and changes to a regimen introduced one at a time.[12] For pediatric doses, the most concentrated form of liquid medication usually is preferable so that smaller volumes are needed. Further, it is helpful for physicians to be aware of the palatability of different medications when a choice can be made. In some cases, generic drugs may be preferable to reduce the cost of the treatment. Issues of access to prescribed therapies should be addressed during the original encounter. Lastly, newer drugs or drug delivery systems including sustained-release medications and insulin pumps may improve compliance among certain patients.

SUMMARY

Successful treatment of pediatric illness often depends on compliance with a therapeutic regimen; unfortunately, noncompliance is common among pediatric patients. The issue of compliance in pediatrics includes the extent and consequences of the problem, factors related to noncompliance, and potential strategies for improving compliance. An understanding of this complicated issue requires consideration of many factors involving the patient, the family, the physician, and the regimen itself.

Pediatricians should consider noncompliance as a potential problem with all patients in order to provide them the best possible care. The differential diagnosis in a child unresponsive to therapy should include a compliance-oriented history that indicates whether the child has taken the medication. Improving compliance requires a multifactorial approach that involves providing accurate, concise, and understandable information to families, addressing health-related beliefs, improving communication between physicians and families, and simplifying and individualizing the treatment. Ideally, all patients requiring sustained therapy should receive compliance monitoring, with consistent follow-up and support from the health care team. Barriers to compliance should be identified early in the course of therapy to allow for timely intervention and to minimize negative consequences.

REFERENCES

1. Ambrose PG, et al: On patient compliance with medication doses (letter), *Pediatr Ann* 26:649, 1997.
2. Becker MH, Drachman RH, Kirscht JP: A new approach to explaining sick-role behavior in low-income populations, *Am J Public Health* 64: 205, 1974.
3. Bender B, et al: Psychological factors associated with medication nonadherence in asthmatic children, *J Asthma* 35:347, 1998.
4. Bergman AB, Werner RJ: Failure of children to receive penicillin by mouth, *N Engl J Med* 268:1334, 1963.
5. Borgsdorf LR, Maino JS, Knapp KK: Pharmacist-managed medication review in a managed care system, *Am J Hosp Pharm* 51:772, 1994.
6. Boulet L: Perception of the role and potential side effects of inhaled corticosteroids among asthmatic patients, *Chest* 113:587, 1998.
7. Canada AT: The pharmacist and drug compliance. In Sackett DL, Haynes RB, editors: *Compliance with therapeutic regimens*, Baltimore, Md, 1976, Johns Hopkins University Press.
8. Carr A: Editorial. *Br J Gen Pract* 40:358, 1990.

9. Cassata DM: Health communication theory and research: an overview of the communication specialist interface. In Nimmo D, editor: *Communication yearbook II*. New York, 1978, ICA.
10. Celano M, et al: Treatment adherence among low-income children with asthma, *J Pediatr Psychol* 23:345, 1998.
11. Dajani AS: Adherence to physicians' instructions as a factor in managing streptococcal pharyngitis, *Pediatrics* 97:976, 1996.
12. Dunbar JM, Stunkard AJ: Adherence to diet and drug regimen. In Levy R, et al, editors: *Nutrition, lipids, and coronary heart disease,* New York, 1979, Raven Press.
13. Elling R, Whittemore R, Green M: Patient participation in a pediatric program, *J Health Hum Behav* 1:183, 1960.
14. Feinstein AR, et al: A controlled study of three methods of prophylaxis against streptococcal infection in a population of rheumatic children, *N Engl J Med* 260:697, 1969.
15. Fotheringham MJ, Sawyer MG: Adherence to recommended medical regimens in childhood and adolescence, *J Paediatr Child Health* 31:72, 1995.
16. Gordis L, Markowitz M, Lilienfeld AM: Studies in the epidemiology and preventability of rheumatic fever. IV. A quantitative determination of compliance in children on oral penicillin prophylaxis, *Pediatrics* 43: 173, 1969.
17. Hanchak NA, et al: Patient misunderstanding of dosing instructions, *J Gen Intern Med* 11:325, 1996.
18. Haynes RB: A critical review of the "determinants" of patient compliance with therapeutic regimens. In Sackett DL, Haynes RB, editors: *Compliance with therapeutic regimens,* Baltimore, 1976, Johns Hopkins University Press.
19. Haynes R, Taylor D, Sackett, D: *Compliance in health care,* Baltimore, 1979, John Hopkins University Press.
20. Hussar DA: Importance of patient compliance in effective antimicrobial therapy, *Pediatr Infect Dis J* 6:971, 1987.
21. Janz NK, Becker MH: The health belief model: a decade later, *Health Educ Q* 11:1, 1984.
22. Korsch BM, Gozzi EK, Francis V: Gaps in doctor-patient communication. I. Doctor-patient interaction and patient satisfaction, *Pediatrics* 42:855, 1968.
23. Legorreta AP, et al: Compliance with national asthma management guidelines and specialty care: a health maintenance organization experience, *Arch Intern Med* 158:457, 1998.
24. Lewis CE, Michnich M: Contracts as a means of improving patient compliance. In Barofsky I, editor: *Medication compliance: a behavioral management approach,* Thorofare, NJ, 1977, Charles B Slack.
25. Ley P: Primacy, rated importance, and the recall of medical statements, *J Health Soc Behav* 13:311, 1972.
26. Ley P, et al: A method for increasing patients' recall of information presented by doctors, *Psychol Med* 3:217, 1973.
27. Litt IF, Cuskey WR: Compliance with medical regimen during adolescence, *Pediatr Clin North Am* 27:3, 1980.
28. Maiman LA, et al: Improving pediatricians' compliance-enhancing practices: a randomized trial, *Am J Dis Child* 142:773, 1988.
29. Rapoff MA, Barnard MU: Compliance with pediatric medical regimens. In Cramer JA, Spilker B, editors: *Patient compliance in medical practice and clinical trials,* New York, 1991, Raven Press.
30. Rokart JF, Hofmann PB: Physician and patient behavior under different scheduling systems in a hospital outpatient department, *Med Care* 7:463, 1969.
31. Sackett DL, et al: Helping patients follow the treatments you prescribe. In *Clinical epidemiology: a basic science for clinical medicine,* Boston, 1991, Little, Brown and Co.
32. Sczupak CA, Conrad WF: Relationship between patient oriented pharmaceutical services and therapeutic outcomes of ambulatory patients with diabetes mellitus, *Am J Hosp Pharm* 34:1238, 1977.
33. Teach SJ, Lillis KA, Grossi M: Compliance with penicillin prophylaxis in patients with sickle cell disease, *Arch Pediatr Adolesc Med* 152:274, 1998.
34. Thatcher Shope J: Medication compliance, *Pediatr Clin North Am* 28:5, 1981.

14 The Art of Consultation

Henry M. Seidel

The major purpose of consultation is to gain assistance in the diagnosis, treatment, or management of a patient's problem, as well as to reassure the patient and family. A practitioner often wants similar reassurance, sometimes for legal reasons. Unfortunately, an insecure practitioner may hesitate to ask for consultation for fear of being thought incompetent. "Going it alone" is not always in the patient's best interest. That interest cannot be compromised by someone who does not recognize the limits of individual knowledge and competence in a time when omniscience is beyond anyone's capacity. Trust in the relationship between the practitioner and patient and family is essential; it usually is reinforced, not undermined, by appropriate consultation. Patients and parents appreciate and respond to a practitioner's candor in defining the areas of his or her expertise and in stating limitations. Sound communication maintains trust, whatever the consultant contributes, and requires the role of each participant in the process to be clearly defined. These fundamental principles apply, whether the practice arrangement of the referring physician and the consultant is a health maintenance organization, a large group practice, or a fee-for-service setting. The primary question must always be, "What will serve the best interests of the patient?"

A consultation is not a referral. The physician who requests a consultation is not intending to transfer care to another physician or even, necessarily, to share care with another physician. In some circumstances, a referral or a transfer of care may be appropriate. More often, a sharing of care serves the best interests of the patient.

PRIMARY CARE PROVIDERS

The primary care provider is responsible for arranging a consultation. There is no need to be personally acquainted but it is well to know and be assured of the consultant's education and experience. The ultimate value depends in large part on how skillfully it is managed by that practitioner. The need for consultation often arises during the stress of an acute illness, a time when the family and patient may react to the suggestion with increased anxiety about the gravity of the illness. This anxiety can be tempered by acknowledging it and by putting any underlying fears in appropriate and honest context. In addition, problems in choosing a consultant can be anticipated if there is frank discussion of skills, personalities, and cost. It is generally best to avoid being too specific about what the consultant might say or recommend. There must be leeway for flexible decision making.

The information given to the consultant by the referring physician provides the basis for a successful response. Any behavioral, emotional, social, and economic factors that can influence decision making should be made clear. Problems must be stated concisely, and individual responsibilities for the patient's continuing care should be arranged according to the competence, knowledge, and particular skills of the physicians involved. The primary care provider orchestrates the entire process and must be available to keep all participants fully informed to maintain their optimal contributions. The consultant must clearly understand the goals of the interaction and that the primary care provider's role in the decision-making process is not abdicated. The time at which the patient returns to the primary care physician must be clearly defined. The consultant may need to continue contact with the patient, however, and these visits often may parallel primary care visits. When the relationship with the consultant ends, the primary care physician must ensure follow-up care.

NONPHYSICIAN HEALTH PROFESSIONALS

Over the past several decades the work of the primary pediatrician has been increasingly complemented by that of nonphysician health professionals. The team of health workers may include nurses, nurse practitioners, and physician assistants; physical, occupational, and speech therapists; educational, developmental, and clinical psychologists; audiologists; social workers; and nutritionists. The pediatrician is responsible for understanding the resources provided by these professionals, referring patients to them when indicated, and maintaining effective communication among all involved.

The rules for communication are the same as those that govern consultation with another physician. Three-way interaction is essential when the patient requires care that is not within the competence of the pediatrician or that demands time that the pediatrician does not have. The nonphysician health professional takes on all the responsibilities of any consultant, including that of maintaining open and respectful communication.

CONSULTANTS

The patient and family often are understandably anxious about the unresolved problem presented to the consultant. Concerns about illness and practical considerations of cost must be understood. The consultant should avoid demeaning

BOX 14-1

REASONS FOR CONSULTATION WITH PHYSICIANS AND NONPHYSICIANS IN A VARIETY OF HEALTH AND MEDICAL DISCIPLINES

1. Uncertainty in diagnosis
2. Confirmation of diagnosis
3. Specific skill required for diagnostic process, for example:
   a. Pediatric subspecialist—to perform a variety of diagnostic techniques
   b. Radiologist—to consider all the "imaging" modalities and to select them appropriately
   c. Endoscopist—to see a lesion and perform a biopsy
   d. Surgeon—to explore and remove a lesion, to obtain a biopsy specimen, or to correct a problem
   e. Pathologist—to interpret the nature of the tissue removed
   f. Psychologist, psychiatrist, and mental health counselor—to search for more subjective insights
   g. Teacher and social worker—to discover aspects of patient and family life unknown to the referring physician
4. Uncertainty as to appropriate management or therapy, or both
5. Specific skill required for therapy or management, or both, for example, the variety of surgical disciplines
6. Reassurance for the patient and family or the primary pediatrician, for example:
   a. Reassurance as to the diagnosis (even in the face of certainty)
   b. Reassurance as to a suggested course of action
7. Assistance in long-term follow-up and management of chronic illness, for example:
   a. Physical therapist
   b. Occupational therapist
   c. Rehabilitationist
   d. Schoolteacher

BOX 14-2

GUIDELINES FOR REQUESTING A CONSULTATION

- Be precise in stating your goals for the consultation and the information you need.
- Do not be so rigid in your goals that the consultant is deprived of flexibility in decision making.
- Be aware of uncertainty in the patient and family and in yourself, and be prepared to take every step necessary to resolve it.
- Keep the needs of the patient and family sharply in mind, and keep them well informed and active in the decision-making process.
- Clarify the extent to which you want only to consult or to which you want to refer and share in the care of the patient; do not abdicate your role in decision making.
- Do not abdicate your responsibilities for keeping informed, coordinating information, and maintaining continuity and communication with all the persons involved; this, of course, requires precise and detailed record keeping.

BOX 14-3

GUIDELINES FOR PROVIDING A CONSULTATION

- Be precise and prompt in providing information, using language appropriate to each of the persons involved; different professionals have different jargon, but patients have variable understanding of jargon, most often none at all.
- Keep the patient and family informed but not without parallel or prior information to the referring physician.
- Be available for sharing, but not usurping, the privilege of care for a child who is referred by someone more specifically experienced in the care of adults.
- Keep thorough records and always provide the referring physician with a detailed consultation note; do not rely solely on spoken communication, whether in person or on the telephone.
- Define information with your own observations; accept the word of others only in rare circumstances.
- Be wary of "off-the-cuff" corridor or telephone consultation; when there is the least uncertainty, see the patient.

the primary practitioner because any hint of incompetence or error, verbal or nonverbal, can destroy trust among all participants. Sometimes hindsight, new information, or superior knowledge might prompt a criticism of past management. This must be constructive and must be discussed without hesitancy with the referring physician in private. Health care decision making should, however, tolerate disagreement; many times two or more valid approaches to a problem are possible. Nevertheless, when there is evidence of possible incompetence, the needs of the patient always come first. This is a circumstance that demands honesty and delicacy and, at times, a difficult step—the provision of information to responsible authorities in hospitals, medical societies, and licensing boards. Indeed, once the consultant agrees to consultation, legal responsibility in all its dimensions is assumed. For that matter, the referring physician shares the same responsibility if there is evidence of incompetence in the behavior of the consultant. For everyone involved, failure to fulfill the necessary obligations, for instance, of communication, should be directly confronted.

The consultant cannot rely solely on the observations of others. Information should be obtained independently because the answer to a puzzle may lie in a retaken history, a discriminating observation during the physical examination, or a reevaluation of laboratory data. Reconstruction, reinterpretation, and careful attention to detail are critical.

The consultant must make recommendations promptly, either in person, by e-mail or by telephone. Findings and recommendations must be documented on the hospital chart or in the consultant's office file and also in a letter to the referring practitioner. All information shared with the patient and family must also be made available to the primary physician in timely fashion. If the patient and family circumvent the primary physician and seek additional advice without his or her knowledge, an awkward or threatening situation for the primary care provider could result. The consultant must be sensitive to this while still holding the patient's needs paramount.

The pediatrician who is asked to consult should be aware that many physicians who ask for consultation may not have the necessary education and training for continuing management of a given child's problem. One should be sensitive to this possibility and to the delicate issue that arises from a perception of competition between pediatricians and family practitioners. The reality here is far less than the supposition; nevertheless, it cannot be ignored. Again, the patient's needs must remain paramount, and the consulting pediatrician must be prepared to share care and to accept a transfer of responsibility without usurping that responsibility inappropriately.

Cost Containment

Second opinions have been suggested, particularly when surgery is being considered, as a means of ensuring an appropriate and perhaps cost-saving decision. Ideally, only necessary surgery is performed, and the expectation is that a second opinion will ensure this. There is no certainty, however, that the second opinion is more valid if it contradicts the first. An obvious absurdity can result if the patient is subjected to the opinion of a third expert to overcome a tie vote. This can be avoided if the rules of consultation are scrupulously observed and if the consultant is objective. Referring physicians should take care that no conflict of interest exists between them and the clinicians they consult. Further opinions rarely are necessary when a primary physician and a consultant communicate well with each other and, above all, keep the patient fully and appropriately informed. Recommendations made by the consultant are not binding and may be rejected by the patient and family and referring physician. They need not be compelled to yield to a consultant and all should retain the privilege of being involved in the final decision. The consultation process does lose value if it is diluted by too many opinions, so the referring physician must see that balance is maintained. Thus, optimal patient care requires the orchestrating hand of the primary pediatrician while a variety of individuals contribute their special skills to understanding and solving the patient's problems. Certainly, should the consultant's advice be rejected after clear and open discussion with everyone concerned, the reasoning underlying the entire process from the beginning to end must be clearly documented. Unhappily, the courts, often wrongly, give greater weight to the consultant in a legal proceeding.

A CAVEAT

The consultative process can be abused. Used in excess and without clear need, it can confuse the patient, add to cost, and depersonalize individual care. What Peter Berczeller has characterized as "management by committee" underlies much of a resident's experience in recent years, as more and more people are involved in the continuing management of one person's problems. Judicious self-reliance is no longer as often the tempering factor it must be if a mature clinician is to develop. *Judicious* is an important word. One must respect one's limits. That is achievable without surrendering the responsibility to orchestrate and to keep the consideration of the patient "whole."

Boxes 14-1 to 14-3 outline situations in which a practitioner may decide that a consultation would be in the best interests of the patient and family.

SUGGESTED READINGS

Balint M: *The doctor, his patient, and the illness,* New York, 1972, International Universities Press.

Berczeller PH: The malignant consultation syndrome, *Hosp Pract* 15:33, 1991.

Bursztajn H, et al: *Medical chances: how patients' families and physicians can cope with uncertainty,* New York, 1981, Delacorte Press/Seymour Lawrence.

Drutz JE: The pediatrician hospital consultant, *Pediatr Rev* 13:125, 1992.

Howard BJ: The referral role of pediatricians, *Pediatr Clin North Am* 42: 103, 1995.

Manian FA, Janssen DA: Curbside consultations: a closer look at a common practice, *JAMA* 275:145, 1996.

Nazarian LF: On consulting and being consulted, *Pediatr Rev* 13:124,1992.

Tumulty PA: *The effective clinician,* Philadelphia, 1973, WB Saunders.

Wilde JA, Pedroni AT Jr: The do's and don'ts of consultations, *Contemp Pediatr* 8:23, 1991.

15 Assessing the Medical Literature

S. Michael Plaut

Two studies published the same year in the same journal reported on the relationship between marijuana smoking and testosterone levels in young adult men.[4,5] One study reported a statistically significant dose-related relationship between these two variables; the other could find no relationship. What is a practitioner to make of this discrepancy in results? Perhaps the answer lies in the methods used in the two studies. The first study used retrospective self-reports of marijuana smoking in the subjects' normal environment. In the second study, testosterone levels were measured before, during, and after the smoking of standardized, government-issued "joints" in a controlled institutional environment. Can either of these methods be considered inherently better than the other? Both studies used certain screening devices to minimize suspected extraneous factors that might affect the results. However, were all such factors accounted for? In dealing with a value-laden topic about which the reader may have some prejudices, the interpreter must ask whether personal feelings color his or her interpretation of the data. Thus, a number of factors, including logistical and methodological limitations, the possibility of human bias, and a practitioner's knowledge of the field and its technology, are involved in the appropriate interpretation of a scientific study.

IMPORTANCE OF CRITICAL EVALUATION

"The physician," writes Dykes,[3] "will be equipped to allow the public access to high quality medical care only to the extent that he has been able to keep up with and to grasp the import of advances in the science of medicine." To maintain currency in his or her field, the practitioner must maintain a level of dissatisfaction with the status quo in clinical medicine and a commitment to the idea that science itself "depends for its vitality on a milieu that fosters vigorous, open dissent."[3] Beveridge wrote, "Nothing could be more damaging to science than abandonment of the critical attitude and its replacement by too ready acceptance of hypotheses put forward on slender evidence."[1] This chapter addresses factors important to the critical evaluation of research data, as well as guidelines useful for interpreting those data.

Limitations of Individual Studies

No matter how well conceived and designed a study is and regardless of how effectively its results are communicated, certain necessary limitations must be taken into account in interpreting its value.

Scope and feasibility. As implied by the discussion of the previous two studies, certain decisions must be made in designing a study—decisions that eventually define the nature and extent of the study's usefulness. The investigator may opt for the natural conditions of a field study or for the higher level of control afforded by a laboratory or institution. Although a heterogeneous subject population allows greater generalization from the results, a homogeneous sample tends to reduce variability in the data; thus, fewer subjects are required to obtain conclusive results. Although an investigator may wish to observe many aspects of a phenomenon, the number of variables that can be accounted for will be limited by factors such as the investigator's breadth of expertise, the amount of blood or tissue that can be collected, a subject's ability to concentrate for long periods when completing questionnaires, or the possibility that measurement of one variable might influence the reliability of another.

Relevance and application. Because an investigator must set limits when designing a study, these limits must extend to the interpretation and applicability of the data. For example, although human studies may be considered more relevant than animal studies for clinical purposes, animal studies have the advantage of allowing a measure of manipulation and control that only rarely is possible with human subjects. Any one study can investigate only a relatively small facet of the larger conceptual problem it attempts to address. Thus, the ultimate value of any study depends on replication of the findings in different research settings and synthesis of these findings into a comprehensive picture of the field of study.

Medium of presentation. Review papers and books are the best sources of comprehensive summaries of research findings. However, although such sources have the advantage of a longer perspective on a field of study, they do not have the currency of the journal article or meeting presentation. Besides being current, a journal article has the additional advantages of procedural detail and peer review before publication. Although information presented at a scientific meeting or in a professional "throwaway" publication has a shorter time lag, it often has not undergone thorough peer review. Additionally, articles in peer-reviewed electronic journals are likely to be more trustworthy than self-published papers on the Internet. Thus, a practitioner must consider the source of the information in evaluating its scientific merit or practical relevance.

Human Element in Research

A second major consideration when assessing scientific literature is the individual contribution each participant makes to the research process. As suggested in the aforementioned marijuana studies, cultural or personal values probably color an individual's approach to a research area. In addition, researchers may respond to real or implied institutional pressures to produce a certain quantity of research output. Such pressures may affect many aspects of the research process, from the choice of a research question based on expediency, to excessive haste in publishing the results. An investigator's emotional investment in his or her research may be especially high in areas that might be considered "faddish" or controversial or that reflect a strong theoretical or cultural bias. Examples in developmental research include the areas of mother-infant bonding, hyperactivity, and intelligence testing. Even at best, the knowledge of a researcher, reviewer, or reader is finite, and this limitation may become most apparent in dealing with multidisciplinary issues. As Dykes has written, "Physicians must recognize the fallibility of even our species' greatest intellects. . . . The biases of eminent men are still biases."[3]

Subjective factors may influence the evaluation of research in many ways; a few common examples are given here.

Dichotomous thinking. Practitioners often tend to oversimplify their thinking about natural phenomena by placing the phenomena in categories rather than on continua. Thus, mental illness has either a behavioral or a biological origin, adult traits are determined either genetically or environmentally, and diseases are either physical or psychosomatic. A practitioner may be inclined to think of research subjects as being either normal or abnormal, depending on the issue in question. Although such categorization often is useful or even necessary, few biological questions have a simplistic, all-or-nothing answer. It usually is more fruitful to think in terms of the degree to which each of several factors may interact to influence a phenomenon, rather than attempting to attribute the cause exclusively to one factor or another.

Overemphasis on results and applications. An author's interest in publication or a reader's interest in application often may lead him or her to be "data oriented" in conducting or evaluating research. The value of a study, however, can be determined only by examining the methods used to gather the data. Factors such as the validity of operational definitions, the proper use of controls, the choice of subject population, and the use of suitable methods and procedures for collecting and analyzing data are critical to appropriate interpretation of results.

Conformance to expectations. Claude Bernard once said that "men who have excessive faith in their theories or ideas are not only ill-prepared for making discoveries; they also make poor observations."[1] Although research papers often are written as though the results obtained were exactly as predicted in the introduction, this rarely is the case. Many scientific discoveries are made by the alert, open-minded observer of an unexpected finding. Bernard further admonishes the scientist to forget his or her hypothesis once the study begins, and the reader of a paper should do the same. As mentioned earlier, it is only by challenging one's expectations and assumptions that any scientific field can be advanced.

Assumed attributes of design. Readers of research papers sometimes assume that certain attributes of scientific studies are universally desirable, such as using control or comparison groups of subjects, randomizing procedures, and using large numbers of subjects. However, none of these procedures is necessarily of service to the research question being asked. For example, a hypothesis about the relationship between two characteristics (e.g., nutritional status and school performance) of a given subject population does not need a control group to be tested adequately, *unless* the prediction is that the relationship between those characteristics is not of the same magnitude in another subpopulation, as defined by age, race, sex, or other relevant qualities. However, the absence of a control group also means that the group studied cannot necessarily be considered *distinctive* based on a single study. Nutritional status may be found to be related to school performance in a group of children with diabetes, but this cannot be considered uniquely characteristic of such children unless children without diabetes are studied similarly.

Belief in technical complexity. Studies often appear more credible when highly technical procedures are described in detail. However, simply because a study employs a standardized questionnaire or test to measure some aspect of social interaction or because a computer is used to analyze data does not necessarily mean that the methods used were appropriate to the research question or that the data derived from these procedures led to valid conclusions.

Excessive skepticism toward the research process. Because they are aware that human frailties and technical limitations are real elements of the research process, some practitioners may become hypercritical of all research results. It should be apparent, however, that the cause of biomedical science would not be served either by total acceptance or total rejection of all scientific endeavor. A spirit of openness and curiosity and a healthy skepticism toward scientific thinking are necessary no matter whose work the practitioner evaluates. This kind of attitude can make science both exciting and productive.

Influence of socially validated standards. It also is important to realize that many of the practices of science are determined, at least in part, by social standards within the broad community of scientists or within society itself. Thus, what is now considered unethical scientific practice might not have been so 30 or 40 years ago. Other socially validated standards include authorship practices, expectations for frequency of publication, levels of statistical significance that define the reliability of data, and even the use of statistical criteria for interpreting data. These practices not only vary with the passage of time and social events but also differ among various scientific specialties.

USEFUL KNOWLEDGE AND SKILLS

The preceding section emphasized the attitudinal aspects of effective research critique. Certain knowledge and skills also are extremely useful for evaluating research results competently.

Content and Methods

An important characteristic of research is that it builds on the thinking and findings of the past. Therefore, some knowledge of the literature of the field in question will help the reader determine whether the rationale for a given study and the techniques and procedures used are based on current practices, controversies, or interpretations.

Minimizing bias and "confounds." Probably the greatest number of errors made in interpreting data derive from a poor understanding of the importance of instituting good operational definitions and control procedures and accounting for confounded variables in conducting any research. For example, in the study by Kolodny et al[4] mentioned earlier, any statement made about differences in testosterone levels between users and nonusers of marijuana had to account for the possibility that users and nonusers of marijuana may have used other substances to a different extent than did nonusers of marijuana, inasmuch as such substances also might alter levels of testosterone. Without accounting for this possible confound, it would be difficult to attribute any difference between the groups to marijuana use per se. Thus, by taking a good history, the investigator can control for the possible effect of substances other than that under study. In addition, because this study was based on reported use of "street variety" marijuana, the operational definition of marijuana necessarily included any impurities that might be contained in the joints smoked by the study subjects.

Data presentation and analysis. Another frequent impediment to interpretation of scientific findings is difficulty understanding and interpreting statistical terms and test results. For example, the concept of variance is basic to an understanding of the quantitative expression of data, yet it often is overlooked in their interpretation. Nonetheless, as illustrated in Fig. 15-1, a practitioner's interpretation of the difference between two means must depend on the spread of individual data points around those means. The more dispersed the data are around the mean, the less certain the practitioner can be about the distinction between groups of subjects. Beveridge[1] has suggested that practitioners try to learn at least enough about statistical methods to maintain some respect for them and to know when to consult someone else. A course in basic statistics, coupled with hands-on problem solving, will help the practitioner feel more at ease with these concepts and methods.

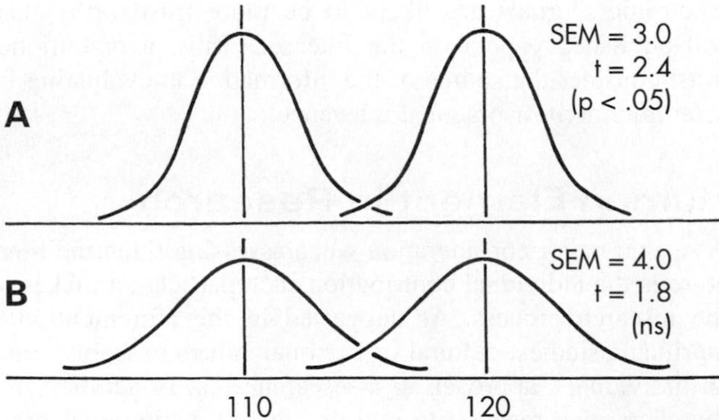

Fig. 15-1 The importance of variance in determining the significance of a difference between means using the *t* test. Once *t* is computed, a table is consulted to determine whether it meets the criterion for significance. **A**, The smaller variance, or standard error of the mean (SEM), leads to a larger *t* value and thus to the conclusion that a difference between means of that magnitude could have occurred by chance less than once in 20 times *($p<0.05$)*. This is not the case in **B**, even though the means are the same, because the variances (SEMs) are too large. Thus, the difference is considered not significant *(ns)*.

(From Plaut SM: Psychosocial aspects of scientific investigation. In Balis GU, et al, editors: *The psychiatric foundations of medicine: dimensions of behavior,* London, 1978, Butterworth.)

Literature search techniques. For some clinicians, reviewing scientific literature involves reading the journals to which they subscribe and attending professional meetings. However, if a clinician wishes to pursue any area of research in greater depth, he or she should have some knowledge of the most advanced techniques for keeping up with and researching specialized literature. In addition to a number of publications that can be found in medical libraries or obtained by subscription (e.g., *Current Contents, Index Medicus,* and *Science Citation Index*), an increasing number of computer search services are available that can be invaluable for gaining a historical perspective or maintaining a current awareness in any field. Such services are accessible not only through libraries but also through web-based programs such as *Grateful Med,* from which one can search a number of databases from any computer that has a modem and an Internet browser. With such programs it is possible not only to search the literature but also to obtain abstracts and authors' addresses and to order reprints of articles.

Scientific communication. It is easier to assess the value of a paper or presentation realistically if the practitioner has some appreciation for the processes by which scientific data are disseminated. Learning how to prepare a good paper or presentation can help a clinician assess the quality of others' work. Some knowledge of the screening processes involved in selecting research reports for presentation or publication also is useful. For example, journals typically submit their papers to a more rigorous peer review process than do scientific meeting program committees, and the extent of peer review that a report undergoes varies somewhat, even within those two spheres.

Nature of the research process. Finally, intensive involvement with a research project can go a long way toward acquainting the clinician with both the technical and the human aspects of the research process. The value of supervised research training early in a career cannot be overemphasized. If such an experience is not possible, participation in a research methodology course or journal club can provide some guided experience in critical evaluation of research reports. A third but less effective alternative is reading in some of the aforementioned areas.

EVALUATION GUIDELINES

A research study should be timely, reflecting a knowledge of current developments in its field of interest and using current methodology. Usually, authors need not provide a comprehensive review of the literature. Rather, they should demonstrate in either the introduction or discussion that the study accounts for relevant knowledge, issues, and controversies related to the topic of interest.

Method

The study's stated purpose, the definitions of variables and terms, the methods and procedures used, the reporting of data, and the interpretation of results all should show a logical consistency. One of the marijuana studies was based on the use of street marijuana, which could have contained impurities, preventing the investigator from conclusively attributing any effects to marijuana per se. The other used joints manufactured and standardized specifically for the study, resulting in a more specific operational definition of the independent variable, marijuana. If a practitioner wishes to apply the results of these studies, he or she must consider which of the two operational definitions is more relevant to his or her purpose. Which is relevant: whether smoking marijuana itself affects testosterone levels in a controlled, institutional setting, or whether the experience of using marijuana in more customary situations is related to levels of this hormone? Each of these questions is more relevant for certain readers and for certain purposes of application or further investigation.

An important and oft-stated rule of thumb for writing the methods section of a paper is that it should, according to Day,[2] "provide enough detail that a competent worker can repeat the experiments . . . . The cornerstone of the scientific method requires that your results, to be of scientific merit, must be reproducible; and, for the results to be adjudged reproducible, you must provide the basis for repetition of the experiments by others." A complete presentation also makes it easier to evaluate the timeliness, relevance, and effectiveness of the methods and procedures used.

Results

Authors sometimes tend to present only the results of statistical tests, as though the only intent of the study were to report the difference between two groups of subjects or a relationship between two variables. It is important that sufficient descriptive data be presented so that the reader can see the data on which these statistical tests were performed. However, journals' space limitations require that authors make some judgments as to which data are best presented in graphs, tables, or text, or not at all. The practitioner's primary concern should be that the questions addressed by the study are reflected appropriately in the data presented and that any interpretation of results is supported by the actual presentation of relevant data. At times there may be relatively subtle aspects of data presentation that the reader should consider. For example, if an author reports relative changes in the scores of two groups of subjects over time as the percentage of an initial value, the practitioner should expect that the author also will provide some information about the initial values themselves. If a group of children performed extremely well on an achievement test, it might not be appropriate to expect that an experimental training program would improve their scores on that particular test.

Statistical Analysis

The following three factors should be considered in evaluating the use of statistical methods.

Relevance to the research question. The statistical methods used should reflect the nature of the question asked by the study. For example, if an author were to predict a systematic relationship between body weight and blood pressure in a group of young adolescents, dividing the children into two discrete groups of body weight and comparing the mean blood pressures for each by use of a *t* test would not provide the most sensitive method for exploring this question. A correlational technique that takes into account the individual weights and blood pressures of the children would be a more sensitive and appropriate way to proceed.

Conformance to underlying assumptions. Appropriate use of any statistical test is based on certain assumptions about the data. For example, certain tests require that the data approximate a normal, or gaussian, distribution; that the number of observations exceeds a certain level; or that two groups of data being compared be independently acquired. If a test that is used to analyze a body of data does not meet its underlying assumptions adequately, inappropriate conclusions may result.

Use of appropriate documentation. If the statistical tests used are not as widely known as, for example, the chi-square, *t* test, or Pearson correlation, the author should provide a reference to the source of the test used. Noting that a particular computer was used to analyze the data is not acceptable documentation. The work of a computer is no more effective than the program it is asked to follow, and the program itself must reflect an appropriate statistical method. Finally, the reader should expect the author to identify all tests used and, in most cases, to report actual results. The simple assertion that "the difference was significant ($p < 0.05$)" does not allow the reader to address the statistical issues outlined here.

Discussion

The reader should determine whether the interpretation of results is consistent with and limited to the data presented. Were conclusions based on data that were either not presented or ambiguous? Does the author generalize inappropriately to populations that have different characteristics from those of the one observed? Sound data and clear thinking usually result in a logical, concise interpretation. As mentioned previously, a scientist's effectiveness often is related to alertness to the unexpected finding and a willingness to consider various alternative explanations for a phenomenon. Regardless of whether the author of a paper considers such alternatives, the reader should be as alert to what is not included in the discussion section as to what is. As Beveridge[1] has said, "The most difficult mental act of all is to rearrange a familiar bundle of data, to look at it differently and escape from the prevailing doctrine."

SUMMARY

In assessing medical literature, the practitioner must remember that any study's value is limited by certain technical considerations and that every aspect of research is affected somewhat by the psychosocial milieu of both researcher and audience. Good scientific pursuit and effective critique require an understanding of these facts, a conscious effort to look at relationships in new and unexpected ways, and a certain level of technical knowledge in the area of research methodology. Conscientious, competent evaluation of research does not simply serve clinicians and their patients; ultimately, it enhances the quality of published research and clinical practice.

REFERENCES

1. Beveridge WIB: *The art of scientific investigation,* ed 3, New York, 1957, Vintage.
2. Day RA: *How to write and publish a scientific paper,* ed 5, Phoenix, 1998, Oryx.
3. Dykes MHM: The physician: the key to the clinical application of scientific information, *JAMA* 237:239, 1977.
4. Kolodny RC, et al: Depression of plasma testosterone levels after chronic intensive marihuana use, *N Engl J Med* 290:872, 1974.
5. Mendelson JH: Plasma testosterone levels before, during and after chronic marihuana smoking, *N Engl J Med* 291:1051, 1974.

SUGGESTED READINGS

Feinstein AR: *Clinical epidemiology: the architecture of clinical research,* Philadelphia, 1985, WB Saunders.

Fletcher RH, Fletcher SW, Wagner EH: *Clinical epidemiology: the essentials,* ed 3, Baltimore, 1996, Williams & Wilkins.

part [illegible]

Principles of Patient Care

[illegible] ection and [illegible]

17 Prevention of Disease

18 [illegible]

19 Nutrition
[illegible] and Requirements
[illegible] Feeding of Infants and Children

[illegible] Immunizations

19 Identification of Developmental [illegible] Delays and the Early Intervention System

20 [illegible]
[illegible]
[illegible] Tests
[illegible]
[illegible] Contraception
[illegible]
[illegible]
Six Screening [illegible]
Seven [illegible] Drugs
Eight Use of Drugs [illegible]
Child Care in Screening
Nine Language and Speech Assessment
Ten Hearing Screening
Eleven Vision Screening
Twelve [illegible]
Thirteen Developmental Surveillance and Intervention
Fourteen Psychosocial Screening

21 Counseling Families on Health Lifestyles

22 Family Systems Approach to the Care of Children

23 Prevention of Disease
One Prevention of Dental Caries
Two Injury Control
Three Preventive Cardiology
Four Adolescent [illegible]
Five Prevention of Smoking

part three

Principles of Patient Care

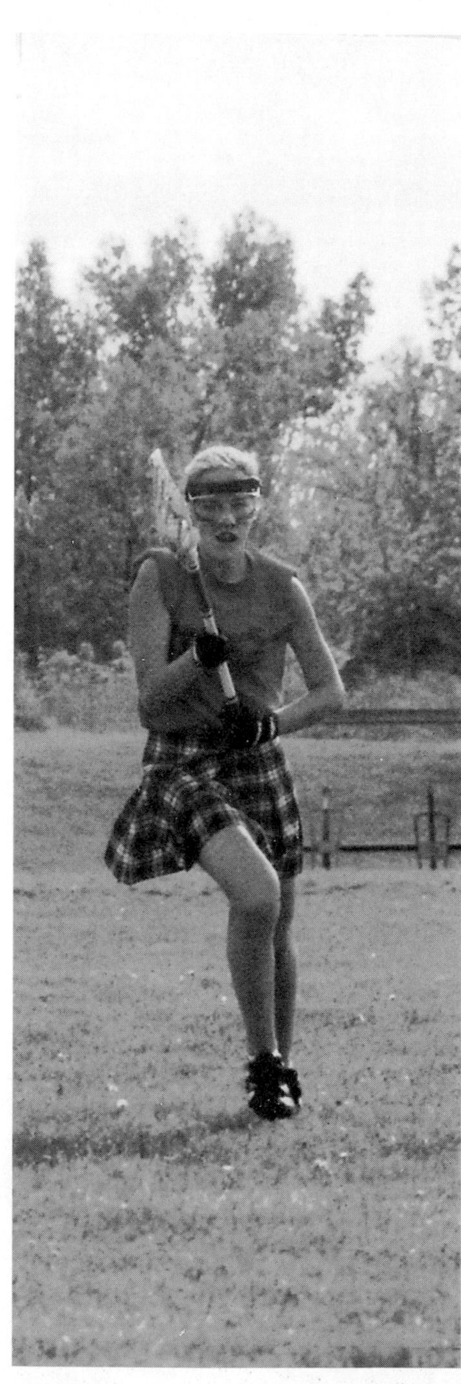

section one

Prevention of Disease

section two

Treatment of Disease

section three

Management of Chronic Illness

16 Anticipatory Guidance

Howard R. Foye, Jr.

Anticipatory guidance is the key to achieving two of the primary goals of pediatric care: promoting health and preventing disease. Providing anticipatory guidance in primary care is challenging because of the range and complexity of appropriate issues, the enormous individual differences among normal children and their families, and the limited time available in health supervision visits. Except for time constraints, these challenges can be the greatest source of interesting variety and rewarding physician-patient interactions in the practice of primary pediatric care.

Three major activities are involved in anticipatory guidance: (1) gathering information, (2) establishing a therapeutic alliance, and (3) providing education and guidance. Many discussions of anticipatory guidance focus only on the third element. Without the first two, however, education and guidance often are misguided or ineffective.

GATHERING INFORMATION AND ESTABLISHING A THERAPEUTIC ALLIANCE

Gathering information through careful history-taking and observation is a prerequisite if the pediatrician is to understand and respect the unique qualities of the child and family. Effective anticipatory guidance, like any teaching, should begin with an understanding of the student's knowledge base, preconceptions, and motivation; guidance is effective to the extent that it is targeted to the individual. A therapeutic alliance between the parents and the physician, based on mutual trust and respect, is another prerequisite for effective anticipatory guidance. Besides enhancing the effectiveness of teaching, this alliance can be a powerful source of emotional support. By listening respectfully, sympathizing with the parents' frustrations, and reinforcing effective parenting positively, the pediatrician can help the parents gain a sense of competence and confidence in their parenting. As the child develops, it becomes increasingly important to establish a therapeutic alliance directly with the child. This relationship is crucial to support and anticipatory guidance as the child becomes more independent.

Box 16-1 outlines information that should be gathered before anticipatory guidance is provided. The two major categories are information about the *child* and information about the *child's environment*. Traditional pediatric health care focuses on the child, particularly on issues of promoting physical health, preventing disease, detecting and treating disorders, and monitoring for attainment of developmental milestones. More recently, pediatric health care has broadened its focus to include issues of behavior and the environment in which the child is developing. The list is imposing, particularly with the time limitations of primary care visits, but at least brief attention must be given to these areas to target anticipatory guidance appropriately. Prior knowledge of the child and family obviates the need to survey all these topics at each visit, although frequent updates are important.

Some fundamental principles about the prerequisites for anticipatory guidance need to be highlighted:

1. The parents and child must be given the opportunity to express their concerns at the beginning of every visit; the pediatrician's agenda for the visit will not get their attention until the physician has addressed *their* agenda.
2. Because it is important to develop a good relationship with the child as well as the parents, the pediatrician should interact warmly with the child at each visit. Even if only briefly, the physician should greet, talk, and play with the child before proceeding to more threatening procedures such as a physical examination and immunizations.
3. The pediatrician always should inquire about how things are going for the parents. Particularly in today's society of fragmented families, parenting can be lonely and demanding. To be a good nurturer, a person needs to be nurtured. The physician should take advantage of every opportunity to compliment the parents and to encourage them to save time for themselves and each other. By supporting the parents and helping them support each other, the pediatrician indirectly can help them nurture their child.
   Two questions that bear frequent repeating are:
   What do you and your child enjoy doing together?
   Is there enough time for spontaneity—for listening to your child and for doing what the child wants to do with you?

PROVIDING EDUCATION AND GUIDANCE

With the information outlined in Box 16-1, the pediatrician is in a position to provide anticipatory guidance that is more focused on the unique qualities and needs of each family. Table 16-1 suggests topics for anticipatory guidance by age.

BOX 16-1

PERTINENT INFORMATION FOR ANTICIPATORY GUIDANCE

A. Information about the *child*
  1. *Concerns:* expressed by parent or child
  2. *Health:* current status and follow-up of past problems
  3. *Routine care:* feeding, sleep, and elimination
  4. *Development:* evaluated by school performance or with standardized tests (e.g., Denver Developmental Screening Test,[6] Early Language Milestone Scale[3])
  5. *Behavior:* temperament and interaction with family, peers, and others

B. Information about the child's *environment*
  1. *Family composition* (at home)
  2. *Caregiving schedule:* who and when
  3. *Family stresses:* (e.g., work, finances, illness, death, moving, marital and other relationships)
  4. *Family supports:* relatives, friends, organizations, material resources
  5. *Stimulation* in the home
  6. *Stimulation/activities* outside the home, (e.g., preschool/school, peers, organizations)
  7. *Safety*

It is, of course, impossible to cover all of the issues listed at each visit. A reasonable goal at each health supervision visit would be to at least ask an open-ended question about each of the general categories—for example, health, safety, nutrition, development/behavior, child care, and family. That will give the family an opportunity to guide the discussion to specific topics of interest to them. Discussion of a small number of salient topics for them is likely to be much more helpful than a rapid, rote checklist approach to anticipatory guidance.

One way to expand the scope of your anticipatory guidance with a very small commitment of time is to use preprinted handouts. The American Academy of Pediatrics publishes an extensive variety of patient education materials. These materials provide a very efficient way to present standard information that you may want to provide to all of your families. To avoid littering your parking lot with handouts, it is wise to introduce the material during your conversation with the family, emphasizing why you feel the topic is important. Preprinted handouts, of course, are only a supplement, not a substitute for personal discussion with the family.

Many potentially important topics may be overlooked if anticipatory guidance is limited to topics linked to specific ages. Topics that may be among the most important at any age and, therefore, always worthy of consideration include:

1. *Family stresses* (e.g., single parenthood, divorce, separation, moving, illness, death, unemployment)
2. *Temperament*[8]
3. *Hurried children*[4]—tight schedules and pressure to achieve and grow up fast
4. *Self-esteem*—development of a sense of competence[9]

The lists in Table 16-1 should not limit the pediatrician's scope but merely serve as examples and reminders. Much anticipatory guidance will follow from information gathered at the beginning of the visit, including new concerns of the parent or child and follow-up of old problems.

The following sections supplement information in Table 16-1 by briefly discussing the major developmental tasks of each period and related issues of anticipatory guidance. For each age period after birth, the major developmental tasks are described for each of three broad categories of development: socioemotional development, cognitive development, and physical/motor development.

Prenatal Visit

The family's developmental tasks in the period before delivery involve planning and preparing for the birth and early care of the infant. The main goal of the prenatal visit is to begin the development of a therapeutic alliance with the family. Specific objectives include learning about the family's health and social history and discussing their plans and concerns about the remainder of the pregnancy, labor, delivery, and early child care. Other objectives include a discussion of the nature of the pediatrician's working relationship with the family and details about how the practice functions.

Newborn Visits

During the newborn period, the major developmental tasks for infants involve the transition to the extrauterine environment. The major tasks for parents include bonding and learning to respond appropriately to the emotional and physical needs of their infant. The objectives of newborn pediatric care include assessing the infant's physical status, behavioral individuality, and caregiving environment at home; managing health problems; and promoting bonding and parenting competence and confidence.

Up to 6 Months

The major developmental tasks in the first 6 months include caregiver-infant reciprocity[2] (socioemotional development); attention to events in the external environment (cognitive development); and rapid growth and visually guided manipulation with the hands (physical/motor development).

Reciprocity is a term used to describe the achievement of mutually satisfying and predictable interactions between an infant and a caregiver. The development of reciprocity is influenced both by the clarity and predictability of the cues provided by the infant and by the caregiver's sensitivity, responsiveness, and predictability. This is an important period of learning for all participants in these interactions. Learning is more difficult when the infant is irritable or unpredictable or when the caregiver's responsiveness is hindered by fatigue, depression, or distractions caused by family stress. The following anticipatory guidance may be helpful: (1) anticipatory teaching about the normal unpredictability of feeding and sleeping schedules and the frequency of unexplained episodes of crying in the first few months, (2) discussion of the parenting of infants who have various temperaments, and (3) discussion and counseling about issues that may be inter-

Table 16-1 Topics of Anticipatory Guidance

Prenatal and Newborn

Prenatal visit

1. *Health:* pregnancy course; worries; tobacco, alcohol, drug use; hospital and pediatric office procedures
2. *Safety:* infant car seat, crib safety
3. *Nutrition:* planned feeding method
4. *Child care:* help after birth, later arrangements
5. *Family:* changes in relationships (spouse, siblings), supports, stresses, return to work

Newborn visits

1. *Health:* jaundice, umbilical cord care, circumcision, other common problems, when to call pediatrician's office
2. *Safety:* infant car seat, smoke detector, choking, keeping tap water temperature below 120° F (48.8° C)
3. *Nutrition:* feeding, normal weight loss, spitting, vitamin and fluoride supplements
4. *Development/behavior:* individuality, "consolability," visual and auditory responsiveness
5. *Child care:* importance of interaction, parenting books, support for primary caregiver
6. *Family:* postpartum adjustments, fatigue, "blues," special time for siblings

First Year

Up to 6 months

1. *Health:* immunizations, exposure to infections
2. *Safety:* falls, aspiration of small objects or powder, entanglement in mobiles that have long strings
3. *Nutrition:* supplementing breast milk or formula, introducing solids, iron
4. *Development/behavior:* crying/colic, irregular schedules (eating, sleeping, eliminating), response to infant cues, reciprocity, interactive games, beginning eye-hand coordination
5. *Child care:* responsive and affectionate care, caregiving schedule
6. *Family:* return to work, nurturing of all family relationships (spouse and siblings)

6-12 months

1. *Safety:* locks for household poisons and medications; gates for stairs; ipecac; poison center telephone number; outlet safety covers; avoiding dangling cords or tablecloths; safety devices for windows/screens; toddler car seat when infant reaches 20 pounds; avoiding toys that have small detachable pieces; supervise child in tub or near water
2. *Nutrition:* discouraging use of bottle as a pacifier or while in bed; offering cup and soft finger foods (with supervision); introducing new foods one at a time
3. *Development/behavior:* attachment, basic trust versus mistrust, stranger awareness, night waking, separation anxiety, bedtime routine, transitional object
4. *Child care:* prohibitions few but firm and consistent across caregiving settings; defining discipline as "learning" (not punishment)
5. *Family:* spacing of children

Second Year

1-2 years

1. *Health:* immunizations
2. *Safety:* climbing and falls common; supervising outdoor play; ensuring safety caps on medicine bottles; noting dangers of plastic bags, pot handles hanging over stove, and space heaters
3. *Nutrition:* avoiding feeding conflicts (decreased appetite is common); period of self-feeding, weaning from breast or bottle; avoiding sweet or salty snacks
4. *Development/behavior:* autonomy versus shame/doubt, ambivalence (independence/dependence), tantrums, negativism, getting into everything, night fears, readiness for toilet training, self-comforting behaviors (thumb sucking, masturbation), speech, imaginative play, no sharing in play, positive reinforcement for desired behavior
5. *Child care:* freedom to explore in safe place; day care; home a safer place to vent frustrations; needs show of affection, language stimulation through reading and conversation
6. *Family:* sibling relationships, parents modeling of nonaggressive responses to conflict (including their own conflict with their toddler)

Preschool

2 to 5 years

1. *Health:* tooth brushing, first dental visit
2. *Safety:* needs close supervision near water or street; home safety factors include padding of sharp furniture corners, fire escape plan for home, and locking up power tools; should have car lap belt at 40 pounds and bike helmet; should know (a) name, address and telephone number, (b) not to provoke dogs, and (c) to say "no" to strangers
3. *Nutrition:* balanced diet; avoiding sweet or salty snacks; participating in conversation at meals

Continued

Table 16-1 Topics of Anticipatory Guidance—cont'd

Preschool—cont'd

2 to 5 years—cont'd

4. *Development/behavior:* initiative versus guilt; difficulty with impulse control and sharing; developing interest in peers, high activity level; speaking in sentences by age 3; speech mostly intelligible to stranger by age 3, reading books; curiosity about body parts; magical thinking, egocentrism
5. *Child care/preschool:* needs daily special time with parents, bedtime routine; talking about day in day care; limiting TV watching with child, reprimanding privately, answering questions factually and simply; adjusting to preschool, kindergarten readiness
6. *Family:* chores, responsibilities

Middle Childhood

5 to 10 years

1. *Health:* appropriate weight; regular exercise; somatic complaints (limb and abdominal pain, headaches); alcohol, tobacco, and drug use; sexual development; physician and child dealings (more direct)
2. *Safety:* bike helmets and street safety; car seat belts; swimming lessons; use of matches, firearms, and power tools; fire escape plan for home; saying "no" to strangers
3. *Nutrition:* balanced diet, daily breakfast, limiting sweet and salty snacks, moderate intake of fatty foods
4. *Development/behavior:* industry versus inferiority, need for successes, peer interactions, adequate sleep
5. *School:* school performance, homework, parent interest
6. *Family:* more time away but continuing need for family support, approval, affection, time together, and communication; family rules about bedtime, chores, and responsibilities; guidance in using money; parents should encourage reading; limiting TV watching and discussing programs seen together; teaching and modeling nonviolent responses to conflict
7. *Other activities:* organized sports, religious groups, other organizations, use of spare time

Adolescence

Discuss with adolescent

1. *Health:* alcohol, tobacco, and drug use, health consequences of violence, dental care, physical activity, immunizations
2. *Safety:* bike and skateboard helmet and safety, car seat belts, driving while intoxicated, water safety, hitchhiking, risk taking
3. *Nutrition:* balanced diet, appropriate weight, avoiding junk foods
4. *Sexuality:* physical changes, sex education, peer pressure for sexual activity, sense of responsibility for self and partner, OK to say "no," preventing pregnancy and sexually transmitted diseases, breast and testes self-examination
5. *Development/relationships:* identify versus role confusion, family, peers, dating, independence, trying different roles, managing anger other than with verbal and physical attacks
6. *School:* academics, homework
7. *Other activities:* sports, hobbies, organizations, jobs
8. *Future plans:* school, work, relationships with others

Discuss with parents

1. *Communication:* allowing adolescents to participate in discussion and development of family rules; needs frequent praise and affection, time together, interest in adolescent's activities
2. *Independence:* parent and child ambivalence about independence; expecting periods of estrangement; promoting self-responsibility and independence; still needs supervision
3. *Role model:* actions speak louder than words—parents provide model of responsible, reasonable, nonviolent, and compassionate behavior

fering with the caregiver's ability to provide a responsive environment for the infant.

The major cognitive developmental task for the infant in this period involves a shift from activities centered on the body (e.g., sucking) to a greater interest in the external environment. At first this is manifested by increasing visual and auditory attention to external events. Then, from 4 to 6 months of age, the infant's ability to guide the grasp and manipulation of objects visually progresses rapidly.

6 to 12 Months

The major developmental tasks of the 6- to 12-month-old infant include attachment,[1] basic trust versus mistrust[5] (socioemotional development); object permanence, early means-end relationships[7] (cognitive development); and mobility (physical/motor development).

The concepts of *attachment* and *basic trust* are similar. Basic trust develops in the first year to the extent that an infant learns that the caregiver is a predictable and reliable provider of essential physical and emotional needs. Trust in this most important aspect of the external environment, the primary caregiver, is believed to result in more confident exploration of the wider environment during the second year, when autonomy becomes the major socioemotional issue. Attachment theorists refer to this as *exploration from a secure base.* An infant who is insecurely attached (who mistrusts more than trusts) because of unpredictable or unreliable caregiving in the first year will more likely be inhibited in exploring the environment. The insecurely attached infant also is more likely to be clinging and demanding as a result of insecurity about the caregiver's availability. These behaviors may lead to the erroneous conclusion that the infant is too "attached" to the caregiver. It is important to remember, however, that most infants go through a period of separation anxiety toward the end of the first year, when clinging behavior increases. Also, some infants who temperamentally are more timid or socially withdrawn may have an extended period of "clinginess."

Object permanence means that the infant now understands that objects continue to exist even when they are not present in the immediate physical environment. Calls for an absent primary caregiver often are the earliest evidence that the infant has developed this cognitive ability. Separation anxiety and night waking also may be manifestations of this new achievement. A budding understanding of means-end relationships is apparent in the infant's ability to remove a barrier or to use a second object to retrieve a toy that is out of reach. Another manifestation may be the infant's association of the coat closet with Mommy's departure and, therefore, the bitter protests that occur when the mother approaches the closet.

Increasing mobility has many implications for anticipatory guidance, particularly regarding issues of safety.

1 to 2 Years

The major developmental tasks of the 1- to 2-year-old include autonomy versus shame and doubt[5] and ambivalence regarding dependence and independence (socioemotional development); exploration, early language, "pretend" play (cognitive development); and ambulation and slower growth (physical/motor development).

The issue of autonomy is at the heart of "the terrible twos," which actually start during the second year of life. This period is characterized by frustrating, dramatic behavioral shifts from stubborn independence ("I want to do it myself" and "no" to most parental requests) to infantile clinging and dependence. Parents often wish that their child were both more independent and less independent at the same time. The wild fluctuations are related to the child's newly acquired walking and climbing skills, as well as his or her eagerness to explore, which often outstrips the cognitive ability to anticipate danger or surprise. The brazen explorer quickly can be reduced to a tearful clinger to mommy's skirt.

The second year is a very exciting time for cognitive development. The developing ability to understand and to use language is a manifestation of the child's cognitive ability to use symbols for objects. By age 2, the child's play becomes a theater for imitating past events and demonstrating a budding ability to think symbolically and creatively.

A decline in the growth rate in the second year is the cause of one of the most frequent parental concerns in this period: "He eats like a bird." Explaining normal growth and intake usually reassures the parents.

Preschool: 2 to 5 Years

The major developmental tasks of the preschool period include initiative versus guilt,[5] mastery—for example, toilet training—and peer interactions with true sharing (socioemotional development); speech, deferred imitation, and imagination (cognitive development); and steady growth and increasing coordination (physical/motor development).

The initiative that characterizes this period is demonstrated in widening interactions with the physical environment and with people outside the family. Good parenting involves giving the child opportunities to exercise initiative and to experience mastery over new challenges, while ensuring close supervision to provide necessary support and encouragement and to prevent harm. An overprotective or restrictive caregiving environment may result in fear or guilt and may inhibit initiative and the developing sense of self-mastery. A caregiving environment that pushes the child too hard toward "independence" may not provide enough supervision and support to allow the child to master the developmental tasks of this period.

During the preschool period, language develops so remarkably that it is easy to forget that the preschooler's thinking often is still illogical. It is characterized by an egocentrism that cannot comprehend a perspective other than the child's own and assumes that other people have seen and experienced exactly what the child has. It also is characterized by magical thinking—the blurring of fantasy and reality. Wishes, dreams, and actual events are not clearly distinguished. These logical limitations may help explain the common occurrence of irrational fears and exasperating misunderstandings between parent and child. A wish that a new sibling would go away may be a frightening source of guilt and self-blame when the new infant is hospitalized. The child may think that wishing made it happen. Careless comments by a parent also may be a source of anxiety for a child who cannot distinguish a threat from reality.

Middle Childhood: 5 to 10 Years

The major developmental tasks of middle childhood include industry versus inferiority[5] (socioemotional development); concrete logical thinking,[7] basic functions of mathematics, and classification of objects (cognitive development); and preadolescence (physical/motor development).

This is the period when the pediatrician should increasingly engage the child directly in discussions and anticipatory guidance. By the end of this period, some physicians already are spending part of each visit alone with the child.

Middle childhood is the period when critical appraisal of a child's abilities begins in earnest. Although preschool children (and their parents) frequently compare themselves with their age mates, comparisons become much more quantitative and official in middle childhood. Tests and opportunities for public humiliation in school are unending. Even when teachers are careful to avoid overt comparisons, the children know how they measure up. After-school activities, particularly sports, often are highly competitive. It is easy to understand how a child may develop a sense of inferiority, particularly in a culture that so emphasizes being number one, as if anything else is not good enough.

The socioemotional task of industry (i.e., motivation to succeed through work) requires that the child experience success. Lack of success in tasks leads to a feeling of inferiority, discouragement, and giving up. This is an important issue for anticipatory guidance, because parents also may have accepted the notion that the child is not good at anything. Some creative thinking must be done to provide successful experiences for each child so that lack of motivation does not rob the child of his or her potential.

Adolescence

The major developmental tasks of adolescence include identity versus role confusion[4] (socioemotional development), abstract and hypothetical thinking[5] (cognitive development), and puberty (physical/motor development).

Adolescence frequently is described as comprising three stages. Early adolescence (roughly 10 to 13 years of age) is the period of most rapid physical growth and sexual development. Because of the rapid changes, many children are preoccupied with their bodies and with comparing themselves with their peers. In addition, they begin to separate from their parents, frequently challenging parental authority. During middle adolescence (roughly 14 to 17 years of age), preoccupation with physical changes lessens. This period is characterized by intense involvement with peers, conflicts over independence with parents and, often, sexual exploration. Late adolescence (roughly 18 to 21 years of age) is characterized by increased concern over future plans, including college studies and career plans. Social skills are more advanced, and many adolescents are involved in committed, intimate relationships.

LITERATURE FOR PARENTS AND CHILDREN

Literature for parents and children's books frequently are valuable supplements to discussions with the pediatrician about topics of anticipatory guidance. Often, practitioners lack sufficient time to discuss an issue in depth in the office. One alternative is to begin a discussion in the time available and then suggest a pertinent reference. Literature references for the parents and child are listed at the end of the chapter; however, follow-up is crucial. Perhaps the next regular visit is soon enough, but it is always appropriate to invite the family to call or to make an appointment if family members wish to discuss further questions sooner. Of course, sometimes a definite follow-up visit or referral should be scheduled immediately.

A note of caution is warranted about recommending books. Some parents have a tendency to overintellectualize parenting—to place too much reliance on specific "expert" advice that is not individualized to their family. Good literature for parents points out that specific advice needs to be tailored to the unique qualities of the child and the parents and to the environment in which they live. Good parenting involves more than general knowledge about children and behavior management; it also involves sensitivity and responsiveness to the special qualities of each child and self-awareness about how the parent's feelings and events in the environment influence interactions with the child. Written advice alone, therefore, is not sufficient. The parents must interpret and modify the advice to fit their situation. Some can do this themselves; many will benefit from anticipatory guidance by the pediatrician.

REFERENCES

1. Bowlby J: *Attachment,* New York, 2000, Basic Books.
2. Brazelton TB, Koslowski B, Main M: The origins of reciprocity: the early mother-infant interaction. In Lewis M, Rosenblum L, editors: *The effect of the infant on its caregiver,* New York, 1974, John Wiley & Sons.
3. Coplan J: Evaluation of the child with delayed speech or language, *Pediatr Ann* 14:203, 1985.
4. Elkind D: *The hurried child: growing up too fast too soon,* ed 2, Reading, Mass, 1989, Addison-Wesley.
5. Erikson E: *Childhood and society,* thirty-fifth anniversary edition, New York, 1993, WW Norton.
6. Frankenburg W, Sciarillo W, Burgess D: The newly abbreviated and revised Denver Developmental Screening Test, *J Pediatr* 99:995, 1981.
7. Ginsburg H, Opper S: *Piaget's theory of intellectual development,* ed 3, Englewood Cliffs, NJ, 1990, Prentice-Hall.
8. Thomas A, Chess S, Birch H: *Temperament and behavior disorders in children,* New York, 1968, New York University Press.
9. White R: Motivation reconsidered: the concept of competence, *Psychol Rev* 66:297, 1959.

SUGGESTED READINGS

Brazelton TB: Anticipatory guidance, *Pediatr Clin North Am* 22:533, 1975.

Casey P, Sharp M, Loda F: Child-health supervision for children under 2 years of age: a review of its content and effectiveness, *J Pediatr* 95:1, 1979.

Chamberlin R, Szumowski E, Zastowny T: An evaluation of efforts to educate mothers about child development in pediatric office practices, *Am J Public Health* 69:875, 1979.

Committee on Psychosocial Aspects of Child and Family Health, American Academy of Pediatrics: Guidelines for health supervision. II, Elk Grove Village, Ill, 1988, The Academy.

Prothrow-Stith D: *Deadly consequences,* New York, 1991, Harper Collins.

The following professional texts contain extensive, annotated bibliographies of parent and child literature on a wide variety of topics (health and development):

Dixon S, Stein M: *Encounters with children: pediatric behavior and development,* ed 3, Chicago, 1999, Mosby.

Sahler OJ, McAnarney E: *The child from three to eighteen,* St. Louis, 1981, Mosby.

Parents may find the following books particularly helpful:

American Academy of Pediatrics: *Caring for Your Baby and Young Child: Birth to Age 5,* ed 5, New York, 1998, Bantam Books.

American Academy of Pediatrics: *Caring for Your School-Age Child: Ages 5 to 12,* New York, 1995, Bantam Books.

American Academy of Pediatrics: *Caring for Your Adolescent,* New York, 1991, Bantam Books.

Brazelton TB: *Touchpoints: the Essential Reference,* Reading, Mass, 1994, Addison-Wesley. This is an engaging and insightful review of development, with a particular emphasis on emotional and behavioral development from the prenatal period through the first 3 years. It is as sensitive to parents as it is to children. I recommend it most highly.

Brazelton TB: *Working and Caring,* Reading, Mass, 1992, Addison-Wesley. A wonderful book for parents trying to balance working and child care—honest and positive.

Elkind D: *All Grown Up and No Place to Go: Teenagers in Crisis,* Reading, Mass, 1997, Addison-Wesley. This is a provocative and insightful discussion of adolescence today.

Schmitt B: *Your Child's Health: the Parents' Guide to Symptoms, Emergencies, Common Illnesses, Behavior and School Problems,* New York, 1991, Bantam Books. This book provides brief, well-organized information on a wide variety of pediatric topics. A very good quick reference for parents' questions.

17 Nutrition

one Nutritional Requirements

Gilbert B. Forbes

To live, to grow, and to thrive, human beings must take in nutrients from their environment. Before birth these are supplied by the mother; thereafter, they must be ingested. If too little is provided, the infant or child will not grow and may become ill; too much may lead to toxicity or obesity. Nutritionists have tried for decades to define the optimum intakes for various nutrients; a few are known, yet for most the only data available are in the form of educated guesses. In an attempt to cover the maximum conceivable need (because individuals vary in size, there may be individual differences in requirements), quasiofficial bodies such as the National Academy of Sciences have recommended generous allowances of most nutrients. Although this would provide for the upper extremes of need, in effect it advises most of the population to eat more than they need. Dietary surveys among healthy individuals thus show that the diets of many people do not satisfy the listed recommended dietary allowances. Perhaps this is just as well, inasmuch as overnutrition now is a greater problem in this country than undernutrition, and there is concern over the possibility that the former may shorten the life span.

Nutritional requirements can be considered on the basis of age, body size, growth rate, physiological losses (as in menstruation and lactation), and caloric intake. The following discussion deals primarily with the normal child; for the most part, situations that call for special nutritional advice are dealt with in other chapters.

Note should be taken of the contribution of food technology to the modern nutritional scene: the pasteurization of milk, the addition of certain vitamins and minerals to some foods, alterations in milk composition to serve the needs of young infants better, hypoallergenic formulas, and the special formulas for infants who have certain inborn errors of metabolism (e.g., phenylketonuria). All this has made it possible to feed the majority of infants most satisfactorily. An undesirable consequence has been a decline in breast-feeding; although of minor nutritional importance in Western society, this decline may be disadvantageous in poor countries and in depressed areas where sanitation is inadequate and the supply of animal protein is meager. However, interest in breast-feeding has revived in recent years in all societies.

ENERGY

Energy Metabolism

The body continuously expends energy, in the form of heat and work. Body temperature must be maintained, physical activity provided for, and the processes of digestion, cellular transport, and tissue synthesis supported. The unit of energy generally employed in metabolism is the kilocalorie (kcal),* usually designated simply as a *calorie* (Cal). Foods have approximately the following energy equivalents when burned in the body:

1 g protein = 4 calories (protein is 16% nitrogen)
1 g carbohydrate = 4 calories
1 g fat = 9 calories

It is axiomatic that the body cannot exist on only one or even two of these sources of energy, so it is fortunate that nature has provided a mixture of the three in many foods. Satisfactory, palatable diets for infants and children (and adults, too) provide 8% to 15% of total calories from protein and 30% to 50% each from fat and carbohydrate.

Energy intake is put to five broad uses:

1. *Resting metabolic rate* (RMR), also known as *resting energy expenditure* (REE) (formerly *basal metabolic rate* [BMR]). This term refers to energy expenditure at rest in the fasting state. On a body weight basis, the resting metabolic rate (RMR) is higher in infants than in adults, primarily because (1) infants' surface area to weight ratio is higher, (2) a certain amount of infants' "basal" energy is used for growth, and (3) the relative size of the viscera and brain (the most metabolically active organs in the body) is considerably greater in infants. During the first year of life the RMR is about 55 Cal/kg/day; thereafter this value diminishes gradually to the adult level of about 25 to 30 Cal/kg/day. Because adipose tissue has a low metabolic rate, the RMR *per kilogram of body weight* is lower in obese individuals than in thin ones and in women compared with men. However, the RMR bears a linear relationship to *lean weight* in adolescents and adults.
2. *Requirement for growth.* The synthesis of tissue obviously requires energy. The exact amount is not known, but studies of young children recovering from malnutrition and

*A kilocalorie is the amount of heat required to raise the temperature of 1 kg of water by 1° C (from 14.5° to 15.5° C); it equals 1000 small calories. Some would like to replace this with another unit of energy, the *joule* (equivalent to 10^7 ergs), which physical scientists commonly use. One kilojoule (kJ) equals 0.239 kcal; to convert kilocalories to kilojoules, multiply by 4.18.

Table 17-1 Calories (kcal) Expended per Hour by Adults

Activity	Calories Men	Calories Women
Sleeping	65	54
Sitting quietly	83	69
Walking (3 miles/hr)	220	180
Swimming, tennis	400	300
Rowing	450+	360+

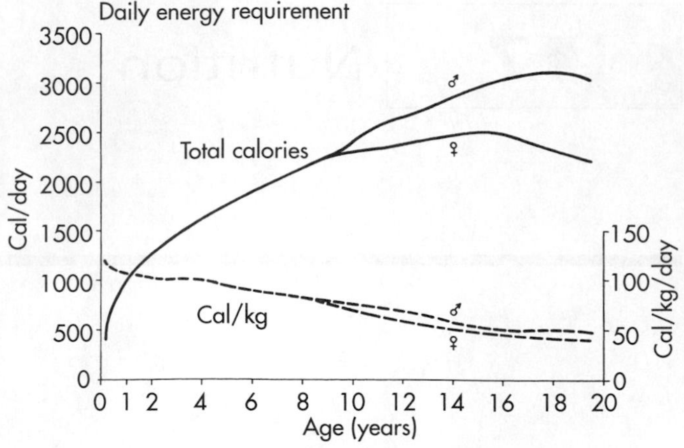

Fig. 17-1 Daily energy requirement as a function of age and sex.

studies of intentionally overfed adults show that 4 to 8 extra calories are required for each gram of weight gain. During the first 4 months of life, one third of the total caloric intake is used for growth. By the end of the second year of life, this has dropped to 1% to 2% of calories.

3. *Energy lost in excreta.* Some nitrogen is excreted in the urine, and feces contain both protein and fat. It is estimated that such losses constitute about 10% of the energy intake of the normal diet.
4. *Thermic effect of feeding* (formerly *specific dynamic action*). Resting metabolism rises somewhat after a meal, especially after a generous protein intake, and may not return to the baseline for several hours. The amount of energy dissipated in this manner is estimated to be 5% to 10% of total calories ingested.
5. *Requirement for physical activity.* Studies of adults show that sedentary men require about 2700 Cal/day and very active men, 4000; for women, these values are 2000 and 3000 Cal/day, respectively. Thus, very active people need 1½ times more food. Although estimates of this sort are not available for infants and children, casual observation confirms that physical activity varies from person to person. Some infants are more restless than others, and, obviously, the energy expenditure of high school athletes is different from that of their spectator friends. Because a major portion of the total energy expenditure is directly proportional to body weight, large persons expend more energy in a given task and at rest.

Table 17-1 lists energy expenditures for adults (these values would apply to late adolescents as well) for various activities. The total daily energy requirement as a function of age and sex is depicted in Fig. 17-1. These data are based on reports by the Food and Nutrition Board of the National Academy of Sciences and the World Health Organization. The diagram shows the estimated average requirement. Note the sex difference both in total calories and calories per kilogram during adolescence. This is due to (1) boys' greater lean weight and (2) their greater physical activity. The values for individuals 19 to 20 years of age equal those for young adults.

In this context, it is instructive to consider the growth of the lean body mass (LBM) inasmuch as this represents the bulk of the body's metabolically active tissue, whereas the adipose tissue component is relatively inert. The data shown in Fig. 17-2 are based on total body potassium measurements.* Note that the LBM growth curve differs from that of total body weight, because the latter includes a variable proportion of fat. The adolescent growth spurt in LBM is considerably greater for boys than for girls. It should be obvious that an adolescent boy has a greater need for calories and for many nutrients, particularly calcium and nitrogen. Indeed, in the midst of his adolescent growth spurt, a boy's need for iron to provide growth of blood volume and muscle mass may equal that of a postmenarchal girl.

Fig. 17-1 shows the *average* energy requirement. Larger individuals need more calories, both for maintenance and for a given degree of physical activity; smaller people need less. This amounts to 18 to 20 calories a day for each kilogram of weight difference. Under normal circumstances, appetite is a good indicator of energy need. In situations of abnormal growth, either too little or too much, this chart can help the pediatrician determine whether the stated intake of food is appropriate and thus whether food intake could be a contributing factor.

Low-birth-weight neonates need a generous intake of calories (i.e., 130 to 150 Cal/kg/day) to provide for "catch-up" growth, and their inadequate fat stores demand that feeding be started as soon after birth as possible.

One additional point is worth noting: If calories are obtained from a variety of foods, an adequate intake of calories usually ensures an adequate intake of essential nutrients. Therefore, calories should be the first item evaluated in assessing a dietary history.

Pregnancy and Lactation

The large number of teenage pregnancies demands that pediatricians and child health personnel be aware of the extra energy requirements for pregnancy and lactation. Studies of chronically undernourished poverty groups have shown that birth weight and the chances of infant survival can be improved by providing additional calories during pregnancy; it now generally is admitted that a weight gain of 10 to 13 kg is desirable. Weight gain during pregnancy, as well as the prepregnancy weight, influences birth weight. The extra energy cost to the mother is estimated at 150 to 300 Cal/day throughout pregnancy, depending on how much she curtails her physical activity. Although based on adults,

*One of the naturally occurring isotopes of potassium (^{40}K) is radioactive, and the body contains enough of this isotope to allow its measurement by specially designed scintillation counters. Because potassium is found only in lean tissue, LBM can be estimated.

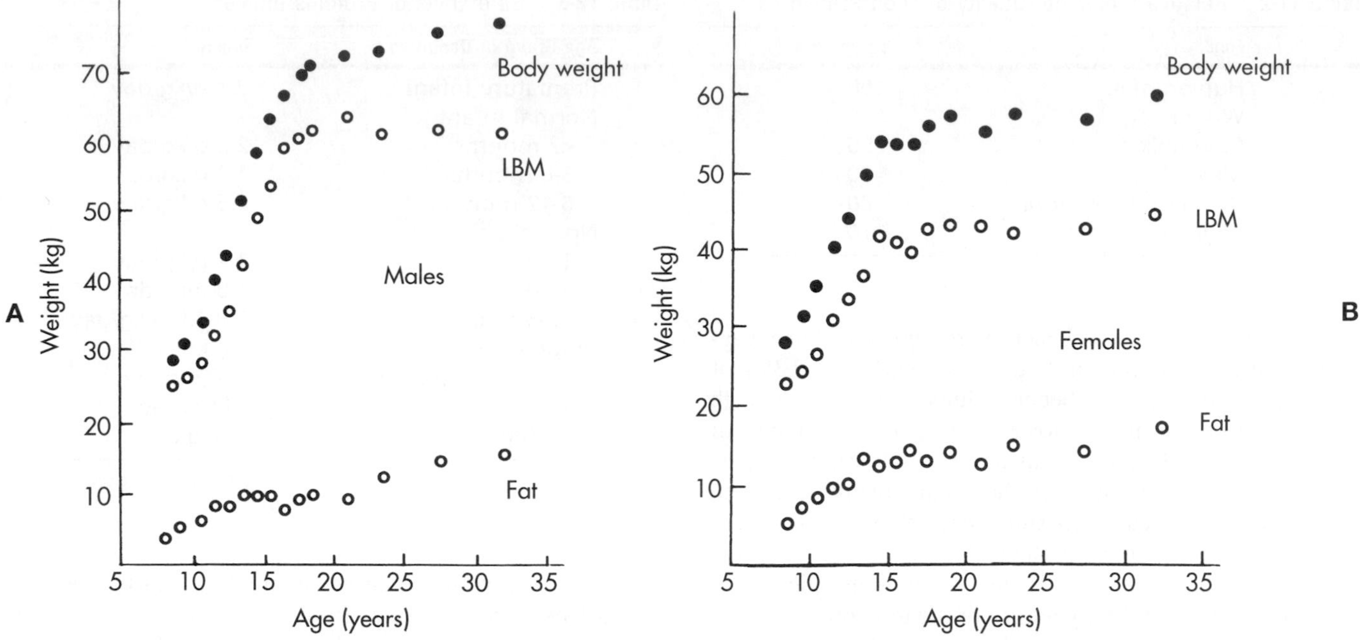

Fig. 17-2 Mean body weight and estimated lean body mass *(LBM)* and fat by ^{40}K counting for 604 males **(A)** and 467 females **(B)** ages 8 to 35 years.

these figures should pertain equally well to the pregnant teenager.

Lactation requires even more energy. Each deciliter of milk produced contains 72 calories, and milk production is said to be 80% efficient; thus 90 extra calories must be ingested by the mother for each deciliter of milk produced. A total milk production of 850 ml/day, therefore, requires an extra 760 calories. An underweight mother should be urged to get more than this, whereas the well-nourished mother needs less—perhaps only an extra 500 Cal/day—because she can draw on her generous fat stores.

PROTEIN

Proteins are high-molecular-weight polypeptides that serve many functions in the body. Enzymes are proteins, as are antibodies and some hormones; hemoglobin, plasma albumin, and the contractile elements of muscle also are proteins. All proteins are composed of some 20 amino acids, in varying proportions; the function of a particular protein is governed by the sequence of amino acids within the molecule. Of these amino acids, nine cannot be synthesized by the body; therefore they are known as *essential amino acids*—histidine, isoleucine, leucine, lysine, methionine, phenylalanine, threonine, tryptophan, and valine. There are indications that cystine and taurine may be essential for low-birth-weight infants; these essential amino acids must be supplied in food.

As with energy, the body needs a constant supply of protein; during growth, new tissue must be synthesized because *all* tissues (even bone and adipose tissue) contain protein. Even during adult life there is a constant turnover of protein, with some nitrogen being lost in the urine even on a protein-free diet and during fasting. There is a protein requirement for growth and maintenance, and this is an unremitting requirement because the body has no storage site for protein. An inadequate supply results in a slowing of growth, a compromise of many body functions, and the wasting of muscle; in severe deprivation, impaired resistance to infection, reduced mentality, and even death may result.

Ingested protein first must undergo hydrolysis, a process begun in the stomach and carried to partial completion in the upper small intestine, mainly by pancreatic enzymes. The resultant amino acids and small peptides then are transported by specific metabolic processes (which themselves involve special proteins) into the interior of the intestinal mucosal cells (the peptide bonds having been split at the brush border), and the amino acids are absorbed into the portal blood.

The end products of protein metabolism appear in the urine mainly as urea, the deaminated amino acids being either converted to carbohydrate and fat or burned to carbon dioxide and water.

Biological Quality

The variable amino acid composition of food proteins leads to variations in the efficiency with which they supply the body's needs. The methods for estimating the biological quality of a given protein include tests on animals, observation of the growth of children on differing diets, nitrogen balance studies on adult volunteers, and a chemical score based on the amino acid content. Although these do not always yield the same result, the biological quality of the proteins in various food groups generally is agreed upon. In Table 17-2, the two sources with the highest quality protein (human milk and whole egg) are arbitrarily assigned a score of 100. Simply stated, a child must ingest more of a low-quality protein to achieve proper nutrition and the desired growth rate. The low quality of vegetable proteins is due to relative deficiencies of one or more essential amino acids. For example, wheat is low in lysine, corn is low in lysine and tryptophan, rice is low in lysine and threonine, and beans are low in methionine. Commercial formulas based on processed

Table 17-2 Relative Biological Quality of Food Protein

Food	Score
Human milk	100
Whole egg	100
Cow milk	95+
Meat	80+
Processed soy flour	80+
Vegetable proteins	50-70

Table 17-3 Safe Level of Proteins Intake*

Age Group or Condition	Intake
Premature Infant	3-4 g/kg/day
Normal Infant	
<2 months	2.2 g/kg/day
3-6 months	1.9 g/kg/day
6-12 months	1.5 g/kg/day
Normal child	
1-3 yr	1.2 g/kg/day
3-10 yr	1.0 g/kg/day
Adolescent	0.8-1.0 g/kg/day
Pregnancy	
Second trimester	+6 g/day
Third trimester	+11 g/day
Lactation	+17 g/day

*Based on high biological quality proteins: milk, eggs, meat. Add 20% to 50% for vegetable proteins.

soy flour have proved satisfactory for infants. Some vegetables are so low in protein (e.g., cassava has only 0.35 g of protein per 100 Cal) that it becomes impossible to eat enough to meet the protein need. However, a judicious mixture of vegetables can yield a most satisfactory result. Strict vegetarians have survived in apparent health for many years, and tests of suitable vegetable mixtures have shown good results in the treatment of protein malnutrition.

Generally speaking, it is wise to include some animal protein in the diet; even if only a third of the total protein intake comes from this source, the risk of a specific amino acid deficit becomes negligible.

Requirement

There are many problems in estimating the precise protein requirement for any age; indeed, estimates for early infancy are based on the average intake of human milk by infants who appear to be thriving. Table 17-3 represents a composite of estimates by the National Academy of Sciences (NAS) and the World Health Organization (WHO). Although protein can be limited in the diets of infants and children in poorer nations, the vast majority of Americans have access to sufficient quantities of high-quality protein. Fig. 17-3 illustrates the concept of the protein:energy ratio of the diet, with the two oblique lines defining the limits of this ratio, here expressed as a percentage of total calories from protein. The upper oblique line is based on cow's milk, in which 20% of the calories are supplied by protein (i.e., protein energy: total energy = 0.2); a ratio higher than this would probably never be needed. The lower oblique line is based on human milk, in which 7% of calories are from protein (i.e., the ratio is 0.07); the fact that human infants can grow and thrive on this rather low-protein food testifies to its adequacy. If energy intake is adequate and the protein:energy ratio of the diet falls between these limits, protein intake will be satisfactory. The only truly protein-deficient foods are the fruits; potatoes, rice and whole grains have a ratio of about 0.08, whereas legumes, meat, and eggs all have protein:energy ratios of 0.2 or more. Indeed, the much beloved peanut butter and jelly sandwich has a protein energy:total energy ratio of 0.14, whereas the equally favored hamburger (21% fat) on a bun has a ratio of 0.27.

A diet comprised of items from each of the four basic food groups (dairy products; meat, eggs, and legumes; fruits and vegetables; and grains) that also meet the individual child's energy requirement should provide an adequate amount of protein. There is no evidence that high-protein diets promote growth, enhance athletic performance, or improve the outcome of pregnancy. Indeed, premature infants who have a high relative growth rate thrive on milk formulas that provide 8% to 10% of their calories from protein; severely malnourished infants can also recover on similar diets. Protein quality is obviously important. The lower oblique line in Fig. 17-3 is based on high-quality protein, like that in foods such as milk, meat, and eggs. For diets that consist largely of vegetables, in which proteins are only about two-thirds as efficient as the high-quality protein sources, the slope of this line should be increased to about 11%. The average American diet provides about 15% of total energy from protein.

It is important to note that the protein requirements (per kilogram of weight) of a young infant are relatively high compared with those of the older child or adult. High-quality protein is important for young infants, and a reasonable intake of milk ensures that is achieved. However, there is no particular advantage to providing protein in excess of actual need, inasmuch as the excess cannot be stored and therefore is metabolized as an energy source and appears in the urine as urea and amino acids. Studies of infants recovering from severe malnutrition have shown that satisfactory recovery can be achieved at protein intakes as low as 2.5 g/kg. In fact, there is serious doubt that diets really high in protein are needed under any circumstances save those associated with abnormal protein losses (e.g., as with extensive burns or gastrointestinal disease).

Several groups require special consideration, as Table 17-3 shows. The rapid growth rate of low-birth-weight newborns demands a protein intake of 3 to 4 g/kg during the early months of life. Lactating women need an extra supply: 850 ml of human milk contains 10 g of protein; under the assumption that protein utilization is only 60% efficient, the mother should receive an extra 17 g of protein daily. The extra demand for protein during pregnancy is appreciable but not great; the body of the term newborn contains about 400 g of protein, to which should be added the 500 g contained in the placenta, gravid uterus, and breasts and in the expanded blood volume. Most of this increased need for protein occurs during the latter half of pregnancy.

Excessive amounts of protein (5 g/kg or more) can lead to toxicity. The concentration of blood urea nitrogen rises, the urine may contain albumin and casts and, if water intake is low, the excessive renal solute load leads to an increase in

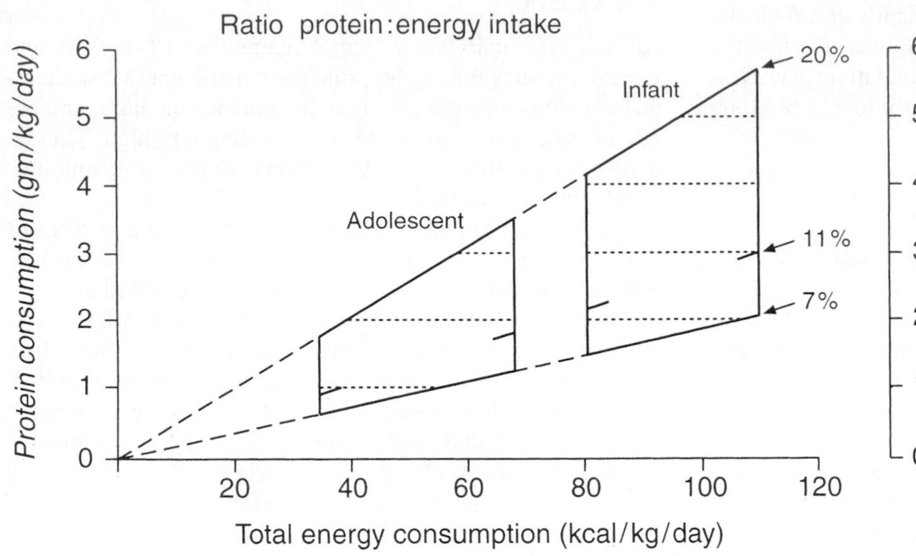

Fig. 17-3 Ratio of protein intake to energy intake for normal infants and adolescents. The trapezoids define the usual range of energy intake and the stated limits for the percentage of energy from protein. The ratio represents that of calories from protein to total calories (not grams of protein to total calories). The dotted lines define protein intake per unit body weight.

(Modified from Appelbaum M, Astier-Dumas M, editors: *L' alimentation des adolescents,* Paris, 1988, Maison de la Chemie, Sante' du CIDIL.)

obligatory renal water excretion and to dehydration; that plus the increased thermic effect of food can result in fever, the so-called protein fever.

FAT

Fat is a constituent of all body tissues. The term *fat* is applied to a heterogeneous group of low-molecular-weight compounds that contain fatty acids and that have in common the property of being soluble in solvents such as chloroform and ether. Neutral fats, or triglycerides, are fatty acid esters of glycerol. They serve the functions of energy storage and insulation against the cold and provide a cushion for internal organs. This depot fat accounts for about 14% of body weight in term newborns and 10% to 30% in adults. Fig. 17-2 shows that body fat content varies with age and sex. Obese individuals may have as much as 50% fat.

The high energy content of adipose tissue (composed of fat-laden adipocytes and a connective tissue stroma) is due to two factors: the high caloric value of fat itself (which has the energy equivalent of gasoline), and the fact that, unlike protein and carbohydrate, fat deposition is not accompanied by an increase in tissue water. This makes for efficient energy storage; indeed, a moderately thin adult can survive fasting for at least a month, and the very obese have survived for as long as 250 days. Newborn animals (including humans) and adult hibernators have a special adipose organ—brown fat—that supplies energy quickly in response to cold.

Fatty acids are classified according to the number of double bonds in the hydrocarbon chain. *Saturated fat* contains a relatively small percentage of fatty acids having double bonds, and *polyunsaturated fat* contains a high percentage of fatty acids having such bonds. Generally, the former have higher melting points and thus a firmer consistency at room temperature (compare lard and corn oil). Fats of vegetable origin tend to be more unsaturated than those of animal origin; human milk fat is less saturated than cow milk fat. In addition to neutral fats, there are other fats. Some contain phosphorus or galactose, which are essential components of tissue. Some—the lipoproteins—are linked to protein; these contribute to the stability of cell membranes and serve in combination with proteins and polysaccharides as structural components of cells (lysozymes and myelin sheaths are examples).

Except for linoleic, linolenic, and arachidonic acids, the multitude of fats found in the body can be formed from protein or carbohydrate precursors. Although symptoms and signs of essential fatty acid deficiency (dermatitis and impaired growth and lipid transport) have been observed under experimental conditions and in patients fed parenterally for long periods, the requirement is low—only 1% to 2% of total calories—thus, such deficiencies have not been described under natural circumstances. Essential fatty acids are precursors of an important series of compounds, the prostaglandins. Cholesterol, which is a sterol and not a fat in the true sense, plays an important role in metabolism. It is a precursor of bile acids, vitamin D, adrenocortical steroids, and sex hormones. It is synthesized in the body and thus is present in foods of animal origin, and its absorption by the intestine is facilitated by a high-fat diet. Diets high in fat and cholesterol are thought to accelerate the process of atherosclerosis.

Fat digestion occurs in the upper small intestine by the action of pancreatic and intestinal lipases, which split off two fatty acids from glycerol. The 2-monoacyl glycerol residue combines with bile salts to form micelles (which, incidentally, incorporate fat-soluble vitamins and cholesterol), which act to dissolve the free fatty acids and are taken up by the mucosal cells. Here the triglycerides are reconstituted and released into the lymph as chylomicrons. Short- and medium-chain fats (12-carbon chains or less) are handled differently; these are hydrolyzed by the brush border of mucosal cells, and the resultant fatty acids are released into the portal vein.

Fat exists in several forms in plasma: as triglycerides, free fatty acids, lipoproteins, and phospholipids. Fatty acids are a source of energy for muscle, and they can be esterified by adipocytes to form depot fat; they also can be synthesized in liver and adipose tissue from dietary carbohydrate precursors.

Unsaturated fatty acids that have a double bond at the third carbon from the methyl terminal (alpha-linolenic acid is one such omega-3 fatty acid) are present in significant amounts in marine fish oils. These fatty acids and their derivatives reduce platelet aggregation and appear to retard the progress of atherosclerosis. Fish-eating populations have less atherosclerotic disease and also have slightly longer bleeding times.

CARBOHYDRATES

As the name implies, carbohydrates are a series of compounds composed of carbon, hydrogen, and oxygen. They generally are classified into three groups: monosaccharides, which contain five or six carbon atoms (e.g., glucose and fructose); disaccharides, which have 12 carbon atoms (e.g., sucrose and lactose); and polysaccharides, which are high-molecular-weight polymers (e.g., glycogen and starch are examples). Their main function is to supply energy, although certain specialized forms are involved in antigen-antibody reactions. Deoxyribonucleic acid (DNA) and ribonucleic acid (RNA) both contain a five-carbon sugar (deoxyribose and ribose, respectively); glucose and galactose are essential constituents of tissues such as collagen and cerebrosides; and the various glycoproteins have specialized functions.

Some tissues, such as muscle, can use fatty acids as a prime source of energy, but the brain derives most of its energy from glucose. In theory, the body can exist without dietary carbohydrate (CHO) because it can be formed from protein and fat; however, diets that are very low in CHO (less than 5% of calories) quickly lead to excessive combustion of fat and a rise in fatty acid and ketone body levels in the blood, and thus to acidosis. This is what occurs when a ketogenic diet is used to treat epilepsy.

Monosaccharides require no digestion. Disaccharides are hydrolyzed in the upper small intestine by specific enzymes. Digestion of starch begins in the mouth (salivary amylase) and is carried to completion in the intestine by the action of pancreatic amylase and specific disaccharidases in the brush border of the jejunal epithelial cells. The resultant mixture of simple sugars, principally glucose, is taken into the mucosal cells and then into the portal circulation. In the liver, fructose and galactose are converted to glucose; some glucose is released to the general circulation, and some is stored as glycogen. The entry of glucose into cells of all types, save brain cells, is facilitated by the action of insulin. The level of blood glucose is maintained by the combined action of pituitary and adrenal, as well as pancreatic, hormones.

Diets very high in monosaccharides or disaccharides may cause diarrhea, and consuming these sugars (particularly sucrose) in a physical form that adheres to the teeth promotes dental caries. Generally, the proportions of protein, CHO, and fat in the diet can vary considerably without metabolic or nutritional risk. The limits are rather wide: protein, 8% to 20% of calories; CHO, 15% to 60% of calories; and fat, 25% to 60% of calories. Contrary to widespread belief, obesity is *not* the result of an abnormal distribution of calories among these three dietary components (e.g., starches are no more "fattening" than fat); rather, it is the *total* caloric intake that is at fault. There is evidence that high-fat diets, particularly those that provide large amounts of saturated fats and cholesterol, can be detrimental to health; however, an excess of total calories and a sedentary lifestyle also are important in this regard.

WATER

All tissues contain water (dental enamel has 1% to 2%), and for most tissues this is the principal constituent. Most chemical reactions take place only in an aqueous medium, and the rate of water turnover in the body is relatively high. Thus, it is no accident that most edible foods contain large amounts of this dietary essential.

Water is continuously lost from the body by a number of routes. There is an obligatory loss in urine because the kidney has a limited capacity to produce a concentrated urine. In children and adults this limit is about 1400 mOsm/L,* corresponding to a specific gravity of about 1.040. Thus, diets high in solutes, which are largely excreted in the urine (nitrogen, sodium, phosphorus), call for a large urine volume. It should be noted that very young infants are able to achieve a urine concentration of only 700 mOsm/L. Water also is lost continuously from the lungs and skin in the absence of sweating, the so-called insensible water loss, the amount of which is roughly proportional to the RMR. Such losses amount to about 10 ml/kg/day in an adult and 30 ml/kg/day in an infant. Water loss through sweating varies with the environmental temperature and humidity and with physical activity. Under extreme conditions an adult can lose 500 ml/hr through sweating.

Daily fecal water loss amounts to about 150 ml in an adult and 10 ml/kg in an infant.

Besides food and drink, the body has its own source of water. The burning of fat and CHO produces carbon dioxide (CO_2) and water (H_2O), the so-called water of oxidation (100 g of fat yields 107 ml of H_2O and 100 g of glucose yields 60 ml). For an adult, this amounts to about 300 ml/day and for an infant, about 90 ml/day. Fig. 17-4 depicts the overall water economy for the average infant and the average adult. It is apparent that the infant is at greater risk from water deprivation inasmuch as infants' water turnover is much larger—about 16% of total body water each day, compared with about 6% per day in adults. Likewise, infants are at greater risk from conditions that accelerate water loss (e.g., vomiting and diarrhea), from heat stress, and from diets that provide excessive amounts of solute for urinary excretion (high protein, high salt). It is no accident that human milk has a high ratio of water to solute.

MINERALS

The diet must provide the minerals that are essential components of body tissues. A deficiency of these minerals leads to diminished growth and to disease, and excessive intakes may result in toxicity. Table 17-4 provides information on the functions, dietary sources, and requirements for minerals for which requirements have been estimated. Except for iron and fluoride, a well-balanced diet provides a satisfactory intake of minerals. Iron deficiency now is the most common nutritional deficiency in the United States. Attempts to improve this situation have been made through iron fortification

*An osmole is the molecular weight in grams of an osmotically active particle, whether it be a nonionized compound such as glucose or urea or an ion such as Na^+ or Cl^-. A milliosmole (mOsm) is one thousandth of an osmole.

of cereal products and infant formulas. Fluoride is added to the drinking water in many communities, as well as to toothpastes.

It should be mentioned here that the average American diet provides a generous amount of salt, to the point that some nutritionists are concerned about this as a possible factor in the pathogenesis of hypertension.

Besides those listed in Table 17-4, a number of minerals are known to be essential for animals and presumably for humans. These are chloride, chromium, manganese, molybdenum, nickel, silicon, tin, and vanadium. Deficiencies of these minerals are unlikely except with protracted parenteral feeding or, in the case of chloride, with excessive vomiting.

VITAMINS

As the word itself implies, vitamins are necessary for proper tissue function and thus for growth. These compounds act as cofactors for a number of enzymes. Most cannot be synthesized in the body and so must be supplied in the diet. Exceptions to this rule include vitamin D (activation of skin sterols by sunlight) and vitamin K (synthesized by intestinal bacteria). Small amounts of vitamin B_{12} are manufactured by intestinal bacteria, and some niacin is produced by conversion from tryptophan, but not in quantities sufficient to meet requirements. Vitamin deficiencies result in disease, and excessive intakes may lead to toxicity. The story of the discovery of the relationship of certain diseases to dietary inadequacies, of the presence of certain "vital amines" in trace amounts of food, and of the elucidation of their chemical structures and metabolic functions is a fascinating one, as well as being intimately associated with the development of modern nutritional science.

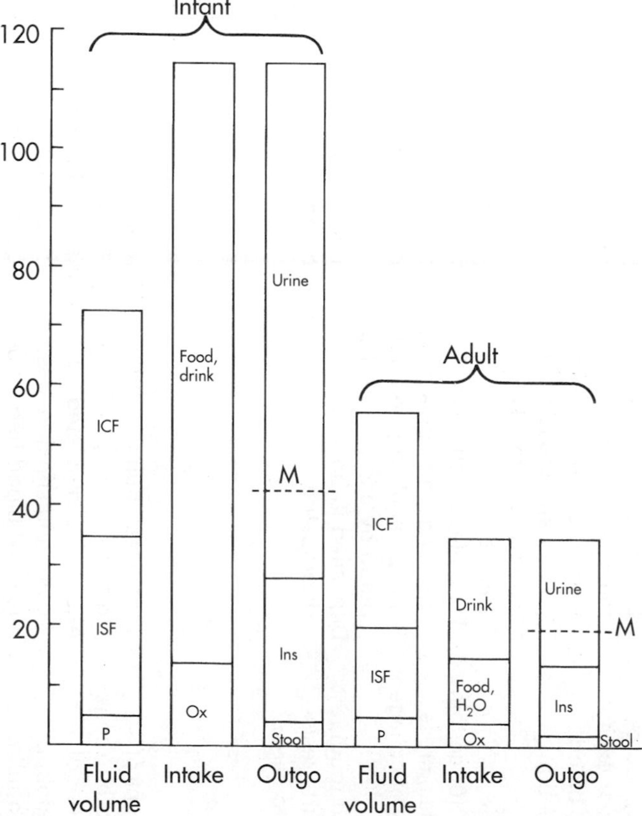

Fig. 17-4 Comparisons of body fluid volumes (percentage of body weight) and daily intake and outgo of water (ml/kg) for an infant and an adult. The values shown are averages and vary somewhat with the method used and the subject's fat content. *Dashed line (M),* Value for minimal water expenditure; *P,* plasma volume; *ISF,* interstitial fluid volume; *ICF,* intracellular fluid volume; *Ox,* water of oxidation; *Ins,* insensible water loss.

(From Farmer T, editor: *Pediatric neurology,* ed 3, New York, 1983, Harper & Row.)

Table 17-5 lists the vitamins known to be important for humans, including the chemical name, function, estimated dietary requirement, dietary sources, and toxicity level.

It should be noted that certain foods are fortified with vitamins. By law, vitamin D must be added to milk, and vitamins now are added to many commercial infant formulas, to certain cereal products, to some breads, to fruit substitute drinks, and to other foods. Vitamin products are sold widely. As a result, overt vitamin deficiencies now are rare in the United States. Nevertheless, infants and children are at greater risk than adults because their requirements are proportionally greater, and thus dietary deficiency results in disease more quickly.

Recent claims have been made that massive intakes of vitamin C and the B complex will protect against respiratory tract infection and atherosclerosis and will ameliorate abnormal behavior and poor school performance. Such claims for *megavitamin therapy* and *orthomolecular treatment* are without merit.

A daily intake of 400 μg of folic acid, started before conception and continued during pregnancy, has been associated with a significant decrease in the incidence of neural tube defects (see Table 17-5). For women who have borne an infant who has such a defect, a daily intake 10 times greater (i.e., 4 mg), begun before conception, is recommended.[1]

NUTRITION IN THE UNITED STATES TODAY

Of the many factors that bear on today's nutritional scene, none has had a greater impact than *food technology* and *sanitation.* These modern developments have resulted from combined actions of government, industry, nutritional scientists, and physicians.

Before the turn of the century, the greatest hazards to infant health were infection and improper food. The whole history of infant nutrition is one of attempts to devise a satisfactory milk for babies who could not be fed at the breast. It was the realization in the past that raw cow milk was not a satisfactory food for young infants that led the fortunate few to employ wet nurses for their young.

The following features of raw cow milk render it less than suitable for young infants. *Bacterial contamination* arises from several sources: the cow herself (tubercle bacilli, streptococci [mastitis is common in high-producing herds], and *Brucella* organisms) and the various humans who handle the milk, any one of whom may add bacteria to the milk from respiratory or cutaneous foci. Lack of suitable refrigeration in former days (or in some areas still) accentuated the problem.

Cow milk contains about three times as much protein as

Table 17-4 Nutritionally Important Minerals

Mineral	Function	Physiology	Effects of Deficiency	Effects of Excess	Daily Requirement	Sources
Calcium	Structure of bone, ion transport across cell membranes, neuromuscular excitability, blood coagulation	Absorption aided by vitamin D and parathyroid hormone (PTH), hindered by phosphate; PTH facilitates release from bone, thyrocalcitonin inhibits; gravity and muscle tension needed for skeletal stability	Osteoporosis only with severe deficiency, muscle paralysis, or malabsorption	Hypercalciuria with excessive vitamin D, and immobilization	Infants—400-600 mg Adolescents—600-700 mg Pregnancy (latter half), lactation—1000-1200 mg	Milk, cheese, green leafy vegetables, beans, canned salmon
Copper	Cofactor for certain enzymes, cross-linking of collagen	Plasma level 110 μg/dl, mostly as ceruloplasmin; intestinal absorption hindered by excessive zinc	Anemia, osteoporosis, defective myelination	None, except with massive ingestion	0.5-2 mg	Liver, meats, grains
Fluoride	Bone and tooth structure, resistance to caries	Deposited in bone as fluorapatite	Tendency for dental caries	4-8 mg/day—mottled teeth 20+ mg/day for long periods—osteosclerosis Large doses—acute poisoning	1 mg/L in drinking water	Seafoods, many municipal water supplies
Iodine	Constituent of thyroid hormone	Concentrated in thyroid gland	Simple goiter, endemic cretinism	Iodism	40-150 μg	Seafoods, iodized salt
Iron	Constituent of hemoglobin, myoglobulin, enzymes	Absorption regulated by gastrointestinal mucosa, level of blood hemoglobin; menstrual loss averages 0.7 mg/day	Anemia: if severe, cardiac failure, poor growth, lethargy	Hemosiderosis, poisoning by medicinal iron	Infants—1 mg/kg Adolescents—10-18 mg	Liver, whole grains, eggs, legumes, meat

Magnesium	Cofactor for enzymes, neuromuscular excitability	Principal cation of intracellular fluid	Tetany, hypocalcemia	Poisoning from medicinal magnesium (intravenous or intramuscular)	Infants—4 mg/kg	Meat, cereals, milk
Phosphorus	Constituent of phospholipids, ATP, nucleic acids; intermediary metabolism	Absorption regulated by vitamin D, dietary calcium, PTH; latter affects renal excretion	Muscle weakness; dysesthesia; rickets in premature infants	In newborn, hypocalcemia	Infants—two thirds of calcium requirement All others—same as calcium requirement	Most foods
Potassium	Cellular transport, CHO and protein metabolism, membrane potential in muscle and nerve	Principal cation of intracellular fluid; regulation by adrenocortical steroids	Muscle weakness, abdominal distention, cardiac failure, alkalosis	Cardiac failure	1.5-2 mEq/kg	All foods
Selenium	Constituent of glutathione peroxidase	Interaction with vitamin E, heavy metals	Cardiomyopathy; muscle degeneration (animals)	Animals—"blind staggers"	Adults—50-200 µg	Seafood, liver, meat
Sodium	Osmotic pressure, cellular transport, extracellular fluid volume	Principal cation of extracellular fluid; regulation by adrenocortical hormones	Weakness, dehydration	Edema; CNS irritability if severe	2 mEq/kg	Most foods
Zinc	Constituent of enzymes	Absorption impaired by diet high in calcium, fiber	Growth failure, hypogonadism, reduced taste acuity	None except with massive ingestion	Children—6 mg Adults—15 mg	Meat, especially pork, whole grains, nuts, cheese

Table 17-5 Nutritionally Important Vitamins

Vitamin	Characteristics	Biochemical Action	Effects of Deficiency	Effects of Excess	Daily Requirement	Food Sources
Vitamin A (retinol); 1 IU = 0.3 μg retinol	Fat soluble, heat stable; bile necessary for absorption, specific binding protein in plasma; stored in liver	Component of visual purple; integrity of epithelial tissues, bone cell function	Night blindness, xerophthalmia, keratomalacia, poor growth, impaired resistance to infection	Hyperostosis, hepatomegaly, alopecia, increased cerebrospinal fluid pressure	Infants—300 μg Adolescents—750 μg Lactation—1200 μg	Milk fat, eggs, liver
Provitamin A (beta-carotene); one sixth the activity of retinol	Converted to retinol in liver, intestinal mucosa			Carotenemia		Dark green vegetables, yellow fruits and vegetables, tomatoes
Biotin	Water soluble; synthesized by intestinal bacteria; deficiency with large intake of egg *white*, total parenteral nutrition	Coenzyme	Dermatitis, anorexia, muscle pain, pallor	Unknown	Unknown	Liver, egg yolk, peanuts
Cobalamin (vitamin B_{12})	Slightly soluble in water, heat stable only at neutral pH, light sensitive; absorption (ileum) dependent on gastric intrinsic factor; cobalt a part of the molecule	Coenzyme component; red blood cell maturation; CNS metabolism	Pernicious anemia, neurological deterioration	Unknown	1-2 μg	Animal foods only; meat, milk, eggs
Folacin (group of compounds containing pteridine ring, *p*-aminobenzoic and glutamic acids)	Slightly soluble in water, light sensitive, heat stable; some production by intestinal bacteria; ascorbic acid involved in interconversions; interference from oral contraceptives, anticonvulsants	Tetrahydrofolic acid (the active form): synthesis of purines and pyrimidines, and methylation reactions	Megaloblastic anemia	Only in patients with pernicious anemia not receiving cobalamin	Infants—60 μg Adolescents—200 μg Pregnancy—400 μg	Liver, green vegetables, cereals, oranges
Niacin (nicotinic acid, nicotinamide)	Water soluble, heat and light stable; availability from corn enhanced by alkali; synthesized in the body from tryptophan (60 : 1), some by intestinal bacteria	Component of coenzymes I and II (NAD, NADP); many enzymatic reactions	Pellagra: dermatitis, diarrhea, dementia	Nicotinic acid (not the amide): flushing, pruritus	6.6 mg/1000 Cal	Meat, fish, whole grains, green vegetables
Pantothenic acid	Water soluble, heat stable	Component of coenzyme A; many enzymatic reactions	Observed only with use of antagonists; depression, hypotension, muscle weakness, abdominal pain	Unknown	Unknown—estimated at 5-10 mg	Most foods
Vitamin B_6 (pyridoxine, pyridoxal, pyridoxamine)	Water soluble, heat and light labile; interference from isoniazid; pyridoxal is the active form	Cofactor for many enzymes	Dermatitis, glossitis, cheilosis, peripheral neuritis; infants—irritability, convulsions, anemia	Polyneuropathy	Infants—0.2-0.3 mg Adults—1-2 mg	Liver, meat, whole grains, corn, soybeans

[illegible]	Water soluble, light labile, heat stable; synthesis by intestinal bacteria (?)	Cofactor for many enzymes	Photophobia, cheilosis, glossitis, corneal vascularization, poor growth	Unknown	0.6 mg/ 1000 Cal	Meat, milk, eggs, green vegetables, whole grains
Thiamine (vitamin B_1)	Heat labile; absorption impaired by alcohol; requirement a function of CHO intake; synthesis by intestinal bacteria	Coenzyme for decarboxylation, other reactions	Beriberi; neuritis, edema, cardiac failure; hoarseness, anorexia, restlessness, aphonia	Unknown	0.4 mg/ 1000 Cal	Liver, meat, milk, whole grains, legumes
Ascorbic acid (vitamin C)	Easily oxidized, especially in presence of copper, iron, high pH; absorption by simple diffusion	Exact mechanism unknown: functions in folacin metabolism, collagen biosynthesis, iron absorption and transport, tyrosine metabolism	Scurvy	Massive doses may lead to temporary increase in requirement	Infants— 10-20 mg Adolescents— 30 mg	Citrus fruits, tomatoes, cabbage, potatoes, human milk
Vitamin D (D_2—activated calciferol; D_3—activated dehydrocholesterol); 1 IU = 0.025 μg	D_2 from diet, D_3 from action of ultraviolet light on skin; hydroxylated sequentially in liver and kidney to form 1,25-dihydroxycholecalciferol, the active compound; regulated by dietary calcium and PTH; now called a hormone; anticonvulsant drugs interfere with metabolism	Formation of calcium transport protein in duodenal mucosa; facilitates bone resorption and phosphorus absorption	Rickets, osteomalacia	Hypercalcemia, azotemia, poor growth, vomiting, nephrocalcinosis	Infants— 10 μg (400 IU) Others— 2.5-10 μg (100-400 IU)	Fortified milk, fish liver, salmon, sardines, mackerel, egg yolk, sunlight; human milk not an adequate source
Vitamin E; 1 IU = 1 mg alpha-tocopherol acetate	Stored in adipose tissue, transported with beta-lipoproteins; absorption dependent on pancreatic juice and bile (iron may interfere); requirement increased by large amounts of polyunsaturated fats	Antioxidant; role in red blood cell fragility	Hemolytic anemia in premature infants; otherwise, no clear-cut deficiency syndrome in humans	Unknown	Infants— 4 mg Adolescents— 15 mg	Cereal seed oils, peanuts, soybeans, milk fat, turnip greens
Vitamin K (naphthoquinones)	Fat soluble, bile necessary for absorption, synthesis by intestinal bacteria	Blood coagulation: factors II, VII, IX, X	Hemorrhagic manifestations	Water-soluble analogs only: hyperbilirubinemia	Newborn— single dose of 1 mg; thereafter 5 μg/day Older infants and children— unknown	Cow milk, green leafy vegetables, pork liver

human milk, and it is this high protein content (a large fraction of which is casein) that accounts for the formation of tough, voluminous curds on gastric acidification and thus leads to *impaired digestibility.* According to casual observation, formula-fed infants have larger stool volumes than do breast-fed babies. The sum total of solutes available for renal excretion is 2½ times higher in cow milk than in human milk, and this *high solute load* calls for a higher obligatory urine volume; thus the infant is at greater risk from hot weather. For the newborn, the high phosphorus content of cow milk is one factor in the pathogenesis of neonatal hypocalcemia. Raw cow milk supplies barely enough *ascorbic acid* (21 mg/L) to prevent scurvy, and unfortunately, the process of pasteurization destroys about half the vitamin present. A few infants are *allergic* to cow milk protein and suffer gastrointestinal disturbances or eczema as a result.

Modern technology has overcome these difficulties. Pasteurization, combined with mandated refrigeration, has virtually eliminated bacterial contamination; evaporated milk and commercial infant formulas are sterile and keep well without refrigeration. Heat treatment also improves digestibility, and diluting the milk with water and adding carbohydrate to restore the caloric content reduces the solute load.

Industry also has modified modern cow milk formulas by adding ascorbic acid, vitamin D, and iron, reducing the phosphorus content, developing hypoallergenic milks based on soybean and hydrolyzed casein, reducing the sodium and protein content, and substituting vegetable fat for milk fat. Some commercial infant formulas contain added vitamin E and B complex and nucleotides, some are free of lactose (this sugar might not be tolerated by babies who have gastrointestinal disorders), and others contain hydrolyzed protein as a source of nitrogen. This wide variety of infant formulas makes it possible to feed every baby satisfactorily by formula from nonhuman sources. Modern technology has wrought a change of unprecedented magnitude in infant welfare.

However, these technological advances have two disadvantages: cost, and the decline in breast-feeding. Cost is a problem for poor Americans and a major stumbling block to the exportation of food technology to poverty-stricken nations. Moreover, the more advanced the technology, the higher the cost. For example, a mother who nurses her 2- to 3-month-old infant needs only to drink an extra pint of pasteurized milk each day to satisfy the additional calcium and protein requirements, plus eat an extra two slices of bread and one potato (or 10 g of butter) to complete the caloric need, together with giving her baby vitamin D drops every day. Using an evaporated milk-water-Karo syrup formula also is inexpensive (additional vitamin C is needed), whereas the cost of a commercial ready-to-feed formula complete with added vitamins is considerably greater.

The ease and convenience of formula feeding have led inevitably to a decline in breast-feeding in our society and even in some developing countries. There is some evidence of an immunological advantage in human milk and for better absorption of iron, zinc, and fat; furthermore, the lack of contamination and the psychological benefit that may accrue with nursing are clear advantages. It is appropriate, therefore, to encourage breast-feeding in situations in which sanitation is poor, refrigeration is lacking, and cost is critical. It is encouraging to note that many more mothers have chosen to nurse their babies in recent years. However, it should be remembered that human milk contains very little vitamin D; thus nurslings must be given this vitamin, and mothers should be advised to eat a well-balanced diet.

Governmental regulations, public health activities, food technology, and governmental assistance are of the utmost importance to the modern nutritional scene. Municipal water supplies are now pure, and pasteurization is a uniform requirement for the sale of cow milk commercially. Dairy cattle are tested for tuberculosis and brucellosis, and those that have mastitis are removed from milk production. Other measures include inspection of food handlers and meats, inspection of restaurant kitchens, codes for infant formulas shipped from one state to another, and codes for canned foods. The result is that diseases such as typhoid fever, bovine tuberculosis, trichinosis, botulism, and staphylococcal food poisoning now are rare.

Modern agricultural practices, food processing, and distribution services, have resulted in the widespread availability of reasonably priced, palatable, attractively displayed, high-caloric foods, with the result that many of our citizens, be they children or adults, find it easy to eat more than they need. It is no wonder that obesity is so prevalent.

Many studies have shown the deleterious effects of severe infection, particularly gastroenteritis, on nutrition (vitamin turnover increases, and nitrogen balance becomes negative). The high prevalence of infantile malnutrition in developing countries is due in part to the occurrence of repeated infections. The Food and Drug Administration (FDA) was formed in 1938; this agency has the authority to regulate, among other things, food quality, food labeling, use of food additives, and vitamin fortification. The Federal Trade Commission (FTC) monitors advertising claims. These measures have resulted in better, cleaner, and more wholesome food. One of the most dramatic improvements was effected by the mandatory addition of vitamin D to milk, which has led to virtual elimination of dietary-deficiency rickets in this country.

Food assistance programs are now fairly widespread. These include school lunch programs, the food stamp program, the program for women, infants, and children (WIC) and, in reality, the farm subsidy program. As a result, families that have limited financial means can augment their otherwise meager food supply. Millions of people are receiving food stamps, and about a half million are enrolled in the WIC program.

Finally, local, state, and federal governments play an important role in providing free or low-cost health care for poor people and salaries for school and public health nutritionists and for helping to defray the cost of special foods for children who have certain diseases, such as phenylketonuria.

The result of these efforts, both industrial and governmental, is that with but one exception (iron-deficiency anemia), overt nutritional deficiency now is uncommon in the United States, and obesity and dental caries have become the most prevalent nutritional conditions.

Two quasiofficial organizations have published recommendations for nutritional allowances (*not* requirements): the Food and Nutrition Board of the National Academy of Sciences–National Research Council (NAS) and the Food and Agricultural Organization (FAO) of the United Nations.

The former organization publishes a series of pamphlets at roughly 5-year intervals that include a listing of recommended dietary allowances (RDAs) for people of all ages. These are based on knowledge of actual requirements, to which is added a generous "safety factor" to account for supposed individual variation in requirements and for variations in food quality. Except for calories, the "recommended" amounts all are in excess of actual need for the average individual; however, dietary surveys reveal that a sizable proportion of the population consumes less of many nutrients than the NAS recommends. The FAO recommendations are closer to actual requirements for protein, calcium, and a number of vitamins (see WHO *Handbook*); unfortunately, this list of nutrients is not as complete as the one published by the NAS.

POSSIBLE ROLE OF INFANT AND CHILD NUTRITION IN ADULT HEALTH

Generally, the nutritional status of infants and children today is reasonably good. Some experts say our biggest challenge is the adult—that is, whether current infant feeding practices are compromising their health and longevity.

Several facts have been established. An intake of fluoride in early life, at a time when dental enamel is forming, results in a long-term diminution of the dental caries rate. It is known that a high intake of sucrose, particularly in solid, sticky foods, predisposes a person to dental caries; thus, early learning of food habits that minimize the consumption of such foods should be beneficial.* Childhood obesity tends to persist into adult life, and this obesity shortens life span; therefore, attempts to prevent childhood obesity are important. Severe malnutrition in *early life* may impair intellectual performance† and should be avoided through procedures such as early feeding of premature infants, use of intravenous alimentation in certain critical situations, and early requests for medical advice and treatment of diseases that compromise nutrition during infancy.

The most challenging question relates to atherosclerosis and its cardiac and cerebral consequences. (This discussion forgoes consideration of the inherited abnormalities of lipoprotein metabolism associated with early-onset arterial disease.) Arterial changes (the fatty streaks) appear in childhood, and by age 20 an appreciable percentage of men already have atherosclerotic plaques. The dietary components that have been considered as possible factors in initiating or intensifying this aging process are total calories, animal protein, saturated fats, and cholesterol. Cross-cultural surveys of adult autopsies reveal that any or all of these factors may be at fault; there also is some evidence that "postcoronary" adults who limit their intake of calories, saturated fat, and cholesterol have a better prognosis. The possible preventive role of fish has been mentioned earlier; however, certain species now are contaminated with mercury and polychlorinated hydrocarbons and therefore should not be eaten.

Experiments conducted many years ago showed that rats fed (from weaning) an amount of food equal to about two thirds of their usual intake lived much longer and had less arterial disease and fewer tumors that those fed ad libitum. These results have been confirmed by Ross,[3] who states, "The effects of chronic restriction in food intake on laboratory animals have been so apparent that it is difficult to avoid concluding that no environmental factor so decisively reduces the rate or expression of the aging process," and, "The mechanisms through which nutrition influences the aging processes are already operative during the *youthful stage* of life [italics mine]." If dietary restriction is postponed until maturity, the benefits are not as great.

Recent surveys show that Americans' average protein intake is at least twice the estimated requirement, that average milk consumption is about a pint a day, that solid food supplements are offered to infants at a very early age, and that obesity is prevalent; thus the results of the animal experiments are worth serious consideration. Berry[1] makes this cogent comment: "Throughout the world the State does not accept the responsibility to protect its individuals from overnutrition" as it does to minimize undernutrition. It is of interest that strict vegetarians are leaner and have lower levels of serum lipids and lower blood pressures than do nonvegetarians.

Some students of nutrition claim that there is evidence that modern refined foods have a deleterious effect, in that their consumption favors the incidence of diverticulosis and colonic tumors. These individuals advocate a diet that is higher in fiber, such as whole-grain cereals, bran, and raw vegetables. Others caution against an excess of dietary fiber because this may interfere with the absorption of certain minerals.

Committees of the U.S. Senate and of the American Heart Association suggest that it would be advantageous for everyone to reduce his or her intake of saturated fats, refined sugar, salt, and cholesterol while proportionally increasing the amount of complex carbohydrates, and to balance energy intake with energy expenditure. These "dietary goals" should apply to children (but *not* infants) as well as to adults.

"WELL-BALANCED" DIET

Consumption of a variety of foods is the best protection against nutritional deficiency. Except for the first few months of life, when milk is the principal, if not the sole food, the daily diet should include items from each of the following general food groups, known in nutritional circles as "the basic four": (1) meat, fish, poultry, eggs, (2) dairy products (milk, cheese, milk products), (3) fruits and vegetables, and (4) cereals. The U.S. Department of Agriculture has depicted

*Statements by manufacturers reveal a generous consumption of sucrose. For the United States, this amounts to about 50 kg per capita per year, equivalent to 125 g, or 500 calories, per day. Furthermore, this figure has remained fairly constant over the past 50 years.

†There is reasonable evidence of such an effect when malnutrition occurs in the early months of life, and particularly when it is prolonged. In late infancy and childhood the effect has not been demonstrated clearly, probably because brain maturation is well on its way to completion. Nor has nutritional deprivation during pregnancy been shown to impair intellectual performance of the offspring. The effect of malnutrition per se is very difficult to study because it is almost always accompanied by cultural or emotional disadvantages.

these as a food "pyramid," with high-frequency foods placed at the bottom.

Today, the term *junk food* often is heard in reference to prepared foods high in refined carbohydrate and low in protein and vitamins, full of so-called empty calories. These foods do supply energy, and one cannot help thinking of the simpler life of previous generations, when foods of similar composition (e.g., apple pie, cake with thick frosting, jellied preserves, and home-canned fruits) were consumed freely, without opprobrium, their production considered the hallmark of a successful housewife.

Vegans, the colloquial term for strict vegetarians, should be counseled by a nutritionist because their diet is devoid of vitamin B_{12} and is likely to be low in calcium. Grains and vegetables must be chosen so as to include all the essential amino acids.

All those who follow "fad diets" of one sort or another and those who limit their food intake voluntarily in an effort to lose weight also should receive nutritional guidance, inasmuch as such diets may lack one or more essential nutrients. There are now reports of growth failure in adolescents who consume low-fat diets, for such diets usually are too low in calories.

REFERENCES

1. Berry WTC: Nutrition in a health service. In McLaren DS, Burman D, editors: *Textbook of paediatric nutrition,* New York, 1976, Churchill Livingstone.
2. Rosenberg IH: Folic acid and neural-tube defects: time for action? *N Engl J Med* 327:1875, 1992.
3. Ross MH: Nutrition and longevity in experimental animals. In Winick M, editor: *Nutrition and aging,* New York, 1976, John Wiley & Sons.

SUGGESTED READINGS

American Psychiatric Association Task Force: *Megavitamins and orthomolecular therapy in psychiatry,* Washington, DC, 1973, The Association.

Barness L, editor: *Pediatric nutrition handbook,* ed 3, Elk Grove Village, Ill, 1985, American Academy of Pediatrics.

Burkitt DP, Walker ARP, Painter NS: Dietary fiber and disease, *JAMA* 229: 1068, 1974.

Fomon SJ: *Infant nutrition,* ed 2, Philadelphia, 1974, WB Saunders.

Food and Nutrition Board, National Academy of Sciences: *Recommended dietary allowances,* ed 10, Washington, DC, 1989, The Academy.

Forbes GB: Food fads: safe feeding of children, *Pediatr Rev* 1:207, 1980.

Forbes GB: *Human body composition: growth, aging, nutrition, and activity,* New York, 1987, Springer-Verlag.

Grand RJ, Sutphen JL, Dietz WH, editors: *Pediatric nutrition,* Boston, 1987, Butterworth.

Hytten FE, Leitch I: *Physiology of human pregnancy,* ed 2, Oxford, 1971, Blackwell Scientific.

Klein PS, Forbes GB, Nader PR: Effects of starvation in infancy (pyloric stenosis) on subsequent learning abilities, *J Pediatr* 87:8, 1975.

Leaf A, Weber PC: Cardiovascular effects of *n*-3 fatty acids, *N Engl J Med* 318:549, 1988.

Lechtig A, et al: Maternal nutrition and fetal growth in developing countries, *Am J Dis Child* 129:553, 1975.

McCann ML, Schwartz R: The effects of milk solute on urinary cast excretion in premature infants, *Pediatrics* 38:555, 1966.

McKigney JI, Munro HN, editors: *Nutrient requirements in adolescence,* Cambridge, Mass, 1976, MIT Press.

Mertz W: The essential trace elements, *Science* 213:1332, 1981.

Pike RL, Brown ML: *Nutrition: an integrated approach,* ed 2, New York, 1975, John Wiley & Sons.

Rush D, Davis H, Susser M: Antecedents of low birth weight in Harlem, New York City, *Int J Epidemiol* 1:393, 1972.

Sacks FM, et al: Plasma lipids and lipoproteins in vegetarians and controls, *N Engl J Med* 292:1148, 1975.

Stein Z, et al: *Famine and human development,* New York, 1975, Oxford University Press.

Tsang RC, Nichols BL, editors: *Nutrition during infancy,* Philadelphia, 1988, Hanley & Belfus.

Walker WA, Watkins JB, editors: *Nutrition in pediatrics,* ed 2, Hamilton, Ontario, 1996, BC Dedkham.

Waterlow JC, Alleyne GAO: Protein malnutrition in children. In Anfinsen CB Jr, Edsall JT, Richards FM, editors: *Advances in protein chemistry,* vol 25, New York, 1971, Academic Press.

World Health Organization: Energy and protein requirements. Report of a Joint FAO/WHO/UNU expert consultation, Tech Rep Series 724, Geneva, 1985, WHO.

two Feeding of Infants and Children

Marvin S. Eiger

Infant nutrition should be considered a holistic enterprise. After the initial physical examination and the pronouncement of normality in her new offspring, the mother's primary concern becomes how she will nourish her infant. During pregnancy, maternal good health, a carefully supervised dietary intake, and adequate rest ensure proper nutrition of the fetus. This symbiotic union persists once infant and mother become two separate beings, and adequate nutrition for the infant becomes a more purposeful procedure, the details of which absorb much of the mother's time and energy during the first 6 to 12 months of the infant's life. This is the period of most rapid extrauterine growth, during which infants double their birth weight in the first 6 months and triple it by the twelfth month. Food during this period satisfies both physical and emotional growth, and the setting in which it is provided is of paramount importance to the infant, whose oral orientation translates food into ego satisfaction. Thus, the practice of infant feeding cannot be based solely on what type of milk the infant should receive. Numerous other factors must be considered.

Most infants appear to grow normally and maintain a satisfactory state of health despite variations in nutritional management. The goal of infant nutrition is to produce an adequately (but not overly) nourished child whose diet is readily digestible, with all the essential nutrients provided through a reasonable distribution of calories derived from protein, fat, and carbohydrate. Because the pattern and content of feeding in infancy strongly affects dietary habits later in life, considerable care must be given to constructing the early dietary milieu.

Based on studies of nutritional requirements in infancy, reasonable dietary recommendations for full-term infants are: 7% to 16% of calories from protein, 30% to 55% from fat, and the remainder from carbohydrate.[6] Human milk provides approximately 7% of calories from alpha-lactalbumin, a more bioavailable protein that is absorbed almost entirely by the infant, 55% from mostly saturated fat containing all the essential fatty acids needed by the infant, and 38% from lactose. Current ongoing research indicates that the high content of saturated fat of human milk is nature's method of programming the breast-fed infant to metabolize fats more efficiently, thereby decreasing the risk of adult coronary disease. Most commercially prepared cow milk-based formulas in the United States are modeled after human milk and provide 9% to 15% of calories from a less bioavailable protein, beta-lactoglobulin, which is responsible for the increased gastric curd tension and the large protein loss in the stool of the artificially fed infant. Cow milk formulas contain 45% to 50% of their caloric density mostly from polyunsaturated fats and the remainder from carbohydrate, usually lactose.

With the possible exceptions of vitamin D, iron, and fluoride, the infant fed breast milk from a healthy mother receives more than adequate nutrition without further supplementation for at least the first 6 months of life. Thus, from a physiological and teleological point of view, the maxims "breast is best" and "human milk is for humans, cow milk is for cows" are unchallengeable. Only in the past 50 years or so has there been any question as to whether a mother would breast-feed her baby. With the advent of pasteurization, dependable refrigeration, and production of formulas from cow milk, alternatives have been provided. Thus, the decision to breast-feed depends on: the customs of the community, lifestyle, the mother's personality, and the attitudes of the obstetrician, pediatrician, and family.

In 1997, the American Academy of Pediatrics (AAP), in its strongest policy statement ever, advised pediatricians and other child health clinicians of the importance and the need to recommend breast-feeding over formula feeding.[1] The AAP's policy, recommending human milk as ideal nutrition and the preferred method of feeding for all infants, including premature and sick newborns, states that breast-feeding should begin within the first hour postpartum and that exclusive nursing should be continued without supplementation for approximately the first 6 months, after which solids may be added while nursing is continued through the first year and beyond by mutual consent of mother and baby. Breast-feeding, best initiated immediately after delivery by continuous rooming-in and nursing on cue, should be evaluated by a trained observer within the first 24 to 48 hours. Mother and baby should be observed for proper latch-on technique, infant weight and general health should be assessed 2 to 4 days after discharge, and both should be followed closely by the pediatrician for the first 6 weeks until breast-feeding is well-established. The pediatrician, while remaining sensitive to the mother's own feelings and needs, must be aware of the advantages of human milk over cow milk for infant feeding and encourage mothers to breast-feed.

COMPARISON OF HUMAN MILK AND COW MILK

Milk is the primary source for satisfying nutritional needs during the entire first year of life. Solid foods are unnecessary for most infants until 6 months of age. Therefore, it is essential that the physician be knowledgeable about the composition of human milk and cow milk. The manufacturers of infant formulas constantly attempt to modify cow milk to produce a product comparable to human milk. It is of interest that the growth rates of the human infant and the calf are different. An infant takes two to three times longer than a calf to double its birth weight. Inasmuch as cow milk contains 3.5 g of protein per deciliter to human milk's 1.1 g, a ratio of 3 : 1, the symmetry of nature is satisfied. (See Table 17-6 and Appendix C, Tables C-14 and C-15, for further comparisons of human milk and various cow milk formulas.)

Besides the larger amount of protein in cow milk than in human milk, the proteins in the two milks have qualitative differences. The percentage of casein, as compared with whey proteins (lactalbumin and lactoglobulins), is higher in cow milk. Both proteins have high biological value, but casein causes higher curd tension in the infant's stomach and, thus, must be treated by homogenization, heating, and acidification for better digestion.

The fat of cow milk (butterfat) contains predominantly saturated fatty acids and is less well digested by infants than is the fat of human milk, which contains monounsaturated fatty acids such as oleic acid and polyunsaturated fatty acids such as essential linoleic acid. The fat composition in human milk allows for excellent fat and calcium absorption and ensures that all essential fatty acids are provided. Human milk, in contrast to cow milk, is rich in lipase, which when added to intestinal lipase, aids in the rapid splitting of free fatty acids from triglycerides to ensure quick absorption. It has been shown that free fatty acids are the most important sources of energy for the young infant, and the lipase in human milk makes these free fatty acids available rapidly, even before digestion with intestinal lipase begins.

Lactose is present in higher concentrations in human milk than in the milk of any other mammal. Lactose is split into glucose and galactose. Galactose is synthesized into galactolipid, which is an essential component of the central nervous system in mammals. In most commercial formulas, lactose is provided as the carbohydrate in a percentage similar to that found in human milk.

The total ash content of human milk (0.2%) is less than one third that of cow milk (0.7%); this provides a greater margin of safety for renal excretion during illness in early infancy.

BREAST-FEEDING VERSUS ARTIFICIAL FEEDING

Many studies indicate that breast-fed infants develop fewer gastrointestinal infections, respiratory illnesses, and allergic reactions than do artificially fed infants.[4,7,8,9,11] These differences are most striking in the developing countries, where poor sanitary practices prevail. However, breast-feeding affords a large degree of protection against illness to infants in the developed countries as well. This protection is based on the presence of secretory antibodies in colostrum; the bifidus factor in human milk, which promotes the development of the characteristic intestinal microflora of *Lactobacillus bifidus;* and other host factors in mature milk, primarily secretory IgA (Table 17-7). Each year researchers add more defensive factors found in breast milk to this list of properties. The infant acquires maximum protection against infection if exclusive breast-feeding, without solid foods, is offered until at least 6 months of life.

The immunological advantages of breast milk are most evident during the infant's first half year, but protection against many pathogens does endure through the toddler

Table 17-6 Comparison of Nutrients in Formulas and Mature Human Milk

Component (per dl)	Recommended Daily Dietary Allowances (0-6 Months)	Human Milk—Values Variable	"Humanized" Formulas: Enfamil with Iron	Similac with Iron	SMA	Evaporated Milk; 1:1 Dilution	Evaporated Milk 13 oz, Water 19 oz, Carbohydrate 1 oz	Whole Milk 3.5% Fat
Calories (kcal)	117 kcal/kg	67-75	67	68	67	69	67	66
Protein (g)	2.2 g/kg	1.1	1.5	1.6	1.5	3.5	2.8	3.5
Fat, total (g)	Not listed	4.5	3.7	3.6	3.6	3.8	3.0	3.5-3.7
Saturated		2.2	1.2	1.4	1.6	2.4	1.9	2.2
Unsaturated		2.3	2.5	2.2	2.0	1.4	1.1	1.3
Cholesterol (mg)	Not listed	7-47	1.4	1.6	3.3	10-34	8-28	10-35
Carbohydrate (g)	Not listed	6.8 Lactose	7 Lactose	7.1 Lactose	7.2 Lactose	4.8 Lactose	7.0 Lactose Sucrose	4.9 Lactose
Calcium (mg)	360	34	55	58	44	126	100	118
Phosphorus (mg)	240	14	46	43	33	102	81	92
Sodium (mg)	Not listed	16	28	25	16	60	48	50
Potassium (mg)	Not listed	51	69	75	56	152	122	137
Magnesium (mg)	60	4	4	4	5	12	10	12
Iron (mg)	10	0.05	1.2	1.2	1.3	0.05	0.04	0.05
Copper (μg)	Not listed	40	60	40	50	Estimate 30	Estimate 20	30
Zinc (mg)	3	0.3-0.5	0.4	0.5	0.4	0.3-0.5	0.2-0.4	0.3-0.5
Iodine (μg)	35	3	7	10	7	5	4	5
Vitamin A (IU)	1400	200	170	250	264	185	150	140
Thiamine (mg)	0.3	0.016	0.05	0.07	0.07	0.03	0.02	0.17
Riboflavin (mg)	0.4	0.036	0.06	0.1	0.1	0.19	0.16	0.17
Niacin (mg)	5	0.1	0.8	0.7	0.7	0.1	0.1	0.1
Pyridoxine (mg)	0.3	0.01	0.04	0.04	0.04	0.04	0.03	0.06
Folacin (mg)	0.05	0.005	0.01	0.005	0.005	0.005	0.004	0.005
Vitamin B_{12} (μg)	0.3	0.03	0.2	0.2	0.1	0.08	0.06	0.4
Vitamin C (mg)	35	4	5	6	6	0.5	0.4	1
Vitamin D (IU)	400	2	42	40	42	Fortified 40	Fortified 32	Fortified 42
Vitamin E (IU)	4	0.2	1.3	1.5	1	0.04	0.03	0.04
Vitamin K (μg)	Not listed	1.5	6	9	5.8	Estimate 6	Estimate 5	6

Data from Fomon SJ: *Infant nutrition,* ed 2, Philadelphia, 1980, WB Saunders; and the Committee on Dietary Allowances: *Recommended dietary allowance,* ed 9, rev ed, Washington, DC, 1980, National Academy of Sciences.

period. Breast-feeding offers greatest protection against diarrheal disease and against serious respiratory disease (wheezing, bronchitis, bronchiolitis, pneumonia) rather than uncomplicated respiratory tract infections. Bottle-feeding increases the risk of otitis media and of hospitalization for bacterial infections, septicemia, and meningitis.[4]

Breast-fed infants have been shown to have a lower incidence of allergic diseases when foreign food antigens are avoided for the first 6 months of life.[5] In one study of more than 20,000 infants, those who were fed artificially were seven times as likely to develop eczema as those who were completely breast-fed.[9] The first 6 months is the period in which infants' passively acquired transplacental antibodies are being replaced with their own; thus, lack of exposure to foreign food antigens in the breast-fed infant presumably results in a reduced frequency of allergic reactions. Infants are never allergic to their mother's milk, whereas allergy to cow milk does occur.

An infant can digest human milk much more easily than the milk of other mammalian species. Breast milk forms softer curds in the infant's stomach than does cow milk and is assimilated more rapidly. Although it contains less protein than formulas made from cow milk, virtually all the protein in breast milk is used by the infant, whereas a large amount of the protein in formula is passed in the stool. A breast-fed infant rarely gets diarrhea and rarely becomes constipated because breast milk does not form hard stools in the intestinal tract.

Breast milk has no synthetic compounds, no preservatives, and no artificial ingredients. It is always available at the right temperature and the right consistency. Suckling at the breast is good for the infant's tooth and jaw development. Nursing technically is different from artificial feeding in that the bottle-fed infant does not have to exercise the jaws so energetically, inasmuch as light suckling alone produces a rapid flow of milk. Bottle-fed infants use their tongue in a manner quite opposite that of the breast-fed baby; the flow of milk through the rubber nipple is produced by a tongue-thrusting motion with each suck while the infant's lips create a negative pressure in the oral cavity, thus suctioning milk from the bottle.

Table 17-7 Host Resistance Factors in Human Milk

Components	Proposed Mode of Action
Growth factor of *L. bifidus*	*L. bifidus* interferes with intestinal colonization of enteric pathogens
Antistaphylococcal factor	Inhibits staphylococci
Secretory IgA and other immunoglobulins	Protective antibodies for the gut and respiratory tract
C4 and C3	C3 fragments have opsonic, chemotactic, and anaphylatoxic activities
Lysozyme	Lysis of bacterial cell wall
Lactoperoxidase-H_2O_2-thiocyanate	Killing of streptococci
Lactoferrin	Kills microorganisms by chelating iron
Leukocytes	Phagocytosis
	Cell-mediated immunity—production of IgA, C4, C3, lysozyme, and lactoferrin

The breast-fed baby places the tongue over the lower jaw, where it remains throughout the nursing session, and draws the nipple by suction well into the mouth, elongating it to three times its normal length and extending it to the junction between the hard and soft palates. The elongated nipple rests in a trough formed by the U-shaped tongue. As each suckling cycle is initiated, the infant's jaws compress the milk sinuses just under and proximal to the areola, pinching off a bolus of milk and propelling it toward the posterior pharynx by a peristaltic, wavelike motion. This rollerlike movement, which begins at the anterior tip of the tongue and progresses toward its base, effectively strips the milk bolus from the proximal portion of the nipple out toward its tip, where it exits into the infant's mouth and is swallowed (Fig. 17-5). The jaw muscles are thus strenuously exercised, encouraging the development of well-formed jaws and straight, healthy teeth.[18]

Because of this fundamental difference between suckling at the breast and sucking on a bottle or pacifier, a very young infant (under 6 weeks of age) should be fed exclusively on the breast lest "nipple confusion" occur. This is a development that may ensue in some young infants, full-term as well as preterm, whereby too early introduction of a rubber nipple, and the tongue-thrusting that it requires to control rapid milk flow, prevents the necessary conditioning mechanism essential to the development of proper suckling technique. Suckling at the breast is not instinctual in humans, as it is in other mammals; rather, it is a learned response for both mother and baby, and in the early weeks, much time, attention, and support must be devoted to this educational process.

Perhaps most important, although most nebulous, are the psychological benefits the infant derives from breast-feeding.[13] Factors such as the more intimate interaction between the breast-feeding mother and child and the more immediate satisfaction of the nursing baby's hunger seem to augur healthier mental development. The infant also gains a sense of security from the warmth and closeness of the mother's body. Breast-feeding eliminates the practice of bottle propping; the infant, of necessity, must be drawn close at each feeding. Although the bottle-feeding mother also can show her love for her baby by holding and cuddling the baby at feeding times, in actual practice she may do less of this, and of course she cannot duplicate the unique skin-to-skin contact between the nursing mother and her infant. Montagu[14] states, "The breast-feeding relationship constitutes the foundation for the development of all human social relationships, and the communications the infant receives through the warmth of the mother's skin constitute the first of the socializing experiences of his life." Babies gain a sense of well-being from secure handling, and mothers who nurse their infants successfully often seem more confident in managing them. Whether the woman who is sure of her maternal abilities is more likely to breast-feed—or whether the experience itself infuses her with self-confidence—is difficult to determine. Mothers who nurse may be better able to soothe their babies when they are upset, perhaps because the very

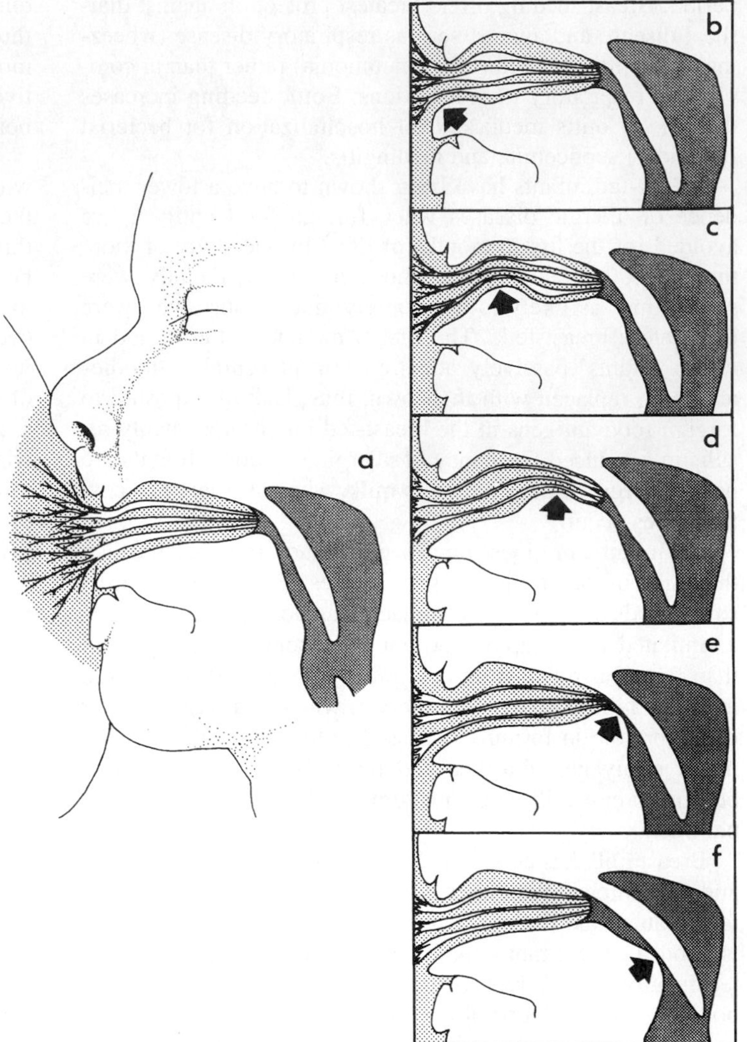

Fig. 17-5 Complete "suck" cycle. **a,** The infant's jaws compress the sinuses, and the nipple is drawn into the mouth with the tip at the junction of the hard and soft palates; the tongue is cradling the nipple. **b,** The lower jaw constricts the nipple base, pinching off the milk bolus, and the anterior tip of the tongue begins a wavelike motion. **c,** The rollerlike tongue action moves milk posteriorly. **d** and **e,** A wave of compression pushes the milk into the oropharynx, where it is swallowed. **f,** The jaw lowers, allowing the milk to flow into the nipple base again as the next "suck" cycle begins.

(From Woolridge MW: *Midwifery* 2:166, 1986.)

act of putting them to the breast is such a comfort to them that the mother does not have to search for other methods of reassurance.

The mother also gains distinct benefits from breast-feeding. These include (1) stimulation, by early suckling, of oxytocin secretion, which fosters uterine contractions and rapid placental expulsion, inhibits postpartum hemorrhaging, and hastens postpartum uterine involution; (2) the mood-ameliorating effect of prolactin secretion, which stimulates milk production and has been referred to as the "mothering hormone,"[3] convenience, obviating the need to prepare formula, sterilize nipples and bottles, and refrigerate formula when traveling; (4) economy; (5) esthetics—breast-fed infants smell better because the odor of both bowel movements and regurgitated milk is less offensive than that of bottle-fed infants; (6) decreased risk of postpartum thromboembolism, premenopausal breast cancer,[15] ovarian cancer, and osteoporosis, and (7) emotional satisfaction and a sense of fulfillment.

The "nursing couple," mother and baby, forge an especially close and interdependent relationship. The baby depends on the mother for sustenance and comfort, and the mother looks forward to feeding times to gain a pleasurable sense of comfort with her infant and a period of rest and relaxation during her busy day. Because of this unique relationship, many women consider the nursing months among the most fulfilling of their lives.

A mother should not breast-feed unless she is fully convinced that she wants to. In most instances the wishes of the baby's father affect the decision to breast-feed inasmuch as the extended family has been replaced by the nuclear family, and he has become the nursing mother's chief support system. For most women, nursing is accomplished easily; however, if for any reason the desire to breast-feed is lacking or poorly supported, initiating or continuing nursing may be difficult and may produce emotional strains that could disrupt the mother-child-father relationship. Physicians should support the mother completely whether her decision is to nurse, not to nurse, or to discontinue nursing, regardless of their personal opinions on the matter.

For a working mother, breast-feeding requires a great deal of patience, development of time-saving routines, and cooperation at the workplace, where privacy for expressing milk and storage facilities should be available. Many large corporations are recognizing this need and realizing the economic and psychological advantages of enabling nursing mothers to

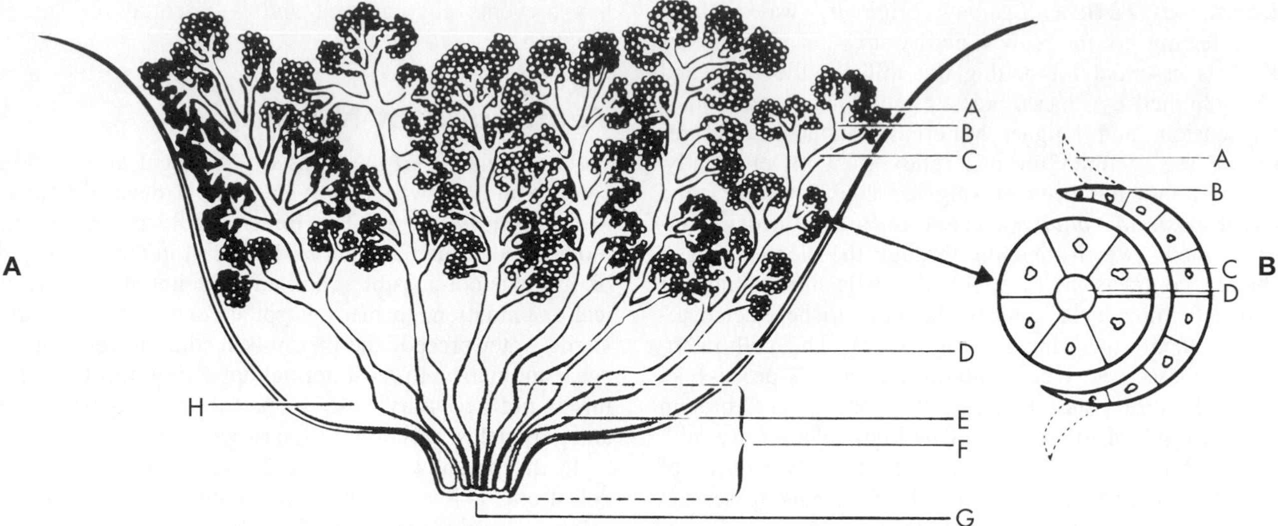

Fig. 17-6 **A,** Diagram of the breast as a "forest of trees." With full development of the uterine-menstrual cycle, groups of gland-secreting cells (alveoli) bud from the small ducts (ductules). The alveoli secrete milk under the influence of prolactin, a hormone of the pituitary gland. *A,* Alveolus; *B,* ductule; *C,* duct; *D,* lactiferous duct; *E,* lactiferous sinus; *F,* ampulla; *G,* nipple pore; *H,* areolar margin. **B,** Diagram of an alveolus. Gland-secreting cells are arranged in a circle around the ductule opening. The alveolus is surrounded by a contractile cell. When suckling begins, this cell, under the influence of oxytocin from the pituitary gland, contracts and squeezes the milk into the duct system; this reflex is called *letdown. A,* Uncontracted myoepithelial cell; *B,* contracted myoepithelial cell; *C,* gland-secreting cell; *D,* ductule opening.

(From Applebaum RM: *Pediatr Clin North Am* 17:205, 1970.)

return to work early. Lightweight, efficient, easy-to-use electric pumps can be rented inexpensively over the long term and can be left at the workplace so that milk can be expressed, refrigerated, and taken home for the infant's next-day feeding. If expressed milk is to be used within 48 hours, it may be placed in the refrigerator; if frozen immediately after collection and kept in the freezer, it should be used within 6 months. Although the breast-feeding routine may be more challenging for the working mother, a sympathetic family and physician and access to various support systems will help her to continue nursing.[16]

BREAST-FEEDING

Basis of Lactation

Successful breast-feeding depends on a strongly motivated mother, a healthy infant who has a strong suckling impulse, and a physician who is confident and competent in his or her knowledge of the anatomy of the mammary gland, the composition of human milk (see Table 17-6), and the physiology of lactation.

Directly beneath and behind the areola is a group of milk pools, or lactiferous sinuses, that with proper "latch-on," the nursing infant's jaws compress, squeezing milk into and along the pores of the nipple. The nipple itself is merely a spout through which the milk is conducted into the infant's mouth and should not itself be traumatized by the infant's jaws. The sinuses are widened parts of the lactiferous ducts, of which there are 15 to 20, each emptying into the nipple. At their proximal ends within the breast, the ducts branch off into smaller canals, called *ductules.* At the end of each ductule is a grapelike structure composed of a cluster of tiny, rounded, saclike alveoli, in which the milk is made. The ducts and the alveoli are surrounded with myoepithelial cells that contract (in response to oxytocin), squeezing the milk into and through the entire duct system, finally ending up in the sinuses. Clusters of alveoli compose the lobules, which are bound together by connective tissue, richly interwoven with blood vessels and lymphatics into the 15 to 20 lobes in each breast. Each lobe is connected to one duct, and each duct empties into one opening on the nipple (Fig. 17-6).

Physiology of Lactation

Successful lactation is a simple process, the result of reflex interactions between the nursing couple; it is based on the simultaneous occurrence of two reflexes, the prolactin (or milk secretion) reflex and the "letdown" (or milk ejection) reflex.

Prolactin reflex. When the infant suckles at the breast, the maternal *anterior pituitary* gland is stimulated, via the vagus nerve and the hypothalamus, to secrete the hormone prolactin, which acts on the breast alveoli to produce milk. Prolactin secretion, and thus the production of breast milk, is totally determined by the frequency and duration of infant suckling on the breast Until the milk supply is well established, which normally takes 3 to 6 weeks of exclusive breast-feeding without supplementation with either water or formula, the breasts require stimulation on an average of 8 to 12 times each 24-hour period.

Letdown reflex. *Letdown* originally was a dairy term, referring to the cow's ability to "let down" her milk. It is essential for getting the milk to the baby and can be inhibited by illness, breast engorgement, pain, emotional tension, and fatigue. Maternal confidence and reassurance are required for this reflex to work efficiently. After the infant has been nursing for 2 to 3 minutes, the maternal *posterior pituitary* gland releases oxytocin, another hormone, which traveling through the bloodstream to the breast, contracts the myoepithelial cells surrounding the alveoli and milk ducts, causing the milk to be ejected toward the lactiferous sinuses (Fig. 17-7). The cell membranes of the secretory cells rupture during this process, so larger and more concentrated fatty globules and protein particles are added to the milk. This high-calorie fatty milk is called "hindmilk"; it constitutes the final two thirds of the volume of milk during each individual nursing session and is added to the previous one third of "foremilk" produced during the height of the earlier prolactin secretion phase. Thus, a vigorous letdown reflex increases the caloric content of the milk and, by forceful ejection, refills the milk sinuses with the rich, creamy "hindmilk" that ensures rapid weight gain when the infant obtains it regularly. Ensuring adequate drainage of milk through an effective letdown reflex prevents engorgement and is essential for successful lactation.

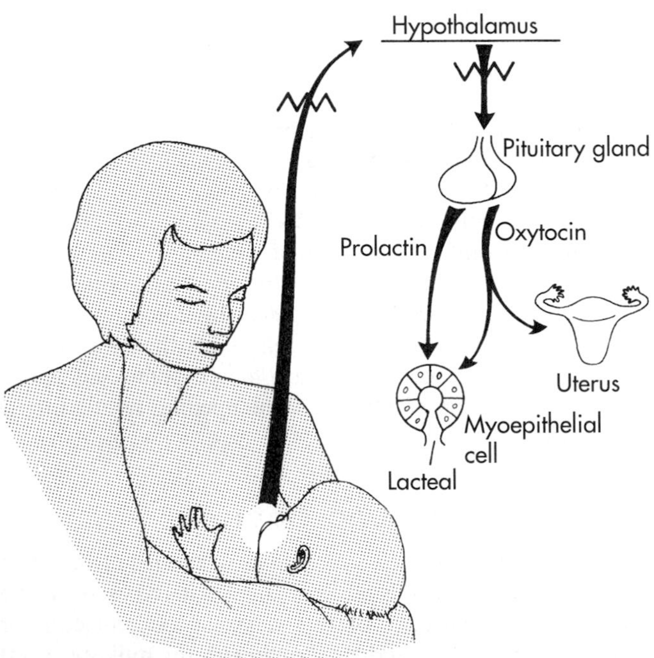

Fig. 17-7 Diagrammatic outline of the ejection reflex arc. The infant's suckling stimulates mechanoreceptors in the nipple and areola that send stimuli along nerve pathways to the hypothalamus, which in turn stimulates the posterior pituitary to release oxytocin. The bloodstream carries the oxytocin to the breast and the uterus. In the breast, oxytocin stimulates the myoepithelial cell to contract and eject milk from the alveolus. Prolactin, which is secreted by the anterior pituitary gland in response to the infant's suckling, effects milk production in the alveolus. Stress, such as pain or anxiety, can inhibit letdown, whereas the sight or cry of an infant can stimulate it.

(From Lawrence RA: *Breastfeeding: a guide for the medical profession,* ed 5, St Louis, 1999, Mosby.)

Technique of Nursing

Early stimulation of the breasts by frequent nursing will encourage milk flow and provide a rapid development of an adequate milk supply. The infant should be placed on the mother's abdomen and put to the breast in the delivery room or, if this is not possible, soon after the initial newborn physical examination. In many hospitals one or two feedings of sterile water precede the first milk feeding to rule out esophageal anomalies. In most normal-appearing, full-term infants, this is not necessary; also, it may lead to nipple confusion and may delay initiation of breast-feeding.

In the first few days after delivery, the breast produces colostrum, a low-fat, high-protein milky fluid rich in fat-soluble vitamins and antibodies. Colostrum sustains the newborn until the "real" milk comes in; it is replaced by transitional milk by the third or fourth day, and by 10 days to 2 weeks postpartum the mature milk appears. The breast-fed baby is a hungry baby who cries often to be fed; this is a normal response that occurs at 1- to 3-hour intervals in the first 4 to 6 weeks of life. Because breast milk is more digestible than cow milk, a breast-fed infant's stomach empties more rapidly. Therefore, breast-fed babies require feeding more often than bottle-fed babies (8 to 12 feedings in 24 hours versus 6 for a bottle-fed baby).

Optimal breast-feeding is *"demand" feeding*. Maximal milk production occurs when engorgement is reduced and the breast is emptied frequently by the infant. A breast emptied of milk will *quickly* produce more, and a natural state of equilibrium is established between the mother and the infant.

Successful breast-feeding can be thwarted by an overrigid hospital administrator's concern for a germ-free environment and tight nursing and medical staff regulations, which can be extremely inconvenient for the nursing couple. The optimal physical and emotional health of mothers and infants often demands changes in many traditional hospital procedures. Demand feeding of the nursing infant ideally is effected by a complete rooming-in program. The infant should be with the mother for as long as possible to allow the mother to become acquainted with her new infant and to become accustomed to her baby's natural eating and sleeping rhythms.

A comfortable position, either sitting or lying, is essential for successful nursing. The cradle position, the hold used most commonly, is best accomplished with the mother sitting in an armless chair, the leg on the side on which she is nursing resting on a footstool, and a pillow on her lap supporting the forearm on which her baby is resting. Her infant should be facing her directly, his stomach against hers, his head in line with his body, his neck in the bend of her elbow, with her hand on his buttocks so that he is pulled up close, with his face almost touching the breast. The mother's free hand then grasps her breast in the C-hold: thumb on top and well behind the areola, index finger opposite, below, and again well behind the areola, with the other three fingers supporting the breast from underneath. In this position the infant's mouth directly opposes the nipple, which the mother should stroke patiently against the infant's lower lip until the baby's mouth opens quite wide to accept the nipple (rooting reflex); at this point the mother pulls the baby's head firmly onto the breast, inserting the nipple deep into his mouth and allowing him to close his jaws over the base of the nipple for proper and effective latch-on (Fig. 17-8). When feeding on the first side is complete, the mother breaks the suction by placing her fifth finger gently into the corner of the infant's mouth before transferring him to the other breast.

An effective latch-on, or attachment of the baby to the breast, is essential for efficient and painless initiation of lactation. Although breast-feeding is a natural process, it is the result of the transmission to the new mother of a generationally accumulated experience that is to a great extent lacking in our modern, technologically oriented Western society, in which the extended family has been replaced by its inadequate nuclear counterpart and wherein the central hospital nursery severely interferes with the necessary interaction between mother and infant.[13] The latch-on is not instinctual, and the new mother must be taught by trained, knowledgeable personnel, in the immediate postpartum hours, how to perform it properly. Breast-feeding should not be painful, even at the beginning, and with the correct latch-on technique it will be comfortable for the mother, allowing an effective letdown and early, rapid establishment of a rhythm of frequent draining and filling of the breasts, which is essential to building a dependable milk supply.

No time limit should be imposed on nursing on each breast, even in the early days, because the infant's jaws will not traumatize the nipple if the mother uses the correct latch-on technique.[12] In the first few weeks, however, the baby should be encouraged to suckle both breasts at each nursing session, and the breast used last at the previous feeding should be used first at the next feeding. The mother should be taught to listen for her infant's swallowing sounds (short, sighing-like noises), rather than observing the suckling, as an indication that her baby is removing milk from her breast. The ideal ratio is no more than one to two sucks per swallow. After the first few weeks, when the milk supply is adequate, an older, thriving infant may desire to remain on one breast throughout the entire feeding to obtain the benefits of the rich, satiety-producing hindmilk, and the mother should be told that this is acceptable so long as the breasts are alternated at ensuing feeding sessions.[17]

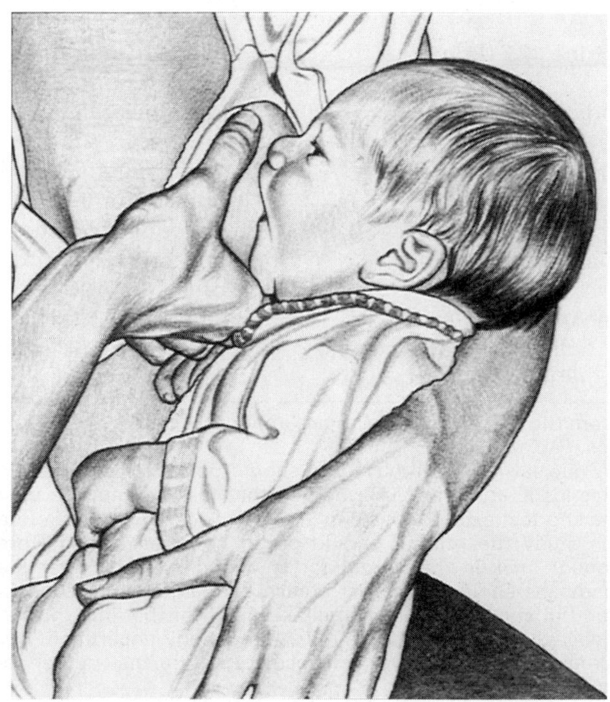

Fig. 17-8 Correct latch-on position: The baby faces the mother directly, his stomach against hers, his head, which is kept in line with his body, resting in the crook of his mother's arm. The mother uses the C-hold to support her breast.

(From Eiger MS, Olds SW: *The complete book of breastfeeding,* ed 3, New York, 1999, Workman, Bantam.)

Breast-fed babies may lose up to 10% of their birth weight, but the initial weight loss can be decreased markedly by immediately initiating nursing in the delivery suite, by allowing frequent, unrestricted demand feeding sessions with mother and baby rooming-in together, by avoiding supplementation with either water or formula, and with the constant support of trained medical and nursing personnel. Attention must be given in the early weeks to the adequacy of the buildup of the maternal milk supply. The infant younger than 1 month of age who is ingesting sufficient mother's milk is never constipated and should be having at least four or more stools per 24-hour day. Fewer than that number, even if the infant is wetting frequently, is a danger sign of intestinal dysfunction or of inadequate breast milk intake and intervention is needed. Close follow-up is in order for breast-fed infants who lose more than 5% to 7% of their weight or who have other risk factors (e.g., early hospital discharge, feeding-related jaundice, maternal history of previous breast surgery, or birth by cesarean section). In the early weeks, bottle supplementation should be used rarely because of the physiological differences between suckling the breast and sucking the bottle and the consequent risk of nipple confusion. Many new and exciting techniques have been developed to increase an insufficient milk supply. Formula supplementation at the breast with a nursing supplementer in addition to the use of an electric breast pump to provide breast stimulation is available to tide the infant over, without undermining the development of the suckling mechanism, until the mother's milk supply increases.

Drugs in Breast Milk

All drugs that a lactating woman ingests appear in the breast milk, usually in amounts that do not approximate the concentration in the mother's plasma. The total amount excreted into the milk after a single maternal dose is a function of time and nursing frequency; for most drugs, the amount is less than 1% to 2% of the maternal dose.[2] Reasonable concern exists about the effect on the nursing infant of substances the mother ingests. The effect on the infant is determined by the volume of milk ingested, the amount absorbed from the intestine, the activity of the drug, the infant's sensitivity to and tolerance of the specific substance, the cumulative effect of chronicity of maternal therapy with the particular drug, and the infant's size and maturity. Maternal dosing immediately after a nursing session minimizes the entry of the substance into the milk at the next feeding, inasmuch as the peak maternal plasma level of the drug follows the curve of peak milk

Table 17-8 Drugs Contraindicated during Breast-Feeding

Drug	Reason for Concern
Bromocriptine	Suppresses lactation; may be hazardous to the mother
Cocaine	Cocaine intoxication
Cyclophosphamide	Possible immune suppression; unknown effect on growth or association with carcinogenesis; neutropenia
Cyclosporine	Possible immune suppression; unknown effect on growth or association with carcinogenesis
Doxorubicin*	Possible immune suppression; unknown effect on growth or association with carcinogenesis
Ergotamine	Vomiting, diarrhea, convulsions (doses used in migraine medications)
Lithium	One-third to one-half therapeutic blood concentration in infants
Methotrexate	Possible immune suppression; unknown effect on growth or association with carcinogenesis; neutropenia
Phencyclidine (PCP)	Potent hallucinogen
Phenindione	Anticoagulant; increased prothrombin and partial thromboplastin time in one infant; not used in the United States

From the Committee on Drugs, American Academy of Pediatrics: *Pediatrics* 93:137, 1994.
*Drug is concentrated in human milk.

production. Short-acting preparations should be prescribed, if possible, rather than long-acting formulations. Data rapidly are becoming available to guide practitioners' recommendations to mothers regarding the drugs they can take without fear of affecting their babies adversely.[3]

The factors that affect the appearance of a drug in breast milk are its lipid solubility, its pK_a, its protein-binding ability, and the pH of the milk. Unionized drugs that have a high lipid solubility are transported better than ionized ones. The concentration of a drug in breast milk depends on the volume of mammary alveolar cells and the concentration of unbound drug in the mother's plasma. Drugs usually pass through membranes by passive diffusion, depending on the concentration gradient and their lipid solubility. The pH of breast milk is approximately 7.0 and that of plasma is approximately 7.4; therefore, weak acids usually have low milk/plasma ratios, whereas weak bases are likely to have high ratios. Most drugs for which specific information is available can be grouped into categories relating to their potential effect on the nursing infant (Tables 17-8 through 17-12). Steroids, when taken in large doses over time by the mother, can suppress growth and interfere with endogenous steroid production in the infant. Infants who have a glucose-6-phosphate dehydrogenase (G6PD) deficiency may suffer hemolysis from ingesting nalidixic acid, sulfonamides, and other oxidant drugs in breast milk. Chronic salicylate ingestion by the mother can produce hemorrhagic problems in her breast-feeding infant.

Antibiotics usually do not produce acute adverse effects in

Table 17-9 Drugs of Abuse: Contraindicated during Breast-Feeding*

Drug	Reason for Concern
Amphetamine†	Irritability, poor sleeping pattern
Cocaine	Cocaine intoxication
Heroin	Tremors, restlessness, vomiting, poor feeding
Marijuana	Only one report in the literature; no effect mentioned
Nicotine (smoking)	Shock, vomiting, diarrhea, rapid heart rate, restlessness; decreased milk production
Phencyclidine	Potent hallucinogen

From the Committee on Drugs, American Academy of Pediatrics: *Pediatrics* 93:137, 1994.
*The AAP's Committee on Drugs strongly believes that nursing mothers should not ingest any of the compounds listed in this table. Not only are they hazardous to the nursing infant, but also they are detrimental to the mother's physical and emotional health. Obviously, this list is not complete; nursing mothers should not ingest *any* drug of abuse, even if no adverse reports are found in the literature.
†Drug is concentrated in human milk.

Table 17-10 Radioactive Compounds Requiring Temporary Cessation of Breast-Feeding*

Drug	Recommended Period of No Breast-feeding
Copper 64 (^{64}Cu)	Radioactivity in milk present at 50 hr
Gallium 67 (^{67}Ga)	Radioactivity in milk present for 2 wk
Indium 111 (^{111}In)	Very small amount present at 20 hr
Iodine 123 (^{123}I)	Radioactivity in milk present up to 36 hr
Iodine 125 (^{125}I)	Radioactivity in milk present for 12 d
Iodine 131 (^{131}I)	Radioactivity in milk present for 2-14 d, depending on study
Radioactive sodium	Radioactivity in milk present for 96 hr
Technetium-99m (^{99m}Tc), ^{99m}Rc macroaggregates, ^{99m}Tc O4	Radioactivity in milk present for 15 hr to 3 d

From the Committee on Drugs, American Academy of Pediatrics: *Pediatrics* 93:137, 1994.
*A nuclear medicine physician should be consulted before a diagnostic study is performed so that the radionuclide with the shortest excretion time in breast milk can be used. Before the study the mother should pump her breasts and store enough milk in the freezer for feeding the infant; after the study she should pump her breasts to maintain milk production but should discard all milk pumped for the time that radioactivity is present in the milk. A radiology department can screen milk samples for radioactivity before the mother resumes nursing.

Table 17-11 Drugs Whose Effect in Nursing Infants Is Unknown but May Be of Concern

Psychotropic drugs (those listed in the Antianxiety, Antidepressant, and Antipsychotic categories) are of special concern when given to nursing mothers for long periods. Although there are no case reports of adverse effects in breast-feeding infants, these drugs appear in human milk and thus conceivably could affect short-term and long-term functioning of the central nervous system.

Drug	Reported or Possible Effect
Antianxiety	
Diazepam	None
Lorazepam	None
Midazolam	—
Perphenazine	None
Prazepam*	None
Quazepam	None
Temazepam	—
Antidepressants	
Amitriptyline	None
Amoxapine	None
Desipramine	None
Doxepin	None
Duthiepin	None
Fluoxetine	—
Fluvoxamine	—
Imipramine	None
Trazodone	None
Antipsychotic	
Chlorpromazine	Galactorrhea in the mother; drowsiness and lethargy in the infant
Chlorprothixene	None
Haloperidol	None
Mesoridazine	None
Chloramphenicol	Possible idiosyncratic bone marrow suppression
Metoclopramide*	None described; dopaminergic blocking agent
Metronidazole	In vitro mutagen; may discontinue breast-feeding 12-24 hr to allow excretion of dose when the mother is given single-dose therapy
Tinidazole	See metronidazole

From the Committee on Drugs, American Academy of Pediatrics: *Pediatrics* 93:137, 1994.
*Drug is concentrated in human milk.

breast-fed infants (see Chapter 31, Antimicrobial Therapy). However, continuous ingestion of the aminoglycosides may alter an infant's intestinal flora, affect some immune mechanisms adversely, and predispose the infant to hypersensitivity. Tetracycline ingestion through breast milk has not been reported to cause mottled teeth in breast-fed infants, even when tetracyclines are found in high concentrations in breast milk, probably because the calcium complexing of tetracyclines in breast milk interferes with their absorption by the infant.

Table 17-12 Drugs Associated with Significant Effects on Some Nursing Infants (Should Be Given with Caution to Nursing Mothers)

Drug	Reported Effect
5-Aminosalicylic acid	Diarrhea (one case)
Aspirin (salicylates)	Metabolic acidosis (one case)
Clemastine	Drowsiness, irritability, refusal to feed, high-pitched cry, neck stiffness (one case)
Phenobarbital	Sedation; infantile spasms after weaning from milk containing phenobarbital, methemoglobinemia (one case)
Primidone	Sedation, feeding problems
Sulfasalazine (salicylazo-sulfapyridine)	Bloody diarrhea (one case)

From the Committee on Drugs, American Academy of Pediatrics: *Pediatrics* 93:137, 1994.
When possible, the blood concentration in the infant should be measured.

Lactating mothers must always be aware that anything they ingest may pass into their milk and have an undesirable effect on their infant. Physicians, dentists, and paramedical personnel responsible for prescribing drugs should be informed that the mother is breast-feeding so that care can be taken in prescribing a drug compatible with the nursing baby. Should it be necessary to prescribe a medication that is incompatible with breast-feeding, a reasonable, safe alternative almost always can be substituted. Nursing should never be terminated arbitrarily because of the need for maternal therapy. If breast-feeding must be stopped temporarily, a breast-pumping regimen to maintain the mother's milk supply and the continuous support of the family and sympathetic medical personnel will allow it to be resumed successfully. Over-the-counter (OTC) medications taken for a short time rarely present problems for the nursing baby, but caution should be exerted in their administration.

Complications of Breast-Feeding

The complications of nursing usually pertain to difficulties the mother experiences, but occasionally an infant will become seriously ill for a prolonged period and will be unable to nurse adequately. During brief illnesses in which feeding at the breast is not possible, the breast can be emptied periodically during maternal-infant separation with an electric breast pump and the infant fed the expressed breast milk through a nursing supplementer or a bottle, depending on the baby's age and maturity.

Sore, cracked nipples need not occur if careful attention is paid to the correct latch-on technique, proper positioning, and prevention of engorgement. Pain on latch-on is a signal that the baby must be removed from the breast and the proper latch-on sequence repeatedly attempted until a pain-free attachment is accomplished. Mothers should be aware that breast-feeding is a pleasurable experience and that the adage that "if it hurts, then it is wrong" is valid. If nipple trauma does occur, treatment consists of nipple exposure, relief of engorgement by frequent feeding or mechanical pumping, avoidance of any creams or ointments because the nipple pores are easily blocked and the areolar tissue easily macerated, and application to the sore nipple of the mother's own expressed breast milk, coupled with instruction in proper positioning and latch-on.

Incomplete emptying of a portion of the breast can easily lead to a plugged duct in that area. Nursing mothers should palpate their breasts regularly to become aware of the appearance of full areas, which when found should be treated with breast massage and by specific positioning of the infant on that breast in order to empty the suspicious area frequently and effectively.

Breast engorgement and plugged ducts, when unresolved, can quickly lead to mastitis, which is *not* a contraindication to continued nursing. Even if fever, breast tenderness, and erythema develop, there is ample evidence that administering antibiotics and continuing nursing—because it relieves engorgement and thus ensures drainage of the affected areas—will prevent many cases of mastitis from progressing to breast abscesses, which then may require surgical incision. The infant who nurses on the infected breast does *not* become ill and is in *no* danger. Feeding from the affected breast may be discontinued temporarily just after surgical drainage, but breast-feeding can be resumed from that breast after the wound has healed.

Concomitant with the resurgence of breast-feeding in the 1980s has been a rapid expansion of knowledge in the field of lactation; a new specialist, the lactation consultant, armed with innovative intervention techniques, has emerged to aid the physician in diagnosing and treating problems of the nursing couple. Lactation consultants certified by the International Board of Lactation Consultant Examiners are identified by the degree IBCLC (International Board-Certified Lactation Consultant) as individuals who have acquired in-depth knowledge and special skills to help mothers with breast-feeding problems. A busy pediatrician who may be unable to devote the required amount of attention to these time-consuming, common, and often urgent problem-solving needs of nursing mothers benefits his or her patients by referring them to a certified lactation consultant. The lactation consultant has clarified the concept of "insufficient milk syndrome," which actually is a composite of maternal and infant etiological factors that usually are correctable with supportive professional management.

ARTIFICIAL FEEDING

If bottle-feeding is chosen, or if breast-feeding is not feasible or successful, the infant will still thrive on an artificially prepared formula. Commercially prepared formulas for normal infants are modifications of whole cow milk that approximate the composition of human milk. Thus, the "humanized" formulas compare favorably with breast milk in their content of protein, carbohydrate (lactose), and saturated and unsaturated fats. Special formulas are available for milk-intolerant infants and for those who have specific malabsorptive problems (see Appendix C).

Feeding Schedule

When bottle-feeding is used, a demand schedule should be encouraged, as with the breast-fed infant. Bottle-fed babies should be fed only as much as they desire, although maternal pressure may subtly urge them to empty the bottle. This should be discouraged inasmuch as overfeeding at this age may establish a pattern of eating that eventually will result in obesity. Because the gastric emptying time of bottle-fed babies is longer, they require less frequent feedings than do breast-fed babies. An artificially fed infant usually shows a greater weight gain than a breast-fed infant. There is no evidence that this increased weight gain is desirable; indeed, it probably is not.

Whether breast- or bottle-fed, an infant who is fed on demand will adjust intake to needs for growth. The following patterns, with some variation, usually are established:

Age (mo)	Number of feedings per 24 hours
Birth-1	6-8
2-6	4-5
7-10	3-4
11-12	3

Age (mo)	Ounces per feeding
1	2-4
2	5
3	5-6
4	6-7
5-12	8

It should be noted that during the second or third month of life, most infants eliminate the night feeding.

Preparation of Formula

In the United States, most artificial feeding with cow milk is accomplished with proprietary formulas prepared commercially and supplied as "ready to feed" or "easy to mix" in presterilized bottles and cans. The ready-to-feed formulas are supplied with attached nipples in 4-, 6-, and 8-ounce disposable bottles and in 1-quart cans. Ready-to-feed formulas offer convenience to mothers who must travel with their infants and often are used as complementary and supplementary feedings for breast-fed babies, but they are too expensive for most families to use every day. Easy-to-mix, concentrated formulas are supplied in 13-ounce cans of liquid, which are mixed with equal amounts of water, and in 6-ounce cans of powder, which are mixed with appropriate amounts of water, usually in a 1 : 2 ratio.

In some parts of the United States and the rest of the world, the cost of commercially prepared formula is too high for mothers who cannot or choose not to breast-feed, and a home-prepared formula is used.

Calculation of the ingredients needed for a home-prepared infant formula made from whole cow milk (20 Cal/oz) or evaporated milk (44 Cal/oz) is based on four principles: (1) all formulas should contain milk, water, and carbohydrate and have an energy content of approximately 20 Cal/oz; (2) full-term infants require 110 to 120 Cal/kg and 150 to 180 ml of fluid per kilogram each day; (3) 2 ounces of evaporated

BOX 17-1

PREPARATION AND TERMINAL STERILIZATION OF INFANT FORMULA

Preparation

1. Measure the prescribed number of ounces of hot water into a clean quart pitcher.
2. Stir in the carbohydrate. Measure powdered sugar with a standard-size tablespoon and level each spoonful with a table knife.
3. Add the prescribed number of ounces of milk to the formula and stir to mix well.
4. Pour the formula into clean nursing bottles.
5. Put nipples and caps on the bottles, leaving the caps loose.

Sterilization

1. Put the bottles of formula on a rack in the sterilizer or deep kettle. Caps should be loose, not screwed on tightly. Put about 3 inches of water in the sterilizer, and cover.
2. Bring the water to a boil over moderate heat, then allow to boil gently (with the sterilizer still covered) for 25 minutes.
3. Remove the sterilizer from the heat. Leave it closed (do not even lift the lid) until the side of the sterilizer has cooled enough so that you can touch it with the palm of your hand.
4. Open the sterilizer. Then cool the bottles gradually, adding a small amount of cool water to the hot water in the sterilizer. (Gradual cooling prevents "skimming," which frequently causes nipple clogging.)
5. Remove the cooled bottles and screw the caps tight.
6. Store the bottles of formula in the refrigerator.

milk (EM) or 4 ounces of whole milk (WM) per kilogram are required each day; and (4) most infants require feeding five or six times every 24 hours. According to these principles, a 24-hour supply of formula for a 10-pound (4.5 kg) baby would consist of approximately 500 calories and 750 ml. The amount of EM required would be 10 ounces (300 ml),* which would provide 440 calories. The balance of fluid required (450 ml) would be made up with water, and the balance of 60 calories would be supplied with carbohydrates (e.g., table sugar, 60 Cal/tbsp; Karo, 60 Cal/tbsp; and Dextri-Maltose, 30 Cal/tbsp). The formula, then, would consist of 10 ounces of evaporated milk, 15 ounces of water, and 1 to 2 tablespoons of carbohydrate (depending on the kind used). The 25 ounces of formula would contain 500 calories, or 20 Cal/oz, and would be divided into five or six bottles, each containing 4 to 5 ounces. When larger amounts of formula are needed or when whole milk is used, the four formula principles can be met by either of the following mixtures: 13 ounces of EM, 19 ounces of water, and 120 calories (2 to 4 tablespoons) of carbohydrates; 23 ounces of WM, 9 ounces of water, and 180 calories (3 to 6 tablespoons) of carbohydrates. These formulas would meet the needs of a baby weighing 6 kg or more. A fifth principle of artificial feeding is that babies rarely require more than 1 quart of formula per 24 hours.

The method of mixing formulas described previously assumes that a full 24-hour supply will be prepared. Single 8-ounce feedings (3 ounces of EM, 5 ounces of water, and 30 calories of carbohydrate) or fractions thereof can be mixed, based on the amount the baby usually takes.

Depending on where the family lives, the mother may need to be instructed to prepare her infant's formula under aseptic conditions or to use terminal sterilization; milk is a rich culture medium, and significant contamination may result if neither of these methods is used in areas where the purity of the water supply is sometimes questionable. However, in most urban areas with safe water systems, sterilization is unnecessary. Box 17-1 presents, in instructional form, a step-by-step method of preparing and sterilizing infant formulas. This process should be followed when well water is used and when organism counts in tapwater are too high. Aseptic methods of preparing single feedings or 24-hour supplies of formula also can be used under these circumstances. With these methods, the water, bottles, nipples, and utensils must be boiled beforehand. Refrigerating prepared formula reduces the number of bacteria found in contaminated bottles. Realistically, as Kendall, Vaughn, and Kusakcioglu[10] and others have shown, fewer than 50% of mothers can prepare a sterile formula by using either method. If a pediatrician suspects that a mother is unlikely to use aseptic or terminal sterilization techniques, a presterilized proprietary formula or single-feeding mixture should be used. It probably is wise to use some form of sterile formula preparation during the first 4 months of life.

Although most mothers warm their infant's bottle before feeding, there is no evidence that babies prefer their milk warmed. Parents should be cautioned to avoid warming baby bottles in microwave ovens, which can result in overheating of the formula and can cause esophageal burns on ingestion. In addition, steam can form inside the bottle, causing an explosion.

VITAMIN SUPPLEMENTS

Except for vitamin K, most infants have adequate vitamin stores from birth until rapid postnatal growth ensues at 10 to 14 days of life; vitamin supplementation should begin by that time. Most commercially prepared formulas have an adequate vitamin content; therefore, except for babies who have special needs, infants given these formulas do not need additional vitamins. Although human milk can be expected to satisfy the recommended requirements for vitamins A, C, and E and the B vitamins, it may be advisable to provide breastfed infants a preparation containing the minimum daily requirement of vitamin D if the mother's vitamin D intake is

*For ease of calculation, 1 ounce is considered to contain 30 ml.

inadequate or if the mother's or infant's exposure to sunlight is limited.

Infants fed home-prepared formulas should receive supplemental vitamins (A, C, and D) as well as iron and fluoride. These are available commercially in a combination liquid (TRI-VI-FLOR with Iron), of which 1 ml is given orally by dropper daily.

FLUORIDE SUPPLEMENTS

All children older than 6 months of age living in areas that lack adequate fluoridation of the water supply should receive daily fluoride supplements because fluorides have been demonstrated to inhibit the development of dental caries (see Table 23-1 for fluoride supplemental dosage schedule).

IRON SUPPLEMENTATION IN INFANCY

The AAP's Committee on Nutrition recommends that during the first year of life, infants should have an iron intake of 1 mg/kg/day to a maximum of 15 mg/day to prevent the development of iron-deficiency anemia. Milk, both human and cow, is deficient in iron. Commercial formulas are supplemented with 8 to 12 mg of iron/liter. Breast-fed infants need not receive this amount of iron with their vitamin supplements because the small amount of iron in breast milk is almost completely bioavailable to the nursing infant; thus, breast milk provides sufficient iron until the sixth month of life. However, an iron preparation should be administered to the breast-fed infant who has low iron stores or anemia.

WEANING

Weaning customs vary considerably around the world. In many countries, babies routinely are nursed well into the second and sometimes the third year of life. The 1997 policy statement on breast-feeding of the American Academy of Pediatrics recommends nursing ideally for at least a year and as long thereafter as mother and child desire to continue. Both the World Health Organization and UNICEF recommend breast-feeding for at least 2 years. The emotional benefits that a mother and baby derive from breast-feeding are just as great at 9 months or at 1 year or even later. The age at which the infant is weaned from the breast should be based on a mutual decision between mother and infant. Child-led weaning is commonly practiced throughout the world; however, in the United States, various social and cultural factors, unfortunately, tend to dictate earlier weaning than in other countries. Mothers who are having a gratifying breast-feeding experience and who are made aware of the nutritional, immunological, and emotional benefits their nursing infants enjoy throughout and even beyond the breast-feeding period will want to continue as long as possible, and it behooves the pediatrician to urge them to do so. If weaning occurs when the infant is younger than 12 months of age, cow milk formula should be provided in a bottle or cup. The older infant may be weaned directly to whole milk from a bottle or cup.

The process of weaning should be gradual and should begin with substituting one breast-feeding with a bottle or cup feeding, usually at the midday meal. Once the bottle or cup is accepted, other breast-feedings are similarly eliminated and replaced gradually over a period of 1 to 4 weeks. The mother's milk supply will diminish during this time, as the stimulus of regular emptying of the breast is removed. However, many mothers are able to continue one or two daily breast-feedings over several months, should they so choose.

Occasionally, because of an illness in the mother or infant or the development of a complication of nursing, it is necessary to discontinue breast-feeding abruptly. To diminish the mother's discomfort, she should be instructed to wear a tight breast binder, reduce her fluid intake, and apply ice packs to her breasts. The administration of 20 mg of stilbestrol orally each day for 3 days is effective in reducing her discomfort and in "drying up" her milk supply but is seldom necessary. Whenever possible, weaning should not be instituted during very warm weather because some babies will initially refuse any feeding other than breast milk for as long as 24 to 48 hours. A formula-fed infant can be weaned from a bottle to whole cow milk from a cup by 12 months of age.

Skim milk should not be given to infants until they reach at least 2 years of age because, at a time when milk serves as the major source of food, skim milk would provide too few calories, an excessive protein intake, and an inadequate amount of essential fatty acids.

FEEDING SOLID FOODS

Introduction to Solid Foods

From a developmental point of view, there are cogent reasons why solids should not be added to the infant's diet before 4 to 6 months of age. When a solid object such as a spoon or a tongue depressor is introduced between the lips of a young baby, she purses her lips, raises her tongue, and pushes against the object vigorously (extrusion reflex). By 4 to 6 months the behavior changes so that when a spoon is inserted between the lips, they part, the tongue depresses, and food placed in the mouth is drawn to the back of the pharynx and swallowed. Thus, the physiologically appropriate time to begin feeding solids is somewhere between 4 and 6 months. It should be noted once again that the 1997 policy statement of the American Academy of Pediatrics recommends that solid food not be initiated until after 6 months.[1] Somewhat later, at about 7 to 9 months of age, rhythmic biting movements begin, even in the absence of teeth; foods requiring some chewing may be added to the diet at this time.

Schedule for Solid Foods

An appropriate regimen for introducing solid foods begins with grains and fruits. Rice cereal appears to be the least allergenic of the cereals and thus should be offered first. Progression through vegetables, meats, and eggs can be accomplished in the following manner:

5-6 mo	Cereals and fruits
6-7 mo	Meats and vegetables
7-8 mo	Egg yolk
8-9 mo	Egg white

To ensure an adequate amount of protein, fat, and carbohydrate during the sixth to twelfth months, infants should be offered and should consume no more than an average of 28 ounces of milk each day in addition to their quota of solids. An example of an infant diet in this age group follows:

Breakfast	Cereal and milk
Midmorning snack	Cup of orange juice
Lunch	Meat, yellow or green vegetables, fruit, milk
Midafternoon snack	Cup of orange juice or milk
Dinner	Cottage cheese or yogurt, egg, vegetable, fruit, and milk
Bedtime	Milk

Solid foods may be prepared easily from fresh ingredients and pureed by use of a food grinder or blender, or commercially prepared baby foods may be used.

In late infancy and particularly during the toddler period (12 to 30 months), a normal physiological decline in appetite occurs, paralleling the decrease in growth rate. The parents should be made aware both of this normal decline in interest in food, particularly at meal times, and of the concomitant reduction in milk intake, which may drop to 16 ounces a day by 24 to 36 months of age. By 4 to 7 years of age the appetite normally increases, as does the growth rate. The intake of *total* calories increases rapidly during the first year of life, then less rapidly to about age 4, and then rapidly again. The average full-term infant, by 7 to 10 days of life, will consume approximately 300 calories; thereafter, the first-year increment is nearly 600 Cal/day, the second-year increment nearly 275 Cal/day, the third- and fourth-year increments nearly 100 Cal/day, and the fifth- to seventh-year increments nearly 130 to 140 Cal/day. Thus, despite a decrease in appetite, the actual *intake of calories* does not decrease during the preschool period, and growth patterns remain satisfactory.

PRUDENT DIET FOR THE SCHOOL-AGE CHILD AND THE ADOLESCENT

The diet of a school-age child and an adolescent should be similar to that of an active adult; however, the extra caloric needs created by the period of rapid growth should be taken into account. Dietary habits and food preferences are closely linked with early associations and family influences. *Children will eat what they see their families eat.* Parents must be told that their infants and young toddlers, when they become older children and adults, will crave salt and sugar in their foods if that is what they have been accustomed to in early life. Basically, preparing foods without additives for infants and young children will ensure adequate nutrition and lay the groundwork for sound eating habits in later life.

The pediatrician is in a position to educate entire families in ways to eat more healthful foods in an attempt to prevent obesity and atherosclerosis. Physicians need to know the facts about good nutrition if they are to effect changes in the lifetime habits of families that involve consuming fewer calories and less fat, salt, and refined sugars.

The American Health Association has endorsed a prudent diet for the child and adolescent, which in simplified form has the following requirements:

A high-quality protein with every meal
Milk (preferably skimmed) with vitamin D added and other low-fat dairy products
Vegetables high in vitamin A
Fruits for vitamin C
Whole-grain or enriched breads or cereals
Vegetable oils high in polyunsaturated fats
Meat—four servings per week of 4 ounces each
Fish (a good source of polyunsaturated fats)—one to two times a week
Poultry (low fat)—one to two times a week
Dark green, leafy, or deep yellow vegetables—at least four times a week, preferably once a day
Eggs—a maximum of four a week

A prudent diet thus limits the use of fatty meats, high-fat dairy products, eggs, and hydrogenated shortenings and promotes the consumption of fish and the substitution of polyunsaturated vegetable oils and margarines for butter, lard, and other saturated fats.

REFERENCES

1. American Academy of Pediatrics Work Group on Breastfeeding: Breastfeeding and the use of human milk, *Pediatrics* 100:1035, 1997.
2. Berlin CM: Drugs and chemicals in breast milk, personal communication, June 26, 1989.
3. Committee on Drugs, American Academy of Pediatrics: The transfer of drugs and other chemicals into human milk, *Pediatrics* 93:137, 1994.
4. Cunningham AS, Jelliffe DB, Jellife EFP: Breast-feeding and health in the 1980s: a global epidemiological review, *J Pediatr* 118:659, 1991.
5. Eiger MS, Olds SW: *The complete book of breastfeeding,* ed 3, New York, 1999, Workman, Bantam.
6. Fomon SJ: *Infant nutrition,* ed 2, Philadelphia, 1980, WB Saunders.
7. Goldman AS: The immune system of human milk: antimicrobial, anti-inflammatory, and immunomodulating properties, *Pediatr Infect Dis J* 12:664, 1993.
8. Goldman AS, Smith CW: Host resistance factors in human milk, *J Pediatr* 82:1082, 1973.
9. Grules CG, Sanford HN: The influence of breast and artificial feeding on infantile eczema, *J Pediatr* 9:223, 1936.
10. Kendall N, Vaughn VC, Kusakcioglu A: Study of preparation of infant formulas, *Am J Dis Child* 122:215, 1936.
11. Lawrence RA: *Breastfeeding: a guide for the medical profession,* ed 5, St Louis, 1999, Mosby.
12. L'Esperance C, Frantz K: Time limitation for early breastfeeding, *J Obstet Gynecol Neonatal Nurs* 14:114, 1985.
13. Lozoff B, et al: The mother-newborn relationship: limits of adaptability, *J Pediatr* 91:1, 1977.
14. Montagu A: *Touching: the human significance of the skin,* New York, 1971, Harper & Row.
15. Newcomb PA, et al: Lactation and reduced risk of premenopausal breast cancer, *N Engl J Med* 330:82, 1994.
16. Olds SW: *The working parents' survival guide,* New York, 1983, Bantam.
17. Woolridge MW: Colic, "overfeeding," and symptoms of lactose malabsorption in the breast-fed baby: a possible artifact of feed management? *Lancet* 2:382, 1988.
18. Woolridge MW: The anatomy of infant sucking, *Midwifery* 2:166, 1986.

SUGGESTED READINGS

Auerbach KG, Riordan J: *Breastfeeding and human lactation,* Boston, 1993, Jones & Bartlett.

Bennett I, Simon M: *The prudent diet,* Port Washington, NY, 1973, David White.

Briggs G, Freeman R, Yaffe S: *Drugs in pregnancy and lactation,* ed 2, Baltimore, 1986, Williams & Wilkins.

Eiger MS, Olds SW: *The complete book of breastfeeding,* ed 3, New York, 1999, Workman, Bantam.

Eiger MS, Rausen AR, Silverio J: Morbidity of breast-fed vs bottle-fed infants, *Clin Pediatr* 23:9, 1984.

Winikoff B, Baer EC: The obstetrician's opportunity: translating "breast is best" from theory to practice, *Am J Obstet Gynecol* 138:105, 1980.

18 Immunizations

Sharon G. Humiston • Lance E. Rodewald • Peter G. Szilagyi

Vaccine-preventable diseases have left a legacy of suffering that must not be forgotten. We should remember our progress from a time when smallpox eradicated entire human communities to a time when humans eradicated wild smallpox. We also should remember that although in recent years we have made marked progress, there are children in this country and many children elsewhere who die when they lose their very personal battles with vaccine-preventable diseases.

Vaccination is one of the most important achievements in pubic health in the twentieth century. The most salient feature of this achievement is decreased disease levels. Compared with prevaccination-era disease levels, the current U.S. disease levels are from 97% to 100% lower. Recent immunization successes include the first-ever interruption of indigenous measles and rubella transmission in the United States in 1994 and the elimination of wild-type polio from the Western hemisphere, declared in 1994. Routine childhood vaccination is one of the few health care interventions that saves both lives and dollars; compared with a no-vaccination program, routine vaccination saves from $29 (for MMR vaccination) to $2 (for hepatitis B vaccination) for every dollar spent.

The primary reason for the record low disease incidence is record high immunization coverage levels—an achievement by the health care system that was accomplished during a period of increasing complexity in the immunization schedule. In 1996, the Childhood Immunization Initiative vaccination coverage goals for the U.S. were met. These goals included 90% immunization coverage levels for the most important doses of the recommended vaccines. Tables 18-l and 18-2 show the disease rates, immunization coverage levels, and benefit-to-cost ratios of the routine vaccines per dose administered. These successes were due largely to major efforts by private and public health care providers. Sustaining success will require even greater effort because the process of vaccinating children is becoming increasingly complicated as the number of vaccines and vaccine combination choices increases.

THE VACCINES

Principles of Vaccination

Live versus inactivated vaccines. Currently available vaccines are either live or inactivated.

Live vaccines include live, attenuated viruses (MMR, OPV, vaccinia, varicella, yellow fever); live, attenuated bacteria (BCG); and recombinant bacteria (oral typhoid). Inactivated vaccines include:

- inactivated viruses (IPV, hepatitis A, influenza, rabies)
- inactivated whole bacteria (whole-cell pertussis, typhoid, cholera, plague)
- inactivated subunits (acellular pertussis, hepatitis B, split-virus influenza, typhoid Vi, Lyme disease)
- toxoids (diphtheria, tetanus)
- polysaccharides (unconjugated—pneumococcal, meningococcal, or conjugated—Hib and pneumococcal)

Live vaccines replicate in the body. Live injected vaccines usually induce immunity through a single dose. Inactivated viruses do not replicate in the body and generally require three or more doses to immunize the patients completely. Live vaccines are susceptible to vaccine failure caused by circulating antibodies, including remaining maternal antibodies in infants, while inactivated vaccines are not susceptible to acquired antibodies passively.

Spacing and timing

THE ROUTINE SCHEDULE. In 1995, the routine vaccination schedule was harmonized among the American Academy of Pediatrics (AAP), the American Academy of Family Physicians (AAFP), and the Centers for Disease Control and Prevention (CDC) Advisory Committee on Immunization Practices (ACIP). The harmonized schedule is allowed to change once a year; updated versions are published annually in *Pediatrics,* usually in January. A copy of an always-current harmonized schedule is available from the CDC and at http://www.cdc.gov/nip. Fig. 18-1 shows the year 2000 recommended harmonized schedule.

The result of the harmonization was not necessarily a simplification of the schedule. Rather, the schedule was changed to reflect allowable differences in vaccination scheduling so that offices could most easily accommodate routine vaccination into their well-child care schedule.

INTERVALS BETWEEN DIFFERENT VACCINES NOT ADMINISTERED SIMULTANEOUSLY. It is safe and effective to use all vaccines simultaneously, provided that vaccines are not combined within a single syringe. There are no contraindications to giving any two different routine childhood vaccines at the same visit. In fact, there are no contraindications to simultaneous administration of any vaccines except cholera and yellow fever (which must be separated by at least 3 weeks).

Vaccines that are not administered simultaneously may be given without regard to intervals, with one exception: Live injected vaccines (e.g., MMR and varicella) that are not administered simultaneously should be separated by at least

Table 18-1 Incidence of Vaccine-Preventable Diseases

Disease	Maximum Cases	1997 Cases	% Change	1997 Vaccination Coverage Levels*
Diphtheria	206,939	5	−99.99	81%
Measles	894,134	135	−99.99	91%
Mumps	152,209	612	−99.59	–
Polio (wild-type, paralytic disease)	21,269	0	−100	91%
Rubella	57,686	161	−99.72	–
Congenital rubella syndrome	20,000†	4	−99.98	–
Tetanus	1560‡	43	−97.24	81%
H. Influenzae§ invasive disease (<5 yr of age)	20,000†	242	−98.79	93%
Pertussis	265,269	5519	−97.92	81%

From *MMWR* 46:1265, 1997, and *MMWR* 47:547, 1998.
*Estimated vaccination coverage among children ages 19 to 35 months for ≥4 doses of DTP/DtaP/DT, ≥1 of a measles-containing vaccine, ≥3 of Hib vaccine; United States, National Immunization Survey, 1997.
†Estimated.
‡Mortality.
§Includes invasive disease caused by non–type b *Haemophilus influenzae.*

Table 18-2 Benefit/Cost Analysis of Commonly Used Vaccines

Vaccine	Direct Medical Savings*	Direct and Indirect Savings*
DTP	$ 6.0	$30.1
MMR	$16.3	$21.3
OPV	$ 3.4	$ 6.1
Hib	$ 1.4	$ 2.2
Hepatitis B	$ 0.5	$ 2.0
Varicella	$ 0.9	$ 5.4

From Centers for Disease Control and Prevention.
*Per dose administered.

4 weeks. This "4-week separation rule" is intended to reduce the theoretical risk of interference from the first vaccine on the later vaccine. If, for example, varicella is given 1 week after an MMR, the varicella vaccine should be repeated or serological testing should be used to confirm seroconversion.

Providers, parents, and no doubt, children prefer fewer injections. As a consequence of increasing the number of diseases that can be prevented through vaccination, the number of required injections has increased dramatically. The number of combination vaccines is likely to increase, which will reduce the number of injections. Until that time, however, all vaccines for which the child is eligible should be offered whenever possible. This strategy not only keeps the child on schedule but also it prevents an additional, unnecessary office visit—a benefit to busy parents.

MINIMUM AGE AND INTERVALS BETWEEN DIFFERENT DOSES OF A MULTIDOSE VACCINE. Vaccine doses that are given too early in life or too soon after a previous dose may be ineffective. Table 18-3 shows the earliest acceptable ages of administration of the routinely recommended childhood vaccines and the minimum spacing between their doses.

Specific questions about the minimum spacing between vaccinations are the questions most commonly asked of the National Immunization Program information hotline. Providers frequently ask whether to count a vaccine dose given at an interval shorter than the minimum interval. For example, should a child who received two DTaP vaccines within fewer than 28 days be revaccinated? Was the first dose valid if a child received an MMR vaccination before 12 months of age? The ACIP is now reexamining its stand on these issues. At present, ACIP considers a vaccination invalid if the vaccine dose was incorrect, an inappropriate route of administration was used, or the interval between doses in a series was too short. Steps should be taken to prevent these errors from occurring, and it should be remembered that vaccination is a safe procedure, even if the child is overvaccinated. Overvaccination with live vaccines is without consequence (except for the rare allergic reaction) because the extra vaccine virus will not infect an already immune person. Overvaccination with inactivated vaccines might cause an increase in local reactions if antibody levels are high.

Prolonged intervals between doses of a multidose vaccination series do not diminish vaccine effectiveness. Series never need to be restarted because of prolonged intervals.

LATE-START OR INTERRUPTED SCHEDULE. Some children start routine vaccination late. The recommended compressed, "catch-up," or "accelerated" immunization schedule for such children is derived from the minimum intervals for the routine vaccinations. There are two accelerated schedules—one for children younger than 7 years of age and another for children 7 to 12 years of age who were not vaccinated previously. These are available in the AAP *Red Book* or from the CDC's National Immunization Program (NIP) (at 1-800-232-2522).

The presentation of a new patient whose vaccination status is unknown presents a challenge. In this situation, it is important to determine whether any immunization record exists for the child and, if so, to obtain a copy of the record or a report from the previous provider. If no record can be found, the vaccination series should be restarted using the accelerated schedule.

INTERVALS BETWEEN LIVE INJECTED VACCINES AND ANTIBODY-CONTAINING BLOOD PRODUCTS. Live injected vaccines (e.g., MMR and varicella vaccines), which have to replicate in the body to induce immunity, are compromised by circulating antibodies against the vaccine. Live oral vaccines (OPV and rotavirus) replicate in the gut and, therefore, are not affected by circulating antibodies. Inactivated vaccines are not affected by circulating antibodies and can be administered without regard to the relative timing of the administration of immune globulin-containing products.

MMR and varicella vaccine doses given 14 days *before* immune globulin-containing products are administered have time to replicate and are effective. When live injected vaccines are given *after* antibody-containing blood products, the situation is more complex. The specific immune globulin–containing product and its dose dictate the waiting period necessary before a valid dose of a live injected vaccine is given. MMR and varicella vaccination should be delayed from 3 months to 11 months, depending on the specific immune globulin preparation administered. Details of the appropriate waiting period can be found in the ACIP's General Recommendations on Immunization at http://www.cdc.gov/nip and in the AAP's *Red Book*.

Vaccinations administered in foreign countries. Determining the immunization status of foreign-born children or other children who have been partially or completely vaccinated in another country can be difficult. Vaccines differ, their abbreviations differ, and vaccination age criteria differ. The immunization status needs to be determined for all such children and special attention paid to the rest of the family in the case of recent immigration.

The first assumption to make is that the vaccines administered in other countries were as potent as those available in the United States. Then it becomes a matter of determining which vaccines were administered and whether the doses qualify as valid doses when considering the minimum ages of administration and the minimum time intervals between doses. Determining which vaccines were administered can be difficult because the standard abbreviations recorded in hand-held vaccination records are different from those used in the United States. Assistance can be obtained from your state immunization program or from the CDC's National Immunization program by calling 800-232-2522 or via e-mail at nipinfo@cdc.gov. Once the vaccine types are determined, Table 18-3 can be used to determine which doses are valid and which, if any, need to be repeated.

Variation in vaccination strategies creates a problem for clinicians caring for internationally adopted children as well as recent immigrants. Although there has been evidence that the documented vaccination status of foreign adopted children is not always accurate, the current recommendation when interpreting the vaccination status of international adoptees is that documented vaccinations (that include the doses and dates of administration) are acceptable proof of vaccination.

Contraindications and precautions

ANAPHYLACTIC ALLERGY. Anaphylactic type allergy to a vaccine or a vaccine component is a contraindication to further vaccination with that vaccine.

ENCEPHALOPATHY. Encephalopathy following a previous dose of a pertussis-containing vaccine is a contraindication to further vaccination with a pertussis-containing vaccine.

MINOR, ACUTE ILLNESSES. Some children will be ill at the time of a scheduled vaccination visit, and some children being seen at illness visits will be in need of vaccination. These two circumstances differ in important ways. Illness visits usually are short visits focused on diagnosis and treatment rather than on prevention and frequently are attended by a partner of the child's usual provider. To be overdue for a vaccination at an illness visit, a child generally will have to have missed a previously scheduled well-child visit. In contrast, children who happen to be ill at a well-child visit are at least attending a preventive visit that was initiated to vaccinate the child and to provide other preventive services. The two circumstances have the common dilemma of forcing the clinician to decide whether to recommend vaccination. This decision requires two types of clinical judgments: (1) whether it is safe to vaccinate the ill child, and (2) the likelihood that the child, if not vaccinated at the visit, will return for a scheduled vaccination.

Guidelines such as the AAP's *Red Book* and the ACIP's recommendations are available to help the clinician determine the safety of vaccinating an ill child. As a general rule, minor illnesses, including upper respiratory tract infections, otitis media, and diarrheal illnesses, whether or not febrile, are not valid contraindications to vaccination. A second, perhaps more difficult, consideration is whether minor vaccine side effects such as fever will cause diagnostic confusion during the follow-up period for the illness—a problem that may be especially difficult in situations involving very young infants.

Guidelines are not available to help the clinician determine the likelihood that the child will return for a scheduled vaccination visit. Although past appointment-keeping behavior will help in the judgment, it is not completely reliable. Predictive models have not been found that reliably determine the likelihood that a child will keep a preventive-visit appointment.

Because vaccinating children who have minor illnesses is safe and effective and because it may be unclear whether a child will be brought back for an appointment, it is best to err on the side of vaccinating the ill child, especially if he or she has missed previous preventive-care visits. This does involve additional effort by the clinician, but it will probably pay off in having patients who are better vaccinated. Table 18-4 shows a comparison of valid and invalid contraindications, and can be used as a guide to decision making.

IMMUNOCOMPROMISE. Immunocompromised children and their close contacts require individual attention. In general, live vaccines cannot be used in immunocompromised individuals, because of the potential for severe or fatal reactions from uncontrolled replication of the vaccine virus. Because inactivated vaccines cannot replicate, they are safe for use in immunocompromised children, but such children may have a diminished immune response to these vaccines.

Children who have congenital immunodeficiency, leukemia, lymphoma, or generalized malignancy should not receive live vaccines. Persons receiving treatments that cause immunosuppression—for example, alkylating agents, antimetabolites, and radiation therapy—also should not receive live vaccines. Persons receiving continuous, daily, large doses of corticosteroids—the equivalent of 2 mg/kg of prednisone per day—should not receive live virus vaccines. Live vaccine use is not contraindicated if the corticosteroid is aerosolized (as in asthma inhalers) or topical, nor if it is given on an alternate day, short course (fewer than 14 days),

Recommended Childhood Immunization Schedule United States, January - December 2000

Vaccines[1] are listed under routinely recommended ages. Bars indicate range of recommended ages for immunization. Any dose not given at the recommended age should be given as a "catch-up" immunization at any subsequent visit when indicated and feasible. Ovals indicate vaccines to be given if previously recommended doses were missed or given earlier than the recommended minimum age.

Age ▶ / Vaccine ▼	Birth	1 mo	2 mos	4 mos	6 mos	12 mos	15 mos	18 mos	24 mos	4-6 yrs	11-12 yrs	14-16 yrs
Hepatitis B[2]	Hep B (bar: Birth–2 mos)											
			Hep B (bar: 1–4 mos)			Hep B (bar: 6–18 mos)					(Hep B)	
Diphtheria, Tetanus, Pertussis[3]			DTaP	DTaP	DTaP		DTaP[3] (bar: 15–18 mos)			DTaP	Td (bar: 11–16 yrs)	
H. influenzae type b[4]			Hib	Hib	Hib	Hib (bar: 12–15 mos)						
Polio[5]			IPV	IPV		IPV[5] (bar: 6–18 mos)				IPV[5]		
Measles, Mumps, Rubella[6]						MMR (bar: 12–15 mos)				MMR[6]	(MMR[6])	
Varicella[7]						Var (bar: 12–18 mos)					(Var[7])	
Hepatitis A[8]									Hep A[8]-in selected areas (bar: 24 mos–12 yrs)			

Approved by the Advisory Committee on Immunization Practices (ACIP), the American Academy of Pediatrics (AAP), and the American Academy of Family Physicians (AAFP).

On October 22, 1999, the Advisory Committee on Immunization Practices (ACIP) recommended that Rotashield (RRV-TV), the only US-licensed rotavirus vaccine, no longer be used in the United States (MMWR Morb Mortal Wkly Rep. Nov 5, 1999;48(43):1007). Parents should be reassured that their children who received rotavirus vaccine before July are not at increased risk for intussusception now.

1 This schedule indicates the recommended ages for routine administration of currently licensed childhood vaccines as of 11/1/99. Additional vaccines may be licensed and recommended during the year. Licensed combination vaccines may be used whenever any components of the combination are indicated and its other components are not contraindicated. Providers should consult the manufacturers' package inserts for detailed recommendations.

2 **Infants born to HBsAg-negative mothers** should receive the 1st dose of hepatitis B (Hep B) vaccine by age 2 months. The 2nd dose should be at least 1 month after the 1st dose. The 3rd dose should be administered at least 4 months after the 1st dose and at least 2 months after the 2nd dose, but not before 6 months of age for infants.
Infants born to HBsAg-positive mothers should receive hepatitis B vaccine and 0.5 mL hepatitis B immune globulin (HBIG) within 12 hours of birth at separate sites. The 2nd dose is recommended at 1 month of age and the 3rd dose at 6 months of age.
Infants born to mothers whose HBsAg status is unknown should receive hepatitis B vaccine within 12 hours of birth. Maternal blood should be drawn at the time of delivery to determine the mother's HBsAg status; if the HBsAg test is positive, the infant should receive HBIG as soon as possible (no later than 1 week of age).
All children and adolescents (through 18 years of age) who have not been immunized against hepatitis B may begin the series during any visit. Special efforts should be made to immunize children who were born in or whose parents were born in areas of the world with moderate or high endemicity of hepatitis B virus infection.

3 The 4th dose of DTaP (diphtheria and tetanus toxoids and acellular pertussis vaccine) may be administered as early as 12 months of age, provided 6 months have elapsed since the 3rd dose and the child is unlikely to return at age 15 to 18 months. Td (tetanus and diphtheria toxoids) is recommended at 11 to 12 years of age if at least 5 years have elapsed since the last dose of DTP, DTaP, or DT. Subsequent routine Td boosters are recommended every 10 years.

4 Three *Haemophilus influenzae* type b (Hib) conjugate vaccines are licensed for infant use. If PRP-OMP (PedvaxHIB or ComVax [Merck]) is administered at 2 and 4 months of age, a dose at 6 months is not required. Because clinical studies in infants have demonstrated that using some combination products may induce a lower immune response to the Hib vaccine component, DTaP/Hib combination products should not be used for primary immunization in infants at 2, 4, or 6 months of age unless FDA-approved for these ages.

5 To eliminate the risk of vaccine-associated paralytic polio (VAPP), an all-IPV schedule is now recommended for routine childhood polio vaccination in the United States. All children should receive four doses of IPV at 2 months, 4 months, 6 to 18 months, and 4 to 6 years. OPV (if available) may be used only for the following special circumstances:

1. Mass vaccination campaigns to control outbreaks of paralytic polio.
2. Unvaccinated children who will be traveling in <4 weeks to areas where polio is endemic or epidemic.
3. Children of parents who do not accept the recommended number of vaccine injections. These children may receive OPV only for the third or fourth dose or both; in this situation, health care professionals should administer OPV only after discussing the risk for VAPP with parents or caregivers.
4. During the transition to an all-IPV schedule, recommendations for the use of remaining OPV supplies in physicians' offices and clinics have been issued by the American Academy of Pediatrics (see *Pediatrics*, December 1999).

6 The 2nd dose of measles, mumps, and rubella (MMR) vaccine is recommended routinely at 4 to 6 years of age but may be administered during any visit, provided at least 4 weeks have elapsed since receipt of the 1st dose and that both doses are administered beginning at or after 12 months of age. Those who have not previously received the second dose should complete the schedule by the 11- to 12-year-old visit.

7 Varicella (Var) vaccine is recommended at any visit on or after the first birthday for susceptible children, ie, those who lack a reliable history of chickenpox (as judged by a health care professional) and who have not been immunized. Susceptible persons 13 years of age or older should receive 2 doses, given at least 4 weeks apart.

8 Hepatitis A (Hep A) is shaded to indicate its recommended use in selected states and/or regions; consult your local public health authority. (Also see *MMWR Morb Mortal Wkly Rep*. Oct 01, 1999;48(RR-12); 1-37).

Fig. 18-1 Recommended childhood immunization schedule, United States, January-December 2000. Approved by the Advisory Committee on Immunization Practices (ACIP), the American Academy of Pediatrics (AAP), and the American Academy of Family Physicians (AAFP).

Table 18-3 Minimum Age for Initial Vaccination and Minimum Interval Between Vaccine Doses, by Type of Vaccine

Vaccine	Minimum Age for Dose 1[a]	Minimum Interval from Dose 1 to 2[a]	Minimum Interval from Dose 2 to 3[a]	Minimum Interval from Dose 3 to 4[a]
DTP/DTaP (DT)[b]	6 wk	4 wk	4 wk	6 months
DTP-Hib	6 wk	4 wk	4 wk	6 months
Hib (primary series)				
HbOC	6 wk	4 wk	4 wk	[c]
PRP-T	6 wk	4 wk	4 wk	[c]
PRP-OMP	6 wk	4 wk	[c]	
Polio[d]	6 wk	4 wk	4 wk[e]	[f]
MMR	12 months[g]	4 wk		
Hepatitis B	Birth	4 wk	8 wk[h]	
Varicella	12 months	4 wk		

From Atkinson W, et al: *Epidemiology and prevention of vaccine-preventable diseases,* ed 5, Department of Health and Human Services, Centers for Disease Control and Prevention, 1999.
[a]These minimum acceptable ages and intervals may not correspond with the optimal recommended ages and intervals for vaccination. See tables 3 to 5 in the Advisory Committee on Immunization Practices' (ACIP) *General recommendations on immunization.*
[b]The number of doses of diphtheria and tetanus toxoids should not exceed six *each* before the seventh birthday.
[c]The booster dose of Hib vaccine that is recommended following the primary vaccination series should be administered no earlier than age 12 months *and* at least 8 weeks after the previous dose of Hib vaccine. See tables 3 and 4 of the ACIP's *General recommendations on immunization.*
[d]All-IPV, sequential IPV/OPV, or all OPV.
[e]Unvaccinated adults who expect to be at increased risk of exposure to poliovirus need IPV. If they have longer than 2 months but less than 3 months before protection is needed, 3 doses of IPV should be administered at 4-week intervals.
[f]In an all-IPV or all-OPV schedule, if the third dose is given after the third birthday, the fourth (booster) dose is not needed.
[g]Although the age for measles vaccination may be as young as 6 months in outbreak areas where cases are occurring in children younger than 1 year of age, children initially vaccinated before their first birthday should be revaccinated at 12 to 15 months of age, and an additional dose of vaccine should be administered at the time of school entry or according to local policy. Doses of MMR or other measles-containing vaccines should be separated by at least 4 weeks.
[h]This final dose is recommended at least 4 months after the first dose and no earlier than those infants 6 months of age.

or if the child is on a physiological replacement schedule. For vaccination of bone marrow transplant patients, the *Red Book* should be consulted. Notably, children who have *asymptomatic* HIV infection may receive MMR and varicella vaccines, but children who have symptomatic HIV infection should not receive either of these vaccines. People with immunocompromise limited to humoral immunodeficiency (e.g., IgA deficiency) also may be routinely vaccinated with varicella vaccine.

The only vaccine contraindicated for a person living with an immunocompromised household contact is OPV. Inactivated polio vaccine should be substituted for OPV. MMR and varicella vaccines also should be given if indicated.

PREGNANCY. Pregnant women should not receive live injected vaccines because of the theoretical risk of fetal damage. Pregnant women may receive inactivated vaccines such as hepatitis B, Td, and influenza vaccines. If polio protection needs boosting during pregnancy, OPV is the preferred vaccine.

PREMATURITY. Preterm infants should be vaccinated by using the routine schedule and the standard doses of vaccine. Exceptions to this are: (1) premature infants who remain hospitalized should not receive live oral vaccines until discharged and of the appropriate age and (2) to maximize vaccine efficacy, infants weighing fewer than 2000 g and whose mothers are hepatitis B surface antigen negative should not receive hepatitis B vaccine until they reach a body weight of 2000 g. Infants whose mothers' hepatitis B surface antigen status is positive should receive the vaccine. If the mother's hepatitis B surface antigen is unknown, hepatitis B immune globulin should be given within 12 hours of birth regardless of weight.

Universal Childhood Vaccines

This section describes the individual vaccines that are recommended for routine administration to all healthy children and the vaccines that are recommended for targeted administration. Travel-related vaccines will not be described in this chapter, but details on these vaccines can be obtained through the CDC at (404) 332-4559, in the *Yellow Book Online* at http://www.cdc.gov/travel, and in the AAP's *Red Book.*

Diphtheria, tetanus, pertussis (DTaP) vaccine. DTaP is the recommended form of the oldest combination vaccine, DTP, which is a combination of diphtheria toxoid, tetanus toxoid, and acellular pertussis vaccine. Vaccination against tetanus and diphtheria has been highly successful. For example, the prevaccination annual incidences of tetanus and diphtheria were more than 1500 and 200,000, respectively. In 1996, zero cases of tetanus and only four cases of diphtheria were reported (none in children younger than 5 years of age). Pertussis has been a more recalcitrant disease, with more than 5000 cases reported in 1995. However, that is still a decrease of 98% from the prevaccination incidence of more than 250,000 cases annually.

DTaP is licensed for all of the preschool doses. Currently, no pertussis vaccine is licensed for children older than 7 years of age. Unfortunately, pertussis is not uncommon in older children and adults, who represent a reservoir for the bacteria and a continuing source of danger for young children. This clearly is problematic because younger children have the greatest morbidity and mortality from the disease.

DTaP, DTP, or DTP/Hib vaccines should arrive at the office unfrozen and should be refrigerated upon arrival at a temperature of 2° to 8° C. The shelf life is up to 1 year. The

Table 18-4 Guide to Contraindications and Precautions to Immunizations

Vaccine	True Contraindications and Precautions	Not True (Vaccines May Be Given)
General for All Vaccines (DTP/DTaP, IPV, MMR, Hib, Hep A, Hep B, Var, PPV, Flu)	Anaphylactic reaction to a vaccine contraindicates further doses of that vaccine Anaphylactic reaction to a vaccine constituent contraindicates the use of vaccines containing that substance Moderate or severe illnesses with or without a fever	Mild to moderate local reaction (soreness, redness, swelling) following a dose of an injectable antigen Fever following a prior vaccine dose Mild acute illness with or without low-grade fever Current antimicrobial therapy Convalescent phase of illnesses Prematurity (same dosage and indications as for normal, full-term infants) Recent exposure to an infectious disease History of penicillin or other nonspecific allergies or family history of such allergies Pregnancy of mother or household contact Unvaccinated household contact
DTP/DTaP	Encephalopathy within 7 days of administration of previous dose of DTP/DTaP Precautions[a] Fever ≥40.5° C (105° F) within 48 hours after vaccination with a prior dose of DTP/DTaP and not attributable to another identifiable cause Collapse or shocklike state (hypotonic-hyporesponsive episode) within 48 hr of receiving a prior dose of DTP/DTaP Seizures within 3 days of receiving a prior dose of DTP/DTaP (see footnote 2[b] regarding management of children with a personal history of seizures at any time) Persistent, inconsolable crying lasting ≥3 hours, within 48 hours of receiving a prior dose of DTP/DTaP Guillain-Barré syndrome (GBS) within 6 wk after a prior dose[c]	Temperature of <40.5° C (105° F) following a previous dose of DTP/DTaP Family history of convulsions[b] Family history of sudden infant death syndrome (SIDS) Family history of an adverse event following DTP/DTaP administration
IPV	Anaphylactic reaction to neomycin, streptomycin, or polymyxin B Precaution[a] Pregnancy	
MMR[g]	Anaphylactic reaction to neomycin or gelatin Pregnancy Known immunodeficiency (hematological and solid tumors, congenital immunodeficiency, long-term immunosuppressive therapy, HIV infection with evidence of severe immunosuppression) Precautions[a] Recent (within 3-11 months, depending on product and dose) administration of a blood product or immune globulin preparation Thrombocytopenia[e] History of thrombocytopenic purpura[e]	Tuberculosis or positive PPD Simultaneous tuberculin skin testing[d] Breast-feeding Pregnancy of mother or household contact of vaccine recipient Immunodeficient family member or household contact Asymptomatic HIV infection Allergic reaction to eggs[f] Nonanaphylactic reactions to neomycin

Continued

Table 18-4 Guide to Contraindications and Precautions to Immunizations—cont'd

Vaccine	True Contraindications and Precautions		Not True (Vaccines May Be Given)
Hib	None		
Hep A	Anaphylactic reaction to alum or (*for Havrix only*) 2-phenoxyethanol		Immunodeficiency
Hep B	Anaphylactic reaction to baker's yeast		Pregnancy
Varicella[g] (Var)	Anaphylactic reaction to neomycin or gelatin Pregnancy Known immunodeficiency (hematological and solid tumors, congenital immunodeficiency, long-term immunosuppressive therapy, symptomatic HIV)		Immunodeficiency in a household contact Household contact with HIV Pregnancy in the mother or other household contact of the recipient
	Precautions[a]	Recent (within 5 months) IG administration[h] Family history of immunodeficiency[i]	
Pneumococcal (PPV and PCV)	None		
	Precautions[a]	Pregnancy	
Influenza (Flu)	None		Pregnancy Breast-feeding
	Precautions[a]	Anaphylactic reaction to eggs	

Modified from the Minnesota Department of Health.

[a]Precautions, though not outright contraindications, indicate a need to weigh the risks and benefits of giving specific vaccines under specific circumstances. Administer the vaccine if the benefits outweigh the risks (e.g., during an outbreak or for foreign travel). Withhold the vaccine if the risks outweigh the benefits. Whether and when to administer DTP/DTaP to children with proven or suspected underlying neurological disorders should be decided on an individual basis. Although there is no evidence that any live vaccine (including rubella) causes birth defects, it is prudent on theoretical grounds to avoid vaccinating pregnant women with live virus vaccines. Inactivated vaccines should be administered to pregnant women for whom they are indicated.

[b]DTP/DTaP and convulsions: Consider giving acetaminophen or ibuprofen before administering DTP/DTaP and thereafter every 4 or 6 hours for 24 hours for children with a personal history of convulsions or such history in siblings or parents.

[c]DTP/DTaP and GBS: The decision to give additional doses of DTP/DTaP should be based on consideration of the benefit of further vaccination versus the risk of recurrence of GBS. For example, completion of the primary series in children is justified.

[d]MMR and TB testing: Because measles vaccination may temporarily suppress tuberculin reactivity, give MMR vaccine after, or on the same day, as TB testing. If, however, MMR was given recently, postpone the TB test for 4 to 6 weeks. If giving MMR simultaneously with tuberculin skin test, use the Mantoux test and not multiple puncture tests, because the latter require confirmation if positive, which would have to be postponed 4 to 6 weeks.

[e]MMR and thrombocytopenia: When deciding whether to vaccinate, consider the benefits of immunity to measles, mumps, and rubella versus the risk of recurrence or exacerbation of thrombocytopenia, either following vaccination or from natural infections of measles or rubella. In most instances, the benefits of vaccination greatly exceed the potential risks and will justify giving MMR, particularly in view of the even greater risk of thrombocytopenia following measles or rubella disease. However, if a prior episode of thrombocytopenia occurred within approximately 6 weeks after a previous dose, it might be prudent to avoid a subsequent dose.

[f]MMR and egg allergy: Recent data suggest that most anaphylactic reactions to measles- and mumps-containing vaccines are associated with hypersensitivity, not to egg antigens, but to other components of the vaccines. Because the risk of anaphylactic reactions after administration of measles- and mumps-containing vaccines in persons who are allergic to eggs is extremely low and skin testing with vaccine is not predictive of allergic reactions to these vaccines, skin testing and desensitization are no longer required before administration of MMR vaccine to persons who are allergic to eggs.

[g]MMR and varicella: Administer MMR and varicella vaccines to healthy children older than 12 months of age either on the same day or ≥28 days apart.

[h]Varicella and IG: Do not give varicella vaccine for at least 5 months after administration of blood (except washed red blood cells), or plasma transfusions, immune globulin, or VZIG. Do not give immune globulin or VZIG for 3 weeks following vaccination unless the benefits exceed those of the vaccination. A patient who receives IG within 3 weeks of varicella vaccine will need to either be revaccinated 5 months later or tested for immunity 6 months later and revaccinated if seronegative.

[i]Varicella and immunodeficiency: Varicella vaccine should not be given to a member of a household with a family history of immunodeficiency until the immune status of the recipient and other children in the family is documented.

This guide is based on recommendations of the Advisory Committee on Immunization Practices (ACIP) and those of the Committee on Infectious Diseases (*Red Book* Committee) of the American Academy of Pediatrics (AAP). Sometimes these recommendations vary from those contained in the manufacturers' package inserts. For more detailed information, providers should consult the published recommendations of the ACIP, AAP, the American Academy of Family Practice (AAFP), and the manufacturers' package inserts. Questions should be directed to the Minnesota Immunization Hotline at (612) 676-5100 or (800) 657-3970. Website: www.health.state.mn.us/divs/dpc/adps/adps.htm.

vials must be shaken vigorously before withdrawing the individual doses.

The vaccine is administered intramuscularly by using a dose of 0.5 ml. Children older than 7 years of age in need of tetanus toxoid should receive adult-type Td, which contains a lower dose of diphtheria toxoid, to minimize adverse reactions.

Acellular pertussis vaccine has replaced whole-cell pertussis vaccine as the recommended vaccine against whooping cough. The acellular pertussis vaccine is as immunogenic but has fewer adverse side effects than the whole-cell vaccine. Because the licensed acellular pertussis vaccines contain different components, one should complete the pertussis vaccination series with vaccine from the same manufacturer. When this is not feasible, it is not necessary to revaccinate individuals with the same manufacturer's product to complete the vaccination series. The series can be finished with any of the acellular vaccines. Similarly, DTaP can be used to complete an immunization series started with DTP.

Adverse reactions to diphtheria and tetanus toxoids include: (1) local reactions, such as redness and induration, (2) nodule at the injection site, and (3) Arthus-type hypersensitivity reactions. Mild adverse reactions to DTaP include (1) local reactions of redness, swelling, induration, and tenderness and (2) systemic reactions of drowsiness, vomiting, crying, and low-grade fever. Moderate to severe reactions include high fevers of 40.5° C (105° F) or more, persistent and inconsolable crying of more than 3 hours' duration, hypotonic-hyporesponsive episodes, and febrile seizures. All of these reactions occur much less frequently with DTaP than with DTP, and all are believed to occur without permanent sequelae.

Contraindications to DTaP vaccination include an anaphylactic reaction caused by a previous dose and encephalopathy within 7 days of a previous dose. Precautions to DTaP include a convulsion within 3 days of a previous dose; persistent, severe, inconsolable screaming or crying for 3 or more hours within 48 hours of a previous dose; collapse or shock-like state within 48 hours of a previous dose; and a temperature of 40.5° C (105° F), unexplained by another cause, within 48 hours of a previous dose.

Hepatitis B vaccine. Vaccination with hepatitis B vaccine prevents hepatitis B and its complications, which include hepatocellular cancer. Thus, hepatitis B vaccine is the first anticancer vaccine. In the United States there are an estimated 200,000 to 300,000 new hepatitis B infections annually, with 20,000 to 30,000 new carriers per year. Risk factors for hepatitis B infection are lifestyles, occupations, or environments in which contact with blood from infected persons occurs frequently.

The strategy of targeting hepatitis B vaccination toward high-risk persons failed to control the disease. In 1991, the targeted strategy was replaced with universal infant vaccination, which was, in turn, augmented with universal adolescent vaccination in 1996. In addition, current control measures include (1) prenatal testing of pregnant women to identify newborn infants in need of immunoprophylaxis and household contacts in need of vaccination, and (2) vaccination of high-risk adults. It should be remembered that children and adolescents who have not yet been vaccinated should be vaccinated at the earliest opportunity. For the next several years, the most common reason for lack of vaccination will be because the children were born before the adoption of universal infant vaccination against hepatitis B. Thus, this population represents a cohort of children at risk who need to be vaccinated.

Two recombinant hepatitis B vaccines are licensed for use in the United States. Both are made by inserting the gene for hepatitis B surface antigen protein into baker's yeast. The altered yeast produces large quantities of hepatitis B surface antigen, which then is purified.

The vaccine should arrive at the office with a refrigerant, but unfrozen. It should be refrigerated upon arrival and stored at 2° to 8° C. The vaccine should not be frozen. The shelf life is up to 3 years.

A vaccination series started with one manufacturer's product can be completed with the other manufacturer's product. The seroconversion rate is greater than 95% for infants, children, and adolescents receiving all three doses. The vaccine is 80% to 100% effective at preventing infection.

A three-dose schedule is recommended for active immunization. For routine infant immunization, the initial dose can be given in the hospital, postnatally. The *minimum* intervals between doses include:

Between the first and second doses	1 month
Between the second and third doses	2 months
Between the first and third doses	4 months

The third dose should be administered at the time or after the infant turns 6 months of age. For infants, children, and adolescents, the dose is 0.5 ml of either the pediatric formulation of Recombivax HB or Engerix B.

A contraindication to the administration of hepatitis B vaccine is a serious allergic reaction to a prior dose of hepatitis B vaccine. The most common adverse event following hepatitis B vaccine is pain at the injection site. Mild systemic complaints, including fatigue, headache, and irritability, occur in fewer than 20% of children. Low-grade fever occurs in up to 6.4% of children. Serious systemic adverse events and allergic reactions are rare.

HIGH-RISK GROUPS FOR HEPATITIS B. High-risk groups include Alaskan Natives, American Asian and Pacific Islanders, and children of immigrants or refugee families from countries having high rates of hepatitis B infection. Special efforts should be made to bring these children in for vaccination.

BABIES BORN TO HEPATITIS B SURFACE ANTIGEN POSITIVE MOTHERS. All pregnant women should be screened for hepatitis B surface antigen (HBsAg), and the results of the test should be known by the time of delivery so that perinatal transmission can be prevented by a combination of hepatitis B vaccination and administration of hepatitis B immune globulin (HBIG). The regimen is approximately 95% effective in preventing transmission.

Infants born to HBsAg positive women should receive a dose of hepatitis B vaccine and a dose of HBIG (at a different injection site) within 12 hours of birth. The second dose of vaccine should be given at 1 to 2 months of age, and the third dose should be given at 6 months of age. If born to an HbsAg positive mother, preterm infants weighing less than 2000 g at birth require a total of four doses of vaccine—the dose given shortly after birth with the HBIG and three more doses—starting just before hospital discharge (if the infant weighs 2 kg or more) or at approximately 2 months of age.

Infants born to mothers who were not tested for HBsAg should receive an initial dose of hepatitis B vaccine within 12 hours of birth. The mother should be tested immediately, and if she tests positive, the baby should receive HBIG within 7 days.

The *Red Book* or ACIP guidelines should be consulted for dose volumes and additional details for this critical preventive measure.

LOW-BIRTH-WEIGHT INFANTS. Hepatitis B vaccination should be postponed if an infant is born to an HBsAg negative woman and weighs fewer than 2000 g. Low-birth-weight infants whose mother's surface antigen status is positive or unknown should receive immediate vaccination and HBIG, as previously described.

THIMEROSAL. Thimerosal is a mercury-based preservative found in many inactivated vaccines packaged in multidose vials. Because of concerns about whether vaccination with thimerosal-containing vaccines constitutes a significant exposure for infants, thimerosal has been removed from some infant vaccines. At least one brand of every vaccine does not contain thimerosal as a preservative. If hepatitis B vaccine free of thimerosal preservative is *not* available, then infants should be vaccinated with thimerosal-containing vaccine, but the age of vaccination varies with the infant's level of risk for contracting hepatitis B infection, as follows:

- Infants of mothers who are HBsAg positive or untested at the end of pregnancy should receive the vaccine at birth
- Infants of mothers who are HBsAg negative, but in a high-risk group should receive the vaccine at birth to 2 months of age
- Infants of low-risk mothers who are HBsAg negative should receive the vaccine at 2 months of age

Haemophilus influenzae type b vaccine. The near-elimination of invasive Hib disease in the United States is a success story that happened within the careers of most practicing primary care providers. In the prevaccination era, an estimated 20,000 cases of invasive Hib disease occurred annually. The most recent surveillance data show that the annual number of cases decreased by 99%.

The Hib vaccines in use today are conjugated vaccines in which the polysaccharide component of the capsule (polyribosylribitol phosphate [PRP]) is bonded chemically to a protein carrier to enhance immunogenicity (especially in infants) and response to booster doses. Available vaccines vary by the carrier protein to which PRP is bonded. Carriers include diphtheria toxoid (PRP-D), a *Neisseria meningitidis* outer membrane protein complex (PRP-OMP), a mutant diphtheria toxin (HbOC), and tetanus toxoid (PRP-T). Hib vaccine has high efficacy—approximately 97% following three doses.

Hib vaccines should arrive in insulated containers to prevent freezing. They should arrive not frozen and should be refrigerated immediately and stored between 2° and 8° C. Freezing reduces potency. Shelf life is up to 2 years. Stability after reconstitution should be determined by consulting the manufacturer's package insert.

The differences among the vaccines result in slightly different administration schedules. The most important difference is that the PRP-D product is only for use in children between 15 and 59 months of age. Hib vaccine also is marketed in several combination vaccines, including separate combinations with DTaP and hepatitis B vaccines. The schedule for Hib vaccination is complicated because different brands of Hib vaccine require different numbers of doses and because the number of doses depends on the age at which the series is started. The package insert should be consulted for product-specific dosing schedules. It is acceptable practice to complete the series with a different Hib product from the product used to start the Hib vaccination series.

Adverse events following Hib vaccination are unusual. Between 5% and 30% will have a local reaction consisting of swelling, redness, or pain. Systemic adverse events such as fever are uncommon.

The only contraindications to Hib vaccination are previous history of anaphylaxis resulting from prior Hib vaccination or moderate to severe concurrent illness.

Polio vaccine. Polio vaccination has been so successful that "wild type" paralytic polio has been eliminated from the Americas. The peak annual incidence of paralytic polio in the United States was 21,269 cases. Since 1979, the only remaining cause of polio in the United States is vaccine-associated paralytic polio (VAPP) among recipients of oral polio vaccine or their close contacts. During America's primary reliance on OPV, 5 to 10 cases of VAPP occurred each year.

There are two licensed products for polio vaccination: enhanced-potency, inactivated polio vaccine (IPV, or Salk vaccine) and oral polio vaccine (OPV, or Sabin vaccine). IPV is administered subcutaneously (or intramuscularly) with a dose of 0.5 ml. IPV is the only type of polio vaccine that can be used for immunocompromised individuals. It consists of formaldehyde-killed polio virus. OPV, in contrast, is a live, attenuated vaccine that is administered orally.

IPV should arrive at the office unfrozen and should be refrigerated between 2° and 8° C. The shelf life is up to 18 months. The product comes as 10-dose vials or single-dose ampules. OPV is no longer manufactured for use in the United States.

For either IPV or OPV, a total of four polio vaccinations is required before school entry—three doses in the primary series and one supplementary dose. If an all-IPV or all-OPV schedule is used and the third dose is administered after the child's fourth birthday, no supplemental dose is indicated.

To reduce the incidence of vaccine-associated paralytic polio (VAPP) and to assure the public that the safest vaccines are recommended, beginning in January 2000, ACIP recommended an all-IPV series. OPV, which is no longer manufactured for use in the United States, should be used if a previously unvaccinated child is traveling to a polio-endemic country in fewer than 4 weeks, if parents of a child with 2 doses of IPV refuse to allow further injections, or if there should be an outbreak of paralytic polio.

Adverse effects following OPV are limited to VAPP. Approximately one third of VAPP cases occur in healthy OPV recipients; another one third occur in contacts of OPV recipients, and another third occur in immunocompromised individuals. No serious adverse effects have been reported following IPV.

Rotavirus. Rotavirus, the most common cause of severe diarrhea in infants and young children in the United States, is estimated to account for about 50,000 hospitalizations each year among children younger than 5 years old. Rotavirus also accounts for about 500,000 physician visits each year; 10 to 40 children die each year from rotavirus disease.

In prelicensure studies, a live oral rotavirus vaccine, known as *RRV-TV* (rhesus rotavirus tetravalent), was 49% to 68% effective in preventing any rotavirus diarrhea and 64% to 91% effective in preventing severe diarrhea. It was licensed for use in the United States on August 31, 1998, but even before that, in June 1998, the ACIP recommended routine immunization of all full-term infants. It was known that temperature of ≥38° C (100.4° F) attributable to the vaccine occurred in 3% to 25% of vaccine recipients, usually 3 to 5 days after the first dose, but during post-marketing surveillance the possibility of a more serious side effect, intussusception, arose. Consequently, the CDC in July 1999 announced its recommendation to postpone further use of rotavirus vaccine while studies progressed and, in October 1999, announced its recommendation that the vaccine "no longer be given for infants in the United States" because of a positive association with intussusception.

Several other rotavirus vaccine formulations are in development, but it is not known when or if any of these will be licensed for use. Until that time, secondary prevention measures, especially the proper use of oral rehydration solution, is urged.

Measles, mumps, rubella (MMR) vaccine. The MMR vaccine is a combination of three live, attenuated vaccines that together protect against measles, mumps, and rubella. The purpose of the measles and mumps vaccines is to protect against those specific diseases; the purpose of the rubella vaccine is to prevent congenital rubella syndrome by preventing the occurrence of rubella (which, itself, is a mild disease) in the general population, thereby preventing its spread to susceptible pregnant women. The incidence of measles in the prevaccination era has been reduced more than 99%, from 894,134 cases to fewer than 500 per year. Mumps and rubella incidences also have been reduced by more than 99%.

One strain of measles vaccine is available—the Moretan strain, which is grown in chick fibroblast culture. It initially was licensed in 1968. Highly immunogenic, a single dose causes seroconversion in more than 95% of recipients vaccinated at age 15 months or later. For mumps, a single strain of vaccine (Jeryl Lynn) is available. It was licensed in 1967 and causes a seroconversion rate of more than 90%. And, for rubella, a single strain of vaccine is available (RA 27/3). Created by passage through human diploid fibroblasts and licensed in 1979, it causes seroconversion in more than 95% of recipients.

MMR vaccine should arrive at the office in an insulated container at a temperature <10° C. It should be refrigerated upon arrival and stored between 2° and 8° C (never frozen). The shelf life is up to 2 years; the expiration date is marked on the vials. Upon reconstitution, the vaccine should be stored in a dark place between 2° and 8° C, and must be used within 8 hours.

The AAP and ACIP both recommend administration of two 0.5-ml doses of MMR vaccine subcutaneously—one at 12 to 15 months of age and the second before elementary school entry. The purpose of the second dose is to immunize children who failed to respond to the initial dose of MMR; the recommendation to give a second dose was made in 1989 because of the persistence of epidemics of measles among schoolchildren who had received the then recommended single dose.

Because MMR is composed of live, attenuated vaccines, the non–allergy-related side effects to its administration are delayed for roughly 5 to 12 days. From the measles vaccine, 5% to 15% of recipients get a fever, 5% get a rash, fewer than 1 in 30,000 get thrombocytopenia, and fewer than 1 in 1 million get encephalopathy. From mumps vaccine, there are rare reports of parotitis. From rubella vaccine, 10% of recipients get a rash. Joint pain after vaccination is common in adult recipients but not among children. Transient arthritis occurs in fewer than 1% of children recipients.

Contraindications to MMR vaccination include the following:

- A history of anaphylaxis following exposure to neomycin or gelatin
- An impairment of the immune system resulting from cancer or its treatment, immunodeficiency diseases, or immunosuppressive therapy; however, asymptomatic HIV infection is not a contraindication to receipt of MMR
- Pregnancy

Varicella vaccine. In the prevaccination era, almost everyone acquired varicella, resulting in approximately 4 million cases per year. However, disease surveillance did not start until 1991; thus, exact incidence figures are not available. Varicella is responsible for approximately 9000 hospitalizations and 100 deaths per year. The majority of the hospitalizations occur among previously healthy children and adolescents, and almost half of the deaths occur among children and adolescents.

A single product is licensed today, which is the Oka strain, a live, attenuated vaccine developed in the early 1970s in Japan. Seroconversion rates are 97% for children 12 months to 12 years of age and 78% to 82% for older children. It is not known whether immunity is lifelong, but the current data are promising. The efficacy of the vaccine is approximately 70% for preventing any varicella disease and greater than 95% for preventing severe varicella disease. Breakthrough infection rates are less than 1% per year for children and 4.1% per year for adolescents and adults. Thus, parents should be told of the possibility of breakthrough infection and that any breakthrough illness generally is very mild. Although it is not known for certain, varicella vaccination will probably reduce the life-time incidence of herpes zoster.

Varicella vaccine has stringent cold chain and storage requirements. The vaccine should arrive at the office frozen, having been shipped in dry ice (which should still be present in the shipping container). It should be maintained in a freezer or a refrigerator/freezer that has separate doors for the refrigerator and the freezer compartments. The shelf life of vaccine properly handled is 18 months. After reconstitution, the vaccine must be administered within 30 minutes.

The CDC Advisory Committee on Immunization Practices recommends vaccination against varicella before entering child care or school for all healthy children who do not have a reliable history of varicella disease. The recommended dose is 0.5 ml injected subcutaneously. For children 12 months to 13 years of age, a single dose is recommended. For children beyond their thirteenth birthday who have neither a history of the disease nor of previous varicella vaccination, two doses are recommended, separated by 4 to 8 weeks. Varicella vaccine may be given simultaneously with MMR, but if not given on the same day, at least 28 days must elapse between administration of the two.

There are several contraindications and precautions for varicella vaccination. Although individuals who have asymptomatic HIV or a pure humoral immunodeficiency may safely receive varicella vaccine, other immunocompromised individuals cannot be vaccinated against varicella. Children receiving more than 14 days of high-dose corticosteroids should not receive varicella vaccine until 1 month has elapsed after discontinuing steroid therapy. Pregnancy is a contraindication, and at least 1 month should elapse between vaccination and conception. A history of anaphylactic reaction to the vaccine components (e.g., gelatin and neomycin) is a contraindication. The vaccine manufacturer recommends discontinuing salicylate therapy for 6 weeks after vaccination for the theoretical risk of Reye's syndrome.

Adverse reactions to varicella vaccine include (1) local complaints such as pain, soreness, redness, and swelling, which occur in 19% of young children and 24% to 33% of adolescents; (2) a varicella-like rash at the injection site, which occurs within 2 weeks in 3% of first-dose recipients; and (3) a varicella-like rash at non-injection sites, which occurs within 3 weeks in 4% to 6% of children.

Conjugate pneumococcal vaccine. *Streptococcus pneumoniae* (pneumococcus) is one of the remaining major causes of serious infectious childhood diseases. Each year in the United States, *S. pneumoniae* causes 3000 cases of meningitis, 50,000 cases of bacteremia, 125,000 cases of pneumonia requiring hospitalization, a far greater number of cases of outpatient pneumonia, and 4 million cases of otitis media.

The currently available, pure polysaccharide pneumococcal vaccine effectively prevents invasive pneumococcal disease, but only in those 2 years of age and older. Unfortunately, the highest incidence of invasive pneumococcal disease is in children younger than 2 years of age for whom the pure polysaccharide vaccine is not licensed. The emergence of antimicrobial resistance has increased the concern about pneumococcus and the desire for a pneumococcal vaccine for infants and toddlers.

The pneumococcal conjugate vaccine (PCV) is analogous to the Hib conjugate vaccine, in which a protein is joined to the polysaccharide. It contains seven serotypes that account for most of the invasive pneumococcal disease. Thus, it is called *PCV7.* Prelicensure studies of the conjugate vaccine indicate a high efficacy against invasive disease, 10% reductions in acute otitis media, and reductions in nasopharyngeal carriage of the bacteria. For these reasons, the ACIP now recommends that all children <24 months of age and high-risk children 24 to 59 months old be immunized with PCV7.

High-risk medical conditions include sickle cell disease, asplenia, HIV infection or other immunocompromising conditions, and chronic disease (e.g., cardiopulmonary disease except asthma, chronic liver disease, or diabetes mellitus). Blacks, Native Americans, and Native Alaskans also are considered to be at high risk. Vaccination should be considered for other children younger than 59 months old, with priority given to children who have had frequent or complicated acute otitis media during the previous year, are economically or socially disadvantaged, or attend group day care.

PCV7 is administered intramuscularly as a 0.5-ml dose. Administration should begin at 2 months, but not earlier than 6 weeks of age. The recommended interval between the subsequent two doses is 2 months; the minimum interval is 6 weeks. The booster dose should be given at 12 to 15 months of age.

Recommended schedules vary with age and risk factors as shown in Table 18-5.

Currently available studies show that severe local reactions have been uncommon. Monitoring systems for severe systemic adverse reactions are being augmented to include the new vaccine.

Table 18-5 Pneumococcal Conjugate Vaccine Schedule According to Risk Factors

Risk	Age When Series Starts	Schedule
Healthy, including Alaskan Natives* and American Indians*	≤6 months	3-dose primary series plus booster
	7-11 months	2-dose primary series plus booster
	12-23 months	2 doses (no booster)
	>23 months	1 dose (no booster)
Asplenia* or HIV-positive*	>23 months	2 doses (no booster)
Chronic illness* or immunocompromise*	>23 months	1 or 2 doses (no booster)
Status/post bone marrow transplant	No age limit	2 or 3 doses starting at 12 months following transplant

*Children who are Alaskan Native or American Indian or have asplenia, HIV, chronic illness, or immunocompromise AND who are 24 to 59 months of age AND who have received their PCV7 should receive a single dose of pure polysaccharide vaccine subsequently. The recommended interval between the conjugate and the polysaccharide vaccine is 2 months and the minimum interval is 6 weeks.

Contraindications to PCV7 include anaphylaxis allergy to the vaccine or its components and moderate to severe acute illness. It appears that technological breakthroughs in vaccine development offer the possibility of preventing one of the major scourges affecting young children—pneumococcal disease. It will be up to primary care clinicians to ensure that this new vaccine is administered effectively, on a timely basis, to all eligible children. It is hoped that pneumococcal disease may go the route that Hib has gone—from daily battles by patients and clinicians whose patients have potentially life-threatening illnesses caused by this organism to the sanctuary of history books.

Vaccines for Defined Populations

Children who have certain chronic illnesses, such as asthma, cardiopulmonary disease, and sickle cell disease, require additional vaccines to those recommended routinely. To ensure that these high-risk children are vaccinated appropriately, the primary care practitioner should establish a system for tracking their immunization needs and status. Vaccines recommended for children who have a chronic illness are mentioned in this section on targeted vaccines.

Influenza virus vaccine. Current influenza vaccines consist of highly purified, egg-grown, inactivated influenza virus subtypes. The composition is changed periodically to protect against viral strains expected during the winter influenza virus season. The split-virus vaccines, which consist of either purified surface antigens or subviral particles prepared by disrupting the virus membrane, are the only type that can be administered to children younger than 13 years of age. Either split-virus vaccines or whole-virus vaccines can be administered to older children. Immunity after vaccination lasts only 1 year.

The vaccine is administered intramuscularly in an age-dependent dose and schedule as follows:

- Children 6 months to 8 years of age require two doses the first time they receive influenza vaccine, with single annual doses thereafter; only the split-virus vaccine is licensed for this age group
- Children 9 to 12 years of age require only one dose annually; only the split-virus vaccine is licensed for this age group
- Children 13 years of age and older require only one dose annually; *both* the split and whole-cell vaccines are licensed for this age group

For the two-dose regimen, a one-month minimum interval is recommended.

Influenza vaccine should arrive at the office unfrozen and should be refrigerated immediately upon arrival. The vaccine should be stored between 2° and 8° C; shelf life is up to 18 months.

Annual influenza vaccination in the fall of each year is recommended for children who have the following conditions: asthma and other chronic pulmonary diseases, significant cardiac disease, immunosuppressive conditions, HIV infections, sickle cell disease and other hemoglobinopathies, and long-term aspirin use. Other high-risk conditions for which vaccination is recommended include diabetes mellitus, chronic renal disease, chronic metabolic disease, and others that may compromise immunity. It is recommended that close contacts of individuals who have high-risk medical conditions should receive the vaccine to reduce the latter's exposure to influenza. Vaccination is also recommended for women who will be in the second or third trimester of pregnancy during influenza season.

Influenza vaccine rarely causes systemic or febrile reactions. Local reactions, including soreness, redness, and induration at the site of the injections, occur in fewer than 30% of vaccinees. Immediate hypersensitivity reactions, such as hives, angioedema, allergic asthma, or anaphylaxis, occur rarely after influenza vaccination.

Valid contraindications to influenza vaccination include severe allergic reaction to a previous dose of influenza vaccine or to a vaccine component such as eggs.

Pure polysaccharide pneumococcal vaccine. (Refer also to the discussion of conjugate pneumococcal vaccine on p. 210.)

Pneumococcal vaccination provides protection against invasive disease caused by *Streptococcus pneumoniae,* a potentially life-threatening disease among children who have certain chronic conditions. Although a major cause of adult mortality, pneumococcal disease is also a cause of childhood meningitis, pneumonia, and otitis media. The pure polysaccharide pneumococcal vaccine consists of purified capsular polysaccharide antigen from 23 types of the pneumococcal bacteria. The vaccine is given by intramuscular or subcutaneous injection. Unlike the conjugate pneumococcal vaccine, this vaccine does not alter the pneumococcal carriage rate, nor does it protect children younger than 2 years of age.

Pure polysaccharide pneumococcal vaccine should arrive at the office unfrozen and should be refrigerated immediately upon arrival. The vaccine should be stored between 2° and 8° C. Shelf life is up to 2 years.

Use of the pure polysaccharide pneumococcal vaccine is recommended for children older than 59 months of age who have conditions that place them at increased risk of systemic pneumococcal infection and for revaccination of certain youths who received the conjugate pneumococcal vaccine. For older children undergoing splenectomy or chemotherapy initiation, vaccination should occur more than 2 weeks before splenectomy or the start of chemotherapy. One revaccination is recommended after 3 to 5 years.

Adverse events following vaccination include mild local effects in about 50% of recipients, fever or severe local reactions in fewer than 1%, and severe allergic reactions in approximately 5 out of 1 million doses. A contraindication to vaccination is serious allergic reaction to a prior dose of pneumococcal vaccine. Information is insufficient about the safety of vaccinating pregnant women with pneumococcal vaccine to recommend vaccination of pregnant women. Therefore, women who have high-risk conditions should be vaccinated before pregnancy.

Hepatitis A vaccine. Hepatitis A vaccine is a relatively newly licensed weapon against a disease that, until recently, was only prevented through hygienic measures and passive immunization with immune globulin. Two products currently are licensed for children ages 2 to 18 years; both are inactivated viral vaccines made by using human fibroblasts. The vaccine is given by intramuscular injection. Depending on the particular vaccine and age of the recipient, a two-dose schedule or a three-dose schedule is used. Hepatitis A vaccine has an efficacy rate of greater than 90% after the first dose has been administered and approximately 100% after the second dose.

The vaccine should arrive unfrozen and should be stored at temperatures between 2° and 8° C. The shelf life is up to 3 years.

Hepatitis A vaccine is recommended for non-outbreak preexposure use among the following groups:

1. Children, ages 2 years and older, in communities that have a high incidence of hepatitis A (Arizona, Alaska, Oregon, New Mexico, Utah, Washington, Oklahoma, South Dakota, Idaho, Nevada, and California), as well as children in communities or counties where the average annual hepatitis A rate during 1987-97 was at least 20/100,000 population. (Routine vaccination also should be considered for children 2 years of age and older who live in Missouri, Texas, Colorado, Arkansas, Montana, Wyoming, and other communities or counties in which the incidence is lower, but still at least 10/100,000.)
2. People at increased risk of hepatitis A infection because they travel or work in countries of high to intermediate endemicity, have homosexual sex with males, use illegal drugs, work with hepatitis A–infected primates or laboratory specimens, or take clotting-factor concentrates
3. People with chronic liver disease

Hepatitis A vaccine should not be given to individuals who have a history of hypersensitivity to the vaccine or its components such as alum and phenoxyethanol. Serious adverse events have not been associated with hepatitis A vaccination. The most frequent side effects are local reactions, including soreness at the injection site.

Lyme disease vaccine. Lyme disease is a tick-borne zoonosis caused by a spirochete, *Borrelia burgdorferi.* Since 1982, when national surveillance began, the annual number of cases has increased to more than 12,000. Although Lyme disease has been reported in almost all states, it occurs primarily in the Northeast, mid-Atlantic states, upper north-central region, and several areas of northwest California. People who have had tick contact in endemic areas are at greatest risk; tick avoidance and protection with clothing and insect repellents containing DEET are very helpful in preventing this disease. (See Chapter 233, Lyme Disease.)

Lyme disease usually begins with a characteristic rash (erythema migrans) and nonspecific systemic symptoms, but it can be asymptomatic. Within days or weeks of the initial rash, signs of early disseminated infection can appear in various organ systems, including neurological (e.g., meningitis, neuropathy), musculoskeletal (e.g., arthralgias, arthritis), or rarely, cardiac (e.g., myocarditis, arrhythmias). Weeks to months after infection, late disseminated Lyme disease can occur involving chronic neurological or musculoskeletal symptoms. The diagnosis can be established on clinical or serological grounds. Antibiotic therapy usually is effective in the early stages.

The first licensed Lyme disease vaccine is genetically engineered and is composed of lipoprotein OspA, an outer-surface protein of the spirochete. Studies have suggested that the vaccine induces human antibodies that then are digested by the tick. The antibodies reduce the number of *B. burgdorferi* spirochetes residing in the tick's gut and, thus, the size of the inoculum. The vaccine is administered intramuscularly at 0.5 ml. Three doses are given—after the initial dose, a second is given 1 month later and the third 11 months after the second dose. Optimally, the second and third doses should be administered in the spring around March, several weeks before the beginning of spirochete transmission season.

Phase III trails of the current vaccine demonstrated a three-dose efficacy of 76% against definite Lyme disease and 100% against asymptomatic infection (i.e., positive serology without symptoms). Although there were no serious adverse reactions in the large placebo-controlled trial, local reactions included injection site soreness (24%) or redness and swelling (<2%); systemic reactions included myalgias and flu-like symptoms (3%). Vaccine recipients were more likely than controls to report arthralgia or myalgia within 30 days of vaccination, but not after 30 days.

The clinician needs to decide which patient should receive Lyme disease vaccine. This decision is based on an assessment of the individual's risk, which is a function of (1) the density of ticks (which varies by location and season), (2) the prevalence of *B. burgdorferi* in local ticks, and (3) the extent of the individual's contact with ticks. At this time, Lyme disease vaccine is not licensed for children younger than 15 years of age because safety and immunogenicity have not been established in this age group. The recommendations of the Advisory Committee on Immunization Practices for persons 15 to 70 years of age include:

- Persons who reside, work, or "recreate" in areas of moderate to high risk should consider vaccination if their exposure is frequent or prolonged; may consider vaccination if their exposure is infrequent; and need not receive vaccination if their exposure is minimal
- Persons who reside, work, or recreate in areas of no or low risk need not receive vaccination
- Travelers to areas of moderate to high risk should consider vaccination if frequent or prolonged exposure is anticipated

Vaccine administration and specific issues regarding vaccination in unusual circumstances are discussed in the May 28, 1999, issue of *MMWR.*

IMMUNIZATION DELIVERY SYSTEMS: FROM VACCINE ARRIVAL TO PATIENT DEPARTURE

Standards for Pediatric Immunization Practices

Standards for Pediatric Immunization Practice came into being in 1992. Endorsed by private and public health organizations, these standards express the importance of immunizing within the context of comprehensive child health care and the need for improvements in present childhood immunization practices. The standards are listed in Table 18-6.

There is a major, new thrust to protect adolescents from vaccine-preventable diseases. The strategy for protecting adolescents is targeted at children in the age range of 11 to 12 years and includes: (1) establishing routine preventive care visits to the primary care provider, (2) vaccinating those who

Table 18-6 Standards of Pediatric Immunization Practices

Standard 1	Immunization services are *readily available.*
Standard 2	There are *no barriers* or *unnecessary prerequisites* to the receipt of vaccines.
Standard 3	Immunization services are available *free* or for a minimal fee.
Standard 4	Providers utilize all clinical encounters to *screen* and, when indicated, *immunize* children.
Standard 5	Providers *educate* parents/guardians about immunization in general terms.
Standard 6	Providers *question* parents/guardians about *contraindications* and, before immunizing a child, *inform* them in specific terms about the risks and benefits of the immunizations their child is to receive.
Standard 7	Providers follow only true *contraindications.*
Standard 8	Providers administer *simultaneously* all vaccine doses for which a child is eligible at the time of each visit.
Standard 9	Providers use accurate and complete *recording procedures.*
Standard 10	Providers *co-schedule* immunization appointments in conjunction with appointments for other child health services.
Standard 11	Providers *report adverse events* following immunization promptly, accurately, and completely.
Standard 12	Providers operate a *tracking system.*
Standard 13	Providers adhere to appropriate procedures for *vaccine management.*
Standard 14	Providers conduct semiannual *assessments* of immunization coverage levels and review the immunization records of the patients they serve.
Standard 15	Providers maintain up-to-date, easily retrievable *medical protocols* at all locations where vaccines are administered.
Standard 16	Providers operate with *patient-oriented* and *community-based* approaches.
Standard 17	Vaccines are administered by *properly trained* individuals.
Standard 18	Providers receive *ongoing education* and *training* on current immunization recommendations.

From Centers for Disease Control and Prevention: Standards for pediatric immunization practices, *MMWR* 42(No RR-5), 1993.

have had no previous varicella vaccination (or history of disease) against varicella, (3) vaccinating with MMR those who have a history of only a single dose of MMR, (4) vaccinating with hepatitis B vaccine those not previously vaccinated against hepatitis B, (5) providing a booster dose of Td, (6) providing other vaccines (influenza, pneumococcal polysaccharide, and hepatitis A) indicated for certain high-risk adolescents, and (7) providing other preventive care measures as described in the Guidelines for Adolescent Preventive Services (GAPS). Some states are enacting regulations requiring adequate vaccination of adolescents for school entry. (See the listing of suggested readings at the end of this chapter to obtain GAPS documentation.)

Optimizing Immunization Levels in a Practice

Office-based assessment of immunization levels. Most clinicians overestimate the immunization coverage levels of their patients. However, by systematically assessing vaccination coverage levels and procedures, clinicians can determine any problem with their coverage levels or vaccination procedures. Assessment of immunization coverage levels has been shown to be effective at improving practice procedures and coverage levels; practice-based assessment tools are available from the AAP, state immunization programs, and the CDC.

The standard assessment package available from the CDC is the Clinic Assessment Software Application (CASA), which is a computer program that runs in a Microsoft Windows environment. Conducting a CASA assessment is a 1- to 2-day process that involves selecting a representative sample of the practice patients and entering their immunization histories (and, optionally, their visit histories to identify missed opportunities) into CASA. The program then prints an assessment report that identifies the practice's immunization coverage levels for 12- and 24-month-old children, missed opportunities for simultaneous administration of vaccines, children who started their immunization series late, and children who dropped out of the practice (those who started their vaccinations at the office but failed to complete them). Most state immunization programs are willing to provide assistance to those conducting CASA-based assessments of practices enrolled in the Vaccines for Children's Program (VFC). Less extensive assessments also are available.

Immunization records. Immunization records that are available at the time of the visit and from which one can easily determine immunization status are essential to good immunization rates. Active medical records should reflect who actually is in the practice. Charts of people who have moved or are going elsewhere for services should be clearly marked accordingly or removed; charts should not be "archived" simply because a patient has not presented for a prolonged time. All those who provide immunizations should communicate with each other quickly and reliably (e.g., telephone, e-mail) to ensure that each knows of the immunizations given at the other's site.

Clinician's recommendation. The importance of the primary care practitioner's recommendations needs to be emphasized. Several studies have shown that this recommendation about vaccination decisions greatly influences parental preference—parents strongly tend to follow the recommendations and advice of their children's primary care practitioner. The challenge to the clinician is to inform the parents so that they can share in the decision making.

Patient reminders and recall. The most effective intervention to improve immunization coverage levels among a practitioner's patients is to operate a recall system to bring children who are behind in their immunizations into the office for vaccination. A recall system does not need to be complicated or even computerized to be effective—simple card-file tickler systems work very well. In addition to operating a recall system, an office routine should be established to remind patients of upcoming appointments. Parental forgetfulness is the most common reason for missed appointments.

A simple method to set up a tickler file is to obtain a card file that has monthly dividers. Within each month, the patients are arranged alphabetically by name. The cards record the immunization history of the patient and are filed according to the date of the next vaccination appointment. New cards are created whenever a new patient (newborn infant or transfer) is added to the practice. As a patient is vaccinated, the vaccines administered are recorded on the card and the card is refiled into the month of the next vaccination appointment. At the end of the month, the remaining cards in the file identify the patients who should have been vaccinated during the month but who were not vaccinated. This forms the list of patients who need to be recalled into the practice for vaccination. After the routine vaccinations for the first 2 years of life are provided, the card is removed from the file. Recording the vaccination history on the cards is optional, but it does provide a double check on the vaccination status.

As an adjunct to operating a recall system, charts of children who missed vaccination appointments should be "flagged" to indicate that the children are overdue for vaccines (and which vaccines are needed). This simple task will facilitate identification and vaccination of "past due" children when they come to the office for an acute care visit.

Clinician reminders and recall. Provider reminders and recall messages are communications from health care personnel (or computers) to health care practitioners that for individual clients, routine immunizations are due soon (reminders) or past due (recall). They have been found to increase immunization levels when used alone or in combination with related strategies such as providing education or recalling patients.

Storage

Proper vaccine storage is essential because improper storage may destroy the vaccine potency in such a way that would not be noticed by the clinician, resulting in vaccine failure from administration of ineffective vaccine. All vaccines need to be stored either refrigerated or frozen, with varicella vaccine requiring the coldest storage, at 5° F (–15° C). Refrigerators that have open freezers set within the refrigerator (such as dormitory-style refrigerators) are not capable of sustaining such low temperatures. The other vaccine that requires freezing is OPV, which is quite sensitive to increased temperature.

Specific instructions on vaccine storage are discussed in the section on vaccines. They also can be found in the manufacturer's package insert or from the document "Vaccine Management," which is available from the CDC National Immunization Program (1-800-232-2522) and at http://www.cdc.gov/nip. If the potency of any vaccine is in question, the quality control officer at the vaccine's manufacturer should be notified.

Reconstitution

To save time, some practitioners reconstitute and draw into syringes the vaccines that will be used for an office session. Because this practice has not been proven to keep a vaccine's potency, it should be discouraged. Some vaccines are very sensitive to storage time and conditions after reconstitution. For example, varicella vaccine must be used within 30 minutes of reconstitution, making the practice of reconstitution ahead of time impractical. The shelf life of prepared vaccine will vary by vaccine type; thus, the individual package inserts should be consulted to determine the maximal allowable time between preparation and administration. Because acceptable shelf lives will vary by manufacturer, it is important to consult the package insert to determine the maximum allowable time between reconstitution and administration of specific vaccines. General guidelines on the shelf life of prepared doses are available in the publication "Vaccine Management," available at http://www.cdc.gov/nip.

Assessment of an Individual's Immunization Record

The assessment of every child's immunization status during each office visit is an important contributor to a successful office immunization practice. Numerous studies have shown that failure to vaccinate at all encounters is due to lack of assessment of the vaccination status of the children being seen at all office visits, including follow-up visits and acute care visits.

Ideally, a system to assess all children being seen should be established in every primary care clinician's office. An example of a systematic method is to have the staff responsible for checking children into examination rooms also check the immunization status and record the results on the encounter form attached to the medical chart.

Because the vaccination schedule is changing continuously and has considerable allowance for variation in practice style, the decision makers for an office practice should meet periodically to determine the schedule they will use to immunize their patients. This office-approved schedule should then form the basis for assessing immunization status. For example, the fourth dose of DTaP is recommended to be administered to those between 15 and 18 months of age, but it may be given at 12 months of age (provided at least 6 months have elapsed since the third dose was given). The practice's decision makers might determine that the children in their practice would benefit from administration of the fourth dose of DTaP as early as 12 months of age. Such a decision would translate into adding an additional injection with the 12-month MMR and varicella vaccinations. Generally, the earlier in life that vaccines are administered (within acceptable guidelines), the greater the time that individuals are protected from disease. However, one schedule does not fit all practices—which is why there is an allowance for variation.

Vaccine Risk and Benefit Communication

Vaccine safety. A core ingredient to the success of any immunization program is the assurance to parents, clinicians, and patients that the safest and most effective vaccines are recommended and used. Because immunization is recommended for all healthy children, it is held to a higher standard of safety than are curative services. Without widespread public support for routine vaccination, the protection of all children through vaccination is jeopardized. Examples in which decreasing public support resulting from concerns about vaccine safety led to epidemics of vaccine-preventable disease, including the British, Japanese, and Swedish experiences with declining pertussis vaccination in the early 1980s. In these situations, declining vaccination rates led to large epidemics of pertussis, with its concomitant morbidity and mortality. The United States, in contrast, did not have significant decreases in coverage during this time, most likely because of widespread support among practitioners and their professional organizations.

Extremely low rates of vaccine-preventable disease (as a result of high vaccination coverage levels) have made vaccine-related adverse events more common than the diseases. Thus, the very success of vaccination programs have made it more challenging to maintain the confidence of parents and providers in the high degree of safety and efficacy of the recommended vaccines. Oral polio vaccination serves as an example. OPV served as the workhorse of global polio eradication for almost four decades and the United States' primary reliance on it has led to an incidence of zero cases of indigenously acquired wild type polio since 1979. As the incidence of wild polio decreased, the rare, but steady occurrence of vaccine-associated paralytic polio (VAPP) became intolerable. To ensure the public that the safest vaccines are recommended, the ACIP and AAP have shifted to a primary reliance on IPV.

In addition to the vaccine manufacturers, who conduct internal quality control and post-marketing surveillance, two federal agencies have primary responsibility for ensuring the safety of vaccines—the Food and Drug Administration's (FDA) Center for Biologics Evaluation and Research (see http://www.fda.gov/cber) and the CDC. In the prelicensure phase of vaccine development, vaccines are tested in animals. If those tests show no significant adverse events, a series of three or four phases of human testing is conducted. The initial two phases of safety trials are small, with sample sizes between 20 and several hundred individuals. Unless severe reactions or a lack of effectiveness becomes apparent during the first two phases, the trials are expanded in Phase III to include several hundred to several thousand people. These trials assess both safety and efficacy. Only after successful completion of this testing can a manufacturer apply for a product license for the vaccine and an establishment license for the manufacturing plant. Phase IV testing is the postlicensure surveillance of many thousands of individuals to look for specific adverse events. In addition, manufacturers must submit samples of each vaccine lot and the results of their own tests for potency, safety, and purity to the FDA before release.

Over the past 10 years, there have been only three vaccine recalls.

A problem with prelicensing testing of vaccines for safety is that the number of people exposed to the vaccine in the three phases of FDA testing is too small to detect adverse events that happen less frequently than approximately one in 10,000 vaccinations. Given the U.S. birth cohort size of 4 million, one can readily see the need for implementing postlicense surveillance to detect rare adverse events. This challenge is met through passive and active surveillance mechanisms. The passive surveillance method is the Vaccine Adverse Event Reporting System (VAERS), which is administered jointly by the FDA and the CDC. Surveillance is conducted through the Vaccine Safety Datalink Project, which is administered by the CDC.

VAERS was created in response to the National Childhood Vaccine Injury Act of 1986, which requires practitioners to report certain events following vaccination. Table 18-7 shows the events that should be reported through VAERS. Reporting forms are available from the FDA, the CDC, and the Internet at http://www.cdc.gov/nip or http://www.fda.gov/cber. Reports also can be made over the telephone by calling 1-800-822-7967. In addition to collecting data on required reportable events, VAERS collects reports of any adverse events that a clinician or parent thinks might be associated with vaccination. Thus, it is used to identify adverse events previously unrecognized.

VAERS has some shortcomings as an epidemiological tool for determining potential causality between vaccination and adverse event. For example, VAERS only accepts reports about vaccinated individuals. Thus, there is no control group for comparing rates of specific events to determine if the event occurs more frequently following vaccination than it occurs normally. VAERS receives a large number of reports (more than 10,000 per year), making data verification problematic. To augment the ability of VAERS to identify candidate vaccination-related adverse events for determination of causality, the Vaccine Safety Datalink Project was developed. This project is a form of active surveillance in which the membership of four large health maintenance organizations is monitored intensively through electronic billing and encounter files. These files contain vaccination histories and clinical information recorded for each health care encounter. More than 500,000 children younger than 6 years of age are monitored through this project. Information about the Vaccine Safety Datalink Project can be found at http://www.cdc.gov/nip.

The combination of (1) intensive, on-going, active and passive surveillance for adverse events associated with vaccination, (2) improvement of vaccines and vaccination programs through use of the surveillance data, and (3) effective risk communication to parents and clinicians based on the best available evidence is essential to meet the high expectations of the safety and effectiveness of childhood vaccines recommended routinely.

Screening for contraindications. One of the most important steps in the immunization process is screening for contraindications and documenting screening results. A screening questionnaire for children and teen immunization and another for adult immunization are available from the Immunization Action Coalition, which can be reached at (651) 647-9009 or on the Internet at http://www.immunize.org.

Table 18-7 National Childhood Vaccine Injury Reporting System*

Vaccine	Adverse Event†	Interval from Vaccination to Onset of Event‡
I. Tetanus toxoid-containing vaccines (e.g., DTaP, DTP, DT; Td, or TT)	A. Anaphylaxis or anaphylactic shock	0-7 days
	B. Brachial neuritis	0-28 days
	C. Any acute complication or sequela (including death) of above events	No limit
	D. Events described in manufacturer's package insert as contraindications to additional doses of vaccine	No limit
II. Pertussis antigen-containing vaccines (e.g., DTaP, DTP, P, DTP-Hib)	A. Anaphylaxis or anaphylactic shock	0-7 days
	B. Encephalopathy (or encephalitis)	0-7 days
	C. Any acute complication or sequela (including death) of above events	No limit
	D. Events described in manufacturer's package insert as contraindications to additional doses of vaccine	No limit
III. Measles, mumps, and rubella virus–containing vaccines in any combination (e.g., MMR, MR, M, R)	A. Anaphylaxis or anaphylactic shock	0-7 days
	B. Encephalopathy (or encephalitis)	0-15 days
	C. Any acute complication or sequela (including death) of above events	No limit
	D. Events described in manufacturer's package insert as contraindications to additional doses of vaccine	No limit
IV. Rubella virus–containing vaccines (e.g., MMR, MR, R)	A. Chronic arthritis	0-42 days
	B. Any acute complication or sequela (including death) of above event	No limit
	C. Events described in manufacturer's package insert as contraindications to additional doses of vaccine	No limit
V. Measles virus–containing vaccines (e.g. MMR, MR, M)	A. Thrombocytopenia purpura	0-30 days
	B. Vaccine-strain measles viral infection in an immunodeficient recipient	0-6 months
	C. Any acute complication or sequela (including death) of above events	No limit
	D. Events described in manufacturer's package insert as contraindications to additional doses of vaccine	No limit
VI. Polio live virus–containing vaccines (OPV)	A. Paralytic polio	
	in a nonimmunodeficient recipient	0-30 days
	in an immunodeficient recipient	0-6 months
	in a vaccine-associated community case	No limit
	B. Vaccine-strain polio viral infection	0-30 days
	in a nonimmunodeficient recipient	0-6 months
	in an immunodeficient recipient	No limit
	in a vaccine-associated community case	No limit
	C. Any acute complication or sequela (including death) of above events	No limit
	D. Events described in manufacturer's package insert as contraindications to additional doses of vaccine	
VII. Polio inactivated virus–containing vaccines (e.g., IPV)	A. Anaphylaxis or anaphylactic shock	0-7 days
	B. Any acute complication or sequela (including death) of above event	No limit
	C. Events described in manufacturer's package insert as contraindications to additional doses of vaccine	No limit
VIII. Hepatitis B antigen-containing vaccines§	A. Anaphylaxis or anaphylactic shock	0-7 days
	B. Any acute complication or sequela (including death) of above event	No limit
	C. Events described in manufacturer's package insert as contraindications to additional doses of vaccine	No limit
IX. *Hemophilus influenzae* type b polysaccharide vaccines (unconjugated, PRP vaccines)§	A. Early-onset Hib disease	0-7 days
	B. Any acute complication or sequela (including death) of above event	No limit
	C. Events described in manufacturer's package insert as contraindications to additional doses of vaccine	No limit

Table 18-7 National Childhood Vaccine Injury Reporting System*—cont'd

Vaccine	Adverse Event†	Interval from Vaccination to Onset of Event‡
X. *Hemophilus influenzae* type b polysaccharide conjugate vaccines§	A. No condition specified for compensation	Not applicable
	B. Events described in manufacturer's package insert as contraindications to additional doses of vaccine	No limit
XI. Varicella virus–containing vaccine§	A. No condition specified for compensation	Not applicable
	B. Events described in manufacturer's package insert as contraindications to additional doses of vaccine	No limit
XII. Any new vaccine recommended by the Centers for Disease Control and Prevention for routine administration to children, after publication by the Secretary, Health and Human Services, of a notice of coverage.	A. No condition specified for compensation	Not applicable
	B. Events described in manufacturer's package insert as contraindications to additional doses of vaccine	No limit

*Effective March 24, 1997.
†Taken from the Reportable Events Table (RET), which lists conditions reportable by law (42 USC 300aa-25) to the Vaccine Adverse Event Reporting System (VAERS), including conditions found in the manufacturer's package insert. In addition, individuals are encouraged to report *any* clinically significant or unexpected events (even if they are not certain the vaccine caused the event) for *any* vaccine, whether or not it is listed on the RET. Manufacturers are also required by regulation (21 CFR 600.80) to report to the VAERS program all adverse events made known to them for any vaccine. VAERS reporting forms and information can be obtained by calling 1-800-822-7967.
‡Taken from the Vaccine Injury Table (VIT) used in adjudication of claims filed with the National Vaccine Injury Compensation Program. Claims may also be filed for a condition with onset outside the designated time intervals or a condition not included in the table. Information on filing a claim can be obtained by calling 1-800-338-2382 or through the Division of Vaccine Injury Compensation's home page: http://www.hrsa.dhhs.gov/bhpr/vicp.
§The effective date of coverage is August 6, 1997 (P.L. 105-34).

Informing parents and using the Vaccine Information Statements. Before vaccinating a child, the provider has a duty to tell the parents about the benefits and risks of vaccination. In addition to state requirements concerning informed consent, the federal government requires all U.S. health care clinicians who administer any routinely recommended childhood vaccine to provide a copy of the relevant Vaccine Information Statement. This statement must be the most recent version produced by the CDC, and it must be given to the child's legal representative before administration of each dose of the vaccine. (For the purposes of this requirement, "legal representative" is defined as a parent or other individual who is qualified under state law to consent to the immunization of a minor.)

To fulfill the duty to warn, the provider should do the following: (1) provide copies of the Vaccine Information Statement, which are available through state health departments and through the Immunization Action Coalition (http://www.immunize.org) or CDC (http://www.cdc.gov/nip), (2) discuss the information contained within the sheets, (3) answer any parental concerns or questions, and (4) document appropriately (see the facing page).

If a parent declines the recommended vaccination for the child, the clinician should discuss the consequences and document persistent refusal in the chart. Many clinicians require the refusing parent to indicate this decision in writing with a signature because there have been several lawsuits over failure to vaccinate when a person acquires a vaccine-preventable disease. It is important to listen to concerns and to work with parents to find ways to maximize their children's immunizations.

Many parents will have questions that are not answered by the brief Vaccine Information Statements. Additional information for parents can be obtained from the CDC. Also, information is available to help clinicians answer parents' questions. Examples are the publications "Six Common Misconceptions about Vaccination and How to Respond to Them" and "Parent's Guide to Childhood Immunization." The former is intended for clinicians; the latter is intended for parents. Both can be obtained by contacting the CDC at 1-800-232-2522.

Counseling on reporting adverse events. The parent should be told to report any suspected vaccine-associated side effects to the clinician. Although the majority of vaccine-related minor side effects can be handled over the telephone, it may be necessary to see the child for an accurate diagnosis. The timing of the problem relative to the vaccination can help sort out vaccine-related fever, for example, from a new, unrelated febrile illness. MMR-caused fever happens more than a week after vaccination; fever from inactivated vaccines occurs the same or next day.

Significant side effects also should be reported to the national Vaccine Adverse Effects Reporting System (VAERS). Reporting forms are available from state immunization programs, from the National Immunization Program at http://www.cdc.gov/nip, from the FDA at http://www.fda.gov/cber, and over the telephone at 1-800-822-7967. Table 18-7 lists the adverse events that always should be reported through VAERS; however, any event that might be related to vaccination should be reported. About 85% of vaccine adverse event reports concern relatively minor events, such as ordinary fevers or redness and swelling at the injection site. The remaining 15% describe serious events, such as seizures, high fevers, life-threatening illnesses, or deaths. The reports of serious events, of course, are of greatest concern to the FDA and the CDC and receive the most careful scrutiny.

Reports to VAERS do not affect practitioner liability—the National Childhood Vaccine Injury Act of 1986 provides liability protection for practitioners through the Vaccine Injury Compensation Program.

Counseling on handling adverse events. One of the most common questions for parents is about how to handle common adverse events. The most common adverse events after administration of inactivated vaccines are local reactions that can be prevented or treated with over-the-counter medicine such as acetaminophen or ibuprofen. The Immunization Action Coalition produces a useful hand-out for parents called "After the Shots . . . What to Do if Your Child Has Discomfort" that can be downloaded from their website (http://www.immunize.org).

Vaccine Administration

Site and route of injection. Injected vaccines are either administered intramuscularly or subcutaneously. Recommended sites of intramuscular injection are the anterolateral aspect of the thigh and the deltoid muscle. Because of the potential to injure the sciatic nerve, the buttock should not be used for routine injection. For infants, the thigh is preferred, although if needed to accommodate several injections (and if sufficient muscle mass is present), the deltoid can be used. For toddlers, the thigh can be used, but a longer needle may be needed than that for infants. For adolescents, the deltoid is preferred.

Injection pain control. Parental (and, presumably, child) satisfaction with routine immunization can be enhanced by use of injection pain control measures. Most providers give acetaminophen to reduce fever after immunization with vaccines that cause febrile reactions, such as DTP. However, few providers use measures to reduce injection pain to the child. At least two products have been reported to be effective: EMLA cream, which requires about 45 minutes to elapse between application and vaccination, and Vapocoolant spray, which has been shown in a randomized, controlled trial to supply equivalent pain control without the need to wait 45 minutes before vaccination. Several nonpharmological methods are effective in reducing pain from vaccination. These include physical pressure (firm pressure to the injection site before and after injection), distraction techniques (e.g., "blowing away the pain" with a pinwheel), interactional techniques (involving parents), and hypnosis (see Chapter 27, Self-Regulation Therapies: Hypnosis and Biofeedback).

Vaccination Documentation

For each vaccination given, the following must be documented: (1) the vaccine type, (2) the date of the vaccination, (3) the vaccine manufacturer and lot number, (4) the name and address of the health care practitioner, (5) the date printed on the Vaccine Information Statement (VIS) provided to the parent, and (6) the date the VIS was given. There may be additional state laws regarding vaccination documentation. Many providers also require parental signature before vaccination, although this is not a federal requirement.

Parents should be provided with a vaccination record. Portable records facilitate immunization status assessment at sites away from the office, such as child care, schools, and WIC clinics (the Special Supplemental Nutrition Program for Women, Infants, and Children), and reduce the problem of "immunization record scattering" by providing information to new providers. They also are useful for "opportunistic" vaccinations given during visits to hospital emergency rooms or to health care clinicians other than the patient's primary care physician.

A NATIONAL PERSPECTIVE ON IMMUNIZATION

Barriers to Immunization

Although national vaccination coverage levels among children are at a record high, there still are approximately 1 million children, ages 19 to 35 months, who are only partially vaccinated—that is, usually missing one or two of the recommended vaccine doses. In addition to being incompletely protected from vaccine-preventable diseases, these underimmunized children also are underutilizers of primary care—for example, they are less likely to be screened adequately for anemia and lead exposure, and they are less likely to have completed the recommended number of well-child care visits. Thus, underimmunized children are a high-risk group that can and should be targeted for improvement in their preventive care.

Why are some children incompletely vaccinated? A great deal of research was conducted during the 1990s to answer this question. In addition to the barrier of poverty and its associated factors, three potentially changeable barriers have been described consistently. They are as follows:

1. The cost of routine vaccination can result in referral from the medical home to a health department clinic, with resulting delayed vaccination and potential record scattering.
2. Parents generally want their children protected through vaccination but do not know the vaccination status of their children, and err on the side of believing that their child is up-to-date.
3. Health care practitioners believe in vaccination for their patients but seldom assess their performance on immunization delivery, seldom operate information systems to identify patients in need of vaccination or recall undervaccinated patients into the office, and frequently miss opportunities to vaccinate at visits other than well-child care visits.

Changes in the financing of vaccination services by the Vaccines for Children Program (described in the following section) and state-based health insurance reform have reduced the financial barrier to parents and practitioners. However, the remaining barriers amount to an information gap that needs to be filled by use of either community- or "provider"-based information systems that can identify and recall children in need of vaccination. Provider-based information systems are known to be effective, even if they are simple tickler file systems as described on p. 214, as long as they allow the office to track children through the early vaccination years. The Standards for Pediatric Immunization Practices were developed to address these issues. Endorsed by all major groups of professionals that care for children, including the American Academy of Pediatrics, the American Academy of Family Physicians, and the American Nurses Association, the standards were created in 1992. Key features of the standards are in Table 18-6 and are discussed in the section on immunization delivery systems. Copies of the standards also are available at http://www.cdc.gov.nip.

Vaccine Financing

The cost of vaccines increased dramatically in the 1980s, resulting in increased referrals to health department clinics for routine vaccination. To reduce the cost barrier to parents and providers (who usually purchase the vaccines "up front"), several vaccine financing reforms have been instituted. Some states enacted regulations requiring insurance companies to cover the cost of routine vaccination services; some states became "universal purchase" states that purchase vaccine for all providers, public and private; and the federal government started the Vaccines for Children Program (VFC).

VFC is an entitlement program that provides free vaccine for children who have no health insurance, children who receive Medicaid, and children who are Alaskan Natives or Native American. Children who have commercial health insurance that does not cover vaccination must be referred to a federally qualified health center to receive the free VFC vaccine. Health care providers enrolled in VFC benefit from the program because they do not have to pay for VFC vaccine and because they are allowed to charge a state-determined fee for the administration of the vaccines, a fee larger than previous Medicaid vaccine administration fees. The VFC program has been shown to reduce the rate of referral from private practitioners to health department clinics for immunizations.

Details on the VFC program can be obtained from the state immunization program or from the National Immunization Program at its Internet home page (http://www.cdc.gov/nip). Currently, there are more than 50,000 practitioners enrolled in the program. Because VFC vaccine is purchased from the manufacturer at a lower price than is privately purchased vaccine, it is important for the practice to ensure, in a systematic way, that only VFC-eligible children receive VFC-purchased vaccine. Accountability methods vary from state to state, and they are specified upon enrollment in the VFC program.

Linkages to WIC

The U.S. Department of Agriculture's Special Supplemental Nutrition Program for Women, Infants, and Children (WIC) can play an important role in preschool immunization programs because WIC has access to approximately 44% of the infant birth cohort. Also, strong evidence exists showing that linkage between WIC and immunizations raises immunization coverage without harming WIC enrollment. Because WIC eligibility is based in part on income and low income is associated with underimmunization, WIC participants are at higher risk for underimmunization than are non-WIC participants. WIC linkage for preschool children is analogous to the school-based vaccination status assessment of children entering school. Although several WIC linkage strategies are being tested, the strongest available evidence supports a three-step approach: (1) assessment of each child's immunization status via a documented immunization history as frequently as possible, (2) referral of every underimmunized child to his or her practitioner, and (3) the requirement of more frequent visits to the WIC clinic until the child is up-to-date on immunizations.

Primary care clinicians can facilitate local WIC linkages by referring WIC-eligible children to the WIC program, promoting the use of handheld immunization records, and being prepared to receive referrals back from WIC for children not up-to-date on their immunizations.

Exemptions to School-Entry Requirements

Children having valid, long-term medical contraindications to specific vaccines should have this information documented in the medical record in a prominent place. If the charting system includes a designated area for vaccination history, the information should be placed in that area so that a practice partner seeing the child for an illness visit will not administer a contraindicated vaccine to the child. Parents of children who have medical contraindications should be provided a list of the contraindicated vaccines, educated about the reason for the contraindication, and counseled about the duration of the contraindication (e.g., lifelong versus "3 months after chemotherapy"). All states provide exemption from school-entry vaccination requirements for children who have valid medical contraindications.

Certain religions forbid vaccination, and almost all states recognize this by allowing religious exemption from school-entry vaccination laws. In addition, some states allow exemption from vaccination for philosophical reasons—that is, the parents do not have a religious contraindication to vaccination, but they are philosophically opposed to vaccination. The decision by a parent to exempt their child from vaccination should not be taken lightly. Clinicians should help parents understand the critical importance of high vaccination coverage to protect not only the vaccinated children but also those children who cannot be vaccinated because of medical or religious reasons. For example, failure to vaccinate healthy children jeopardizes children who have cancer who cannot receive some vaccines by increasing their chances of exposure to vaccine-preventable, communicable diseases.

Policy Committees

Two major advisory bodies provide the strongest influence over technical issues regarding U.S. childhood vaccination policy—the Advisory Committee on Immunization Practices (ACIP), which advises the Centers for Disease Control and Prevention, and the Committee on Infectious Diseases of the American Academy of Pediatrics (COID, commonly called "the Red Book Committee"). The ACIP meets three times a year and consists of experts in clinical medicine, infectious diseases, and public health, as well as liaison and ex-officio representatives from a large, diverse group of organizations, including the AAP and the AAFP. It establishes preferred immunization schedules, indications and contraindications for vaccination, and strategies for disease prevention. Guidelines from the ACIP are available on the Internet at http://www.cdc.gov/nip and are published in the *MMWR*.

The COID consists of 12 voting-member pediatricians (most have expertise in infectious diseases) and liaison representatives from external organizations, including the CDC, the FDA, and the National Institutes of Health. The COID establishes vaccination recommendations, including indications and contraindications for vaccination and vaccination schedules, that are geared toward practicing pediatricians. Surveys have shown that pediatricians are more aware of the COID recommendations than of the ACIP recommendations and that they obtain most immunization information from the AAP. The recommendations of the COID are published in *Pediatrics* and in the *Red Book Committee Report,* which is published every 3 years. The ACIP, the AAP, and the AAFP recently have harmonized their recommended immunization schedule to minimize confusion and maximize the impact of new recommendations.

Recommendations in this chapter were derived from the ACIP and the COID recommendations. Because recommendations change as new information becomes available and because the amount of detail and supporting information supplied in this chapter is limited by space, it is important that the clinician obtain ACIP and COID recommendations to use as an office reference.

In addition to the two technical advisory committees, additional policy guidance is obtained from other national advisory groups, including the National Vaccine Advisory Committee (NVAC) and the Advisory Commission on Childhood Vaccines (ACCV). The ACCV is an advisory commission to advise to the Secretary of Health and Human Services regarding the National Vaccine Injury Compensation Program, which provides compensation for certain vaccine-related injuries or deaths. The ACCV also provides advice on the Vaccine Injury Table, which determines compensation for specific vaccine-related injuries, and the Vaccine Information Statements, which clinicians use to inform parents of the benefits and risks associated with routine vaccination. The commission holds four open meetings per year and consists of nine members: three health professionals; three members from the general public (two of whom had children injured by vaccines); three attorneys; and several liaison members from other governmental and nongovernmental agencies.

The NVAC advises the Department of Health and Human Services on the optimal prevention of infectious diseases through immunizations and on means to prevent adverse reactions to vaccines. It is concerned with availability and supply of vaccine and with research to enhance the safety and efficacy of vaccines. The 15-member committee holds open meetings three times a year. The committee consists of individuals engaged in vaccine research, members of parent organizations concerned with immunizations, representatives of health departments, and representatives of other governmental agencies, including the FDA, the CDC, and the Health Care Financing Administration. The NVAC writes reports and position statements on such topics as barriers to childhood immunizations, immunization registries, and adult immunization.

AN INTERNATIONAL PERSPECTIVE ON IMMUNIZATION

Vaccine-preventable diseases do not recognize national borders. After indigenous transmission of measles was interrupted in the United States, all domestic measles cases were linked directly to an imported case. Most imported cases have been from European countries or Japan, where measles vaccination coverage levels are below U.S. levels and measles still circulates in the population. In addition to variation in vaccination coverage across countries, there is a great deal of variation among countries in the selection of diseases to be vaccinated against. For example, Mexico started vaccinating against rubella in 1998 and is doing so by using a strategy of immunizing preschool children with measles-rubella vaccine. Thus, most immigrants from Mexico have not been vaccinated against rubella. The failure of pathogens to recognize national borders, combined with the variation in vaccines used by different countries, creates a situation in which some countries are reservoirs of vaccine-preventable disease that can spread to other countries.

The implications in the variation in vaccines recommended by different countries goes beyond strictly domestic concerns. The growing gap between developed and developing countries in the vaccines in routine use concerns those involved in the health care of children. During the 1980s, the gap was narrow because of the tremendous successes of the World Health Organization's Expanded Programme on Immunization, which included BCG, OPV, DTP, hepatitis B, and measles vaccines. Globally, 80% of children are estimated to receive the primary childhood vaccination series with BCG, OPV, DTP, and measles, averting a total of more than 3 million deaths. However, since the late 1980s, developed countries have been protecting their children from more diseases than have developing countries. Hib and varicella vaccines are seldom offered in developing countries even though they have significant morbidity and mortality from the diseases. Introducing new vaccines into developing countries is being pursued, despite the challenges for financing international vaccination programs.

The global polio eradication program is on track to be completed on or shortly after the year 2000, relieving forever the tremendous suffering caused by that disease. An important additional benefit of the polio eradication program is the creation of a network of immunization programs that can deliver other vaccines, such as MMR. Other vaccine-preventable diseases are being considered for eradication.

GREAT EXPECTATIONS FOR THE FUTURE OF VACCINATION

Until the late 1980s, routine childhood vaccination had been a field marked by slow, but steady progress. Since that time (and into the foreseeable future), routine vaccination has been anything but routine. Driven by major advances in biotechnology, the performance of childhood immunization, in terms of disease prevention, has been remarkable. However, this increased performance has come at the cost of increased complexity, including more choices among vaccines and combinations of vaccines and a more complex and rapidly changing immunization schedule. For example, combination vaccines allow prevention of diseases with fewer injections; however, the presence of non-overlapping, noncomplementary vaccines (e.g., DTaP-Hib and Hib-HepB) makes the choice of which vaccines to purchase difficult.

Advances in biotechnology will continue to bring new combination vaccines, vaccines against additional diseases, improvements in existing vaccines, and more changes in the routine vaccination schedule. There currently are more than 20 vaccines at various stages of development and testing. More combination vaccines will lead to greater complexity in the short term, but eventually these combinations will produce protection from disease with fewer injections. Also, they will facilitate vaccination against newly preventable diseases by "piggybacking" new vaccines onto accepted and fully implemented vaccines—for example, by including hepatitis A vaccine in a combination vaccine.

Licensing new vaccines against diseases that previously were not vaccine-preventable is one of the more exciting aspects of these advances. Vaccines against herpes simplex and chlamydia will be available eventually. An important vaccine for infants will be one against respiratory syncytial virus, because RSV is a leading cause of infant hospitalization.

Just as vaccine technology is changing, so is the U.S. immunization delivery system. For example, a greater proportion of immunizations are now given in the private sector than a decade ago. This privatization of immunization delivery is being driven by the need for efficiency, changes in the financing of vaccines, changes in the health care industry, and parental preferences. On average, health department clinics generally see a more impoverished population of children than do private practitioners. Therefore, as the health department clinics are being used less frequently for referral of children who have no insurance coverage for immunizations, the private sector will care for an increasing share of high-risk patients.

Much has been accomplished since 1796 when Edward Jenner inoculated James Phipps with cowpox, terming the procedure *vaccination* (after the word *vacca* for cow). The future is bright for children to live free of many vaccine-preventable diseases. By combining technological advances of vaccines with aggressive delivery of immunizations by primary care clinicians and public health practitioners, our health care system will ensure healthier lives for our children.

SUGGESTED READINGS

Advisory Committee on Immunization Practices: General Recommendations on Immunization: Recommendations of the Advisory Committee on Immunization Practices, *MMWR* 43(No RR-1), 1994. (This is a valuable resource that contains ACIP recommendations. The general recommendations are updated periodically; the latest version can be obtained through the CDC and at http://www.cdc.gov/nip. Other vaccine- and disease-specific recommendations by the ACIP also are available at no charge.)

American Academy of Pediatrics, Pickering LK, editor: *Red Book 2000: Report of the Committee on Infectious Diseases,* ed 25, Elk Grove Village, Ill, 2000, American Academy of Pediatrics. (This book contains general recommendations on immunization, specific information on diseases and the vaccines, and numerous tables that succinctly provide valuable information for the clinician. It is an indispensable resource that should be in every immunizing practice.)

American Medical Association: *AMA guidelines for adolescent preventive services* (GAPS), Baltimore, 1994, Williams and Wilkins.

Atkinson W, et al: *Epidemiology and prevention of vaccine-preventable diseases,* ed 6, Department of Health and Human Services, Centers for Disease Control and Prevention, 2000. (This is an excellent book that discusses the diseases, their epidemiology, and the vaccines. Included as appendices are key immunization resources. The book is available from the Public Health Foundation at (toll-free) 1-877-252-1200 or 1-800-41-TRAIN. The text also is available at http://www.cdc.gov/nip.

Centers for Disease Control and Prevention: *Assessing vaccination levels of the 2-year-old population,* US Department of Health and Human Services, 1995. (A description of the CDC-recommended method for determining a clinic's vaccination coverage rates. Available from the CDC.)

Centers for Disease Control and Prevention: *Manual for the surveillance of vaccine-preventable diseases,* Atlanta, 1996, CDC. (This is the manual for state health departments that describes the national vaccine-preventable disease surveillance system.)

Centers for Disease Control and Prevention: *Six common misconceptions about vaccination and how to respond to them,* US Department of Health and Human Services, 1996. (A helpful, but brief article for clinicians to assist in parent education. Available from the CDC and at http://www.cdc.gov/nip.)

Centers for Disease Control and Prevention: *Vaccine management: recommendations for handling and storage of selected biologicals,* US Department of Health and Human Services, 1996. (Available from the CDC and http://www.cdc.gov/nip.)

Centers for Disease Control and Prevention: Vaccine-preventable diseases: improving vaccination coverage in children, adolescents, and adults: a report on recommendations of the Task Force on Community Preventive Services, *MMWR* 48(No RR-8), 1999.

Humiston SG, Good C: *Vaccinating your child: questions and answers for the concerned parent,* Atlanta, 2000, Prentice Publications.

Immunization Action Coalition: *Needle tips.* (This is a periodical that is published every 6 months by the Immunization Action Coalition. It contains timely and extraordinarily user-friendly information of interest to all who provide immunizations. A free subscription can be obtained by writing to IAC, 1573 Selby Avenue, St Paul, MN 55104, by calling 651-647-9009, or by browsing www.immunize.org.)

Institute of Medicine: *Adverse events associated with childhood vaccines:* Washington, DC, 1994, National Academic Press. (A comprehensive look at the evidence regarding adverse events and childhood vaccination.)

Plotkin S, Orenstein W: *Vaccines,* ed 3, Philadelphia, 1999, WB Saunders. (This is a comprehensive textbook on vaccines and the diseases they prevent.)

19 Identification of Developmental Delays and the Early Intervention System

Ruth K. Kaminer • Susan Vig

A fundamental screening principle states that positive findings must be followed by appropriate evaluations and treatment. Therefore, when a pediatrician identifies a child who has delayed development, that child needs to be connected to the early intervention system. The importance of early intervention as a national concern has been reflected in recent federal legislation. The Amendments to the Education of the Handicapped Act (Part H of PL 99-457), enacted by Congress in 1986 and subsequently incorporated into the Individuals with Disabilities Education Act (IDEA) of 1989, gave the states the option of participating in the early intervention system, and all 50 states chose to do so. The legislation requires participating states to develop a coordinated, comprehensive, multidisciplinary system of early intervention services for young children (birth to 3 years) and their families. The 1997 Amendments to IDEA (PL 105-17 Part C) have prioritized the provision of services in natural environments. This means that services should be offered, when possible, in the home and in community settings, such as child care facilities, in which children who have no disabilities participate.

Key components of the legislation include a definition of developmental delay, a comprehensive "child find" and referral system, a public awareness program, policy regarding personnel standards, and procedural safeguards to ensure protection of confidentiality and the rights of families to due process. In each state a lead agency is designated to administer, supervise, and monitor early intervention programs and activities; most states have assigned these roles to the Department of Education or the Department of Health. Early intervention legislation requires a comprehensive, multidisciplinary evaluation to determine the needs of children and families. After evaluation, family members and professionals work together to develop an Individualized Family Service Plan (IFSP) that describes services, supports, and coordination of services to be provided for the child and family.

Pediatricians play an important role in this process by identifying and serving children who have developmental delays. Good pediatric practice embodies the principles on which the IDEA legislation is based—a family orientation and an awareness of the need to support a child's future independent functioning. Pediatricians have learned that any factor affecting a child's functioning affects the parents and family, regardless of whether the cause of such limitations is known.

The pediatrician's role in identifying and serving children who have developmental delays may be interpreted narrowly or broadly, depending to some extent on the physician's training, interest, and level of comfort (see Chapter 20 [Thirteen], Developmental Surveillance and Intervention). However, minimal expectations include screening for developmental delays by routinely asking the parents during health maintenance visits about their concerns, judiciously using appropriate, validated screening instruments, and referring children whose development is questionable or delayed for evaluation and services. Routine screening of vision and hearing in preschoolers is an accepted part of health maintenance.

For those pediatricians who have a greater interest in developmental disabilities, other roles include participating with other professionals in multidisciplinary evaluations of the child's delay, helping the parents understand the child's strengths and weaknesses, interpreting medical information for early intervention providers, and monitoring the outcomes of any interventions. Parents need and value the support of their pediatrician in dealing with the possibility or reality of developmental delay in their child.[2]

Once children are known to the early intervention system, the pediatrician's role shifts from identifying delays to monitoring the child's progress and giving parents guidance. Parents tend to have the unstated expectation that the intervention will correct the developmental delay. This may occur in some instances but is not universally true. After dealing with the stress of identifying the delay, parents often need the period of optimism that starting intervention provides. However, the pediatrician needs to be aware and needs to make the parents aware that some developmental problems will persist and will require different kinds of intervention at different ages.

The pediatrician's role of monitoring the progress of children receiving early intervention services includes asking parents for an update on the child's functioning, learning what progress has been achieved, and what the current intervention goals are. Changes in the child's functioning may require a change in types of intervention. For example, in the first year of life, former prematures frequently manifest abnormalities of tone and asymmetries in motor function, for which physical and occupational therapy are prescribed. These problems tend to improve by 1 year of age, only to be replaced by newly identified delays in language or cognition, which require language therapy or special education services. Ongoing contact with the child enables the pediatrician to determine that some delays have resolved and to identify others that have emerged. Sharing this information with parents helps them to obtain and understand modifications in the child's intervention program.

Although many pediatricians are involved in identifying, evaluating, referring, and managing children who have developmental delays, the following barriers, which may prevent some pediatricians from getting involved in these roles, have been noted.

1. *Reluctance to identify developmental delays because the physician has to confront the parents with the possibility of these delays*

Just as pediatricians share the parents' enjoyment of their children's developmental progress, they share their distress when it becomes necessary to question the adequacy of that progress. Some parents wait for the pediatrician to voice the concerns they have begun to feel, and they interpret the physician's silence as an indication that no problem exists. By routinely questioning parents about development and behavior at all contacts and observing the child's development along with the parent, the pediatrician creates a comfortable atmosphere for discussing concerns identified either by the parents or the pediatrician.

2. *Questioning the efficacy of early intervention*

A pediatrician who is convinced that early intervention will help a child and family is more likely to try to identify a child who needs this service. Current literature contains well-designed studies documenting the efficacy of early intervention in improving children's developmental outcomes. The Infant Health and Development Program, an extensive eight-site clinical trial for low-birth-weight infants, demonstrated such an impact. Children who had participated for 3 years with their families in this comprehensive early intervention program, which provided health, developmental, and family services, had higher mean IQs and fewer maternally reported behavior problems at corrected age 36 months than did controls.[3] Follow-up at age 8 years showed intervention-related advantages in cognitive and academic skills for the heavier low-birth-weight premature children.[5] Follow-up studies of economically disadvantaged children have shown that daily participation in intensive, center-based early intervention is associated with a higher IQ, stronger school achievement, and fewer failing grades at age 12.[6] In general, the best developmental outcomes have been associated with early intervention programs that are comprehensive, involve the family as well as the child, and focus on strengthening the parent-child relationship.[1] The two groups that appear to benefit most are children who have biological risk factors and are growing up in adverse circumstances and all children who have mild degrees of developmental delay.

3. *Concerns about overidentifying delays, upsetting the family, and subjecting the child to unnecessary evaluations*

Sensitive exploration of possible delays harms neither the parents nor the child, whereas avoiding the issue may be detrimental. Evaluation is a way of gaining a better understanding of the child and, when necessary, may serve as a ticket into the system of developmental services.

4. *Time pressures*

The increasing pressure to see patients in shorter time slots and the limitations on the number of health care maintenance visits by some managed care systems significantly affect the pediatrician's ability to address developmental issues. It takes time to elicit the child's current developmental function by parent interview or observation, and it takes time to talk to the parent about delays or deviations and to achieve consensus on a plan of action. These tasks are uniquely a pediatrician's role because there is no other professional involved in the lives of children whose opinion and recommendations carry the same authority as that of the pediatrician. Several strategies may enable a busy pediatrician to address developmental issues. These include using short parent questionnaires for parents who are literate, such as the Child Development Review,[4] or training the office nurse or another staff member to perform developmental screening. The most effective method is scheduling a separate appointment for developmental screening by the pediatrician when developmental concerns are identified on regular visits. Some early intervention systems will reimburse participating pediatricians for performing developmental screenings.

5. *Lack of familiarity with resources and service systems*

Pediatricians may not have the time to be involved in the early intervention system; however, they must inform themselves on how to connect their patients and families to this system so that the children may obtain services to which they are entitled. Literature for patients can be obtained from state or county health departments that describe early intervention programs and should be available in the pediatrician's office. Most medical school-affiliated pediatric departments have specialists in developmental disabilities who are a useful resource for evaluation and referral to publicly funded services.

It is painfully common for clinicians evaluating children who have developmental disabilities to hear from parents that the pediatrician reassured them about the child's delay by saying "he'll outgrow it." Although children may outgrow various problems, a physician always should investigate the parents' concerns thoroughly before reassuring them. Without careful screening and monitoring of the development of all children, only those who have more severe delays are likely to be identified. There is evidence that early intervention may make the most critical difference in the development, behavior, and success of children whose delays are mild.

REFERENCES

1. Bennett FC, Guralnick MJ: Effectiveness of developmental intervention in the first five years of life, *Pediatr Clin North Am* 38:1513, 1991.
2. Committee on Children with Disabilities, American Academy of Pediatrics: Pediatrician's role in the development and implementation of an Individualized Education Plan (IEP) and/or an Individualized Family Service Plan (IFSP), *Pediatrics* 89:340, 1992.
3. The Infant Health and Development Program: Enhancing the outcomes of low-birth-weight, premature infants, a multisite, randomized trial, *JAMA* 263:3035, 1990.
4. Ireton HR: Child Development Review. Minneapolis, 1990, Behavior Science Systems.
5. McCarton CM, et al: Results at age 8 years of early intervention for low-birth-weight premature infants: the Infant Health and Development Program, *JAMA* 277:126, 1997.
6. Ramey CT, Ramey SL: Effective early intervention, *Ment Retard* 30:337, 1992.

20 Screening

one General Considerations

Paul H. Dworkin

Because of their access to young children and families, pediatric providers are well positioned to participate in the early detection of childhood problems and conditions. Within the context of child health supervision, screening refers to the process of testing whole populations of children at various set ages to detect those at high risk for significant, unexpected deviations from normal. The emphasis is on distinguishing between children at high and low risk for certain problems, rather than on diagnosing such conditions. This typically involves the application of rapidly administered tests, examinations, or other procedures.

Several factors have contributed to an increase in the number of conditions for which screening currently is recommended or mandated. Research has better delineated the adverse effects of certain childhood conditions, such as the neurobehavioral and intellectual deficits associated with moderate lead poisoning and iron-deficiency anemia. Technological advances, such as the development of automated equipment to measure auditory brainstem response for the diagnosis of hearing loss in young infants, have enabled affected individuals to be distinguished more effectively from those nonaffected following an abnormal screening test. Changing morbidity within pediatric practice has emphasized the importance of the early identification of behavioral, developmental, and psychosocial problems and suggests the need for revised screening policies for certain conditions such as tuberculosis. Societal changes, including demands for confidentiality of test results, concerns with the stigma associated with certain diagnoses, and legislative mandates requiring early intervention for children who have developmental problems and other chronic conditions, have influenced the scope and content of screening programs. The continuing debate over health care reform, with its emphasis both on primary prevention and cost containment, has contributed to an increased scrutiny of screening practices.

Despite the time-honored tradition of performing screening tests during child health supervision visits, the effectiveness of many such practices is uncertain. The U.S. Congress Office of Technology Assessment, in a critical review of the value of child health supervision services, concluded that the only cost-effective and cost-saving screening procedure is newborn testing for metabolic disorders.[16] Because recommendations for screening practices typically are determined by a combination of limited scientific data, empiricism, and good intentions, they often provoke considerable debate. Recent examples include the following:

- The 1993 recommendation of the U.S. Department of Health and Human Services that all infants be screened for sickle cell disease regardless of race or ethnic background[14]
- The 1993 National Institutes of Health Consensus Statement, which recommended screening of all infants for hearing impairment within the first 3 months of life and preferably before discharge from the hospital newborn nursery[11]
- The 1997 recommendation by the Centers for Disease Control and Prevention that universal screening for elevated blood lead levels be limited to areas with at least 27% of housing built before 1950 and to populations in which the percentage of 1- and 2-year-olds who have elevated blood lead levels is at least 12%[3]

The goal of this chapter is to review the criteria by which conditions are judged appropriate for screening and tests are selected for use in screening programs. Examples of screening recommendations that have generated debate and controversy illustrate the extent to which conditions and tests fulfill such criteria. In addition, screening is compared with other approaches to early detection during child health supervision services.

CRITERIA FOR CONDITIONS TO BE SCREENED

Conditions are judged appropriate for the screening process if they fulfill certain well-accepted criteria:

1. *The condition must have significant morbidity or mortality with serious consequences if not detected early on and remediated.* Recommendations for universal lead screening have been supported by evidence that some adverse effects may occur at blood lead (BPb) levels as low as 10 μg/dl in children. (However, some critics of universal screening emphasize the lack of conclusive evidence that BPb levels less than 20 μg/dl at age 1 year cause a clinically important decrease in intelligence and an increase in behavioral problems by the time of school entry.) The adverse effects of early sensorineural hearing loss on language development and subsequent academic achievement and on social and emotional development are cited to support recommendations for universal screening for hearing impairment among infants.
2. *The condition must be sufficiently prevalent to justify the cost of screening programs.* Determining the true prev-

alence of certain conditions is difficult. For example, recommendations for universal lead screening were influenced by data indicating that 17% of all American preschool children have BPb levels greater than 15 μg/dl. However, more recent surveys from various parts of the country found that only 2% to 10% of children have BPb levels greater than 10 μg/dl.[7]

3. *The screening program must include the entire population, especially those at particular risk for the condition.* Screening programs optimally are implemented within a comprehensive system of preventive child health care directed at the entire population. The lack of access of many young children and families to child health supervision services and a medical home is well recognized. Disadvantaged children at increased risk for conditions such as iron-deficiency anemia, lead poisoning, and tuberculosis are less likely to receive recommended screening tests because of their limited access to health care.
4. *Diagnostic tests must enable affected individuals to be distinguished from nonaffected persons or those who are "borderline."* Screening should be performed only for conditions that can be diagnosed with certainty. Concerning universal screening for hearing impairment in infants, some have criticized the test that measures evoked otoacoustic emissions (EOAEs) because the results may be affected by fluid or debris in the middle or external ear. In the past, auditory brainstem response (ABR) equipment available in hospitals was considered difficult to operate and time consuming, and test results were difficult to interpret.[2]
5. *The condition, after detection, must be treatable or controllable.* Developmental screening is based on the premise that identification will result in intervention that will benefit the child. Although the benefits of early intervention for children who have physical handicaps (e.g., sensory impairment, Down syndrome, cerebral palsy) or delayed speech or language are reasonably well established, only limited evidence supports the benefits of early identification and intervention for young children who have learning disabilities and mild mental retardation. Although blood lead can be reduced by house dust control, whether such intervention benefits children who have initial BPb levels less than 20 μg/dl is uncertain.
6. *Detection and treatment during the asymptomatic stage must improve prognosis, and early treatment must have significant advantage.* Newborn screening for phenylketonuria (PKU) clearly is beneficial, because early treatment prevents later brain damage and neurological impairment. Similarly, prophylactic penicillin has been shown clearly to reduce both morbidity and mortality from pneumococcal infections in infants who have sickle cell anemia. Screening for cystic fibrosis has been supported by evidence that treatment before the development of severe pulmonary disease may increase the chance and duration of survival.
7. *Adequate resources must be available for the definitive diagnosis and treatment of disorders identified by screening.* A major criticism of the Early Periodic Screening, Diagnosis and Treatment (EPSDT) component of Medicaid has been the failure to ensure that all children whose findings on screening are suspect receive appropriate diagnostic and treatment services. The lack of adequate diagnostic and therapeutic resources for developmental, behavioral, and psychosocial problems hampers efforts at early identification. This lack of resources has raised concerns about the ethics of screening for developmental, behavioral, and psychosocial problems.[13] Universal screening for hearing impairment in infants is problematic for some, because follow-up diagnostic testing and treatment of hearing loss are difficult to carry out in rural or remote areas.
8. *The cost of screening must be outweighed by the savings in suffering and alternative expenditure that would occur if the condition were not diagnosed until the symptomatic stage.* Costs of screening programs must include not only the direct cost of the procedures themselves but also the cost of diagnostic evaluation, monitoring, and intervention as a consequence of screening, as well as the costs of false-positive and false-negative results. For example, the cost of universal screening for hearing impairment in infants has been estimated to be $200 million per year.[2] In contrast, the lifetime economic cost of a single case of congenital deafness is estimated to exceed $1 million.[12] Screening for developmental delay defies simple cost-benefit analysis, and the cost of screening has yet to be justified by either the savings in alternative expenditures (such as special educational programs or services) or a quantifiable lessening of anxiety or suffering. Furthermore, such screening is not without risks, such as the dangers of labeling and creating a self-fulfilling prophecy.

CRITERIA FOR SCREENING TESTS

Widely accepted criteria exist for judging specific tests appropriate for use in screening programs:

1. *Tests must be simple, practical, convenient, and safe.* That newborn babies who have cystic fibrosis have abnormally high levels of immunoreactive trypsin (IRT) in serum has been the basis for a screening test for this disorder. The relative ease and simplicity of performing EOAE testing facilitates universal screening for hearing impairment in infants. However, the decrease in specificity of this test during the first 24 hours of life poses logistical problems in that early discharge may necessitate a second screening on an outpatient basis.[1]
2. *Tests must be acceptable, with assurance of informed parental consent and confidentiality of findings.* Children should not be subjected to screening procedures without prior parental approval. Informed parental consent includes a discussion of potential false-positive and false-negative findings, the possible need for time-consuming and often expensive follow-up evaluations, and the anxiety generated by positive screening results. Confidentiality of screening results must be maintained, because positive findings for disorders such as HIV infection and sickle cell disease may be socially stigmatizing and result in discrimination by insurance companies and potential employers.
3. *Tests must be accurate and reliable.* Although anodic stripping voltimetry and graphite furnace atomic absorption spectroscopy may yield BPb results having a ±4 μg/dl accuracy, some 10% to 20% of clinical laboratories

do not meet proficiency standards.[7] Furthermore, capillary screening may include skin contamination that falsely elevates BPb.

Although a wide variety of developmental screening tests are used in health programs during infancy and early childhood, all suffer to varying degrees from problems of reliability and validity and from the need for well-established norms. The validity of screening tests consists of two components: sensitivity, the proportion of individuals who have a disorder whose test result is positive; and specificity, the proportion of individuals who haven't the disorder whose test is negative. Of particular clinical importance is the probability of an individual having the disorder when the test is positive—the test's positive predictive value—as well as the probability of not having the disorder when the test is negative—negative predictive value. The predictive value of a test depends greatly on the prevalence of the disorder in the population being tested. The low prevalence of approximately 1 to 3 of every 1000 otherwise healthy newborns being born deaf contributes to the reported low specificity of EOAE testing alone, and favors a two-step screening system with EOAE combined with ABR testing.[1]

4. *Tests should be economical.* The costs of newborn screening for metabolic disorders such as congenital hypothyroidism, galactosemia, and maple syrup urine disease are minimal, because such tests are incorporated within established screening programs for PKU. The cost of screening for such rare disorders in isolation would be prohibitive.
5. *Tests should lend themselves to easy interpretation.* Screening test results may be complex. For example, reports of screening for sickle cell disease should include the hemoglobin phenotype and the diagnostic possibilities associated with the phenotype. The screening program must ensure the availability of appropriate education and genetic counseling for parents.

ALTERNATIVE APPROACHES TO EARLY DETECTION

Early detection is considered desirable for certain conditions that do not fulfill criteria for screening. For example, neither the types of developmental delays for which screening is performed nor the screening tests themselves fulfill standard criteria for acceptance.[4] Nonetheless, early identification of and intervention for developmental delays are goals of child health supervision. Alternative approaches to early detection should be considered for such conditions.

Selective Screening

Selective as opposed to universal screening may be performed for certain conditions. For example, reported differences in BPb levels between children living in urban and suburban areas have been cited to support a strategy of geographical targeting.[7] An approach to more selective lead screening is the use of a five-item questionnaire to identify children who are at increased risk and therefore should receive BPb testing.[3]

Screening programs may target a specific racial or ethnic group that has an increased prevalence of a particular disorder. For example, screening programs for Tay-Sachs disease target Ashkenazi Jews. However, selective screening undoubtedly will fail to identify certain affected individuals. For example, screening programs targeting a specific racial or ethnic group will not identify all infants who have sickle cell disease, because it is not possible to define an individual's racial or ethnic background reliably by surname, self-report, or physical characteristics. Because prophylactic administration of penicillin has been demonstrated to reduce morbidity and mortality in children who have sickle cell anemia, universal screening of all newborns is recommended, regardless of race or ethnic background.[14]

High Risk Register

Before 1994, the Joint Committee on Infant Hearing favored the use of a register to identify infants at risk for hearing impairment. The Registry listed those conditions that place a newborn at increased risk for hearing loss, for example, a family history of hearing loss, anomalies of the head and neck, and a birthweight less than 1500 g. Listing these high-risk factors in the form of a questionnaire and asking parents to complete the form after delivery was followed by ABR screening for infants considered at risk. Because risk-factor screening identifies only 50% of infants who have significant hearing loss, the Joint Committee recommended in 1994 the option of evaluating all infants before discharge from the newborn nursery.[9] More recently, the American Academy of Pediatrics Task Force on Newborn Hearing endorsed the implementation of universal newborn hearing screening.[1]

Questionnaires

A limited number of questionnaires have been developed to aid in the early detection of children's behavioral, emotional, and psychosocial problems. Parents may be asked to complete these brief questionnaires before meeting with the pediatric provider. Examples include the *Pediatric Symptom Checklist (PSC),* designed for screening the emotional well-being of school-age children in pediatric practice,[8] and a self-administered questionnaire for structured psychosocial screening.[10] Results from small-scale validation studies have been encouraging and suggest that such questionnaires deserve further study to assess their value in pediatric office practice.

Surveillance

The approach currently practiced by primary care pediatricians to the early detection of developmental problems is most consistent with the process termed "developmental surveillance." Surveillance is a flexible, continuous process whereby knowledgeable professionals observe children during the provision of child health supervision.[4] The components of developmental surveillance include eliciting and attending to parents' concerns, obtaining a relevant developmental history, observing children accurately and informatively, and sharing opinions and concerns with other relevant professionals, such as preschool teachers. Parent-completed developmental questionnaires, such as the *Parents' Evalua-*

tion of Developmental Status (PEDS) and the *Ages and Stages Questionnaire (ASQ),* also may be used to involve parents in the monitoring of their infants' and children's development.[6,15] To improve the accuracy of surveillance, pediatric providers may choose to supplement their subjective impressions occasionally by administering a test such as the *Denver II* or may selectively use such a test as a "second-stage" screening instrument when suspicions arise.[5]

REFERENCES

1. American Academy of Pediatrics Task Force on Newborn and Infant Hearing: Newborn and infant hearing loss: detection and intervention, *Pediatrics* 103:527, 1999.
2. Bess FM, Paradise JL: Universal screening for infant hearing impairment: not simple, not risk-free, not necessarily beneficial, and not presently justified, *Pediatrics* 93:330, 1994.
3. Centers for Disease Control and Prevention: *Screening young children for lead poisoning. guidance for state and local public health officials,* Atlanta, 1997, US Department of Health and Human Services, Public Health Service, Centers for Disease Control and Prevention.
4. Dworkin PH: British and American recommendations for developmental monitoring: the role of surveillance, *Pediatrics* 84:1000, 1989.
5. Frankenburg WK, et al: The Denver II: a major revision and restandardization of the Denver Developmental Screening Test, *Pediatrics* 89:91, 1992.
6. Glascoe FP: *Collaborating with parents. using parents' evaluations of developmental status to detect and address developmental and behavioral problems*, Nashville, 1998, Ellsworth & Vandermeer Press.
7. Harvey B: Should blood level screening recommendations be revised? *Pediatrics* 93:201, 1994.
8. Jellinek MS, Murphy JM: The recognition of psychosocial disorders in pediatric office practice: the current status of the pediatric symptom checklist, *J Dev Behav Pediatr* 11:273, 1990.
9. Joint Committee on Infant Hearing: *1994 position statement*, Elk Grove Village, Ill, 1994, American Academy of Pediatrics.
10. Kemper KJ: Self-administered questionnaire for structured psychosocial screening in pediatrics, *Pediatrics* 89:433, 1992.
11. NIH Consensus Statement: Early identification of hearing impairment in infants and young children, 11:1, 1993.
12. Northern JL, Downs MP: *Hearing in children*, Baltimore, 1991, Williams & Wilkins.
13. Perrin EC: Ethical questions about screening, *J Dev Behav Pediatr* 19: 350, 1998.
14. Sickle Cell Disease Guideline Panel: *Sickle cell disease: screening, diagnosis, management, and counseling in newborns and infants*, Clinical practice guideline number 6, Rockville, Md, 1993, US Department of Health and Human Services, Public Health Service, Agency for Health Care Policy and Research.
15. Squires JK, Nickel R, Eisert D: Early detection of developmental problems: strategies for monitoring young children in the practice setting, *J Dev Behav Pediatr* 17:420, 1996.
16. United States Congress, Office of Technology Assessment: *Healthy children: investing in the future*, OTA-H-345, Washington, DC, 1988, US Government Printing Office.

SUGGESTED READINGS

Dworkin PH: Detection of behavioral, developmental, and psychosocial problems in pediatric primary care practice, *Curr Opin Pediatr* 5:531, 1993.

Frankenburg WK: Periodic screening, *Adv Pediatr* 20:149, 1973.

Meisels SJ, Provence S: *Screening assessment: guidelines for identifying young disabled and developmentally vulnerable children and their families*, Washington, DC, 1989, Zero to Three/National Center for Clinical Infant Programs.

Whitby LG: Screening for disease: definition and criteria, *Lancet* 11:819, 1974.

two The Physical Examination as a Screening Test

Robert A. Hoekelman

The physical examination is a composite of individual screening tests that assesses the structure and, in part, the function of the human body. It includes a series of specific measurements, as well as many objective observations, that the examiner makes by using the senses of sight, smell, hearing, touch, and occasionally, taste. Judgments as to the normality or abnormality of these measurements and observations are then made based on predetermined standards. The methodology for conducting the physical examination and some of the standards of normality are discussed in Chapter 8, The Pediatric Physical Examination.

When performed on a healthy child as part of a well visit, the physical examination is more of a screening test than it is when it is performed as one aspect of the evaluation of a specific complaint. The physical examination is an extremely sensitive and specific screening test for some conditions (e.g., strabismus, umbilical hernia, and dental caries), but not for most others. The yield from all or parts of the physical examination varies with the prevalence of abnormal conditions in the population screened. For instance, tonometric and proctoscopic examinations are not performed for infants and children except under unusual circumstances, whereas auscultation of the heart and lungs and otoscopic examination are performed routinely.

In the screening of healthy children, certain parts of the physical examination ordinarily need to be performed only once to determine the presence or absence of a specific condition (e.g., undescended testicle, choanal atresia, or color blindness). Once height, weight, head circumference, and blood pressure initially have been determined to be in the normal range for the infant's or child's age, they are highly unlikely to become abnormal without specific signs or symptoms that bring the child to the physician's attention. Nevertheless, they need to be measured periodically. Other procedures, however, do require repeated performance inasmuch as illnesses are acquired and many congenital or genetically determined conditions may not be evident on examinations performed early in life (e.g., pyloric stenosis, scoliosis, patent ductus arteriosus, and Marfan syndrome). Indeed, a normal finding may be only an assurance of normality for very brief periods (e.g., absence of an abdominal mass, presence of normal mobility of the tympanic membrane, or normal skin turgor).

There is a yield from the physical examination beyond the determination of normality or abnormality. Certain benefits accrue from "a laying on of hands" in terms of strengthening the physician-patient-parent relationship. The thoroughness, deftness, gentleness, and consideration shown to the patient by the physician in conducting the examination can be as reassuring as the results of the examination itself.

Pronouncement by the physician that the examination results show no abnormal findings and the child is normal may lead the parents to sense that all is well, even though many aspects of health and normality cannot be confirmed simply by the child's "passing" a physical examination. Periodic examinations also may lead the parents to cease using their own powers of observation and judgment regarding their children's health and often to delay seeking care for observed deviations from normal because the examination is scheduled in the near future. On the other hand, parents may misinterpret the meaning of variations in normal findings discovered in the routine physical examination (e.g., the innocent heart murmur), which can cause undue alarm and far-reaching consequences.

The actual yield of abnormal findings (not known to be present beforehand) on routine, periodic physical examinations of presumably well children is extremely small (1.5% in infants during their first year,[1] 2.5% in preschool children,[5] and 4% in primary school children[10] and high school students[9]). Because most of these findings are minor and can be detected by other means, periodic routine physical examinations of well children is considered to be an inefficient use of medical personnel and of little value from a case-finding (screening) perspective.[3,6]

Many of the elements of the physical examination—specifically, determination of height, weight, head circumference, vital signs, and hearing and visual acuity—involve measurements that physicians usually delegate to others. These are apt to yield more in terms of early detection of disease than are the remaining elements of the physical examination. However, specific conditions at certain ages might go unrecognized by parents or teachers or might remain undiscovered through routine screening measures but are detectable on the physical examination:

Cataract
Congenital heart disease
Congenital hip dysplasia
Cryptorchism
Genetic syndromes
Glaucoma
Lymphadenopathy
Scoliosis
Strabismus
Tumors (benign and malignant)

Screening generally is believed to be important in two of these conditions: congenital hip dysplasia (CHD) during infancy and scoliosis during late childhood and early adolescence. However, a study conducted in Birmingham, England, casts serious doubts on the effectiveness of screening for CHD in terms of reducing the frequency of late discovery and poor outcome of the anomaly; it suggests that the screening tests used (the Barlow and Ortolani maneuvers) and early management of "unstable" hips by holding them in an extended and flexed position may in themselves cause CHD.[7] Studies of ultrasound screening for CHD among newborns who have repeat ultrasonographic examinations throughout infancy indicate that the Barlow and Ortolani maneuvers can lead to false-negative results and that positive ultrasound results in the neonatal period are not highly predictive of eventual CHD requiring treatment.[2]

Although screening for scoliosis has a low yield—2 in 100 children require follow-up and 2 in 1000 require active treatment[8]—it generally is regarded as a cost-effective screening test despite the large numbers of children who are referred, based on screening, for radiographic assessment and orthopedic consultation. The use of moiré topography (a photographic technique that defines the body contours) as a secondary screening procedure may reduce the number of these referrals.[4]

For the 10 diagnoses listed above and the amount of medical time spent on the physical examination, we need to ask two questions. First, in which of these 10 conditions will waiting until signs and symptoms of the disease become evident to the parents, with the ensuing delay in making the diagnosis, change the outcome? Second, can those elements of the physical examination that must be performed to detect these conditions be taught adequately to persons other than physicians, that is, in a way that ensures a sufficiently high degree of sensitivity and specificity?

The frequency with which physical examinations for purposes of screening need to be performed in infants and children should reflect the risk of abnormality that each child runs. That risk is determined by a number of variables that must be assessed by the physician. The risk is not the same for all children; therefore, the scheduling of physical examinations for the purpose of screening depends on the patient. For the well child at low risk, "screening" physical examinations probably need to be performed only at birth, 1 and 6 months, and 1, 2, 5, 10, and 14 years of age.

REFERENCES

1. Anderson FP: Evaluation of the routine physical examination of infants in the first year of life, *Pediatrics* 45:950, 1970.
2. Castelein RM, Sauter AJM: Ultrasound screening for congenital dysplasia of the hip in newborns: its value, *J Pediatr Orthop* 8:666, 1988.
3. Del Mar CB, Miller IS: Are child surveillance clinics worthwhile? *Lancet* 2:1334, 1987.
4. Editorial: School screening for scoliosis, *Lancet* 2:378, 1988.
5. Hoekelman RA: A summer Head Start medical program, Rochester, NY, 1969: implications for change, *JAMA* 219:730, 1972.
6. Kennedy FD: Have school-entry medicals had their day? *Arch Dis Child* 63:1261, 1988.
7. Knox EG, Lancashire RJ: Effectiveness of screening for congenital dislocation of the hip, *J Epidemiol Community Health* 41:283, 1987.
8. Renshaw TS: Screening school children for scoliosis, *Clin Orthop* 229: 26, 1988.
9. Rogers KD, Reese G: Health studies—presumably normal high school students. I. Physical appraisal, *Am J Dis Child* 108:572, 1964.
10. Yankauer A, Lawrence R: A study of periodic school medical examinations. II. The annual increment of new "defects," *Am J Public Health* 46:1553, 1956.

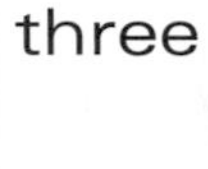

three Recognition of Genetic-Metabolic Diseases by Clinical Diagnosis and Screening

Nancy E. Braverman and Ada Hamosh

This is a time of rapid progress in the identification of human genes, including genes in which mutations cause disease, or a predisposition to it. Consequently, there is an increased number of disorders for which genetic testing is currently available. Many of these tests will be used only when clinical suspicion is aroused. Prompt diagnosis of genetic disease is important for two reasons. First, therapeutic interventions are now available for some genetic disorders. Early therapy will result in a better outcome for a number of conditions. Second, diagnosis is followed by genetic counseling, which informs parents about recurrence risk and future reproductive options.

In the first part of this section, we consider early clinical manifestations of inherited metabolic disorders and how they should be evaluated by primary care clinicians. In the second part, we consider population-wide screening—that is, testing without regard to occurrence in a family.

SUSPECTING METABOLIC DISEASE

Although the inborn errors of metabolism individually are rare, their collective incidence is not: About 1 in 1000 live births and about 1 in 5 sick full-term newborns who have no risk factors for infection and 1 in 100 children who have a serious medical problem will have a metabolic disease.[4,36] Thus, over the course of practice, a pediatrician can expect to see several patients who have these disorders. The primary care physician often will be the first person to evaluate these children and should be familiar with the clinical presentations and how to proceed with the initial laboratory evaluation. Formal diagnosis and treatment usually are done in consultation with a specialist.

The first disorders of metabolism to be identified were specific enzyme defects in major catabolic or biosynthetic pathways in cells. Their symptoms result from the buildup of toxic precursors and/or the inability to produce a necessary product. With recent advances in understanding cellular processes, we are recognizing defects in transport proteins,[25] membrane proteins,[20] organelle assembly,[68] intracellular processing and trafficking,[24,40] and many other biological processes that result in biochemical disturbances with clinical expression. A scheme for classifying these disorders is presented in Table 20-1.

Diagnostic suspicion that a patient has a metabolic disorder does not require comprehensive knowledge of the various biochemical pathways involved. These disorders have typical clinical presentations, specific historical clues, and pertinent findings on clinical examination that should lead to their consideration. Furthermore, some of the laboratory tests that are obtained routinely in ill children can help to determine the presence of metabolic disease.

Characteristic Presentations

Many common pediatric illnesses present with similar signs and symptoms. Such high-risk scenarios are considered by symptom complex and age in this section and in Table 20-2. Unfortunately, metabolic disease often is not considered until other disorders are excluded. Diagnostic delay is particularly common for metabolic disorders that have a nonacute presentation, especially when slow development is the major initial finding. For optimal outcomes, metabolic disease should be included in the earliest differential diagnosis.

Acute or recurrent episodes of illness. Serious acute illness in a previously well newborn or recurrent episodes of illness in a child are classic presentations of metabolic disease. The disorders characterizing this group include aminoacidopathies, organic acidemias, urea cycle defects, and disorders of fatty acid oxidation and carbohydrate metabolism.

NEONATAL PRESENTATIONS. Sudden deterioration of a full-term normal neonate within the first few days of life is a hallmark of metabolic disease. Many infants remain symptom-free for the first 24 hours of life. When feeding begins, toxic metabolites accumulate, vomiting may occur, and the infant becomes increasingly lethargic. Neurological abnormalities, respiratory distress, and shock highlight the progression of many severe illnesses in a neonate who has a limited repertoire of responses. The differential diagnosis often includes sepsis, congenital heart disease, neurological insults, gastrointestinal obstruction, and metabolic disease.

The clinician should pay particular attention to the possibility of metabolic disease when risk factors for infection are absent or when the infant deteriorates in spite of antibiotic therapy. The documentation of infection, however, or cardiomyopathy or brain abnormalities does not exclude underlying metabolic disease. Serious infection occurs in metabolically debilitated patients; for example, untreated infants who have galactosemia are at higher risk for developing *Escherichia coli* sepsis.[51] Cardiomyopathies develop in several categories of metabolic disease, including disorders of fatty acid oxidation and may present during infancy.[75] Metabolic crisis may result in diffuse cerebral swelling and stroke. Seizure activity predominates in certain disorders; others are associated with developmental brain abnormalities.[70]

Some disorders (peroxisomal defects, disorders of pyruvate metabolism, and respiratory chain defects) present within the first 24 hours of life. They may be associated with dysmorphic features and congenital abnormalities. Hydrops is an unusual presentation of some lysosomal storage diseases.[86]

The infant who has a metabolic disorder also may present less fulminantly within the first few months of life with poor feeding, recurrent vomiting, and generalized hypotonia. Infants who have hereditary tyrosinemia type I present with liver dysfunction and can deteriorate rapidly.[73] In one third of patients who have inborn errors of metabolism, disease does not become apparent clinically until childhood or even later.

LATE-ONSET PRESENTATIONS. These are more variable and frequently involve precipitating factors, such as diet and illness. In some, mutations in the responsible genes encode a protein with more residual activity than in patients with neonatal presentations. Associated findings of poor growth, developmental delay, or other underlying chronic abnormalities often are observed; however, illness resulting from a metabolic disorder also can occur acutely in a previously well individual. Toddlers who have medium chain acyl-CoA dehydronase (MCAD) deficiency typically present acutely. Some patients who have urea cycle defects had late-onset presentations.[10,30,84] These presentations involve neurological symptoms and include encephalopathy, psychiatric symptoms, ataxia, and strokelike episodes. Recovery may be slow, with permanent or transient neurological dysfunction. Nongenetic diagnoses usually considered include Reye's syndrome, toxic ingestion, and encephalitis. In those children who present with recurrent vomiting, lethargy, and

Table 20-1 Classification of Genetic-Metabolic Disorders

Biochemical Pathways	Subgroups	Examples
Amino acid catabolism		Phenylketonuria, homocystinuria, tyrosinemia, maple syrup urine disease, nonketotic hyperglycinemia
	Amino acid transport	Lysinuric protein intolerance, cystinuria
	Urea cycle disorders	Ornithine transcarbamylase deficiency (X-linked), citrullinemia, arginosuccinic aciduria
Organic acid metabolism		Propionic acidemia, methylmalonic acidemia, isovaleric acidemia, glutaric acidemia 1, biotinidase deficiency
Fatty acid oxidation		SCAD, MCAD, LCAD
	Fatty acid transport disorders	Carnitine transport defect, carnitine palmitoyl transferase deficiencies
Carbohydrate metabolism	Carbohydrate intolerances	Galactosemia, hereditary fructose intolerance
	Disorders of glycogen breakdown (glycogen storage disorders)	*Hepatic forms:* glucose-6-phosphatase deficiency (GSD 1), debrancher enzyme deficiency (GSD 3) *Muscle form:* muscle phosphorylase deficiency (GSD 5) *Lysosomal form:* Pompe's disease (GSD 2)
	Disorders of glucose catabolism (glycolysis) and synthesis (gluconeogenesis)	Pyruvate dehydrogenase deficiency, pyruvate carboxylase deficiency, fructose diphosphatase deficiency
Protein glycosylation		Carbohydrate-deficient glycoprotein syndromes
Organelles	**Subgroups**	**Examples**
Peroxisomal disorders	Disorders of peroxisome assembly	Zellweger syndrome, neonatal adrenoleukodystrophy, infantile Refsum disease, rhizomelic chondrodysplasia punctata
	Single enzyme defects	X-linked adrenoleukodystrophy
Lysosomal storage disorders	Lysosomal enzyme deficiencies	*Mucopolysaccharidoses:* Hurler/Scheie (MPS 1), Hunter (MPS 2, X-linked), Sanfilippo (MPS 3) *Sphingolipidoses:* Tay-Sachs, Krabbe, metachromatic leukodystrophy, Niemann-Pick, Gaucher, Fabry (X-linked) *Glycoprotein degradation:* mannosidosis, fucosidosis
	Disorders of lysosomal enzyme transport	*Mucolipidoses:* I-cell disease (ML 2)
Mitochondrial disorders	Defects in respiratory chain complexes	Leigh syndrome (one of several causes), primary lactic acidoses, multiple acyl-CoA dehydrogenase deficiency (glutaric acidemia 2) *Mitochondrial encoded defects:* MELAS, MERRF (maternal inheritance)

All disorders are autosomal recessive unless otherwise noted.
LCAD, Long chain acyl-CoA dehydrogenase deficiency; *MCAD,* medium chain acyl-CoA dehydrogenase deficiency; *SCAD,* short chain acyl-CoA dehydrogenase deficiency; *MPS,* mucopolysaccharidosis; *GSD,* glycogen storage disease; *ML,* mucolipidosis, *MELAS,* mitochondrial encephalomyopathy, lactic acidosis, strokelike episodes; *MERRF,* myoclonic epilepsy, ragged red fibers.

dehydration resembling a viral illness, each episode is protracted, and improvement often requires parenteral fluids. Patients who have methylmalonic acidemia and maple syrup urine disease can present later on in this fashion. Recurrent crisis of fever, vomiting, and diarrhea associated with dysmorphic features is found in mevalonic aciduria.[35] The recurrence of similar episodes of illness is characteristic to metabolic disease. Abdominal pain, vomiting, and evidence of pancreatitis (e.g., elevated serum amylase) occurs in about 8% of patients who have organic acidemia and may be the presenting finding. Organic acidemias constitute a significant proportion of otherwise unexplained pancreatitis in children.[43]

Neuropsychological regression. Neuropsychological regression is a characteristic feature of lysosomal storage disorders such as Tay-Sachs disease. Typically a child demonstrates either normal development or slow developmental progress and then loses developmental milestones. Progressive deterioration ensues at variable ages and rates.

Table 20-2 High-Risk Scenarios for the Consideration of Metabolic Disorders

Clinical Picture	Disorders to Consider
Acute illness in a previously normal newborn	Aminoacidopathies, organic acidemias, urea cycle defects, galactosemia
Neonatal seizure disorder	Pyridoxine-dependent seizures, nonketotic hyperglycinemia, sulfite oxidase deficiency
Recurrent episodic illness (lethargy, vomiting, ataxia, encephalopathy, strokelike episodes, myopathy, "near miss" SIDS)	Aminoacidopathies, organic acidemias, urea cycle defects, defects in fatty acid metabolism, disorders of carbohydrate metabolism, mitochondrial disorders
Neurological regression	Lysosomal storage disorders, X-linked adrenoleukodystrophy
Chronic, progressive symptomology (poor feeding, poor growth, slow development, neurological and other organ system dysfunction)	Aminoacidopathies, organic acidemias, disorders of carbohydrate metabolism; mitochondrial and peroxisomal diseases

Certain associated physical findings can narrow the differential diagnosis in this group.

Chronic, progressive symptoms. Metabolic disease can affect any of the major organ systems chronically and progressively without episodes of acute illness.

Historical Clues

Dietary history. For disorders in which protein catabolism is defective (amino acid and organic acid disorders), high protein intake precipitates symptoms such as vomiting, lethargy, and coma. An infant who vomits, who improves on glucose feeding, and in whom vomiting recurs within a few days of reinstitution of milk feeding could have a metabolic disease. The history may reveal the onset of illness upon weaning from breast milk, which has a lower protein content than commercial formulas, or the association of illness with high protein meals. Some older patients are found to be protein avoiders who limit their protein intake. Carbohydrate intolerances manifest with the introduction of fructose (fruit juices) in hereditary fructose intolerance[8] or lactose (human or cow milk) in galactosemia.

Response to infection, fever, and fasting. Obtaining a history of unusual lethargy during mild illness or intolerance of fasting is a significant historical clue for metabolic disease. Infections, fever, and fasting result in an overall catabolic state.[18] Under these conditions, disorders involving impaired glucose production and fatty acid catabolism are exacerbated, and endogenous protein catabolism may precipitate expression of amino acid and organic acid disorders. Glycogen storage disease may present within the first few months of life, when time between feedings is lengthened. Disorders of fatty acid oxidation classically present during an episode of intercurrent illness with prolonged fasting.[7] Immunizations, which may produce mild illness in normal children, can cause metabolic decompensation in children who have inborn errors of metabolism. Immunization should not be avoided in children who have metabolic disorders; rather, they should be followed carefully after immunization. Flu vaccines are recommended yearly at some genetic centers.

Adverse reactions to anesthesia and surgery. Other situations that stress metabolic systems, such as general anesthesia and surgery, can precipitate illness in patients who have metabolic disease. Patients who have homocystinuria are prone to thromboembolism upon the administration of high osmolar contrast dyes and during surgery.[59] Some patients who have myopathy are at risk of developing malignant hyperthermia when given halothane.[41]

Family history. It is essential to obtain a thorough family history for all patients suspected of having metabolic disease. The majority of these disorders are inherited in an autosomal recessive fashion. Parental consanguinity, similarly affected siblings, or early death of a sibling increases the likelihood of autosomal recessive disease. However, consanguinity is uncommon in this country, and nuclear families are small. Thus, a negative family history does not exclude the possibility of a metabolic disorder. Some autosomal recessive metabolic disorders are found at higher frequency in certain ethnic groups. The finding of similarly affected male relatives on the maternal side is consistent with X-linked disorders. Disorders of the mitochondrial genome show an exclusively maternal pattern of inheritance.

Pertinent Physical Findings

Metabolic disease affects multiple organ systems and produces a variety of physical findings. Table 20-3 lists common signs, including classic radiological findings. Some general themes exist. In the disorders that present with episodic illness, significant findings may be present or exacerbated only during the acute illness. Neurological abnormalities and vomiting predominate in episodic presentations, but hepatomegaly, cardiomyopathy, and muscle weakness also can be present, as in disorders of fatty acid oxidation. Tachypnea and hyperpnea often are overlooked as signs of metabolic acidosis or respiratory alkalosis.

Other disorders feature a characteristic pattern of findings that develop over time. Coarse facial features, corneal clouding, hepatosplenomegaly, macrocephaly, and skeletal changes suggest mucopolysaccharidoses, disorders of glycoprotein degradation, and mucolipidoses.[27] The constellation of alopecia, chronic dermatitis, ataxia, and seizures is seen

Table 20-3 Pertinent Clinical Findings in Genetic-Metabolic Disorders

System	Findings
Neurological	Encephalopathy
	Strokelike episodes
	Macrocephaly
	Developmental delay
	Ataxia
	Choreoathetosis
	Dystonia
	Hypotonia or hypertonia
	Seizures
	Myoclonus
	Deafness
	Brain malformations
Ophthalmological	Cataracts
	Corneal opacities
	Macular cherry red spot
	Lens dislocation
	Retinal pigmentary changes
Respiratory	Tachypnea
	Hyperpnea
Cardiovascular	Cardiomyopathy
	Pericardial effusion
	Rhythm disturbance
	Thrombosis
Abdominal	Hepatomegaly
	Cirrhosis
	Jaundice
	Splenomegaly
	Nephrolithiasis
	Renal Fanconi syndrome
	Renal cysts
	Pancreatitis
Muscular	Hypertrophy
	Myopathy
	Myalgias
	Recurrent myoglobinuria
Skin	Eczematous rash
	Ichthyosis
	Photosensitivity
	Angiokeratomas
Hair	Sparse
	Brittle, dry
Skeletal	Scoliosis
	Kyphosis
	Joint contractures
	Dysostosis multiplex
	Epiphyseal calcifications
Other	Dysmorphic features
	Coarse facial features

with biotinidase deficiency.[94] Lens dislocation, long extremities, and vascular occlusion secondary to thrombosis are found in homocystinuria.[66] When physical examination reveals abnormalities in more than one organ system, metabolic disease should be suspected.

Initial Laboratory Evaluation

Routine laboratory investigations can provide useful diagnostic clues. The key laboratory abnormalities in many of these disorders are metabolic acidosis, hypoglycemia with or without ketosis, and hyperammonemia. The particular combination present can help predict which biochemical pathway is affected and thus which group of disorders to consider.[92] Metabolic acidosis is assessed routinely by reviewing serum electrolytes for bicarbonate level and blood gas for pH. If the serum bicarbonate level is low, the anion gap is calculated [Na—(HCO_3 + Cl)]. An increased anion gap (greater than 16) with a normal chloride concentration reflects the presence of unmeasured anions, such as organic acids, lactate, and ketones.[23] These compounds accumulate in amino acid and organic acid disorders. Accumulation of lactic acid predominates secondary to defects of the mitochondrial respiratory chain, multiple carboxylase deficiency, and some disorders of carbohydrate metabolism.[80] A nongenetic cause of lactic acidosis is severe tissue hypoxia. A normal anion gap with an elevated chloride concentration reflects bicarbonate wasting secondary to intestinal dysfunction or renal tubular defects. It is important to note that a normal blood pH does not rule out a mild metabolic acidosis, because neutrality is maintained by various buffer systems. Low serum sodium concentration with normal or high serum potassium suggests the salt-losing form of congenital adrenal hyperplasia.

Hypoglycemia occurs either because of a primary defect in the generation of glucose (disorders of glycogen breakdown and gluconeogenic pathways) or because of toxic interference with these pathways (organic acidemias). Carbohydrate depletion or impaired glucose metabolism stimulates lipid catabolism, providing ketones as an alternative fuel and resulting in ketosis. Hypoglycemia without significant ketosis is the hallmark for disorders of fatty acid oxidation in which the pathway is blocked before the formation of ketones[35] or for excessive insulin secretion. Hyperglycemia occasionally is seen in organic acidemias.[71]

Ammonia is produced normally from protein catabolism and detoxified in the liver through the urea cycle. Ammonia levels are elevated in urea cycle disorders and also in some of the organic acidemias, disorders of fatty acid oxidation, and liver disease. Hyperammonemia induces central hyperventilation, resulting in respiratory alkalosis.[10]

Low uric acid levels, which often escape attention, are present consistently in molybdenum cofactor deficiency and disorders of purine catabolism but also may be secondary to renal tubular defects.[5] Leukopenia and thrombocytopenia have been found in patients who have organic acidemias. Patients who have methylmalonic acidemia develop evidence of renal dysfunction.[7]

A recommended primary laboratory evaluation is delineated in Table 20-4. Ancillary tests that may provide additional clues also are listed. When the results suggest a metabolic disorder, more specific testing is done. These secondary tests often are available on site or through an experienced reference laboratory; they are shown in Table 20-5. In disorders that have episodic symptoms, laboratory values may be abnormal only at the time of acute illness. Furthermore, partial treatment with intravenous fluids, transfusions, or dietary changes can mask abnormalities. Drug metabolites can result in false positives.[6] By testing for metabolic disease early in the course of illness, diagnostic results are more likely to be obtained. A practical approach consists of collecting specimens (urine, heparinized plasma, spinal fluid) early, stor-

Table 20-4 Initial Blood and Urine Tests for Suspected Genetic-Metabolic Disorders

Blood Tests	Abnormal Finding	Disease
Blood gases, electrolytes	Metabolic acidosis, elevated anion gap	Organic acidemias, maple syrup urine disease, disorders of carbohydrate metabolism, mitochondrial defects
	Respiratory alkalosis	Urea cycle defects
Glucose	Low with ketosis	Disorders of carbohydrate metabolism, organic acidemias
	Low without ketosis	Fatty acid oxidation defects
Ammonia	High	Urea cycle defects, organic acidemias, fatty acid oxidation defects, nongenetic disorders that have significant liver dysfunction
Lactate, pyruvate	High	Disorders of carbohydrate metabolism, respiratory chain defects, severe tissue hypoxia
Uric acid	High	Glycogen storage disorders, fatty acid oxidation defects, organic acidemias
Urea nitrogen	Low	Urea cycle disorders
Liver transaminases	High	Tyrosinemia, galactosemia, hereditary fructose intolerance, fatty acid oxidation defects
Phosphate	Low	Hereditary fructose intolerance, fructose 1,6 diphosphatase deficiency
Creatine kinase	High	Primary carnitine defects, fatty acid oxidation disorders, mitochondrial myopathies, muscular dystrophies
Blood count	Neutropenia, thrombocytopenia	Organic acidemias
Urine Tests	**Abnormal Finding**	**Disease**
Odor (assess by opening a closed container left at room temperature for 3 hours)	Sweaty feet, musty, tomcat urine, maple syrup*	Organic acidemias, aminoacidopathies
Ketones—essential test whenever hypoglycemia is documented	Positive	Organic acidemias, maple syrup urine disease, disorders of carbohydrate metabolism
Reducing substances (requires urine glucose determination for interpretation)	Positive with glucose, galactose, fructose	Galactosemia, hereditary fructose intolerance

*See Chapter 160, Odor (Unusual Urine and Body).

ing them frozen, and sending them later for analysis, if warranted.

Treatment

Treatment of metabolic disease can be divided into two categories: acute therapy and chronic management.

Acute therapy. In treatment during episodes of metabolic decompensation (before or after the diagnosis has been established), the ill child is approached as usual, with attention paid to respiratory, cardiovascular, fluid, and neurological status. Intake of all potentially offending compounds (protein, lactose, fructose) is stopped, and further catabolism is inhibited by providing high caloric intake. Caloric supplements should include 60 calories/kg/day from glucose to prevent proteolysis.[32] Bicarbonate is useful in cases of severe acidosis. If a vitamin-responsive disorder is suspected, a trial of vitamin cofactors (cobalamin, biotin, thiamin, riboflavin, pyridoxine, and folate) can be instituted. Carnitine may be added in organic acidurias and disorders of fatty acid oxidation to promote excretion of toxic metabolites.[4] Hyperammonemia is treated with intravenous phenylacetate, sodium benzoate, and arginine, which help detoxify and remove ammonia.[10] These medications can be obtained through contact with a specialist in inherited metabolic diseases. Progressive hyperammonemia, or comatose states secondary to hyperammonemia or other toxic metabolites, requires prompt institution of hemodialysis.[69] Acute therapy (as well as chronic treatment) should be managed in consultation with a physician skilled in treating metabolic disease. Careful monitoring of laboratory parameters and clinical status is required, with attention being given to complications that may occur secondarily to the biochemical abnormalities and therapy.

Chronic management. Long-term therapy is disease specific and involves several strategies. To reduce the accumulation of toxic metabolites, the intake of offending

Table 20-5 Specific Laboratory Tests for Genetic-Metabolic Disorders

Type	Diseases
Blood	
Quantitative plasma amino acids	Aminoacidopathies, abnormalities also found in organic acidemias and disorders of carbohydrate metabolism
Carnitine levels (total, free, and esterified), acylcarnitine profile	Disorders of fatty acid metabolism
Very long chain fatty acids, plasmalogens, phytanic acid	Peroxisomal disorders
Urine	
Quantitative amino acids	Specific amino acid transport defects, Fanconi's syndrome
Organic acids	Organic acidemias
Oligosaccharide thin layer chromatography	Lysosomal disorders of glycoprotein degradation
Screens (ferric chloride, dinitrophenylhydrazine, sulfite oxidase, mucopolysaccharide spot)	Aminoacidopathies, organic acidemias, mucopolysaccharidoses (frequent false positives and negatives)
Spinal Fluid	
Amino acids (glycine)	Nonketotic hyperglycinemia (requires simultaneous plasma amino acids)
Enzyme Assays	
Blood, skin, or other tissue	Required for diagnosis of all lysosomal storage disorders, definitive diagnosis of most metabolic disorders

Note: In the event the child dies before a definitive diagnosis is made, a small piece of muscle and liver should be quick frozen and held at –70° C. A skin biopsy for cultured fibroblasts should be obtained premortem.

compounds is limited to the minimal amount needed for growth and development. This often requires an artificial diet that includes special formulas and caloric supplementation. Regular monitoring of amino acids and other laboratory values is required so that adjustments can be made to optimize the diet for each individual patient. For some disorders, the offending compound is nonessential and can be eliminated entirely from the diet. When the enzyme defect involves binding of a cofactor (usually a vitamin) or defective synthesis of the cofactor itself, therapy centers on dietary supplementation of the cofactor. Other strategies include the stimulation of alternative biochemical pathways to detoxify and remove the offending substance.[50] In hereditary tyrosinemia type I, treatment with the drug nitro trifluoromethylbenzoyl cyclohexanedione (NTBC) blocks the formation of succinylacetone, a toxic compound.[72] Administration of the aminothiol, cysteamine, to patients who have cystinosis reduces their lysosomal storage of cystine.[24] In disorders that are accompanied by fasting intolerance, treatment consists of frequent meals, which may require the use of complex carbohydrates such as cornstarch between meals to allow prolonged absorption of glucose and nocturnal nasogastric feeding.[58]

Other therapeutic approaches have utilized provision of the missing product. Mannose supplements are given to children who have some forms of cystic fibrosis transmembrane conductance regulator,[25] and cholesterol is being provided to patients who have Smith-Lemli-Opitz syndrome.[63] None of these interventions constitutes a cure, and most are only partially successful in alleviating clinical symptoms. With better understanding of the pathophysiology of these disorders, better therapies will become available. Liver and bone marrow transplantations have been done in several disorders, with mixed results.[44] Enzyme and gene replacement therapies are being developed for some disorders, and in utero gene therapy is being explored.[87,97]

Illustrative Case

The following case is included to illustrate some of the principles discussed in the previous sections.

J.S. was the full-term product of a normal pregnancy and delivery. His birth weight was 3.2 kg. The infant was started on a cow milk formula and discharged on day 2 of life without incident. From days 2 to 8, anorexia, lethargy, and vomiting became progressively worse. The formula was changed to a soy base, without clinical improvement. On day 8 the mother noted respiratory difficulties. There was no history of fever. Examination at this time revealed a dehydrated, hypothermic infant who had a weak suck and cry. Tachypnea and tachycardia were present. Perfusion was decreased in the distal extremities, but blood pressure was normal. Oxygen saturation was 98% by pulse oximetry. The abdomen was soft, without apparent hepatosplenomegaly or renal enlargement. The remainder of the examination was normal. Family history revealed two normal sisters and no history of early infant deaths or parental consanguinity. The initial clinical impression was that of a septic infant. Intravenous fluids and antibiotics were given, and the infant was warmed. Initial laboratory evaluation revealed the following: WBC, 3500; platelets, 192,000; venous blood gases, pH 7.03, PCO_2 31, PO_2 98; electrolytes, Na 146, K 4.4, Cl 103, HCO_3 5 (anion gap 38); glucose, 25 mg/dl; urine, pH 5; ketones 2+ (obtained after rehydration); spinal fluid, normal chemistries and cell counts; chest radiograph, right upper lobe pneumonia.

The primary diagnosis was sepsis with aspiration pneumonia. All cultures were negative, but this was thought to be the result of antibiotic administration just before the obtaining of cultures. The hospital course was protracted, requiring several days for the acidosis to improve on IV fluids containing bicarbonate. Persistent vomiting and severe acidosis recurred upon reintroduction of formula feedings. A barium swallow test did not reveal gastrointestinal obstruction. On day 14 of life the infant became increasingly lethargic, and laboratory investigation showed the following: WBC, 4300; platelets,

7800; arterial blood gases, pH 7.1, PCO_2 33, PO_2 97; electrolytes, Na 141, Cl 103, HCO_3 9 (anion gap 29); glucose, SO mg/dl; ammonia, 191 uM; urine, ketones 4+.

The infant was transferred to a tertiary care hospital for diagnosis and management of suspected metabolic disease. Plasma amino acids showed elevated glycine, and measurement of urine organic acids revealed elevated levels of propionic acid and methylcitrate. These findings are suggestive of propionic acidemia.[49] The defective enzyme is propionyl CoA carboxylase, a biotin-dependent enzyme. The enzyme defect was confirmed later on tissue samples. The patient responded to intravenous fluids with appropriate amounts of glucose provided through a central line. He was not responsive to a trial of megavitamin therapy with biotin. With clinical and laboratory improvement, oral feedings were instituted first with a glucose polymer solution and then advanced to a low-protein diet supplemented with a special formula deficient in the precursors of propionic acid: valine, isoleucine, methionine, threonine, and odd chain fatty acids. If the patient had not improved quickly or had continued to deteriorate, hemodialysis would have been indicated for urgent removal of toxic metabolites.

Discussion. Several indicators of metabolic disease were overlooked in the initial presentation of this patient. A history of acute illness in a normal newborn represents a typical high-risk scenario for the consideration of metabolic disease. The initial laboratory findings provide further evidence consistent with metabolic disease: metabolic acidosis with an elevated anion gap, hypoglycemia, and ketosis. Ketosis, an unusual finding in a neonate, indicates metabolic disease in this age group. Recurrence of symptoms when milk feedings were resumed also is characteristic. The elevated ammonia level finally led to the suspicion of an underlying metabolic disorder. Ammonia levels should be determined in the initial evaluation of a lethargic infant. Poor response to therapy also should have prompted an investigation for metabolic disease. If this possibility was considered in the primary differential diagnosis, plasma amino acid and urine organic acid levels would have been measured early on, providing a diagnosis and more timely institution of therapy.

SCREENING FOR GENETIC AND METABOLIC DISORDERS

Certain disorders for which treatment is effective are asymptomatic until too late for effective intervention. This is the case, for instance, for phenylketonuria (PKU); although nonspecific signs occasionally appear early in infancy (such as eczema), by the time that developmental delay is apparent, the infant has sustained irreversible damage. For other disorders, such as galactosemia and maple syrup urine disease, symptoms appear early, but the diagnosis often is delayed. This also is the case in some infants who have congenital hypothyroidism (CH). Newborn screening can accelerate the diagnosis, provided that specimens are analyzed quickly and abnormal results are reported promptly. A *sine que non* of newborn screening is that the prognosis can be improved by the prompt institution of therapy. Accumulated experience with screening has demonstrated that the outcome is not always as good as anticipated, and for some disorders a few infants may be started on therapy unnecessarily.

A few single-gene conditions manifest only after exposure to environmental agents that are not harmful to most people in the doses encountered. Screening for such susceptibilities could result in treatment that ameliorates the harmful effects or warns people at risk to avoid exposure. Among people who develop cancer (retinoblastoma and breast and colon cancer have been studied the most thoroughly), a small proportion (fewer than 10%) has inherited alleles at single loci that greatly increase their susceptibility to malignant transformation as a result of spontaneous or environmentally induced mutations of other genes. The benefits of screening the entire population for these genetic susceptibilities remain to be established. (In conjunction with genetic counseling, tests should be made available to high-risk cancer families, usually as part of investigational protocols.) Recent claims of inherited risk factors for complex disorders such as Alzheimer's disease need thorough assessment before population screening is even considered. Genetics plays a role in adult-onset coronary artery disease. Cholesterol screening is discussed in another part of this chapter.

Most single-gene disorders are not treatable, but those at risk for them, as well as heterozygous carriers, can be detected by genetic tests. Carrier testing before pregnancy provides couples the option of avoiding the conception (by adoption, artificial insemination of donor sperm, or in the case of X-linked disorders, ovum donation or surrogacy) of children who have severe, untreatable, inherited disorders, such as Tay-Sachs or thalassemia. Carrier testing early in pregnancy by chorionic villi sampling or amniocentesis provides couples the option of avoiding the birth (by selective abortion) of a similarly affected child. Prenatal cytogenetic and biochemical testing can avoid, respectively, the birth of children who have Down syndrome or neural tube defects.

Primary health care clinicians will be involved increasingly with neonatal, carrier, and prenatal screening and presymptomatic testing for adult-onset disorders. In some cases, the clinician will inform patients about the availability of tests and will counsel them about having the test and, when they decide to be tested, about the meaning of the results.

False Positives and False Negatives

Very few people being screened, whether newborns, nonpregnant women, or pregnant women, will be at risk of disease in themselves or their offspring. Except for DNA tests, many of the techniques used in screening yield positive results in the absence of the condition of interest. These false positives frequently occur more often than the condition of interest in the population being screened. The immunoreactive trypsinogen (IRT) test used in a few places to screen newborns for cystic fibrosis (CF) yields over five times as many false positive as true positive results. Because the blood phenylalanine concentration may exceed normal levels only minimally in infants who have PKU during the first few days of life, the cutoff for phenylalanine elevations (and other metabolites) must be set lower than the minimum phenylalanine concentration needed to establish a diagnosis of

PKU. Consequently, false-positive results often will exceed true positive results.

On average, using current methodology, more than 50 false positives are identified for every confirmed case.[47] For congenital adrenal hyperplasia, more than 200 false positives occur for every true positive.[47] When the screening test entails enzyme assays, as for one type of testing for galactosemia and for biotinidase deficiency, heat denaturation (by prolonged mailing time in hot weather or letting samples dry on a radiator) greatly increases the percentage of false positives. When DNA tests are performed appropriately for single-gene disorders, false-positive results seldom are encountered. For multifactorial disorders, however (such as colon cancer or Alzheimer's disease), in which a single-gene mutation increases the risk of disease but is insufficient to cause it, positive DNA test results do not always mean that disease will occur. Other factors, mostly unknown, also play a role.

False-negative results are a problem with DNA as well as with more traditional tests. In the case of DNA tests, they occur when the test does not detect all of the different mutations capable of causing disease.

Early discharge of healthy newborns before 24 hours of age increases the number of infants who have false-negative and false-positive test results. Infants who have PKU have near-normal levels of phenylalanine in cord blood, and adequate exposure to exogenous protein is required to develop a high phenylalanine level. Similarly, when quantitation of blood galactose is used to screen for galactosemia, galactosemic infants must have consumed sufficient amounts of galactose-containing human milk or cow milk formula to accumulate galactose. Approximately 10% of infants who have congenital hypothyroidism (CH) will have normal thyroxine levels when screened early, and most of these also have normal thyroid-stimulating hormone (TSH) levels.[11] When TSH is used as the initial screening test (common in European countries but not in the United States), as many as 25% of infants discharged early may have elevated levels.[21] In screening for congenital adrenal hyperplasia, samples collected before 36 hours of age are much more likely to yield false-positive elevations of I 70H-progesterone than are samples collected after 48 hours.[2]

Although the chance of misclassification is greater the earlier an infant is screened, most infants (but not all) who have the disorders for which screening usually is provided will be detected when tested after 24 hours of age. In view of difficulties of guaranteeing that a screening test will be performed soon after discharge, no infant should be discharged from the newborn nursery, even if younger than 24 hours old, without first being screened. Raising the threshold value to reduce the number of false positives or lowering it to reduce the number of false negatives for infants screened before 48 hours has the problem of increasing, respectively, the number of false negatives and false positives. Using a different value for infants screened early or late requires the laboratory to treat the two groups of infants separately. The best solution is not to discharge infants until they are at least 48 hours old.

False-positive and false-negative test results are both dangerous and costly. Parents of infants who have false-positive test results may become anxious until the result is proven to be false; even then anxiety may linger in a small number of parents, particularly if their infants had low Apgar scores.[83] The parent-child relationship could be influenced adversely as a result of this stress in the neonatal period.

With a high false-positive rate, more infants require follow-up testing, which adds to the cost of screening. The affected infants missed by screening suffer severely, usually at great cost to their families and society. Health care clinicians have been found financially liable for infants missed by screening. No clinician should ever assume that an infant who has symptoms of a disorder for which screening was performed could not have that disorder.

Screening tests can give erroneous results because of the presence of other substances that interfere with the analysis. Most important for DNA-based screening is the presence of a donor's blood products as the result of recent transfusion. Certain antibiotics can interfere with the bacterial inhibition assays used in newborn screening.

In the absence of rigorous quality control programs, of which there are few in the United States, laboratory error probably is the most common cause of false-positive and false-negative newborn screening test results. Errors include misidentification of specimens and failure to transmit the results properly, as well as erroneous assays.

Newborn Screening

All states and Puerto Rico and the Virgin Islands routinely screen newborns for PKU (1 in 14,000 live births) and CH (1 in 3300 live births).[47] Forty-five states screen for sickle cell anemia (more than 1 in 400 live births of blacks)[16] and other hemoglobinopathies and 43 for galactosemia (about 1 in 59,000 live births).[47] Fewer than half of the states screen for maple syrup urine disease (less than 1 in 100,000 live births),[61] homocystinuria (less than 1 in 100,000 live births),[61] biotinidase deficiency (about 1 in 80,000 live births),[47] and congenital adrenal hyperplasia (1 in 20,000 live births),[47] and CF (I in 3200 white live births).[33] Because states differ in the tests that are required, it is incumbent on health care practitioners to be familiar with the policies of their own state. In at least one state, physicians were not notified when new tests were introduced. Whether this contributed to the failure of a few of them to act when notified of a positive test result is unknown, but their failure to act could have resulted in an infant's death.[52] Physicians should document screening test results and any follow-up on the child's medical record.

Because screening tests can be falsely negative, practitioners should not place undue faith in a negative result. A repeat test, or a more definitive one, should be obtained for infants who have suspicious findings. Because of the problem of false-positive test results, treatment should not be started merely based on one positive screening test result. Consultation with someone experienced in the evaluation of metabolic disorders is highly recommended. When treatment is indicated, the response may vary; careful monitoring and expert evaluation are needed. Furthermore, consultation is reassuring to the family.

Some infants may escape screening. The largest group are infants born at home. They should be screened at their first visit for pediatric care. Sick infants transferred from one hospital to another fall through the cracks when each hospital believes that the other did screening. If any doubt exists, the receiving hospital should rescreen the baby.

Screening for PKU and CH is cost effective. The addition of other tests from which infants will benefit usually involves only marginal cost increments. The economics of sickle cell screening depends on the proportion of infants at high risk in a state's population. Centralization of laboratories and more stringent regulations for quality control reduce laboratory error, increase cost effectiveness, and reduce cost to the patient.

Phenylketonuria. Infants who have PKU show few signs until they develop mental retardation, which may not be appreciated until the second year of life and is irreversible. Screening early in infancy, followed by prompt administration of a low phenylalanine diet, is the only way to improve the outcome of those born with the condition. Evidence shows that intellectual performance correlates with the age at which dietary treatment is started and with the success of dietary control.[38] Studies to confirm positive test results should be performed quickly to permit the initiation of the low phenylalanine diet as soon as possible and no later than the third week of life.

The American Academy of Pediatrics recommends that every infant in the United States be screened before discharge from the nursery but that infants initially screened before 24 hours of age should be rescreened before the third week of life. Premature and sick infants should be screened by the seventh day.[16] A few states recommend that all infants have a second screen between 2 and 4 weeks of age, and a few infants who have PKU with negative first test results have been detected by the repeat screen. The second screen costs much more per infant who has PKU detected than the first screen.

In addition to the predominant phenylalanine hydroxylase deficiency, defects in the synthesis or regeneration of biopterin cofactors for the conversion of phenylalanine to tyrosine also result in positive screening test results and clinical disease. Dietary restriction of phenylalanine is insufficient to prevent mental deterioration and seizures in these infants. The use of biopterin or neurotransmitter precursors offers some hope of improving the outcome. Infants who have these disorders will be identified by neonatal screening for PKU; they represent fewer than 3% of all infants who have hyperphenylalaninemia. Tests for these variant forms should be performed in any infant who persistently has elevated blood phenylalanine levels, even in the moderate range of 10 to 20 mg/dl while on a normal diet.

Congenital hypothyroidism. See also Chapter 223, Hypothyroidism. The etiology of CH is multiple and complex, including transplacental passage of maternal antibodies that interfere with fetal thyroid development or thyroid function.[21] Maternal antibodies also can cause transient hypothyroidism. Mothers receiving antithyroid medication (propylthiouracil) also may have babies who have transient hypothyroidism. Genetic factors are suggested in families that have more than one affected infant, although such findings do not rule out environmental or maternally acquired etiologies. For unknown reasons, females are twice as likely to have CH as males, and the birth prevalence is somewhat higher in Hispanics and Native Americans than in whites or Asians, in whom it is higher than in blacks.[54]

Infants who have the most profound deficiencies of thyroxine, usually as a result of thyroid agenesis, are more likely to have symptoms in the neonatal period, of which persistent jaundice, feeding difficulty, and lethargy are most frequent.[21,28] Nevertheless, even infants who have agenesis may be asymptomatic when they are examined as part of the evaluation of their abnormal screening test result. Placental transfer of thyroxine (T_4) and some fetal production of T_3 in the brain may explain this. The 10% of infants who have CH that is found on a second screen (in states that screen twice) are less often symptomatic and have lesser elevations of TSH. Negative newborn screening test results are no guarantee against hypothyroidism developing in infancy or childhood.

The incidence of CH detected by neonatal screening is higher than by clinical diagnosis in the prescreening era. This suggests either that infants who have milder disease escaped diagnosis or that some infants being diagnosed today do not really have CH. Because of this latter possibility, the need to ensure that CH persists in equivocal cases, as discussed below, is important.

In most laboratories in the United States, T_4 is measured on the screening specimen, and if it is low, thyroid-stimulating hormone (TSH) is measured on the same specimen. If the TSH is elevated and the findings are confirmed on another specimen, treatment with thyroxine is started. Most infants who persistently have low T_4 levels but who have normal TSH levels will prove on further study to have normal free T_4 concentrations and thyroid-binding globulin deficiency; they do not require treatment. A few infants who have low T_4 and normal TSH levels have pituitary gland failure, but it is encountered much less frequently than thyroid-binding globulin deficiency. Occasionally an infant who has initial low T_4 and normal TSH levels will have a delayed rise in TSH level and symptoms of hypothyroidism. If an infant has an initial low T_4 level and a normal TSH level, TSH should be retested if symptoms appear.

The motor and cognitive development of infants who have CH at 7½ years of age correlates with the age at which thyroxine treatment is started.[46] Although the vast majority of infants treated early have IQs in the normal range,[21] many of them are at the low end compared with matched controls,[46] with approximately a 5- to 10-point loss in IQ. When 48 adolescents who had CH diagnosed by newborn screening were compared with matched controls, the CH patients had persistent deficits in visuospatial abilities, memory, and attention, which were correlated with severity of early hypothyroidism.[69] Attention deficits were even seen in a group of 28 10-year-olds who had less severe CH (T_4 greater than 40 nmol/L).[78]

The need for long-term thyroid replacement can be assumed if scans or other studies reveal absent or ectopic thyroid or goiter caused by an enzyme defect. In the absence of these findings but when low T_4 and elevated TSH levels indicated the need for early treatment, a test of continued need for thyroid replacement therapy should wait until the child is between 3 and 4 years of age. At that time, thyroid replacement therapy should be discontinued for 30 days or until signs and symptoms of CH appear. At that time, serum should be obtained for T_4 and TSH assays. If the results are normal, no further treatment is needed. Such transient cases usually are those in which the TSH level was elevated only moderately (20 to 100 μU/ml) in the newborn period.

Sickle cell anemia. Because of a randomized controlled trial demonstrating that penicillin prophylaxis reduces the incidence of pneumococcal infections in sickle cell anemia[26] and a call for universal screening of newborns from the Agency for Health Care Policy and Research,[1,43] states have added sickle cell to their newborn screening programs.[16] Before screening was initiated, approximately 10% of infants in the United States who had sickle cell disease died by 10 years of age, most from pneumococcal sepsis.[48] The effectiveness of screening in reducing morbidity and mortality depends on ensuring that infants detected by screening are referred to a continuing source of care from which they can receive prophylactic penicillin and their parents can learn how to manage situations that increase the chance of sickle cell crises. As yet there is no specific treatment for sickle cell anemia.

The tests used for screening—hemoglobin electrophoresis, isoelectric focusing, and HPLC—will reveal hemoglobinopathies in addition to sickle cell anemia, not all of which are symptomatic. The test also identifies infants who have sickle trait who will remain healthy. However, a couple who delivers an infant who has sickle cell trait may be at risk for having an infant who has sickle cell anemia if both partners are carriers of the sickle cell gene. A screening program will have 40 times more carriers to notify than parents of infants who have sickle cell anemia, raising the costs of the program. The purpose of notifying the parents of a trait is to determine, by offering to have them both tested, whether they are both carriers and, consequently, at 25% risk of having an affected offspring with each subsequent pregnancy. They then can be offered prenatal diagnosis in any future pregnancies. The infant who has trait, who triggers this process, has nothing to gain from it. Moreover, in the vast majority of couples who have an infant with tralt, only one partner will be a carrier, and the couple will not be at risk. An Institute of Medicine panel recommended that parents be informed that newborn screening might provide information about their future risks of having a child with a serious hemoglobinopathy and be given the opportunity of requesting the results.[3]

Galactosemia. In contrast to PKU, serious manifestations of classic galactosemia occur soon after milk feedings are started. Consequently, the diagnosis can be, and often is, made clinically before screening test results are reported. The prompt administration of a lactose-free diet in the newborn will save the lives of patients who have this disorder, but it may not prevent retardation or other developmental problems, including a high incidence of ovarian failure. The age of starting the galactose-free diet is not associated significantly with the magnitude of developmental delay, physical growth, or speech problems.[19,88]

It is not certain that all infants who have galactosemia found by screening would have developed symptoms had they not been started on a lactose-free diet. Some infants discovered by screening have variant forms of galactosemia, in which residual amounts of galactose-1-phosphate uridyl transferase, the enzyme that is absent in classic cases, are found. Although infants who have some of these variants have acute neonatal symptoms, they generally are milder than in the classic cases. Other infants manifest no symptoms. Whether they are less likely to have long-term manifestations, such as developmental delay, is not clear.

We have much to learn about the pathogenesis of galactosemia and the development of effective therapy. Until we do, the value of neonatal screening for galactosemia is questionable, although classical galactosemia is lethal if untreated. The principal goal is to ensure prompt intervention in those who have early onset of symptoms whose lives are threatened. These infants can be diagnosed clinically.

Maple syrup urine disease. Infants who have the classic form of maple syrup urine disease (MSUD) usually show signs within 2 weeks of birth. The course can be fulminant and rapidly fatal, but early treatment can prevent or ameliorate the acute symptoms. If the special diet (low in branched-chain amino acids) is started very early, the long-term outcome can be good. One of the problems with routine screening is the inherent delay in obtaining results. A specimen collected on day 2 may not be reported back until day 10. By that time, most infants who have the classic form will be severely ill or dead. Starting the special diet usually will save those infants still alive at this point, but the outcome often will be marred by mental retardation and neurological problems.

Sometimes confirmation of a diagnosis of MSUD in sick infants can be accelerated by contacting the laboratory responsible for performing newborn screening; a positive result may have been obtained already. Often, the laboratory will process the specimen more quickly when it receives a special request. Infants known to be at risk because of a previously affected family member or because of North American Mennonite descent should have definitive testing (quantitative plasma amino acids) in the second day of life with immediate initiation of diet for affected individuals to ensure the best possible outcome. Lapse into coma is associated with a drop of up to 40 IQ points in this condition.

The enzyme that is defective in MSUD is complex,[65] and multiple different mutations have been characterized. Except in a North American Mennonite community, where one mutation accounts for a high prevalence of the condition, several different mutations have been found.[62] Many patients are compound heterozygotes. As a result of screening and the immediate institution of the special diet, it has been difficult to establish genotype-phenotype relations. Some infants started on the diet may have forms of the disorder that would have appeared only later in infancy or childhood with episodes of ataxia, failure to thrive, and mild ketoacidosis, particularly following infection or high protein ingestion.

Congenital adrenal hyperplasia. In 21-hydroxylase deficiency, which accounts for more than 90% of those who have congenital adrenal hyperplasia (CAH), and in 11-hydroxylase deficiency, accounting for about 5% of cases, cortisol production is impaired. As a result of the deficiency, feedback inhibition of adrenocorticotropic hormone (ACTH) is lacking, and cortisol precursors, including those that have androgenic activity, are overproduced.

In girls, ambiguous genitalia should permit clinical diagnosis in the neonatal period. Because the diagnosis is not always made, however, screening could increase recognition of females, permitting them to be raised as girls. The diagnosis is much more difficult to establish in newborn males. About two thirds of infants who have 21-hydroxylase deficiency are salt losers; they may suffer severe dehydration and vascular collapse accompanied by hyponatremia during the first 3 weeks of life. In a large retrospective cohort analysis, unscreened males who had salt-losing CAH were diagnosed at the median age of 26 days versus 12 days for screened males.[9] Males who had simple virilizing CAH were detected only in the screened cohort.[9] Several different mutations in the gene for 21-hydroxylase have been found. The presence of salt losing depends on the particular mutation, but a complete genotype-phenotype correlation has not been established.[64]

By accelerating the diagnosis and instituting mineralocorticoid therapy promptly, screening can prevent life-threatening episodes in males and females. Salt-losing crises, however, often can occur before the results of screening are known. Screening also offers an advantage to affected boys who do not lose salt; steroid therapy will prevent virilization, rapid early growth, and premature closure of the epiphyses with resultant short adult stature.

The observation of more living females than males who have this autosomal recessive disorder suggests that males may die in the neonatal period before they are diagnosed.[82] Through screening, an almost equal number of males and females are detected, and the birth prevalence is considerably higher than by clinical diagnosis.[64]

17-Hydroxyprogesterone is increased in the blood in both 21- and 11-hydroxylase deficiency and is measured by the screening test. Examined retrospectively, laboratory or administrative error has accounted for the handful of false negatives. When these are excluded, the test detects more than 98% of infants who have CAH.[64] About 30 false-positive results occur for every infant who has a true positive result. In females, the presence of ambiguous genitalia establishes a true positive, but in the absence of such findings and in most males, additional studies are needed. Measuring serum electrolytes is the most important immediate follow-up to determine the presence of salt loss, which should prompt immediate mineralocorticoid treatment.

Symptom-free adults who have genetic variant forms of 21-hydroxylase deficiency have been identified. The possibility arises, therefore, that clinical problems will not develop in all symptom-free infants who have a confirmed deficiency, unambiguous genitalia, and no salt losing.

Prenatal diagnosis in high-risk females is possible. Prenatal administration of dexamethasone orally to the mother at or before 10 weeks' gestation prevents or reduces intrauterine virilization in most infants. Dexamethasone is safe for both the mother and the fetus.[13]

Biotinidase deficiency. Biotin is a cofactor of a number of carboxylases. Its availability through recycling is reduced in inherited deficiencies of biotinidase. The manifestations and age of onset of biotinidase deficiency vary, possibly because of differences in the degree of enzyme deficiency and the amount of biotin available to the infant. Symptoms usually appear between 2 weeks and 3 years. Ataxia, alopecia, hearing loss, decreased vision, optic atrophy, and seizures have been observed. It is not known yet whether some infants who have the disorder remain free of symptoms and, consequently, how many of the infants detected by screening would develop symptoms if left untreated. In view of the recent observation that significantly more infants found by screening have higher levels of residual biotinidase than those diagnosed clinically,[34] it seems possible that not all infants discovered by screening will ever develop symptoms. Nevertheless, the treatment—providing supplemental biotin—is simple and inexpensive. Although biotin reverses some of the symptoms after they appear, this is not always true for the hearing and visual impairments and developmental delay.[95] Moreover, it is by no means clear that clinical diagnosis always will be made expeditiously. Infants treated as a result of screening have so far remained symptom-free.

Cystic fibrosis. Immunoreactive trypsinogen (IRT) is elevated in the blood of most newborns who have cystic fibrosis (CF).[31] Colorado and Wisconsin currently are performing the test, with second-tier DNA testing for common cystic fibrosis transmembrane conductance regulator (CFTR) mutations in infants who have elevated IRTs. This methodology decreases the rate of false positives identified by IRT screening alone, but may miss up to 10% of CF patients who do not carry a common mutation on either allele. In Wisconsin, a long-term randomized controlled trial is being conducted to determine whether neonatal detection improves the health of children who have CF. Preliminary findings indicate that early identification and intervention prevent malnutrition. However, whether infants discovered by screening ultimately will be better off nutritionally remains to be established.[22] In Australia, one study showed improved nutritional status and pulmonary function in 10-year-olds identified by newborn screening when compared with the prior 3-year birth cohort.[93] Given the significant advances in life expectancy and treatments available, this historical comparison may not be valid. Controversy is considerable over the use of newborn screening for CF. There is no treatment yet available that prevents the clinical manifestations, but earlier therapy may ameliorate the condition.

Homocystinuria. Although vitamin B_6-dependent forms of homocystinuria are treated easily and effectively and account for about 50% of cases, newborn screening will not detect all affected infants.[67] The detection rate after the first week of life, using tests that measure blood or urine homocystine, will be higher than that of neonatal screening, which detects hypermethioninemia. In view of this, as well as the rarity of the disorder, newborn screening by bacterial inhibition assay is hard for some to justify. Others suggest lowering the blood methionine cutoff to 1 mg/dl to decrease the false-negative rate.[66]

New Techniques in Newborn Screening

Tandem mass spectrometry is able to quantitate accurately multiple amino acids, organic acids, and metabolites of fatty acid oxidation from dried blood on filter paper.[74] The advent of this technique could broaden the scope of newborn screening while dramatically decreasing (by two orders of magnitude) the false-positive rates.[14,72] It also would decrease the false-negative rates for homocystinuria.[15] Medium chain CoA dehydrogenase deficiency has an incidence of 1 in 10,000 to 14,000 in the white population and a 25% initial decompensation fatality rate. However, it is easily treated by avoiding fasting and catabolism and by instituting carnitine supplementation and intravenous glucose during intercurrent illness. Newborn screening for this disorder makes sense.[76] For many of the other disorders that would be identified by tandem mass spectrometry, no fully effective treatment exists, and few data suggest that early intervention would affect outcome. However, undiagnosed infant deaths would decrease, and the availability of prenatal diagnosis in subsequent pregnancies for at-risk families would increase.

Equipment costs are very high for this methodology, but after that the cost per sample is quite low. Regionalization probably would be required and may be politically difficult, given the state-based nature of public health. Ethically, one has to balance the value of current prospective therapies with the psychosocial burden imposed by the early diagnosis of disorders affecting the quality and length of life.

Screening for Genetic Susceptibilities

In a few genetic conditions, disease is likely to appear only in certain environments. Screening of infants or young children provides warning that certain exposures will be harmful and should be avoided. If harmful exposures occur, awareness of the genetic susceptibility could speed appropriate management. In the United States, no state currently screens newborns for such genetic susceptibilities. This may reflect a lack of confidence in the ability of the health care system or parents to ensure that the harmful exposures will be avoided. Screening workers or prospective employees for genetic susceptibilities (including the two conditions discussed below), in which the harmful agent may be encountered on the job, is of interest to some employers.[37]

Glucose-6-phosphate dehydrogenase deficiency. A number of different alleles result in this X-linked genetic susceptibility. The usual manifestations are hemolytic anemia accompanied by jaundice and hemoglobinuria. Approximately 10% of black males inherit the mild A form. Except for some sulfur compounds (e.g., sulfamethoxazole), the drugs that trigger reactions seldom are used in the United States (e.g., primaquine), although some may develop hemolysis following heavy exposure to naphthalene (moth balls). In the more severe Mediterranean variant (but only occasionally in the A variant), hemolytic anemia (favism) is encountered following ingestion of fava beans, a staple of diets in many Mediterranean countries. The initiation of a newborn screening program for glucose-6-phosphate dehydrogenase (G6PD) deficiency in Sardinia, together with more education about the deficiency, was associated with a marked decline in the occurrence of favism and the need for blood transfusions.[57]

Alpha$_1$-antitrypsin deficiency. Individuals who have severe alpha$_1$-antitrypsin (AT) deficiency, usually the result of inheriting Z alleles from both parents, are at increased risk of chronic obstructive pulmonary disease (COPD), although in population-based surveys many people who have severe deficiency remain asymptomatic throughout life.[77] Those who have the deficiency and who smoke are likely to encounter pulmonary problems between 20 and 40 years of age, approximately 15 years earlier than nonsmokers.[96] Not all nonsmokers who have AT deficiency get COPD. Severe AT deficiency accounts for about 1% of all COPD. Presymptomatic screening could alert those who have AT deficiency to the especially harmful consequences of smoking. Treatment of AT-deficient, emphysematous adults with human AT elevated their serum and lung AT levels but did not improve their pulmonary function.[39] Whether such treatment would prevent COPD remains to be established.

Because adolescents who have AT deficiency have normal pulmonary function,[91] screening of newborns or young children is of questionable value in improving outcome. A pilot program involving 200,000 newborns in Sweden was stopped when pediatricians reported adverse psychological effects on parents and on the parent-child relationships. Both short- and long-term effects were confirmed in a systematic study. In addition, although parents were told of the harm of exposing their children who had AT deficiency to cigarette smoke, there was as much parental smoking as in a control group.[56]

About 10% of infants who have AT deficiency develop cholestasis, and 2% to 3% later develop cirrhosis. There is no specific treatment or known means of preventing the liver manifestations, although human milk may be protective.[85] Consequently, newborn screening would not be expected to alter the prognosis. AT deficiency should be included in the differential diagnosis of persistent jaundice in young infants. Screening adolescents or young adults might be of benefit.

Carrier Screening

Carrier screening is undertaken for severe untreatable inherited disorders to provide those identified as carriers with options for avoiding the conception or birth of affected children. Carrier screening for Tay-Sachs disease has resulted in a significant decrease in the disease in many Jewish communities.[42] Carrier screening for thalassemia in Sardinia[12] and elsewhere in the Mediterranean basin has lowered its incidence. Most American couples found by carrier screening to be at risk of having a child who has sickle cell anemia decide not to terminate the pregnancy.[53] With nondirective counseling, they may not view the disorder as severe as do those at risk of having children who have Tay-Sachs or thalassemia.

School-based screening programs for sickle cell and Tay-Sachs carriers probably recruit a much higher proportion of the at-risk population than do community programs or office or clinic screening programs. However, they may lead to the stigmatization of students identified as carriers unless all those being screened understand the reasons for the screening and the significance of the results. Nor is it clear that adolescents whose carrier status is identified will retain this information or act on it when they consider having children.[98] If prenatal diagnosis of a condition is available and abortion of an affected fetus acceptable, there is less reason to offer screening before mating. Couples could be screened before the woman becomes pregnant or early in pregnancy, although the latter may require more expensive testing and preclude certain options, such as artificial insemination of sperm from a donor who is not a carrier.

It now is possible to detect approximately 90% of the mutations responsible for cystic fibrosis in Caucasian populations. Questions have been raised about the merits of carrier screening, because not all mutations can be discovered and the prognosis of the disorder is improving steadily.[60] A number of pilot programs have explored consumer interest in carrier screening.[81]

Screening young women to determine if they are carriers of X-linked disorders, such as fragile X syndrome, hemophilia, and Duchenne muscular dystrophy, is becoming technically feasible with DNA analysis. Because of new mutations, not all births of infants who have these disorders could potentially be avoided.

Prenatal Screening

Practitioners who provide care to the young usually do not have primary responsibility for managing pregnancies; however, they often will have prior contact with the mother and the father and can contribute to the parents' understanding of the indications for screening in pregnancy. They also may be contacted by obstetricians to assist in counseling or in anticipation of high-risk newborns. A review of prenatal genetic diagnosis for pediatricians has been published.[17] Only prenatal screening tests are discussed in this chapter.

Neural tube defects. Folate supplementation of bread products was begun recently when it became apparent that women of child-bearing age did not recognize the need for periconceptional folate supplementation.[45] Maternal serum screening of alpha-fetoprotein (AFP) between the fifteenth and twenty-first weeks of pregnancy provides women an opportunity to avoid the birth of most infants who have anencephaly and open spina bifida by prenatal diagnosis and abortion or, if they chose to carry to term, of possibly improving the outcome. Identifying fetuses affected with open spina bifida before delivery permits prelabor cesarean section, which may improve their sensorimotor function.[55]

The maternal serum AFP test is capable of detecting 90% of fetuses that have anencephaly and about 80% of those that have open spina bifida.[89] For every true positive result, however, approximately 30 women who do not have affected fetuses will have false-positive results. In women who have elevated maternal serum AFP, sonographic examination is needed to determine the accuracy of the gestational age estimate; the normal maternal serum AFP concentration is highly dependent on gestational age. If sonography confirms the gestational age, amniotic fluid is obtained by amniocentesis. If the amniotic fluid AFP is elevated, the likelihood of an open neural tube defect exceeds 90%. Further assurance that a defect is present is obtained by performing acetylcholinesterase determinations[90] and high-detail (level 2) ultrasound. Although high-level ultrasound performed by expert sonographers detects most fetuses that have open spina bifida, it should not replace AFP screening.

Down syndrome. Until recently, prenatal diagnosis for Down syndrome (DS) was offered routinely only to pregnant women 35 years and older. The lower risk to younger women of having a fetus with DS and the risk to the fetus of chorionic villi sampling or amniocentesis, as well as the costs, could not justify testing all pregnant women. Nevertheless, most infants who have DS are born to women younger than 35 years of age. In 1984, an association between low concentrations of maternal serum alpha-fetoprotein (MSAFP) and DS in pregnant women regardless of their age was reported, but only about 20% of infants who had DS born to women younger than 35 years were detected.

The detection rate has now substantially improved by measuring human chorionic gonadotropin, which is elevated in pregnancies that have DS (but not trisomy 18), and unconjugated estriol, which is reduced (as well as MSAFP) in pregnancies that have DS. When measurements of these three substances are combined with the maternal age, women can be provided an estimate of their risk of having DS. Currently, risks greater than 1 in 190 to 1 in 270 (depending on the center) are the basis for offering amniocentesis for chromosome analysis. Using this protocol, it is possible to detect almost 60% of pregnancies that have DS. For every pregnancy in which DS is diagnosed, 37 amniocenteses in women found not to have a DS fetus must be performed. More than 80% of pregnant women younger than age 35 years who were at high risk accepted amniocentesis, but only 59% of women 35 and older did.[29]

AVAILABILITY OF SCREENING TESTS

Health departments usually can provide information about newborn screening and hemoglobinopathy screening. Community groups for sickle cell anemia, thalassemia, Tay-Sachs disease, and cystic fibrosis often know where carrier screening for these conditions can be obtained. The Alliance of Genetic Support Groups (www.geneticalliance.org) also can provide information. Genetests (www.genetests.org), operating out of the University of Washington in Seattle, maintains an up-to-date list of laboratories providing DNA tests as well as some biochemical tests.

ETHICAL AND LEGAL ISSUES IN SCREENING

In view of the reproductive implications of most genetic screening tests, as well as respect for the autonomy of individuals, agreement is widespread that genetic screening, with the possible exception of newborn screening, requires informed consent.[3] The disclosure should include the nature of the disease; the probability that the condition will occur; the nature, benefits, and risks of the interventions should the result be positive (including pregnancy termination in the case of prenatal screening); the probability of test error; and other possible deleterious effects.

Some have argued that newborn screening for incurable disorders—for instance, Duchenne muscular dystrophy (DMD), fragile X syndrome, or cystic fibrosis (CF) (for which the benefits of newborn screening have not been fully established)—is appropriate, because the prompt diagnosis affords parents the opportunity of avoiding the birth of another affected child. Others have argued that the infant found to be affected by newborn screening derives no benefit from the test and may even be harmed—for instance, interference with parental bonding.[3] With current DNA test technology, some of those at high risk of having affected children can be identified by carrier screening either before or early in pregnancy. Couples at risk then have the opportunity of avoiding the conception or birth of any affected offspring, whereas only second or additional affected children can be avoided by newborn screening.

Third parties, such as insurers and employers, may have an interest in learning the results of genetic tests, for instance, to deny employment or health insurance coverage to those who have positive results. It is widely agreed that test results should not be released to such third parties without explaining to the screenee, or his or her parents in the case of newborn screening, the implications of obtaining consent and releasing the results. Except in very unusual circumstances, health care practitioners are not obliged to notify relatives of a patient who has a positive test result, but who refuses to inform relatives that they are at risk.[3]

One reason for screening newborns in hospitals is that they are a captive population. Unless screening confers a benefit not otherwise attainable, such a reason is ethically suspect. For disorders for which treatment is effective only before symptoms appear, and when those symptoms appear early in childhood, newborn screening does confer a benefit not otherwise attainable. This is not true for conditions that manifest later in childhood, or not until adulthood, and for which intervention in infancy or childhood is of no proven benefit. This issue is likely to emerge if and when it becomes possible to screen for genetic predispositions to cancer and, perhaps, other mainly adult-onset disorders. Telling children or their parents that they are at risk for a late-onset condition for which intervention after childhood is adequate could alter child-rearing patterns and generate considerable anxiety. In some cases, parents and their children might differ on having the child screened. Older children should be informed of such screening and assent to it.

FUTURE OF GENETIC SCREENING

The Human Genome Project continues to increase the identification of genes that play a role in disease. The major advances of DNA technology make it possible to test a small specimen containing nucleated cells for genetic variants that increase the risk of many different disorders. The ethical and legal challenges to this multiplex testing may prove more difficult than the technological hurdles. The different disorders that might be included in multiplex testing will be markedly different in their age of onset, their severity, and in the interventions available to treat, ameliorate, or avoid their occurrence. How will prospective subjects of testing, or their parents, be able to decide whether they want any or all of the tests available?

The discovery of genes that play a role in complex (polygenic or multifactorial) disorders holds great appeal, but much needs to be learned of the role of alleles at these loci in the general population, as well as in high-risk families, before screening is even considered.

Many mutations of a single gene are capable of causing or predisposing to disease. One drawback of current DNA technology is not being able to detect all of these mutations or to distinguish mutations that result in disease from those that do not. Advances in DNA technology will overcome these problems. In addition, it will be possible to examine gene products in readily accessible cells by amplifying the protein synthesized by the gene of interest and examining its structure or function. Alterations in structure or function are likely to indicate the presence of more disease-causing or susceptibility-conferring mutations than could DNA analysis.

Intensive efforts are being made to isolate fetal cells from maternal circulation to be able to perform prenatal diagnosis without placing the fetus at risk.[79] If feasible, it will be possible to use fluorescent DNA probes to determine the presence of extra chromosomes (as in Down syndrome) on the fetal cells as well as to perform DNA analysis for disease-causing mutations. Within a few years, this technique might make the screening of every fetus for several congenital and hereditary disorders feasible. Once again, the ethical and legal issues may be more difficult to solve than the technical issues.

The marked expansion of genetic testing and screening has increased commercial interest in manufacturing test reagents and providing genetic testing services. Health care clinicians can expect pressures from companies offering tests to provide these services. Unfortunately, tests can be made available without adequate assessment of their safety and effectiveness. Practitioners would do well to go beyond material in the lay press and in company-sponsored brochures before offering these tests to their patients.

REFERENCES

1. Agency for Health Care Policy and Research, Sickle Cell Disease Guideline Panel: *Sickle cell disease: screening, diagnosis, management, and counseling in newborns and infants*, Rockville, Md, 1993, US Department of Health and Human Services.
2. Allen DB: Newborn screening for congenital adrenal hyperplasia in Wisconsin, *Wis Med J* 92:75, 1993.
3. Andrews LB, et al: *Assessing genetic risks: implications for health and social policy*, Washington, DC, 1994, National Academy of Sciences Press.
4. Arn P, Valle D, Brusilow S: Inborn errors of metabolism: not rare, not hopeless, *Contemp Pediatr* 5:47, 1988.
5. Arnold GL, et al: Molybdenum cofactor deficiency, *J Pediatr* 123:595, 1993.
6. Bachmann C, et al: Pitfalls in amino acid and organic acid analysis: 3-hydroxyproprionic aciduria, *Eur J Pediatr* 153(suppl l):23, 1994.
7. Baumgarter ER, Viardot C: Long-term follow-up of 77 patients with isolated methylmalonic acidaemia, *J Inherit Metab Dis* 18:138, 1995.
8. Berghe G: Inborn errors of fructose metabolism, *Annu Rev Nutr* 14:41, 1994.
9. Brosnan PG, et al: Effect of newborn screening for congenital adrenal hyperplasia, *Arch Pediatr Adolesc Med* 153:1272, 1999.
10. Brusilow SW, Maestri NE: Urea cycle disorders: diagnosis, pathophysiology, and therapy, *Adv Pediatr* 43:127, 1996.
11. Buist NRM, Tuerck JM: The practitioner's role in newborn screening, *Pediatr Clin North Am* 2:199, 1992.
12. Cao A, et al: Thalassemias in Sardinia: molecular pathology, phenotype-genotype correlation, and prevention, *Am J Pediatr Hemat-Oncol* 13: 179, 1991.
13. Carlson AD, et al: Congenital adrenal hyperplasia: update on prenatal diagnosis and treatment, *J Steroid Biochem Mol Biol* 69:19, 1999.
14. Chace DH, et al: Use of phenylalanine-to-tyrosine ratio determined by tandem mass spectrometry to improve newborn screening for phenylketonuria of early discharge specimens collected in the first 24 hours, *Clin Chim* 44:2405, 1998.

15. Chace DH, et al: Rapid diagnosis of homocystinuria and other hypermethioninemias from newborns' blood spots by tandem mass spectrometry, *Clin Chim* 42:349, 1996.
16. Committee on Genetics: Newborn screening fact sheets, *Pediatrics* 98: 473, 1996.
17. Committee on Genetics: Prenatal genetic diagnosis for pediatricians, *Pediatrics* 93:1010, 1994.
18. Dixon M, Leonard JV: Intercurrent illness in inborn errors of intermediary metabolism, *Arch Dis Child* 67:1387, 1992.
19. Donnell GN: Clinical aspects and historical perspectives of galactosemia. In Donnell GN, et al, editors: *Galactosemia: new frontiers in research*, Washington, DC, 1993, US Department of Health and Human Services.
20. Drumm ML, Collins FS: Molecular biology of cystic fibrosis, *Mol Genet Med* 3:33, 1993.
21. Dussault JH: Neonatal screening for congenital hypothyroidism, *Clin Lab Med* 13:645, 1993.
22. Farrell PM, et al: Nutritional benefits of neonatal screening for cystic fibrosis. Wisconsin Cystic Fibrosis Neonatal Screening Study Group, *N Engl J Med* 337:963, 1997.
23. Foreman JW: Acid-base physiology in health and disease. In Cohn RM, Roth KS, editors: *Metabolic disease: a guide to early recognition*, Philadelphia, 1983, WB Saunders.
24. Freeze HH: Disorders in protein glycosylation and potential therapy: tip of an iceberg? *J Pediatr* 133:593, 1998.
25. Gahl WA, Schneider JA, Aula PP: Lysosomal transport disorders: cystinosis and sialic acid storage disorders. In Scriver CR, et al, editors: *Metabolic and molecular basis of inherited disease*, New York, 1995, McGraw-Hill.
26. Gaston MH, et al: Prophylaxis with oral penicillin in children with sickle cell anemia: a randomized trial, *N Engl J Med* 314:1593, 1986.
27. Gieselmann V: Lysosomal storage diseases, *Biochim Biophys Acta* 1270: 103, 1995.
28. Grant DB, et al: Congenital hypothyroidism detected by neonatal screening: relationship between biochemical severity and early clinical features, *Arch Dis Child* 67:87, 1992.
29. Haddow JE, et al: Prenatal screening for Down's syndrome with use of maternal serum markers, *N Engl J Med* 327:588, 1992.
30. Hale DE, Bennett MJ: Fatty acid oxidation disorders: a new class of metabolic diseases, *J Pediatr* 121:1, 1992.
31. Hammond KB, et al: Efficacy of statewide neonatal screening for cystic fibrosis by assay of trypsinogen concentrations, *N Engl J Med* 325:769, 1991.
32. Hamosh A: Inherited metabolic diseases in the newborn. In Rosenstein BJ, editor: *Primary care of the newborn*, St Louis, 1992, Mosby.
33. Hamosh A, et al: Comparison of the clinical manifestation of cystic fibrosis in black and white patients, *J Pediatr* 132:255, 1998.
34. Hart PS, et al: Comparison of profound biotinidase deficiency in children ascertained clinically and by newborn screening using a simple method of accurately determining residual biotinidase activity, *Biochem Med Metabol Biol* 48:41, 1992.
35. Hoffmann GF, et al: Clinical and biochemical phenotype in 11 patients with mevalonic aciduria, *Pediatrics* 91:915, 1993.
36. Holtzman NA: Inherited metabolic disease. In Hoekelman RA, editor: *Principles of pediatrics: health care of the young*, New York, 1978, McGraw-Hill.
37. Holtzman NA: *Proceed with caution: predicting genetic risks in the recombinant DNA era,* Baltimore, Md, 1989, The Johns Hopkins University Press.
38. Holtzman NA, et al: Effect of age at loss of dietary control on intellectual performance and behavior of children with phenylketonuria, *N Engl J Med* 314:593, 1986.
39. Hubbard RC, et al: Biochemical efficacy and safety of monthly augmentation therapy for α_1-antitrypsin deficiency, *JAMA* 260:1259, 1988.
40. Jaeken J, Hagberg B, Stronime P: Clinical presentation and natural course of the carbohydrate deficient glycoprotein syndrome, *Acta Paediatrica Scandinavica Suppl* 375:6, 1991.
41. Johnson C, Edleman KJ: Malignant hyperthermia: a review, *J Perinatol* 12:61, 1992.
42. Kaback M, et al: Tay-Sachs disease: carrier screening, prenatal diagnosis, and the molecular era: an international perspective, 1970-1993, *JAMA* 270:2307, 1993.
43. Kahler S, et al: Pancreatitis in patients with organic acidemias, *J Pediatr* 124:239, 1994.
44. Kelly DA: Organ transplantation for inherited metabolic disease, *Arch Dis Child* 71:181, 1994.
45. Knowledge and use of folic acid by women of childbearing age—United States, 1995 and 1998, *MMWR Morb Mortal Wkly Rep* 48:325, 1999.
46. Kooistra L, et al: Motor and cognitive development in children with congenital hypothyroidism: a long-term evaluation of the effects of neonatal treatment, *J Pediatr* 124:903, 1994.
47. Kwon C, Farrell PM: The magnitude and challenge of false-positive newborn screening test results, *Arch Pediatr Adolesc Med,* in press, 2000.
48. Lane PA, Eckman JR: Cost-effectiveness of neonatal screening for sickle cell disease, *J Pediatr* 120:162, 1992.
49. Lehnert W, et al: Propionic acidaemia: clinical, biochemical, and therapeutic aspects. *Eur J Pediatr* 153(suppl l):568, 1994.
50. Levy HL: Nutritional therapy in inborn errors of metabolism. In Desnick RJ, editor: *Treatment of genetic diseases*, New York, 1991, Churchill Livingstone.
51. Levy HL, et al: Sepsis due to *E. coli* in neonates with galactosemia, *N Engl J Med* 297:823, 1977.
52. Listernick R, Frisone L, Silverman BL: Delayed diagnosis of infants with abnormal neonatal screens, *JAMA* 267:1095, 1992.
53. Loader S, et al: Prenatal hemoglobinopathy screening. IV. Follow-up of women at risk for a child with a clinically significant hemoglobinopathy, *Am J Hum Genet* 49:1292, 1991.
54. Lorey FW, Cunningham GC: Birth prevalence of primary congenital hypothyroidism by sex and ethnicity, *Hum Biol* 64:531, 1992.
55. Luthy DA, et al: Cesarean section before the onset of labor and subsequent motor function in infants with meningomyelocele diagnosed antenatally, *N Engl J Med* 324:662, 1991.
56. McNeil TF, Sveger T, Thelin T: Psychological effects of screening for somatic risk: the Swedish α_1-antitrypsin experience, *Thorax* 43:505, 1988.
57. Meloni T, Forteleoni G, Meloni GF: Marked decline of favism after neonatal glucose-6-phosphate dehydrogenase screening and health education: the Northern Sardinian experience, *Acta Haematol* 87:29, 1992.
58. Moses SW: Pathophysiology and dietary treatment of the glycogen storage diseases, *J Pediatr Gastroenterol Nutr* 11:155, 1990.
59. Mudd SH, et al: The natural history of homocystinuria due to cystathionine B-synthase deficiency, *Am J Hum Genet* 37:1, 1985.
60. National Institutes of Health: Statement from the workshop on population screening of the cystic fibrosis gene, *N Engl J Med* 323:70, 1990.
61. National screening status report: *Infant Screen* 17:5, 1994.
62. Nobukuni Y, et al: Heterogeneity of mutations in maple syrup urine disease (MSUD): Screening and identification of affected E1α and E1β subunits of the branched-chain α-keto-acid dehydrogenase multienzyme complex, *Biochim Biophys Acta* 1225:64, 1994.
63. Opitz JM, de la Cruz F: Cholesterol metabolism in the RSH/Smith-Lemli-Opitz syndrome: summary of an NICHD conference, *Am J Med Genet* 50:326, 1994.
64. Pang S, Clark A: Congenital adrenal hyperplasia due to 21-hydroxylase deficiency: newborn screening and its relationship to the diagnosis and treatment of the disorder, *Screening* 2:105, 1993.
65. Peinemann F, Danner DJ: Maple syrup urine disease 1954 to 1993, *J Inherit Metab Dis* 17:3, 1994.
66. Peterschmitt MJ, Simmons JR. Levy HL: Reduction of false negative results in screening of newborns for homocystinuria, *N Engl J Med* 341:1572, 1999.
67. Pyeritz RE: Homocystinuria. In Beighton P, editor: *Heritable disorders of connective tissue*, St Louis, 1993, Mosby.
68. Raymond GV, Moser HW: Clinical diagnosis and therapy of peroxisomal diseases. In: Applegarth DA, Dimmick JE, Hall JG, editors. *Organelle diseases: clinical features, diagnosis, pathogenesis and management*, London, 1997, Chapman and Hall.
69. Rovet JF: Congenital hypothyroidism: long-term outcome, *Thyroid* 9:74 1, 1999.

70. Rutledge SL, et al: Neonatal hemodialysis: effective therapy for the encephalopathy of inborn errors of metabolism, *J Pediatr* 116:125, 1990.
71. Saudubray JM, Charpentier C: Clinical phenotypes: diagnosis/algorithms. In Scrivner C, editor: *Metabolic and molecular basis of inherited disease*, New York, 1995, McGraw-Hill.
72. Schulze A, Kohlmueller D, Mayatepek E: Sensitivity of electrospray-tandem mass spectrometry using the phenylalanine/tyrosine-ratio for differential diagnosis of hyperphenylalaninemia in neonates, *Clin Chim Acta* 283:15, 1999.
73. Schwarzenberg SJ, Sharp HL: Pediatric gastroenterology: update on metabolic liver disease, *Pediatr Clin North Am* 43:27, 1996.
74. Seashore MR: Tandem spectrometry in newborn screening, *Curr Opin Pediatr* 10:609, 1998.
75. Servidei S, Bertini E, DiMauro S: Hereditary metabolic cardiomyopathies, *Adv Pediatr* 41:1, 1994.
76. Seymour CA, et al: Newborn screening for inborn errors of metabolism: a systematic review, *Health Technol Assess* 1:1, 1997.
77. Silverman EK, et al: Variability of pulmonary function in alpha-1-antitrypsin deficiency: clinical correlates, *Ann Intern Med* 111:982, 1989.
78. Simons WF, et al: Educational progress, behaviour, and motor skills at 10 years in early treated congenital hypothyroidism, *Arch Dis Child* 77:2 19, 1997.
79. Simpson JL, Elias S: Isolating fetal cells from maternal blood: advances in prenatal diagnosis through molecular technology, *JAMA* 270:2357, 1993.
80. Sue CM, et al: Neonatal presentations of mitochondrial metabolic disorders, *Semin Perinatol* 23:113, 1999.
81. Tambor ES, et al: Offering cystic fibrosis carrier screening to an HMO population: factors associated with utilization, *Am J Hum Genet* 55:626, 1994.
82. Thompson R, Seargeant L, Winter J: Screening for congenital adrenal hyperplasia: distribution of 17 alpha-hydroxyprogesterone concentrations in neonatal blood spot specimens, *J Pediatr* 114:400, 1989.
83. Tluczek A, et al: Parents' knowledge of neonatal screening and response to false-positive cystic fibrosis testing, *J Dev Behav Pediatr* 13:181, 1992.
84. Touma EH, Charpentier C: Medium chain acyl-CoA dehydrogenase deficiency, *Arch Dis Child* 67: 142, 1992.
85. Udall JN, et al: Liver disease in α_1-antitrypsin deficiency: a retrospective analysis of the influence of early breast- vs bottle-feeding, *JAMA* 253:2679, 1985.
86. Ullrich K: Screening for lysosomal disorders, *Eur J Pediatr* 153(suppl 1):538, 1994.
87. Valle D: Treatment and prevention of genetic disease. In Wilson JD, editor: *Harrison's principles of internal medicine*, New York, 1994, McGraw-Hill.
88. Waggoner DD, Donnell GN, Buist NRM: Long-term prognosis in galactosemia: results of a survey of 350 cases. In Donnell GN, et al, editors: *Galactosemia: new frontiers in research*, Washington, DC, 1993, US Department of Health and Human Services.
89. Wald NJ, Cuckle HS: Open neural-tube defects. In Wald J, editor: *Antenatal and neonatal screening*, Oxford, 1984, Oxford University Press.
90. Wald N, Cuckle H, Nanchahal K: Amniotic fluid acetylcholinesterase measurement in the prenatal diagnosis of open neural tube defects, *Prenat Diagn* 9:813, 1989.
91. Wall M, et al: Long-term follow-up of a cohort of children with alpha-1-antitrypsin deficiency, *J Pediatr* 116:248, 1990.
92. Ward JC: Inborn errors of metabolism of acute onset in infancy, *Pediatr Rev* 11:205, 1990.
93. Waters DL, et al: Clinical outcomes of newborn screening for cystic fibrosis, *Arch Dis Child Fetal Neonatal Ed* 80:Fl, 1999.
94. Werler MM, Shapiro S, Mitchell AA: Periconceptional folic acid exposure and risk of occurrent neural tube defects, *JAMA* 269:1257, 1993.
95. Wolf B, Heard GS: Biotinidase deficiency, *Adv Pediatr* 38:1, 1991.
96. Wulfsberg EA, Hoffmann DE, Cohen MM: Alpha 1-antitrypsin deficiency: impact of genetic discovery on medicine and society, *JAMA* 271:217, 1994.
97. Zanjani ED, Anderson WF: Prospects for in utero human gene therapy, *Science* 285:5436, 1999.
98. Zeesman S, et al: A private view of heterozygosity: eight-year follow-up study on carriers of the Tay-Sachs gene detected by high school screening in Montreal, *Am J Med Genet* 18:769, 1984.

SUGGESTED READINGS

American Academy of Pediatrics Committee on Genetics: Newborn screening fact sheets, *Pediatrics* 98:473, 1996.

American Academy of Pediatrics Committee on Genetics and American Thyroid Association: Newborn screening for congenital hypothyroidism: recommended guidelines, *Pediatrics* 80:745, 1987.

Consensus conference: Newborn screening for sickle cell disease and other hemoglobinopathies, *JAMA* 258:1205, 1987.

Holtzman NA: *Proceed with caution: predicting genetic risks in the recombinant DNA era*, Baltimore, 1989, The Johns Hopkins University Press.

Holtzman NA, Leonard CO, Farfel MR: Issues in antenatal and neonatal screening and surveillance for hereditary and congenital disorders, *Annu Rev Public Health* 2:219, 1981.

March of Dimes Birth Defects Foundation: *International directory of genetic services*, White Plains, NY, 1986, The Foundation.

National Center for Education in Maternal and Child Health: *State treatment centers for metabolic disorders*, Washington, DC, 1986, The Center.

New England Regional Genetics Group Prenatal Collaborative Study of Down Syndrome Screening: combining maternal serum alpha-fetoprotein measurements and age to screen for Down syndrome in pregnant women under age 35, *Am J Obstet Gynecol* 160:575, 1989.

Rhoads GG, et al: The safety and efficacy of chorionic villus sampling for early prenatal diagnosis of cytogenetic abnormalities, *N Engl J Med* 320: 609, 1989.

Scriver CR, et al: *The metabolic basis of inherited disease*, ed 7, New York, 1995, McGraw-Hill.

four Cardiovascular Screening

Michelle Ann Grenier and Perry Santos Nemecheck

Proposed screening methodologies in the pediatric population that may be used to identify existing cardiovascular disease as well as identifying those patients who are predisposed to cardiovascular disease as an adult are outlined in this chapter. In a 1988 national survey of primary care providers, the identification and management of cardiovascular diseases varied greatly. The survey was repeated in 1998 and indicated some improvement in these practices; however, the survey's conclusions were that practitioners needed to be educated further regarding the National Heart, Lung, and Blood Institutes (NHLBI) screening and treatment guidelines.[14]

In this section, recent guidelines are discussed, with suggestions for screening disorders for which guidelines have not yet been formally developed. Blood pressure abnormalities, lipid disorders, athletic participation and risk for sudden death, cardiac effects of psychotropic medications, structural or other heart disease associated with specific genetic disorders, and exposure to known cardiotoxins all require evaluation by screening techniques.

BLOOD PRESSURE SCREENING

The benefits of controlling high blood pressure have been documented by many studies over the years.[24] Cardiac risk factors in children are additive; the more risk factors for cardiac disease in an individual, the more likely that individual will develop long-term sequelae of cardiac disease.[2] The result of high blood pressure of any etiology, whether secondary to other disease states such as renovascular disease or essential hypertension, is end-organ (heart, kidney, brain) damage. Complications of hypertension may be avoided by the appropriate reduction of blood pressure through diet and exercise modification, medication, and control of secondary disease states.[24] Therefore, routine screening of blood pressure in the pediatric age group may serve to identify children who have actual hypertension and those at risk for hypertension in adulthood, thereby allowing intervention and reducing the overall morbidity and mortality of this pervasive and potentially devastating disease. The role of mass blood pressure screening, its cost effectiveness, and its role in identifying individuals who will develop hypertension in adulthood remain unclear.

Children whose disease states are associated with secondary hypertension are frequently identified through routine examinations for their primary disease processes, obviating the role for mass screening in identifying this small subpopulation of pediatric patients. Children who have a strong family history of acquired heart disease and sudden death may be selectively screened. The Task Force on Blood Pressure in children recommends annual blood pressure measurements beginning at 3 years of age.[30] A thorough discussion of high blood pressure in infants, children, and adolescents is provided in Chapter 146.

LIPID ABNORMALITIES

Despite the identification of risk factors, the low-fat diet revolution, the fitness craze, as well as the implementation of antilipid medications and public education, coronary artery disease (CAD) remains a leading cause of medical expenditure and death in the United States.[6,21] Several studies have documented that atherosclerosis begins in childhood and progresses through adulthood,[2] with the ultimate outcome being symptomatic CAD with its associated morbidity and mortality. A universal approach to the prevention of CAD through diet and lifestyle modification is advocated, and the American Academy of Pediatrics (AAP) and the Expert Panel on Blood Cholesterol in Children and Adolescents of the National Cholesterol Education Program (NCEP) have given specific recommendations regarding the selective screening. The NCEP recommends that children who have known risk factors for CAD may be screened as young as 2 years of age, although adolescent cholesterol levels are more likely to correlate with adult lipid levels. Further details regarding the diagnosis and treatment of lipid abnormalities are available in Chapter 23 (Three), Preventive Cardiology.

OBESITY

Although there are no specific standards for obesity screening, pediatric patients are routinely plotted on the national height and weight charts. Obesity is a well-known risk factor for cardiovascular disease and is linked to dyslipidemia, elevated blood pressure, and increased left ventricular mass.[7] Therefore, its presence should be addressed. Primary prevention of obesity through screening by height and weight is imperative.

Obesity is excess adipose tissue, the normal values of which vary by gender (postpubertal females greater than males) and age (12% body fat at birth and 25% body fat at 5 months of age, decreasing to 15% to 18% body fat during puberty). The standards for defining obesity have not been well established. Although anyone plotted with height for weight greater than the seventy-fifth percentile may be considered obese, one must be cautious in excluding those individuals who have excess lean body mass (muscle). There are numerous measures of obesity, but a standard definition for adults and adolescents is a body mass index (weight in kilograms divided by height in meters squared) greater than or equal to 30 kg/m^2 or greater than or equal to 130% ideal body weight for height.[7]

The prevalence of obesity is rising,[7] and screening should be routine in most primary care office visits. The obese child should be managed adequately through a behavioral modification program, understanding of emotional needs, and nutritional counseling for the family. Physical activity should be encouraged rather than excessive television watching and playing computer games. The AAP Committee on Sports Medicine and Fitness has published guidelines for the promotion of healthy weight-control practices in young athletes.[3]

ATHLETIC PARTICIPATION AND SCREENING FOR SUDDEN DEATH

In the United States each year, 300,000 sudden deaths occur (defined as an unexpected death occurring in an otherwise healthy individual under the age of 55 years).[16] Although few sudden deaths occur in people younger than age 20 years (1.3 to 8.5 per 100,000 patient years), two thirds of these cases are attributed to a primary cardiac cause.[16] Although very few young people die of sudden death because of cardiac disease, when one does, it is a tragic and well-publicized event. The devastation associated with sudden death in those younger than 20 years has prompted the screening sports physical examination.

Classification of Exercise

The screening sports physical examination takes into account the athlete's musculoskeletal, respiratory, and cardiovascular systems.

Competitive sports can place an athlete with a cardiovascular abnormality at medical risk because of an increase in work load on the heart or stress on the vascular system caused by increases in blood flow and pressure and increased body temperature. This may be reflected in an increased risk for sudden death, life-threatening cardiovascular alterations or disease progression.[19]

Although exercise may be classified as either dynamic or static, most forms of exercise have components of each.[19] Dynamic exercise is rhythmic and involves small contractions of muscles and movements of joints; static exercise involves development of large intramuscular force, with a small change in muscle length and little joint movement. Each form of exercise exacts differing demands on the cardiovascular system; dynamic exercise causes a volume load on the left ventricle; static exercise induces a pressure load. The potential athlete should be questioned about the type of exercise in which he or she plans to participate in order to determine the type of load to the heart. Various forms of exercise are known to produce muscular/anatomical changes within the left ventricle.

Family and Personal History

One of the best predictors of the risk of sudden death or cardiovascular disease is the family history. Anyone who has a strong family history of cardiac disease or sudden death must be screened more intensely. Sudden death has been associated with the following:

- Hypertrophic cardiomyopathy, which may cause arrhythmia or myocardial ischemia
- Congenital heart disease, either previously repaired or as yet to be diagnosed
- Congenital or acquired valve diseases, particularly aortic stenosis and mitral valve prolapse
- Specific syndromes, such as Marfan disease, which is associated with mitral valve prolapse and aortic root dissection secondary to ongoing root dilation
- Congenital or acquired coronary disease (anomalous coronary arteries or early atherosclerosis)
- History of myocarditis or dilated cardiomyopathy
- Systemic hypertension
- Arrhythmias, particularly the long QT syndrome.

Nonspecific screening questions that might give the practitioner some clues include the following questions:

Have you or anyone in your family ever

- Fainted during or shortly after exercise?
- Experienced seizures or seizure-like episodes?
- Had chest pain with exertion?
- Experienced deafness?
- Noticed feelings of heart racing or jumping up into neck or out of chest?
- Been unable to keep up with peers or fatigue easily?
- Been diagnosed with myocarditis or rheumatic heart disease?
- Been diagnosed as having high cholesterol, high blood pressure, or early heart attacks or strokes?

Most patients can answer these questions, which can give a great deal of insight into specific cardiac diseases warranting further screening.

The Child Who Has Chest Pain

Because of its implication in adults, chest pain in children, although mostly a benign occurrence, can be very frightening. Rare, life-threatening causes of chest pain exist in children, including cardiomyopathy, dysrhythmia, and unidentified structural heart disease, all of which require immediate evaluation, treatment, and subspecialty consultation. Noncardiac causes of chest pain include asthma, gastroesophageal reflux, and costochondritis. Chest pain also may be caused by drug ingestion (e.g., cocaine). The most common diagnosis causing chest pain in children is "idiopathic," and the symptoms typically are chronic.[15] Subspecialty consultation is warranted, but laboratory testing tends to not be cost effective.[15] In general, these children may be screened for cardiac disease, but their families primarily require reassurance.

Specific Recommendations

The AAP Committees on Sports Medicine and Fitness have issued specific recommendations for sports participation, including guidelines for children and adolescents who have mitral valve prolapse and a cardiac dysrhythmia.

Specialized Testing

Hypertrophic cardiomyopathy has been identified as the primary cause of sudden cardiac death in young, competitive athletes accounting for about one third of all fatal cases in the United States.[17] The cost effectiveness of screening all young people for hypertrophic cardiomyopathy has remained controversial. A recently published prospective study screening 33,735 young athletes in Italy showed that the national screening program, in place in Italy for more than 20 years, suggests that hypertrophic cardiomyopathy is an uncommon cause of sudden death, but that the identification and disqualification of affected athletes before participation may have prevented many sudden deaths.[4]

The cost of screening echocardiograms for every young competitive athlete in the United States would be prohibitive. It currently is recommended that athletes who have a suspicious medical or family history of cardiac disease or suspicious findings on physical examination undergo more thorough evaluation by a pediatric cardiologist.

The 12-lead electrocardiogram is an excellent and relatively inexpensive screening tool. Although less sensitive and specific than other forms of cardiac testing, when combined with a thorough history and physical examination, it provides additional assistance in screening.

PROLONGATION OF THE QT INTERVAL

One abnormality that presents insidiously and appears to be diagnosed more frequently is the prolonged QT syndrome.

Patients who have the prolonged QT syndrome are at high risk of sudden death through the sudden development of a form of ventricular tachycardia known as *torsades de pointes*, a rapidly degenerative and unstable rhythm. These patients have been labeled incorrectly as having seizure activity, which causes delays in reaching the proper diagnosis. Commonly used medications such as erythromycin may prolong the QT interval further, and anything inducing a rapid surge of epinephrine, such as a loud noise or a frightening movie, may trigger an episode of torsades.

Sudden Infant Death Syndrome

Prolongation of the QT interval has been implicated in the sudden infant death syndrome (SIDS).[25] It has been proposed that the prolonged QT interval is a result of developmental abnormalities of cardiac sympathetic innervation and may present as sudden death, particularly in the first week of life.[25] This study of 34,442 infants demonstrated a strong association of prolongation of QT interval and sudden death in the first week of life. This study suggests that mass neonatal electrocardiographic testing, to detect a prolongation of the QT interval may be appropriate as a means of detecting infants who are at risk for SIDS.[25] Many investigators believe that further studies must be conducted to support or refute this suggestion.[10,12,13,18,26-28]

Screening Before Medication Use

A number of medications are known to prolong the QT interval. Cisapride (Propulsid), a drug used frequently in the neonatal population, is known to prolong the QT interval, and it is presently recommended that an electrocardiogram be performed before starting this medication. The report of at least seven deaths in children associated with the use of tricyclic antidepressants prompted screening before the start of psychotropic medications and the generation of guidelines by the American Heart Association.[11] Although the exact cause of death in these children remains unknown, tricyclic antidepressants can cause prolongation of the PR interval, an increase in the QRS duration, and prolongation of the QTc. Serotonin reuptake inhibitors have minimal cardiovascular effects, and the stimulants such as methylphenidate and clonidine affect only blood pressure, not the conduction system.

Screening for the use of psychotropic medications involves taking a very thorough history, and paying attention to symptoms of syncope, near-syncope, and palpitations.[11] The family history should focus on deafness, seizures, and sudden death. Patients should be advised to discuss the use of additional medications, including over-the-counter drugs that might interact with prescribed psychotropics. Terfenadine (Seldane), when used in combination with antifungal agents, has caused sudden death.[11] Electrocardiographic monitoring is recommended for tricyclic antidepressants and antipsychotics such as the phenothiazines, butyrophenones, and diphenylbutylpiperidine.[11] Blood pressure monitoring is advocated only for clonidine use.

FETAL ECHOCARDIOGRAPHY

Ultrasound screening of fetuses for suspected congenital heart disease is widely practiced, but its impact on overall outcome still is controversial. Most infants who are diagnosed in utero with chromosomal anomalies or congenital syndromes undergo fetal echocardiography because they may have some form of congenital heart defect. A study of the prenatal diagnosis of congenital heart disease and Down syndrome done in Great Britain demonstrated only a small effect on the use of pediatric cardiology services.[1] However, the prenatal diagnosis of congenital heart disease, especially if it is complex, allows for delivery at a tertiary care center where pediatric cardiology services are available immediately. The cost effectiveness of fetal echocardiography is yet to be determined.

Molecular and Genetic Testing

"Genetic approaches have succeeded in defining the molecular basis of an increasing array of heart diseases, such as hypertrophic cardiomyopathy and the long-QT syndromes, associated with serious arrhythmias."[24] These techniques are no longer just research tools, but evolving clinical tools to be used in conjunction with more formal clinical screening techniques. An example has been published as a consensus report of the Europen Working Group on Arrhythmias.[24]

Individuals who have known syndromes, chromosomal anomalies, metabolic and storage disorders, and neuromuscular disorders should be screened for cardiac defects. The list is long, but examples might include individuals who have Marfan syndrome (aortic root dilatation and mitral valve prolapse), Noonan's syndrome (pulmonary valve stenosis and hypertrophic cardiomyopathy), trisomy 18 (ventricular septal defects and redundant valves), methylmalonic aciduria (dilated cardiomyopathy), Pompe's disease (hypertrophic and dilated cardiomyopathy), and Duchenne or Becker muscular dystrophy (dilated cardiomyopathy). The presence of these defects necessitates screening for cardiac disorders to allow for comprehensive care and improved quality of life.

Exposure to Cardiotoxins

A population of pediatric patients exposed to cardiotoxins should be screened for cardiac defects. These cardiotoxins may be immunologically or infectiously induced (as in children who have vertically transmitted human immunodeficiency virus, or HIV) or a side effect of therapy (such as oncological treatments). Although a variety of causes exist for secondary cardiovascular diseases, few guidelines are established for screening for and monitoring cardiac disease. For example, although it is established that patients who have muscular dystrophy will ultimately develop cardiomyopathy, no firmly established guidelines are in place for screening and monitoring them.

However, published screening and monitoring guidelines do exist for cardiovascular disease associated with HIV exposure in children.[8] The spectrum of cardiac disease associated with HIV infection includes asymptomatic left ventricular dysfunction, cardiomyopathy, myocarditis, pericarditis, endocarditis, cardiac malignancy (rare), and abnormalities of heart rate, rhythm, and blood pressure.[8] Although not all children go on to develop cardiovascular disease, particularly if they were HIV exposed rather than HIV infected, at least one screening echocardiogram is recommended.[8] Because asymptomatic left ventricular dysfunction is the most common form of cardiac disease that may progress to cardiomyopathy, an echocardiogram is more sensitive and specific for detecting most HIV cardiac disease in children than are a physical examination, a chest radiograph, or an electrocardiogram. Children who are actively infected with symptomatic HIV disease are screened and followed more closely.

Treatment of childhood cancer has become so successful that by the year 2010, an estimated 1 of every 250 adults (ages 20 to 45 years) in the United States may be a survivor of malignant disease in childhood or adolescence.[9] Successful cancer treatment modalities such as anthracycline and radiation therapy have been associated with cardiomyopathy, asymptomatic left ventricular dysfunction, and other cardiovascular diseases and with known cardiovascular risk factors such as obesity and dyslipidemia.[5,9,20] The successful treatment of childhood cancer creates one of the largest populations of young adults with the potential for premature cardiovascular disease. A longitudinal study to evaluate cardiovascular risk factors in long-term survivors of childhood cancer is currently being conducted[22] to provide guidelines for formalized cardiovascular screening and monitoring procedures.

As medical therapies become more efficacious and many more children who have genetic syndromes and metabolic, infectious, musculoskeletal, and neoplastic diseases survive into adulthood, cardiovascular disease (as the result of the natural history of their disease or the side effects of their treatment) may become more prevalent.

SUMMARY

Screening for cardiovascular diseases allows early intervention that may prevent future cardiac-related morbidity and mortality. Screening procedures must be easy to implement, relatively noninvasive, and cost effective. As our knowledge base increases regarding the natural history and outcome of diseases as well as the long-term effects of treatments, there will be a more intense need for screening and monitoring to afford early intervention.

REFERENCES

1. Abu-Harb M, et al: Antenatal diagnosis of congenital heart disease and Down's syndrome: the potential effect on the practice of pediatric cardiology, *Br Heart J* 74:192, 1995.
2. Berenson GS, et al: For the Bogalusa Heart Study. Association between multiple risk factors and atherosclerosis in children and young adults, *N Eng J Med* 338:1650, 1998.
3. Committee on Sports Medicine and Fitness: Promotion of healthy weight-control practices in young athletes, *Pediatrics* 97:752, 1996.
4. Corrado D, et al: Screening for hypertrophic cardiomyopathy in young athletes, *N Eng J Med* 339:364, 1998.
5. Delbecque-Boussard L, et al: Nutritional status of children with acute lymphoblastic leukemia: a longitudinal study, *Am J Clin Nutr* 65:95, 1997.
6. Diehl HA: Coronary risk reduction through intensive community-based lifestyle intervention: the Coronary Health Improvement Project (CHIP) experience, *Am J Cardiol* 82:83T, 1998.
7. Gidding SS, et al: Understanding Obesity in Youth: A statement for health care professionals from the Committee on Atherosclerosis and Hypertension in the Young of the Council on Cardiovascular Disease in the Young and the Nutrition Committee, American Heart Association Writing Group, *Circulation* 94:3383, 1996.
8. Grenier MA, Lipshultz SE: Clinical manifestations of HIV infection: cardiac problems. In Zeichner SE, Read JS, editors: *Handbook of pediatric HIV care*, Philadelphia, 1999, Lippincott Williams & Wilkins.
9. Grenier MA, Lipshultz SE. Epidemiology of anthracycline cardiotoxicity in children and adults, *Semin Oncol* 25:72, 1998.
10. Guntheroth WG, Spiers PS: Prolongation of the QT interval and the sudden infant death syndrome, *Pediatrics* 103:813, 1998.
11. Gutgesell H, et al: Cardiovascular monitoring of children and adolescents receiving psychotropic drugs: a statement for healthcare professionals from the Committee on Congenital Cardiac Defects, Council on Cardiovascular Disease in the Young, American Heart Association, *Circulation* 99:979, 1999.
12. Hodgman JE, Siasi B: Prolonged QTc as a risk factor for SIDS, *Pediatrics* 103:814, 1998.
13. Hoffman JIE, Lister G: The implications of a relationship between prolonged QT interval and the sudden infant death syndrome, *Pediatrics* 103:815, 1998.
14. Kimm SY, et al: National trends in the management of cardiovascular disease risk factors in children: second NHLBI survey of primary care physicians, *Pediatrics* 102:E50, 1998.
15. Kocis KC: Chest pain in pediatrics, *Pediatr Clin North Am* 46:189, 1999.
16. Liberthson RR: Sudden death from cardiac causes in children and young adults, *N Engl J Med* 334:1039, 1996.
17. Maron BJ, et al: Sudden death in young, competitive athletes: clinical, demographic and pathological profiles, *J Am Med Assoc* 276:199, 1996.
18. Martin RJ, Miller MJ, Redline S: Screening for SIDS: a neonatal perspective, *Pediatrics* 103:812, 1998.
19. Mitchell JH, Haskell WL, Raven PB: Classification of sports, *J Am Coll Cardiology* 24:845, 1994.
20. Parsons SK, et al: Aspariginase-associated lipid abnormalities in children with acute lymphoblastic leukemia, *Blood* 89:1886, 1997.
21. Pearson TA, Swan HJ: Lipid lowering: the case for identifying and treating the high-risk patient, *Cardiol Clin* 14:117, 1996.
22. Personal communication May 1999, Lipshultz SE, NIH funded proposal.
23. Priori SG, et al: Genetic and molecular basis of cardiac arrhythmias: impact on clinical management parts I and II, *Circulation* 99:518, 1999.
24. Ramsay LE, et al: The rationale for differing national recommendations for the treatment of hypertension, *Am J Hypertension* 11:79S, 1998.
25. Schwartz PJ, et al: Prolongation of the QT interval and the sudden infant death syndrome, *New Engl J Med* 338:1709, 1998.
26. Shannon DC: Method of analyzing QT interval can't support conclusions, *Pediatrics* 103:819, 1998.
27. Southall DP: Examine data in Schwartz article with extreme care, *Pediatrics* 103:819, 1998.
28. Tonkin SL, Clarkson PM: A view from New Zealand: comments on the prolonged QT theory of SIDS causation, *Pediatrics* 103:818, 1998.
29. Update on the 1987 task force report on high blood pressure education program. National High Blood Pressure Education Program Working Group on hypertension control in children and adolescents, *Pediatrics* 98:649, 1996.

five Screening for Anemia

Robert F. Reiss

Screening for anemia in infants and young children should be undertaken at 6 to 12 months and again at 2 years of age, because at these ages the more common congenital anemias and iron-deficiency anemia may become apparent.

Office-based pediatricians generally screen for anemia by determining the whole blood hemoglobin concentration, using blood obtained by skin puncture. This procedure has replaced determination of the microhematocrit procedure by centrifugation of capillary tubes, because this procedure was considered to pose a biohazard because of the creation of blood aerosols and bloody glass fragments when the capillary tubes broke during centrifugation.

The whole blood hemoglobin concentration can now be measured quickly, simply, and accurately in the physician's office. Small portable photometers are available that measure the hemoglobin concentration in a drop of blood. The 1-minute procedure consists of allowing the drop to flow into a small cuvette and subsequently inserting the cuvette into the photometer and reading the digital display on the instrument. Ongoing quality control is simple and consists of reading the display after inserting a control cuvette supplied with the photometer. The hemoglobin concentration determined by this method is compared with reference values obtained from age-matched normal children. Infants and children found to have a hemoglobin concentration less than the lower reference level (2 standard deviations below the population mean) are defined as anemic.

Determination of anemia through these simple screening tests must be confirmed and further information about the morphological characteristics of the patient's blood cells obtained before deciding on further diagnostic workup. These data usually are obtained by submitting a venous blood sample to the hematology laboratory for a complete blood count (CBC) and microscopic examination of a Wright-stained peripheral blood smear.

A CBC can be performed on small samples of EDTA-anticoagulated blood by the modern electronic particle counters. These instruments not only measure the red cell count, mean corpuscular volume (MCV), and whole blood hemoglobin concentration directly, but also calculate the hematocrit, mean corpuscular hemoglobin (MCH), and mean corpuscular hemoglobin concentration (MCHC). In addition, they measure the total white blood cell and platelet counts directly. Finally, modern cell counters perform white cell differential and reticulocyte counts.

Based on the reticulocyte count and the red cell indices (MCV, MCH, and MCHC), the anemia can be presumptively categorized according to mechanism as either (1) hypoproliferative (inappropriately low reticulocyte count for the degree of anemia) or (2) hemolytic (significantly increased reticulocyte count) and by its principal morphological features as (1) microcytic, usually hypochromic (decreased MCV and MCHC), (2) normocytic, usually normochromic (normal MCV and MCHC), or (3) macrocytic (increased MCV). The interpretation of the reticulocyte count and red cell indices and their use in the classification of anemias are discussed fully in Chapter 117, Anemia and Pallor.

Examination of the peripheral smear for red cell size and the degree of cell hemoglobin content permits validation of the indices by determining whether these mean values are representative of a rather monomorphic cell population or of multiple cell populations. The finding of a wide disparity of red cell sizes on the smear is known as anisocytosis and is reflected in an increased red cell volume distribution width (RDW), an additional red cell index reported by the newer cell counters. In addition, the finding of numerous grayish-staining (polychromatophilic) macrocytes, a feature known as polychromasia, suggests increased reticulocytosis. Finally, the red cells themselves may have specific morphological abnormalities of diagnostic significance (e.g., sickled red cells and red cell fragments), or the smear may contain abnormal numbers of types of white cells or platelets, which often helps explain the etiology of the anemia.

With only modest formal training and subsequent ongoing experience, the practicing physician can gain considerable expertise in the interpretation of peripheral blood smears. Acquisition of this skill permits office examination of a smear of a blood drop from a skin puncture. This information, together with that gained from a physical examination and history, including family history of anemia, permits an initiation of specific diagnostic testing at the time the venous CBC sample is submitted to the hematology laboratory.

Among the most common anemias detected in such screening programs are those that have microcytic indices resulting from defects in hemoglobin synthesis. The vast majority of these are due to iron deficiency and thalassemia trait. Although it has been observed that the RDW tends to be increased in the former and normal in the latter, the definitive differential diagnosis will rest on the results of iron studies, free erythrocycte porphyrin measurements, and in older children, hemoglobin A2 levels.

Congenital hemolytic anemias are characterized by increased reticulocytosis, usually have normocytic and normochromic indices, demonstrate polychromasia, and often have diagnostically important red cell morphological abnormalities in the peripheral smear.

The finding of a microcytic anemia and the suspicion of iron deficiency require a search for a source of blood loss, including gastrointestinal bleeding and intestinal parasites. In the absence of evidence for blood loss, iron replacement therapy can be initiated, pending the results of definitive laboratory tests. Increased polychromasia in the peripheral smear after 5 to 7 days and a subsequent rise in whole blood hemoglobin concentration confirm the diagnosis of iron-deficiency anemia and require the continuation of treatment to replace tissue stores.

In summary, performance of the whole blood hemoglobin concentration and examination of the peripheral smear from a drop of whole blood can be office procedures that not only detect the presence of anemia but also often permit its preliminary classification and facilitate expeditious determination of its etiopathogenesis. Finally, the availability of these office tests allows the treating physician to monitor the patient's response to therapy.

SUGGESTED READINGS

Bessman JD, Gilmer PR, Gardner FH: Improved classification of anemias by MCV and RDW, *Am J Clin Pathol* 30:322, 1983.

Yip R, Johnson C, Dellman PR: Age-related changes in laboratory values used in the diagnosis of anemia and iron deficiency, *Am J Clin Nutr* 39:427, 1984.

six Screening for Lead Poisoning

Michael L. Weitzman

Childhood lead poisoning represents one of the great pediatric public health success stories in the United States. It now is very rare for a child to suffer from acute lead encephalopathy. Virtually no children in the United States die from this disease, and most pediatricians have never seen a child who has overt symptoms resulting from this condition. Despite these successes, large numbers of children continue to have levels of exposure that affect their health negatively, requiring continued efforts in the areas of screening, public education, and removal of sources of lead.

EPIDEMIOLOGY OF CHILDHOOD LEAD POISONING

Blood lead levels of children in the United States have been reduced remarkably. Whereas the mean blood lead level of children 1 to 5 years of age was 15 μg/dl between 1976 and 1980, it was 2.7 μg/dl between 1991 and 1994. These changes were accompanied by declines in the prevalence of blood levels of 10 μg/dl or greater from 88.2% to 8.9%, and in the prevalence of levels above 25 µg/dl from 9.3% to 0.5%. An estimated 890,000 children, however, still have blood lead levels of 10 µg/dl or greater, a level high enough to have adverse neurocognitive effects.[7]

Although individuals of all ages can get lead poisoning, blood lead levels tend to peak in those between 1 and 3 years of age, and they vary inversely with family income. Because living in impoverished homes is linked so closely to increased exposure to lead, Medicaid enrollment is an excellent marker for elevated blood lead levels: 60% of children whose blood lead levels are at least 10 µg/dl and 83% of those whose levels are at least 20 µg/dl are enrolled in Medicaid. All children enrolled in Medicaid are required by federal regulation to be screened for elevated blood lead levels at 1 and 2 years of age.[8]

Children may be exposed to lead in water, food, soil, toys, ceramics, and multiple other sources. Parents whose clothing becomes contaminated with lead at work may inadvertently bring lead home on their clothing. Occupations at high risk for "take home exposures" include those involving battery production or repair, the making of pottery, smelting, printing, paint contracting, and working on a firing range, in a brass foundry, or on demolition and renovation of outdoor structures. There also are a number of hobbies that can place children at risk, such as making lead fishing sinkers or bullets, collecting lead figurines, spending time at indoor firing ranges, and making ceramic pottery. In certain cultures, such as several from Latin America and Southeast Asia, a number of home remedies such as azarcon or greta can serve as sources of lead poisoning. Lead glazed ceramic dishes and containers also can lead to lead poisoning, especially if acidic foods such as salad dressings or citric acid juices are served on, or stored in them. These sources should be sought when children who are recent immigrants are poisoned.

For most, however, lead-contaminated interior and exterior household paint that has chipped, pealed, or chalked in their primary residences or in homes of relatives, babysitters, or child care providers remains the most common and the most concentrated source of their exposure. The older the house, the more likely it is to contain lead-based paint; the less affluent the family, the more likely this paint is to be in disrepair. Housing built before 1950 poses the greatest danger of exposure.

ADVERSE HEALTH EFFECTS

Lead has numerous adverse health consequences. Most of our concern, however, has to do with its adverse neurocognitive effects. An impressive array of studies have identified a series of subtle but potentially serious alterations of children's neurocognitive functioning associated with lead exposure at levels believed previously to be innocuous.[1,3-5] It is important to note that no evidence exists of a threshold for the toxic effects of lead—that is, negative cognitive effects—appear to occur at levels as low as 10 µg/dl. The magnitude of the effect of blood lead on IQ is estimated to be in the range of a loss of 2 to 3 IQ points for each 10 µg/dl increase in blood lead. In addition to effects on IQ, many studies have identified adverse effects on other aspects of children's functioning, including attention, vigilance, language development, the transfer of information from short-term to long-term memory, aggression, and antisocial or delinquent behaviors.

SCREENING FOR ELEVATED BLOOD LEAD LEVELS

Screening is essential to the prevention of childhood lead poisoning, the goal being to identify children who need individual interventions to reduce their blood lead levels. Screening is accomplished by measuring blood lead levels. A capillary blood sample collected by finger stick is acceptable, but because of the potential for contamination by lead deposits on the skin, capillary specimens that have lead values of greater than 10 µg/dl should be confirmed with a venous sample.

In 1991, the CDC issued new lead screening guidelines[6] for the first time since 1985, including the following:

1. Children were now to be considered to have elevated blood lead levels if their levels were 10 µg/dl or higher rather than 25 µg/dl
2. Screening was to be accomplished by using blood lead levels rather than free erythocyte porphyrin (FEP) levels because the FEP is very insensitive at blood lead levels below 35 µg/dl
3. Universal screening was recommended for all children 12 to 36 months of age
4. The risk for lead poisoning was to be assessed by using lead screening questionnaires that would guide decisions about the age to begin screening and the frequency of screening
5. Environmental assessment and intervention were to be considered at blood lead levels of 20 µg/dl or higher

The most controversial of these recommendations was the one calling for universal screening. Numerous articles and commentaries appeared in medical journals contesting the use of this recommendation. Some also began to describe anecdotal experiences with what was called "lead hysteria," which was the supposed phenomenon of excessive parental anxiety about subsequent cognitive functioning among children who had mild elevations in blood lead levels. Not only was it questioned whether this anxiety was warranted but also ill effects of such parental anxiety were proposed. No empirical data existed to guide clinicians in ways to allay parental anxiety or to reduce such lead burdens in children.

In 1995, almost 50% of the pediatricians in the United States reported not screening all children in their practices.[2] Even more disturbing was that although children covered by Medicaid are three times as likely as children not covered by Medicaid to have elevated lead levels (and Congress had passed a law in 1989 requiring lead screening of all Medicaid-insured children), a 1998 government report indicated that 81% of Medicaid children had never been screened.[8] This report also showed that 65% of a sample of Medicaid-insured children who were identified as having elevated blood lead levels had never been screened beforehand. Thus, despite a national policy aimed at screening all children, even the majority of high-risk children were not being screened.

Since the 1991 CDC lead screening guidelines were issued, a number of studies have demonstrated that questionnaires aimed at identifying high-risk children have reasonably good screening characteristics in terms of sensitivity, specificity, and negative predictive values. Because of concerns about the implementation of universal screening, the documentation of markedly diminishing rates of elevated blood lead levels among children who were screened, and evidence that high-risk children could be identified before screening, the CDC issued new guidelines for screening in 1997. These guidelines advise state health officials to devise systems to facilitate targeted screening. Within the state or locale for which recommendations are made, it was advised that child health care professionals use blood lead tests to screen children ages 1 and 2 years (and children 3 to 6 years of age who have not been screened previously) who are found to have potentially high levels of exposure by meeting one of the criteria in Box 20-1.

In addition, health care professionals were encouraged to identify children who should be screened because of their increased risk of being exposed to less usual sources, such as risks associated with various parental occupations or hobbies. In the absence of a statewide plan or other formal guidelines from public health officials, universal screening for virtually all young children, as was called for in the 1991 CDC guidelines, was again encouraged. Similarly, whenever a parent or a health care professional suspects that a child is at risk for lead exposure, the child should be screened with a blood lead test, regardless of health department recommendations or responses to questionnaires.

Follow-up of Positive "Screens"

Children whose blood lead screening test is less than 10 µg/dl at 1 year of age should be rescreened at 2 years of age. A change in the child's potential exposures or if the parent or primary care professional is concerned that the child is at heightened risk, may necessitate rescreening the child earlier. If at the 2-year screen the blood lead level again is less than 10 µg/dl and the child's potential exposures have not increased, the child should not be subjected to subsequent screening.

Children with blood lead values of 10 to 19 µg/dl. If a venous sample confirms that the child does have an elevated blood lead level, parents are counseled on ways to diminish ongoing exposure (Box 20-2). Children whose blood lead levels are between 10 and 14 µg/dl should be retested every 3 months; those whose levels are between 15 and 19 µg/dl should be retested every 2 months.

Children with blood lead values of 20 to 44 µg/dl. Children whose blood lead levels are in this range are described as having moderately elevated blood lead levels; they require both medical and environmental intervention. If the confirmatory venous lead level is 20 µg/dl or greater, the child should have (1) a medical evaluation, consisting of a detailed medical, nutritional, developmental, and environmental history, and a complete physical examination; (2) a

BOX 20-1

RECOMMENDATIONS FOR LEAD SCREENING IN THOSE AT RISK

- Child resides in a Zip code area in which at least 27% of housing stock was built before 1950 or 12% or more of children have blood lead levels ≥10 µg/dl.
- Child receives services from public assistance programs for the poor, such as Medicaid or the Supplemental Food Program for Women, Infants, and Children (WIC).
- Child's parent or guardian answers "yes" or "don't know" to any of the following three questions:
  1. *Does your child live in or regularly visit a house that was build before 1950?* This question could apply to a facility such as a home child-care center or the home of a babysitter or relative.
  2. *Does your child live in or regularly visit a house built before 1978 that has had renovations or remodeling within the past 6 months?*
  3. *Does your child have a sibling or playmate who has or did have lead poisoning?*

Data from The Centers for Disease Control and Prevention: *Screening young children for lead poisoning: guidance for state and local public health officials,* Atlanta, 1997, US Department of Health and Human Services, Public Health Service.

BOX 20-2

AVOIDING LEAD HAZARDS IN THE HOME

Cover leaded paint that is chipping or peeling.
Move cribs, playpens, furniture, and play areas away from chipping or peeling paint.
Wet-mop floors and wet-clean window sills and window wells with a high-phosphate detergent.
Avoid dry dusting or sweeping.
Wash children's hands, toys, and pacifiers regularly.
Use cold water for cooking; run tap water for 2 to 3 minutes every morning before using.
Repair deteriorated window panes in house and on porches.
Replace old windows.
Remove paint in old homes (only by trained contractors).
Families must be out of their homes during paint removal.
Postabatement cleanup, preferably by professional housecleaners, is essential.
Relocate the family to lead-safe housing.

Data from The Centers for Disease Control and Prevention: *Preventing lead poisoning in young children: a statement by the Centers for Disease Control,* Atlanta, 1991, US Department of Health and Human Services.

laboratory evaluation of iron status, including a hematocrit and mean corpuscular volume (MCV), and either a ferritin level or iron and iron binding capacity levels; (3) an environmental inspection, and where indicated, environmental intervention to diminish or curtail further exposure to lead; and (4) case management to ensure that the needed counseling and medical, nutritional, and environmental interventions are provided quickly and effectively.

The medical evaluation identifies signs and symptoms of lead poisoning that are very unusual at this level. The developmental assessment is conducted to see if the child is in need of early intervention services, although it is very unlikely that blood lead levels in this range would result in demonstrable delays. Concerns about inattention and hyperactivity should prompt referral for early intervention services.

Nutritional assessment is conducted to identify eating patterns that may result in increased absorption of lead from the gastrointestinal tract, such as iron deficiency, low calcium intake, or infrequent meals. Many children whose blood lead levels are in this range are eligible for WIC support and should be referred. If the child is iron deficient, iron supplements should be prescribed.

Such children require home inspections, usually performed by local public health departments, to identify sources of lead exposure. Abatement of lead-based hazards and subsequent dust control are the cornerstones of treatment for children whose blood lead levels are in this range. Families should be counseled to (1) have lead-based paint abatements performed by a properly licensed contractor and, if possible, with supervision of the local health department; (2) relocate children and pregnant women to another site while abatement is being performed; and (3) have a thorough cleanup of dust before allowing children to reinhabit the home. The use of chelating agents for children whose blood lead levels are less than 25 μg/dl is not indicated. Children whose blood lead levels are in this range should have blood lead tests repeated weekly or monthly (the higher the blood lead levels, the more frequently the child should be retested).

Children with blood lead values of 45 μg/dl or higher. The clearest management strategies exist for children in this category. Children whose blood lead screens are 45 to 59 μg/dl should be retested with venous blood within 48 hours; those whose are 60 to 69 μg/dl should be retested within 24 hours; and those whose are at least 70 μg/dl should have a venous blood lead level conducted on an emergency basis. There is broad consensus that such children must be removed from sources of lead in their environments and receive chelation therapy, as described in Chapter 293, Poisoning.

REFERENCES

1. Agency for Toxic Substances and Disease Registry: *The nature and extent of lead poisoning in children in the United States: a report to Congress,* Atlanta, 1988, US Department of Health and Human Services
2. Campbell JR, et al: Screening for elevated blood lead practices among United States' pediatricians, *Pediatrics* 98:372, 1996.
3. National Research Council: *Measuring lead exposure in infants, children, and other sensitive populations,* Washington, DC, 1993, National Academy Press.
4. Needleman HL, Gatsonis CA: Low-level lead exposure and the IQ of children, *JAMA* 263:673, 1990.
5. Schwartz J: Low-level lead exposure and children's IQ: a meta-analysis and search for a threshold, *Environ Res* 65:42, 1994.
6. The Centers for Disease Control and Prevention: *Preventing lead poisoning in young children: a statement by the centers for disease control,* Atlanta, 1991, US Department of Health and Human Services.
7. The Centers for Disease Control and Prevention: *Screening young children for lead poisoning: guidance for state and local public health officials,* Atlanta, 1997, US Department of Health and Human Services, Public Health Service.
8. United States General Accounting Office: *Medicaid: elevated blood led levels in children,* General Accounting Office/Health, Education and Human Services Division-98-78, Washington DC, February 1998.

seven Screening for Drugs

Deborah E. Campbell and Kathy Silverman

The use of psychoactive drugs is associated with potential somatic and behavioral consequences in all individuals; however, a series of health issues have particular relevance to those providing health care to the pediatric population. These serious concerns regarding drug abuse express themselves at both ends of the pediatric spectrum and relate to the impact of drug abuse on the developing fetus and the developing adolescent. The widespread use of psychoactive drugs and the frequent association of such use with perinatal and adolescent morbidity and mortality have engendered extensive debate about public health measures to minimize the consequences of this behavior. Among the measures that have been promulgated are recommendations for criminal prosecution, incarceration, and forced rehabilitation of drug abusers, and in particular, pregnant substance users.

In addition, as a result of improved methods of detecting drugs and their metabolites in body fluids, mass screening of pregnant women, newborns, and adolescents has been proposed. This has caused controversy within the pediatrics, obstetrics, and bioethics communities. Although much can be gained from the early detection of substance use in pregnant women, infants, and adolescents, both ethical and practical considerations suggest caution before imposing drug screening on unwilling patients and parents. An additional caution relates to the discriminatory fashion in which such screening often is carried out. Although drug abuse is encountered across all cultural, ethnic, and socioeconomic groupings, experience indicates that both screening initiatives and punitive responses are applied more often to disadvantaged and minority populations.

ANALYTICAL TECHNIQUES

Several techniques can be used to detect the metabolites of drugs of abuse in urine, serum, hair, nails, and meconium. In general, the less expensive and less complex methods generate a greater incidence of false-positive and false-negative results than do more costly and sophisticated tests. Such methods range from simple spot tests, which can be performed in the physician's office, to gas chromatography/mass spectrometry (GC/MS) tests, which require highly technical and expensive equipment.

Color or spot tests are screening techniques used to detect specific drugs, such as salicylates or ethanol, that often are undiscovered by broad spectrum analysis. A specific color change occurs when a reagent is mixed with urine that contains the suspected drug. The color change may be observed visually or identified spectrophotometrically. The advantages of spot testing are that it is inexpensive and easy to perform, and its results are available immediately. The disadvantages are that other substances can cross react with the reagent to produce the same color changes as the suspect psychoactive drug, leading to a false-positive result. In addition, spot tests are not highly sensitive, requiring a high concentration of the drug to yield a positive result.

Other screening tests include thin-layer chromatography (TLC) and immunoassays. The drug screening methodologies employed most commonly in clinical practice are the immunoassays. These tests are available at most laboratories and are reasonably accurate and affordable.[25] Included among the immunoassays are the enzyme multiplied immunoassay technique (EMIT); the kinetic interaction of microparticles in solution (KIMS); the cloned donor immunoassay (CEDIA); the radioimmunoassay (RAI); and the fluorescence polarization immunoassay (FPIA). All the immunoassays share a common mechanism; a specific antibody reacts with the drug being tested to produce a product that can be measured. The advantages of immunoassays are that they test for almost all drugs of abuse; the test results are rapidly available; and because of broad cross-reactivity, the tests are able to identify a class of drugs rather than a specific drug. Disadvantages are that false-positive tests do occur; thus, positive results need to be confirmed by more sophisticated techniques.

Confirmation techniques that are used to substantiate positive screening results include gas chromatography (GC), gas chromatography/mass spectrometry (GC/MS), high performance liquid chromatography (HPLC), liquid chromatography/mass spectrometry (LC/MS), and a variety of other methods. GC/MS is both sensitive and specific and is considered the "gold standard" for identifying drugs of abuse in urine. Because of its cost and complexity, it is not used for screening.[25]

The length of time that test results will remain positive subsequent to use varies with the drug, the extent of its abuse, and the sensitivity of the test employed. With the immunoassay techniques, most drugs can be detected for at least 2 to 3 days after their last use. The metabolites of phencyclidine (PCP), however, may be detected for up to 1 week, and cannabinoids can be found for up to 3 to 4 weeks in heavy users. Among neonates the detection of drug metabolites in urine is limited because of dependence on the degree of transplacental passage; the time of the last maternal drug intake; and time when the infant's urine was collected.

In prospective studies, urine testing alone fails to identify approximately 50% of drug-exposed infants. Consequently, other specimens, such as meconium and hair, have been suggested for analysis as a means to optimizing drug detection. Several recent reviews summarize toxicological screening, specimen analysis, and implications for clinical care of the infant.[6,16,28]

SPECIMENS FOR ANALYSIS

Urine

Urine is the specimen most commonly used for toxicological analysis. The duration of drug detection in urine depends on many variables, including the route and frequency of ingestion, the timing and amount of the last dosage, and the individual's intrinsic physiology. The latter determines the rate of drug metabolism and excretion. In neonates, the detection of drug metabolites in urine depends not only on the time of the last maternal drug ingestion, but on urine collection and storage practices, as well. Maternal abstinence from drug use for several days before delivery or the inability to obtain a urine sample from the infant soon after birth contributes to false-negative results. As noted previously, urine testing alone misses nearly 50% of drug-exposed infants.

Another factor that diminishes the utility of urine as an optimal specimen for testing relates to cross-reaction among immunoassays for opiates and amphetamines. Several over-the-counter and herbal preparations produce false-positive enzyme or radioimmunoassay tests.[16] A pregnant woman may be taking medications that either contain a drug (codeine) or metabolize the drug to a reacting substance (e.g., ephedrine, benzphetamine). Tests for opioids are among the most difficult to interpret, even using both screening and confirmatory tests. Opioids are found in a variety of medications including antitussives, paregoric, codeine, and hydrocodone (Percocet), as well as in foods containing poppy seeds. Immunoassays for opiates do not distinguish between morphine, codeine, or their common glucuronide conjugates. Breast-feeding[15] and passive inhalation of marijuana and crack also have been documented as sources for positive urine tests.[6,17,28]

Meconium Analysis

Meconium has been widely investigated as an alternate to urine for drug testing in the neonate. Meconium begins to form in the fetal gut at 18 to 20 weeks' gestation. Drug accumulation in meconium occurs either through direct deposition via the biliary tree or through fetal ingestion of amniotic fluid. Drug metabolites are tightly bound to cell fragments in the meconium, impeding their diffusion. Meconium, therefore, should reflect in utero exposure during the second and third trimesters. Ostrea et al[24] and others[8,20,21] have demonstrated the improved detection of metabolites of commonly abused drugs (cocaine, opiates, and cannabinoid) in meconium, reporting rates of in utero drug exposure three to four times greater than maternal self-report and 25% greater than urine testing alone. In a recent publication, Ostrea demonstrated substantial exposure of neonates to xenobiotic agents, including food additives, local anesthetics, and other prescribed and over-the-counter medications in addition to drugs of abuse.[23]

Meconium testing has been shown to have a 93% sensitivity and 83% positive predictive value. Meconium testing has been used as a tool in various prevalence studies. However, screening test results must be confirmed by GC/MS because false-positive rates of up to 43% have been reported.[20,25] The National Institute on Drug Abuse (NIDA) has concluded that although it is reasonable to quantify drugs and their metabolites in meconium, it is inappropriate to equate these results with dosage exposure. The use of meconium for mass screening has been debated. However, although meconium testing is becoming more readily available, it remains more expensive and time consuming to perform than urine testing.

Hair Analysis

Hair samples may be analyzed for the presence of drugs.[16,19] Exposure to a drug results in incorporation of the substance into the hair follicle, cuticle, and hair shaft. The drug remains in the hair until it is replaced, offering a greater window for detection—much broader than either urine or meconium testing. Testing of newborn hair to document in utero exposure remains an investigational tool. Hair grows during the third trimester in the neonate. Analysis of a sample of hair at birth would reflect maternal drug use during the last trimester. It has been purported that sectional analysis of hair may help determine the timing and duration of substance use.

Hair analysis is technically more involved than that of urine or meconium. The validity and interpretability of the data are questionable at this time, because several factors currently preclude valid use of this testing method. The mechanisms by which drugs enter the hair have not yet been elucidated. Furthermore, the effect of environmental contamination, chemical treatment, or color pigmentation and the racial, ethnic, gender, and age (newborn versus adult) differences in the accumulation of drug in hair have yet to be determined. Confirmation of positive test results by gas chromatography-mass spectroscopy requires larger amounts of hair, in some instances necessitating shaving the infant's head.

ISSUES AND CONTROVERSIES

The major issues concerning drug screening do not relate to the expense of the testing, the accuracy of the results, or the number of days that testing will show a positive reaction. Rather, the controversies center on the ethical and practical implications of such screening procedures. Seeking evidence of substance abuse differs greatly from other screening procedures, in which patient and physician share a mutual concern in detecting a condition previously unknown to either.

PERINATAL ISSUES

It has been estimated that approximately 10% of infants born in the United States have been exposed to illicit drugs in utero. The 1996 National Pregnancy and Health Survey,[22] conducted in the 48 contiguous states, reported a 5.5% overall prevalence of illicit prenatal substance abuse.In addition, approximately 20% of women reported alcohol consumption during pregnancy, and a similar percentage admitted tobacco use.[2,18] Other investigators have found that 8% to 12% of women acknowledged illicit substance use within the month preceding their delivery.[2,18] Use of other substances (alcohol, tobacco, and prescribed or over-the-counter drugs) is far more common but difficult to quantify.

The greatest concern regarding perinatal drug exposure involves the potential teratogenic and developmental effects of particular drugs: alcohol, marijuana, opiates, and cocaine/crack. Drug-exposed infants are more likely to suffer a range of health and developmental problems and require prolonged neonatal hospitalization because of low birth weight and prematurity, neonatal abstinence syndromes, and birth complications. Many of these children need long-term developmental support and habilitative care for the remediation of cognitive and behavioral sequelae.*

Patterns of maternal drug use have changed during the past 2 decades. In the 1980s the use of crack and cocaine during pregnancy increased dramatically. Since the mid to late 1990s, there has been a shift, with decreasing cocaine and crack use concurrent with a resurgence of heroin abuse (particularly among adolescents) and regional increases in methamphetamine use. When substance abuse is associated with perinatal morbidity and mortality, it often is difficult to ascribe causality to a particular agent. Pregnant substance abusers frequently are polysubstance users, typically reporting tobacco and alcohol use in conjunction with illicit substances. The high prevalence of substance use among innercity minority populations adds confounding factors related to lifestyle, environment, and resources. However, not all infants experience detrimental effects from perinatal drug exposure. Genetic and maternal characteristics, differences in the chemical structure of drugs, and patterns of use interact to influence fetal vulnerability.†

Continuing parental drug abuse after the infant's birth is a significant concern and has been associated with (1) increased frequency of physical abuse of their infants, (2) diversion of limited family resources and involvement in criminal activity to enable them to buy drugs, (3) high risk for mental and physical illness, and (4) postnatal passive exposure of the infant to substances.[6,18,27,28]

IMPLICATIONS OF DRUG TESTING IN NEWBORNS

It is well recognized by clinicians that it is important to identify substance-abusing women in the prenatal and postpartum periods as a means to facilitate appropriate treatment and follow-up and to optimize the health and developmental well-being of the child. Screening for substances of abuse is a useful adjunct in the assessment of both the pregnant woman and the infant. Self-reporting alone has been shown to seriously underrepresent actual illicit substance use during pregnancy. Reliance on the use of laboratory tests in response to self-report or clinical suspicion of in utero substance exposure also underestimates the prevalence of drug exposure. This has resulted in the recommendation by some that universal screening be conducted.

The issue of universal or mandatory screening for drugs of abuse has engendered significant debate about the punitive consequences affecting the mother, infant, and family.[7] A 1991 report of state maternal and newborn drug testing and reporting policies identified 13 states that have mandatory reporting of drug-exposed infants.[1] Three states required notification of criminal justice agencies, and 10 mandated child abuse/neglect reports to be filed. Controversies surround the ethical and practical implications of universal screening pro-

*References 5, 9, 11, 12, 27, 28.

†References 5, 11, 12, 17, 27, 28.

cedures. Three ethical principles—beneficence, autonomy and justice—should guide the physician and health care giver to act in the best interest of the patient. In the case of the substance-abusing woman, these principles must be applied not only to the woman but also to her fetus or infant and family as well. This can create conflicts when the best interests of the mother may conflict with her infant's interests. Maternal confidentiality is juxtaposed against the infant's right to protection from harm. The uncertainty in defining which specific women and fetuses are affected by drug use during pregnancy, the intense reaction by society to punish women who use illicit drugs while ignoring the serious impact of licit substances such as tobacco and alcohol on the fetus, and the documented discrimination against poor and minority women in the enforcement of sanctions are critical issues to be addressed.

Mandatory or coerced testing of pregnant women stands in contrast to traditional adherence to ethical principles of informed voluntary consent for all physician-patient interactions. Similarly, testing a neonate for the presence of drugs is, in fact, an assessment of maternal drug use. Thus, many find it ethically difficult to justify testing either the baby or the mother without appropriate consent. Identical concerns have been raised regarding testing for human immunodeficiency virus, and most jurisdictions forbid such testing without informed parental consent.

A second concern is that the practice of screening mothers for drugs may cause pregnant women to delay or to avoid prenatal care. Fear of detection and punitive consequences associated with the identification of illicit substance abuse are viewed as bases for the premise that mandatory screening will inhibit use of prenatal care services.

Finally, some concern exists regarding how best to use the information gathered from drug screening. There would be little concern if it were used only to provide support services to families in difficulty and to facilitate drug abuse treatment. Unfortunately, this is not the case in many areas of the country, particularly in those communities in which drug abuse is common. Often the mandatory or voluntary reporting of positive findings to child protective agencies results in (1) punitive actions that, although motivated by the presumed best interest of the infant, separate the mother and her newborn, and (2) occasionally in other interventions that do not serve the needs of the family or the child well. This is of particular concern owing to evidence of racial and cultural biases that make it more likely that, despite similar rates of substance abuse, black women and poor women are more likely to be reported to state authorities than are others.[10]

For a condition to warrant a screening initiative, it must meet several criteria: (1) the disorder must cause substantial mortality, morbidity, or suffering; (2) screening tests must be safe, effective, simple, reliable, practical, valid, and of reasonable cost; and (3) treatment for the condition must be efficacious, available, accessible, and easy to comply with, and early treatment must be more effective than later treatment.[14]

Mass screening for drugs of abuse during the perinatal period is problematic for several reasons. First, all available screening tests have limitations in terms of sensitivity, specificity, and cost. The limited number of existing drug treatment programs and lack of comprehensive services for pregnant and parenting women who have young children preclude the offer of appropriate services to all identified substance abusing women. Furthermore, neurodevelopmental and behavioral outcome data for infants born to recreational substance users have not consistently demonstrated deficits beyond those environmental factors that are a proxy for poverty and low maternal education. Even among heavy substance users, data conflict with regard to infant and childhood outcomes.*

The National Institute on Drug Abuse recommends use of maternal self-report and validated biological markers to guide testing. The American Academy of Pediatrics (AAP) opposes universal neonatal laboratory screening for illicit drugs.[2-4] However, AAP guidelines stipulate that these infants and children require a clearly identified medical home, comprehensive care, and ongoing developmental surveillance with periodic developmental screening and assessment. The AAP also recommends that every newborn evaluation have a comprehensive medical and psychosocial history, including specific information regarding maternal drug use. Infants born to mothers who have clinical indicators of drug use should be screened. Social indicators such as low income, race, and ethnic origin are not sufficient reasons for selective screening. When clinical indicators are present and the screening test results are positive, caretakers have the opportunity to intervene positively for the benefit of the family and the infant. These interventions include the following:

1. Exercise influence for early enrollment of the mother and father in comprehensive local drug treatment centers.
2. Observe the infant carefully for signs of drug withdrawal and initiate early treatment upon the occurrence of symptoms.
3. Discourage breast-feeding, which can cause the infant further toxicity.
4. Monitor the infant for signs of central nervous system and renal dysfunction, including the use of central nervous system and renal ultrasound testing, when indicated.
5. Involve parents in parenting and family support programs that guide, support, and coordinate services to optimize parent-child interactions and child health and developmental outcomes.

Recommended guidelines for newborn urine drug screening are shown in Box 20-3.

Screening for drug abuse with informed voluntary consent or when clinically indicated in a particular newborn (with parental or court-ordered consent) is not at issue. What is debated vehemently is the routine screening of all newborns or their mothers without consent, and it must be viewed as ethically questionable because of its unproved benefits and its potential to affect other aspects of perinatal care adversely.

ADOLESCENT ISSUES

More than 80% of high school seniors have had some experience with alcohol; more than 50% report use during the previous month, and nearly 5% report drinking daily. Nearly 50% of high school seniors report some lifetime use of marijuana, with approximately 20% of these adolescents using marijuana at least once per month.[4,13,26] Although fewer

*References 6, 9, 11, 12, 15, 17, 28.

BOX 20-3

GUIDELINES FOR NEWBORN URINE DRUG SCREENING

1. The following neonates should have urine sent for toxicology screens:
   a. Neonates of mothers who have admitted histories of substance abuse
   b. Neonates of mothers who have a past or present history of maternal drug use
   c. Neonates whose mothers exhibit behaviors indicative of substance abuse during labor or delivery. These include drug-related or bizarre behaviors, such as slurred speech, unsteady gait, inappropriate affect, and/or confusion
   d. Neonates who evidence symptoms of drug intoxication or withdrawal (i.e., sneezing, jitteriness, irritability, high-pitched cry, seizure, or other neurological symptoms).
2. The following neonates may also have urine sent for toxicology upon assessment and review by a physician:
   a. Neonates of mothers with no prenatal care
   b. Neonates not delivered in-hospital
   c. Cases of abruptio placenta
   d. Cases of congenital syphilis or those whose mother has had a positive syphilis screening test (e.g., VDRL, RPR, FTA)

Reproduced with permission from the Division of Neonatology, Department of Pediatrics, Albert Einstein College of Medicine, Montefiore Medical Center, Bronx, New York.

young people abuse opiates, cocaine/crack, and other drugs, the spectrum of abuse of psychoactive drugs emerges as a leading cause of direct or indirect death among adolescents and also is a cause of major morbidity and social and educational disruption.

There may be a great temptation to screen all youths for substance abuse, both to intercede on their behalf and to diminish the effects of drug abusers on society. A ruling by the United States Supreme Court (Veronia School District 47J, *Petitioner v. Wayne Acton;* June 26, 1995) held that random drug screening of students participating in interscholastic sporting events was constitutional. Although the Court, in that same opinion, cautioned "against the assumption that suspicionless drug testing will not readily pass constitutional muster in other contexts," the decision, at a minimum, facilitated drug screening of high school athletes and opened the door for consideration of even wider application of drug screening programs. Despite this permissive court ruling and other arguments in favor of the random drug testing of adolescents, ethical and practical concerns remain regarding routine, nonconsensual drug screening of adolescents.[3]

Although parental consent most often is sufficient for performing any procedure in the younger child who lacks the capacity to make informed judgments, parental permission alone is not sufficient for performing diagnostic or therapeutic procedures on competent adolescents. Despite the temptation to apply a different ethical standard to adolescents when investigating the potential for drug abuse, it is treacherous to adhere to principles of informed consent only when such adherence is convenient or expedient.

Beyond ethical issues are concerns regarding the effect on the physician-adolescent relationship inherent in the practice of nonconsensual (and even secretive) screening for drugs—such a practice would not remain secret for long. The major concerns are the following:

1. Adolescents who use drugs know they are using drugs and, wishing to keep that behavior a secret from their physician and parents, would not seek care if involuntary screening were a part of that care.
2. Adolescents would abstain from drug use for the few days necessary to produce a clean and deceptively reassuring urine specimen.
3. Pediatricians would not be willing to collect urine specimens under direct observation to prevent the adulteration or substitution techniques available to knowledgeable young drug abusers.
4. The information gained from such involuntary screening would not add sufficiently to the knowledge acquired from interview to justify the risk of establishing an adversarial relationship with the teenager.

Certainly, requisites for consent and voluntary screening may be waived when there is reason to doubt competency or when information gathered by interviewing the parent or adolescent suggests that the adolescent is out of control or at high risk to self and others. However, both ethical and practical questions strongly indicate that routine involuntary screening of all adolescents is not essential. The advancing technology of drug screening should be applied selectively to monitoring the therapeutic progress of known drug abusers and to testing young persons who have been identified as being at special risk for drug abuse.

REFERENCES

1. American Academy of Pediatrics: *Drug exposed infants. Status of state laws and legislative initiatives,* Elk Grove Village, Ill, American Academy of Pediatrics, Division of State Government Affairs, March 1994.
2. American Academy of Pediatrics Policy Statement: Drug-exposed infants (RE9533), *Pediatrics* 96:364, 1995.
3. American Academy of Pediatrics Policy Statement: Testing for drugs of abuse in children and adolescents (RE9628), *Pediatrics* 98:305, 1996.
4. American Academy of Pediatrics Policy Statement: Tobacco, alcohol, and other drugs: the role of the pediatrician in prevention and management of substance abuse (RE9801), *Pediatrics* 101:125, 1998.
5. Brown JV, et al: Maternal drug use during pregnancy: are preterm and full-term infants affected differently? *Dev Psychol* 34:540, 1998.
6. Buchi K: The drug-exposed infant in the well-baby nursery, *Clin Perinatol* 25:335, 1998.
7. Campbell DE, Fleischman AR: Ethical challenges in medical care for the pregnant substance abuser, *Clin Obstet Gynecol* 35:803, 1992.
8. Casanova OG, et al: Detection of cocaine exposure in the neonate, *Arch Path Lab Med* 118:988, 1994.
9. Chasnoff IJ, et al: Prenatal exposure to cocaine and other drugs: outcome at four to six year, *Ann NY Acad Sci* 846:314, 1998.
10. Chasnoff IJ, Landress HJ, Barrett ME: The prevalence of illicit drug or alcohol use during pregnancy and discrepancies in mandatory reporting in Pinellas County, Florida, *N Engl J Med* 322:1202, 1990.
11. Day N, et al: The effect of prenatal marijuana exposure on the cognitive development of offspring at age three, *Neurotoxicol Teratol* 16:169, 1994.
12. Eyler FD, et al: Birth outcome from a prospective, matched study of prenatal crack/cocaine use: I. Interactive and dose effects on health and growth, *Pediatrics* 101:229, 1998.

13. Flannagan P, Kokotailo P: Adolescent pregnancy and substance use, *Clin Perinatol* 26:185, 1999.
14. Frankenburg WK: Selection of diseases and tests in pediatric screening, *Pediatrics* 54:612, 1974.
15. Howard CR, Lawrence RA: Breast-feeding and drug exposure, *Obstet Gynecol Clin North Am* 25:195, 1998.
16. Kwong TC, Shearer D: Detection of drug use during pregnancy, *Obstet Gynecol Clin North Am* 25:43, 1998.
17. LaGasse LL, Seifer R, Lester BM: Interpreting research on prenatal substance exposure in the context of multiple confounding factors, *Clin Perinatol* 26:39, 1999.
18. Millard DD: Toxicology testing in neonates, *Clin Perinatol* 23:491, 1996.
19. Moeller MR, Fey P: Simultaneous determination of drugs of abuse (opiates, cocaine and amphetamine) in human hair by GC/MS and its application to a methadone treatment program, *Forensic Sci Int* 63:185, 1993.
20. Moore C, Lewis D, Leikin J: False-positive and false-negative rates in meconium drug testing, *Clin Chem* 41:1614, 1995.
21. Moore C, Negrusz A, Lewis D: Determination of drugs of abuse in meconium, *J Chromatogr B Biomed Sci Appl* 713:137, 1998.
22. National Institute on Drug Abuse: *National pregnancy & health survey*, Rockville, Md, 1996, National Institutes of Health.
23. Ostrea EM Jr, et al: Spectrum of gestational exposure to illicit drugs and other xenobiotic agents in newborn infants by meconium analysis, *J Pediatr* 133:513, 1998.
24. Ostrea EM Jr, et al: Drug screening of newborns by meconium analysis: a large-scale, prospective, epidemiologic study, *Pediatrics* 89:107, 1992.
25. Schwartz JG, et al: Accuracy of common drug screen tests, *Am J Emerg Med* 9:166, 1991.
26. Schwartz RH: Adolescent heroin use: a review, *Pediatrics* 102:1461, 1998.
27. Smeriglio VL, Wilcox HC: Prenatal drug exposure and child outcome, *Clin Perinatol* 26:1, 1999.
28. Wagner CL, et al: The impact of prenatal drug exposure on the neonate, *Obstet Gynecol Clin North Am* 25:169, 1998.

eight Use of Urinalysis and the Urine Culture in Screening

George J. Schwartz

Examination of the urine is a simple and efficient office procedure that may provide clues to specific renal abnormalities or more generalized diseases. A midstream clean-catch specimen is most reliable for this purpose. A first morning specimen tends to be the most reproducible, because it is more concentrated and less affected by recent fluid intake. The value of screening is warranted only if the identified conditions would benefit from early diagnosis and treatment.

Urinalyses and urine cultures have been used to screen children and adolescents for proteinuria, hematuria, glucosuria, and bacteriuria. The value of screening clearly is warranted in symptomatic children: glucosuria (diabetes mellitus), leukocyte esterase or nitrites (urinary tract infection), heavy proteinuria (nephrotic syndrome or other significant renal disease), or blood (reddish-brown urine of glomerulonephritis) can help the pediatrician diagnose and manage the pathologic condition.

However, the rationale for screening urinalyses in asymptomatic children remains controversial. Several principles need to be considered in screening for abnormalities in the urinalysis. First, screening should identify conditions that will benefit from early diagnosis and treatment. Second, screening should be reliable and accurate. Third, screening should be only for conditions that can be diagnosed with certainty—that is, with a high sensitivity (ability to detect true positive results) and with few false negatives. Fourth, identified positives should be followed up with appropriate evaluation and treatment. Fifth, a screening test should be cost effective for the individual and the general population. The cost effectiveness of mass urine screening depends on the total monetary and psychosocial cost of performing the screening test compared with the value of early detection in ameliorating or preventing subsequent progression of disease. Of significance is a study by Dodge et al,[4] who determined a cumulative occurrence of bacteriuria, proteinuria, and hematuria (i.e., having one or more of these findings) to be 6475 cases per 100,000 children ages 6 to 12 years. This occurrence (6.5%) greatly exceeds the number of children expected to have significant morbidity from progressive renal disease and is 1000 times the point prevalence of pediatric end stage renal disease (7 cases per 100,000 population).[25] Murakami et al[15] found that the incidence of asymptomatic hematuria was more than 10 times the prevalence of chronic renal diseases in Japanese children.

Such findings reflect the high degree of sensitivity and the lack of specificity (ability to detect true negative results) of current urine tests in detecting significant renal or urinary tract disease in symptom-free children. Several studies[6,8,14] reveal rather high rates (10% to 20%) of abnormalities on initial urinalysis screen, but 80% to 90% of these abnormalities are transient. In contrast, in a 1988 report,[12] extensive urine screening of symptom-free school children in Japan detected 65% to 80% of the diagnosed cases of IgA and non-IgA mesangial proliferative glomerulonephritis and membrano-proliferative glomerulonephritis. Many of these cases showed only mild glomerular lesions, and they were asymptomatic, indicating the identification of the early stages of renal disease. Although the early discovery of a symptom-free child who has renal disease may prove to be important, the cost effectiveness to society of mass screening remains unproved; each case could require hundreds of dollars for further examination. In otherwise healthy children, a single complete urinalysis performed before school entry should be sufficient screening for health maintenance purposes; a test with a positive result should be repeated one or two more times before an extensive evaluation is contemplated. Confirmation by using alternative methods, including microscopic analysis of the urine, should be considered.

Screening has enabled the early detection of acute, chronic, and hereditary glomerulonephridites, as well as urinary tract infection, obstructive uropathy, left renal vein entrapment syndrome, hypercalciuria, urolithiasis, renal proximal tubular dysfunction, and renal tumors. The American Academy of Pediatrics (AAP) now recommends that a complete urinalysis be performed at 5 years of age and then repeated during adolescence[1] (see Chapter 4, Child Health Supervision).

PROTEINURIA

Proteinuria is detected most easily by the dipstick method, which makes use of a plastic strip to which is affixed the indicator, tetrabromophenol blue. The presence of protein causes a change in color from yellow to blue-green that is proportional to the amount of protein present; albumin causes the indicator to change color more readily than do other proteins. False-positive findings can occur in alkaline urine (pH greater than 6.5) or in urine contaminated by skin antiseptics such as chlorhexidine or benzalkonium chloride. The small quantity of protein that healthy persons excrete normally is not usually detected by this method.

A urine sample is considered positive for protein if it registers at least 1+ (30 mg/dl) in a urine with specific gravity less than 1.015 or greater than or equal to 2+ if the specific gravity is greater than 1.015. Proteinuria is considered to be persistent if the dipstick is positive for at least two of three random urines collected at least 1 week apart.[17] An alternative qualitative turbidometric method precipitates all types of protein in acid. Sulfosalicylic acid is convenient, is cheap, and has a long shelf life; it is more accurate for urine that has an alkaline pH. Proteinuria often is confirmed quantitatively by measuring protein and creatinine concentrations and computing a protein creatinine ratio: Significant proteinuria is considered when the ratio is greater than 0.2.[5] (The clinical approach to children who have proteinuria is discussed in Chapter 163, Proteinuria.)

The prevalence rate for proteinuria in the symptom-free pediatric population varies, depending on the degree and frequency of proteinuria that is considered abnormal. Gutgesell[6] found the prevalence of proteinuria to be 6.3% in 2309 symptomatic and asymptomatic children who made their first visit to a neighborhood clinic. Screening was performed by a dip-and-read strip; 1+ or greater on a single urine specimen was the criterion for proteinuria. However, on retesting, only 0.65% had persistent proteinuria. When Silverberg[20,21] applied a more stringent criterion for proteinuria (2+ or greater on two urinalyses) to more than 50,000 school children, they found the prevalence to be only 0.45% for boys and 1.6% for girls.

Several investigators have noted a direct relationship of proteinuria to age during childhood, the incidence peaking at adolescence and then declining rapidly only to rise progressively thereafter into adulthood.[4,15] Furthermore, proteinuria is more common at each age in girls during childhood, with the occurrence rates in boys lagging 3 to 5 years behind. It has been hypothesized that these gender differences are due to the earlier onset of adolescence in girls. No differences in prevalence have been noted by ethnic group or socioeconomic level.

The prevalence of proteinuria (alone or in combination with glucosuria or hematuria) determined by urinalysis on routine hospital admission has been reported to be 2.5%,[8] which is similar to values in outpatient studies. When the criteria were made more stringent by requiring two consecutive abnormal urinalysis results only from patients who were afebrile and not menstruating, the prevalence decreased to 0.6%. The influence of such clinical factors must be considered when any data on the prevalence of proteinuria are considered.

Because more than 75% of symptom-free patients found to have protein in a single urinalysis will have normal urine on repeat testing, the value of this screening as part of well-child health care has been questioned. Furthermore, of those having several positive random urinalysis results, 60% will have orthostatic proteinuria, a diagnosis that is not considered to be a harbinger of clinically significant renal disease. In a 20-year follow-up study of young men who had persistent orthostatic proteinuria, none developed renal insufficiency, including those who had nonspecific glomerular abnormalities on renal biopsy.[22] Regular follow-up, however, remains important for these children so that changes in the pattern of protein excretion or the appearance of hematuria can be detected and appropriately investigated. Follow-up care of children determined by screening tests to have proteinuria has shown spontaneous resolution in more than 40% of cases within 4 years and an incidence of identifiable renal disease in only 1 child per 1000 children screened.[4] Clearly, if hematuria is excluded, children who have proteinuria are not likely to have overt renal disease. Vehaskari and Rapola[27] biopsied 28 children who had the highest protein excretion rates after identifying them from 8954 classmates by school screening; no definite morphological renal disease was identified. Furthermore, large studies have shown that children who have been identified by screening as having renal disease are usually known by their parents and physicians to have renal disease (e.g., nephrotic syndrome).

In contrast to the generally benign prognosis of isolated proteinuria, Yoshikawa et al[31] reported 53 children who were examined retrospectively after being biopsied for asymptomatic fixed isolated proteinuria. They found that 47% had significant glomerular changes (focal segmental glomerulosclerosis, IgA nephropathy, mesangial proliferative glomerulonephritis, and membranous glomerulonephritis), which appeared to progress with time to chronic renal impairment. In Silverberg's studies, approximately 9% of children screened to have isolated proteinuria had evidence of pyelonephritic scarring.[20,21] Although some children who have proteinuria may have an abnormality that requires no additional management (e.g., a hypoplastic kidney), others may have diseases that heretofore were not treatable but are now commonly, and often successfully, managed by pediatric nephrologists (e.g., focal glomerulosclerosis or IgA nephropathy). Most children who have significant renal disease have other signs and symptoms (e.g., edema, poor weight gain, or hypertension) that cause them to seek medical care and thus be identified even in the absence of screening programs.

The high sensitivity and low specificity of screening for proteinuria can produce undue anxiety in patients and parents and direct the practitioner to perform more invasive testing, which often provides no new information. Such screening may not only detract from the overall well-being of the population, but may be costly to families and their health maintenance organizations. Kaplan et al[10] estimate that approximately $200 is spent to evaluate the proteinuria, before referral to a pediatric nephrologist. In addition, false-positive screening will cause anxiety and discomfort in many patients and their parents because of the extensive subsequent evaluation.[10]

Currently, there is less enthusiasm for mass screening for proteinuria in symptom-free children. On the other hand, many isolated cases of significant renal disease without symptoms have been associated solely with proteinuria. It is concluded that a satisfactory compromise for the health of children is to screen a first morning urine at 5 years of age.[2,10,13] The use of the first morning urine prevents the identification of children who have orthostatic proteinuria. However, in the case of persistent proteinuria, a meticulous examination of fresh urinary sediment should precede any additional laboratory evaluation.[2,13]

The general lack of utility in screening symptom-free patients, however, does not apply to children who have symptoms. Urinalysis is an important tool in evaluating the child who has renal symptoms and also should be employed in patients who have vague signs and symptoms, such as failure to thrive, or recurrent diarrhea, inasmuch as some renal diseases may present in such nonspecific ways.

HEMATURIA

Not every brown, red, pink, or orange urine indicates hematuria. Urine can be colored by beets, blackberries, lead, urates, bile pigments, diphenylhydantoin, pyridium, desferoxamine mesylate, porphyrins, phenothiazines, phenolphthalein, *Serratia marcescens* infection, myoglobin, and hemoglobin.[30] The commercially available dipstick tests turn blue when oxidized by peroxide in a reaction catalyzed by hemoglobin or myoglobin in the urine; the dipstick is highly sensitive for hematuria, reacting to as few as three red blood cells per high power field (RBCs/hpf).

False-positive tests for blood in the urine may result from the presence of contaminating oxidizing cleansing agents (e.g., povidone-iodine or hypochlorite) or microbial peroxidases. False-negative tests result from the presence of large amounts of a reducing agent such as ascorbic acid. A positive dipstick result for blood does not discriminate between hemoglobin and myoglobin; differentiation requires spectrophotometric analysis. Furthermore, the dipstick test does not differentiate hemoglobinuria from hematuria or give clues to whether the blood originates from the upper or lower urinary tracts. (For these questions, the microscopic examination of the centrifuged urine sediment is essential [Chapter 143, Hematuria].) For this purpose, 10 to 15 ml of freshly voided urine is centrifuged in a conical tube at 1500 rpm for 5 minutes, the supernatant decanted, and the sediment resuspended in the remaining urine and pipetted onto a slide for microscopic examination. One should examine 5 to 10 high-powered fields (at 40×); an average of at least 5 RBCs/hpf is considered significant.

Hematuria can originate from the kidney or urinary tract; localization of the source of bleeding can facilitate the diagnosis. The presence of RBC casts usually indicates a glomerular etiology, as does the presence of other cellular casts and renal tubular cells. In addition, associated proteinuria (more than 2+) suggests glomerular bleeding. Brownish or tea-colored urine also suggests glomerular bleeding, whereas red or pink urine usually comes from the lower urinary tract. Clots usually indicate bladder or ureteral bleeding.

Examination of the morphology of these RBCs by phase contrast microscopy (achieved on standard microscopes by "racking down" the condenser or reducing the transmitted light) can help to differentiate glomerular from lower urinary tract bleeding. Dysmorphic (deformed) RBCs are likely to be glomerular in origin; eumorphic (uniform and normal) RBCs are likely to be from the lower urinary tract.[18]

The prevalence of microscopic hematuria in an ambulatory setting ranges from 2% to 6% when a single urinalysis is abnormal[4] to about 1% when more than one urinalysis is positive.[26] However, in fewer than 0.5% of these cases, the hematuria persists longer than 6 months.[4,26] The annual incidence of new cases (defined as at least 5 RBCs/hpf) is 0.4%.[4] No consistent trends exist for the age, gender, and race dependence of hematuria. The prevalence of hematuria (alone or in combination with glucosuria or proteinuria) in children admitted to the hospital for medical illnesses in one study was 5.3%. When sources of false positivity (fever or menstruation) were eliminated and the criteria were made more stringent by the requiring of two consecutive abnormal specimens, the prevalence decreased to 2.2%.[8]

Few of the children detected in screening programs to have hematuria are found to have significant renal or urological disease. However, isolated hematuria persisting for longer than 6 months is likely to be associated with renal disease if the family history of hematuria is positive in a first-degree relative or if the patient has had at least one episode of gross hematuria.[23] The most likely diagnoses in these cases are Alport's syndrome (hereditary nephritis) and IgA nephropathy. In addition, the finding on screening of both hematuria and proteinuria markedly increases the chances of having renal disease. In a review of studies of screened symptomless microhematuria, IgA nephropathy was found in 2% to 21% of biopsies, and other glomerular lesions were much less frequent.[3] The most common nonglomerular finding was asymptomatic urinary tract infection (4.8% to 6.0%), and less commonly were ureteropelvic junction obstruction and reflux nephropathy. In another follow-up study of children referred for isolated hematuria, 20% were found to have hypercalciuria; in 72% of those, urolithiasis developed 2 to 15 years after presentation.[24] Also, 14% developed a more serious glomerulopathy 2 to 17 years after presentation; in each of these children, proteinuria was associated with the hematuria more than 2 years after onset. Two thirds of the glomerulopathies were membrano-proliferative glomerulonephritis or hereditary (Alport) nephropathy, and 2% developed a 50% or greater reduction in glomerular filtration rate (GFR) over a 2- to 17-year follow-up.

Thus, although screening for hematuria also is limited by high sensitivity and low specificity, there is potential value in identifying patients at risk for renal disease. An examination of the first morning urine at age 5 years is recommended.[2,10,13] However, in the case of persistent microscopic hematuria, a careful examination of fresh urinary sediment should precede any additional laboratory evaluation.[2,13] Renal ultrasonography and serum C3 levels also would be recommended in this circumstance.

GLUCOSURIA

Urinary glucose can be detected by glucose oxidase-impregnated dipsticks. Normally, all of the filtered glucose is reabsorbed by the proximal tubules, and glucose is not detectable in the urine when the plasma glucose is less than 180 mg/dl. Glucosuria is seen most commonly when the filtered load of glucose is increased as a result of hyperglycemia in diabetes mellitus. Less often there is a defect in proximal tubular reabsorption that may be selective, as in renal glucosuria, or as part of a more generalized proximal tubular dysfunction, as in Fanconi's syndrome. Measurement of blood glucose will differentiate among these conditions. Glucosuria also is seen in the latter stages of tubular destruction of focal segmental glomerulosclerosis; in this condition, the urinalysis usually also shows heavy proteinuria and hematuria, and the urinary sediment contains renal tubular cells and casts.

Screening for glucosuria reveals a prevalence that is less than 0.1%.[6,20,21] However, in large populations, it is likely that 10 to 50 previously undetected cases of diabetes mellitus per 100,000 children will be identified. Rarer cases of renal glucosuria, Fanconi's syndrome, and other tubular dysfunction also will be found. The cost effectiveness, however, is rather low, and it is likely that the glucosuric diabetics would soon present with symptoms to the pediatrician. Therefore, it can be recommended only that well children be screened once at age 5 years for glucosuria.

BACTERIURIA

Bacteriuria is defined as growth of more than 100,000 bacteria/ml in at least two consecutive urine specimens seen in a child who has no symptoms at a regular checkup. The prevalence of asymptomatic bacteriuria in school-age children is 1% to 2% in girls and 0% to 0.1% in boys.[11,19,20,21]

On the dipstick, detection of the esterases of polymorphonuclear leukocytes or the nitrites generated by gram-negative organisms from nitrates will detect nearly all urines that have significant bacteriuria, but the specificity is only 69%.[29] When both leukocytes esterase and nitrite tests are positive, sensitivity (proportion of true positives labeled as positive) and specificity (proportion of true negatives labeled as negative) for bacteriuria are about 95%. On the other hand, if both leukocyte esterase and nitrite tests are negative, urinary tract infection is virtually excluded.

Extensive investigations of asymptomatic or covert bacteriuria in school girls have shown that nontreatment does not influence the episodes of symptomatic urinary tract infection, renal growth, or glomerular filtration rate in normal or scarred kidneys.[7,16,28] Furthermore, treatment of the asymptomatic bacteriuria may be associated with a greater risk for pyelonephritis because of the development of more pathogenic and resistant organisms. However, because the number of pyelonephritic episodes has been well correlated with the development of renal scarring,[9] the importance of preventing repeated bouts of pyelonephritis cannot be overemphasized.

On the other hand, screening of school girls reveals that as many as 15% of those who have asymptomatic bacteriuria have renal scarring, and 33% or so may have vesicoureteral reflux.[16,19] The severity of vesicoureteral reflux correlates with renal scarring. Unfortunately, antibiotic treatment does not prevent further renal scarring or restore poor renal growth. Children who have renal scarring are certainly considered at risk for the development of hypertension and renal insufficiency.

With the use of renal sonography in asymptomatic bacteriuric children, most renal scarring, when present, can be demonstrated, and those at risk for chronic renal disease and hypertension can be identified readily. Therefore, it is recommended that pediatricians screen at age 5 years for leukocyte esterase and nitrites. Positive results should be confirmed by urine cultures. Persistent bacteriuria should be pursued with a careful history as to renal and urinary tract symptomatology, examination of growth and blood pressure, and probably a renal ultrasound to determine those at risk for progressive renal disease. Asymptomatic bacteriuria should not be treated; however, a diagnosis of acute pyelonephritis requires antibiotic therapy and renal evaluation (see Chapter 273, Urinary Tract Infections).

REFERENCES

1. American Academy of Pediatrics, Committee on Practice and Ambulatory Medicine: Recommendations for preventive pediatric health care, *Pediatrics* 96:373, 1995.
2. Arant BS Jr: Screening for urinary abnormalities: worth doing and worth doing well, *Lancet* 351:307, 1998.
3. Benbassat J, et al: Symptomless microhaematuria in schoolchildren: causes for variable management strategies, *Q J Med* 89:845, 1996.
4. Dodge WF, et al: Proteinuria and hematuria in schoolchildren: epidemiology and natural history, *J Pediatr* 88:329, 1976.
5. Ettenger RB: The evaluation of the child with proteinuria, *Pediatr Ann* 23:486, 1994.
6. Gutgesell M: Practicality of screening urinalysis in asymptomatic children in a primary care setting, *Pediatrics* 62:103, 1978.
7. Hansson S, et al: Untreated bacteriuria in asymptomatic girls with renal scarring, *Pediatrics* 84:964, 1989.
8. Hermansen MC, Blodgett FM: Prospective evaluation of routine admission urinalyses, *Am J Dis Child* 135:126, 1981.
9. Jodal U: The natural history of bacteriuria in childhood, *Infect Dis Clin North Am* 1:713, 1987.
10. Kaplan RE, et al: Screening dipstick urinalysis: a time to change, *Pediatrics* 100:919, 1997.
11. Kemper KJ, Avner ED: The case against screening urinalysis for asymptomatic bacteriuria in children, *Am J Dis Child* 146:343, 1992.
12. Kitagawa T: Lessons learned from the Japanese nephritis screening study, *Pediatr Nephrol* 2:256, 1988.
13. Linshaw MA, Gruskin AB: The routine urinalysis: to keep or not to keep; that is the question, *Pediatrics* 100:1031, 1997.
14. Mitchell N, Stapleton FB: Routine admission urinalysis examination in pediatric patients: a poor value, *Pediatrics* 86:345, 1990.
15. Murakami M, et al: Urinary screening of elementary and junior high-school children over a 13-year period in Tokyo, *Pediatr Nephrol* 5:50, 1991.
16. Newcastle Covert Bacteriuria Research Group: Covert bacteriuria in schoolgirls in Newcastle upon Tyne: a 5-year follow-up, *Arch Dis Child* 56:585, 1981.
17. Norman ME: An office approach to hematuria and proteinuria, *Pediatr Clin North Am* 34:545, 1987.
18. Rizzoni G, et al: Evaluation of glomerular and nonglomerular hematuria by phase-contrast microscopy, *J Pediatr* 103:370, 1983.
19. Savage DC: Natural history of covert bacteriuria in schoolgirls, *Kidney Intl* 4:S90, 1975.
20. Silverberg DS: City-wide screening for urinary abnormalities in schoolgirls, *Can Med Assoc J* 109:981, 1973.
21. Silverberg DS: City-wide screening for urinary abnormalities in schoolboys, *Can Med Assoc J* 111:410, 1974.
22. Springberg PD, et al: Fixed and reproducible orthostatic proteinuria: results of a 20-year follow-up study, *Ann Int Med* 97:516, 1982.
23. Trachtman H, et al: Isolated hematuria in children: indications for a renal biopsy, *Kidney Intl* 25:94, 1984.
24. Turi S, et al: Long-term follow-up of patients with persistent/recurrent isolated haematuria: a Hungarian multicentre study, *Pediatr Nephrol* 3:235, 1989.
25. US Renal Data System: USRDS 1999 Annual Data Report; Chapter VIII: Pediatric End-Stage Renal Disease, *National Institutes of Health, National Institute of Diabetes and Digestive and Kidney Diseases*, 1999.
26. Vehaskari VM, et al: Microscopic hematuria in schoolchildren: epidemiology and clinicopathologic evaluation, *J Pediatr* 95:676, 1979.
27. Vehaskari VM, Rapola J: Isolated proteinuria: analysis of a school-age population, *J Pediatr* 101:661, 1982.

28. Verrier Jones K, et al: Glomerular filtration rate in schoolgirls with covert bacteriuria, *Br Med J* 285:1307, 1982.
29. Wiggelinkhuizen J, et al: Dipstick screening for urinary tract infection, *S Afr Med J* 74:224, 1988.
30. Yadin O: Hematuria in children, *Pediatr Ann* 23:474, 1994.
31. Yoshikawa N, et al: Asymptomatic constant isolated proteinuria in children, *J Pediatr* 119:375, 1991.

nine Language and Speech Assessment

Hiram L. McDade and Elaine M. Frank

Each child who enters school is assumed to possess a fully developed system of spoken language skills. It is upon this system that the foundation for teaching higher levels of communication is built. The late talker, the 3-year-old whose speech is unintelligible, or the child who has a limited vocabulary or word-finding difficulties invariably becomes identified by second or third grade when he or she needs special assistance in reading, spelling, writing, and mathematics.

Often, early remedial services are not provided for these children because of a "wait-and-see" attitude among health professionals. Actually, Johnny, who didn't begin talking until he was 2 years old, and whose speech could not be understood until he was 4 years old, never really outgrew his problem. It simply was manifested in other channels of language learning. The literature is compelling regarding the relationship between failure in reading and writing in the primary grades and a history of earlier communication difficulties.[1,7] In a 5-year follow-up study of 3-year-old children, as many as 40% of those diagnosed as having preschool articulation/phonological disorders were receiving some type of special education by third grade.[9] Furthermore, of the various skills assessed on standardized intelligence tests, the items most predictive of later academic performance are language based. For this reason, assessment of any child's readiness for school must give primary consideration to the adequacy of his or her general communicative abilities.

Because of the variability in the ages at which "normal" children achieve spoken language milestones, the fundamental question confronting the health professional is this: "Is the child I am examining, who appears to be slow in speech or language development, simply at the low end of the normal continuum (and presumably will catch up without professional assistance), or is this a child who is at risk for later learning difficulties?" Nurses and primary care physicians are the only trained professionals who routinely see young children before school entry. Speech-language pathologists, occupational therapists, and other early interventionists see these children only after a problem is suspected and a referral is made. Consequently, this accessibility to young children carries with it a responsibility: that of making early and appropriate referrals to those specialists trained to perform comprehensive evaluations.

HEARING ASSESSMENT

Because normal speech and language development requires an intact auditory system, a hearing assessment is an integral part of any developmental screening. However, children who have recurrent otitis media frequently pass pure-tone screenings for two reasons: (1) the resultant hearing loss usually is intermittent, and (2) the test signals often are presented at increased levels to compensate for the noise level of the examination room. Thus, hearing screenings are inadequate follow-up procedures for children who have been diagnosed as having persistent or serous otitis media. Such children require full audiological testing.[3] More recently, tympanometry has become a routine component of hearing assessments.[4] Coupled with the results of a pure-tone screening, tympanograms help identify a potential conductive component (middle ear problems) that otherwise might be missed.

SPEECH AND LANGUAGE DEVELOPMENT

As in other developmental areas, obtaining a thorough history is an important step in assessing a child's oral communication skills. Because the emergence of certain critical speech and language abilities follows a relatively stable timetable, a child's competency may be compared with these norms, either by history or by direct observation. The purpose of such "screenings" (formal or informal) is not to diagnose but to identify those in need of further testing. Consequently, children who fail to measure up to normative data should be referred to a speech-language pathologist. Such a referral provides two benefits: (1) children found to be deficient in speech and language abilities are ensured early intervention, and (2) children whose developmental status remains uncertain may be reassessed at appropriate intervals. For the latter group, the evaluation provides objective baseline data that allow the examiner to measure the child's rates of progress over time.

The acquisition of first words (at approximately 12 months of age) is the initial evidence of a child's language development. In general, children who are still nonverbal at 18 months of age should be referred for further testing.[2] However, a word of caution about the achievement of this developmental milestone: In their eagerness for and anticipation of the child's development of speech, parents frequently interpret the utterances "mama" and "dada" as meaningful words. These vocalizations usually are merely a function of the child's advanced babbling stage, and if the examiner accepts them as words, a spuriously low age level will be assigned to the acquisition of first words (e.g., 6 or 8 months). For this reason, more detailed information should be obtained by asking the parents how old their child was when he or she first spoke words other than "mama" or "dada."

The emergence of two-word phrases is a significant milestone in language learning. It is at this stage that the rudimentary rules of grammar are first evidenced. The term *grammar* here refers to (1) syntax, or the rules that govern how words may be combined to form phrases and sentences, and (2) morphology, which determines how the sounds that make up a word may be altered to modify its meaning, such as plural, possession, and verb tense.[2] As a child develops the ability to combine words (through the acquisition of syntax), the meaning of each utterance becomes more apparent, making the child a better communicator. Normal children, as young as 18 months of age, begin producing two-word combinations. A child who has failed to achieve this milestone by 24 months of age should be referred for further testing.

By age 3 years, most children have a spoken vocabulary of more than 500 words. In addition, their grammatical skills have developed to the point where they routinely speak in three- and four-word sentences. At this age the basic rules of morphology are fine tuned. Plural, possessive, and past tense forms of words are beginning to be mastered, and use of pronouns such as *I, me, you,* and *mine* is common. Three-year-olds demonstrate an appropriate understanding of *why* questions, indicating an appreciation of cause and effect. The speech of a 3-year-old is highly intelligible, and despite frequent mispronunciations, a stranger has no difficulty understanding the child. In short, 3-year-olds have the capacity to carry on a reasonable conversation with an adult.[6]

The language of 4-year-olds approaches adult competency with respect to grammatical skills. Unlike 2- and 3-year-olds, 4-year-olds speak in complete sentences. Rarely are words omitted from the four- and five-word sentences that these children typically produce. Although 4-year-olds do not have as many different ways to say the same things as do older children, they usually have at least one way to express all thoughts and desires. The vocabulary of a 4-year-old also is quite extensive. By this age most children can recognize and name several colors, count to 10 by rote, understand the prepositions *in, on, under, beside, in front*, and *in back* (but not *behind* until age 5), and answer complex questions, such as "How much?," "How long?," and "What if?"

By age 5 years, children have developed most of the language-based concepts that are important for schooling. They can sort and classify objects by category, name all the basic colors, and understand the concept of time (which allows them to answer *when* questions) and the concept of numbers up to 10 integers. Their articulation skills also are developed fully by age 5. Any residual mispronunciations at this point represent disordered speech and should prompt immediate referral to a speech-language pathologist (see Chapter 96, Stuttering).

INTELLIGIBILITY OF SPEECH

In the course of normal development, it is common for children to mispronounce certain sounds or to have difficulty producing particular words. The mastery of sounds in the language is a gradual process that takes place over a period of 3 to 4 years. Unfortunately, many children whose speech is disordered are not identified as such until later years, because their deviant articulation patterns occur during a time when adults expect a certain amount of mispronunciation. Differences exist, however, between normal and disordered speech, even as early as 2 to 3 years of age. Our tolerance for mispronunciations during this developmental period often prevents us from discerning these differences. The speech-language pathologist is specifically trained to determine if the pattern of misarticulation exhibited by a particular patient is common for normal children his or her age or indicates disordered speech and, thus, is not likely to be self-corrected.

One important factor the health professional should consider is the child's intelligibility. Young children who are acquiring a sound system normally are understood easily, despite their frequent misarticulations.[6] That is, regardless of how noticeable their speech errors are, normal children have little trouble communicating, even with unfamiliar listeners. In contrast, a child who is unintelligible, or whose parents report difficulty understanding his or her speech, is exhibiting a pattern of misarticulation that is not part of normal development.[2] Such a child is less likely to outgrow the problem and thus requires thorough evaluation to determine the need for speech therapy.

ACQUIRED SPEECH AND LANGUAGE DISORDERS IN CHILDREN

Acquired brain injury in children and adolescents may result in significant speech or language dysfunction. Acquired communication disorders frequently occur secondary to an open or closed traumatic brain injury (TBI), anoxia, or cerebral infection. TBI is by far the leading cause of brain injury among children; each year, 150,000 to 200,000 children are hospitalized for this condition. Falls are the most common cause of injury, followed by bicycle accidents, motor vehicle accidents, and child abuse. Open head injuries from gunshot wounds have increased among children and adolescents.[5]

Among children who have a TBI, studies have reported a high rate of risk taking, limited judgment, and learning problems. Contrary to previous thought, young children (birth to age 4 years) who experience a brain injury have a poorer prognosis for normal communicative function than school-age children or adolescents. A brain injury often interferes with acquisition of new knowledge and skills. Older children have the advantage of knowledge acquired before the brain injury.[8]

TBI can result in a focal or, more often, a diffuse brain injury (see Chapter 286, Head Injuries). The TBI sequelae presents speech, cognitive-language, and swallowing problems. The language problems may include disorganized, tangential, wandering discourse; imprecise language; word-retrieval difficulties; disinhibited, socially inappropriate language with ineffective use of contextual cues; restricted output and lack of initiation; difficulty comprehending extended language in spoken or written form and detecting main ideas; difficulty understanding abstract language including indirect or implied meaning; and inefficient verbal learning due to reduced memory ability.[8] Because these problems are different from the grammatical difficulties typical of children who have developmental problems, they frequently are misunderstood and are not seen as being symptomatic of a language disorder. Speech disturbances can include apraxic speech, characterized by difficulty initiating and programming speech, or dysarthric speech resulting from paralysis or paresis of oral or pharyngeal musculature. This muscle weakness may contribute to a secondary swallowing or dysphagia disorder.

Standardized testing may not be sensitive to the communicative-intellectual effects of TBI. Insightful clinical evaluation of speech and language function is essential in determining the need for rehabilitative or specialized educational intervention. Although a positive correlation between initial indices of severity (including the Glasgow coma scale and the length of coma) and the long-term outcome is relatively strong, individual outcomes may vary. Children who have a mild head injury and only a short-term loss of consciousness may require minimal medical intervention but still may experience interruption in normal cognitive functioning. Behavioral changes, including easy fatigability, inconsistent performance, and slow processing, often are evident. Children who have a more severe head injury may require intensive speech and language inpatient rehabilitation and outpatient follow-up.

Therapeutic intervention goals may be rehabilitative or compensatory. Rehabilitation of attention, awareness, perception, memory, learning, organization, social cognition, problem solving, and general executive system functioning are necessary for cognitive processing and language functioning. Compensatory techniques may include memory devices, organizational patterning, or referent cues. Stimulating speech programming and muscular strengthening may improve oral communication, or compensatory techniques may be required in the form of augmentative communicative devices (e.g., communication boards or computerized speech). Successful educational reentry for children who have a TBI should include assistance in school programming and inservice for family, teachers, other school personnel, and the child's peers. Children whose TBI is significant need continued monitoring through successive developmental stages to achieve maximum functional ability and academic success.

REFERENCES

1. Aram D, Ekelman B, Nation J: Preschoolers with language disorders: 10 years later, *J Speech Hear Res* 27:232, 1984.
2. Berko Gleason J: *The development of language,* New York, 1993, Macmillan.
3. Bess F: *Audiology: the fundamentals,* Baltimore, 1990, Williams & Wilkins.
4. Martin F: *Introduction to audiology*, ed 4, Englewood Cliffs, NJ, 1991, Prentice-Hall.
5. National Institute of Disability and Rehabilitation Research: National Pediatric Trauma Registry: a progress report, *Rehabilitation Update* Summer/Fall, 1993.
6. Owens R: *Language development*, ed 3, Columbus, Ohio, 1992, Merrill.
7. Silva P, Williams S, McGee R: A longitudinal study of children with developmental language delay at age three: later intelligence, reading and behavior problems, *Dev Med Child Neurol* 29:630, 1987.
8. Ylvisaker M: Communication outcome following traumatic brain injury, *Semin Speech Lang* 13:239, 1992.
9. Zimmerman D, McDade H, Montgomery A: The relationship between preschool speech problems and later school performance, *ASHA Leader* 3:108, 1998.

ten Auditory Screening

David R. Cunningham

JUSTIFICATION

Routine screening for hearing loss is justified based on the prevalence of this disorder in both the general pediatric population and in at-risk groups. The prevalence of profound sensorineural hearing loss in the well-baby population is 1 in 1000 births. This estimate, however, fails to account for the greater prevalence of sensorineural hearing loss among infants at risk for developmental disabilities and the greater number of well-babies who have mild, moderate, or severe sensorineural hearing loss than who are profoundly deaf. Adjusting the prevalence rate for infants at risk for developmental disabilities and for well babies who have lesser degrees of sensorineural hearing loss yields a prevalence of approximately 7 babies who have hearing loss for every 1000 births.[12] (Compare this with 1 in 14,000 who have phenylketonuria at birth.) By 2 years of age, 1 in 25 children will have a mild to moderate (20 to 50 decibel) hearing loss resulting from ear disease. Nearly 20% of public school children in disadvantaged neighborhoods fail auditory screening tests.

The first 18 to 24 months of life are crucial for the acquisition of normal speech and language. Undetected hearing loss in this period of life leads to irreparable communicative and learning problems. Early intervention in the form of audiological management, otological treatment, amplification, parental counseling, and special education is vitally important. Regular hearing screening for toddlers and school-age children is important not only because of the seriousness of the medical sequelae of active otopathology but also because of the negative consequences that even mild (15 to 20 decibel) hearing loss (either conductive or sensorineural) has for language growth, academic success, and behavioral development.

GOALS

The goal of auditory screening programs is to identify hearing loss cost efficiently as early as possible, regardless of its degree. The screening strategies must have high sensitivity and specificity to reduce both false-positive and false-negative rates. The methods of achieving this goal are adjusted for each age group. In the early 1990s, infant screening programs were designed to identify primarily those neonates who had profound sensorineural hearing loss. Current techniques and technologies make it feasible to detect not only severe and profound hearing loss but also milder degrees of hearing loss.

In the toddler and preschool periods, the screening protocol is modified to identify otopathology (especially otitis media with effusion), milder conductive hearing loss, as well as unnoticed acquired or progressive sensorineural hearing impairment. Routine periodic auditory screening of school-age children is designed to maintain educationally optimal hearing. Although the method of screening children in the school-age group has not changed significantly in the last decade or so, there is a far greater awareness of and sensitivity to the effects of hearing loss on skills development and educational achievement. Clinicians must be especially vigilant for those children who are academic underachievers. These children may have no peripheral hearing loss but may exhibit signs of a specific auditory learning disorder. The following discussion addresses feasible, reliable, and cost-efficient auditory screening protocols in three age groups.

NEONATAL AND EARLY INFANT PERIOD

Much of the information presented in this section is available in greater detail in the NIH Consensus Statement on Early Identification of Hearing Impairment in Infants and Young

Children published by the National Institutes of Health in 1993.[10] This panel recommends that auditory screening be implemented for *all* infants, those both of high and low risk, within the first 3 months of life, but preferably before discharge from the hospital nursery. The panel emphasizes that comprehensive intervention and management for those infants identified as having hearing loss must be an integral part of a universal screening program.

The NIH panel rejects the notion of using a "high-risk register" to limit the number of infants screened. Screening only those who satisfy one or more high-risk factors identifies only 50% of infants who have significant hearing loss.[3,9,14] Failure to identify the remaining 50% of children who have hearing loss results in an unacceptably late age of diagnosis and intervention.

The NIH panel recommends that evoked otoacoustic emissions (EOAE) and auditory brainstem response (ABR) audiometry be used as the screening tools. EOAE should be used to screen all newborns.[13] Those who pass the EOAE screen are discharged from the process; those who fail the EOAE screen are given a second stage, or confirmatory, screen, using ABR. Babies who pass the ABR screen are discharged but should be "flagged" for rescreening within 3 to 6 months. Babies who fail the ABR screen are referred for a complete diagnostic evaluation, the purpose of which is to determine the type and degree of hearing loss and to initiate a remediation program for the child and family.

The acoustic stimulus for ABR screening should include the frequency band important for speech recognition. The most important portion of the "speech frequency range" lies between approximately 500 Hertz (Hz) and 4 kilohertz (kHz). Acoustic "clicks," which generate their primary energy in the 2 kHz to 4 kHz region, often are used as stimuli in large-scale infant screening programs. (Although it also is possible to use tone pips or tone bursts to obtain more frequency-specific responses, these acoustic stimuli generally are used in comprehensive audiological evaluations rather than in screening programs.) The "pass" criterion for ABR infant screening is a response from both ears at intensity levels of 40 dB (decibels) referenced to normal hearing level (NHL), that is, 40 dB NHL. Infants who pass the ABR screen but who are at risk for progressive hearing loss should be monitored audiologically periodically throughout the preschool years.[11]

The largest study to date to report on the feasibility of using EOAE as an infant screening method is the Rhode Island Hearing Assessment Project (RIHAP).[21] By the end of 1993, more than 23,000 infants had been screened by using "transient" EOAE. EOAE screening of all infants in the regular care and special care nurseries yielded an average "pass" rate of 91.6%. The sensitivity for transient EOAE was 100%; its specificity was 82%. This is compared with sensitivity and specificity rates for ABR of approximately 94% and 89%, respectively. Thus, the two screening technologies are complementary when used in a two-stage screening protocol.

Transient EOAE are low-intensity sounds produced by the cochlea in response to acoustic clicks. They are by-products of normal cochlear function. EOAE appear to be associated with the motility of the outer hair cells, which seem to be responsible for "amplifying" low-level sounds within the cochlea. This mechanical response creates motion patterns within the cochlear duct that are transmitted outward from the cochlea and through the middle ear. Motion of the tympanic membrane, which normally occurs in response to sound, now produces sound that can be detected in the ear canal by a sensitive microphone.[5] EOAE are recorded by using a computer averaging technique similar to ABR instrumentation. Because transient EOAE tend not to occur in people who have peripheral hearing loss greater than about 30 dB HL,* they appear to serve as a valuable method for identifying those who have normal or near-normal peripheral hearing sensitivity. Research is ongoing to discover the optimal EOAE stimulus/response patterns and pass/fail criteria for large-scale neonatal screening programs. Another type of EOAE, the "distortion-product" EOAE, is under investigation as a possible screening tool.

Approximately 10% of all babies tested will fail EOAE screening. It is a rapid, highly sensitive, cost-effective method of identifying those infants who have normal hearing and limiting the size of the population that is carried over to the second stage ABR screening protocol. Northern and Hayes[12] report that using a two-stage EOAE-ABR screening protocol will result in only 1.7 infants who have normal hearing being referred for a complete diagnostic evaluation for every baby who has hearing loss (based on a prevalence rate of 6 hearing-impaired infants per 1000 births).

Bess and Paradise[1] and Paradise[15] have questioned the validity and predictive value of the two-stage EOAE-ABR screening protocol recommended by the NIH. Using a prevalence rate of 1 hearing-impaired infant per 1000 births, Bess and Paradise calculated that nearly 10 infants who have normal hearing would be referred for full diagnostic evaluations for every baby who has a hearing loss. They argue that the NIH protocol would result in an unacceptably high overreferral rate. Their conclusions do not appear to have wide support in the professional community, and their prevalence rate estimate (1:1000) generally is regarded as too low in that it applies only to those infants who are profoundly deaf and not to those who have lesser degrees of handicapping hearing loss.[12] Indeed, much evidence supports the NIH EOAE-ABR auditory screening consensus statement in literature from the United States and abroad.[2,7,8,17-21]

Although the NIH panel endorses the two-stage EOAE-ABR infant auditory screening protocol, they recognize that adopting its recommendations will take time. Additionally, they acknowledge that many infant screening programs already are in place that use only ABR (either automated or conventional) as a screening tool. Some of these existing screening programs use ABR technology only for NICU babies or for babies who have one or more at-risk "indicators" associated with congenital or acquired conductive or sensorineural hearing loss. The panel encourages all centers to adopt the two-stage EOAE-ABR protocol as soon as possible but would encourage existing programs to continue using the

*HL refers to hearing level referenced to American National Standards Institute (ANSI) 33:6, 1989; Specifications for Audiometers.

BOX 20-4

INDICATORS FOR NEONATAL SENSORINEURAL OR CONDUCTIVE HEARING LOSS TESTING*

1. Family history of hereditary childhood sensorineural hearing loss
2. In utero infection such as cytomegalovirus, rubella, syphilis, herpes, or toxoplasmosis
3. Craniofacial anomalies, including those who have morphological abnormalities of the pinna and ear canal
4. Birth weight less than 1500 g (3.3 lb)
5. Hyperbilirubinemia at a serum level requiring exchange transfusion
6. Ototoxic medications, including but not limited to the aminoglycosides used in multiple courses or in combination with loop diuretics
7. Bacterial meningitis
8. Severe depression at birth with Apgar scores of 0 to 4 at 1 minute or 0 to 6 at 5 minutes
9. Prolonged mechanical ventilation lasting 5 days or longer (e.g., persistent pulmonary hypertension)
10. Stigmata or other findings associated with a syndrome known to include a sensorineural or a conductive hearing loss

*For use when universal newborn screening (NIH consensus model) is not available.

ABR-only protocol in the interim. The Joint Committee on Infant Hearing recommends that screening programs based on at-risk indicators continue to provide screening services to those infants identified by use of those indicators.[7]

Erenberg et al,[4] writing for the Task Force on Newborn and Infant Hearing of the American Academy of Pediatrics, endorses the implementation of universal newborn hearing screening but defers a recommendation as to the preferred method. The indicators for neonatal sensorineural or conductive hearing loss testing are listed in Box 20-4. These indicators might be used to reduce the size of the population screened by using ABR until universal screening of infants by using EOAE and ABR is achieved.

Not all hearing loss in infancy or early childhood will be present at birth or acquired before the baby is discharged from the hospital. Such hearing loss may be acquired as a result of other medical conditions or from progressive hereditary etiologies. Clinicians must be vigilant for the possibility of these situations. The indicators shown in Box 20-5 will help identify those infants and very young children who should be monitored carefully for hearing loss and re-evaluated as necessary to rule out acquired or progressive hearing loss.

A comprehensive universal infant auditory screening program has a number of administrative elements. Parents and caregivers should be offered educational materials pertaining to the signs and symptoms of hearing loss in infants and toddlers. This should include an overview of speech, language, and auditory developmental milestones by age in months. Parental concern about a baby's hearing or speech-

BOX 20-5

INDICATORS FOR POSTNEONATAL SENSORINEURAL OR CONDUCTIVE HEARING LOSS TESTING*

1. Parental concern regarding hearing, speech, language, or developmental delay
2. Bacterial meningitis and other infections associated with sensorineural hearing loss
3. Head trauma associated with loss of consciousness or skull fracture
4. Stigmata or other findings associated with a syndrome known to include sensorineural or conductive hearing loss
5. Ototoxic medications including but not limited to chemotherapeutic agents, or aminoglycosides used in multiple courses or in combination with loop diuretics
6. Recurrent or persistent otitis media with effusion for at least 3 months
7. Family history of hereditary childhood hearing loss
8. History of in utero infection such as cytomegalovirus, rubella, syphilis, herpes, or toxoplasmosis
9. Neurofibromatosis type II and neurodegenerative disorders
10. Persistent pulmonary hypertension in the newborn period
11. Anatomical deformity and other disorders that affect eustachian tube function

*Health conditions that may develop and require hearing evaluations every 6 months until age 3 years (infants 29 days to 3 years old).

language development is justification for an audiological evaluation. Data amassed in large-scale infant auditory screening programs should be forwarded to a central repository for analysis and tracking of those children who are suspected of having hearing loss. In states where auditory screening programs are mandated by law, these data are managed by agencies such as the public health department and the commission for handicapped children. Infant screening programs generally are supervised by audiologists or neonatologists associated with the hospital nurseries. The actual screening (EOAE and ABR protocols) may be carried out by well-trained nursing personnel or closely monitored paraprofessionals or volunteers. Per-patient cost always is a consideration in large-scale screening programs. Each hospital needs to determine its costs based on personnel, time, supervisory and training needs, durable equipment purchases, expendable supplies, test interpretation services, report preparation, and overhead.

PRESCHOOL PERIOD

The primary goal of screening in the 2- to 5-year-old period is the detection of medically remediable otopathology associated with a very mild (less than 15 dB HL) to moderate (approximately 40 dB HL) conductive hearing loss. The screening focuses on this objective on the assumption that more severely handicapping hearing losses will have been found by 2 years of age. The principal cause of hearing loss in this age range is otitis media, a pathology capable of producing subtle, but significant, auditory learning disorders and permanent middle ear damage.[11]

Auditory screening of preschoolers often is performed at the time of well-child visits to the primary physician's office, Head Start programs, child care centers, preschool programs, or kindergartens. Although the screening procedures might differ from site to site depending on the availability of equipment and trained personnel and on the level of background noise in the screening environment, the "ideal" protocol would include four elements: (1) pure tone hearing screening, (2) acoustic immittance testing (tympanometry), (3) otoscopic inspection of the ear canal (as performed by the supervising professionals), and (4) an elicitation of parental/caregiver concern about the child's hearing and speech and language development. See Chapter 141, Hearing Loss, for additional discussion of office-based auditory screening.

Northern and Downs[11] described the following procedure for conducting pure tone auditory screening for preschool-age children.

Play-conditioning procedure for testing the 3- and 4-year-old child

1. Have available a peg board, a ring tower, plain blocks, or other simple toys that appeal to young children.
2. With headphones on your ears, take a block (or peg) and hold it up to one ear as if listening. Make believe you hear a sound, say "I hear it," and put the block on the table.
3. Put the phones on the child's ear and hold his or her hand with the block up to the child's ear.
4. Present a 50 dB tone at 1000 Hz and guide the child's hand to build the block tower. Repeat once or twice and then see if he or she can do it alone. If he or she can, go on.
5. Decrease the hearing level to 20 dB and repeat the test. If the child responds, go on to the other frequencies (2000 and 4000 Hz) and repeat the procedure. Praise him or her for each correct response. After each presentation, place another block in the child's hand.
6. Switch to the opposite ear and repeat the test, starting at 4000 Hz, then to 2000 Hz and 1000 Hz.

A criterion for referral is failure to respond to 20 dB HL at any frequency in either ear or failure on immittance screening (tympanometry). Children who fail the "screen" should be retested in 2 weeks. If the rescreen also is failed, the child should be referred for a comprehensive audiological evaluation.

Screening children younger than 3 years of age presents a greater challenge to the busy clinician. Tympanometry generally is tolerated well by this group of children and should be done routinely. Auditory screening, however, is more problematic in that it requires the tester to be not only skillful in the presentation of auditory stimuli, but also familiar with the developmental hierarchy of auditory alerting and localization behaviors in young children. During the 4- to 24-month period, behavioral responses to quiet noisemakers include alerting, orienting toward the acoustic stimuli, crude head-turning for visual observation of the noisemakers, and finally brisk and precise localizing of the source of the acoustic stimuli by the time the child is 24 months of age. The 2- to 3-year-old who has normal hearing should have no difficulty localizing a sound source in any plane around the head. The absence of a localization response constitutes a failed screening test, as does a positive tympanometric test. Those who fail the screen and those whose caregivers express concern about hearing or speech and language development should be referred for a complete audiological evaluation.

Tympanometry is (1) an essential element of a screening protocol for the preschool group and (2) an objective method of determining the status of the tympanic membrane and the middle ear mechanism. Tympanometry can reliably detect the presence of middle ear effusion and eustachian tube dysfunction that often is a precursor to otitis media with effusion (OME). Tympanometry is especially helpful in detecting OME in children who "pass" the auditory screen because their hearing loss is so slight.

The American Speech-Language-Hearing Association (ASHA) has published guidelines pertaining to tympanometric screening for hearing loss and middle ear disorders,[6] but these are more appropriate for large-scale screening programs than for "screening" at periodic intervals in the physician's office. For this reason, a discussion of the ASHA guidelines will be presented in the subsequent section on strategies for screening the school-age population. A scaled-down but rational approach to "in-office tympanometric screening" is required. The practitioner or his or her assistant can perform basic tympanometric measurements on all preschool-age children as part of routine examinations. Fig. 20-1 describes the five major tympanogram types.

Easy-to-use, automated tympanometers can discriminate between normal and abnormal middle ear systems reliably and inexpensively. Children whose tympanometric screening reveals one or more of the following "fail" criteria should be examined more fully in the physician's office or referred for a complete audiological evaluation:

1. Normal tympanic membrane–ossicular compliance with middle ear pressure that is less than -200 mm H_2O (type C tympanogram often associated with eustachian tube dysfunction)
2. Significantly reduced or completely absent tympanic membrane–ossicular compliance with normal equivalent ear canal volume, that is, 1.0 cm^3 (type B tympanogram often associated with middle ear fluid accumulation)
3. Abnormally large equivalent ear canal volume, that is, 1.0 cm^3 and "flat" tympanogram (associated with either tympanic membrane perforation or patent tympanostomy tube)

This "in-office" screening protocol, combining an auditory test and basic tympanometry along with otoscopy and special attention to the child's speech and language development, will identify those patients who require more exhaustive evaluations.

SCHOOL-AGE PERIOD

The principal goal of screening programs for school-age populations is the maintenance of educationally optimal hearing. The secondary goal is the detection of otopathology. The physician should use the screening protocol described for 3- to 5-year-olds in the preschool section above for school-

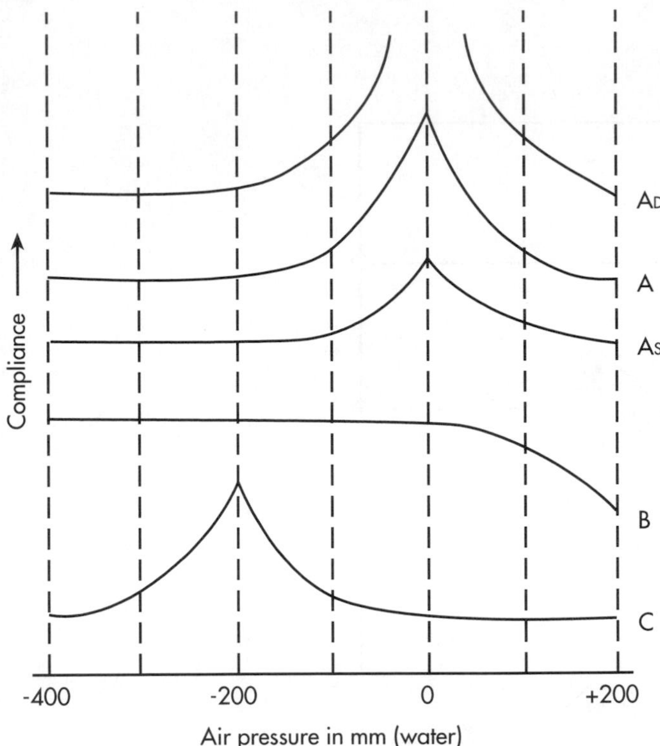

Fig. 20-1 Five typical tympanograms illustrating various conditions of the middle ear. Type A shows normal pressure-compliance functions and is typical of normal middle ears. Type AS curves are like the A curves but are much shallower and are associated with stiffness of the stapes, the smallest of the middle ear bones. Type AD curves are much deeper than the normal type A curves and are symptomatic of interruptions in the chain of bones or flaccidity of the eardrum membrane. Type B shows no pressure setting at which the eardrum membrane becomes most compliant and suggests fluid in the middle ear space. Type C shows the eardrum membrane to be most compliant when the pressure in the ear canal is negative, suggesting that the pressure within the middle ear is below atmospheric pressure.

(From Martin FN: *Introduction to audiology*, ed 4, 1991, Prentice-Hall, Inc.)

age patients who have come to the office for annual physical examinations or with otological complaints. This "in-office" procedure combines screening audiometry, tympanometry, and otoscopy and paying special attention to speech and language milestones.

What follows, however, is an explanation of a large-scale screening protocol for school-age populations, as conducted in the school (or public health facility) itself. Although the primary care physician may be called on as a consultant to these mass screening efforts, the actual management and implementation of school-based programs generally are conducted by a supervising audiologist and trained paraprofessionals or volunteers. The large-scale screening of school-age populations for hearing impairment and middle ear disorders presented here is based on the recommendations of the Working Group on Acoustic Immittance Measurements and the Committee on Audiologic Evaluation of the American Speech-Language-Hearing Association.[6] The screening protocol includes four sources of data: history, visual inspection of the ear canal, identification audiometry, and tympanometry.

History

A request for basic otological/audiological information can be obtained from the parents or caregivers (in advance) in a letter sent to them explaining the purpose of the screening program. A recent history of otalgia or otorrhea is sufficient cause for immediate medical referral.

Otoscopy

The following conditions merit medical referral without further audiological/tympanometric screening: structural defects of the ear, head, or neck; inflammation, blood, effusion, excessive cerumen, tumors, or foreign body in the ear canal; or eardrum appearance consistent with active middle ear disease, that is, abnormal color, bulging eardrum, fluid line or bubbles, perforation, or retraction. Tympanometry should not be performed when a tympanostomy tube is in place at the time of screening.

Audiometric Screening

The school-age screening protocol is given in Fig. 20-2, and the referral criteria are shown in Box 20-6.

Pure-tone stimuli presented at 20 dB HL[16] with frequencies of 1 kHz, 2 kHz, and 4 kHz should be used. Failure to respond to any frequency in either ear constitutes a screening failure. A second on-site rescreen or a rescreen at a later date is recommended. A second failure indicates the need for a more exhaustive evaluation.

Low Static Admittance

Peak admittance (Ya) is the total acoustic immittance of both the ear canal and the lateral surface of the tympanic membrane. Peak admittance is measured in millimhos, a unit that indicates the ease with which sound pressure waves flow through the outer and middle ear. A peak admittance value less than 0.2 millimhos associated with an abnormally large physical volume in front of the measuring probe is evidence of a tympanic membrane perforation and warrants immediate medical referral.

Equivalent ear canal volume is an estimated measure of the air medial to the probe tip and is measured in cubic centimeters (cm^3). An equivalent ear canal volume that exceeds 1.0 cm^3 in the presence of a "flat" tympanogram is evidence of a tympanic membrane perforation and merits a medical referral. (Note: Low static admittance, in isolation, may or may not be associated with a middle ear disorder; a rescreening in 4 to 6 weeks is recommended before these children are referred for medical evaluation.)

Abnormally Wide Tympanometric Width (TW)

Sometimes referred to as "tympanometric gradient," this metric is used to describe the shape of the tympanogram in the vicinity of the peak and is measured in units of air pres-

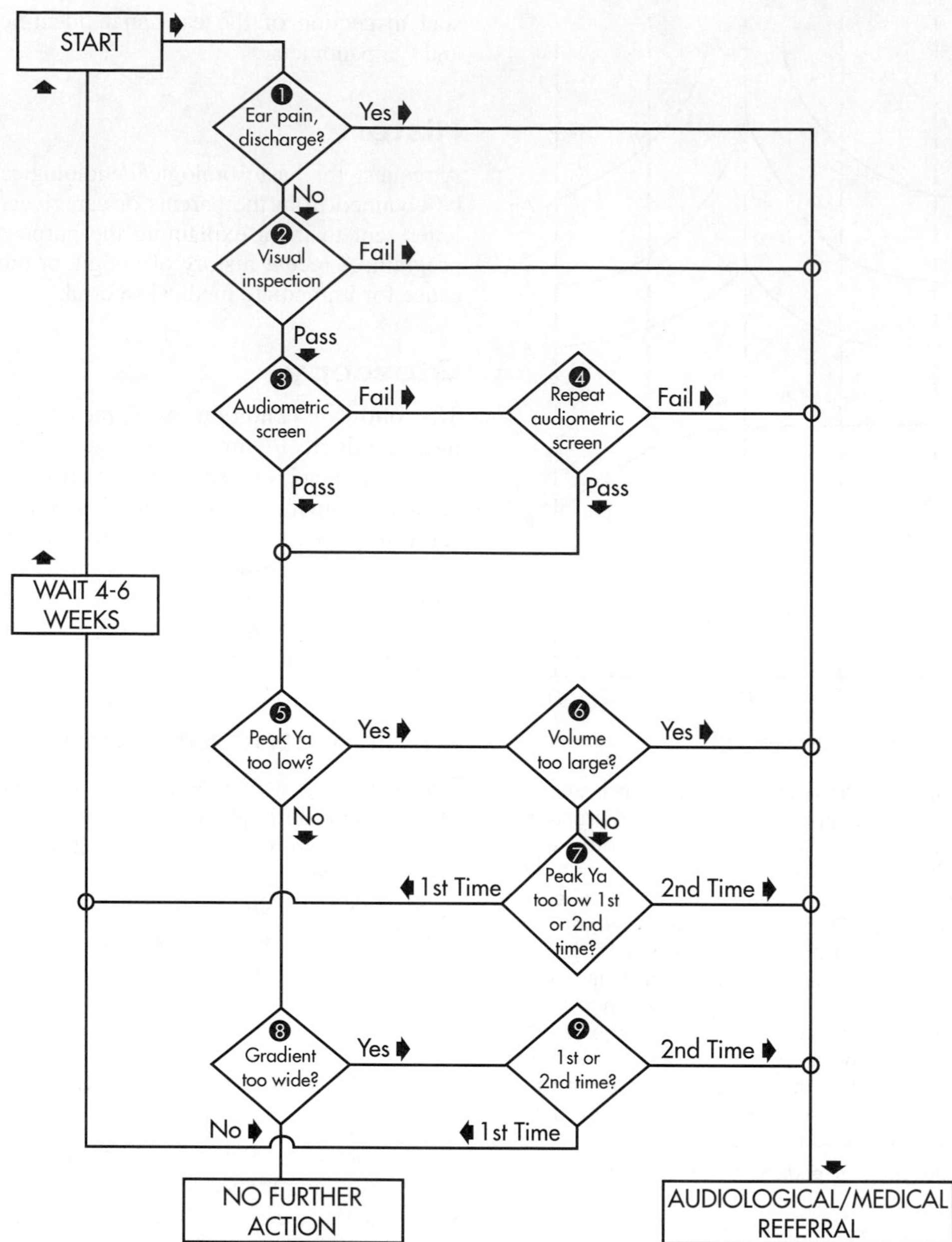

Fig. 20-2 Flow chart for determining the need for audiological/medical referral incorporating case history, visual inspection, pure-tone audiometry, and tympanometry. Each numbered box is discussed in the text. The flowchart represents the logic used to determine the need for referral. It does not indicate the order of test procedures.

(From American Speech-Language-Hearing Association: *ASHA* 32(suppl 2):21, 1990. Reprinted by permission.)

BOX 20-6

REFERRAL CRITERIA

I. History
- A. Otalgia
- B. Otorrhea

II. Visual Inspection of the Ear
- A. Structural defect of the ear, head, or neck
- B. Ear canal abnormalities
  1. Blood or effusion
  2. Occlusion
  3. Inflammation
  4. Excessive cerumen, tumor, foreign material
- C. Eardrum abnormalities
  1. Abnormal color
  2. Bulging eardrum
  3. Fluid line or bubbles
  4. Perforation
  5. Retraction

III. Identification Audiometry

Fail air conduction screening at 20 dB HL at 1, 2, or 4 kHz in either ear; these criteria may require alteration for various clinical settings and populations.

IV. Tympanometry
- A. Flat tympanogram and equivalent ear canal volume (Vec) outside normal range
- B. Low static admittance (peak Y) on two successive occurrences in a 4- to 6-week interval
- C. Abnormally wide tympanometric width (TW) on two successive occurrences in a 4- to 6-week interval

From American Speech-Language-Hearing Association: Guidelines for screening for hearing impairment and middle-ear disorders, *ASHA* 32 (suppl 2):21, 1990. Reprinted by permission.

sure called dekapascals (daPa). (Note: 1 daPa = 1.02 mm of water pressure.) A TW greater than 150 daPa is suggestive of middle ear disease in children. Those who have an abnormally wide TW and no other findings should be rescreened in 4 to 6 weeks and referred for medical evaluation only if they fail the second screen.

REFERENCES

1. Bess FH, Paradise JL: Universal screening for infant hearing: not simple, not risk-free, not necessarily beneficial, and not presently justified, *Pediatrics* 98:330, 1994.
2. Bonfils P, Uziel A, Pujol R: Screening for auditory dysfunction in infants by evoked oto-acoustic emissions, *Arch Otolaryngol Head Neck Surg* 114:887, 1988.
3. Elssman S, Matkin N, Sabo M: Early identification of congenital sensorineural hearing impairment, *Hear J* Sept 1987, p 13.
4. Erenberg A, et al: American academy of pediatrics task force on newborn and infant hearing. Newborn and infant hearing loss: detection and intervention, *Pediatrics* 103:527, 1999.
5. Glattke TJ, Kujawa SG: Otoacoustic emissions, *Am J Audiol* 1:29, 1991.
6. Guidelines for screening for hearing impairments and middle-ear disorders, *ASHA* 32(suppl 2):17, 1990.
7. Joint Committee on Infant Hearing: 1993 position statement, *Pediatr* 95:152, 1995.
8. Kennedy C, et al: Otoacoustic emissions and auditory brainstem responses in the newborn, *Arch Dis Child* 66:1124, 1991.
9. Mauk GW, et al: The effectiveness of high-risk characteristics in early identification of hearing impairment, *Ear Hear* 12:312, 1991.
10. NIH Consensus Statement: Early identification of hearing impairment in infants and young children, 11:1, March 1-3, 1993, Office of Medical Applications of Research, National Institutes of Health, Federal Bldg Room 618, Bethesda, Md 20892.
11. Northern JL, Downs MP: *Hearing in children*, ed 4, Baltimore, 1991, Williams & Wilkins.
12. Northern JL, Hayes D: Universal screening for infant hearing impairment: necessary, beneficial, and justifiable, *Audiology Today* 6:10, 1994.
13. Norton S: *Infant screening/pediatric testing with otoacoustic emissions*, Richmond, Va, April 27, 1994, American Academy of Audiology.
14. Pappas DG: A study of the high-risk registry for sensorineural hearing impairment, *Head Neck Surg* 91:41, 1983.
15. Paradise JL: Universal newborn hearing screening: should we leap before we look? *Pediatrics* 103:670, 1999.
16. Specifications for audiometers: ANSI S3.6-1969, New York, 1970, American National Standards Institute.
17. Stevens J, et al: Click evoked otoacoustic emissions compared with brainstem electric response, *Arch Dis Child* 64:1105, 1989.
18. Stevens J, et al: Click evoked otoacoustic emissions in neonatal screening, *Ear Hear* 11:128, 1990.
19. Uziel A, Piron J: Evoked otoacoustic emissions from normal newborns and babies admitted to an intensive care baby unit, *Acta Otolaryngol Suppl* 482:85, 1991.
20. White KR, et al: Neonatal hearing screening using evoked otoacoustic emissions: the Rhode Island hearing assessment project. In Bess FH, Hall J, editors: *Screening children for auditory function*, Nashville, Tenn, 1992, Bill Wilkerson Center Press.
21. White KR, Behrens TR, editors: The Rhode Island hearing assessment project: implications for universal newborn hearing screening, *Seminars in Hearing* 14:1, New York, 1993, Thieme.

eleven Vision Screening

Richard C. Wasserman and Alex R. Kemper

RATIONALE

Adequate vision is important for everyone, especially young children. Amblyopia, a permanent uncorrectable vision loss, is a major threat to vision that is preventable when detected in early childhood. During development, the visual cortex must receive focused images from both eyes to "learn" how to see. Conditions that interfere with the normal visual image during this time, such as strabismus, certain refractive errors, or cataracts, can lead to amblyopia if not identified and corrected.

The earlier these conditions are identified and treated, the more likely and the more easily amblyopia can be prevented. Amblyopia is unlikely to be prevented after 9 years of age, and the goal is to detect amblyogenic conditions before 5 years of age.

From a public health standpoint, screening for vision problems is readily justified on the following counts:

- Vision problems pose a threat to children's current and future well-being.
- Vision problems are common. Between 5% and 10% of preschool-age children and more than 10% of school-age

children have abnormal vision. Amblyopia is the leading cause of monocular blindness in adults younger than 70 years old.[5]
- Vision problems are likely to go undetected without screening.
- Screening tests are available that are inexpensive and that reliably and accurately identify those who have or are at risk for vision problems.
- Efficacious treatments for vision problems are readily available.
- Early diagnosis and treatment confer significant advantages in outcome for many vision problems (e.g., congenital cataracts, strabismus, amblyopia).
- Overall, the benefits of early diagnosis and treatment of vision problems justify the costs of screening.

GOALS

The goals of vision screening are (1) to identify deficits in vision or conditions that ultimately could threaten vision before they otherwise would be discovered and (2) to ensure that appropriate diagnostic and therapeutic referrals are made so that conditions threatening vision are ameliorated. To achieve the first goal, the practitioner and staff must learn the appropriate vision screening techniques and procedures and then apply them systematically in their practice. To achieve the second goal, the practitioner must structure the primary care encounter so that screening results are communicated accurately to parents, appropriate referrals are made (when indicated), and proper follow-up is achieved.

Appropriate vision screening techniques and procedures vary in some degree for infants and toddlers (younger than age 3 years), preschool children (3 to 5 years), and school-age children and adolescents. The practitioner's physical examination provides some of the elements of vision screening, especially in infants and toddlers, but vision is tested more efficiently by ancillary personnel and apart from the physical examination. Children who have developmental disabilities often are at increased risk for vision problems and may require special expertise for assessment. Criteria for referral are discussed below.

INFANTS AND TODDLERS

Physical Examination

The eyes are first examined as part of the newborn examination and should be assessed subsequently at each health supervision visit. As part of the examination, the eyes should be inspected for any structural abnormalities. The red reflex is evaluated for abnormality or asymmetrical appearance through an ophthalmoscope. After an infant can fixate on an object, generally by 3 months of age, the corneal light reflections should be tested by using a penlight held in midline 12 inches in front of the eye (Hirschberg test). Asymmetry of the light's reflection on the two corneas suggests strabismus. The examiner should assess ocular motility by having the child "follow" a brightly colored object or toy. The cover/uncover test detects movement of each eye when the other is covered and then uncovered. Such movement suggests either a unilateral visual defect or an ocular muscle weakness in the eye that moves. See Chapters 171, Strabismus, and 179, Visual Disturbance, for more detailed discussions of the physical examination of the eyes.

Formal Screening

See Table 179-1 for methods used to screen for visual acuity at various ages.

Photorefractive screening is a new technology based on the interpretation of photographic images of the eyes for conditions that potentially could lead to amblyopia. The validity and reliability of this screening strategy in primary care practices as yet are unclear.

Special Circumstances

Infants whose circumstances or family history place them at special risk for visual problems, such as preterm infants at risk for retinopathy of prematurity, those who have a family history of congenital eye problems, or those who have genetic (e.g., trisomy 21) or acquired problems (e.g., cerebral palsy) that place their eyes at risk should be evaluated by an ophthalmologist.

Parents sometimes give a history of asymmetry of the child's eyes when none can be demonstrated at the visit. Because some problems of muscle imbalance are manifest only when the child is fatigued, it is wise to pay attention to such a history and refer to a specialist if these complaints are persistent. A family history of amblyopia, a "lazy eye," or "crossed eyes" confers a higher risk of problems and should prompt consideration of referral.

PRESCHOOL CHILDREN

Physical Examination

Inspection, red reflex, corneal light reflection, ocular motility, and the cover/uncover test should be performed at each health supervision visit.

Formal Screening

Testing for visual acuity should be attempted beginning at age 2½ years (see Table 179-1), and an interpretable result should be achieved by age 4 years. It is reasonable to have a child who is uncooperative or inconsistent in responses return for a repeat test. Repeated failure to achieve an interpretable test result may be an indication of a visual problem.

At this age, the simpler tests of acuity that do not rely on knowledge of letters are the most acceptable. Many such tests are available.[1,2] The Lea chart has become popular because children may have an easier time identifying the four symbols (apple, circle, square, and house) on this test than some of the other tests.[4] In general, these tests are available for testing from a distance of 10 and of 20 feet. At 10 feet, children are less likely to become distracted by other activities in the immediate environment.

Testing for binocular vision (stereoacuity) is not a substitute for assessing visual acuity, but it is a very useful adjunct and sometimes will identify a child whose vision problems have been missed on physical examination and acuity testing.

Acceptable tests for this age group include the Random Dot E test and the Stereo Fly test.

Vision testing machines may be accepted by older children.

Special Circumstances

Children at high risk for poor vision, as discussed previously, should be referred if satisfactory results cannot be obtained on screening.

SCHOOL-AGE CHILDREN AND ADOLESCENTS

Physical Examination

Eyes should be inspected and the red reflex, corneal light reflex, ocular motility, and cover/uncover tests should be performed at each health supervision visit.

Formal Screening

Once a child knows the alphabet, the Snellen letters on a wall chart are appropriate for visual acuity screening. For school-age children and adolescents, vision testing machines that combine acuity testing with tests of binocular vision are readily accepted and require less office space.

Special Circumstances

School difficulties may be a presenting symptom of visual problems, and all children who have such troubles should have their vision evaluated if not done recently. Although the prevention of amblyopia becomes less of a concern with increasing age, the overall prevalence of vision problems increases steadily over time; therefore, children should continue to be tested at health supervision visits.

PERSONNEL AND EQUIPMENT

Nonprofessional personnel who have a high school education can be trained to administer all of these formal tests. The equipment necessary for most of these tests is readily available from medical supply houses and is inexpensive. Vision not tested with testing machines requires a well-lighted environment with at least 10 feet of available space. Vision testing machines require less space but are expensive.

REFERRAL

When strabismus or amblyopia is suspected, the child should be referred to an ophthalmologist who is skilled in working with young children.

A child who has a structural abnormality of the eye or its movements, any asymmetry or abnormality of the red reflex, any asymmetry of the corneal reflections, aversion to the occlusion of one eye, or any movement of the eyes on the cover/uncover test should be referred.

Preschool children failing to pass a visual acuity test in either or both eyes at the 20/40 level or who display a two-line discrepancy between the eyes (e.g., 20/20 and 20/40) should be referred. In addition, any child who cannot be tested successfully by age 4 years after repeated attempts should be referred. School-age children and adolescents who fail to pass at the 20/30 level in either or both eyes should be referred. In addition, children who have developmental disabilities who cannot be tested successfully should be referred.

Children of any age who fail a test of binocular vision should be referred.

IMPROVING VISION SCREENING AND ITS OUTCOMES

The primary care practice and clinic settings, because they provide continuity of care, remain ideal places to carry out vision screening. Practitioners need to screen, systematically, *all* of the children whom they see for health supervision visits. They should record and communicate the results of the screening to parents, and make sure that follow-up and referral appointments are made and kept. Currently, rates of screening are suboptimal, and many children whose visual testing is abnormal never receive evaluation by an eye care specialist.[3,6]

As in any screening program, a proportion of children will fail vision screening but have a normal ophthalmologic evaluation. False-positive tests are a feature of all screening programs and should not discourage practitioners from screening. Vision screening examinations will detect the overwhelming proportion of children who have treatable vision problems; practitioners must ensure that these cases are detected and treated properly.

REFERENCES

1. American Academy of Pediatrics Committee on Practice and Ambulatory Medicine, Section on Ophthalmology: Eye examination and vision screening in infants, children, and young adults, *Pediatrics* 98:153, 1996.
2. Barker J, Barmatz H: Eye function. In Frankenburg WK, Camp BW, editors: *Pediatric screening tests*, Springfield, Ill, 1975, Charles C Thomas.
3. Campbell LR, Charney E: Factors associated with delay in diagnosis of childhood amblyopia, *Pediatrics* 87:178, 1991.
4. Hered RW, Murphy S, Clancy M: Comparison of the HOTV and Lea Symbols charts for preschool vision screening, *J Pediatr Ophthalmol Strabismus* 34:24, 1997.
5. Simons K: Preschool vision screening: rationale, methodology and outcome, *Surv Ophthalmol* 41:3, 1996.
6. Wasserman RC, Croft CA, Brotherton SE: Preschool vision screening in pediatric practice: a study from the pediatric research in office settings (PROS) network, *Pediatrics* 89:834, 1992.

SUGGESTED READINGS

American Academy of Ophthalmology: *Amblyopia: preferred practice pattern* San Francisco, 1997, The Academy.

Trobe JD: *The physician's guide to eye care,* San Francisco, 1993, American Academy of Ophthalmology.

twelve Sickle Cell Conditions

Charles F. Whitten

Two distinctly different types of sickle cell conditions exist: (1) sickle cell disease (primarily sickle cell anemia, sickle cell-hemoglobin C disease, and sickle cell-beta-thalassemia disease) and (2) sickle cell trait, the benign "carrier" state (see Chapter 117, Anemia and Pallor). As with all health problems, screening for sickle cell conditions is justifiable only if those whose screening tests are positive receive some beneficial service. Beneficial services and the methodology for providing them exist for both types of sickle cell conditions.

Screening is of value with respect to the sickle cell diseases, although they are incurable. No established procedures exist for preventing the episodic complications or the progressive damage to tissues. Because of splenic dysfunction, children who have sickle cell disease are prone to the development of bacterial infections, particularly by *Streptococcus pneumoniae,* which can proceed to septicemia and death ("sudden death") in a matter of hours. The level of red blood cell fetal hemoglobin is high enough for the first several months to prevent intravascular sickling and the resultant manifestations of sickle cell disease. After that time, although intravascular sickling is present, overwhelming bacterial infections leading to death can occur before the onset of characteristic symptoms that result in the diagnosis of sickle cell disease. A study conducted by the National Institutes of Health has demonstrated clearly the value of twice daily oral administration of penicillin in preventing pneumococcal infections and death in young children who have a sickle cell condition.[3] Based on results of that study, participants in an NIH consensus conference[2] recommended that all newborns be screened for hemoglobinopathies and that penicillin be given for the first 5 years of life to those who have sickle cell disease.

Subsequently the Agency For Health Care Policy and Research's Sickle Cell Panel recommended that infants who had documented or suspected sickle cell anemia or sickle cell-beta-thalassemia should be started on oral prophylactic penicillin as soon as possible, but no later than 2 months of age.[1] Furthermore, prophylaxis should be continued until at least 5 years of age.

APPROACH TO SCREENING

Given the scope of the problem, the consensus conference participants further recommended that state governments mandate newborn screening for hemoglobinopathies and that effective follow-up service programs be established. As of January 1999, 35 states required sickle cell newborn screening; in 15 states screening was voluntary.

For screening to be effective in reducing morbidity and mortality from infections, several services must accompany screening of newborns:

1. A repeat test must be performed when the infant is 2 to 3 months old, because the newborn test results are only presumptive unless the hemoglobin genotypes of the biological parents are known. The fetal and sickle hemoglobin (FS) pattern that is present if the newborn has sickle cell anemia may also be found if the newborn has sickle cell hereditary persistence of fetal hemoglobin, which is not a disease. Also, when an FS pattern is detected, it is possible that a small amount of normal adult hemoglobin (hemoglobin A) is present but not detected. The presence of small amounts of normal adult hemoglobin containing F and S hemoglobin is characteristic of sickle cell-beta-thalassemia disease at birth.
2. Parents must be taught the manifestations of sickle cell disease.
3. Parents must be told why penicillin prophylaxis is necessary and how they should respond if the early signs and symptoms of infection or acute splenic sequestration (another cause of sudden death) should occur. Symptoms include nasal congestion, cough, fever, lassitude, anorexia, pallor, and enlargement of the spleen.
4. Emergency rooms must be prepared to respond appropriately when a child who has sickle cell disease manifests the aforementioned signs and symptoms. For example, in addition to receiving appropriate emergent medical care eventually, which consists of parenteral antibiotics (for infections) and transfusions (for acute splenic sequestration), they must be evaluated immediately. Children who have pneumococcal septicemia have died in emergency rooms while waiting to be seen by a physician.
5. Children must receive 125 mg of penicillin twice daily, beginning early—when they are 2 months old—and always by the time they are 3 months old. The dosage must be increased to 250 mg twice daily when they are 3 years old and continued until their fifth birthday.
6. The maintenance of penicillin prophylaxis must be monitored regularly.
7. Efforts must be made to ensure that potential barriers to the maintenance of penicillin prophylaxis (e.g., transportation for monitoring of parental compliance in administering penicillin, and paying for penicillin) are removed.
8. Children must receive polyvalent pneumococcal vaccine at 2 and 5 years of age and every 5 years thereafter.

Voluntary sickle cell organizations in many communities have trained counselors and social workers who can assist in the provision of the necessary services, some of which are difficult for physicians to provide.

In those states that do not mandate hemoglobinopathy screening during the newborn period, it is incumbent upon physicians to screen all of their infants who are at risk for sickle cell disease early enough to enable affected infants to be started on penicillin prophylaxis by the time they are 3 months old.

The recommendation of penicillin prophylaxis is, of course, not restricted to children whose disease is detected through newborn screening. All children younger than age 5 years who are diagnosed as having sickle cell disease should be placed on penicillin prophylaxis immediately.

The identification of sickle cell disease in the newborn period has other benefits. A high percentage of adults who have sickle cell disease are not self-sufficient economically—that is, they depend on public assistance or their families for support despite the only limitations with respect to employment being heavy manual labor and the potential for frequent attacks of pain that result in a high level of absenteeism. Considerable evidence exists that this discrepancy between potential for a person to be employed and that person's ability to gain and retain employment is the result of poor adjustment to the disease.

Thus, the early identification of sickle cell disease in infants provides an opportunity for health care providers to begin to work with parents during their child's infancy to help them and their children make appropriate lifestyle adjustments to the disease. This attitude might be stated simplistically: persons who have a sickle cell disease are to be treated as being ill only when they are experiencing a manifestation of the disease; at all other times they are to be treated as though they are well.

With respect to the second sickle condition, sickle cell trait, it needs to be recognized that individuals who have this condition rarely have related health problems and so usually do not discover their sickle cell trait other than through screening. These persons, however, have the potential (25% chance in each pregnancy) for having a child who has one of the sickle cell diseases if the other parent has a gene for one of the relevant hemoglobinopathies. Unless they are made aware of this potential, they may have children who have a sickle cell disease that they might have chosen not to have or they may suffer emotional and adjustment problems through lack of preparation for handling the difficulties associated with these illnesses. Thus, the purpose of screening for sickle cell trait is to provide counseling that enables those counseled to make informed decisions that they believe are in their best interest with respect to marriage and childbearing.

Screening for sickle cell trait, therefore, is only of benefit for children who are approaching the childbearing age—a time at which information regarding marriage and reproduction is relevant. At that time the services consist of providing substantive information on the nature of sickle cell conditions, the risk of having a child who has sickle cell disease, and the available reproductive options.[4] Traditionally, this is termed *counseling,* but the process really is one of education, because persons should not be advised as to what they should do, but simply informed of consequences and the options available to them.

The physician should present a balanced picture of sickle cell anemia when "counseling" individuals who have sickle cell trait. Presentations that underplay the potential severity can influence persons to chance having a child who has sickle cell anemia whom they would not have had if they had been informed accurately. Presentations that fail to indicate the spectrum of severity and the potential for individuals who have sickle cell anemia to live satisfying lives can influence individuals not to take the risk despite their strong wishes to have children.

The physician should not assume that the differences between sickle cell trait and sickle cell anemia are understood among the laity. Thus, when some individuals are told that they have sickle cell trait, they may believe that their health status is threatened, a belief that can generate severe anxiety and apprehension.

The physician should not depict sickle cell trait as a disease. Other than the rare occurrence of hematuria, it has not been documented that sickle cell trait has any influence on health status under usual physiological circumstances. Although the risk of intravascular sickling is theoretical if oxygen is deprived sufficiently during surgery, there is no reason to assume that competent surgeons and anesthesiologists would handle oxygen-deprived persons who have sickle cell trait differently from those whose hemoglobin patterns are normal.

The physician should inform those being counseled that sickle cell anemia can be diagnosed prenatally by DNA analysis of cells obtained by chorionic villus sampling at about 9 weeks and by amniocentesis at about 15 weeks. This allows them to ascertain the status of their fetus and to decide whether they wish to continue or terminate the pregnancy if sickle cell anemia is present. For those parents who find termination of pregnancy an acceptable option, the availability of prenatal diagnosis enables them to have their own biological children without the possibility of having a child who has sickle cell anemia. Before prenatal diagnosis was available, parents had to forego having children if they wished to avoid having a child with sickle cell anemia.

As stated previously, reproductive decisions relative to the sickle cell gene should be based entirely on the potential parents' informed judgment as to what is in their best interest.

As indicated, the optimum time for sickle cell testing is at birth, a procedure that if practiced universally would lead to a population that would not require testing at any other time. However, because an at-risk population exists that to a large extent has not been screened for sickle cell conditions either through mandatory newborn testing programs or testing by their health care providers, it is important to decide when the unscreened should be tested for sickle cell disease.

For sickle cell trait, inasmuch as the sole purpose of screening is to enable personal marriage and reproductive decisions, the procedure should be deferred until just before the child-bearing age is reached. It is of no value, for example, for an 8-year-old to be tested for sickle cell trait.

For sickle cell diseases, because the purpose is to provide comprehensive care, it is not necessary to screen the population after the age of 5 years, because by that age manifestations of the disease invariably will have led to the diagnosis, and the danger of developing pneumococcal septicemia has become remote.

Although from a programmatic standpoint the optimal timing for screening for sickle cell diseases and sickle cell trait is different, all of the screening methods identify both types of conditions. Thus, in screening newborns for sickle cell disease, newborns with sickle trait are identified. This potentially is advantageous because it means that at least one and possibly both parents have sickle cell trait, which results in a highly cost beneficial detection of couples who have sickle cell trait at a time when they are having children. Among black people, the incidence of sickle cell trait couples is approximately 1 in 144, whereas if a newborn has sickle cell trait the probability of both parents having sickle cell trait is 1 in 12.

In addition to implementing services that achieve the benefits of screening, it is equally important to institute policies, procedures, and practices that avoid potential harmful outcomes. One of these is the exposure of nonpaternity. Instances in which the putative father is not the biological father will be discovered in genetics screening in all racial groups, and this information can traumatize and even destroy previously stable families.

When a father is told that the child he thought was his is not, this is highly likely to have a negative effect on his relationship with his partner and the child, particularly when the child has a chronic illness. The impaired relationship with the child might extend throughout a lifetime. This can be avoided to a large extent in newborn screening programs.

Unless it is essential for the treatment of the child or for the provision of reproductive counseling, the parents need not be tested when the child has a sickle cell disease. In most instances the diagnosis is clear and the parents can be told which genes they have collectively; the service providers do not need to know which parent carries which gene. Obviously, if the parents request testing, it should be done. Similarly, if the newborn has one of the hemoglobinopathy traits, the mother should be tested for the purposes of reproductive counseling. If the mother does not have the trait in question, she can be told that the father does. It is not necessary to confirm this by testing the alleged father. On the other hand, if the mother has the trait, the father then can be tested with impunity, because a source of the child's gene has been identified.

If the providers in a given program feel morally compelled to give all fathers their results (which means that in some cases presumed fathers will become aware that they are not the biological fathers), they must implement informed consent procedures that give mothers sufficient information for them to decide whether they wish to take the risk of disclosing nonpaternity when they agree to parental testing.

Newborn screening for sickle cell conditions with the current methods also detects the presence of other hemoglobinopathies that generally do not require immediate intervention because of morbidity or mortality. Given that the racial mix and thus the incidence of the various hemoglobinopathies vary from state to state, each state must determine how this information is handled.

Several methods currently are used to screen newborns for sickle cell disease: hemoglobin electrophoresis (cellulose acetate followed by citrate agar), ion exchange chromatography, isoelectric focusing, and high-performance liquid chromatography. The methodology to be used in central laboratories for statewide programs should be selected after careful consideration of the advantages and disadvantages of each.

In the past the solubility test has been used in screening programs conducted by voluntary sickle cell organizations and by individual physicians. It is simple and inexpensive but should not be used for primary screening. Although the solubility test identifies accurately all who have inherited the sickle hemoglobin gene, it will not detect individuals who have inherited the gene for hemoglobin C. Hemoglobin C occurs in about 2% of the black population and gives a negative solubility test result, leading individuals screened by this procedure to assume that they cannot have a child who has a sickle cell disease. However, a black person who has hemoglobin C trait whose partner is black has approximately an 8% chance of the partner having sickle cell trait. In this situation a 25% chance exists in each pregnancy for the child to have sickle cell-hemoglobin C disease, a condition that is accompanied by the same symptoms found in sickle cell anemia, although it tends to be a milder disorder.

Screening programs, therefore, should use one of the other aforementioned tests (rather than the solubility test), all of which will detect hemoglobin C trait, as well as hemoglobin C disease. Individuals who have hemoglobin C disease may have a mild hemolytic anemia.

REFERENCES

1. Agency for Health Care Policy and Research, Sickle Cell Disease Guideline Panel: *Sickle cell disease: screening, diagnosis, management and counseling in newborns and infants*, Pub No 93-0562, Rockville, Md, 1993, US Department of Health and Human Services.
2. Consensus Conference: Newborn screening for sickle cell disease and other hemoglobinopathies, *JAMA* 258:1205, 1987.
3. Gaston MD, et al: Prophylaxis with oral penicillin in children with sickle cell anemia, *N Engl J Med* 314:1593, 1986.
4. Whitten CF, Thomas J, Nishiura EN: Sickle cell trait counseling: evaluation of counselors and counselees, *Am J Hum Genet* 33:802, 1981.

thirteen Developmental Surveillance and Intervention

Rune J. Simeonsson and Nancy West Simeonsson

Although the significance of early intervention for infants and young children whose development is delayed or at risk is well established, effective identification of such children represents a continuing challenge for pediatricians. At issue is the need for identification procedures and tools sufficiently sensitive to detect significant variations in development and yet practical and efficient in clinical contexts. Screening tests have been recommended as the major approach to identification, but their use has been employed less than universally because of concerns about training, time demands, and the utility of findings.[7] Other issues that may limit screening by pediatricians include concerns about managed care restrictions, lack of support staff, and referral sources.[32] The cost of screening as a limiting factor has been addressed by Glascoe, Foster, and Wolraich,[17] who have shown that the use of parents' concerns about their child's development is the most cost-beneficial approach for pediatricians. A problematic result of this limited use and increased reliance on clinical judgment among pediatricians has been an underidentification of developmental, behavioral, or emotional problems in early childhood.[15] This is at a time when pediatricians increasingly are likely to be confronted with developmental problems, reflected by the growth of early intervention programs.[24] Pediatricians now are more likely to experience demands for activities related to screening and assessment of developmental problems[8] and contact with schools about children's readiness to learn.[10]

In response to these challenges, Dworkin[9] has advocated for developmental surveillance as an alternative approach, defined as a "flexible, continuous process that is broader in scope than screening, whereby knowledgeable professionals perform skilled observations of children throughout all encounters during child health care." This approach is comprehensive and encompasses monitoring of development and identifying and assessing potential delays. As such, it is consistent with the recommendation by the American Academy of Pediatrics[2] (AAP) for continuity of comprehensive care, as embodied in the monitoring guidelines for preventive pediatric care (see Chapter 4, Child Health Supervision). Of particular relevance is the significance attached to the early years, evident in the recommendation for six visits in the first year of life and five visits from 1 through 4 years of age. Also relevant is the integration of effort that can be achieved by attending to the domains of the medical history, sensory screening, and developmental and behavioral guidance for both parent and child. Developmental assessment requires familiarity with developmental processes and capitalizes on opportunities for observations in all encounters with children. The results can yield information about developmental progress and provide a base for referral, parent counseling, and intervention.

ELEMENTS OF DEVELOPMENTAL SURVEILLANCE

Developmental surveillance should be integrated into the pediatric examination with a complete assessment of physical characteristics and laboratory studies[11]; it involves (1) a thorough history and knowledge of environmental influences, (2) familiarity with normal development, and (3) awareness of the relative significance of developmental indicators.

History

Obtaining a good history begins with a review of the family history, with particular attention to behavioral and developmental indicators. Details of the pregnancy, delivery, and perinatal period contribute indexes to identify children at risk. Understanding the influence of the environment on development, which includes nutrition, illness, and medication history, as well as social and psychological variables, is important in developmental assessment. The quality of the parent-child interaction, the nature and availability of developmental stimulation, and the composition of the social environment are important data to obtain from parents and other caregivers, including grandparents and child care and preschool providers.[10]

Developmental Perspective

The importance of developmental surveillance is based on the conviction that patterns of development observed in the earliest years of life are sequential and, therefore, predictable (see Chapter 19, Identification of Developmental Delays and the Early Intervention System). Biological maturation stimulates, as well as reflects, developmental changes in interaction with the environment. Developmental assessment of children, therefore, requires a perspective encompassing quantitative and qualitative aspects of development. A normative perspective views development as a sequence of milestones achieved at specific ages. In one way or another, most measures of development encompass milestones across the major streams of development of language, motor, problem solving, and psychosocial skills. Development also can be seen as a series of critical tasks to be mastered within certain stages of life, such as infancy, early childhood, middle childhood, and adolescence. Other developmental perspectives can be derived from stage-based theories, such as Erikson's theory of psychosocial stages or Piaget's stages of cognitive growth (see Chapter 52, Theories and Concepts of Development as They Relate to Pediatric Practice).

A basic synthesis of developmental tasks and Piaget's cognitive stages reveals the first 18 to 24 months as a period in which the infant reacts to and acts upon the physical and social environment through sensation and motor activity. This is expressed in a sequence of skills leading to independent mobility and the control involved in feeding, elimination, exploration, and initial symbol use in gestures and speech. These characteristics of infancy change in the toddler and preschool period to increasingly sophisticated language production, coordination of gross and fine motor movements for games and play, and increased awareness and conformity to peer and adult demands.

The preschooler's awareness of physical and social reality, however, is constrained by intuitive and self-referenced perceptions. As the child reaches school age, a qualitative cognitive shift occurs, in which understanding no longer remains unidimensional and self-referenced but can integrate several dimensions and alternative perspectives. This is reflected in the child's ability to reason logically and to classify, and perform operations necessary for academic skills.

Relative Significance of Developmental Indicators

Effective assessment requires an awareness of the relative importance of specific achivements at different points in development. In the newborn period for example, organization of behavioral states is a crucial dimension.[25] Indices of development, such as acquisition of symbolic representation, speech, and fine motor coordination, particularly in a young child, have greater prognostic significance than does acquisition of gross motor skills. The developmental points at which communication skills emerge are perhaps the most useful clues in determining normal development. Second in importance, and closely related to speech, are appropriate social behaviors. Delayed or atypical communication and social behaviors are highly significant in identifying children at risk in terms of developmental delays. A particular priority for the pediatrician is increased alertness to emotional and behavioral difficulties.

Although such difficulties may reasonably be identified in school-age children, the task is more difficult with infants. The availability of measures to assess temperament or behavioral style in infants and toddlers, including a recent description by Medoff-Cooper, Carey, and McDevitt[26] on the assessments of infants younger than 4 months of age, suggests that this task can be made easier. The environment clearly plays an important role in mediating the child's behavior and development. A variety of measures are available to assess the environment, and their use can help to identify situational contexts in which stimulation and support for the child may be indicated.

A final consideration is an emphasis on *rate as a principle* in developmental surveillance. Observations and assessments should be made on two or more occasions to determine the trajectory of development. This is necessary to rule out transient delays attributable to normal variation, situational factors, or the influence of illness or fatigue. Although developmental levels can be assessed adequately with most young children, predicting ultimate outcome, particularly intellectual competence, is hazardous and should be avoided. Individual variations from developmental norms may be transient and, at first, simply should indicate the need for more comprehensive evaluation.

APPROACHES TO DEVELOPMENTAL SURVEILLANCE

For the practitioner invested in developmental surveillance, at least three complementary approaches can be used:(1) clinical observation, (2) parental involvement, and (3) screening tests.

Clinical Observation

Developmental assessment is crucial in the preschool years because growth and development in this period are particularly rapid, the pediatrician has a central role in the lives of children and their families, and qualitative developmental markers in the form of signs and symptoms can be observed clinically. As Rapin[34] noted, no gold standard exists for making developmental diagnoses, and the pediatrician needs to draw on clinical observations of sign, symptoms, and screening results. These signs and symptoms can serve as indicators of at-risk status and developmental delay as well as of general school readiness. Of importance are those signs and symptoms of developmental functions associated with the identification of risk status or developmental delay. The publication of the *Diagnostic and Statistical Manual for Mental Disorders in Primary Care (DSM-PC)* represents an important tool to differentiate sign and symptoms in terms of normal variations, problems, and disorders.[37]

In typical usage, the terms *sign* and *symptom* are used diagnostically in regard to features or characteristics based either on objective or subjective criteria, respectively. With reference to developmental delay, consideration of signs and symptoms is complicated by several qualifications: (1) their significance is relative to development (timing); (2) their significance often is a function of temporal qualities (frequency, duration); and (3) they may be either common to developmental delay in general or associated with specific disorders.

Several issues are of value for the pediatrician to consider in this regard. One is the significance of rhythmic patterns such as body rocking and head rolling. In an early study, Kravitz and Boehm[23] found that the onset, pattern, and decline of rhythmic movements serve to document developmental delay. Another issue is the value of motor milestones. Allen and Alexander[1] found that the serial screening of motor milestones in preterm infants revealed that 18% have cerebral palsy at 1½ to 2 years of age. A final issue pertains to signs and symptoms in emotional development, a difficult but important domain to consider. Minde's[31] comprehensive view of symptoms of behavioral abnormalities in children younger than 36 months is a valuable resource in this regard. Major developmental domains and representative signs and symptoms are summarized in Box 20-7.

Petersen, Kube, and Palmer[33] have proposed that although developmental delay is used frequently to identify young children in pediatric practice in need of close survaillence, it should be seen as a chief complaint rather than as a diagnosis. Identification lies in documenting discrepancies in rate of development across key domains, yielding a profile. This is consistent with Aylward's[3] caution to consider congruence across developmental areas and integrative rather than isolated functions in the identification of delay. Although criteria may vary, age discrepancies of 25% or more or scores 2 or more standard deviations below the mean on a developmental measure are assumed typically to be indicative of developmental delay. In this context, a 20-month-old child whose mental, motor, or other domain of development resembles that of a 15-month-old or younger would be identified as developmentally delayed.

Identification of developmental delay is achieved more readily in some domains than in others. In domains for which age norms are available (e.g., motor, mental), the identification can be supported objectively through motor and mental scales. In other domains (e.g., social, behavioral), clinical judgment may serve as the primary basis for identification. Recognizing the central role of clinical reasoning in developmental assessment, Glascoe and Dworkin[15] have proposed that systematic attention to the process of impression formation can improve the accuracy of monitoring development.

Parental Involvement

The increasing importance of parental involvement is evident in pediatric practice[21] and reflects changing views of patient care and early intervention legislation (Public Law 99-457)[6] (see Chapter 19, Identification of Developmental Delays and the Early Intervention System). In addition to detailing the child's history, parental contribution to developmental assessment can be enhanced productively and efficiently. An initial activity is to determine the expectations of parents about the purpose, nature, and form of developmental assess-

BOX 20-7

DEVELOPMENTAL DELAY OR ATYPICAL FEATURES: REPRESENTATIVE SIGNS AND SYMPTOMS BY DOMAINS

Motor Domain
Hypertonicity or hypotonicity
Delayed creeping and walking
Poor coordination

Mental Domain
Delayed or atypical play
Delayed or atypical use of objects
Delayed development of symbolic skills

Communication and Language Domain
Articulation and production errors
Immature speech
Absent or delayed speech

Social and Emotional Domain
Lethargy
Anxiety
Sleep difficulties
Depression
Social withdrawal
Selective attention deficits

Behavioral Domain
Rhythmic habit patterns
Stereotypical behavior
Variable threshold level
Altered activity level

ment. This can serve not only to document the extent of expectations and their realism but also to alert providers to significant areas of concern.[35]

Increasing evidence also exists for the value of involving parents directly in assessing their child in terms of rating child characteristics and gathering observational data. Glascoe and Sandler[19] have shown that simply asking parents to estimate their child's developmental age can serve as a sensitive and specific "screen." Given the opportunity and appropriate format, parents can make reliable and valid judgments about the nature of their child's ability-disability profile.[4]

In addition to the approaches just mentioned, parents also can use various observation techniques (e.g., diary, interval, and time sampling) to record the frequency, duration, and pattern of a particular problem (e.g., enuresis or temper tantrums). Glascoe[13] has shown that solicitation of specific concerns about their child's development yields very useful information. Of interest are related findings showing that such concerns vary in intensity both as a function of stage of development and the child's underlying impairment.[20] Used individually or in combination, they constitute effective ways to involve parents in developmental screening.

Selected Screening Tests

The crux of developmental assessment is to differentiate the child who has a significant developmental problem from the one who manifests variations within a normal pattern. Appropriate measures can assist a clinician to identify developmental problems in infancy, and the preschool physical examination provides an excellent opportunity to predict school performance. Developmental status of most preschool children can be assessed validly and efficiently by use of the physical examination and selected surveillance measures (Table 20-6).

The *Denver Developmental Screening Test*,[12] including its most recent version (*Denver II*), is used widely and is shown in Fig. 20-3. It differs from the prior *DDST* with an increase of items from 105 to 125, particularly items pertaining to language (86%). The age scale of the test form conforms to the AAP's Health Supervision Visit Schedule, the norms have been updated and restandardized, and ratings of behavioral characteristics are included. The *Denver II* also enables identification of significant subpopulation differences attributable to race, gender, maternal education, and place of residence (rural, semirural, urban). It is easy to administer (see sample test materials, Fig. 20-4), covers the age range of birth to 6 years, and has strong interrater and test-retest reliability. Only a few test items are needed, and instructions for administration of items, shown in Fig. 20-5, are printed on the back of the test form (see Fig. 20-3). More detailed administration and scoring instructions are given in the *Denver II* manual, which must be used to administer the test accurately.

Although the *DDST* is a well-established tool to monitor development in pediatric settings, concerns exist about its screening accuracy in that standard scoring yielded high sensitivity but low specificity.[16] These concerns have led Meisels[27] and Glascoe et al[16] to caution its use and interpretation in general screening efforts. Similar concerns have been raised about the *Developmental Profile-II,* another tool recommended for pediatric screening.[14] This underscores the importance of attending to the larger issue of quality control relative to the purpose and method of screening. This issue is particularly significant for children who have mild or at-risk conditions often confounded by situational factors of poverty or minority status.[30]

Screening tools are subject to misuse in surveillance; this mandates care to ensure that common pitfalls are avoided and that tools meet criteria for specificity and sensitivity. As indicated, screening could encompass vision, hearing, expressive and receptive language, cognitive development, school readiness, self-awareness, and social awareness. Screening instruments, therefore, should be selected in terms of their purposes and incorporated in the pediatric visit. Screening measures having acceptable specificity and sensitivity include the *Early Screening Inventory (ESI),* the *Battelle Developmental Inventory Screening Test,*[6,28] and the *Child Development Inventory.*[22]

With continuing interest in the need for efficient surveillance, new screening measures are being developed. Sturner, Funk, and Green[36] for example, have shown that a brief procedure *(Simultaneous Techniques for Acuity and Readiness Testing, START)* can be incorporated into routine pediatric procedures with strong evidence of concurrent validity. Monitoring of linguistic and auditory status is also a domain in which screening of development in preterm infants has been found to be effective.[5]

For technical information (validity, specificity) on these and other screening instruments, see Meisels[28] and Glascoe, Martin, and Humphrey.[18] (See also Appendix D, Common Psychological and Educational Tests.)

Table 20-6 Selected Surveillance Measures

Instrument	Age (yr)
Early Infancy Temperament Questionnaire	0-4 mo
Infant Monitoring System	0-3
Denver Developmental Screening Test	0-6
Battelle Developmental Inventory Screening Test	1-8
Minnesota Child Developmental Inventory (MCDI)	6 mo-6 yr
Toddler Temperamental Scale	1-3
Peabody Picture Vocabulary Test-Revised (PPVT-R)	2-adult
Early Screening Inventory (ESI)	3-6
Minnesota Preschool Screening Inventory (MPSI)	3½-5½
School Readiness Survey	4-6
Behavioral Style Questionnaire	4-7

DEVELOPMENTAL SURVEILLANCE AND PRIMARY PEDIATRIC CARE

Diagnosis

For those children whose developmental course is of sufficient concern to warrant one or more of the assessments described above, several outcomes are likely to involve primary pediatric care. One of these is the identification

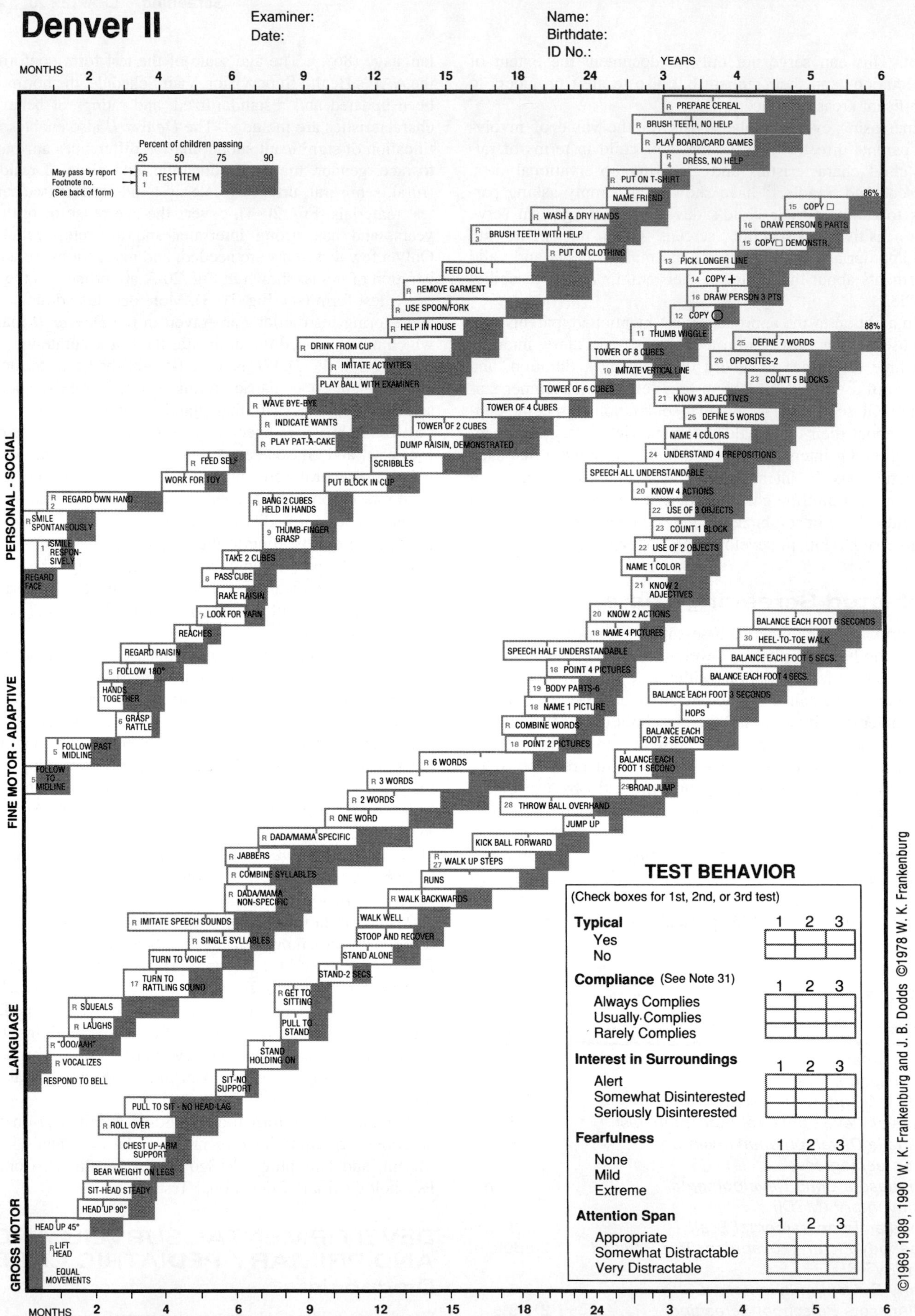

Fig. 20-3 Testing kits, test forms, and reference manuals (which must be used to ensure accuracy in administration of the test) for the DDST may be ordered from Denver Developmental Material, Inc., P.O. Box 6919, Denver, CO 80206-0919.
(Reprinted with permission from William K. Frankenburg.)

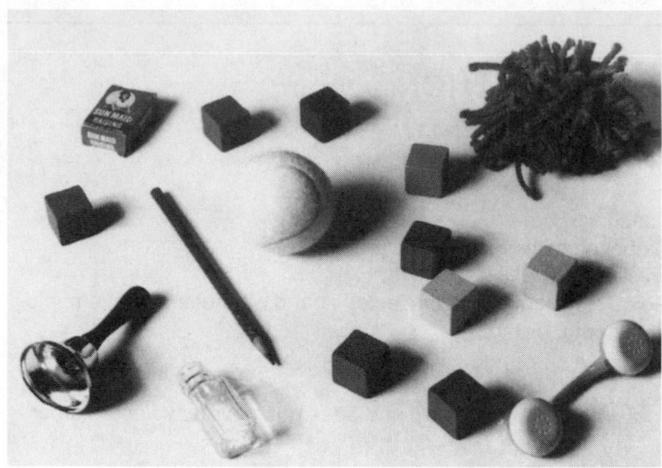

Fig. 20-4 Testing materials used in administering the *Denver Developmental Screening Test.*

of developmental delay or disorder. Although these diagnoses have come into wide use with the early intervention mandate, the definitions may vary substantially from state to state.

In general, however, developmental delay is defined as a condition in which functional aspects of the child's development are significantly delayed relative to the expected age-specific level of development. A typical criterion for developmental delay is a discrepancy of 25% or more from the expected rate in one or more domains of development. In references to standardized values, discrepancies of 1½ to 2 standard deviations also may be used. Signs and symptoms reflective of delays in functional development lead to an initial diagnosis of developmental delay. This diagnosis is either confirmed or dismissed after a consideration of the history, signs and symptoms, and associated etiological factors. In clinical contexts, "developmental delay" is a diagnostic label usually restricted to the preschool child in that neither the presenting characteristics nor assessment procedures are as specific as with older children. In the absence of findings associated with a specific developmental or behavioral disorder, the term *developmental delay* is used to define preschool children's eligibility for intervention.

Atypical Development

Screening for emotional and behavioral problems is challenging in that indicators of atypical behavior may vary as a function of cultural expectations and values. Behavior that might evoke concern in a middle-class environment may not be considered inappropriate in a lower-class environment (see Chapter 74, School Behavioral Problems).

Identifying psychological problems in young children is not without difficulty. Merritt et al[29] have noted that the diagnosis of behavioral and emotional problems by pediatricians is only 25% to 33% of true prevalence rates. Caregiver-completed questionnaires and checklists, as well as interview responses, may lack accuracy, particularly when there may be reluctance to reveal a problem. The reading level of some instruments may be inappropriate for many parents, yielding questionable results. The use of psychological tests and formal observation may not be an assessment option for most practitioners, given the need for specialized training and the administration time involved.

Presented with these challenges, the pediatrician who wishes to screen for psychological problems should work with mental health professionals to identify effective and efficient methods (see Chapter 20 [Fourteen], Psychosocial Screening). In a study of school-age children, Merritt et al[29] have shown that maternal completion of behavior checklists in primary care pediatrics enhanced the accuracy of screening children who have behavioral and emotional problems. The presence of echolalia; repetitive, stereotypic mannerisms; withdrawn, uncontrollable, self-destructive or abusive behavior; poor or absent eye contact; and limited social communication suggest the need for referral to a psychologist or a psychiatrist. Alone or in combination, these characteristics may reflect a variety of emotional and behavioral disturbances, ranging from acting out and testing of limits to expressions of psychopathological conditions. Identification of children for referral and intervention can be facilitated by the recent availability of two classification documents, *Diagnostic Classification of Mental Health and Developmental Disorders of Infancy and Early Childhood*[38] and the *Classification of Child and Adolescent Mental Diagnoses in Primary Care.*[37]

Erratic or Discrepant Development

Some children demonstrate wide gaps in developmental skills. Most notably, they may experience difficulty with fine or gross motor coordination, understanding or producing language, and encoding or decoding letters and numbers. The child's developmental profile may reflect a wide range of skills that include some average abilities. A modality or functional deficit is suggested when a discrepancy of one third or more is observed in developmental skills between one area and others; such a discrepancy should be the basis for referring for further assessment and possible intervention by developmental specialists. These discrepancies may signal sensory deficits or specific disabilities involving cognitive functioning, indicating the need for focused diagnostic evaluations.

Referral

If significant speech, motor, or other developmental deficits are noted, referral to allied health specialists can provide parents and health care professionals a realistic assessment of the child's needs and the development of specific plans for habilitation. Referral to psychologists should be made when comprehensive evaluation of the child's cognitive or affective functioning is indicated. The psychologist or educational specialist also can document the nature of the child's academic skills. Such information is a valuable base for parental understanding and involvement in interventions for the child.

It is important not to lose sight of the necessity of the primary care practitioner's advocacy when referral is made (see Chapter 83, Consultation and Refereral for Behavioral and Developmental Problems). To avoid potential problems in the referral process, the information and interventions desired from the consultant should be defined clearly. Sensitivity to environmental or situational factors is particularly sig-

DIRECTIONS FOR ADMINISTRATION

1. Try to get child to smile by smiling, talking or waving. Do not touch him/her.
2. Child must stare at hand several seconds.
3. Parent may help guide toothbrush and put toothpaste on brush.
4. Child does not have to be able to tie shoes or button/zip in the back.
5. Move yarn slowly in an arc from one side to the other, about 8" above child's face.
6. Pass if child grasps rattle when it is touched to the backs or tips of fingers.
7. Pass if child tries to see where yarn went. Yarn should be dropped quickly from sight from tester's hand without arm movement.
8. Child must transfer cube from hand to hand without help of body, mouth, or table.
9. Pass if child picks up raisin with any part of thumb and finger.
10. Line can vary only 30 degrees or less from tester's line.
11. Make a fist with thumb pointing upward and wiggle only the thumb. Pass if child imitates and does not move any fingers other than the thumb.

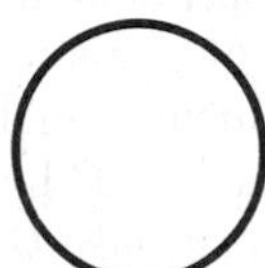

12. Pass any enclosed form. Fail continuous round motions.

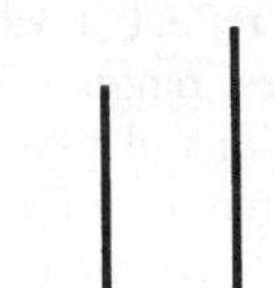

13. Which line is longer? (Not bigger.) Turn paper upside down and repeat. (pass 3 of 3 or 5 of 6)

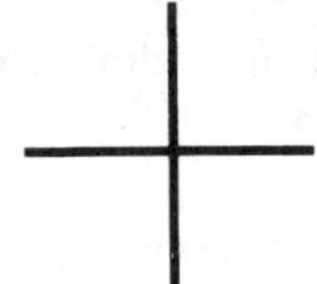

14. Pass any lines crossing near midpoint.

15. Have child copy first. If failed, demonstrate.

When giving items 12, 14, and 15, do not name the forms. Do not demonstrate 12 and 14.

16. When scoring, each pair (2 arms, 2 legs, etc.) counts as one part.
17. Place one cube in cup and shake gently near child's ear, but out of sight. Repeat for other ear.
18. Point to picture and have child name it. (No credit is given for sounds only.) If less than 4 pictures are named correctly, have child point to picture as each is named by tester.

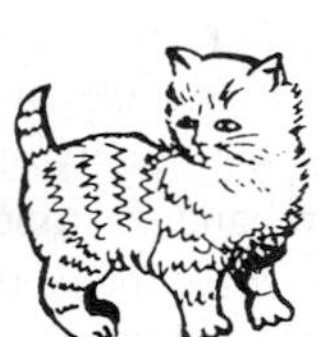
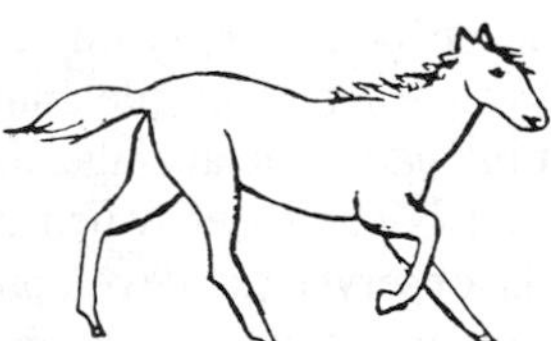
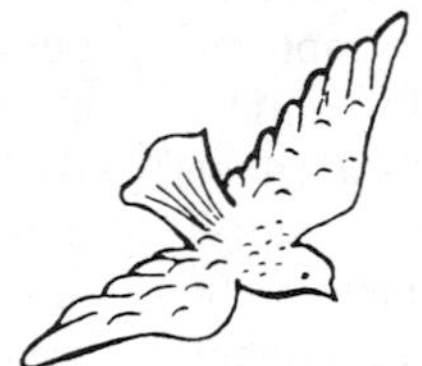
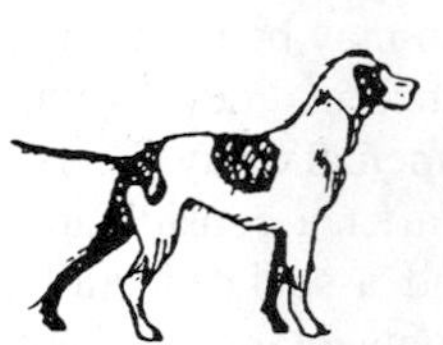
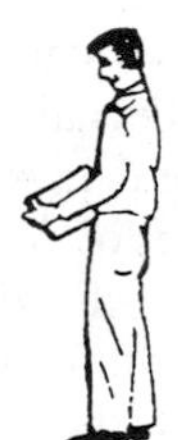

19. Using doll, tell child: Show me the nose, eyes, ears, mouth, hands, feet, tummy, hair. Pass 6 of 8.
20. Using pictures, ask child: Which one flies?... says meow?... talks?... barks?... gallops? Pass 2 of 5, 4 of 5.
21. Ask child: What do you do when you are cold?... tired?... hungry? Pass 2 of 3, 3 of 3.
22. Ask child: What do you do with a cup? What is a chair used for? What is a pencil used for? Action words must be included in answers.
23. Pass if child correctly places and says how many blocks are on paper. (1, 5).
24. Tell child: Put block **on** table; **under** table; **in front of** me, **behind** me. Pass 4 of 4. (Do not help child by pointing, moving head or eyes.)
25. Ask child: What is a ball?... lake?... desk?... house?... banana?... curtain?... fence?... ceiling? Pass if defined in terms of use, shape, what it is made of, or general category (such as banana is fruit, not just yellow). Pass 5 of 8, 7 of 8.
26. Ask child: If a horse is big, a mouse is __? If fire is hot, ice is __? If the sun shines during the day, the moon shines during the __? Pass 2 of 3.
27. Child may use wall or rail only, not person. May not crawl.
28. Child must throw ball overhand 3 feet to within arm's reach of tester.
29. Child must perform standing broad jump over width of test sheet (8 1/2 inches).
30. Tell child to walk forward, heel within 1 inch of toe. Tester may demonstrate. Child must walk 4 consecutive steps.
31. In the second year, half of normal children are non-compliant.

OBSERVATIONS:

Fig. 20-5 Instructions printed on the back of the *DDST* form for administering some of the items contained in the *Denver Developmental Screening Test*.
(Reprinted with permission from William K. Frankenburg.)

nificant in monitoring the course of treatment for children identified as being hyperactive or having attention deficits.

Referral for evaluation and diagnosis should be predicated on knowledge that intervention services and resources are available. Services and resources for infants and young children who have developmental problems may take the form community programs as well as private providers. Familiarity with available specialized resources for children who have disabilities and their families is essential if comprehensive management is to be developed and implemented.

Management

The pediatrician's role in the management of children who have developmental delays differs somewhat from that taken in the management of most illnesses. Cure with a return to normality usually is not achievable. Most of the professionals consulted about the child's assessment and treatment are nonmedical. Pediatricians who must inform parents of the presence of a chronic and disabling condition should consider their initial approach carefully (see Chapter 11, Communication with Parents and Patients). This information should be shared in a quiet, private consultation with both parents present whenever possible. Sufficient time should be allocated to allow a complete and unhurried sharing of both information and feelings. Clarifying the parents' perceptions early on is important. More often than not, the pediatrician will discover that the news confirms long-standing parental suspicions. In such instances, the parents are likely to be relieved that someone finally is taking them seriously. Support by the physician will do much to form a therapeutic alliance.

Information given to the parents should be as complete and honest as the pediatrician is capable of providing; withholding information only builds mistrust. The pediatrician should be careful to minimize the use of technical terminology and provide developmental diagnoses if they apply. If the parents react negatively, the pediatrician should avoid arguments or attempts to convince. The parents' perspective on their child's status can evolve in the context of an understanding relationship with a pediatrician. For children who have a specific diagnosis or who simply are at risk for developmental delay, management involves monitoring progress and being supportive of the child and family. Management of children who have specific disorders (e.g., cerebral palsy, autism) involves similar activities, with the addition of specific medical or allied interventions as indicated.

Because of the complex needs of many children who have developmental problems, it is highly desirable that assessment and management be integrated into an overall plan for the child's care. Such an overall plan is implicit in the requirements of the Individualized Family Service Plan (IFSP) for young children and the Individualized Education Plan (IEP) for school-age children as defined in the reauthorization of the Individuals with Disabilities Education Act (IDEA). Particularly important is establishing lines of communication and accountability on behalf of the family raising a child who has developmental problems. Given that care for the child and family may involve contacts with an array of professionals in health and related fields, the pediatrician is the logical coordinator of services. Advocating for the child and family is essential to the therapeutic process and the promotion of the child's potential.

REFERENCES

1. Allen MC, Alexander GR: Using motor milestones as a multistep process to screen preterm infants for cerebral palsy, *Dev Med Child Neurol* 39:12, 1997.
2. American Academy of Pediatrics: Recommendations for preventive pediatric health care, *Pediatrics* 81:466, 1988.
3. Aylward GP: Conceptual issues in developmental screening and assessment, *J Dev Behav Pediatr* 18:340, 1997.
4. Bailey DB, et al: Reliability of an index of child characteristics, *Dev Med Child Neurol* 35:806, 1993.
5. Belcher HM, et al: Using the clinical linguistic and auditory milestone scale for developmental screening in high-risk preterm infants, *Clin Ped* 36:635, 1997.
6. Blackman JA, Healy A, Ruppert ES: Participation by pediatricians in early intervention: impetus from Public Law 99-457, *Pediatrics* 89:98, 1992.
7. Casey PH, Swanson M: A Pediatric perspective of developmental screening in 1993, *Clin Ped* 32:209, 1993.
8. Dobos AE, Dworkin PH, Bernstein BA: Pediatricians' approaches to developmental problems: has the gap been narrowed? *J Dev Behav Pediatr* 15:34, 1994.
9. Dworkin PH: Developmental screening—expecting the impossible? *Pediatrics* 84:619, 1989.
10. Dworkin PH: Ready to learn: a mandate for pediatrics, *J Dev Behav Pediatr* 14:192, 1993.
11. First LR, Palfrey JS: The infant or young child with developmental delay, *N Engl J Med* 330:478, 1994.
12. Frankenburg WK, et al: The Denver II: a major revision and restandardization of the Denver Developmental Screening Test, *Pediatrics* 89:91, 1992.
13. Glascoe FP: Parents' concerns about children's development: Prescreening techniques or screening test? *Pediatrics* 99:522, 1997.
14. Glascoe FP, Byrne KE: The usefulness of the developmental Profile-II in developmental screening, *Clin Ped* 32:203, 1993.
15. Glascoe FP, Dworkin PH: Obstacles to effective developmental surveillance: errors in clinical reasoning, *J Dev Behav Pediatr* 4:344, 349, 1993.
16. Glascoe FP, et al: Accuracy of the Denver-II in developmental screening, *Pediatrics* 89:1221, 1992.
17. Glascoe FP, Foster M, Wolraich ML: An economic analysis of developmental detection methods, *Pediatrics* 99:830, 1997.
18. Glascoe FP, Martin ED, Humphrey S: A comparative review of developmental screening tests, *Pediatrics* 86:547, 1990.
19. Glascoe FP, Sandler H: Values of parents' estimates of children's developmental ages, *J Pediatr* 127:831, 1995.
20. Hodapp RM, et al: Maternal emotional reactions to young children with different types of handicaps, *J Dev Behav Pediatr* 13:118, 1992.
21. Hutchison T, Nicoll A: Developmental screening and surveillance, *Br J Hosp Med* 39:22, 1988.
22. Ireton H, Glascoe FP: Assessing children's development using parents' reports, *Clin Ped* 34:248, 1995.
23. Kravitz H, Boehm JJ: Rhythmic habit patterns in infancy: their sequence, age of onset, and frequency, *Child Dev* 42:399, 1971.
24. Levy SE, Hyman SL: Pediatric assessment of the child with developmental delay, *Ped Clin North Am* 40:465, 1993.
25. Majnemer A, Mazer B: Neurologic evaluation of the newborn infant: definition and psychometric properties, *Dev Med Child Neural* 40:708, 1998.
26. Medoff-Cooper B, Carey WB, McDevitt SC: The early infancy temperament questionnaire, *J Dev Behav Pediatr* 14:230, 1993.
27. Meisels SJ: Can developmental screening tests identify children who are developmentally at risk? *Pediatrics* 83:578, 1989.
28. Meisels SJ: Developmental screening in early childhood: the interaction of research and social policy, *Ann Rev Public Health* 9:527, 1988.

29. Merritt KA, et al: Screening for behavioral and emotional problems in primary care pediatrics, *J Dev Behav Pediatr* 14:340, 1993.
30. Miller JE: Developmental screening scores among preschool-aged children: the roles of poverty and child health, *J Urban Health* 75:135, 1998.
31. Minde K: Behavioral abnormalities commonly seen in infancy, *Can J Psychiatry* 33:741, 1988.
32. Minkovitz C, Mathew MB, Strobino D: Have professional recommendations and consumer demand altered pediatric practice regarding child development? *J Urban Health* 75:739, 1998.
33. Petersen MC, Kube DA, Palmer FB: Classification of developmental delays, *Semin Pediatr Neurology*, 5:1, 1998.
34. Rapin I: Physicians' testing of children with developmental disabilities, *J Child Neurol* 10:S11, 1995.
35. Simeonsson RJ, et al: Family involvment in multidisciplinary team evaluation: professional and parent perspectives, *Child Care Health Devel* 21:199, 1995.
36. Sturner RA, Funk SG, Green JA: Simultaneous technique for acuity and readiness testing (START): further concurrent validation of an aid for developmental surveillance, *Pediatrics* 93:83, 1994.
37. Wolraich ML, Felice ME, Drotar D, editors: *The classification of child and adolescent mental diagnoses in primary care*, Elk Grove, Ill, 1996, American Academy of Pediatrics.
38. Zero to Three: National Center for Infants, Toddlers, and Families: *Diagnostic classification of mental health and development disorders of infancy and early childhood (Diagnostic classification: 0-3)*, Washington, DC, 1994.

SUGGESTED READINGS

Carey WB: Clinical use of temperament data in pediatrics, *J Dev Behav Pediatr* 6:137, 1985.

Drillien CM, Pickering RM, Drummond MB: Predictive value of screening for different areas of development, *Dev Med Child Neurol* 30:294, 1988.

Dworkin PH: Detection of behavioral, developmental, and psychosocial problems in pediatric primary care practice, *Curr Opin Pediatr* 5:531, 1993.

Frankenburg WK: Preventing developmental delays: is developmental screening sufficient? *Pediatrics* 93:589, 1994.

Kaplan BJ, et al: Physical signs and symptoms in preschool-age hyperactive and normal children, *J Dev Behav Pediatr* 8:305, 1987.

Meisels SJ, Provence S: *Screening and assessment: guidelines for identifying young disabled and developmentally vulnerable children and their families*, Washington, DC, 1989, National Center for Clinical Infant Programs.

fourteen Psychosocial Screening

Steven Schlozman and Michael S. Jellinek

THE NEED FOR PSYCHOSOCIAL SCREENING

Recent estimates have suggested that roughly 12% of American children[20,23] suffer from psychosocial difficulties that include significant functional impairments and psychiatric disorders defined by the fourth edition of the *Diagnostic Statistical Manual of Mental Disorders (DSM-IV)*. Beyond mental health concerns, psychosocial issues in primary care have multiple secondary consequences. Psychosocial dysfunction is both a major risk factor for accidents, the most common cause of death in pediatric patients, and perhaps a marker to identify parents who use substances or suffer from depression. Incidents such as fires, falls from windows, drowning, and motor vehicle accidents all are more common among children who have higher rates of psychosocial stressors.[3,15,17] *DSM-IV* diagnoses do not take into account developmental expectations and corresponding functional assessments. Thus, the pediatrician is served best by broadly screening for psychosocial dysfunction rather than focusing exclusively on psychiatric diagnoses.

Despite a high prevalence of psychosocial and psychiatric difficulties encountered by children and adolescents, multiple studies have shown that the majority of these problems are not detected by primary care physicians.[5,6,10,24,25] Potential reasons for this lack of recognition include time limitations, hesitancy among practitioners to attach possibly stigmatizing labels to children, the absence of widely available screening procedures, lack of adequate training regarding psychosocial issues, and limited resources for referral and treatment. The theoretical benefits of managed and consistent quality assurance are being overshadowed by pressures of productivity that have decreased the number of minutes per patient and by barriers to referral. However, in principle, managed care should encourage referral by emphasizing screening and quality, and perhaps, lower costs over time.

Increasing Recognition

Obtaining a comprehensive psychosocial history is time consuming and inefficient. Currently, some children are recognized because of parental complaints of overt behavioral problems or school referral. Less obvious problems, such as dysfunction stemming from divorce or depression, often are identified in the primary care setting. The goal of psychosocial screening is to provide methods in harmony with pediatric primary care for early, efficient, and effective recognition of developing psychosocial problems.

A number of strategies may increase effective recognition of psychosocial difficulties. Careful attention to developmental aspects of the child's life, such as the child's family, friends, school, play, and mood will help the pediatrician assess the child's overall function.[11] Despite the obvious time involved, face-to-face interviewing, in which high-risk issues are discussed with the patient and family, offers many advantages. The physician can address key issues directly, communicating to the family the importance of psychosocial issues, thus increasing the likelihood that the family will consider these issues appropriate to bring to the physician's attention.

Raising questions face-to-face builds trust; examples of clinically relevant questions are available through the American Academy of Pediatrics' *Guidelines for Health Supervision* and the Public Health Service manual *Bright Futures*.[7] Topics mentioned in both documents include instructions such as the following:

- At intake, ask all parents for a family history of psychiatric disorder (e.g., depression and substance use).
- At annual visits, ask about parental discord and marital stability.
- For newborns, assess parental coping, family support, and maternal depression.
- For toddlers, ask about the child's autonomy and the ability to "separate."
- For early school-age children, ask about social functioning.
- For adolescents, ask parents about their child's autonomy, and ask the adolescent about mood and substance use.

Because of the time constraints inherent in a face-to-face approach, alternative strategies have been developed to screen more efficiently for psychosocial difficulties. The *Achenbach Child Behavior Checklist (CBCL)* is the most studied and best validated behavioral screening device available for children ages 4 to 16 years.[1] The *CBCL* is completed by the child's parents and is divided into two distinct item groups: behavior problems and school competency. Although the results of the *CBCL* are reliable and valid, the main drawbacks to the use of this instrument include length of administration (more than 100 items requiring about 20 minutes of the parent's time), as well as some complexity in methods for scoring and interpreting the results of the questionnaire.

A possible and less cumbersome alternative to the *CBCL* is the *Pediatric Symptom Checklist (PSC)*, a 35-item survey also given to the parents and requiring only a few minutes to complete (http://healthcare.partners.org/pcc).[4,12] In addition, the results of the *PSC* can be score scored quickly with 2 points assigned to each question answered "often," 1 point assigned to each answered "sometimes," and 0 points assigned to each answered "never." Administration and scoring commonly take 3 to 5 minutes. A score greater than 28 suggests a 70% likelihood that the child has significant psychosocial difficulties; scores less than 28 suggest a greater than 95% likelihood that the child has no substantial psychosocial problems. Thus, if the parents complete the *PSC* in the waiting room and have it scored by a receptionist or clinical assistant, the pediatrician can quickly recognize and more closely evaluate significant psychosocial issues. However, although the *PSC* works well in adolescent populations, it is somewhat hampered in this age group by the parents' limitations in correctly assessing through a questionnaire their child's intrapsychic state. Specifically, some parents will not know that their child is depressed because he or she appears to be in reasonable spirits and functioning well; thus, the *PSC* will, in this circumstance, yield a false-negative result. Despite this difficulty, because the *PSC* primarily assesses function, it still yields efficient and important information that can direct further inquiry.

The issue of identifying the adequately functioning but depressed teenager can be addressed by having *The Beck Depression Inventory* completed by the adolescent. Twenty percent or more of teenagers have scores that raise concerns, using this screening instrument.[2,14]

Clinical Perspectives

As stated earlier, formal psychiatric diagnoses do not always take into account important developmental and functional assessments. For example, family discord may lead to school phobia or oppositionality in young children but to depression and substance abuse in adolescents. A more holistic nosology is available through the *Diagnostic and Statistical Manual of Mental Disorders,* primary care version *(DSM-PC)*, a manual defining psychosocial issues within a developmental context.[26]

The *DSM-PC* discusses a broad range of problems, some of which are consistent with formal psychiatric diagnoses, as well as many issues that are clinically relevant in spite of not meeting full *DSM-IV* criteria. Problems are grouped into three main categories: normal variation, problems, and disorders. *Normal variation* allows for different temperaments, personalities, and developmental paths among healthy children. *Problems* refer to a broad range of issues that may not meet formal criteria for a discrete psychiatric disorder. For example, the *DSM-PC* recognizes that while a child's anxious reaction to divorce may be a normal and expected developmental response, the child still might be in need of support and services during this difficult time. Finally, *disorders* refers to those conditions that meet *DSM-IV* criteria for a psychiatric disorder.

Psychosocial difficulties also should be assessed for the severity of the impairment in functioning. Although conditions such as psychosis or serious suicidal ideation clearly are severe, other problems, such as depression or anxiety, are quite variable in their severity. Not all cases of depression, for example, need specialized treatment, although some depressed children require an aggressive and multimodal approach and even hospitalization.

An assessment of severity includes the following three items[9]:

1. Symptoms—number, frequency, duration, and places where the symptoms are experienced
2. Functioning—developmental impact on functioning in key areas such as family, friends, school, activities, and self esteem
3. Burden of suffering—intensity of suffering, duration, limitations on family activities, danger to self and others, and intrusion into developmental tasks or daily activities

Finally, it is important to note that a number of biological and environmental factors may be protective against the risk of adversity leading to serious psychosocial problems. Table 20-7 outlines both protective and risk factors for psychosocial difficulties.[9] Although each risk factor carries potential impact, studies have suggested that the number of moderate risk factors can have a cumulative effect on a child's dysfunction greater than any one severe risk factor. Children facing three or more risk factors have a very high likelihood of psychosocial problems.[11] Individual risk factors that have special significance include single parent households and poverty.[11]

The issue of poverty deserves special mention. Although numerous studies have connected low social-economic status with increased risk of psychosocial dysfunction,[8,16,18] research has suggested that pediatricians tend to address a larger proportion of psychosocial concerns in highly educated families than in less educated families. One potential explanation for this discrepancy is that more-educated parents might feel more comfortable bringing psychosocial issues to their pediatrician's attention, whereas less-educated families might not realize that the pediatrician's office is appropriate for psychosocial inquiries. In addition some studies have shown that middle- to upper-class parents tend to overreport their children's psychosocial problems, whereas lower-class parents tend to underreport. These findings demonstrate the need for a careful and systematic review of psychosocial issues in all patients within a pediatric practice.

The Brief Evaluation

As outlined above, many psychosocial problems will be elucidated through focused interviewing, the *CBCL*, or the *PSC*.

Table 20-7 Children's Well-Being: Risk and Protective Factors

	Protective Decreased Impact of Stress	Risks Increased Impact of Stress
Health	Good health	Chronic disease/ill health
Temperament	e.g., Pleasant mood	e.g., Negative mood; irritable
Cognitive status	Normal IQ (particularly verbal)	Learning disability/low IQ
Emotional health	Good mental health function	Pre-existing emotional disorder
Sociability	Good peer relations	Poor peer relations
Child reaction to stress	Perceives stress as limited; does not blame self	Perceives continued threat; blames self
Quality of attachment	High quality, high continuity; securely attached	Low quality, discontinuous; ambivalent, insecurely attached
Parent competence	Competent	Incompetent
Family resources	Adequate economic resources	Poverty/discrimination
Quality, stability, safety of environment	Adequate, stable, safe	Inadequate, unstable, unsafe
Family relationships	Good communication, little conflict	Poor communication, much conflict
Emotional and physical health of caregivers	Caregivers in good emotional and physical health	Mental illness or physical illness in caregivers
Availability/access to community resources	High access	Low access

In addition, patients might present with a definite psychosocial complaint, often mentioned by parents or the school. At this point, the clinician should attempt to elaborate the symptoms, further defining the nature of the complaint. Risk factors and developmental concerns should be considered, and the child's daily functioning should be examined. A number of guidelines will be helpful in this process[9]:

1. For younger children, observe them and direct questions to the parents
2. For school-age children, use confirmatory questions, if possible, without parents being present
3. For adolescents, perform a separate interview with the patient alone. Assess important issues such as substance use and depression. Inquire about sexual relations. Consider parental functioning, especially abuse, depression, substance use
4. Review relevant risk factors, as well as potentially protective factors
5. Assess safety, paying special attention to potential accidents, suicidal ideation, and risk-taking
6. Complete a severity estimate based on to the *CBCL* and the *PSC* formats, ranking the current issue as mild, moderate, or severe

Once the foregoing information is gathered, the presenting complaint should be categorized as either a normal variation that requires no further action or a problem that requires consideration Many issues can be followed at the primary care level, often with comanagement by mental health professionals or school personnel. Other more serious problems require outside referral for evaluation by a specialist and, possibly, ongoing treatment. The most severe cases often require emergency referral.

Treatment

All psychosocial difficulties require services beyond support and guidance, and pediatricians should use whatever community resources are available (e.g., the child's extended family, parent support groups, local clubs and teams, and school guidance and personnel). Some more serious issues call for referral and comprehensive treatment. In these instances, the clinician should attempt to integrate all areas of the child's functioning into the treatment plan. Potential treatments include individual and family therapy, out-of-home services such as hospitalization, partial- and day-treatment programs, or foster care, and the appropriate use of medications. In situations involving key issues such as substance abuse, focused treatment often is helpful. Where learning disorders are suspected, psychological testing and recommended learning strategies should be implemented. The goal of such multimodal treatments is to take into account all of the developmental and functional aspects of the child's difficulties.

CONCLUSION

The changes in pediatric practice created by managed care constraints make psychosocial screening and referral for appropriate treatment increasingly difficult. For the majority of children in the United States, mental health services are carved out of pediatric care with financial incentives that discourage referral and comprehensive treatment.[13] These carved-out companies limit the role of psychiatrists primarily to medication management, creating an environment increasingly overfocused on psychotropic administration at the expense of alternative treatments.[13,19,21,22] Furthermore, capitation may be an additional disincentive to referral to specialty services.

However, innovative practices may be able to provide adequate treatment in spite of the current health care insurance climate. For example, some pediatricians are bringing mental health professionals into their practices to provide consultation and services. Some large group practices may be able to offset costly treatments with preventive methods such as divorce or adolescent focus groups. It remains paramount that psychosocial difficulties be detected early and treated efficiently and effectively. To this end, the primary care pediatrician is in an ideal setting to provide crucial screening and to initiate important treatments.

REFERENCES

1. Achenbach TM: *Manual for the child behavior checklist/4-18 and 1991 profile*, Burlington, Vt, 1991, University of Vermont Department of Psychiatry.
2. Beck AT, et al: An inventory for measuring depression, *Arch Gen Psychiatry* 45:561, 1961.
3. Bijur PE, Stewart-Brown S, Butler N: Child behavior and accidental injury in 11,966 preschool children, *Am J Dis Child* 140:487, 1986.
4. Bishop SJ, et al: Psychosocial screening in pediatric practice: a survey of interested physicians, *Clin Pediatr* 30:142, 1991.
5. Costello EJ: Primary care pediatrics and child psychopathology: a review of diagnostic, treatment, and referral practices, *Pediatrics* 78:1044, 1986.
6. Costello EJ, Janiszewski S: Who gets treated? factors associated with referral in children with psychiatric disorders, *Acta Psychiatr Scand* 18:523, 1990.
7. Green M, editor: *Bright futures: guidelines for health services of infants, children and adolescents,* Arlington, Va, 1994, National Center for Education in Matemal and Child Health.
8. Hack S, Jellinek MS: Historical clues to the diagnosis of the dysfunctional child and other psychiatric disorders in children, *Pediatr Clin North Am* 45:25, 1998.
9. Jellinek MS: Approach to the behavioral problems in children and adolescents. In Stern TA, Herman JB, Slavin PL, editors: *The MGH guide to psychiatry in primary care,* New York, 1997, McGraw Hill.
10. Jellinek M: The present status of child psychiatry in pediatrics, *N Engl J Med* 306:1227, 1982.
11. Jellinek M, et al: The Pediatric Symptom Checklist: support for a role in a managed care environment, *Arch Pediatr Adolesc Med* 149:140, 1995.
12. Jellinek MS, et al: Use of the Pediatric Symptom Checklist to screen for psychosocial problems in pediatric primary care: a national feasibility study, *Arch Pediatr Adolesc Med* 153:254, 1999.
13. Jellinek M, Little M: Supporting child psychiatric services using current managed care approaches: you can't get there from here, *Arch Pediatr Adolesc Med* 152:321, 1998.
14. Kashani JH, et al: Utility of the Beck Depression Inventory with clinic-referred adolescents, *J Am Acad Child Adolesc Psychiatry* 29:278, 1990.
15. Kemp A, Silbert J: Childhood accidents: epidemiology, trends and prevention, *J Accid Emerg Med* 14:316, 1997.
16. Kleinman RE, et al: Hunger in children in the United States: potential behavioral and emotional correlates, *Pediatrics* 101:E3, 1998.
17. Larrison JO, Aurelius G: Accidents in childhood: relation to psychosocial conditions and mental development, *Acta Paediatricia* 85:285, 1996.
18. Lipman EL, Offord DR, Boyle MH: Relation between economic disadvantage and psychosocial morbidity in children [see comments], *CMAJ* 151:431, 1994.
19. Murphy JM, et al: Screening for psychosocial dysfunction in pediatric practice: a naturalistic study of the Pediatric Symptom Checklist, *Clin Pediatr* 31:660, 1992.
20. Office of Technology Assessment: *Children's mental health: problems and services—a background paper,* Washington, DC, 1986, Office of Technology Assessment.
21. Pincus HA, et al: Prescribing trends in psychotropic medications: primary care, psychiatry, and other medical specialties, *JAMA* 279:526, 1998.
22. Schreter RK: Coping with the crisis in psychiatric training, *Psychiatry* 60:1, 1997.
23. Schwartz-Gould M, Wunsch-Hitzig MA, Dobrenwend B: Estimating the prevalence of childhood psychopathology: a critical review, *J Am Acad Child Psychiatry* 20:462, 1998.
24. Sharp L, et al: Psychosocial problems during child health supervision visits: eliciting, then what? *Pediatrics* 89:619, 1992.
25. Starfield B: Behavioral pediatrics and primary health care, *Pediatr Clin North Am* 29:377, 1982.
26. Woiraich ML, editor: *The classification of child and adolescent mental diagnoses in primary care: Diagnostic and Statistical Manual for Primary Care (DSM-PC) Child and Adolescent Version,* Elk Grove Village, Ill, 1996, American Academy of Pediatrics.

21 Counseling Families on Healthy Lifestyles

R. Joseph Jopling

A "healthy lifestyle" is the product of numerous decisions a person must make about health-related fitness, diet, and psychosocial issues that allow the individual to maximize his or her genetic potential for a healthy life.[14]

Many people have misguided notions about these components. Health-related fitness, for example, is related neither to athletic ability nor to physical appearance. The decline in health-related fitness parameters among children, adolescents, and young adults in the United States is well documented,[36] and the relationship between those parameters and many preventable diseases of adulthood has been strongly suggested, if not proved.* The problem is pervasive and has seemed refractory to change. This chapter suggests how primary care physicians can discuss the problem with their patients and then help them devise a healthy lifestyle plan for the whole family.

HEALTHY LIFESTYLE PARAMETERS AND PREVENTABLE DISEASES

Cardiovascular diseases (myocardial infarction, hypertension, and stroke), obesity, and some types of cancer (e.g., lung and colon cancer) not only are major sources of morbidity and mortality but also they are thought to be preventable, at least in part, by lifestyle changes.[30,33] A lifestyle is learned in childhood and tends to become more difficult to change as the individual grows older. Therefore, the younger the patient, the more easily lifestyle changes can be made, and the more likely it is that those changes will help prevent, or at least reduce, the effects of the above-mentioned diseases later in life. It should be easier and more cost effective to prevent inherently active children from becoming sedentary adults than to try to change this habit once adulthood has been reached.[33]

Most experts agree that the decline in healthy lifestyle parameters correlates directly with an increase in the risk factors for cardiovascular disease such as obesity, hypertension, high serum cholesterol, smoking, psychosocial stress, and physical inactivity. Sometimes the tale is best told in numbers.

Obesity. Sixty percent of adults are overweight, and more than 25% are obese (more than 20 pounds overweight); 20% of children are now considered overweight (body mass index [BMI] greater than the 95th percentile), a significant increase in just 10 years.[10,45]

Hypertension. Ten percent of adults and 5% of children are considered hypertensive. This statistic, coupled with those for obesity, is particularly sobering because the risk of dying of cardiovascular disease appears to be greater in the families of children who are persistently obese, especially those who have persistent high blood pressure.[4]

High serum cholesterol. Ten percent to 20% of adults have high serum cholesterol levels; however, this is not just a disease of adulthood—the problem begins in childhood. Atherosclerotic fatty streaks have been found in children as young as age 3 years. By age 22, anywhere from 45% to 77% of individuals may have evidence of atherosclerosis.[47]

Smoking and psychosocial stress. Most cigarette smokers begin smoking before age 20, and psychosocial stress is more intense and more prevalent at earlier ages than ever before.

Physical inactivity. An epidemiological study reported in 1987 by the Centers for Disease Control and Prevention (CDC) has shown that physical inactivity is as strong a risk factor for coronary heart disease as are the traditional risk factors (smoking, hypertension, and high serum cholesterol).[30] Even more important, physical inactivity was shown to be three to six times more prevalent than any other risk factor. Only 20% of adults exercise adequately, and 60% do not exercise at all. One of the national health objectives for Healthy People 2000 is to decrease by 15% the proportion of persons ages 6 years or older who are inactive during their leisure time. Unfortunately, the numbers are actually edging up from 28.7% in 1992 to 29.4% in 1994. Several factors seem to make matters worse: rural location (especially in the South), lower educational level, and lower socioeconomic status.[36]

Only 36% of schoolchildren have daily physical education classes. The 1984 National Children and Youth Fitness Study found that only 66% of children and adolescents 10 to 17 years of age were participating in physical activity at the recommended level.*[40]

Not surprisingly, the U.S. Public Health Service's 1990 goal of having more than 90% of schoolchildren participating

*References 6, 19, 21, 22, 25, 47.

*To meet the recommended level, the children had to be exercising three or more times a week for 20 minutes or longer per session, at an activity that was likely to be pursued as an adult, that used 60% or more of cardiorespiratory capacity, and that involved large muscle groups in dynamic contraction (e.g., walking, swimming, or cycling).

in physical activity at the recommended level was not met, and budgetary constraints in school systems across the country pose a definite risk of a decline in participation as we enter the new millennium. Even when offered, physical education classes often emphasize team sports rather than individual lifelong activities (i.e., aerobic activities that can be done alone, such as walking, jogging, swimming, or cycling).

Aggravating the problem of inactivity is that children in the United States average 25 hours a week watching television, often while munching some type of unhealthy snack food.

Physical inactivity is not a recently identified issue. As early as the 1940s, Kraus and Hirschland[18] recognized a health-related physical fitness problem. When their findings for American children were compared with those for European children, American children were found to be significantly less fit than their European counterparts. In an effort to change that trend, the President's Council on Youth Fitness was formed, known today as the President's Council on Physical Fitness and Sports. In 1988, Kraus reported that fewer than 50% of the children who took the council's fitness test passed. Only 60% of boys 6 to 12 years of age and 30% of girls 6 to 17 years of age could do more than one chin-up; similarly, only 64% of boys and 50% of girls ages 6 to 12 could run or walk a mile in fewer than 10 minutes.[17]

As mentioned previously, almost all experts agree that the best way to resolve these fitness problems is to change people's lifestyles. One of the best ways to accomplish this is to develop a program for the whole family. This program should focus on cardiorespiratory endurance, strength and endurance of the large-muscle groups, flexibility, body composition, a healthy diet, and development of stress management techniques and improved communication skills (Box 21-1).

BOX 21-1

COMPONENTS OF A HEALTHY LIFESTYLE

Cardiorespiratory Endurance

Cardiorespiratory endurance is achieved by performing any one of a number of aerobic exercises while maintaining the heart rate at 60% to 80% of a calculated maximum for at least 30 minutes at a time, at least three times a week, for at least 6 consecutive months.

Muscle Strength and Endurance

Leg muscle strength enables a person to perform aerobic exercise. Abdominal muscle strength aids in proper breathing technique and helps protect the lower back. Upper body strength is important to overall muscle balance and aids in many everyday activities.

Flexibility

Flexibility helps prevent musculoskeletal injuries and makes a person feel more spry. Without warm-up and cool-down stretching periods, an exercise program can lead to loss of flexibility.

Body Composition

Baseline and follow-up measurements of body composition (ratio of fat to muscle) is one of the best methods of tracking progress in health-related fitness. Using only body weight or the height-to-weight ratio can be misleading in assessing the fitness level.

Healthy Diet

A diet high in carbohydrates, low to moderate in protein, low in fat, and moderate in total calories is essential to any fitness program.

Stress Management/Communication Skills

In today's fast-paced world, techniques for managing stress and improved communication skills have become increasingly important components of good health.

Modified from Jopling RJ: *Pediatr Rev* 10:141, 1988.

CARDIORESPIRATORY ENDURANCE

Cardiorespiratory endurance is best achieved by performing aerobic exercise for at least 30 minutes per session while maintaining the heart rate at 60% to 80% of a calculated maximum. The minimum exercise time thought to be needed for an aerobic effect initially was 15 minutes, and then 20 minutes; now it is 30 minutes. The American College of Sports Medicine now recognizes three 10-minute episodes of physical activity in a day to be as beneficial as one 30-minute episode. This certainly allows for more flexibility in designing any physical activity program for all members of the family. An inactive person should start at whatever level and duration of continuous activity he or she can tolerate safely and gradually work up to 30 minutes.

In the adult literature, whenever a positive relationship is found between exercise and a decline in serum cholesterol, the correlate seems to be that the more vigorous and sustained the exercise, the greater its effect.[10] This implies that "more is better" with regard to intensity, but as with duration, the recommendations for intensity level have changed. Initially, exercise physiologists proposed that a person had to reach a target heart rate to achieve an aerobic exercise threshold that led to improved aerobic fitness. Most exercise physiologists and cardiologists now believe that unless an individual already is relatively fit, it is a mistake even to discuss target heart rates. Initially, it is much more important to stress becoming physically active at any level and then begin to increase that level gradually.[1] Borg[2] has proposed a "perceived exertion" scale as an adequate measure of heart rate, a concept that has been validated more than once.[7] A common rule of thumb for finding the proper intensity is to exercise at least enough to perspire while maintaining the ability to carry on a conversation.

For those ready to use the heart rate as a guide, the recommendation is that a person who has been relatively active should aim for a target rate of about 60% when starting an aerobic exercise program. It is unwise at any time to exceed 80% of the maximum heart rate. People who are already active and who want more specific information should consult published guidelines for heart rates during exercise (Table 21-1). It cannot be overemphasized that these numbers are based on suggestions for training athletes and should not be thought of as hard-and-fast rules. Gradually warming up before exercising and cooling down afterward help to ensure

Table 21-1 Suggested Training Heart Rates*

Age (yr)	Heart Rate (beats/min) Maximum	80%	60%
5-9	220	176	132
10	210	168	126
11	209	167	125
12	208	166	125
13	207	165	124
14	206	165	123
15	205	164	123
16	204	163	122
17	203	162	122
18	202	162	121
19	201	161	121
20	200	160	120
22	198	158	118
24	196	157	117
26	194	155	116
28	192	154	115
30	190	152	114
32	189	151	113
34	187	150	112
36	186	149	111
38	184	147	110
40	182	146	109
45	179	143	107
50	175	140	105
55	171	137	102
60	160	128	96
65	150	120	90

From Jopling RJ: *Pediatr Rev* 10:141, 1988.
*These numbers are taken from a variety of sources and are suggested guidelines initially developed for training athletes. Individuals will vary. If the target heart rate seems too hard to maintain, a lower one should be accepted; conversely, if the target heart rate does not seem high enough to produce a sweat, the individual should work harder.

a safe workout by allowing muscles, joints, and the cardiovascular system to adapt to the changes of exercise. The optimal times to stretch, and thereby to help maintain flexibility, are just after the warm-up and cool-down periods.

When talking about intensity, the pediatrician should discuss overuse syndromes and well-meaning adults who put undue pressure on children. Exercising to the point of pain should be discouraged because it eventually leads to injury and can exacerbate a previous chronic injury. It is important to emphasize that "slow but sure" most often achieves the goal when trying to make long-term changes. Before starting any type of exercise program, adults over age 40 or those who have a family history of cardiovascular disease should see their physician.

Exercising at least three times a week helps to maintain an aerobic fitness level; exercising five times a week usually ensures a change in a person's aerobic fitness level. These training guidelines are well established for adults, and although there is less documentation for children, they have been applied to children as young as age 6. Most people need a commitment of at least 6 months to any exercise program (and some more than 12 months) to see any significant changes in the parameters of their health-related fitness. The reverse also is true in that the positive changes gained from physical activity are lost if the activity is not maintained. Some of the benefits and risks of physical activity are presented in Table 21-2.[29]

Numerous activities can qualify as aerobic (Box 21-2). Brisk walking deserves special mention because it is an aerobic activity that can be done by almost everyone right from the beginning of any fitness program. Few exercises enable a family to exercise as a unit and at the same time allow all of the members to achieve an aerobic intensity level, but walking at a brisk pace usually can be done at the same time by all, or at least by most, family members. It can be done around the neighborhood for convenience or as a hike for

Table 21-2 Benefits and Risks of Physical Activity

System and Benefit	Surety Rating*	Risk	Surety Rating
Cardiovascular			
Blood pressure	2+	Cardiac arrest	2+
Improved serum lipid profile	1+		
Smoking cessation/prevention	0+		
Weight control	2+		
Independent effect	2+		
Psychological			
Improved affect	1+	Exercise addiction	1+
Increased self-esteem	2+		
Positive personality change	0		
Improved cognition	0		
Musculoskeletal: Prevention of postmenopausal bone loss	2+	Amenorrhea/bone loss	2+
		Trauma	2+
Central nervous system: Improved sleep	0		
Endocrine: Decreased risk of type II diabetes	0	Decreased libido	0
Gastrointestinal tract: Increased colonic motility	0	Diarrhea	1+

From Phelps JR: *West J Med* 146:200, 1987.
*The surety rating is derived from a review of the literature and is a subjective judgment of Dr. Phelps. The ratings indicate: *0*, the current literature presents mixed data claiming benefit or risk; *1+*, most but not all data in the literature support the claim; *2+*, data in the current literature establish the benefit or risk.

BOX 21-2

SUGGESTIONS FOR FITNESS ACTIVITIES*

Brisk walking
Cycling
Swimming
Aerobic exercise class
Dancing
Basketball
Tumbling
Skating
Playground activities
Cross-country skiing
Racquet sports
Jogging
Hiking
Soccer
Jumping rope
Strength training
Volleyball
Stretching
Martial arts
Tag games
Other ______________

NOTE: Stretch before and after every activity. For a more balanced fitness program, include activities for stomach muscles (modified sit-ups) and upper body muscles (push-ups/pull-ups).

From the Governor's Family FUN Award Program, Utah Governor's Council on Health and Physical Fitness, Salt Lake City, Utah.
*Minimum of 30 minutes daily.

variation. If inclement weather is a problem, one can walk inside a shopping mall or a gym.[15]

Jump ropes, stationary bicycles, cross-country ski machines, and rowing machines are reasonable investments to ensure a family access to aerobic exercise day or night year round. With a little insistence, one of these activities could replace snacking as the activity that accompanies TV viewing most frequently.[15]

LARGE-MUSCLE STRENGTH AND ENDURANCE

Large-muscle strength and endurance are related to aerobic exercise in two ways: large-muscle groups usually are the ones used in aerobic activities, and repetition of the large-muscle relaxation-contraction cycle for a sufficient length of time increases the mitochondrial mass of the muscle tissue and thus increases the amount of aerobic enzymes per unit of tissue mass. Muscle contraction tends to occlude local circulation when the muscle is contracting at greater than 30% of its maximum capacity. As muscles become stronger, they can perform more work before interfering with local circulation and therefore stay aerobic longer whether performing intense exercise or everyday activities.

Abdominal muscles help in proper breathing and protect the lower back muscles. The safest way to strengthen the abdominal muscles is to increase gradually the number of modified sit-ups one can do. Modified sit-ups are done with the knees flexed and the feet on the floor or with the lower legs resting on the seat of a chair. The lumbar spine is kept in contact with the floor during the sit-up (Fig. 21-1).

Upper body strength also is important because it is helpful in everyday activities and balances the person's overall fitness. Push-ups, modified push-ups, pull-ups, or flexed arm hangs are easy ways to improve upper body strength (see Fig. 21-1). If free weights or weight machines are used to strengthen muscles, relatively low weights and a high number of repetitions (20 or more) are recommended for health-related fitness because this regimen will develop muscle endurance strength rather than muscle bulk.

FLEXIBILITY

Flexibility helps prevent musculoskeletal injuries and makes a person feel more spry. Stretching at the end of the warm-up period can help prevent injury during exercise; stretching at the end of the cool-down period can help prevent muscles from tightening after exercise, which reduces flexibility and increases muscle soreness.

Static stretching involves stretching a muscle group to the point at which a sense of tightness first is felt, holding the stretch for 20 to 30 seconds, and then releasing the stretch. This is repeated several times for each muscle group being stretched. Ballistic stretching, which involves bouncing during the stretch, can be dangerous because it can lead to muscle or tendon damage.

The book *Stretching* by Bob Anderson (Shelter Publications, Bolinas, California) is an excellent resource for information about stretching. Its many illustrations of the techniques for everyday stretches and sports-specific stretches can be referred to for patient education. Fig. 21-2 shows some examples of everyday stretches.

BODY COMPOSITION

Before any health-related fitness program is started, the percentage of body fat should be measured or the BMI calculated, and these values should be rechecked regularly to help assess progress. Determining body composition is a more accurate reflection of health-related fitness than is using weight or weight-to-height percentile comparisons. The weight and height percentile comparisons of growth charts do not take body habitus into consideration. A muscular or large-framed person who has a low percentage of body fat may have a weight percentile greater than his or her height percentile.

When first starting a fitness program, a person actually may gain weight, although the percentage of body fat will be the same or even lower. This phenomenon is explained by muscle being denser than fat; therefore, as a person starts to exercise, muscle may be added faster than fat is lost, which would make for an overall weight gain. This seems to be especially true for individuals who are not very active before starting an exercise program.

Hydrostatic (underwater) weighing is considered the most accurate way to measure body composition; it has a 1% to 3% error factor. It also is the most inconvenient method. Using skin calipers is much more convenient and with practice can approach a 3% to 5% error factor. Methods using laser techniques are becoming more reliable and in time may become the most commonly used method of measuring the percentage of body fat. Whatever method is used, the final numbers are most helpful when comparing a person's progress over time, much as growth charts or blood pressure charts are used to follow a particular patient's trend over 6 months or longer.

The BMI is based on the calculation of kilograms per meter squared.[11] This number is plotted on a percentile graph based on the person's age and gender and compared with figures for others of the same age and gender (Table 21-3, Figs. 21-3 and 21-4). The BMI is recommended when hydrostatic or skin caliper methods are not available for the determination of the percentage of body fat.

When skin calipers are used, the more skin sites measured, the more accurate the final determination of percentage of body fat. The triceps and calf are the sites most often used by school systems when mass testing is done and for that reason should be used if only two sites are selected. The proper techniques for using skin calipers can be found in many references. Fig. 21-5 presents a graph of suggested ranges for the body fat percentage of the triceps and calf sites. Percentile graphs for age and gender for triceps and subscapular measurements were determined a number of years ago in England.[44]

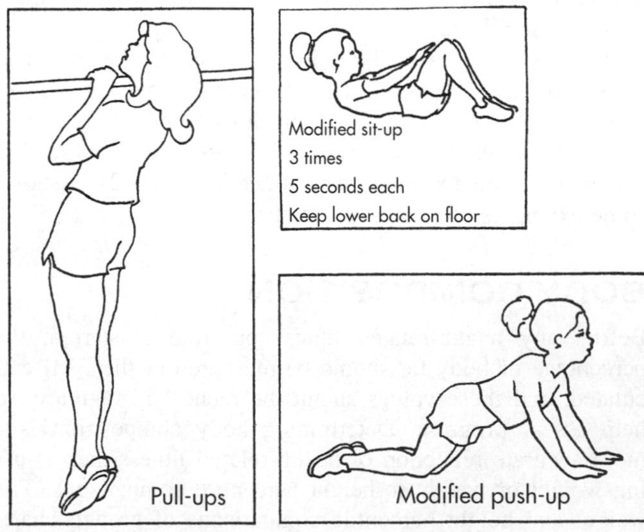
Modified sit-up
3 times
5 seconds each
Keep lower back on floor
Pull-ups
Modified push-up

Fig. 21-1 Suggested exercises to increase muscular strength.

(From "Youth Fitness," an educational handout from Ross Laboratories.)

HEALTHY DIET

Sustaining weight loss and improving health-related fitness parameters are difficult if not impossible without making use of a proper diet as well as routine exercise.[3] It would seem logical that to lose weight, a person must make sure that the total caloric intake for one day is less than the total caloric output for that day. However, it must be emphasized that crash diets and ketogenic diets are essentially starvation diets and are impossible to sustain and usually lead to the person going back to overeating and poor dietary choices. This cycle usually is attempted repeatedly and hence the term *yo-yo diet*. This cycle leads to loss of muscle tissue while sparing fat tissue.

Proper dietary recommendations are fairly simple. Unfortunately, fewer than 40% of children 2 to 19 years of age met the U.S. Department of Agriculture's recommendations for dietary intake.[26] For growing children and adolescents, a safe and practical starting point is to worry less about total calories and more about total dietary fat. Simply following the proportions and servings of the Food Guide Pyramid is a good recommendation for most patients. Table 21-4 shows the total number of calories recommended per day in relation to age in years. It has been shown that even when the total number of calories remains unchanged, eating the largest meal of the day at breakfast instead of at night helps people lose weight. Other dietary recommendations include increasing dietary fiber, reducing the use of salt in the diet, and increasing daily water intake. Some specific suggestions for improving dietary habits are listed in Box 21-3 and in Fig. 21-6.

Carbohydrates should be the main source of calories. Current recommendations for carbohydrates in relation to total daily calories range from 55% to 70%. Complex carbohydrates, such as those found in fruits, vegetables, legumes, and whole-grain cereals, are preferable to the refined carbohydrates found in candy.

For adults and for children over age 2 years, it is recommended that no more than 30% of total daily calories come from fats, with vegetable fats (except palm oil and coconut oil) recommended over animal fats.[20] How much fat is appropriate for the diet of a child younger than 2 years of age is still controversial. The American Academy of Pediatrics (AAP) currently recommends 30% to 40% to ensure adequate fat for myelinization of the nervous system.[27] Although most dietary recommendations start after age 5 years, some experts believe that as early as 2 years of age is an appropriate time to begin to expand children's taste experience to foods lower in fat. When fat is removed from the diet, energy levels fall; therefore, moderation in fat reduction is important for children. The AAP recommendation of whole milk from 1 to 2 years of age, 2% milk from 2 to 5 years of age, and skim milk after 5 years of age is enough to make a significant difference in the amount of fat in most children's diet.[28] All age groups would do well to be given low-fat luncheon meats.[38] (For a detailed review of the role of dietary cholesterol in cardiovascular disease, refer to Kwiterovich.[19])

Protein should make up the remaining 15% to 20% of the total daily caloric intake. Fish and poultry, because they have a lower percentage of fat than many cuts of beef and pork, are considered safer from a cardiovascular standpoint.

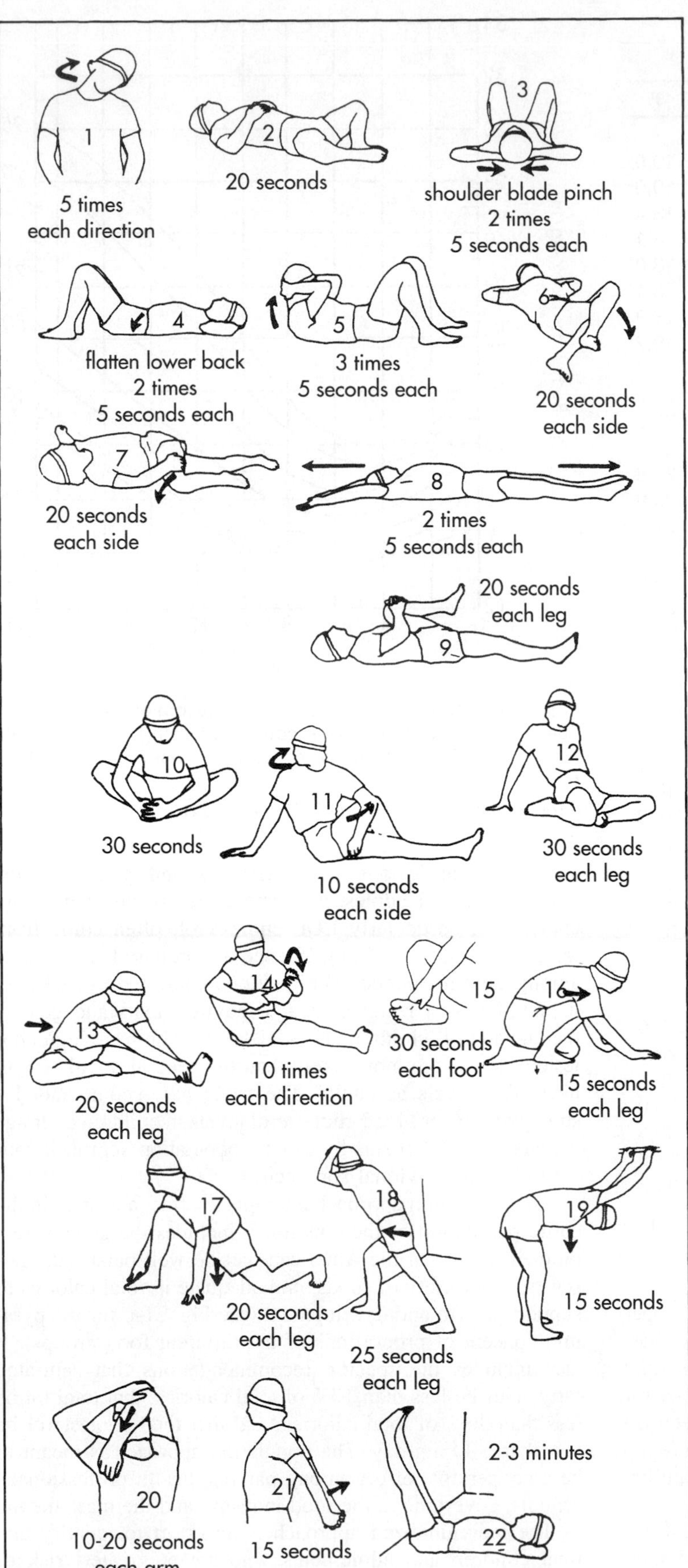

Fig. 21-2 Everyday stretches—approximately 10 to 15 minutes. These stretches should be done every day to fine-tune the muscles. This is a general routine that emphasizes stretching and relaxing the muscles used more frequently during normal day-to-day activities. In simple tasks of everyday living, the body often is used in strained or awkward ways, creating stress and tension. A kind of muscular rigor mortis sets in. Setting aside 10 to 15 minutes every day for stretching will offset this accumulated tension so that the body can be used with greater ease.

(From Anderson B: *Stretching,* Bolinas, Calif, 1980, Shelter Publications [Random House].)

Table 21-3 Percentile Values of Body Mass Index*

Age (yr)	5	10	25	50	75	90	95
Males							
1	14.6	15.4	16.1	17.2	18.5	19.4	19.9
2	14.4	15.0	15.7	16.5	17.0	18.4	19.0
3	14.0	14.6	15.3	16.0	17.0	17.8	18.4
4	13.8	14.4	15.0	15.8	16.6	17.5	18.1
5	13.7	14.2	14.9	15.5	16.3	17.3	18.0
6	13.6	14.0	14.7	15.4	16.3	17.4	18.1
7	13.6	14.0	14.7	15.5	16.5	17.7	18.9
8	13.7	14.1	14.9	15.7	17.0	18.4	19.7
9	14.0	14.3	15.1	16.0	17.6	19.3	20.9
10	14.2	14.6	15.5	16.6	18.4	20.3	22.2
11	14.6	15.0	16.0	17.2	19.2	21.3	23.5
12	15.1	15.5	16.5	17.8	20.0	22.3	24.8
13	15.6	16.0	17.1	18.4	20.8	23.3	25.8
14	16.1	16.6	17.7	19.1	21.5	24.4	26.8
15	16.6	17.1	18.4	19.7	22.2	25.4	27.7
16	17.2	17.8	19.1	20.5	22.9	26.1	28.4
17	17.7	18.4	19.7	21.2	23.4	27.0	29.0
18	18.3	19.1	20.3	21.9	24.0	27.7	29.7
19	19.0	19.7	21.1	22.5	24.4	28.3	30.1
Females							
1	14.7	15.0	15.8	16.6	17.6	18.6	19.3
2	14.3	14.7	15.3	16.0	17.1	18.0	18.7
3	13.9	14.4	14.9	15.6	16.7	17.6	18.3
4	13.6	14.1	14.7	15.4	16.5	17.5	18.2
5	13.5	14.0	14.6	15.3	16.3	17.5	18.3
6	13.3	13.9	14.6	15.3	16.4	17.7	18.8
7	13.4	14.0	14.7	15.5	16.7	18.5	19.7
8	13.6	14.2	15.0	16.0	17.2	19.4	21.0
9	14.0	14.5	15.5	16.6	18.0	20.8	22.7
10	14.3	15.0	15.9	17.1	19.0	21.8	24.2
11	14.6	15.3	16.2	17.8	19.8	23.0	25.7
12	15.0	15.6	16.7	18.3	20.4	23.7	26.8
13	15.4	16.0	17.1	18.9	21.2	24.7	27.9
14	15.7	16.4	17.5	19.4	21.8	25.3	28.6
15	16.1	16.8	18.0	19.9	22.4	26.0	29.4
16	16.4	17.1	18.4	20.2	22.8	26.5	30.0
17	16.9	17.6	18.9	20.7	23.3	27.1	30.5
18	17.2	18.0	19.4	21.1	23.7	27.4	31.0
19	17.5	18.4	19.8	21.4	24.0	27.7	31.3

(Columns 5–95 are under the spanning header "Percentile".)

*National Health and Nutrition Examination Survey, 1971 to 1974 (NHANES I).

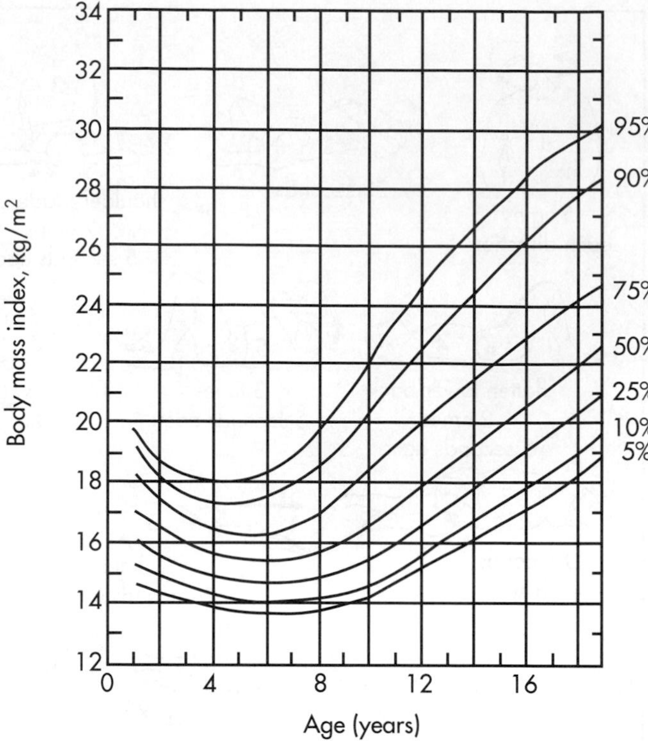

Fig. 21-3 Body mass index for white males ages 1 to 19 years. The percentiles were computed using data from the First National Health and Nutrition Examination Survey, 1971 to 1974.

(From Hammer LD, et al: *Am J Dis Child* 145:259, 1991.)

A new concept in understanding and following proper nutrition has been presented in the books *Nutripoints* (Vartabedian and Matthews) and *The New American Diet* (Conners and Conners). These are two excellent books for families seeking a more extensive reference on diet (see Suggested Readings). Recommending the counsel of a registered dietitian is important in some cases, such as familial hyperlipidemia.

In 1991, the Report of the Expert Panel on Blood Cholesterol Levels in Children and Adolescents[27] stated that: (1) high levels of serum total cholesterol, low-density lipoprotein (LDL) cholesterol, very-low-density lipoprotein (VLDL) cholesterol, and low levels of high-density lipoprotein (HDL) cholesterol are linked to the extent of early atherosclerotic lesions in adolescents and young adults; (2) children and adolescents who have an elevated serum cholesterol, particularly LDL cholesterol, often come from families that have a high incidence of coronary heart disease among adult members; (3) high blood cholesterol aggregates in families as a result of shared environments and genetic factors; and (4) children and adolescents who have high cholesterol levels are more likely than the general population to have high levels as adults. The panel has recommended a strategy to lower blood cholesterol levels in children over age 2 years and adolescents by using a population approach coupled with an individual approach.

The population approach attempts to effect a change in the entire population of the country. It includes the general recommendation that the American diet be well balanced, chosen from a variety of foods, and adequate in total calories to support growth and development (see Fig. 21-6 for the pyramid concept of proportions of the different food groups). It also includes the specific recommendations that saturated fatty acids be less than 10% of total calories, that total fat be less than 30% of total calories, and that total cholesterol be less than 300 mg/day. The population approach is meant to be a cooperative effort among parents, health professionals, schools, government, the food industry, and the mass media.

The individualized approach is an effort to identify and treat children and adolescents who are at greatest risk of having high serum cholesterol as adults and at subsequent risk of coronary heart disease. The panel recommends using a family history of high serum cholesterol as the basis for obtaining a serum cholesterol value for people under age

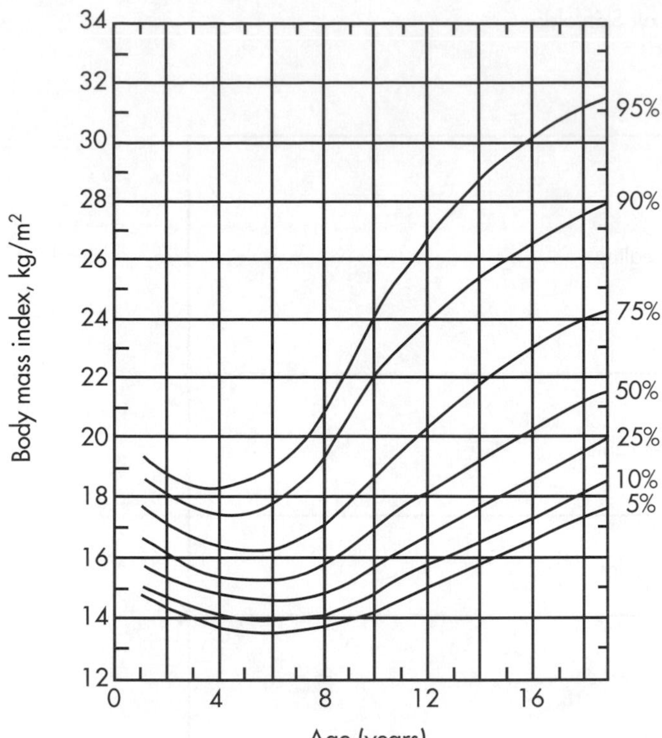

Fig. 21-4 Body mass index for white females ages 1 to 19 years. The percentiles were computed using data from the First National Health and Nutrition Examination Survey, 1971 to 1974.

(From Hammer LD, et al: *Am J Dis Child* 145:259, 1991.)

20 years. Specifically, the panel suggests screening of children and adolescents whose parents or grandparents, at age 55 or younger, underwent diagnostic coronary arteriography and were found to have atherosclerosis. The panel also suggests screening a child or adolescent if (1) the parents or grandparents, at age 55 or younger, suffered a documented myocardial infarction, angina pectoris, peripheral vascular disease, cerebrovascular disease, or sudden cardiac death, and (2) one parent has had a blood cholesterol level of 240 mg/dl or higher. Finally, the panel suggests screening when the family history is unknown, particularly if other risk factors are present. For individuals older than age 20 years, obtaining a baseline serum cholesterol level is recommended, followed by repeat serum cholesterol determinations every 5 years.

Potential for error exists in this screening format,[9,31,46] which has led some to propose mass screening, beginning as early as age 2 years. However, mass screening also has several potential problems[12]:

1. The tracking of individuals from children who have high cholesterol levels to adults who have high cholesterol levels has enough variation to make exact prediction for any one person more difficult than expected.
2. Overzealous use of low-fat diets and cholesterol-lowering drugs can have significant side effects.
3. Serious psychological consequences may result in children labeled "at risk" for an early death.
4. "Labeling" can affect insurability and employment opportunities.

STRESS MANAGEMENT/ COMMUNICATION SKILLS

The psychological components of a healthy lifestyle actually are fairly familiar topics to pediatricians. They have been presenting aspects of stress management, behavior modification, and improved communication skills for years when they discuss a wide variety of anticipatory guidance topics with parents and patients.

Stress management is incorporated because many of the diseases targeted for prevention are related to psychological stress. Common examples of stress management techniques include deep breathing, ascending muscle relaxation, body awareness, positive mental imagery, meditation, priority setting, time management, and even the simple body stretches mentioned earlier. Examples of family activities that can aid in stress management are listed in Box 21-4. The book *Handbook of Stress: Theoretical and Clinical Aspects* (see Goldberger and Breznitz under Suggested Readings) is an extensive reference on stress management.

COMPLIANCE

The most important factor in the ultimate success or failure of all lifestyle changes is compliance; compliance is the basis of success or failure in any effort at prevention or intervention by medical care providers. The keys to compliance are multiple. The first is gaining knowledge of a new concept through education by the medical provider. Next, the patient must be persuaded of the concept's importance by gaining a positive attitude toward the new concept. The implementation of the new concept begins through methods suggested by the medical provider. Finally, the motivation to adopt the new concept on a long-term basis comes through repeated reinforcement and tracking of the new behavior.[23,24,34] The first step is to establish rapport by listening carefully as the concerns of the patient and family are discussed. Involvement of the patient and parents should be elicited by developing a plan based on the common understanding of the issues of the visit. The plan is implemented by offering the family opportunities to learn new behaviors, develop new experiences, and modify their environment.[14] Realistic goals should be set that are achievable by incremental change. The plan is evaluated by identifying strategies for tracking the patient's progress. Teaching the patient (when possible), and the family about the problem may be motivation enough for starting a change in lifestyle. Long-term compliance, however, is more difficult. The physical and mental benefits of the program may provide a self-sustaining motivation, as they become noticeable. It is during the gap between starting a program and reaching a point at which the benefits are tangible (as early as the third month or as late as the twelfth month) that the dropout rate is greatest. The average dropout rate in the first 6 to 12 months of starting a fitness program frequently is 50% or higher.[39] As was stated earlier, the beneficial changes achieved through any health-related fitness program are not sustained if the program is discontinued; this is why it is important that the family comprehend the concept of a lifestyle change.

Many factors have been studied in efforts to solve the compliance problem. Some of the important findings in an adult survey included scheduling of the time, accessibility to

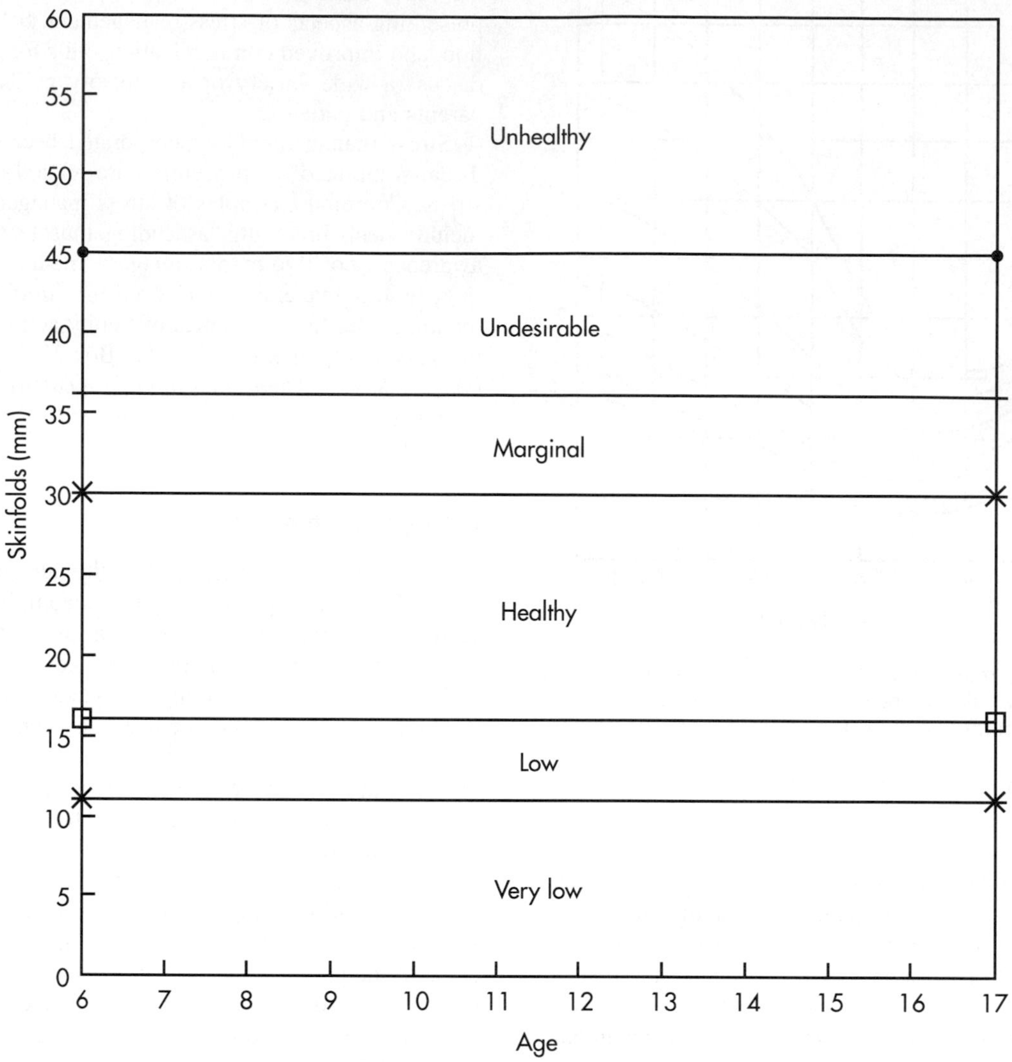

Fig. 21-5 Skinfold measurement ranges for the triceps and calf combination.

(Modified from Lohman TG: Appraising and monitoring body composition. In Eisenman PA, Johnson SC, Benson JE, editors: *Coaches' guide to nutrition and weight control,* Salt Lake City, 1990, Human Kinetics Publishers.)

Continued

facilities, weather, time of year, and an interested friend or family member.[37] In a survey of children and adolescents with diabetes who participated in an exercise program, the most important factors involved with compliance were enthusiastic leadership, individual attention, and parental support.[35] It also has been shown that children of physically active parents are more physically active themselves.[25] A study on the prevention of progression to severe obesity by use of family therapy showed some effectiveness when the program was started in childhood (before age 11 years).[8] Therefore, the help of a motivated and involved adult is essential for children to acquire positive lifestyle habits. That role is most likely to be filled by one or both parents. The next most likely individual may be a teacher or organization leader (Scouts, YMCA/YWCA, or church).

A study of previously sedentary adults showed that subjects who exercised at home were more likely to achieve long-term compliance than those who attended exercise classes if both groups received the benefit of planning and encouragement from experts.[16] The same study showed that the home-based group tended toward moderation in intensity. Two thoughts arise from that study. One is that the convenience of home is certainly important; the second is that many people may not stay with an exercise program because either they themselves or well-meaning trainers push them too hard.

By instructing the patient and family to keep a daily log of all areas of lifestyle changes and to return with the log in 1 month, the physician can provide an incentive to comply and a basis for discussion at the follow-up visit. For example, if one day the patient walked for 30 minutes, participated in a family meeting, and had broiled skinless chicken (instead of hamburgers) for one of the day's meals, that person could write the following on his or her individual calendar: *F* (for

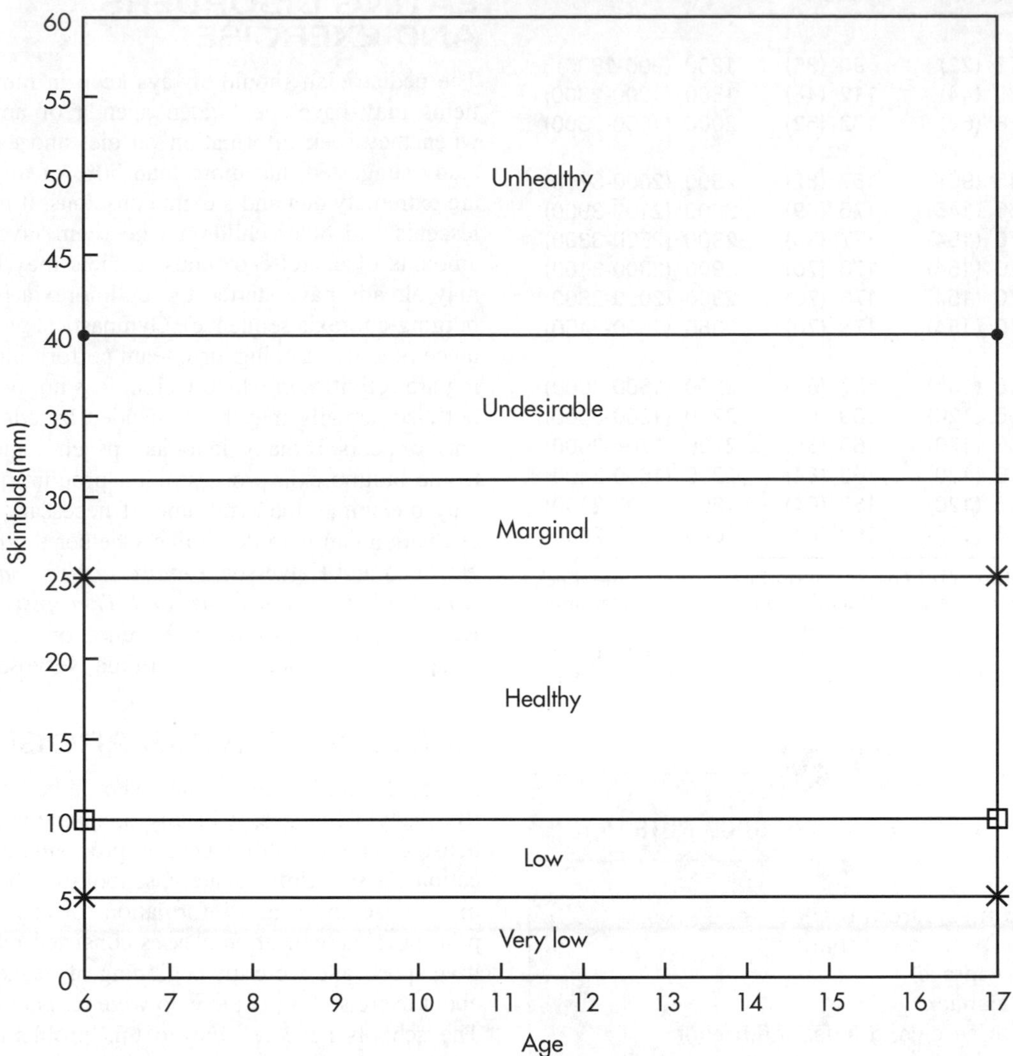

Fig. 21-5, cont'd For legend see opposite page.

fitness): walked 30 minutes; *U* (for unity, or family communication): had a family meeting; *N* (for nutrition): ate broiled skinless chicken. Everyone needs motivation and encouragement to stay with any lifestyle change, and one of the keys to achieving this is to make the process fun. This is important for adults, but it is critical for children. Spelling out FUN on the calendar helps reinforce the importance of making the program enjoyable.

Use of age- and time-appropriate rewards is essential. For example, the family could go out for frozen yogurt (instead of ice cream) if one week's goal is met; each family member could buy a desired article of clothing if one month's goal is met; and a family vacation to a favorite spot could be the reward if a 6- or 12-month goal is met. Each family member should be allowed to help decide what reward is important for him or her.

Varying the selection of exercise activities makes for a more interesting exercise program and helps prevent overuse injuries, both of which will aid in compliance. For example, one could walk twice a week, ride a stationary bike twice a week, and play games at the park as part of a family outing once a week.

For many individuals as well as families, lack of time to begin or maintain a fitness program is a major obstacle. A good starting point is to divide the day into 30-minute increments, then make the program a priority to be worked into one of those increments. Specific suggestions for getting in the desired exercise time include getting up 30 minutes earlier in the morning, taking 30 minutes of the lunch break, or allotting 30 minutes after dinner. It now is evident that even three 10-minute episodes of activity over the day may be as beneficial from a health standpoint as one 30-minute activity.

It obviously would behoove the pediatrician to be familiar with antismoking techniques and strategies.[13] Evidence shows that pediatricians are the physicians most commonly in touch with adolescents and are among the most likely to be able to help convince the adolescent of the importance of smoking cessation. One of the best windows of opportunity

Table 21-4 Recommended Total Daily Calories* (Moderate Activity Level)

Group and Age (yr)	Weight (kg [lb])	Height (cm [in])	Energy Needs (kcal [range])
Children			
1-3	13 (29)	90 (35)	1300 (900-1800)
4-6	20 (44)	112 (44)	1800 (1300-2300)
7-10	28 (62)	132 (52)	2000 (1650-3300)
Males			
11-14	45 (99)	157 (62)	2500 (2000-3700)
15-18	66 (145)	176 (69)	3000 (2100-3900)
19-22	70 (154)	177 (70)	2900 (2500-3300)
23-50	70 (154)	178 (70)	2900 (2300-3100)
51-75	70 (154)	178 (70)	2300 (2000-2800)
76+	70 (154)	178 (70)	2050 (1650-2450)
Females			
11-14	46 (101)	157 (62)	2200 (1500-3000)
15-18	55 (120)	163 (64)	2200 (1200-3000)
19-22	55 (120)	163 (64)	2200 (1700-2500)
23-50	55 (120)	163 (64)	2200 (1600-2400)
51-75	55 (120)	163 (64)	1900 (1400-2200)
76+	55 (120)	163 (64)	1600 (1200-2000)

Modified from the Food and Nutrition Board: *Recommended Dietary Allowances,* ed 10, Washington, DC, 1989, National Academy of Sciences, National Research Council.
*These recommendations may vary significantly up or down for specific sports and for very active children and adolescents.

BOX 21-3

SUGGESTIONS FOR PRACTICING GOOD NUTRITION

Develop a weekly meal plan
Eat balanced meals from the four food groups
Bake, boil, or broil rather than fry
Reduce sugar intake
Eat fruit for a snack
Use high-fiber cereals, grains, and breads
Use low-fat dairy products
Eat more chicken and fish
Eat low-fat meals
Cut use of butter and gravies in half
Do not add salt to food
Do not add sugar to food
Eat more raw and fresh fruits and vegetables
Drink more water
Place a copy of the Food Guide Pyramid on the refrigerator door for visual reinforcement of good nutrition

Modified from the Governor's Family FUN Award Program, Utah Governor's Council on Health and Physical Fitness, Salt Lake City, Utah.

for pediatricians to help any parent who smokes is when the child has just been diagnosed with any illness that is made worse by passive inhalation of smoke. Although a very recalcitrant problem, the best chance for success lies in a combination approach of behavior modification and pharmacotherapy. The basic classifications of over-the-counter and prescription medications include various dosages of nicotine in transdermal patches, chewing gums, nasal spray, or oral inhaler, and bupropion in oral tablets.

EATING DISORDERS AND EXERCISE

The pediatrician should always keep in mind that some patients may have the hidden agenda of an eating disorder when they seek information on diet and exercise. A recent study suggested that more than 50% of all adolescent girls are extremely diet and weight conscious, if not phobic.[5] Adolescents and older children who seem involved in unusual amounts of exercise or unusual diets may be at risk for or may already have started the bulimorexia process (bulimia-purging-anorexia sequence). Gymnastics, wrestling, long distance running, dancing, drill team performing, and cheerleading are activities in which weight loss not only is encouraged but also actually may be demanded by adult sponsors, parents, or peers. If the patient has a psychological susceptibility to the bulimorexia process, adult prodding or peer pressure may precipitate the syndrome. If necessary, a psychological evaluation can help determine whether the patient is at risk. Newman and Halverson's *Anorexia Nervosa and Bulimia: A Handbook for Counselors and Therapists* (see Suggested Readings) is an extensive reference on this topic (see also Chapter 102, Anorexia and Bulimia Nervosa).

SPECIFIC FITNESS PROGRAMS

Although health-related fitness should be based first on family lifestyle changes, it ideally is supplemented by comprehensive school health education programs and physical education classes. Unfortunately, school may be the only source of exercise and health information for any one child. In the past, physical education classes consisted mainly of competitive sports and were the beginning of negative connotations about exercise for people who were less athletically inclined. The schools have recognized this problem and have been making efforts to emphasize enjoyable "lifetime" physical activities for all children.

Totally new ideas are needed from schools and the community at large. Schools could sponsor physical activities and/or study halls during the after-school period before most parents get home, which may help prevent latchkey children from developing the problem behaviors that have been described in this group.[32] (See Chapter 66, Latchkey Children: Children in Self-Care.) Sports programs for young people can accomplish the same goal and should be supported by the community.

Health-related fitness programs for schools and families already are available in a variety of forms. Box 21-5 lists some of these programs, as well as addresses for obtaining further information. This list is not meant to be all encompassing, nor is it necessarily an endorsement of the programs mentioned.

The concept of comprehensive health education deserves special mention. Some programs in various parts of the country address all the factors mentioned earlier, as well as topics such as sex education, drug abuse education, and decision-making skills, all packaged for grades K through 12. To help

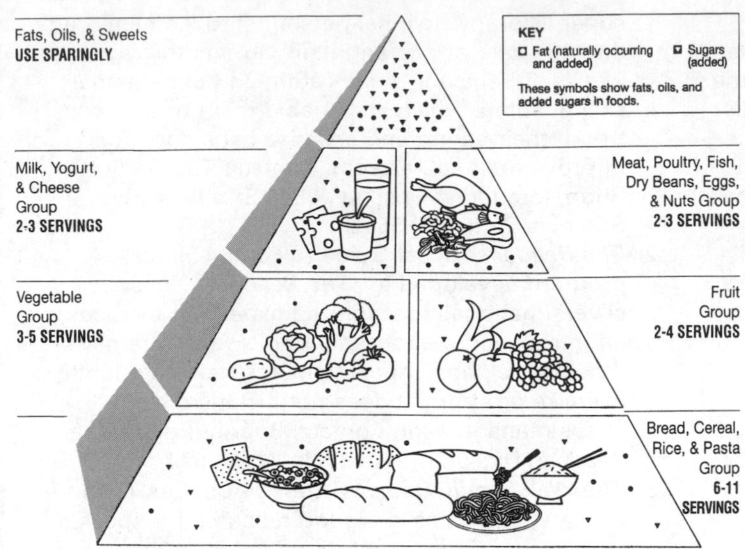

Fig. 21-6 The U.S. Department of Agriculture's Food Guide Pyramid emphasizes foods from the five food groups shown in the three lower sections of the pyramid. Each of these food groups provides some, but not all, of the nutrients a body needs. Foods in one group cannot replace those in another, and no one food group is more important than any other.

BOX 21-4

SUGGESTED FAMILY ACTIVITIES FOR STRESS MANAGEMENT

Keep a family calendar
Keep a family job list
Hold a family meeting
Have a family game night
Attend a health fair
Read together
Keep a stress diary
Get involved in service projects
Set aside meditation and quiet time
Prepare a meal together
Keep a journal
Engage in family outdoor adventures
Have a family picnic
Get adequate sleep
Cut television time in half
Discuss family budgeting
Attend cultural events
Play new games together

Modified from the Governor's Family FUN Award Program, Utah Governor's Council on Health and Physical Fitness, Salt Lake City, Utah.

local school boards implement comprehensive school health programs in their districts, the National School Boards Association has established a Comprehensive School Health Programs Database. It identifies districts that have health education issues similar to those of districts seeking program models. See Box 21-5 for more information and an address for the database.

OPPORTUNITIES FOR DISCUSSING HEALTH-RELATED FITNESS

One of the best times to broach the topic of health-related fitness is a consultation for a specific problem (e.g., obesity, reactive airway disease). At these times the parent and/or patient may be especially receptive to specific therapeutic or preventive measures.[41,42] Obesity is especially difficult to treat without the team approach, which usually is offered through various hospitals and private clinics. Preventive health care visits such as well-child checkups, camp physicals, and sports preparticipation physicals are some of the other physician visits that promote discussion of this topic. The kindergarten checkup often is the last time a pediatrician can count on seeing a patient for a preventive health care visit, and it probably is the earliest age at which a program that includes exercise recommendations can be introduced. Thus, it should be considered as a time to discuss a healthy lifestyle.

Height, weight, and blood pressure measurements can be obtained easily and can be plotted on an age- and gender-appropriate graph before the patient sees the pediatrician on any of the above-mentioned visits. BMI or skin caliper measurements can be determined with relative ease and proficiency by the nurse or examining physician. This information then can be compared with age- and gender-appropriate graphs to be used as a baseline for future reference and can serve as the basis for introducing this topic to the patient and parents.

The pediatrician usually cannot impart all the information needed to begin changing a family's lifestyle in the 20 or 30 minutes generally allotted for preventive health care visits. It is important to remember to introduce the topics of discussion personally by quickly going over the major points already listed in a brochure that the patient or parent can take home, to make specific suggestions to get the family started, and to set up a follow-up visit for 2 to 4 weeks later. At the

BOX 21-5

EXAMPLES OF HEALTH-RELATED FITNESS PROGRAMS

School Programs

1. The Comprehensive School Health Programs Database. An information source and a network, the database contains information on 150 school districts that have at least one of the elements of a comprehensive school health program and that are actively working on additional elements. The database can provide information on which districts have particular program elements, as well as statistics on the characteristics of each district and the staffing of the health program. It also provides the names of people in the programs to contact. For the database, contact: Comprehensive School Health Programs Project, National School Boards Association, 1680 Duke St., Alexandria, VA 22314; telephone: 1-703-838-6717.
2. "Feeling Good". A program that appears to be the most extensive in depth (it covers all the areas mentioned in this chapter and more) and in breadth (books are available for children from kindergarten through high school, for parents, and for administrators). The emphasis in the exercise segment is on noncompetitive cardiovascular movement through "fun" games. A "homework" section helps to get families involved. Contact: Charles T. Kuntzleman, Ph.D., Fitness Finders, 133 Teft Road, Spring Arbor, MI 49283.
3. "Know Your Body". A plan developed as a school-based program that focuses on teaching decision-making skills in the areas of nutrition, exercise, and preventing smoking. The program has been used in all socioeconomic settings. Contact: The American Health Foundation, 320 East 43rd St., New York, NY 10017.
4. "Growing Healthy". A comprehensive school-based program that covers many areas, including exercise and nutrition. Contact: The National Center for Health, 30 East 20th St., New York, NY 10016.

Personal and Family Programs

1. The Body Shop. A program originally developed at a hospital in Minnesota and now marketed to other hospitals. It calls for intense, direct adult supervision by hospital personnel to lead children 8 to 18 years of age and their parents through 10 weeks of behavior modification and experiential skill building, which will enable them to take control of their eating and exercise behaviors and to improve their self-esteem. Contact: The Body Shop, Methodist Hospital, 6500 Excelsior Blvd., St. Louis Park, MN 55426.
2. *The Reader's Digest* Guide to Family Fitness. A program developed for *The Reader's Digest* by several nationally recognized experts. It includes an introduction, information on testing a family's fitness level, and suggestions for starting a family exercise program. It does not include diet or stress management. Contact: Reprint Editor, The Reader's Digest, Pleasantville, NY 10570.
3. *The Well Family Book.* Written by Charles T. Kuntzleman, Ph.D., this is a good resource for specific examples of fitness, nutrition, and stress management for families. Contact: Here's Life Publishers, P.O. Box 1576, San Bernardino, CA 92402.
4. "Shapedown." A weight-loss program of diet and exercise that uses behavior modification techniques and is available in versions for three age groups—6 to 8, 9 to 12, and 13 to 18. The program includes a 200-page section for parents, "Guide to Supporting Your Child," which is based on setting weekly goals. This program is offered at approximately 400 medical centers, health maintenance organizations, and clinics in various parts of the country. The fee is $200 for a program lasting 12 to 16 weeks. Contact: Balboa Publishing; telephone: 1-415-453-8886.
5. Publications from the American Academy of Pediatrics. "Better Health Through Fitness," a brochure for teens ($20/100 copies), and *Sports Medicine: Health Care for Young Athletes,* a comprehensive manual on physical fitness ($35 for AAP members, $40 for nonmembers), both are available from the American Academy of Pediatrics, P.O. Box 927, Elk Grove Village, IL 60009. For information on these and other AAP publications on fitness, call 1-708-981-7389.

follow-up visit, the daily log can be reviewed, measurements can be repeated, and the program can be reinforced and clarified.

Primary care physicians could try to collaborate with the local school system to create a "health-related fitness profile" for all the children in that particular school system.[43] Certainly, school-based physicians have an automatic voice with their school's administrators. The school can test the students in the areas of cardiovascular endurance capacity (1 mile run), muscle strength and endurance (flexed arm hang/pull-ups in 1 minute and sit-ups in 1 minute), and flexibility (sitting on the floor and reaching as far as possible past the feet). The child's pediatrician or school personnel could measure body composition (triceps and calf skin caliper measurements), height, weight, and blood pressure. When the child's test results are known, the child's physician, or one appointed by the school, could work with the parents and teachers to improve any one of the child's deficient areas (details on specific programs already available are given in Box 21-6).

With all the problems facing medicine today, is all of this actually important enough to take up a pediatrician's time? Can we financially afford to take all of the time that is necessary to educate our patient population, to fight for insur-

BOX 21-6

SPECIFIC PROGRAMS FOR DEVELOPING A HEALTH-RELATED FITNESS PROFILE*

1. Physical Best program of the American Alliance for Health, Physical Education, Recreation and Dance (AAHPERD), 1900 Association Drive, Reston, VA 22091.
2. President's Physical Fitness Award Program of the President's Council on Physical Fitness and Sports, Washington, DC 20001.
3. The Fitness Gram of the Institute for Aerobics Research, the Aerobics Center, 12330 Preston Road, Dallas, TX 75230.

*These programs apply national standards according to age and gender.

ance reimbursement, and to encourage schools to include this topic in their curriculum? Some believe that the answers await longitudinal studies yet to be done, but most professionals in the areas of medicine, nutrition, and exercise believe that adopting a healthy lifestyle can enhance the quality and duration of life within the framework of any one person's genetic potential for health.

REFERENCES

1. Blair SN, Kohl HW: Physical activity or physical fitness: which is more important for health? *Med Sci Sports Exerc* 20(suppl):S8, 1988.
2. Borg GAV: A category-ratio perceived exertion scale: relationship to blood and muscle lactates and heart rate, *Med Sci Sports Exerc* 15:523, 1983.
3. Brownell KD, Nelson Steen S: Modern methods for weight control: the physiology and psychology of dieting, *Physician Sports Med* 15:122, 1987.
4. Burns TL, Moll PP, Lauer RM: Increased familial cardiovascular mortality in obese schoolchildren: the Muscatine Ponderosity Family Study, *Pediatrics* 89:262, 1992.
5. Casper RC, Offer D: Weight and dieting concerns in adolescents: fashion or symptom? *Pediatrics* 86:384, 1990.
6. Consensus Conference: Lowering blood cholesterol to prevent heart disease, *JAMA* 253:2080, 1985.
7. Dunbar CC, et al: The validity of regulating exercise intensity by ratings of perceived exertion, *Med Sci Sports Exerc* 24:94, 1992.
8. Flodmark CE: Prevention of progression to severe childhood obesity in a group of obese schoolchildren treated with family therapy, *Pediatrics* 91:880, 1993.
9. Garcia RE, Moodie DS: A case for routine cholesterol surveillance in childhood, *Pediatrics* 84:751, 1989.
10. Geitmaker SL, Dietz WH: Increasing pediatric obesity in the United States, *Am J Dis Child* 141:535, 1987.
11. Hammer LD, et al: Standardized percentile curves of body mass index for children and adolescents, *Am J Dis Child* 145:259, 1991.
12. Hoekelman RA: A pediatrician's view: cholesterol mania, *Pediatr Ann* 19:229, 1990 (editorial).
13. Irons TG, Kennay RD: Let's get parents to stop smoking, *Contemp Pediatr* 3:107, 1988.
14. Jopling RJ: Health-related fitness as preventive medicine, *Pediatr Rev* 10:141, 1988.
15. Jopling RJ: Let's make fitness a family affair, *Contemp Pediatr* 4:23, 1992.
16. King AC, et al: Group- vs home-based exercise training in healthy older men and women: a community-based clinical trial, *JAMA* 266:1535, 1991.
17. Kraus H: Unfit kids: a call to action, *Contemp Pediatr* 5:18, 1988.
18. Kraus H, Hirschland RP: Minimum muscular fitness tests in schoolchildren, *Res Q* 25:178, 1954.
19. Kwiterovich PO Jr: Biochemical, clinical, epidemiologic, genetic, and pathologic data in the pediatric age group relevant to the cholesterol hypothesis, *Pediatrics* 78:349, 1986.
20. LaRosa J, Finberg L: Preliminary report from a conference titled "Prevention of adult atherosclerosis during childhood," *J Pediatr* 112:317, 1988.
21. Lauer RM, Clarke WR: Childhood risk factors for high adult blood pressure, *Pediatrics* 84:633, 1989.
22. Lipid Research Clinics Population Studies Data Book, vol 1, *The prevalence study,* US Department of Health and Human Services, National Institutes of Health Pub No 80-1527, Washington, DC, 1980, US Government Printing Office.
23. Martin AR, Coates TJ: A clinician's guide to helping patients change behavior, *West J Med* 146:751, 1987.
24. McCann DP, Blossom HJ: The physician as a patient educator: from theory to practice, *West J Med* 153:44, 1990.
25. Moore LL: Parents' physical activity levels and those of their young children, *J Pediatr* 118:215, 1991.
26. Munoz KA, et al: Food intakes of US children and adolescents compared with recommendations, *Pediatrics* 100:323, 1997.
27. National Cholesterol Education Program: Report of the Expert Panel on Blood Cholesterol Levels in Children and Adolescents, NIH Pub No 91-2732, Washington, DC, 1991, US Department of Health and Human Services.
28. Peterson S, Sigman-Grant M: Impact of adopting lower-fat food choices on nutrient intake of American children, *Pediatrics* 100:380, 1997.
29. Phelps JR: Physical activity and health maintenance: exactly what is known? *West J Med* 146:200, 1987.
30. Powell KE, et al: Physical activity and the incidence of coronary heart disease, *Annu Rev Public Health* 8:253, 1987.
31. Resnicow K, Cross D: Are parents' self-reported total cholesterol levels useful in identifying children with hyperlipidemia?: an examination of current guidelines, *Pediatrics* 92:347, 1993.
32. Richardson JL: Relationship between after-school care of adolescents and substance use, risk taking, depressed mood, and academic achievement, *Pediatrics* 92:32, 1993.
33. Rippe JM: The health benefits of exercise, *Physician Sports Med* 15: 115, 1987.
34. Rogers, EC: *Diffusion of innovations,* ed 4, New York, 1995, Free Press.
35. Rowland TW: Motivational factors in exercise training programs for children, *Physician Sports Med* 14:122, 1988.
36. Self-reported physical inactivity by degree of urbanization—United States, 1996, *MMWR* vol 47/no 50:1097, Dec. 25, 1998.
37. Shepard RJ: Motivation: the key to fitness compliance, *Physician Sports Med* 13:88, 1985.
38. Sigman-Grant M: Dietary approaches for reducing fat intake of preschool-age children, *Pediatrics* 91:955, 1993.
39. Song TK, Shepard RJ, Cox M: Absenteeism, employee turnover and sustained exercise participation, *J Sports Med Phys Fitness* 22:392, 1983.
40. Status of the 1990 physical fitness and exercise objectives, *MMWR* 34:521, 1985.
41. Strong WB: You are a preventive cardiologist: the scope of pediatric preventive cardiology, *Am J Dis Child* 143:1145, 1989.
42. Strong WB, Dennison BA: Pediatric preventive cardiology: atherosclerosis and coronary heart disease, *Pediatr Rev* 9:303, 1988.
43. Strong WB, Wilmore JH: Unfit kids: an office-based approach to physical fitness, *Contemp Pediatr* 5:33, 1988.
44. Tanner JM, Whitehouse RH: Revised standards for triceps and subscapular skinfolds in British children, *Arch Dis Child* 50:142, 1975.
45. Troiano RP, Flegal KM: Overweight children and adolescents: description, epidemiology, and demographics, *Pediatrics* 101, Part 2:497, 1998.
46. Wadowski SJ, et al: Family history of coronary artery disease and cholesterol: screening children in a disadvantaged inner city population, *Pediatrics* 93:109, 1994.
47. Webber LS, et al: Cardiovascular risk factors from birth to 7 years of age: the Bogalusa Heart Study, *Pediatrics* 80:767, 1987.

SUGGESTED READINGS

Anderson B: *Stretching,* Bolinas, Calif, 1980, Shelter Publications (Random House).

Connor SL, Connor WE: *The New American diet,* New York, 1986, Fireside Books (Simon & Schuster).

Dietz WH, Robinson TN: Assessment and treatment of childhood obesity, *Pediatr Rev* 14:337, 1993.

Dishman RK: *Exercise adherence: its impact on public health,* Champaign, Ill, 1990, Human Kinetics Publishers.

Eisenman PA, Johnson SC, Benson JE: *Coaches' guide to nutrition and weight control,* Champaign, Ill, 1990, Human Kinetics Publishers.

Fish HT, Fish RB, Golding LA: *Starting out WELL: a parents' guide to physical activity and nutrition,* Champaign, Ill, 1989, Human Kinetics Publishers.

Goldberger L, Breznitz S: *Handbook of stress: theoretical and clinical aspects,* New York, 1982, Free Press (Macmillan).

Jopling RJ: Getting families to "eat right," *Contemp Pediatr* 9:97, 1992.

Linder CW, DuRant RH: Exercise, serum lipids, and cardiovascular disease: risk factors in children, *Pediatr Clin North Am* 29:1341, 1982.

Newman P, Halverson P: *Anorexia nervosa and bulimia: a handbook for counselors and therapists,* New York, 1983, Van Nostrand Reinhold.

Rogers EM: *Diffusion of innovations,* New York, 1995, The Free Press (Simon & Schuster).

Rowland TW: *Exercise and children's health,* Champaign, Ill, 1990, Human Kinetics Publishers.

Suskind RM, Varna RN: Assessment of the nutritional status of children, *Pediatr Rev* 5:195, 1984.

Vartabedian RE, Matthews K*: Nutripoints: the breakthrough point system for optimal nutrition,* New York, 1990, Harper & Row.

22 Family Systems Approach to the Care of Children

William L. Coleman

The family context is the domain of pediatricians. The family is the most central and enduring influence on children. Children affect their families, and families affect their children. Today the well-being of children and adolescents more often is affected adversely by psychosocial morbidity than by medical illness. The importance of parenting issues and psychosocial-behavioral problems has increased in pediatric practice with the rapid pace of social changes affecting families.[9]

To understand and work with families in his or her practice, the pediatric clinician needs knowledge and communication skills not often taught in most residency programs or continuing medical education courses. Furthermore, working with families is an intensely human experience that, in addition to knowledge and skills, requires a strong desire to support the family and a willingness to help the family resolve the painful feelings they are experiencing. Pediatricians are child advocates, but they need to broaden this concept and become child and family advocates to be most effective.

The purpose of this chapter is to enhance the pediatrician's skills, via a family systems approach, in the assessment and management of behavioral-psychosocial problems.

THE BIOPSYCHOSOCIAL MODEL AND FAMILY SYSTEMS CONCEPTS

The Biopsychosocial View

To better understand the biopsychosocial model and family systems concepts, it is helpful first to describe the biomedical model. Traditionally, illness and problems have been divided into those that have biological or physical causes and those that have psychosocial causes. This dichotomy characterizes the biomedical model that focuses on the child, the disease, and the pediatrician as the powerful healer. But this model ignores important aspects of illness and health, limits our understanding of symptomatology, interferes with a correct or complete diagnosis, and reduces the likelihood of optimal treatment.

A family systems approach is an integral part of the biopsychosocial model that is based on the interaction of the biological and psychosocial factors.[5] Psychosocial forces influence the adaptation of the child and family to an illness or stress regardless of etiological factors. The biopsychosocial model proposes that all the elements (biological, individual, family, community) affect each other in ways that influence health and illness. It emphasizes the integrity of disease (physical and emotional), the whole patient (body and mind), and the family-social context.

The biopsychosocial model has been demonstrated to be the most effective approach to child health and well-being.[7] It emphasizes that psychosocial forces affect health and illness as much as biological factors. Family, environmental, and psychosocial stresses can cause medical illness, injuries, and mental illness. Medical and emotional problems in any family member affect all family members. Pediatricians must be able to assess the stresses in and on families; all families need help, not just those who are most disadvantaged or at risk.

The concept of "contextual pediatrics" is also an integral aspect of the biopsychosocial model.[6] It advocates a vision of the child, the family, and the community as a "seamless continuum." Pediatricians must move from individual child health to family contextual child health, and the family is the most immediate context of the child. The focus of child care is the child in the context of the family.

Family Systems Concepts

Family systems concepts envision the family as a set of connected relationships. Everything that happens to a child occurs, at some level, within the family and always affects the family. Everything that affects the family always affects the child.

Family members, in or out of the pediatrician's office, behave much like the individual pieces of a mobile—that is, each is capable of independent behavior, but each is connected to another; therefore, any movement by a single member influences and changes the movement of the group as a whole. Visualize a mobile with four or five pieces suspended from the ceiling, gently moving in the air. The whole is in balance, steady yet moving.[4] A breeze catching only one piece of the mobile immediately influences the movement of every piece (some more than others), and the pace picks up, with some pieces unbalancing themselves and moving about chaotically for a time. Gradually the whole exerts its influence on the errant piece(s), and balance is restored. Notice also the changeability regarding closeness and distance among the pieces and the importance of vertical hierarchy; they describe the behavior and relationships among individuals in a family.[4] The concept of homeostatic balance within a system is most important here—balance and movement, movement and balance.[1]

Family systems approaches should not be confused with family counseling. Family systems approaches are built on the mobile model. The pediatrician uses this perspective and family interviewing techniques to help the family find solutions to their problems; for example, improving communication, changing behavioral interaction patterns, reestablishing an appropriate hierarchy and parent-child boundaries, improving their ability to adapt and problem solve, and respecting the rights and needs of both the family and the individual members. Family counseling is more in the biomedical tradition, with the pediatrician as expert providing advice and other treatment. For the majority of mild to moderate psychosocial problems encountered in primary care pediatrics, a combination of family systems approaches and family counseling is often very effective.

SUITABLE PROBLEMS FOR A FAMILY SYSTEMS APPROACH

Psychosocial-behavioral problems may be classified by three general levels of severity and/or complexity. Level I problems are predictable and mild and/or represent variations of normal development. They usually resolve with conventional wisdom and generic advice of the biomedical model, specifically the 5 Rs: Reassurance (emotional support), Recipes (parenting advice), Reading (education), Resources (parent support groups, state and national associations), and Ritalin (various medications).

Level II problems are suitable for family systems approaches in the office. They may be: (1) a Level I problem that has failed to resolve, recurs, or intensifies (e.g., noncompliance, complicated ADD, sibling rivalry, sleep disorders); (2) child problems that have an apparent psychosocial etiology (e.g., chronic somatic complaints, school refusal, parent-child conflict); or (3) parent problems (e.g., parental disagreement over discipline, parent feeling overwhelmed and unappreciated, parental depression). Level II problems generally entail two characteristics: relationship issues (e.g., child-parent, parent-parent) invariably emerge as a major, if not the major issue; and children often present as the "symptomatic patient" or the "identified patient" of a disturbed or stressed (not necessarily dysfunctional) family system.

Again, Level II problems are not exclusive and often are discovered to be part of, or evolve from, a Level I problem—for example, the emotional and family interaction complications of ADD. Consequently, Level II problems often require both Level I interventions (e.g., medication, advice) and Level II interventions (family systems approaches). The inexperienced pediatrician initially should select simple problems and families that appear to be competent, caring, and capable of working together. Common examples of Level II problems are listed in Box 22-1.

Level III characterizes families that have long-standing, intense, complex, and/or multiple problems—for example, child abuse, domestic violence, alcoholism. These families should be referred to the appropriate professionals and agencies, and the primary care clinician can still treat and follow the child, communicate with the other professionals, and continue to advocate for the child and family.

THE FAMILY INTERVIEW

Who Should Attend the Family Meeting?

It is not always practical or necessary for the entire family to attend a family meeting. Family interviewing may be successful with only the parent and the child. If it becomes apparent that other members are needed, they should be invited to the next meeting.

BOX 22-1

SELECTED LEVEL II PROBLEMS

1. Any Level I problem that is not resolving or is intensifying
2. Poor compliance with medical regimens
3. Risky behaviors (unsafe sexual behavior, truancy, dropping out of school)
4. Vulnerable child syndrome and overprotected child
5. Significant parent disagreement/conflict about parenting style that negatively affects the child
6. School refusal/separation anxiety
7. Punitive parenting, including constant threats or use of corporal punishment
8. Family communication-interactive patterns that discourage expressions of affection, acceptance, and approval and result in diminished self-esteem
9. Intense parent-child conflict, including a poor "fit" between child and parent temperaments
10. Emotional problems in the child or in a family member that affects the child
11. Chronic pain complaints (abdominal pain, headache)
12. Family stresses (losses, changes, transitions); for example, divorce, formation of stepfamily, death of or illness in a loved one, diagnosis of a developmental delay
13. When a referral is needed and the family does not understand or is hesitant
14. When a parent brings a child in repeatedly for minor complaints, especially in the evening
15. When the problem appears to center on family relationships and interactions
16. When the family is stuck and feels hopeless/helpless
17. When the pediatrician is confused
18. Whenever the pediatrician feels a family systems approach is appropriate

Scheduling

The initial visit should be at least 30 minutes. Follow-up visits should be 20 minutes. Most problems can be resolved with three to six visits.

Engaging the Family: Forming a Therapeutic Alliance

Forming a therapeutic alliance between the pediatrician and *each member* of the family, also known as *joining,* is the first step of a family interview. The greeting begins with introductions, handshakes, and smiles. Children should be addressed by name, not "your son," "he," or "she," and parents by formal names or titles. A few minutes of social conversation allow the pediatrician to establish personal contact with each member and overcomes the patient's normal tendency to feel nervous and hesitant. This is especially important for the first interview.

Once in the room, the members are invited to sit where they wish. Their seating arrangement itself may reveal something about family relationships. The pediatrician also needs keen observational skills, noting both what family members say and how they communicate. The "what" is the "content," the subject and issues they talk about. The "how" is the "process," the way members interact verbally and nonverbally—for example, body movements, facial expressions, affect, tone of voice, seating arrangement, eye contact.

Working with the Family: Five Family Interviewing Techniques

The five selected family interviewing techniques are (1) problem definition within a family context, (2) ABC, (3) exception questions, (4) goal definition and negotiation, and (5) scaling questions. These techniques help achieve the general goals of the family interview, which are to obtain an initial brief assessment of the problem within the family context, to help the family define their goals, and to help them develop their solutions with the guidance of the pediatrician. The "movement" of the interview(s) should be from problem to solutions, using the problem mainly as a "launching pad" for solutions. Unhappy families tend to resemble one another and share some common problems, whereas happy families tend to be happy by developing their own unique solutions; therefore, the emphasis of the interviews should be on solutions.

Because there often is no "one way" or "right way" to resolve these problems, the pediatrician needs to determine the best approach by using wisdom and experience and by observing the family and following their lead. The interview, however, usually begins with a brief problem discussion, but too much problem talk becomes repetitious, instills a sense of blame and hopelessness, and often discourages the family from returning for another visit. Furthermore, the interview should never end on "problem" talk but on a hopeful note. The pediatrician can compliment them on their willingness to meet as a family and their ability to speak openly and can note any progress already achieved by the end of the visit. As the word "problem" often implies blame, psychopathology, or incompetence, the pediatrician should use words such as "issue" or "concern" with the family.

Problem definition within a family context. Families expect to discuss the problem, usually a child-centered complaint. The pediatrician should respect the parents' stated concern and let them tell their story, even if the pediatrician thinks the "real" problem lies within the family. The pediatrician must work with the subjective experience of the family. The initial problem description itself should be brief. More time should be devoted to assessing the family and social contexts in which the problems arise—for example, members of the household (including nonbiological family members), recent stresses, losses, and changes (their influence on the child and the family), and the marital-social situation of the parents. The family history (e.g., medical and emotional illness, behavioral or learning problems, substance abuse) is critical and provides an opportunity for psychosocial intervention.[10]

Antecedent behavior consequence. Antecedent behavior consequence (ABC) is a method for eliciting a brief description of the problem that illustrates the interactive context or the relationship aspects, while still respecting the family's need to describe the problem. The ABC interview technique illustrates the circular cause and effect pattern of the interaction, minimizes the blame-the-victim (child or parent) notion, and provides brief and specific descriptions of the behaviors and feelings within the context in which they arise.

The pediatrician should invite both the parent and child to describe each of the ABC components in order for the pediatrician and each of them to hear the others' perceptions and interpretations of the behaviors and emotions—to get both sides of the story.

A is an antecedent event. The parent's request or command, communication style, and affect may be the "trigger" events in a parent-child interaction. Where did the problem take place? What else was happening? What exactly did the parent say? How did she communicate? What was the tone of voice? What were the parent's and child's perceptions?

B is behavior. The child's behavioral and emotional response to the parent's request is usually the complaint—for example, "She never listens." The child's behavior and affect are described. What exactly did the child do or say? What were the child's feelings? How were they expressed? Did the child hear or understand the parent's command? What were the child's and parent's perceptions?

C is consequences. The parent's behavioral and emotional responses to the child's behavior represent its consequences. These responses reveal much about the parent's parenting style, and they shape the child's behavior. What are the parent's behaviors and affect? What exactly did the parent say or do? What were the child's and parent's perceptions and interpretations?

The pediatrician might have the parent and child describe one more circular, interaction pattern to reinforce the relationship aspects of the problem and ultimately of the solution.

Exception questions. Exception questions follow naturally after the problem discussion. They are exceptions to the problem questions. They are intended to determine what is right, what is working, when were things better, and what made them better. Exceptions suggest their own solutions for parent and child.[2] For example, after definition of the problem within the family context or the ABC, the pediatrician might ask, "What has helped in the past?" "When were things better?" "How were they different?" "What helped?"

To proceed from a focus on the problem to the solution, the pediatrician should illustrate the interactive context of past successes by asking the parent and child to describe what each was doing and what the other was doing when things were better (the exception times). This encourages the two to discuss positive events, share good feelings, and discuss solutions and past successes instead of problems. "When things were better, what were you doing?" "What was mom doing?" "What were you feeling?" "How was mom feeling?" "How did you know she was feeling better?" Exception questions also can be asked at the end of a meeting to instill a sense of hope and competence.

Goal definition and negotiation. Goal definition and negotiation allows the family to discuss positive feelings and behaviors and what they want to achieve, and highlights the interactive context of solutions. Ideally, goals should be defined by the end of the first interview, because a family meeting, especially the first one, should not end with talk about the problem. Discussing the progress toward the goal is another way to end the meeting on a positive note. Well-defined goals lead to well-defined solutions. The pediatrician might ask, "What would you like to see happen as a result of coming here?" "What would tell you that you don't need to come and see me anymore?" "So suppose things were better, what would be happening?" "If you could make a wish, what would you be doing?" "What would mom (dad, sibling) be doing?"

Every member should state his or her goal; then the pediatrician should help the family negotiate and agree upon a realistic and meaningful goal. The goal must be described as a desired behavior or the start of something new, not as the absence or end of something undesired—for example, talking politely to each other instead of no more yelling.[3]

Scaling questions. Scaling questions, like the others, may be asked at any time. They help the family members assess their current hope, confidence, or competence. They encourage members to rate their progress toward their goal.[4] The pediatrician might ask, "On a scale of 1 to 10, with 1 being the worst things have been, like when we first met (when you called for an appointment), and 10 being the best things could be (when you are at your goal), where are you now between 1 and 10?"

Scaling questions also allow each member to state his or her own present position and to appreciate others' positions. They also can help each member define a behavior—for example, strengths, past successes, and exceptions that helps achieve their goal. "What would you need to do to go from a 5 to a 6?" "How would you know you are at a 6?"

Finally, scaling questions highlight the interactive process of the family. The pediatrician might ask, "How would your son know that you are at a 6?" "What could you do to help your son go from a 7 to an 8?" "How would you feel when your mother is at 6?" "How would your mother act when she sees you at an 8?" "Would you like to have more of that?"

FURTHER TRAINING

Pediatric clinicians who wish to incorporate family systems approaches into their practices should get some extra training. Knowledge and training in family-oriented pediatric care may be obtained at various academic medical centers (departments of pediatrics and psychiatry), meetings of professional societies and academies (e.g., Society for Developmental and Behavioral Pediatrics, Ambulatory Pediatric Association, and American Academy of Pediatrics), and family therapy training centers.[8] Obtaining guidance and advice from a mentor or supervisor is highly advised.

SUMMARY

Every child is part of a family. The family influences the child and the child influences the family, as illustrated by the mobile. Psychosocial problems of children and families present increasingly to pediatric clinicians. Most of these problems require a family systems approach, which is a family-centered method designed to resolve behavioral, relationship, and interaction problems. Many of these problems present to pediatricians at the early and mild stage of severity. By selecting simple problems, and caring and competent families (especially already known to the care provider), these problems can be dealt with by the use of family systems approaches (viewing the problem in a family context and using brief, family-interviewing techniques). Other traditional interventions also may be needed.

REFERENCES

1. Allmond BW: Health care management of the family: the family as the focus of treatment in pediatrics. In Hoekelman RA, et al, editors: *Primary pediatric care,* ed 2, St Louis, 1992, Mosby.
2. Coleman WL: Family-focused pediatrics: solution-oriented techniques for behavioral problems, *Contemp Pediatr* 14:121, 1997.
3. Coleman WL, Howard BJ: Family-focused behavioral pediatrics: clinical techniques for primary care, *Pediatr Rev* 16:448, 1995.
4. Coleman WL, Stein MT, Epstein RM: "We've tried everything and nothing works": family centered pediatrics and clinical problem-solving, *J Dev Behav Pediatr* 18:114, 1997.
5. Engel GL: The biopsychosocial model and medical education, *N Engl J Med* 306: 802, 1982.
6. Green M, editor: *Bright futures: guidelines for health supervision of infants, children, and adolescents,* Arlington, VA, 1994, Maternal and Child Health Bureau.
7. Haggerty RJ, Roghmann KJ, Pless IB: *Child health and the community,* ed 2, New Brunswick, NJ, 1993, Transaction Publishers.
8. Tanner JL: Training for family-centered pediatric care, *Pediatr Clin North Am* 42:193, 1995.
9. Young KT, et al: Listening to parents: a national survey of parents with young children, *Arch Pediatr Adolesc Med* 152:255, 1998.
10. Zuckerman B: Family history: a special opportunity for psychosocial intervention, *Pediatrics* 87:740, 1991.

SUGGESTED READINGS

Allmond BW, Tanner JL: *The family is the patient,* Baltimore, 1998, Williams and Wilkins.

Berg IK: *Family-based services,* New York, 1994, Norton.

Coleman WL, Taylor EH: Family-focused pediatrics: issues, challenges, and clinical methods, *Pediatr Clin North Am* 42:1, 1995.

Doherty W, Baird M: *Family therapy and family medicine,* New York, 1983, Guilford.

McDaniel S, Campbell TL, Seaburn DB: *Family-oriented primary care,* New York, 1990, Springer-Verlag.

23 Prevention of Disease

one Prevention of Dental Caries

Robert J. Berkowitz and Pamela K. Den Besten

Dental caries is one of the most common bacterial infections afflicting children and adolescents. The disease may be defined as a localized, progressive destruction of tooth structure by bacterial activity. The occurrence of dental caries is related to critical interrelationships among the tooth, dietary carbohydrate, saliva, and specific oral bacteria. The decay process is initiated by demineralization of the outer tooth surface as a result of organic acids formed during bacterial fermentation of dietary carbohydrates. Simultaneously, saliva functions as a remineralizing and buffering solution to counter the effect of demineralization. Should bacterial-derived demineralization exceed saliva's remineralization and buffering capacity, caries lesions form. Incipient lesions first appear as opaque white spots; with progressive loss of tooth mineral, cavitation occurs.

During the past three to four decades, dental research has had significant impact on the prevention of dental caries. Accordingly, this chapter provides information regarding the etiology and prevention of this infectious disease.

ETIOLOGY

Microbial Factors

Studies in laboratory animals have clearly demonstrated that dental caries can be characterized as an infectious and transmissible disease. In such models, the infection is quite specific and usually involves a group of oral streptococci collectively designated mutans streptococci. Strains of these species isolated from dental plaque and caries lesions in humans routinely exhibit a high level of pathogenicity when tested under the optimal conditions of the rodent model. The cariogenicity of these bacteria relates to their ability to synthesize insoluble dextrans from dietary sucrose. These extracellular dextrans mediate attachment of mutans streptococci to one another and the tooth surface. In addition, their acidogenic and aciduric characteristics significantly contribute to their odontopathic potential. Implications for the involvement of mutans streptococci in human dental caries also come from clinical studies that demonstrate a positive correlation between caries activity and the degree of infection with these organisms. The etiological potential of mutans streptococci in human dental caries is also illustrated by its preferential association with the initial caries lesion or "white spot." Clinical studies regarding the bacteriology of "radiation" caries further demonstrate that a significant increase in oral mutans streptococci levels routinely precedes the onset of dental caries. Accordingly, several investigators have used salivary levels of mutans streptococci to predict caries risk. Collectively, the evidence indicates that mutans streptococci are a primary etiological agent in human dental caries.[3]

One important approach toward prevention of dental caries is to reduce intraoral levels of mutans streptococci. Epidemiological, chemotherapeutic, and immunological strategies are currently under investigation.

Salivary Factors

Observations in desalivated experimental animals and xerostomic humans clearly indicate that saliva is the primary host defense against dental caries. The relationship between salivary gland hypofunction and dental caries is related to several factors. First, the physical flow of saliva augmented by the activity of the oral musculature removes a large number of bacteria from the teeth. Second, saliva possesses multiple antibacterial systems. A group of salivary proteins, lysozyme, lactoferrin, and lactoperoxidase, working in conjunction with other salivary components has an immediate effect on oral bacteria, interfering with their ability to replicate or killing them directly. Salivary peroxidase exerts an anticaries effect through a mechanism that reduces the acidogenic potential of cariogenic bacteria. Saliva can also interfere with bacterial attachment by means that involve molecular interactions. The ability to inhibit bacterial attachment is a major characteristic of the secretory IgA system. In addition to antibodies, saliva contains a variety of macromolecules that interfere with bacterial attachment via several mechanisms that include aggregation, masking of bacterial adhesions, and competition for attachment sites. Finally, saliva has properties that directly protect the tooth surface from demineralization. Salivary bicarbonate, phosphate, and histidine-rich peptides diffuse into plaque and act directly as buffers. In addition to helping to counter plaque acidity, saliva helps protect the teeth from demineralization via a mechanism termed *remineralization.* Remineralization is defined as the deposition of salivary minerals into enamel defects. The presence of fluoride in trace quantities is critical to the remineralization process. Fluoride enhances enamel crystal growth, and hence, makes remineralization more rapid and effective. Because remineralization is promoted by the frequent introduction of a low concentration of fluoride into the mouth, the small amount of fluoride in fluoridated drinking water is sufficient to promote remineralization.[4]

Salivary hypofunction may be a consequence of a variety of factors, including (in part): radiotherapy when the salivary glands are within the radiation ports; chronic administration of anticholinergic or parasympatholytic drugs; and salivary gland disease (e.g., Sjögren's syndrome). Accordingly, such patients should be referred for aggressive caries preventive measures.

Table 23-1 Daily Fluoride Supplement Dosage Schedule

	Concentration of Fluoride in Drinking Water (ppmF)*		
Age	**<0.3**	**0.3-0.6**	**>0.6**
Birth-6 mo	0	0	0
6 mo-3 yr	0.25 mg	0	0
3 yr-6 yr	0.5 mg	0.25 mg	0
6 yr-16 yr	1.0 mg	0.5 mg	0

**ppmF,* Parts per million fluoride (1 mg of fluoride per liter of water = 1 ppmF).

Fluoride dosage regimen accepted by the American Academy of Pediatrics, American Academy of Pediatric Dentistry, and the American Dental Association (1994).

Dietary Factors

Most dietary sugars, carbohydrates, and starches are readily metabolized to organic acids by mutans streptococci and are termed *cariogenic substrates*. Multiple investigations in humans and laboratory animals demonstrate that frequent and prolonged oral exposure to cariogenic substrates facilitates dental caries activity.[2,9] Stated differently, it is not how much "sugar" you eat but how you eat "sugar" that determines the "sugar's" relative cariogenic potential. For example, the cariogenic potential of apple juice contained in a nursing bottle that is sampled throughout the night or nap times, or both, is quite different from that of the same volume of apple juice consumed at a single meal. Similarly, sugars contained in food products retained orally for a long time are more cariogenic than those in food products retained for short times.

PREVENTION

Fluoride

Water fluoridation. The relationships among natural water fluoride concentrations, caries prevalence, and enamel fluorosis were determined in classic epidemiological studies by H. Trendley Dean in the 1930s and 1940s. It was through these studies, as well as subsequent community trials with artificial water fluoridation, that the level of 1 ppm fluoride in drinking water was determined as optimal for caries prevention, with a minimal risk of fluorosis. Later, the recommendation for an optimal level of water fluoridation was refined to a range of 0.7 to 1.2 ppm fluoride, depending on the amount of water intake as a function of the annual average maximum daily air temperature in a community. Since these early studies, fluoridation of public water supplies has proven to be the most effective, convenient, and economical measure available to prevent dental caries.[5]

Fluoride supplements. The dramatic reduction in caries susceptibility in populations drinking fluoridated water led to recommendations to administer fluoride as a dietary supplement for those who did not receive it in their drinking water. Fluoride was assumed to have a systemic mode of action resulting in the formation of a more caries-resistant enamel structure, leading to the conclusion that fluoride supplements should mimic previous estimates of dietary fluoride intake. Fluoride supplements, therefore, were proposed for the period during which teeth were developing.

More recent research has shown that the most important mechanism by which fluoride results in caries prevention is the topical effect. Fluoride promotes salivary remineralization of demineralized enamel. This effect is enhanced by exposing the teeth frequently to relatively low levels of fluoride, as occurs with drinking fluoridated water.[1] The realization that systemic fluoride ingestion is not the major mechanism of action of fluoride in caries prevention and reports on increased dental fluorosis have lead to a reassessment of fluoride supplementation recommendations.

Dental fluorosis is a hypomineralization of enamel that occurs when higher than optimal levels of fluoride are ingested during the period of enamel formation. Fluorosis may vary from very mild to severe. Very mild to mild cases appear as chalky whitening of the enamel; severe fluorosis presents as mottled enamel that is pitted and brown in color. Recent reports have shown a trend toward a higher prevalence of dental fluorosis, relative to historical data from earlier studies. This increase in the prevalence of fluorosis was found to correlate with the ingestion of fluoride from sources other than drinking water, including fluoride supplements and fluoridated toothpaste.[6] Accordingly, because fluoride's major mechanism of caries prevention is topical, coupled with the increased prevalence of enamel fluorosis, the Council on Dental Therapeutics of the American Dental Association has endorsed a new fluoride supplementation schedule (Table 23-1). In this regard, fluoride supplements are not recommended prenatally or during the first 6 months of life. In addition, breast-fed infants residing in optimally fluoridated communities should not receive fluoride supplements.

As indicated in Table 23-1, dosage is based on the patient's age and fluoride content of the water supply. The fluoride level of a water supply can usually be obtained by calling the local water board. Should the patient use a private water supply, a fluoride analysis is indicated. The patient's parent should be instructed to use a plastic container for the water specimen (a glass container may impair the accuracy of the fluoride assay). No fluoride prescription should be written for more than 120 mg of fluoride. Even if a child ingested the entire supply, probably only mild gastric upset would ensue. However, in such an event, a poison control center should be contacted immediately.

Fluoride dentifrice. Fluoride-containing dentifrices are highly effective in preventing dental decay. However, before age 6 years, children tend to swallow rather than expectorate toothpaste, and nearly all of the ingested fluoride is absorbed, primarily from the small intestine. Furthermore, fluoride dentifrice constitutes approximately 95% of all dentifrice sold. The ingestion of fluoride-containing toothpaste is responsible for the strong association between early use of fluoride dentifrice and increased risk of dental fluorosis. To reduce the risk of dental fluorosis from toothpaste ingestion, a pea-sized amount of toothpaste should be used in brushing a young child's teeth. In this regard, toothpaste should be dispensed by the parent.

Fluoride rinses. Fluoride rinses containing 0.05% fluoride have been shown to be highly effective in reducing dental decay. These products are available without a prescription and should be recommended for children older than 6 years of age at risk for dental decay because of conditions such as compromised salivary flow rates, orthodontic therapy, and a high caries experience. They are not recommended for children younger than 6 years of age because of their inability to expectorate properly, resulting in excessive fluoride ingestion.

Oral Hygiene

Thorough daily brushing and flossing of the teeth helps prevent dental caries and periodontal disease. Parents should receive professional instruction regarding oral hygiene techniques for children. Clinical studies demonstrate that most children 8 years of age and younger do not have the hand-eye coordination required for adequate oral hygiene; accordingly, parents must assume responsibility for oral hygiene. The degree of parental involvement should reflect the child's level of competency.

Sealants

Excellent oral hygiene and optimal fluoride exposure have minimal effect in preventing dental caries in the pits and fissures on the occlusal (biting) surfaces of the posterior teeth. The use of sealants has been shown to be effective in the prevention of pit and fissure caries.[7] Sealants are plastic coatings that are applied professionally to the occlusal surfaces of the posterior teeth. A survey conducted by the National Institute of Dental Research indicated that relatively few schoolchildren in the United States have sealants on their teeth.[8] Unfortunately, regardless of proven clinical efficacy, the use of sealants is not routine in the prevention of dental caries.

Diet

Decreasing the frequency of cariogenic substrate ingestion prevents dental caries. Parents and children should be encouraged to avoid between-meal snacks that contain cariogenic substrates. The use of gum, candy, and soft drinks containing sugar substitutes (mannitol, sorbitol, xylitol, and aspartame [with precautions]) is an effective approach for the child who has a "sweet tooth." Chewing "sugarless" gum has been proven clinically to enhance salivary flow rate and, in turn, neutralize plaque pH. In addition, infants should be weaned by 1 year of age to eliminate their risk for nursing bottle caries (Fig. 23-1). Otherwise, bedtime and naptime nursing bottles should contain only water. Finally, sweetened elixirs of medications used on a chronic basis result in an increase in oral exposure to cariogenic substrates, thereby increasing caries risk. Patients exposed to this risk factor should be referred for aggressive caries preventive measures.

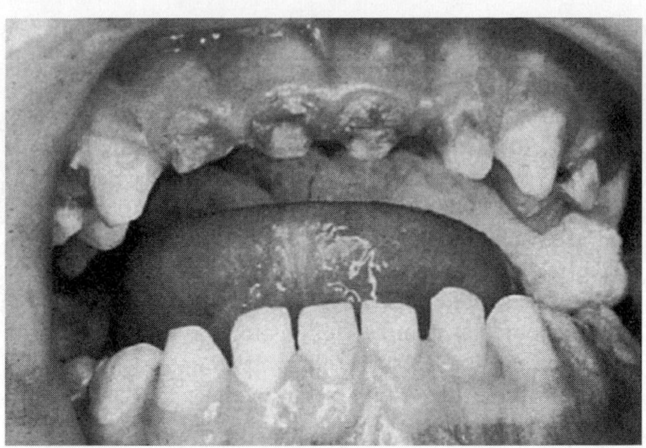

Fig. 23-1 Nursing bottle caries in a 2½-year-old child.

New Approaches

New approaches for caries prevention are being sought. These include improved fluoride delivery vehicles and new formulations that enhance the anticaries efficacy. The use of fluoride varnishes that can be painted on the teeth are now available in the United States. Dentifrice formulations that have mineral additives intended to improve the remineralizing ability of fluoride are being evaluated. Also, antimicrobial agents such as chlorhexidine are being used alone and in combination with fluoride. The use of laser treatments of tooth enamel is being evaluated for its ability to increase caries resistance alone and in combination with fluoride.

REFERENCES

1. Beltran ED, Burt BA: The pre- and posteruptive effects of fluoride in the caries decline, *J Pub Health Dent* 48:233, 1988.
2. Bibby B: Influence of diet on the bacterial composition of plaques. In Stiles HM, Loesche WJ, O'Brien TC, editors: *Microbiol aspects of dental caries,* vol 2, London, 1976, Information Retrieval.
3. Loesche WJ: Role of *Streptococcus mutans* in human dental decay, *Microbiol Res* 50:353, 1986.
4. Mandel ID: The functions of saliva, *J Dent Res* 66(special issue):623, 1987.
5. Newbrun E: Effectiveness of water fluoridation, *J Pub Health Dent* 49(special issue):279, 1989.
6. Pendrys DG: Dental fluorosis in perspective, *J Am Dent Assoc* 122:63, 1991.
7. Ripa LW: The current status of pit and fissure sealants: a review, *J Can Dent Assoc* 51:367, 1985.
8. Sealant use low, *Am Dent Assoc News* 20:24, 1989.
9. Van Houte J: Dental caries, *Int Dent J* 30:305, 1980.

two Injury Control

Modena Hoover Wilson

By many measures injury is the most significant health problem of childhood and adolescence. Injury *control* includes (1) preventing events that might cause injury; (2) diminishing the likelihood or severity of injury, even though events with injury-causing potential occur; and (3) minimizing the effects of the injury, once it occurs, through state of the art emergency response, medical care, and rehabilitation. This section concentrates on the first two parts of injury control—those classically thought of as injury *prevention*—and describes the role of the pediatrician in the clinical setting in ensuring injury prevention. It highlights the critical opportunity to prevent injury by providing counseling about injury and injury prevention to children and families. Pediatricians can assume effective roles for injury prevention at many additional levels—for example, with schools, communities, local health departments, and state and national agencies and legislatures. Successful injury control demands active advocacy outside the pediatrician's office.

Although the number of unintentional injury deaths during childhood has been decreasing, as a result in part to the hard work of pediatricians and public health professionals, the number of injury deaths compared with deaths from other causes is still high (Table 23-2). Although the leading causes of injury death vary by age group (Table 23-3), events involving motor vehicles, firearms, fires, suffocation, and drowning are important in every age group.

Deaths may be the most often noted injury statistic, but injury results in many other problems, including acute morbidity, short- and long-term disability, and high medical care costs. The causes of nonfatal injury encompass those that cause fatal injury, but falls, burns, poisonings, fights, sports, and recreational activities (including play) are more prominent causes of nonfatal injury than they are of fatalities. For almost all types of injury, males are at greater risk than are females. This increased risk has yet to be explained fully but may accrue from a number of factors, including innate behavioral differences, societal expectations, and exposure. Children living in poverty are more likely to suffer serious and fatal injury of many types than are advantaged children, and injury risk varies by geographical factors as well.

Successful clinical prevention is based on a clear understanding of the principles of injury prevention and on sound counseling skills.

PRINCIPLES OF INJURY CONTROL

Events leading to injury are, for the most part, predicable and preventable. They should not be thought of as "accidents," if that word implies a sense of helpless victimization. The focus should be on preventing the disease—the injury. Sometimes, prevention is achieved through eliminating injury-producing events—for example, building divided highways to reduce vehicular crashes. Sometimes, prevention is achieved by eliminating injury even though the event takes place (e.g., protecting child passengers by restraining them in car safety seats).

Energy is the "germ" leading to the disease injury. When energy affects the body acutely at a damaging level, injury results. For most pediatric injuries, the energy is mechanical,

Table 23-2 Injury Deaths Compared with All Deaths by Age Group U.S. Children and Adolescents, 1995

Age Group	<1	1-4	5-9	10-14	15-19	0-19
Unintentional injury	761	2249	1598	1916	6598	13,122
Suicide	–	–	7	330	1890	2227
Homicide	311	452	157	404	3262	4586
Undetermined	57	45	11	35	154	302
All injury	1129	2746	1773	2685	11,904	20,237
All deaths	29,583	6393	3780	4816	15,089	59,661
Percent of all deaths that are due to injury	4%	43%	47%	56%	79%	34%*

Data from National Center for Health Statistics. Abstracted from Appendix A. Committee on Injury and Poison Prevention, American Academy of Pediatrics: *Injury prevention and control for children and youth,* 1997.
*Sixty-four percent of deaths of persons ages 1 to 19 years are due to injury.

Table 23-3 Numbers and Rates of Injury Deaths by Age and Event U.S. Children and Adolescents, 1995

	Age in Years											
	<1		1-4		5-9		10-14		15-19		0-19	
Event	N	R	N	R	N	R	N	R	N	R	N	R
Motor vehicle traffic	172	4.5	703	4.5	854	4.4	1104	5.8	5107	28.3	7040	10.5
Firearms	8	*	97	0.6	107	0.6	641	3.4	4432	24.5	5285	7.0
Poisoning	19	*	47	0.3	21	0.1	45	0.2	348	1.9	480	0.6
Falls	20	0.5	42	0.3	28	0.1	36	0.2	145	0.8	271	0.4
Suffocation	424	11.0	200	1.3	91	0.5	211	1.1	512	2.8	1438	1.9
Drowning	74	1.9	557	3.5	229	1.2	246	1.3	461	2.6	1567	2.1
Fires/burns	78	2.0	488	3.1	249	1.3	115	0.6	84	0.5	1014	1.5
Cutting/piercing	4	*	18	*	7	*	38	0.2	256	1.4	323	0.4

Data from National Center for Health Statistics. Abstracted from Appendix A. Committee on Injury and Poison Prevention, American Academy of Pediatrics: *Injury prevention and control for children and youth,* 1997.
R, Deaths per 100,000 population.
*Rate is lower than 0.1.

but thermal, chemical, and electrical energy also are agents of injury. To prevent injury, energy must be kept away from the child, or the forces must be spread out over time and/or space so that they do not reach damaging levels. The former is well illustrated by building a bicycle path as an alternative to riding amidst motor vehicles. The latter is illustrated by the protection provided by a helmet in a fall from a bicycle. The helmet mitigates the forces reaching the brain, even though the fall has occurred.

Injury control strategies may be categorized in a number of ways. With respect to timing, they can apply before the event *(pre-event phase),* during the event *(event phase),* or after the event *(post-event phase).* For example, the pediatrician in the office might recommend *against* buying a walker or *for* turning down the water heater (pre-event), *for* using a car safety seat (event), and *for* CPR training (post-event).

With respect to the involvement of the child who needs protection (or the child's parent), strategies can be active or passive. Active strategies require involvement every time protection is needed. Seat belts in automobiles are a good example. Passive (or automatic) strategies protect whether or not the person needing protection is mindful of the need and takes appropriate action. Airbags to protect adolescent drivers are a good example. Both active and passive strategies can be quite successful when employed, but passive strategies, when they exist, often are favored over active strategies. Because active strategies require compliant behaviors on the part of individuals, there is always a risk that they will not be fully employed. It often is the case that active strategies are least likely to be adopted by the persons at greatest risk.

Injuries often have been classified as unintentional or intentional; this dichotomy has been useful in many ways. It is well to keep in mind, however, that the volitional contribution to human behavior is not always clear cut. Intent probably assorts along a continuum. Additionally, strategies that prevent unintentional injury (e.g., locking up firearms or turning down the hot water heater) may also prevent some intentional injuries. For these reasons and because injuries result from both, injury control efforts often address both intentional and unintentional injury. Nevertheless, some blatant forms of intentional injury—for example, child abuse and child and adolescent suicide and homicide—are so important as causes of pediatric morbidity and mortality that they demand focused attention. Violence prevention has become an explicit goal of injury control for the pediatrician.

Pediatricians can attempt to persuade individuals to decrease their risk of injury through educational efforts with individuals or groups. Injury control advocates have additional strategies at their disposal. These include media campaigns, legislation, and regulation and litigation, as well as environmental, design, and cultural change. For most types of injury, multiple strategies will need to be applied.

ANTICIPATORY GUIDANCE

A structured review of the literature has provided evidence of positive outcomes following injury prevention counseling as part of health supervision. It should be noted, however, that the evidence base for the effectiveness of injury control counseling is stronger in some areas than in others, prompting continual calls for additional research, improvements in counseling, and investment in more automatic injury control strategies.

Even though injury control counseling has become a cornerstone of pediatric prevention, it can be daunting, not only because of the time and expertise it requires but also because of its breadth. Injury risk is so universal and the sources of possible injury so diverse that a pediatrician cannot counsel on all possible risks. A group of injury control experts based their priorities on severity of the injury, frequency with which the injury occurs, and the availability of environmental strategies.[2] Pediatricians will want to be sensitive to the individual circumstances of patients and families as well. For instance, farm families may need advice that city families do not, and vice versa. Knowing that a family has a boat or a backyard pool prompts a specialized discussion of drowning risk. In another example of the need to customize anticipatory guidance, counseling a family who has two automobiles about car safety seats poses a different set of issues than does counseling a family who relies on taxis for transportation; yet car passenger safety is a high priority for both.

The American Academy of Pediatrics (AAP) recommends that parents be given advice by the pediatrician about a number of injury issues organized by age of the child (Box 23-1).[3] The AAP also provides a number of tools to facilitate counseling, including age-specific survey instruments to assess risk and handouts for families, as part of The Injury Prevention Program (TIPP).[6]

COUNSELING TECHNIQUE

Counseling about any injury control topic requires both technical expertise and counseling skill. In addition to the TIPP materials cited in the previous discussion, a number of resources are listed at the end of this section that can provide a pediatrician with the knowledge for advising parents (and communities) about injury prevention.

Counseling technique is not specific to injury prevention but can be adapted from the literature on prompting and supporting heath behavior change. A strategy, designed around the pneumonic SAFE, which has been used to help pediatricians move through the parts of patient counseling, is given in Box 23-2.

VIOLENCE PREVENTION

A complete discussion of violence prevention is contained in Chapter 23 (Four), Violence Prevention. Recognition of the pediatrician's role in violence prevention is growing.[4] A pediatrician has many opportunities to affect the likelihood that children will become victims or perpetrators of violence throughout the course of ongoing care of the child.[5] A number of these opportunities are listed in Box 23-3; the list is likely to get longer. Where violence prevention is concerned, it is well to remember that, as is true for injury control as a whole, the problems are too large and complex to be addressed completely by pediatric practice, even of the highest quality. This, on the other hand, does not relieve us of the responsibility to act within the practice arena. Injury is too significant a health problem to ignore.

BOX 23-1

TOPICS RECOMMENDED BY THE AMERICAN ACADEMY OF PEDIATRICS FOR OFFICE-BASED INJURY PREVENTION COUNSELING

Infants and Preschoolers

Traffic safety: Appropriate use of child safety restraints

Burn prevention: Smoke detectors, hot water temperature no higher than 125° F

Fall prevention: Window and stairway guards and gates, avoiding walker use

Poison prevention: Storage of poisons, child-resistant containers, ipecac

Drowning prevention: Emptying buckets, supervising baths, fencing pools, not relying on swimming lessons

School-Age Children

Traffic safety: Seat belt use, avoiding riding on ATVs and in the beds of pickup trucks, safe pedestrian practices, helmets for biking, protective equipment for roller blading and skateboarding

Water safety: Swimming lessons but no swimming alone; personal flotation devices for boating

Sports safety: Safety equipment, physical conditioning

Firearm safety: Keeping firearms out of the home or at least keeping firearms unloaded and locked separately from locked ammunition

Adolescents

Traffic safety: Seat belt use, role of alcohol in motor vehicle crashes, helmets for biking and motorcycling, protective equipment for roller blading and skateboarding

Water safety: Role of alcohol in water-related injuries; personal flotation devices for boating

Sports safety: Safety equipment, physical conditioning

Firearm safety: Keeping any firearms in the home unloaded and locked separately from locked ammunition

Modified from Committee on Injury and Poison Prevention, American Academy of Pediatrics: Office-based counseling for injury prevention, *Pediatrics* 94:566, 1994.

BOX 23-2

SAFE COMMUNICATION FRAMEWORK

Communication Skills	Description
Solicit information	Ask parent (or child) what parent (or child) knows, does, and is concerned about regarding a specific safety topic
Advise	Explain safety practices Provide information on how to perform practices
Focus on risks and barriers	Help parent (or child) understand injury risk Acknowledge barriers to safety practices Help parent (or child) to problem solve
Encourage adherence	Negotiate a commitment Reinforce intentions and efforts Plan to follow-up

From Gielen A, et al: The Johns Hopkins SAFEHome Project (MCJ-240638). Funded by the Maternal and Child Health Bureau (Title V, Social Security Act), Health Resources and Services Administration, Department of Health and Human Services. The Johns Hopkins Schools of Public Health and Medicine.

BOX 23-3

OPPORTUNITIES FOR VIOLENCE PREVENTION DURING THE COURSE OF PEDIATRIC PRACTICE

Refer to effective parenting support programs

Suspect and report child maltreatment

Recognize signs of domestic violence and offer assistance

Counsel about limiting TV viewing and avoiding other violent entertainment

Counsel about child discipline and offer effective alternatives to corporal punishment

Promote school readiness and literacy skills

Recognize behavioral problems early and intervene

Diagnose and treat attention deficit/hyperactivity disorder

Arrange appropriate treatment for children who have mental health problems

Detect school problems and intervene

Counsel about avoiding drugs and alcohol

Help children/adolescents rehearse nonviolent problem-solving strategies

Diagnose drug and alcohol abuse and intervene

Counsel about elimination and/or safe storage of firearms in the home

Screen for adolescent depression and intervene

REFERENCES

1. Bass JL, et al: Childhood injury prevention counseling in primary care settings: a critical review of the literature, *Pediatrics* 92:544, 1993.
2. Cohen LR, et al: Pediatric injury prevention counseling priorities, *Pediatrics* 99:704, 1997.
3. Committee on Injury and Poison Prevention: Office-based counseling for injury prevention, *Pediatrics* 94:566, 1994.
4. Rivara F, Farrington D: Prevention of violence: role of the pediatrician, *Arch Pediatr Adolesc Med* 149:421, 1995.
5. Task Force on Violence, American Academy of Pediatrics: The role of the pediatrician in youth violence prevention in clinical practice and at the community level, *Pediatrics* 103:173, 1999.
6. TIPP, The Injury Prevention Program: *A guide to safety counseling in office practice,* Elk Grove Village, Ill, American Academy of Pediatrics.

ADDITIONAL RESOURCES

Publications

Baker SP, et al: *The injury fact book,* ed 2, New York, 1992, Oxford University Press.

Baker SP, et al: *Injury to children and teenagers: state-by-state mortality facts,* Baltimore, 1996, The Johns Hopkins Center for Injury Research and Policy.

Committee on Injury and Poison Prevention, American Academy of Pediatrics: *Injury prevention and control for children and youth,* Widome MD, editor, Elk Grove Village, Ill, 1997, American Academy of Pediatrics.

Committee on Injury and Poison Prevention, American Academy of Pediatrics: Selecting and using the most appropriate car safety seats for growing children: guidelines for counseling parents, *Pediatrics* 97:761, 1996.

Wilson MH, et al: *Saving children: a guide to injury prevention,* New York, 1991, Oxford University Press.

Telephone Numbers

National Highway Traffic Safety Administration, 800-424-9393.

US Consumer Product Safety Commission, 800-638-2772.

Websites

American Academy of Pediatrics: www.aap.org/ (For policy statement and updates, media messages, and other resources).

Harborview Injury Prevention and Research Center: www.depts.washington.edu/hiprc/ (For information on childhood injury and systematic reviews of injury prevention strategies).

National Center for Injury Prevention and Control at the CDC: www.cdc.gov/ncipc/ (For injury data and prevention information).

three Preventive Cardiology

Thomas J. Starc, Kathleen McGrath, and Steven E. Lipshultz

ATHEROSCLEROSIS

Atherosclerosis continues to be a leading cause of death and disability in the United States. Although myocardial infarction, stroke, and other clinical manifestations of atherosclerosis usually appear in the mature adult, there is mounting evidence that their pathogenesis begins much earlier. Furthermore, epidemiological studies suggest that atherosclerosis is not an inevitable consequence of aging but rather an acquired disease with well-described risk factors.

Although many risk factors for heart disease remain beyond the control of the individual, some, such as hypercholesterolemia and level of physical activity, are modifiable, and at least one, smoking, is completely avoidable. A goal of primary care practitioners is the prevention of disease, and it is hoped that focusing on risk factors in children ultimately will lead to a decline in morbidity and mortality resulting from atherosclerosis. Risk factors for adult coronary heart disease are being identified increasingly during childhood, and scientifically based recommendations to begin prevention in childhood are being developed. Because the process of atherosclerosis and habits that influence the risk of heart disease begin early in life, it is appropriate also to initiate preventive measures during childhood.[12,29]

Well-established risk factors for atherosclerosis include hypertension, smoking, elevated LDL-cholesterol, decreased HDL-cholesterol, diabetes mellitus, advancing age, male gender, and a family history of premature heart disease.[23,26] Other risk factors being investigated include hypertriglyceridemia, sedentary lifestyle, and obesity. Primary prevention in childhood should include attention to established risk factors that can be eliminated or minimized.

In their classic study of combatants dying in the Korean War, Enos, Beyer, and Holmes showed that young American soldiers had a 77% incidence of coronary arterial lesions, whereas such abnormalities were virtually nonexistent among young Korean soldiers.[9] Recent studies from the Bogalusa Heart Study[4] and the Pathobiological Determinants of Atherosclerosis in Youth (PDAY) study group[16] have demonstrated that risk factors such as cholesterol and smoking contribute to the formation of atherosclerosis in a graded manner and that these findings are present in children and young adults before the onset of clinical heart disease.

Total cholesterol is the combination of low-density lipoprotein cholesterol (LDL-cholesterol), high-density cholesterol (HDL-cholesterol), and very low-density cholesterol (VLDL-cholesterol). LDL-cholesterol may be viewed as the atherogenic lipoprotein, while HDL-cholesterol has a protective effect against coronary heart disease. Plasma cholesterol levels are influenced by dietary fat and cholesterol and by the individual's ability to synthesize and degrade cholesterol. Severe or familial hypercholesterolemia secondary to a defect in the LDL-cholesterol receptor occurs in approximately 1 in 500 individuals. Children who have this defect commonly have LDL-cholesterol values of 200 to 300 mg/dl. These children inherit the receptor defect from an affected parent and have a strong predilection for heart disease as young adults. There are more than 200 different mutations of the LDL receptors that result in clinical disease of premature atherosclerosis. Approximately 50% of men who have this disease will have a myocardial infarction by age 50 years and 75% to 85% by age 60 years. Approximately 50% of women will develop ischemic heart disease by age 60. Fortunately, recent studies suggest that even in these high-risk patients, treatment will decrease the incidence of heart disease.[25]

In 1991, the National Cholesterol Education Program (NCEP) suggested a number of guidelines for the prevention of heart disease in children.[19] Although most authorities agree that prevention of heart disease is a laudable goal, the optimal methods of prevention have remained controversial regarding such fundamental questions as at what age to begin screening, who actually should be screened, and how ultimately to treat those individuals who have elevated cholesterol levels.[11,21] As has occurred with the adult guidelines, the pediatric NCEP guidelines undoubtedly will be revised as more information regarding treatment of hypercholesterolemia is accrued.

RECOMMENDATIONS FOR CHOLESTEROL SCREENING

The NCEP suggested two separate approaches to hypercholesterolemia in children: a broad, population-based approach and an individual patient approach. The panel suggested that all children older than 2 years of age consume a diet that is relatively low in fat (e.g., 30% of calories from fat and 10% from saturated fat). Universal screening of all children is not recommended despite the awareness that cholesterol testing based on family history would miss a substantial number of hypercholesterolemic children.[7,27] The NCEP guidelines suggest cholesterol testing of children older than 2 years of age whose parent or grandparent has or had premature coronary heart disease, defined as younger than 56 years of age. Heart disease includes a history of documented myocardial infarction, angina pectoris, peripheral vascular disease, cerebrovascular disease, or sudden cardiac death. In addition, children who have a parent with hypercholesterolemia (≥240 mg/dl) also should be screened. Children whose parental history is unknown or unobtainable, especially if they have other risk factors, also may be screened to identify those in need of nutritional advice.

For children who have a family history of premature heart disease, the NCEP suggested obtaining a lipid profile including total cholesterol, HDL-cholesterol, triglycerides, and LDL-cholesterol. For children who have a family history of hypercholesterolemia and no history of early heart disease, the NCEP suggested initial screening by measuring total cholesterol only.

RECOMMENDATIONS FOR TREATMENT

Most of our information regarding the risk of heart disease in adults is based on LDL-cholesterol; therefore, recommendations in children are based on LDL-cholesterol values. Absolute "normal" values for cholesterol are unknown, and the treatment values are based on percentile ranks of children in the United States. Total cholesterol ≥200 mg/dl and LDL-cholesterol ≥130 mg/dl represent values above the 95th percentile for children and are designated as high. Total cholesterol <170 mg/dl and LDL-cholesterol <110 mg/dl represent values below the 75th percentile and are acceptable. Values between these limits are borderline (Table 23-4).

If a child is found to have a high or borderline cholesterol value, the test should be repeated. Management should be based on the average of at least two lipoprotein levels using the following general strategy:

Acceptable (LDL-cholesterol <110 mg/dl): Repeat cholesterol analysis in 5 years and follow a moderately low-fat diet.

Borderline (LDL-cholesterol 110 to 129 mg/dl): Follow a Step 1 Diet, provide advice regarding other risk factors, and reevaluate in 1 year.

High (LDL-cholesterol ≥130 mg/dl): Before dietary or medical treatment, a history detailing use of drugs such as isotretinoin (Accutane), steroids, and alcohol should be obtained to identify any secondary cause of hypercholesterolemia. These children also should be screened for other secondary causes of elevated cholesterol such as liver, thyroid, and renal disease (Table 23-5).

The initial dietary treatment guidelines suggest a Step I diet intake of approximately 30% of calories from fat and 10% from saturated fat (Table 23-6).[10,19] This diet has been shown to be safe and efficacious in the management of children who have hypercholesterolemia.[30] Care must be taken to ensure adequate calories so that the child is not deprived of caloric intake in an attempt to decrease fat intake. In contrast to adults, the majority of children who have hypercholesterolemia are not overweight. Restriction of calories is not the primary treatment for hypercholesterolemia for children, as it is often for adults.

For children whose LDL-cholesterol remains >130 mg/dl, a Step 2 diet with approximately 30% of calories from total fat and less than 7% of calories from saturated fat is advised. Compliance with a Step 2 diet often is improved by having

Table 23-4 Classification of Total and LDL-Cholesterol Levels in Children and Adolescents from Families with Hypercholesterolemia or Premature Cardiovascular Disease

Category	Total Cholesterol (mg/dl)	LDL-Cholesterol (mg/dl)
Acceptable	<170	<110
Borderline	170-199	110-129
High	≥200	≥130

From National Cholesterol Education Program: Report of the Expert Panel on Blood Cholesterol Levels in Children and Adolescents, *Pediatrics* 89:525, 1992.

Table 23-5 Causes of Secondary Hypercholesterolemia

Exogenous
- Drugs—corticosteroids, isotretinoin (Accutane), thiazides, anticonvulsants, beta blockers, anabolic steroids, certain oral contraceptives
- Alcohol
- Obesity

Endocrine and Metabolic
- Hypothyroidism
- Diabetes mellitus
- Lipodystrophy
- Pregnancy
- Idiopathic hypercalcemia

Storage Diseases
- Glycogen storage diseases
- Sphingolipidoses

Obstructive Liver Diseases
- Biliary atresia
- Biliary cirrhosis

Chronic Renal Diseases
- Nephrotic syndrome

Others
- Anorexia nervosa
- Progeria
- Collagen disease
- Klinefelter's syndrome

From National Cholesterol Education Program: Report of the Expert Panel on Blood Cholesterol Levels in Children and Adolescents, *Pediatrics* 89:525, 1992.

the family meet with a nutritionist trained in management of hyperlipidemia in children. Drug treatment with binding resins such as cholestyramine or colestipol is suggested for those children older than 10 years of age who have LDL-cholesterol >190 mg/dl and a family history of premature atherosclerosis. Other medications such as HMG CoA-reductase inhibitors are not recommended routinely for children.

The cholesterol screening and treatment guidelines can be initiated safely by a primary care practitioner (Figs. 23-2 to 23-4) who has an interest in nutrition and the prevention of heart disease. A review of family history, evaluation for secondary causes of hyperlipidemia, and dietary treatment should be initiated by the primary care clinician. In addition, identification of children who have risk factors for coronary heart disease should lead to screening of other family members, including the parents, because many of these risk factors tend to cluster in families. Children who have severe

Table 23-6 Characteristics of American Heart Association Step 1 and Step 2 Diet

Nutrient	Step 1	Step 2
Calories	Adequate for normal growth	Same
Total fat	≤30% of calories	Same
Saturated fat	<10% of calories	≤7%
Polyunsaturated fat	Up to 10% of calories	Same
Monounsaturated fat	Remainder of fat calories	Same
Carbohydrates	About 55% of calories	Same
Protein	About 15%-20% of calories	Same
Cholesterol (mg/day)	<300	<200

Data from National Cholesterol Education Program: Report of the Expert Panel on Blood Cholesterol Levels in Children and Adolescents, *Pediatrics* 89:525, 1992.

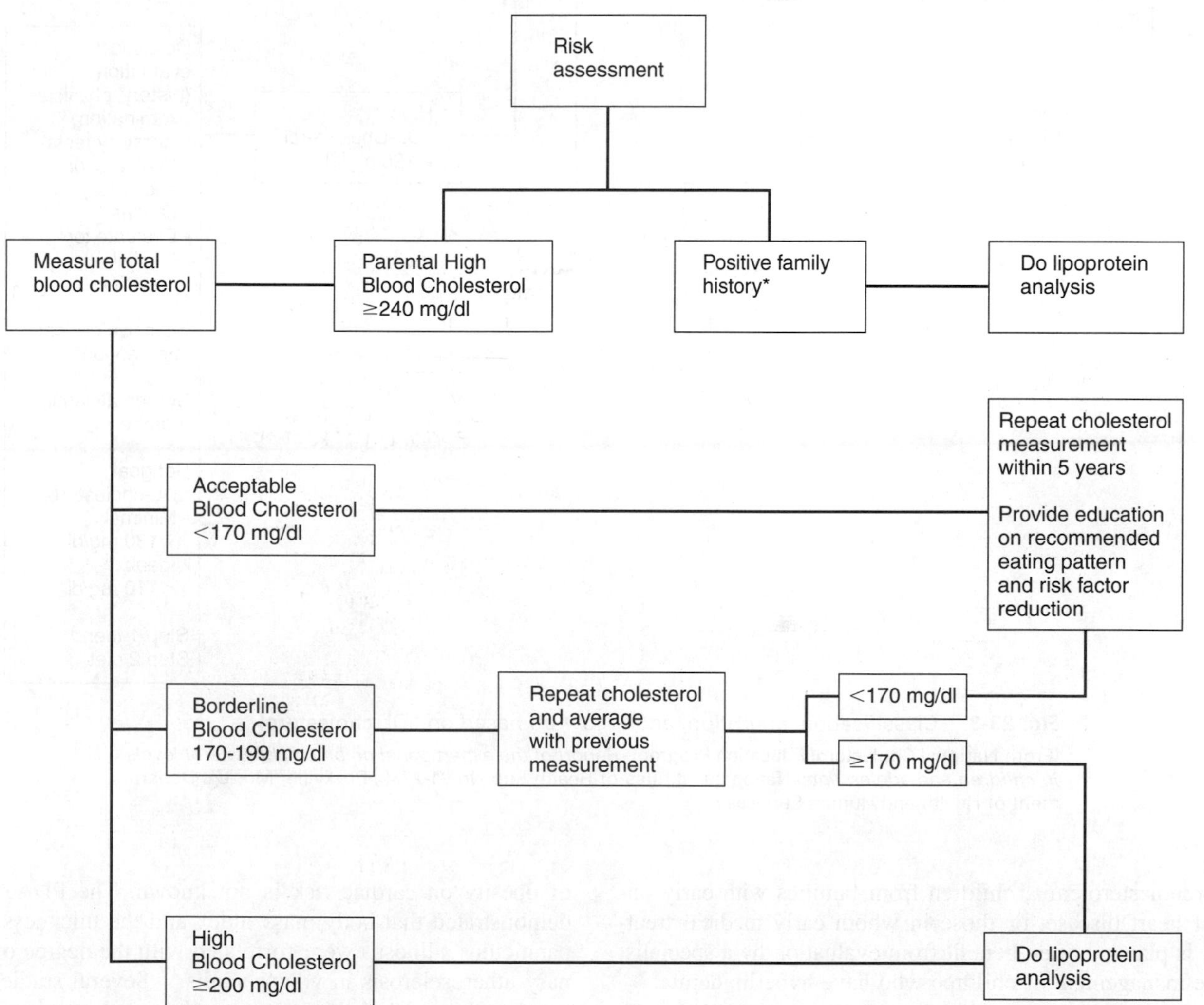

*Defined as a history of premature (before age 55 years) cardiovascular disease in a parent or grandparent.

Fig. 23-2 Risk assessment.
(From National Cholesterol Education Program: *Report of the expert panel on blood cholesterol levels in children and adolescents,* National Institutes of Health Pub No 91-2732, Rockville, Md, US Department of Health and Human Services.)

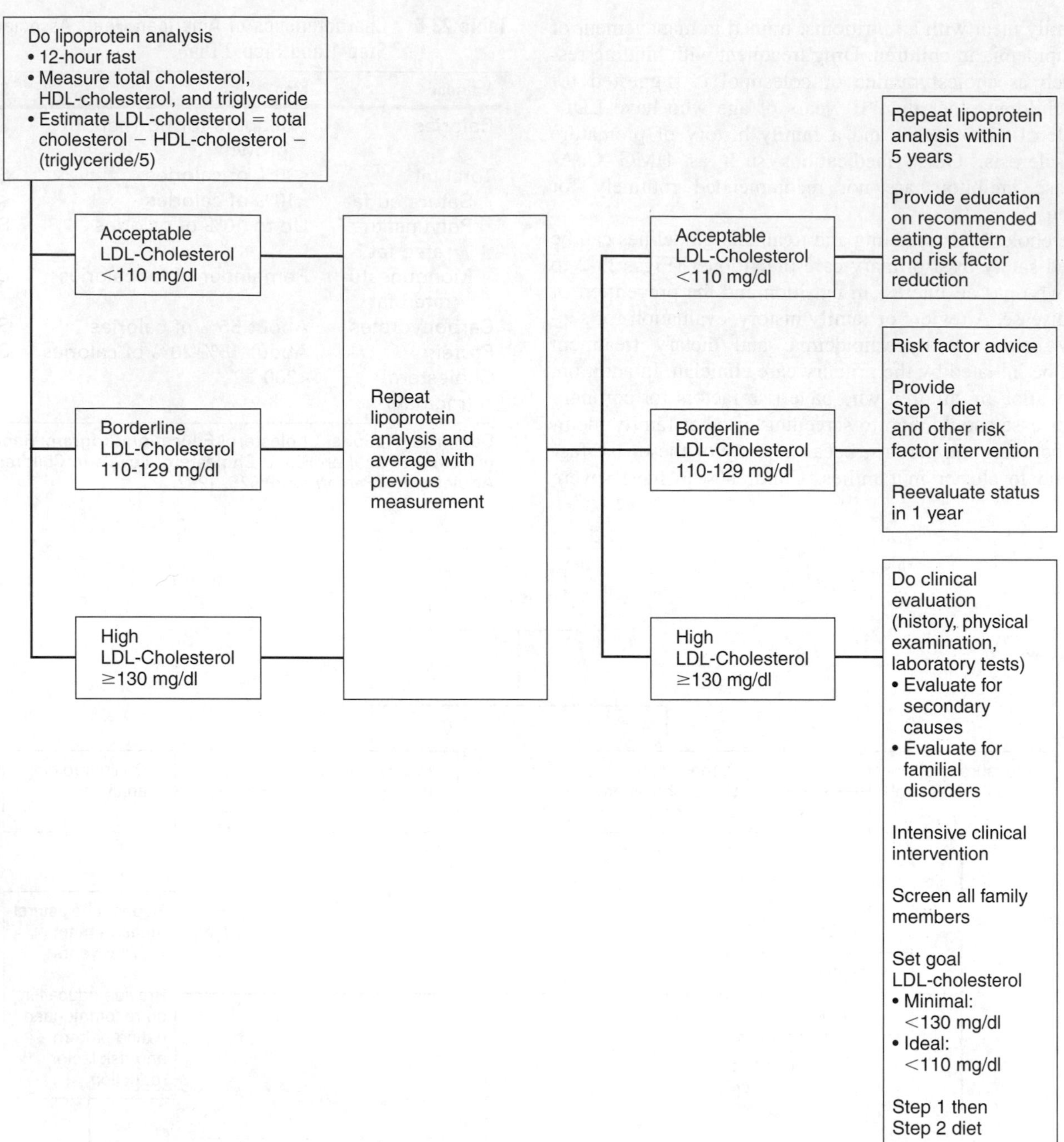

Fig. 23-3 Classification, education, and follow-up based on LDL-cholesterol.

(From National Cholesterol Education Program: *Report of the expert panel on blood cholesterol levels in children and adolescents,* National Institutes of Health Pub No 91-2732, Rockville, Md, US Department of Health and Human Services.)

hypercholesterolemia, children from families with early onset of heart disease, or those in whom early medical treatment is planned often benefit from evaluation by a specialist in the management of children who have hyperlipidemia.

OBESITY AND PHYSICAL ACTIVITY

Obesity increases the risk for heart disease through its association with abnormalities such as altered lipids, hypertension, and glucose intolerance, and possibly through other, as yet undefined, mechanisms.[13,15] The magnitude of the effect of obesity on cardiac risk is not known. The PDAY study demonstrated that body mass index and the thickness of the panniculus adiposus were correlated with the degree of coronary atherosclerosis in young adults.[17] Several studies have suggested a relationship between the level of obesity and abnormal lipid profiles.[2,3]

The prevalence of obesity in the United States has increased in both boys and girls of all races so that it now is the most common nutritional disorder in children and adolescents.[14] Among children ages 6 to 11 years, the prevalence of obesity increased from 5.2% in surveys during the years 1963 to 1964 to 10.8% during 1988 to 1991. Similar in-

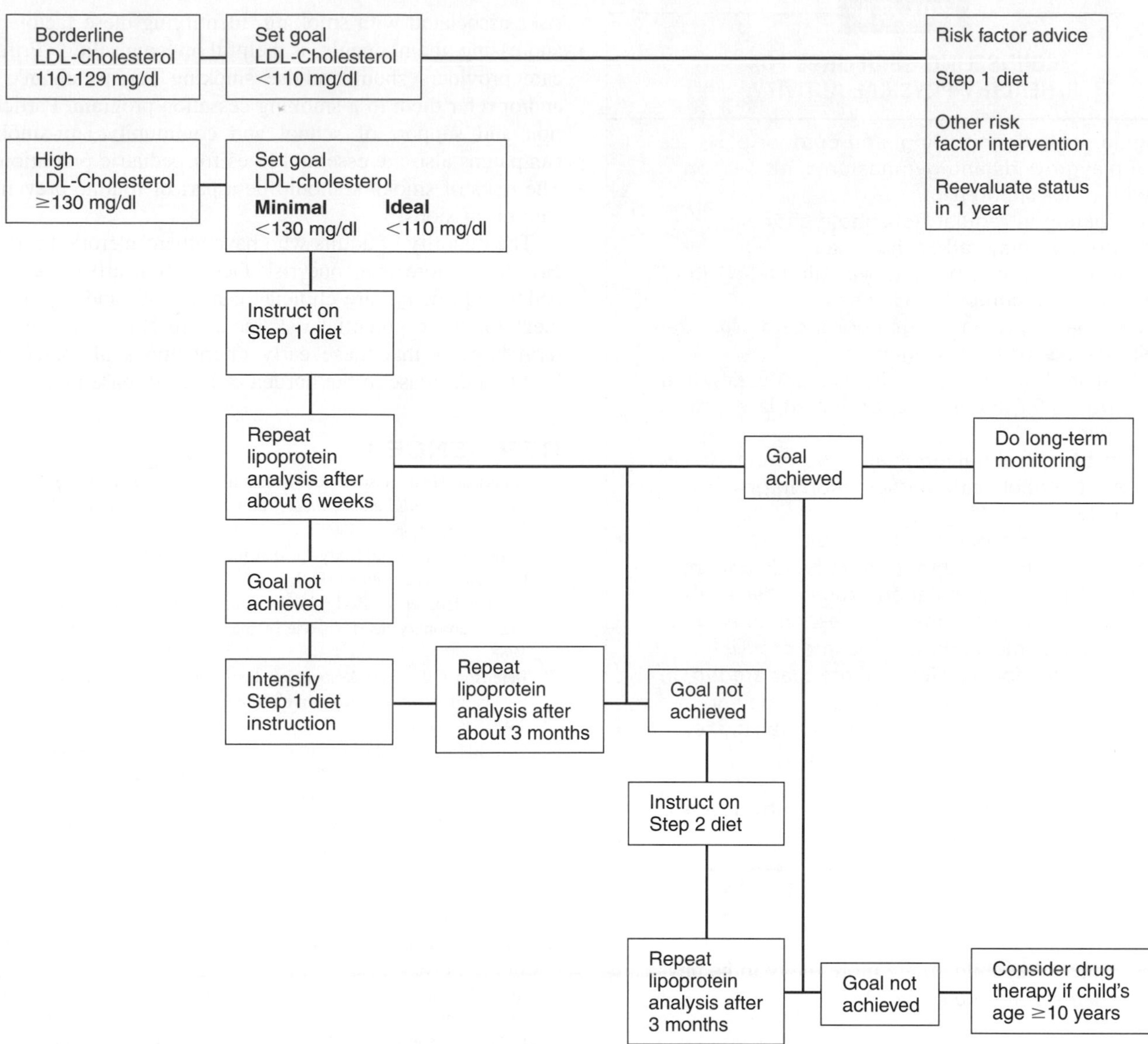

Fig. 23-4 Diet therapy.

(From National Cholesterol Education Program: *Report of the expert panel on blood cholesterol levels in children and adolescents,* National Institutes of Health Pub No 91-2732, Rockville, Md, US Department of Health and Human Services.)

creases were seen in children ages 12 to 17.[28] Blacks and Hispanics have a higher incidence of obesity compared with whites, although the effects of confounding variables such as education and income level are not understood fully.[6,24] Although genetic factors are important in the etiology of obesity, environmental factors also play a role, suggesting that intervention by the medical establishment may be important. No universally accepted definition of obesity exists; however, a reasonable approach would be to identify children who have a body mass index (kg/m^2) greater than the 85th percentile as "overweight" and those who have a body mass index greater than the 95th percentile as "obese." One approach suggests that these patients should be screened for hypertension, orthopedic complaints, hypoventilation, and abnormalities of lipids and glucose metabolism.[12] The need for additional endocrinological evaluation should be made on a case by case analysis. No single treatment program for children has been proven to be uniformly successful. A combination of dietary and exercise therapy with behavioral modification and family counseling is sometimes needed.

The role of physical activity in preventing or ameliorating other risk factors such as obesity, hyperlipidemia, and hypertension has been recognized increasingly over the past several years. Furthermore, higher levels of physical activity have been associated with decreased rates of heart disease above and beyond those associated with changes in known cardiac risk factors.[5,22] Children in the United States have become more sedentary in recent decades; some of these changes are attributed to increased television and computer use and a decrease in physical education programs in schools. The combination of decreased physical activity and increased caloric intake undoubtedly contributes to the increase in obesity. The goal of health care professionals should be to encourage children to make physical activity a part of their daily routine (Box 23-4).[1] Children and their families should be encouraged to be physically active, and

BOX 23-4

COUNSELING GUIDELINES FOR HEALTHY PHYSICAL ACTIVITY

Regular walking, bicycling, and outdoor play; use of playgrounds and gymnasiums; interaction with other children
Participation in regular household chores
Emphasis on play rather than exercise
Fewer than 2 hours per day watching television, videos, and computer activities
Weekly participation in age-appropriate organized sports, lessons, clubs, games
Daily school or child care physical education that includes 20 minutes of coordinated large muscle exercise
Access to school buildings and community facilities that enable safe participation in physical activity
Extracurricular programs in schools and community recreation centers to meet needs and interests of specific populations such as racial and ethnic minority groups, females, persons who have disabilities, and low-income groups
Opportunities for physical activity that are fun, increase confidence, and involve friends and peers
Regular family outings that involve walking, cycling, swimming, and other recreation
Positive role modeling for a physically active lifestyle by parents, other caretakers, physicians, and school personnel

Data from Anderson AJ, et al: *Arterioscl* 8:88, 1988.

studies suggest that children are more likely to be physically active if their parents are active.[18]

SMOKING

The evidence that cigarette smoking is a risk factor for cardiovascular disease is overwhelming. Studies as early as 1940 determined a relationship between coronary artery disease and tobacco use.[8] A task force formed in 1996 "considered proven" that smoking increases the risk for cardiovascular disease. In addition to negative effects on lipid levels, tobacco usage is associated with decreased exercise capacity, increased platelet aggregation, increased incidence of respiratory illness, low-birth-weight deliveries, and increased infant mortality. In addition, exposure to passive smoking has been linked with changes in risk factors for coronary artery disease in children. Neufeld et al found a relationship between passive smoking and reduced HDL-cholesterol in children who have high-risk lipid profiles.[20]

Adolescents are the largest growing population of smokers. The risk of starting to smoke increases from ages 12 to 16 years. Preventing smoking, therefore, lies in the realm of pediatric practice. Children whose parents or siblings smoke are at an increased risk of beginning to smoke. Other factors that may play a role in predicting children at risk for smoking include peer influence, less educated parents, independence and rebelliousness, and decreased concerns about the health risks associated with smoking. Identifying these factors and addressing them openly is helpful in counseling. Primary care providers should advise smoking parents about risks and/or refer them to a smoking cessation program. Participation and support of school and community anti-smoking campaigns also are essential roles for pediatric practitioners. The risks of smoking should be a part of routine preventive care discussions.

The majority of adults who have atherosclerotic heart disease have more than one risk factor for heart disease. The pediatric primary care clinician can identify and begin treatment for these potential risk factors in children. The long-term hope is that these early interventions ultimately will lead to a decrease in the burden of heart disease in adult life.

REFERENCES

1. American Heart Association: Scientific position: *Exercise (physical activity) and children in heart and stroke A-Z Guide*, http:www.//americanheart.org.
2. Anderson AJ, et al: Body fat distribution, plasma lipids, and lipoproteins, *Arterioscler* 8:88, 1988.
3. Barakat HA, et al: Body fat distribution, plasma lipoproteins and the risk of coronary heart disease of male subjects, *Int J Obesity* 12:473, 1988.
4. Berenson GS, et al: Association between multiple cardiovascular risk factors and atherosclerosis in children and young adults, *N Engl J Med* 338:1650, 1998.
5. Blair SN, et al: Influences of cardiorespiratory fitness and other precursors on cardiovascular disease and all-cause mortality in men and women, *JAMA* 276:205, 1996.
6. Brussard BA, et al: Prevalence of obesity in American Indians and Alaska natives, *Am J Clin Nutr* 53:1535S, 1991.
7. Dennison BA, et al: Parental history of cardiovascular disease as an indication for screening for lipoprotein abnormalities in children, *J Pediatr* 115:186, 1989.
8. English JP, Willus FA, Berkson J: Tobacco and coronary disease, *JAMA* 13:1327, 1940.
9. Enos WF, Beyer JC, Holmes RH: Pathogenesis of coronary artery disease in American soldiers killed in Korea, *JAMA* 158:912, 1953.
10. Fisher EA, Van Horn L, McGill HC for the Nutrition Committee: Nutrition and Children, *Circulation* 95:2332, 1997.
11. Garber AM: Cholesterol screening should be targeted, *Am J Med* 102: 26, 1997.
12. Gidding SS: Preventive pediatric cardiology, *Pediatr Clin North Am* 46:253, 1999.
13. Gidding SS, et al: Understanding obesity in youth, *Circulation* 94:3383, 1996.
14. Gortmaker SL: Increasing obesity in childhood, *Am J Dis Child* 141: 535, 1987.
15. Kaplan NM: The deadly quartet: upper-body obesity, glucose intolerance, hypertriglyceridemia and hypertension, *Arch Intern Med* 149:1514, 1989.
16. McGill HC Jr, et al: Relation of glycohemoglobin and adiposity to atherosclerosis in youth: Pathobiological Determinants of Atherosclerosis in Youth (PDAY) Research Group, *Arterioscler Thromb Vasc Biol* 15:431, 1995.
17. McGill HC, et al: Effects of serum lipoproteins and smoking on atherosclerosis in young men and women, *Arterioscler Thromb Vasc Biol* 17:95, 1997.
18. Moore LL, et al: Influence of parents' physical activity levels on activity levels of young children, *J Pediatr* 118:215, 1991.
19. National Cholesterol Education Program: Report of the Expert Panel on Blood Cholesterol Levels in Children and Adolescents, *Pediatrics* 89: 525, 1992.
20. Neufeld EJ, et al: Passive cigarette smoking and reduced HDL cholesterol levels in children with high-risk lipid profiles, *Circulation* 96:1403, 1997.

21. Newman TB, Browner WS, Hulley SB: The case against childhood cholesterol screening, *JAMA* 264:3039, 1990.
22. Paffenbarager RSJ, et al: The association of changes in physical activity level and other lifestyle characteristics with mortality among men, *N Engl J Med* 328:538, 1993.
23. Pasternak RC, et al: Task force 3: spectrum of risk factors for coronary heart disease, *J Am Coll Cardiol* 27:978, 1996.
24. Pawson IG, Martorell R, Mendoza FE: Prevalence of overweight and obesity in US Hispanic populations, *Am J Clin Nutr* 53:1522S, 1991.
25. Scientific Steering Committee on behalf of the Simon Broome Register Group: Mortality in treated heterozygous familial hypercholesterolaemia: implications for clinical management, *Atheroscler* 142:105, 1999.
26. Stamler J, et al: Relationship of baseline major risk factors to coronary and all-cause mortality, and to longevity: findings from long-term follow-up of Chicago cohorts, *Cardiology* 82:191, 1993.
27. Starc TJ, et al: Family history fails to identify many children with severe hypercholesterolemia, *Am J Dis Child* 145:61, 1991.
28. Troiano RP, et al: Overweight prevalence and trends for children and adolescents: the National Health and Examination Surveys, 1963-1991. *Arch Pediatr Adoles Med* 149:1085, 1995.
29. Williams C: Prevention of coronary artery disease. In Gewitz MH, editor: *Primary pediatric cardiology,* Armonk, NY, 1995, Futura Publishing.
30. Writing Group of the DISC Collaborative Research Group: Efficacy and safety of lowering dietary intake of fat and cholesterol on children with elevated low-density lipoprotein cholesterol, *JAMA* 273:1429, 1995.

four Violence Prevention

Robert D. Sege

UNDERSTANDING VIOLENCE

Most peer violence in the United States results from conflicts between friends, acquaintances, or intimate partners. Estimates of stranger violence range from 6% to a maximum of 40%. Published estimates from the Department of Justice and from primary care and emergency room surveillance projects indicate that violence of all levels of severity is a result of conflicts between persons who know each other, often quite well. Although physicians traditionally have viewed patients as the victims, this new insight suggests that the distinction between victim and perpetrator is more fluid and varied than previously thought. From a public health perspective, the conclusions from years of research is dramatically simple: young people who fight get hurt.

Thus, primary prevention in pediatrics must focus beyond preventing a child from becoming a victim; it must help the child learn the importance of nonviolent problem-solving skills and attitudes. The development of these skills and attitudes begins in infancy. Effective, nonviolent discipline is one key to developing resilient children who can resist being drawn into violence.

VIOLENCE IS LEARNED

In the 1980s, Patterson proposed a model, based on an extensive review of the literature, that accounted for the developmental progression of antisocial behavior.[7] Antisocial behavior begins with coercive or inadequate parenting in early childhood. Children whose parents are unable to set effective limits, particularly where extensive use of corporal punishment is used, develop dysfunctional behavior patterns in interactions with their peers and with adult authorities, including teachers. These children, then, have behavioral problems even before they enter school.

In school, the children are both rejected by "normal" peers and have difficulties academically. In later childhood and adolescence, these ostracized children find each other and form peer groups that reward violence and antisocial behavior. The result of this cycle, which began in early childhood, is juvenile delinquency.

More recent descriptions of growing up in violent urban settings have reiterated the importance of peer relationships but stressed the central role that being willing to fight plays in establishing social hierarchy.[3] Boys, in particular, need to establish themselves as courageous fighters early in life or else they fear that they will be picked on. Nevertheless, the majority of the young men growing up in these communities have figured out how to avoid participating in violence. Their resilience begins early in life.

This model provides a focus for interventions in the pediatric office. In 1999, the AAP task force on youth violence endorsed a similar, far-reaching model that traces the origins of violent behavior to earliest childhood.[2] Although many social and environmental factors place children at high risk for violence, countervailing resilience factors, many beginning in early childhood, help to reduce the risk. The following discussion contains practical advice for addressing these issues in the office.

WITNESSING VIOLENCE: DOMESTIC VIOLENCE

The greatest risks for infants and toddlers revolve around the family, particularly domestic violence and child abuse. One of the goals of the pediatrician in speaking with families of new babies can be to assess family functioning, including the risks of domestic violence. Pediatricians suspicious that the patient's mother has been the victim of spousal abuse should ask her directly: Have available in the office information concerning battered women's advocates or shelters.[1] Many offices place small cards with relevant telephone numbers in the restroom, so that this information can be obtained discretely.

WITNESSING VIOLENCE: TELEVISION VIOLENCE

American children spend more time watching television than any other activity except sleep—more time than they spend going to school. While watching television, they observe an enormous amount of violence; the average child will "see" more than 10,000 deaths resulting from violence before completing high school.

Television violence differs from real-life violence in quality as well as quantity. On television, violence is used by both heroes and villains and generally is viewed as socially acceptable behavior in TV land. Although adults feel competent to separate fiction from reality, research suggests that even adults exposed to television violence have a more negative view of society and feel more hopeless and alienated than do less frequent viewers. Those adults who rely on television as their major news source, for example, feel less safe in their homes and neighborhoods than do other adults.

Children, because they have more difficulty separating facts from fantasy, are even more likely to be affected by television violence. The American Psychological Association, in reviewing hundreds of research studies, has concluded that exposure to television violence is a major risk for children.[5] Children who view television are more likely to experience violence as victims or aggressors and are much less likely to intervene in tense situations, as bystanders, to reduce the likelihood of violence.

Television and its influence on children is discussed further in Chapter 69, Children, Adolescents, and the Media.

VIOLENCE IN URBAN MINORITY COMMUNITIES

Ethnographic research conducted in some of America's poorest urban neighborhoods has identified another pattern of violence, in which fighting and the willingness to fight are key components of a broader protective strategy for coping with extremely dangerous environments. The following is variously called the "sucker" phenomenon or the "Code of the Streets": Young people have observed that suckers, unable to defend themselves, are likely prey to multiple and repeated attacks. Parents also understand this phenomenon and encourage their children to "stand up for themselves" by becoming able fighters.[3] Other parents adopt protective strategies that keep their children out of harm's way in the first place, often by enrolling them in supervised after-school programs or keeping them safely in the house, watching television, rather than risking participation in the street culture.

In counseling patients in these communities, physicians need to be aware of this logic and refrain from offering unrealistic or counter-productive advice. Nevertheless, in discussions with most young people, we need to remember that these same communities also contain nonviolent problem solvers who are well known to the their classmates. Thus, the validity of the code of the streets need not prevent individual children and adolescents from avoiding violent injuries through avoiding the culture of violence.

PRIMARY PREVENTION: ANTICIPATORY GUIDANCE

Young Children

During infancy and early childhood, patterns of behavior and family interactions are established. The proper role of the pediatrician is to ameliorate risk factors and reinforce those factors that protect the child from harm. In this age group, the following topics should be addressed to the parents during anticipatory guidance: (1) reduction in exposure to violence, including both domestic violence and television violence, and (2) teaching appropriate, nonviolent methods of discipline (violence-free parenting). Because patients and families see their physicians often during this age period, there are multiple opportunities for brief, focused interventions. Our research has demonstrated the effectiveness of focused guidance during early childhood.

Violence-free parenting: effective parenting without corporal punishment. As children enter the second year of life, patterns of discipline become established in families. Developmentally, this is an age when children typically are separating emotionally and cognitively from their parents, a time of potential stress in the family. Several lines of research evidence suggest that there is a link between the use of corporal punishment and the subsequent use of violence by children as they grow up. The AAP issued a policy statement in 1998 advocating that pediatricians counsel families in the use of alternatives to corporal punishments.

Many families, however, believe in the need for corporal punishment. A direct challenge to family beliefs is unlikely to lead to successful behavior change. Instead, the pediatrician may realize several things about families who use corporal punishment. First, most of the parents who use corporal punishment do not like to hit their children. This results in an erratic pattern of punishment, as parents end up using threats and cajoling to avoid spanking. Second, these same parents often believe that there are some children who "don't need to be spanked." One appropriate goal for guiding these families is to teach them effective techniques for discipline that will allow their children to be among those who do not "need" to be spanked.

Most importantly, many parents have little knowledge of other effective alternatives to corporal punishment. Faced with a choice of spanking a child or letting him "run wild," many parents will opt for corporal punishment. The goal for anticipatory guidance at this age, therefore, is to describe and endorse specific effective behavioral techniques to help discipline children.

Maintaining toddler discipline is understood best from the child's perspective: toddlers gain power over their world by being able to understand what is happening and predict what will happen next. Maintaining a schedule for children—for example, bedtimes, naptimes, mealtimes, bath time, and play time—helps give the child this feeling of mastery.

Toddlers crave parental attention. The best kind of attention, of course, is parental praise for good behavior. In the absence of this positive reinforcement, toddlers may feel ignored and misbehave simply to grab the attention of their parents. The parental misperception that children who are praised will become self-centered and egotistical blocks the effective use of parenting and parental attention for good behavior. Parents can be told very simply to tell their child, "I love it when you do . . . "

Of course, there are times when a child's misbehavior necessitates negative consequences. The most effective simple negative reinforcement technique for parents to use is "time out" from positive reinforcement. Parents can be taught that time-outs can be used judiciously, in the background of positive reinforcement, and consistently whenever the child has certain behavior patterns that need to be stopped. Children should be placed in time-out for approximately 1 minute per year of age. Parents should explain clearly to the child why the time-out was deserved and ignore the child during the time-out. Longer explanations and discussions should be deferred until things have calmed down.

School Age

As children get older, the external influences of their behavior become more important. This is the age when television has an enormous impact. It also is the age when children begin dealing with playground fights and bullying.

Bullying. Bullying prevention is an important task for school administrators. Bullying—the repeated infliction of harm on younger, smaller, or less powerful peers—is a nearly universal problem for school-age children. Severe and even lethal bullying has been described in the United Kingdom, Japan, and Scandinavia, as well as in the United States. Bullies usually are larger and stronger (among boys) or more socially powerful (among girls) than are their victims. Typically, bullies will begin the school year by trying to pick on several children. Those children who become singled out as targets are weaker, physically and emotionally, and unable to strike back either physically or verbally. Although bullying is a problem of school-age children, the negative behaviors often happen outside of school supervision: before school, after school, or at recess. Thus, classroom teachers often are unaware of the problem and almost always are unable to solve it without significant support from their administrators.

Bullying has severe adverse consequences for both bully and victim. Victims may be hurt physically, often cannot concentrate on their studies, and develop poor self-esteem. Recent news reports suggest that several perpetrators in school shootings in the United States were victims of bullies, and their lethal outbursts may have resulted from the effects of being bullied.

Children who are bullies, in contrast, often feel powerful and effective. They typically come from chaotic households, and their parents feel ineffective in controlling their behavior. Often, bullies do not experience effective limit-setting at home. In the long term, the outcome for bullies is poor: by age 30, they are more likely to be incarcerated and less likely to be employed, married, or in other stable adult relationships than their peers.

Olweus has developed an effective anti-bullying program in Scandinavia, where it has led to a dramatic reduction in bullying.[6] Reports in the United States suggest that it also may be effective here. Anti-bullying programs begin with information gathering. Students, who are asked to complete anonymous surveys, are quite willing to report to school administrators where and when bullying usually occurs. Active efforts to control bullying occur on three levels: in the school building and grounds, in the classroom, and with individual students.

Schoolwide interventions focus on two issues: ensuring a safe physical environment and endorsing and coordinating classroom activities. To ensure a safe physical environment, staff monitoring is improved before and after school and at lunch, and any architectural or landscaping changes needed to improve supervision are made. A schoolwide assembly is convened in which it is announced that bullying will not be tolerated anywhere in the school environment and that all necessary steps will be taken to control it.

Classroom teachers lead discussions with their students. These discussions identify roles of bullies, victims, and bystanders and establish that bullying behavior will not be tolerated. The students themselves are helped to generate rules to prevent bullying and to prevent the social isolation of victims. The students agree to (1) report bullying behavior, and (2) resist attempts by the bullies to ostracize their victims. Successful anti-bullying programs work, in part, by mobilizing the large number of bystanders. In so doing, they make bullies less respected and accepted by their peers and, thereby, reduce the allure of bullying.

Individual measures reinforce the anti-bullying messages. When bullies are identified, the child receives a stern message from the principal, and the principal also speaks with the child's parents. Parents are told of the possible short- and long-term consequences for their child, and a social worker or guidance counselor is assigned to work with them on setting appropriate and enforceable behavioral limits at home.

Television. The AAP Committee on Communications has recommended that pediatricians counsel families to reduce the amount of television viewing by young children. Pediatricians should counsel parents to:

- Limit television viewing to 2 hours or fewer per day
- Monitor the content of the programs their children watch, restricting access to especially violent programs
- Discuss television programming and news with their children
- Not place a television set in the child's bedroom

Adolescents

Adolescents are affected disproportionately by violence.[4] This has long been a major concern of urban teens and parents, and the recent outbreak of school violence has led to a much broader concern in American society. Pediatricians have several clear roles to play in working with their adolescent patients to reduce the risk of violence: (1) screening all adolescents to identify those at high risk, (2) preventing reinjury to injured adolescents, and (3) referring high-risk or traumatized adolescents for appropriate treatment. See also Chapter 112, Violent and Aggressive Behavior.

Screening

VIOLENCE HISTORY. Teenagers can be asked directly about their experiences with violence, using the acronym FISTS (Box 23-5).

FIGHTING. Ask about the teen's last fight and about the number of fights he or she has been in in the past 12 months. Those teens who have been in more than one physical fight in the preceding 12 months are at increased risk of violence-related injury.

INJURIES. A review of medical records of teens seriously injured or killed through violence usually reveals previous episodes of injuries that required medical attention. Multiple or serious previous injuries may indicate an increased risk of future injury.

SEXUAL VIOLENCE. Teen-dating violence is both a serious problem in itself and a harbinger of future domestic violence.

THREATS. Previous threats with a weapon indicate that the patient is at future risk of weapons-related injury, either through the circumstances that led to the original threat or

BOX 23-5

TAKING A VIOLENCE HISTORY ADOLESCENTS AND YOUNG ADULTS (FISTS)

Fighting: When was your last pushing/shoving fight? How many fights have you been in in the past month? Year?

Injuries: Have you ever been injured in a fight? Has anyone you know been injured in a fight? Has anyone you know been injured or killed?

Sexual violence: What happens when you and your boyfriend or girlfriend have an argument? Have you ever been forced to have sex against your will?

Threats: Have you ever been threatened with a knife? A gun?

Self-defense: How do you avoid getting in fights? Do you carry a weapon for self-defense?

Alpert E, Sege R, Bradshaw Y: Interpersonal violence and the education of physicians, *Acad Med* 72(suppl):S41, 1997.

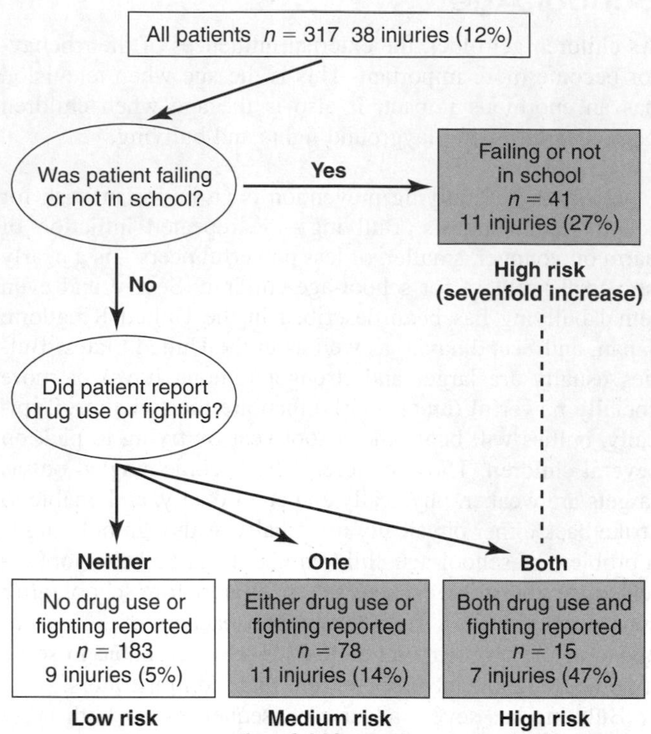

Fig. 23-5 Classification of patients into high, medium, and low risk for future violence-related injury.
(From Sege RD, et al: *J Adolesc Health* 24:395, 1999.)

because these young people are far more likely to arm themselves than are those who have never been threatened directly.

SELF-DEFENSE. Those young people who have learned to de-escalate situations of conflict (or to avoid them altogether) deserve praise and encouragement. On the other hand, those teens who arm themselves in self-defense are at extremely high risk, as discussed above. (See Bullying, p. 319.)

Risk factor screening

A second, broader set of risk factors influences the likelihood of serious violence-related injury. Problem teen behaviors tend to cluster, as a result of both intrapersonal and social factors. As shown in Fig. 23-5, analysis of office-based risk factor screening has identified three classes of risk. Young people in school who report neither drug use nor fighting to their primary care provider are at low risk of violence-related injuries.[8] Those who are in school and are passing their courses, but who report either fighting or drug use, are at medium risk—approximately 3 times that of low-risk students. Those adolescents who are failing school, already dropped out of school, or report both fighting and drug use are at about a sevenfold increased risk for future violence-related injury than are low-risk students.

COUNSELING AND REFERRAL FOR ADOLESCENTS AT INCREASED RISK. Intervention for these patients identified as being at increased risk for violence-related injuries through either screening approach must be tailored to fit both the degree of risk and the individual circumstances of each child. Those at low risk deserve acknowledgment of their success at avoiding this problem, particularly noting that it often takes courage to walk away from a fight. Teens at moderate risk need to hear that the risks are real and individual: "You are strong and healthy. However, I am worried about your telling me that you have been in several fights this year." Basic information concerning techniques for defusing particularly tense situations should be discussed. Teens who carry weapons, have left school, or otherwise are at high risk deserve intense social service or psychological intervention. Adolescent health providers need to maintain a roster of appropriate community-based referral agencies or individual counselors for these children and emphasize the importance of follow-up to both the patient and parents.

Following a fight (secondary prevention)

Patients who have been hurt in a fight are at high risk for further violence either as the victim of another violence-related injury or by attempting to exact revenge on the assailants. The immediate need after an injury is for crisis intervention. Ask the patient: "Is the fight over? Do you feel safe leaving here? If the fight is ongoing, is there someone who can mediate?" If the situation is volatile, the patient and family should be referred to social services or, occasionally, the police. At a minimum, parents and patients should be advised of the risk of serious injury and that successful injury prevention involves learning how to de-escalate conflicts.

Following a serious injury, the following steps have been advocated:

- Have the child tell you about the problem. Allow the narrative to flow freely, avoiding judgments. This allows for feelings about revenge to be expressed and offers an opportunity to learn of the patient's perspective before offering advice.
- Evaluate the youth's other risks: Does he or she carry a weapon? Does he or she use alcohol or other drugs? Is the youth involved in a gang?
- Discuss with the patient the known risk factors for violence, including that most violent injuries occur between friends or acquaintances and often involve alcohol or

drugs. Weapons-carrying *increases* the risk of serious injury by encouraging the patient to take unnecessary risks and by encouraging his or her opponent to "draw first."

- Develop a plan to stay safe after leaving the hospital or clinic. Does he or she have a relative with whom to stay who lives out of the neighborhood? Do the police need to be involved?
- Discuss conflict-avoidance strategies. This discussion can start with the particular incident involved and may need to be continued on subsequent visits. Health care professionals need to respect the patient's need not to be labeled as a "sucker" by peers.
- Refer to other services, including psychology or social work. For many patients, this may involve reaching out to church members, recreation departments, or mentoring programs.

Advocacy

As is apparent from the previous discussion, youth violence, although a serious health risk, is a complex social problem that requires broad-based public action. Pediatricians, in addition to caring for their own patients, often are able to influence public debate in areas that affect child health. The AAP and other organizations have advocated for social policies that benefit children.

Those pediatricians who serve as school consultants have a critical role to play. School boards and principals should be advised of the importance of age-appropriate violence prevention programs. A number of successful school programs have been developed and are available for adaptation and use in other schools. Primary schools can focus on adequate supervision of playgrounds, teaching and modeling nonviolent problem-solving skills, and implementing effective anti-bullying programs. Middle schools have several proven anti-violence and conflict resolution curricula available that can be incorporated into health education programs. Successful high school programs may involve the use the school health clinics to provide services to students who have problems of violence, drug abuse, or pregnancy. Schools have successfully developed peer education programs to help reinforce these areas of concern. Peer mediation, which allows students another, formal venue for resolving conflict, has been widely adopted and appears to be quite successful, both in school and in the communities in which the students live.

Media violence recently has received greater public attention, in part due to concerted efforts by pediatricians and child psychologists to call attention to the dangers of excess exposure to media violence. In addition to counseling individual families, many pediatricians have provided testimony at public hearings or endorsed community TV "tune-out" weeks.

Despite a general reduction in traumatic injury and death, child and adolescent deaths caused by firearms continue to soar. Individual families can be counseled that the safest home for children is one without handguns and that any guns present in the home should be locked and unloaded. State and federal regulations now under consideration would mandate the provision of trigger locks and prevent the marketing of certain kinds of weapons. Physician testimony and endorsement by medical professional organizations have helped push forward these initiatives.

SUMMARY

Adolescent peer violence is a major cause of death and disability for American children. Although the problem has complex social roots and requires multifaceted solutions, pediatricians have important roles to play. Primary prevention of violence begins with anticipatory guidance for parents of infants and toddlers. Secondary prevention involves the identification, counseling, and referral of high-risk patients and should be a part of a standard care for older children and adolescents. Finally, pediatricians can advocate for school policies and state and federal legislation to reduce the risk of violence for children.

REFERENCES

1. Alpert E, Sege R, Bradshaw Y: Interpersonal violence and the education of physicians, *Acad Med* 72(suppl):S41, 1997.
2. American Academy of Pediatrics Task Force on Violence: The role of the pediatrician in youth violence prevention in clinical practice and at the community level, *Pediatrics* 103:173, 1999.
3. Canada G: *Fist, stick, knife, gun: a personal history of violence in America*, Boston, 1995, Beacon Press.
4. Centers for Disease Control and Prevention: *Mortality trends, causes of death, and related risk behaviors among US adolescents,* Atlanta, 1995.
5. Donnerstein E, Slaby RG, Eron LD: The mass media and youth aggression. In Eron LD, Gentry JH, Schlegel P, editors: *Reason to hope: a psychosocial perspective on violence and youth,* Washington, DC, 1996, American Psychological Association.
6. Olweus D: *Bullying at school*, Oxford, UK, 1993, Blackwell Publishers.
7. Patterson GR, DeBaryshe D, Ramsey E: A developmental perspective on antisocial behavior, *Am Psychol* 44:331, 1989.
8. Sege R, et al: Ten years after: examination of adolescent screening questions that predict future violence-related injury, *J Adolesc Health* 24:395, 1999.

five Prevention of Smoking

C. Andrew Aligne

SMOKING AS A PEDIATRIC DISEASE

Cigarette smoking is the single most common cause of premature death and disability in the United States.[6] Although much of the attention about tobacco use has been focused on adults, smoking also is a pediatric disease: Most smokers start as minors, and passive smoking is an important preventable cause of death and disease among young children.[1,27] Moreover, these are problems that are becoming increasingly widespread. The prevalence of current cigarette smoking among U.S. high school students is above 36%, and more than 42% of children are exposed regularly to tobacco smoke.[11,34] Tobacco companies have continued ingenious and extremely aggressive marketing campaigns, many of which have been aimed directly at children; these have increased the initiation of cigarette smoking over the past decade.[10,29,33,36] Thus, we can expect to see a rise in the num-

BOX 23-6

DISEASES ASSOCIATED WITH PASSIVE SMOKING

Perinatal: Fetal loss, prematurity, low birth weight, perinatal death, difficulty with breast-feeding
Infancy: Sudden infant death syndrome
Pulmonary: RSV bronchiolitis; development and exacerbation of asthma; exacerbation of cystic fibrosis; pneumonia; reduced lung function
Upper respiratory: Acute and chronic otitis media; irritation of the eyes, nose, and throat; tonsillitis; upper respiratory infections
Allergic: Allergic rhinitis; atopic eczema
Growth: Decreases in linear growth of 1 to 2 cm
Intellectual development: Missed school days, lower scores on intelligence tests, grade retention in school
Behavioral problems: Decreased attention span; hyperactivity; aggressiveness
Miscellaneous: Fire injuries; future active smoking
Adult health effects: Cardiovascular disease; lung cancer

ber of today's children who will become adult smokers. As a result, there will be even more children born exposed to parents who smoke.

Passive Smoking

Tobacco smoke is a poisonous mixture of more than 4000 substances, including known carcinogens and toxins such as benzene and carbon monoxide.[8] Although filter tips on cigarettes can reduce the toxicity of the "mainstream smoke" delivered directly to the active smoker, they do nothing to reduce the toxicity of what is released from the burning end of the cigarette to nonsmoking bystanders. Indeed, this "sidestream smoke" generally has higher concentrations of harmful compounds than does mainstream smoke.[52] In addition, children are more vulnerable than adults to such exposures because of their smaller size, higher metabolic rate, and on-going development. Multiple studies over the past few decades have provided overwhelming evidence of the hazards of both active and passive smoking.* Even the tobacco industry's research shows that active and passive smoking are harmful.[4,24] Box 23-6 lists conditions that have been found to be associated with children's exposure to environmental tobacco smoke.

Reliable data exist that allow one to calculate the impact of parental smoking for the following tobacco-related causes of pediatric death: low birth weight (LBW), sudden infant death syndrome (SIDS), respiratory syncytial virus (RSV) bronchiolitis, and fire injuries. Little direct information is available regarding smoking-related deaths for children; passive smoking is not listed as an official cause on death certificates. However, using published determinations of the relative risk (RR) for having disease if one is exposed to tobacco, and the proportion of children exposed to tobacco P(E), it is possible to calculate the attributable risk (AR)—that is, the fraction of cases of disease that would not have occurred had no one in the population been exposed. Using the AR and the known national incidence of various pediatric illnesses, one can determine the number of annual cases attributable to passive smoking.

Women who smoke during pregnancy, compared with nonsmokers, have almost twice the risk of delivering a low-birth-weight infant.[17] Low birth weight accounts for half of all infant deaths and significant long-term morbidity for many of the survivors. Maternal smoking contributes to approximately 5% of perinatal deaths (less than 1 month old), or 2800 deaths per year. SIDS is the leading cause of death in infants between 1 month and 1 year of age, resulting in more than 5500 deaths per year. The AR fraction for smoking is 36%, which is equivalent to almost 2000 cases of SIDS each year. RSV bronchiolitis is the leading cause of lower respiratory infection in infants and young children; it leads to 4500 deaths each year; the AR to smoking for cases of RSV is 25%, leading to approximately 1100 deaths annually. Fire and burn injuries are the third leading cause of death for children. Neglected cigarettes kill more Americans than any other cause of fire, and cigarette-related paraphernalia such as matches and lighters cause ignition in another 33% of all fires that kill children under age 5 years. Approximately 200 pediatric fire-deaths annually are related to smoking. Adding up the numbers just cited yields a total of approximately 6000 excess childhood deaths annually. Hence, parental smoking has been estimated to kill more preschool children than motor vehicle crashes, poisonings, drownings, gunshots, bicycle accidents, and all other unintentional injuries combined.[1,17]

Primary pediatric care practitioners are the only medical professionals who come into contact routinely with nonsmokers at high risk of becoming smokers (i.e., preadolescents); thus, they are in an excellent position to try to prevent smoking. These clinicians also may be the only medical professionals in routine contact with parents of young children, because healthy young adults rarely visit physicians. Thus, because of their regular contact with young children and their families, pediatricians have the opportunity to intervene against both active and passive smoking.

Many physicians have self-defeating beliefs regarding smoking-related anticipatory guidance, such as that smokers do not welcome such questioning, that it is not the pediatrician's responsibility to discuss the parents' behavior, that there is no time for discussing smoking, or that there is nothing to offer if someone says that he or she wants to quit.[20,21] Physicians should document smoking at all health supervision visits; however, many of them are not doing so: Only 11% in one study routinely recorded smoking information on charts.[19,21] However, studies of parents' attitudes reveal that more than 85% of smoking mothers who were bringing their child to a pediatrician reported that they would welcome, or at least not mind, their child's physician asking them about tobacco use.[20,26] Most smoking parents would like to quit but have been addicted to nicotine since childhood.[27] Perhaps the most critical times to intervene are at the prenatal visit or directly after a baby's birth, because it is very common for women who abstain from smoking during pregnancy to resume after the baby is born.[39,53,56]

*References 3, 12, 14-17, 31, 37, 43-47, 52.

"Red flags." Certain medical complaints represent "red flags" that should prompt the pediatrician to address passive smoking. For example, visits for recurrent otitis or hospitalizations for asthma constitute opportunities to reinforce the link between smoking and the child's illness. Inquiries should be nonaccusatory. Any discussions of smoking should communicate that it is an addictive behavior that harms the smoker and those around him, and that you are offering encouragement and help to stop this addiction. Congratulate nonsmokers, including those who have quit smoking. Many options are available for helping people to quit smoking. Although there is little evidence for effective cessation programs for teens, it generally is recommended that strategies found to have some effectiveness in adults be used for adolescents. Young people who do start smoking can become addicted to tobacco very quickly, and some may want to stop smoking.[33,35] Basic cessation counseling involves the "four As": Ask about smoking at every opportunity; advise all smokers to quit; assist the smoker to stop; arrange follow-up.[35,48,53] The effectiveness of such counseling is enhanced by medical therapies such as nicotine replacement and by organizational factors including reminders in patients' charts.[30,40-42]

Reducing children's exposure. For parents who are unwilling or unable to quit, efforts must be directed toward reducing children's exposure to tobacco smoke.[7] Absorption of tobacco smoke by children is a function of the number of cigarettes smoked around the child and the proximity of the smokers, and a dose-response relationship has been noted between exposure and health effects.[13,25] Thus, even reduction of smoking (as opposed to complete cessation) will benefit the child.[54] Smoking should not be allowed inside the home or other places in which the child spends significant amounts of time (including automobiles). If a family member insists on smoking indoors, he or she should smoke as far away from the child as possible, perhaps going under a kitchen exhaust fan or by an open window.[32]

Preventing Initiation

The optimal solution to the problem of tobacco-related disease in children, adolescents, and adults would involve preventing the *initiation* of smoking.[38] Almost all smokers start before adulthood: The peak age of onset is 12 to 16 years, with the majority of smokers starting by age 14 and almost all by age 20.[22,23,28] Thus, anticipatory guidance regarding cigarettes should begin *before* age 12 years. There is some evidence that clinician advice against tobacco use is associated with decreased smoking initiation among young people: Youths to target are those who are poor, white, female, having trouble in school, and living with relatives or friends who smoke.[55] Discussing attitudes with pre-teens about smoking may reveal incorrect perceptions, which can be countered with facts: For example, children tend to believe that smoking is more prevalent than it really is and that quitting is easier than it really is.[18] On the other hand, children often do have correct knowledge of the health effects of smoking, but this does not appear to influence smoking initiation behavior strongly.[50]

The AAP has recommended that pediatricians abstain from smoking, promote a smoke-free environment in public places, support community anti-smoking programs, and cancel subscriptions to waiting-room magazines that advertise tobacco.[2] Comprehensive public health interventions that have been used to try to reduce smoking at a population level include increased cigarette taxes, mass media anti-cigarette campaigns, school programs, and increased enforcement of laws restricting the sale of tobacco to minors. Studies of statewide programs in Oregon, California, and Massachusetts indicate that an adequately funded, comprehensive tobacco control strategy including both increased excise taxes and mass media programs can reduce tobacco use quickly and substantially.[9] Support for such measures should help to decrease the prevalence of cigarette smoking in the United States and prevent the suffering it causes in people of all ages. It should be noted that even as the domestic market becomes more restricted, U.S. tobacco companies have become increasingly successful in capturing the market abroad, so that smoking is becoming a global epidemic.[5]

CONCLUSION

Smoking is a legitimate concern of pediatricians because it is a behavior that almost always starts during childhood and because children are innocent victims of passive smoking. Pediatricians can take many steps to help reduce the suffering caused by parental and youth smoking. As clinicians, they can screen for, document, and discuss both active and passive smoking behaviors, and they can offer (or refer for) help with smoking cessation, reduction, or abstinence. As citizens, they can advocate for effective population-level tobacco control measures in their communities and beyond. Reduction not only of overall smoking prevalence but also of youth smoking and childhood passive smoking are recognized as national health priorities.[51] Moreover, prevention of smoking initiation by future parents is primary prevention of passive smoking. Our goal should be a tobacco-free environment for all children.[2,49]

REFERENCES

1. Aligne CA, Stoddard JJ: Tobacco and children: an economic evaluation of the medical effects of parental smoking, *Arch Pediatr Adolesc Med* 151:648, 1997.
2. American Academy of Pediatrics, Committee on Substance Abuse: Tobacco-free environment: an imperative for the health of children and adolescents, *Pediatrics* 93:866, 1994.
3. Anderson HR, Cook DG: Passive smoking and sudden infant death syndrome: review of the epidemiological evidence, *Thorax* 52:1003, 1997.
4. Barnes DE, et al: Environmental tobacco smoke: the Brown and Williamson documents, *JAMA* 274:248, 1995.
5. Bartecchi CE, MacKenzie TD, Schrier RW: The global tobacco epidemic, *Sci Am* 272:44, 1995.
6. Bartecchi CE, MacKenzie TD, Schrier RW: The human costs of tobacco use (1), *N Engl J Med* 330:907, 1994.
7. Beeber SJ: Parental smoking and childhood asthma, *J Pediatr Health Care* 10:58, 1996.
8. Brownson RC, et al: Environmental tobacco smoke: health effects and policies to reduce exposure, *Annu Rev Public Health* 18:163, 1997.
9. Centers for Disease Control: Decline in cigarette consumption following implementation of a comprehensive tobacco prevention and education program—Oregon, 1996-1998, *MMWR* 48:140, 1999.

10. Centers for Disease Control: Incidence of initiation of cigarette smoking—United States, 1965-1996, *MMWR Morb Mortal Wkly Rep* 47:837, 1998.
11. Centers for Disease Control: Tobacco use among high school students—United States, 1997, *MMWR Morb Mortal Wkly Rep* 47:229, 1998.
12. Charlton A: Children and passive smoking: a review, *J Fam Pract* 3:267, 1994.
13. Chilmonczyk BA, et al: Association between exposure to environmental tobacco smoke and exacerbations of asthma in children, *N Engl J Med* 328:1665, 1993.
14. Cook DG, Strachan DP: Health effects of passive smoking. 3. Parental smoking and prevalence of respiratory symptoms and asthma in school age children, *Thorax* 52:1081, 1997.
15. Cook DG, Strachan DP: Parental smoking, bronchial reactivity and peak flow variability in children, *Thorax* 53:295, 1998.
16. Cook DG, Strachan DP, Carey IM: Health effects of passive smoking. 9. Parental smoking and spirometric indices in children, *Thorax* 53:884, 1998.
17. DiFranza JR, Lew RA: Morbidity and mortality in children associated with use of tobacco products by other people, *Pediatrics* 97:560, 1996.
18. Epps RP, Manley MW: A physician's guide to preventing tobacco use during childhood and adolescence, *Pediatrics* 88:140, 1991.
19. Fiore MC, et al: Smoking status as the new vital sign: effect on assessment and intervention in patients who smoke, *Mayo Clinic Proceedings* 70:209, 1995.
20. Frankowski BL, Secker-Walker RH: Advising parents to stop smoking: opportunities and barriers in pediatric practice, *Am J Dis Child* 143: 1091, 1989.
21. Frankowski BL, Weaver SO, Secker-Walker RH: Advising parents to stop smoking: pediatricians' and parents' attitudes, *Pediatrics* 91:296, 1993.
22. Gilpin EA, et al: Smoking initiation rates in adults and minors: United States, 1944-1988, *Am J Epidemiol* 140:535, 1994.
23. Giovino GA, et al: Surveillance for selected tobacco-use behaviors—United States, 1900-1994, *MMWR CDC Surveill Summ* 43:1, 1994.
24. Glantz SA, et al: *The cigarette papers,* Berkeley, Calif, 1996, University of California Press.
25. Irvine L, et al: What determines levels of passive smoking in children with asthma? *Thorax* 52:766, 1997.
26. Kahn RS, et al: The scope of unmet maternal health needs in pediatric settings, *Pediatrics* 103:576, 1999.
27. Kessler DA: Nicotine addiction in young people, *N Eng J Med* 333:186, 1995.
28. Kessler DA, et al: The Food and Dug Administration's regulation of tobacco products, *N Engl J Med* 335:988, 1996.
29. Kluger R: *Ashes to ashes: America's 100-year cigarette war, the public health, and the unabashed triumph of Philip Morris,* New York, 1996, Alfred A. Knopf.
30. Lancaster T, et al: Training health professionals in smoking cessation, *Cochrane Database of Systematic Reviews* Issue 2, 1999.
31. MacKenzie TD, Bartecchi CE, Schrier RW: The human costs of tobacco use (2), *N Engl J Med* 330:975, 1994.
32. Murray AB, Morrison BJ: The decrease in severity of asthma in children of parents who smoke since the parents have been exposing them to less cigarette smoke, *J Allergy Clin Immunol* 91:102, 1993.
33. Pierce JP, Gilpin EA, Choi WS: Sharing the blame: smoking experimentation and future smoking-attributable mortality due to Joe Camel and Marlboro advertising and promotion, *Tob Control* 8:37, 1999.
34. Pirkle JL, et al: Exposure of US population to environmental tobacco smoke: the Third National Heath and Nutrition Examination Survey, 1988 to 1991, *JAMA* 275:1233, 1996.
35. Raw M, McNeill A, West R: Smoking cessation guidelines for health professionals: a guide to effective smoking cessation interventions for the health care system, *Thorax* 53:S1, 1998.
36. Redmond WH: Effects of sales promotion on smoking among US ninth graders, *Prev Med* 28:243, 1999.
37. Samet JM, Lewit EM, Warner KE: Involuntary smoking and children's health, *Future Child* 4:94, 1994.
38. Selected cigarette smoking initiation and quitting behaviors among high school students—United States, 1997, *MMWR* 47:386, 1998.
39. Severson HH, et al: Reducing maternal smoking and relapse: long-term evaluation of a pediatric intervention, *Prev Med* 26:120, 1997.
40. Silagy C, Ketteridge S: Physician advice for smoking cessation, *Cochrane Database of Systematic Reviews* Issue 2, 1999.
41. Silagy C, et al: Nicotine replacement therapy for smoking cessation, *Cochrane Database of Systematic Reviews* Issue 2, 1999.
42. Smith TA, et al: Nicotine patch therapy in adolescent smokers, *Pediatrics* 98:659, 1996.
43. Spitzer WO, Lawrence V, Dales R: Links between passive smoking and disease: a best-evidence synthesis. A report of the working group on passive smoking, *Clin Invest Med* 13:17, 1990.
44. Strachan DP, Cook DG: Health effects of passive smoking. 1. Parental smoking and lower respiratory illness in infancy and early childhood, *Thorax* 52:905, 1997.
45. Strachan DP, Cook DG: Health effects of passive smoking. 4. Parental smoking, middle ear disease and adenotonsillectomy in children, *Thorax* 53:50, 1998.
46. Strachan DP, Cook DG: Health effects of passive smoking. 6. Parental smoking and childhood asthma: longitudinal and case-control studies, *Thorax* 53:204, 1998.
47. Strachan DP, Cook DG: Health effects of passive smoking .5. Parental smoking and allergic sensitization in children, *Thorax* 53:117, 1998.
48. The Smoking Cessation Clinical Practice Guideline Panel and Staff: The Agency for Health Care Policy and Research Smoking Cessation Clinical Practice Guideline, *JAMA* 275:1270, 1996.
49. Torrens PR, Lynch BS, Bonnie RJ: Growing up tobacco free, *JAMA* 273:1326, 1995.
50. Tyas SL, Pederson LL: Psychosocial factors related to adolescent smoking: a critical review of the literature, *Tob Control* 7:409, 1998.
51. US Department of Health and Human Services: *Healthy people 2000: national health promotion and disease prevention objectives,* DHHS Pub No PHS 91-50213, Washington, DC, 1991.
52. US Environmental Protection Agency, Office of Health and Environmental Assessment: *Respiratory health effects of passive smoking: lung cancer and other disorders,* EPA/600/6-90/006F, Washington, DC, 1992.
53. United States Preventive Services Task Force: Counseling to prevent tobacco use. In *Guide to clinical preventive services,* ed 2, Alexandria, Va, 1996, International Medical Publishing.
54. Wahlgren DR, et al: Reduction of environmental tobacco smoke exposure in asthmatic children: a 2-year follow-up, *Chest* 111:81, 1997.
55. Wahlgren DR, et al: Predictors of tobacco use initiation in adolescents: a two-year prospective study and theoretical discussion, *Tob Control* 6:95, 1997.
56. Wall MA, et al: Pediatric office-based smoking intervention: impact on maternal smoking and relapse, *Pediatrics* 96:622, 1995.

24 The Ill Child

Marianne E. Felice • Stanford B. Friedman

Although great strides have been made in the prevention, diagnosis, and treatment of childhood illnesses in the past half century, children continue to become ill. Illnesses today, however, are different from those of former years. For example, children now have chronic illnesses that in the past were fatal, and they now have fatal diseases that in the past were not known. Sick children and their families continue to consume a major portion of the pediatrician's time, talents, and energy. It is important that the specific knowledge and skills of pediatricians reflect the changing patterns of childhood disease.

A discussion of the management of the ill child must encompass a variety of topics, including the degree and duration of illness, hospitalization and the medical delivery system, family support systems, the emotional components of physical illness, and finally, the plight of the dying child.

THE ACUTELY ILL CHILD

Treatment at Home

Whenever possible, the acutely ill child should be treated at home surrounded by a familiar environment and tended to by a responsible, caring adult who knows the child well. Fortunately, this is the usual case, rather than the exception, because most youngsters are only mildly to moderately ill for a brief period and have their parents, extended family members, or reliable, familiar baby-sitters to tend to them. The pediatrician, however, should not always presume that adults are in attendance. When deciding whether to treat a child at home, the physician should specifically seek answers to the following questions: Who will assume responsibility for the child during the illness? Is a telephone easily available? Are medical facilities relatively nearby? Above all, do the parents understand the nature of the child's illness and the instructions that have been given? The answer to the last question should be verified by having one or both parents repeat the instructions to the physician.

In two-parent households, fathers should be encouraged to participate in their children's health care. Often mothers assume full responsibility for the children's health and fathers are ignored; thus, fathers often cannot support either the mother or the child. This leaves the mother in the difficult position of having not only to tend to the child but also to repeat the physician's explanations and directions to her husband, a situation that can be the source of misunderstanding, misinterpretation, and resentment for both parents. When a child has a significant illness, the pediatrician should encourage *both* parents to bring the child to the physician whenever possible, and the physician should relate directions and explanations to both parents simultaneously. In this way parents can share the task of caring for their sick child and support each other.

Few families conform to the traditions of a wage-earning father and a stay-at-home mother. Among married couples who have children under 18 years, both parents work outside the home in 64% of these families.[2] About 77% of women who have children ages 6 to 17 years are in the work force[14]; 71% of all single mothers are employed.[2] The proportion of children being reared by fathers alone is about 20%.[2] Consequently, physicians always should be aware of and sensitive to the household composition and problems, particularly in giving directions concerning at-home care. For example, single-parent fathers may be new to the primary caretaker role; surrounded by experienced mothers in the pediatrician's office, they may feel uncomfortable. They may be unsure of details concerning the child's birth or immunizations. This parent may need more detailed information than do other parents about the treatment of an acute illness. Working mothers may feel caught between the demands of their job and the demands of their sick child and feel guilty about asking the physician for advice. Physicians will serve the child's needs best by being attuned to these psychosocial and societal issues.

Treating an ill child offers an opportunity for the pediatrician to teach parents about medications. If a drug is prescribed, the physician should name the drug and explain why it is being given and what side effects should be anticipated. Antibiotic therapy frequently results in low compliance; parents begin to give antibiotics to their child and then stop when the child starts to feel better, usually after 24 to 48 hours of treatment.[16] Parents may need to be told that many types of infections require a full course of antibiotic therapy. When a medication is discontinued by a physician before all the liquid, pills, or capsules are finished, the parents should be advised about what to do with the unused portion. For example, those medications that decompose with time, such as tetracycline, should be discarded; other medications, such as antihistamines, may be used again at a later date. Parents also should be taught which over-the-counter drugs they should have available, such as acetaminophen for children and ipecac syrup, and how to use them. Physicians also can educate parents by teaching them the proper administration of medications. The familiar "1 teaspoon 4 times a day" may result in varied quantities of medicine being administered if careful directions are not given. Some parents may need practical hints for helping a child take an unpalatable medicine—for example, crushing a tablet in applesauce.

In most families there is a tradition of myths and home remedies for common acute illnesses, and parents often turn to these ideas when their children are ill. Again, this provides the opportune time for parent education. For example, when talking to the parents of a child who has an upper respiratory tract infection, the physician can explain that the youngster did not "catch cold" because of failure to wear galoshes in the rain. In explaining the management of fever, a physician may wish to emphasize certain *do nots* in an effort to dispel misconceptions: *Do not* give enemas to bring down fever; *do not* give cold baths to bring down fever (see Chapter 25, Management of Fever). Some myths and home remedies are peculiar to certain communities and cultures, and each pediatrician should become familiar with the traditions of the locality (see Chapter 12, Cultural Issues in Primary Pediatric Care).

In this age of widespread immunization programs, issues of contagion often are neglected. Parents should be informed of the infectious nature of certain childhood illnesses in order to protect other siblings, pregnant relatives, and elderly persons. The most common examples are protecting pregnant relatives from rubella or warning those taking steroids or immunosuppressive drugs to avoid contact with children who have chickenpox.

Acutely ill children at home often pose problems for the parents caring for them. Parents unaccustomed to seeing their normally active toddler listless may feel compelled to entertain the child without realizing that the child may need rest and may not be in the mood for entertainment. On the other hand, many parents may try to restrain a child and insist on bed rest when the child feels well enough to play. Parents need to be reminded that children restrict their own activity when they are ill. Parents also have a tendency to overfeed a sick child, and they must be reassured that if a child drinks an appropriate amount of fluids, this is sufficient intake during a brief illness.

It is natural for parents to become anxious when their children are ill; this anxiety may result in frequent telephone calls to the pediatrician. The pediatrician may perceive such calls as unneeded and annoying without appreciating how frightened parents may be. New parents in particular require support during their child's illnesses, and the pediatrician should teach parents patiently when it is and is not appropriate to call. The pediatrician should not frighten parents into not calling and reporting on their child's progress. When a physician decides to treat a child at home, arrangements should be made for a follow-up check, either in terms of a telephone conversation or another office visit, and the importance of such follow-up visits should be explained and emphasized to the parents.

Indications for Hospitalization

It is not always feasible or safe to treat an acutely ill child at home; hospitalization may become necessary. Whom to hospitalize and when to hospitalize are not always clear-cut. But, in the last decade, there has been a definite trend toward decreased hospitalizations for children.[14] Children who are critically or seriously ill are obvious candidates for inpatient care. Children who are not seriously ill also must be considered for hospitalization if the circumstances at home are such that the child will not receive adequate care. Some hospitalizations, however, can be averted by the utilization of available community resources such as public health nurses, homemaker services, and medical home care programs. Such alternative arrangements not only may be far more economical but also will allow the child and parents to remain in their home.

It sometimes is necessary to hospitalize children for diagnostic workups. Most diagnostic procedures can be accomplished on an outpatient basis and should be done so as often as possible. Occasionally, children require numerous or complicated tests or clinical observation, and it may be more efficient to admit them for a few days for evaluation. When this is necessary, the pediatrician should schedule the admission carefully, keeping the hospital stay as short as possible; the pediatrician, for example, should postpone an admission from Friday to Monday if no tests or only a few tests can be performed over the weekend. In this age of health care reform,[16] admissions to or discharges from hospitals often are monitored or authorized by clerical staff who may not be trained in pediatric issues and who are instructed to follow guidelines designed for cost containment and not optimal care. Pediatricians always should ensure that decisions concerning a child's health are based on the child's medical needs and not on financial restraints.

Some children require elective surgical procedures. The pediatric literature has reflected an emphasis on the timing of these procedures based on the observation that between the ages of 4 and 7 years, children seem to be dramatically concerned about body integrity. Psychiatrists refer to this as *mutilation anxiety* or *castration anxiety.* Some authorities have recommended that elective surgery not be done during these particular years of psychosocial development. In actual clinical practice, however, it usually is not feasible to postpone surgical procedures for 3 to 4 years. An alternative approach is to delay surgery only long enough to explain to the child what is going to happen to him or her. This should be explained gradually, using age-appropriate language, and the parents should be the primary supportive resources.[15]

Unfortunately, children sometimes are admitted to the hospital primarily for the convenience of the physician. After receiving a call from the parents at night, the pediatrician may have the child admitted at a late hour and attended by a pediatric house officer on call, thus avoiding having to examine the child at that time. The pediatrician should look into the "real" reason for ordering the hospitalization and avoid doing so for personal convenience.

Care of the Child in the Hospital

When a child is admitted to the hospital, the child and the family become enmeshed in an unfamiliar and often frightening web known as the medical delivery system. To the lay person, hospital activities are unpredictable, and families lack control over this environment. In such a milieu both the child and the parents may express their fear in several ways. For instance, the child may cry and be uncooperative. The child is afraid of separation from the parents, of pain, of the unfamiliar environment and strange people, and of the unknown. Parents may become hostile or agitated or may constantly question the health team. They realize that their child's care is being usurped from them, and they fear that they no longer can care for or protect their child. They, too, are afraid of the strange people and the unknown environment.

There may be no facilities for parents on the pediatric floor, not even a waiting area. Nevertheless, the supportive role of the parents in helping their child get well must be emphasized, and the parents should be assured that they are needed and welcomed on the pediatric floor. In fact, in recent years, many health facilities for children have espoused the concept of family-centered care, which emphasizes the need for collaboration between health care professionals and parents in meeting the health care needs of children.[5,21] This particularly is true for children who have chronic illness who may have frequent admissions to the hospital and have interactions with many health care professionals.[8] In the complicated network of hospital personnel who encounter the youngster, the parents should have one person consistently available to them for communication about their child's care. This person, usually the primary care physician, should report at least daily to the parents and more often if the child is critically ill. Whenever possible, information should be given to both parents at the same time. They then have the opportunity to ask questions, and neither parent needs to interpret the physician's remarks to the other.

It is common for a youngster to have one or even multiple consultants during hospitalization. It is vital that the child and the parents be notified that a consultation has been requested and the reasons for it explained. Communication between the pediatrician and the consultant should be made clear before the consultant sees the child so that the parents do not receive conflicting or confusing reports. The following case vignette illustrates the confusion that can occur in the process of consultation:

Gary was an obese 10-year-old admitted to the hospital for a diagnostic workup of recent "spells" consisting of dizziness and falling down. The degree of consciousness after each episode was unclear. On the day of hospital admission, Gary appeared to vacillate between a state of near coma and insensitivity to pain and aggressive fighting behavior. The physical examination disclosed no abnormal findings. All study results were negative except those of an equivocal electroencephalogram. Neurological consultation was requested without Gary's or his parents' knowledge. The neurologist told the mother that Gary probably had a form of seizure disorder and that medication would be recommended to the pediatrician. The nurses noted that Gary seemed quiet and did not play with other children, and a child psychiatric consultation was requested. Because the pediatrician feared the mother would object to psychiatry, she was simply told that "another doctor" would be talking to her son. The child psychiatrist arrived on the ward and introduced himself to the mother as a psychiatrist. The mother said that she was confused. While the psychiatrist talked to Gary, the mother was told to wait in the hall until the interview was over. A few minutes later the mother went to the nurses' station and demanded to see her son's pediatrician, who was paged but did not answer. The child psychiatrist returned to the mother and said that Gary appeared to be depressed and that he would return the next day to take the boy to the playroom to complete the evaluation. The mother began shouting at the nurses about the quality of care in the hospital.

Problems illustrated by the above vignette can be avoided easily if before the consultant sees the patient, the primary care physician and the consultant decide together who will discuss the consultant's findings with the child and the family (Fig. 24-1). Just as it is important for the pediatrician to communicate with parents, it is necessary for the pediatrician to communicate with the child in a developmentally appropriate manner, no matter what the child's age. This communication may take the form of actions rather than words. For example, it is more comforting for a toddler to be held for reassurance than to hear words of reassurance. When speaking to a child, the pediatrician should remember to sit down at the child's eye level and use age-appropriate words to ensure that the child understands what is to be done and to allow the child an opportunity to ask questions. To help the youngster trust hospital personnel, procedures should be explained honestly. If a child is to have blood drawn, for instance, and asks whether it will hurt, the pediatrician should admit that it will hurt for a few moments. All painful procedures should be performed as quickly and gently as possible. Often it is appropriate to perform any painful procedures in a special treatment room so that the ward or hospital room is not associated with unpleasant experiences.

Children who must undergo surgery should have the surgical procedure explained to them.[15] The physician can use a doll and a bandage to show where the patient's bandage will be. Children should be told where they will be when they awaken and who will be there. If a child is expected to be returned to an intensive care unit after major surgery, the nurses from that unit should visit the child before the surgery so that the child will feel more at ease in the new surroundings after surgery.

In preparation for anesthesia the child should be forewarned about the anesthesia mask and the odor of the gas. Many physicians find that the presence of parents during the induction and recovery phases of anesthesia helps to alleviate much of the fear and fantasy for both parents and child.

It generally is accepted that children admitted to hospitals should be placed in pediatric units designed especially for children and staffed by personnel trained to care for children. In large children's centers, children may be assigned to wards

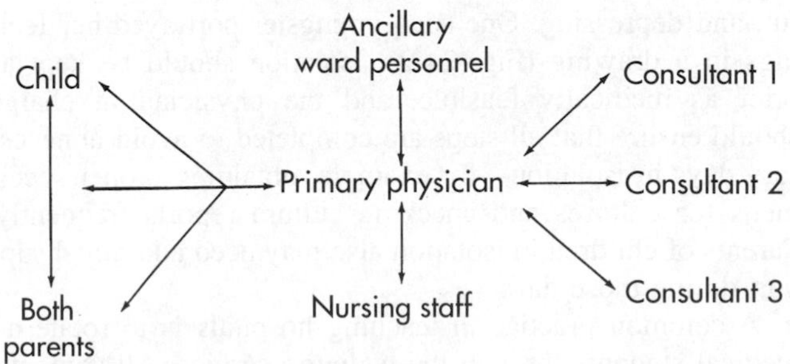

Fig. 24-1 Relationship between the primary care physician and all consultants.

by age and type of medical problem; in community hospitals, children usually are assigned to wards according to age alone; and in smaller hospitals children of all ages may be assigned to one pediatric ward. Any of these arrangements is appropriate. Many hospitals have no facilities for adolescent patients, and teenagers are admitted to the adult wards. For a few older adolescents this may be acceptable, but for younger adolescents and for some older ones, such an arrangement may be detrimental to their emotional health. Whenever possible, adolescents should be placed together in a setting designed for their needs.[6]

For young children in particular, separation from parents is painful. In these instances, rooming-in arrangements are strongly recommended until the child adjusts to the hospitalization. In fact, rooming-in may result in a shorter hospital stay for the child and lower anxiety for both child and parents. This practice reinforces the benefits of parental involvement in a child's care.[4] The issues of visiting hours and who may visit are important in pediatrics. Policies regarding these issues should be based on what is best for the child and the family and not on what is most convenient for the hospital personnel.

The question of whether it is more beneficial for a child to have a private room than to be with other children often is raised. The answer depends on the patient's particular needs and illness. Parents often believe that their child will receive better care if placed in a private room; if this is not true, the pediatrician should communicate this to the parents. Generally, children should have as much contact with other children as is medically feasible.

When hospitalized, children often regress in development, commonly in toilet training. Parents need reassurance that this phenomenon may occur because of the strange and frightening hospital environment. Neither children nor adolescents are accustomed to using medical terminology to describe urination and defecation; thus, they may hesitate to express these needs to nurses. Parents can be invaluable in clarifying these terms to their children. It is important to respect a child's or an adolescent's need for privacy in completing his or her toilette, in dressing or undressing, or in being examined. Hospital personnel should be sensitive to a child's embarrassment and pull curtains around the bed when the child is undressing or draw a sheet over the child's naked genitalia when the abdomen is being examined in full view of the hall. Although isolation may be medically necessary, pediatric personnel must remember that it does affect the child. Children in isolation receive fewer visits from the nurses. When someone does come into the room, the visitor is gowned and often masked. This can be frightening, stressful, and depressing. One such youngster portrayed her feelings in a drawing (Fig. 24-2). Isolation should be kept as brief as medically feasible, and the physician in charge should ensure that all steps are completed to avoid unnecessary days in isolation—for example, obtaining proper specimens for cultures and checking culture reports frequently. Parents of children in isolation also may need additional support during those days.

A common practice in teaching hospitals is to rotate all medical students through the pediatric service. All students, regardless of their career interests, are then taught pediatric procedures (e.g., starting IVs, drawing blood, performing spinal taps, and aspirating bone marrow) by practicing on young patients. Although students interested in pediatrics must learn these procedures, they will have ample opportunity to do so as first-year house officers. Pediatric teaching programs should be reevaluated to determine whether *all* students need to master pediatric procedures and if alternative methods are available to acquire these skills, such as the use of mannequins and animal models. Current New York State Department of Health regulations severely limit medical student involvement in performing these procedures. It is likely that other states will follow suit.

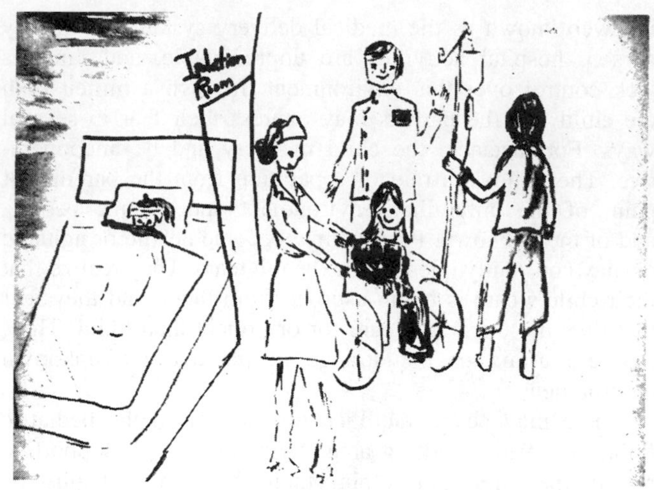

Fig. 24-2 Drawing by a 13-year-old girl in isolation.

Siblings of Hospitalized Children

When a child is hospitalized, siblings should not be neglected by the parents.[10] Some children resent the attention being paid to the hospitalized child and begin to misbehave at home. Other children, particularly those of school age, are confused by their brother's or sister's absence from home and may even fantasize that they caused the hospitalization in some way. Parents may need to be reminded that *all* the children should be informed of their sibling's hospitalization and told the reason for it. It sometimes helps the children at home to feel included and needed if each one has a special chore to do for the hospitalized youngster—for example, feeding the patient's goldfish or painting a picture to decorate the hospital room. Whenever practical, the nonhospitalized siblings should speak to their hospitalized brother or sister by telephone and be encouraged to visit the hospital. Siblings told that the hospitalized child has a minor problem (e.g., anemia or the flu) when indeed the medical situation is serious or potentially fatal may be psychologically vulnerable in later life when they have these same minor medical problems.

Activities for the Young Patient

A major component of a child's life is school. School-age children admitted to the hospital miss their usual classroom instruction.[1,22] Obviously, children who are critically or seriously ill cannot be expected to study, but children who are convalescing should be given as much schooling as possible to prevent their falling too far behind their peers. If a child is hospitalized for a short time (i.e., 7 to 10 days), the parents can serve as liaison between the classroom and the child and can work with the child's teacher to ensure that the youngster keeps abreast of classes. Children whose anticipated hospitalization is for a longer period should receive instruction through the school system as soon as possible by a hospital or home tutor. In many school systems, hospital instruction cannot be requested until the child has been out of school for 6 weeks or more. This is too much time for a child to miss school work; whenever possible, the physician should protest such a policy.

Another valuable component to any child's life is play. For the hospitalized child, play also is important, and most pediatric floors are well stocked with age-appropriate toys and games. A structured activities program now is common in most pediatric wards and is known by various names in different hospitals—for example, the child-life program, play program, or children's activities program. Physicians should make use of a child-life program in caring for their patients and welcome the observations made of the child at play. Such observations often can add insight to a child's progress or lack of progress in the hospital. Children should be encouraged to act out or "draw out" their feelings about their illness or hospitalization. Where there are structured activities, as many children as possible should participate. Youngsters who have intravenous lines should have the tubing anchored in such a way that walking is possible. Children in traction or restricted to bed often can have their beds moved to the playroom so that they too can take part in the activities.

While recuperating from a long illness in the hospital, children should be able to receive "leave" or passes. Pediatric health care personnel sometimes neglect the importance of children attending significant and meaningful events in their lives, such as a school occasion or a family celebration. Often a child can be allowed to leave the hospital for a few hours without detriment to his or her health, particularly for the adolescent struggling to maintain peer group acceptance during the illness.

Patients, parents, and members of a hospital staff are partners in the healing process. Each has rights and responsibilities (Box 24-1). The primary care physician, as the patient's advocate and a member of the hospital staff, should ensure that all concerned understand and respect these rights and responsibilities.

Indications for Discharge from the Hospital

It sometimes is as difficult to decide when to discharge children from the hospital as it is to decide when to admit them. Children should not be kept in the hospital unnecessarily, but what constitutes an unnecessary length of time is not always clear. Fortunately, most children are admitted for a given symptom, diagnosed, treated, and then sent home within a brief period. Some children require extended convalescence with minimal nursing care; for these children, alternatives to traditional hospitalization should be sought, such as convalescent homes for children, hospitals for children with chronic illnesses, and visiting nurse programs. If parents are expected to perform nursing tasks for the child at home, such as injections, gavage, or dressing changes, they should be taught the procedure gradually, and the child should be discharged only when the parents and physician both feel comfortable that proper care can be given at home. Again, public health nurses can be invaluable in helping such families.

Often children are admitted to the hospital having suspected primary psychosocial problems, such as those caused by child abuse. In these cases, social work consultation should be requested as early as possible so that the child will not spend extra days in the hospital while such a consultation and disposition are implemented. Pediatric health care personnel must be innovative and imaginative to minimize the length of hospitalization and to encourage comprehensive rehabilitation of the child.

THE CHRONICALLY ILL CHILD

Chronically ill children pose many issues for pediatric health care personnel.[20] Sometimes these youngsters have complex medical problems and thus require the services of several physicians or clinics. They may have psychosocial problems concomitant with or as a result of their illness.[7] They often require frequent checkups and characteristically have thick medical records. Their families need and deserve much support, understanding, and guidance concerning the disease and its effect on the total family.[23,24] Finally, children who have a chronic disease evoke a vast array of feelings in the staff members who work with them. These feelings often are ignored, suppressed, or displaced.

The number of children who have chronic illnesses is increasing rapidly, as advances in technology are enabling physicians to change the natural history of many diseases and prolong life.[14,17] This advancement, however, has resulted in some new problems. For example, before the era of antibiotics, children who had cystic fibrosis usually died before adolescence; now these patients often live to young adulthood and beyond. When adolescents, they usually depend on several medications simultaneously and may resent this dependence. Boys who have cystic fibrosis nearly always are sterile; adolescent girls who have it must grapple with their fears of having children when their own life expectancy is so uncertain. Therefore, physicians must focus on the psychosocial and psychosexual problems related to these issues of sterility and pregnancy.

Effects of Chronic Illness on the Child's Development

How a chronic illness influences a child's development is contingent on several questions. Was the child born with the illness? Is the illness inherited, or was it acquired? How old was the child when the illness was acquired or when it was diagnosed? The importance of these answers relates to children's beginning development of a body image, even in infancy. Five-month-old infants explore their own bodies, including their fingers, toes, genitalia, and faces, and they incorporate their findings into their developing self-images. By the age of 2 or 3 years, these youngsters have some concept of their own bodies that they identify as "mine." If in their exploration they discover that an arm or a leg is absent or that they have some other abnormality, they incorporate that abnormality into their self-image. Later, at age 3, 4, or 5 years, they begin to compare their body with other children's bodies and recognize that they are different from other children. The child growing up with an abnormality appears to be better adjusted and more accepting of his or her self-image than the child who acquires a disability during later years.

After children who have a chronic illness or physical deformity have accepted their self-image, they must learn to cope with their peers' perceptions.[3] Young children are adaptive and generally will play with other children to the best of their abilities despite their deformities. Although youngsters can be cruel and tease one another about their differences, usually children accept other children, particularly if the disabled children accept themselves. Parents, however, often become anxious about their disabled or chronically ill children being in the presence of "normal" children and may try to shield them from their peers. Physicians should reassure and support the parents so that the child is given the opportunity to relate to normal peers.[9]

Children whose disabilities are visible often receive more attention and support than do children with "hidden" ones. For example, the child who has rheumatoid arthritis and visibly swollen joints and difficulty moving may evoke much support from family, teachers, and friends. On the other hand, the child who has juvenile diabetes, whose disability is not visible, may not receive similar support.

A major problem for children who have chronic illnesses is the difficulty that physicians and parents have in allowing them to develop independence. Parents tend to overprotect their chronically ill child,[11] and physicians contribute to that overprotectiveness by emphasizing restrictions. It is helpful to both parents and child if the physician lists those activities the child *should* do as well as those activities that he *should not* do.

When treating a chronically ill child over several years,

BOX 24-1

RIGHTS OF PATIENTS AND PARENTS

You have the right, consistent with law, to:

1. Understand and use these rights. If for any reason you do not understand or you need help, the hospital must provide assistance, including a translator.
2. Receive treatment without discrimination as to race, color, religion, gender, national origin, disability, sexual orientation, or source of payment.
3. Receive considerate and respectful care in a clean and safe environment free of unnecessary restraints.
4. Receive emergency care if you need it.
5. Be informed of the name and position of the doctor who will be in charge of your care in the hospital.
6. Know the names, positions, and functions of any hospital staff involved in your care and refuse their treatment, examination, or observation.
7. A no smoking room.
8. Receive complete information about your diagnosis, treatment, and prognosis.
9. Receive all the information that you need to give informed consent for any proposed procedure or treatment. This information shall include the possible risks and benefits of the procedure or treatment.
10. Receive all the information that you need to give informed consent for an order not to resuscitate. You also have the right to designate an individual to give this consent for you if you are too ill to do so. If you would like additional information, please ask for a copy of *"Do Not Resuscitate Orders: A Guide for Patients and Families."*
11. Refuse treatment and be told what effect this may have on your health.
12. Refuse to take part in research. In deciding whether to participate, you have the right to a full explanation.
13. Privacy while in the hospital and confidentiality of all information and records regarding your care.
14. Participate in all decisions about your treatment and discharge from the hospital. The hospital must provide you with a written discharge plan and written description of how you can appeal your discharge.
15. Review your medical record and obtain a copy of your medical record, for which the hospital can charge a reasonable fee. You cannot be denied a copy solely because you cannot afford to pay.
16. Receive an itemized bill and explanation of all charges.
17. Formulate an advance directive and appoint a health care proxy.
18. Participate in the consideration of ethical issues that arise in your care.
19. Complain without fear of reprisals about the care and services you are receiving and to have the hospital respond to you and, if you request it, issue a written response. You first should speak to the nurse or doctor caring for you and, if you remain dissatisfied, to Patient Relations. If you are not satisfied with the hospital's response, you can complain to the state health department. The hospital must provide you with the health department phone number.

If you have any questions about your rights, please speak with a staff member, especially the doctor or nurse caring for you.

Modified from University of Rochester Strong Memorial Hospital Medical Center, Statement on patients' rights, Rochester, NY, April, 1993.

the physician can attend to vocational planning for the youngster, either personally or through staff members. Each child should be encouraged to develop socially and intellectually as completely as possible, but the physician also must recognize a child's limitations and encourage realistic aspirations. One problem peculiar to pediatricians is their reluctance to terminate the physician-patient relationship when a youngster reaches adulthood, particularly if the pediatrician has cared for the child from infancy. Whenever possible, chronically ill children, on reaching adulthood, should be transferred to internists or family practitioners; such a transfer supports the patient's striving for independence. The patient should be prepared for this change over several visits.

Effects of Chronic Illness on the Family

The parents of chronically ill children often feel guilty about their child's illness. If a child has an inherited disorder, both parents may scrutinize their family backgrounds to see how the disease was inherited. If the illness is acquired, the parents may feel that they did not protect their child adequately from getting the disease. If an infant is born having a congenital but not inherited disorder, the mother may become obsessed about her prenatal activities and wonder if some action of hers caused the disorder.

Guilt often leads to anger (Fig. 24-3). Guilt feelings cause discomfort, and the parents become angry at feeling uncomfortable. This anger may be directed toward the physician who initially diagnosed the child's illness, toward each other, toward themselves, and even toward the afflicted child. In this age of widespread communication, parents, siblings, and even the child who has a specific illness, may turn to the Internet for information on a particular disease topic. In some cases, this helps in learning about a child's illness. In other cases, families may receive erroneous information. Clinicians should provide written materials about a chronic illness when possible and suggest reliable sources for additional information.

The marital relationship between parents of a chronically ill child may either improve remarkably or disintegrate shortly after the illness is diagnosed. Being told that one's youngster has a chronic illness is a crisis and imposes stress on most marriages. If the marriage is stable and the parents are mutually supportive, the marital bonds grow stronger. If the marriage is unstable, the child's illness serves as a final stress that may sever marital ties.

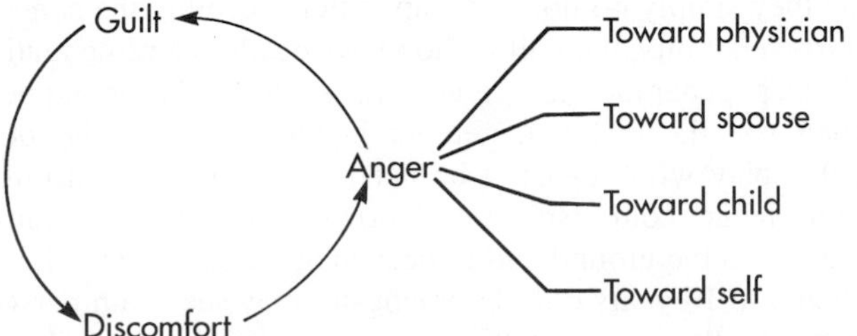

Fig. 24-3 Parental guilt over a child's illness often leads to anger.

To the family, the monetary cost of having a child with a chronic illness may be astounding,[5] in which case the parents will need help finding financial aid. Most families are not able to carry the financial burden of their child's illness alone, but they may be too proud to ask for help. Physicians should be sensitive to these needs and offer their help or the services of their staff whenever possible.

To society, the cost of children who are chronically ill can be immeasurable.[14] These children often require expensive medications and repeated hospitalizations, and some require long-term institutional care.

The siblings of children who have a chronic illness also require attention.[10] Siblings often worry about whether they will have the same disease if it is congenital or inherited. If the disorder is inherited and they have been spared, they often feel guilty. If the disease is acquired, these children may think or fantasize that their brother or sister did something to deserve the illness. Often in sibling rivalry a child may wish that the brother or sister were dead. When that brother or sister acquires an illness, the sibling may then feel tremendous guilt and responsibility for "causing" the illness. The primary physician caring for the child who has a chronic illness should always inquire as to the health, well-being, and psychological state of the youngster's siblings and may be able to provide insight to the parents concerning the siblings' behavior. Direct contact with the sibling(s) may be appropriate for counseling.

The Medical Delivery System

Children who have chronic illnesses often receive fragmented health care. Frequently, a primary care physician suspects an illness and requests a consultation at a children's hospital or service, where the child is taken, a workup completed, and a diagnosis made. The child then is assigned to a specialty clinic, returning regularly for care. Usually, this clinic is attended by full-time staff specialists, but at each visit the child is seen by a different house officer who does not know or recognize either the child or the family. The contribution to the overall care by the primary care physician who referred the child originally often is ignored.

Whether a child who has a chronic illness should receive care from specialty clinics or from a primary care physician may be controversial. Often a child can be seen once or twice a year at the specialty clinic and have other checkups through the regular pediatrician. This arrangement is suitable if communication is good between the specialist and the primary care physician. During adolescence, children who have chronic illnesses often continue to be treated in pediatric clinics, where they now feel uncomfortable, and their dependency is reinforced. Whenever possible, adolescents should be treated in a setting designed for teens.[6] If this is not possible, it may be appropriate to have adolescents treated by adult medical groups, if those physicians are sensitive to the issues of development.

When to hospitalize the chronically ill child is a difficult question to answer. Usually the parents are able to cope with innumerable medical problems at home simply through years of experience. Hospitalization often takes on special meaning to the child who is a regular visitor to the physician or hospital; the child may view hospitalization as being followed by death if the reasons for hospitalization are not explained carefully.

Pediatricians and their staff must be aware of their own emotional responses to the chronically ill child. This child, more than any other youngster, is able to evoke mixed feelings and frustration in the staff. The staff members often are angry while caring for the child, frustrated because their patient does not get better. Often the care of a chronically ill child involves several consultants, and each consultant may give different messages to the child and the family. Complicated cases, especially those involving mental retardation, often are rejected by all members of the medical delivery system. When such children are hospitalized, they and their families frequently spend much time in the admissions office while house officers and administrative clerks decide where the children belong. The 15-year-old mentally retarded patient who has cerebral palsy may be rejected by the staff responsible for adolescent care because the patient looks like an 8-year-old child; the same patient may be rejected by the ward for school-age children because the child "is really an adolescent."

Counseling

Chronically ill children and adolescents and their parents should have opportunities to receive counseling.[9,18] Usually, parents need this help early in the disease, shortly after it is diagnosed. Youngsters generally need this assistance as they approach adolescence. Not all chronically ill children and their parents will require counseling, but all should be given this option.

Usually the counseling can be provided by a sensitive and understanding physician willing to spend time with the family. Social workers and psychologists also are resources for handling these problems and can work closely with the physician who cares for the child. A group of adolescents who have similar problems may wish to meet regularly with an interested physician or staff member to share their common problems. In many areas, parents of chronically ill children meet to support one another.

Role of the School

Children who have chronic illnesses frequently are absent from school because of their illness, clinic or physician visits, or hospitalization. Absence from school should be minimized. In some communities children who have chronic illnesses attend special schools, particularly when they are severely disabled. However, many children whose chronic illnesses are moderately severe attend regular schools. According to Public Law 94-142, children must receive (1) education in the least restricted environment compatible with their condition and (2) related services to facilitate their education. In either situation the school should be made aware of the children's medical problems.

Teachers may be helpful as objective observers of a child's condition. When medications are changed, teachers can be instructed to look for untoward side effects. With the parent's and child's permission, a physician may contact the school and notify the teacher, principal, or school nurse of changes in a youngster's illness. Often parents prefer to communicate this information themselves. Not all teachers are medically knowledgeable, and they may welcome information the medical profession can give them about a youngster in their classroom. In this way the school system and the medical system can collaborate to benefit the chronically ill youngster.

THE DYING CHILD

To care for the dying child properly, the physician must recognize that children have different concepts about death that depend on many factors, including chronological age, cognitive development, other experience with death, and religious and cultural beliefs. All these factors should be considered when caring for the dying child.

Developmental Aspects of Death

To understand a child's concept of death, it is useful to apply Piaget's theory of sequential cognitive development[20] (Table 24-1). Infants and toddlers (2 years of age or younger) are in the *sensorimotor* stage of cognitive development. They learn through their senses (seeing, hearing, touching, and tasting), and they use their advancing motor skills to find new objects and experiences to see, hear, touch, or taste. Although young infants are developing language, they essentially are preverbal, and the word *death* has no meaning for them. As they realize differences in individuals around them, however, infants can experience separation from loved ones (parents) and "know" the feelings of separation anxiety.

The next stage of cognitive development, described as *preoperational,* is characteristic of most children between 2 and 6 years of age. In this stage of development children have verbal skills but cannot yet think logically. Thus, the preschooler has a very limited concept of death. By age 2 to 6 years youngsters generally have had some contact with death; a pet or a grandparent may have died. It is believed that these young children consider death a reversible phenomenon, as demonstrated in movies and television. For example, it is common to see a cartoon character flattened like a pancake with a steamroller and the next moment up and about and racing down the road. Such activity is completely plausible in the mind of the preschooler.

The school-age child 6 to 12 years old usually is in the *concrete operational* stage, when logical thought about the physical world is developing. Children's concepts of death undergo many changes during this time. For example, by the age of 6 to 8 years, the youngster often views death as a prolongation of sleep: Dead people's eyes are closed as though they were asleep; therefore they must be asleep, and they simply do not wake up. After accepting the concept of irreversibility, the child who views death as a prolongation of sleep generally asks questions such as: What happens when you die and you get put in the ground? Who does Jackie play with? Doesn't he need some cookies and milk? Won't he get cold? Isn't it dark down there? How can somebody be in the ground and in heaven at the same time? Later, when 8 to 10 years old, the youngster may see death personified, usually as a monster who sneaks in at night and kills the living. This fantasy often is "substantiated" by movies and television.

Table 24-1 Development of the Concept of Death

Range (years)	Piagetian Developmental Stage	Concept of Death	Approximate Age
0-2	Sensorimotor *Preverbal* Reflex activity Purposeful activity Rudimentary thought	Expresses discomfort with separation	Infancy
2-6	Preoperational *Prelogical*	Uses word *dead* but only to distinguish "not alive"	3 yr
	Development of representational or symbolic language	Limited notion; may express no personal emotion but may associate death with sorrow of others	4 yr
	Initial reasoning	Avoids dead things; imagines death as a personified being; believes he or she will always live, only other people (especially older ones) die	5 yr
		Associates death with "old age"; may be violent and emotional about death, including representations (e.g., magazine pictures), or may display intense curiosity about dead things	6 yr
6-12	Concrete operational *Logical*	Morbid interest in details (e.g., graveyards, coffins, possible causes); seeks answers through observation of decomposition, etc.; suspects he himself may die	7 yr
	Problem-solving restricted to physically present, real objects that can be manipulated	Less morbid, more expansive: interested in what happens after death; accepts, without emotion, that he too will die	8 yr
	Development of logical functions (e.g., classification of objects)	Understands logical and biological (e.g., absence of pulse) essentials of death; can accept full and rational explanation of death process	9-10 yr
12+	Formal operational *Abstract* Comprehension of purely abstract or symbolic content Development of advanced logical functions (e.g., complex analogy, deduction)	Meaning of death appreciated, but reality of personal death not accepted	Adolescence

From Sahler OJZ, Friedman SB: *Pediatr Rev* 3:160, Nov 1981.

The final stage of cognitive development, known as the *formal operational* stage, is marked by the ability to understand and verbalize abstract concepts. Sometime during adolescence, usually by the midpoint, the teenager is able to perceive the concept of death as an irreversible phenomenon. This recognition may occur at the same time that most adolescents begin to deal with various philosophies, such as those concerning the purpose of life and the meaning of existence. Sometime in late adolescence or early adulthood, most people begin to grapple with the concept of their own death.[17]

Children, as well as adults, have fears concerning death; frequently, physicians do not recognize or acknowledge these fears. Dying children, whose concept of death is poorly defined, exhibit a fear of abandonment and are concerned that while they are dying their parents will leave them alone. The child who is terminally ill and has experienced innumerable medical tests and studies usually is more afraid of bodily harm than of death. How much children know about their impending death is not completely understood, but children may be more aware of the seriousness of their illnesses than adults realize.

In managing the care of the dying child, medical personnel and parents must be aware that in addition to the normal developmental concepts of death, a child's perceptions can be affected by other experiences with death: the death of a sibling, a parent, or a grandparent. How the family reacted to the death of another family member may be reflected in the dying child's behavior. The child who has seen a torturous death of a very sick grandparent or sibling may be more frightened of the pain or bodily harm associated with dying than of death itself. Children from religious families also will be influenced by the family's religious attitude toward death.

The Family of the Dying Child

Parents of terminally ill children typically react to the information that their child has a fatal illness with initial disbelief and shock, which may take days or several weeks to subside. This disbelief may not necessarily be intellectual denial. The parents usually can accept the diagnosis intellectually but cannot absorb the full emotional impact. Parents may desire a second opinion, as a result of denial or in the hope that the diagnosis is incorrect. They can be warned that these feelings may occur.

After the initial disbelief and shock, the parents frequently experience anger.[17] The anger may be directed toward the physician who made the diagnosis, toward staff members caring for the child, toward each other, or toward themselves for not having protected their child from contracting the terminal illness. After anger, parents may experience the "bargaining" stage when they say to themselves, "If I give up such and such, perhaps my child will be cured." After going through the bargaining stage, parents generally feel depressed and only then perhaps begin to deal with their feelings about the illness. Some parents actually grieve over the loss while their child is still alive, particularly if they are parents of children who have leukemia at the terminal stages of the disease.

As part of their "anticipatory grieving," some parents have experienced what may be described as the *Lazarus syndrome*. A child is expected to die and is quite ill, and the parents actually grieve as though the death had already taken place, psychologically preparing themselves for it. The child then recovers unexpectedly and the parents are not always equipped psychologically to deal with the child. The physician can help the parents deal with their feelings at this time.

The marriage of parents who have a terminally ill or dying child often is stressful. In traditional two-parent families it may be typical for the husband to support his wife emotionally early in the course of their child's illness and to make the important family decisions, thus allowing his wife to experience more emotion than he. In fact, the husband truly may feel the impact of the diagnosis only some days or weeks later, when his wife no longer needs such intensive support. In some instances, of course, these roles are reversed. Parents' support for each other is extremely important for the child, for the parents themselves, and for the other siblings. When children are hospitalized, mothers may be more comfortable than fathers in caring for them. Because of their inexperience in caring for a child and their work schedules, fathers may spend significantly less time with the child in the ward and have little contact with the physician. The mother then has to tell the father what the physician has said. Also, both parents may work. In estranged families, one parent may shoulder major responsibility for the child and feel little support from the other parent, or the other parent may feel "left out" of decision making and resent the former spouse or the physician, or both. To avoid such a situation, the physician should inform both parents about their child's condition, preferably at the same time.

The siblings of the dying child often are ignored by the parents and the physician. To decide what to tell siblings and how to tell them, parents must take into account their children's ages, development, and experiences. They should be told that their brother or sister is dying, but with words that are in a manner that is comfortable for the family. They should be made to feel that they still are part of the family and can help deal with this family crisis. If the siblings are old enough, issues such as heredity or contagion should be brought up to reassure them that they themselves do not have the same illness.

The parents also may ask for help coping with extended family members and deciding what to tell grandparents, aunts, and uncles. What information parents give depends on the relationship with family members and how close they feel to them. All family members, however, should be told the same thing so that they do not hear conflicting information. Parents also should be warned that extended family members and neighbors may unintentionally add more stress to their lives. Relatives may say things such as "Johnny can't have leukemia, he looks too healthy," or they may send newspaper and magazine articles that contradict what the physician has told the family. Well-meaning grandparents or relatives may not allow the parents to lead normal lives when their child is terminally ill or shortly after their child's death. They may make statements such as "How can you have a party when one of your children is dying?" or "How can you go away on a trip when your son just died a few months ago?" If parents are forewarned of these possibilities, they may be better equipped to deal with them.

The role of religion in helping families deal with a dying child also must be considered. Ministers, priests, and rabbis can be greatly supportive to the parents and the dying child, and religious families often contact their pastor for help. In some hospitals there is a ministry devoted to dying patients and their families, and even though these clergy may not be of the same faith as the family, they can be of help to them. Most studies and written discussions to date concerning terminally ill children have been about parents of children whose deaths followed a terminal illness. Parents who lose a child suddenly or unexpectedly may not respond to the child's death in the same manner as parents who have had time to prepare themselves psychologically for the loss. They often experience disbelief that can last for several weeks. Parents may deny the death of the child for some time and often dream of the deceased youngster. Parents who endure the sudden, unexpected loss of a child experience intense, disruptive, and at times, almost intolerable grief reactions.

Death by accident deserves special attention because the parents or an older sibling may feel indirectly responsible for the death. The resulting guilt may persist, particularly if the accident might have been prevented by better judgment or supervision by the parent or sibling responsible for the child's safety. Guilt arising under such circumstances often is not resolved by the usual grief process.

The Medical Delivery System

Open communication should be maintained among the staff members caring for the dying child to determine ahead of time who will be responsible for telling the parents that the child is dying or has died. When a child has multiple consultants, the physician with the closest rapport with the family and the child should inform the parents of the death.[4] This responsibility should be shouldered by the primary care physician and not left to an unfamiliar intern.

How to tell parents that their child has died is another concern. In talking about the diagnosis of terminal illness or about death, privacy for the parents and the physician is needed. Most physicians are sensitive to parents' needs, yet often parents are told about the diagnosis or the death in the hallways and in the presence of other people. By *sitting down* with the parents, the physician assures the parents that he or she plans to spend some time with them and is not eager to leave as soon as possible. The physician should keep explanations as simple as possible. Parents often complain that they do not understand the medical situation. What they primarily want is only enough information to comprehend the situation, to understand the recommendations of the physician, and to know what is expected of them as parents.

The parents should be spoken to every day, and the same information usually should be repeated several times because they may not hear what the physician says the first time. The various details of the illness should be conveyed in a series of discussions rather than all at once. During these discussions the parents can be forewarned about the questions they may be asked by relatives and friends, and they also can be told to anticipate the desire to shift to a different hospital or a different physician. Then if and when they actually have these feelings, they will be relieved to know that this is what their physician had expected.

Staff members who care for a dying child often are depressed, and the morale of the nurses, house staff, and medical students suffers. On "losing" a child, the staff may experience feelings of failure and loss; often it is desirable for them to meet to discuss a child's death as soon as possible after the event. Blame should not be placed by one group of professionals on another; rather, a supportive attitude should be maintained by those in charge. Staff members in intensive care nurseries and other intensive care units are particularly susceptible to feelings of depression and low morale. To be constantly in the presence of severely ill children and to cope with the reactions of strained parents is stressful; therefore, the programs of such units always should include outlets for emotional release and discussion of feelings concerning the death of infants and youngsters.

Whenever medically appropriate, permission for a postmortem examination should be obtained. This request should come from the physician who has the closest rapport with the family, and the responsibility should not be shifted from attending physician to house staff to student. Ideally it would be best not to ask for the autopsy at the same time that the physician is informing the parents of their child's death. Unfortunately, the postmortem examination must be done within a brief time after death, and the time the parents first learn of their child's death may be the only chance that the physician has to ask the parents. Regardless of when the subject is broached, the physician should be as frank as possible, explain the reasons for the postmortem examination, and reassure the parents that mutilation and maiming will not result.

Follow-up after Death

The physician should meet with the parents within 1 to 2 weeks and again 2 to 3 months after the child's death, giving the parents an opportunity to ask the physician those questions they did not think to ask earlier or that have been raised by others. Parents often relive the illness and repeat questions they had asked previously to assure themselves that their understanding of the child's disease was correct. As one mother said, "Talking later put a period on the whole episode." The physician also has the opportunity to see how the parents and siblings are adjusting. When a postmortem examination is performed, the physician should meet with the parents as soon thereafter as possible to convey the results to them. Such actions assure the parents that the physician still cares about them and their adaptation to the stress of their child's death.

A family naturally grieves after a child has died, and the physician should support the grief reaction.[12] Lindemann[13] classically describes the process of mourning in detail, distinguishing features of acute grief such as frequent sighing respirations, waves of somatic distress, exhaustion, and digestive symptoms. The period of mourning cannot be sharply defined because there are marked differences among individuals. In general, however, feelings related to the loss are intense for 3 to 4 months after the death of a child. Birthdays, the date of the child's death, and holiday seasons all may remind parents of their loss and even years later may be associated with renewed periods of grieving. In the normal mourning process, however, parents return more or less to their previous level of psychological and social functioning approximately 4 to 6 months after their child's death.

After parents have lost a child through death, they may wonder whether they should have another child. After discussing this possibility with the parents, the physician generally can recommend that they have another child but should also forewarn them that the new baby is not to be a replacement. A phenomenon previously described as the *replacement child syndrome* occasionally occurs in which parents attempt to have another child as soon as possible after the death of a child and to make the new child into the one who has died.[19] In some extreme cases the same name is given to the second child. A sensitive physician who maintains contact with the parents can help them avoid this potential problem and realize that no child can truly replace another and that a subsequent child might be emotionally damaged in the attempt.

Everyone involved finds caring for dying children difficult and painful. The parents and siblings of these children need support from the physician during the terminal illness as well as after the death, and pediatric staff members, particularly nurses and house officers, need opportunities to express their feelings of failure and loss when an infant or child dies.

REFERENCES

1. Bossert E: Stress appraisals of hospitalized school-age children, *Child Health Care* 23:33, 1994.
2. Bureau of Labor Statistics: *Labor force statistics from the Current Population Survey, 1997 and 1998,* Washington, DC, 1999, Department of Labor.
3. Chin DG, et al: Elementary school-age children's developmental understanding of the causes of cancer, *J Dev Behav Pediatr* 19:397, 1998.
4. Cooley WC, McCallister JW: Putting family-centered care into practice, *J Dev Behav Pediatr* 20:120, 1989.
5. Feldman HM, Ploof D, Cohen WI: Physician-family partnerships: the adaptive practice model, *J Dev Behav Pediatr* 20:111, 1999.
6. Fisher M: Adolescent inpatient units, *Arch Dis Child* 70:461, 1994.
7. Gartstein MA, et al: Psychosocial adjustment of children with chronic illness: an evaluation of three models, *J Dev Behav Pediatr* 20:157, 1999.
8. Garwick AW, et al: Families' recommendations for improving services for children with chronic conditions, *Arch Pediatr Adolesc Med* 152: 440, 1998.
9. Hausenstein EJ: The experience of distress in parents of chronically ill children: potential or likely outcome? *J Clin Child Psychol* 19:356, 1990.

10. Janus M, Goldberg S: Sibling interactions and empathy among siblings of chronically ill children: maternal versus children's reports, *J Dev Behav Pediatr* 15:296, 1994.
11. Jellinek MS: Managed care: good or bad news for children? *J Dev Behav Pediatr* 15:273, 1994.
12. Kubler-Ross E: *On death and dying,* New York, 1969, Macmillan.
13. Lindemann E: Symptomatology and management of acute grief, *Am J Psychiatry* 101:141, 1944.
14. Maternal and Child Health Bureau: *Child health USA '96-97,* DHHS Pub No HRSA-M-DSEA-97-48, Washington, DC, 1997, US Department of Health and Human Services.
15. McGraw T: Preparing children for the operating room: psychological issues, *Can J Anaesth* 41:1094, 1994.
16. Palmer D, Boucher H: Parents' and physicians' views on antibiotics, *Pediatrics* 99(6):E6, 1997. URL: http://www.pediatrics.org/cgi/content/fall/99/6/e6.
17. Perrin EC, et al: Issues involved in the definition and classification of chronic health conditions, *Pediatrics* 91:787, 1993.
18. Phipps S, Srivastava DK: Approaches to the measurement of depressive symptomatology in children with cancer: attempting to circumvent the effects of defensiveness, *J Dev Behav Pediatr* 20:150, 1999.
19. Poznanski EO: The "replacement child": a saga of unresolved parental grief, *J Pediatr* 81:1190, 1972.
20. Sahler OJZ: Grief and bereavement. In McAnarney ER, et al, editors: *Textbook of adolescent medicine,* Philadelphia, 1992, WB Saunders.
21. Shelton TL: Family-centered care in pediatrics practice: when and how? *J Dev Behav Pediatr* 20:117, 1999.
22. Stein RE, Westbrook LE, Silver EJ: Comparison of adjustment of school-age children with and without chronic conditions: results from community-based samples, *J Dev Behav Pediatr* 19:267, 1998.
23. Thyen U, et al: Impact of long-term care of children assisted by technology on maternal health, *J Dev Behav Pediatr* 19:273, 1998.
24. Warfield ME, et al: Adaptation during early childhood among mothers of children with disabilities, *J Dev Behav Pediatr* 20:9, 1999.

25 Management of Fever

Henry M. Adam

There is a long history, at least in Western cultures, of viewing fever both as a response to illness and as a disease in itself. Hippocrates perceived fever as a defense mounted by the body against an underlying disorder; the Galenic and medieval traditions understood fever to be a means of restoring balance among the humors by burning off an excess of phlegm (water) with yellow bile (fire).[29] On the other hand, the writers of the Gospels saw fever itself as the disease that Jesus "rebuked," miraculously curing Simon's mother-in-law.[21,23]

This "double vision" regarding fever has persisted despite our relatively sophisticated understanding of the physiology of temperature control, still blurring how we as physicians and as parents see the febrile child. Although our science teaches us that fever, as part of the inflammatory response, is only a sign or symptom of the real pathological process, we seem to have the need to "treat" fever with a drug and a sponge, as if it were the noxious culprit itself. Fever, as opposed to hyperthermia, rarely poses a threat to a child's well-being; in fact, the argument has been made that as an energy-expensive phenomenon, it is not likely to have weathered evolution without conferring some survival benefit.[15] Considering that fever is the most common signal of illness in children, serving as the chief complaint for as many as a third of all pediatric office visits, we would do well to clarify our approach to its management distinct from the illnesses that cause it.

FEVER AND THERMOREGULATION

Fever is a regulated elevation of body temperature, mediated by the anterior hypothalamus, that occurs in response to any insult that stimulates the body's inflammatory defenses.[22] Like a thermostat, the hypothalamic *set-point* controls the temperature the body tries to maintain. Some provocation, in children most commonly a viral infection, induces macrophages to release low—molecular-weight proteins called cytokines, among them interleukin-1 and interleukin-6 and probably tumor necrosis factor, that function as *endogenous pyrogens*. They circulate to the anterior hypothalamus, where by increasing local levels of prostaglandin E_2, they induce a rise in the set-point.[15,41] With the body's thermostat now "up-regulated," several mechanisms come into play to bring the *core temperature* (defined as the temperature of blood within the pulmonary artery[19]) up to the new set-point. Because the core temperature, even as it begins to elevate, is lower than the thermostat setting, a person developing fever feels chilled. Physiologically, the body's response is to generate more internal heat, setting skeletal muscles to shivering and stimulating cellular metabolism while minimizing heat loss to the environment by vasoconstricting the skin and turning off sweat glands. The one strategy is analogous to heating up the furnace, the other to closing the windows.

Hyperthermia, on the contrary, is an unregulated rise in core temperature to a level above the hypothalamic set-point, either from overproduction of heat (thyroid storm), a reduced ability to dissipate heat (a bundled-up baby), or as with heat stroke from overexertion on a hot and humid day, a combination of the two.[35] The body's response to hyperthermia is in fact the opposite of its response when a fever is induced: Instead of an initial chill, intense flushing ensues as blood vessels in the skin vasodilate and sweat glands activate in an attempt to lose as much heat as possible to the outside. The furnace is burning out of control; the only strategy is to try to open the windows wide.

Whereas hyperthermia may raise body temperature to dangerous, even deadly, levels, fever appears to be a homeostatic process, physiologically regulated within benign limits. DuBois[11] first noted how unusual it was even for patients who had an untreated serious infection to have fever exceeding 106° F (41.1° C). Two studies, one retrospective[27] and the other prospective,[28] that looked at large numbers of children who came to emergency departments were consistent in finding that in only 0.05% of visits did the child have a temperature of 106° F or higher. Although the pediatric literature is conflicting about whether a temperature greater than 106° F (frequently called *hyperpyrexia*) is a marker for particular risk for serious underlying infection,[1,6,27,28,38] no study suggests that the elevated temperature itself poses a threat to an otherwise healthy child except in the extraordinarily rare event that fever exceeds 107° F (41.7° C). In fact, a child who has a temperature greater than 106° F is likely to have an element of hyperthermia, such as dehydration, in addition to fever. Evidence is accumulating that as an intrinsic feature of the febrile response, the body releases *endogenous cryogens*—peptides that counterbalance pyrogens and modulate how high the hypothalamus sets its thermostat.[15]

Vasopressin and melanocyte-stimulating hormone, as well as some of the cytokines that also may act as pyrogens, appear to help limit the height fever generally can reach.[15]

As a centrally regulated response to an inflammatory insult, fever may well serve as a helpful component of the body's acute phase reaction. A growing number of studies are demonstrating that fever is an adaptive response widely present in the animal kingdom, among cold-blooded as well as warm-blooded species.[5,9,15,43] At least some species of fish and lizards, when infected, move to a warmer part of their environment, thus raising their body temperatures. This behaviorally induced fever has demonstrable survival benefit, which can be negated with antipyretic agents that lower temperature and increase mortality.[5,9,43] Fever can retard the growth and reproduction of many invasive pathogenic microorganisms, both bacterial and viral, and it appears to lower the amount of iron available to invading bacteria, many of which have a greater iron requirement at higher temperatures.[16] Among its other effects on human physiology, fever enhances neutrophil migration and the production of superoxides; it promotes T-cell proliferation and increases the release and activity of interferon.[15,30] Interestingly, some of fever's apparently beneficial stimulation of immunological function may be reversed at very high temperatures, in the hyperpyretic range.[20]

Unfortunately, no conclusive experimental information is available to prove that fever benefits humans clinically in the course of an infection, and some data suggest that at least within the context of endotoxemia, the metabolic cost of fever contributes to mortality. But in a teleological sense, its metabolic cost argues for fever generally playing some protective role in the infected host; a process that results in a 7% to 10% increase in energy expenditure for every 1° C rise in temperature is not likely to have persisted so widely in nature, among invertebrates, fish, amphibians, and reptiles, as well as among birds and mammals, for so many millions of years without conferring some survival advantage.[14,15]

FEVER PHOBIA

If, then, fever itself only rarely poses a threat to a child and may even be of benefit, why are parents and pediatricians so generally aggressive about treating it? Schmitt[33] coined the phrase "fever phobia" when he described the prevalence of misunderstanding about fever among parents bringing their children to an inner city clinic. He found that 58% of parents defined fevers below 102° F (39° C) as "high," and 16% actually believed that if left untreated, fever could rise to 110° F (43.3° C) or higher. Almost every parent thought fever could cause harmful side effects, with 46% fearing permanent brain damage. Given these responses, it is not surprising that 63% of all the parents worried "lots" about the harm fever might cause their children and that 56% gave an antipyretic agent for a temperature within the normal range. For temperatures below 102° F (38.9° C), 85% of parents treated with a drug and 62% with sponging.

The population Schmitt described consisted mainly of medically indigent, poorly educated families. Kramer, Naimark, and Leduc[18] essentially repeated Schmitt's study in a private practice with middle-class parents. Almost 50% defined temperatures in the normal range as fever; 43% thought that temperatures below 104° F (40° C) could be dangerous, and 15% believed that untreated fevers could rise above 107.6° F (42° C). Death, brain damage, and stroke were among the complications of fever these educated parents feared, with 20% believing that such complications could occur at temperatures below 104° F and 95% believing that they could occur below 107.6° F. One in five of these parents would treat normal temperatures, and virtually all (97%) would treat a temperature below 104° F.

It is no wonder that the use of medication to treat fever is so widespread. The English, for example, administer an estimated 68 million child-days of antipyretic drugs each year.[32] Fifty percent of the parents in Schmitt's study[23] stated that physicians or nurses were their most important source of information about fever. This claim was given credence by a survey of members of the American Academy of Pediatrics in Massachusetts,[24] in which two of three believed fever itself can pose a danger to children, and 25% of the responding physicians cited death and brain damage as potential complications of fever as low as 104° F (40° C). Almost three fourths of the pediatricians always or often recommended treatment for fever, two thirds of them for temperatures under 102° F (38.9° C). It may be the children who swallow the medicine, but the therapy seems aimed more at the anxiety of their parents and physicians than at any real danger fever holds for them.

DEFINITION AND MEASUREMENT

As would be expected with any physiological parameter, no single normal value represents the gold standard for body temperature. Rather, a range of normal values must take into account variations from person to person, fluctuations that reflect both a circadian pattern and age-related differences, and disparities arising from the method and site of temperature measurement. A reading of 98.6° F (37° C) traditionally has been considered the "norm"; however, the average mean daily oral temperature, measured every 6 hours for 41 to 108 days, of nine healthy young adult volunteers was 97.9° F (36.61° C), with a range of 97.5° to 98.4° F (36.41° to 36.9° C).[9] Young children tend to have higher normal body temperatures than older children or adults, yet infants in the first month or two of life are less likely than older children to develop fever with an infectious illness. Normally, body temperature is higher in the late afternoon and early evening than late at night or early in the morning, with a swing of as much as 3° F (1.7° C).[10,14,24,26] Probably the temperature cited most frequently as defining fever is 100.4° F (38° C), measured rectally. However, given all the variables that affect a particular person's body temperature, any specific number used to define fever is arbitrary.

The measurement of fever is discussed fully in Chapter 136, Fever.

MANAGEMENT

The management of fever rightly begins well before a child becomes febrile. As a first step, we pediatricians must recognize the part we have played in creating "fever phobia" in our patients' parents. Our almost ritualistic dependence on measuring a child's temperature, even at routine encounters in which illness is not an issue, as well as our readiness to recommend antipyretic therapy for any elevation of temperature, certainly must confuse parents when we tell them not to worry about fever itself. Offering counseling about fever when a child already is ill is not as likely to be effective as introducing the subject routinely in the course of a health maintenance visit.[7,31] We need to explain that fever is one of the body's natural responses and not a threat in itself and that temperature will not spiral out of control to dangerous heights without treatment other than sensible care (e.g., maintaining hydration and not overbundling).[12] In identifying the underlying illness as the possible danger to the child, we would do well to educate parents about the symptoms and behaviors that should alert them to trouble and signal the need for medical attention.

Hyperthermia is different from fever, posing a real and immediate threat to any child suffering from heat illness. Successful treatment depends on restoring the core temperature to normal as rapidly as possible. Antipyretic agents, which work by lowering the hypothalamic set-point, are not helpful because the set-point already is below a rising body temperature that has escaped regulation; physical cooling is the mainstay of therapy.[35]

Treating fever, on the other hand, is a question of judgment. If the source of the fever poses a threat, obviously it must be addressed specifically. But intervening against fever per se should be a decision individualized to each febrile child. By far the most common reason for treating fever is that it makes the child uncomfortable. Although on an evolutionary scale fever surely must be beneficial, its benefit during the course of an acute illness is not so well proven as to override concern for the child's comfort. The decision to treat for comfort's sake ought not to be based on any particular temperature threshold, but on how the child looks and behaves; many children tolerate fevers to 104° F (40° C) without apparent ill effect, whereas others become cranky and restless with a temperature barely above 100.4° F (38° C). In some cases, concern for a child's comfort may have to be balanced against the usefulness of a fever's pattern or persistence when making a diagnosis. At least one study[17] has even suggested that acetaminophen's efficacy in improving a febrile child's comfort is more presumption than fact. In a randomized, double-blind, placebo-controlled trial of 225 children 6 months to 6 years of age who had acute fever, those treated with acetaminophen were somewhat more active and alert than the control group but were no different in mood, comfort, appetite, or fluid intake. The acetaminophen group's fever and other symptoms lasted as long, and at the end of the trial parents were unable to tell with any reliability whether their child had received the drug or the placebo.

Particularly when comfort is the issue for an infant in the first few months of life, two factors weigh against routine use of medication for fever. The half-lives of all available antipyretics are significantly prolonged early in infancy, making inadvertent overdosage more of a problem. With their larger surface area relative to volume, infants also are more responsive to physical interventions that reduce body heat, such as removing clothing and blankets, keeping the room temperature moderate, and improving air circulation.

Some also believe that reducing fever with a dose of antipyretic can distinguish children who appear ill only because they are febrile from children who have a seriously threatening infection. In fact, neither the magnitude of fever reduction nor a child's clinical appearance after receiving antipyretic medication can reliably distinguish serious from trivial infectious disease.[2,40]

Although fever itself is benign in an otherwise healthy child who has a self-limited viral illness, the metabolic stress it entails may be more than an already compromised child can tolerate. Increased oxygen consumption and insensible water loss, along with tachycardia and tachypnea, can further threaten a child who is significantly anemic, septic, or in shock, as well as a child rendered vulnerable by cardiac, pulmonary, renal, or any other systemic disease that strains homeostasis. Fever also may exacerbate an acute brain injury, either infectious or traumatic, and its effect on the sensorium may be confounding in a child who has a neurological disorder.

More troublesome is defining the role of antipyretic medication in preventing febrile seizures. Children most at risk for febrile seizures (those 3 months to 3 years of age) are also the children who most frequently have self-limited viral illnesses. Urging parents to treat their young children's every fever with an antipyretic agent likely will promote fever phobia, as well as an unwarranted fear of the risk a febrile seizure poses. Undeniably a convulsive episode in a young child is terribly frightening, but only very rarely is it dangerous.[25] Aggressive attention to the possibility of a seizure with any fever will only magnify the anxiety parents already feel about both—and without any convincing evidence the strategy will work. The relationship between fever and seizures is neither clear nor predictable. Parents often are not aware that their child has a fever until after the seizure has occurred. Some children "seize" with low-grade fever and not again when their temperature is high. The lower the child's temperature with the first febrile seizure, the greater the risk of a second seizure[4]; this makes it more difficult for parents to have a sense of control because lower fevers are harder to detect. Parents overcall fever when they use palpation,[3] which may lead either to excessive dosing with an antipyretic drug or confirmatory rectal probes that become part of too many children's routine. Lastly, it has even been questioned whether around-the-clock administration of acetaminophen or ibuprofen can prevent recurrence of febrile seizures.[34,42] Although no approach seems perfect, a reasonable compromise might be to use antipyretics prophylactically only for the approximately 3% of children who have had a first febrile convulsion, where the risk for recurrence is 1 in 3.[4] Even then, parents deserve reassurance that another seizure is neither their fault nor a real threat to their child's well-being. In fact, the threat may come from the treatment if prophylaxis becomes too aggressive. The use of alternating antipyretics, given every 2 hours, has worked its way into practice without real evidence to give it support but certainly with the potential to generate more toxic reactions.

If a fever is to be treated beyond routine attention to hydration and ambient conditions, the most sensible approach follows from understanding how the brain controls the body's temperature. When the hypothalamic set-point rises, fever follows. Acetaminophen and nonsteroidal antiinflammatory drugs (NSAIDs), particularly aspirin and ibuprofen, are all effective antipyretic agents because they lower the hypothalamic set-point back toward normal by inhibiting the synthesis of prostaglandin E_2.

In most circumstances aspirin should not be the drug of choice for children because of its reported association with Reye's syndrome.[8,37] Whether this association is unique to aspirin or generic to NSAIDs, which all have similar modes of action, remains unclear. When reducing fever is the principal concern, acetaminophen has the advantage of a long record of safety; it has almost no side effects, other than allergic reactions, unless ingested in toxic amounts (more than 140 mg/kg), which is at least tenfold greater than its therapeutic dose (10 to 15 mg/kg).[39] Children younger than age 6 years, the group most frequently febrile, are significantly less susceptible than older children and adults to liver destruction, the major toxicity of acetaminophen poisoning.

At its optimal dose (10 mg/kg) ibuprofen reduces fever as effectively as acetaminophen, and because its duration of action is moderately longer, it can be given every 6 hours rather than every 4 hours.[13,44] However, there is a cost to ibuprofen's less frequent dosing; typically of antiinflammatory agents, it can cause gastritis and gastrointestinal bleeding, and it inhibits platelet function. The clinical situation determines whether ibuprofen's suppression of inflammation is a benefit or potentially an undesirable side effect. In a child febrile with rheumatoid disease, ibuprofen offers relief that acetaminophen cannot; a child whose fever arises from infection may well do better with the inflammatory response left intact. Other NSAIDS, with properties and side effects similar to ibuprofen's, are coming on the market. Naproxen is already available in a pediatric suspension; although it is approved only for use in children over the age of 2 years for treatment of juvenile arthritis, it will doubtlessly be used as an antipyretic too. Because of its relatively long half-life, naproxen can be given twice daily, at a dose of 5 mg/kg.

As an alternative to medication, physical cooling can lower the body temperature of a febrile child, but the physiology of fever explains why the result may paradoxically make the child feel worse. With fever the hypothalamic thermostat is set above normal, dictating that the body generate heat. Whereas acetaminophen or NSAIDs push the thermostat back down, damping the impulse to produce heat, physical measures such as sponging work the opposite way; in effect, they open the windows to let heat escape without adjusting the thermostat at all. As cooling begins, the hypothalamus senses wider divergence between its own set-point and the body's actual temperature; to close the gap, it sends out the directive to generate still more heat, with muscular shivering and a rise in the general metabolic rate. Aside from how uncomfortable the child may feel, with the set-point remaining high once the sponging is finished, the temperature is likely to renew its climb.

Of course, under some circumstances physical cooling has a place. Some fevers that warrant intervention clinically may not respond to antipyretic drugs, as in a neurologically impaired child whose temperature control is aberrant. If an underlying illness gives special urgency to reducing the metabolic stress that comes with a fever, the combination of an antipyretic medication and cooling not only works more quickly than either alone[36] but also makes physiological sense; while cooling physically draws heat off, the drug lowers the set-point to avert a rebound temperature rise. The same holds for the rare fever high enough to be a concern itself or for a fever that is complicated by some element of hyperthermia. When sponging a child, tepid water (about 90° F [32° C]) probably is best. It sets a moderate but effective gradient down from body temperature, rather than the precipitous decline colder water would induce, and it is less likely to distress the child who has a shivering response. Alcohol solutions have no place at all in the management of a febrile child because alcohol can be absorbed through the skin.

Hippocrates saw it right when, without the insights of our science, he somehow appreciated fever as part of the body's natural defense. Often, we do best to let nature have its way.

REFERENCES

1. Alpert G, Hibert E, Fleisher GR: Case control study of hyperpyrexia in children, *Pediatr Infect Dis J* 9:161, 1990.
2. Baker RC, et al: Severity of disease correlated with fever reduction in febrile infants, *Pediatrics* 83:1016, 1989.
3. Banco L, Veltri D: Ability of mothers to subjectively assess the presence of fever in their children, *Am J Dis Child* 138:976, 1984.
4. Berg AT, et al: A perspective study of recurrent febrile seizures, *N Engl J Med* 327:1122, 1992.
5. Bernheim HA, Kluger MJ: Effect of drug-induced antipyresis on survival, *Science* 193:237, 1976.
6. Bonadio WA, et al: Relationship of fever magnitude to rate of serious bacterial infections in infants aged 4-8 weeks, *Clin Pediatr* 30:478, 1991.
7. Casey R, et al: Fever therapy: an educational intervention for parents, *Pediatrics* 73:600, 1984.
8. Committee on Infectious Diseases, American Academy of Pediatrics: Special report: aspirin and Reye syndrome, *Pediatrics* 69:810, 1982.
9. Covert JB, Reynolds WW: Survival value of fever in fish, *Nature* 267:43, 1977.
10. Dinarello CA, Wolff SM: Pathogenesis of fever in man, *N Engl J Med* 298:607, 1978.
11. DuBois EF: Why are fever temperatures over 106° F rare? *Am J Med Sci* 217:361, 1949.
12. Fruthaler GJ: Fever in children: phobia and facts, *Hosp Pract* (Off/Ed) 20(11A):49, 1985.
13. Kauffman RE, Sawyer LA, Scheinbaum ML: Antipyretic efficacy of ibuprofen vs acetaminophen, *Am J Dis Child* 146:622, 1992.
14. Kluger MJ: Fever, *Pediatrics* 66:720, 1980.
15. Kluger MJ: Fever revisited, *Pediatrics* 90:846, 1992.
16. Kluger MJ, Rothenberg BA: Fever and reduced iron: their interaction as a host defense response to bacterial infection, *Science* 203:374, 1979.
17. Kramer MS, et al: Risks and benefits of paracetamol antipyresis in young children with fever of presumed viral origin, *Lancet* 337:591, 1991.
18. Kramer MS, Naimark L, Leduc DG: Parental fever phobia and its correlates, *Pediatrics* 75:1110, 1985.
19. Lorin MI: Measurement of body temperature, *Semin Pediatr Infect Dis* 4:4, 1993.
20. Lorin MI: Rational, symptomatic therapy for fever, *Semin Pediatr Infect Dis* 4:9, 1993.
21. Luke, 4:38-39.
22. Mackowiak PA: Concepts of fever, *Arch Intern Med* 158:1870, 1998.
23. Matthew, 8:14-15.
24. May A, Bauchner H: Fever phobia: the pediatrician's contribution, *Pediatrics* 90:851, 1992.
25. Maytal J, Shinnar S: Febrile status epilepticus, *Pediatrics* 86:611, 1990.
26. McCarthy PL: Fever in infants and children. In Machowiak PA, editor: *Fever: basic mechanisms and management,* New York, 1991, Raven Press.
27. McCarthy PL, Dolan TF: Hyperpyrexia in children, *Am J Dis Child* 130:849, 1976.
28. Press C, Fawcett NP: Association of temperature greater than 41.1° C (106° F) with serious illness, *Clin Pediatr* 24:21, 1985.
29. Richards DW: Hippocrates and history: the arrogance of humanism. In Bulger RJ, editor: *Hippocrates revisited,* New York, 1973, Medcom Press.
30. Roberts NJ Jr: Impact of temperature elevation on immunologic defenses, *Rev Infect Dis* 13:462, 1991.
31. Robinson JS, et al: The impact of fever health education on clinic utilization, *Am J Dis Child* 143:698, 1989.
32. Rylance GW, et al: Use of drugs by children, *Br Med J* 297:445, 1988.

33. Schmitt BD: Fever phobia: misconceptions of parents about fevers, *Am J Dis Child* 134:176, 1980.
34. Schnaiderman D, et al: Antipyretic effectiveness of acetaminophen in febrile seizures: ongoing prophylaxis versus sporadic usage, *Eur J Pediatr* 152:747, 1993.
35. Simon HB: Hyperthermia, *N Engl J Med* 329:483, 1993.
36. Steele RW, et al: Evaluation of sponging and of oral antipyretic therapy to reduce fever, *J Pediatr* 77:824, 1970.
37. Surgeon General's advisory on the use of salicylates and Reye syndrome, *MMWR* 31:289, 1982.
38. Surpure JS: Hyperpyrexia in children: clinical implications, *Pediatr Emerg Care* 3:10, 1987.
39. Temple AR: Pediatric dosing of acetaminophen, *Pediatr Pharmacol* 3:321, 1983.
40. Torrey SB, et al: Temperature response to antipyretic therapy in children: relationship to occult bacteremia, *Am J Emerg Med* 3:190, 1985.
41. Ushikubi F, et al: Impaired febrile response in mice lacking the prostaglandin E receptor subtype EP3, *Nature* 395:281, 1998.
42. Van Stuijvenberg M, et al: Randomized, controlled trial of ibuprofen syrup administered during febrile illnesses to prevent febrile seizure recurrences, *Pediatrics* 102:E51, 1998.
43. Vaughn LK, Bernheim HA, Kluger MJ: Fever in the lizard *Dipsosaurus dorsalis, Nature* 252:473, 1974.
44. Walson PD, et al: Comparison of multidose ibuprofen and acetaminophen therapy in febrile children, *Am J Dis Child* 146:626, 1992.

26 Management of Acute Pain in Children

Myron Yaster • Sabine Kost-Byerly
Rita S. Khandwala • Lynne G. Maxwell

We must all die. But that I can save (a person) from days of torture, that is what I feel as my great and ever new privilege. Pain is a more terrible lord of mankind than even death itself.

ALBERT SCHWEITZER, M.D.

I will use my power to help the sick to the best of my ability and judgment; I will abstain from harming or wronging any man by it.

HIPPOCRATES

Even when their pain is obvious, children frequently receive either no treatment or inadequate treatment for pain or painful procedures.[18,20] The common "wisdom" that children neither respond to nor remember painful experiences to the same degree as do adults simply is untrue.[3] Unfortunately, even when physicians decide to treat children in pain, they rarely prescribe potent analgesics or adequate doses because of their overriding concern that children may be harmed by the use of these drugs. This is not at all surprising because physicians are taught throughout their training that potent analgesics cause respiratory depression, cardiovascular collapse, depressed levels of consciousness, vomiting, and with repeated use, addiction. Rarely, if ever, are the appropriate therapeutic uses of these drugs, or rational dosing regimens, discussed.

Nurses are taught to be wary of physicians' orders (and patients' requests) as well. The most common prescription order for potent analgesics, "to give as needed" *(pro re nata, "prn"),* has come to mean "to give as infrequently as possible." The prn order also means that either the patient must ask for pain medication or the nurse must identify when a patient is in pain. This is particularly difficult when dealing with children because it may be impossible for the very young to tell us when or where they hurt. Many children withdraw or deny their pain in an attempt to avoid yet another terrifying and painful experience—the intramuscular injection, or "shot." Finally, several studies have documented the inability of nurses and physicians to identify and treat pain correctly even in postoperative pediatric patients.[19]

PAIN NEUROPHYSIOLOGY

The physiology of pain is very complex and is more than simply the transmission of pain from peripheral receptors to the brain.[17] It probably is understood best in terms of Wall and Melzack's "gate theory of pain," which can be summarized as follows.[23] Beginning with the site of active tissue damage, such as a fracture or surgical incision, and ending with the perception of pain that follows lies a complex series of physiological events, collectively termed *nociception.* Nociception can be divided into four processes: *transduction, transmission, modulation,* and *perception.* After an injury, peripheral pain receptors transmit sensory information to the spinal cord through relatively small diameter (A delta and C) sensory nerves whose cell bodies are located within the dorsal root ganglia. A delta fibers are associated with sharp, well-localized pain, whereas C fibers are associated with dull, burning, diffusely localized pain. The C fibers also include efferent sympathetic nerve fibers that increase the sensitivity of peripheral pain receptors. In the periphery, local release of prostaglandins, serotonin, bradykinin, norepinephrine, hydrogen ion, potassium ion, and substance P (a peripheral pain transmitter) can increase the responsiveness of the peripheral receptors to painful stimuli. *Transduction* refers to this process in which noxious stimuli are translated into electrical activity at the sensory nerve endings. Pharmacological manipulations of these local factors by prostaglandin inhibitors (e.g., aspirin, acetaminophen, or ibuprofen) or substance P blockade (capsaicin) can thereby blunt the transmission of pain.

The pain receptor impulse is *transmitted* to the dorsal horn of the spinal cord, where diverse synapses occur with essentially all incoming sensory input. In the dorsal horn of the spinal cord, interneurons are activated and release multiple neurotransmitters, including substance P, an 11-amino acid peptide pain transmitter. Alternatively, the pain impulse may be *modulated*—that is, it may either be reduced in intensity, completely inhibited, or augmented. Modulation occurs both between interneurons, as well as via pathways of descending inhibition originating in the thalamus and brainstem. Perhaps the most important of these sites is the dorsal horn of the spinal cord. In the dorsal horn, inhibitory neurotransmitters including norepinephrine, serotonin, gamma-aminobutyric acid (GABA), glycine, and enkephalin block the release of substance P, glutamate, and other excitatory neurotransmitters and modulate ascending transmission of painful stimuli. Descending fibers also "synapse" at the interneurons to inhibit or modulate sensory input related to an injury via the release of neuropeptides. Of these neuropeptides, the opioid peptides (e.g., endorphins and enkephalins) are the best known and most extensively studied. Indeed, the identification of a variety of opioid receptors in the dorsal horn of the spinal cord explains the effects of intrathecal and epidural opioid administration in the management of pain. Finally, stimulation of large-diameter peripheral nerve fibers can block painful information effectively from the periphery as well. This is the underlying principle behind transcutaneous electrical nerve stimulation (TENS).

If unblocked, pain reception is transmitted to the brain through the classic spinothalamic and spinoreticular nerve pathways. Several areas within the brain may further modulate or abolish pain transmission, including the brainstem's medial and lateral reticular formations, the medullary raphe nuclei, the periaqueductal gray matter, the thalamus, and the cerebral cortex. Binding of either endogenous or pharmacologically administered opiates to receptors in these central locations initiates the modulation of pain transmission.[16] The gate theory, therefore, depends not only on peripheral stimulation and transmission of pain but also on modulation of the transmission within the spinal cord and higher central nervous system structures. Finally, *perception* is the result of the application of the nociceptive information upon the existing psychological framework. It is the experience of pain, both emotional and sensory in character. That experience then changes the framework itself and thereby affects subsequent painful experiences.

Thus, pain or the transmission of pain receptor impulses requires intact neuroanatomical pathways from the peripheral origin of pain to the central nervous system. These pathways and receptors develop in early fetal life and essentially are mature and completely developed by birth.[2] The development of descending pathways for inhibiting pain receptor neurons and interneurons in the dorsal horn of the spinal cord and within the brainstem occurs during the final third of gestation and is completed during infancy and early childhood.

Pain management, therefore, can best be understood or designed in terms of afferent pain pathways and descending pain modulation pathways. Pain can be relieved by (1) reducing the sensory input from damaged tissue (by prostaglandin inhibitors or local anesthetics administration), (2) modulating the transmission of the pain receptor input to the central nervous system (by TENS, pharmacological opioid administration, or the administration of local anesthetics), and (3) altering the patient's emotional responses to such actual or perceived sensory input (by antidepressants, hypnotics, or amnestics). However, before one can treat pain effectively, one must be able to measure accurately and assess pain as well as the therapies used in treating it.

PAIN ASSESSMENT

The International Association for the Study of Pain (IASP) defines pain as "an unpleasant and emotional experience associated with actual or potential tissue damage, or described in terms of such damage."[15] Pain is a subjective experience; operationally it can be defined as "what the patient says hurts" and exists "when the patient says it does." Infants, preverbal children, and children between the ages of 2 and 7 years (Piaget's "preoperational thought stage") may be unable to describe their pain or their subjective experiences. This has led many to conclude that children do not experience pain in the same way as do adults. Clearly, children do not have to know or be able to express the meaning of an experience to have the experience. On the other hand, because pain is essentially a subjective experience, it is becoming increasingly clear that the child's perspective of pain is an indispensable facet of pediatric pain management and an essential element in the specialized study of childhood pain. Indeed, pain assessment and management are interdependent; one is essentially useless without the other. The goal of pain assessment is to provide accurate data about the location and intensity of pain as well as the effectiveness of measures used to alleviate or abolish it.

Valid, reliable instruments exist to measure and assess pain in children older than age 3 years.[7] These instruments, which measure the quality and intensity of pain, are "self-report measures" and make use of pictures or word descriptors to describe pain. Pain intensity or severity can be measured in children as young as 3 years by using picture scales—for example, (1) Wong's "smiley" face scale, which has a smiling face on one end; a distraught, crying face on the other; and several gradations in between; or (2) the "Oucher" scale, a two-part scale that has vertical numerical gradations (0 to 100) on one side and six photographs of a young child on the other (Fig. 26-1).[7,25] Pain has been assessed in infants and newborns by measuring physiological responses to painful stimuli; typically, blood pressure, heart rate, heart rate variability, vagal response, and levels of adrenal stress hormones are measured.[13] Alternatively, behavioral approaches have used facial expression, body movements, and the intensity and quality of crying as indices of response to painful stimuli. Finally, it is important to define the location of pain accurately. This is accomplished readily by using either dolls, other figures, or drawings of body outlines, both front and back.

PAIN MANAGEMENT

Nonopioid (or "Weaker") Analgesics

The "weaker" or "milder" analgesics, of which acetaminophen (Tylenol), salicylate (aspirin), ibuprofen (Motrin), and ketorolac (Toradol) are the classic examples, constitute a heterogenous group of drugs that commonly are used to treat mild to moderate pain (Table 26-1). The nonsteroidal antiinflammatory drugs (NSAIDs) provide pain relief primarily by blocking peripheral prostaglandin production, whereas acetaminophen primarily provides pain relief by blocking central prostaglandin production. These analgesic agents are administered enterally via the oral and rectal routes and parenterally (ketorolac) via the intravenous or intramuscular routes. The NSAIDs are particularly useful for inflammatory, bony, or rheumatic pain. Unfortunately, regardless of dose, the nonopioid analgesics reach a "ceiling effect" above which pain cannot be relieved by these drugs alone. Indeed, because of this, these weaker analgesics often are administered in combination with other more potent opioids such as codeine, oxycodone, or hydrocodone.

Aspirin, one of the oldest and most effective nonopioid analgesics, has largely been abandoned in pediatric practice because of its possible role in Reye's syndrome, its effects on platelet function, and its gastric irritant properties. Despite these problems, choline-magnesium trisalicylate (Trilisate) is being used increasingly in pediatric pain management, particularly in the management of postoperative pain and in the child who has cancer. Choline-magnesium trisalicylate is a unique aspirin-like compound that does not bind to platelets and therefore has no effect on platelet function. It is a convenient drug to give to children because it is available in both liquid and tablet form and is administered only twice a day

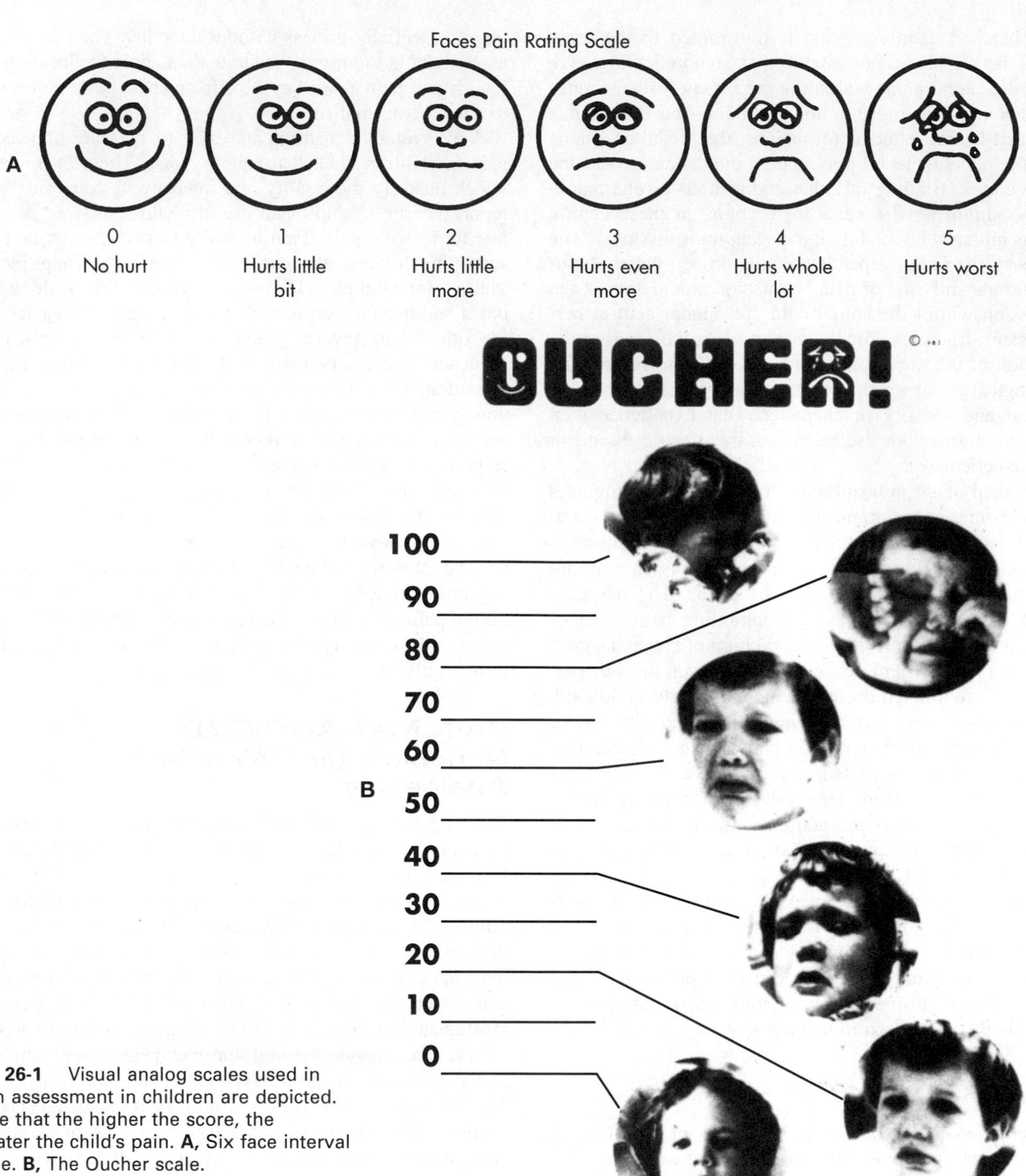

Fig. 26-1 Visual analog scales used in pain assessment in children are depicted. Note that the higher the score, the greater the child's pain. **A,** Six face interval scale. **B,** The Oucher scale.

(**A** from Wong DL, Hockenberry-Eaton M: *Wong's essentials of pediatric nursing,* ed 6, St Louis, Mosby, 2001. **B** Courtesy Dr. Judith Beyer.)

(see Table 26-1). The association of salicylates with Reye's syndrome limits its use, even though the risk of developing this syndrome postoperatively or in cancer is extremely remote. The NSAIDS most commonly used for pain management in children are ibuprofen and ketorolac.

The nonopioid analgesic used most commonly in pediatric practice remains acetaminophen. Unlike aspirin and the NSAIDs, acetaminophen has minimal, if any, antiinflammatory activity. Acetaminophen is unique in that it blocks prostaglandin synthesis centrally and not peripherally, which accounts for its antipyretic, as well as analgesic, properties and why it does not interfere with platelet aggregation. The antipyretic effect is believed to be exerted via the hypothalamus, yet the analgesic effect may be mediated spinally. When administered in normal doses (10 to 15 mg/kg, PO or PR every 4 hours; 30 to 40 mg/kg when administered rectally as a single [loading] dose, follow-up rectal doses are 10 to 15 mg/kg), acetaminophen has very few serious side effects.[28] It is an antipyretic, and like all other NSAIDs, takes about 40 to 60 minutes to provide effective analgesia. Dosage guidelines

Table 26-1 Dosage Guidelines for Commonly Used Nonsteroidal Antiinflammatory Drugs (NSAIDs)

Generic Name	Brand Name	Dose (mg/kg); Frequency	Maximum Adult Daily Dose (mg)	Comments
Salicylates	Aspirin—many brands (e.g., Bayer, Bufferin, Anacin, Alka-Seltzer)	10-15 q 4 h	4000	Inhibits platelet aggregation, GI irritability, Reye's syndrome
Acetaminophen	Many brand names (e.g., Tylenol, "aspirin-free," Panadol, Tempra)	10-15 q 4 h	4000	Lacks antiinflammatory activity
Ibuprofen	Many brand names (e.g., Motrin, Advil, Medipren)	6-10 q 6-8 h	2400	Available as an oral suspension
Naproxen	Naprosyn	5-10 q 12 h	1000	Available as an oral suspension
Indomethacin	Indocin	0.3-1.0 q 6 h	150	Commonly used in NICUs to close a patent ductus arteriosus
Ketorolac	Toradol	0.2-0.5 q 6 h	150	May be given IV, IM, or PO
Choline-magnesium trisalicylate	Trilisate	8-10 q 8-12 h	3000	Does not bind to platelets; see "Salicylates" above

for the nonopioid analgesics used most commonly are listed in Table 26-1.

Opioids

Terminology. The terminology used to describe potent analgesic drugs is constantly changing. They commonly are referred to as "narcotics" (from the Greek *narco,* "to deaden"), "opiates" (from the Greek *opion,* "poppy juice," for drugs derived from the poppy plant), "opioids" (for all drugs that have morphine-like effects, whether synthetic or naturally occurring), or euphemistically as "strong analgesics" (when the physician is reluctant to tell the patient or the patient's family that opioids are being used).[27,29] We prefer the term *opioid* and use it throughout this chapter. The discovery of endogenous endorphins and opioid receptors has necessitated the reclassification of these drugs into agonists, antagonists, and mixed agonist-antagonists based on their receptor-binding properties.

The differentiation of agonists and antagonists is fundamental to pharmacology. A neurotransmitter is defined as having agonist activity, whereas a drug that blocks the action of the neurotransmitter is an antagonist. By definition, receptor recognition of an agonist is "translated" into other cellular alterations, whereas an antagonist occupies the receptor without initiating the transduction step. Morphine and related opiates are agonists; drugs that block the effects of opiates, such as naloxone, are designated antagonists.

Opioids interact with specific receptors that are distributed widely throughout the central nervous system. Different effects, sensitivities, and anatomical localization have been ascribed to these various receptors. Although there are as many as eight different opioid receptors, three are of major importance in terms of pain management. These are designated as the mu, delta, and kappa receptors. The mu receptor and its subspecies and the delta receptor are related to analgesia, respiratory depression, euphoria, and physical dependence. Morphine is 50 to 100 times weaker at the delta than at the mu receptor. By contrast, the endogenous opiate-like neurotransmitter peptides known as enkephalins tend to be more potent at delta than at mu receptors. The kappa receptor, located primarily in the spinal cord, is related to spinal analgesia, miosis, and sedation. The sigma receptor is responsible for the psychotomimetic effects observed with some opiate drugs, particularly the mixed agonist-antagonist drugs. These effects include dysphoria and hallucinations.

A number of studies suggest that the respiratory depression and analgesia produced by opiates involve different receptor subtypes. These receptors change in number in an age-related fashion and can be blocked by naloxone. Zhang and Pasternak,[31] working with newborn rats, showed that 14-day-old rats are 40 times more sensitive to morphine analgesia than are 2-day-old rats.[31] Nevertheless, morphine depresses the respiratory rate in 2-day-old rats to a greater degree than in 14-day-old rats. Thus, the newborn is particularly sensitive to the respiratory depressant effects of the opioids in what may be an age-related receptor phenomenon. Obviously, this has important clinical implications for the use of opioids in the newborn (see p. 346).

Myths and misconceptions concerning opioids. Despite the confusion of terminology and the plethora of available drugs, it is essential to realize that at *equipotent* analgesic doses, all commonly used opioids produce similar degrees of respiratory depression, sedation, euphoria, nausea, biliary tract spasm, and constipation. Mixed agonist-antagonist drugs such as pentazocine (Talwin), nalbuphine (Nubain), and butorphanol (Stadol) produce significantly less respiratory depression and biliary spasm than do pure agonist drugs such as morphine. However, they also are significantly less potent analgesics than are the pure agonists and reach a "ceiling" above which no further analgesia can be achieved. Furthermore, they can reverse previously induced opioid analgesia and should never be used in patients who are long-term users (or addicts) of opioids. Although an enormous number of opioids are available for clinical use, each with some purported advantage (typically "more effective," "less respiratory depression," or "less addiction" potential), the drugs listed in Table 26-2 are those used most commonly.

Opioids usually are administered at fixed intervals despite enormous variability in patient response. It is not uncommon for doctors to order doses that are too small and at intervals that are too long for individual patient needs (Fig. 26-2). Furthermore, nurses often delay administering opioids for several reasons: unfamiliarity with the child's pain symptoms, demands of other patients, fear of addiction, and difficulty in finding the keys to the locked narcotic cabinet. Rational use of opioids requires a flexible, patient-oriented approach to allow for variability in individual pain and tolerance, as well as both the beneficial and adverse effects of the particular drug being used. Increasingly, an alternative approach utilizes patient-controlled analgesia (PCA) devices, in which patients can administer small amounts of an analgesic whenever they feel a need for more pain relief. This technology allows patients to titrate drug to effect and because only the patient can self-administer a dose of opioid, the potential for overdosage is minimized. In adults, adolescents, and children older than 6 years of age, intravenous PCA has become commonplace (see discussion of PCA on p. 350).

Morphine

Morphine (from Morpheus, the Greek god of sleep) is the standard for analgesia against which all other opioids are compared. When small doses, 0.1 mg/kg (IV, IM), are administered to otherwise unmedicated patients in pain, analgesia usually occurs without loss of consciousness. The relief of tension, anxiety, and pain usually results in drowsiness and sleep. Older patients suffering from discomfort and pain usually develop a sense of well-being or euphoria after morphine administration. Interestingly, when morphine is given to pain-free adults, they may show the opposite effect, namely dysphoria and increased fear and anxiety. Mental clouding, drowsiness, lethargy, and an inability to concentrate and sleep may occur after morphine administration, even in the absence of pain. Less advantageous central nervous system effects of morphine include nausea and vomiting, miosis, and at high doses, seizures. Seizures are a particular problem in the newborn because they may occur at commonly prescribed doses (0.1 mg/kg). The nausea and vomiting that are seen with morphine administration are due to stimulation of the chemoreceptor trigger zone in the brainstem.

Morphine (and all other opioids at equipotent doses) depresses respiration, principally by reducing the sensitivity of the brainstem respiratory centers to arterial carbon dioxide content. Infants younger than 1 to 2 months of age are particularly sensitive to this depression. *Indeed, this is of such great concern that the use of any opioid in children younger than 2 months of age must be limited to a monitored, high-surveillance unit.* Possible explanations for this increased sensitivity include differences in opiate receptors (see p. 345), the blood-brain barrier, and pharmacokinetics.

Way, Costley, and Way suggested that an incomplete blood-brain barrier (as demonstrated in newborn rats) allows greater penetration of morphine to central nervous system receptor sites.[24] Presumably this would allow more drug to enter the central nervous system and produce a more profound effect. Several studies have demonstrated a prolonged elimination half-life (6.8 versus 2.9 hours) and decreased clearance (6.3 versus 23.8 ml/kg/min) of morphine in infants younger than 1 month of age when compared with older

Table 26-2 Commonly Used Mu Agonist Drugs

Agonist	Equipotent IV Dose (mg/kg)	Duration (hr)	PO Absorption (%)	Comments
Morphine	0.1	3-4	20-40	• May cause seizures in newborns; also in all patients at high doses • Causes histamine release, vasodilation, so avoid in patients with asthma and in circulatory compromise • MS Contin; 8-12 h duration
Meperidine	1.0	3-4	40-60	• Catastrophic interactions with monoamine oxidase (MAO) inhibitors • Tachycardia; negative inotrope • Metabolite produces seizures • **Not recommended for routine analgesic therapy** • Low dose (0.25 mg/kg) stops shivering
Methadone	0.1	6-24	70-100	• Can be given IV even though the package insert says SQ or IM
Fentanyl	0.001	0.5-1		• Bradycardia; minimal hemodynamic alterations • Chest wall rigidity (>5 µg/kg rapid IV bolus). R_x naloxone, succinylcholine, or pancuronium • Oral transmucosal preparation 10 µg/kg
Codeine	1.2	3-4	40-70	• PO only • Prescribe with acetaminophen
Oxycodone (Tylox)	0.1	3-4	60-80	• PO only, less nauseating than codeine • Usually prescribed with acetaminophen

infants and adults. Nevertheless, the half-life of elimination and clearance of morphine in children older than 1 month is similar to adult values. Thus, infants younger than 1 month of age will attain higher serum levels that will decline more slowly than those in older children and adults, which may account for the increased respiratory depression seen in this age group. Conversely, based on its relatively short half-life (2.9 hours), one would expect older children and adults to require morphine supplementation every 2 to 3 hours when being treated for pain, particularly if the morphine is administered intravenously. This has led to the recent use of continuous infusion regimens of morphine and PCA (see p. 350), which maximize pain-free periods (see Fig. 26-2).

Although morphine produces peripheral vasodilation and venous pooling, it has minimal hemodynamic effects in normal, euvolemic, supine patients. The vasodilation associated with morphine is due primarily to its histamine-releasing effects. Significant hypotension may occur if sedatives such as diazepam are administered concurrently with morphine. Otherwise, it produces virtually no cardiovascular effects when used alone. It will cause significant hypotension in hypovolemic patients; its use in trauma, therefore, is limited.

Morphine (and all other opioids at equipotent doses) inhibits intestinal smooth muscle motility. This decrease in peristalsis and increase in sphincter tone explains the historical use of opioids in the treatment of diarrhea as well as its "side effect" when treating chronic pain, namely, constipation. In fact, laxatives should be prescribed for patients expected to be treated with opioids for more than 2 or 3 days. Obviously, morphine will potentiate biliary colic by causing spasm of the sphincter of Odi and should be used with caution in patients who have, or are at risk for, cholelithiasis (e.g., sickle cell disease). Finally, to minimize the complications associated with the administration of intravenous morphine (or any opioid), bedside titration of the dose should be instituted until the desired level of analgesia is achieved.

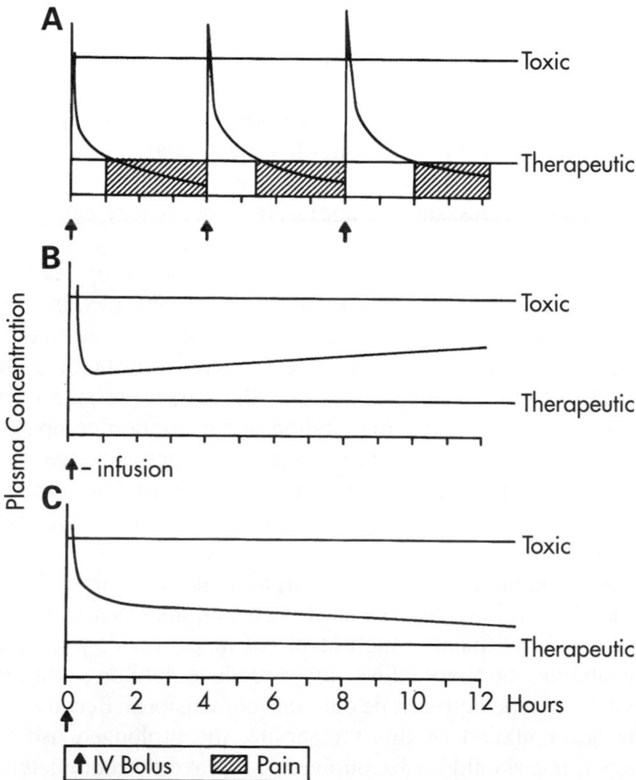

Fig. 26-2 Simulated blood concentration-dose relationships for opioids by different administration regimens. **A,** IV bolus administration of morphine sulfate (elimination half-life, 4 hours) every 4 hours. **B,** IV bolus administration of morphine sulfate followed by continuous IV infusion. **C,** IV bolus infusion of methadone (elimination half-life, 19 hours). Note the absence of pain periods in **B** and **C.** (*Arrows,* time of IV bolus administration.)

Morphine and most mu agonists (meperidine, methadone, and fentanyl) are biotransformed in the liver before excretion. Many of these reactions are catalyzed in the liver by microsomal mixed-function oxidases. Morphine primarily is glucuronidated into two forms—an inactive form, morphine-3-glucuronide, and an active form, morphine-6-glucuronide. Both glucuronides are excreted by the kidney. In patients who have renal failure, the morphine 6-glucuronide can accumulate and cause toxic side effects, including respiratory depression. This is important to consider not only when prescribing morphine but also when administering other opioids that are metabolized into morphine, such as methadone and codeine.

Finally, only about 30% of an orally administered dose of morphine reaches the systemic circulation. In the past, this led many to believe that morphine was ineffective if administered orally. This is not true and was the result of failing to provide sufficient morphine. When converting a patient's intravenous morphine requirements to oral maintenance, one needs to multiply the intravenous dose by 3 to 4. Oral morphine is available as a liquid in various concentrations (as much as 20 mg/ml), as a tablet—MSIR (morphine sulfate immediate release), available in 15- and 30-mg doses, and as a sustained-release preparation (MS Contin and Oramorph tablets, and Kadian "sprinkle capsules"), which may be opened and sprinkled on applesauce. Because it is so concentrated, the liquid is particularly easy to administer to children and severely debilitated patients. Indeed, in terminal patients who cannot swallow, liquid morphine will provide analgesia when simply dropped into the patient's mouth (see Table 26-2).

Fentanyl

Because of its rapid onset and brief duration of action, fentanyl has become a favored analgesic for short procedures, such as bone marrow aspirations, fracture reductions, suturing of lacerations, endoscopy, and dental procedures. Fentanyl is approximately 100 times more potent than morphine (the equianalgesic dose is 0.001 mg/kg, [see Table 26-2]) and largely is devoid of hypnotic or sedative activity. Its ability to block painful stimuli with concomitant hemodynamic stability is excellent and makes it the drug of choice for trauma, cardiac, or intensive care unit patients. Furthermore, in addition to its ability to block the systemic and pulmonary hemodynamic responses to pain, fentanyl also prevents the biochemical and endocrine stress (catabolic) response to painful stimuli that may be so detrimental in the seriously ill patient. Fentanyl does have a serious side effect—namely, the development of chest wall rigidity after rapid infusions of 0.005

mg/kg or greater. This may make ventilation difficult or impossible. Chest wall rigidity can be treated with either muscle relaxants, such as succinylcholine or pancuronium, or with naloxone.

Fentanyl is a highly lipophilic drug and penetrates all membranes rapidly, including the oral mucosa and skin. Indeed, this has made transmucosal and transdermal preparations of this drug possible. Fentanyl is eliminated rapidly from plasma as the result of its extensive uptake by body tissues. Its pharmacokinetics differ between newborn infants and children and adults. The total body clearance of fentanyl is greater in infants 3 to 12 months of age than in children older than 1 year or adults (18.1 ± 1.4, 11.5 ± 4.2, and 10.0 ± 1.7 ml/kg/min, respectively), and the half-life of elimination is longer (233 ± 137, 244 ± 79, and 129 ± 42 minutes, respectively). The prolonged elimination half-life of fentanyl from plasma has important clinical implications. Repeated doses of fentanyl for maintenance of analgesic effects will lead to accumulation of fentanyl and its ventilatory depressant effects. Very large doses (0.05 to 0.10 mg/kg, as used in anesthesia) may be expected to induce long-lasting effects because plasma fentanyl levels would not fall below the threshold level at which spontaneous ventilation occurs during the distribution phases. On the other hand, the greater clearance of fentanyl in infants older than 3 months produces lower plasma concentrations of the drug and may allow these children to tolerate more drug without respiratory depression.

Because fentanyl is extremely lipophilic, it can be readily absorbed across any biological membrane, including the skin. Thus, it can be given painlessly by new, nonintravenous routes of drug administration, including the transmucosal (nose and mouth) and transdermal routes. The transdermal route is used frequently to administer many drugs, including scopolamine, clonidine, and nitroglycerin, over long periods. A selective semi-permeable membrane patch with a reservoir of drug allows for the slow, steady state absorption of drug across the skin. Transdermal fentanyl is ***contraindicated*** for *acute* pain management and is applicable only for patients who have chronic pain (e.g., cancer) or in opioid-tolerant patients. The use of this drug delivery system for acute pain has resulted in the death of an otherwise healthy patient. Additionally, the safety of this drug delivery system is compromised even further because fentanyl will continue to be absorbed from the subcutaneous fat for almost 24 hours after the patch is removed. Even when transdermal fentanyl is appropriate, the vehicle imposes its own constraints: The smallest "denomination" of fentanyl "patch" delivers 12.5 μg of fentanyl per hour. Patches *cannot* be physically cut in smaller pieces to deliver less fentanyl, which often limits usefulness in smaller patients.

On the other hand, the transmucosal route of fentanyl administration is extremely effective for acute pain relief and heralds a new era in the management of acute pain in children. In this novel delivery technique, fentanyl is manufactured in a candy matrix (Fentanyl Oralet) attached to a plastic applicator (it looks like a lollipop); as the child sucks on the candy, fentanyl is absorbed across the buccal mucosa and is absorbed rapidly into the systemic circulation in 10 to 20 minutes. If excessive sedation occurs, the fentanyl "lollipop" is removed from the child's mouth. The Fentanyl Oralet has been approved by the Federal Drug Administration for use in children for premedication before surgery and for procedure-related pain (e.g., lumbar puncture, bone marrow aspiration). When administered by this route, fentanyl, given in doses of 10 to 15 μg/kg is effective within 20 minutes and lasts approximately 2 hours. Approximately 25% to 33% of the given dose is absorbed. Thus, when administered in doses of 10 to 15 μg/kg, blood levels equivalent to 3 to 5 μg/kg IV fentanyl are achieved. The major side effect, nausea and vomiting, occurs in approximately 20% to 33% of patients who receive it. This product is available only in hospital (and Surgicenter) pharmacies and like all sedative/analgesics, requires vigilant patient monitoring. It is best used in opioid-experienced patients (e.g., burn patients, trauma victims) who undergo repeated painful procedures. In these patients, the incidence of nausea is much less than in opioid-naive patients.

Meperidine

Meperidine (Demerol) is a synthetic opioid used most commonly in children as either a premedicant for anesthesia (or sedation) or as a treatment for postoperative pain. It is a potent analgesic that has pharmacokinetic properties similar to those of morphine. Meperidine is a mu agonist that binds to opioid receptors in the central nervous system and can produce analgesia, sedation, euphoria, dysphoria, miosis, and respiratory depression. At equianalgesic doses (1.0 mg/kg [see Table 26-2]), there is little quantitative difference between meperidine and morphine in producing these effects. It stimulates the chemoreceptor trigger zone in the brainstem to the same degree that morphine does and thereby may produce either nausea, vomiting, or both. Its effects on respiration and on gastrointestinal motility are similar to those of all the other mu-agonist opioid analgesics; thus, it is a potent respiratory depressant and antitussive. Meperidine depresses intestinal smooth muscle motility and exerts a spasmogenic effect on intestinal smooth muscle. Some studies suggest that meperidine exerts less of an effect on the biliary tract, including the common bile duct, than does morphine. Other studies dispute this. Indeed, there is *no* evidence to substantiate the belief that at *equianalgesic* doses, biliary tract pressure rises to a lesser extent after meperidine administration compared with morphine. Thus, there is no reason to prescribe meperidine preferentially for patients at risk for, or who are experiencing, biliary colic pain (e.g., sickle cell vasoocclusive crisis).

Meperidine differs from morphine in that large doses (toxic levels) may produce slow waves on the electroencephalogram. Additionally, high levels of meperidine's principal metabolite, normeperidine, may produce tremors, muscle twitches, hyperactive reflexes, and convulsions. Because of the accumulation of this metabolite, the prolonged use of meperidine should be discouraged, if not avoided completely. Meperidine when administered at low doses (0.25 to 0.5 mg/kg) intravenously, has the unique property of abolishing shivering; it will stop shivering regardless of its cause (e.g., transfusion or drug [amphotericin] reactions, hypothermia, and so on).

Meperidine is effective whether administered orally or parenterally. The drug is extremely well absorbed from the gastrointestinal tract and has a bioavailability of approximately 50%, making it among the most popularly prescribed oral opioids. It is available in both liquid (syrup) and tablet form, the usual dose being 1 to 2 mg/kg. Typically, it can exert analgesic effects within 15 to 30 minutes of oral administration and achieves peak plasma concentrations within 1 to 2 hours of ingestion. Intramuscular injection provides a more rapid onset of analgesia (approximately 10 minutes) and reaches a peak effect within 60 minutes of administration. Obviously, plasma concentrations may vary markedly after intramuscular injection, based on an individual patient's state of peripheral perfusion.

In the past, meperidine was administered intramuscularly for moderate to severe pain or as part of a "lytic," sedative cocktail (meperidine, promethazine, and chlorpromazine). Currently, intramuscular administration of analgesics is not recommended for children, nor is the use of the lytic cocktail. *In fact, the lytic cocktail is considered to be an archaic and dangerous sedative combination.*

Methadone

Primarily thought of as a drug to treat (narcotic) addicted patients, methadone increasingly is being used for postoperative pain relief and to treat intractable pain. It is noted for its slow elimination, very long duration of effective analgesia, and high oral bioavailability.

Methadone has the longest half-life of elimination ($t_{1/2}$ beta) of any of the commonly available opiates and provides 12 to 36 hours of analgesia following an intravenous injection. In children (ages 1 to 18 years), the $t_{1/2}$ beta of methadone averages 19.2 hours and the clearance averages 5.4 ml/min/kg. Pharmacokinetically, children are indistinguishable from young adults. Finally, because methadone is extremely well absorbed from the gastrointestinal tract and has a bioavailability of 80% to 90%, it is extremely easy to convert intravenous to oral dosing regimens.

Because a single intravenous dose of methadone can achieve and sustain a high drug plasma level, it is a convenient way to provide prolonged analgesia without requiring an intramuscular injection (see Fig. 26-2). Indeed, when administered either orally or intravenously, it may be viewed as an alternative to the use of continuous intravenous opioid infusions. Berde et al recommend "loading" patients with an initial dose of intravenous methadone, 0.1 to 0.2 mg/kg, and then titrating in 0.05 mg/kg increments.[6] Supplemental methadone can be administered in 0.05 to 0.1 mg/kg increments by slow intravenous infusion every 6 to 12 hours as needed.

Codeine, Oxycodone, and Hydrocodone

Codeine, oxycodone (the opioid in Tylox and Percocet), and hydrocodone (the opioid in Vicodin and Lortab) are opioids that frequently are used to treat pain in children and adults, particularly for less severe pain or when patients are being converted from parenteral to enteral opioids (see Table 26-2).[28] Morphine is used commonly in regimens for chronic pain (e.g., cancer). Codeine, oxycodone, and hydrocodone are administered most commonly orally, usually in combination with acetaminophen (Tylox, Percocet, Vicodin, Lortab, Codeine No. 1, 2, 3, and 4), or aspirin.

In equipotent doses, codeine, oxycodone, hydrocodone, and morphine are equal both as analgesics and respiratory depressants. In addition, these drugs share with other opioids common effects on the central nervous system including sedation, respiratory depression, and stimulation of the chemoreceptor trigger zone in the brainstem. Indeed, the latter is particularly true for codeine. Codeine is very nauseating; many patients claim they are "allergic" to it because it so commonly induces vomiting. There are far fewer nausea and vomiting problems with oxycodone. Indeed, because of this, oxycodone or hydrocodone are now the preferred oral opioids. Despite surgical folklore, at equipotent doses all opioids delay gastric emptying and can increase biliary tract pressure. Indeed, meperidine offers no advantage over other opioids in this regard, even though it frequently is prescribed for its presumed lack of effect on the sphincter of Odi. Finally, codeine (like all mu-agonist opioids) has potent antitussive properties and is prescribed commonly for this effect.

Codeine, hydrocodone, and oxycodone have a bioavailability of approximately 60% following oral ingestion. The analgesic effects occur as early as 20 minutes following ingestion and reach a maximum at 60 to 120 minutes. The plasma half-life of elimination is 2.5 to 4 hours. Codeine undergoes nearly complete metabolism in the liver before its final excretion in urine. Approximately 10% of codeine is metabolized into morphine; it is this 10% that is responsible for codeine's analgesic effect. Interestingly, approximately 10% of the population cannot metabolize codeine into morphine; in these patients, codeine will have no analgesic effects.

Oral codeine, hydrocodone, and oxycodone almost always are prescribed in combination with either acetaminophen or aspirin (Tylenol and codeine elixir, Percocet, Tylox, Vicodin, Lortab).[28] Typically, codeine is prescribed in a dose of 0.5 to 1 mg/kg. Elixirs, which are available in virtually every pharmacy, contain 120 mg acetaminophen and 12 mg codeine per teaspoon (5 ml). If prescribing codeine, the premixed combination compound is recommended for most children. When prescribed as a single agent, codeine is not readily available in liquid form at most pharmacies and is almost twice as expensive as the combined form. Furthermore, acetaminophen potentiates the analgesia produced by codeine and allows the practitioner to use less opioid and yet achieve satisfactory analgesia. Codeine and acetaminophen also are available as "numbered" tablets—for example, Tylenol No. 1, 2, 3, or 4. The number refers to how much codeine is in each tablet. Tylenol No. 4 has 60 mg codeine, No. 3 has 30 mg, No. 2 has 15 mg, and No. 1 has 7.5 mg. Although it is an effective analgesic when administered parenterally, intramuscular codeine has no advantage over morphine or meperidine. Intravenous administration of codeine is associated with serious complications including apnea and severe hypotension, probably secondary to histamine release. Therefore, the intravenous administration of this drug in children is not recommended.

Hydrocodone is prescribed in a dose of 0.05 to 0.1 mg/kg. The elixir is available as 2.5 mg/5 ml combined with acetaminophen 167 mg/5 ml. As a tablet, it is available in hydrocodone doses between 2.5 to 10 mg, combined with 500 to 650 mg acetaminophen. Oxycodone is prescribed in a dose of 0.05 to 0.1 mg/kg. Unfortunately, the elixir is not available in most pharmacies. When it is, it comes as 1 mg/ml. In tablet form, oxycodone is commonly available as Tylox (500 mg acetaminophen and 5.0 mg oxycodone) and as Percocet (325 mg acetaminophen and 5 mg oxycodone). *In all "combination preparations," one should beware of inadvertently administering an hepatotoxic acetaminophen dose when increasing doses for uncontrolled pain.*[28] Toxicity may result from a single dose, from repeated ingestion of large doses (e.g., in adults, 7.5 to 10 g daily for 1 to 2 days, children 60 to 420 mg/kg/day for 1 or more days), or from chronic ingestion of smaller amounts.

Oxycodone also is available without acetaminophen in a sustained-release tablet for use in chronic pain. Like all time-release tablets, it must *not* be ground up and therefore cannot be administered through a gastric tube. Like sustained-release morphine, sustained-release oxycodone is for use only in opioid-tolerant patients who have chronic pain, *not* for routine postoperative pain. In patients with rapid GI transit, sustained-release preparations may not be absorbed at all; liquid methadone may be used as an alternative.

Opioid Antagonists

A discussion of opioid analgesics would be incomplete without mentioning the opioid antagonists. As mentioned previously, a drug that blocks the action of a neurotransmitter is an antagonist. By definition, receptor recognition of an agonist is "translated" into other cellular alterations, whereas an antagonist occupies the receptor without initiating the transduction step. Naloxone is a pure opioid antagonist that has virtually no agonist activity. It antagonizes the effects of the pure agonist drugs, such as morphine, as well as the mixed agonist-antagonist drugs, such as butorphanol. It is the most commonly used opioid antagonist in clinical practice.

Naloxone is extremely potent and nonselective in its opioid reversal effects. It reverses not only the sedation, respiratory depression, and gastrointestinal effects of the opioid agonists but also the analgesia. Indeed, the antagonism of opioid agonist effects must be accomplished with great caution, particularly in patients who have been receiving prolonged opioid therapy, who exhibit opioid dependence, or who are in extreme pain because it may be accompanied by overt withdrawal symptoms. Occasionally a life-threatening "overshoot" phenomenon may occur in these patients, with the development of tachypnea, tachycardia, hypertension, nausea and vomiting, and sudden death. In healthy young adults this phenomenon may be accompanied by the onset of pulmonary edema. Indeed, it is prudent to employ mechanical ventilation as a safer treatment for opioid-induced respiratory depression in dependent patients or patients in severe pain. Obviously, the magnitude of the withdrawal syndrome depends on the dose of naloxone administered as well as on the degree of the patient's physical dependence and needs. On the other hand, when naloxone is administered to patients who have not received opioids, it produces minimal to no effects (except in patients in shock) and has no inherent properties that induce physical dependence or tolerance.

Naloxone metabolizes rapidly in the liver (conjugation with glucuronic acid) and is best given parenterally because of its rapid first-pass extraction through the liver after oral administration. After intravenous administration it reverses opioid effects virtually instantaneously. Unfortunately, it has a plasma half-life of elimination of only 60 minutes and a duration of action that is much shorter than the agonists it is used to antagonize ("reverse"). Therefore, when naloxone is used to reverse opioid-induced respiratory depression, patients must be monitored for return of the depression on the basis of the half-life of the opiate agonist. This may require repeat intravenous doses, intramuscular (depot) injection, or a continuous intravenous infusion of naloxone.

Naloxone is supplied as a parenteral solution (1.0 mg/ml, 0.4 mg/ml, or 0.02 mg/ml). The usual initial dose in children (and adults) is 0.01 to 0.10 mg/kg given intravenously. If an intravenous route is not available, naloxone may be administered intramuscularly or subcutaneously. Doses as low as 0.001 to 0.002 mg/kg may be effective at antagonizing opioid-induced respiratory depression (or other unwanted side effects such as pruritus or biliary spasm) without reversing analgesia. If the initial dose of naloxone does not result in the desired degree of clinical improvement, subsequent doses of 0.02, 0.04, 0.08, and 0.1 mg/kg may be administered in a step-wise manner. The highest doses, 0.1 mg/ml, are used to treat cardiopulmonary arrest. When used to antagonize neonatal respiratory depression (from opioids administered to the mother in labor), the usual initial dose is the same dose as used in older children (0.01 mg/kg of the 0.02 mg/ml solution).

Patient-Controlled Analgesia

Because of the enormous individual variations in pain perception and opioid metabolism, fixed doses and time intervals make little sense when administering opioids. Based on the pharmacokinetics of the opioids, it should be clear that intravenous boluses of morphine or meperidine may need to be given at intervals of 1 to 2 hours to avoid marked fluctuations in plasma drug levels (see Fig. 26-2). Continuous intravenous infusions can provide steady analgesic levels and are preferable to intramuscular injections; however, they are not a panacea because the perception and intensity of pain is not constant. Indeed, the most common method of opioid administration in adults and children is intramuscular injection. It is well known that children will suffer in silence and underreport their level of pain rather than ask for yet another painful stimulus, namely, the "shot." Thus, rational pain management requires some form of titration to reach the desired effect whenever an opioid is administered. To give patients some measure of control over their pain, demand analgesia, or patient-controlled analgesia (PCA), devices have been developed. These are microprocessor-driven pumps with a button that the patient presses to self-administer a small dose of opioid.

PCA devices allow patients to administer small amounts of an analgesic whenever they feel a need for more relief. The opioid, usually morphine, is administered either intravenously or subcutaneously. The dosage of opioid, number of boluses per hour, and the time interval between boluses (the "lock-out period") are programmed into the equipment to allow maximum patient flexibility and sense of control with minimal risk of overdosage (Table 26-3). Generally, because patients know that if they have severe pain they can obtain

Table 26-3 Intravenous Patient-Controlled Analgesia (PCA) Treatment Guidelines

Drug (concentration mg/ml)	Basal Rate Range (mg/kg/hr)	Bolus Rate Range (mg/kg)	Lock-out Interval Range (minutes)	Number of Boluses/hr Range
Morphine (1.0)	0.01-0.03	0.01-0.03	5-10	2-6
Fentanyl (0.01 in children <20 kg; 0.05 in children >20 kg)	0.0005 (0.5 μg)	0.0005-0.001 (0.5-1.0 μg)	5-10	1-6
Hydromorphone (0.2 in children <50 kg; 0.5-1.0 in children >50 kg)	0.003-0.005 (3.0-5.0 μg)	0.003-0.005 (3.0-5.0 μg)	5-10	2-6

relief immediately, many prefer dosing regimens that result in mild to moderate pain in exchange for fewer side effects such as nausea or pruritus. Typically, morphine is prescribed as a 20 μg/kg/bolus, at a rate of 5 boluses/hour, with a 6- to 8-minute lock-out interval between each bolus (see Table 26-3). Variations include larger boluses (30 to 50 μg/kg), and shorter time intervals (5 minutes) between boluses. Hydromorphone has fewer side effects than morphine and often is used when pruritus and nausea complicate morphine PCA therapy. The PCA pump computer stores within its memory the number of boluses the patient has received and the number of attempts the patient has made at receiving boluses. This allows the physician to evaluate how well the patient understands the use of the pump and provides information to program the pump more efficiently. Many PCA units allow low "background" continuous infusions (morphine, 20 to 30 μg/kg/hour) in addition to self-administered boluses. This sometimes is called "PCA-Plus." A continuous background infusion is particularly useful at night and often provides more restful sleep by preventing the patient from awakening in pain. It also increases the potential for overdosage. Although the literature on pain does not support the use of continuous background infusions, it has been the experience of some physicians that continuous background infusions are essential when IV (or epidural) PCA is prescribed.

PCA requires a patient who has enough intelligence and manual dexterity and strength to operate the pump. Thus, it was limited initially to adolescents and teenagers, but the lower age limit at which this treatment modality can be used continues to fall. In fact, any child able to play Nintendo (age 5 to 6 years) can operate a PCA pump. Difficulties with PCA include its increased costs, patient age limitations, and the bureaucratic (physician, nursing, and pharmacy) obstacles (protocols, education, storage arrangements) that must be overcome before its implementation. Contraindications include inability to push the bolus button (weakness, arm restraints), inability to understand how to use the machine, and a patient's desire not to assume responsibility for his or her own care.

Intrathecal/Epidural Opioid Analgesia

The presence of high concentrations of opioid receptors in the spinal cord makes it possible to achieve analgesia, in both acute and chronic pain, by using small doses of opioids administered in either the subarachnoid or epidural spaces. By bypassing the blood and the blood-brain barrier, small doses of agonist are effective because they can reach the receptor by the "back-door."[9] Indeed, cerebrospinal fluid (CSF) opioid levels, particularly for morphine, are several thousand times greater than those achieved by the parenteral route (see below). These high levels produce the profound and prolonged analgesia that accompanies intrathecal/epidural opioid administration.

The passage of epidurally administered agonists across the dura into the CSF depends on the lipid solubility of the drug. Additionally, once in the CSF, opioids must pass from the water phase of the CSF into the lipid phase of the underlying neuraxis to reach the receptor. This, too, depends on lipid solubility. Hydrophilic agents such as morphine will have a greater latency and duration of action than more lipid-soluble agonists such as fentanyl. On the other hand, the lipid-soluble agonists produce more segmental analgesia with less rostral spread than do the less lipid-soluble agonists.

Even when administered caudally, epidural morphine has been shown to provide effective postoperative analgesia after abdominal, thoracic, and cardiac surgery. Krane, Tyler, and Jacobson[11] reported that 0.03 mg/kg of caudal-epidural morphine is equally effective as 0.1 mg/kg in providing postoperative analgesia, although the higher dose provides a significantly longer duration of analgesia (10.0 ± 3.3 versus 13.3 ± 4.7 hours, respectively).[11] The incidence of side effects was the same in both groups, although one patient receiving 0.1 mg/kg developed late respiratory depression. Therefore, these investigators suggest starting with the lower dose when using this technique. Whether even lower doses are effective is unknown.

Spinal opiates produce analgesia without altering autonomic or neuromuscular function. Additionally, both light touch and proprioception are preserved. Thus, unlike local anesthetics, spinal opioids allow patients to ambulate without developing orthostatic hypotension. Common side effects of intrathecal/epidural opioids include segmental pruritus, urinary retention, nausea and vomiting, and respiratory depression. These side effects occur with greater frequency when opioids are administered intrathecally as opposed to epidurally. Except for urinary retention, adverse side effects can be reversed with maintenance of adequate analgesia through the use of a low-dose (0.001 to 0.002 mg/kg) naloxone infusion. Pruritus and nausea also can be treated with intravenous or oral diphenhydramine (Benadryl), 0.5 to 1.0 mg/kg, or hydroxyzine (Vistaril, Atarax). Urinary retention has not been a reported complication in children because the majority of pediatric patients studied to date have had bladder catheters as part of their postoperative management regimen.

Although rare, respiratory depression is a major risk when intrathecal/epidural opioids are used. Attia et al[4] demonstrated that the ventilatory response to carbon dioxide is depressed for as long as 22 hours after the administration of 0.05 mg/kg of morphine epidurally. Nichols et al[14] demonstrated, in children between 3 months and 15 years of age, significant depression of the ventilatory response to carbon dioxide for up to 18 hours after intrathecal morphine administration (0.02 mg/kg). The greatest respiratory depression correlated with the highest CSF morphine levels (2863 ± 542 ng/ml), which occurred 6 hours after administration. This depression persisted despite a fall in CSF morphine levels 12 (641 ± 219 ng/ml) to 18 (223 ± 152 ng/ml) hours later. This confirms the clinical impression that respiratory depression usually occurs within the first 6 hours after the administration of epidural or intrathecal morphine but may occur as long as 18 hours afterward.

In clinical practice, respiratory depression occurs most commonly when IV or IM opioids have been administered to supplement the intrathecal opioid. The risk of respiratory depression can be minimized if smaller doses of supplemental opioids are used or through the epidural use of shorter-acting, more lipid-soluble agents (fentanyl, sufentanil), which produce more segmental analgesia, with little rostral spread. On the other hand, because of its shorter duration of action, fentanyl and sufentanil are being administered increasingly by continuous epidural infusion, either alone or in combination with very dilute bupivacaine (1/16%, [0.0625 mg/ml]) or lidocaine (3 to 5 mg/ml) solutions. Typically, the epidural solution contains 1 to 5 μg/ml of fentanyl and is administered at rates ranging between 0.5 and 1.0 μg/kg/hr. This provides effective analgesia for both postoperative, acute, and chronic medical (e.g., cancer, sickle cell anemia) pain. Higher doses usually result in pruritus.

Regardless of the opioid and route of administration, a regular system of monitoring for respiratory depression is required. Clinical signs that predict impending respiratory depression include somnolence, small pupils, and small tidal volumes. Oxyhemoglobin saturation monitoring ("pulse oximetry"), especially in the first 24 hours of instituting this therapy, is essential.

LOCAL ANESTHETIC AGENTS AND TECHNIQUES

Pharmacology and Pharmacokinetics of Local Anesthetics

The local anesthetics are tertiary amines and are of two types: either "esters" (e.g., tetracaine [Pontocaine], procaine [Novocain], chloroprocaine [Nesacaine], cocaine) or "amides" (lidocaine [Xylocaine], prilocaine, bupivacaine [Marcaine, Sensorcaine])[30] (Table 26-4). Both the ester and amide local anesthetics are weak bases that block nerve conduction primarily at the sodium channel when they are in their ionized (cation) form. To reach the sodium channel, the local anesthetic must cross the nerve membrane, and only the nonionized (base) form of the drug can do this. How much drug is available to cross the nerve membrane depends on the pKa of the drug and the pH of the fluid surrounding the nerve; the lower the pKa of the drug, the more nonionized drug is available to cross the nerve membrane at physiological pH. For example, 28% of lidocaine exists in the base form at pH 7.4 compared with only 2.5% for chloroprocaine, because the pKa of these drugs are 7.9 and 9.0, respectively. Acidosis and hypercapnia, by significantly affecting tissue drug uptake, also increase the toxicity of local anesthetics. Indeed, studies in rats have shown that both hypercapnia and acidosis drastically lower the convulsive threshold of local anesthetics and elevate total plasma and tissue concentrations of drug.

The standard of local anesthetic potency is Cm, or the minimum concentration of local anesthetic necessary to block impulse conduction along a given nerve fiber. A variety of factors affect Cm, including fiber size and degree of myelination of the nerve to be blocked, pH, local calcium concentration, and the rate at which a nerve is stimulated. Relatively unmyelinated fibers such as the A delta and C fibers carry pain receptive information and have a lower Cm than do heavily myelinated fibers that control muscle contraction. Because of the lower Cm, less local anesthetic is necessary to block the transmission of pain than is necessary to produce muscle paralysis. Thus, one can block pain sensation and not motor function by using dilute concentrations of local anesthetics. In fact, concentrated local anesthetic solutions (e.g., 2% lidocaine versus 1%) increase the quality of sensory blockade only minimally. On the other hand, a concentrated local anesthetic will increase the incidence of motor blockade and systemic toxicity. (Concentrated solutions of local anesthetics can be diluted with *preservative-free* normal saline.) Furthermore, because the process of myelinization of the central nervous system is not completed until approximately 18 months after birth, Cm may be reduced in younger children. Thus, newborns and infants may develop complete analgesia and even motor blockade when even dilute concentrations of local anesthetics are used.

Other factors also influence the quality and duration of a nerve block, such as the addition of a vasoconstrictor to the anesthetic mixture, the use of mixtures of local anesthetics, and the site of drug administration. Vasoconstrictors, particularly epinephrine, frequently are added to local anesthetic solutions. Epinephrine decreases the rate of vascular reabsorption of local anesthetic from the site of administration and thereby lengthens the duration of sensory blockade. By causing local vasoconstriction, epinephrine also reduces

Table 26-4 Comparative Pharmacology of Local Anesthetics

Classification	Potency*	Onset	Duration after Infiltration (min)
Esters			
Procaine	1	Slow	45-60
Chloroprocaine	4	Rapid	30-45
Tetracaine	16	Slow	60-180
Amides			
Lidocaine	1	Rapid	60-120
Mepivacaine	1-2	Slow	90-180
Bupivacaine	4-8	Slow	240-480
Etidocaine	4-8	Slow	240-480
Prilocaine	1	Slow	60-120

*Related to procaine (for esters) and lidocaine (for amides).

bleeding at sites of injury. Interestingly, epinephrine also improves the intensity of anesthesia achieved and increases the effectiveness of dilute concentration of local anesthetics. *Epinephrine should never be injected into areas supplied by end arteries, such as the penis or digits.* Injection of an epinephrine-containing solution into these areas may lead to tissue ischemia or necrosis. Finally, epinephrine most commonly is added to local anesthetic solutions in concentrations of 0.005 mg/ml (1:200,000).

The site of an injection also alters the duration of a nerve block, depending on the nerve's anatomy, differences in the rate of drug absorption, and the amount of drug deposited. Bupivacaine, for example, has a 4-hour duration when injected epidurally but a 10-hour duration when injected into the brachial plexus.

Toxicity

The systemic effects of local anesthetics are determined by the total dose of drug administered and by the rapidity of absorption into the blood. This belies the idea of accepted "maximum" doses of these drugs, because even small fractions of the accepted "maximum" dosages of local anesthetics will produce toxic systemic effects if the local anesthetic is injected intraarterially or intravenously or into any highly vascular location (Table 26-5). In general, peak absorption of local anesthetic depends on the site of the block. The order of absorption from highest to lowest is as follows:

intercostal, intratracheal > caudal/epidural > brachial plexus > distal peripheral > subcutaneous

Peak local anesthetic blood levels are related directly to the total dose of drug administered, regardless of the injection site or the volume of solution used. Thus, the most dilute concentration of a local anesthetic should be used. At recommended clinical dosages, plasma levels usually remain well below recognized toxic concentrations. A continuum of toxic effects exists and depends on the rapidity of rise and the total plasma concentration achieved after drug administration. Mild side effects (tinnitus, light-headedness, visual and auditory disturbances, restlessness, muscular twitching) occur at low plasma concentrations; severe side effects (seizures, arrhythmias, coma, cardiovascular collapse, respiratory arrest) occur as plasma levels increase.

Cardiovascular and central nervous system toxicity occur rarely in children after administration of a local anesthetic. The hemodynamic response to regional anesthesia, even after fairly extensive epidural blockade (cutaneous analgesia below T4 to T5 dermatome, the nipple line) is minimal among children compared with adults. Convulsions are rarely noted because they may be masked or the seizure threshold may be increased by the use of sedatives, particularly the benzodiazepines. Alternatively, children may be less sensitive to the toxic effects of local anesthetics than are adults; however, this is unlikely, because several animal studies have demonstrated no significant differences in the sensitivity to the toxic effects of local anesthetics between newborn and adult animals.

The treatment of toxic responses to local anesthetics is the same as for any emergency, namely, maintaining a patent *a*irway, ensuring adequate *b*reathing, and supporting *c*irculation—in other words, the ABCs. Patients who seize for even brief periods become acidotic and have ineffective ventilation. Thus, emergency airway and resuscitative equipment must be available for immediate use before the administration of any local anesthetic agent (Box 26-1). Finally, bupivacaine as a cause of arrhythmias and cardiovascular collapse is particularly worrisome because the cardiovascular collapse has been relatively refractory to treatment. The ventricular arrhythmias caused by bupivacaine that precede the cardiovascular collapse may be treated effectively with intravenous phenytoin or bretylium.[12]

Drug allergy is very uncommon with amide local anesthetics but does occur with the ester family of drugs. Usually, a previous history of allergies to local anesthetics or to suntan lotions that contain PABA can be obtained. However, local anesthetic allergy is rare and often is attributed mistakenly to adverse experiences occurring during dental anesthesia. In the dentist's office, many patients experience tachycardia and a sense of flushing and dizziness following nerve root infil-

Table 26-5 Suggested Maximal Doses of Local Anesthetics (mg/kg)*

Drug (Concentration)†	Caudal/Lumbar Epidural	Peripheral‡	Subcutaneous‡
Esters			
Chloroprocaine (1.0% infiltration) (2%-3% epidural)	8-10§	8-10§	8-10§
Procaine	NR	8-10§	8-10§
Amides			
Lidocaine (0.5%-2.0%) (0.5%-1.0% infiltration) (1%-2% peripheral, epidural, subcutaneous) (5% spinal)	5-7§	5-7§	5-7§
Bupivacaine (0.0625%-0.5%) (0.125%-0.25%)	2-3§	2-3§	2-3§
Prilocaine (0.5%-1% infiltration) (1%-1.5% peripheral) (2%-3% epidural)	5-7§‖	5-7§‖	5-7§‖

*These are suggested safe upper limits; direct intraarterial or intravenous injection of even a fraction of these doses may result in systemic toxicity or death.
†Concentrations are in mg percent; e.g., a 1% solution contains 10 mg/ml.
‡Epinephrine should never be added to local anesthetic solution administered in the area of an end artery (e.g., penile nerve block).
§The higher dose is recommended only with the concomitant use of epinephrine 1:200,000.
‖Total adult dose should not exceed 600 mg. Should be used with caution in neonates.
NR, Not recommended.

BOX 26-1

EMERGENCY DRUGS AND EQUIPMENT REQUIRED FOR SEDATION AND ADMINISTRATION OF LOCAL ANESTHETIC

I. Personnel
   A. The practitioner performing the procedure
   B. A qualified person to monitor and administer drugs
      1. Training in basic life support (CPR)
      2. Knowledge of emergency cart inventory
II. Equipment for intravenous access
   A. Catheters (various sizes)
   B. Administration sets
   C. Fluids
      1. Lactated Ringer's solution
      2. D5W + NaCl (0.2%, 0.45%, 0.9%)
III. Emergency cart
   A. Suction (large-bore device, e.g., Yankauer suction device)
   B. Oxygen and oxygen delivery system
   C. Airway
      1. Oral airways (various sizes)
      2. Masks (various sizes)
      3. Laryngoscope and appropriate size blades
      4. Endotracheal tubes (various sizes)
      5. Stylets
   D. Drugs
      1. Epinephrine
      2. Bicarbonate
      3. Atropine
      4. Lidocaine, bretylium
      5. Calcium
      6. Glucose
      7. Naloxone, physostigmine
      8. Anticonvulsants (thiopental, diazepam, or midazolam)
IV. Monitoring equipment*
   A. ECG
   B. Sphygmomanometer
   C. Pulse oximeter

Modified from American Academy of Pediatrics Committee on Drugs: *Pediatrics* 89:1110, 1992.
*Monitoring equipment should be available, particularly if the child is sedated for the procedure.

tration with procaine and epinephrine. This usually is caused by direct intravascular injection of epinephrine and does not mean that the patient is allergic to local anesthetics.

Pharmacokinetics

The ester local anesthetics are metabolized by plasma cholinesterase. Neonates and infants up to 6 months of age have less than half of the adult levels of this plasma enzyme. Clearance thereby may be reduced and the effects of ester local anesthetics prolonged. Amides, on the other hand, are metabolized in the liver and bound by plasma proteins. Neonates and young infants (younger than 3 months of age) have reduced liver blood flow and immature metabolic degradation pathways. Thus, larger fractions of local anesthetics are unmetabolized and remain active in the plasma than in the adult. More local anesthetic is excreted in the urine unchanged. Furthermore, neonates and infants may be at increased risk for the toxic effects of amide local anesthetics because of lower levels of albumin and alpha-1 acid glycoproteins, which are proteins essential for drug binding. This leads to increased concentrations of free drug and potential toxicity, particularly with bupivacaine. On the other hand, the larger volume of distribution at steady state seen in the neonate for these (and other) drugs may confer some clinical protection by lowering plasma drug levels.

The metabolism of the amide local anesthetic prilocaine is unique in that it produces oxidants that can lead to the development of methemoglobinemia. This occurs in adults who are given doses of prilocaine greater than 600 mg. Because premature and full-term infants have decreased levels of methemoglobin reductase, they are more susceptible to methemoglobinemia. An additional factor rendering newborns more susceptible to methemoglobinemia is the relative ease by which fetal hemoglobin is oxidized compared with adult hemoglobin. Unfortunately, this may limit the use of an exciting new topical local anesthetic, EMLA (eutectic mixture of local anesthetics), in the newborn. Nevertheless, a single dose is safe and has been shown to be effective in the management of newborn circumcision.

REGIONAL ANESTHETIC TECHNIQUES

Subcutaneous Injection

Subcutaneous infiltration of the skin with a local anesthetic solution is the regional ("local") anesthetic technique performed most commonly in pediatric practice. Local anesthetics, particularly lidocaine, are commonly injected subcutaneously before the performance of many painful medical and surgical procedures to minimize procedure-related pain. Examples of procedures that benefit from prior local anesthetic infiltration include repair of minor surgical wounds (traumatic lacerations or deliberate incisions, e.g., before a cutdown for venous access), insertion of an arterial or an intravenous catheter (e.g., routine percutaneous intravenous access or cardiac catheterization), bone marrow aspiration, thoracostomy tube placement, and lumbar puncture. When used in this way, the local anesthetic agent blocks nerve conduction at the most terminal branches of the sensory nerves.

Local anesthetic infiltration of traumatic lacerations requires special attention. Commonly, the wound is dirty and requires extensive scrubbing and irrigation. The local anesthetic should be injected through intact skin adjacent to the wound before the wound is cleaned (Fig. 26-3). Alternatively, the peripheral nerve supplying the injured area more proximally should be blocked, because smaller amounts of local anesthetic are used and it requires fewer injections.

Because local anesthetics are manufactured at a pH of 4 to 5 and are administered by injection, they are painful in and of themselves. This pain can be minimized by using buffered anesthetic solutions and small needles. Buffering a local anesthetic solution, such as lidocaine or bupivacaine, with sodium bicarbonate (9 ml of lidocaine combined with 1 ml of bicarbonate, or bupivacaine 29 ml with 1 ml bicarbonate) may make the injection painless and shorten the onset of

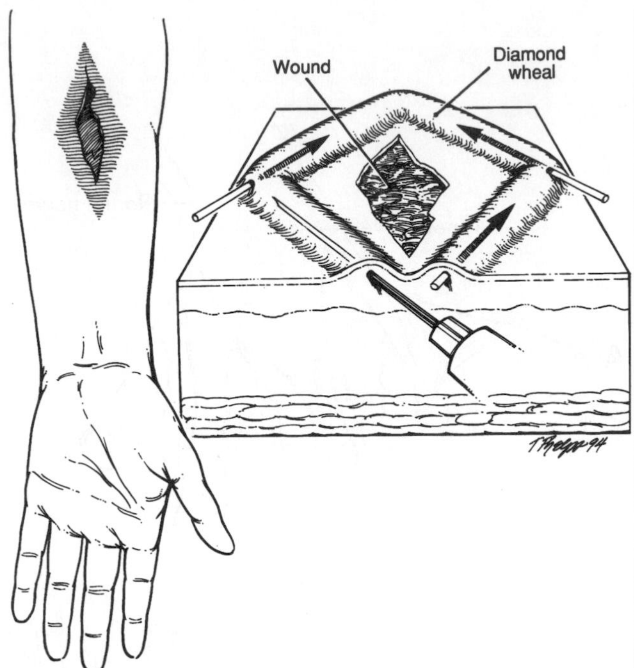

Fig. 26-3 Technique of infiltration of local anesthetic.

analgesia.[5,26] Local anesthetics are not manufactured with buffer because the buffering affects the shelf life of the drug. Obviously, using small-gauge needles affects the amount of pain produced when infiltrating local anesthetics. Either 26- or 30-gauge needles should be used and the local anesthetic should be injected immediately as the needle punctures the skin. Finally, the pain of local anesthetic injection can be minimized further by not aspirating first, by warming the solution to be injected, and by injecting slowly.

Topical Local Anesthetic Techniques

TAC solution. A useful and increasingly popular topical anesthetic mixture for laceration repair is known by its acronym, TAC. This solution consists of a mixture of tetracaine, epinephrine (adrenalin), and cocaine. A stock solution is prepared in the pharmacy by mixing 7 g of cocaine, 300 mg of tetracaine (15 ml of a 2% solution), 30 mg of epinephrine (30 ml of a 1:1000 solution), and saline to bring the total volume to 60 ml. The resulting mixture can be kept refrigerated and dispensed as needed. This method of topical anesthesia avoids the use of a local anesthetic injection. It is most effective when used on lacerations of the face and scalp and less effective on lacerations of an extremity. It does not penetrate unbroken skin well. Typically, a 3-ml solution of TAC provides analgesia for an approximately 3-cm-long laceration. Half of the solution is instilled directly into the wound; the other half is applied to a gauze pad held on the wound surface for 10 to 15 minutes. Blanching of the surrounding tissue indicates effective penetration. Failure to keep the TAC solution in contact with the wound surface for 10 to 15 minutes usually accounts for most cases of TAC's ineffectiveness and provides inadequate analgesia. In the 10% to 25% of patients in whom TAC is not completely effective, the subsequent injection of lidocaine required to complete the procedure is much less painful. Use of TAC also avoids the swelling and distortion of the wound edges that may be caused by injections. This painless method of application enhances patient compliance and results in briefer suturing times for minor lacerations. Gloves must be worn by all personnel coming into contact with TAC solution because it can cause vasoconstriction even in intact skin.

Because this mixture contains very high concentrations of its components, toxicity is a major concern.[10] Three milliliters of TAC contains the equivalent of 1.5 ml of 1 : 1000 epinephrine and 350 mg cocaine, the latter being unique among local anesthetics because of its sympathomimetic actions. It impairs the reuptake of catecholamines at adrenergic nerve endings and blocks muscarinic cholinergic receptors, resulting in the promotion of hypertension and cardiac dysrhythmias, the most common causes of toxic deaths resulting from cocaine abuse. In the central nervous system, cocaine affects transmission by several monoamines such as norepinephrine, serotonin, dopamine, and tryptophan. Toxic reactions include dysphoria, anxiety, convulsions, and fever and do not necessarily correlate with blood levels.

Although some systemic absorption of cocaine occurs with the proper use of TAC, toxic reactions usually result from the rapid systemic absorption after unintentional contact with mucosal membranes. Case reports have documented prolonged seizures when TAC was applied to the buccal mucosa and death when excess solution dripped into the nares and mouth from a sponge that was applied to the upper lip.[10] Other fatalities and neuropsychological reactions have been reported, leading some to condemn the use of this solution.

In addition, because of its mechanism of monoamine oxidase action, cocaine should not be used concurrently with tricyclic antidepressants or monoamine oxidase (MAO) inhibitors (which also inhibit the reuptake of catecholamines at nerve endings) or in patients who have hypertension or cardiac conduction disturbances. Finally, because of its systemic absorption, patients should be advised that urinary drug screens for cocaine and its metabolites will be positive for 48 to 72 hours after an application of TAC.

Interactions among the components of TAC have been suspected of enhancing the potential for toxic reactions. Cocaine and epinephrine both act at adrenergic receptors; cocaine and tetracaine both compete for plasma cholinesterase for metabolism. Thus, attempts to reduce the toxic potential of the mixture have focused on removing one of the components. However, use of either tetracaine alone, tetracaine with epinephrine, or cocaine alone was found to be far less effective than the complete mixture. Alternative solutions include lidocaine-epinephrine-tetracaine (LET) and bupivacaine-norepinephrine (BN).

The most serious local adverse reaction is ischemia of end-arterial tissues caused by the potent vasoconstrictive properties of TAC. Thus, it should not be applied to the digits, nose, pinna of the ear, penis, or a skin flap. Despite concerns about serious toxicity, during the past decade, TAC, LET, and BN have continued to enjoy widespread use when used selectively and prudently.

EMLA cream. EMLA (eutectic mixture of local anesthetics) cream, a topical emulsion composed of prilocaine and lidocaine, produces complete anesthesia of intact skin after application. Unfortunately, for best effect, EMLA cream must be applied and covered with an occlusive dressing (such as Saran wrap) for 60 to 90 minutes before a procedure is performed. This limits its use in the emergency room or office unless the site is prepared well in advance of anticipated use. Furthermore, if the procedure is a venipuncture, multiple sites must be prepared, in case the initial attempt is unsuccessful.

Unfortunately, the effectiveness of EMLA cream (like all other methods) in reducing pain depends on who makes the assessment. Soliman et al[21] studied the efficacy of EMLA cream compared with injected lidocaine at reducing the pain associated with venipuncture. Both an observer and a physician performing the procedure judged pain relief to be virtually complete in both groups. The children involved in the study were not so sanguine and were equally dissatisfied with both methods, particularly if the needle used for venipuncture was visible to them. Thus, despite two observers feeling that the child was pain-free, the child's cooperation with venipuncture did not improve. Therefore, it is not clear whether the delay involved in the use of EMLA (60-minute wait for effect) is justified. On the other hand, EMLA may be more effective in children accustomed to frequent medical procedures (e.g., oncology patients) or for procedures in which the child cannot see the needle, such as lumbar puncture or bone marrow aspiration. It also has been used quite effectively for newborn circumcision.

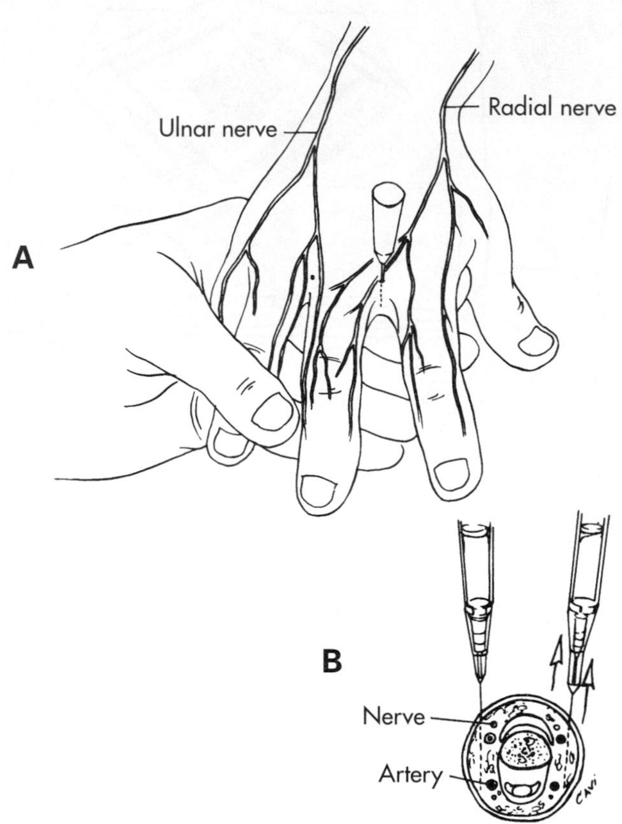

Fig. 26-4 Anatomy of the digital nerves of the hand and of the digital nerve block. **A,** A 25-gauge needle is inserted between the heads of the metacarpals (or metatarsals) on either side of the digit to be anesthetized. Both dorsal and ventral branches are blocked by continuously injecting during advancement of the needle from the dorsal surface to the palm. **B,** One can see the anatomical relationship of the digital nerves and arteries at the level of the metacarpal head in this cross section view.

Peripheral nerve blocks. As mentioned previously, emergency airway and resuscitative equipment, as well as individuals trained in using it, must be available for use before the performance of a peripheral nerve block. Additionally, if a patient is to be sedated during a nerve block, one member of the health care team must be responsible for the patient's overall well-being.[1] This person is responsible for monitoring vital signs, assessing the adequacy of the airway, and alerting other members of the health care team if a problem is occurring (see Box 26-1).

Digital nerve blocks. The digital nerve block provides excellent anesthesia for surgery performed on either the fingers or toes. It particularly is useful for incision and drainage of an abscess (paronychia). The alternative, local anesthetic infiltration, may fail because the acidic pH of infected tissue may not allow the active (nonionized base) form of the local anesthetic to reach the nerve membrane.

PERFORMANCE OF THE DIGITAL NERVE BLOCK. Digital nerve block is performed similarly for both the fingers and toes. Each digit is supplied by two pairs of nerves (palmar and dorsal), which travel on either side of that digit (Fig. 26-4). *Epinephrine-free* local anesthetic (0.5 to 1.0 ml) is injected between the metacarpal (or metatarsal) heads on either side of the digit. The 25-gauge needle is kept perpendicular to the plane of the hand or foot and advanced from the dorsal to the palmar surface. Local anesthetic is injected continuously. Aspiration before injection is unnecessary because the volume of local anesthetic is small.

Complications are few. Obviously, the digital nerve block should never be performed when there is any question of the digit's blood supply. Indeed, even when epinephrine is not used, the most serious complication of this block is caused by the use of too large a volume of local anesthetic. A large volume within a closed fascial space may result in vascular compression ("compartment" syndrome).

Penile nerve block. Although routine circumcision of newborns has been condemned by various groups, it remains a common practice. Active campaigns by pediatricians and obstetricians to discourage the procedure in the newborn period has resulted in increasingly large numbers of older children being presented for this surgery. These older children obviously require general anesthesia for their surgery. In both the newborn and older child, the penile nerve block can be used either for complete anesthesia or for postoperative pain relief. The efficacy and safety of this block for newborn circumcision has been demonstrated in several studies and requires very little time to perform (<60 sec).[13] This extremely safe and effective block should be performed *routinely* before newborn circumcision. In both the older child and the newborn, postoperative analgesia also can be provided by the topical application of 2% lidocaine jelly.[22]

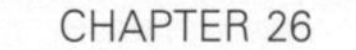

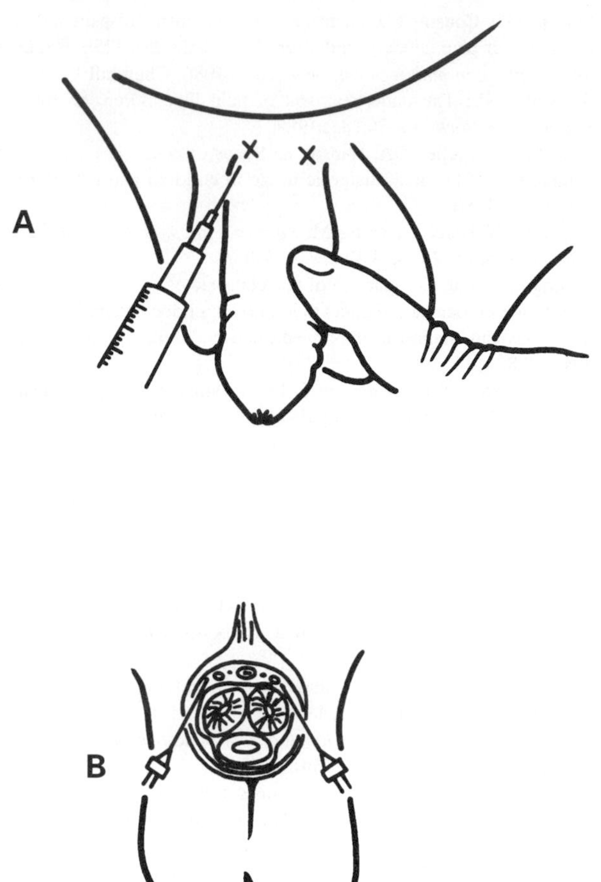

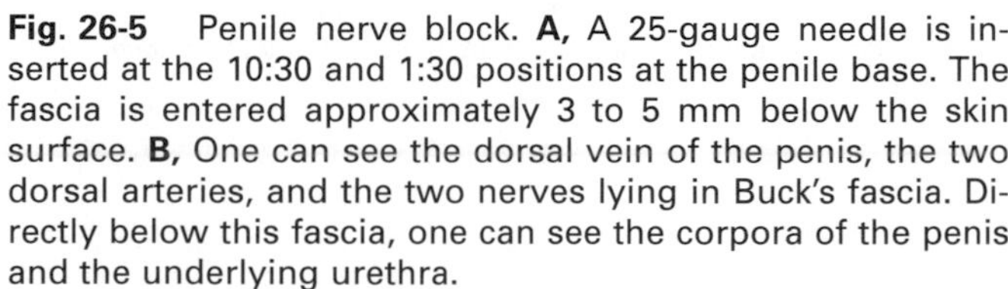

Fig. 26-5 Penile nerve block. **A,** A 25-gauge needle is inserted at the 10:30 and 1:30 positions at the penile base. The fascia is entered approximately 3 to 5 mm below the skin surface. **B,** One can see the dorsal vein of the penis, the two dorsal arteries, and the two nerves lying in Buck's fascia. Directly below this fascia, one can see the corpora of the penis and the underlying urethra.

(From Maxwell LG, et al: *Obstet Gynecol* 70:415, 1987.)

PERFORMANCE OF THE PENILE NERVE BLOCK. In the newborn, 0.8 ml of 1% lidocaine and in older children from 1 to 3 ml of 0.25% bupivacaine are used.[13] Peak plasma lidocaine levels in the newborn average less than 0.6 µg/ml. In either case, it is vital that *epinephrine-free solution* be used because the artery supplying the penis is an end artery and vasoconstriction by epinephrine can cause catastrophic consequences. The dorsal nerves of the penis (Fig. 26-5) lie on either side of the dorsal artery and vein of the penis. They are deep to Buck's fascia but are superficial with respect to the skin at the penile base. The child should be placed in a restraining papoose and given a pacifier soaked in a 27% dextrose solution (a packet of table sugar in 10 ml of water). Following aseptic preparation of the skin, two injections of local anesthetic solution are made by using either a 25- or 26-gauge needle. The anesthetic solution is injected at the 10:30 and 1:30 positions at the penile base just beneath Buck's fascia. This fascia is approximately 3 to 5 mm below the skin surface. Alternatively, a single midline injection may be used. In this technique the needle is advanced to the lower surface of the pubic symphysis in the midline. Local anesthetic (approximately 1 to 3 ml) is injected slowly as the needle is withdrawn. As the needle passes through Buck's fascia, the local anesthetic is spread to both sides, anesthetizing the nerves. Broadman et al described a ring block of the penile base in which no attempt was made to inject below Buck's fascia.[8] Complications are rare.

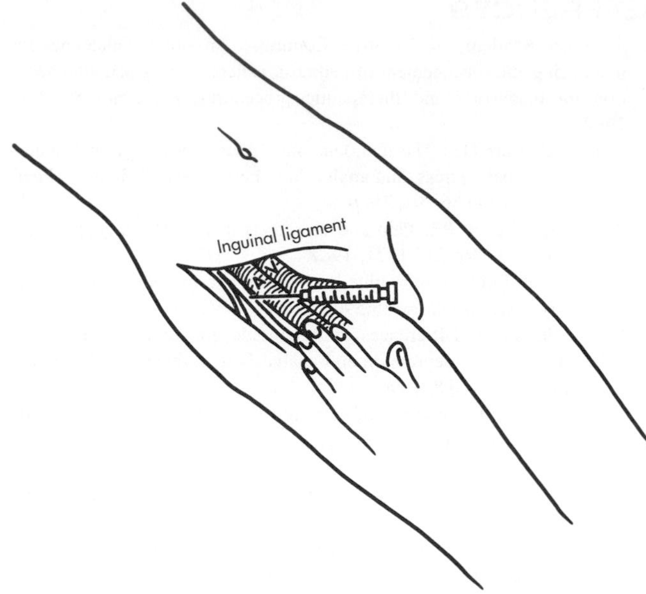

Fig. 26-6 Femoral nerve block. After placing a skin wheal, the physician's nonoperative hand compresses the femoral artery and nerve against the underlying tissue and bone immediately below the inguinal ligament. A 22- or 25-gauge needle then is inserted perpendicularly, approximately ½ to 1 cm lateral to the pulsation of the femoral artery ***(A)*** into the perineural fascia of the femoral nerve.

(From Yaster M, et al, editors: *The handbook of pediatric pain management and sedation,* Mosby, St Louis, 1997.)

Femoral nerve block. The femoral nerve block (L2, 3, 4) is the quickest, easiest, and most effective technique for relieving the pain of a femoral shaft fracture. The femoral nerve block provides fracture patients with adequate anesthesia for the application of traction as well as for the necessary (and usually painful) manipulations that occur during radiological examinations. The duration of analgesia for bupivacaine without epinephrine is 3 hours, and peak plasma levels of bupivacaine average less than 1 µg/ml.

PERFORMANCE OF THE BLOCK. Following aseptic preparation of the skin, a 22- or 25-gauge needle is inserted perpendicularly, approximately 3 to 5 mm lateral to the pulsation of the femoral artery at the level of the inguinal ligament (Fig. 26-6). The needle is inserted to a depth clearly deeper than the artery. The feeling of penetration of the fascia over the nerve (a distinct "pop") helps in judging the depth of penetration. Following a negative aspiration for blood, 5 to 10 ml of local anesthetic solution (0.25% bupivacaine with 1:200,000 epinephrine) is injected. Local anesthetic solution then is injected in a fanlike manner lateral and deep to the femoral artery. The dose of 0.25% bupivacaine used is 1 ml/kg, up to 10 ml.

REFERENCES

1. American Academy of Pediatrics Committee on Drugs: Guidelines for monitoring and management of pediatric patients during and after sedation for diagnostic and therapeutic procedures, *Pediatrics* 89:1110, 1992.
2. Anand KJ, Carr DB: The neuroanatomy, neurophysiology, and neurochemistry of pain, stress, and analgesia in newborns and children, *Pediatr Clin North Am* 36:795, 1989.
3. Anand KJ, Hickey PR: Pain and its effects in the human neonate and fetus, *N Engl J Med* 317:1321, 1987.
4. Attia J, et al: Epidural morphine in children: pharmacokinetics and CO_2 sensitivity, *Anesthesiology* 65:590, 1986.
5. Bailey PL, et al: Differences in magnitude and duration of opioid-induced respiratory depression and analgesia with fentanyl and sufentanil, *Anesth Analg* 70:8, 1990.
6. Berde CB, et al: Comparison of morphine and methadone for prevention of postoperative pain in 3- to 7-year-old children, *J Pediatr* 119:136, 1991.
7. Beyer JE, Wells N: The assessment of pain in children, *Pediatr Clin North Am* 36:837, 1989.
8. Broadman LM, et al: Post-circumcision analgesia: a prospective evaluation of subcutaneous ring block of the penis, *Anesthesiology* 67:399, 1987.
9. Cousins MJ, Mather LE: Intrathecal and epidural administration of opioids, *Anesthesiology* 61:276, 1984.
10. Dailey RH: Fatality secondary to misuse of TAC solution, *Ann Emerg Med* 17:159, 1988.
11. Krane EJ, Tyler DC, Jacobson LE: The dose response of caudal morphine in children, *Anesthesiology* 71:48, 1989.
12. Maxwell LG, Martin LD, Yaster M: Bupivacaine-induced cardiac toxicity in neonates: successful treatment with intravenous phenytoin, *Anesthesiology* 80:682, 1994.
13. Maxwell LG, et al: Penile nerve block for newborn circumcision, *Obstet Gynecol* 70:415, 1987.
14. Nichols DG, et al: Disposition and respiratory effects of intrathecal morphine in children, *Anesthesiology* 79:733, 1993.
15. Pain terms: a list with definitions and notes on usage. Recommended by the IASP Subcommittee on Taxonomy, *Pain* 6:249, 1979.
16. Pasternak GW: Multiple morphine and enkephalin receptors and the relief of pain, *JAMA* 259:1362, 1988.
17. Phillips GD, Cousins MJ: Neurological mechanisms of pain and the relationship of pain, anxiety, and sleep. In Cousins MJ, Phillips GD, editors: *Acute pain management,* New York, 1986, Churchill Livingstone.
18. Schechter NL: The undertreatment of pain in children: an overview, *Pediatr Clin North Am* 36:781, 1989.
19. Schechter NL, Allen DA, Hanson K: Status of pediatric pain control: a comparison of hospital analgesic usage in children and adults, *Pediatrics* 77:11, 1986.
20. Schechter N, Berde C, Yaster M: *Pain in infants, children, and adolescents,* Baltimore, 1993, Williams & Wilkins.
21. Soliman IE, et al: Comparison of the analgesic effects of EMLA (eutectic mixture of local anesthetics) to intradermal lidocaine infiltration prior to venous cannulation in unpremedicated children, *Anesthesiology* 68: 804, 1988.
22. Tree-Trakarn T, Pirayavaraporn S, Lertakyamanee J: Topical analgesia for relief of post-circumcision pain, *Anesthesiology* 67:395, 1987.
23. Wall PD, Melzack R: *Management of pain,* New York, 1985, Churchill Livingstone.
24. Way WL, Costley EC, Way EL: Respiratory sensitivity of the newborn infant to meperidine and morphine, *Clin Pharmacol Ther* 6:454, 1965.
25. Wong DL, Hockenberry-Eaton M: *Wong's essentials of pediatric nursing,* ed 6, St Louis, Mosby, 2001.
26. Yaster M, et al: Hemodynamic effects of primary closure of omphalocele/gastroschisis in human newborns, *Anesthesiology* 69:84, 1988.
27. Yaster M, Deshpande JK: Management of pediatric pain with opioid analgesics, *J Pediatr* 113:421, 1988.
28. Yaster M, et al, editors: *The handbook of pediatric pain management and sedation,* St Louis, 1997, Mosby.
29. Yaster M, Maxwell LG: Opioid agonists and antagonists. In Schechter NL, Berde CB, Yaster M, editors: *Pain in infants, children, and adolescents,* Baltimore, 1993, Williams & Wilkins.
30. Yaster M, Tobin JR, Maxwell LG: Local anesthetics. In Schechter NL, Berde CB, Yaster M, editors: *Pain in infants, children, and adolescents,* Baltimore, 1993, Williams & Wilkins.
31. Zhang AZ, Pasternak GW: Ontogeny of opioid pharmacology and receptors: high and low affinity site differences, *Eur J Pharmacol* 73:29, 1981.

27 Self-Regulation Therapies: Hypnosis and Biofeedback

Laurence I. Sugarman

Hypnosis and biofeedback training are primary strategies for helping children and adolescents change maladaptive psychophysiological responses. Necessarily patient-centered, these methods allow young people, motivated by their innate desires for novelty, autonomy, and mastery, to use their imagination to enhance coping. By integrating self-regulation skills training into a developmentally appropriate program of health supervision and problem-oriented clinical encounters, child health care practitioners invest repeatedly in their young patients' coping ability.[34] This recurring "stress-immunization" may have benefits into adulthood, particularly with respect to health and prevention.

HYPNOSIS

The term *hypnosis* was coined (from the Greek *hypnos*) in the early 1800s by the English physician James Braid, who researched the physiological phenomena attributed to mesmerism. Braid recognized that these phenomena were not a manifestation of "animal magnetism" but of the imagination of the patient in a state of so-called nervous sleep.[30,35] Nearly 200 years later, there are many definitions of hypnosis and little consensus within the field as to what characterizes it. There currently is no unified theory of hypnosis. The theoretical bases divide into two main currents: (1) hypnosis is a form of dissociation, an interference with or loss of familiar associative processes, and (2) hypnotic responding is a socio-cognitive construct derived not from an altered state of consciousness but from "an interrelated set of ideas that provide guidelines concerning how hypnotists and hypnotized subjects are supposed to act and feel while enacting their respective roles in those social situations defined as hypnotic."[23] It is likely that both dissociative and socio-cognitive aspects are keys to the complex set of interactions called hypnosis.

A practical operational definition is that hypnosis is a *process* by which an individual narrows and intensifies his or her focus of attention and heightens his or her responsivity to ideas and suggestions for changing an identified physical or psychological problem. Viewed this way, hypnotic processes are a part of our daily life. We are aware that narrowly focused, intensified attention facilitates physical and psychological responses. For instance, we will salivate while imagining a favorite food, become tachycardic and tachypneic while reading an exciting portion of a mystery novel, and rehearse mentally for performances. Thus, hypnosis is a naturally occurring experience that involves the purposeful, instinctive, or spontaneous intensification of concentration that facilitates adaptation to psychophysiological stressors.

Hypnotherapy takes place when a health care professional, trained in clinical hypnosis, helps a patient use his or her hypnotic capacity in therapy. Therapeutic teaching in hypnosis may involve (1) development of imagery as a metaphor to help change symptoms, (2) suggestions for changing behavior, and (3) exploration of feelings and relationships. It long has been observed that there is an enhanced aptitude for transforming the idea received into action in hypnosis. The purpose of hypnosis in therapy is to foster the mental activity that allows change to occur.

The notion that "hypnotists" magically exert "mind control" over passive subjects is learned from the mass media, fairy tales, cartoons, and those who attempt to use hypnosis for entertainment. This belief is not only incorrect but impedes the success of these strategies. To teach self-regulation skills, these misconceptions need to be dispelled for colleagues, parents, and patients. This misconception reflects a sociocultural wish that such an external force or a "hypnotist" can magically solve our problems. In actuality, hypnosis augments the patient's own abilities. In hypnosis, children and adolescents are more willful, mentally active, and aware of themselves than in usual states of awareness. Hypnosis is not sleep. Hypnosis is not magic. All hypnosis is *self-hypnosis*.

There are, as yet, no unique physiological properties that characterize the hypnotic state or "trance." When young people use hypnosis, they tend to lower their level of autonomic nervous system arousal, relax skeletal muscles, increase α-frequency range electroencephalographic activity, increase peripheral skin temperature, and decrease electrical skin conductance (or electrodermal activity [EDA]) through sweat glands. There is some variation to this pattern. While children elevate their skin temperature when engaged in imagined activities, their heart rate and EDA can increase with stimulating imagined activities and decrease with relaxation.[21] These physiological characteristics also are seen when people meditate, pray, or engage in other mind-body techniques. The eventual development of objective physiological criteria that delineate hypnosis may be contingent on the clarification of those clinical behaviors that can be defined as uniquely hypnotic.

Nevertheless, a variety of behaviors and alterations in perception have been associated with hypnosis. These hypnotic phenomena (Box 27-1) can be used strategically in hypnotherapy. For example, a child who is anxious, fearful, and in

BOX 27-1

COMMON HYPNOTIC PHENOMENA

- Rapport
- Ideosensory activity
- Ideomotor activity
- Hallucination
- Dissociation
- Time distortion
- Induced dreams
- Catalepsy
- Depersonalization
- Memory modification
- Amnesia

BOX 27-2

CHARACTERISTICS COMMON TO SELF-HYPNOSIS AND BIOFEEDBACK TRAINING

- Cultivation of a lower state of arousal
- Enhanced and narrowed focus of attention
- Facilitation of a sense of curiosity
- Facilitation of imagery/fantasy abilities
- Development of an internal locus of control
- Fostering of themes of empowerment and self-mastery, both concretely and metaphorically
- Reinforcement of awareness of mind-body linkages
- Enhanced access to unconscious information
- Heightened suggestibility

pain with a laceration of the hand may use an *induced dream* to imagine playing with friends in a comfortable, enjoyable place, leaving body sensations behind (*dissociation*) and imagining that the injured hand has a thick glove on it (*ideosensory activity*), thereby diminishing sensory awareness of pain (*hallucination*) and anxiety while the laceration is sutured. Although many of these same phenomena, such as relaxation, enhanced therapeutic rapport, and time distortion, can occur within a clinical context that is not explicitly labeled as "hypnotic," they seem to be enhanced in hypnosis.

BIOFEEDBACK TRAINING

Biofeedback training lends precision and validation to self-regulation strategies. It employs electrical or mechanical devices to provide dynamic information (or "feedback") about a specific physiological function to the patient, enabling the patient to learn how to change the physiological process by changing his or her thinking and behavior.[33] The responses measured most commonly are peripheral temperature, electromyography (EMG), and electrodermal activity (EDA). The latter two modalities increase with sympathetic tone and decrease with relaxation. Muscle tension and migraine headaches have been well documented to respond to biofeedback protocols, often utilizing peripheral skin temperature or EMG.[2] Ano-rectal manometry and EMG have been shown to assist in the sensory discrimination necessary to resolve encopresis.[28,30] Although not commonly understood as biofeedback, nocturnal enuresis alarm devices are highly effective.[1,4] Autonomic nervous system disorders such as Raynaud's disease and reflex sympathetic dystrophy can be treated effectively with biofeedback modalities that cultivate enhanced sympathetic nervous system control (peripheral skin temperature, heart rate, breathing pattern).[2,33] Electroencephalographic (EEG) biofeedback in which patients learns to increase β–activity and suppress τ-activity is being explored as a treatment strategy for children who have attention deficit disorders.[22]

INTEGRATION OF STRATEGIES

Self-hypnosis and biofeedback share several common characteristics, listed in Box 27-2. Four "application paradigms" integrating biofeedback and self-hypnosis with children and adolescents have been described: (1) biofeedback can be applied for the purpose of teaching and strengthening one's awareness of the mind-body link; (2) specific markers of a given individual's stress responses can be determined in a "physiological stress profile," utilizing advanced biofeedback instrumentation that simultaneously responds to different physiological variables; (3) for some young people, hypnotic imagery, suggestions, and metaphors can enhance biofeedback training; and, conversely, (4) biofeedback tools can be used to facilitate the lowered state of arousal, narrowly focused attention, and as an ego-strengthening technique that can motivate one to explore and better engage in hypnotherapy.[3] There are no controlled studies indicating that one self-regulation method is superior to another for a given problem. Rather, it is likely that the most appropriate strategy stems from the interplay between the young person's capabilities and needs and the practitioner's flexibility, creativity, skill, and training.

TRAINING AND SKILL DEVELOPMENT

Similar to other methods in patient care, including prescribing diet or medication, physical therapy, or using adaptive equipment, the integration of self-regulation skill training into primary care requires expertise. Clinicians must understand each methodology and its limitations, gain experience in the art and science of its use, and know their patients' needs and abilities.

The practitioner beginning education in self-regulation skills training should enroll in a basic workshop sponsored by the Society for Developmental and Behavioral Pediatrics (SDBP),* the Society for Clinical and Experimental Hypnosis (SCEH),† the American Society for Clinical Hypnosis (ASCH),‡ or at a university school of medicine or a department of psychology. The Association for Applied Psychophysiology and Biofeedback (AAPB) sponsors training and certification programs in biofeedback.§ Following this

*Contact SDBP, Noreen M. Spota, Administrative Director, 19 Station Lane, Philadelphia, PA 19118.

†Contact SCEH, 2201 Haeder Road, Suite 1, Pullman, WA 99163.

‡Contact ASCH, 33 West Grand Avenue, Suite 402, Chicago, IL 60610.

§Contact AAPB, 10200 West 44th Avenue, Suite 304, West Ridge, CO 80033.

training, practitioners should apply their new skills to limited areas of treatment. Recent literature specific to these areas of application should be reviewed. Ongoing self-evaluation is vital. Faculty and peers should critique videotaped patient encounters. Intermediate and advanced workshops afford the practitioner the opportunity to hone skills and focus on specific problems of children. ASCH sponsors programs for Certification of Training in Clinical Hypnosis and an advanced level of training: Approved Consultant in Clinical Hypnosis.

The American Board of Medical Hypnosis (ABMH)* is the only organization in the United States sanctioned by the SCEH and the ASCH to certify competency in medical hypnosis. This is the highest credentialing available for physicians skilled in hypnosis. Applicants must be licensed physicians in good standing with active board certification in their specialty, have a minimum of 5 years of clinical hypnosis experience, and meet the requirements established by ASCH for Approved Consultant status. The three-part examination includes written, oral, and practical clinical demonstration.

It is crucial that the practitioner restrict self-regulation skill training to those patients whose problems lie within their therapeutic expertise. The initial role of hypnosis or biofeedback as part of the treatment plan for chronic conditions (e.g., asthma and migraine) should be established at the outset, though its potential usefulness need not be limited. A careful medical evaluation is necessary when self-regulation strategies are included as primary or adjunctive treatment of a disorder. In one study of children referred for hypnotherapy, 20% had a previously undiagnosed biological etiology for their condition.[29] Olness and Kohen have suggested indications and contraindications for self-regulation therapy with children[28] (Box 27-3).

Successful application of self-regulation strategies depends in large part on the practitioner's understanding of his or her young patient's developmental level, learning abilities, and the family context of the youngster's problems. Younger children will respond best to concrete suggestions, become animated with open eyes, and may be comfortable with their parents' presence during hypnotic imagery. In contrast, adolescents often will require suggestions for relaxation, require prompting to use mental imagery, and often will be inhibited by their parents' attendance.[18]

With hypnosis training, practitioners learn to be sensitive to the pace and tone of their language and actions, modifying them to reinforce the young person's innate abilities. Directive phrases such as "I want you to," "you should," and "you will" usually are perceived as parental and do not facilitate self-control. Distraction techniques, such as pinching the contralateral arm while an injection is given, may diminish awareness of the needle momentarily, but do not teach the child about his or her own potential for self-regulation, nor do they enhance trust and rapport. Semantics must support a child's curiosity and mastery by emphasizing that they are in control of the process, as in, "You know, it's neat how you didn't know that you already know how to help your arm feel numb so the needle poke can't bother you."

*Contact ABMH, Donald F. Lynch, Jr., M.D., Sentara Cancer Institute, 600 Gresham Drive, Norfolk, VA 23510.

BOX 27-3

INDICATIONS AND CONTRAINDICATIONS FOR SELF-REGULATION THERAPY WITH CHILDREN

Self-regulation therapy methods are indicated if:
- A child is responsive to hypnotic suggestions
- The problem has been demonstrated to be treatable with hypnosis or biofeedback
- The therapist has a positive relationship with the child
- The child is motivated to remedy the problem
- No iatrogenic harm is foreseen from using such methods

Self-regulation therapy methods are contraindicated if:
- They would lead to physical endangerment
- They might aggravate existing problems or create new ones
- They are used for "fun" or entertainment
- The problem could be addressed more effectively and appropriately through a different method (e.g., medication or family therapy)

These general skills of understanding the social and developmental context of a child's problem, performing thorough medical evaluations, knowing the limits of one's expertise, being responsive to the child's feedback, and using therapeutic language carefully are well within the primary care practitioner's expertise. Although all may not be inclined to spend the time and effort required to learn these skills, those who do are rewarded by enriched experience in pediatric practice. The child health practitioner trained in hypnotherapeutic methods grows increasingly sensitive to the value of language in therapy, the connections between the child's state of mind and physiological response, and the benefits to the child of joining in therapy.[25,34,35]

INTEGRATING HYPNOSIS AND BIOFEEDBACK INTO PEDIATRIC PRACTICE

Hypnosis and biofeedback training have been used with success for a variety of problems encountered commonly in general pediatric practice (Box 27-4). Although many reports are anecdotal, in prospective, controlled, randomized, clinical trials, hypnosis has reduced juvenile migraine severity and frequency more effectively than placebo or medication,[31] decreased the severity of asthma,[14] diminished antiemetic medication use in children receiving chemotherapy for cancer,[9] and shortened children's postoperative hospital stays.[19]

In a series of 505 pediatric encounters using hypnotherapy for enuresis, headaches, other recurrent pain, and a variety of other problems, 83% of children and adolescents had more than a 50% reduction in symptoms; 50% showed complete resolution. There was an inverse correlation between success and the number of visits, with most children acquiring usable skills by the second visit. Less suc-

BOX 27-4

PEDIATRIC PROBLEMS THAT RESPOND TO SELF-REGULATION THERAPIES

Anxiety associated with procedures or illness
Asthma
Attention deficit disorders
Cerebral palsy
Conditioned nausea and vomiting
Diabetes mellitus
Dysfluencies
Encopresis
Enuresis
Habit coughs
Insomnia
Irritable bowel syndrome
Migraine syndromes
Nail biting
Nightmares
Pain associated with acute problems (injuries, procedures)
Pain associated with chronic disease (malignancy, hemophilia, sickle cell disease)
Performance anxiety
Pruritus
Psychogenic seizures
Reflex sympathetic dystrophy
Thumb sucking
Tongue thrusting
Tourette's syndrome
Trichotillomania
Warts

cessful children were more likely not to have practiced self-hypnosis and to have been reminded by their parents to practice more. Parental reminders may have negated the autonomy required for success in self-regulation. Successful children noted a "spillover effect" of self-efficacy into other life challenges.[16]

When self-regulation strategies are learned for either adjunctive or primary therapy, it is useful to follow a protocol.[35] During an initial visit for the problem, the following elements should be explored:

- The history, physical findings, and laboratory evaluation
- The therapy to date and its efficacy
- The limitations imposed on the youngster by his or her symptoms
- A method for understanding symptom intensity (a scale from 1 to 10, a visual analog scale)
- The significance of the symptoms for the family
- The child's likes, dislikes, and fears
- The child's and family's understanding of concepts in self-regulation therapy

After gathering these data, the practitioner can explain how "thinking and feeling affect our bodies" and that people regulate these subconsciously. Examples include:

- How our brain takes care of us even during sleep (an especially useful example for children who have nocturnal enuresis)
- How a youngster can "turn off his parent's voice" when focusing his attention on a television show or video game (meaningful when parents have been frustrated by their inability to change a child's habit behavior)
- How a sleeping mother can remain asleep despite the familiar sounds of cars at night but awakens to the cries of her baby (a reassuring illustration for parents)[8]

A brief example of relaxation and mental imagery or demonstration of biofeedback devices can close the session. This experience demystifies the process and stimulates curiosity. The practitioner can provide written materials on hypnotherapy[34] and biofeedback, and the youngster can be handed a personal calendar for recording symptom frequency, intensity, and therapy before the next visit.

The timing of the next encounter depends on the characteristics of the symptom and its meaning for both the child and family. Self-monitoring is reviewed while the symptom is described further and reframed. Self-hypnosis or biofeedback training is started and intensified by using appropriate imagery and biofeedback devices and by reinforcing the patient's ability with ego-strengthening suggestions. After this, the young person's understanding of the experience is assessed. The practitioner can explain to the youngster that as in other learning, practicing self-hypnosis or biofeedback will enhance symptom control. Follow-up is important, whether by telephone, letter, or more visits. No studies have been done that investigate the correlations among follow-up interval, method, and outcome.

In all cases, the teaching of self-regulation strategies is a process in which the clinician helps the young patient realize and use his or her ability to change maladaptive conditioned psychological and physiological responses. The clinician does not act upon the patient to produce change. The patient is not hypnotized in the office as the sole therapy. Instead, the clinician acts as a coach, teacher, and facilitator who empowers the patient to help him- or herself. With the clinician's expertise, the patient explores self-management techniques for therapeutic change and then takes that learning out of the office to exercise, apply, and generalize.

Tools in Self-Regulation Therapies

Breathing control is a fundamental method of focusing and relaxation. Pinwheels, hanging mobiles, balloons, and wands for blowing bubbles encourage the child to breathe with purpose and control.[6,7] Pop-up books, puppets, stuffed animals, and dolls provide means for distraction and imagery. They also can be the child's allies during procedures.[18]

Favorite recorded stories and songs can be played during procedures on an audio cassette player that has headphones.[18] This is an often unexpected and enjoyable way for older children and adolescents to focus and narrow their attention quickly. When practical, patients may bring their own cassettes in preparation for a procedure. Hypnosis sessions in the office also can be recorded for home use.

Videotapes of other youngsters using self-hypnosis can demonstrate efficiently the technique. Written informed consent must be obtained before videotaping youngsters for this purpose. It is the author's experience that young people are pleased with the opportunity to act as teachers.

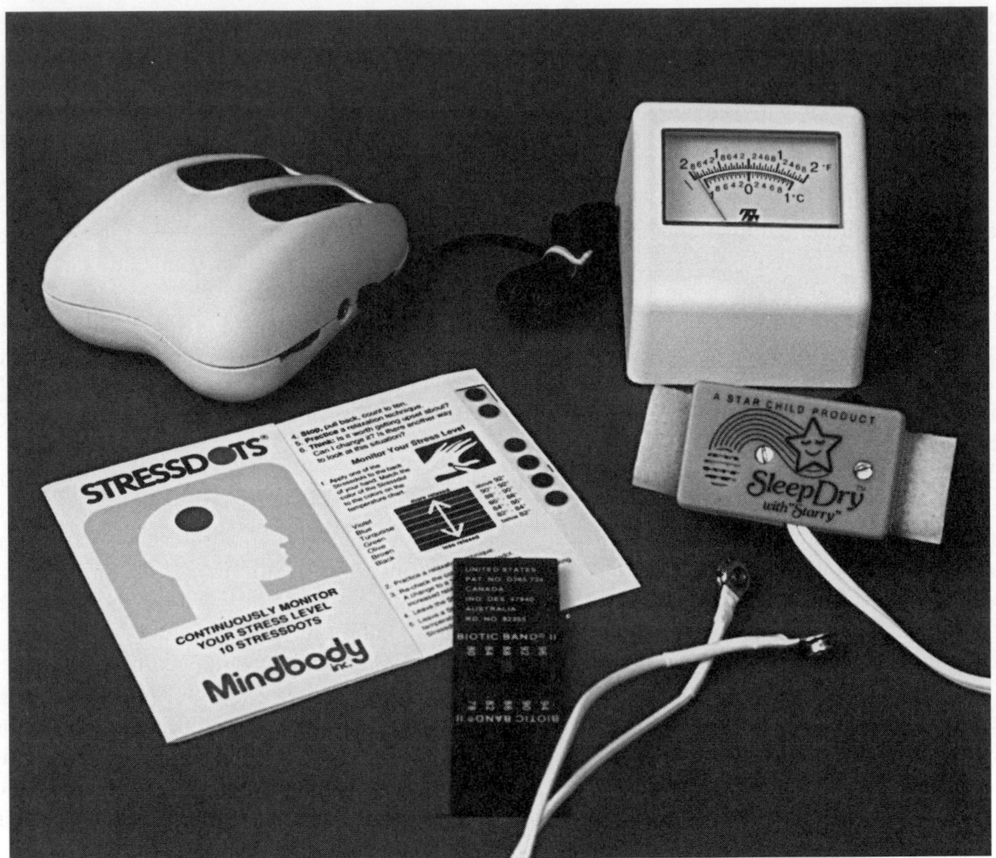

Fig. 27-1 Biofeedback devices (clockwise from top left): (1) GSR/TEMP-2 Biofeedback System, (2) peripheral temperature meter, (3) StarChild Sleep Dry enuresis alarm, (4) Biotic Band II, and (5) Stressdots.
(Photograph by William Rhinehart.)

Among those videotapes produced for this purpose (and for the education of health care professionals) are "No Fears, No Tears,"*"No Fears, No Tears—13 Years Later,"† and "Imaginative Medicine: Hypnosis in Pediatric Practice."‡ The first two video productions illustrate the use of self-management techniques for children who have cancer and reviews the lessons they learned as they are interviewed 13 years later. The latter video documentary explores the range of applications of hypnotic techniques in a general pediatric practice.

During periodic health supervision visits, the clinician can casually make the physical examination an exploration of mind-body linkages. Young patients can be made cognizant of their own heart rate or respiratory rate by palpation, self-auscultation with a stethoscope, or simply by being asked to "feel" or "notice" their heart beating or each breath. This focused self-awareness inevitably results in a change in pulse and respiratory rates that the practitioner can ratify with a statement such as, "Isn't it *interesting* how you *slow* your [*heartbeat* or *breathing*] simply by *paying attention* to it?" Ensuing suggestions can lead to a decrease in autonomic arousal. The relaxation that results from this intensification of awareness can alleviate tension and facilitate comfort during a subsequent abdominal, pelvic, or rectal examination. The clinician acts as the biofeedback instrument, allowing the patient to learn physiological self-regulation to cope with the common stress of a physical examination.

Various inexpensive biofeedback devices are available and practical for use in the pediatric office (Fig. 27-1). The Biotic Band II and Stressdots display peripheral skin temperature as color changes in a liquid crystal medium. Analog-display temperature devices are more expensive and more accurate and can be combined with EDA monitors. EDA devices such as the GSR/TEMP 2 Biofeedback System come with instructional materials for the patient and practitioner.* For home enuresis monitoring, the Sleep Dry comes with excellent instructions for parents as well as a motivational "Star Chart" on which to track progress.† The wireless Potty Pager has a vibrating buzzer that can be worn day or night.‡

*Available from Magic Lantern Film Distributors, Vancouver, B.C., Canada; telephone 1-604-273-8111.
†Available from Leora Kuttner, Ph.D., Suite 204, 1069 West Broadway, Vancouver, B.C. V6H-1E5, Canada.
‡Available from Laurence I. Sugarman, M.D., 2233 Clinto Avenue South, Rochester, NY 14618.

*These devices are available from Bio-Medical Instruments, Inc., 2387 East Eight Mile Road, Warren, MI 48091; telephone 1-800-521-4640.
†StarChild/Labs, P.O. Box 404, Aptos, CA 95001-0404; telephone 1-408-662-2659.
‡Ideas for Living, Inc., 1285 N. Cedarbrook, Boulder, CO 80304; telephone 1-303-440-8517.

More complex computer-based biofeedback devices are available. These systems allow the patient to see multiple channels of physiological processes simultaneously on a computer screen. Child-friendly displays engage the child in games such as basketball, automobile racing, or the changing of artwork on the computer screen. Although the operation of this equipment requires advanced training, it can be worthwhile because it appeals to children, allowing them, literally, to engage in video games for their bodies.

Computer-based biofeedback games for home use are being developed. The MindBody Game,* for example, employs an EDA sensor plugged into the microphone port of a personal computer to demonstrate for children how their feelings and thoughts create changes in the body. Children choose one of four fierce-looking animal figures on the computer monitor and are prompted by a young person's voice to relax and imagine and thereby lower their EDA. The computer software processes the decreasing EDA and, in turn, displays an ever-softening facial expression of the chosen animal. A recorded young person's voice offers praise and encouragement throughout the game. This experience demonstrates for children that their thoughts and emotions affect their bodies and others as well. With a laptop or notebook computer, this device can be brought into the examination room during patient encounters.

Applications of Hypnosis and Biofeedback for Pediatric Pain

Because the experience of pain is subjective, it can be altered. Hypnoanalgesia has long been reported to be a successful component of pain management. In 1843, John Elliotson reported the use of hypnoanalgesia for surgery.[5] The advent of effective chemical anesthesia in the late 1800s and, later, medical analgesics, relegated hypnotic methods to occasional use. However, the value of hypnoanalgesia as adjunctive and primary therapy is reemerging as case reports and studies document its effectiveness in reducing procedural pain, augmenting operative anesthesia, and reducing the frequency and severity of recurrent or chronic pain syndromes.[28] For young people who have acute or recurrent pain, the value of self-regulation strategies rests in the ability to facilitate the patient's mastery and self-efficacy in the face of potentially disabling discomfort.

Acute pain. Acute pain influences the child's perception. Already in a heightened state of awareness, the young person's attention is intensely focused and is often more responsive to suggestions for comfort. No lengthy explanation of self-regulation in hypnosis is required. It is necessary only to capture the child's intensified attention, establish therapeutic rapport, and convey the confidence that the situation will improve. For example, one might say, "You are smart to come to the doctor (or emergency room) when part of you is hurt so that we can help you begin to get it better," or "I bet that arm really hurts right now . . . and, when it's all better, you can be proud of how well you helped it heal."[11]

One can facilitate the child's search for comfort in a variety of ways. By asking the child where he or she would rather be, the clinician can suggest multisensory imagery to help the child dissociate from the painful experience. For example, "You can certainly enjoy your birthday party in your mind while I sew up this cut. Can you *see* [visual imagery] all the presents? Do you *hear* [auditory imagery] your friends and family singing? Would you tell me when you make a wish and *feel* [tactile imagery] yourself *blowing* [breathing suggestions] out all the candles? Can you *smell* [olfactory imagery] the kind of cake you are having? Does it *taste* [gustatory imagery] good?" The youngster may find comfort in the cognitive mastery of knowing he or she can change sensation with relaxation and breathing, as in "It is good to discover that you can change how your stomach feels with your breathing . . . that's right . . . simply breathing out helps your stomach relax . . . and the more you notice your breathing, in . . . then out . . . the more comfortable you can get . . . as if you are breathing out the discomfort as it comes . . . then it goes." Some children cope best by focusing on the cause of the pain and its manifestations, thereby altering the experience. One may ask the child to notice "how bright and red and healthy your blood is" and "It is good that the skin here tells you when it is hurt; it sends messages up wires to your brain," and "there probably have been other times when you have had something hurt (and then gotten better!). On a scale of 0 to 10, how does this compare to those?" Young patients in pain can be taught quickly to raise their finger temperature, lower their heart and respiratory rates, or decrease their EDA by using portable biofeedback units during examinations, injections, insertion of intravenous lines, radiographic procedures, or the cleaning and suturing of wounds.

Several hypnotic techniques for acute pain management have been described by Kuttner,[17] Kohen,[11] and Olness et al.[31] Used in acute settings, these methods decrease the young person's anxiety, and increase comfort, self-control, and cooperation, leading to increased self-efficacy and mastery. The following clinical vignette illustrates the use of relaxation and mental imagery for acute procedural pain and anxiety:

Fourteen-year-old Scott is in an outpatient clinic for IV placement and chemotherapy. He tries to appear calm as a nurse reports that he is a "difficult stick" and has a history of multiple attempts for IVs because "he clamps down." The following encounter takes place:

Clinician: Hi, Scott. I'm Dr. _______________ How's it going?

Scott: OK . . . I guess (shrugs).

C: And you aren't sure, huh? What are you *going to do* here today?

S: Get vincristine . . . if they ever get this IV in me.

C: It *has* felt like they never get it into the vein?

S: Well, they do get it in, but then my vein gets tight and it doesn't work.

C: I see. That's *what has happened before*. So . . . what do *you do* to *make the veins stay loose*?

S: (Rolls eyes) I don't know. What are you talking about?

*Contact Me2, Limited, 7609 Mountain Park Drive, Concord Township, Ohio 44060; telephone 440-354-8364; or at their website: www.me2Ltd.com.

C: Well, you already keep *those* veins open and loose almost all of the time so the blood can move through them easily, right? They really don't spend much time getting tight at all. Most of the time the veins are loose. Usually that happens even better when people *breathe deeply and feel relaxed and comfortable* . . . OK?

S: (Staring at the veins on the back of his hand, shrugs) I guess so.

C: Sure. *You may not have even known that you already know how to do that.* Now you do. You can keep breathing *comfortably* and *deeply* to keep the veins *relaxed* . . . and *open* . . . and *loose* (slow words, pacing breathing with Scott for a few breaths). Right. So . . . are you ready, in a moment, to *do it on purpose* this time so those veins do well?

S: Yeah . . . If it will work.

C: You can *learn more* about how to *make it work,* and I will help you. Is it a deal?

S: OK.

C: Good. While you keep on keeping your breathing comfortable, imagine a place you'd rather be than here . . . simply let it come to mind . . . some place where you feel really relaxed, loose, and comfortable . . . just the way your veins will be. Let me know if that's OK and *when* you do, notice that letting *me know* helps make you *even more comfortable.*

S: (Nods head, eyes begin to close)

C: Good. As you imagine that place more and more, you can notice what your eyes see there . . . what it feels like to be there . . . what sounds come to your ears there while you enjoy yourself . . . there. Because I have noticed that you look really comfortable and relaxed . . . you probably have to . . . .right?

S: Yeah, I'm lying by the pool.

C: You sure are. With every breath, you can use your mind to be more there and less here. (His eyes close but he keeps reopening them) You can leave your eyes open or closed—whatever helps you to relax and imagine the best. You may have already noticed that the more your mind is there, the less things bother you here.

S: (Nods head, eyes stay closed)

C: Good . . . You just use your mind this way to keep the veins nice and loose, so the IV slides right into the vein and then that vein stays nice and loose and open. You can nod . . . again . . . and let us know that you're ready for the IV.

S: (Nods head after 30 seconds. His fingers flex and respiration increases as the nurse prepares the hand for the IV.)

C: That's fine. You are doing a great job there by the pool. Simply notice your breathing . . . That's all that really matters . . . The veins can stay loose as you breathe in and out, as you let yourself go a little more there with each breath. You can let that hand get looser and looser and sink right down into the table . . . Nice . . . You are making your veins just fine with your breathing and imagining. Just keep doing it. Here it goes . . . .

(IV perforates vein that collapses)

S: (Opening eyes abruptly) I CAN'T DO IT! IT'S NOT GOING TO WORK!! I HATE THIS!!!

C: Sure you can, Scott. YOU are doing great; WE missed the vein. We'll find another vein. You can *go right back* to where you were.

S: But it ALWAYS goes like this!

C: Only if *you decide* it does. You are already helping it go better by relaxing and imagining. You are doing a great job. You are the boss of how well you do . . . and the more you practice the better you will get, right?

S: I guess so.

C: You *know* so. So . . . I'm ready if you are.

S: OK. Let's do it.

C: That's right! Let me know when you are ready.

S: (Closes eyes, breathes deeply and slowly, and visibly relaxes.) I'm there.

(IV is placed successfully)

C: (After) Nice job, Scott. How did you do?

S: It worked?

C: Of course. You did it.

S: That was cool. I hardly paid attention to it this time. Like . . . I knew what was happening . . . but I didn't let it bother me.

C: Or your veins! Now you know how you do that. Give yourself a pat on the back. I'd like to thank your veins, personally. So take these good feelings with you. Can you go back to the pool or wherever else you imagine next time you do the IV or another procedure?

S: Yeah . . . I think so . . .

C: You can go back to that place in your mind whenever you'd like, by taking nice deep breaths or by doing whatever you need to do to get there. You're the boss.

S: Thanks.

C: You're welcome. Thank *you.*

Chronic and recurrent pain. Chronic and recurrent pains differ from acute discomfort in that they are more disabling. The person who has chronic or recurrent pain learns that when the pain starts, it worsens, and even when it is relieved, it returns. This intensifies the young person's anxiety and sense of despair, magnifies the perception of pain, and often leads to depression. Teaching self-regulation to children and adolescents who have chronic and recurrent pain requires that the therapist help them reduce both the severity of pain and the negative expectancy that accompanies it.

Self-hypnosis is taught and practiced to reduce anxiety and to create positive expectancy. Using the young person's own descriptions of the pain and the limitations that it causes, the clinician helps him or her develop a hypnotic experience during which he or she may imagine experiencing that "throbbing, dark blue glob that feels like a headache becoming softer and changing slowly to a lighter color," or "skiing on that mountain with a strong, healthy, comfortable leg that has completely healed." It is most important that the imagery be of the child's own choosing and not prescribed. During this experience, ego-strengthening suggestions for mastery, positive outcome, and reminders that "the more you practice, the better and easier it will get" help the child or adolescent develop his or her ability for self-control. A symptom and hypnosis practice diary can help the child and practitioner monitor progress and modify the hypnotic exercise as needed.

The next clinical example demonstrates the use of hypnosis and biofeedback for recurrent pain.

Twelve-year-old Marissa has suffered recurrent, disabling twice-monthly migraine headaches for 3 years despite a thorough neurological evaluation and multiple medication regimens. An excellent student, she enjoys drawing and playing computer games. She wants to be an artist when she grows up. At the pediatrician's office, she agrees to play a computer game in which she changes the color patterns on a computer screen by raising her finger temperature and lowering her EDA while relaxing. She chooses to imagine herself painting in her own art studio. She remarks that learning she can creatively change how her temperature and sweat glands work with her imagination is "cool." The clinician explains that practicing the exercise of painting in her studio and feeling this same way when she does this exercise at home can help her reduce the frequency and intensity of her headaches. She views a portion of a video documentary about other adolescents who have used self-regulation to treat their migraine headaches successfully. After two more visits to reinforce her learning and monitor her headache diary, Marissa has been headache-free for 2 months. She explains that she imagines that she is in her studio and the headache is a drawing that she paints over and turns into something else. She adds that she has used the same self-hypnotic method to help her fall asleep at night, control anger and frustrations, and better focus her attention for tests at school. She admits that she "really does not need to practice anymore because it has become automatic." Finally, she asks if she can return to the office occasionally "just to play the computer game."

Chronic and recurrent pain, especially when there is no clear biological etiology, may be symptomatic of significant psychopathology, including posttraumatic stress disorder, sexual and physical abuse, and depression. The youngster's somatic symptoms may be protecting him or her from more severe psychological pain. If the presenting symptom is serving a protective psychological purpose, hypnotic techniques may be ineffective, and contraindicated, without psychotherapeutic intervention directed at the underlying psychological condition. It is vital that primary care pediatricians carefully reevaluate their approach to self-regulation training for children and adolescents who have persistent symptoms, obtaining appropriate mental health consultation.

Applications for Habit Disorders

Children often develop habits that are frustrating and worrisome to themselves and to family members. These include problems such as nail biting, thumb-sucking, habit coughs, hyperventilation, hair pulling, and tongue rolling or thrusting. Some habits begin with a normal physiological response, such as cough associated with a respiratory infection that becomes conditioned. In addition to these habitual behaviors, nocturnal enuresis, transient tic disorders, and sleep disorders can be treated similarly with self-regulation training constituting adjunctive or primary therapy.[13,15,28] In a series of 35 patients, Kohen has reported that hypnosis training can reduce medication use and increase self-control for young people who have Tourette's syndrome.[12]

If a child wishes to eliminate a problematic habit, the most practical approach to these behaviors is to teach a self-management method that emphasizes mastery and control. It is imperative for the pediatrician to ascertain whether the problem is of more concern to the parent than to the child. The child's motivation for change is a primary factor in learning self-regulation therapies for his or her habit. Parents who try to control their child's habit often unintentionally motivate the child to continue with the habitual behavior as an expression of autonomy. Therefore, it is important to take the time to communicate to the parents that they must disengage from the problem as much as possible and not remind the child to practice the exercise in self-regulation. In fact, this therapeutic approach can become an exercise in helping parents change *their* habit of reminding the child.

As always, the training approach must take into account the child's interests, likes, learning style, and fears. In the following case, the history emphasizes what he or she will be able to do better when he or she has changed the habit. Descriptors of what the habit feels like (for example, the "tickle" that precedes the cough tic), its triggers, activities that are associated with an increase or decrease in habitual behavior, as well as previous efforts to control the habit, shed light on the young person's perception of the problem and imply that there are factors that the patient can use for control (for example, learning to decrease the "tickle" preceding the cough). These factors gathered from the interview form the basis for the imagery and metaphors that are incorporated in the youngster's hypnotic experience and learning.

Often the use of adjunctive biofeedback provides graphic evidence to the child that he or she can control a body response such as EDA or peripheral temperature. After establishing that the child is motivated and capable of changing the habit, an exercise in self-regulation is developed with and for the child to use instead of the habit. The following vignette illustrates one approach:

Ten-year-old Anna has had a troubling dry cough for 8 months, ever since an episode of "choking" on a potato chip at school. After that episode, it took her a month to feel comfortable swallowing solid foods, but the "tickle" in her throat has never gone away. Anna loves playing with friends, riding her bicycle, playing with the home computer, and singing. The latter activity has been limited by her cough, and she has quit the school chorus. Ordinarily an outgoing child, her parents have noticed that she has lost some confidence in herself. The cough (and the "tickle") does not bother her in sleep and when she is concentrating on reading or watching TV. Evaluations by a gastroenterologist, otorhinolaryngologist, and pulmonologist have revealed no organic pathology. Medications have not helped her.

Anna agrees that the tickle and cough vary with her attention. The clinician suggests that "in a way you do not know yet, the computer we call the brain helps you to control the cough." She learns a relaxation and imagery exercise in which she imagines herself riding her bicycle and singing. The more vividly she imagines the less she feels the tickle. In hypnosis, Anna says that the singing feels soothing to her throat, "like butterscotch." She agrees to practice this exercise twice daily, to record the time of her practice on a calendar, and to assign a number on a scale of 0 to 10 for the intensity of the tickle in her throat.

Two weeks later she proudly displays her calendar and exclaims that the cough has decreased by half. Her mother concurs. Anna is asked to show the clinician her hypnotic exercise while fingertip monitors record her EDA activity and temperature. The biofeedback software allows Anna to choose the type of audiofeedback she would prefer. She picks chimes with tones that play down a continuous scale as she lowers her EDA. During the 12-minute exercise, Anna imagines, listens to the audio output from the computer, and does not cough. As she finishes the exercise, she says, "I knew I could do it!" The clinician suggests that Anna can use the exercise to remind herself that she always has the ability to control the cough and feeling in her throat.

One month later, the cough is gone. Anna explains that she always carries her music with her. She says that she can tune into the "Anna Station" on the radio in her mind whenever she wants to feel sure of herself.

Applications for Chronic Disease

The essence of introducing self-regulation strategies for children who have chronic disease is to facilitate a sense of mastery and partnership in treatment. The medications and varied, repeated procedures brought to bear upon young people who have cancer, diabetes, asthma, and cystic fibrosis, for example, carry with them an implicit message that such external therapies are required because the young patient is ineffective in staying healthy. Children and adolescents who live with chronic disease may benefit from learning that they *do* have innate abilities to diminish pain, anxiety, and physiological components of stress responses.

Much of the literature on self-regulation strategies with children who have chronic diseases focuses on benefits in children who have cancer.[9,10,20,26] Hypnosis has been shown to relieve pain and anxiety during the multiple procedures that these youngsters undergo, and it is most effective when introduced early, before conditioned responses become fixed.

Jacknow et al followed, prospectively, a group of 20 children who had a variety of malignancies through two courses of chemotherapy while providing adjunctive hypnosis training to half of them. Those who used hypnosis had significantly less prn anti-emetic medication use and less anticipatory nausea. The hypnosis group showed a stable medication use from the first to second course of chemotherapy. This demonstrates less conditioned reliance on medication or, perhaps, more personal mastery. With the second round of chemotherapy, however, those who had not learned hypnosis had a doubling of their medication usage. This could be interpreted as a loss of control.[9]

Similarly, children who have a chronic disease such as asthma can learn to change the conditioned response of anxiety engendered by an exacerbation of their disease. Episodes of wheezing often are associated with a self-reinforcing cycle of increasing anxiety leading to more dyspnea that, in turn, worsens anxiety. By practicing self-hypnosis, including imagery of relaxed, mucus-free, patent airways and enjoyable activities, young patients can learn that the onset of wheezing constitutes a hypnotic suggestion from their own lungs to exercise hypnosis and reverse the progression of panic and anxiety. The patient can use a home peak expiratory flow rate monitor as a biofeedback device before and after self-hypnosis to validate the reduction in airway resistance. Kohen demonstrated that children who learned self-hypnosis as adjunctive therapy for their asthma had fewer missed school days, emergency department visits, and decreased symptom severity than did controls.[14]

In the office, self-regulation can be introduced to youngsters who have acute exacerbations of asthma by using a pulse oximeter to show them that they can lower their heart rate and raise their oxygen saturation. This can be supported and intensified by patient-centered language and embedded suggestions (italicized), such as, "You can notice how *much better you are making* your breathing tubes as *you help* the oxygen in your blood go up and that heart rate slow down . . . and isn't it *good to know* that *you are helping yourself get better* as you *make it change*?" Although such monitoring instruments are used, in acute settings, primarily to inform clinicians of the patient's physiological status, they can be transformed, simply by the use of empowering therapeutic language, into biofeedback tools that serve the child's or adolescent's needs for self-control and comfort.

Parents of children who have a chronic, complex disease are often very concerned, protective, and enmeshed with their children and their treatments. It is important that the practitioner clarify that the success with self-regulation strategies rests in the child's drive for autonomy. For this reason it is recommended that the child be taught self-regulation without the parents present. It can be explained that these skills must be learned first by the child and, once mastered, taught to parents by the child. Often, parents are relieved to know that their children have this ability to help themselves and that the clinician has faith in that ability. With very young or severely ill children, parents and children can be taught self-hypnosis as a team, helping them to find comfort together.[28]

The following clinical example illustrates these principles:

Six-year-old Jonathan suffers from frequent and recurrent exacerbations of asthma and is on appropriate medical and environmental therapy, resulting in frequent visits to the emergency department, which Jonathan hates and fears. His parents report increasing family anxiety with each episode of wheezing. Jonathan asks for more and more "breathing treatments" (inhaled albuterol), thinking that they can prevent trips to the hospital. Using a pulse oximeter in the office, Jonathan learns that he can slow his heart rate by relaxing and speed it up by simply thinking about "fun stuff," because he is "the boss" of his body. The clinician, Jonathan, and his mother draw a picture of Jonathan's respiratory tract. Jonathan draws cool, blue, soothing air coming down his breathing tubes and says, "That's what it is like when I make them comfortable."

Sitting on his mother's lap and staring at his drawing, the two talk together about the feelings associated with relaxed, open, comfortable, happy breathing tubes. They agree to practice and draw together daily in the evening "to keep those breathing tubes feeling good." Jonathan agrees to monitor his albuterol use on a calendar and put a sticker on the calendar days that he needs no extra "puffs."

Three weeks later, there have been no hospital visits. He has stickers on more than half of the days and says, "sometimes I pretend about my breathing without my Mom." Twice as he began to wheeze, he grabbed the metered dose inhaler containing albuterol but did not use it because he "calmed those breathing tubes down and made them happy."

RESEARCH AND THE FUTURE

Training in self-regulation has been demonstrated to be effective therapy for a variety of pediatric biobehavioral disorders. These mind-body techniques that promote self-regulation represent an emerging discipline that has promising implications for preventive health care and research in physiology. While the precise pathways by which self-regulation strategies mediate therapeutic change are as yet unknown, so are the limits of their potential benefits. These methods are not a panacea for all psychophysiological disorders. One must maximize medical therapy and make appropriate psychological referrals.

There are three broad directions for future research: (1) clarifying the roles of self-regulation strategies for biobehavioral disorders and defining their efficacy; (2) elaborating the implications of self-regulation training for preventive care and health care economics; and (3) elucidating the mechanisms by which the mind effects physiological change.

The majority of research in pediatric self-regulation therapies has focused on new applications in the form of case reports. Several hypnotic susceptibility scales have been developed for use with children. None has proven to be predictive of outcome in clinical settings, because the average child scores high. Few controlled studies show increased medication efficacy, and none demonstrates prolonged survival as a result of biofeedback training or hypnotherapy. Larger series that have standardized regimens reported in the mainstream literature will be required to elucidate the therapeutic roles of self-regulation methods. Practitioners need direction regarding indicators of success, choice of techniques, duration of effect, and measures of efficacy.

Ripe opportunities for discovery lie in the preventative potential of self-hypnosis and biofeedback. Incorporating self-regulation training in well-child care and as part of anticipatory guidance can form the basis for teaching lifelong coping strategies in health and disease. Training children to condition relaxation before tests in school, as well as musical and athletic performance, may foster the development of adults who meet challenges with more poise and competence. It is conceivable that teaching self-regulation skills to youngsters at risk for familial disease such as hypertension, asthma, and attention deficit/hyperactivity disorder may delay their onset or diminish morbidity. Assessing each youngster's ability to use self-regulation skills on hospital admission would allow nursing and medical staff to facilitate training and enhance both the child's and family's comfort and response to therapy. Certainly, such training could reduce the amount of medications used for treatment as well as the sociocultural dependence on stress-reducing drugs.

Exciting breakthroughs are being made in our understanding of the mechanisms by which psychological processes affect the autonomic, immune, and endocrine systems.[32] In structured settings, children have the ability to vary salivary immunoglobulin A content and increase neutrophil adherence compared with matched controls who have had no self-regulation training.[27] In another experimental design, children who have asthma were shown to have cholinergically mediated airway reactivity in response to emotional stimuli.[24]

These paths of discovery are intertwined. Methods for self-regulation therapy in childhood asthma, for example, have great preventative potential while shedding new light on the neurophysiological mediators of reactive airways. This research direction can forge new coalitions between physiologist, psychologist, subspecialist, and primary care practitioner—all aligned to rediscover and facilitate each child's innate ability to engage the future with equanimity.

REFERENCES

1. Butler RJ, Forsythe WI, Robertson J: The body-worn alarm in the treatment of childhood enuresis, *Br J Clin Pract* 44:237, 1990.
2. Culbert TP, Kajander RL, Reaney JB: Biofeedback with children and adolescents: clinical observations and patient perspectives, *J Dev Behav Pediatr* 17:342, 1996.
3. Culbert TP, Reaney JB, Kohen DP: "Cyberphysiologic" strategies for children: the clinical hypnosis/biofeedback interface, *Int J Clin Exp Hypn* 42:97, 1994.
4. Devlin JB, O'Cathain C: Predicting treatment outcome in nocturnal enuresis, *Arch Dis Child* 65:1158, 1990.
5. Elliotson J: *Numerous cases of surgical operations without pain in the mesmeric state,* Philadelphia, 1843, Lea and Blanchard.
6. French GM, Painter EC, Coury DL: Blowing away shot pain: a technique for pain management during immunization, *Pediatrics* 93:384, 1994.
7. Gall JC: The art of examining a child: use of naturalistic methods in the pediatric physical examination, *Ericksonian Monogr* 7:69, 1990.
8. Gardner GG: Parents: obstacles or allies in child hypnotherapy? *Am J Clin Hypn* 17:44, 1974.
9. Jacknow DS, et al: Hypnosis in the prevention of chemotherapy-related nausea and vomiting in children: a prospective study, *J Dev Behav Pediatr* 15:258, 1994.
10. Jacobs E, Pelier E, Larkin D: Ericksonian hypnosis and approaches with pediatric hematology oncology patients, *Am J Clin Hypn* 41:139, 1998.
11. Kohen DP: Applications of relaxation/mental imagery (self-hypnosis) in pediatric emergencies, *Int J Clin Exp Hypn* 34:283, 1986.
12. Kohen DP: Coping with the stress of Tourette syndrome in children and adolescents: use of self-hypnosis techniques, *Aust J Clin Exper Hypn* 23:145, 1995.
13. Kohen DP: Management of trichotillomania with relaxation/mental imagery (self-hypnosis): experience with five children, *J Dev Behav Pediatr* 17:5, 328, 1996.
14. Kohen DP: Relaxation/mental imagery (self-hypnosis) for childhood asthma: behavioral outcomes in a prospective, controlled study, *Hypnos* 22:132, 1995.
15. Kohen DP, et al: Sleep-terror disorder in children: the role of self-hypnosis in management, *Am J Clin Hypn* 34:233, 1992.
16. Kohen DP, et al: The use of relaxation/mental imagery (self-hypnosis) in the management of 505 pediatric behavioral encounters, *J Dev Behav Pediatr* 1:21, 1984.
17. Kuttner L: *A child in pain: how to help, what to do,* Point Roberts, Washington, 1996, Hartley and Marks.
18. Kuttner L: Helpful strategies in working with preschool children in pediatric practice, *Pediatr Ann* 20:120, 1991.
19. Lambert SA: The effects of hypnosis/guided imagery on the postoperative course of children, *J Dev Behav Pediatr* 17:307, 1996.
20. LeBaron S, Hilgard JR: *Hypnotherapy of pain in children with cancer,* Los Altos, Calif, 1984, William Kaufmann.
21. Lee LH, Olness KN: Effects of self-induced mental imagery on autonomic reactivity in children, *J Dev Behav Pediatr* 17:323, 1996.
22. Lubar JF: Discourse on the development of EEG diagnostics and biofeedback for attention-deficit/hyperactivity disorders, *Biofeedback Self Regul* 16:201, 1991.
23. Lynn SJ, Rhue JW, editors: *Theories of hypnosis: current models and perspectives,* New York, 1991, Guilford Press.
24. Miller BD, Wood BL: Psychophysiologic reactivity in asthmatic children: a cholinergically mediated confluence of pathways, *J Am Acad Child Adolesc Psychiatry* 33:1236, 1994.
25. Mize WL: Clinical training in self-regulation and practical pediatric hypnosis: what pediatricians want pediatricians to know, *J Dev Behav Pediatr* 17:317, 1996.
26. Olness KN: Imagery (self-hypnosis) as adjunctive therapy in childhood cancer: clinical experience with 25 patients, *Am J Pediatr Hem/Onc* 3:313, 1981.
27. Olness K, Culbert TP, Uden D: Self-regulation of salivary immunoglobulin A by children, *Pediatrics* 83:66, 1989.
28. Olness KN, Kohen DP: *Hypnosis and hypnotherapy with children,* ed 3, New York, 1996, Guilford Press.
29. Olness K, Libbey P: Unrecognized biologic bases of behavioral symptoms in patients referred for hypnotherapy, *Am J Clin Hypn* 30:1, 1987.
30. Olness K, MacParland F, Piper J: Biofeedback: a new modality in the treatment of children with fecal soiling, *J Pediatr* 96:505, 1980.
31. Olness KN, et al: Prospective study comparing propranolol, placebo, and hypnosis in management of juvenile migraine, *Pediatrics* 79:593, 1987.
32. Rossi EL: *Psychobiology of mind-body healing: new concepts of therapeutic hypnosis,* New York, 1986, WW Norton.
33. Schwartz MS, editor: *Biofeedback: a practitioner's guide,* New York, 1995, Guilford Press.

34. Sugarman LI: Hypnosis in a primary care pediatric practice: developing skills for the new morbidities, *J Dev Behav Pediatr* 17:300, 1996.
35. Sugarman LI: Hypnosis: teaching children self-regulation, *Pediatr Rev* 17:5, 1996.

SUGGESTED READINGS

Haley J: *Uncommon therapy: the psychiatric techniques of Milton H. Erickson, M.D.*, New York, 1993, WW Norton.

Hammond DC, editor: *Handbook of hypnotic suggestions and metaphors*, New York, 1990, WW Norton.

Olness K (guest editor): Biofeedback therapy, *Pediatr Ann* 20:113, 1991.

Olness KN, Kohen DP: *Hypnosis and hypnotherapy with children*, ed 3, New York, 1996, Guilford Press.

Rossi EL: *Psychobiology of mind-body healing: new concepts of therapeutic hypnosis*, New York, 1986, WW Norton.

Schwartz MS, editor: *Biofeedback: a practitioner's guide*, New York, 1995, Guilford Press.

28 Complementary and Alternative Medical Therapies

Kathi J. Kemper

As more and more Americans turn to complementary and alternative medical (CAM) therapies for themselves and their children, pediatricians are being asked a variety of questions for which their formal training may not have prepared them:

- Is this herb safe to use for my child's condition?
- Do you think acupuncture might help my child's allergies?
- I'd like to try massage to help my child's asthma; can you refer me to a pediatric massage therapist?
- My grandmother recommended hot, spicy foods for my baby when she has a cold. What do you think?

Pediatricians need not be expert in every form of complementary and alternative therapies to be able to help answer questions such as these. Nor do pediatricians need to throw out all they've learned about critical thinking and evidence-based medicine to begin to understand some of the values that drive families' choices. But pediatricians do need to be aware of the trends, the remedies their patients are using, some of the theories behind CAM practices, something about the professional practices of CAM providers, how to talk with families to elicit a complete history of the different therapies they might be using for their child, and where to turn for additional information.

EPIDEMIOLOGY

Increasing numbers of children and families are turning to complementary and alternative medicine (CAM). The percentage of American adults using CAM increased from 34% in 1990 to 42% in 1997, and out-of-pocket expenditures increased 45% during this same period.[7,9] In fact, the annual number of outpatient visits in the United States to CAM providers now exceeds the number of outpatient visits to mainstream physicians. And the amount of money spent out of pocket for CAM care exceeds the amount spent out of pocket for all U.S. hospitalizations.[8] Despite the increased use and payment for CAM services, patients were no more likely to discuss their use of CAM in 1997 than they were in 1990; the majority of patients did not talk with their physicians about their use of CAM therapies.

The percentage of general pediatric patients using CAM was approximately 11% in 1994 and increased to approximately 20% in 1997.[33] The percentage is substantially higher for children and families faced with chronic, recurrent, or fatal conditions such as rheumatoid arthritis, asthma, and cancer.[17,34] For children and adolescents facing these conditions, rates of CAM use range from 30% to more than 70% depending on age, acculturation, and access to services.[4]

Although many physicians are concerned that families who use CAM may be dissatisfied with mainstream medical care and fear they may abandon effective therapies in favor of unproved alternatives, data do not support these concerns. For the most part, families seek therapies that are consistent with their values, world view, and culture, and they seek care from therapists who respect them as individuals and who offer them time and attention.[1,27] Families continue to value highly the care they receive from compassionate, comprehensive primary care pediatricians. And they seek additional information on healthy lifestyles, dietary supplements, and environmental therapies over which they may exert some control.[20] They also seek care from CAM therapists who offer personal attention, hope, time, and therapies consistent with their culture and values. Families who seek out complementary and alternative medical therapies rarely abandon their pediatrician, but they may not feel comfortable discussing those therapies if they perceive the pediatrician to be antagonistic or judgmental toward them.

The professional CAM therapists most often sought out by families include chiropractors, acupuncturists, naturopaths, homeopaths, and massage therapists.[32] The CAM therapies sought most often include prayer and spiritual healing, vitamins, minerals, herbs and other dietary supplements, special diets, and mind/body techniques such as relaxation training, hypnosis, and biofeedback.

DEFINITIONS OF CAM

Alternative medicine refers typically to therapies that generally are not taught at American medical schools, not provided in hospitals, lack evidence of effectiveness, and are not reimbursed by third-party payers.[8] Because of changes in practice and emerging research, this definition is problematic. Many therapies formerly considered alternative, such as acupuncture and hypnosis, are now part of the range of therapies offered in pediatric settings, including children's hospitals. More than half of American medical schools now offer courses on alternative therapies.[39] New evidence is emerging on the safety and effectiveness of a wide range of dietary supplements, massage, and other therapies. As a result of both science and public pressure, increasing numbers of third-party payers reimburse families for services once considered to be alternative.

Complementary therapies are those that are used in conjunction with mainstream medical therapies. Examples that have found their way into conventional medical settings include massage, support groups, guided imagery, biofeedback, and hypnosis.[29] These therapies do not necessarily replace medical regimens for cancer, depression, prematurity, or other serious medical problems, but they are offered to support the patient and family.

Folk medicine refers to therapies that families or group members provide as part of a family or cultural tradition. Examples include chicken soup for upper respiratory infections, "cold" foods for "hot" illnesses, and particular religious or ritual healing practices such as cupping, coining, and sand painting.[30,31]

Integrative medicine refers to the practice of integrating complementary and alternative medical therapies into mainstream practice, based on scientific evidence of their safety and effectiveness.[22] Pediatricians who incorporate chamomile, ginger, and other home remedies in their advice about treatments for common pediatric conditions such as colic and nausea may be said to practice integrative medicine.[21]

Holistic medicine is closely related to contextual pediatrics or comprehensive care. It simply refers to care of the whole patient—body, mind, emotions, spirit, and relationships—in the context of the patient's values, beliefs, culture, and community. Examples include screening for depression and alcohol use in family members,[23] promoting housecleaning to reduce allergic symptoms, and promoting literacy via the pediatric clinic.[26]

These various definitions include an implicit recognition of the primary importance of treating the patient as an individual rather than as a constellation of symptoms. They also recognize the primary role of the family in providing care and place the pediatrician in the role of counselor, teacher, and advice-giver rather than a role akin to a general giving orders in a battle. Family-physician relationships are viewed as partnerships rather than hierarchically. Such changes mirror societal and cultural changes reflecting values of individual rights (e.g., civil rights, women's rights) and the growing educational levels and access to information that characterize modern society.

EFFECTIVENESS AND SAFETY

Effectiveness and safety are paramount in evaluating any therapy for children. Pediatricians recognize that mainstream therapies have varying effectiveness depending on the individual child, condition, and therapy and depend to some extent on variations in the environment, the quality of care, and access to services. For example, although surgery is the safest and most effective therapy for some conditions (e.g., appendicitis), it is neither the safest nor the most effective therapy for the common cold, migraine headaches, or attention deficit disorder. Medications used to reduce the symptoms of upper respiratory infections in adults have no proven benefit on children's cold symptoms.

Research on the effectiveness of complementary and alternative medical therapies may focus on the therapy itself (e.g., the effectiveness of chamomile tea in treating neonatal colic) or on the therapist who provides care (e.g., the process of care provided by homeopaths, chiropractors, or massage therapists).[22] Outcomes of interest may include effects on standard measures of morbidity and mortality, side effects, and costs and may also include broader outcomes such as satisfaction with care, sense of self-efficacy, cultural identity, and effects on the environment.

BOX 28-1

INTEGRATIVE APPROACH TO THERAPIES

Biochemical Therapies
- Medications
- Vitamins and minerals
- Dietary supplements (e.g., herbs, amino acids, hormones)

Lifestyle Therapies
- Diet (e.g., vegetarian, low fat, high fiber, avoidance of sensitivities, macrobiotic)
- Exercise (aerobic, weight training, yoga)
- Environment (light, vibration, music, aromas, magnets, media, social)
- Mind-body (hypnosis, biofeedback, meditation, counseling, support groups)

Biomedical
- Massage and bodywork
- Chiropractic and other spinal adjustments
- Surgery and transfusions

Bioenergetic
- Acupuncture
- Therapeutic Touch, Reiki, Healing Touch
- Prayer and ritual
- Homeopathy

Regardless of the focus of research, fairness demands that similar therapies for similar conditions be evaluated by similar standards (Box 28-1). Double-blind, randomized, controlled trials are well-established means of evaluating medications and should be used to evaluate other biochemical therapies such as vitamins, minerals, and other dietary supplements (herbs and vitamins). Double-blind trials are not feasible for evaluating the impact of lifestyle changes such as diet (e.g., breast-feeding, vegetarianism, or macrobiotics), exercise (e.g., swimming or yoga), environment (e.g., phototherapy, white noise, aromatherapy), or mind-body therapies (e.g., psychotherapy, support groups, hypnosis, biofeedback, or meditation). It simply is impossible to "blind" families as to whether they are breast-feeding, exercising, or relaxing. Trials of biomechanical therapies such as chiropractic and massage should be judged by standards similar to trials of new surgical techniques.

Studies regarding therapies that are based on substantially different world views, such as traditional Chinese medicine or homeopathy, require sensitivity and creativity. Mainstream researchers evaluating therapies for migraine headaches obviously avoid including patients who have brain tumors and sinus infections because these conditions have different etiologies, even though patients suffering from them may present with recurrent headaches. Similarly, conditions that may have one diagnosis in mainstream medicine may have multiple different diagnoses within different healing traditions, depending on patient and environmental factors that may seem irrelevant to a mainstream researcher.

Many complementary and alternative medical therapies recommend a very broad approach to treatment, including diet, dietary supplements, prayer, environmental changes, and others. Attempting to reduce such a comprehensive approach to a single intervention would be akin to evaluating the effectiveness of treating a sprained ankle with rest alone, omitting ice, compression, and elevation from the treatment model.

Given the central role of culture and values, the emphasis on changes in lifestyle, the values of therapy, and the time and attention provided by holistic healers, the placebo effect undoubtedly plays at least as much of a role in complementary therapies as it does in mainstream medicine.[25] Given the enormously helpful potential of placebos in eliciting positive psychological, neurological, and immunological effects in a variety of health conditions, this is a rich area for research.[6] Because many conditions are self-limited, relying on the patient's own ability to heal rather than on a specific biomedical therapy, the reliable elicitation of the placebo effect represents a vital key to safe and effective therapeutic interventions.[2,36]

COMPLEMENTARY AND ALTERNATIVE MEDICAL PROFESSIONALS

Patients and families may well be confused about the proliferating diversity of professional providers (Box 28-2). One of the most common questions is the difference between medical doctors (MDs) and doctors of osteopathy (DOs). Unlike in England, in the United States, an osteopath is a fully licensed and trained physician and surgeon like an MD, with the addition of training in osteopathic manipulation. To be licensed in the United States, DOs must graduate from one of 16 osteopathic medical schools accredited by the Bureau of Professional Education of the American Osteopathic Association. Like MDs, training is 4 years long, followed by a 1- to 6-year residency training program in general or subspecialty areas. All must pass an unlimited physician and surgeon licensing examination and seek licensing in any state. Like MDs, DOs may practice in fully accredited, licensed hospitals and medical centers and have the right to prescribe drugs and perform surgery.

Osteopathic philosophy is explicitly holistic. Osteopaths believe in an interdependent, synergistic model of human functioning—the whole is greater than the sum of the parts—and that the mind and spirit are equally as important as the body. Osteopathic training focuses on maintaining and promoting resilience and coping in the face of stress and a strong emphasis on health promotion and disease prevention. These ideals are embraced by many medical doctors as well.

Both MDs and DOs are considered mainstream physician practitioners. There were approximately 35,000 DOs in the United States in 1998, with the number expected to rise to 45,000 by the year 2000.

The number of non-physician clinicians graduating from professional training doubled between 1992 and 1997. The per capita supply of these clinicians is expected to increase 150% between 1995 and 2005.[5] Many of these non-MD clinicians care for children.

BOX 28-2

CAM PROFESSIONALS

Licensed in 10 or More States
- Licensed acupuncturist (LiAc)
- Doctors of chiropractic (DC)
- Naturopathic doctor (ND)
- Licensed massage therapist (LMT)

Licensed in Fewer Than 10 States (or No Professional License)
- Homeopathic practitioners
- Therapeutic Touch practitioners
- Reiki healers
- Herbalists
- Aromatherapists

Doctors of Chiropractic

Chiropractors are the CAM therapists used most often by adults and children in the United States and Canada. Chiropractors are licensed in all 50 states, and Medicare and most major insurance carriers cover professional chiropractic care. In 1998, there were more than 50,000 doctors of chiropractic in the United States; the number of licensed chiropractors is expected to double by 2010. In many ways, then, chiropractic is more of a mainstream than alternative form of health care.[19]

Many chiropractors, particularly members of the International Chiropractic Association, have begun promoting regular chiropractic care for children as an essential part of pediatric health promotion. The concept of "family chiropractic" became widespread during the 1990s; chiropractors began to hold mass screenings in public schools and community settings. Surveys estimate that 20 million pediatric visits to chiropractors occurred in 1993, increasing to more than 30 million pediatric visits by 1998. Children and adolescents typically account for 10% to 20% of all visits to chiropractors.

Chiropractors treat many more patients per week than do most other CAM providers. The average number of visits is 120 to 150 per week, with initial visits lasting 45 minutes and follow-up visits lasting 15 to 20 minutes. Patients are scheduled for follow-up visits two to three times weekly for acute conditions. Nearly half of chiropractor fees are covered by third-party payers.

Most chiropractic schools now offer courses in pediatric care. Chiropractors tend to take fewer radiographs for children, to use lighter force when making adjustments, and to use a device called an activator to make adjustments. Chiropractors also use special pediatric tables or treat the children in their parents' laps. Only about one third of chiropractors actively recommend childhood immunizations.

In addition to health promotion, many chiropractors claim to treat otitis media, asthma, allergies, infantile colic, and enuresis. Randomized trials to evaluate these claims are rare, but no comparison studies have demonstrated that chiropractic is as or more effective than mainstream treatments for these common pediatric conditions. Nor have studies demonstrated chiropractic's effectiveness in preventing mild or serious pediatric disorders. On the other hand, acute significant adverse effects from chiropractic adjustments are very rare, and the rate of malpractice claims against chiropractors is much lower than the rate of suits against medical doctors.[35]

The chiropractic community itself is sharply divided into two main camps. The International Chiropractic Association promotes chiropractic as essential to health promotion and is opposed to mandatory childhood immunizations. The American Chiropractic Association tends to focus on treatment of low back pain and other musculoskeletal disorders and to include exercise, dietary, and nutritional supplement counseling among their therapeutic maneuvers.

Licensed Acupuncturists (LiAc)

There are approximately 11,000 practicing acupuncturists in the United States, and the number is expected to reach 21,000 by the year 2005.[5] Acupuncture is one of the CAM therapies endorsed and recommended most frequently by physicians. The NIH Consensus conference on acupuncture concluded that acupuncture was effective in treating several kinds of pain and nausea in adults. Among major teaching hospitals that have a pediatric pain service, nearly one third offer acupuncture therapy to treat chronic pain in children.[40]

Acupuncture is one component of traditional Chinese medicine. It is based on the theory of a vital energy, or Chi (Qi), that circulates through the body in channels called meridians. When the flow of vital energy is blocked or disrupted, there is disease; when the flow is balanced, harmonized, and restored, the patient returns to health. The energy flow can be affected by stimulating specific points along the energy meridians. Thus, acupuncture is one way of restoring the balanced, harmonious flow of the Chi, or vital energy. Approximately 80% of licensed acupuncturists also recommend dietary changes, herbs, and other supplements and changes in lifestyle, exercise, rest, and relationships to enhance health.

Although acupuncturists are licensed in more than 20 states, there is no formal licensure or certification for practicing pediatric acupuncture. Most acupuncturists who treat children use special techniques, including non-needle methods of stimulating point-heat, magnets, lasers, and vigorous massage or tapping. Many use the gentler Japanese style rather than the more vigorous Chinese style of acupuncture. Fewer than 10% of acupuncturists see three or more pediatric patients weekly; most acupuncturists rarely treat children.

Most American acupuncturists are now American trained. They typically see 30 to 60 patients weekly, with initial visit lengths of 90 minutes and follow-up visit lengths of 60 minutes. For acute conditions, visits usually are recommended two to three times weekly for 2 to 3 weeks, reducing to one to two weekly for 2 to 3 weeks and then less often until no longer needed. Benefits, when achieved, are nearly always notable within the first five treatments. Acupuncture visits rarely are covered by insurance; the majority of patients pay out of pocket for acupuncture services unless a physician acupuncturist provides those services.

Naturopathic Doctors (NDs)

Naturopathic medicine grew out of the German spa movement in the nineteenth century. It is based on the belief that the body has a strong, innate power to heal and that symptoms reveal the body's attempt to achieve a whole state in the face of internal and external challenges. Treatment is focused not on individual symptoms so much as on restoring the whole person to healthy balance and resilience. Like mainstream physicians, naturopaths try to help patients avoid unhealthy habits such as smoking, excessive use of alcohol, and illicit drugs. Their focus on health promotion includes attention to a healthy diet (free of pesticides, herbicides, antimicrobials; low in fat; high in fiber and micronutrients), exercise, rest, and a positive mental and emotional state enhanced by meditation, imagery, and counseling. Naturopathic therapies also include hot and cold baths, steam baths, dietary supplements such as herbs and vitamins, and massage. Some naturopaths also incorporate elements of chiropractic, acupuncture, homeopathy, and midwifery into their practices.

In 1997, there were an estimated 1900 naturopathic doctors (NDs) in the United States, with a threefold growth anticipated by 2012. Fewer than 15 states currently license NDs, but the number is expected to grow substantially upon citizen demand. There are four accredited schools of naturopathy in the United States—in Washington, Oregon, Arizona, and Connecticut. Training is 4 years in length. There is a national certifying examination, the Naturopathic Physician Licensing Examination (NPLEX). Internship and residency are not required. Visit lengths are typically about 60 to 90 minutes for an initial visit and 30 to 45 minutes for a follow-up visit. Third-party coverage of ND services varies by state, but the majority of pediatric care is paid out of pocket by families.

Only about one third of NDs report having specific pediatric training. Little or no training is provided for the recognition of potentially serious pediatric problems (e.g., febrile neonates) or standard safety counseling (e.g., car seats, smoke detectors, hot water temperature). However, similar to patients of family practitioners, children and adolescents account for about 20% to 30% of the patient loads of NDs. Some families rely on their ND as a source of primary care. Only 20% of naturopaths recommend childhood immunizations, and a small percentage are opposed to immunizations.

Licensed Massage Therapists and Bodyworkers

Massage is the type of bodywork most familiar to physicians. There are hundreds of types of bodywork and massage, but the four major categories practiced in the United States are Swedish massage (long, gliding strokes, kneading, and stroking), deep tissue massage (e.g., Rolfing and Hellerwork), pressure point techniques (e.g., shiatsu and acupressure), and movement integration (e.g., Feldenkrais and Alexander techniques). Nearly every cultural group in the world has an historical tradition of massage therapy.

Training and licensure for massage are variable. Some states license massage within the field of health; others include it in the entertainment category. Some states require a certifying examination; others regulate massage by municipality rather than at the state level. The largest professional national organization of bodyworkers is the American Massage Therapy Association. Membership requires training in an accredited school and hundreds of hours of supervised practice. Massage therapists focus primarily on muscles and connective tissues and do not perform spinal adjustments.

Although most massage schools provide very little training in pediatrics and most massage therapists rarely treat children, there is substantial and growing evidence that massage helps children and adolescents who suffer from a wide range of conditions. It can enhance the growth rate of premature infants, reduce the severity of asthma in school-age children, and ease suffering from anxiety and depression in adolescents hospitalized for psychiatric disorders.[10,11,13,15,17] Massage also is helpful in relieving pain, reducing edema, improving circulation, loosening tight joints, decreasing levels of stress-hormones, enhancing endogenous levels of serotonin, and enhancing an overall sense of relaxation and well-being.[12,14]

In some hospitals, nurses and physical therapists provide massage therapy for children. Sadly, with the drive toward increased reliance on billable medications and decreased use of non-billable personal services, massage therapy appears to have moved from a mainstream to an alternative therapy in modern hospitals.

CAM THERAPIES PROVIDED BY PHYSICIANS, NURSES, AND PARENTS

Homeopathy

Almost 2 million visits to homeopathic practitioners were made in the United States in 1997. Retail sales of homeopathic remedies were estimated at $250 million in the United States and $1.15 billion worldwide in the late 1990s. Homeopathic remedies were rated second following chiropractic therapy as the CAM therapies most commonly used by children in 1994. An estimated 12,000 homeopaths practice in the United States; of these, about 50% are lay practitioners, 35% are chiropractors, about 10% are physicians, and the rest are naturopaths, nurses, and other health professionals.[38]

Homeopathy is a system of medical treatment invented in the 1800s by a German physician, Samuel Hahnemann. Currently, homeopathy is popular in Europe, Russia, India, and South America.[3] Homeopathy is based on two principles: (1) the Law of Similars or "like cures like" and (2) the Law of Dilutions. The Law of Similars *(similia similibus curantur)* means that a remedy that would cause a symptom in a healthy person is used to treat the same symptom in a sick person. For example, a homeopathic remedy for poison ivy (rhus toxicum) might be used to treat a child suffering from eczema. Although pediatricians might reasonably be concerned about dangerous sounding homeopathic remedies such as rhus toxicum, nux vomica, and belladonna, serious side effects from homeopathic treatment are incredibly rare, far less common than side effects from standard medications.

Homeopathy's gentleness and safety are attributable to its second principle—the Law of Dilutions (*doses minimae*, or potentiation through dilution). This law says that the more the remedy is diluted, the more powerful it becomes. For regular medicines and herbs, we know that, in general, the larger the dose, the more powerful the effects. But in homeopathy, the most powerful remedies are the ones that have been diluted over and over again hundreds, thousands, and even millions of times. Homeopaths believe that these very dilute remedies contain an energy, or information, that is used by the patient to heal his or her symptoms. Most mainstream physicians believe that there are no active molecules of the remedy left in the solution and that the remedies are nothing more than placebos, triggering the patient's psycho-neuro-immunological healing systems.

As expected in a European-originated therapy, nearly all homeopaths in the United States (like chiropractors and naturopaths) are white. Visit lengths are long—typically 90 minutes for an initial visit and 30 to 45 minutes for a follow-up visit. Visits also are scheduled frequently—every 4 to 6 weeks. Insurance coverage for homeopathic care varies by state, carrier, and the professional status of the practitioner. Homeopathic services provided by physicians and chiropractors are much more likely to be covered than are services provided by non-physicians. In addition to homeopathic remedies, many practitioners who engage in this therapy also discuss and recommend dietary therapies, dietary supplements, and relaxation techniques. Typically, about 20% to 30% of a homeopath's patient load are pediatric and adolescent patients.

Regardless of one's view of the theoretical basis for its effectiveness, homeopathic remedies have been evaluated in several randomized controlled trials, with several studies documenting statistically significant improvement for patients who have common conditions such as allergic rhinitis and diarrhea. As mainstream physicians and nurses grow uncomfortable with the side effects of modern medications, more and more are turning to homeopathy as a safe alternative therapy. Homeopathic remedies are available over the counter and through mail order catalogs and the Internet without a prescription. Almost anyone can claim to be a homeopathic practitioner.

Therapeutic Touch/Reiki

Therapeutic Touch and Reiki are two kinds of bioenergetic therapy in which the healer transmits an invisible healing energy through his or her hands to help patients. They are both nonreligious forms of "laying on of hands" healing.

Despite its name, Therapeutic Touch is performed most typically without actually touching the patient. This therapy was invented in the 1970s by a nursing professor at New York University, Dolores Krieger, and a lay healer, Dora Kunz. Based on their observations of numerous religious healers, they distilled the process into five steps (not requiring a specific religious faith or belief) that a healer could use to help patients. These are:

1. Having a clear and conscious *intent* to be helpful and heal

2. Being *centered* in a peaceful state of mind
3. Using the hands to *assess* the patient's energy (typically moving the hands 1 to 3 inches away from the body in a slow downward sweep from the head to the toes)
4. Using the hands to help *restore* the patient's energy to a balanced, harmonious, peaceful state (again, slowly moving the hands a few inches away from the body)
5. Releasing the patient to complete his or her healing process while the healer returns to his or her own centered, peaceful state of mind

Nurses and other health professionals in more than 80 countries have received training in Therapeutic Touch from its founders. It currently is taught in nursing schools across the United States. Nursing practice in many hospitals, including children's hospitals, includes policies and procedures for performing Therapeutic Touch. There are no national certifying examinations, and no states currently license Therapeutic Touch practitioners.

Few studies have evaluated the effectiveness of Therapeutic Touch in treating children.[18] Studies of adults report that Therapeutic Touch helps reduce pain and anxiety, enhancing sleep and a sense of well-being. A few preliminary studies suggest that it may promote wound healing.[37] Side effects are rare. Costs vary depending on whether the practice is provided as part of routine nursing care or through an independent practice.

Reiki is a similar practice, growing out of a Japanese tradition. Reiki practitioners are trained by a Reiki master through a sort of apprenticeship and spiritual/energetic initiation. Reiki practice relies on a belief in an invisible energy that may be transmitted from healer to patient through intention and focus via hands placed on particular parts of the patient's body. In some cases, Reiki healers do long-distance healing in which the patient is visualized and energy is sent through intention rather than through transmission by direct physical contact. There are no national certifying examinations, no state licensure, and no studies evaluating its effectiveness in treating children. There are no reported side effects.

Guided Imagery/Biofeedback

Guided imagery, hypnosis, and biofeedback have moved from alternative therapies into mainstream medical practice. Physicians, psychologists, social workers, and other mainstream health professionals use them. Training is available through workshops sponsored by the Society for Behavioral and Developmental Pediatrics, among other places. These techniques have proven useful in treating a wide range of pediatric conditions—from pain to behavioral problems—and in promoting optimal performance. They are discussed in detail in Chapter 27, Self-Regulation Therapies: Hypnosis and Biofeedback.

Herbs and Dietary Supplements

Families of children and adolescents increasingly turn to herbs, vitamins, minerals, and other dietary supplements to promote health (Table 28-1). Although pediatricians may

Table 28-1 Commonly Used Herbal Therapies

Herb	Common Uses
Aloe	Burns, minor wounds, skin irritations, aphthous stomatitis, constipation, gastric and duodenal ulcers
Astragalus	Immune booster
Calendula	Skin soother
Cascara	Constipation
Cayenne	Topical treatment for pain, postherpetic neuralgia, nasal spray for migraines and cluster headaches
Chamomile	Sedative, colic, antiinflammatory, antispasmodic
Clove oil	Teething pain
Coffee	Stimulant, attention deficit-hyperactivity disorder, bronchodilator
Dandelion	Mild diuretic; liver tonic
Dill	Antispasmodic, colic, decrease flatulence
Echinacea	Immune stimulation, antiinflammatory
Ephedra (ma huang)	Vasoconstriction; allergy, upper respiratory infection; asthma; appetite suppressant
Evening primrose oil	Eczema, premenstrual syndrome
Feverfew	Migraine headaches, rheumatoid arthritis
Garlic	Antimicrobial, cholesterol lowering
Ginger	Antiemetic, antinausea
Ginkgo	Enhance blood flow past clogged arteries; prevent memory loss; marketed to treat attention deficit-hyperactivity disorder
Ginseng	Stimulant, enhance endurance and performance, adaptogen
Hawthorn	Cardiac stimulant; enhance cardiac contractility
Hops	Sedative
Kava kava	Anxiolytic
Lavender	Sedative
Licorice	Antiinflammatory, demulcent
Milk thistle	Hepatoprotection; cirrhosis, hepatitis
Oats	Antipruritic; eczema, varicella
Pine bark extract	Antioxidant promoted to treat attention deficit-hyperactivity disorder
Rhubarb root	Constipation, chronic renal failure
Saint John's wort	Depression, antiviral
Skullcap	Sedative
Slippery elm bark	Demulcent; pharyngitis
Tea tree oil	Antimicrobial; acne; minor skin infections, including fungal and yeast infections
Thyme	Antimicrobial; colds, sore throats; cough; expectorant
Valerian	Sedative

BOX 28-3

CAUTIONS ABOUT HERBS AND DIETARY SUPPLEMENTS

1. Product *purity* is questionable; there is potential for misidentification and contamination with
   - pesticides
   - herbicides
   - pharmaceuticals
   - heavy metals
   - excipients such as alcohol

   particularly for products imported from developing countries
2. *Reliability* of products is uncertain; there is great variability in concentration of active ingredients within plants by the parts used, growing conditions, processing, and storage
3. *Effectiveness* of active ingredients in children often is not studied
4. *Safety and toxicity for short-term use* in children is often unknown
5. *Safety and toxicity for chronic use* in children is often unknown
6. Unknown *interactions* with other medications and treatments
7. Unknown *metabolism* in children who have renal, hepatic, and other disorders
8. Cost of products is not necessarily related to quality, purity, or concentration of active ingredients

counsel patients and families routinely about multivitamins, iron, calcium, folate, and fiber and may include discussions of specific nutrients for patients who have specific diseases (e.g., fat-soluble vitamins for cystic fibrosis; B_6 for certain seizure disorders), they may be less familiar and less comfortable with the wide range of supplements now marketed to children and families.[21]

Multivitamins and minerals, particularly chelated, colloidal, and other forms of these products are promoted for children suffering from autism, Down syndrome, and other serious developmental disabilities. Fish oils and antioxidants and herbs are marketed for children who have attention deficit-hyperactivity disorder. Magnesium and a variety of Asian herbs are sought as a natural approach to asthma management.[24] Adolescents spend money on dietary supplements to lose weight, build strength, enhance moods, and clear skin blemishes.

Despite their ubiquitous presence and the conventional wisdom that herbs and other dietary supplements are safe because they are natural, pediatricians should caution about potential toxicities from these products (Box 28-3). Physicians know that natural products can have potent physical effects—digitalis, morphine, curare, hemlock, amanita mushrooms, and tobacco, to name a few. Some effects are quickly obvious with one dose (acute toxicity); others occur over years of accumulated exposure (chronic toxicity) (Table 28-2).

LIFESTYLE RECOMMENDATIONS: DIET, EXERCISE, ENVIRONMENT

Because diet is something that families can control, particularly for very young children, it is one of the lifestyle therapies of most interest to families who pursue alternative and complementary approaches. Many parents choose to put their child on restrictive diets, omitting possible allergens and other sensitizers such as wheat, dairy products, strawberries, shellfish, corn, soy, and peanuts, unaware of the potential deficiencies such restrictions may cause. Others, for religious, ethical, or health reasons, choose to follow vegetarian, macrobiotic, and other special diets. As concerns about antibiotic resistance and environmental impacts grow, more and more Americans avoid foods produced on "factory" farms in favor of organic meats and produce.

Pediatricians regularly discuss diet with families during routine health supervision visits. From promoting breastfeeding to managing diabetic diets, pediatricians have experience and expertise in nutritional therapies. Physicians are well aware of the impact of specific dietary changes on conditions ranging from anemia and anorexia to obesity and constipation. Yet, families frequently turn to other health professionals, including nutritionists, naturopathic doctors, chiropractors, and licensed acupuncturists, about specific foods and may consult with lay advisers within their cultural communities as well.

Pediatricians also talk about *exercise* during well child care. Although we advocate more active lifestyles, we may be less familiar with the use of specific therapies for specific conditions. Yoga, for example, may be particularly useful for children who have asthma.[24]

As with diet and exercise, environment is another topic frequently covered by pediatricians during the course of routine well child care. Whether we're addressing environmental allergens, the presence of guns in the home, the use of child restraints in automobiles, the availability of books, or testing for lead, we're always aware, at least unconsciously, that the environment has an enormous impact on children's health.

Environmental manipulations are part of routine pediatric advice for treating as well as preventing disease: phototherapy for jaundice, white noise and vibration for colic, music to reduce stress, cold to minimize pruritus—all are part of mainstream medical therapies. Despite familiarity with a great range of environmental strategies for promoting health and treating disease, pediatricians may be less aware of the complementary and alternative therapies that are environmentally based: crystals, lights, sounds, magnets, ionizers, aromatherapies, radionics devices, and others are heavily marketed as safe, effective treatments for children. There are few data evaluating these claims. However, most appear to be benign to everything except the pocketbook.

SUMMARY

Pediatricians are increasingly faced with families who use and ask about complementary and alternative medical therapies and therapists. Such use is particularly high among children faced with chronic or incurable conditions. Pediatricians need to be sensitive to families' values and cultural practices that promote these kinds of therapies and need to be knowl-

Table 28-2 Selected Herbal Toxicities: Acute and Chronic

Acute	
Herb	**Potential Toxicity**
Aconitum species Monkshood Wolfsbane	• CNS: paresthesia, muscular weakness, dizziness, ataxia, seizures, and coma • Cardiac: bradycardia, hypotension, rhythm disorders • GI: nausea, vomiting, and hypersalivation
Artemisia absinthium Wormwood	• CNS: restlessness, vertigo, tremors, agitation, seizures, and headache • GI: vomiting, cramping • Renal: rhabdomyolysis and renal failure
Atropa belladonna Deadly nightshade	• Cardiac: tachycardia and respiratory depression • Hyperthermia, mydriasis, urinary and bowel retention, restlessness
Digitalis purpurea Foxglove	• CNS: stupor, confusion, visual disorders, headache, depression, psychosis, hallucinations • Cardiac: rhythm disorders • GI: nausea, vomiting, and anorexia
Ephedra sinica Ma huang Mexican or Mormon or Miner's tea Desert herb	• CNS: dizziness, restlessness, headaches, anxiety, hallucinations, tremors, seizures, psychosis, strokes • Cardiac: hypertension, cardiomyopathy, myocardial infarction, arrhythmias, and hypertension • GI: nausea and vomiting
Lobelia inflata Lobelia	• CNS: anxiety, headache, dizziness, tremors, seizures, paresthesias, euphoria • Cardiac: arrhythmias, bradycardia, transient increase in blood pressure, decreased respiratory rate (in an overdose, lobeline may cause hypotension) • GI: nausea, vomiting, abdominal pain, and diarrhea • Diaphoresis, muscle fasciculations, and weakness • Dermatitis
Mentha pulegium Pennyroyal	• CNS: delirium, dizziness, convulsions, seizures, paralysis, encephalopathy, and coma • GI: nausea, vomiting, abdominal pain, hepatitis • Renal: renal failure and HTN • Shock and disseminated intravascular coagulation • Uterine contractions
Pausinystalia yohimbe Yohimbe	• CNS: dizziness, headache, anxiety, insomnia, tremors, hallucinations, nervousness, paresthesia • Cardiac: palpations, tachycardia, hypertension • GI: diarrhea, vomiting • Hypothermia, salivation, mydriasis
Phytolacca americana Pokeweed American nightshade	• CNS: dizziness, somnolence, headache, seizures • Cardiac: hypotension, tachycardia, respiratory depression • GI: nausea, vomiting, diarrhea, hemorrhagic gastritis • Lymphocytosis
Sanguinaria canadensis Blood root	• CNS: depression, dyspnea, and respiratory paralysis • GI: nausea, vomiting, diarrhea
Stramonium folium Jimsonweed	• CNS at high doses: restlessness, mania, hallucinations, delirium • Overdose: tachycardia, mydriasis, flushing, dry mouth, decreased sweating, miction, constipation
Viscum album Mistletoe	• Cardiac: bradycardia, angina, change in blood pressure • GI: nausea, vomiting, diarrhea • Allergic reactions, miosis, mydriasis, chills, fever, headaches • Coma

Continued

Table 28-2 Selected Herbal Toxicities: Acute and Chronic—cont'd

	Chronic
Herb	**Potential Toxicity**
Artemisia absinthium Wormwood	• CNS: restlessness, vertigo, tremors, agitation, seizures, and headache • GI: vomiting, stomach and intestinal cramps • Renal: rhabdomyolysis and renal failure
Glycyrrhiza radix Licorice	• CNS: ptosis, headache • Cardiac: dysrhythmias, hypertension • Myoglobulinemia (rare) • Myopathy and edema • Syndrome of pseudoprimary hyperaldosteronism leading to a mineralocorticoid-like effect
Kombucha tea A mixture of yeast and bacteria fermented in black tea and sugar	• Cardiac: cardiovascular collapse and respiratory distress • GI: hepatotoxicity, abdominal cramping, and anorexia • Metabolic acidosis • Dermatitis
Larrea divaricata Chaparral	• GI: liver damage, e.g., hepatitis • Renal: possible renal cystic disease • Fatigue and gastritis
Symphytum species Comfrey, Boneset, Blackwort, Slippery root	• GI: hepatic veno-occlusive disease, cirrhosis • Pulmonary disease
Teucrium chamaedrys Germander	• Centrilobular hepatic necrosis

BOX 28-4

HOW TO TALK WITH PATIENTS ABOUT COMPLEMENTARY AND ALTERNATIVE THERAPIES

1. DO talk about the different kinds of therapies families may have tried to help their child.
2. Do NOT wait for families to bring it up.
3. Ask in an open-minded, nonjudgmental fashion. Avoid using potentially pejorative terms such as "unproved," "unconventional," or "alternative."
4. Elicit further information with questions about specific therapies. For example,
   - have you tried any HERBAL therapies, such as Echinacea or ginkgo?
   - have you tried any DIETARY therapies, such as avoiding wheat or milk?
   - have you sought care from any OTHER HEALTH PROFESSIONALS such as acupuncturists or chiropractors?
5. Elicit the values, beliefs, and influences that led parents to these therapies. For example,
   - suggested by family members?
   - consistent with their religious, spiritual, or cultural beliefs?
   - value of natural or organic approaches?
   - fear of side effects of mainstream treatments?
6. Whenever possible, join with the parents and support their decision to pursue avenues that may help their child; be an ally rather than a tyrant.
7. Ask how well the family thinks the therapies worked or didn't work BEFORE offering your opinion.
8. Offer to talk with other therapists involved in the child's care to maintain coordinated, comprehensive care.
9. Offer to learn more to help answer the family's questions.
10. Offer families additional information and resources to address their questions about alternative and complementary therapies.

edgeable in answering families' questions about the safety and effectiveness of these types of care. A structured approach may be useful to discussing such issues with families (Box 28-4). For additional information, a growing number of books and publications are available (see Suggested Readings).

REFERENCES

1. Astin JA: Why patients use alternative medicine: results of a national study, *JAMA* 279:1548, 1998.
2. Benson H, Friedman R: Harnessing the power of the placebo effect and renaming it "remembered wellness," *Annu Rev Med* 47:193, 1996.
3. Berman BM, et al: Physicians' attitudes toward complementary or alternative medicine: a regional survey, *J Am Board Fam Pract* 8:361, 1995.
4. Breuner CC, Barry PJ, Kemper KJ: Alternative medicine use by homeless youth, *Arch Pediatr Adolesc Med* 152:1071, 1998.
5. Cooper RA, Henderson T, Dietrich CL: Roles of nonphysician clinicians as autonomous providers of patient care, *JAMA* 280:795, 1998.
6. de Saintonge D, Herxheimer A: Harnessing placebo effects in health care, *Lancet* 344:995, 1994.
7. Eisenberg D, et al: Trends in alternative medicine use in the United States, 1990-1997, *JAMA* 280:1569, 1998.
8. Eisenberg DM, et al: Unconventional medicine in the United States: prevalence, costs, and patterns of use, *N Engl J Med* 328:246, 1993.
9. Elder NC, Gillcrist A, Minz R: Use of alternative health care by family practice, *Arch Fam Med* 6:181, 1997.
10. Field T: Stimulation of preterm infants, *Pediatr Rev* 10:149, 1988.
11. Field TM: Adolescents with attention deficit hyperactivity disorder benefit from massage therapy, *Adolescence* 33:103, 1998.
12. Field T, et al: Burn injuries benefit from massage therapy, *J Burn Care Rehabil* 19:241, 1998.
13. Field T, et al: Children with asthma have improved pulmonary functions after massage therapy, *J Pediatr* 132:854, 1998.
14. Field T, et al: Juvenile rheumatoid arthritis: benefits from massage therapy, *J Pediatr Psychol* 22:607, 1997.
15. Field T, et al: Massage and relaxation therapies' effects on depressed adolescent mothers, *Adolescence* 31:903, 1996.
16. Field T, et al: Massage reduces anxiety in child and adolescent psychiatric patients, *J Am Acad Child Adolesc Psychiatry* 31:125, 1992.
17. Grootenhuis MA, deGraaf-Nijkerk JH, Wel MVD: Use of alternative treatment in pediatric oncology, *Cancer Nurs* 21:282, 1998.
18. Hughes PP, Meize-Grochowski R, Harris CN: Therapeutic touch with adolescent psychiatric patients, *J Holist Nurs* 14:6, 1996.
19. Kaptchuk TJ, Eisenberg DM: Chiropractic: origins, controversies and contributions, *Arch Intern Med* 158:2215, 1998.
20. Kaptchuk TJ, Eisenberg DM: The persuasive appeal of alternative medicine, *Ann Intern Med* 129:1061, 1998.
21. Kemper KJ: Seven herbs every pediatrician should know, *Contemp Pediatr* 13:79, 1996.
22. Kemper KJ, Cassileth B, Ferris T: Holistic pediatrics: a research agenda, *Pediatrics* 103:902, 1999.
23. Kemper KJ, et al: Family psychosocial screening: should we focus on high-risk settings? *J Dev Behav Pediatr* 15:336, 1994.
24. Kemper K, Lester M: Alternative asthma therapies: an evidence based review, *Contemp Pediatr* 16:162, 1999.
25. Linde K, et al: Are the clinical effects of homeopathy placebo effects? A meta-analysis of placebo-controlled trials, *Lancet* 350:834, 1997. (Published erratum appears in *Lancet* 351:220, 1998.)
26. Needlman R, et al: Clinic-based intervention to promote literacy: a pilot study, *Am J Dis Child* 145:881, 1991.
27. Neuberger J: Primary care: core values. Patients' priorities, *BMJ* 317: 260, 1998.
28. NIH Consensus Conference on Acupuncture: Acupuncture, 1998, *JAMA* 280:1518, 1998.
29. Olness K: Hypnosis and biofeedback with children and adolescents: clinical, research, and educational aspects. *J Dev Behav Pediatr* 17:299, 1996.
30. Pachter L: Practicing culturally sensitive pediatrics, *Contemp Pediatr* 139:54, 1997.
31. Pachter LM: Culture and clinical care: folk illness beliefs and behaviors and their implications for health care delivery, *JAMA* 271:690, 1994.
32. Spigelblatt L: Alternative medicine: a pediatric conundrum, *Contemp Pediatr* 14:51, 1997.
33. Spigelblatt L, et al: The use of alternative medicine by children, *Pediatrics* 94:811, 1994.
34. Stern RC, Canda ER, Doershuk CF: Use of nonmedical treatment by cystic fibrosis patients, *J Adolesc Health* 13:612, 1992.
35. Studdert DM, et al: Medical malpractice implications of alternative medicine, *JAMA* 280:1610, 1998.
36. Turner JA, et al: The importance of placebo effects in pain treatment and research, *JAMA* 271:1609, 1994 (review).
37. Turner JG, et al: The effect of therapeutic touch on pain and anxiety in burn patients, *J Adv Nurs* 28:10, 1998.
38. Ullman D: Homeopathy and managed care: manageable or unmanageable, *J Altern Complement Med* 5:65, 1999.
39. Wetzel MS, Eisenberg DM, Kaptchuk TJ: Courses involving complementary and alternative medicine at US medical schools, *JAMA* 280: 784, 1998.
40. Yuan-Chi Lin: Complementary and alternative medical therapies offered by pediatric pain treatment services. Presented at the 1999 Pediatric Academic Societies meeting, San Francisco, May 4, 1999.

SUGGESTED READINGS

Bratman S: *The alternative medicine sourcebook,* Los Angeles, 1997, Prima Publishing.

Cassileth BR: *The alternative medicine handbook,* New York, 1998, WW Norton.

Fugh-Berman A: *Alternative medicine: what works,* Media, Pa, 1997, American Health Consultants.

Kemper KJ: *The holistic pediatrician,* New York, 1996, Harper Collins.

Micozzi M, editor: *Fundamentals of complementary and alternative medicine,* New York, 1996, Churchill Livingstone.

29 Fluid Therapy

Regulation of body water, solute concentration, and acid-base parameters is critical to the preservation of health in humans. Virtually every disease process results in some alteration of input, output, or amount of water or solute needed. At the same time, powerful homeostatic mechanisms are at work that make severe electrolyte or fluid imbalances uncommon. Although a thorough understanding of these aspects of physiology is important to enable physicians to approach the care of their patients rationally, recognition of a few basic principles will allow for management of the vast majority of patients in a relatively simple fashion. This chapter reviews the homeostatic mechanisms that enable the human body to maintain relative stability despite large fluctuations of intake, metabolism, and excretion. It also addresses how primary care physicians can intervene when these homeostatic mechanisms fail.

one Theory: Body Fluid, Electrolyte Concentration, and Acid-Base Composition

Julius G. Goepp and Alice D. Ackerman

BODY FLUID COMPARTMENTS

The entire body mass is composed of total body water (TBW) and body solids (fat, skeletal muscle, and cellular solids). Traditionally, TBW has been viewed as a composite of intracellular fluid (ICF) and extracellular fluid (ECF).[31] ECF is composed of intravascular fluid (plasma) and interstitial fluid (ISF). Although further subdivisions of extravascular fluid have been devised, it is sufficient for the purposes of most clinical situations to view the body fluid compartments as depicted in Fig. 29-1.

The size of the body's fluid compartments changes significantly in the first year of life. TBW comprises about 75% of infant TBW and approximates the adult figure of 60% by 1 year of age.

SOLUTE CONCENTRATIONS

Clinically, one measures the amount of the various electrolyte concentrations and other solute particles found in the plasma. Most solutes are electrically charged particles. In plasma, sodium is the major cationic (positively charged) particle, with smaller concentrations of calcium, magnesium, and potassium present. To maintain electroneutrality, an equal number of anionic (negatively charged) particles needs to be present. These primarily are chloride, bicarbonate, and protein. However, there also are the unmeasured anions that constitute the "anion gap"—phosphate, sulfate, and various organic acids.

The composition of ICF is different from that of plasma. Potassium is the major intracellular cation, followed by magnesium and a relatively small amount of sodium. The major intracellular anions are organic phosphates and proteins, with smaller concentrations of bicarbonate and sulfate. The exact composition of intracellular contents is difficult to determine and probably varies substantially from one tissue type to another.

The large concentration gradient of electrically charged particles between ECF and ICF is maintained by active transport mechanisms found in cell membranes. The gradient is critical to the maintenance of various cellular functions, such as nerve conductance, muscle movement, and secretory processes. Disturbances of the delicately maintained gradient result in rapid and profound disruption of cellular function.

OSMOLALITY AND OSMOTIC PRESSURE

Another parameter that is critical to maintenance of normal cellular function is osmolality, a measure of the amount of dissolved solids in the various fluid compartments. Water will flow along an osmotic gradient from areas of low osmolality to areas of high osmolality. Osmolality is determined by the number of molecules in solution, independent of their size. Again, both active and passive transport mechanisms are involved in the maintenance of normal plasma and intracellular osmolality.

By far the most substantial contribution to normal plasma osmolality is made by sodium and its associated anions. Under most circumstances the plasma osmolality is approximately equivalent to twice the concentration of plasma sodium. However, under unusual circumstances or for precision, the osmolality can be calculated using the following formula:

$$\text{Osmolality (mOsm/kg body water)} = 2\ [\text{Na}]\ \text{mEq/L} + [\text{Glucose}]\ \text{mg/dl}/18 + [\text{BUN}]\ \text{mg/dl}/28$$

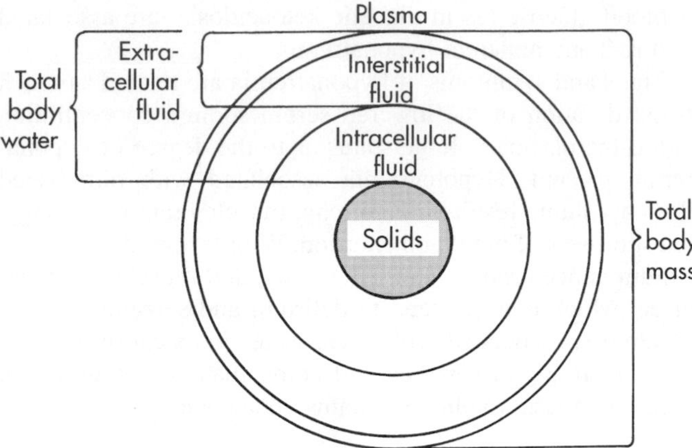

Fig. 29-1 Fluid compartments of the body.

CONTROL OF BODY FLUID VOLUME AND OSMOLALITY

Both plasma volume and osmolality remain nearly constant despite wide variations of water and solute intake. Control of osmolality and volume can be viewed as two separate but related mechanisms involved in a thirst-regulating hypothalamus-pituitary-kidney feedback system that works to adjust intake or output of water rapidly in response to changes, however minor, in plasma osmolality. The feedback mechanism hinges on the action of antidiuretic hormone (ADH) on the kidney's distal and collecting tubules to increase renal reabsorption of water.

Thirst and Antidiuretic Hormone

Thirst is regulated by plasma osmolality. Normal adults begin to experience thirst at plasma osmolality levels of 290 mOsm/kg, with profoundly increasing intensity as the osmolality reaches 300 to 305 mOsm/kg. At this point the person consumes large amounts of water (assuming free access, which is not the case with infants and young children) until plasma osmolality is brought back below the thirst threshold level. Secretion of ADH occurs at a lower threshold than that for thirst and is initiated (thus inhibiting renal water loss) at a plasma osmolality level above 280. With rising osmolality, ADH secretion increases, so changes in osmolality as small as 2.9 mOsm/kg effect a measurable increase in ADH release. Maximum antidiuresis usually occurs at around the same osmolality level responsible for initiation of the thirst mechanism just described. The ADH mechanism is far more sensitive than that of thirst, but drinking is the only physiological way to replace large losses of fluid. When osmolality levels fall below 280, ADH secretion is inhibited, enabling the kidney to secrete a high volume of dilute urine. The thirst mechanism is repressed simultaneously.

TOTAL BODY FLUID HOMEOSTASIS

In addition to the primary factors regulating water intake and output, other organs contribute to fluid gain or loss and must be considered when trying to understand TBW homeostasis. In health, these organs or systems work together to preserve the integrity of the child; in disease, however, any or all systems may either malfunction individually or lose the ability to compensate for the instability of another system.

The gastrointestinal (GI) tract is responsible for the digestion and absorption of nutrients—calories (in the form of fat, carbohydrate, and protein), vitamins, minerals, and water—and the excretion of food-derived waste products, including water. Control of intestinal secretion and absorption depends heavily on ion concentrations in plasma, ICF, and the intestinal lumen. Numerous diseases may inhibit adequate intake or stimulate large losses.

The evaporative water loss of sweat makes the skin the major organ of temperature regulation. The lungs also excrete water and may provide some component of temperature control. In addition to responding to alterations in ADH release, the kidneys adjust their water output to meet the requirements of the solutes they secrete. Finally, certain of the endocrine glands contribute to water needs and excretion by altering the metabolic rate, the systemic blood pressure, or other metabolic and physiological parameters.

CONTROL OF INDIVIDUAL SOLUTE CONCENTRATIONS

Sodium

As noted on p. 380, sodium is the major osmotically active cation in plasma. The total body content of sodium approximates 60 mEq/kg, but almost 43% of this is contained in bone, most of which plays almost no role in daily regulation of sodium concentration. The majority of the remainder is concentrated in the interstitial and plasma fractions, with only a small amount in the intracellular space.

Sodium homeostasis results from the balance of sodium intake and excretion. Intake is controlled by dietary habits, and although there may be some higher central regulation for sodium intake as there is for thirst (many patients who lose salt seem to develop a craving for sodium), it appears to be poorly developed and has not yet been localized. The typical American adult's diet contains 100 to 170 mEq of sodium per day; the amount of sodium in the infant's diet varies according to the formula or breast-milk feedings he or she receives. Most of the dietary sodium is absorbed actively in the jejunum. Aldosterone secretion increases gastrointestinal sodium absorption.

Sodium excretion is controlled primarily by the kidneys but also by the GI tract and skin. Although a large amount of sodium is presented to the kidneys during glomerular filtration, almost 99% of it is reabsorbed in the kidney tubules. In conditions of severe sodium depletion, volume depletion, or both, the amount reabsorbed may increase to nearly 100%; in cases of sodium and water overload, it may decrease to approximately 90%. The renin-angiotensin-aldosterone system, when stimulated by decreased renal blood flow, facilitates a greater degree of sodium reabsorption in the distal convoluted tubules and collecting ducts through the action of aldosterone at those sites.

Hypernatremia and hyponatremia are conditions usually tied closely to changes in the extracellular volume and are discussed fully in the clinical sections on dehydration and fluid overload in this chapter. However, a brief overview of associated conditions is included here.

Hypernatremia (serum sodium ≥150 mEq/L) may follow dehydration if there is a greater loss of water than sodium. These losses may occur through the lungs, skin, stool, or urine (especially in the presence of diabetes insipidus). Another important, although infrequent, cause of hypernatremia in young children is the overuse of commercial enema preparations containing high concentrations of phosphate and sodium. Elevated sodium content of breast milk has been implicated as a cause of hypernatremia in breast-fed infants.[16]

Signs and symptoms of hypernatremic dehydration may be difficult to interpret accurately, and the severity of dehydration may not be apparent based on physical examination alone. ECF volume remains relatively well preserved; therefore, shock is unlikely, even with marked loss of body water, and skin turgor and perfusion may remain close to normal. Notable hypernatremia results in marked changes in central nervous system (CNS) function, especially if the electrolyte disturbance occurred rapidly (in a few hours), which is common in small children. Affected infants exhibit marked irritability alternating with severe lethargy—the hallmark of acute hypernatremia. Seizures may occur and may be followed by coma if the condition is not diagnosed and adequate therapy is not initiated. In addition, elevation of the serum sodium concentration may lead to skeletal muscle rigidity and hyperactive deep-tendon reflexes. In small children, one may observe fever, emesis, and respiratory distress when the onset is acute.

Hyponatremia (serum sodium <130 mEq/L) occurs whenever body sodium stores are diluted or depleted. It more often is related to failure to excrete adequate amounts of water than to simple overhydration; however, in small infants the intake of hypotonic formulas or breast milk low in sodium may lower the plasma sodium concentration substantially. Although less common than isotonic or hypernatremic dehydration, hyponatremic dehydration occurs in approximately 10% of cases of acute diarrhea and most often is encountered because large stool losses are replaced with solutions containing little or no sodium. Any situation that increases the secretion of ADH may be associated with low serum sodium concentrations. This is seen in patients who have the syndrome of inappropriate antidiuretic hormone secretion (SIADH) resulting from CNS disease, pneumonia,[4] or meningitis.[25] Addison's disease and congenital adrenal hyperplasia are associated with excessive loss of sodium in the urine and with retention of potassium. Children who have obstructive uropathy and progressive renal failure are less able to reabsorb sodium from their renal tubules; therefore, they sustain large sodium losses and may exhibit mild dehydration with a borderline or low serum sodium concentration. Children treated with vasopressin or 1-deamino-8-D-arginine vasopressin (DDAVP) may develop iatrogenic hyponatremia,[2,27] as may children receiving diuretic therapy. The administration of enemas low in saline concentration also may result in hyponatremia. An excessive loss of sodium and water occurs in individuals suffering from heat-related illnesses. The serum sodium concentration reported by the laboratory may be artificially low in the presence of marked hyperlipidemia and hyperproteinemia. Highly elevated concentrations of blood glucose (as in diabetic ketoacidosis) are associated with real and apparent hyponatremia.

Signs and symptoms of hyponatremia are related as much to the duration of the lowered serum sodium concentration and to the plasma volume status as to the degree of hyponatremia present. Hyponatremia associated with diminished plasma volume results in anorexia, muscle cramps, lethargy, and shortness of breath on exertion. With further decreases in sodium concentration, nausea, emesis, and muscle weakness ensue, which may proceed to delirium and seizures.[4,29] Hyponatremia associated with acute water intoxication is more likely to result in seizures and coma than in conditions in which the plasma volume remains unchanged.

Potassium

Unlike sodium, only a small fraction of total body potassium is present in the intravascular and extracellular spaces. The total potassium content is approximately 50 mEq/kg body weight, with concentrations of intracellular and extracellular potassium of 145 mEq/L and 4 to 5 mEq/L, respectively.[31]

The majority of potassium absorption occurs in the proximal portions of the GI tract. It is excreted in the colon in exchange for sodium. Increased potassium loss results from diarrhea or overuse of laxatives. Elevated levels of plasma aldosterone also increase potassium excretion from the GI tract, the skin (losses here are relatively minimal), and the kidneys. Urinary excretion of potassium results from tubular secretion rather than glomerular filtration. Aldosterone acts at the level of the distal tubule to foster sodium reabsorption and potassium secretion. Thus, sustained hypovolemic states result in enhanced renal potassium losses. Potassium frequently shifts between the intracellular and extracellular spaces, mediated mostly by alterations in the serum acid-base status. An increase in extracellular potassium concentration occurs with systemic acidosis. Alkalosis leads to movement of potassium into the cell.

Cardiac toxicity is the most significant effect of hyperkalemia. Electrocardiographic changes may be seen, such as elevation and peaking of T waves, depression of ST segments, disappearance of P waves, heart block, and ventricular tachycardia or fibrillation.[24] The most severe effects are not seen until the serum potassium concentration is greater than 8 mEq/L. Most frequently the clinical findings in hypokalemia include muscle weakness and ileus. There also may be cardiac effects exhibited on the electrocardiogram by low voltage, flattening of the T waves, depression of ST segments, prominence of U waves, arrhythmias, and asystole. However, these effects usually are not seen until the serum potassium concentration falls below 2.0 mEq/L. Hypokalemia also may inhibit renal concentrating ability and worsen any existing hypochloremic alkalosis.

Other Ions

Concentrations of chloride, calcium, magnesium, and phosphorous also are critical to maintenance of cellular function, but their role in typical fluid disturbances is relatively minor and will not be discussed here. The remaining ion of interest is bicarbonate (HCO_3^-), which is crucial in the acid-base mechanism. Bicarbonate is a part of the major buffer system found in plasma, which is responsible for the close maintenance of a normal pH in the face of widely varying conditions. Control of HCO_3^- is the result of interactions between its plasma concentration and those of carbon dioxide (CO_2) and water. The concentrations of these components, and thus control and maintenance of pH, are affected by the function of the kidneys and the lungs. In metabolic acidosis, when plasma pH falls in the face of poor tissue perfusion or increased acid production, the kidney retains bicarbonate ion, while the lungs increase their elimination of CO_2 by increasing minute ventilation, driving the system toward higher pH. In respiratory acidosis, usually induced by excessive CO_2 production or inadequate elimination by the lungs, the kidney responds by retaining bicarbonate ion. Conversely, with respiratory alkalosis, in the case of increased minute ventilation and excessive CO_2 losses, the kidney excretes increased amounts of bicarbonate ion, lowering plasma pH.

In most situations requiring fluid therapy, a metabolic acidosis prevails as the result of diminished tissue perfusion. Attention to the pH and buffering characteristics of fluids administered is important, but more important still is the administration of sufficient amounts of isotonic fluids that will result in rapid reexpansion of the ECF. The resulting enhanced tissue perfusion, elimination of tissue acids, and restoration of end-organ function in turn will shut off the acidosis.

two Fluids and Electrolytes in Clinical Practice

Julius G. Goepp and Alice D. Ackerman

MAINTENANCE REQUIREMENTS

As described in previous sections, the body's numerous homeostatic mechanisms combine to orchestrate a complex balance between gains of water and electrolytes (ingested, administered, or internally generated) and obligatory losses (through the kidneys, lungs, skin, and GI tract). Fortunately, the human organism is adaptable and in health can adjust easily to most conditions of excess and can tolerate limitations to a point. However, to support vital functions, maintain health, and encourage adequate growth, the body must be supplied with water, electrolytes, nutrients, and vitamins. This section deals predominantly with water and solute requirements; other nutritional necessities for health maintenance are discussed in Chapter 17 (One), Nutritional Requirements.

Knowledge of fluid and salt needs is helpful in everyday pediatric practice but becomes most important in situations in which the physician is responsible for the child's intake. Notably, these situations occur when parenteral fluids are administered to a child who is unable to drink or who has experienced major losses in addition to his or her usual excretion of water and solutes. Furthermore, familiarity with basic requirements is important when physicians attempt to determine why a child loses weight or "fails to thrive." Before one can approach fluid therapy for any of the previously described circumstances, it is essential to understand the child's needs under usual conditions and then adjust the intervention to meet his or her altered requirements.

Water

Traditionally, water requirements have been calculated by one of three methods: body weight, body surface area, or metabolic rate. Water need per unit of body weight changes dramatically with age and size and, therefore, is not very useful. Body surface area once was thought to correlate well with both metabolic expenditure and fluid needs, but this subsequently has been shown not to be the case, especially in small babies during the newborn period and in children between 6 months and 3 years of age. Additionally, surface area is determined by comparing height and weight with a nomogram, which is cumbersome and depends on accurate measurements (height is notoriously difficult to measure in young children and infants). Use of the metabolic rate to calculate fluid requirements is attractive because it is based on physiological principles and is a constant number: approximately 100 ml (1 deciliter [dl]) of water is needed for every 100 calories consumed.[26] Using an average child who has a metabolic rate midway between normal activity and basal metabolic rate as a standard, one derives a fluid requirement based on calorie expenditure that is quite simple and can be calculated from body weight (Fig. 29-2). This results in a maintenance water requirement of 100 ml/kg/day for each of the first 10 kg, 50 ml/kg/day for each additional kilogram from 11 to 20, and 20 ml/kg/day for each subsequent kilogram. When converting to an hourly fluid rate, the simplest approximation is 4 ml/kg/hour for the first 10 kg, 2 ml/kg/hour for the next 10, and

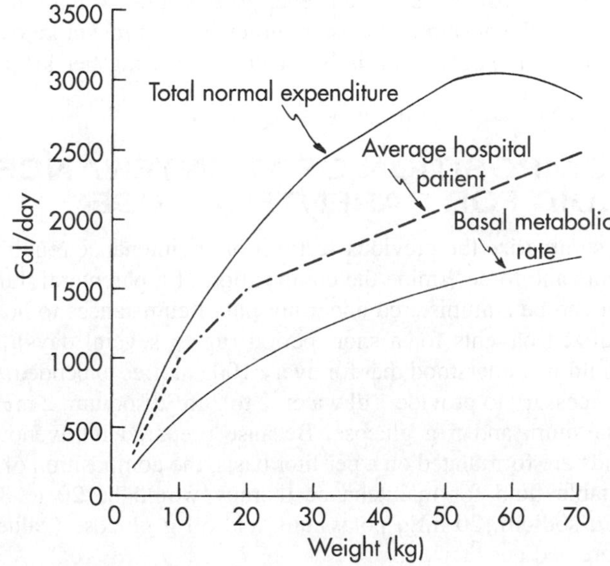

Fig. 29-2 Metabolic requirements of the average hospitalized patient. The center line represents calculated caloric requirements for average hospitalized patients. See text for explanation of the three sections of the curve.

(From Winters RW, editor: *The body fluids in pediatrics,* Boston, 1973, Little, Brown. Modified from Segar WE: *Pediatrics* 19:823, 1957.)

1 ml/kg/hour for each additional kilogram. This would result, for example, in an hourly maintenance rate of 32 ml/hour for an 8-kg infant (4 ml/kg × 8 kg), 50 ml/hour for a 15-kg toddler (4 ml/kg × 10 kg = 40 ml, plus 2 ml/kg × 5 kg = 10 ml), and 70 ml/hour for a 30-kg child (4 ml/kg × 10 kg = 40 ml, plus 2 ml/kg × 10 kg = 20 ml, plus 1 ml/kg × 10 kg = 10 ml). This simple approach will meet maintenance fluid requirements for most children and should be adjusted up or down depending on factors such as rate of insensible fluid losses (tachypnea, burns) or decreased fluid excretion (renal failure).

Electrolytes

The maintenance requirement of sodium for the average infant is between 2 and 3 mEq/100 Cal; potassium is closer to 2 mEq/100 Cal. Because sodium and potassium are supplied routinely in the form of chloride salt, the infant or child receives between 4 and 5 mEq/100 Cal of chloride ion, although the absolute chloride requirement probably is very small. Conversely, renal excretory ability is such that this amount of chloride does not present any particular hardship under normal conditions.

Calories

For short-term administration of parenteral fluids, little consideration usually is given to trying to replace caloric expenditure calorie per calorie. Rather, the reason for adding calories in the form of dextrose to parenteral fluids is to prevent ketosis and the breakdown of endogenous protein. In the average hospitalized patient this requires that approximately 25% of caloric expenditure be provided with an intravenous solution that contains glucose; therefore the aim should be 25 Cal/100 Cal expended energy. Because each gram of dextrose provides 4 calories, 5 g of dextrose per 100 calories expended provides sufficient energy. For infants and small children, the absolute glucose requirement to prevent ketosis and overt hypoglycemia is between 4 and 6 mg per kg per minute.

COMPOSITION OF MAINTENANCE FLUID FOR PARENTERAL USE

To summarize the previous sections on maintenance requirements and to determine the composition of a parenteral fluid that can be administered under normal circumstances to hospitalized patients for a short period (up to several days), it should be understood that for every 100 calories expended, it is necessary to provide 1 dl water, 2 to 3 mEq sodium, 2 mEq potassium, and 5 g glucose. Because prepared intravenous fluids are formulated on a per liter basis, the composition of a suitable fluid for maintenance therapy would be 20 to 30 mEq sodium, 20 mEq potassium, and 50 g glucose (values expressed per liter).

Values of sodium in parenteral fluids usually are expressed as a fraction of "normal saline solution." Normal saline (NS) is a 0.9% solution of sodium chloride that provides 154 mEq of sodium per liter of solution. The prepared solutions available most commonly contain either "half-normal" saline (77 mEq of sodium per liter) or "quarter-normal" saline (38 mEq of sodium per liter). Because of the body's ability to excrete any excess sodium, a solution containing quarter-normal (or 0.225%) saline is an acceptable preparation. This usually is formulated with 5% glucose (50 g/L); to each liter one can add 20 mEq of potassium, yielding a solution that is slightly hypertonic (compared with plasma), with an osmolarity of 386 mOsm/L, but that is hypotonic with respect to sodium. It is possible to add sodium in any desired concentration to a liter of 5% dextrose in water if the need arises, but usually this is unnecessarily time consuming and expensive.

ADMINISTRATION

Once the appropriate concentration of each solute in the parenteral fluid has been determined, the solution is administered at a rate of 100 ml/100 Cal of expected energy expenditure through a peripheral vein (extremity or scalp). Procedures for gaining vascular access in children are described in Appendix B, Special Procedures. Although not a new method, the technique of administering fluids and medications into the bone marrow (intraosseous infusion) recently has been demonstrated to be safe and effective in providing volume replacement and resuscitation drugs in an emergency. It may be used in infants and children when intravenous access cannot be obtained rapidly. Techniques for performing this procedure also are found in Appendix B. Any solution that can be given intravenously may be given via the intraosseous route.

WHEN MAINTENANCE IS NOT ADEQUATE

In the preceding sections, a rational approach was developed for supplying children with maintenance fluids. Based on the physiology of the illness, the needs of any given child may differ considerably from these "maintenance" requirements. However, the calculations presented remain valid over a wide range of situations if used as a base to which unusual losses are added. Any and all of the organs normally involved in water homeostasis may be included: water lost through the GI tract in the form of diarrhea; massive renal excretion of water in diabetes mellitus or diabetes insipidus or following the administration of osmotic or other diuretics; excessive sweating caused by autonomic instability, fever, or high ambient temperature; and an increased loss of lung water with hyperpnea from any cause, including hyperpyrexia. Processes that normally do not contribute to water loss also may be involved, such as massive vomiting, losses through a nasogastric tube, and acute blood loss. In addition, increased demands for fluids exist in various conditions of elevated metabolic rate (e.g., thyrotoxicosis), in situations that create large shifts in the body's fluid compartments (usually of the vascular space), and in many perioperative conditions (third spacing) that if uncorrected may produce shock. Persistence of any of these abnormal conditions in the absence of adequate fluid intake leads to water or electrolyte deficits or both. The purpose of replacement fluid therapy is to determine a rational approach to body water and electrolyte restoration. Additionally, the fluid administration scheme so devised has to take into consideration the ongoing losses that persist beyond the institution of parenteral fluid therapy and provide appropriate replacement of these lost fluids.

Fluids sometimes need to be supplied in amounts below those estimated for the average hospitalized patient. Any child who has a diminished urine output because of renal failure does not require as much free water as his or her normal counterpart. Children who are placed in mist tents or maintained on ventilators lose less water through their lungs and should have a lower estimate made of insensible water loss. Children whose activity levels are below those predicted for most bedridden patients (e.g., those in coma or who are paralyzed) expend fewer calories and therefore require less water (see Fig. 29-2; water requirement is closer to that for the basal metabolic rate).

ESTIMATION AND CORRECTION OF DEFICITS AND ONGOING LOSSES

The best way to estimate fluid and electrolyte deficits is to determine how much fluid has been lost from each body compartment, the electrolyte concentration of the lost fluid, and the period over which such losses have occurred. In most situations, however, therapy must be initiated before all of these data can be collected. In addition, volumes of diarrheal or emetic losses may be extremely difficult to measure.

The first step in the evaluation of a child who has a fluid and electrolyte deficit is to determine the degree of total body volume that has been lost. Although fluids and electrolytes are lost from all body compartments, the intravascular volume status is the most immediately relevant. Children who have sustained severe losses of intravascular (circulating) fluid volume are at risk for shock, which may result in irreversible organ system damage and death if not addressed promptly.

Table 29-1 contains a systematic approach to the estimation of fluid losses. Typically, a child may be categorized as mildly, moderately, or severely dehydrated according to clinical findings (the term *dehydration* is used here in its most common sense, meaning losses of fluid volume. Technically, dehydration refers only to pure water losses, a condition almost never seen clinically). Attention should be given to the immediate replacement of the estimated fluid losses via the oral, intravenous, or intraosseous routes, depending on the child's overall clinical status. Even before a formal calculation is made, an initial fluid bolus of 20 ml/kg over 20 to 30 minutes should be given to any child who appears to be severely dehydrated or in shock.

When calculating the final amount of fluid to be replaced, one should use either a recent normal weight, if available, or one may calculate the deficit based on an average (50th percentile) weight for the child's age. Formerly, fluid replacements were administered over a 24-hour period, with the aim of restoring half of the deficit in the first 8 hours of therapy and the second half in the subsequent 16 hours. It now is apparent that faster rates of fluid repletion are both more effective and simpler and that complicated formulas for calculating fluid and electrolyte replacements are not necessary. In most cases, dehydration of a mild to moderate degree may be managed on an outpatient basis, often without the use of intravenous therapy at all. In general, one should aim to replace the entire calculated deficit in the initial 4 to 6 hours of treatment.[8] This more rapid treatment hastens the restoration of circulating fluid volume, speeds the excretion of tissue acids and ketones that are the result of diminished end-organ perfusion, and contributes to the more rapid resolution of compensatory mechanisms such as renal sodium retention and potassium losses.

Similarly, it traditionally has been taught that serum electrolytes must be determined before or concomitant with the initiation of fluid therapy. More recent evidence has led to the

Table 29-1 Signs and Symptoms Related to Degree of Dehydration*

	Degree of Dehydration		
Parameter	**Mild**	**Moderate**	**Severe**
Weight loss (%)†	3-5 (2-3)	10 (6-9)	15 (≥10)
Skin color	Pale	Gray	Mottled
Skin turgor	May be normal	Decreased	Tenting
Mucous membranes	Slightly dry	Dry	Dry, parched, collapse of sublingual veins
Eyes	Probably normal	Decreased tears	Sunken, absence of tears, soft globes
CNS	Normal	Irritable	Lethargic
Pulse			
Quality	Strong	Somewhat decreased	Distal pulse not palpable
Rate	Probably normal	Somewhat increased (orthostatic changes)	Markedly tachycardic
Capillary refill	Normal (<2 seconds)	2-4 seconds	>4 seconds
Blood pressure	No change	Orthostatic decrease	Decreased while supine
Urine	Probably normal or slightly decreased volume	Elevated specific gravity, decreased volume	Less than 0.5 ml/kg/hr over past 12-24 hr; may be anuric

*Table is most useful for situations involving isotonic dehydration. (See text for adjustments needed for other forms of dehydration.)
†Percentage of weight loss listed applies to infants younger than 1 year of age. In older children and adults, dehydration becomes more notable with smaller losses of water (these values are listed in parentheses).

conclusion that in the vast majority of cases, electrolyte determinations do not add useful information to management.[1] The exceptions to this rule include a child who has a severely abnormal mental status (irritable or lethargic), seizures, or clinical signs of hypo- or hypernatremia. Furthermore, isotonic saline (0.9% or "normal" saline) should be the initial fluid of choice in virtually all instances, until a specific electrolyte abnormality is detected that mandates a more hyper- or hypotonic solution. It should be remembered that regardless of measured serum sodium concentration, a child who is significantly dehydrated usually has a net deficit of *total body sodium*, so that even a hypernatremic child (as determined by the serum concentration of sodium) will benefit by the initial administration of isotonic saline.

Fluid volume for initial rehydration should be based on calculated or estimated healthy weight. After an initial bolus administration of 20 ml/kg over 20 to 30 minutes, the child should be reevaluated. If evidence of shock persists, repeated boluses should be administered, with reevaluation after each bolus. When heart rate and capillary refill time have returned to normal, the rate of fluid administration may be reduced to an amount calculated to replace the remaining deficit over 4 to 6 hours. In a healthy child who has normal kidneys, this usually may be accomplished safely by the administration of half normal saline (77 mEq of sodium per liter).

THERAPEUTIC APPROACH TO SPECIAL SITUATIONS

Shock (see also Chapter 296)

Severe plasma volume deficit, with actual or impending cardiovascular collapse, is a life-threatening pediatric emergency, requiring *immediate* action; initial therapy is as stated previously—replacing the intravascular volume depletion with normal (0.9%) saline. Hemorrhagic shock, which must be considered with any history of trauma or any possible internal source of bleeding (e.g., a known peptic ulcer or other gastrointestinal disease that might lead to acute blood loss), must be treated with administration of packed red blood cells. This is because administering additional electrolyte solutions to a patient who has an already diminished hematocrit decreases oxygen-carrying capacity further and may result in irreversible damage to vital organs (especially the heart and brain). Therefore, most hospital blood banks keep a fairly ready supply of type O blood, which should be infused as rapidly as possible once the diagnosis of hemorrhagic shock has been considered. A sample of the patient's blood (obtained before transfusion) should be sent to the blood bank so that a properly matched unit of donor blood can be obtained without delay in case it is needed for further therapy. Also, if the patient's blood type is known, type-specific non–cross-matched blood, which carries less risk than the use of O non–cross-matched blood, may be administered. While awaiting the arrival of blood from the blood bank, normal saline solution should be given, as noted previously. The use of colloid-containing plasma expanders such as albumin or dextran remains controversial and probably provides no benefit over the use of a crystalloid solution unless the shock is the result of protein loss. Additionally, if the shock is cardiogenic, administration of albumin may worsen pulmonary edema. In sepsis, where volume depletion is caused by leaky capillaries and exudation of plasma into extravascular spaces, fresh-frozen plasma may be useful (because it also replaces many clotting factors) and sometimes is used in combination with other fluids.

Shock in babies and small children is associated almost invariably with depletion of glycogen stores. Thus, hypoglycemia often may be present. Administration of 2 to 4 ml/kg of a 25% dextrose solution will correct hypoglycemia and improve the results of further resuscitation efforts. For this reason, rapid bedside determination of blood glucose concentration always should be part of the initial evaluation of the infant or child in shock (current or impending).

Serious Electrolyte Abnormalities

Although most patients who are dehydrated may be managed with the empirical administration of normal saline, and without measurement of serum electrolytes, special situations exist in which more attention must be given to electrolyte status. Clinically, these situations will become apparent if a child demonstrates signs associated with hyper- or hyponatremia (see the following discussion) or if signs of dehydration do not resolve in response to standard management. In this section, we discuss specific electrolyte abnormalities.

Sodium. The pediatric electrolyte aberrations encountered most commonly relate to sodium balance, and they ordinarily occur with dehydration. The clinical conditions of hyponatremia and hypernatremia, which involve abnormalities of both the patient's volume status and plasma osmolality, are discussed in the section. When significant electrolyte disturbances are evident, efforts must be made to determine the cause of the disturbance, and any factors that may tend to perpetuate it so that they can be addressed in the treatment plan.

HYPONATREMIA. Hyponatremia usually is associated with hypotonicity. When it is not, the clinician must suspect either artifactual lowering of the serum sodium such as with hyperlipidemia and hyperproteinemia, as described earlier, or the presence of an osmotically active substance such as glucose or mannitol.[30] These compounds cause a shift of intracellular water into the extracellular space to restore osmotic neutrality, thereby lowering effective serum sodium by 1.6 mEq/L for every 100 mg/dl rise in serum glucose or mannitol concentration. Such situations are associated almost universally with preservation of intravascular volume (except in some extreme cases of diabetic ketoacidosis) and often are apparent from the history, physical examination, or a few simple laboratory tests.

The most common clinical situation leading to hyponatremia is volume loss, usually caused by diarrhea, in which the child has lost fluid with a sodium concentration higher than that of the serum. If ongoing diarrheal losses are replaced with hypotonic fluids, hyponatremia will develop, even if the volume deficit is not great. Sodium-rich fluid also is lost from the intravascular space when ascites or other abnormal accumulations of fluid occupy a body cavity. This phenomenon is known as *third spacing*.

When volume status is normal, one must consider situations that lead to a combination of sodium loss with water intake sufficient to maintain usual hydration. Such negative sodium balance can result from severe restriction of sodium intake or profound loss of sodium through the skin, GI tract, or kidneys (salt-losing nephropathy or diuretic use).

Mild hyponatremia (serum sodium 128 to 134 mEq/dl) with normovolemia or hypovolemia usually is undetectable clinically and can be managed by providing isotonic sodium solutions with adequate fluid administration, thereby allowing excretion of water at an appropriate rate. When there are simultaneous large deficits of both water and saline solution, it is important to replace both effectively; the usual normal saline solution is sufficient at the outset.

Severe total body potassium depletion, sometimes overlooked, may lead to persistent hyponatremia. Because potassium is the major intracellular cation, sodium ions enter the cells to replace potassium ions to provide electroneutrality; therefore, the concentration of sodium in the extracellular space may fall. Potassium then must be supplied to allow the restoration of normal sodium balance.

More rapid correction of the sodium deficit may be necessary with serious symptoms (seizures), which may accompany a large or precipitous decline in serum sodium concentration. Rapid correction can be achieved through the administration of 3% saline solution (containing 500 mEq of sodium per liter), which allows rapid replacement of sodium without infusing a large volume of water.[23] Administration of 10 to 12 ml/kg of 3% saline over 1 hour will provide rapid and temporary relief of signs of severe hyponatremia by elevating the serum sodium level rapidly.

Osmotic equilibrium is established rapidly once intravascular tonicity is restored, because sodium is distributed quickly throughout all body fluid compartments. Intravenous administration of hypertonic sodium chloride solutions is not without risk to the patient, however, especially one who has cardiac or renal disease. Such infusions cause a rapid shift of water into the intravascular space and may lead to acute volume overload. This therapy, therefore, must be reserved for potentially life-threatening situations, and the child must be monitored closely throughout the infusion. Demyelination syndromes have been noted in adults because of rapid reversal (a rise of more than 12 mEq/L in 24 hours) of longstanding or chronic hyponatremia.[4]

When hyponatremia exists with *expanded* vascular volume, the most likely cause is excessive secretion of ADH, which may occur because of increased intracranial pressure, severe pneumonia, or the stress of certain surgical procedures. SIADH is diagnosed based on laboratory and physical examination data and requires the presence of hyponatremia with normal or increased intravascular volume (the diagnosis *cannot* be made if the patient has an inadequate intravascular volume) and a urine osmolality that is less than maximally dilute. Sodium excretion in the urine is variable but usually is higher than expected for the level of serum sodium concentration. Treatment of this disorder, whatever the cause, consists of fluid restriction and not sodium administration, unless the patient is convulsing. Some authors have urged the simultaneous use of a potent diuretic such as furosemide, which is expected to induce the loss of more water than sodium.[20] In most cases, however, fluid restriction remains the safest and most efficacious mode of therapy. Once the sodium concentration returns to near normal, moderate fluid restriction (generally to two thirds of maintenance requirements) may need to be continued, usually for at least 24 hours, but sometimes for as long as the underlying disorder continues.

HYPERNATREMIA. As with decreased serum sodium concentration, hypernatremia may occur with overhydration, dehydration, or normal hydration. However, unlike hyponatremia, an elevated serum sodium level *always* is associated with hypertonicity.

Hypernatremia associated with overhydration generally is an iatrogenic problem created by (1) administering intravenous or oral solutions with high salt content and (2) not providing the requisite free water. Patients treated with large amounts of sodium bicarbonate for metabolic acidosis also are at risk of developing marked hypernatremia (there is approximately 1 mEq of sodium for every milliliter of bicarbonate solution administered). Occasionally, when infant formulas are being mixed, mistakes occur that result in markedly hypertonic solutions that may induce particularly severe hypernatremias. These patients are at risk of developing obvious signs of plasma volume overload, including hypertension, congestive heart failure, and pulmonary edema.

Under such circumstances, administration of additional fluid is risky and may prove fatal. The most rational approach is to limit sodium and water input and attempt to induce sodium loss to a greater extent than water. This may be accomplished by the use of a potent loop diuretic such as furosemide, which will induce a net sodium loss if the child's renal function is adequate. One concurrently must watch closely for the development of dehydration because it is impossible to predict precisely how much water and sodium will be lost. Generally, some portion of the induced urine output (50% to 75%) should be replaced with intravenous fluid that is slightly hypotonic (i.e., 66% or 75% normal saline solution) until normal hydration and tonicity have been achieved. In patients who have severe hypernatremia (ordinarily considered as a serum sodium value greater than 160 mEq/L), serious complications may occur if the sodium concentration falls too rapidly. This action produces marked shifts of extracellular water to the intracellular space and results in cellular swelling. This is most worrisome in the CNS because cerebral edema may occur, which may lead to seizures, coma, or death. Therefore, when the serum sodium value is high and is accompanied by overhydration, the preferred therapeutic approach is to restrict sodium and water, thus permitting a spontaneous diuresis to occur. Serum electrolyte values must be monitored every few hours. If the patient has substantially decreased renal function, hemodialysis or peritoneal dialysis should be considered, especially in the presence of hypertension or pulmonary edema.

Hypernatremia associated with decreased plasma volume is encountered frequently in pediatric practice. It is caused most commonly by acute gastroenteritis that induces relatively larger losses of water than sodium. Although these children may have severe hypernatremia, their total body sodium content usually is depleted; they, therefore, present quite a therapeutic challenge.

Patients who have this condition need to be evaluated carefully. The physician must consider all the aspects of dehydration previously discussed but must remember that because ECF volume is relatively well preserved, he or she may seriously underestimate the severity of the plasma volume loss. Even with significant fluid losses, these children rarely have signs of incipient vascular collapse. When using the signs and symptoms of dehydration shown in Table 29-1 to determine the degree of dehydration, if the serum sodium concentration is greater than 155 mEq/L, another 3% to 5% should be added to the weight loss in predicting the degree of dehydration.

Fluid therapy of hypernatremic dehydration is not nearly as straightforward as for other types of dehydration because the risk of creating major fluid shifts and cerebral edema is great. One cannot simply try to remove sodium because a decrease in the plasma tonicity without an increase in plasma water may induce circulatory collapse. Therefore, a cautious rehydration scheme must be developed.

Instead of being rehydrated over a short period, as with isonatremic or hyponatremic dehydration, the child who has a serum sodium greater than 155 mEq/L should have his or her fluid deficit replaced over 48 to 72 hours. It is *not* possible to calculate the actual amount of sodium lost. The physician should estimate the water deficit (based on weight and clinical signs) and plan to replace that volume evenly over 48 to 72 hours. The solution used should be slightly hyponatremic (containing 100 to 120 mEq of sodium per liter). Glucose should be added so that the solution is not hypotonic. As soon as the urine output is judged to be adequate, potassium should be added to the intravenous solution to correct the potassium deficit and to preserve the intracellular osmolality, thus helping to prevent intracellular edema. It is particularly important to monitor serum electrolyte concentrations, serum osmolality, and urine output and osmolality as frequently as possible. Although one needs to avoid a persistent elevation of the serum sodium concentration, it also is important to ensure a slow, steady decline in the serum sodium and osmolality levels.[9] Decreases in serum tonicity should be limited to a rate of 5 mOsm/hr. Serum sodium concentration should fall at a rate no more rapid than 0.5 mEq/L/hour. In many cases it is feasible to add up to 40 mEq of potassium per liter to the infused solution and reduce its sodium concentration to 50 mEq/L.

Sometimes, no matter how carefully hypernatremia is handled, seizures ensue during the rehydration period. They usually can be managed successfully by infusing a solution slightly more hypertonic than the one being given (i.e., normal saline or lactated Ringer's solution). If the seizures are particularly severe, or if there is evidence of brain herniation, the use of a hypertonic agent such as mannitol may be required. Unfortunately, the diuresis induced by mannitol may worsen the dehydration substantially. Also, mannitol should *not* be used if urine output has not been established.

A relatively uncommon cause of hypernatremia is diabetes insipidus, which usually presents as hypernatremia with a normal plasma volume. This presupposes an intact thirst mechanism and that the patient has access to the large volume of water required to replace renal losses. Such is not the case for small babies and certain other patients who have diabetes insipidus and hypernatremic dehydration. Large renal losses of free water may occur because of deficient ADH (central or pituitary diabetes insipidus) or impairment of the normal renal response to the hormone (nephrogenic diabetes insipidus).

In infants and children the most common cause of central diabetes insipidus is a brain tumor, such as a craniopharyngioma. The syndrome also may follow intracranial surgical procedures or trauma. Other causes include CNS diseases of vascular, infectious, or granulomatous origin or histiocytosis. The familial form of central diabetes insipidus accounts for fewer than 1% of all cases. Probably 50% of adult patients who have diabetes insipidus remain classified as *idiopathic;* that percentage is much lower in children.

Nephrogenic diabetes insipidus may be evident as a congenital disorder, but more commonly it is secondary to renal failure (particularly that caused by obstructive uropathy) or to electrolyte disorders, drug ingestions, or sickle cell disease. Laboratory findings in diabetes insipidus usually include a moderate to marked hypernatremia (depending on how adequately the lost fluid volume has been replaced) and dilute urine, usually produced in large volumes. Clinically, these patients exhibit a tremendous thirst (often craving ice-cold water) and, as already mentioned, usually show signs of normal hydration. The laboratory differentiation between central and nephrogenic diabetes insipidus is unnecessary when the cause is apparent (e.g., after surgical removal of a craniopharyngioma) but in other situations is essential to help guide the therapeutic approach. This generally is determined by performing a "water deprivation test."

Potassium

HYPOKALEMIA. Symptoms of hypokalemia were discussed in the sections on solute homeostasis. A low serum potassium concentration seldom represents an emergency unless cardiac effects are seen, and this does not occur typically until the serum potassium level is less than 2 mEq/L. In patients receiving digitalis preparations, however, a combined cardiac toxicity may ensue, and the typical T wave changes and arrhythmias of hypokalemia may occur at serum potassium levels closer to normal. Other patients at risk of exhibiting an exaggerated response to mild hypokalemia include those who have an acid-base disturbance or other ionic aberration that may create a cardiac conduction disturbance by substantially altering the flux of ions between the intracellular and extracellular spaces. At particular risk of developing such alterations are children receiving long-term diuretic therapy. Hypokalemia may occur following large losses of potassium from the GI tract during treatment for diabetic ketoacidosis and as a manifestation of hyperaldosteronism.

When emergency therapy for hypokalemia is necessary (in the situations just mentioned and in the preoperative patient who has a serum potassium concentration less than 3.5 mEq/L), intravenous potassium repletion should be implemented. This is accomplished either by increasing the concentration of potassium ion in the fluids given intravenously (maximum of 80 mEq/L) or by administering a bolus of potassium into a central vein. The maximum amount of potassium that may be given is 1 mEq/kg over a 1-hour period (with the physician at the bedside and continuous electrocardiographic monitoring), but generally it is safer to deliver only 20% or 25% of that amount and to repeat the dose as necessary to raise the concentration to a safe level. In nonemergent circumstances, enteral potassium supplementation is safer and very effective.

HYPERKALEMIA. Substantial elevations of serum potassium concentration are encountered most frequently with renal failure or systemic acidosis, combined with an increased intake of potassium or a rapid breakdown of tissue or blood products.

When the potassium concentration reaches 8 mEq/L or more, or if characteristic electrocardiographic abnormalities are noted at any potassium concentration, the child is in grave danger of cardiac toxicity. Such a patient should have continuous electrocardiographic monitoring, and immediate steps should be taken to protect the heart from the effects of severe hyperkalemia. The first priority is the infusion of intravenous calcium, 0.2 ml/kg of 10% calcium chloride given over 2 to 5 minutes.[3] This should be followed by the administration of sodium bicarbonate (2 to 3 mEq/kg given within a 30-minute period) to raise the serum pH level and help move the potassium into cells, thereby decreasing (transiently) the intravascular potassium concentration. Simultaneously or immediately following the above steps, a mixture of glucose and insulin should be infused, which also induces movement of potassium ions from the extracellular to the intracellular spaces. This accelerates the usual process by which glucose moves into the cells and is converted to glycogen. A dose of 2 ml/kg of a 25% glucose solution is given along with 1 U/kg of regular insulin. This solution may be administered over 30 minutes and repeated as necessary. Serum glucose concentration must be monitored closely during and following therapy.

Salbutamol, a selective beta-2 agonist, has been used successfully to reduce temporarily serum potassium levels in neonates[7,10] and children.[11] It may be administered intravenously or by nebulization. The parenteral form is not yet available commercially in the United States.

Once lifesaving measures have been instituted, attention must be given to removing potassium from the body. One of the most effective means of accomplishing this is with hemodialysis or peritoneal dialysis. One or the other should be initiated without delay in patients who have hyperkalemia accompanied by congestive heart failure and volume overload. The other mechanism used commonly for removing potassium from the body is to bind potassium in the GI tract by using an exchange resin such as sodium polystyrene sulfonate (Kayexalate).[13,15] This usually is introduced through a retention enema that contains sorbitol. One can expect a decline in serum potassium of 1 mEq/L for each g/kg of resin introduced. The dose is calculated based on the severity of the hyperkalemia, with a maximal adult dose of 60 g. Caution should be used in patients who have renal failure, because sodium is absorbed as potassium is excreted, and each gram of resin contains 4.1 mEq of sodium; hypernatremia and hypervolemia may result. Additionally, one must monitor the patient for the development of hypocalcemia and hypomagnesemia. Metabolic alkalosis may result from repeated polystyrene sulfonate enemas. When hyperkalemia becomes a chronic but not life-threatening problem, the best approach is to restrict dietary potassium and administer potassium-losing diuretics concomitantly.

SPECIAL SITUATIONS REQUIRING FLUID THERAPY

Fluid Therapy of the Neonate

The provision of adequate fluid replacement therapy for newborn infants depends on perinatal alterations in body composition and the infant's size and gestational age. Hydration of sick premature babies who weigh less than 1500 g is beyond the scope of this chapter. See Chapter 49, Critical Neonatal Illnesses.

TBW content decreases progressively throughout gestation and the first year of postnatal life. This is accompanied by increases in the body's content of protein and fat. Shrinkage of the ECF compartment accounts largely for the decrease in TBW. In the first few days of extrauterine life, both term and premature babies normally lose up to 10% of their body weight. Although this is considered a physiological reduction, failure to replace such losses may lead to substantial dehydration.

All newborns show a progressive increase in their metabolic rate. The metabolic rate for full-term infants approximates 32 Cal/kg/day at birth and reaches close to 43 Cal/kg/day within 3 days. Following this, there is a slow, steady increase over the first 2 weeks of life. Premature infants maintain a higher metabolic rate than full-term babies, even when they achieve a similar weight.

In addition to the baseline metabolic expenditure of calories, newborns use energy with cold, stress, and muscular activity. The growth rate is rapid during this period, and the average newborn requires 25 to 35 Cal/kg/day for growth. Therefore, the total caloric need of an infant older than 3 days is between 100 and 125 Cal/kg/day.

Water requirements are governed by losses through the skin, respiratory tract, and kidneys. Evaporative losses through the skin generally average 20 to 30 ml/kg/day; respiratory losses account for approximately 15 ml/kg/day. Both parameters are affected by ambient humidity, and respiratory losses actually may be reduced by 50% with provision of high humidity to the baby's immediate environment.

The newborn's kidneys are limited in their ability to concentrate urine because of the relative shortness of the loops of Henle and the absence of a notable concentration gradient. Thus, they are able at best to excrete urine with an osmolality that approaches 300 mOsm/kg. As the solute load increases, the free water requirement rises; thus, for a formula-fed infant, urinary water loss may be as high as 120 ml/kg/day. However, the average range probably is closer to 60 to 75 ml/kg/day.

Electrolyte requirements for infants have not been fully established, but they seem to tolerate a fairly wide range of electrolyte provisions. Fluids that have been used successfully yield between 1 and 3 mEq of sodium per 100 calories per day; this has become the recommended starting range for maintenance fluid therapy.

When preparing a maintenance parenteral fluid formula for newborns, it is important to ensure adequate monitoring, which will indicate whether fluid estimates have been adequate. It also is important, especially with the sick neonate, to record weights once or twice a day and to record intake, output, vital signs, urinary osmolality, electrolyte concentrations, and other indications of optimum cardiac and respiratory homeostasis frequently. Frequent changes may be needed; therefore, the physician must never become "locked into" a particular formula but rather must apply the basic rules of fluid therapy to the situation logically and be ready to compensate for failing systems or increasing losses when necessary.

Fluid Therapy for Burns

Children who have partial or full-thickness burns over significant amounts of their total body surface area (BSA) present major challenges for fluid management. Damage to the integrity of skin poses the immediate threat of enormous and uncontrolled increases in fluid loss from the circulation by means of transudate. Too little fluid early in the course of therapy may produce fatal hypovolemia and electrolyte disturbances; excessive fluids later in the course expose the child to the dangers of congestive heart failure and pulmonary edema. In the days to weeks following a major burn, the risk of infection rises dramatically, further threatening the child's ability to maintain appropriate fluid homeostasis. In this section, we outline an immediate approach to the management of a burned child. Reference should be made to other sources for a more thorough description of the calculation of body surface area and of the finer points of fluid management. See also Chapter 299, Thermal Injuries.

The Parkland formula provides a useful starting point for fluid therapy in burns. This requires the administration of 4 ml of fluid per kilogram per percentage of BSA burned during the first 24 hours, giving 50% of the total in the first 8 hours. Some centers prefer to administer the initial resuscitation fluids more rapidly and therefore provide the first half of the first day's requirement in the initial 2 to 4 hours of care.[17] A balanced salt solution such as lactated Ringer's solution should be used. *Glucose should not be given.* Severe burns induce a marked outpouring of catecholamines and steroids, which raises the serum glucose concentration and renders the child relatively resistant to insulin. Exogenously administered glucose concentrates in the burned area, increasing the likelihood of infection. The need for glucose is determined best by measuring the blood glucose frequently, especially in young children.

Although the initial rate of intravenous fluid administration is guided by the Parkland formula, one should ensure that sufficient fluid is given to maintain a urine output of 0.5 to 2.0 ml/kg/hr. In this situation, more is not better, because too much fluid worsens peripheral edema, delays healing, and may lead to heart failure when the extravasated liquid begins to resorb.[14] The best indicator of optimum fluid therapy is a normal cardiac output. However, a pulmonary artery catheter must be placed to measure cardiac output accurately. Blood pressure, heart rate, and weight measurement may be helpful in estimating cardiac output indirectly, but each of these can be affected by a number of other factors. Maintenance requirements should be added to the daily fluids suggested by the Parkland formula in children who have burns of less than 30% BSA and in all infants.

Colloid (such as plasma or 5% albumin) generally is withheld until 24 hours after the burn has occurred, although some authors advise the use of colloid in the initial resuscitation phases.[5,6] Because children show some evidence of earlier healing of the capillary bed, colloid may be useful at 12 to 18 hours. The usual dose is 0.5 ml/kg/% of burned BSA given over 24 hours, with D_5W added to reach a total of approximately 50% of the previous day's requirement. Measuring electrolyte concentrations carefully and frequently (especially potassium, because with burns there can be massive losses of this ion through the kidneys) determines whether and how much electrolyte solution is necessary.

After the first several days a fluid rate of an amount close to maintenance may be sufficient (at approximately 72 hours maximum resorption of edema has taken place). If the burn is of major proportions, parenteral nutrition or early enteral feeding should be initiated once the electrolyte balance is stable.[5,12] Attention also must be paid to the social and psychological needs of the child and the family. Recovery from a major burn injury is slow, is fraught with complications, and leaves substantial scars. If the child's emotional well-being is not tended to adequately, the psychological scars may outweigh any physical disability that results.

Hydration of the Ambulatory Patient: Alternatives to Parenteral Fluid Therapy

It is fairly common practice for pediatricians in the United States to recommend oral fluids for young patients who have mild diarrhea or vomiting. Such therapy has been suggested for many years on totally empirical grounds, and most physicians have urged the use of a dilute solution that contains sodium and potassium in concentrations of 30 and 20 mEq/L, respectively, and 5% to 7% glucose. When diarrhea leads to moderate or severe dehydration, or if substantial emesis accompanies the illness, the standard teaching had dictated hospitalization of such children and "resting" the GI tract with the use of parenteral therapy, as outlined in previous sections.

Through the efforts of scientists working with the World Health Organization (WHO) in an effort to curb the large diarrhea-associated mortality seen in developing countries, data concerning gastrointestinal function in diarrhea have been accumulated.[21,22]

Sodium absorption in the small intestine depends on the presence of glucose or small neutral amino acids such as glycine or alanine. Likewise, the absorption of glucose is enhanced by the presence of sodium salts. Movement of salt and glucose across the mucosal border is accompanied by an influx of water and other electrolyte concentrations. Maximum rates of absorption are achieved when (1) sodium and glucose are present in a 1:1 to 1:2 molecular ratio, (2) glucose concentration is between 110 and 140 mmol (2% to 2.5% solution), and (3) sodium concentration is not substantially less than that of normal jejunal fluid.

Based on this and other information, WHO derived a formula for use with all patients who have diarrheal illness regardless of its cause. It contains 90 mmol of sodium, 20 mmol of potassium, 30 mmol of bicarbonate, 80 mmol of chloride, and 111 mmol of glucose per liter. This formulation provides a solution that has an osmolality of 331 mOsm/L. When given ad lib to patients who have diarrhea, it corrects dehydration rapidly and can return electrolyte concentrations to the normal range regardless of the presence of hyponatremia or hypernatremia on initial evaluation. Large field studies have documented its successful use in patients who have ongoing emesis. There has been no evidence to suggest that the use of such fluid prolongs the duration of diarrhea; just the reverse appears to be the case. In addition, children given this oral rehydration therapy (ORT) seem to tolerate resumption of a regular diet earlier than those treated solely with intravenous fluids. Use of a solution that has lower osmolality (224 mOsm/L) has been shown to result in superior water absorption and patient weight gain.[18]

In 1985, the American Academy of Pediatrics (AAP) Committee on Nutrition published recommendations for the use of the WHO solution or similar solutions in developed countries.[10] These guidelines were strengthened and amplified in 1996 in the form of Practice Parameters.[1]

The Committee concluded that the WHO oral rehydration solution (WHO-ORS) is appropriate for use in both rehydration and maintenance phases. The fluid should be dispensed with an appropriate-size container to avoid mixing errors; after rehydration, children should be given the ORS on a 1:1 basis with fluid low in sodium content, such as breast milk or water, to avoid potential hypernatremia.

Preparations that meet WHO and AAP guidelines, as indicated above, are available commercially. Because such preparations are available ready to use, the bicarbonate found in the WHO powder has been replaced with citrate.[21] Studies have documented equivalent efficacy of the two bases in correcting the mild acidosis that accompanies mild to moderate diarrhea. Most of the large-scale evaluations that have been performed in developed countries have excluded the use of ORS in patients in shock who are treated initially with intravenous fluids.[19,28] Despite considerable efforts to develop a "super ORS," most evidence suggests that the standard WHO solution, accompanied by early return to normal diet and sufficient access to free water, is still the best overall therapy.

In summary, oral rehydration therapy provides a cost-efficient approach to the problem of childhood diarrhea for the patient who is able to drink, is not in shock, and has a relative or other responsible person who can understand the instructions for using the ORT formula. Such a therapeutic approach avoids the hospitalization of a child and the consequent disruption in the lives of the family members. This treatment approach eliminates the potential complications of intravenous therapy. See also Chapter 124, Diarrhea and Steatorrhea, and Chapter 278, Dehydration.

When to Refer

Abnormal electrolytes refractory to fluid therapy
Seizure or encephalopathy
Inability to rehydrate by chosen means (oral or intravenous)

When to Hospitalize

Failure to rehydrate completely in 6 hours
Persistent abnormal mental status
Inability of parent to maintain hydration at home

REFERENCES

1. American Academy of Pediatrics: Practice parameter: the management of acute gastroenteritis in young children, *Pediatrics* 97:424, 1996.
2. Beach PS, Beach RE, Smith LR: Hyponatremic seizures in a child treated with desmopressin to control enuresis: a rational approach to fluid intake, *Clin Pediatr* 31:566, 1992.
3. Broner CW, et al: A prospective, randomized, double-blind comparison of calcium chloride and calcium gluconate therapies for hypocalcemia in critically ill children, *J Pediatr* 117:986, 1990.
4. Cheng JC, et al: Symptomatic hyponatremia: pathophysiology and management, *Acute Care* 14-15:270, 1988-1989.
5. Derganc M: Present trends in fluid therapy, metabolic care, and prevention of infection in burned children, *Crit Care Med* 21:S397, 1993.
6. Gomez-Cia T, Roa L: A burn patient resuscitation therapy designed by computer simulation (BET). Part 2. Initial clinical validation, *Burns* 19:332, 1993.
7. Greenough A, et al: Salbutamol infusion to treat neonatal hyperkalemia, *J Perinat Med* 20:437, 1992.
8. Hirschhorn N: The treatment of acute diarrhea in children: an historical and physiological perspective, *Am J Clin Nutr* 33:637, 1980.
9. Jacobson J, Bohn D: Severe hypernatremic dehydration and hypokalemia in an infant with gastroenteritis secondary to rotavirus, *Ann Emerg Med* 22:1630, 1993.
10. Mauer AM, et al: American Academy of Pediatrics Committee on Nutrition: use of oral fluid therapy and posttreatment feeding following enteritis in children in a developed country, *Pediatrics* 75:358, 1985.
11. McClure RJ, Prasad VK, Brocklebank JT: Treatment of hyperkalemia using intravenous and nebulised salbutamol, *Arch Dis Child* 70:126, 1994.
12. McDonald WS, Sharp CW Jr, Deitch EA: Immediate enteral feeding in burn patients is safe and effective, *Ann Surg* 213:177, 1991.
13. Meyer I: Sodium polystyrene sulfonate: a cation exchange resin used in treating hyperkalemia, *ANNA J* 20:93, 1993.
14. Murison MS, Laitung JK, Pigott RW: Effectiveness of burns resuscitation using two different formulae, *Burns* 17:484, 1991.
15. Noerr B: Sodium polystyrene sulfonate (Kayexalate), *Neonatal Netw* 12:77, 1993.
16. Peters JM: Hypernatremia in breast-fed infants due to elevated breast milk sodium, *J Am Osteopath Assoc* 89:1165, 1989.
17. Puffinbarger NK, Tuggle DW, Smith EI: Rapid isotonic fluid resuscitation in pediatric thermal injury, *J Pediatr Surg* 29:339, 1994.
18. Rautanen T, et al: Randomised double-blind trial of hypotonic oral rehydration solutions with and without citrate, *Arch Dis Child* 70:44, 1994.
19. Rautanen T, el-Radhi S, Vesikari T: Clinical experience with a hypotonic oral rehydration solution in acute diarrhoea, *Acta Paediatr* 82:52, 1993.
20. Rossi NF, Cadnapaphornchai P: Disordered water metabolism: hyponatremia, *Crit Care Clin* 5:759, 1987.
21. Salazar-Lindo E, et al: Bicarbonate versus citrate in oral rehydration therapy in infants with watery diarrhea: a controlled clinical trial, *J Pediatr* 108:55, 1986.
22. Santosham M, et al: Oral rehydration therapy for acute diarrhea in ambulatory children in the United States: a double-blind comparison of four different solutions, *Pediatrics* 76:159, 1985.
23. Sarnaik AP, et al: Management of hyponatremic seizures in children with hypertonic saline: a safe and effective strategy, *Crit Care Med* 19:758, 1991.
24. Satlin LM, Schwartz GJ: Disorders of potassium metabolism. In Ichikawa I, editor: *Pediatric textbook of fluids and electrolytes*, Baltimore, 1990, Williams & Wilkins.
25. Shann F, Germer S: Hyponatremia associated with pneumonia or bacterial meningitis, *Arch Dis Child* 60:963, 1985.

26. Simmons CF, Ichikawa I: External balance of water and electrolytes. In Ichikawa I, editor: *Pediatric textbook of fluids and electrolytes*, Baltimore, 1990, Williams & Wilkins.
27. Smith TJ, et al: Hyponatremia and seizures in young children given DDAVP, *Am J Hematol* 31:199, 1989.
28. Tamer AM, et al: Oral rehydration of infants in a large urban US medical center, *J Pediatr* 107:14, 1985.
29. Wattad A, Chiang ML, Hill LL: Hyponatremia in hospitalized children, *Clin Pediatr* 31:153, 1992.
30. Weisburg LS: Pseudohyponatremia: a reappraisal, *Am J Med* 86:315, 1989.
31. Winters RW, editor: *The body fluids in pediatrics*, Boston, 1973, Little Brown.

30 Blood Products and Their Uses

Eva G. Radel

The ability to separate blood into its components, store them appropriately, and administer them as needed has resulted in markedly improved supportive care, particularly in the areas of oncology and neonatology. However, the unfortunate occurrence of blood-transmitted acquired immunodeficiency syndrome (AIDS) has made the medical profession and the public aware of the hazards of blood products, and in some cases, has led to excessive fear of transfusion. As a result, the indications for transfusion have been reassessed, transfusion policies have become more conservative, and more effort is being devoted to a search for alternatives to the use of blood products.

GENERAL INDICATIONS FOR BLOOD TRANSFUSION

The general indications for transfusion of blood or blood products are (1) restoration of blood volume when it has been acutely depleted, (2) restoration of oxygen-carrying capacity, (3) restoration of a particular blood component (cellular or humoral) to a level allowing adequate function, (4) replacement or supplementation of an abnormally functioning component with a normal one, and (5) replacement after removal of large amounts of plasma or blood cells (exchange transfusion or apheresis).

The circulating amount of a blood component almost never has to be restored to the normal range; instead, the goal should be a level that will correct pathological processes and allow normal physiological functioning for the patient's current condition. In deciding whether component replacement is necessary, physicians should ask themselves two questions: (1) Is it essential to correct the particular deficit immediately through replacement? and (2) Is there another method that would restore an adequate physiological state? The necessary component should be administered selectively, if possible. An increasing number of non-blood-product medications, such as erythropoietin, granulocyte colony-stimulating factor (G-CSF, filgrastim), interleukin-11 (opreleukin), and desmopressin (DDAVP), are available for some situations in which previously only blood components could be used. Clinical trials are in progress for the development of red cell substitutes.[34]

BLOOD DONORS AND HANDLING OF BLOOD PRODUCTS

In recent years, public demand has been high for directed donations from family members and friends; this allows an individual to avoid receiving blood from routine donors, whom many consider unsafe. However, a higher incidence of hepatitis B and C has been found among first-time directed donors than among volunteer donors.[22] In addition, there is a risk of graft-versus-host disease (GVHD) developing in immunocompetent blood recipients who have been transfused with blood products from relatives who are homozygous for one of the patient's HLA haplotypes. The risk is greatest for donors who are first-degree relatives. This problem can be prevented by irradiating all blood products from blood relatives.[15]

All possible precautions must be taken to avoid clerical errors when drawing and labeling blood specimens to be used for cross-matching blood, as well as when starting transfusions. Mislabeling tubes and administering blood to the wrong patient are the most common causes of severe hemolytic transfusion reactions. Blood products also must be stored and handled properly. Once blood has been taken out of the blood bank, it should be used promptly and not refrigerated. If administration will be delayed, the blood should be returned to the blood bank immediately. Improper refrigeration can cause blood to freeze, resulting in lysis of the red cells, hemoglobinuria, and poor response to transfusion.

RED BLOOD CELL TRANSFUSIONS

In some situations (e.g., exchange transfusions, massive bleeding), use of whole blood is desirable. However, most blood banks no longer store whole blood and have only packed red blood cells (PRBCs) available. These can be reconstituted, if indicated, with saline, albumin (or another colloid), or fresh-frozen plasma (FFP). FFP rarely is needed in these situations, and using it exposes the recipient to risks similar to those of receiving another unit of blood. RBC preparations are described in Table 30-1.

Acute Blood Loss

Acute loss of more than 20% of the blood volume should be managed by volume replacement with fluids, and loss of more than 30% to 40% usually requires transfusion of PRBCs. If the patient is actively bleeding, rapid administration may be necessary.[20]

Massive bleeding involving the loss and replacement of more than one blood volume in several hours can give rise to some unique problems.[9] The mortality in this situation has been about 40%. A bleeding tendency may develop partly as a result of dilution, but more importantly, as a result of a consumption coagulopathy that is related at least in part to the presence of shock. Acidosis and hypothermia

Table 30-1 Red Blood Cell Preparations

Product	Preparation	Hematocrit (%) or Cell Count	Volume/Unit (ml)	Indications/Comments
Whole blood	450 ml blood, plus anticoagulant	40%	500	Massive bleeding, exchange transfusion
Packed RBCs	Centrifuged or sedimented to remove about two thirds of plasma	55%-80%	250-350	Most RBC transfusions
Buffy coat–depleted RBCs	Centrifuged to remove white cell layer	90% Contains 15%-30% of original WBCs	200	Chronically transfused patients; patients who have severe febrile reactions
Washed RBCs	Several manual and automated techniques available to remove plasma; must be used within 24 hr	90% Contains <1% of original plasma, <10% of WBCs	200	Repeated febrile and allergic reactions
Frozen RBCs	Frozen in glycerol, thawed, and washed; must be used within 24 hr of thawing; 10%-15% loss of original RBCs	Contains <0.025% of original plasma, 1%-5% of original WBCs and platelets	200	Rare blood types, multiple severe febrile/allergic reactions, IgA deficiency, autologous blood donations

also can result in increased bleeding. Platelet transfusions should be given if the platelet count is below 75,000/μl, and FFP is indicated if the prothrombin time and/or partial thromboplastin time are (is) greater than 1.5 times normal. Occasionally, cryoprecipitate can be helpful in replacing fibrinogen.

Restoration of Oxygen-Carrying Capacity

Transfusion often is recommended for a variety of indications to improve oxygen delivery in anemic patients, but frequently there is no scientific basis for such recommendations. The patient's general clinical condition is very important when determining the need to correct mild degrees of anemia. Transfusions often are given to small premature newborns or to older children who are critically ill and have cardiovascular compromise. The indications in these situations are controversial.[2,25,33] Careful consideration must be given to the risks of transfusion versus those of a low hemoglobin concentration. In many situations, treating the underlying cause of the anemia can avert the need for transfusion.

The volume of PRBCs given for anemia usually is about 10 ml/kg (15 to 20 ml/kg in the premature infant[25]), which can be given over 2 to 3 hours to a patient who is clinically stable. With very severe chronic anemia, the risk of congestive heart failure from transfusion may be greater than the risk of treating the patient medically. In this situation the volume transfused should be no more than 4 to 5 ml/kg given over 4 hours, and a diuretic may be needed. If the anemia must be corrected rapidly (e.g., for emergency surgery), a partial exchange transfusion can be done.

Chronic Transfusion

Several precautions that are not relevant to a patient receiving short-term transfusions are advisable for a child who is likely to undergo repeated and prolonged transfusion therapy:

1. *Red cell phenotyping:* For black patients, typing for several common red cell antigens should be done to prevent transfusion of blood containing antigens against which the recipient is likely to form antibodies. This has been a particular problem for patients who have sickle cell disease.[26]
2. *Leukocyte depletion:* Because most "minor" transfusion reactions are caused by leukocytes or plasma proteins, patients who are transfused frequently should receive leukocyte-reduced red cells.
3. *Hemosiderosis:* Serum ferritin should be monitored, and chelation therapy may be required.
4. *Hepatitis:* Although the incidence of hepatitis transmission has been reduced markedly by routine donor screening, hepatitis B vaccine should be given to individuals likely to receive repeated transfusions. Hepatitis A vaccine also is advisable.

Surgery

Individuals who have significant anemia develop more complications from surgery and anesthesia. In the past, a hematocrit of 30% (10.2 g/dl hemoglobin) was recommended as the minimum requirement for patients undergoing anesthesia. However, recent observations indicate that otherwise healthy adults may tolerate hematocrit values as low as 17.6% (6 g/dl hemoglobin).[20] However, such low values would be problematic for infants and children. The extent of surgery, the likelihood of massive blood loss, and coexisting factors such as impaired pulmonary function or inadequate cardiac output must be considered when deciding about a transfusion. The combination of anemia and hypovolemia must be avoided.

There has been an increasing tendency to use autologous blood donations for elective surgery. This has been done successfully in adolescents, children, and even in infants as young as 3 months old.[16,28] The largest experience has been in orthopedic procedures that are associated with significant blood loss, in cardiac surgery, and in prospective bone marrow donors. Several phlebotomies can be performed over a period of a few weeks just before surgery, or the process can be carried out over a longer period, and the blood can be frozen and stored. Formulas are available to calculate the amount of blood to be phlebotomized and the amount of anticoagulant to be used in children.[31] Another approach to blood conservation during surgery is normovolemic hemodilution: Whole blood is removed and anticoagulated, volume is replaced with lactated Ringer's solution or other fluid to lower the hematocrit to 20% to 25%, and the blood is reinfused if the hematocrit drops to less than 15% or at the end of the procedure.[28] Salvaging blood intraoperatively as well as postoperatively, collecting it with special equipment, and reinfusing it is an additional technique used to reduce the use of banked donor blood.[8,28] The administration of erythropoietin beginning 1 to 2 weeks preoperatively also has been shown to reduce the requirement for blood transfusion during surgery.[21] These procedures can be combined with added efficacy.

Special Circumstances in Red Blood Cell Transfusion

Newborns. Maternal blood is used, if possible, to cross-match blood for the infant's transfusion. However, the blood used should be ABO-specific for the baby or type O with a low titer of isoagglutinins. If the infant is Rh-negative, the blood should be Rh-negative as well. An infant who has hemolytic disease of the newborn, whether for simple transfusion or exchange transfusion, should receive blood that does not contain the antigen to which the mother is sensitized. With ABO incompatibility, the blood should be type O.

With a small premature infant who is transfused frequently, it no longer is considered necessary to perform a cross-match procedure for each transfusion unless plasma, platelets, or granulocytes have been administered. Many blood banks now designate certain blood units, which are drawn into four small bags, to be used for repeated transfusions for specific neonates to limit the number of donor exposures. Stored blood has been shown to be as safe and effective as fresh blood in most situations.[6,24]

Sickle cell disease. Patients who have sickle cell disease often are transfused to replace cells capable of sickling in the circulation with cells that are more deformable and will not participate in a vasoocclusive process. The blood used should be from sickle-negative donors. These patients have a high incidence of developing red cell antibodies; this can be decreased by matching for specific antigens that are prevalent in the white population, from which most donors come, and are absent more frequently in black individuals.[26] Some investigators have advocated erythrocytapheresis instead of simple transfusion for patients who require chronic transfusions to limit hemosiderosis.[11] The disadvantages of this approach are increased exposure to donor units and increased cost.

Potential bone marrow transplant recipients. Children who may require bone marrow transplantation should not be given blood products from genetically related family members because it may lead to sensitization to HLA antigens and subsequent bone marrow rejection. In addition, cytomegalovirus (CMV) infection must be avoided (see section on immunosuppressed patients below).

Immunosuppressed patients. This category includes (1) patients being treated for a malignancy, (2) bone marrow or organ transplant recipients, (3) premature infants weighing fewer than 1250 g and other severely ill neonates, (4) fetuses receiving intrauterine transfusions, and (5) children who have severe congenital immune deficiency disorders. These children are susceptible to graft-versus-host disease (GVHD) because of their failure to eliminate viable lymphocytes from the transfused blood. Leukodepletion does not prevent this complication. Irradiation of all blood products with a minimum of 25 Gy is recommended for these children.[32]

CMV infection also is a risk in neonates and potential bone marrow transplant recipients. If the child (or the mother of a newborn) does not already have antibodies to CMV (indicating preexisting infection), then blood products from CMV-seronegative donors should be given. If this is not possible, then the product should be administered with a leukofilter that can remove 99.9% of the white cells.[13] CMV-negative blood also should be given to pregnant females who are seronegative.

PLATELET TRANSFUSION

Platelet transfusions are useful primarily in situations in which there is a lack of production of platelets by the bone marrow. If thrombocytopenia is due to peripheral destruction, transfusion is unlikely to raise the platelet count significantly. Spontaneous hemorrhage usually does not occur with a platelet count above 10,000/mm^3, although in the past it often was standard procedure to maintain the count above 20,000/mm^3. Patients who have chronically low platelet counts are less likely to bleed spontaneously than are those whose platelets are diminishing rapidly. Coexistent fever or a coagulation disorder may predispose patients to bleeding at somewhat higher platelet counts. Traumatic or surgical bleeding may require platelet counts above 50,000/mm^3, and neurosurgical or ophthalmological procedures may warrant platelets above 100,000/mm^3. For small premature infants, many neonatologists prefer to maintain platelet counts above 50,000/mm^3 if the infant is stable and above 100,000/mm^3 if ill.[14] Dysfunctional platelets (e.g., those that may result from a congenital platelet disorder, after extracorporeal perfusion, or after massive blood replacement) also may result in bleeding at somewhat higher platelet count levels.

The half-life of transfused platelets is about 24 hours under normal circumstances, but survival may be shortened by fever or infection, platelet antibodies, splenomegaly, massive bleeding, or any condition that results in peripheral destruction or consumption of platelets. Variations in donor platelet count and collection or storage techniques, as well as increased manipulation of platelets, also may result in decreased platelet recovery.[17]

Platelets are not cross-matched for transfusion, but ABO-compatible platelets should be used when possible. If Rh-positive platelets must be given to an Rh-negative individual, then Rh immune globulin should be administered to prevent sensitization of the body's immune system by contaminating RBCs. For patients who need a single transfusion or a brief period of platelet transfusions, random donor platelets are satisfactory. For patients who have a malignancy or aplastic anemia, who likely will require repeated platelet transfusions, single donor (apheresed) platelets are preferable (Table 30-2). Patients who have aplastic anemia and require frequent platelet transfusions have a high incidence of alloimmunization and may benefit from having a limited number of designated platelet donors who are apheresed regularly. For patients who have malignancies or are immunosuppressed, the precautions recommended above for red blood cell transfusions should be followed. Patients who have become refractory to random donor platelets and who are not candidates for bone marrow transplantation may benefit from receiving platelets from family members who are at least partly HLA-matched. Unrelated but HLA-matched donors also may be good platelet donors for such individuals.

GRANULOCYTE TRANSFUSIONS

White blood cells (WBCs) are the most difficult blood cellular components to transfuse because of problems with yield, recovery, and complications. The use of granulocyte transfusions has been controversial; some centers use them regularly and others rarely. Studies have shown conflicting results and have been difficult to compare and interpret, both in neonatology and oncology. Bacterial sepsis that is unresponsive to appropriate antibiotic therapy in a severely neutropenic patient is the major indication.[23] Newborns who have sepsis and absolute neutrophil counts less than 3000/mm^3 also may be given granulocytes.[14] Febrile reactions and pulmonary infiltrates often are seen with granulocyte transfusion and may be associated with alloimmunization to both HLA antigens and granulocyte-specific antigens. Simultaneous administration of granulocytes and amphotericin has been implicated in severe pulmonary decompensation with intraalveolar hemorrhage and should be avoided.[5] CMV transmission is a risk (see p. 395).

EXCHANGE TRANSFUSION AND THERAPEUTIC APHERESIS

One unit of whole blood is equivalent to approximately twice the blood volume of a full-term neonate (i.e., a double volume exchange) and will replace about 85% of the infant's RBCs. PRBCs can be reconstituted with FFP. The blood used

Table 30-2 White Cell, Platelet, and Whole Plasma Preparations*

Product	Preparation	Cell Count or Content	Volume/Unit (ml)	Indications and Comments
Random donor platelets	Separated from single whole-blood units	5 to 7 × 10^{10} platelets/unit	40 to 50	Infants, short-term need. 1 unit/10 kg increases platelet count by 50,000
Single donor platelets	Collected by apheresis	Equivalent to 6 to 8 random units	200 to 400 may be divided in two bags	Patients who require multiple transfusions
Apheresed granulocyte concentrates	Varying techniques to increase donor neutrophil count and yield	0.5 to 3 × 10^{10}/unit	500	Contains RBCs, must be ABO-compatible; must be used within 24 hr of collection
Fresh-frozen plasma	Whole plasma	1 unit of coagulation factors/ml	200 to 220 or 600 (pheresed)	Multiple factor deficiency; DIC: reversal of warfarin effect; HUS or TTP; unknown coagulation defect; deficiency of factors II, V, VII, X, XI, or XIII. Contains all plasma factors; not virus-inactivated
Solvent-detergent FFP	Pooled whole plasma	1 unit of coagulation factors/ml	200	Same as above, but virus-inactivated.† Low levels of high-molecular-weight VWF multimers

*For plasma products used to treat coagulation deficiencies, see Chapter 214, Hemophilia and Other Hereditary Bleeding Disorders, Table 214-1.
†Virus attenuation processes may not inactivate parvovirus, hepatitis A, and possibly other viruses.
DIC, Disseminated intravascular coagulation; *F,* factor; *FFP,* fresh-frozen plasma; *HUS,* hemolytic-uremic syndrome; *TTP,* thrombotic thrombocytopenic purpura; *VWF,* von Willebrand factor.

should be fewer than 3 to 5 days old, and the recommendations for transfusion of newborns (see p. 395) should be followed. Although manual exchange transfusion often is done in older children for a variety of indications, this can be difficult and time-consuming. Automated cell separators simplify the process, and some can be adapted for use in young children. Whole blood is removed, plasma, platelets, leukocytes, and red cells are separated, and the desired component is removed. Except with erythrocytapheresis, the red cells are returned to the patient. Volume can be replaced with saline, albumin, or FFP.[30]

Erythrocytapheresis (partial exchange transfusion) may be done for polycythemia in neonates or in older children who have cyanotic heart disease by using volume replacement with saline or albumin. The volume of exchange can be calculated as follows:

$$\text{Volume exchanged} = \text{Total blood volume} \times (\text{Observed hematocrit} - \text{Desired hematocrit})/\text{Observed hematocrit}$$

In sickle cell disease, red cells may be removed and replaced with normal ones. An exchange of one red cell volume (70 ml/kg × hematocrit) will reduce the hemoglobin S (Hb S) to about 35%. The RBCs should be reconstituted with albumin or FFP, and an additional RBC infusion can reduce the Hb S level further.[31] The final hematocrit should not be greater than 30% to 35%. Leukocytapheresis may be done for patients who have leukemia and very high WBC counts to reduce viscosity and leukostasis until chemotherapy takes effect. Plasma exchange can be done for thrombotic thrombocytopenic purpura or hemolytic-uremic syndrome by using FFP for replacement. Many autoimmune disorders and other related conditions also have been treated with plasmapheresis, using albumin for replacement.

PLASMA PRODUCTS

Plasma products used to treat coagulation disorders are described in Table 214-1 in Chapter 214, Hemophilia and Other Hereditary Bleeding Disorders. Commercial lyophilized coagulant concentrates have the advantage of being assayed so that the physician knows exactly how much of a desired factor is being administered. Several very effective methods for inactivating viruses have made commercial concentrates much safer in recent years, although some viral agents such as parvovirus and hepatitis A still cause concern. Recently, FFP that has been treated to inactivate viruses (solvent detergent-FFP) has become available.[12] This product is advisable for individuals who are likely to require repeated infusions. Indications for FFP administration include: (1) active bleeding or prophylaxis for an invasive procedure in patients who have a congenital or acquired coagulation defect for which no specific concentrate is available or, in an emergency, until the specific defect is identified; (2) massive transfusion (see p. 393); (3) urgent reversal of warfarin; (4) hypercoagulable state resulting from deficiency of a plasma protein factor when rapid correction is necessary; and (5) plasma exchange for thrombotic thrombocytopenic purpura or hemolytic-uremic syndrome.

Albumin

Albumin is available as a 5% or 25% solution, the latter being advantageous for patients who have hypoproteinemia and need large amounts of albumin and who would get a much larger sodium load with the larger volume needed, using the less concentrated product. Albumin is fractionated from pooled plasma and is pasteurized to inactivate viruses.

Immune Globulin

Two types of immune globulin preparations are available, one for intramuscular (IM) administration and another for intravenous (IV) use. Special products prepared from individuals who have high titers for specific infectious agents (varicella-zoster, hepatitis, and tetanus) also are available for IM administration. Intravenous gamma globulin (IVGG) is used to treat hypogammaglobulinemia, idiopathic thrombocytopenic purpura (ITP), Kawasaki disease, and a variety of immune disorders. Recently, an association of renal failure with the administration of IVGG has been described in adults.[1] IV anti-Rh gamma globulin (WinRho) also can be used to treat ITP in Rh-positive patients.[27]

Anticoagulants

Pediatric patients who have thrombotic disease are more likely than adults to have a congenital deficiency of one of the natural anticoagulants (antithrombin III [ATIII], protein C, or protein S) or an abnormal coagulant protein (factor V Leiden or prothrombin 20210). ATIII concentrate is available, and protein C is awaiting Federal Drug Administration approval for use in the United States.

COMPLICATIONS OF TRANSFUSION

Immediate Hemolytic Transfusion Reaction

Severe, immediate hemolytic transfusion reactions almost always are related to ABO-incompatibility and clerical errors, such as incorrect labeling of a blood specimen tube sent to the laboratory for cross matching, or administration of another patient's unit of blood. An acute onset of fever and chills may be accompanied by nausea, abdominal and lower back pain, dyspnea, and hypotension. Renal failure, disseminated intravascular coagulation (DIC), and shock may rapidly ensue. If such a reaction is suspected, the transfusion must be stopped at once. Blood from the patient should be sent to the blood bank immediately, together with the remainder of the unit of donor blood or the empty bag and any attached blood tubing. A rapid screening test can be performed by obtaining a blood specimen (with care taken to avoid artificial hemolysis) and centrifuging it; pink, red, or brown plasma indicates intravascular hemolysis. At the same time, a urine sample should be checked for the presence of hemoglobin. If there is evidence of a hemolytic reaction, good venous access should be established and the patient transferred to an intensive care unit for close monitoring, aggressive fluid administration, possible administration of dopamine, and supportive care. Treatment of DIC and renal dialysis may be needed, and blood components should be given as indicated.[4]

Delayed Hemolytic Transfusion Reaction

Delayed reactions may develop 3 to 21 days after transfusion in patients who may have had prior sensitization to red cell antigens with titers too low to be detected before the recent transfusion. An anamnestic reaction may increase antibody production so that hemolysis ensues, and the patient becomes anemic, with or without hyperbilirubinemia and hemoglobinuria. Usually, no specific therapy is required, but an additional transfusion may be needed.

Febrile Transfusion Reaction

Fever is the most common transfusion reaction, occurring most often in patients who are multiply transfused and those who receive platelet transfusions. The fever usually is associated with antibodies directed against leukocytes or with cytokines in the blood product.[10] The onset usually occurs 30 minutes to 2 hours after the transfusion is begun, and the patient also may have chills. If the reaction is mild and the patient has been multiply transfused and has had previous febrile reactions, it is not necessary to stop the transfusion, but it should be slowed. In more severe reactions, temporary interruption or discontinuation of the transfusion is indicated. If chills and back or abdominal pain accompany the reaction, the transfusion must be stopped immediately and the precautions for a hemolytic transfusion reaction taken. Treatment with acetaminophen and, for more severe reactions, corticosteroids is helpful; for future transfusions, pretreatment may prevent such reactions. If they continue to occur, leukodepleted blood should be used.

Allergic Reactions

The etiology of urticarial reactions usually is not clear, although they may be associated with antigens in donor plasma. The plasmas of allergic donors also may result in an allergic reaction if the recipient is exposed to the corresponding antigen. Individuals who have congenital IgA deficiency have a 20% to 25% incidence of antibodies directed against IgA. These patients may develop severe anaphylactic reactions to any blood product containing plasma proteins.[18] Anti-IgA antibodies also may develop in normal individuals and result in urticarial or anaphylactic reactions. People who have repeated minor allergic reactions should be pretreated with an antihistamine; corticosteroids may be used if more severe reactions have occurred. Frozen washed RBCs may be effective and may be available from IgA-deficient donors. Urticarial reactions cannot be prevented by leukodepletion.

Transfusion-Transmitted Infections

Routine screening of donors for antibodies to the human immunodeficiency virus (HIV) has been in effect in the United States since 1985, when 27 per 100,000 donations were found to be HIV positive. Currently it has been estimated that failure to detect HIV in a donor might occur in only about 1 in 500,000 donations.[7,19] The greatest danger is posed by products containing pooled plasma that have not been treated for virus inactivation.

Groups at risk for CMV infection have been discussed earlier in this chapter. Individuals who have been infected carry the virus in their leukocytes indefinitely. In a normal recipient, infection is asymptomatic or associated with a mild, mononucleosis-like illness 3 to 4 weeks after transfusion. Epstein-Barr virus (EBV) also can be transmitted by transfusion but has less clinical significance than CMV.

Routine screening of blood donors for hepatitis B has reduced the incidence to 1 in 60,000 units (usually resulting from donation during the incubation period). In the United States, donor blood has been tested for antibody to hepatitis C virus since 1990. This agent previously was the major cause (90%) of non-A, non-B transfusion-associated hepatitis, but is now estimated to have a transmission risk of about 1 in 100,000.[19] Other viruses that may be transmitted by transfusion include hepatitis G (not known to cause disease), hepatitis A, parvovirus, human T-cell leukemia virus I (HTLV-I), and HTLV-II.[8] Donors are now screened for the latter two viruses.

There has been much concern in recent years about the possible transmission of new variant Creutzfeldt-Jakob disease and other prion-induced diseases by blood transfusion.[29] Although this has never been documented, fear has led to the recall of various blood products, occasionally resulting in nationwide shortages.

Malaria and babesiosis also can be transmitted by contaminated blood. The latter resembles malaria and is a problem only for patients who have undergone a splenectomy or who are immunocompromised. Bacterial contamination of blood is quite rare but is associated most often with transfusion of platelets.

REFERENCES

1. Ahsan N: Intravenous immunoglobulin induced-nephropathy: a complication of IVIG therapy, *J Nephrol* 11:157, 1998.
2. Bifano EM, Curran TR: Minimizing donor blood exposure in the neonatal intensive care unit: current trends and future prospects, *Clin Perinatol* 22:657, 1995.
3. Cahill MR, Lilleyman JS: The rational use of platelet transfusions in children, *Semin Thromb Hemost* 24:567, 1998.
4. Capon SM, Goldfinger D: Acute hemolytic transfusion reaction, a paradigm of the systemic inflammatory response: new insights into pathophysiology and treatment, *Transfusion* 35:513, 1995.
5. Chanock SJ, Gorlin JB: Granulocyte transfusions: time for a second look, *Infect Dis Clin North Am* 10:327, 1996.
6. Cohen A, Manno C: Transfusion practices in infants receiving assisted ventilation, *Clin Perinatol* 25:97, 1998.
7. Goodnough LT, et al: Transfusion medicine. First of two parts—blood transfusion, *N Engl J Med* 340:438, 1999.
8. Goodnough LT, et al: Transfusion medicine. Second of two parts—blood conservation, *N Engl J Med* 340:525, 1999.
9. Harvey MP, et al: Massive blood transfusion in a tertiary referral hospital: clinical outcomes and haemostatic complications, *Med J Aust* 163: 356, 1995.
10. Heddle NM, et al: The role of the plasma from platelet concentrates in transfusion reactions, *N Engl J Med* 331:625, 1994.
11. Hilliard LM, et al: Erythrocytapheresis limits iron accumulation in chronically transfused sickle cell patients, *Am J Hematol* 59:28, 1998.
12. Horowitz B, et al: Virus inactivation by solvent/detergent treatment and the manufacture of SD-plasma, *Vox Sang* 1(74 suppl):203, 1998.

13. Lane TA: Leukocyte reduction of cellular blood components: effectiveness, benefits, quality control, and costs, *Arch Pathol Lab Med* 118:392, 1994.
14. Manno CS: What's new in transfusion medicine? *Pediatr Clin North Am* 43:793, 1996.
15. McMilin K, Johnson RL: Transfusion-associated graft-versus-host disease, *Trans Med Rev* 7:37, 1993.
16. Murray DJ, et al: Transfusion management in pediatric and adolescent scoliosis surgery: efficacy of autologous blood, *Spine* 22:2735, 1997.
17. Rintels PB, et al: Therapeutic support of the patient with thrombocytopenia, *Hematol Oncol Clin North Am* 8:1131, 1994.
18. Sandler SG, et al: IgA anaphylactic transfusion reactions, *Transfus Med Rev* 9:1, 1995.
19. Schreiber GB, et al: The risk of transfusion-transmitted viral infections: the Retrovirus Epidemiology Donor Study, *N Engl J Med* 334:1685, 1996.
20. Simon TL, et al: Practice parameter for the use of red blood cell transfusions: developed by the Red Blood Cell Administration Practice Guideline Development Task Force of the College of American Pathologists, *Arch Pathol Lab Med* 122:130, 1998.
21. Spence RK: Emerging trends in surgical blood transfusion, *Semin Hematol* 34(suppl 2):48, 1997.
22. Starkey JM, et al: Markers for transfusion-transmitted disease in different groups of blood donors, *JAMA* 262:3452, 1989.
23. Strauss R: Granulocyte transfusion therapy, *Hematol Oncol Clin North Am* 8:1159, 1994.
24. Strauss RG: Practical issues in neonatal transfusion practice, *Am J Clin Pathol* 107:S57, 1997.
25. Strauss RG: Red blood cell transfusion practices in the neonate, *Clin Perinatol* 22:641, 1995.
26. Tahhan HR, et al: Antigen-matched donor blood in the transfusion management of patients with sickle cell disease, *Transfusion* 34:562, 1994.
27. Tarantino MD, et al: Treatment of childhood acute immune thrombocytopenic purpura with anti-D immune globulin or pooled immune globulin, *J Pediatr* 134:21, 1999.
28. Thompson HW, Luban NL: Autologous blood transfusion in the pediatric patient, *J Pediatr Surg* 30:1406, 1995.
29. Turner ML, Ironside JW: New-variant Creutzfeldt-Jakob disease: the risk of transmission by blood transfusion, *Blood Rev* 12:255, 1998.
30. Urban C, et al: Feasibility of peripheral blood stem cell (PBSC) and peripheral blood mononuclear cell (PBMNC) separation in children with a body weight below 20 kg, *Med Pediatr Oncol* 29:115, 1997.
31. Walker RH: *Technical manual,* ed 11, Bethesda, Md, 1993, American Association of Blood Banks.
32. Webb DK: Irradiation in the prevention of transfusion associated graft-versus-host disease, *Arch Dis Child* 73:388, 1995.
33. Wilson SM, et al, editors: *Improving transfusion practice for pediatric patients,* Arlington, Va, 1991, American Association of Blood Banks.
34. Winslow RM: New transfusion strategies: red cell substitutes, *Annu Rev Med* 50:337, 1999.

31 Antimicrobial Therapy

Blaise L. Congeni

The use of antimicrobial agents to treat diseases caused by bacteria is part of the day-to-day practice of pediatrics. Antimicrobial therapy has advanced and continues to advance at a rate unparalleled in medicine; even experts on infectious diseases have trouble staying abreast of new agents and their pharmacology and pharmacodynamics. Developing a rationale for the use of antimicrobial agents should help prevent overuse and allow consistent evaluation of the merits and drawbacks of new antimicrobial agents. For the practitioner, it is more important to know how to use a limited number of antimicrobial agents well than to have a meager knowledge of many.

APPROACH TO ANTIMICROBIAL THERAPY

Three important questions should be answered before antimicrobial therapy is begun: (1) where is the infection (anatomical site), (2) what pathogens usually cause infections at this site, and (3) which antimicrobial agents, given by what route of administration, will achieve effective concentrations at that site? The answers to the first two questions usually are addressed critically by the practitioner. However, selection of an antimicrobial agent is more likely to be based on a "bug-drug" relationship than on knowledge about the ability to achieve an effective concentration at the site of infection.

The anatomical site of most bacterial infections can be identified by a combination of historical information and findings on physical examination. When the site of infection is more obscure, diagnostic studies such as roentgenograms, radionucleotide scans, computed tomography (CT) scans, magnetic resonance imaging (MRI), and ultrasound evaluation often are helpful.

Based on the site of infection and the patient's age, habitat, history of exposures, and clinical signs and symptoms, the pediatrician usually can develop a list of potential bacterial pathogens. Knowing the site of infection and possible causative agents helps the clinician to decide what (if any) specimens should be cultured for bacteria, as well as whether the laboratory should be alerted to use special culture media or techniques. Selecting an antimicrobial agent based on its ability to achieve effective concentrations at the site of infection requires a working concept of what an effective concentration is. To define an "effective concentration," it first is necessary to review some of the basic pharmacodynamics of antimicrobial agents.

PHARMACODYNAMICS/ PHARMACOKINETICS

The term *pharmacodynamics* describes the relationship between the serum concentration of the drug and its pharmacological and the toxicological effects. *Pharmacokinetics,* on the other hand, describes the absorption, distribution, and elimination of drugs. Clinicians most often are interested in the relationship between drug concentration and the antimicrobial effect, the interrelationship between pharmacokinetics and pharmacodynamics. Once administered, an antimicrobial agent initially is distributed throughout the intravascular volume and the extracellular fluid of tissues with high perfusion rates. The drug enters tissues that are not highly perfused at a slower rate. Some antimicrobial agents, such as the beta-lactams, are distributed only in extracellular fluid, whereas others distribute intracellularly as well[9] (rifampin, trimethoprim-sulfamethoxazole [TMP-SMX]).

Correlation of Drug Concentration and Clinical Effect

During the past decade, a great deal has been learned concerning the interaction between serum concentrations and bacterial killing. During this time, a number of investigators have proposed that antibiotics could be divided into two different groups based on their pattern of bactericidal activity.[2] The first group of agents exhibits a greater rate and extent of bactericidal activity the higher the drug concentration. These agents exhibit *concentration-dependent killing.* Aminoglycosides, fluoroquinolones, and metronidazole exhibit this type of bactericidal activity for anaerobic bacteria. In contrast, other antibiotics demonstrate bactericidal activity that is independent of drug concentration as long as the concentration exceeds four times the minimum inhibitory concentration (MIC). These agents demonstrate minimal concentration-dependent killing, but instead, their bactericidal activity depends on the time of exposure. Time-dependent agents include the beta-lactam antibiotics, vancomycin, clindamycin, and the macrolides.[2]

Postantibiotic Effect

Part of the explanation for the pharmacodynamic division of antibiotics into time- and concentration-dependent killing is explained by the postantibiotic effect (PAE). For some antibiotics, continued suppression of bacterial growth occurs even after concentrations of the agent have declined below levels sufficient to inhibit growth, a PAE. All antimicrobial agents exhibit PAEs in vitro when susceptible gram-positive bacteria are exposed to them. Prolonged PAEs for gram-negative bacteria are observed only after exposure to antibiotics that inhibit protein synthesis or nucleic acid synthesis.[2] A notable exception is the carbapenems, which produce prolonged PAEs with strains of *Pseudomonas aeruginosa*.

Relationship of Pharmacokinetic and Pharmacodynamic Parameters and Efficacy

Practical implications result from the application of the aforementioned pharmacodynamic and pharmacokinetic principles. For time-dependent agents, organisms begin to regrow once the serum concentration of the agent has fallen below the MIC. Consequently, the most effective regimens will allow for drug concentrations at the site of infection to be above the MIC for as large a part of the dosing interval as possible. In general, a cure of 85% to 100% can be anticipated when the drug concentration exceeds the MIC for at least 40% of the dosing interval for time-dependent agents such as beta-lactams.

This information has implications for clinical practice. Some investigators have suggested that for infections such as endocarditis or osteomyelitis, more time above the MIC may be required for clinical cure. Serum bactericidal activity is used to monitor pediatric patients who have acute hematogenous osteomyelitis. Peak levels traditionally have been used, but based on this model, at least one group of investigators has suggested that serum bactericidal activity at trough concentrations may correlate better with cure.[2] In other words, a trough serum bactericidal concentration may be a more accurate reflection of the portion of the dosing interval during which the drug concentration was above the MIC.

The implications for the use of concentration-dependent drugs in clinical practice also are significant. Based on this model, infrequent dosing of concentration-dependent agents such as aminoglycosides and fluoroquinolones makes better sense. During the 1990s, a number of studies have reported equal or superior clinical efficacy when the entire aminoglycoside dose is given as a single daily dose. This allows for a single peak concentration at least tenfold higher than the MIC. Although considerable debate continues, toxicity does not appear to be increased, and some investigators have suggested that toxicity actually is dependent more on the length of time the drug is present in drug-sensitive tissues (e.g., the kidney or inner ear) rather than on the highest concentration attained in the serum at any point.

Minimal Inhibitory and Minimal Bactericidal Concentrations

An antimicrobial agent's activity against a particular bacterium in vitro is expressed as the agent's minimal inhibitory concentration (MIC) or minimal bactericidal concentration (MBC). To determine the MIC, bacteria are grown in broth to a concentration of 100,000 (10^5) microorganisms per milliliter. The broth containing the bacteria, which is clear to the naked eye, is then placed in a series of test tubes, and a decreasing amount of antimicrobial agent is added to each test tube. The broth containing the bacteria and antimicrobial agent is incubated overnight and then examined for visible turbidity, since turbidity represents bacterial growth. The test tube with the smallest concentration of antimicrobial agent that remains clear to the naked eye represents the MIC. To determine whether the antibiotic is bactericidal, the tubes that remained clear are quantitatively subcultured onto agar plates. After overnight incubation, bacterial colonies are counted. Each colony represents one bacterium that survived, or one colony-forming unit (CFU). The smallest amount of antibiotic that results in the death of 99,900 (99.9%) of the original 100,000 microorganisms per milliliter inoculum (a 1000-fold reduction) is the MBC. MIC and MBC results are reported in micrograms of antimicrobial agent per milliliter of broth required to inhibit or kill the microorganism, respectively.

Serum Inhibitory and Bactericidal Titers

Antimicrobial activity in vivo can be approximated by determining the inhibitory or bactericidal titers. Although the test usually is performed using serum, it can be done with most body fluids that are clear, except urine. The test is performed by growing organisms to 10^5 CFU per milliliter of broth, as in determining the MIC. However, instead of adding known concentrations of antimicrobial agent to each test tube, serial twofold dilutions of serum (or other body fluids) are added to sequential tubes (i.e., undiluted serum is added to the first tube, serum diluted 1:2 to the second tube, 1:4 to the third, and so on). After incubation overnight, the tubes are examined for visible turbidity; the most dilute sample that has no visible turbidity is the serum inhibitory titer. To determine if the bacteria are being killed, the broth is cultured quantitatively as for the MBC, and the most dilute specimen that results in the death of 99.9% of the original inoculum is the serum bactericidal titer.

Tolerance

Tolerance to an antimicrobial agent describes the situation in which organisms are inhibited by the normal concentration of a bactericidal agent but require much higher concentrations of the agent to achieve a bactericidal effect. The clinical significance of tolerance is still controversial, but it appears that this phenomenon may be important with infections that require bactericidal activity to effect a cure.[6]

Bacteriostatic Versus Bactericidal

Most infections in children do not require a bactericidal antimicrobial agent. In general, bactericidal agents are needed for optimal treatment of bacterial endocarditis, meningitis, and osteomyelitis. The effectiveness of bacteriostatic agents depends on the host's ability to opsonize and phagocytize bacteria that have been inhibited; thus, bactericidal agents usually are necessary to treat bacterial infections in a neutropenic host.

Role of the Laboratory in Antimicrobial Therapy

For the vast majority of bacterial infections treated in the ambulatory setting, little or no laboratory testing is necessary to use antimicrobial agents rationally. For example, otitis media is the most common infection of children that is treated with antimicrobial agents in the ambulatory setting. The site of infection is identified by physical examination. The bacterial pathogens that cause otitis media have been well established, and several antimicrobial agents have been shown to produce a clinical and microbiological cure when given orally. Only if empirical therapy fails does it become necessary to perform a tympanocentesis to obtain a specimen for isolating the bacteria and performing antibiotic susceptibility tests. Likewise, by knowing the usual pathogens and their susceptibility to antimicrobial agents, the practitioner can manage common infections such as impetigo, cellulitis, cervical adenitis, local abscesses, and conjunctivitis without obtaining specimens for culture.

Culture and Susceptibility

When the usual therapy fails, when the patient is more seriously ill or is immunocompromised, or when the clinical situation is unusual, the first step is to obtain appropriate specimens to culture for bacterial pathogens. When bacterial pathogens are isolated from a normally sterile specimen, antimicrobial susceptibility is tested. Susceptibility is tested by either determining the MIC as described previously or by using the disk diffusion method.

In the disk diffusion method, a culture plate is inoculated with the bacteria to be tested, and paper disks containing standardized concentrations of antimicrobial agents are placed on the surface of the culture medium. The culture plates are incubated, and the moisture from the medium allows the antimicrobial agents to diffuse out of the paper disks. The farther from the disk the diffusion reaches, the lower the concentration of antimicrobial agent. If the bacteria are inhibited by the antibiotic, a zone around the disk forms in which the bacteria do not grow. The zone of inhibition is measured after overnight incubation and, based on its diameter, the organism is determined to be "susceptible" or "resistant" to the antimicrobial agent. A report of "intermediate" or "indeterminant" should be interpreted to mean that the microorganism is resistant or that the MIC should be determined. The diameter of the zone of inhibition has been correlated to MIC determinations so that "susceptible" actually means that the MIC will be equal to or less than a certain concentration of the antimicrobial agent.

When an organism is reported to be susceptible by disk, it means that 95% of the strains of this bacteria are inhibited by concentrations of the antimicrobial agent that can be achieved in the serum if the antimicrobial agent is given at the usual dose by the usual route of administration for an infection with that organism. This concentration is called the *MIC_{95}*. The MIC_{95} of selected antimicrobial agents for bacteria reported as susceptible by disk are listed in Table 31-1. Clearly, the site of infection, the proposed antibiotic's activity against the pathogen, and the concentration of the antibiotic that can be achieved at the site of infection all must be considered.

For example, "susceptible to ampicillin" has very different meanings, depending on the organism being tested. When gram-negative organisms or enterococci are reported as being susceptible to ampicillin (see Table 31-1), it means that 95% of these organisms are inhibited by serum concentrations of 8 μg/ml or less of ampicillin.[11] For gram-positive cocci, susceptible means that 95% are inhibited by serum concentrations of 0.2 μg/ml or less or 40 times less ampicillin than it takes to inhibit gram-negative enterics.[11] For *Haemophilus influenzae,* susceptible means that it takes serum concentrations of 2 μg/ml or less to inhibit 95% of all strains.[11] Unless the MIC has been determined for the individual isolate, the clinician must assume that MIC_{95} must be achieved at the site of infection to inhibit the isolate.

SPECIFIC ANTIBACTERIAL AGENTS

Because of the large number of antimicrobial agents currently available, several usually are equally effective for a given infectious disease. The antimicrobial agents preferred by a practitioner reflect the drugs' cost and availability as well as the physician's training and local practices. In general, it is far better to know how to use a small number of antimicrobial agents well than to know all of the possible alternatives. Table 31-1 presents the antimicrobial agents physicians use most frequently and selected pharmacological and pharmacodynamic information about them. This table is intended to serve as an example of the information a practitioner should have at hand when using antimicrobial agents; the specific antimicrobial agents that should be used for selected infections are discussed later in this chapter, following some general information about classes of antimicrobial agents.

Penicillins

Mechanism of action. Although the general mechanism of action of penicillins is to inhibit cell wall synthesis, precisely how they do this is unknown. Current evidence, however, points to inhibition of transpeptidation. Most bacteria have penicillin-binding proteins (PBP) in their cell membranes. There are a number of PBP, and the number and type vary from bacteria to bacteria. The activity of penicillins generally correlates with the number of high-affinity PBP the organism has.

Bacterial resistance. Bacterial resistance to penicillins can be based on three principal mechanisms: enzymatic degradation, reduced penetration of the agent to the target site, and alteration in the PBP.[22] Inactivation of the penicillin as a result of degradation caused by a penicillinase produced by the bacteria has been the most common mechanism of resistance for this class of agents. Beta-lactamase enzymes hydrolyze the beta-lactam ring. A variety of beta-lactamases have been identified and are classified based on substrate preference. Beta-lactamases have been produced by both gram-positive and gram-negative organisms, and production of these enzymes has been mediated by either plasmid or chromosomal mechanisms.

Table 31-1 Dosage, Peak Serum Concentrations, and MIC_{95} for Selected Antimicrobial Agents

Antimicrobial Agent	Route of Administration	Age: <1 Wk* (<2000 g) mg/kg/Dose/Interval	Age: 1 Wk-1 Mo* (<2000 g) mg/kg/Dose/Interval	Age: >1 Mo mg/kg/Dose/Interval	Age: Adult Dose† g/Dose/Interval	Peak Serum Concentration (μg/ml)	Susceptibility (MIC_{95})(μg/ml)‡
Penicillin G	IV	50,000 U q8h (50,000 U q12h)	50,000 U q6h (50,000 U q8h)	25,000-50,000 U q4-6h	25,000-50,000 **U/kg** q4-6h	400	≤0.01 *L. monocytogenes* ≤2
Procaine penicillin	IM	50,000 U q24h (50,000 U q24h)	50,000 U q24h (50,000 U q24h)	25,000-50,000 U q12-24h	25,000-50,000 **U/kg** q12-24h	5-6	≤0.1
Benzathine I penicillin	IM	50,000 U; 1 dose (50,000 U; 1 dose)	50,000 U; 1 dose (50,000 U; 1 dose)	50,000 U; 1 dose	2.4×10^6 U; 1 dose	0.2	≤0.1
Penicillin V	PO	Not recommended	Not recommended	6.25-12.5 q6h	0.25-0.5 q6h	3-5	≤0.1
Ampicillin	IV IM	25-50 q8h (25-50 q12h)	25-50 q6h (25-50 q8h)	25-75 q4-6h	1-2 q4-6h	40 8	Gram negative ≤8 Streptococci ≤0.1 *H. influenzae* ≤2
Amoxicillin	PO	Not recommended	Not recommended	10-15 q8h	0.25-0.5 q8h	4.7-7.5	As for ampicillin
Nafcillin	IV	20 q8h (25 q12h)	37.5 q6h (25 q8h)	25-50 q6h	0.5-1.5 q4-6h	11	≤1
Methicillin§	IV	25-50 q8h (25-50 q12h)	25-50 q6h (25-50 q8h)	—	—	—	—
Dicloxacillin	PO	Not recommended	Not recommended	3-6.25	0.25-0.5 q6h	15-18	≤1
Mezlocillin	IV IM	75 q12h (75 q12h)	75 q8h (75 q8h)	50-75 q4-6h	3-4 q4-6h	200-300 15	≤64
Cefazolin	IV IM	20 q12h (20 q12h)	20 q8h (20 q12h)	8.3-25 q6-8h	0.5-1.5 q6-8h	188	≤8
Cephalexin	PO	Not recommended	Not recommended	6.25-12.5 q6h	0.25-1 q6h	8-40	≤8
Cefoxitin	IV IM	Not recommended	Not recommended	20-26.6 q4-q6h	1-2 q4-q6h or 3 q8h	110-125	≤8
Cefotaxime	IV	50 q12h (50 q12h)	50 q8h (50 q8h)	25-50 q6h	1-2 q4-q12h	1 g 40 2 g 80-90	≤8
Ceftriaxone	IV IM	50 q24h (50 q24h)	50-80 q24h (50 q24h)	50 q24h CNS: 80 q24h	0.5-2 q24h	1 g 150 1 g 50	≤8
Ceftazidime	IV IM	30 q8h (50 q12h)	50 q8h (50 q8h)	25-50 q6h	0.5-2 q8-12h	1 g 85 1 g 34	≤8

*Doses and intervals shown in parentheses are for infants with a birth weight <2000 g; doses and intervals shown without parentheses are for infants with a birth weight >2000 g.
†Maximum recommended dose (units other than grams are in **boldface**).
‡μg/ml of the antimicrobial required to inhibit isolate reported to be susceptible to disk diffusion method.
§Methicillin is preferred for newborns when kernicterus is a concern.

Continued

Table 31-1 Dosage, Peak Serum Concentrations, and MIC_{95} for Selected Antimicrobial Agents—cont'd

Antimicrobial Agent	Route of Administration	Age: <1 Wk* (<2000 g) mg/kg/Dose/Interval	Age: 1 Wk-1 Mo* (<2000 g) mg/kg/Dose/Interval	Age: >1 Mo mg/kg/Dose/Interval	Age: Adult Dose† g/Dose/Interval	Peak Serum Concentration (μg/ml)	Susceptibility (MIC_{95})(μg/ml)‡
Amikacin	IV	10 q12h	10 q8h	5 q8h or 7.5 q12h	5 **mg/kg** q8h or 7.5 **mg/kg** q12h	20-40	≤16
	IM	(7.5 q12h)	(7.5 q8h)			20	
Gentamicin	IV	2.5 q12h	2.5 q8h	1-2.5 q8h	1-1.7 **mg/kg** q8h	4-10	≤4
	IM	(2.5 q12h)	(2.5 q8h)			7	
Tobramycin	IV	2 q12h	2 q8h	1-2 q8h	1-1.7 **mg/kg** q8h	4-14	≤4
	IM	(2 q12h)	(2 q8h)			4	
Trimethoprim-sulfamethoxazole (TMP-SMX)	PO IV	Not recommended	Not recommended	3-6 TMP/15-30 SMX q12h 5 TMP/25 SMX q6h for pneumocystosis	0.16 TMP/0.8 SMX q12h	2-4/80-100	≤2/38
Sulfisoxazole	PO	Not recommended	Not recommended	30-37.5 q6h	0.5-1 q6h	40-50	≤100 (urinary tract infection only)
Erythromycin estolate	PO	10 q12h (10 q12h)	10-12.5 q8h (10 q8h)	10 q8h or 15 q12h	0.25-0.5 q6h	4.2	≤0.5
Erythromycin ethylsuccinate	PO	10 q12h (10 q12h)	10 q8h (10 q8h)	10 q6h	0.25-0.5 q6h	1.5	≤0.5
Clindamycin	PO	5 q8h	5 q6h	2.5-7.5 q6h	0.15-.45 q6h	2.5-3.6	≤0.5
	IV	(5 q12h)	(5 q8h)				
Chloramphenicol	IV	25 q24h	25 q24h	12.5-18.75 q6h	12.5-25 **mg/kg** q6h	19	*H. influenzae* ≤4
	PO	(25 q24h)	(25 q24h)	18.75-25 q6h (meningitis)		25	Others ≤12.5
Tetracycline	IV	Not recommended	Not recommended	Children >8 yr	0.25-0.5 q6h	8	≤4
	PO			6.25-12.5 q6h		4	
Vancomycin	IV	15 q12h (10 q12h)	10 q8h (10 q8h)	10-15 q6h	15 **mg/kg** q12h or 6.5-8 **mg/kg** q6h	30-40	≤5
Metronidazole	PO	7.5 q12h	15 q12h	5-12 q8h	7.5 **mg/kg** q6h	11.5	≤4
	IV	(7.5 q12h)	(7.5 q12h)	7.5 q6h		20-25	
Rifampin	PO	Not recommended	Not recommended	10-20 q24h	0.6 q24h	7	≤1

Occasionally, resistance is mediated by failure of the penicillin to reach the site of infection. Some bacteria are resistant because, as a result of shape or electronic charge, penicillin cannot reach the binding site.

During the past decade, alteration in PBP has become an important mechanism of resistance. This is the mechanism of resistance responsible for methicillin resistance seen with *Staphylococcus aureus*. This mechanism also is responsible for the reduced susceptibility of *Streptococcus pneumoniae* to beta-lactams and other antimicrobics. Use of beta-lactamase–stable agents under these circumstances is not effective; however, the antimicrobial activity of beta-lactams and other classes of antimicrobics will vary from agent to agent.

Classification. Based on their specific antibacterial activity, penicillins can be classified loosely as (1) natural, (2) penicillinase-resistant, (3) amino, (4) antipseudomonad, and (5) extended-spectrum. The practitioner should be well versed in the use of one penicillin from each class, as presented in this chapter in the section on use of selected penicillins.

Pharmacological properties. Penicillins vary greatly in absorption after oral administration, with penicillin V, amoxicillin, cloxacillin, and dicloxacillin having the greatest absorption. Food reduces the absorption of oxacillin and dicloxacillin but not of penicillin V or amoxicillin. Procaine penicillin G and benzathine penicillin G are absorbed slowly after intramuscular injection and are given every 12 to 24 hours and every 15 to 20 days, respectively. Penicillins are excreted by renal tubular cells and have a very short half-life, ranging from less than 30 minutes to slightly more than 1 hour. Penicillins are distributed to most areas of the body if inflammation is present. However, they are poorly lipid soluble and do not enter the central nervous system (CNS) well, even if inflammation is present. Penicillins do not enter cells well. Passage of penicillins from the serum of a pregnant woman to her fetus depends on the degree of protein binding present; little of highly protein-bound penicillins reaches the fetus.

Side effects. The most important adverse reactions to penicillins are caused by hypersensitivity; they range from skin rashes to anaphylaxis. Anaphylactic reactions to penicillin are IgE mediated and occur in about 1 of every 500 courses of treatment (0.2%); about 1 of every 100,000 courses results in a fatality (0.001%).[3] The morbilliform rashes seen during therapy with penicillins probably are IgM mediated and often disappear even when therapy is continued. Less common reactions include serum sickness, exfoliative dermatitis, and Stevens-Johnson syndrome.

Penicillin desensitization. When it is deemed important to use penicillin in a patient who may have an anaphylactic reaction, immunotolerance to penicillin can be achieved by starting with very small doses. An effective protocol is to administer 5 U of penicillin G intracutaneously, in the forearm, and then, at 60- to 90-minute intervals, increase the dose to 10, 100, 1000, 10,000, and 50,000 U. If the intradermal doses are tolerated, IV penicillin can be instituted.

Use of selected penicillins (see Table 31-1). The natural penicillins listed in Table 31-1 are penicillin G (aqueous, procaine, and benzathine) and penicillin V. These antimicrobial agents are most active against both aerobic and anaerobic gram-positive cocci, *Neisseria meningitidis, Neisseria gonorrhoeae, Fusobacterium* species, *Eikenella* species, *Listeria monocytogenes,* and *Borrelia burgdorferi.* Penicillins still are the mainstay of treatment for infections caused by group A beta-hemolytic streptococci, group B streptococci, *Streptococcus pneumoniae, N. meningitidis,* and *L. monocytogenes.* Penicillin also is the drug of choice for acute infections with *B. burgdorferi* (Lyme disease) in children and for infections caused by anaerobes normally found in the mouth.

The potassium salt of penicillin G usually is used and is almost exclusively given intravenously. When given intramuscularly, aqueous penicillin G is excreted very rapidly; when given by mouth, it is poorly absorbed. Either procaine or benzathine preparations are used for intramuscular administration. It must be remembered, however, that very low serum concentrations are achieved with these preparations; they can be used only for exquisitely sensitive organisms and generally should not be used to treat CNS infections. Procaine penicillin can be used in a newborn to treat neurosyphilis. Penicillin V is well absorbed from the gastrointestinal tract and, therefore, is preferred for oral administration. Peak serum concentrations and MIC_{95} equivalents for susceptibility by disk are listed for individual penicillins in Table 31-1.

Ampicillin has the same general activity as penicillin, but it also is active against *Escherichia coli, Proteus mirabilis, Salmonella* species, and *Shigella* species and is more active against group D streptococci and *L. monocytogenes.* Amoxicillin differs from ampicillin in molecular composition only by the presence of a hydroxyl group. Because amoxicillin is absorbed much better than ampicillin, peak serum concentrations of amoxicillin after oral administration are equal to those achieved with an equivalent dose of ampicillin given intramuscularly. The antimicrobial activity of amoxicillin is virtually identical to that of ampicillin, except that it is not useful in the treatment of shigellosis; because of the increased absorption of amoxicillin, less drug is available in the intestinal tract.

Several fixed combination, beta-lactam/beta-lactamase inhibitors are available. Beta-lactamase inhibitors include clavulanic acid, sulbactam, and tazobactam. Four agents currently are available: amoxicillin-clavulanate (Augmentin), ampicillin-sulbactam (Unasyn), ticarcillin-clavulanate (Timentin), and piperacillin-tazobactam (Zosyn). Piperacillin-tazobactam does not have a pediatric indication for its use. The beta-lactamase inhibitor extends the activity of the beta-lactam to include some organisms that produce beta-lactamase. Amoxicillin/clavulanate, for example, is active against beta-lactamase producing *Staphylococcus aureus, H. influenzae, N. gonorrhoeae,* and *Moraxella catarrhalis* that otherwise would be resistant to amoxicillin. The MIC for *E. coli, Klebsiella* species, *Proteus* species, and *Bacteroides fragilis* ranges from 8 to 16 µg/ml. This combination is no more active than amoxicillin for *Streptococcus pneumoniae* strains that are resistant to penicillin. Ampicillin in a fixed combination with sulbactam is marketed as Unasyn for intravenous use only. The activity of ampicillin-sulbactam is similar to that of ampicillin-clavulanate, and this agent frequently is used in adults and children for respiratory infections and infections in which anaerobes are likely to be pathogens, such as intraabdominal or intraoral infections. Safety and efficacy for intraabdominal infections in pediatric patients have not been established. Ticarcillin-clavulanate (Timentin) and piperacillin-tazobactam (Zosyn) utilize a beta-lactam that is an extended-spectrum penicillin with antipseudomonal activity, thereby extending the spectrum of these fixed combinations further. These agents would be more appropriate for infections in which gram-negative organisms, including *Pseudomonas,* are thought to be pathogens.

Nafcillin is one of several penicillinase-resistant penicillins used primarily to treat infections caused by *S. aureus.* Most strains of *S. aureus* are inhibited by concentrations of 2 to 3 μg/ml. Because nafcillin is highly protein bound, methicillin is preferred for newborns when the possibility of kernicterus is a concern, because the amount of albumin for binding bilirubin will be diminished. Absorption of nafcillin from the gastrointestinal (GI) tract is erratic; it should not be given orally. Dicloxacillin is absorbed from the GI tract more consistently and is a good oral agent for treating *S. aureus* infections. The oral suspension of dicloxacillin has a very bitter taste, which can create problems with compliance.

Several antipseudomonad and extended-spectrum penicillins currently are available. In general, *Pseudomonas* infections should be treated with a combination of one of these agents plus an aminoglycoside, both for synergy and to reduce the emergence of resistant bacteria. A possible exception to this rule is for the treatment of a urinary tract infection caused by *Pseudomonas aeruginosa.* Mezlocillin has the antipseudomonad activity of carbenicillin and ticarcillin, plus it is more active against enterococci, *Klebsiella* species, *H. influenzae,* and *B. fragilis.* It is important to remember that a report of "susceptible to mezlocillin" means that concentrations as high as 64 μg/ml will be needed to inhibit 95% of the strains tested; this is compensated for by the high serum concentrations achieved when the drug is given intravenously (the peak serum concentration is 300 μg/ml after an intravenous dose of 4 g).

Cephalosporins

Mechanism of action. Like penicillins, cephalosporins are beta-lactam antibiotics that interfere with cell wall synthesis. However, the precise mechanism is not known, and the effects of cephalosporins on bacteria range from lysing the organism to producing bacteria that have unusual morphologies.

Bacterial resistance. Bacterial resistance to cephalosporins can arise if the cephalosporin is inactivated by beta-lactamase, if it is unable to reach antibiotic-binding proteins, if the bacteria does not have appropriate binding sites, or if tolerance develops (see the previous discussion of penicillins).

Classification. In the past two decades, more new cephalosporins have been introduced for general use than any other type of antimicrobial agent.[10] Currently, ceftriaxone and cefotaxime are two of the agents used most commonly for the empirical therapy of the febrile infant. The usual classification system for cephalosporins is based on antibacterial activity and is divided into first, second, and third generations (Box 31-1). Some experts recently have added a fourth generation. This classification system appears more useful for parenteral agents and may result in very dissimilar agents being grouped together. In general, the first-generation cephalosporins have good activity against gram-positive cocci except enterococci, coagulase-negative staphylococcal species, and methicillin-resistant *S. aureus;* they have limited activity against gram-negative organisms except *E. coli, Klebsiella pneumoniae,* and *P. mirabilis.* Activity of these agents against Enterobacteriaceae is unpredictable; the clinician should be guided by in vitro susceptibility testing. Organisms susceptible to one cephalosporin of this class are generally susceptible to all. The second-generation cephalosporins have the general activity of the first generation but are somewhat more active against gram-negative organisms, including *H. influenzae.* Third-generation cephalosporins are more active than second-generation drugs against gram-negative organisms but are less active against some gram-positive organisms, especially *S. aureus,* than are the first-generation drugs.

Pharmacological properties. Because of the number of cephalosporins and the wide variations in pharmacology, each drug should be considered individually.

Side effects. The side effects seen with cephalosporins generally are those seen with penicillins. Hypersensitivity reactions are the most common side effects. Although immunological studies have shown about a 20% cross-reactivity between penicillins and cephalosporins, in practice

BOX 31-1

CEPHALOSPORINS

First Generation
Cefadroxil*
Cefazolin
Cephalexin*
Cephalothin
Cephapirin
Cephradine†

Second Generation
Cefaclor*
Cefamandole
Cefmetazole
Cefonicid
Cefotetan
Cefotiam
Cefoxitin
Cefprozil*
Cefuroxime
Cefuroxime axetil*

Third Generation
Cefepime
Cefixime*
Cefmenoxime
Cefoperazone
Cefotaxime
Cefpiramide
Cefpodoxime proxetil*
Ceftazidime
Ceftibutin*
Ceftizoxime
Ceftriaxone
Moxalactam

*Oral
†Oral and parenteral.
All others are parenteral.

only 5% to 10% of persons who have hypersensitivity reactions to penicillins have them with cephalosporins. In general, if a patient has had only a nonurticarial rash as the manifestation of penicillin hypersensitivity, it is safe to use cephalosporins. For patients who have had urticaria or an anaphylactic reaction in response to penicillins, cephalosporins should be used with great caution or not at all. Less common side effects with cephalosporins are nephrotoxicity (cephaloridine should not be used), diarrhea, alcohol intolerance, and bleeding.

Use of selected cephalosporins

FIRST-GENERATION CEPHALOSPORINS. First-generation cephalosporins are used to treat infections caused by gram-positive cocci when penicillin cannot be used, to treat infections caused by methicillin-sensitive *S. aureus,* and to provide coverage against *E. coli, K. pneumoniae,* and *P. mirabilis.* Cefazolin is preferable to cephalothin because it has greater activity against *E. coli* and *Klebsiella* species, achieves higher peak serum concentrations, and has a longer half-life. The peak serum concentration of cefazolin after a dose of 1 g given intravenously is 188 μg/ml; the serum half-life is 1½ to 2 hours. Susceptible by disk means that 95% of the bacteria tested are inhibited by 8 μg/ml or less. The longer half-life compared with antistaphylococcal penicillins, nafcillin, or cephalothin makes cefazolin a particularly attractive agent for patients who are not hospitalized. Cefazolin can be given three times a day compared with the other agents, which require dosing four times a day. Cephalexin (Keflex) is a first-generation cephalosporin that can be given orally. A peak serum concentration of 16 μg/ml can be achieved with a dose of 0.5 g. The antibacterial activity of cephalexin is similar to that of cefazolin. Cefadroxil achieves peak serum concentrations and has antimicrobial activity similar to that of cephalexin but is excreted more slowly, allowing administration at 12- to 24-hour intervals.

SECOND-GENERATION CEPHALOSPORINS. Based on activity, second-generation cephalosporins should be divided further into two separate groups. The true cephalosporins of the second generation include cefuroxime and cefamandole.

Cefuroxime was used widely in pediatrics for the treatment of infection when gram-positive cocci such as *S. aureus* and *H. influenzae* were considered as likely pathogens. Many of these infections are now treated with the third-generation cephalosporins, ceftriaxone or cefotaxime, because of improved penetration into the cerebrospinal fluid and because of the possibility of *S. pneumoniae* as a pathogen in these circumstances. Cefuroxime is the only second-generation cephalosporin that achieves therapeutic concentrations in cerebrospinal fluid (CSF). For a time, cefuroxime was advocated as single-drug therapy for bacterial meningitis in infants and children older than 2 months of age. However, cefuroxime does not sterilize the CSF as rapidly as does ampicillin plus chloramphenicol or selected third-generation cephalosporins and should not be used to treat meningitis. Cefuroxime can be used when parenteral coverage for both *S. aureus* and *H. influenzae* is desirable in a patient who has no CNS infection.

The second-generation cephamycins include cefoxitin, cefotetan, and cefmetazole. These agents are rarely used in pediatrics because more suitable agents are available. Cefoxitin is highly resistant to beta-lactamases and is more active against anaerobes, especially *B. fragilis,* than are other cephalosporins. It is not as active as other second-generation cephalosporins against *H. influenzae* and Enterobacteriaceae, nor is it as active against gram-positive cocci as are first-generation cephalosporins. Cefotetan is more active against aerobic gram-negative bacilli than cefoxitin but is less active against aerobic gram-positive cocci. Cefmetazole appears to be more active against *S. aureus* than are either cefoxitin or cefotetan but is less active than cefotetan against Enterobacteriaceae and less active than cefoxitin against *B. fragilis.*[5] Because of its activity against anaerobes plus some gram-positive and gram-negative aerobes, cefoxitin has proved useful in the treatment of pelvic inflammatory disease and lung abscesses. The peak serum concentration after a dose of 1 g given intravenously is about 22 μg/ml; and the serum half-life is about 50 minutes. Susceptible by disk means that the MIC_{95} for the organism is 8 μg/ml or less. Use of cefoxitin declined dramatically in the 1990s because of the development of safer, more effective agents. Fixed-combination beta-lactam/beta-lactamase inhibitors including Unasyn are more active against anaerobes and have better activity against gram-positive cocci, including *S. aureus.* Metronidazole and carbapenems also are more active against anaerobes. Consequently, these agents are preferred in clinical situations in which cefoxitin may have been used in the past.

Second-generation cephalosporins available for oral administration include cefaclor (Ceclor), cefuroxime axetil (Ceftin), cefprozil (Cefzil), and loracarbef (Lorabid). Loracarbef technically is a carbecephem rather than a cephalosporin.[19] These agents are used primarily as the second- or third-line agents to treat upper respiratory infections (e.g., otitis media or sinusitis) in patients who have failed less expensive first-line agents such as amoxicillin. The structure and spectrum of activity of loracarbef are very similar to those of cefaclor.

THIRD-GENERATION CEPHALOSPORINS. The third-generation cephalosporins are more active than even the first- or second-generation drugs against gram-negative organisms, but these agents are less active against *S. aureus.* Cefotaxime and ceftriaxone are the most active of the cephalosporins against *S. pneumoniae,* including many strains that are resistant to penicillin as well as other streptococci.

Third-generation cephalosporins can be thought of as those that have a role in treating *Pseudomonas* infections and those that do not. Cefotaxime and ceftriaxone do not have activity against *P. aeruginosa.* Cefotaxime, the first third-generation cephalosporin to be used widely in the United States, is still useful clinically. Ceftriaxone is very similar to cefotaxime in antibacterial activity but has a much longer half-life. Both cefotaxime and ceftriaxone are active against most gram-positive aerobes except enterococci and *L. monocytogenes.* Neither is active against methicillin-resistant *S. aureus* or coagulase-negative staphylococci. Both are active against most gram-negative aerobic bacteria, except for *Pseudomonas* species. The diacetyl breakdown product of cefotaxime also has a broad range of activity, but specific activity is less than that of cefotaxime itself. The peak serum concentration after IV administration of 1 g of cefotaxime is about 40 μg/ml, compared with 150 μg/ml for ceftriaxone.

The serum half-life of cefotaxime is about 1 hour, compared with 8 hours for ceftriaxone. Because ceftriaxone is excreted slowly, a peak serum concentration of 50 μg/ml is achieved in adults after a dose of 0.5 g is given intramuscularly. Susceptible by disk means that the MIC_{95} of either drug for the bacteria tested is 8 μg/ml or less.

The two third-generation cephalosporins that have good antipseudomonad activity are cefoperazone and ceftazidime. Ceftazidime is more active than cefoperazone against *Pseudomonas* in vitro but is less active than cefotaxime against gram-positive organisms. Whether ceftazidime should be used as a single agent to treat *Pseudomonas* infections still is controversial. In adults, the peak serum concentration of ceftazidime after 1 g is given intravenously is 85 μg/ml; the serum half-life is about 1 hour and 48 minutes. About 90% of *Pseudomonas* isolates are inhibited by 8 μg/ml or less of ceftazidime.

Three third-generation cephalosporins currently are available for oral use; they are cefixime (Suprax), cefpodoxime proxetil (Vantin), and ceftibuten (Cedax).[19] Cefixime and ceftibuten have a similar spectrum; consequently, they are grouped together. They have limited activity against some gram-positive cocci such as *S. pneumoniae* and no activity against *S. aureus*. Both are active against the gram-negative bacilli responsible for most urinary tract infections. Because *S. pneumoniae* coverage is incomplete, these agents are recommended only as second-line agents for the treatment of otitis media, and only if treatment with an antimicrobial that has good antipneumococcal activity fails when used alone. Both of these agents are active against *Streptococcus pyogenes* and can be used for pharyngitis. The usual dose of cefixime is 8 mg/kg/day given as a single dose; the usual dose of ceftibuten is 9 mg/kg/day given once daily or divided into two equal doses.

Cefpodoxime proxetil has a spectrum of activity for gram-negative microorganisms that is similar to those of other oral third-generation cephalosporins. Cefpodoxime, however, has good activity against gram-positive cocci, including *S. pneumoniae, S. pyogenes,* and *S. aureus*. Cefpodoxime achieves higher tissue concentrations in the lungs and tonsils than do other cephalosporins. The usual dosage is 5 mg/kg every 12 hours, with a maximum dose of 400 mg/day for otitis media and 200 mg/day for pharyngitis or tonsillitis. Although the oral third-generation cephalosporins are effective in treating bacterial pneumonia, otitis media, tonsillitis, and pharyngitis, equally effective and less expensive alternatives are available.

FOURTH-GENERATION CEPHALOSPORINS. Currently, cefepime (Maxipime) is available for use in individuals older than 2 months. This agent tentatively has been classified as a fourth-generation cephalosporin. Available only for parenteral use, it is unique compared with other cephalosporins because of its broad spectrum of activity against both gram-positive cocci, including *S. aureus, S. pneumoniae,* and *S. pyogenes,* as well as most aerobic gram-negative bacilli, including *P. aeruginosa*. This agent has a half-life of 2 hours, which permits dosing twice daily at 100 mg/kg/day. It has been used primarily in adults for the treatment of pneumonia and febrile neutropenia. Although it appears to penetrate into the cerebrospinal fluid, it does not have an indication for the treatment of meningitis.

Other Beta-Lactam Antibiotics

Three other beta-lactam antibiotics—imipenem, meropenem (carbapenems), and aztreonam (monobactam)—have a limited role in the treatment of bacterial infections in children. Imipenem and meropenem have an extremely broad range of activity that covers most gram-positive organisms, including enterococci, *Listeria* species, and methicillin-susceptible staphylococci, including coagulase-negative staphylococci. Strains of *S. pneumoniae* that demonstrate intermediate or high levels of resistance to penicillin are frequently susceptible to these agents. Imipenem and meropenem also inhibit most Enterobacteriaceae, *P. aeruginosa,* and *Pseudomonas maltophilia,* as well as most anaerobic bacteria.

Because imipenem is rapidly destroyed by a renal peptidase, it is supplied in a fixed combination with a dehydropeptidase inhibitor called *cilastatin*. In adults, 500 mg of imipenem with cilastatin given intravenously produces an average peak serum concentration of 33 μg/ml; the serum half-life is about 1 hour. The MIC_{95} of bacteria susceptible by disk is 4 μg/ml or less. Imipenem's broad spectrum of antimicrobial activity seldom is required in clinical practice.

The major risk factor that has somewhat limited the usefulness of the carbapenems is seizure activity. The risk of seizures appears to be somewhat lower with meropenem compared with imipenem. Consequently, carbapenems should be used with caution in patients who have associated risk factors that may increase the likelihood of seizures, such as renal failure and CNS conditions, including meningitis.

Imipenem recently has been licensed for use in patients as young as 1 week of age. Meropenem, however, does not have an indication for use in children under 12 years of age. Given the broad spectrum of activity, these agents occasionally are useful in resistant infections with *S. pneumoniae,* mixed infections, including those caused by anaerobes, and in febrile neutropenic patients.

Aztreonam, a monobactam, has little activity against gram-positive or anaerobic bacteria because these bacteria have little PBP 3, which is the primary binding site for aztreonam. On the other hand, aztreonam is very active against Enterobacteriaceae (MIC, 0.5 μg/ml or less) and moderately active against *P. aeruginosa* (MIC, 16 μg/ml or less). In adults, 1 g of aztreonam given intravenously results in a peak serum concentration of about 125 μg/ml; the serum half-life is 1 hour and 42 minutes. Susceptible by disk means that the MIC_{95} will be 8 μg/ml or less. There is very little experience with the use of aztreonam in children.

Aminoglycosides

MECHANISMS OF ACTION. It is known that aminoglycosides inhibit bacterial protein synthesis, but a second mechanism appears to be necessary to explain bacterial killing, and this second mechanism is not yet known. Protein synthesis is inhibited through interaction with bacterial ribosomes at the interface between the smaller and larger ribosome subunits.

BACTERIAL RESISTANCE. There are three known mechanisms of bacterial resistance to aminoglycosides. The first, ribosomal resistance, is known to occur only with streptomycin, when alteration in the protein of the smaller ribosomal subunit results in inability to bind streptomycin.

The most common mechanism of resistance is the production of enzymes that inactivate the aminoglycosides. Because aminoglycosides are similar in structure, certain enzymes can inactivate more than one aminoglycoside. The capacity to produce aminoglycoside-inactivating enzymes is inherent among gram-negative aerobic bacteria and seldom occurs by induction. The number and types of enzymes vary among places and populations. As an aminoglycoside becomes used more widely, bacteria that produce inactivating enzymes become more prevalent. The ability to produce inactivating enzymes can be carried by plasmids and transferred among gram-negative bacteria. Amikacin appears to be an unsuitable substrate for many of these inactivating enzymes; consequently, amikacin may be active against some organisms resistant to other aminoglycosides, including gentamicin and tobramycin.

The third mechanism of resistance is bacterial impermeability to aminoglycosides. This mechanism is not very common, and it has been observed that permeability mutants generally are not very virulent. When an organism is susceptible to tobramycin or gentamicin (or both) but is resistant to amikacin, the amikacin resistance must be based on amikacin's inability to enter the organism. This must be the reason because the only enzyme produced by gram-negative organisms that inhibits amikacin also inhibits tobramycin and gentamicin.

PHARMACOLOGICAL PROPERTIES. Aminoglycosides are absorbed poorly or not at all after oral administration. Absorption after intramuscular administration is excellent, with the peak serum concentration occurring 30 to 90 minutes after administration. The serum concentration after intravenous administration over 20 to 30 minutes is about the same as after intramuscular administration. Aminoglycosides do not cross cell membranes well and, therefore, achieve poor concentrations inside most cells except renal tubular cells, which actively transport these agents. In general, only low concentrations of aminoglycosides are achieved in the CNS, eyes, biliary tract, or prostatic fluid. Aminoglycosides do enter synovial fluid well.

Because aminoglycosides are excreted by glomerular filtration, care must be taken to adjust the dosage for patients who have renal failure. After filtration, some of the aminoglycoside is reabsorbed by the proximal renal tubular cells; this reabsorption probably plays a role in nephrotoxicity caused by these drugs. By convention, the drug is infused over a 30-minute period, and the peak serum concentration is measured 30 minutes after the infusion is completed. With intramuscular administration, the peak serum concentration is measured 1 hour later. Because the therapeutic-to-toxic index is very low for aminoglycosides, the serum concentration should be monitored closely.

SIDE EFFECTS. The two most common side effects of aminoglycosides are ototoxicity and nephrotoxicity. Ototoxicity generally is considered to be reversible and is caused by destruction of the outer hair cells in the organ of Corti and possibly is related to the concentration of aminoglycoside in the endolymph or perilymph that bathes these cells. The relationship between serum concentrations and the development of ototoxicity remains unclear.[22] Some investigators have suggested that elevated trough concentrations predispose a patient to ototoxicity. Others have recently postulated that once-daily dosing of aminoglycosides may actually reduce the likelihood of ototoxicity by reducing drug accumulation in the inner ear.

Hearing loss generally begins at higher frequencies than those commonly used for conversation. Consequently, routine screening of hearing may be useful in patients at risk for auditory ototoxicity such as those who have cystic fibrosis and are receiving repeated courses of aminoglycosides. Vestibular toxicity is another manifestation of ototoxicity that is thought to be irreversible and can be very disabling. Transient elevations in aminoglycoside concentrations probably do not affect hearing.

Nephrotoxicity is manifested as a decrease in the glomerular filtration rate. As with ototoxicity, the relationship between serum concentrations and the development of nephrotoxicity is not completely understood. Nephrotoxicity generally is mild and reversible. Associated risk factors are frequently found in patients who have nephrotoxicity, including taking other medications and suffering concurrent illnesses. Again, some investigators have suggested that the risk of nephrotoxicity is reduced by administering the entire daily aminoglycoside dose once a day. Both ototoxicity and nephrotoxicity seem to occur less often in children than in adults. Nonetheless, it is important to monitor the serum concentration to make sure it is both safe and therapeutic, especially when dosed two or three times daily.

Aminoglycosides also can cause neuromuscular paralysis, particularly when given along with curare-like drugs, in the presence of botulin toxin, and in patients who have myasthenia gravis. Neuromuscular paralysis usually does not occur if aminoglycosides are given intramuscularly and when they are given intravenously within 30 minutes. Neuromuscular paralysis can be treated by the administration of calcium.

USE. Streptomycin, the first aminoglycoside used clinically, is used almost exclusively to treat tuberculosis, but it also is used to treat tularemia, plague, and brucellosis. Neomycin is used primarily to reduce the number of bacteria in the large bowel. It is given by mouth, and very little reaches the bloodstream.

Three aminoglycosides—gentamicin, tobramycin, and amikacin—currently are used systemically to treat serious infections caused by gram-negative aerobic bacteria. In general, there is no evidence that one of these aminoglycosides is clinically superior to another in the treatment of susceptible bacteria. Tobramycin is more active against *P. aeruginosa* than is gentamicin or amikacin, but differences in its clinical effectiveness have not been observed. Tobramycin and amikacin are somewhat less nephrotoxic than gentamicin. As previously stated, amikacin is susceptible to inactivation by one aminoglycoside-inactivating enzyme, whereas tobramycin and gentamicin are inactivated by at least six enzymes. Thus, organisms are less likely to be resistant to amikacin than to either tobramycin or gentamicin. Because amikacin is less toxic on a weight basis, a larger dose is given and a higher peak serum concentration is achieved. With a dose of 7.5 mg/kg of amikacin given intravenously, the peak serum concentration averages 38 μg/ml. At a dose of 2 mg/kg of tobramycin or gentamicin, the peak serum concentration ranges from 3 to 12 μg/ml. All three drugs have a serum half-life of 2 to 2½ hours. The MIC_{95} of amikacin for bacteria reported susceptible by disk is 16 μg/ml or less; the MIC_{95} of gentamicin or tobramycin is 4 μg/ml or less.

Once-daily dosing of aminoglycosides has been found to have several advantages over dosing every 8 to 12 hours. The pharmacodynamic model presented earlier suggests that because aminoglycosides kill in a concentration-dependent manner, once-daily dosing should offer more rapid and effective killing of bacteria.[2] Once-daily dosing results in a higher peak serum concentration, an acceptably low trough concentration, and possibly a lower incidence of nephrotoxicity and ototoxicity. Dosing once daily also facilitates more convenient administration and reduces costs. Gentamicin and tobramycin are dosed at 4 to 7 mg/kg/day, producing a peak serum concentration that ranges from 10 to 20 μg/ml and a trough concentration below 2 μg/ml. Actually, the serum concentration will be below the MIC for a substantial portion of the dosing interval. Amikacin is dosed at 15 mg/kg/day, with a resulting peak serum concentration of 54 μg/ml and a trough concentration below 5 μg/ml. Monitoring serum concentrations in patients receiving once-daily dosing generally is accomplished by obtaining a single serum sample 6 hours after the dose. A nomogram is available that then enables the physician to decide whether that dose is administered most appropriately once a day, every 36 hours, or once ever other day.[14] Despite studies showing an efficacy equivalent to divided daily doses, once-daily administration of aminoglycosides has not become widespread in pediatrics. It appears that a majority of adult patients, however, are treated using a single daily dose. Some investigators have cautioned that once-daily dosing should not be used for patients who have enterococcal endocarditis, who are newborns, or who are febrile and neutropenic.

Sulfonamides and trimethoprim

MECHANISMS OF ACTION. Sulfonamides inhibit bacterial growth by reducing bacterial synthesis of folic acid, resulting in a decrease in bacterial nucleotides. Trimethoprim inhibits bacterial dihydrofolate reductase, which is the step in folic acid synthesis that follows the one inhibited by sulfonamides. The combination of trimethoprim and sulfamethoxazole results in a synergistic, sequential blockage of folic acid.

BACTERIAL RESISTANCE. Resistance to sulfonamides can be based on overproduction of substrate by the bacteria or a change in enzyme structure to one that has diminished sulfonamide binding. Trimethoprim resistance also may be caused by a decline in the bacteria's capacity to bind the drug or to a change in dihydrofolate reductase. Resistance to both drugs can result if an organism develops decreased permeability to the drugs. Resistance occurs less often when the combination trimethoprim-sulfamethoxazole (TMP-SMX) is used.

PHARMACOLOGICAL PROPERTIES. The sulfonamides currently used in the United States, either alone or in combination with trimethoprim, are sulfisoxazole (Gantrisin), sulfamethoxazole, and sulfadiazine. Sulfonamides usually are given orally, but intravenous preparations of sulfadiazine and sulfisoxazole are available. These sulfonamides are quickly and completely absorbed from the stomach and small intestine. Sulfonamides are distributed throughout the body, including the CSF. They readily cross the placenta and are found in fetal blood. Sulfonamides are partially metabolized in the liver, and free drug metabolites are excreted by glomerular filtration.

Trimethoprim also usually is given orally and is readily absorbed. It is well distributed throughout the body, with the CSF concentration reaching about 40% of the serum concentration. Excretion is primarily by renal tubular secretion.

SIDE EFFECTS. A wide variety of toxicities are associated with sulfonamides, ranging from GI upset, headache, and rash to serum sickness and hepatic necrosis. Severe hypersensitivity reactions can occur, such as toxic epidermal necrolysis, Stevens-Johnson syndrome, erythema nodosum, vasculitis, and anaphylaxis. Blood cell disorders, including aplastic anemia, granulocytopenia, thrombocytopenia, and leukopenia, have been attributed to sulfonamides. Patients who have glucose-6-phosphate dehydrogenase (G6PD) deficiency are at heightened risk for aplastic anemia. Sulfonamides should not be taken during the last month of pregnancy because they cross the placenta and compete for bilirubin-binding sites, increasing the risk for kernicterus. All the side effects associated with sulfonamides can occur with trimethoprim as well, the most common being GI upset and hypersensitivity reactions. With prolonged use, trimethoprim can interfere with folate metabolism, resulting in a megaloblastic anemia. This can be prevented by administering folinic acid.

USE OF TRIMETHOPRIM-SULFAMETHOXAZOLE AND SELECTED SULFONAMIDES. The combination of trimethoprim and sulfamethoxazole was introduced initially to treat urinary tract infections. However, because of its wide range of antibacterial activity, it has proved useful in a number of bacterial infections. Gram-positive organisms susceptible to TMP-SMX include both coagulase-positive and coagulase-negative staphylococci, *S. pneumoniae,* enterococci, *Listeria* species, and *S. pyogenes.* However, TMP-SMX is not as effective as penicillin in the treatment of *S. pyogenes.* Many strains that are methicillin resistant are susceptible to TMP-SMX. TMP-SMX also is inhibitory for a wide range of gram-negative aerobic organisms, including *E. coli, Klebsiella* species, *Salmonella* species, *Shigella* species, *H. influenzae,* and *N. meningitidis.*

Trimethoprim-sulfamethoxazole is useful in the treatment of acute urinary tract infections and for long-term bacterial suppression in patients who have chronic or recurrent urinary tract infections, respiratory tract infections, otitis media, sinusitis, prostatitis, orchitis, and epididymitis. TMP-SMX is the drug of choice for treating *Pneumocystis carinii* infections and has proved effective in preventing *P. carinii* infection in children who have malignancies. Many adults infected with the human immunodeficiency virus (HIV) do not tolerate TMP-SMX well. To date, however, this has not been a major problem in HIV-infected infants. The peak serum concentrations for both drugs, reached about 2 hours after an oral dose, average 2 μg/ml for trimethoprim and 60 μg/ml for sulfamethoxazole. After repeated doses the peak serum concentration of trimethoprim approaches 9 μg/ml. The MIC_{95} for bacteria susceptible to the combination is 2 μg/ml or less for trimethoprim and 38 μg/ml or less for sulfamethoxazole. However, the combination usually is synergistic in vivo.

Sulfisoxazole is used primarily to treat acute urinary tract infections or to effect long-term suppression in patients who have chronic or recurrent urinary tract infections. Sulfadiazine is effective prophylaxis for close contacts of patients who have *N. meningitidis* infections if the strain is known to be susceptible (see Chapter 291, Meningococcemia). The peak serum concentrations after an oral dose of 2 g range from 30 to 60 μg/ml for sulfadiazine, 40 to 50 μg/ml for sulfisoxazole, and 80 to 100 μg/ml for sulfamethoxazole.

Topical sulfonamides are used primarily in two settings. Ophthalmic preparations of sulfacetamide are used to treat acute conjunctivitis and as adjunctive therapy in the treatment of trachoma. Silver sulfadiazine is used in the topical treatment of burns. In this combination, the sulfadiazine serves principally as a vehicle for the release of silver ions, which have an antibacterial effect.

Macrolides and Azalides: Erythromycin, Clarithromycin, and Azithromycin

Mechanism of action. Macrolides inhibit RNA-dependent protein synthesis at the step of chain elongation.

Bacterial resistance. Bacteria that lack the appropriate binding site are resistant to erythromycin, as are bacteria that are less permeable to the drug.

Erythromycin

PHARMACOLOGICAL PROPERTIES. A number of erythromycin preparations are available for oral administration. Erythromycin base is destroyed by gastric acid and, therefore, is useful only when given as an enteric-coated tablet. Pediatric preparations use the ester or ester salt derivatives of erythromycin because they are acid stable, soluble, and tasteless. Preparations vary in their rate and degree of absorption from the GI tract. The best absorbed is the estolate ester, which results in a peak serum concentration of about 4 μg/ml. The ethylsuccinate and stearate preparations produce peak serum concentrations that range from 0.4 to 1.9 μg/ml when given at a dose equivalent to the ester. Erythromycin is distributed throughout the body and persists in tissue longer than in the blood. Therapeutic concentrations are reached in middle ear fluid, paranasal sinuses, tonsils, and pleural fluid, but not the CSF, even when the meninges are inflamed. Limited data suggest that entry into synovial fluid is poor.

Erythromycin's route of elimination is not clear. A small percentage of a dose of erythromycin can be found in the urine, and erythromycin is known to be concentrated in and excreted with bile. However, most of an administered dose cannot be recovered.

SIDE EFFECTS. The most common side effect of erythromycin is GI upset characterized by abdominal pain, nausea, vomiting, or diarrhea. Erythromycin actually is used primarily to promote gastrointestinal motility in some adults. Allergic reactions occur but are relatively uncommon. Cholestatic hepatitis occurs after treatment with the estolate ester but can be seen with any of the preparations. This side effect has been seen primarily in adults. The better absorption characteristics of the estolate preparation of erythromycin probably outweigh the slight risk of cholestatic hepatitis in children.

USE. Erythromycin has a broad range of antibacterial activity and is the drug of choice for infections caused by *Mycoplasma pneumoniae, Legionella* species, *Corynebacterium diphtheriae, Bordetella pertussis, Chlamydia trachomatis,* and *Campylobacter jejuni*. Erythromycin is an alternative drug for the treatment of streptococcal and staphylococcal infections and as prophylaxis for syphilis, urinary tract infections, rheumatic fever, and bacterial endocarditis. The MIC_{95} of erythromycin required to inhibit bacteria reported as susceptible by disk is 0.5 μg/ml or less. Lactobionate and gluceptate preparations are available for parenteral administration but are not used often. The peak serum concentration after intravenous administration is about equal to that achieved when estolate is given by mouth.

Clarithromycin

PHARMACOLOGICAL PROPERTIES. Clarithromycin is stable in gastric acid and is well absorbed from the GI tract; further, its bioavailability is not affected by food.[7,13] A peak serum concentration of 4 to 5 μg/ml is reached in 2½ to 3 hours, and concentrations in middle ear fluid and lung tissue exceed serum concentrations. The major route of excretion is in bile, but about one third of an administered dose can be recovered in the urine. A metabolite of clarithromycin, 14-hydroxyclarithromycin, achieves a serum concentration that is about 60% that of clarithromycin and is about twice as active against *H. influenzae*.

SIDE EFFECTS. Clarithromycin causes much less gastric upset than does erythromycin, but diarrhea (6% of cases), vomiting (6%), abdominal pain (3%), and nausea (1%) are the most common side effects. Pediatric patients frequently complain that the suspension is unpalatable and leaves an unpleasant aftertaste.

USE. Clinical trials have demonstrated efficacy in the treatment of otitis media, pharyngitis, skin and soft-tissue infections, *Mycobacterium avium* complex (MAC) infections, and *Helicobacter pylori* infections. In general, clarithromycin can be used for infections traditionally treated with erythromycin. Because of the activity of its 14-hydroxy breakdown product, clarithromycin may prove useful in *H. influenzae* infections.

Azithromycin

Azithromycin differs structurally from erythromycin and clarithromycin by having a 15-member rather than a 14-member ring.[7,21] Because of its unique structure, azithromycin has a much larger volume of distribution, a longer half-life, and greater penetration at the cellular level. In vitro studies show equivalent antimicrobial activity for gram-positive cocci and atypical pathogens, including *Mycoplasma*. Azithromycin is more effective against *H. influenzae* than erythromycin or clarithromycin. Because of its volume of distribution and longer half-life, once-daily dosing is appropriate, and short-course therapy for streptococcal pharyngitis (i.e., 5 days) is recommended.

The macrolide antibiotics may interact with other drugs by inducing cytochrome P-450. Commonly used drugs that may interact include theophylline, zidovudine, cimetidine, and most anticonvulsants. Because azithromycin does not induce formation of cytochrome P-450, drug-to-drug interactions do not occur with this formulation.

Clindamycin

MECHANISM OF ACTION. Clindamycin shares binding sites with erythromycin and chloramphenicol on the 50S ribosomal subunit and interferes with protein synthesis by inhibiting the transpeptidation reaction.

MECHANISMS OF RESISTANCE. The mechanisms of bacterial resistance are the same as for erythromycin.

PHARMACOLOGICAL PROPERTIES. Clindamycin usually is given orally, but preparations for intramuscular and intravenous administration are available. About 90% of a dose of clindamycin is absorbed after oral administration, and peak serum concentrations are reached in 1 hour and are dose dependent. Clindamycin palmitate (oral suspension) and clindamycin phosphate (preparation for intravenous administration) are inactive but are hydrolyzed rapidly in vivo to the active free base. Clindamycin is well distributed throughout the body except for the CSF. Clindamycin is one of the few antimicrobial agents that is concentrated in polymorphonuclear neutrophils. The serum half-life of clindamycin is about 2 hours and 24 minutes. Most clindamycin is metabolized in the liver to products that have variable antibacterial activity. Antibacterial activity in the bile and GI tract is very high and results in a dramatic decline in sensitive bowel flora.

SIDE EFFECTS. The most highly publicized side effect of clindamycin is the occurrence of colitis secondary to the toxin of *Clostridium difficile* (pseudomembranous colitis). This complication now has been associated with many other antimicrobial agents and seems to occur less often in children than in adults. Other side effects include allergic reactions, rashes, and minor elevations in transaminase concentrations.

USE. Clindamycin is highly active against most gram-positive aerobic bacteria and most anaerobic bacteria. The major clinical use of clindamycin is the treatment of anaerobic infections. Clindamycin is used routinely when intraabdominal spillage of fecal material has occurred, and it also is used to treat anaerobic bronchopulmonary infections. When used for the treatment of intraabdominal infections, it generally is given along with an aminoglycoside. Clindamycin also is used as alternative therapy for groups A and B streptococcal infections and as oral therapy to complete a course of antibiotics for *S. aureus* osteomyelitis. Under these circumstances, clindamycin is an especially attractive alternative in patients who are allergic to beta-lactams. Many stains of penicillin-resistant *S. pneumoniae* remain susceptible to clindamycin in the United States. Consequently, clindamycin occasionally has been used in this clinical circumstance. Clindamycin does not enter the CSF in useful concentrations. A peak serum concentration of 2.5 to 3.6 μg/ml is achieved about 1 hour after oral administration, and a concentration of 6 to 9 μg/ml can be reached after intravenous infusion. The MIC_{95} of clindamycin for bacteria reported as susceptible by disk is 0.5 μg/ml or less.

Chloramphenicol

MECHANISM OF ACTION. Like erythromycin and clindamycin, chloramphenicol binds to the 50S ribosomal subunit and inhibits protein synthesis.

BACTERIAL RESISTANCE. Mechanisms of resistance include (1) bacterial production of an acetyltransferase that inactivates chloramphenicol and (2) inability of chloramphenicol to enter bacteria.

PHARMACOLOGICAL PROPERTIES. Chloramphenicol can be given orally as the free base or as chloramphenicol palmitate, which is hydrolyzed in the intestine to free base. Because chloramphenicol is extremely bitter, oral palmitate suspension is given to patients who cannot take capsules containing free base. The intravenous preparation is chloramphenicol succinate, which also is hydrolyzed to free base. Because the palmitate is hydrolyzed more completely than the succinate, its peak serum concentration generally is higher after oral administration. Chloramphenicol distributes well throughout the body, including the brain and CSF. Chloramphenicol is conjugated by the liver and excreted in an inactive form in urine.

SIDE EFFECTS. The major side effects of chloramphenicol are dose-related bone marrow suppression, which is reversible; aplastic anemia, which is idiosyncratic and usually fatal; and gray-baby syndrome. Gray-baby syndrome was first described and occurs most commonly in infants, but it has been reported in all age groups. The syndrome, which is characterized by cyanosis, circulatory collapse, and death, occurs when the chloramphenicol concentration becomes very high.

USE. Chloramphenicol's importance in the treatment of infectious diseases has waxed and waned since its introduction in the late 1940s. Because of its side effects, practitioners have tended to use alternative antimicrobial agents whenever possible. However, because of its antibacterial and pharmacological properties, it often must be included to optimize treatment. With the introduction of the third-generation cephalosporins, use of chloramphenicol in the United States has declined sharply. Formerly, chloramphenicol frequently was considered the drug of choice to treat brain abscesses, bacterial meningitis in infants and children older than 2 months of age, typhoid fever, and salmonellosis. Currently, metronidazole frequently is selected for anaerobic coverage in brain abscesses, ceftriaxone or cefotaxime for bacterial meningitis, and either TMP-SMX or ceftriaxone to treat typhoid fever and salmonellosis. Although chloramphenicol, rather than tetracycline, is considered by many to be the drug of choice for rickettsial infections in children younger than 8 years, some experts continue to consider tetracyclines to be the drug of choice for children who have rickettsial disease or ehrlichiosis regardless of their age. Chloramphenicol frequently is active against vancomycin-resistant enterococci and frequently is included in regimens to treat such infections. Data are limited concerning use of chloramphenicol in ehrlichiosis, but some studies have suggested that it may be less effective or ineffective in the treatment of human granulocytic ehrlichiosis in contrast to monocytic ehrlichiosis. Tetracycline use in children younger than 8 years generally is precluded because of its well-known side effects. Some experts recommend tetracycline when the benefits and the risks of its use are weighed. These are considered more fully under the discussion of tetracyclines.

When chloramphenicol must be used, the peak serum concentration should be measured after four or five doses to ensure that the concentration is safe and therapeutic and that the drug is not accumulating in the patient. A complete blood count and differential count should be done twice a week while the patient is receiving chloramphenicol to check for dose-related bone marrow suppression. The peak serum concentration is reached 1 to 2 hours after oral or intravenous administration and averages 25 μg/ml (PO) and 19 μg/ml IV.[11] The serum half-life of chloramphenicol is about 4 hours. The MIC_{95} of chloramphenicol for bacteria reported as susceptible by disk is 4 μg/ml or less for *H. influenzae* and 12.5 μg/ml or less for other organisms. Although chloramphenicol is bactericidal for *H. influenzae, S. pneumoniae,* and *N. meningitidis,* it is bacteriostatic for most other bacteria. When used with a beta-lactam to treat organisms inhibited only by chloramphenicol, antagonism may occur.[16]

Tetracycline

MECHANISM OF ACTION. Tetracycline binds to the 30S ribosomal subunit and blocks aminoacyl-tRNA binding to the receptor site; this inhibits protein synthesis.

BACTERIAL RESISTANCE. Tetracycline's entry into bacterial cells is energy dependent; resistance usually is based on interference with entry into the cell. In general, tetracycline is not altered by resistant bacteria.

PHARMACOLOGICAL PROPERTIES. A number of analogs of tetracycline have been produced, but the range of antibacterial activity is similar for each. The semisynthetic analogs, minocycline and doxycycline, are the most active tetracyclines but are used less often than are other tetracyclines because they are considerably more expensive.

Tetracycline has a broad spectrum of activity that includes inhibition of *Streptococcus* species, *Neisseria* species, *E. coli,* and many common anaerobic bacteria. Tetracyclines are well absorbed from the intestinal tract, and the peak serum concentration is achieved 1 to 3 hours after oral administration. Tetracycline distributes in varying concentrations throughout most of the body, with concentrations in synovial fluid, urine, and the maxillary sinuses approaching the serum concentration, whereas the CSF concentration reaches only 10% to 20% of the serum concentration.

SIDE EFFECTS. The side effects of tetracycline essentially preclude its use in children younger than age 8 years and in pregnant women. Tetracycline causes a permanent gray-brown to yellowish discoloration of the teeth and can be associated with hypoplasia of the enamel. Skeletal growth can be depressed when the drug is given to premature infants. Although bone and tooth defects are associated with the total dose of tetracycline given and occur more often after repeated courses, it is safest to avoid using the drug during pregnancy and in young children. Although these side effects generally preclude the use of tetracycline in children younger than 8 years, for rickettsial diseases and ehrlichiosis, some experts continue to consider doxycycline the drug of choice because the usual duration of therapy is only 7 to 10 days and staining of teeth is related to the total dose received.[16] Doxycycline is less likely to stain teeth than are other tetracyclines. In addition, tetracyclines are effective against both rickettsial diseases or ehrlichiosis, but chloramphenicol may not be (see p. 412). Other side effects of tetracycline are allergic reactions and skin toxicity.

USE. For individuals older than age 8 years, tetracycline is considered the drug of choice for brucellosis, chlamydial infections, lymphogranuloma venereum, epididymitis, granuloma inguinale, infections with spirochetes (Lyme disease, relapsing fever, leptospirosis), pelvic inflammatory disease, plague, prostatitis, and rickettsial infections. Tetracycline also is an effective alternative drug for many other infectious diseases.

In adults, the peak serum concentrations after oral administration of 500 mg of tetracycline or 200 mg of doxycycline or minocycline are 4 μg/ml, 2.5 μg/ml, and 2.5 μg/ml, respectively. The peak serum concentration is reached 1 to 3 hours after administration. The serum half-life of tetracycline is 8 hours, compared with 16 hours for minocycline and 18 hours for doxycycline. Intravenous administration of tetracycline results in a peak serum concentration about twice that achieved when the same dose is given by mouth. The MIC_{95} of tetracycline for bacteria reported as susceptible by disk is 4 μg/ml or less.

Vancomycin

MECHANISM OF ACTION. Vancomycin inhibits cell wall synthesis during the second stage by inhibiting formation of peptidoglycan. This is in contrast to beta-lactams that inhibit cell wall synthesis during the final stage by binding to the penicillin-binding proteins, which are enzymes crucial to the formation of the cell wall.

BACTERIAL RESISTANCE. To date, no cross-resistance between vancomycin and other antimicrobial agents has been observed. However, enterococci resistant to vancomycin (and all other approved antimicrobial agents) have become a clinical problem in some regions. As the use of vancomycin increases, the number of resistant bacteria probably will increase.

PHARMACOLOGICAL PROPERTIES. Vancomycin is absorbed minimally after oral administration and is given orally only to treat pseudomembranous colitis caused by the toxin of *C. difficile*. Most experts prefer to use metronidazole for this indication because increased use of vancomycin has been associated with a marked increase in resistance of commonly encountered gram-positive organisms. After intravenous administration, vancomycin is distributed throughout the body, except for the aqueous humor of the eye and the CSF when the meninges are not inflamed. A bactericidal concentration can be achieved in the CSF in cases of meningitis caused by susceptible organisms. Sometimes, vancomycin must be administered intraventricularly to treat meningitis adequately with or without ventriculitis. Vancomycin is excreted unchanged in the urine by glomerular filtration. It, therefore, is important in certain circumstances to monitor the serum concentration and adjust the dosage based on renal function. (See the following discussion.)

SIDE EFFECTS. When vancomycin initially became available for clinical use, commercial preparations contained as much as 20% of another substance, and its use was limited because of its toxicity. Currently available preparations are more highly purified and less toxic. The most common side effects are fever, chills, and pain at the injection site or, less often, flushing and tingling of the face, neck, and thorax (red neck syndrome). These side effects can be avoided largely by infusing vancomycin slowly in a large volume of fluid. Reports of ototoxicity and nephrotoxicity caused solely by vancomycin have been difficult to confirm. Furthermore, the relationship of toxicity to serum concentrations remains controversial. In the pediatric population, it appears that ototoxicity and nephrotoxicity are uncommon, and no clear correlation between serum concentrations and toxicity has been proven. Consequently, many experts now recommend that *routine* monitoring of vancomycin levels is unnecessary. Routine monitoring also seems to offer little relative to establishing a therapeutic dose. In children who have no underlying conditions, levels in the "therapeutic range" almost invariably are achieved.[20] Many experts feel that it would be reasonable to monitor vancomycin serum concentrations under the following circumstances: (1) patients who have changing renal function as established by changes in serum creatinine, (2) patients receiving doses in excess of 40 mg/kg/day, and (3) neonates and patients who have cancer, or are receiving other nephrotoxic drugs such as aminoglycosides.

USE. In recent years, infections caused by methicillin-resistant *S. aureus,* coagulase-negative staphylococci (e.g., *Staphylococcus epidermidis*), and ampicillin-resistant enterococci have become major indications for the use of vancomycin as the drug of choice. Vancomycin is active against most aerobic gram-positive cocci, including most *Streptococcus* species and *L. monocytogenes* and, in combination with streptomycin or gentamicin, is synergistic against enterococci. Many anaerobic streptococci also are susceptible to vancomycin, whereas most gram-negative bacteria are resistant. Some methicillin-resistant staphylococci have demonstrated tolerance to vancomycin killing, and rifampin or TMP-SMX must be added to kill bacteria. Vancomycin is the drug of choice to treat serious infections with methicillin-resistant staphylococci or coagulase-negative staphylococci and to treat enterococcal endocarditis in patients allergic to penicillin. Patients who have staphylococcal infections that are methicillin susceptible could be treated with an antistaphylococcal penicillin. Patients who have bacterial endocarditis caused by a methicillin-resistant *S. aureus* cleared their bacteremia slowly when treated with vancomycin compared with using an antistaphylococcal penicillin in patients who have methicillin-sensitive *S. aureus* endocarditis.[8]

The initial dose of vancomycin should be a full therapeutic dose, even in patients in renal failure. Subsequent doses and intervals should be adjusted to achieve a peak serum concentration of 30 to 40 μg/ml. The MIC_{95} of vancomycin for bacteria reported as susceptible by disk is 5 μg/ml or less.

A concentration of 20 μg/ml of vancomycin in a heparin flush or hyperalimentation solution has been shown to prevent line-related infections in premature infants[18] and children who have cancer in whom tunneled central venous catheters have been placed.[17]

Metronidazole

MECHANISM OF ACTION. After being taken up by bacteria, metronidazole is reduced to intermediate products that are toxic to the bacteria; the organism then releases inactive end products.

BACTERIAL RESISTANCE. Resistance to metronidazole develops infrequently. It has been associated with decreased entry of the drug into bacteria and a decreased rate of reduction once in their cells.

PHARMACOLOGICAL PROPERTIES. Metronidazole is active against most anaerobic bacteria, *Treponema pallidum, H. pylori, Campylobacter fetus, Gardnerella vaginalis, Actinobacillus, Actinomycetem comitans, Capnocytophaga,* and *Trichomonas vaginalis,* as well as certain parasites. After oral administration, metronidazole is absorbed rapidly and completely, with the peak serum concentration being proportional to the dose administered. Metronidazole is distributed well throughout the body, including the CNS and the aqueous humor of the eyes. The serum half-life is about 8 hours. After being metabolized, metronidazole is excreted primarily in the urine.

SIDE EFFECTS. The most common side effect of metronidazole is GI upset. Metronidazole also has been associated with CNS dysfunction (seizures, encephalopathy, ataxia) and peripheral neuropathy, and it can potentiate the effects of warfarin and cause a disulfiram reaction when alcohol is consumed. A major concern with the use of metronidazole has been its carcinogenic potential. Although rats and mice that have received metronidazole for a long period have shown an increase in neoplasms, mutagenicity for human cells has not been demonstrated in vitro, and follow-up studies on women who received metronidazole for trichomonal infections have shown that they did not have an increased frequency of tumors up to 10 years later.

USE. Originally introduced to treat *T. vaginalis,* metronidazole also has proved to be effective in the treatment of amebiasis and giardiasis. More recently, it has gained widespread use in the treatment of anaerobic bacterial infections; it is not effective in treating actinomycosis or *Propionibacterium acnes* infections. Metronidazole also is not optimally effective in the treatment of anaerobic lower respiratory tract infections, perhaps because of the presence of aerobic bacteria; the outcome generally is good if penicillin or ampicillin is given concomitantly.

The peak serum concentration achieved in adults after 0.5 g of metronidazole is given orally averages 11.5 μg/ml; after an intravenous dose of 0.5 g, the serum concentration ranges from 20 to 25 μg/ml. The MIC_{95} of metronidazole for susceptible bacteria usually is 4 μg/ml or less. Most diagnostic microbiology laboratories do not test anaerobic bacteria routinely for susceptibility.

Rifampin

MECHANISM OF ACTION. Rifampin works by inhibiting DNA-dependent RNA polymerase at the B subunit, preventing chain initiation but not elongation.

BACTERIAL RESISTANCE. Bacterial resistance to rifampin develops rapidly by mutation of the DNA-dependent RNA polymerase. The rates of mutation are so high that they preclude use of rifampin as monotherapy except for very short courses of prophylaxis.

PHARMACOLOGICAL PROPERTIES. Rifampin usually is administered orally and is completely and rapidly absorbed, with the peak serum concentration achieved 1 to 4 hours after ingestion. An intravenous form of rifampin also is available. Rifampin is distributed throughout the body, deacetylated by the liver, and excreted in the bile. The serum half-life is 2 to 5 hours early in therapy, but it declines over time because of increased biliary excretion. Rifampin also can enter phagocytes and kill viable intracellular organisms, which may explain why rifampin is better able to enter and sterilize abscesses than are other antimicrobial agents.

SIDE EFFECTS. When rifampin is given daily, the most common side effects are a mild, self-limited rash and mild GI complaints. When rifampin is used intermittently at high individual doses, a flulike syndrome with fever, aches, and chills develops in up to 20% of patients. Because rifampin crosses the placenta and teratogenic effects have been observed in rodents, it should not be used during pregnancy except in severe cases of tuberculosis. Patients or parents should be warned that urine, feces, saliva, and tears may turn a red-orange color while they are taking the drug. The patient should not wear contact lenses while on rifampin therapy, because the lenses can become permanently discolored.

USE. Rifampin is extremely active against a wide range of organisms. Most strains of *S. aureus* and coagulase-negative staphylococci are exquisitely sensitive to rifampin, which also is active against most other gram-positive cocci. *H. influenzae, N. meningitidis,* and *N. gonorrhoeae* are exquisitely susceptible to rifampin, but other aerobic gram-negative pathogens are less so. Rifampin also is active against *Legionella* species and *Mycobacterium tuberculosis.*

Despite its widespread use for treating tuberculosis and as prophylaxis for *N. meningitidis* and *H. influenzae,* no pediatric preparation of rifampin is available. Instructions for preparing a suspension for pediatric use are detailed in the *Physicians' Desk Reference.*[15] Internationally, rifampin is used most commonly to treat tuberculosis and leprosy. Rifampin also is recommended for prophylaxis of close contacts of patients who have meningococcal disease and for household contacts of children who have systemic *H. influenzae* type b disease. When another antimicrobial agent is used with rifampin for the last 4 days of treatment of group A beta-hemolytic streptococcal infections, the microbiological failure rate falls to almost zero. Rifampin in combination with other antistaphylococcal agents has been used to treat severe staphylococcal infections such as *S. aureus* endocarditis, osteomyelitis, and CSF shunt infections caused by coagulase-negative staphylococci.

The peak serum concentration of rifampin after oral administration of 600 mg to an adult or 10 mg/kg to a child averages 7 μg/ml. Because of rifampin's long half-life, the peak serum concentration and bioavailability are better if the drug is given once a day. The MIC_{95} of bacteria reported as susceptible by disk to rifampin is 1 μg/ml or less.

INITIAL THERAPY OF SELECTED ACUTE INFECTIONS

In most clinical situations, the physician must decide which antimicrobial agent or agents to use before the offending organism has been positively identified through culture results, serological tests, or microscopic examination of material obtained from the infected site. The practitioner should consider the following points before starting treatment:

- The patient's age and immune status
- Whether concomitant disease is a factor
- The patient's history of exposure to infectious agents
- Current or recent administration of antimicrobial agents
- The findings on physical examination

Appropriate specimens for bacterial and viral cultures and specimens for serological tests and microscopic examinations should be obtained before antimicrobial therapy is started, and specific adjunctive, supportive therapy should be instituted concomitantly. Table 31-2 lists the most likely offending organisms and the antimicrobial agent or agents that could be used empirically for various diagnoses under these circumstances. Local susceptibility patterns and other special circumstances always should be considered.

PROPHYLAXIS

Antimicrobial agents can be given to prevent colonization, to eradicate carriage, to prevent bacteria that colonize one body site from causing disease at a usually sterile site, or to prevent bacteria that have been introduced into a usually sterile site from causing disease. In general, an antimicrobial agent that has the narrowest spectrum that is effective against the most likely pathogen or pathogens should be used at the lowest dosage and for the shortest period that will prevent infection. Prophylaxis also should be restricted to situations in which it is known to be effective and in which the risk of infection exceeds the potential risks of the antimicrobial agent or the emergence of resistant bacteria. Specific bacterial pathogens for which prophylaxis has proved effective are shown in Table 31-3, and clinical situations in which prophylactic antimicrobial agents might be effective are listed in Table 31-4. The reader is referred to the *Red Book* (Report of the Committee on Infectious Diseases, American Academy of Pediatrics) for triannually updated recommendations for prophylaxis in specific situations, such as prevention of bacterial endocarditis.[16]

ANTIMICROBIAL THERAPY FOR VIRAL, FUNGAL, AND PARASITIC INFECTIONS

Currently, there are only a limited number of agents and a limited number of indications for systemic treatment of viral, fungal, and parasitic infections in the United States; thus, most primary care pediatricians are unlikely to be familiar with the use of these agents. Therefore, it is recommended that the pediatrician consult a specialist in pediatric infectious diseases before treating a patient with these drugs. The antiviral drugs available currently, along with their indications and dosages, are presented in Table 31-5; antifungal drugs (and their dosages and adverse reactions) are listed in Table 31-6. Treatment of parasitic infections is discussed in Chapter 246, Parasitic Infections, and in the AAP's *Red Book 2000,* in the *Pocketbook of Pediatric Antimicrobial Therapy,*[12] and in *The Medical Letter Handbook of Antimicrobial Therapy.*[1]

Text continued on p. 422

Table 31-2 Initial Empirical Therapy for Selected Infections*

Clinical Diagnosis	Most Likely Offending Organisms	Antimicrobial Agents
Meningitis	**Neonate:** group B streptococci, *E. coli, L. monocytogenes*	Ampicillin and cefotaxime (or ceftriaxone)
	Child: *S. pneumoniae, N. meningitidis, H. influenzae* type b	Ceftriaxone or cefotaxime (plus vancomycin if *S. pneumoniae* is suspected)
Brain abscess	Streptococcal species, anaerobes, *S. aureus*	Penicillin and metronidazole (plus nafcillin if *S. aureus* is suspected [plus cefotaxime or ceftriaxone if gram-negative bacilli are suspected])
Orbital cellulitis	Streptococcal species, *S. aureus, H. influenzae* type b	Ceftriaxone or cefotaxime plus clindamycin or nafcillin
Epiglottitis	*H. influenzae* type b	Ceftriaxone or cefotaxime
Pneumonia (lobar or segmental)	**Neonate:** group B streptococci, *S. aureus,* gram-negative organisms	Ampicillin plus an aminoglycoside
	Child: *S. pneumoniae, H. influenzae* type b, *S. aureus, S. pyogenes, M. pneumoniae*	Penicillin, nafcillin, or erythromycin
Infective endocarditis	*Streptococcus viridans, S. aureus*	Nafcillin and an aminoglycoside
Acute diarrhea (fecal WBC present)	*Salmonella, Shigella* species	If patient is systemically ill, very young, or immunocompromised, cefotaxime or ceftriaxone
Abdominal sepsis	Anaerobes, aerobic enterics, enterococci	Clindamycin, aminoglycoside, and ampicillin (Unasyn and Timentin are suitable alternatives)
Urinary tract infection	**Acute:** *E. coli, Klebsiella* species	Gentamicin or trimethoprim/sulfamethoxazole (TMP-SMX)
	Chronic: *E. coli, Proteus* species, *Pseudomonas* species	Await culture and sensitivity results
Osteomyelitis	**Neonate:** group B streptococci, *S. aureus, S. pyogenes, S. pneumoniae*	Nafcillin and an aminoglycoside
	Child: *S. aureus, S. pyogenes*	Nafcillin
Pyogenic arthritis	**Neonate:** group B streptococci, *S. aureus, S. pyogenes, N. gonorrhoea*	Nafcillin and an aminoglycoside (or cefotaxime)
	Child: *H. influenzae* type b (<5 yr), *S. aureus, S. pyogenes, N. gonorrhoea*	Ceftriaxone or cefotaxime (test MIC for *S. aureus*) plus nafcillin
Suspected sepsis	**Neonate:** group B streptococci, *L. monocytogenes,* gram-negative enteric organisms	Ampicillin and an aminoglycoside (or cefotaxime)
	Infant (1-6 wk): as for neonate plus as for child	Ampicillin and ceftriaxone
	Child: *S. pneumoniae, H. influenzae* type b, *N. meningitidis*	Ceftriaxone
Compromised Host		
Fever only	*S. aureus, E. coli, Pseudomonas* species	Cefotaxime or aminopenicillin
Pneumonia	As under pneumonia above, and *P. carinii, Candida albicans,* other fungi	As under pneumonia above plus TMP-SMX; if patient's condition deteriorates, broncho-alveolar lavage (BAL) or lung biopsy is needed to direct therapy
Shock (sepsis without source)	**Neonate:** group B streptococci, enterics	Ampicillin and an aminoglycoside
	Child: *N. meningitidis, S. pneumoniae*	Ceftriaxone or cefotaxime

*For most clinical diagnoses, an acceptable alternative choice of antibiotics could be proposed.

Table 31-3 Antimicrobial Prophylaxis Against Specific Pathogens

Pathogen	Disease to Be Prevented	Antimicrobial Agent	Dose	Duration of Therapy
Bacteria				
Bordetella pertussis	Secondary cases of pertussis in household contacts	Erythromycin estolate (some experts will recommend azithromycin)	40-50 mg/kg/day in 4 doses (not to exceed 2 g/day)	14 days
*Chlamydia trachomatis**	Urogenital infections in exposed individuals	Doxycycline (>8 yr) **or**	200 mg/day in 2 doses	7 days
		azithromycin (adolescents) **or**	1 g	1 dose PO
		erythromycin	40-50 mg/kg/day in 4 doses (not to exceed 2 g/day)	7 days
*Corynebacterium diphtheriae**	Diphtheria in unimmunized contacts	Benzathine penicillin **or**	*<30 kg:* 600,000 U *>30 kg:* 1.2 million U	1 dose IM
		erythromycin	40-50 mg/kg/day in 4 doses (not to exceed 2 g/day)	7 days
Haemophilus ducreyi	Urogenital infection in exposed persons	Ceftriaxone	250 mg	single dose
		Azithromycin	1 g	single dose
		Amoxicillin-clavulanate	125 mg in 4 doses	7 days
		Ciprofloxacin	500 mg in 2 doses	3 days
Haemophilus influenzae	Secondary cases of systemic infection in close contacts <1 yr of age and in children 12-47 mo who are not fully immunized	Rifampin	*≤1 mo:* 10-20 mg/kg *>1 mo:* 20 mg/kg (maximum 600 mg)	Once a day for 4 days
Mycobacterium avium complex	Infection in HIV-infected host	Clarithromycin, azithromycin, rifabutin	*Adult:* 300 mg *Pediatric:* 5 mg/kg	Once a day for life
Mycobacterium tuberculosis	Overt pulmonary or metastatic infection	Isoniazid	10-20 mg/kg (not to exceed 300 mg)	Once a day for 9 days
Neisseria gonorrhoeae	Gonococcal infection in exposed individuals, including newborns whose mothers have gonorrhea	Ceftriaxone **or**	125 mg	1 dose IM
		cefixime **or**	400 or 800 mg	1 dose PO
		ofloxacin (≥18 yr)	400 mg	1 dose PO
Neisseria meningitidis	Meningococcemia in exposed susceptible individuals	Rifampin	*≤1 mo:* 5-10 mg/kg *>1 mo:* 10 mg/kg (maximum 600 mg)	q12h for 4 doses
		Ceftriaxone	*≤12 yr:* 125 mg	1 dose IM
			≥12 yr: 250 mg	1 dose IM
		Ciprofloxacin *(≥18 yr)*	500 mg	1 dose PO
Streptococcus pneumoniae	Fulminant pneumococcal infection in individuals with asplenia or sickle cell disease	Penicillin V	125 mg	2 times/day for life

Modified from Peter G, et al, editors: *1997 Red Book: Report of the Committee on Infectious Diseases,* ed 24, Elk Grove Village, Ill, 1997, The American Academy of Pediatrics.
*Efficacy of treatment has not been established.

Continued

Table 31-3 Antimicrobial Prophylaxis Against Specific Pathogens—cont'd

Pathogen	Disease to Be Prevented	Antimicrobial Agent	Dose	Duration of Therapy
Group A streptococcus	Recurrent rheumatic fever	Benzathine penicillin **or**	1.2 million U	Every 4 wk
		penicillin V **or**	125-250 mg	2 times/day
		sulfadiazine	*<27 kg:* 0.5 g	Once a day for life
			>27 kg: 1 kg	Once a day for life
Group B streptococcus	Neonatal infection	Ampicillin	*Mother:* 2 g IV given intrapartum, followed by 1 g q4h until delivery	
			Infant: 50 mg/kg IM q12h for 2 days	
Treponema pallidum	Syphilis in exposed individuals	Benzathine penicillin	2.4 million U	1 dose IM
*Vibrio cholerae**	Cholera in close contacts	Tetracycline or trimethoprim-sulfamethoxazole	250 mg q6h (>8 yr)	3 days
			5 mg/kg as trimethoprim 2 times/day	3 days
*Yersinia pestis**	Plague in household contacts or individuals exposed to pneumonic disease	Tetracycline (>8 yr) **or**	15 mg/kg/day in 4 doses	7 days
		sulfonamide	40 mg/kg/day in 4 doses	7 days
Parasites				
Plasmodium species (malaria)	Overt infection in endemic areas	Chloroquine	5 mg/kg base once a week (maximum 300-mg base), beginning 2 wk before entering endemic area, while in area, and for 6 wk after leaving area	
Viruses				
Herpes simplex	Recurrent genital lesions	Acyclovir	800-1000 mg/day in 2-5 doses	1 year
HIV	Congenital infection	Zidovudine	*Mother:* 100 mg in 5 doses initiated at 14-34 weeks of gestation intrapartum until delivery	
			Infant: 2 mg/kg/day in 4 doses initiated 8-12 hours after birth	Until 6 weeks of age
Influenza A	Influenza in individuals at risk of complications	Amantadine	*1-9 yr:* 2-4.4 mg/kg q12h (maximum 150 mg/day)	Duration of influenza outbreak
			>9 yr: 100 mg q12h	
Varicella-zoster	Varicella in persons at risk of complications	Acyclovir	80 mg/kg/day in 4 doses	5 days
Other				
Pneumocystis carinii	Pneumonia in a compromised host	Trimethoprim-sulfamethoxazole	5 mg trimethoprim/25 mg sulfamethoxazole	Once a day while patient is undergoing chemotherapy

Modified from Peter G, et al, editors: *1997 Red Book: Report of the Committee on Infectious Diseases,* ed 24, Elk Grove Village, Ill, 1997, The American Academy of Pediatrics.

Table 31-4 Clinical Situations in which Prophylaxis with Antimicrobial Agents Has Proved Effective

Body Site	Infection to Be Prevented	Agents	Recommended Dosage
Conjunctivae	Neonatal gonococcal ophthalmia	1% silver nitrate, 0.5% erythromycin, 1% tetracycline, penicillin	Applied topically once shortly after delivery
Abnormal heart valve	Bacterial endocarditis (e.g., after dental extraction)	Penicillin, ampicillin	*Standard-risk patients, oral procedures:* penicillin V, 2 g PO, then 1 g 6 hours later; *high-risk patients, dental, or all patients, GU or GI tract procedures:* ampicillin, 2 g IM or IV plus gentamicin, 1.5-2 mg/kg 30 min before and 8 hours after procedure
Surgical wound	Serious postoperative wound infection	Appropriate for expected contaminants	See Kaiser AB: *N Engl J Med* 315: 1129, 1986[4]
Middle ear	Recurrent otitis media	Sulfisoxazole	40-50 mg/kg given q12h during winter and spring
		Amoxicillin	5-10 mg/kg given q12h during winter and spring
Urinary tract	Recurrent infection	Trimethoprim/ sulfamethoxazole	2 mg TMP and 10 mg SMX/kg once daily
		Nitrofurantoin	1-2 mg/kg once daily Duration: months to years, depending on clinical situation
Human/animal bite wound*	Wound infection, cellulitis	Penicillin V	25-50 mg/kg/day, given q6-8h for 5-7 days
		Amoxicillin/clavulanate	40 mg of the amoxicillin component/ kg/day given q8h for 5-7 days

Modified from Peter G, et al, editors: *1997 Red Book: Report of the Committee on Infectious Diseases,* ed 24, Elk Grove Village, Ill, 1997, The American Academy of Pediatrics.
*Efficacy of treatment has not been established.

Table 31-5 Antiviral Drugs for Non-HIV Infections

Generic (Trade Name)	Indication	Route	Normal Recommended Dosage
Acyclovir* (Zovirax)	Genital herpes simplex virus (HSV) infection, first episode	PO IV	1200 mg/day in 3 divided doses for 7-10 days† 15 mg/kg/day in 3 divided doses for 5-7 days
	Genital HSV infection, recurrence	PO	1000-1200 mg/day in 3-5 divided doses for 5 days†
	Recurrent genital HSV episodes in patient with frequent recurrences:		
	Chronic suppressive therapy	PO	400-1200 mg/day in 2-3 divided doses for as long as 12 continuous months†
	HSV in immunocompromised host (localized, progressive, or disseminated)‡	IV PO	15-30 mg/kg/day in 3 divided doses for 7-14 days 1000 mg/day in 3-5 divided doses for 7-14 days†
	Prophylaxis of HSV in immunocompromised HSV-seropositive patient‡	PO IV	600-1000 mg/day in 3-5 divided doses during risk period† 15 mg/kg/day in 3 divided doses during risk period

Modified from Pickering LK, et al, editors: *Red Book 2000: Report of the Committee on Infectious Diseases,* ed 25, Elk Grove Village, Ill, 2000, The American Academy of Pediatrics.
*Dose should be reduced if the patient's renal function is impaired.
†In children, oral dose of acyclovir should not exceed 80 mg/kg/day.
‡As of June 1994 the drug had not been licensed for this use or was investigational.

Continued

Table 31-5 Antiviral Drugs for Non-HIV Infections—cont'd

Generic (Trade Name)	Indication	Route	Normal Recommended Dosage
Acyclovir* (Zovirax) —cont'd	HSV encephalitis	IV	30 mg/kg/day in 3 divided doses for a minimum of 14-21 days
	Neonatal HSV‡	IV	60 mg/kg/day in 3 divided doses for 14-21 days
	Varicella or zoster in immunocompromised host	IV	*Children <1 yr:* 30 mg/kg/day in 3 divided doses (some experts also recommend this dosage for children ≥1 yr)
		IV	*Children ≥1 yr:* 1500 mg/m²/day in 3 divided doses for 7-10 days
	Zoster in immuno-competent host‡	IV	Same as for zoster in immunocompromised host
		PO	4000 mg/day in 5 divided doses for 5-7 days for patients ≥12 yr†
	Varicella in immuno-competent host	PO	80 mg/kg/day in 4 divided doses for 5 days; maximum dose is 3200 mg/day
Amantadine (Symmetrel)	Influenza A: treatment and prophylaxis	PO	*>20 kg:* 100 mg/day in 1 or 2 divided doses for duration of exposure
			<20 kg: 5 mg/kg/day in 1 or 2 divided doses for duration of exposure
Cidofovir	Cytomegalovirus (CMV) retinitis	IV	Induction: 5 mg/kg once with probencid with hydration Weekly maintenance: 3 mg/kg once with probencid and hydration
Famciclovir	Genital HSV infection	PO	For adolescents, 750 mg/day in 3 divided doses for 7-10 days
	Episodic recurrent genital HSV infection	PO	For adolescents, 250 mg/day in 2 divided doses for 5 days
	Daily suppressive therapy	PO	For adolescents, 250-500 mg/day in 2 divided doses for 1 yr, then reassess for recurrence of HSV infection
Foscarnet* (Foscavir)	CMV retinitis in patients with acquired immunodeficiency syndrome	IV	180 mg/kg/day in 3 divided doses for 14-21 days, then 90-120 mg/kg once a day as maintenance dose
Ganciclovir* (Cytovene)	Acquired CMV retinitis in immunocompromised host	IV	10 mg/kg/day in 2 divided doses for 14-21 days; for long-term suppression, 5 mg/kg/day for 5-7 days/wk
	Prophylaxis for CMV in high-risk host	IV	10 mg/kg/day in 2 divided doses for 1 wk, then 5 mg/kg/day in 1 day dose for 100 days
Oseltamivir phosphate (Tamilfu)	Influenza A and B treatment	PO	For persons ≥18 years of age: 75 mg twice a day for 5 days
Ribavirin (Virazole)	Treatment of respiratory syncytial virus (RSV) infection	Aerosol	Given by a small particle generator, in a solution of 6 g in 300 ml of sterile water (20 mg/ml), for 12-20 hours/day for 1-7 days or 6 g in 100 ml of sterile water for 2 hr 3 times/day; longer treatment may be necessary for some patients
Rimantadine (Flumadine)	Influenza A: treatment and prophylaxis	PO	*>20 kg:* 100 mg/day in 1 or 2 divided doses for duration of exposure
			<20 kg: 5 mg/kg/day in 1 or 2 divided doses for duration of exposure
Valacyclovir	Genital HSV infection	PO	For adolescents, 2 g/day in 2 divided doses for 7-10 days
	Episodic recurrent genital HSV infection	PO	For adolescents, 1 g/day in 2 divided doses for 5 days
	Daily suppressive therapy for (HSV) infection	PO	For adolescents, 500-1000 mg once daily for 1 y, then reassess for recurrences
Zanamivir	Influenza A and B treatment	Inhalation	For persons ≥12 years of age 10 mg inhaled twice a day for 5 days with a special breath-activated plastic inhaler

Modified from Pickering LK, et al, editors: *Red Book 2000: Report of the Committee on Infectious Diseases,* ed 25, Elk Grove Village, Ill, 2000, The American Academy of Pediatrics.

Table 31-6 Recommended Doses of Parenteral and Oral Antifungal Drugs

Drug	Route	Dose (Per Day)	Adverse Reactions*
Amphotericin B	IV	0.25-0.5 mg/kg (after test dose†) initially, increase as tolerated to 0.5-1 mg/kg; infuse as single dose over 2-3 hr 0.5-1 mg/kg weekly for suppressive therapy in HIV-infected patients with cryptococcosis or histoplasmosis	Fever, chills, phlebitis, renal dysfunction, hypokalemia, anemia, cardiac arrhythmias, anaphylactoid reaction, hematological abnormalities
	Intrathecal (IT)	0.025 mg, increase to 0.5 mg twice weekly	Radiculitis, sensory loss, foot drop
Amphotericin B lipid complex (ABLC)	IV	5 mg/kg infused over 2 hr	Fever, chills, other reactions associated amphotericin B, but less nephrotoxicity; hepatotoxicity
Amphotericin B cholesteryl sulfate complex (ABCD)	IV	3-6 mg/kg infused at a rate of 1 mg/kg/hr	Fever, chills, other reactions associated with amphotericin B, but less nephrotoxicity; hepatotoxicity
Liposomal amphotericin B lipid complex (AmBisome)	IV	5 mg/kg infused over 1-2 hr	Fever, chills, other reactions associated with amphotericin B, but less nephrotoxicity; hepatotoxicity
Clotrimazole (troches)	PO (topical)	10 mg tablet 5 times/day (dissolved slowly in the mouth)	Nausea, vomiting, increase in serum transaminase
Fluconazole	IV PO	*Children‡:* 3-6 mg/kg/day *Adults:* 200 mg once, followed by 100 mg/day for oropharyngeal, esophageal candidiasis; 400 mg once, followed by 200-400 mg/day for cryptococcal meningitis (200 mg/day for maintenance in patients with acquired immune deficiency syndrome [AIDS])	Rash, nausea, abdominal pain, diarrhea, headache, possibly hepatotoxicity
Flucytosine	PO	50-150 mg/kg in 4 doses at 6-hr intervals (adjust dosage with renal dysfunction)	Bone marrow suppression; renal dysfunction can lead to drug accumulation; nausea, vomiting, increases in transaminases, blood urea nitrogen (BUN), and creatinine
Griseofulvin	PO	Ultramicrosize: 5-10 mg/kg/day, single dose; maximum dose, 750 mg Microsize: 10-20 mg/kg/day divided in 2 doses; maximum daily dose, 1000 mg	Rash, leukopenia, proteinuria, paresthesia, GI symptoms, mental confusion
Itraconazole	PO	*Children:* 5-10 mg/kg/day as a single dose or in 2 doses *Adults:* 100-200 mg once or twice daily	Nausea, epigastric pain, headache, edema, hypokalemia, increased serum aminotransferase, hypertension, adrenal insufficiency
Ketoconazole	PO IT	*Children:* 3.3-6.6 mg/kg, once daily§ *Adults:* 200-400 mg once daily 20 mg per dose for 3-7 days	Rash, anaphylaxis, nausea, vomiting, abdominal pain, fever, gynecomastia, thrombocytopenia, hepatoxicity, and depression of endocrine function (dose dependent, reversible); should not be given concurrently with the antihistamine terfenadine
Nystatin	PO	*Infants:* 200,000 U 4 times/day, after meals *Children and adults:* 400,000-600,000 U 3 times/day	Nausea, vomiting, diarrhea, rash

Modified from Pickering LK, et al, editors: *Red Book 2000: Report of the Committee on Infectious Diseases,* ed 25, Elk Grove Village, Ill, 2000, The American Academy of Pediatrics.
*See the package insert or the listing in the current edition of the *Physicians' Desk Reference,* Montvale, NJ, Medical Economics.
†Test dose is 0.1 mg/kg, with a maximum dose of 1 mg/kg.
‡The daily dose has not been established for children ≤2 yr.
§Efficacy has not been established for children. A small number of children 3 to 13 years of age have been treated safely with this dose.

REFERENCES

1. Abramowicz M, editor: Drugs for parasitic infections, *Med Lett* 1/2/98.
2. Craig WA: Pharmakokinetic/pharmacodynamic parameters: rationale for antibacterial dosing of mice and men, *Clin Infect Dis* 26:1, 1998.
3. Idsoe O, et al: Nature and extent of penicillin side reactions with particular reference to fatalities from anaphylactic shock, *Bull World Health Organ* 38:159, 1968.
4. Kaiser AB: Antimicrobial prophylaxis in surgery, *N Engl J Med* 315: 1129, 1986.
5. Karam GH, Sanders CV, Aldridge KE: Role of newer antimicrobial agents in the treatment of mixed aerobic and anaerobic infections, *Surg Gynecol Obstet* 172(suppl):57, 1990.
6. Kim KS: Clinical perspectives on penicillin tolerance, *J Pediatr* 112: 509, 1988.
7. Klein JO: Clarithromycin: where do we go from here? *Pediatr Infect Dis J* 12:S148, 1993.
8. Levine DP, Fromm BS, Reddy BR: Slow response to vancomycin or vancomycin plus rifampin in methicillin-resistant *Staphylococcus aureus* endocarditis, *Ann Intern Med* 115:674, 1991.
9. Moellering RC Jr, editor: Proceedings of symposium, tissue-directed antibiotic therapy, *Am J Med* 91(suppl 3A):1S, 1991.
10. Molavi A: Cephalosporins: rationale for clinical use, *Am Fam Physician* 43:937, 1991.
11. National Committee for Clinical Laboratory Standards: *Performance standards for antimicrobial disk susceptibility tests,* ed 3, Wayne, Pa, 1984, The Committee.
12. Nelson JD: 1998-1999 *Pocketbook of pediatric antimicrobial therapy,* ed 13, Baltimore, 1998, Williams & Wilkins.
13. Neu HC: The development of macrolides: clarithromycin in perspective, *J Antimicrob Chemother* 27(suppl A):1, 1991.
14. Nicolau DP, et al: Experience with a once-daily aminoglycoside program administered to 2,184 patients, *Antimicrob Agents Chemother* 39: 650, 1995.
15. *Physicians" Desk Reference,* ed 54, Montvale, NJ, 2000, Medical Economics.
16. Pickering LK, editor: *Red Book 2000: Report of the Committee on Infectious Diseases,* ed 25, Elk Grove Village, Ill, 2000, The American Academy of Pediatrics.
17. Schwartz C, et al: Prevention of bacteremia attributed to luminal colonization of tunneled central venous catheters with vancomycin-susceptible organisms, *J Clin Oncol* 8:1591, 1990.
18. Spafford PS, et al: Prevention of central venous catheter-related coagulase negative staphylococcus sepsis in neonates, *J Pediatr* 125:259, 1994.
19. Stamos JK, Yogev R: Oral cephalosporins: the newest of the new, *Contemp Pediatr* 10:28, 1993.
20. Thomas MP, Steele RW: Monitoring serum vancomycin concentrations in children: is it necessary? *Pediatr Infect Dis J* 17:351, 1998.
21. Whitman MS, Tunkel AR: Azithromycin and clarithromycin: overview and comparison with erythromycin, *Infect Control Hosp Epidemiol* 13: 357, 1992.
22. Yu VL, Merigan TC, Barriere SL, editors: *Antimicrobial therapy and vaccines,* Baltimore, 1999, Williams and Wilkins.

SUGGESTED READINGS

Donowitz GR, Mandell GL: Beta-lactim antibiotics, *N Engl J Med* 318:419, 1988.

Kucers A, Bennett N: *The use of antibiotics,* ed 4, Philadelphia, 1987, JB Lippincott.

Mandell GL, Douglas RG Jr, Bennett JE, editors: *Principles and practice of infectious diseases,* ed 4, New York, 1995, Churchill Livingstone.

Moellering RC, editor: Antibacterial agents: pharmacodynamics, pharmacology, new agents, *Infect Dis Clin North Am* 3:375, 1989.

32 Minimally Invasive Surgery

George W. Holcomb III

Minimally invasive surgery (MIS) is an attempt to achieve the same results as open surgery but with added benefits such as fewer days of hospitalization, reduced discomfort, faster return to regular activities, and improved cosmesis. The two primary techniques employed in MIS are laparoscopy (MIS in the abdomen) and thoracoscopy (MIS in the chest).

The technology for widespread application of MIS in patients has become refined only recently for application to a broad spectrum of diseases. Over the past few years, its use in children has increased significantly. The purpose of this chapter is to introduce the principles of MIS in pediatric patients and to describe indications for its use.

PRINCIPLES

The basic principle of MIS is the use of 3- to 10-mm incisions through which hollow tubes (cannulas) are inserted into a body cavity such as the abdomen or thorax. A telescope, similar to the ones employed for esophagoscopy, bronchoscopy, and cystoscopy, is introduced through one of the cannulas for visualization. The telescope is attached to a camera, which also is connected to one or several video monitors. By placing instruments through the hollow cannulas and by observing their manipulation on the video monitor, it is possible to perform various surgical procedures.

Laparoscopy requires that the abdomen be distended to develop an adequate space to perform the procedure. If the abdomen is not distended, the underlying abdominal visceral and intestinal organs are at risk for injury. However, in the chest, with intubation of the contralateral mainstem bronchus and desufflation of the ipsilateral lung, adequate working space is obtained and insufflation is usually unnecessary.

The number of incisions required for a laparoscopic procedure usually is proportional to the difficulty of the procedure. For example, diagnostic laparoscopy may require only a single incision. This usually is placed in the umbilicus because the incision can be hidden well and results in a satisfactory cosmetic appearance. In infants, a 3-mm incision is all that is needed for diagnostic laparoscopy because a 3-mm cannula and telescope can be inserted with adequate visualization. In children, whether of preschool, elementary school, or high school age, a 5-mm telescope provides excellent visualization.

For procedural laparoscopies such as appendectomy and cholecystectomy, two and sometimes three other incisions are required. For appendectomy a 5-mm incision customarily is placed in the left lower abdominal quadrant and a 3-mm incision in the suprapubic area. Therefore, by using a total of three incisions, including one in the umbilicus, laparoscopic appendectomy usually can be performed. For cholecystectomy, an additional cannula is needed for retraction.

As the complexity of the laparoscopic procedure increases, more cannulas may be needed for retraction. Procedures such as fundoplication and splenectomy usually require four and sometimes five small incisions.

Thoracoscopic operations necessitate three incisions. One incision is employed for insertion of the telescope, one for placement of an instrument for retraction, and another as the working port for the surgeon. The position of the thoracoscopic incisions should be individualized according to the disease process. For instance, placement of the incisions for evaluation of an anterior mediastinal mass would be different from that for a posterior mediastinal mass.

Different instruments have been developed specifically for laparoscopic and thoracoscopic procedures. Vascular ligation usually is accomplished with endoscopic clip appliers by using stainless steel clips or by endoscopic staplers similar to those used with open surgical procedures. Other instruments such as curved dissectors, scissors, grasping forceps, and cautery also are standard for both laparoscopic and thoracoscopic operations.

DIAGNOSTIC LAPAROSCOPY

Diagnostic laparoscopy is performed easily in infants and children and can be quite useful in evaluating certain surgical problems (Box 32-1). It has been used since 1991 at Children's Hospital-Vanderbilt University Medical Center (CH-VUMC) for evaluation of boys who have a nonpalpable testis.[31] The vexing question facing surgeons who treat boys who have a nonpalpable testis is the uncertainty of its location. It is known that some nonpalpable testes have atrophied during in utero descent into the scrotum. However, in others, the descent of the testis has been arrested within the abdomen or in the upper inguinal canal, accounting for the testis not being palpable (Fig. 32-1). It is in this latter group that orchiopexy can be technically difficult because of the very short length of the testicular artery and vein. Thus, when shortened, these vessels are the limiting factor regarding whether the testicle can be brought into the scrotum. If their length is insufficient and the testicle is placed forcefully in the scrotum with undue tension, vascular spasm will result in ischemia and testicular infarction.

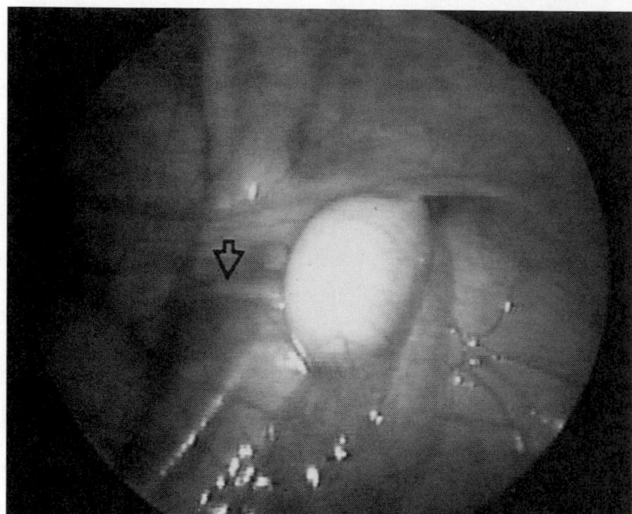

Fig. 32-1 Diagnostic laparoscopy was used in this 18-month-old infant who had a nonpalpable right testis. An intraabdominal testis was identified at laparoscopy. Note the vas deferens *(open arrow)* as it is coursing toward the intraabdominal testis.

(From Holcomb GW III: *Pediatr Ann* 22:678, 1993.)

BOX 32-1

INDICATIONS FOR DIAGNOSTIC LAPAROSCOPY IN CHILDREN

Nonpalpable testes
Contralateral patent processus vaginalis
Chronic abdominal pain
Diagnostic evaluation for appendicitis
Evaluation of possible traumatic injury
Evaluation of infants who have ambiguous genitalia
Staging evaluations in children who have cancer

To overcome the problem of short testicular vessels in a child who has an intraabdominal testis, the Fowler-Stephens orchiopexy was developed. The basic principle of this procedure is that with division of the testicular artery and vein, the testicle will be nourished through collateral vessels along the vas deferens. Because the vas deferens originates in the pelvis and has a lengthy course along the lateral pelvic wall into the inguinal canal, it usually is of sufficient length to reach into the scrotum. The success rate for a Fowler-Stephens orchiopexy when performed as a single stage varies between 50% to 70%.[3]

A more favorable experience with a two-stage approach was reported by Ransley et al in 1984 in which the testicular vessels were divided at the first stage followed by orchiopexy several months later.[54] The rationale for this approach is that initial ligation of the testicular vessels allows augmentation of the collateral vessels and thereby improves the chances that the collateral vasculature will be sufficient to nourish the testis. In 1988, this initial vascular ligation using laparoscopy was described by Bloom.[4] Following that report, several other investigators have described successful endoscopic ligation of the testicular vessels in an attempt to enhance the vasal collaterals before Fowler-Stephens orchiopexy.[5,10,11,23,31]

Diagnostic laparoscopy is performed on boys with a nonpalpable testis as an outpatient procedure by using a 3- or 5-mm umbilical incision to determine if an intraabdominal testis exists. When there is no evidence of an intraabdominal testis but viable testicular vessels and a vas deferens are seen entering the inguinal canal, inguinal exploration is required. In this circumstance, either a very small, atrophic testicular remnant is encountered in the canal and should be excised, or a small testicle is found and orchiopexy is performed. However, if there is no laparoscopic evidence of an intraabdominal testis and the testicular vessels clearly end before entering the inguinal canal (Fig. 32-2), an inguinal exploration is unnecessary. At diagnostic laparoscopy, however, if an intraabdominal testis is found and the testicular vasculature appears too short for performance of a tension-free orchiopexy, one option is to ligate the testicular vessels through a 5-mm contralateral midabdominal incision through which an endoscopic clip applier is inserted for ligation of the vessels (Fig. 32-3). As mentioned previously, this will allow augmentation of the collateral vasculature along the vas deferens and, it is hoped, will enhance the success of a second-stage orchiopexy several months later. Another option is to perform a laparoscopic orchiopexy by dividing the testicular vessels and mobilizing the intraabdominal testis. The testis then is brought through the abdominal cavity over the pubic tubercle, through the subcutaneous tissue, and anchored in the hemiscrotum. For teenagers who have an intraabdominal testis, laparoscopic orchiectomy is preferred because there is little evidence to suggest that this gonad will have adequate testicular function. This also can be performed by using a 5-mm contralateral midabdominal incision and a 3-mm ipsilateral lower abdominal incision.

Diagnostic Laparoscopy for Contralateral Inguinal Hernia

Diagnostic laparoscopy also is used in infants and children to evaluate the contralateral inguinal region in those who have a known unilateral inguinal hernia. The reason for diagnostic laparoscopy in this setting is to identify patients who need contralateral exploration while undergoing anesthesia for a unilateral hernia repair. An alternative technique, popular in the past, would be routine blind contralateral inguinal exploration for the same purpose. However, there is a negative exploration experience of 40% to 60% in several series in which such contralateral inguinal exploration has been used.* For this situation, diagnostic laparoscopy can be performed by using a 3-mm telescope and cannula and requires approximately 5 to 10 minutes of additional operating time. With this information, the surgeon knows with certainty which contralateral inguinal region needs exploration and which does not (Figs. 32-4 and 32-5).

Other Indications

Another indication for diagnostic laparoscopy in the pediatric patient is evaluation for chronic abdominal pain. Previously,

*References 17, 23, 37, 65, 68, 74.

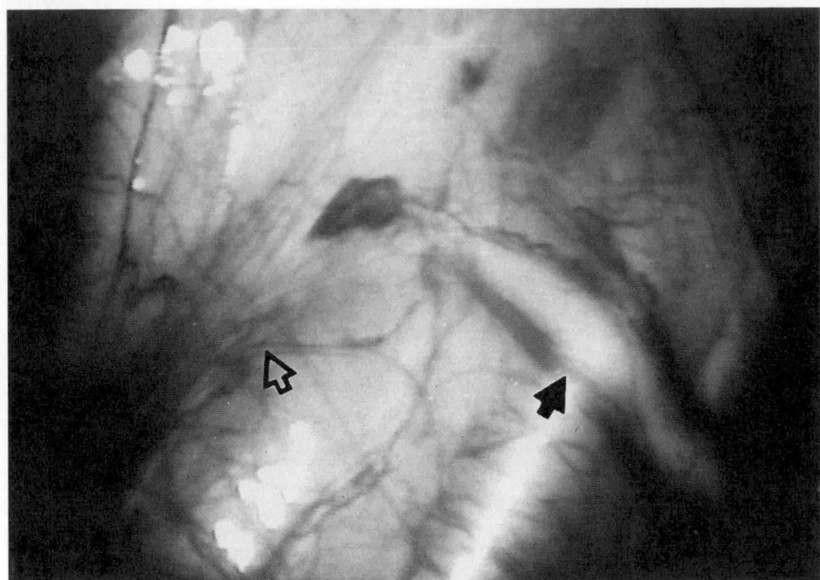

Fig. 32-2 This operative photograph depicts a blind-ending vas deferens *(solid arrow)* and testicular vessels *(open arrow).*

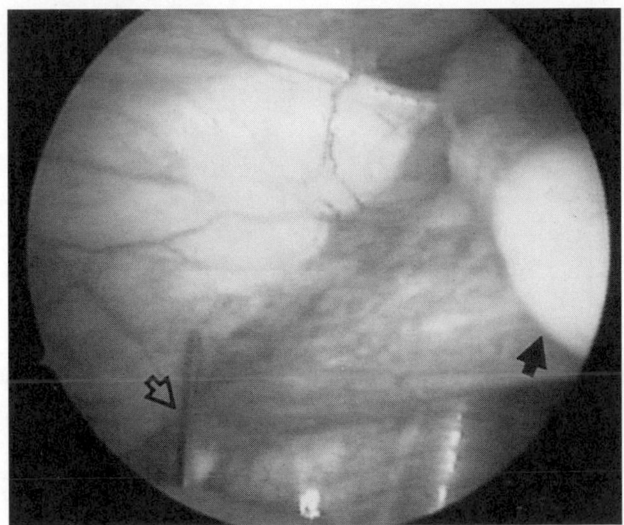

Fig. 32-3 The testicular vascular leash appeared to be short and could not reach into the scrotum in this boy who had a nonpalpable right testis. Therefore, a two-stage Fowler-Stephens orchiopexy was performed. At laparoscopy, the initial stage was accomplished by endoscopically placing a clip *(open arrow)* across the testicular vessels. Note the testicle *(solid arrow)* on the right side of the photograph.

(From Holcomb GW III: *Pediatr Ann* 22:678, 1993.)

laparotomy often was required despite multiple radiographic and physical examinations in selected circumstances when abdominal pain recurred. The incidence of positive findings accounting for the etiology of the pain varies among pediatric surgeons. Stafford[75] has presented his experience in Philadelphia with 20 patients. In that report, 60% of the children were free of abdominal pain 3 months after laparoscopic evaluation and management, which included appendectomy and lysis of adhesions.

Other indications include diagnostic evaluation for patients who have appendicitis, evaluation of traumatic injury in children in whom radiographic evaluations are equivocal, and evaluation of infants who have ambiguous genitalia.

Laparoscopy also is being used to evaluate resectability and for staging when the radiographic evaluations are not diagnostic in children who have cancer. Rather than performing an extensive initial laparotomy, this evaluation can be performed endoscopically. If resectability is possible, an open laparotomy can be performed; otherwise, treatment with adjuvant therapy is initiated and followed later by either repeat laparoscopy or laparotomy, depending on the results of radiographic studies. In a review of institutions participating in Children's Cancer Group (CCG) protocols, 24 children were found to have undergone laparoscopy as part of their surgical management for a variety of indications. Included were evaluations for possible metastatic tumor or recurrent disease, consideration of a new mass for suspected cancer, and evaluation of hepatoblastoma for resectability. In addition, second-look laparoscopy was performed in four patients following chemotherapy to evaluate if resection was now possible. Five patients underwent diagnostic staging laparoscopy, including four who had Hodgkin's disease. No complications were noted within this group of patients undergoing laparoscopy for evaluation of their cancer.[32]

PROCEDURAL LAPAROSCOPY

Cholecystectomy

Laparoscopic cholecystectomy has become the preferred technique for removing the gallbladder in adults. Descriptions of its use in children, however, have been limited to small series because cholelithiasis and gallbladder disease are much less prevalent in children than in adults.[26,30,49,50,72] The incidence of cholelithiasis, however, has increased dramatically in the past two decades, and gallstones should now be considered in the differential diagnosis of every child or adolescent who has vague or colicky upper abdominal pain, particularly those who are at risk.

The percentage of children who have cholelithiasis caused by hemolytic disease is likely to be greater in institutions that have an active pediatric hematology program than in hospitals that do not. The early reports of cholelithiasis in children indicate that most patients who have gallstones

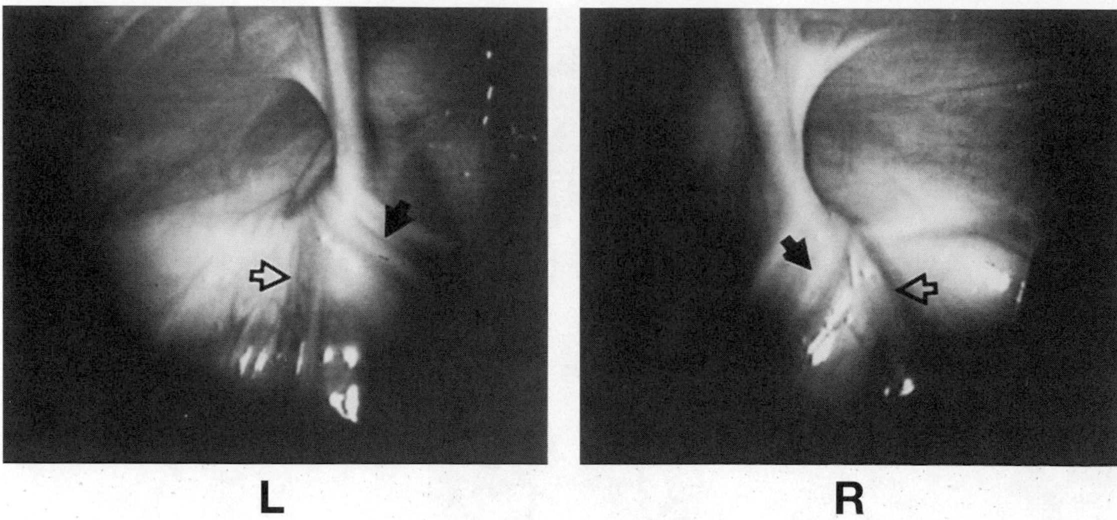

Fig. 32-4 This 3-year-old child had a known right inguinal hernia *(right)*. At laparoscopy, an equally large left inguinal hernia was documented *(left)*. Note the vas deferens *(solid arrow)* and the testicular vessels *(open arrow)* coursing through the internal opening of the hernia sac.

(From Holcomb GW III: *Pediatr Ann* 22:678, 1993.)

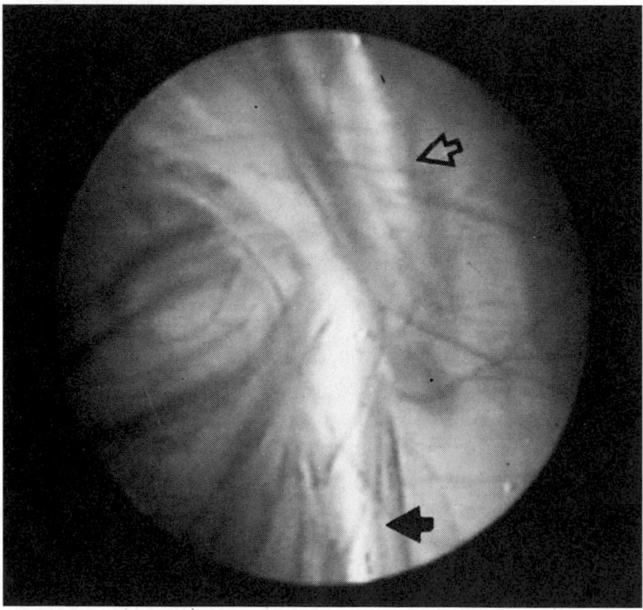

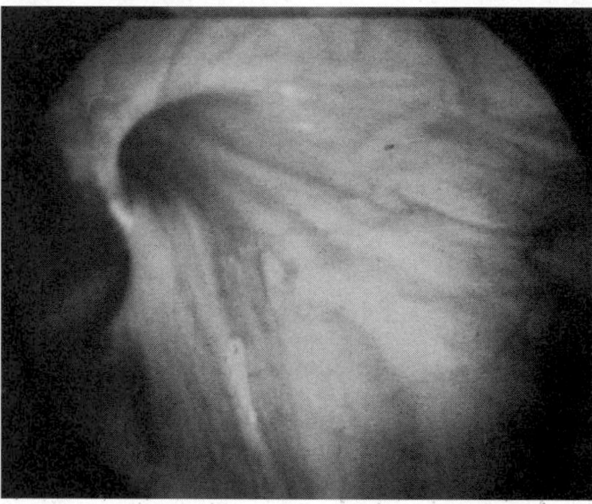

Fig. 32-5 This 6-month-old infant had a known right inguinal hernia *(right)*. However, at laparoscopy there was no evidence of a hernia on the left side *(left)*, and unnecessary contralateral exploration was avoided. The vas deferens *(solid arrow)* and testicular vessels *(open arrow)* are seen best on the left side.

(From Holcomb GW III: *Pediatr Ann* 22:678, 1993.)

have associated hemolytic disease. In fact, the diagnosis usually was not considered in children who did not have hemolysis.[18,38,70] However, in two earlier reports from our institution, the growing incidence of nonhemolytic cholelithiasis has been emphasized and recently observed by other investigators.*

For laparoscopic cholecystectomy, four cannulas are required. Three 5-mm incisions and one 10-mm incision are used (Figs. 32-6 and 32-7). Following isolation of the cystic duct, cholangiography will identify the cystic and common ducts correctly and help prevent inadvertent injury to these structures in small patients (Fig. 32-8). After completion of the cholangiogram, the gallbladder is dissected from its liver bed and extracted through the 10-mm cannula.

One hundred twenty children ranging in age from 25 months to 19 years underwent laparoscopic cholecystectomy at CH-VUMC between June 1990 and December 1998.[29] Twenty-four children had hemolytic disease. The mean age was 9.9 years, the median age 13 years. Twenty-three patients presented initially with complications of cholelithiasis (acute cholecystitis [8], jaundice and pain [6], gallstone pancreatitis [5], and acute biliary colic [4]). The remaining 97 children underwent elective laparoscopic cholecystectomy, with a mean postoperative stay of 1 day and no complications.

*References 1, 13, 24, 26, 27, 56.

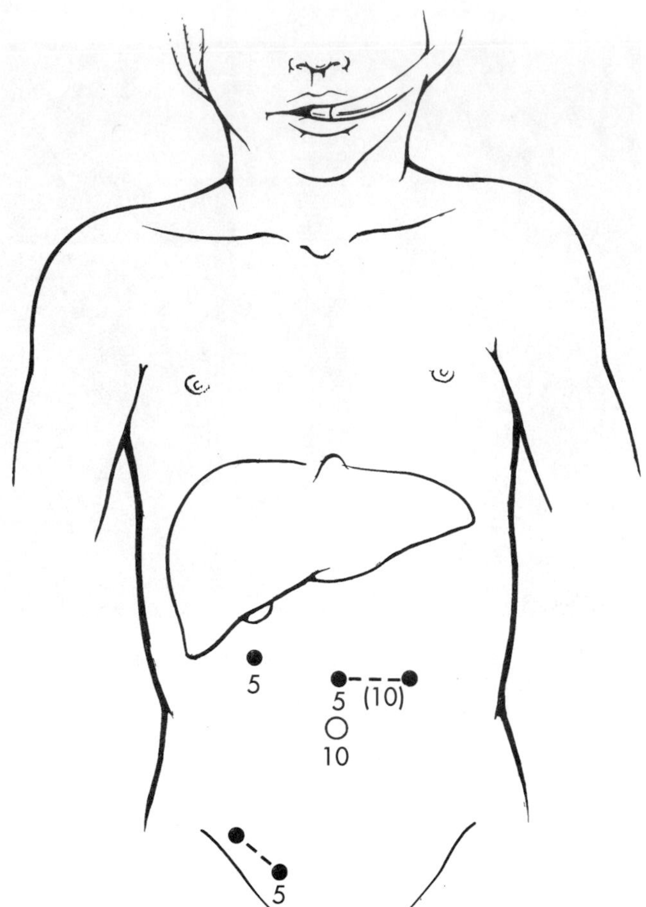

Fig. 32-6 Placement of the ports for laparoscopic cholecystectomy depends on the size of the patient. The 5-mm epigastric port should be placed laterally in small children. In addition, the right lower port can be placed in the inguinal crease in smaller children.

(From Holcomb GW III: *Semin Pediatr Surg* 2:159, 1993.)

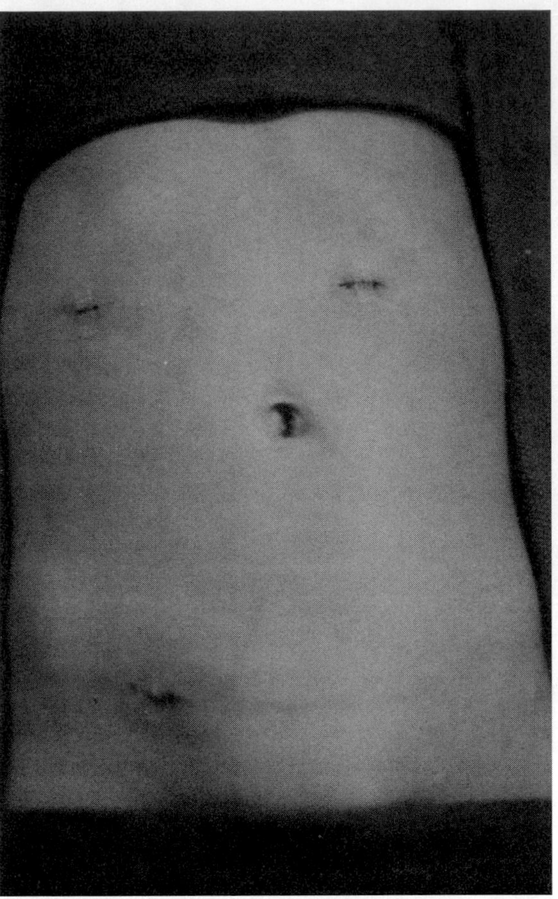

Fig. 32-7 The cosmetic result following laparoscopic cholecystectomy is seen in this 4-year-old patient. A 10-mm cannula was placed through the umbilicus. The other three incisions are 5 mm in length.

Appendectomy

Appendicitis is a common pediatric surgical problem. In 1980, Leape and Ramenofsky[43] reported the use of diagnostic laparoscopy to reduce the number of appendectomies in which a noninflamed appendix was removed. Three years later, Semm[71] described incidental laparoscopic appendectomy during gynecological procedures but did not think that laparoscopy should be employed for the acutely inflamed appendix. However, with the evolution in laparoscopic technology, this approach is being used increasingly to treat acute appendicitis in children (Fig. 32-9).

A three-cannula technique is used, with a 10- or 12-mm cannula being placed in the umbilicus. A 5-mm cannula is located in the left lower abdominal quadrant and a 3-mm cannula in the suprapubic region (Fig. 32-10). A 5-mm telescope then is inserted through the left lower quadrant cannula for visualization. The working port is the umbilical port and is 10 or 12 mm in size for removal of the enlarged appendix. Either endoscopic clips or an endoscopic stapler is used to ligate the mesoappendix (Fig. 32-11). Pre-tied ligatures on the stapler are used to ligate the base of the appendix. The appendix is removed through the umbilical port.

Laparoscopic appendectomy appears to be the preferential approach in certain selected circumstances (Box 32-2). For thin children younger than 7 or 8 years of age, an appendectomy generally can be performed, through a 15-mm right lower abdominal incision, with minimal morbidity and brief hospitalization. However, in older children in whom a longer incision is required, the laparoscopic approach is preferred because of reduced postoperative discomfort. Also, in obese children who require a long incision for exposure, in athletes who desire a quick return to participation in their athletic activity, and in adolescent females in whom the differential diagnosis between gynecological or appendiceal origin is not completely clear, the laparoscopic approach has advantages over the open approach.

One area of controversy is the child who has suspected or known perforation. It has been estimated that 30% of children who develop appendicitis are perforated before an appendectomy is performed. Therefore, management of suspected perforative appendicitis is a frequent pediatric surgical dilemma. One advantage of the laparoscopic approach in this situation is the opportunity for a more thorough irrigation and debridement of the abdominal cavity than can be performed through a small right lower quadrant incision. On the other hand, these patients may require 5 to 8 days of hospitaliza-

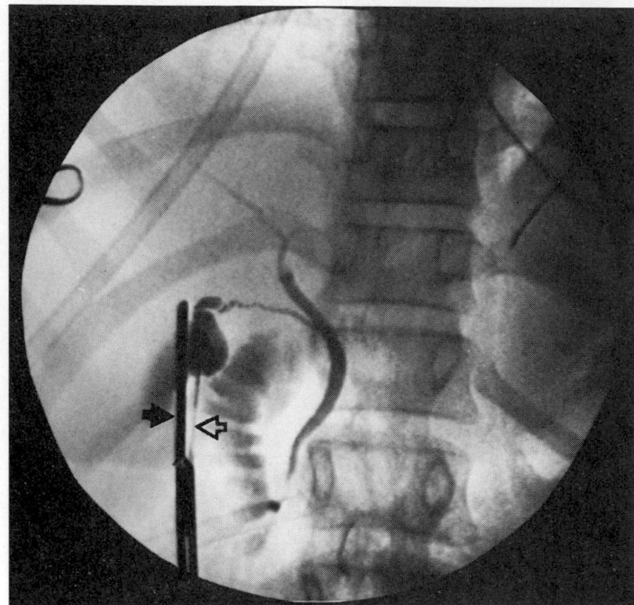

Fig. 32-8 Cholangiography is now being performed by using fluoroscopy. The cholangioclamp *(solid arrow)* is placed across the infundibulum of the gallbladder, and a sclerotherapy needle *(open arrow)* is inserted into the infundibulum. A small, long cystic duct is seen to enter the common bile duct, with free flow of dye into the duodenum. There is no evidence of choledocholithiasis.

(From Holcomb GW III, et al: *J Pediatr Surg* 29:900, 1994.)

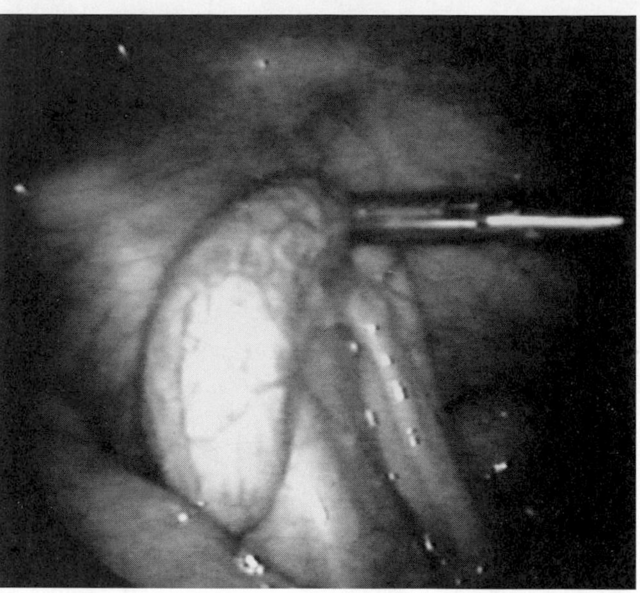

Fig. 32-9 The operative photograph depicts an acutely inflamed, distended appendix.

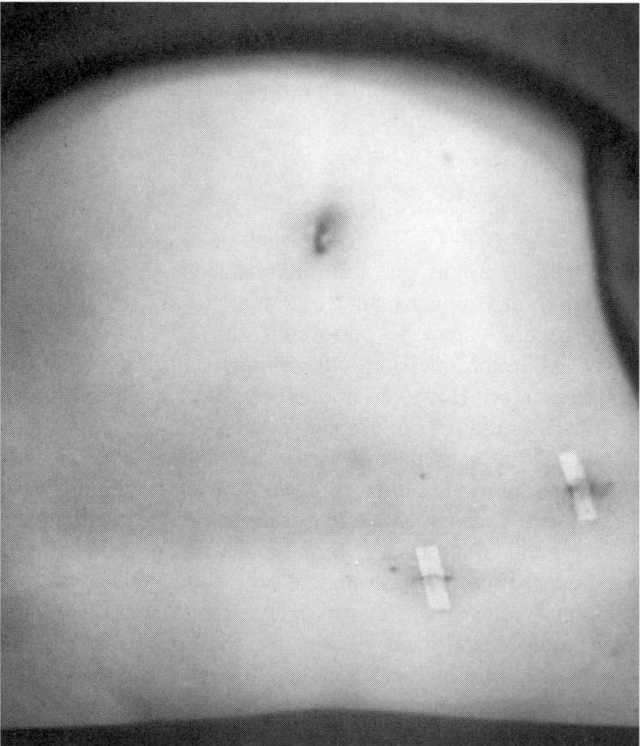

Fig. 32-10 This postoperative photograph depicts the location of the cannulas used in the three-port technique for laparoscopic appendectomy in a 14-year-old girl. A 10- or 12-mm cannula is inserted through the umbilicus for laparoscopic visualization and insertion of an endoscopic stapler. A 5-mm cannula is placed in the left lower quadrant, and a 3-mm port is situated in the suprapubic area.

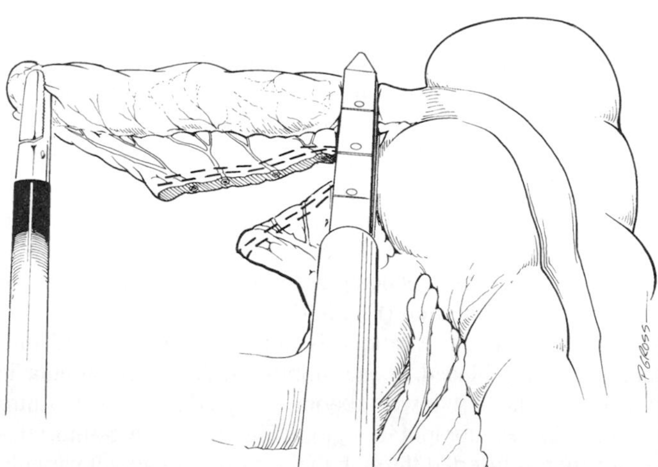

Fig. 32-11 The mesoappendix has already been divided with the stapler, and the proximal appendix is now being ligated and divided with an endoscopic stapler.

(From Holcomb GW III: *Laparosc Surg* 1:145, 1993.)

BOX 32-2

SELECTED INDICATIONS FOR LAPAROSCOPIC APPENDECTOMY IN CHILDREN

Patient older than 8 to 10 years
Obese patient
Athletes
Adolescent females whose diagnosis is unclear

tion to recover from the complications of perforation, including sepsis and ileus; therefore, reduced hospitalization is not an advantage of the laparoscopic route. In addition, laparoscopic management for perforated appendicitis usually requires longer operating time than for nonperforated appendicitis; therefore, the cost of the operative procedure itself is increased. If the initial management is nonoperative (intravenous fluids and antibiotics), an interval appendectomy 6 to 8 weeks later can be performed laparoscopically as an outpatient procedure.

Splenectomy and Fundoplication

The laparoscopic approach in many medical centers is becoming the preferred approach for fundoplication and splenectomy in children. Advantages of the laparoscopic technique for these two procedures include reduced discomfort compared with that of an upper abdominal incision and reduced respiratory complications. Also, resulting postoperative ileus is minimized by the laparoscopic approach. Finally, the endoscopic procedure has a cosmetic advantage.

The principles of the endoscopic procedure are very similar to those of the open operation.[45,46,77] For splenectomy, three 5-mm incisions are required, as well as a 15-mm one through which the spleen is extracted (Fig. 32-12). The peritoneal attachments to the spleen are divided, exposing the splenic vessels and pancreas within the hilum of the spleen. The vessels can be ligated by using endoscopic clips before division or by placing an endoscopic stapler across the vessels for ligation and division. Following mobilization of the spleen within the abdominal cavity, it is placed in a reinforced nylon bag. The neck of the bag is exteriorized through the largest incision, and the resulting splenic tissue is morcellated or diced into small pieces until the entire sac can be removed from the abdomen.

In a recent case-controlled study by Rescorla, Breitfeld, and West,[57] 50 patients undergoing laparoscopic splenectomy were compared with 32 patients having open splenectomy. The patients were similar in age, weight, indications for surgery, and estimated blood loss during the procedure. Although laparoscopic splenectomy required a longer operative time (115 versus 83 minutes), the need for postoperative intravenous narcotic was less, the total narcotic dosage was lower, length of hospital stay was shorter, and average total hospital charges in the laparoscopic group compared with the open group were lower. There were no deaths or major complications in either group.

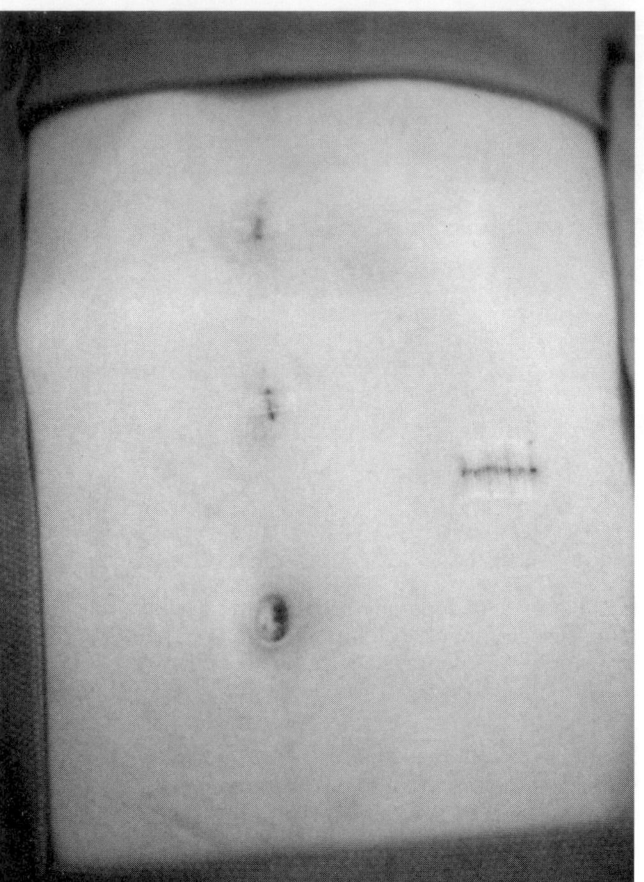

Fig. 32-12 This postoperative photograph demonstrates the incisions used for laparoscopic splenectomy. Two 5-mm incisions are situated in the midline of the upper abdomen, and one 5-mm incision is placed in the umbilicus. Through the 15-mm left midabdominal incision, the neck of the laparoscopic bag is exteriorized and the spleen removed in small pieces.

Fundoplication

Fundoplication in children is a commonly performed operation, which usually is required in three distinct groups: neurologically impaired infants, neurologically normal infants who have associated conditions (apnea/near-SIDS event, esophageal atresia/fistula), and neurologically normal older children who have gastroesophageal reflux refractory to medical management.

For laparoscopic fundoplication, five cannulas (3 and 5 mm) are required. The gastric fundus is mobilized, the diaphragmatic crura are approximated as in the open procedure, and fundoplication usually is performed with nonabsorbable sutures. Either a complete (Nissen) (Fig. 32-13) or partial (Thal, Toupet) fundoplication can be performed. A gastrostomy can be established if required, either endoscopically (percutaneous endoscopic gastrostomy) or laparoscopically at the time of fundoplication.

Georgeson recently reported his experience with 389 consecutive pediatric patients over 5 years requiring laparoscopic fundoplication with or without gastrostomy.[15] In the first 10 patients, the operative time required was 3 hours but was slightly over 1 hour for the last 50 patients, indicating the learning curve for the operation. Equivalent results with

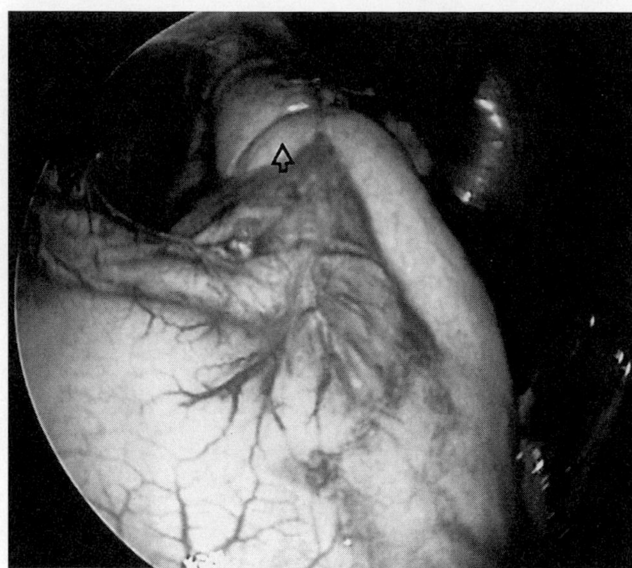

Fig. 32-13 This operative photograph demonstrates a complete Nissen fundoplication *(open arrow)*. The gastric fundus is wrapped 360 degrees around the esophagus.

less postoperative pain for those undergoing the laparoscopic operation were noted when patients undergoing the laparoscopic and open fundoplication were compared. Rothenberg has published his experience with 220 consecutive laparoscopic fundoplications in infants and children with similar results.[63] The average time to discharge following laparoscopic fundoplication was 1.6 days. He and other colleagues recently reviewed their experience with 56 patients who had severe steroid-dependent reactive airway disease and medical refractory gastroesophageal reflux who underwent laparoscopic Nissen fundoplication.[66] The mean operative time in this group was 62 minutes. Fifty of the 56 patients had been weaned off oral steroids at the time of publication; four others had a greater than 50% decrease in their dosage.

Other Indications

Other indications for procedural laparoscopy in children include laparoscopic gastrostomy without fundoplication, assistance with insertion and removal of ventriculo-peritoneal shunts, gonadectomy for intergender abnormalities, ovarian cystectomy, and testicular vein ligation for management of varicoceles. In addition, the laparoscopic approach for endorectal pull-through in newborns and young children who have Hirschsprung's disease recently has been popularized. In a combined publication from six pediatric surgical centers, the experience with 80 patients over the past 5 years was presented.[16] The age at surgery ranged from 3 days to 96 months, with the average duration of the surgical procedure being 2.5 hours. Most of the patients passed stool and flatus within 24 hours of surgery; the average time for discharge was 3.7 days. From this combined report, it is apparent that the technique can be learned quickly, and consistently good results can be achieved at many centers.

A small number of patients have undergone laparoscopic adrenalectomy for pheochromocytoma and hyperplasia.[9,47] Also, laparoscopic pyloromyotomy is becoming increasingly popular. Although satisfactory outcomes have been achieved with the open operation, the results have been consistently as good with the laparoscopic approach, with the added benefit of an improved cosmetic appearance to the abdominal wall.

A final area of potential application for this evolving technology is fetoscopic surgery. Physicians at The Fetal Treatment Center at the University of California in San Francisco have pioneered fetoscopic techniques in research animals for repair of fetal cleft lip and creation of a vesicocutaneous fistula for managing obstructive uropathy.[12] They also have performed fetoscopic repair of large congenital diaphragmatic hernias.[19] Yng and Adzick recently have reported their clinical application for fetoscopic surgery in more than 150 cases.[79]

THORACOSCOPY

In 1976, Rodgers and Talbert[61] first described the use of thoracoscopy in children. They reported nine children who required pulmonary or pleural biopsy. However, only a few pediatric surgeons were persuaded initially to use this approach. As the technique of laparoscopy has become refined, interest in the application of endoscopy to thoracic conditions also has blossomed. It now is being used extensively for a variety of conditions.

Principles of Technique

The patient's position on the operating table depends on the site of pathology. Unlike laparoscopy, in which the patient is placed supine, the patient is placed in the lateral decubitus position similar to that used in open thoracotomy. For lesions located in the anterior mediastinum, the patient is placed in a modified lateral decubitus position, allowing the ipsilateral lung to fall posteriorly, resulting in improved visualization of the anterior mediastinum. For posterior mediastinal masses, the patient is placed in an exaggerated decubitus position and the lung is allowed to fall forward, which improves access to the posterior mediastinum (Fig. 32-14).

If possible, it is helpful to collapse the ipsilateral lung to improve visualization and increase the working space within the thoracic cavity. Unlike the abdominal cavity, which is distended with carbon dioxide to achieve improved visualization and enlarge the working space, the thoracic cavity is rigid and does not expand with insufflation. Therefore, insufflation usually is not required but may be used selectively to compress the lung when selective intubation of the contralateral lung is not possible. The ipsilateral lung may be collapsed in older children by selected intubation of the contralateral mainstem bronchus and in younger children by insertion of a Fogarty catheter down the ipsilateral bronchus.

Indications

Indications for thoracoscopy in children are different from those in adults (Box 32-3). In adults, the most compelling reason is the evaluation or treatment of pleural effusions and pleural masses. However, the most frequent indication in children is for the evaluation of mediastinal masses.[58] Both

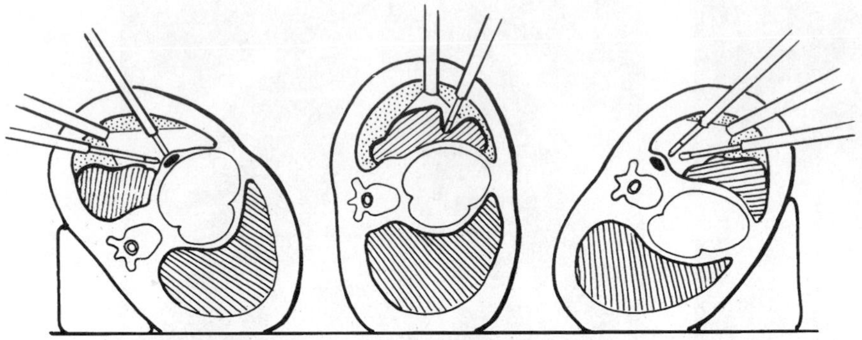

Anterior lesions: relative face up — Lung biopsy: lateral decubitus — Posterior lesions: relative face down

Fig. 32-14 Patient positioning for the thoracoscopic approach to mediastinal and pulmonary lesions in children is important. The relative positions of the three cannulas are also illustrated for these lesions.

(From Rodgers BM: Thoracoscopy. In Holcomb GW III, editor: *Pediatric endoscopic surgery,* Norwalk, Conn, 1993, Appleton & Lange.)

BOX 32-3

COMMON INDICATIONS FOR THORACOSCOPY IN CHILDREN

- Biopsy of mediastinal mass
- Lung biopsy for diagnosis
- Evacuation of empyema
- Pleural mass biopsy
- Resection of pulmonary bleb (recurrent pneumothorax)

the anterior and posterior mediastinum are readily available for endoscopic visualization, especially if the patient is positioned properly. Biopsy of anterior mediastinal masses and resection of benign posterior mediastinal masses can be performed. In addition, small neuroblastomas located in the posterior mediastinum may be amenable to resection in selected circumstances. Diagnostic accuracy for thoracoscopy in children who have mediastinal masses has ranged from 88% to 100%.[35,62,69]

Another frequent indication for thoracoscopy in children is the diagnosis of diffuse or localized pneumonia. Included in this patient population are those who are immunocompromised with diffuse interstitial pneumonia and those who have localized pneumonic processes not responding to appropriate antibiotic therapy. Diagnostic accuracy has been more than 90% in reported series.[33,59] Most of the morbidity in pediatric thoracoscopy occurs in immunocompromised patients who have diffuse parenchymal involvement. In one report, two patients required transfusion; however, an open procedure was not necessary. The 30-day mortality was 11%, although the procedure itself was not thought to have influenced the deaths of these critically ill children directly.[60] No mortality has been reported in patients who have localized inflammatory processes who undergo thoracoscopic biopsies.[33,60,62]

The most common use for thoracoscopy at CH-VUMC has been for the evaluation and treatment of pleural diseases, with a focus on early surgical intervention for children who have empyema for evacuation and debridement of the pleural space.[21,22] At CH-VUMC, 27 children have undergone thoracoscopic debridement and decortication between 1993 and 1999 without complications or recurrence of disease. Other pediatric surgeons have had similar good results (Figs. 32-15 and 32-16).[14,34,39,48,53]

Thoracoscopy is being used increasingly in children for management of recurrent pneumothoraces. The entire visceral pleural surface can be examined and bullous disease identified. Usually, a fibrin peel is visualized that has been caused by an inflammatory response from the ruptured bulla. The bulla can be resected by using the endoscopic stapler or a pretied surgical ligature. Recurrent pneumothoraces are seen frequently in children who have cystic fibrosis. Thoracoscopy is ideal for this fragile patient population. Tribble, Selden, and Rodgers[76] reported on five patients with cystic fibrosis who were undergoing thoracoscopic management. They also performed pleurodesis in these patients by dusting the pleural surface with dry talc or by using mechanical abrasion. Although the use of talc has been successful in most cases, using this substance in patients who have cystic fibrosis who later may be candidates for lung transplantation is controversial.

Thoracoscopy also is advantageous for localized or diffuse pleural-based masses in children in whom malignancy is suspected. Thoracoscopic biopsy can be performed, obviating the need for an open thoracotomy for diagnosis. In a review of patients undergoing thoracoscopy for suspected cancer by the Children's Cancer Group (CCG), 60 patients underwent 63 thoracoscopic operations. For the 51 operations in which either a wedge resection or biopsy was possible thoracoscopically, diagnostic tissue was obtained in all but one patient.[32] A similarly good experience has been reported at St. Jude's Children's Hospital.[55] In 64 procedures, thoracoscopy yielded a successful diagnosis in 90% of the cases. Conversion to open thoracotomy was necessary in 11 patients.

The thoracoscopic approach in children is being used for numerous other indications. It has been described in conjunction with placement of cerebral spinal fluid shunts in children, diaphragmatic plication, azygos vein cannulation, and repair of Bochdalek hernia, as well as evaluation for traumatic injury.* It also has been useful for division of vascular rings and ligation of patent ductus

*References 2, 8, 28, 36, 73, 78.

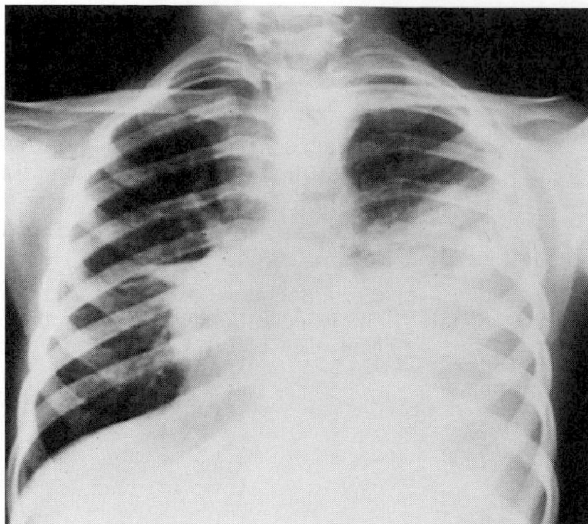

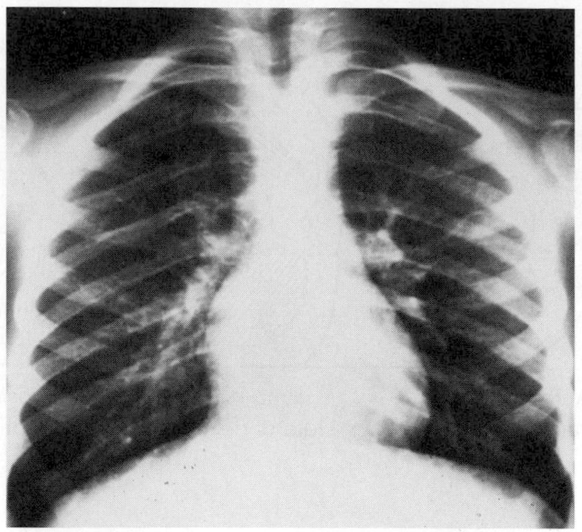

Fig. 32-15 A 6-year-old girl presented with fever, respiratory distress, and a large left thoracic empyema *(left)*. Following thoracoscopic debridement and evacuation of her left pleural space, she was discharged on the fifth postoperative day. A chest radiograph *(right)* 1 month postoperatively documents almost complete resolution.

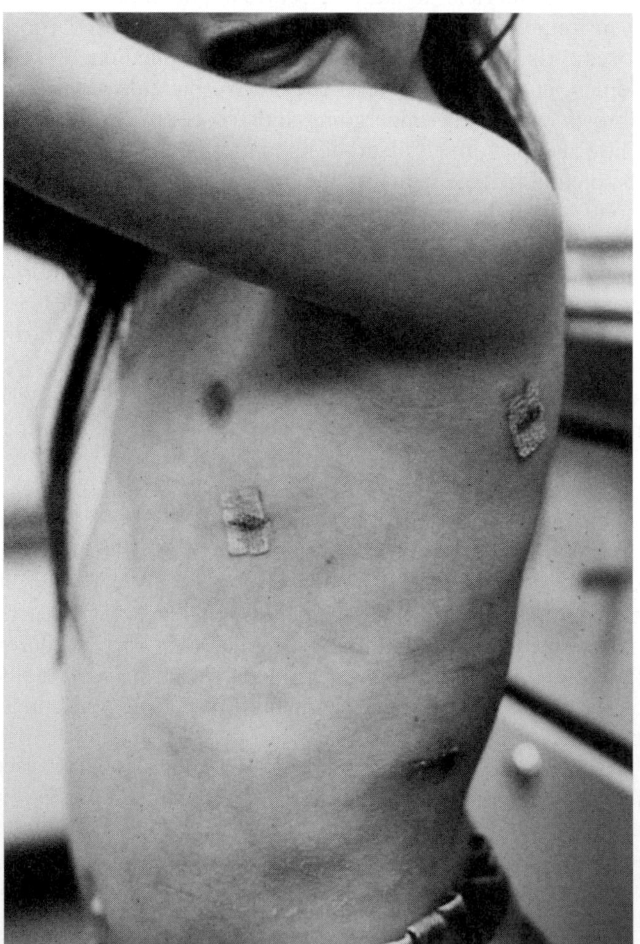

Fig. 32-16 Postoperative photograph of the 6-year-old girl described in Fig. 32-15. Note the three small incisions for her thoracoscopic procedure.

arteriosus.[7,20,41,42,44] In a recent presentation of 100 children undergoing thoracoscopic lung resection, Rothenberg described seven patients who underwent pulmonary lobectomy or segmental resection.[64]

Anterior Thoracoscopic Release, Diskectomy, and Fusion

Recently, pediatric thoracic surgeons and spine surgeons have gained an experience with video assisted thoracoscopic diskectomy and fusion for correction of scoliosis.[6,25,40,51,67] Between 1995 and 1999, 40 patients at CH-VUMC underwent thoracoscopic release, diskectomy, and fusion before posterior fusion and instrumentation. Bleeding from an intercostal vessel in one patient was the only serious complication; it required transfusion but not conversion to thoracotomy. The anticipated operation was completed in all patients, which allowed further correction of severe scoliosis than would have been possible with the posterior operation alone. The primary benefit of this approach is reduced operative time as well as reduced postoperative discomfort compared with an anterior thoracotomy. In two additional patients, anterior instrumentation was performed thoracoscopically, which obviated the need for posterior instrumentation and fusion.

Minimally Invasive Repair for Pectus Excavatum

In 1998, Nuss et al reported a 10-year experience with the minimally invasive approach for a correction of pectus excavatum.[52] Since that initial report, many pediatric surgeons have embraced it as the ideal operation for correction of this condition. With this novel approach, a curved steel bar is inserted under the sternum through a 2.5-cm incision in each lateral chest wall between the anterior axillary and posterior axillary lines. Selection of the appropriate intercostal space depends on the nadir of the pectus excavatum deformity because it is important to situate the bar directly under the most prominent point of the defect. A long, curved clamp is advanced slowly across the mediastinum anterior to the heart and directly posterior to the sternum until it emerges through the contralateral intercostal space. The tunnel that is created by passage of the curved clamp is enlarged slowly. Once the tract is wide enough, a 1.5-cm wide and 2-mm thick steel bar is grasped by the clamp and pulled beneath the sternum. The bar initially is passed under the sternum, with the convexity facing posteriorly but is rotated with the convexity facing anteriorly once it is in the desired position, thereby raising the sternum and anterior chest wall. It is important to secure the bar to the lateral chest wall muscles and ribs with heavy sutures. Occasionally a second bar is required for those patients who have a long and deep deformity; this bar is situated cephalad or caudal to the first one, as needed. If two bars are required, a cross bar stabilizing device may be used to connect the ends of each bar, one to the other, so that the bars will be stable and will not slip. The bar(s) usually are left in place for 2 years and are removed as an outpatient procedure.

This approach is advantageous because a midline chest incision, which often results in hypertrophic scarring postoperatively, is not required, and the operative time is reduced from approximately 5 hours to 2 hours. However, application of this technique probably should be reserved for those patients who have a symmetrical excavatum deformity; a combined excavatum/carinatum deformity will result in a more prominent carinatum deformity postoperatively when the excavatum portion has been corrected. Because this approach takes less time to perform than the traditional open operation, it is rapidly becoming the procedure of choice for correction of severe pectus excavatum deformities (see also Chapter 247, Pectus Excavatum and Pectus Carinatum).

THE FUTURE

At some point, almost every operation will likely be performed utilizing a minimally invasive approach. However, as pediatric surgeons learn these new endoscopic operative techniques, it will be necessary to apply this approach judiciously and selectively as more complex operations are entertained.

REFERENCES

1. Bailey PV, et al: Changing spectrum of cholelithiasis and cholecystitis in infants and children, *Am J Surg* 158:585, 1989.
2. Bax NM, van der Zee DC: Thoracoscopic guided percutaneous cannulation of the azygos vein in children, *Surg Endosc* 10:863, 1996.
3. Bloom DA: Two-step orchiopexy with pelviscopic clip ligation of the spermatic vessels, *J Urol* 145:1030, 1991.
4. Bloom DA, Ayers JWT, McGuire EJ: The role of laparoscopy in the management of nonpalpable testes, *J Urol* 94:465, 1988.
5. Bloom DA, Ritchey ML, Manzoni G: Laparoscopy for the nonpalpable testis. In Holcomb GW III, editor: *Pediatric endoscopic surgery*, Norwalk, Conn, 1993, Appleton & Lange.
6. Burgos J, Rapariz JM, Gonzalez-Herranz P: Anterior endoscopic approach to the thoracolumbar spine, *Spine* 23:2427, 1998.
7. Burke RP, et al: Video-assisted thoracoscopic vascular ring division in infants and children, *J Am Coll Cardiol* 25:943, 1995.
8. Chen MK, Schropp KP, Lobe TE: The use of minimal access surgery in pediatric trauma: a preliminary report, *J Laparoendosc Surg* 5:295, 1995.
9. Clements RH, Goldstein RE, Holcomb GW III: Laparoscopic left adrenalectomy for pheochromocytoma in a child, *J Pediatr Surg* 34:1408, 1995.
10. Diamond DA, Caldamone AA: The value of laparoscopy for 106 impalpable testes relative to clinical presentation, *J Urol* 148:632, 1992.
11. Elder JS: Laparoscopy for the nonpalpable testis, *Semin Pediatr Surg* 2:168, 1993.
12. Estes JM, Adzick NS, Harrison MR: Fetoscopic surgery. In Holcomb GW III, editor: *Pediatric endoscopic surgery,* Norwalk, Conn, 1993, Appleton & Lange.
13. Frexes M, Neblett WW III, Holcomb GW Jr: Spectrum of biliary disease in childhood, *South Med J* 79:1342, 1986.
14. Gandhi RR, Stringel G: Video-assisted thoracoscopic surgery in the management of pediatric empyema, *J Soc Laparoendosc Surg* 1:251, 1997.
15. Georgeson KE: Laparoscopic fundoplication and gastrostomy, *Semin Laparosc Surg* 5:25, 1998.
16. Georgeson KE, et al: Primary laparoscopic-assisted endorectal colon pull-through for Hirschsprung's disease, *Ann Surg* 229:678, 1998.
17. Gilbert M, Clatworthy HW: Bilateral operations for inguinal hernia and hydrocele in infancy and childhood, *Am J Surg* 97:255, 1959.
18. Hagberg B, Svennerholm L, Thorén L: Cholelithiasis in childhood, *Acta Chir Scand* 123:307, 1962.
19. Harrison MR, Albanese C, Jennings R: *Repair of diaphragmatic hernia in utero: from open fetal surgery to fetendo clip* (video presentation), American Pediatric Surgical Association, Rancho Mirage, Calif, 1999.
20. Hines MH, et al: Video-assisted thoracoscopic ligation of patent ductus arteriosus: safe and outpatient, *Ann Thorac Surg* 66:853, 1998.
21. Hoff SJ, et al: Parapneumonic empyema in children: decortication hastens recovery in patients with severe pleural infections, *Pediatr Infect Dis J* 10:194, 1990.
22. Hoff SJ, et al: Postpneumonic empyema in childhood: selecting appropriate therapy, *J Pediatr Surg* 24:659, 1989.
23. Holcomb GW III: Laparoscopic evaluation for a contralateral inguinal hernia or a nonpalpable testis, *Pediatr Ann* 22:678, 1993.
24. Holcomb GW Jr, Holcomb GW III: Cholelithiasis in infants, children, and adolescents, *Pediatr Rev* 11:268, 1990.
25. Holcomb GW III, Mencio GA, Green NE: Video-assisted thoracoscopic diskectomy and fusion, *J Pediatr Surg* 32:1120, 1997.
26. Holcomb GW III, Olsen DO, Sharp KW: Laparoscopic cholecystectomy in the pediatric patient, *J Pediatr Surg* 26:1186, 1991.
27. Holcomb GW Jr, O'Neill JA Jr, Holcomb GW III: Cholecystitis, cholelithiasis and common duct stenosis in children and adolescents, *Ann Surg* 191:626, 1980.
28. Holcomb GW III, Smith HP: Laparoscopic and thoracoscopic assistance with CSF shunts in children, *J Pediatr Surg* 30:1642, 1995.
29. Holcomb GW III, et al: Laparoscopic cholecystectomy in children: lessons learned from the first 100 patients, *J Pediatr Surg* 34:1236, 1999.
30. Holcomb GW III, et al: Laparoscopic cholecystectomy in infants and children: modifications and cost analysis, *J Pediatr Surg* 29:900, 1994.
31. Holcomb GW III, et al: Laparoscopy for the nonpalpable testis, *Am Surg* 60:143, 1994.
32. Holcomb GW III, et al: Minimally invasive surgery in children with cancer, *Cancer* 76:121, 1995.
33. Janik JS, Nagaraj HS, Groff DB: Thoracoscopic evaluation of intrathoracic lesions in children, *J Thorac Cardiovasc Surg* 83:408, 1982.
34. Kern JA, Rodgers BM: Thoracoscopy in the management of empyema in children, *J Pediatr Surg* 28:1128, 1993.
35. Kern JA, et al: Thoracoscopic diagnosis and treatment of mediastinal masses, *Ann Thorac Surg* 56:92, 1993.
36. Kern JA, et al: Thoracoscopy: a potential role in the subacute management of patients with thoraco-abdominal trauma, *Chest* 104:27, 1992.
37. Kiesewetter WB, Oh KS: Unilateral inguinal hernias in children: what about the opposite side? *Arch Surg* 115:1443, 1980.
38. Kirtley JA, Holcomb GW Jr: Surgical management of diseases of the gallbladder and common duct in children and adolescents, *Am J Surg* 111:39, 1966.

39. Klena JW, et al: Timing of video-assisted thoracoscopic debridement for pediatric empyema, *J Am Coll Surg* 187:404, 1998.
40. Kokoska ER, Gabriel KR, Silen ML: Minimally invasive anterior spinal exposure and release in children with scoliosis, *J Soc Laparoendosc Surg* 2:255, 1998.
41. Laborde F, et al: A new video-assisted thoracoscopic surgical technique for interruption of patent ductus arteriosus in infants and children, *J Thorac Cardiovasc Surg* 105:278, 1993.
42. Laborde F, et al: Video-assisted thoracoscopic surgical interruption: the technique of choice for patent ductus arteriosus. Routine experience in 230 pediatric cases, *J Thorac Cardiovasc Surg* 110:1681, 1995.
43. Leape LL, Ramenofsky ML: Laparoscopy for questionable appendicitis: can it reduce the negative appendectomy rate? *Ann Surg* 191:410, 1980.
44. Le Bret E, Folliguet TA, Laborde F: Videothoracoscopic surgical interruption of patent ductus arteriosus, *Ann Thorac Surg* 64:1492, 1997.
45. Lobe TE, Schropp KP, Lunsford K: Laparoscopic Nissen fundoplication in childhood, *J Pediatr Surg* 28:358, 1993.
46. Lobe TE, Schropp KP, Rogers DA: Laparoscopic management for inguinal and hiatal hernia (Nissen fundoplication). In Holcomb GW III, editor: *Pediatric endoscopic surgery,* Norwalk, Conn, 1993, Appleton & Lange.
47. Lopoo JB, et al: Laparoscopic adrenalectomy in children, *Pediatr Endosurg Innovative Tech* 2:107, 1998.
48. Merry CM, et al: Early definitive intervention by thoracoscopy in pediatric empyema, *J Pediatr Surg* 34:178, 1999.
49. Moir CR, Donohue JH, VanHeerden JA: Laparoscopic cholecystectomy in children: initial experience and recommendations, *J Pediatr Surg* 27:1066, 1992.
50. Newman KD, et al: Laparoscopic cholecystectomy in pediatric patients, *J Pediatr Surg* 26:1184, 1991.
51. Newton PO, et al: Anterior release and fusion in pediatric spinal deformity: a comparison of early outcome and cost of thoracoscopic and open thoracotomy approaches, *Spine* 22:1398, 1997.
52. Nuss D, et al: A 10-year review of a minimally invasive technique for the correction of pectus excavatum, *J Pediatr Surg* 33:545, 1998.
53. Patton RM, Abrams RS, Gauderer MW: Is thoracoscopically aided pleural debridement advantageous in children? *Am Surg* 65:69, 1999.
54. Ransley PG, et al: Preliminary ligation of the gonadal vessels prior to orchidopexy for the intra-abdominal testicle: a staged Fowler-Stephens procedure, *World J Urol* 2:266, 1984.
55. Rao BN: Present day concepts of thoracoscopy as a modality in pediatric cancer management, *Int Surg* 82:123, 1997.
56. Reif S, Sloven DG, Lebenthal E: Gallstones in children: characterization by age, etiology and outcome, *Am J Dis Child* 145:105, 1991.
57. Rescorla FJ, Breitfeld PP, West KW: A case controlled comparison of open and laparoscopic splenectomy in children, *Surgery* 124:670, 1998.
58. Rodgers BA: Thoracoscopy. In Holcomb GW III, editor: *Pediatric endoscopic surgery,* Norwalk, Conn., 1993, Appleton & Lange.
59. Rodgers BM: Thoracoscopy in children, *Poumon-Coeur* 37:301, 1981.
60. Rodgers BM, Moazam F, Talbert JL: Thoracoscopy in children, *Ann Surg* 189:176, 1979.
61. Rodgers BM, Talbert JL: Thoracoscopy for diagnosis of intrathoracic lesions in children, *J Pediatr Surg* 11:703, 1976.
62. Rogers DA, et al: Thoracoscopy in children: an initial experience with an evolving technique, *J Laparoendosc Surg* 2:7, 1992.
63. Rothenberg SS: Experience with 220 consecutive laparoscopic Nissen fundoplications in infants and children, *J Pediatric Surg* 33:274, 1998.
64. Rothenberg SS: Thoracoscopic lung resection in children, *J Pediatr Surg* 35:271, 2000.
65. Rothenberg RE, Barnett T: Bilateral herniotomy in infants and children, *Surgery* 37:947, 1955.
66. Rothenberg SS, et al: Laparoscopic fundoplication to enhance pulmonary function in children with severe reactive airway disease and gastroesophageal reflux disease, *Surg Endosc* 11:1088, 1997.
67. Rothenberg S, et al: Thoracoscopic anterior spinal procedures in children, *J Pediatr Surg* 33:1168, 1998.
68. Rowe MI, Copelson LW, Clatworthy HW: The patent processus vaginalis and the inguinal hernia, *J Pediatr Surg* 4:102, 1969.
69. Ryckman FC, Rodgers BM: Thoracoscopy for intrathoracic neoplasm in children, *J Pediatr Surg* 17:521, 1982.
70. Seiler I: Gallbladder disease in children, *Am J Dis Child* 99:662, 1960.
71. Semm K: Endoscopic appendectomy, *Endoscopy* 15:50, 1983.
72. Sigman HH, et al: Laparoscopic cholecystectomy: a treatment option for gallbladder disease in children, *J Pediatr Surg* 26:1181, 1991.
73. Silen ML, et al: Video-assisted thoracic surgical repair of a foramen of Bochdalek hernia, *Ann Thorac Surg* 60:448, 1995.
74. Sparkman RS: Bilateral exploration in inguinal hernia in juvenile patients, *Surgery* 51:393, 1962.
75. Stafford PW: The evaluation of chronic abdominal pain in children: a role for diagnostic laparoscopy? Third International Congress on Endoscopy and Laparoscopy in Children, Munster, Germany, Feb 1-2, 1994 (abstract).
76. Tribble CG, Selden RF, Rodgers BM: Talc poudrage in the treatment of spontaneous pneumothoraces in patients with cystic fibrosis, *Ann Surg* 204:677, 1986.
77. Tulman S, et al: Pediatric laparoscopic splenectomy, *J Pediatr Surg* 28:689, 1993.
78. Van Smith C, Jacobs JP, Burke RP: Minimally invasive diaphragm plication in an infant, *Ann Thora Surg* 65:842, 1998.
79. Yng EY, Adzick NS: Fetoscopy, *Semin Laparosc Surg* 5:31, 1998.

33 Physical Disability and Chronic Illness

Gregory S. Liptak

DEFINITION AND DEMOGRAPHICS

Children who have chronic health conditions and physical disabilities (frequently termed *children who have special health care needs*) are those who have or are at increased risk for a chronic, physical, or developmental condition and who also require health and related services of a type or amount beyond that required by children generally.[16] Chronic disabling conditions include (but are not limited to) asthma, bronchopulmonary dysplasia, cystic fibrosis, congenital heart disease, diabetes mellitus, hemophilia, HIV infection, cerebral palsy, meningomyelocele, inflammatory bowel disease, renal failure, epilepsy, cancer, juvenile arthritis, and red cell disorders (such as sickle cell disease).

Although each condition taken individually is uncommon, taken together they affect approximately 5% to 15% of all children and constitute an important part of pediatric practice.[10,21] Over the past 20 years disease-specific survival rates have improved dramatically; however, many of these survivors have severe limitations of activity and function.[14]

COMMON CHARACTERISTICS

Although these children differ from each other in various ways, they and their families share common characteristics, which are shown in Box 33-1.[10] A widely held generalization is that 85% of the issues with which children and families must deal are common to all chronic conditions, whereas 15% of the issues are specific to the child's particular condition.

The negative impact of a chronic condition, which can manifest as behavioral problems and psychopathology, such as depression, poor socialization, and family disruption,[5,24] is worsened at all periods of development by low socioeconomic status.[9]

DEVELOPMENTAL CONSIDERATIONS

In addition to understanding the medical condition and commonalties cited above, the health care provider caring for a child who has a chronic disability also must understand the interactions between the condition and the developing child and family.[19]

Infancy

Conditions that affect the physical appearance of an infant, such as cleft lip and palate or hydrocephalus, can affect the bonding and attachment between child and caretakers.[12] In addition, once a chronic condition has been diagnosed, the parents will begin to grieve for the lost "normal" child. This bereavement includes shock, denial, anger, sadness/depression, guilt, and anxiety. Parents may go through these stages of mourning at any time in the child's development, especially during transitions—for example, when the child begins kindergarten or the family moves to a new community.[25] One parent may be primarily experiencing one set of feelings such as guilt while another experiences feelings such as anger. This makes communication between them difficult and decreases their ability to support each other. This grief also may interfere with their ability to become attached to the chronically ill child. Parents may direct their feelings of anger toward the pediatrician or seek multiple opinions because of their denial of the diagnosis and prognosis that has been made.

The behavior of pediatricians during this period can have a major influence on the family's acceptance of their disabled child. The words that are used and the actions that are shown, such as holding the infant or encouraging the parent to do so, can improve acceptance. Discussion of parental feelings and counseling about financial assistance and community support can be invaluable to improving the family's coping abilities.

Whenever a pediatrician informs a family of the presence of a chronic disability in their child, care must be taken to ensure that the family understands the condition and that their needs (including those of siblings) are met.[20] Start with an open-ended question such as, "How are you feeling?" or "What have you been told so far?" and listen nonjudgmentally, even to negative opinions and feelings. This requires the ability to listen, without providing false reassurances or premature suggestions (before the family feels that they understand the import of their child's condition or have received empathy from the physician). Such news often leads to very strong emotions. Acknowledge them with a statement such as, "This must be absolutely awful for you." Ask about the care they are receiving, such as, "Is there anything we are doing or not doing that worries you?" Review the information you've discussed, identify a plan for the next contact

BOX 33-1

COMMON FEATURES OF CHRONIC DISABILITY IN CHILDHOOD

Child
- Chronic, often unpredictable course
- No cure
- Pain and discomfort
- Restricted growth and development
- Frequent hospitalizations and outpatient visits
- Painful, embarrassing treatments
- Inability to participate in peer activities
- Daily burden of care

Family
- Loss of "ideal" child
- Daily burden of care
- Expense (financial, time)
- Lost opportunities
- Neglected siblings
- Confusing systems of health and other care
- Social isolation

Community
- Poor understanding of chronic illness
- Inconsistent policies and funding
- Inadequate facilities (including barriers to access)
- Poor communication and coordination within the health care system and with other agencies

and for future care. Patience and repetition of information often are required, as is sensitivity to verbal and nonverbal communication.

Preschool

The normal development of preschool children includes the achievement of a sense of autonomy and initiative. One way that children show autonomy is by literally walking away. If a child is physically disabled and cannot walk or is bedridden because of illness, he or she cannot express autonomy by walking away and must express it in some other way. This may manifest as negative verbal behavior or disobedience.[8] Allowing the child to show autonomy in acceptable ways—for example, by having the child choose clothing or food items on a menu or the arm into which the intravenous line will go—can lessen the occurrence of unacceptable behaviors.

The demands of the chronic condition placed on the family, as well as feelings of sympathy for the child (e.g., "She has suffered enough") may make consistent limit-setting difficult for parents and can lead to behavior problems in the child. One parent (often the mother) may become overinvolved with the child, thus blurring normal family relationships. The father may become isolated from health care decisions or the care of the child, a process that is promulgated by the typical Monday through Friday, 9:00 AM to 5:00 PM office hours of most pediatricians and paternal work schedules. Efforts should be made to alter physician and parent schedules to include both parents in discussions of treatment and prognostications. Encouraging parents to achieve a balance in their roles as parents, spouses, and workers by helping them find support in the community (e.g., for spending time as a couple away from the children) can help families cope.

Referring a young child to an early intervention program may provide support for the family and educational and therapeutic treatments that will assist the child's development. It also may encourage the family to increase their contact with their child. Legislation, such as the Individuals with Disabilities Education Act, is increasing the availability of preschool programs for children at risk for developmental delay.[2] Unfortunately, day care and nursery programs for children with disabilities who are not at risk for developmental delay, such as those who have asthma, are woefully insufficient to meet the demand.

Young children are especially vulnerable to the effects of separation that occur when they are hospitalized. The pediatrician should encourage rooming-in for parents during hospitalizations, as well as frequent visits from all family members. This includes helping the family obtain transportation, child care, or other nonmedical services.

The pediatrician needs to be aware of the child's temperament, as well as his or her abilities and motivations. Children who are intense, persistent, irregular in day-to-day rhythm, and negative in mood can be especially difficult for families, even without the added stress of a chronic illness.[6] Providing insight to families about the nature of their child's temperament can decrease their guilt and can provide them with more effective ways of coping with their child's behavior.

School Ages

Previous problems with autonomy and initiative may manifest upon school entry and thereafter. The dependent, disabled child may have serious difficulty separating from his or her parents to attend school. Separation anxiety can affect the parents, who may impose unreasonable restrictions on their child's activities or who may have unreasonable expectations of their child's abilities.

Some chronic conditions such as hydrocephalus, cerebral palsy, lead toxicity, or brain injury impair the child's cognitive or motor abilities directly. Other conditions, such as cyanotic heart disease and sickle cell anemia, which do not affect the brain directly, also have been shown to impair cognition. Children who have chronic conditions often miss more school than do other children.[7] These features of chronic illness can hinder a child's ability to achieve a sense of industry at school. A wide array of educational and health-related services is mandated by the Individuals With Disabilities Education Act (IDEA) and Section 504 of the Rehabilitation Act, which require children from ages 3 years to 21 years to receive an appropriate education in an inclusive, least restrictive environment (see Chapter 39, The Chronically Ill and Disabled Child in School). These laws authorize the provision of services such as physical therapy, occupational therapy, speech therapy, audiology, transportation, psychological services, assistive technology, social work services, and nursing services. Taking children away from their classrooms to perform these services, however, may affect their academic performance and socialization adversely. IDEA also entitles every child to a written Individualized Education Plan (IEP); parents are guaranteed the right to question decisions about placement and the right to due process in settling differences.

According to social learning theorists,[3] a child's conviction that he or she can execute successfully a behavior required to produce a certain outcome (self-efficacy) determines how much effort will be expended in that activity. Because chronically disabled children may look or act different from others, they frequently are rejected by peers despite their best efforts at socialization. Their repeated lack of success in this regard will lead to decreased efforts in the development of social relations (learned helplessness) and may produce deviant social and personality development as they grow older. Children who have learning disabilities as part of their chronic condition and are unable to learn the "rules" of socialization may also be rejected by peers. Children who are deficient in physical and self-help skills have been shown to have fewer coping skills and more difficulty establishing satisfactory social relations than their peers.[4]

If the child's teacher or the school nurse is not knowledgeable about the child's condition, the child's care at school may be impaired. The pediatrician should inform and regularly update school personnel about the child's condition and expectations for achievement. Providing a written assessment of the child's needs and a plan for the school to follow during an emergency and clarifying roles and responsibilities can greatly decrease the discomfort of school personnel, improve communication, and enhance care.[18] Parents also should be encouraged to collaborate with school personnel.

During this period the pediatrician can encourage the child to increase his or her responsibility to manage the chronic condition—for example, the child can be made responsible for ensuring that medications and treatments are received as scheduled and can keep a diary of illness-related events.

Adolescence

Chronic disabilities can affect the social and emotional development of the adolescent profoundly. Issues of major concern during this period are shown in Box 33-2. The presence of a chronic condition significantly increases the risk for behavior problems and psychiatric disorders such as depression. The pediatrician should be aware of the signs and symptoms of depression, which may be subtle, including a sad or flat affect, loss of interest in usual activities, lowered self-esteem, social withdrawal, impaired school work, fatigue, and irritability. Behavioral problems and emotional distress are not directly correlated with the physiological severity of the condition, however. Children who are marginally affected—for example, those who have low-level spina bifida or minimal arthritis—may have greater difficulty adjusting during adolescence than those more severely affected.[23] Minimally affected children may not be able to identify with the world of "normals" because they cannot accomplish many normal activities (such as running or achieving continence), nor would they identify with the world of the severely impaired individual, such as a child in a wheelchair.

BOX 33-2

ISSUES OF SPECIAL RELEVANCE FOR ADOLESCENTS

- Physical appearance (actual and perceived)
- Social isolation
- Sexual development
  - Physical maturation, including onset of puberty
  - Heterosexual relationship ideations
  - Sexual behavior and contraception
- Vocational planning
- Genetic counseling

The adverse effects of chronic conditions are modified by the gender of the child as well as by socioeconomic status.[8] For example, delayed sexual maturation is more likely to lead to depression and social isolation in boys than in girls.

Adolescents develop a sense of identity by emulating role models. Adolescents with disabilities often have few role models. The normative values for concepts such as "beauty," which assail adolescents through the print media and television, often are widely discrepant from their own self-images. The lack of role models, isolation from peers, poor self-image, and a pervasive culture that stresses physical appearance make the development of a positive identity difficult at best.

The pediatrician should address the issues outlined in Box 33-2 and address the feelings of the adolescent related to his or her self-concept and condition. Most authorities recommend that the adolescent be evaluated by the pediatrician without the parents present in order to build a trusting relationship that inspires independence.

SYSTEMS OF CARE

The goal for the management of the child who has chronic disabilities should be to *achieve maximum functioning*. For example, the goal of a specific orthopedic intervention should be to help a child walk, not to straighten his or her feet. It is ironic that the specialization that has improved the health and longevity of children who have chronic conditions has resulted in fragmentation of care within the health care system. Also, communication between medical personnel and other agencies, such as the educational and legal systems, often is inadequate. Access to services still is difficult for many families, especially those who have no health insurance, and preventive services may be unavailable.[11,22] This has resulted in duplication of some services and gaps in others. Managed care has the potential to improve coordination of services; however, it also may reduce access to specialty physicians and to other professional services, including behavioral medicine and social work.[1]

Case Management

Achieving optimum functioning requires an organized, coordinated approach to care, which is embodied in the concept of case management.[13] Comprehensive case management includes (1) *assessing needs*—identifying and assessing the needs of the child and family, including their financial needs[15]; (2) *planning comprehensive care*—planning and arranging for medical and nonmedical services; (3) *facilitating and coordinating services* (including training community providers); (4) *following up*—monitoring services and patient progress; and (5) *empowering*—counseling, educating, training, and supporting the child and family. Successful implementation requires knowledge of the child, the family, and the community in which they function.

Possible case managers for children who have chronic conditions have been suggested, including the primary care physician, the specialty program, the community health nurse, and governmental programs. However, any professional who cares for a child who has special health care needs must ensure that *someone* is providing this service. Without it these children will receive less than optimum care, and families will face an even greater burden.

The pediatrician who attends the child who has a chronic condition can foster the child's development and functioning in the community. Achieving this goal requires knowing the needs of the child's family and the resources in the community. This does not necessitate the provision of all services by that single provider. It does, however, require time, which frequently is not reimbursed; thoughtful coordination of effort; support of other professionals; and advocacy.

SUMMARY

The physician who cares for the child or adolescent who has a physical disability or chronic condition is in a particularly advantageous position to foster the child's psychological development. He or she can do this both at the time of the "informing" interview[17] with the parents and throughout the patient's infancy, childhood, and adolescence. Even when the physician is not in a position to carry out this process directly, his or her support of others, such as social workers, psychiatrists, and psychologists, in their interactions with the parents and the child will help the parents to recognize the importance of psychosocial issues in their child's development. In this way, it may be possible to reduce the high prevalence of behavioral and emotional problems that reflect maladaptation to a physical disability or chronic illness.

When to Refer

1. Whenever the child and family need more care coordination than can be provided by the primary care health provider
2. Whenever the child or family requires specific interventions such as financial counseling or mental health services
3. When a child has a complex condition that would benefit from tertiary care

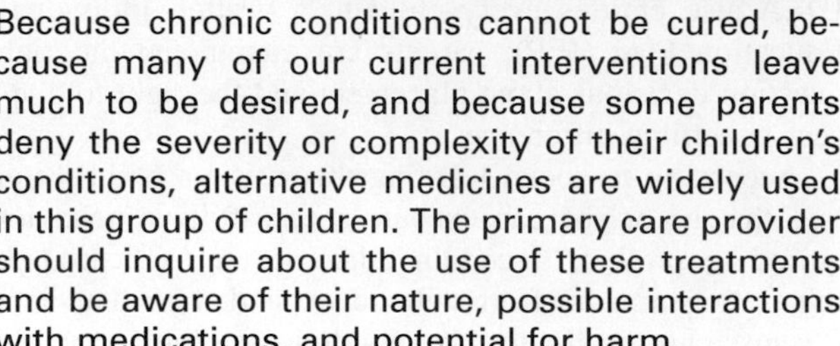

Use of Alternative Medicine

Because chronic conditions cannot be cured, because many of our current interventions leave much to be desired, and because some parents deny the severity or complexity of their children's conditions, alternative medicines are widely used in this group of children. The primary care provider should inquire about the use of these treatments and be aware of their nature, possible interactions with medications, and potential for harm.

REFERENCES

1. American Academy of Pediatrics: Managed care and children with special health care needs: a subject review, *Pediatrics* 102:657, 1998.
2. American Academy of Pediatrics: The role of the pediatrician in prescribing therapy services for children with motor disabilities, *Pediatrics* 98:308, 1996.
3. Bandura A: *The social foundations of thought and action: a social theory,* Englewood Cliffs, NJ, 1986, Prentice Hall.
4. Breitmayer BJ, et al: Social competence of school-aged children with chronic illnesses, *J Pediatr Nurs* 7:181, 1992.
5. Cadman D, et al: Chronic illness, disability and mental and social well-being: findings of the Ontario Child Health Study, *Pediatrics* 75:805, 1987.
6. Carey WB: Temperament issues in the school-aged child, *Pediatr Clin North Am* 39:569, 1992.
7. Charlton A, et al: Absence from school related to cancer and other chronic conditions, *Arch Dis Child* 66:1217, 1991.
8. Eiser C, et al: Adjustment to chronic disease in relation to age and gender: mothers' and fathers' reports of their childrens' behavior, *J Pediatr Psychol* 17:261, 1992.
9. Gortmaker SL, et al: Chronic conditions, socioeconomic risks, and behavioral problems in children and adolescents, *Pediatrics* 85:267, 1990.
10. Hobbs N, Perrin JM, Ireys HT: *Chronically ill children and their families,* San Francisco, 1985, Jossey-Bass.
11. Jessop DJ, Stein RE: Providing comprehensive health care to children with chronic illness, *Pediatrics* 93:602, 1994.
12. Klaus MG, Kennell JH, Klaus PH: *Bonding: building the foundations of secure attachment and independence,* Reading, Mass, 1995, Addison-Wesley.
13. Martinez NH, Schreiber ML, Hartman EW: Pediatric nurse practitioners: primary care providers and case managers for chronically ill children at home, *J Pediatr Health Care* 5:291, 1991.
14. McCormick MC, Gortmaker SL, Sobol AM: Very low birthweight children: behavior problems and school difficulty in a national sample, *J Pediatr* 117:687, 1990.
15. McManus MA, Newacheck P: Health insurance differentials among minority children with chronic conditions and the role of federal agencies and private foundations in improving financial access, *Pediatrics* 91:1040, 1993.
16. McPherson M, et al: A new definition of children with special health care needs, *Pediatrics* 102:137, 1998.
17. Myers BA: The informing interview: enabling parents to "hear" and cope with bad news, *Am J Dis Child* 137:572, 1983.
18. Palfrey JS, Haynie M, Porter SN: *Children assisted by medical technology in educational settings: guidelines for care,* Boston, 1989, Project School Care, The Children's Hospital.
19. Revell GM, Liptak GS: Understanding the child with special health care needs: a developmental perspective, *J Pediatr Nurs* 6:258, 1991.
20. Sahler OJ, et al: Sibling Adaptation to Childhood Cancer Collaborative Study: the association of sibling adaptation with maternal well-being, physical health, and resource use, *J Dev Behav Pediatr* 18:233, 1997.
21. Stein RE, Silver EJ: Operationalizing a conceptually based noncategorical definition: a first look at US children with chronic conditions, *Arch Pediatr Adolesc Med* 153:68, 1999.

22. Stein R, Jessop DJ, Riessman CK: Health care received by children with chronic illnesses, *Am J Dis Child* 137:225, 1983.
23. Wallander JL, et al: Children with chronic physical disorders: maternal reports of their psychological adjustment, *J Pediatr Psychol* 13:197, 1988.
24. Weiland SK, Pless IB, Roghmann KJ: Chronic illness and mental health problems in pediatric practice: results from a survey of primary care providers, *Pediatrics* 89:445, 1992.
25. Worthington RC: Models of linear and cyclical grief: different approaches to different experiences, *Clin Pediatr* 33:297, 1994.

34 Mental Retardation

Thomas J. Kenny • Jennifer Willoughby

The prevalence of mental retardation is such that all primary care physicians will confront it frequently. In 1992, the American Association on Mental Retardation (AAMR) adopted a new definition of mental retardation, as follows:

> Mental retardation refers to substantial limitations in present functioning. It is characterized by significantly subaverage intellectual functioning, existing concurrently with related limitation in two or more of the following applicable adaptive skill areas: communication, self-care, home living, social skills, community use, self-direction, health and safety, functional academics, leisure, and work. Mental retardation manifests before age 18 years.[16]

Considerable controversy surrounds this new definition. Critics point out that it could increase the number of persons identified as mentally retarded, in that the definition is less exact and raises the IQ cutoff to 75 from the previous 70. Others note that the 10 areas of adaptive behavior specified in the diagnosis are difficult to define and measure.[17] Jacobson believes that the new diagnosis expands the social or political aspects of the problem, which can be seen as humanistic, but it does so at the expense of science: "Foundation in science has been replaced by referendum and affirmation."[10] For the purposes of this chapter and to keep the focus on the issues that concern the primary care physician, we will simplify the definition and stress the broader elements that are shared by the old and new definitions.

It is noteworthy that in both definitions, subaverage general intellectual functioning and deficits in adaptive behavior must coexist for diagnostic criteria to be fulfilled.[8] *Subaverage intelligence* has been defined as a score that is at least two standard deviations below the mean on a standardized intelligence test. This statistically based definition indicates that 2.5% of a given population will be classified as mentally retarded; in the United States this definition encompasses about 5 million individuals. Actually, however, the number of individuals who are identified as being mentally retarded at any given time is far lower.[19] *Adaptive behavior* means the effectiveness or degree with which individuals meet the standard of personal independence and social responsibility expected of their age or cultural group. Thus, it is possible that a given individual could be considered mentally retarded in one setting (or one age group) but not at another age or in another environment—one that is perhaps less competitive or more relaxed, permissive, and accepting. Such a circumstance is much more likely to occur with "educable" or mildly retarded persons, who account for 75% of the total population of those who are or may be retarded.

In the old definition, the AAMR defined four official levels of mental retardation (Table 34-1); the new definition eliminates these levels, despite a strong feeling that significant differences are associated with the levels of retardation. In the old definition, mild retardation (encompassing those who are educable) is the most prevalent and is significantly more so among persons of lower socioeconomic status. In this group the incidence of overt neurological problems and multiple handicaps is not markedly elevated. In fact, no specific etiology is identified for 75% to 80% of those at this level. In contrast, the more pronounced types of retardation, although less common, are found equally across all socioeconomic groups. These more markedly disabled individuals are more likely to be identified early, are more likely to have an identifiable etiology and diagnosis, and are more likely to have other overt neurological handicaps (e.g., seizures, cerebral palsy).[14,15,18]

The 10 areas of adaptive behavior listed in the AAMR definition are similar to those the federal government adopted in defining developmental disabilities. In PL-100-146, the Developmental Disabilities Bill of Rights and Assistance Act amendments of 1987, the law defines seven areas of life function—thinking, economic self-sufficiency, communication, locomotion, capacity for independent living, self-care, and motivation; deficiencies in three or more of these functions caused by physical or verbal impairment that occurred before 22 years of age constitute a developmental disability. Studies have demonstrated that this definition tends to include only some of those persons who would fit the AAMR categorical definition. Because such definitions often dictate eligibility criteria for services, the disparity may create problems for some children in states that have adopted the federal definition.[3]

A number of causal factors have been linked with mental retardation. In most cases, particularly in the mildly retarded range, specific etiological mechanisms are unknown. Risk of mental retardation is associated with a number of contributing social and physiological factors that have been linked to developmental outcome. In recent years, children known to have one or more of these risk factors have been monitored in an effort toward early identification of delays. Various early intervention programs have been designed to stimulate these children and to offset or modify the effects of deleterious social and physiological factors. These programs have demonstrated varying degrees of success and have not always had the broad and long-lasting effects that theorists predicted. However, they appear to affect developmental outcome positively.[14,18]

Table 34-1 Official Levels of Mental Retardation and Some Developmental Characteristics*

Level and Title	IQ Range	Estimated Percentage of Total Retarded	Adaptive and Developmental Characteristics: Preschool Age 0-5 (Maturation and Development)	School Age 6-20 (Training and Education)	Adult ≥21 (Social and Vocational Adequacy)
1. Profound	<20	5	Gross retardation; minimum capacity for functioning in sensorimotor areas; may need nursing care	Some motor development present; may respond to minimum or limited training in self-help	Some motor and speech development; may achieve very limited self-care; may need nursing care
2. Severe	20-35		Poor motor development; minimal speech; able to profit from training in self-help; little or no expressive skills	Can talk or learn to communicate; can be trained in elemental health habits; can profit from systematic habit training	May contribute partially to self-maintenance under complete supervision; can develop self-protection skills to a minimum useful level in controlled environment
3. Moderate	36-51	20	Can talk or learn to communicate; has poor social awareness; has fair motor development; profits from training in self-help; can be managed with moderate supervision	Can profit from training in social and occupational skills; unlikely to progress beyond second-grade level in academic subjects; may learn to travel alone in familiar places	May achieve self-maintenance in unskilled or semiskilled work under sheltered conditions; needs supervision and guidance when under mild social or economic stress
4. Mild	52-68	75	Can develop social and communication skills; minimal retardation in sensorimotor areas; often not distinguished from normal until later age	Can learn academic skills up to approximately sixth-grade level by late teens; can be guided toward social conformity; "educable"	Can usually achieve social and vocational skills adequate to minimum self-support but may need guidance and assistance when under unusual social or economic stress

*Definition of mental retardation: "Significantly subaverage general intellectual functioning existing concurrently with deficits in adaptive behavior and manifest during the developmental period."

Often it is not possible to confirm a diagnosis of mental retardation during the newborn period; Down syndrome (with an incidence of 1 in 800 births) and primary microcephaly are two exceptions. In most other clinical circumstances the diagnosis of retardation is first suspected because the child does not reach developmental milestones when expected rather than because of any specific positive findings. Because developmental differences in early childhood can be difficult to assess, the physician's responsibility in this regard can be burdensome.

Individuals who are mildly mentally retarded frequently are not identified as such during the preschool years. The first real concern about their developmental status may be raised when they encounter academic problems.[12] After leaving school many of these individuals are assimilated into society. They may obtain jobs, raise families, and be self-sufficient, at least to some degree. Mildly retarded individuals may demonstrate their disabilities most prominently in the academic area and may function quite well in nonacademic activities. Some observers have even charged that mildly retarded children are "manufactured" by the school system. Speech and language problems are characteristic of persons who are mentally retarded. Usually the greater the degree of retardation, the higher the incidence and the more marked the degree of speech problems. It is estimated that about 50% of mildly retarded persons and more than 95% of severely retarded persons have speech problems; about 50% of profoundly retarded persons are nonverbal.

PHYSICIAN'S ROLE

The primary care physician has a four-part role in the care of the person who is mentally retarded: (1) identification and diagnosis; (2) provision of continuous, comprehensive health care; (3) counseling; and (4) case management and advocacy. The most effective way to identify children at risk for mental retardation is to assess developmental status at each health care visit. This assessment should include a history of motor, language, and social development. A screening tool that measures cognitive and behavioral development also can be useful. One standard tool for such screening is the *Denver Developmental Screening Test*, presented in Chapter 20 (Thirteen), Developmental Surveillance and Intervention. Repeated studies have demonstrated that this instrument is highly effective and easily administered. Another option is to use the combined vision/developmental screening procedure developed by Sturner,[24] which is both brief and valid.

After identification, the physician's role in health care remains important. Although there is no specific medical treatment for most types of mental retardation, children who are mentally retarded are at increased risk for many medical problems. For example, the child who has Down syndrome is at risk for congenital heart disease, thyroid dysfunction, visual problems, obesity, and leukemia. As a group, mentally retarded persons have a higher incidence of delayed speech development, decreased visual acuity, and seizures. Therefore, it is vital that the physician provide comprehensive health care to the affected youngster or see that it is provided.

The third role of the physician involves counseling parents of the child who is mentally retarded. Simple, clear, effective communication with the parents about their child and issues of mental retardation is needed. A frequent issue the physician may face pertains to the developmental course of mental retardation. This is one of the most difficult and frequently asked questions by parents. It is difficult to predict developmental outcome for any individual child who is mentally retarded, except for those children who are functioning within the range of severe to profound retardation. Parents especially may benefit from anticipatory guidance to help them adjust to the transitions they may face in the future regarding developmental milestones and life skills. Issues that may necessitate anticipatory guidance by various professionals cover the entire lifespan. They include (1) toilet training, (2) peer relations, (3) puberty, (4) sexual relationships, and (5) job training. The physician who feels uncomfortable in addressing any of these issues should refer parents to health professionals who can address them. Sexual development and related behaviors are often difficult areas for parents to face. Specific issues, such as the management of menstruation or the general problems of adolescence can be difficult to deal with in young persons who are mentally retarded. They have normal sex drives, but their more limited, social heterosexual contacts provide fewer reasonable outlets for these feelings.

The parent or professional who has concerns in these areas should contact local agencies, including the local Association for Retarded Citizens (ARC), that are likely to have a spectrum of help available. Possibilities include educational programs and appropriate literature. Two very useful books for parents or professionals are Kempton's *A Teacher's Guide to Sex Education for Persons with Learning Disabilities*[13] and Monat's *Sexuality and the Mentally Retarded.*[20] A more recent book by Monat, *Understanding and Expressing Sexuality: Responsible Choices for Individuals with Developmental Disabilities,*[21] has information relating to the issue of AIDS as well as a helpful directory of resources.

The fourth role for the physician is that of case manager or advocate. The physician, therefore, should be ready to refer the child for appropriate evaluations (including psychological evaluation) to establish basic data about the child's developmental status, especially in the areas of cognition and social skills. The results of this evaluation should help the physician and parents plan for the child's needs; thus, the child should be evaluated as early as possible. A reasonably accurate assessment usually can be conducted when the child is about 2 years of age, and a comprehensive evaluation should be performed before the child starts school.

The primary care physician's role in care coordination has increased dramatically with the increasing number of mentally retarded children who do not live in institutions and remain with their families until adulthood. Health care for children who are mentally retarded often does not exceed the level of care necessary for children who do not have disabilities. Mentally retarded children require allied health, educational, and family support services, which the physician is in a unique position to coordinate.[9]

Other evaluations that may be necessary include those for speech and language development and audiometric evaluation. In addition, ophthalmological and neurological consultations frequently are indicated.

BEHAVIORAL PROBLEMS

As a group, mentally retarded persons have a greater incidence of behavioral problems than do those in the general population. Foale[7] found the incidence of psychoneurosis in retarded persons to be twice that of the general population. Pervasive emotional problems such as psychosis and autism also are more frequent among retarded children.[11,18] In an excellent review of the prevalence of psychopathology in people who are mentally retarded, Borthwich-Duffy[4] cited studies estimating the range from less than 10% to more than 80%. The more severely retarded person often has poor communication abilities and frequently has increased motor activity (i.e., hyperactivity). Mentally retarded persons also tend to have short attention spans. Their behavior tends to be impulsive, repetitive, or stereotypical, and they are at increased risk of engaging in self-stimulatory or self-injurious behaviors.

Mildly retarded children have many of the characteristics of children who have an attention deficit disorder. They usually are overactive, have a poor attention span, and are impulsive; they also tend to be aggressive and to "act out" their frustrations. Management of these problems is similar to that for nonretarded children. Medications such as methylphenidate hydrochloride (Ritalin) or dextroamphetamine sulfate (Dexedrine) can be useful if used judiciously and monitored carefully. Behavior management techniques have been demonstrated to be effective. A number of books can be used by parents to develop behavior management programs, including *Parents Are Teachers* by Wesley Becker,[1] and Gerald Patterson's book, *Families: Application of Social Learning to Family Life.*[22]

Cromwell[5] sees the behavior of retarded persons as a consequence of the frustration related to the many failures they experience. He proposes that this causes the retarded person to (1) perform in a new situation below the level of his or her constitutional ability, (2) be less likely to be motivated by failure, and (3) be less likely to try harder after a minor failure—that is, to give up more easily. Cromwell, thus, describes the retarded child as a "failure-avoider" as opposed to a "success-striver."

MANAGEMENT

Current trends in the management of mentally retarded persons will require increased services from the primary care physician. Improved medical care has extended the life span of such people, which has resulted in a greater need for ongoing health maintenance by the physician as well as for expanded efforts in case management, especially in the psychosocial area. Managed care and the pressures associated with that system present a challenge to the primary physician in terms of finding the time and the means to provide for the mentally retarded patient. It is a challenge that must be met if we are to provide optimal care for this population.

The current emphasis on "deinstitutionalization" and "normalization" of living experiences requires a comprehensive and sustained social support system. More attention must be devoted to vocational training and the development of occupational opportunities. The deinstitutionalization effort necessitates helping the family and the mentally retarded person prepare for alternate living arrangements. Greater numbers of mentally retarded persons are moving into group homes and apartments in the community, which requires a support system that meets their physical, social, and occupational needs.[6] Available data on the effectiveness of such programs are conflicting but suggest that much remains to be done to facilitate the optimum adjustment of mentally retarded persons and to match settings to individual needs.[2,14,23] The physician can help the family and the child prepare for entry into this system of independent living and working.

Acknowledgment

This chapter is dedicated to Raymond L. Clemens, M.D., Emeritus Professor of Pediatrics, University of Maryland School of Medicine, who died in July 1998. He was co-author of the original chapter in the first edition of this book and devoted his career to the field of behavioral and developmental pediatrics.

REFERENCES

1. Becker WC: *Parents are teachers: a child management program,* Champaign, Ill, 1971, Research Press.
2. Birenbaum A, Re M: Resettling mentally retarded adults in the community: almost 4 years later, *Am J Ment Defic* 31:323, 1979.
3. Boggs E, Henney RL: *A numerical and functional description of the developmental disabilities population,* Philadelphia, 1979, EMC Institute.
4. Borthwich-Duffy SA: Epidemiology and prevalence of psychopathology in people with mental retardation, *J Consult Clin Psychol* 62:17, 1994.
5. Cromwell RL: Personality evaluation. In Baumeister A, editor: *Mental retardation: appraisal, education, and rehabilitation,* Chicago, 1967, Aldine.
6. Eyman RK, Arndt S: Life-span development of institutionalized and community-based mentally retarded residents, *Am J Ment Defic* 86:342, 1982.
7. Foale M: The special difficulty of high-grade mental defective adolescents, *Am J Ment Defic* 60:867, 1956.
8. Grossman HJ: *Classification in mental retardation,* Washington, DC, 1983, The American Association on Mental Deficiency.
9. Guralnick MJ, Bennett FC: *The effectiveness of early intervention for at-risk and handicapped children,* Orlando, Fla, 1987, Academic Press.
10. Jacobson J: Mental retardation: definition, classification, and systems of support, *Am J Ment Retard* 98:539, 1994.
11. Jacobson J: Problem behavior and psychiatric impairment within a developmentally disabled population. I. Behavior frequency, *Appl Res Ment Retard* 3:121, 1982.
12. Kappelman M, Kenny T, Clemmens R: Mild mental retardation: clinical characteristics in early and late identification, *Md Med J* 23:83, 1974.
13. Kempton W: *A teacher's guide to sex education for persons with learning disabilities,* North Scituate, Mass, 1975, Duxburg Press.
14. Landesman-Dwyer S: Living in the community, *Am J Ment Defic* 86:223, 1981.
15. Lazar I, Darlington RB: Lasting effects of early education, *Monogr Soc Res Child Dev* 47:1, 1982.
16. Luckasson D, et al: *Mental retardation: definition, classification, and systems of supports,* Washington, DC, 1992, American Association on Mental Retardation.
17. MacMillan DZ, Gresham FM, Lipnstein GN: Conceptual and psychometric concerns about the 1992 AAMR definition of mental retardation, *Am J Ment Retard* 98:325, 1993.
18. McKey RH, et al: Impact of Head Start on children, families, and communities, Pub No (OHDS) 85-31193, Washington, DC, 1985, Department of Health and Human Services.
19. Mercer J: The myth of 3% prevalence. In Tarjan G, Eyman RK, Meyers CE, editors: *Sociobehavioral studies in mental retardation,* Monograph No 1, Washington, DC, 1973, The American Association on Mental Deficiency.
20. Monat RK: *Sexuality and the mentally retarded,* San Diego, 1982, College-Hill Press.
21. Monat-Haller RK: *Understanding and expressing sexuality: responsible choices for individuals with developmental disabilities,* Baltimore, 1992, Paul H Brookes.
22. Patterson GR: *Families: application of social learning to family life,* Champaign, Ill, 1975, Research Press.
23. Reiss S: Psychopathology and mental retardation: survey of a developmental disabilities mental health program, *Ment Retard* 20:128, 1982.
24. Sturner RA, et al: Simultaneous screening for child health and development: a study of visual/developmental screening of preschool children, *Pediatrics* 65:614, 1980.

SUGGESTED READINGS

Clarke ADB, Clarke AM: Research on mental handicap, 1957-1987: a selected review, *J Ment Defic Res* 31:317, 1987.

Hill BK, Lakin KC, Bruininks RH: Trends in residential services for mentally retarded people, 1977-1982, *J Assoc Persons Severe Handicap* 9:243, 1984.

State MW, King B, Dykens E: Mental retardation: a review of the past 10 years: II. *J Am Acad Child Adolesc Psychiatry* 31:1669, 1997.

35 Children Assisted by Medical Technology

Laurie J. Glader • Judith S. Palfrey

Primary care pediatricians frequently find themselves in the position of caring for children assisted by technology. Providing care for this population is ripe with challenges and rewards. Complete care includes management of certain common medical, psychosocial, and educational issues.

SCOPE OF THE CHALLENGE

Over the past two decades advances in pediatric medical and surgical techniques have allowed children who have chronic illness and disabilities to live longer, more functional lives.[12] Children who have spina bifida, congenital heart disease, and leukemia live at least twice as long as they did a few decades ago. Children who have cystic fibrosis have a sevenfold higher chance of surviving to age 21 than previously.[18] Extremely premature infants and children who have congenital anomalies also are surviving longer.[17]

Prolonged survival and improved function in children who have chronic illness and disabilities are due, in part, to an increasing reliance on the use of medical technologies. Such technologies include oxygen therapy, ventilators, tracheostomies, central venous lines, urinary bladder catheterization, renal dialysis, urostomies, enterostomies, and gastrostomy tubes.[10,24,28] As a result, a new population of children who have special health care needs has evolved—children assisted by medical technology. By definition, these are children who have a chronic condition that requires daily assistance by a medical device to replace or augment a bodily function in order to sustain life.[13,26] Examples of such conditions include an 18-year-old boy who has a high cervical cord injury and is ventilator dependent; a 2-year-old girl who has spastic quadriplegic cerebral palsy and a gastrostomy tube; and a 1-year-old boy who has a craniofacial abnormality and a tracheostomy. Usually, such conditions require daily regular monitoring by trained personnel.

Estimates of the number of children assisted by medical technology are sparse. A study in Massachusetts indicated the prevalence rate to be 1 to 2 per 1000 children.[19] Other resources only provide ranges of estimates of the size of the population nationwide.[13]

Although some advances in medical care over the past 20 years have led to an increase in the use of the technologies enumerated above, other developments have resulted in reduced need for these same technologies. For example, with the availability of bovine surfactant, the prevalence of bronchopulmonary dysplasia is decreasing, resulting in decreased use of oxygen and ventilators among premature infants.[1] Advances in injury prevention have led to a decrease in devastating accidents that can result in the need for assistive technology.[3] On the other hand, reproductive technology has led to a rise in multiple gestation births, which are associated with increased risk of prematurity and cerebral palsy.[22] Ease in placement of percutaneous gastrostomy tubes[11] and improved nutritional outcomes for children who have complex medical issues may result in an increase in this technologically assisted population.

Children assisted by technology are becoming increasingly visible in the community as they leave tertiary care medical centers to live at home.[15] Home care improves quality of life and overall development and enhances parents' sense of control over their child's care. Additionally, increases in home care may reduce health care costs by avoiding lengthy and complex hospitalizations. The primary care clinician undoubtedly will have several patients assisted by technology in his or her practice and needs to develop the skills necessary to provide good medical care, as well as effective advocacy, for these children.

ETIOLOGY

Within this population, the need for technology is variable. In part, this is because the range of disabilities is broad. Etiologies include chronic illness, genetic syndromes, congenital anomalies, problems associated with prematurity, and sequelae of injury, infection or illness. At times, the diagnosis is unclear. Additionally, children assisted by technology vary in the age at which they develop need for assistance and by whether the need is transient or permanent.[13]

Some technologies are used temporarily to enhance or replace a physiological function until the child is old enough to undergo corrective surgery or "outgrows" the need. Children born with severe congenital malformations of the head and neck, such as those who have Pierre Robin syndrome, lymphatic malformations, or craniosynostosis syndromes, frequently need their airways protected via tracheotomies for several months to years; many subsequently are able to be decannulated. Infants who have necrotizing enterocolitis may require enterostomies that are closed within a few months or a year. Children unable to eat by mouth because of anatomical problems such as esophageal atresia may require gastrostomy tubes for several months until their atresia has been repaired. Children on long-term parenteral chemotherapy frequently have central venous lines that are removed once their course of chemotherapy is completed. Continuous ambulatory peritoneal dialysis may be used by a small child who is awaiting a renal transplant.

Other technologies are necessary for long-term use by children who will never gain the function that the technology provides. A gastrostomy tube may be required as a result of dysphagia secondary to severe neuromuscular involvement in cerebral palsy. Children who have neurogenic bladders from myelodysplasia or cervical cord injury require bladder catheterization several times daily. Children who have AIDS are being treated increasingly with feeding tubes and central venous lines for hyperalimentation.[4] Children who have high cervical spinal cord injuries or muscular dystrophy may require permanent ventilatory assistance.

PSYCHOSOCIAL ISSUES

The psychosocial issues facing children assisted by medical technology and their families are the same as those encountered by children who have other forms of chronic illness.[17] Children who are dependent on medical technology may or may not be obviously "different" from their peers as a result of their underlying condition. Some technology is relatively easy to conceal, such as enterostomies, gastrostomy tubes, and central venous lines; ventilators are not. Being different from one's peers is especially stressful for adolescents. Issues concerning body image, independence, and self-identity may be exacerbated for those assisted by medical technology.

For younger children, assistance by medical technology does not seem to be as stigmatizing. However, the underlying condition or the technology may make participation in regular childhood activities difficult. For instance, the child who has a tracheostomy may not be able to play in a sandbox or use glitter unless the tracheostomy is covered by an appropriate device. For some children, dependence on caregivers may hamper development of independence and interpersonal skills.

As children assisted by medical technology have moved out of tertiary care centers and into their homes, familial stress levels have increased.[21] Mothers of children assisted by technology have impaired health related to pain, social functioning, and mental health and demonstrate substantially more depressive symptoms than mothers of children who are not assisted by technology.[27] Parental burnout occurs as a result of physical and emotional exhaustion. Other family members are affected as well. Issues such as the lack of privacy, the pure physical burden of the care involved, anxiety, sleep deprivation, lack of recreational opportunities, and increased financial burdens all compound the stress. For those who have ventilator-assisted children, burnout appears to increase with the duration of ventilator use.[23]

Parents of children assisted by technology at times have ambiguous roles. On the one hand, they are expected to develop expertise at caring for their child's complex medical needs. On the other hand, they are expected to defer to the advice of multiple professionals. They need respite and advocacy. Unfortunately, achieving respite in this population is not always easy. Many barriers to child care exist. Directors of private child care programs report being able to manage mild physical disabilities such as asthma, diabetes mellitus, hearing deficits, epilepsy, and visual problems. Far fewer report being able to manage more complex children who rely, for example, on ventilators or wheelchairs.[9]

As the population of children assisted by medical technology who go to school increases, adults and children in the community are more exposed to the child who is "different." Teachers may be frightened by medical conditions with which they are not familiar. Procedures once only done in hospitals are now being done in schools, which seems to highlight the child's problems. The term *medically fragile* serves to increase anxiety about the stability and oddness of children whose medical needs are complex. Playmates and peers may not understand the equipment used or the child's need for privacy to perform some procedures, such as catheterization.

MANAGEMENT

The primary care pediatrician discovers both challenges and rewards in caring for a child assisted by medical technology. In addition to providing routine pediatric well-child care targeted toward sustaining physical health, the pediatrician must work with the child's parents to provide family-centered care to foster growth and development.[12] Such care is described in the "medical home" model by the American Academy of Pediatrics put forward in 1992.[2]

In 1995, the Committee on Children with Disabilities published guidelines for home care of children with chronic disease, placing special emphasis on the importance of a home health care team.[6] Ideally, such a team places the parents at the head, working closely with the primary care physician. Other team members include consulting physicians, nurses, rehabilitative therapists, child development specialists, educators, a nutritionist, and community service representatives such as home care agencies, equipment vendors, and early intervention workers. A team approach, with the primary care physician in the role of case coordinator, allows for the most complete, efficient, and sensitive care of the child. This team approach also is probably cost effective, reducing duplication and fragmentation of services because the model encourages communication between the physician and all other team members. Pediatricians may receive assistance from pioneering programs focused on streamlined, family-centered care of children who have special health care needs. The Pediatric Alliance for Coordinated Care is such a program based at Children's Hospital in Boston.

The pediatrician often is called on to advocate for optimal school placement of children assisted by technology. The federal mandated Individuals with Disabilities Education Act (IDEA, 1990) and Supreme Court rulings, including *Tatro v. Irving School District* (1984) and *Garrett v. Cedar Rapids* (1999), create opportunities for children assisted by technology to participate more fully in school settings. Children who have special health care needs may require special instruction, classroom arrangements, equipment, therapies, and care. In all cases, the child should have access to an appropriate, safe educational placement that allows for the least restrictive environment possible.[20]

The primary care pediatrician, thus, is involved in many aspects of the life of a child assisted by technology. He or she constantly evaluates the appropriateness of home care for the child; coordinates the child's health care, services, and schooling; and often assists in ordering equipment. Portability of equipment is of paramount importance so that the child may go to school, social events, doctor appointments, and so on. Finally, the primary care pediatrician spends substantial time teaching the child and family about the child's medical condition, treatments available, and relevant technical care.[15,25]

Specific medical management revolves around the child's underlying condition and issues pertinent to the technology used. Children assisted by mechanical ventilators require frequent monitoring of their respiratory status. A high level of home nursing care may be necessary to maintain good pulmonary "toilet."[16] A child who has a tracheostomy may be more prone to respiratory infections secondary to organisms bypassing the defense mechanisms of the upper airway, as well as the slightly increased risk of aspiration of secretions and food around the tracheostomy tube (especially if the tube is uncuffed). He or she may be at risk for the tracheostomy becoming plugged if secretions are not humidified adequately. Reactive airway disease may result from frequent aspiration or contact with airborne particles that are normally filtered through the nasopharynx. Accidental decannulation could be life threatening, depending on the degree of tracheolaryngeal stenosis.[8] Caretakers must be trained in changing tracheostomy tubes. Children assisted by technology are often vulnerable to respiratory decompensation in the setting of infection. For children who meet criteria, palivizumab (Synagis) is an intramuscular immunoglobulin treatment now available for passive protection against respiratory syncytial virus. It is given as a series of monthly injections during the viral season.[7]

For a child who has a gastrostomy tube (G-tube), gastroesophageal reflux often is a confounding issue. This especially is true for children who have a neuromuscular impairment, such as cerebral palsy. Gastrostomy feedings result in improved weight gain and possibly better developmental outcome; however, for the child who has severe spastic quadriplegic cerebral palsy, aspiration pneumonia and severe esophagitis are risks associated with reflux of the gastrostomy feedings. Children who have G-tubes but do not have fundoplications frequently require prokinetic agents and H_2 blockers to manage the reflux. If a gastrostomy tube falls out or is pulled out, it must be replaced within a few hours because of the risk of the gastric stoma and gastrointestinal tract closing. All children receiving specialized home nutritional therapy should be followed by a nutritionist.

Central venous catheters provide excellent access for frequent blood drawing and administration of parenteral nutrition or chemotherapy. However, they are sites for infection and thrombosis, both of which can be life threatening. Fevers require investigation. Central venous lines can break or become plugged with blood clots, requiring surgical replacement or chemical thrombolysis.

PROGNOSIS

The prognosis for children assisted by technology depends largely on the underlying medical condition. Consider the following examples. Children who have Pierre Robin syndrome and have a tracheostomy and a G-tube placed at birth likely will not need either by 1 to 2 years of age and will go on to enjoy "normal" good health.[5] The use of technology gives their mandibles time to grow while preserving normal cognitive functioning. Children who have spina bifida require clean intermittent catheterization four or five times daily and are likely to need this for the rest of their lives. However, the risk of developing end-stage renal disease from recurrent infections is significantly lower than when this therapeutic approach is not instituted.[14] A ventilator-dependent adolescent who has had high cervical cord trauma requires permanent ventilator support but may be able to hold a job. Adolescents and young adults who have muscular dystrophy and anterior horn cell disease may live for several years with ventilator assistance.

CONCLUSION

Children assisted by medical technology are a relatively new subgroup of the chronically ill and disabled patients. As advances in surgical techniques and technology applications continue, technologies such as gastrostomy tubes, tracheotomies, central venous catheters, and ventilators will continue to be used for this small group of children, both temporarily and chronically. The goal of these technologies should be to enhance the quality of life for the children and their families. The medical focus should be on maximizing capabilities while minimizing disabilities. Primary care pediatricians have the opportunity to coordinate and manage the care of these children who require frequent contact with specialists and tertiary care medical centers, but who must thrive at home and in the community.

Acknowledgment

Rewritten in fond memory of Marilynn Haynie, M.D., who authored the original chapter and dedicated her life to the care of children with special health care needs.

REFERENCES

1. Abman SH, Groothius JR: Pathophysiology and treatment of bronchopulmonary dysplasia: current issues, *Pediatr Clin North Am* 41:277, 1994.
2. Ad Hoc Task Force on Definition of the Medical Home: The medical home, *Pediatrics* 90:774, 1992.
3. Bass JL, et al: Childhood injury prevention counseling in primary care settings: a critical review of the literature, *Pediatrics* 92:544, 1993.
4. Beaver BL, et al: Surgical intervention in children with human immunodeficiency virus infection, *J Pediatr Surg* 25:79, 1990.
5. Bull MJ, et al: Improved outcome in Pierre Robin sequence: effect of multidisciplinary evaluation and management, *Pediatrics* 86:294, 1990.
6. Committee on Children with Disabilities: Guidelines for home care of infants, children, and adolescents with chronic disease, *Pediatrics* 96:161, 1995.
7. Committee on Infectious Diseases and Committee on Fetus and Newborn: Prevention of respiratory syncytial virus infections: indications for the use of palivizumab and update on the use of RSV-IGIV, *Pediatrics* 102:1211, 1998.
8. Duncan BW, et al: Tracheostomy in children with emphasis on home care, *J Pediatr Surg* 27:432, 1992.
9. Fewell R: Child care for children with special needs, *Pediatrics* 91:193, 1993.
10. Gauderer ML: Gastrostomy techniques and devices, *Surg Clin North Am* 72:1285, 1992.
11. Gauderer ML: Percutaneous endoscopic gastrostomy: a ten-year experience with 220 children, *J Pediatr Surg* 26:288, 1991.

12. Hostler SL: Family-centered care, *Pediatr Clin North Am* 36:1545, 1991.
13. Kirk S: Families' experiences of caring at home for a technology-dependent child: a review of the literature, *Child Care Health Dev* 24: 101, 1998.
14. Klose AG, Sackett CK, Mesrobian HG: Management of children with myelodysplasia: urological alternatives, *J Urol* 144:1446, 1990.
15. Liptak GS: Home care for children who have chronic conditions, *Pediatr Rev* 18:271, 1997.
16. Mallory GB, Stillwell PC: The ventilator-dependent child: issues in diagnosis and management, *Arch Phys Med Rehab* 72:43, 1991.
17. Morbidity and Mortality Weekly Reports Centers for Disease Control Surveillance Summaries, 39:19, 1990.
18. Newacheck PW, Taylor WR: Chronic childhood illness: prevalence, severity, and impact, *Am J Public Health* 82:364, 1992.
19. Palfrey JS, Haynie M, Porter S: Prevalence of medical technology assistance among children in Massachusetts in 1987 and 1990, *Public Health Rep* 109:226, 1994.
20. Palfrey JS, et al: Project School Care: integrating children assisted by medical technology into educational settings, *J School Health* 62:50, 1992.
21. Patterson JM, Leonard BJ, Titus JC: Home care for medically fragile children: impact on family health and well-being, *J Dev Behav Pediatr* 13:248, 1992.
22. Petterson B, et al: Twins, triplets and cerebral palsy in births in West Australia in the 1980s, *BMJ* 307:1239, 1993.
23. Quint RD, et al: Home care for ventilator-dependent children: psychosocial impact on the family, *Am J Dis Child* 114:1238, 1990.
24. Selzman AA, Elder JS, Mapstone TB: Urologic consequences of myelodysplasia and other congenital abnormalities of the spinal cord, *Urol Clin North Am* 20:485, 1993.
25. Storgion SA: Care of the technology-dependent child, *Pediatr Ann* 25: 677, 1996.
26. Task Force on Technology-Dependent Children: Fostering home and community-based care for technology-dependent children, Washington, DC, 1988, Maternal and Child Health Task Force.
27. Thyen U, et al: Impact of long-term care of children assisted by technology on maternal health, *Develop Behav Pediatr* 19:273, 1998.
28. Toder DS, McBride JT: Home care of children dependent on respiratory technology, *Pediatr Rev* 18:273, 1997.

SUGGESTED READINGS

Berger S, et al: Caring for the graduate from the neonatal intensive care unit, *Pediatr Clin North Am* 45:701, 1998.

Cardoso P: A parent's perspective: family-centered care, *Child Health Care* 20:258, 1991.

Lantos JD, Kohrman AF: Ethical aspects of pediatric home care, *Pediatrics* 89:920, 1992.

Perrin JM, Shayne MW, Bloom SR: Home and community care for chronically ill children, New York, 1993, Oxford University Press.

36 Cystic Fibrosis

Jeffrey M. Ewig • Juan C. Martinez

Cystic fibrosis (CF), the most common lethal inherited disease of the white population, follows an autosomal recessive mode of inheritance. Carriers are asymptomatic. The majority of CF patients are white (95%), with an estimated incidence of 1 in 3100.[16] This disease occurs among all races, with an estimated incidence of 1 in 14,000 live black births and 1 in 11,500 live Hispanic births.[16] The main characteristics are recurrent pulmonary infection, pancreatic insufficiency, increased salt loss in sweat, and male infertility.

Cystic fibrosis was first described as a clinicopathological entity in 1938.[2] Since then the survival rate has improved steadily as a result of better nutritional support and antibiotic therapy. The major cause of death is from respiratory insufficiency secondary to chronic recurrent pulmonary infection and inflammation. The median age of survival is approximately 31 years, with males having a slight survival advantage. It has been a decade since the discovery of the CF gene and its protein product, and as expected, this has led to an improved understanding of the pathophysiology of this debilitating disease and active research into novel therapeutic approaches. Because pulmonary disease is the major cause of death (>95%), this chapter focuses on this aspect of CF.

RESPIRATORY PATHOPHYSIOLOGY AND MANIFESTATIONS

The CF gene was identified in 1989.[26,45,47] It consists of 250 kilobases located on the long arm of chromosome 7. It codes for a 1480 amino acid protein product known as the cystic fibrosis transmembrane conductance regulator (CFTR). The most common mutation in North America and Europe is a deletion of three base pairs, resulting in the deletion of phenylalanine (F) at position 508 (ΔF_{508}). This deletion is present in approximately 70% of whites who have CF; however, more than 700 mutations have been identified. Certain populations (e.g., Ashkenazi Jews) have a relatively low frequency of ΔF_{508} and a high frequency of other mutations. This factor must be considered when screening individual patients and when devising larger scale screening programs. The mutations have been grouped into "classes" based on the main reason for reduced CFTR function. Class 1 mutations cause no protein product to be formed (e.g., stop codons). Class 2 mutations lead to improper trafficking through the endoplasmic reticulum and premature protein degradation, with little or no CFTR detectable at the cell membrane. The ΔF_{508} mutation is a class 2 mutation. In class 3 mutations, CFTR is found in the cell membrane; however, it is insensitive to activation and, therefore, nonfunctional. Class 4 mutations affect the rate of ion flow or the amount of time the chloride channel remains open and results in partial chloride channel function. Class 5 mutations lead to reduced amount of functional CFTR at the cell surface. Class 6 mutations affect CFTR's ability to regulate other ion channels.[36,40] Mutations may belong in more than one class. Mutations in class 4 and 5 often are associated with pancreatic sufficiency, but there is no correlation between severity of pulmonary disease and genotype.[23] Variability in pulmonary severity in relation to genotype has been attributed to several factors, including alternative genes, which may compensate partially for defects in CFTR, environmental factors such as cigarette smoke, and differences in therapy and/or compliance.[56]

Current understanding about the pathophysiology of CF continues to focus on the role of CFTR as a cAMP-regulated chloride channel in the apical cell membrane; however, other functions, such as the acidification of intracellular organelles and regulation of other ion channels, may be important in the pathogenesis.[3] The consequence of the genetic defect is abnormal electrolyte transport. This may alter the volume or composition of the airway surface fluid (ASF). Classic teaching of CF pathophysiology focused on reduced volume or dehydrated secretions. Chloride secretion from the apical respiratory epithelial cell to the airway lumen is impaired, and sodium reabsorption from the airway lumen is increased two to three times the normal amount. Water passively follows sodium away from the airway lumen, leading to dehydration of airway secretions, making them more viscous and more difficult to clear, thus predisposing the patient to infection. An alternative theory is that the abnormally high sodium composition of ASF in CF patients may impair local respiratory defense mechanisms.[52] Respiratory epithelia express bacteriocidal factors, or defensins, as a first line of antimicrobial defense. Human beta defensin-1 (hBD-1) is a salt sensitive, bacteriocidal factor expressed throughout respiratory epithelia in the lung.[22] The bacteriocidal ability of hBD-1 is reduced markedly at high salt concentrations, which appear to exist in the CF ASF. This may be an important factor in the initiation of infection. Because of difficulties in measurement, however, the exact composition of the ASF, whether hypernatremic or hyponatremic, remains controversial.[30]

The CFTR defect may lead to an increase in receptors or adhesins on epithelial cells and/or mucin for pathological bacteria. Epithelial injury appears to increase exposure of epithelial cell receptors. This mechanism probably contributes to the maintenance, rather than the initiation, of infection. The most common initial bacterial isolates in the first years of life are *Staphylococcus aureus* (SA) and *Haemophilus influenzae*.[1] By contributing to airway inflammation, epithelial injury, and altered production of mucus, SA colonization may create an environment favorable to *Pseudomonas aeruginosa* (PA) adherence and colonization. Over time, PA becomes the prominent bacterial pathogen in CF, with a prevalence of 60%.[34] The mucoid variant rarely is found in non-CF patients, and its presence strongly suggests the diagnosis of CF.

The host systemic immune response to PA is intact, if not excessive. Certain features of the host-microbe relationship contribute to the ability of PA to evade host defense in CF. PA exoproducts promote colonization and impair local host defense. The expression of these exoproducts may be increased in hyperosmolar conditions that *may* exist in the lungs of CF patients.[6] It is not PA, but the immune-mediated inflammatory response that is responsible for the progressive lung damage of CF. PA exoproducts stimulate the recruitment of neutrophils. Neutrophil and PA elastase overwhelm the host antiprotease defense and injure the respiratory epithelium directly. In addition, elastase excess interferes with host defense by cleaving IgG, thus rendering phagocytosis ineffective.[15] The elastase imbalance leads to further recruitment of neutrophils, perpetuating the cycle of inflammation and lung destruction. There is decreased production of the antiinflammatory cytokine, IL-10, and elevated levels of proinflammatory cytokines. Levels of glutathione may be regulated by CFTR. Glutathione is important in lung antioxidant defense. Reduced levels in CF ASF may increase susceptibility of the lung to oxidative damage.[40] Another important consequence of the influx of neutrophils is the release of large amounts of DNA and actin from damaged and disintegrating cells, which greatly increases the viscosity of airway secretions. Chronic bronchopulmonary infection and airway inflammation lead to progressive lung damage, dysfunction, and death.

Some patients are colonized with other organisms, such as *Burkholderia cepacia*, *Alcaligenes xylosoxidans*, and *Stenotrophomonas maltophilia*. *B. cepacia* can cause a virulent pneumonia, sepsis, and an accelerated decline in pulmonary function.

Recurrent and persistent lower respiratory tract infection leads to the symptoms of chronic cough, bronchiectasis, hemoptysis, and pneumothorax. Classically, cough is productive of purulent sputum that is worse on arising in the morning or following activity; however, some patients may have intermittent symptoms and a nonproductive cough. Physical findings may include an increased anteroposterior diameter of the thorax, persistent crackles or wheezing, and digital clubbing.

The upper respiratory tract commonly is involved as well. Between 10% to 20% of patients have nasal polyps, often multiple and recurrent, that require surgical removal if associated with refractory sinusitis or severe nasal obstruction. Chronic pansinusitis is present radiographically in 90% to 100% of patients; the degree of symptomatology from sinus disease varies among patients. Surgery often helps relieve symptoms, but the results are usually not long lasting.

GASTROINTESTINAL MANIFESTATIONS

Pancreatic exocrine insufficiency is present in 85% to 90% of patients. Inspissated secretions lead to pancreatic duct obstruction, progressive pancreatic damage, and reduced secretion of digestive enzymes and bicarbonate, leading to malabsorption of protein, fat, and fat-soluble vitamins (A, D, E, and K). Presenting symptoms and signs include frequent bulky, greasy stools; failure to thrive; rectal prolapse; hypoproteinemia; edema; and delayed puberty. Droplets of fat may be seen in the stool. Because of the increased fat content, stools often are malodorous. Presentation caused by vitamin deficiency alone is rare but does exist and includes bleeding diathesis from vitamin K deficiency. One or more of these manifestations may be the initial presenting symptom and should prompt referral for a sweat test, even in the absence of pulmonary symptoms. Pancreatic sufficiency is associated with an improved prognosis. Supplementation with pancreatic enzymes, fat-soluble vitamins, and increased caloric intake are the mainstays of therapy for pancreatic insufficiency.

Insulin deficiency is thought to be the primary cause of CF-related diabetes (CFRD). The incidence of CFRD increases with age: Estimates of prevalence are 3% in children ages 5 to 9 years, 11% in ages 10 to 19 years, and 15% in patients older than 20 years of age.[38] A prediabetic insulin-deficient state exists, which may be affected by individual patient factors such as degree of illness severity, malnutrition, and other mitigating factors.[37] Identifying impaired glucose tolerance is important because it may influence prognosis.[33] Clinically significant reduction in weight parameters and pulmonary function have been noted up to 4 years before the development of diabetes.[33] Oral glucose tolerance testing should be considered for patients who have inadequate weight gain or weight loss despite aggressive nutritional intervention, significantly delayed progression of puberty, or unexplained polydipsia and polyuria. Patients can be categorized as having either impaired glucose tolerance or CFRD, based on results of fasting blood glucose tests and oral glucose challenge. Management is similar to that for non–CF-related diabetes, except for avoiding caloric restriction. Insulin therapy is recommended for patients who have CFRD.

Meconium ileus syndrome is associated almost exclusively with CF and is the presenting symptom in 7% to 20% of newborns who have CF. Extremely viscid meconium causes intestinal obstruction and occasionally is complicated by volvulus, atresia, and/or meconium peritonitis. The presence of meconium ileus seems to be related to intestinal gland involvement rather than to pancreatic insufficiency. Infants who have meconium ileus and survive beyond 6 months of age have the same prognosis as other CF patients. Patients who have complicated meconium ileus who require surgical intervention may have a higher incidence of long-term surgical intestinal complications.[21] Meconium plug syndrome is more common in CF, but it is less specific for CF than is meconium ileus.

Some patients suffer from recurrent episodes of crampy abdominal pain with partial or complete bowel obstruction known as *distal intestinal obstruction syndrome* (DIOS). The etiology of DIOS includes some combination of pancreatic insufficiency, inspissated intestinal secretions, undigested food residues, fecal stasis, and dehydration. This syndrome must be distinguished from other causes of acute abdomen, including cholecystitis, pancreatitis, and appendicitis. Intussusception occurs in 10% of patients. The diagnosis of CF should be considered in patients who have intussusception after infancy or recurrent episodes. Rectal prolapse is present in approximately 20% of patients and usually occurs before CF is diagnosed (before pancreatic enzyme replacement therapy).

Recently, some patients have developed colonic strictures (fibrosing colonopathy) that seem to be associated with large quantities of pancreatic enzyme supplements. This diagnosis should be considered in patients who present with evidence of obstruction, bloody diarrhea, or chylous ascites.[4] Current recommendations are to limit the dose of pancreatic enzyme supplementation to fewer than 10,000 units of lipase per kilogram per day or 2500 units of lipase per kilogram per meal.[17]

HEPATOBILIARY MANIFESTATIONS

Liver disease in cystic fibrosis can be quite heterogeneous. The spectrum of involvement can range from neonatal cholestasis to hepatic steatosis, or focal biliary or multilobular cirrhosis. CFTR protein in non-CF patients normally is expressed along intrahepatic and extrahepatic bile duct canaliculi.[8] Inspissated secretions and altered chemical properties of bile alter flow, creating biliary obstruction and eventual hepatocyte damage, although this progression is found inconsistently. Estimates of clinically significant hepatic disease, defined as significant hepatic fibrosis with liver dysfunction, range from 13% to 17%. Meconium ileus may be a risk factor for development of liver disease.[10] It is believed that the manifestations of liver disease in CF may represent a continuum, with cholestasis representing early lesions and multilobular cirrhosis at the severe end.[54] Identification of liver disease is difficult because of the lack of obvious clinical symptoms. The main screening tools are a careful examination of the liver and spleen for signs of organomegaly and yearly liver function tests, including serum AST, ALT, alkaline phosphatase, GGT, and bilirubin. Persistently elevated levels (more than 6 months) suggest probable clinically significant liver disease and the need for a more complete evaluation, including ultrasonography and referral to a pediatric gastroenterologist who has experience in CF.[54] Although no treatment can prevent liver disease progression, the tertiary bile salt ursodeoxycholic acid (URSO) is thought to improve bile flow and has shown promise of curbing progression in patients who have primary biliary cirrhosis.[11,41] Liver disease is the third leading cause of death among patients who have CF.*

*CF Foundation Patient Registry Data, 1997.

OTHER MANIFESTATIONS

The elevated electrolyte concentration of sweat is present in 99% of patients and formed the basis for the diagnostic sweat test. The abnormally functioning chloride channel reduces the amount of chloride and sodium normally reabsorbed from the resorptive duct and leads to elevated levels of these ions in sweat compared with normal patients. Excessive chloride loss has led to the development of hypochloremic metabolic alkalosis, especially in infants and young children who cannot regulate their salt intake independently.

The majority of male patients (98%) have obstruction of the vas deferens with resultant azoospermia and sterility. Although fertility in females is decreased because of thickened cervical mucus, many women who have CF are able to have children. Pregnancy is well tolerated in women who have good pulmonary function but may accelerate pulmonary decline in those who have moderate to severe disease.

DIAGNOSIS

Often, pediatricians fail to consider the diagnosis after infancy. Although 70% of patients are diagnosed in the first year of life, almost 10% are diagnosed after the first decade, occasionally in adulthood.[16] It is important to realize that there is no such thing as a child who "looks too healthy" to have CF. Other misconceptions are that CF is such a rare disease that it is not a diagnostic consideration or that the patient *must* have pancreatic insufficiency to be diagnosed. Pediatricians often hesitate to refer a child for a sweat test for fear of alarming the parents about the possibility that their child might have a fatal disease. To the contrary, once parents become educated about CF, they often become quite angry about delays in the diagnosis and lose faith in the pediatrician as a primary caretaker for that child and/or other non-CF siblings. One should strongly consider referring children for a sweat test if they have any of the following symptoms: chronic/recurrent pulmonary infection, wheezing or productive cough, clubbing, positive sputum cultures for SA or PA (especially mucoid PA), failure to thrive, malnutrition, or malabsorption. For a more complete list of indications for a sweat test, see Table 36-1.

Early recognition of CF avoids costly diagnostic workups. The diagnosis of CF is confirmed or ruled out in 98% of patients by a sweat test (quantitative pilocarpine iontophoresis). The two sample collection methods approved by the United States Cystic Fibrosis Foundation are the Gibson-Cooke procedure and the macroduct sweat collection system. Adequate sweat collection using these methods is 75 mg and 15 μl, respectively. Alternative sweat test procedures have a high incidence of false-positive and false-negative results and should not be used.[48] The sweat test should be done at a CF center to avoid erroneous results from inexperienced laboratories. Sweat chloride levels greater than 60 mEq/L in the presence of signs or symptoms suggestive of the disease confirm the diagnosis. Testing in the first few weeks of life can be performed successfully; however, results occasionally may be unreliable because of low sweat rates.

Positive tests at this time should be confirmed, and negative tests should be repeated without hesitation if sus-

Table 36-1 Indications for Sweat Testing

Respiratory	Gastrointestinal	Other
Lower Respiratory	Meconium ileus	Aspermia
Chronic cough	Meconium plug	Absent vas deferens
Recurrent/chronic pneumonia	Intestinal atresia	Metabolic alkalosis
Recurrent wheezing	Prolonged jaundice	Salty taste to skin
Atelectasis	Malabsorption	Salt crystals on skin
Bronchiectasis	Steatorrhea	Positive family history
Clubbing	Edema and hypoproteinemia	Hypoprothrombinemia
Colonization with mucoid PA	Failure to thrive	
Hemoptysis	Rectal prolapse	
Pneumothorax	Recurrent intussusception	
Upper Respiratory	Recurrent pancreatitis	
Nasal polyps	Recurrent intestinal obstruction	
Pansinusitis	Cirrhosis	
	Cholecystitis	

picion about the diagnosis persists. Some patients who have typical clinical symptoms of CF and repeatedly borderline sweat chloride levels (40 to 60 mEq/L) have been reported. In these cases, mutational analysis is indicated. Although mutational analysis has high specificity for confirming the diagnosis of CF, it has poor sensitivity because current mutational analysis screens for only 80% to 85% of the 700 CF mutations.[48] Electrical potential patterns from sodium and chloride ion movement across nasal airway epithelial cells are very different in CF patients than in normal patients and their determination (nasal potential difference measurements) may be helpful in diagnosing CF if the mutational analysis also is nondiagnostic (only one mutation identified), but this testing currently is available only in a few centers.

PSYCHOSOCIAL

Patients who have CF should be followed up by their general pediatrician and at a CF center that offers a multidisciplinary approach to this complex disease. The team includes the CF specialist, a nurse, a social worker, a nutritionist, a respiratory therapist, and a geneticist. The CF specialist, usually a pulmonologist, is able to optimize current medical treatment, enter patients into ongoing clinical trials, and alert patients appropriately to the most recent and relevant developments in the field. Although all team members provide emotional support, the nurse and social worker have major input in this regard. Social workers help the patients and families through the various stages of the disease from diagnosis to adulthood—hospital admissions, pulmonary deterioration, genetic counseling, and death. Social workers are invaluable in helping families cope with the emotional and financial burden of CF. The nutritionist may be able to give valuable insights to maximize caloric intake and optimize pancreatic enzyme use.

Patients often are referred to a CF center after having a positive result on a sweat test at an institution that is not a CF center. After learning of a positive sweat test result, the pediatrician should contact a CF specialist who will make every effort to see the patient and family within a day or two to evaluate the child and confirm the diagnosis. Despite increasing publicity, many parents of newly diagnosed patients have not heard of the disease. The initial approach to the family at the CF center is crucial. Cystic fibrosis is presented as a chronic disease primarily involving the lungs and digestive tract. The genetic basis of CF is explained, and the parents are told clearly that no one is to blame, nor is there any way to have prevented its occurrence. Issues of life expectancy are discussed, and survival into adulthood with current treatment and the hope of further improvements given the rapid progress in CF research is emphasized. The goal is to paint a picture of cautious optimism. Genetic counseling and prenatal diagnosis should be offered to the parents and other close family members. All siblings should have sweat testing to rule out CF. If the result is negative, they have a two-thirds risk of being a carrier; absolute carrier status can be determined by genetic analysis.

Parents will forget most of this initial discussion; various aspects should be reintroduced at regularly scheduled clinic visits. In the past, all newly diagnosed patients were hospitalized for medical treatment and to help the family adjust to the diagnosis; currently, this decision is individualized. If the decision is made to forego admission, frequent follow-up and telephone contacts are made to ensure appropriate understanding of the disease. Appropriate reading materials are provided to the family, and they are encouraged to meet, for emotional and practical support, other families of patients who have CF who are coping well. Often, after diagnosis and treatment with dietary supplementation, pancreatic enzymes, and/or antibiotics, patients do well and have a "honeymoon" phase. Many parents may deny the presence of CF or think that the major sequelae will somehow skip over them. "My child is no different from other children; he just needs to take some pills before he eats," is a common theme of denial. The first hospitalization for a pulmonary exacerbation or first sputum culture positive for *Pseudomonas aeruginosa* (PA), therefore, may have the same devastating impact on the family as the initial diagnosis.

During late childhood and adolescence the responsibility for care should be transferred gradually to the patient. Genetic and vocational counseling are mandatory. Most men

(98%) who have CF are sterile; however, this topic is not discussed often by the family. The difference between sterility and penile virility (not impaired in CF) needs to be addressed. Adult males contemplating fatherhood should have a semen analysis. Female fertility is only mildly impaired, and most women who have CF are capable of bearing children. They need to be counseled concerning the risk of having a child who has CF, the role of genetic screening of their spouse for the most common mutations, the availability of prenatal screening, and the potential negative effects of a pregnancy to their health.

GENETICS

Accurate prenatal diagnosis and carrier status have been a goal of caretakers and affected families for many years. In the early 1980s prenatal diagnosis was limited to analysis of microvillar intestinal enzymes (reduced activity caused by transient meconium ileus in utero). A high rate of false-positive and false-negative results limited use to families at high risk. The discovery of DNA markers tightly linked to the CF gene further improved prenatal diagnosis through linkage analysis. In most families, linkage of these markers can be followed and restriction fragment length polymorphisms (RFLPs) of affected and unaffected chromosomes analyzed. With this technique, virtually all families can receive accurate information. The major limitation of linkage analysis is that a sample of DNA from the affected patient who has CF must be available. Cloning of the CF gene has improved genetic screening, even in families in whom no DNA is available from the index case. Current prenatal testing involves the use of one or more molecular genetic techniques, including direct detection of the most common known mutations. Carrier screening of the general population is limited by the large number of CF mutations.

MANAGEMENT

The management of the patient who has CF can be categorized as standard therapy, treatment of respiratory complications, and novel approaches targeted toward various stages of the pathophysiological process.

Standard Therapy

Once acquired, PA infection rarely is eradicated. This longstanding dogma is being reexamined. Aggressive antibiotic therapy with inhaled colistin and oral ciprofloxacin at the time of the first positive culture for PA has been shown to reduce chronic PA infection and slow deterioration in lung function when compared with historical controls.[18] Additional prospective studies are needed to confirm these findings and define optimal antibiotic regimens.

Once chronic infection occurs, patients have periods of relative stability, with intermittent "exacerbations" of disease. Pulmonary exacerbations often have a subacute presentation. Triggers are multifactorial and include viral or bacterial infection and exposure to allergens, airway irritants, and pollutants. Classic signs of lung infection such as fever, leukocytosis, and chest radiograph changes usually are absent; the condition often is diagnosed based on subjective findings (Box 36-1). Management includes some combination of antibiotics, chest physiotherapy (CPT), bronchodilators, and nutritional support. Pulmonary exacerbations are treated with a combination of intravenous antibiotics (an aminoglycoside and a penicillin derivative) effective against PA for approximately 10 to 14 days. Recommended doses are higher for CF patients because of their higher clearance rates for many antibiotics and the difficulty in achieving adequate drug levels in their pulmonary secretions. Some patients appear to have equivalent results from home or hospital treatment; however, others may not do as well on outpatient parenteral therapy. Differences in patient motivation, adherence and quality of CPT, and nutritional support are some of the variables that may account for these differing outcomes.[5] Decisions regarding inpatient or outpatient therapy should be made on an individualized basis. Ciprofloxacin used orally is effective for milder exacerbations; however, acquired bacterial resistance is not uncommon. Frequent need for treatment with ciprofloxacin often signals the need for parenteral antibiotic therapy.

BOX 36-1

PULMONARY EXACERBATION: SIGNS AND SYMPTOMS*

Change in sputum volume, color, and appearance
Deterioration in pulmonary function test results
Increased cough, dyspnea, and tachypnea
New chest examination findings
New chest radiographic findings
Fever
Fatigue
Decreased exercise tolerance
Decreased appetite
Weight loss

*Often insidious onset.

Aerosolized tobramycin in high concentrations when used every other month reduces the risk of hospitalization and increases pulmonary function compared with placebo.[44] No significant increases in resistant organisms were seen in this 6-month study, although this remains a possible concern with long-term use. Transient tinnitus and voice alteration were minor adverse effects seen in a small number of patients. Recommendations are to consider this therapy for patients who have moderate to severe lung disease (FEV_1 between 25% to 75% predicted) who are infected with PA.

Daily prophylactic therapy with an anti-SA antibiotic is no longer recommended because a multicentered, double-blind, placebo-controlled study using cephalexin did not demonstrate any advantage in the treatment group. Patients in the treatment group had a higher incidence of PA infections, suggesting that daily use of anti-SA antibiotics may predispose patients to the acquisition of PA.[34] Anti-SA antibiotics are used intermittently for mild exacerbations when SA is isolated from respiratory secretions.

Prevention of disease in CF patients is essential in routine health care maintenance. Parents should be warned about the dangers of second-hand smoke. In addition to routine immunizations, all CF patients should be vaccinated yearly for influenza virus.

Chest physiotherapy (CPT) continues to be a component of therapy for lung disease. The rationale is that the airway secretions of CF are difficult to expectorate and that these techniques facilitate clearance of mucus. Unfortunately, CPT is one of the most time-consuming aspects of therapy and constitutes a frequent area of noncompliance. Alternative methods, such as the forced expiration technique, use of a positive expiratory pressure mask, self-positional drainage, use of mechanical percussors, high-frequency chest wall oscillation (ThAIRapy Vest, American Biosystems, St. Paul, Minnesota), and the Flutter device have been developed to meet the need for patient independence. Currently, CPT is individualized to meet the patient's needs.

Wheezing and airflow obstruction are major features of CF. Nebulized beta agonists are used most often before CPT to augment mucociliary clearance. Cystic fibrosis patients who have classic symptoms of asthma benefit from the use of bronchodilators. Although the rationale for the use of bronchodilators (BD) seems clear, many patients have an inconsistent response to BD.[39] Some patients may have a paradoxical response to BD because of the collapse of bronchiectatic central airways and reduced cough efficacy. Frequent evaluation of pulmonary function is necessary to ensure optimum bronchodilator use.

In an attempt to reduce the inflammatory response that is responsible for progressive lung damage, various antiinflammatory agents are being assessed, including corticosteroids, ibuprofen, and antiproteases.[35] High-dose, alternate-day prednisone (2 mg/kg qod) was associated with unacceptable side effects (cataracts, growth retardation, and glucose intolerance) in a multicenter trial. The group of patients that received a lower dose (1 mg/kg qod) showed a mild improvement in pulmonary status; however, adverse effects developed after 24 months.[14] High-dose inhaled corticosteroids have been shown to induce a small reduction in bronchial hyperresponsiveness in a short-term trial.[55] Longer-term studies are needed to establish the effect of inhaled corticosteroids on airway inflammation and long-term outcomes. At present, inhaled corticosteroids are recommended for patients who have CF and classic asthma symptoms. High-dose ibuprofen when taken consistently over 4 years slowed significantly the progression of lung disease without serious adverse effects.[31] Adequate dosing with pharmacokinetic studies to verify therapeutic blood levels and close monitoring for adverse effects (gastrointestinal bleeding, peptic ulcers, and renal toxicity) are essential. Ibuprofen should be discontinued temporarily during intravenous aminoglycoside therapy, based on case reports suggesting enhanced renal toxicity when the two are used together.[32]

Large amounts of DNA released from neutrophils add greatly to the viscosity of mucus. Recombinant human DNase (Pulmozyme) by inhalation has been shown to reduce rates of respiratory tract infection and improve pulmonary function and patient perception of well-being.[20,42] No allergic or anaphylactic responses were seen; voice alteration is a potential, self-limited side effect. The currently recommended dosage is 2.5 mg/day, using one of the nebulizer systems studied during clinical trials (Hudson T/Updraft II Nebulizer/Pulmo-aide DeVilbiss Compressor, Marquest Alcorn II Nebulizer/Pulmo-aide DeVilbiss Compressor, Pari LC Nebulizer/Pari Proneb Compressor). Pulmozyme should not be mixed with other drugs in the nebulizer.[43] The response to Pulmozyme is heterogeneous. Still unknown is what impact, if any, Pulmozyme has on disease progression. Patients who have purulent airway secretions should have a trial of Pulmozyme for 3 to 6 months, with continued use based on clinical response.[51]

Therapy for Pulmonary Complications

Pneumothorax (PTX) is caused most often by rupture of subpleural blebs through the visceral pleura; 5% to 8% of patients eventually will experience a PTX. The incidence increases with disease severity and age. Pneumothorax should be suspected in patients who present with sudden onset of chest pain and respiratory distress. Every CF patient who has a PTX, even if asymptomatic, should be hospitalized for a minimum of 24 hours. A chest tube should be inserted if the PTX is greater than 20% of the hemithorax volume or if the patient is symptomatic. A large PTX is managed best initially by letting the lung slowly expand without applying suction in order to reduce the incidence of reexpansion pulmonary edema. Removal of the chest tube is recommended for PTX that resolves with simple chest tube drainage. Excision of blebs and a limited surgical pleurodesis (production of adhesions) are recommended for most patients who persistently leak air. Chemical pleurodesis with quinacrine or tetracycline should be reserved for high-risk surgical candidates. Pleurodesis is not an absolute contraindication for lung transplantation; however, for those patients experiencing a PTX while on a transplant list, the transplant team should be contacted before pleurodesis in initiated.[50]

Blood streaking of sputum is common (50% to 60%) and requires no specific treatment. Major hemoptysis (240 ml/24 hr or 100 ml/day × 3 to 7 days) may be life threatening because of asphyxiation or, more rarely, exsanguination. The bleeding usually is from dilated and tortuous bronchial (systemic) arteries and often is associated with pulmonary infection. Hemoptysis should be differentiated from bleeding originating from other sites (gastrointestinal, upper airway). Drugs that interfere with coagulation should be discontinued, and any coagulation defects should be corrected. An episode of major hemoptysis does not change the long-term prognosis. The major risk is during the acute bleeding. Although the bleeding may respond to bedrest and antibiotics, bronchial artery embolization is indicated for major hemoptysis. This procedure should be performed by an interventional radiologist at a facility that has personnel who have experience with this procedure.

Lung transplantation is a final option for patients who have end-stage pulmonary disease. Suitable candidates for referral are patients who have a FEV_1 <30% of predicted.[27] Earlier referral for females and pediatric patients should be considered because of their increased risk for mortality at this level of lung function.[57] The procedure is heart-lung or double lung transplantation. The 3-year survival rate of 60% is similar to that among non-CF patients. Early complications include sepsis and technical complications, including bronchial dehiscence/stenosis, bleeding, and primary graft failure. Long-term morbidity and mortality is increased by the development of infection and bronchiolitis obliterans.[57]

Novel Therapeutic Approaches

The newer understanding of CFTR function is leading to a variety of novel potential therapeutic approaches. The common goal to all approaches is to get sufficient levels of functional, or partially functional, CFTR to the cell surface, thereby improving ASF volume and/or composition toward normal, with resulting lessening of symptoms or slowing down the progressive lung destruction. Initially, the major emphasis focused on gene replacement therapy. The advantages in CF are several. The airways are a good target for aerosolized gene replacement therapy. In vitro studies suggest that gene replacement of 7% to 10% of cells is sufficient to correct the ion transport abnormalities.[46] If successful gene transfer were possible, a cure might be achieved without complete knowledge of CFTR function.[56] A variety of approaches to gene replacement are being investigated.[9] Some vectors for gene transfer (adenovirus, liposomes) do not integrate into the host genome and are likely to have only a transient effect, requiring multiple reapplications. Adenovirus vectors are limited by the immune response, and liposomes are limited by inefficiency of transfer.[46] The use of adeno-associated virus as a vector offers the potential for longer-lasting treatment, because the gene product is incorporated into the host genome; however, random integration raises concerns of carcinogenesis.[46] Many questions of safety, efficacy, and cell type requiring treatment need to be addressed. Early phase I trials are under way.

The characterization of CF mutations into classes (see the section on respiratory pathophysiology and manifestations on p. 448) is leading to treatment approaches in a genotype-specific manner. Recent in vitro studies have demonstrated that certain aminoglycoside antibiotics, such as G-418 and gentamicin, can suppress premature stop mutations (class 1) and produce full-length, functional CFTR.[24] Clinical trials are under way in patients who have class 1 mutations.

In patients who are homozygous for ΔF_{508}, CFTR is "trapped" intracellularly. In certain experimental conditions, mutant ΔF_{508} CFTR has partial chloride channel function once at the cell surface. A variety of chemical "chaperones" that may enable more partially functional CFTR to reach the cell surface before degradation in the endoplasmic reticulum (class 2) is being investigated. The drug CPX binds to the first nucleotide binding fold of the ΔF_{508} mutation, facilitating trafficking to the cell surface.[7,56] Phase I trials are under way. Buphenyl (phenylbutyrate) appears to increase ΔF_{508} CFTR expression, thereby overwhelming the degradation abilities of the endoplasmic reticulum, resulting in increased expression at the cell surface.[49] Dose escalation and safety trials are under way.

Some CFTR mutations have residual function at the cell surface (class 4) that may be increased by the use of phosphatases or a combination of a beta agonist and a phosphodiesterase inhibitor.[12,25]

Chloride channels other than CFTR may be candidates for manipulation to restore the ASF toward normal. Attempts to alter ion transport with amiloride, a sodium channel blocker that blocks the reuptake of sodium from the airway surface, have shown a slowed rate in decline of vital capacity, reduced sputum viscosity, and increased mucociliary clearance.[28] Chloride secretagogues, such as ATP and UTP, may be useful in correcting the ionic environment toward normal after pretreatment with amiloride.[29]

Antimicrobial peptides that are not inhibited by the high salt concentration in the ASF of CF patients are being developed in the hopes that they will augment host defense and delay the onset of infection with typical CF pathogens.

A specific defect in essential fatty acid metabolism, independent of nutritional status, resulting in increased levels of arachidonic acid (AA) and low levels of docosahexaenoic acid (DHA) has been described recently.[19] Administration of a modified form of DHA corrected the imbalance and reversed the CF disease manifestations in CF mice. This effect appears to be DHA specific. Supplementation with other fatty acids either separately or in addition to DHA worsened the pancreatic pathology. Patients are warned to avoid current DHA formulations available in health food stores because they are combined with other fatty acids and may be detrimental. A modified form of DHA is under development to allow trials for optimal dosing and minimize gastrointestinal side effects. These trials are expected to start in the year 2000.

The discovery of the gene also has led to the development of animal models[13,53] that should help in evaluating the multiple therapeutic approaches mentioned above.

SUMMARY

Most current CF therapy has involved the treatment of preexisting disease. Although the life expectancy of CF patients has improved steadily, it is clear that new approaches to therapy are necessary to achieve further significant improvement in patient survival. The discovery of the CF gene has led to an evolving concept and understanding of the pathophysiology of the disease and an explosion in research and promising therapeutic modalities. The accessibility of the target tissue by the aerosol route makes the possibility of genetic transfer feasible. The approach to CF will represent a model approach for other genetic diseases in the future.

REFERENCES

1. Abman SH, et al: Early bacteriologic, immunologic, and clinical courses of young infants with cystic fibrosis identified by neonatal screening, *J Pediatr* 119:211, 1991.
2. Anderson DH: Cystic fibrosis of the pancreas and its relation to celiac disease: a clinical and pathological study, *Am J Dis Child* 56:344, 1938.
3. Barasch J, et al: Defective acidification of intracellular organelles in cystic fibrosis, *Nature* 352:70, 1991.
4. Borowitz DS, et al: Use of pancreatic enzyme supplements for patients with cystic fibrosis in the context of fibrosing colonopathy, *J Pediatr* 127:681, 1995.

5. Bosworth DG, Nielson DW: Effectiveness of home versus hospital care in the routine treatment of cystic fibrosis, *Pediatr Pulmonol* 24:42, 1997.
6. Cacalano G, et al: Production of *Pseudomonas aeruginosa* neuraminidase is increased under hyperosmolar conditions and is regulated in genes involved in alginate expression, *J Cline Invest* 89:1866, 1992.
7. Cohen BE, et al: 8-cyclopentyl-1,3-dipropylxanthine and other xanthines differentially bind to the wild-type and ΔF_{508} mutant first nucleotide binding fold (NBF-1) domains of the cystic fibrosis transmembrane regulator, *Biochemistry* 36:6455, 1997.
8. Cohn JA, et al: Localization of the cystic fibrosis transmembrane conductance regulator in human bile duct epithelial cells, *Gastroenterology* 105:1857, 1993.
9. Collins FS: Cystic fibrosis: molecular biology and therapeutic implications, *Science* 256:774, 1992.
10. Colombo C, et al: Analysis of risk factors for the development of liver disease associated with cystic fibrosis, *J Pediatr* 124:393, 1994.
11. Colombo C, et al: Scintigraphic documentation of an improvement in hepatobiliary excretory function after treatment with ursodeoxycholic acid in patients with cystic fibrosis and associated liver disease, *Hepatology* 15:677, 1992.
12. Delaney SJ, Wainwright BJ: New pharmaceutical approaches to the treatment of cystic fibrosis, *Nat Med* 2:392, 1996.
13. Dorin JR, et al: Cystic fibrosis in the mouse by targeted insertional mutagenesis, *Nature* 359:211, 1992.
14. Eigen H, et al: A multicenter study of alternate-day prednisone therapy in patients with cystic fibrosis, *J Pediatr* 126:515, 1995.
15. Fick Jr RB: Pathogenesis of the *Pseudomonas* lung lesion in cystic fibrosis, *Chest* 96:158, 1989.
16. FitzSimmons SC: The changing epidemiology of cystic fibrosis, *J Pediatr* 122:1, 1993.
17. Fitzsimmons SC, et al: High dose pancreatic enzyme supplements and fibrosing colonopathy in children with cystic fibrosis, *N Engl J Med* 336:1283, 1997.
18. Frederiksen B, Koch C, Hoiby N: Antibiotic treatment of initial colonization with *Pseudomonas aeruginosa* postpones chronic infection and prevents deterioration of pulmonary function in cystic fibrosis, *Pediatr Pulmonol* 23:330, 1997.
19. Freedman SD, et al: A membrane lipid imbalance plays a role in the phenotypic expression of cystic fibrosis in cftr (-/-) mice, *Proc Natl Acad Sci U S A* 96:3995, 1999.
20. Fuchs HJ, et al: Effect of aerosolized recombinant human DNase on exacerbations of respiratory symptoms and on pulmonary function in patients with cystic fibrosis, *N Engl J Med* 331:637, 1994.
21. Fuchs JR, Langer JC: Long term outcome after neonatal meconium ileus obstruction, *Pediatrics* 101:E7, 1998.
22. Goldman MJ, et al: Human beta-defensin-1 is a salt-sensitive antibiotic in lung that is inactivated in cystic fibrosis, *Cell* 88:553, 1997.
23. Hamosh A, Corey M: Correlation between genotype and phenotype in patients with cystic fibrosis, *N Engl J Med* 329:1308, 1993.
24. Howard M, Frizzell RA, Bedwell DM: Aminoglycoside antibiotics restore CFTR function by overcoming premature stop codons, *Nat Med* 2:467, 1996.
25. Kelley TJ, et al: Activation of endogenous ΔF_{508} cystic fibrosis transmembrane conductance regulator by phosphodiesterase inhibition, *J Clin Invest* 98:513, 1996.
26. Kerem B, et al: Identification of the cystic fibrosis gene: genetic analysis, *Science* 245:1073, 1989.
27. Kerem E, et al: Prediction of mortality in patients with cystic fibrosis, *N Engl J Med* 326:1187, 1992.
28. Knowles MR, et al: A pilot study of aerosolized amiloride for the treatment of lung disease in cystic fibrosis, *N Engl J Med* 322:1189, 1990.
29. Knowles MR, et al: Activation by extracellular nucleotides of chloride secretion in the airway epithelia of patients with cystic fibrosis, *N Engl J Med* 325:533, 1991.
30. Knowles MR, et al: Ion composition of airway surface liquid of patients with cystic fibrosis as compared with normal and disease-controlled subjects, *J Clin Invest* 10:2588, 1997.
31. Konstan MW, et al: Effect of high dose ibuprofen in patients with cystic fibrosis, *N Engl J Med* 332:848, 1995.
32. Kovesi TA, Swartz R, MacDonald N: Transient renal failure due to simultaneous ibuprofen and aminoglycoside therapy in children with cystic fibrosis, *N Engl J Med* 338:65, 1998.
33. Laning S, et al: Influence of the development of diabetes mellitus on clinical status in patients with cystic fibrosis, *Eur J Pediatr* 151:684, 1992.
34. Marshall BC, Samuelson WM: Basic therapies in cystic fibrosis: does standard therapy work? *Clin Chest Med* 19:487, 1998.
35. McElvaney NG, et al: Modulation of airway inflammation in cystic fibrosis: in vivo suppression of interleukin-8 levels on the respiratory epithelial surface by aerosolization of recombinant secretory leukoprotease inhibitor, *J Clin Invest* 90:1296, 1992.
36. Mickle JE, Cutting GR: Clinical implications of cystic fibrosis transmembrane conductance regulator mutations, *Clin Chest Med* 19:443, 1998.
37. Moran AM: Diabetes and glucose intolerance in cystic fibrosis, *New insights into cystic fibrosis*, 5:winter, 1997.
38. Moran A, et al: Abnormal glucose metabolism in cystic fibrosis, *J Pediatr* 133:10, 1998.
39. Pattishall EN: Longitudinal response of pulmonary function to bronchodilators in cystic fibrosis, *Pediatr Pulmonol* 9:80, 1990.
40. Pilewski JM, Frizzell RA: Role of CFTR in airway disease, *Physiol Rev* 79(suppl):S215,1999.
41. Poupon RE, et al: Combined analysis of randomized controlled trials of ursodeoxycholic acid in primary biliary cirrhosis, *Gastroenterology* 113: 884, 1997.
42. Ramsey BW, et al: Efficacy and safety of short-term administration of aerosolized recombinant human deoxyribonuclease in patients with cystic fibrosis, *Am Rev Respir Dis* 148:145, 1993.
43. Ramsey BW, et al: Consensus conference: practical applications of Pulmozyme, *Pediatr Pulmonol* 17:404, 1994.
44. Ramsey BW, et al: Intermittent administration of inhaled tobramycin in patients with cystic fibrosis, *N Engl J Med* 340:23, 1999.
45. Riordan JR, et al: Identification of the cystic fibrosis gene: cloning and characterization of complementary DNA, *Science* 245:1066, 1989.
46. Robinson CB: Is DNA destiny? A cure for cystic fibrosis, *Clin Chest Med* 19:527, 1998.
47. Rommens JM, et al: Identification of the cystic fibrosis gene: chromosome walking and jumping, *Science* 245:1059, 1989.
48. Rosenstein BJ: What is a cystic fibrosis diagnosis? *Clin Chest Med* 19:423, 1998.
49. Rubenstein RC, Zeitlin PL: A pilot clinical trial of oral sodium 4-phenylbutyrate (buphenyl) in ΔF_{508}-homozygous cystic fibrosis patients, *Am J Respir Crit Care Med* 157:484, 1998.
50. Schidlow DV, Taussig LM, Knowles MR: Cystic Fibrosis Foundation Consensus Conference Report on pulmonary complications of cystic fibrosis, *Pediatr Pulmonol* 15:187, 1992.
51. Shah PL, Hodson ME: The overuse or underuse of dornase alfa, *Curr Opin Pulm Med* 3:410, 1997.
52. Smith JJ, et al: Cystic fibrosis airway epithelia fail to kill bacteria because of abnormal airway surface fluid, *Cell* 85:229, 1996.
53. Snouwaert JN, et al: An animal model for cystic fibrosis made by gene targeting, *Science* 257:1083, 1992.
54. Sokol RS, Durie PR for the Cystic Fibrosis Foundation Hepatobiliary Disease Consensus Group: Recommendations for management of liver and biliary tract disease in cystic fibrosis, *J Pediatr Gastroenterol Nutr* 28:S1, 1999.
55. Van Haren EHJ, et al: The effects of the inhaled corticosteroid budesonide on lung function and bronchial hyperresponsiveness in adult patients with cystic fibrosis, *Respir Med* 89:209, 1995.
56. Zeitlin PL: Therapies directed at the basic defect in cystic fibrosis, *Clin Chest Med* 19:515, 1998.

57. Zuckerman JB, Kotloff RM: Lung transplantation for cystic fibrosis, *Clin Chest Med* 19:535, 1998.

SUGGESTED READINGS

Berger HA, Welsh MJ: Electrolyte transport in the lungs, *Hosp Pract* March 1991, p 53.

Fiel SB: Clinical management of pulmonary disease in cystic fibrosis, *Lancet* 341:1070, 1993.

Koch C, Hoiby N: Pathogenesis of cystic fibrosis, *Lancet* 341:1065, 1993.

Marshall BC, Samuelson WM: Basic therapies in cystic fibrosis: does standard therapy work? *Clin Chest Med* 19(3):487, 1998.

Pilewski JM, Frizzell RA: Role of CFTR in airway disease, *Physiol Rev* 79(suppl):S215,1999.

Tizzano EF, Buchwald M: Cystic fibrosis: beyond the gene to therapy, *J Pediatr* 120:337, 1992.

37 Muscular Dystrophy

Richard T. Moxley III

The muscular dystrophies represent a group of slowly progressive inherited diseases that usually have a very specific pattern of muscle wasting and weakness (Tables 37-1 to 37-4). These disorders occur infrequently in childhood; a busy pediatrician may follow only a few patients during his or her career. However, breakthroughs in molecular biology have provided direct genetic tests for these diseases and have created opportunities for the pediatrician to recommend and coordinate family counseling and prenatal testing. Primary care physicians play important roles by coordinating care with specialists in neuromuscular disease, by helping with genetic testing, and by monitoring patients for the various complications of these muscular dystrophies.

Duchenne dystrophy is the most common muscular dystrophy in childhood, and major advances have been made in its diagnosis and treatment. For these reasons, this chapter focuses on Duchenne dystrophy. However, Tables 37-1 to 37-4 provide useful information about other muscular dystrophies that occur in childhood, and the last section of the chapter includes a short commentary on these other muscular diseases, as well as suggestions for further reading on these disorders.

DUCHENNE DYSTROPHY

Duchenne dystrophy is a slowly progressive muscle-wasting disease marked by symptoms that develop before age 5 years. Early in its course, Duchenne dystrophy affects the proximal hip and shoulder girdle muscles as well as the anterior neck and abdominal muscles.[6,12,21,29] The symptoms arise from an absence or extreme deficiency of a large cytoskeletal protein, dystrophin, that attaches to the inner surface of the muscle fiber membrane as a part of a complex of glycoproteins.* Dystrophin also is part of the inner membrane structure of smooth and cardiac muscle and of certain cells in the central nervous system and in specialized connective tissues, such as the myotendinous junctions.[1] This distribution of dystrophin corresponds closely to those tissues that have major clinical manifestations in Duchenne dystrophy.

The mechanism by which dystrophin deficiency causes dysfunction in some muscle groups while sparing others is a puzzle. Some have speculated that dystrophin protects and strengthens the muscle membrane to withstand the stresses of repeated muscle contractions and that it helps prevent excessive influx of calcium and to speed effective repair of tears in the muscle membrane that occur with vigorous exercise.[1,7,12] But this puzzle still remains: Why do heavily used muscles, such as the extraocular and laryngeal muscles or the gastrocnemius muscles, maintain their strength despite the lack of dystrophin? Some researchers have wondered if another large cytoskeletal protein, such as utrophin, can take the place of dystrophin and help maintain muscle function.[7,10,13,36] Further research is in progress to clarify the role that such alternative proteins may play in rescuing muscle fibers from destruction in diseases involving dystrophin deficiency. The findings will help in developing new strategies for treatment.

Genetics

The gene for dystrophin in the Xp21 region is among the largest known, occupying 1% of the entire X chromosome.[1,7,12,33] It contains 79 exons, and five different promoters control production of isoforms that are cell-type specific (e.g., muscle, cerebral cortex, Purkinje, glial, and Schwann cells).[1,7,12,33] Large deletions occur in 60% to 65% of cases of Duchenne dystrophy and in an even higher percentage of cases of Becker dystrophy (a later onset X-linked dystrophy also caused by a deficiency of dystrophin).[1,7,12,33] In addition to large deletions, smaller point mutations occur in approximately 30% of patients who have Duchenne dystrophy and 15% of those who have Becker dystrophy.[12,32] No consistent relationship has been established between clinical severity (Duchenne dystrophy versus the milder Becker dystrophy) and the size of the gene mutation. However, deletion of the first muscle exon and the adjoining muscle promoter region appears to produce two somewhat consistent phenotypes—cases that have either mild muscle involvement or cases that have mild muscle involvement but severe cardiomyopathy.[12,32]

Clinical Presentation and Course

As outlined in Table 37-1, Duchenne dystrophy typically manifests between 2 and 4 years of age. Parents notice weakness of forward head flexion that persists beyond infancy, accompanied by slowed motor development. Patients demonstrate progressive gluteal and shoulder girdle muscular weakness, leading to a widened stance, lumbar lordosis, forward thrusting of the abdomen, and winging of the scapulae. Patients never run normally and usually put their hands on their knees to arise from the floor (Fig. 37-1) and to assist in climbing steps. These patients have difficulty keeping up with their peers, which becomes more apparent as they enter

Text continued on p. 463

*References 1, 7, 11, 32, 33, 36.

Table 37-1 Muscular Dystrophies in Childhood: Symptoms, Genetics, and Diagnostic Testing

	Duchenne Dystrophy	Becker Dystrophy	Myotonic Dystrophy
Onset	Before age 5 yr typically between 2 and 4 yr	After age 5; can begin in adult life	Infancy, childhood, or adult life
Initial symptoms	Cannot run or keep up with peers; can take only one step at a time	Fatigue or marked thigh weakness; trouble climbing steps; occasional calf or thigh cramps; patients can ambulate beyond age 15 yr	*Congenital form:* floppy infant; poor suck; weak respiratory effort; talipes *Childhood form:* bifacial weakness; slurred speech; impaired hearing; mental retardation
Incidence	1:3500 of male births	1:35,000 of male births	1:8000 of all births
Genetics	X-linked recessive/XP21 region of gene for dystrophin	X-linked recessive/XP21 region of gene for dystrophin	Autosomal dominant chromosome 19
Gene lesion	Absence of dystrophin	Marked deficiency of dystrophin	Abnormal expansion of CTG trinucleotide repeat in 3′ nontranslated region of a gene coding for a serine/threonine kinase
Serum CPK	10× above normal	5-10× above normal	Normal or 2-5× above normal
Electrodiagnostic testing	Normal nerve conduction; myopathic EMG	Normal nerve conduction; mildly myopathic EMG	Normal nerve conduction; myotonic discharges present in children and adults, but often absent in infants (EMG should be performed on the mother)
Muscle biopsy	Active myopathy, absence of dystrophin, severe reduction in dystrophin-associated proteins	Moderately active myopathy, absence or deficiency of dystrophin, reduction in dystrophin-associated proteins	Increased central nuclei, atrophy of type I fibers, ringbinden and subsarcolemmal masses
Leukocyte DNA testing	If suspicion is high, perform DNA screening first. If leukocyte DNA testing is negative, perform muscle biopsy. DNA is screened for deletions (60%-70% have them); if deletion is found, deletion tests are performed in at-risk family members; if no deletion is found, linkage analysis can be used to screen the family if muscle biopsy shows deficiency/absence of dystrophin	Same as Duchenne dystrophy	If this diagnosis is suspected, a Southern blot analysis is done to identify an abnormally large expansion of CTG repeats in the DM gene; if the Southern blot test is normal, a polymerase chain reaction test is done to search for smaller expansions of the repeat; most childhood cases show very abnormal CTG repeat enlargements (e.g., 500-4000 repeats), whereas normal alleles have 5-30 repeats

Facioscapulohumeral Dystrophy	Fukuyama-Type Congenital Muscular Dystrophy	Congenital Muscular Dystrophy: Primary Deficiency of Merosin	Emery-Dreifuss Muscular Dystrophy
Rare cases in infancy, occasionally in childhood, usually in adult life	Infancy	Infancy	Middle to late childhood
Congenital form (rare): bifacial weakness; sometimes ophthalmoparesis; occasionally, floppy; deafness *Childhood form (more common):* mild facial weakness and weakness of scapular fixator muscles	Floppy infant, slow improvement up to 6-8 yr, then a decline	Floppy, contractures	Mild elbow contractures and mild weakness of triceps, biceps, and scapular fixator muscles; occasionally as isolated cardiomyopathy
1:20,000 of all births	1:18,000 of all births	Unknown	1:100,000 of all births
Autosomal dominant, most cases localize to chromosome 4	Autosomal recessive, chromosome 9, q31-33 region for most cases	Autosomal recessive, chromosome 6q22-23 region, laminin $\alpha 2$ gene	X-linked recessive form Xq28 and autosomal dominant form 1q21.3
Deletion of a variable quantity of 3.3kb tandem repeats at 4q35	3kb insertion in 3′ noncoding region of gene encoding fukutin. Mutation causes instability of mRNA for fukutin. Fukutin probably helps to stabilize the muscle membrane	Complete (or partial) loss of merosin (laminin $\alpha 2$) in both muscle and skin	X-linked form involves gene for emerin and dominant form gene for lamins A and C. Emerin and lamins A and C are attached to nuclear membrane. Their functions are not yet known
2-5× above normal	>10× above normal	>10× above normal	5-10× above normal
Normal nerve conduction; EMG occasionally myopathic, often within normal limits	Normal nerve conduction; myopathic EMG	Normal nerve conduction; myopathic EMG	Normal nerve conduction; EMG often normal in early stages
Variable changes, often shows moderately active myopathy	Active myopathy, dystrophin, sarcoglycans, and dystroglycans normal. Partial deficiency of merosin (laminin $\alpha 2$)	Active myopathy. Typically, complete loss of merosin with preservation of dystrophin and the associated glycoprotein complex	Increased variation in fiber size; areas of fiber atrophy; increased connective tissue
DNA analysis available to identify the 3.3 kb deletions noted above. Should perform before obtaining muscle biopsy if clinical suspicion is high	Not yet available commercially	Not yet available commercially	Not yet available commercially

Table 37-2 Muscular Dystrophies in Childhood: Complications and Treatment

	Duchenne Dystrophy	Becker Dystrophy	Myotonic Dystrophy
Muscle weakness	Treatment with prednisone slows or stabilizes muscle strength; lightweight long-leg bracing maintains ambulation in later stages	No controlled studies of prednisone treatment; bracing is helpful in late stages	No specific therapy; braces for foot drop; children usually can participate in gym in school
Respiratory problems	Forced vital capacity is monitored (in later stages, atelectatic pneumonitis is common); colds are treated aggressively; if signs of respiratory failure develop, nasal/oral ventilation should be considered	Uncommon until late stages; management then is as with Duchenne dystrophy	For congenital cases, ventilary care often is needed; the prognosis for survival is very poor if the patient is ventilator dependent >4 wk; other management is as for Duchenne dystrophy
Cardiac problems	Occasionally, cardiomyopathy leads to congestive heart failure—afterload-reducing therapy often helps; the role of digoxin is uncertain; patient should be monitored for intracardiac clots	Occasionally, severe cardiomyopathy develops; treatment is the same as for Duchenne dystrophy	Occasionally, tachyarrhythmias or heart block develops in childhood forms, and pacemaker treatment is indicated
Orthopedic problems	Achilles tendon contractures respond to stretching in early stages, later tendon release surgery often is necessary; contractures at the hips, knees, elbows, and wrists usually develop after the patient becomes wheelchair bound; scoliosis often develops when patients stop ambulating, and spinal stabilization surgery helps maintain use of the arms and preserves pulmonary reserve	Uncommon; contractures are much less common than in Duchenne dystrophy	Talipes deformity requires treatment with stretching and orthotic support; occasionally, surgery is necessary
Nervous system problems	Increased incidence of cognitive and behavioral problems; some patients improve with small doses of methylphenidate	Uncommon	Mental retardation is common, especially in congenital cases, and special classroom care is needed; hearing deficits are common and may require hearing aids; facial weakness, dysarthria, and hearing problems exaggerate the impression of mental retardation
Gastrointestional problems	Constipation is common, especially late in the disease; careful dietary monitoring, stool softeners, and good water intake (urine specific gravities 1.007-1.010) usually are effective; occasionally acute gastric dilation occurs; it resolves over 2-3 days with NG tube decompression of the stomach and intravenous hydration	Uncommon	Spastic colon–type complaints with abdominal pain are common; occasionally, these symptoms improve with antimyotonia therapy with mexiletine; eating small portions at each meal diminishes tendency to aspirate

Facioscapulohumeral Dystrophy	Fukuyama-Type Congenital Muscular Dystrophy	Congenital Muscular Dystrophy: Primary Deficiency of Merosin	Emery-Dreifuss Muscular Dystrophy
No specific treatment; patients should avoid lifting with arms fully extended and abducted; braces are sometimes needed	No specific treatment; bracing and physical therapy are useful in some patients	Same as Fukuyama-type congenital muscular atrophy	No specific treatment; skeletal muscle weakness often is relatively mild compared with cardiac problems and does not limit function
Uncommon	As with Duchenne dystrophy; patients often succumb to respiratory failure late in childhood or in early teens	Same as Fukuyama-type congenital muscular atrophy	Mild other than symptoms related to cardiac dysfunction
Uncommon	Uncommon	Uncommon	Frequent cardiac conduction defects; atrial paralysis, cardiac arrest, and sudden death are common; pacemaker treatment and preventive therapy for cardiac emboli often are necessary
Occasionally, knee effusion and low-back pain develop secondary to weakness; conservative care measures are effective; in late stages some surgeons have reported good results with procedures to stabilize the scapula; surgery is uncommon	Contractures develop in 70% of patients by 3 months of age at the ankles, knees, and hips	Contractures, especially feet and hips	Contractures, especially in the elbows and ankles, occur early and respond somewhat to physical therapy; surgical release of Achilles tendon may be necessary; some patients develop a rigid spine syndrome, for which there is no effective therapy
Uncommon; in rare cases, the infant-onset form of the disease occurs in association with hearing loss and/or retinal disease	Generalized or focal seizures occur in most patients; anticonvulsant therapy is necessary; mental retardation is common; most patients have microcephaly, as well as polymicrogyria, pachygyria, and heterotopias, in the brain on postmortem examination	Mental retardation common; MRI of head shows increased signal from white matter on T2 weighted images; occipital agyria	Due only to stroke from heart block or cardiac emboli
Uncommon	Uncommon	Uncommon	Uncommon

Table 37-3 Autosomal Dominant Forms of Limb Girdle Muscular Dystrophy (LGMD)

	LGMD 1A	LGMD IB	LGMD 1C	LGMD 1D
Onset	Late teens and adult life	Childhood to early adult life	Around age 5 yr	Teens and adult life
Genetics	Chromosome 5q22-24; gene unknown	Chromosome 1q12-21; no gene identified	Chromosome 3p25; gene for caveolin; mutations alter scaffolding domain of the protein	Chromosome 6q23; no gene identified
Serum CPK	Normal or 2-5× normal	Normal or 2-5× normal	Often >10× normal	2-5× normal
Muscle biopsy	Fiber size variation; moth-eaten fibers; increased internal nuclei; occasional necrotic and regenerating fibers	Fiber size variation; increased internal nuclei; mild endomysial fibrosis; occasional necrotic and regenerating fibers	Similar findings to LGMD 1A and LGMD 1B; absence or deficiency of caveolin 3 on immunocytochemistry	Similar findings to LGMD 1A and LGMD 1B
Clinical features	Proximal weakness; occasional dysarthria; slow progression; Achilles tendon contractures; may show anticipation	Cardiac conduction disturbances prominent; proximal weakness; slow progression; may be allelic to autosomal dominant locus for Emery-Dreifuss dystrophy	Proximal weakness; calf hypertrophy; muscle pain on exertion; variable progression	Cardiac conduction disturbances prominent; proximal weakness; problems worse in males

LGMD 1 indicates the general code for autosomal dominant inheritance. The letters A, B, C, and D indicate the specific forms of dominantly inherited LGMD.

Table 37-4 Autosomal Recessive Forms of Limb Girdle Muscular Dystrophy (LGMD 2A-2F)

	LGMD2A—Calpainopathy	LGMD 2B—Dysferlinopathy	LGMD 2C-2F—Sarcoglycanopathy
Onset	Usually 8-15 yr; occasionally during adult life	Late teens	Majority in childhood; infrequently in adult life
Genetics	Mutations in CAPN3 gene; chromosome 15q15; homozygous null mutations tend to cause more severe clinical picture than missence mutations; no gender difference; mutation causes absence/deficiency of calpain 3; physiological function of calpain 3 is unknown	Mutations in gene for dysferlin; chromosome 2p13; cause absence/deficiency of dysferlin; the function of dysferlin is unknown	Mutations occur in genes encoding the specific sarcoglycans: 17q21 α sarcoglycan (LGMD 2D); 4q12 β sarcoglycan (LGMD 2E); 13q12 γ sarcoglycan (LGMD 2C); 5q33-34 δ sarcoglycan (LGMD 2F)
Serum CPK	Often >10× normal	Marked elevation 10-100× normal	Usually 2-5× normal
Muscle biopsy	Fiber size variation; mild endomysial fibrosis; occasional necrotic and regenerating fibers	Findings similar to Duchenne dystrophy but normal dystrophin staining; deficiency or absence of dysferlin	Findings similar to Duchenne or Becker dystrophy but almost normal dystrophin staining; specific sarcoglycan staining necessary to reveal absence/deficiency of sarcoglycans
Clinical features	Proximal weakness; scapulohumeral wasting; hip abductors spared; calf hypertrophy rare; respiratory complications often severe; cardiac problems not reported	Proximal or distal lower extremity weakness with mild scapular stabilizer weakness; unable to rise on tiptoes	Proximal weakness with shoulder girdle initially greater than pelvic girdle involvement; variable progression from mild to severe; occasional cases of cardiomyopathy; respiratory complications common in later stages

LGMD2 indicates the general code for autosomal recessive inheritance. The letters A, B, C, and D indicate the specific forms of recessively inherited LGMD.

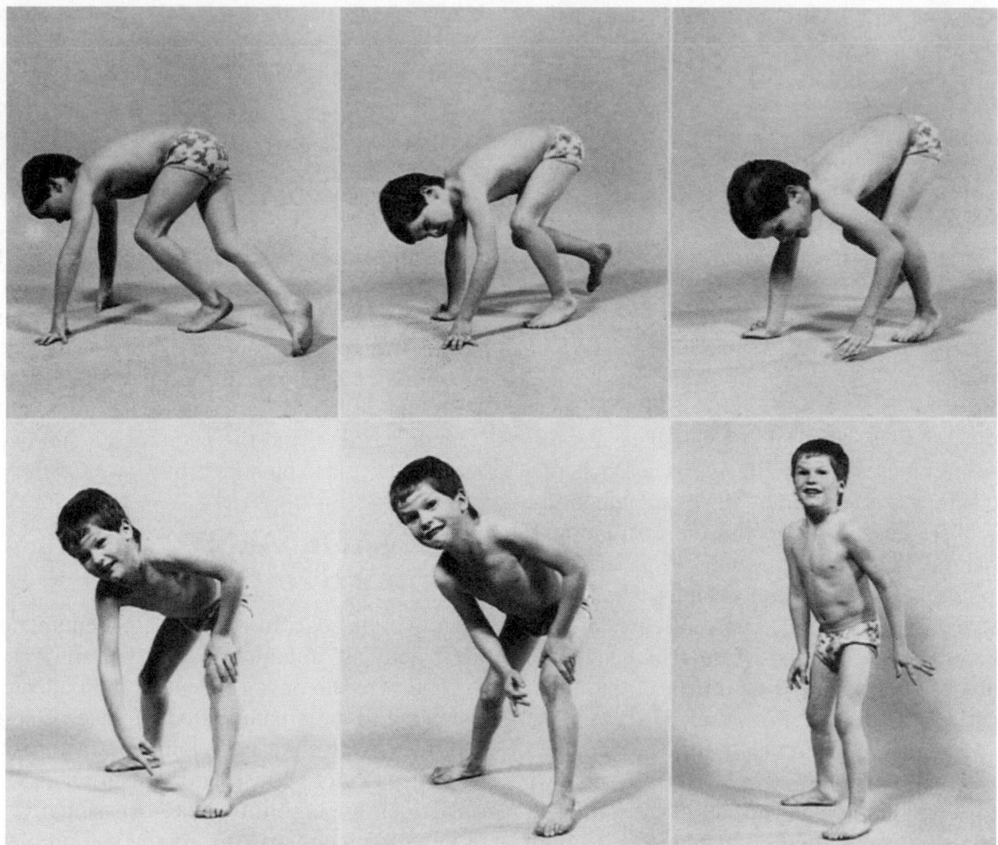

Fig. 37-1 A boy who has Duchenne muscular dystrophy demonstrates the sequence of maneuvers that constitutes Gowers sign. The child pushes off the floor with all four extremities, then prepares to push up by moving this hands along the floor closer to the feet, and finally placing the hands on the thighs and pushing up to the erect position. The maneuver is necessary primarily because of marked weakness of the hip extension.
(From Swaiman KF: *Pediatric neurology principles and practice,* ed 2, St Louis, 1994, Mosby.)

nursery school and kindergarten. Often the teacher observes a problem and helps the parents decide to bring the child to the pediatrician. It becomes clear that their son has a real problem and is not just normally clumsy and that poor motivation is not the cause for his tendency to fall easily and for his complaints of tiredness and calf cramps. A busy pediatrician has to be sensitive to the protean nature of these early complaints in Duchenne dystrophy.

Because Duchenne dystrophy has an increased frequency of mild cognitive deficits,[12] the patient may appear to be mentally retarded, and the pediatrician may not consider Duchenne dystrophy. Because of the gradual development of hip and knee extensor weakness in mid-childhood, patients often toe-walk to use the power of the gastrocnemius to help stabilize knee extension. Reliance on the calf muscles during ambulation contributes to the hypertrophy of the calf muscles that is so typical for most patients who have Duchenne dystrophy. However, the pattern of walking in these patients and the presence of a dull intellect sometimes can lead to the incorrect diagnosis of cerebral palsy, delaying effective treatment.

A careful history almost always distinguishes patients who have Duchenne dystrophy from those who have other conditions that cause proximal weakness without sensory findings in childhood. Hypothyroidism usually has more generalized symptoms, as does carnitine deficiency. Blood tests can exclude these two conditions from the differential diagnosis. Neither causes the marked elevation of creatine kinase that occurs in Duchenne dystrophy. Variants of spinal muscular atrophy and early-onset cases of facioscapulohumeral dystrophy (FSHD) may resemble Duchenne dystrophy. Hypertrophy of the calf muscles may be a feature of either condition. Spinal muscular atrophy produces no elevation or only a mild rise in creatine phosphokinase (CPK); FSHD causes only a mild to moderate elevation. As outlined in Table 37-1, electrodiagnostic testing and subsequent muscle biopsy are the appropriate diagnostic tests to establish the diagnosis of Duchenne dystrophy. Muscle biopsy also will help distinguish among many of the recently described autosomal dominant and autosomal recessive forms of limb girdle muscular dystrophy (LGMD) that sometimes have a close clinical similarity to Duchenne dystrophy (Tables 37-3 and 37-4).

Other, more acute conditions, such as childhood myasthenia gravis and inflammatory myopathy, usually are not confused with Duchenne dystrophy. The more rapid evolution of weakness, along with the presence of ptosis, ophthalmoparesis, and facial weakness, distinguish myasthenia gravis from Duchenne dystrophy. The more generalized weakness that occurs in inflammatory myopathy, along with a skin rash, helps to separate these patients from those who have Duchenne dystrophy. In rare cases, chronic demyelinating polyneuropathy may be confused with Duchenne dystrophy, but the absence of ankle reflexes, more generalized weakness, a more rapid course, and abnormally slowed nerve conduction identify these patients.

The combination of a careful history and judicious use of the tests outlined in Table 37-1 will establish the diagnosis of Duchenne dystrophy in virtually all cases. In rare cases, a "floppy" infant will have a markedly elevated serum CPK level, and physicians will wonder if the baby has a variant of Duchenne dystrophy. Newborns or infants who have Duchenne dystrophy do have a marked elevation of creatine kinase, but they are not floppy infants. Some other problem must be present as well, if a Duchenne dystrophy patient is floppy. Floppy infants who have a markedly elevated creatine kinase usually do not have Duchenne dystrophy. If such a patient does not have an infectious, toxic, or metabolic disorder that causes muscle destruction to account for the marked elevation of serum CPK, usually he has one of the two relatively rare childhood muscular dystrophies noted in Tables 37-1 and 37-2. These diseases are the severe childhood autosomal recessive forms of congenital muscular dystrophy. The workup and treatment of these disorders are summarized in Tables 37-1 and 37-2, and the reader may wish to consult other reviews for more detailed discussion of these conditions.[25,41,42,44] Other recent reviews provide a thorough commentary on muscle diseases that fit into the broad category of congenital myopathies.[3,14] Certain congenital myopathies may be marked by floppiness, but these infants do not have significantly elevated creatine kinase levels.[3,14]

Evaluation and Workup

Once the physician suspects the possibility of Duchenne (or Becker) dystrophy, it is helpful to measure the serum CPK. A marked elevation (tenfold or more above normal) excludes most other disorders and strongly suggests the diagnosis of Duchenne dystrophy. At this point it is appropriate to raise with the parents the possibility that the child has a muscular dystrophy. However, it is important to refer the patient for further evaluation by a neurologist skilled in the care of patients who have neuromuscular disease. It also is useful to mention that the neuromuscular specialist may want to perform other diagnostic tests, such as electromyography, a nerve conduction evaluation, and a muscle biopsy. A detailed discussion of the natural history of Duchenne dystrophy or of the procedures for screening the mother and other at-risk family members for carrier status can be postponed; this discussion is best initiated after the neurological consultation and after specific diagnostic information is available (see Table 37-1; Fig. 37-2). The neuromuscular specialist should assume responsibility for the initial description of the course of Duchenne dystrophy and should discuss the treatment options. Fig. 37-2 outlines the flow chart that neurologists typically follow to arrive at a diagnosis of Duchenne dystrophy. It emphasizes the helpful role of initial leukocyte DNA screening for deletions or duplications in reaching a diagnosis.

In patients suspected of having Duchenne dystrophy in whom DNA testing fails to demonstrate specific deletions or duplications, the absence of dystrophin on the muscle biopsy specimen establishes the diagnosis. If DNA testing reveals a deletion, it can be used to identify any women in the family who are carriers.[12,43] If deletions are not detected and dystrophin is absent on the muscle biopsy specimen, linkage analysis can be used to identify carriers. This analysis involves more extensive DNA testing of family members and is more expensive.

If the biopsy tissue shows an absence of dystrophin, the neurologist should discuss the results with the patient and parents, and the primary care physician should arrange a referral for genetic counseling. This aids development of a coordinated care plan for the patient and family. The geneticists can discuss different options for preventive therapy with female carriers, and the pediatrician and neuromuscular specialist can focus on supportive care for the patient.

MANAGEMENT

Supportive Care

The overall goals in managing patients who have Duchenne dystrophy are to maintain ambulation for as long as possible, to optimize the development of the patient's cognitive abilities, and to anticipate the occurrence of complications, such as excessive weight gain, joint contractures (especially of the Achilles tendons), respiratory insufficiency, scoliosis, gastrointestinal hypomotility, and occasionally, cardiomyopathy. Table 37-2 summarizes the principal problems and treatment options.

The patient and his family need to work closely with the physicians, school teachers, physical educators, and physical and occupational therapists to develop an individualized care plan for the patient for each stage of his disease. Early in the illness the patient usually can play with his peers in most activities, but by the first or second grade some adaptation of physical education requirements becomes necessary. The natural history of Duchenne dystrophy predicts that the patient will become wheelchair bound between 10 and 12 years of age.[6] Often, lightweight long-leg bracing is helpful at this stage to prolong weight bearing and ambulation, both of which delay the development of joint contractures and scoliosis. Contractures and scoliosis both develop when the patient becomes wheelchair bound. They do not appear at a specific age but depend on the patient's functional status. Once contractures begin to develop, usually at the ankles and elbows (flexion), it is important to obtain physical therapy (PT) and occupational therapy (OT) consultations. Follow-up care can be coordinated with PT and OT, and patients usually can receive this care in their schools. Once significant heel cord contractures develop, it also is useful to obtain an orthopedic consultation. The orthopedist can help guide the timing of the use of long-leg bracing and can discuss the possible need for surgery to lengthen the Achilles tendons. The orthopedic care, PT, OT, and neurological care often are coordinated by the neuromuscular specialist and typically are provided in a clinic financed partly by the Muscular Dystrophy Association (MDA).

Although MDA clinics provide an excellent opportunity to offer multiple services to patients, the role of the primary care physician remains critical. The pediatrician usually provides routine care of upper respiratory infections, as well as

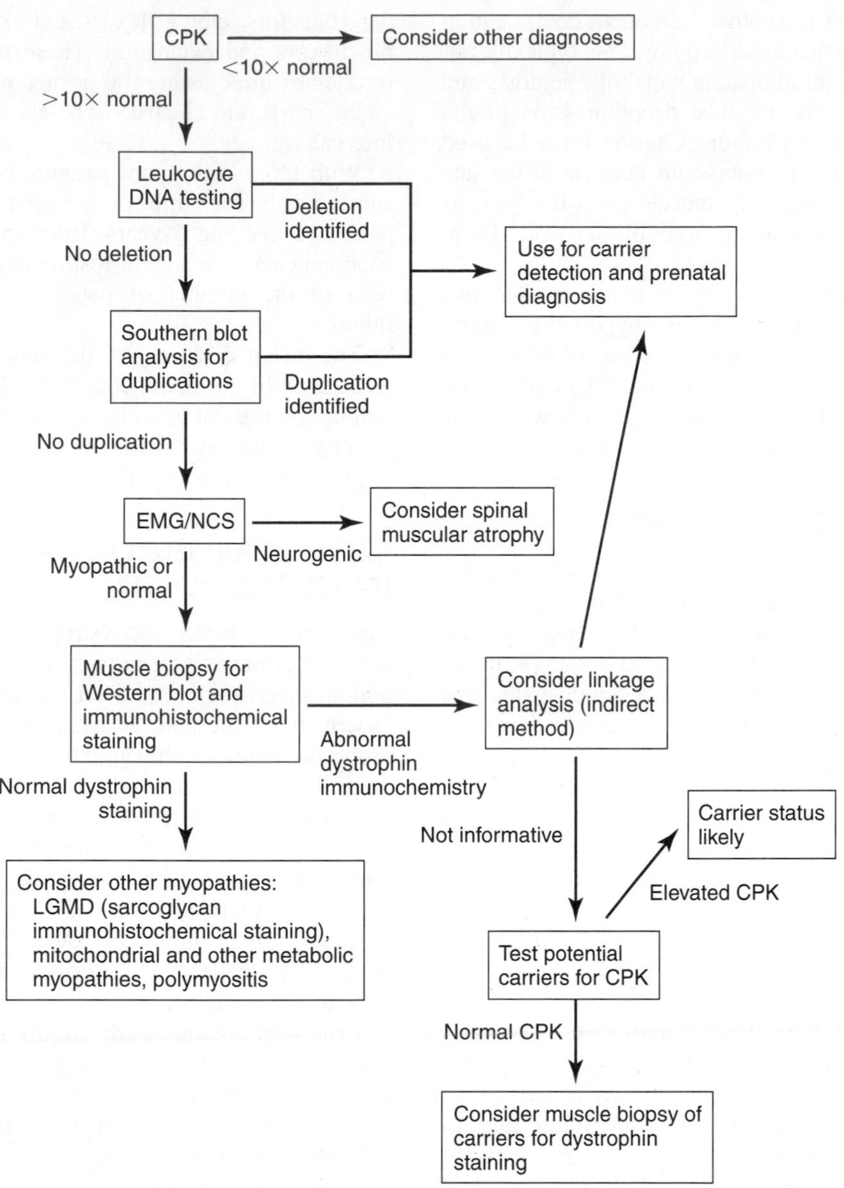

Fig. 37-2 Flow chart outlining diagnostic tests for a boy suspected of having Duchenne dystrophy without a family history of this disorder.

treatment for other common medical problems. In the middle and late stages of Duchenne dystrophy, minor medical problems can provoke major complications. A mild cold may lead to atelectatic pneumonitis and acute respiratory insufficiency. Such a problem, if treated aggressively, is fully reversible. Even chronic constipation can produce respiratory compromise in the later stages of Duchenne dystrophy, because of abdominal distention and upward pressure on the diaphragm. An effective regimen to maintain regular bowel movements becomes very important in routine care. Respiratory insufficiency often develops in the late stages of Duchenne dystrophy. Forced vital capacity declines, usually into the range of 600 to 1000 ml. One recent review describes the management options, which include nasal ventilation rather than positive pressure ventilation via tracheostomy.[34] Ventilatory care usually is coordinated among the pediatrician, neuromuscular specialist, pediatric pulmonologist, and the patient and his family. All have to participate if the treatment plan is to be effective. Considerable discussion is necessary to educate the patient and family at this stage and to help to decide which options are most appropriate for them. Often, physicians and nurses who have special training in neuromuscular diseases are the individuals who educate the family, and the roles of the pediatric pulmonologist and pediatrician have to be tailored to each medical care setting.

Occasionally, in the late stages of Duchenne dystrophy, patients develop cardiomyopathy.[12,13,32] A chest roentgenogram reveals a dilated heart, and the cardiac ejection fraction falls to 10% to 20% of normal. Heart failure often is exacerbated by coexisting respiratory insufficiency. In all these cases, simultaneous ventilatory support must be considered if the patient and his family have decided to pursue a vigorous course of treatment. The heart failure is difficult to manage, and afterload reduction therapy often is more effective than digoxin. Occasionally, ventricular and/or atrial clots are present, and long-term anticoagulant therapy is necessary.

Acute gastric dilation is another infrequent complication in the late stages of Duchenne dystrophy. This typically occurs in association with an idiopathic metabolic acidosis and responds rapidly to nasogastric tube decompression of the stomach and intravenous hydration. Caution must be used with intravenous repletion of potassium because in the late stages of the disease the patient's muscle mass is considerably diminished and is not available to buffer an acute rise in extracellular potassium.

The cause of the gastric dilation is unknown, but this problem, as well as the chronic intestinal hypomotility (constipation), probably results from the deficiency of dystrophin in the smooth muscle of the gastrointestinal (GI) tract. Good hydration, a balanced dietary intake, and regular bowel habits are the mainstays of treatment for these problems.

PREDNISONE TREATMENT

The only effective therapy for Duchenne dystrophy is prednisone. Double-blind, randomized, controlled studies have shown that prednisone in a daily dose of 0.75 mg/kg maintains muscle strength and function for at least 18 to 36 months[16,17,20,21,29] These studies also have demonstrated that daily treatment is more effective than alternate-day therapy.[16,29] Some benefit occurs at doses as low as 0.3 mg/kg/day,[17,20] and prolonged improvement of strength has occurred at doses ranging from 0.5 to 0.6 mg/kg/day.[17] The mechanism responsible for the beneficial effect of prednisone is unknown. However, there are several clues about the process involved. The increase in strength begins to develop after only 10 days of treatment[20] and reaches a maximum response after 3 months of therapy.[20,21,29] Muscle mass increases 10% after 3 months of prednisone treatment,[20,29,38] and the rate of muscle breakdown declines in association with maintenance of a normal rate of muscle protein synthesis.[38] One investigation compared the efficacy of 12 months of azathioprine immunosuppressive therapy with that of prednisone; no beneficial effect occurred with azathioprine.[20] This result argues against the possibility that an immunosuppressive effect accounts for the improvement in muscle strength with the use of prednisone.

Patients have been treated with prednisone at only a small number of specialized neuromuscular centers.[16,17,20,21,29] Prednisone treatment preferably is monitored by or coordinated with one of these centers. The protocols for monitoring side effects and for assessing muscle strength and function have been published previously.[17,20,21,29] The most common side effects are excessive weight gain, mood disturbances (more aggressive, more tearful), and cushingoid facial appearance.[16,17,20,21,29] More serious side effects (compression fractures of the spine, high blood pressure, GI bleeding, severe infections, or diabetes) are uncommon. Some patients have developed small, dot-shaped cataracts; others, as expected, have had decreased linear growth, which probably has helped maintain ambulation.

To allow monitoring for the development of side effects, patients are seen every 3 months for weight, blood pressure, pulse, and forced vital capacity checks, urinalysis, and assessment of neuromuscular functioning. At each visit the patient undergoes timed function tests (time needed to travel 30 feet, to arise from supine to standing position, and to climb four standard steps) and a muscle strength evaluation (shoulder abductors, elbow flexors and extensors, knee extensors, hip flexors and extensors). These measures help guide the physicians in adjusting the dosage of prednisone. The blood count and serum electrolyte levels are measured at 6-month intervals.

With close follow-up, patients have been kept stable or showed only very mild progression of muscle weakness for periods exceeding 5 years. Even in the late stages, prednisone appears to maintain respiratory muscle power and has reduced the number of patients who develop respiratory failure.

The recent discovery of the gene in Duchenne dystrophy and the ability to manufacture small segments of DNA containing the normal gene for dystrophin has raised hopes that direct gene therapy, either by local injection or by viral vector, will prove feasible. Research is in progress.

OTHER MUSCULAR DYSTROPHIES IN CHILDHOOD

Myotonic dystrophy, or dystrophica myotonia (DM), is due to an abnormal enlargement of a trinucleotide repeat in the 3′ nontranslated region of the DM gene on chromosome 19.* Discovery of the gene has led to the development of gene probes to identify both symptomatic and asymptomatic carriers.[39] Genetic counseling and prenatal testing now can be done with a high degree of accuracy, an important advance in preventive therapy.[22,37,39] One article provides a detailed review of management of the problems that occur in the neonatal and childhood forms of DM.[31] Other reports include comments about the complications that occur when patients receive anesthetics and describes the problems involved in pregnancy and delivery.[22,24,27,28,31]

Facioscapulohumeral dystrophy is not common in childhood and usually does not pose significant management problems. Many are optimistic that the gene for this disease soon will be isolated from its localization on chromosome 4.[40] DNA testing is now available.[35] This disease is reviewed in detail in a recent text.[40]

The infant-onset congenital muscular dystrophies are rare disorders and already have been mentioned in the discussion of the differential diagnosis of Duchenne dystrophy. For more detailed discussion of these diseases, the reader should refer to the recent literature on genetic and neuromuscular diseases.[25,41,42,44]

Emery-Dreifuss muscular dystrophy is a rare X-linked[8,30] and occasionally, autosomal dominantly transmitted disorder[4,15] that is clinically and genetically distinct from but occasionally confused with Becker dystrophy. It can have severe cardiac complications that require urgent treatment. These cardiac symptoms may prompt medical evaluation before the muscle weakness or contractures. For this reason, it has been included in Tables 37-1 and 37-2. For more detailed discussion of this disease, the reader should consult recent reviews.[15,30]

Tables 37-3 and 37-4 outline the recently discovered forms of autosomal dominant[9] and autosomal recessive[7,9,11,36] forms of limb girdle muscular dystrophy (LGMD). These disorders have been included in this chapter

*References 2, 5, 18, 19, 23, 26.

to emphasize the number of different primary muscle diseases that can present in childhood or in the teens and on superficial evaluation resemble Duchenne dystrophy. Unlike Duchenne dystrophy, most of the forms of LGMD are more slowly progressive. It would be inappropriate to give the same prognosis for one of these disorders that one would give for Duchenne dystrophy. The autosomal dominant forms (LGMD 1A through LGMD 1D)[9] are especially uncommon, as are certain of the autosomal recessive forms of LGMD 2A and LGMD 2B.[7,9,11,36] However, the sarcoglyconopathies (LGMD 2C through 2F) probably account for more than 10% of patients who have a limb-girdle pattern of muscle weakness who have normal staining for dystrophin on their muscle biopsy.[11] The sarcoglycans are glycoproteins associated with dystrophin and other muscle membrane-associated proteins. Their relationship to specific forms of limb girdle muscular dystrophy and to the different theories about the pathomechanism of these different disorders is discussed in recent reviews.[7,9,11,36] The various forms of LGMD are important to consider in referring children to the neurologist. Knowledge that there are a variety of uncommon muscular dystrophies with different prognoses will help parents and patients understand that different tests may be necessary to establish a specific diagnosis, a prognosis, and a plan of treatment.

REFERENCES

1. Ahn AH, Kunkel LM: The structural and functional diversity of dystrophin, *Nat Genet* 3:283, 1993.
2. Ashizawa T, Anvret M, Baiget M: Characteristics of intergenerational contractions of the CTG repeat in myotonic dystrophy, *Am J Hum Genet* 54:414, 1994.
3. Bodensteiner JB: Congenital myopathies, *Muscle Nerve* 17:131, 1994.
4. Bonne G, et al: Mutations in the gene encoding lamin A/C cause of autosomal dominant Emery-Dreifuss muscular dystrophy, *Nat Genet* 21: 285, 1999.
5. Brook JD, et al: Molecular basis of myotonic dystrophy: expansion of a trinucleotide (CTG) repeat at the 3′ end of a transcript encoding a protein kinase family member, *Cell* 68:799, 1992.
6. Brooke MH, et al: Clinical investigation in Duchenne dystrophy. II. Determination of the "power" of therapeutic trials based on the natural history, *Muscle Nerve* 6:91, 1983.
7. Brown RH Jr: Dystrophin-associated proteins and the muscular dystrophies, *Ann Rev Med* 48:457, 1997.
8. Buckley A, Dean J, Mahy I: Cardiac involvement in Emery-Dreifuss muscular dystrophy: a case series, *Heart* 82:105, 1999.
9. Bushby K: Making sense of the limb-girdle muscular dystrophies, *Brain* 122:1403, 1999.
10. Deconinck N, et al: Expression of truncated utrophin leads to major functional improvements in dystrophin-deficient muscles of mice, *Nat Med* 3:1216, 1997.
11. Duggan DJ, et al: Mutations in sarcoglycan genes in patients with myopathy, *N Engl J Med* 336:618, 1997.
12. Engel A, et al: Dystrophinopathies. In Engeland AG, Franzini-Armstrong C, editors: *Myology: basic and clinical*, ed 2, vol 2, New York, 1994, McGraw-Hill.
13. Fanin M, et al: Could utrophin rescue the myocardium of patients with dystrophin gene mutations? *J Mol Cell Cardiol* 31:1501, 1999.
14. Fardeau M, Tome FM: Congenital myopathies. In Engeland AG, Franzini-Armstrong C, editors: *Mycology: basic and clinical*, ed 2, vol 2, New York, 1994, McGraw-Hill.
15. Fatkin D, et al: Missense mutations in the rod domain of the lamin A/C gene as causes of dilated cardiomyopathy and conduction-system disease, *New Engl J Med* 341:1715, 1999.
16. Fenichel GM, et al: A comparison of daily and alternate-day prednisone therapy in the treatment of Duchenne muscular dystrophy, *Arch Neurol* 48:575, 1991.
17. Fenichel GM, et al: Long-term benefit from prednisone therapy in Duchenne muscular dystrophy, *Neurology* 41:1874, 1991.
18. Fu YH, et al: An unstable triplet repeat in a gene related to myotonic muscular dystrophy, *Science* 255:1256, 1992.
19. Fu YH, et al: Varying expression of myotonin-protein kinase mRNA and protein levels in the adult form of myotonic dystrophy, *Science* 72:971, 1993.
20. Griggs RC, Moxley III RT, Mendell JR: Prednisone in Duchenne dystrophy: a randomized, controlled trial defining the time course and dose response, *Arch Neurol* 48:383, 1991.
21. Griggs RC, et al: Duchenne dystrophy: randomized, controlled trial of prednisone (18 months) and azathioprine (12 months), *Neurology* 43: 520, 1993.
22. Harper PS: Myotonic dystrophy as a trinucleotide repeat disorder: a clinical perspective. In Wells RD, Warren ST, editors: *Genetic instabilities and hereditary neurological diseases*, San Diego, 1998, Academic Press.
23. Jansen G, et al: Gonosomal mosaicism in myotonic dystrophy patients: involvement of mitotic events in (CTG)n repeat variation and selection against extreme expansion in sperm, *Am J Hum Genet* 54:575, 1994.
24. Joseph JT, et al: Congenital myotonic dystrophy pathology and somatic mosaicism, *Neurology* 49:1457, 1997.
25. Kondo-Iida E, et al: Novel mutations and genotype-phenotype relationships in 107 families with Fukuyama-type congenital muscular dystrophy (FCMD), *Hum Mol Genet* 8:2303, 1999.
26. Mahadevan M, et al: Myotonic dystrophy mutation: an unstable CTG repeat in the 3′ untranslated region of the gene, *Science* 255:1253, 1992.
27. Martinello F, et al: Clinical and neuroimaging study of central nervous system in congenital myotonic dystrophy, *J Neurol* 246:186, 1999.
28. Martorell L, et al: Somatic instability of the myotonic dystrophy (CTG)n repeat during human fetal development, *Hum Mol Genet* 6:877, 1997.
29. Mendell JR, et al: Randomized, double-blind six-month trial of prednisone in Duchenne's muscular dystrophy, *N Engl J Med* 320:1592, 1989.
30. Morris G, Manilal S: Heart to heart: from nuclear proteins to Emery-Dreifuss muscular dystrophy, *Hum Mol Genet* 8:1847, 1999.
31. Moxley III RT: Myotonic dystrophy. In Vinken PJ, et al, editors: *Handbook of clinical neurology*, New York, 1992, Elsevier Science.
32. Muntoni F, et al: Deletions in the 5′ region of dystrophin and resulting phenotypes, *J Med Genet* 31:843, 1994.
33. Nobile C, et al: Exon-intron organization of the human dystrophin gene, *Genomics* 45:421, 1997.
34. Normand M, et al: Management of respiratory problems in neuromuscular disease. In Lane RJM, editor: *Handbook of muscle disease*, New York, 1996, Marcel Dekker.
35. Orrell RW, et al: Definitive molecular diagnosis of FSH dystrophy, *Neurology* 52:1, 1999.
36. Ozawa E, et al: From dystrophinopathy to sarcogylcanopathy: evolution of a concept of muscular dystrophy, *Muscle Nerve* 21:421, 1998.
37. Redman JB, et al: Relationship between parental trinucleotide CTG repeat length and severity of myotonic dystrophy in offspring, *JAMA* 269:1960, 1993.
38. Rifai Z, Welle S, Moxley III RT: Effect of prednisone on protein metabolism in Duchenne dystrophy, *Am J Physiol* 268:67, 1995.
39. Shelbourne P, et al: Direct diagnosis of myotonic dystrophy with a disease-specific DNA marker, *N Engl J Med* 328:471, 1993.
40. Tawil R, Griggs RC: FSH dystrophy. In Karpati G, Griggs RC, Hilton-Jones D, editors: *Disorders of voluntary muscle*, ed 7, Cambridge, UK, Cambridge University Press (in press).
41. Tome F: The saga of congenital muscular dystrophy, *Neuropediatrics* 30:55, 1999.
42. Voit T, et al: Preserved merosin M-chain (or laminin-alpha 2) expression in skeletal muscle distinguishes Walker-Warburg syndrome from Fukuyama muscular dystrophy and merosin-deficient congenital muscular dystrophy, *Neuropediatrics* 26:148, 1995.
43. Voskova-Goldman A, et al: DMD-specific FISH probes are diagnostically useful in the detection of female carriers of DMD gene deletions, *Neurology* 48:1633, 1997.
44. Yoshioka M, Kuroki S: Clinical spectrum and genetic studies of Fukuyama congenital muscular dystrophy, *Am J Med Genet* 53:245, 1994.

38 Cerebral Palsy

Gregory S. Liptak

The cerebral palsies are a heterogeneous group of conditions classified according to the type and distribution of motor abnormality. They are defined as a group of *disorders of movement and posture caused by a nonprogressive lesion of the developing brain.*[3] Although the cerebral palsies are neither distinct neuropathological nor etiological conditions, their clinical classification is important because it determines the child's functional status, treatment, and prognosis.[26,37]

EPIDEMIOLOGY

The incidence of cerebral palsy is about 2 to 2.5 cases per 1000 live births in developed countries. Although some variation has been described, the incidence has generally remained stable over the past 20 years.[23,31,35,44] In a survey of 156,000 newborn infants, 28% of the 192 cases of cerebral palsy that occurred among them occurred in children born weighing less than 1500 g; 20% occurred in children born weighing between 1500 and 2500 g. Children born weighing less than 1000 g constituted 0.2% of the survivors but accounted for 8% of the children who had cerebral palsy.[12]

Cerebral palsy has a major impact on the lives of children. For example, in a national survey, 59% of children who had cerebral palsy attended a special school, compared with 0.5% of those who did not have cerebral palsy. Use of health care services is much higher, too; in the 12 months before the survey, children who had cerebral palsy (compared with those who did not) had 16 visits to a physician (versus 3), 29 hospital episodes per 100 children (versus 4), and 108 hospital days per 100 children (versus 20).[5]

ETIOLOGY AND PREDICTION

Since Little's description[28] in 1862 of the influence of prematurity and abnormal birth on the development of spasticity and developmental delay, health care providers have attributed the cause of cerebral palsy to these perinatal events. However, in 1897 Freud[20] argued that it was impossible to identify the timing or nature of the events that caused cerebral palsy and that many factors operating in the prenatal, perinatal, and postnatal periods could damage the infant's brain.

A definite cause cannot be identified for most cases of cerebral palsy, and when a cause can be identified, it usually is of prenatal origin.[34] Intrapartum events play a limited role[48] and often are influenced by a preexisting abnormality.[5,7,32] Neither sophisticated fetal monitoring nor a higher rate of cesarean sections has reduced the occurrence of cerebral palsy.[33] Isolated risk factors such as fetal bradycardia, neonatal acidosis, intraventricular hemorrhage in the absence of periventricular leukomalacia, and low Apgar scores taken in isolation are poor predictors of cerebral palsy, especially in full-term infants. However, a low birth weight (2000 g or less), periventricular leukomalacia (necrosis of white matter near the lateral ventricles), hydrocephalus, congenital malformations, and newborn encephalopathy (recurrent seizures, hypotonia, coma) all are associated with cerebral palsy.[25]

In about 10% of children who have cerebral palsy, the etiology of the condition is thought to be postneonatal (after 28 days).[6] The most common of these causes are infections (e.g., meningitis and encephalitis), asphyxia, and accidental injury. In some cases cerebral palsy may be prevented by devising strategies to reduce the occurrence of injuries during childhood and by measures to minimize periventricular leukomalacia in premature infants, such as improving circulation and countering the effects of excitatory neurotransmitters.

CLASSIFICATION AND DIAGNOSIS

Cerebral palsies may be classified according to the type and distribution of motor abnormality (Box 38-1). This classification system can be simplified into three categories: spastic (involving the pyramidal tracts), athetoid (involving the extrapyramidal tracts), and mixed (involving both). Spasticity is defined as velocity-dependent passive resistance of muscle to stretch. It is associated with neurological signs including hyperreflexia, clonus, extensor plantar response, cocontractures, abnormal postural control, and weakness. These abnormalities impair normal movements, such as gait and the manipulation of objects, in complex ways. Diplegia is defined as greater involvement of the legs than the arms, quadriplegia as an equal involvement of all four limbs, hemiplegia as involvement of one side of the body, and double hemiplegia as greater involvement of the arms than the legs. Dyskinesia includes the involuntary movements of athetosis and chorea, which are most pronounced when the child initiates a movement, as well as dystonia. Dysarthria commonly occurs with dyskinesia. Ataxia involves incoordination of movement and impaired balance and may be associated with an intention tremor. Children who have mild ataxia appear to have normal coordination but are apraxic—that is, they are unable to initiate acts such as hopping, skipping, or buttoning. Because the fibers in the corticospinal tract that control the legs

BOX 38-1

CLASSIFICATION OF CEREBRAL PALSY

Spastic
- Diplegic
- Quadriplegic
- Hemiplegic
- Double hemiplegic

Athetoid
- Dyskinetic
  - Hyperkinetic
  - Dystonic
- Ataxic

Mixed

are closest to the ventricles, mild periventricular leukomalacia or hydrocephalus is most likely to lead to spastic diplegia. Children who have spastic quadriplegia generally have more extensive lesions, and they are more likely to be mentally retarded (64% have an IQ below 50) and have seizures (56%) than are children who have other kinds of cerebral palsy.[17] Children who have spastic quadriplegia also are more likely to have feeding difficulties, severe joint contractures, and scoliosis.

Each form of cerebral palsy can be caused by a multitude of conditions, and a single etiological factor (e.g., meningitis) can lead to different forms of cerebral palsy. Therefore, a direct link between the type of cerebral palsy and its etiology cannot be established without using diagnostic evaluations such as ultrasonography or magnetic resonance imaging (MRI).

Early and Differential Diagnosis

Although the brain lesion in cerebral palsy is not progressive, the clinical signs change, especially in the first several years of life. Abnormal patterns emerge as the damaged nervous system matures. For example, the child who is destined to have spastic quadriplegia often will be hypotonic in early infancy. At 6 months of age, as his tone increases, he may develop adduction of the thumb (palmar thumb) followed in a month or two by scissoring of the legs when he is held upright. By 9 months of age, he may have diffuse spasticity and hyperactive deep tendon reflexes. Dyskinetic patterns generally are not obvious until about 18 months of age. Ataxia, as opposed to the incoordination and motor delay of mental retardation, may not be apparent until even later. In a study of 1726 children from 5 urban school districts, the mean age at which cerebral palsy was diagnosed was 10 months.[36]

Early diagnosis of cerebral palsy is aided by a history of an abnormal pregnancy, labor, delivery, or neonatal period or by the occurrence of a serious acute illness and trauma. The diagnosis is further aided by evaluation of the child's primitive reflexes (e.g., the asymmetrical tonic neck response), postural responses (righting the head when tilted to the side), muscle tone, motor milestones, and neurobehavioral responsiveness.[4] Early signs that suggest cerebral palsy include difficulty feeding because of abnormal oral-motor patterns (tongue thrusting, tonic bite, oral hypersensitivity), irritability, and delayed milestones such as head control. Exaggerated or persistent infantile reflexes such as the asymmetrical tonic neck response, hyperreflexia, and asymmetry may be seen. Delayed milestones, primitive or exaggerated reflexes, abnormal muscle tone, abnormal posture, and an abnormal neurological examination suggest the diagnosis of cerebral palsy.

A diagnosis of cerebral palsy implies that no active disease is present and that the disorder is in the brain. The differential diagnosis includes neurodegenerative disorders, inborn errors of metabolism, developmental or traumatic lesions of the spinal cord, severe neuromuscular disease, movement disorders, spinocerebellar degeneration, neoplasms, hydrocephalus, and subdural hematoma. Repeated examination is necessary to rule out a degenerative condition. Recurring subclinical seizures or adverse reactions to anticonvulsants may worsen the clinical condition of children who have cerebral palsy. Hypotonia in association with weak muscles and depressed tendon reflexes suggests a neuromuscular disease. Extrapyramidal signs in early infancy or marked worsening during periods of illness also makes the diagnosis of cerebral palsy suspect. If a child diagnosed as having dyskinetic cerebral palsy has symptoms that worsen significantly as the day progresses, Dopa-responsive dystonia should be considered.[24] This rare but treatable form of dystonia may begin with toe-walking and difficulties with gait, and it responds dramatically to administration of levodopa. There usually is no history of a preexisting condition that would be consistent with cerebral palsy. Other rare inborn errors of metabolism such as arginase deficiency and glutaric aciduria may mimic cerebral palsy. However, these conditions cause progressive deterioration, whereas cerebral palsy does not. If a child has a parent who has "cerebral palsy" and has late-onset spastic diplegia with no preceding history of prenatal or neonatal problems, then hereditary spastic diplegia may be the etiology.[19]

ASSOCIATED DISORDERS

Table 38-1 lists disabilities and impairments associated with cerebral palsy. All types of language abnormality may be encountered, from aphasia to poor articulation. Abnormal speech may be related to hearing, intelligence, experience, language development, the integration of motor mechanisms of the oropharynx, and coordination of breathing patterns. Nearly 75% of individuals who have cerebral palsy are cognitively impaired. About 60% are mentally retarded (mildly so in about one third of cases and moderately or worse in another third). In the remainder, who function in the normal range, specific learning disabilities such as visual-spatial impairment are common. Impaired mobility also is common and may result from spasticity with or without joint contractures and scoliosis. Self-care and hygiene may be impaired by gross motor and fine motor abnormalities and problems such as drooling. Defects in gastrointestinal functioning and growth are common. In general, physical growth is inhibited.[43] Many of these patients fail to thrive, especially those who have dyskinesia or spastic quadriplegia. Feeding difficulties caused by oropharyngeal incoordination and recurrent vomiting occur and may be associated with aspiration and

Table 38-1 Disabilities and Impairments Associated with Cerebral Palsy in Children and Possible Interventions

Disability/Impairment	Possible Intervention	Possible Consultation
Impaired communication	Augmentative communication aids	Speech therapist, audiologist
Impaired cognition	Early intervention, special education program	Education specialist, psychologist, school advocate
Impaired mobility	Orthoses (braces), walker, wheeled mobility	Orthopedist, orthotist, physical therapist, specialty program, gait laboratory
Spasticity	Medications, selective dorsal rhizotomy, intrathecal baclofen, botulinum toxin injection	Orthopedist, neurodevelopmental specialist, physiatrist, neurologist
Joint contractures	Range of motion, orthoses, surgery	Physical therapist, orthopedist, orthotist
Scoliosis	Orthoses, surgery	Orthopedist, orthotist
Impaired self-care and hygiene	Assistive technological devices, home modifications, training	Occupational therapist, rehabilitation engineer
Drooling	Scopolamine patch, surgery	Otolaryngologist
Sexual functioning	Education, adaptive devices	Gynecologist, urologist, psychologist
Impaired nutrition/feeding	Education, monitoring, medical evaluation, medication, surgery	Nutritionist/dietitian, gastroenterologist, speech therapist, occupational therapist
Dental caries, malocclusion	Repair of caries, orthidonture	Dentist, pedodontist, orthodontist
Seizures	Medication, surgery	Neurologist
Impaired vision or hearing	Assistive device, surgery	Ophthalmologist, otolaryngologist
Impaired access to care	Financial counseling, care coordination, transportation	Financial counselor, care coordinator, specialty program
Adverse effects on family	Parent support group, counseling, support	Social worker, psychologist, specialty program, care coordinator
Impaired transition to adulthood	Counseling, adult-oriented health care, care coordination, transportation, recreation, vocational services	Internist, family physician, care coordinator, vocational specialist, independent living specialist, attorney, psychologist

gastroesophageal reflux. Dental disease (malocclusion and caries) is common. Seizures are common, as are impaired vision and hearing. Roughly 40% of these children develop seizures, which most often have their onset in the first 2 years of life. Oculomotor anomalies include strabismus, refractive error, and nystagmus. Behavioral problems are five to eight times more likely to occur in children who have cerebral palsy than in their uninvolved peers.[29]

Sociocultural risk factors have a profound effect on development and interact with biological risk factors. Perinatal and other biological risk factors that can lead to intellectual impairment do not have the same detrimental consequences for middle- or upper-class children as they do for poor children.

Children who have cerebral palsy have much in common with children who have other chronic conditions. Cerebral palsy is a lifelong disorder with no cure. The treatments used, such as bracing, often are difficult and sometimes embarrassing. Children who have cerebral palsy often appear different from their peers and have restricted physical development, which makes them unable to engage in peer-related activities. Many children who have cerebral palsy experience pain and physical discomfort as well as psychological distress. Access to care may be a problem. These children visit numerous health care professionals and require services from others such as those in the educational and social services fields. Characteristically, communication is poor within the health field and among professionals and agencies in different arenas. Policies affecting chronically ill children often are erratic. For example, the rules in one county for obtaining money from the state's program for children with physical disabilities may be very different from those in another county.

For the family, cerebral palsy means the loss of the ideal child—the loss of a dream. This may lead to mourning characterized by denial, anger, guilt, sadness, and depression. In addition, care of a child who has cerebral palsy may be extraordinarily expensive. The burden of daily care falls on the family, and families may feel isolated because of the lack of understanding of cerebral palsy in the community. Siblings may be neglected and have behavioral and other problems. Facilities such as play areas and public facilities (transportation, libraries) often are inaccessible to wheelchair users. Schools may be inaccessible to children who have special mobility needs or may be unable to provide the "adapted" facilities that they require. Because cerebral palsy is considered a *pediatric problem,* transition to adulthood is difficult because physicians who care for adults, social service agencies, and other health care personnel are unfamiliar with the care of adults who have cerebral palsy.

INVESTIGATION

Neuroimaging techniques such as ultrasonography, computed tomography (CT), and magnetic resonance imaging (MRI) have increased our understanding of the structural abnormalities associated with cerebral palsy and may help clarify the timing of a lesion.[45,46] Neuroimaging may demonstrate periventricular leukomalacia, postischemic necrosis, cerebral dysgenesis, hydrocephalus, porencephaly, tumor, prenatal ischemic injury, or leukodystrophy. The information gained with brain imaging, although usually not helpful in directing therapy, can be useful to the physician in explaining (or demonstrating) the specific cause of a child's cerebral palsy to the parents. The electroencephalogram (EEG) is an important part of the diagnosis and management of associated seizures; continuous EEG monitoring with videography may help differentiate seizures from other movement disorders. The presence of dysmorphic features may trigger a search for a chromosomal abnormality. However, an increase in minor congenital anomalies is common in cerebral palsy in the absence of any apparent genetic cause for them. Evaluation of complications such as altered gait and feeding disorders may require special diagnostic studies, such as gait analysis and videofluoroscopic swallowing studies.

INTERVENTION

Pathophysiological abnormalities of the brain such as leukomalacia lead to impairments such as spasticity. Spasticity then leads to alterations in functioning, for example, shortened stride length, which leads to disabilities, (e.g., a slow gait). The disabilities may lead to adverse social consequences, or handicaps, (e.g., inability to use public transportation).[9,22] Adults who have cerebral palsy have identified communication skills, self-care activities, and mobility as the three most important functional outcomes of care. The goals of intervention are to prevent adverse functional outcomes, disabilities, and handicaps. Thus, although spasticity occurs, muscle relaxation or surgery around a joint will not be worthwhile if it does not improve the child's ability to function.

Table 38-1 lists some possible interventions and referrals to address the complications of cerebral palsy. No single professional can fulfill the multiple medical, social, psychological, educational, and therapeutic needs of a child who has cerebral palsy.[15] Comprehensive management requires a multidisciplinary team, such as those found in a specialty program, whose members instruct and support parents to enable them to achieve maximal potential for self-help and care for their child and to understand their child's ability and potential for development. The Individuals With Disabilities Education Act (IDEA) mandates access to early intervention services for infants at risk for handicapping conditions. These services include special education; physical, occupational, and speech therapies; adaptive equipment; training for mobility and living skills; and communication. The therapies may not change the basic disorder significantly.[38] However, the therapists may help the families by teaching them how to position and handle their child, by providing more opportunity for play and learning, and by facilitating feeding and the parent/child relationship. Whether or not formal early intervention services are provided, the family should have early professional support to help them cope with the crisis of diagnosis.[16]

The care provided should be integrated. For example, children whose legs are spastic often have dorsiflexion at the ankle, flexion at the knee, and flexion and adduction of the hip. Repair of only one or two of these problems may leave the child unimproved or worse off—all three problems must be addressed. Gait analysis using videography, EMG, and sensors has improved the orthopedic care given to these children. After orthopedic surgery, therapy should be started to maximize range of motion and skills.

Medications are used to reduce spasticity (e.g., diazepam, oral baclofen, tizanidine, and dantrolene), but all have potential adverse effects. No controlled studies have documented improvement in functioning from these medications. Selective dorsal rhizotomy and intrathecal baclofen can reduce spasticity and increase range of motion, and some patients' sitting and gait may improve functionally.[1,21,30,39] Intramuscular botulinum toxin has been used in children who have functional spasticity to reduce spasticity in individual limbs.[10,11,41] Although reduction in spasticity can be accomplished with these treatments, they cannot improve selective motor control, difficulties with balance, and weakness. Recent interventions to strengthen muscles using strength training have shown promise in improving functioning.[13] Various casting and splinting techniques that may maintain muscle length and inhibit increased tone may be helpful. In many cases, orthopedic procedures such as tenotomies, tendon releases, and transfers are necessary to address the soft tissue and bony problems that occur.

Drooling has been managed with scopolamine, which is available as a transdermal patch and as a tablet,[27] glycopyrrolate,[2] and surgery of the salivary glands.[8] Because children who have cerebral palsy are at increased risk for nutrition and feeding problems, careful monitoring of their physical growth is critical. Reliable measures of height or length in children who have cerebral palsy often are impossible to obtain because of the scoliosis, fixed joint contractures, involuntary muscle spasms, and poor cooperation stemming from cognitive deficits. Tibial length has been used as a proxy for height. Evaluation of the child whose growth is impaired includes evaluation of dietary intake for calories and content, and evaluation for gastroesophageal reflux (using pH probe, endoscopy with biopsy, or barium swallow or radionuclide gastric emptying study). A clinical feeding evaluation includes assessment of the child's seating and posture during "feeds" as well as assessment of the swallowing mechanism, which can be aided by a videofluoroscopic swallow study using foods of different consistencies.[47] The assistance of feeding specialists is invaluable in this evaluation. Treatment options may include providing special seating devices to maintain the child in an upright, neutral position, or insertion of a gastrostomy tube with or without fundoplication. This usually improves weight gain and general health but may not improve longitudinal growth. The primary care physician should act as an advocate to ensure that a child who has cerebral palsy has access to first-rate care. In addition to the individual child and family, advocacy includes ensuring that the community provides access to services so that disabilities do not become handicaps.

PROGNOSIS

More than 90% of infants who have cerebral palsy survive into adulthood. Those who are so severely affected that they cannot move their extremities or bodies voluntarily are at increased risk for early death.[18,40] Prognostication before the child's second birthday may be difficult, except at the extremes of involvement. In general, the prognosis for functioning is related to the clinical type of cerebral palsy, pace of motor development, evolution of infantile reflexes, intellectual abilities, sensory impairment, and emotional-social adjustment.[42] Patients who sit unsupported by 24 months of age and crawl by 30 months of age are more likely eventually to walk independently.[14] Most of those who first sit between 3 and 4 years of age walk only with aids or braces or have restricted functional ambulation. Retention of obligatory primitive reflexes at 18 months of age makes independent ambulation unlikely. Virtually all children who have hemiplegia learn to walk, as do many who have athetosis or ataxia. Those who walk before age 2 years are more likely to have a normal or borderline IQ. Individual achievement is related to many factors, such as intelligence, physical functioning, ability to communicate, and personality attributes. The availability of training, jobs, sheltered employment, and counseling is a major factor in the adjustment of affected adults. A supportive family and the availability of specialist medical care are other important factors.

Long-term planning and preparation are required to help these patients make the transition from adolescence to adulthood, particularly when a patient has multiple needs. A variety of assistive technologies, such as switches that improve the individual's ability to control the environment, computers, and small electric motors, which may replace some motor activities, are available. Speech synthesizers, symbol charts, or spelling boards can enhance an individual's ability to communicate effectively. Simple environmental enhancements, such as ramps or accessible showers, and assistive devices, such as a pencil holder or mouth-activated switch, can improve the quality of life dramatically for individuals who have cerebral palsy. The 1997 amendments to IDEA require that children who have disabilities be assessed for the utility of assistive devices and be given the support needed to utilize them effectively. Gaining access to these services requires coordination of care, knowledge of the resources available in the community, referral to experts, and financial assets. The physician who cares for patients who have cerebral palsy is obliged to ensure that these services are available both to the patient and the family.

When to Refer

In the United States, all infants who have cerebral palsy who are from birth to 3 years of age should be referred to an early intervention program.

All children who have moderate or severe cerebral palsy should be referred to an interdisciplinary clinic, if one exists. If not, they should be referred to an orthopedist, physical therapist, and someone (developmental pediatrician, neurologist, pediatric rehabilitation specialist) who can manage spasticity. Children who have cerebral palsy and seizures should be referred to a neurologist.

Use of Alternative Medicine

A number of therapies such as cranio-sacral massage, Adeli suit for spasticity, and hyperbaric oxygen have been touted as beneficial for the treatment of children who have cerebral palsy. However, none of them has been studied by using rigorous controlled trials and thus should be regarded as experimental. Because many of the conventional therapies are ineffective in treating the symptoms of cerebral palsy and no cure exists, families often turn to alternative therapies, including herbal medications. The primary care provider should inquire about the use of these treatments and be aware of their nature, possible interactions with medications, and potential for harm.

When to Hospitalize

Some children who have cerebral palsy aspirate food or saliva into their lungs; others have inadequate nutrition. Therefore, they are more susceptible to acute illnesses such as pneumonia and are likely to become more ill with these illnesses. They should be hospitalized if they are severely ill or cannot be managed at home. They should be hospitalized for most major surgeries too, such as complex orthopedic procedures.

REFERENCES

1. Albright AL, Cervi A, Singletary J: Intrathecal baclofen for spasticity in cerebral palsy, *JAMA* 265:1418, 1991.
2. Bachrach SJ, Walter RS, Trzcinski K: Use of glycopyrrolate and other anticholinergic medications for sialorrhea in children with cerebral palsy, *Clin Pediatr* (Phila) 37:485, 1997.
3. Blair E, Stanley FJ: Issues in the classification and epidemiology of cerebral palsy, *Ment Retard Devel Disabil Res Rev* 3:184, 1997.
4. Blasco PA: Primitive reflexes: their contribution to the early detection of cerebral palsy, *Clin Pediatr* (Phila) 33:388, 1994.
5. Boyle CA, Decoufle P, Yeargin-Allsopp M: Prevalence and health impact of developmental disabilities in US children, *Pediatrics* 93:399, 1994.
6. Boyle CA, et al: Prevalence of selected developmental disabilities in children 3-10 years of age: the Metropolitan Atlanta Developmental Disabilities Surveillance Program, 1991, *MMWR CDC Surveill Summ* 45:1, 1996.
7. Brann AW: Factors during neonatal life that influence brain disorder. In Freeman JM, editor: *Prenatal and perinatal factors associated with brain disorders,* NIH Pub No 85-1149, Washington, DC, 1985, US Government Printing Office.
8. Burton MJ: The surgical management of drooling, *Dev Med Child Neurol* 33:1110, 1991.
9. Butler C, et al: Evaluating research in developmental disabilities: a conceptual framework for reviewing treatment outcomes, *Dev Med Child Neurol* 41:55, 1999.
10. Calderon-Gonzalez R, et al: Botulinum toxin A in management of cerebral palsy, *Pediatr Neurol* 10:284, 1994.
11. Corry IS, et al: Botulinum toxin A in the hemiplegic upper limb: a double-blind trial, *Dev Med Child Neurol* 39:185, 1997.
12. Cummins SK, et al: Cerebral palsy in four northern California counties, births 1983 through 1985, *J Pediatr* 123:230, 1993.

13. Damiano DL, Abel MF: Functional outcomes of strength training in spastic cerebral palsy, *Arch Phys Med Rehabil* 79:119, 1998.
14. daPaz AC Jr, Burnett S, Bragga LW: Walking prognosis in cerebral palsy: a 22-year retrospective analysis, *Dev Med Child Neurol* 36:130, 1994.
15. Davis DW: Review of cerebral palsy. Part II: Identification and intervention, *Neonatal Netw* 16:19, 1997.
16. Diamond M: Rehabilitation strategies for the child with cerebral palsy, *Pediatr Ann* 15:230, 1986.
17. Edebol-Tysk K: Epidemiology of spastic tetraplegic cerebral palsy in Sweden. I. Impairment and disabilities, *Neuropediatrics* 20:41, 1989.
18. Eyman RK, et al: Survival of profoundly disabled people with severe mental retardation, *Am J Dis Child* 147:329, 1993.
19. Fink JK: Advances in hereditary spastic paraplegia, *Curr Opin Neurol* 10:313, 1997.
20. Freud S: *Infantile cerebral paralysis* (1897) (Translated by Russin LA), Coral Gables, Fla, 1968, University of Miami Press.
21. Gerszten PC, Albright AL, Barry MJ: Effect on ambulation of continuous intrathecal baclofen infusion, *Pediatr Neurosurg* 27:40.
22. Goldberg MJ: Measuring outcomes in cerebral palsy, *J Pediatr Orthop* 11:682, 1991.
23. Hagbery B, et al: The changing panorama of cerebral palsy in Sweden, *Acta Paediatr Scand* 78:283, 1989.
24. Iivanainen M, Kaakkola S: Dopa-responsive dystonia of childhood, *Dev Med Child Neurol* 35:362, 1993.
25. Kuban KC, Leviton MD: Cerebral palsy, *N Engl J Med* 330:188, 1994.
26. Levine MS: Cerebral palsy in children over 1 year: standard criteria, *Arch Phys Med Rehabil* 61:385, 1980.
27. Lewis DW, et al: Transdermal scopolamine for reduction of drooling in developmentally delayed children, *Dev Med Child Neurol* 36:484, 1994.
28. Little WJ: On the influence of abnormal parturition, difficult labour, premature birth, and asphyxia neonatorum on the mental and physical conditions of the child, especially in relation to deformities, *Transactions of the Obstetrical Society of London* 3:293, 1862.
29. McDermott S, et al: A population-based analysis of behavior problems in children with cerebral palsy, *J Pediatr Psychol* 21:447, 1996.
30. McLaughlin JF, et al: Selective dorsal rhizotomy: efficacy and safety in an investigator-masked randomized clinical trial, *Dev Med Child Neurol* 40:220, 1998.
31. Meberg A, Broch H: A changing pattern of cerebral palsy: declining trend for incidence of cerebral palsy in the 20-year period 1970-89, *J Perinat Med* 23:395, 1995.
32. Miller G: Minor congenital anomalies and ataxic cerebral palsy, *Arch Dis Child* 64:557, 1989.
33. Nelson KB: The neurologically impaired child and alleged malpractice at birth, *Neurol Clin* 17:283, 1999.
34. Nelson KB, Ellenberg JH: Antecedents of cerebral palsy: multivariate analysis of risk, *N Engl J Med* 315:81, 1986.
35. O'Shea TM, et al: Trends in mortality and cerebral palsy in a geographically based cohort of very low birth weight neonates born between 1982 to 1994, *Pediatrics* 101:642, 1998.
36. Palfrey JS, Singer JD, Walker DK: Early identification of children's special needs: a study in five metropolitan communities, *J Pediatr* 111: 651, 1987.
37. Palisano R, et al: Development and reliability of a system to classify gross motor function in children with cerebral palsy, *Dev Med Child Neurol* 39:214, 1997.
38. Palmer F: Evaluation of developmental therapies in cerebral palsy, *Ment Retard Develop Rev* 3:145, 1997.
39. Peacock WJ, Staudt LA: Spasticity in cerebral palsy and selective posterior rhizotomy procedure, *J Child Neurol* 5:179, 1990.
40. Plioplys AV, et al: Survival rates among children with severe neurologic disabilities, *South Med J* 91:161, 1998.
41. Russman BS, Tilton A, Gormley ME Jr: Cerebral palsy: a rational approach to a treatment protocol, and the role of botulinum toxin in treatment, *Muscle Nerve Suppl* 6:S181, 1997.
42. Sala DA, Grant AD: Prognosis for ambulation in cerebral palsy, *Dev Med Child Neurol* 37:1020, 1995.
43. Samson-Fang L, Stevenson RD: Linear growth velocity in children with cerebral palsy, *Dev Med Child Neurol* 40:689, 1998.
44. Stanley FJ, Watson L: The cerebral palsies in Western Australia: trends, 1968 to 1981, *Am J Obstet Gynecol* 158:89, 1988.
45. Sugimoto T, et al: When do brain abnormalities in cerebral palsy occur? An MRI study, *Dev Med Child Neurol* 37:285, 1995.
46. Volpe JJ: Value of MR in definition of the neuropathology of cerebral palsy in vivo, *AJNR* 13:79, 1992.
47. Wright RE, Wright FR, Carson CA: Videofluoroscopic assessment in children with severe cerebral palsy presenting with dysphagia, *Pediatr Radiol* 26:720, 1996.
48. Yudkin PL, et al: Assessing the contribution of birth asphyxia to cerebral palsy in term singletons, *Paediatr Perinat Epidemiol* 9:156, 1995.

39 The Chronically Ill and Disabled Child in School

Michael L. Weitzman • Nienke P. Dosa • Gregory S. Liptak

Nearly one third of children in the United States have a chronic physical condition, and approximately 5% have limitations in age-appropriate activities as a result of chronic illness or disability.[14] Although these children have the same basic educational and developmental needs as their healthy peers, a significant minority have a range of problems that may interfere with their school performance or require special medical services in school. Collaborative efforts among school personnel, health professionals, and families enhance the health, education, and development of such children and should be the basis for addressing their needs in school.

In the past, children who have chronic conditions often were isolated from healthy children in schools or were taught at home, thus being deprived of crucial social contacts and a broad educational experience. Several laws now ensure that all children have access to education in the least restrictive environment. Public Law 94-142, the Education For All Children Act of 1975, ensures a free and appropriate public education for children who have disabilities. The law was amended in 1990 by Public Law 101-476 and now is known as the Individuals with Disabilities Education Act (IDEA). The Education of the Handicapped Act Amendment, passed in 1986, provides early intervention services from birth to 2 years, 11 months of age, if children have an established disability, developmental delay, biological risks such as low birth weight and/or prematurity, or environmental risks such as having a teen mother or parent abusing a substance. Under these laws, children and parents are entitled to therapeutic, "related" services such as occupational, physical, vision, and hearing therapy; family support; social services; mental health services; educational intervention; and case management services, even if the child is not receiving special education. Children identified as disabled are required to have a written service plan: an Individual Family Service Plan (IFSP) for children birth through 2 years of age or an Individual Education Plan (IEP) for children ages 3 through 21 years. Some states now also require an Individualized Transition Plan (ITP) for adolescents to address vocational, independent living, and insurance issues by age 15. All such plans must be reviewed annually. Involvement in formulating them is an opportunity for the pediatrician to coordinate a child's educational program with a medical treatment plan and to help families and children review beneficial services to which they are entitled. Purvis[16] presents an excellent overview of relevant public laws.

PROBLEMS OF CHILDREN WHO HAVE CHRONIC HEALTH CONDITIONS IN SCHOOL

School provides a child with academic skills and multiple experiences critical to emotional and social development. The school-related problems and concerns that all children have can be exacerbated for a child who has a chronic health condition or disability. The child's condition may require frequent and, occasionally, long absences; illness and medications may affect cognitive functioning; and physical limitations may restrict participation in school activities. These obstacles, when combined with inappropriate expectations of teachers and parents and altered interactions with peers, can provide formidable impediments to academic achievement, psychosocial development, and vocational placement.

Medical Issues

The primary school-related goal for the pediatrician who cares for children who have chronic conditions is to ensure a safe environment. Specific issues such as transportation, special equipment and backup, and emergency plans need to be identified. Additional issues, such as notification of the parents if the child's health status changes in school, responsibility for monitoring the child's health in school, and the role of the physician need to be determined. For children who have severe or complex conditions, especially those who are dependent on technology (see Chapter 35, Children Assisted by Medical Technology), a formal process of entry into school should be followed, including early notification of the school and discussion with school administrators of the condition and needs.[15] The physician helps develop and approve a formal health care plan, created in collaboration with the family and the child, school administration, and other health care personnel. The physician also can make recommendations regarding the program, placement, and staffing and can participate in the training of school personnel. Excellent guides for the training of school personnel who care for children who have chronic conditions are available.[11] Box 39-1 lists the components of an emergency plan; Box 39-2 lists specific guidelines for a child who has a chronic condition in school.

School Achievement

Although the majority of children who have chronic health conditions do not have academic difficulties, as a group they are about 1.5 times as likely to repeat a grade and 2.5 times

BOX 39-1

COMPONENTS OF AN EMERGENCY PLAN FOR A CHILD WHO HAS A CHRONIC CONDITION IN SCHOOL

1. Names, addresses, and telephone numbers of family and caretakers
2. Emergency phone numbers
   Ambulance
   Home care company
   Utility companies
   Hospital
   Emergency department
   Primary care physician
   Specialists
3. Child-specific emergency plan
4. Other school personnel to contact

BOX 39-2

COMPONENTS OF CHILD-SPECIFIC GUIDELINES

1. Important personnel
2. Background information:
   Conditions
   Medical history
   Special health care needs
   Baseline status
   Medications
   Diet
   Technological aids
   Transportation needs
3. Procedures required
4. Equipment
5. Child-specific techniques
6. Special considerations and precautions (e.g., latex allergy)
7. List of possible problems—observation, reason, action
8. Daily log

as likely to receive special education compared with healthy children.[12] This risk may be present in the earliest school years, as evidenced by children who have these conditions being significantly more likely than their healthy peers to repeat kindergarten or first grade.[10] The transition from home to kindergarten and from high school to independent living can be particularly stressful for such children and their families. Pediatricians can help such families by providing applicable anticipatory guidance at times of transition.

In some cases, school difficulties are due to direct effects on neurocognition or to visual or auditory impairments. Medical treatment, such as intrathecal chemotherapy and cranial irradiation, and certain medications, such as steroids, may impair cognitive functioning. For the majority of children who have chronic health conditions, however, these are not significant concerns. Many face academic adversity because of the social and psychological consequences of their condition. "Chains of adversity"[17] can occur when the individual's physical impairments initiate a sequence of disadvantageous outcomes. For example, depression may have a profound negative effect on school functioning. Diminished expectations and lower self-esteem, fatigue, pain, and preoccupation with symptoms that often accompany chronic conditions can be associated with a decreased self-efficacy that may develop into a "learned helplessness" that results in diminished expectations and efforts. This may be complicated by altered parental expectations that involve many aspects of the "vulnerable child syndrome" (see Chapter 75, School Absenteeism and School Refusal). Failure to understand these psychosocial complications can lead to expectations that are unreasonably high or detrimentally low.

Children who have chronic health conditions often have increased school absences, which may lead to significant educational disadvantage (see Chapter 75, School Absenteeism and School Refusal). Homebound teaching often becomes available only when a child misses 2 to 4 weeks of school, yet most children who have chronic conditions have frequent, intermittent absences. Pediatricians can encourage parents and teachers to help children disadvantaged by absences from falling behind in school work and can advocate that a child be made eligible for homebound teaching without the usual waiting period. Homebound teaching has significant limitations, however, and school attendance should be encouraged whenever possible.

Job Achievement and Independent Living

For the majority of children who have chronic health conditions, expectations for participation in the work force as adults should be no different from the expectations for their healthy peers. Yet many fail to participate fully in society once they become young adults. High school graduation rates for those who have disabilities are lower than for those who have no disabilities, and of those who graduate, fewer go on to college. Many of them have specialized vocational needs, and many enter workshops as young adults. Vocational rehabilitation, a federally funded, state-operated program, helps many others. Because most vocational services do not become available until candidates are 18 years old, prevocational skills, including social skills training and independent living planning, should be included in a child's IEP or ITP during the high school years.

Adolescents "transitioning" to adulthood often face loss of insurance coverage and uncertainty regarding independent living arrangements. It is essential that schools encourage attention to future employment and independent living from the earliest stages of the child's academic experience. Parental support is essential; studies have demonstrated the importance of role models for the successful transition to adulthood by adolescents who have chronic conditions.[8,9,11,13]

COLLABORATION OF SCHOOL STAFF AND HEALTH PROFESSIONALS

Collaboration among school-based educational and health personnel, community-based providers, and parents is essential in the management of the chronically ill child in school. It is only through well-coordinated efforts that educators are aware of the child's medical needs and that health providers are aware of the child's learning needs.

Pediatricians provide direct medical care and guidance about medical issues and play a vital role as advocates for their patients who have chronic conditions. The American Academy of Pediatrics has a number of extremely useful statements regarding ways in which pediatricians can assist children who have chronic conditions in the school.[1-7] As the professional who knows the child medically and psychosocially, the pediatrician can encourage academic achievement and socialization and help anticipate major transitions in a child's educational career. Familiarity with a child's individualized service plan is a prerequisite for effective primary care of the child who has a chronic health condition.

Teachers need to know the implications of the child's medical condition for school performance. Lack of such information can result in misunderstanding of the child's medical condition, which can lead to denial of services, misinterpretation of behaviors, or undue restrictions or expectations. With adequate information, teachers can foster not only academic achievement but also social competence. They can implement recommendations and provide ongoing evaluation of a child's progress. Their input is central to the individualized service plan and invaluable to comprehensive medical management.

The *school nurse* usually coordinates health services in the school. In most school districts the nurse is responsible for contacting physicians and parents about a child's medical needs. In the case of children who have chronic health conditions, the nurse's role as liaison among community health providers, educators, and parents often forms the core of collaborative efforts to meet these children's medical needs. The role of the school nurse and models of school health services are discussed in greater detail in Chapter 71, School Health Education. Also, the number of *school-based health care clinics* is growing rapidly, especially in medically underserved areas. Most have a multidisciplinary staff (e.g., a physician, nurse practitioner, social worker, and health educator); their potential contribution to the care of children who have chronic conditions should not be overlooked.

REFERENCES

1. American Association of Pediatrics Committee on Children with Disabilities: Children with health impairments in schools (RE9191), *Pediatrics* 86:636, 1990.
2. American Association of Pediatrics Committee on Children with Disabilities: Pediatrician's role in the development and implementation of an Individual Education Plan (IEP) and /or an Individual Family Service, (IFSP) (RE9242), *Pediatrics* 89:340, 1992.
3. American Association of Pediatrics Committee on Children with Disabilities: The role of the pediatrician in implementing the Americans with Disabilities Act: a subject review (RE9623), *Pediatrics* 98:146, 1996.
4. American Association of Pediatrics Committee on Children with Disabilities: Role of pediatrician in prevocational and vocational education of children and adolescents with developmental disabilities (RE6065), *Pediatrics* 78:529, 1986.
5. American Association of Pediatrics Committee on Children with Disabilities and Committee on Psychosocial Aspects of Child Health and Family Health: Psychosocial risks of chronic health conditions in childhood and adolescence (RE9338), *Pediatrics* 92:876, 1993.
6. American Association of Pediatrics Committee on Injury and Poison Prevention. School Bus Transportation of Children with Special Needs *(RE9401), Pediatrics*, 1994, 93:129-130.
7. American Association of Pediatrics Committee on Sports Medicine: *Sports medicine: health care for young athletes,* ed 2, Evanston, III, 1991, The Academy.
8. Blum RW, et al: Family and peer issues among adolescents with spina bifida and cerebral palsy, *Pediatrics* 88:280, 1991.
9. Burroughs TE, et al: Research on social support in adolescents with IDDM: a critical review, *Diabetes Educ* 23:438, 1997.
10. Byrd RS, Weitzman M: Predictors of early grade retention among children in the United States, *Pediatrics* 93:481, 1994.
11. Cadman D, et al: Children with chronic illness: family and parent demographic characteristics and psychological adjustment, *Pediatrics* 87:884, 1991.
12. Gortmaker S, et al: Chronic conditions, socioeconomic risks, and behavioral problems in children and adolescents, *Pediatrics* 85:267, 1990.
13. La Greca AM: Peer influence in pediatric chronic illness: an update, *J Pediatr Psychol* 17:775, 1992.
14. Newachek PW, et al: An epidemiologic profile of children with special health care needs, *Pediatrics* 102:117, 1998.
15. Palfrey JS, Haynie M, Porter SN: *Children assisted by medical technology in educational settings: guidelines for care,* Boston, 1989, Project School Care, The Children's Hospital.
16. Purvis P: The public laws for education of the disabled: the pediatrician's role, *J Dev Behav Pediatr* 12:327, 1991.
17. Rutter M: Pathways from childhood to adult life, *J Child Psychol Psychiatry* 30:23, 1989.

part four

The Reproductive Process

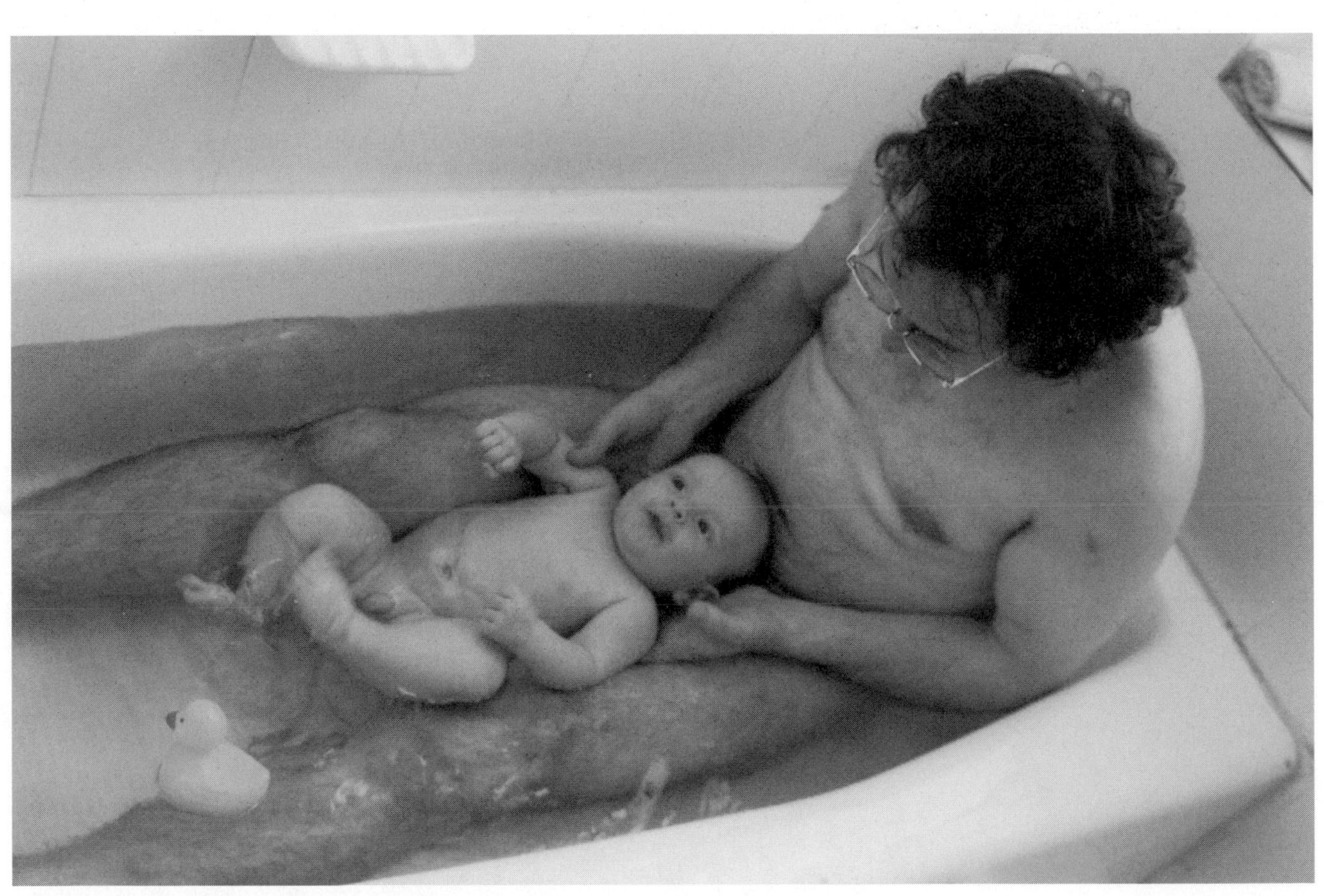

40 Approaches to Genetic Diseases

Marvin E. Miller

Physicians who care for children need to be aware of how genetic diseases and congenital malformations can be diagnosed, which individuals are at increased risk for these disorders, and the various laboratory tests available to help determine the diagnosis. For almost 30 years chromosome analysis has made accurate diagnosis of most chromosomal disorders possible. More recently, application of molecular genetics has resulted in remarkable advances in the diagnosis of common genetic diseases. The alpha- and beta-hemoglobin genes, the cystic fibrosis gene, and the dystrophin gene have been cloned and sequenced, which permits molecular diagnosis of the various hemoglobinopathies, cystic fibrosis, and Duchenne muscular dystrophy. Significant advances also have been made in prenatal diagnosis of congenital malformations and genetic disease through amniocentesis, chorionic villus sampling, maternal serum alpha-fetoprotein screening, and ultrasound. However, despite all these scientific and technological advances, the family history and an understanding of the types of genetic disease and their inheritance patterns still form the foundation for the diagnosis of genetic disease.

TYPES OF GENETIC DISEASE

The human genome consists of 23 pairs of nuclear chromosomes and a much smaller mitochondrial genome. The nuclear chromosomes consist of 22 pairs of autosomes that are the same for males and females and a sex chromosome pair that is different in the two sexes. Females have two X chromosomes (XX); males have one X chromosome and one Y chromosome (XY). There are about 50,000 genetic loci in the human genome. The X chromosome contains several thousand loci and thus is similar to the autosomal chromosomes. The Y chromosome, however, contains only one or perhaps only a few genetic loci that determine male gonadal differentiation.

The 24 different nuclear chromosomes (22 autosomes, X, and Y) can be readily distinguished from each other by their size, centromere location, and banding pattern. Each of the 22 autosomes is designated by a number. Chromosomal disorders can be diagnosed by a karyotype, which is a photographic enlargement of the chromosomes arranged by their numbered pairs.

One chromosome of each chromosomal pair is inherited from the father; the other chromosome of that pair is inherited from the mother. Thus, at each genetic locus an individual has two genes, which more properly are called *alleles.*

Genetic disorders can be divided into four categories:

1. *Chromosomal disorders,* which involve an excess or a deficiency of chromosomal material
2. *Mendelian disorders,* which involve an abnormality (mutation) at a single genetic locus in one or both of the alleles at that locus
3. *Polygenic disorders,* which involve mutations at two or more genetic loci
4. *Multifactorial disorders,* which involve mutations at one or more genetic loci that interact with an environmental factor, such as exposure to a drug, an infectious agent, or a xenobiotic (a foreign substance)

The mitochondrial genome recently has been sequenced and encodes a number of genes that have been associated with specific disorders.

Chromosomal Disorders

Chromosomal abnormalities occur in 0.5% of newborns; almost all arise from meiotic nondisjunction (i.e., abnormal splitting of homologous chromosomes so that one daughter cell receives both and the other receives none) in one of the parental gametes (sperm and egg). This produces a fertilized egg with a chromosomal number that is different from the normal diploid number of 46 chromosomes, a condition called *aneuploidy* (i.e., any numerical deviation from the normal 46-chromosome human karyotype). Most aneuploidy abnormalities have 47 chromosomes, such as trisomy 13, 18, and 21. Although the etiology of nondisjunctions is unclear, there is an association with advanced maternal age in some chromosomal disorders, such as in the autosomal trisomies. This association is the reason that prenatal diagnosis with amniocentesis is offered to pregnant women 35 years of age and older. The recurrence risk for aneuploidy abnormalities is small—1% or less.

The karyotypes of parents who have had a child with an aneuploidy abnormality are normal and thus need not be obtained. However, parents who have had a child with an unbalanced karyotype, in which 46 chromosomes are present but additional material is attached to another chromosome (duplication) or is deleted from one chromosome (deletion), should have their karyotypes determined. In these situations, one of the parents could be a "balanced" carrier and at increased risk for having another child with a chromosomal abnormality.

A recent advance in the diagnosis of chromosomal disorders is fluorescence in situ hybridization (FISH). This technology utilizes fluorescent-labeled DNA probes that bind to a specific complementary DNA region on a particular chromosome. A FISH probe designed for a specific region of an autosome will give two signals when the cell is scored under the microscope, because there normally are two chromosomes for each autosomal chromosome, and the specific recognition segment of DNA is normally present on both chromosomes. FISH is especially suited for the detection of chromosomal microdeletions that are too small for detection by a conventional karyotype. A number of microdeletion syndromes have been described and characterized, using FISH in which a specific FISH probe is used when the clinical suspicion of the particular microdeletion syndrome is suspected.

A list of microdeletion syndromes in which FISH can be used for diagnosis is given in Table 40-1. Noteworthy is the recently described entity CATCH-22 (*c*ongenital heart disease, *a*bnormal facies, *t*hymic aplasia, *c*left palate, *h*ypocalcemia, 22=22q11 microdeletion). This microdeletion syndrome encompasses DiGeorge syndrome, velocardiofacial syndrome, and some individuals who have isolated conotruncal defects, and it should be considered in the differential diagnosis of any individual who has any of the five clinical features of CATCH.

Mendelian Disorders

There are four mendelian, or single-gene, inheritance patterns: autosomal dominant, autosomal recessive, X-linked recessive, and X-linked dominant (Table 40-2). Determination of the pattern involved is based on whether the genetic locus is on an autosome or on the X chromosome and whether a single dose of the mutant allele causes the disease (dominant) or a double dose of the mutant allele causes the disease (recessive). There are no known Y-linked human diseases.

Autosomal dominant inheritance. Individuals who have an autosomal dominant disorder have one normal (N) and one abnormal (A) or mutant allele at the genetic locus in question. Thus, an affected individual has the genotype of NA and has a 50% chance of passing the N allele and a 50% chance of passing the A allele to each child. Because an affected person's mate almost always has two normal alleles (NN) at the same locus, there is a 50% chance that their children will inherit the A allele and thus have the disorder.

Pedigrees of autosomal dominant disorders often show successive generations of affected individuals in which affected children have an affected parent. An individual who has an autosomal dominant condition, however, sometimes can have normal parents who do not have the condition,

Table 40-1 Microdeletion Syndromes

Syndrome	Clinical Features	Chromosome Region
Langer-Gideon syndrome	Sparse hair, bulbous nose, multiple exostoses, loose skin	8q24.1
Prader-Willi syndrome	Hypotonia, obesity, mental retardation	15q11
Angelman syndrome	Seizures, mental retardation, paroxysms of laughter, ataxia, jerky movements	15q11
Miller-Dieker syndrome	Lissencephaly, mental retardation	17p13.3
Williams syndrome	Characteristic facies, loquacious personality, hypercalcemia	7q11.23
CATCH-22	CATCH (see above)	22q11

Table 40-2 Characteristics of Mendelian Inheritance Patterns

	Autosomal Dominant	Autosomal Recessive	X-Linked Recessive	X-Linked Dominant
Sex	M = F	M = F	Only M	F > M (2:1)
Genotype of affected individual	AN	AA	X^AY	X^AY; $X^A X^N$
Generations affected	Successive	Single	Successive; through carrier females	Successive
Recurrence risk for parents with affected child	50% if parent affected; negligible if parents unaffected	25%	25% if mother is carrier; negligible if new mutation	If M affected, all daughters affected; no sons affected If F affected, 50% offspring affected
Male-to-male transmission	Yes	NA	No	No
Other features	Advanced paternal age with new mutations in some disorders; variable expressivity	Consanguinity sometimes found	—	Rare inheritance pattern

A, Abnormal allele on autosomal chromosome; *F,* female; *M,* male; *N,* normal allele on autosomal chromosome A; *NA,* not applicable; *X,* abnormal allele on X chromosome.

which illustrates the concept of a *new mutation*. In this situation the risk of the normal parents having another affected child is negligible, whereas there is a 50% risk that the person who has the new mutation will have an affected child.

Achondroplasia is a well-documented autosomal dominant condition that most likely represents new mutations; 90% of affected individuals are born to parents of normal stature. Advanced paternal age has been associated with new mutations in a number of autosomal dominant conditions, including achondroplasia, Apert syndrome, and myositis ossificans.

On average, equal numbers of males and females are affected; male-to-male transmission also occurs. These two characteristics help distinguish autosomal dominant inheritance from X-linked recessive inheritance. In X-linked inheritance, females almost never are affected and male-to-male transmission cannot occur (see the section on X-linked recessive inheritance, below).

Variable expressivity is another feature of some autosomal dominant disorders in which a spectrum of clinical manifestations can appear in affected individuals. This principle is illustrated in the autosomal dominant condition of Marfan syndrome, in which any combination of the following can occur: musculoskeletal abnormalities, including long, thin fingers; high arched palate; pectus excavatum; pes cavus; and scoliosis; the eye abnormality of dislocated lenses; and cardiac abnormalities, including mitral valve prolapse and a dilated aortic root.

Autosomal recessive inheritance. Individuals who have an autosomal recessive disorder have two mutant alleles at the genetic locus in question; thus, they have the genotype AA and are homozygous for the mutant allele. Most individuals, however, are homozygous for the normal allele (NN) at this locus, although the occurrence of the heterozygote or carrier (NA) can be as high as 5% for some common autosomal recessive disorders such as cystic fibrosis. Persons who have the NA genotype are entirely normal and show no evidence of the disease in question.

Couples who have had a child with an autosomal recessive condition are both carriers (NA) of one abnormal allele; the other allele is normal. Each parent has a 50% chance of passing the A allele to subsequent children. Thus, the probability that both will pass on the A allele to produce an affected child is 50% × 50%, which is 25%. On average, equal numbers of males and females are affected. Pedigrees almost always show the disease confined to one sibship without transmission of the disease from generation to generation. The probability that an affected individual will have an affected child is negligible because the mate of this individual also would have to be a carrier of the same abnormal allele, which is relatively unlikely. Consanguinity sometimes is found in pedigrees of autosomal recessive diseases, especially in very rare conditions, because inbreeding increases the likelihood of two individuals having the same mutant allele at a genetic locus that they can pass on to their children.

X-linked recessive inheritance. X-linked recessive disorders are caused by a mutation at a genetic locus on the X chromosome. Because females have two X chromosomes, it is highly unlikely that they will have mutant alleles at a given locus on both X chromosomes. Males, however, have only one X chromosome; if they inherit an X chromosome from their mother with a mutation at a disease-associated locus, then they will have the disease. Thus, females rarely are affected with X-linked recessive disorders; for all practical purposes, only males are affected. Males can inherit an X-linked disorder from a carrier female, or the X chromosome that the mother passes on can mutate and give rise to the disorder.

Male-to-male transmission in X-linked recessive inheritance never occurs because the genetic locus is on the X chromosome, and a man has to pass the Y chromosome, not the X chromosome, to his male child. The sons of carrier females have a 50% chance of being affected with an X-linked recessive disorder; the daughters of carrier females have a 50% chance of being carriers. In those X-linked conditions in which males can reproduce, such as hemophilia, none of the male children of affected fathers will be affected, but all female children will be carriers.

X-linked dominant inheritance. X-linked dominant inheritance is a rare type of inheritance pattern. Twice as many females are affected as males, there is no male-to-male transmission, and all female children of affected males are affected.

Polygenic and Multifactorial Inheritance

Because it is difficult to distinguish between polygenic and multifactorial inheritance in human genetic diseases, they will be discussed together. These disorders are characterized by a recurrence risk that is greater for the development of the disorder than the general population's risk, but that clearly is lower than that of the 25% autosomal recessive or 50% autosomal dominant mendelian disorders.

Table 40-3 lists some of these disorders, with general population frequency and recurrence risk if a couple already has had an affected child. These disorders are important in pediatrics because they are common and because many are associated with significant morbidity and mortality. It has been difficult to define the specific genetic loci and environmental factors that cause these disorders. Etiological heterogeneity is one explanation for the observation of an intermediate risk after a couple has an affected child. This means that there could be distinctly different causes of the same clinical phenotype. For example, some cases of congenital heart disease may result from an environmental cause such as a congenital

Table 40-3 Polygenic/Multifactorial Diseases

Disorder	General Population Frequency (%)	Recurrence Risk After One Affected Child (%)
Neural tube defects	0.1	4
Congenital heart disease	0.6	3
Cleft lip ± palate	0.1	4
Juvenile diabetes	0.1	4

Table 40-4 Populations at Increased Risk for Specific Genetic Diseases

Population	Disease	Disease Frequency/10,000 Births
Black	Sickle cell	20
Ashkenazi Jew	Tay-Sachs	3
Mediterranean	Beta-thalassemia	20
Southeast Asian	Alpha-thalassemia	20
White	Cystic fibrosis	5
Inuit	Congenital adrenal hyperplasia	20

infection, whereas others may result from a single gene disorder such as Holt-Oram syndrome. Thus, the recurrence risk for each is different. In the former case, the risk would be negligible; in the latter, which is an autosomal dominant disorder, it would be 50% if a parent is affected.

Mitochondrial Disorders

Mitochondrial DNA is inherited maternally. The hallmark of mitochondrial inheritance is that disease transmission is never through the father and is always through the mother or occurs as a fresh mutation. Examples of mitochondrial disorders include the MELAS (*m*itochondrial *e*ncephalomyopathy with *l*actic *a*cidosis and *s*trokelike episodes) syndrome, the MERRF (*m*yoclonic *e*pilepsy and *r*agged-*r*ed *f*ibers) syndrome, and Leber's hereditary optic neuropathy.

FAMILY HISTORY

A family history should be part of the medical record of every pediatric patient. It should consist of a three-generation pedigree that shows the age and state of health of all living individuals and the age and cause of death of all deceased individuals (see Fig. 7-1, p. 63, with accompanying text). Spontaneous and induced abortions should be listed, as well as stillbirths. The ethnic backgrounds of both sides of the family should be noted, as should consanguinity, if present.

As shown in Table 40-4, certain ethnic groups have an increased incidence of disease-associated alleles and, thus, are at increased risk for some genetic diseases. Consanguinity increases the risk that a child will be homozygous for a disease-associated allele and, thus, for autosomal recessive diseases. For example, first-cousin matings have a twofold greater risk (4% to 6%) for a congenital disorder, compared with the background risk of unrelated matings (2% to 3%).

PRENATAL SCREENING

Amniocentesis

Amniocentesis is the process of removing amniotic fluid from the amniotic cavity by a needle puncture through the abdominal wall and anterior portion of the uterus. It is a safe procedure that typically is performed at about 16 weeks of gestation, although it can be done as early as 12 to 13 weeks. The amniotic fluid contains fetal cells that can be karyotyped or used for biochemical and DNA analysis.

The most common indication for amniocentesis is advanced maternal age because older mothers are at increased risk for chromosomal disorders. Pregnant women 35 years of age and older are offered amniocentesis and fetal chromosome analysis as part of their prenatal care. Couples who have a child who has a chromosomal abnormality or who are balanced translocation carriers also should be offered amniocentesis and fetal karyotyping.

Couples who have had a child who has a genetic disease may choose to have amniocentesis if the condition can be diagnosed by enzyme analysis of fetal cells or by biochemical analysis of amniotic fluid. For example, Hurler syndrome, an autosomal recessive disorder that has a 25% recurrence risk, causes severe mental retardation; most affected children die by adolescence. The disease is caused by a lack of production of the enzyme iduronidase. The disorder can be diagnosed by determining the iduronidase activity in fetal cells obtained by amniocentesis.

Molecular genetics has paved the way for prenatal diagnosis of some of the more common and severe genetic disorders. DNA analysis of fetal cells obtained from amniocentesis can be used to diagnose cystic fibrosis, Duchenne muscular dystrophy, sickle cell anemia, beta-thalassemia, and alpha-thalassemia. Couples who have a child who has one of these disorders have a 25% risk of having another affected child. Because DNA diagnosis is highly accurate, many couples who have an affected child choose to have amniocentesis and DNA analysis in subsequent pregnancies.

Amniotic fluid also can be analyzed for alpha-fetoprotein, which is significantly elevated in neural tube defects. The alpha-fetoprotein concentration usually is determined when an amniocentesis is performed for advanced maternal age. Couples who are at increased risk for having a baby with a neural tube defect may choose to have amniocentesis, including the determination of alpha-fetoprotein, as well as fetal ultrasound. Couples who have had a baby with a neural tube defect are at increased risk for having another child with this defect; other risk factors are maternal diabetes and maternal use of valproic acid during pregnancy.

Chorionic Villus Sampling

Chorionic villus sampling (CVS) is another technique for procuring fetal tissue that can be used for chromosomal, biochemical, or DNA analysis. Fetal tissue is obtained transcervically by means of a catheter that can retrieve small pieces of chorionic villus. The procedure is relatively safe, although there is not as much experience with CVS as with amniocentesis. Because CVS can be performed earlier in a pregnancy, couples who are extremely anxious about having a child with a particular condition may choose to undergo CVS rather than amniocentesis.

Ultrasound

Significant advances in fetal ultrasound have resulted in the diagnosis of many congenital abnormalities during pregnancy. These conditions include major central nervous system abnormalities (hydrocephalus, anencephaly, myelomeningocele, and holoprosencephaly), gastrointestinal abnormalities (duodenal atresia and diaphragmatic hernia), many types of congenital heart disease, genitourinary abnormalities (polycystic kidney disease and hydronephrosis), and many types of skeletal disorders. Ultrasound has been helpful to couples who have had children who have congenital abnormalities and who want reassurance that subsequent children will be unaffected.

Maternal Serum Analyte Screening

The first maternal serum analyte that was discovered to be useful in the prenatal detection of congenital malformations and genetic disease was alpha-fetoprotein. Elevated levels of maternal serum alpha-fetoprotein screening (MSAFP) are associated with an increased risk for open neural tube defects. Although the test is not as accurate as amniotic alpha-fetoprotein determination, it requires only a maternal blood specimen. If the levels are high, ultrasound or amniocentesis and amniotic alpha-fetoprotein analysis can be considered. Recently, low levels of MSAFP have been associated with Down syndrome; however, this association is weak and the test was not designed to detect Down syndrome. The addition of two other maternal serum analyte measurements, unconjugated estriol and human chorionic gonadotropin, with MSAFP can detect up to 60% of cases of Down syndrome born to mothers younger than 35 years of age. A maternal serum analyte profile that is very low in all maternal serum analyte compounds is associated with an increased risk for trisomy 18. Pregnant women are now offered maternal serum analyte testing routinely.

It should be noted that prenatal screening for genetic diseases is designed to provide accurate information about the likelihood of a child being affected by one of these diseases. Parents are advised of the consequences of such an outcome so that they may make an informed decision as to whether they wish to continue the pregnancy.

NEWBORN SCREENING

All states have mandatory newborn screening programs. Although the tests vary from state to state, all states test for phenylketonuria and congenital hypothyroidism because they are relatively common, easily treated, and cost effective. Some states mandate testing for maple syrup urine disease, homocystinuria, cystic fibrosis, hemoglobinopathies, biotinidase deficiency, congenital adrenal hyperplasia, and galactosemia. Tandem mass spectrometry is a technology that has been used recently in some newborn screening programs because of its ability to detect not only inborn errors of amino acid metabolism but also fatty acid oxidation defects, the most important of which is medium chain acyl-CoA dehydrogenase deficiency. The results of newborn screening tests usually are available 1 to 2 weeks after an infant is discharged from the hospital; the pediatrician always should ascertain that the newborn screening test has been performed and is normal. Obviously, any abnormal values or borderline-normal should be investigated further with retesting.

DNA-BASED DIAGNOSIS OF GENETIC DISEASES

Molecular genetic advances now allow for DNA-based diagnosis of several common pediatric genetic disorders and have changed the diagnostic evaluations of these conditions.

Fragile X Syndrome

Fragile X syndrome used to be diagnosed in the laboratory by cytogenetic-based evaluation of cells for the fragile X chromosome. The gene for fragile X syndrome was characterized in 1992 and has been called FMR-1 (fragile X mental retardation syndrome; the 1 designates the first X-linked mental retardation gene to be characterized). A novel form of mutation has been found in affected individuals who have fragile X syndrome in which the trinucleotide repeat CGG (cytosine-guanine-guanine) is amplified in the FMR-1 gene. Males and females who have fragile X syndrome have more than 230 copies of the CGG repeat; normal individuals have fewer than 50 copies. Carrier females have between 50 and 230 copies.

Laboratory evaluation of an individual suspected of having fragile X syndrome because of autism, mental retardation, or the physical features of fragile X syndrome (large testes, large ears, a prominent jaw) should be done with the DNA-based test and not the more expensive and less reliable cytogenetic-based test.

Duchenne Muscular Dystrophy

Duchenne muscular dystrophy (DMD) has been diagnosed by muscle biopsy. In 1987 the gene that causes DMD was characterized and named dystrophin. About two thirds of cases of DMD are from large intragenic deletions in the dystrophin gene that can be detected by the molecular methods of either Southern blotting or polymerase chain reaction. In most cases, DMD can be diagnosed by using DNA-based methods and thus avoiding a muscle biopsy. In cases in which there is no deletion, a muscle biopsy is required.

Spinal Muscular Atrophy

The gene for spinal muscular atrophy (SMA) was characterized in 1995. Microdeletions of this gene are a common cause of SMA, and DNA-based diagnosis is now possible.

Cystic Fibrosis

In 1989, the gene for cystic fibrosis was characterized and found to encode for a transmembrane protein of epithelial cells that controls chloride transport; this gene was named CFTR (cystic fibrosis transmembrane regulator). One common mutation has been found at the CFTR locus, which accounts for about 70% of the CF alleles in the white population; it has been named ΔF_{508} (deletion of a phenylalanine residue at the 508 position of CFTR). It now is possible to perform mutational analysis on individuals to determine their genotype at the CFTR locus. This approach commonly is used in families that have had cystic fibrosis, particularly to determine the carrier status of at-risk individuals. Typically, a panel of CF alleles is evaluated, which will detect 85% to

Table 40-5 Common Genetic Disorders

Disorder	Manifestation	Frequency/10,000 Births
Chromosomal		
Trisomy 21	Congenital heart disease, Brushfield spots, short hands, clinodactyly, simian crease, hypotonia, dysmorphic facies	16
Trisomy 18	Congenital heart disease, small for gestational age (SGA), clenched fist, rocker-bottom foot, dysmorphic facies	3
Trisomy 13	Congenital heart disease, SGA, polydactyly, holoprosencephaly, dysmorphic facies	2
XO (Turner's syndrome)	Congenital peripheral edema, webbed neck, short stature, primary amenorrhea	3
XXY (Klinefelter's syndrome)	Behavior problems, small testes, infertility, clinodactyly	5
Autosomal Recessive		
Sickle cell disease	Anemia, infection	20 (Black)
Beta-thalassemia	Anemia	20 (Mediterranean)
Cystic fibrosis	Failure to thrive, malabsorption, cough, recurrent pneumonia	5 (White)
Autosomal Dominant		
Familial hypercholesterolemia	Family history of early coronary artery disease	20
Neurofibromatosis	Café-au-lait spots	3
X-Linked Recessive		
Fragile X	Mental retardation, large testes, dysmorphic facies	5
Duchenne muscular dystrophy	Muscle weakness, pseudohypertrophy of calf	1

90% of CF alleles. The initial diagnostic test for cystic fibrosis in an individual suspected of having the disease still is the sweat chloride test. In situations in which it is difficult to obtain sweat, such as in very young infants, or in equivocal sweat tests, mutational analysis of CFTR may be especially helpful.

Fragile X syndrome, DMD, and cystic fibrosis all can be diagnosed prenatally with great accuracy by using molecular genetic techniques on a chorionic villus sample or on amniocytes obtained by amniocentesis.

Other Genetic Diseases

The human genome project is providing knowledge about human genes that is being translated rapidly into increasing capabilities for DNA diagnosis of genetic diseases. To this end, the human genome project has supported the establishment of HELIX, a computer-based registry of laboratories that provide molecular diagnosis for specific genetic diseases. Thus, any family that has a genetic disease may be interested in the availability of DNA diagnosis for confirmation of diagnosis or for evaluation of individuals at risk. Provision of DNA-based diagnosis should be through a genetic counselor or medical geneticist because issues of interpretation, follow-up, and confidentiality are best managed by such experienced individuals.

In genetic diseases where a single disease allele accounts for the vast majority of disease alleles, molecular diagnosis is inexpensive and much easier than if a large panel of disease mutations needs to be tested or if an entire gene has to be sequenced. Three clinical presentations exemplify this. In the evaluation of the infant who has nonketotic hypoglycemia, medium chain acyl-CoA dehydrogenase (MCAD) deficiency needs to be considered, and there is one very common MCAD disease allele, G-985, which can be tested easily by molecular methods. In the evaluation of the child who has an unexplained vascular thrombosis, resistance to activated protein C [APC] needs to be considered. Factor V Leiden is the most common cause of resistance to APC, and Factor V Leiden accounts for some 14% of vascular thrombosis events in children. In the evaluation of nonsyndromic hearing loss in children, abnormalities of the connexin 26 gene account for the majority of these cases, and there is one common connexin 26 disease allele, 35delG, which can be tested easily. The common disease alleles—G-985 in MCAD deficiency, Factor V Leiden in APC resistance, and 35delG in nonsyndromic hearing loss—can be tested easily and inexpensively.

SCOPE OF PEDIATRIC GENETIC DISORDERS

It is beyond the intent of this chapter to describe in any detail the numerous genetic diseases. Table 40-5 lists some of the more common genetic disorders that manifest in children. Two excellent references that may help pediatricians to establish a genetic diagnosis or a dysmorphology syndrome are Jones' *Smith's Recognizable Patterns of Human Malformation*[1] and McKusick's *Mendelian Inheritance in Man.*[2]

REFERENCES

1. Jones KL: *Smith's recognizable patterns of human malformation*, ed 4, Philadelphia, 1988, WB Saunders.
2. McKusick VA: *Mendelian inheritance in man*, ed 10, Baltimore, 1992, Johns Hopkins University Press.

SUGGESTED READINGS

Gelehrter TD, Collins FS, Ginsburg D: *Medical genetics*, ed 2, Baltimore, 1998, Williams and Wilkins.

Johns DR: Mitochondrial DNA and disease, *N Engl J Med* 333:638, 1995.

41 Contraception and Abortion

Eric A. Schaff

There are 3.0 million unintended pregnancies each year in the United States, which represent 48% of all pregnancies. An unintended pregnancy has significant consequences socially, physically, and financially for an unprepared teenager, her family, and the community. The rate of unintended pregnancies in the United States is in modest decline but continues to be higher than in other developed countries. Pediatricians are particularly attuned to preventive public health measures that decrease morbidity, and can play an important role in preventing unintended pregnancies. Standard interventions include family planning information for all teenagers and help in choosing and accessing contraceptive methods with emergency contraception as backup for sexually active teens. Advocacy also is needed to make contraceptives more available, affordable, and covered by health insurance.

Teenagers who are sexually abstinent need encouragement and reassurance regarding the importance of their decision. To improve compliance with contraception, pediatricians need to ensure confidentiality. They also must assess their patients' understanding of the effectiveness, benefits, and risks of the chosen method; their concerns about becoming pregnant; and their motivation to use the method selected.

Significant advances have been made in early abortion services. Detection of early pregnancy has been simplified by inexpensive, home and office pregnancy tests that are positive 4 weeks after the last menstrual period. The transvaginal sonogram has assumed an increasing role in normal and ectopic pregnancy detection. These technologies have allowed much earlier surgical abortions to be performed. Medical abortion with methotrexate combined with misoprostol is currently available, and mifepristone (formerly known as RU 486) combined with misoprostol is expected to be available in 2000.

This chapter provides information basic to the pediatrician's task of providing reproductive health care to teenagers.

CONTRACEPTION

In general, all contraceptive methods are highly effective when used correctly, and their benefits outweigh their health risks. When considering a contraceptive method, the short- and long-term medical risks and financial costs should be compared with the risks and costs associated with not using the method—that is, an unintended pregnancy.

Hormonal Methods

Hormonal methods have many features in common that include their mechanism of action, effectiveness, advantages, disadvantages, and side effects. These methods prevent pregnancy by three mechanisms: (1) suppressing luteinizing and follicle-stimulating hormones, thereby inhibiting ovulation; (2) thickening cervical mucus, making it less penetrable by sperm; and (3) altering the endometrium, making it less receptive to implantation of a fertilized ovum. Inhibiting ovulation is the primary mechanism of action of hormonal methods, but ovulation is not always inhibited. When used correctly, these methods are more than 99% effective in preventing pregnancy and are reversible when stopped. All hormonal methods should be started within 5 days of the onset of a normal menses to ensure that the teen is not pregnant and that ovulation will be suppressed during the first month. When possible, oral contraceptives should be started on the first Sunday following the onset of menses.

Menses usually are lighter, shorter in duration, and sometimes absent. These methods are associated with less dysmenorrhea, less benign breast disease, less pelvic inflammatory disease (because of the thickened cervical mucus), and less ovarian and endometrial cancer.[2] The progestin-only methods (progestin-only oral contraceptives, 3-month injectable, and 5-year implant) are not associated with venous thromboembolic events, which is a risk of estrogen use.

Informed counseling is key to initial management of side effects. Side effects such as breakthrough vaginal bleeding, nausea, headaches, bloating, hair loss, mood changes, and irritability are likely to resolve spontaneously after several menstrual cycles. Weight gain caused by an increase in appetite can be countered by good eating habits. Persistent mood changes or depression will require stopping the hormonal method. These methods do not protect against sexually transmitted diseases (STDs), and the use of condoms must be encouraged.

Oral contraceptives. After almost four decades of availability, decreases in estrogen and progestin concentrations have made oral contraceptives ("the Pill") extraordinarily safe, effective (<1% annual use pregnancy rate), and popular. The combination pill consists of a synthetic estrogen and progesterone. A progesterone-only pill, often referred to as the "mini-pill," is slightly less effective (97%) and is indicated for women with a contraindication to estrogen use.

All low-dose combination pills consist of only one estrogen, ethinyl estradiol (20 to 35 μg/day). Synthetic progestins are more varied but derive from either estranes or gonanes. Estranes were marketed first and consist of norethindrone or compounds that convert to norethindrone. Gonanes consist of norgestrel/levonorgestrel, norgestimate, and desogestrel. The latter two have the advantage of being potent progestins that have fewer androgenic side effects. They also increase high-density lipoprotein, which is protective against atherosclerosis, and have a slightly longer half-life, which theoretically makes vaginal spotting and pregnancy less likely if the patient forgets to take a pill.

ADVANTAGES. Besides the advantages in common with the other hormonal methods, oral contraceptive use is associated with predictable menses, a rapid return to fertility after stopping, and lower cost.

DISADVANTAGES. The disadvantages of oral contraceptive use include (1) need for daily compliance; (2) eversion of columnar epithelium of the cervix, possibly explaining the increased risk of chlamydia infection resulting from its attraction to these cells and, theoretically, increasing the risk of papillovirus infection; (3) decreased effectiveness of some antibiotics (e.g., rifampin and doxycycline) and anti-seizure medications (e.g., phenobarbital and phenytoin); (4) possible increased risk of breast cancer in women younger than age 35[3]; and (5) increased risk of rare venous thromboembolic disease. For women between 20 and 24 years of age, the incidence of venous thromboembolic events increases from 3.2/100,000 for non-users of oral contraceptives to 9.7/100,000 for oral contraceptive users.[14]

PRESCRIBING ORAL CONTRACEPTIVES. Before prescribing oral contraceptive pills, one should be certain that there are no contraindications to their use; these include a history of venous thromboembolism, active liver disease, and a current pregnancy. Pills should be prescribed cautiously for teenagers who have mild hypertension, diabetes, renal disease, epilepsy, hemorrhagic disorders, immune deficiency disease, and sickle cell disease. A baseline blood pressure should be obtained. A general physical examination and pelvic examination are recommended for routine health maintenance and to rule out pregnancy. There are few other findings on physical examinations of healthy young women that contraindicate prescribing oral contraceptives.

Considerable flexibility exists regarding which brand of oral contraceptive pills to prescribe. Most commonly, a 28-day cycle pack (21 days of active hormones and 7 days of placebo) is used. Despite claims by manufacturers, clinical differences among brands of low-dose pills are minimal regardless of whether the hormones are fixed (monophasic) or varied (triphasic) throughout the month. Clinicians can choose any one of the following in prescribing oral contraceptives: (1) an inexpensive generic brand, (2) a low-estrogen preparation containing 20 μg of ethinyl estradiol, (3) a weak progestin such as norethindrone, or (4) a new-generation progestin that has weak androgenic effects (norgestimate or desogestrel). To improve compliance, it is important to prescribe a sufficient number of 28-day packs to avoid "running out of pills." The first few months should serve to identify any health concerns or problems the patient may identify in taking the pills. Following this, 12-month supplies should be prescribed to increase compliance.

Oral contraceptive pills typically are started on the Sunday after a normal menstrual period begins. If the period begins on Sunday, then the first pill is taken that day. The correct start ensures that the teen is not pregnant and increases the likelihood of suppressing ovulation that month. The pill should be taken at the same time each day. Taking pills before bedtime may cause less nausea during the day. If one pill is forgotten (particularly during the first 7 days that are needed to suppress ovulation), it should be taken as soon as it is remembered. If two pills are missed, two pills should be taken each day for 2 days, and a barrier birth control method should be used for the next week. If more than two pills are missed, another contraceptive method should be used and another pill pack should be started on the first Sunday after the next menses begins. Withdrawal bleeding usually occurs on day 2 or 3 after the last pill is taken.

If mild side effects do not resolve after several cycles, the brand can be changed to another containing a different progestin. If menstruation does not occur, the pills should be continued and a pregnancy test obtained for reassurance and to detect the rare pregnancy.

Progesterone-only injections and implants. As many as 10% to 15% of female teenagers report using depo-medoxyprogesterone acetate (DMPA; Depo-Provera). Although available "off-label" for two decades in the United States, it received formal U.S. Food and Drug Administration (FDA) approval in a 150-mg dose in 1992.

Depo-Provera is an injectable progestin that provides 12 weeks of effective contraceptive protection plus an additional 1-week "grace" period (for a total of 13 weeks). It requires vigorous shaking to suspend all the particles, and is given deep intramuscularly in either the deltoid or upper outer quadrant of the gluteal muscle. The site should not be massaged because it may increase the rate of absorption and metabolism, and thereby decrease effectiveness.

The Norplant System is a long-acting, 5-year hormonal method consisting of six match-size (2.4 mm in diameter and 34 mm in length), flexible capsules made of Silastic, a soft, rubberlike material. The progestin levonorgestrel, which also is found in some common birth control pills, is continuously released from the capsules over the next 5 years, providing a 99% pregnancy protection rate. Unfortunately, the number of new users has decreased significantly because of negative publicity generated around unfounded lawsuits related to side effects.

Norplant capsules are placed just under the skin in the inside area of a woman's upper arm. The capsules are inserted under local anesthesia (using about 6 ml of lidocaine) in an 85-degree fanlike pattern through a single 3-mm puncture to allow entry of the manufacturer's capsule-implanting trocar. No sutures are necessary. The implanted capsules are minimally visible but can be palpated. After 5 years, the capsules should be removed and, if desired, another set of capsules inserted. Approximately 20% of women with implanted capsules have them removed each year for a variety of personal and health reasons, most commonly, irregular bleeding. They, of course, have to be removed if the woman wishes to become pregnant.

ADVANTAGES. The unique advantages of these progesterone-only injectable and subdermal implant methods include (1) long-acting protection, (2) avoidance of estrogen and, therefore, the risk of venous thromboembolic disease, (3) lack of interference with breast-feeding, (4) possible reduction in the incidence of seizures and sickling episodes with Depo-Provera use, (5) continued effectiveness of antibiotics and anti-seizure medicines with Depo-Provera, and (6) amenorrhea in up to 50% of women after the first year of Depo-Proverause and an even higher percentage of women thereafter.

DISADVANTAGES. The disadvantages of these medicines include (1) the need for either repeated injections every 3 months or minor surgery for insertion and removal of the implants, (2) local reactions such as infection or tenderness at the site of the subdermal implant, (3) hypo-estrogen state with Depo-Provera that causes a reversible decrease in bone density, (4) delay in clearance of Depo-Provera for as long as 12 months, and (5) rare reports of reversible pseudotumor cerebri (headaches, blurred vision, and papilledema) with the implants that necessitates their removal.

The initial cost of the implants is high—$390 plus the insertion fee. However, the lack of any additional costs before removal of the implants makes this method reasonably cost effective. The Norplant Foundation provides free kits for low-income women. Depo-Provera costs about $35 per injection plus the office visit fee.

Managing side effects is important in supporting continued use of these methods. Irregular vaginal bleeding can be managed by offering a 28-day cycle of oral contraceptive pills. With support, implant continuation rates in the first year can be more than 90%.[6]

Emergency contraception. Emergency contraception (EC) is the *only* treatment available to prevent unintended pregnancy after unprotected intercourse. The two EC methods are emergency use of oral contraceptive pills containing either progestin only or combined progestin and estrogen, and an intrauterine device (IUD). In 1999, progestin-only emergency contraceptive pills (ECPs), also called postcoital, or "morning-after," contraception, received FDA approval. High-dose estrogen ECPs received FDA approval in 1997. It has been estimated that more than 50% of the current abortions in the United States could be avoided by widely available ECPs. Unfortunately, emergency contraception has been mislabeled by some as an abortifacient, and the abortion controversy has prevented more widespread acceptance. ECPs do not cause an abortion of an established pregnancy.

ECPs are indicated when other methods fail, when no other contraception is used, or when rape occurs. Specifically packaged products (PlanB is the progestin-only and Preven is the estrogen/progesterone combination) are less confusing for users and providers. One strategy to increase access to ECPs is to give a prescription in anticipation of an unprotected intercourse.[4] It may give extra confidence to teens who rely on condoms. Ideally, *teenagers who want to avoid an unintended pregnancy should keep one dose of an ECP available for emergency use.*

ECPs reduce the risk of pregnancy by 75% to 88%.[12,13] For example, if 100 women have unprotected intercourse in the second or third week of their cycle, 8 will become pregnant without emergency contraception, but 1 will become pregnant using progestin ECPs (88% reduction) and 2 will become pregnant using combined ECPs (75% reduction). If a current pregnancy is possible, a pregnancy test should be performed before the ECPs are taken.

Progestin-only pills are slightly more effective and cause less nausea. Two doses of one PlanB pill are taken 12 hours apart. Ethinyl estradiol (50 μg) and norgestrel (0.5 mg) tablets, now packed as Preven or the 28-day pack of Ovral, are available. Two doses of two tablets of Preven or Ovral are taken 12 hours apart.[14] Alternatively, other ECP brands use two doses of four tablets (LoOvral, Nordette, Levlen, Levlite, Levora, Triphasyl, Trivora, and Tri-Levlen), or two doses of five tablets (Alesse). The doses should be taken at convenient times (e.g., 8 PM and 8 AM). Nausea (50%) and vomiting (20%) may occur and may require anti-nausea treatment. If nausea and vomiting are problematic, the second dose may be inserted with a finger high into the vagina to be absorbed through the vaginal mucosa. Breast tenderness, irregular bleeding, fluid retention, and headaches occasionally occur. Thereafter, if the patient is so inclined, oral contraceptives can be started on the first Sunday after the onset of the next menstrual period or one pill daily after taking the ECPs. If menses are delayed, the teen should be instructed to return for a pregnancy test.

The IUD can be used for emergency contraception within 5 days of unprotected intercourse and is more than 99% effective. It can be left in place for up to 10 years or be removed at the next menstrual period. This method may be ideal for the young woman wanting long-term contraception and not at risk for STDs that might cause an ascending infection and infertility.

Barrier Methods

Teenagers interested in barrier methods should feel comfortable about touching their genitals and be able to plan ahead for intercourse. The extra lubrication associated with these methods may be a benefit.

Condoms. Condom use has increased because of the HIV epidemic. Latex condoms work by containing the ejaculate. Condoms are effective in pregnancy prevention and in reducing the spread of all STDs, including HIV. Making condoms readily available increases their use.[5,11] Even if teenagers prefer a hormonal birth control method as their primary method for preventing pregnancy, they should be encouraged to *use condoms if they are at risk for sexually transmitted infections.*

Condoms are (1) inexpensive, (2) available over the counter, (3) a means to involve the male in sharing responsibility for contraception, (4) lubricated, (5) associated with minimal side effects, and (6) simple to use. If a condom breaks, ECPs can be used as backup.

The disadvantages of condoms are (1) the diminished genital sensation, (2) the need to place the condom prior to any penile-perineal contact, and (3) the lack of 100% protection against STDs.

Lubricated latex condoms with or without the spermicidal nonoxynol-9 offer the best protection. "Natural" condoms (made from lamb intestine) provide significantly less protection because of their greater permeability to viruses and, therefore, are not recommended. Condoms should be placed on the erect penis just before any vaginal, anal, or oral contact. To prevent condom breakage, condoms should

(a) not be stored in warm places (e.g., a wallet) for long periods, (b) not be lubricated with oil-based lubricants such as Vaseline, and (c) not be reused. To avoid accidental spillage, teens should be instructed that the penis should be removed shortly after ejaculation while holding the rim of the condom on the base of the penis. If spillage occurs or a condom breaks, the female can use emergency contraception.

Diaphragm, female condom, and cervical cap. The diaphragm is a thin, rubber, 6.5- to 8-cm dome that is inserted into the vagina. It covers the cervix and blocks sperm from entering. It must be used with a spermicidal contraceptive jelly whose active ingredient is nonoxynol-9. When used correctly and consistently, the diaphragm's effectiveness can be quite high, although the annual use failure rate ranges from 6% to 16% when used alone. It also offers some protection from STDs and has minimal side effects. A diaphragm is a reasonable choice for a motivated teenager who wants to avoid taking contraceptive hormones. The disadvantages of the diaphragm include (1) the skill needed for placement, (2) the need to leave it in place 6 hours after intercourse, (3) the need for a second application of spermicidal jelly if intercourse is repeated after 6 hours, and (4) the increased risk of vaginitis and urinary tract infections. Disadvantages for the health care provider include keeping a set of diaphragm rings for sizing available, as well as learning and maintaining the skill to fit one when the requests are likely to be few.

The female condom is available but not widely used. It is made from polyurethane, with two flexible polyurethane rings. One ring is placed inside the vagina to cover the cervix, similar to a diaphragm; the open ring remains on the outside to protect the perineum from STDs. The female condom, which costs about $2.50, should not be used concomitantly with latex condoms, nor should it be reused.

The cervical cap is a thimble-shaped rubber device that fits over the cervix and can be left in place for continuous protection up to 48 hours. Its advantages and rates of effectiveness are similar to those of the diaphragm. Disadvantages include (1) the skill needed for insertion and removal (significantly more than that for the diaphragm), (2) the association of cervical dysplasia in the early months of use, and (3) the inability to fit the cervix of some women.

Spermicidals: vaginal foam, vaginal sponge, and vaginal suppository. Vaginal foam, sponges, and suppositories contain nonoxynol-9, which has in vitro and in vivo protective properties against some STDs. These methods are relatively simple, effective, and inexpensive and can be obtained without a prescription. They have an 18% to 28% annual use pregnancy rate when used alone. The spermicidals are important complementary methods (1) when used with condoms, (2) when intercourse is infrequent, and (3) when used as a backup for other birth control methods.

The vaginal sponge, which first is moistened with water, can be inserted several hours before intercourse and remains effective for 24 hours. Suppositories must be in the vagina at least 10 to 15 minutes before intercourse to allow them to dissolve.

Natural Family Planning

Natural family planning methods include (1) charting of menstrual cycles on the calendar, (2) recording basal body temperatures, and (3) monitoring cervical mucus to detect when ovulation occurs. Advantages include (1) the lack of side effects, (2) acceptance by religious groups opposed to hormonal and barrier methods, (3) knowledge gained about reproductive physiology, and (4) its practicality when there are barriers to accessing other methods. Disadvantages for teenagers include their irregular menstrual cycles, which make predicting ovulation difficult, the high degree of motivation required for effective use, and a 20% annual failure rate.

Intrauterine Device

Advances in the IUD (with copper wire containing levonorgestrel) has made this method highly effective and increasingly attractive.[9] Exactly how the method works is not known. It probably irritates the endometrium, making it unsuitable for implantation of a fertilized egg. The IUD is about 99% effective at preventing pregnancy, making it one of the most effective methods. The IUD is indicated for women interested in highly effective, nonhormonal, long-term, and reversible contraception. Once in place, it requires no effort for continued effectiveness and has no additional costs.

The IUD has traditionally not been offered to teenagers because of their increased risk for STDs and the fact that an IUD can provide a conduit for bacteria-causing pelvic inflammatory disease with its associated infertility. There has been a resurgence in interest in this method for a subset of teenagers at low risk for STD. A marked decline in IUD use has been due to its high initial costs as a result of the expenses incurred by pharmaceutical companies in defending the large number of lawsuits related to IUD use.

SUCTION CURETTAGE

Approximately 35% to 40% of pregnant teenagers in the United States choose abortion (suction curettage). Surgical abortion is greater than 99% effective and serious complications in the first 3 months of pregnancy are rare.[1] Unfortunately, mortality rates remain high in developing countries where there continues to be a great need for safe, legal, and accessible abortion services.[8]

Complications of abortion can include excessive bleeding, infection, perforation of the uterus, and adverse anesthetic events. The earlier the abortion is performed, the safer it is. Unfortunately, teens are more likely than older women to delay an abortion. The reasons cited most often by teens for choosing an abortion are how having a baby will negatively affect their lives, financial concerns, and feeling that they are not mature enough to have a child.

Most young teenagers involve their parents in these decisions. Some states require parental consent or notification for a minor to obtain an abortion. In these states, a minor who does not want to involve her parents must be able to obtain a judicial or administrative bypass.

Suction curettage initially was used only in first-trimester pregnancies. With additional experience, gynecologists have used variations of this procedure for up to 20 weeks' gestation. In the first trimester, this procedure involves placement of misoprostol or laminaria 6 to 24 hours earlier, local paracervical anesthesia, dilation of the cervix with metal or plastic dilators, and introduction of a cannula of appropriate size to remove the pregnancy by suction curettage. Surgical abortion before 7 weeks had been discouraged in the past because of increased complication rates. Now, with highly sensitive pregnancy tests and transvaginal sonography, the risks of early abortions are no greater than they are for those performed after 7 weeks of gestation. The advantages of a handheld, manual vacuum aspiration syringe in early pregnancy are its low cost, portability, relative ease of use, and lack of machine noise.

MEDICAL ABORTION

Mifepristone (formerly known as RU 486, the "French abortion pill") is available in as many as 11 European countries and China and should be available in the United States in 2000. Mifepristone blocks the action of progesterone, causing the cervix to soften and a pregnancy to detach from the endometrium. The second required medication, misoprostol, is a synthetic prostaglandin used to prevent stomach ulcers but also causes the uterus to contract and a pregnancy to be expelled. Oral mifepristone (from 200 to 600 mg), followed in 48 hours by either oral misoprostol 400 μg or vaginal misoprostol 800 μg is more than 95% effective in inducing an abortion in women who are up to 8 weeks pregnant.[10]

Methotrexate and misoprostol have been studied for medical abortion in the United States since the mid-1990s. Methotrexate blocks folic acid in DNA synthesis, thereby preventing the division of embryonic cells. It is slower acting and slightly less effective than mifepristone. Approximately 65% of women will have a complete abortion at 1 week, 85% at 2 weeks, and 90% to 95% by 4 weeks. Methotrexate (50 mg/m^2) given intramuscularly (considered a low dose compared with treatments for cancer) followed in 5 to 6 days by misoprostol (800 μg) given vaginally is currently recommended for women who are up to 7 weeks pregnant.[7] Misoprostol may be repeated if needed. Neither drug has FDA approval for this indication but may be used "off-label."

There are few medical contraindications for a medical abortion. They include liver or renal disease, a bleeding disorder, and allergies to the medications. The most common reason women choose a medical abortion is to "avoid" a surgical abortion. Relative contraindications for a medical abortion include teenagers who (1) are extremely ambivalent about their decision; (2) are unwilling to have a suction curettage, which is necessary because of the teratogenicity of both methotrexate and misoprostol, if the method fails; (3) have a low tolerance for pain or bleeding; (4) lack access to an emergency phone or transportation; and (5) lack support during misoprostol vaginal insertion if not performed in the physician's office.

The advantages of low-dose methotrexate include its safety, availability, low cost, and relative ease of use. Mifepristone has a consistent bleeding response within hours of using the second medication, misoprostol. The disadvantages of methotrexate include its higher failure rate (up to 10%), the delay of up to 4 weeks until a complete abortion occurs in about 10% of women, and its teratogenicity if the pregnancy continues. Mifepristone will be more expensive than methotrexate and its use will be closely regulated by the FDA. Other disadvantages of both regimens include (1) the side effects of nausea, vomiting, and diarrhea; (2) severe cramping; (3) unexpected heavy or persistent bleeding requiring suction curettage in 2% to 4% of patients; and (4) continuing pregnancies requiring suction curettage in up to 2% of women. Clinicians offering medical abortion must be able to perform or have access to 24-hour emergency suction curettage.

SUMMARY

Sexually active teenagers are at high risk for an unintended pregnancy. Current contraceptive methods are highly effective and safe. Hormonal methods have important noncontraceptive benefits such as the reduced risks of ovarian cancer. Emergency contraception is a new tool to reduce unintended pregnancies. Pediatricians can ensure that sexually active teenagers have easy access to ECPs for backup when another method fails or none was used. Medical abortion is new and may decrease delays in teenagers seeking abortion who are fearful of a surgical abortion. Pediatricians can expand their role in meeting the reproductive health care needs of their teenage patients.

REFERENCES

1. Abortion surveillance: preliminary analysis—United States, *MMWR* 47: 1025, 1035, 1998.
2. Beral V, et al: Mortality associated with oral contraceptive use: 25 year follow up of cohort of 46,000 women from Royal College of General Practitioners' oral contraception study, *BMJ* 318:69, 1999.
3. Brinton LA, et al: Modification of oral contraceptive relationships on breast cancer risk by selected factors among younger women, *Contraception* 55:197, 1997.
4. Glasier A, Baird D: The effects of self-administering emergency contraception, *N Engl J Med* 339:1, 1998.
5. Guttmacher S, et al: Condom availability in New York City public high schools: relationships to condom use and sexual behavior, *Am J Public Health* 87:1427, 1997.
6. Levine AS, et al: Subdermal contraceptive implant (Norplant) continuation rates among adolescents and adults in a family planning clinic, *J Pediatr Adolesc Gynecol* 9:67, 1996.
7. National Abortion Federation: *Guidelines for the use of methotrexate and misoprostol for early abortion,* National Abortion Federation, Washington, DC, html://www.prochoice.org, 1998.
8. Odlind V: Induced abortion: a global health problem, *Acta Obstet Gynecol Scand* (suppl) 164:43, 1997.
9. Pasquale S: Clinical experience with today's IUDs, *Obstet Gynecol Surv* 51(12 suppl):825, 1996.
10. Schaff EA, et al: Mifepristone 200 mg and vaginal misoprostol for induced abortion, *Contraception* 59:1, 1999.
11. Schuster MS, et al: Impact of a high school condom availability program on sexual attitudes and behaviors, *Fam Plann Perspect* 30:67, 88, 1998.
12. Task Force on Postovulatory Methods of Fertilization Regulation: Randomized controlled trial of levonorgestrel versus the Yuzpe regimen of combined oral contraceptive for emergency contraception, *Lancet* 352: 428, 1998.
13. Trussell J, Ellertson C, Stewart F: The effectiveness of the Yuzpe regimen of emergency contraception, *Fam Plann Perspect* 28:58, 87, 1996.
14. World Health Organization Technical Report 877, Geneva, Switzerland: World Health Organization, 1998.

SUGGESTED READING

Hatcher RA, et al: *Contraceptive technology,* ed 17, New York, 1998, Ardent Media.

42 The Fetus at Risk

George A. Little • Emily R. Baker

Pediatricians, as primary care specialists and as subspecialist neonatologists, consult and work collaboratively with obstetrical providers in preconception counseling, fetal risk identification, and peripartum decisions. They assume primary responsibility for resuscitation, stabilization, and ongoing care of the neonate from the moment of birth. Years ago, pediatricians first saw their newborn patients in the nursery, but only after the events of pregnancy and delivery.

Knowledge of fetal health includes appreciation of the interaction of the fetus with the mother, father, health professionals, and society. There are now many examples of the ability of fetal medicine, as part of preconception and prenatal care, to prevent or treat problems and to improve outcomes.

Prospective parents and professionals have good reason to be concerned about the immediate and long-term effects of agents or processes on the fetus. Infections such as rubella can result in fetal loss or multisystem disease. The magnitude and seriousness of manifestations of maternal alcohol consumption, tobacco use, or substance abuse during pregnancy may be evident in the infant's physical appearance or behavior in the neonatal period and throughout the infant's life span. Furthermore, problems may not appear until a subsequent generation. The effects of diethylstilbestrol (DES), once given to mothers for threatened abortion, did not manifest until the appearance of clear cell carcinoma of the vagina in female offspring 10 to 20 years later.[26]

Growth and development are as much a key to fetal medicine as they are to pediatrics, of which study of the fetus is merely the first installment. One must regard human growth and development as a continuum that begins with conception (Fig. 42-1). This chapter depicts some of the normal physical and interactive aspects of fetal existence, followed by a discussion of selected pathophysiological states that may affect that existence adversely.

FETAL LIFE SPAN

Clinicians use menstrual dating when describing the course of human pregnancy, beginning with the first day of the last menstrual period. Others use conceptual dating and a timeline that begins with conception or approximately 2 weeks after the last menstrual period. Occasional confusion arises when the differences between these two conventions are not appreciated. Furthermore, clinicians discuss pregnancy in terms of portions of weeks, such as 36 0/7 or the beginning of the thirty-sixth week. A pregnancy can thus be 37 completed weeks (36 7/7) or in the thirty-eighth week (38 0/7), when it is considered to be at term. This concept is similar to a child not being 1 year old until his or her first birthday on the 366th day of life.

The normal human pregnancy lasts 36 to 40 weeks from fertilization or 38 to 42 weeks from the last menstrual period (by menstrual dating). Fetal development begins at fertilization, when a sperm combines with an oocyte to form a zygote. The fetal life span is defined here in the broad sense to include the entire gestational interval (Fig. 42-2). The human product of conception technically becomes a fetus at the end of the eighth postfertilization week and remains so until birth.

Development proceeds from conception to birth in three stages: (1) the ovum, zygote, and blastocyst; (2) the embryo; and (3) the fetus. The conceptus, or product of conception, comprises all the structures that develop from the zygote, both embryonic (the embryo or fetus) and extraembryonic (the membranes and the placenta).

The stage of the ovum, zygote, and blastocyst, illustrated in Fig. 42-2, begins with fertilization, wherein a single haploid sperm (23 chromosomes) penetrates the oocyte (immature haploid female ovum with 23 chromosomes). This usually takes place within the ampulla of the fallopian tube. The fertilization process is complicated and takes up to 24 hours after initial penetration by the sperm before the genetic material from the two haploid cells fuses to form a diploid cell, the *zygote,* with a full complement of genetic material (called the *stage of syngamy*).

The preembryo consists of the developing cells, produced by division of the zygote, and lasts until the formation of the "primitive streak," approximately 14 days after the beginning of fertilization. The preembryonic stage has been of special interest clinically and ethically, because it is possible to sustain human preembryos in vitro for up to 6 to 9 days after fertilization.

Preembryo development, during the interval before implantation in the uterine lining, includes a series of morphological changes. Progression proceeds from blastomeres, or individual cells, to a tightly compacted group of cells called the *morula*. The blastocyst, a mass of cells having a fluid-filled inner cavity, appears at about 4 days after syngamy. Early mitotic divisions lead to totipotential cells that are able to produce all the products of conception. It is during this time that "twinning" becomes possible; by approximately day 7, differentiation leads to cells becoming individualized. The multicellular blastocyst with a trophectoderm and an in-

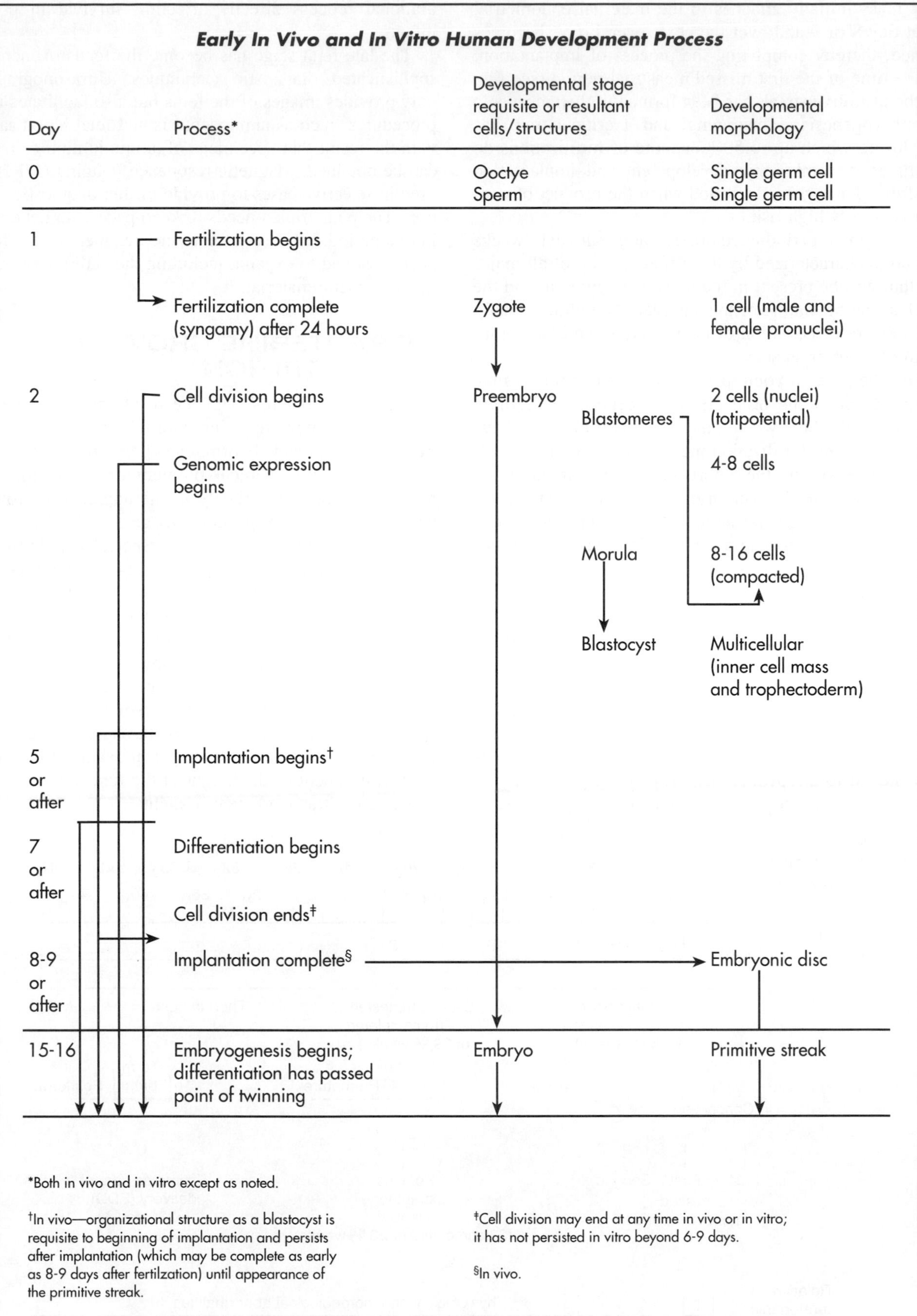

Fig. 42-1 Fetal and child development begins with fertilization and is similar in vivo and in vitro for 6 to 9 days.
(From American College of Obstetricians and Gynecologists Preembryo Research: *History, scientific background, and ethical considerations,* ACOG Committee Opinion No 136, Washington, DC, 1994, ACOG.)

ner cell mass initially attaches to the maternal endometrial lining at day 8 or 9 and over the next several days becomes embedded, thereby completing the process of implantation.

By the time of the first missed menstrual period (see Fig. 42-2), the primitive streak has been formed in the embryonic disk, embryogenesis is beginning, and a critical time has passed during which up to 50% or more of fertilizations do not complete preembryonic development and implantation successfully. Thus, this is a period when the product of conception is at very high risk.

The *embryonic* period encompasses approximately weeks 3 to 8 and is characterized by the differentiation of all major organs that will be present in the fetus, the newborn, and the adult. Near the beginning of this interval, the mother usually becomes aware of cessation of menstruation, and laboratory tests can confirm pregnancy.

During the preembryonic period, adverse conditions may cause the death of the products of conception. This often occurs around the time when a menstrual period would have been expected, and fertilization may not be recognized. Adverse influences during the embryonic period can cause severe interruptions in the pattern of system development, resulting in major congenital anomalies in a surviving fetus. The embryo is recognizable as humanoid toward the end of this period; malformations, such as those of the limbs, resulting, for example, from maternal ingestion of thalidomide, are readily identifiable.

The *fetal* stage, the longest of the three stages of the fetal life span, ends with delivery. Growth in size is the most apparent change during this interval, but maturation of organ systems and bodily processes is equally important. The high incidence and problems of premature birth make the degree of organ and enzyme system maturation of compelling interest to the pediatrician. The development of pulmonary surfactant is probably the single most important maturational process directly affecting survival in premature infants.

The late fetal stage has become the focus of increasingly sophisticated diagnostic techniques. Ultrasonography not only provides images of the fetus but also facilitates invasive procedures, such as amniocentesis and fetal blood sampling, with the result that specimens of amniotic fluid or fetal cells can be obtained. Magnetic resonance imaging (MRI) can be used in selective cases to provide further diagnostic information. The pediatrician needs to keep pace with developments in this period, because intrauterine treatment of the fetus appears destined to expand, including the addition or modification of genetic material.

INTRAUTERINE GROWTH AND NUTRITION

The physician dealing with the newborn must have a firm conceptual framework of intrauterine growth to evaluate and treat the normal and abnormal newborn effectively. In particular, the common clinical problem of prematurity can be managed more appropriately if one appreciates growth patterns as they relate to gestational age.

The growth rate of the fetus is especially rapid from 12 to 16 weeks of gestation and again during its final months. Both of these rapid-growth phases are associated with events of immediate concern to the practitioner. By the end of the sixteenth week after fertilization, the size and activity of the fetus have reached the point that many multiparous and some primiparous women are able to feel fetal motion ("quickening"). This can be a valuable marker when assessing fetal age and well-being. The late-growth phase can be monitored by several means, especially physical examination, including the measurement of the height of the fundus above the symphysis and ultrasound measurements.

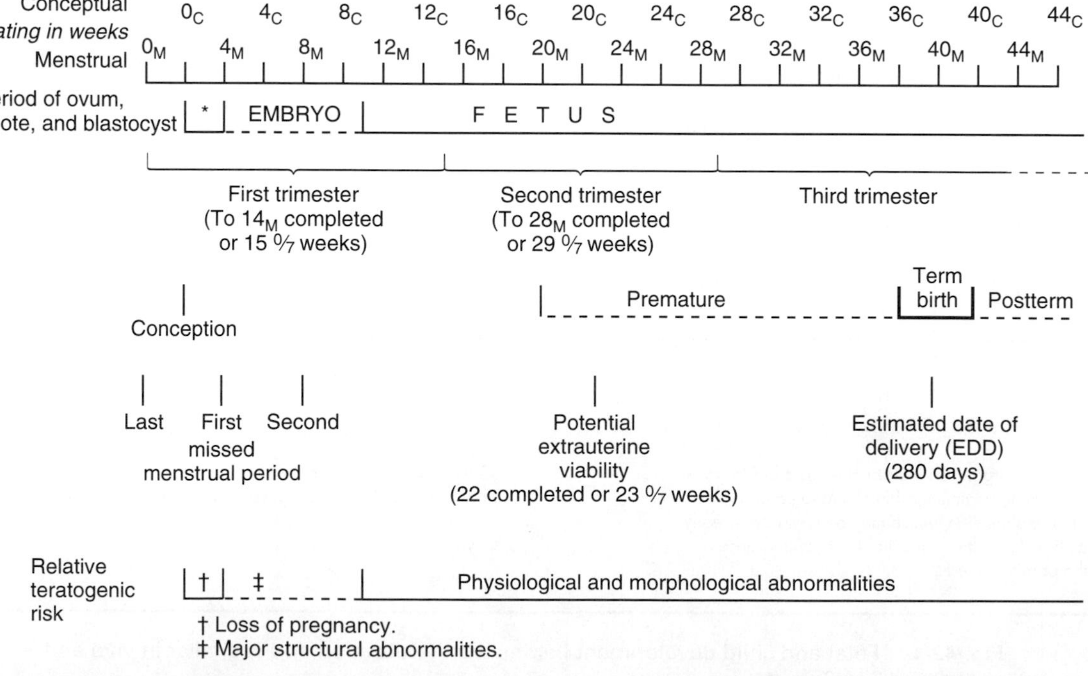

Fig. 42-2 Fetal life span by conceptual and menstrual dating. Note timing of important events and relative teratogenic risk.

The period from 8 to 12 weeks after fertilization begins with a fetus whose head makes up almost half of the total length. By 12 weeks the total length has doubled, but the head represents a smaller proportion. The 12- to 16-week interval is characterized by extremely rapid growth in length. In the 17- to 20-week interval growth slows somewhat, but extremities assume their relative proportions. The 21- to 25-week interval after fertilization is characterized by significant gains in both length and weight.

Twenty-one weeks after fertilization, or 23 weeks from the last menstrual period, represents an extremely important milestone, because the threshold for extrauterine viability is currently recognized as occurring at approximately 23 weeks (menstrual dating), with neonatal intensive care necessary to sustain that potential.[11,17]

Many studies have attempted to quantify fetal growth through the use of postnatal data. Such growth curves, derived from measuring infants born at varying gestational ages, can give an approximation of intrauterine growth, but they have shortcomings. The baseline population is, by definition, abnormal, because the babies were born before term. In addition, the population of premature live births is very difficult to standardize for factors such as race, parity, socioeconomic status, maternal smoking, and maternal disease states.

Despite all this, intrauterine growth curves derived from postnatal data can be of great clinical assistance. The Colorado Intrauterine Growth Charts (Fig. 42-3) are among the better known. They provide percentiles of intrauterine growth for weight, length, and head circumference. In addition, a weight-to-length ratio is shown. From weight and length data, a ponderal index can be derived to depict proportionality. The growth curves in Fig. 42-3 were derived from a population of hospital-born and nonhospital-born infants who had mixed racial backgrounds and were living at an altitude of 5000 feet. Intrauterine growth curves derived from live births in other populations show significantly different values, particularly at some of the higher percentiles. However, the basic sigmoid shape of the curve persists. A few investigators have questioned the sigmoid shape of the growth curve as artifactual because it is based on the inaccuracies of menstrual dating. They suggest that when ultrasound dating is used, the curves become linear. With the use of growth curves and ultrasound, fewer pregnancies now are delivered at 43 and 44 weeks' gestation.[18]

Intrauterine growth curves for the last trimester of pregnancy can be very helpful in both fetal and neonatal medicine. One cannot assume without reservation that intrauterine growth is a steady process; it is conceivable that growth occurs in bursts of undetermined length. However, monitoring individual fetuses for growth against the baseline of an intrauterine growth scale can be helpful.

Fetal nutrition can be conceptualized in basic parameters that are familiar to the pediatrician. As with the child, two basic processes are under way: accretion of substance for growth of new tissues and oxidation or energy production for metabolism. Growth and development occur as a continuum from fetal to extrauterine existence, but the physiology of nutrition for that continuum changes abruptly at birth when the principal fetal organ for respiration and nutrition (the placenta) gives way to other organs and systems.

Glucose is a primary nutrient for the fetus, with its transplacental passage providing material for energy and for contributions to the fetal carbon pool. Initially, tissue growth is the main location for carbon and other constituents, with the 20-week fetus having little or no fat and about 90% water in its body composition. By term, fetal body water has decreased to about 76%, a figure high by adult standards; fat, a material of high carbon content, approximates 16%. These

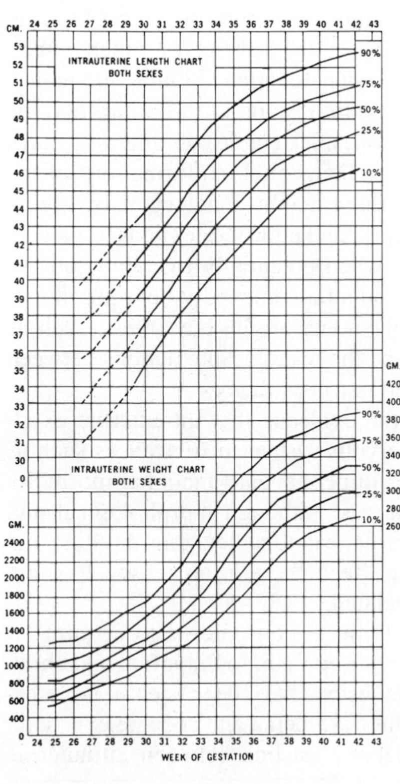

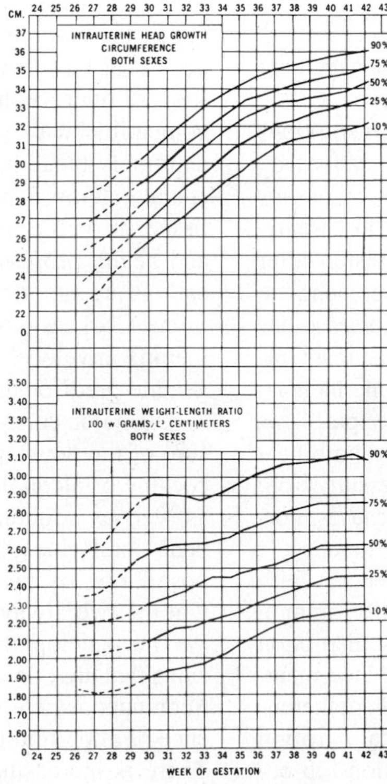

Fig. 42-3 Colorado Intrauterine Growth Charts. These charts were developed from measurements of babies after birth. They remain useful as a means for determining relative growth status of a baby compared with a reference population.

(From Lubchenco LO, et al: *Pediatrics* 37:403, 1966.)

observations, coupled with the instability of neonatal glucose metabolism, when the baby is stressed by infection or other problems, should reinforce the importance of glucose metabolism in the perinatal period and particular respect for the relatively depleted stores of energy in the small premature infant.

Amino acids, both essential and nonessential, are important as the building blocks of fetal protein synthesis. The uptake of essential amino acids through the placenta seemingly serves as a basic requirement for growth, yet the fetal ability to synthesize nonessential amino acids leaves the point unclear. Maternal nutritional state and placental function are crucial to fetal well-being and growth, whereas in the neonate, amino acids and nitrogen originate with digestion of milk and uptake through the portal venous route.[6]

The clinician dealing with the newborn must consider the prior fetal nutritional state. Fortunately, when the digestive system of the neonate is unable to function at a level sufficient to provide energy and growth, today's physicians have the knowledge and technology available to approximate the fetal nutritional state. Total parenteral nutrition effectively returns the baby to the fetal state, where all necessary nutrients, including essential and trace substances, enter directly into the circulation. Although this can be maintained for reasonable intervals, such therapy does have complications, including infection and liver disease, making very long-term parenteral nutrition of the child much more problematic than it is for the fetus.

FETAL SYSTEM FORMATION AND MALFORMATION

Teratology is the study of the etiology, development, structure, and classification of fetal abnormalities. Modern prenatal diagnosis provides information about the presence of structural abnormalities in a large portion of cases well before birth. The pediatrician and other health care providers must be prepared to discuss the teratological process with parents; that discussion increasingly includes management during pregnancy and the peripartum period.

The vast majority of major malformations and disruptions of system function can be categorized as being caused by genetic or intrauterine factors, maternal conditions, and drugs or other agents. Genetic factors have their origin in parental cell lines or in aberrations of initial cellular division after fertilization and are discussed in Chapter 40, Approaches to Genetic Diseases. Evaluation of risk for genetic disease has advanced rapidly as the techniques for prenatal diagnosis (including fetal cell and tissue sampling) have become increasingly sophisticated. Intrauterine factors include problems such as uterine abnormalities, amniotic bands, and umbilical cord or placental abnormalities. Mechanical pressure from uterine constraint (as in severe oligohydramnios) causes morphological changes categorized as a deformation sequence. If otherwise normally developing tissue is disrupted, as with the damage caused by amniotic bands from early amnion rupture, the resulting damage is categorized as a disruption sequence.[21] Maternal medical conditions that produce metabolic imbalance, such as diabetes mellitus and phenylketonuria (PKU), are teratogenic. The effect of maternal nutrition is of major concern, especially because the relationship between folic acid deficiency and neural tube defects now is well regognized.[13] Drugs and other agents are a major concern, because of the recognition that practically any drug is potentially teratogenic and the observation that chemical, radiation, or infectious agents may vary in degree of expression, depending on genetic predisposition or gestational age at the time of insult. (See the section on maternal nutrition, familial environment, and lifestyle on p. 505.)

The major systems are discussed in the following sections, with attention drawn to the gestational time of origin of the major types of abnormalities.

Central Nervous System

The central nervous system (CNS) starts from an ectodermal origin at about day 18 of gestation; development continues through delivery and long after birth. It is susceptible to teratogenic agents throughout the embryonic and fetal periods and is most susceptible during the first half to two thirds of the embryonic period.

The original neural plate develops into a neural tube that has cranial and caudal ends. The neural tube walls develop to become the brain and spinal cord; the inner part evolves into the ventricles of the brain and the central canal of the spinal cord. Brain development is very complex and passes through stages of a forebrain, midbrain, and hindbrain, with subsequent development of the cerebrum, midbrain structures, pons, and cerebellum. Cells that originally separated from the neural plate and became the neural crest develop into cranial, spinal, and autonomic ganglia, as well as the autonomic nervous system and chromaffin tissue, especially the adrenal medulla.

Malformations of the CNS confront the clinician frequently. Some of these defects are among the most grotesque, such as the anencephalic baby or infants who have very large encephaloceles. Application of life-supportive technology, in the form of assisted ventilation and nutrition, to babies who have such problems has been the subject of much public debate, as has the issue of organ donation.[35] Other anomalies, such as microcephaly or cystic lesions in the brain, may be compatible with life for variable lengths of time but carry extremely bleak prognoses. Congenital malformations of the spinal column, especially those that have defects in overlying tissue, also pose major moral and ethical dilemmas to parents and health professionals, when potentially treatable complications are superimposed on a fundamentally poor prognosis. Some CNS lesions are of known origin, but others, such as meningomyelocele, may be the result of interactions between genetic predisposition and extrinsic factors.

Of major concern is the evidence that intrauterine exposure of the developing nervous system to substances such as cocaine or alcohol results in permanent functional morbidity as well as structural changes. Although morphological and behavioral changes often appear together, thus inviting the postulation of cause and effect, there is no reason to think that the two always are related.

The developing fetal brain is now known to acquire lesions that are clinically very important to the infant and child. Spontaneous hemorrhagic lesions have been seen in the presence of alloimmune thrombocytopenia and cocaine exposure. There is increasing evidence of a link between intrauterine infection, premature rupture of the membranes, and increased risk of periventricular leukomalacia.[2,34]

Cardiovascular System

The cardiovascular system is the first to function, with a rudimentary blood circulation beginning in the third week. Initially, two tubes fuse to form a single tube that evolves into the four-chambered heart and great vessels. By the end of the fourth or fifth week, partitioning of the chambers is completed, with two atria and two ventricles. Equally complex is the initial formation of a truncus arteriosus, aortic sac, and aortic arches, which evolve by the eighth week into a fetal circulatory pattern. This system undergoes changes in flow patterns during adjustment to extrauterine existence.

Schematic representations of the process whereby the initial pair of tubes forms a single tube with subsequent twisting and formation of chambers and very complex vascular structures—some of which become atretic whereas others become dominant—can help in understanding spatial relationships and the reasons specific lesions develop. The lymphatic system, which develops in a similar time frame, is seen initially somewhat later than the cardiovascular system. The lymphatics have connections with the venous side of the developing cardiovascular system. Malformations of the cardiovascular system occur in approximately 7.5 of 1000 live births. The critical period for teratogenic effects terminates relatively early in the intrauterine period, but the process of formation is so complex that a multitude of possibilities for maldevelopment exists. The degree of severity varies considerably.

Some structural malformations, such as the patent foramen ovale type of atrial septal defect, may be functional only when another pathological condition exists. The patent ductus arteriosus (PDA) as a pathological entity occurs when closure fails after birth; in the fetal state, PDA is normal. Use of nonsteroidal antiinflammatory agents by pregnant women in the third trimester can cause premature closure of the ductus ateriosus and cardiac failure. Early malrotation of the fused cardiac tubes can result in dextrocardia. This can occur with an otherwise normal heart and great vessel structures and may not be a clinical problem if complete situs inversus of the viscera also is present. Dextrocardia without situs inversus often is a major problem because of a tendency for associated complex intrinsic abnormalities.

Intracardiac malformations, such as septal defects, are very common, especially in the ventricle. Complex problems, with formation of the great vessels evolving from an inappropriate partitioning of the truncus arteriosus, also are fairly common. Coarctation of the aortic arch is an example of a malformation that may be some distance from the heart itself. Manifestations of malformations can occur in utero and are believed in some instances to result in large-for-gestational-age infants. In severe and relatively rare instances, they can produce a form of nonimmune hydrops fetalis.

The physiology of cardiac function in the fetus is basically different from that in the infant, child, and adult. The fetal circulation has several parallel circuits, rather than the series (or sequence) circuitry that is established after the closure of physiological shunts during or shortly after birth (Fig. 42-4). The fetal heart has lower myocardial compliance and ventricular ability to increase stroke work. Increases in heart rate or filling pressure cause little increase in cardiac output.[10]

The pediatrician, pediatric cardiologist, and neonatologist increasingly are becoming involved with cardiac dysfunction before birth. The evaluation of fetal well-being includes that of cardiac status, with the result that problems such as cardiac arrhythmia or cardiac failure can be detected in utero. Fetal echocardiography can detect specific structural defects, with the interval from 18 to 24 weeks optimal for such an evaluation. Pregnant women who are themselves healthy are admitted to hospitals for treatment of fetal cardiovascular disease; maternal digitalization to treat fetal cardiac arrhythmias is an example of fetal treatment via the maternal and placental circulations.

Musculoskeletal System

Formation of the musculoskeletal structures becomes grossly apparent in the embryo by at least the fourth week, when limb buds—first the upper and subsequently the lower—become obvious. Muscle structures originate from mesoderm, much of which arises directly from the somites. Bone evolves from mesoderm that undergoes a process of chondrification. Cardiac muscle and other smooth muscles have a different origin in the splanchnic mesoderm of the primitive gastrointestinal tract. The origin of some muscles, such as those of the iris and extrinsic eye, is unclear. The limb buds elongate while forming bone and large-muscle masses. A process of rotation and growth, in which upper and lower extremities rotate in different directions, results in the muscle groupings and dermatome patterns of the child and adult.

Malformations of the limbs are relatively common; otherwise, skeletal and muscular abnormalities are rare. The health professional providing newborn care often is struck by the significant attention paid by parents to the extremities, particularly the hands of newborns. For this reason, relatively minor defects can have major emotional significance. Polydactyly or syndactyly are among the more common human malformations.

Many limb abnormalities are genetic in origin, but some malformations result from genetic predisposition interacting with environmental factors. The thalidomide deformities were a specific and perhaps relatively isolated example of limb teratogenesis.

Gastrointestinal System

The alimentary tract, developing from a primitive anlage seen initially at the fourth week, has three main divisions: foregut, midgut, and hindgut. Each of these has its own specific blood supply in the celiac, superior mesenteric, and inferior mesenteric arteries. Because development of each tract can be traced, abnormalities of the individual divisions are seen. The foregut, from the pharynx to the insertion of the common bile duct, develops into various structures, including the intestine and the liver and pancreas. Midgut structures include all the small intestines (except for the duodenum proximal to the insertion of the common bile duct) plus the cecum, appendix, ascending colon, and about two thirds of the proximal transverse colon. The midgut structures go through a complex rotation during development, whereby an

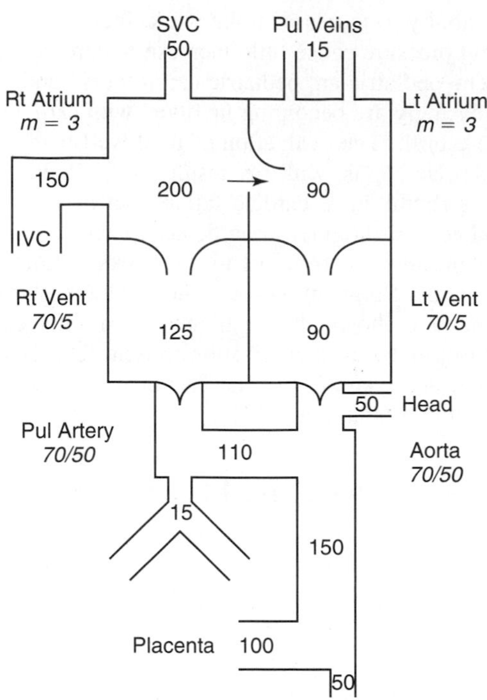

Fetal circulation in parallel

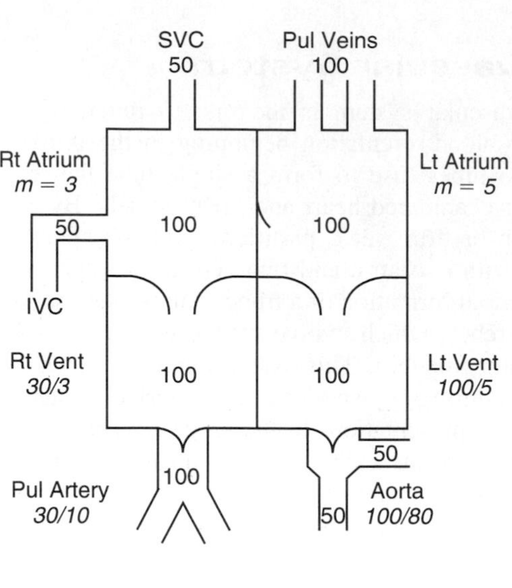

Extrauterine circulation in series

Fig. 42-4 In the fetus, blood follows several routes, with a small portion going to the lungs. Oxygenated and nonoxygenated blood is admixed in the fetus, and the placenta serves as the fetal organ of respiration. The risk of expression of cardiovascular disease differs before and after birth because of changes in structure and flow. The numbers inside the diagram represent blood flow (rate) and numbers in italics, pressure.

(From Flanagan MF, Yeager SB, Weindling SN: Cardiac disease. In Avery GB, et al, editors: *Neonatology,* Philadelphia, 1999, JB Lippincott.)

initial loop develops outside the fetal abdomen and rotates approximately 90 degrees at that time. At approximately the tenth week, these midgut intestinal structures return to the abdomen and go through a further complex rotation of 180 degrees, leading to the final anatomical relationships of the intestine. Hindgut structures include the transverse, descending, and sigmoid colon and rectum through the final portion of the anal canal, which develops from an anal pit. The cloaca (the early expanded end of the hindgut) and tissues of other origin form the perineal structures.

Alimentary tract malformations are fairly common and often are associated with other anomalies. The foregut has an initial tracheoesophageal common origin, with subsequent separation. Tracheoesophageal fistulas resulting from errors in formation of the tracheoesophageal septum occur in four basic patterns (see Chapter 49, Critical Neonatal Illnesses); early detection is important to prevent extensive aspiration pneumonitis. Errors of midgut development and malrotation lead to many problems, the most spectacular of which is the lack of return of the bowel to the abdominal cavity, with a resultant omphalocele. Other malrotation presentations include acute intestinal obstruction and ischemia in utero or at varying lengths of time after birth, often after initial feedings. Malformations of the intestinal tube in the form of stenosis, duplication, or atresia are of unclear origin but may result from problems with recanalization or from a compromised vascular supply. Hindgut malformations occur most commonly at the most distal portion, resulting in atresia, stenosis, membranous obstruction, or imperforate anus. Many other intestinal malformations can be seen. Of special interest is Meckel's diverticulum (an outpouching in the ileum), representing the remnant of the yolk stalk.

Respiratory System

Respiratory system formation is noteworthy for development that begins at approximately 26 days and goes on long after birth. Initial cell lines arise on the floor of the primitive pharynx and produce a laryngotracheal tube. Endoderm of this tube becomes the lining and glands of the lower respiratory system; connective tissue and cartilage of the respiratory system arise from splanchnic mesoderm.

Further growth of the endotracheal tube results in two lung buds that divide further into two sections on the left and three on the right; these correspond to the adult lobes. Branching continues after this point to form the pulmonary segments. At approximately 5 to 7 weeks after fertilization, a pseudoglandular period exists during which there is major growth of the bronchi and terminal bronchioles.

During the canalicular period beginning at 13 weeks and continuing to approximately 25 weeks, bronchioles and alveolar ducts develop, and significant vascularization occurs. From 24 weeks until birth, terminal sacs arise and become alveoli. These initially are lined by a cuboidal epithelium, which changes to a squamous form at about 26 weeks of gestation. Alveolar development continues through early childhood.

Surfactant is not produced until alveoli are formed. Complex cell types lining the alveoli have been described. A vacuolated cell, the type II pneumocyte, appears to have a secretory function and to be involved in alveolar stabilization through the elaboration of surfactant.

Anatomical malformations of the pulmonary parenchyma are unusual but include many dysplastic and cystic abnormalities. Because of the nature of fetal respiration, in which gas exchange is not occurring in the lung, these usually are not problematic until after birth. Abnormalities in development of the diaphragm, the most common of which is diaphragmatic hernia, are most common on the left and often are associated with severe restriction of lung development on one or both sides. Some babies who have diaphragmatic hernia develop pulmonary hypertension, a complication that includes elevated vascular resistance similar to that seen in the fetal state.

The pediatrician often is confronted with neonatal respiratory problems closely related to the formative and maturational status of the lung. For example, at 22 to 25 weeks' gestation, alveolar formation may not be advanced to the point of being able to support life for a limited time, even when exogenous surfactant, mechanical ventilation, and other interventions of present-day neonatal intensive care are utilized. This situation is encountered in the extremely low-birth-weigh infant, or "micropremie," and is basically a problem of pulmonary immaturity rather than prematurity. Whether respiratory distress syndrome is present after the birth of a premature baby depends largely on the functional cellular maturity of the infant's lungs. Treatment includes administration of exogenous surfactant until endogenous production occurs. (See Chapter 49, Critical Neonatal Illnesses.)

Hematopoietic System

Initial red cell formation is seen as early as day 14 after conception, when cells containing embryonic hemoglobin arise from the endothelium of primitive vessels of the yolk sac. Hematopoiesis within the embryo begins in the liver at approximately the sixth week. The liver is the most active site of hematopoiesis for the early part of the fetal life span. The bone marrow assumes the primary role at about the sixth month, and other sites, especially the spleen and lymph nodes, play a contributory role.

Fetal hemoglobin (Hb F) predominates for much of intrauterine existence and under normal circumstances is seen to a small degree in early infancy. Beginning at about the third month, some hemoglobin A (Hb A) is present (5% to 10%), and the proportion of Hb A to Hb F increases rapidly from about 35 weeks to term, when blood is approximately 50% to 65% Hb F. Hb F has an increased oxygen affinity compared with Hb A; this probably is the result of a differing action of 2,3-diphosphoglycerate (2,3-DPG), which facilitates oxygen saturation in the intrauterine environment. Blood group antigens are familial in their determination and can be identified as early as the second month of fetal life. Platelets also are seen at approximately the second month. The presence of hematopoietic abnormalities is important for the clinician to recognize. In the first place, certain hemoglobinopathies may result in intrauterine disease. Alpha-thalassemia results in hemoglobin Bart (tetrameric gamma chains), which has a very high oxygen affinity, resulting in intrauterine distress from tissue hypoxia and nonimmune hydrops fetalis. There are several other significant hemoglobinopathies (e.g., homozygous and heterozygous beta thalassemia) and structurally abnormal hemoglobins, such as HbS and HbC. Polymerase chain reaction (PCR) analysis of DNA from samples obtained by amniocentesis is now possible without the risks associated with attempts at direct fetal blood sampling. Hemolytic anemia secondary to maternal-fetal blood group incompatibilities and transplacental passage of antibody is an immune disease; however, it has a marked effect on hematopoiesis, resulting in erythroblastosis fetalis and extensive proliferation of hematopoietic tissue. Fetal thrombocytopenia may be primarily of fetal origin, or it may be associated with some form of extrinsic agent or process, such as immune antibody of maternal origin or intrauterine infection. Many fetal intrauterine hematological manifestations are part of disease processes involving other systems.

Percutaneous umbilical blood sampling (PUBS) (see p. 505) is clinically useful in many fetal hematological disorders. For example, PUBS can be used to diagnose thrombocytopenia and to administer platelet transfusions or for exchange transfusions in the fetus who has severe blood group isoimmunization.

Immune System

Immune system components function very early in fetal life, with some parts present as early as the eighth week and with a total rudimentary system capability by the twelfth week. Activation usually does not occur before birth. The cellular immune system originates in liver or spleen stem cells that migrate to the thymus at about the eighth week. These T cells enter the bloodstream and are distributed to the body, mainly to the lymph nodes and spleen. The antibody immune system generates IgM in lymphoid tissues as early as the eleventh week and IgG at about the twelfth week. IgA, IgD, and IgE are seen in the fetus in small amounts toward the end of pregnancy. Current thinking suggests that specific immunoglobulin synthesis occurs in stem cells or B cells. Passive transfer of maternal antibody has been demonstrated very early in fetal life. Maternal IgG is detectable as early as the fortieth day, and practically all cord IgG is maternal in origin, arising from both passive and active enzymatic transplacental passage. IgM is not transferred passively. The complement system has some fractions present during the embryonic period at the eighth week, and by 12 to 14 weeks of gestation a considerable complement fraction is present. Malformations of the fetal immune system, either of familial or developmental origin, have been described and have contributed to an understanding of the adult system.

Abnormalities are believed to exist in all parts of the immune system, and it is important that clinicians understand the basic possibilities because of the fetal and neonatal diseases that result. Fetal graft-versus-host reactions have been documented after intrauterine transfusions. Congenital infections activate the immune system, with an elevated cord IgM level possibly being evidence of such infections. Fetal IgM is usually not present until the third trimester. At term, IgM and IgA are detectable but at levels much less than in the adult. Transplacental antibody passage with effects on the fetus, as seen in isoimmunization (erythroblastosis fetalis), is the classic clinical example of fetal disease resulting from activation of a maternal immune system response.

Urogenital System

A close interrelationship exists between the development of two basic systems: the urinary (or excretory) system and the genital (or reproductive) system. There are three separate excretory organs in the human embryo: the pronephros, the mesonephros, and the metanephros. The metanephros appears at approximately the fifth week after fertilization, functions 2 to 3 weeks later, and remains as the permanent kidneys. The other two systems involute, with the mesonephros remaining as a few ducts in the male genital tract and as a vestigial remnant in the female. The final excretory system has two main divisions. The entire collecting system from the kidney to the bladder originates from the ureteric bud; nephrons arise from the mesodermic-metanephric mass. The kidney tissue appears originally in the early pelvic region and ascends into the abdomen. The bladder develops from the urogenital sinus and splanchnic mesenchyme. Excretory system function is present by approximately the ninth week; theoretically, contributions to amniotic fluid are possible at this time and become the major component later in gestation.

The prospective phenotype of the genital system is determined at fertilization. However, there is an indifferent stage of genital development ending at approximately the seventh week, with the gonads showing specific sexual characteristics. By the twelfth week after fertilization, the genitals are distinctly male or female. The Y chromosome appears to be responsible for the differentiation of testes. Masculinizing hormones from the testes stimulate development of mesonephric ducts into genital components and result in the external genitals forming a penis and scrotum. Feminization of the external genitalia seemingly occurs in the absence of androgens. Gonadal tissue has its origin in the lateral abdominal wall, with the testes descending into the scrotum late in fetal life.

Malformations of the urogenital system are relatively common and result in a myriad of morphological and microscopic manifestations. Some entities, such as renal agenesis, result in intrauterine manifestations, including oligohydramnios, and in morphological changes in the fetus. Other problems may present in the immediate neonatal period. For example, renal abnormalities that result in cystic lesions of the kidneys initially may be detected in the newborn period as abdominal masses found on physical examination or as abnormalities in renal function. Malformations in the vascular supply to the kidneys or the collecting system result in congenital problems such as obstructive uropathy that predispose the person to renal disease, manifesting in infancy and childhood. Malformations arising from problems of formation of the urogenital sinus and urachus may be severe, as in extrophy of the bladder or, less obviously, as in fistulae between perineal structures.

Abnormalities of kidney function can develop in utero. Maternal exposure to angiotensin-converting enzyme (ACE) inhibitors in the second and third trimester can cause renal failure and severe oligohydramnios without structural abnormalities.

Malformations of the genitals also can be complex in origin. Those resulting from errors in the sex-determining mechanism can result in hermaphrodites but are rare. Errors in sexual differentiation, producing pseudohermaphrodites, are somewhat more common. The presence of neonatal ambiguous genitalia is a true medical emergency, because congenital adrenal hyperplasia, which is characterized by fetal androgen excess and masculinization of the female fetus is accompanied by a deficiency of cortisol, leading to salt-wasting and shock. See Chapter 29, Fluid Therapy.

Special Considerations

Certain situations of fetal formation and malformation deserve special mention. The special senses, specifically those of the eyes and ears, are very sensitive to teratogenic activity and result in profound effects on the developing infant and child. Eye formation begins at the fourth week and proceeds very rapidly, especially through the sixth week. Malformations of the eye and ear may be associated with errors in genetic material; some syndromic conditions have readily identifiable eye and ear malformation patterns. Intrauterine infections, particularly rubella, can affect the eye and inner ear. Errors in position or morphology of the external ear often are associated with other malformations.

Malformations of the face and palate are of major concern. These have their origin in the embryonic branchial apparatus from which the face, pharynx, and attendant structures develop. Cleft lip often is associated with cleft palate but arises from distinctly different origins. Difficulties in these areas are probably of mixed genetic and environmental causation. The branchial arch merging in the formation of palate structures is most susceptible to teratogenic factors between 6 and 10 weeks of gestation.

FETUS, MOTHER, AND FAMILY

The fetus influences the mother and family physically and emotionally. Although expectations regarding conception and childbearing vary, the most positive situation is one of physical reproductive readiness and a wanted pregnancy. Psychological factors involved in the decision to become pregnant are extremely complex and heavily influenced by the reproductive instinct. More than 50% of all pregnancies in the United States, and a much higher portion of teenage and unmarried pregnancies, are unintended, but not necessarily unwanted, at conception.[36] Psychosocial situations that detract from optimum health before conception should be interpreted as the beginning of potential fetal risk.

Many maternal and familial situations of unfortunate familiarity to the physician provide a negative start for the fetus. A common example is pregnancy in the younger adolescent, who is both physically and emotionally immature and who may well not have a stable interpersonal relationship with her male partner. Postconceptual factors interact once fertilization occurs, with a progression of biochemical, physical, and emotional changes that influence the mother, father, and family. Poverty has a profound impact on the physical, emotional, and cognitive well-being of children, adolescents, and adults. These effects can be mitigated by health and social programs such as Medicaid and WIC.[7,27]

These postconceptual changes, some subtle and some not, permanently alter the parents' lifestyle. New situations demand behavioral adaptations and a process of coping. If the coping process is successful, major developmental progress has been made, especially by the mother; this usually is true to a lesser extent in the father and to varying degrees in people further removed. But if attitudes and the coping process are unsatisfactory, in certain situations an adoption or abortion might be considered.

The first missed menstrual period, an overt sign of change to many women, does not occur until after the stage of the dividing zygote essentially is complete. By the time of the second missed menstrual period, the embryonic stage is half over (see Fig. 42-2). Although the zygotic stage is relatively unaffected by teratogens, the embryonic stage is one of very high risk. Maternal and familial habits potentially injurious to the fetus are difficult to alter under any circumstances and are even more so when the mother does not yet know that she is pregnant. Pregnancy often is not confirmed in the present medical system until after the second missed menstrual period.

The customary use of trimesters as a means of dividing pregnancy into three intervals of equal length of particular personal or medical significance is considered imprecise by obstetricians and is discouraged for clinical situations. Previous generalizations are no longer applicable, such as the statement that viability is associated with the third trimester (see Fig. 42-2). Nonetheless, the trimester concept remains in common usage in discussions of the progression of pregnancy and its influence.

The first trimester may be the most important phase of adjustment to the fetal presence. Many physical symptoms such as fatigue, nausea, headache, and changes in emotional status may reflect emotional tension. However, there also are complex interactions of psychological stress and physiological change that can involve the autonomic nervous system, produce discomfort, and alter lifestyle.

The second trimester usually is marked by less overt signs of physical and emotional adjustment. System development in the fetus basically is complete, and major growth is occurring. This leads to the phenomenon of "quickening," when a woman feels fetal movements for the first time at about week 18 to 20 in the primigravida; in the multigravida, such movement may be felt 1 to 2 weeks earlier. Quickening undoubtedly represents a major milestone in the relationship between a mother and her fetus. This is the first overt or direct sign of independent fetal activity. Quickening can provide some information about gestational age. For some women it also serves as a milestone after which abortion is less acceptable.

The third trimester is marked by an acceleration of the fetal alteration of lifestyle. Maternal physical activity, previously undertaken easily, may become increasingly difficult. Sexual activity between parents may be subject to changes or even cessation. Preparation for delivery becomes more of a part of everyday life; childbirth education, financial planning, and other aspects of preparation and emotional adjustment should be in progress. Initially in the third trimester the maternal emotional state is oriented largely toward the fetus; however, as labor and delivery approach, a mother's concern, and very often the father's, may center more on maternal well-being.

FETUS, HEALTH PROFESSIONAL, AND SOCIETY

Great concern over the influence of factors such as smoking, alcohol consumption, radiation, and pesticides on the fetus is supported by many studies, and research continues to expand the database. Societies that advocate preconception care and the introduction of employment, nutritional, and lifestyle changes for women as soon as they miss a period (or preferably before conception), surely are enlightened in their advocacy of improved fetal and pregnancy outcomes.

Amniocentesis, chorionic villus, and percutaneous umbilical cord sampling represent procedures of major interest to individuals and society because they enable physicians to detect conditions incompatible with what is considered normal human existence. Moral and ethical concerns over these procedures are related to those associated with abortion generally. The debate over legalized abortion has brought to the fore concerns about the legal and interpersonal status of the fetus. Health professionals are embroiled in this debate, especially over whether a practitioner of perinatal medicine can personally oppose abortion by not mentioning all alternatives to patients.

Viability, or the capability of a fetus to assume an independent extrauterine existence, is a concept that demands attention and thought. We do know that 23 (22 completed weeks) weeks from the last menstrual period is the time at which some fetuses, if born into an environment in which neonatal intensive care is available, can survive. The role of the family in decision-making, especially that with regard to the extent of intervention for a baby born at the threshold of viability, is a matter of great interest. In particular, the frequency of somber modes of survival need to be presented sensitively. Parents and pediatricians have advocated that between 22 and 24 weeks parental wishes should be recognized and followed.[11,17]

The clinician must be aware of the close approximation of potential viability and gestation limits on legal abortion in the context of significant variations in clinical estimates of fetal age. The Supreme Court decision *(Roe v. Wade)* has been interpreted to support legal abortion until 24 weeks, a point previously thought to be the threshold for extrauterine viability, but menstrual dating by history and physical examination is only accurate within a range of 2 to 4 weeks. Confirmation of such dating by ultrasound examination improves the precision of dating to approximately 10%, so that a variation of 2 weeks still is possible in the late second trimester. Of course, dating in the first trimester is associated with a smaller margin of error.

THE IDENTIFICATION AND MANAGEMENT OF FETAL AND MATERNAL RISK

Any factor that increases the possibility of adverse pregnancy outcome contributes to risk. Medical risk includes physiological, nutritional, obstetrical, and genetic factors. Psychosocial risk includes psychological, social, environmental, and behavioral factors and personal habits. These two broad categories of risk often act concurrently, and individual risks may overlap, accompany, or follow each other. The relationship between risk factors and adverse outcome may be obvious, as with a specific toxic agent such as mercury; more often, however, risk is both subtle and cumulative.

Preconception Care

Health before pregnancy has become increasingly recognized as an important determinant of pregnancy outcome. Preparation for pregnancy should begin before conception, including assessment of risk and preventive or therapeutic intervention, including change of behavior. Box 42-1 illustrates the general categories and some specific problems that should be addressed in preconceptional care.

The concept of care before conception is related to, but not the same as, family planning; much more is involved than merely spacing of pregnancies. Wider acceptance of this concept within society may have a major effect on the outcome of pregnancy in such specific populations as adolescents. The role of the pediatrician in preconception and interconception care recently has been emphasized.[23]

Prenatal Care

A report entitled *Caring for Our Future: The Content of Prenatal Care* published by the U.S. Department of Health and Human Services (HHS) in 1989 defines the three basic components of prenatal care as (1) early and continuing risk assessment, (2) health promotion, and (3) medical and psychosocial interventions and follow-up.[8]

Previous discussion has emphasized that during the prenatal period the fetus is undergoing rapid and continuous growth and development. Anything that jeopardizes that process must be recognized as a fetal risk factor and assessed. Major contributors to fetal risk are listed in Box 42-2.

There is little doubt that prenatal care is associated with healthier babies and mothers. Much of the original interest in and emphasis on prenatal care involved pregnancy-induced hypertension (PIH) and the use of periodic blood pressure determinations. Standardized schedules (with details such as number and timing of visits, procedures, and studies) are available. In addition, the aforementioned HHS report offers

BOX 42-1

PRECONCEPTION CARE INVENTORY

- Medical history
  - Reproductive
  - Family
  - Genetic
  - Current medications
  - Substance use, including alcohol, tobacco, and illicit drugs
  - Abuse, physical and emotional
  - Environmental exposures
- General physical examination
- Immunization when indicated (rubella, hepatitis B)
- Screening
  - Sexually transmissible infections depending on risk assessment
  - Genetic disorders based on racial and ethnic background and family history (sickle hemoglobinopathies, beta-thalassemia, alpha-thalassemia, Tay-Sachs disease, cystic fibrosis, fragile X syndrome, Duchenne muscular dystrophy)
- Counseling
  - HIV prevention and testing
  - Abstention from tobacco and alcohol
  - Folic acid supplementation when attempting pregnancy and during first trimester
  - Good control of preexisting medical conditions such as diabetes, hypertension

Modified from *Guidelines for perinatal care,* ed 4, Elk Grove Village, Ill, and Washington, DC, 1997, American Academy of Pediatrics, American College of Obstetricians and Gynecologists.

BOX 42-2

MAJOR CONTRIBUTORS TO FETAL RISK

Genetic
- Chromosome abnormalities
- Inherited traits

Maternal-Familial Environment and Lifestyle
- Socioeconomic status
- Social environment
- Physical environment
  - Radiation
  - Teratogens
- Nutrition
- Smoking or secondary exposure to smoke
- Drugs or alcohol abuse
- Lack of prenatal care

Maternal Reproductive Capability and Health
- Age, weight, height
- Reproductive tract abnormalities
- Maternal medical disorders
  - Cardiac
  - Respiratory
  - Renal
  - Hematological (e.g., sickle cell disease)
  - Metabolic (e.g., diabetes, thyroid disorders, phenylketonuria)
  - Epilepsy
- Emotional status

Placenta and Membrane Disorders
- Implantation (abdominal, tubal, previa)
- Vessel and cord complications
- Abruption
- Premature rupture of membranes (PROM) and infection

Maternal-Fetal Unit
- Multiple gestation
- Obstetrical complications
  - Malposition and malpresentation
  - Cephalopelvic disproportion
- Abnormal fetal growth and gestation
- Isoimmunization (erythroblastosis fetalis)
- Intrauterine infections
- Pregnancy-induced hypertension

suggestions, including the addition of preconception care, to traditional prenatal care.

Assessing Fetal Status Before Labor

The clinician is obligated to make every effort to identify risk and practice expectant fetal medicine. Pediatricians must be familiar with the basic principles of techniques used to gather information. Family and reproductive history, fetal structure and growth, heart rate, and amniotic fluid and fetal blood analyses provide the basis for the majority of these methods. Some are noninvasive, have been part of obstetrical practice for years, and provide statistically valid information—for example, history taking and the measurement of uterine size. They are used to screen the need for other investigative techniques, such as those discussed below.

Fetal activity. The duration, amplitude, and frequency of fetal movement after quickening and in the third trimester can provide important information about fetal well-being. An inactive fetus may be chronically compromised, and the rapid onset of inactivity in a previously active fetus can be ominous. Daily assessment of fetal movement has some value as a test of fetal well-being. Obstetricians often ask women to report if they perceive fewer than 10 fetal movements in a 2-hour period of close observation ("kick counts"). Change in fetal activity does not predict specific fetal abnormalities but warrants follow-up with more standardized nonstress tests of fetal well-being.

Fetal heart rate. The normal fetal heart rate (FHR) settles in the range of 120 to 160 beats/min by the final trimester and is monitored easily by a Doppler device (after 10 weeks), a fetoscope (after 20 weeks), and a stethoscope (after 28 weeks). During labor, continuous electronic fetal monitoring is used widely but has not been shown conclusively to be more efficacious than intermittent auscultation, despite many large studies.

Bradycardia, especially fewer than 100 beats/min, is of concern because of an association with acute or chronic distress. Explanation for its presence must be sought. The list of possible causes is long and includes many that have a poor outcome, such as placental insufficiency. An intrinsic fetal cause, heart block, is not as ominous. Tachycardia usually occurs as an autonomic response to stimulation and can indicate fetal normality. It also may be associated with a maternal condition, such as pyrexia. Intrinsic fetal arrhythmias, such as supraventricular tachycardia, can result in secondary manifestations, including hydrops fetalis.

Uterine size. The uterus and the products of conception are monitored closely at each prenatal visit. Measurements of fundal height above the symphysis are obtained and plotted; the umbilicus is reached by 20 to 22 weeks. Deviations from the expected curve may indicate a number of abnormal and high-risk states.

Fundal height at a level greater than expected may be the result of a miscalculation of dates, with the pregnancy being further along than anticipated. Another relatively straightforward cause of unexpectedly large uterine size is multiple pregnancy. Conversely, fetal causes of smaller than expected uterine size include pregnancy less advanced than anticipated and many problems that lead to intrauterine growth retardation (IUGR).

The amniotic fluid volume deviations, oligohydramnios or polyhydramnios, may be detected initially by abnormal uterine size or fundal height. Confirmation and further study by ultrasonography should follow, because imaging by ultrasound can estimate more precisely the volume of fluid present and assess fetal structures.

Under normal circumstances, amniotic fluid volume increases until 36 weeks and then decreases. Oligohydramnios thus can be associated with both postterm and postmature pregnancies. The pediatrician also needs to be alert to those fetal situations in preterm pregnancies in which oligohydramnios occurs, inasmuch as this may be associated with a number of disease processes, including IUGR and renal abnormalities with severely compromised urinary excretion. Renal agenesis (Potter's syndrome) or dysplasia and structural and functional renal problems may not become evident until after birth.

Polyhydramnios may result from maternal problems, such as diabetes, or from fetal causes. The pediatrician immediately should suspect fetal and neonatal abnormalities of the upper gastrointestinal tract, such as esophageal obstruction, because the normal circulation of amniotic fluid is interrupted on the absorptive side of the loop in these conditions. The baby will require special attention at birth and probable surgical intervention. Central nervous system and neuromuscular abnormalities, such as myotonic dystrophy, impair fetal swallowing and cause polyhydramnios.

Ultrasonography. Clinical ultrasound has had a profound effect on all aspects of perinatal medicine. A transducer, acoustically linked to the skin surface by a gel, transmits ultrasonic vibrations, and the returning sound echoes are processed electronically to produce a two-dimensional image. New technology is now allowing production of three-dimensional images.[31]

Two- and three-dimensional images are used to evaluate fetal size and morphology. Doppler ultrasound is used to measure velocity of blood flow in fetal and maternal blood vessels.[25] Color Doppler depicts local flow by color encoding an estimate of the mean Doppler frequency shift at a particular position, thereby demonstrating direction and velocity of blood flow. This is useful in evaluating fetal heart structure. Power Doppler ultrasound is a technique that encodes the amount of blood flow in color. Its usefulness includes evaluation of placental abnormalities.

Although no clinically untoward effects of clinical ultrasound have been documented in humans, potential structural and functional biological effects have been hypothesized. Doppler ultrasound theoretically has greater potential for harm because of the continuous, rather than pulsed, wave and the amount of time in use. The U.S. Food and Drug Administration, together with the American Institute of Ultrasound in Medicine and other organizations, has developed standards for safe information display.

Controversy continues about the usefulness of and indications for routine prenatal ultrasound examination; a number of large clinical studies provide conflicting results. An American College of Obstetricians and Gynecologists (ACOG) "practice pattern review" developed the following conclusions: specificity of ultrasound fetal anomaly survey is high (99%), sensitivity varies widely and depends on clinical setting and professional skill, uncertainty exists whether the outcome of pregnancies with fetal anomalies is improved, and in low-risk pregnancy, routine ultrasound use is not associated with lower perinatal mortality or morbidity, nor fewer unnecessary interventions. The conclusion is that ultrasound should be performed for specific indications only in low-risk pregnancy.[32]

A National Institutes of Health consensus development conference in 1984 concluded that, when there is an accepted medical indication, ultrasound improves pregnancy outcome, and listed a large number of specific risk situations. Routine screening, identification of fetal gender, parental education, and parental desire to see their fetus were not considered appropriate, because of possible risk and ethical concerns. It is estimated that approximately 70% of pregnancies undergo ultrasound examination.

Ultrasound evaluations are a very important part of evaluation of fetal well-being. Measurements of fetal growth pattern and distribution and amniotic fluid volume are important observations. A fetus for which biometric parameters are concordant and within acceptable range for gestational age and for which amniotic fluid volume is normal has a low risk of adverse outcome, such as stillbirth. While the sensitivity varies with the type of birth defect and the skill of the operator, ultrasound can detect many birth defects. Ultrasound also is being used as a noninvasive tool to detect minor markers of trisomy 21.

Fetal surgery. Fetal surgery is a controversial intervention that has attracted considerable medical and public interest. Pediatric care practitioners should be aware of the general level of activity in this field, since they may be consulted by families in their practices. The media and increasingly the worldwide web serve as informants about possible interventions, often without adequate attention to status of investigation and outcomes.

Fetal risk identification through accurate and timely prenatal diagnosis by ultrasound in conjunction with fetal sampling techniques and technical ability to intervene surgically though endoscopic or open techniques has resulted in attempts to correct fetal lesions that interfere with normal development. Fetal problems, theoretically amenable to surgical correction with resultant continued development in utero, include diaphragmatic hernia, cystic adenomatoid malformation, urinary obstruction (urethral valves), twin-twin transfusion syndrome resulting from placental vascular abnormalities, aqueductal stenosis, and myelomeningocele. Select situations such as congenital diaphragmatic hernia without liver herniation have been subject to randomized controlled studies of intervention and outcome evaluation. Risks and benefit evaluation of fetal surgery should include the mother as well as the fetus.[1]

Maternal serum screening. An increasingly valuable technique of perinatal risk assessment involves maternal serum screening for markers that correlate with risk of specific outcomes. Essentially all pregnant women in the United States are offered testing for detection of neural tube defects and trisomy 18 and 21. Analysis commonly includes alpha feto-protein, unconjugated estriol, and human chorionic gonadotrophin ("triple markers"). The sensitivity of detection of spina bifida is approximately 80%, with a 3% to 5% false-positive rate. Ultrasound sensitivity for open neural tube defect is 90% to 95%. Women who have unexplained elevated serum alpha feto-protein are at risk for adverse pregnancy outcomes other than neural tube defects, including intrauterine growth retardation and stillbirth. The sensitivity of a triple marker study panel for trisomy 21 is 60%, with a false-positive rate of 5% to 6%. Women whose "screens" are positive are offered amniocentesis and often accept the procedural risk to achieve a definitive diagnosis. Other maternal serum and urine markers are under study, as are innovations involving combinations of marker studies and techniques such as transvaginal ultrasound measurement of nuchal lucency, a marker for aneuploidy.

Amniocentesis. Amniotic fluid bathes the fetus, is swallowed by the fetus, and contains fetal cells, urine, and other substances, including pulmonary surfactant. The technique for obtaining a specimen of this fluid by percutaneous aspiration has been made more successful by the use of ultrasonography.

Diagnostic amniocentesis at 14 to 18 weeks of gestation, in conjunction with ultrasonography, confirms placental localization, fetal size, and gestational age, in addition to providing information obtained from fluid analysis. Evaluation of fetal cells through karyotyping can detect chromosomal abnormalities before potential extrauterine viability, so that termination can be considered. Fluorescent in-situ hybridization (FISH) studies are available, which produce results for some aneuploidies within only a few days, as opposed to the 10- to 21-day requirement for standard metaphase karyotype analysis. Molecular genetic studies on DNA extracted from fetal cells are expanding so rapidly that the pediatrician is advised to contact a prenatal diagnostic center to determine if prenatal testing has become available for a specific disorder.[30]

Chorionic villus sampling. Chorionic villus sampling (CVS) involves ultrasound-directed aspiration of trophoblastic tissue surrounding the gestational sac during the first trimester. The approach can be transcervical or abdominal. CVS usually is performed at 10 to 12 completed gestational weeks, thereby providing information significantly earlier than does amniocentesis.

Studies of the safety and efficacy of CVS have found a slightly higher rate of pregnancy loss and procedure failure than midtrimester amniocentesis. Some centers have higher rates of loss with transcervical than with transabdominal CVS. It generally is accepted that CVS requires more professional experience than does amniocentesis. The advantage of CVS is more rapid and earlier diagnostic information, allowing more time for consultation and intervention, including abortion. The disadvantages of CVS include the slightly higher loss rate, lack of information about neural tube defect, and the possible need for later amniocentesis to clarify CVS results or to diagnose neural tube defect. In recent years, controversy has existed concerning possible limb reduction defects associated with CVS. The procedure usually is not performed before 10 weeks in an effort to minimize this risk.

Percutaneous umbilical blood sampling (PUBS or cordocentesis). Direct aspiration of fetal blood by means of a needle placed transabdominally through maternal skin and into a fetal blood vessel is another technique facilitated by ultrasound that has improved fetal diagnosis and therapy significantly. Sampling is possible from about 17 weeks to term with greater apparent safety than with other techniques. Fetoscopy has a complication rate of 4% to 5%, fetal scalp sampling requires labor and cervical dilation, and placental aspiration results in contamination with maternal blood in more than 50% of attempts.

Common diagnostic indications for PUBS are the need for rapid fetal karyotype and evaluation of fetal isoimmune hemolytic disease. The main treatment is transfusion for fetal anemia. The PUBS technique is useful because it provides immediate fetal blood specimens for study of hemoglobin, platelets, blood gases, blood typing, and other parameters in the same fashion as studies in the neonate. Risk is a concern, with fetal loss a possibility. Currently, this is a technique that requires sophisticated technology and expertise.

Nonstress and contraction stress tests. Tests that record fetal heart rate (FHR) and the presence, absence, or temporal sequence of uterine contractions are used extensively. The FHR is driven by neurogenic reflex mechanisms similar to those seen in newborns.

The nonstress test (NST) observes FHR patterns by continuous fetal monitoring before the onset of labor. The interrelationship between FHR and fetal movement or spontaneous uterine contractions is observed. Such testing can begin at 26 to 28 weeks but usually is performed closer to term. NST is indicated for patients at risk for uteroplacental insufficiency and fetal death. It is repeated once or twice weekly. A normal or "reactive" NST is defined by a normal baseline heart rate (120 to 160 beats/min), moderate variability (5 to 20 beats/min), two or more accelerations of at least 15 seconds duration, and a 15-beats/min peak above baseline in a 20-minute period.[16] A nonreactive or abnormal NST is defined as one that does not meet these standardized criteria and may actually show decelerations. The test has a false-positive rate for prediction of adverse fetal outcome of approximately 80%.

The contraction stress test (CST), or oxytocin challenge test (OCT), uses oxytocin-stimulated uterine contractions and records the FHR response. The NST is used more commonly; the CST is employed by some physicians only after a nonreactive (abnormal) NST result. The presence of repeated late decelerations is considered problematic. Interpretations can be difficult, and there are relative and absolute contraindications for performing CST, in addition to a false-positive rate of approximately 50%. Interpretation requires experience. Nipple stimulation rather than oxytocin challenge is used by some practitioners to induce uterine contractions.

Fetal biophysical profile. Fetal well-being can be assessed through the use of multiple parameters identified on ultrasound. Items such as muscle tone, body movement, breathing movement, amniotic fluid volume, and results of the NST can be identified and a score derived in a fashion similar to that for determining an Apgar score.

The biophysical profile probably has a lower false-positive rate than the CST and has been found to have a reasonable correlation with fetal blood gas scores. Some investigators have found the combination of amniotic fluid volume assessment and NST to have equivalent performance as a biophysical profile.

MATERNAL NUTRITION, FAMILIAL ENVIRONMENT, AND LIFESTYLE

Many authorities have pointed to socioeconomic status and social environment as causes of fetal risk. Delineation of specific influences is difficult, but poverty undoubtedly is important, as are nutrition and hygiene. Intrauterine infection is more frequent in mothers of lower socioeconomic status. Emotional influences on fetal wastage have been discussed; the possibility that medical or socioeconomic deprivation contributes as well cannot be discounted.

Maternal Nutrition

Maternal nutritional disorders represent a definite risk to the fetus, including situations in which gross deprivation is not apparent. The supply of substrate to the fetus for growth originates with the maternal circulation and passes through an interface with fetal tissue at the placenta. Placental insufficiency can result in intrauterine growth retardation (IUGR) that is not of maternal origin. The relation between maternal and fetal nutrition is complex. Maternal dietary changes usually do not directly or rapidly influence fetal well-being; thus, the positive or negative effects of changes in maternal nutrition are not recognized easily. Maternal weight is an important but not overriding concern.

Traditionally, two types of nutritional deficiency have been conceptualized: general caloric or energy-related deficiency states and specific deficiencies. Deprivation of maternal caloric intake to the point where fetal growth is markedly impaired also may be associated with specific deficiencies. If maternal caloric deprivation is severe, fertility is decreased.

Women whose prepregnancy weight is below standard for height tend to have babies whose weight is less than expected. Women who are obese tend to have babies of higher weight. Problems such as hyperemesis gravidarum can be sufficient to result in fetal caloric deprivation. The expression during reproductive years of eating disorders that often start during late childhood and adolescence, such as anorexia, is a possible fetal risk.

Specific deficiencies are well recognized; their risk to the fetus can be reduced through public health and individual clinical interventions. Vitamin deficiency has been of interest, and problems such as congenital beriberi (lack of thiamin) and infant calcium disorders (maternal vitamin D lack) are of historic interest and decreasing incidence. Recent studies have confirmed that neural tube defects can be reduced by consuming folic acid, with the best protection being achieved when 0.4 mg is ingested from at least 1 month before conception through the first month of pregnancy.

Minerals are a major concern in pregnancy. Iodine deficiency is said to be the most common cause of preventable mental deficiency in the world; treatment during pregnancy protects the fetal brain, with later treatment being much less beneficial to neurological status.[38] Zinc deficiency also may be associated with anomalies. Maternal anemia caused by reduced availability of iron is well known; the fetus and infant, as a result, can have low iron stores, making the infant susceptible to iron deficiency if intake after birth is inadequate.

Environmental factors, such as radiation, chemicals, and drugs, affect all socioeconomic classes. Radiation exposure in mammals causes fetal death, growth retardation, and congenital malformation, with the central nervous system commonly affected. The relationship between embryonic or fetal irradiation and carcinogenesis is unclear. Effects are both dose and rate related. Death during the preimplantation period, malformation during early organogenesis, and cell deletion and hypoplasia during fetal life form a general pattern in animal studies. Guidelines exist for limiting radiation to the embryo and fetus during occupational exposure or elective diagnostic techniques; however, dilemmas often arise as a result of lack of foreknowledge about pregnancy, nonelective medical evaluations, and emotional factors. When necessary, a radiation physicist should be consulted.

Chemicals in the environment are of natural and synthetic origin, with the latter being of greater concern. Certain substances, such as pesticides and mercury, have received publicity, with more study of other potential environmental toxins needed. Many agents potentially are more toxic to the embryo, fetus, and neonate than to older children and adults.

Mercury exposure is a major issue in environmental health, in large part because of its toxicity to the brain and especially the more susceptible fetal brain. Mercury is common in the environment in small amounts and occurs in three forms: the metallic element, inorganic salts, and organic compounds. Exposure to predatory fish is the primary exposure, and local fish advisory bans are available from the U.S. Environmental Protection Agency. Women planning pregnancy, and those pregnant or breast-feeding, as well as children younger than 15 years of age, have been advised not to eat swordfish or shark. Thimerosal, a mercury-containing preservative used since the 1930s in many vaccines, has recently been the subject of concern and controversy,[3] resulting in its no longer being used in vaccines (see Chapter 18, Immunizations).

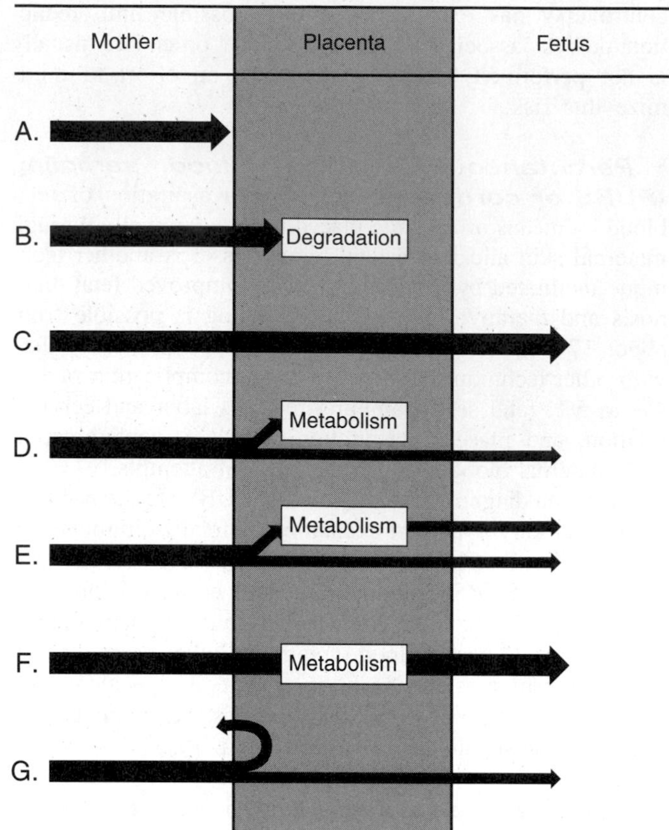

Fig. 42-5 Maternofetal transport patterns and the role of the placenta, a fetal organ with active metabolic activity. **A** illustrates a placental barrier with minimal uptake or transfer (e.g., succinylcholine, highly charged quaternary compounds). **B** represents active placental uptake and degradation without transfer as seen with insulin; **C** represents placental uptake and transfer without significant change as with bilirubin. In **D,** the placenta is actively involved in uptake, partial use, and transfer (oxygen, glucose, amino acids, free fatty acids). **E** represents uptake, partial metabolism, and transfer (cyclosporine). In **F,** the placenta actively modifies during transfer (25-hydroxyvitamin D_3). In **G,** carrier-coupled uptake occurs with release of ligand to the fetus and regeneration of carrier on the maternal side (transferrin-iron).

(From Pridjian G: Feto-maternal interactions: placental physiology and its role as a go-between. In Avery GB, et al, editors: *Neonatology,* Philadelphia, 1999, JB Lippincott.)

Drugs and Other Substances

Drug use during pregnancy is extensive and may be on the rise. The physician must be concerned about all types: legitimate (nonprescription and prescription), social, illegal, and abusive. All health care professionals, especially the primary care physician, should recognize that the concept of the placenta as an effective toxic-substance barrier between maternal and fetal circulation has been discarded.

Maternal-fetal pharmacology is complex (Fig. 42-5), with the placenta serving as an organ of exchange. Placental diffusing capability or permeability of the simple variety is operative for many substances; energy-utilizing transport also is important. Virtually all drugs in the maternal circulation should be assumed to cross the placenta, and all should be considered potentially teratogenic. The risk to the fetus depends on a number of factors, including concentration, length of exposure, and when exposure occurs during gestation.

Therapeutic agents, both prescribed and nonprescribed, may be taken before pregnancy is recognized, thereby placing the products of conception at risk during the period of organogenesis in early gestation. An important benefit of preconception or interconception care is the opportunity to identify medication uses that are necessary, such as anticonvulsants, or desirable, such as nonnarcotic analgesics, and monitor or modify exposure. Examples of problems include fetal hydantoin syndrome and the potential effects on the mother and fetus of aspirin, including clotting abnormalities and disruption of prostaglandin synthesis.

Many of the therapeutic agents indicated during the

course of pregnancy and delivery require judicious use, because of known and potential risks. Antimicrobials are necessary when treating maternal conditions, such as urinary tract or gynecological infections, but must be used with the knowledge that well-recognized fetal problems can result, such as bone and dental dysplasias associated with fetal tetracycline exposure and the potential hearing loss of fetal aminoglycoside toxicity. Cardiovascular medications that cross the placenta readily, such as digitalis, can be used to treat the fetus and can cause fetal problems. Pediatricians need to know the effects of obstetrical drugs on the fetus, including narcotics, oxytocin, and magnesium sulfate, which can cause depressed respiration, hyperbilirubinemia, and hypotonia, respectively. Socially used and abused drugs are very well known to pediatricians for their deleterious effect on the fetus, newborn, child, and adult. Mothers who smoke have babies who are smaller than those of nonsmokers by an average of 200 g. Varied active agents in smoke, such as carbon monoxide and nicotine, have physiological effects; although studies to document long-term negative neurodevelopmental outcomes have given mixed results, the clear medical consensus is that smoking must be considered a health hazard for the fetus and newborn. Maternal alcohol consumption is associated with fetal alcohol syndrome (FAS) and should be discouraged during pregnancy in all trimesters, although it is difficult to demonstrate deleterious effects from small amounts consumed.

Addictive drug use during pregnancy creates major medical and societal problems of seemingly increasing and endlessly complex proportions. Many, if not most, users have lifestyles that include factors, such as poor nutrition or lack of prenatal care, that present significant background risk regardless of the addictive agent. Heroin is known to reach the fetus soon after maternal use, with intrauterine dependency and withdrawal recognized. Cocaine is considered to be responsible, directly or indirectly, for many admissions to neonatal intensive care units. It can result in problems such as placental abruption that compromise the fetal and neonatal cardiovascular and neurological systems. Investigative efforts to characterize and quantify long-term neurodevelopmental effects are ongoing (see Chapter 50, Prenatal Drug Abuse and Neonatal Drug Withdrawal Syndrome).

Identification of environmental and lifestyle risk relies largely on the maternal medical history. When specific factors such as radiation or chemical exposure are detected, assessment of fetal well-being, especially its growth and morphology, may be helpful. In many situations, however, decisions to continue or terminate pregnancy are made based on nebulous possible fetal effects, involve parental emotions and values, and require compassionate, nondirective counseling in addition to the presentation of available scientific knowledge.

Maternal Reproductive Capability and Health

Certain maternal factors result in fetal risk regardless of the nature of the products of conception. Pregnancy can produce physiological changes in the mother that may complicate preexisting maternal conditions, thereby jeopardizing the fetus. For example, mothers who have asymptomatic cardiac disease when nongravid may decompensate with pregnancy.

Maternal biological factors such as age, weight, height, race, parity, and previous obstetrical history affect fetal risk directly. Perinatal mortality increases at the extremes of maternal age; one large observational study determined the lowest risk to be in the 16- to 19-year range.[4] However, such observations should not be taken to encourage adolescent pregnancies; pregnancy in those younger than age 16 has definite associated risks, and pregnancy throughout the teen years is associated with medical and social morbidity. Newborn weight and height are related to maternal nutrition, socioeconomic status, and other variables, which may jeopardize the fetus by increasing the incidence of prematurity or intrapartum complications. Race is a complex factor that includes socioeconomic considerations; some congenital anomalies and medical conditions may be racially predisposed. Congenital maternal reproductive tract abnormalities frequently are associated with fetal wastage via spontaneous abortion or prematurity. Cervical incompetence occurs in 1 of 500 to 600 pregnancies and can result in premature delivery. The interval between pregnancies is an important contributor to the risk of low birth weights.

Maternal medical disorders carry a significant risk to both fetus and mother. Cyanotic congenital heart disease in a mother clearly is related to fetal problems, including intrauterine growth retardation and prematurity. Elective abortion is a consideration if maternal cardiac decompensation later in the pregnancy is anticipated. Asthma can threaten mother and fetus but commonly is well-controlled with medication. Tuberculosis demands aggressive management of maternal disease with attention to potential fetal exposure to drugs. Pregnancy in women who have cystic fibrosis presents the fetus with a variety of medications, maternal pulmonary insufficiency, and possible nutritional deficiency.

Preexistent and new-onset renal disease can occur during pregnancy. The fetal risk increases markedly in the presence of maternal proteinuria, impaired renal function, and hypertension. The latter can result in placental changes leading to intrauterine growth restriction (IUGR). Adverse fetal outcome from urinary tract infection relates primarily to the risk of premature birth. Successful pregnancy is possible in women who have had kidney transplantation, with the best outcomes seen among women who have good, stable renal function; time since transplantation of at least 2 years; and no evidence of rejection. Some risks are associated with exposure to immunosuppressants, such as corticosteroids, but they do not prohibit a good outcome.

Maternal hematological problems are very common. In developing countries, anemia has been demonstrated to correlate with low birth weight; the effect of moderate maternal iron deficiency on the fetus is unclear. Some hemoglobinopathies can increase fetal mortality and morbidity profoundly, either as a result of maternal health status or of fetal disease. Pregnant patients who have sickle cell disease require close attention. Immune sensitization problems (Rh, ABO) are discussed on pp. 510 and 511 and in Chapter 48, Common Neonatal Illnesses.

Maternal metabolic disorders can be significant for the fetus. The interaction of mother and fetus seems limitless; compounds are metabolized actively on both sides of the placenta; fetal organogenesis and development may be affected, and fetal end organs may respond to maternal abnormalities. Two conditions, diabetes and thyroid disorder, deserve special mention.

Diabetes in pregnancy causes a myriad of fetal complications, including stillbirth, increased frequency of congenital anomalies, macrosomia (a large-for-gestational-age [LGA] state characterized by an increase in fat but not in total body water), and conversely, growth retardation in a small number of infants. Evidence suggests that fetal pulmonary and neurological maturity may be delayed in these pregnancies. In addition, obstetrical problems, including preeclampsia, hydramnios, and intrapartum complications, resulting from excessive size, increase risk further. As discussed previously, glucose is a primary metabolite of the fetus. Pregnancies complicated by diabetes probably cause fluctuations in maternal-fetal glucose, with resultant fetal hyperinsulinism and hypoglycemia. These fetuses have an increase in pancreatic islet tissue leading to fetal hyperinsulinism, which may be associated with a growth hormone effect that results in macrosomia. Severe maternal diabetes, especially when complicated by prepregnancy vascular disease, may result in small fetuses rather than macrosomia, because of placental insufficiency and fetal nutritional deficit. Close control of maternal diabetes results in a better overall perinatal outcome.[22]

Maternal thyroid disease is much less common than diabetes but also has profound fetal effects. Fetal thyroid function appears by 12 weeks of gestation; thyroxine and triiodothyronine probably can cross the placenta in small amounts in either direction. Classic cretinism, a reflection of maternal and fetal hypothyroidism, includes obvious fetal neurodevelopmental problems and is a result of endemic iodine deficiency or autoimmune maternal thyroiditis. Evidence is accumulating that maternal hypothyroidism, even when subclinical, interferes with normal fetal brain development and may be prevented by maternal screening and treatment.[20] Abortions, stillbirths, anomalies, and prematurity can be associated with hypothyroidism. Hyperthyroidism, when untreated, increases fetal wastage. Its treatment, however, carries a definite fetal risk, because antithyroid drugs may affect the fetal thyroid, and surgical intervention carries an operative risk to fetus and mother. Postoperative treatment with thyroid replacement therapy may minimize fetal complications.

Although seizure disorders are common, their course during pregnancy is difficult to predict with certainty. The status of approximately half of those affected is unchanged, and of the remaining number, half improve and half become worse. Status epilepticus is an emergency for the mother and fetus, but unfortunately there appears to be an increased incidence of congenital anomalies among infants of mothers who have seizures, even after cessation of anticonvulsant medication. Some anticonvulsants, such as trimethadione and valproic acid, are clearly teratogenic. Phenytoin has been linked with a fetal hydantoin syndrome, although the actual incidence is much debated. Phenobarbital, carbamazepine, phenytoin, and other medications have a broad-based impact on fetal enzymatic systems; they are associated with vitamin K–dependent coagulation factor deficiency in neonates. Many perinatologists recommend additional supplementation of vitamin K in the last month of pregnancy. Women who have epilepsy have an approximately 1 in 40 chance that their children will develop the same condition.

Seizures that appear de novo in pregnancy must be evaluated thoroughly. Eclampsia usually manifests with other signs and symptoms but is associated with a high incidence of fetal and neonatal complications (see the section on pregnancy-induced hypertension at the end of this chapter).

Maternal emotional status presents too complex a relationship with physical and familial status to be used as a specific fetal risk factor in most situations. Whether maternal emotional illness, not related to pregnancy, can affect the fetus directly is unclear. Pregnancy-caused or pregnancy-aggravated crises leading to abortion, drug abuse, or poor maternal nutrition can generate obvious fetal consequences.

Placenta and Membrane Disorders

The placenta and associated membranes are tissues on which the fetus depends for respiration, nutrition, protection, and other functions. Manifestations of placental disease are diverse, severe, and include fetal death, as well as distress, hypoxia, shock, anemia, polycythemia, infection, congenital anomalies, and neoplasia.

The implantation site is normally in the upper uterus but may be in the lower segment, in the tubes, or rarely, in the abdominal cavity. Maternal anatomical factors may contribute to abnormal implantations. Abdominal and tubal (ectopic) pregnancies are potential disasters for both mother and fetus; except for a rare surviving abdominal fetus, fetal wastage is nearly uniform, and maternal mortality and morbidity are common.

Placenta previa is associated with multiparity and places the fetus at risk in the event of hemorrhage; premature delivery, often by cesarean section, is necessary. Abruption of the placenta often is associated with maternal problems, including preeclampsia, hypertension, renal disease, and multiparity. Sudden fetal demise may occur after an extensive placental separation; lesser degrees of separation can result in hypoxia and acute fetal stress. Bleeding from placenta previa and abruption is usually maternal but can be fetal and sufficient to cause fetal hypovolemia and anemia.

Cord abnormalities are unusual but may have severe consequences. A short umbilical cord may be complicated by abruption. True knots are unusual, but they do occur and can cause fetal stress. Vasa previa and velamentous insertion are difficult to identify before labor but can result in distress and fetal exsanguination. A circumvallate placenta is associated with fetal growth restriction. Vascular abnormalities within the main placental structure occur rarely; fetal risk in monochorionic multiple pregnancies includes the possibility of twin-to-twin transfusion syndrome, in which arteriovenous vascular anastomoses result in blood flow between the fetuses and in severe circulatory problems for recipient or donor or both.

A vascular abnormality of the cord observed in 1% of pregnancies is a two-vessel cord with but a single umbilical artery, rather than the normal two. Current evidence suggests that anomalies are associated with a two-vessel cord.[9,37] The risk of associated abnormalities, including fetal growth retardation, renal abnormalities, and aneuploidy, approximates 7%.

Premature, or prolonged, rupture of membranes (PROM) is a major contributor to perinatal mortality and morbidity. It often is defined as rupture that occurs an hour or more before onset of labor; it is usually spontaneous but may be accidental during an examination or artificially induced to precipitate labor. Regardless of classification, the perinatal care team must be aware that an inevitable process of increased fetal risk begins soon after rupture and that prospective treatment protocols are desirable. Most protocols stipulate evaluation and treatment in relation to the time since rupture. Most authorities consider 18 hours after rupture of the membranes to be the beginning of accelerated risk.

The primary cause of fetal and maternal morbidity and mortality in PROM is sepsis. At term, labor occurs within 24 hours of rupture in 80% of pregnancies; in preterm pregnancies, labor begins within 24 hours in fewer than 50%. Prolonged rupture of membranes, with 24 hours or more elapsed between rupture and delivery, is much more common in preterm pregnancies. The cause of spontaneous rupture often is not clear and, except for entities such as an incompetent cervix, there is no statistical correlation with prior risk factors.

The frequency and degree of inflammation of membranes, cord, or fetus vary directly with time and onset of labor. Infection apparently ascends to the fetus through the cervix, with labor accelerating the process. Antibiotics given before delivery are of uncertain value in providing effective maternal treatment but do prevent some cases of sepsis in the fetus and newborn. This is particularly true of chemoprophylaxis strategies for prevention of group B streptococcal infection.

A dilemma in fetal risk management occurs in the PROM pregnancy that is significantly preterm. The fetus in this situation is at risk not only from infection but also from premature birth and its complications, especially respiratory distress syndrome (RDS). On the other hand, it is debated whether PROM results in an acceleration of fetal lung maturity that decreases the risk of RDS. The clinician has available prepartum agents (corticosteroids) that seem to accelerate pulmonary maturity in certain situations and improve postpartum status overall in certain populations. A 1994 National Institutes of Health (NIH) Consensus Development Conference recommended antenatal treatment with corticosteroids for fetuses between 24 and 32 weeks that have premature rupture of membranes.[14]

An increasing body of knowledge suggests an increased risk of neurological sequelae among babies born prematurely after PROM. An increased incidence of periventricular leukomalacia and cerebral palsy seems to be at least associated with, if not caused by, chorioamnionitis. It is unknown at present whether immediate induced vaginal delivery or cesarean section delivery with preterm PROM will decrease these risks.

Maternal-Fetal Unit

Fetal risk and poor perinatal outcome frequently are associated with pathophysiological processes in which both mother and fetus play an integral role. Causality in some situations is well understood, as in, for example, isoimmunization, but there also are situations, such as toxemia, in which causality is not yet clear.

Premature birth. Prematurity and its complications are the prime contributors to perinatal mortality and morbidity. Only birth asphyxia challenges this entity as the most common indication for prompt, skilled intervention. The problems of prematurity and low birth weight are similar but not identical (see Chapter 45 [Three], Recovery Period).

The prevention and management of premature birth has been and remains the primary objective of perinatal care providers. Prematurity probably is multifactorial in origin, and its causes likely will remain unclear for the foreseeable future, inasmuch as the precise mechanisms that cause normal labor have yet to be elucidated. Many of the factors listed in Box 42-2 as contributors to fetal risk precipitate adverse outcomes directly or indirectly through premature birth.[19]

Pharmacological intervention. Tocolysis, or inhibition of uterine activity, is therapy directed at preventing premature birth once labor has begun. Pharmacological agents have been used with this intent for some time, but with minimal success.

The theoretical basis for the use of beta-mimetic drugs as tocolytics is their inhibitory effect on uterine contractions through activation of beta-adrenergic receptors. Beta-adrenergic receptors are subdivided into beta-1 and beta-2 groups, with the latter dominant in blood vessels and the uterus. Isoxsuprine hydrochloride, a derivative of catecholamine; ritodrine hydrochloride; and terbutaline sulfate have been used and are believed to be effective in depressing uterine contractions. A beta-mimetic that has a narrow impact on only the uterus has yet to emerge. Thus, maternal and fetal or neonatal side effects do occur, with cardiovascular, pulmonary, and metabolic complications documented. For example, neonatal hypoglycemia is a recognized complication of isoxsuprine therapy.

Calcium antagonists also may be useful in the future but as yet are unproved. Magnesium sulfate is no more effective than other agents but is used commonly because of a better maternal side effect profile than the beta-adrenergic agents. Prostaglandin synthetase inhibitors may have a future role, but their use at present cannot be recommended, because of their potential vasoactive effect on the fetus, especially on the ductus arteriosus.

Tocolytic therapy continues to be controversial; however, such intervention appears beneficial in some preterm labors, especially between 26 and 33 weeks of gestation.[24] A major benefit to be gained from a relatively short delay of preterm delivery through tocolysis or other interventions is a time interval long enough (24 to 48 hours) to allow administration of corticosteroids for the enhancement of fetal lung maturity and maternal antibiotics for group B streptococcal sepsis prophylaxis.

Prevention of prematurity. Certain authorities, especially Papiernik et al[28] in France and Creasy[12] in the United States, have documented and promoted comprehensive programs to prevent prematurity through alteration of patient and professional behavior. Key to such efforts is the identification of the risk factors associated with prematurity. Subsequent interventions to alter risk might be medical, but social and behavioral interventions may be equally important. Unfortunately, studies of such interventions have had mixed results.

For patients who have had previous idiopathic preterm birth, screening for bacterial vaginosis in early pregnancy and treatment with oral antibiotics has been associated with a significant decrease in risk of subsequent preterm birth. Theoretically, bacterial vaginosis promotes upper genital tract colonization, which triggers early parturition.

Health professionals can play a major role in such preventive programs because they ensure that the need for intervention is documented and that intervention occurs. In addition to management of specific medical problems, alterations in lifestyle, work environment, and behavior patterns may be necessary. Good prenatal care and early work leave may be very important. Countries where such policies exist, such as Sweden, have low prematurity rates but it is unclear whether this is an association or a contributing relationship.

Multiple gestation. Multiple gestation is relatively common (twins occur naturally in about 1 in 88 births) and increases fetal risk. These risks range from those that are placental in origin, such as twin-to-twin transfusion, to fetal malformations that are rare, as in conjoined twins, to the much more frequent problems of prematurity and obstetrical complications. Multiple gestation is one of the three most common causes of prematurity. Complications of labor and delivery markedly increase the risk of hypoxia or trauma, with the second-born twin being more susceptible to damage than the first. The incidence of multiple gestation has recently and remarkably increased, because of the application of newer reproductive technologies to treat infertility.

Obstetrical complications. Obstetrical complications jeopardize the fetus, the most dire manifestation being intrapartum fetal demise. Even the most ideally healthy fetus is at increased risk during labor and delivery. Stress to the fetus may be documented retrospectively by low Apgar scores, poor recovery after birth, and subsequent complications. A fetus chronically compromised by adverse factors, such as diabetes in pregnancy, may be compromised further by obstetrical problems.

Abnormal presentations, such as breech and transverse lie, greatly increase fetal risk, as does cephalopelvic disproportion (a mismatch between the maternal pelvis and the fetal head). Malproportion can be predominantly fetal, as in congenital hydrocephalus, or maternal when congenital pelvic bone abnormalities exist.

Abnormal growth and gestation. Discrepancies between fetal growth and gestation often are manifestations of an underlying disease process but may occur without apparent cause. A general discussion of intrauterine growth and nutrition, including growth curves, was introduced earlier (see Fig. 42-3). Regardless of cause, discrepancies in growth and gestation often can result in such severe risk to the fetus as to be more worrisome than the underlying problem. Postmaturity occurs much less frequently than prematurity but presents increased risk to the fetus. Continued growth in utero increases the risk of macrosomia and birth trauma. Placental insufficiency may result in the development of hypoxia and acidosis during labor that manifests as fetal distress, poor Apgar scores, and perinatal hypoxic encephalopathy. Meconium passage is common and poses a risk of meconium aspiration syndrome (MAS). It may also signal peripartum infection.[29]

Deviations of growth and gestation can be cumulative for fetal risk. The premature infant also affected by intrauterine growth retardation tolerates intrauterine stress poorly, may manifest RDS or gestationally related apnea after birth, and is at risk for the development of hypoglycemia. New information is emerging about the long-term effects of fetal growth retardation. Fetal nutritional adaptations to placental insufficiency may persist through adulthood, since there is an increased risk of coronary artery disease and chronic hypertension among adults who were born with IUGR.[5] The clinician should appreciate that evaluation of the fetus or newborn by birth weight and gestational age can provide specific information that facilitates diagnosis and treatment.

Isoimmunization. Isoimmunization is a disease of the maternal-fetal unit that is decreasing in incidence because of successful efforts to prevent Rh disease with Rho globulin (RhoGAM). Passage into the maternal circulation of fetal red cells, which possess antigens not present in the mother, stimulates production of antibodies. Maternal antibodies of the IgG class cross the placenta, resulting in a hemolytic process in the fetus that can be severe. Variations on this basic theme occur. The initial isoimmunization can occur with blood transfusions, with spontaneous or induced abortion, or with the first or subsequent pregnancy. Small amounts of red cell antigen contained in blood measuring 1 ml or less (especially if repeated) can cause an antibody response even in normal pregnancies. Sensitization risk is increased by complications such as preeclampsia or cesarean section.

Rh incompatibility is associated with a variable but often severe sensitization that can cause stillbirth, massive fetal erythropoiesis or erythroblastosis, anemia, hydrops fetalis, and other systemic manifestations. Hyperbilirubinemia occurs in the newborn and to a lesser degree in utero, where the maternal liver clears bilirubin.

The incidence of fetal Rh disease varies with the prevalence of Rh negativity. This genetically determined state is not often documented in Asians and Native Americans; however, it occurs in 15% of whites, resulting in the possibility of approximately 9% of their pregnancies involving an Rh-negative woman carrying an Rh-positive fetus. With successful prophylaxis by RhoGAM, the incidence of D-antigen isoimmunization is decreased, but isoimmunization still occurs in response to a number of other red cell antigens, including c, C, e, E, Kell, Kidd, and Duffy. These "minor" antigens can cause very serious hemolysis. Some patients even acquire more than one hemolytic antibody.

Since the delineation of the cause of Rh sensitization, a wide range of diagnostic and therapeutic methods has become available that make Rh incompatibility treatment a paradigm for intensive perinatal care. Today's routine proce-

Table 42-1 Maternal-Fetal Infections: the TORCH Acronym

Infection	Agent	Comment
T—Toxoplasmosis	Protozoa	Transplacental passage; mild maternal illness, variable fetal or neonatal manifestations; maternal antibody test available
O—Other	Virus, bacteria, parasite	HIV, *Listeria,* syphilis, gonococcus, group B streptococcus, varicella-zoster, malaria
R—Rubella	Virus	Prototype for transplacental viral infections; severe and chronic fetal or neonatal disease; antibody test and immunization available
C—Cytomegalovirus	Virus	Transplacental passage, ubiquitous agent; broad spectrum of fetal or infant manifestations
H—Herpes simplex	Virus	Rare transplacental passage, usual intrapartum transmission from maternal genitalia; severe neonatal disease; antiviral treatment available

Modified frorn Nahmias AJ: *Hosp Pract* 9:5, 1974.

dures for the disease include initial screening for the presence of isoimmunization and for Rh-negative women who are still candidates for prevention with RhoGAM. If hemolytic antibody is detected, maternal serum levels and amniotic fluid analysis can assess the possibility of severe fetal illness. Amniotic fluid can now be analyzed by PCR-DNA analysis to determine fetal blood type and the risk of hemolytic disease. When a high hemolytic risk is detected, fetal blood sampling via the percutaneous umbilical route (see p. 505) can make an accurate assessment and provide a means to administer an in utero blood transfusion. The timing of delivery includes consideration of fetal health, the possibility of in utero treatment, and the degree of prematurity. Immediate, aggressive neonatal intensive care, including exchange transfusion and cardiopulmonary support, may be indicated.

Incompatibilities of the ABO system result from the presence of maternal anti-A or anti-B antibodies when the fetus' blood type is group A or B and the mother's is group O. Severe hemolysis is much less common, even though ABO incompatibility potentially is present in about 20% of pregnancies. Fetal erythrocytes appear to have fewer antigenic loci, and maternal antibody appears in IgA, IgM, and IgG forms, with only the latter crossing the placenta. These facts may explain why ABO isoimmunization usually is of greater concern in the newborn than in the fetus. Stillbirths and hydrops fetalis are rare, but prolonged neonatal hyperbilirubinemia occurs frequently.

Intrauterine Infections

Our understanding of the scope of the problem of intrauterine infections and its fetal effects has broadened considerably but probably is far from complete. Expression ranges from fetal loss from spontaneous abortion and stillbirth through severely debilitating congenital anomalies resulting from teratogenic effects, to subtle systemic manifestations, including those of the central nervous system, not detected until later in childhood when problems with higher cerebral function and behavior become manifest.

The important infectious agents include viruses, bacteria, spirochetes, and protozoa. The route for infection varies with the agent and can be transplacental, ascending through the cervix, with or without the rupture of membranes (which provide an imperfect protective cover), as well as through direct contact with the fetus during passage through the birth canal.

The pediatric practitioner needs to have a basic appreciation for the variety of intrauterine infectious agents and the pathophysiological processes and clinical problems they invoke. Table 42-1 is a modification of the TORCH acronym that has served well for several decades. Since it was originally derived, however, newer knowledge has emerged concerning the intrauterine manifestations of *Parvovirus* B-19 infection (fetal hydrops and death) and the complexities of human immunodeficiency virus.

Human immunodeficiency virus (HIV). Fetal, intrauterine, and peripartum considerations are but a small part of the story of this agent; a complete discussion appears in Chapter 219, Human Immunodeficiency Virus Infection and Acquired Immunodeficiency Syndrome. Given the magnitude of the HIV/AIDS problem and that of the three predominant modes of transmission in the United States (sexual contact, percutaneous contact with contaminated sharps, and fetal or infant contact with an infected mother), two involve reproduction, the pediatrician must know the specifics of transmission and intervention. Our newly developed ability to decrease vertical transmission from mother to fetus makes universal screening of pregnant women for HIV imperative, despite complaints regarding "invasion of privacy." The fetus can be infected in utero, although the exact timing is uncertain; other possibilities for transmission include transplacental or peripartum, as well as postpartum (through breast-feeding). The timing of the expression of disease in children is variable and thought to be determined by whether the infection was acquired before delivery or during parturition. Without antiviral therapy, approximately 25% of babies born to HIV-infected women will become infected themselves. The use of antepartum, intrapartum, and postpartum zidovudine decreases the risk of congenital infection to 8%. Even further decreases in transmission may be associated with multiple-agent antiretroviral therapy and by cesarean section delivery or vaginal delivery within 4 hours postrupture of membranes.[33] Whether cesarean section delivery is protective for fetuses of women who have low viral loads is uncertain.[15] Newborns discovered to be at risk should be continued on antiretroviral agents until their infective status becomes clarified.

Rubella. Rubella virus is recognized as a potent teratogen. Infections during the first trimester result in approximately 20% of fetuses being severely damaged or malformed, with second-trimester involvement damaging 10%. Third-trimester infection has presented few clinical problems. The expression of rubella syndrome is variable. Manifestations of first-trimester fetal disease can be severe (e.g., abortion, stillbirth, and severe rubella syndrome). Severe rubella syndrome includes growth retardation, eye defects (cataracts and microphthalmia), congenital cardiac defects, deafness, thrombocytopenic purpura, hepatosplenomegaly, bone lesions, pneumonitis, and cerebral defects (microcephaly, encephalitis, mental retardation, and spastic quadriplegia). Infections in the second trimester are variable and tend to be less severe.

The high fetal risk and potentially devastating consequences of intrauterine rubella have stimulated aggressive efforts to prevent maternal rubella. Congenital rubella is a reportable disease. Vaccination of children between the ages of 1 and 12 years is routine. Administration of vaccine to women of childbearing age has been controversial because of concern of possible vaccine effects on the developing fetus. However, a registry of cases in which women received vaccine within 3 months of conception has found no cases of congenital rubella syndrome. Vaccine virus was cultured from fetal and placental tissue, but teratogenic effects were not seen. Preconception counseling should include rubella serotesting to determine the need for vaccination before conception occurs.

Cytomegalovirus (CMV) infections. The cytomegaloviruses may be the most common cause of congenital infections, occurring in somewhat fewer than 1% of births. This group of viruses is widespread and produces various apparent and inapparent infections in the general population: 3% to 5% of pregnant women have this virus in their cervical canal or urine. Fetal infection usually occurs transplacentally.

The fetal disease has been called *cytomegalic inclusion disease* (CID) because of the large inclusion-bearing cells found in urine and many organs. Severe CID includes hepatosplenomegaly, microcephaly, cerebral calcifications, mental and motor manifestations, and chorioretinitis. Reviews suggest that expression of intrauterine infections is variable and that full recognition of incidence is yet to come. Serological tests for CMV are available and can provide presumptive evidence for infection; however, reliability is not as good as with rubella titers, and a vaccine is not available.

Herpes simplex virus infections. Herpes simplex virus (HSV) infections in humans result from two strains, types 1 and 2, each with distinct serotypes yet some cross-reactivity. Perinatal disease usually is associated with type 2, although type 1 is more common in the general population. Type 2 HSV produces genital lesions and is transmitted sexually in most instances. Herpetic disease in the fetus or newborn is relatively rare but can be devastating. Transmission occurs by direct contact at birth or by ascending transcervical infection after rupture of the membranes. Transplacental infection early in pregnancy with fetal manifestations similar to those of CMV infection has been documented but apparently is rare.

Newborn manifestations of intrapartum contact are well known. They range from vesicular lesions of the skin to encephalitis and severe systemic disease, with a mortality of more than 90% without treatment and severe central nervous system morbidity in those who survive. Expression probably is linked to primary versus recurrent maternal disease, being more intense in the former.

A major recent development is the success of antiviral agents in the treatment of systemic herpes infection—in particular, encephalitis. Early diagnosis and treatment are essential. Prevention is desirable and possible. (See the discussion of herpes infections in Chapter 217.) Current recommended management for a pregnant mother who has genital lesions is a cesarean birth to prevent fetal inoculation by passage through the birth canal. This should be performed within 4 hours of rupture of the membranes, if possible.

Toxoplasmosis. Toxoplasmosis is caused by an intracellular protozoan parasite, *Toxoplasma gondii*. Infection is widespread, is congenital or acquired, and varies in expression from almost asymptomatic to generalized and fatal. The fetus is at risk for death when the infection occurs early in pregnancy or may be born with fully developed disease indicative of a long intrauterine course. Chorioretinitis, cerebral calcification, hydrocephalus or microcephaly, hepatosplenomegaly, and a host of systemic manifestations are observed. Long-term sequelae, especially involving the central nervous system, are present in the majority of infants who have severe infection and who survive.

It is believed that pregnant women become infected through exposure to cat feces or incompletely cooked meat. Prevention of toxoplasmosis in pregnancy is possible by careful handwashing after changing cat litter, gardening, or handling raw meat. The incidence of the perinatal disease is higher in certain locales.

Detection of toxoplasma antibody by a reference laboratory can document the onset of infection, if IgM antibody appears, coupled with a rise of IgG antibody in paired samples over at least 2 weeks. Antibody levels can remain high for years; unchanging elevated levels indicate old infection. Infection before pregnancy appears to prevent congenital disease, but there is a single report of congenital infection with maternal disease that preceded conception. If toxoplasmosis is suspected by serology, amniotic fluid can be tested by using PCR for toxoplasma. Treatment with pyrimethamine and sulfadiazine is effective in decreasing the severity of congenital infection. Congenital toxoplasmosis may be inapparent at birth and not recognized until later in infancy or early childhood. See Chapter 246, Parasitic Infections.

Other intrauterine infections. Fetal syphilis is caused by transplacental passage of *Treponema pallidum*. Fetal infection has been thought not to occur before the eighteenth week of gestation, but this is subject to dispute. Pregnancy in a woman who has primary- or secondary-stage disease may terminate in stillbirth. Other manifestations vary from presentation in the newborn to those appearing in the first 2 years of life or later. In general, the earlier the onset of infection, the more severe the lesions. Severe fetal infection manifests in early infancy by osteochondritis and periostitis, rhinitis (snuffles), rash, and mucosal fissures, or patches. Premarital and prenatal screening for syphilis, in conjunction with antibiotic treatment, has decreased the incidence of intrauterine disease effectively, especially that with the more severe or classic manifestations. Unfortunately, a resurgence occurred in the late 1990s. Recently trained clinicians have not had the experience in recognizing congenital syphilis that many of their older colleagues have had, sometimes resulting in a delayed diagnosis. Detection of disease during pregnancy and treatment with penicillin will arrest development of the fetal disease. (See Chapter 262, Sexually Transmitted Diseases.)

Listeria monocytogenes is a gram-positive bacillus that probably plays an important role in overall fetal wastage. Incidence varies widely. Fetal death may occur after a relatively mild systemic maternal disease. Listeria chorioamnionitis can be diagnosed by amniocentesis, and successful antibiotic treatment is possible. Neonatal manifestations include systemic disease at birth or a delayed appearance as meningitis in the second to fifth week of life, with a characteristic monocellular cerebrospinal fluid.

Group B streptococcal (GBS) disease has many similarities in presentation to that of *Listeria* and is a more common problem (see Chapter 49, Critical Neonatal Illnesses). Infection is acquired by exposure to organisms during parturition. Maternal immune status and bacterial subtype are important determinants of virulence. The Centers for Disease Control and Prevention, the American College of Obstetricians and Gynecologists, and the American Academy of Pediatrics have proposed prophylactic regimens; debate continues over which to use. One regimen involves ascertaining maternal colonization status at 36 weeks' gestation by culture and treating all colonized women as labor commences. Another protocol treats only women in labor who have a risk factor such as prolonged rupture of membranes, preterm labor, fever or systemic manifestations, or a previous child who had GBS disease, whether their GBS status be positive or unknown.

All neonatal services should have a structured approach to identifying and treating patients at risk for, or manifesting, GBS disease in its two dominant modes of presentation—a fulminant hemorrhagic pneumonitis in the first hours after birth or neonatal meningitis that appears a few days or weeks after birth.

Other known intrauterine infections include agents of all known classes: undoubtedly, many others are yet to be discovered. Many viruses can cause fetal infection, including varicella, coxsackie virus, mumps, rubeola, echovirus, hepatitis, and others. *Mycoplasma pneumoniae* also is an important perinatal agent, and malaria is a significant fetal threat in many areas of the world.

Assessment of fetal well-being in suspected intrauterine infection follows the precepts mentioned above. Serological tests have been alluded to in the discussion of individual entities and will be helpful, as in rubella. Unfortunately, although diagnostic certainty often is quite satisfactory for the newborn, it is less reliable for the fetus.

Pregnancy-induced hypertension. Hypertension of pregnancy is a major contributor to fetal risk. A group of diseases seen only in pregnancy and presenting with acute and chronic manifestations of hypertension, edema, and proteinuria may be lumped together in this category. *Preeclampsia* is another term for the basic process, which can be severe; when convulsions or coma occur, *eclampsia* is present. Chronic hypertensive vascular disease with pregnancy is believed by many to be a separate disease state that can have superimposed toxemic manifestations.

Spontaneous premature labor of uncertain etiology occurs frequently in all hypertensive gestations. Premature birth is increased further in incidence because early delivery frequently is elected on maternal or fetal indication. As the severity of the disease increases, and particularly when eclampsia develops, stillbirth and maternal death become much more frequent. Intrauterine growth retardation is seen in a third of perinatal deaths associated with toxemia. From the fetal viewpoint, this disease process presents a bleak perspective; fetal stress is significant, and labor and delivery are often premature and timed for maternal relief rather than for fetal well-being. Neonatal complications are many and severe.

Successful perinatal management of maternal hypertension relies heavily on early detection during prenatal care. When the process is discovered, intensive perinatal care may be necessary, with anticonvulsants, especially magnesium sulfate, a mainstay of therapy. Severe preeclampsia is a significant maternal threat and may lead necessarily to a decision to deliver a premature baby. Careful maternal and fetal surveillance, including assessment of fetal well-being by nonstress testing, biophysical profile, amniotic fluid volume determinations, Doppler studies of umbilical blood flow, and ultrasound studies of fetal growth are all part of proper expectant management.

REFERENCES

1. Albanese CT, Harrison MR: Surgical treatment for fetal disease: the state of the art, *Ann N Y Acad Sci* 847:74, 1998.
2. Alexander JM, et al: Clinical chorioamnionitis and the prognosis for the very low birth weight, *Obstet Gynecol* 91:725, 1998.
3. American Academy of Pediatrics, Committee on Infectious Diseases: Thimerosal in vaccines: an interim report to clinicians, *Pediatrics* 104: 570, 1999.
4. Amini SB, et al: Births to teenagers: trends and obstetric outcomes, *Obstet Gynecol* 87:668, 1996.
5. Barker DJ: The long-term outcome of retarded fetal growth, *Clin Obstet Gynecol* 40:853, 1997.
6. Battaglia F, Meschia G: *An introduction to fetal physiology,* Orlando, Fla, 1986, Academic Press.
7. Brooks-Gunn J, Duncan GJ: The effects of poverty on children, *Future Child* 7:55, 1997.
8. *Caring for our future: the content of prenatal care,* Report of the Public Health Service Expert Panel on the Content of Prenatal Care, US Public Health Service, Washington, DC, 1989, Department of Health and Human Services.
9. Chow JS, et al: Frequency and nature of structural abnormalities with single umbilical arteries, *J Ultrasound Med* 17:765, 1998.
10. Clyman RI, Heymann MA: Fetal cardiovascular physiology. In Creasy RK, Resnik R, editors: *Maternal-fetal medicine,* ed 4, Philadelphia, 1999, WB Saunders.
11. Committee on Obstetric Practice, American College of Obstetricians and Gynecologists; Committee on Fetus and Newborn, American Academy of Pediatrics: *Perinatal care at the threshold of viability,* Washington, DC, and Elk Grove, Ill, 1995.
12. Creasy RK: Preterm birth prevention: where are we? *Am J Obstet Gynecol* 168:4, 1223, 1993.
13. Czeizel AE, Dudas I: Prevention of the first occurrence of neural-tube defects by periconceptional vitamin supplementation, *N Engl J Med* 327:1832, 1992.

14. *Effect of corticosteroids for fetal lung maturity on perinatal outcomes,* Consensus Development Conference Statement, March 1994, National Institutes of Health.
15. Elective cesarean-section versus vaginal delivery in prevention of vertical HIV-1 transmission: a randomised clinical trial, *Lancet* 353:1035, 1999.
16. Electronic fetal heart rate monitoring: research guidelines for interpretation, National Institute of Child Health and Human Development Research Planning Workshop, *Am J Obstet Gynecol* 179:560, 1997.
17. Fetus and Newborn Committee, Canadian Paediatric Society; Maternal-Fetal Medicine Committee, Society of Obstetrics and Gynaecologists of Canada: Management of the woman with threatened birth of an infant of extremely low gestational age, *Can Med Assoc J* 151:547, 1994.
18. Gardosi J: Routine ultrasound is the method of choice for dating pregnancy, *Br J Obstet Gynaecol* 105:933, 1997.
19. Goldenberg RL, Rouse DJ: Medical progress: prevention of preterm birth, *N Engl J Med* 339:313, 1998.
20. Haddow JE, et al: Maternal thyroid deficiency during pregnancy and subsequent neuropsychological development of the child, *N Engl J Med* 341:549, 1999.
21. Jones KL: *Smith's recognizable patterns of human malformation,* ed 4, Philadelphia, 1988, WB Saunders.
22. Kios SL, Buchanan TA: Current concepts: gestational diabetes mellitus, *N Engl J Med* 341:23, 1749, 1999.
23. Klerman L, et al: Interconception care: a new role for the pediatrician, *Pediatrics* 93:327, 1994.
24. Korenbrot CC, Alto LH, Laros RK Jr: The cost effectiveness of stopping labor with beta-adrenergic treatment, *N Engl J Med* 310:691, 1984.
25. Martinoli C, et al: Power Doppler sonography: clinical applications, *Eur J Radiol* 27:S133, 1998.
26. Mittendorf R, Herbst AL: DES exposure: an update, *Contemp Pediatr* 11:59, 1994.
27. Moss N, Carver K: The effect of WIC and Medicaid on infant mortality in the United States, *Am J Public Health* 27:S133, 1998.
28. Papiernik E, et al: Prevention of preterm babies: a perinatal study in Haguenau, France, *Pediatrics* 76:154, 1985.
29. Piper JM, et al: Meconium: a marker for peripartum infection, *Obstet Gynecol* 91:741, 1998.
30. Prenatal genetic diagnosis for pediatricians, American Academy of Pediatrics, Committee on Genetics, *Pediatrics* 93:1010, 1994.
31. Riccabona M, et al: Three-dimensional ultrasound: display modalities in obstetrics, *J Clin Ultrasound* 25:157, 1997.
32. Routine ultrasound in low-risk pregnancy: ACOG practice pattern, No 5, Washington, DC, 1997, American College of Obstetricians and Gynecologists.
33. Sperling RS, et al: Maternal viral load, zidovudine treatment, and the risk of transmission of human immunodeficiency virus type 1 from mother to infant, *N Engl J Med* 553:1621, 1996.
34. Spinillo A, et al: Obstetric risk factors for periventricular leukomalacia, *Br J Obstet Gynaecol* 105:865, 1988.
35. Stumpf DA, et al: The infant with anencephaly: the Medical Task Force on Anencephaly, *N Engl J Med* 322:669, 1990.
36. *The best intentions: unintended pregnancy and the well-being of children and families,* Committee on Unintended Pregnancy, Institute of Medicine; Brown SS, Eisenberg L, editors; Washington, DC, 1995; National Academy Press.
37. Thummala MR, et al: Isolated single umbilical artery anomaly and the risk for congenital malformations: a meta-analysis, *J Pediatr Surg* 33: 580, 1998.
38. Xue-Yi C, et al: Timing of vulnerability of the brain to iodine deficiency in endemic cretinism, *N Engl J Med* 331:1739, 1994.

SUGGESTED READINGS

American College of Obstetricians and Gynecologists Preembryo Research: *History, scientific background, and ethical considerations,* ACOG Committee Opinion No 136, Washington, DC, 1994, ACOG.

Beckman DA, Brent RL: Mechanisms of known environmental teratogens: drugs and chemicals, *Clin Perinatol* 13:649, 1986.

Chalmers I, Enkin M, Keirse M, editors: *Effective care in pregnancy and childbirth,* Oxford, 1989, Oxford University Press.

Dorris M: *The broken cord,* New York, 1989, Harper & Row.

Fetal research and applications: a conference summary, Institute of Medicine, Washington, DC, 1994, National Academy Press.

Hauth JC, Merenstein GB: *Guidelines for perinatal care,* ed 3, American Academy of Pediatrics, American College of Obstetricians and Gynecologists, Washington, DC, 1997.

Hetzel BS: Iodine deficiency and fetal brain damage, *N Engl J Med* 331: 1770, 1994.

Moore KL, Persaud TVN: *The developing human: clinically oriented embryology,* ed 5, Philadelphia, 1993, WB Saunders.

Report of the Human Embryo Research Panel, National Institutes of Health, Bethesda, Md, 1994, NIH.

section two **Perinatal Medicine**

43 Perinatal Medicine

one Overview

Nicholas M. Nelson

PERINATAL MEDICINE

The sharper inflection of the general and continuing downward trend in neonatal mortality in the United States beginning around 1970 (Fig. 43-1) has engendered much discussion because it is chronologically coincident with the rise of modern perinatal-neonatal medicine. This field has been characterized by a level of intense obstetrical and pediatric collaboration on the needs of the fetus and newborn.

Fig. 43-2 shows that much of this progress has been achieved through better management of the obstetrical aspects of the perinatal period, particularly near or at term gestation. This has been associated with a reciprocal rise to prominence of premature labor (which precipitates immature but genetically sound fetuses) as the major unyielding problem of modern obstetrics. If that issue were resolved, most neonatologists could retire from active duty and instead observe and support the progress of geneticists, teratologists, and others in addressing the unyielding bedrock problems of congenital malformations and heritable diseases.

Scientific and technological advances (Table 43-1) have formed a necessary, but not yet sufficient, foundation for this achievement. Just as the entrepreneur must have channels for the distribution of his or her product from factory through dealership to consumer, neonatal and perinatal care clinicians must establish ways to identify the high-risk target populations likely to need special care, then bring patients so identified to the best site for delivering such services, inasmuch as multidisciplinary human services are not distributed as easily as manufactured products.

Meeting this requirement has necessitated the assessment of the risk of perinatal morbidity and mortality as far in advance of the anticipated risk event as possible (Box 43-1 and Tables 43-2 to 43-4). Pregnant women identified as being at risk for having a complicated pregnancy, labor, or delivery (about 15% of the total) are managed best under the supervision of staff at a level II (Specialty-Obstetrics) or level III (Subspecialty-Perinatology) facility. In some locales, about 50% of these high-risk mothers are delivered safely in their own community (Basic or level I) hospital following consultation with a perinatologist. Nearly 1 in 15 of these patients probably will have an unanticipated stillbirth, and of the 80% of pregnant women identified initially as being at low risk, about 1 in 30 will develop an unanticipated problem during pregnancy (e.g., toxemia, vaginal bleeding, or premature labor) and require referral. The delivered infant also may develop unanticipated problems requiring referral, but most neonatal morbidity and mortality risk factors (e.g., maternal age, diabetes, abortion, gestational age, or birth weight) can be anticipated well before delivery.

Although the obstetrician or perinatologist is concerned first with the mother, the near-total conquest of maternal mortality in developed countries has allowed him or her to focus at least equal attention on fetal health, both prepartum and intrapartum (Tables 43-5 and 43-6).

Fetal growth and, therefore, accurate gestational age, is now monitored by abdominal ultrasound techniques with considerable accuracy (even to the point of identifying "catch-up" growth in some growth-retarded fetuses) by measuring the fetal crown-rump length (at 6 to 12 weeks) and, later, the biparietal diameter (at 14 to 26 weeks). The frequency and degree of fetal breathing movements also are used as indices of fetal well-being. The perinatologist uses a Doppler-shift measuring device to assess fetal heart rate patterns when seeking evidence of healthy variability in the basal fetal heart rate in association with normal fetal movements (nonstress test). If such variability is lacking (nonreactive nonstress test), or if there is evidence of fetal growth failure, the perinatologist may want to stress the fetoplacental unit by mimicking labor, using sufficient oxytocin to produce at least three uterine contractions within 10 minutes. A positive test result, indicating uteroplacental insufficiency, is one in which two thirds of the induced contractions are followed by a late (10-second delay) deceleration of the fetal heart rate. This evidence then is weighed against that of fetal pulmonary maturity and the availability of neonatal special care, among other factors, in deciding whether to continue or terminate the pregnancy. When assessing fetal health, many practitioners likewise consult the mother regarding fetal activity. Indeed, some have incorporated her observations into a simple and effective plan for surveillance, despite an acknowledged lack of reproducibility of such observations.

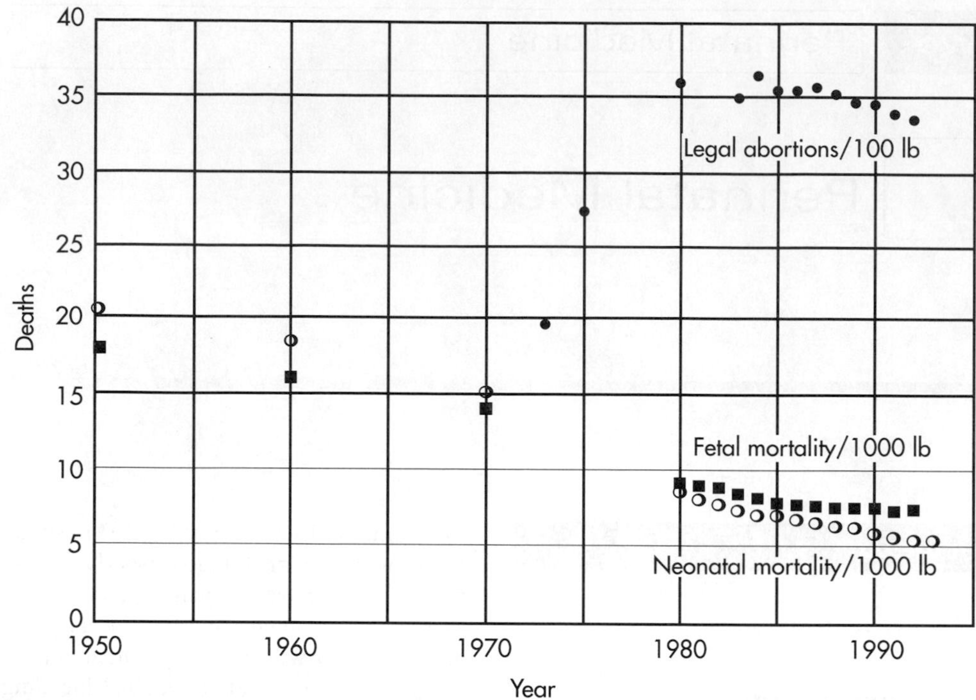

Fig. 43-1 Fetal and neonatal mortality in the United States. *lb,* Live births.

(Data from Health, United States, 1994. US Department of Health and Human Services, Public Health Service, Centers for Disease Control, National Center for Health Statistics, Hyattsville, Md, 1995, DHHS Pub No [PHS] 95-1232.)

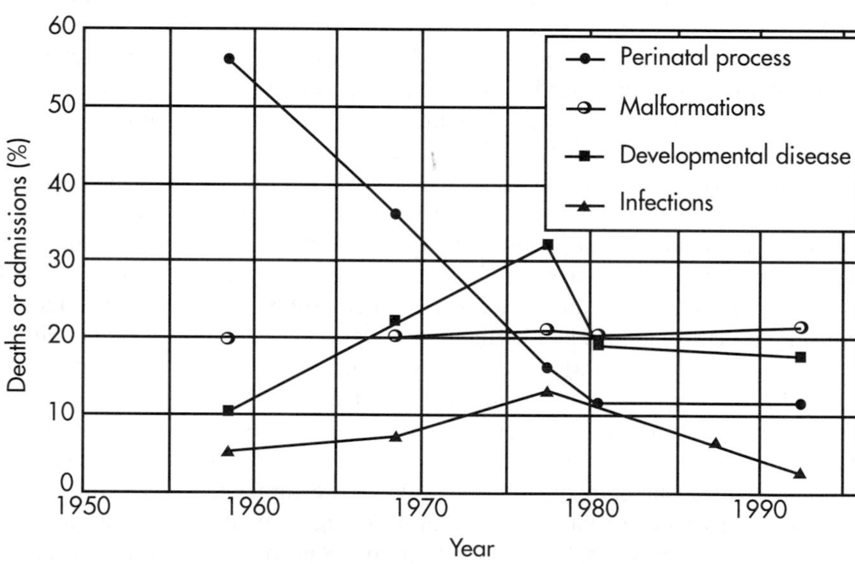

Fig. 43-2 Incidence and fatality rates of certain perinatal conditions. Experience at Milton S. Hershey Medical Center, Hershey, Pennsylvania (1973-1987), the United Kingdom (1950-1970), and the United States (1980-1992). *HMD,* Hyaline membrane disease.

(Modified from Vulliamy DG: *The newborn child,* ed 2, Boston, 1967, Little, Brown.)

Table 43-1 Advances in Perinatal-Neonatal Medicine

	Mortality/1000 Live Births					
Years	**Fetal**	**Neonatal**	**Basic Science**	**Obstetrics**	**Anesthesia**	**Pediatrics**
1940-1950	18	21	Blood grouping, antibiotics	Elimination of maternal mortality		Umbilical venous catheterization, exchange transfusion
1950-1960	16	18	Human karyotyping, surfactant, blood gas measurements, pulmonary function tests	Elimination of mid forceps and high forceps	Apgar score, local anesthesia	Phototherapy
1960-1970	15	15	Lecithin/sphingomyelin ratio, shake test, ultrasound	Liberalized abortion practices, RhoGAM, fetal heart rate monitoring		Umbilical artery catheterization, regionalization of care
1970-1980	10	10	Rubella vaccine, steroid induction of surfactant	Liberal use of cesarean section, deferred labor, regionalization of care, stress testing	Constant positive airway pressure, positive end-expiratory pressure	Total parenteral nutrition
1980-1990	6	6	Prostaglandins cause of onset of labor (?)	Real-time fetal ultrasound	High-frequency ventilation	Neonatal ultrasound, surfactant replacement
1990-2000	7	5	Artificial pulmonary surfactant	Arrest premature labor (?)		Extracorporeal membrane oxygenation (ECMO), nitric oxide (NO)

BOX 43-1

HEALTH SCREENING FOR WOMEN OF REPRODUCTIVE AGE

- Reproductive awareness
  - Pregnancy prevention counseling
  - Preconception and nutrition counseling (e.g., folate intake)
- Medical diseases (counsel regarding future pregnancy effects)
  - Diabetes mellitus
  - Hypertension
  - Epilepsy
  - Other chronic illness
- Infectious diseases (counsel, test, or refer)
  - STD, including HIV
  - Hepatitis B (immunize if at high risk)
  - Rubella (immunize if nonimmune)
- Teratogens/genetics (counsel regarding future pregnancy effects)
  - Hemoglobinopathy
  - Medication and vitamin use (e.g., retinoic acid)
  - Self or prior child who had congenital defect
  - Family history of genetic disease (e.g., phenylketonuria)
  - Environmental exposure at home or workplace
- Behavior (counsel regarding future pregnancy effects)
  - Alcohol use
  - Tobacco use
  - Illicit drug use (e.g., heroin, cocaine)
- Social supports
  - Extended family
  - Safety (e.g., domestic violence)
  - Personal resources (e.g., income, housing, transportation)

From American Academy of Pediatrics and the American College of Obstetricians and Gynecologists: *Guidelines for perinatal care,* ed 4, Elk Grove Village, Ill, 1997, The Academy.
HIV, Human immunodeficiency virus; *STD,* sexually transmitted disease.

Table 43-2 Risk Factors Associated with Spontaneous Preterm Labor and Birth

Pregnancy	Risk Factors
Past	Preterm birth
	Midtrimester spontaneous abortion
	Known uterine anomaly
	Exposure to diethylstilbestrol
	Incompetent cervix
Present	Hydramnios
	Second or third trimester bleeding
	Preterm labor
	Preterm premature rupture of membranes
	Multiple gestation
	Preterm cervical dilation:
	≥2 cm (multipara)
	≥1 cm (primipara)
	Prepregnancy weight <115 pounds
	Age <15 years

From American Academy of Pediatrics and the American College of Obstetricians and Gynecologists: *Guidelines for perinatal care,* ed 4, Elk Grove Village, Ill, 1997, The Academy.

NEONATAL MEDICINE

The major problems faced in neonatal special care units are indicated in the typical experiences shown in Fig. 43-2. Problems of the perinatal process include birth trauma, asphyxia, and aspiration. Developmental diseases include prematurity, immaturity, and respiratory distress syndrome. Overall survival is exquisitely sensitive to gestational age (Fig. 43-3), and respiratory distress (resulting from surfactant deficiency) often imposes an added burden that can be fatal.

The major intellectual advance in neonatal medicine during the latter half of the twentieth century probably has been the description of the appropriately grown (or inappropriately grown) infant (Fig. 43-4). Once grasped, this concept enhances the practitioner's approach to the newborn patient by focusing attention on those problems most likely to be encountered in the patient experiencing normal growth, undergrowth, or (more rarely) overgrowth. This approach depends critically on assessing gestational age accurately; in this assessment, the fetal sonographic data, physical examination, and the mother's opinion should be accorded approximately equal weight. Note also, in Fig. 43-3, that overall mortality decreases by approximately 50% with each biweekly advance in gestation beyond the onset of viability (currently around 24 weeks of gestation).

Some have questioned the wisdom and even the morality of investing precious societal resources in the effort to achieve the survival of infants weighing fewer than 1500 or 1000 g at birth, in whom the incidence of chronic and crippling diseases (e.g., necrotizing enterocolitis and bronchopulmonary dysplasia) and crushing disappointments (e.g., intraventricular hemorrhage and attendant neurological catastrophe) begins to rise dramatically. These critics should study the data in Table 43-7 and be challenged to present 28% to 54% normal survivors of comparably devastating illnesses occurring at any other stage in life. Similarly criticized in 1913 regarding his efforts on behalf of marasmic infants in New York City's foundling hospitals, Dr. L. Emmett Holt, Sr., insisted, "These infants are *not* unfit, they are merely unfortunate!" Nonetheless, it would appear that 23 to 24 weeks of gestation is the current floor for fetal viability, regardless of birth weight.

REGIONALIZATION OF CARE

The advent of neonatal intensive care around 1960 presaged and somewhat catalyzed similar developments in obstetrics in such a manner that around 1975, neonatally oriented pediatricians and fetally oriented obstetricians began engaging in close daily therapeutic collaboration over the needs of their patients. This and other forces led to the development of subspecialty boards of examiners in each discipline and culminated in the joint production in 1983 (by the American Academy of Pediatrics [AAP] and the American College of Obstetricians and Gynecologists [ACOG]) of *Guidelines for Perinatal Care,*[1] supplanting the AAP's preceding 5-yearly revisions of *Standards and Recommendations for Hospital Care of Newborn Infants.* The current version of this publication properly celebrates recent achievements in lowering perinatal mortality (see Figs. 43-1 to 43-3), particularly in the under-1500-g birth weight group, and codifies many of the means that have brought it about, especially the process of regionalization in perinatal health care. This process is defined as a systems approach in which program components in a geographical area are defined and coordinated.

The phrase *defined and coordinated* implies more centralized planning than historically was the case. Rather, pioneering efforts in improving neonatal mortality were undertaken spontaneously and separately in Montreal, Toronto, New York, Denver, San Francisco, Boston, and many other sites beginning around 1960. These efforts attracted the attention of obstetricians, pediatricians, primary care physicians, parents, medical equipment developers, and later, hospital boards of trustees, partly because they were glamorous, but mostly because they were successful. In a process of healthy and natural self-selection, hospitals began to identify themselves as providing what has come to be known as (Basic: Level I, Specialty:Level II, or Subspecialty:Level III) perinatal-neonatal care. Given the size, demographics, and medical history of North America, a certain amount of natural geographical coalescence was inevitable. Also, given the tendency for medical personnel to congregate in attractive urban and suburban environments, compounded by a certain amount of entrepreneurial spirit, some conflict over turf and duplication of services was equally inevitable—especially under a system of unlimited reimbursement in the United States that automatically paid back to hospitals nearly every dollar expended (cost reimbursement).

The prospective hospital payment system (diagnosis-related group [DRG]) inaugurated in the United States in July 1984 has not yet reversed unnecessary proliferation of perinatal services, despite their being expensive and many of the most needy consumers lacking medical insurance. The perinatal effects of "managed care," however, are now becoming more clear. There are pressures from HMOs to maintain all patients within the premium-paying base and to deliver mothers in an efficient and streamlined manner (some characterize these as "drive-by deliveries"). Although the establishment of supra-regionalized databases (e.g., the Vermont-Oxford or NICHD Networks) can obviate some of

Table 43-3 Early Pregnancy Risk Identification and Consultation

Risk Factor	Recommended Consult
Medical history/condition	
Asthma	
Symptomatic (on medication)	OBG
Severe (multiple hospitalizations)	MFM
Cardiac disease	
Cyanotic, prior MI, aortic stenosis, primary pulmonary hypertension, Marfan syndrome, prosthetic valve, or ≥ AHA Class II	MFM
Other	OBG
Diabetes mellitus	
Class A-C	OBG
≥ Class D	MFM
Drug/alcohol use/abuse	OBG
Epilepsy (on medication)	OBG
Family history of genetic problems	MFM
Down Sx, Tay-Sachs, other	
Hemoglobinopathies	MFM
Hypertension	
Chronic, with renal/heart disease	MFM
Chronic, without renal/heart disease	OBG
Prior pulmonary embolus/deep vein thrombosis	OBG
Psychiatric illness	OBG
Pulmonary disease	
Severe obstructive or restrictive	MFM
Moderate	OBG
Renal disease	
Chronic, creatinine ≥3 w/wo hypertension	MFM
Chronic, other	OBG
Requirement for prolonged anticoagulation	MFM
Severe systemic disease	
Obstetrical history/conditions	
Age ≥35 years at delivery	OBG
Cesarean delivery (prior classical or vertical incision)	OBG
Incompetent cervix	OBG
Prior fetal structural/chromosomal abnormality	MFM
Prior neonatal death	OBG
Prior fetal death	OBG
Prior preterm delivery or preterm PROM	OBG
Prior low birth weight (<2500 g)	OBG
Prior 2nd trimester pregnancy loss	OBG
Uterine leiomyomata or malformation	OBG
Initial laboratory tests	
HIV	
Symptomatic or low CD4 count	MFM
Other	OBG
Rh (CDE) or other blood group	MFM
Isoimmunization (excluding ABO, Lewis)	OBG
Initial examination	
Condylomata (extensive)	OBG

From American Academy of Pediatrics and the American College of Obstetricians and Gynecologists: *Guidelines for perinatal care,* ed 4, Elk Grove Village, Ill, 1997, The Academy.
AHA, American Heart Association; *MFM,* subspecialist in maternal/fetal medicine; *MI,* myocardial infarction; *OBG,* obstetrician-gynecologist; *PROM,* premature rupture of membranes; *Sx,* syndrome; *w/wo,* with/without.

Table 43-4 Ongoing Pregnancy Risk Identification and Consultation

Risk Factor	Recommended Consult
Medical history/conditions	
Drug/alcohol use/abuse	OBG
Proteinuria (≥2+ by catheter /wo UTI)	OBG
Pyelonephritis	OBG
Severe systemic disease adversely affecting pregnancy	OBG
Obstetrical and history/conditions	
Hypertension (diastolic ≥90 mm Hg /wo proteinuria)	OBG
Fetal growth restriction suspected	OBG
Fetal anomaly suspected on ultrasound examination	
Anencephaly	OBG
Other	MFM
Fetal demise	OBG
Gestational age 41 wk	OBG
Gestational diabetes mellitus	OBG
Herpes, active lesions 36 wk	OBG
Hydramnios by ultrasound	OBG
Hyperemesis, persisting beyond first trimester	OBG
Multiple gestation	OBG
Oligohydramnios by ultrasound	OBG
Preterm (<37 weeks) labor, threatened	OBG
Premature rupture of membranes	OBG
Vaginal bleeding ≥14 weeks	OBG
Examination/laboratory findings	
Abnormal MSAFP (low or high)	OBG
Abnormal Pap test	OBG
Anemia (hematocrit <28%, unresponsive to Fe-Rx)	OBG
Condylomata, extensive	OBG
HIV	
Symptomatic or low CD4 count	MFM
Other	OBG
Rh (CDE) or other blood group	MFM
Isoimmunization (excluding ABO, Lewis)	OBG

From American Academy of Pediatrics and the American College of Obstetricians and Gynecologists: *Guidelines for perinatal care,* ed 4, Elk Grove Village, Ill, 1997, The Academy.
Fe-Rx, Iron therapy; *MFM,* subspecialist in maternal/fetal medicine; *MSAFP,* maternal serum alpha-fetoprotein; *OBG,* obstetrician-gynecologist; *UTI,* urinary tract infection; */wo,* without.

Table 43-5 Assessment of Fetal Health—Prepartum

	Biochemical	Biophysical
Genome	Karyotype by chorionic villus sampling*	
Well-being	Alpha-fetoprotein	Electronic monitoring of fetal heart rate
	Conjugated estriol	Nonstress test
	Human chorionic gonadotropin	Oxytocin challenge test
	Fetal blood sampling from cord vessels*	Ultrasound monitoring of fetal breathing
Maturity	Renal and muscular by amniotic creatinine*	Ultrasound monitoring of crown-rump length (early) and fetal biparietal diameter (late)
	Pulmonary by amniotic lecithin/sphingomyelin ratio,* shake test*	
Semiqualitative		Maternal notation of fetal activity ("kick count")

*Invasive procedure.

the educational and professional difficulties of such de-regionalization, the restraints upon traditions of choice have begun to chafe. Patients (now called consumers) are just beginning to add demands for freer perinatal choices to the "Patient's Bill of Rights" that both political parties are happily and expensively "marking up" for them. Hence, the de-regionalizing effects of managed care may be reversing under consumer pressures. The question remains as yet unresolved, however, whether Americans, finally, are willing to pay for these demands.

Regionalization of perinatal services has been remarkably effective in reducing perinatal mortality and has now been embraced officially as policy by the two most pertinent professional groups—the AAP and ACOG. How the concept develops in a given geographical area begins with the definition of the pregnant patient's status and needs by her primary care practitioner as she enters the health care system. That definition, once displayed against local availability of the requisite services (and the consultative permissiveness of her HMO), helps her physician determine the level of the institution that can serve her needs best. The guiding concept is "risk identification, care in a setting appropriate to the level of risk, and transport when necessary."[1]

To the physician in a given local community who would contend that the infant in respiratory distress or the laboring woman having ineffectual contractions is "within my level of competence," the proper response is, "Agreed, but is the problem within your level of availability?" A patient's medical outcome is not affected by the expertise of the physician who is not present. The particular set of medical and surgical skills employed most frequently by the perinatologist and neonatologist was learned by nearly every general obstetrician and pediatrician during his or her residency. However, the neonatologist and perinatologist are hospital-based and have no medical commitment other than the high-risk pregnant mother or sick newborn; it is these attentions of time (as well as expertise) that have been the most important factors in reducing perinatal mortality.

Thus, based on the presumption that appropriate expertise is constantly available at each institutional level, the AAP-ACOG *Guidelines*[1] for institutional responsibility are shown in Table 43-8. These guidelines imply and demand a high level of bidirectional and tridirectional communication, education, and, where necessary, transportation (including return transportation of the infant to his or her hospital of birth, once the need for intensive care has subsided). Education and communication frequently diminish the need for transporting the infant.

Table 43-6 Assessment of Fetal Health—Intrapartum

Observation	Significance
Monitoring of fetal heart rate during and after uterine contractions (stages I, II)	
Early deceleration	Compression of fetal head
Variable deceleration	Compression of umbilical cord
Late deceleration	Uteroplacental insufficiency
Sampling of fetal scalp pH (stage II)	Anticipate postpartum difficulties if pH <7.20

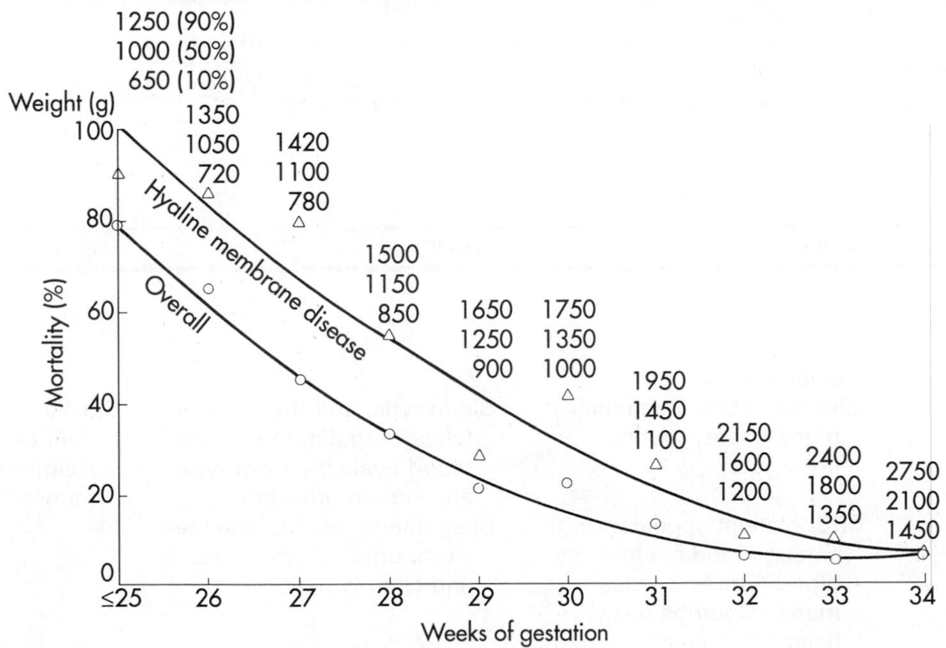

Fig. 43-3 Neonatal mortality in 1114 admissions at Milton S. Hershey Medical Center (1976-1980), caused by hyaline membrane disease and overall factors. The 90th, 50th, and 10th percentiles for grams birth weight at each week of gestation are taken from the Denver data.

(From Battaglia FC, Lubchenco LO: *J Pediatr* 71:159, 1967.)

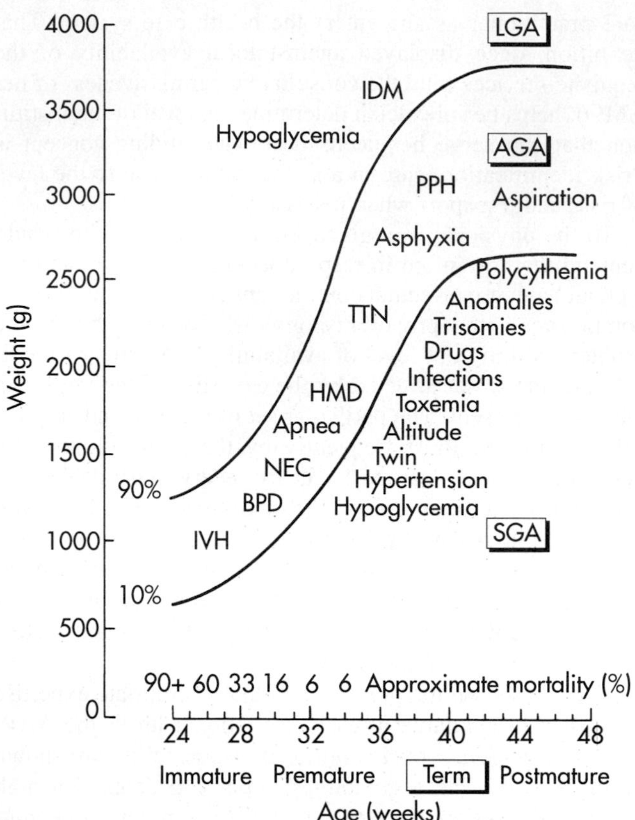

Fig. 43-4 Specific perinatal clinical entities encountered frequently in the three major developmental channels: (1) large for gestational age *(LGA)*, (2) appropriate for gestational age *(AGA)*, and (3) small for gestational age *(SGA)*. Expected approximate overall mortality is superimposed on the abscissa. *IDM,* Infant of a diabetic mother; *IVH,* intraventricular hemorrhage; *BPD,* bronchopulmonary dysplasia; *NEC,* necrotizing enterocolitis; *HMD,* hyaline membrane disease; *TTN,* transient tachypnea of the newborn; *PPH,* persistent pulmonary hypertension or persistent fetal circulation.

(From Battaglia FC, Lubchenco LO: *J Pediatr* 71:159, 1967.)

Some primary care practitioners may feel that taking responsibility for a Basic:Level I unit provides insufficient professional gratification or challenge. They should inspect the experience (Table 43-9) from a large and unselected maternal population and note how many of the problems listed they are likely to encounter in their own primary care practice. They also should note how many of these conditions they *alone* have the first opportunity to prevent or correct. Indeed, many feel that the major portion of the recent reduction in perinatal mortality is attributable solely to improved monitoring of the fetus, better timing of the termination of the threatened pregnancy, and careful attention to the oxygen, thermal, and nutritional needs of the "large" 1500- to 2500-g infant.

Moreover, there are stirrings within obstetrics that presage a likely future move from a hospital-based emphasis upon the third trimester toward a more ambulatory and family-centered emphasis upon preconception that gives promise of treating pregnancy as something other than an annoying complication of sexual activity. Currently, it is believed that nearly 50% of all pregnancies are unplanned and that, worse, many of these are unwanted, leading to high rates of legal abortions (see Fig. 43-1). The great challenge for American medicine (specifically, primary care) is to diminish the former statistic while eliminating the latter.

Table 43-7 Neurological Outcome among Very Low–Birth-Weight Infants: Results from a 2-Year Follow-Up Study

Outcome	90 Infants, 501-1000 g (%)	201 Infants, 1001-1500 g (%)
Normal	27.8	53.7
Impaired	7.8	10.0
Died	60.0	23.9
Lost to follow-up care	4.4	12.4

Data from Hack M, Fanaroff AA, Merrkatz IR: *N Engl J Med* 301:1162, 1979.

Table 43-8 Perinatal Care Programs—Ancillary Services*

Services	Level I	Level II	Level III
Laboratory (microtechnique for neonates)			
Within 15 min	Hematocrit		
Within 1 hr	Glucose, BUN, creatinine, blood gases, routine urinalysis	Blood type, and Rh, electrolytes, coagulation studies, blood available from type and screen program	Special blood and amnotic fluid tests (creatinine, lecithin/sphingomyelin ratio, shake, karyotype)
Within 1-6 hr	CBC, platelet appearance on smear, blood chemistries, blood type and cross-match, Coombs test, bacterial smear	Coagulation studies, magnesium, urine, electrolytes, and chemistries	
Within 24-28 hr	Bacterial cultures and antibiotic sensitivity	Liver function tests, metabolic screening	
Within hospital or facilities available	Viral cultures		All laboratory facilities available

*All ancillary services listed for level I nurseries should be available at level II and III nurseries, and those listed for level II nurseries should be available at level III nurseries.

Continued

Table 43-8 Perinatal Care Programs—Ancillary Services*—cont'd

Services	Level I	Level II	Level III
Radiography and Ultrasound	Technicians on call 24 hr/day available in 30 min Technicians experienced in performing abdominal, pelvic, and obstetrical ultrasound examinations Professional interpretation available on 24-hr basis Portable radiograph and ultrasound equipment available to labor and delivery rooms and nurseries	Experienced radiology technicians immediately available in hospital (ultrasound on call) Professional interpretation immediately available Portable radiograph equipment Ultrasound equipment may be in labor and delivery or nursery areas Sophisticated equipment for emergency GI, GU, or CNS studies available 24 hr/day	Computed tomography Magnetic resonance imaging
Blood Bank	Technicians on call 24 hr/day, available in 30 min, for routine blood banking procedures	Experienced technicians immediately available in hospital for blood banking procedures and identification of irregular antibodies Blood component therapy readily available	Resource center for network Direct line communication to labor and delivery area and nurseries

Table 43-9 Morbidity among Premature Infants*

Causes	Percent Affected	Causes	Percent Affected
Metabolic		**Hematological**	
Acidosis	43	Hemoglobin (outside 10-21 g/dl range)	64
Glucose (outside 40-150 mg/dl range)	26	Platelets (<100,000/mm^3)	11
Calcium (<7 mg/dl)	24	TOTAL	75
Body temperature on admission (<96° F [<36° C])	24	**Infection**	
Sodium (outside 130-150 mEq/L range)	15	Premature rupture of membranes	25
TOTAL	132†	Localized systemic	16
Cardiorespiratory		Sepsis	5
Asphyxia at birth (Apgar 0-6)	54	TOTAL	46
Apnea	29	**Gastrointestinal**	
Respiratory distress syndrome	20	Hyperbilirubinemia (>12 mg/dl)	12
Patent ductus arteriosus	19	Necrotizing enterocolitis	11
Bronchopulmonary dysplasia, air leak	10	Cholestatic jaundice	10
TOTAL	132	TOTAL	33
		Neurological—Convulsions	5

Data from Usher RH: The special problems of the premature infant. In Avery GB, editor: *Neonatology,* ed 3, Philadelphia, 1987, JB Lippincott.

*Data from 110 preterm infants (<34 weeks of gestation) from an unselected maternal population.

†Cumulative frequencies may exceed 100% because of multiple occurrences.

REFERENCE

1. American Academy of Pediatrics and the American College of Obstetricians and Gynecologists: *Guidelines for perinatal care*, ed 4, Elk Grove Village, Ill, 1997, The Academy.

two Perinatal Transport

George A. Little

Primary, secondary, and tertiary perinatal care cannot always be provided in the same place. The primary care provider functions within a system in which risk assessment, appropriate referral and movement of pregnant women and babies, when necessary, is commonplace and expected. For outcomes to be optimized, risks associated with transport must be minimized.

In the United States, well over 90% of births occur in hospitals. Most out-of-hospital births occur in birthing centers or as planned home events. Unanticipated transport of a pregnant woman or recently delivered mother and baby is necessary on occasion; emergency-response teams must be prepared to respond and provide care. The much more common perinatal event involves evaluation, stabilization, and ongoing care during the interval patients are being moved to another facility.

HISTORICAL PERSPECTIVE

The early literature regarding perinatal transport describes the transfer of stable, pregnant women to hospitals, but little mention is made of critically ill newborns. With the development of regional centers for the care of premature infants and the diminished mortality and morbidity at these centers, transfer of neonatal patients became increasingly important. Early transport services were primitive by today's standards, involving the use of equipment such as wood or tin boxes heated with hot water bottles. In 1948, the New York City Department of Health and Hospitals instituted a service staffed by five nurses to transport infants to centers caring for premature infants; Denver instituted a similar program at about the same time.

With the emergence of improved critical care capability and perinatal regionalization, transport services became increasingly sophisticated. The Canadian Pediatric Society published the first manual devoted to neonatal transport in the early 1970s[9] at a time when North American pediatricians were debating aspects of neonatal transport.[3] Later in the decade the benefits of maternal and neonatal transport were documented, while concerns and risks were evaluated.[1,6] The American College of Obstetricians and Gynecologists' and the American Academy of Pediatrics' technical advisory committees since then have assumed an active role in supporting and standardizing transport.[7,10]

CURRENT STATUS

There are three types of perinatal transport: maternal-fetal, neonatal, and return (or back) transport of the neonate and/or mother. Maternal-fetal transport is initiated for an identified high-risk condition in the mother (e.g., poorly controlled diabetes, preeclampsia) or for fetal risk (e.g., premature rupture of membranes at less than 34 weeks of gestation or omphalocele documented by prenatal ultrasound). The concept of maternal-fetal transport evolved more slowly than that of neonatal transport. Issues in the establishment of maternal-fetal transport have included uncertainty about the level of risk, cost containment, and the reluctance of local physicians to refer patients. With increasing documentation favoring maternal-fetal transport,[6,7] many hospitals that have neonatal intensive care units (NICUs) now receive the majority of their neonates in utero.

Maternal-fetal transports often use local ambulances and health professionals. Studies clearly show that babies born in the same hospital as the location of their neonatal intensive care have the best outcomes.[6,7] Most clinical situations necessitate attendance during transport by a professional such as the referring physician, nurse-midwife, or obstetrical nurse in case delivery occurs en route. An important exercise of judgment to minimize risk involves deciding when not to undertake maternal transport, deliver the baby, and utilize neonatal transport. Such decisions are not easy and must be individualized. Maternal-fetal and neonatal transports that originate at a community hospital and do not involve the center transport team are known as *one-way transports*.[1] These transports can shorten the time it takes for the patient to arrive at the regional center. In less acute situations, when little or no risk of delivery en route is involved, the pregnant patient may be referred and be responsible for her own travel. In all situations, direct communication between the referring physician and the physician who will be attending the patient at the regional center is mandatory before departure.

Neonatal transports are initiated by the referring physician, usually a primary care provider. Most often the physician calls the regional center to ask for transport when a problem is identified after birth; however, the request may be made before the birth. For example, if a woman who is at 28 weeks of gestation arrives at the hospital in active labor and delivery is imminent, nurses and physicians should consider requesting the regional center's transport team to be present for the delivery or to arrive soon thereafter. The *two-way transport,* in which an ambulance and team from the regional center travel to the community hospital to pick up the neonate, is the most common type of neonatal transport. Some community hospitals have the equipment and trained personnel necessary for one-way transports to their regional center.

The request for a neonatal transfer to the regional center should prompt the initiation of an established protocol that immediately alerts the provider of the transport vehicle, the transport personnel, and the responsible neonatologist. Telephone communication with the referring physician enables the regional center's neonatologists to define a plan for stabilizing the infant and meeting his or her immediate needs. Depending on the capabilities of the local hospital, this plan may include studies and interventions such as placing an arterial or a venous catheter, expanding fluid volume, determining serum electrolytes and blood gases, obtaining appropriate roentgenograms, and initiating antibiotic or oxygen therapy. Communication should be continuous to allow for management changes according to a neonate's needs. The regional center's transport team usually assumes responsibility for care of the infant on their arrival at the community hospital but works closely with the referring physician, who should be present when the team arrives. Samples of maternal and umbilical cord blood, roentgenograms, and copies of records should accompany the newborn to the regional center. The transport team should obtain the placenta for examination.

Optimal transport of a newborn is best achieved when stabilization of the newborn is as complete as possible before departure to the referral NICU.

Parents should have the opportunity to see, touch, and if possible, hold their newborn before transport and to receive information from the transport team members about how to communicate with regional center personnel. A brochure listing names of center personnel and telephone numbers can be helpful. A photograph of the baby taken before transport can be a comfort for the parents during the stressful period of separation from their infant. A telephone call soon after arrival at the neonatal unit from the transport team to the parents and the referring physician is important to bring them up to date on the neonate's status. NICU personnel should make subsequent contact with the parents or the referring physician at least daily and more frequently if the neonate's condition is critical.

It often is possible to transfer the mother to the postpartum floor of the tertiary center so that she can be close to her newborn. Parents should be encouraged to visit the NICU at any hour to see, touch, and hold their baby and to participate in his or her care as soon as possible. Perinatal care clinicians are aware that parental grief and stress reactions develop when a pregnancy is abnormal and that parents may express their grief verbally or behaviorally. Transport and distance add to their stress.

Return transport is indicated as soon as the infant can be treated appropriately at the community hospital and the services of a regional center are no longer needed to ensure the best possible outcome. The timing of the return depends on the facilities and the capabilities of the home community hospital. For example, the baby may be growing well but still require special care such as gavage feedings, monitoring for occasional apneic episodes, or completion of antibiotic therapy. Communication between the hospital staffs with the parents regarding plans for return transport must be established well before the return is scheduled. An NICU nurse who can discuss the neonate's problems and needs with the nursing staff of the community hospital should accompany the neonate on the return transport to ensure the greatest continuity of care. A return transport places the infant in his or her own community near the parents and frees space and resources at the regional center for treatment of other critically ill newborns. A specific benefit is the return of direct responsibility for the infant's care to the primary care physician. Unfortunately, payors do not always recognize that return transport is part of optimal care and have resisted payment for interhospital care.

TRANSPORT VEHICLES

Improved technology of two types, the vehicle itself and the mobile equipment used to stabilize and treat in transit, has expanded transport capability and alternatives. Discussions of transport include comparisons of the advantages and disadvantages of alternatives.[2,10] Specially equipped ground ambulances ensure optimum care during transport and are adequate for distances of up to 300 miles. When distances are great or when physical barriers or time are problematic, air transport has advantages. Fixed-wing aircraft have the speed and space for distances from several hundred to more than a thousand miles and can be pressurized. Rotary-wing aircraft (helicopters) are being used increasingly, with their obvious advantages of speed and ability to land near the sites of care but have internal environmental concerns such as space, noise, and vibration. Prior planning and an appropriate decision-making process at the time of transport, which takes into consideration the needs of the patient and the safety of the crew, are indicators of a well-managed transport service.

PERSONNEL

The transport team must have the capability to stabilize the infant at the referring hospital and provide care during each phase of the journey. Traditionally, the team consists of an experienced physician and a neonatal nurse. More recently, programs have used a specially trained neonatal nurse practitioner as the primary transport specialist. An emergency care nurse, a respiratory therapist, or an emergency medical technician also may complement the team. Administrative personnel responsible for interfacility patient transfer are important to successful completion of the mission.

An NICU nurse, preferably the newborn's primary care nurse, usually accompanies the newborn on the return transport to communicate the neonate's current status, including the feeding routine, the presence of apneic episodes, and any special family problems, to the receiving nurse at the community hospital.

The importance of primary care physicians in the care of the neonate cannot be overemphasized. The identification of the newborn at risk, the initial resuscitation and stabilization of the newborn, the communication with the regional center before transport and thereafter, and the management of the neonate on return from the regional center are their special responsibilities (Table 43-10).

EQUIPMENT

Neonatal transport equipment should be adequate to provide full intensive care and should include a transport incubator, a portable ventilator, an oxygen mixing and measuring system, a cardiorespiratory monitor, blood pressure monitors, infusion pumps, and essential drugs and supplies such as chest tubes. All electrically powered equipment should have "stand-alone" capability, with batteries as an alternative power source. Batteries must have sufficient longevity for the duration of the transport, should electricity not be available. Critical care equipment should be adaptable to 12- and 24-volt DC as well as 110-volt AC power for use in a hospital or an ambulance so that excessive use of batteries can be avoided.

MANAGEMENT

Perinatal transport involves 24-hour availability of a service able to provide critical care en route that also is situated uniquely at the interface between primary and referral care. Administration of such a service needs to be appropriate and properly supported.

Collection of data, evaluation, and quality improvement

Table 43-10 Physician Responsibility in Perinatal Transport

Physician Base	Maternal-Fetal Transport (MFT)	Neonatal Transport	Return Neonatal Transport
Referring	Understand benefits of MFT Identify high-risk situations at earliest moment Communicate with regional center Assume proper transport including appropriate professional accompaniment Assume care of the patient on return to the community	Understand benefits of neonatal transport Identify problems and initiate communication with regional center Initiate stabilization of the infant and provide appropriate therapy until transport team arrives, then assist the transport until departure Provide appropriate documentation, including hospital record, maternal and cord blood, and roentgenograms Participate in case discussion at follow-up conferences	Assess local resources and provide optimal neonatal care at community hospital Accept the infant in transfer as soon as medically indicated Understand importance and support of continuity of care, including parental participation
Receiving	Educate regional physicians about benefits of MFT Establish and maintain a 24-hour telephone consultation and referral system Establish and maintain data collection for evaluation and educational purposes Provide tertiary care for the mother and the fetus Maintain communication with community health care practitioners Discuss the case with local physicians at all stages, including a follow-up conference and case-based transport conferences	Educate regional physicians on benefits of neonatal transport Establish and maintain a 24-hour telephone consultation referral system Ensure immediate availability of an experienced transport team Assess responsibility for the infant at community hospital and direct the continuing stabilization process before transport Communicate with the family and their physicians at all stages of care Discuss case with local physicians in a follow-up conference and case-based transport conferences	Maintain knowledge of local hospital capabilities Communicate with local physicians, nurses, and parents in anticipation of transfer Provide documentation, including a written discharge summary, to accompany the patient

are important components of a transport service just as they are for clinical activities that are geographically located in the hospital. Data and information collected appropriately and made available as a resource by administration can be used to advance care through education and quality improvement.

EDUCATION

The responsibility of the regional perinatal center does not end with the successful transport and treatment of the patient. Comprehensive regional perinatal care requires that referral centers assume direct responsibility for the continuing education of perinatal care professionals in their region.[4,5] These activities should include didactic presentations and the distribution of related printed materials.

Case-based transport conferences at the community hospital can be educationally effective.[5,8] These conferences also should involve physicians and nurses from the regional center to promote interaction with referring community hospital staff members. Open discussion of all aspects of care, including management at the community and referral center levels, is important. Such discussion facilitates development of improved clinical skills, decision making, and continuity of care.

REFERENCES

1. Boehm FH, Haire MF: One-way transport: an evolving concept in patient services, *Am J Obstet Gynecol* 134:484, 1979.
2. Bose CL: The transport environment. In MacDonald MG, Miller MK, editors: *Emergent transport of the perinatal patient,* Boston, 1989, Little, Brown.
3. Chance GW, O'Brien MJ, Swyer PR: Transportation of sick neonates, 1972: an unsatisfactory aspect of medical care, *Can Med Assoc J* 109: 847, 1973.
4. Committee of Perinatal Health: *Toward improving the outcome of pregnancy: the 90s and beyond,* White Plains, NY, 1993, March of Dimes Birth Defects Foundation.
5. Frank JE, et al: The New Hampshire Perinatal Program: twenty years of perinatal outreach education, *J Perinatol* 19:3, 1999.

6. Harris TB, Isamen J, Giles HR: Improved neonatal survival through maternal transport, *Obstet Gynecol* 52:294, 1978.
7. Interhospital care of the perinatal patient. In Hauth JC, Merenstein GB, editors: *Guidelines for perinatal care,* ed 4, Elk Grove Village, Ill, and Washington, DC, 1997, American Academy of Pediatrics and American College of Obstetricians and Gynecologists.
8. Philip AGS, Little GA, Lucey JF: The transport conference as a teaching strategy: evaluation in the Vermont/New Hampshire regional perinatal program, *Perinatatology/Neonatology* 8:63, 1984.
9. Segal S, editor: *Manual for the transport of high-risk infants: principles, policies, equipment, techniques,* Vancouver, 1972, Canadian Pediatric Society.
10. Task Force on Interhospital Transport, American Academy of Pediatrics: *Guidelines for air and ground transport of neonatal and pediatric patients,* Elk Grove Village, Ill, 1999, American Academy of Pediatrics.

SUGGESTED READINGS

Avery GB, Fletcher MA, MacDonald MG, editors: *Neonatology: pathophysiology and management of the newborn,* ed 5, Philadelphia, 1999, JB Lippincott.

Budin P: *The nursling: the feeding and hygiene of premature and full-term infants*, London, 1907, CEEPI, Ltd (translated by WJ Maloney).

Clifford SH: Postmaturity with placental dysfunction; clinical syndrome and pathological findings, *J Pediatr* 44:1, 1954.

Curran JS: Birth-associated injury, *Clin Perinatol* 8:111, 1981.

Davis JA, Dobbing J, editors: *Scientific foundations of pediatrics*, ed 2, Baltimore, 1982, University Park Press.

Fanaroff AA, Martin RJ, editors: *Neonatal-perinatal medicine: diseases of the fetus and infant,* ed 6, St Louis, 1997, Mosby.

Klaus MH, Fanaroff AA, editors: *Care of the high-risk neonate*, ed 4, Philadelphia, 1993, WB Saunders.

Ledger WJ: Bacterial infections complicating pregnancy, *Clin Obstet Gynecol* 21:455, 1978.

Lubchenco LO: *The high risk infant,* Philadelphia, 1976, WB Saunders.

Lubchenco LO, et al: Intrauterine growth as estimated from liveborn birthweight data at 24 to 42 weeks gestation, *Pediatrics* 32:793, 1963.

Monheit AG, Resnik R: Cesarean section: current trends and perspectives, *Clin Perinatol* 8:101, 1982.

Painter MJ, Bergman I: Obstetrical trauma to the neonatal central and peripheral nervous system, *Semin Perinatol* 6:89, 1982.

Parmalee AH: *Management of the newborn,* ed 2, Chicago, 1959, Mosby.

Taeusch HW, Ballard RA: *Avery's diseases of the newborn,* ed 7, Philadelphia, 1998, WB Saunders.

von Reuss AR: *The diseases of the newborn,* New York, 1922, William Wood.

Vulliamy DG: *The newborn child,* ed 5, New York, 1982, Churchill Livingstone.

44 Sequelae to Infertility

Edith A. McCarthy • Peter A.M. Auld

Infertility rates in industrialized countries have been rising for three decades, mostly as a result of couples delaying childbirth. From 1988 to 1995 the number of American women of childbearing age who suffered from fertility problems increased by 25%, from 4.9 million to 6.1 million.[12] With this increase in infertility have come astounding advances in the field of reproductive medicine. Since 1978, when the world's first successful human pregnancy after in vitro fertilization (IVF) was achieved,[23] the clinical management of infertility has been completely transformed by the array of new medicines and assisted reproductive technologies (ART) now available. Some milestones in fertility medicine have included:

1978: Louise Brown, the first "test tube baby," is born in Britain.[23]

1984: The first infant created from a donor egg is born in the United States; the first infant born from a frozen embryo is born in Australia.[12]

1986: A surrogate mother in New Jersey, Mary Beth Whitehead, sues to keep the baby. In a landmark case, she loses the battle for custody but wins visitation rights.

1993: The only living sextuplets in the United States are born.

1994: A postmenopausal woman in Italy uses donor eggs and her husband's sperm to give birth at age 62.

1997: The world's first living septuplets are born—four boys and three girls—after the mother received fertility drugs.[11]

1998: The world's first set of octuplets are born alive but premature, again owing to fertility agents; one infant died in the newborn period.

1999: A woman in New York who underwent IVF gives birth to two boys, one black and one white, as a result of an embryo mix-up.[25]

1999: In California, an infant is born after sperm was harvested from the deceased father and used to fertilize the egg of the mother via IVF, raising ethical questions over whether a man must consent to be a father.[1]

In the United States alone, more than 3200 live deliveries per year result from IVF procedures.[22] By 1999, more than 33,000 babies were born in the United States via IVF.[12] Thus, many couples who once were considered barren are now experiencing the miracle of childbirth. However, while the soaring advances in reproductive technologies have offered new hope to childless couples and new opportunity to couples wanting to postpone childbearing, they also have uncovered a number of ethical and legal dilemmas. Rates of multiple births have been increased dramatically by ART, resulting in increased rates of prematurity with all of its inherent complications. A recent report from the Centers for Disease Control[3] showed an increased incidence of low birth weight associated with an increased rate of multiple births, highest among whites—especially older and better educated women. This is because they are the principal consumers of IVF. This statistic is best explained by IVF not being covered by insurance in most states in the United States. Therefore, assisted reproduction of high quality, which costs nearly $8000 per *attempt,* is only accessible to those who have adequate financial means. An equally disturbing fact is that assisted reproduction is one of the least regulated medical specialties in the United States. In fact, fertility clinics in the United States are not required to be licensed, as they are in most of Europe. As stated by Gladys White, executive director of the National Advisory Board on Ethics in Reproduction, "The U.S. has some of the best and some of the worst infertility centers in the world."[12]

This chapter aims to inform the primary care physician about the problem of infertility, as well as the current treatments for infertile couples, including IVF and other modes of assisted reproduction. The risks and complications of such interventions, their expected outcomes, and their inherent ethical considerations as they relate to patients presenting to the primary care physician will be presented.

INFERTILITY

A couple is considered infertile only after unprotected intercourse for a period of more than 12 months has failed to result in pregnancy. Primary infertility, as seen in 30% of infertile women, indicates that the female partner has never achieved a pregnancy; secondary infertility, as seen in 70% of infertile women, implies that a previous pregnancy was achieved, regardless of outcome. It is important to distinguish infertility, or a reduced potential for pregnancy, from sterility, in which case there is no chance for pregnancy. Most childless couples younger than age 43 years who are having problems conceiving are infertile but not sterile.

Approximately 8.4% of women ages 15 to 44 in the United States have impaired fecundity,[18] and the great majority of these women and their partners seek the assistance of a physician specializing in fertility medicine. It is the responsibility of these reproductive endocrinologists not only to determine the cause of infertility but also to counsel the infer-

BOX 44-1

CAUSES OF INFERTILITY

Ovulation problems
Tubal infertility
Sperm problems
Age-related factors
Unexplained infertility
Uterine problems
Endometriosis
Previous tubal ligation
Previous vasectomy
Infertility associated with immunological problems

tile couple about realistic expectations and their prognosis for future fertility. This can be a challenge in today's era of multimedia coverage of the advances in fertility medicine, which serves to raise patient expectations to new, and occasionally, insurmountable, heights.

The most common causes of infertility are listed in Box 44-1. The cause of infertility is sought by performing a basic infertility evaluation, which includes a history, physical examination, semen analysis, and blood tests including follicle-stimulating hormone (FSH), luteinizing hormone (LH), prolactin, testosterone, estradiol, progesterone, 17-OH progesterone, thyroxine, thyroid stimulating hormone (TSH), lupus anticoagulant, anticardiolipin, and complete blood count (CBC).[2] Hysterosalpingogram and laparoscopy are indicated only if necessary to evaluate the anatomy of the endometrial cavity of the uterus and the fallopian tubes.

TREATMENT OF INFERTILITY

Appropriate treatment depends in large part on the determined cause for infertility.

Ovulation Induction

Ovulation induction, which utilizes ovary-stimulating drugs, has been used traditionally for women who have anovulation and oligo-ovulation, for whom ovulation induction improves the chance for conception each month by increasing the number of eggs that will ovulate. More recently, ovulation induction has been used before intrauterine insemination in IVF cycles to enhance the number of embryos for transfer. The first successful human IVF pregnancy by Steptoe and Edwards[23] followed retrieval of a single oocyte in a spontaneous menstrual cycle. Although this approach permits the natural selection of a mature ovum by endogenous mechanisms, the clinical inefficiency of single embryo transfer led to disappointing pregnancy rates. Furthermore, natural cycle IVF is a cumbersome technique, requiring around-the-clock monitoring to detect the onset of the endogenous LH surge and often mandating oocyte harvest in the middle of the night. Therefore, subsequent attempts at IVF have utilized superovulation protocols in an effort to enhance both success rates and efficiency of IVF. Some of the agents used include clomiphene citrate, either alone or in combination with human menopausal gonadotropin (HMG) and FSH to enhance multifollicular recruitment and increase the number of embryos for transfer. This combination of two agents results in improved pregnancy rates relative to clomiphene alone. Cycle monitoring consists of serial sonographic follicular measurements and daily estradiol determinations. Once follicular diameter exceeds 14 mm, around-the-clock LH monitoring is performed to detect the onset of a possible LH surge. HCG is administered when the follicles attain a mean diameter of at least 18 mm, and oocyte retrieval is performed 34 to 36 hours later. Other superovulation protocols include pure gonadotropins, pulsatile GnRH, and adjunctive GnRH agonists.

Artificial Insemination with Donor Sperm, Intrauterine Insemination

For many years, artificial insemination with donor sperm (AID), intrauterine insemination (IUI) was the only available treatment for male factor infertility. Today, IUI is indicated also for idiopathic or unexplained infertility and also to bypass cervical abnormalities. When IUI is combined with ovarian hyperstimulation, the chance of achieving a pregnancy is increased compared with IUI alone.

Intracytoplasmic Sperm Injection

Intracytoplasmic sperm injection (ICSI) is one of the reproductive techniques that represents a true revolution in assisted reproduction. ICSI involves the insertion of a *single spermatozoon*, selected by a trained embryologist, based on its morphology and motility, into the cytoplasm of an oocyte, thereby bypassing all of the inherent obstacles for penetrating the oocyte, such as the zona pellucida. ICSI currently is the treatment of choice for male factor infertility and for couples who have experienced previous IVF failures. Significant concerns have been raised over the possibility of adverse effects resulting from the ICSI technique, such as chromosomal abnormalities, congenital malformations, and mental retardation (see p. 530, Long-Term Outcome).

In Vitro Fertilization and Related Assisted Reproductive Technologies

The year 1978 marked the beginning of a new era in the treatment of infertility with the advent of IVF. IVF was originally developed to treat women who had absent or irreparable fallopian tubes, but use of this procedure has since expanded widely to treat many other etiologies of infertility, including tubal obstruction and/or pelvic adhesions, endometriosis, male factor infertility, and immunological and/or idiopathic infertility. *A woman's age is the single most important variable affecting success rates after IVF.* Pregnancy rates drop precipitously and miscarriage rates rise in women older than 40 years of age because of a lack of ovarian reserve. IVF has become employed so widely that it now is a simple outpatient procedure that utilizes ovulation induction, ultrasound-guided oocyte retrieval techniques, followed by in vitro insemination, and transcervical embryo transfer 2 to 3 days after retrieval. The procedure can be performed under sedation without the need for general anesthesia. Pregnancy rates generally are expressed as either clinical or delivered pregnancies per retrieval or embryo transfer procedure, although per-embryo implantation rates may be more indicative of a program's efficiency. Multiple pregnancies may be reduced, particularly triplets, by reducing the number of eggs or embryos transferred to two, when egg or embryo quality is high.

Related assisted reproductive technologies include zygote intrafallopian transfer (ZIFT), gamete intrafallopian transfer (GIFT), embryo cryopreservation, and oocyte/embryo micromanipulation. The advantage of GIFT and ZIFT over conventional IVF is that the clinical pregnancy rates are comparable to the natural fecundity of the population at large, as opposed to pregnancy rates in IVF, which generally have been lower. However, these procedures have a drawback in that two successive invasive operations are required: oocyte retrieval and tubal replacement of either oocytes and spermatozoa, two-pronuclear oocytes, or cleaved embryos. Tubal replacement is carried out by direct access to the oviducts via the uterine cervix.

Embryo freezing, or cryopreservation, has made a small but important contribution to overall pregnancy rates by enabling patients to use excess eggs and embryos; this use of frozen embryos, however, has raised new ethical and legal considerations. The use of donor eggs has made a small contribution to achieving pregnancy in women who have absent or inappropriate eggs and has increased the chance of conception in women older than 40 years. Micromanipulation of sperm and eggs has enabled fertilization and conception when sperm are defective in quantity or quality. Preimplantation genetic diagnosis (PGD) via sampling of cells in early embryos may be used in selecting chromosomally normal embryos in IVF procedures or in couples at risk for recessive genetic disease. The availability of this technique raises concerns over future use of gender selection for frivolous reasons, such as family balance, with resultant elective abortion if the desired gender is not obtained.

RISKS/COMPLICATIONS

IVF and the related ART outlined above are not without risks and complications, both obstetrical and perinatal. The 1991 U.S. IVF Registry recorded overall clinical pregnancy and delivery rates of 19.1% and 15.25%, respectively, resulting from 20,914 oocyte retrievals.[7] Approximately 20% of IVF pregnancies are lost, most as first trimester spontaneous abortions, although this number exceeds 50% in women older than 40 years.[7] The rate of loss after IVF exceeds that for spontaneous conceptions for a number of reasons, including the adverse endometrial impact of high ratios of estradiol to progesterone, as well as an increased incidence of genetically abnormal oocytes and embryos after ovulation induction, in an inherently higher risk population. The 1991 IVF Registry also reported a 5.5% rate of ectopic pregnancies, compared with the 1% risk in the general population.[22]

The most frequent complication of IVF is multiple gestation. In 1991, approximately 30% of IVF pregnancies were multiple gestations, with 25.0% twins, 4.8% triplets, and 0.2% higher-order multiple gestations.[22] Multifetal pregnancies are at increased risk for preterm delivery or miscarriage and have the potential for significant sequelae in the offspring, including in utero fetal death, low birth weight, and major permanent handicaps such as cerebral palsy, necrotizing enterocolitis, chronic seizure disorders, and developmental delay, to name a few. Multifetal pregnancy reduction (MFPR) offers an alternative to couples who have high-order multiple gestations but poses an ethical/religious dilemma for many couples. Several series comparing obstetrical outcome data from quintuplets or quadruplets reduced to twins and nonreduced multiple births suggest that the obstetrical outcome of pregnancies following reduction is improved compared with the data from nonreduced pregnancies. Even a reduction from triplet to twin decreases the chance of a very early prematurity and short-term morbidity. Although multifetal pregnancy reduction reduces the number of babies taken home by a couple, it increases the proportion of surviving infants without complications. Unfortunately, no information is yet available from a prolonged follow-up in any study to demonstrate an improvement in the long-term outcome of the survivors.

LONG-TERM OUTCOME

The first child conceived through the use of IVF is now 20 years of age. Since then, thousands of scientific papers have been published on various aspects of IVF, but very few reports address perinatal complications and long-term follow-up of IVF children. Most of the existing reports present reassuring data, but because of faults in methodology, are insufficient to conclude that IVF undoubtedly has no detrimental effect on the growth or the motor and psychological development of the children conceived with this technique. The main problem of IVF remains the high rate of multiple pregnancies leading to pediatric complications related to their high rate of perinatal adverse outcome. Poor outcome measures, such as growth and development, are more likely related to the effects of multiple births than to the IVF procedure itself.

Growth and Development

The first report on long-term outcome of IVF children was made by Mushlin et al in 1985, using the Bayley Scales and *Denver Developmental Screening Test* to evaluate 33 of their 52 children ages 12 to 37 months.[14] These authors concluded that no particular abnormalities were observed in the IVF children. In 1989, similar results were presented by the group from Norfolk, which compared the follow-up of 110 IVF children with a control group of spontaneously conceived children. The children were ages 13 to 30 months.[13] Once again, no difference was found between the two groups of children for congenital malformations or neurological and psychomotor evaluations made with the Bayley Scales. Brandes et al[5] in 1992 compared a group of 116 IVF children ages 12 to 14 months with a control group of non-IVF children, matched for birth weight, gestational age, rank of the pregnancy, mode of delivery, gender, age, and socioeconomic status of parents. Again, no difference was found between the groups; however, a correlation was found between the multiple births and a lower developmental index on the Bayley and Stanford-Binet. The most recent IVF follow-up study to date was performed by Saunders et al in 1996,[20] in which they followed a group of 314 children ages 22.5 to 25.5 months, comparing them with a control group matched for the number of children and term and date of birth. These authors also found no difference between the two groups of children for malformations, growth, and neurological development. Scholastic performance was evaluated in a cohort of 422 children ages 6 to 13 years,in which no deficiency in school performance was observed for the IVF children.[16] One study actually found the IVF children to have, globally, a slightly higher average developmental index.[6] With regard to the outcome of IVF children coming from frozen/thawed embryos, only one study exists, by Sutcliffe et al,[24] in which the test results were slightly lower than average for IVF children from cryopreserved embryos. This study, however, did not take prematurity into account, which was twice as high in the IVF group. Also, there was a 4-month difference in the mean age of the two groups at the time of evaluation.

Psychological Consequences

Indeed, most of the studies published on the follow-up of IVF children are reassuring, although insufficient to eliminate any slight adverse effects on the well-being of IVF children. For example, many questions have been raised about the psychological consequences of IVF on the children: Will an unnatural (cold) conception fail to engender a good (warm) relationship between parents and children? Will the medical specialist be seen as a "third" parent, thus interfering with the parent-child relationship? Will the "real" child of these infertile parents have difficulties meeting expectations created by the "fantasy" child? If a donor egg is used, who is the biological mother?

IVF infants might be seen as very different but also very precious, which may create, subsequently, overprotective parents who have highly elevated expectations. Some researchers have found that IVF children exhibit a high level of psychomotor development, which apparently is due to the elevated social status and high motivation of IVF parents.[6]

The most extensive study of psychological development, carried out by Golombok et al,[10] compared families who had an IVF child, families who had a child conceived after donor insemination, adoptive families, and normally fertile families. The psychological development of the children, ages 4 to 8 years, was assessed from three perspectives: mother, child's teacher, and child. Overall, the various measures of the study children's psychological development yielded no significant differences among the four groups. Of interest, the IVF families scored higher on open expression of affection by the mother and quality of parent-child interaction.

The main problem of IVF remains the high rate of multiple pregnancies. Twins and triplets very often are preterm babies, and we know that prematurity can lead to developmental problems. In the case of higher-order multiple pregnancies, the social and psychological consequences for the parents may lead, as well, to psychological problems for the children.[9] It can be concluded that although the parent-child relationship in IVF families seems equal if not better than in "spontaneous child families," the psychological consequences of IVF on children are not yet established.

Congenital Malformations

Are congenital anomalies increased with ART? Available data provide no indication that congenital anomalies are increased in ART pregnancies. In fact, offspring resulting from IVF show the same 2% to 3% anomaly rate as the general population.[21] However, one area remains controversial—the nearly 1% prevalence of chromosomal aberrations in children born after assisted reproduction through ICSI.[4] Several reports of increased de novo sex-chromosomal polysomy in ICSI pregnancies highlight potential concerns. This increased incidence of chromosomal aberrations may result from the ICSI procedure itself or it may be linked to a defined subgroup of males who have impaired semen samples. Interestingly, it has been observed that all de novo sex-chromosomal aberrations were found after spermatozoa had been used from men with extreme oligoasthenoteratozoospermia (i.e., concentration 0.1 to 4.6×10^6/ml; normal morphology 0% to 40%; progressive motility 0% to 18%).[4] With respect to visually evident major congenital anomalies, several investigators, including Palermo et al, have demonstrated that the incidence of congenital malformation in ICSI-generated offspring was actually within the range observed with standard IVF—that is, 2.3%.[17] This is reassuring, especially for males suffering from male factor infertility, for whom ICSI represents the only hope to achieve fertilization without the need for donor sperm.

ETHICAL/LEGAL/SOCIAL CONSIDERATIONS

Although all these new techniques have offered more reproductive choices for the infertile, they also have created complex ethical and legal issues. Indeed, almost every clinical advance in assisted reproduction has led to unforeseen dilemmas. For example, in ICSI, the male factor infertility, which necessitated ICSI in the first place, may actually be caused by a genetic defect, which the father may then pass unknowingly onto his son. Another sensitive issue is that of posthumous reproduction. With the advent of assisted reproduction and the availability of such techniques as stimulated ejaculation, microsurgical epididymal sperm aspiration, and testicular sperm extraction, widows now can request sperm collection and insemination with a dead husband's sperm even without his consent or prior knowledge.[8] This raises many ethical, practical, and legal questions concerning legitimacy, inheritance, and rights of the donor, the gestating woman, prospective rearing parent(s), and any children who may result. Another controversial issue is that of egg freezing. When clinics freeze test-tube embryos for later use, what happens if that use never takes place? If the parents divorce or die, who gets custody of the embryos? And what happens to leftover embryos when the parents are done having children? In the United States, clinics request parents to specify how they want unused embryos handled. Some will donate them to other infertile couples or to scientists for research; others have them destroyed for fear of creating offspring for whom they have no knowledge or follow-up. However, many individuals and religious institutions consider these embryos to be human beings and their disposal equivalent to murder.

Egg freezing has allowed women who are nearing menopause to freeze their own eggs, rather than use a donor's genetically foreign eggs, for later use to conceive and give birth. This advent has increased the number of older women who now want to give birth. Some 100 women ages 50 years and older have borne children in the United States, and so have many more in other countries. Some ethicists believe that this is not fair to the child and that "We're designing orphans by choice," as stated by John Paris, professor of bioethics at Boston College and a Jesuit priest.[12] For this reason, only a handful of the hundreds of fertility clinics in the United States will treat women 50 years and older. The ethics committee of the American Society for Reproductive Medicine has issued guidelines stating, "infertility should remain the natural characteristic of menopause."[8] However, these guidelines are voluntary, and no law prevents physicians from treating any woman who requests it. Indeed, assisted reproduction is among the least regulated medical specialties in the United States. Licensing is not even required of fertility clinics in the United States.

Furthermore, there is the matter of fiduciary responsibility. In most of the world, IVF is covered by national health insurance. Private insurers in the United States, by contrast, often refuse to pay for it. Because each attempt costs $8000 to $10,000, patients often risk multiple births to avoid having to pay for a second visit. Eight states now mandate IVF coverage, but in most of the United States, high-quality assisted reproduction is available only for those who have the financial means.

Beyond the issues of affordability and fairness and concerns about aging mothers and disposing of frozen embryos, a single ethical question underlies all assisted reproduction: Have we the right, as physicians, to "play God" by intervening in this most basic of biological functions? According to Dr. Zev Rosenwaks, director of the Center for Reproductive Medicine and Infertility at The New York Presbyterian Hospital/Cornell Medical College, "playing God" is an unfair description of assisted reproduction. He states with regard to the tens of thousands of infertile couples who have been helped by fertility medicine, "All of us in medicine are facilitators, trying, essentially, to put things back to the way they work in nature."[19]

In conclusion, many complex medical and ethical issues surround the work of reproductive endocrinology. That tens of thousands of infertile couples continue to seek relief from their "barrenness" and have heightened expectations to have a child one day points to the conclusion that fertility medicine continues to make advances every day and is here to stay. The obstetrical and neonatal outcomes, particularly for multiple births, show that reducing the proportion of multiple pregnancies should be a goal of centers undertaking IVF and embryo transfer. Furthermore, ethical and legal guidelines affecting new reproductive technologies should be developed to protect all participants only when the need for regulation is clear. Such guidelines and possible legislation where appropriate should be established worldwide, with contributions from the medical and scientific community at large.

REFERENCES

1. A birth spurs debate on using sperm after death, *NY Times,* March 27, 1999.
2. Advanced Fertility Center of Chicago, website http://www.advancedfertility.com, 1998.
3. Bartletz L: Personal communication, Centers for Disease Control/Division of Reproductive Health, April 28, 1999 re: Impact of multiple births on low birth weights in Massachusetts, *MMWR* vol 48, no 14, April 16, 1999.
4. Bonduelle M, et al: Incidence of chromosomal aberrations in children born after assisted reproduction through intracytoplasmic sperm injection, *Hum Reprod* 13:781, 1998.
5. Brandes JM, et al: Growth and development of children conceived by IVF, *Pediatrics* 90:424, 1992.
6. Cederblad M, et al: Intelligence and behaviour in children born after in vitro fertilization treatment, *Hum Reprod* 11:2052, 1996.
7. Davis OK, Rosenwaks Z: In vitro fertilization. In Adashi EY, Rock JA, Rosenwaks Z, editors: *Reproductive endocrinology, surgery, and technology,* Philadelphia, 1996, Lippincott-Raven.
8. Ethics Committee of the American Society for Reproductive Medicine: *Ethical considerations of assisted reproductive technologies,* 1998, The Society.
9. Garel M, et al: Psychological consequences of having triplets: a 4-year follow-up study, *Fertil Steril* 67:1162, 1997.
10. Golombok S, et al: The European study of assisted reproduction families: family functioning and child development, *Hum Reprod* 11:2324, 1996.
11. Klotzko AJ: Medical miracle or medical mischief? The saga of the McCaughey septuplets, *Hasting Cent Rep* 28:5, 1998.
12. Lemonick MD: Special report: The new revolution in making babies. A host of breakthroughs—from frozen eggs to borrowed DNA could transform the treatment of infertility, but tampering with nature can be risky, *Time,* pp 40+, Dec 1, 1997.
13. Morin N, et al: Congenital malformations and psychological development in children conceived by IVF, *J Pediatr* 115:222, 1989.
14. Mushlin DN, et al: Children of IVF, *J Clin Obstet* 12:865, 1985.
15. Oliviennes F, Tine-Brissaud S: Long-term follow up of ART children including psychological aspects. In Kempers RD, et al, editors: *Fertility and reproductive medicine,* New York, 1998, Elsevier Science BV.
16. Oliviennes F, et al: Follow up of a cohort of 422 children aged 6 to 13 years conceived by in vitro fertilization, *Fertil Steril* 67:284, 1997.
17. Palermo MD, et al: Evolution of pregnancies and initial follow-up of newborns delivered after intracytoplasmic sperm injection, *JAMA* 276: 1893, 1996.
18. Rosenwaks Z: The Center for Reproductive Medicine and Infertility of the New York Hospital-Cornell Medical Center, website http://www/ivf.org/, March 9, 1999.
19. Rosenwaks Z: Personal communication, The New York Presbyterian Hospital/Cornell Medical Center, Feb 23, 1999.
20. Saunders K, et al: Growth and physical outcome of children conceived by in vitro fertilization, *Pediatrics* 98:688, 1996.
21. Simpson JL: Are anomalies increased after ART and ICSI? In Kempers RD, et al, editors: *Fertility and reproductive medicine,* New York, 1998, Elsevier Science BV.
22. Society for Assisted Reproductive Technology, American Fertility Society: Assisted reproductive technology in the United States and Canada: 1991 results from the Society for Assisted Reproductive Technology generated from the American Society Registry, *Fertil Steril* 59:956, 1993.
23. Steptoe PC, Edwards RG: Birth after reimplantation of a human embryo. *Lancet* 2:366, 1978.
24. Sutcliffe A, et al: Outcome in children from cryopreserved embryos, *Arch Dis Child* 72:290, 1995.
25. Yardley J: Health officials investigating to determine how woman got the embryo of another, *NY Times,* March 31, 1999.

part five

The Newborn

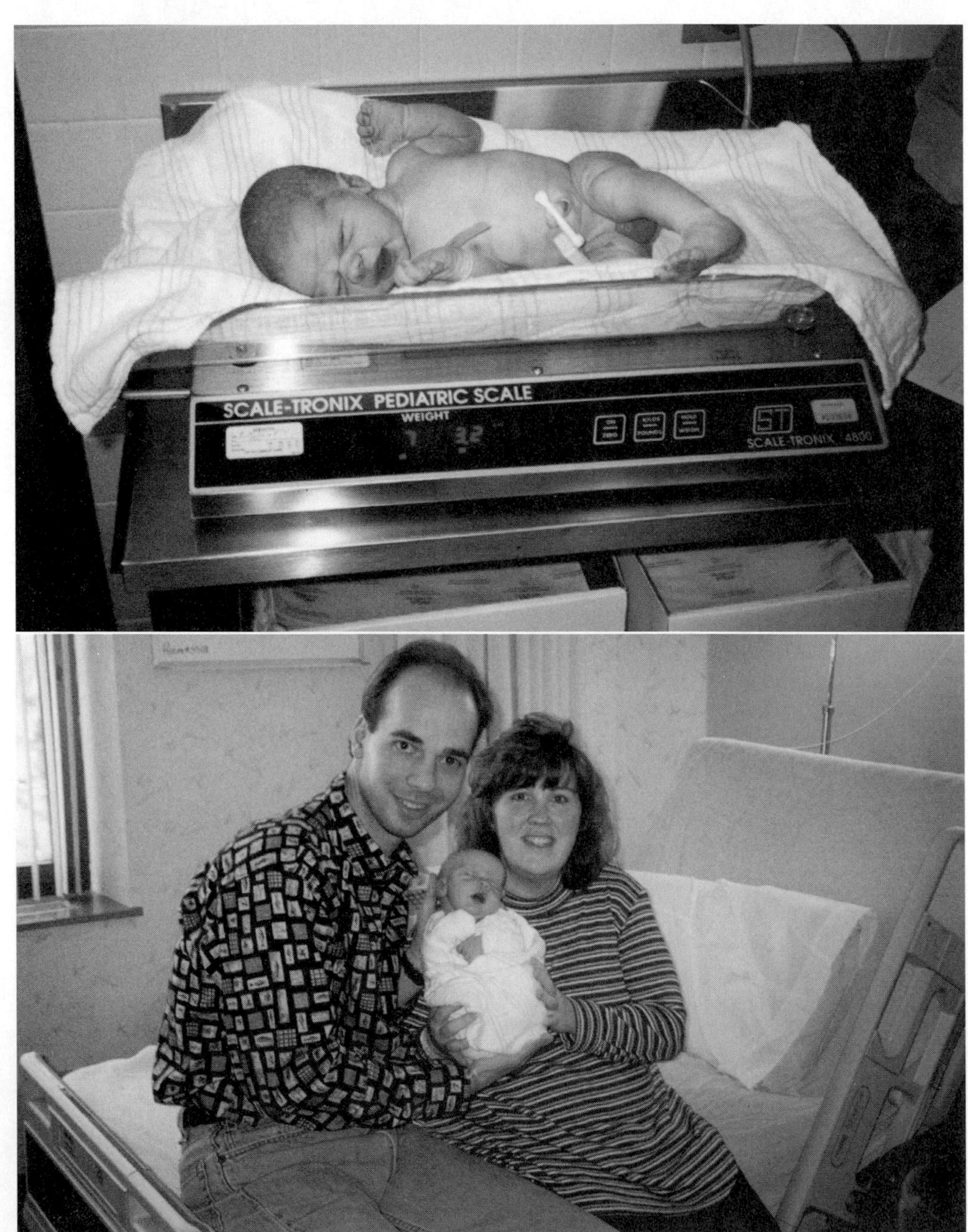

45 Neonatal Adaptations

The fundamental objective of that component of pediatric practice that involves neonatal adaptations is the healthy transition of the fetus from intrauterine to extrauterine life. The most effective strategy for achieving this objective calls for the physician to enlist the parents (as well as the extended family) in a continuous collaboration designed to stimulate, form, and enhance their developing parenting skills.

It often has been noted, accurately, that no human activity of comparable responsibility is undertaken more often with so little preparation or training than is parenthood. Somewhere in the past millennia, humans, as a species, appear to have lost many of those instinctual elements of parenting behavior so clearly designed to foster thriving survival of their young—elements that we observe daily, for example, in the parenting behavior of house pets. The possible role of the health professions in contributing to this loss of skills is a matter outside the scope of this chapter, but evidence is found throughout this textbook (e.g., failure to thrive and the abused child) to support the contention that many pediatric problems stem from the misfortune of a child's being unwelcome on arrival. Conversely, there are few better guarantees for a child's health or even for optimal adjustment to ill health than that his or her birth be happily and lovingly anticipated by both parents—a blessing that far outweighs any material support, public or private. Equally blessed are the obstetrician and pediatrician who have the good fortune to work with parents motivated by such love to seek and sustain their child's health. The best tactic for optimizing parenting skills is a staged approach to anticipatory guidance and problem management, marked by continuing obstetric-pediatric collaboration extending throughout gestation and the puerperium (Table 45-1). Each stage typically is pursued in a different site, addresses different processes, pursues different objectives, requires different observations, and may require different interventions.

one Peripartum Considerations

Maureen M. Gilmore and Nicholas M. Nelson

The management of the peripartum stage (from 0 to 40 weeks of gestation) occurs principally in the obstetrician's office but also in the community hospital's prenatal, labor, and birth classes, as well as its high-risk pregnancy clinics. The main biological processes supervised are organogenesis in the first trimester and maternal and fetal nutrition in the second and third trimesters (focusing on more strictly obstetrical concerns in the third trimester). The embryo is largely unavailable for scrutiny in the first trimester, but chiefly through amniocentesis and ultrasonography, it becomes accessible during the second trimester, when its activity, breathing, growth, and general well-being can be observed. Medicine has developed a considerable capability to diagnose structural defects, particularly during the last trimester—a capability nearly as sophisticated as that for diagnosing genetic defects in the second trimester. However, our ability to repair specific genotypic or phenotypic defects in utero still is rudimentary. The fundamental decision to be made concerning a pregnancy so threatened is whether the parents want termination before the threshold of viability (currently around 24 weeks' gestation) or as far beyond that threshold as is consonant with reasonable fetal health.

More and more often specialists are deciding that a fetus threatened by any of several conditions (e.g., intrauterine growth retardation, uteroplacental insufficiency, hemolytic disease, maternal diabetes, hydronephrosis, hydrocephalus, and ileal atresia) stands a better chance for effective intervention by early delivery and management in a neonatal intensive care unit than by continuing in utero much beyond the stage of fetal pulmonary maturation (about 32 weeks).

In developed nations for more than 50 years, birth has taken place nearly exclusively in the hospital, to which most attribute the near-total conquest of maternal deaths from labor and delivery. However, the benefits for the term infant, the mother-infant pair, and the nuclear family increasingly have been called into question. Such things as overly rigid hospital "routines," established under the rubric of safeguarding the mother and infant (and often serving only to maximize hospital efficiency and staff convenience), and use of the newborn nursery glass to separate the infant and parents (with occasional excursions out for breast-feeding) had generally depersonalized the central human event that is birth.

Since the mid 1980s, the medical profession has yielded significantly on its more rigid stances regarding the management of the birth process. Now, fathers in labor classes and delivery rooms, infants and mothers rooming-in, breast-feeding (with hospital support from lactation consultants), and "birthing rooms" (née delivery rooms) have become common. These advances still are almost exclusively applied in the hospital, making it more homelike. Maternal mortality remains near zero, with perinatal (fetal plus neonatal) mortality approaching the zero level, provided that gestation has proceeded beyond about 36 weeks. Of more recent concern is the drive by HMOs for early discharge, such that term infants

Table 45-1 Management of the Newborn*

Stage	Age	Obstetrics	Pediatrics
Prenatal	0-40 wk	*****	*
Birth	0-1 hr	****	**
Recovery	1-8 hr		***
Adjustment	8-48 hr		****
Establishment	48 hr-6 wk		*****

*Asterisks indicate the degree of involvement of obstetricians and pediatricians in decisions of management.

now are being sent home in 1 to 2 days ("drive-by" births), often a critical period for establishing breast-feeding and teaching parents the routine care of their newborn.

The current major challenges remaining are the unsolved problems of premature labor and a rapidly rising rate of cesarean section deliveries. Should electronic fetal monitoring and cesarean birth (which now accounts for more than 20% of all deliveries in some hospitals) be regarded as merely the current medical means of dehumanizing the birth process or as instruments of fetal salvation?

NEWBORN TRANSITION: CHANGES IN RESPIRATION AND CIRCULATION

The most immediate biological processes involved in transition are the non-negotiable demands placed on the newborn for successful conversion from placental to pulmonary respiration and from fetal to mature circulation. Also in transition is the infant's ability to support its metabolic needs (for maintaining body temperature and creating new tissue) through its own gastrointestinal, endocrine, and genitourinary systems, rather than those systems of the mother via the placenta.

The first breaths at birth (the fetus actually has been "breathing" in utero for some weeks) are taken in response to many stimuli—new sounds, light, chilling (from 98.6° to 71.6° F [37° to 22° C]), pressure, and probably pain. This "sensory overload," which has been compared to that of weightless astronauts returning from orbit, modulates the fundamental respiratory regulation by the chemoreceptors in the carotid and aortic bodies and by the medullary centers.

Every normal labor is, to a degree, an asphyxiating event, because each uterine contraction interrupts umbilical venous flow. This brief and intermittent asphyxia often is reflected in simultaneous and brief slowing of the fetal heart rate. Indeed, many infants at cesarean delivery not preceded by labor are notably slow to take their first breath until submitted to that ultimate asphyxiating event, the clamping (or natural constriction) of the umbilical cord vessels. If excessive prenatal hypoxia (as from placental infarction) or intranatal hypoxia (as from a "nuchal," or knotted, umbilical cord) occurs, agonal or preagonal responses may well lead to passage of meconium, aspiration, and inspissation in utero.

As the fetal thorax is compressed by passage through the birth canal and the head emerges on the perineum, a small amount of fetal lung liquid may be expressed through the upper airways to the exterior. As the chest wall recoils to its natural proportions after emergence of the thorax, some small amount of air then may be drawn into the airways, thus establishing an air-liquid interface. Next, the first breaths and cries are taken, and the airless (but liquid-filled) alveoli begin to establish air-liquid interfaces under the counterforces of elevated surface tension tending toward atelectatic collapse. The lung usually is expanded within the first few breaths. It is the special function of pulmonary surfactant (a phospholipoprotein complex, produced by alveolar pneumocytes) to reduce surface tension at the air-liquid interface, thus promoting alveolar stability.

Once the lung is expanded, its vascular resistance (as high as the systemic resistance in utero) begins to decline rapidly. This occurs as pericapillary alveolar pressure diminishes and arteriolar resistance relaxes, under the influence of the rapid rise in PaO_2 from the normal fetal level of about 25 torr to that of the newborn (about 80 torr). Pulmonary blood flow (only about 5% of total cardiac output in utero) increases vastly with subsequent return to the left heart. The left atrium, receiving this increased pulmonary venous return, begins to distend its walls to their compliant limits, and left atrial pressure rises to exceed that of the right (which is decreasing with diminishing umbilical venous return); consequently, the foramen ovale (basically a one-way flutter valve barring egress from the left atrium) functionally closes. Meanwhile, the placental circulation (formerly a low-resistance shunt during fetal life) shuts down, as the umbilical vessels are either constricted naturally or clamped artificially.

Birth converts the systemic circulation to one of higher total vascular resistance than that of the pulmonary circulation. Blood returning to the right side of the heart from the superior and inferior venae cavae (SVC and IVC) now preferentially flows through the pulmonary circulation. During fetal life, the right ventricular output had bypassed the high-resistance pulmonary circulation, as two thirds of this fetal blood crossed the foramen ovale directly into the left atrium. The remainder passed through the right ventricle into the main pulmonary artery, then across the ductus arteriosus to the aortic isthmus (shunting from the right to the left circulation). The coronary and carotid vessels, which come directly off the aorta, were bathed with the best-oxygenated blood available to the fetus—that from the umbilical vein (which crosses the liver through the ductus venosus, coursing to the IVC and the right atrium). However, upon reversal of the pulmonary and systemic vascular resistances after birth, blood returning from the lungs to the left atrium is pumped by the left ventricle to the aortic root, where again it confronts an open ductus arteriosus. Now with a higher systemic than pulmonary resistance, blood preferentially passes through the ductus from left to right to recirculate through the lungs. Within the first 1 to 2 days after birth, the circulation, thus, is "transitional," in that the foramen ovale is functionally closed, while the ductus arteriosus is still partially open and is allowing some recirculation of blood from the left to the right circulatory systems through the lungs. Moreover, during this period the volume and pressure load on the left ventricle nearly triples compared with that of fetal life, during which the right ventricle was dominant in both load and size and both ventricles worked "in parallel," connected by shunts at the foramen ovale and the ductus arteriosus.

The terminal phase in conversion of the fetal circulatory pattern to the neonatal pattern is marked by closure of the ductus arteriosus in a process of interaction between the increasing oxygen content of the blood coursing through it and decreasing levels of circulating or local tissue prostaglandins. This usually occurs by 24 to 48 hours of age, when early systolic murmurs at the base of the heart often are heard, presumably related to ductal closure.

OBSERVATIONS DURING AND IMMEDIATELY AFTER LABOR AND DELIVERY

Observations during the perinatal period should be directed toward ensuring fetal well-being. The progress of labor can be evaluated by intermittent vaginal examinations. Fetal heart rate monitoring is used to follow fetal status during labor, through either acoustic or electronic means. Any nonreassuring tracings require physician assessment and may indicate intervention. After full cervical dilation, the fetal scalp becomes available for microsampling of fetal blood gases; the pH is a more reliable indicator of hypoxia than is oxygen tension under these circumstances. At delivery the cord blood becomes available for the same purpose, and both arterial and venous cord gases should be analyzed if possible.

Immediately after delivery, the infant should be assessed to establish the success of oxygenation throughout labor. The Apgar score (see Table 8-1) is useful for evaluating the infant's status at birth and in initial transition.

PHYSICAL EXAMINATION

With an uncomplicated delivery of a low-risk fetus, the responsibility for the delivery room examination of the newborn falls most often to the obstetrical team performing the delivery. With a high-risk delivery, resuscitation if required and the initial delivery room assessment normally are in the hands of the pediatrician in attendance.

Every infant should receive a brief and "directed" physical examination in the delivery room (if possible, before formal introduction to the parents). Ideally, this is done on a radiant warmer with floodlight illumination, a means for promoting maximum visibility while preventing chilling. The objectives of this examination are threefold:

1. To seek evidence of obstetrical trauma (e.g., shoulder dystocia, forceps marks or abrasions, clavicular fracture)
2. To evaluate unanticipated gross congenital anomalies
3. To assess gestational age

Most of the important information at this stage is gathered by careful observation, along with brief palpation and auscultation. Prophylactic eye ointment and vitamin K also may be given. A full physical assessment, with an emphasis on the points listed in Box 45-1, can be completed in the nursery or neonatal intensive care unit (NICU). Obstetrical situations in which the physician should be especially wary of possible delivery trauma are listed in Table 45-2.

The infant who is to be presented to his or her parents as "normal" will display several important characteristics. Such an infant has good flexor muscle tone, is properly reactive to tactile stimuli, is "pink" in midface and trunk by about 5 minutes of age (but still may have acrocyanosis), has a perforate anus and unambiguous genitalia, and has a closed neural tube and palate. Auscultation of the chest and palpation of the abdomen are normal. (See the description of the physical examination in Chapter 45 [Two], Physiological Status of the Healthy Infant.)

Infants who are tachycardic or who have grunting respirations and flaring alae nasi at about 10 minutes of age may be regarded with some suspicion but not yet alarm, because much fetal lung fluid (about 20 ml/kg) must be absorbed into the circulation. If air entry into the lungs is satisfactory, the outlook may well be sanguine. The heart examination may reveal an early systolic murmur that merits continuing observation. The second sound usually is single until increasing pulmonary blood flow leads to its normal splitting some hours later.

Apart from sharing in the parents' joy and relief, the primary physician's remaining time in the delivery room might be devoted to study of the placenta, which usually is available for inspection about the time the initial examination of the infant is completed. The placenta should be searched for gross areas of infarction, marginal separation, velamentous insertion of vessels, meconium staining, and purulence, as clues to the infant who may be pallid (from occult blood loss) or subsequently septic. The cord vessels (two arteries and one vein) also should be confirmed as normal because there appears to be an association between the presence of a single umbilical artery and other anomalies, most of which are obvious (e.g., trisomies). Pathological examination of the placenta should be requested in any high-risk delivery or if the placenta appears abnormal in any way.

INTERVENTIONS AT BIRTH

Placental Transfusion

The obstetrician's management of the placenta and umbilical cord determines the extent of the placental transfusion at delivery, which is the major factor affecting a newborn's blood volume in the first few days of life. Some obstetricians clamp the umbilical cord immediately, which will maintain a stable hematocrit in the range of 48% to 51% during the first few days. Others wait until the pulsations have ceased, and some prefer to wait until the infant has breathed and cried *or* placental artery pulsations have ceased (whichever is later). If the infant is held at or below the level of the introitus and placenta with the cord unclamped, a maximal "placental transfusion" of blood (nearly 75 to 100 ml in term deliveries) will occur within about 3 minutes.

Perinatal scientists have not yet achieved consensus on the proper management of this placental transfusion. A placental transfusion may increase the neonate's blood volume by 25% to 50% and have adverse effects, including documented increases in blood pressure and cardiac load. It has been suggested that there may be a reduced incidence of respiratory distress syndrome (RDS) after cesarean delivery. Thus, it remains unclear whether the "extra" blood provides an advantage or whether the volume presented by such transfusion presents a significant cardiopulmonary disadvantage. Recollecting that the primeval delivery posture probably placed the mother on her knees or in a squatting position, so as better to attend the infant and afterbirth *before* the cord was cut, may suggest nature's (as opposed to medicine's) intent in the matter.

BOX 45-1

ASSESSMENT IN DELIVERY ROOM OR SHORTLY THEREAFTER

A. General
   1. Whole
      a. Proportions
      b. Symmetry
      c. Facies
      d. Gestational age (approximate)
   2. Skin (color, subcutaneous tissue, imperfections, bands, and birthmarks)
   3. Neuromuscular
      a. Movements
      b. Responses
      c. Tone (flexor)

B. Head and neck
   1. Head
      a. Shape
      b. Circumference
      c. Molding
      d. Swellings
      e. Depressions
      f. Occipital overhang
   2. Fontanelles, sutures
      a. Size
      b. Tension
   3. Eyes
      a. Size
      b. Separation
      c. Cataracts
      d. Colobomas
   4. Ears
      a. Placement
      b. Complexity
      c. Preauricular tags or sinuses
   5. Mouth
      a. Symmetry
      b. Size
      c. Clefts
   6. Neck
      a. Swellings
      b. Fistulas

C. Lungs and respiration
   1. Retraction
   2. Grunt
   3. Air entry (breath sounds)

D. Heart and circulation
   1. Rate
   2. Rhythm
   3. Murmurs
   4. Sounds

E. Abdomen
   1. Musculature
   2. Bowel sounds
   3. Cord vessels
   4. Distention
   5. Scaphoid shape
   6. Masses

F. Genitalia and anus
   1. Placement
   2. Testes
   3. Labia
   4. Phallus

G. Extremities
   1. Bands
   2. Digits (number and overlapping)

H. Spine
   1. Symmetry
   2. Scoliosis
   3. Sinuses

Table 45-2 Obstetrical Situations in Which Delivery Trauma May Occur

Type of Injury	Normal Vertex	Cesarean	Premature	Precipitate	Difficult		
					Breech Extraction	Large Infant	High Midforceps
Hemorrhage							
Cerebral							
Subdural							X
Subarachnoid				X	X	X	X
Intraventricular			X				
Abdominal							
Liver					X	X	
Spleen					X	X	
Adrenal gland					X	X	
Cutaneous, presenting part	X				X		
Conjunctival	X						
Fracture or Dislocation							
Clavicle						X	
Humerus					X		
Femur					X		
Skull							X
Nerve Injury							
Brachial plexus						X	
Spinal cord					X		
Facial	X						
Laceration		X					

Preparation in the Delivery Room

Perinatal depression can arise as the result of an intrauterine or intrapartum problem, during which the fetus becomes hypoxic and hypercapnic and may develop metabolic acidosis. In the delivery room, the result of perinatal depression (whatever its cause) is that the infant fails to initiate adequate respiration or that respirations simply are insufficient to provide adequate gas exchange. The sine qua non of its management is to provide immediate ventilatory assistance.

Planning for Resuscitation

Organization and preplanning are essential to ensure appropriate action for a high-risk delivery and, more importantly, for an unanticipated problem. The "disaster plan" for delivery room resuscitation should be the primary responsibility of a physician and should be reviewed periodically. The labor and delivery staff should maintain, display, and refer to a list of maternal and fetal complications that require the presence in the delivery room of a professional qualified specifically in newborn resuscitation (Box 45-2).

Equipment Required

All equipment should be checked at regular intervals, as well as just before any delivery, for readiness and appropriate function. Is a radiant warmer available and turned on? Is the laryngoscope light bright? Does the bag and mask ventilation system provide adequate flow and pressure, free of leaks? Is appropriate suction equipment present? A list of suggested equipment is provided in Box 45-3.

Personnel

Proper resuscitation cannot be performed alone. It is best if two people (e.g., physician and nurse) are solely responsible for the infant's care directly after birth. For an elective cesarean birth at term, which does not itself define a high-risk delivery, qualified caretakers skilled in neonatal resuscitation should be present; the obstetrician and anesthesiologist are committed to the mother's needs and may not be immediately available themselves to assess the newborn and to perform any necessary resuscitation.

Apgar Score

The Apgar score is useful for describing the infant's status soon after birth and in initial transition. The score includes a grading of neuromuscular reactivity (muscle tone and reflex irritability), as well as of heart rate, respiration, and color. The Apgar score should be determined 1 and 5 minutes after birth (see Table 8-1). If the 5-minute score is less than 7, additional scores should be obtained every 5 minutes up to 20 minutes, unless and until two successive scores of 8 or higher are attained. It is crucial to realize that the most serious decisions for resuscitation of the neonate in the delivery room are made within the first minute or two. Thus, Apgar scores reflect the success of any resuscitation but are not meant to direct the interventions required. Ideally, a person not directly involved in the resuscitation (e.g., a nurse) should compile the Apgar score.

BOX 45-2

PERINATAL CONDITIONS THAT INCREASE THE RISK OF NEONATAL ASPHYXIA

Antepartum Conditions

1. Diabetes
2. Toxemia
3. Hypertension
4. Rh sensitization
5. Previous stillbirth or neonatal death
6. Third trimester bleeding
7. Maternal infection
8. Polyhydramnios
9. Oligohydramnios
10. Postterm gestation
11. Multiple gestation
12. Intrauterine growth retardation

Intrapartum Conditions

1. Operative delivery
    a. Cesarean section
    b. Midforceps delivery
2. Breech or other abnormal presentation
3. Premature labor
4. Ruptured membranes (>24 hr)
5. Chorioamnionitis
    a. Maternal fever, tachycardia, or both
    b. Ruptured membranes (>24 hr)
    c. Tender uterus
    d. Foul-smelling amniotic fluid
6. Prolonged labor (>24 hr)
7. Fetal distress
    a. Fetal tachycardia (>160 beats/min)
    b. Fetal bradycardia (<120 beats/min)
    c. Persistent late decelerations
    d. Severe variable decelerations without baseline variability
    e. Scalp pH $\leq$7.25
    f. Meconium-stained amniotic fluid
    g. Cord prolapse
8. General anesthesia
9. Narcotics administered during labor
10. Abruptio placentae
11. Placenta previa

Initial Resuscitation Procedure

Fig. 45-1 outlines the initial steps.

1. *Temperature control*. Immediately after delivery, the infant should be placed under a previously heated radiant warmer and completely dried with prewarmed towels to prevent excessive evaporative heat loss.
2. *Suctioning*. Suctioning is not essential for all infants; however, if necessary, it should be gentle. In particular, vigorous suctioning of the posterior pharynx must be avoided because this frequently produces significant bradycardia via vagal stimulation. If the amniotic fluid is meconium-stained, the mouth and pharynx should be suctioned thoroughly by the obstetrician, using a DeLee trap. (See the section on meconium aspiration on p. 544.)
3. *Establishing respiration*. A normal infant should breathe within a few seconds of delivery and establish regular,

BOX 45-3

EQUIPMENT REQUIRED FOR RESUSCITATION

Ventilation
1. Oxygen source—oxygen, warmed and humidified
2. Suction—De Lee suction trap, wall suction with adjustable pressure gauge; suction catheters; sizes 6, 8, 10, 12 Fr
3. Ventilation bag—500-ml self-inflating type with reservoir (capable of delivering 100% oxygen) or 500-ml anesthesia type
4. Face masks—infant sizes, premature and term
5. Laryngoscope—blade sizes 0 and 1, spare batteries, and bulbs
6. Endotracheal tubes—sizes 2.5, 3, and 3.5 mm with plastic adapters attached
7. Soft metal stylets for endotracheal tubes
8. Stethoscope
9. Feeding tube—8 Fr tubes to evacuate stomach contents

Temperature Control
1. Evaporation—warm towels
2. Conduction—mattress covered with prewarmed towels
3. Convection—air conditioning turned down; delivery room temperature 75° F (23.9° C) minimum
4. Radiation—radiant warmer

Circulation and Biochemical Resuscitation
1. Umbilical catheterization tray
2. Drugs and volume expanders

Other
50-ml syringe with three-way stopcock and 21-gauge butterfly needle for evacuation of pneumothorax

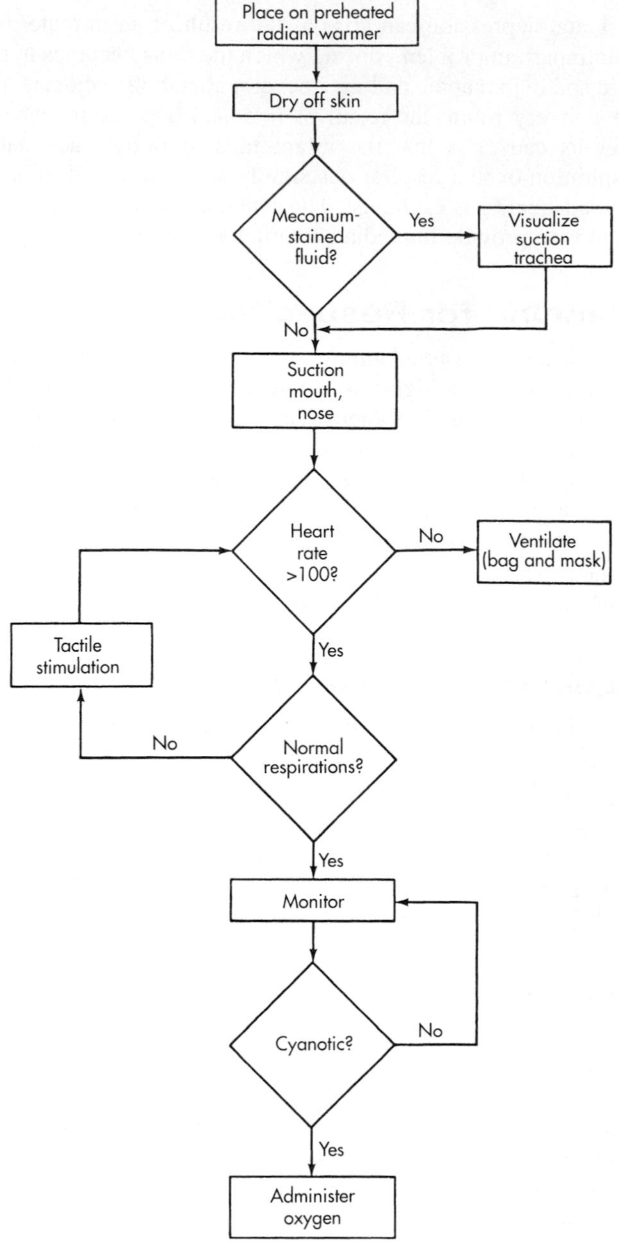

Fig. 45-1 Protocol for initial steps in resuscitation of an infant in the delivery room.

(Modified from Klaus MH, Fanaroff AA: *Care of the high-risk neonate*, ed 4, Philadelphia, 1993, WB Saunders.)

effective respirations by 1 minute after birth. Any infant, regardless of gestation, who is not breathing spontaneously and whose heart rate is less than 100 beats/min requires immediate ventilation. Fig. 45-2 provides a flow chart for positive pressure ventilation.

Positive Pressure Ventilation

Positive pressure ventilation via bag and mask, when performed correctly, will provide adequate ventilation for most infants. The few infants in whom it should not be used include those who have a known diaphragmatic hernia and those depressed infants who have thick meconium. In addition, it may be very difficult to achieve adequate lung expansion by means of bag and mask ventilation in small premature infants whose lungs have reduced compliance. *These exceptional cases require endotracheal intubation.*

Critical to the success of bag and mask ventilation are an airtight facial seal and a nonobstructed airway. Position the infant supine with the neck slightly extended and place the mask over the mouth and nose, being careful to avoid pressure on the eyes. While holding the mask in place, use at least one finger to hold the chin to the edge of the mask (Fig. 45-3). This actually should elevate the angle of the jaw, bringing the tongue forward and opening the airway. The neck must *not* be hyperextended, because hyperextension narrows the airway.

There are two kinds of bags: the flow-inflating *anesthesia bag*, which requires continual gas flow to inflate, and the *self-inflating (Ambu) bag*, which remains inflated with or without gas flow. The latter is the more convenient to use, particularly for less experienced resuscitators. The self-inflating bags must be fitted with an oxygen reservoir to deliver high concentrations of oxygen (90% to 100%). The

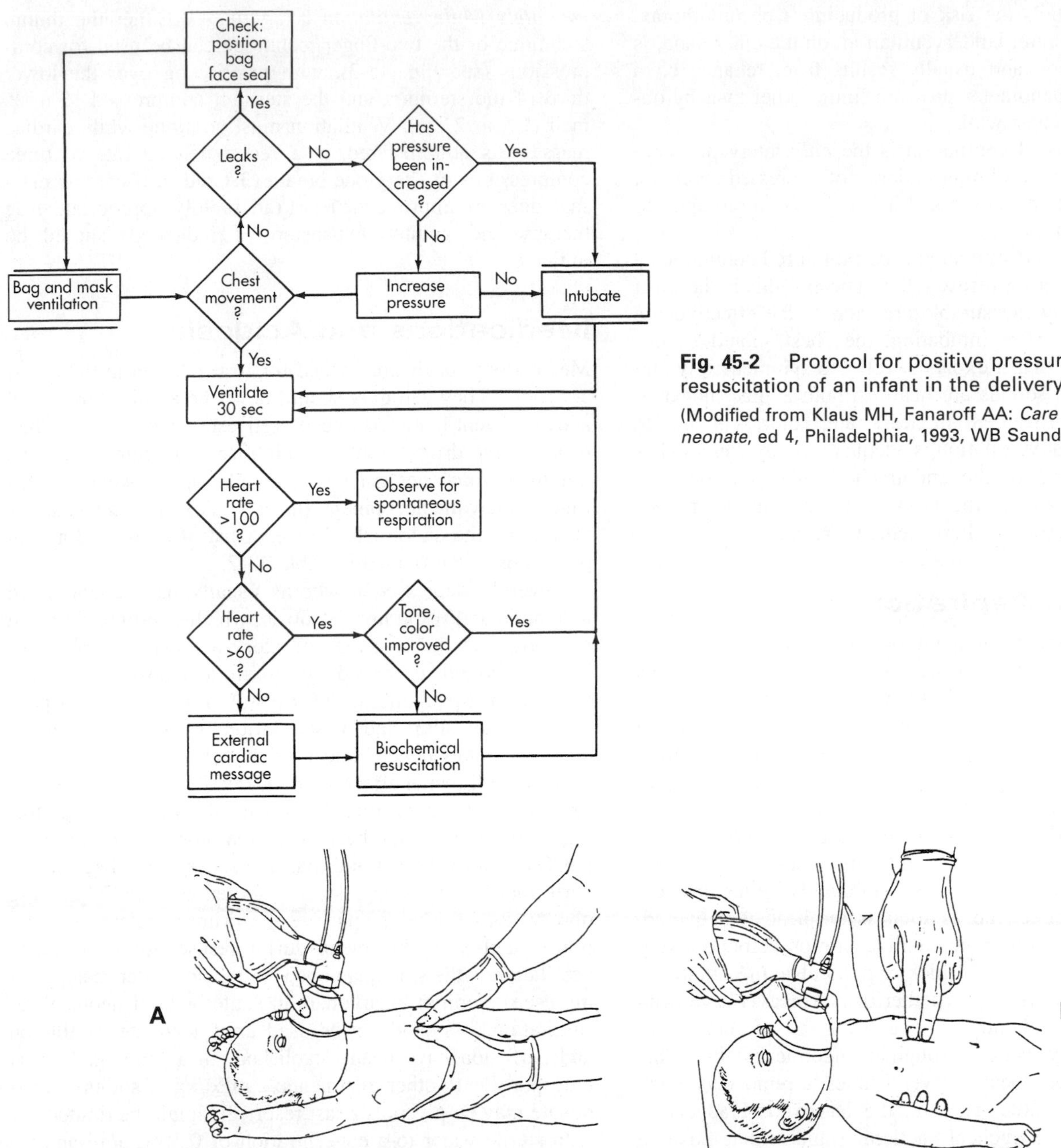

Fig. 45-2 Protocol for positive pressure ventilation in resuscitation of an infant in the delivery room.
(Modified from Klaus MH, Fanaroff AA: *Care of the high-risk neonate*, ed 4, Philadelphia, 1993, WB Saunders.)

Fig. 45-3 Technique for bag and mask ventilation, with **A,** chest compressions using the thumb method, and **B,** chest compressions via the two-finger method.
(Used with permission of the American Academy of Pediatrics, from Bloom RS, Cropley C, American Academy of Pediatrics and American Heart Association: *Textbook of neonatal resuscitation*, ed 2, Elk Grove Village, Ill, 1994, The American Academy of Pediatrics.)

absence of a reservoir allows mixing with room air and limits oxygen delivery to only 40%, a level inadequate for delivery room resuscitation. Also, the valve assembly in most self-inflating bags permits oxygen flow *only when the bag is being compressed*; thus, these bags cannot be used to provide free-flowing oxygen to the baby's face.

With a good seal and successful ventilation, the chest should rise and fall while the infant's heart rate and color rapidly improve. If this does not occur, the infant's position, the seal between mask and face, and the pressure being used should be checked. Any continued inability to obtain adequate chest movement by bag and mask ventilation despite repositioning mandates endotracheal intubation.

Whether ventilation is provided via mask or endotracheal tube, *the appropriate inflating pressure is that which is required to expand the chest and improve gas exchange.* It is not determined solely by reference to a manometer. If the manometer indicates that high pressures are necessary to expand the chest, the possibilities of airway obstruction, severe RDS, or hypoplastic lungs should be considered. Although overinflation entails the risk of producing a pneumothorax, this is relatively rare. Underventilation, on the other hand, is far more common and usually results from reliance on a predetermined manometer pressure limit, rather than by observation of the chest wall.

Effective assisted ventilation is the *only* intervention required for the overwhelming majority of depressed neonates. With few exceptions, depressed infants respond promptly to adequate ventilation.

The infant's heart rate should be monitored continuously by an assistant during resuscitation, because this is the most useful and readily measurable criterion of the effectiveness of resuscitation. After intubation, the chest should be observed to ensure that it expands well and symmetrically and that equal breath sounds are heard in both axillae (not over the apices). Improvement in heart rate, color, and muscle tone confirms that ventilation is adequate. If any doubt exists about the position of the endotracheal tube, it should be checked by visualizing the larynx directly with a laryngoscope or by obtaining a chest roentgenogram.

Meconium Aspiration

Meconium staining of the amniotic fluid is taken as evidence of possible significant fetal hypoxia, acute or chronic. This should alert the attending physician to the potential need for aspiration of meconium from the nasopharynx and trachea before the first few breaths. Note that with significant stress in utero, an infant may already have had the opportunity to aspirate and inspissate that viscous material into the airways, increasing the risk for meconium aspiration syndrome.

When the amniotic fluid is meconium-stained, the nares and pharynx should be suctioned thoroughly by the obstetrician, using a DeLee trap as soon as the head is delivered. This is done to prevent meconium aspiration before delivery of the shoulders. If there is thick or particulate meconium, or if the infant is in distress, whether or not breaths have been taken, the larynx should be visualized and meconium removed directly by suction through an endotracheal tube. This procedure may be repeated several times to remove as much meconium as possible, clearing the larynx. If bradycardia occurs, discontinue tracheal suctioning and initiate positive pressure ventilation. Guidelines for endotracheal tube sizes and suction catheters are provided in Table 45-3.

External Cardiac Massage

If the heart rate is less than 60 beats/min or does not increase above 80 beats/min after effective ventilation with 100% oxygen, chest compressions should be instituted immediately while ventilation is continued. Either the thumb technique or the two-finger technique can be used for compressions (see Fig. 45-3), with positioning over the lower third of the sternum, and the sternum compressed ½ to ¾ inch (1.5 to 2 cm). Ventilation must continue while cardiac massage is administered, at a recommended rate of three compressions to every one breath (3:1 ratio). If cardiac massage does not improve the heart rate rapidly, appropriate drug therapy and volume expansion (if indicated) should be initiated.

Table 45-3 Guidelines for Endotracheal Tubes and Suction Catheters

Infant's Weight (kg)	Endotracheal Tube Internal Diameter (mm)	Depth of Insertion from Upper Lip (cm)	Suction Catheter Size (Fr)
1	2.5	7	5
2	3	8	6
3	3.5	9	8

Medications and Acidosis

Medications *rarely* are needed for resuscitation in the delivery room. They certainly should never be administered until adequate ventilation has been well established. If possible, resuscitative drugs should be administered centrally via the umbilical vein after emergent cannulation. However, if this route is unavailable, epinephrine and naloxone can be administered via the endotracheal tube. A list of drugs and appropriate doses is provided in Table 49-2.

Severely depressed newborns usually have a combined metabolic and respiratory acidosis, which is properly treated by correcting the cause. Respiratory acidosis, the result of hypoventilation, is treated by intermittent positive pressure ventilation. Metabolic acidosis results from prolonged poor tissue oxygenation and accumulation of lactic acid. Some experimental evidence indicates that metabolic acidosis has a specific detrimental effect on myocardial function in the hypoxic heart. However, it also has been shown that the performance of the ischemic heart is related more closely to tissue $PaCO_2$ than to the pH and that nonischemic cardiac muscle performance also is depressed by increases in $PaCO_2$. These observations further emphasize the primary role of ventilation in acid-base adjustments during resuscitation—adequate ventilation is the sine qua non. There is no evidence supporting use of sodium bicarbonate in acute or brief neonatal resuscitation. It should not be used until adequate ventilation and perfusion have been established. In a prolonged arrest unresponsive to other treatments, 2 mEq/kg of sodium bicarbonate may be given as a last resort. It should be diluted 1:1 with sterile water to a concentration of 0.5 mEq/ml and infused slowly over at least 2 minutes.

Hypovolemia

Most asphyxiated neonates are not hypovolemic. Moreover, it is important to recognize the potential hazards (e.g., intracranial hemorrhage) involved in overzealous volume expansion, particularly in the preterm infant. On the other hand, certain conditions (e.g., vasa previa, abruptio placenta, fetal-maternal bleeding) may produce significant hemorrhage from the fetoplacental unit. Compression of the umbilical cord during labor also may be associated with hypovolemia. If significant hypovolemia is suspected (clinical signs of shock are usually not apparent until 20% to 25% of the blood volume has been lost), small infusions of volume expanders (10 to 20 ml/kg) may be given (see Table 49-2). In very low–birth-weight preterm infants, these infusions should be given over a minimum of 30 minutes. The infant's response should be assessed after each infusion, and volume expansion should be discontinued as soon as tissue perfusion is adequate.

Respiratory Depression Caused by Narcotics

Narcotic drugs occasionally are used to relieve maternal labor pain; these are able to cross the placenta. Respiratory depression caused by narcotics given within 4 hours of delivery can be managed by assisted ventilation alone. However, if respiratory depression persists despite adequate assisted ventilation, naloxone (0.1 mg/kg) may be given. The narcotic effects may persist longer than that of the naloxone, with a duration of action of 1 to 4 hours. Thus, close observation is required, and repeated doses of naloxone may be necessary. In a narcotic-addicted mother, who may be using other illicit drugs as well, naloxone should be avoided because it may precipitate severe seizures in the neonate.

Acknowledgment

We would like to acknowledge the contributions of M. Jeffrey Maisels to earlier editions of this section.

two Physiological Status of the Healthy Infant

Maureen M. Gilmore and Nicholas M. Nelson

Throughout fetal life the placenta is at once the necessary and sufficient organ for respiration, nutrition, metabolism, excretion, and immune defense, whereas certain endocrine functions (likely including growth itself), as well as the events of parturition, require more active fetal effort. The fetal lung, intestines, liver, kidney, thymus, and even the brain have no functional assignment, other than to grow, differentiate, and be ready to assume function at birth. Thus, it is perfectly possible for nature to carry many of her human "experiments" to term with no kidneys, intestines, liver, lungs, or brain. However, a fetal circulatory system, comprising pump and "exchange" vessels (capillaries), is necessary very early in gestation for all placental mammals, although a single ventricle will do.

CIRCULATORY SYSTEM

The major cardiorespiratory events that attend birth (see Chapter 45 [One], Peripartum Considerations) sever the connections between the *parallel* greater (i.e., systemic) and lesser (i.e., pulmonary) circulations by closing the foramen ovale and ductus arteriosus, thus terminating the shunt of blood through them. This results in a circulatory pathway now in *series* from right ventricle to pulmonary vasculature to left ventricle to systemic vasculature, and guarantees that 100% of cardiac output (rather than about 5%, as in the fetus) passes through the lungs. This, perhaps paradoxically, results in a decrease in load on the right ventricle, because pulmonary vascular resistance diminishes concomitantly with an increase in left ventricular (LV) load. This LV load is created by an increased volume of blood returning from the lungs, as well as removal of the low-resistance placental shunt at birth. Ultimately, the pulmonary circulation converts to a high-flow, low-resistance circuit, while the systemic circulation converts to a lower-flow, higher-resistance circuit, relative to their states in utero. The right ventricular predominance characteristic of fetal and early neonatal life begins to give way to the left ventricular dominance of later life. These events are most obvious in the changing QRS and T vectors on an electrocardiogram of the developing infant's heart over the first 1 to 2 weeks after birth.

In the young infant, these alterations in hemodynamics set the conditions that place the two ventricles (especially the left) high on their respective function curves—that is, producing relatively high cardiac outputs but with little further reserve for emergencies.

The infant myocardium appears to be less able than that of the adult to sustain tension against the loads imposed by high volume (preload) or high pressure (afterload). This may result from a level of sympathetic innervation that, as yet, is incomplete, even by term gestation, so that myocardial beta-receptors are insufficiently stimulated. In neonates, and especially in a premature newborn, there appears to be a degree of parasympathetic/sympathetic innervational imbalance with parasympathetic dominance. With marked imbalance, bradycardia can occur. Moreover, in preterm infants the myocardium has less contractile mass (because of greater water content), less distensibility of the ventricles, and less force generated, compared with more mature infants.

Moreover, for a time the pulmonary arterioles retain their thick fetal musculature, which renders them supersensitive to any vasoconstrictive stimuli, such as hypoxia. In the first days after birth, the condition known as persistent pulmonary hypertension of the newborn (PPHN; formerly "persistent fetal circulation") is characterized by such pulmonary vasoconstriction. In PPHN, blood shunts right to left across the anatomically still open foramen ovale and ductus arteriosus to produce cyanosis and a general picture quite difficult to distinguish clinically from true cyanotic congenital heart disease.

HEMATOPOIETIC SYSTEM

Certainly the earliest fetal organ function to become established, hematopoiesis originates in the yolk sac (0 to 2 months), switches to the liver (2 to 6 months), and finally, the bone marrow (6 to 9 months). The ontogeny of the hemoglobin chains is such that at birth fetal hemoglobin (Hb F) is dominant. In response to the chronic hypoxic state that is fetal life (with an average oxygen tension of 22 to 25 mm Hg), hepatic (initially) and then renal production of erythropoietin (Epo) is stimulated. Epo is the growth factor that stimulates production of red blood cells to maximize oxygen-carrying capacity. At birth the red cell mass is at a maximum (hematocrit of 55% to 65%), beyond which increasing blood viscosity would so impede blood flow as actually to diminish oxygen transfer. With birth, normal physiological reduction of this red cell mass begins, with breakdown of some of these young red cells and release of hemoglobin, thus adding to the infant's bilirubin load. Oxygen transfer from placenta to red cells in the relatively hypoxic fetus is aided by hemoglobin F, which displays greater affinity for oxygen than does adult hemoglobin (Hb A), and a reduced affinity for its reciprocally binding coenzyme, 2,3-diphosphoglycerate (DPG). Immediately after birth the concentration of DPG rises sharply, and the oxygen affinity of the infant's blood appropriately falls, because now, after birth, the infant is operating at an oxygen pressure of about 70 to 100 mm Hg (rather than at 25 mm Hg). These two factors allow the infant's red cells to give up the bound oxygen that is carried to the peripheral tissues of the newly born (and now better-oxygenated) body.

The multiple components of reliable hemostasis (blood vessel constriction, platelet aggregation, the coagulation cascade, and clot lysis) are largely present in the term newborn. However, the hemostatic system is dynamic and will mature further postnatally. In a healthy newborn, the somewhat decreased platelet aggregation and lower levels of some clotting factors are considered physiological, unless complications of bleeding or thrombosis occur. For example, the vitamin K–dependent factors (II, VII, IX, and X) are present but at levels 30% to 50% lower than those of adults. Without vitamin K at birth, they may decline even further, to as low as 5% to 20% of adult levels, and pose the risk of hemorrhagic disease of the newborn. The clotting factor levels gradually increase and approach adult levels by 6 months of age.

RESPIRATORY SYSTEM

During fetal life the infant's respiratory system, made up of gas-exchanging alveoli and air-conducting pathways, prepares developmentally to take on (very quickly after ligation of the cord) the awesome responsibility for gaseous metabolism assumed previously by the placenta.

From very early in gestation through about 35 to 36 weeks of gestation, the alveoli, complete with their integrated perfusing blood supply, develop from "glandular" to bronchiolar to more acinar structures. At about 24 weeks, the alveolar type II pneumocytes are present and begin to elaborate a complex of phospholipids and proteins, (i.e., pulmonary surfactant) and store it for the moment of the first breaths of life. This surfactant is spread in a thin layer over the alveolar epithelium to stabilize the alveoli by diminishing the surface tension established at the air-liquid interface. Absorption of fetal lung liquid occurs during the first hour of life, principally through the lymphatics, after the lungs have fully expanded and as the lungs are going through the vascular transition described in the previous section. Disruptions or slowing of this process of liquid resorption probably play a role in the condition called *transient tachypnea of the newborn.*

By the time of birth at term, the neuromuscular and skeletal apparatus that constitutes the thoracic bellows (ribs, intercostal muscles, and diaphragm) has had considerable intrauterine practice at breathing through a paroxysmal form of rapid panting (oscillatory movement of only very small amounts of amniotic fluid in the airways). These paroxysms (at least in fetal sheep) temporally coincide with episodes of "active sleep" (see Chapter 45 [Three], Recovery Period). The only significant inefficiency of the thoracic bellows occurs during active or rapid eye movement (REM) sleep, when there is widespread inhibition of motor neurons, particularly those responsible for ongoing intercostal muscle tone. Consequently, the chest wall becomes relatively less fixed and stiff (i.e., more "compliant," like a loose-fitting glove). The tendency of the underlying expanded lung to collapse is less opposed by a firm chest wall than is the case in quiet sleep; the descending diaphragm, thus, is able to pull the lower rib cage counterproductively inward during inspiration ("paradoxical" respiration). Therefore, the mechanical situation for an infant's lung is a bit more tenuous than is the case for an adult—specifically, the infant's lung tends to operate at a level rather close to its "collapse volume." Increasing inspiratory muscle tone and laryngeal tone during expiration must counteract this tendency.

Nonetheless, the newborn's ability to ventilate and perfuse his or her alveoli and thereby permit exchange of carbon dioxide for oxygen within them is more than sufficient and quite on par with that of an Olympic runner. Indeed, the reason for the characteristic mild hypoxemia of the newborn (arterial PO_2 of 70 to 90 mm Hg) is not that arterialization of venous blood within the lung is imperfect, but rather that a certain amount of right-to-left "fetal" shunting of desaturated venous blood continues to occur across the foramen ovale and ductus arteriosus in the first hours and days. Likewise, the hypocapnia typical of neonatal life (arterial PCO_2 of 35 mm Hg) may result from a progesterone-mediated lowering of the respiratory center's threshold for carbon dioxide or may simply reflect the prolonged fluid volume expansion of fetal life, in the form of lowered serum and cerebrospinal fluid bicarbonate levels.

RENAL FUNCTION

It has been suggested that the perinatal kidney emerges at birth from a primeval, water-rich swamp into an extrauterine desert. This is because the fetus and newborn infant in the first few days behave in many ways as does a chronically volume-expanded patient, with decreased tubular resorption of water and sodium, bicarbonate, glucose, and phosphate, leading to "wasting" into the fetal urine. The teleological and metaphysical question arises whether the fetus sustains such polyuria to maintain amniotic fluid volume. This question has not been answered clearly, but certainly the fetus that has renal agenesis (Potter's syndrome) exists in an intrauterine environment with tremendously reduced amniotic fluid (called *amnion nodosum,* to describe profound oligohydramnios).

Renal vascular resistance, like that of the lung, is great in utero and is associated with a low renal blood flow (RBF) rate of only 2% to 4% of fetal cardiac output. After birth, RBF achieves a 5% value by 12 hours and 10% by the end of the first week. The estimated RBF in older children and adults is 20% to 25% of cardiac output. The postnatal improvement in RBF is associated with decreased renal vascular resistance and increased systemic blood pressure. The glomerular filtration rate (GFR) also is reduced in utero and in newborns, doubling over the first 2 weeks after birth. A number of hormones and vasoactive substances are involved in regulation of these maturational processes.

The neonate is undergoing a rather rapid physiological reduction of the expanded extracellular fluid (ECF) volume; thus, the fluid requirements of the healthy term newborn infant are not as great in the first 1 to 2 days after birth.

DIGESTIVE SYSTEM

The newborn at term is neuromuscularly equipped to create the intraluminal pressure gradients that constitute a sufficient peristalsis for movement of an ingested feeding from mouth to rectum. These pressure gradients begin in the oropharynx in the form of swallowing, which requires cooperative intermingling of motor and sensory effectiveness throughout the hindbrain (cranial nerves IX, X, and XII) working in concert with the midbrain (cranial nerves V and VII). Although gastrointestinal motility immediately postpartum may appear uncoordinated by adult standards, it nevertheless is extremely effective in moving swallowed air from mouth to rectum by 2 to 4 hours of age. By histological criteria, all the requisite structures (e.g., microvilli) for efficient absorption of nutrients from the small bowel appear to be in place by the time of birth at term. The biochemical necessities for absorption also appear to be satisfied for digestion of carbohydrates (amylase, lactase, other disaccharidases) and proteins (gastric acid and pepsin, trypsin, and other pancreatic peptidases).

Fat absorption, on the other hand, is more tenuous, particularly for the preterm newborn. Lipase and bile salts are present by term, and their rate of functional appearance is a linear function of gestational age. Additional lipases are present in maternal breast milk, and it appears that this can compensate for the low levels of pancreatic lipases produced by preterm infants. Breast milk seems to have the optimum ratio of unsaturated to saturated fatty acids and the optimum distribution of carbon chain lengths of saturated fatty acids for digestion.

The microbiological sterility of the gut in utero begins to change immediately after birth. Gut colonization proceeds through invasion of the mouth and anus by ambient microorganisms, which reflect both the maternal and neonatal environments. Aerobic organisms will appear within the first few hours; anaerobes follow within hours thereafter.

HEPATIC FUNCTION

During fetal life, most hepatic duties are assumed by the maternal liver via the placenta. Indeed, most fetal blood flow returning from the placenta is actually shunted through the liver via the ductus venosus, which collapses after birth (as umbilical and placental venous return collapses), thus forcing perfusion of the liver by the portal circulation. In midgestation, the liver is functioning mainly as a hematopoietic organ.

After birth, the stores of glycogen accumulated by the liver in utero are rapidly depleted, consumed to supply energy until effective oral feeding is established. Stored fat is next used as an energy source, once the liver glycogen stores have become depleted. Liver and cardiac glycogen and the energy these stores contain are the likely basis for the newborn's greater resistance to hypoxia.

Throughout life the major function of the liver is to produce proteins—the plasma proteins (albumin and globulins), enzymes, and clotting factors. In a healthy newborn, these anabolic functions are present, though further postnatal maturation will occur over the first weeks. However, because of this, many drug or other detoxifying reactions under enzymatic control are slower in infants, leading to prolonged half-lives for many drugs compared with adults.

The best known example of this enzymatic torpor in the newborn is the conjugation of free bilirubin (lipid soluble) with glucuronic acid to form excretable (water-soluble) indirect bilirubin diglucuronide. The reaction is controlled by glucuronyl transferase, an enzyme whose activity is diminished at birth (which accounts in part for the common occurrence of "physiological" jaundice in newborns) but which rises rapidly to adult levels thereafter.

IMMUNE SYSTEM

The B-cell function of antibody production develops relatively late in fetal life. Moreover, the bacteriologically sterile fetus normally receives no stimulus from foreign antigens to produce antibodies. Why maternal cells leaking into the fetus are not soon rejected as immunological invaders is one of the great mysteries of reproductive biology. In any case, the only significant antibody level normally mounted at birth is IgG, passively obtained transplacentally from the mother. However, the infant shortly will (or should) receive a good deal of IgA and macrophages from the mother's colostrum and breast milk. These facts can be diagnostically useful, in that elevations of cord blood IgM may be taken as evidence for preexisting (long enough to mount an antibody response) intrauterine infection.

Cellular immunity (T-cell function) is largely intact in a newborn and, along with the borrowed maternal IgG, is the bedrock of the young infant's immune competence. Phagocytosis is depressed, however, and in the face of large bacterial inocula, sometimes critically so. The problem is that although the newborn's macrophages and neutrophils are quite capable of ingestion and digestion, the particles and bacteria to be attacked are insufficiently opsonized by the low serum complement levels. Thus, although the infant's system inevitably must learn to deal with microorganisms through exposure, it would be most prudent to arrange that all such exposures occur in moderation.

ENDOCRINE SYSTEM

The thyroid gland is operative early in fetal life and by term has stored sufficient triiodothyronine (T_3) and thyroxine (T_4) to enable the infant's metabolism to sustain him or her against thermal and nutritional stress, by virtue of the miniature thyroid storm precipitated by the birth process.

The parathyroid gland is similarly functional but perhaps not robustly so. The relatively high serum calcium level of fetal life drops rapidly at birth from about 11 to 8.5 mg/dl as phosphorus rises, and yet apparently does not elicit a reactive resorption of bone to defend serum calcium or enhanced excretion of phosphorus. Precise explanations are not at hand but may deal in part with a high ingested phosphorus load, especially in the infant who is fed cow milk-based formula.

The adrenal cortex of the healthy infant is quite capable of mounting a suitable glucocorticoid and mineralocorticoid response to stress. The adrenal medulla (and the paraspinal chromaffin organ of Zuckerkandl) is almost totally devoted to the production of norepinephrine (an alpha-agonist) rather than to epinephrine (an alpha- and beta-agonist). Perhaps these organs sense that the heart is near the peak of its function curve and may not be able to respond to much further beta-stimulation without decompensation. In addition, norepinephrine is the facilitator of thermogenesis within dark adipose tissue ("brown fat"), an important factor in helping infants maintain their body temperature after birth.

In the pancreas, the hormones insulin and glucagon produced by the islet cells are functional at birth, although in the case of insulin, somewhat sluggishly released. Equally important, the receptors for these hormones in body tissue are present and functional.

NEUROLOGICAL SYSTEM

Through most of the last half of fetal life, glial and neuronal cells differentiate in the paraventricular germinal matrix. The neuronal axons develop dendrites that, through a prolonged process of arborization, develop many thousands of synapses. Through neuronal migration these neurons are distributed throughout the neuraxis (cord, hindbrain, midbrain, forebrain) in the form of compact nuclei, looser reticular formations, or the laminated sheets (six in all) of the cerebral gray matter.

The axonal pathways are formed when neurons and glial cells are combined and become myelinated. This occurs differentially (caudad to cephalad), so that at birth the forebrain and midbrain are still largely unmyelinated. Although unmyelinated pathways have slower conduction times, the shorter interneuronal and neuromuscular distances in the newborn result in reflex arcs not much different in duration of action from those of adults.

The behavior of reflexes is influenced significantly by the state of consciousness. Proprioceptive reflexes, which generate postural body tonus, are abolished during active REM sleep, which strongly inhibits motor neurons. Similarly, quiet sleep diminishes the exteroceptive reflexes whose efferent arcs come from skin, retinal, and aural receptors, rather than from the muscle stretch receptors of proprioception.

The higher cortical functions are continuing to be investigated through both biophysical and psychological techniques. It appears that newborn humans are a great deal more involved with and occasionally manipulative of their environment and caregivers than previously supposed.

three Recovery Period

Nicholas M. Nelson

The most complex modern surgical procedure is unlikely to equal the physiological strain upon an infant during a normal birth—massive head trauma, asphyxiation, massive blood transfusion with cardiopulmonary bypass, and often resuscitation, all followed by major hypothermic insult—no wonder the infant cries! Clement Smith[2] has called this "the Valley of the Shadow of Birth," but it is a normal event experienced by every human being (just as is death) and may be regarded as the disease from which *nearly* everyone recovers. However, where should the "recovery room" be?

Important observations need to be made in these first few hours, and it is not easy in either home or hospital (however homelike) to make them without untoward medical intrusion on what many would wish were more of a private family affair. The solution is to begin early in pregnancy to build toward expanding the parents' "family" to include the hospital's perinatal personnel to the point that it becomes almost immaterial whether these observations are made in the mother's room or in a contiguous recovery room (observation nursery).

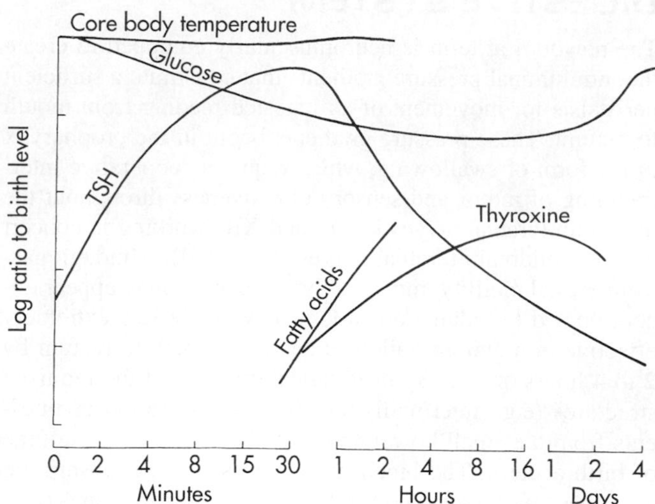

Fig. 45-4 Metabolic changes at birth. Data are shown as the approximate log (value at time/value at birth), which ranges from 0 *(bottom tic)* to 1 *(top tic)*. *TSH,* Thyroid stimulating hormone.

(Data from Smith CA, Nelson NM: *The physiology of the newborn infant,* ed 4, Springfield, Ill, 1976, Charles C Thomas.)

CONVERSION FROM PLACENTAL TO ORAL ENERGY ASSIMILATION

The eviction from the womb that is birth may be compared, metabolically speaking, to forceful ejection from one's warm and friendly neighborhood "pub" into the cold, midwinter streets—naked and without a free lunch. The sober adult in such circumstances would immediately seek clothing—not out of civilized modesty but from a primal necessity to prevent excessive loss of body heat through convection, by surrounding the skin with layers of insulating dead air. He or she simultaneously would vasoconstrict his or her skin ("blue with cold"—acrocyanosis), shiver to produce muscular heat, and begin to generate an increased amount of chemical heat by releasing thyroxin (to energize all cells) and catecholamines (to release the energy stored in fat by its lipolysis into glycerol and free fatty acids). The newborn baby does precisely the same (but does not shiver) and with at least as great efficiency (Fig. 45-4).

Thoughtful medical attendants to the newborn will supply warm clothing (or warmth by radiant warmer, incubator, or other thermal device) and arrange the ambient temperature so that minimal thermal energy demands (the "neutral temperature," Fig. 45-5) are made upon the infant, who must concentrate most of his or her stored energy investment on the principal continuing task of growth and development, at least until ingestion, digestion, and excretion are well established.

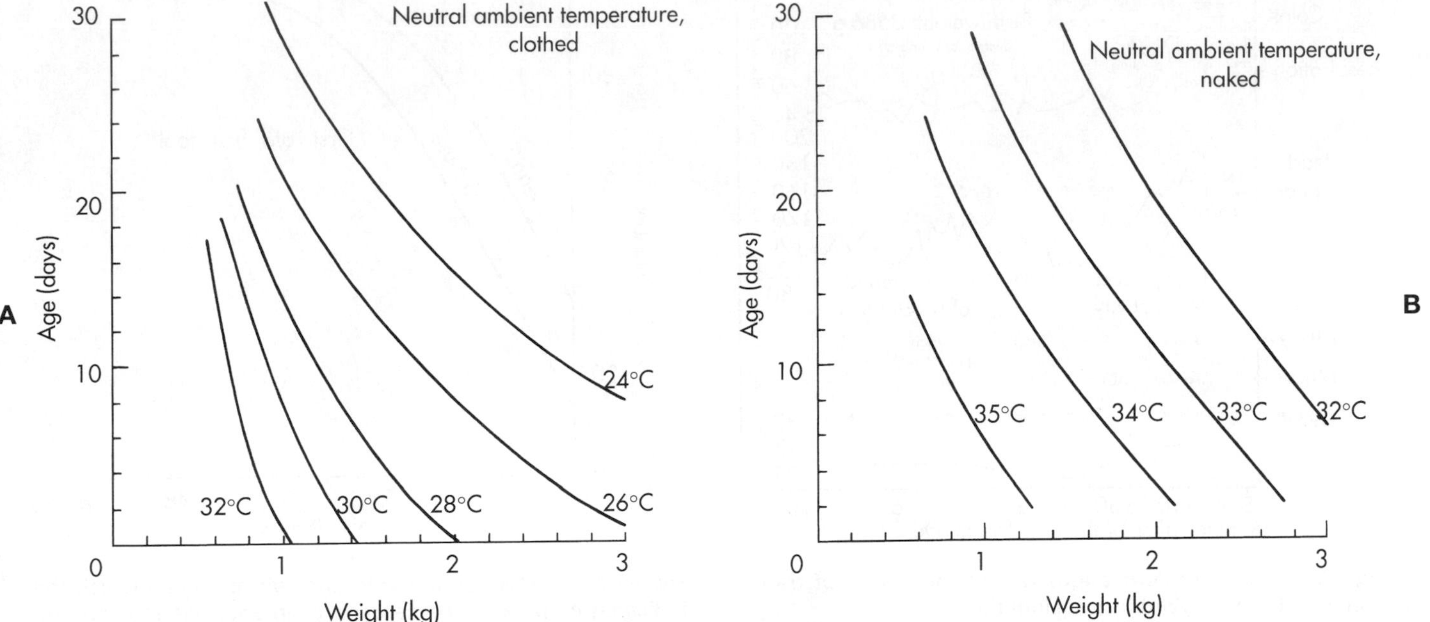

Fig. 45-5 Neutral ambient temperature for clothed **(A)** and naked **(B)** infants of varying postpartum age and weight. The neutral temperature is that ambient temperature at which energy expenditure to maintain body temperature is minimal (e.g., a naked 1-kg infant at age 10 days requires an ambient temperature of about 94.1° F (34.5° C) for minimal energy expenditure to defend body temperature).

(Data from Scopes JW, Ahmed I: *Arch Dis Child* 41:417, 1966.)

TRANSITION AND ESTABLISHMENT OF VITAL FUNCTION

The infant's behavioral status during the initial hours of recovery have been characterized clinically as alert (0 to 30 minutes), then unresponsive (30 minutes to 2 hours), and finally, reactive (2 to 8 hours), as shown in Fig. 45-6, during which time the infant displays signs of general sympathetic discharge (tachycardia, tachypnea, and vasomotion) and then parasympathetic discharge (peristalsis), probably in response to the sensory overload that attends birth, particularly chilling. The onset of peristalsis heralds the first defecation and micturition, the timing of which should be carefully noted, because untoward delay in either (Fig. 45-7) may signal significant gastrointestinal or genitourinary abnormalities.

With a normal birth, the pediatrician is likely to make first physical acquaintance with the newborn in the nursery rather than in the delivery room. Therefore, after a period of observation by the nursery ("recovery room") staff, those elements calling for special surveillance (Table 45-4) need to be gleaned from the obstetrical history and brought to the pediatrician's attention as a confirmation of previous alerts from the obstetrical staff.

Even in the absence of such obstetrical markers of high risk for neonatal morbidity, observers in the nursery should always assume that every infant harbors clinically occult congenital anomalies or birth trauma that may have escaped detection in the initial (delivery room) or subsequent detailed (nursery) physical examination, until the passage of time gradually documents without error, the establishment of certain vital functions (Table 45-5).

During this period of stabilization, the following elements are observed most closely: body temperature, skin color, heart rate, blood pressure, peripheral circulation, respiratory rate and type of effort, muscle tone, body activity, and apparent behavioral state (Box 45-4).

MATURATIONAL, BEHAVIORAL, PHYSICAL, AND NEUROLOGICAL EXAMINATIONS

As in all of pediatrics, the components of a physician's thinking about a normal or abnormal infant are very much structured around the baby's growth and development compared with accepted norms. In later infancy and childhood, the required time dimension (the *x*-axis of growth charts) is measured in months or years, and the origin is fixed with certainty (date of birth). Practicing these principles is more difficult in the perinatal period because time is measured in weeks and the date of conception cannot be fixed with any real certainty. Nonetheless, fetal and neonatal examinations of many infants from many different populations by many observers have produced a number of acceptable norms and have standardized the assessment of gestational age.

Assessment of Gestational Age

The combined assessment of neuromuscular maturity (presented in instructional form in Box 45-5) and certain physical features of genitalia, ears, skin, breast, plantar creases, and hair have proved to be a reliable means for estimating gestational age (Fig. 45-8). Further corroboration may be sought

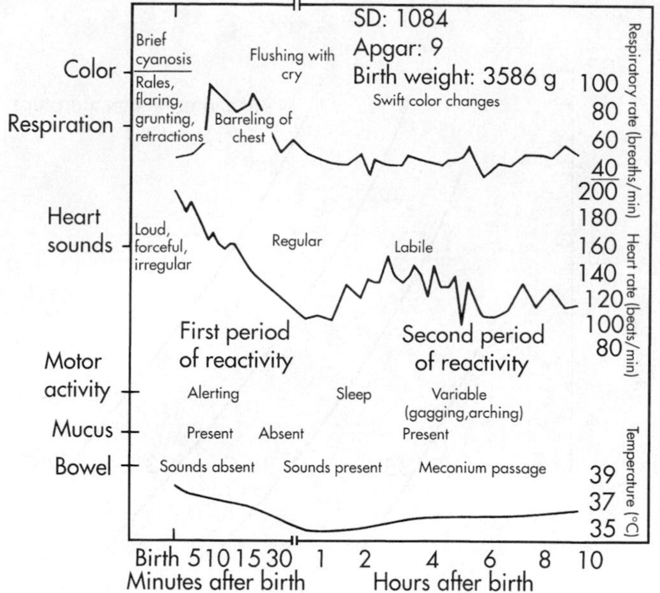

Fig. 45-6 Autonomic changes during the period of transition after birth. *SD,* Subject designation.

(From Desmond MM, Rudolph AJ, Phitaksphraiwan P: *Pediatr Clin North Am* 13:656, 1966.)

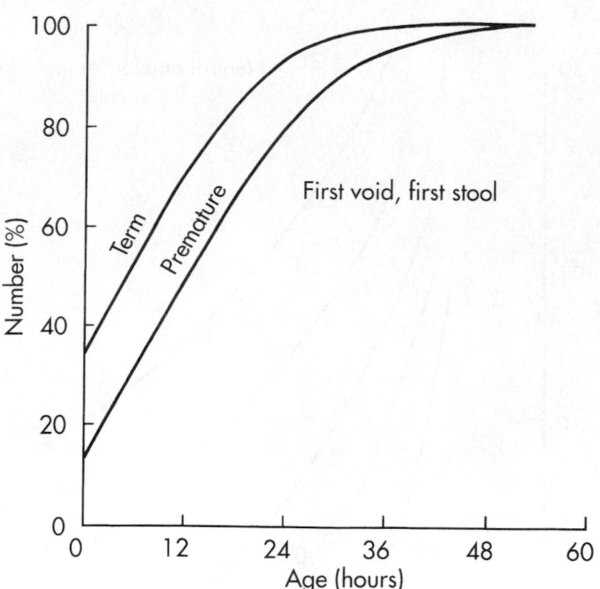

Fig. 45-7 First stool and void after birth: age by which the indicated cumulative percentage of infants has stooled and voided.

(Data from Sherry SN, Kramer I: *J Pediatr* 46:158, 1955, and Kramer I, Sherry SN: *J Pediatr* 51:373, 1957.)

Table 45-4 Levels of Surveillance of the Newborn Based on the Obstetrical History

	Level of Surveillance		
History	**Normal**	**Alert**	**Alarm**
Pregnancy			
Surveillance	Registered during first trimester	Unregistered during second trimester	Unregistered and in labor
Genetic disease	None known	In family	In sibling of fetus
Uterine volume		Polyhydramnios	Oligohydramnios
Fetal movement		Increased	Decreased
Biochemical		Decreased estriol levels	Increased alpha-fetoprotein
Biophysical		Positive oxytocin challenge test	Uterine ultrasound abnormality
Maternal disease		Diabetes and hypertension	Active tuberculosis
Rupture of membranes		<36 wk	
Labor	36-42 wk	<36, >42 wk	<34 wk
Delivery			
Vaginal		"Difficult" breech	
Cesarean	Elective (repeat)	Elective (initial)	Emergency
Fetus	Apgar 8-10	Apgar 4-7, visible congenital anomaly	Asphyxia (Apgar <4) and hydrops fetalis

Table 45-5 Levels of Surveillance of the Newborn Based on Vital Functions

	Level of Surveillance		
Vital Function	**Normal**	**Alert**	**Alarm**
Respiration	Paradoxical (during active sleep)	Periodic tachypnea or retractions	Apnea, bradycardia, grunting, or gasping
Circulation	Acrocyanosis and heart rate 110-165 beats/min	Tachycardia, hypertension, or cardiac murmur	Central cyanosis, bradycardia, hypotension, enlarged heart, or pallor
Metabolism	Body temperature 95.9° to 99.5° F (35.5° to 37.5° C)	Hyperthermia	Hypothermia
Digestion	Drooling or "transitional" stools	Spitting	Vomiting or diarrhea
Excretion		No voiding (>24 hr) and no stooling (>24 hr)	Dribbling stream
Behavior	Alert, unresponsive, reactive, startle, or sneeze	Hyperactive, jittery, or yawning	Coma or convulsions

BOX 45-4

OBSERVATION POINTS DURING RECOVERY

"Hands Off"	"Hands On"
Behavioral state	Heart rate
Quiet sleep	Muscle tone
Active sleep	Body temperature
Quiet alert	Blood pressure
Active awake	Blood sugar
Skin color	
Peripheral circulation	
Body activity	
Suck activity	
Respiratory effort	
Respiratory rate	

by examining the vascularity in the anterior capsule of the lens (Fig. 45-9). Thus, armed with a working knowledge of gestational age, in comparison with birth weight against established norms (e.g., the Colorado Intrauterine Growth Charts), the examiner next should judge whether the infant is large, appropriate, or small for his or her gestational age (LGA, AGA, and SGA, respectively) and thus become appropriately alerted to diagnostic possibilities (see Fig. 43-4).

Behavioral Assessment

Although not often part of the routine surveillance of the normal newborn infant, a Brazelton score determined by a skilled observer of newborn behavior has proved to be a reproducible and valid means of evaluating infant behavior (Box 45-6) and of detecting behavioral changes imposed by birth injury or maternal analgesics.

Through this and other means, it recently has become apparent that term newborns regularly indulge in considerably more environmental interaction (and even manipulation) than heretofore suspected; they prefer human faces to other faces, listen to high-pitched voices, and respond to speech cadences; they are soothed by resumption of the intrauterine "position of comfort," and they can smell their mother's milk.

How much of this behavioral display may be available for viewing depends on the infant's behavioral "state," which includes several states of sleep, variously graded on a scale of 4 points (awake, active sleep, indeterminate sleep, and quiet sleep) or 6 points (awake-crying, awake-active, quiet-alert, drowsy, rapid eye movement [REM] sleep, and deep sleep). They are at their most competent behaviorally in the quiet-alert state and at their most interesting physiologically in REM sleep (Fig. 45-10). During REM sleep, for instance, breathing becomes irregular and "paradoxical," as intercostal muscle tone collapses (thus weakening the chest wall) to allow the diaphragm to pull the thorax inward during its inspiratory descent.

General Physical Examination

As is implicit from the preceding discussion, the newborn's first formal and complete physical examination (Fig. 45-11)

BOX 45-5

TECHNIQUES FOR ASSESSMENT OF NEUROMUSCULAR MATURITY

Posture

With the infant supine and quiet, score as follows:
- Arms and legs extended = 0
- Slight or moderate flexion of hips and knees = 1
- Moderate to strong flexion of hips and knees = 2
- Legs flexed and abducted, arms slightly flexed = 3
- Full flexion of arms and legs = 4

Square Window

Flex the hand at the wrist (exert pressure sufficient to get as much flexion as possible); do not rotate the wrist. Measure and score the angle between the hypothenar eminence and the anterior aspect of the forearm according to Fig. 45-8.

Arm Recoil

With the infant supine, fully flex the forearm for 5 seconds, then fully extend by pulling the hands and releasing. Score the reaction according to the following:
- Remains extended or random movements = 0
- Incomplete or partial flexion = 1
- Brisk return to full flexion = 2

Popliteal Angle

With the infant supine and the pelvis flat on the examining surface, use one hand to flex the leg on the thigh and then fully flex the thigh; use the other hand to extend the leg. Score the angle attained as in Fig. 45-8.

Scarf Sign

With the infant supine, take the infant's hand and draw it across the neck and as far across the opposite shoulder as possible (assistance to the elbow is permissible by lifting it across the body). Score according to the location of the elbow:
- Elbow reaches beyond the opposite anterior axillary line = 0
- Elbow reaches to the opposite anterior axillary line = 1
- Elbow is between opposite anterior axillary line and midline of thorax = 2
- Elbow is at midline of thorax = 3
- Elbow does not reach midline of thorax = 4

Heel-to-Ear Maneuver

With the infant supine, hold the infant's foot with one hand and move it as near to the head as possible without forcing it. Keep the pelvis flat on the examining surface. Score as in Fig. 45-8.

From Amiel-Tison C: *Arch Dis Child* 43:89, 1968; and Dubowitz LMS, Dubowitz V, Goldberg C: *J Pediatr* 77:1, 1970.

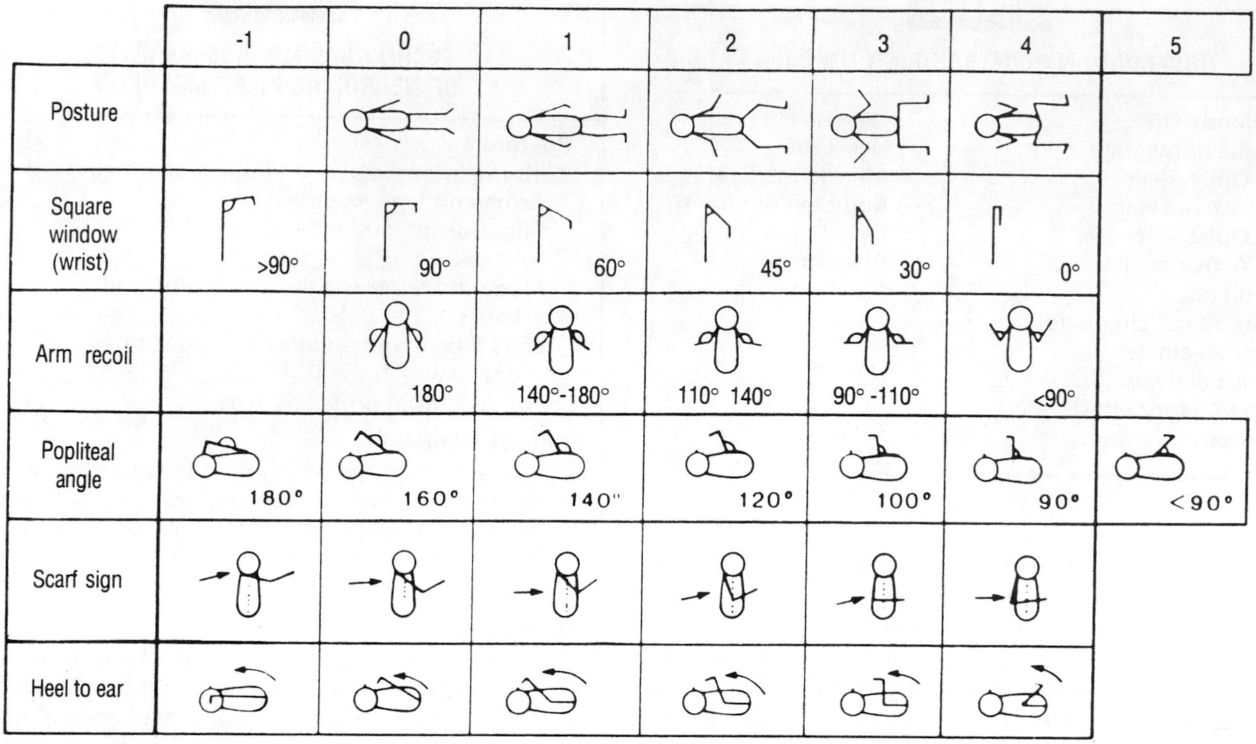

	-1	0	1	2	3	4	5
Posture							
Square window (wrist)	>90°	90°	60°	45°	30°	0°	
Arm recoil		180°	140°-180°	110° 140°	90° -110°	<90°	
Popliteal angle	180°	160°	140°	120°	100°	90°	<90°
Scarf sign							
Heel to ear							

Physical Maturity	-1	0	1	2	3	4	5
Skin	sticky friable transparent	gelatinous red, translucent	smooth pink, visible veins	superficial peeling &/or rash, few veins	cracking pale areas rare veins	parchment deep cracking no vessels	leathery cracked wrinkled
Lanugo	none	sparse	abundant	thinning	bald areas	mostly bald	
Plantar surface	heel-toe 40-50 mm:- 1 <40 mm: -2	>50 mm no crease	faint red marks	anterior transverse crease only	creases ant. 2/3	creases over entire sole	
Breast	imperceptible	barely perceptible	flat areola no bud	stippled areola 1-2 mm bud	raised areola 3-4 mm bud	full areola 5-10 mm bud	
Eye/Ear	lids fused loosely: -1 tightly: -2	lids open pinna flat stays folded	sl. curved pinna: soft: slow recoil	well-curved pinna: soft but ready recoil	formed & firm instant recoil	thick cartilage ear stiff	
Genitals male	scrotum flat, smooth	scrotum empty faint rugae	testes in upper canal rare rugae	testes descending few rugae	testes down good rugae	testes pendulous deep rugae	
Genitals female	clitoris prominent labia flat	prominent clitoris small labia minora	prominent clitoris enlarging minora	majora & minora equally prominent	majora large and minora small	majora cover clitoris & minora	

Maturity Rating

score	weeks
-10	20
-5	22
0	24
5	26
10	28
15	30
20	32
25	34
30	36
35	38
40	40
45	42
50	44

Fig. 45-8 Assessment of gestational age in weeks, using a combination of neuromuscular and physical maturity criteria. The box on the top describes methods used to assess neuromuscular maturity. The assessment is quickly and easily performed because the box includes measures of physical maturity and of passive but not active tone. Physical maturity is most accurately assessed in the minutes or hour or so after birth. The score for each item is indicated at the top of the vertical column. However, neuromuscular maturity may be spuriously retarded in an asphyxiated neonate or in a neonate obtunded by anesthetic agents or drugs. Thus, the neuromuscular maturity rating should be repeated after a day or two. The sum of the scores on all the items of physical and neuromuscular maturity provides an estimate of maturity in weeks *(see lower right)*.

(From Ballard JL: *J Pediatr* 119:417, 1991.)

POINTS	0	1	2	3	4
BREAST SIZE		< .5 cm	> .5 cm < 1 cm	> 1 cm	
FOOT CREASES		faint red marks ant. half	faint red marks >ant half indent. <ant 1/3	indent >ant. 1/3	deep indent. >ant 1/3
EAR FIRMNESS	soft easily folded no recoil	soft easily folded slow recoil	cartilage thin in places ready recoil	definite cartilage extend. to periph. immediate recoil	
LENS					
wks	27-28	29-30	31-32	33-34	>35

Total Score	Gestational Age Weeks
1	28
2	29
3	29½
4	30½
5	31

GESTATIONAL AGE

For scores >5: Score + 26 = weeks gestational age (example: score = 6 (+ 26) = 32 weeks gestational age).

Fig. 45-9 Rapid assessment of gestational age.
(Modified from Narayan I, et al: *Pediatrics* 69:27, 1982; and Hittner H, et al: *J Pediatrics* 9:455, 1977.)

BOX 45-6

BRAZELTON BEHAVIORAL SCALE

Environmental Interactions	Motor Processes
Alertness	Activity
Consolability	Defensive reactions
Cuddliness	Hand-to-mouth movement
Orientation	Maturity
Stress responses	Reflex
Skin color lability	Tone
Startle reaction	**Physiological State**
Tremulousness	Habituation to stimuli
	Self-quieting

occurs during the period of transition in a setting of continuous and intense scrutiny by both the delivery room and nursery staffs, not to mention the parents. Moreover, observations and interventions overlap considerably during the nursery stay.

The nursing staff observes the vital signs (Fig. 45-12), which now can include blood pressure, as conveniently measured by oscillometric or Doppler devices. The most cooperative infant is one who is 1 to 2 hours postprandial, in the quiet-alert behavioral state, and examined under thermal conditions not too far from his or her neutral thermal environment (see Fig. 45-5). The infant's general appearance will have been noted during the assessment of gestational age, but particular attention should now be directed to his or her apparent nutritional state (especially subcutaneous tissue and muscle mass) and postural tone. The more mature the infant, the greater the flexor tone displayed as part of the resting posture.

Much of the normal (or normal variant) findings of the newborn's physical examination are presented in Chapter 8, The Pediatric Physical Examination; here we focus on those aspects that should raise the suspicion of abnormality. Nevertheless, those portions of Chapter 8 that deal with the physical examination of each of the organ systems under the heading "Newborn" also should be consulted.

The skin and its appendages (Table 45-6). The naked infant should be observed most carefully for skin color; pallor, jaundice, and cyanosis may each become an indication for alarm, depending on the time of onset, dura-

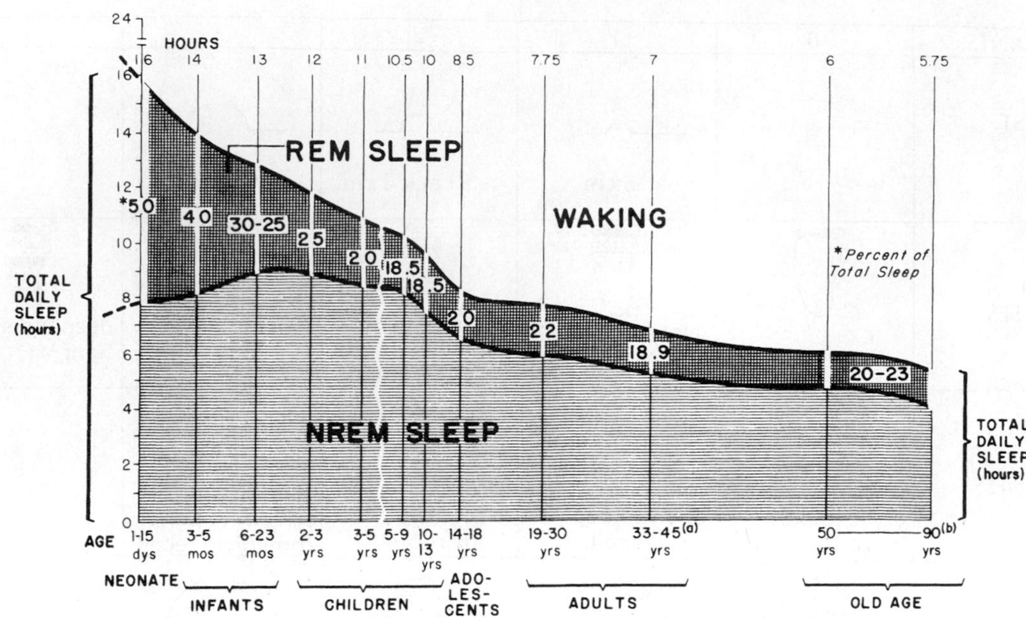

Fig. 45-10 Graph showing changes (with age) in total amounts of daily sleep, daily rapid eye movement (REM) sleep, and percentage of REM sleep. Note sharp diminution of REM sleep in the early years. REM sleep falls from 8 hours at birth to less than 1 hour in old age. The amount of nonrapid eye movement (NREM) sleep throughout life remains more constant, falling from 8 hours to 5 hours. In contrast to the steep decline of REM sleep, the quantity of NREM sleep is undiminished for many years. Although total daily REM sleep falls steadily during life, the percentage rises slightly in adolescence and early adulthood. This rise does not reflect an increase in amount; it is caused by the fact that REM sleep does not diminish as quickly as total sleep.

(From Rofftvarg HP, Muzio JN, Dement WC: *Science* 152:604, 1966.)

NEONATAL RECORD (2)—NURSERY

BIRTH

BORN AT HOSPITAL	CITY	STATE
TIME	DATE	REFERRING PHYSICIAN M.D.
LMP	EDC	GESTATIONAL AGE WKS / VIT K_1 GIVEN AT HRS OF AGE

INTERVAL HISTORY

NURSERY EXAMINATION

DATE	TIME	AGE HRS	WGT GMS	SEX	RACE
LENGTH CMS	BIP CMS	SKULL CMS	CHEST CMS	ABDOMEN CMS	
[KEY ✓= NORMAL, 0 = ABSENT, X = ABNORMAL]		EFFECTS OF FETAL POSTURE		GENERAL APPEARANCE	
SKIN	SC TISSUE	FACIES	MASSES	SPLEEN	HIPS
VERNIX	EDEMA	EYES	THORAX	KIDNEYS	CNS-REFLEXES
PALLOR	NODES	EARS	BREATHING	CORD	CRY
ICTERUS	HEAD	NARES	LUNGS	ANUS	TONE
CYANOSIS	FONTANELLES	MOUTH	HEART	GENITALIA	PARALYSIS
BIRTHMARKS	SUTURES	NECK	ABDOMEN	SKELETON	MORO
BRUISING	CPHLHMTOMA	THYROID	LIVER	CLAVICLES	GRASP

GESTATIONAL AGE ASSESSMENT = WEEKS

ABNORMAL FINDINGS

IMPRESSION

SIGNED M.D.

Fig. 45-11 Data relevant to the neonatal physical examination.

NEWBORN NURSING ASSESSMENT

Admission: Date ______ Time ______ Birth: Date ______ Time ______ Weight ______ Length ______ Head ______
Gestation: By Dates ______ By Dubowitz ______ AGA/LGA/SGA ______
Relevant OB History

Ears & Eyes — $AgNO_3$ 1% Crede ☐ 2 gtts each eye

Nose — Nares Patent: By occlusion ☐ catheter ☐

Mouth

Skin

Head

Chest

Abdomen, Umbilical Vessels

Genitals — Anus Patent: By appearance ☐ catheter ☐

Extremities, Skeleton

Nervous System

Activity

Transitional TPR

Time		Comments	Initials	General Comments
				Signature:

Six Hour Assessment

Skin ______
Chest ______
Abdomen ______
Nervous System ______
Activity ______

Comments:

Signature: ______

Fig. 45-12 Nursing surveillance of a normal newborn infant.

Table 45-6 Levels of Surveillance of the Newborn Based on the Examination of the Skin and Its Appendages

	Level of Surveillance		
Characteristic	**Normal**	**Alert**	**Alarm**
Color (age of occurrence)			
Cyanosis	Acrocyanosis (<12 hr)	Central (<1 hr)	Central (>1 hr)
Jaundice	>24 hr	18-24 hr	<18 hr
Pallor			>30 min
Epidermis	Dermatoglyphics	Excoriations	Sloughing
Hair	Lanugo	Lumbosacral tuft and scalp defect	
Texture	Soft and moist	Dry and scaling	Thickened and crusting
Vascular pattern	Harlequin, mottling (cold)	Persistent mottling	
Cysts	Milia and Epstein pearls		
Papules	Acne and miliaria		
Desquamation	Delicate scaling (>2 days)	Peeling (<2 days)	Denuded sheets (anytime)
Hemangiomas	Telangiectatic (forehead, lids, lips, and nape)	Telangiectatic (trigeminal) and angiomatous (few)	Angiomatous (multiple)
Hemorrhage	Petechiae (head or upper body)	Petechiae (elsewhere)	Ecchymoses and purpura
Macules	Mongolian spots	Café-au-lait spots (fewer than 6)	Café-au-lait spots (6 or more) and "mountain ash" leaf
Pustules	Erythema toxicum		Large and dermal
Vesicles			Any
Nodules		Subcutaneous fat necrosis	Sclerema

tion, and intensity. Excoriations of the epidermis can be a normal result of long fingernails, but when observed in a yawning or "jittery" baby, they also may indicate neonatal abstinence syndrome (withdrawal from maternal narcotics; see Chapter 50, Prenatal Drug Abuse and Neonatal Drug Withdrawal Syndrome). A lumbosacral tuft of hair may point to pilonidal sinus, diastematomyelia, or teratoma, and it should be established that a scalp defect is not accompanied by other signs of trisomy 18. The skin's texture normally is soft and moist ("as a baby's bottom") at term, but it lacks fullness of subcutaneous tissue in a preterm infant and is dry, cracked, or peeling in a vernix-deprived postmature or undergrown infant. The skin is grotesquely thickened and crusted ("collodion baby") in various rare types of ichthyosis. An apparently normal phenomenon of vascular reactivity is the mottled ("marbled") vascular pattern of dilated venules in the (usually chilled) newborn. When persistent, this mottled cutis marmorata may be associated with trisomy 18 (see Chapter 40, Approaches to Genetic Diseases) or trisomy 21 (see Chapter 204, Down Syndrome: Managing the Child and Family). A phenomenon of the late neonatal period (1 month) is *acne* (true comedo), seen mostly over the cheeks and chin as tiny, coalescing, erythematous papules that usually disappear over a few weeks.

The clay-colored and greasy vernix caseosa that covers the healthy term newborn at birth evaporates almost magically within hours after birth and is sparse to absent in a postmature infant, whose superficial epidermal layers are often cracked and peeling. However, this is quite different from the full-thickness denudation that marks the scalded skin syndrome of staphylococcal sepsis.

Probably the most common tumors in humans (or, certainly, in infants), hemangiomas range from the telangiectatic ("capillary") nevi, or "salmon patch," so common on the lids, forehead, and nape ("stork bite") of the newborn to the multiple or massive and often grotesque angiomatous ("cavernous") lesions. Diffuse neonatal hemangiomatosis is the rare but fatal maximum expression of this spectrum, often marked by cardiac failure to manage the vast volume overload presented by multiple arteriovenous fistulas, often in major organs, such as the liver and brain. Between these extremes is Sturge-Weber syndrome (venous angiomatosis of leptomeninges, atrophic cerebral cortex, buphthalmos, seizures, hemiparesis, and mental retardation), suggested by an ipsilateral facial port-wine stain in the trigeminal distribution. However, the linkage of cerebral and cutaneous venous angiomatosis is not firm, because many children who have a *port-wine stain* have perfectly normal cerebral function.

A cutaneous hemorrhage in any form is justifiable cause for concern that some form of bleeding diathesis may be at hand. Yet some petechiae (and subconjunctival hemorrhages) may well be observed within the superior vena caval drainage system after a normal vertex delivery, as an expression of the significant pressure differentials to which the fetus is subject upon rupture of the forewaters.

The very common, completely mysterious, and completely benign perifollicular eruption known as erythema toxicum ("flea-bite dermatitis") appears on the second or third day of life as 1- to 3-mm white or pale yellow papules or pustules on a small erythematous but uninflamed base. They can become much larger and even confluent, risking confusion with bacterial pyoderma; however, smears of the sterile contents of these lesions reveal eosinophils rather than neutrophils. The infants are well, and the pustules resolve simultaneously within hours to days.

Vesicles may be associated with benign conditions (e.g., transient neonatal pustular melanosis) but always must raise concern that a serious disease is involved, whether infectious (e.g., herpes, syphilis, toxic epidermal necrolysis) or inherited (e.g., epidermolysis bullosa or incontinentia pigmenti). These lesions demand expert consultation.

Nodules are perhaps the least common primary cutaneous lesion seen in newborns. Subcutaneous fat necrosis (pseudosclerema) appears in the first few days as localized areas of induration over the buttocks, cheeks, or back, with blotchy, reddened overlying skin. Its definitive cause is unknown, but it is attributed to poor perfusion caused by cold stress or asphyxia, and it resolves spontaneously over weeks to months. Sclerema neonatorum is a presumably related process of induration in adipose tissue, formerly seen in hypothermic and usually moribund premature infants.

For further information about skin lesions of the neonate, see Chapter 46, Skin Lesions of the Neonate.

The head and neck (Table 45-7). Caput succedaneum is subcutaneous edema over the presenting part of the head; it is far more common than cephalohematoma, is usually situated over the occiput, and crosses suture lines. Caput tends to feel soft and lacks a well-defined outline, but it is not fluctuant (as is a cephalohematoma). The edema is most pronounced at birth and subsides within 2 or 3 days. It is particularly common after delivery by vacuum extraction.

Cephalohematoma, on the other hand, is a subperiosteal collection of blood and as such is bounded by suture lines. It occurs in full-term healthy babies, most often in the parietal region. Cephalohematoma may not be obvious at birth but may increase in size over the first few hours or days of life, giving rise to a firm mass with a well-defined edge. The center of the swelling may liquefy, giving a feel of fluctuance or an erroneous impression of a depressed skull fracture. The mass occasionally calcifies and persists for weeks to months. Complications include hyperbilirubinemia and underlying skull fracture, the latter being associated with about 20% of cephalohematomas.

A subgaleal hemorrhage sometimes is mistaken for cephalohematoma. However, the subgaleal space is not limited by suture lines, and the blood tends to collect in dependent positions. Moreover, the space is large; thus, a newborn may lose a large amount of blood, leading to hyperbilirubinemia and anemia or even shock.

Molding refers to the overriding of sagittal, coronal, or lambdoid sutures in a normal newborn delivered vaginally from the vertex position. Molding serves as benign testimony to the forces of labor, not shared by the infant delivered by cesarean section or from the breech position; the latter often is characterized by a pronounced occipital "overhang" in the skull contour. The molded head often is irregular in shape, with the parieto-occipital region prominent; the forehead tends to slope backward. Molding is especially likely to be seen in first babies, in a large infant after prolonged labor, or with an element of cephalopelvic disproportion. The abnormal skull features usually return to normal by 5 or 6 days after birth.

A large anterior fontanelle should alert the examiner to the possibility of a defect in membranous bone formation (e.g., achondroplasia, hypophosphatasia, or cretinism) or increased intracranial pressure. Small or absent fontanelles, if associated with a misshapen skull or facies, may indicate a number of cosmetically threatening but treatable bony abnormalities, such as Crouzon's disease or craniosynostosis, although the latter usually is not evident in the immediate neonatal period. The uninformed observer often is too willing to attribute a unilateral facial palsy to "misapplied" forceps, which may leave a temporary blade mark over the eye or cheek. Most such infants actually have a shoulder that tucks neatly under the ear (and into the stylomastoid foramen) of the palsied side. In any case, these palsies tend to resolve quickly after birth.

Two of the most threatening observations to be made of the skull are also two of the most subtle: (1) the examiner must listen specifically for a bruit, which may indicate a cerebral arteriovenous fistula, and (2) positive transillumination ("candling") of the head (using a flashlight in a darkened room or a high-intensity "Chun gun" beam in a lighted room) may be the only clinical indication of hydranencephaly—massive liquefaction of cerebral tissue.

After noting the presence of a retinal red reflex and palpebral fissures of normal size, the examiner also should ensure that the eyes do not have a mongoloid slant (as in Down syndrome) and that the iris is present, because of the high correlation between Wilms' tumor and aniridia. An enlarged or cloudy cornea may be the only visual indication of congenital glaucoma.

A high-arched palate, described as a frequent accompaniment of many complex malformation syndromes, usually is simply short and hypoplastic. An observation of macroglossia should stimulate the search for other signs of cretinism or Beckwith-Wiedemann syndrome, whereas micrognathia suggests, among other things, Treacher Collins and Pierre Robin

Table 45-7 Levels of Surveillance of the Newborn Based on the Head and Neck Examination

	Level of Surveillance		
Location	**Normal**	**Alert**	**Alarm**
Skull	Caput succedaneum, molding, or occipital overhang	Cephalohematoma, craniotabes, large fontanelle, or forceps mark	Craniosynostosis, transillumination, or bruit
Facies		Hypoplasia or palsy	
Eyes		Mongoloid slant	Aniridia and enlarged cornea
Nose		Nasal obstruction	
Mouth		High-arched palate or macroglossia	Cleft palate and/or lip or micrognathia
Ears		"Simple" structure or low set	
Neck	Rotation ±90 degrees	Dimple or webbing	

syndromes. Although cleft lip or palate may occur singly, the examiner should determine whether other signs of trisomy 13 are present (i.e., low-set or malformed ears, webbed neck, scalp defects, microphthalmia, and micrognathia). Similarly, any ear that apparently is low-set (i.e., whose upper attachment to the scalp is below an imaginary line connecting the inner and outer canthi and extended to the occiput), particularly if the foldings of pinna and tragus appear "simplified," should prompt a search for bilateral renal agenesis (Potter's syndrome) and other markers of genetic disease (e.g., webbed neck, "rocker-bottom" feet, or a hypoplastic and incurved fifth digit).

The neck should be freely rotatable and free of dimples or masses, which could suggest a thyroglossal duct cyst (midline) or branchial cleft cyst (anterolateral).

The chest (Table 45-8). Apart from inspecting the newborn's breasts for engorgement or discharge, the thoracic wall is observed closely so as to characterize respiration. Paradoxical respirations are those in which inspiratory efforts are accompanied by protuberance of the abdomen and a sinking in of the lower ribs as the diaphragm descends, unopposed by adequate intercostal muscle tone. Although this phenomenon is characteristic of normal active (REM) sleep in the newborn, it also can signify abnormal respiration. Inspiratory retractions of the lower sternum and intercostal spaces, particularly if accompanied by the use of accessory respiratory muscles (alae nasi and sternocleidomastoids), imply a decrease in lung compliance (stiffening), often caused by atelectasis or accumulation of fluid within the lung. Expiratory grunting (actually, an explosive Valsalva maneuver) is the hallmark of loss of alveolar volume and is displayed most frequently in pediatric experience by the small premature infant whose lungs are atelectatic shortly after birth because of insufficient amounts of stabilizing pulmonary surfactant (i.e., respiratory distress syndrome). However, other causes of respiratory distress (e.g., transient tachypnea, meconium aspiration, and congenital pneumonia) may be impossible to distinguish clinically based on the physical characteristics alone.

Diminished auscultatable air entry on inspiration is difficult to evaluate during quiet breathing. However, when observed in situations in which greater respiratory effort is seen yet not heard, this means that the tidal volume of airflow is reduced, potentially because of atelectasis or airway obstruction. When bowel sounds are clearly audible within the chest, especially the left hemithorax and particularly when accompanied by a displacement of heart sounds to the right, a diaphragmatic hernia must instantly be ruled out by chest roentgenogram, regardless of whether respiratory distress is obvious.

Indeed, although its use cannot be advocated routinely for newborns who do not have symptoms, the chest roentgenogram should be the diagnostic supplement of first resort in the assessment of an ill infant. If it is used, maximum advantage should be extracted from it, particularly by inspecting those areas of prime interest last; this policy prevents many embarrassing omissions of such "incidental" findings as a fractured clavicle or rib, a hemivertebra or spina bifida, or a paralyzed diaphragm. The character of the lung parenchyma should be noted, as well as the presence or absence of fluid or effusion, an "air bronchogram," or a distinct cardiac border (an indistinct border signifies lack of alveolar air). In an infant who has any cardiovascular symptoms, the examiner should be especially careful to estimate the cardiac size and determine if the vascularity of the lung fields is oligemic, normal, or plethoric.

The physician should be concerned by a cardiac impulse that lifts rather than taps at the examining palm or fingertips, because this implies a more generously developed left ventricle than should be the case at the immediate conclusion of fetal life, during which the right ventricle is dominant in both pressure and volume work. Any diminishment of peripheral pulses (especially femoral) is evidence of impeded left ventricular outflow (e.g., coarctation of the aorta) and demands measurement of blood pressure in all four extremities. Sinus

Table 45-8 Levels of Surveillance of the Newborn Based on the Chest Examination

	Level of Surveillance		
Characteristic	**Normal**	**Alert**	**Alarm**
Respiration		Paradoxical, periodic, or retractions	Apnea, expiratory grunt, flaring alae nasi, stridor
Auscultation		Diminished air entry	Bowel sounds
Chest roentgenogram		Enlarged heart	Oligemia or plethora
Cardiac			
Impulse	Tapping	Heaving, lifting	
Pulses	Full	Decreased	Absent (femoral) and lag (cardiac-radial)
Rate and rhythm	110-165, sinus arrhythmia	Sinus bradycardia	Persistent sinus tachycardia
Sounds	"Tick-tock"	S_2 widely split	S_2 fixed split
Murmurs	Systolic (<24 hr)	Systolic (>24 hr)	Diastolic
Electrocardiograph (QRS)			
Vector	+35 to +180 degrees		0 to −90 degrees; −90 to −180 degrees
Amplitude			
V_1	Rs	Rs	rS
V_6	qrS	qRs	qRs

Table 45-9 Levels of Surveillance of the Newborn Based on Examination of the Abdomen

	Level of Surveillance		
Characteristic	**Normal**	**Alert**	**Alarm**
Shape	Cylindrical	Scaphoid	Distended
Muscular wall	Diastasis recti		Absent
Umbilicus	Amniotic navel or cutaneous navel	Exudation or leakage, granuloma, hernia, inflammation, or less than 3 cord vessels	Gastroschisis, omphalitis, or omphalocele
Liver	Smooth edge, 2-3 cm below ribs	>3 cm below ribs	Enlarged
Spleen	Nonpalpable	<1 cm below ribs	Enlarged
Kidneys	Lobulated or palpable (lower poles)	Horseshoe	Enlarged

bradycardia may be precipitated, presumably by vagal reflex, during suctioning or other stimulations of the nasopharynx. Some immature infants may sustain alarming but transient episodes of bradycardia with no apparent stimulus (or symptoms, including apnea), but bradycardia is seen most often during the episodes of prolonged apnea so common in a premature newborn. Indeed, many authorities believe that cardiac (rather than cardiorespiratory) monitoring is a perfectly adequate means of monitoring vital signs in the newborn special care unit. Unameliorated paroxysmal auricular tachycardia can lead to cardiac exhaustion and failure.

The normal tick-tock quality of infant heart sounds results from the near-equal duration of systole and diastole. The high (but subsiding) pulmonary vascular resistance of the first hours and days of life normally accentuates the intensity of the pulmonary component of the second heart sound (S_2), at first difficult to distinguish from the preceding aortic component. However, as pulmonary vascular resistance decreases (and, hence, pulmonary flow increases), the "splitting" of S_2 widens, because closure of the pulmonary valve is delayed by the longer time required to eject the increased right-sided stroke volume. Similarly, the widened and "fixed split" in the S_2 of critical pulmonary stenosis denotes the increased time required to force blood past the obstructed outflow tract of the right ventricle.

An acute and undistracted ear may often (about 20% to 30% of the time) hear transient systolic ejection murmurs at the base of the heart during the first day, presumably associated with flow through the closing ductus arteriosus. Later-developing murmurs have more significance because the increasing resistance (and pressure) differential between the pulmonary and systemic circulations allows the expression of murmurs caused by increasing flow across abnormal connections (e.g., septal defects) between the two circulations. Systolic ejection murmurs heard early (even in fetal life) and that persist throughout the neonatal period may well result from flow across a stenotic valve (i.e., pulmonary or aortic stenosis). Diastolic murmurs should alarm the examiner whenever heard, but they are rarely solitary. See Chapter 142 for a more detailed discussion of heart murmurs.

Apart from specific diagnostic aid regarding the type and probable origin of an arrhythmia, the electrocardiogram, like the chest roentgenogram, is a helpful supplement to the physical examination in assessing the volume (preload) and pressure (afterload) presented to the ventricles. Indeed, knowledge of three major data points alone—whether the right or left ventricle is electrically dominant, whether plethora or oligemia of the pulmonary vasculature is seen on a chest roentgenogram, and whether cyanosis is present or absent clinically, with application of a suitable diagnostic algorithm ("recipe" for systematic assessment of clinical data)—can narrow the likely cardiac diagnosis to two or three entities before echocardiographic or catheter confirmation and without reference to murmurs. For instance, the "adult progression" of precordial QRS complexes (rS in V_1, qRs in V_6) suggests an abnormally dominant left ventricle (or abnormally diminished right ventricle). Combined with cyanosis and oligemic lung fields, these data might well suggest pulmonary atresia. See Chapter 119, Cardiac Arrhythmias, and Chapter 198, Congenital Heart Disease, for more detailed discussion of these subjects.

The abdomen (Table 45-9). A significantly distended abdomen is usually distinctly tense and accompanied by signs of obstruction (vomiting, no stool). The traditional scaphoid (empty) abdomen of a diaphragmatic hernia perhaps is more the exception than the rule, depending on the amount of intestinal gas. Generally, the normal infant abdomen is pleasingly round, soft, and full in the flanks. It often appears to lack a muscular wall, until it becomes rigid during the expiratory phase of crying (or, less fortunately, it displays the "prune belly" appearance of truly absent abdominal musculature).

Although drainage of clear liquid from the navel can accompany a simple (and cauterizable) umbilical granuloma, the examiner must be careful not to miss a urachal fistula. The grosser umbilical malformations (omphalocele and gastroschisis) are impossible to miss and demand immediate intervention. Any sign of inflammation must be watched closely; however, use of "triple dye" for cord care may so discolor the skin (while exerting bacteriostatic action) that inspection becomes quite difficult. Finding less than the normal complement of one large-diameter, thin-walled central vein and two smaller-diameter, thicker-walled arteries at about the 4-o'clock and 8-o'clock positions (facing the infant) in the freshly cut surface of the umbilical cord (best done in the delivery room) should alert the examiner to the likelihood of other developmental anomalies, especially genitourinary ones.

Detection of true enlargement of either the liver or the spleen must be regarded with suspicion. The upper borders of both organs should be located by percussion before conclu-

Table 45-10 Levels of Surveillance of the Newborn Based on Examination of the Perineum

Location	Level of Surveillance: Normal	Alert	Alarm
Anus	Coccygeal dimple		Imperforate, fistula, patulous
Female			
Clitoris		Enlarged, hooded	
Vulva	Bloody secretion, edema, gaping labia, or hymenal tags		Hydrometrocolpos
Male			
Gonad	Edema, hydrocele	Bifid scrotum	Cryptorchidism, inguinal hernia
Phallus	Phimosis	Chordee, hypospadias	Microphallus

Table 45-11 Levels of Surveillance of the Newborn Based on Examination of the Musculoskeletal System

Characteristic	Level of Surveillance: Normal	Alert	Alarm
Fetal posture	Flexor, position of comfort	Frank breech	Extensor
Hand	Webbing	Cortical thumb, overlapping fingers, short, incurved little finger	Polydactyly, syndactyly
Foot	Dorsiflexion 90 degrees, plantar flexion 90 degrees, abduction or adduction of forefoot 45 degrees, inversion or eversion of ankle 45 degrees	Decreased range of motion	Fixed
Extremities	Tibial bowing		Constriction bands, amputation
Neck	Rotation ±90 degrees		
Joints		Reluctance to use	Subluxation (hips), contracture

sions are drawn about enlargement, because they are easily displaced downward by the diaphragm under a lung often distended during the early hours after birth by several "wet lung" conditions (e.g., transient tachypnea).

The kidneys are easier to evaluate at this time than perhaps at any subsequent period in life because the infant abdomen offers little resistance to a gentle yet deep bimanual paraspinal exploration, which should easily yield the impression of at least the (often lobulated) lower poles of the kidneys. Any apparent malformation or enlargement should be confirmed immediately by ultrasonographic examination, as should any frank intraabdominal mass.

The perineum (Table 45-10). Examination of the perineum is straightforward and mainly involves ensuring that the anus is patent and puckers, that the male phallus is well formed and accompanied by palpable gonads, and that the female vaginal vault is patent and contains no extraneous tissues. An incorrect assignment of gender is extremely difficult to retract; therefore, any initial ambiguities must be carefully and courageously faced with the parents while the ambiguities are explored.

The musculoskeletal system (Table 45-11). All late fetuses spend considerable periods in one rather cramped position of "comfort," which can be easily and visibly restored during the nursery examination by enfolding the infant's feet, tibias, and femurs with gentle pressure placed on the soles of the feet. Everything then seems to fall magically into place as it was in utero, and the infant becomes soothed (and the origin of the tibial torsion of infancy becomes obvious). Given current obstetrical trends away from vaginal delivery of the breech presentation, the splayed and extended legs (and hematomas and edema of the buttocks and perineal parts) of the frank breech delivery are increasingly rare. Although a dominantly extensor posture of the extremities is characteristic of the premature infant (and a fundamental part of gestational age assessment by physical examination), its appearance in a newborn at term should suggest significant neuromuscular abnormality.

A certain amount of digital webbing can be familial and normal, but true syndactyly and polydactyly are common in many complex congenital syndromes of malformation; they also occur singly. Similarly, although normal infants frequently (but transiently) manipulate their digits into strange positions, a persistent and almost obligatory grasping of the thumb within the "fisted" fingers suggests the cortical thumb of corticospinal tract malformation. A shortened, curved little finger (clinodactyly), just as a "simple" ear, can be a general marker of genetic disease. The foot that can display the normal range of motion outlined in Table 45-11 cannot be a clubfoot, whereas one more restrained may be. General joint contractures (arthrogryposis) suggest neuromuscular disease, but an infant's reluctance to use a normal-appearing joint suggests trauma. However, subluxated hips are a congenital defect that must be treated forthwith.

The nervous system. Recent discoveries regarding the behavior of newborns, particularly their responses to visual and auditory stimuli, have made it clear that it is no longer appropriate to consider them, at least in their quiet-alert state, as "thalamic" animals. The exteroceptive reflexes (rooting, grasping, plantar, and superficial abdominal), involving touch receptors, are emphasized in the quiet-alert state, whereas the proprioceptive reflexes (deep tendon, Moro, and ankle clonus) are accentuated during quiet sleep.

Depressive changes in mental status, if occurring early (at younger than 1 to 2 days of age), are related most often to the birth process (oxygenation, trauma, or drugs); if they occur later, metabolic processes are probably involved. For instance, an infant who is normal at birth but days later (after digestion of milk and assimilation of its protein and carbohydrate) develops lethargy, stupor, coma, or convulsions (and may have a peculiar odor of, say, maple syrup) might very well have an inborn error of metabolism.

The less flexor and symmetrical the posture, the less wise it is to accept a term infant as neurologically normal. It can be difficult to distinguish between neuromuscular tone and neuromuscular strength as being responsible for the "floppy" baby who slides between the examiner's opposing palms in upright suspension or who droops over the examiner's uplifting palm in ventral suspension. Beyond the purely neuromuscular causes of hypotonia (hypoxic, metabolic, or genetic encephalopathies; traumatic, toxic, and infectious myelopathies and neuropathies; and congenital, structural, and metabolic myopathies) can lurk a bewildering and poorly understood array of connective tissue, endocrine, and totally idiopathic causes of floppiness.

The jittery, tremulous baby is a common sight in nurseries, and such movements occasionally raise concern that the infant may be sustaining a convulsion. However, unlike "jitters," a true seizure tends to be asymmetrical and stimulus insensitive. The tremors of jitteriness are precipitated most often by noise or motion and usually can be obliterated, unlike the seizure, by manual restraint of the involved limb.

The most useful and diagnostically informative reflexes to be elicited from the newborn are listed in Table 45-12. As in most other aspects of the neurological examination, the reflex responses are normally symmetrical and tend to diminish in intensity (habituate) on repetition. Because of the newborn's slow nerve conduction relative to that of the adult, sensory responses can be quite slow. Yet a definite response to a pinprick, and certainly to more noxious stimuli, must be elicitable from all areas of the body.

Table 45-13 should make clear that all the cranial nerves, possibly excluding the olfactory, are easily tested in a newborn. The visual and auditory responses require the most patience and equipment (including, if necessary, formal evaluation of evoked electroencephalographic potentials); yet one dealing with a seeing and hearing infant can gain considerable confidence in the baby's possession of those abilities by

Table 45-12 Levels of Surveillance of the Newborn Based on Examination of the Nervous System

	Level of Surveillance		
Characteristic	**Normal**	**Alert**	**Alarm**
State	Awake: crying, active, quiet-alert Asleep: active, indeterminate, quiet	Hyperalert, lethargic	Stupor, coma
Motor			
Posture	Flexor, symmetrical	Extensor, asymmetrical	Obligatory, decerebrate
Tone	Obtuse popliteal angle	Limp in upright suspension	Limp in ventral suspension
Movement	All extremities, nonrepetitive, random, symmetrical	Jitteriness, tremor	Seizures
Reflexes	Deep tendon, grasp, Moro, placing and stepping, sucking, tonic neck	Asymmetrical, does not habituate	Absent
Sensory	Pinprick response slow (2-3 sec)	Pinprick response equivocal	No response

Table 45-13 Levels of Surveillance of the Newborn Based on Examination of the Cranial Nerves

	Level of Surveillance		
Cranial Nerves	**Normal**	**Alert**	**Alarm**
Forebrain: II	Fix and follow (visual evoked potential)	Equivocal (arc <60 degrees)	No response
Midbrain: III, IV, VI, and VIII	Pupillary response, "doll's eye" response	Unequal, disconjugate, nystagmus	Absent, fixed position
Hindbrain			
VIII	Auditory evoked potentials, evoked otoacoustic emissions	Diminished	No response
V, VII, and XII	Sucking	Weak	Unequal
IX and X	Swallowing	Uncoordinated	
XI	Sternocleidomastoid muscles	Weak	

presenting a red ball or human face to determine his or her ability to fix and follow and a human voice or loud noise to assess aural attention.

Interventions: Measures to Ensure the Integrity of the Newborn

Measures to ensure the integrity of a newborn infant are enumerated in Box 45-7 and are straightforward. Although effective for the prophylaxis of gonorrheal ophthalmitis, 1% silver nitrate uniformly produces a brief chemical conjunctivitis (which may distress uninformed parents), and any drops spilled on the skin will discolor it temporarily. For these reasons, the antibiotic ointments have gained favor as prophylactic agents.

Apart from strictly cosmetic issues, skin and cord care is addressed to controlling the rate at which and the microorganisms with which the infant's skin will become colonized, as it inevitably must. Previous efforts to prevent establishment of a staphylococcal flora through use of hexachlorophene baths and the like were doomed to failure. The current emphasis is on permitting controlled colonization with what one hopes are benign bacterial strains. This is complemented by rigidly excluding any staphylococcal "carriers" from contact with the newborn and by minimal handling of the infant by all involved in his or her care. However, because it affords a direct route to the bloodstream, excessive infestation of the cord stump is discouraged with application of a bacteriostatic agent.

Premature rupture of the membranes places the fetus at risk for ascending *amnionitis* and the physician in a quandary as to just how aggressively to approach prevention or treatment of what often may turn out *not* to be a problem. Many find it helpful to be guided by the presence of leukocytes or bacteria (usually dead or otherwise nonculturable) in the gastric aspirate or ear canal. More recently, and under the threat of continuing serious perinatal group B streptococcal (GBS) infections, the recommendation has arisen to attempt prevention by intrapartum antimicrobial prophylaxis of those women identified as being at increased risk for transmission of GBS to their infants.[1]

Hypoglycemia is sufficiently common and threatening that it must be aggressively sought out and treated. Occult hemorrhage is less common, but failure to detect and treat it can be instantly tragic.

BOX 45-7

INITIAL CARE OF THE NEWBORN DESIGNED TO DETECT OR AVERT DIFFICULTIES DURING THE NEONATAL PERIOD

At Delivery

Cord blood—*saved* for possible ABO typing, Rh typing, or Coombs test

Identification of infant as belonging to mother

At Nursery Admission

If not previously done in the delivery room:
- Eye care—1% silver nitrate drops or 1% tetracycline or 0.5% erythromycin ointments
- Hemorrhagic prophylaxis—0.5 to 1 mg vitamin K_1 oxide (phytonadione [Pholloquinone]), administered parenterally

Subsequent Care

Skin care—"dry"(after initial cleansing with sterile water and cotton sponges)

Cord care—triple dye or bacitracin ointment

Diagnostic Care

If indicated by:
- Premature rupture of membranes
- Temperature instability
- Small or large for gestational age
- Pallor

Then:
- Search for leukocytes and bacteria in gastric aspirate
- Perform blood glucose screen
- Obtain hemogram (hemoglobin, hematocrit, red blood cell count, white blood cell count, differential)

REFERENCES

1. Prevention of perinatal group B streptococcal disease: a public health perspective, *MMWR Morbid Mortal Wkly Rep* 45 (RR-7):1, 1996.
2. Smith CA: The valley of the shadow of birth, *Am J Dis Child* 82:171, 1951.

four Adjustment Period

Kathleen L. Gifford and Nicholas M. Nelson

The next sequential but overlapping stage in management of the newborn is that of replacing the maternal-fetal unit with the mother-infant pair; this pairing encompasses tactile and emotional factors, as well as biological and nutritional concerns. Beyond this, and as important as the obvious processes of feeding, stooling, burping, and weighing, are the mystical, magical, and arguable processes of "bonding" and extending the family to include father, brothers and sisters, and grandparents, as well as medical personnel. Much of this already will have been achieved during a properly managed pregnancy, but reinforcement is always in order.

ONSET OF ORAL NUTRITIONAL INTAKE AND PARENTING

The first few days (or hours, in hospitals practicing early discharge) are devoted largely to mutual patterning by mother and child, as their schedules for sleeping, eating, relaxing, and playing begin to mesh. This prolonged and productive process seems easier and certainly more natural if managed in a rooming-in setting, whether at home or in the hospital.

As the new or experienced mother establishes or refines her skills at mothering during this period, she should expect and receive from hospital personnel nothing but the warmest, most enthusiastic support, regardless of how many tiresome and routine deliveries were managed that day without morbidity or death. In teaching hospitals these personnel often include young pediatric house officers who typically are terrified by (and therefore avoid) the daily duty of confidently answering the normal questions of normal mothers about their normal infants. The place to learn this aspect of the art of medicine is not in a book, but in the mother's room.

OBSERVATIONS AND EXAMINATION

Although in the absence of specific symptoms no particular examination of the infant is called for, the processes of feeding, growing, and excreting are monitored with particular care—the amount (of formula) ingested, the amount regurgitated, the quality and strength of sucking, the frequency and type of stooling and voiding, and the daily weight gain or loss.

A loss of 6% to 8% of birth weight is expected over the first 3 or 4 days, largely because of normal fluid shifts but also because of the decreased oral (as opposed to placental) fluid and nutritional intake in the first days of life. This weight loss tends to be somewhat more pronounced and prolonged in a nursing infant. Weight usually begins to increase after the fourth day, and the birth weight should be regained by 1 to 2 weeks of age; however, the outline offered here is purposefully vague, because there is much normal variation.

FEEDING

The decision for breast-feeding or bottle-feeding will best have been made by the unpressured mother well before her delivery (see Chapter 17 [Two], Feeding of Infants and Children). Her decision should be supported without undue proselytizing in either direction. On the other hand, the mother who is undecided can be apprised, without prejudice or commitment, of the advantages of nursing (simplicity, certainty, safety, nutritional quality, as well as immunological and economic superiority).

A strictly biochemical comparison of breast and formula feeding is presented in Table 17-6, wherein it is noted that breast milk is lower in protein, higher in fat, lower in calcium, and much lower in phosphorus. The various commercial formulas have been fortified with vitamins (particularly vitamin D), and a nursing infant probably should not need to receive vitamin supplementation, assuming a healthy mother consuming an adequate diet. Although a well-mothered, well-fed normal infant in North America can expect to receive adequate nutritional iron by the appropriate age (4 to 6 months) as his or her diet expands to include fortified cereals, meats, and egg yolks, it is unfortunate that not all infants are nutritionally so blessed. In addition, many if not most of these latter babies are probably not breast-fed. In any case, the recommendation has been made and implemented that all infant formulas be supplemented with iron to improve infant health (similar to the fluoridation of water). There seems to be little question that both forms of supplementation have been effective passive supports for the public health. Iron supplementation for the nursing infant is optional but probably wise for those older than 6 months of age, especially in the form of iron-fortified baby cereals.

ESTABLISHMENT OF LACTATION

Human milk is the ideal food for human infants, and breast-feeding is the most natural and practical way to feed a baby. It is emotionally satisfying, provides the closest possible contact between mother and infant, and should produce a unique sense of fulfillment. Unfortunately, breast-feeding in the Western world is no longer universal, and mothers who want to nurse their infants require guidance and emotional support. At no time is this more important or the mother more receptive than in the immediate postpartum period. However, the psychological and physical preparation for nursing should begin well before delivery, with information about nursing and a detailed discussion of its benefits.

Given an uncomplicated delivery and a vigorous infant, the baby should be nursed within the first hour of life during the first stage of transition, when he or she is alert and shows an interest in sucking. "Test feeds" of water are unnecessary because patency of the esophagus can be confirmed on examination in the nursery. Babies should be nursed on demand and no less than eight times a day to ensure establishment of adequate lactation; some infants require nursing as often as every 2 hours. This is normal and, thus, is to be encouraged. Frequent nursing (more than eight times a day) has been shown to reduce serum bilirubin levels in the newborn, produce good milk "letdown," and help prevent breast engorgement.

A schedule of 5 minutes on each breast for each feeding the first day, 5 to 10 minutes on each breast for each feeding the second day, and 10 to 15 minutes on each breast for each feeding thereafter is said to prevent nipple soreness, although satisfactory data to support this contention are lacking. However, it has been shown that most infants can empty a breast in about 7 minutes, so additional sucking, however pleasant for either or both parties, is nonnutritive and may lead to sore nipples. These time limits are not sacrosanct, and mothers should be encouraged not to nurse "by the clock." To ensure adequate emptying and stimulation of both breasts, the mother should be instructed to alternate the breast with which she begins each feeding.

Good technique involves washing the hands, finding a comfortable position and support, using the rooting reflex (placing the infant's cheek against the warm, naked breast, which stimulates him or her to turn the face into the breast) to encourage the baby's grasp of the entire nipple and areola, and gently breaking suction by putting a finger in a corner of the baby's mouth.

An explanation of the anatomy and physiology of lactation and suckling helps the mother respond naturally to the process and avoid complications. Hormonal changes immediately after delivery enhance the process that provides colostrum. The production of milk occurs secondary to the release of prolactin and oxytocin in response to a number of stimuli, including the tactile stimulus of the suckling infant. In fact, the milk ejection (letdown) reflex and the release of oxytocin occur in most women before actual suckling begins, and further release of oxytocin follows in response to the suckling. Oxytocin causes the smooth muscle cells around the alveolar cells (milk glands) to contract, leading to a release of milk, which flows via the ducts into the lactiferous sinuses (milk pools) situated behind the areola. The release of oxytocin is readily affected by the mother's emotional state and her ability to relax before and during nursing.

The letdown reflex is of utmost importance because its failure can lead to congestion, engorgement, a diminished milk supply, and a hungry baby. Mothers recognize the letdown when they feel a tingling sensation in the breasts or start to leak milk from the unused breast. To encourage letdown, mothers should practice relaxing in a quiet room and should feed their infant on demand. Warm showers, warm compresses, and warm beverages also may be helpful.

Technique

When the infant grasps the nipple, the tongue pulls it into the mouth and presses it against the palate. This brings the lactiferous sinuses into a position where they are accessible to pressure from the gums and facial muscles. It is the baby's pressure on these sinuses and *not* the sucking that squeezes milk from the breast and is necessary for adequate emptying.

Establishing a good nursing pattern should be the major goal during the first few weeks; supplementation with formula or water, which disrupts this pattern, should be avoided. Offering a bottle confuses the infant, diminishes his or her desire to suckle, and may cause the mother concern about her ability to provide adequate nutrition. Contrary to popular belief, water supplementation does not lower serum bilirubin levels in a breast-fed baby.

Common Complications

Sometime during the first 24 hours postpartum the mother is likely to complain of a "lazy" baby who refuses to suckle. She can be reassured that her baby does not require large amounts during the first day. Despite lack of vigorous suckling, each session at the breast provides experience in position and technique for both mother and child. By the second day the baby's appetite and technique should begin to improve.

Mothers often develop sore nipples when the baby begins to suckle with vigor, but this can be prevented or minimized by feeding the baby on demand and by good technique (Box 45-8).

Sometime between 48 and 96 hours postpartum, when true (i.e., noncolostrum) milk production starts, most mothers experience some degree of engorgement caused by venous and lymphatic stasis in the breast tissue and the presence of milk in the alveolar cells (and therefore merit congratulatory reassurance that milk production has begun). This lasts for several days and diminishes as the breast adjusts to the nursing pattern. Frequent suckling is the most effective means of preventing and treating engorgement and helps ameliorate discomfort by relieving pressure from the presence of milk. A badly engorged breast prevents the baby from drawing the nipple well into the mouth and makes nursing difficult. Manual or mechanical expression of a little milk before nursing, sufficient to soften the breast and extend the nipple, allows the infant to grasp it easily.

Special Situations

Inverted nipples. Nongraspable or nonprotractile nipples may be manipulated in the prenatal or postpartum periods to loosen adhesions and improve protractility. A breast pump, stretching techniques, milk cups, and nipple shields will draw the nipples out so that the infant can grasp them.

BOX 45-8

AID FOR SORE NIPPLES

1. Air-dry nipples after each feeding.
2. Change bra and breast pads when they become moist.
3. Clean nipples with water only. Excessive soap dries the nipples.
4. Nurse every 2 hours, but for only 5 to 7 minutes on each breast, and offer the least sore nipple first.
5. Apply a small amount of breast cream, anhydrous lanolin, or hydrophilic ointment to the nipples after each feeding. (The efficacy of this therapy is questionable.)
6. Change the baby's nursing position to alter the mouth-to-nipple pressure points.
7. As a last resort, use a nipple shield for 24 to 48 hours to allow for healing before commencing the toughening process again.

Cesarean section. The processes of postoperative recovery require only slight variations in the initial breast-feeding routine. Comfort techniques, analgesics, and appropriate positioning help improve the nursing experience.

Twins. Mothers can produce sufficient milk for twins and sometimes for triplets. The babies may be fed either simultaneously or separately.

Jaundice. Breast-feeding has been associated with an increased incidence of jaundice in the first week of life. The increase in the bilirubin level generally is small and of no clinical importance. Frequent nursing (at least eight times a day) may ameliorate this problem. If the bilirubin level approaches 20 mg/dl ("true" breast milk jaundice syndrome), nursing should be interrupted for 24 to 48 hours, the mother pumping her breasts in the interim. Invariably the serum bilirubin level declines, and breast-feeding can be resumed. The mother needs positive support and reinforcement to reassure her that it is desirable and safe for her to continue nursing. After breast-feeding is resumed, the bilirubin level may rise slightly, but it rarely returns to the previous concentration.

Prematurity. Premature infants often thrive on their mother's breast milk and can suckle adequately at the breast by about 34 weeks of gestation. Expressed breast milk can be given to the more premature infant. To succeed, the mother needs instruction in breast pumping and milk collection, accompanied by continued support and a strong personal motivation. The milk from the mother of a premature infant has a higher protein content than that from the mother of a full-term infant. Thus, the infant's own mother's milk is more desirable than either pooled or "banked" breast milk.

Cleft lip and palate. Nursing may be difficult when a cleft in the lip or palate prevents the infant from maintaining sufficient suction to seal the nipple in the mouth. If the infant has a cleft lip but intact palate, the mother's soft breast tissue should help occlude the cleft and improve the seal. However, a palatal cleft complicates the infant's attempt to press the nipple against the palate and "milk" it. In the case of a unilateral cleft, placing the nipple may avoid this problem. Highly motivated mothers have maintained breast-feeding by holding the nipple in place, by manually expressing directly into the infant's mouth, or by pumping the breasts and then bottle-feeding the expressed milk.

Additional Concerns

Additional concerns about breast-feeding include the following:

1. Milk may leak for several months; this can be controlled by applying pressure to the nipple and using an absorbent, not plastic, breast pad.
2. During the first weeks, engorgement diminishes as the baby's demands increase. Thus, the mother may be concerned about a lack of milk. Reassurance, a discussion of supply and demand, and an explanation of physiology will help.
3. The baby is getting enough milk when six or seven moderately wet diapers must be changed each day.
4. A periodic replacement bottle may be offered after the first 2 to 3 weeks, but only after consistent feeding patterns and a steady milk supply have been established.
5. A plugged milk duct is seen as a small, tender lump in the breast that persists after a feeding. Massage, frequent feedings, and cleansing of caked milk from the nipple usually resolve this problem.
6. Mastitis produces flu-like symptoms and a reddened, tender area on one or both breasts. It should be treated with rest, warm compresses to the affected breast, frequent nursing to prevent stasis, and antibiotics (if symptoms persist). Left untreated, mastitis can progress to a breast abscess, requiring surgical drainage and discontinuation of feeding at the affected breast until it heals.

Vitamins, Iron, and Fluoride

Whether the diet of breast-fed infants needs to be supplemented with vitamins, iron, and fluoride is controversial. However, based on the estimated needs of growing infants, many feel it wise to provide additional vitamin D and iron, especially in the case of the "high-risk" infant. Because the fluoride content of breast milk is low, fully breast-fed infants also require supplemental fluoride.

Maternal Medication and Diet

Almost all drugs ingested by the mother are excreted in breast milk, but very few in amounts large enough to be hazardous to the infant (see Tables 17-8 through 17-12). To minimize risk, however, maternal drugs should be avoided whenever possible. If maternal medication is absolutely necessary, the *infant should be nursed before each dose*. The mother requires a well-balanced diet during pregnancy, plus approximately 200 calories in high-protein food while breast-feeding. The nursing period is no time for "crash" or fad dieting.

Acknowledgment

We would like to acknowledge the contributions of M. Jeffrey Maisels to earlier editions of this section.

five Establishment of Equilibrium

Nicholas M. Nelson and Dennis M. Super

In this final phase of management of the newborn, the practitioner pursues the twin objectives of completing the infant's perinatal adjustments and integrating the mother-infant pair into an ongoing program for their health supervision. Precisely where this begins or is implemented (hospital, home, private office, or clinic) varies with local facilities, resources, and expectations, but the principal expectation to be instilled before discharge is that continuing health supervision is the best guarantee for maintaining the healthy process already begun.

In these later days of the infant's hospital course, jaundice is especially sought out and, if excessive (more than 10 to 12 mg/dl total bilirubin), investigated. In addition, the various requirements for statewide screening programs (e.g., phenylketonuria and hypothyroidism) need to be fulfilled and a decision reached (not imposed) concerning the *circumcision* of a baby boy.

The benefits of neonatal circumcision remain controversial in North America. In the United States, more than 70% of male infants are circumcised, whereas in Europe, neonatal circumcision is rare.[16] Proponents state that neonatal circumcision reduces the risk of urinary tract infections (UTI) in the first year of life, as well as sexually transmitted diseases (STD) and penile carcinoma in adulthood; that it prevents balanoposthitis, phimosis, and paraphimosis; that it has a lower anesthetic risk than does circumcision performed later in life; and that it eliminates the need for penile hygiene. Opponents state that it subjects the neonate to additional stress and that the procedure has a definite complication rate. They also argue that proper penile hygiene will prevent phimosis, paraphimosis, balanoposthitis, and penile cancer and that the foreskin reduces the risk of meatal stenosis by protecting the delicate urethral meatus from the irritation of soiled diapers. In 1999, the American Academy of Pediatrics Task Force on Circumcision, using an "evidence-based" approach, stated that even though there are "potential medical benefits" from newborn male circumcision, the data are insufficient to recommend the routine practice of the procedure.[2]

The best evidence supporting newborn male circumcision is the association of an increased risk of UTI in the uncircumcised neonate.[13,16,18] The strength of this association is difficult to confirm, owing to methodological problems in these retrospective studies—the frequency and method of urine collection, the inclusion of patients who have comorbidities, and failure to control for breast-feeding.[2] Even though the reported risk of UTI during the first year of life is four- to tenfold greater among the uncircumcised, the absolute risk, nevertheless, is relatively low; the operative ratio is 195 neonatal circumcisions to each hospitalization for infant male UTI.[13] A possible biological explanation for this association may be that the urethra of the uncircumcised newborn male is readily colonized with uropathogenic organisms, in contrast to the urethra of a circumcised infant.[17] An alternative to circumcision in preventing infantile urinary tract infections may be to foster more natural colonization of the infant's urethra with nonuropathogenic maternal bacteria by promoting strict rooming-in of mother and baby, by encouraging breast-feeding, or by active colonization of the baby with his mother's nonpathogenic, anaerobic intestinal flora.[15] Further studies should determine which of these interventions may best prevent urinary tract infections.

The complication rate for newborn male circumcision is almost 2% and includes hemorrhage, postcircumcision infection, wound dehiscence, and strangulation of the glans from a tight plastic bell.[6] The frequency of complications that require hospitalization, or may even be life-threatening, is almost 0.2%. These complications include hemorrhage, systemic infections, and denudation of the shaft of the penis.[6,18] Other reported complications include penile lacerations, postcircumcision phimosis, urethral cutaneous fistula, penile amputation, transient hypoxia, and death.[8] The contraindications to neonatal circumcision because of increased risk for complications are (1) any type of congenital anomaly (especially hypospadias), (2) bleeding diathesis, (3) prematurity, and (4) any neonatal illness.

The physician should perform a circumcision only after a complete physical examination has been done and after the child has urinated. Circumcision should be delayed until after the first day of life because the infant may not have recovered fully from the stress of delivery. Also, some illnesses may take time to become clinically evident during the neonatal period.

Infants undergoing elective circumcision without analgesia feel pain, as evidenced by increases in heart rate, respiratory rate, blood pressure, and plasma cortisol levels.[1] After the procedure, these infants also are more irritable and display altered behavior that may last for up to a day.[10] Hence, the clinician should consider analgesia for the neonate in the same way as one would for an older patient.[1] Some methods of relieving pain include a dorsal penile nerve block, subcutaneous ring block (infiltration of the foreskin with 1% lidocaine), topical anesthesia (30% lidocaine in an acid mantle base or an eutectic mixture of 2.5% lidocaine and 2.5% prilocaine), and a pacifier saturated with 24% sucrose solution.[3,7,9,10,14] Local infiltration with lidocaine produces better analgesia than either a dorsal penile nerve block or topical anesthesia.[9,10] Special care is needed in administering analgesia to neonates because of the prolonged pharmacological half-lives in infants, increased skin permeability, and susceptibility to apnea (opiates). Some of the potential rare side effects of these medications include allergic reactions, intravascular injection of local anesthetics (irritability, lethargy, convulsions, bradycardia, hypotension, and cardiac arrest), and methemoglobinemia (prilocaine).[4] In addition, a hematoma from a dorsal penile nerve block could compromise the blood supply to the penis, resulting in gangrene of the glans.

The parents' desire for their son to be circumcised should be discussed during a prenatal visit during which they can reflect calmly and rationally on the risks and benefits of the procedure.[2] If they decide against circumcision, physicians should include proper foreskin hygiene in their anticipatory guidance during subsequent health maintenance visits. Once the foreskin is easily retracted, the parents should be instructed to retract it gently each day, to wash the glans and foreskin with soapy water, and to dry the area thoroughly.[11]

Perhaps no wiser words have ever been spoken on the subject of infant circumcision than the following:

> My dear C.,
>
> Your patient, C.D., at age 7 months, has the prepuce with which he was born. You ask me, with a note of persuasion in your question, if it should be excised. Am I to make this decision on scientific grounds or am I to acquiesce in a ritual that took its origin at the behest of that arch-sanitarian Moses?
>
> If you can show good reason why a ritual designed to ease the penalties of concupiscence amidst the sand and flies of the Syrian deserts should be continued in this England of clean bed linen and lesser opportunity, I shall listen to your argument, but if you base your argument on anatomical faults, then I must refute it.
>
> The anatomists have never studied the form and evolution of the preputial orifice. They do not understand that Nature does not intend it to be stretched and retracted in the Temples of the Welfare Centres or ritually removed in the precincts of the operating theatres. Retract the prepuce and you see a pin-point opening, but draw it forward and you see a channel wide enough for all the purposes for which the infant needs the organ at that early age. What looks like a pin-point opening at 7 months will become a wide channel of communication at 17. Nature is a possessive mistress, and whatever mistakes she makes about the structure of the less essential organs such as the brain and stomach, in which she is not much interested, you can be sure that she knows best about the genital organs.[12]

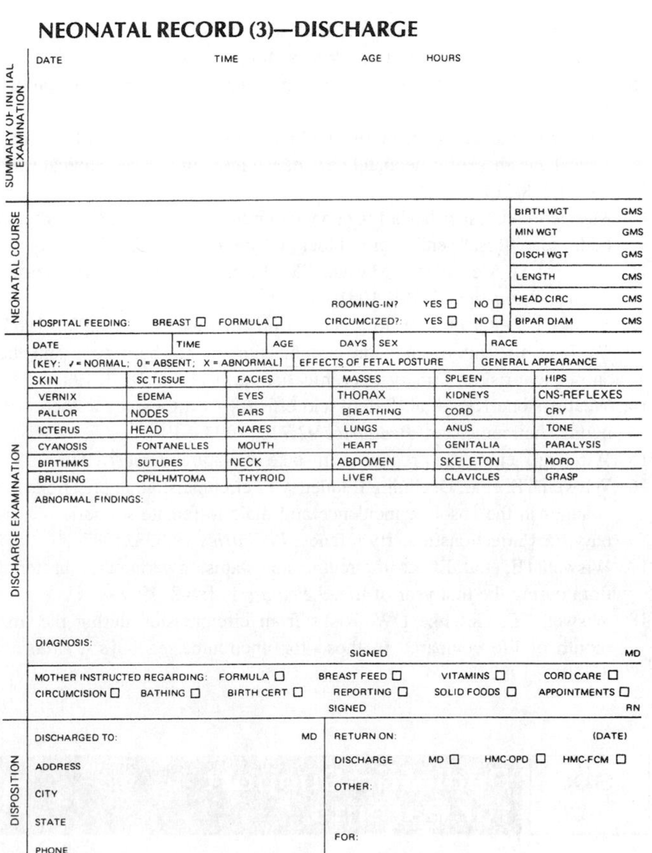

NEONATAL RECORD (3)—DISCHARGE

SUMMARY OF INITIAL EXAMINATION

DATE TIME AGE HOURS

NEONATAL COURSE

BIRTH WGT GMS
MIN WGT GMS
DISCH WGT GMS
LENGTH CMS
HEAD CIRC CMS
BIPAR DIAM CMS

ROOMING-IN? YES ☐ NO ☐
HOSPITAL FEEDING: BREAST ☐ FORMULA ☐ CIRCUMCIZED?: YES ☐ NO ☐

DISCHARGE EXAMINATION

DATE | TIME | AGE DAYS | SEX | RACE

[KEY: ✓ = NORMAL; 0 = ABSENT; X = ABNORMAL] | EFFECTS OF FETAL POSTURE | GENERAL APPEARANCE

SKIN	SC TISSUE	FACIES	MASSES	SPLEEN	HIPS
VERNIX	EDEMA	EYES	THORAX	KIDNEYS	CNS-REFLEXES
PALLOR	NODES	EARS	BREATHING	CORD	CRY
ICTERUS	HEAD	NARES	LUNGS	ANUS	TONE
CYANOSIS	FONTANELLES	MOUTH	HEART	GENITALIA	PARALYSIS
BIRTHMKS	SUTURES	NECK	ABDOMEN	SKELETON	MORO
BRUISING	CPHLHMTOMA	THYROID	LIVER	CLAVICLES	GRASP

ABNORMAL FINDINGS:

DIAGNOSIS:
SIGNED MD

MOTHER INSTRUCTED REGARDING: FORMULA ☐ BREAST FEED ☐ VITAMINS ☐ CORD CARE ☐
CIRCUMCISION ☐ BATHING ☐ BIRTH CERT ☐ REPORTING ☐ SOLID FOODS ☐ APPOINTMENTS ☐
SIGNED RN

DISPOSITION

DISCHARGED TO: MD
ADDRESS
CITY
STATE
PHONE

RETURN ON: (DATE)
DISCHARGE MD ☐ HMC-OPD ☐ HMC-FCM ☐
OTHER:
FOR:

Fig. 45-13 Data relevant to the entire neonatal course that should be conveyed from the hospital of birth to the physician assuming responsibility for continuing health supervision.

Despite such wisdom and its frequent reiteration, many parents expect, some insist on, and not a few physicians and hospitals seem too anxious to support the continuing North American cultural ritual of circumcision.[5]

On the day of discharge a careful physical examination needs to be repeated, particularly emphasizing the baby's behavioral state, the appearance (or disappearance) of any cardiac murmurs, and a close inspection of the umbilical cord. These findings and a recapitulation of the infant's progress since birth need to be recorded in a form (Fig. 45-13) easily transmissible to the physician or facility assuming responsibility for the infant's continuing care.

By 2 to 3 weeks of age, weight gain should be well established, the mother's breast milk abundantly flowing, and the infant's real impact on the household readily apparent.

REFERENCES

1. American Academy of Pediatrics, Committee on Fetus and Newborn, Committee on Drugs: Neonatal anesthesia, *Pediatrics* 80:446, 1987.
2. American Academy of Pediatrics, Report of the Task Force on Circumcision: Circumcision Policy Statement, *Pediatrics* 103:686, 1999.
3. Benini F, et al: Topical anesthesia during circumcision in newborn infants, *JAMA* 270:850, 1993.
4. Berde CB: Toxicity of local anesthetics in infants and children, *J Pediatr* 122:S14, 1993.
5. Brown MS, Brown CA: Circumcision decision: prominence of social concerns, *Pediatrics* 80:215, 1987.
6. Gee WF, Ansell JS: Neonatal circumcision: a 10-year overview with comparison of the Gomco clamp and the Plastibell device, *Pediatrics* 58:824, 1976.
7. Herschel M, et al: Neonatal circumcision; randomized trial of a sucrose pacifier for pain control, *Arch Pediatr Adolesc Med* 152:279 1998.
8. Kaplan GW: Complications of circumcision, *Urol Clin North Am* 10: 543, 1983.
9. Lander J, et al: Comparison of ring block, dorsal penile nerve block and topical anesthesia for neonatal circumcision: a randomised clinical trial, *JAMA* 278:2157, 1997.
10. Masciello AL: Anesthesia for neonatal circumcision: local anesthesia is better than dorsal penile nerve block, *Obstet Gynecol* 75:834, 1990.
11. Osborn LM, Metcalf TL, Mariani EM: Hygienic care in uncircumcised infants, *Pediatrics* 67:365, 1981.
12. Spence J: Letter of 1950 to a general practitioner, *Lancet* 2:902, 1964.
13. To T, et al: Cohort study on circumcision of newborn boys and the subsequent risk of urinary-tract infection, *Lancet* 352:1813, 1998.
14. Weatherstone KB, et al: Safety and efficacy of a topical anesthetic for neonatal circumcision, *Pediatrics* 92:710, 1993.
15. Winberg J, et al: The prepuce: a mistake of Nature? *Lancet* 1:598, 1989.
16. Wiswell TE, et al: Declining frequency of circumcision: implications for changes in the absolute incidence and male-to-female sex ratio of urinary tract infections in early infancy, *Pediatrics* 79:338, 1987.
17. Wiswell TE, et al: Effect of circumcision status on periurethral bacterial flora during the first year of life, *J Pediatr* 113:442, 1988.
18. Wiswell TE, Geschke DW: Risks from circumcision during the first month of life compared to those for uncircumcised boys, *Pediatrics* 83:1011, 1989.

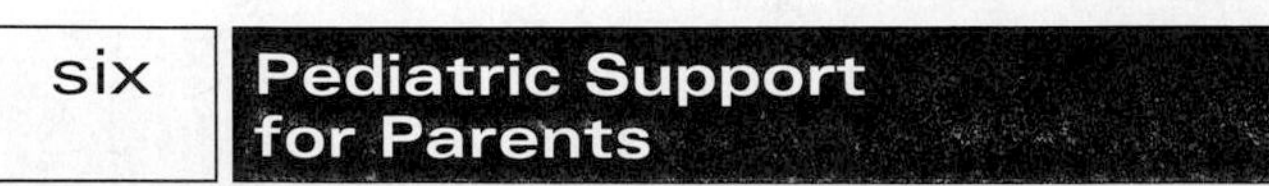

six Pediatric Support for Parents

John H. Kennell and Marshall H. Klaus

Experiences during pregnancy, labor, and delivery and events shortly after birth may greatly affect an infant's later development. We explore here what is known about this period in the life of the infant, the parents, and the family and emphasize what interventions may aid in the maturation of the family.

It has been a challenge to assess which factors determine the parenting behavior of human beings and how pediatric support can alter the process. Parents' actions and responses toward their infant derive from a complex combination of their own genetic endowment, the way the baby responds to them, the long history of interpersonal relations within their own families and with each other, their experiences in this or previous pregnancies, the practices and values of their respective cultures, and—probably most important—how each was raised by his or her own mother and father. The mothering or fathering behavior of each woman and man, their ability to tolerate stress, and their need for support may differ greatly and will depend on a mixture of all of these factors. Strong evidence for the importance of the effect of the mother's own mothering on her caretaking comes from an elegant 35-year study by Engel, Reichsman, and Harvey[8] that documented the close correspondence between how Monica (an infant who had a tracheoesophageal fistula) was fed during the first 2 years of life, how she then cared for her dolls, and how as an adult she fed her own four children.

Fig. 45-14 represents our current conception of the major influences on parenting behavior and the resulting disturbances that we postulate as arising from them.

Although the effects of these particular determinants once were thought to be fixed and unchangeable, it has been observed that their impact may be altered, both favorably and during the experience of birth. Parenting behavior and the parent-child relationship also may be influenced significantly by factors such as the parents' observations of attitudes, statements, and practices of the nurses and physicians in the hospital, whether the mother is alone for short periods during her labor, whether the mother and father are separated from their infant in the first few days of life, the infant's nature and temperament, and whether the infant is healthy, sick, or mal-

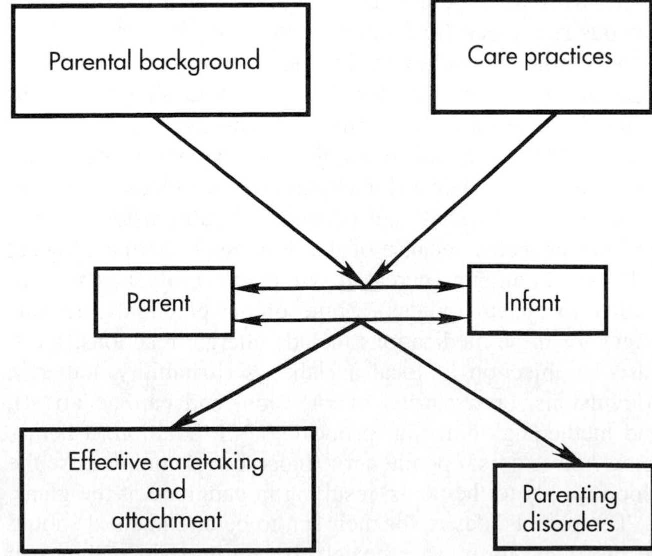

Fig. 45-14 Major influences on parent-infant attachment and the resulting outcomes.

(From Klaus MH, Kennell JH: *Parent-infant bonding*, ed 2, St Louis, 1982, Mosby.)

formed. Included under parent disorders are the following: (1) child abuse and neglect, (2) nonorganic failure to thrive, (3) vulnerable child syndrome, (4) disturbed parent-child relationship, and (5) some developmental and emotional problems among high-risk infants.

The following questions are helpful in focusing on the special needs of each member:

1. How long have you lived in this area, and where do most of your family live?
2. How often do you see your mother and other close relatives?
3. Has anything happened to you in the past (or do you have any condition) that causes you to worry about pregnancy or the baby?
4. What was your husband's reaction to your becoming pregnant?
5. What other responsibilities do you have outside the family?

It also is important to inquire about how the pregnant woman herself was mothered: Did she have a neglected, deprived infancy and childhood, or did she grow up in a warm, intact family?

In addition to those who received inadequate or disturbed mothering in their own early life, other mothers who have special needs are single, young, or adoptive parents. We will consider the needs of all these women who have healthy full-term newborns, together with those of healthy parents from "normal" backgrounds.

INFANT STATE

For parents to begin to understand and meet their infant's needs, it is important that they understand the infant's differing states of consciousness. The "state" or "pattern" of behavior refers to the infant's overall level of functioning at any given time, ranging from deep sleep to wakefulness, activity, or crying (Box 45-9). These six states can be differentiated by physiological measurements, including respiration, heart rate, eye movements, and electromyography, or by behavioral observation.

BOX 45-9

LEVELS OF FUNCTIONING FOR INFANTS

Six Infant States

1. Deep sleep—Eyes closed, no movement, very regular respiration
2. Active sleep—REM*: eyes closed but move in sleep; very irregular respiration; moves arms, legs, and body during sleep
3. Drowsy—Waking up or going to sleep
4. Quiet alert—Looks at parent's face and eyes, follows sound and parent's face
5. Active alert—Looking around the room but not at faces; gross movements, no crying
6. Crying—(Vocalization)

From Wolff PH: *Psychosom Med* 21:110, 1959.
*REM, Rapid eye movement.

These states appear to form a continuum that differs qualitatively and with distinct types of organization. They are relatively stable and recur in regular cycles during the day and night. Practically every behavior and body function of the newborn depends on his or her state and on the stability and control of this state. Cognitive functions in the newborn period, for instance, can be assessed in the quiet-alert state. Each of these six states is accompanied by quite specific and individual behaviors. In the *quiet-alert state,* which is very similar to conscious attention in adults when they are listening closely to us, babies rarely move. Their eyes are wide open and bright, and they can look eye to eye. In this state they can follow a red ball, select pictures they prefer, and even imitate their mother's facial expression. Right after birth, within the first hour of life, normal infants have a prolonged period of quiet-alertness, averaging 40 minutes, during which they can look directly at their mother's and father's face and respond to voices. It appears to be a perfect time to meet their parents. In this state, motor activity is suppressed and all of the baby's energy seems to be channeled into seeing and hearing.

LABOR AND DELIVERY FOR PARENTS OF NORMAL FULL-TERM INFANTS

A review of ethnographical material has shown that in 127 of 128 representative, nonindustrialized societies, another woman was present with the mother during labor—in only one society did the mother labor alone. The significance of this almost universal custom of support has been revealed in seven randomized, controlled studies, which have shown that the presence of a supportive woman companion (a *doula*) during labor and delivery reduced the cesarean delivery rate 50%, reduced length of labor by 25% (and oxytocin use by 40%), and reduced pain medication by 30%, the need for forceps by 40%, and requests for epidurals by 60%.[10-12,14,15,18,20] In one study, mothers who had received doula support shortly after birth were awake most of the time, and when they were with the newborns after delivery, they showed more affectionate interaction with their babies than did mothers who had no doula.[28]

We believe that supportive management of labor and delivery should adhere to the following principles:

1. The less anxiety the mother experiences during delivery, the better will be her immediate relationship with her baby. Thus, she, her husband, or other support person should visit the maternity unit to see where labor and delivery will take place and to learn about delivery routines. What will happen should be presented in detail, realistically but tactfully, if not covered previously in a childbirth class.
2. It is essential that parents be involved in the many decisions associated with labor and birth. A birth "plan" should be developed in the third trimester.
3. The mother and father ought to have one experienced woman for guidance and reassurance (midwife, nurse, or doula) who is present at the mother's side throughout labor and birth to help the couple.[20] *No woman should ever "labor" alone.*

4. Once delivery has been completed, it is important for the mother to have a few moments to regain her composure before she proceeds to the next task. It is best not to present her with her baby before drying and examining the infant briefly (1 to 3 minutes) to confirm that he or she is completely normal and before the mother indicates that she is ready to take her baby; it should be her decision.
5. It is valuable for the mother, father, and infant to be together for at least 1½ hours.[5] The mother and father usually never forget these significant and exciting shared experiences. It helps some parents to begin the process of attaching themselves to the infant. We emphasize that this should be a private, "executive" session and that many normal parents take many days to fall in love with their infants.
6. The mother and father should stay together continuously or have long periods together in the days after birth. The postpartum period should be a time when the mother interacts with her infant, becoming acquainted and gaining confidence in her own abilities. It is suggested that the infant stay in the mother's bed or in a small bassinet at the mother's side (Fig. 45-15). After a cesarean delivery it will be painful for the mother to pick up, feed, and manage her infant without assistance. The father or another family member should be encouraged to stay with the mother throughout the day to provide this assistance. Help at home with household tasks is especially valuable.
7. Whenever possible, infants who require additional heat in an incubator should be allowed to remain with the mother, and phototherapy for hyperbilirubinemia should take place in the mother's room. A mother may become extremely anxious about the health of her baby when they are apart and is reassured by the baby's presence.[35]
8. Breast-feeding mothers should be encouraged to feed their babies during the first hour and then on demand. This can mean between 8 and 18 feedings in a 24-hour period. Studies by DeCarvalho[5,6] reveal that women who feed this often in the first 14 days are more successful at breast-feeding, have a larger milk output at 2 weeks, have minimum nipple soreness, and have infants who have significantly lower bilirubin levels than do women who nurse fewer than eight times a day in the first 2 weeks.
9. After giving birth, the mother needs the emotional support of close contact with her husband or chosen companion, as well as with her children, especially those younger than 3 years of age. Even under a policy of early discharge 24 to 48 hours after delivery, sadness on separation from husband and children may compel a woman to leave the hospital before she is ready physically. The first few days usually go more smoothly for the siblings and mother if they have had daily visits during the hospitalization.
10. We strongly recommend that nurses, physicians, and other maternity staff consistently be optimistic and avoid criticism in their interaction with new mothers. In the postpartum period, even a perfectly normal woman may be extremely sensitive to physicians' and nurses' opinions and statements about her baby or herself.

THE INFANT BREAST CRAWL

One of the most exciting observations made in our era is the discovery that the newborn has the ability to find his mother's breast all on his own and decide for himself when to take his first feeding. So as not to remove the taste and smell of the mother's amniotic fluid, it is necessary to delay washing the baby's hands. The baby uses the taste and smell of the amniotic fluid on his hands to make a connection with a certain oily substance on the nipple related to the amniotic fluid. The infant usually begins with a time of rest and quiet alertness, during which he rarely cries and appears to take great pleasure in looking at his mother's face. Soon after birth, the newborn begins making mouthing movements, sometimes with lip smacking; shortly after, saliva begins to pour down onto his chin. When placed on the mother's abdomen, babies maneuver in their own ways to reach the nipple. They often use stepping motions of their legs to move forward, while to go horizontally to the nipple, they use small push-ups, lowering one arm first in the direction they want to

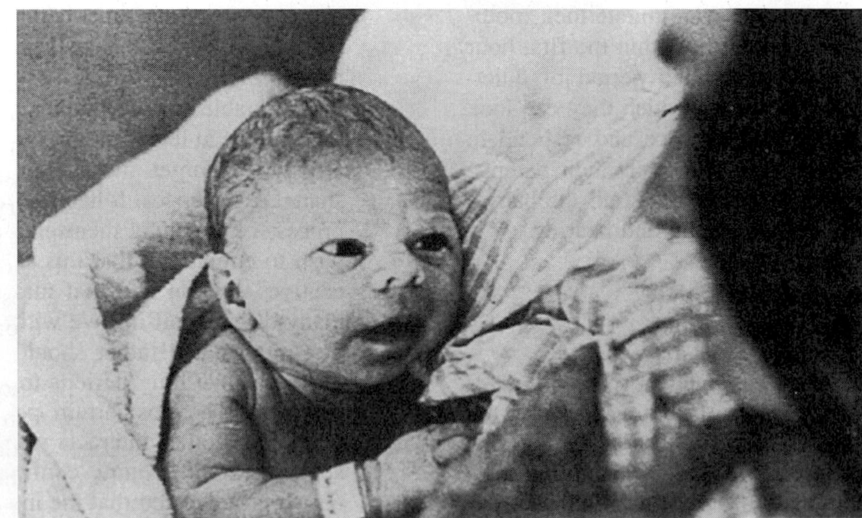

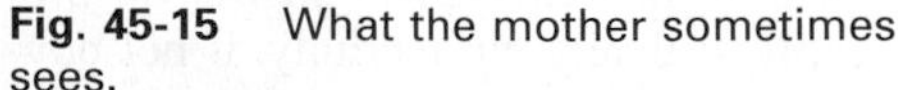

Fig. 45-15 What the mother sometimes sees.

(From Klaus MH, Kennell JH: *Parent-infant bonding,* ed 2, St Louis, 1982, Mosby.)

go. These movements are interspersed with short rest periods and take effort and time. Parents find patience well worthwhile as they wait and observe their infant on her first journey. Repeated mouthing and sucking of the hands and fingers is commonly observed. With a series of push-ups and rest periods, she makes her way to the breast completely on her own, placing her lips on the areola of the breast.[34] She now begins to suckle effectively and closely observes her mother's face. This sequence is helpful to the mother as well, because the massage of the breast induces a large oxytocin surge into her bloodstream, which helps contract the uterus, expelling the placenta and closing off many of its blood vessels, thus reducing bleeding. The stimulation and suckling also helps in the manufacture of prolactin, and the suckling enhances closeness and bonding between the mother and baby. Mother and baby appear to be carefully adapted for these moments together. Eons ago this adaptation may have served to save the mother's life and thereby that of her baby.

To allow this first intimate encounter, we strongly urge that the injecting of vitamin K, applying of eye ointment, washing, and any measuring of the infant's weight, height, and head circumference be delayed for at least an hour and a half. More than 95% of all full-term infants are normal at birth. In a few moments they could be easily evaluated to ensure that they are healthy. They can then, after thorough drying, be safely placed on their mother's abdomen if their parents wish.

The odor of the nipple appears to guide the infant to the breast.[30] If the right breast is washed with soap and water, the infant will crawl to the left breast, and vice versa. If both breasts are washed, the infant will go to the breast that has been rubbed with the amniotic fluid of the mother. The special attraction of the newborn to his mother's amniotic fluid may reflect the time in utero when, as a fetus, it swallowed the liquid. It appears that amniotic fluid contains some substance that is similar to some secretion of the breast, though not the milk. Amniotic fluid on the infant's hands probably also explains part of the interest in sucking the hands and fingers. This early hand-sucking behavior is reduced markedly when the infant is bathed before the crawl.

Stepping reflexes help the newborn push against her mother's abdomen to propel her toward the breast. Pressure of the infant's feet on the abdomen may also help in the expulsion of the placenta and in reducing uterine bleeding. The ability to move her hand in a reaching motion enables the baby to massage the nipple. Taste, smell, and vision all help the newborn detect and find the breast. This scenario may take place in a matter of minutes, or within 30 to 60 minutes, but it is all within the capacity of the newborn. It appears that human young, like other baby mammals, know how to find their mother's breast. In one group of mothers who did not receive pain medication and whose babies were not taken from them during the first hours of life for a bath, vitamin K administration, or application of eye ointment, 15 of 16 babies were observed to make this trip on their own and begin to suckle effectively.[24]

Swedish researchers have shown that the normal infant, when dried and placed nude on the mother's abdomen and then covered with a blanket, will maintain his or her body temperature as adequately as do elaborate, high-tech heating devices that usually separate the mother and the baby. The same researchers found that when the infants are skin-to-skin with their mothers for the first 90 minutes after birth, they cry hardly at all compared with infants who were dried, wrapped in a towel, and placed in a bassinet.[3] It seems likely that each of these features—the crawling ability of the infant, the decreased crying when close to the mother, and the warming capabilities of the mother's body—are adaptive and evolved genetically more than 400,000 years ago to help preserve the infant's life.

STUDIES OF A SENSITIVE PERIOD

The question of whether additional time for close contact between the mother and her full-term infant in the first minutes and hours of life can alter the quality of the mother-infant bonding over time has been the subject of numerous studies and extensive debate. Because hospital practices recently have been altered based on these studies, it is essential to explore their design, ecology, and outcome measures. Thirteen separate studies have looked at the effect of additional mother-infant contact in the first hour of life, with contact after this period being similar in both the experimental and the control groups.[19] In 9 of the 13 studies, differences in the behavior of both mother and infant were noted in the experimental group.

In six of those nine studies[29] breast-feeding was more successful and continued for a significantly longer period for mothers who had contact that involved suckling their babies in the first hour after birth than for those whose suckling occurred later. It is difficult to know whether it was the early contact per se or, more specifically, the early suckling that altered the length of time that these mothers continued to breast-feed. It may be argued that the length of time of breast-feeding is not a valid assessment of the strength of the mother-infant bond because breast-feeding is determined to a great extent by culture.

When additional time is given for close mother-infant contact after the first 8 hours following delivery, differences in later mothering behavior also occur. In a study of 301 mothers, O'Connor et al[23] noted that increasing the time by 12 hours (6 hours on days 1 and 2) reduced the number of mothering disorders that lead to child abuse and there were 10 such occurrences in the control group, but only 2 in the group of mothers who received extra time with their infants (Table 45-14). Using a similar design, Siegel et al[26] studied a

Table 45-14 Relationship Between Extended Early Mother-Infant Contact and Child Abuse and Neglect

Study	Number of Subjects	Number of Cases
O'Connor et al[23] (1980)		
Extended contact	134	2
Control	143	10*
Siegel et al[26] (1980)		
Extended contact	97	7
Control	105	10

Modified from Klaus MH, Kennell JH: *Parent-infant bonding,* St Louis, 1982, Mosby.
*$p < 0.05$.

group of primiparous and multiparous mothers and found differences in parenting at 4 and 12 months, and 10 versus 7 infants experienced mothering disorders. A woman was defined as having a mothering disorder if her infant had been abused or neglected, had nonorganic failure to thrive, was abandoned, or was given up for an unplanned adoption. When these two studies are put together in a meta-analysis, there is a suggestion that extended contact and rooming in lead to a reduction in child abuse ($p = 0.054$). Larger studies are required to confirm this finding.

Feelings of love for the infant are not necessarily instantaneous with initial contact. Many mothers have shared with us their distress and disappointment that they did not experience the feelings of love for their baby in the first minutes or hours after birth. It should be reassuring for them to learn of the following study of normal, healthy mothers in England. MacFarlane, Smith, and Garrow[21] asked 97 Oxford mothers, "When did you first feel love for your baby?" The replies were as follows: during pregnancy, 41%; at birth, 24%; first week, 27%; and after the first week, 8%.

A review of a representative ethnographical sample shows that 183 of 186 nonindustrial societies expect mothers and babies to "nest" together for days or weeks after delivery (a rooming-in equivalent); virtually none permits the degree of separation that has been routine in maternity hospitals in many "developed" nations. This early rooming-in usually is followed by extensive mother-infant contact and prolonged, frequent breast-feeding during the early months. This almost universal practice of protecting and supporting the mother-infant pair together in the first weeks has evolved over thousands of years. Does it have significance for the industrialized societies of today, particularly in view of the widespread shift to early hospital discharge and the absence of a public health nursing system of support for mothers and infants and of legislated maternity or paternity leave with pay in the United States?

In 1957, Winnicot[35] made remarkably perceptive observations that appear to describe what we call the "sensitive period." He proposed that a healthy mother goes through a period of "primary maternal preoccupation" that "gradually develops and becomes a state of heightened sensitivity during, and especially toward the end of, the pregnancy. It lasts for a few weeks after the birth of the child." According to Winnicott, "The mother who develops this state . . . provides a setting for the infant's constitution to begin to make itself evident . . . and for the infant to . . . become the owner of the sensations that are appropriate to this early phase of life." He notes further that this is true only if a mother is sensitized in the way described and can identify with her baby's needs and thus be better able to meet them.

Several studies[25,32] have shown that when the father is more supportive of the mother, she evaluates her maternal skills more positively and is more effective in feeding her baby. But it also might be the case that competent mothers generally elicit more positive evaluation and support from their husbands; therefore, it is important to avoid fitting the data to expectations. However, the facts seem to indicate that increased paternal contact and involvement at the time of early infancy can provide important benefits to the newborn, to the mother, and to the father himself.[13,25,37] For this reason it seems particularly important to support and encourage both parents during labor, delivery, and the postpartum period. It also is beneficial to provide for early and extended mother-infant contact, especially for single and teenage parents.

Anisfeld and Lipper[2] have reported that mothers who have poor social supports (i.e., two or more of the following: unmarried, on public assistance, not a high school graduate, no father or other support person in the delivery room) showed greatly reduced affectionate interaction with their infants when they received routine care that separated the mother and infant after delivery. On the other hand, mothers from the same background who were given their infants for the first hour showed a high level of affectionate interaction, even higher than mothers who had better social supports. At the 3-month checkup, 69% of mothers with low social support who had early infant contact returned with their infants for the scheduled appointment, in contrast to 26% in the group of women who had received only routine care.

No studies specifically have considered the effects of the early or delayed contact between infants and adoptive parents. Most adoptive parents, of course, achieve a satisfactory attachment to their infant, but this may take extra time, effort, patience, and motivation. Based on the evidence now available, we believe that parents and adoptive infants should be brought together as soon as possible after birth and that the adopted parents should be encouraged to take over full responsibility for care and planning for the infant, just as other parents do.

THE PARENTS OF A SICK, PREMATURE, OR HIGH-RISK INFANT

When talking to the parents of an infant in the neonatal intensive care unit (NICU) or to the mother before her first NICU visit, it is best to describe what the infant looks like and how the infant will appear physically to the mother. Rather than talking about the chances of survival, rates, or percentages, we stress that most babies survive despite early and often worrisome problems. There is no need to emphasize problems that may occur in the future; however, we do try to anticipate common developments (e.g., the need for phototherapy for jaundice in small premature infants). The following guidelines may be helpful:

1. A mother's room arrangements should be adjusted to her needs—does she or does she not wish to be with other mothers who have healthy, full-term infants?
2. If at all possible, mother and infant should be kept near each other, and the mother should be able to visit whenever she wishes.
3. It is best to talk with the mother and father together, whenever possible. At least once a day, discuss with the parents how the infant is doing; talk with them at least twice a day if the infant is critically ill. It is necessary to find out what the mother believes is going to happen and what she has read about the problem. Any discussion should move at her pace.
4. The physician should not relieve his or her own anxiety by unburdening to the parents; once mentioned, for instance, the thought of death or brain damage can never be erased completely.
5. During the mother's first NICU visit, a chair should always be nearby so that she can sit down. A nurse can

stay at her side during most of the visits, describing in detail the procedures being carried out.

6. It is important to remember that feelings of love for the baby are often elicited through eye-to-eye contact. Therefore, if an infant is under bilirubin lights, the lights should be turned off and the eye patches removed so that the mother and infant can see each other.
7. It may be possible to enhance normal attachment behavior as late as several days or weeks after birth by permitting a special "nesting" period of 2 or more days and nights of close physical contact, with privacy and virtual isolation during which the mother provides complete care for her small infant, with help and nursing support readily available.[15] Because providing care enhances maternal attachment, it is best to involve the mother in tasks appropriate for the infant's condition as early as possible (e.g., stroking the baby's extremities to reduce apnea and enhance weight gain, changing the diaper, or assisting with nasogastric feedings).

Allowing a mother to hold the infant skin to skin for prolonged periods in the hospital appears to have beneficial effects.[33] It has been shown in several trials that if the usual precautions are taken, such as hand washing, there is no increase in the infection rate or problems in oxygenation, apnea, or temperature control. Although the most significant medical benefit appeared to be increased success of maternal lactation, several studies showed that the mother's own confidence in her caretaking improved along with an eagerness for discharge, and many women reported feeling an increased closeness to the infant compared with a control group of mothers.

Another approach for the mother who is severely distressed emotionally after the birth of a small premature infant is to alter the responses of the developing infant, an area of intense study by Als et al.[1] In a series of creative studies, they demonstrated that their individualized nursing care plans for high-risk, low-birth-weight infants, which took into account the babies' behavioral and environmental needs, altered the infants' outcome remarkably. The babies' requirements for light, sound, positioning, and nursing care were developed only after a detailed behavioral assessment.

In four randomized trials using the preceding procedure, infants receiving individualized behavioral management required fewer days on a respirator and fewer days on supplemental oxygen; their average daily waking time was increased; they were discharged many days earlier; and they also had a lower incidence of intraventricular hemorrhage. In addition, their behavioral development after discharge progressed more normally, and their parents more easily developed ways of sensing their needs and responding and interacting with them pleasurably. Parents have an easier time adapting to premature infants who are more responsive.

Minde et al[22] have reported a randomized trial in which parents of premature infants who participated in self-help groups rated themselves as being more competent in infant care measures, as visiting their infants more often, and as more often touching, talking to, and looking at their infants *en face*. This interest in the infant persisted in the home until at least 3 months after discharge.

At the Ramon Sarda Mother and Infant Hospital in Buenos Aires, Argentina,[16] an exemplary program has been developed, based on extensive research of premature infants and their parents. The program applies those features that have been shown to enhance the attachment of mothers to sick and premature infants and reduced or removed factors, such as mother-infant separation, that interfere with it. Mothers are invited to stay at the Residence for Mothers when discharged from the obstetrical unit. The poorer mother usually stays until her baby is discharged. Beds and meals are provided. The mothers rest and are well fed, and collectively they make up a community with common concerns—their children's premature birth or illness. There are formal and informal group meetings to develop maternal abilities and to teach mothers how to care for special infants. At the human milk bank, a mother extracts colostrum and breast milk to be given to her infant. The mother has access to the NICU, with no time restrictions. She is involved in the care of her infant, usually from the time of admission. She learns from experience by sharing ideas and by "imitating" within the group of resident mothers.

In contrast to most neonatal intensive care centers, the poor mothers living in the residence usually develop a solid relationship with their infants and the hospital (Fig. 45-16). This is shown by the excellent rate of breast-feeding, contin-

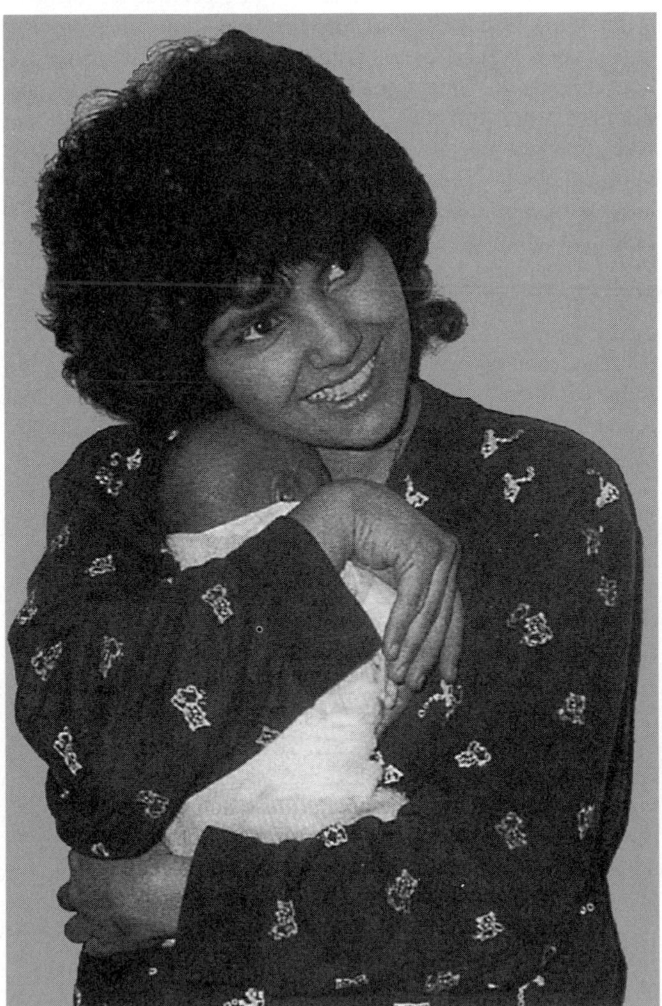

Fig. 45-16 A mother who has lived in the Residence for Mothers and cared for her premature infant from birth.

(From Klaus MH, Kennell JH. *Parent-infant bonding*, ed 2, St Louis, 1982, Mosby.)

uous attendance at follow-up evaluations, and the disappearance of preventable diseases or problems such as malnutrition and diarrhea, and child abuse, neglect, or desertion.

Further emphasizing the importance of the home and family in the final outcome is a very large, randomized, well-carried-out trial (985 premature infants) in centers in the United States.[9] The study demonstrated that a comprehensive program with weekly home visits in the first year of life, group meetings for the mothers during all 3 years, and daily attendance by the child at a developmental center from 1 to 3 years of age resulted in a significant improvement in intelligence quotient (IQ) scores, as well as reports by mothers of fewer developmental problems.

It is important to remember that more than half the variance in IQ can be accounted for by social conditions such as parental occupation, education, minority status, anxiety, and mental illness. As we improve the social conditions for the entire population, we will significantly improve the outcome for the low-birth-weight infant.

THE PARENTS OF AN INFANT WHO HAS A CONGENITAL ANOMALY

Although previous investigators[4,7,31] agree that the birth of an infant who has a congenital malformation often precipitates major family stress, Solnit and Stark's conceptualization[27] of parental reactions is most valuable. They note that the malformed infant is a distortion of the ideal infant that was dreamed of and planned for. The parents must first mourn the loss of the normal child they had expected before they can become fully attached to their living, defective infant. This significant aspect of adaptation may take many months. Parental reactions to the birth of a child who has a congenital malformation appear to follow a predictable course (Fig. 45-17). Most parents experience initial shock, disbelief, and a period of intense emotional upset (including sadness, anger, guilt, and anxiety), followed by a period of gradual adaptation that is marked by a lessening of intense anxiety and emotional reaction. This adaptation is characterized by an increased satisfaction and ability in caring for the baby.

These stages in parental reaction are similar to those reported in other crises, such as having a terminally ill child. The intense emotional turmoil described by parents who have produced a child who has a congenital malformation is a period of crisis (defined as "an upset in a state of equilibrium caused by a hazardous event that creates a threat, a loss, or a challenge for the individual"[7]). During such crises, a person is unable, at least temporarily, to respond with his or her usual problem-solving activities.

The sequence of parental reactions to the birth of a baby who has a malformation differs from that following the death of a child in one important respect: The mother and father must become attached to their living but damaged child. The task of becoming attached to the malformed infant and providing his or her physical care can be overwhelming for parents at just the time around birth when they are physiologically and psychologically depleted. The mother's initiation of the relationship with her child is a major step in reducing the anxiety and emotional upset associated with the trauma of birth.

Our assessment and practice in this area includes:

1. The parents' mental picture of the anomaly may often be far more severe and distorted than the actual defect. Any delay in seeing and touching the baby greatly heightens this anxiety. Therefore, we suggest bringing the baby to both parents when they are together as soon after delivery as possible.
2. Parents should not be given tranquilizers, which tend to blunt responses and slow adaptation to the problem.
3. Parents who become very involved, by trying to find out what the best corrective procedures are, and who ask many questions about the care of their baby and his or her abnormality often adapt best. We are most concerned about parents who ask few questions and who appear stunned or overwhelmed by the problem.
4. It is best to move at the parents' pace. If the physician moves too quickly, he or she runs the risk of "losing" the parents along the way. It is beneficial to ask the parents how they view their infant. We try to show parents one problem at a time or wait until several can be put together logically.

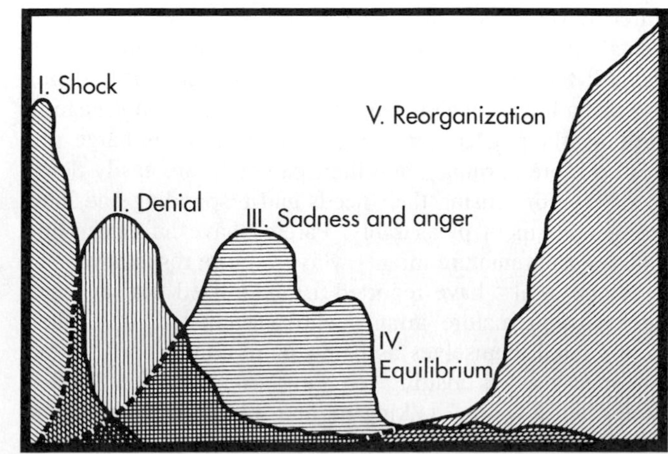

Fig. 45-17 Hypothetical model of the sequence of normal parental reactions to the birth of a child with congenital malformations.
(From Drotar D, et al: *Pediatrics* 56:710, 1975.)

5. Each parent moves through the process of shock, denial, sadness, anger, guilt, and adaptation at his or her own pace. If they are unable to talk with each other about the baby, their own relationship may be disrupted. During our discussions with parents, we ask the mother how she is doing, how she feels the father is doing, and how he feels about the infant. We then reverse the questions and ask the father how he is doing and how he thinks the mother is progressing. Thus, they start to think not only about each other but also about their own adaptation. Often, communication between the parents improves after one or two of these sessions. Some couples who did not seem to be close previously may move closer together over the next weeks and months. As with any painful experience, the parents may emerge much stronger after they have gone through the ordeal together.

STILLBIRTH OR NEONATAL DEATH

When the diagnosis of a stillbirth is established in utero, both parents should be fully informed and the events surrounding labor and delivery thoroughly explained. As much as possible, an atmosphere of understanding and mutual support should be established between the bereaved parents and the medical staff.

Many have emphasized the importance of establishing the stillborn infant's identity. A death without a body that has been seen by a family member seems unreal. Grief after stillbirth is susceptible to distortion because there are no postpartum experiences with the baby to remember, and the infant often is perceived as someone who did not exist, a person without a name. This sense of nonexistence is exaggerated in women who are heavily sedated or anesthetized during delivery and thereby are deprived of the memories necessary for normal grief. The infant's identity can best be established if the bereaved parents are encouraged to look at, touch, and hold their child.

Parents first may find the idea of holding a dead baby abhorrent, but once the baby is dead, there is no need to rush. We have found that parents frequently change their minds; to facilitate this, we may keep the baby on the delivery floor for a few hours. Parents who have held their stillborn infant or dead neonate report that this was a meaningful experience that they "never would have wanted to miss."

We gradually have come to appreciate that almost no baby is so deformed that the parents will not benefit from viewing the infant, if they so wish. It often is possible to present such babies (e.g., a baby who has anencephaly) to parents, using receiving blankets in such a way as to minimize any shock that might arise on seeing the malformation.

If a mother loses an infant any time after she has felt movement, she usually goes through a long period of intense mourning. To help with the mourning process after a neonatal death or stillbirth, mothers should be encouraged to see and handle the infant after death, in privacy, if they desire. Some parents choose to hold the dying baby when intensive resuscitation efforts are no longer appropriate. Some mothers have cleaned, diapered, and dressed their dead baby. At first one might think that it is only good to remember the baby as a normal, active infant, but it is important for parents to see the dead infant, so that they have clear, visual proof that the baby really died. Also, if the baby had been rushed away right after birth, it is particularly valuable for the mother and father to see that they really did produce a baby who was normal in most respects. Many mothers report having lost a baby in the past and wishing for years that they could have seen, touched, handled, or even just seen a picture of the baby before he or she was taken away. Most have had none of these opportunities. If the mother is still confined in another hospital, there should be no reason that the infant's body cannot be held until the mother is discharged and ready to see the baby and participate in the funeral. The experience of seeing and holding a stillborn infant may temporarily deepen the sadness of both parents, but it provides concrete memories that will facilitate a normal mourning. It is highly desirable to obtain a photograph of every stillborn infant or liveborn infant who dies, even if the parents do not wish to see it at the time.

Our general plan is to meet with the parents at least three times after a neonatal death or stillbirth. The first time is right after the death. At this moment they are so overwhelmed that they are unable to hear or retain anything other than the event of the death. However, we describe the details of the mourning process in simple terms. For example, we explain to the parents that they may have physical symptoms, such as chest pains. Waves of intense sadness may come over them for the first few weeks, but these gradually diminish after 6 months and stop after 1 year. At times the parents may find themselves angry with each other and their friends and may feel guilty about the death of their infant, believing that actions they could have taken would have saved the infant or prevented the illness. At times they may imagine that they see their baby alive and hence believe that they are going crazy.

We meet with the parents together for a second time (sometimes with their own parents), usually within the first 3 days but at least within the first week. At this meeting it is much easier to review the grieving process. It is helpful for the parents to understand what the usual reactions are so that they will not worry that they are ill. The most important action is to listen and then listen again. We stress that the parents meet with us together to maintain rapport and communication. The third meeting with the parents occurs 3 to 6 months after the death. We meet with them to ensure that their grieving is progressing normally and that there is no persistently high level of mourning or other sign of pathological grief. If such symptoms are noted during the interview, we refer the parents to a psychiatrist.

Our attendance, over three decades, at monthly meetings of parents who have experienced a perinatal loss has shown the great value of parents supporting, understanding, and listening to other parents who have experienced a similar loss. This monthly little window into the lives of bereaved parents has progressively broadened our own view of the "normal" range and duration of mourning reactions. Helping parents through these experiences is, to be sure, taxing and difficult, but it is a rewarding aspect of being a physician.

REFERENCES

1. Als H, et al: Individual developmental care for the very low-birth-weight preterm infant, *J Am Med Assoc* 272:853, 1994.

2. Anisfeld E, Lipper E: Early contact, social support, and mother-infant bonding, *Pediatrics* 72:79, 1983.
3. Christensson K, et al: Temperature, metabolic adaptation, and crying in healthy, full-term newborn babies cared for skin to skin or in a cot, *Acta Paediatr* 81: 488, 1992.
4. Daniels LL, Berg GM: The crisis of birth and adaptive patterns of amputee children, *Clin Proc Child Hosp DC* 24:108, 1968.
5. DeCarvalho M, Klaus MH, Merkatz RB: Frequency of breast-feeding on early milk production and infant weight gain, *Am J Dis Child* 136: 737, 1982.
6. DeCarvalho M, et al: Effect of frequent breast-feeding on early milk production and infant weight gain, *Pediatrics* 72:307, 1983.
7. Drotar D, et al: The adaptation of parents to the birth of an infant with a congenital malformation: a hypothetical model, *Pediatrics* 56:710, 1975.
8. Engel GH, Reichsman F, Harvey VT: Infant feeding behavior of a mother gastric fistula fed as an infant: a 30-year longitudinal study of enduring effects. In Anthony EJ, Pollock GH, editors: *Parental influences in health and disease*, Boston, 1985, Little, Brown.
9. Gross R, et al: Enhancing the outcomes of low-birth-weight premature infants, *JAMA* 263:3035, 1991.
10. Hemminnki E, et al: A trial on continuous human support during labor: feasibility, interventions, and mothers' satisfaction, *J Psychosom Obstet Gynecol* 11:239, 1990.
11. Hodnett ED, Osborn R: Effect of continuous intrapartum professional support on childbirth outcomes, *Res Nurs Health* 12:289, 1989.
12. Hofmeyer GJ, Nikodem VC, Wolman, WL: Companionship to modify the clinical birth environment: effects on progress and perceptions of labour and breast-feeding, *Br J Obstet Gynaecol* 98:756, 1991.
13. Keller WD, Hildebrandt KA, Richards M: Effects of extended father-infant contact during the newborn period, *Infant Behav Dev* 8:337, 1985.
14. Kennell JH, et al: Labor support: what's good for mother is good for baby, *Pediatr Res* 25:15, 1989.
15. Kennell JH, Klaus MH: Interventions in the premature nursery: impact on development, *Pediatr Clin North Am* 29:1263, 1982.
16. Kennell JH, Klaus MH: The perinatal paradigm: is it time for a change? *Clin Perinatol* 15:801, 1988.
17. Kennell JH, et al: Continuous emotional support during labor in a US hospital, *JAMA* 265:2197, 1991.
18. Klaus MH, et al: Effects of social support during parturition on maternal and infant morbidity, *Br Med J* 293:585, 1986.
19. Klaus MH, Kennell JH, Klaus PH: *Bonding*, Reading, Mass, 1995, Perseus.
20. Klaus MH, Kennell JH, Klaus PH: *Mothering the mother: how a doula can help you have a shorter, easier, and healthier birth*, Reading, Mass, 1993, Perseus.
21. MacFarlane AA, Smith DM, Garrow DH: The relationship between mother and neonate. In Kitzinger S, Davis JA, editors: *The place of birth*. New York, 1978, Oxford University Press.
22. Minde K, et al: Self-help groups in a premature nursery: a controlled evaluation, *J Pediatr* 96:933, 1980.
23. O'Connor S, et al: Reduced incidence of parenting inadequacy following rooming-in, *Pediatrics* 66:176, 1980.
24. Righard L, Alade MO: Effect of delivery routines on success of first breast-feeding, *Lancet* 344:989, 1994.
25. Rödholm M: Effects of father-infant postpartum contact on their interaction 3 months after birth, *Early Hum Dev* 5:79, 1981.
26. Siegel E, et al: Hospital and home support during infancy: impact on maternal attachment, child abuse and neglect, and health care utilization, *Pediatrics* 66.1 83, 1980.
27. Solnit AJ, Stark MH: Mourning and birth of a defective child, *Psychoanal Study Child* 16:523, 1961.
28. Sosa R, et al: The effect of a supportive companion on perinatal problems, length of labor, and mother-infant interaction, *N Engl J Med* 303: 597, 1980.
29. Sosa R, et al: The effect of early mother-infant contact on breast-feeding, infection, and growth. In *Breast-feeding and the mother*, Ciba Foundation Symposium 45 (new series), Amsterdam, 1976, Elsevier.
30. Varendi H, Porter RH, et al: Does the newborn find the nipple by smell? *Lancet* 344:989, 1994.
31. Voysey M: Impression management by parents with disabled children, *J Health Soc Behav* 13:80, 1972.
32. Westbrook MT: The reactions to childbearing and early maternal experience of women with differing marital relationships, *Br J Med Psychol* 51:191, 1978.
33. Whitelaw A, et al: Skin-to-skin contact for very low-birth-weight infants and their mothers: a randomized trial of "kangaroo care," *Arch Dis Child* 63:1377, 1988.
34. Widström AM, et al: Gastric suction in healthy newborn infants: effects on circulation and developing feeding behavior, *Acta Paediatr* 76:566, 1989.
35. Winnicott DW: *The child, the family, and the outside world*, New York, 1964, Penguin Books.
36. Wolff PH: Observations on newborn infants, *Psychosom Med* 21:110, 1959.
37. Yogman MW: Development of the father-infant relationship. In Fitzgerald HE, Lester BM, Yogman MW, editors: *Theory and research in behavioral pediatrics*, vol 1, New York, 1980, Plenum Press.

SUGGESTED READINGS

American Academy of Pediatrics and the American College of Obstetricians and Gynecologists: *Guidelines for perinatal care*, ed 4, Washington, DC, 1997, The American Academy of Pediatrics.

American Academy of Pediatrics and the American Heart Association: *Textbook of neonatal resuscitation*, ed 2, Dallas, 1994, American Heart Association.

Avery GB, editor: *Neonatology: pathophysiology and management of the newborn*, ed 4, Philadelphia, 1999, JB Lippincott.

Bloom RS, Cropley C, American Academy of Pediatrics, and American Heart Association: *Textbook of neonatal resuscitation*, ed 2, Elk Grove Village, Ill, 1994, The Academy.

Eiger MS, Olds SN: *The complete book of breast feeding*, ed 3, New York, 1999, Workman.

Fanaroff AA, Martin RJ, editors: *Neonatal-perinatal medicine*, ed 6, St Louis, 1997, Mosby.

Jones KL: *Smith's recognizable patterns of human malformation*, ed 5, Philadelphia, 1997, WB Saunders.

Klaus MH, Fanaroff AA, editors: *Care of the high-risk neonate*, ed 4, Philadelphia, 1993, WB Saunders.

Polin RA, Fox WW, editors: *Fetal and neonatal physiology*, ed 2, Philadelphia, 1998, WB Saunders.

Seidel HM, Rosenstein BJ, Pathak A: *Primary care of the newborn*, ed 2, St Louis, 1997, Mosby.

Volpe JJ: *Neurology of the newborn*, ed 3, Philadelphia, 1995, WB Saunders.

46 Skin Lesions of the Neonate

Marvin E. Miller • Julian J. Trevino

Birthmarks are common, and many newborn babies exhibit some type of skin lesion that may arouse parental concern. Fortunately, the overwhelming majority of these skin lesions are benign. It is important for the practicing physician who evaluates newborns to be familiar with these benign birthmarks and also to recognize the much less common birthmarks that may indicate a significant underlying condition. Listed in Table 46-1 are the birthmarks discussed in this chapter and their approximate frequency in newborns.

SKIN LESIONS

Transient Lesions

Several common, transient skin abnormalities occur in the newborn.[5,6,9] Because they are self-limited, no medical treatment is indicated.

Milia. Milia are multiple, 1- to 2-mm, pearly white papules found on the forehead, cheeks, and nose. When found on the oral mucosa, they are called *Epstein pearls.* Milia are found in about 50% of newborns and represent cystic inclusions of keratin and sebaceous material in the pilosebaceous apparatus. They disappear spontaneously during the first month of life and require no treatment.

Miliaria. Miliaria, or neonatal "prickly heat," are 1- to 2-mm, clear, thin-walled vesicles (miliaria crystallina) or erythematous macules with central papules, pustules, or vesicles (miliaria rubra). They are very fragile and rupture when light pressure is applied. Miliaria result from eccrine duct occlusion and sweat retention. These lesions occur when an infant is placed in a warm and humid environment; they disappear when a dry and cooler environment is provided or when the infant is dressed in lighter clothing. Topical medications should not be used because they often exacerbate these lesions.

Erythema toxicum. Erythema toxicum consists of erythematous macules, papules, and pustules. Erythema toxicum is seen in 50% of full-term newborns but only rarely in premature babies. The lesions can be seen on any part of the body except the palms and soles. They usually appear at 1 to 2 days of age and rarely are present at birth or after 5 days. The lesions persist for several hours to as long as a few days. Smears of the papular contents show numerous eosinophils but no organisms. The cause of erythema toxicum is unknown. These babies are well while they have the lesions, and no treatment is necessary.

Transient neonatal pustular melanosis. Transient neonatal pustular melanosis is a benign, self-limiting disorder that is present in 4% of black and 0.3% of white newborns. The lesions are superficial vesicopustules that rupture easily to leave a collarette of white scales around a central pinhead-size macule of hyperpigmentation. This hyperpigmentation remains for several weeks to several months. The clusters of lesions are seen most often on the forehead, under the chin, on the back of the neck, on the lower back, and on the shins. The palms and soles are affected infrequently.

The pustules last from 1 to 2 days, but cultures of the lesions are sterile, and smears of the pustules show cellular debris with variable numbers of neutrophils. Small numbers of eosinophils sometimes are present but never in such abundance as in erythema toxicum. Babies who have transient neonatal pustular melanosis are healthy, and no treatment is needed.

Nevi

Nevi constitute a group of common birthmarks that result from the local proliferation of any of the following three major cell types that make up the skin[1,2,5,8,9]:

1. Cells that line the vascular channels of either capillaries (hemangiomas) or lymph vessels (lymphangiomas)
2. Cells that produce pigment (pigmented nevi)
3. Cells from the epidermis (epidermal nevi), including those that make keratin or those that compose the epidermal appendages

Vascular Nevi

Vascular nevi can be divided into two groups: hemangiomas and vascular malformations.[2] Hemangiomas are benign vascular neoplasms that have both an initial growth phase and a subsequent involutional phase. Malformations are permanent structural lesions comprised of veins, arteries, or capillaries, with no tendency to involute spontaneously.

Salmon patch (nevus simplex, telangiectatic nevus). The salmon patch is the most common vascular lesion of infancy and is found in about 40% of all

Table 46-1 Birthmarks and Their Frequency[1,6,9]

Birthmark	Frequency
Transient Lesions	
Milia	50%
Miliaria	Common
Erythema toxicum	50%
Transient neonatal pustular melanosis	Uncommon
Nevi	
Vascular nevi	
Salmon patch	40%
Flat hemangiomas	0.3%
Raised hemangiomas	3%
Hemangiomas associated with malformation syndromes	Rare
Lymphangiomas	Uncommon
Hyperpigmented lesions	
Café-au-lait spots	Common*
Pigmented nevi	Common*
Mongolian spots	Common*
Hypopigmented lesions	Uncommon
Epidermal nevi	Uncommon
Miscellaneous	
Cutis marmorata	Common
Birthmarks from delivery trauma	Common
Cutis aplasia	Rare
Purpura	Rare

*There is a significant difference in the frequency of hyperpigmented lesions between black and white newborns; the frequency of café-au-lait spots, 12% versus 0.3%; pigmented nevi, 20% versus 2%; and Mongolian spots, 90% versus 10%, respectively.

newborns. This lesion is flat and light pink, with poorly defined borders; it commonly is seen on the nape of the neck (nevus nuchae), glabella, forehead, upper eyelids, or the nasolabial region. The salmon patch is not a true nevus because there is no actual proliferation of vascular elements, which is seen in the flat hemangiomas. Histopathological examination of the salmon patch reveals distended dermal capillaries, representing a persistent, localized fetal capillary bed that usually matures into the normal vasculature.

Within the first year of life, 95% of salmon patches fade, although portions can persist, particularly those found on the nape of the neck. Salmon patches are not associated with any malformation syndromes. No treatment is necessary, and parents can be reassured that the salmon patch is a benign lesion that almost always will fade and disappear. Some will reappear during childhood and adulthood momentarily associated with anger or embarrassment, particularly nevus nuchae.

Flat hemangiomas (nevus flammeus). The flat hemangioma, or port-wine stain, is similar in appearance to the salmon patch but is darker and has a deep red or purplish red hue. Port-wine stains usually involve the face or the extremities and usually, but not always, are unilateral. These stains commonly are present at birth and grow in proportion to the child's growth. Microscopic examination shows proliferation of dilated dermal capillaries. Although port-wine stains usually are an isolated defect, facial lesions may be associated with ocular and intracranial involvement (Sturge-Weber syndrome), while extremity lesions can be associated with bony and soft-tissue hypertrophy (Klippel-Trenaunay-Weber syndrome). Port-wine stains do not resolve over time and tend to darken and thicken with age. The pulsed-dye laser is the treatment of choice for port-wine stains in infants and children. Lesions can be camouflaged by waterproof cosmetic formulations such as Covermark or Dermablend.

Raised hemangiomas. The raised hemangiomas are benign hamartomas of proliferating vascular endothelium. Clinically, fully developed hemangiomas range from soft, bright red, lobulated nodules (superficial or "strawberry" hemangiomas) to purplish-blue, poorly defined tumors involving the deeper, subcutaneous tissue (deep or cavernous hemangiomas). Many lesions are "mixed," containing features of both superficial and deep lesions.

Raised hemangiomas may be present at birth but more commonly become apparent within the first weeks of life; 90% are noted by 1 month of age. Most raised hemangiomas begin as small well-demarcated macules or papules with telangiectasia, often surrounded by an area of pallor. Rapid growth produces red, raised, well-defined tumors that are lobulated and compressible, although they usually do not blanch. Raised hemangiomas can occur on any part of the body; about 38% occur on the head and neck and 29% on the trunk (80% of affected individuals have an isolated lesion; 20% have more than one).

Hemangiomas grow rapidly during the first 6 months of life and then begin to involute by 15 months of age. Most strawberry hemangiomas grow to 3 to 4 cm in diameter, with some as small as a few millimeters and others as large as 20 cm. At least 90% of raised hemangiomas resolve by 9 years of age without treatment. Although various modes of treatment have been used to remove raised hemangiomas, the rational approach is to let these lesions regress on their own because the cosmetic appearance is much better than those treated by surgery or radiotherapy. Parents should be reassured that time is the best treatment for the majority of these lesions.

Life-threatening hemangiomas that impinge on vital structures such as the eye, esophagus, or trachea are rare but require aggressive therapy to reduce the size of the tumor and to relieve the compromise of the vital structure. Until recently, corticosteroid therapy was the only medical approach to reduce the size of large hemangiomas.[9] Laser therapy and interferon alfa-2a are two promising new therapeutic modalities in the treatment of life-threatening hemangiomas.[3,4] Laser therapy also is being used to treat flat and raised hemangiomas of the skin for cosmetic reasons.[4]

The vast majority of hemangiomas are not associated with other malformations. However, infants who have extensive facial or lumbosacral hemangiomas require careful evaluation and imaging studies to exclude the presence of significant underlying abnormalities. There are several malformation syndromes in which port-wine stains or raised hemangiomas are seen; the features of these syndromes are listed in Table 46-2.

Lymphangiomas. Lymphangiomas are much less common than hemangiomas; sometimes elements of both are found in one lesion. Lymphangiomas usually manifest as (1) a cluster of circumscribed gelatinous papules 2 to 4 mm in diameter, containing clear lymph fluid (lymphangioma cir-

Table 46-2 Malformation Syndromes Associated with Congenital Hemangiomas[2,5]

Condition	Nature of Hemangioma	Other Features
Sturge-Weber syndrome	Large, flat hemangioma over face; usually involves ophthalmic branch of trigeminal nerve; usually unilateral	Seizures Glaucoma Mental deficiency
Kasabach-Merritt syndrome	Usually large cavernous hemangiomas, although small ones have been reported	Thrombocytopenia from platelet sequestration
Klippel-Trenaunay-Weber syndrome	Large, flat hemangioma on an extremity	Hemangioma overlies area of soft tissue and bone overgrowth Macrocephaly
Diffuse neonatal hemangiomatosis	Multiple hemangiomas that can involve skin and internal organs	High-output cardiac failure; poor prognosis

cumscription); (2) a larger cavernous nodule (cavernous lymphangioma); or (3) a large mass (cystic hygroma). There is no satisfactory treatment. Surgical removal can be attempted, but recurrences are common.

Hyperpigmented nevi. Several common hyperpigmented lesions manifest at or shortly after birth. As shown in Table 46-1 and demonstrated in the discussions that follow, black newborns have a greater frequency of each of the three common hyperpigmented lesions than do white newborns.

Café-au-lait spots. Café-au-lait spots are flat, sharply bordered, uniformly light brown pigmented lesions of varying shape. They usually are present at birth or develop shortly thereafter. An isolated café-au-lait spot has no medical implications. However, the presence of multiple café-au-lait spots that have smooth (rather than ragged) borders is diagnostic of neurofibromatosis, and such individuals are susceptible to the complications of this genetic condition. A striking difference has been noted in the frequency of café-au-lait spots in white versus black newborns. Only 0.3% of the former will have one café-au-lait spot, as opposed to 12% of the latter; 1.8% of black newborns will have three or more café-au-lait spots without evidence of neurofibromatosis during follow-up care or by family history. Thus, the finding of several café-au-lait spots in a black newborn is not, in itself, indicative of neurofibromatosis.

Café-au-lait spots are not always present at birth and may appear during infancy. Histologically, café-au-lait spots result from increased melanogenesis in a group of melanocytes and thus are not true nevi. In adults, more than six café-au-lait spots greater than 1.5 cm in diameter are diagnostic of neurofibromatosis. In children who have neurofibromatosis, however, the café-au-lait spots may be fewer in number and smaller in size because the spots increase in number and size over time. Thus, among children younger than 5 years of age, the finding of five café-au-lait spots greater than 0.5 cm in diameter is strongly suggestive of neurofibromatosis. Café-au-lait spots also can be seen in McCune-Albright syndrome (polyostotic fibrous dysplasia and pubertal precocity), but the café-au-lait spots in this condition are larger and have irregular borders.

Pigmented nevi (pigmented moles, melanocytic nevi, neurocellular nevi). Pigmented nevi are very common in adults (most adults have an average of 30 lesions), and many people call them birthmarks because they believe they were born with them. However, this usually is not the case because almost all pigmented nevi are acquired and do not appear until later in infancy; some do not appear until adolescence. Only 2% of white newborns and 20% of black newborns are born with pigmented nevi. Congenital pigmented nevi range in appearance from small light brown or tan, uniformly pigmented macules or papules to extensive raised lesions with variation in thickness and pigmentation that may involve segments of the trunk or extremities ("bathing trunk" or "garment" nevus). The lifetime risk of melanoma in these giant nevi is approximately 5%. The incidence of malignant change in smaller lesions is not well established. There are no firm guidelines as to when a congenital pigmented nevus should be removed, although the giant congenital nevi are usually removed surgically in infancy. Prophylactic excision of smaller congenital nevi is controversial; however, the lesions should be examined periodically and biopsied if suspicious changes occur, such as enlargement, induration, or deepening of pigmentation.

Mongolian spots. Mongolian spots are large, flat, diffuse, and poorly circumscribed areas of blue-gray or blue-green pigmentation located over the buttocks or lumbosacrum. This is the most common of all birthmarks in darker-skinned races and is present in more than 80% of Asian, Native American, and black newborns. It is seen in fewer than 10% of white newborns. The natural history of Mongolian spots is benign, with most disappearing by late childhood. They result from pigment-producing cells in the dermis. When a similar-appearing lesion is seen in the periorbital region, it is called a *nevus of Ota;* when seen on one side of the neck and shoulder, it is referred to as a *nevus of Ito*.

Hypopigmented lesions. Hypopigmented lesions are uncommon in newborns; their presence may be the first sign of a more serious condition. There are two important neurocutaneous conditions (phacomatoses) in which hypopigmented areas that appear at birth or in early infancy usually are found—tuberous sclerosis and hypomelanosis of Ito. It is important for the physician to recognize these conditions because of the likelihood of some neurological dysfunction.[7]

Almost 90% of individuals who have tuberous sclerosis will have one or more oval, linear, or more characteristically, ash leaf-shaped hypopigmented macules. These can range in size from a millimeter to several centimeters in diameter and are always present at birth or in early infancy. They almost always are the first manifestation of tuberous sclerosis; later features include developmental delay, seizures, cutaneous angiofibromas (adenoma sebaceum), and intracranial calcifications.

Hypomelanosis of Ito (incontinentia pigmenti) is a recently described and poorly understood condition in which irregular swirls and whorls of hypopigmentation appear at birth or in infancy. Like tuberous sclerosis, the association with neurological abnormalities such as developmental delay and seizures is high. In addition, ocular and musculoskeletal abnormalities can be seen.

Epidermal nevi. Epidermal nevi are skin lesions appearing at birth or in the first few weeks of life. They are composed of aggregates of epithelial cells (keratinocytes) or cells of any of the epidermal appendages (apocrine, eccrine, sebaceous gland, or hair follicle). Although lesions of mixed histology are common, there usually is one predominant cellular element.

The verrucose nevus represents a proliferation of the epidermal cells and their product, keratin. These lesions are raised, yellow-brown, velvety or rough and warty, and often pigmented. They usually are found as a cluster of linear papules on the limbs. Extensive forms of epidermal nevi can involve large areas of the trunk and extremities and can be associated with abnormalities of the eyes, central nervous system, cardiovascular system, and skeletal system (epidermal nevus syndrome). The tendency to develop benign or low-grade malignant tumors within epidermal nevi is small. Surgical excision is the most effective treatment.

Sebaceous nevi are elevated yellow or orange plaques found on the face and scalp. Surgical excision is the treatment of choice because benign or malignant tumors (including basal cell carcinoma) can arise within sebaceous nevi after puberty.

Miscellaneous Lesions

The physician should be familiar with several other congenital skin abnormalities.[5,9]

Cutis marmorata. Cutis marmorata is a reticulated bluish mottling of the skin, which is the normal newborn response to chilling. When the infant is warmed, the cutis marmorata disappears. The tendency may persist for several months, and usually there is no medical significance. However, cutis marmorata may be a persistent feature in the dysmorphic conditions of Cornelia de Lange's syndrome, congenital hypothyroidism, or in Klippel-Trenaunay-Weber syndrome, trisomy 18, and trisomy 21.

Birthmarks from delivery trauma. Birthmarks from the mechanical trauma of forceps or suction are common. Ecchymoses of the face where forceps have been placed often are distressing to parents. The marks themselves will disappear, but when they are present, the physician should be certain that no neurological deficit in ocular or facial muscle function is present. Suction marks on the vertex of the scalp almost always are seen when suction is used to augment delivery. These are benign and indicate no underlying brain lesions. The parents should be reassured that they will disappear.

Cutis aplasia. Cutis aplasia is a congenital absence of skin that occurs most commonly on the vertex of the scalp. The lesion appears as a punched-out ulcer that may be "weeping" or covered by a thin membrane. The defect may include the absence of subcutaneous tissue and underlying bony structures. Management is directed at prevention of infection until healing is complete. Cutis aplasia can be seen in any one of several settings. First, it can be transmitted as an autosomal dominant condition with variable expression; thus, a family history is important. Second, it can be an isolated lesion that has an unremarkable family history. Third, it can be seen in association with other birth defects such as brain malformation, limb anomalies, and gastrointestinal defects; in this group, a vascular origin is likely. Scalp defects also can be seen in infants who have trisomy 13. Management is directed at prevention of infection until healing is complete. Once healed, the lesion may be excised surgically to correct the scarring alopecia. For medicolegal reasons, it is important to recognize cutis aplasia as an intrauterine event that is not related to birth trauma or forceps delivery.

Purpura. Purpura are flat, bluish purple lesions of variable size that represent subcutaneous bleeding and can be present at birth. If they are very small, they are called *petechiae;* if large areas are involved, they are called *ecchymoses.* The differential diagnosis of neonatal purpura includes congenital infection, coagulation defects, autoimmune disorders, and hemangioma with platelet trapping (Kasabach-Merritt syndrome).

REFERENCES

1. Alper J, Holmes LB, Mihm MC Jr: Birthmarks with serious medical significance: nevocellular nevi, sebaceous nevi, and multiple café-au-lait spots, *J Pediatr* 95:696, 1979.
2. Easterly N: Cutaneous hemangiomas, vascular stains, malformations, and associated syndromes, *Curr Probl Dermatol* 7:65, 1995.
3. Ezekowitz RA, Mulliken JB, Folkman J: Interferon alfa-2a therapy for life-threatening hemangiomas of infancy, *N Engl J Med* 326:1456, 1992.
4. Garden LM, Bakus A, Paller AS: Treatment of cutaneous hemangiomas by the flashlamp-pumped pulsed dye laser: prospective analysis, *J Pediatr* 120:555, 1992.
5. Hurwitz S: *Clinical pediatric dermatology,* ed 2, Philadelphia, 1993, WB Saunders.
6. Jacobs AH, Walton RG: The incidence of birthmarks in the neonate, *Pediatrics* 58:218, 1976.
7. Orlow SJ: Congenital and genetic disorders associated with hypopigmentation, *Curr Probl Dermatol* 6:157, 1994.
8. Salmon JK, Friedin IJ: Congenital and genetic disorders of hyperpigmentation, *Curr Probl Dermatol* 5:148, 1995.
9. Weinberg S, Hoekelman RA: *Pediatric dermatology for the primary care practitioner,* New York, 1978, McGraw-Hill.

SUGGESTED READINGS

Wagner AM: Lumps and bumps in childhood, *Curr Probl Dermatol,* 8:137, 1996.

Wagner AM, Hansen RC: Neonatal skin and skin disorders. In Schachner A, Hansen RC, editors: *Pediatric dermatology,* ed 2, New York, 1995, Churchill Livingstone.

47 Signs and Symptoms of Neonatal Illness

Kristi L. Watterberg

The term *clinical signs* refers to objective evidence of disease, whereas the term *symptoms* refers primarily to subjective descriptions. The newborn and infant, although unable to verbalize complaints, are able to relay information in ways that are equally informative to the astute clinician. The recognition of neonatal illness, therefore, relies primarily on the correct interpretation of objective findings. The clinical assessment of newborn infants emphasizes the basic skills of assessment. Much of the information relevant to evaluating the health of a newborn or infant can be obtained simply by looking, without palpation or auscultation. The determination of vital signs and growth measurements provides further clues to health status. Although it is not possible to get a history directly from the newborn infant, one must not underestimate the diagnostic value (and courtesy) of speaking with the parents and reviewing the maternal chart.

In this chapter, signs commonly noted in full-term newborns are described and correlated with more specific clinical diagnoses. In most cases, more information related to specific diagnoses can be found in subsequent chapters. The material is organized in the fashion by which most newborns and infants actually are monitored in the normal newborn nursery.

VITAL SIGNS

Heart Rate

Abnormalities of the heart rate (HR) or rhythm are quite common in the newborn period and, if isolated, usually are benign. In some instances these abnormalities first may be noted prenatally or during labor and delivery. During the first few days of life, the normal heart rate is from 120 to 160 beats/min. Abnormalities of heart rate fall into two main groups: tachycardia (HR greater than 180 beats/min) or bradycardia (HR less than 80 beats/min). The initial evaluation of heart rate or rhythm abnormalities includes a 12-lead electrocardiogram (ECG) and "rhythm strip."

Tachycardia

Sinus tachycardia. The differential diagnosis of a narrow QRS complex tachycardia is between sinus tachycardia and paroxysmal supraventricular tachycardia (SVT). Sinus tachycardia most often can be differentiated from SVT on the following basis: (1) the heart rate usually is less than 200 beats/min, (2) the beat-to-beat interval varies, and (3) vagal stimulation slows the heart rate gradually. Sinus tachycardia is a common manifestation of a wide variety of both physiological and pathological factors. It may be caused by an elevated temperature, providing an early warning of infection or inappropriate environmental heat regulation. It also may be a sign of the newborn's attempt to increase cardiac output in response to situations such as severe anemia, congestive heart failure, or shock.

Supraventricular tachycardia. Supraventricular tachycardia (SVT) usually is associated with a more rapid heart rate (220 to 320 beats/min) than is seen with sinus tachycardia. P waves may or may not be visible, preceding the narrow QRS complexes. Newborns can tolerate this rate for variable periods but often have associated irritability, poor feeding, tachypnea, and poor perfusion. Although SVT is associated with structural anomalies less than 20% of the time, newborns who have SVT need an echocardiographic assessment of this possibility. Other causes include underlying abnormalities of the conducting system, such as Wolff-Parkinson-White syndrome (WPW), and conditions that increase myocardial irritability, such as infectious or metabolic cardiomyopathies.

Ventricular tachycardia. Ventricular tachycardia is an unusual problem in the newborn period. When seen, it usually is associated with severe underlying electrolyte disturbances or structural heart disease. The ECG usually shows wide QRS complexes. By definition, it is abnormal and potentially life threatening.

Bradycardia

Sinus bradycardia. Sinus bradycardia is the most common form of slow heart rate seen in the neonatal period. The heart rate usually is less than 80 beats/min, with a well-formed P wave preceding each QRS complex. The episodes usually are transient and associated with feeding or sleeping. The heart rate speeds up readily with stimulation. Persistent bradycardia not responding to stimulation should be evaluated further. Abnormalities occasionally associated with persistent sinus bradycardia include increased intracranial pressure, hypoxemia, and hypothyroidism.

Congenital heart block. Congenital heart block, on the other hand, is diagnosed on ECG by varying degrees of incoordination between atrial and ventricular depolarizations. The most serious form of congenital heart block is third-degree block (complete atrioventricular [A-V] dissociation). Approximately 30% of infants who have a complete A-V dissociation will have underlying structural heart disease (e.g., atrial septal defect, corrected transposition). It frequently is caused by connective tissue disorders in the mother and may be the first manifestation of the maternal disease. The heart rate usually is in the range of 50 to 80 beats/min, and the newborn frequently is asymptomatic, whereas symptomatic newborns usually have rates of less than 50 beats/min.

Irregular Heart Rate

The most common cause of irregular heart rate in the newborn is an extrasystolic arrhythmia, such as premature atrial or ventricular contractions. Both should be considered benign in the absence of underlying cardiac disease and if they disappear with increasing sinus heart rate (i.e., upon stimulation of the newborn). They usually disappear within a few days or weeks. Newborns who have very frequent extra beats or extra beats associated with cardiopulmonary symptoms deserve further evaluation to rule out electrolyte abnormalities or cardiomyopathies.

Blood Pressure

It is unusual to have blood pressure (BP) abnormalities as isolated findings in neonatal illness. Low blood pressure (systolic pressure less than 60 mm Hg for a full-term infant) most often is associated with tachycardia and signs of poor cardiac output. Hypertension (systolic BP greater than 90 mm Hg; diastolic BP greater than 60 mm Hg) also is unusual in the otherwise healthy newborn infant. Coarctation of the aorta often is diagnosed by the combination of increased blood pressure in the upper extremities with low blood pressure and/or poor pulses in the lower extremities. Renal vascular occlusion also may manifest initially as persistently elevated blood pressure; this especially should be considered if the newborn or older infant has had umbilical artery catheterization. Determination of serum electrolytes, as well as evaluation of renal structure and perfusion, often is helpful in evaluating the infant whose blood pressure is persistently elevated.

Temperature

Meticulous attention to the thermal status of the newborn is a hallmark of good newborn care. The increased relative surface area characteristic of newborns makes them extremely sensitive to environmental conditions, especially immediately after delivery when they are wet. The infant should be dried carefully and placed in a heat-gaining environment until stabilized and should not be bathed until thermal stability is ensured. Term infants should be dressed and blanketed and the room temperature maintained at 24° C to 26.5° C (75.2° F to 79.7° F) in the normal newborn nursery.

In the sick infant, fluctuations in body temperature (T) are more common than is stable pyrexia; therefore, persistent hyperthermia more than 37.5° C axillary usually is a manifestation of poor environmental heat control. One clue to whether a fever is disease-related is the core-to-leg temperature (rectal-to-midthigh temperature) gradient. A rectal temperature more than 1° to 2° C greater than midthigh temperature suggests a disease-related fever.

Hypothermia is a prominent finding in neonatal illness, especially sepsis. Hypothermia caused by the environment increases the metabolic demands on the newborn and can have disastrous consequences, including metabolic acidosis, pulmonary hypertension, and hypoxemia.

Respiration

Given the dramatic physiological changes associated with transition from the aqueous fetal environs to the air-breathing newborn state, it is not surprising that respiratory compromise is common in the newborn period. Abnormalities in both respiratory rate and the quality of respiratory effort are associated with neonatal illness. The normal respiratory rate of the term newborn is 40 to 60 breaths/min.

Tachypnea

Infants commonly attempt to increase their minute ventilation through increases in respiratory rate. Tachypnea is defined as a respiratory rate of more than 60 breaths/min. A primary pulmonary cause of tachypnea is suggested by the presence of other signs of respiratory distress, including expiratory grunting, nasal flaring, inspiratory crackles, or rales. Evaluation of neonatal respiratory distress includes chest roentgenography, which should be considered part of the physical examination of the sick newborn and which may well lead to a specific diagnosis. For example, this study may reveal a congenital malformation (such as a diaphragmatic hernia or cystic adenomatoid malformation) or a pneumothorax. Inserting a nasogastric tube before obtaining the chest roentgenogram may be helpful. The diagnosis of tracheoesophageal fistula (with a proximal esophageal pouch and a distal fistula) should be suspected when copious oral secretions and tachypnea are associated with a roentgenogram showing the nasogastric tube coiled in the proximal esophagus.

Transient tachypnea. Transient tachypnea of the newborn (TTN) is the most common cause of neonatal tachypnea in the term infant and probably represents delayed clearing of the normal fetal lung fluid. TTN is especially common following cesarean section delivery without labor. The onset is at birth; typically, gradual improvement is noted with resolution generally occurring by 3 to 5 days of age. Because TTN can be difficult to distinguish from other entities, such as pneumonia or aspiration, the clinician must maintain a high index of suspicion for these possibilities.

Pneumonia. Congenital pneumonia is an ominous cause of respiratory distress in the infant, and group B beta-hemolytic streptococcus probably is the most frequent pathogen. Often the clues to the diagnosis are subtle, and death can result even if the infant is treated promptly. Concerns over this possibility greatly influence our prompt response to all newborns in respiratory distress.

Aspiration syndrome. Aspiration syndromes also are relatively common. This category includes both blood and amniotic fluid aspirations. A newborn who has aspiration pneumonitis typically has a barrel-shaped, hyperexpanded chest and rapid, shallow respirations. If the aspirated amniotic fluid is meconium stained, clinical management may become especially difficult. In addition, pulmonary "air leaks," such as pneumothorax or pneumomediastinum, often accompany aspiration pneumonitis. In the case of suspected meconium aspiration, attention also should focus on determining why the infant passed meconium in the first place (e.g., resulting from asphyxia or sepsis). Often the answer to this question has a greater bearing on the baby's long-term outcome than does the aspiration itself.

Spontaneous pneumothorax. Spontaneous pneumothoraces are relatively common occurrences in otherwise healthy infants and also may manifest initially as tachypnea. Usually, auscultation of the lungs helps in the clinical diagnosis because decreased breath sounds may be noted over the involved lung. In addition, the chest may be hyperresonant to percussion on the side of the air leak. The diagnosis is confirmed by transillumination and chest roentgenogram. Treatment is dictated by the degree of cardiopulmonary compromise.

Metabolic acidosis. Metabolic acidosis may elicit an increase in respiratory rate as the baby attempts to provide respiratory compensation. An arterial blood gas analysis will assist in the recognition of this possibility. The differential diagnosis of metabolic acidosis is extensive and can be divided broadly into two groups: bicarbonate wasting (most commonly in the urine) or acid gain. Lactic acidosis signifies either tissue hypoxia (most commonly) or an inborn error of metabolism. Other circulating acids (e.g., pyruvic or methylmalonic acid) may cause a metabolic acidosis as a sign of an inborn error of metabolism.

Irregular Respiration

Apnea. In contrast to breathing too rapidly, some ill infants may breathe too slowly or not at all. Apnea is defined as the cessation of air flow and may result from decreased respiratory drive, airway obstruction, or a combination of the two (mixed apnea). Symptomatic (prolonged) apnea is defined as apnea lasting for 20 seconds or longer or as shorter periods of apnea associated with cyanosis, marked pallor, hypotonia, or bradycardia. A wide variety of disorders display the common sign of apnea, so this sign deserves a meticulous search for cause. Symptomatic apnea never is a normal finding in the term or near-term (more than 35 weeks' gestation) infant. Perhaps the most ominous cause is *infection;* however, any metabolic disturbance or airway anomaly may result in apnea. Certain drugs administered to the mother, especially narcotics and magnesium sulfate, also may depress the newborn's respiratory drive. Although specific antidotes may be available in certain instances (e.g., naloxone for narcotic depression), the first treatment is to ensure adequate ventilation.

Periodic breathing. Periodic breathing is a breathing pattern in which three or more respiratory pauses lasting longer than 3 seconds are separated by less than 20 seconds of respiration. Most commonly, periodic breathing is normal, especially in infants born prematurely. However, it also may be a manifestation of instability of the brainstem respiratory control center, a condition induced by disease.

GROWTH

Body Weight

One of the first questions asked by new parents is, "How much does my baby weigh?" The answer to this question may give the clinician valuable clues to the health of the infant. Abnormalities in growth may reflect effects of fetal nutrition, environmental toxins, systemic infections, chromosomal or syndromic influences, or family heritage. The adequacy of growth usually is assessed by comparing a newborn's measurements with normal values obtained from published standards. This involves accurate determination of gestational age so that the appropriate standards can be used. The gold standard for determination of gestational age is good obstetrical dating; physical examination of the newborn may confirm the age. (See Chapter 45, [Three] Recovery Period.)

Macrosomia. The term *macrosomia* refers to a newborn whose weight places him or her above the ninetieth percentile, compared with other newborns of similar gestational age (large for gestational age, or LGA). Newborns born to mothers who have either preexisting or gestational diabetes often are macrosomic. This is believed to represent the effects of increased fetal insulin levels, which result from exposure to a chronically elevated blood glucose level. Acute complications may include hypoglycemia, hyperbilirubinemia, hypocalcemia, and polycythemia. Preexisting maternal diabetes, but not gestational diabetes, also is associated with an increased incidence of congenital anomalies. Macrosomia may also result from intrinsic hyperinsulinemia, resulting from unusual disorders characterized by early onset of hypoglycemia and elevated glucose requirements. The best known of these uncommon problems is Beckwith-Wiedemann syndrome. Infants who have this syndrome also have macroglossia and may have an omphalocele. Macrosomic newborns may be difficult to deliver and thus predisposed to birth trauma. *All macrosomic infants should be considered to be at high risk for hypoglycemia and should have careful monitoring of blood glucose concentrations.*

Microsomia. Microsomia (small for gestational age, or SGA), on the other hand, most often is defined as a birth weight below the tenth percentile compared with other newborns of the same gestation. Other growth measurements, such as length or head circumference, may or may not be similarly affected. Asymmetrical growth retardation (underweight for length and head circumference) often suggests a problem extrinsic to the baby, such as decreased uteroplacental blood flow, whereas symmetrical growth retardation suggests either a long-standing cause or a problem intrinsic to the infant, such as a congenital viral infection or a chromosomal abnormality. Of note is that certain ethnic groups (e.g., East Asian) have newborns who "plot" as being small compared with normal American standards but are appropriate relative to other infants of their heritage. Microsomic infants may have hypoglycemia because glycogen and fat stores often are very minimal. Therefore, *all microsomic infants should be considered to be at high risk for hypoglycemia and should have careful monitoring of blood glucose concentrations.*

Head Growth

Macrocephaly. Newborns whose head circumference exceeds two standard deviations above the mean, or the ninety-seventh percentile, are said to be macrocephalic. It is critical to search for evidence of neurological impairment. Macrocephaly may be caused by volume increases in any of the normal components of the cranial vault—namely brain, blood, or cerebrospinal fluid. Increases in the cerebrospinal fluid compartment, either intraventricular or external to the ventricles around the surfaces of the brain, are referred to as *hydrocephalus*. This finding often is associated with a rapid rate of increase in the head circumference. The shape of the cranium may give clues as to whether fluid collections are intraventricular (frontal bossing) or external to the brain (biparietal enlargement). Hydrocephalus may or may not be a progressive finding and is relatively easily diagnosed by cranial ultrasonography or computed tomography.

Increases in brain volume also may be noted. This may represent either a normal brain (as in benign familial megalencephaly), accumulation of abnormal metabolic products (e.g., lipidoses, mucopolysaccharidoses), a generalized growth disorder (e.g., achondroplasia), or in rare cases, tumors.

Blood collections either in or around the brain may result in macrocephaly. Auscultation of the head may reveal a bruit, which is a sign of an arteriovenous malformation. Intracranial hemorrhage is an unusual primary cause of increased head size but frequently leads to hydrocephalus.

Microcephaly. Microcephaly refers to a head circumference less than the third percentile. It is an ominous finding and often indicates a severe underlying abnormality of brain growth or development or both, caused either by primary brain dysgenesis or by secondary insults such as teratogens, an infection, or hypoxic-ischemic encephalopathy.

Body Length

Abnormally short or long newborns usually fit into the classification of the connective tissue or skeletal disorders. Unfortunately, body length is one of the most notoriously inaccurate measurements made in the nursery but, if done carefully, can be accurate. If a newborn's length seems inappropriate, further measurements, such as long bone or upper-to-lower segment ratios, may be beneficial, along with a skeletal survey.

TONE, POSTURE, AND ACTIVITY

The normal term infant assumes a flexed posture of all limbs and, when awake, is active on gentle stimulation. Limbs often move in an alternating fashion. When pulled to sit, the head should be righted, then held in the same plane as the rest of the body for several seconds. Muscle tone is evaluated best by passive limb manipulation.

Hypertonia

Hypertonia can be a prominent manifestation of hypoxic-ischemic brain injury, meningitis, or intracranial hemorrhage. Arching of the back (opisthotonos) is a manifestation of extensor hypertonia.

Hypotonia

Hypotonia perhaps is the most common motor abnormality noted in the neonatal period. Any acutely ill infant may demonstrate some degree of mild hypotonia. Most often hypotonia is associated with at least some degree of weakness, although significant disproportion may be noted. The hypotonic newborn often assumes a "spread-eagle" posture, with little to no resting limb flexion. Certain patterns of tone and weakness are associated with specific disorders.

Increased Activity

Increased activity clearly is a subjective finding, based to a great extent on the past clinical experiences of the observer. Unfortunately, an important diagnostic consideration in our society is neonatal abstinence syndrome (drug withdrawal). The importance of recognizing this syndrome cannot be overemphasized. If drug withdrawal is suspected, the newborn's behavior can be monitored with a neonatal abstinence scoring system (see Seidel et al, Suggested Readings). The syndrome usually is diagnosed by the demonstration of illicit drugs in the newborn's urine or meconium stool. (See Chapter 50, Prenatal Drug Abuse and Neonatal Drug Withdrawal Syndrome.)

Decreased Activity

Decreased activity may represent the effects of pharmacological agents administered in the peripartum period, such as narcotics or magnesium sulfate. Both of these agents also may result in transient but significant respiratory depression. An underlying neurological abnormality also needs to be considered. An inborn error of metabolism should be suspected in any infant who initially seemed to have normal activity but then developed decreasing levels of activity and responsiveness. As always, sepsis remains a possibility in any newborn who persistently has decreased activity.

Jitteriness

Jitteriness is defined as rhythmical tremors of equal amplitude and probably is the most common involuntary movement of the healthy infant. The movements of jitteriness (or tremors) are provoked easily in susceptible neonates by external stimuli, such as handling or loud noise, and can be stopped simply by holding the affected extremity gently. Although tremors usually occur in healthy infants, jitteriness may be caused by hypoglycemia, hypocalcemia, or perinatal asphyxia, and these diagnoses should be investigated. In addition, neonatal jitteriness may be seen in association with maternal use of marijuana, cocaine, and narcotics.

Seizures

Seizures in the newborn rarely occur as dramatic, well-organized, symmetrical, generalized tonic-clonic episodes. More frequently, seizure episodes appear as focal abnormalities or as subtle findings such as repetitive staring, blinking, or sucking movements. Because seizures in the newborn usually are a sign of an underlying abnormality, including primary central nervous system disease, systemic illness, or metabolic abnormality, they must be diagnosed and treated as relative medical emergencies.

COLOR

Cyanosis

Peripheral cyanosis involving the hands and feet (acrocyanosis) is a common normal finding in the first 1 to 2 days of life. In contrast, persistent central cyanosis always is abnormal. The ability to detect it clinically, however, depends on the skill of the observer. Therefore, whenever central cyanosis is suspected, the oxygen saturation of arterial hemoglobin should be monitored with a pulse oximeter to confirm the diagnosis. The data obtained from the saturation monitor are useful *only* when the instrument accurately senses the heart rate. When the oximeter is consistently tracking the arterial pulse and when the baby is quiet, oxygen saturation should be at least 90% while breathing room air. Additional valuable information can be obtained by monitoring arterial oxygen saturation in the right arm and comparing it with saturation in a lower extremity. A right-to-left shunt at the level of the ductus arteriosus will result in desaturated blood in the lower extremities. Cyanosis resulting from a respiratory origin usually occurs with associated signs of respiratory distress. *Cyanosis without respiratory distress suggests an anatomical right-to-left shunt caused by a congenital cardiac anomaly.* (See Chapter 198, Congenital Heart Disease.) This right-to-left shunt can be confirmed by finding little or no increase in pO_2 (pO_2 less than 100) with administration of 100% oxygen. In rare instances, cyanosis may be caused by an abnormal hemoglobin, such as methemoglobin.

Jaundice

Visible jaundice in the first 24 hours of life is abnormal and usually suggests an increase in red blood cell destruction and production of bilirubin. Hemolysis on an immune or an infectious basis occurs most frequently. Inherited red cell membrane and enzymatic defects are less common problems that often are difficult to diagnose in the first few days of life. Aggressive treatment aimed at keeping levels of indirect bilirubin from climbing too rapidly is important in preventing the central nervous system complications of hyperbilirubinemia. Although some degree of jaundice is normal in healthy newborns, elevation of the direct, or conjugated, fraction of bilirubin is not. Levels of direct bilirubin persistently above 1.5 mg/dl require further evaluation, including but not limited to assessments of liver function.

Petechiae/Purpura

Petechiae are pinpoint hemorrhages into the skin that do not blanch with pressure, whereas purpura are larger, nonblanching areas of bleeding into the skin. Petechiae may appear on the presenting part for a vaginal delivery without signifying an underlying pathological condition. Extensive, generalized petechiae, on the other hand, may be the initial manifestation of an underlying platelet abnormality. The differential diagnosis includes infectious, immunological, hematological, and a myriad of miscellaneous causes.

Pallor

The term *pallor,* or *paleness,* describes a decrease in the normal rosy skin color of the white newborn. It may result from anemia or a generalized vasoconstriction.

Anemia. Anemia that appears in the newborn (hematocrit less than 45%) may have multiple causes, which can be subdivided into two main categories: excessive loss or destruction of red blood cells (e.g., acute or chronic hemorrhage, hemolysis) or inadequate red cell production (red cell hypoplasia). The first group is much more common. Diagnostic evaluation includes assessment of cardiovascular stability, because acute blood loss may cause hypotension, tachycardia, and poor perfusion, with delayed capillary refill. Determination of central hematocrit, red blood cell indices, indices of red blood cell production, and adequacy of other blood cell lines (white blood cells, platelets) may give other clues. The detection of acid-stable fetal hemoglobin in maternal blood (Kleihauer-Betke test) is diagnostic of fetal bleeding into the maternal circulation (fetomaternal hemorrhage). Anemia in the newborn is discussed more thoroughly in Chapter 117, Anemia and Pallor.

Vasoconstriction. Pallor caused by vasoconstriction may represent a normal response to cold stress, which requires attention to thermoregulatory management. On the other hand, this finding may be a clue to underlying hemodynamic compromise most commonly related to hypovolemia or cardiac dysfunction. In this case, pallor often accompanies tachycardia, weak pulse, and low blood pressure. A history of blood loss (or a tight nuchal cord resulting in occult blood loss) during delivery may provide an additional clue to the diagnosis of hypovolemia; a therapeutic response to volume expansion confirms this diagnosis. If cardiac dysfunction is the underlying cause, then other physical findings may be present, including a "gallop" heart rhythm, pulmonary rales, and hepatomegaly. In this situation, volume expansion actually may exacerbate the problem. A chest roentgenogram may help differentiate between these two causes of pallor.

Plethora

Plethora usually is caused by polycythemia, and a venous hematocrit reading of more than 65% confirms the diagnosis. Polycythemia occurs more frequently among infants who are postmature, who demonstrate intrauterine growth retardation, or who are born to mothers who smoke or have diabetes or preeclampsia. Twin-to-twin transfusion and chromosomal anomalies (e.g., trisomies 13, 18, and 21) are other causes. The main clinical concern related to polycythemia is that a high hematocrit often is associated with an elevated blood viscosity, which may impede tissue blood flow. Therefore, a wide variety of clinical signs also may be associated with plethora, including respiratory distress and cyanosis, central nervous system (CNS) signs, poor feeding, hypoglycemia, and many others. The treatment for symptomatic polycythemia is a partial exchange transfusion aimed at decreasing the hematocrit to approximately 50% and thus eliminating hyperviscosity.

SOUNDS

Crying

Abnormalities of an infant's cry have long been recognized as markers for a variety of neonatal disorders. More recently, advances in electronics have enabled investigators to characterize individual cry patterns. High-pitched cries may herald CNS abnormalities, whereas hoarse or low-pitched cries can be associated with upper airway abnormalities.

Breathing

Noisy breathing often is a clue to underlying airway problems and is associated with clinical evidence of increased work of breathing. Inspiratory stridor implicates extrathoracic airway obstruction caused by entities such as laryngomalacia, laryngeal web, and vocal cord trauma or paralysis. Accurate diagnosis requires direct visualization of the larynx and upper airway by someone trained in airway management of the newborn. Less invasive methods of evaluation include fluoroscopy or measurement of air flow-volume loops. Expiratory grunting often is noted in infants who have poorly compliant lungs and represents a compensatory maneuver that increases end-expiratory lung volume. Expiratory stridor and wheezing implicate intrathoracic obstruction involving the small and midsize airways.

ODORS

The astute clinician uses all senses in the evaluation of newborns, including the sense of smell. Inborn errors of metabolism often are associated with unusual odors of the urine or of the infant. Although individual inborn errors of metabolism are rare, as a group they are not uncommon. Unusual odors have been described, for example, as mustiness (phenylketonuria), sweaty feet (isovaleric acidemia), and maple syrup (maple syrup urine disease). Screening of urine and plasma for specific metabolic compounds provides an initial step toward diagnosis. See Chapter 20 (Three), Recognition of Genetic-Metabolic Diseases by Clinical Diagnosis and Screening, and Chapter 160, Odor (Unusual Urine and Body).

ABDOMINAL DISTENTION

Although mild gastric distention can be a normal finding, moderate distention that persists or is associated with other systemic signs of illness should be evaluated. Abdominal distention can result from gas, fluid, or an abdominal mass. See Chapter 113, Abdominal Distention.

Gaseous Distention

Gaseous distention can be diagnosed by hyperresonance to percussion. Functional decreases in bowel motility (ileus) can accompany a wide variety of systemic illnesses in the neonate. Usually there is no associated tenderness. Mechanical bowel obstruction often is associated with bilious emesis and delayed passage of stools. Free intraabdominal air resulting from a perforated viscus usually is accompanied by signs of peritonitis, which may include erythema of the abdominal wall, marked tenderness to palpation, and absence of bowel sounds.

Fluid Distention

Intraabdominal fluid is diagnosed by a fluid wave on palpation or by shifting dullness to percussion. Hemoperitoneum occasionally is noted after a difficult delivery or in association with disorders characterized by massive splenomegaly (e.g., erythroblastosis). Urinary ascites occasionally is noted in association with obstructive uropathy. The most common cause of fluid distention (ascites) is transudation, resulting from conditions such as hemolytic disease, congestive heart failure, or nonimmune hydrops.

Distention Caused by Abdominal Mass

Urogenital. Most abdominal masses in the newborn are urogenital in origin. Palpation of the abdomen may give clues as to location and consistency; however, the preferred method for diagnosis is an abdominal ultrasound examination. Flank masses (either unilateral or bilateral) usually are caused by cystic dysplasia of the kidneys or by hydronephrosis. Cystic ovary may appear as a lower abdominal mass in female infants.

Hepatomegaly. Hepatomegaly also may appear as an enlargement of the abdomen. The liver may normally be palpable 2 cm below the right costal margin, with the upper border typically percussed at the fifth intercostal space. Liver enlargement can be seen with a wide variety of systemic illnesses, including infections, primary hepatic disease, congestive heart failure, hematological disorders, storage disorders, trauma, and in rare cases, tumors. For more information, see also Chapter 145, Hepatomegaly.

Splenomegaly. The tip of the spleen occasionally may be palpable in normal infants during the first days of life. A prominent spleen may be associated with congenital viral infection, inborn errors of metabolism, or more commonly, with the increased extramedullary hematopoiesis noted with hemolytic disease. For more information, see also Chapter 170, Splenomegaly.

Adrenal hemorrhage. Massive adrenal hemorrhage may manifest as a flank mass in a stressed infant after a difficult delivery. Risk factors include macrosomia, breech presentation, and perinatal asphyxia.

Gastrointestinal enteric duplication cysts. Gastrointestinal enteric duplication cysts may be palpable and can lead to bowel obstruction. Intrauterine meconium peritonitis may result in formation of a palpable pseudocyst. An olive-size mass in the epigastrium can be caused by the hypertrophied pylorus of pyloric stenosis. (See Chapter 255, Pyloric Stenosis.)

Tumor. Wilms' tumor, neuroblastoma, and congenital mesoblastic nephromas are uncommon; however, their usual presenting sign is abdominal swelling or a palpable abdominal mass. See Chapter 193, Cancers in Childhood.

INTAKE AND OUTPUT

Feeding Problems

Oral feeding, although often taken for granted, represents a very complicated neuromotor process involving coordination of sucking, swallowing, and breathing. Indifference to feeding may be noted in conjunction with other systemic illnesses. As a result, difficulties in feeding are seen in association with a wide variety of disorders. Although this group of disorders is nonspecific, it commonly is seen in newborns born prematurely or in those who have CNS and neuromuscular disorders. Less commonly, the cause may be an anatomical abnormality, such as tracheoesophageal fistula.

Oliguria

More than 90% of infants void by 24 hours of age and 99% do so by 48 hours; they maintain adequate output thereafter (>1 ml/kg/hr). Failure to pass urine by 48 hours suggests either primary renal dysfunction or obstructive uropathy. For more information, see also Chapter 186, Anuria/Oliguria.

Polyuria

Polyuria is uncommon in the newborn. It is considered pathological when the infant is unable to achieve normal total body water and electrolytes because of persistent passage of unconcentrated urine. Most commonly this represents renal tubular dysfunction, as can be seen after acute tubular necrosis or in association with a partial obstruction of the renal collecting system. Less common causes include other renal parenchymal disease and inadequate antidiuretic hormone response. For more information, see also Chapter 162, Polyuria.

Hematuria/Hemoglobinuria

Red urine usually indicates hematuria; however, other possible causes include the presence of hemoglobin, uric acid, or porphyrins. Examination of a freshly voided urine sample will aid in the diagnosis. If intact red blood cells are detected, extraurinary sources (e.g., rectal or vaginal bleeding) must be excluded. If red cell or other types of renal casts are present, then parenchymal kidney disease is the likely cause. The differential diagnosis of hematuria in the newborn includes asphyxial kidney injury (e.g., acute tubular necrosis, cortical necrosis), renal vascular accident (e.g., renal vein thrombosis), obstructive uropathy, cystitis, nephritis, or underlying coagulopathy. For more information, see also Chapter 143, Hematuria.

Hemoglobinuria is seen most commonly in association with intravascular hemolysis. Urate crystals may give a reddish orange cast to the urine in infants who otherwise are healthy.

Proteinuria

A small amount of protein normally may be detected in the urine of healthy newborns; however, most term newborns excrete less than 25 mg in 24 hours. If excessive proteinuria is suspected, then a timed urine collection should be obtained. Proteinuria may be seen in association with nearly any form of renal disease. For more information, see also Chapter 163, Proteinuria.

Delayed Passage of Meconium

Most term infants (94%) pass their first meconium stool by 24 hours of age; 99% pass meconium by 48 hours. Delays in passage may represent significant underlying bowel pathology, including Hirschsprung's disease, atresias, meconium ileus, or meconium plug syndrome.

Melena/Hematochezia

The most common source of blood in the newborn infant's stool is maternal blood swallowed at delivery. These infants typically are not ill. This cause can be diagnosed quickly at the bedside by the Apt-Downey test for the presence of adult hemoglobin. Neonatal gastrointestinal (GI) hemorrhage may be acute and life threatening or may be detected only in trace amounts by stool heme testing. GI hemorrhage may be the presenting sign of a generalized bleeding disorder, such as vitamin K deficiency, disseminated intravascular coagulation, thrombocytopenia, or hereditary coagulopathy. Upper GI trauma, such as from vigorous suctioning or placement of a nasogastric tube, usually results only in occult blood in the stool; lower GI pathology typically results in more obvious hematochezia. The differential diagnosis includes, but is not limited to, peptic ulcers, necrotizing enterocolitis, malrotation and volvulus, Meckel's diverticulum, and intussusception. Hematochezia with mucus may result from infectious enteritis, which can be diagnosed by appropriate cultures.

Vomiting

Although spitting up small amounts of formula occurs frequently in otherwise healthy newborns, large or persistent emesis may herald underlying pathological conditions. Vomiting of non-bile-stained fluid usually represents anatomical or functional obstruction at or above the first portion of the duodenum. Causes include esophageal atresia, gastric web, pyloric stenosis, or severe gastroesophageal reflux (GER). Anatomical obstruction should be ruled out before linking the diagnosis of vomiting to GER alone. Obstruction below the opening of the bile duct may produce bilious vomiting. This may result from a functional ileus caused by systemic disease (such as hypokalemia, adrenal hyperplasia, or elevated intracranial pressure) or may represent a structural abnormality (e.g., atresia or malrotation with volvulus). Diagnostic tests start with anteroposterior and horizontal beam abdominal roentgenograms.

Diarrhea

Diarrhea is the passage of frequent stools. Newborn infants may have up to five or six stools per day, especially if breast-fed. Persistent passage of watery stools, however, is abnormal and may be a sign of enteric or systemic disease.

Gastroenteritis. Bacterial gastroenteritis is unusual in the newborn period; however, nursery epidemics, as well as isolated cases, do occur. The diagnosis is suggested by the presence of blood and mucus in the stools and is confirmed by appropriate cultures. Viral gastroenteritis, especially that caused by rotavirus, has been described in newborns.

Lactose intolerance. Lactose intolerance is a very common cause of diarrhea in the newborn. Stools are watery and test positive for reducing sugars. The diagnosis is suggested further when these findings resolve after a lactose-free formula is begun. Most commonly, this represents a transient lactase deficiency. Therefore, lactose-containing formula can be reinstituted after several weeks.

Other causes. Other, less common causes of diarrhea include phototherapy, neonatal abstinence syndrome, thyrotoxicosis, and other specific malabsorption syndromes, such as cystic fibrosis.

OTHER FINDINGS ON EXAMINATION

Leukokoria

Leukokoria literally means white pupil and is not a normal finding in the newborn. The observation of a white pupil requires immediate, further evaluation by an ophthalmologist experienced in examining newborns. The most common cause is a cataract, of which nearly 50% have diagnosable and potentially treatable causes. Other causes include persistent hyperplastic primary vitreous, cicatricial retinopathy of prematurity, retinal dysplasia, tumor (retinoblastoma), glaucoma, and numerous other conditions.

Red Eye

Ophthalmia neonatorum, or neonatal conjunctivitis, often manifests as a red eye with exudate (see Chapter 168, Red Eye). The cause is chemical (silver nitrate or antibiotic drops), bacterial, viral, or chlamydial in nature. All cases should be examined thoroughly with appropriate culture and sensitivity studies performed and appropriate therapy instituted promptly, especially when the eyelids are markedly swollen and a purulent discharge is present, most likely representing infection with *Neisseria gonorrhoeae.*

Heart Murmur

A large number of normal, healthy newborns have a soft, short systolic murmur heard in the first few days of life, relating to ductal closure. The absence of a murmur, on the other hand, does not eliminate the diagnosis of a serious cardiac anomaly. Falling pulmonary vascular resistance over the first few days of life also affects the presence and the quality of the murmur. A significant murmur heard on the first day of life is more likely to be caused by an obstructive lesion, such as aortic stenosis, pulmonic stenosis, or coarctation of the aorta. A significant murmur first heard after the day of birth suggests a shunt lesion, such as a patent ductus arteriosus or ventricular septal defect. Loud, persistent systolic murmurs, especially if accompanied by other cardiopulmonary findings, require further evaluation. For more information, see also Chapter 142, Heart Murmurs, and Chapter 198, Congenital Heart Disease.

Acknowledgment

The author wishes to acknowledge the contribution of Keith J. Gallaher to earlier editions of this chapter.

SUGGESTED READINGS

Fanaroff AA, Martin RJ: *Neonatal-perinatal medicine: diseases of the fetus and infant,* ed 6, St Louis, 1997, Mosby.

Jones KL: *Smith's recognizable patterns of human malformation,* ed 5, Philadelphia, 1997, WB Saunders.

Klaus MH, Fanaroff AA: *Care of the high-risk neonate,* ed 4, Philadelphia, 1993, WB Saunders.

Long WA: *Fetal and neonatal cardiology,* Philadelphia, 1990, WB Saunders.

Parker S, et al: Jitteriness in full-term neonates: prevalence and correlates, *Pediatrics* 85:17, 1990.

Seidel HM, Rosenstein BJ, Pathak A: Primary care of the newborn, ed 2, St. Louis, 1997, Mosby

Volpe JJ: *Neurology of the newborn,* Philadelphia, ed 3, 1995, WB Saunders.

48 Common Neonatal Illnesses

Charles Palmer • Dennis J. Mujsce

APNEA

Newborn infants must establish and maintain regular respiration immediately following umbilical cord clamping and disruption of placental gas exchange. Irregularities of respiration such as apnea, however, occur frequently among premature infants and less commonly among term infants. In contrast to adults, both premature and term neonates demonstrate a biphasic response to a reduction of inspired oxygen concentration and hypoxemia. An initial transient increase in ventilation is followed by a sustained depression of ventilation. Additionally, neonates who experience hypoxia may respond in a blunted fashion to progressive levels of carbon dioxide accumulation. Term infants establish a mature response to hypoxia after the first week of life; preterm infants born before 33 weeks' gestation respond abnormally to hypoxia and hypercapnia into the second month of postnatal life.[12]

Apnea is defined as a transient cessation of respiratory airflow. The three types of apnea that have been described are central, obstructive, and mixed. Central apnea, which is characterized by the total absence of respiratory effort, is due to a cessation of rhythm generation by brainstem respiratory neurons. During obstructive apnea, the respiratory effort is ineffective, as a result of partial or complete obstruction of the upper airway. Mixed apnea contains both central and obstructive components. A typical mixed apnea may begin with a short central apnea, but progressive declines of heart rate and arterial saturation occur during the subsequent airway obstruction that results from a loss of muscle tone of the pharynx. Short (<15 seconds) central apnea can be normal at all ages. Pathological apnea is defined as a prolonged (>20 seconds) respiratory interruption or a shorter period associated with cyanosis, marked pallor, hypotonia, or bradycardia.[13] Apnea of prematurity is defined as pathological apnea in a premature infant. Periodic breathing is defined as a breathing pattern in which three or more respiratory pauses of more than 5 seconds' duration are separated by fewer than 20 seconds of respiration.

Apnea occurs predominantly during active (REM) sleep in both term and preterm infants. It is uncommon for prolonged apnea to be observed during quiet sleep, when respiratory rhythm is regular and tidal volume varies little. Other respiratory variations associated with REM sleep include asynchronous breathing (chest and abdomen move in opposite directions), reduced functional residual capacity (FRC), hypoxemia, attenuated responses to hypercapnia and hypoxia, and increased incidence of periodic breathing.

Apnea of prematurity usually starts after the first day of life and resolves when the infant grows to 37 weeks' gestation, but occasionally may persist to 44 to 48 weeks postconceptual age. Apnea is very common in preterm infants and reflects the immaturity of the respiratory system. These infants do not have the benefit of fully developed brainstems, peripheral nervous systems, peripheral and central chemoreceptors, mechanical stretch receptors, respiratory muscles (diaphragm, intercostals, upper airway), or chest wall mechanics. Although most apnea of prematurity is benign, prolonged apneic periods can lead to significant hypoxemia and bradycardia. Extremely premature infants experience central apnea that is more frequent, longer, more likely to cause hypoxemia, and more persistent than those born closer to term. Apnea of prematurity previously was thought to consist largely of central apnea, but it now is recognized that mixed and obstructive types of apnea are at least as common and problematic in the premature population.[7]

Although uncomplicated idiopathic apnea of prematurity is common, apnea also may be symptomatic of an underlying disorder, even in the preterm infant. Some infants are thought to experience apnea because of gastroesophageal reflux, but the available evidence does not conclusively support this common perception. Specific causes for apnea that warrant investigation include the following:

1. Septicemia (e.g., meningitis or necrotizing enterocolitis)
2. Impaired oxygenation, hypoxemia, severe anemia, and shock or marked systemic to pulmonary circulatory shunt (e.g., patent ductus arteriosus)
3. Metabolic disorders (e.g., hypoglycemia, hypercalcemia, hyponatremia, hypernatremia, and hyperammonemia)
4. Drugs administered to the mother or to the baby (e.g., narcotics or central nervous system depressants, prostaglandin E_1)
5. Central nervous system disorders (e.g., intracranial hemorrhage, seizures, hypoxic-ischemic injury, or congenital malformations of the brain)
6. Thermal instability (i.e., a rapid increase or decrease of temperature)
7. Postoperative status following general anesthesia

Investigation for an underlying cause should be pursued vigorously whenever apneic episodes: (1) occur within 24 hours of delivery, (2) occur in infants born after 36 weeks of gestation, (3) require vigorous resuscitation, (4) are preceded by or are associated with marked cyanosis, and (5) become more frequent and increase in severity.

The preterm infant should be monitored for apnea; because bradycardia usually follows mixed and obstructive apnea, heart rate monitoring also should be included. A cardiac monitor is important because obstructive apnea does not trigger the most commonly used respiratory monitor, which relies on changes in chest wall electrical impedance. Pulse oximetry is monitored routinely in the neonatal intensive care unit but usually is not necessary following discharge. Home monitors that track both respiration and heart rate are available for rental from vendors of durable medical equipment. Home monitoring likely is not necessary for premature infants who are thriving and have not experienced a significant apneic event for at least 8 days.[6] Before discharging an infant on a home monitor, caretakers should be instructed properly in the use of the device, as well as in cardiopulmonary resuscitation. It also is extremely important that parents are instructed to place their infants to sleep in the supine position ("back to sleep"), as is consistent with the current recommendations of the American Academy of Pediatrics (AAP).[2]

Treatment of neonatal apnea always should begin with an assessment of its underlying cause. Once treatable causes are ruled out, several treatments are available for apnea of prematurity, with selection of the appropriate therapy based on the frequency and severity of the problem. Treatments for apnea currently include the following:

1. Tactile stimulation. Gentle tapping on the infant's heel usually suffices. A pulsating water bed or rhythmically moving mattress has been used for recurrent episodes, but this generally is ineffective for persistent apnea.
2. Pharmacological intervention with methylxanthines (theophylline or caffeine), which acts on the brainstem to produce central stimulation. A loading dose of theophylline (5 mg/kg) is followed by maintenance therapy at 1 to 2 mg/kg/dose (two to three times a day). Caffeine citrate usually is given as a 20 mg/kg loading dose orally, followed by 5 mg/kg/day.
3. Continuous positive airway pressure by nasal prongs. This may ameliorate mixed and obstructive type apneas. The method of action may include an increased functional residual capacity (FRC) with consequent alteration of stretch receptor influence on respiratory timing, as well as keeping the upper airways open. The nasal prongs can be cumbersome, however, interfering with oral feeding and parental bonding, as well as traumatizing the nares.
4. Small increases in inspired oxygen from 21% to 25%, with monitoring of oxygenation to maintain the arterial oxygen pressure (PaO_2) between 50 and 90 mm Hg. Care must be taken to avoid hyperoxia. This therapy is not recommended to reduce the incidence of benign periodic breathing or short central apnea.
5. Endotracheal intubation with positive end-expiratory pressure may be required briefly in some cases.

When pharmacological therapy is used, age-related variations in theophylline metabolism necessitate the monitoring of the plasma theophylline concentration, which does not have a large margin of safety. The concentration required for apnea is less than that required for bronchodilation; thus, levels should be maintained between 5 to 10 μg/ml. Because caffeine, in contrast, has a broad therapeutic index, its concentration usually does not need to be monitored, if given in the prescribed dose. Physicians who administer methylxanthines should be aware that hepatic metabolism of these drugs is slowed by macrolide antibiotics, such as erythromycin, and by intercurrent viral illnesses. The toxicity of theophylline is related to its serum level; clinical manifestations usually begin with tachycardia, succeeded by jitteriness, irritability, and signs of gastrointestinal dysfunction. No long-term sequelae of methylxanthine therapy have been documented.

The term *apnea of infancy* applies to the occasional infant who has an unexplained respiratory pause for at least 20 seconds or a shorter respiratory pause associated with bradycardia, cyanosis, pallor, and/or marked hypotonia. The term generally refers to infants who are greater than 37 weeks' postconception at the onset of pathological apnea.

An apparent life-threatening event is an episode that is frightening to the infant's observer and characterized by some combination of apnea (central or obstructive), color change (cyanosis or pallor), marked change in muscle tone (usually marked limpness), choking, or gagging. The observer may fear that the infant has died, and these incidents should be investigated for an underlying cause, especially gastroesophageal reflux, a tracheoesophageal fistula, or possible seizures. When the particular causal diagnosis is in question, the simultaneous recording of respiratory electrical impedance, nasal air flow, esophageal pH, and the electrocardiogram for prolonged periods ("pneumograms") can document the occurrence of apnea and bradycardia. After diagnostic evaluation of an apparent life-threatening event, the patient should be discharged home with a cardiorespiratory monitor.

The outcome of apnea of prematurity usually is good, provided appropriate monitoring and treatment are ensured to prevent long periods of hypoxia. Apnea of prematurity and periodic breathing are not linked to sudden infant death syndrome (SIDS) risk, but the relationship of apnea of infancy to SIDS is less clear. Among apneic newborns and infants, pneumograms cannot predict which infants will require resuscitation to terminate a subsequent apneic spell. Compared with a control group, however, infants who have apnea of infancy have significantly higher respiratory and heart rates.

HYPERBILIRUBINEMIA

Hyperbilirubinemia occurs commonly during the first week of life. It usually is physiological, and appropriate management includes reassurance, with avoidance of unnecessary investigations and maternal-infant separation. Occasionally, hyperbilirubinemia is symptomatic of an underlying pathological condition. These cases need identification and an etiological workup. Select cases may require specific management to prevent the harmful effects of excessive unconjugated bilirubin on the central nervous system.

Physiological Jaundice

Clinical jaundice is visible at serum bilirubin levels of approximately 5 to 7 mg/dl (85 to 120 µmol/l). Approximately 50% of all normal newborns and a higher percentage of premature infants appear jaundiced during the first week of life. Nearly all newborns have some degree of mild hyperbilirubinemia that disappears after a few days; this transient hyperbilirubinemia has been called *physiological jaundice*. Mechanisms involved in producing physiological jaundice include an interaction between an increased load of bilirubin (from increased red cell mass) and a decreased ability of the newborn liver to clear bilirubin. The clinician can recognize the presence of physiological jaundice by certain criteria. It is evident clinically after the first 24 hours of life. It peaks between days 3 and 5, and in normal full-term infants it does not rise higher than 12.7 to 12.9 mg/dl.[11] The bilirubin is almost all unconjugated. Jaundice usually is not detectable after 10 days. Deviation from this physiological pattern generally signifies a pathological process and requires special investigations to define a cause.

Breast-Feeding and Jaundice

Breast-feeding has been associated with increased levels of bilirubin and prolongation of hyperbilirubinemia. The association between breast-feeding and jaundice in the healthy, full-term newborn can be considered in terms of two categories: (1) the jaundice that is associated with breast-feeding and (2) true breast-milk jaundice.

Jaundice associated with breast-feeding. Prolonged hyperbilirubinemia in association with breast-feeding occurs in about 30% of breast-fed babies. Frequent feeding may reduce the incidence of hyperbilirubinemia, so breast-feeding should not be withheld. An association between decreased frequency of nursing and higher bilirubin levels has been found. Hence, breast-feeding mothers should be encouraged to nurse their infants as frequently as possible. If it appears that the bilirubin concentration will rise above 20 mg/dl, feeding should be stopped temporarily for 48 hours and then be resumed.

True breast-milk jaundice. The syndrome of true breast-milk jaundice, in which the bilirubin concentration rises progressively from the fourth day of life, reaching a maximum of 10 to 30 mg/dl (171 to 153 µmol/l) by 10 to 15 days, develops in approximately 1% to 2% of breast-fed neonates. If breast-feeding continues, the bilirubin may continue to rise before declining after about 4 to 10 days to reach normal levels by 3 to 12 weeks of age. Finally, if breast-feeding is interrupted at any stage, the bilirubin concentration declines markedly within 48 hours. With resumption of nursing, bilirubin concentrations may rise moderately by 1 to 3 mg/dl/day but usually do not reach the previous level.

If breast-feeding needs to be withheld temporarily, mothers should be given enthusiastic support and encouraged to resume breast-feeding after a 48-hour interruption. They also should be encouraged to maintain lactation by breast pump or manual expression, to provide ample formula feedings, and to expose their baby to ultraviolet light.

Pathological Jaundice

Pathological jaundice refers to a pattern of hyperbilirubinemia that falls outside the limits defined for physiological jaundice. It may occur earlier, last longer, or reach higher levels. In these cases, jaundice should be regarded as symptomatic of an underlying pathological condition. The following criteria, modified from Maisels,[11] help identify pathological hyperbilirubinemia:

1. Clinical jaundice in the first 24 hours of life
2. Total serum bilirubin concentrations increasing by more than 5 mg/dl/day (85 µmol/l/day)
3. Total serum bilirubin concentrations exceeding 12.9 mg/dl (221 µmol/l) in full-term infants or 15 mg/dl (257 µmol/l) in premature infants
4. Direct (conjugated) serum bilirubin concentration exceeding 1.5 to 2 mg/dl (25 to 34 µmol/l)
5. Clinical jaundice persisting for more than 1 week in full-term infants or 2 weeks in premature infants

Deviations from these guidelines should be investigated.

In certain patients, jaundice will reach levels above 12.9 mg/dl, and a higher level may be tolerated before special investigations are initiated. In one study, only 6% of infants admitted to a well-baby nursery had serum bilirubin levels that exceeded 12.9 mg/dl. Serum bilirubin levels above 12.9 mg/dl were significantly associated with breast-feeding, maternal diabetes, oxytocin-induced labor, prematurity, Asian race, and male gender. In these patients, a peak bilirubin level of 15 mg/dl can be tolerated as the upper range of normal before investigation is warranted. In the absence of these listed considerations, however, values higher than 12 mg/dl should be used as the level at which jaundice should be investigated.[11]

Causes of pathological jaundice in the neonate. The newborn who has jaundice should have total and direct (conjugated) bilirubin estimated as soon as jaundice is diagnosed. Physiological jaundice first is evident clinically after 48 hours. That which occurs during the first 24 hours usually is caused by an excessive load of bilirubin, resulting from hemolysis caused by maternal antibodies to fetal red cell ABO or Rh antigens. Nonimmune causes of hemolysis also should be considered, including hereditary spherocytosis and deficiency of glucose-6-phosphate dehydrogenase (G6PD).

Infants of mothers who have diabetes are prone to increased bilirubin production, as are patients who have increased intrahepatic circulation of bilirubin secondary to small or large bowel obstruction. Clearance of bilirubin also can be hindered in premature infants by breast-feeding and by certain inborn errors of metabolism, such as hypothyroidism. Essential investigations for nonphysiological jaundice include (1) serum bilirubin concentration, including a determination of the direct bilirubin if jaundice is prolonged; (2) blood typing of both mother and infant; and (3) direct Coombs test on the infant. A peripheral blood smear for red cell morphology, reticulocyte count, and hematocrit is optional. An increased direct bilirubin level exceeding 1.5 to 2 mg/dl (or one third of the total serum bilirubin) requires further diagnostic evaluation. This should proceed rapidly because patients who have biliary atresia (a possible cause of elevated direct bilirubin) require early surgical intervention for optimal outcome.

The presence of pathological jaundice should provoke a review of the maternal and infant history and a thorough examination of the infant. A family history of jaundice or liver disease and a maternal history of illness, diabetes, or drug ingestion during pregnancy should be excluded. The labor and delivery history should be reviewed for documentation of oxytocin administration, delayed cord clamping, and vacuum extraction, because these may lead to increased red cell mass and thus an elevated serum bilirubin level from hemolysis. The maternal history should be evaluated further for evidence of bacterial or viral infection (fever, premature rupture of membranes), and the mother's blood needs to be analyzed for ABO and Rh blood groups and the presence of isoantibodies. Any maternal history of hepatitis or family history of anemia or G6PD deficiency should be noted.

The infant who has nonphysiological (pathological) jaundice (especially if jaundice is prolonged or associated with an elevated direct fraction) should be examined carefully for signs of sepsis such as lethargy, temperature instability, a change in feeding pattern, cutaneous petechiae, and poor capillary perfusion. Signs of extramedullary hematopoiesis, including hepatosplenomegaly, may reflect a congenital infection. The presence of a hematoma, extensive bruising, plethora, polycythemia, or ingested maternal blood may provide an additional hemoglobin source, producing an elevated serum bilirubin level.

Conjugated hyperbilirubinemia. An increase in direct (conjugated) bilirubin greater than 1.5 to 2 mg/dl (or more than 33% of the total serum bilirubin concentration) almost always is pathological. Causes include liver inflammation and congenital obstruction to bile flow. Hepatitis can be caused by sepsis, intrauterine infection, inborn errors of metabolism (alpha$_1$-antitrypsin deficiency, galactosemia), or pyloric stenosis and upper gastrointestinal obstruction (e.g., annular pancreas). Inflammation of the liver and cholestasis also can be produced by prolonged parenteral nutrition.

Cholestasis in the infant also can result from biliary atresia, either intrahepatic or extrahepatic, a choledochal cyst, or inspissated bile. The presence of bile pigment in the stool or duodenal aspirate excludes complete biliary atresia, but such patients should be examined carefully for signs of hepatosplenomegaly (which would support a congenital infection), and the urine should be cultured so that a urinary tract infection can be excluded; blood cultures should be drawn to exclude septicemia. An ultrasound examination of the liver can demonstrate the presence of a choledochal cyst and dilated biliary structures. Bile flow also can be evaluated by radioisotopes excreted through the hepatobiliary system. Finally, a liver biopsy and cholangiogram may be necessary to determine the specific pathology.

Patients who have conjugated hyperbilirubinemia should be investigated at a referral center where facilities permit full investigation of this disorder. The Kasai procedure of hepatic enterostomy (portoenterostomy) can improve bile drainage for patients who have extrahepatic biliary atresia; the earlier the procedure is performed, the better the results. Thus, every effort should be made to arrive at an early diagnosis and to begin appropriate intervention.

Treatment of Neonatal Hyperbilirubinemia

The reemergence of kernicterus. Observations made some 30 years ago established a strong association between severe (hemolytic) hyperbilirubinemia and the clinical syndrome of kernicterus among patients who have erythroblastosis fetalis. *Kernicterus* refers to the finding at autopsy of yellow discoloration and neuronal degeneration of the brain, particularly in the basal ganglia, hippocampus, and cerebellum. Survivors often manifest severe neuropathological sequelae, including athetoid cerebral palsy, deafness, and failure of upward gaze. Kernicterus was not seen in full-term infants if the serum bilirubin concentration was maintained below 20 mg/dl (342 μmol/l). Despite the regrettable absence of randomized clinical trials, a serum unconjugated bilirubin level of 20 mg/dl has been adopted widely as the maximum acceptable for full-term infants who have hemolytic jaundice. Levels above this are reduced by exchange transfusion; this practice has diminished the incidence of kernicterus dramatically. However, in the past decade, kernicterus has reemerged, with more than 30 cases reported in term and near-term infants in 10 of the United States since 1990. It is believed that this reemergence is a direct and unfortunate consequence of decreasing the length of postnatal hospitalization.[9]

The precise mechanism of bilirubin neurotoxicity is not known. Animal and human experiments demonstrate that hyperbilirubinemia can disrupt neurotransmission, producing lethargy, disturbances in the cry, and impairment of the brainstem auditory-evoked response, even at levels of serum bilirubin below 20 mg/dl. These changes, however, are reversible and may not reflect permanent neuronal injury. Theoretically, bilirubin must be "free" (from binding with albumin) to cross the blood-brain barrier. Animal studies have shown that when the normal blood-brain barrier is disrupted by exposure to hyperbilirubinemia, both bound and unbound bilirubin can cross it. Recent studies have shown that in addition to imparting a yellow color to the brain tissue, disruption of the blood-brain barrier in the presence of hyperbilirubinemia also can impair cellular energy metabolism. Other experiments indicate that acidosis exacerbates bilirubin neurotoxicity further.

Although both exchange transfusion and phototherapy can lower serum bilirubin effectively, the indications for their use remain hotly debated. Except for the infant who has hemolytic jaundice, most current recommendations for use of these therapies have developed out of a general consensus that has not yet been validated by the properly designed randomized clinical trials of "evidence-based medicine."

Assessment of jaundice. The clinical assessment of jaundice is unreliable, especially if ambient lighting is low and the infant already has received phototherapy, which bleaches the skin. Recently, devices for the transcutaneous measurement of bilirubin have been tested clinically. They use reflectance measurements on the skin to determine the amount of yellow color present. Although these transcutaneous measurements correlate well with serum bilirubin levels, they do not reflect them precisely enough to be used in making decisions about transfusions or phototherapy. They may become a useful tool to determine when a laboratory corroboration of serum bilirubin is needed.[5]

The "Practice Parameter for the Management of Hyperbilirubinemia in the Healthy Newborn Infant," published in 1994 by the AAP,[3] recommends that serum bilirubin be measured in any infant noted to be jaundiced by visual assessment in the first 24 hours after birth and that "follow-up should be provided to all neonates discharged less than 48 hours after birth by a health care professional . . . within 2 to 3 days of discharge." Recently, nomograms have been developed using hour-specific total serum bilirubin (TSB) measurements to predict subsequent bilirubin levels. According to their nomograms, if TSB at 20 to 28 hours of age is less than 5 mg/dl, the likelihood of developing a TSB greater than 17mg/dl within the next week is zero.[9]

Phototherapy. Phototherapy lowers serum bilirubin levels and may reduce the need for exchange transfusion. No data exist, however, to indicate that phototherapy used to lower serum bilirubin will enhance developmental outcome. As a general guideline, phototherapy may be started at a bilirubin level 5 mg/dl lower than the threshold level for exchange transfusion. For ABO incompatibility, phototherapy can be started when there is evidence of a rapidly rising bilirubin level, as defined by an increase of 0.5 mg/dl/hour or more. The routine use of phototherapy for ABO incompatibility is not necessary because hyperbilirubinemia develops in only a minority of these infants, even when the Coombs test is positive.

For healthy full-term newborns between 24 and 72 hours of age who have no hemolysis, phototherapy should start at a total serum bilirubin level between 15 to 20 mg/dl (260 to 340 μmol/l), and an exchange transfusion should be performed if the bilirubin level reaches 20 to 25 mg/dl (340 to 430 μmol/l) despite intensive phototherapy (the lower level of bilirubin is used for the 24 hour-old infant and the higher level for the relatively older infant).[3] For infants of low birth weight, phototherapy often is started at 5 mg/dl below the exchange threshold. Some authorities use phototherapy prophylactically for newborns weighing less than 1500 g because the exchange threshold recommended is lowered in proportion to birth weight. An exchange should be performed at a total serum bilirubin level of 13 to 16 mg/dl (220 to 275 μmol/l) for infants weighing less than 1500 g, 16 to 18 mg/dl (275 to 300 μmol/l) for infants weighing between 1500 and 1999 g, and 18 to 20 mg/dl (300 to 340 μmol/l) when the birth weight is between 2000 and 2499 g. These recommendations represent ranges currently used in neonatal intensive care units and do not take into account all possible situations.

Bilirubin absorbs light maximally in the wave lengths near 460 nm (the blue-green visible spectrum) and undergoes molecular isomerization. The photo-isomers are hydrophilic and are excreted directly into bile and urine. Although blue light delivers the optimal wave length for phototherapy, it also obscures the infant's skin color and unfortunately can induce headaches and nausea among nursing staff. This problem can be alleviated by combining three or four "special blue" narrow-spectrum lamps (Westinghouse 20W F20T12BB) with daylight lamps placed on the outside of the phototherapy unit.

To achieve the maximum therapeutic effect from phototherapy, it is necessary to provide the highest intensity irradiance over the largest surface area of the baby. The response to phototherapy increases with irradiance until a saturation point is reached at an irradiation of approximately 25 to 30 $\mu W/cm^2/nm$ in the blue spectrum. Because irradiance is inversely proportional to the square of the distance from the light source, free-standing phototherapy units should be as close to the baby as possible without incurring the risk of burn. If the intent is to provide intensive phototherapy, this may be as close as 15 to 20 cm from the infant.

Another way to improve phototherapy is to increase the surface area exposed. This can be achieved by removing the diaper, surrounding the infant by more than one bank of lights, placing reflective material strategically, and also by placing the infant on a fiberoptic phototherapy blanket. The infant should be kept well hydrated, preferably with milk, because it inhibits the enterohepatic circulation and, thereby, facilitates the excretion of bilirubin.

Phototherapy can be discontinued when bilirubin levels fall below 14 to 15 mg/dl in full-term infants. A rebound of less than 1 mg/dl (17 μmol/l) can be expected, provided that the infant does not have hemolytic disease. Additional follow-up of serum bilirubin is necessary if phototherapy is discontinued before 3 to 5 days of age, when bilirubin levels normally peak in full-term newborns, or if the infant has (or is suspected of having) hemolytic disease.

Whenever phototherapy is used, serum bilirubin measurements must be monitored because the skin is bleached by phototherapy, making it an unreliable indicator of the degree of jaundice. Side effects of phototherapy include increased insensible water loss, frequent loose stools, occasional abdominal distention, lethargy, and skin erythema. Skin erythema can be reduced by placing an acrylic plastic shield between the patient and the light source. This is used to filter out damaging ultraviolet and infrared rays. Patients who have an elevated conjugated (bound) bilirubin level and who receive phototherapy develop a dark green-brown discoloration ("bronze baby").

Because retinal damage has occurred in animals during phototherapy, the infant's eyes must be shielded with opaque patches. These patches need constant attention to ensure that they do not obstruct the nostrils. No long-term harmful complications of phototherapy have been identified.

Home phototherapy. Equipment designed for delivering phototherapy in the home is available. This service was developed to reduce costs of hospitalization and to prevent separation of the mother and infant. The service is appreciated especially by lactating mothers because it facilitates continuation of breast-feeding. The physician should limit the use of home phototherapy to infants who have the following characteristics (as amended from the recommendations outlined by the Committee on Fetus and Newborn of the AAP[4]):

1. Full-term, older than 48 hours, and otherwise healthy
2. Serum bilirubin concentrations greater than 14 mg/dl but less than 18 mg/dl
3. No elevation in direct-reacting (conjugated) bilirubin
4. No pathological causes of hyperbilirubinemia

A candidate for home phototherapy should have caretakers who can follow instructions regarding use of the equipment, correct application of eye patches, and provision of adequate hydration. Therapy should be under the supervision of a physician who should contact the caretakers daily and ensure that arrangements are made for serum bilirubin to be measured at least every 12 to 24 hours. The committee suggests that the newborn be removed from phototherapy during feedings and diaper changes and when the parents are asleep. Phototherapy should be discontinued once the serum bilirubin concentration falls below 14 mg/dl. If phototherapy is discontinued before 5 days of age, the serum bilirubin concentration should be remeasured 12 to 24 hours after cessation of phototherapy because a rebound in bilirubin concentration may occur.

Exchange transfusion. Bilirubin can be toxic to the central nervous system under certain circumstances. Thus far, the association between increasing levels of serum bilirubin concentration below 20 mg/dl and developmental outcome in both full-term and preterm infants remains unresolved. A recent literature review concluded that hyperbilirubinemia below 25 mg/dl in full-term infants (who have no hemolysis) does not cause significant cognitive, neurological, or hearing impairment. Accordingly, for well, healthy full-term newborns who have no hemolysis, exchange transfusion should be performed only if, despite intensive phototherapy, the bilirubin level remains between 25 and 29 mg/dl (425 to 500 μmol/l). For sick full-term infants or those in whom hemolysis is likely, an exchange transfusion should be performed at significantly lower total serum bilirubin levels of 17 to 22 mg/dl (290 to 375 μmol/l).[3,10]

The diagnosis of hemolysis often is difficult without the advantage of special investigations. An infant who has hyperbilirubinemia within 24 hours of birth should be considered hemolytic or ill and is not to be regarded in the same category as a well infant. A negative Coombs test does not rule out nonimmune causes of hemolysis. For instance, the diagnosis of G6PD deficiency requires an awareness of genetic background and should be considered in geographical regions where the disease is prevalent and in certain ethnic groups, including Sephardic Jews or families of Middle Eastern, Nigerian, Chinese, or Mediterranean origin. In cases of G6PD deficiency, clinical jaundice often manifests initially after the first 24 hours of life, which is relatively late for the immune causes of hemolysis.

Much concern has been expressed regarding the risk of kernicterus in sick, low-birth-weight infants. Yellow-stained brain tissue has been reported at autopsy among premature neonates in whom the serum bilirubin concentrations were below 10 mg/dl. In premature infants, serum bilirubin levels alone do not predict kernicterus accurately. Thus, decisions regarding the initiation of phototherapy and exchange transfusion should include consideration of possible risk factors contributing to bilirubin neurotoxicity, such as acidosis, hypoglycemia, and birth asphyxia, as well as those factors that promote delivery of bilirubin to the brain, such as displacement of bilirubin from albumin-binding (unconjugated bilirubin) or impairment of the blood-brain barrier.

Bilirubin normally binds tightly with the serum protein albumin in a one-to-one molar ratio, because there is only one primary binding site per molecule of albumin. If the molar concentration of bilirubin exceeds the molar concentration of albumin, unbound bilirubin can distribute beyond the intravascular albumin space, cross the blood-brain barrier, and produce neurotoxicity. Accordingly, unconjugated (unbound) bilirubin is a better predictor of long-term neurological outcome among jaundiced infants than is the conjugated (bound) bilirubin concentration.

Theoretically, the binding sites for bilirubin on albumin are saturated when a molar ratio of 1.0 is reached. This occurs when the bilirubin/albumin ratio is 9.0 (bilirubin expressed in mg/dl divided by albumin in g/dl). Thus, the lower the serum albumin level, the lower the bilirubin level required to reach saturation. Albumin levels are lower among sick and among premature infants. In addition to the absolute level of bilirubin, consideration must be given to the compounds that can compete with bilirubin for the albumin-binding sites. Sepsis and hemolysis reduce binding affinity, whereas free fatty acids, sulfonamides, and diuretics all compete for bilirubin-binding sites on albumin. Some authorities have recommended using the bilirubin/albumin ratio as an indirect surrogate for the unbound bilirubin concentration. In 1994, Ahlfors[1] showed that if the bilirubin/albumin ratio was greater than 6.7, there was a greater than 65% chance of having a serum-unbound bilirubin level of greater than 20 μmol/L. When the bilirubin/albumin ratio reaches 8.0, approximately 95% of neonates will have more than 20 nmol/l of unbound bilirubin in the serum and nearly 90% will have an abnormal auditory brainstem response. Recommended exchange transfusion criteria extend over a broad range of total serum bilirubin levels at all gestational ages. Some authorities recently have recommended considering the bilirubin/albumin ratio to assist in the decision whether to do or delay an exchange transfusion. Accordingly, when the bilirubin/albumin ratio is added to help fine-tune established exchange transfusion criteria, a decision to perform an exchange transfusion is recommended if the bilirubin/albumin ratio exceeds 7 and is not declining upon intensive phototherapy. (The technique for performing an exchange transfusion is presented in Appendix B, Special Procedures.)

THE INFANT OF THE MOTHER WHO HAS DIABETES

Maternal diabetes during pregnancy encompasses a range of metabolic disturbances involving carbohydrate intolerance with an elevation of serum glucose levels. Included in considering the infant of the diabetic mother (IDM) are both the infant and the mother who has long-standing insulin-dependent diabetes and who manifests glucose intolerance only during pregnancy (gestational diabetes).

Maternal hyperglycemia imposes a continuous glucose loadup on the fetus because glucose readily crosses the placenta. In the face of continuing hyperglycemia, the fetal pancreatic islet cells undergo hypertrophy and hyperplasia, and the fetus produces large amounts of insulin from about 12 to 14 weeks of gestation. This hyperinsulinemia stimulates the intracellular transport of glucose and is the main mechanism of diabetic fetopathy. This produces infants who have enlarged and immature organs.

The reported incidence of gestational diabetes varies from 0.15% to 12.3%. The highest prevalence rates are found among young black women. It now is recognized that all pregnant women should be screened for gestational diabetes at least once during the course of their pregnancy. The screening procedure consists of a 50-g glucose load that is administered orally followed by a venous plasma glucose assessment 1 hour later. A serum glucose level of 140 mg/dl (7.8 mmol/l) or greater is considered a positive finding. This screening procedure has a sensitivity of 79% and a specificity of 11% for all pregnant women. A positive screening test result should be corroborated by a formal oral glucose tolerance test.

Control of maternal diabetes is important to the outcome of the fetus. Mothers who have diabetes under good metabolic control before conception have a spontaneous abortion rate approximating that of the general population, whereas women who have poorly controlled diabetes have a significantly higher rate of pregnancy loss at all stages of gestation; pregnancy loss correlates directly with the degree of hyperglycemia and with glycosylated hemoglobin levels in the first trimester. When adequate control of diabetes is not achieved, the pediatrician often must deal with complications among infants of affected mothers. These complications include congenital malformations, birth injury, neonatal asphyxia, hypoglycemia, respiratory distress, polycythemia, hyperbilirubinemia, hypocalcemia, and renal vein thrombosis.

Structural Abnormalities

At birth, the IDM may have the classic appearance ("Campbell Soup baby") of being large for gestational age (with plump, plethoric cheeks) and lethargic. The head appears small because adipose tissue is concentrated around the trunk. Occasionally the infant is appropriately grown or even small for gestational age and is at great risk for teratogenesis, with major organ system malformation. The major defects occur within four systems: central nervous, cardiovascular, urinary tract, and gastrointestinal.

The caudal regression syndrome comprises the classic central nervous system abnormality. This syndrome consists of absence or maldevelopment of the sacrum and coccyx, with hypoplastic femurs, dislocated hips, and defects in the tibias and/or fibulas. It occurs in 0.5% of diabetic pregnancies. Neural tube defects also are reported more frequently among IDMs, as are hydrocephaly and microcephaly.

The incidence of congenital heart disease in IDMs is five times that of the general population. The most common malformations are septal defects, transposition of the great vessels, coarctation of the aorta, and situs inversus. The IDM also is susceptible to a cardiomyopathy secondary to asymmetrical septal hypertrophy from glycogen deposition in the myocardium. Hypertrophic changes may occur in the ventricular septum or in the subaortic valve area to produce a self-limiting idiopathic hypertrophic subaortic stenosis. Treatment with digoxin or other inotropic agents worsens the obstruction, but myocardial wall tension can be decreased with propranolol. Cardiomegaly with or without congestive heart failure can be seen on chest roentgenogram and may reflect prior hypoxia, hyperglycemia, hypocalcemia, or current hypertrophic cardiac disease.

Management

The pediatrician should be prepared to resuscitate the IDM, especially because delivery may be complicated by vigorous attempts to deliver a large infant vaginally. Thus, birth injury commonly is encountered in the macrosomic infant; this takes the form of shoulder dystocia and associated fracture of the clavicle or humerus, or brachial plexus injury. Because polycythemia and hyperviscosity are common complications in the IDM, the umbilical cord should be clamped early to prevent an excessive placental transfusion.

Hypoglycemia. The hypoglycemia that occurs in the IDM largely is related to fetal hyperinsulinemia and can be aggravated by maternal hyperglycemia immediately before delivery. Hypoglycemia in the infant usually occurs within the first 1 to 3 hours of age, and the diagnosis is based on a blood glucose determination below 30 mg/dl (1.7 mmol/l) in term infants or below 20 mg/dl (1.1 mmol/l) in preterm infants. Hypoglycemia often manifests no symptoms because newborns are able to use alternative substrates, such as ketone bodies. Blood glucose screening should begin within the first hour of delivery and continue at least hourly for 6 hours; if the baby is stable, the screening is continued less frequently for the first 3 days. Glucose levels can be monitored in drops of whole blood obtained from heel pricks by using a glucose oxidase enzyme method (Chemstrip or Dextrostix). If the infant shows symptoms or if the glucose screen shows a level of less than 45 mg/dl, the blood glucose should be measured chemically.

Expectant management of the IDM should include an intravenous glucose infusion begun as early as possible, despite lack of symptoms. These infants, in addition to having hyperinsulinemia, are further unable to produce glucose because they lack the normal neonatal surge in circulating free fatty acids, as well as having depressed glucagon levels. They should receive an infusion of glucose via peripheral vein at a dose of 4 to 6 mg/kg/min to establish and maintain normal blood glucose levels. Because it can be difficult to cannulate peripheral veins in fat babies, the umbilical vein may provide convenient access, provided that the catheter is placed within the ductus venosus or in the inferior vena cava (with radiological confirmation). Symptomatic hypoglycemia can be prevented by this management, and feeding should be initiated within the first 2 to 6 hours of life if the cardiorespiratory status allows it. Small feedings, starting with 5% glucose in water followed (importantly) by advancement to milk formula or breast milk, can be provided every 2 hours. Infusion of glucose can be tapered once feeding is established and the patient's condition is stable.

Symptomatic hypoglycemia can have a wide range of clinical manifestations that include jitteriness, tremors, seizures, apathy, apnea, difficulty in feeding, and an abnormal cry. Because these symptoms may be caused by other life-threatening conditions, such as sepsis and asphyxia, it is imperative that the diagnosis of symptomatic hypoglycemia be confirmed by a blood glucose determination and that the symptoms promptly disappear after parenteral glucose administration. Symptomatic hypoglycemia warrants immediate treatment with an intravenous infusion of a 10% to 12.5% glucose solution that delivers 6 mg/kg/min. The response to treatment should be monitored every 15 minutes until the blood glucose level has normalized. Treatment should not be instituted with a rapid infusion of 25% to 50% glucose, because of its high osmolality and because it also will stimulate insulin secretion, resulting in "rebound" hypoglycemia. If hypoglycemia persists, despite glucose infusion of 12 mg/kg/min, glucagon administered intramuscularly (0.3 mg/kg) generally will maintain the blood glucose at normal levels for 2 to 3 hours.

Refractory hypoglycemia can be treated with hydrocortisone (5 mg/kg/day divided into three doses), which usually will stabilize the glucose level. The physician should ensure that hypoglycemia has not been induced by inappropriate treatment with a hypertonic glucose infusion and that an umbilical arterial catheter does not deliver glucose above the level of the diaphragm, because this circumstance may stimulate pancreatic insulin secretion. In rare cases, refractory hypoglycemia is caused by hyperinsulinism accompanying disorders of the pancreas.

The IDM is at increased risk for several other neonatal problems. Among these is respiratory distress syndrome, which may be caused by an inhibition of surfactant production secondary to fetal hyperinsulinemia. The synthesis of phosphatidylcholine and phosphatidylglycerol (PG) is inhibited in the IDM. Monitoring of fetal lung maturity during the diabetic pregnancy calls for the assessment of both the amniotic fluid lecithin/sphingomyelin (L/S) ratio and the amniotic PG. An L/S ratio of less than 2:1 indicates a high potential risk for respiratory distress syndrome. Owing to the delay in the appearance of PG among IDMs, the usually adequate L/S ratio of 2:1 does not completely ensure a low risk for respiratory distress syndrome, because low PG itself also is associated with respiratory distress syndrome, despite a normal L/S ratio. Therefore, an amniotic PG measurement also should be obtained, in addition to the L/S ratio; in the absence of a biochemical assay for PG, an L/S ratio greater than 3:1 generally correlates with an adequate PG level.

The IDM also is prone to respiratory distress from causes other than surfactant deficiency (hyaline membrane disease). The infant is at increased risk for transient tachypnea of the newborn, which can be related to such conditions as asphyxia, hyperglycemia, retained lung fluid, congestive heart failure, and polycythemia. The incidence of physiological hyperbilirubinemia is increased in the IDM (see previous section). Management should include the usual modalities of phototherapy and exchange transfusion.

Chronic intrauterine hypoxia often occurs in the IDM. This stimulates erythropoietin production, resulting in an increased incidence of polycythemia (central hematocrit above 65%) and hyperviscosity. In addition, the IDM is susceptible to an excessive placental transfusion at delivery. Because this adds to the polycythemia, the cord, as previously mentioned, should be clamped immediately after delivery of the body to minimize further postnatal placental transfusion.

The appropriate treatment for polycythemia and hyperviscosity is a partial exchange transfusion. This consists of the removal of the patient's blood and replacing it with an isovolemic expander, usually 5% albumin or saline. Most authors agree that such treatment of polycythemia should be begun only when clinical signs become detectable, such as arterial and venous thromboses, pulmonary hemorrhage, apnea, lethargy, transient tachypnea (with evidence of interlobar fluid on chest roentgenogram), jitteriness, and hypoglycemia. There also may be signs of impending congestive heart failure and necrotizing enterocolitis. Patients who have central hematocrit values in excess of 65% and who display the foregoing symptoms should receive a partial exchange transfusion. The indications for treatment in symptom-free patients who have hematocrit values below 65% to 70% are not pressing. When the central hematocrit is above 70% to 75% at less than 12 hours after birth, it also is best to treat with a partial exchange transfusion, even in the absence of symptoms.

TRANSIENT TACHYPNEA OF THE NEWBORN

Transient tachypnea of the newborn (TTN) refers to one of the most common causes of respiratory distress in the neonatal period. It is believed to be caused by a delay in the absorption of the normal fetal lung fluid. Between 2 and 6 hours after birth, tachypnea, grunting, chest wall retractions, and (often) cyanosis in room air develop. Typically the symptoms are mild and resolve within 72 hours after birth. The term *wet lung* refers to the same condition.

The fetal lung secretes fluid that fills the airways. During vaginal delivery, some of this fluid is squeezed out of the major airways, but the remainder takes between 2 and 6 hours to be reabsorbed from the alveoli. This fluid passes into the interstitial space and then into the perivascular lymphatics and venules. According to hypothesis (the Starling equilibrium), this resorption can be impeded by (1) decreased capillary or lymphatic oncotic pressure (e.g., low serum protein, often found in premature infants), (2) increased capillary or lymphatic hydrostatic pressure (e.g., hypervolemia and polycythemia, which may occur with delayed cord clamping), (3) increased alveolar or interstitial fluid osmotic pressure, or (4) decreased alveolar or interstitial fluid hydrostatic pressure.

Thus, as normal lung fluid is being absorbed during the first 4 hours of life, mild respiratory symptoms may be accepted as a variant of normal; TTN should not be diagnosed unless symptoms persist or progress beyond 4 hours. Infants born by cesarean section are not subjected to a thoracic squeeze and the resultant expulsion of lung fluid that occurs during passage through the birth canal. Consequently, with increased lung fluid present, these infants commonly manifest mild transient tachypnea. Birth asphyxia and premature labor also predispose to TTN.

TTN usually occurs in the more mature preterm infant (34 to 37 weeks) and in term infants born by cesarean section. Tachypnea usually persists beyond the first few hours, peaks by 6 to 36 hours, and resolves in 5 or 6 days. The clinical picture is characterized by signs of air-trapping with widening of the anteroposterior diameter of the chest. The liver often is palpable well below the right costal margin because it is pushed down by pulmonary hyperaeration. Tachypnea shortly after birth in the full-term or more mature preterm infant must be differentiated from pneumonitis (e.g., meconium aspiration and bacterial infection), air leak (e.g., pneumothorax and pneumomediastinum), pulmonary vascular congestion resulting from congestive heart failure or polycythemia, and the respiratory restriction imposed by congenital diaphragmatic hernia or cystic adenomatoid malformation of the lung. Last, tachypnea in the face of a normal-appearing chest roentgenogram may be symptomatic of a central nervous system disorder (such as drug withdrawal) or a metabolic derangement (such as acidosis, hyperthermia, or hypoglycemia).

Newborns who have mild TTN usually do not need more than 40% oxygen to maintain adequate oxygenation (PaO_2 of 50 to 70 mm Hg), but the severity may vary and rarely may require intermittent positive pressure ventilation for respiratory failure. TTN is nonprogressive, and supplemental oxygen usually is not necessary for longer than 1 to 3 days. Treatment of the excess lung water is not required. Because bacterial pneumonia cannot practically be excluded from the initial diagnostic presentation as a primary cause or secondary complication, many feel that antibiotics should be given after blood cultures have been obtained. Oral feedings should be suspended, because the ability to suck and swallow may be impaired by the respiratory difficulty. Intravenous fluids should be minimized to equal only insensible fluid losses and to maintain serum glucose concentration.

The radiological changes of transient tachypnea are characteristic and help to differentiate it from hyaline membrane disease. According to Wesenberg[14]:

> The earliest radiographs usually are taken at age 2 to 6 hours, when the tachypnea becomes evident clinically. In infants having the most lung fluid, the initial radiographs show a pattern of diffuse bilateral alveolar edema with concomitant hyperaeration of the lungs, sternal retraction, and an "air bronchogram" effect. In the next 8 to 10 hours, there is progressive clearing of the alveoli, with some patients developing a bilateral granular or miliary pattern suggestive of hyaline membrane disease. This is a transitory stage, usually lasting only several hours. The lung fields remain hyperaerated. The pulmonary vascularity becomes prominent during this stage. This then progresses to complete clearing of the alveoli, with congestive pulmonary vascularity secondary to interstitial edema and engorged perivascular lymphatics. Occasionally, a small amount of pleural fluid is present. The lower lobes are last to clear. The clearing pattern of the lung fluid is thus from peripheral to central and from upper to lower lung fields. By 48 to 72 hours, the chest radiographs are within normal limits.

Occasionally the fetus may inhale a small amount of amniotic fluid into the already fluid-filled upper airway. Amniotic fluid has more protein than does fetal lung fluid, and the increased protein concentration lowers the oncotic gradient between the alveoli and the pulmonary lymphatics. Amniotic fluid also contains desquamated cellular debris and lanugo.

After delivery, this debris is transported into the alveoli and may produce a syndrome indistinguishable from TTN. Such aspiration of amniotic fluid occurs more frequently in breech deliveries because the thoracic squeeze occurs while the head is still within the uterine cavity and the cord is compressed between the infant and the mother's pelvic brim. These asphyxiated infants are more likely to gasp in utero and inhale their amniotic fluid. If the fetus has passed meconium, it also will be inhaled into the upper airway. Such aspiration of meconium must be prevented because it can cause a life-threatening pneumonitis, usually accompanied by severe pulmonary air trapping, respiratory failure, and pulmonary hypertension.

Therefore, when delivery is imminent and thick (particulate) meconium is present in the amniotic fluid, attendants should prepare to suction the oropharynx of the infant as soon as the head delivers and before the first breath; immediately after delivery of the infant the trachea also should be suctioned with an endotracheal tube to clear the meconium.

Intrauterine passage of meconium increases with advancing gestation to a frequency as high as 30% by 42 weeks. In addition to meconium aspiration, postmature infants (older than 42 weeks of gestation) are at risk for hypoglycemia and intrauterine asphyxia as a result of uteroplacental insufficiency. These three potential problems should be anticipated in postmature infants. Hyperaeration may persist for 4 to 5 days in infants who aspirate clear amniotic fluid.

LOW BIRTH WEIGHT

The most common causes of low birth weight are prematurity and intrauterine growth retardation.

Prematurity

Accurate assessment of gestational age is critical to the appropriate care of the mildly to moderately premature infant, because knowledge of gestational age guides management, helps one to anticipate potential problems, and provides a standard by which to assess developmental changes related to postconceptional age (gestational age at birth plus postnatal age). Traditionally, many problems of the premature infant have been related to the more easily and accurately measured birth weight rather than to gestational age because, for a large population of appropriately grown infants, the two are closely related. In the individual patient, however, the use of birth weight alone may lead to overestimating or underestimating potential problems often related to immaturity. Considering only newborns who are appropriately grown for gestational age (AGA), a birth weight of 1700 g may be associated with a gestational age of 30 to 35 weeks; yet a baby who weighs 2500 g at birth may have a gestational age of 33.5 to 39 weeks. Thus, the infant born weighing more than 1700 or even more than 2500 g still may be at significant risk for perinatal problems that relate to prematurity, not size.

Standard criteria have been developed to assess gestational age in the first 3 days after birth. Physicians who care for newborns must become skilled in the use of these methods because maternal dates may not be accurate and birth weight per se may not accurately reflect the perinatal problems likely in the individual patient; the frequency of most neonatal problems decreases as gestational age increases.

Premature infant: birth weight of 1700 g or more. Despite the major physiological differences between infants of equal birth weight but of different gestational age, most countries maintain neonatal mortality statistics according to birth weight. Thus, in what follows, we consider the gestational age of the infant who weighs 1700 g or more. For the fetus whose gestation has progressed 32 to 38 weeks, a small risk remains for development of severe neonatal problems related to prematurity (e.g., hyaline membrane disease, persistent patent ductus arteriosus, necrotizing enterocolitis, sepsis and pneumonia, symptomatic apnea, and intracranial hemorrhage). Fortunately, however, the problems of the premature infant beyond 32 to 33 weeks of gestation and weighing more than 1700 g most often are not severe or life threatening and are limited mainly to simple apnea, hyperbilirubinemia, and an inability to feed orally, or to maintain body temperature outside an incubator. Management of these infants ordinarily is well within the competence of most primary care facilities (i.e., level I or level II nurseries). Nonetheless, physicians who accept responsibility for the care of these infants must be aware that the signs of more serious disorders should be recognized promptly, if they are to be managed optimally.

The cause of premature onset of labor should be determined, inasmuch as a small portion of cases may occur because of placental abruption, a multiple gestation, or a uterine abnormality. Spontaneous and premature rupture of membranes has been associated with an increased incidence of neonatal infection. The risk of neonatal septicemia increases when membranes have been ruptured for longer than 24 hours.

Obstetrical management of the preterm fetus that has had its membranes ruptured prematurely can be assisted by daily fetal "biophysical profile" assessment. The first manifestations of impending fetal infection usually are a "nonreactive, nonstress test" result and the absence of fetal breathing movements. Loss of fetal movements and fetal tone are later and more ominous signs of fetal infection. A poor fetal biophysical profile in patients whose membranes have ruptured prematurely may be an early predictor of fetal infection and can help determine obstetrical management.

Management of infants born after prolonged rupture of membranes should include careful observation for subtle signs of infection such as lethargy, poor feeding, hyperthermia, hypothermia, early hyperbilirubinemia, jitteriness, poor skin perfusion, diarrhea, or abdominal distention as a result of ileus. Prematurity may mask some signs of the nonspecific origin of sepsis.

Examination of placentas from a large group of premature infants frequently reveals evidence of chorioamnionitis. Therefore, clinical signs of amnionitis, such as uterine tenderness or maternal fever, indicate the need to obtain a culture specimen from the neonate and to initiate antibiotic treatment. Prophylactic antibiotics administered to the mother before delivery will not treat fetal infection effectively and actually may impair accurate cultures of the newborn (false-negative culture results). Any clinical sign of infection in a premature newborn warrants cultures of blood and cerebrospinal fluid, followed by treatment with appropriate antibiotics. It is the usual practice to culture blood, cerebrospinal fluid, and urine specimens and treat with ampicillin and gentamicin for 2 to 3 days while definitive culture results are pending. When careful cultures are done under research conditions of the amniotic fluid during preterm labor, there is a high incidence of positive cultures. Blood cultures of the newborn infant rarely are positive, however. This could be due to the influence of partial treatment by maternally administered antibiotics or to the limitations of small volumes sampled for culture. The clinician must be alert for signs of sepsis in the newborn that would warrant a full course of antibiotic therapy. Significant systemic signs of infection, such as pneumonia, seizures, apnea, or shock, may mandate active treatment of sepsis for 7 to 10 days, even in the absence of positive culture results.

Recent studies suggest that when a newborn, especially if premature, is exposed to an infected environment (such as chorioamnionitis or amniotic fluid infection), the fetus develops an inflammatory response associated with increased inflammatory cytokines in the blood. This fetal inflammatory response is associated with an increased risk for severe neonatal morbidity, including cerebral palsy and chronic lung disease.[8]

Certain laboratory tests are helpful in the diagnosis of chorioamnionitis. A Gram stain of a gastric aspirate taken before the first feed, showing more than five cells per high-powered field and the presence of organisms, indicates chorioamnionitis, but not necessarily fetal infection. Inspection of the placenta may reveal cloudiness of the amniotic membranes, but histopathological examination of the placenta is the definitive diagnostic standard. Vasculitis of the fetal vessels is associated with increased risk of brain injury.

Management. For infants whose birth weight is between 1700 and 1900 g (less than 36 weeks), respiration and heart rate should be monitored during the first 10 days at least, because there is some risk of apnea. Some preterm infants may present with respiratory distress syndrome (RDS) from surfactant deficiency (hyaline membrane disease) and require surfactant replacement therapy. Currently, exogenous surfactant is administered via an endotracheal tube to newborns receiving mechanical ventilation, who have the typical radiological appearance of RDS and require endotracheal intubation and mechanical ventilation. For these infants, it is important to provide surfactant early and provide adequate continuous positive airway pressure. Patients who have RDS should be referred to a neonatal intensive care unit where treatment can be provided.

Until consistent weight gain is established, these preterm infants should remain in incubators kept at the "neutral temperature" to maintain body heat and to prevent excessive caloric expenditure. Some newborns in this weight range may grow rapidly in a bassinet, but they are exceptions to the rule.

Management of feedings and fluids is the most important aspect of care for the healthy, mildly to moderately premature infant. Feedings can be initiated within the first 24 hours after birth in the infant who is stable and has experienced no preceding perinatal distress or birth asphyxia (which may have compromised intestinal perfusion). During the first 8 hours of life, little is to be gained by initiating feeds with sterile water. Breast milk or dilute proprietary formula may be given orally or by a gastric tube in an initial volume of 2 to 4 ml/kg every 3 hours. Newborns whose gestational age is less than 34 weeks are fed initially by nasogastric tube. Proprietary formulas that have a 60:40 whey:casein ratio more closely resemble human milk and are better suited for the preterm infant. Unmodified cow milk is not suitable to the preterm newborn because its predominant casein content is not well tolerated.

Breast milk may be fed to any preterm newborn whose mother wishes to do so and who can supply it. The milk is collected individually into a sterile container after careful washing of the breast and nipple. When possible, the milk is given immediately to the infant. Otherwise it is refrigerated for up to 24 hours and either used or immediately frozen. Once full-volume feedings are well tolerated, breast milk needs to be fortified with carbohydrate, protein, and essential minerals to provide optimal nutrition for the growing premature newborn. Special powdered preparations for breast milk fortification are available that, when added to breast milk, bring up the caloric density to that of standard premature formulas (80 kCal/dl).

If feeding must be delayed or is not well tolerated, 10% dextrose in 25% normal saline should be infused intravenously. Fluid and caloric intake should be calculated daily, and growth measurements of length, weight, and head circumference should be plotted weekly so that caloric intake can be assessed adequately. Feeding volumes should be increased slowly from 60 to 80 ml/kg/day but only if tolerated without emesis or without there being increasing gastric residual volumes before feedings. A total fluid volume of 150 to 180 ml/kg/day or 100 to 120 kcal/kg/day should be reached by 7 days of age. Fluid requirements depend largely on environmental conditions. The newborn receiving phototherapy, for instance, may well require increased fluid.

When the newborn is ready to progress from tube to oral feeding, the tube may be retained for an extra 12 to 24 hours to measure gastric residuals. A residual of more than 3 to 4 ml immediately before the next feeding suggests intolerance; this situation may require a reduction in the feeding volume, but only after systemic illness is carefully considered and excluded. Abdominal distention or bile-stained gastric drainage from a properly positioned gastric tube (not in the duodenum) warrants immediate cessation of feedings and evaluation of the intestinal tract of infants who are at risk of developing necrotizing enterocolitis. The stool should be examined for macroscopic and microscopic blood. Microscopic blood (positive occult blood test result) may not in itself suggest a pathological condition unless it becomes more severe or represents a recent change.

Although coordination of sucking and swallowing develops around 33 to 34 weeks of gestation, the care of each infant should be managed individually and cooperatively between physician and nurse. The nurse experienced at feeding premature infants helps guide the infant's tolerance of the workload imposed by oral feeding. No more than 30 minutes ordinarily should be spent coaxing an infant to take a feeding if he or she lacks sufficient endurance to persist in sucking. Infants should be cuddled comfortably and securely in the feeder's lap; great benefit can be derived from cuddling and close body contact during feeding. The bottle should be held so that air rises in the upturned bottle and the infant sucks in milk and not air through the nipple. The bottle should never be propped unattended for a young infant.

Patients are discharged from the hospital when they can maintain body temperature in a bassinet, feed sufficiently on demand, and show evidence of normal growth.

The overall prognosis for the premature infant between 33 and 38 weeks of gestation is good. At this age, there is an inherently lower incidence and better tolerance of severe neonatal problems. For the healthy premature newborn weighing more than 1700 g, survival and outcome approach those of full-term infants. Intellectual function generally is normal.

The Infant Who Is Small for Gestational Age

The infant whose birth weight is at or below the tenth percentile for gestational age is considered small for gestational age (SGA). Poor fetal weight gain results from aberrant maternal, placental, or fetal circumstances that restrain growth. Other categories in which these infants may be placed include light-for-date, intrauterine growth retardation, and dysmaturity. These infants show an increase in perinatal mortality (both fetal and neonatal) that is four to eight times that of the appropriately grown infant of equal gestational age.

Early diagnosis of SGA is difficult, and most patients are diagnosed after birth. A high index of suspicion, accompanied by serial physical examinations, during which progressive growth of the uterine fundus is palpated through the abdominal wall, aids early diagnosis. A fundal height less than 4 cm or less than that for the estimated gestational age suggests poor intrauterine growth. This clinical impression can be confirmed by careful fetal ultrasound examination. Ideally, serial ultrasound measurements of fetal growth parameters should be obtained. The head/abdominal ratio (as defined by the head circumference divided by the abdominal circumference) is used to detect asymmetrical (abdomen undergrown relative to head) forms of intrauterine growth retardation. The normal head/abdominal ratio is approximately 1 from 32 to 36 weeks and less than 1 from 36 weeks to term.

Etiological factors. Growth of the fetus is determined by genetic, nutritional, and environmental factors. Fetal factors that can compromise growth potential include (1) congenital abnormalities, (2) congenital infections—for example, toxoplasmosis, rubella, cytomegalovirus, herpes, and syphilis (TORCH infections), (3) chromosomal defects, and (4) inborn errors of metabolism. Inherent fetal conditions usually result in early growth retardation and an actual reduction in the number of fetal cells. These patients appear symmetrically growth retarded (head and abdomen equally undergrown). Maternal factors include low maternal weight (less than 50 kg), poor weight gain during pregnancy, and chronic maternal disease, especially conditions that produce hypoxemia or reduce placental blood flow (e.g., chronic hypertension, preeclampsia, toxemia, cyanotic congenital heart disease, and sickle cell disease). Drug ingestion, including alcohol, cigarette smoke, and heroin, can affect the quality of fetal growth adversely. Phenylketonuria often results in decreased fetal growth and microcephaly; thus, the maternal diet must be controlled strictly during pregnancy.

During the third trimester, less than adequate maternal-placental transport becomes the major growth-limiting factor, despite normal fetal growth potential. Optimal fetal growth depends on the placenta for nutrient and gaseous exchange. The placenta promotes fetal growth by actively transporting amino acids and synthesizing chorionic somatomammotropin, which is responsible for mobilizing maternal substrate for the fetus. Diminished placental function thus will affect total nutrient and gaseous transfer adversely, resulting in fetal

BOX 48-1

FACTORS ASSOCIATED WITH POOR INTRAUTERINE GROWTH

Maternal

1. Prepregnancy weight <50 kg
2. Poor nutrition; poor weight gain during pregnancy; socioeconomic factors
3. Maternal illness:
   a. Associated with uterine ischemia: hypertensive vascular disease, preeclampsia, diabetes mellitus, sickle cell anemia, autoimmune vasculitis
   b. Associated with chronic hypoxia: cyanotic congenital heart disease, high altitude
4. Drug ingestion:
   a. Drugs that affect fetal growth directly, e.g., ethanol, methadone, heroin
   b. Drugs that inhibit placental blood flow (nicotine)
5. Multiple gestation, primiparity, grand multiparity

Placental

1. Villitis associated with congenital infections (TORCH infections)
2. Ischemic villous necrosis or infarction
3. Chronic separation (abruptio placentae)
4. Diffuse fibrinosis
5. Abnormal insertion
6. Umbilical vascular thrombosis

Fetal

1. Syndromes associated with diminished birth weight (e.g., Cornelia de Lange syndrome, Potter's disease, anencephaly, and dwarfism)
2. Metabolic disorders (inborn errors of metabolism)
3. Chromosomal disorders: trisomies 13, 18, 21; XO
4. Congenital infections: TORCH infections, malaria, varicella

growth retardation. Placental insufficiency is associated classically with postmaturity; it, therefore, is understandable that placental abnormalities, such as chronic abruption, infarction, single umbilical artery, and multiple fetuses, affect the transfer of fetal nutrients directly during the third trimester. Box 48-1 lists factors associated with poor intrauterine growth.

Clinical presentation. The SGA infant may be "symmetrically" growth retarded in some cases; in others, birth weight may be reduced relatively more than length and head circumference. Fetuses subjected to third-trimester "starvation" may be of normal length but appear wasted at birth. The skin is parchmentlike, and the head appears too large for the body. These infants are asymmetrically growth retarded. These various presentations offer some insight into etiological factors because symmetrical growth retardation usually implies a more chronic problem—for example, chromosomal or congenital infection.

If based on physical criteria alone, gestational age assessment of the SGA infant may be misleading. Because less vernix is produced in these infants, the skin is exposed continuously to amniotic fluid and will begin to desquamate after birth. Creases on the sole of the foot are more mature and breast tissue markedly reduced as a result of diminished estriol levels. Ear cartilage also may be diminished. In contrast, neurological criteria are affected less by intrauterine growth retardation than are physical criteria, inasmuch as organ maturation continues despite diminished somatic growth. Moreover, stress in utero may even promote the maturation of some organ systems, such as the lung. This may explain why respiratory distress syndrome is less frequent among SGA infants.

BOX 48-2

NEONATAL PROBLEMS IN INFANTS OF LOW BIRTH WEIGHT

Preterm

Respiratory distress syndrome
Patent ductus arteriosus
Retinopathy of prematurity
Hyperbilirubinemia
Necrotizing enterocolitis
Intraventricular hemorrhage

Small for Gestational Age

Perinatal asphyxia
Meconium aspiration
Polycythemia

Common to Both Groups

Fasting hypoglycemia
Temperature instability
Hypocalcemia

Because the SGA infant is prone to perinatal asphyxia and its sequelae, optimal management should begin with antenatal assessment. Expert resuscitation must be provided for these infants in the delivery room, with strict attention paid to the prevention of possible meconium aspiration, because decreased placental reserve and decreased cardiac glycogen stores put the fetus at risk for perinatal asphyxia. The fetus should be delivered if at or near term, but even earlier if tests of placental function, such as stress and nonstress monitoring, indicate fetal compromise. When gestational age is unknown, the risks of preterm birth can be defined by assessing pulmonary maturity with the use of amniocentesis (lecithin/sphingomyelin ratio). Occasionally, maternal disease will necessitate delivery of a preterm, growth-retarded infant who will be prone to all the complications of both immaturity and growth retardation (Box 48-2).

The SGA newborn, especially when showing evidence of third-trimester wasting with low ponderal index, is more prone to fasting hypoglycemia because of decreased glycogen stores and impaired gluconeogenesis. Thus, blood glucose values must be determined frequently in the first few days after birth. Hourly recordings are recommended in the first 4 hours of life. Thereafter, if the newborn is stable, measurements of blood glucose levels can be spaced more widely. If asymptomatic hypoglycemia occurs (whole blood glucose concentrations less than 30 mg/dl during the first 3 days in term or 20 mg/dl in preterm newborns), a glucose infusion of 4 to 8 mg/kg/min should be started. If symptomatic hypoglycemia—especially concomitant with seizure activity—has occurred, an intravenous bolus of 10% dextrose in water at 200 mg/kg (2 ml/kg) should be given, followed by constant infusion of glucose. As a consequence of their increased metabolic rate, these infants often need a higher caloric intake.

Attention to thermoregulation is required because decreased subcutaneous fat stores impair conservation of body heat. This is important in delivery room management where these patients frequently are compromised by perinatal asphyxia. Radiant heat and warm, dry towels will help to maintain the newborn's body temperature during neonatal resuscitation.

A thorough examination for clinical stigmata of congenital infection is indicated in all SGA babies, as is appropriate screening for intrauterine infection. This should include estimation of total IgM and a urine culture for cytomegalovirus. A urine and (especially) stool "screen" for illicit drugs may provide evidence of maternal drug exposure otherwise denied. Because chronic fetal hypoxia stimulates erythropoietin production, polycythemia and hyperviscosity also should be excluded.

Prognosis. The growth and developmental outcome for the SGA infant depend on the cause of the growth failure. The prognosis is poorest for infants who have congenital infections, chromosomal disorders, and severe congenital abnormalities. Intellectual development in the remaining infants depends on the presence or absence of adverse perinatal events, in addition to the specific etiological factors of the growth retardation. Even when perinatal problems are minimal, the SGA infant may have developmental handicaps. Developmental problems should be looked for beyond infancy and may not become manifest until 2 to 5 years of age or even later. Term SGA infants may exhibit little difference in developmental quotient during infancy, but their school performance is poor, in part because of behavioral and learning disabilities. SGA infants who demonstrated decreased fetal head growth earlier than 26 weeks of gestation have diminished developmental quotients in infancy. SGA infants, however, are a heterogeneous group; in some follow-up studies of both term and preterm SGA infants, they have compared well developmentally with appropriate-for-gestational-age (AGA) infants. Perhaps this discrepancy in developmental outcome is related to obstetrical and early neonatal management and to the quality of home care and parental involvement.

With regard to postnatal growth, the cause of the intrauterine growth retardation and the time of its onset during gestation will dictate the infant's growth potential. Newborns who have early-onset intrauterine growth retardation (because of an intrauterine infection, teratogen, or chromosomal abnormality) will remain small throughout life. Those who have late-onset, third-trimester, intrauterine growth retardation, however, may show evidence of catch-up growth in the first 6 months of life and usually catch up to their AGA counterparts.

REFERENCES

1. Ahlfors CE: Criteria for exchange transfusion in jaundiced newborns, *Pediatrics* 93:488, 1994.
2. American Academy of Pediatrics: Positioning and sudden infant death syndrome (SIDS): update (RE9647), *Pediatrics* 98:1216, 1996.
3. American Academy of Pediatrics: Practice parameter for the management of hyperbilirubinemia in the healthy term newborn, *Pediatrics* 94:558, 1994.
4. American Academy of Pediatrics, Committee on Fetus and Newborn: Home phototherapy, *Pediatrics* 76:136, 1985.
5. Dai J, Parry DM, Krahn J: Transcutaneous bilirubinometry: its role in the assessment of neonatal jaundice, *Clin Biochem* 30:1, 1997.
6. Darnell RA, et al: Margin of safety for discharge after apnea in preterm infants, *Pediatrics* 100:795, 1997.
7. Finer NN, et al: Obstructive, mixed and central apnea in the neonate: physiologic correlates, *J Pediatr* 121:943, 1992.
8. Gomez R, et al: The fetal inflammatory response syndrome, *Am J Obstet Gynecol* 179:194, 1998.
9. Johnson L, Bhutani VK: Guidelines for management of the jaundiced term and near-term infant, *Clin Perinatol* 25:555, 1998.
10. Maisels MJ: Jaundice. In Avery GB, Fletcher MA, MacDonald MG, editors: *Neonatology: pathophysiology and management of the newborn,* ed 4, Philadelphia, 1994, JB Lippincott.
11. Maisels MJ: Jaundice in the newborn, *Pediatr Rev* 3:305, 1982.
12. Martin RJ, et al: Persistence of the biphasic ventilatory response to hypoxia in preterm infants, *J Pediatr* 132:960, 1998.
13. National Institutes of Health Consensus Development Conference Statement in Infantile Apnea and Home Monitoring, NIH Pub No 87-2905 6:3, 1986.
14. Wesenberg RL: Wet lung disease and aspiration of clear amniotic fluid. In Wesenberg RL, editor: *The newborn chest,* Hagerstown, Md, 1973, Harper & Row.

SUGGESTED READINGS

Cornblath M: Hypoglycemia. In Nelson NM, editor: *Current therapy in neonatal-perinatal medicine,* vol 2, Philadelphia, 1990, BC Decker.

Dickinson JE, Palmer SM: Gestational diabetes: pathophysiology and diagnosis, *Semin Perinatol* 14:2, 1990.

Kliegman RM, Hulman SE: Intrauterine growth retardation: determinants of aberrant fetal growth. In Fanaroff AA, Martin RJ, editors: *Neonatal-perinatal medicine: disease of the fetus and infant,* ed 4, St Louis, 1987, Mosby.

Lawrence S, Yeomans ER, Rosenfeld CR: Intrauterine growth retardation: pediatric aspects. In Nelson NM, editor: *Current therapy in neonatal-perinatal medicine,* vol 2, Philadelphia, 1990, BC Decker.

Maisels MJ: Hyperbilirubinemia. In Nelson NM, editor: *Current therapy in neonatal-perinatal medicine,* vol 2, Philadelphia, 1990, BC Decker.

Meyer BA, Palmer SM: Pregestational diabetes, *Semin Perinatol* 14:12, 1990.

Vintzileos AM, Campbell WA, Nochimson DJ: Premature rupture of the membranes. In Nelson NM, editor: *Current therapy in neonatal-perinatal medicine,* vol 2, Philadelphia, 1990, BC Decker.

49 Critical Neonatal Illnesses

Maureen M. Gilmore • Keith H. Marks

For the physician who is called on to treat the newborn in a critical situation, it is important to be able to make a clear assessment and diagnosis, if possible, institute immediate treatment for stabilization, and plan for continuing consultation in caring for the patient. Errors or omissions may result in permanent damage or death. Thus, recognition and immediate resuscitation of a baby in distress require an organized plan for the actions of immediately available and qualified personnel, supported by the proper equipment.

The emergence throughout the Western world of regionalized systems for neonatal care has played a crucial role in the overall improvement in neonatal outcome. It also has made it possible and desirable for almost all critically ill infants to be cared for in a tertiary care neonatal center. Assuming that most primary care physicians embrace this approach, the following discussion deals mainly with those conditions that require recognition, initial management, and stabilization preceding the transport of infants to such centers. Safe and efficient transport of an infant likewise requires an organized approach.* See Chapter 43 (Two), Perinatal Transport.

The resources available at the hospital of birth will determine the need for transport. In general, neonatal transport should be considered when those resources immediately available (equipment, support services, clinical expertise, and availability of the attending physician) are inadequate to deal with the infant's current or anticipated medical and surgical problems. Note, however, that the decision to transfer a newborn should be made only *after* consultation with the neonatologist at the receiving hospital so that bed availability can be confirmed and preparations undertaken.

STABILIZATION

Certain basic laboratory investigations should be performed on every critically ill infant (Box 49-1); every hospital should be capable of performing these tests rapidly. The data gathered may help narrow the differential diagnosis (e.g., the chest roentgenogram reveals evidence of pneumothorax or of cardiomegaly; the hematocrit reading indicates polycythemia associated with respiratory distress) and guides appropriate intervention.

By far the most frequent reason for referral of an infant to a neonatal intensive care unit (NICU) is the onset of respiratory distress soon after birth. Such infants most often demonstrate tachypnea, retractions, expiratory grunting, nasal flaring, cyanosis, or some combination of these signs. However, they may show only apnea or tachypnea. An approach to the differential diagnosis of respiratory distress is shown in Box 49-2.

In some cases the suddenness and severity of the infant's distress make it apparent that immediate referral to an ICU is necessary. In others, the major challenge to the primary care clinician is to separate those infants whose respiratory distress or cyanosis may be only transient and are likely to improve from those whose condition almost certainly will deteriorate and necessitate further investigation and intervention.

Changes in clinical status can occur with frightening rapidity; thus, constant vigilance is necessary to anticipate and prevent potentially disastrous deterioration. Infants who have respiratory failure require immediate referral to a neonatal center. *Respiratory failure is imminent or actual when any of the following signs are present:*

- Increasing tachypnea, retractions, and grunting
- Persistent tachycardia with minimal variability in the heart rate
- Apnea
- Poor peripheral perfusion (shock)
- Congestive heart failure
- Cyanosis unresponsive to the administration of oxygen at greater than 40%
- Rising $PaCO_2$, falling pH, and falling PaO_2

Any infant who is cyanotic and does not respond to the administration of oxygen requires immediate attention. Central cyanosis should never be disregarded in the hope that it will disappear. Such infants inevitably get worse, and their cyanosis requires urgent investigation and treatment. Many cyanotic infants also have significant respiratory distress, so their referral is all the more mandatory. Others, however, may appear merely "dusky" and not suffer from respiratory distress yet, thus inviting an unwise expectant temporization before eventual emergent transfer. By definition, cyanosis reflects the presence in the circulation of at least 3 g of reduced (desaturated) hemoglobin. *Central* cyanosis (as opposed to *peripheral,* or acrocyanosis) implies cyanosis of the lips, tongue, and oral mucous membranes. Because cyanosis is produced by a definitive amount (not relative concentration) of desaturated hemoglobin, it may be detected even at high arterial oxygen saturations, should the total hemoglobin concentration be sufficiently elevated (polycythemia). In other words, polycythemic infants actually may have normal PaO_2 levels yet be clinically cyanotic. Conversely, when the hemo-

*This is discussed in detail in American Academy of Pediatrics and the American College of Obstetricians and Gynecologists: *Guidelines for perinatal care,* ed 4, Elk Grove Village, Ill, 1997, American Academy of Pediatrics.

BOX 49-1

LABORATORY INVESTIGATIONS TO BE PERFORMED ON ALL ACUTELY ILL NEWBORN INFANTS

Venous or arterial hematocrit
Rapid reagent strip glucose screening (Dextrostix or Chemstrip)
Quantitative laboratory blood glucose level
Portable chest roentgenogram
Measurement of O_2 saturation by pulse oximetry
Arterial (or arterialized capillary*) PaO_2, $PaCO_2$, and pH
White blood cell count and differential
Blood culture
Response of infant's PaO_2 and SaO_2 to breathing oxygen

*These measurements are unreliable in the presence of shock or when the PaO_2 exceeds 50 to 60 mm Hg.

globin concentration is low, as in severe anemia, significant central cyanosis may not be apparent visually, despite substantial arterial desaturation. *The following are immediate investigations required in all cyanotic infants:*

Chest roentgenogram
Pulse oximetry—measurement of O_2 saturation
Arterial blood gases—measurement of PaO_2, $PaCO_2$, and pH
Hyperoxia test—increase in PaO_2 or O_2 saturation when breathing 100% oxygen
Complete blood count (CBC)—hemoglobin and hematocrit
Blood glucose levels
Echocardiogram

Any infant who is cyanotic and whose PaO_2 does not respond promptly to the administration of 100% oxygen should be referred immediately to a tertiary care center for treatment. Such infants are likely to have *cyanotic congenital heart disease, persistent pulmonary hypertension* (formerly called persistent fetal circulation), or *severe respiratory disease.*

The initial approach to all critical situations is similar—namely, to establish and maintain vital functions. Thus, the *maintenance of oxygenation, perfusion, blood glucose levels, and body temperature is the cornerstone of successful initial management.*

Ventilation

Most importantly, *oxygen should be provided in whatever concentration (including 100%) is necessary to keep the baby pink.* The legacy from the 1950s and '60s of the alleged association between hyperoxia and retinopathy of prematurity (ROP) continues to haunt us. However, no clear relation between *brief* periods (several hours) of hyperoxia (PaO_2 levels greater than 150 mm Hg) and ROP has ever been documented. Moreover, recent data suggest that there may be an association of ROP with episodes of hypoxemia (PaO_2 less than 40 mm Hg). Thus, although historically the necessity for avoiding hyperoxia has been emphasized, it may be equally, if not more important, to avoid periods of hypoxia, as well as of compromised perfusion.

Degrees of visible "pinkness" cannot be used to estimate PaO_2 levels reliably; therefore, actual measurements of arterial blood gases or oxygen saturation by pulse oximetry are necessary for optimal management. Pulse oximetry is simpler and more reliable than capillary blood gas measurement. Supplemental oxygen should be given sufficient to maintain the baby's PaO_2 within the range of the normal newborn (50 to 100 mm Hg) or the oxygen saturation (SaO_2) to greater than 90%. Oxygen should be warmed, humidified, and delivered by using an oxygen hood. The infant should be given assisted ventilation if, despite breathing 100% oxygen, cyanosis persists, the PaO_2 is less than 50 mm Hg, or the SaO_2 is less than 90%.

The early use of nasal continuous positive airway pressure (CPAP) at 5 to 7 cm H_2O pressure may obviate the subsequent need for mechanical ventilation. However, mechanical ventilation, preferably through an endotracheal tube, is indicated if respiratory failure is evidenced by recurrent apnea, $PaCO_2$ greater than 50 to 60 mm Hg (and rising), pH less than 7.25, with a rising $PaCO_2$, or PaO_2 less than 50 mm Hg in 70% to 100% oxygen.

BOX 49-2

CAUSES OF RESPIRATORY DISTRESS IN THE NEWBORN

Pulmonary Causes

Common
Hyaline membrane disease
Transient tachypnea of the newborn (TTN)
Meconium aspiration
Primary pulmonary hypertension

Occasional
Pulmonary hemorrhage
Pneumonia
Pneumothorax
Pulmonary dysmaturity

Rare
Airway obstruction
- Choanal atresia

Space-occupying lesion
- Diaphragmatic hernia
- Cysts
- Tumors

Nonpulmonary Causes

Cerebral
Hemorrhage
Edema

Metabolic
Acidosis
Hypoglycemia
Hypothermia

Hematological
Hypovolemia
Acute blood loss
Twin-to-twin transfusion
Hyperviscosity

Should someone skilled in infant intubation not be immediately available, bag and mask ventilation must be used.* The bag used must be capable of delivering 100% oxygen (see section on positive pressure ventilation in Chapter 45 [One], Peripartum Considerations, and Fig. 45-3 for the technique of bag and mask ventilation). An orogastric tube must be placed to prevent gastric distention.

The correct management of respiratory acidosis is ventilation, not "buffering" with intravenous (IV) sodium bicarbonate. Among preterm infants who have severe respiratory distress syndrome, it invariably is necessary to perform endotracheal intubation (see Appendix B, Special Procedures, for the technique to be used) to ensure adequate ventilation. Intubation also allows the application of positive end-expiratory pressure (PEEP), which is critical to maintaining adequate oxygenation by overcoming atelectasis. The instillation of exogenous pulmonary surfactant via the endotracheal tube can reduce the severity of some pulmonary diseases underlying respiratory failure.

Perfusion

Infants who are in shock have a low effective circulating blood volume and show all the signs of poor perfusion: paleness, mottled skin, and poor capillary filling. Adequate capillary filling is present when normal pink color returns within 3 seconds after pressing the skin. In practice, capillary filling time has only limited accuracy in newborns, and the information must be interpreted with caution. Recent studies suggest that in older infants and children, capillary refill is a highly unreliable measurement and almost totally dependent on ambient room temperature. In the premature infant who is several hours to days old, and in a controlled thermal environment, delay in capillary filling may be useful in the assessment of peripheral perfusion. In normal full-term infants who are much more acrocyanotic in the first several hours, a prolonged capillary refill time may be present.

The infant in shock also frequently has cyanosis, tachycardia, and acidosis, but may or may not have low blood pressure. The blood pressure (BP) should be determined by the oscillometric technique (e.g., DinaMap [Critikon, Inc.]). Table 49-1 shows normal systolic and diastolic BP levels for newborns at various birth weights. The oscillometric method, used carefully, is quite accurate for the noninvasive determination of arterial BP. Two important conditions must be met: (1) the width of the cuff must be at least 50% to 60% of the limb circumference, and (2) the infant must be quite still during the measuring of BP to prevent motion artifact in the readings. The physician should note, however, that many infants, despite severe underperfusion, may maintain normal BP by means of vasoconstriction. *Thus, a normal BP by no means rules out the diagnosis of shock* (hypoperfusion of the peripheral tissues).

Hypovolemia is the single most important cause of shock and always should be considered when metabolic acidosis exists. Shock is treated by expanding the circulating blood volume by use of 10 to 20 ml/kg of normal saline solution over 5 to 10 minutes. If necessary, packed red blood cells also may be given.

Table 49-1 Blood Pressure in Newborns

	Systolic (mm Hg)		Diastolic (mm Hg)	
Birth Weight (g)	5%	95%	5%	95%
1000	35	58	16	36
1500	40	62	19	39
2000	43	67	22	41
2500	48	70	25	43
3000	50	73	28	48
3500	54	78	30	49
4000	58	81	31	51

Data from Versmold HT, et al: *Pediatrics* 67:607, 1981.

Metabolism

Blood glucose concentration should be determined on all sick infants by a semiquantitative screening technique (Dextrostix or Chemstrip). If the screening test indicates a blood glucose level less than 45 mg/dl, quantitative laboratory analysis of blood glucose should be performed. Documented hypoglycemia (quantitative blood glucose level of less than 40 mg/dl) is treated by a continuous IV infusion of 10% dextrose in water solution. An initial IV bolus of 2 to 3 ml/kg should be given slowly over about 5 minutes and the infusion then continued at a rate of 5 ml/kg/hr—this provides 8 mg/kg/min of glucose. Another Dextrostix test should be performed within 15 minutes. If the blood glucose level remains persistently low, 12.5% or 15% dextrose in water solution should be infused. If there still is no response, hydrocortisone (1 to 2 mg/kg IV) should be given every 12 hours (see the discussion of persistent neonatal hypoglycemia on p. 604).

All sick infants, particularly those of very low birth weight (<1500 g), require meticulous attention to *thermoregulation*. The body temperature should be maintained in the neutral thermal environment (see Fig. 45-5). If a warmer bed is not available, these newborns should be swaddled in plastic wrap or similar insulating material.

Most sick infants have some degree of *ileus* and should not be fed by mouth. All require IV fluids. An appropriate IV solution is 0.2% saline in 10% dextrose in water, administered initially at a rate of 60 to 70 ml/kg/day for term infants and 80 to 100 ml/kg/day for preterm infants. Adjustments to this rate of fluid administration may be required if the infant has hypoglycemia or evidence of gastrointestinal obstruction, when large amounts of fluid may be lost into the bowel lumen.

Metabolic acidosis occurs when organic acids (e.g., lactic acid) accumulate in tissues that are hypoxemic or underperfused. Other causes are loss of bicarbonate (which does not occur in the first hours or days of life) and some rare inborn errors of metabolism. The proper treatment of metabolic acidosis is directed to its cause rather than to its effect (i.e., adequate oxygenation and perfusion should be provided rather than an infusion of bicarbonate). The administration of sodium bicarbonate should be limited to those very few infants in whom metabolic acidosis is not self-corrected by the time the PaO_2 is normal and adequate perfu-

*Meconium-stained amniotic fluid and diaphragmatic hernia are two situations in which bag and mask ventilation should not be used; endotracheal intubation should be used in those conditions (see the discussion of congenital diaphragmatic hernia [CDH] on p. 609 of this chapter.)

sion has been attained. Respiratory acidosis is, by definition, an elevation of the $PaCO_2$ with a normal bicarbonate level and, therefore, can be treated only by the use of assisted ventilation; bicarbonate administration is not indicated in this situation.

SPECIFIC MEDICAL CONDITIONS

Ambiguous Genitalia

The finding of ambiguous genitalia must raise the suspicion of congenital adrenal hyperplasia (CAH), which can produce convincing masculinization of the female external genitalia, leading to unfortunate (and difficult to retract) misassignment of sex in the delivery room. Therefore, CAH should be suspected in all infants whose genitalia are ambiguous, as well as in all those who are vomiting, are dehydrated, or fail to thrive in the first weeks of life.

Congenital adrenal hyperplasia. Congenital adrenal hyperplasia (CAH) is a group of inherited autosomal recessive disorders caused by the absence of essential enzymes in the pathways for synthesis of cortisol and aldosterone. The interruption of the normal negative-feedback systems stimulates excessive release of ACTH and overactivity in the biosynthetic steps preceding the block, with a resultant accumulation of androgenic steroids. The most common variety is 21-hydroxylase deficiency. This presents in affected females as virilization at birth, including clitoral hypertrophy and variable fusion of the labia minora. *These masculinized girls, tragically, may be misdiagnosed as males who have hypospadias and cryptorchidism.* Diagnosis is confirmed by serum and urinary electrolyte patterns, hormonal measurements, and occasionally, karyotyping. Prompt recognition of this problem is more challenging in males, who may not be diagnosed before an adrenal crisis, which usually occurs in the second week of life. A salt-losing adrenal crisis is manifest clinically by vomiting and poor weight gain, and biochemically by low serum sodium and high serum potassium levels. It can progress to vascular collapse.

A salt-losing crisis demands urgent therapy with IV saline, glucose, and hydrocortisone. Elevation of the plasma 17-hydroxyprogesterone level confirms the diagnosis of 21-hydroxylase deficiency. Cortisol is the drug of choice for replacement of glucocorticoid action in adrenal insufficiency. Acutely, in the face of hyponatremia and hyperkalemia, desoxycorticosterone (DOCA), 1 mg/day IM, is indicated. Hydrocortisone (Solu-Cortef) is given as a 50-mg/m^2 IV bolus, with another 50 to 100 mg/m^2 placed in the IV maintenance solution. Should the patient decompensate further, 5% albumin (10 ml/kg) should be given. The use of morphine, barbiturates, or other sedatives is contraindicated. Potassium should not be added to any of the IV fluids. A prompt and complete endocrinological evaluation and maintenance therapy are required for these infants. The aims of long-term management are to suppress the hyperplastic adrenal glands and provide replacement hydrocortisone and a salt-retaining steroid such as fludrocortisone (Florinef).

Drug Withdrawal Syndrome

Infants born to mothers who are users of narcotics have withdrawal symptoms in the first days of life. When the symptoms include severe irritability and tremors (which prevent normal feeding), vomiting and diarrhea, seizures, hypothermia or hyperthermia, or severe tachypnea, treatment is indicated (see Chapter 50, Prenatal Drug Abuse and Neonatal Drug Withdrawal Syndrome).

Hydrops Fetalis

The care of Rh-negative women likely to deliver infants who have severe erythroblastosis should be managed exclusively in perinatal centers capable of the full range of obstetrical and neonatal intensive care. The successful management of these previously doomed infants demands a comprehensive team approach that includes intensive monitoring and vigorous treatment of asphyxia, acidosis, hypoglycemia, hypothermia, effusions, and edema. Intubation and mechanical ventilation frequently are required.

Hypoglycemia*

The maintenance of a normal blood glucose concentration in the newborn is important because glucose is the primary energy substrate for the brain. Thus, hypoglycemia may result in central nervous system (CNS) damage. Newborns have brain weights that are greater in relation to body weight than is the case in adults and thus are at greater risk from the effects of hypoglycemia. Long-term follow-up studies regarding the neurological impairment of infants who have had symptomatic hypoglycemia as newborns indicate that *hypoglycemia represents a critical situation for the newborn.* This requires that all nurseries have a plan to screen newborns for hypoglycemia and to institute immediate therapy when it is diagnosed.

Glucose should be monitored on all premature infants and newborns who are either large for gestational age (LGA) or small for gestational age (SGA) until the plasma glucose is stable within the normal range.

Any infant, term or preterm, who has a Dextrostix determination of blood glucose of 45 mg/dl or less should have an immediate quantitative blood glucose level (glucose oxidase method) determined in the laboratory. Infants who have (1) a whole blood glucose level of less than 35 mg/dl in the first 24 hours or less than 40 mg/dl thereafter or (2) a plasma glucose level of less than 40 mg/dl in the first 24 hours or less than 45 mg/dl thereafter require immediate intervention and subsequent glucose monitoring.

Transient neonatal hypoglycemia. CNS abnormalities—for example, septo-optic dysplasia associated with agenesis of the septum pellucidum, malformation of the optic chiasma, agenesis of the corpus callosum, and growth hormone deficiency—all can cause transient neonatal hypoglycemia. Other causes include being SGA or LGA, asphyxia, anoxia, respiratory distress syndrome, sepsis, cold injury, prolonged starvation, hydrops fetalis, and abrupt cessation of IV glucose solution. Infants of diabetic mothers (IDMs), as well as those whose mothers have been given certain drugs (e.g., propranolol), also are prone to develop symptomatic transient hypoglycemia as newborns. Finally, this difficulty

*See also Chapter 289, Hypoglycemia.

may develop in some infants without apparent predisposing causes.

Persistent neonatal hypoglycemia. Any of the following conditions can give rise to persistent hypoglycemia in the newborn:

1. Pancreatic defects
   a. Hyperinsulinism
   b. Beta-cell hyperplasia
   c. Beckwith-Wiedemann syndrome
   d. Nesidioblastosis
   e. Islet cell adenoma
   f. Focal adenomatosis
   g. Microadenomatosis
   h. Idiopathic leucine sensitivity
2. Hereditary defects of carbohydrate metabolism
   a. Glycogen storage diseases
   b. Deficiencies of enzymes important to gluconeogenesis
   c. Other enzyme defects (e.g., galactosemia, hereditary fructose intolerance)
3. Hereditary defects in amino acid and organic acid metabolism
   a. Maple syrup urine disease
   b. Propionic acidemia
   c. Methylmalonic aciduria
   d. Tyrosinosis
   e. 3-hydroxy-3-methylglutaric aciduria
   f. Glutaric aciduria type II
4. Hereditary defects of fat metabolism
   a. Systemic carnitine deficiency
   b. Carnitine palmitoyl transferase deficiency
5. Hormone deficiencies
   a. Congenital hypopituitarism
   b. Hypothalamic abnormalities that lead to diminished production of growth hormone, cortisol, adrenocorticotropic hormone (ACTH), glucagon, thyroid hormone, and catecholamines

Although the clinical manifestations of neonatal hypoglycemia are varied, they may include episodes of tremor (jitteriness), apnea, cyanosis, irregular respirations, hypotonia, twitching, sweating, hypothermia, weak cry, refusal to feed, eye rolling, and seizures. For all infants at increased risk for hypoglycemia, it is common practice to estimate the plasma glucose concentration by Dextrostix as soon as possible after birth, at 2 hours, and again at 4 to 6 hours of age. It is advisable to monitor blood glucose levels frequently until the plasma glucose is stable within the normal range and oral milk feedings have been well established. In the event of a confirmed blood glucose reading of less than 45 mg/dl, the infant who can feed orally should be started immediately on a feeding of 5% to 10% glucose, followed by breast milk or standard formula feedings at intervals of 2 to 3 hours. The blood glucose level should be monitored before each feeding. Adequate glucose concentrations usually can be maintained by this regimen; however, if plasma glucose values remain below 40 mg/dl, an IV infusion of 10% dextrose should be started to provide 5 to 8 mg/kg/min of glucose. For infants who may not yet feed orally, an IV 10% dextrose bolus of 2 to 3 ml/kg/dose may be given, and they are similarly started on a continuous 10% dextrose infusion. On rare occasions when hypoglycemia persists despite such an infusion of glucose, hydrocortisone may need to be administered at intervals of 12 hours (1 to 2 mg/kg/dose IV or IM). On this regimen the blood glucose level in most infants should stabilize rapidly. The IV infusion of glucose can be tapered after 48 hours and the hydrocortisone therapy gradually eliminated during the subsequent 4 to 5 days. Should the hypoglycemia persist for more than 72 hours on this regimen, other causes must be sought (see Chapter 289, Hypoglycemia).

Meningitis

For a discussion of meningitis, see Chapter 235, Meningitis.

Pneumothorax

Spontaneous pneumothorax occurs in 0.5% to 2% of all newborns, but with much greater frequency among infants who have severe respiratory distress syndrome (RDS) or aspiration pneumonia. The clinical diagnosis is suspected when an infant shows signs of respiratory distress with breath sounds decreased on one side. This physical sign, however, may be very difficult to elicit, particularly in the small premature infant. A more reliable technique, therefore, is to transilluminate the chest with a high-intensity fiberoptic light. Increased lucency on one side of the chest suggests the presence of a pneumothorax. Ultimately, however, the gold standard for diagnosis is the chest roentgenogram, which reveals lucency in one hemithorax, partial collapse of the lung, and displacement of the mediastinum to the opposite side of the chest. Indeed, a roentgenogram of the chest should be part of the routine assessment of all ill newborns.

In a full-term infant, a small pneumothorax that produces only mild distress may require no therapy other than observation. On the other hand, in an infant who is severely distressed and has cyanosis or bradycardia (signs of cardiovascular compromise from a tension pneumothorax), immediate evacuation of the accumulated intrathoracic air is essential. This is performed by inserting an 18- or 20-gauge angiocatheter through the chest wall in the midclavicular line at the second or third intercostal space. The stylet is removed and the catheter connected to an airtight stopcock and a 30-ml syringe, using small extension tubing. As the catheter is advanced into the chest, negative pressure is applied, removing the air collection. This procedure, which may at first appear intimidating, actually is relatively simple and safe. Because the intercostal blood vessels course along the inferior border of each rib, by inserting the angiocatheter over its superior rim there is no danger of producing a hemorrhage. Furthermore, the presence of the pneumothorax tends to prevent inadvertent puncture of the lung. Even if a lung puncture or a hemorrhage does occur, rarely is either severe.

Persistence of a significant pneumothorax requires insertion of a chest tube, although an angiocatheter secured in place may be used as a temporary device for transporting the baby to a neonatal ICU. If an angiocatheter or a chest tube is in place, it should be connected to underwater drainage. If no underwater seal is available, a one-way Heimlich flutter valve may be used (Bard-Parker No. 3460).

Respiratory Distress

For a discussion of respiratory distress, see Chapters 47, Signs and Symptoms of Neonatal Illness, and 48, Common Neonatal Illnesses.

Seizures

For a complete discussion of neonatal seizures, see Chapter 260, Seizure Disorders.

Shock and Sepsis

Shock may be defined as an acute hemodynamic disturbance that causes significant generalized reduction of capillary blood flow throughout the body, with consequent decreased tissue perfusion and anoxia. If prolonged, this leads to a generalized impairment of cellular function. The major causes of shock in the newborn are hypovolemia, sepsis, severe congestive heart failure with low cardiac output (e.g., the hypoplastic left heart syndrome [see Chapter 198, Congenital Heart Disease]), and rarely, endocrine failure (hypoadrenocorticism) (see also Chapter 296, Shock).

Hypovolemic shock. Shock caused by hypovolemia in the newborn is attributable most often to hemorrhage, caused by (1) obstetrical accidents or malformations of the placenta and cord, (2) occult hemorrhage from the fetus into the maternal circulation or into a twin fetus, and (3) internal hemorrhage (Box 49-3).

A second mechanism is loss of fluid and electrolytes, which may cause dehydration sufficient to reduce the circulating blood volume and result in hypovolemic shock similar to that caused by actual hemorrhage. Causes in the neonate include fluid losses in severe diarrhea or vomiting, inadequate intake of fluid and electrolytes (particularly with the use of potent diuretics), or inadequate replacement of large insensible water losses from the very premature infant.

Loss of plasma (rather than whole blood) from the circulatory system is a third mechanism that at times can be severe enough to cause hypovolemic shock (e.g., the exudation of severe extensive peritonitis, necrotizing enterocolitis, or gastroschisis).

The relation between cardiac output and hypovolemia depends not only on the amount of blood or fluid lost but also on the rate of that loss; during slow (chronic) bleeding compensatory mechanisms come into play for which there is insufficient time if the bleeding is acute. Clinical signs of shock may not become apparent until 10% to 25% of the blood volume has been lost, if that loss is sufficiently slow. The immediate reaction of the body to oligemia from acute, unreplaced blood loss is to maintain circulation to vital areas (brain, heart, adrenal glands, and lungs). This occurs by vasoconstriction of less vital vessels in the skin, muscles, and splanchnic bed, sacrificing perfusion to these areas. Initiated by powerful sympathetic reflexes that stimulate the release of circulating epinephrine, this compensatory mechanism increases the peripheral resistance and raises the blood pressure but decreases the tissue perfusion. This emergency increase in peripheral sympathetic activity is manifest clinically by tachycardia and rapid, shallow, irregular respirations, as well as by pale, cool skin that frequently appears mottled because capillary filling is slow. The low peripheral venous pressure presents clinically as collapsed peripheral veins; thus, it may be more difficult to introduce an intravenous catheter. A central umbilical catheter may need to be inserted to provide fluids and nutrition.

Reflexes from pressure receptors initially maintain total body perfusion to some extent in early shock by increasing cardiac output. If oligemia is mild, circulating blood volume may be restored partially by absorption of fluid from interstitial tissues and gradual replacement of red cells. The blood pressure is reasonably well maintained; this state is known as

BOX 49-3

TYPES OF HEMORRHAGE IN THE NEWBORN

Obstetrical Accidents and Malformation of the Placenta and Cord
- Rupture of a normal umbilical cord
  - Precipitous delivery
  - Entanglement
- Hematoma of the cord or placenta
- Rupture of an abnormal umbilical cord
  - Varices
  - Aneurysm
- Rupture of anomalous vessels
  - Aberrant vessel
  - Velamentous insertion
  - Communicating vessels in multilobed placenta
- Incision of placenta during cesarean section
- Placenta previa
- Abruptio placentae

Occult Hemorrhage Before Birth
- Fetoplacental
  - Tight nuchal cord
  - Cesarean section
  - Placental hematoma
- Fetomaternal
  - Traumatic amniocentesis
  - Following external cephalic version, manual removal of placenta, or use of oxytocin
  - Spontaneous
  - Chorioangioma of the placenta
  - Choriocarcinoma of the placenta
- Twin-to-twin transfusion
  - Chronic
  - Acute

Internal Hemorrhage
- Intracranial
- Giant cephalohematoma, subgaleal, or caput succedaneum
- Adrenal
- Retroperitoneal
- Ruptured liver, ruptured spleen
- Pulmonary

Iatrogenic Blood Loss
- Blood sampling

Modified from Oski FA, Naiman JL: *Hematological problems in the newborn,* ed 3, Philadelphia, 1982, WB Saunders.

compensated oligemic shock. However, when blood volume loss exceeds this compensation, blood pressure falls to produce what is known as *uncompensated oligemic shock.* With the decrease in venous return and consequent decreased cardiac filling, poor cardiac output results eventually in a further drop in blood pressure. Ischemic damage to the myocardium then may produce myocardial failure, which further reduces cardiac output and aggravates the fall of arterial blood pressure. In this state the infant usually will display gasping respirations and an altered state of consciousness. The peripheral pulses are weak, and the blood pressure is low or unobtainable.

Diagnosis. In the evaluation of acute blood loss from the fetus at the time of delivery, the bleeding site, appearance of the blood, signs of blood loss, and evidence for disordered hemostasis all should be considered. The sites and common causes of bleeding are listed in Box 49-3.

Factors in the obstetrical history that should arouse suspicion of hemorrhage include placenta previa, abruptio placentae, and antepartum hemorrhage occurring in the third trimester. A mandatory part of establishing a diagnosis is careful examination of the placenta and cord, looking for clots or a site of blood loss. A traumatic delivery should arouse suspicion of possible internal bleeding (e.g., intracranial hemorrhage, ruptured liver or spleen, or retroperitoneal hemorrhage). Hemorrhage into the adrenal glands and subcapsular hematoma of the liver or spleen may manifest as enlarging abdominal masses.

The appearance and intensity of signs and symptoms depend on the amount and rate of bleeding. If hemorrhage is repeated or chronic, anemia develops slowly. The fetus will have developed hemodynamic compensation, so there may be only pallor noted, and the blood pressure can be normal. After acute hemorrhage, the infant appears ill, pale, and hypotonic, with gasping and signs of shock. The hemoglobin concentration and hematocrit often are normal initially, not reflecting the magnitude of blood loss. Generally, 20% of blood volume lost acutely produces signs of shock, and the hemoglobin level drops within 3 hours of the "bleed."

Capillary hemoglobin (Hb) and hematocrit (Hct) levels may be misleadingly high because of peripheral sludging and stasis, so these levels should be determined only on *central* venous or arterial blood samples, obtained as blood is drawn for cross-matching. Over the first 12 to 24 hours of life, Hb levels must be followed closely to observe the expected fall as hemodilution occurs.

Fetomaternal hemorrhage is diagnosed by demonstrating the presence of fetal red cells in the maternal circulation (Kleihauer-Betke test). A twin-to-twin transfusion should be suspected when a Hb difference of greater than 5 g/dl exists between identical twins.

The metabolic response to acute blood loss also depends on the degree of the hemorrhage. If recruitment of extracellular fluid and contraction of the great veins are sufficient to compensate for the loss of circulating blood volume, the metabolic response will be slight and signs and symptoms transient. With further blood loss, the increased glycolysis and lipolysis are manifested by increased blood glucose, fatty acid, and lactate levels in the blood. A respiratory alkalosis can be detected in the arterial blood gas levels, and decreased urinary sodium and volume are noted. With marked blood loss, severe lactic acidosis and oliguria occur.

Treatment. Optimal treatment of shock has four main goals:

1. *Ensure adequate ventilation and oxygenation.* Poor tissue perfusion results in anoxia and anaerobic metabolism with metabolic acidosis, which may be aggravated in the presence of hypoxia. Therefore, 100% oxygen should be administered and an adequate airway ensured. An endotracheal tube may be necessary for intermittent positive pressure ventilation.
2. *Restoring the circulating blood volume by transfusion.* Treatment should be directed toward restoration of cardiac output and tissue perfusion to prevent the ongoing effects of continuing anoxia. If significant hypovolemia is suspected, it should be treated with repeated small infusions of volume expanders given by IV push over 5 to 10 minutes (10 to 20 ml/kg). Packed red blood cells, type O, Rh-negative and cross-matched against the mother's blood, are best to use but may not be readily available. For unanticipated shock in the delivery room, the infant's own heparinized placental blood may be used in an emergency. This is obtained from the umbilical cord after sterilization with a solution of 1% iodine and 70% alcohol. Blood is withdrawn into a 20-ml syringe (containing 1 ml of 50 U/ml heparin) and administered using a filter from an IV blood administration set. Alternatively, normal saline may be used. The volume expander infusions should be discontinued only when tissue perfusion is markedly improved. This may be determined by the response of the infant to restoration of a satisfactory circulatory blood volume: the pulse rate should come down; the skin should become pink, warm, and dry, with capillary refill of less than 2 seconds; the urinary volume should increase; the central venous pressure should rise to normal; and the blood pressure should rise also.
3. *Improve cardiac function with chest compressions and appropriate drugs when indicated.** If the heart rate is less than 80 beats/min and does not increase to normal with ventilation, chest compressions should be instituted at a rate of three compressions to one ventilation (90 chest compressions per minute). In general, because of infants' responsiveness to adequate ventilation with 100% oxygen, drug therapy rarely is necessary for resuscitation in the delivery room. When medications are needed, they should not be administered until adequate ventilation has been established. The preferred route for drug administration in the delivery room is the umbilical vein. However, epinephrine and naloxone also can be administered through an endotracheal tube (Table 49-2).
4. *Stop the hemorrhage.* Acute hemorrhage and concurrent disseminated intravascular coagulation (DIC) re-

*This is discussed in detail in Bloom RS, Cropley C, American Academy of Pediatrics, and American Heart Association: *Textbook of neonatal resuscitation*, ed 2, Elk Grove Village, Ill, 1994, American Academy of Pediatrics.

Table 49-2 Medications for Neonatal Resuscitation

Medication	Concentration to Administer	Preparation (ml)	Dosage/Route*	Total Dose/Infant			Rate/Precautions
Epinephrine	1:10,000	1	0.1-0.3 ml/kg	**Weight (kg)**	**Total ml**		Give rapidly. May dilute with normal saline to 1-2 ml if giving ET
				1	0.1-0.3		
				2	0.2-0.6		
			IV or ET	3	0.3-0.9		
				4	0.4-1.2		
Volume expanders	Whole blood	40	10 ml/kg	1	10		Give over 5-10 min
	5% albumin		IV	2	20		
	Normal saline			3	30		
	Lactated Ringer			4	40		
Sodium bicarbonate	0.5 mEq/ml	20	2 mEq/kg		**Total dose (mEq)**	**Total ml**	Give *slowly,* over at least 2 min
		or		1	2	4	
	(4.2% solution)	two 10-ml prefilled syringes	IV	2	4	8	Give only if infant being effectively ventilated
				3	6	12	
				4	8	16	
Naloxone hydrochloride	0.4 mg/ml	1	0.25 ml/kg		**Total ml**		
				1	0.25		
			IV, ET, IM, SQ	2	0.50		
				3	0.75		
				4	1.00		Give rapidly, IV, ET preferred
	1.0 mg/ml	1	0.1 ml/kg	1	0.1		
				2	0.2		
			IV, ET, IM, SQ	3	0.3		
				4	0.4		
Dopamine	$\frac{6 \times \text{Weight (kg)} \times \text{Desired dose } (\mu g/kg/min)}{\text{Desired fluid (ml/hr)}}$ = mg of dopamine per 100 ml of solution		Begin at 5 μg/kg/min (may increase to 20 μg/kg/min if necessary) IV		**Total μg/min**		Give as a continuous infusion using an infusion pump
				1	5-20		Monitor HR and BP closely
				2	10-40		Seek consultation
				3	15-60		
				4	20-80		

From Bloom RS, Cropely C, American Academy of Pediatrics, and American Heart Association: *Textbook of neonatal resuscitation,* ed 2, Elk Grove Village, Ill, 1994, American Academy of Pediatrics.
**ET,* Endotracheal; *IM,* intramuscular; *IV,* intravenous; *SQ,* subcutaneous.

quire volume support and replacement of clotting factors. An infant who has a ruptured liver generally appears to be well for 24 to 48 hours, but then suddenly goes into shock, coinciding with the gradually swelling hematoma finally rupturing the hepatic capsule and causing hemoperitoneum. Gastrointestinal hemorrhage, splenic rupture, or intracranial hemorrhage also can lead to significant shock. All of these situations may require surgical intervention, after volume resuscitation and treatment of DIC.

Acute or massive hemorrhage most prominently affects the general circulation, but virtually all vital organs (lungs, kidneys, liver, gut, muscle) may be affected by impaired perfusion. Less frequently considered, but often altered, are body chemical composition, the hormonal settings that control fluid, fuel, and electrolyte balance, neurological function, circulating inflammatory mediators, and the antibacterial defense systems.

After resuscitation, an infant may become irritable and have involuntary muscular movements, often resulting from electrolyte abnormalities. Many of these infants suffer hypoglycemia, hypokalemia, and hypocalcemia in the first days after birth. They often require 10% dextrose IV to keep blood glucose levels above 40 mg/dl, as well as additional calcium gluconate (200 to 400 mg/kg/24 hr).

Increased pulmonary capillary permeability or "capillary leak" often persists, even after perfusion pressure is restored to normal. Thus, transient pulmonary edema with worsening respiratory distress should be anticipated and monitored closely with arterial blood gases. The infant may suffer increased susceptibility to pulmonary infection after a major hemorrhage, which increases pulmonary insufficiency. The effect of severe hemorrhage on the gastrointestinal tract also is significant: Small ulcerations may occur in the stomach and progress to necrotic ulcers; alterations in the distribution of blood flow combined with the general decrease in blood flow, producing ischemic injury to the mucosa, can result in enterocolitis. The liver often is damaged by severe hemorrhage; jaundice with an elevation of liver enzymes is a frequent finding; and centrilobular necrosis with fatty infiltration of the liver is found at autopsy. Disorders of hemostasis with bleeding are common after hemorrhagic shock and generally are associated with consumption of coagulation factors caused by disseminated intravascular coagulation.

Septic shock. Septic, or "warm," shock is characterized by vasodilation of peripheral vessels with the loss of peripheral resistance, a fall in blood pressure, poor tissue perfusion, diminished venous return, and reduced cardiac output. Damage to the capillary endothelium results in an increase in capillary permeability, edema, and loss of fluid from the intravascular space into the extravascular tissues, resulting in hypovolemia and a shocklike state. A direct toxic effect on the heart with cardiac failure may occur, as well as toxic effects in other vital organs noted above.

The most common bacteria that cause septic shock in neonates include *group B streptococci* and the gram-negative rod, *Escherichia coli* (which may produce endotoxic shock). The onset of respiratory distress or apnea, though nonspecific, together with shock in full-term or preterm infants, ominously heralds group B streptococcal disease. Signs include low blood pressure, congested mottled skin, and the effects of the toxin on other vital organs. An underlying illness, such as peritonitis or necrotizing enterocolitis, may modify the vascular response because of superimposed hypovolemia. The physician should suspect disseminated herpes simplex virus type 2 (HSV-2) infection in infants in whom an acute shocklike state develops within 7 to 10 days after delivery, particularly when there is a history of exposure to primary maternal genital HSV-2 infection.

The diagnosis of neonatal septicemia ultimately depends on a positive blood culture, but cerebrospinal fluid and urine cultures also should be obtained, particularly if signs appear after the first 24 hours of age. Indirect evidence of the presumptive diagnosis of overwhelming sepsis includes abnormally elevated or depressed neutrophil and band counts with thrombocytopenia. Abnormal coagulation studies indicating DIC and generalized bleeding may complicate septic shock.

Treatment for presumed neonatal septicemia must be instituted immediately after appropriate diagnostic studies have been performed, including blood, cerebrospinal fluid, and urine cultures. Broad-spectrum antibiotics must be administered before even initial identification of the responsible microorganism. The choice of antibiotics depends on the location of the infection, as well as on the timing of the onset of septic shock. When the presumed septicemia occurs within the first 48 to 72 hours of life (congenital infection), antibiotic coverage with ampicillin and gentamicin (or cefotaxime) most often is used. In late-onset sepsis, secondary to hospital-acquired infection, a penicillinase-resistant penicillin or vancomycin should be given in combination with an aminoglycoside such as amikacin or gentamicin. Once the specific pathogen has been identified, antibiotic coverage should be narrowed based on susceptibility of that organism in vitro.

Although correct antibiotic therapy is the key to successful management of neonatal septic shock, comprehensive supportive measures also are essential, as in other types of shock. This includes increasing the circulating blood volume by transfusion of packed red blood cells or normal saline as necessary. An attempt to improve cardiac function and vasomotor tone with use of cardiotonic drugs may be required. Careful monitoring of fluid balance is necessary, with measurements of intake and output recorded and surveillance of electrolyte status. Gastric dilation, increased gastric secretion, and ileus are common in sepsis; the stomach and bowel should be decompressed to prevent aspiration. In severe, overwhelming sepsis the infusion of granulocytes or gammaglobulin, use of an exchange transfusion, or administration of G-CSF (granulocyte colony-stimulating factor) may be effective, although more knowledge needs to be gained in this area.

Some acutely ill infants, particularly those who are in shock or are septic, may have a simultaneous problem defined recently as the systemic inflammatory response syndrome (SIRS). Inflammatory mediators such as tumor necrosis factor and various interleukins are released, which exacerbate local inflammation and cause systemic effects as well (e.g., vasodilation, fever, increased capillary leak, and pain). If left unchecked, this can progress to multiple organ dysfunction, which carries a high mortality. Infants who have severe sepsis should be transferred to a tertiary care center once stabilized.

Shock resulting from hypoadrenocorticism. In the neonatal period, bilateral adrenal hemorrhage after a traumatic delivery can lead to shock from blood loss and adrenal insufficiency. A mass may be palpable in each flank and visible on abdominal ultrasound examination. The disorder occurs most often in large infants who have had a traumatic delivery. It must be differentiated from renal vein thrombosis, which is associated with gross hematuria, whereas with adrenal hemorrhage the hematuria usually is microscopic. Infants who have unilateral adrenal hemorrhage do not have symptoms of adrenal insufficiency, but they may still experience shock from blood loss.

Congenital adrenal hyperplasia (CAH, see discussion on p. 603), when severe and associated with a salt-losing syndrome, can develop profound hyponatremia with vascular collapse. Thus, CAH must be considered in all infants whose genitalia are ambiguous, as well as in those who are vomiting, dehydrated, or fail to thrive in the first 2 weeks of life. Treatment involves expanding the circulating volume with isotonic saline and subsequently administering glucocorticoids and mineralocorticoids.

SPECIFIC SURGICAL CONDITIONS

Cardiogenic Shock

Cardiogenic shock usually is associated with underlying severe congestive heart failure, with low cardiac output states secondary to an obstruction of the left ventricular outflow tract, such as severe coarctation of the aorta or hypoplastic left-heart syndrome. (See Chapter 198, Congenital Heart Disease.) Because there is no output from the left ventricle, the venous blood returning to the left atrium must pass through the atrial septum to the right atrium. The smaller the atrial opening, the greater the pulmonary venous hypertension and congestion—hence the earlier the appearance of symptoms. These infants generally have poor pulses (although they may be normal early in life), mild to moderate cyanosis, characteristic mottling of the skin, and hepatomegaly. Mechanical ventilation and sedation usually are required for stabilization. Diagnosis is made by clinical, radiographic, and echocardiographic procedures. This is followed rapidly by cardiac catheterization and surgery in selected infants. Prostaglandin E_1 (0.05 μg/kg/min IV) should be infused to maintain the patency of the ductus arteriosus (to bypass the obstructed left ventricular outflow) before surgical correction of the lesion.

Congenital Diaphragmatic Hernia

Congenital diaphragmatic hernia (CDH) occurs in 1 in 2200 live births; most defects (90%) are present on the left side. The infant may manifest only mild respiratory distress initially, but more commonly may be profoundly distressed, with severe cyanosis that is unresponsive to ventilation. The diagnosis should be suspected if the infant has a flat or scaphoid abdomen and bowel sounds are heard in the chest. Infants who have a left CDH will have heart sounds displaced to the right. The diagnosis is confirmed easily by a chest roentgenogram. A large-bore (10 or 12 Fr) orogastric tube is inserted into the stomach immediately and placed to low continuous suction in order to decompress the air in the herniated bowel and reduce compression of the lung. All these infants should be given 100% oxygen initially, because they are at high risk for persistent pulmonary hypertension. If respiratory distress is significant, endotracheal intubation and intermittent positive pressure ventilation must be performed. This is one of the few situations in which bag and mask ventilation and nasal continuous positive airway pressure (CPAP) are contraindicated because these force gas into the intestinal tract, thus increasing distention of the intestine that lies within the thorax and compromising pulmonary function further. Transport to a tertiary care center, preferably one that has ECMO (extracorporeal membrane oxygenation) capability, should be arranged while the infant is being stabilized.

Esophageal Atresia and Tracheoesophageal Fistula

The diagnosis of esophageal atresia with or without a tracheoesophageal fistula (TEF) should be suspected whenever there is a history of polyhydramnios during the pregnancy (because amniotic fluid cannot be swallowed by the fetus). Eight types of these anomalies have been described and are illustrated in Fig. 49-1. More than 85% of these infants have a type A lesion, with a blind proximal esophageal pouch and a fistulous connection from the distal esophagus to the trachea. Type B is the next most common and is distinguished from type A by absence of air in the intestinal tract on roentgenogram. In types A, B, and C the infant is unable to swallow secretions, giving rise to the clinical presentation of excessive oral secretions, with or without aspiration pneumonia soon after birth. The diagnosis is suspected when a nasogastric (NG) tube cannot be passed into the stomach and the contents aspirated. It is confirmed by a roentgenogram of a radiopaque NG tube curled up in the short, blind esophageal pouch. These infants should be kept with the head up (45-degree angle) and a Replogle tube inserted into the upper esophageal pouch with continuous suction. If a Replogle tube is not available, a large-bore (10 to 12 Fr) catheter will suffice. Immediate transfer to a regional NICU is mandatory for definitive diagnostic testing and surgical correction of the defect.

A flat or gasless abdomen suggests an esophageal atresia without TEF. Rarely, when a TEF is proximal to the esophageal atresia (types D and E), severe aspiration is likely to occur soon after birth. Those infants who have the H-type fistula (type F) may have minimal symptomatology initially but subsequently develop respiratory distress with feedings or manifest recurrent pneumonias.

Gastroschisis or omphalocele. Infants who have gastroschisis or an omphalocele may suffer from severe evaporative fluid loss and hypothermia. They are best managed by placing the entire body below the shoulders in a bowel bag (a clear sterile plastic bag). A drawstring permits the bag to be tightened at the level of the axillae, preventing both heat and fluid loss. A gently applied moist sterile gauze dressing is safe and protects the exposed bowel. Most importantly, the infant should be placed in a side-lying position with the bowel supported in "neutral tension" to avoid intestinal ischemia. A large-bore (10 to 12 Fr) orogastric tube should be inserted and continuous suction applied to decrease intestinal distention. Intravenous fluids should be adminis-

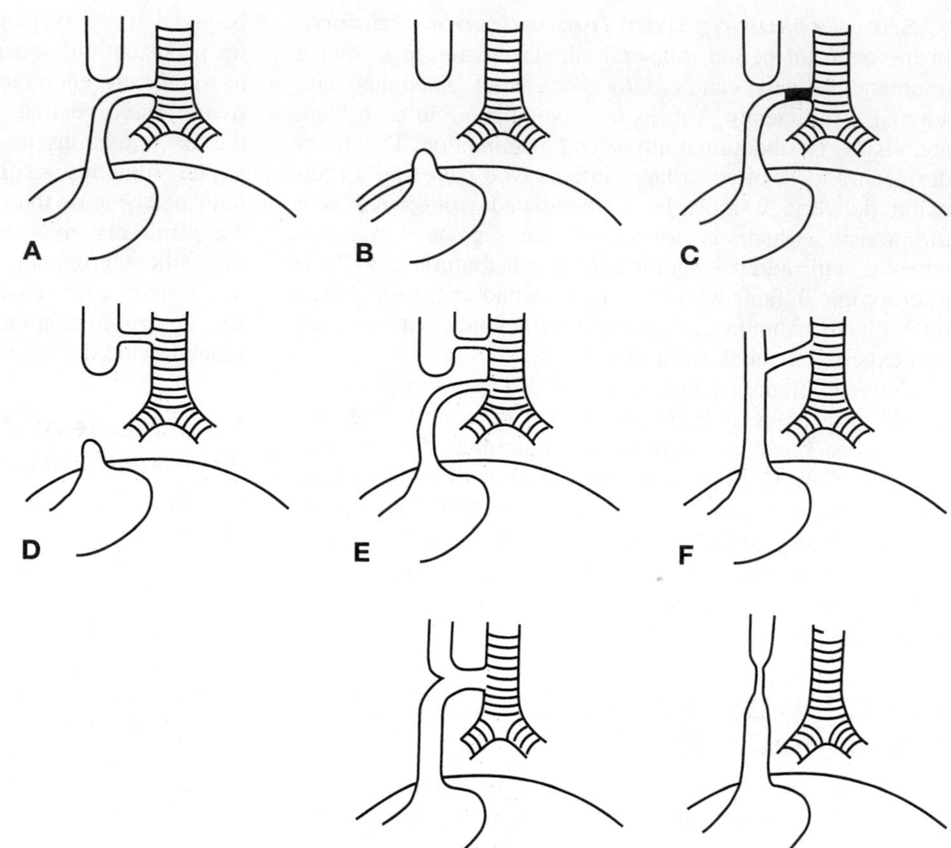

Fig. 49-1 Types of esophageal atresia and stenosis with and without tracheoesophageal fistula.
(From Taeusch HW, Ballard RA, editors: *Avery's diseases of the newborn,* ed 7, Philadelphia, 1988, WB Saunders.)

tered at 1.5 times maintenance, and broad-spectrum antibiotics started. The baby then should be transported in the above-described position to a tertiary care pediatric facility for definitive pediatric surgical evaluation and corrective surgery.

Necrotizing Enterocolitis

Necrotizing enterocolitis (NEC) is a potentially life-threatening gastrointestinal disease and one of the most common reasons for emergent abdominal surgery in the neonatal period. Nearly 90% of infants affected with NEC are low-birth-weight preterm infants. The exact etiology and pathogenesis of NEC remain unclear. The clinical presentation is quite variable. Infants with NEC are classified according to modified Bell's criteria. Infants with suspected NEC (grade I) present with feeding intolerance, abdominal distention, occult blood in stool, ileus, and nonspecific signs such as temperature instability, apnea, and/or bradycardia. Definite ("medical") NEC (grade II) includes the signs and symptoms of grade I, plus metabolic acidosis, abdominal tenderness, and pneumatosis intestinalis (air) in areas of bowel wall seen on abdominal films. Advanced ("surgical") NEC (grade III) involves seriously ill neonates with intact bowel, or bowel wall perforation with free air or intrahepatic air noted on abdominal films (see Fig. 113-1), and signs of peritonitis. These infants are acutely ill, often with marked respiratory and metabolic acidosis, bradycardia, hypotension, DIC, and sepsis. They require ventilation, intravenous antibiotics, fluid and electrolyte and blood product resuscitation, and transport to a tertiary center for pediatric surgical evaluation and intervention, usually with resection of the affected bowel.

Acknowledgment

We would like to acknowledge the contributions of M. Jeffrey Maisels to earlier editions of this chapter.

SUGGESTED READINGS

American Academy of Pediatrics and American College of Obstetricians and Gynecologists: *Guidelines for perinatal care*, ed 4, Elk Grove Village, Ill, 1997, American Academy of Pediatrics.

Avery GB, Fletcher MA, MacDonald MG, editors: *Neonatology: pathophysiology and management of the newborn,* ed 4, Philadelphia, 1994, JB Lippincott.

Bloom RS, Cropley C, American Academy of Pediatrics, and American Heart Association: *Textbook of neonatal resuscitation*, ed 2, Elk Grove Village, Ill, 1994, American Academy of Pediatrics.

Fanaroff AA, Martin RJ, editors: *Neonatal-perinatal medicine*, ed 6, St Louis, 1997, Mosby.

Nelson NM, editor: *Current therapy in neonatal-perinatal medicine*, ed 2, Philadelphia, 1990, BC Decker.

Taeusch HW, Ballard RA, editors: *Avery's diseases of the newborn*, ed 7, Philadelphia, 1998, WB Saunders.

50 Prenatal Drug Abuse and Neonatal Drug Withdrawal Syndrome

Enrique M. Ostrea, Jr. • Mary Anne Tan-Laxa

The problem of drug abuse has reached epidemic proportions during the past two decades, increasing not only in the number of drug users but also in the types of drugs abused. In 1996, the National Household Survey on Drug Abuse estimated that approximately 13 million Americans were current illicit drug users, a figure that represents 6.1% of the population 12 years of age and older.[77] The use of marijuana alone was most common (54%), whereas use of marijuana and some other illicit drugs was 23% and use of other illicit drugs without marijuana was also 23%. Equally alarming was the proportion of drug users among women of childbearing age (15-44 years) or who were pregnant. Among women of childbearing age, 10% were nonpregnant, current illicit drug users while 3.2% of users were pregnant. The type of substance abused varied (1.6% for marijuana, 0.5% for cocaine or crack, 0.2% for hallucinogens, 0.3% for heroin, 0.2% for stimulants, 16.1% for alcohol, and 20.3% for cigarettes). These prevalence rates for illicit drug use were obtained exclusively from maternal interviews and, therefore, are highly underestimated, because of significant underreporting of drug use by these women. In one study, an estimate of drug use among pregnant women varied from 0.4% to 27% where drug use was detected by maternal history, urine toxicology, or both. But when meconium drug analysis, which is a more sensitive method for drug testing, was employed, a prevalence rate of 44% of illicit drug use was found in a study population in contrast to 11% by maternal self-report.[53,69]

Most drugs ingested by the pregnant woman, whether licit or illicit, readily cross the placenta into the fetal circulation. There is very little barrier to the passage of drugs across the placenta or to its biotransformation in the placenta.[55] Thus, the fetus is chronically exposed to the drugs that the pregnant woman uses throughout gestation. This can lead to a number of complications in the pregnancy or in the infant, including a high incidence of stillbirths, meconium-stained amniotic fluid, premature rupture of the membranes, maternal hemorrhage (abruptio placenta or placenta previa), and fetal distress.[43,46] In the newborn infant, mortality as well as morbidity are high—for example, a high incidence of asphyxia, prematurity, low birth weight, infections, pneumonia, congenital malformations, cerebral infarction, drug withdrawal, and increased risk of acquired immunodeficiency disease.[9,10] Long-term sequelae in the infants also have been reported, which include some delays in physical growth and mental development, sudden infant death syndrome, and learning disabilities.[11,83,84] In this chapter, we discuss one specific complication of the infant who is antenatally exposed to drugs—the neonatal drug withdrawal syndrome, referred to by some as the "neonatal abstinence syndrome."

As tolerance or addiction to drugs develops in the pregnant woman, passive dependence on the drug also develops in her fetus. Two major theories about the etiology of withdrawal have been postulated. The theory of disuse hypersensitivity postulates that a drug may depress certain neural systems and render their targets hypersensitive to their usual stimuli, with an increase in binding sites for the drugs. When the depressant drug is removed, the withdrawal syndrome occurs as a result of rebound hypersensitivity of the affected targets. Morphine, for instance, has been shown to inhibit activation of nonadrenergic cells in the brainstem. Thus, chronic morphine exposure results in an increase in the number of brainstem adrenergic-binding sites. When morphine is withdrawn, the withdrawal syndrome occurs as a consequence of adrenergic hypersensitivity.[1,85] The theory of alternate pathways states that a drug may depress a primary neural pathway; as a result, alternate pathways, normally of minor activity, become prominent in an attempt to compensate. When the drug is removed, both the primary and alternate pathways are operative in an additive fashion and cause the withdrawal syndrome.[79]

Withdrawal of the infant from drugs may occur in utero or soon after birth. In utero withdrawal manifests as an increase in fetal movement or activity, increase in catecholamine levels in the amniotic fluid,[87] or signs of fetal distress—for example, meconium staining of the amniotic fluid. Thus, it is not safe for the pregnant addict to undergo rapid withdrawal, as can occur in detoxification, because this will lead to withdrawal in her fetus and its concomitant complications.

DRUGS ASSOCIATED WITH NEONATAL WITHDRAWAL SYNDROME

Drug withdrawal in the mother and infant can occur from gestational exposure to narcotics or nonnarcotic hypnosedatives (Box 50-1) because addiction to both groups of drugs can occur. However, some important differences exist in the addiction to these agents and between the mother and her infant[49]: First, unlike narcotics, the development of addiction in adults (mother) to nonnarcotic hypnosedatives requires prolonged and continuous use of large and partially incapacitating doses of the drugs, usually over months or years, par-

BOX 50-1

DRUGS THAT CAN CAUSE WITHDRAWAL IN THE NEONATE

A. Narcotics or opiates:
  1. Morphine
  2. Codeine
  3. Heroin
  4. Methadone
  5. Propoxyphene (Darvon)
  6. Pentazocine (Talwin)
  7. Meperidine (Demerol)
  8. Oxycodone (Percodan, Tylox, and Percocet)
  9. Morphine (Dilaudid)
  10. Fentanyl (Immovar, Sublimaze)

B. Nonnarcotic hypnosedatives:
  1. Barbiturates
  2. Nonbarbiturate sedatives and tranquilizers:
    a. Bromides
    b. Chloral hydrate
    c. Chlordiazepoxide (Librium)
    d. Diazepam (Valium)
    e. Ethchlorvynol (Placidyl)
    f. Glutethimide (Doriden)
  3. Alcohol (ethanol)

C. Stimulants:
  1. Cocaine
  2. Amphetamine and congeners
  3. Nicotine
  4. Phencyclidine
  5. Marijuana

D. Inhalant (volatile substance) drugs:
  1. Paint solvents
  2. Lacquers
  3. Glues

ticularly if the drugs are taken orally. On the other hand, passive addiction in the neonate to nonnarcotic hypnosedative can occur, even at therapeutic doses taken by the mother during pregnancy. For instance, maternal use of phenobarbital for epilepsy may not cause addiction in the mother to the drug but can induce passive addiction in her fetus. Second, the manifestations of withdrawal from nonnarcotics are frequently more intense in the adult or infant compared with withdrawal from narcotics, particularly the more frequent occurrence of convulsions. Third, withdrawal from narcotics in the infant is observed commonly within the first 3 postnatal days, because of the short half-life of narcotics. In contrast, withdrawal from the nonnarcotics (e.g., phenobarbital) may occur 7 to 21 days after birth, because of the slow clearance of the drug in the infant. Last, unlike narcotic addiction, neonatal addiction to nonnarcotic hypnosedatives is induced often by physicians who treat the mother, not realizing that the drugs are addicting to her fetus.

Addiction by the adults to a large number of central nervous system (CNS) stimulants also can occur. These include cocaine, amphetamines and their congeners, indolealkylamines (e.g., LSD, psilocin), phenylethylamines (mescaline, peyote), cannabinoids, inhalants (solvents and aerosols), and phencyclidines. Neonatal withdrawal to some of these drugs has been described, although it is likely that the abnormalities described in the infants reflect the continued drug effects rather than manifestations of withdrawal.

Neonatal drug withdrawal can be strictly iatrogenic, caused by the abrupt withdrawal of opioids administered for analgesia and sedation.[26] A withdrawal syndrome from volatile substances also has been described.[78]

Narcotics

The term *narcotics,* or opiates, refers to a family of natural or synthetic drugs that have morphine-like pharmacological actions. These include the natural opiates (e.g., morphine and codeine) and the synthetic opiates (e.g., heroin, methadone, propoxyphene [Darvon], pentazocine [Talwin], nalbuphine [Nubain], buprenorphine [Buprenex], butorphanol [Stadol], meperidine [Demerol], oxycodone [Percodan, Tylox, and Percocet], hydromorphone [Dilaudid], and fentanyl [Immovar and Sublimaze]). As previously mentioned, extended use of narcotics, even in therapeutic doses, can result in addiction in the mother and infant, which is characterized by psychological, as well as physical, dependence on the drug.

Barbiturates

Although barbiturates have been used in clinical medicine for more than 50 years, their addiction potential was recognized only recently. It may be the frequent association in the adult of barbiturate use with alcohol that prevented the earlier recognition of the addicting potential of the barbiturates.[15] The ability of barbiturates to abolish withdrawal from alcohol may partly explain this.

Barbiturates are classified based on their duration of action as ultrashort, intermediate, and long-acting. The intermediate-acting barbiturates are those abused most frequently—for example, secobarbital (Seconal), pentobarbital (Nembutal), amobarbital (Amytal), and butabarbital (Butisol). The abuse of the long-acting barbiturates (e.g., phenobarbital) is not as common as the abuse of the shorter-acting forms. However, phenobarbital is involved most frequently with nonnarcotic abstinence in the newborn because it frequently is used for insomnia, for the relief of anxiety, as an anticonvulsant, or for sedation in toxemia of pregnancy.

Passive acquisition by the fetus of physical dependence on barbiturates can occur after prolonged intrauterine exposure to the drug.[15,35] Barbiturates readily cross the placenta and establish high levels in both maternal and cord blood. Relatively high levels of barbiturates have been found in the fetal brain, liver, and adrenals.[61] The manifestations of barbiturate withdrawal in the neonate are similar, regardless of which barbiturate was actually used by the mother. However, the time of onset of withdrawal may differ. Withdrawal from intermediate-acting barbiturates occurs within a day after birth[56] but about 3 to 7 days after birth in the case of the long-acting barbiturates.[15]

Barbiturates are metabolized principally by the liver, although a significant portion may be excreted unchanged by the kidney. In adults, for instance, up to 30% of the total dose of phenobarbital ingested is excreted in the urine in unchanged form.[73] The half-life in infants of prenatally administered phenobarbital is almost twice that in the adult and varies inversely with the extent of the prenatal exposure to phenobarbital.[36] The prolonged half-life of phenobarbital in the neonate is secondary to a lower glomerular filtration rate and to a decreased capacity of the neonatal liver to metabolize drugs.

As previously mentioned, withdrawal from barbiturates can occur in infants even at therapeutic, nonaddicting maternal doses. Withdrawal from phenobarbital has been reported in an infant born to an epileptic mother receiving phenobarbital at a dose of 60 mg/day.[15] An awareness of the possibility of late-onset withdrawal, especially after exposure to long-acting barbiturates, should alert one to follow these infants closely during their first 2 weeks of life.

Benzodiazepines

Chlordiazepoxide (Librium) and diazepam (Valium) are used widely for their hypnosedative effects. Abuse of these drugs and dependence on them have both been reported in adults. During pregnancy, benzodiazepines cross the placenta with relative ease, resulting in significant levels of the drug in the serum and tissue of the fetus.[24]

An acute withdrawal syndrome in the newborn infant from chlordiazepoxide and diazepam has been described.[4,65] In the former, chlordiazepoxide withdrawal was diagnosed in a set of twins born to a mother who used chlordiazepoxide at a dose of 20 mg/24 hr during the second and third trimesters of her pregnancy.[4] The withdrawal occurred on the twenty-first day of life and consisted of severe irritability and coarse tremors.

Three cases of presumptive neonatal withdrawal from diazepam also have been reported.[65] Withdrawal occurred within 2½ to 6 hours after birth and consisted of tremors, irritability, hypertonicity, vigorous sucking, vomiting, and diarrhea. In all cases, phenobarbital was effective in controlling the withdrawal in the infant, although the drug had to be administered for a prolonged period.

Alcohol

Ethanol is an anxiolytic analgesic that has a depressant effect on the CNS.[59] It is rapidly absorbed by diffusion in the mucosa of the stomach (20%) and intestines (80%). The absorption rate is not affected by the pregnancy, but blood alcohol levels may be higher in pregnancy. Alcohol usually is cleared from the blood stream within 1 hour in adults and 2 hours in newborns. Approximately 95% is metabolized by the liver and 5% eliminated by the kidneys and lungs. Ethanol is metabolized to acetaldehyde and then to acetate. Acetaldehyde is more toxic than ethanol itself.

Infants "withdraw" from alcohol, but this rarely is noted because the withdrawal may be mistaken for narcotic or other drug withdrawal. The withdrawal from ethanol occurs early (within birth to 12 hours of life), because of its short half-life, and may manifest as abdominal distention, opisthotonus, convulsions, tremors, hypertonia, apnea, and cyanosis. The infants are irritable, sleep restlessly, and engage in exaggerated mouthing behavior.[13,67]

STIMULANTS

Neurobehavioral abnormalities have been observed in infants born to mothers who have abused a class of stimulants during pregnancy—for example, cocaine, methamphetamine, and phencyclidine. The manifestations are similar to those observed in narcotic and nonnarcotic withdrawal. However, it is likely that these manifestations represent drug effects rather than withdrawal.

Cocaine

Neurobehavioral abnormalities, such as tremulousness, irritability, hypertonicity, high-pitched cry, abnormal sleep pattern, and sometimes, seizures, have been observed in infants who have been exposed prenatally to cocaine[23,29,44,71] and are similar to the manifestations of withdrawal from opiates. It is difficult to separate the overlapping effects of cocaine and opiate withdrawal, because it is not uncommon for the addicted woman to abuse both drugs. The effect of multiple drug abuse on withdrawal is controversial. In two reports, no difference was observed in the severity of withdrawal in infants born to mothers who have used both cocaine and methadone or either singly,[19,68] whereas one report noted higher abstinence scores in infants exposed to both drugs compared with one.[28] In general, the CNS manifestations in the cocaine-exposed infants are significantly milder than those observed in narcotic withdrawal. Abnormalities in cardiorespiratory patterns (increased episodes of apnea, periodic breathing),[74] electroencephalogram (EEG) (bursts of sharp waves and spikes),[19] and neonatal behavior as assessed by the Brazelton score (impairment of orientation, motor and state regulation)[23,29,44,71] also have been described. Again, these abnormalities may be manifestations of the drug's stimulant effect, rather than withdrawal.

Marijuana

Marijuana is the illicit drug used most widely among women of childbearing age in the United States.[77] Tetrahydrocannabinol (THC) is highly bound to the lipoprotein fraction in the blood. THC crosses the placenta within minutes of administration. The concentrations of THC in maternal and fetal sera are essentially identical.[51]

Most studies do not show a significant effect of prenatal marijuana use on fetal growth or weight.[86] There is an equivocal relationship between prenatal marijuana use and neurobehavioral outcome of the offspring. Prenatal marijuana exposure has been associated with increased fine tremors in the infant, accompanied by exaggerated and prolonged startles, both spontaneous and in response to mild stimuli; poorer visual but not auditory stimuli habituation[27]; decreased ability to regulate state; and disrupted sleep patterns.[72] Elevated serum norepinephrine levels have been observed among these infants.[45] Other reports have found no altered neurobehavioral patterns in marijuana-exposed offspring.[32,66]

Nicotine

Nicotine is considered the compound primarily responsible for the pharmacological effects of smoking. It is absorbed readily from the lungs, almost with the same efficiency as intravenous administration, and is distributed rapidly throughout the body. Nicotine is metabolized principally in the liver to its two principal metabolites, cotinine and

3′ p-hydroxyconiine. These metabolites have been measured in meconium. The highest concentrations were found in infants whose mothers were heavy smokers (more than two packs a day). Of interest, equivalent amounts of cotinine were found in the meconium of infants whose mothers were passive smokers compared with mothers who smoked one pack a day.[54] This illustrates the significant amount of exposure of the mother to nicotine secondary to passive smoking.

Tobacco is used widely by women of childbearing age. Data from the 1995 and 1996 National Household Survey on Drug Abuse show that 63.1% of pregnant women had smoked tobacco in their lifetime, 29% had smoked tobacco in the past year, and 20.3% were current smokers. Most of the current smokers were ages 26 to 44 years.[77]

Several studies have investigated the impact of cigarette smoking during pregnancy on newborn behavior and on later child development.[70] Offspring of mothers who smoked during pregnancy have been observed to perform less well on the Brazelton Neonatal Behavioral Assessment Score in items such as habituating to sound or orienting to a voice, compared with the offspring of nonsmoking mothers. Other studies indicate poorer performance with head turning and sucking, lower visual alertness, more crying, tremors, and startles, and increased lability of color. Most of the studies, however, do not demonstrate a clinically significant effect on neonatal behavior that can be attributed to maternal cigarette smoking alone.[7,21]

Phencyclidine

Phencyclidine (PCP) was first introduced as a dissociative anesthetic, but its clinical use was discontinued after reports of adverse effects that included agitation, confusion, delirium, and persistent hallucinations. It remains a popular drug of abuse because of its hallucinogenic and sedative effects. Phencyclidine has strong, centrally mediated effects in animals and humans and influences many different neuronal systems. It inhibits the uptake and increases the release of monoamines in the brain, interacts with cholinergic and serotonergic systems, and antagonizes the neuronal stimulation caused by the excitatory amino acid *N*-methyl-D-aspartate.

The prevalence of PCP abuse during pregnancy has not been established firmly because most reports have come from urban areas and could not be generalized nationally. In 1983, a study reported that 12% of a random sample of 200 newborns had measurable quantities of PCP in their cord blood.[38] In 1995 and 1996, about 2.6% of pregnant women admitted having used PCP in their lifetime, while 0.2% admitted having used it in the past year.[77]

Early case reports of PCP-exposed newborns showed abnormal neurobehavioral findings in the infants. These included irritability, tremors, hypertonicity, poor attention, bizarre eye movements, staring spells, hypertonic ankle reflexes, and depressed grasp and rooting reflexes.[8,31,76] One of the most characteristic features in infants is a sudden and rapid change in level of consciousness, with lethargy alternating with irritability. The behavior of these newborns has been attributed to PCP intoxication, rather than to withdrawal.[62]

Amphetamines

The amphetamines are a group of chemically related sympathomimetic amines that have both CNS stimulant and peripheral actions. The potential for abuse is very strong because of their psychic effects, which include a decreased sense of fatigue, wakefulness, alertness, mood elevation, self-confidence, and often, euphoria and elation.

Methamphetamine is the methylated derivative of amphetamine and is prepared through the reduction of ephedrine or pseudoephedrine. The ease of its synthesis, its availability and affordability, and a prolonged "high" have made it an increasingly popular drug of abuse. "Ice," the smokable form of methamphetamine, is claimed to produce an intense euphoria.

An infant born to a woman addicted to amphetamine manifests with diaphoresis, episodes of agitation alternating with lassitude, miosis, and vomiting.[63] Infants exposed to both cocaine and methamphetamine are described as having abnormal sleep patterns, tremors, poor feeding, hypertonia, sneezing, a high-pitched cry, frantic fist sucking, tachypnea, loose stools, fever, yawning, hyperreflexia, and excoriation.[48]

Inhalant (Volatile Substance) Abuse

Neonatal withdrawal from volatile substances has been described recently.[78] Approximately 12,000 infants are born each year to mothers who have abused volatile substances during pregnancy. The principal products abused are paint solvents, lacquer, and glue. Toluene and other hydrocarbons may be present in the solvent. A characteristic chemical odor in the neonate or mother is noted that can persist for several days, because the lungs are a major route for excretion, and the substances, being highly lipophilic, are excreted slowly. The typical manifestations in the infant include excessive and a high-pitched cry, sleeplessness, tremors, hypertonia, and poor feeding. Metabolic acidosis also has been described[78,82]; it occurs within the first 24 hours of life, and two different patterns are observed. The common form is transient and resolves spontaneously or after a single dose of sodium bicarbonate. The other type is more persistent and lasts for 1 to 2 weeks and requires treatment with repeated doses of sodium bicarbonate or Shohl's solution (Bicitra). The cause of the metabolic acidosis is not known, although it may be secondary to the acid load of toluene metabolite or from renal tubular acidosis.

ONSET AND DURATION OF NEONATAL DRUG WITHDRAWAL

The onset of withdrawal is common within the first 72 hours after birth, usually within the first 24 to 48 hours. In a few instances the onset may appear soon after birth if the drug has a short half-life or if the mother already has begun to experience withdrawal while in labor. Reports of withdrawal occurring after the first or second week have been observed in drugs that have a longer half-life (e.g., phenobarbital).[15] Among narcotics, delayed manifestations of withdrawal, sometimes as late as 6 weeks, have been observed with methadone.[37]

The onset and severity of the withdrawal is affected by a number of factors, among which are the amount of maternal drug use, such as seen with methadone,[57] the timing of the last dose before delivery, the use of anesthesia or analgesia in the mother during labor, the maturity and nutrition of the infant, and the metabolism and excretion of the drugs and their metabolites.[17,36,50]

Neonatal withdrawal from narcotics usually peaks by about the third day of postnatal life and subsides by the fifth to seventh day. The duration of withdrawal is related to its severity.[57] If drugs are used to treat the withdrawal, relapse may occur if treatment is discontinued abruptly. It should be noted that although withdrawal manifestations diminish in intensity within the first week after birth, they do not disappear completely. The tremors and irritability may persist for as long as 8 to 16 weeks.

NEONATAL NARCOTIC WITHDRAWAL

The prototype of drug withdrawal in the neonate is withdrawal from opiates. The manifestations are multisystemic and involve the central nervous, respiratory, gastrointestinal, vasomotor, and cutaneous systems (Box 50-2).

BOX 50-2

THE MANIFESTATIONS OF NEONATAL DRUG WITHDRAWAL SYNDROME

A. Central nervous system signs:
 1. Hyperactivity
 2. Hyperirritability—excess crying, high-pitch outcry
 3. Increased muscle tone
 4. Exaggerated reflexes
 5. Tremors
 6. Sneezing, hiccups, yawning
 7. Short, nonquiet sleep
 8. Fever
B. Respiratory signs:
 1. Tachypnea
 2. Excess secretions
C. Gastrointestinal signs:
 1. Disorganized, poor sucking
 2. Vomiting
 3. Drooling
 4. Sensitive gag
 5. Hyperphagia
 6. Diarrhea
 7. Abdominal cramps
D. Vasomotor signs:
 1. Stuffy nose
 2. Flushing
 3. Sweating
 4. Sudden, circumoral pallor
E. Cutaneous signs:
 1. Excoriated buttocks
 2. Facial scratches
 3. Pressure-point abrasions

Central Nervous System

Neurological signs predominate and appear early. Findings are those of CNS excitability, such as hyperactivity, irritability, tremors, and hypertonicity. Occasionally, fever may accompany these increased neuromuscular activities.

Hyperactivity manifests as almost incessant movements of the extremities. When the infant is supine and unrestrained, movements assume a jerky, purposeless, "en masse" nature, apparently perpetuated by unchecked proprioceptive stimuli. When placed in the prone position, the infant's motor behavior becomes more organized. There are crawling movements, which actually may lead to the infant's displacement from the crib, and other motions such as chin lifting, head movement from side to side, chest elevation, and hand-to-mouth activity. The latter usually quiets the infant, indicating the usefulness of pacifiers.

Hyperirritability manifests as an almost incessant shrill, high-pitch crying. The infant's tone is exaggerated, sometimes assuming an opisthotonic position. This makes the infant hard to hold, because of its failure to mold to the body of the holder. Tremors and myoclonic jerks are frequent and sometimes are sustained. To distinguish from seizures, tremors can be abolished by restraint of the tremulous extremity. The reflexes of the infant, such as Moro, traction response, weight bearing, placing, stepping, crawling, and Landau, are all exaggerated. The infant's response to stimuli, such as sound and light, also is disproportionately increased.

Electroencephalographic tracings on the addicted neonate may be abnormal and show high-frequency dysynchronous activity suggestive of CNS irritability. The prevalence of seizures is estimated to be between 5% and 21% in infants manifesting narcotic withdrawal.

In premature infants, the neural hyperexcitability is more episodic. The infants appear restless and overactive for short periods and then lapse into periods of lethargy and inactivity. Sustained tremors are not usually seen in premature infants until they reach the gestational age when tone is present in the upper and lower extremities. Sweating, which is seen in the full-term infant, also is not observed in preterm infants.[18]

The normal patterns of active and quiet sleep periods in the infant also are disturbed, with a significant decrease in sleep from a normal 3 to 4 hours to less than 1 hour. Heroin- and methadone-addicted infants also have fewer periods of quiet sleep.[64] Initially, these observations were thought to be related to withdrawal. However, because these abnormal sleep patterns persist beyond the period of withdrawal, they might be the result of the addiction process itself, rather than to the general distress secondary to withdrawal, and may be secondary to the direct effects of chronic opiate exposure on the opiate receptors in the brain involved in the regulation of sleep.[60]

Cardiorespiratory Signs

Abnormalities in ventilation have been described in infants withdrawing from narcotics, including longer and increased frequency of apneic episodes and periodic breathing. During withdrawal, these infants also may also exhibit tachypnea, with concomitant respiratory alkalosis.[31] Morphine has been shown in animals to have a dual action on fetal breathing—apnea, followed by tachypnea. It is postulated that the dual action of morphine is secondary to the effects of the drug concentration and to the effects of the drug on two different sites involved in the control of respiration. After a bolus of morphine, its initial high concentration causes respiratory depression and apnea. As the drug is metabolized, the lower concentration is associated with stimulation of respiration, hence the tachypnea. Morphine is found to be inhibitory to the respiratory neurons in the medulla and to the neurons located more rostrally that act to inhibit respiration.

Abnormal heart rate tracings associated with elevated serum creatine phosphokinase were noted to be significantly different in infants of drug-dependent mothers compared with nonexposed infants.[58] In addition, these changes were more intense among infants who had moderate to severe withdrawal. The elevated serum CPK is postulated secondary to the excess muscular activity of infants undergoing withdrawal.

Other physiological alterations include elevated systolic blood pressure, an increase in plasma renin activity, and elevated catecholamine levels.[80] In one report, these conditions persisted for 21 days postdelivery, which suggests increased beta-adrenergic activity.[20]

Gastrointestinal Signs

The suckling of the infant is disorganized and poorly coordinated with swallowing.[57] Both suckling rate and nutrient consumption are low.[39] Frequently, milk drools around the corners of the infant's mouth. The infant appears incessantly hungry, which when unfulfilled, leads to mounting agitation, persistent crying, hyperactivity, and exhaustion. The poor nutrient intake and increased caloric expenditure from hyperactivity may be responsible for the significant weight loss seen in these infants. Vomiting and diarrhea also are often observed. This can lead to dehydration, electrolyte imbalance, and excoriations around the buttocks.

Vasomotor Signs

Significant vasomotor instability manifests as a stuffy nose, flushing, mottling, sweating, and episodes of sudden, circumoral pallor.

Cutaneous Signs

Because of hyperactivity, facial scratches and abrasions on pressure points may be observed on the infant's skin. Excoriations of the buttocks can occur if diarrhea is present.

NEONATAL WITHDRAWAL FROM NONNARCOTIC DRUGS

Withdrawal from nonnarcotic drugs is essentially similar to narcotic withdrawal. However, convulsions are observed more frequently in the former. On the other hand, infants born to mothers who have abused stimulants during pregnancy (e.g., cocaine, amphetamines) also may manifest tremors, irritability, a high-pitched cry, and abnormal sleep patterns during the neonatal period. However, these probably are manifestations of drug effects rather than withdrawal.

PERSISTENCE OF DRUG WITHDRAWAL

Withdrawal signs in infants who have narcotic withdrawal may persist for as long as 8 to16 weeks of age. The manifestations consist of irritability, tremors, hypertonicity, sneezing, hiccups, and regurgitation but generally are milder than those of the initial withdrawal. The persistence of drug withdrawal is related directly to the initial severity; it is more prolonged in those who had severe withdrawal. Infants treated for withdrawal also show a prolonged withdrawal period. Thus, drug treatment may ameliorate the manifestations of withdrawal, but it does not shorten its duration. It is important that the mother be made aware that her infant's symptoms of withdrawal may persist for weeks after discharge from the nursery. The unwary mother also may misinterpret her infant's irritability as hunger and then overfeed, which can lead to diarrhea and vomiting. The mother also should be instructed on how to reduce the infant's discomfort by swaddling and cuddling. She should be reassured that signs of withdrawal will subside eventually without the use of medications. In most instances, the mother who is well informed can cope with the situation successfully.

DIAGNOSIS

The diagnosis of drug withdrawal is based on the clinical manifestations and the verification of fetal drug exposure. However, identifying drug exposure in an infant is not easy, because there is significant underreporting of maternal drug use because of fear of the consequences stemming from such an admission. Even with maternal cooperation, information regarding the type and extent of drug usage often is inaccurate.[53] Similarly, many of the drugs to which the fetus is exposed in utero do not produce immediate or recognizable effects.[37] Numerous laboratory tests are used commonly to detect drug exposure in the infant. These include toxicological analysis of the infant's urine, hair, and meconium for drugs. Urine screening can have a high false-negative rate because only the results for infants who have had recent exposure will be positive. Meconium drug testing is more likely to identify infants of drug-abusing mothers than is infant urine testing.[51-53,69,71]

DIFFERENTIAL DIAGNOSIS

Withdrawal from narcotic and nonnarcotic drugs needs to be distinguished from other entities such as hypoglycemia, hypocalcemia, hypomagnesemia, sepsis, meningitis, subarachnoid hemorrhage, infectious diarrhea, and intestinal obstruction. Blood chemistry, cerebrospinal fluid, and radiographic studies and cultures should be performed as indicated by the clinical circumstances.

Infants whose mothers are on tricyclic antidepressants or lithium may exhibit manifestations similar to those of withdrawal, such as irritability, tachycardia, respiratory distress, sweating, and convulsions.[22,75,81] Likewise, maternal use of phenothiazines (e.g., chlorpromazine) may induce extrapyramidal dysfunctions in the newborn such as tremors, facial grimacing, increased muscle tone, cog-wheel rigidity, increased reflexes, and torticollis, all of which can resemble the withdrawal syndrome.[33,41] The history, as well as identification of the offending drug's metabolites in the infant's serum or urine, are necessary to establish the diagnosis.

ASSESSMENT OF THE SEVERITY OF NEONATAL DRUG WITHDRAWAL

The manifestations of withdrawal can range in severity from none or mild to severe. It has been shown that neither the infant's gender, race, or Apgar score nor the mother's age, parity, or duration of heroin intake correlate with the severity of the infant's withdrawal.[50] Likewise, control of the environment to reduce the amount of light or noise in the nursery does not improve the severity of withdrawal.[50] Because adults undergoing withdrawal experience abdominal cramps, palpitation, nausea, and other discomforts, it is possible that the same discomforts also are experienced by the infant, which may abolish any potential benefits from stimuli (light or noise) reduction in the nursery. It also has been shown in infants withdrawing from methadone that the severity of the infant's withdrawal correlates significantly with the methadone dose of the mother.[50] Neonatal withdrawal tends to be more intense if the mother was on 20 milligrams or more of methadone per day before delivery.

After birth, the infant of a drug-dependent mother should be observed closely for withdrawal and for the possibility of treatment with drugs. However, only 25% of infants who exhibit withdrawal will need drug treatment.[57] The rest are managed conservatively with success. This includes swaddling the infant, placing it in a prone position, and cuddling it more often. Swaddling, particularly with the infant's extremities flexed and hands placed before its mouth, enhances the infant's hand-to-mouth facility, which is soothing. A similar soothing action can be achieved with a pacifier.

The frequency of diarrhea and vomiting should be noted and the infant's weight checked at least every 8 hours. The temperature, heart rate, and respiratory rate should be taken every 4 hours. Laboratory examinations to detect serum electrolyte or pH imbalance should be done, as indicated.

The severity of the withdrawal can be assessed clinically by several scoring systems.[25,42,49] One of these[49] evaluates the infant's need for drug treatment and focuses on manifestations of withdrawal that are life threatening—for example, irritability, tremors (convulsion), weight loss, vomiting, diarrhea, and tachypnea (Table 50-1).

SUPPORTIVE TREATMENT OF DRUG WITHDRAWAL

The care of drug withdrawal in the neonate primarily is supportive. Appropriate measures include swaddling to decrease sensory stimulation and frequent small feedings of hypercaloric (24 cal/oz) formula to supply the additional caloric requirements, as well as observation of sleeping habits, temperature stability, weight gain loss, and change in clinical status that might suggest another disease process. Daily caloric intake should provide the 150 to 250 cal/kg required for proper growth in neonates suffering withdrawal.[2]

PHARMACOLOGICAL TREATMENT OF DRUG WITHDRAWAL

The decision to use pharmacological agents to treat withdrawal is based on the assessment of the severity of withdrawal. In the system of clinical assessment shown in Table 50-1, drugs are used to treat withdrawal if there is present any severe criterion or moderate degree of vomiting, diarrhea, or weight loss.

The drugs that are used to treat drug withdrawal in the infant are listed in Table 50-2. As a rule, drug selection should match the class of agent withdrawn. Thus, for opioid withdrawal, narcotics are the drugs of choice, whereas for nonnarcotic withdrawal, nonnarcotic hypnosedatives (e.g., phenobarbital) are preferred. Although the neurological manifestations of narcotic withdrawal may be controlled successfully by a nonnarcotic agent, the alleviation of other, non-CNS manifestations of withdrawal (e.g., diarrhea) are treated more effectively with narcotics.

Paregoric, a tincture of opium (laudanum) and methadone, are the narcotics used most commonly to treat neonatal opiate withdrawal. However, the use of paregoric has declined with recognition of the potential toxic effects of some of its ingredients.[2] Besides camphor, a potent CNS stimulant, par-

Table 50-1 Assessment of the Clinical Severity of Neonatal Drug Withdrawal Syndrome

	Mild	Moderate	Severe
Vomiting	Spitting up	Extensive vomiting for 3 successive feedings	Vomiting associated with imbalance of serum electrolytes
Diarrhea	Watery stools <4 times/day	Watery stools 5-6 times/day for 3 days; no electrolyte imbalance	Diarrhea associated with imbalance of serum electrolytes
Weight loss	<10% of birth weight	10%-15% of birth weight	>15%
Irritability	Minimal	Marked, but relieved by cuddling or feeding	Unrelieved by cuddling or feeding
Tremors or twitching	Mild tremors when stimulated	Marked tremors or twitching when stimulated	Convulsions
Tachypnea	60-80/min	80-100/min	>100/min and associated with respiratory alkalosis

From Ostrea EM: Infants of drug-dependent mothers. In Burg FD, Ingelfinger JR, Wald ER, editors: *Gellis & Kagan's current pediatric therapy,* vol 14, Philadelphia, 1993, WB Saunders. Reprinted with permission.

Table 50-2 Common Drugs Used to Treat Neonatal Drug Withdrawal Syndrome

Drugs	Dosage
Narcotics	
Paregoric	3-6 drops every 4-6 hr, po
Laudanum (0.4%)	3-6 drops every 4-6 hr, po
Methadone	0.05-0.1 mg/kg every 6 hr, po Increase dose by 0.05 mg/kg until withdrawal signs are controlled
Nonnarcotics	
Phenobarbital	3-6 mg/kg/day in divided doses, every 6 hr, po
Chlorpromazine	2-3 mg/kg/day in divided doses every 6 hr, po

egoric contains isoquinolone derivatives (noscapine and papaverine), which are antispasmodics. It also contains a high concentration of ethanol (44% to 46%), a CNS depressant, and anise oil, which may cause habituation. Laudanum is the preferred drug for neonatal narcotic withdrawal. *Caution:* Laudanum, USP is available only as a 10% solution that contains 1.0% morphine. Laudanum must first be diluted twenty-fivefold to a concentration of 0.4% to reduce its morphine content. At this dilution, the recommended initial dose of 0.4% laudanum is 2 drops/kg (0.1 ml/kg) with feedings every 4 hours. The dose may be increased by 2 drops/kg every 4 hours as needed to control withdrawal. After the infant has stabilized for 3 to 5 days, the dose should be decreased gradually without altering the frequency of administration. Marked decreases in dosage or abrupt discontinuance of the drug should be avoided for risk of relapse.

If methadone is used, initial doses of 0.05 to 0.1 mg/kg may be given every 6 hours, with increases of 0.05 mg/kg until withdrawal signs are controlled. Thereafter, methadone may be given every 12 to 24 hours and discontinued after weaning to a daily dose of 0.05 mg/kg per day.[3]

Nonnarcotic hypnosedatives are used to treat neonatal withdrawal from nonnarcotic drugs (Table 50-2). The drugs that are used commonly are phenobarbital and chlorpromazine. Barbiturates can be used to treat withdrawal from nonbarbiturates (including alcohol) or vice versa. Although chlorpromazine is not a nonnarcotic hypnosedative, its ability to treat withdrawal may be due to its ability to suppress REM sleep, which is exaggerated during withdrawal.[16] Diazepam has not been used commonly, because of reported side effects such as bradycardia and respiratory depression.

During the treatment of withdrawal, attention also should focus on the nutrition and fluid and electrolyte balance of the infant, particularly if vomiting, diarrhea, hyperpyrexia, and hyperhidrosis are present. Appropriate intravenous fluids may be required to correct deficits or prevent the occurrence of imbalances.

The aim of treatment with drugs is to render the infant comfortable, but not obtunded. Thus, the drug should be titrated, starting with the smallest recommended dose and increased accordingly, until the desired effect is achieved. Once the infant has become asymptomatic for 3 to 5 days, the drug can be slowly tapered in dose until completely discontinued. The total detoxification period can last for 2 to 3 weeks. After discontinuance of the drug, the infant should be observed for a day or two for possible recurrence of the withdrawal (rebound phenomenon). Once the infant is discharged from the nursery, the mother should be informed that some mild jitteriness and irritability may still persist for as long as 8 to 16 weeks.

Neonatal abstinence syndrome can occur as well in infants who receive narcotics for analgesia or sedation (iatrogenic neonatal abstinence syndrome). The guidelines for effective weaning of infants from opioids are not well established. It is recommended that all patients in the neonatal intensive care unit who have received opioids for more than 3 to 5 days be systematically weaned from the opioid while being regularly evaluated for signs of withdrawal.[26]

COMPLICATIONS

The complications in neonatal drug withdrawal are related to the severity of the withdrawal. Biochemical aberrations in the serum electrolytes and pH and dehydration may occur secondary to vomiting and diarrhea. Weight loss may be profound not only because of excess fluid losses but also because of poor oral intake. Aspiration pneumonia may occur secondary to vomiting and to incoordinate sucking and swallowing. Respiratory alkalosis can occur because of tachypnea. Convulsions may be present and are observed more frequently in withdrawal from nonnarcotic drugs. The use of naloxone in the delivery room is contraindicated in infants whose mothers are known to be opioid-dependent. Administration of naloxone may result in neonatal seizures because of abrupt drug withdrawal.[5] However, in the absence of a specific history of opioid abuse, naloxone treatment remains a reasonable option in the delivery room management of a depressed infant whose mother recently has received a narcotic. However, the physician should be prepared to treat withdrawal in the delivery room.

OTHER SUPPORTIVE MEASURES

The addicted woman has some serious impediments to a successful mothering role. She has meager past mothering experience on which to rely; often there is little or no support from a father or husband, because she frequently is single, and finally, the neurobehavioral abnormalities and withdrawal in her infant prevent gratifying feedback that she wishes to experience with her infant. Thus, the mother and child should have early and repeated contacts. Staff personnel also should have repeated contacts with the mother to discuss the infant's condition and to assure her that with control of withdrawal manifestations, the infant will feed more vigorously and respond better to maternal ministrations.

Should there be plans to place the infant in foster care, the infant will need, in the interim, human contact and should receive stimulation through regular handling and fondling by staff professionals.

BREAST-FEEDING

Most drugs taken by the mother will cross into her breast milk. The concentration of illicit drug(s) in the breast milk will depend on the amount and time of drug intake by the mother. There also is the danger of transmission of the human immunodeficiency virus (HIV) through the breast milk; thus, breast-feeding is not recommended in a mother who is HIV positive.[47]

For the infant whose mother has continued to use illicit substances throughout pregnancy, breast-feeding is likely to be unsafe. For the woman who is in treatment for substance abuse and who is abstinent at the time of delivery, postpartum breast-feeding support, close monitoring of the mother for relapse and of the infant for adequate weight gain, as well as frank discussions concerning the risks posed by exposure to illicit substances through breast milk are essential.[34]

Methadone treatment in the mother is compatible with breast-feeding; no adverse effects have been reported in nursing infants when the mother is on a methadone dose of 20 mg/day or less.[6,14] The suggestion has been made that the mother should take the dose of methadone after the evening feeding and that she supplement breast-feeding with a bottle at the next feeding.[40] Moderate use of alcohol, cigarettes, or caffeine is compatible with breast-feeding.

DECISIONS REGARDING THE INFANT'S CAREGIVER

The ability of the drug-addicted woman to provide adequate care for her infant has often been questioned. Frequently, these women are denied their rights and responsibility to care for their infants based on an unstable home and lifestyle and emotional and psychological weaknesses. Current evidence suggests that this practice may be counterproductive. A study that determined the outcome of such infants based on the type of caregiver[12] showed that the outcome (growth, development, and frequency of medical illnesses and child abuse) of infants cared for by their own mother with the help of a caregiver (either a husband or relative) was better than in foster care. Thus, with appropriate guidance and supervision and the presence of a supportive person, the addicted mother is capable of providing adequate care for her infant, particularly if she is highly motivated. Although a high incidence of medical problems suggestive of child abuse (cigarette burns or hematoma) has been observed in infants born to drug-dependent mothers, these have occurred in situations in which the infant was cared for exclusively by the mother, and very few occurred in infants whose mothers had help available. Thus, it is important that a support person be available at home to help the mother in the care of her infant and to prevent child abuse or neglect.

SOCIAL/PROTECTIVE SERVICE REFERRAL AND FOLLOW-UP

All infants of drug-dependent mothers should have a social service referral to assess the adequacy of parenting and care of the infant at home. The discharge of the infant to the mother's care, with the help of a support person, is the primary objective, unless serious conditions dictate otherwise. The discharge of the infant to a person other than the mother (foster parent) or an agency should be attempted only when it is apparent that the infant will be neglected, poorly cared for, or abused. Most mothers hesitate to admit to drug use during pregnancy because of fear that their infants will be taken away from them. They should be assured otherwise; in fact, they should be encouraged to be responsible for the primary care of their infant. The social worker and physician also should advise the mother regarding the availability of medical and social services in the community, including substance abuse counseling and family planning.

As part of child protection laws operative in many states, infants born to drug-dependent mothers are considered as potentially abused and are required by law to be reported to a child protection agency. The agency usually requires a positive drug screen in the infant before any action can be taken to separate the mother and infant. Maternal admission to the use of illicit drugs during pregnancy is not sufficient to generate the child protection agency referral, because the mother subsequently can deny her admission. The precautionary measures in the referral are helpful when the intent is to ensure the adequacy of care of the infant at home. But, when punitive measures are taken against the mother, the referral can become counterproductive.

The infant of the drug-dependent mother is at risk for many long-term problems. These include child abuse and delay in physical, mental, and motor development, as well as learning disabilities. The infant also is at risk for ongoing exposure to illicit drugs in the household, as a result of accidental ingestion or passive exposure, particularly to crack cocaine. Follow-up of these infants should be planned, not only to assess their medical well-being but also to ascertain the occurrence of such complications and to initiate appropriate interventions.

REFERENCES

1. Aghajanian GK: Tolerance to locus coeruleus neurons to morphine and suppression of withdrawal response by clonidine, *Nature* 276:186, 1978.
2. American Academy of Pediatrics and Committee on Drugs: Neonatal drug withdrawal, *Pediatrics* 101:1079, 1998.
3. Anand KJ, Arnold JH: Opioid tolerance and dependence in infants and children, *Crit Care Med* 22:334, 1994.
4. Athinarayanan P, et al: Chlordiazepoxide withdrawal in the neonate, *Am J Obstet Gynecol* 124:212, 1976.
5. Bloom RS, Cropley C: *Textbook of neonatal resuscitation,* Elk Grove Village, Ill, 1990, American Heart Association/American Academy of Pediatrics.
6. Briggs GG, Freeman RK, Yaffe SJ: Methadone. In Mitchell CW, editor: *Drugs in pregnancy and lactation,* Baltimore, 1994, Williams and Wilkins.
7. Butler NR, Goldstein H: Smoking in pregnancy and subsequent child development, *Br Med J* 4:573, 1973.
8. Chasnoff IJ, et al: Phencyclidine: effects on the fetus and neonate, *Dev Pharmacol Ther* 6:404, 1983.
9. Chasnoff IJ, Hatcher R, Burns WJ: Polydrug and methadone addicted newborns: a continuum of impairment, *Pediatrics* 70:210, 1982.
10. Chasnoff IJ, et al: Perinatal cerebral infarction and maternal cocaine use, *J Pediatr* 108:456, 1986.
11. Chavez CJ, et al: Sudden infant death syndrome among infants of drug-dependent mothers, *J Pediatr* 95:407, 1979.
12. Chavez CJ, Ostrea EM: Outcome of infants of drug-dependent mothers based on the type of caregiver, *Pediatr Res* 11:375A, 1977.
13. Coles CD, et al: Neonatal ethanol withdrawal: characteristics in clinically normal, nondysmorphic neonates, *J Pediatr* 105:445, 1984.
14. Committee on drugs and the American Academy of Pediatrics: The transfer of drugs and other chemicals into human milk, *Pediatrics* 93: 137, 1994.

15. Desmond MM, et al: Maternal barbiturate utilization and neonatal withdrawal symptomatology, *J Pediatr* 80:190, 1972.
16. Dinges DF, Davis MM, Glass P: Fetal exposure to narcotics: neonatal sleep as a measure of nervous system disturbance, *Science* 209:619, 1980.
17. Doberczak TM, Kandall SR, Friedmann P: Relationship between maternal methadone dosage, maternal-neonatal methadone levels, and neonatal withdrawal, *Obstet Gynecol* 81:936, 1993.
18. Doberczak TM, Kandall SR, Wilets I: Neonatal opiate abstinence syndrome in term and preterm infants, *J Pediatr* 118:933, 1991.
19. Doberczak TM, et al: Neonatal neurologic and electroencephalographic effects of intrauterine cocaine exposure, *J Pediatr* 133:354, 1988.
20. Dube SK, et al: Urinary catecholamines, plasma renin activity and blood pressure in newborns: effects of narcotic withdrawal, *Dev Pharm Ther* 3: 83, 1981.
21. Dunn HG, et al: Maternal cigarette smoking during pregnancy and the child's subsequent development. II. Neurological and intellectual maturation to the age of 6.5 years, *Can J Public Health* 68:43, 1977.
22. Eggermont E: The adverse influence of imipramine on the adaptation of the newborn infant to extrauterine life, *Acta Pediatr Belg* 26:197, 1972.
23. Eisen LN, et al: Perinatal cocaine effects on neonatal stress behavior and performance on the Brazelton Scale, *Pediatrics* 88:477, 1991.
24. Erkkola R, Kangas L, Pekkarinen A: The transfer of diazepam across the placenta during labour, *Acta Obstet Gynecol Scand* 52:167, 1973.
25. Finnegan LP: Neonatal abstinence. In Nelson NM, editor: *Current therapy in neonatal-perinatal medicine,* Philadelphia, 1990, BC Decker.
26. Franck L, Vilardi J: Assessment and management of opioid withdrawal in ill neonates, *Neonatal Network* 14:39, 1995.
27. Fried PA: Marijuana use during pregnancy: consequences for the offspring, *Sem Perinatol* 15:280, 1991.
28. Fulroth R, Phillips B, Durand D: Perinatal outcome of infants exposed to cocaine and/or heroin in utero, *Am J Dis Child* 143:905, 1989.
29. Gingras JL, et al: Maternal polydrug use including cocaine and postnatal infant sleep architecture: preliminary observations and implications for respiratory control and behavior, *Early Hum Dev* 43:197, 1995.
30. Glass L, et al: Effect of heroin withdrawal on respiratory rate and acid-base status of the newborn, *N Engl J Med* 286:746, 1972.
31. Golden NL, Kuhnert BR, Sokol RJ, et al: Neonatal manifestations of maternal phencyclidine exposure, *J Perinat Med* 15:185, 1987.
32. Hayes JS, Dreher MC, Nugent JK: Newborn outcomes with maternal marihuana use in Jamaican women, *Pediatr Nurs* 14:107, 1988.
33. Hill RM, Desmond MM, Kay JL: Extrapyramidal dysfunction in an infant of a schizophrenic mother, *J Pediatr* 69:589, 1966.
34. Howard C, Lawrence R: Breastfeeding and drug exposure, *Obstet Gynecol Clin North Am* 25:195, 1998.
35. Isbell H: Addiction to barbiturates and the barbiturate abstinence syndrome, *Ann Intern Med* 33:108, 1950.
36. Jalling B, et al: Disappearance from the newborn of circulating prenatally administered phenobarbital, *Eur J Clin Pharmacol* 6:234, 1973.
37. Kandall SR, Gartner LM: Late presentation of drug withdrawal symptoms in newborns, *Am J Dis Child* 127:58, 1974.
38. Kaufman KR, et al: Phencyclidine in umbilical cord blood: preliminary data, *Am J Psychiatry* 140:450, 1983.
39. Kron R, et al: Neonatal narcotic abstinence: effects of pharmacotherapeutic agents and maternal drug usage on nutritive sucking behavior, *J Pediatr* 88:637, 1976.
40. Lawrence RA: *Breastfeeding: a guide for the medical profession,* ed 4, St. Louis, 1994, Mosby.
41. Levy W, Wisniewski K: Chlorpromazine causing extrapyramidal dysfunction in newborn infant of psychotic mother, *N Y State J Med* 74:684, 1974.
42. Lipsitz PJ: A proposed narcotic withdrawal score for use with newborn infants, *Clin Pediatr* 14:592, 1975.
43. MacGregor SN, et al: Cocaine use during pregnancy: adverse perinatal outcome, *Am J Obstet Gynecol* 157:686, 1987.
44. Mayes LC, et al: Neurobehavioral profiles of neonates exposed to cocaine prenatally, *Pediatrics* 91:778, 1993.
45. Mirochnick M, et al: Elevated plasma norepinephrine after in utero exposure to cocaine and marijuana, *Pediatrics* 99:555, 1997.
46. Neerhof M, et al: Cocaine abuse during pregnancy: peripartum prevalence and perinatal outcome, *Am J Obstet Gynecol* 161:633, 1989.
47. Oleske J, et al: Immune deficiency syndrome in children, *JAMA* 249: 2345, 1983.
48. Oro AS, Dixon SD: Perinatal cocaine and methamphetamine exposure: maternal and neonatal correlates, *J Pediatr* 111:571, 1987.
49. Ostrea EM: Infants of drug dependent mothers. In Berg FD, Ingelfinger JR, Wald ER, editors: *Current pediatric therapy,* Philadelphia, 1993, WB Saunders.
50. Ostrea EM, Chavez CJ: Perinatal problems (excluding neonatal withdrawal) in maternal drug addiction: a study of 830 cases, *J Pediatr* 94:292, 1979.
51. Ostrea EM, Subramanian MG, Abel EL: Placental transfer of cannabinoids in humans: comparison between meconium, maternal and cord blood sera. In Chesner G, Consroe P, Musty R, editors: *Marijuana: an international research report: proceedings of the Melbourne Symposium on Cannabis,* Series 7. Canberra, 1987, Australian Government Publishing Service.
52. Ostrea EM, et al: Drug screening of meconium in infants of drug-dependent mothers: an alternative to urine testing, *J Pediatr* 115:474, 1989.
53. Ostrea EM, et al: Drug screening of newborn infants by meconium analysis: a large-scale prospective epidemiologic study, *Pediatrics* 89: 107, 1992.
54. Ostrea EM, et al: Meconium analysis to assess fetal exposure to active and passive maternal smoking, *J Pediatr* 15:474, 1994.
55. Ostrea EM, et al: The effect of chronic maternal drug addiction on placental drug (xenobiotic) metabolism, *Dev Pharmacol Ther* 12:42, 1989.
56. Ostrea EM Jr: Neonatal withdrawal from intrauterine exposure to butalbital, *Am J Obstet Gynecol* 143:597, 1982.
57. Ostrea EM Jr, Chavez CJ, Strauss ME: A study of factors that influence the severity of neonatal narcotic withdrawal, *J Pediatr* 88:642, 1976.
58. Ostrea EM Jr, et al: Abnormal heart rate tracings and serum creatine phosphokinase in addicted neonates, *Neurotoxicol Teratol* 9:305, 1987.
59. Pietrantoni M, Knuppel RA: Alcohol in pregnancy, *Clin Perinatol* 18: 93, 1991.
60. Pinto F, et al: Sleep in babies born to chronically heroin-addicted mothers: a follow-up study, *Drug Alcohol Depend* 21:43, 1988.
61. Ploman L, Persson BH: On the transfer of barbiturates to the human fetus and their accumulation in some of its vital organs, *J Obstet Gynecol Br Empire* 64:706, 1957.
62. Rahbar F, et al: Impact of intrauterine exposure to phencyclidine (PCP) and cocaine on neonates, *J Natl Med Assoc* 85:349, 1993.
63. Ramer CM: The case history of an infant born to an amphetamine-addicted mother, *Clin Pediatr* 13:596, 1974.
64. Reddy A, Harper R, Stern G: Observations on heroin and methadone withdrawal in the newborn, *Pediatrics* 48:353, 1971.
65. Rementeria JL, Bhatt K: Withdrawal symptoms in neonates from intrauterine exposure to diazepam, *J Pediatr* 90:123, 1977.
66. Richardson GA, Day NL, Taylor P: The effect of prenatal alcohol, marijuana and tobacco exposure on neonatal behavior, *Infant Behav Dev* 12:199, 1989.
67. Robe LB, Gromisch DS, Iosub S: Symptoms of neonatal ethanol withdrawal, *Curr Alcohol* 8:485, 1981.
68. Rosen TS, Johnson HL: Children of methadone-maintained mothers: follow-up to 18 months of age, *J Pediatr* 101:192, 1982.
69. Ryan RM, et al: Meconium analysis for improved identification of infants exposed to cocaine in utero, *J Pediatr* 125:435, 1994.
70. Saxton DW: The behavior of infants whose mothers smoke in pregnancy, *Early Hum Dev* 2:363, 1978.
71. Scafidi FA, et al: Cocaine-exposed preterm neonates show behavioral and hormonal differences, *Pediatrics* 97:851, 1996.
72. Scher MS, et al: The effects of prenatal alcohol and marijuana exposure: disturbances in neonatal sleep cycling and arousal, *Pediatr Res* 24:101, 1988.
73. Sharpless SK: The barbiturates. In Goodman LS, Gilman A, editors: *The pharmacological basis of therapeutics,* London, 1970, MacMillan.

74. Silvestri JM, et al: Effect of prenatal cocaine on respiration, heart rate, and sudden infant death syndrome, *Pediatr Pulmonol* 11:328, 1991.
75. Stothers J: Lithium toxicity in the newborn, *Br Med J* 3:233, 1973.
76. Strauss AA, Modaniou D, Bosu SK: Neonatal manifestations of maternal phencyclidine (PCP) abuse, *Pediatrics* 68:550, 1981.
77. Substance Abuse and Mental Health Services Administration (1997a) National Household Survey on Drug Abuse: *Main findings 1995,* DHHS Pub No (SMA) 95-3127, Washington, DC, US Government Printing Office.
78. Tenenbein M, et al: Neonatal withdrawal from maternal volatile substance abuse, *Arch Dis Child* 74:F204, 1996.
79. Volpe JJ: Teratogenic effects of drugs and passive addiction. In Volpe JJ, editor: *Neurology of the newborn,* ed 3, Philadelphia, 1995, WB Saunders.
80. Ward SL, Schuetz S, Wachsman L: Elevated plasma norepinephrine levels in infants of substance-abusing mothers, *Am J Dis Child* 145:44, 1991.
81. Webster PAC: Withdrawal symptoms in neonates associated with maternal antidepressant therapy, *Lancet* 2:318, 1973.
82. Wilkins-Haug L, Gabow PA: Toluene abuse during pregnancy: obstetric complications and perinatal outcomes, *Obstet Gynecol* 77:504, 1991.
83. Wilson GS: Clinical studies of infants and children exposed prenatally to heroin, *Ann N Y Acad Sci* 562:183, 1989.
84. Wilson GS, et al: The development of preschool children of heroin-addicted mothers: a controlled study, *Pediatrics* 63:135, 1979.
85. Wuster M, Schultz R, Herz A: Opioid tolerance and dependence: re-evaluating the unitary hypothesis, *Trends Pharmacol Sci* 6:64, 1985.
86. Zuckerman B, et al: Effects of maternal marijuana and cocaine use on fetal growth, *N Engl J Med* 320:762, 1989.
87. Zuspan FP, et al: Fetal stress from methadone withdrawal, *Am J Obstet Gynecol* 122:43, 1975.

51 High-Risk Follow-up

Dennis J. Mujsce • Nicholas M. Nelson

Discharge from the neonatal intensive care unit (NICU) does not terminate the problems faced by high-risk infants, their families, medical care professionals, and our society. Although the special needs of seriously ill neonates usually abate during the course of hospitalization, their follow-up home care often remains formidable. These survivors have markedly higher rates of serious illness, rehospitalization, and death in the first years of life than do infants who did not need intensive care. Graduates of neonatal intensive care also are more likely to demonstrate developmental delays, behavioral difficulties, and other significant neurological sequelae. Care of a high-risk infant at home may create large demands on time, energy, and money. Unfortunately, many of these infants are discharged to severely disadvantaged homes, which are poorly equipped to manage a healthy infant, much less one who has such extensive needs.

CHARACTERISTICS OF HIGH-RISK INFANTS

The term *high risk* can be applied appropriately to any infant who experiences an unusual perinatal course, demonstrates a greater than normal likelihood of morbidity or mortality, or requires other than standard newborn care. Recognizing an infant's high-risk status is the important first step toward anticipating defined problems and providing optimal care.

Population

Premature neonates. The cornucopia for high-risk infants is the premature population. Over the past four decades, mortality related to birth weight has been reduced remarkably in this group.[20] In 1960, for newborns weighing fewer than 1500 g, the mortality rate was 70%; for those weighing fewer than 1000 g, it was 90%. By 1985, those figures had been cut to 30% and 50%, respectively.[32] Survival rates for extremely low-birth-weight infants continued to improve during the latter half of the 1980s and the early 1990s. Neonatal intensive care units of this era reported approximately 60% survival of infants who had birth weights between 500 and 800 g and 85% survival of infants weighing 800 to 999 g at birth.[34,37] Unfortunately, the advances in neonatal care that improved these survival rates did not eradicate all of the serious sequelae that handicap NICU survivors. Furthermore, the number of infants born weighing fewer than 1500 g (50,000 annually in the United States) has not declined significantly during the past decade. As a result, larger numbers of both well and handicapped infants from this high-risk population are being seen in follow-up clinics today.

Other neonates. Although premature birth and its attendant complications contribute most heavily to the high-risk pool, numerous other causes of neonatal morbidity and mortality (Box 51-1) are now being treated in the NICU. Indeed, expanded diagnostic and therapeutic capabilities (Box 51-2) allow aggressive management of a growing number of disorders, some of which were once considered fatal. Survivors of these newborn conditions may well have long-term follow-up needs that equal or exceed those of the tiniest premature infants.

Special Needs

Each high-risk infant is an individual who brings a unique mix of problems and needs to the health care system. All these patients require standard well-baby care, but few will move smoothly and quickly through a pediatric office or clinic because they represent extraordinary medical illnesses, treatments, and altered family dynamics that demand considerable time and attention. Physicians who care for high-risk infants, therefore, must be prepared to allocate a disproportionate amount of effort to this minority of patients.

Comprehensive care of these infants often is best accomplished as a team effort involving the follow-up group of the tertiary care center and the infant's own primary care physician. To be effective members of the high-risk follow-up team, however, all health care professionals need to become familiar with many treatments that originally were confined to the hospital. Such therapies now include the administration of supplemental oxygen, home ventilator support, tracheostomy care, gastrostomy and nasogastric tube feedings, intravenous hyperalimentation, peritoneal dialysis, and home apnea monitoring. In addition to such technical forms of therapy, physicians also are called on to stay abreast of the wide range of medications and services now incorporated into outpatient care of high-risk infants. Finally, the physician must understand the disease processes themselves, so that significant changes or deterioration of an infant's condition can be detected and addressed promptly. Perhaps most important, the primary health care professional must recognize subtle impairments of motor development, cognition, and behavior that can appear beyond the neonatal period and affect the infant's quality of life adversely.

BOX 51-1

MAJOR NEONATAL ILLNESSES TREATED IN THE NICU

Sepsis and meningitis
Altered growth and gestation
- Infants of extremely low birth weight (<1000 g) and gestation (<28 weeks)
- Severe intrauterine growth retardation

Pulmonary disorders
- Respiratory distress syndrome (hyaline membrane disease)
- Meconium aspiration syndrome
- Pneumonia
- Congenital diaphragmatic hernia
- Pulmonary hypoplasia

Cardiovascular disorders
- Acyanotic heart diseases (e.g., hypoplastic left-heart syndrome, coarctation of aorta)
- Cyanotic heart disease (e.g., transposition of great arteries, pulmonary atresia)
- Arrhythmias and heart blocks
- Persistent pulmonary hypertension

Renal/genitourinary disorders
- Obstructive uropathy
- Renal dysplasias

Gastrointestinal disorders
- Necrotizing enterocolitis (NEC)
- Biliary atresia
- Malformations (e.g., gastroschisis, omphalocele, bowel atresias, Hirshsprung's disease)

Central nervous system (CNS) disorders
- Developmental anomalies (e.g., hydrocephalus, Arnold-Chiari malformation, neural tube defect)
- Hypoxic-ischemic encephalopathy
- Intracranial hemorrhage
- Seizures

Endocrine disorders and inborn errors of metabolism
Genetic and chromosomal disorders

BOX 51-2

CURRENT NICU TREATMENTS

Diagnostic Modalities
Cardiac catheterization and angiography (heart, blood vessels)
Computed tomography
Magnetic resonance imaging
Nuclear medicine scans (renal, hepatobiliary)
Positron emission tomography (brain)
Real-time and Doppler ultrasonography (brain, heart, abdomen)

Therapeutic Interventions
Medical management
Conventional and high-frequency ventilation
Exogenous surfactant administration
Nitric oxide therapy (pulmonary hypertension)
Cardiovascular drugs
- Vasopressor agents (dopamine, dobutamine, epinephrine)
- Prostaglandin E_1 infusion (to maintain ductus arteriosus patency)
- Indomethacin (to close ductus arteriosus)

Immunoglobulin and antibiotic therapy (infection)
Steroid therapy (bronchopulmonary dysplasia)

Surgical management
Extracorporeal membrane oxygenation (diaphragmatic hernia, pulmonary hypertension)
Cardiopulmonary bypass, hypothermic circulatory arrest (cardiac repair)
Dialysis and hemofiltration (renal failure)
Subspecialty surgical procedures
- Neurosurgical (ventriculoperitoneal shunt, closure neural tube defect)
- Cardiac (repair and palliation of congenital heart defects)
- Gastrointestinal (repair of congenital and acquired disorders)
- Genitourinary (correction of urinary obstruction)
- Otolaryngology (tracheostomy, repair of airway anomalies)

Organ transplantation (biliary atresia)

DISCHARGE PLANNING

Follow-up care begins with discharge planning, one of the least dramatic but most important aspects of the high-risk infant's neonatal hospitalization. Continued success of even the most spectacular NICU story requires a comprehensive plan at the time of discharge that has been developed specifically for each individual infant.

The first step is to identify infants who will benefit from high-risk follow-up. Opinions vary, but Box 51-3 lists some conditions that most agree warrant special attention after discharge. Besides these infants, who can be followed up best by primary care practitioners working cooperatively with high-risk clinics, many neonates who have specific problems (e.g., imperforate anus, congenital heart defects, ventriculoperitoneal shunts) require services now available only in subspecialty clinics at regional medicine centers. Follow-up care for these babies is achieved best through collaboration of the primary care physician and the appropriate subspecialists.

Development of a discharge plan early in the infant's hospitalization helps to ensure that discharge occurs at the appropriate time, that all the infant's needs will be met, and that parental anxiety is kept to a minimum. Parents require a great deal of time and repetition of explanations and instructions to assimilate all the necessary information. Logistical barriers to the exchange of information (e.g., early discharge of the mother and large distances separating the family from the infant in the tertiary care center) make early communication imperative. A truly multidisciplinary plan must be formulated, one based on the opinions of parents and family, social workers, nurses, neonatologists, subspecialists, and the infant's primary care physician. Communication among these groups is achieved best when it is done continuously throughout the neonatal hospitalization and not left to become a last-minute item for discussion before discharge.

A primary goal of discharge planning is to ensure

a smooth transition of the infant's care from the well-staffed, specialized NICU to the home, where adequate support mechanisms have been put in place. A successful discharge plan must outline the support network clearly, must match the infant's needs with appropriate resources, and must define the responsibilities of all follow-up participants precisely. An effective plan is kept as simple as possible to prevent delay, absences, duplication, or fragmentation of necessary services. Sound discharge planning also must provide for continual reevaluation of the plan itself and for alternative measures to be taken in the event of unforeseen emergencies. The timing of the actual discharge will depend on the readiness of the infant, the family, the home, and the follow-up team. Therefore, each component must be assessed thoroughly before discharge.

The majority of contemporary neonatal staffs no longer insist on achievement of a minimum body weight for safe discharge, provided the infant's medical problems have been stabilized and several criteria met.[4] The infant should maintain body temperature competently while in a bassinet, feed regularly by mouth (or gastrostomy tube in selected cases), maintain consistent growth, and breathe regularly without frequent or severe apnea. The mother and other caretakers must demonstrate appropriate care-taking skills, and the home environment must be proved adequate. Implementation of early discharge planning and community-based follow-up services has been shown to reduce the length of NICU hospitalization significantly.[5,27] Recent pressures to reduce health care costs further and provide more services in an ambulatory setting have challenged these "traditional" criteria for discharge of high-risk preterm infants. For example, insurers are investigating the feasibility of managing convalescing premature infants at home, rather than in the NICU or step-down nursery. Care at home might include an incubator to maintain a thermoneutral environment, nasogastric tube feedings, and electronic surveillance of the heart and respiratory rates. Insurance providers are contracting with home nursing agencies to assist the parents in administering care to the infant, to assess the infant's condition, and to provide feedback to the responsible physician. Although the average premature infant is discharged at an adjusted age of 36 to 37 weeks, some NICUs are discharging stable infants routinely as early as 34 weeks corrected gestational age. Increasingly, primary care physicians, the "gatekeepers" of tomorrow's health care system, will be expected to manage these high-risk infants as they are discharged from the NICU, earlier on.

Most NICU patients are discharged directly to the care of their parents, but stable, high-risk infants increasingly are being transferred from distant, tertiary care centers to a local "level II" NICU or nursery near their home for further treatment before being sent home. Proximity to home allows the parents and extended family to bond with the infant, to perform routine care-taking procedures, and to participate in medical management. These internursery transfers reduce health care costs and open NICU beds for new acutely ill patients. In this scenario, the receiving health care professionals must share responsibility for discharge planning with the referring NICU staff.

BOX 51-3

CRITERIA FOR NEONATAL HIGH-RISK FOLLOW-UP PROGRAMS

- Birth weight <1500 g or gestation <28 weeks
- Severe intrauterine growth retardation (birth weight <10% for gestation)
- Persistent pulmonary hypertension requiring nitric oxide or extracorporeal membrane oxygenation
- Bronchopulmonary dysplasia
- Symptomatic perinatal asphyxia, persistently abnormal neurological examination
- Hydrocephalus/microcephaly
- Intracranial hemorrhage/periventricular leukomalacia
- Meningitis and sepsis
- Symptomatic hypoglycemia
- Hyperbilirubinemia requiring exchange transfusion
- Medical management requiring specialized services or insufficient primary care follow-up
- Inadequate home resources to manage without close supervision/intervention

GOALS OF HIGH-RISK FOLLOW-UP

The benefits of a comprehensive follow-up program are important to the health care system, as well as to the patients and families it serves. Longitudinal studies of high-risk patients are the gold standard source for information to guide and gauge the effectiveness of NICU care. Educators, politicians, and policymakers at all levels require such follow-up data to allocate funds and resources based on the special medical and educational needs of NICU graduates. Parents, of course, need the best information available to understand what may lie in store for their child and family and to plan their lives accordingly. Although short-term neonatal mortality and morbidity can be estimated from acute NICU statistics, many effects of neonatal intensive care are appreciated only through the data gathered in long-term follow-up studies. Such effects include later mortality and health problems, incidence of rehospitalization, neurodevelopmental outcome, academic achievement, and quality of life. Longitudinal follow-up of NICU graduates over years also allows caregivers to identify the impact of evolving neonatal therapies and the effects of advancing postneonatal age on high-risk infants. Earlier studies searching for abnormalities that are classically discovered before 2 years of age, such as cerebral palsy, gross developmental delay, and seizures, identified these major sequelae in 10% to 20% of very low-birth-weight (VLBW) infants. Approximately 50% to 60% of the VLBW population may have abnormal outcomes, however, if more subtle problems such as learning disabilities are added to the list of sequelae.[29] Indeed, a significant proportion of infants weighing less than 1000 g at birth (extremely low birth weight [ELBW]) who test normally during infancy demonstrate abnormal neurodevelopment when reassessed in early childhood.[7] Subsequent reports demonstrated a rising incidence of cerebral palsy in VLBW survivors (<1500 g) as neonatal practice was being refined (and more premature infants were surviving) from 1967 to 1985 in Australia,[41] Great Britain,[36] and Sweden.[22] More recent studies show that the incidence of cerebral palsy in extremely premature infants born at 23 to 25 weeks' gestation or weighing fewer than 750 g at birth has stabilized around 10% to 20%. Despite this, the overall rate of disability caused by retardation, behavioral and attention difficulties, poor school performance, and visual impairment appears to have increased as these tiniest infants survived in greater numbers during the past decade.[10,21] Behavioral and academic problems also have been reported in a significant percentage (40% to 50%) of patients who have survived extracorporeal membrane oxygenation without major neurological disabilities.[17] Such findings have obvious implications for those treating pregnant women and neonatal patients, as well as the caretakers and educators of these surviving children.

Although such programs are responsible for our understanding of neonatal outcomes, parents often are reluctant to return with their infants to high-risk follow-up programs for a variety of real or perceived reasons. Examples commonly cited include extra cost, inconvenience, time away from the job, distance between the home and clinic, a previous unpleasant NICU experience, fear of uncovering new abnormalities, and the conviction that the clinic staff benefits more from the visit than does the infant or family. Primary care physicians, concentrating on immediate infant care needs, may unintentionally reinforce the belief that little is to be gained from return visits to the follow-up clinic. Such clinic "dropouts" can skew outcome figures seriously. One report found that only 4.4% of "easy to review" patients were severely disabled; in the "hard to review" group, the figure was 35%![45]

Most medical students and pediatric residents learn about management of acute neonatal problems in the NICU, but few receive sufficient exposure to a structured high-risk follow-up program. They may fail to realize that each critically ill infant is a person who is part of a family, and they may have little understanding of what happens to the infant and family after discharge from the NICU. Most recently graduated pediatricians regard their residency training as their primary source of information about the care of high-risk infants. Therefore, a residency curriculum that encourages and guides house staff in attending a high-risk clinic should produce better prepared pediatricians.

Thriving high-risk infants who are brought to the follow-up clinic for return visits can rejuvenate the morale of NICU personnel, who spend long, stressful hours attending sick infants whose outcome is uncertain. Infants who return with medical or developmental issues, on the other hand, remind the staff that the family's work may begin in earnest when they are discharged from the security of the NICU. Additionally, this forum is a good opportunity to review instructions, dispel misconceptions, and address the new questions that invariably crop up once the parents have brought their infant home.

ORGANIZATION OF HIGH-RISK FOLLOW-UP

In some clinics, the neonatologists and other staff who cared for the infants in the NICU maintain a strong presence in the follow-up program; in other facilities, outpatients are "transitioned" to teams that specialize in high-risk follow-up. When an organized neonatal follow-up program is not available, the infant is discharged from the NICU directly to his or her primary care physician without scheduled high-risk follow-up. Thus, primary care physicians should be aware of any local public health, community, and ancillary health services available (Box 51-4) and should use them to the benefit of their high-risk patients.

Successful strategies for high-risk follow-up all have several elements in common. First, each infant has an individual discharge plan specifically tailored to provide routine pediatric care while attending to his or her particular needs. Second, continuity of care is maintained when the infant is discharged home and different people assume new roles in the infant's ongoing care. Third, all those participating in the follow-up plan make sure that the other team members are kept up to date. Each must understand his or her role and who holds coordinating responsibility for the infant's care.

The Neonatal Intensive Care Unit

Because the NICU staff has weeks or months to become familiar with the infants it manages, it generally is in the best position to identify the patient's needs, initiate discharge planning, and ensure that the required components of the follow-up team are in place. Responsibility for identifying an infant as being at high risk is assumed by the infant's primary nurse, the neonatologist, a discharge planner, or a neonatal follow-up coordinator. High-risk infants are identified as quickly as possible, and the benefits and logistics of the comprehensive follow-up program are discussed with the parents. Early discussion with the parents is essential, for it allows them to contribute to and understand the objectives of the follow-up plan.

As the day of discharge from the NICU approaches, neo-

BOX 51-4

RESOURCES AVAILABLE TO FAMILIES OF HIGH-RISK INFANTS

Ancillary Health Care Services
Dietitians and nutrition specialists
Home health equipment and services vendors
Home nursing services
Physical, occupational, and hearing and speech therapy
Social services

Community Resources
Churches and religious organizations
Community health nurses
Departments of public health
County and state financial support programs
Early intervention programs
Hospice and respite services
Parental support groups
Schools and special educational programs
Specialized foster care parents

Family Support Network
Extended family
Significant friends

natal staff members must be satisfied that the infant's condition is stable and that the family is capable of assuming his or her care. Any major medical problems either should have been resolved or stabilized. Medication regimens should be rechecked to determine that each has been simplified to the extent possible, that all dosages are correct, that the parents have obtained the necessary medications and can administer them capably, and that adverse reactions or side effects have been explained to the parents. The final days of hospitalization also provide time to ensure that all necessary testing has been completed (e.g., hematocrit and other appropriate laboratory testing, hearing screening, ophthalmological examination for retinopathy of prematurity, head ultrasonography, and state-mandated or optional newborn metabolic screening). The infant's medical history is reviewed with family members, their questions are answered, and any residual concerns are addressed. Parents require a clear understanding of any issues or areas of concern at this point, but it also is helpful to highlight positive aspects of the infant's progress and to be reassuring when possible.

Unfortunately, evidence persists that when many infants leave the NICU, their parents do not have a good understanding of what has transpired or of what they can expect. The primary care physician also sometimes is placed at a disadvantage because he or she has not received timely telephone updates from the NICU staff, nor appropriate written documentation such as a concise narrative summary of the NICU hospitalization. Even with the practitioner's busy schedule, the telephone (and electronic mail) can be invaluable tools for exchanging information. Such a call allows each party to participate in discharge planning and to discuss issues of concern; it also provides an opportunity to update the primary care physician on new treatments, fosters a feeling of collaboration, and encourages future discussion. Despite the availability of such avenues of communication, 55% of pediatricians in one survey believed that they had been inadequately informed about the NICU discharge status of their high-risk patients before the first office visit.[25]

High-Risk Follow-up Programs

High-risk neonatal follow-up clinics are not meant to provide primary care or in any way to replace the community physician. Indeed, most high-risk clinics prefer to work in conjunction with the infant's primary care physician, assisting wherever possible and offering supplemental services. A typical neonatal high-risk follow-up schedule might include an initial visit 2 to 6 weeks after the infant's discharge, followed by visits at 6 months, 1 year, and 2 years of age. Fewer programs follow NICU graduates beyond this age, but it is becoming increasingly important to track the outcomes of these children as they become a growing constituency of the school-age population. The strengths of a neonatal high-risk clinic include its multidisciplinary composition and its links to other health care resources. During a clinic visit an infant may be evaluated by any combination of the following: neonatologists, nurses, nutritionists, physical therapists, social workers, developmental specialists, and child psychologists. Using this team of experts allows a look beyond the child's more immediate medical problems to such long-range issues as infant development and behavior, family stresses, and financial problems.

Subspecialty Clinics

Among the services neonatal patients and their illnesses attract into the NICU are cardiology, neurology, endocrinology, genetics, hematology, surgery, orthopedics, urology, cardiothoracic surgery, neurosurgery, otolaryngology, and ophthalmology. Dietitians, physical therapists, audiologists, nurses specializing in wound care, and many others also participate in the care of NICU patients. The neonatal high-risk follow-up clinic is a natural coordinating center for the efforts of these individuals and their communication with the primary care physician and parents. It is extraordinarily beneficial to the family when follow-up care can occur in single rather than multiple visits.

Ancillary Health Services

A number of nonphysician personnel can enhance, considerably, the care given high-risk infants in the NICU and in their homes.

Neonatal nurses, who bond with the infants they care for day after day, develop relationships with the families that persist beyond the day of discharge. Social workers are consulted frequently in the NICU, because families of high-risk infants often are high risk in nature themselves. Single-parent households, young and uneducated parents, an inadequate home environment, unemployment and financial stress, child abuse and neglect, drug abuse, and other difficulties that have major implications for the well being of discharged infants may exist. These problems often are magnified during the course of NICU hospitalization and can become formidable obstacles during the discharge process.

Physical and occupational therapists and feeding specialists strengthen follow-up and enhance the quality of life for high-risk infants. Physicians may rely on therapists to perform serial assessments of gross and fine motor development, reflexes, muscle tone, strength, range of motion, posture, ambulation, feeding abilities, phonation, and adaptational skills. After a thorough evaluation, these therapists are able to counsel parents and physicians, suggest management strategies, and instruct parents in how to perform specific therapies at home. As treatment proceeds, the therapists should participate in the reevaluation of both the patient and the treatment.

Commercial home health care companies are burgeoning, and all physicians need to be familiar with and use them. They supply a wide range of services and home health care equipment that are especially appropriate for high-risk infants. Examples of such home resources include intravenous nutrition and medications, feeding tubes, home oxygen supplies, ventilators, pulse oximeters, apnea monitors, and suction machines. The use of any home equipment must be explained to parents, who must be instructed in its use, and must be backed by 24-hour maintenance and service. These companies also must employ professionals who have experience in pediatrics who can go into the home and participate in physical assessment of the infant and parental education at the physician's direction. These companies rely on physician referrals and usually are conscientious about reporting problems within the home or changes in the infant's condition. Thus, they can serve as an essential local link of expertise between the high-risk follow-up staff and the primary care physician.

Community Resources and Public Health Services

A comprehensive review of all community resources and public health services is beyond the scope of this chapter, but knowledge of regionally available programs will assist the physician in the management of high-risk infants. Such programs include visits from community health nurses or special services for children, special educational programs, early intervention programs with evaluation and rehabilitation, respite or hospice care, and financial assistance for food, supplies, and medical needs. In considering community resources, the physician should not neglect friends, relatives, parental support groups, and individuals who are of religious or social significance to the family. Foster care families that specialize in the care of medically complex children can occasionally act as a bridge between the NICU and placement in a more permanent home. Physicians should learn to take advantage of these types of resources because they can affect the immediate health and long-term development of their patients significantly.

Parents of High-Risk Infants

By necessity, the parents of a high-risk infant become immediate members of the follow-up team. These are the people with the heaviest emotional investment in their baby; ultimately, they will assume the greatest share of the caretaking responsibilities. A major prerequisite for adequate parenting (sadly, not always satisfied) is that the parents have a genuine interest in the infant and his or her well being. Once it is established that this basic requirement has been fulfilled, the neonatal staff must begin the rigorous preparation that these parents need.

During the hospitalization, the parents should have developed a reasonable idea of their infant's illnesses, symptoms, treatments, and prognoses. This information provides the groundwork for the observational skills the parents will use in the home to monitor their infant's medical condition. Because they will have the most extensive contact with the baby, the parents must be capable of detecting any deterioration or significant alteration in their infant's health and bringing these findings to medical attention. Parents who will be expected to administer medications must demonstrate understanding and competence regarding dosages, timing, routes of administration, adverse effects, and precautions. Parents of infants who are discharged with special equipment (e.g., nasal cannula oxygen and home apnea monitors) must be completely and explicitly schooled in their use. They also must understand what to do and whom to notify when malfunctions occur.

Parents often are required to learn certain basic or even "high-tech" nursing functions, as well as cardiopulmonary resuscitation. Nonetheless, time spent demonstrating how to feed, bathe, dress, and simply enjoy their baby will enhance the quality of care rendered and boost the parents' self-esteem. The neonatal team also should ascertain whether the parents can procure food, clothing, a car seat, and a crib for their infant and if they have access to a telephone and transportation.

Although these requirements must be fulfilled before an infant is discharged from the NICU, it is equally important to ensure that circumstances do not deteriorate over time after discharge. The primary care physician must assume principal responsibility for continued monitoring of these aspects of the infant's family and home.

The Primary Care Physician

The distribution of high-risk infant survivors is such that any primary care practitioner today can expect to be called upon to manage these infants. Whether that involvement begins during or subsequent to the NICU stay is very much a function of local custom and geography relative to the NICU, as well as the practitioner's interest, training, and available time.

The primary care practitioner often plays a fundamental role in the family's assimilation and translation of the information onslaught presented by personnel encountered in the NICU or subsequent visits to the high-risk follow-up clinic. As the health care clinician who may have known the family before and after the added stress of its high-risk infant, the primary care physician is the natural case manager for this child. Under this circumstance, the practitioner must serve as the link between the family and the NICU and its follow-up staff.

MEDICAL MANAGEMENT OF HIGH-RISK INFANTS

A comprehensive presentation of common and critical neonatal illnesses and treatments is provided in Chapters 48 and 49. The review presented here concentrates on VLBW infants, weighing less than 1500 g, and ELBW infants, weighing less than 1000 g, and their diverse problem lists. When appropriate, the issues pertaining to the management and follow-up of critically ill term infants are addressed.

Primary Health Care Considerations

In addition to monitoring the identified medical problems of high-risk infants, primary care physicians must promote normal growth and development, anticipate normal age-appropriate problems, and educate parents about routine pediatric issues, just as they do with their low-risk patients. For example, the parents should receive anticipatory counseling about preventing injuries, because they may not realize initially that their NICU graduate eventually will encounter the same hazards as other children. In fact, evidence suggests that VLBW survivors are more likely to encounter serious accidental and intentional injury than their full-term counterparts. Likewise, pediatricians need to emphasize that infants must be secured adequately whenever traveling by automobile. All states now enforce seat belt laws, which were meant to prevent the hundreds of deaths and many thousands of injuries suffered by children each year in the United States as the result of automobile accidents. Parents taking VLBW infants home need to know that most infant restraint systems are marketed for babies weighing more than 7 pounds. Some of these devices may be inappropriate for tiny infants because they do not provide enough support of the head and neck when the infant is seated upright. In this scenario, the infant's head may fall forward, causing partial airway obstruction that may be followed by arterial desaturation and bradycardia. Most NICUs now require demonstration that the infant will remain stable in his or her car seat for at least the duration of the longest anticipated drive before discharge occurs. Alternative devices exist that allow for safe automobile transportation of small infants in a recumbent position if they are unstable in a sitting position. Any medical equipment also must be secured; if an apnea monitor has been recommended for the infant, it should function properly during any automobile travel. Helpful guidelines are available from the American Academy of Pediatrics' Committee on Accident and Poison Prevention.

Growth

Growth, an exquisitely sensitive marker of health, must be monitored and documented frequently. Weight, length, and head circumference must be measured and plotted against "adjusted postnatal age" (postnatal age in weeks less the number of weeks the infant was born prematurely) on appropriate growth curves. Although there are specific growth charts for sick, tiny premature infants while they are in the NICU, these generally are not required after an infant is discharged; standard growth charts are suitable. Weight should be plotted against the infant's adjusted postnatal age until 24 months of age, after which time thriving premature infants generally follow the same weight curves as children who were born at term. Significant upward or downward deviations from expected weight gain may indicate excess fluid retention or inadequate caloric intake relative to metabolic demands, respectively. Length should be similarly corrected for prematurity until the infant is 3 years of age; head circumference (as an indicator of brain growth) should be plotted against corrected age until 18 months of age.

Although not entirely predictive, correlation does exist between growth failure and neurodevelopmental delays.[39] Head circumference is a particularly important, but sometimes neglected, growth variable that can help determine the neurodevelopmental prognosis of high-risk infants. Investigators assessing ELBW survivors at 6 years of age noted that these infants had a smaller head circumference than that of a term control group and that microcephaly correlated with functional neurological disabilities.[44] Conversely, achievement of a normal head circumference by 8 months of age is a predictor of normal psychosocial development at age 3 years.[19]

Many premature infants at discharge are smaller than the third growth percentiles for adjusted postnatal age, either because of intrauterine growth retardation or because of serious neonatal illness. "Catch-up growth" should be expected and promoted in most of these infants in the first year of life. Generally, head circumference reaches a normal percentile first, followed by length, and finally by weight. Catch-up growth is maximal between 36 to 44 postconceptual weeks, with most infants beginning to grow along their new growth curve by 6 to 12 months. One small study, however, suggested that ELBW infants exhibit catch-up growth through childhood and adolescence.[24] This desirable finding has not been replicated in other studies of ELBW infants or premature infants who had intrauterine growth restriction, where continued impairments of growth were present at 36 months of age.[12,42,43] Although exceptions exist, significant future catch-up growth should not be anticipated in a premature infant of birth weight appropriate for gestational age who does not achieve at least the third percentile by 3 years of adjusted age.

Nutrition

The American Academy of Pediatrics (AAP) recommends breast milk as the feeding of choice for all infants, including premature infants. To achieve 1800 to 2000 g of body weight, premature infants require calorically dense (24 to 27 Cal/ounce) feedings, which can be achieved with specialized "premature formulas" or (preferably) mother's breast milk fortified by calories, minerals, and vitamins. The AAP's Committee on Infant Nutrition believes that after the infant has attained a weight of 2000 g, breast milk alone is a practical, nutritionally adequate source of nutrition that has immunological properties that may reduce the incidence of respiratory and gastrointestinal infections. Because many growing premature infants who otherwise fulfill discharge criteria still weigh less than 2000 g and are not fully competent at breast-feeding, it is becoming increasingly common to supplement breast-feeding with bottle feedings of calorically dense infant formula at the time of discharge. This supplementation may continue for weeks to months until the infant is thriving and breast-feeding well. Mothers who opt not to breast-feed may use standard infant formula after normal growth has been demonstrated and the baby's weight exceeds 2000 g. Certain infants, such as those who are growing poorly, have severe osteopenia, or whose fluids must be restricted, may benefit from the increased calcium/phosphorus content and caloric density (22 to 24 Cal/ounce) of formula for premature infants until they reach 44 to 48 weeks of postconceptual age. Commercially available 22 Cal/ounce formulas have been designed specifically to support the nutritional needs of growing premature infants during the months following their discharge from the NICU. Breast-fed infants who are well enough to be discharged from the NICU should receive standard amounts of vitamins A, D, and C, with fluoride added. The need for vitamin E supplementation usually diminishes after 6 to 8 weeks of postnatal age, by which time the risk of hemolytic anemia has passed. Despite the osteopenia common to acutely ill premature infants, most ultimately will undergo normal bone development on the usual amounts of calcium and phosphorus found in standard lactose-based infant formulas. Formula-fed premature infants should receive 2 to 3 mg/kg/day of supplemental elemental iron from 6 to 8 weeks of postnatal age until approximately

6 months of age. Some believe that infants whose birth weight is less than 1000 g may benefit from supplementary doses of iron approaching 4 mg/kg/day until they are 1 year old. Finally, dietary advances in premature infants should be based on their actual, rather than "adjusted," postnatal age.

The feeding of high-risk infants should be normalized as much as possible, but there are many qualifying conditions that deserve consideration. Infants who have experienced particularly severe cardiopulmonary difficulties and suboptimal nutrition may be discharged on electrolyte, mineral, or vitamin supplements. Some infants, such as those who have intrauterine growth restriction or bronchopulmonary dysplasia, have such a high metabolic rate that their bodies demand 120 to 150 Cal/kg/day for sustained growth. Ironically, many infants who have the highest caloric requirements also have the misfortune of requiring fluid restriction. In others, a structural or functional short-bowel syndrome (secondary to conditions such as necrotizing enterocolitis, gastroschisis, bowel atresia, malrotation, meconium ileus, or Hirschsprung's disease) can seriously limit enteral caloric intake. Loss of gastrointestinal surface area because of such diseases or their surgical treatment also can limit absorption of other important nutrients, such as vitamins and minerals. In many cases, the amount and composition of the infant's feedings will require continual reevaluation and alteration. Protein, fat, and carbohydrate can be added to breast milk or formula to provide a more calorically dense feeding. Caloric densities as high as 30 Cal/ounce can be achieved, but care must be taken to prevent unwanted gastrointestinal or renal effects as a result of inordinate amounts of any one of these sources of calories. If the infant's enteral diet will not be sufficient to support acceptable growth, intravenous total parenteral nutrition should be instituted. This route for nutrition is quite demanding and usually requires a central venous catheter and occasional laboratory monitoring. More importantly, it demands profound parental commitment, as well as a qualified team responsible for designing and monitoring the nutritional strategy and working with the primary care physician.

Aside from monitoring growth variables, the primary care physician should review details of the infant's feeding habits and monitor for signs of gastroesophageal reflux or other feeding difficulties. Graduates of the unnatural NICU environment who have experienced prolonged periods of nasogastric or endotracheal intubation, as well as insufficient amounts of nonnutritive sucking, can be notoriously difficult feeders. Parents often need much reassurance, coaching, and support in this regard; referral to a qualified feeding specialist or lactation consultant occasionally is indicated. The physician also should inquire about stooling and voiding patterns, because these may be clues to underlying conditions, such as malabsorption or colonic stricture (secondary to previous episodes of necrotizing enterocolitis).

Immunizations

In general, immunization schedules for high-risk premature infants do not differ from those recommended for term infants by the AAP Committee on Infectious Disease. Dosages generally should not be reduced, divided, or delayed to correct for prematurity.[26] Moreover, these recommendations are updated continuously; thus, primary care practitioners must stay abreast of revisions as they occur.

Hepatitis B is common in high-risk pregnancies, and any infant born to a mother who is seropositive for hepatitis B surface antigen (or whose hepatitis B status is unknown) is a candidate for prophylactic therapy. Such infants should receive hepatitis B immunoglobulin intramuscularly within the first 12 hours of life and hepatitis B vaccine intramuscularly within the first day. The hepatitis B vaccine should be repeated at 1 month and again at 6 months. The AAP currently recommends that all infants receive hepatitis B vaccine on the first day of life, at 1 to 2 months of age, and again at 4 to 6 months of age.

Certain chronically ill high-risk infants, such as patients who have bronchopulmonary dysplasia or congestive heart failure, should be vaccinated annually against influenza. In the fall, before the influenza season begins, infants generally are given two doses of split-virus vaccine intramuscularly at least 4 weeks apart. The desired immunological protection is best achieved, however, when vaccination is initiated in infants who are older than 6 months of age.[18]

Recommendations for immunoprophylaxis against respiratory syncytial virus (RSV) have been developed by the AAP Committee on Infectious Diseases and the Committee on Fetus and Newborn for premature infants and those who have chronic lung disease. Immunoprophylaxis against RSV is currently achieved with monthly intramuscular injections of recombinantly produced monoclonal antibody ("Synagis") throughout the RSV season. Before Synagis was available, immunoprophylaxis required monthly intravenous infusions of a human immunoglobulin preparation rich in antibodies against RSV ("RespiGam"). This time-consuming therapy exposed patients to large fluid boluses and human blood products. Although Synagis generally is the preferred method of providing immunity against RSV, RespiGam should be considered in significantly immunocompromised infants who may warrant broader antibody coverage. The AAP recommends protection against RSV with Synagis in the following groups: infants younger than age 2 years who have chronic lung disease and received therapy for their lung disease less than 6 months before RSV season; infants born at or less than 28 weeks' gestation who are younger than 1 year old; infants born at 29 to 32 weeks' gestation who are younger than 6 months old; and infants born at more than 32 weeks who have additional risk factors for RSV (e.g., bronchopulmonary dysplasia and congestive heart failure).

Other Primary Care Issues

As with any other children, pediatricians should screen NICU graduates for common problems such as anemia, lead intoxication, and tuberculosis. Sadly, they also must maintain awareness of the risks of HIV infection, especially among those who have disordered lifestyles. Infant behavior, development, and sleep patterns frequently are areas of intense concern and stress for parents of high-risk infants who had a lengthy stay in an NICU. Finally, all health care professionals must guard against the chronic environmental insults of malnutrition, poor hygiene, abuse, and neglect. High-risk infants appear to be more likely than others to suffer these insults.

Rehospitalization

The path back to the hospital may be well worn during the first year or two after discharge from the NICU: 25% to 50% of VLBW infants will require rehospitalization during their first year of life.[8,13,30] Common reasons for rehospitalization include disorders of growth and nutrition (especially after necrotizing enterocolitis) and surgical procedures such as herniorrhaphies, ventriculoperitoneal shunt revision, and patent ductus arteriosus ligation. Especially wearing are the rehospitalizations during winter for RSV and other respiratory infectious diseases that often plague children receiving home oxygen therapy for residual bronchopulmonary dysplasia. Even when one considers more mature and less critically ill neonatal graduates of community NICUs, these infants demonstrate a 20% higher rehospitalization rate than do healthy term newborns.[11] Rehospitalizations seriously weaken the resolve and decimate the morale of even the most robust family networks; they are considerably more oppressive for the often dysfunctional "nonfamilies" in which many high-risk infants live.

Specific Neonatal Problems

Hearing. The high-risk infant's situation is fraught with opportunities to sustain significant sensorineural hearing loss. Insults that can affect hearing include asphyxia, hyperbilirubinemia, meningitis, and TORCH infections (*T*oxoplasma, *r*ubella, *c*ytomegalovirus, *h*erpes simplex virus), as well as frequent exposure to aminoglycoside antibiotics. The NICU environment itself often can be a loud, unwanted, noxious stimulus during critical periods of development of the premature infant's auditory systems. Moderate to profound hearing loss is two to five times more likely to develop in high-risk infants than in the general population of children. In addition to premature infants and those who experience the conditions just listed, a hearing evaluation is warranted for infants who have craniofacial anomalies or a family history of hearing deficits. The usual behavioral-observational pace of ascertaining whether a child hears is simply too slow to be of much help in this assessment. Accordingly, the development of brainstem auditory evoked response (BAER) testing, an electroencephalographic technique, is especially helpful in meeting the challenge of evaluating infants younger than 6 months of age.[3,31] These examinations usually are performed before the infant is discharged from the NICU, but reassessment may be necessary. The efficacy of universal hearing screening guidelines is being evaluated nationwide. See Chapter 20 (Ten), Auditory Screening.

Vision. The retina of a 23- to 24-week fetus delivered prematurely is essentially devoid of any vascular supply. Orderly vascularization from the optic nerve to the periphery of the retina normally occurs in utero between 25 and 35 weeks' gestation. During an NICU hospitalization, the expected development of these blood vessels can be interrupted by numerous potential insults, including increased ambient light, higher levels of oxygen in circulating blood, and altered metabolism of the retina itself. Instead of branching normally, blood vessels grow in a very disorganized and aggressive fashion, leading to abnormal vascular shunts. The acute form of this process, known as *retinopathy of prematurity* (ROP), is graded in severity from stage I to stage III+. The advanced, end-stage progression of this disorder was seen more commonly decades ago and was referred to as *retrolental fibroplasia* (RLF). The renaming of retrolental fibroplasia to retinopathy of prematurity has served to emphasize that this is more a developmental than an iatrogenic phenomenon. Indeed, as ELBW (<1000 g) infants increasingly survive, their risk for the development of some degree of ROP is about 50%, regardless of the amount of supplemental oxygen needed to treat their pulmonary disease. This risk falls to less than 5% as the birth weight advances beyond 1500 g. The so-called second epidemic of RLF (the original episode occurred during the 1950s) recently reported is attributable to the increasing survival of the ELBW infant who is at maximum developmental risk for ROP.[16] The pathogenesis of ROP is multifactorial, but the greatest risk for this disease remains immaturity of the retinal vascularization.

The current approach to managing ROP is one principally of close ophthalmological surveillance (indirect ophthalmoscopic examination under pupillary dilation by the pediatric ophthalmologist) and early intervention with laser surgery if the disease threatens to advance beyond the reversible early stages to irreversible, cicatricial RLF. Cryosurgery previously was the therapy for advanced ROP, but laser surgery has proved to be faster, less traumatic, and more effective.[35] Most VLBW infants will need continuing ophthalmological evaluation to ascertain retinal maturity, monitor for the resolution of ROP, and look for the refractive errors and problems of ocular alignment so commonly found in the VLBW population. Although visual function has been preserved with both cryotherapy and laser surgery,[33] as many as one third of premature infants (even without ROP) will experience significant ocular disorders.[23] Severe brain injury, such as periventricular leukomalacia, can lead to profound visual deficits via the mechanisms of cortical blindness and oculomotor disturbances.[6]

Bronchopulmonary dysplasia. Bronchopulmonary dysplasia (BPD) is the frustrating outcome for 20% to 30% of the VLBW survivors of hyaline membrane disease; its incidence is inversely related to gestational age and birth weight. The necessary ingredients are pulmonary immaturity (including surfactant deficiency and immature immunological/antioxidant systems), increased alveolar oxygen concentration, and the "barotrauma" imposed by prolonged periods of artificial ventilation at high airway pressures. BPD also can develop in extremely immature infants who have not had preceding hyaline membrane disease. The pathophysiological behavior of BPD is similar to that of chronic obstructive pulmonary disease (COPD) seen in later life. These behavioral features include (1) "reactive" small airway disease, characterized by increased resistance to gas flow through the airways; (2) consequent "air-trapping" and mismatching of deoxygenated pulmonary blood flow with deoxygenated (rather than freshly oxygenated) alveolar gas; and (3) increased vascular resistance and right-sided heart strain. Just as in adult emphysema, the gas-exchanging hallmark is one of hypercapnia and hypoxemia. The former usually is compensated by bicarbonate retention via the kidneys; the latter can be palliated with an enriched oxygen environment. Treatment is similar to that for other reactive airway diseases (e.g., asthma) and currently involves bronchodilators, diuretics, physiotherapy, and, increasingly, steroids. The primary care practitioner who assists in the home care of these infants needs to help the family deal with home oxygen therapy (chiefly by nasal cannula), apnea monitoring (impedance monitor), and pulse oximetry. These therapies typically are required for 4 to 6 months of life, as the pulmonary parenchyma and vasculature remodel, but infrequently can stretch through the first years of life in severe BPD. Serial chest roentgenograms, electrocardiograms, and echocardiography can be helpful in detecting early cor pulmonale during this period. It is essential that patients who have BPD receive enough calories daily (often in the face of fluid restriction) to support adequate growth and activity. During this trying time, the infant can be expected to be particularly susceptible to respiratory infections, especially respiratory syncytial virus. Exposure to such infections should be minimized wherever possible, and rehospitalization should be quickly considered for possible respiratory support, should such prevention not succeed. The chest roentgenogram may normalize by about 2 years of age, but abnormalities of the small airways are detectable by certain pulmonary function tests well into adolescence. The degree of residual pulmonary abnormalities seen later in childhood is related more to the degree of prematurity than to the duration of artificial ventilation therapy.[14] Severe BPD also predisposes high-risk infants to later disturbances of feeding, cognition, and motor function.[15,38,40]

Developmental delays. Despite the numerous insults that affect premature infants during their stay in the NICU, a happy developmental outcome for most VLBW infants weighing more than 1000 g at birth can be expected. Those complications that generate potentially devastating neurodevelopmental outcomes include intraventricular hemorrhage, porencephaly, periventricular leukomalacia, and advanced cicatricial ROP. The development of significant BPD may itself be a marker of poor neurodevelopmental outcome, even where no specific injury to the brain can be documented. The current biological threshold for reasonable expectation of a healthy viability appears to be about 25 weeks of gestation and a birth weight of 750 g, if the infant is appropriately grown for gestational age.[1,20] Major disabilities (mental retardation, cerebral palsy, hydrocephalus, seizure disorders, sensorineural impairments) can be expected in about 30% of surviving infants below this threshold.[29] A recent study exploring the limits of viability reports intact survival rates of 2%, 21%, and 69% for infants born at 23, 24, and 25 weeks' gestation, respectively.[1]

Even the more horrendous developmental disabilities, once sustained, tend to be stable rather than progressive. However, infants who have hydrocephalus and have shunts in place are susceptible to shunt malfunction and infection. These events may dictate that the neurosurgeon share with the primary care physician the role of maintaining the shunt. Indeed, the ongoing management of shunts in these children is a paradigm for the multidisciplinary approach required to best serve all multiply disabled children. The government also plays a role in the multidisciplinary approach. Public Law 94-142 (Education for All Handicapped Children, 1975) stipulated the provision of special education within the school system for disabled children; this law was extended by Public Law 99-457 (1986) to include infants and preschool children. It, therefore, supports the extension of appropriate early intervention services directly to NICU graduates as they are enrolled in high-risk follow-up clinics.

Apnea/bradycardia. Pathological apnea has been defined operationally as a cessation of respiration for at least 20 seconds or as a briefer episode of apnea that is associated with bradycardia, cyanosis, pallor, or loss of muscle tone. Brief respiratory pauses, as well as frank periodic breathing, are normal respiratory patterns of preterm infants. The severity and frequency of these immature respiratory patterns are related inversely to gestational age; these cardiopulmonary events usually disappear as premature infants approach 34 to 36 weeks of adjusted postnatal age. Current evidence suggests that premature infants who achieve 7 to 8 days without an apnea alarm are not likely to experience another prolonged apnea, thus making them candidates for discharge without a home apnea monitor.[9] In many cases, however, otherwise thriving premature infants now are discharged from the NICU to their homes to continue the same sort of cardiorespiratory monitoring that characterized their NICU stay. The family monitors the infant's heart rate, respiration (impedance pneumography), and pulse oximetry (occasionally) until respiratory function matures, as documented by 2 to 3 alarmless months of monitoring. The most recent Consensus Statement by the National Institutes of Health does not endorse the use of "pneumograms" to decide when home apnea monitoring can be discontinued safely. Impedance pneumography is the method that is used most commonly to monitor respiration, but this technology is imperfect, and frequent false alarms occur because of poor signal quality. These false alarms can cause anxiety and fatigue within families, who sometimes discontinue the monitor prematurely because of frustration. Monitors with built-in memory units are available that allow professionals trained in the field of infant apnea to evaluate any events that occur at home. Parents usually are reassured that the apnea alarms are artifacts, but true exacerbation of apnea is sometimes identified, prompting the parents to seek medical attention. Some evidence exists that the use of home monitors that have memory capability allows for the rejection of artifactual events and can shorten the duration of home monitoring.

For some years, much emotion but little information has swirled around the presumption that infantile apnea (long or short) is related to sudden infant death syndrome (SIDS, see Chapter 269). Parents (but not their physicians) may be excused for confusing a very large population of normal premature infants with the very different and immensely smaller population of infants at true risk for SIDS. These latter infants include the siblings of infants who died of SIDS and babies who have suffered an acute life-threatening event (ALTE) characterized by sudden apnea, pallor or cyanosis, limpness, and unconsciousness. Infants who suffer from severe bronchopulmonary dysplasia also appear to be at substantially increased risk of SIDS. The infant who has an ALTE merits particular investigation to rule out gastroesophageal reflux, upper airway obstruction, seizure disorder, sepsis, metabolic disorders, intracranial injury, or other remedial disorders before he or she automatically is placed on a regimen of home apnea monitoring. More than a decade of such monitoring efforts appears not to have prevented many SIDS deaths; however, many episodes of less severe apnea may have been prevented.[2,28]

All health care professionals should be familiar with and promote the AAP Policy Statement "Infant Positioning and SIDS." These guidelines recommend the nonprone, preferably supine sleeping position for healthy infants, as well as the removal of all soft surfaces and gas-trapping objects from the bed. There may be some cases, such as infants who have severe gastroesophageal reflux or airway anomalies, in which a prone sleeping position is indicated. Premature infants previously spent most of their NICU hospitalization in the supine position, but this practice has been abandoned in favor of a more "developmentally kind" approach. Neonatal patients now spend much of their time nested in side-lying or prone positions, and parents witness the calming effect this has on their infants. As discharge approaches and the family is educated about the "Back to Sleep" recommendations of the AAP, the NICU staff must make certain that parents understand the rationale behind the proposed change in sleeping position and know how to position the infant properly for sleep at home.

SUMMARY

As difficult as the VLBW infant may have been to care for within the protective shell of the NICU, the challenge presented to the family does not slacken quickly after discharge. These children are more expensive, more temperamentally "difficult," and often perceived as more vulnerable than is a child of term birth. The emotional and fiscal burdens they present often are unloaded on a shaky family structure. Primary care physicians must remain a vital member of the multidisciplinary team that is required to care for VLBW infants, as well as NICU graduates who have other significant neonatal diagnoses. Much hard work is required from all members of the (inpatient and outpatient) team to optimize the health, growth, development, and happiness of high-risk infants discharged from the NICU. The happy photographic "rogues' gallery" of NICU graduates that adorns the entrance to most such units bears smiling testimony to the level of success that can be anticipated to reward this effort.

REFERENCES

1. Allen MC, Donohue PK, Dusman AE: The limit of viability: neonatal outcome of infants born at 22 to 25 weeks' gestation, *N Engl J Med* 329:1597, 1993.
2. American Academy of Pediatrics' Committee Statement, Task Force on Prolonged Infantile Apnea: Prolonged infantile apnea 1985, *Pediatrics* 76:129, 1985.
3. American Academy of Pediatrics' Joint Committee on Infant Hearing: Position statement 1982, *Pediatrics* 70:496, 1982.
4. Brooten D, et al: A randomized clinical trial of early hospital discharge and home follow-up of very-low-birth-weight infants, *N Engl J Med* 315:934, 1986.
5. Casiro OG, et al: Earlier discharge with community-based interventions for low birth weight infants: a randomized trial, *Pediatrics* 92:128, 1993.
6. Cioni G, et al: Cerebral visual impairment in preterm infants with periventricular leukomalacia, *Pediatr Neurol* 17:331, 1997.
7. Collin MF, Halsey CL, Anderson CL: Emerging developmental sequelae in the 'normal' extremely low birth weight infant, *Pediatrics* 88:115, 1991.
8. Cunningham CK, McMillan JA, Gross SJ: Rehospitalization for respiratory illness in infants of less than 32 weeks' gestation, *Pediatrics* 88: 527, 1991.
9. Darnall RA, et al: Margin of safety for discharge after apnea in preterm infants, *Pediatrics* 100:795, 1997.
10. Emsley HC, et al: Increased survival and deteriorating developmental outcome in 23 to 25 week old gestation infants, 1990-4 compared with 1984-9, *Arch Dis Child* 78:F99, 1998.
11. Escobar GJ, et al: Rehospitalization in the first two weeks after discharge from the neonatal intensive care unit, *Pediatrics* 104:e2, 1999.
12. Finnstrom O, et al: Neurosensory outcome and growth at three years in extremely low birthweight infants: follow-up results from the Swedish national prospective study, *Acta Paediatrica* 87:1055, 1998.
13. Furman L, et al: Hospitalization as a measure of morbidity among very low birthweight infants with chronic lung disease, *J Pediatr* 128:447, 1996.
14. Galdès-Sebaldt M, et al: Prematurity is associated with abnormal airway function in childhood, *Pediatr Pulmonol* 7:259, 1989.
15. Giacola GP, et al: Follow-up of school-age children with bronchopulmonary dysplasia, *J Pediatr* 130:400, 1997.
16. Gibson DL, et al: Retinopathy of prematurity-induced blindness: birth weight-specific survival and the new epidemic, *Pediatrics* 86:405, 1990.
17. Glass P, et al: Neurodevelopmental status at age five years of neonates treated with extracorporeal membrane oxygenation, *J Pediatr* 127:447, 1997.
18. Glezen WP, et al: Influenza virus infection in infants, *Pediatr Infect Dis J* 16:1065, 1997.
19. Hack M, Breslau N: Very-low-birth-weight infants: effects of brain growth during infancy on intelligence quotient at 3 years of age, *Pediatrics* 77:196, 1986.
20. Hack M, Fanaroff AA: Outcomes of extremely-low-birth-weight infants between 1982 and 1988, *N Engl J Med* 321:1642, 1989.
21. Hack M, et al: School-age outcomes in children with birth weights under 750 g, *N Engl J Med* 331:753, 1994.
22. Hagberg B, et al: The changing panorama of cerebral palsy in Sweden, *Acta Paediatr Scand* 78:283, 1989.
23. Hebbandi SB, et al: Ocular sequelae in extremely premature infants at 5 years of age, *J Pediatr Child Health* 33:339, 1997.
24. Hirata T, Bosque E: When they grow up: the growth of extremely low birth weight (≤1000 gm) infants at adolescence, *J Pediatr* 132:1033, 1998.
25. Hurt H: Continuing care of the high-risk infant, *Clin Perinatol* 11:3, 1984.
26. Khalak R, Pichichero ME, D'Angio CT: Three-year follow-up of vaccine response in extremely preterm infants, *Pediatrics* 101:597, 1998.
27. Kotogal UR, et al: Description and evaluation of a program for the early discharge of infants from a neonatal intensive care unit, *J Pediatr* 127: 285, 1995.
28. Light MJ, Sheridan MS: Home monitoring in Hawaii: the first 1000 patients, *Hawaii Med J* 48:304, 1989.
29. McCormick MC: Long-term follow-up of infants discharged from neonatal intensive care units, *JAMA* 261:1767, 1989.
30. Mutch L, et al: Secular rehospitalization of very-low-birth-weight infants, *Pediatrics* 78:164, 1986.
31. Nield TA, et al: Unexpected hearing loss in high-risk infants, *Pediatrics* 78:417, 1986.
32. Office of Technology Assessment: Neonatal care for low-birth-weight infants: costs and effectiveness, Health Technology Case Study 38, Pub No OTA-HCS-38, Washington, DC, 1987, US Government Printing Office.
33. O'Keefe M, O'Reilly J, Lanigan B: Longer-term visual outcome of eyes with retinopathy of prematurity treated with cryotherapy or diode laser, *Br J Ophthalmol* 82:1246, 1998.

34. O'Shea MT, et al: Survival and developmental disability in infants with birth weights of 501 to 800 grams, born between 1979 and 1994, *Pediatrics* 100:982, 1997.
35. Pearce IA, et al: Three year visual outcome for treated stage 3 retinopathy of prematurity: cryotherapy versus laser, *Br J Ophthalmol* 82:1254, 1998.
36. Phavoah P, et al: Birth-weight-specific trends in cerebral palsy, *Arch Dis Child* 65:602, 1990.
37. Piecuch RE, et al: Outcome of extremely low birth weight infants (500 to 999 grams) over a 12-year period, *Pediatrics* 100:633, 1997.
38. Reilly S, Skuse D, Ximena P: Prevalence of feeding problems and oral motor dysfunction in children with cerebral palsy: a community survey, *J Pediatr* 129:877, 1996.
39. Saigal S, et al: Follow-up of infants 501 to 1500 gm birth weight delivered to residents of a geographically defined region with perinatal intensive care facilities, *J Pediatr* 100:606, 1982.
40. Singer L, et al: A longitudinal study of developmental outcome in infants with bronchopulmonary dysplasia and very low birth weight, *Pediatrics* 100:987, 1997.
41. Stanley F, Watson L: Trends in perinatal mortality and cerebral palsy in Western Australia, 1967 to 1985, *Br Med J* 304:1658, 1992.
42. Strauss RS, Dietz WH: Effects of intrauterine growth retardation in premature infants on early childhood growth, *J Pediatr* 130:95, 1997.
43. Sung I, Vohr B, Oh W: Growth and neurodevelopmental outcome of very low birth weight infants with intrauterine growth retardation: comparison with control subjects matched by birth weight and gestational age, *J Pediatr* 123:618, 1993.
44. Teplin SW, Burchinal M, Johnson-Martin N: Neurodevelopmental, health and growth status at age 6 years of children with birth weights less than 1001 grams, *J Pediatr* 118:768, 1991.
45. Wariyar UK, Sam R: Morbidity and preterm delivery: importance of 100% follow-up, *Lancet* 1:387, 1989.

SUGGESTED READING

Taeusch HW, Yogman MW: *Follow-up management of the high-risk infant,* Boston, 1987, Little, Brown.

part six

Psychosocial Issues in Child Health Care

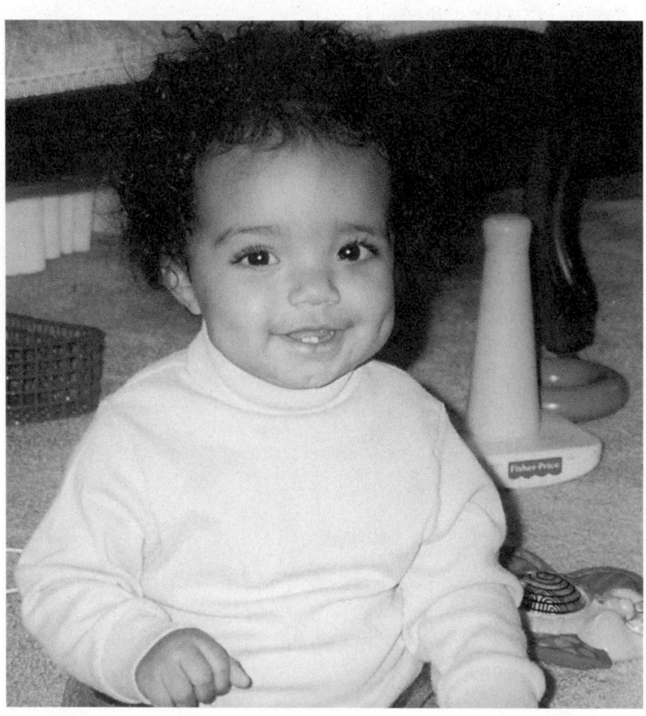

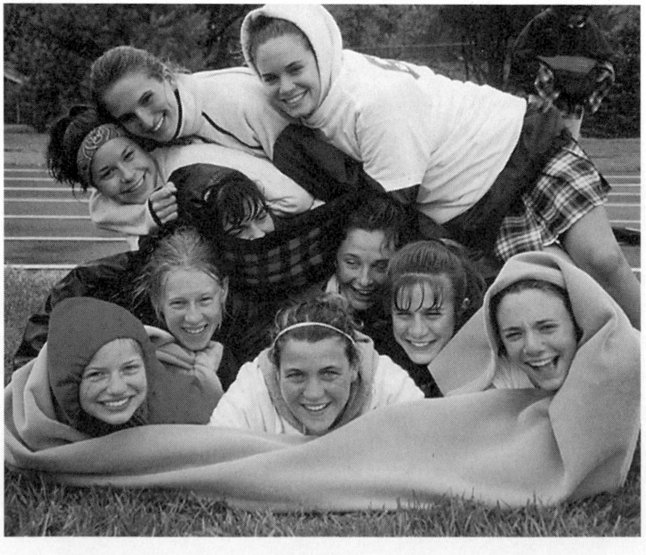

section one

Psychological Development

section two

The Family

52 Theories and Concepts of Development as They Relate to Pediatric Practice

Olle Jane Z. Sahler • Beatrice L. Wood

This chapter focuses on the psychological development of the child from fetal life through adolescence. For the purposes of this discussion, *psychology* is defined as that branch of science devoted to the study of emotion, cognition, and social conduct. Because the individual is part of a larger psychosocial-biological system, this chapter incorporates discussions of the effects on development of heredity, environmental influences, and biological maturation. Finally, the development of moral judgment is examined as an example of how understanding of a specific concept reflects the child's psychosocial cognitive stage.

No unified developmental theory, by itself, explains all the behaviors that can be observed in any particular child. Thus, we present several theories that, taken collectively, enable us to understand and interpret behaviors common to a particular developmental age. With this framework it becomes possible to interpret a child's behavior to parents in a developmental context and to devise strategies that can help children and their families cope effectively with common stressful situations.

The ever-developing personality style and cognitive functioning of the pediatric patient require continual reevaluation and renegotiation of any treatment regimen, regardless of whether a child's problem is physical or the result of a combination of physical and emotional elements. However, this very fluidity and malleability often make it possible to intervene substantively with a child when it would be impossible with an adult. The practitioner's ability to help rechannel and refocus the child's emotional energy along more constructive paths before undesirable habits or other maladaptive behaviors become fixed is one of the rewards of working with children. Primary prevention is a realistic goal. Conversely, the child's relatively unformed and fragile sense of self is particularly vulnerable to outside influences that might have little or no effect on the adult. Thus, the practitioner has an obligation to evaluate the social network surrounding the child to identify and help eliminate impediments to the child's realization of his or her fullest potential. In this context, the practitioner, as developmentalist, can become a knowledgeable and effective advocate for someone who is too young, too inexperienced, and too politically naive to speak as an independent individual.

FACTORS THAT INFLUENCE PSYCHOLOGICAL DEVELOPMENT

It is now generally accepted that the nature-nuture debate is moot. Asking whether a behavioral phenomenon is due to heredity *or* environment misses the point. Instead, current research supports an integrated perspective that appreciates the complex interplay among genetic factors and environmental conditions (family, peers, and social group) in shaping the individual throughout development. In recent years the field of behavioral genetics has contributed greatly to the development of theoretical models and methods that permit more sophisticated investigations. We are now better able to address the issue of *how* (rather than if) heritable predispositions interact with environmental factors to influence the developmental trajectory. Key new constructs and methods include gene-environment correlation, gene-environment interaction, and shared and nonshared environment.

Genetic and Environmental Contributions to Intelligence: Familial, Twin, and Adoptive Studies

Intelligence, or general cognitive ability, is a strong determinant of developmental outcome. As defined in our culture, intelligence is a composite of specific abilities, including verbal ability (use of language), quantitative ability (use of numbers), spatial ability (discrimination of objects in space), disembedding (separation of an element from its background), analytical ability (problem solving), reasoning (formulation and testing of hypotheses), and mastery of concepts (abstract notions). Individuals neither are born with all these skills, nor are these skills all learned during infancy. Rather, skills are acquired gradually over a period that extends through adolescence and into adulthood. Thus, the concept of the intelligence quotient (IQ) or the ratio of the cognitive maturational age (MA) to the chronological age (CA),

$$IQ = MA/CA \times 100$$

has become a popular device for comparing the abilities of a particular child with those of other children at a similar age. Although test interpretations and score distributions vary somewhat, IQs in the range of 90 to 110 usually are considered average. The most widely used tests are composed of subscales that measure both verbal and performance intelligence (see Appendix D).

What determines intelligence? Correlations among pairs of individuals show that similarity of IQ scores depends on the closeness of the genetic relationship. The correlation of IQ scores for randomly selected pairs of individuals is 0.00. The correlation for cousins is about 0.15. For half siblings, who have just one parent in common, the correlation is about 0.30. For full siblings who have both parents in common, the correlation is about 0.45; this correlation is similar to that between parents and offspring. Scores for fraternal twins correlate about 0.60 and for identical twins about 0.85. Husbands and wives correlate about 0.40, providing evidence for assortative (nonrandom) mating.[33]

However informative, these methods do not disentangle genetic and environmental contributions. For example, consider parents and offspring. Parents in a family study are "genetic-plus-environment" parents in that they share both heredity (through genetic transmission) and environment (living situation, experiences, resources) with their offspring.

Adoption studies are the most direct way to distinguish genetic from environmental sources of family resemblance. Adoption results in "genetic" (birth) parents and "environmental" (adoptive) parents. Resemblance between birth parents and their adopted-away offspring directly assesses the genetic contribution to parent-offspring resemblance. Resemblance between adoptive parents and children directly assesses the environmental contribution to parent-offspring resemblance. In these studies, "genetic" siblings are full siblings adopted apart early in life into different homes; "environmental" siblings are genetically unrelated children adopted early in life into the same adoptive home. Patterns of correlations among these variously genetically related pairs are submitted to statistical path analyses and model fitting to determine which genetic-environmental models best fit the data.

Fig. 52-1 summarizes adoption results for general cognitive ability. "Genetic" parents and offspring and "genetic" siblings significantly resemble each other, even though they are adopted apart and do not share family environment. As can be seen, genetics accounts for about half of the resemblance in cognitive ability for "genetic-plus-environmental" parents and siblings. The other half of familial resemblance appears to be explained by family environment, assessed directly by the resemblance between adoptive parents and adopted children and between adoptive siblings. About half of the environmental influence appears to be accounted for by shared environmental factors.

The effects of shared environment on cognitive ability decrease during childhood to negligible levels by adolescence; the heritability of general cognitive ability increases during the life span.[33] This is a prime example of the relative nature of the index of heritability. That is, the relative contributions of genetic factors and environmental factors change reciprocally throughout the life span. This means that genetic effects are *not* set in stone from the moment of conception.

Family studies of specific cognitive abilities show greater genetic contribution for verbal and spatial abilities than for perceptual speed and memory.[10] In contrast, a review of 10 twin studies of creativity yielded average twin correlations of 0.61 for identical twins and 0.50 for fraternal twins, indicating only modest genetic influence.[30] Clearly, genetic factors contribute to cognitive abilities, but environmental influences also are important.

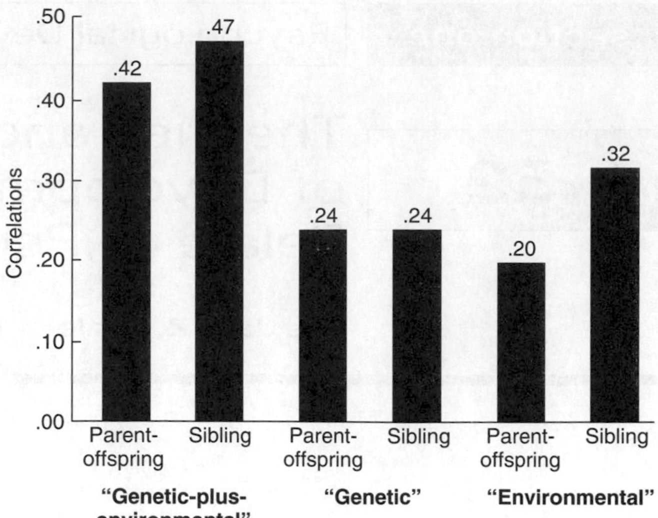

Fig. 52-1 Adoption data indicate that family resemblance for cognitive ability is due both to genetic resemblance and to environmental resemblance. "Genetic" relatives refer to genetically related relatives adopted apart. "Environmental" relatives refer to genetically unrelated individuals adopted together.

(From Loehlin JC: *Am Psychol* 44:1285, 1989.)

Shared and Nonshared Environment

Genetics studies continue to point to the importance of the environment as directly contributing to developmental outcomes. Environment also plays an important indirect role through correlation and interaction with genetic factors in shaping development. For children and adolescents, most environmental influences come from the family, school, and peer systems.

Family. The family is the first social unit to which the child belongs. Because family structure is highly variable (e.g., two heterosexual parents, single-parent, same-sex parents, communal), we define "family" functionally as "that group of people, living together or in close contact, who take care of one another and provide guidance for their dependent members." Membership in a family helps to ensure that the child is physically and emotionally nurtured. The ultimate goal of the family is to produce an autonomous adult who can "individuate" from the family of origin and live a meaningful and generative life.

Traditional approaches to studying the relationship between a child's environment and his or her development assumed that children in the same family experience or "share" similar environmental influences, such as opportunities for learning and child rearing attitudes. It was assumed that the shared family environment is a major determinant of the degree of similarity among family members. In fact, however, behavioral genetic research consistently shows that family resemblance for various attributes is almost entirely due to shared heredity rather than shared family environment. For example, shared family environment plays a negligible role in the development of personality and psychopathology and has little effect on rates of alcoholism in males, on attitudes, and even on body weight. Only a few possible exceptions have been found, such as conduct disorder in adolescence[34] and sociability and self-reliance in adolescence.[35]

Behavioral genetics research also reveals that siblings are surprisingly different from one another, despite their upbringing in the "same" family environment. In a study of personality, Scarr and Grajek[40] assert, "Lest the reader slip over these results, let us make explicit the implications of these findings: upper middle-class brothers who attend the same school and whose parents take them to the same plays, sporting events, music lessons, and therapists, and use similar child rearing practices on them are little more similar in personality measures than they are to working class or farm boys, whose lives are totally different." Other studies confirm that siblings are strikingly different from one another in personality and also in cognitive function and psychopathology—far more different than expected, given their genetic relatedness.[20] One factor that may contribute to sibling dissimilarity is the *difference* in the set of experiences (nonshared environment) siblings undergo, both within and outside the family. For example, within families, siblings differ in how they perceive parental affection, parenting practices, and sibling relationships; outside the family, siblings experience different relationships with teachers and peers. Definitions and estimated contributions of shared and nonshared environment are contained in Box 52-1.

Although family environment may not contribute in major ways to the *resemblance* of family members with respect to psychological or behavioral attributes, such factors are likely to determine developmental outcome by contributing to *differences* among family members through *nonshared* influences. Recent research indicates that family relationships (marital, parent-child, and sibling) also play essential and unique roles in mediating or moderating genetic influences contributing to adolescent outcomes.[35]

Sibling relationships are a pervasive feature of family life. Moreover, sibling relationships are likely to endure over the life span. Behavioral genetics research studies siblings in two ways. First, sibling research has been a central tool (as described above) for drawing inferences about the extent of genetic and environmental influences on psychological development. Second, research using these techniques has, with a few exceptions, shown that siblings in the same family are different from one another on many measures of developmental outcome. The next step is to determine which aspects of environment make siblings different.

BOX 52-1

SHARED AND NONSHARED ENVIRONMENT

Shared Environment

This refers to all environmental factors that contribute to similarity among family members on some measured attribute.

Nonshared Environment

This refers to all environmental factors that contribute to dissimilarity among family members on some measured attribute.

Estimating Shared and Nonshared Environment

A direct test of *shared family environment* is resemblance among adoptive relatives. Why do genetically unrelated adoptive "siblings" correlate about 0.25 for general cognitive ability in childhood? The answer must be "shared family environment," because adoptive siblings are unrelated genetically. Identical twins provide a direct test of *nonshared environment*. Because they are identical genetically, differences within pairs of identical twins can only be due to nonshared environment. Genetic designs incorporating siblings varying in genetic relatedness also permit indirect estimates of nonshared environment. First, heritability is estimated by comparing correlations of pairs of identical twins, fraternal twins, full sibs, half sibs, and adoptive or step sibs. Shared family environment is estimated as family resemblance *not* explained by genetics. Nonshared environment is the rest of the variance (which also includes measurement error).

The gene-environment dialectic. Reiss et al[35] have recently reported the results of a study assessing 720 adolescents, their closest-in-age sibling, and their caregivers at two points in time: early and late adolescence. The adolescent outcomes studied were competency (cognitive and social competence, self worth) and psychological compromise (depression and antisocial behavior). The genetic contribution to outcomes was estimated by using path analytical techniques in a design that compared "pairs" of siblings with varying levels of genetic relatedness (identical and fraternal twins, full sibs, half sibs, and blended sibs). The study focused on family environmental factors and assessed marital, parent-child, and sibling relationship variables. Parent-child relationships were assessed separately for mothers and fathers by using parent and child report and observer rating of family dyadic interactions during conflict resolution discussions.[35]

Parents reported that they treat their children similarly, particularly when monitoring behavior. Parents also reported that the siblings treat one another similarly. In the siblings' eyes, parents treat them each differently, and they treat each other differently. Raters of family process tended to agree more with the children, suggesting that siblings, despite living in the same family, experience different parent-child and sibling relationship environments.[35] Furthermore, the data show strong associations between the quality of these nonshared aspects of various relationship environments and such domains of adolescent adjustment as antisocial behavior, depressive symptoms, sociability, autonomy, and self-worth. Negativity and parent-child conflict were associated with poor adjustment; in contrast, warm nuturant relationships were associated with positive adjustment.

The father-child relationship was as important as the mother-child relationship in predicting adjustment. The quality of the sibling relationship was also associated with most of these domains of adjustment, in the expected direction. Parent monitoring of the child had more complex parent-specific (mother versus father) associations with outcome. Fathers and mothers make different contributions to the adjustment of their children. The most notable effect of shared environment was on sociability. In this instance, the most important environmental factors appeared to be school and peers.[35]

Genetic factors have been found to account for more than 50% of the variance among measures of adolescent adjustment. Previous psychosocial studies have found comparably sized influences of family process (i.e., environmental effects) on adolescent adjustment. How can these potentially contradictory findings be reconciled? The Reiss study[35] discovered that parent-child relatedness factors, which were associated strongly with a range of outcome from antisocial behavior to social responsibility, also were influenced by genetic factors. In fact, about half of all differences among families in parent-adolescent conflict can be attributed to genetic differences among the adolescents, suggesting potentially important genetic-environment interplay. It is possible that genetically influenced characteristics in the adolescent evoke parental responses that in turn contribute to psychosocial outcomes for the adolescent.

This interplay of heredity and environment in which genotype-environment correlation and interaction occur is described in Box 52-2. The methodology and findings of the Reiss study[35] will likely serve as a model for genetically informed psychosocial research. Such research will enable new insights into the complex interplay of genetic and environmental influences on the developmental trajectory of children and have important clinical implications for pediatricians who provide anticipatory guidance.

Shared and nonshared environments are not limited to family environments. Experiences outside the family, such as in school and with peers, also can be shared or not shared by siblings.[29]

School. The two basic functions of school are education and socialization. For some children, the first regular and routine experiences outside the home are provided by attending school.

In its role as an agent of socialization, school provides a graded transition from the circumscribed environment of the home to the world at large. The most crucial social goals of early schooling are the facilitation of individuation from the family, control of gross motor activity to achieve decorum in the classroom, mastery of the skills necessary to read and write, and promotion of qualities that promote the educational process, such as cooperation, completion of tasks, and respect for others.

During the late elementary grades, competition and achievement become prominent aspects of school life. In elementary school, the results of school achievement tests are influenced strongly (about 60%) by the shared environment and influenced modestly (about 30%) by genetic factors. However, later in the school years, the contribution from genetic influence increases in importance and that from shared environment decreases. This same phenomenon is seen for cognitive ability in general.[33]

Peer group. Peers model behavior, help determine value systems, and provide the security of group identity. Children have their first recognizable peer interactions at about 6 months of age. At this time, infants placed together look at, approach, and explore one another for a few seconds.[19] These interactions increase in duration and complexity as the child matures. Reciprocal social play emerges at about 1 year of age; social pretend play appears at about age 2 years. Most children have developed a characteristic way of relating to peers, independently seeking friendships and engaging in social activities by about age 3 years. Early friendships are based on proximity (the child next door).

BOX 52-2

INTERPLAY OF HEREDITY AND ENVIRONMENT

It is likely, given the complexity of the developmental process, that genetic and environmental contributions are interrelated. There are two principal ways of understanding how genetic and environmental factors operate together: genotype-environment correlation and interaction.

Genotype-Environment Correlation

Three types of genotype-environment correlation are commonly described: passive, evocative, and active.[32,39,41]

Passive genotype-environment correlation results simply from each parent sharing 50% of his or her genes with their children and parents providing the environment in which their children live. Therefore, any correlation between the child's genotype and the environment may occur because the environment provided by the parents also is correlated with the parents' genotypes. Passive genotype-environment correlation is likely to be most important in infancy and early childhood, when the parent is the primary source of environmental influences. When the child's genotype evokes a response from the environment, *evocative* genotype-environment correlation is said to have occurred. For example, a child who has a difficult temperament is likely to elicit responses from others that signal anger or frustration.

Active genotype-environment correlation occurs when individuals actively seek out environments that are correlated with their genotype. Using the same example of difficult temperament, a child who is difficult and aggressive may be more likely to select peers who are also aggressive, increasing their likelihood of fitting in, but also of increasing their problem behaviors.

Genotype-Environment Interaction

In a gene-environment interaction, a genetic factor expresses itself more readily in some environments than in others. For example, a study of couples at genetic risk for alcohol abuse indicated that only couples with marital dysfunction actually succumbed to the genetic predisposition.

Later, the classroom is the major source of friends. Finally, friendships become defined by mutual interests.

Friendship becomes more enduring as children grow older.[5] Friendships perceived as intimate are most likely to endure, and good friends tend to be of similar age, gender, and peer status. A key determinant of friendship formation appears to be common interests. Self-disclosure of feelings and private thoughts as well as shared activities contribute to the bond between friends.

During adolescence the peer group may be more influential than the family in determining social activities and values. In some instances, adolescents deliberately choose a peer group that has values antithetical to those of their parents. This process of strong group identification coupled with conflict with parents helps them individuate from the family—a major goal of late adolescence.

Temperament and Attachment: a Classic Example of Genetic and Environmental Interplay

Pioneering investigators such as Thomas and Chess[46,47] identified a complex system of idiosyncratic differences in the responsiveness of infants and young children to their environment. These individual tendencies have been shown to be stable from early infancy through early adulthood. This collection of nine behavioral attributes has been labeled *temperament:* (1) activity level, (2) rhythmicity, (3) approach/withdrawal from a new stimulus, (4) adaptability, (5) intensity of reaction, (6) threshold of responsiveness, (7) mood, (8) distractibility, and (9) attention span and persistence. These temperamental traits lead to parental perceptions that a particular child is "easygoing" or "difficult." Such judgments are based on the parents' observations of how the child responds to various environmental stimuli and on the degree to which the child is self-sufficient in achieving contentment.

The concept has been refined through empirical validation studies. Currently, constructs of temperament emphasize psychophysiological reactivity[22] and self-regulation, particularly of arousal level and emotion.[36,37] There is strong support for the heritability of temperament and even personality,[15,28] although only about half of the influence seems to be of genetic origin. Thus, even the so-called innate or constitutional characteristics of temperament also are influenced by environmental factors.

Chess and Thomas[8] suggested that the "match" of a child's temperamental style with the demands and expectations of the child's environment influence functional outcome, with mismatches being associated with increased risk of behavioral and emotional disorders. For example, quiet, easygoing parents may have an energetic, excitable child whom they want to be like themselves because that is their expectation for appropriate child behavior. This situation is even more likely to arise if the child has a quiet sibling whose disposition is similar to that of the parents.

It has been suggested that temperament influences the quality of attachment between a parent and child.[11] For example, an anxious parent may respond defensively ("He doesn't like me") to an infant who is highly emotionally reactive or prone to distress, leading to insecure parent-child attachment. Such findings lend support to Chess and Thomas' "goodness of fit" model.[8] Although to date there have been no formal behavioral genetics studies examining the nature of the genetic-environmental interplay between temperament and attachment, these phenomena are likely candidates for gene-environment correlation and interaction studies in the future.

Practical "take-home" messages for parents and pediatricians

1. Each child is the product of complex interrelationships between genetic and environmental influences.
2. Family, school, and peers play key roles in determining developmental outcomes.
3. The quality of the relationships between parent and child and between siblings influences adjustment.
4. Both parents play important roles in determining developmental outcomes.
5. Similarities in siblings are due to heredity; differences are due to nonshared environment.
6. Siblings' experiences with their parents are different (nonshared environment), even if parents believe they treat all their children the same way.
7. Sibling dyads experience each other differently (nonshared environment), whereas parents think siblings behave reciprocally with one another.

General advice: Identify, appreciate, and encourage each child's individual strengths. Address weaknesses and challenging behavior with warmth and nurturance. Minimize negativity and conflict. Support siblings in being kind to one another.

Temperment and Psychobiological Stress

Although stress has long been recognized as a risk factor for mental and physical illness in adults, only recently has it been recognized as a risk factor for childhood morbidity as well.

Temperament appears to be an important determinant of individual vulnerability to stress, which carries with it increased risk for various childhood diseases.[6] Studies have documented a pattern of physiological hyperreactivity, consisting of elevated heart rate, sympathetic adrenomedullary activation, and a rise in plasma cortisol or corticotropin levels, among both behaviorally inhibited infant monkeys[44] and human children.[22] These characteristics of psychobiological reactivity persist into later periods of development and are related to social withdrawal in group settings. Developmental studies focused on cardiovascular responsivity suggest that exaggerated reactivity is at least partly determined genetically and persists into adult life,[13] possibly contributing to an increased risk of cardiovascular disease and other chronic health problems.[6]

Psychobiological hyperreactivity also has been implicated in the development of subsequent anxiety disorders.[21] In addition, Miller and Wood[29] found that emotional and physiological reactivity was related to the degree of airway compromise induced in certain children who have asthma who were exposed to emotional challenge under laboratory conditions. These findings suggest that certain temperamental patterns place some children at risk for later health problems if they grow up in stressful environments or if they have a particular physiological vulnerability (e.g., asthma).

In a similar vein, Porges[34] identified and documented the importance of parasympathetic (vagal) activation in moderating the impact of stress on the individual. He demonstrated that high-risk preterm newborns have lower vagal tone than do full-term newborns and that these differences are related to later dimensions of clinical risk, such as poor weight gain, inability to respond to stimuli, and lack of attention. This work suggests that children who were high-risk preterm newborns may be more vulnerable to stress-related physical or emotional illnesses later in life.

The influence of stress on the organism's ability to mount an effective immune response is well documented.[1,9] Research with infant primates indicates that the nutritional and psychological effects of separation from the mother may have long-lasting effects on some immune responses. These findings suggest that the quality of parent-child attachment may have significant implications for the physical well-being of the child.

In addition to impeding adaptation, psychobiological reactivity also can enhance adaptation. For example, children who have greater elevations of cortisol in response to stressors such as academic examinations, hospitalization, and surgery tend to be children who are more competent with peers, more involved in their school work, more positive and cooperative in the clinic, and more realistic in their appraisals of the importance of the stressor.[17] Interestingly, studies attempting to correlate level of anxiety and degree of distressed behavior among both infants and older children have been inconclusive.

Both risks and benefits are associated with particular temperamentally based individual differences in psychobiological reactivity. Some children are unusually shy and withdrawn or emotionally reactive. High psychobiological reactivity is not abnormal, nor necessarily prodromal for any abnormal physical or emotional condition (see Barr[4] for a discussion of "normal"). Rather, children who have such a temperament might best be considered as highly sensitive individuals who will thrive in facilitating environments but who will be more vulnerable when stressed. It most likely is the interaction of temperament and environment that will determine the child's developmental outcome, not one factor or the other alone.

THEORIES OF DEVELOPMENT

Even bizarre behavior is understandable when we know the developmental basis for a child's actions. Because no single theory explains all aspects of psychological development, it has become customary to examine behavior from several perspectives. Typically, these include emotional, cognitive, and social development.

Each approach has its own vocabulary and set of assumptions and hypotheses. It is noteworthy, however, that each of these perspectives relies on the presence of certain primitive instinctual behaviors that are operative at birth and later modified by the environment. Given our original definition of psychology as the study of emotion, cognition, and social conduct, we immediately see that each theory is incomplete; taken collectively, however, they complement each other.

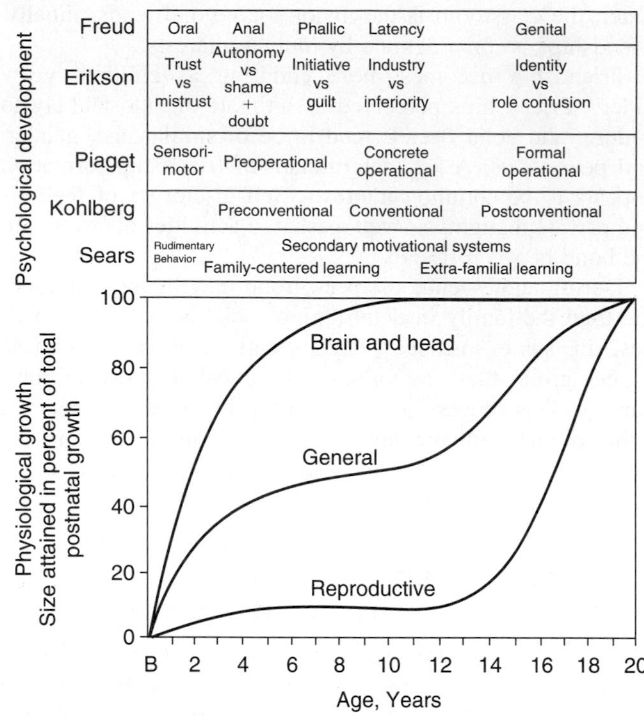

Fig. 52-2 Psychological and physiological growth and development.

(*Top,* from Sahler OJZ, McAnarney ER: *The child from three to eighteen,* St Louis, 1981, Mosby. *Bottom,* modified from Tanner JM: *Growth at adolescence,* ed 2, Oxford, England, 1962, Blackwell Scientific Publications, Ltd.)

Fig. 52-2 provides a summary of physical and psychological development from these perspectives from childhood through young adulthood.

Psychodynamic Theory

Freud and psychosexual development. The theory of psychosexual development is derived from Freud's retrospective analysis of childhood behaviors he thought contributed to the neuroses for which his patients, as adults, were seeking treatment. Based on the content of memories supplied by his patients, Freud theorized that personality formation results from intrapsychic struggles experienced by an individual during maturation. This particular approach and the theoretical framework derived from it are limited in that (1) objective observations of current behavior are lacking and (2) heavy emphasis is placed on explanations for the development of undesirable adult behaviors rather than on behavior in general. Despite these shortcomings, Freud and his work have had a formidable influence on generations of developmental psychologists.[19]

The family triad of mother-father-child and, in particular, the early mother-child dyad were central to Freud's interpretations of later adult behaviors. Although pediatric psychology currently focuses largely on the individual in relation to a broader social unit than the family and on coping mechanisms (positive management strategies in stressful situations) rather than on defense mechanisms (often interpreted as negative management strategies), elements of Freudian theory are represented in a variety of other major developmental theories. Similarly, Freud's discussions of both conscious and unconscious motivations provide a unique framework for understanding observable behavior.

The total personality as conceived by Freud consists of three motivating forces: the id, the ego, and the superego. The *id* is the foundation of the personality; its aim is to avoid pain, find satisfaction or pleasure, and maintain constancy in the midst of internal or external disturbance.

The *ego,* that part of the personality most visible to the external world, is the intermediary system between the id and reality; it provides the individual an accurate perception of what exists in the environment. On some occasions, fulfillment of pleasure as desired by the id may be suspended by the ego in acknowledgment of reality.

The *superego* is the moral function of the personality; it is concerned with strivings for perfection rather than for pleasure or for responses that reflect reality. Freud further divided the superego into the *ego ideal,* the conception of what is morally good, and *conscience,* the conception of what is morally bad. To the superego, thought is synonymous with action; therefore, feelings of guilt or satisfaction may be experienced merely by thinking something "bad" or "good." Clinically, this conceptualization has relevance to psychosomatic illness, which is considered in this theoretical framework to be an example of pain or dysfunction resulting from the superego's displeasure with the individual.

Although behavior can be motivated by the drive to fulfill a variety of needs (e.g., food, sleep), the major motivational system according to the psychosexual theory of development is *libido,* which is based in the instinctual (sexual) drive to preserve the species. Satisfaction of the sexual instinct is derived from stimulation or manipulation of both genital and nongenital body regions that have been called *erogenous zones.* Three primary erogenous zones, each with its associated vital need and presented in the chronological order in which each gains prominence, are (1) the mouth and eating, (2) the anus and elimination, and (3) the genitalia and reproduction. According to Freud, the action an individual takes to reduce tension (derive pleasure) in an erogenous zone may or may not actually fulfill the vital need associated with that area (e.g., both eating and nonnutritive thumb-sucking produce pleasure in the oral area).

Activities involving the erogenous zones may bring the child into conflict with the parents. The resulting frustrations and anxieties associated with these conflicts lead to the development of a number of adaptive maneuvers or defense mechanisms, such as repression, regression, denial, projection, intellectualization, and sublimation. Resolution of the conflict associated with a given stage allows the individual to progress to the next developmental stage. Freud conceptualized five psychosexual stages: oral, anal, phallic, latency, and genital. Full maturation of psychosexual development is thought to occur in late adolescence or early adulthood with the establishment of a stable heterosexual relationship.

Erikson and psychosocial development. Whereas Freud focused on the intrinsic development of the individual, especially as it is shaped by the mother-father-child relationship, Erikson focused on the development of the individual within the wider context of his or her historical-cultural-social milieu.[12] For Erikson, unconscious motivation (id) exists, but it is the process of socialization (learning how to be an accepted and productive member of society) that is key to development and determines outcome.

Unlike Freud, Erikson studied individuals and their families within the spheres of their everyday lives and at a particular moment in their cultural history. Also, unlike Freudian theory, Erikson's theory focuses with optimism on an individual's potential for mastery by successfully resolving developmental crises, rather than with pessimism on the potential for dysfunction from persistent psychological conflict.

Erikson conceptualized eight ages in human life. These represent a reformulation and extension of Freud's five psychosexual stages of development. However, whereas psychosexual theory postulates that the individual attains full developmental maturity at entry into the genital stage during adolescence or young adulthood, psychosocial theory postulates that developmental change occurs throughout the life cycle. The first six Eriksonian ages are easily associated with their corresponding Freudian stages: basic trust versus basic mistrust (oral), autonomy versus shame and doubt (anal), initiative versus guilt (phallic), industry versus inferiority (latency), and the combination of identity versus role confusion and intimacy versus isolation (genital). The last two Eriksonian ages, generativity versus stagnation and ego integrity versus despair, deal with the specific developmental transitions of middle and old age.

Cognitive-Intellectual Theory

Piaget and cognitive development. Cognition is defined as the means by which an individual accumulates organized knowledge about the world and uses that knowledge to solve problems and modify behavior. Whereas psychodynamic theories are concerned primarily with issues of motivation as a force for change, cognitive-intellectual theory is centered on the process of acquiring and using knowledge.

According to Piagetian theory, cognitive development is the result of neurophysiological maturation, environmental stimulation, experience, and continual internal cognitive reorganization. Two major principles form the framework for Piaget's theory: (1) all species tend to organize or order their activities hierarchically and (2) all species tend to adapt through assimilation (incorporating new information into already existing ideas about the world) and accommodation (changing ideas about the world in response to new knowledge). For example, when infants are handed a set of small blocks for the first time, they are likely to bite or shake them. That is, they assume the new objects are similar to familiar objects (e.g., nipples and rattles). This is an illustration of assimilation. Once children discover that blocks can be used to build a tower, they change their behavior and stack the blocks each time they are presented. This is an illustration of accommodation.

Piaget's theory is premised on a stepwise, ordered sequence of learning in response to experience. He defined four discrete stages from birth to adulthood: sensorimotor, preoperational, concrete operational, and formal operational. The exact chronological age at which certain abilities are attained depends on factors such as individual differences in physiological functioning, experience, and environment. Transitional periods, during which children exhibit some but not all characteristics of the next stage of thinking, exist between developmental stages. Targeted teaching during these times may result in rapid acquisition of new cognitive skills characteristic of the next stage.

Learning Theory

Learning theory is an outgrowth of behaviorism, or stimulus-response psychology. Following are some basic principles of learning theory:

1. Behavior is learned; however, genetic factors and innate, involuntary reflexive behaviors influence this learning.
2. All types, patterns, and combinations of behavior can be learned as long as they are not incompatible physically.
3. Behavior can be conditioned.
4. Behavior can be shaped.
5. Behavior is learned through reinforcement, which may be internal or external and positive or negative.
6. Learning results from many independent processes, including observation and imitation.

Behavior can be conditioned in two ways. In the process of *classical conditioning*, discovered by the Russian physiologist Pavlov, a reflex response associated in nature with one stimulus can be modified in such a way that it can be evoked by another stimulus. In Pavlov's original experiment, reflexive salivation in a dog at the sight of food could be induced eventually by the sound of a ringing bell, which over a period of time was "paired" with eating. (Interestingly, the saliva evoked by the ringing bell differs slightly in chemical content from naturally occurring saliva.)

In the process of *instrumental conditioning*, a nonreflexive behavior is learned because it is reinforced positively. For example, a rat in a cage might, by chance, depress a lever. If a pellet of food is released each time this occurs, the rat will "learn" to depress the lever and will do so with increasing frequency, especially when hungry.

Several features of conditioned behavior are important clinically. Conditioned behavior can be *extinguished,* or unlearned, if it is not reinforced; it can be *inhibited,* or counteracted, if it is followed by negative reinforcement; it can be *partially reinforced* by inconsistent or random reinforcement; it can be *generalized* so that similar stimuli will elicit the same response; and it can be made *discriminatory* so that by selective reinforcement only one specific stimulus elicits the response.

Reinforcement is the key element in learning theory. According to this theoretical framework, an individual can be motivated to perform a certain behavior because of the positive effect (reward) derived from it. Furthermore, an individual can be motivated *not* to perform a certain behavior because of the negative effect (punishment) derived from it or because some other behavior gives more benefit. Thus, giving a neutral response (not reinforcing, ignoring) or reinforcing a behavior negatively leads to the behavior being extinguished. A consistent response, whether it is positively or negatively reinforcing, leads to the most rapid learning.

Shaping is the process of molding a given behavior to be more like a desired behavior. This is accomplished by positively reinforcing successive approximations of the desired behavior. A classic example of this has been described by Baldwin in his recounting of the work of B.F. Skinner[3]:

> When Skinner wanted to teach a pigeon to hit a ping pong ball through a pair of goal posts by pecking at it, he did not wait until the pigeon just happened to do so. He began by reinforcing the pigeon whenever it was within a certain distance of the ball. The pigeon gradually learned to stay close to the ball. The experimenter then reinforced the pigeon only when it was close to the ball and looking in the ball's direction; thus, he taught the pigeon to keep its eye on the ball. In the next stage, the experimenter required the pigeon to peck at the ball to receive reinforcement. Finally, the pigeon was required to peck the ball through the goal posts.

Social learning theory is that specialized area of behaviorism that stresses the dyadic nature of human behavior. Thus, the child is in constant interaction with the environment and other individuals in that environment. The child's response to an environmental stimulus acts as a stimulus itself, thus evoking a response from the environment or persons in that environment, and so on.[42]

At another level, however, learning also can occur indirectly through observation and imitation of others who are having the actual experience. In *observational learning* the individual watches others and modifies his or her behavior in accord with the reinforcements others receive. *Imitative learning* is rooted in the process of identification (Freud). The child imitates a desired model (e.g., mother or father) and is positively reinforced with rewards that either are internal (being proud of oneself) or external (being praised by others). Both observational and imitative learning are particularly common in social groups.

If individuals learn by observational imitation, then modeling (demonstrating) is a particularly important way to elicit a particular behavior. Models can be used to demonstrate everything from simple one-step behaviors to entire lifestyles (role models). Children and youth observe the behaviors of others and, based on how much they wish to identify with these others, will imitate their actions. The adage "actions speak louder than words" may have preceded the formulation of learning theory by centuries, but it still is the most profound basis for explaining behaviors that persist within families over generations, despite parental admonitions to the contrary. For example, modeling helps explain successive generations of child or spouse abuse. If children observe such behaviors in their parents, their earliest teachers, they will come to believe that abuse is normal and acceptable. Intervention aimed at altering child-rearing practices, for example, is difficult because change requires not only learning new behaviors but also questioning the teaching of those to whom we have been taught to have a strong allegiance (our parents).

RELATIONSHIP BETWEEN PHYSIOLOGICAL AND PSYCHOLOGICAL DEVELOPMENT

In this section we examine the child developmentally at different chronological ages. A basic premise of most developmental theories is that reflexive, instinctual behavior is the foundation for all future behaviors. A second premise is that psychological development and physiological maturation occur simultaneously and are interdependent.

Several important principles of physical development that bear directly on psychological development can be summarized as follows:

1. Development is a continuous process that begins at conception. Birth is merely an event in the natural course of development that signals the individual's readiness to cope independently with the environment.
2. Although the developmental sequence is relatively fixed, developmental rates vary considerably and different systems mature at different times.
3. Development of both involuntary (autonomic) and voluntary (motor) activity is related to maturation of the nervous system.
4. Certain primitive reflexes (e.g., stepping, grasping) must be "lost" before the corresponding voluntary (e.g., walking, holding) movement is acquired.
5. Development occurs cephalocaudally.

Pregnancy

The bonds of parent-child attachment that eventually form are initiated during pregnancy. According to Ainsworth,[2] attachment is a long-lasting emotional tie between one person and another that persists even when they are apart. Although the emotions of attachment are complex and vary from time to time, in general, positive feelings toward the other person predominate, and attachment is thought of as implying affection or love.

"Precursors of attachment" are physical and psychosocial changes that occur in couples anticipating the birth of their child. These changes have been researched best in pregnant women, but studies of men suggest that expectant fathers also experience emotional changes and share many of the same feelings as expectant mothers.[31] Examples of such behavior include changes in social patterns because of fatigue, alterations in economic planning (e.g., less disposable income), and the accumulation of various material goods, such as a crib and baby clothes. On another level, many expectant parents report a heightened sense of responsibility to keep the mother (and therefore the fetus) well and fit (e.g., abstaining from tobacco, drugs, or alcohol) and to protect the father (e.g., reducing risky behavior). Planning for the future of someone who will depend totally on them becomes a major preoccupation of the pregnant couple.

During pregnancy a woman experiences two types of developmental change: physical and emotional changes within herself and the growth of the fetus. The woman faces two adaptive tasks: acceptance of the pregnancy and perception of the fetus as an individual.

Most women report strong emotional swings from positive to negative anticipation; frequently they feel ambivalent about the pregnancy. Perceiving the fetus as an individual usually commences with the first sensation of fetal movement, or "quickening." If the original reaction to the pregnancy was predominantly negative (unplanned, unwanted), many women report heightened acceptance and noticeable changes in attitude when fetal movement is first felt. After quickening, women usually begin to have fantasies about the physical and personality characteristics they hope or fear the child will have.[23]

Most likely every couple has some fantasies, regardless of how carefully they attempt to avoid them. Gender preference probably is the most common,[38] but inherent in all individuals is the wish to have children who will be a credit to them, carry on tradition, excel in some activity, and be attractive, well-adjusted, and healthy. As the time of delivery approaches, this last concern, to have a healthy baby, increases in importance. Thus, should a child be born with a congenital defect, life threatening or not, the parents actually suffer the loss of their "expected" child, and some time may pass before they can reorganize their expectations and fully accept their child.

Birthing Process

Data relating to the birthing process suggest that mothers who are relaxed during labor and who have a supportive person (husband, family member, friend) assisting them are likely to have a shorter labor and to be more alert and interactive with their infant on first sight.[43] Being unconscious during birth does not appear to cause rejection of the infant, although systematic studies in this important area are lacking. What is known, however, is that the more difficult the labor, the less likely the mother is to breast-feed.

Certain delivery procedures and administration of anesthetics can affect both the mother and child at birth. For example, an infant who is physiologically depressed because of a narcotic given during delivery to the mother is more likely to respond poorly on initial contact or during feedings and thus be less stimulating to the mother.

Research on the behavior of fathers toward the newborn has shown that engrossment, absorption, and preoccupation with the infant occur in men as well as in women. A sense of increased self-esteem also has been reported among new fathers.[16,31,48]

Immediate Postpartum Period

The interval immediately after birth has been called the *maternal sensitive period*[23] and is characterized by reciprocal mother-infant interaction. The mother supplies touch, eye-to-eye *(en face)* contact, high-pitched voice, heat, and odor; the infant supplies eye-to-eye contact, odor, and entertainment, and if breast-feeding, stimulates maternal production of prolactin and oxytocin.

The mother's behaviors match certain infant needs. For example, the female voice is naturally high pitched, and the mother consciously makes it more so. This fits the infant's sensitivity and attraction to speech in the high-frequency range. The mother's odor also appears to affect the infant. It has been found that infants can discriminate their own mother's axillary odor[7] and the smell of their own mother's breast milk from that of other women.

The infant's reflexive behaviors (suckling, clinging) are care-eliciting—that is, they serve to bring the caregiver closer to the child and help to maintain physical and emotional contact between them by mutual reinforcement. In turn, parental reinforcement behaviors (feeding, fondling) in response to the child's care-eliciting behaviors lead to further suckling and clinging. In this way the infant's innate behaviors and the responses they generate in the caregiver initiate the attachment process.[25]

Certain factors inhibit the development of attachment. For example, the provocative stimulus of the young infant's intense gaze is missing if the child is blind. Variations of normal behavior, such as an infant who stiffens rather than clings on being held, may be a response to caregiver anxiety or a manifestation of a "difficult" temperament. A psychological impediment to attachment is the tendency of some parents to identify their own or another's undesirable traits in the infant.

Infancy

The period of infancy, which extends from birth to 24 months of age, is divided most logically at 12 months. The first year is marked by tremendous physical growth and the development of rudimentary skills, culminating in the ability to walk several steps unassisted and to speak three to six intelligible words.

The second year is characterized by skill refinement. Some children can pedal a tricycle and speak in relatively complete, although syntactically poor, sentences. Infants also learn that other individuals inhabit their world and that these individuals, most notably family members, come, go, and return. Lastly, they learn that they have a will and can manipulate their environment purposefully.

Emotional maturation is intricately interwoven with somatic growth. Of the many changes taking place, two principal psychological tasks are mastered during infancy: attachment (first year) and separation (second year).

Attachment does not depend on the infant's perceiving the attachment figure as separate from self. It actually is facilitated by the newborn's earliest perception of the caregiver as an extension of self.[2] Indeed, bonding, an early manifestation of attachment, usually is discussed with reference to mother-child interactions in the newborn period.[23] The recognition of potential impediments to bonding (use of anesthesia, separation of mother and infant) has led to major changes in obstetrical and newborn care. However, true attachment is such an important element for successful growth and development that it is "overdetermined," that is, many opportunities, over time, are available to facilitate and cement the formation of attachment, not only with the mother but with the father and other significant caregivers as well.[26]

Interestingly, it has been found that as the infant becomes able to discriminate between caregivers, the infant's expectations for the father's behavior are different from those for the mother; fathers do, in fact, act differently, providing less rhythmic and more exciting physical and auditory stimulation.[26,27] Despite such differences in interaction, attachment between the infant and any consistent caregiver is strengthened by continued mutual reinforcement.

If we assume that object permanence (the object is out of sight but not out of mind) is a prerequisite for the formation of true attachment, it probably does not occur before 6 to 8 months of age. At this age, the infant and caregiver can derive enough positive reinforcement from each other that periods of being apart do not interrupt the essential tie; true attachment is considered to have taken place when the bond remains strong despite periods of absence.

Separation is a direct extension of attachment. Without attachment, there is no separation; rather, there merely is movement from one more or less contiguous relationship to another. Just as positive affect usually is associated with attachment, negative affect usually is associated with separation.

Separation anxiety occurs after the child becomes able to recognize and discriminate among individuals. It is manifested by distress when the attachment figure is not present. Closely allied with separation anxiety is stranger anxiety, or fear of someone unfamiliar to the infant. A stranger, however, almost always is reasonably well tolerated when a familiar, safe caregiver also is present.

Psychosexual Development: Oral and Anal Stages

In Freudian or psychosexual terms, the child younger than 12 months of age is considered to be in the *oral stage* of development, so called because the mouth is the primary source of tension and pleasure. Satisfaction of hunger, as well as many comforting measures (e.g., finger-sucking and mouthing), center on stimulation of the mouth.

The mouth has at least five primary modes of functioning that, in analytical theory, are prototypes for certain later personality types: (1) taking in (acquisitiveness), (2) holding on (tenacity), (3) biting (destructiveness), (4) spitting out (rejection), and (5) closing (negativism). The theory proposes that the extent to which any of these traits becomes part of the mature personality depends on the amount of anxiety or frustration the individual experienced with a particular function. For example, abrupt weaning may lead to a strong tendency to hold onto things; or children who are oral-aggressive and bite with their teeth may become adults who are oral-aggressive and "bite" with sarcasm.

During the second year of life the infant moves into the *anal stage* of psychosexual development. Tensions arise in the anal region as the result of accumulated fecal material; expulsion brings relief. It is hypothesized that as a consequence of experiencing a pleasant reduction in tension from elimination, the infant may use this action to reduce tension arising in other parts of the body. Thus, expulsive elimination is considered the prototype for emotional outbursts, temper tantrums, rages, and other primitive discharge reactions.

Usually, during the second to fourth year of life, involuntary expulsive reflexes are brought under voluntary control through a set of experiences known as toilet training. This usually is the first critical experience the child has with discipline and external authority. Toilet-training methods and caregiver attitudes about defecation, cleanliness, control, and responsibility are thought to leave indelible imprints on the child's development. For example, if the training method is strict and punitive, the child may react by soiling intentionally. When older, the child may react to authority figures by being messy, disorderly, or irresponsible.

Psychosocial Development: Basic Trust Versus Basic Mistrust and Autonomy Versus Shame and Guilt

The first psychosocial task, occurring early during the first year, is developing a sense of basic trust and overcoming a sense of mistrust. According to Erikson, to do this the young infant needs to experience a mutually satisfying relationship based on familiarity, regularity, and predictability.

The development of trust initially requires a feeling of physical comfort, which then promotes emotional comfort. If this feeling of comfort is achieved, the infant becomes trusting (i.e., anticipates receiving support and assistance) even in new environments. If, however, the infant experiences physical discomfort or is uncertain about whether needs will be met because of past unpredictability, new experiences elicit apprehension and mistrust. Thus, developing a sense of confidence in the well-intentioned motives of others is the foundation for developing trusting future relationships and anticipating success in new endeavors.

Basic trust is mutual and, according to Erikson,[12] "implies not only that one has learned to rely on the sameness and continuity of the outer providers, but also that one may trust oneself and the capacity of one's own organs to cope with urges and that one is able to consider oneself trustworthy enough so that the providers will not need to be on guard lest they be nipped."

The second Eriksonian stage of psychosocial development, autonomy versus shame and doubt, is analogous to the anal stage of Freudian psychology. It begins in infancy but is not realized fully until toddlerhood. Erikson notes that muscular maturation during this time is an important element for experimentation with two simultaneous sets of social modalities, holding on and letting go.

With increasing control over both self and the environment, the child begins to experiment with manipulation and control. Some attempts are successful and others not. The manner in which successes and failures are met by caregivers helps determine how freely children express themselves. "From a sense of self-control without loss of self-esteem comes a lasting sense of good will and pride; from a sense of loss of self-control and of foreign over-control comes a lasting propensity for doubt and shame."[12]

Cognitive Development: Sensorimotor Period

According to Piagetian theory, the child from birth to approximately age 2 years is in the *sensorimotor stage*, manifested by sensory exploration, purposeful movement, manipulation of the environment, and imitation. Although the infant largely is preverbal throughout most of this period, instrumental language (use of words to indicate needs or identify objects) develops toward the end of this phase.

The sensorimotor period can be divided into six stages:

- Stage 1: Modification of reflex activity through experience (e.g., rooting evolves into active searching for the nipple)
- Stage 2: Anticipation (e.g., make sucking movements at the sight of the bottle)
- Stage 3: Imitation (e.g., clapping hands when someone else within sight claps)
- Stage 4: Purposeful action (e.g., removing an obstacle to a goal)
- Stage 5: Production of novel behaviors (e.g., trying new methods to remove an obstacle to a goal)
- Stage 6 (transition phase): Thinking about problems, imitating an absent model from memory, and using words to designate ongoing events, immediate desires, or objects in view. In addition, the child has a well-developed sense of object permanence—that is, he or she will look for a vanished object even if it has been displaced. Thus, the child appears to understand that things exist independently of the self

Social Learning Development: Rudimentary Behavior Phase

The social learning theorists describe infancy as the period during which basic needs are met and initial learning takes place within the intimate environment of the home. Positive reinforcement in the form of attention (feeding, comforting) is the predominant mode used by the family to shape the infant's behavior. Reflexive activities (grasping in response to a parental finger in the infant's palm) are rewarded (parent plays with the infant's hand, talks, and coos, therefore giving attention). In time, true grasp is learned and is followed by lifting the arms as a signal to be played with or to be held. In this way a naturally occurring primitive reflex evolves into a purposeful activity.

A further step takes place during later infancy, when the child begins to modify behavior in response to signals that are not directly or immediately physically rewarding (e.g., a smile rather than actually being held). Sensitivity to nonphysical cues is the foundation for the social component of human learning. In Freudian and Eriksonian terms, such responsiveness to the environment and acknowledgment that we are only part of it are indicators of ego development.

Toddlerhood and Preschool Age (2 to 5 Years)

During the toddler stage, the growth rate slows, personality develops further, and important strides are made in cognitive ability. Bowel and bladder control usually evolve during the third year, although the range extends from 15 months to 4 years and sometimes beyond. What the child can do physically influences his or her perception of self, which in turn influences social development and independence. The positive feedback loop of testing leading to success, leading to confidence, leading to further testing is particularly significant during this stage of rapid achievement of milestones.

Psychosexual development: phallic stage. According to Freud, the preschool-age child derives pleasure from self-stimulation of the genitalia. This masturbatory drive is different from the sexual drive of the genital stage characteristic of adolescence and adulthood, even though the same erogenous zone is involved. The basic innocence of masturbation in both boys and girls deserves repeated emphasis, especially to parents who may be highly concerned or disturbed by it.

Another hallmark of the phallic stage is intense attachment to the parent of the opposite sex and hostility toward the same-sex parent. This situation has been called the *Oedipal complex* after the mythological Greek character who killed his father and married his mother. The sex-specific rivalries are the Oedipal conflict (boys) and the Electra conflict (girls).

Before the phallic stage the mother is the primary love object for both boys and girls. During the phallic stage the boy develops a more intense relationship with his mother and becomes rivalrous with his father for his mother's attention. Conversely, the girl begins to pursue her father, relying on him to be her ally against the mother. Such behavior can be consternating to the family if the parents do not appreciate the universality of such alliances. Conflict resolution begins when the child recognizes the futility of his or her desires and, instead of wishing to take the place of the same-sex parent, moves in the direction of trying to become more like him or her. This process, by which boys desire to become more like men in their self-concept and girls desire to become more like women, has been called *identification.* It includes the incorporation of many of the same-sex parent's qualities into the child's own personality.

Freud assumed that all people are constitutionally bisexual and that the tendencies of both sexes are inherited by each child. Furthermore, he also hypothesized that a child experiences some degree of identification with each parent. Ultimately, the degree of masculinity or femininity that the child displays in later life depends on the relative strengths of his or her innate masculine or feminine tendencies, the degree to which these tendencies are rewarded or inhibited, and the strength of identification with each parent.

This stage has resolved completely when incorporation of parental qualities (internalization of parental controls) is sufficient for what Freud has called *superego formation***,** or the development of conscience. The child develops a rudimentary sense of right and wrong based on instruction and modeling by the parents.

Psychosocial development: initiative versus guilt. In Eriksonian terms, children of this age are in the initiative versus guilt stage and are moving into a larger social environment in which they are able to initiate new activities. Occasionally, the sense of personal autonomy they developed previously is challenged or frustrated by the autonomous activity of others. The ensuing conflict may lead to a sense of guilt for having gone too far in striving for initiative. This sense of guilt is overcome by learning self-modulation through the development of a conscience that reflects parental and societal values. Thus, children begin to learn to put personal and social needs into perspective and to modify the one to be in concert with the other.

Cognitive development: preoperational period. Extending from 2 to 7 years of age, the preoperational period, as defined by Piaget, is distinguished by the appearance of representational language and rudimentary reasoning. Problem solving during this period is intuitive rather than logical, and the children cannot explain their reasoning strategies.

The thought processes of the preoperational child are limited by centration (inability to consider several aspects or dimensions of a situation simultaneously), syncretism (the tendency to group several apparently unrelated things or events into a confused whole), juxtaposition (failure to perceive the real connection among several things or events), irreversibility (inability to understand successive changes or transformations), egocentrism (perception of the world only from his or her own point of view and the belief that he or she is the origin of all actions in the world), and magical thinking (equation of thought and fantasy with action, feeling that a wish can cause some external event).

The thought content of the preoperational child is influenced by animism (the belief that inanimate objects are alive as people are alive), artificialism (all things are made for a purpose), and participation (some continuing connection or interaction exists between human actions and natural processes).

Social learning development: secondary motivational systems and family-centered learning. As the child moves into the environment, more individuals become available to model and reinforce behavior. In addition, punishment is introduced as an agent for modifying the child's behavior. Discipline that is either too prescriptive or too indulgent can produce a child who has little internal sense of responsibility for personal actions. In the first instance, the child relies on the environment to provide all cues about what is or is not acceptable. In the latter instance, excessive indulgence makes it difficult for the child to learn how to distinguish right from wrong actions.

Negative attention-seeking behaviors are common at this age. They arise most often when the child is frustrated by persistent lack of attention (such as might occur if a new infant is born into the family, diverting parental time and attention away from the preschooler). Frustration at not receiving positive reinforcement for good behavior may lead to bad behavior that demands attention, even though it is negative. Although some children fear the punishment they receive for their behavior, such punishment is preferred to feeling neglected or unimportant.

School Age (6 to 12 Years)

Freud called the developmental stage between the end of toddlerhood and the onset of adolescence *latency* to describe the relatively quiescent period of sexual activity between the resolution of the Oedipal conflict and the emergence of the sexual drives of adolescence. Actually, the child's sexual drive is not really latent (dormant) at all. However, it is channeled differently.

During latency there is no qualitative change in the external genitalia, which retain their infantile appearance. Lack of observable physical change and low levels of sexually oriented drive do not mean that children are uninterested in sex, especially sex differences. Curiosity is common among 5- to 7-year-old children of both genders. Because children have been taught to keep themselves clothed in the presence of others, "playing doctor" becomes a way of satisfying natural curiosity. Girls and boys of middle latency often "kiss and run"; snapping the bra strap of a more developed girl is common in late latency. Intense "crushes," especially those focused on an unattainable idol, occur regularly. Parents sometimes need reassurance that these practices represent normal behavior.

The first major task of the latency-age child is to enter school and achieve independence from home. Teachers, first as parent surrogates and then as independent role models and authority figures, help set expectations and goals for behavior and achievement.

The 6-year-old child has the ability to perform most rudimentary gross and fine motor tasks. Therefore, latency is the time when skills are refined. Progress is tested less by the acquisition of new skills than by the rapidity and accuracy with which old skills are performed.

Indeed, skill plays a critical part in the development of the emerging personality. For the agile or athletic child, playing games and being a member of a team bring pleasure and friendship. For the physically inept child, little positive reinforcement is gleaned from these activities, and the individual may need to be directed to other areas of strength. Some children can turn to books or the arts and receive praise from parents and teachers. However, the group's emphasis, especially among boys, is on athletic prowess. The 8-year-old boy experiences tremendous pressure to play sports well; if he is clumsy, he can be at a decided disadvantage in making and keeping friends.

The child who cannot excel in sports or schoolwork is a prime candidate for developing acting-out behavior. For this child, like the toddler who is displaced by a new baby in the family, attention (usually reprimand) comes primarily from negative attention-seeking behaviors. The boy becomes "famous" among his friends, who marvel at his ability to get into trouble and his bravado about inviting punishment.

In previous generations, girls often were categorized as belonging to one of two groups during latency. The first group comprised girls known as *tomboys*. These girls tend to be more physically mature or skilled than boys their age, making them athletically competitive. The second group was made up of girls who tend to enjoy activities and games that revolve around playing house and other more strictly "feminine" activities (see Chapter 86, Cross-Sex Behavior and Gender Identity Disorder).

In more recent time, social roles have become less categorized and restrictive for both boys and girls. In addition, a new value system for social roles has emerged that encourages both athleticism in girls (e.g., Title IX legislation that mandates equal support for male and female sports) and relational interests in boys.

Psychosexual development: latency. Freud has described the latency stage as that period during which previously active libidinal and aggressive drives of the Oedipal stage become latent, and a truce is established between the id and the ego. At the beginning of latency, the superego (conscience) becomes more firmly internalized. The outlook of the latency-age child is black and white; notions about good and bad are clear and absolute and follow the guidelines set by the family.

Psychosocial development: industry versus inferiority. Erikson[12] has called the latency period the *age of industry versus inferiority*, stating that the child

> has mastered the ambulatory field and the organ modes. He has experienced a sense of finality regarding there being no workable future within the womb of his family and thus becomes ready to apply himself to given skills and tasks, which go far beyond the mere playful expression of his organ modes or the pleasure in the function of his limbs. He develops a sense of industry—that is, he adjusts himself to the inorganic laws of the tool world. He can become an eager and absorbed unit of a productive situation. To bring a productive situation to completion is an aim that gradually supersedes the whims and wishes of play.

According to Erikson, the potential danger to the child at this stage lies in acquiring a sense of inadequacy or inferiority. If the child does not believe that he or she has adequate tools or skills, becoming a successful member of the group may be impossible. Failure to become a member of the group may result in withdrawal into the family and social isolation.

Systematic instruction occurs in all cultures during this time, although not all learning takes place in school. In fact, perhaps the greatest amount is learned from older children, who are perceived as "touchable" heroes. Society's contribution is to support "questing," provide guidance, and praise achievements.

Cognitive development: concrete operational stage. Piaget characterized cognitive processes in the latency-age child as concrete operational. The child is able to take an external point of view, use logic, and be objective. Thinking becomes dynamic, decentralized, and reversible. It also becomes possible to "conserve" or to recognize that certain changes (e.g., physical rearrangement) do not necessarily alter other properties (e.g., quantity) of a substance. In Piaget's classic experiment, a clay ball is rolled into (i.e., becomes) a clay sausage. If the child can think about the transformation in such a way as to appreciate that shape does not alter quantity, the child is described as able to conserve. Conservation is the result of the child's ability to focus on several aspects of a problem or situation at one time and relate them. Thus, in the ball-sausage experiment, the child who can conserve *mass* can understand the reciprocity of length and width.

A child in the early concrete operational period can solve a problem only if the elements of the problem are physically present and often they must be actually manipulated. By the late concrete operational period, the child can solve problems of space and time; can conserve substance, quantity, weight, and volume; and can classify objects into hierarchical systems. Physical manipulation remains helpful but is not essential to problem solving.

Social learning development: secondary motivational systems and extrafamily learning. Beginning with the child's entrance into school, the values and customs of people outside the family become increasingly important. Dependency on the family must be unlearned; instead, the child must learn to act independently and in compliance with expectations made by nonfamily members of the larger social group. Admiration and approval reinforce socially acceptable behaviors. If desirable behaviors are not reinforced consistently or if the only attention the child receives is through socially unacceptable behaviors, undesirable behaviors will be learned at this stage just as they were at earlier ages within the home. Thus, the basic principles of learning are independent of the individual's age and setting.

Adolescence and Young Adulthood

The term *adolescence* is derived from the Latin *adolescere* (to grow up) and refers to the psychological, biological, and sociological aspects of development that occur during the second decade of life. *Puberty* refers to the condition of becoming sexually mature and being capable of sexual reproduction.

The age of onset of puberty has varied considerably over the centuries, a phenomenon known as the *secular trend*.[45] For example, earlier maturation was noted over a period of 150 years during the nineteenth and early twentieth centuries but reached a plateau in American teenagers beginning in the 1960s. Reasons for such changes have been related to a variety of environmental factors such as nutrition and global temperature cycles.

Adolescence usually is divided into three stages: early, middle, and late. During early adolescence most of the individual's physical and emotional energy is centered on physical change and its consequences. During middle adolescence the focus is on separation from parents, and during late adolescence on preparation for an adult identity.

Important gender-specific differences exist in both the timing of growth and final adult size. The female growth spurt occurs about 2 years earlier than the male growth spurt, but the final adult height of women is less than that of men because of their shorter growth period. Muscle growth appears to be influenced primarily by androgenic stimulation. Thus, the mature man has greater muscle mass and strength than the mature woman.

Increase in body size and maturation of neuronal pathways contributes to the child's and adolescent's increasing ability to perform complex motor tasks. Large muscles develop before small muscles. Therefore, younger children are more skillful in activities involving gross motor movements than they are in activities requiring fine motor coordination. In early adolescence, differential bone and muscle growth can result in transient increases in awkwardness, particularly in gross motor functioning. During middle and late adolescence, the growth rate slows over time, leading to greater stability in body proportions; motor awkwardness gradually decreases.

Throughout infancy and childhood, circulating levels of pituitary follicle-stimulating hormone and luteinizing hormone are low. Although growth of both the internal and external genitalia parallels increases in body size, the genitalia retain their infantile appearance and function. For reasons that are not completely clear but that may be related to critical body weight, the hypothalamus becomes less sensitive to negative feedback from circulating gonadotropin. As a result, luteinizing hormone-releasing factor is produced and gonadotropin secretion is enhanced, rising progressively toward adult levels. This marks the onset of puberty.

Pubertal change can be divided into three stages. During the first, prepubescence (prepuberty), the gonadotropin and sex steroid levels remain low; however, secondary sexual characteristics begin to appear. In girls, the earliest sign of sexual maturation is widening of the pelvic girdle. This is followed by breast and pubic hair development and the onset of the height spurt. In boys, testicular growth precedes penile growth, development of pubic hair, and the onset of the height spurt.

During the second stage, pubescence (puberty), the reproductive organs (primary sexual characteristics) become functional, and the secondary sexual characteristics become more evident. The last stage, postpubescence (postpuberty), includes a 1- to 2-year period of relative reproductive infertility. Skeletal growth is completed during this time.

Psychosexual development: the genital stage. According to Freudian theory, sexual impulses reemerge during adolescence, marking the onset of the genital stage. Whereas pleasure seeking through oral, anal, and genital stimulation was the aim of the infantile form of sexuality, during puberty another sexual aim arises: reproduction.

During early adolescence there is thought to be a partial recrudescence of the Oedipal conflict, or a regression to the psychosexual stage characteristic of the preschool child. This may occur because the adolescent feels safer expressing new and confusing sexual feelings within the familiar environment of the family. However, the adolescent recognizes that emotional closeness to the parent of the other gender is both unrealistic and unacceptable. The adolescent also has learned from experiences during the phallic stage that real competition with the parent of the same gender is hopeless.

Eventually the adolescent seeks independence from both parents, not just the parent of the same gender. In some cases a period of significant alienation from the family may be necessary to gain sufficient distance for independence to be attained. During the resolution of the parent-child conflict of the genital stage, the boy completes his (adult) identification with his father by choosing a female partner. Similarly, the girl completes her (adult) identification with her mother by seeking a male partner. Thus, full sexual maturity, in Freudian terms, is attained when feelings directed toward the parent of the other gender are transferred successfully to a love object that is not taboo.

In addition to whatever sexual overtones may be associated with movement into the genital stage, the process of renewed competition with the parent of the same gender also provokes questioning of the behavior, values, and judgments of the parent. To explain this phenomenon, it is important to recall that resolution of the Oedipal phase in early childhood brought with it acceptance of the parental value system and a desire to be like the parent. The value system that was accepted, however, was rudimentary because the child was not cognitively capable of fully understanding such concepts as intent and competing priorities. For example, the preoperational child cannot understand that although behavior may be modified depending on the situation, such modifications do not necessarily impair the basic underlying value system. That is, for the young child, judgments are black and white.

However, as becomes evident in the study of cognitive growth during adolescence, the ability to understand hypothetical situations and to argue both for and against a given point of view renders the teenager's previous value system inadequate to deal with larger moral and philosophical issues. However, rather than turn to the parent for explanation and clarification, the adolescent assumes that the parents' value system is exactly as he or she conceived of it as a young child (e.g., parents of adolescents often comment, "My teenager thinks I don't know anything"). Thus, the adolescent turns to peers or adults outside the family, looking for a new, expanded set of values. In this process the adolescent is likely to reject the parents' values. Interestingly, however, the value system the individual eventually develops is more like than unlike that of the parents. This is, perhaps, best illustrated by Mark Twain's comment: "When I was 14, I thought my father was the stupidest man alive. When I was 21, I was amazed by how much he had learned in 7 years."

The genital stage is the longest phase in the psychosexual developmental framework, lasting from adolescence to senility, when regression to the pregenital stage is thought to be common. However, attainment of the genital stage does not preclude continuing to derive pleasure from satisfaction of pregenital as well as genital drives. In addition, the personality constructs and defense mechanisms developed during the pregenital stages continue as part of the individual's permanent character structure and are manifested throughout life.

Psychosocial development: identity versus role confusion and intimacy versus isolation. Identity formation is thought by many to involve answering three questions: Who am I as a physical being? Who am I as a sexual being? Who am I as a vocational being? Of these, the major focus of this phase of development in Eriksonian terms is the task of choosing an identity (i.e., selecting a role to play within the adult community).

The process of identity formation begins in early adolescence. The individual becomes determined to be just like the other members of his or her peer group, which often is a continuation of a latency-age "chum" group. Frequently cruel in its exclusion of others, the "in" group, or clique, attempts to establish its identity as a separate social unit. The rigid structure of the group provides security for individual members to identify and fulfill particular roles without feeling confused.

Thus, as adolescents move out of the known environment of family into the world, they pass through a transitional phase as members of closely knit peer groups. In much the same way parents did, the group defines acceptable and unacceptable behavior. However, to facilitate separation from family, the rules and values of the group the adolescent chooses often are different from, if not antithetical to, those of the family. In this way teenagers seek to demonstrate that they are their own persons, doing their "own thing" (see Chapter 91, Peer Relationship Problems).

Part of developing identity is (1) recognizing personal strengths and weaknesses, (2) aspiring to goals that are realistic and attainable, and (3) working toward those goals. The potential danger is never achieving clarity of role; closely allied is having too many roles (identity diffusion) or choosing a role without exploring options (identity foreclosure).

Some adolescents choose a negative identity (i.e., an identity counter to that suggested by society) because they see conformity as the route to being a nonentity. The positive role of the individual who has a negative identity can be social change. In such situations, even though overcoming the inertia of the status quo may require great energy and commitment, such deviance can have such a major effect on social mores that the individual perceives the effort as worthwhile. For example, many of the characteristics of the hippie of the late 1960s could be found in conventional youth by the mid 1970s. Similarly, the antiwar sentiments of young people ostracized in the 1970s became common in the 1980s. For those who advocated such changes, assuming an identity outside the mainstream may have appeared to be the only option for changing the system. The danger of assuming a counterculture identity, however, is permanent ostracism: never achieving sufficient reintegration to effect desired change or to derive a satisfying sense of self from society.

During late adolescence and young adulthood, the individual moves into the stage of intimacy versus isolation. Once personal identity becomes established, the young adult is eager to fuse his or her identity with that of another: to develop intimacy or the capacity to commit oneself to a partnership despite personal sacrifice and compromise. Although often thought of in sexual terms, intimacy includes close friendships, inspiring teacher-student relationships, and other affiliations in which personal vulnerability and true glimpses of the self are permitted. The antithesis of intimacy, in Eriksonian terms, is the state of *distantiation*, or isolation from or the destruction of those who appear to be a danger to oneself or to one's intimate relations (i.e., prejudices against those who are unfamiliar or foreign and thus threatening).

True genitality, a term borrowed from Freud, develops during this phase. Erikson believed that to be of lasting social significance, true genitality should include a heterosexual love relationship that ultimately produces children.

The danger of this adolescent/young adult phase is selection of an inappropriate partner for reasons of expediency rather than for fulfillment of mutual purposes.

Cognitive development: formal operational period. Beginning in early adolescence and extending throughout adulthood, the period of formal operations is distinguished by the ability to use abstract thought. Characteristics of formal operational thought include flexibility, complex reasoning, and hypothesis formation.

Not all adolescents or all adults apply formal operational thinking to all aspects of reality, nor are they "formal operational" under all conditions and circumstances. Rather, use of formal operations often is restricted to cognitive functioning in areas of particular personal interest or professional concern and is applied most productively at times of low stress and anxiety. In addition, there are gender-specific differences. For example, females are more likely than males to apply formal operations to interpersonal matters; males are more likely to apply formal operations to scientific matters.

The development of formal operational or abstract thought allows the adolescent to understand certain moral, political, and philosophical ideas for the first time. With the emergence of the ability to deal with concepts such as liberty and justice, adolescents become preoccupied with social, religious, and political issues. Because they can conceive of the ideal, be it society, religion, or family, they become aware of the contradictions, falsehoods, and shortcomings embedded in their previously accepted beliefs.

Adolescents can think about thinking; they understand the thought processes of others and wonder how individuals see them and what these individuals really think about them. A belief that others may dwell on or constantly evaluate their appearance and behaviors results in the egocentrism or self-centeredness particularly characteristic of the early and middle adolescent. Self-consciousness is a direct reflection of this self-centeredness. As formal operational thinking becomes better established, the individual begins to distinguish between personal preoccupation and the thoughts of others. Once this distinction can be made, the adolescent is able to enter into an intimate emotional relationship with others.

Stress, such as illness, can profoundly impair the individual's ability to use higher-order cognitive skills. Thus, cognitive regression frequently accompanies the general physical and emotional regression seen in a hospitalized child. Such phenomena as magical thinking ("my wish equals action") or egocentrism ("my action caused some external unrelated event") are common. The ability to think futuristically about the potential consequences of current actions also can be impaired. Conversely, long-term illness can result in increased learning and adult-like understanding of related issues. Because this can occur in children of all ages, it is not unusual for children who have long-term, fatal malignancies, for example, to have an understanding of body function or a conception of death that is surprisingly mature. This finding is in keeping with Piaget's premise that cognitive functioning is highly dependent on experience.

Social learning development: secondary motivational systems and extrafamilial learning. As the individual matures, the nature and scope of interactions with others broaden. Reinforcement of rudimentary behaviors becomes less critical as socially acceptable behaviors become habitual. Rewards and punishments are based more on internal than external controls. Thus, the adolescent is able to enter into relationships based on the mutuality of needs of two or more independent people.

SPECIFIC DEVELOPMENTAL ISSUES

Research that has focused on the development of the child's understanding of certain concepts has provided the opportunity for practical application of developmental theory. The development of moral judgment is presented as an example.

Development of Moral Judgment

Parents often ask pediatricians why a child appears to have little concept of right and wrong or why irreconcilable conflicts arise between a parent and child or between two children, even though the solution seems straightforward to the parent. Many parents feel frustrated when they must resort to time-out or the threat of no bedtime story to induce their children to do what is "right." Most parents would prefer to use logic or rely on some higher moral authority to persuade the child. Although this eventually becomes possible, the wise clinician knows that one of the reasons the "terrible twos" are terrible is precisely because reason and reasoning are beyond the cognitive capabilities of the typical preschooler.

How, then, do children learn right from wrong? It is clear that children's moral judgments are qualitatively different from those of adults. Furthermore, the ability to make moral judgments based on an internal rather than external value system evolves through a series of steps. A useful way to provide anticipatory guidance is to put the development of moral thinking into a framework that helps parents think in terms of stages. This approach not only provides a basis for current behavior but also demonstrates how growth is occurring, although rarely as quickly as parents wish.

Kohlberg[24] has pioneered this field, basing his model on the cognitive-intellectual principles described by Piaget. According to Kohlberg's theory, thinking about moral issues depends on the individual's general cognitive stage of development. He also suggests that there is a "cultural universality" to the sequencing of moral development, although the chronological ages at which certain stages appear differ in different cultures; within a culture, they may depend on particular social experiences. Kohlberg's scheme describes three overall levels of moral judgment: preconventional (premoral), conventional, and postconventional (principled). Each level is subdivided further into two stages: level I, stages 1 and 2; level II, stages 3 and 4; and level III, stages 5 and 6.

In the discussion that follows, these stages are presented and then related to the Freudian, Eriksonian, and social learning theory stages that occur simultaneously. These associations among theories illustrate the variety of simultaneously occurring events and challenges children experience that shape how they will respond to situations that require judgment about appropriate behavior.

Level I. The *preconventional level* is characteristic of children in the sensorimotor and preoperational periods of cognitive development, in the oral and anal stages of psychosexual development, and the trust versus mistrust and autonomy versus shame and doubt stages elaborated by Erikson. Judgments about right and wrong are determined by the external physical consequences of the actions: by whether the actions elicit punishment or rewards.

In stage 1, moral judgment is based on the principle of punishment and obedience. The child depends entirely on the external cues of the caregiver for decisions about right and wrong behavior, and compliance is motivated by a desire to obtain love and nurturance. In stage 2, the child is able to take some responsibility for satisfying personal needs but behaves out of a sense of pleasing himself or herself primarily and others secondarily. That is, stage 2 behavior is instrumental and relativistic. Fairness, reciprocity, and sharing are based on pragmatism ("I help you; you help me") rather than on loyalty or gratitude.

In early level I, behavior first is conditioned and then shaped by positive reinforcement and nonreinforcement (withholding attention). Restraint and redirection are other successful strategies for modifying behavior. Late in this stage, punishment is introduced as a form of negative reinforcement. Because the child lacks experience to understand that some behaviors (e.g., sucking on an electrical cord) could have lasting negative consequences, punishment (e.g., yelling, spanking) may be used to denote the potentially serious outcome of that behavior. Thus, the child learns not to suck on electrical cords, not because of understanding the consequence of being electrocuted, but to avoid the consequence of being verbally or physically reprimanded.

Level II. At the conventional level, moral judgments are based on (1) receiving praise and (2) following the rules. Unlike judgments characteristic of level I, those characteristic of level II can function independently of any actual physical consequences of the action.

Stage 3 behavior is that which pleases or helps others, who then show their approval by designating the child a "good boy" or a "nice girl." Stage 4 behavior, based on the principles of "law and order," is determined by respect for authority and the rules of the social group, which are seen as unchangeable. That is, rules are "concrete" (fixed and independent of circumstance or situation).

In Freudian and Eriksonian terms, this level develops in concert with resolution of the Oedipal conflict and occurs during the stages of initiative versus guilt and industry versus inferiority.[18] Thus, children learn to sublimate their own immediate aims and to incorporate the values of others. Desire to be like the parent helps the child to internalize parental qualities that please others. With this process comes the emergence of the superego, or conscience. Similarly, in Eriksonian terms, the child learns to modulate both wishes and behavior to please others. Part of pleasing others is to play by the rules: construct products, attend to learning, and refine skills: to become a person who is seen as being industrious.

According to social learning theory, the child who is moving into the community learns through observation and imitation of an increasingly large pool of individuals who act as models. Conformity to rules and respect for authority are particularly important attributes for successful participation in large group activities and, therefore, are strongly reinforced as socially acceptable behaviors.

Level III. At this level, moral judgments are based on personal conformity to principles that are seen as valid apart from social authority and convention. This level of reasoning requires full formal operational thinking.

In stage 5, sometimes known as the social contract or legalistic stage, the individual recognizes that personal rights and standards exist but that such personal values and opinions are relative. Procedural rules for reaching consensus are exercised; laws are recognized as changeable to meet the needs of the common good rather than as rigid and inflexible. Stage 6 judgments are based on broad abstract moral principles (e.g., the Golden Rule) rather than on concrete moral imperatives (e.g., the Ten Commandments). Universal principles of justice, reciprocity, equality of human rights, and respect for human dignity are applied to moral decision making.

Again, striking similarities exist in the way Kohlberg conceptualizes this stage and the major characteristics identified in the genital stage of Freudian theory and the identity versus role confusion stage of Eriksonian theory. Thus, knowledge of and respect for oneself as an individual allow the adolescent/young adult to engage in mutual and reciprocal relationships with other people (the basis of "true genitality" as well as of "identity" and "intimacy").

Finally, in terms of social learning theory, participation in broad extrafamilial learning systems in which the motivations for behavior are secondary and derived from nonimmediate reinforcement permits the individual to obtain satisfaction from behavior that is conducive to some higher social goal, even though it may be unsatisfying personally in the short term. Certainly there can be little argument that the ability to delay gratification, or even suffer personally, is a key element if adherence to such stage 6 principles as justice and equality is to be successful.

In keeping with other general developmental theorists, Kohlberg states that individuals who have attained certain levels of moral judgment still have available to them, and occasionally use, lower levels of judgment.[26] He has called this regression a *judgment of ease* as opposed to a *judgment of preference,* because he assumes that individuals would, under all circumstances, prefer to use the highest level of moral reasoning available to them. Kohlberg also suggests that the motivation for a given behavior may not always be clear from the behavior itself. For example, if the driver of a car decelerates to the speed limit when a police car appears ahead, such behavior may represent a judgment of ease based on stage 1 (obedience and punishment) reasoning or higher order stage 4 (law and order) reasoning. (Interestingly, it is possible that someone operating at stages 5 or 6 might not slow down at all if traffic were light and the driving conditions excellent, arguing that speed limits are arbitrary and the spirit of the law [safe driving] and not the letter of the law [55 mph speed limit] is the more valid ethic on which to base behavior.)

Although the Kohlberg model provides a reasonable framework for understanding moral development in general, its applicability is limited by its reliance on boys and men as the major subject pool from which his observations were drawn. Gilligan[14] and others who have studied girls and women have questioned whether the intense focus on competitiveness and the following of rules is as valid in the development of moral reasoning and judgment in females as it may be in males. Indeed, it has been suggested that compared with boys, girls are more pragmatic about rules, more contextual in their application (e.g., factoring relational variables into the reasoning process to promote harmony within the group), and more adaptable to innovation. These characteristics of female decision making are thought to reflect society's traditional tendency to socialize girls so that they will view "playing the game" as subordinate to keeping friends, a tradition that, in the past, has placed them at substantial disadvantage when seeking the time-honored male version of corporate success. However, the trend in current American society is toward less gender role stereotyping. Although the influence on both male and female moral judgments remains to be seen, the effects of some recent changes in corporate structure, especially in the direction of such management strategies as shared decision making, are already evident.

"IT'S JUST A STAGE"

Although, theoretically, children and adolescents achieve biopsychosocial maturity in a predictable fashion, in reality, human variability and dissonance between growth and development make predictions about a given individual difficult, frustrating, and challenging. When the pediatrician can offer reassurance about the temporary nature of a particular undesirable or anxiety-provoking stage of development, children and their families often are better able to cope, knowing that minor changes in parenting expectations or interpersonal relationships will result in better adjustment to the current stage and smoother transition to the next stage.

Although the spectrum of variability is broad, not all deviations from average expected development are normal. The greatest challenge to the practitioner is to distinguish between adequate, although not necessarily perfect, development and true dysfunction. Passing a situation off as merely "a stage" is justified only when the true limits of acceptable behavior for that stage are clearly understood, the reasons for the behavior can be explained in such a way that the parents or child can understand what they are experiencing and why, and appropriate guidance to help them master the stage is provided.

REFERENCES

1. Ader R, Felton DL, Cohen N: *Psychoneuroimmunology*, ed 2, San Diego, 1991, Academic Press.
2. Ainsworth MDS: Object relations, dependency, and attachment: a theoretical review of the infant-mother relationship, *Child Dev* 40:969, 1969.
3. Baldwin AL: *Theories of child development*, New York, 1967, John Wiley & Sons.
4. Barr RG: Normality: a clinically useless concept—the case of infant crying and colic, *J Dev Behav Pediatr* 14:264, 1993.
5. Berndt TJ, Hawkins JA, Hoyle SG: Changes in friendship during a school year, *Child Dev* 57:1284, 1986.
6. Boyce WT, Barr RG, Zeltzer LK: Temperament and the psychobiology of childhood stress, *Pediatrics* 90:483, 1992.
7. Cernoch JM, Porter RH: Recognition of maternal axillary odor by infants, *Child Dev* 56:1593, 1985.
8. Chess S, Thomas A: *Origins and evolution of behavior disorders: from infancy to early adult life*, New York, 1984, Brunner/Mazel.
9. Coe CL, et al: Early rearing conditions alter immune responses in the developing infant primate, *Pediatrics* 90:505, 1992.
10. DeFries JC, et al: Familial resemblance for specific cognitive abilities, *Behav Genet* 9:23, 1979.
11. Eder R, Mangelsdorf SC: The emotional basis of early personality development: implications for the emergent self-concept. In Hogan R, Johnson J, Briggs S, editors: *Handbook of personality psychology*, Orlando, Fla, 1994, Academic Press.
12. Erikson EH: *Childhood and society*, ed 2, New York, 1963, WW Norton.
13. Falkner B, Ragonesi S: Psychosocial stress and reactivity as risk factors of cardiovascular disease, *J Am Acad Child Adolesc Psychiatry* 25:779, 1986.
14. Gilligan C: *In a different voice: psychological theory and women's development*, Cambridge, Mass, 1982, Harvard University Press.
15. Gottesman II: Heritability of personality: a demonstration, *Psychol Monogr* 77 (No 9, Whole No 572), 1963.
16. Greenberg M, Morris N: Engrossment: the newborn's impact upon the father, *Am J Orthopsychiatry* 44:520, 1974.
17. Gunner MR: Reactivity of the hypothalamic-pituitary-adrenocortical system to stressors in normal infants and children, *Pediatrics* 90:491, 1992.
18. Hall CS: *A primer of Freudian psychology*, New York, 1954, World.
19. Hay D, Nash A, Pedersen J: Interactions between 6-month-old peers, *Child Dev* 54:557, 1983.
20. Hetherington EM, Reiss D, Plomin R: *Separate social worlds of siblings: the impact of nonshared environment on development*, Hillsdale, NJ, 1994, Lawrence Erlbaum.
21. Hirshfeld DR, et al: Stable behavioral inhibition and its association with anxiety disorder, *J Am Acad Child Adolesc Psychiatry* 31:103, 1992.
22. Kagan J, Reznick JS, Snidman N: The physiology and psychology of behavioral inhibition in young children, *Child Dev* 58:1459, 1988.
23. Klaus MH, Kennell JH: *Parent-infant bonding*, ed 2, St Louis, 1982, Mosby.
24. Kohlberg L: Moral development. In Sills DL, editor: *International encyclopedia of the social sciences*, New York, 1968, Macmillan.
25. Korner AF: The effect of the infant's level of arousal, sex, and ontogenetic stage on the caregivers. In Lewis M, Rosenblum LA, editors: *The effect of the infant on its caregiver*, New York, 1974, John Wiley & Sons.
26. Lamb ME: Father-infant and mother-infant interaction in the first year of life, *Child Dev* 48:167, 1977.
27. Lamb ME: The role of the father: an overview. In Lamb ME, editor: *The role of the father in child development*, New York, 1981, John Wiley & Sons.
28. Loehlin JC, Rowe DC: Genes, environment, and personality. In Caprara G, Van Heck GL, editors: *Modern personality psychology: critical reviews and new directions*, New York, 1992, Harvester Wheatsheaf.
29. Miller BD, Wood BL: Psychophysiologic reactivity in asthmatic children: a cholinergically mediated confluence of pathways, *J Am Acad Child Adolesc Psychiatry* 33:1236, 1994.
30. Nichols RC: Twin studies of ability, personality, and interests, *Homo* 29:158, 1978.
31. Parke RD: Perspectives on father-infant interaction. In Osofsky JD, editor: *Handbook of infant development*, New York, 1979, John Wiley & Sons.
32. Plomin R, DeFries JC, Loehlin JC: Genotype-environment interaction and correlation in the analysis of human behavior, *Psychological Bulletin* 84:309, 1977.
33. Plomin R, et al: *Behavioral genetics*, ed 3, New York, 1997, WH Freeman.
34. Porges SW: Vagal tone: a physiologic marker of stress vulnerability, *Pediatrics* 90:498, 1992.
35. Reiss D, et al: *The relationship code: deciphering genetic and social influences on adolescent development*, Cambridge, Mass, 2000, Harvard University Press.
36. Rothbart MK, Derryberry D: Development of individual differences of temperament. In Lamb ME, Brown AL, editors: *Advances in developmental psychology*, vol 1, Hillsdale, NJ, 1981, Lawrence Erlbaum.
37. Rothbart MK, Posner MJ: Temperament and the development of self-regulation. In Hartlage H, Telzrow CG, editors: *The neuropsychology of individual differences: a developmental perspective*, New York, 1985, Plenum Press.
38. Rubin JZ, Provenzano FJ, Luria Z: The eye of the beholder: parents' views on sex of newborns, *Am J Orthopsychiatry* 44:512, 1974.
39. Scarr S: Developmental theories for the 1990s: development and individual differences, *Child Dev* 63:1, 1992.
40. Scarr S, Grajek S: Similarities and differences among siblings. In Lamb ME, Sutton-Smith B, editors: *Sibling relationships: their nature and significance across the life span*, Hillsdale, NJ, 1982, Lawrence Erlbaum.
41. Scarr S, McCartney K: How do people make their own environments: a theory of genotype-environment effects, *Child Dev* 54:424, 1983.
42. Sears RR: A theoretical framework for personality and social behavior, *Am Psychol* 6:476, 1951.
43. Sosa R, et al: The effect of a supportive companion on perinatal problems, length of labor, and mother-infant interaction, *N Engl J Med* 303:597, 1980.
44. Suomi SJ: Genetic and maternal contributions to individual differences in rhesus monkey biobehavioral development. In Krasnagor N, editor: *Psychobiological aspects of behavioral development*, New York, 1988, Academic Press.
45. Tanner JM: *Fetus into man: physical growth from conception to maturity*, Cambridge, Mass, 1978, Harvard University Press.
46. Thomas A, Chess S: An approach to the study of sources of individual differences in child behavior, *J Clin Exp Psychopathol Q Rev Psychiatry Neurol* 18:347, 1957.
47. Thomas A, Chess S: *Temperament and development*, New York, 1977, Brunner/Mazel.
48. Yogman MW: Development of the father-infant relationship. In Fitzgerald H, et al, editors: *Theory and research in behavioral pediatrics*, New York, 1980, Plenum.

53 Mental Health of the Young: An Overview

William R. Beardslee • Julius B. Richmond

Advances in knowledge of child development, gained through the in-depth study of healthy infants and children, as well as through observations of deviations or delays in development, have provided the pediatrician with the conceptual framework needed to deal effectively with the mental health needs of children. Recent advances within child psychiatry also have contributed substantially, including, for example, the development of reliable, standardized interview instruments, a criterion-based diagnostic system (*Diagnostic and Statistical Manual-IV* of the American Psychiatric Association), and the description of the epidemiology of a number of childhood mental disorders. Based on a series of well-conducted efficacy studies, evidence that there are good treatments for many of the major mental disorders of childhood is increasing. Interest also is growing in ascertaining how best to translate these research findings into broadscale programs that reach all children—that is, in public health terms, the transition of efficacy studies to effectiveness studies and then to large-scale programs.[12] A more sophisticated understanding of the prevalence and nature of neurodevelopmental and neuropsychiatric difficulties also has substantially expanded the information available to the pediatrician. An expanding knowledge base in the neurosciences, including molecular biology and molecular genetics, already has strengthened our understanding of the etiology and treatment of childhood psychiatric disorders and undoubtedly will continue to expand in the years to come. For example, in both Tourette's syndrome and childhood depression, evidence of interference with neurotransmitter function leading to the behavioral manifestations of the disorder is established. Recent findings emphasize the plasticity of development and point to the need to understand the interactions of both biological factors and environmental influences at each stage across the course of childhood.[3]

Advances in the development of preventive and therapeutic agents over the past 40 years have brought about major reductions in infant mortality and childhood morbidity and mortality. No longer is the practicing pediatrician's time consumed by rickets, scurvy, or the acute infectious diseases such as measles, pertussis, diphtheria, and poliomyelitis. Rather, more time and energy are available to focus on the prevention of disease and the early detection and care of children who have chronic disorders, including developmental disabilities.

In addition, the past decade has been characterized by an increasing awareness by organized consumers of the desirability of high-quality child health and child care services. Pressure from communities for improved child health services has increased, a concern reflected in the development of programs such as Head Start; early periodic screening, diagnosis, and treatment (EPSDT) for Medicaid-eligible children; and community mental health centers. The new approaches to more comprehensive services for children with handicaps also reflect intensified community sophistication, such as the Education for All Handicapped Children Act (Public Law 94-142), which emphasizes the need to "mainstream" such children. Public Law 99-457 has mandated adequate services for younger children with handicaps.

Recently, attention to cost effectiveness and the need for broadening the base of medical and psychiatric coverage to include all Americans also has led to a reexamination of the service delivery system. An initial report from the Carnegie Foundation[2] has emphasized the need for a wide array of services for children, as has current interest in the expansion downward of the Head Start Program to include youngsters 0 to 3 years of age. In general, the need to prepare children for entrance to kindergarten has received attention. There also is greater awareness of the need for partnerships with communities and parents for the success of such initiatives. This interest in child health in the early years undoubtedly will result in an effort to reorganize services and generate local initiatives to reflect local needs and priorities. The emphasis increasingly will be on the enhancement of health and the prevention of disease. Thus, competence in the assessment and guidance of growth and development needs to be among the pediatrician's clinical skills.

The pediatrician must have a firm grasp of the child development field. Piaget's work[8] provides the most useful framework within the cognitive sphere because of its emphasis on the child's actions as necessary for the acquisition of knowledge and on the predictable sequence of stages through which a child passes in developing intelligence. Skinner's work[14] in the area of behavioral modification and its applications has proved valuable both in helping children to learn and in suggesting ways to manage difficult or troublesome symptoms. Several workers in the area of early infant and child behavior, including Thomas, Chess, and Birch,[15] have helped to focus attention on the importance of temperament as an early influence. Expansion of developmental frameworks to include moral development[6] and interpersonal development[13] have contributed further to the understanding of normal development. In addition, large-scale epidemiological studies have provided valuable data about prevalence and incidence of both physical and mental disorders.[7] See also Chapter 52, Theories and Concepts of Development as They Relate to Pediatric Practice.

The work of Erikson[4] probably provides the best integrative framework through which pediatricians can understand the different factors shaping the mental health of the child and then best meet the needs of their patients. Erikson stresses the importance of all three major factors—biological, intrapsychic, and cultural—in the child's mental health. He sees the child as going through a series of stages in development and formulates the essential task or critical area to be mastered for each stage. Thus, as one example, the dilemma for the very young infant is basic trust versus mistrust; firm patterns for the solution of this dilemma must be successfully established for the infant to develop in a healthy way. As another example, the dilemma for the adolescent is identity versus role diffusion. Youths in this stage must come to understand their own physical endowments, experiences, and opportunities in a way that allows them to function in the world and have a sense of certainty about themselves. Specifically, youths must come to grips with three areas: (1) relationships with others, both sexual and nonsexual; (2) independence from family; and (3) choice of work or career. Familiarity with each stage, both with its task and the signs of its successful resolution, provides the pediatrician with knowledge of the principles of child mental health. More generally, it is useful for the pediatrician in working with families to conceptualize the developmental challenge and the resources available in the child, the family, and the community, at a particular developmental stage. Then, the pediatrician will be able to recognize that a developmental stage has either been successfully accomplished or requires from a pediatrician either remedial or preventive intervention.

Common to a series of recent investigations of youngsters at risk because of poverty or parental mental illness or other stressors is the finding that no matter how great the risk, a significant number of children turn out to do well and, indeed, function very effectively.[5] Rutter has indicated a variety of conceptual areas to be reviewed in studying the sources of resiliency and looking for explanations.[11] These include genetic effects, individual differences, particularly the role of temperament, inner psychological processes, and the role of influences outside of the home, especially the schools. Two characteristics of resilient youngsters across studies are the involvement in close confiding human relationships and the capacity to take action outside of the home, in school, extracurricular activities, religious and community organizations, and work or other age-appropriate developmental venues. Of particular relevance to pediatric practice are a number of studies of resilient individuals that have emphasized the importance of the way these individuals understand themselves and what they have accomplished—their capacity for self-reflection and the ability to use that self-reflection to inform planning for the future—in short, self-understanding.[1] This self-understanding involves adequate appraisal of the stresses to be dealt with, realistic assessment of the capacity to act, and actions congruent with the assessment, and has characterized people in such diverse circumstances as survivors of cancer, civil rights workers, and children of parents who have an affective disorder. The recognition and characterization of resilient behavior in pediatric practice in high-risk families is important and emphasizes the need to assess a child or family's strengths and capacities to adapt to an adversity.[9] Often, the ability to mount an effective intervention depends on the recognition of strengths at the individual family and community levels and the mobilization of resources to enhance those strengths.[5]

Increasing attention has been paid to the prevention of mental disorder and psychological difficulty in addition to the treatment of disorder once it occurs. This requires an understanding of the developmental pathways of both psychopathology and healthy development and the positioning of interventions at the times of greatest likelihood of success—for example, enhancing the bond between caregiver and child early in life or assisting in developmental transition in adolescence. A number of well-validated preventive strategies exists that can contribute strongly to the mental health of children across the life span.[7]

Knowing the cultural and psychological background of a child's family is important for understanding the mental health needs of that child. The emotional climate in which a child is reared reflects the personality development of the parents or parent substitutes. Therefore, the pediatrician must know about the developmental background of each parent and the immediate environmental factors that are significant in the child's life. Because different families impose different roles on children, it is important for the pediatrician to know how the child fits into the family constellation. Just as the physiological structure and function of an infant have determinants that antedate birth, the practices and attitudes that determine how the child will be cared for have comparable antecedents. The pediatrician may develop an understanding of these factors as they become apparent during the prenatal period or after birth, as he or she comes to know the family as a unit.

The pediatrician can regard the family as carrying the "chromosomes" that perpetuate the culture and also that form the cornerstone of emotional development. Cultural influences are like a mainstream with many tributaries: Each varies from time to time in depth, rate of flow, and course; the mainstream is modified by its tributaries, but also influences them.

In the United States many variations exist in cultural patterns relating to childbearing attitudes and practices. These are determined in part by geographical, religious, educational, social, and economic backgrounds. For example, in some communities a great premium is placed on the first child being male. Religious backgrounds definitely tend to influence the size of families. Higher educational backgrounds of parents have been correlated with a later childbearing age and with limitation in family size.

The relative rapidity of social movement tends to confuse young parents in terms of their basic group identification. Also, increasing educational opportunities usually generate upward social mobility for many young parents. The pediatrician should know how much parents identify with their old and how much with their new social grouping and its culture. Either of these identifications (usually some of both) involves some reintegration on the part of the parents, who may require professional assistance. Over the past 50 years, the number of different, distinct cultures has increased. There is growing awareness of the need to tailor interventions individually to a particular culture, and the strategies required to do so also have expanded.[10]

Furthermore, more and more changes in the structure of the American family have occurred—among them, an increase in the number of single-parent families, a rise in the number of children and families living in poverty, and an expansion of the number of children being raised by relatives and adoptive parents. Another important factor is lack of availability of extended family either to help in child rearing or to provide the necessary child developmental knowledge. For all these reasons, parents, grandparents, and other caregivers rely more and more on pediatricians for guidance about child rearing.

The pediatrician should learn to adjust his or her cultural background and attitudes toward childbearing and child rearing with the cultural backgrounds and attitudes of parents who seek advice. It then becomes easier to understand that there is no right attitude or practice. A certain practice may be effective for one family and yet its objectives fail with another. Thus, the pediatrician can help by being objective rather than judgmental in viewing the family. This requires the capacity to observe, listen, and as a consequence, understand.

The pediatrician can develop an objective attitude by remembering that it is the culture, and not the physician, that, within certain limits, defines mental health. For example, Erikson[4] and others have pointed out that children brought up in one Native American culture might not be considered capable of performing the developmental tasks required of children in another tribe living in a different climate with significantly different cultural demands. Many similar cross-cultural comparisons can be made. Although the pediatrician generally deals with more subtle contrasts, they nevertheless are real and significant for each family. In a country of people who have such varied origins and so much educational, social, economic, and geographical movement, it is unlikely that any one stable tradition of child rearing practices will emerge in the next several decades. Therefore, the objective in each instance is to help each family attain its goal in child rearing uniquely and effectively.

Schools, families, child care centers, and hospitals all are concerned with the mental health of children. The pediatrician can combine medical findings with observations of children within their families and perceptions of larger cultural influences to evaluate and meet the mental health needs of children. The evaluation of psychological health is a vital part of the comprehensive pediatric assessment of children. Such evaluations provide the basis for helping parents become more effective in rearing their children through helping them to articulate and realize their own goals for them. Because of the increasing numbers of health professionals and disciplines that work with children, the pediatrician's role has become even more integrative. He or she is the one who brings together the different disciplines and different kinds of knowledge—biological, psychological, and social—in a comprehensive understanding of the treatment for the child.

When the pediatrician approaches the management of illness as one aspect of the total care of the child and is interested in the interpersonal relations between the pediatrician and family, each child can provide an intriguing study. The pediatrician also has the opportunity to help foster the psychological development of the child. In this regard, and in dealing with the child and parents, the pediatrician's attitudes, interest, and curiosity about human behavior and relations are important, probably more so than formal knowledge in this area. The pediatrician's receptivity and alertness in recognizing psychologically charged situations will extend, condition, or limit his or her effectiveness in the care of many children.

Assuming the primary responsibility for all physical and medical care of the child also provides pediatricians with responsibility and opportunity to learn about and care for the psychological and mental health needs of children. Pediatricians who wish to provide total care should be interested in children not only in intellectual terms but also in emotional terms. Those pediatricians are in a unique position from which to encourage wholesome attitudes of child rearing during each contact with the family. Concomitantly, they can detect unwholesome attitudes and disturbances early in a child's life and endeavor to provide a more favorable setting for the child through interviews and counseling with the parents. In situations of severe distress, the pediatrician may decide that more extensive psychological treatment through psychotherapy or other means is needed and make a referral for psychiatric consultation. But fundamentally, he or she remains the key professional who evaluates the overall health of the child comprehensively, including the child's mental health, while serving as the central person in the parents' eyes for counseling and guidance.

REFERENCES

1. Beardslee WR: The role of self-understanding in resilient individuals: the development of a perspective, *Am J Orthopsychiatry* 59:266, 1989.
2. Carnegie Task Force: *Starting points: meeting the needs of our youngest children: the report of the Carnegie Task Force on meeting the needs of our youngest children,* New York, 1994, Carnegie Corporation of New York.
3. Eisenberg L: The social construction of the human brain, *Am J Psychiatry* 152:1563, 1995.
4. Erikson EH: *Childhood and society,* ed 2, New York, 1963, WW Norton.
5. Glantz MD, Johnson JL, editors: *Resilience and development,* New York, 1999, Kluwer Academic/Plenium Publishers.
6. Kohlberg L: Stage and sequence: the cognitive-developmental approach to socialization. In Goslin D, editor: *Handbook of socialization theory and research,* Chicago, 1969, Rand McNally.
7. Mrazek PJ, Haggerty RJ, editors: *Reducing risks for mental disorders: frontiers for preventive intervention research,* Report of the Committee on Prevention of Mental Disorders, Division of Biobehavioral Sciences and Mental Disorders, Institute of Medicine, Washington, DC, 1994, National Academy Press.

8. Piaget J: *The origins of intelligence in children*, New York, 1963, WW Norton.
9. Richmond JB, Beardslee WR: Resiliency: research and practical implications for pediatricians, *J Dev Behav Pediatr* 9:157, 1988.
10. Rogler LH: The meaning of culturally sensitive research in mental health, *Am J Psychiatry* 146:296, 1989.
11. Rutter M: Meyerian psychobiology, personality development, and the role of life experiences, *Am J Psychiatry* 143:1077, 1986.
12. Schorr LB: *Common purpose: strengthening families and neighborhoods to rebuild America,* New York, 1997, Anchor Books, Doubleday.
13. Selman RL, Watts CL, Schultz LH: *Fostering friendship*, New York, 1997, Aldine de Gruyter.
14. Skinner BF: *Science and human behavior,* New York, 1953, Macmillan.
15. Thomas A, Chess S, Birch H: *Temperament and behavior disorders in children,* New York, 1968, New York University Press.

SUGGESTED READINGS

Richmond JB: An idea whose time has arrived, *Pediatr Clin North Am* 22:517, 1975.

Richmond JB: Child development: a basic science for pediatrics, *Pediatrics* 39:649, 1967.

54 Foster Care and Adoption

Moira Szilagyi

In an ideal world, every child would be reared by nurturing and caring birth parents. But for many children, the world is far from ideal, and children who cannot reside with their birth families need to be cared for in alternative settings. Such care may be provided informally by their extended family, neighbors, or friends. Alternatively, such children may be removed from or surrendered by their families to social agencies and placed in foster care and/or adopted. Foster care is intended to be a temporary respite for a family in crisis, with the ultimate goal of reunification of the child and family; adoption is a permanent joining of a child to a new family. Many of the children adopted in the United States are adopted out of the foster care system; others are adopted privately, and some are adopted internationally, often out of another country's child welfare system. Emotional and health issues for foster and adopted children often overlap; because most pediatricians will encounter such children in their practices, familiarity with the themes, issues, and mandates of both systems is imperative.

FOSTER CARE

In the United States, about 520,000 children reside in foster care on any given day.[17,18] They are, by and large, the children of the indigent, and their lives, before placement, were riddled by violence and neglect. Removed from, or abandoned by their families, these children were placed in a system intended to nurture and repair them, while facilitating the rehabilitation of their families. In reality, foster care has become a system of last resort for our most vulnerable children and intransigent families.

Foster care is a system in crisis. The system remains crushed by huge caseloads, families that have multiple intractable problems, and complex and often conflicting bureaucratic, legal, and ethical demands. It is underfunded and understaffed. The system also is in transition, because recent legislation has shifted the balance from parental rights toward the best interests of the child, with the goal of reunification now offset by the need to "transition" a child into an appropriate, permanent family setting as quickly as possible.

History of the Foster Care System

The foster care system is a twentieth-century institution rooted in England's Elizabethan Poor Laws of 1601, which evolved out of the dedicated efforts of many individuals to improve the lot of destitute and abandoned children. Designed to protect children previously left to their own resources, the charity of the community, or warehoused in institutions, foster care is founded in the beliefs that society has a responsibility for such children and that children fare best when reared in nurturing, family-based settings.

Government funding and regulation of the foster care system in the United States is relatively recent. As part of the Social Security Act of 1935, Aid to Dependent Children provided economic support to widowed parents left with young children. Beginning in the1960s, amendment of Title IV-A of the Social Security Act allowed states to use federal matching funds to support Aid to Families with Dependent Children (AFDC) eligible children placed in foster care. Over the next several decades, the population of children in foster care expanded rapidly because of increased admissions and longer placements. The burgeoning costs of the system and the recognition that separating children from their families almost always is traumatic led to several attempts at reform. In 1980, the Adoption Assistance and Child Welfare Act, PL-96-272, mandated states to provide broader services (such as counseling, day care, parenting education, and drug rehabilitation) to avert the removal of children from their birth families. Agencies were mandated to conduct semiannual case reviews and to develop permanency plans within 18 months of placement. Adoption subsidies were funded, so that marginal family income would be less of a barrier to the adoption of children out of foster care.

After enactment of PL-96-272, the size of the foster care population diminished transiently. Unfortunately, in the past two decades, the number of children in foster care has increased dramatically, as a surge in parental substance abuse has offset the impact of earlier reforms. Late 1990s welfare reform initiatives are expected to increase admissions further to foster care, as funding for preventive services and public assistance is curtailed. Recent data suggest that while more women of child-bearing age have entered the work force, the number of children living in the poorest of poor families has increased, because "safety net" services have shrunk. Such services sometimes are the only barrier to the complete dissolution of a destitute, multi-problem family.

The Adoption and Safe Families Act (ASFA) of 1997 was enacted by Congress to address a number of issues. Previously, the focus on reunification and parental rights placed some children at considerable risk of injury, neglect, or prolonged stays in foster care. ASFA shifted the emphasis in child welfare toward the health and safety of the child and more timely permanency planning. States now are obligated to pursue termination of parental rights for any child who has been in foster care for 15 of the prior 22 months, although continuing efforts at reunification may occur. Furthermore, the state is not obligated to reunify families and children when a parent has behaved violently toward any one of their children. Although the full impact of this legislation is yet to be realized, the number of adoptions out of foster care has increased dramatically.

Epidemiology

Families whose children reside in foster care generally are impoverished, living on the fringes of society and having few social supports.[1,2] Many experience multiple social stressors, including single parenthood, lack of education, unemployment, substance abuse, mental or physical health problems, domestic violence, and criminal justice involvement. Many birth parents are disturbed emotionally, and some (less than 10%) are mentally retarded. In the 1990s, the incidence of parental addiction to drugs or alcohol, especially crack cocaine, rose dramatically. About one third of birth parents admit to being abused or neglected as children; about the same number spent time in foster care. About one third have abused their own children physically or sexually or have failed to protect them from abuse by others. In about 70% of cases, removal of a child occurs after prolonged involvement with social service agencies, including Child Protective Services, after preventive strategies have been exhausted and the child's health and safety are at imminent risk.

Admission to foster care is and should be difficult. Almost all children entering foster care are placed involuntarily by court order, either because of child abuse and neglect (about 70%), or by the juvenile justice system as PINS (Person in Need of Supervision) or JD (Juvenile Delinquent) placements (27%). Only 3% are placed voluntarily by families temporarily unable to care for them; these usually are children who have a catastrophic medical illness or a severe behavioral disturbance.[17]

The immediate reasons for placement in foster care have changed in recent decades. In the past, economic hardship and child abandonment were the primary reasons for placement. Although poverty remains the pervasive factor underlying foster care placement, child neglect and abuse have become the predominant reasons cited for removal of a child (70% of cases). The surge in parental substance abuse (more than 80% of children entering foster care in Monroe County, NY, have a parent who abuses drugs and/or alcohol) and the resulting impairment in parenting behavior are blamed for this trend. Parental mental health problems, incarceration, and abandonment of the child continue to be factors leading to placement.

Less than 5% of admissions to foster care occur because of a parent or child's physical health problems. Women who are infected with the human immunodeficiency virus (HIV) who are in declining health and without family resources may place their children. Some stabilization in the numbers of HIV-infected infants entering foster care has occurred because of improved health outcomes of mothers, although these women by and large do not avail themselves of prenatal antiviral therapy. HIV-infected children also sometimes are placed when their families can no longer care for them.

Exact numbers of children in foster care are difficult to ascertain. Daily, approximately 520,000 children reside in foster care, but many more "cycle" through the system annually. According to government statistics, the foster care population increased by 80% between 1981 and 1991, with most of the increase occurring after 1986. Indeed, between 1986 and 1991, the population of children younger than age 5 years mushroomed by 110% in large cities, resulting in a downward shift in the average age. Although the genders are represented fairly equally in foster care, there is a dramatic preponderance of children of black and mixed racial heritage in out-of-home care, reflecting, in part, their preponderance in the poorer segments of our society. Unaccompanied refugee minors, especially from Cuba and Haiti, represent a very small proportion of the total foster care population.[23]

The Foster Care System

The foster care system, simple in its conception of providing needy children with nurturing families, has become a complex bureaucracy.[1] Federal legislation determines patterns of funding and regulatory guidelines, but responsibility for the structure and implementation of foster care programs resides with state social service agencies, which delegate daily management to county or private child welfare agencies.

Each foster care program retains responsibility for hiring and training caseworkers and foster families. Casework positions are entry-level jobs in most child welfare agencies, requiring no more than 2 years of college education; the professional demands are more commensurate with masters' level social work skills. Foster care caseworkers are advocates for the biological family and must undertake a "diligent effort" to rehabilitate the parent(s), ensuring the accessibility of whatever educational or service resources are necessary (such as housing, counseling, medical care, or drug and alcohol rehabilitation) for reunification. They also must coordinate educational, developmental, medical, and mental health services for the children. When birth parents are noncompliant or unable to undertake the tasks necessary for reunification, caseworkers have the delicate task of supporting them through the process of developing an alternate permanency plan and enabling the child to develop secure attachments and a sense of belonging in a different family than the family of origin. Caseworkers also recruit, train, monitor, annually recertify, and investigate minor complaints about foster homes.

Caseworkers also must develop a working familiarity with the legal system, in particular, the family court and the juvenile justice system. Within 72 hours of removal of a child from his or her birth home, the caseworker must prepare a petition for the court documenting the reasons for the removal. Many children are returned to their birth homes if the court finds insufficient basis for the removal. The caseworker must return to court at intervals to provide ongoing documentation for the continuation of placement and to detail her or his own efforts at permanency planning.

The court may appoint a law guardian to represent the child's interests in unclear situations. In some states, the court also may appoint a CASA (court-appointed special advocate) worker to advocate on behalf of the child in particularly difficult cases. As trained volunteers who are not attorneys, CASA workers devote many hours to investigating the child's circumstances for presentation to the court. Most children in foster care, however, do not have a designated advocate, except for the caseworker, who is regarded more accurately as the case manager for the entire family.

Legally, parents retain guardianship of their children residing in "the care and custody" of the county commissioner of social services. Guardianship can be terminated only as part of a separate legal process, in which the commissioner then becomes the child's legal guardian until the child either reaches the age of majority or is adopted. Sometimes, parents choose to surrender their children for adoption; more often, parental rights are terminated (TPR) involuntarily, after a parent has failed all efforts at reunification. The TPR process used to take years, during which time dual, but conflicting, efforts at reunification and alternative permanency planning occurred. The time constraints imposed by ASFA legislation on beginning the TPR process and the focus on the child's health and safety will shorten, it is hoped, the time between placement and TPR (and, thus, adoption) for children for whom reunification is not an option.

The Child in Foster Care

Foster care for the child is a world fraught with uncertainty, upheaval, and losses.[19,23] Children often are removed under urgent circumstances from all that is familiar to them. For a child, their family, no matter how dysfunctional in society's terms, is the center of their world. Separated from parents, the child also is removed from all that is familiar. The system is literally thrust upon the child. Agencies may first place children in a shelter or an emergency foster home, pending the availability of a traditional foster home. Most homes are kind and welcoming, but unfamiliar to the child. Within the first few days, the child meets a variety of strangers, from child protective and foster care caseworkers to police officers, physicians, and members of the foster home. There is little privacy, and most children, grieving the loss of their home and family, uncertain when they will see them again and afraid to ask questions, feel alone, isolated and out of control of their lives. Children often are wary the first several weeks, termed the "honeymoon period," but then, as they adjust, they begin to act out their anger, frustration, and sadness. The honeymoon period is viewed by most child welfare professionals as a time of emotional shut-down for an overwhelmed and confused child.

Children removed from their families spend varying lengths of time in foster care. Although many children (about 50%) cycle through foster care in weeks to months, about 10% to 20% remain in the system for years, as their families repeatedly fail to meet the goals set for reunification and resist other permanent options. The largest determinant of length of stay (LOS) is the biological family's level of cooperation with the individualized case plan for their child(ren), although it has been documented that minorities, older children, and children who have developmental disabilities are almost twice as likely to remain in care.[15] The average LOS in the foster care system has declined from its high of just over 5 years to about 2 years, attributed in part to increased efforts at reunification, greater dependence on relatives as resources, and more intensive permanency planning.

Longer stays in foster care are associated with reduced likelihood of reunification and an increased number of placements. Changes in foster care placement are almost always traumatic for children, because each one involves a loss, reinforcing feelings of rejection and worthlessness. About 50% will experience more than one foster care placement, with about 25% having three or more placements. Reasons for disrupted placements vary, but most frequently a child's behavior problems are beyond the skills of a particular foster parent or deteriorate to the point where the child needs a higher level of care. Less often, foster parents may retire, become ill or die, or move out of a child's county of residence. About 20% of all foster homes close each year, with 50% of them closed by child welfare agencies for providing inadequate care.

For the child who remains in foster care, even in a stable placement, there are major issues with which to contend. Although consistent visitation with the biological family is the best predictor of reunification, visits are laden with difficulty for the child. The tenor of the parent-child relationship is variable. Children who have been abused or severely neglected by their parents may not feel safe, even in a supervised visitation setting. Birth/foster parents attempt to sabotage the relationship of the child with the other set of parents. Parents may visit inconsistently, which is confusing and frightening for children. When the parent does come, the visit ends with the child reliving the initial separation from the parent. When the parent fails to show up, feelings of rejection and abandonment are reinforced. Visitation usually progresses through stages, beginning with visits supervised by caseworkers in a neutral setting; visits then take place in the parent's home for more extended periods and eventually become unsupervised.

Uncertainty, powerlessness, and guilt pervade the life of the child in foster care. Such children often deny awareness of the reason for placement, and younger children may blame themselves for the disruption of their families. Children do not know how long they will be in care, whether their parent will show for visits, or when their parent will get out of jail or rehabilitation. Most children worry about the well-being of their parents. Birth parents may make promises they do not or cannot keep. Children, sometimes, are discharged from foster care or moved between placements with the same abruptness they entered care. Other children tease them about being in foster care, contributing to their already poor self-regard and sense of alienation. Younger children and infants quickly form attachments to foster parents and may view their seldom-seen birth parent as a stranger.

For children whose families will never be able to resume their care, the process of terminating parental rights can create significant conflict. Termination of rights severs the child's legal ties to the birth family, but not their emotional ties, and the child may be torn between conflicting loyalties to the birth and adoptive families. If the parent surrenders the child, the child may view this as the ultimate rejection. Behavior problems often escalate around the time that children are freed for adoption and the adoption process is begun in earnest.

In the past decade, there has been a greater than 300% increase in the numbers of children placed in "kinship care" (foster care that is provided by a relative who has become certified as a foster parent) and relative resource care (relatives not certified as foster parents but with whom children are placed and who receive public assistance monies to help with their care).[10] For relatives whose income is marginal, certification includes eligibility for foster care stipends, which usually exceed the monies available through public assistance for the child's care. Placement with a relative is believed to be advantageous for the child because it maintains the child within the larger family of origin and is associated with fewer placement disruptions. In one study, children were half as likely to be abused or neglected when placed with a relative versus a nonrelative, although concern remains that relative resource homes are monitored less rigorously than are certified foster homes.[10]

Foster Families

Foster families are the unsung heroes of the foster care system.[19,23] Most are warm, caring, dedicated individuals who open their homes to society's most difficult and fragile children, taking them into their own families and nurturing them through multiple crises. Although foster parents vary in the education and skills they bring to caring for children, they are, in general, motivated by religious conviction, altruism, or personal need. They tend to be "child-centered," often having raised children of their own, and see foster care as a mission because of their love for children. They usually are married, of middle or lower middle income, from tradition-rich backgrounds, deeply religious, and have a fairly open definition of whom constitutes family. About 5% of foster families have specialized training or skills and act as resources for severely emotionally disturbed or medically fragile children. Many states now have designated skilled homes that provide care for children who have HIV infection or other complex medical problems.

Reimbursement rates for foster families vary widely. Families are paid a daily "board rate" for each child. The rate, set by individual states, is determined by the child's age, health needs, and the complexity of the parenting tasks. Average board rates for uncomplicated children hover around $300 per month and are expected to cover food, shelter, personal needs, recreation, and most transportation and educational costs. Many agencies reimburse for some transportation (involving medical or mental health visits) and pay an additional stipend for clothing. The highest foster family board reimbursements are for children who have extremely complex medical issues or severe behavioral and emotional problems, and may exceed $1000 per month. About 30% of children in foster care, mostly adolescents, reside in residential or group home placements, the most costly form of care. Residential placement costs may exceed $40,000 per child per year.

Recruitment and adequate training of suitable foster families are two of the most compelling tasks facing child welfare agencies. Agencies provide potential foster parents with education in the areas of child development, child abuse and neglect, behavior problems, discipline, safety, and their roles in relation to the agency and birth families, but the training is minimal. Agencies lack the staff to scrutinize foster homes adequately, and annual recertification is less rigorous than the original certification process.

Boundaries are blurred in the foster care system, in terms of authority, responsibility, and accountability. Foster families retain the bulk of the daily responsibility but are accountable to caseworkers, the legal system, and the birth family for the child's care. Foster parents may feel excluded from planning on the child's behalf, because birth parents retain legal custody, child welfare agencies generate permanency plans, and courts make placement decisions. However powerless, foster families remain the individual child's strongest advocate.

Foster parents often have only limited information about children in their care. Placement in a foster home often is regarded as the only necessary therapeutic intervention a child needs, and agencies vary widely in the amount of guidance they provide to foster parents. Foster families may be overwhelmed, and placements may fail when foster families feel isolated in dealing with a child's complex behavioral and emotional problems. Because there are shortages of foster homes in many areas, particularly large urban centers, most homes maintain the maximum number of children allowed under regulations, further stressing the foster family's emotional resources.

Foster families, like children in foster care, experience multiple separations and losses, as children enter and leave their homes, often for a living situation they deem unsuitable. Relationships with birth families range from adversarial to mutually supportive. Foster parents often bear the brunt of a child's anger over a failed parental visit or a parent's phone call. They may feel scrutinized, but simultaneously unsupported, by the system, and they sometimes are accused of child abuse or neglect by an angry child or parent.

It is the foster family to which the system turns for adoption when reunification is no longer considered an option, and it usually is the foster family who does adopt the child. Some families choose to retain a child as a long-term foster care placement either because they are too old to adopt, the child is not freed for adoption, or the child chooses against adoption. The impact of AFSA legislation on long-term foster care as a placement option has yet to be realized.

Birth Families

Removal of a child also is traumatic for the birth parent. For some, the shock of the removal is sufficient to precipitate improved parenting behaviors, resulting in speedy reunification. About 50% of children in foster care are returned to their birth families within 6 months. For other families, even the removal of a child does not alter ingrained patterns of substance abuse, violence, and child neglect.

Parents, while battling addiction and poverty, often have to contend with feelings of guilt, powerlessness, inadequacy, anger, frustration, and resentment when their children are removed. Although they retain legal custody, their contact with their children is constrained, with only several hours of supervised visitation per week. Parents may fail to show up for visitation, whether because of guilt, the pain of separation, fear of confronting their child(ren), or barriers such as illness and transportation.

Although one of the goals of the foster care system is reunification and caseworkers are mandated to provide a range of services supporting this goal, some parents become locked in an adversarial relationship with the system, resentfully refusing all help offered. In the past, some effectively abandoned their children to the system, maintaining contact just sufficient to prevent termination of their rights. Many of these same parents refused to surrender their children for adoption, even when it was clear that reunification was not an option. ASFA legislation has made it easier to terminate parental rights in such situations. This legislation also reinforces the concept of "open adoptions," believed to benefit the child by providing some ongoing limited contact with the family of origin.

Outcomes for Children in Foster Care

As already noted, about 50% of children are returned to a parent or relative within the first 6 months of placement. Of the remainder, 30% eventually are returned to the family of origin; unfortunately, there is about a 20% to 30% recidivism rate in the first year after reunification.

About 15% to 20% of children in foster care eventually are adopted; more than 90% of these are adopted by their foster families. About 10% of adoptive foster families are relatives. Almost all adoptions out of foster care involve some subsidy, which reflects the county-of-residence board rate at the time of the adoption. Subsidy continues until the child reaches 18 years of age.

About 5% of all children in the United States grow up in the foster care system. Most are adolescents who have no hope of reunification with their families; others are children considered difficult to adopt by virtue of their medical or behavioral problems or are older minority children awaiting adoptive placement. Studies indicate that even older adolescents in foster care continue to hope for adoption. About 20,000 children per year "age out" of foster care's independent living programs; many leave the system without any permanent family resource, while some maintain some contact with their family of origin or their foster family. Most adolescents age out at 18 years, although some states allow adolescents to remain in care until 21 years of age. A small percentage (3% of adolescents) are lost to care through elopement, and a similar number become involved with the criminal justice system or are placed in long-term residential care.

HEALTH CARE ISSUES AND RECOMMENDATIONS FOR CHILDREN IN FOSTER CARE

Children in foster care represent a highly vulnerable, medically complex population, suffering high rates of chronic medical illness, developmental disabilities, educational disorders, and behavioral, emotional, and mental health problems.[14,20,25] In general, for older infants and children, these conditions predate placement. Prenatal drug exposure, poor maternal nutrition, and poor prenatal care predispose to a higher incidence of premature and small-for-gestational age infants. Postnatally, psychosocial deprivation, poor nutrition, and failure to attend to the child's health care and developmental needs exacerbate problems. Limited use of preventive health services, fragmentation of health care, and underimmunization are typical of children entering foster care, and 70% have a history of neglect, physical abuse, and/or sexual abuse.

Studies of the health status of the foster care population have yielded fairly bleak results. Approximately 80% have at least one chronic medical condition, with about 25% of all children in care having three or more chronic problems. The diagnoses encountered most commonly are listed in Table 54-1.[14,20] Respiratory problems affect about 18% of children in foster care, with asthma being the diagnosis encountered most commonly (15%); the high prevalence is attributed partially to a higher incidence of premature birth and attendant lung disease and partially to the concentration of the foster care population in urban settings. About 10% of children in foster care have short stature, with an additional 6% to 10% of infants and toddlers meeting criteria for failure to thrive. At the other extreme, about 15% of children in foster care meet the criteria for obesity. Hematological disorders, mostly attributable to anemia, are present in about 20% of children. Dermatological diagnoses are reported, especially atopic dermatitis, acne, and seborrhea. Burn scars or scars from physical abuse are encountered commonly (10% to 15% of children younger than 12 years). Visual and hearing impairment, recurrent otitis media, gastroesophageal reflux, neurological disorders (varying from mild motor delay to seizures and cerebral palsy), and congenital anomalies are more prevalent than in the general pediatric population. Sexually transmitted and other infectious diseases also are commonly encountered. About 8% of children in foster care are "high-cost" patients, because they are technology-dependent, multiply disabled, and/or heavy users of ancillary services.

Once children enter foster care, their overall health does

Table 54-1 Common Medical Diagnoses for Children in Foster Care in Oakland, California

Diagnosis	Percentage
Growth failure	43%
Height <5%	23%
Weight <5%	15%
Head circumference <5%	19%
Failue to thrive	9%
Infections/parasites	17%
Recurrent otitis media	10%
Congenital infections	8%
Hematological, any	21%
Neurological, any	30%
Respiratory, any	18%
Asthma	15%
Gastroesophageal, any	15%
Gastroesophageal reflux	8%
Encopresis	3%
Genitourinary, any	10%
Enuresis	7%
Skin, any	23%
Congenital anomaly	8%

Modified from Halfon N, Mendones A, Berkowitz G: *Arch Pediatr Adolesc Med* 149:386, 1995.

not appear to improve; this is attributed to multiple issues. The transient nature of the population makes it very likely that they will continue to have multiple health care providers. There is an almost universal lack of medical information at admission, and identifying prior health care providers is cumbersome and often fruitless. Neither caseworkers nor foster parents have the level of knowledge necessary to serve as the medical case manager, yet that is whom the system relies on to perform this complex task. Inadequate care management underlies the pattern of inadequate, fragmented, sometimes redundant care received.[12,24] The reliance on Medicaid limits access to care because of inadequate financing, delays in payment, and limited numbers of medical subspecialists willing to accept Medicaid patients. Medicaid managed care may increase access to medical subspecialists but significantly reduce mental health access. Complex issues of consent and confidentiality limit access, delay evaluations and treatment, and confound communication among professionals.

Recommendations for Optimizing Health Care for Children in Foster Care

In light of these complexities, recommendations for optimizing health care for children in foster care include the following:[4,6,9]

1. The pediatrician should establish a relationship with the foster care agency. The caseworker is the case manager; establishing methods of communication and information exchange will facilitate the child's health care.
2. The caseworker should obtain appropriate releases of information and medical consents from the birth family and make copies available to the primary care practitioner. The pediatrician should become familiar with the foster care agency's guidelines regarding consent and confidentiality. Whenever possible, a signed consent to provide medical treatment should be obtained, but care should not be withheld pending signed consents because providing care in the absence of consent is deemed less harmful than withholding care. Certain adolescent health issues, such as pregnancy, sexually transmitted diseases, birth control, and substance abuse are governed by separate confidentiality laws in most states.
3. As much prior health history as possible should be gathered. The caseworker, again, will be invaluable in this respect, although that person also may be stymied by a dearth of prior records. The caseworker and the physician's office should attempt to access records from other professionals, including the prenatal and perinatal histories, developmental history, growth curves, immunization records, and risk factors for HIV and other vertically transmitted infections. For older children, additional information also should include any chronic illnesses, medications, allergies, and educational and mental health problems. One should be aware that there may be a paucity of such information because the child may not have received adequate services before foster care or may have had multiple providers, none of whom has a complete record.
4. Children entering foster care should have a series of health care encounters over the first 2 months, because they are in crisis and multiple visits often reveal more than one isolated evaluation. It is recommended that children entering foster care have an initial medical screen within 72 hours to document growth parameters, signs and symptoms of abuse or neglect, and the presence of acute or chronic illness. Children should have a comprehensive medical evaluation within 30 days of placement, including recommended screening tests, HIV risk assessment, and developmental and behavioral screening. A follow-up to this visit should occur within another 30 to 60 days, as the adjustment to foster care is nearly complete by then, and further issues may be identified.
5. Well-child care should follow AAP guidelines between birth and 2 years of age (see Fig. 4-1), although it is reasonable to do monthly evaluations on children younger than 6 months and to add a 21-month-old preventive visit. After age 2 years, children should have a comprehensive medical visit at least every 6 months until age 6 years and at least annually thereafter, although some experts recommend semiannual visits for all children in foster care. Comprehensive preventive health care in the foster care population requires diligent effort on the part of the physician. Longer appointment slots and a tracking system are strongly suggested. Ideally, the agency should inform the practitioner about changes in placement and casework assignment and any referrals made by the caseworker. The health care practitioner should communicate with the caseworker about the assessment and recommended plan at each health care encounter.
6. Approximately 70% of children and adolescents entering foster care have been physically abused, sexually abused, or neglected. Screening for signs and symptoms of abuse and neglect at the time of admission is essential in this high-risk population. Physicians should be familiar with the signs and symptoms of abuse and neglect; children who may have been sexually abused should be referred to a center specializing in child sexual abuse to avoid the trauma of repeated interviews and examinations. Any concern about the adequacy of parenting in a foster home should be addressed with the foster care agency, and a heightened awareness for issues of abuse and neglect in the foster home is encouraged. *Inadequate weight gain in a foster home often is the first sign of neglect.*
7. Children in foster care have a high prevalence of dental problems, especially caries and malocclusion. Changes in placement may result in a lapse in dental care, so continued monitoring of dentition and reminders to foster parents about the importance of routine dental care are important. Referral for dental care should begin at age 1 year.
8. Children in foster care tend to be underimmunized, even compared with other poor children, and every health encounter should be viewed as an opportunity to immunize a child in foster care. Varicella vaccine should be withheld until the child's HIV status is known to be negative. Children in foster care should be universally immunized against hepatitis B. The population is transient, the children are at high risk for vertically transmitted infection,

and adolescents are at risk because of sexual practices. A baseline hepatitis screen should be performed on all children older than 11 years of age before beginning the immunization series.

9. Underutilization of routine preventive health care services implies a deficiency of screening for lead, iron-deficiency anemia, and tuberculosis exposure. Many children in care reside in or have resided in older housing, and pica is a commonly encountered behavioral issue in this population, increasing the risk for elevated plasma lead levels. Poor nutrition before foster care places children at risk for iron-deficiency anemia. Thus, clinicians should obtain plasma lead levels and screen all children younger than 6 years for anemia at least annually. Adolescent females also should have annual hemoglobin screening. Universal tuberculosis screening is recommended, using the Mantoux test at admission and every 3 to 5 years thereafter while in foster care. Hemoglobin electrophoresis in at-risk children who have no documentation of sickle-cell screening at birth should be considered.
10. Maternal lifestyles during pregnancy, including substance abuse and promiscuity, place children in foster care at increased risk for a variety of vertically transmitted infectious diseases, including HIV, hepatitis B and C, congenital syphilis, and herpes. Every child placed in foster care should have an rapid plasma reagin (RPR) and hepatitis C antibody screen. Up to 80% of young children placed in foster care are at high risk for HIV infection,[7] but fewer than 10% are screened, because of the complexities of risk assessment, the obtaining of informed consent, and issues of confidentiality; these guidelines vary from state to state. Some agencies use risk-assessment tools to determine a child's risk for HIV infection, although the accuracy of such tools depends on the birth parent's availability and veracity. In general, the biological parent retains the right to consent to testing or not, unless the child has been freed for adoption or parental rights have been terminated. Agencies vary in their policies regarding consent procedures when a parent declines screening but the child meets high-risk criteria. Identification of children who are HIV-positive is critical to appropriate medical management (including Pneumocystis pneumonia prophylaxis), modification of the immunization schedule, and early anti-retroviral therapy. The practitioner should understand the HIV policies of the agency that has custody of the child.
11. Adolescents in foster care also represent a high-risk group for HIV infection, usually because of unprotected sex with multiple partners. In general, adolescents in care may give consent for HIV testing, unless they are cognitively impaired. Confidentiality laws vary, but in some states the adolescent has the right to designate who has access to HIV-related information; in others, social service agencies and their representatives have access to such data on any child in their care and custody, including adolescents.
12. Approximately 60% of preschool children in foster care have a developmental disability,[8] especially language disorders, and poor social-adaptive and delayed fine-motor skills. Older children have higher rates of educational disorders, including learning disabilities, behavioral disorders, and limited cognitive ability, such that upward of 40% qualify for special education services. Many are placed in special education settings for emotional rather than for cognitive concerns, as severe attentional difficulties, poor impulse control, and aggressive behaviors often preclude placement in a regular classroom. Children younger than 5 years of age should have a formal developmental evaluation within 3 months of admission to foster care and should have developmental screening at admission and at each well-child care visit, with follow-up evaluations as indicated. The high prevalence of language disorders (50% to 60% of preschool children) implies that universal hearing and speech evaluations of toddler and preschool children may be beneficial in identifying children who would benefit from special educational services. Older children who are not performing at grade level should be referred in a timely manner for an educational evaluation. The primary care practitioner should maintain contact with the case manager for developmental and/or educational services and obtain copies of all evaluations.

Table 54-2 Common Mental Health Diagnoses in Children in Foster Care

Problem	Percentage of Population
Conduct disorder	30%-52%
Oppositional defiant disorder	17%-35%
Attention deficit disorder	18%-32%
Anxiety disorders	7%-19%
Depressive disorders	2%-9%

Modified from Stein E, et al: *Can J Psychiatry* 39:344, 1994.

13. Mental health care is the single overwhelming health care need of most children in foster care.[13,21] The prevalence of a severe disturbance ranges from 35% to 85%. Children in foster care use both inpatient and outpatient mental health services at rates 15 to 20 times that of other children of similar backgrounds who are not in foster care, but are still believed to be underserved. Conduct disorder, oppositional defiant disorder, attention deficit/hyperactivity disorder, attachment, and anxiety disorders are the mental health diagnoses cited most commonly for children in foster care (Table 54-2). Experienced professionals in foster care believe that the prevalence and severity of mental health disabilities have increased dramatically in the past decade. Preplacement issues, such as prenatal drug exposure, poor maternal nutrition, inappropriate parenting, and abuse and neglect during early childhood, all contribute to the poor emotional health of children in foster care. Entry to foster care, instead of remediating emotional disorders, may exacerbate them because of the trauma of separation from families and the emotional turmoil of living as a child in an uncertain world. Physicians should screen for emotional and behavioral issues at admission and at each preventive health care visit. Every child in foster care older than age 2 years should have a full mental health evaluation within 3 months of placement. Children who have identified mental health and/or behavioral

problems should be referred appropriately for mental health services. All children in foster care have to deal with issues of ongoing separation and loss as well as their feelings of anger, sadness, rejection, powerlessness, alienation, and guilt. Even children who do not appear initially to need mental health services should be rescreened at intervals to assess changes in their emotional well-being. Foster parent questionnaires can be used to elicit information about behavioral and emotional health. Some of the behaviors addressed include fire-setting, animal cruelty, hyperphagia, hoarding, serious sleep disorders, and self-injurious behaviors. There are junctures in foster care that affect the emotional well-being of children, including inconsistent parental visitation, resumption of regular visits after a prolonged lapse, cessation of visitation, incarceration of a parent, illness of a foster parent, and being freed for adoption. Resumption of lapsed counseling or increased frequency of counseling visits are beneficial at these critical junctures.

14. Many foster families have a wealth of child-rearing experience, but the clinician should not presume that their knowledge about child development, behavior, discipline, and safety are adequate. Anticipatory guidance should be a routine part of well-child care and should include issues specific to foster care, such as behavior problems related to visitation and the permanency planning process, significant sleep disorders, confused loyalties, attachment, violence, and coercion. Adolescents should be counseled about high-risk behaviors.
15. All medical information should be shared with the child's caseworker and foster parents in appropriate lay language. The caseworker is responsible for communicating the information to the birth parents, in the likely event they were not present at the medical visit. If possible, the practitioner should provide a written summary of each medical encounter, respond to caseworker requests for semiannual summaries needed for adequate case management (Uniform Case Review), and assume the role of medical advocate when necessary.

Standards for health care of children placed in out-of-home care were published by the Child Welfare League of America and the American Academy of Pediatrics in 1988.[6] Unfortunately, many states have only broad guidelines governing the provision of health services to children in foster care, and there are multiple barriers to translating those guidelines into accessible, effective, and efficient health care. These barriers include inadequate funding, insufficient caseworker and foster family knowledge, limited understanding of the foster care experience by health professionals, and blurred boundaries over where the responsibility lies for health care management for this complex population. District II (New York State) of the American Academy of Pediatrics published a more detailed set of standards in 1999, which defines the parameters for health care more clearly for this complex population and describes the essential components of health care management.[5]

ADOPTION

Adoption is believed to be the most beneficial outcome for a child who cannot remain with his or her family of origin, because in the process of forming a new legal family, it creates a sense of stability and belonging unmatched by any other form of substitute care. Outcome studies have shown almost uniformly positive results despite the type of adoption: infant adoption, adoption out of foster care, special-needs adoption, transracial adoption, or international adoption. Adoption is difficult to study because there is no centralized adoption registry and no imposed uniform set of rules or regulations. Many areas of controversy exist in adoption, including the establishment of a national adoption registry, regulation of international and independent adoptions, transracial adoption, open adoption and the conflict between the adoptee's need for family history and connectedness to their family of origin, and the birth parent's right to confidentiality.

Epidemiology

Exact numbers of children residing in adoptive homes are difficult to determine because there is no centralized adoption registry.[26] As of 1993, it was believed that there were about 1 million children living with adoptive parents, so that 2% to 4% of American families are adoptive families. These numbers, however, are completely unreliable. The most accurate numbers probably exist for international adoptions, which are monitored by the U.S. Immigration and Naturalization Service; there also is some accounting for children adopted each year out of the foster care system. Although *all* adoptions must be approved by a court, courts do not track the numbers or types of adoptions upon which they rule.

Although children may be adopted under various circumstances, there are only two types of legal adoption—agency (which may be public or private) and independent (nonagency). Independent adoptions, which constitute about 20% of the total, are arranged privately between two individuals with only a legal intermediary. For example, stepparents often adopt the biological children of their spouse, or individuals may adopt children within their extended family to prevent future custody issues. About two thirds of newborn adoptions are handled independently. Public and private agencies account for about 40% and 30% of adoptions, respectively. Agencies arrange adoptions for children in the foster care system, who are most often adopted by their foster families, although some agencies may locate adoptive families outside the system. Public agencies often have the most "special needs" children to place—children who are older, who are of minority status, or who have behavioral, mental health, or medical problems. International adoptions are facilitated by private agencies.

Scant information exists on children who are adopted. Most of the information we do have relates to adoption out of foster care or international adoption. It is estimated that at any given time more than 20,000 children are awaiting adoptive placement or living in nonfinalized adoptive homes in the United States. Children adopted out of foster care tend to be older (less than 7% are adopted under age 1 year), and the median age for adoption out of foster care is close to 5 years, with an approximate 4-year wait between placement in foster care and adoption. ASFA legislation is expected to reduce this waiting time significantly. Sixty percent of children adopted out of foster care are white, 23% are black, and about 10% are Hispanic. Sixty percent of children adopted out of foster care fit the definition of "special needs."

Children adopted through international adoption are younger and most often infants or young toddlers. The countries of origin have shifted over the past decade, with Romanian-born children no longer readily available. Increasing numbers of children come from China, Russia, Korea, and South America. The shift has been driven by the recognition that some countries mandate better care for their young charges than others, so that the children are less likely to have unrecognized or unreported developmental or health issues at the time of adoption.

Information on the numbers of women who voluntarily relinquish their children for adoption is limited, although it has declined in recent decades despite the increase in out-of-wedlock births. There also is only limited information about adoption-seekers, including the numbers of individuals seeking to adopt who complete adoption, average waiting times, or why some individuals "drop out" of the adoption process. Data are scarce on the numbers of disrupted adoptions (those in which the child is removed from the home before the legalization of the adoption) and adoptive dissolution (in which a legalized adoption is broken). Both of these engender particularly heart-rending situations for both the child and the adoptive parents.

Transracial Adoption

The transracial adoption debate is a multifaceted and complex one.[11] Professional social work and community standards have long supported a policy of placing children in ethnically similar homes, deeming it to be "in the child's best interest," because it supposedly preserves the child's cultural heritage, thereby minimizing cultural discontinuity and ethnic-identity issues for the child. States have used this policy to proscribe transracial placements in all but extreme cases. The practical outcome of this approach has been a flood of minority children awaiting placement in a limited number of minority adoptive homes. Legislation enacted by Congress in 1996 prohibits the use of race as the sole determining factor in the selection of an adoptive or foster family, although race may be one factor considered among others. The intent of the legislation was to achieve some balance between the best interests of the child, which lie in having a stable family structure, preferably of similar cultural heritage, and the interests of the community in preserving minority families and culture.

International Adoption

The foster family care system as it exists in the United States, Canada, Great Britain, and a few other countries, such as Korea, is an unusual solution to the problem of unwanted, abandoned, and destitute children throughout the world. Korea has a well-regarded foster family care system, subsidized by adoption fees, in which families are well screened, well paid, and limited to one child per family. Most countries, however, rely on orphanages, run by the government or charitable organizations, to care for their destitute children. Such institutions range in the quality of the care they provide, staff training, and staff/child ratios. Concern also exists regarding the reliability of information they collect and make available to adoptive families about children.

The number of children adopted into families in the United States from international countries increased from about 7000 in 1990 to more than 11,000 in 1996. Most children now originate from China (3000 per year), Russia (2500 per year), and Korea (1500 per year), along with several hundred per year from Romania, India, and Vietnam. International adoption is risky, complex, and poorly regulated. The adoptive family must simultaneously comply with adoption and immigration regulations, which vary from country to country. Families must also adopt the child in the country of origin and then complete a second adoption process in the United States.

Children available for adoption from foreign countries have much in common with children in the foster care system in our country.[16,22] They are the children of the poor and disenfranchised in their own culture and have often been neglected or abused before placement in their country's dependent care system. For many, the physical abuse and neglect continue after placement. Postinstitutional syndromes, particularly resulting in sensory integration deficits, are common, especially in children adopted from Russia and Romania. Parental drug and/or alcohol abuse is a common issue internationally for children in out-of-home placement, and some children manifest the developmental and behavioral sequelae of prenatal exposure. Failure to thrive, developmental delay, psychosocial dwarfism, fetal alcohol syndrome, and infections are common but may remain undiagnosed until the child arrives in the United States. Despite these issues, most children adopted internationally appear to thrive in their adoptive settings. The lure of international adoption remains strong because families can usually complete the adoption process in a more timely fashion and can adopt a younger child than is possible out of the American foster care system. The opportunity for white families to adopt a white child from Russia or Eastern Europe also appeals to many. Again, implementation of AFSA legislation may make adoption out of the American foster care system more attractive, as time between placement and adoption is reduced and younger children become available for adoption.

Placement with an adoptive family carries some risk for the child also, in that there are limited safeguards in place. Agencies may simply serve as "facilitators" for international adoption, in which case they are not accountable for investigating an adoptive family to assess the appropriateness of the placement and may abrogate any responsibility toward the child once the adoption is complete. Some foreign countries seek to provide some minimal assurance that children are adopted into safe and appropriate settings. For example, Korea forbids adoption except by married couples, and both Thailand and Romania require the adoptive parent to appear in court to complete the adoption. China has fairly restrictive criteria for adoptive families but simultaneously provides minimal, often inaccurate information to prospective parents.

Child and family advocates involved in international adoptions strongly recommend that families work only with reputable licensed adoption organizations, preferably ones that do home studies and remain a resource once the adoption is complete. Families should request any available written documentation and a videotape of the child; while far from perfect, the latter aids in the assessment of the developmental and physical well-being of the child. It also is strongly recommended that adoptive parents travel to the country of origin, both to familiarize themselves with the child's background and culture and to obtain as much information about the child as possible. Although there are many corollaries between children in foster placement and international adoptees, there also are many issues specific to international adoption covered in detailed reviews elsewhere.

HEALTH CARE RECOMMENDATIONS AND ISSUES FOR ADOPTED CHILDREN

Health care issues for children who are adopted depend on the age and circumstances of the child at the time of adoption.[2-4] Adoptive parents of newborn infants should be provided with a family health history and prenatal history for the child. Adoptive parents of older infants and children from within the United States should be provided with these plus a complete health history of the child, including medical, developmental, and mental health history, immunizations, results of any laboratory tests performed, and risk factors for HIV infection. In particular, children who are adopted from the foster care system should have a comprehensive health history available. Children from foster care who have not already had a comprehensive developmental and mental health evaluation, including recommended laboratory tests and screening, should have these done before adoption.

Adoption of children from other countries presents special issues.[16] Often, potential adoptive parents will seek advice from a physician before adopting a child internationally. Families should be encouraged to obtain as much health, developmental, and social history as possible from the agency handling the adoption, should be counseled regarding the variable reliability of such information, and should try to obtain at least a picture, if not a videotape, of the child for review with the physician. The family should be counseled regarding the variability in care across different countries, the potential negative impact of orphanage life on a young child, and the need to repeat any laboratory work at the time of arrival in the United States. Children adopted internationally often are being adopted out of another country's child welfare system and should be regarded as having the same overall risk factors as children coming out of our own child welfare system. Some institutions have falsified children's ages to make them appear younger than they actually are, especially if they are small in size and/or developmentally delayed; health information may be both over- and underreported.

Children adopted from other countries should have a full medical evaluation and developmental assessment shortly after their arrival in the United States.[3,16] Immunization records should be scrutinized carefully, and if any concern exists regarding accuracy, the child should be reimmunized. Vision, hearing, anemia, hepatitis B, syphilis, and lead screening are universally recommended. Tuberculosis screening (using the Mantoux test) also is recommended, but one needs to bear in mind the impact of prior BCG administration on the interpretation of results. HIV risk assessment should be completed, and children at risk should have HIV screening. Children who have poor growth and/or chronic diarrhea should be evaluated for the presence of parasitic disease and lactase deficiency. Physicians knowledgeable about foreign adoption also recommend carefully following the child's developmental progress over the first 6 to 12 months in the United States to assess competencies more accurately. Any lingering concerns about chronological age should be addressed through a bone age and dental examination about 12 months after arrival. Families should be counseled about the transient increased risk of minor acute illnesses after arrival in this country, which results from exposure to unfamiliar pathogens.

Many wonderful resources exist for pediatricians caring for adoptive children and families, including American Academy of Pediatrics policy statements and ADOPTMED, a listserve on the Internet for professionals.

Acknowledgement

The author gratefully acknowledges the children and families with whom she works daily for their inspiration, and the staff of Foster Care Pediatrics for their compassion, dedication, and caring.

REFERENCES

1. Allen M: Crafting a federal legislative framework for child welfare reform, *Am J Orthopsychiatry* 161:610, 1991.
2. American Academy of Pediatrics, Committee on Early Childhood, Adoption and Dependent Care: Families and adoption: the pediatrician's role in supporting communication (RE9240), *AAP News*, February 1992.
3. American Academy of Pediatrics, Committee on Early Childhood, Adoption and Dependent Care: Initial medical evaluation of an adopted child, *Pediatrics* 88:642, 1988.
4. American Academy of Pediatrics, Committee on Early Childhood, Adoption and Dependent Care: Issues of confidentiality in adoption: the role of the pediatrician (RE9405), *Pediatrics* 93:339, 1994.
5. American Academy of Pediatrics, District II, NYS, Task Force on Foster Care Health Care: Fostering health: health care for children in foster care in New York State, A resource manual, *AAP District II*, 1999.
6. Child Welfare League of America: *Standards for health care services for children in out-of-home care,* Washington, DC, 1988, Child Welfare League of America.
7. Cohen FL, Nehring WM: Foster care of HIV-positive children in the United States, *Public Health Rep* 109:60, 1994.
8. Committee on Early Childhood, Adoption and Dependent Care: Developmental issues in foster care for children, *Pediatrics* 91:1007, 1993.
9. Committee on Early Childhood, Adoption and Dependent Care: Health care of foster children, *Pediatrics* 79:644, 1987.
10. Dubowitz H, et al: The physical health of children in kinship care, *Am J Dis Child.* 146:603, 1992.
11. Griffith EH, Duby JL: Recent developments in the transracial adoption debate, *Bull Am Acad Psychiatry Law* 19:339, 1991.
12. Halfon N, Berkowitz G, Klee L: Children in foster care in California: an examination of Medicaid reimbursed health services utilization, *Pediatrics* 89:1230, 1992.
13. Halfon N, Berkowitz G, Klee L: Mental health service utilization by children in foster care in California, *Pediatrics* 89:1238, 1992.
14. Halfon N, Mendones A, Berkowitz G: Health status of children in foster care: the experience of the center for the vulnerable child, *Arch Pediatr Adolesc Med* 149:386, 1995.
15. Horwitz SM, Simms MD, Farrington R: Impact of developmental problems on young children's exits from foster care, *J Dev Behav Pediatr* 15:105, 1994.
16. Jenista JA, Chapman D: Medical problems of foreign-born adopted children, *Am J Dis Child* 141:298, 1987.
17. Schor EL: Foster care, *Pediatr Clin North Am* 35:1241, 1988.
18. Schor EL: Foster care, *Pediatr Rev* 10:209, 1989.

19. Simms MD: Foster children and the foster care system. Part II. Impact on the child, *Curr Prob Pediatr* 21:345, 1991.
20. Simms MD: The foster care clinic: a community program to identify treatment needs of children in foster care, *J Dev Behav Pediatr* 10:121, 1989.
21. Stein E, et al: Psychiatric disorders of children "in care": methodology and demographic correlates, *Can J Psychiatry* 39:341, 1994.
22. Szilagyi M: Medical issues in children adopted from foster care: guide for physicians, *Adoption Med News* 2:1, 1996.
23. Szilagyi MA: The pediatrician and the child in foster care, *Pediatr Rev* 19:39, 1998.
24. Takayama JI, Bergman AB, Connell FA: Children in foster care in the state of Washington: health care utilization and expenditures, *JAMA* 271:1850, 1994.
25. US General Accounting Office: *Foster care: health needs of many young children are unknown and unmet,* Publication GAO/HEHS 95-114, Washington, DC, May 1995.
26. US State Department, Office of Visa Processing: *Significant source countries of immigrant orphans,* (FY 85-FY96), 1996.

INTERNET RESOURCES

Adoptmed, a listserve and resource for medical professionals interested in adoption: Adoptmed@u.washington.edu
American Academy of Pediatrics: www.AAP.org
Court Appointed Special Advocates: www.casanet.org/library
National Adoption Clearinghouse: www.calib.com/naic

55 Changing American Families

Shirley A. Smoyak

Pediatrics is best practiced with a solid groundwork in the family, which includes its biological, cultural, socioeconomic, and demographic dimensions. The family contexts in which infants, children, and adolescents are raised set the patterns for their response to illness and their expectations of caregivers. Families' beliefs about health and illness—what is preventable, what is treatable, what is natural, what is good, and what is to be avoided—are communicated to each new generation, both directly and subtly.

Scientists who attempt to study the family are faced with a peculiar dilemma. Something familiar to all of us growing up in a family somehow eludes the grasp of the scientific method. Because most of us have experienced childhood and adolescence in a family setting, and because most of us as adults create families of our own, the temptation is great to view our experiences as normal and to use them as a standard for understanding others. This ethnocentric tendency leads to assumptions that the familiar must be the correct or better way and that other styles or patterns at best are strange and at worst are wrong or deviant. The "family" is an elusive concept; its shape, character, and functions have been interpreted differently by historians, sociologists, psychologists, and anthropologists.

Privacy about matters of family life has produced what sociologists call *pluralistic ignorance*. Each of us knows what goes on in our own bedrooms and bathrooms and how we handle a sassy 2-year-old at bedtime or an adolescent who comes home drunk or smelling of pot, but we really do not know how the neighbors do it. Systematic, rigorous research on the intimacies of family life is in its infancy, although the study of marriage and the family can be traced back several centuries.

Despite the less-than-adequate funding for research on the family, the literature has grown voluminously. Today there are nearly two dozen professional journals that deal with the family, some specializing in theory and research, some on family issues and policy matters, and many on clinical and therapeutic concerns. Family agendas are addressed at conferences convened by prominent professional associations in the major social science disciplines, and the field is not lacking in newsletters, monographs, audiotapes and videotapes, and books.

This chapter provides an overview of changing patterns of family structure and the associated changes in functions. It attempts to explode some cherished myths about "the American family" and to provide clinicians who treat sick, injured, or well children with a more realistic understanding of families. In this chapter a family will be viewed as a married couple or other group of adult kinsfolk who cooperate economically and psychosocially in bringing up children and who share a common dwelling (see Chapter 63, Family-Centered Care in Pediatric Practice).

FAMILY ORIGINS

According to Gough,[6] "The trouble with the origin of the family is that no one knows." She provides evidence that it is not known *when* the human family originated (probably between 2 million and 10,000 years ago) or whether some kind of embryonic family came before, with, or after the origin of language. Although varying significantly in structure and function, some kind of family exists in all known human societies. "Family" implies several universals: (1) that sexual relations between close relatives are forbidden, (2) that men and women cooperate through a division of labor based on gender, and (3) that marriage is a durable although not necessarily lifelong arrangement. Another universal, that men in general have higher status and authority than the women in their families, has generated much controversy between feminist scholars and other historians. Although feminist writers persuasively have demonstrated the long-standing, erroneous bias of earlier male "scholars," they disagree among themselves about the exact nature of past relationships among men and women in families.

The exact nature of family structure and gender relationships is shrouded in many layers of conjecture and scientific guesswork. Since the beginning of recorded history, no fixed pattern across cultures has been found.[7] Culture, not biology, determines the rules of organization within families. In most primitive, nomadic, communal societies, family descent was traced through the mothers, possibly because maternity could be verified, whereas paternity often was a mystery. Roughly 5000 years ago, when the development of agriculture so drastically changed how people lived and organized themselves, patrilineal groups emerged. As the concept of private property developed, the transfer of such property from father to son influenced not only economic but also social patterns.

Historians of the family, notably Aries,[2] have taught us that much of what we take as familiar and commonplace is a relatively recent invention. Childhood as a concept to us is real; Aries maintains that it did not exist as an idea before the Middle Ages. In medieval days, as soon as a child could live without the constant attention of its mother, he or she was accorded adult status. No institution has been changed so remarkably by modernization as has the family. Until the late eighteenth century, families were primarily economic units. Marriages were arranged to preserve property, and children were a cheap source of labor or a hedge against poverty in old age.

Historically all the work necessary for safety and survival was done within family units. Within the boundaries of the family, functions performed were educating the young; ensuring safety from invaders; praying to God or a superior being; providing nurturance, clothing, and shelter; and caring for the sick, infirm, young, or disabled. Every family textbook includes a discussion of the "erosion of family functions," and it has been popular from time to time to predict the eventual demise of the family as we know it because all the reasons for its existence have been reassigned to institutions outside the family, such as schools, hospitals, welfare boards, and churches.

There actually have been several experiments in alternative forms of living in human groups, but none has survived. Although there is no general societal law that people must live in families, most do. Historical perspectives help in understanding social contexts and institutions. Present patterns, when the observer can see their roots, make more sense. More important, such understanding eliminates or dampens the tendency toward emotionality over issues of intimacy, closeness, and human relationships. Perceptions of American family life are full of myths, such as the belief that a three-generational household is and was the norm. Such beliefs generate a false nostalgia—a longing for what never was. In popularizing an image of the American family as three generations in one household, Norman Rockwell actually did a disservice to the American public—there had never been a time when three generations living in one household was typical. Given the short life span (an expected 49 years at the turn of the century), most parents could not have expected to live with their grandchildren. Although the three-generation family of the past largely was mythical, today more grandparents and great-grandparents are alive than ever before.

For the first time in history families may have four or five generations alive. Children today may have not only living grandparents, but also great-grandparents and perhaps great-great grandparents. This increased longevity poses problems for families that they have never faced before. On a simple level there is the question of what the "layers" of grandparents should be called by their grandchildren. On a more complex level, great economic and psychosocial concern faces middle-aged persons who see their retirement years not as golden but as burdened by financial and social support of several elder generations.

There are two major reasons for the difficulty in tracing accurate patterns and structures for families. First, upper-class or high-status families were grossly overrepresented in the literature. Second, until about the past 60 years, writers tended to describe families as they *should* be, rather than as they really were. This led to what Goode has so aptly labeled "the classical extended family of Western nostalgia."[5] For instance, some accounts of colonial families in America are so steeped in nostalgia that the reader concludes that those times were not so rough at all and that if they were, the close, warm family ties healed all wounds.

Families have turned over many of their previous functions, already noted, to institutions, organizations, and professionals outside the family, but they have maintained the functions of childbearing, primary socialization of children, and psychosocial validation or "refueling" for all their members. This last function, the provision of psychosocial verification, worth, and meaning, probably is the most important. Standards for its performance have increased tremendously in recent years, with the popular press reporting all types of help available to meet increased expectations, from individual psychotherapy and counseling to retreats and renewals, self-help books and groups, and high-priced encounters with marriage and family specialists. At the turn of this century the only interpersonal, behavioral requirement between husbands and wives was that they be civil to each other. The new requirement is that they love one another and continue to express this love unfailingly, even into their elder years. An associated new requirement is for increased intimacy through sexuality. Since those who marry for economic purposes have few reasons to terminate marriage, the current high rate of divorce is an indication that marriage as an economic arrangement is definitely a thing of the past.

The high divorce rates in the United States have been viewed by some as symptomatic of an erosion of the American family and its associated value systems. An alternative view, however, is to interpret these statistics as indicating that Americans today place a higher value on forming *successful* marriages than did earlier generations. The new requirement that marital partners "love each other" carries with it the expectation that irreconcilable differences can be settled by divorce. The consequences of divorce for children is a separate issue and will be discussed later.

"THE AMERICAN FAMILY"

Everyone (even non-Americans) knows what the stereotypical American family is. It is thought to be a white, middle-class mother and father living together in a suburban home with their boy child and girl child (and an optional third child of either sex). The father leaves for work daily and is successful in his career; the mother transforms the house into a home and is not expected to work full time until the last child is in school.

Although this stereotype is changing rapidly, to a great extent it is still thought to be true, even among minorities or those who live in dual-career families or single-parent families. The stereotype excludes more than half the population in the United States today. It is a tribute to American advertising to realize how pervasive this "ideal type" picture is despite the fact that census data provide contradictory evidence. The 1990 census data are presented herein; the reader is reminded that data from the 2000 census (not yet available) will be considerably different.

The old notions of family life span are dysfunctional; many families today change their structures repeatedly by marriage, divorce, and remarriage, interspersed by varying lengths of time alone or as single parents. For instance, in the first half of this century the sequence described was courtship, marriage, childbearing and rearing, "empty nest," retirement, and death of one or both spouses. Today there are many departures from this sequence. Among alternative family forms are unmarried couples living together (with or without children); homosexual couples (with or without children); deliberately childless couples, married or not; single-parent families with either a father or a mother as the parent; middle-aged couples whose divorced adult children return home with their young children; middle-aged couples living in very crowded situations because of the former pattern, and in addition, with their elderly parent or parents living with them; various types of blended families created by divorced or widowed parents remarrying; and group families, in which several unrelated families share a large space. A new structure is grandparents (largely grandmothers) rearing their grandchildren, because the parents are victims of AIDS, incarcerated, or addicted to drugs and/or alcohol. Within each of these various structures the rules of organization for carrying out the chores of daily living differ widely.

Marriage, divorce, widowhood, remarriage, and childbearing patterns have changed dramatically since the 1950s and have altered the size and composition of the American family radically. The biggest change is the increase in single parents. In 1980, one in five babies born had a single mother; in 1993, it was one in three. Of the single mothers giving birth in 1993, 50% were never married. Further, 30% of the single mothers were teenagers. For large numbers of people, marriage is no longer a precondition for procreation. Although many people believe (fostered by the media) that most single mothers are black, the fact is that most are white.[8]

The "trajectory" of women's lives has changed in dramatic ways, influencing childbearing and childrearing practices. Fifty years ago, women finished their education, married, raised a family, and only then considered working outside the home when the nest was empty. Today, women are more likely to delay marriage and family until after a period of work or professional involvement. When they do marry and begin a family, they continue to work since the current economic picture is such that two incomes are needed to sustain a middle class household. This shift has lowered birth rates, increased childless marriage and single parents, and considerably decreased the social stability of children's lives.[8]

As of 1998, 5.5 million American children were living below the poverty line. About 42% of the poor are children; only 10% are elderly.[14] The age group most likely to be crime victims are children 12 to 15 years old. This statistic is a clear indicator of the distressing situations faced by many families, who are unable to carry out a core function of providing a safe haven.

Although marriage was less permanent in the 1990s than ever before, (the number of people divorced rose to 16.7 million in 1993 from 4.3 million in 1970), it still was highly likely that marriage would be part of the future for better than 90% of Americans.[11] For pediatricians, the relevance of these different marital, financial, and living arrangements is that children being raised within them experience very different levels of support and nurturance.

One trend in American families of which most physicians certainly are aware is that families are smaller than they were just a decade ago. They may not be aware, however, that the number of children in families is related to the family's general physical and mental health. The obvious inverse correlation of the more children, the fewer the resources for each reveals some surprises when social class is added. Infant and childhood mortality rates fell for both upper and lower classes when fewer children were born into the families. Young children of large families continue to have more infections, more accidents, and higher overall mortality than do the children of small families, regardless of social class.[12] An only child in a poor family has about the same chance of surviving the first year of life as a child who is born into a professional family but who has four or more siblings. Small families, however, are more prone to violence. One possibility for the increased likelihood of violence in small families is that fewer resources are available when a crisis occurs. For instance, if a single mother of two children younger than 5 years old becomes ill, she is likely to be less tolerant of noise or even simple demands of the children. If they do not sleep, or even if they remain relatively quiet when she is trying to rest, they are more likely to be hit or punished. Divorced fathers, trying to make every moment of their visits count, often lose their tempers and end up verbally or physically abusing their children. Spousal abuse also is more common in smaller than in larger families.

CHANGING FAMILY STRUCTURES AND FUNCTIONS

Although the myth of the American family as a married couple with two or more children, the father as breadwinner, and the mother as homemaker remains an ideal type in popular media, the demographic reality is very different. The 1990 census revealed that just over one third of all families (37%) consisted of a married couple with children, regardless of the number of children or the employment status of the wife; only 20% of married couples fit the popular stereotype.[1,14]

The Census Bureau distinguishes between a "household" and a "family." Households consist of units occupied by persons. A household may consist of one person living alone or several people sharing the dwelling. A family is two or more persons related by birth, marriage, or adoption who reside together. Relatives who may be involved with the family very integrally, but who do not share the dwelling, are not counted. Although 70% of U.S. households contain a family unit, family composition is quite diverse. Families include married couples with and without children, single-parent families headed by a woman or a man, siblings living together, and many other arrangements. Just under half of all families have children, but their structures, the number of generations, and the number of people in each generation varies considerably.

Hodgkinson, who holds the distinction of being regarded as "America's demographer" states that " . . . Americans are totally uninterested in youth issues, even though foreigners often observe that we are 'eating our corn' and that our greatness as a nation will decline if we ignore our youth."[8] In 1970, 34% of our society was younger than 18 years of age; by 1990, this age group had decreased to 26%. Only one household in four had a child in the public schools. Although pediatricians would find the following fact astounding, the average American adult can go for an entire week without significant contact with a child younger than age 18 years.

Although more than 80% of stepfamilies are white, the odds of being in a stepfamily are double for blacks. Estimates are that a third of all Americans are stepparents, stepchildren, stepsiblings, or some other member of a stepfamily.

Single-parent families doubled between 1970 and 1991, when nearly one in eight families was headed by a single parent. Women are five times more likely to be the single parent than men, and blacks are almost three times more likely than whites to be single parents. Single parents rearing children head one in five white families, one in three Hispanic families, and six in 10 black families. About 50% of America's children will spend some time in a one-parent family, mostly as a consequence of divorce.

Twenty-five percent of homeless individuals are in family units. Of these, 60% are children, 32% are their parents (overwhelmingly single mothers), and 8% are couples that have no children.

Another new pattern is the increasing involvement of grandparents in childrearing. Adult children, both divorced and married, when faced with tough economic times are doubling up households by returning to their parents' homes. This trend is more likely in minority families. In 28% of households, grandparents become the sole caretakers of the children, with neither parent present. The absent parent may be the victim of AIDS, or incarcerated, or addicted to drugs and/or alcohol. With increased longevity, these grandparents may also be responsible for their parents. The so-called sandwich generation has moved up one generation.[13]

In past generations, pediatricians were surprised if anyone other than the child's mother brought the child for visits to the office or was the caretaker during minor and major crises. Today pediatricians encounter grandmothers, grandfathers, fathers, and even babysitters in increasing numbers. Pediatricians accustomed to dealing with mothers face the challenge of adjusting their psychosocial style as they encounter men as caretakers.

Although contraception has been available to teens, the increase in birth rates among women under 20 is rising steadily. In 1970, there were 21 births per 1000 unmarried teenagers; by 1993, this rate had doubled. However, teenagers account for fewer than a third of all unmarried mothers, black teenagers for fewer than 12%. Out-of-wedlock childbearing has risen fastest among women age 20 and older. Furthermore, married women are having fewer children, thus inflating the share of out-of-wedlock births.

Working mothers are creating pressures for social change both inside and outside the family. The willingness of men to adjust their priorities and to shift energies from work to family is critical for producing the expected "home as haven." Their unwillingness to change in the direction of more family involvement often produces stress, even chaos, for their wives and children. Chapman[3] has analyzed the effects of fathers' changing roles and functions as breadwinners and homemakers. In 1991, 58% of mothers who had children younger than 6 years were employed full time. In 1960, the figure was 20%.[7] In 1994, two thirds of preschool children and three fourths of school-age children had mothers who worked outside the home. As Chapman studied the contributions of children to household chores, she also discovered that husbands/fathers continue to contribute less effort than what their spouses desire.[3]

THE DEMOGRAPHICS OF DIVERSITY

In the twenty-first century, schools and health care practitioners will face the challenge of delivering care to children of many cultures and faiths. By 2010, whites will account for only about 9% of the world's population, compared with 17% in 1997. Thus, whites will have become the world's smallest ethnic minority. These worldwide changes will be felt in the United States, as immigration patterns continue to shift. The European influence is already history; only 15% of current immigrants are European. South and Central America and Asia are the most widely represented in immigration statistics. People of color are the new immigrants and continue to have population growth; the white fertility rate has declined to 1.7 children per woman. By 2030, most of our school-age children will be "minority," as will most Americans by 2050.[9]

Like the world, the white population in the United States is concentrated in the northern half and is rich, well educated, and declining in number. The southern half is ethnically diverse, younger, poorer, and less well educated. Yet more than 90% of the population growth is in the South.[8]

The youngest children in America are the most diverse. Although 26% of all Americans are non-white, 37% of schoolchildren are. The world comprises 215 nations, and every one of them has someone living in the United States. Another trend that will have significant effects is the increasing tendency for intermarriages among the diverse ethnic groups. In fact, it will be impossible to "check the box" in future census questionnaires to accurately capture racial heritage. Intermarriage has dramatically altered older, out-of-date conceptions of black, white, red, or yellow as racial "colors."

DISTINGUISHING "NORMAL" FROM "ABNORMAL" FAMILIES

Clinical theory about dysfunctional families has not kept pace with the dramatic changes that have occurred in family structures and associated functions and ways of living. As Walsh[16] points out, "Most clinical theory explicitly or implicitly upholds the ideal model of the family as intact, with father as primary wage-earner and instrumental leader and mother as primary parent, homemaker, and socioemotional caretaker." However, fewer than 20% of American families fit this pattern. Still, deviation from this standard is regarded in much of the literature as unquestionably pathogenic. Current textbooks used in the clinical training of health professionals virtually ignore alternative arrangements as possibly being more normative. Even when divorce or separation are acknowledged as occurring in half the marriages, the normal sequence of dissolution of ties, emotional upset, management of stress, and adaptations to community demands are not given appropriate consideration.

According to Walsh, clinicians thus lack knowledge about what is and is not normal in family life.[16] She describes two types of errors frequently made: the first is to identify mistakenly as pathological a family pattern that is normal; the second is to assume normality because of failure to recognize a dysfunctional pattern. An example of the first error is the reaction of a clinician, reared in a family in which adults did not demonstrate affection openly and children were supposed to follow the directions of adults, who encounters a family that is noisy, affectionate, and open in expressions of joy and anguish. This clinician, seeing the solicitous concern of a mother for her child—to the point of her bringing homemade lasagna to her hospitalized child—might view this behavior as enmeshment or symbiosis instead of normal caring. Of course, clinicians do not always assume that what they experienced at home was normal. Some, instead, see their own upbringing as departing from normal and then apply this view to the families they see; when they encounter a family like their own, they view it suspiciously and diagnose the behavior as pathological.

An example of the second error, according to Walsh, is acceptance of the myth that healthy families are free of conflict. Such a view would preclude the clinician from exploring further an assertion by a couple that they have not disagreed in 20 years of marriage. What is common also may be accepted as normal. For instance, noncustodial fathers are so frequently cut off from their children after a divorce that clinicians may fall into the trap of seeing this as normal and, thus, fail to explore ways that the father and his children might be together.

Pediatricians who feel uncomfortable about exploring the psychosocial aspects of their patients' families miss opportunities to suggest repairs and to help families rethink destructive relationships. Recent research demonstrates a positive association between continued supportive contact with the noncustodial parent and long-term adjustment of children. Such contact also affects the custodial mothers positively. Even when previous contact had negative consequences, continuing paternal detachment produces poorer functioning and more symptomatic behavior, especially in boys. Fathers who had negative relationships with their children before divorce have been able, in many cases, to develop improved relationships after divorce. Citing several long-term studies, Walsh[16] concludes that a clinical imperative in cases of nonparticipating parents is to assess and build the coparenting alliance in postdivorce families.

The degree to which pediatricians feel comfortable in adding psychosocial exploration to their "history taking" or ongoing assessments of treatment depends on the messages they received from their mentors or subsequent attempts to change practice habits, which might come from colleagues or the families themselves. Some are reluctant to suggest that psychiatric consultation be sought, even when there is clear evidence of the need either in the child or in the parent. Some are reluctant to discuss behavior that is willful or that reflects a lifestyle rather than an illness. Drug and alcohol abuse are examples of problems that, even when noticed, are not mentioned by many clinicians.

Early research in family behavior tended to overrepresent white, Anglo-Saxon, Protestant, middle-class families. Comparative studies have included the differences in structures and styles of relating among varied ethnic groups.[10] Other recent studies focus on alternative family forms, such as single-parent and blended family systems. Wallerstein[15] has contributed an insightful and clinically relevant study of the children of divorce, tracing the lives of families 5 to 10 years after breakup. An emergent theme is that no single pattern distinguishes well-functioning from pathological families. Something that looks like intrusiveness to a less-than-careful observer may simply be caring, expressed in a particular ethnic style. Also, no single family structure is "healthier" than other arrangements. If the stresses and the available resources are more or less equivalent, children in single-parent families or children raised by a homosexual couple can do just as well as those in families having two biological parents.

Walsh[16] cautions that "too often, families with the same presenting problem are presumed to have a similar dysfunctional style, when research, albeit limited to date, reveals a good deal of diversity among families with similarly diagnosed members." Clinicians need to remind themselves that there is no one-to-one correspondence between symptom and system. In the past, rigid application of theories, unsubstantiated by adequate research, created additional strains for families who already were burdened by caring for a sick child. For instance, about 40 years ago, it was fairly popular to remove children who had asthma from their families as a therapeutic strategy; this was called a "parentectomy," the reasoning being that overinvolved, enmeshed emotionality between parent (mostly mothers) and child precipitated asthma attacks. Just as there is no single pattern that demarcates a normal family clearly, families cannot be typed by the diagnosis of a family member, whether that is asthma or alcoholism or cancer. Keeping in mind that families are tremendously complex and that a wide array of variables is operative at any moment prevents jumping to faulty conclusions. A better stance is to form a tentative hypothesis and then engage the family in its mutual exploration.

Increasingly, residents in family medicine programs are being taught to use family genograms as a part of the history taking and assessment. This technique would also provide valuable data for pediatricians. A three-generation genogram can be completed within 20 minutes and is well worth the time and effort when weighing these against the gains in information. The genogram information can be focussed on physical or psychosocial targets and provide clues to both physical symptoms and dysfunctional behavior.[13] Day-Salvatore, the well-known geneticist, makes the point that genograms and a carefully executed history significantly improve the diagnostic process. When histories are not taken thoroughly, important facts about relatives and earlier illnesses are overlooked.[4]

CHANGING SOCIALIZATION NORMS

Generations ago parents simply bore and raised children, with almost no input from strangers and generally little, depending on ethnicity, from extended family members. Today there are specialists for every dimension of these functions, from how to be healthy in pregnancy to how to respond to an adolescent's bad manners. Americans generally are the greatest consumers of advice on children and health in the world. Depending on their social class and culture, parents choose different authorities to consult. The appropriate resource for parents' questions is determined very much by their social group, their level of education, and their general sense of assuredness about parenting. All of us, parents or not, tend to hear and believe what we *want* to hear and believe. Most parents measure the advice not against a standard of good research but rather against a more pragmatic one of whether the advice giver is trustworthy or has a track record of sensible prior advice.

Fifty years ago no profession identified as one of its functions how to teach parents to be parents. Parents were supposed to know how to be good parents either intuitively or because they learned it from growing up in large extended families. Today, advice, counseling, and teaching about parenting are considered part of the work of pediatricians, pediatric nurse practitioners, child study specialists, health educators, child psychologists, and behavior modifiers. Courses on effective parenting can be found in high school, college, and graduate school curricula, as well as on public television. Failure at socialization might be treated by an educational course or by a stay at a psychiatric hospital; some parents still see the military as a solution for offspring who fail to adopt parental values and norms. When a younger child behaves badly in the classroom or resists going to school entirely, the tendency now is to treat this as a "system" difficulty and to use a range of strategies to involve the parents in some type of parenting program. There even are programs for parents whose teenagers abuse drugs or alcohol and for other comparable sibling support groups.

Two revolutions currently face families. One revolution is under way inside families, where changes in sex roles, resulting in increased participation in the work force, are challenging traditional marital rules. Wives who work two jobs every day, one outside the home and one inside the home, resent the noninvolvement of their husbands in the tasks necessary to make a house a home. The second revolution is going on outside the family, where unmarried people now can experience the privacy, dignity, and authority (and sometimes the loneliness) of living in their own home. There now is a choice available, and some adults are choosing not to live within a family.

The first revolution is creating significant pressure to change the normative order between husbands and wives, with fathers being much more involved in homemaking and childrearing and mothers being more involved with careers and contributing economically to families. Changes in how family roles and rules are carried out, departing drastically from the traditional norms, produce "new families." Further, the diversity of styles and traditions encountered with the changing demographic patterns demand taking new approaches and new strategies for problem-solving. Even if the parents are from the same cultural background, their children will be encountering diversity in the classroom settings and inviting children reared by different norms into their homes.

The second revolution, in which adults choose not to marry and instead to live independently away from families, produces the alternative of "no family at all." Although the outcomes are different, both revolutions have the same origin—our social priorities valuing the workplace over the home. Men, while acknowledging the importance of families and the necessity to do family tasks to provide a comfortable environment, do not see themselves as the primary workers in this arena. Women increasingly spend more of their time and energy on issues in the workplace rather than on family matters. These new directions are leading to a generation of children who know less and less about what it takes to run a family, whether that includes inside tasks such as cleaning and meal preparations, or outside chores such as lawn-cutting or snow removal. The allocation of their energies mirrors that of their parents: they spend more time on school work, after-school activities, friends, and recreation than on domestic responsibilities.[3]

FAMILY TIES

Sagan[12] has suggested that the real reason we live longer is related directly to changes in how children are treated within families rather than to advances in medicine and science. It is well known that life expectancy has risen dramatically in most societies over the past few centuries. As recently as 1900, the typical American lived only 49 years, and one child in five died in infancy. Today, the life expectancy for Americans is 75 years, and infant mortality has declined to less than 1 in every 170 births. Both physicians and the public credit modern medicine for these bold achievements, assuming almost reflexively that people who lack expert medical care die earlier and that providing more care is the key to longer life. Sagan's plea is that we look more carefully at these assumptions, which largely are unfounded. He provides compelling data for our rethinking of the assumptions we tend to make about the relationship between our efforts at health care on the one hand and our actual health on the other. He shows that although America spends more on health care than does any other nation in the world, in many respects Americans are not actually healthier. He does not deny that modern medicine has accomplished much that is of great value, such as alleviating suffering and developing useful surgical treatments for illnesses or trauma, but he shows clearly that neither saving individual lives nor alleviating suffering has contributed to overall life expectancy. Most therapy is not aimed directly at prolonging life, nor do the vast majority of missed medical appointments endanger life. He reminds the reader that too often what physicians do is not necessary or is based on poor research or no research at all and that they prescribe too many medications, often without justification for their use.

Life expectancy has increased spectacularly during the late nineteenth and twentieth centuries. There is no question that sanitation and nutrition have been beneficial. Neither of these, however, accounts fully for the leaps in longevity. Sagan attributes family ties as the key variable in longevity, suggesting that it is impossible to trace the hardiness of modern people directly to improvements in medicine, sanitation, or diet. He sees an alternative explanation for our increased life expectancy, one that has less to do with these developments than with changes in our psychological environment. Growing up and living surrounded by scarcity and ignorance and constant loss is to endure a special misery—that which is a consequence of forces beyond one's control. A kind of personal powerlessness prevails, in which one's best efforts are not enough to ward off disaster. There is ample evidence that such a sense of helplessness often is associated with apathy, depression, and death—whether in laboratory animals or in prisoners of war. The reader is reminded of Martin Seligman's classic experiments with dogs, which resulted in the concept of learned helplessness as an explanation for why animals and human beings give up, endure pain, and die rather than act to prevent pain and death. People in poverty now share a feature of most premodern societies.

Modernization, with its associated community supports such as fire departments, building codes, social insurance, and emergency medical care, cushions most of us from physical, psychic, and economic disaster. These supports have created circumstances in which few of us feel utterly powerless or unable to take control over our lives. We generally feel like the masters of our own destinies, "and that, in itself, leaves us better equipped to fight off disease."[12]

A sense of personal efficacy and self-esteem is an outcome of changed family system values and practices. Until the late eighteenth century, families primarily were economic units. Marriages were arranged to preserve property, and children were regarded as cheap labor. Beating and whipping were commonplace, even among royalty, as approved tools to teach or extract conformity and obedience. During the Enlightenment the standards and goals of child rearing began to change. Philosophers argued, eloquently and at length, that if children were to survive in a disorderly and unpredictable world, they could not rely passively on traditional authority. They needed reasoned judgment. To develop such judgment children needed affection and guidance rather than harsh, unreasoned discipline and brute force. Gradually, as these ideas took hold, childhood came to be recognized as a special stage of life.[2] Affection and nurturing replaced obligation and duty as the cohesive elements among family members.

Childhood mortality fell as a direct consequence of families having fewer children. Starting with the upper classes, families came to see that children had needs of their own and did not exist to serve the family. This revolutionary idea resulted in curtailing the numbers of births. Children were seen as individuals in their own right, to be paid attention to and nurtured rather than always to do for others. As lower classes also had fewer children, mortality fell among them as well. Family size is an excellent predictor of childhood survival, even today. Children in small families are strengthened by the extra nurturance and resources available to them; several studies of infants in institutions during World War II and after demonstrated that infants who receive only physical care do not survive.

The new field of psychoneuroimmunology is pursuing the connections between emotional and physical health. Whatever the mechanism that produces greater physical health during periods of emotional well-being needs to be understood. Affection and security may be thought of as natural vaccines. Children who receive consistent love and attention—who grow up in situations in which self-reliance and optimism are nurtured and expected—are better equipped to survive.

THE FUTURE

The future of the family cannot be predicted without placing it squarely in its social context. The trends toward equality of the sexes within families and the larger society certainly have increased self-esteem for women but may cause new stresses for both men and women. Careful watching of morbidity and mortality trends will provide clues to the effect of this important social movement. Divorce rates have leveled, and marriage again is gaining in popularity. The number of dual-career or dual-job marriages and unions is growing each year. Although such arrangements improve the family's economic assets, child care becomes complex and costly, especially in the preschool years. Considering recent trend analyses and surveys, it seems likely that the following future directions for American families might be possible:

1. Increasing value will continue to be placed on human potential, tenderness and warmth, and psychosocial needs being met, rather than on material pursuits. Human well-being will be a primary goal for families, rather than economic well-being.
2. The trend toward decreasing numbers of children per family will continue and will result in greater attention being paid to parent-child relationships and an increased use of professionals as parenting advisers.
3. Neighborhoods will reemerge along with increased numbers of community support systems.
4. Extended families will gain the attention of researchers, as will grandparent-grandchild relationships.
5. The new American ideal—strength without domination—will gain impetus and influence in socialization patterns of families.

The challenge for pediatricians will be to keep abreast of changes in family patterns and dynamics and to use this knowledge in providing humanistically oriented and enlightened patient care and advice regarding parenting.

REFERENCES

1. Ahlburg DA, DeVita CJ: New realities of the American family, *Pop Bull* 47:2, 1992.
2. Aries P: *Centuries of childhood,* New York, 1962, Random House.
3. Chapman V: Working hard or hardly working? An examination of children's household contributions in the 1990s, doctoral dissertation, Princeton, NJ, 1994, Princeton University.
4. Day-Salvatore, D: The Genome Project: Family Systems Perspective, lecture, Family Health Science, 20 October 1999, Robert Wood Johnson Medical School, Piscataway, NJ.
5. Goode WJ: *World revolution and family patterns,* New York, 1963, The Free Press.
6. Gough K: The origin of the family. In Skolnick A, Skolnick J, editors: *Family in transition: rethinking marriage, sexuality, child rearing and family organization,* Boston, 1986, Little, Brown.
7. Hareven T: American families in transition: historical perspectives on change. In Walsh F, editor: *Normal family processes,* New York, 1982, Guilford.
8. Hodgkinson H: *Bringing tomorrow into focus: demographic insights into the future,* Washington, DC, 1996, Center for Demographic Policy, The Institute for Educational Leadership.
9. Hodgkinson H: The demographics of diversity, *Principal,* September 1998, pp 27-32.
10. McGoldrick M, Pearce J, Giordano J, editors: *Ethnicity and family therapy,* New York, 1982, Guilford.
11. *New York Times:* Birthrate for unwed women up 70% since '83, study says, p 1 and A8, July 20, 1994.
12. Sagan L: Family ties: the real reason that people are living longer. In *Annual editions: Health, 1989-1990,* Guilford, Conn, 1989, Dushkin Press.
13. Smoyak S: Systems theory as a model to understand families. In Burgess A: *Psychiatric nursing: promoting mental health,* Stamford, Conn, 1997, Appleton and Lange.
14. U.S. Census Bureau, 1998.
15. Wallerstein J: *Second chances: men, women, and children a decade after divorce,* New York, 1989, Ticknor & Fields.
16. Walsh F: The clinical utility of normal family research, *Psychotherapy* 24:496, 1987.

56 Gay- and Lesbian-Parented Families

Melanie A. Gold

American family structures are changing. The traditional structure of a married couple—a working father, homemaker mother, and one or more children—no longer describes the majority of American families. According to the 1990 U.S. Census, 37% of U.S. families consist of a married couple who have children; only 7% of those families report a pattern in which the father works and the mother stays home full time.[13] Alternative forms of family are quite diverse. For example, unmarried couples live together with or without children. Single mothers and fathers, step-parents, and "blended" families can be created by divorce, death, and remarriage. Gay men and lesbian women can form stable families with or without children. Children can flourish in various family environments as long as these include adequate nurturance and guidance for optimal development.

Current estimates suggest that there are about 5 million lesbian mothers, 3 million gay fathers, and 6 to 14 million children of gay or lesbian parents in the United States. These figures probably underestimate the true total because many gay and lesbian parents are reluctant to reveal their sexual orientation. Gay- and lesbian-parented families themselves exist in a wide range of constellations. Until recently the majority of gay men or lesbian women became parents in the context of a heterosexual relationship before they recognized or acknowledged their homosexuality. Such parents may continue to live with their heterosexual spouse and their children, or they may divorce and live as single parents or form stable relationships with a gay or lesbian partner. These parents may have full or joint custody or regular visitation with their children.

As gay men and lesbian women choose increasingly to "come out" in their youth, growing numbers are becoming parents in the context of an ongoing homosexual relationship. Gay men may father children through arrangements with friends or surrogates, and lesbian women may become parents by using insemination techniques with a known or unknown donor. When the donor is known, he may or may not have an acknowledged, active role as the child's parent. Gay men and lesbian women also can become parents by adoption or foster parenting. In most states only one member of the same-sex couple may be designated the child's legal parent, by birth or adoption. This convention results in formidable obstacles to both parents' having legal status consistent with their joint parental responsibilities.

RESEARCH ON CHILDREN WHO HAVE HOMOSEXUAL PARENTS

Research on children reared by homosexual parents has been limited by small sample sizes, non-random subject selection, a narrow range of demographic variables, and lack of long-term follow-up. The majority of studies were not "double-blinded" and have been done by gay researchers, who may be perceived as being biased. Most research has focused on demonstrating the absence of a pathological situation rather than on elucidating patterns of strength and resilience.

Much of the earlier research has been on children whose gay or lesbian parents divorced after a heterosexual marriage. For the children who have lived through parental discord, separation, and divorce, these experiences may be of more concern to them and have greater effect on their emotional and social development than the sexual orientation of their parents. Consciously planned families are different from those that occur from the loss of a parent or through divorce. During the 1990s, more research has become available on children conceived in the context of lesbian relationships. However, data are still scant for children raised from infancy by gay men.

A 1992 review by Patterson[10] found that children who have gay or lesbian parents did not differ from children who have heterosexual parents in terms of psychological health and social relationships. Patterson reviewed 12 studies whose sample sizes ranged from 12 to 56 children whose parents were gay or lesbian and equal numbers of children who had heterosexual parents. No differences were found in the development of sexual or gender identity or gender role behavior between children who had homosexual parents and those who had heterosexual parents. Adolescent sexual orientation was similar, with about 5% to 8% of teenagers in both groups reporting homosexual attraction or behavior. No differences were found in personality characteristics, locus of control, moral maturity, intelligence, or the incidence of psychiatric disturbance or behavioral problems.

These studies also report that children whose mothers are part of a lesbian couple spend more time with their mothers' male friends and relatives and have more contact with their biological fathers than do children whose mothers are heterosexual and single. Children do not become confused or have difficulty relating to two same-sex parents but will easily create names to address their same-sex parents (e.g., Daddy and Papa, or Mommy Sue and Mommy Jane), just as they do routinely to identify grandparents and other relatives. Children growing up having homosexual parents have been shown to be more tolerant of diversity in general and more open to discussions on topics such as sexuality and interpersonal relationships than children having heterosexual parents. Children in a gay- or lesbian-parented family are less likely to be victims of parental sexual or physical abuse than are children in a heterosexual-parented family.[9]

In 1996, Allen and Burrell[1] conducted a meta-analysis summarizing the available quantitative literature comparing the impact of heterosexual and homosexual parents on the children. The analyses examined parenting practices, the emotional well-being of the child, and the sexual orientation of the child. The results demonstrate no differences between heterosexual and homosexual parents regarding any of these measures.

A longitudinal study of 25 young adults from lesbian families and 21 young adults raised by heterosexual single mothers revealed that those raised by lesbian mothers functioned well in adulthood in terms of psychological well-being and of family identity and relationships.[12] No significant differences were found between young adults from lesbian and heterosexual mothers in the quality of their relationship with their mother and father. However, young adults brought up by lesbian mothers were significantly more positive about their mother's unconventional relationships than were those raised by single heterosexual mothers. Those adults from lesbian family background were no more likely to remember general teasing or bullying by their peers than were those from heterosexual single-parent homes. However, those from lesbian families were more likely to recall having been teased about being gay or lesbian themselves. No significant difference was found between young adults from lesbian and heterosexual single-parent homes in the proportion who had experienced same-gender attraction. However, those from lesbian households were more likely to have been involved in a same-gender sexual relationship than those from a heterosexual singe-parent household. Likewise, those from a lesbian household were more likely to consider the possibility of becoming involved in a same-gender sexual relationship. Having a lesbian mother appeared to widen the adolescent's view of what is acceptable sexual behavior to include same-gender sexual relationships.

Although those from lesbian families were more likely to explore same-gender sexual relationships, particularly if their childhood family environment was characterized by an openness and acceptance of lesbian and gay relationships, the large majority of children who grew up in lesbian families identified their sexual identity as heterosexual. Of the 25 adults raised by lesbian mothers, 2 identified themselves as lesbian compared with none of the adults raised by heterosexual mothers. This group difference did not reach statistical significance. No significant associations were found between same-gender sexual interest in adulthood and the number of years raised in a heterosexual household, the mother's warmth to the child, the child's contact with the father, the child's gender role behavior, the quality of the child's peer relationships, the quality of the mother's relationship with her female partner, the mother's contentment with her sexual identity, the mother's political involvement, or the mother's attitude toward men.[7]

Brewaeys et al[3] conducted a comparative study investigating family relationships and the emotional and gender development of children raised in lesbian families who were conceived through donor insemination compared with children in heterosexual families who were either conceived naturally or by donor insemination. The quality of the couples' relationships and the quality of the mother-child interaction did not differ between lesbian families and the two types of heterosexual families. The quality of interactions between the social (nonbiological) mother and the child in lesbian families was superior to that between the father and child in both groups of heterosexual families. Children raised in lesbian mother families were well adjusted, and their gender role development did not differ from that of children raised in either of the two groups of heterosexual families.

Chan, Raboy, and Patterson[5] assessed lesbian couples and heterosexual couples whose children were conceived via donor insemination. Assessments included measures of parental adjustment and relationship satisfaction and measures of their children's' adjustment, using the Child Behavior Checklist and the Teacher Report Form. The study revealed that all the children were developing normally and that their adjustment was unrelated to family structural variables such as maternal sexual orientation. These results held true for teacher reports as well as parent reports. Parents' sexual orientation was unrelated to teacher reports of the children's behavior problems. Parents who were experiencing high levels of parenting stress and higher levels of interparental conflict, and lower levels of love for each other had children who exhibited more behavioral problems by both parental and teacher reports. The best predictor of teachers' reports of child behavior problems was nonbiological parents' parenting distress. Among families headed by couples, children were rated as being better adjusted when their parents reported greater relationship satisfaction, higher levels of love, and lower interparental conflict.

A study by Golombok, Tasker, and Murray[8] compared children raised in fatherless families from infancy with either heterosexual or lesbian mothers with those raised within a family where the father was present. Children from single-mother families experienced greater warmth and interaction with their mothers and were more securely attached to their mothers than children raised in families that had a father present. Children raised without fathers experienced themselves to be less cognitively and physically competent than their peers from father-present families. There were no differences identified between families headed by lesbian and single heterosexual mothers, except for greater mother-child interaction in lesbian mother families. Although there were no differences in terms of frequency of discipline disputes between father-absent and father-present families, there were significantly more severe disputes in single-mother homes compared with father-present homes. There were no differences in the seriousness of disputes found between lesbian and heterosexual mother families. There also were no significant differences in levels of anxiety or depression or visits to mental health professionals between young adults from lesbian and heterosexual single-parent homes.

Children growing up with gay fathers have been studied less extensively than those having lesbian mothers. In a review of the literature that included more than 20 studies, Bozett[2] compared characteristics of parenting among gay and heterosexual fathers and found no differences between the two groups in problem solving, providing recreation for children, or encouraging autonomy. Gay fathers were found to be less traditional, to demonstrate greater nurturance, and to have more investment in their paternal role and to view it more positively than did heterosexual fathers. Gay fathers who have disclosed their homosexuality to their children tended to be less authoritarian and to use less corporal punishment with their children than did gay fathers living with wives. Gay fathers who did not have physical custody of their children maintained contact with them more consistently than did divorced or separated heterosexual fathers.

SOCIAL RELATIONSHIPS AND DISCLOSURE

It is important for all children, especially as they reach school age, to develop a wide range of relationships outside their nuclear family. Children who have gay or lesbian parents may be assumed to be homosexual and experience stigmatization by peers when their parents' sexual orientation becomes known. Casper, Schultz, and Wickens[4] described the conflict raised for children who have gay or lesbian parents when the dominant cultural values reflected in the school define "family" in ways that are different from what the children experience in their own homes. This discrepancy may be distressing to children and add to their social isolation and uncomfortable relationships with peers. Gay and lesbian parents frequently fear that school staff will treat their children differently if they disclose their sexual orientation and family constellation. As a result, many parents help children to learn "differential disclosure"—to be open about their parents' homosexuality to some people but not to others—so that harassment and social isolation can be minimized. Parents should understand that both secrecy and disclosure represent potential burdens for their children.

Pediatricians and other health professionals can act as intermediaries between the family and the school to help make the educational environment more supportive. They can talk to child care providers and teachers and can encourage schools to include information about diverse family structures in their libraries and curricula. Pediatricians also can encourage families to develop a social support network in the interest of their children. In many larger cities, an active network of gay and lesbian parents work to create an environment of peer support in which their children feel accepted and less "different" than they may in their other social contexts. Parent-child discussion or play groups, "story hours," and periodic communal meals have helped some parents and children seeking mutual support.

LEGAL ISSUES

There is a growing trend toward legal security of parental rights for gay and lesbian parents. Still, in most states only one parent in a same-sex couple can be a child's legal parent, and ambiguity in laws governing custody, compounded by vast differences in state laws, have left decisions in the hands of individual judges. Despite court precedents declaring that parents cannot be deprived of child custody based solely on parental sexual orientation, a heterosexual parent still is more likely than a homosexual parent to be granted custody and visitation rights unless the heterosexual parent is unavailable or obviously unfit.

Because courts have continuing legal authority to "protect" children until they reach majority (18 years of age), questions of custody can be reopened in any state in which the child resides, leaving the family vulnerable if they move to another state. If a court finds it to be in the child's "best interest," it can remove the child from the home if parental custody is challenged (e.g., by a former spouse or grandparents), particularly when a parent's homosexuality was unknown in a previous custody decision.

In the frequent circumstance that only one of the same-sex couple is legally recognized as a child's parent, the pediatrician should clarify how responsibility for medical decisions and consent for treatment for the child will be shared. In the event of serious illness, injury, death, or voluntary separation of the legal parent, a prior written agreement giving the other parent power of attorney in making medical decisions for the child is necessary.

In general, when gay and lesbian couples first contemplate raising a child together, they should agree in writing on issues concerning child custody, support, and consent for treatment. Curry, Clifford, and Leonard[6] give guidelines for writing agreements that specify parental rights and responsibilities. Without a written agreement, a nonbiological/nonadoptive parent may have difficulty proving his or her status as the child's parent. Fig. 56-1 contains a sample of an Authorization to Consent to Medical, Surgical, or Dental Examination or Treatment of a Minor.

ISSUES IN PROVIDING PEDIATRIC CARE

Pediatricians should convey their support of all forms of caring families and not assume that all parents are heterosexual. Pediatricians who care for children who have gay or lesbian parents should communicate trust and respect, be sensitive and aware of the special needs, expectations, and concerns of these parents, and focus on the family's strengths and resources as they pertain to the child's care and development. Pediatricians should be wary of giving unintentional signals of negative feelings toward homosexuality, which can interfere with the supportive and helpful role expected by parents. Those physicians who cannot reconcile their personal beliefs with their professional obligation to provide supportive, understanding, and respectful care to gay- and lesbian-headed families should recognize this limitation and refer these families to a physician who can meet their needs.

Gay or lesbian parents may choose not to identify their sexual orientation to their pediatrician. They may worry that latent homophobia or bias in professional and nonprofessional staff will jeopardize the care their children receive or that the pediatrician will not honor their confidentiality, particularly if the parents are concerned about legal challenges to their custody rights. Pediatricians should discuss consent for medical care and clarify in writing any power of attorney granting the nonbiological/nonadoptive parent the right to make medical decisions. They should discuss issues of confidentiality with parents—with whom parents will confide and from whom will they withhold disclosure of their family

I, ______________, being the parent with legal custody of
(name of custodial parent)

______________, born ______________, hereby authorize
(name of minor) (date of birth of minor)

______________ into whose care ______________
(name of nonbiological parent) (name of minor)

has been entrusted, to consent to any x-ray, examination, anesthetic,

medical, or surgical diagnosis, or treatment and hospital care to be

rendered to ______________ under the general or specific
(name of minor)

supervision and upon the advice of a physician or surgeon licensed

to practice medicine in any state of the United States, or to consent

to an x-ray, examination, anesthetic, dental or surgical diagnosis, or

treatment and hospital care to be rendered to ______________
(name of minor)

by a dentist licensed to practice dentistry in any state of the United

States. This authorization is valid from ______________ until
(starting date)

______________.
(ending date)

Dated: ______________ Signature: ______________
(custodial parent)

Dated: ______________ Signature: ______________
(nonbiological parent)

Notarization: ______________ Date: ______________

Fig. 56-1 Authorization to Consent to Medical, Surgical, or Dental Examination or Treatment of a Minor.

(Modified from Curry H, Clifford D, Leonard R: *A legal guide for lesbian and gay couples,* ed 7, Berkeley, Calif, 1993, Nolo Press.)

structure (e.g., school officials and hospital and office personnel).

Pediatricians should create a safe and inclusive environment for same-sex parents and their children. Part of creating that environment entails an awareness among professional and nonprofessional staff about issues of concern to lesbian and gay parents and the problems presented by homophobia, heterosexism, and bias. Discussion of nontraditional family structures can be facilitated by evidence of the pediatrician's acceptance of diverse families (Box 56-1). Questions on standardized office intake forms using gender-neutral terms such as "parent" or "family member" (instead of mother/father), pictures of diverse families in the waiting room, and brochures, books, and magazines that acknowledge same-sex parents, communicate the pediatrician's availability to assist *all* families in their parenting challenges. Pediatricians can create and implement a policy against lesbian and gay slurs, jokes, and put-downs in the office, which might hurt or offend patients, parents, and staff. Such office modifications also will help adolescents questioning their sexual orientation to discuss their concerns with the pediatrician.

As with any family, the pediatrician should discuss the parents' histories, as individuals and as a couple, and their plans for partnership in the care of their children. Knowledge about the family provides the pediatrician with valuable information in helping parents to care for their children. Asking questions sensitively about each parent's family background, perhaps including the creation of a genogram, helps to establish a fuller understanding of the family's sometimes complex relationships.

BOX 56-1

QUESTIONS TO CLARIFY THE FAMILY CONSTELLATION

Is there anything about your family that would be helpful for me to know?
Who are the adults who make up your family?
Who are the important people in your child's life?
Who lives at home? What is your relationship with each child caretaker?
By what name does your child call each family member?
Who are the other important members of your family or support system who help care for your child?
Do you share parenting responsibilities with anyone else?
Who helps you with parenting?
Is there anyone else who participates in parenting?
Do(es) the biological parent(s), if not part of the current constellation, have any involvement in child care?
Which of your child's caretakers can give legal consent for medical care?
Do any of your child's biological relatives have any medical conditions?

Pediatricians in communities in which there are many gay- or lesbian-headed families may want to know more about the specific concerns and issues surrounding these families. This perspective can be achieved by talking to friends, a spouse or partner, or members of the gay or lesbian communities; attending relevant continuing medical education courses; reading professional literature on the effect of family structure and sexual orientation on child development; attending gay or lesbian support groups; and reading both fiction and nonfiction that address issues about homosexuality and gay and lesbian parenting.

Medical Access and Experiences of Gay and Lesbian Parents

Perrin and Kulkin[11] investigated the experiences of gay and lesbian parents in obtaining pediatric care for their children. Of the 255 questionnaire surveys returned, 77% reported that their pediatrician knew of their sexual orientation and family constellation, nearly all (96%) having made it a point to inform the pediatrician at the initial visit. Nevertheless, many parents reported fears related to their pediatric care, including that their child's health care might suffer, that there might be potential negative implications for custody and adoptive decisions, that negative attitudes might be transmitted to their children, and that any difficulties their children might have would be attributed to the parents being gay. Indeed, several parents described experiences in which their family constellation had been presumed to be the etiology of their child's growth failure or behavioral and school difficulties. As many as 40% of parents reported problems such as exclusion of the nonbiological parent from the evaluation and treatment process and explicit insensitivity to particular family involvements in clinics, emergency departments, and hospitals.

This study included primarily white, middle-class, suburban, and urban parents. Lesbian and gay parents who are poor, live in rural areas, or are members of a racial or ethnic minority are likely to have less choice in the selection of a pediatrician and thus may be faced with the dilemma of working with a health care provider who may be insensitive or unsympathetic to their family constellations. Pediatricians should recognize that gay and lesbian parents, even those who are open about their orientation, may have a number of fears that should be addressed. Pediatricians also should work within hospitals to change policies that exclude nonbiological/nonadoptive parents from participating in their child's medical care.

Physician Advocacy

There is no evidence to suggest that children raised by gay or lesbian parents will develop abnormally or be maladjusted. Nevertheless, because of the extent of homophobia and bias, these children may be faced with criticism and isolation, which may affect their self-esteem. Pediatricians have an opportunity, and perhaps responsibility, to help change social attitudes and restrictive legal codes that are damaging to gay and lesbian parents and their children. Pediatricians should be informed community resources and may choose to be available as consultants to gay or lesbian support groups. They may be able to foster community understanding by participating in parent-teacher association meetings and various community programs. They can learn which programs are receptive and supportive of alternative family lifestyles and can provide guidance to gay and lesbian parents regarding child care and school selection. Pediatricians also can provide a bibliography of books for children and parents and a list of local and national resource groups. Above all, pediatricians have the opportunity and the responsibility to support and advise all families in achieving their maximal nurturing potential.

Acknowledgment

The author wishes to acknowledge the contribution of Ellen C. Perrin in the third edition of this textbook to the original chapter on this subject.

REFERENCES

1. Allen M, Burrell N: Comparing the impact of homosexual and heterosexual parents on children: meta-analysis of existing research, *J Homosex*, 32:19, 1996.
2. Bozett FW: Gay fathers: a review of the literature, *J Homosex* 18:137, 1989.
3. Brewaeys A, et al: Donor insemination: child development and family functioning in lesbian mother families, *Hum Reprod* 12:349, 1997.
4. Casper V, Schultz S, Wickens E: Breaking the silences: lesbian and gay parents and the schools, *Teachers College Record* 94:109, 1992.
5. Chan RW, Raboy B, Patterson CJ: Psychosocial adjustment among children conceived via donor insemination by lesbian and heterosexual mothers, *Child Dev* 69:443, 1998.
6. Curry H, Clifford D, Leonard R: *A legal guide for lesbian and gay couples,* ed 7, Berkeley, Calif, 1993, Nolo Press.
7. Golombok S, Tasker F: Do parents influence the sexual orientation of their children? Findings from a longitudinal study of lesbian families, *Dev Psych* 32:3, 1996.
8. Golombok S, Tasker F, Murray C: Children raised in fatherless families from infancy: family relationships and the socioeconomic development of children of lesbian and single heterosexual mothers, *J Child Psychol Psychiatry* 38;783, 1997.
9. Jenny C, Roesler JA, Poyer KL: Are children at risk for sexual abuse by homosexuals? *Pediatrics* 94:41, 1994.
10. Patterson CJ: Children of lesbian and gay parents, *Child Dev* 63:1025, 1992.
11. Perrin EC, Kulkin H: Pediatric care for children whose parents are gay or lesbian, *Pediatrics* 97:629, 1996.
12. Tasker F, Golombok S: Adults raised as children in lesbian families, *Am J Orthopsychiatry* 65:203, 1995.
13. US Bureau of the Census Current Population Report: Series P20, No 486, 467, *Statistical Abstract of the U.S.: 1992*, ed 112, 1992, Washington, DC, the Bureau.

SUGGESTED READINGS

Gold MA, et al: Children of gay or lesbian parents, *Pediatr Rev* 15:354, 1994.

Martin A: *The lesbian and gay parenting handbook: creating and raising our families,* New York, 1993, Harper Collins.

Parks CA: Lesbian parenthood: a review of the literature, *Am J Orthopsychiatry* 68:376, 1998.

Tasker FL, Golombok S: *Growing up in a lesbian family: effects on child development*, New York, 1997, The Guilford Press.

NATIONAL ORGANIZATION

Family Pride Coalition (formally known as the Gay and Lesbian Parents Coalition International [GLPCI]), PO Box 34337, San Diego, CA 92163 Telephone: (619) 296-0199. Website: www.familypride.org. This national organization can assist physicians and families in locating local support and information in their own or neighboring communities. It also provides an extensive reference list of books, articles, and videotapes for a nominal fee.

57 Child Abuse and Neglect

Howard Dubowitz • Martin A. Finkel

In 1997, 45 of every 1000 children were reported to child protective services (CPS) nationwide for possible maltreatment, representing more than 3 million children.[25] Between 1988 and 1997 there was a 41% increase in reports. Approximately 10% of the reports investigated by CPS are made by physicians.[24] In community surveys, approximately 3% of parents report using very severe violence (e.g., hitting with fist, burning, using gun or knife) against their child in the prior year.[26] Studies suggest that as many as one in three girls and one in six boys have been sexually abused.[6] Over the past few years, the number of CPS reports nationwide has decreased. This decrease most likely is due to changes in policies regarding how reports are recorded; many states have coded cases as family problems rather than as abuse, creating the appearance of a decrease in the incidence of maltreatment. Furthermore, reported cases reflect only the tip of the iceberg; child abuse and neglect usually occurs behind closed doors and often is not detected.

There can be serious sequelae for maltreated children, ranging from subtle neurological signs to death. In 1997, 1185 children died because of maltreatment.[25] Approximately half the fatalities resulted from neglect, usually children left unsupervised and dying in fires or by drowning. Since 1985, there has been a 34% increase in child fatalities attributable to child maltreatment. In part, this dramatic increase may be attributable to the development of statewide child death review teams and more skilled investigations. The 1997 federal Child Abuse Prevention and Treatment Act (CAPTA) mandates that states review all child deaths. Other effects of maltreatment include cognitive and language delays, poor social skills, diminished self-esteem, aggressive behavior, and serious emotional problems. Preliminary research suggests that abused and neglected children may have impaired brain growth and development. There are many potential negative effects of child maltreatment, which may be long term.

Pediatricians typically enjoy trusting relationships with their patients' families and do not have the stigma often associated with the child welfare and mental health systems. Thus, they are in a position to be knowledgeable about children and their family's situation and their strengths and difficulties and are able to intervene appropriately. They may be the only professionals in contact with preschoolers. Every state has a law mandating pediatricians to report suspected maltreatment to a designated public agency. Failure to do so may lead to legal action or professional censure.

DEFINITIONS

A consensus in defining abuse and neglect has been elusive. However, it generally is agreed that *abuse* refers to acts of commission and *neglect* to acts of omission. Debate surrounds whether potential harm (or endangerment) should be included in the definition, as well as actual harm. The federal model definition (a guideline for states) does include endangerment. Including potential harm allows consideration of consequences that may be uncertain or that may only appear later.

Physical abuse includes severe beatings, shaking, scalding, and an uncommon form of abuse termed *Munchausen by proxy,* wherein a parent induces or feigns illness in a child to attract medical care. Given that corporal punishment is widely accepted in the United States, what is the threshold for defining abuse? One approach is to discourage all hitting (and provide preferable alternatives) and to consider any injury beyond immediate redness of the skin as abuse. In addition, acts of severe violence (e.g., throwing a rock at a child) are abusive even if no injury ensues, because there is significant risk of harm.

Sexual abuse has been defined as "the involvement of dependent, developmentally immature children and adolescents in sexual activities which they do not fully comprehend, to which they are unable to give consent, or that violate the social taboos of family roles."[13] The spectrum of sexually abusive activities that children experience include exposure to sexually explicit materials, oral-genital contact, genital-to-genital contact, and genital-to-anal contact. See Chapter 68, Sexual Abuse of Children.

Child neglect refers to omissions in caregiver obligations to provide adequate child care in the areas of health, education, supervision, physical needs (e.g., clothing, food), and emotional support, with abandonment being the most severe form of neglect. Most state laws exclude cases in which these needs are unmet because of poverty. In many states, the threshold for CPS accepting a report of neglect is very high, requiring actual harm to the child.

An alternative view to focusing on caregiver behavior is to consider the basic needs of children (i.e., adequate food, clothing, shelter, health care, education, and nurturance*); neglect occurs when one of these needs is not met*, whatever the reasons. This broader perspective encompasses the role of caregivers as well as other factors (e.g., lead in the environment, lack of access to health care, costs of medications) that may contribute to the neglect of children. This perspective requires broad strategies in addressing such contributing factors.[5]

Emotional abuse has been difficult to define, impeding its diagnosis and posing problems for intervention. Emotional abuse includes verbal abuse and belittlement and acts that terrorize a child. The manifestations of emotional abuse (e.g., low self-esteem) are frequently not overt or specific to abuse. Although this form of abuse may be extremely harmful to children, CPS seldom becomes involved in these cases. The emotional aspect of all forms of maltreatment may be the most damaging, particularly in the long term.

The 1997 National Committee on the Prevention of Child Abuse's 50-state survey of reported cases found the following distribution of types of maltreatment: neglect 54%, physical abuse 22%, sexual abuse 8%, emotional abuse 4%, and other types 12%.[25]

ETIOLOGY

Child abuse and neglect generally have been understood to result from parental or caregiver acts of commission or acts of omission, respectively. This is a limited and often inaccurate view. There is no single cause of child maltreatment; rather, there are multiple and interacting contributory factors.[18,26] The following are examples of these factors at four different levels. At the *individual* level a child's difficult temperament or a parent's poor impulse control may increase the risk of physical abuse. At the *familial* level, spousal abuse or desertion by a father poses risks for children. Influential *community* factors include stressors such as dangerous neighborhoods or the lack of recreational facilities. There also are broad *societal* factors that may contribute to maltreatment; examples include the broad acceptance of corporal punishment and violence explicitly portrayed in the media.

There are resources that can help protect children against abuse and neglect. These include a parent's recognition of a problem and interest in seeking help; a supportive grandparent; a concerned pediatrician; good, affordable child care; and a federal program to make fathers pay child support. Child abuse and neglect result from the complex interplay among many positive and negative factors. For example, a single mother who has a colicky baby and who recently lost her job is at high risk for maltreatment, but a loving grandmother may be a protective influence. A good understanding of what is contributing to the abuse or neglect, as well as the family's strengths, is key to intervening effectively.

SCREENING (BOX 57-1)

The *review of systems* is a standard part of child health supervision. This screening interview should briefly probe the psychosocial situation of the child and family, including a few questions pertaining to such areas as the parent's feelings about the child, problems with the child and how the parents cope with them, the interspousal relationship, substance abuse, supports and stresses, and recent changes in the family's circumstances. Such questions may be introduced by saying: "I am interested in helping every child to be in a safe environment. It's not easy being a parent. There are some problems lots of families have, so I'm asking everyone these questions." Beginning with questions regarding the use of bicycle helmets and the presence of smoke alarms and smokers in the homes, more sensitive areas can be broached gradually. Many providers may feel uncomfortable probing these areas, but they have enormous implications for the safety of children. Sample questions are as follows:

"Do you sometimes have trouble getting enough food for your family?"
"Do you sometimes find you need to hit or spank (child's name)?"
"Have you talked with (child's name) about preventing sexual abuse ("OK" and "not OK" touching)?"
"Have you felt that you or anyone at home should cut down on their drinking?"
"Is anyone harassing you, making you afraid, or physically hurting you?"

It also is recommended that some of the review of systems be asked directly of the child.

Sample questions include the following:
"How do you get punished?"
"Are you sometimes hungry, and there's no food at home?"
"Is anyone giving you a hard time at home?" If yes, "how so?"

If a response to any of these questions emerges as a "red flag," clarification is needed. In addition to screening for potential problems, strengths (e.g., good family ties and emotional support) also should be explored. In some instances, there should be a referral to appropriate professionals for further evaluation and management.

Direct observation of parent(s) and children and their interaction can reveal useful information about their affect, functioning, and relationship and can provide cues for further evaluation For example, does a parent appear involved in the child's issues? Does the child seem afraid of the parent and reluctant to talk forthrightly? How does the parent discipline the child? Does the relationship between them appear warm and comfortable or tense and hostile?

BOX 57-1

SCREENING FOR CHILD MALTREATMENT

Expanded Review of Systems

Ask *parent* about:
- Coping with child, discipline
- Any concerns about possible abuse
- Possible domestic violence
- Meeting child's basic needs (e.g., health care, food)
- Risk factors for maltreatment (e.g., depression, substance abuse)

Where possible, ask *child* as well about discipline, hunger, other concerns

Direct Observation

Note the behavior of parent(s) and child and their interactions (e.g., interested, warm, hostile, suspicion of substance abuse)

PREVENTION (BOX 57-2)

Even though more than 40 years have elapsed since the "battered child" was first described, most efforts in pediatrics continue to be *after* abuse and neglect have occurred. Greater attention to prevention is needed desperately. Pediatricians can help prevent child maltreatment in a number of ways.[4] Anticipatory guidance during child health supervision visits may be valuable in assisting parents cope with the challenges of raising children. This support can enhance their competence and confidence, diminishing the likelihood of child abuse and neglect. For example, empathy for a parent struggling with difficult child behavior and practical guidance on discipline may prove valuable. Or, referring a family to food benefit programs may help ensure adequate nutrition.

Screening, with an expanded review of systems and direct observations, should alert clinicians to family difficulties that might lead to maltreatment. Effective screening must be followed by careful evaluation and helpful interventions. An array of interventions may be appropriate. More frequent office visits could be scheduled to offer support and counseling. Other key family members could be invited to attend and valuable informal supports encouraged. Practices could arrange parent groups through which problems and solutions are shared. Pediatricians need to recognize their limitations and when other professional intervention is indicated. Knowledge of community resources for referral is essential.

Good health education helps ensure that children receive the care they need. Clear communication, written treatment plans, practical and affordable regimens, and guidance on what to expect and when to seek help should enhance adherence to the recommended treatment and prevent medical neglect. Furthermore, prevention requires addressing the problems that contribute to abuse and neglect such as the lack of supportive resources for families in some communities or the lack of health insurance.

DIAGNOSIS (BOX 57-3)

Pediatricians frequently must decide whether a child's injury is inflicted. To differentiate with some degree of certainty, an understanding of the manifestations of trauma and the context in which maltreatment occurs is essential. Before reaching a conclusion, it is necessary to consider alternative explanations for the injury. A careful evaluation is needed when physical or behavioral signs or symptoms suggest maltreatment. A thorough history, including comprehensive psychosocial information, an examination, and appropriate laboratory and radiological studies are needed. Past medical history may reveal several noninflicted injuries suggestive of poor supervision, injuries that raise suspicions of abuse, or inadequate adherence to medical recommendations. If one is not the child's primary care practitioner, it helps to get that person's impressions of the family.

Just as pediatricians are accustomed to viewing subspecialists as consultants, so should they consider physician experts in child maltreatment, social workers, police officers, and mental health colleagues as consultants. Interdisciplinary evaluation is valuable in determining whether maltreatment has occurred, as well as the needs of the child and family. For example, law enforcement officers or CPS workers who have visited the home may provide useful information on the circumstances surrounding the injury and insight into the functioning of a family. Such information can help assess the likelihood of maltreatment and the risk of further abuse or neglect.

When attempting to find out what has happened to a child, it is important to do so nonjudgmentally and empathically. It may be necessary to control one's outrage at a child's maltreatment. Pediatricians should be nonaccusatory and nonconfrontational. It is the pediatrician's responsibility to consider all available information objectively to explain an injury. Maintaining a position as a concerned, helping professional who has a mandate to protect children will serve the child's and family's interests best. Most maltreated children are not removed from their caregivers; if they are, the placement usually is temporary. Thus, it is important to maintain a constructive relationship with the family, while also following statutory requirements to report suspected maltreatment.

When obtaining a history, it is advisable to interview the parents and the child separately. In a supportive and safe environment, children frequently can explain how their injuries occurred. The physical finding may be nonspecific; therefore, the history is extremely important. A history that does not explain an injury reasonably is key to determining abuse. Caregivers may attempt to avoid providing any history, stating that they did not witness the injury and do not

BOX 57-2

PRACTICAL STEPS FOR PREVENTION OF CHILD MALTREATMENT

- Anticipatory guidance
- Health education
- Screening (as in Box 57-1)
- More frequent office visits
- Involvement of other key family members
- Parent groups
- Facilitation of referrals

BOX 57-3

"RED FLAGS" SUGGESTING INFLICTED INJURY

- Injuries not explained adequately
- A pattern to the bruises
- Bruising in nonambulatory infants
- Multiple injuries in various stages of healing
- Subdural hematoma, retinal hemorrhages, complex skull fractures
- Burns in glove/stocking pattern, "doughnut" burn of buttocks
- Duodenal hematoma, ruptured/lacerated internal organs
- Fractures of the metaphyses, posterior ribs, spinous processes

know how an injury occurred; this may be true. Despite great skill on the part of all involved professionals, how an injury occurred may never be known.

Just as great care must be used when obtaining a history, the physical examination must be comprehensive and meticulous, with detailed and legible documentation. Whenever possible, documentation should be supplemented by photography to create a permanent and objective record of an injury, enabling a second opinion.

Cutaneous Manifestations of Maltreatment

The skin is the first line of protection that absorbs the impact of trauma. The location, age, shape, and pattern of a bruise help determine its cause. Bruises over hard bony surfaces such as the shin and forehead generally are noninflicted (i.e., accidental); in contrast, injuries to soft or padded areas such as the buttocks or cheeks, as well as to the axilla, neck, and groin, are more likely to have been inflicted. Circumferential marks around wrists, ankles, and the neck may result from squeezing, grabbing, or the using of a ligature. These injuries usually are inflicted.

There should be an attempt to date the injury based on its physical appearance and corroborate this information with the history. As blood breaks down, contusions change color, providing a rough guide to the age of the injury. Previous published tables need to be revised.[21] If the bruise is red, it is very likely to be less than a week old. If it is blue, it is likely to have occurred within the past week. If it is yellow or green, the injury is probably more than 24 to 48 hours old. Hence, an explanation for a red bruise caused by an injury that occurred 2 weeks earlier would be very worrisome.[22] However, as these time frames indicate, there is a great deal of overlap in relating the color of a bruise to its duration; thus, color cannot be used in dating bruises with any degree of certainty.

Some injuries have distinct configurations that suggest a hand or implements such as belt buckles, electrical cords, hangers, switches, paddles, or hot metal objects. Injuries that have clearly delineated borders suggest abuse.[12] A pair of bruises on one or both arms strongly suggests that the child was vigorously gripped and squeezed. In one study, 2.2% of infants, not yet walking with support, had evidence of bruising. When bruises are present in infants younger than 9 months of age, abuse should be considered before accepting other explanations.[23]

Clearly, bruises can result from causes other than trauma and abuse. Contusions and erythema can be seen following the cultural practices of "coining" and "cupping" in the treatment of illness.[9] These cultural practices should probably not be considered maltreatment; clearly, the context is quite different. Mongolian spots can be confused with bruises; there should be no tenderness, and their appearance does not change in days. If an underlying bleeding disorder is suspected as the cause of easy bruising, a platelet count, prothrombin time, partial thromboplastin time, and a bleeding time should be obtained. However, the pattern of the bruising and location of the bruises generally are distinctive when caused by abuse as opposed to a coagulopathy. Some children may have a bleeding disorder *and* be abused. Henoch-Schönlein purpura (HSP) is the most common vasculitis seen in young children and may be confused with inflicted trauma. Lacerations seldom result from abuse.

Bite Marks

The oval impression of a pair of crescentic bruises following a bite varies depending on the location, degree of force, and movement of the jaw and victim.[8] A bite by a child younger than approximately 8 years of age who does not have permanent teeth has a distance of less than 1 inch between the canines. Thus, it generally can be determined if a bite was inflicted by a young child or an adult. A forensic odontologist may be consulted to assist in documenting and preserving bite mark evidence. Police photographers are capable of photographing these injuries precisely for their size for later study to identify the person who bit the child.[29] When access to forensic consultation is not readily available, all suspected bite marks should be photographed; a ruler or a known object such as a dime should be included in the photograph for sizing purposes.

Burns

Burns can be challenging to determine their origin. In one study, 86% of 507 burns in children were considered accidental, 6% of suspicious cause, and 8% due to abuse. Burns involving both hands, legs, or arms were more likely to be of concern than single-extremity burns.[2] Burns generally are categorized as flame, scald, electrical, chemical, or thermal. Hot liquids are the most common cause of burns. Scalding burns generally are of two types: immersion and splash. An immersion burn pattern that has a stocking and glove distribution, and burns of the buttocks and perineum with or without the "doughnut" pattern (circle of burned skin from hot water, with the central area spared where child was pressed down against the cooler tub) strongly suggest abuse. Splash patterns are seen most commonly in noninflicted injuries. Liquids naturally flow downward, and as they flow they cool; thus, the most proximal burned area tends to be more severe and broader than the most distal burned area, conferring an "arrowhead" pattern. The depth of a burn is a function of the temperature, exposure time, and thickness of the exposed skin.[15] Water at a temperature of 150° F may cause a second-degree burn in 1.5 seconds, whereas water at 120° F may take 5 minutes.[10] Burns from hot objects such as curling irons, hot plates, radiators, steam irons, metal grids, hot knives, and cigarettes generally are distinct and mirror in configuration the implement that was used. When children accidentally brush against such objects, the burns generally are superficial and not extensive. Second-degree burns must be differentiated from blistering skin disorders that can mimic burns. For example, impetigo may be confused with a cigarette burn. The diameter of a cigarette is 7 to 8 mm; impetiginous lesions tend to vary in size and may exceed the diameter of a cigarette burn.

In the case of hot water burns, concluding whether the injury was inflicted will depend on the history and the pattern of the burn. A scene investigation conducted by specially trained investigators can provide valuable information (e.g., hot water heater temperature setting to determine the likelihood that a child was burned in the manner described), but such investigations are rarely performed.

Skeletal Trauma

Fractures strongly suggestive of inflicted injury in children younger than 2 years of age are classic metaphyseal lesions, posterior rib fractures, and fractures of the scapula, sternum, and spinous processes.[14] These fractures all require substantial force (twisting, rotating, and shearing), which do not occur from minor falls or routine handling of a child. Rib and sternal fractures rarely result from cardiopulmonary resuscitation.[7] These fractures usually are caused by the violent compression and shaking of a young child's thorax.

Clavicular, femoral, supracondylar humeral, and distal extremity fractures in children older than 2 years are most likely noninflicted unless they are multiple or accompanied by other stigmata of abuse. It used to be thought that spiral fractures of the femur in young children were very suspicious for abuse. This still holds for infants who are not yet walking. However, with increasing mobility and running, toddlers can fall with enough rotational force to cause a spiral, femoral fracture. Nevertheless, abuse must be considered.

The differential diagnosis of fractures includes osteogenesis imperfecta, metabolic and nutritional disorders (such as scurvy and rickets), renal osteodystrophy, osteomyelitis, congenital syphilis, and neoplasia. Multiple fractures in various stages of healing should be considered to be child abuse until proven otherwise.[14]

A skeletal survey should be obtained in children younger than age 3 years who have a fracture. If the survey is negative but concern of an occult injury remains, a radionucleotide bone scan is recommended.[20] A scan generally will be positive within 24 to 48 hours after an injury and will remain positive throughout the stage of callous formation. In corroborating the history and the injury, the age of the fracture can be crudely estimated.[14] Soft-tissue swelling generally subsides in 2 to 21 days. Periosteal new bone can be seen as early as 4 days after injury, but up to 21 days later. Loss of definition of the fracture line occurs between 10 and 21 days. Soft callus on a long bone can first be observed 10 days after an injury. Hard callus is evident between 14 and 90 days. Remodeling of bone can continue until epiphyseal closure. These time frames are shorter in infancy and longer when the child's nutritional status is poor or there is a chronic underlying disease. Fractures of flat bones such as the skull cannot be aged.

Central Nervous System Injury

Of all inflicted injuries, those to the central nervous system (CNS) result in the most significant morbidity and mortality.[3] Injury results from direct impact, asphyxia, or shaking (shaken-baby syndrome). The term *inflicted head trauma* is used for this group of CNS injuries. Direct trauma may be the result of punching, slapping, or the child's head being struck against a hard surface. Choking and suffocation result in asphyxial (hypoxic) injury, often with minimal external signs. Shaking can result in a constellation of injuries that are intracranial and intraocular (particularly retinal hemorrhages). A fall from a height of 4 feet or less by children younger than 2 years of age rarely results in a skull fracture. Any skull fracture associated with retinal hemorrhages is very suspicious for abuse. "Raccoon eyes" may be observed in association with subgaleal hematomas following traction on the hair and scalp. Bruises from attempted strangulation may be visible on the neck. The differential diagnosis of an infant presenting with a CNS injury includes noninflicted trauma and spontaneous bleeds of vascular anomalies. Radiographs are best to identify skull fractures. CT scans are best suited for screening CNS injury and for detecting cerebral edema and subarachnoid hemorrhages; an MRI is of greatest value for identifying and dating parenchymal injury and subdural hematomas.

In inflicted head injury, the history commonly related by the caregiver is one of insidious onset of symptoms or that the infant appeared fine before suddenly presenting with severe symptoms (e.g., not breathing). Lucid periods following severe head injuries rarely are seen following noninflicted trauma (e.g., motor vehicle accidents) and are unlikely to be present following severe shaking.[17,28] Severe CNS injury in the absence of a credible account of a major accident must be considered inflicted until proved otherwise. In a study of children younger than 3 years of age in whom the diagnosis of inflicted head trauma was initially missed, 28% were reinjured.[11]

Retinal hemorrhages are a significant marker of inflicted head trauma. Resuscitation and severe noninflicted head trauma rarely result in retinal hemorrhages.[19,27] Direct trauma to the orbital region may result in corneal abrasions, subconjunctival hemorrhages, globe fractures, and orbital edema. Orbital edema and globe fractures may lead to an altering of the visual axis and amblyopia. Anterior chamber injuries such as a hyphema reflect severe direct trauma.[15] Indirect trauma may lead to retinal or vitreous hemorrhages, most commonly the result of "shaken-baby syndrome." Retinal hemorrhages usually resolve within a week or two, whereas vitreous hemorrhages may persist and can help to approximate when the injury occurred.[16] The postmortem examination may demonstrate patterns of posterior orbital hemorrhage and intraorbital optic nerve injury, helping to differentiate noninflicted head injury from shaken baby syndrome. The presence of ocular injury (e.g., optic nerve injury, retinal hemorrhage), CNS injury, and skeletal trauma strongly suggests shaken baby syndrome.

Visceral Injuries

Although only 5% of physically abused children have intraabdominal injuries, 90% of blunt abdominal trauma in children is inflicted. Abdominal trauma is the second most common cause of death in abused children. Children most vulnerable to blunt trauma are those younger than 3 years of age because of the limited protection afforded by their small rib cages, relatively large abdomens, and lax muscle tone. Infants who were crying before the blunt trauma may have swallowed large volumes of air, increasing the potential for intestinal perforation at the time of impact. In blunt trauma to the abdomen, the hollow viscera, liver, pancreas, adrenal gland, kidneys, and mesentery are all vulnerable to injury.

Children who have a ruptured viscus with associated bleeding may present with nonspecific complaints or with signs and symptoms of an acute abdomen. Most children who have sustained intraabdominal trauma do not have external injuries.

When solid viscera are injured, bleeding may result from trauma to the organ or from shearing of the vascular supply. Duodenal hematomas are virtually diagnostic of inflicted blunt trauma in young children, unless they follow bicycle or motor vehicle accidents. Bilious vomiting in the absence of fever or peritoneal irritation suggests a duodenal hematoma.

Laboratory and radiological evaluation can help to define the nature and extent of injury. Liver enzymes and serum amylase help to identify hepatic and pancreatic trauma. An elevated CPK and myoglobin reflect muscular trauma. Acute renal failure in the absence of direct renal trauma may be secondary to myoglobin. Serial hematocrits help determine the degree of blood loss, a urinalysis helps to screen for renal trauma, and testing stool for occult blood screens for bowel trauma. Plain films of the abdomen or a gastrointestinal series of radiographs using water-soluble radiopaque dye are valuable in identifying hollow viscus injury. A computed tomography (CT) scan with both oral and intravenous contrast media is of value in assessing solid visceral injuries. Renal and pancreatic trauma can be assessed readily with ultrasound.

Orofacial Injuries

Injuries to the head, neck, and oral cavity are commonly seen in physically abused children. Fractures of the facial bones and subluxation of the mandible are far less common. In cases of significant trauma, a dentist should be consulted to assist in managing the obvious injuries and detecting the possible subtle injuries such as fractured teeth. Soft-tissue injuries to the upper lip or the frenulum are seen in force feeding but also can occur when a toddler trips with a hard object in his or her mouth. The forceful introduction of sharp objects or hot or caustic liquid into a child's mouth may result in intraoral lacerations or mucosal injury.[1]

Blunt trauma to the ear manifests with subperichrondral hematoma and intracranial injury caused by the rotational acceleration of the head. Noninflicted trauma to the forehead, lower lip, chin, and nose are common in toddlers and should be differentiated from inflicted injuries. A slap to the face also can be emotionally and physically traumatic. Chronic dental neglect may result in multiple caries, eating difficulties, chronic pain, and periodontal infection.

Behavioral Manifestations of Child Maltreatment

Many emotional and behavioral effects have been associated with child maltreatment. These include depression, anger, poor self-esteem, developmental delays, poor cognitive abilities and poor school performance, and aggressive and delinquent behavior. None of these problems is specific to child abuse or neglect. Consequently, pediatricians encountering children who have such problems should consider the *possibility* of maltreatment, but be cautious not to jump to conclusions. Some maltreated children appear to cope well, without apparent behavioral problems. This does not preclude the possibility of problems occurring later on.

Manifestations of Child Neglect

The manifestations of child neglect are varied. For example, infants of depressed mothers who are emotionally unresponsive to their needs might not feel securely attached and may be very anxious in unfamiliar situations. Older children who are neglected emotionally might be sad, withdrawn, and depressed. Inadequate supervision of children and youth may contribute to their risk-taking behavior.

Neglect of physical needs may be quite apparent.[5] Inadequate food might manifest as hunger and poor growth. Inadequate clothing may be obvious when, for example, children lack appropriate clothing for cold weather. Poor hygiene similarly may be overt. Recurrent noninflicted injuries or ingestions suggest that poor supervision may be a factor. Inadequate or delayed health care also may be a problem.

Inadequate education is another form of neglect. This may present as a child who is not enrolled in or attending school, and who is not being home-schooled. The risks of exposure to second-hand smoke, especially for children who have respiratory diseases, can be considered to be neglect (see Chapter 23 [Five], Prevention of Smoking). Similarly, the failure to use bicycle helmets and car seat restraints clearly involves potential harm to children, as does access to a loaded firearm.

REPORTING

State laws mandate pediatricians to report *suspected* child abuse or neglect to the designated public agency. It remains a judgment call whether the level of suspicion transcends the threshold for reporting. A physician does not need to be certain that maltreatment has occurred to make a report; reasonable suspicion is adequate. Consultation from an interdisciplinary team expert in child maltreatment or from CPS may be very helpful in making this decision.

Reporting child maltreatment is never easy (Table 57-1). Parental inadequacy or culpability is at least implicit, and considerable anger may result. Pediatricians should inform families directly of the report, supportively and sympathetically. It can be explained as an effort to clarify the situation and provide help, or as a professional (and legal) responsibility. It is useful to explain what the ensuing process is likely to entail (e.g., a visit from a CPS worker and sometimes, a police officer) and what will *not* happen (e.g., that their child will be removed from their care).

Although CPS traditionally provides services when abuse or neglect has been substantiated, CPS also may have "voluntary" services for supporting a variety of family needs, such as food, shelter, homemaker services, and child care.

LEGAL ISSUES

Whenever a physician is involved in a case of possible abuse or neglect, there is the potential for legal involvement, although only a small percentage of cases is tried in court. It is important to be aware of the nuances of differentiating inflicted from noninflicted injury, to describe the findings, and to interpret them for the court. The astute diagnostician who

Table 57-1 Common Issues for Pediaticians When Faced with a Potential Case of Child Abuse or Neglect

Issue	Considerations
Unsure of the diagnosis	Law requires reporting *suspected* maltreatment All the data should be weighed and the likelihood of maltreatment assessed; consultation should be obtained Terms such as "probable" or "possible" may be used
Discomfort involved confronting parents	One should convey concerns forthrightly and compassionately and avoid being confrontational The goal is to protect the child and help the family
Collaboration with public agencies	One should recognize agencies' resources (e.g., to visit home) and work with them
Prefers to handle the matter alone	This assumes an immense responsibility and liability; better to report to and work with agencies
Neglect is less serious than abuse	Morbidity and mortality caused by neglect are substantial
Cases are so time consuming	Time demands often are unavoidable One needs to adjust practice, as for other complex cases
Reluctant to testify	This is understandable; see references on documentation and legal system Consult with expert colleague in this field The legal system *can* protect children Most cases do *not* require medical testimony

explains the basis for the diagnosis clearly should not feel intimidated by the adversarial court system.

Most physicians provide their opinion in their capacity as the treating physician. This is important because much of what the child tells the physician (i.e., "hearsay") may be admissible in criminal court proceedings as one of the few exceptions to hearsay rules of evidence. A requirement for admissibility of these out-of-court statements is that the patient understands that they are being examined for diagnosis and treatment. A simple explanation of this and documentation in the medical record will help ensure admissibility of a child's statements.

Documentation is crucial to the admissibility of all evidence. Verbal evidence in cases of child abuse may be as important as physical evidence. Both the questions asked and the responses must be recorded verbatim. This allows objective interpretation of the degree of suggestibility and the content of the verbal evidence. Questions preferably should be open-ended (e.g., "Tell me what happened") and not leading (e.g., "Did your dad hurt you?"). A comprehensive and legible record may diminish the need to testify.

Pediatricians may be called to testify before a grand jury, which in many states is a preliminary step to indictment. It is an opportunity for the prosecution alone to present their case. A grand jury indictment implies that there is sufficient evidence to justify a trial, and it determines what charges will be filed. If the case proceeds to trial, most pediatricians who then testify do so to provide details of the medical history and examination findings. The court determines whether the physician can testify as an expert, thus allowing the physician to provide an opinion as to the likelihood of abuse. Frequently, a physician who is an expert in child maltreatment will be asked to interpret the findings for the court.

A subpoena often is the physician's first notice of the need for involvement in the legal system. Different subpoenas are generated on behalf of the state, the child, or the defendant. When a subpoena is received, one should consult with the person who issued the subpoena for help in preparing for trial. Prosecutors and the court generally respect and accommodate the time constraints of physicians.

Any information a physician has should be considered privileged and confidential. Confidential information should be disclosed only when the client or legal guardian consents or a subpoena requires such disclosure. Each state varies as to specific laws concerning confidentiality and reporting responsibility in suspected child abuse and neglect. Physicians need to know their state's statutes regarding confidentiality and reporting. In the pretrial process of "discovery," both the prosecutor and the defense attorney have an opportunity to learn what evidence the other possesses. The defense attorney may contact the examining physician directly to discuss the case as part of discovery. The physician is not legally obligated to comply unless the request is accompanied by a subpoena. During cross examination, failure to have met with the defense attorney if previously requested may be used to demonstrate a lack of objectivity. It is well to note that the defense is responsible for representing the accused; the interests of the child are secondary. This is the essence of the adversarial process.

Lastly, all reporting statutes supersede any ethical duty to protect confidentiality. As long as the physician's statutory obligation to report suspected abuse and neglect is made in good faith, he or she is immune from both civil and criminal liability.

TREATMENT

The specific treatment depends on the specific problems contributing to a child's maltreatment, as well as the consequences. The following are important general principles. Pediatricians are naturally responsible for helping address any medical problem. It usually is helpful to approach problems of neglect by beginning with less intrusive interventions. For example, if an infant's failure to thrive is due to an error in the mixing of the formula, parent education and perhaps a visiting nurse should be the initial strategy. At the same time, ensuring a child's safety is paramount. Therefore, severe failure to thrive requires hospitalization, and if the contributing factors are particularly serious (e.g., a psychotic mother), out-of-home placement may be needed. Thus, in situations in which less intrusive efforts have not succeeded or in which the circumstances of the maltreatment are severe, a report to CPS should be made. Primary care practitioners can be a valuable liaison between the family and the public agencies, and they should make every effort to remain involved after reporting to CPS. Families typically are under great duress following a report, and the involvement of the different professionals and agencies can be very confusing. With more frequent office visits, practitioners can offer support and guidance.

In families in which maltreatment occurs, the parents may need to be nurtured before they are able to nurture their children. Therefore, it is important that a treatment plan consider the needs of the family. The use of informal supports such as family members, neighbors, and friends (e.g., inviting the father or a grandparent to an office visit) should be encouraged. Families also may benefit from other professional interventions (e.g., family therapy), and practitioners can help with referrals.

The importance of concrete needs should not be overlooked. Accessing nutrition programs, obtaining health insurance, and helping with housing can make a valuable difference. The problems contributing to child maltreatment often require long-term professional support and monitoring; there are few "quick fixes."

ADVOCACY

Advocacy should target the factors contributing to child maltreatment. At the *individual* level, explaining to a parent that a "hyper" toddler is behaving normally albeit being a challenge, and the child is "not out to get you" is advocating on behalf of that child. Encouraging a mother to seek help dealing with a violent spouse, saying "you and your life are very important," is advocacy on behalf of someone feeling powerless.

Pediatricians advocate on behalf of *families* when they try to enhance the functioning of families. Encouraging the involvement of fathers in child care, strengthening ties with extended family, and referring for family therapy all are forms of advocacy. Remaining involved after reporting to protective services and helping to ensure the implementation of appropriate interventions is another.

In the *community,* practitioners can be influential advocates for resources for children and families. These may include parenting programs, services for battered women and their children, and recreational facilities. Other efforts might attempt to combat violence in a neighborhood or the sale and use of drugs. Pediatricians have many opportunities to share their special knowledge of children's physical, developmental, and emotional needs. Pediatricians can participate as members of local multidisciplinary child abuse review teams or local or state child death review teams, or as advisors to organizations interested in preventing child abuse. Engaging in such activities provides opportunities to understand better the issues concerning child maltreatment and to help improve the system for securing safe and nurturing environments for children.

Finally, pediatricians can advocate at the *state* and *national* levels for policies and programs that benefit children and families. Such efforts include contacting one's congressperson or supporting effective advocacy groups. Child maltreatment is a complex problem that has no easy solutions. Enough is known, however, that interested professionals can make a difference.

REFERENCES

1. Ambrose JB: Orofacial signs of child abuse and neglect: a dental perspective, *Pediatrician* 16:188, 1989.
2. Andronicus M, et al: Burns: non-accidental burns in children, *Burns* 24:552, 1998.
3. Bonnier C, Nassogne MC, Evard P: Outcome and prognosis of whiplash shaken infant syndrome: late consequences after a symptom-free interval, *Dev Med Child Neurol* 37:973, 1995.
4. Dubowitz H: Pediatrician's role in preventing child maltreatment, *Pediatr Clin North Am* 37:989, 1990.
5. Dubowitz H, editor: *Neglected children: research, practice and policy,* Thousand Oaks, Calif, 1999, Sage Publications.
6. Faller KC: *Understanding child sexual maltreatment,* Newbury Park, Calif, 1990, Sage Publications.
7. Feldman KW, Brewer DK: Child abuse, cardiopulmonary resuscitation and rib fracture, *Pediatrics* 73:339, 1984.
8. Furners J: A general review of bite mark evidence, *Am J Forensic Med Pathol* 2:49, 1981.
9. Gellis S, Feingold M: Cao gio, pseudo-battering in Vietnamese children, *Am J Dis Child* 130:857, 1976.
10. Hobbs CJ: When burns are not accidental, *Arch Dis Child* 61:357, 1986.
11. Jenny C, et al: Analysis of missed cases of abusive head trauma, *JAMA* 281:621, 1999.
12. Johnson CF, Sahuers J: Injury variables in child abuse, *Child Abuse Negl* 9:207, 1985.
13. Kempe CH: Sexual abuse: another hidden pediatric problem, *Pediatrics* 62:382, 1978.
14. Kleinman PK: *Diagnostic imaging of child abuse,* Baltimore, 1998, Mosby.
15. Levin AV: Ocular manifestations of child abuse, *Ophthal Clin North Am* 3:249, 1990.
16. Massicotte SJ, et al: Vitreoretinal traction and perimacular retinal folds in eyes of deliberately traumatized children, *Ophthalmology* 98:1124, 1991.
17. Nashhelesky MB, Dix JD: The time interval between lethal infant shaking and onset of symptoms: a review of the shaken baby syndrome literature, *Am J Forensic Med Pathol* 16:154, 1995.
18. Newberger CM, Newberger EH: The etiology of child abuse. In Ellerstein NS, editor: *Child abuse and neglect: a medical reference,* New York, 1981, John Wiley & Sons.
19. Odum A, et al: Prevalence of retinal hemorrhages in pediatric patients after in-hospital cardiopulmonary resuscitation: a prospective study, *Pediatrics* 99:e3, 1997.
20. Pickett WJ, et al: Comparison of radiologic and radionucleotide skeletal surveys in battered children, *South Med J* 76:207, 1989.
21. Schwartz AJ, Ricci LR: How accurately can bruises be aged in abused children? Literature review and synthesis, *Pediatrics* 97:254, 1996.
22. Stephenson T, Biales Y: Estimation of the age of bruising, *Arch Dis Child* 74:53, 1996.
23. Sugar NF, Taylor JA, Feldan KW: Bruises in infants and toddlers: those who don't cruise rarely bruise, *Arch Pediatr Adolesc Med* 153:399, 1999.
24. US Department of Health and Human Services, US Advisory Board on Child Abuse and Neglect, Third Report: *The continuing child protection emergency: a challenge to the nation,* Washington, DC, 1993.

25. Wang CT, Daro D: *Current trends in child abuse reporting and fatalities: the results of the 1997 Annual Fifty State Survey,* Prevent Child Abuse America, Chicago, 1998.
26. Wauchope BA, Straus MA: Physical punishment and physical abuse of American children. In Straus MA, Gelles RJ, editors: *Physical violence in American families: risk factors and adaptions to violence in 8145 families,* New Brunswick, NJ, 1990, Transaction Publishers.
27. Wilkinson WS, et al: Retinal hemorrhage predicts neurologic injury in the shaken baby syndrome, *Arch Opthalmol* 107:1472, 1989.
28. Willman KY, et al: Restricting the time of injury in fatal inflicted head injuries, *Child Abuse Negl* 21:929, 1997.
29. Wright FD: Photography in bite mark and patterned injury documentation, *J Forensic Sci* 43:877, 1998.

SUGGESTED READINGS

American Medical Association: *Diagnostic and treatment guidelines on child physical abuse and neglect,* Chicago, 1992, AMA.

Cicchetti D, Carlson V, editors: *Child maltreatment,* New York, 1989, Cambridge University Press.

Ludwig S, Kornberg AE, editors: *Child abuse—a medical reference,* New York, 1992, Churchill Livingstone.

Myers JEB: *Legal issues in child abuse and neglect,* Newbury Park, Calif, 1992, Sage Publications.

Reece RM, editor: *Child abuse—medical diagnosis and treatment,* Philadelphia, 1994, Lea & Febiger.

58 Child Custody

Elizabeth Meller Alderman

Child custody arrangements at the time of a divorce have evolved over a long period, being a judicial issue only since the early nineteenth century. Changes in child custody laws reflect the social mores of the times. This chapter reviews the history of child custody statutes, different custody arrangements, and the role of mediation. The pediatrician often is called to court to assess the family and child's situation in determining custody arrangements and, thus, should be familiar with these aspects of family law.

HISTORY

Roman law dictated that the wife and children were under the absolute control of the father. This also was the case in feudal England, British common law, and courts in the United States until the nineteenth century. With the advent of developmental and psychological studies of infants and children that highlighted the importance of the mother-child bond, the concept of *parens patriae,* or judicial consideration of the best interest of the child, became the law. Both parents received equal consideration in cases of child custody.

The "tender years doctrine" subsequently evolved and was first introduced in the United States in the 1900s. This interpretation of the law gave custodial preference to the mother because of the perceived notion that mothers were the best caretakers for young children. The growing women's rights movement also advocated for maternal custody. However, this concept has fallen out of favor in the past 20 years, with laws forbidding discrimination based on gender and because it violates the father's rights. Thus, according to judicial standards, the pendulum has swung back. The best interests of the child now are given the greatest consideration. Current laws and court decisions try to preserve the parenting rights of both parents and provide for their ongoing commitment.

Over the past three decades the total number of children younger than age 18 years involved in a divorce has tripled; 50% of first marriages end in divorce; and 75% of black children in families in which both parents were previously married experience divorce before age 18 years, and this is true for 38% of Americans of European descent.[6] This increased divorce rate has forced the courts, as well as pediatricians and mental health professionals, to evaluate the impact of different custody arrangements on children and adolescents. Additionally, new considerations in awarding child custody have surfaced as lifestyles and the definition of family have changed. In most cases, both parents have joint legal custody, but the primary physical residence is with the mother.[6] However, fathers are now more likely to demand a greater role in the child's life. Issues that may have impeded a parent receiving custody in the past, such as sexual orientation, parental health, psychiatric history, lifestyle, religion, and cohabitation out of wedlock, now are being scrutinized. Grandparents and nonbiological parents also may wish to obtain some degree of custody or visitation privileges.

CUSTODY ARRANGEMENTS

Many different custody or parenting arrangements exist. *Sole custody* had been the traditional settlement in the past and still exists if one parent deserts a family or is judged to be unfit or if the parents cannot agree on what is best for the child. The custodial parent is legally responsible for all major decisions regarding the child.

Split custody, in which each parent assumes custody of one or more of their children, rarely is awarded. This arrangement usually is not made because it is considered to be important to keep children together to provide consistency and mutual support.

Joint custody, which encompasses either joint legal or joint physical custody, is the most common arrangement and occurs in 80% to 90% of all custody arrangements.[3] Joint legal custody is the most popular and allows both parents equal responsibility in important decisions regarding the child's life. One parent is awarded physical custody of the child, with the other receiving liberal visiting privileges. In 80% of the cases, the children's primary residence is with the mother. Joint physical custody provides for the child to live with both parents for significant amounts of time, but not simultaneously.

The majority of states in the United States have enacted joint custody laws.[4] Some states have ordered joint custody as the preferred arrangement; others have the legal assumption of joint custody if agreed upon by both parents. Advocates of joint custody, such as fathers' rights activists and family mediators, believe that children living solely with mothers have less paternal contact and that mothers are overburdened physically and financially if they are the sole caretakers.

Research examining whether joint physical custody is preferable to sole custody has shown mixed results. Joint custody provides the best continuity for the child with both the parents. Parents in joint custody arrangements have better cooperation with former spouses and greater financial resources than those who obtain sole custody.

Joint custody is a more expensive option, as each parent must provide full physical facilities for the child. Joint physical residence is best if parents are cooperative and have minimal conflict. This custody arrangement may be detrimental if conflict over child-rearing and discipline arise and children get caught in the middle.[6] Also, as children grow older, especially during adolescence, their primary residence may need to be reevaluated. At that point, the adolescent's wishes need to be respected.

Most parents demonstrate high satisfaction with joint custody. Success of such an arrangement depends on geographical proximity, valuing the other parent as the child's parent, lack of guilt, and low levels of anger.

Contrary to popular belief, only a small percentage of child custody decisions are made in the courtroom; most cases are settled by attorneys and clients or go to mediation. Those cases that do go to court result from different motivations. A parent may wish to establish the incompetency of the other in a public forum such as the courtroom. Custody of the child may be a way to seek revenge on a former spouse or fulfill a parent's emotional needs after the divorce. From a financial standpoint, the parent providing child support may wish to have full custody to have greater control over the child's life, as well as decreased support payments. In addition, a continued court battle may allow former spouses to maintain a relationship although their marriage has been dissolved. Child custody may become a bargaining chip in a divorce settlement. Unfortunately, some parents use desperate measures, such as allegations of child abuse, to obtain custody of a child. If abuse does exist, it is important for the courts to know of it. However, if it is an unfounded allegation, it will lengthen the proceedings and could cause undue emotional harm to an already fragile family constellation.

In the past decade the legal system has moved away from litigation and toward mediation as a method of resolving child custody disputes. In fact, many states have statutes that mandate mediation as the first step in determining child custody to facilitate communication and conflict resolution and encourage exploration of all alternatives to reach a compromise that is acceptable to both parties. The benefits of mediation are that (1) the needs of both parties are heard, (2) the spouse feels more competent because a third party (lawyer or judge) is not relied on to arrive at a decision, (3) it is less expensive, and (4) the process is shorter. Mediated settlements usually are stable because they have been obtained by consensus rather than mandated from the courts.

Mediation encourages parental cooperation and, thus, better outcomes for children. Usually this increased parental satisfaction translates to better compliance with mediated agreements. Studies have shown that with successful mediation, there is less risk of relitigation and increased communication between parents.[5] Benefits of mediation also include greater involvement with children and greater compliance with visitation by noncustodial parents. In terms of long-term effects, these parents also have more frequent communication during the period following the dispute.

The majority of couples who use mediation are able to reach a mutually acceptable agreement, which usually is joint custody. The key variables that predict successful conflict resolution are commitment, communication, and the experience of the mediator. A situation of great conflict, such as allegations of child abuse or domestic violence, is less likely to be resolved by mediation. Mediation also is not appropriate if a spouse has a serious psychiatric illness or is mentally retarded.

THE ROLE OF THE PEDIATRICIAN

The pediatrician may be asked by the attorney to evaluate the family and by the court to help determine the best custody arrangement. In fact, evaluation by a health or mental health professional is one of the most influential factors considered by judges in disputed child custody cases. There are several considerations in determining the best custody arrangement: health, safety, and welfare of the child; maintenance of a consistent living arrangement; quality of the parent-child relationship; degree to which a parent has been a caretaker; the child's preference; the parent's physical and mental health; styles of parenting and discipline; conflict resolution; and the parent's ability to provide emotional support for the child. Practical factors include location of the child's school, the parent's work schedule and location, parental finances, and availability of social support systems.[1] It is important for the health professional to consider all aspects of a child's life. This should be done by interviewing the child and the parents and observing their interactions. The physician also may need to gather information from the child's school, friends of the family, relatives, and other community organizations with which the family is involved. Medical records also could be very important.

The pediatrician needs to know the exact custody arrangements. As the child's health care provider, the pediatrician must clarify who has the right to medical information regarding the child and who can give consent for medical treatment and who must be informed about the child's medical needs. Also, if there is joint physical custody, both parents must be instructed to coordinate health care regimens for the child.[2]

The pediatrician should reassess custody situations periodically; the child's needs may change as he or she changes physically and developmentally. The physician may need to refer some children and families for psychological support. The pediatrician also can offer developmentally appropriate advice to parents who are helping their child cope with divorce and a new living situation.

REFERENCES

1. American Academy of Child and Adolescent Psychiatry: Practice parameters for child custody evaluation, *J Am Acad Child Adolesc Psychiatry* 36:57S, 1997.
2. American Academy of Pediatrics: The pediatrician's role in helping children and families deal with separation and divorce, *Pediatrics* 97:119, 1994.
3. Binder RL: American Psychiatric Association resource document on controversies in child custody: gay and lesbian parenting, transracial adoptions, joint versus sole custody, and custody gender issues, *J Am Acad Psychiatry Law* 26:267, 1998.
4. Coller DR: Joint custody: research, theory, and policy, *Fam Process* 27: 459, 1988.
5. Dillon PA, Emery RE: Divorce mediation and resolution of child custody disputes: long-term effects, *Am J Orthopsychiatry* 66:131, 1996.

6. Emery RE, Coiro MJ: Divorce: consequences for children, *Pediatr Rev* 16:306, 1995.

SUGGESTED READINGS

American Psychiatric Association Task Force on Clinical Assessment in Child Custody: *Child custody consultation,* American Psychiatric Association, 1400 K Street NW, Washington, DC, 20005, 1988.

Brems C, et al: Assessment of fairness in child custody decisions, *Child Abuse Negl* 19:345, 1995.

Cancian M, Meyer DR: Who gets custody? *Demography* 35:147, 1998.

Emery RE: *Marriage, divorce and children's adjustment,* London, 1988, Sage.

Emery RE: *Renegotiating family relationships: divorce, child custody and mediation*, New York, 1994, Guilford.

Griffith DB: The best interest standard: a comparison of the state's *parens patriae* authority and judicial oversight in best interests determinations for children and incompetent patients, *Issues Law Med* 7:283, 1991.

Hlady LJ, Gunther EJ: Alleged child abuse in custody access disputes, *Child Abuse Negl* 14:591, 1990.

Kappelman MM, Black J: Children of divorce: the pediatrician's responsibility, *Pediatr Ann* 9:50, 1980.

Kunin CC, Ebbesen EB, Konecni VJ: An archival study of decision-making in child custody disputes, *J Clin Psychol* 48:564, 1992.

Wallerstein JS, Kelly JB: *Surviving the breakup: how children and parents cope with divorce,* New York, 1980, Basic Books.

59 Children of Divorce

Michael L. Weitzman

Approximately 1 million children experience divorce in the United States each year.[9] For adults, divorce is second only to the death of a spouse or a parent in terms of its intensity as a stressor and the length of time required to adjust to it.[10] It often produces anger and a sense of failure for parents; conflicted loyalties, guilt, grief, and anxiety for children; and concern on the part of all about whether the children will suffer long-term harm. Most children of divorce experience it, at the least, as a potent transient stress. Many accommodate to their new circumstances successfully, but a substantial percentage suffer long-term negative effects. Many of the problems of these children and their families can be anticipated, prevented, or alleviated by thoughtful and timely intervention.

FAMILY CHANGES PRECIPITATED BY DIVORCE

In most cases, both parents are awarded joint legal custody, but the children's primary physical residence is with their mother in more than 80% of cases.[9] Divorce often has devastating financial consequences for these children and their mothers, and children in postdivorce families are four times as likely to live in poverty compared with children overall. A significant number of divorced mothers have fewer financial and personal resources to direct toward the children, and many take on new employment arrangements. This may result in new child care arrangements for younger children, older children taking care of themselves or siblings for greater parts of the day, and curtailment of certain activities because of expense or parental time constraints.

For nonresidential parents, who most often are fathers, problems range from what to do with children on visiting days to profound concern about the emotional consequences for their children. Some fear that their children will abandon them, some have unrealistic expectations about the kind of relationship they will have with their children, and some believe divorce deprives them of the right to exercise authority and discipline the children. Much public attention has deservedly gone to issues of failed child support, nonresidential fathers who do not visit, and the economic plight of single-parent households. In addition, the importance of long-term paternal involvement in a meaningful and unconflicted relationship with their children cannot be overstated.

Stages of Divorce

The period immediately before and after the separation is referred to as the *acute stage,* characterized by maximal turmoil, and generally lasts up to 2 years. The family then moves into the *transitional stage,* which is characterized by more controlled changes. The final stage is the *postdivorce stage,* when major family restructuring ceases.

During the acute stage, all family members are confronted with disruptions of their expectations, relationships, and support systems. Parents may be depressed, may be preoccupied with personal concerns, and evidence diminished parenting abilities. During this stage, two events appear to be most stressful to most children: learning about the divorce and the actual departure of a parent. The first year after divorce is the year of maximal negative behavior by children and the poorest parenting by parents. The apparent intensity of a child's reaction to this stage, however, does not predict long-term adjustment. Initially, many parents make fewer demands on the children, communicate less effectively, are less affectionate, and have difficulty disciplining children. In a significant minority of divorces, the troubled relationship between parents continues indefinitely. These are the cases in which children have the greatest incidence of postdivorce maladjustment.[1,2,4,7-9]

The *transitional stage* is marked by new undertakings for the single-parent household and more stability than the acute stage. Children must accommodate to their parents' new relationship with each other, to new friends, and often to new romantic partners of one or both parents. During this stage, children often are concerned about the well-being of and their relationship with the nonresidential parent. Visitation patterns tend to have become more stable, whether or not they are acceptable to all parties. The major exception to the general pattern of increased stability is the family in which the parents still are actively in conflict, either informally with each other and the children or formally through the legal system.

In the *postdivorce stage,* relative stability is achieved. The family may still be headed by one parent, or a step-parent may now be present. Remarriage does not convey automatic stability but requires new adjustments as a result of the reawakening of unresolved issues and conflicts and to new roles in the new family.

EFFECTS OF DIVORCE ON CHILDREN

A substantial literature demonstrates small, but detectable negative emotional, cognitive, social, and physical effects, both short-term and long-term, of divorce.

Initial Effects

Initial responses are greatly influenced by the developmental level of the child, the level of parental conflict, and the emotional, cognitive, and economic support available to the child. Preschoolers, ages 2 to 5 years, initially tend to manifest regressive behaviors that can be highly stressful for parents, such as sleep disturbances, temper tantrums, separation anxiety, loss of bowel and bladder control, and increased need for parental attention. School-age children, 5½ to 12 years of age, may experience sadness, grief, or intense anger at one or both parents. School performance and peer relationships may deteriorate, and phobias may emerge among both early and late school-age children. The adolescent of divorcing parents finds himself or herself without the expected home base from which to move away. This may result in insecurity, loneliness, and depression, which may be overtly or covertly expressed in diminished school performance, school failure, truancy, violent and nonviolent criminal behavior, substance use, eating disorders, or sexual promiscuity.

Long-Term Effects

Recent studies reveal long-lasting effects of parental divorce in a significant minority of cases.[1,2,4,7-9] Adults who experienced divorce as children tend to score lower on a variety of indicators of psychological, interpersonal, and socioeconomic well-being. Although the majority of adults who experienced divorce as children appear to do well, as a group overall they have higher rates of depression, job changes, premarital pregnancies, and divorce themselves; this is especially true if they were exposed to prolonged parental conflict, although parental absence and economic declines also have lasting negative effects.

TASKS FOR THE CHILDREN OF DIVORCE

Children of divorce have several specific tasks on which they work simultaneously and with varying degrees of success.[11] Mastery of these tasks is greatly facilitated by support and cooperation of both parents.

Accepting the Divorce's Permanency

This task requires the child to accept the reality of the divorce despite tendencies to deny the dissolution of the family and fears of abandonment. These tendencies and fears may persist, leading to repeated efforts by children to persuade their parents to reconcile, even after one or more has remarried.

Regaining a Sense of Direction

Immediately following a divorce, many children experience emotional and behavioral difficulties, and many seem to lose interest in school, friends, and leisure time activities. Generally, the return to more typical activities for the child takes about 1 year. If this has not occurred within this period, then referral of the child or family for psychotherapy may be indicated. Children who are better adjusted before the marital break-up, those who are not enmeshed in a prolonged battle between the parents, and those who are supported in their efforts to understand their feelings are better able to accomplish this task.

Dealing with Loss and Feelings of Rejection

Departure of a parent through divorce is experienced by children of all ages as a major assault on their self-esteem and sense of security. Children may believe that they are responsible for the divorce, therefore must be "bad," and consequently believe that they are at risk for further abandonment. Older children, appreciating that the departing parent is exercising a choice to leave, often feel anger as well as other negative aspects of grief. This results in a complex interplay of negative emotions and their consequences. Long-term follow-up studies indicate that this important task may never be accomplished by a significant number of individuals who experienced divorce as children.[11]

Forgiving the Parents

This is most often a task for older children. It requires the ability to appreciate the parents' need to separate as being more important than any reason to stay together, including the desires of the children. The child must overcome grief over the loss of the intact family, as well as the anger and resentment generated by the resulting changes in his or her life.

Resolving Issues of Relationship

Divorce often leaves children fearful and unable "... to reach, sustain, and support the personal vision that love, mutual understanding, and constancy are expectable components of human relationships. Perhaps the major developmental task posed by divorce is this: to achieve realistic hope regarding future relationships and the enduring ability to love and be loved."[10] This has been shown to be a difficult task that has not been resolved in a significant number of adults who experienced divorce as children.

CUSTODY

Chapter 58, Child Custody, contains a detailed discussion of the range of custody arrangements and the pediatrician's role in determining what sorts of arrangements are in the child's best interest. If the noncustodial or nonresidential parent has not abandoned the family and wants to remain involved with the children, it is essential that the custodial or residential parent not attempt to sabotage this relationship.

REMARRIAGE

One of the most common outcomes of divorce is remarriage. In many cases, it restores a secure, two-parent environment, and it may provide children with a model of a loving, caring adult relationship. It also has the potential of creating new tensions and stresses. When one parent remarries, the other may fear that the children will abandon him or her for the new step-parent. Many children feel as if they are betraying one parent if they form a close relationship with the other parent's new spouse, and many continue to wish for a parental reunion.

THE PEDIATRICIAN'S ROLE

The pediatrician can help the family anticipate, prevent, or address some of the many problems that frequently accompany divorce. He or she can help families by providing anticipatory guidance, counseling for problems as they arise, and assessing and referring children and family members for more extensive or detailed psychosocial intervention when needed. Parents and courts also may ask that pediatricians offer expert witness testimony when custody is questioned; there are a number of useful and practical review articles on pediatrician's roles.[3,5,6]

If the parents are not otherwise receiving counseling, the pediatrician may offer to meet with one or preferably with both of them to facilitate cooperation regarding child-related issues, such as helping the parents formulate an approach to informing the children about the divorce. Parents should be encouraged to try to avoid placing the child in the difficult position of which parent to believe or side with when the two most significant adults in his or her life have widely differing views. They also should be informed that behind many of their questions, children are asking "Do you still love me and can I trust you?" It should be suggested that parents be "concrete" about the children's future—where they will live, who will care for them, where the nonresidential parent will live, and how often he or she will visit.

Both before and after the divorce children need reassurance that they are not unique in having the feelings they are having and that there is nothing wrong with feeling this way. They also should be encouraged to ask questions and express feelings, and they should be brought to see that it is useless to expend a great amount of energy hoping their parents will be reunited. In addition, the pediatrician can help by encouraging visitation with the nonresidential parent. If a child does not wish to visit, parents should be informed that he or she should not be made to feel guilty, and the offer to visit soon should be extended. Persistent refusals to visit the nonresidential parent may suggest that the child is enmeshed in parental difficulties, siding with the residential parent, or that the residential parent may be using the child to hurt the nonresidential parent. Visits for well-child care and for acute illnesses can be used routinely to screen children's adjustment and to assess the need for further counseling by the primary care practitioner or for referral for individual or family therapy.

REFERENCES

1. Amato P: Life-span adjustment of children to their parents' divorce, *Future Child* 4:143, 1994.
2. Amato P, Keith B: Parental divorce and the well-being of children: a meta-analysis, *Psychol Bull* 110:26, 1991.
3. American Academy of Pediatrics: The pediatrician's role in helping children and families deal with separation and divorce. Committee on Psychosocial Aspects of Child and Family Health, *Pediatrics* 94:119, 1994.
4. Chase-Lansdale P, Cherin A, Kiernan K: The long-term effects of parental divorce on the mental health of young adults: a developmental perspective, *Child Dev* 66:1614, 1995.
5. Emery R: *Renegotiating family relationships: divorce, child custody, and mediation,* New York, 1994, Guilford.
6. Emery R, Coiro M: Divorce: consequences for children, *Pediatr Rev* 16:306, 1995.
7. Emery R, Forehand R: Parental divorce and children's well-being: a focus on resilience. In Haggerty RJ, et al: *Risk and resilience in children,* London, 1994, Cambridge University Press.
8. Fincham F: Child development and marital relations, *Child Dev* 69:543, 1998.
9. Shiono P, Quinn L: Epidemiology of divorce, *Future Child* 4:15, 1994.
10. Wallerstein JS: Children in divorce: stress and developmental tasks. In Garmezy N, Rutter M: *Stress, coping and development in children,* New York, 1983, McGraw-Hill.
11. Zill N, Morrison D, Coiro M: Long-term effects of parental divorce on parent-child relationships, adjustment, and achievement in young adulthood, *J Fam Psychol* 7:91, 1993.

60 Child Care and Early Education Programs

Susan S. Aronson

USE AND TYPES OF SUPPLEMENTAL CARE

By the time 4- to 5-year-old children in the United States are ready to enter school, 80% have received care regularly in a nonmaternal arrangement. Many families use more than one type of care for the same child or for siblings during the same day, for different days, and for different parts of the year.[19] The primary child care arrangements used by employed mothers are shown in Fig. 60-1. Of the 24 million school-age children whose parents are in the work force or are in education programs themselves, only 1.7 million are enrolled in before- and/or after-school arrangements. An estimated 5 million school-age children provide self-care while their parents work or are attending classes.[4,19]

Out-of-home child care facilities are classified as small-family child care homes (six or fewer children in the caregiver's home), large-family child care homes (7 to 12 children in a caregiver's home that has more than one caregiver), and center-based care (child care centers, nursery schools, and other nonresidential group care facilities). Any of these arrangements may be used for part-day, part-week, or seasonal care. The names given to out-of-home child care programs do not define the type of service provided or the professional competence of the staff who work there. Any type of child care may involve safe or hazardous environments. The staff may be loving or neglectful, culturally attuned or incompatible, skilled or incompetent.

Increasing use of nonparental care parallels the rise in labor force participation by mothers of young children. Mothers are working outside the home for the same reasons that men work outside the home: economic gain, personal satisfaction, and societal recognition. The majority of single parents need to work to support their families. Both employed and stay-at-home parents use child care at times when their activities do not lend themselves to keeping their children with them. Although children spend many hours with caregivers other than their parents, the time that employed fathers and mothers spend with their children has not decreased. By reducing their time for personal activities, employed fathers are spending more time with their children and doing more household chores than was the case 20 years ago.[7] Employed married mothers have preserved the time they spend with their children by decreasing personal time despite spending more hours on the job. Nevertheless, mothers carry the primary child care responsibility. In two-parent families in which both parents are employed, 83% of mothers (versus 22% of fathers) say that they are more likely than their parenting partner to take off from work to care for an ill child or to keep a child's medical appointment.[3]

REGULATION, ACCREDITATION, AND QUALITY OF CARE

Many facilities that serve young children are regulated by states through facility licensing and teacher certification. In most states, some facilities are exempt from regulation. Unregulated facilities may include those that have only a few children; have part-day or part-year operations; and are operated by religious organizations or by public schools. Regulatory control varies widely from state to state. The requirements may be stringent or lax. Inspections may be scheduled or unannounced, superficial or highly professional, conducted only on complaint, or done annually or more often. Because of the rapidly increasing number of child care facilities in most communities, inadequate staffing of licensing agencies is common. Regulations set the "floor" for legal operation; voluntary accreditation addresses issues of program quality. Although accreditation is gaining ground, the number of accredited programs still is small. The accreditation process usually requires compliance with regulations, additional self-study, and peer-validation to meet accreditation criteria. Studies of quality in accredited facilities find many deficiencies, but accredited facilities generally are of better quality than those that are not accredited.[14]

The largest national early care and education member organizations involved in accreditation of caregivers and child care facilities are The National Association for the Education of Young Children, The National Association of Family Child Care, The National Child Care Association, and The National School-Age Child Care Alliance. These organizations use standardized assessment tools for accreditation and evaluation of quality in child care. Many researchers use the Early Childhood Environment Rating Scale (ECERS),[11] Infant/Toddler Childhood Environment Rating Scale (ITCERS),[12] and the Family Day Care Rating Scale (FDCRS)[10] developed by Harms and Clifford at the University of North Carolina.

All of the accreditation and evaluation tools emphasize adult-child interactions and arrangement of the facility for learning and social support of the child and family. Most ask the observer to assess health and safety, but the evaluation tools have few items that focus on specific facility hazards and risky health practices. Making useful health and safety observations in child care facilities requires an understanding

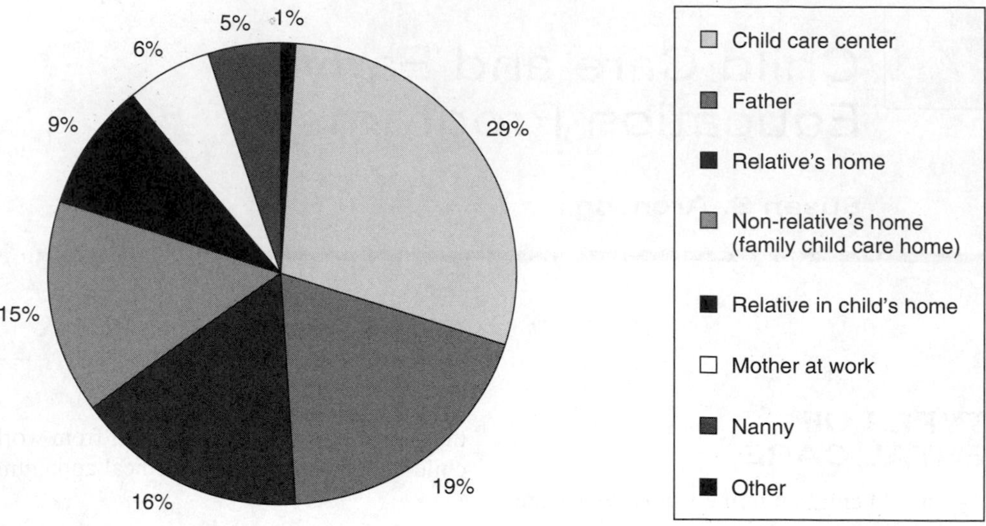

Fig. 60-1 Primary child care arrangement for preschool children whose mothers are employed.

(Data from U.S. Bureau of the Census: Internet update of current population reports, series P70-62. Table A. Primary child care arrangement used for preschoolers by families with employed mothers: selected years, 1977 to 1994. Internet release: January 14, 1998.)

of child care operations, as well as knowledge of and an ability to recognize common hazards and risky practices found in this setting.

Group size and staff:child ratio are related to the quality of care; Table 60-1 shows the recommended limits. Except in small-family child care homes, each group should have at least two caregivers. Because a particular slot in a child care setting might be occupied by different children at different times of day or different days of the week, parents should know the number and ages of children in care at any one time and throughout the duration of their child's stay in child care. One small-family home caregiver (without an assistant) should not care for more than six children, including no more than two children younger than 2 years of age. These numbers include the caregiver's own children younger than 6 years of age. If any child younger than 3 years of age is in care, no more than four children younger than 6 years of age should be in care. If only children younger than 2 years of age are in care, no more than three children, including those of the caregiver, should be in care. In large-family child care homes that have two or more caregivers caring for no more than 12 children, no more than three children younger than 2 years of age should be in care.

In a home setting with only one caregiver, reliable and familiar back-up arrangements should exist for emergencies and times when the caregiver cannot work. Families should check the background of caregivers for reliable references to confirm that the caregiver is mature and experienced in working with young children in situations that have limited supervision.

Young children need consistent caregivers during the day and from day to day. Intimate, familiar, warm, interactive, and trusting relationships are essential for healthy development. In group care, quality of care improves when each child is assigned to a specific caregiver who provides most of that child's daily routines and comforts the child during times of stress. Also, primary caregiver assignments help foster supportive relationships between the child's caregiver and parents. For in-home care, care in a family child care home, or in a center, the relationship between the caregiver and the parent is a complex mixture of important roles: extended family, teacher, and employee.

Table 60-1 Child:Staff Ratio and Group Size

Age	Child:Staff Ratio*	Maximum Group Size
Birth-12 mo	3:1	6
13-30 mo	4:1	8
31-35 mo	5:1	10
3 yr	7:1	14
4 yr	8:1	16
5 yr	8:1	16
6-8 yr	10:1	20
9-12 yr	12:1	24

From American Public Health Association and the American Academy of Pediatrics: *Caring for our children, national health and safety performance standards: guidelines for out-of-home child care programs,* Washington, DC, 1992, the Association.
*When there are mixed age groups in the same room and no infants or toddlers, the child:staff ratio and group size should be consistent with the age of most of the children. When infants or toddlers are in the mixed age group, the child:staff ratio and group size for infants and toddlers should prevail.

The curriculum of an early childhood education and care program should encourage children to be involved in learning. Children need a variety of experiences, including independent and group play, gross and fine motor activities, reading and language development, music, and art. The daily schedule of activities should include going outdoors once or twice a day, alternating quiet and active play, more child-initiated than adult-initiated activities, and planned transitions between activities. TV and video watching should be monitored and limited. Except for older school-age children who are able to move around the community on their own, children always should be under direct adult supervision.

Although research has identified the elements of quality child care and their relationship to child outcomes, recent studies find most care provided in the United States is mediocre to poor. Each situation must be evaluated in terms of how it meets the needs of the child. Although many pediatricians recommend in-home care for infants and toddlers, a national study of child care in home-based settings found more than one third of such programs to be of such low quality that they were likely to harm children's development.[7]

To foster improved health, safety, and quality in child care, the federal Maternal and Child Health Bureau funded state projects to implement the goals of the Healthy Child Care America Campaign (HCCA). Launched in 1995 and staffed nationally by the American Academy of Pediatrics, HCCA has the following goals:

- Safe, healthy child care environments
- Up-to-date routine preventive services for children
- Appropriate care for children who have special health needs
- Health professionals as consultants for medical, mental, nutritional, and oral health in child care
- Health education for families, children, and child care staff

Because few child care programs have a nurse on staff, most seek health and safety advice from public health professionals, from the health providers of children enrolled in the program, or from no one. Generally, child care providers remove hazards and follow safe practices called to their attention, if they have the means. Health consultants for child care must understand the constraints of child care program operations to engage in collaborative, constructive problem solving.

CHILD CARE WORK FORCE

Employed caregivers are mostly females who are better educated than the general population, but who are paid at or below poverty wages and have few or no benefits. Although the amount of preparation varies widely, the average education for child care workers is 2 years of college. College-level preparation for a career in early childhood education focuses on child development and curriculum design and may include some basic facts about child health and safety. Child care work is physically and mentally demanding. With low wages and few benefits, 39% of child care center teachers and 52% of assistant teachers leave their jobs each year. Pay is lower and turnover higher among regulated caregivers who use their own homes as a child care facility. Unregulated providers earn still less, and little is known about them.[14,23]

In addition to traditional academic degrees, caregivers may obtain nationally standardized and validated experience-based credentials as child care teachers and home-based providers. The national organizations of early childhood professionals describe their service as "child care" or "early care and education." Although the terms "day care" and "babysitting" persist, these older terms imply a passive role inconsistent with the intellectual and physical challenges involved in competent care of young children.

Many directors of center-based early care and education programs have a master's degree or higher. In some states, caregivers are not required to have any early childhood training before they start taking care of children. The vast majority of continuing education for caregivers is at entry level. Increasingly, caregiver training articulates with higher education, degree programs in which caregivers become skilled professionals. Career development training for early childhood educators has been shown to improve their competence for work in programs for infants to school-age children and for children who have special needs.[16]

State regulations generally address two types of training requirements for caregivers: preservice training before unsupervised assignment to a given role and ongoing training while employed. The most common type of requirement is for ongoing training in child development and curriculum planning for caregivers. Many states require first-aid training for at least one person in the facility. The majority of states require CPR training, although this requirement makes little sense. Except for children who have specific cardiac problems, and in the event of drowning in cold water, cessation of cardiac function does not occur until respiratory failure causes irreversible and devastating brain damage. Therefore, except when these two situations are likely, caregivers need training in handling minor injuries and respiratory resuscitation for children, not full CPR courses. The training should address the circumstances of an emergency in group care, not just the needs of the injured child.

PSYCHOSOCIAL OUTCOMES

Psychosocial Outcomes for the Child

Data show that exclusive early maternal care is not required for optimum later performance of children. Promotion of exclusive early maternal care in the face of changing cultural norms feeds maternal guilt and fosters public ambivalence about child care as a necessary family support service. The majority of children thrive in a variety of reasonably nurturing child care arrangements.

Both the quality of the child care arrangement and what the family believes about the appropriateness of their child care are strong determinants of the impact of child care arrangements on the child.[7] Data on behavioral and cognitive outcomes for thousands of children assessed in the National Longitudinal Survey of Youth affirm the results of smaller studies: Long-term child development is not affected adversely when mothers of infants and older children work. In fact, for single mothers and low-income families, early parental employment may affect child development positively by increasing family income.[13]

In a comprehensive longitudinal child care study by the National Institutes of Child Health and Human Development (NICHD), researchers assessed children and their child care arrangements at frequent intervals from birth through their elementary school years. During infancy, most used more than one type of care, and most were placed in some type of nonparental care by 4 months of age. Children from the lowest and highest income families received care of better quality than those in the middle. The characteristics of high-quality care that were associated with better developmental outcomes for children were smaller group sizes; lower child-adult ratios; sensitive, responsive, and cognitively stimulating caregivers who allowed children to express their feelings and who took their views into account; and safer, cleaner, more stimulating physical environments. Family characteristics such as family income and the mother's education were much stronger predictors of children's outcomes than the amount of time they spent in child care. Low-income mothers who used full-time higher quality care were more likely to be involved positively with their infants than were low-income mothers who cared for their infants only at home or who used lower-quality full-time care. The behavior of children who spent more hours in care was more of a problem at 2 years of age, but by age 3 years, these children had fewer behavior problems and were more cooperative than those who spent less time in group care.[22]

Psychosocial Outcomes for the Family

Good early care and education programs support families. Early childhood professionals serve as extended families for young parents by addressing everyday questions with the cumulative experience and training involved in this career. In many child care programs, parents and staff exchange information about community resources. Good early childhood programs help identify, care for, and refer to health professionals children who have special needs. By modeling and sharing strategies for healthy development of children, competent caregivers foster parent education and confidence. Because they work with children and families daily, early childhood educators can spot atypical behaviors overlooked by parents and not apparent in brief office visits to physicians.

HEALTH RISKS AND OPPORTUNITIES

Infection, Allergy, and Asthma

Close contact in child care facilitates the spread of many respiratory, gastrointestinal, systemic, and skin infections.[21] The incidence of common respiratory disease is nearly doubled for infants in group care compared with those cared for exclusively at home, but this risk decreases as children grow older or spend more time in group care. Because infectious disease is common in all young children, clinicians should not blame every episode of childhood infection on child care participation. By the time children are 3 years of age, there is little difference in the incidence of infectious disease for children in group care compared with those cared for only at home: 3-year-old children who entered care as infants have fewer common respiratory infections than their peers who were never in group care. Also, child care participation from infancy is associated with an observed reduction in allergy, perhaps related to a reduction in the child's exposure to allergens at home. Other factors play a role, too. For example, one study found that children who use pacifiers in child care have an increased risk of acquiring otitis media compared with those who suck their thumbs.[15,17,23]

Although group care makes work force participation by both parents possible, frequent illness of children in child care is a burden for children, parents, employers, and the community. Many diseases that are transmitted in group care can infect others in the community, including caregivers, parents, and family members. The most important infections transmitted to adult contacts of children in group care are hepatitis A, cytomegalovirus, and parvovirus B19.[24]

The risk of infectious disease in group care can be reduced by keeping immunizations up-to-date, caring for children in age cohorts, and practicing good hygiene. Universal use of hepatitis A vaccine in states where the disease is endemic and administration of universally recommended vaccines can control the spread of diseases in child care. Caregivers must pay particular attention to hand washing, diaper changing, and sanitizing of contact surfaces. As in health facilities, these practices must be taught and monitored continuously or they will be ignored. Everyone in child care should practice hand washing at each contact with a body fluid or a surface that is likely to be heavily contaminated, when moving from one child care group to another, and before food handling. Liquid soap, running water, and dry skin lotion must be close at hand to make such frequent hand washing possible. When plumbing costs make separate and accessible hand washing sinks impractical, portable camp-type sinks should be put into use.

Child care workers need advice about treatment and exclusion of ill adults and children. An infected child does not need to be excluded unless the child cannot participate in activities, requires care that exceeds caregiver resources, or puts the other children at increased risk with continued exposure. Children who have diarrhea must be excluded from ordinary child care until their stools are contained by their diapers or by their ability to use the toilet. Some communities have developed programs to care for ill children whose parents must work, but such programs usually require financial subsidy and should be designed to meet the ill child's need for special care. Guidelines for handling specific types of infections and illness in group care are available from the American Academy of Pediatrics and the American Public Health Association.[2,5]

Injury

Children in child care centers have fewer injuries during their hours at the center than do children who receive care only at home. However, children who use child care centers suffer more injuries during the hours they are at home than do children who are cared for only at home. This suggests that time spent at home may involve less supervision by tired parents or more risk-taking behavior by children making the transition from one environment to another. Children in family child care homes have a higher incidence of injury while in child care than do either children in child care centers or those cared for only in their own homes. Table 60-2

Table 60-2 Injury Rates/100,000 Hours by Type of Child Care

Type of Child Care Setting	Number of Injuries Per 100,000 Hours in Care
Child care center	2.18
Care only in child's own home	2.31
Care in own home (for child who also receives care in child care center)	3.40
Care in family child care home	3.95

From Gunn W, et al: *Am J Dis Child* 145:779, 1991.

summarizes the incidence of injury by type of child care arrangement.[9]

Falls from climbing equipment mounted over surfaces that do not absorb impact are associated with the most common and most severe injuries. Grass, carpeting, packed earth or sand, cement, or asphalt are hazardous. Both indoor and outdoor climbing equipment should be installed over cushioning materials, such as 9 to 12 inches of bark mulch or a manufactured pad rated for the maximum fall height. Play equipment should be designed for the size and developmental abilities of the users. Too often, toddlers and preschoolers use play equipment designed for older children. Because many technical issues are involved in the making of safe playgrounds, their certification by a qualified playground inspector is desirable.

Health Promotion

Child care providers have many opportunities to promote healthy medical, dental, and mental health, as well as sound nutrition. All states have regulatory requirements for immunization of children in specified groups. Child health clinicians should check their state's regulation carefully. The best regulations require immunization of all children in any type of group care, according to the annually updated, national schedule jointly published by the American Academy of Pediatrics, the Centers for Disease Control and Prevention, and the Academy of Family Practice. In addition to up-to-date immunizations, some states require that child care providers document that enrolled children are up to date with all routinely recommended screening tests that identify children who have special needs. These requirements make child care providers natural allies of child health professionals. When children are found lacking preventive health services, or lacking health care insurance, child care providers can refer them to community sources for these services.

Interdisciplinary collaboration between early educators and child health professionals improves the quality of care for all children. Early childhood educators need specific instructions from pediatric practitioners to provide appropriate care for children who have special health care needs. Generally, caregivers prefer to have direct written or verbal instructions from the child's clinician instead of secondhand instructions delivered by parents who may not recall or explain clearly what to do. Early childhood educators and health professionals need to develop effective ways to communicate with each other. Both need parent consent to share information about a child, and both have unpredictable, intense workday demands that make extra paperwork or telephone calls burdensome.

ROLES FOR CHILD HEALTH PROFESSIONALS

Child health professionals can support quality education and care for children by:

- Seeking good care and education for their own children
- Asking and advising families about child care arrangements
- Providing telephone advice and written instructions to caregivers of their patients who have special health care needs
- Offering on-site consultation about decisions related to health and safety policies for children in group care to administrators and staff of programs for early care and education in the community
- Advocating social policies that support quality child care and increase access for all young children and families who need such programs
- Advocating policies and business practices to assist families in caring for their children, such as family medical leave, flex-time, and sick leave to care for an ill child

Paying for Child Care

Families face difficult choices. Some parents can work less and thereby accept reduced income and temporarily limited career opportunities to spend more time with their children. Some couples will work split shifts so that they can share child care between them. Some have relatives who provide good care; others have relatives who constantly disagree with the parents about how to care for their children. Some parents buy low-quality, minimally regulated, unregulated, or illegal care. Some leave their children unattended. Many families find the cost of child care beyond their means.

Although the cost of care varied in 1999, full-day care for one child cost families between $4000 and $10,000 per year, equal to tuition and room and board at a public university. Although the public routinely subsidizes college education, the cost of early childhood education is borne primarily by parents.[1] In 1990, the economics department of the University of Colorado at Denver estimated the full production cost for infant care (if caregivers were paid comparable wages) at $1148 per month, the market cost (fees) at $613 per month, and the net cost to parents after income tax credits at $573 per month.[6] Tax credits favor families that have higher incomes. Even though low caregiver wages subsidize child care fees, many low- to middle-income families spend nearly 25% of their income on child care.

The supply of quality child care is greatest in affluent areas where parents can afford to pay and in urban areas where government subsidies increase supply for those living in poverty. Despite recent increases in federal and state funding of child care associated with welfare reform and support for low-income families, subsidized care is available only to a small percentage of those who are eligible for it. Pressed to fund child care as part of welfare-to-work policies, some states now offer incentives for parents to choose low-cost, low-quality child care.

Helping Parents Make Difficult Choices

Often young parents are too stressed to consider the issues of quality and weigh them against the affordability of child care. Convenience and the cost of care are priorities. In many families, wage earners contrast the cost of child care with the mother's income rather than with the earnings of both parents. Even when parents view the cost of child care as a mutual responsibility, the portion of family income spent on child care can be substantial and still grossly insufficient to purchase good care.

Health professionals can focus parents' attention on issues

related to quality care and help parents make the best choices among their alternatives. From the first contact with the family, the child's health history should include information about who will be involved in the child's care when the child is well and ill. For families who want to provide parent-only care, pediatricians can help explore options such as part-time work for both parents and jobs that permit flex-time and working at home. For those who plan to involve others in their child care, they should ask parents about the caregivers' experience, training, and compatibility of the style of caregiving with that of the family; the child-to-staff ratio; the group size; and observations for hazards at the facility where care will be provided. Beginning with the prenatal visit, questions about child care arrangements should be part of the history-taking routine. When asked to complete a health form for a patient's enrollment or continued participation in a child care program, the child health professional can revisit these issues in greater detail. Before commenting on the child care arrangement, the clinician should find out what options the parent has explored and what the parents have observed about how the child care program actually operates. At subsequent visits, one should ask how the child is responding to the child care arrangement.

Many communities have child care resource and referral agencies (R&Rs), where parents can find out about child care. These agencies help to inform parents about what to look for in a child care facility and try to match available child care to family needs. Some R&Rs keep track of vacancies, size of waiting lists, local sources of subsidy, requirements for providers to operate legally, and many other policy issues related to child care. Some also provide training for child care providers. To determine who inspects, how often, and what they check in community child care facilities, pediatricians should call the local child care licensing agency. The most efficient way to locate a state or local R&R is to call the help line of the National Association for Child Care Resource and Referral: Child Care Aware: 1-800-424-2246.

The Child Health Professional as a Parent

No matter how well educated they are, few parents evaluate their child care arrangements objectively. They tend to deny the presence of evident health and safety hazards, even though they will agree that such hazards are intolerable. With high expectations for job performance, many parents who are professionals suppress doubts about the quality of the care that they arrange for their children. Some health professionals prefer in-home care for their own children because these arrangements provide coverage for irregular and long hours. However, competent caregivers who are well-supervised in the home are rare. Many in-home caregivers are culturally incompatible with the family. Some do not communicate well in the family's language. All need close supervision, which is hard to arrange in the isolated setting of a private home.

Parents who are health professionals have a special responsibility as community role models. They should seek good care and help to improve the care they find. Those who employ in-home caregivers should pay fair wages and benefits. In out-of-home care, parents can contribute materially to improving the facility and as advisors and as trainers.

The Child Health Professional as a Program Consultant

Child health professionals can become involved as paid or volunteer program consultants, as advisors on health problems that have implications for the group. A standard medical liability insurance policy may not provide coverage because no physician-patient relationship exists. Some carriers will issue a letter that amends the standard language to indicate that the policy will cover advising a child care program as part of the insured physician's consultative role.

Before becoming a regular child care health advisor, a pediatrician might visit a child care program during the most active time of day (usually early morning until mid-afternoon) to develop a context for the advice one will give. Important information to note includes how well caregivers manage the needs of the group, often the equivalent of triplets, quadruplets, and more, while nurturing each child. A visit helps the child health professional to see health and safety in context and to offer advice relevant to the program being visited. Learning about any other health professionals who are involved with the child care program facilitates working with them and avoiding unnecessary conflicts. Typical questions child care providers ask physicians are, When should a physician's note be required for return to care? How should we deal with a child who won't stop biting? What can we do to reduce our burden for administering medicine during the day? How do we control outbreaks of lice? Why don't physicians keep children up-to-date with their immunizations? Why do doctors make it so difficult for our program to get information we need to provide good care for children who are their patients? Child care providers are very grateful for thoughtful responses to such questions. If asked about care for an individual child who is not a patient, the consultant should suggest contact with that child's pediatrician.

As a consultant, a child health professional can help plan and provide training for child care providers. Often the children's nap time or evening may be the only time when caregivers can participate in training activities. The primary reference is the national standards for health and safety in out-of-home child care.[2] Information about the standards and material for training is accessible through the Internet web sites of the American Academy of Pediatrics (www.aap.org), the National Association for the Education of Young Children (www.naeyc.org), the National Clearinghouse for the Military Child Development Program (www.dticaw.dtic.mil/milchild), the National Child Care Information Center (www.nccic.org), and the National Resource Center for Health and Safety in Child Care (www.nrc.uchsc.edu).

The Child Health Professional as an Advocate for Quality of Care

Without affordable and accessible early education and child care programs of good quality, children will not come to school eager to learn. Good child care can decrease socially disruptive behaviors and build children's self-esteem and competence. The quality of early childhood programs can be improved by systematic planning to set appropriate requirements, good surveillance systems to measure performance, use of surveillance data to design interventions (technical assistance, training, linkages, resource development), ongoing surveillance to determine whether the interventions improve performance, and allocation of societal resources to these activities. Health professionals can be influential in fostering community actions that support parents and improve options for child care. Improving the quality of care involves the roles of providers, parents, consultants, and advocates.

REFERENCES

1. Adams G, Poersch N: *Key facts about child care and early education: a briefing book,* Washington, DC, 1997, Children's Defense Fund.
2. American Public Health Association and the American Academy of Pediatrics: *Caring for our children, national health and safety performance standards: guidelines for out-of-home child care programs,* Washington, DC, 1992, The Associations.
3. Bond J, Galinsky E, Swanberg J: *The 1997 national study of the changing work force*, New York, 1998, The Families and Work Institute.
4. Child Care Bureau: *Out-of-school time school-age care*. Internet data from the Bureau of the Census. http:\\www.acf.dhhs.gov/programs/ccb/faq/school.htm.
5. Committee on Infectious Diseases of the American Academy of Pediatrics: *Report of the Committee on Infectious Diseases*, ed 24, Elk Grove Village, Ill, 1997, American Academy of Pediatrics.
6. Culkin ML, Helburn S, Morris J: Current price versus full cost: an economic perspective. In Willer B, editor: *Reaching the full cost of quality*, Washington, DC, 1990, National Association for the Education of Young Children.
7. Galinsky E, et al: *The study of children in family child care and relative care: highlights of findings,* New York, 1994, The Families and Work Institute.
8. Galinsky E, Goldsmith J, Hardman R: *Employers, families, and education: promoting family involvement in learning*, New York, 1997, The Families and Work Institute.
9. Gunn W, et al: Injuries and poisonings in out-of-home child care and home care, *Am J Dis Child* 145:779, 1991.
10. Harms T, Clifford R: *Family day care rating scale,* New York, 1989, Teachers College Press.
11. Harms T, Cryer D, Clifford R: *Early childhood environment rating scale,* New York, 1980, Teachers College Press.
12. Harms T, Cryer D, Clifford R: *Infant/toddler environment rating scale,* New York, Teachers College Press, 1990.
13. Harvey E: Short-term and long-term effects of early parental employment on children of the National Longitudinal Survey of Youth, *Dev Psychol* 35:445, 1999.
14. Helburn S, editor: *Cost, quality, and child outcomes in child care centers,* Denver, 1995, University of Colorado at Denver Economics Department.
15. Kramer U, Wjst JH, Wichman HE: Age of entry to day nursery and allergy in later childhood, *Lancet* 353:450, 1999.
16. Morgan G, et al: *Making a career of it: the state of the states report on career development in early care and education,* Boston, 1993, The Center for Career Development in Early Care and Education at Wheelock College.
17. Nafstad P, et al: Day care centers and respiratory health, *Pediatrics* 103:753, 1999.
18. National Center for Education Statistics: *Child care and early education program participation of infants, toddlers, and preschoolers.* Statistics in brief, NCES 95-824, Washington, DC, 1995, US Department of Education, Office of Educational Research and Improvements.
19. National Institute on Out of School Time: *Out-of-school time: school-age care,* fact sheet prepared for the White House Conference on Child Care, October 1997.
20. Niemela M, Uhari M, Mottonen M: A pacifier increases the risk of recurrent acute otitis media in children in day care centers, *Pediatrics* 96:884, 1995.
21. Osterholm M, et al: Infectious diseases and child day care, *Pediatr Infect Dis J* 11:S31, 1992.
22. Peth-Pierce R: *The NICHD Study of Early Child Care*, US Department of Health and Human Services, NIH Pub No 98-4318, April 1998.
23. A profile of the child care work force, *Child Care Bulletin*, issue 16, July/August 1997.
24. Reves R, Pickering L: Impact of child day care on infectious diseases in adults, *Infect Dis Clin North Am* 6:239, 1992.
25. Scarr S, Phillips D, McCartney K: Facts, fantasies and the future of child care in the United States, *Psychol Sci* 1:26, 1990.
26. US Bureau of the Census: *Internet update of current population reports, series P70-62*. Internet release: January 14, 1998. www.census.gov/population/socdemo/child/p70-62/Table A.text.

SUGGESTED READINGS

American Academy of Pediatrics, Committee on Early Childhood, Adoption and Dependent Care: The pediatrician's role in promoting the health of patients in early childhood education and/or child care programs, *Pediatrics* 92:489, 1993.

American Academy of Pediatrics: Part-time care for your child. In *Caring for your baby and young child: birth to age 5*, New York, 1993, Bantam Books.

American Public Health Association and the American Academy of Pediatrics: *Caring for our children, national health and safety performance standards: guidelines for out-of-home child care programs*, Washington, DC, 1992, The Associations.

Chehrazi S, editor: *Psychosocial issues in day care*, Washington, DC, 1990, American Psychiatric Press.

Thacker S, et al: Infectious diseases and injuries in child day care, *J Am Med Assoc* 268:1720, 1992.

61 Domestic Violence and the Family

Peter Sherman

Domestic violence is common in the American family. In addition to negative consequences for the victim, the environment created by domestic violence has profound short- and long-term effects upon the well being of children. Because the pediatric setting may be one of the few places where it is safe for the mother to disclose that she is being battered, it is important that pediatricians screen mothers regarding their exposure to domestic violence, because the immediate safety of a child, exposed to domestic violence, may depend on physician intervention. In addition, a child may need evaluation, referral, or treatment for problems that result from living in an environment in which domestic violence occurs.

Domestic violence can be defined as a pattern of behaviors used by an adult to establish and maintain power and control over another adult. These behaviors, which can occur alone or in combination, sporadically or continually, include physical violence, verbal abuse, psychological abuse, nonconsensual sexual behavior, and economic coercion.[6] It can occur in relationships in which the intimate partner is the same sex as the victim. That the abuser has left the relationship does not necessarily mean that the abuse has stopped.

Nearly one third of women experience battering at least once by an intimate partner during their adulthood.[18] One study revealed the yearly incidence for husbands physically assaulting their wives to be 12%.[15] Women of all ethnic backgrounds are equally vulnerable to attack, though there is an increased risk for women 19 to 29 years of age and those whose annual income is below $10,000.[4] It is estimated that 10 million children are exposed to domestic violence each year.[16]

The impact of domestic violence on the health care system is enormous: 36% of women who go to an emergency department because of violence-related injuries are injured by an intimate partner or ex-partner.[5] Among women who have a current partner who go to an emergency department, one of nine are there as a direct result of domestic violence.[1] Despite this, battering is diagnosed infrequently in a medical setting. The use of clinical protocols can greatly improve identification of victims of domestic violence. In one clinical setting, the use of a protocol increased the identification of battering from 6% to 30% of patients.[13] It is important to have protocols in place and ensure that staff are properly trained in their use. Resources for protocols are listed at the end of this chapter.

IDENTIFYING VICTIMS

Although traditionally the identification of adult victims of domestic violence has not been seen as part of the pediatric assessment, this view has been changing. The American Academy of Pediatrics recommends not only that training concerning domestic violence be incorporated into residency and continuing medical education (CME) programs but also that pediatricians should be capable of intervening when necessary.[2] However, most pediatricians have not received adequate training and may not feel adept at making the diagnosis. One study indicated that only 30% of pediatricians working in an emergency department had received such training, and 64% felt that it was not in the "purview" of pediatrics.[20]

Perpetrators often attempt to maintain complete control over a women's life. A woman may be isolated by the perpetrator limiting access to family, friends, community, and social service agencies. It is common for women to report being locked in an apartment or even restrained. Sometimes the pediatric office visit may be the only instance in which a victim is separated from the abuser and able to disclose her condition safely. The pediatrician needs to take advantage of this window of opportunity and intervene.

Examples of the questions that a clinician can ask are given in Box 61-1. In addition to asking particular questions, it is essential to establish an environment of trust and security by communicating concern nonjudgmentally. Additionally, one should look for signs or symptoms of domestic violence such as bruising, depression, anxiety, failure to keep appointments, reluctance to answer questions about discipline, and frequent office visits for complaints not substantiated by the medical evaluation.[2] It may require several visits for a mother to feel safe enough to discuss her situation; thus, the clinician needs to maintain an index of suspicion, not only at the first visit, but during subsequent visits as well.

Children also can be questioned in a developmentally appropriate manner, though they may be reluctant to talk about what they have seen or heard. Children who have been exposed to domestic violence may be more fearful of interactions with clinicians, and it can require several visits to establish a trusting relationship. This may be especially true with male clinicians, because a child may identify all males as being potentially dangerous.

In addition to information that can be elicited by directly interviewing the child, the pediatrician should be alert to

BOX 61-1

QUESTIONS FOR DETECTING PARTNER VIOLENCE

- Are you in a relationship in which you have been physically hurt or threatened by a partner? Have you ever been in such a relationship?
- Are you (have you ever been) in a relationship in which you felt you were treated badly? In what ways?
- Has your partner ever destroyed things you cared about?
- Has your partner ever threatened or abused your children?
- Has your partner ever forced you to have sex when you didn't want to? Does he ever force you to engage in sex that makes you feel uncomfortable?
- We all fight at home. What happens when you and your partner fight or disagree?
- Do you ever feel afraid of your partner?
- Has your partner ever prevented you from leaving the house, seeing friends, getting a job, or continuing your education?'
- You mentioned that your partner uses drugs/alcohol. How does he act when he is drinking or on drugs? Is he ever verbally or physically abusive?
- Do you have guns in your home? Has your partner ever threatened to use them when he was angry?

From American Medical Association: *Diagnostic and treatment guidelines on domestic violence,* 1994.

nonverbal cues. Although nonspecific, they may indicate possible exposure. Examples are: disruptive behavior, aggression toward others and objects, temper tantrums, somatic complaints, withdrawal, passiveness, clinging, and dependent behavior.[19] If the mother is being examined by the physician, the child may go up to and try to "protect" her or may start crying. Children may demonstrate an excessive fear of strangers. One mother was concerned that her 6-month-old appeared anxious around strangers. The clinician recognized that this was not developmentally appropriate; further interview revealed a history of domestic violence.

ASSISTING THE VICTIM AND HER CHILDREN

The most immediate concern of the pediatrician is the safety of the child and family. Violence directed toward the woman may place the child at increased risk of injury or even death.[14] Though the extent of this problem is not well documented, the Department of Justice found that in a cohort of 84 children younger than 12 years of age murdered by a parent, 6 were the unintended consequence of a lethal conflict between parents.[8] It is important to keep in mind that in homicides in which the perpetrator is known, 28% of female victims are murdered by a current or former intimate partner.[4] Given that a relationship is not identified in nearly 30% of the homicide cases, this number, in fact, may be higher.

It is important to have preexisting protocols to be able to respond immediately to a mother who discloses a history of domestic violence. Community contacts should be identified ahead of time so that the family can be moved quickly into a safe environment. Contacts may include the police, domestic violence shelters, social service agencies, or hotlines. An excellent 24-hour national resource for clinicians and victims is 1-800-799-SAFE. Web sites that contain useful information for the clinician are listed in the resource section at the end of this chapter. In some instances it may be necessary to ensure that office personnel are safe, and this may require working with local law enforcement personnel.

A woman may not be ready or willing to leave an abuser. In this case, once it has been determined that any involved children are safe, one should help the mother create a contingency plan. This should include what to do in case of further episodes of battering—that is, how to contact the police or a local domestic violence hotline. She should also be given resources to contact if she decides to leave at a future date, such as local domestic violence shelter telephone numbers. There are concrete things a mother can be told to do regarding family safety. These include having an emergency bag prepared and placed in a safe location that contains clothing, money, identification, and other important papers; developing a code word for help to use with friends; and teaching children how to call for help safely.[11] It may be necessary to counsel the mother without her children present, to prevent a child from inadvertently communicating to the abuser that the victim is seeking help. Queries should be made regarding firearms that are in the household. The presence of firearms, in these situations, increases the risk of homicide,[10] and they should be removed if this can be done safely. Keep in mind that the highest period for risk of injury or death is when the woman attempts to leave. Finally, if the mother is open to mental health counseling, she and her children should be referred to someone who is adept at working with victims of domestic violence.

There are multiple reasons why a woman who is being battered may choose not to leave. Often the batterer creates an atmosphere of financial and emotional dependence or threatens to harm the woman and her children or take custody of the children. Depression and denial also may be important factors. Though this situation may be frustrating to the clinician, it is much more effective to communicate an understanding for a woman's decision and be available to assist when she is ready and able to leave.

CHILD ABUSE AND DOMESTIC VIOLENCE

Living in a household in which domestic violence occurs places a child at increased risk for abuse (see Chapter 57, Child Abuse and Neglect). One study revealed that a father is five times more likely to abuse his children physically when he frequently assaults his wife (three or more times per year), and children face at least double the risk of being abused physically by a mother who is battered, compared with families in which no physical violence occurs.[15] Thus, it is important to query mothers and children about abuse and complete a thorough, unclothed head-to-toe examination to look for signs of abuse. Any suspected abuse must be reported to the appropriate local child welfare agency. In addition, the child should be referred to a pediatric child abuse center or to a pediatrician who specializes in this area.

A child may be injured or even killed when caught between the batterer and mother. It is crucial that all threats made against a woman and her children be taken seriously and a plan created to minimize the threat. This may involve, in addition to contact with domestic violence shelters or agencies, communicating with law enforcement and child welfare agencies and the court system. If children are in immediate danger and their mother is not willing to leave the batterer, a report needs to be made to the local child welfare agency that a child is living in an unsafe environment. Some states go as far as defining a child's witnessing of domestic violence as maltreatment.[12] However, one should explore other options, prior to removing children, to avoid further victimization of a mother.

ISSUES OF TREATMENT

Children also may manifest medical, developmental, and psychological problems; in some instances these problems may be more prevalent than in the general population. Controlled studies have shown an increase in the following: anxiety, social withdrawal, depression, suicidal ideation, aggressiveness, hyperactivity, conduct problems, reduced social competence, school difficulties, truancy, bullying, clinging behaviors, speech disorders, headaches, bed wetting, disturbed sleep, and failure to thrive.[7]

Witnessing violence can be extremely traumatic[19] and being assaulted can result in a child manifesting characteristics of posttraumatic stress disorder. This may include symptoms such as sleep disturbance, difficulty concentrating, flashbacks, and reenactment of the trauma through play. These may interfere with school, social relationships, and emotional development.[3]

It may be difficult to determine what problems are related directly to a child witnessing domestic violence and those that are a result of the impact that domestic violence has on the functioning of a household, such as maternal depression or not being able to attend to children's needs because the abuser constrains the mother's daily activities. Some mothers are overwhelmed with just trying to survive the relationship emotionally and physically. It is very important to connect a child's condition or behavior directly with the domestic violence because a mother may not be aware or deny the impact that it has had on her children. This is especially true in the case of infants and toddlers, where the mother may think that the child is too young to be cognizant of what is occurring. This awareness can be useful in motivating a mother to leave the batterer.

It is important to obtain a thorough medical, developmental, and psychological history of a child who has lived in a household in which domestic violence occurs, regardless of whether the child has witnessed any such events. Because of barriers to medical care, a child may be behind in basic health care maintenance, such as immunizations, as well as have greater subspecialist referral needs. In addition to any developmental evaluation that may be required, one should have a low threshold for referring for psychological evaluation and treatment. This is particularly important when symptoms persist after physician intervention, in cases in which trauma was particularly violent, and where the parent unrealistically minimizes the impact that domestic violence has had on her children.[9]

One needs to keep in mind that in all studies concerning children who witness domestic violence, substantial proportions of children do not demonstrate any measurable negative effects. Although it is not clear what factors promote resilience in a mother and child, it is important that the clinician support and reinforce positive behaviors. Paying attention to only maladaptive behaviors will underestimate strengths and positive coping mechanisms and can lower self-esteem further.[12]

BREAKING THE CYCLE OF DOMESTIC VIOLENCE

Evidence is substantial that children who witness domestic violence are at increased risk as adults for being battered or becoming a batterer.[17] By identifying children who live in households in which domestic violence occurs, creating safe environments, treating and appropriately referring, and enlisting the strengths of mothers and children, it is hoped that this cycle of violence can be halted.

REFERENCES

1. Abbott J, et al: Domestic violence against women: incidence and prevalence in an emergency department population, *JAMA* 273:1763, 1995.
2. American Academy of Pediatrics Committee on Child Abuse and Neglect: The role of the pediatrician in recognizing and intervening on behalf of abused women, *Pediatrics* 101:1091, 1998.
3. Augustyn M, et al: Silent victims: children who witness violence, *Contemp Pediatr* 12:35, 1995.
4. Bachman R, Saltzman L: Violence against women (NCJ-154348), Washington, DC, 1995, Bureau of Justice Statistics.
5. Bureau of Justice Statistics: Violence related injuries treated in hospital emergency departments (NCJ-156921), Washington, DC. 1997.
6. Burnett LB: Domestic violence. In Conrad SA, editor: *Emergency medicine,* 1998, www.emedicine.com.
7. Campbell JC, Lewandowski LA: Mental and physical health effects of intimate partner violence on women and children, *Psychiatr Clin North Am* 20:353, 1997.
8. Dawson J, Langan P: Murder in families, Washington, DC, 1994, Bureau of Justice Statistics.
9. Groves BM: Witness to violence. In Parker B, Zuckerman B, editors: *Behavioral and developmental pediatrics: a handbook for primary care,* Boston, 1995, Little, Brown.
10. Kellerman AL, et al: Gun ownership as a risk factor for homicide in the home, *N Engl J Med* 329:1084, 1993.
11. Knapp JF, Dowd MD: Family violence: implications for the pediatrician, *Pediatr Rev* 19:316, 1998.
12. Magen RH: In the best interests of battered women: reconceptualizing allegations of failure to protect, *Child Maltreatment* 4:127, 1999.
13. McLeer SV, Anwar R: A study of battered women presenting in an emergency department, *Am J Public Health* 79:65, 1989.
14. Nelson KG: The innocent bystander: the child as the unintended victim of domestic violence involving deadly weapons, *Pediatrics* 73:251, 1984.
15. Straus MA, Gelles RJ: *Physical violence in American families: risk factors and adaptations to violence in 8,145 families,* New Brunswick, NJ, 1990, Transaction Publishers.

16. Straus MA: Children as witnesses to marital violence: a risk factor for lifelong problems among a nationally representative sample of American men and women. In Schwarz DF, editor: *Children and violence, report of the twenty-third Ross roundtable on critical approaches to common pediatric problems*, Columbus, Ohio, 1992, Ross Laboratories.
17. Weinstein N, Bobe C, Mandell D: Opening and closing Pandora's box: discussing sensitive topics with children and their families, Children of Alcoholics Foundation, New York, 1998.
18. Wilt S, Olson S: Prevalence of domestic violence in the United States, *JAMA* 51:77, 1996.
19. Wolfe DA, Korsch B: Witnessing domestic violence during childhood and adolescence: implications for the practicing pediatrician, *Pediatrics* 94:594, 1994.
20. Wright JW, Wright RO, Isaac NE: Response to battered mothers in the pediatric emergency department: a call for an interdisciplinary approach to family violence, *Pediatrics* 99:186, 1997.

RESOURCES

Children's Safety Network: Domestic violence: a directory of protocols for health care providers, Newton, Mass, 1992, Education Development Center.

National Domestic Violence Hotline: 1-800-799-SAFE.

Web Sites

American Bar Association Commission on Domestic Violence: http://www.abanet.org/domviol/home.html.

Domestic Violence Information Center: http://www.feminist.org/other/dv/dvhome.html.

Domestic violence: a practical approach for clinicians: http://www.sfms.org/domestic.html.

Family Violence Prevention Fund: http://www.fvpf.org.

US Department of Justice: http://www.usdoj.gov/vawo.

62 Family Interactions: Children Who Have Unexplained Physical Symptoms

John Sargent

Illness and symptoms are physical, psychological, and social events. The family, as the child's primary social context, is affected significantly by a child's physical condition; in turn, the family affects both the child's physical status and psychological well-being.[12] The family, in collaboration with health care providers, is responsible for managing appropriate treatment and promoting the child's psychosocial adaptation. Because of the importance of the family, the investigation and treatment of unexplained physical symptoms should include examination of the interaction between the family and the child.

CHARACTERISTICS OF FAMILIES THAT HAVE CHILDREN WHO HAVE PSYCHOSOMATIC DISORDERS

Liebman, Minuchin, and Baker[5] and Minuchin et al[7,8] investigated the influence of a child's family in maintaining the symptoms of chronic illness and functional physical symptoms. Their work involved children who had recurrent diabetic ketoacidosis and intractable asthma and adolescents who had anorexia nervosa. They studied the patterns of interaction of these families and identified five specific characteristics of family interaction that typified their daily responses and manner of reacting to the child's physical symptoms: (1) enmeshment, (2) overprotection, (3) rigidity, (4) lack of resolving family conflict, and (5) involvement of the symptomatic child in unresolved parental conflict.

Enmeshment refers to an extremely high degree of involvement and responsiveness among family members. Members are exquisitely sensitive to one another, and minor upsets of one individual may lead to rapid attempts of another to restore calm. Relationships can be overly close to the point that individuation and autonomy are sacrificed. Family members report that they feel for one another and that they know what other family members are thinking. Where parents and infants are concerned, enmeshment is an appropriate and necessary quality. However, as a child grows and develops, more distance in family relationships and independence for the child are required. Pathological enmeshment always entails excessive parental involvement for the child's developmental stage. Enmeshment between parents and child also interferes with the child's development of problem-solving skills, because the parents act rapidly to relieve the child's distress rather than require the child to respond to stressful situations. Family members also accommodate viewpoints of others excessively, even when they disagree. Therefore, family cohesion is based on submerged and denied family conflict rather than on negotiation, compromise, and agreement.

A child who has a chronic illness, such as diabetes, may become angry about the need for medical treatment and dietary discretion. Parents in "adaptive" families learn to allow the child to become upset while continuing to require necessary adherence to the treatment regimen. In the pathologically enmeshed family, the parents become upset when the child attempts to deny his or her disease and need to comply with its treatment regimens, and the parents attempt to rationalize their nonadherence to the restrictions of the illness and its treatment.[1] The parents also may carry out illness management tasks that the child can perform. Finally, one or both parents may become so involved with the ill child that they recognize the symptoms before the child does. In sum, these family responses seriously inhibit the child's acceptance of the illness and autonomy in learning to manage and control his or her body.

The *overprotectiveness* seen in these families refers to an overly high degree of concern of all family members for one another. Although the ill child is the most obviously vulnerable member of the family, all members are perceived as vulnerable and in need of protection. Evidence of distress in any one family member induces protective responses from the rest of the family. The father may be perceived as explosive and in need of calming, the mother as depressed and in need of paternalistic support, and the ill child as sick and weak and in need of care and attention. Immature behavior on the child's part is allowed, and any difficulties that the child might experience at school or with peers lead to pity and excuses from the parents. The parents may try to shield the child from unpleasant events, such as medical procedures, even to the child's physical detriment.

The *rigidity* of these families is demonstrated not only in their attempts to deny family problems and to repeat the same ineffective solutions over and over but also in their desire to maintain fixed relationships among one another, even when development or stress requires change. Each family member states steadfastly that he or she cannot alter how he or she or others behave, regardless of the need for change. A mother will report that she cannot bring her husband to the physician's office or hospital no matter how ill the child is. A father will insist that he cannot assist his wife in following through with illness treatment for their child (e.g., giving insulin injections by himself). The child will state that he cannot help his parents understand his feelings about his chronic illness. These protestations of incompetence persist, thereby increasing the overall family stress and leading to a deterioration in the child's condition and further ineffective family responses, resulting in a circular pattern. These families appear to be in a tenuous balance, with any change seen as highly threatening.

Disagreement and conflict exist in all families. However, in those families in which a member has a psychosomatic disorder, to maintain these rigid patterns of extreme closeness and protectiveness, *conflict is denied and therefore unresolved.* Family members contradict themselves to maintain a facade of agreement, and an immediate consensus develops concerning even small issues of disagreement. If a consensus cannot be achieved immediately, distractions occur that dissipate the conflict, or the disagreeing family members avoid one another until the situation calms. There is an air of chronic tension in the family, which is reinforced by avoidance, denial, or outright capitulation by one member. These unresolved disagreements may involve any aspect of family life; however, the physician should note in particular that the parents do not resolve differences of opinion about the ill child and management of his or her disease.[1]

Finally, when conflict occurs between the parents, the ill child becomes involved in the disagreement, distracting attention to himself or herself and thus reducing the disagreement significantly. The balance of harmony and consensus is then restored. The child often is asked to mediate between the parents; at times he or she sides with one parent against the other; at other times the parents unite (leaving their disagreement) either to protect and nurture the sick child or to attack the child and blame him or her for all family troubles. Chronic marital strife is reinforced as more and more disagreements remain unresolved. Yet, often because of the child's illness or symptoms, neither parent leaves the family. The ill child remains highly vigilant to future family disagreements and experiences, increasing stress as family tension persists. It is precisely at the point of parental disagreement and personal stress that the child becomes symptomatic, requiring medical care and sometimes hospitalization. The cycle then begins again.

Thus, the child's participation in parental conflict reduces physical and psychological distress in the parents but induces symptoms in the labile child. The family's patterns of interaction induce symptoms in the child, while the child's symptoms assist the family in maintaining stability. Minuchin et al[7,8] found that these family characteristics occurred in families who had children who had unexplained (functional) physical symptoms, regardless of the child's primary diagnosis. Although all families engage in enmeshed, protective, and conflict-avoiding interactions, some families engage in these patterns inordinately, even when such patterns are unproductive. This does not mean that the family causes the insulin deficiency of diabetes or the reactive airway diathesis of asthma. The physiological differences in these children are specific vulnerabilities that are affected by the family and other factors to become repeatedly symptomatic. Thus, functional or unexplained symptoms become a circular process, reinforced by the child's vulnerability and the family's characteristic patterns of interaction.

Criticisms of this model have pointed out the lack of consistent data supporting the existence of all of these features in families of children who have unexplained physical symptoms.[2,3] Minuchin's description of the family also has been interpreted as blaming parents for the child's physical difficulties and psychosocial problems. These authors have emphasized that the family does not cause the child's symptoms and that unexplained symptoms in a child often cause significant stress for a family and worsen any interactional difficulties a family might have. Further, many of these family relationship characteristics are noted in families that have children who have other emotional and behavioral difficulties. It may be that these relationship characteristics are prominent in families with poor marital cooperation and a child who has a challenging physical, emotional, or behavioral problem.[9,15] This fact further underscores the importance of being aware that the child's problem is not caused by problematic family interaction. It does highlight, though, that for treatment to be effective, family involvement is essential.[9]

Wood[14,16] has suggested that families who have children who have unexplained physical symptoms have two factors that highlight their situation: (1) biobehavioral reactivity among members, which renders them exquisitely sensitive, physically and emotionally, to one another and (2) poor collaboration among parental figures, leading to marked difficulty dealing with the uncertainty, stress, and confusion associated with persistent unexplained physical symptoms.

IMPLICATIONS FOR THE PEDIATRICIAN

Diagnosis

Assessment of the family, including both parents, is essential in evaluating situations in which a child's illness becomes repeatedly symptomatic at home and yet is controlled easily in the hospital.[11,13] The pediatrician should note how family members behave with one another and should question each member directly about his or her impressions of the causes of the child's frequent symptoms. The pediatrician can suggest to family members that they discuss the problem together and can observe their nonverbal responses when other members are talking. The pediatrician will need to pay attention to the process of family interaction, as well as to the content of their statements.

These families typically are well informed about their child's medical condition, and they understand and carry out treatment. However, they often appear helpless and defeated, relating to the physician in a dependent and demanding fashion. Parental overprotectiveness is common, and the enmeshment within the family is demonstrated as parent and child constantly maintain eye contact, speak for each other, and sit very close together. Therefore, the physician often will find it difficult to develop an interdependent relationship with the child. The father also may be devalued and thus may appear disinterested and unsympathetic. The parents may present differing views of the situation, and when asked to reconcile these different perceptions, they are unable to do so. The child often is immature or pseudomature and frequently clings to one parent. He or she usually has limited peer relationships and is the primary focus of parental attention because of the symptoms. The child's lack of insight and general sense of helplessness often are striking. Finally, both family and symptomatic child readily deny psychological difficulties, and all maintain a strongly somatic orientation.

Pediatric Interventions

The pediatrician's primary goal in these situations is to gain the family's trust and collaboration in the evaluation and with treatment. The physician should not challenge the reality of the child's physical symptoms and should ensure that the appropriate medical evaluation is completed. Results of medical evaluations should be presented clearly and directly and with compassion and support. Through honesty and empathy the pediatrician can enlist the family's trust, accept family difficulties, and create, with family and child involvement, a plan for further assessment and treatment that will foster the child's development.

When caring for a physically symptomatic child, the pediatrician, noting significant parental involvement and protectiveness, can help the parents require more independence from their child. If the physician determines that the parents disagree about how to accomplish this and thus are rendered ineffective, he or she can stress the need for them to act cooperatively. The pediatrician also can ensure that the child is participating in school and in activities with peers. Regular follow-up will be necessary to determine if the parents can cooperate and encourage more maturity from their child and also if that maturity leads to improvements in the child's physical condition.[9] If the child improves, the pediatrician will need to watch for signs of marital distress in the parents. He or she then can discuss with the parents the need to resolve their differences either independently or through psychotherapy. Three principles should guide the pediatrician's efforts: (1) attend first to the physical and psychological difficulties of the ill child before attempting to address stress in the marriage directly; (2) in working with the family, develop and maintain an attitude that places responsibility on them to ensure their child's physical and psychosocial adjustment; and (3) pursue regular follow-up care with the family to ensure that progress is maintained.

Referral for family psychotherapy is indicated in situations in which the ill child demonstrates serious emotional and behavioral immaturity or in which his or her illness is so labile that he or she is hospitalized repeatedly, which leads to school absence, further social isolation, and worsening parental concern.[10,11] Referral also is indicated when the parents are unable to decrease overinvolvement and overprotectiveness with the physician's assistance or to develop and carry out cooperative methods of dealing with the ill child. Before referral, the pediatrician must identify the child's physical condition accurately and outline appropriate medical treatment. All physicians involved in the child's care must agree on the diagnosis, treatment, and recommendation for family therapy. The therapist should be familiar and comfortable with family-oriented treatment of serious physical and emotional disorders in children.[10] In the treatment of these disorders, the physician and family therapist collaborate. The therapist can best be introduced to the family as a professional who will help them manage their child's illness or symptoms more effectively and assist them in reducing the stressful effects of the child's symptoms on both child and family. The physician further can state that psychotherapy is a highly important part of treatment and that without psychotherapy the physician will continue to be ineffective in reducing the symptoms. The family should not perceive the referral for psychotherapy as implying blame for their problems. Rather, it can be described as an opportunity for the family and physician to improve the child's condition. Treatment may be aided by assisting the family in understanding the role and impact of physical illness, medical problems, and medical care within their family throughout its history.[6] Awareness of other family concerns about illness, handicap, and death may free the family to attend to this child and his or her problems more effectively. In addition, attending to the specific developmental, emotional, and physical concerns and needs of the child in question leads to more appropriate treatment and more respectful engagement of the family in the treatment.[4]

Pediatrician-Therapist Collaboration

The pediatrician assists the course of psychotherapy by answering the medical questions of the family directly and by informing the family of the improvements that should be achieved through their work with the therapist. Both professionals will need to support each other's efforts and encourage the family to resolve differences straightforwardly with each of them. The physician should avoid answering psychological questions that the family raises and should inform the family that these issues will need to be addressed with the therapist. This support enables the family to work directly with the therapist and resolve any disagreements they may have with him or her straightforwardly. It also prevents the family from pitting the therapist against the physician during treatment. The therapist, in turn, refers any medical questions the family raises to the physician. During the initial phases of family treatment, the child's medical condition may worsen, and short-term emergencies may develop at stressful points during the psychotherapy. Both the therapist and the physician need to be available to the family at these times. By maintaining a mutually supportive relationship and open communication, the pediatrician and the family therapist can assist each other through difficult phases of treatment. Working together, pediatrician, therapist, and family can improve the child's physical and psychological condition dramatically.

REFERENCES

1. Baker L, et al: Psychosomatic aspects of juvenile diabetes mellitus: a progress report, *Mod Probl Paediatr* 12:332, 1975.
2. Coyne JC, Anderson BJ: The "psychosomatic family" reconsidered. I. Diabetes in context, *J Marital Fam Ther* 14:113, 1988.
3. Coyne JC, Anderson BJ: The "psychosomatic family" reconsidered. II. Recalling a defective model and looking ahead, *J Marital Fam Ther* 15:139, 1989.
4. Friedrich WU: A customized approach to the treatment of anorexia and bulimia: In Mikesell RH, Lusterman DD and McDaniel SH, editors: *Integrating family therapy: handbook of family psychology and systems theory,* Washington, DC, 1995, American Psychological Association.
5. Liebman R, Minuchin S, Baker L: The use of structural family therapy in the treatment of intractable asthma, *Am J Psychiatry* 131:535, 1974.

6. McDaniel SH, Hepworth J, Doherty WJ: Medical family therapy with somatizing patients: the co-creation of therapeutic stories, *Fam Process* 34:349, 1995.
7. Minuchin S, et al: A conceptual model of psychosomatic illness in childhood, *Arch Gen Psychiatry* 32:1031, 1975.
8. Minuchin S, Rosman BL, Baker L: *Psychosomatic families: anorexia nervosa in context,* Cambridge, Mass, 1978, Harvard University Press.
9. Nichols MP, Schwartz RC: *Family therapy: concepts and methods,* ed 4, Boston, 1998, Allyn and Bacon.
10. Sargent J: Physician-family therapist collaboration: children with medical problems, *Fam Syst Med* 3:454, 1985.
11. Sargent J: The family and childhood psychosomatic disorders, *Gen Hosp Psychiatry* 5:41, 1983.
12. Sargent J: The sick child: family complications, *J Behav Develop Pediatr* 4:50, 1983.
13. Sargent J, Liebman R: Childhood chronic illness: issues for psychotherapists, *Community Ment Health J* 21:294, 1985.
14. Wood B: Proximity and hierarchy: orthogonal dimensions of family interconnectedness, *Fam Process* 24:487, 1985.
15. Wood BL: A developmental biopsychosocial approach to the treatment of chronic illness in children and adolescents. In Mikesell RH, Lusterman DD, McDaniel SH, editors: *Integrating family therapy: handbook of family psychology and systems theory,* Washington, DC, 1995, American Psychological Association.
16. Wood BL: Beyond the "psychosomatic family": a biobehavioral family model of pediatric illness, *Fam Process* 32:261, 1993.

63 Family-Centered Care in Pediatric Practice

W. Carl Cooley

CHANGING VIEW OF FAMILIES

Pediatricians, like most physicians, have been taught to watch for deviations from normal and to recognize the occurrence of pathology. Pediatric training concentrates on the abnormal functioning of biological or behavioral systems, etiological identification, and the interventions necessary to correct or ameliorate altered function. This is appropriate, to some degree, for there is much to know, and competence is the first expectation that parents have of their child's pediatrician. However, even with its emphasis on the prevention of disease, pediatric practice should extend beyond pathology to embrace and promote the strengths of individual children and families. Advocating for healthy lifestyles, supporting behaviors that protect children from exploitation or abuse, teaching self-care for children who have chronic conditions, and facilitating the development of self-confidence and self-esteem are important pediatric endeavors.

Most children live in the context of families. Family ecology has been portrayed as a homeostatic system in which the interrelationships among the elements (parents, siblings, extended family) exert complex, but to some degree predictable, tensions on each other. The theory of family systems viewed families like biological systems, seeking balance and equilibrium but disturbed by the stresses introduced when one family member is ill, disabled, or behaviorally disruptive. Although helpful in emphasizing the need to attend to the status of all family members, family systems theory and related therapeutic interventions extend to the family the same focus on pathology that has been overemphasized in our approach to individual patients.

Just as pediatricians should identify and nourish sources of strength and resilience in the individual children for whom they care, they must understand families in the same light. Newer research about families who are stressed by poverty, isolation, or raising a child who has a chronic illness has abandoned hypotheses that assume pathological outcomes. Using open-ended, qualitative methodologies, studies have found that most families use healthy strategies to cope with stress, that the characteristics of resilient families can be identified (Box 63-1) and even taught to other families, and that families often identify different stressors than those predicted by clinicians or researchers.[4,6]

Pediatricians can help families by inquiring about major stressors from the family's perspective, coping strategies the family has used in the past, obstacles to coping or stress reduction, and sources of social support (extended family, friends, place of worship) upon which the family relies. Evidence of poor coping with past crises or the absence of social supports is predictive of low resilience and potential breakdown when multiple stressors accumulate.

DEFINITION OF FAMILY

The family is defined in many ways and has taken many forms in contemporary life. The definition of family that we choose not only determines what we mean by family-centered care but also incorporates the values by which we provide pediatric care. The New Mexico Coalition for Children, Youth, and Families developed the following definition of family*:

> "We all come from families. Families are big, small, extended, nuclear, multi-generational, with one parent, two parents, and grandparents. We live under one roof or many. A family can be as temporary as a few weeks or as permanent as forever. We become part of a family by birth, adoption, marriage, or from a desire for mutual support. As family members, we nurture, protect, and influence each other. Families are dynamic and are cultures unto themselves, with different values and unique ways of realizing dreams. Together our families become the source of our rich cultural heritage and spiritual diversity. Each family has strengths that flow from the individual members and from the family as a unit. Our families create neighborhoods, communities, states, and nations."

(See Chapter 55, Changing American Families.) Families who seek pediatric care usually do so in the pursuit of better health for their children. This may mean for the treatment of a worrisome condition (fever, headache, diarrhea), for a better understanding of confusing symptoms, for advice about behavioral or educational problems, or for the prevention of illness. In most instances, families seek reduction of stress and worry about their child. They want reassurance that they are doing the best they can under the circumstances.

However, each family enters the relationship with a pediatrician having its own personal and cultural history, its own set of perceptions about health and health care, and its own expectations about outcomes. It is unlikely that these characteristics will always be the same as those of the physician or in every way consistent with the physician's perceptions and values. Pediatricians must be able to define families in a way that acknowledges and respects their diversity without subordinating responsibility for the well-being of each child.

*From New Mexico Coalition for Children, Youth, and Families and New Mexico Young Children's Continuum, 1990.

BOX 63-1

THE NINE ASPECTS OF RESILIENT FAMILY PROCESS

1. Balancing illness or other stressors with other family needs
2. Maintaining clear family boundaries
3. Developing communication competence
4. Attributing positive meanings to difficult situations
5. Maintaining family flexibility
6. Maintaining a commitment to the family as a unit
7. Engaging in active coping efforts
8. Maintaining social integration
9. Developing collaborative relationships with professionals

Modified from Patterson JM: *Pediatr Ann* 20:492, 1991.

BOX 63-2

THE KEY ELEMENTS OF FAMILY-CENTERED CARE

- Recognizing that the family is the constant in a child's life, while the service systems and personnel within those systems fluctuate
- Facilitating family/professional collaboration at all levels of health care
- Honoring the racial, ethnic, cultural, and socio-economic diversity of families
- Recognizig family strengths and individuality and respecting different methods of coping with stressors
- Sharing with parents complete and unbiased information on a continuing basis and in a supportive manner
- Encouraging and facilitating family-to-family support and networking
- Understanding and incorporating the developmental needs of infants, children, and adolescents and their families into health care systems
- Implementing comprehensive policies and programs that provide emotional and financial support to meet the needs of families
- Designing accessible health care systems that are flexible, culturally competent, and responsive to family-identified needs

From Johnson BH, Jeppson ES, Redburn L: *Caring for children and families: guidelines for hospitals,* Bethesda, Md, 1992, Association for the Care of Children's Health.

FAMILY-CENTERED CARE

In the late 1970s and early 1980s, the child life movement began fostering new ways of caring for children in hospitals. These new methods involved making the hospital experience less threatening by incorporating age-appropriate activities into the hospital environment. Parents are allowed to "room-in" with sick children and be involved in a child's hospital care. The movement acknowledges and responds to the fears and confusion experienced by hospitalized children.

The evolution of these methods eventually led to the formulation of the Elements of Family Centered Care by the Association for the Care of Children's Health in 1987 (Box 63-2).[5] In the same year, the Surgeon General of the United States published his report on children who have special health care needs, which mandated a commitment to family-centered care.[8] Since then, family-centered practice has become the standard of care among many health, mental health, early intervention, and education professionals. The elements outlined in Box 63-2 provide benchmarks against which pediatricians should measure their own behaviors, the organization of their offices, and the operation of the hospitals in which they practice.

During the 1980s a convergence of consumerism, policy developments, and research led to the formulation of a new relationship between pediatric health care professionals and families. The essence of this new relationship is partnership. When families feel like active participants in their children's care, their sense of competence in providing care increases. Characterized by some as empowerment, the process of building a caring partnership between families and professionals is seen by some as being as important as the outcomes of care.[3] Pediatricians can empower families by involving them as partners rather than as passive recipients of care.[2]

PRIMARY CARE SETTINGS

Translating the Elements of Family Centered Care into day-to-day practice in a primary care setting involves thoughtful planning and self-conscious effort.[3] Every pediatric practice should have a mission statement that is displayed clearly in the waiting area. Each practice should design and implement a method of quality assurance and consumer feedback. This may take the form of consumer satisfaction surveys on a periodic basis or comment forms enclosed with bills or other mailings to patients. Some practices may choose to organize a family council that meets periodically to formulate suggestions for physicians and office staff. Because 15% to 20% of the children in any pediatric practice are affected by chronic conditions, efforts should be made to hear the concerns of specific families who experience the added health care needs of such children.

Families who are new to a primary care practice should be offered an initial visit in which family information is gathered and roles and expectations are made explicit. In this process, parents can define their needs for pediatric care, and the physician can explain his or her interpretation of the primary care physician's role. This meeting offers an opportunity to reconcile differences between a family's expectations and a physician's capacities and practice style. When a child is found to have a chronic illness or disability, an explicit redefinition of roles may be necessary to avoid confusion, for example, about the division of responsibility between specialists and primary care providers, about procedures for communication with schools and other agencies, and about the provision of care coordination or case management services.

Physicians in primary care need to be knowledgeable about resources for families in their communities and states. Current information about eligibility and intake procedures is available from state agencies responsible for special services such as clinics for children who have special health care needs, early intervention services, special education, family support services for children who have disabilities, and Medicaid programs and other entitlements. Physicians should be aware of parent support organizations in their state or region and of the availability of parent-to-parent services that link parents of children who have special needs to one another. Most states now are required to have an accessible resource guide for family services under each state's plan for early intervention services.

THE PEDIATRICIAN AS RELIABLE ALLY FOR FAMILIES

Families who cope successfully with challenges, such as the prolonged hospitalization of a prematurely born infant or the occurrence of a disability in a child, usually have a number of strengths in common. Most important among those strengths is access to social support.[7] Families without social supports not only become socially and emotionally isolated but also fail to access tangible aid such as financial assistance and respite care and informational supports that enhance their self-confidence and mastery over their circumstances. The social supports that families require begin with the informal, natural supports of extended family, friends, and community, and extend when necessary to include the formal supports of professionals and social service agencies.[1]

Families who have strong social support systems usually identify individuals among both their formal and informal networks upon whom they depend as resources. The relationships with these resources may be described as reliable alliances, characterized by mutual respect, mutual trust, common goals and visions, sharing of information, and a shared stake in the outcomes. Although families naturally identify those who are reliable allies within their support systems, pediatricians who aspire to this sort of relationship with families not only will provide more effective care but also will nourish themselves in the process.

REFERENCES

1. Cooley WC: The ecology of support for caregiving families, *J Behav Devel Pediatr* 15:15, 1994.
2. Cooley WC: Pediatric training and family-centered care. In Darling R, Peter M, editors: *Families, physicians, and children with special health care needs: collaborative medical education models,* Boston, 1994, Greenwood Press.
3. Cooley WC, McAllister JW: Putting family-centered care in practice: a response to the adaptive practice model, *J Behav Devel Pediatr* 20:120, 1999.
4. Dunst C, Trivette C, Deal A: *Enabling and empowering families: principles and guidelines for practice,* Cambridge, Mass, 1988, Brookline Books.
5. Johnson BH, Jeppson ES, Redburn L: *Caring for children and families: guidelines for hospitals,* Washington, DC, 1992, Association for the Care of Children's Health.
6. Patterson JM: Family resilience to the challenge of a child's disability, *Pediatr Ann* 20:491, 1991.
7. Singer GHS, Irvin LK: Family caregiving, stress, and support. In Singer GHS, Irvin LK, editors: *Support for caregiving families,* Baltimore, 1989, Paul Brookes.
8. *Surgeon General's report on children with special health care needs,* DHHS Pub No HRS/D/MC87-2, Rockville, Md, 1987, United States Department of Health and Human Services.

SUGGESTED READINGS

Brewer EJ, et al: Family-centered, community-based, coordinated care for children with special health care needs, *Pediatrics* 83:1055, 1989.

Fadiman A: *The spirit catches you and you fall down,* New York, 1997, Noonday Press.

Liptak GS, Revell GM: Community physician's role in the case management of children with chronic illness, *Pediatrics* 84:465, 1989.

Sia CCJ: Medical home and child advocacy in the 1990s, *Pediatrics* 90:419, 1992.

64 Health Needs of Parents

Henry M. Seidel

The health needs of parents, like those of children, are determined by physical, social, and emotional factors. Because pediatric practitioners are basically advocates of the child, they do not, as a rule, view the parent in isolation—that is, as an individual who has needs that may not always include the child as a prime factor. It is essential to the care of the child, however, to understand the differing characteristics of the various groupings possible within a family. For example, given a family of three—mother, father, and child—the various "units" include each of them as individuals, the group of three, and the three dyads—mother-father, mother-child, father-child—a total of seven combinations. Thus, a family of four would have 13 such units. The characteristic of a given unit varies with infinite subtlety, depending on the particular combination and the basis of the interaction in which it may be involved at any given time. Therefore, appropriate care of the child requires an understanding of the parent and that parent's own health needs.

Among the physical, social, and emotional needs of the parent, primary care practitioners are most likely to become involved with the emotional. Within their individual practices and in the broader public arena, pediatricians often have acted as "experts," suggesting "principles" to parents regarding their relationship with their children and their life-styles. Too often there is a sense that there is only one approach to a problem. The variety typical of the human experience seems to be ignored. One effect of this advice in recent decades has been a diminution in the self-confidence of parents, a loss of their ability to resort to common sense, and a consequent breach in their composure and naturalness. In the latter part of the twentieth century, their sense of direction often has been confused by the dizzying impact of the audiovisual media and increasing evidence of disruptions in families.

The care of children might be improved if we, as a society, took greater advantage of the resources inherent in the intelligence, humor, and judgment of parents. To work with and presume to advise parents, pediatricians must seek to exploit these resources, putting aside value judgments and the occasional impulse to "preach." Perhaps their major contribution to the health needs of parents can be to make available an objective listening ear and provide the opportunity to achieve, together, a balanced viewpoint.

Determining the extent to which pediatricians should become involved with the health needs of parents is problematic. For example, should pediatric practitioners take care of the sore throat of a child but not of that child's parent? Is it appropriate, when both are in the office, to send the older person off to another setting at the cost of convenience, dollars, and delay? Much of the response will depend on factors such as the following:

- An objective assessment of one's experience and competency. Much in the primary care of the adult requires a technical sophistication that a pediatrician may not be able to invoke with appropriate confidence.
- The circumstance of the particular family and the individual parent's access to care. The burdens of additional cost or an unreasonable wait for care elsewhere should be alleviated if possible. Often transportation is a problem.
- The equipment and the physical setting available. A vaginal complaint in a parent may require resources not readily available, even in the office of a pediatrician who sees many adolescents.
- The practitioner's concern over the possibility of a malpractice action. The risk is greater if the boundaries of one's specialty are extended.

It is practical to limit involvement to those aspects of parental health that are immediately relevant to the child. There is a gray area, an unspoken constraint on going beyond the limits of one's certified area of competence, the constraint imposed by the generally accepted apportionment of medical responsibilities and economic rewards to the various health care specialties. The practitioner then is left to judge the parent's need and decide accordingly. That judgment is easier in the following instances.

THE ADOLESCENT PARENT

The adolescent parent has needs that require total care from a professional who has a sound perspective on the young. A poignant example is that of the teenage, unmarried mother who elects to raise her child and who sees and treats that child as a "baby doll." The professional can provide a sensitive understanding of the interdependencies of that dyad and a ready availability both to the mother when she needs reassurance about her own self-worth when her baby does not behave perfectly and also to the baby when the mother "acts out" in frustration.

THE ABUSED PARENT OF THE BATTERED CHILD

The origins of child abuse are set most often in the socially disorganized childhood experience of the parent. To end the abuse and preserve the family, the parent must be included within the caring and the curing efforts of the professionals involved. The parent should be "gathered in" rather than "referred out" as much as possible. Fragmentation of service to the individuals concerned, with the consequent requirement of a difficult to achieve, sensitive communication among too many persons, lessens the likelihood of successful treatment.

THE PARENTS OF FIRSTBORNS

Anticipatory guidance is a major responsibility of primary care practitioners and reflects a common need in parents, especially those who are parents for the first time. For example, the emotionally nourishing interdependence of the man-woman dyad before the birth of a child easily may be threatened by the mother's diminishing ability to attend to the care and feeding of the father. Resentment and a strain on the bond between the parents may develop.

THE SICK OR POTENTIALLY SICK PARENT

Many instances arise in which pediatricians can extend care to parents as a result of their involvement with the child. Depression in the parent is a good example. If depression can be described as a feeling of helplessness resulting from a wide gap between one's perception of who one is and who one should be, it is easy to understand the stress imposed by child rearing and the role of the pediatrician in reacting sensitively to parental symptoms.

Although depression is discussed more completely in Chapter 107, Mood Disorders in Children and Adolescents, it is important to note here that the impact of maternal mood on infants and children has been well documented. An infant given to extended periods of distressed crying may provide a clue to stress in a mother who needs attention and counseling. Indeed, a wide range of child behaviors (e.g., breath-holding, failure to thrive, many visits to the doctor for hard to define illness, temper tantrums, disturbed sleep) should prompt an inquiry that includes both parents. If they, individually or together, seem to derive no fun from life or pleasure in the child, express unreasonable guilt, find it difficult to make decisions, are withdrawn and without spontaneity, among many other possible clues, the possibility—indeed the probability—of depression should be considered.

Although the day of the house call is past, it still is possible in the office or clinic (without observing the home) to sense the presence of alcoholism or inappropriate dependency on drugs as a problem within some families. In addition, illness detected in the child should alert one to the possibility of a related condition in the parent. Obviously, for genetically determined diseases, access to genetic counseling and discussions aimed at resolving parental guilt must be sought. In fact, a sensitivity to the potential of parental guilt must be a common denominator in the development of a management plan for all childhood illness. Clinical evidence of physical abnormality in a child should initiate appropriate screening for similar findings in the parent. Obvious environmental and genetic examples are tuberculosis, venereal disease, streptococcal disease, lead poisoning, hearing loss, and glucose-6-phosphate dehydrogenase deficiency. The less obvious circumstance includes increased susceptibility to major psychic disturbance in the relatives of children who have phenylketonuria.

PARENTS INVOLVED IN MARITAL CONFLICT OR DIVORCE

Marital conflict is a major source of "morbidity" among children today. Statistically, nearly one divorce occurs for every two marriages each year. There is, on average, one child per divorce; therefore, divorce is a factor in many children's lives. Moreover, because the median duration of marriage is slightly more than 7 years, most divorces affect young children. The father becomes the noncustodial parent most of the time; however, the tendency in this direction has shifted somewhat. In some current arrangements parents attempt to share the care of the child equally.

We must remember that divorce is a process and not a discrete pathological entity to which psychological disturbances in children can be neatly ascribed. It is in the precursors of divorce or prolonged parental conflict that one finds the psychopathological root in the child and the parents. There are competing priorities for the attention of health professionals, who must walk a fine line, recognizing the priority of the child and the imperative that, in serving that priority, they do not "take sides" with one or the other parent. Although they cannot ignore parental need, they must cooperate in the search for an outcome that provides the optimum nurturance for the child with appropriate support for each parent.

Thus, the responsibility that the pediatric practitioner may have to the health needs of parents often is significant and recurrent. The degree of need and the practitioner's consequent involvement may depend on a judgment based on some of the variables already mentioned and on an assessment of the psychosocial competence of the parents involved. There may, at times, be a competition for loyalties. It is likely that most practitioners choose in favor of the child. In this regard, the practitioner would do well to ponder, for example, the content of subpoenaed testimony in a divorce action when each adult has legal representation but the child has none, particularly with the understanding that due process is not extended fully to children in our society. There is a point, then, when the pediatric practitioner must refer the parent elsewhere for medical assistance and emotional support if for no other reasons than the requirement of technical skills or the priority of child advocacy.

SUGGESTED READINGS

Beardslee WR, McMillan HL: Psychosocial preventive intervention for families with parental mood disorders: strategies for the clinician, *J Dev Behav Pediatr* 14:271, 1993.

Green M: Maternal depression: bad for children's health, *Contemp Pediatr 10:28,* 1993.

Guyer B, et al: Annual summary of vital statistics: 1994, *Pediatrics* 96:1029, 1995.

Miller AR, Barr RG, Eaton WO: Crying and motor behavior of 6-week-old infants and postpartum maternal mood, *Pediatrics* 92:551, 1993.

Zuckerman BS, Beardslee WR: Maternal depression: a concern for pediatricians, *Pediatrics* 79:110, 1987.

65 Homelessness and the Family

Peter Sherman • Irwin Redlener

Although homelessness brings to mind the stereotype of a male panhandling on a street corner, in fact, single women and their children now compromise a significant and increasing proportion of this population. It is increasingly likely that pediatricians will encounter patients in their practice who are experiencing or have experienced homelessness. Knowledge of a patient's past and present housing status is important to clinical care in that homelessness can affect the health and psychological and developmental well-being of a child and can present barriers to accessing needed care.

NUMBERS OF HOMELESS

Although it is well substantiated that homelessness is a major problem for many communities, it is not clear how many individuals are homeless in the United States. Estimates are in the range of 1.7 to 3 million per year, with the number varying according to the definition of homelessness and the methodology used to tabulate individuals.[5,6]

There are several estimates of the number of homeless children and adolescents. The Federal General Accounting Office in 1989 reported that there were 68,000 to 100,000 homeless children in the United States on any given night.[7] According to the U.S. Conference of Mayors, in the 29 cities it surveyed in 1996, families that included children made up 38% of the homeless population.[21] In the same year in New York City, 50% of the homeless population consisted of families.

CAUSES OF HOMELESSNESS

When single-parent families were queried about why they were homeless, 28% related it to housing problems, 20% to economic hardship, 31% to family and/or relationship problems, and 14% to drug use or violence.[23] However, to understand system-wide causes of homelessness, it is necessary to step back and examine its roots in poverty, housing shortages, and the current labor market.

A clear and direct correlation exists between poverty and homelessness. The U.S. Department of Housing and Urban Development (HUD) places those families who have incomes less than 50% of the median family income in their community, are renters, and do not receive federal housing assistance in the category of "worst case housing needs."[22] In the past two decades, there has been a large increase in the number of people falling into this category. Between 1979 and 1990 the number of people living below the federal poverty level increased by 41%. Families and children accounted for more than 50% of that increase.[14] In 1995, 21% percent of children in the United States lived in poverty, compared with 14% of children in 1969. Children of color are the most vulnerable, with 66% of Hispanic and 62% of black children, who live in households headed by a female, falling into this category.[9] The proportion and numbers of homeless families mirror these trends.

Poverty is exacerbated by a lack of affordable housing. Between 1973 and 1993, 2.2 million low-rent units were "lost." At the same time, those requiring low-rent housing increased by 4.7 million. This has resulted in the largest shortage of this category of housing on record.[11] The Section 8 housing program, a federal program that subsidizes rental costs for poor families, is unable to address this housing gap, because of cutbacks in funding. Over the past decade federal spending for housing assistance has decreased 78%.[16] Thus, it is no surprise that only 26% of those eligible for assisted housing receive it.[8]

For those who are working, poverty is fueled by a "service" economy that pays low wages and often provides only part-time work, with few or no benefits. Those earning wages below the poverty line went from 12.6% of workers in 1973 to 23.9% in 1993. The percentage of workers earning less than 75% of the poverty line doubled during this same time period.[4] Even though the minimum wage was raised to $5.15/hour in 1997, full-time employment puts a worker at only 83% of the poverty line for a family of three. In 1995, the share of poor children living in a household headed by a full-time, year-round worker, was 21%, the highest level since these data were first collected in 1975.[12] HUD reported that of the families that have children who fall into the category of "worst case housing needs," more than four out of five have earnings that exceed the equivalent of full-time work at minimum wage.[22]

Most importantly, the number of families headed by single women, the population most vulnerable to poverty and becoming homeless, has soared. In 1996, 68% of children lived with two parents, compared with 85% in 1976. In 1996, 24% of children lived with only their mother. This trend has been fueled by rising divorce rates and births to single mothers.[9]

This overall combination of decreasing income and a scarcity of affordable housing coupled with an increase in the number of families headed by single women has created a virtual epidemic of homeless families in the United States.

IMPACT OF HOMELESSNESS ON CHILDREN'S HEALTH AND DEVELOPMENT

Few studies compare the health of homeless children with housed poor children. Therefore, it is not clear whether there is a significant difference in the health of the two populations. In certain important areas there do appear to be quantifiable differences. When parents were asked to rate the health of their children, 13% of homeless children were reported to be in fair or poor health compared with 3.2% of the general pediatric population and 6.5% of those living in poverty. However, 44% of the problems were clustered in 15% of the children.[13]

One study found several areas of significant difference when comparing housed and homeless children; 3.8% of homeless children had a lead level elevated above 30 μg/dl; this occurred only in 1.7% of housed poor children. Inpatient pediatric admission rates were 11.6/1000 for homeless children and 7.5/1000 for housed poor children; 27% of homeless children had delayed immunization compared with 15% of housed children.[1]

Of particular concern is the nutritional status of homeless children. In one study, when parents were asked if their children received enough food, 21% of the homeless families replied that there was insufficient food 4 days or more in the preceding month, because of a lack of money. This occurred in only 7% of housed poor families. Twenty-three percent of the homeless families reported hunger in their children secondary to insufficient food resources compared with 4% of the housed poor. Fourteen percent of the homeless families stated that they ate in a fast food restaurant or convenience store at least four times per week compared with 4% of housed families. Nine percent of the girls were at less than the fifth percentile for weight for height, which is indicative of failure to thrive, and 12% of the children had weight for height greater than 95%, indicative of obesity.[1] Given the importance of adequate nutrition for development in the infant and young child and the risk factors associated with obesity in later life, these are disturbing findings.

Developmental, educational, and psychological outcomes in homeless children are equally worrisome. Homeless children have a higher rate of developmental delay compared with housed poor children. Fifty-four percent of homeless children had at least one area of delay compared with only 16% of housed poor children in one study.[2] The greatest differences were found in the language and personal/social subscales. One study found significant differences between homeless and housed poor children on receptive vocabulary and visual motor development among preschoolers. Yet only 35% of the homeless children were enrolled in an early intervention program compared with 85% of the housed children.[18] A recent report found that 180,000 homeless preschool children did not attend school because of inadequate funding, lack of transportation to school, state noncompliance with federal laws regarding barriers to school enrollment, and long waiting lists for preschool spaces.[15]

School-age children also are at risk. Homeless children have been found to score significantly lower on the revised Wide Range Achievement Test (WRAT-R), a measure of academic achievement,[19] and lower scores on the revised Wechsler Intelligence Scale for Children (WISC-R), which reflects knowledge gained as the result of experience (see Appendix D, Table D-1).[18] In one study, 41% of homeless mothers reported that their children were failing or doing below average school work compared with 23% of housed poor mothers.[3] Because the differences found are related to a lack of knowledge rather than to innate intelligence, these studies suggest that poor school performance may be due to a disruption in schooling secondary to homelessness rather than to innate differences in intelligence. The exact cause of this, whether due to increased prevalence of illness, depression, or school absence, remains to be elucidated.

Evidence that homeless children may suffer disproportionately from behavioral and psychological problems is persuasive. Using the Children's Depression Inventory, one study found the mean score of homeless children to be 10.3, while that of housed children was 8.3. A score of 9 indicates the need for psychiatric evaluation. Thirty-one percent of a group of homeless children, compared with 9% of housed children, scored at a level indicating the need for further evaluation when tested with the Children's Manifest Anxiety Scale.[3] Homeless preschoolers scored significantly higher on the Child Behavior Checklist compared with a group of housed children.[18] This test reflects anxiety, depression, and acting-out behavior.

Clinical Care Issues

Once a family is identified as homeless, the most important issue is ascertaining that they are living in a safe environment. If not, the family should be assisted with making contacts that will enable them to access a local family homeless shelter system, welfare agency, or charitable institution that can provide temporary housing.

All children need a thorough medical, developmental, and psychological history as well as a physical examination to identify medical conditions that result from lack of access to medical care, preceded homelessness, or current homelessness. Particular attention should be paid to health care maintenance, including immunizations and lead testing, as well as to the diagnosis and treatment of chronic medical conditions. Clinic care that is offered to a child while he or she is homeless should be comprehensive, meeting the criteria of a "medical home." This includes not only primary pediatric care, but access to subspecialty care, developmental and psychological evaluation and treatment, medication and medical devices, case management, and 24-hour, 7-day access through an answering service.[17]

Asthma may be overrepresented in some homeless populations. One study determined that of children living in a homeless shelter system, 29% had been diagnosed previously with asthma, and another 9% had symptoms suggestive of asthma.[12] Children often require aggressive treatment, and parents may need comprehensive education to avoid hospitalization, excessive emergency department use, and school absenteeism for their children. The stress of being homeless can be exacerbated in a child who has asthma not sleeping at night or keeping other family members awake because of coughing.

If a family is living in a "shelter," children may present with frequent acute illnesses as a result of living in close quarters with other families. In treating upper respiratory infection, gastroenteritis, otitis media, and tinea, it is helpful to instruct parents about infection control measures in addition to applying standard treatment regimens. Outbreaks of certain illnesses, such as varicella or hepatitis, may require contacting shelter personnel or the local department of health. Frequent otitides along with difficulty in accessing a child's previous medical records should create a low threshold for referring patients for audiological testing or to ENT. It is important when a parent brings in a child who has an acute illness to use this as an opportunity to perform a thorough medical assessment and initiate treatment and referrals. Follow-up can be problematic for homeless families, and any delay in initiating a comprehensive evaluation and treatment may delay further or prevent needed care.

In addition to referrals that need to be made for developmental assessment or psychological problems found in children, it may be necessary to refer parents for counseling. Parental depression, as a result of homelessness, should be addressed so as to optimize the environment needed for a child's well-being. Some families are homeless because of severe parental mental health problems or substance abuse. In addition to parental referral, one must report to a local child welfare agency any suspicion of child neglect or abuse.

One of the most common reasons for a woman and her children becoming homeless is domestic violence (see Chapter 61, Domestic Violence and the Family). One survey that examined homelessness in several cities found that 22% of families were homeless as a result of domestic violence.[10] Among parents who lived with a spouse or partner, 57% of homeless parents gave domestic violence as their sole reason for homelessness.[10] It is important to query women about this issue. Clinicians should be aware of local resources for battered women so that any necessary referrals can be made.

In addition, children who live in an environment of domestic violence are at increased risk for child abuse. One study revealed that a father is five times more likely to abuse his children physically in cases where he frequently assaults his wife (three or more times per year), and children face at least double the risk of being physically abused by a mother who is battered, compared with families where there is no physical violence.[20] Children need to be carefully evaluated for abuse and a report made to a local child welfare agency if child abuse is suspected.

When a family is moving out of a shelter into permanent housing, they often will need assistance in locating medical care in their new community. This involves helping to identify a new medical home and transferring medical records to the new practitioner.

Chronic medical conditions often are not treated properly because a family's mobility results in being cared for by multiple providers. This leads to both over-referral and undertreatment. A child may be referred multiple times to specialists for the same problem, with a diagnostic workup being restarted with each referral. Because of this delay, one often never reaches the point of implementing an adequate treatment plan. It is useful to provide education about these issues while the patient is homeless to allow for the orderly transfer of medical care when the family enters permanent housing.

Long-Term Effects of Homelessness On Women and Children

It is not clear whether the experience of homelessness, in itself, has long-term effects on the health of a child. Although differences in the psychological and developmental characteristics of homeless children compared with housed poor children have been identified, it is not clear whether this is the result of events that occurred prior to or with homelessness.

Although the long-term effects of homelessness on children are not established, it is prudent to provide needed educational, medical, and psychological services to limit the damaging effects of homelessness on children as well as to prevent long-term sequelae that may increase a child's risk for becoming a homeless adult. Many homeless families demonstrate an enormous amount of strength and resilience under adverse conditions. It is as equally important that a clinician, in addition to identifying problems, reinforce these qualities that are crucial to helping a family get through the crisis of being homeless.

REFERENCES

1. Alperstein G, Rappaport C, Flanigan JM: Health problems of homeless children in New York City, *Am J Public Health* 78:1232, 1988.
2. Bassuk EL, Rosenberg L: Psychosocial characteristics of homeless children and children with homes, *Pediatrics* 85:257, 1990.
3. Bassuk EL, Rosenberg L: Why does family homelessness occur? A case-control study, *Am J Public Health* 78:783, 1988.
4. Bristow H: Why the road off the street is not paved with jobs. In Baumohl J, editor: *Homelessness in America,* Phoenix, 1996, Oryx Press.
5. Children's Defense Fund: *The state of America's children: yearbook 1994,* Washington, DC, 1994, Children's Defense Fund.
6. Children's Defense Fund: *The state of America's children: yearbook 1997,* Washington, DC, 1997, Children's Defense Fund.
7. Committee on Community Health Services: Health needs of homeless children and their families, *Pediatrics* 98:789, 1996.
8. Dolbeare CN: Housing policy: a general consideration. In Baumohl J, editor: *Homelessness in America*, Phoenix, Ariz, 1996, Oryx Press.
9. Federal Interagency Forum on Child and Family Statistics: *America's children: key national indicators of well-being,* Washington, DC, 1997, US Government Printing Office.
10. Homes for the Homeless: *Ten cities, a snapshot of family homelessness across America,* New York, 1998, The Institute for Children and Poverty.
11. Lazere E: *In short supply: the growing affordable housing gap,* Washington, DC, 1995, Center on Budget Policy and Priorities.
12. McLean D: Asthma in homeless children, unpublished manuscript, 1999.
13. Miller DS, Lin E: Children in sheltered homeless families: reported health status and use of health services, *Pediatrics* 81:668, 1988.
14. National Coalition for the Homeless: *Homeless families with children,* NCH Fact Sheet #7. www.nch.ari.net, June 1999.
15. National Law Center on Homelessness and Poverty: *Blocks to their future: a report on the barriers to preschool education for homeless children,* Washington, DC, September 1997.
16. Nunez R: *Hopes dreams & promises: the future of homeless children in America,* New York, 1994, Institute for Children and Poverty.
17. Redlener I, Redlener K: System-based mobile primary pediatric care for homeless children: the anatomy of a working program, *Bull New York Acad Med* 71:49, 1994.
18. Rescorla L, Parker R, Stolley P: Ability, achievement, and adjustment in homeless children, *Am J Orthopsychiatry* 61:210, 1991.
19. Rubin DH, et al: Cognitive and academic functioning of homeless children compared with housed children, *Pediatrics* 97:289, 1996.

20. Straus MA, Gelles RJ: *Physical violence in American families: risk factors and adaptations to violence in 8,145 families,* New Brunswick, NJ, 1990, Transaction Publishers.
21. The United States Conference of Mayors: *A status report on hunger and homelessness in America's cities* Washington, DC, 1996, The Conference.
22. US Department of Housing and Urban Development, Office of Policy Development and Research: *Rental housing assistance at a crossroads: a report to congress on worst case housing needs,* 1996.
23. Wood D, et al: Homeless and housed families in Los Angeles: a study comparing demographic, economic, and family function characteristics, *Am J Public Health* 80:1049, 1990.

66 Latchkey Children: Children in Self-Care

Robert D. Needlman

Concern about children in self-care has paralleled the entry of women into the labor force, beginning in World War II. The precise number of "latchkey" children is unknown. Among grade school children, recent estimates have been as low as 7% (1987 U.S. Census) and as high as 44% (1990 Department of Education survey). A 1998 Department of Education study found that 35% of 12-year-olds were in regular self-care after school. The number of adolescents unsupervised between 3 PM and 6 PM may approach 80%.[12] Supervision of younger children by older siblings accounts for a large, unmeasured amount of nonparental care. Often children participate in two or more care arrangements in the same week.[1] Self-care may be more common in communities with higher socioeconomic status (SES), in which both parents are employed outside of the home.[3]

"Latchkey children" remains a stigmatizing term. Even parents who have chosen self-care for their children may be reluctant to disclose that choice to a survey-taker or to their pediatrician. Many parents feel guilty about their decision to work out of the home or attend school and worry about the effects of self-care on their children. A shortage of extended family members, after-school programs, and funds often limits parents' choices.

EFFECTS OF SELF-CARE

Despite the prevalence of self-care and its salience to parents, a thorough literature search found only 27 articles from 1972 through 1999 addressing its effects. Many potential negative effects are unsupported, or inconsistently supported, in this literature. Self-care has not been associated with school absence, obesity, visits to the school nurse, or increased emergency room or hospital use.[20,21] In cross-sectional studies, children's self-esteem, locus of control, peer relationships, and classroom conduct do not differ as a function of self- versus parent-care.[4,11,15] However, a longitudinal study found that greater time in self-care in grades one, three, and five predicted poorer teacher-rated classroom adjustment in grade six.[9] Latchkey status was associated with lower cognitive test scores in a cohort of lower-income girls (but not boys)[21] but was *not* associated with poorer grades, either among suburban third-graders,[17] rural fifth- and seventh-graders,[4] or urban eighth-graders.[3]

The possibility of emotional harm was raised in a 1981 study of low-income children in first through sixth grades in Washington, D.C.[5] Of those unsupervised after school, 30% were fearful and 40% had nightmares, compared with 0% to 2% of those in parental care for each of these symptoms. Children supervised by siblings had intermediate rates of fears and nightmares. Anecdotally, some children reported hiding in closets or bathtubs or playing the television loud to drown out their fears. The finding of increased fears has been replicated in one study, but not in another.[3,11]

Suburban latchkey children grades K through 8 also reported some mild increase in fears, but 80% nevertheless reported that they "liked or loved" the arrangement.[8] Some parents feel that their children gain in self-confidence by taking on the responsibility of self-care. A 1992 study found no difference in children's self-rated competence between self- and parent care, although children in the care of siblings had lower self-rated competence.[2] There is speculation that sibling care may have negative effects on both the caretaking sibling and the one cared for, although firm data are lacking.[10]

Another area of concern is the possibility of increased substance use and other risk-taking behaviors among adolescents in self-care. Here the studies are more consistent. Rates of teen violence, as well as sexual activity, are highest during the after-school hours.[18] The number of hours of self-care per week has been correlated consistently with rates of cigarette, alcohol, and marijuana use among adolescents.[6,7,13,14] The location of self-care also is important, because it reflects the closeness of parental supervision: adolescents unsupervised at friends' homes are more at risk of succumbing to negative peer pressure than those who stay in their own homes. Those who "hang out" with friends without a set location are at greatest risk.[16] Nonpermissive parenting style, family rules prohibiting substance use, and increased supervision (e.g, through required telephone calls) lower, but do not eliminate, the risk associated with self-care.[6,16]

Early adolescents may be particularly vulnerable to the stresses and temptations of self-care. Compared with parent-supervised eighth graders, those in self-care for 11 or more hours per week reported 1.5 to 2 times higher levels of risk-taking, anger, family conflict, peer influence, attendance at parties, and substance use. Moreover, children who had begun self-care during elementary school (rather than junior high) reported further increases in these negative factors, suggesting possible "sleeper effects" of early self-care.[3] For example, among eighth-graders, 11% of the children in parental care reported heavy alcohol use, compared with 19.5% in self-care since junior high school, and 25.5% in self-care since elementary school.[3]

COMMUNITY RESPONSE

Communities have responded to latchkey concerns by providing educational programs to enhance child safety and preparedness, telephone "warm lines" for children who are bored or frightened, and programs that provide educational and recreational stimulation as well as supervision.[8,18] Children who attend after-school programs or participate in extracurricular activities may watch less television, earn higher grades, and be less likely to engage in risk-taking or illegal activities.[11,18,19]

As with preschool child-care, the *quality* of the program probably is an important determinant of its effects. In 1987, only 15% of public schools offered extended-day programs; by 1994, 30% did.[1] However, such programs are projected to meet only 25% of the need in some urban areas by 2002.[18] A $3.2 billion federal program, the Child Care and Development Fund, seeks to expand childcare programs through block grants to states, but relatively little has been earmarked for school-age child care.

THE PEDIATRICIAN'S ROLE

Pediatricians should ask about child care arrangements at every health supervision visit. Parents of school-age and adolescent children are likely to have questions about self-care but may hesitate to bring up the subject. Although the effects of self-care on school-age children remain unclear, parents should be aware of the increased rates of substance use and other risk taking among unsupervised adolescents. The effects are highly variable from individual to individual. Factors to keep in mind include the duration and location of the care (at home, at a friend's home, or in a program; urban, suburban, or rural), the age and personality of the child, and the quality of the parent-child relationship. Tighter parental supervision (e.g., for example, through regular telephone contacts, firm family standards, and clear behavioral expectations) may facilitate successful self-care. Referrals to local "warm" lines and safety training programs also can be helpful.

For parents who are uncomfortable with self-care, pediatricians can provide a list of after-school programs. The National Child Care Information Center (NCCIC, http://nccic.org) maintains computerized links to directories in each state. Child Care Resource and Referral Programs in most states also offer guidance and referrals. The national toll-free number is 1-800-424-2246. Where available programs are inadequate to meet the community's needs, pediatricians should advocate for more and higher quality out-of-school programs for school-age children and adolescents.

REFERENCES

1. Administration for Children and Families—US Department of Health and Human Services: *Out-of-school time: school-age care,* Washington, DC, 1999. (http://www.acf.dhhs.gov/programs/ccb/faq/school.htm).
2. Berman BD, et al: After-school child care and self-esteem in school-age children, *Pediatrics* 89:654, 1992.
3. Dwyer KM, et al: Characteristics of eighth-grade students who initiate self-care in elementary and junior high school, *Pediatrics* 86:448, 1990.
4. Galambos NL, Garbarino J: Identifying the missing links in the study of latchkey children, *Children Today* 12:2, 40, 1983.
5. Long T, Long L: *Latchkey children: the child's view of self-care,* ERIC Clearinghouse on Elementary and Early Childhood Education, Urbana, Ill, ED 211 229, 1981.
6. Mott JA, et al: After-school supervision and adolescent cigarette smoking: contributions of the setting and intensity of after-school self-care, *J Behav Med* 22:35, 1999.
7. Mulhall PF, Stone D, Stone B: Home alone: is it a risk factor for middle school youth and drug use? *J Drug Educ* 26:39, 1996.
8. Padilla ML, Landreth GL: Latchkey children: a review of the literature, *Child Welfare* 68:445, 1989.
9. Pettit GS, Laird RD: Patterns of after-school care in middle childhood: risk factors and developmental outcomes, *Merrill-Palmer Quarterly* 43: 515, 1997.
10. Pettine AR, Lee A: Self-care and deviance in elementary school-age children, *J Clin Psychol* 54:629, 1998.
11. Posner JK, Vandell DL: Low-income children's after-school care: are there beneficial effects of after-school programs? *Child Dev* 65:440, 1994.
12. Reuter R: Opinion/essays: an after-school haven needed, *Christian Science Monitor* July 3, 1998, p 15.
13. Richardson JL, et al: Relationship between after-school care of adolescents and substance use, risk taking, depressed mood, and academic achievement, *Pediatrics* 92:32, 1993.
14. Richardson JL, et al: Substance use among eighth-grade students who take care of themselves after school, *Pediatrics* 84:556, 1989.
15. Rodman H, Pratto DJ, Nelson RS: Child care arrangements and children's functioning: a comparison of self-care and adult-care children, *Dev Psychol* 21:413, 1985.
16. Steinberg L: Latchkey children and susceptibility to peer pressure: an ecological analysis, *Dev Psychol* 22:433, 1986.
17. Vandell DL, Corasaniti MA: The relation between third graders' after-school care and social, academic, and emotional functioning, *Child Dev* 59:868, 1988.
18. Wellesley College Center for Research on Women: *Fact sheet on school-age children's out-of-school time,* Wellesley, Mass, 1998, National Institute on Out-of-School Time (NIOST). (http://www.wellesley.edu/WCW/CRW/SAC/)
19. Westat Inc: *Adolescent time use, risky behavior, and outcomes: an analysis of national data,* Rockville, Md, 1996, US Department of Health and Human Services.
20. Williams RL, Boyce WT: Health status of children in self-care, *Am J Dis Child* 143:112, 1989.
21. Woods MB: The unsupervised child of the working mother, *Dev Psychol* 6:14, 1972.

67 Teaching Parents About Effective Discipline

Ellen C. Perrin

DEFINITION OF DISCIPLINE

The word *discipline* has its root in the Latin word *disciplinare,* which means "to teach." Discipline refers to the structure created by parents to teach their children how they are expected to behave. The term *discipline* often is used in a much more limited fashion to refer only to punishment. Punishment, however, is only a very small part of the total parenting environment that helps children feel safe, capable, and lovable, and helps parents feel effective.

Pediatricians are in an important position to help parents create a constructive pattern of discipline, fostering optimal interaction and teaching. The pediatrician may be the only, or at least the most accessible, professional who knows children and their families during the preschool period. Even later in children's development pediatricians remain important anchors for parents as they negotiate the ever-changing challenges of parenting. Thus, pediatricians have the opportunity (and thereby the responsibility) to help parents in their efforts to provide the best possible context for growth.[1]

The longitudinal role of primary care pediatricians dictates their continuing involvement from initial guidance about effective parenting through help with the management of any serious dysfunction. Pediatricians can empower parents, help them monitor their children's behavior and development, and provide anticipatory guidance and advice about methods to structure the family environment to avoid difficulties.[2,4,5,11,12] Pediatricians also have the opportunity to recognize and advise parents about observed or described problems with children's behavior early in their course, thus preventing more serious behavioral or emotional dysfunction. They also are critical participants in the management of more serious behavioral or emotional dysfunction; some pediatricians may be able to provide some counseling themselves, and all pediatricians can help families by referring them to respected colleagues in the mental health professions (see Chapter 83, Consultation and Referral for Behavioral and Developmental Problems). Effective involvement of their pediatrician before and after referral makes families' work with a mental health professional more likely to be successful.

TIMING OF DISCUSSIONS ABOUT DISCIPLINE

Because effective discipline is so central to parenting, its discussion should be a part of every health supervision visit.[1,4,15] The earliest discussions about discipline can occur within the first few months of life. Parents' attempts to organize the family's schedule around the infant's eating and sleeping routines are among their earliest efforts at defining and agreeing on a set of rules or limits. Another opportunity to help parents discuss and agree on appropriate rules occurs as children become mobile and parents begin to create and maintain safety guidelines. The responsibility to keep their child safe is accepted by parents quite universally, encouraging a discussion of optimal limits that must be set and a structure by which they can be taught and enforced. The pediatrician can point out to parents that in determining methods of keeping their child from falling down stairs, poking objects into electrical outlets, or spilling hot liquids, they have defined their expectations and some of their earliest rules.

When parents recognize that they must discuss and agree on rules to create a safe structure, they begin to recognize their own power in communicating their expectations for their child's behavior. This empowerment is one step along the arduous trail by which parents create a safe, nurturing environment and help their children to learn appropriate standards of adult behavior. Table 67-1 provides some guidelines of other developmental periods when discussion about discipline can be woven usefully into the context of health supervision visits. Useful "trigger" questions can become routine parts of child health supervision visits. Examples of such questions are, "Are you happy with your discipline strategies?" or "Do you have any questions about your child's behavior?"

BASIC PRINCIPLES AND TECHNIQUES

Parents generally want to do what is best for their children. They may be limited by inadequate knowledge of appropriate strategies and techniques, by depression or anxiety, by overwhelming challenges of their own past or present life, anger, or psychopathology. Box 67-1 outlines several basic principles underlying effective discipline.

It is important to remember that each child exists in the context of a complex family that is an interactive system. The behavior of any member of a family affects in complicated ways the behavior of *all* members. A family can be imagined to be carrying out its life on a waterbed: Each time one member moves, complicated ripples and counter-ripples affect the movements of everyone else. It also is important to remember that parents work primarily on intuition and on the basis of their experiences as children. Although parenting is

Table 67-1 Recommended Contexts for Discussions About Discipline at Various Ages

Age	Contexts to Frame Discussions About Discipline
1-4 months	Sleeping and eating schedules/routines
6-9 months	Rules to ensure safety of the environment
12-18 months	Emerging autonomy and independence
2 years	Toileting; perhaps new sibling
3 years	Entering preschool
4 years	Doing household chores
5 years	Entering a more formal school setting
6-12 years	Increasing peer activities and orientation
Adolescence	Observing curfews, guidelines for alcohol use, driving, and sexual behavior

BOX 67-1

UNDERLYING PRINCIPLES OF DISCIPLINE

1. Parents want to do the best they can for their children.
2. Parents learn to parent from their experience as children.
3. Families are complex systems in continuous transaction.
4. Behavior is learned primarily from its consequences.
5. *Something* is keeping the problematic behavior in place.
6. Punishment only teaches children what's *not* OK.

among the most difficult and the most important jobs we have as adults, it is the one for which we have the least training and support. Pediatricians can be very important in providing support for parents, direction to parents' observations, and guidance if they need help.

Basic Parenting Techniques

Several specific strategies can help children to feel loved and capable. The first is "alone time" with the child (Box 67-2). This technique consists of allocating a short period of time, 15 to 30 minutes, that each parent commits to spending with each child on a predictable schedule. During this time the parent and child interact one-on-one, and no interruptions are tolerated. The parent and child engage in an activity that is pleasurable for both of them, and the time allotted to this activity is monitored by an alarm clock or a kitchen timer. This predictable, promised time is not contingent on the child's behavior or on the parent's mood; it occurs at its scheduled time under all circumstances.

Parents also do well to learn to take notice *actively* of their child's admirable behaviors. Parents should attend to and praise their children liberally when they are playing appropriately, relating well with another adult or child, trying to be helpful, or attempting to do what the parent asks. The most effective comments are short, direct verbal messages, preferably referring directly to the parent's feelings rather than the child's behavior. An evaluative statement such as, "You did a good job," admits the possibility that the child will do a bad job the next time. In contrast, statements such as "I really like how you cleaned up that pile of blocks," or "It makes me feel very proud when I see how well you play with Johnny," refer only to the speaker's response to the behavior and do not predict potential criticism. Nonverbal messages are powerful as well, such as a hug, a smile, or a pat on the back.

BOX 67-2

RULES FOR "ALONE TIME"

1. Predictable
2. One-on-one, with *no* interruptions
3. Time marked with a clock or timer
4. Interactive activity the child enjoys
5. Noncontingent on child's behavior or parent's mood

A third strategy involves giving children appropriate choices. In encouraging children to make and take part in appropriate decisions, parents teach them that they are capable of being responsible for their own behavior. The opportunity to make effective choices empowers children and enhances their growth. Choices must be appropriate to the child's developmental abilities, and parents must be careful to offer choices only when there actually are options from which to choose that are all acceptable to the parents. Questions such as, "Do you want orange juice or apple juice?" or "Do you want to wear your sweater or your jacket?" might be appropriate for a preschool child, whereas "Do you want to go to bed?" would not. For an older child, choices might involve choosing clothes to buy or to wear or how to organize bedtime rituals.

SHAPING CHILDREN'S BEHAVIOR

All behavior is learned, shaped primarily by its consequences. Behavior that is reinforced is likely to be repeated; behavior that results in an unpleasant consequence is much less likely to be repeated. Removing reinforcement (i.e., ignoring) of a particular behavior also decreases its frequency. However, even occasional reinforcement prevents the extinction of an undesirable behavior. It also is important to note that what a parent intends as punishment may have some reinforcing characteristics to the child. A common example of this paradox is yelling at or even spanking a child; although these are not pleasant consequences, they do reflect intense emotional involvement on the part of the parent toward the child, which may be valuable to some children. Table 67-2 outlines a summary of the use of behavioral consequences to shape children's behavior.

Table 67-2 Basic Rules for Effective Discipline

Reward behavior you like	Rewards can be tangible or symbolic Rewards should be immediate Hugs and praise are powerful rewards
Use natural and logical consequences as your ally	*Natural* consequences are what would happen if you did nothing *Logical* consequences are those you impose as a reasonable outcome of the specific behavior
Punish behavior you don't like	Take away something the child values or impose something the child dislikes Punishment should be immediate Frequent small punishments are more effective than occasional big ones Spanking is effective only for the moment and has undesirable side effects

Increasing Desirable Behavior

Parents are the most important people in children's lives; pleasing them is an important goal for most children. Furthermore, children, like the rest of us, appreciate being attended to and considered valuable company. Thus, parents' attention, recognition, and praise are important reinforcers of their children's behavior. Behaviors that are rewarded or reinforced are likely to continue and even to increase in frequency.

Parents may reinforce their children's behavior directly or indirectly. Examples of direct reinforcement of behavior are a parent's praise for appropriate play or accomplishment of a task, a planned gift, or a joint activity contingent on the child's completion of a particular assignment. Indirect rewards for a child's good behavior may include a smile on the mother's face as she watches her child create a high tower and take pleasure in knocking it down or overhearing her mother speaking on the telephone with pride about her accomplishments in school.

Decreasing Undesirable Behavior

All human beings learn faster and more effectively when they are rewarded for good behavior than when they are punished for bad. Nevertheless, because all children at some time behave inappropriately, their parents must find a way to indicate that this behavior is not acceptable and to decrease its frequency. Several mechanisms can be used to decrease the likelihood of undesirable behavior. First, parents must check to be sure that they are not inadvertently rewarding behavior they find unacceptable. For example, a child who receives a cookie to head off a temper tantrum or one whose parents feed her each time she awakens during the night is receiving an unintentional reward for behavior the parents would rather see disappear. Similarly, some attempts by parents to punish their children's unacceptable behavior may in some way reinforce it. Even negative attention from parents is better than none at all—"yelling" is at least intense interaction.

Undesirable behavior will diminish if reinforcement for it is withdrawn (i.e., it is ignored) or if it results in an unpleasant consequence, either naturally occurring or imposed by adults in the environment (i.e., it is punished). Common sense and common advice suggest that parents *ignore* the behaviors they do not like. Given enough time, behaviors that are not reinforced will indeed fade.

This approach has two problems. First, ignoring disruptive behavior works only if the behavior is ignored 100% of the time, and this is virtually impossible to do. Second, behaviors that are *intrinsically* rewarding, such as taking cookies from the cookie jar or staying out late at night, will not diminish simply as a result of the parent's ignoring them. Thus, active punishment techniques generally are necessary some of the time to interrupt children's unacceptable behavior.

Active punishment strategies. The most powerful punishments are outcomes that occur naturally as a result of the child's behavior: *natural consequences.* For example, dawdling in the morning results in being late for school; if a child does not eat at mealtime, he or she may be hungry at bedtime; if the goldfish are not fed, they will die. Parents need only refrain from interfering with the natural consequences that follow upon the child's behavior. If no negative consequences would follow naturally, parents can create some that follow logically: *logical consequences.* Scribbling on the wall might result in no crayons for a week or in the assignment of washing the walls; if toys are not put away by a prescribed time, they are removed for several days.

Some unacceptable behaviors require parents to create a more contrived intervention. For example, hitting or biting do not result in any acceptable, immediately occurring, logical, or natural negative consequence; thus, a punishment needs to be imposed. Active punishment can take two forms: (1) privileges or pleasurable activities can be denied the child, or (2) painful, uncomfortable, or undesirable circumstance or activities can be imposed on the child. Examples of the restriction of privileges include decreasing the amount of time the child may watch television, decreasing the number of books a parent will read at bedtime, or forbidding the child to eat dessert with the family. Commonly used methods of imposing undesirable consequences include spanking, requiring certain chores to be done, or requiring separation, such as a "time-out," from family activities.

Corporal punishment. Despite the prevalent experience and beliefs of many parents and pediatricians,[10] spanking and other forms of physical punishment have no place in the discipline of children.[1,7,8] Although spanking may at first appear effective as a result of children's surprise, pain, and fear, it seldom is effective in the long run and is used at great cost.[3,6,14]

Children learn more effectively by watching their parents' behavior than by listening passively to their words. Parents who spank model a type of behavior that they generally do not allow for the child; how can young children understand

BOX 67-3

RULES FOR "TIME-OUT"

1. Offending behavior(s) described in *concrete* statement(s)
2. Maximum of *three* offending behaviors
3. Occurs *immediately* after the behavior occurs
4. Occurs *each time* the behavior occurs
5. Plans and place arranged in *absence* of problematic behavior
6. One minute per year of age, marked with a *timer*
7. Welcome child back to *"time in"* without lecturing

Table 67-3 Systemic Behavior Change Plan (Examples)

Behaviors We Want to STOP	Consequences
Hurting people	Time-out
Whining	Time-out
Throwing food	Dinner is over
Behaviors We Want to SEE MORE OF	**Consequences**
Set table	Star (sticker)*
Read to Susie	Star (sticker)*
Be ready for school by 7:30 AM	Watch TV from 7:30-8:00 PM

*Ten stars (stickers) earns choice of video rental.

that their parents may hit them while they themselves are punished for hitting other children? Furthermore, spanking reduces the opportunities available for using more effective disciplinary strategies.[9]

Physical punishment undermines parents' attempts to maintain effective, cooperative, and nurturing relationships with their children. Children who are spanked learn aggressive and violent forms of conflict resolution based on power and strength. When adults are hit, they feel violated, shamed, hurt, and angry; children, too, will experience these feelings when being hit. That this action and these feelings come from the adults they trust and love most makes them even more destructive. There is evidence that adolescents and adults who were physically punished as children are more likely to accept and engage in violent behavior as adults.[13,14]

Another reason spanking generally is not effective is that most parents are reluctant to spank their children. This reluctance is a result of two factors: (1) parents do not like to hurt their children, and (2) most parents come to recognize that spanking is, at best, inconsistently effective in changing children's behavior. In addition, physical punishment is difficult to modulate. It generally is carried out when the parent is angry and carries with it the risk of excessive anger and unintentional abuse. If parents are reluctant to punish their children, their discipline is likely to be ineffective and frustrating.

Time-out. For maximal effectiveness, a "time-out" should be instituted in a planned and carefully specified manner after it is described to the child (Box 67-3). Two or three particular behaviors should be targeted for time-out. It is helpful to describe them in writing in very concrete and simple terms at a central location (bulletin board, refrigerator door). Subsequently, time-out must be enforced the *first* time and *each* time these behaviors occur. Time-out should be in a particular place and for a short period, marked with a timer. It is critical that there be absolutely no interaction during a time-out. If a sibling teases or talks to the child in time-out, he or she should be placed in time-out as well. Parents must completely ignore attempts at interaction such as whining or "Is my time up yet?" If the child leaves the designated time-out place or is disruptive, the timer is reset for the predetermined amount of time. It is very important that parents remain calm and controlled when supervising time-out—they should reveal neither anger nor sympathy, but treat the time-out as the inevitable consequence of the child's infraction of a predetermined family rule. When the timer rings, the child should be welcomed back into the family's positive interactions.

Rewarding what's good. When creating a systematic solution for difficult behavior problems, parents should simultaneously attend to boosting those behaviors they would prefer. Parents should specify two or three particular behaviors that they appreciate and want to see the child demonstrate more often. These behaviors should be described in writing in concrete, observable terms such as "set the table within 10 minutes after being asked" or "read a book to younger sister." These expectations should not be simply the absence of an undesirable behavior—for example, "don't whine." The child should understand that these activities result in a prearranged reward. Rewards may be tangible, such as a coin or a cookie, or symbolic, such as a star or a sticker on a chart. Symbolic rewards can be accumulated toward a larger tangible prize—for example, 10 stars earns a trip to the ice cream parlor with Dad, or a chance to choose a video rental.

A chart delineating the *forbidden* behaviors and their consequences, and the *desirable* behaviors and their consequences should be posted in a prominent and accessible location. The particular behaviors, rewards, and punishments will differ according to the child's age, the particular issues on which the family chooses to focus, and the kinds of positive and negative consequences the family prefers. An example is provided in Table 67-3.

SUMMARY

It is very important to remember that punishment is never *enough.* At best, punishment teaches children only what behavior is *not acceptable* but cannot teach them what behavior is *desirable.* Thus, punishment should constitute only a small part of an overall disciplinary strategy. Effective discipline results from parents' creation of an environment in which children feel safe by virtue of predictable rules and consequences, lovable as a result of adequate attention and praise, and capable of making decisions and taking responsibility for

BOX 67-4

PREVENTIVE STRATEGIES

1. Empowerment of parents
2. Discipline = *rules* and *consequences*
3. Praise and attention
4. Alone time
5. Effective choices

BOX 67-5

COMMON PITFALLS LEADING TO INEFFECTIVE DISCIPLINE

Inadvertent rewarding of undesirable behavior
Failure to notice and reward desirable behavior
Insufficient "time in"
Inconsistent rules from day to day, situation to situation
Too many punishable behaviors

their own behavior. These basic preventive strategies are outlined in Box 67-4.

Common problems summarized in Box 67-5 include inadvertently rewarding undesirable behavior, failing to notice and reward desirable behavior, a family environment that is so busy or stressed that the child does not experience sufficient positive interaction with the parents ("time in"), and inconsistency in the consequences that follow "good" or "bad" behaviors.

Pediatricians can provide a model for parents, teaching them the importance of empowerment in the context of a respectful and emotionally safe and nurturing environment. They also can teach parents some of the skills that will help their children know that they are lovable, capable, and responsible. In addition, pediatricians can help parents to construct an effective disciplinary structure by suggesting helpful reading materials and/or audio- or videotapes. Some parents will benefit from discussion groups with other parents.

REFERENCES

1. American Academy of Pediatrics: Guidance for effective discipline, *Pediatrics* 101:723, 1998.
2. Christophersen ER: Discipline, *Pediatr Clin North Am* 39:395, 1992.
3. Friedman SB, Schonberg SK, editors: The short- and long-term consequences of corporal punishment, *Pediatrics* 98:803, 1996.
4. Howard BJ: Advising parents on discipline: what works, *Pediatrics* 98:809, 1996.
5. Howard BJ: Discipline in early childhood, *Pediatr Clin North Am* 38:1351, 1991.
6. Larzelere RE: A review of the outcomes of parental use of nonabusive or customary physical punishment, *Pediatrics* 98:821, 1996.
7. Larzelere RE: Moderate spanking: model or deterrent of children's aggression in the family, *J Fam Violence* 1:27, 1986.
8. Larzelere RE, et al: Relationship of spanking and other parenting characteristics to self-esteem and perceived fairness of parental discipline, *Psychol Rep* 64:1140, 1989.
9. McCord J: Unintended consequences of punishment, *Pediatrics* 98:832, 1996.
10. McCormick KF: Attitudes of primary care physicians toward corporal punishment, *JAMA* 267:3161, 1992.
11. Schmitt BD: Discipline: rules and consequences, *Contemp Pediatr* June 1991, p 65.
12. Smith EE, Van Tassel E: Problems of discipline in early childhood, *Pediatr Clin North Am* 29:167, 1982.
13. Straus MA: Discipline and deviance: physical punishment of children and violence and other crime in adulthood, *Soc Probl* 38:133, 1991.
14. Straus MA: Spanking and the making of a violent society, *Pediatrics* 98:837, 1996.
15. Wissow LS, Roter D: Toward effective discussion of discipline and corporal punishment during primary care visits: findings from studies of doctor-patient interaction, *Pediatrics* 94:587, 1994.

HELPFUL BOOKS FOR PARENTS

Brazelton T: *Touchpoints,* Reading, Mass, 1992, Addison-Wesley.

Clark L: *The time-out solution,* Chicago, 1989, Contemporary Books.

Dreikurs R: *Children: the challenge,* New York, 1964, Penguin Books.

Dreikurs R, Grey LA: *Parent's guide to child discipline,* New York, 1970, Hawthorn Books.

Faber A, Mazlish E: *How to talk so kids will listen and listen so kids will talk,* New York, 1980, Avon Books.

68 Sexual Abuse of Children

John M. Leventhal

Although sexual abuse of children has existed for centuries, it has only been in the past 25 years that clinicians have come to recognize the scope of the problem, including its epidemiology, clinical characteristics, approaches to management, and consequences to children and families.

DEFINITION AND EPIDEMIOLOGY

Sexual abuse is defined as the involvement of children or adolescents in sexual activities that they do not fully understand, to which they cannot give informed consent, and that violate the social taboos of families or society.[22] It includes activities such as the sexual touching of a child's genitals by an adult or adolescent, sexual intercourse between an adult and child, the exposing of children to pornography, or involvement of children in prostitution. Sexual abuse should be distinguished from sexual play or exploration by preschool or young school-age children or sexual activities between consenting adolescents.

Child protection laws passed in the 1960s in each state initially required the reporting of cases of suspected abuse or neglect, but shortly after were broadened to include children suspected of being sexually abused. Since 1976, when national statistics of cases reported to each state's child protection agency were compiled, cases of maltreatment (including physical abuse, neglect, and sexual abuse) have increased yearly. When reports of sexual abuse are examined, the most dramatic increase in reports occurred in the 1980s, as a result of increased publicity and increased recognition by parents and clinicians. In the early 1990s, yearly reports of sexual abuse peaked at more than 400,000 cases (representing about 13% of almost 3 million reports of child maltreatment). Since then, the number of reports has decreased to about 225,000 reports in 1997 (representing 7% of all reports). How much of this recent decrease is due to prevention programs that teach young children about sexual abuse, a change in reporting criteria, a decrease in the backlog of cases detected in the1980s, or a true change in the occurrence of the phenomenon is unknown.

Of the cases of suspected sexual abuse reported to protective services, about 37% are considered substantiated, meaning that protective services had enough evidence to believe that sexual abuse occurred. This rate of substantiation for sexual abuse is somewhat higher than for other forms of maltreatment. The failure to substantiate an allegation does not necessarily mean that the abuse did not occur, but rather that protective services does not have enough evidence. About 75% of children evaluated for suspected sexual abuse are female; the age range is from 6 months to 18 years, with a median age of about 8 years.

Although such cases represent those reported to child protective services, an alternative approach to estimating the frequency of the problem has been to interview adults about their childhood experiences of sexual abuse. These studies provide information about a lifetime prevalence. A review of 19 studies conducted on community samples in the United States or Canada since 1980 found that the rates of sexual abuse reported by women were 2% to 62% and by men, 3% to 16%.[18] Finkelhor has suggested that a summary statistic for women of 20% would be reasonable.[18] Because only nine of the studies surveyed men, there was less certainty about a summary statistic for men, but a conservative estimate would be 5% to 10%.[18] The prevalence of sexual abuse reported by adults in different studies varies because of the population studied, the response rate, the number and types of questions asked, the definition of sexual abuse, the age used to define childhood, the accuracy of the adults' memories, and the willingness of the adults to report past events.[24]

Unlike cases of physical abuse or neglect, which are reported much more commonly in families who are poor and have limited education, cases of sexual abuse occur in families from all social classes and educational backgrounds. Perpetrators of sexual abuse are almost all males, and 20% to 25% of them are adolescents. Most children who have been sexually abused know the perpetrator, who may be the father, stepfather, another male relative, family friend, or an adult in the child's community. Although female perpetrators are unusual in most clinical series, these rates may be falsely low because of under-recognition. Approximately 15% of sexually abused children do not know the perpetrator; these victims usually are older children or adolescents who are victims of forceful sexual assault, or rape.

ETIOLOGY

Although clinicians are able to understand how a parent might lose control and physically abuse a child, it is much more difficult to understand how an adult can move from close bodily contact and even sensual feelings toward actually sexually abusing a child. Two prerequisites for sexual abuse to occur include the offender's sexual arousal to children and the willingness to act upon this arousal.[17] Studies have attempted to examine adults' sexual attraction to children. For example, 21% of male college students in an anonymous questionnaire indicated that they felt sexual attraction toward children.[12] Some offenders may focus their attention on children of a certain age or gender; others may find themselves aroused only by children in certain circumstances. Factors that influence the offender's willingness to act on the aroused feelings toward the child include a lack of conscience about such behaviors, a lack of empathy for the child, a belief that such sexual behaviors are acceptable and not harmful to the child, poor impulse control, and the use of drugs or alcohol that might further decrease the ability to control one's behavior.[17] Additional contributors to the likelihood that sexual abuse may occur include the history of the perpetrator (e.g., having experienced sexual abuse during childhood), circumstances that allow the perpetrator to have increased contact with the child (e.g., a mother hospitalized for a lengthy period), and the particular vulnerabilities of the child (e.g., mental retardation).

Children who are sexually abused are often selected because they seem particularly vulnerable or needy. Such children initially may enjoy and appreciate the attention that they receive from the offender, who may begin by giving the child gifts, attention, and special hugs and touches. These behaviors may progress to special secrets and eventually from nonsexual to sexual activities that lead to sexual intercourse. This process has been labeled the "child sexual abuse accommodation syndrome,"[33] which describes five stages that occur in the sexual abuse of children: (1) secrecy; (2) helplessness; (3) entrapment and accommodation; (4) delayed, unconvincing disclosures; and (5) later retraction of the alleged abuse.

CLINICAL MANIFESTATIONS

Like other forms of family violence, sexual abuse of children often occurs in the privacy of a home or in a setting that involves only the abused and abuser, and thus seldom is witnessed by another person. A child who has been sexually abused may have experienced other forms of maltreatment, including physical abuse or neglect, and certainly has been emotionally abused as well.

A clinician's concerns about the possibility of sexual abuse occur because of reports of specific statements made by the child, usually to a parent or other adult, about uncomfortable experiences, such as being touched on the genitalia; reports of specific behaviors of the child, such as sexualized behaviors with a sibling; symptoms, such as encopresis or vaginal discharge or bleeding; or a genital or anal injury noted on physical examination.

Clear statements by the child (or occasionally, accidental direct observations of the sexual abuse) are the best indicators that sexual abuse has occurred. These statements usually are told to a parent or trusted adult, such as a school teacher. Young children, however, may not have the necessary vocabulary to describe what has happened to them. They may use words that the perpetrator used to encourage their participation (e.g., "we played the hugging game") or words that describe their experience of what happened or what it felt like, but are confusing to the adults (e.g., "he stuck a knife in my pee-pee"). Older children may begin by offering a guarded, vague disclosure (e.g., "My uncle kisses too hard"). If the adult reacts in a concerned manner with appropriate exploratory questions, more details may follow. The older child may be embarrassed about what happened, feel partially responsible, have experienced pleasurable feelings, or be concerned about the threats that the perpetrator made (e.g., "If you tell your mother, I will punch you" or "If you tell, you know they will think you are a liar"). Even after a clear disclosure, once the child realizes how upsetting the information is to the family, he or she may retract the statement. Older children also may feel responsible for holding the family together: If the child tells, the father will go to jail, the house will be sold, and everyone will be angry at the child; on the other hand, if nothing is said, the sexual abuse will continue, but at least the family will be saved. Some children consciously or unconsciously sacrifice themselves for their family.

Children who have been sexually abused may demonstrate a variety of symptoms and behaviors. Some may be relatively asymptomatic and be able to function reasonably well in social settings and in school. Many children exhibit nonspecific symptoms, such as sleep problems, generalized anxiety, suicidal gestures, or poor school performance, which are seen in response to other childhood stresses as well. Sexualized behaviors, such as excessive masturbation, the use of adult words associated with sexuality, or simulation of sexual intercourse with another child, animal, or doll are more suggestive of sexual abuse. Other concerning symptoms include vaginal pain, bleeding, or discharge or rectal bleeding. Even a symptom such as a vaginal discharge, however, has a low likelihood of being due to sexual abuse. Several studies of premenarcheal girls who have complained of vaginal discharge have shown that the occurrence of sexual abuse is infrequent (fewer than 5% to 10% of those who have this complaint) and that the most common etiology is poor hygiene.[32]

Approximately 15% to 20% of sexually abused children will have an abnormal genital or anal finding suspicious of sexual abuse. The absence of physical findings, however, does not rule out sexual abuse, because there may have been no injury to the genital area, or if an injury did occur, it may have healed without leaving any physical signs. Even in cases in which the perpetrator has been convicted of sexual abuse, it is unusual for the victim to have had an abnormal examination. For example, in a series of 236 children in which the perpetrators were convicted, only 23% of genital examinations were considered suspicious or abnormal in girls and only 7% of anal examinations were considered so in boys and girls.[2]

Over the past several years, research has defined normal and abnormal genital and anal anatomy in prepubertal children and adolescents; recently, a glossary of terms has been published.[4] Several studies have described the variations in the anatomy of the hymen in female newborns and have concluded that the hymen is present in all normally developed newborns.[8] The appearance of the hymen is often thickened early in life because of the effects of maternal estrogen in utero; in preschool and school-age girls, the hymenal tissue becomes thinner until the effects of estrogen during puberty result in a thickening of the tissue and the development of redundant folds. Studies of normal prepubertal girls have described the shapes of the hymen as crescentic, annular, and fimbriated (or redundant) and have noted the frequency of normal variations, including hymenal mounds, intravaginal ridges, and adhesions of the labia minora.[9,27] These studies have provided data on the means and ranges of the vertical and horizontal diameters of the hymenal orifice in different age groups, the variations in diameter depending on how the genital examination is performed (e.g., separation versus traction of the labia majora),[26] and the width of the posterior hymenal rim.

Children who have been sexually abused may have acute injuries of the genitalia, including acute lacerations, abrasions, or hematomas.[3] Most children who have been sexually abused, however, do not disclose until weeks or months after the occurrence of the abuse. In such children, findings that are considered suspicious or suggestive of past abuse include U- or V-shaped clefts (or notches) of the posterior rim (from 3 o'clock to 9 o'clock) of the hymen, which occur in the healing process after an acute laceration, and attenuation or decreased hymenal tissue posteriorly (<1 mm). These findings should persist when the child is examined in the prone, knee-chest position.[1,3] Scarring, such as of the posterior fourchette, also is indicative of previous trauma.[1,3] Although, in the past, investigators have considered an enlarged horizontal diameter of the hymen of >4 mm to be suspicious of previous sexual abuse in prepubertal children, studies of normal children have indicated that this demarcation is incorrect and that the size of the opening varies with the child's age and different examination techniques,[26] as well as with the child's state of relaxation. A horizontal diameter of >10 mm may concern a clinician about the possibility of sexual abuse but should not by itself be used to make a diagnosis.

Data about normal physical findings in adolescence have been limited; one study compared three groups of adolescent females: (1) those who denied sexual intercourse and used only pads for menses, (2) those who denied sexual intercourse and used tampons, and (3) those who had experienced sexual intercourse.[15] Although there were significant differences in the median horizontal diameters of the hymenal orifice in the three groups (1.2, 1.5, and 2.5 cm, respectively), there certainly was overlap among the groups. In addition, a striking difference among the groups was that of the sexually active teenagers: 81% had a complete cleft (or V-shaped notch) between the 2 o'clock and 10 o'clock positions on the hymenal border compared with 11% in tampon users and 5% in pad users.

Abnormalities of the male genitalia caused by sexual abuse are unusual. Acute abrasions, lacerations, or bruises caused by physical abuse, however, can be seen.

Acute anal findings, such as lacerations resulting from anal penetration or injury, have been noted in sexually abused children, but there have been few systematic studies of perianal findings in chronically abused children. Worrisome findings include thickening of the rugae, distorted anatomy secondary to scarring, and dilation >2.0 cm (when the child is in the prone, knee-chest position and no stool is visible in the rectal ampulla). A study of normal prepubertal children highlighted common normal findings that were noted when the child was examined in the prone, knee-chest position; these included skin tags in the midline, fan-shaped areas in the midline superiorly, perianal erythema, venous congestion, and anal dilation up to 2.0 cm.[28]

Children who have been sexually abused may acquire a sexually transmitted disease (STD).[13] There continues to be controversy about how children acquire such diseases, in part because of the social and legal implications and because of the difficulty in believing that a young child's disease is from sexual contact. The most commonly occurring STDs in sexually abused children are due to *Neisseria gonorrhoeae, Chlamydia trachomatis,* and human papillomavirus (HPV). Each of these organisms can be transmitted perinatally. In a study of young children who acquired chlamydia perinatally and were followed from birth, the organism was recovered from the throat or nasopharynx up to 28 months of age and from the vagina or rectum up to the first birthday.[7] Although few systematic data have been collected regarding the isolation of HPV from a child after exposure to the organism at birth, the range of the incubation period in adults is 3 weeks to about 8 months.[19] Condylomata that are noted in 12- to 24-month-olds are believed to be due to perinatal transmission, but because of the child's age, it is difficult to be certain about the etiology. HPV can be transmitted nonsexually as well, either by autoinoculation if a child has common skin warts or horizontally from nonabusive contact by a person who has common warts. Other diseases, such as syphilis or infection with the human immunodeficiency virus (HIV), also have been reported in victims of sexual abuse.

Female adolescent victims are at risk of pregnancy from sexual abuse.

ASSESSMENT AND DIAGNOSIS

The evaluation of children for suspected sexual abuse should include a history from the parents and child, a physical examination, appropriate laboratory tests, and careful documentation of the findings. In addition, data may be collected from other professionals who know the child and family. This evaluation often is conducted by a multidisciplinary team: A social worker or psychologist interviews the parents and child, and the medical examination is conducted by a physician, nurse practitioner, or physician's assistant. As part of the evaluation, the clinicians should consider alternative explanations, including an unintentional injury (or "accident"), a medical problem, or a false allegation.[10] Because evaluations for suspected sexual abuse usually include the child protection and legal systems, care should be taken to provide an unbiased assessment and one that provides documentation that can be reviewed by professionals outside the medical system.

History

The purpose of the history is to understand what may have happened to the child. This history should include the events that led to the evaluation, the child's health status and level of development, and the family's strengths and weaknesses. The parents (or guardian) should be asked what the child has said, how the child reacted when telling about the abuse, and whom the child told. Information should be obtained about (1) the child's behaviors, such as changes in behaviors or attitudes toward a specific person or situation, recurrent fears or nightmares, or sexualized behaviors; (2) specific symptoms, such as vaginal bleeding or discharge, anal bleeding, constipation, and encopresis; and (3) where the child spends his or her time and who cares for the child. Also, it should be determined who the alleged perpetrator is, the relationship with the child, and the amount of time spent with the child. In preparation for interviewing the child, it is important to know about the child's developmental history—for example, whether there is a language delay.

The family history should include information about the parents' physical and mental health (including a history of sexual abuse during childhood); the health and developmental status of the siblings; the presence of family violence, substance abuse, or recent stresses; and the resources and supports available to the family. It is important to understand how family members view the allegations and how they have reacted. Because allegations that arise during a custody fight between parents are often difficult to sort out, the clinician should determine whether the parents are separated or divorced, the custody arrangements, the kind of visitation schedule, and any dispute about custody or visitation. It is helpful to distinguish whether the allegations of abuse occurred before the separation or divorce, during the process of separation and divorce, or after the divorce had been finalized.

A child who is old enough to be interviewed directly should be asked about what may have happened.[13,25] This interview or series of interviews should be conducted with the child alone, if possible. The interviewer should be comfortable and skilled at interviewing young children about the possibility of sexual abuse, use simple questions, and be aware of the child's nonverbal responses, as well as direct statements. Leading questions, such as "Didn't he touch your pee-pee?" should be avoided, when possible. Nonleading questions are preferable, such as "Can you tell me what happened?" or "Where did he touch you?" Often, however, children are reluctant to talk because of a variety of reasons, including fear and embarrassment; in such cases, questions with forced choice responses, "Was it your mother or father or teacher who did that?" or "Was his pee green or pink or white?" can be helpful.

To help young children, anatomical drawings or anatomically correct dolls can be used. There has been considerable controversy about the sexual nature of the dolls and whether their use suggests to children that they can talk about sex, thus leading to false allegations. Research, however, indicates that few nonsexually abused children respond in sexual ways with the dolls and that the dolls can be helpful to children in describing what happened.[16] Because of the controversy involving the dolls, most interviewers prefer to use them to help the child identify body parts and explain the details of what happened only after the child has indicated verbally that sexual abuse has occurred. Some older children who have difficulty verbalizing acts of sexual abuse may be able to draw pictures of what occurred.

Physical Examination

The purposes of the physical examination are to determine whether there are (1) signs of physical abuse or neglect, (2) anogenital injuries that are consistent with or suggestive of sexual abuse, and (3) conditions that need medical treatment. In addition, the examination provides an opportunity for the clinician to reassure the child and family about the child's physical condition. In premenarcheal girls, the genital examination is performed best in both the supine and prone, knee-chest positions; a speculum is seldom used. To visualize the hymen, two physical examination maneuvers should be used: labial separation (separating and pulling posteriorly at an angle of 45 degrees) and labial traction (gently pinching the labia and pulling out and toward the examiner). Evaluations conducted in specialty centers rely on the use of a colposcope during the anogenital examination to provide five- to thirtyfold magnification and documentation through photographs or video recordings. A study comparing examinations with and without the use of the colposcope indicated that more than 95% of physical findings can be detected without its use.[29] A handheld magnifying lens that provides two-and-a-half- to threefold magnification or an otoscope (without a speculum) can provide reasonably good magnification.

Laboratory Tests

When the child is at risk of acquiring an STD from suspected sexual contact, appropriate tests should be obtained for gonorrhea, herpes simplex, trichomonas, bacterial vaginosis, chlamydia, syphilis, HIV infection, and hepatitis B and C. Tests for gonorrhea and chlamydia should be cultures for the organisms. In many medical settings, however, obtaining swabs for cultures is no longer routine practice because nonculture tests are used, such as tests for the organism's DNA or RNA (e.g., Gen Probe). In such settings, positive results should be confirmed with cultures; negative results need not be. For a child who has a vaginal discharge, additional studies may be done to test for trichomonas or bacterial vaginosis.

Studies have attempted to determine which children should be tested for STDs. For example, in a review of 2731 preteens who had vaginal cultures, 84 (3.1.%) had gonorrhea and 80 of these had a vaginal discharge.[21] No data, however, are available to help determine which children should have cultures taken from all three sites: the genitals, throat, and anus. If the child has evidence of one STD, it is reasonable to conduct a full range of tests for other STDs.

When a child is evaluated within 72 hours of an episode of suspected sexual abuse, appropriate forensic information, such as swabs to detect semen, should be collected.[6] (See Chapter 294, Rape.) In an adolescent, a pregnancy test may be necessary.

Documentation

Documentation of the evaluation should include direct quotations, when appropriate, from the parents and the child and a clear description of the findings from the physical examination, with sketches, if necessary. In many states the information is recorded on a specific form for suspected sexual assault. A videotape of the child's interview and a videotape or photographs of the examination provide additional detailed information; these should be labeled with the date, child's name, physician's name, and the child's medical record number.

DIFFERENTIAL DIAGNOSIS

Conditions that need to be considered in the differential diagnosis depend on the child's symptoms and physical findings.[5] Some of the physical findings that can be seen in sexually abused children also are nonspecific findings, such as erythema of the vulva or introitus. Bruises to the genital or anal area should raise concern about physical abuse, but if bruising is more widespread, medical conditions, such as bleeding disorders, need to be considered. Straddle injuries, which can affect the genitalia, usually are witnessed, so the history is clear. These types of injuries usually are unilateral or anterior and produce obvious bruising and swelling of the external genitalia; it is unusual for such injuries to affect the hymen because of the protection provided by the labia and bones of the pelvis.

An important dermatological condition that may present with genital soreness and subependymal hemorrhages is lichen sclerosus.[5] This condition usually affects the vulva and perianal region and produces an hourglass appearance with areas of subependymal hemorrhage, decreased pigmentation, and tissue friability. Urethral prolapse can present with vaginal bleeding and dysuria, and the abnormalities noted on physical examination might be considered the result of trauma from sexual abuse. Another condition that may be mistaken for sexual abuse is a streptococcal infection that can cause marked redness of the perianal region and a vaginal discharge. For children who have a foul-smelling vaginal discharge, a foreign body should be considered in the differential diagnosis.

A critical challenge for the examiner is to identify abnormalities that are due to trauma from sexual abuse versus normal variations. Recent studies have shown that physicians do not always agree on their descriptions or interpretations of genital findings. For example, Paradise et al used seven simulated cases to compare the assessments of 206 U.S. physicians who considered themselves skilled at examining sexually abused children with the assessments of a panel of experts.[30] Not surprisingly, the most experienced physicians were more likely than the less experienced physicians to agree with the ratings of the expert panel. In a related study,[31] the history provided in a simulated case was noted to have an influence on physicians' interpretations of findings: When the history did not suggest sexual abuse, the physicians (especially those who had little experience) were more likely to consider the examination normal. The opposite effect was found as well: When the history suggested sexual abuse, physicians were more likely to consider the same examination as abnormal.

The possibility of a false allegation also should be considered in the differential diagnosis.[10] Although false allegations seem to occur infrequently, controversy is increasing about the accuracy of young children's memory, under what research circumstances they can be asked leading questions that result in false reports of what happened, and how relevant these studies are to children's reports of sexual abuse.[14] False allegations should be carefully considered if the child has a serious mental health problem, if the child is part of a bitter dispute between the parents (e.g., a custody fight), or if the child's statements lack detail about the event, have important inconsistencies, or appear rote in nature and the child seems minimally affected by telling what happened.

MANAGEMENT AND TREATMENT

Management of children who are suspected of having been sexually abused includes action in three domains: (1) providing appropriate medical care, (2) reporting the case to protective services, and (3) ensuring mental health services for the child and family.

Guidelines for the treatment of STDs are highlighted in Chapter 294, Rape. In addition, counseling may be necessary about the implications of certain infections, such as HPV or HIV. Occasionally, surgical repairs of genital or anal injuries are necessary, and adolescents may need counseling about terminating a pregnancy that was due to sexual abuse. A major purpose of the physical examination is to provide reassurance to the child and family that his or her body is physically intact. When abnormalities are noted on the physical examination, reassurance often can be provided by indicating that these likely will heal and be of little functional importance to the child.

Clinicians who suspect sexual abuse are mandated to report their findings to the state's child protection agency. Because sexual assault is a criminal offense, the local police also participate in the investigation. Issues that need to be considered include: to what extent the child should be interviewed further, by whom, and in what setting; where the child should go to ensure his or her safety; and whether other children in the home need an evaluation.

The period after the child's disclosure can be emotionally upsetting to all involved and especially confusing to the child. Repeated interviews of the child (by well-meaning professionals, such as police or a protective service worker) may upset the child, who may be confused about why so many people are asking questions, embarrassed about talking about private parts, and worried about the family's reactions. Family members may blame themselves for allowing the abuse to happen and be furious at the suspected perpetrator. If the abuser is a relative, the family may be divided, with the child's side believing the child and the abuser's side believing that the abuse could not happen and that the child is lying. If the abuser is in the immediate family, the psychological issues are even more complicated. A mother will have to decide between siding with and supporting her daughter or believing that her daughter lied and supporting her husband. If her husband did sexually abuse their child, the mother may question her ability to protect her child, her own sexuality, and her ability to choose a partner; at the same time, she may be concerned about how the family will be supported with the father in jail.

The clinician can be helpful by maintaining contact with the family, advocating for a reasonable approach by protective services (e.g., having the alleged abuser leave the home rather than place the child in foster care), and helping the family to recognize and discuss the various emotional issues that surface.

In many communities, multidisciplinary investigative teams (MITs) have been developed to provide a rational and coordinated approach to the evaluation of children suspected of having been sexually abused, to minimize the interviewing of the child, and to help the family through the initial period of crisis. Members of the team often include representatives from the local police, prosecutors' office, and protective services, as well as experts in interviewing and examining the child.

Many sexually abused children and their parents need short- or long-term counseling to help come to terms with what happened to the child. Important issues for the child's treatment include self blame for allowing the abuse to happen, the child's sexuality and sexual awareness, poor self-esteem and feelings of powerlessness, and mistrust of adults. For example, school-age and adolescent boys may be very concerned about their own masculinity and whether, because they were abused by an older male, they are gay. At the same time, because of changes in the family (e.g., the child no longer visits the grandfather), the child has to come to terms with the losses created by the disclosure and the upset and anger in the family.

Because sexual abuse of a child is a criminal offense, the child and family often are involved in the criminal justice system. Despite this involvement, however, most cases do not actually result in a trial in criminal court because of a variety of reasons, including lack of clear evidence that abuse has occurred, the young age of the victim, a confession of the perpetrator, or the willingness of the perpetrator to plea bargain for a lighter sentence. In only approximately 3% to 5% of cases, a criminal trial is held in which the child actually testifies. Additionally, sexual abuse cases sometimes are tried (1) in family court when allegations of sexual abuse occur as a part of a divorce or custody proceeding or (2) in juvenile court when protective services is concerned about the child's safety in the home.

PSYCHOSOCIAL CONSEQUENCES

Sexual abuse can have a long-lasting and devastating impact on the development of children, adolescents, and adults.[11,23] Domains of functioning that can be affected include the survivor's emotional state (e.g., depression, anxiety, suicide), sense of self (e.g., feeling worthless or powerless, and viewing one's self as a victim), and relationships with others (e.g., setting poor boundaries, being promiscuous, using inappropriate sexual behaviors, and having lack of trust). Teenage girls and young women appear to be at an increased risk of other mental health problems, such as eating disorders, multiple personality disorders, and posttraumatic stress disorders. They also are more likely to become pregnant at a younger age.

Men who were sexually abused as children are at increased risk for having mental health or substance abuse problems. They also are more apt to perpetrate sexually coercive acts, including victimizing children sexually.[20]

PREVENTION

Attempts to prevent sexual abuse have been directed toward developing programs to teach children, usually at school, about "good" and "bad" touches and what to do if bad touches occur. Children as young as 4- to 6-year-olds are able to learn these concepts and retain them, at least over a short period. In general, evaluations have focused on the children's increased knowledge resulting from participation in a teaching program but have not been able to provide conclusive evidence that such programs actually have resulted in the prevention or earlier recognition of sexual abuse.

REFERENCES

1. Adams JA, Harper K, Knudson S: A proposed system for the classification of anogenital findings in children with suspected sexual abuse, *Adolesc Pediatr Gynecol* 5:73, 1992.
2. Adams JA, et al: Examination findings in legally confirmed child sexual abuse: it's normal to be normal, *Pediatrics* 94:310, 1994.
3. American Academy of Pediatrics, Committee on Child Abuse and Neglect: Guidelines for the evaluation of sexual abuse of children: subject review, *Pediatrics* 103:186, 1999.
4. American Professional Society on the Abuse of Children: *Glossary of terms and the interpretation of findings for child sexual abuse evidentiary exams,* Chicago, 1998, APSAC.
5. Bays J: Conditions mistaken for child sexual abuse. In Reece RM, editor: *Child abuse: medical diagnosis and assessment*, Philadelphia, 1994, Lea & Febiger.
6. Bechtel K, Podrazik M: Evaluation of the adolescent rape victim, *Pediatr Clin North Am* 46:809, 1999.
7. Bell TA, et al: Chronic *Chlamydia trachomatis* infections in infants, *JAMA* 67:400, 1992.
8. Berenson A, Heger A, Andrews S: Appearance of the hymen in newborns, *Pediatrics* 87:458, 1991.
9. Berenson AB, et al: Appearance of the hymen in prepubertal girls, *Pediatrics* 89:387, 1992.
10. Bernet W: False statements and the differential diagnosis of abuse allegations, *J Am Acad Child Adolesc Psychiatry* 32:903, 1993.
11. Briere J: *Child abuse trauma: theory and treatment of the lasting effects,* Newbury Park, Calif, 1992, Sage Publications.
12. Briere J, Runtz M: University males' sexual interest in children: predicting potential indices of pedophilia in a nonforensic sample, *Child Abuse Negl* 13:65, 1989.
13. Bourg W, et al: *A child interviewer's guidebook,* Thousand Oaks, Calif, 1999, Sage Publications.
14. Ceci SJ, Bruck M: *Jeopardy in the courtroom: a scientific analysis of children's testimony,* Washington, DC, 1995, American Psychological Association.
15. Emans SJ, et al: Hymenal findings in adolescent women: impact of tampon use and consensual sexual activity, *J Pediatr* 125:153, 1994.
16. Everson MD, Boat BW: Putting the anatomical doll controversy in perspective: an examination of the major uses and criticisms of the dolls in child sexual abuse evaluations, *Child Abuse Negl* 18:113, 1994.
17. Faller KC: *Understanding child sexual maltreatment,* Newbury Park, Calif, 1993, Sage Publications.
18. Finkelhor D: Current information on the scope and nature of child sexual abuse, *Future Child* 4:31, 1994.
19. Gutman LT, Herman-Giddens ME, Phelps WC: Transmission of human papillomavirus disease: comparison of data from adults and children, *Pediatrics* 91:31, 1993.
20. Holmes WC, Slap GB: Sexual abuse of boys: definition, prevalence, correlates, sequelae, and management, *JAMA* 280:1855, 1998.
21. Ingram DL, et al: Vaginal gonococcal cultures in sexual abuse evaluations: evaluation of selective criteria for preteenaged girls, *Pediatrics* 1997. URL: http://www.pediatrics.org/cgi/content/full/99/6/e8.
22. Kempe CH: Sexual abuse, another hidden pediatric problem: the 1977 C. Anderson Aldrich Lecture, *Pediatrics* 62:382, 1978.
23. Kendall-Tacket TA, Williams LM, Finkelhor D: Impact of sexual abuse on children: a review and synthesis of recent empirical studies, *Psychol Bull* 113:164, 1993.
24. Leventhal JM: Epidemiology of sexual abuse of children: old problems, new directions, *Child Abuse Negl* 22:481, 1999.
25. Leventhal JM, et al: What to ask when sexual abuse is suspected, *Arch Dis Child* 62:1188, 1987.
26. McCann J, et al: Comparison of genital examination techniques in prepubertal girls, *Pediatrics* 85:182, 1990.
27. McCann J, et al: Genital findings in prepubertal girls selected for nonabuse: a descriptive study, *Pediatrics* 86:428, 1990.
28. McCann J, et al: Perianal findings in prepubertal children selected for nonabuse: a descriptive study, *Child Abuse Negl* 13:179, 1989.
29. Muram D: Child sexual abuse: genital findings in prepubertal girls: comparison of colposcopic and unaided examination, *Am J Obstet Gynecol* 160:333, 1989.
30. Paradise JE, et al: Assessments of girls' genital findings and the likelihood of sexual abuse: agreement among physicians self-rated as skilled, *Arch Pediatr Adolesc Med* 151: 883, 1997.
31. Paradise JE, et al: Influence of the history on physicians' interpretations of girls' genital findings, *Pediatrics* 103:980, 1999.

32. Paradise JE, et al: Vulvovaginitis in premenarcheal girls: clinical features and diagnostic evaluation, *Pediatrics* 70:193, 1982.
33. Summit RC: The child sexual abuse accommodation syndrome, *Child Abuse Negl* 7:177, 1993.

SUGGESTED READINGS

Atabaki S, Paradise JE: The medical evaluation of the sexually abused child: lessons from a decade of research, *Pediatrics* 104(suppl):178, 1999.

Behrman RE, editor: Sexual abuse of children, *Future Child* 4:2, 1994.

Finkel MA, DeJong AR: Medical findings in child sexual abuse. In Reece RM, editor: *Child abuse: medical diagnosis and management,* Philadelphia, 1994, Lea & Febiger.

Heger A, Emans SJ, editors: *Evaluation of the sexually abused child: a medical textbook and photographic atlas,* New York, 1992, Oxford University Press.

Kerns DL, guest editor: Establishing a medical research agenda for child sexual abuse, *Child Abuse Negl* 22: 453, 1999.

Krugman RD, Leventhal JM, editors: *Child sexual abuse: report of the Twenty-Second Ross Roundtable on Critical Approaches to Common Pediatric Problems,* Columbus, Ohio, 1991, Ross Laboratories.

McCann J, Kerns DL: *The anatomy of child and adolescent sexual abuse: a CD-ROM atlas/reference*, St Louis, 1999, Intercorp.

69 Children, Adolescents, and the Media

Victor C. Strasburger

The media's influence on children and adolescents is controversial, but it is widely believed to be profound. Considerable evidence suggests that the media contribute to violence in society, early teen sexual activity, teen cigarette and alcohol use, obesity, and other unhealthful conditions and behaviors.[9,10,39] Although not the leading cause of violence, teenage pregnancy, or teen drug use, the media contribute to each of these problems substantially.[36] Clearly, American society would benefit from television programs and movies that are less violent, less sexually suggestive, and contain less smoking, drinking, and alcohol advertising.

TYPES OF MEDIA

Television is the preeminent medium. Children average 17 hours of viewing weekly, beginning as early as age 2 years; preschool children average 28 hours weekly.[28] Including video game and videocassette recorder (VCR) use, teens may spend as many as 53 hours per week in front of the TV or computer screen, although the range of hours is considerable (Table 69-1).[34]

Other media also are important. Adolescents may spend as much time listening to the radio, audiocassettes, or CDs as they do watching TV, but music usually is used as an accompaniment to other activities rather than as a primary activity. More than 50% of all 15- to 16-year-olds surveyed in one study had seen the majority of the most recent, popular, R-rated movies.[22] In addition, Internet usage is increasing annually, with 61% of teens reporting "surfing the Net," and 14% reporting seeing something that they did not want their parents to know about.[33]

Print media (newspapers, magazines, and billboards), through their articles and advertising, have less of an effect on the behavior of children and adolescent than do other media.

WHAT CHILDREN SEE AND HOW IT AFFECTS THEM

A number of content analyses have documented what the average child or teenager views in an average year. All of these studies contain data that are worrisome for those concerned about violence, teenage sexual activity, and teen drug use.

Violence

Children and adolescents view an estimated 10,000 acts of violence per year (Box 69-1).[17] Surprisingly, programming for children actually contains *more* violence than prime-time programming. Of the 10,000 violent acts, 500 or more are high risk: The perpetrator is an attractive role model; the violence is realistic, is portrayed as justified or goes unpunished; or the consequences of the violence are not shown.[17] See also Chapter 23 (Four), Violence Prevention, and Chapter 112, Violent and Aggressive Behavior.

Sex

The average television viewer is exposed to more than 14,000 sexual references and innuendoes a year, of which fewer than 170 deal with abstinence, birth control, or the risk of pregnancy or sexually transmitted disease.[24] The most recent content analysis found that more than two thirds of prime-time shows contain sexual content, but only 9% of incidents include any mention of the risks or responsibilities of sexual activity or the need for contraception (Fig. 69-1).[27] The media can be considered as one potential access point for teenagers for information about contraception.[38]

Drugs

Alcohol, tobacco, or illicit drugs are present in 70% of prime-time television programming, 95% of top-grossing movies, 50% of music videos, and 20% to 25% of all videos.[14,20] Cigarettes seem to be making a big comeback in Hollywood movies: The prevalence of smoking among lead characters is four times the prevalence of people in real life.[35] Even G-rated children's animated films contain high levels of tobacco and alcohol use—more than two thirds of such films in an analysis of children's films from 1937 through 1997.[21]

According to social modeling theory, television exposes children and adolescents to an endless succession of role models, demonstrating potential behaviors to young, sometimes impressionable viewers.[3] Role modeling may be a crucial determinant in whether teenagers begin consuming alcohol or smoking cigarettes.[37] Children and teenagers who view a lot of television tend to think that it depicts real behavior in the real world (or that the real world should conform to television rules).[19] This is the cultivation hypothesis. Clearly, television and other media have the ability to influence young people's attitudes and perceptions about the world, what one group of researchers calls "stalagmite effects—cognitive deposits built up almost imperceptibly from the drip-drip-drip of television's electronic limewater."[5]

Although the impact of media exposure remains a hot topic of both research and debate, 3 to 4 hours a day spent with media displaces other, more active pursuits such as participating in sports, playing with friends, or reading. Most children spend more time watching television than in any other "activity" except for sleeping.[37] By the time today's children graduate from high school, they will have spent 15,000 hours viewing television but only 12,000 in formal classroom instruction. By the time they reach age 70 years, they will have spent 7 to 10 years of their lives in front of the television and other media.[37]

Table 69-1 Adolescents' Media Use*

Medium	Average Use
Television	24 hr/wk ± 14 hr
Music videos	10 hr/wk ± 12 hr
VCR videos	11 hr/wk ± 11 hr
Video games	8 hr/wk ± 12 hr

Modified from Robinson TN, Chen HL, Killen JD: *Pediatrics* 102:54,1998.
**n* = 1533.

BOX 69-1

HIGHLIGHTS OF THE NATIONAL TELEVISION VIOLENCE STUDY*

60% of programs contain violence
66% of children's programs contain violence
71% of violent scenes contain no remorse, criticism, or penalty for violence
25% of scenes involve the use of a gun

Modified from Federman J, editor: *National television violence study*, vol 3, Santa Barbara, Calif, 1998, Center for Communication and Social Policy.
**n*= 10,000 hours of TV examined.

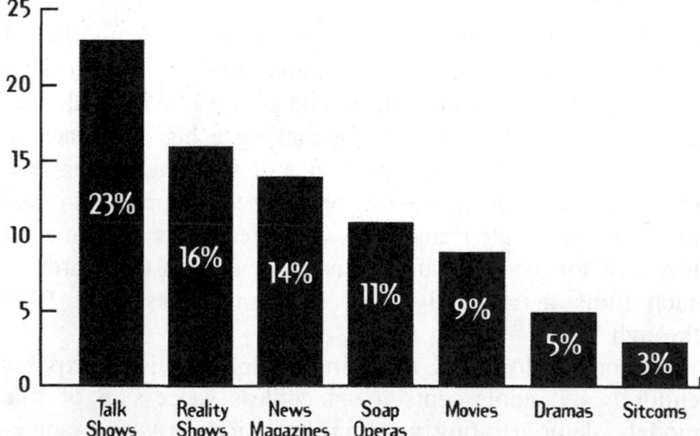

Fig. 69-1 Percent of shows with sexual content that also contain references to the risks and responsibilities of sex, by genre.
(From Kunkel D, et al: *Sex on TV: content and context*, Santa Barbara, Calif, 1999, Henry J. Kaiser Family Foundation.)

VIOLENCE IN THE MEDIA

No area of media effects has been researched as well as the impact of media violence on children and adolescents. More than 1000 studies and reviews have documented potentially harmful effects.[43] The research in this area is so substantial and authoritative that few new studies currently are being conducted.[16]

Studies show that high levels of television viewing are related casually to aggressive behavior and the acceptance of aggressive attitudes (desensitization).[39,43] Related research shows that witnessing violence makes teens more likely to use violence or carry weapons themselves.[13] Television, movies, and computer games allow children and teenagers to witness violence daily, vicariously, on a screen in their own home. In playing many computer-animated games, children take part in and control the killing that takes place every few seconds for hours on end.

Exposure to media violence at young ages (8 years and younger) has been found to be a significant risk factor for adolescent or young adult aggressive behavior and criminal violence.[15] Children appear to develop attitudes about violence at a very young age; these attitudes apparently persist throughout their lives.[15]

American media are problematic in two important ways: (1) movies, television programs, and computer games are rife with portrayals of justified violence (the "good guy" beating up or killing the "bad guy"), and (2) guns are glorified in the media with 25% of all violent episodes on television involving gun play.[17] Research suggests that media violence may contribute to between 5% and 15% of all violence in the United States.[39]

SEX IN THE MEDIA

Whereas 1000 studies address the connection between media violence and aggressive behavior, only 4 studies exist concerning sexual behavior and sexual content in the media.[4,11,30,31] All were conducted more than 10 years ago.

- In a study of 75 adolescent girls, 50% pregnant and 50% not pregnant, the former watched more soap operas before becoming pregnant and were less likely to think that their favorite soap characters would use birth control.[11]
- A study of 391 junior high school students found that those who selectively viewed more sexual content on TV were more likely to have begun having sexual intercourse in the preceding year.[4]
- A study of 326 teenagers showed that those with a preference for MTV had increased amounts of sexual experience in their midteen years.[31]
- Data from the National Surveys of Children revealed that males who watched more TV had the highest prevalence of sexual intercourse. Also, teens who watched

TV apart from their family had a rate of intercourse three to six times higher than those who viewed with their family.[37]

Several other studies show changes in sexual attitudes associated with media use. One study found that heavy exposure to sexual content among 13- and 14 year-olds makes them more accepting of nonmarital sex.[5] Another found that heavy viewing of soap operas and MTV predicts more permissive sexual attitudes among college students.[40] If changes in attitude predict changes in behavior, the media contributes to early teen sexual activity significantly.

DRUGS IN THE MEDIA

Numerous studies document that children under the age of 8 years are developmentally unable to understand the intent of advertisements and tend to believe that all ads are true.[41] Teenagers are capable of understanding the selling intent of television commercials and print media advertising. Alcohol and tobacco manufacturers spend, respectively, $2 billion and $6 billion annually on advertising,[36] but only beer commercials are permitted on television. Although beer advertisers insist that their intent is to promote brand selection, increased consumption is inevitable.

Several studies attest to the power of cigarette and alcohol advertising. In one, Old Joe Camel was found to be as recognizable to 6-year-old children as Mickey Mouse.[18] Among teenagers, a one-to-one correlation exists between advertising expenditures and cigarette brand consumption. Beer advertising targets young people specifically by showing the supposed advantages of being a beer drinker: more friends, greater prestige, more fun, greater sex appeal. They make beer consumption seem like acceptable behavior for adolescents who are under the legal drinking age.

Considerable evidence exists that the media make children more vulnerable to experimentation with alcohol.[23] Although children begin making decisions about alcohol in grade school[42] and are exposed to an average of nearly 2000 beer commercials per year,[38] they lack the adult analytical skills to decode media messages until about the eighth grade.[7] Exposure to beer commercials correlates with brand recognition and positive attitudes toward drinking, and children who enjoy alcohol advertisements are more likely to drink earlier or engage in binge drinking.[2,23] Finally, two longitudinal studies now exist that make a cause-and-effect case for the influence of the media on cigarette and alcohol use.[32,34]

THE ROLE OF THE PEDIATRICIAN

Pediatricians are crucial sources of information for parents and health advocates in their communities and, in league with the American Academy of Pediatrics (AAP), can be agents of change in society as well.

Counseling Parents

According to the AAP, parents should be counseled to limit their children's total media time to no more than 1 to 2 hours a day, to monitor what shows and video games their children use, and to view with them.[9] The media represent an issue of "family values." Research suggests that parents who discuss sensitive issues with their children might be able to prevent early risk-taking behavior.[5] Parents perhaps should be counseled that allowing children or adolescents to have television sets in their bedrooms is unwise (Fig. 69-2).

Media Education

Although parents should be a source of media education to their children, excellent school-based media education programs exist. Such programs have been successful in reducing violence and drug use.[1,25] Computer and video games also may be used for prosocial learning in schools.[12] The United States is one of the few Western nations lacking a comprehensive, school-based, media education program for children.

Advocacy

Pediatricians can have an impact on the government and the entertainment industry regarding the media. The following is a list of some of the issues that pediatricians may want to consider:

- Better funding for public broadcasting. Television originated in the United States, but a distinct lack of related public policy persists. Other countries spend far more money on funding public broadcasting than does the Unites States: The United Kingdom spends $38.56 per capita per year; Canada $32.15; Japan $17.71; and the United States only $1.09.[29] PBS remains the sole consistently high-quality site for nonviolent programming for young children in America and, as such, deserves greater financial support.
- Better enforcement of the Telecommunications Act of 1996 by the Federal Communications Commission (FCC). This law mandates that broadcasters must air 3 hours of core educational programming per week, beginning September 1997.[26] Previous attempts to regulate commercial television have resulted in shows such as "F Troop" and "The Jetsons" being touted as educational programming by broadcasters. The United States

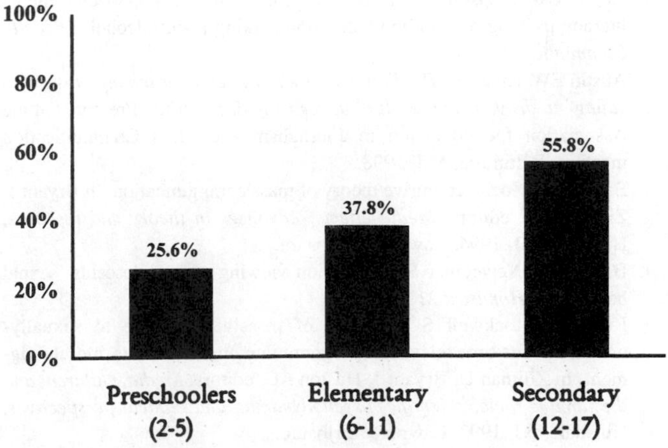

Fig. 69-2 As children age, they are increasingly likely to have a television set in their own bedroom.

(From Stanger JD: *Television in the home: the 1997 survey of parents and children,* Philadelphia, 1997, Annenberg Public Policy Center.)

is unique in not having at least 1 hour of educational programming per channel per day.

- Increased funding for research. Few government agencies or private foundations fund research on the effects of media on children or adolescents. In particular, studies on adolescent sexuality and the media, the use of the Internet, the impact of video games, and the efficacy of media education to prevent early teen sexual activity, violence, and drug use are urgently needed.
- A new governmental report on the impact of the media. The Surgeon General Report on Television was issued in 1972; the National Institutes of Mental Health report was completed in 1982. A year 2005 report is needed that will combine all existing research with a series of recommendations for public policy and future research.
- Stricter regulation of cigarette and alcohol advertising. Tobacco advertising should be banned from all media, and alcohol advertising should be restricted to so-called "tombstone" advertising, in which only the product itself can be displayed, not the qualities the consumer would acquire.[8] The current levels of alcohol and cigarette use by teenagers can be attributable directly to the $8 billion worth of advertising directed at them each year.[38]
- Greater responsibility from the entertainment industry. Hollywood and television networks are unique in extolling their products. However, only a few are good: "To Kill a Mockingbird" is a masterpiece that ennobles us and the old "Cosby Show" displays strong family values.

Yet the entertainment industry continues to deny that any of its movies or television shows can have a negative impact. Again, the research is clear: Media probably contribute to 5% to 30% of violence, early sexual activity, and drug-taking among children and adolescents.[39] Hollywood and television networks need to accept responsibility for what they produce and concentrate on less violent, less sexually suggestive, and less drug-oriented programming.

REFERENCES

1. Austin EW, Johnson KK: Effects of general and alcohol-specific media literacy training on children's decision making about alcohol, *J Health Communic* 2:17, 1997.
2. Austin EW, Knaus C: *Predicting future risky behavior among those "too young" to drink as the result of advertising desirability*. Presented at the Association for Education in Journalism and Mass Communication meeting, Baltimore, Md, 1998.
3. Bandura A: Social cognitive theory of mass communication. In Bryant J, Zillmann D, editors: *Media effects: advances in theory and research,* Hillsdale, NJ, 1994, Lawrence Erlbaum.
4. Brown JD, Newcomer S.: Television viewing and adolescents' sexual behavior, *J Homosex* 21:77, 1991.
5. Bryant J, Rockwell SC: Effects of massive exposure to sexually-oriented prime time television programming on adolescents' moral judgment. In Zillman D, Bryant J, Huston AC, editors: *Media, children, and the family: social scientific, psychodynamic, and clinical perspectives,* Hillsdale, NJ, 1993, Lawrence Erlbaum.
6. Christenson PG, Roberts DF: *It's not only rock 'n' roll: popular music in the lives of adolescents,* Cresskill, NJ, 1998, Hampton Press.
7. Collins WA: Interpretation and inference in children's television viewing. In Bryant J, Anderson DR, editors: *Children's understanding of television: research on attention and comprehension*, New York, 1983, Academic Press.
8. Committee on Communications, American Academy of Pediatrics: Children, adolescents and advertising (policy statement), *Pediatrics* 95:295, 1995.
9. Committee on Communications, American Academy of Pediatrics: Children, adolescents, and television (policy statement), *Pediatrics* 96:786, 1995.
10. Committee on Communications, American Academy of Pediatrics: Media education (policy statement), *Pediatrics* 104:341, 1999.
11. Corder-Bolz C: Television and adolescents' sexual behaviors, *Sex Education Coalition News* 3:40, 1981.
12. Dorman SM: Video and computer games: effect on children and implications for health education, *J School Health* 67:133, 1997.
13. DuRant RH, et al: Intentions to use violence among young adolescents, *Pediatrics* 98:1104, 1996.
14. DuRant RH, et al: Tobacco and alcohol use behaviors portrayed in music videos, *Am J Public Health* 87:1131, 1997.
15. Eron LR: Media violence, *Pediatr Ann* 24:84, 1995.
16. Eron LR: *The problem of media violence and children's behavior,* New York, 1993, The Guggenheim Foundation.
17. Federman J, editor: *National television violence study*, vol 3, Thousand Oaks, Calif, 1998, Sage.
18. Fischer PM, et al: Brand logo recognition by children aged 3 to 6 years, *JAMA* 266:3145, 1991.
19. Gerbner G, et al: Growing up with television: the cultivation perspective. In Bryant J, Zillmann D, editors: *Media effects: advances in theory and research*, Hillsdale, NJ, 1994, Lawrence Erlbaum.
20. Gerbner G, Ozyegin N: *Alcohol, tobacco, and illicit drugs in entertainment television, commercials, news, "reality shows," movies, and music channels*. Report from the Robert Wood Johnson Foundation, March 20, 1997.
21. Goldstein AO, Sobel RA, Newman GR: Tobacco and alcohol use in G-rated children's animated films, *JAMA* 281:1131, 1999.
22. Greenberg BS, Brown JD, Buerkel-Rothfuss N: *Media, sex and the adolescent*, Cresskill, NJ, 1993, Hampton Press.
23. Grube JW: *Alcohol advertising and alcohol consumption: a review of recent research. NIAA tenth special report to Congress on alcohol and health,* Bethesda, Md, 1999, National Institute on Alcohol Abuse and Alcoholism.
24. Harris L, et al: *Sexual material on American network television during the 1987-88 season,* New York, 1988, Planned Parenthood Federation of America.
25. Huesmann LR, et al: Mitigating the imitation of aggressive behaviors by changing children's attitudes about media violence, *J Pers Soc Psychol* 44:899, 1983.
26. Jordan AB: *Children's educational television regulations and the local broadcaster: impact and implementation*, Philadelphia, 1997, Annenberg Public Policy Center.
27. Kunkel D, et al: *Sex on TV: content and context*, Santa Barbara, Calif, 1999, Henry J. Kaiser Family Foundation.
28. Nielsen Media Research, New York, 1998.
29. Palmer EL: *Television and America's children*, New York, 1988, Oxford University Press.
30. Peterson JL, Moore KA, Furstenberg FF Jr: Television viewing and early initiation of sexual intercourse: is there a link? *J Homosex* 21:93, 1991.
31. Peterson RA, Kahn JR: *Media preferences of sexually active teens*. Paper presented at the meeting of the American Psychological Association, Toronto, Canada, August 26, 1984.
32. Pierce JP, et al: Tobacco industry promotion of cigarettes and adolescent smoking, *JAMA* 279:511, 1998.
33. Princeton Survey Research, March 12-16, 1997.
34. Robinson TN, Chen HL, Killen JD: Television and music video exposure and risk of adolescent alcohol use, *Pediatrics* 102:e54, 1998.
35. Stockwell TF, Glantz SA: Tobacco use is increasing in popular films, *Tobacco Control* 6:282, 1997.
36. Strasburger VC: *Adolescents and the media: medical and psychological impact*, Newbury Park, Calif, 1995, Sage.
37. Strasburger VC: Children, adolescents, and the media: five crucial issues, *Adolesc Med State Art Rev* 4:479, 1993.

38. Strasburger VC: "Sex, drugs, rock 'n' roll," and the media: are the media responsible for adolescent behavior? *Adolesc Med State Art Rev* 8:403, 1997.
39. Strasburger VC, Donnerstein E: Children, adolescents, and the media: issues and solutions, *Pediatrics* 103:129, 1999.
40. Strouse JS, Buerkel-Rothfuss NL: Media exposure and the sexual attitudes and behaviors of college students. In Greenberg BS, Brown JD, Buerkel-Rothfuss N: *Media, sex and the adolescent,* Cresskill, NJ, 1993, Hampton Press.
41. Unnikrishnan N, Bajpai S: *The impact of television advertising on children*, New Delhi, 1996, Sage.
42. Wallack L, Cassady D, Grube JW: *TV beer commercials and children: exposure, attention, beliefs and expectations about drinking as an adult,* Washington, DC, 1990, AAA Foundation for Traffic Safety.
43. Willis E, Strasburger VC: Media violence, *Pediatr Clin North Am* 45: 319, 1998.

section three | School Health

70 Overview of School Health and School Health Program Goals

Philip R. Nader

"Health Care is not equivalent to Health. Education is not the same as learning. Health and learning must be defined by more than the current performance of the institutions that claim to serve these ends."

I. ILLICH, *DESCHOOLING SOCIETY*, NEW YORK, 1972, HARPER AND ROW.

Today many economic forces are reshaping the health care system. In addition forces within the educational system reflect an emphasis on traditional academics, but with greater willingness to involve community partners in meeting educational and support needs. Society now places increasing expectations on the school to deal with many of social issues. Similarly, new social problems are being defined as health concerns because of their direct connection with morbidity and mortality. For example, operating a motor vehicle while under the influence of alcohol has a direct economic impact on the health care system, as do the problems of violence in families, among peers, and in schools.

At least two major gaps exist in today's health care system: access to health care and lack of preventive services for youth. School health is rapidly being recognized as a lynchpin for the system to ensure a way to deal with these deficiencies. As with all issues in health care related to youth, this (r)evolution will depend on much larger changes that will sweep school health, along with the tide of reform in the health care system as a whole.

The recent proliferation of school-linked services is a direct outgrowth of these educational, health, and welfare reform movements. They develop most frequently in urban settings and target disadvantaged populations. However, one rural state, Vermont, is developing private-public partnerships to coordinate a wide range of human services for all children and their families.

Historically, school health was initiated to improve health and sanitary conditions in urban schools. A chronology of school health in relation to health care issues and public health is shown in Fig. 70-1.

SCHOOL HEALTH PROGRAM GOALS

The American Academy of Pediatrics' School Health Committee has suggested seven major school health program goals.[2] These goals were adopted by the Institute of Medicine's Report, *Comprehensive School Health: Our Nation's Investment* (1997).[3]

- Goal 1: Ensure access to primary health care
- Goal 2: Provide a system for dealing with critical medical situations
- Goal 3: Provide mandated screening and immunization monitoring
- Goal 4: Provide systems for identifying and solving students' health and educational problems
- Goal 5: Provide comprehensive and appropriate health education
- Goal 6: Provide a healthful and safe school environment that promotes learning
- Goal 7: Provide a system for evaluating the effectiveness of the school health program

Goal 1: Ensure Access to Primary Health Care

For school health programs to be effective, linkages must be formed between the school and the source of primary health care for the child. All pediatric providers might benefit from the ability to link their primary care services to schools for treatment of minor conditions, follow-up and screening, medication administration, immunization delivery systems, the monitoring of school absenteeism, and achievement for selected patients. Major difficulties arise when no regular source of care or insurance coverage exists.

Providers of primary care would be wise to examine ways to use school-based personnel to provide cost-effective services at school sites when it is deemed desirable for a given community. Although a school-based clinic could become a medical home for a family, given no other resources in a community, it would be preferable to develop additional resources so that each family could have an ongoing medical home that would be available over the long term. All school-based services should include provision for 24-hour, 7-day-per-week back-up extending beyond the school day and the school year. Newer systems of managed care need to examine the potential benefits of linking services to families through the schools.

Education Compulsory (Rhode Island) (1840)
Founding of American Medical Association (AMA) (1847)
Shattuck Report (1850)
Smallpox outbreak, New York City (1860)
Metropolitan Board of Health, New York City (1866)
Massachusetts Board of Health (1869)
Smallpox vaccination required for school attendance (1870)
Founding of American Public Health Association (APHA)
Koch Discovery-Age of Bacteriology (1876)
Hygienic Lab (forerunner of National Institutes of Health) (1887)
NYC nurses reduce absenteeism by 50% in several weeks (1902)
Pure Food and Drug Act (1906)
Flesner Report on Medical Education (Carnegie Foundation) (1910)
Joint NEA-AMA Committee on Health Problems (1911)
The Open Air Classrooms (1915)
Welch-Rose Report on Schools of Public Health (Rockefeller Foundation) (1915)
Cardinal Principles of Education (1918)
Maternity and Infancy Act (Sheppard-Towner) (1921)
All states with laws regarding school health, safety, nutrition, health screenings (1921)
Blue Cross Insurance (1929)
School Health Study American Child Health Association (1930)
Social Security Act (Title V and Title VI) (1935)
Astoria Plan (NYC) (1936)
Garfield/Kaiser Prepaid Group Practice (forerunner Kaiser Permanente)
Center for Control of Malaria in War Areas (forerunner of Centers for Disease Control) (1940s)
Kark Community-Oriented Primary Care Clinic—South Africa (1940s)
Hospital Survey and Construction Act (Hill-Burton) (1946)
Separation of primary health services from schools. AMA-NEA, scattered services to indigent populations (1920s-1950s)
Salk Polio Vaccine (1952)
Recognition of social morbidities (1960s)
SHES-School Health Education Study—10 conceptual areas (1960)
Surgeon General's Report on Smoking (1964)
Community Health Centers Program (1964)
Medicare and Medicaid Act (1965)
Health Professions Educational Assistance (1965)
Robert Wood Johnson Foundation Demonstration School Health (1970-1980)
US Health and Nutrition Projects (1970-1980)
Health Maintenance Organization (HMO) Act (1973)
LaLonde Report on Health of Canadians (1974)
Healthy People: Surgeon General's Report on Health Promotion and Disease Prevention (1979)
Medicare Payment Reform (1983, 1989)
Community-Oriented Primary Care (1984)
Health of the Public Program (1985)
DASH-CDC (1988)
The Future of Public Health (Institute of Medicine) (1988)
Healthy People 2000 (1988)
US Preventive Services Task Force: Guide to Clinical Preventive Services (1989)
Healthy Schools, Healthy Communities (1990)
HEDIS-Health Plan Employer Data and Information Set (1993)
Failure of Federal Health Reform (1993-1994)
National Education Goals (1994)
National Congress of the Medicine/Public Health Initiative (1996)
Institute of Medicine Report: Schools and Health (1997)
GWU Comprehensive School Health Initiative (1998)

1850 **Civil War** **1880** **1910** **World War I** **1920** **1930** **Great Depression** **1940** **World War II** **1950** **1960** **Great Society** **1970** **1980** **1990**

Key Health System Issues
Key Health Problems: Professionalism ___ Infrastructure Building ___ Improving Access Cost Control Market Forces Reinventing Government
Infectious Diseases ___ Chronic Diseases ___ Modern Challenges ___
Key Health Strategies:
Quarantine ___ Sanitary Reform ___ Maternal and Child Health Programs ___ Antibiotics ___ Screen and Treat ___ Managed Care ___
Water Systems ___ Pasteurization ___ Personal Hygiene ___ Hospital as Center of Care ___ Categorical Health Programs ___ Healthy Communities ___

Fig. 70-1 Medicine and public health timeline (1840-1998) and school health timeline.

Goal 2: Provide a System for Dealing with Critical Medical Situations

In addition to expected instances of trauma requiring immediate medical attention (e.g., crisis episodes of asthma or seizures), the school health service must be prepared to deal with life-and-death situations of medically fragile children who may be located on school campuses, as well as the unfortunate eruption of violence, shootings and suicide, and community disasters. Trained personnel, standing policies and procedures, and key decision makers need to be identified. Most urban schools have ready access to emergency 911 systems. The American Academy of Pediatrics (AAP) has published suggested guidelines and procedures for school health programs.[1]

Goal 3: Provide Mandated Screening and Immunization Monitoring

Pediatric care providers need to know the required immunizations and screening procedures and also when these are supposed to be carried out in the schools. Guidelines and recommendations vary among the states, and adherence to these regulations varies depending on local resources. Guidelines for establishing screening mandates often are created by the state legislature. Primary care providers can lobby for more reliance on scientific evidence and whether a proposed screening procedure meets scientific criteria for establishing screening programs. These criteria include having a reliable and valid method of screening, as well as having accepted, effective treatment or remediation available to students determined to be in need of services through screening.

Immunizations are required for school attendance in all 50 states. With recent initiatives for improving immunization rates among both school-age and preschool-age children, some schools are providing immunizations directly to school-age children and their preschool siblings. These may be especially important in reaching quality of care standards for immunizations required for the school-age population (such as second measles and hepatitis immunizations).

Goal 4: Provide Systems for Identifying and Solving Students' Health and Educational Problems

An important component of child functioning is academic achievement. Pediatric primary care providers need to inquire routinely about the school progress of their patients.

The completeness and effectiveness of problem identification and solution depend to a large degree on the numbers and quality of school health personnel. The more trained and sophisticated the personnel are, the more they can be expected to achieve. Differentiated staffing with appropriate use of aides, nurses, nurse practitioners, and physician consultant back-up is likely to be the most cost-effective way of responding to the identified needs of a population. Problems may be self-identified by parents and children themselves, or difficulties may be detected through observation in classrooms or consultation with teachers. An analysis of frequent visits to the school health room can identify students who may need attention. Close links to community sources of care for physical and mental health resources are required to develop treatment plans effectively.

Goal 5: Provide Comprehensive and Appropriate Health Education

It is somewhat ironic that the same educational movement that is leading schools to become involved in human services delivery systems is, at the same time, decreasing the already underemphasized role of health education. Health is referred to only obliquely in recent formulations of national educational standards and goals.

Health providers can support schools to enhance health education programs and services. Collaboration and integration with community-wide health promotion efforts are helpful. This espouses the concept that schools cannot do the job alone. Within the school, attempts should be made to relate all aspects of school life with the health program. For example, classroom health curricula need to be integrated with healthful choices in the school nutrition program and activity promotion in the school's physical education program. Schools should be smoke-free environments. Teachers need work-site programs to encourage them to be healthful role models for children and youth. Teachers also need information and skills to communicate and answer children's questions effectively. If they do not know the answers, teachers need to know where to find answers to questions about health.

Human sexuality education programs are needed on a much wider basis than currently are provided to children and youth in this country. Health care providers can help communities see the value of comprehensive health education programs, including education about sexuality. One way to introduce such programs gradually is to develop them jointly with the school. The program can be located in school, but the instruction can be provided by health personnel and teachers. Courses for parents and children will increase acceptability.

Goal 6: Provide a Healthful and Safe School Environment that Promotes Learning

In addition to the environmental aspects of comprehensive school health education mentioned above, other environmental conditions need to be guaranteed. Teachers should be as knowledgeable as possible about principles of child development. Teaching strategies need to be matched to the developmental and cognitive capabilities of children. Research has shown that systems that espouse noncoercive discipline and high academic expectations have the best educational outcomes.

Attention must be given to the physical safety of the school environment. This includes the presence of possible toxic agents, as well as the potential spill-over of neighborhood violence onto school campuses.

Goal 7: Provide a System for Evaluating the Effectiveness of the School Health Program

Because school health programs in the future will be linked more closely to existing and new systems of health care delivery in a community, evaluation will become an integral part of program planning and assessment. A community-needs assessment can determine the needs and resources present in a particular community. The needs assessment should involve all key child health, education, and social services leaders in the community and be broadly based across both private and public sectors. The needs assessment will guide the development of the extent of school-linked or school-based health services to be used.

As mentioned previously, selection of outcome indicators to be measured at periodic intervals will demonstrate to program planners and funders the usefulness of the programs established. It will be important to include outcome indicators for all seven goals for school health programs. Potential outcomes for each goal are listed in Table 70-1. For example, monitoring problem identification and outcomes can be useful by providing rationale and justification for services, as well as assessing needs for additional services.

INTEGRATED SERVICE SYSTEMS

Pediatric primary and secondary care providers need to take an active role in the development and implementation of so-called integrated service systems. These "one-stop" programs propose to streamline and make social, health, and family support services more cost effective and user friendly. Often, these services are placed in (or near) a school and include multiple human services in one easily accessible place. Health services often rank high among perceived needs in these systems. Exactly how to link such programs with the various services, including the great need for mental health services, often presents significant barriers.

The Health-Promoting School

The World Health Organization's Healthy Schools Initiative is addressing school health in many countries around the world. This initiative stresses starting with the school culture and ethos, moving to policy organization and procedures, and then addressing curriculum, teaching, and community involvement. The components in a health-promoting school are illustrated in Fig. 70-2.

Role of the Pediatrician in School-Linked Services

Pediatric primary care providers may serve as consultants to or be directors of comprehensive school-based or school-linked health programs. In these roles, the provider will (1) have had experience in planning, managing, and evaluating systems of care; (2) be knowledgeable about funding and programmatic requirements in both health and education; and (3) be able to establish quality assurance programs. These skills will build on a solid clinical expertise in child and

Table 70-1 Potential Outcome Measures for School Health Program Goals

Goal	Outcome Measure(s)
One: Access to primary care	Number (%) of students who have an identifiable medical care home (ongoing source of primary health care) Decrease in use of emergency departments for nonemergent care
Two: Critical medical situations	Number (%) of staff who have active CPR certification Presence of standing emergency medical orders No preventable deaths Reduction in school accidents
Three: Mandated screening and immunization	Number (%) of vision referrals made, confirmed to need correction, and fitted (using corrective lenses) Number (%) of false-positive screening results (referred but found not to have needed referral) Number (%) referred and not reaching a source of care Number (%) of students up-to-date on required immunizations
Four: Identification/solution of problems	Number (%) of problems identified that are corrected or being dealt with Absenteeism rates; dropout rates Number (%) at risk of academic failure (retention)
Five: Health education	More healthful school lunches (decreased fat and salt) More aerobic/active PE classes Existence of parental programs in health Existence of comprehensive sexual education course(s)
Six: School environment	Smoke-free school No incidents of violence in school Soap, water, paper towels, and toilet paper available
Seven: Evaluation	Existence of a plan for evaluation and publication of an annual report

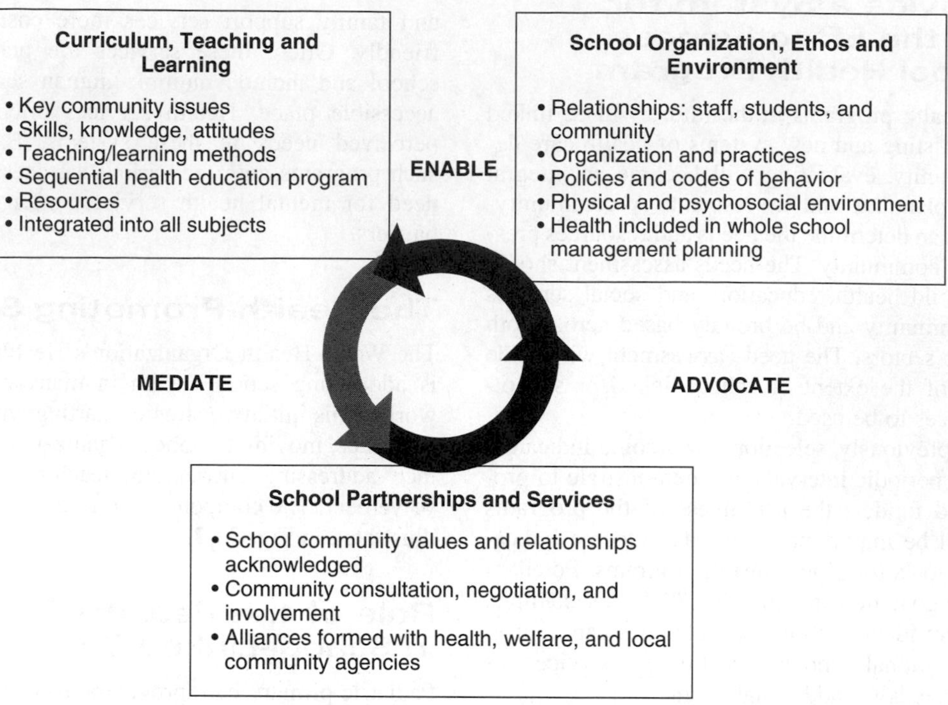

Fig. 70-2 Three components interact dynamically to create a health-promoting school.

youth health issues, as well as firsthand knowledge and expertise with schools and educational systems.

The role of the primary or special care provider requires less expertise in program development and evaluation but does require knowledge of the educational system and how to access the system for the benefit of the patient. These roles may be related to the school by nurse practitioners or other physician-extender personnel who are stationed in or visit the school regularly.

Guidelines for physicians as school consultants have been suggested.[1] Table 70-2 and Boxes 70-1 to 70-3 illustrate examples of activities and suggested guidelines and approaches to be used by primary or secondary care providers interested in working with schools in their locale.

School Health Content for Pediatric Primary Care Providers

First, pediatric clinicians must be current with new approaches and use school-linked human services programs to reach families in need. They should understand the basic principles of community organization and the need for increased public policy support for school-linked preventive care. Second, pediatric clinicians need to be aware of the seven major goals of a comprehensive school health program. Third, they need to be aware of the multitude of health and nonhealth personnel who play key roles. Unless pediatric clinicians are aware of the child development principles from preschool through adolescence, they cannot help implement comprehensive school health programs effectively.

A wide variety of clinical problems are encountered commonly in school health practice, including the following:

1. School attendance and school avoidance problems
2. Psychosomatic complaints
3. Learning problems
4. Attention-related disorders
5. Behavioral and disciplinary problems
6. Medically fragile, technologically dependent students
7. Various communicable diseases, in students and teachers
8. Sexually transmitted diseases, including HIV
9. Substance use and abuse

Because medications, including psychoactive drugs, sometimes are needed to keep children in school and "on task," the clinician must master ways to ensure medication compliance. Standardized procedures for medication administration in schools are available.[2]

Objectives for Educating Physicians in School Health

Many methods of teaching about school health are available. One of the best ways is to expose trainees to experiences in community-based programs. Those responsible for developing educational experiences need to use faculty and staff who have had experience in school health services and schools. Objectives have been developed for medical students, residents, and fellowship trainees in community and school health. They have been published in the American Academy of Pediatrics' manual, *School Health: Policy and Practice*.[2]

CONCLUSION

School health programs are rapidly developing to a point where they may more likely reach their potential in ensuring access to care, as well as provide a good system of preventive health care. Pediatric care providers need to become integral parts of these systems; only in this way will they continue to play a major role in improved health and health educational outcomes for children.

Table 70-2 The Physician's Role in Schools

Clinical Issue/Problem	Examples of Physician's Activities as Child's Primary Health Care Practitioner	Examples of Physician's Activities as Consultant to School or School System
Learning disability	1. Requests teacher's perception of child's learning and behavior; results of individualized testing 2. Shares results of medical evaluation of child with the school 3. Works cooperatively with school personnel and parent(s) to develop educational and behavioral management plan for child (may include school visit) 4. Sets up mechanism for follow-up on behavioral and educational progress of child	1. Serves on district committee to accomplish biannual review of handicapped children's progress 2. Assists in setting up mechanism for providing follow-up behavioral and academic information to physicians who have placed students on psychoactive medication 3. Provides in-service session for classroom teachers on new concepts in attention deficit disorder 4. Advises school board on need for movement training for children who have learning disabilities
Asthma (school-age)	1. Requests school information on absenteeism, visits school nurse, obtains evidence of nonparticipation in physical education activities 2. Sets up mechanism for regular administration of bronchodilator at school 3. Sets up follow-up mechanism for continued monitoring of school attendance, medication-taking compliance, and participation in appropriate physical activities	1. Reviews absenteeism data to identify groups of students who have excessive absences that might be amenable to some intervention 2. Assists curriculum director and nurse in developing educational program for children who have asthma and their parents 3. Helps publicize program and communicates directly with students; solicits primary care physician's input and support for the educational program by reinforcing concepts in their patient visits

From Nader P: *Pediatr Rev* 4:82, 1982.

BOX 70-1

GUIDELINES FOR PHYSICIAN AS CHILD'S CARE PROVIDER

1. Always obtain permission from the parents to communicate with the school and keep them informed of their child's progress.
2. Approach all school personnel as coprofessionals who have skills and interests that complement your expertise and that can provide you with information you do not have. Recognize their interest in helping the children in their charge.
3. When contacting a school for the first time, contact the principal initially.
4. When calling a teacher, find out the best time for him or her to talk.
5. Encourage direct school-parent and parent-school communication.
6. Be willing to attend a school meeting, if necessary, to share information and develop treatment plans.
7. Listen carefully to ascertain the school personnel's main concerns and questions and attempt to respond to them.

BOX 70-2

GUIDELINES FOR PHYSICIAN AS SCHOOL HEALTH CONSULTANT

1. Distinguish between roles of a primary health care practitioner and those of a school consultant.
2. Become aware of laws and regulations affecting schools, including those related to school finance, education for handicapped children, bilingual education, and other educational mandates.
3. Become knowledgeable about the formal and informal decision-making processes in schools regarding "regular" and "special" education of children (including health education).
4. Be a liaison to the rest of the medical community.
5. Establish a contract with the school that defines mutually agreed upon expectations and objectives.
6. Provide a regular report on your consultation to the school district.
7. Attempt to establish relationships with all levels and departments of the school system to permit access from the board and superintendent level to that of the classroom teacher.
8. Become aware of group process dynamics and decision making in groups.

BOX 70-3

A CHECKLIST

State Policies and Programs

Have you apprised yourself of state policies and programs related to comprehensive school health programs?

Have you checked to see whether health outcome objectives exist, and if so, how they are assessed?

Local Policies and Programs

Have you apprised yourself of district policies and programs related to comprehensive school health programs?

Have you determined what health curriculum, textbooks, and materials actually are being used in the schools?

Have you ascertained the following:

- policies and programs that need strengthening?
- serious gaps or deficits?
- opportunities for health professionals to contribute meaningfully?

Influencing Local Policies and Programs

Do you know how the local education system works? Who makes decisions? Who has authority? Who actually does the work?

Do you know who supports (and who is concerned with) various aspects of comprehensive school health programs and their reasons for doing so?

Have you contacted appropriate officials about your ideas and obtained their support for working with schools?

Have you refined your ideas in consultation with key parties—teachers, administrators, school health professionals, public health professionals, school board members, and parents?

Have you provided for periodic progress reports and changed direction or emphasis based on their results?

From National Association of State Boards of Education: *How schools work and how to work with schools,* Alexandria, Va, 1989, The Association.

REFERENCES

1. American Academy of Pediatrics, Committee on School Health: *Guidelines for the administration of medication in school*, Pediatrics 92:499, 1993.
2. American Academy of Pediatrics, Committee on School Health: *School health: policy and practice*, ed 5, Elk Grove Village, Ill, 1993, American Academy of Pediatrics.
3. Institute of Medicine: *Comprehensive school health: our nation's investment*, Washington, DC, 1997, National Academy Press.

SUGGESTED READINGS

Barnett S, Duncan P, O'Connor KG: Pediatricians' response to the demand for school health programming, *Pediatrics* 103:E451-E457, 1999.

Kaplan DW, Calonge BN, Guernsey BP, Hanrahan MB: Managed care and school-based health centers: use of health services, *Arch Pediatr Adolesc Med* 152:25-33, 1998.

Nader PR: A pediatrician's primer for school health activities, *Pediatr Rev* 4:82, 1982.

National Association of State Boards of Education: *How schools work and how to work with schools*, Alexandria, Va, 1989, The Association.

71 School Health Education

Guy S. Parcel • Laura K. McCormick • Sharon S. Cummings

Our increased awareness of the limitations inherent in the curative aspects of health care has made for greater emphasis on the importance of health maintenance and preventive medicine. Through the years health education has been used to help individuals prevent illness and maintain the best state of health possible for them. The underlying assumption has been that an informed public is better prepared to make decisions that will promote health.

Within this framework, health education in the schools has become particularly attractive. Almost all children go to school and while in school constitute a "captive audience." Thus, schools have been suggested as the logical place for children to learn about health and to develop the abilities needed to make effective decisions about health-related behavior. However, it has yet to be demonstrated that schools can meet this objective. As the search continues for ways to improve the effectiveness of school health education, it is becoming increasingly clear that success must involve a cooperative effort between educational and health care personnel. For example, the pediatrician's knowledge of child health and development is much greater than that of most educational personnel in the schools. Therefore, the child health care professional has an essential role in school health education programs. On the other hand, most educational personnel have more refined and effective skills in teaching and a greater opportunity to reach more children than do pediatricians. They also have more time to devote to the process.

Including health education as part of the instructional program in schools is by no means a new concept. Through the involvement of a school nurse or school physician, health education activities have become part of school health services. For example, while screening for vision and hearing, the school nurse can discuss with the children, either individually or in groups, the purpose of the screening and the importance of health care in terms of sight and hearing. The school nurse also could go into the classroom and instruct the students in particular health habits, such as dental health (brushing teeth) or nutrition (good eating habits). When health instruction is incorporated into the curriculum of the regular classroom teacher or the special health education teacher, it is referred to as *curricular health education.* Health education is either integrated into the classroom curriculum or established as a separate curriculum within the total instructional program of the school.

TRENDS IN SCHOOL HEALTH EDUCATION

Early approaches to curriculum development in health education focused primarily on specific types of health problems, particularly those associated with risky or illicit behavior. In the 1950s, it was recognized that drinking had become a serious health and social problem. In an attempt to solve this problem, school personnel were called on to provide instruction, pointing out the dangers and health hazards associated with alcohol consumption. It was assumed that if students knew about these dangers and were told about the health hazards, they would avoid alcohol abuse. Some states went so far as to enact laws requiring public schools to instruct students in the prevention of alcohol abuse.

It has been demonstrated, however, that even when information is presented effectively, it does not necessarily lead to a change in behavior. Many drug education programs were developed that effectively taught the pharmacological aspects, legal penalties, and physical risks of drug abuse; however, evaluations of these programs revealed that they had a limited effect on alcohol abuse and other drug use.[2] Similar results from nutrition and tobacco education programs in the late 1960s, 1970s, and early 1980s further demonstrated the weaknesses of health education programs based primarily on a cognitive approach.[6,18]

This failure reinforced what many educators had been suggesting for years—that health behavior is related not only to knowledge but also to factors such as expectations and values associated with health behavior. It also became apparent that health-related problems could not be resolved effectively on a "crisis" basis; if health problems were to be prevented through education, a means of addressing these problems had to be developed long before they reached a state of crisis. Teaching methods that focus on the learners' attitudes and feelings fall into the realm of *affective education.* Teaching in this area is related more to personal development than to learning facts and concepts. Affective education programs hypothesize that children who feel good about themselves, who can develop effective relationships with others, and who clearly understand what is important to them are less likely to have problems with drug abuse. For the teacher, this approach involves helping students to build self-esteem, to learn interpersonal skills, and to develop effective decision-making and problem-solving techniques.

As an outgrowth of the increased interest in affective education, in the 1970s many school health education programs were expanded or redirected to focus more on attitudes, feelings, and values. Some suggested programs tended to deemphasize the importance of information, whereas others emphasized an integration of cognitive and affective learning. However, a review of affective approaches to preventing substance abuse concluded that, in general, they made no significant impact on substance use.[7]

In the 1980s, school-based interventions were grounded in social learning, which typically involved training students to resist social pressure to engage in unhealthy behavior (e.g., smoking), as well as creating a social environment that encouraged the development of healthy behavior.[14,21]

Social learning methods were expanded to the health education curriculum, which led to development of the *social influences approach*. This approach recognized the importance of preparing students to resist the pressures of an environment that encouraged risk-taking behavior. Teaching strategies in this approach include augmenting students' knowledge about the short-term consequences of risky behavior, training in resisting peer pressure, "inoculation" against mass media messages, establishing normative expectations for healthful behavior, using peer leaders as role models, and having students make a personal commitment to avoid risk-taking behavior or to engage in healthy behavior. These methods have been applied successfully to smoking prevention[19] and drug abuse prevention,[17] and evaluations have indicated a significant effect in reducing risk-taking behavior.

Another approach in school health education from the 1980s is the use of skill development methods to prevent risky behavior. The *skills approach* assumes that a set of social and behavioral skills is essential for making effective decisions about health behavior. Furthermore, if students are able to develop these skills, if they know the consequences of risky behavior, and if they have opportunities to practice these skills, they will be more likely to avoid risk-taking behavior and develop healthier patterns. The skills usually addressed in these types of programs involve decision making, problem solving, communication, and stress management or relaxation. The skills approach has been shown especially effective when applied to smoking; it also has proved effective in other areas of health behavior.[4]

Youth empowerment is a recent model of school health education. The underlying principle of this model is that students must be responsible for identifying and defining the problem to be addressed and determining what action should be taken. Because many of the issues addressed by school health education have roots in community and social problems, the health education process should enable students to recognize these roots and determine appropriate social or community actions to effect positive changes.

Besides the health education curriculum, the concept of school-based health promotion and disease prevention has been expanded to include other components of the school that influence or facilitate healthy behavior.[10] Such programs have been developed to coordinate classroom health instruction with changes in school food services and physical education, thus improving the diet and amount of physical activity of elementary schoolchildren.[14] Efforts also have been made to involve parents and to focus on the family as a critical component in influencing changes in health behavior through school-based programs.[12,19] Linking school-based programs with community programs and agencies also has shown potential for improving the effectiveness of existing programs concerned with promoting healthy behavior and preventing health problems.[16,17,22] In the 1990s, many schools used this multiple component approach to school health education. This approach has been used successfully in an elementary school-based cardiovascular health trial,[11] a community-based alcohol use prevention program for young adolescents,[20] a high school-based intervention to prevent pregnancy and HIV/STD infections,[3] and a middle school-based violence prevention intervention.[9]

The latest multiple component approach for school health education is based on the *comprehensive school health education (CSHE) model*. CSHE programs involve health education; physical education; health services; nutrition services; health promotion for staff; counseling, psychological, and social services; a healthy school environment; and parent and community members' involvement. CSHE programs also involve a set of strategies, activities, and services that provide a sequence of events at each grade level to address each designated content area (e.g., nutrition, safety, substance abuse, chronic disease, infectious disease, mental health, growth and development, and family living). In 1997, the Institute of Medicine published a report written by its committee on CSHE programs in grades K-12.[8] The committee examined the status of school health education programs and made recommendations for the future regarding four topics of school health: education, services, infrastructure, and research and evaluation. Although many components of the CSHE program exist in schools across the country, the committee reported that many programs lack the involvement of critical community stakeholders (e.g., parents, students, educators, health and social service personnel, insurers, and business and political leaders). Additionally, they concluded that one of the most difficult issues to resolve is for CSHE programs to help students obtain access to private-sector services such as preventive and primary health care.

THE PHYSICIAN'S ROLE IN SCHOOL HEALTH EDUCATION

The goal of health education is to help people develop skills and confidence that will enable them to make good choices about their health behavior and about appropriate use of health care resources. If this goal is to be achieved through a school health program, it will require a cooperative effort by health care and educational personnel. In structured classroom activities and in noncurricular health education activities, the physician can contribute to school health education in five distinct ways: (1) by reviewing the content and process of health education for accuracy and age appropriateness, (2) by conducting health education activities for children and parents through the school program, (3) by assisting with the training of personnel involved in health education, (4) by helping to collect data to evaluate the outcomes of health education activities, and (5) by encouraging community support for school health education activities.

The physician can help develop a health education curriculum by identifying the health concerns related to specific age groups. Physicians are aware of the health concerns of and needs expressed by their patients. These concerns and needs can be identified and interpreted for educational personnel in planning health education activities. With the physician's help, critical skills can be identified for the various age groups, and once these skills have been identified, activities can be developed to help children develop them.

Physicians, particularly pediatricians, also can help teachers understand the normal processes of child development and help them identify children's developmental needs. Teachers are required to master a broad spectrum of information related to health behavior, and it is difficult for them to stay current in all these areas. The physician can be especially helpful by alerting teachers to recent information about specific areas of health and by suggesting resources for additional information. There usually is a gap between data generated by the health sciences and the information available for use in instructional programs. The physician can help narrow this gap.

Physicians may be called on to serve as guest lecturers in classrooms. When a teacher is faced with complicated or sensitive material, such as information on HIV or AIDS, contraception and family planning, substance abuse, or specific diseases, the physician may be asked to talk to students. The easiest way for physicians to handle such a request is to visit the classroom. However, there are some obvious drawbacks to this approach. The physician may not be prepared to present the material at a level appropriate for the students, and the physician's time will be limited. A better approach is for the physician to work with the teacher to identify the information students need. Together the physician and teacher can plan an ongoing program that the teacher can then present. In this way, a larger number of students can benefit from the physician's contribution over a longer period.

The time, effort, and resources devoted to the school health education curriculum depend on the priority a school district places on health education. When it comes to health, physicians obviously enjoy considerable influence and prestige in a community. Spending time with school board members and administrators can encourage a high priority for the school health education curriculum. The following section outlines a strategy for physicians and other community members to follow in developing a comprehensive school health education program in their communities.

AN APPROACH TO DEVELOPING HEALTH EDUCATION PROGRAMS

Planning Committees

An initial group consisting of the top school administrators and school staff likely to have responsibility for the health program should be formed to establish the guidelines and process for program planning. Regardless of the level of community enthusiasm and support for health education, school administrators and staff always should be included at the highest levels of the decision-making process to approve and support program development officially. A second group then is organized to develop the program. This program planning group should be made up of administrators, teachers, students, parents, and resource people or consultants from the community and should establish strong communication links with the decision-making group.

Assessment of Needs and Resources

The planning group will need information to determine the scope and direction of the proposed program. Useful information can be obtained from a review of the literature and of programs from other school districts. However, information about the local situation is essential to direct the program toward meeting local needs. Standardized survey questionnaires can be used to measure students' current health knowledge, attitudes, and behaviors. This information can be useful in setting priorities for the program.

Information also should be obtained about the resources available for a health education program. Individuals who have training and experience in health education, in effective educational techniques, in the development of interpersonal skills, and in methodologies of social learning are invaluable resources. It also is important to identify potential sources of funding (local, state, and federal) and available instructional materials and consultants.

Development of Program Goals and Objectives

Goals, the outcomes expected to result from the program, should be realistic and achievable. The goals preferably should be stated in such a way that the extent of their achievement can be measured. For example: (1) at the end of 5 years, the number of youths younger than age 19 arrested for driving under the influence of alcohol or drugs will be reduced by 30%; or (2) at the end of 3 years, the number of youths who begin smoking in the eighth grade will be reduced by 50%. Goals that include statements about "when," "how much," "of what," and "by whom" add specificity that provides more direction and focus for the education program.

The next step is to state specific objectives for each goal by student grade level. Objectives are accomplished by students and, therefore, usually are stated in behavioral terms and address what the student is expected to be able to do as a result of this instruction. For example, the student will be able to (1) demonstrate how to use techniques to resist peer pressure, (2) apply steps in decision making to resolve a conflict about food selection in a social situation, and (3) use relaxation techniques to cope with feelings of stress.

Program Activities

Activities are the experiences that provide the knowledge, skills, practice, reinforcement, and confidence for performing the behaviors stated in the objectives. Activities are linked to objectives and should not be developed until after the specific goals and objectives for the health education program have been identified. Attention also should be given to activities outside the classroom that will support and reinforce classroom learning. Activities for parents, teachers, and other school staff are valuable in providing the social support and environment for reinforcing the learning of new behaviors.

It is helpful to conduct a pilot program in one school or a few schools to test ideas and techniques and to make changes before a districtwide program is implemented. Once a pilot program has worked effectively and has been shown to be acceptable, it usually is easier to implement in other schools in the district. It is essential that the pilot program be evaluated in such a way that components that may require modification can be identified.

Teacher Preparation

In-service training for teachers is essential for implementing a new curriculum. Such training should include attitudinal support for the curriculum and specific teaching skills. Attention also should be given to involving other school personnel who might not teach the curriculum but whose support for it is important. For example, the school principal, nurse, counselor, or social worker should be involved in planning the implementation of the program.

IMPLEMENTATION OF CHANGE

Change in school systems tends to occur slowly, often because of the lack of a systematic approach to effect change. This phenomenon is especially relevant to the introduction of innovative programs to promote school health, an area in which change often needs to occur within several components of the total school program. The model for implementing change in schools has four phases: (1) organizational commitment, (2) change in policies and practices, (3) alteration of roles and actions of staff, and (4) implementation of learning.[13] This model is intended to provide a systematic approach to change that includes school components that support and facilitate behaviors addressed by health education programs in the classroom.

In the first phase, commitment is obtained from key decision-makers in the school system to proceed with the planning of a new or modified health promotion program. A top-down approach would involve school board members, superintendents, and program directors arriving at a decision to commit to the proposed program. The proposal for the new program can come from an agency outside the district, such as a health department or voluntary health agency, or from inside groups, such as curriculum planning committees or task force groups appointed to address specified problems. Commitment usually is obtained through a series of meetings with key decision-makers. These meetings typically involve a written or verbal presentation on the importance of and need for the proposed program. Physicians can provide information to help establish a high priority for proposed health promotion programs.

Commitment also needs to be obtained from a bottom-up, or grassroots, approach, in which the individuals who implement the program (teachers and staff members) are involved in making decisions about planning new or modified programs. One method for obtaining this type of commitment, the "seaside" model (named for a seaside retreat in Oregon), has been implemented in several states. The seaside model involves teams from school districts coming together in a conference to explore their own personal health promotion needs, as well as those of their students. The process involves planning a health promotion program or activity for their district. Recently the seaside model has been expanded to include community representatives. This experience often results in a strong personal and professional commitment for health promotion programs.

Once commitment is demonstrated, a policy-planning group composed of the program directors and key administrators should be established to develop and define policies. The policies then are given to a second planning group to address changes that will be needed in current practices to follow through on the intent of the policies necessary to the new program. This second planning group usually consists of program directors and representatives of teachers and staff members who will be implementing the program.

The third phase focuses on preparing the teachers and staff members to implement the program. In-service training, technical assistance, and monitoring and feedback can be used to alter roles and actions of personnel to implement new programs. Finally, with these changes in place, the school program is ready to provide activities that will help the students develop healthy behavior. Student activities should include classroom instruction, practice in school, practice at home, and reinforcement and social support from the school for practicing the healthy behaviors.

REASONABLE EXPECTATIONS FOR SCHOOL HEALTH EDUCATION

The health professional may expect that, to be effective, health education must influence behavior to reduce the risk of disease or to improve health status. The educator, however, might argue that the role of the school is to increase knowledge and develop critical thinking and not necessarily to change student behavior, which may be greatly influenced by factors outside the classroom. Both perspectives could be considered correct, and each will influence how programs are designed and evaluated.

School health education programs can help students learn about their health. Evaluations of school health education programs have demonstrated their effectiveness in influencing a variety of outcomes, including knowledge, attitudes, health practices, behavior, and physiological factors.[5,15,17,19,22] The program's effect on learning, and eventually on behavior, depends on the quality of the planning and the input of sufficient resources, including teacher training and adequate classroom instructional time.[5] Behavioral change, however, is complex, and simplistic approaches that do not effectively use what has been learned both in research and in the field are unlikely to succeed.

It is unreasonable to expect school-based educational programs alone to influence behaviors that are not supported by the child's larger social environment. For example, how can a child change to a low-fat diet when the other family members continue their same eating patterns? How can an adolescent be expected to avoid the social use of drugs or alcohol when the larger social environment not only supports but also encourages the use of alcohol and drugs? How can an adolescent be expected to prevent an unwanted pregnancy when the appropriate counseling and health services are difficult to find and use? School health education programs should be planned with a consideration of reasonable outcomes and the type of program necessary to accomplish those outcomes.

The CDC's Division of Adolescent and School Health has identified six health risk areas to be targeted by school and community programs: HIV and sexually transmitted diseases, injuries, nutrition, physical activity, alcohol and illicit drug use, and tobacco use. They are supporting this effort by developing a series of guidelines for schools to assist in the planning, implementation, and evaluation of school health programs. The CDC also has supported the American Medical Association (AMA) in the development of the AMA's Guidelines for Adolescent Preventive Services (GAPS),[1] which are designed to set priorities and establish standards for the provision of preventive services by primary care physicians. Although these efforts target different segments of the community (schools and primary care physicians), they have the same long-range goal: improving the health of adolescents. Ultimately, this goal will be realized only when various segments of the community exist within a larger framework of coordinated services.

It is unreasonable to expect that a single unit on health education placed within the total curriculum will accomplish the development of skills needed to adopt healthy behaviors. A comprehensive approach that provides knowledge, the development of skills, and practice in a developmental sequence through each of the grade levels is necessary. It also is important to relate the health education program to other parts of the school curriculum and programs. Students need numerous opportunities to experience personal development, and the social environment of the school should be structured to support students in their practice of decision-making and related skills.

REFERENCES

1. American Medical Association, Department of Adolescent Health: *Guidelines for adolescent preventive services,* Chicago, 1992, The Association.
2. Bangert-Drowns RL: The effects of school-based substance abuse education: a meta-analysis, *J Drug Educ* 18:243, 1988.
3. Basen-Engquist K, et al: The safer choices project: methodological issues in school-based health promotion intervention research, *J School Health* 67:365, 1997.
4. Botvin GJ: Prevention of adolescent substance abuse through the development of personal and social competence. In Glynn T, editor: *Preventing adolescent drug abuse: intervention strategies,* NIDA Research Monograph Series, No 47, Washington, DC, 1983, US Government Printing Office.
5. Connell DB, Turner RR, Mason EF: Summary of findings of the school health education evaluation: health promotion effectiveness, implementation, and costs, *J Sch Health* 55:316, 1985.
6. Contento IR, Manning AD, Shannon B: Research perspectives on school-based nutrition education, *J Nutr Educ* 24:247, 1992.
7. Hansen WB: School-based substance abuse prevention: a review of the state of the art in curriculum, 1980-1990, *Health Educ Res* 7:40, 1992.
8. Institute of Medicine: *Schools & health: our nation's investment,* Washington, DC, 1997, National Academy Press.
9. Kelder SH: The Students for Peace Project: a comprehensive violence-prevention program for middle school students, *Am J Prev Med* 12:22, 1996.
10. Kolbe LJ: Increasing the impact of school health promotion programs: emerging research perspectives, *Health Educ Q* 17:47, 1986.
11. Luepker RV, et al: Outcomes of a field trial to improve children's dietary patterns and physical activity: the child and adolescent trial for cardiovascular health (CATCH), *JAMA* 275:768, 1996.
12. Nader PR, et al: A family approach to cardiovascular risk reduction: results from the San Diego Family Health Project, *Health Educ Q* 16: 229, 1989.
13. Parcel GS, Simons-Morton BG, Kolbe LJ: Health promotion: integrating organization change and student learning strategies, *Health Educ Q* 15:435, 1988.
14. Parcel GS, et al: School promotion of healthful diet and physical activity: impact on learning outcomes and self-reported behavior, *Health Educ Q* 16:181, 1989.
15. Parcel GS, et al: Translating theory into practice: intervention strategies for the diffusion of a health promotion innovation, *Fam Community Health* 12:1, 1989.
16. Pentz MA: Community organization and school liaisons: how to get programs started, *J Sch Health* 56:382, 1986.
17. Pentz MA, et al: A multicommunity trial for primary prevention of adolescent drug abuse, *JAMA* 261:3259, 1989.
18. Perry CL, Kelder SH: Models for effective prevention, *J Adolesc Health* 13:355, 1992.
19. Perry CL, et al: Parent involvement with children's health promotion: a one-year follow-up of the Minnesota home team, *Health Educ Q* 16: 171, 1989.
20. Perry CL, et al: Project Northland: Outcomes of a communitywide alcohol use prevention program during early adolescence, *Am J Public Health* 86:956, 1996.
21. Perry CL, et al: The Child and Adolescent Trial for Cardiovascular Health (CATCH): overview of the intervention program and evaluation methods, *Cardiovasc Risk Factors* 2:36, 1992.
22. US Department of Health and Human Services: Preventing tobacco use among young people: a report of the Surgeon General, Atlanta, 1994, Centers for Disease Control and Prevention.

72 School Readiness

Robert S. Byrd

School readiness is extremely important to the health and well-being of children, and early school performance often predicts and profoundly affects later school success. According to a national survey of kindergarten teachers, 35% of percent of children are not "ready for school," and a fourth of these children (8%) will repeat kindergarten or first grade.[3]

Identifying problems at school entry leaves little time to alter a child's early academic course. Delaying entry is associated with its own problems.[4] Thus, it is imperative that health professionals use their 10 to 20 contacts with children before they start school to continually assess progress and promote readiness. Those children who have successful transitions to school fare better academically, and those whose educational careers are marked by achievement are more likely to lead healthier lives. Persons with a high school education or less have over twice the death rate than those with more than a high school education resulting from chronic disease, injury, and communicable disease.[23]

DIMENSIONS OF READINESS

Children are not simply "ready" or "not ready" for school. The National Educational Goals Panel describes five dimensions to school readiness: (1) physical well-being and motor development; (2) social and emotional development; (3) approaches toward learning; (4) language development; and (5) cognition and general knowledge.[19] Based on a national survey of kindergarten teachers, physical well-being ranked sixth on their list of problems that most restrict school readiness for children. Deficiencies in language was felt to be the most important problem, followed by problems with emotional maturity, general knowledge, social confidence, moral awareness, and finally, physical well-being.[1]

Pediatricians and other child health providers have a special responsibility to address health conditions that may impair school readiness. Aspects of physical health are presented in more detail later in this chapter. Shonkoff summarizes the diverse effects of health problems as follows:

> "Ultimately, the extent to which a child's developing competence and readiness for school is influenced by health factors depends upon a complex interplay among inherent adaptive capacities, the presence and severity of adverse symptoms, and the quality of his or her caregiving and social supports."[20]

The dimension of social and emotional development encompasses early bonding, attachment, self-concept, self-control, and skills in peer relations. To understand the importance of this facet of school readiness, one need only consider some conditions at the extreme: reactive attachment disorder, autism, conduct disorder, or oppositional-defiant disorder. Social competence can be defined as "those skills and behaviors of a child that lead to positive social outcomes with the individuals residing in a given setting and that avoid socially unacceptable responses." Lack of social skills is associated with increased school dropout rates, adolescent and adult mental health problems, and juvenile delinquency.[18]

Approaches toward learning include motivation, perseverance, curiosity, temperament, active versus passive learning styles, initiative, openness to new challenges, imagination, and values. Parents can promote both positive and negative approaches to learning. For example, parents who enjoy reading and share this with their children may pass on their love for reading to their children. Conversely, parents whose literacy skills are limited may pass on their anxieties about reading every time their child sees them struggle with written materials. Negative approaches to learning are not limited to socially and economically disadvantaged children. Use of flashcards and other early drills in reading may not only advance early reading skills but also leave children with little desire to be readers.[20]

Delayed language development is cited most frequently by kindergarten teachers as the problem that most restricts children's school readiness.[1] Language development is more than acquisition of expressive and receptive language skills. The context for language usage also is important. For example, many children are used to parents asking them questions for which the parent already knows the answer. However, children lacking this experience may not know how to respond to a teacher asking them a question that the child knows the teacher should know.

Parents reading to children is one of the most important readiness-promoting activities. Television, although a language medium, has not been shown to promote early language skills and seems to undermine school readiness.[7] The richness of a child's daily language environment can differ by millions of words over the course of the preschool years. The content seems to be more affirming for children in "word-rich" environments and more command oriented or negative among the children living with a paucity of words.[14]

Cognition and general knowledge is the dimension of readiness that receives the most focus by parents who are attuned to preparing their children for school. Parents are more likely than teachers to judge readiness based on basic academic skills, such as knowledge of colors, shapes, numbers, and the alphabet.[26] Some parents believe that the schools will teach children everything that they need to learn and, thus, do little to prepare their children for school. At the other extreme are children in socially advantaged households, some of whom have far too many experiences structured into their lives, many not being developmentally appropriate.[10,11]

There is no universally accepted standard of how much basic knowledge is optimal for school readiness; everyone learns by building on what already is known.[12] A child exposed to an environment in which everything is new has a harder time assimilating what is being taught. Learning by preschool children should be structured so that it is an active process with activities that are developmentally appropriate. Learning should be fun and associated with play for the preschool child to increase basic knowledge while fostering good approaches toward learning.[2]

NEUROBIOLOGICAL AND DEVELOPMENTAL CONSIDERATIONS

Findings from developmental neurobiology support readiness promotion. Infants' brains are one fourth the weight of adults' brains. The infant brain undergoes significant changes in making new synaptic connections and then pruning away connections that are not used.[25] These changes that shape the brain occur largely from birth to about 5 years, or at a time well before formal schooling.

An extreme lack of stimulation results in loss of function. Vision in one eye, for example, can be lost permanently when a congenital cataract obstructs the visual stimulation for a sufficient length of time, even if the anatomical defect is later corrected. Animal models have shown that young animals raised in stimulating environments have greater brain growth than animals raised in less-stimulating environments.[8,15]

Later remediation has to overcome both the deficiencies in a child's experiences and the limitations on brain growth resulting from a lack of developmentally appropriate stimulation. Most often, children are not born with a fixed developmental lesion, but rather their developmental outcomes are the cumulative sum of developmental insults and developmentally enhancing experiences. Data from the Abecedarian Project[17] provide an example of how an effective intervention can ameliorate the effect of multiple developmental insults. Children whose mothers had significant cognitive impairment but who received early educational input from birth through 3 years were shown to have normal IQ scores at age 3 years; on the other hand, children from similar families who did not receive early educational input had IQ scores averaging in the low 70s at age 3 years. This provides strong evidence of our ability to override negative environmental influences on cognitive development.

CLINICAL APPROACHES TO PROMOTING READINESS

A systematic clinical approach to school readiness promotion includes (1) identification of physical conditions, (2) screening for developmental conditions that hinder or impair school readiness, (3) recognition of factors that confer developmental risk, and (4) anticipatory guidance.

Common physical conditions that have been correlated with lack of school readiness include anemia, elevated blood lead levels, passive exposure to tobacco smoke, low birth weight and prematurity, vision and hearing deficits, frequent ear infections, and poor nutrition.[3,24] Children should receive screening at age-appropriate intervals and as warranted by the history or physical examination. Prevention of these conditions obviously is preferable to screening and treatment. In cases in which prevention and treatment do not eliminate the risk for early school problems, early intervention services may ameliorate the risk, as in the case of prematurity. Thus, health supervision in preschool children is a primary aspect of readiness promotion.

Screening for developmental delays, especially language delays, is essential. Although 60% of pediatricians use developmental screening tests, such as the Denver Developmental Screening Test (DDST), only 15% do so routinely (see Chapter 20 [Thirteen], Developmental Surveillance and Intervention). Some offices have incorporated a developmental specialist into their practice.[9] Most child health providers rely on clinical judgment, but this approach alone has not been effective in identifying problems of children who require special education services.[22] Early intervention services have increased as a result of PL 99-457 and should provide developmental assessments for any young child suspected of delays and services for those found to have significant delays. At each well-child visit, assessment of parental concerns and special attention to language delays should guide practitioners in making early referrals.

Assessment of risk for early school problems is an approach that can augment developmental screening. Low birth weight and other perinatal insults increase the risk for early school problems.[3] However, adverse socioeconomic and familial factors play the preeminent role in producing emotional difficulties and diminution in cognitive functioning, except when a child has experienced a severe biological insult. Factors present at birth that may impair the developmental quality of the home environment include poverty, single parent household, low maternal education, teen parent, large family, family history of mental retardation or school problems, and parental mental health problems, such as maternal depression. Other environmental factors that may be evident later but still contribute to developmental risk include family stress and lack of age-appropriate play materials and children's books in the home. The presence of multiple risk factors greatly increases the likelihood of early school problems, and recognition of risk allows for intervention before developmental delays are evident. In addition, when a school-age child is identified as having school problems, preventive efforts should be directed toward any preschool siblings.

Referrals for at-risk children who are not yet failing to meet their developmental milestones are more problematic. With the exception of Head Start, most early intervention services are failure based, requiring children to be sufficiently delayed before they can receive help. The effectiveness of primary care clinicians in promoting school readiness among at-risk children requires collaboration with community services or the development of support services within clinical settings. Although families of at-risk children can be referred to Head Start or other preschool compensatory education programs,[6] these interventions for 4-year-olds are available too late for many at-risk children. Programs for younger children and their families that promote good parenting, language stimulation, and learning through play are available in many communities.

Assisting in finding high quality, developmentally stimulating child care and helping a mother learn to read to her child through referral to adult education programs are useful preventive measures. Although no single universal program meets the myriad of educational needs of at-risk children, pediatricians aware of early childhood resources and adult education services in their communities can make appropriate referrals and help parents provide nurturing and stimulating environments for their children.

Regardless of educational risk or developmental delay, school readiness should be promoted at each health supervision visit. *Bright Futures: Guidelines for Health Supervision of Infants, Children, and Adolescents*[13] includes recommendations for anticipatory guidance that encourage language and literacy development, curiosity, self-esteem, and social skills. The recommendations most applicable to the promotion of school readiness are listed in Box 72-1.

Language mastery is one of the keys to school readiness, and reading to children by parents is one of the most important readiness-promoting activities. Infants learn language interactively from parents who talk, sing, and play with them; who respond to their babbling, engaging them in "conversation" before there are words to speak; and who read to them. The Reach Out and Read program, in which infants to school-age children receive an age-appropriate book at each health supervision visit, while the importance of reading is stressed to parents as part of well child care, provides an effective model for the promotion of practice-based language/literacy.[21] Parenting classes and other programs that encourage language stimulation may also be helpful.

Television viewing does not promote language development and seems to shorten children's attention for classroom situations, where the teacher's face does not change every 7 seconds (as does the image on the TV). Preschoolers in the United States watch an average of 28 hours of television per week; children from families of lower socioeconomic status watch even more. Television viewing by preschoolers limits the time they spend reading, playing with peers, building with blocks, coloring with crayons, cutting with scissors, and most importantly, interacting with caring adults. When discussing TV "limits" during preschool health supervision visits, clinicians can suggest activities that promote cognitive and social development.

Delaying school entry is a common, yet unproven practice aimed at improving a child's readiness for school. Some children deemed unready are denied entry to school and remain in the same environment that failed to foster their readiness. Although the youngest children in a class may evidence some difficulties at school entry, little difference persists by the third or fourth grades.

By adolescence, students who are older than the majority of their classmates have higher rates of parent-reported behavior problems[4] and youth-reported health risk behaviors, including substance use.[5] Some schools have an enrichment rather than a remedial strategy for at-risk students, aimed at bringing all students into the educational mainstream by the end of elementary school and performing at levels appropri-

BOX 72-1

SCHOOL READINESS: ANTICIPATORY GUIDANCE*

- Spend time playing with and talking to your baby during her quiet, alert states (newborn, 1 month)
- Read to the baby (2, 4, 6, 9 months)
- Encourage play with age-appropriate toys (2, 4, 6 months)
- Play music and sing to your baby. Music can contribute to a soothing environment for infants (2, 4, 6, 9 months)
- Encourage the baby's vocalizations. Talk to him during dressing, bathing, feeding, playing, walking, and driving (4, 6, 9 months)
- Provide opportunities for exploration (6, 9, 12, 36 months)
- Encourage language development by reading books to the toddler, singing her songs, and talking about what you and she are seeing and doing together (12, 15, 18, 24 months)
- Limit television and video viewing to less than 1 hour per day of appropriate programs
  - If children are watching TV, parents also should watch along with their children (limiting the use of TV as a babysitter and enhancing the parents' ability to discuss what their children are watching) (12, 15, 18, 24, 36, 48 months)
- Encourage play, which is a way of learning social behavior (15 months)
- Encourage the toddler's autonomous behavior, curiosity, sense of emerging independence, and feeling of competence (15 months)
- Model appropriate language (18, 24 months)
- Appreciate the child's investigatory nature, and do not excessively limit his explorations
  - Guide him through fun learning experiences (24 months)
- To promote a sense of competence and control, invite the child to make choices whenever possible. (The choices should be ones you can live with—e.g., "Red pants or blue ones?") (18, 24 months)
- Encourage interactive reading with the child (36, 48 months)
- Encourage the child to talk with you about her preschool, friends, or observations
  - Answer her questions (36, 48 months)
- Give the child opportunities to make choices (e.g., which clothes to wear, books to read, places to go) (36, 48 months)
- Provide opportunities for the child to socialize with other children in play groups, preschool, or other community activities (36, 48 months)
- Enlarge the child's experiences through trips and visits to parks and other places of interest (48 months)

Data from Green M, Palfrey JS, editors: *Bright futures: guidelines for health supervision of infants, children, and adolescents,* ed 2, Arlington, Va, 2000, National Center for Education in Maternal and Child Health.

*Months shown in parentheses represent the well-child visit(s) at which the anticipatory guidance noted should be provided.

ate to their age group.[16] Unfortunately, most schools set "slower" students on slower paced, remedial tracks, which over time distances them further from their "more ready" peers.

Overcoming the lack of school readiness requires intensive efforts by parents, children, and schools, but even with these efforts, educational outcomes generally are not as good as those of children who begin ready for school.

A 5- to 6-year window of opportunity begins at birth to help enhance children's readiness for school. Developmental assessments help identify children who have developmental delays. Children at risk for school problems can be referred to early childhood programs as a preventive measure. Anticipatory guidance at each health supervision visit can assist parents in enhancing their child's readiness for school. As professionals who consistently assess preschoolers' progress over multiple stages of early development, primary care clinicians can help families prepare their children for school.

REFERENCES

1. Boyer EL: *Ready to learn: a mandate for the nation,* Princeton, NJ, 1991, Carnegie Foundation for the Advancement of Teaching.
2. Bredekamp S, Copple C, editors: *Developmentally appropriate practice in early childhood programs,* revised edition, Washington, DC, 1997, National Association for the Education of Young Children.
3. Byrd RS, Weitzman ML: Predictors of early grade retention among children in the United States, *Pediatrics* 93:481, 1994.
4. Byrd RS, Weitzman M, Auinger P: Increased behavior problems associated with delayed school entry and delayed school progress, *Pediatrics* 100:654, 1997.
5. Byrd RS, Weitzman ML, Doniger AS: Increased drug use among old-for-grade adolescents, *Arch Pediatr Adolesc Med* 150:470, 1996.
6. Campbell FA, Ramey CT: Effects of early intervention on intellectual and academic achievement: a follow-up study of children from low-income families, *Child Dev* 65(2 Spec No):684, 1994.
7. Clarke AT, Kutz-Costes B: Television viewing, educational quality of the home environment, and school readiness, *J Educ Res* 90:279, 1997.
8. Comery TA, et al: Increased density of multiple-head dendritic spines on medium-sized spiny neurons of the striatum in rats reared in a complex environment, *Neurobiol Learn Mem* 66:93, 1996.
9. Developmental specialist in pediatric practice, *Zero to Three Bulletin* June/July 1997.
10. Elkind D: *The hurried child: growing up too fast too soon,* Reading, Mass, 1981, Addison-Wesley.
11. Elkind D: *Miseducation: preschoolers at risk,* New York, 1987, Knopf.
12. Gardner H: *The unschooled mind: how children think and how school should teach,* New York, 1991, Basic Books.
13. Green M, editor: *Bright futures: guidelines for health supervision of infants, children, and adolescents,* Arlington, Va, 1994, National Center for Education in Maternal and Child Health.
14. Hart B, Risley TR: *Meaningful differences in the everyday experience of young American children,* Baltimore, Md, 1995, Paul Brooks.
15. Jones TA, Greenough WT: Ultrastructural evidence for increased contact between astrocytes and synapses in rats reared in a complex environment, *Neurobiol Learn Mem* 65:48, 1996.
16. Levin HM: Educational acceleration for at-risk students. In Huston AC, editor: *Children in poverty: child development and public policy,* New York, 1991, Cambridge University Press.
17. Martin SL, Ramey CT, Ramey SL: The prevention of intellectual impairment in children of impoverished families: findings of a randomized trial of educational daycare, *Am J Public Health* 80:844, 1990.
18. Meisels SJ, Atkins-Burnett S, Nichalson J: Assessment of social competence, adaptive behaviors, and approaches to learning with young children, Working Paper No. 96-18. Washington, DC, 1996, National Center for Education Statistics.
19. National Education Goals Panel: *The National Education Goals Report: Building a Nation of Learners, 1996,* Washington, DC, 1997, Government Printing Office.
20. National Education Goals Panel: Reconsidering children's early development and learning: toward common views and vocabulary (electronic publication), http://www.negp.gov/Reports/child-ea.htm.
21. Needlman R, et al: Clinic-based intervention to promote literacy, *Am J Dis Child* 145:881, 1991.
22. Palfrey JS, et al: Early identification of children's special needs: a study in five metropolitan communities, *J Pediatr* 111:651, 1987.
23. Pamuk E, et al: Socioeconomic status and health chartbook. In *Health, United States, 1998,* Hyattsville, Md, 1998, National Center for Health Statistics, p 90.
24. Pollitt E: Iron deficiency and educational deficiency, *Nutr Rev* 55(4):133, 1997.
25. Purves D, et al: Neural activity and the development of the somatic sensory system, *Curr Opin Neurobiol* 4:120, 1994.
26. West J, Hausken EG, Collins M: Readiness for kindergarten: parent and teacher beliefs, *Statistics in Brief* (NCES 93257), Washington, DC, 1995, US Department of Education, National Center for Education Statistics.

73 Attention Deficit/Hyperactivity Disorder

Karen J. Miller • Esther H. Wender

Attention deficit/hyperactivity disorder (AD/HD) is the most common significant pediatric behavioral disorder. The cluster of behaviors (behavioral syndrome) appears early in a child's life and typically persists throughout childhood and adolescence. The defining behaviors involve a persistent pattern of inattention and/or impulsivity/hyperactivity that is more frequent and severe than typically observed in individuals of the same age and gender. Core symptoms and related problems occur along a continuum and manifest in various combinations and within specific family, academic, and social contexts. The challenge for the clinician is to differentiate primary attention dysfunction from normal variations, inattentiveness resulting from other causes, environmental factors, and the contribution of related disorders. Careful assessment is needed to develop an appropriate treatment plan.

PRESENTING PROBLEMS

Inattention

Children who have difficulty regulating attention processes are often described as having a short attention span and being impersistent and distractible. They may not "stick with" activities requiring sustained concentration. They may daydream or have difficulty shifting from a preferred to a less preferred activity. They do not seem to listen or attend to social cues and often appear immature. They require more supervision and reinforcement than other children. In school, their forgetfulness, disorganization, superficial attention to important details, rapid mental fatigue, and poor management of time lead to markedly inconsistent performance.

Hyperactivity

The young child who has AD/HD may be in constant motion, be jumping about, and be unable to sit still for stories or meals, but may appear glued to the spot for TV or video games. The school-age child often will talk excessively, fidget, or fiddle with anything within reach. Overt hyperactivity tends to decline with age; adolescents may be merely restless. Children who have the inattentive type of AD/HD (see previous paragraph) may appear underactive and sluggish.

Impulsivity

Children who have AD/HD have difficulty inhibiting responses. They become overexcited, grabbing or touching even when told not to. They often are described as noisy, impatient, and overreactive. School work is rushed or incomplete. They frequently interrupt others or act without thinking of consequences. Persistent impulsivity in adolescence can result in serious trouble.

Related Problems

AD/HD often occurs with other disorders and inappropriate behaviors. Children who have AD/HD often have difficulty controlling their emotions and may be easily angered or overly sensitive. They may have difficulty getting along with other children. Some show oppositional, defiant, or negativistic behaviors and are noncompliant. Aggression and antisocial behaviors may occur. Learning problems may indicate an underlying learning disability. (See Differential Diagnosis in this chapter.)

DIAGNOSTIC CRITERIA

The symptom complex associated with AD/HD has been described for more than 100 years, although terminology has changed and controversy continues over definition and boundaries. The 1994 revision of the *Diagnostic and Statistical Manual of Mental Disorders,* fourth edition *(DSM-IV),* defines three subtypes: predominantly inattentive, predominantly hyperactive/impulsive, and combined. The diagnostic behavioral criteria are presented in Box 73-1. Age and gender are not currently taken into account.

Although the new criteria require impairment of functioning in multiple settings, it is unusual for a child to display the same level of dysfunction in all settings or within the same setting at all times. Symptoms typically worsen in situations that require sustained attention and mental effort or that lack intrinsic appeal. They are more likely to occur in group settings. Symptoms may be minimized when the situation provides immediate reinforcement or novelty such as video games or is highly supervised such as at a doctor's visit. Because the symptoms may not be observed directly by the clinician, observations by parents, teachers, and other caregivers are essential.

In primary care settings, symptoms may not present with sufficient frequency or intensity to warrant a diagnosis of AD/HD or may represent only a variation in development. This continuum from normal variation to problem to disorder is recognized in the *Diagnostic and Statistical Manual for Primary Care: Child and Adolescent Version (DSM-PC).* The

BOX 73-1

DIAGNOSTIC CRITERIA FOR ATTENTION DEFICIT/HYPERACTIVITY DISORDER

A. Inattention or hyperactivity-impulsivity
1. Inattention: At least six of the following symptoms of inattention have persisted for at least 6 months to a degree that is maladaptive and inconsistent with the patient's developmental level:
   - Often fails to give close attention to details or makes careless mistakes in school work, work, or other activities
   - Often has difficulty sustaining attention in tasks or at play
   - Often does not seem to listen to what is being said to him or her
   - Often does not follow through on instructions and fails to finish school work, chores, or duties in the workplace (not because of oppositional behavior or failure to understand directions)
   - Often has difficulties organizing tasks and activities
   - Often avoids, expresses reluctance about, or has difficulties engaging in tasks that require sustained mental effort (e.g., schoolwork or homework)
   - Often loses things necessary for tasks or activities (e.g., school assignments, pencils, books, tools, or toys)
   - Often is easily distracted by extraneous stimuli
   - Often is forgetful in daily activities
2. Hyperactivity-impulsivity: At least six of the following symptoms of hyperactivity-impulsivity have persisted for at least 6 months to a degree that is maladaptive and inconsistent with developmental level

Hyperactivity
   - Often fidgets with hands or feet or squirms in seat
   - Often leaves seat in classroom or in other situations in which remaining seated is expected
   - Often runs about excessively in situations when it is inappropriate (in adolescents or adults, may be limited to subjective feelings of restlessness)
   - Often has difficulty playing or engaging quietly in leisure activities
   - Is always "on the go" or acts as if "driven by a motor"
   - Often talks excessively

Impulsivity
   - Often blurts out answers to questions before the questions have been completed
   - Often has difficulty waiting in line or awaiting his or her turn in games or group activities
   - Often interrupts or intrudes on others (e.g., butts into other's conversations or games)

B. Some symptoms that caused impairments are present before age 7 years
C. Some symptoms that cause impairment are present in two or more settings (e.g., at school, work, or home)
D. Evidence of clinically significant impairment in social, academic, or occupational functioning must be clear
E. Does not occur exclusively during the course of a pervasive developmental disorder, schizophrenia, or other psychotic disorder and is not accounted for better by a mood disorder, an anxiety disorder, or a personality disorder

Codes

314.00 Attention Deficit/Hyperactivity Disorder, Predominantly Inattentive Type: If criterion A(1) is met but not criterion A(2) for the past 6 months
314.01 Attention Deficit/Hyperactivity Disorder, Predominantly Hyperactive-Impulsive Type: If criterion A(2) is met but not criterion A(1) for the past 6 months
314.01 Attention Deficit/Hyperactivity Disorder, Combined Type: If criterion A(1) and A(2) are met for the past 6 months
314.9 Attention Deficit/Hyperactivity Disorder, Not Otherwise Specified

From American Psychiatric Association: *Diagnostic and statistical manual of mental disorders,* ed 4, Washington, DC, 1994, The Association.

DSM-PC also outlines relevant differential diagnoses, comorbid conditions, developmental issues, and environmental factors that affect a child's functioning.

PREVALENCE AND ETIOLOGY

The prevalence of AD/HD among school-age children is generally reported to be 3% to 5% with somewhat higher rates when the new criteria are used. The male:female ratio is estimated to be between 3:1 to 6:1. Symptoms of AD/HD emerge in early childhood and continue into adulthood in up to 70% of cases.

Multiple etiologic factors are implicated, with strong evidence for a genetic predisposition that interacts dynamically with the environment to produce the clinical features. Evidence exists that neurotransmitter dysfunction, involving primarily dopamine and norepinephrine, impairs behavioral inhibitory systems. Neuroimaging and neuropsychological studies support the central role of the prefrontal lobes and basal ganglia in AD/HD. No specific diagnostic test is currently available. The diagnosis remains based on characteristic clinical presentations and observable behaviors viewed within a developmental and psychosocial context.

DIFFERENTIAL DIAGNOSIS AND ASSOCIATED CONDITIONS

Differential diagnosis refers to the process of surveying for conditions or factors that might produce behaviors that look like AD/HD, but are not. However AD/HD frequently coexists with other disorders and conditions, and these conditions may be the primary problem, producing symptoms that look like but are not AD/HD. The complexities of these relationships are summarized in Table 73-1.

Comorbidity is common and has substantial impact on functioning, treatment, and prognosis. Symptoms of learning disabilities, behavioral disorders, emotional problems, and AD/HD overlap significantly. Between 10% to 40% of children who have AD/HD have learning disabilities. Oppositional defiant disorder (ODD) is manifested by a pattern of negativistic, hostile interactions (Box 73-2) and occurs in 30% to 60% of children who have AD/HD. The child who has AD/HD and ODD is more likely to develop antisocial behaviors and conduct disorder over time, which increases the risk of substance abuse, delinquency, and other negative outcomes. Depression and anxiety disorders may present with impaired concentration and performance problems, but both of these disorders also may co-exist with AD/HD.

A number of medical conditions, such as fetal alcohol syndrome or other central nervous system disorders, result in learning and attention problems. When children who have these medical conditions have symptoms of inattention and/or hyperactivity/impulsivity that qualify for the diagnosis of AD/HD, they should be treated for both the medical con-

Table 73-1 Differential Diagnosis and Comorbidity

Disorders	Likely to Co-Exist with AD/HD	Likely to Produce Symptoms Similar to AD/HD
Developmental Differences		
Normal variation		x
Mental retardation	x	
Giftedness	x	x
Learning disabilities	x	x
Perceptual/processing disorder	x	x
Language disorders	x	x
Pervasive developmental disorder		x
Fragile X	x	
Medical Disorders		
Sensory impairments		x
Seizure disorders	x	
Sequelae of CNS infection/trauma	x	x
Fetal alcohol syndrome	x	
Lead poisoning	x	
Iron-deficiency anemia		x
Neurodegenerative disorders	x	
Tourette's syndrome	x	
Thyroid disorders	x	x
Substance abuse	x	x
Medication side effects		x
Undernutrition		x
Sleep disorder	x	x
Enuresis and encopresis	x	
Motor coordination disorders	x	
Emotional/Behavioral Disorders		
Depression/mood disorders		x
Anxiety disorders	x	x
Oppositional defiant disorder	x	
Conduct disorder	x	
Obsessive compulsive disorder	x	
Posttraumatic stress disorder		x
Adjustment disorder	x	x
Environmental Disorders		
Child abuse/neglect	x	x
Stressful home environment	x	x
Inadequate/punitive parenting	x	x
Parental psychopathology	x	x
Sociocultural difference	x	
Inappropriate educational setting		x

dition and the AD/HD. Inappropriate parental expectations, inadequate school placement, stressful environments, and adverse psychosocial conditions may either produce behaviors that are mislabeled as AD/HD or increase symptom expression in a child who has AD/HD.

The reciprocal interaction between children and their environment is always important. The presence of a child who has AD/HD appears to increase family stress, feelings of parental incompetence, and marital conflict. However, an increased rate of psychopathology exists in these families based, in part, on a genetic predisposition to the same problems that have affected the child. The causal direction is not always clear. The child's disruptive behavior may precipitate family turmoil, but a dysfunctional family system can contribute to disorganized behavior in a child. Both in home and at school, children who have AD/HD are often highly sensitive to differences in the way they are managed, indicating the important effects of the environment on their behavior.

ASSESSMENT

A comprehensive, developmentally oriented history is essential to define presenting problems, clarify diagnostic issues, identify related problems, and understand the child's academic and psychosocial context (Box 73-3). Input from teachers provides valuable insight because the child's performance can be compared with that of his or her peers.

BOX 73-2

CRITERIA FOR OPPOSITIONAL DEFIANT DISORDER

A. A pattern of negativistic, hostile, and defiant behavior lasting at least 6 months, during which four (or more) of the following are present:
   1. Often loses temper
   2. Often argues with adults
   3. Often defies or refuses to comply with adults' requests or rules
   4. Often annoys people deliberately
   5. Often blames others for his or her own mistakes or misbehavior
   6. Often is touchy or easily annoyed by others
   7. Often is angry and resentful
   8. Often is spiteful or vindictive

   Note: A criterion is considered met only if the behavior occurs more often than is observed typically in individuals of comparable age and developmental level.
B. The disturbance in behavior causes clinically significant impairment in social, academic, or occupational functioning.
C. The behaviors do not occur exclusively during the course of a psychotic or mood disorder.
D. Criteria are not met for conduct disorder, and, if the individual is 18 years of age or older, criteria are not met for antisocial personality disorder.

From the American Psychiatric Association: *Diagnostic and statistical manual of mental disorders,* ed 4, Washington, DC, 1994, The Association.

Questionnaires and behavior rating scales completed by both parents and teachers facilitate data collection and screen for multiple disorders in addition to AD/HD (see list of resources at the end of this chapter). Some of the standardized questionnaires used commonly and developed by Connors have recently been revised. The long form versions of the parent, teacher, and adolescent rating scales include *DSM-IV* criteria. The *Child Symptom Inventory* by Gadow also rapidly screens for multiple disorders. Rating scales are quite useful but indicate only current functioning and may be subject to observer bias.

Sensory, physical, and formal neurological examinations of children who have AD/HD are usually normal, but such assessments provide opportunities to observe the child's behavior, motor coordination, language skills, and social style. Behavioral observations should be interpreted cautiously, because children may show few AD/HD symptoms in this setting. Decisions to perform laboratory studies, such as thyroid screening or electroencephalography, should be based on clinical indications. Lead level and hematocrit screening should be considered in preschool children. Computer-based continuous performance tests cannot be relied on to help

BOX 73-3

ASSESSMENT OF CHILDREN SUSPECTED OF HAVING AD/HD

Parent Interview

Chief concerns
History of core symptoms and related disorders
Medical history
Developmental history
School history
- Remedial or special education or retention
- Development of academic skills
- Classroom functioning

Psychosocial history
- Temperament/personality
- Current emotional status
- Relationships with parents/adults
- Relationships with siblings/peers
- Sociocultural setting and stresses
- Current management strategies

Family history
- AD/HD/behavioral disorders
- Psychiatric disorders
- Academic disorders
- Medical disorders (tics, cardiac, thyroid)

Child interview/observation
Physical/neurological/developmental examination
Laboratory studies (when indicated)
School data (e.g., report cards)
Current teacher report/observations
Psychoeducational evaluation (IQ, achievement)
Behavioral rating scales
Language evaluation (when indicated)
Occupational evaluation (when indicated)
Mental health evaluation (when indicated)

From Miller KJ, Castellanos FX: *Pediatr Rev* 19:373, 1998.

make a diagnosis. Multiple factors affect performance on these tests, and underdiagnosis is common. Referral to a developmental-behavioral subspecialist, a pediatric neurologist, or a mental health professional may be indicated for complex cases.

Information from the school about past and current functioning is essential. Review of school records (report cards, standardized testing) provides valuable information regarding the chronicity of behavioral problems and evidence of a possible learning disorder. If a learning disability is suspected, either the parents or the physician may request individually administered assessments of cognitive ability (IQ) and academic achievement. Language and motor evaluations also may be indicated. Schools are federally mandated to perform appropriate evaluations if a child is suspected of having a disability, such as AD/HD or a learning disorder, that impairs academic functioning.

MANAGEMENT OF AD/HD

Management begins during the assessment process by establishing a team approach, which includes the child, family, physician, school personnel, and others. This "therapeutic alliance" has substantial impact on adherence to recommendations. The characteristics of each child and the stresses and resources within the family, school, and community must be considered when developing a multi-modal treatment plan that integrates behavioral, emotional, academic, and medical interventions.

Behavioral Interventions

Behavioral intervention should include counseling about the effect of AD/HD on behavior and response to discipline. Parents and children must understand that they did not cause this biologically based disorder but are responsible for its management. Information sheets, book suggestions, and referral to parent support groups help accomplish this goal (see list of resources at the end of this chapter). Parents often benefit from referral to a mental health professional for training in basic management strategies and behavior modification. The child may benefit from training in social skills.

Basic management involves providing increased structure, giving clear directions, and using developmentally appropriate parenting techniques. Behavior modification involves the systematic application of specific techniques that target maladaptive behavior patterns at home or school. The most effective programs target a limited number of behaviors and provide prompt feedback, positive and negative consequences, and consistency across settings.

Operant conditioning strategies to modify behaviors include increased positive attention ("catch them being good"), punishment procedures (e.g., time-out) and "selective ignoring." Charts or point systems that track specific behaviors can be useful. Training in social skills involves instructing the child in specific strategies and using behavior modification to reinforce those skills.

Studies show these behavioral interventions can result in short-term improvement in targeted behaviors, but gains appear to be limited by inability to use learned skills independently, lack of maintenance once the intervention is discontinued, and the difficulty that adults have sustaining behavior programs consistently. Behavior management combined with stimulant medication is more effective than behavior management alone, but usually no more effective than stimulant medication alone. However, behavior therapy in a structured setting may permit the use of a lower dose of methylphenidate. Also, the studies that demonstrate the effectiveness of stimulant medication are short term. The favorable effects of behavior management are likely to be more long term, although this has yet to be proven.

Emotional Interventions

Emotional interventions address psychological, emotional, social, and family issues to improve adaptation and psychosocial functioning of children and families. Preservation of self-esteem is a primary goal. Strategies can include "reframing," competency and social development, individual psychotherapy, family or parental therapy, and support groups.

The clinician often can help families caught in negative interaction patterns by reframing problem behaviors ("hyperactivity") or temperament characteristics as positive traits ("high energy") that need to be regulated better. Areas of competence should be developed through hobbies and sports. Individual psychotherapy has not been found to be effective for core symptoms of AD/HD, but it may be indicated to treat low self-esteem, interpersonal issues, demoralization, depression, anxiety, or psychosocial stressors such as parental divorce. Family therapy may be needed to address family dysfunction or facilitate behavior management, especially of adolescents. Therapy for the parents may be indicated in cases of parental psychopathology or marital discord. Participation in support groups is very beneficial for families and individuals, especially the newly diagnosed.

Academic Interventions

Appropriate academic programming, effective classroom management, and good communication with school personnel are crucial. The majority of children who have AD/HD can be served in the mainstream, but some will need tutoring, resource room support, inclusion or blended classes, or self-contained special education. Speech and language therapy may be indicated to address language-processing deficits. Graphomotor, fine motor, or gross motor dysfunctions are common and may require modified expectations or occupational therapy, physical therapy, or adaptive physical education services. Assistive technology, such as computers or calculators, may improve productivity. Modifications may be needed at the classroom level (e.g., assignments written on the board), at the task level (e.g., extended time), or at the individual level (e.g., a private signal when "off-task"). Providing opportunities to develop areas of expertise fosters respect for individual variations among students.

AD/HD is considered a disability under the Individuals with Disabilities Education Act (PL 101-476) and may qualify under the "Other Health Impaired" category for special education or related services. Children who have AD/HD, but who do not require special education services, may qualify for appropriate accommodations within regular education settings under Section 504 of the Rehabilitation Act of 1973, a civil rights legislation that prohibits discrimination against persons who have disabilities. The Americans with Disabilities Act (1990) may provide individuals who have AD/HD with reasonable accommodations in secular private schools, postsecondary education, and the workplace.

Medical Interventions

Medical problems that imitate symptoms of AD/HD or compromise functioning must be identified and treated. Medical illness, drugs used to treat other conditions, or exacerbations of chronic conditions can cause cognitive, behavioral, or academic functioning to deteriorate. Adequacy of sleep, nutrition, and exercise should be reviewed.

When the symptoms of AD/HD are having a significant negative effect on the child's ability to function academically and socially, medication should be considered, at least as a component of the initial treatment. Medication is the only form of treatment that can change the child's ability to control his or her aberrant behaviors, at least in the short term. This improved ability to behave appropriately often has a powerful positive impact on self-esteem, which should be considered as the primary goal of this form of treatment. Psychostimulants continue to be first-line medications for AD/HD. Nonstimulant medications may be appropriate in some cases, but research on this subject is limited. The combination of stimulants with other medications should be approached carefully because of the lack of controlled data.

Stimulant medications. Stimulant medications have been researched extensively for the last 60 years and have been demonstrated to be a safe and highly effective treatment for AD/HD. Stimulant use in the United States has almost tripled in recent years. This increase is due largely to heightened awareness of AD/HD, especially the inattentive subtype, as well as to the increase in treatment of adolescents and adults. In 1995, approximately 2.8% (1.5 million) of youths 5 to 18 years of age in the United States were receiving methylphenidate.

The use of psychotropic medication in children has received a great deal of attention in the popular press. Parents, teachers, or children may have unrealistic fears or excessive expectations concerning these medications. The clinician must provide accurate information; obtain the cooperation of the parents, school, and the child; and carefully monitor treatment response.

Methylphenidate (Ritalin) accounts for more than 80% of stimulant prescriptions. Other stimulants include dextroamphetamine (Dexedrine), pemoline (Cylert), and a combination of amphetamine salts (Adderall) (Table 73-2). Stimulant medications act by increasing the intrasynaptic availability of dopamine and norepinephrine, with resulting enhancement of attention processes, sensitivity to reinforcement, and behavioral inhibitory controls. Stimulants do not have a "paradoxical effect"; individuals who have and who do not have AD/HD show qualitatively similar responses.

Stimulant medications temporarily improve the core symptoms of AD/HD: Attention span is increased, activity level is normalized, and impulsivity is reduced. In school, academic productivity and performance improve. If a child is oppositional and defiant, compliance often is increased, emotional lability reduced, and aggressive behaviors decreased. Therapeutic response varies, and about 70% will respond to the first stimulant tried. If alternative stimulants and a wide range of dosages are tried, the response rate increases to 85% to 90%. However, the response to medication cannot be used as a "test" for AD/HD, because 10% to 30% of those whose AD/HD is appropriately diagnosed do not respond.

Common side effects include transient appetite suppression, weight loss, delay in sleep onset, and rebound hyperactivity when the medication wears off. Medication may slow weight gain and growth velocity slightly, but no evidence exists of effect on adolescent growth or ultimate adult height. If medication-related growth effects are suspected, modifying dosage or scheduling, increasing caloric intake, or increasing medication-free periods may be appropriate. Routine "drug holidays" are unnecessary.

Stimulants should be taken with meals to reduce stomach upset. Insomnia may be managed by structuring bedtime routines, eliminating the afternoon dose, or adding a dose if the child is unable to settle down because of the return of symptoms. A mild hypnotic such as an antihistamine may be beneficial. It is important to obtain baseline assessment of symptoms because sleep and appetite problems are common in children who have AD/HD, before treatment with medication.

Side effects observed less frequently are stomachaches, headaches, moodiness, fatigue, and jitteriness. Tics and dyskinesias may develop when the child is on stimulants, but no evidence exists that stimulants produce permanent tic disorders. About 50% to 60% of children who have Tourette's syndrome also have AD/HD, which often presents 2 to 3 years before the onset of tics. The majority of children who have tics and AD/HD obtain benefit on moderate doses of stimulants without unacceptable worsening of tics. Stimulants do not lower the seizure threshold but may alter blood levels of anticonvulsants. Cardiovascular effects can include minor changes in pulse and blood pressure. Overmedication may result in fatigue, agitation, withdrawn behavior, or a dazed appearance.

No evidence exists that substance abuse results from properly prescribed stimulants in adolescents who have AD/HD. In fact, some evidence suggests that the adolescent who has AD/HD who is appropriately treated with stimulants may be less likely to abuse substances (see Biederman, et al, 1999, in Suggested Readings). The risk of substance abuse in adolescence is increased when conduct disorder is present. If misuse or diversion of methylphenidate or dextroamphetamine by patient, peers, or family is suspected, it may be preferable to prescribe pemoline or nonstimulant medication.

Pemoline is associated with the risk of toxic hepatitis, which may be as high as 3%. Although usually mild and reversible, fulminant liver failure has been observed. The onset of hepatitis cannot be predicted, and the condition may progress rapidly. Recently, the drug manufacturer recommended monitoring of liver function every 2 weeks. However, this is not a mandate, and it is reasonable for clinicians to use their own judgment as to the frequency of testing.

Table 73-2 Stimulant Medications for Attention Deficit/Hyperactivity Disorders

Medication	Dose Schedule	Range*	Onset/Duration	Potential Side Effects/Cautions
Methylphenidate Ritalin or generic 5-, 10-, 20-mg tablets	Initial: 5 mg or 0.3 mg/kg/dose Increase: 2.5 mg to 5 mg weekly Frequency: 2 to 3 doses/day	5 to 80 mg/day 0.3 to 0.8 mg/kg per dose	Onset: 20 to 30 min Duration: 3 to 5 hr	• Anorexia, insomnia, stomachaches, headaches, irritability, "rebound," flattened affect, social withdrawal, weepiness, tics, weight loss, reduced growth velocity • Avoid decongestants • Monitor height, weight, blood pressure, and pulse
Ritalin SR or generic 20-mg sustained-release tablets only	Initial: 20 mg Increase: 20 mg Frequency: 1 or 2 doses/day	20 to 80 mg/day 0.6 to 2 mg/kg per dose	Onset: 60 to 90 min Duration: 5 to 8 hr	• Same as regular MPH. May release unevenly • Should not be chewed or cut in half • 20 mg SR may be equivalent to 12 to 15 mg regular released over 5 to 8 hr
Dextroamphetamine Dexedrine 5-mg tablets Dextrostat 5-, 10-mg tablets Elixir no longer available	Initial: 2.5 to 5 mg (0.15 mg/kg per dose) Increase: 2.5 mg to 5 mg weekly Frequency: 2 to 3 doses/day	2.5 to 40 mg/day 0.15 to 0.4 mg/kg per dose	Onset: 20 to 60 min Duration: 4 to 6 hr	• Anorexia, insomnia, stomachaches, headaches, irritability, "rebound" tics, stereotypies, weight loss, reduced growth velocity • Avoid decongestants • Monitor height, weight, blood pressure, and pulse
Dexedrine Spansules 5-,10-, 15-mg capsules No generic available	Initial: 5 mg in AM (0.3 mg/kg/dose) Increase: 5 mg weekly Frequency: 1 to 2 doses/day	5 to 40 mg/day 0.3 to 0.8 mg/kg per dose	Onset: 60 to 90 min Duration: 6 to 10 hr	• Anorexia, insomnia, stomachaches, headaches, irritability, social withdrawal, weepiness, stereotypies, tics, weight loss, reduced growth velocity • Avoid decongestants • Monitor height, weight, blood pressure, and pulse
Mixed amphetamine salts Adderall 5-, 10-, 20-, 30-mg (Limited data available)	Initial: 2.5 to 5 mg in AM Increase: 2.5 to 5 mg weekly Frequency: 1 to 2 doses/day	2.5 to 40 mg/day?	Onset: 30 min? Duration: 5 to 7 hr?	• Presumed to be similar to dextroamphetamine • Appears to be better tolerated by some
Pemoline Cylert 18.75-, 37.5-, 75-mg tablets 37.5-mg chewable tablets	Initial: 37.5 mg in AM Increase by 18.75 mg weekly Frequency: 1 to 2 doses/day Must be taken daily	18.75 to 112.5 mg/day 2 mg/kg/day	Onset: 2 hr Duration: 7 to 10 hr	• Insomnia, anorexia, stomachaches, irritability, headaches. Choreoathetoid movements • Liver dysfunction. Very rare fulminant liver failure • Monitor height, weight, blood pressure, and pulse • LFTs at baseline should be obtained with regular monitoring

Modified from Miller KJ, Castellanos FX: *Pediatr Rev* 19:373, 1998.
*The high end of these ranges may need to be exceeded in some children. Consultation with a specialist would be prudent in such cases.

Liver function tested every 4 to 6 months is a standard used by many.

Stimulant medication trial management. Appropriate management of medication begins with identification of the specific target symptoms that are expected to improve, discussion of the limitations of medication with the child and parents, and arrangements for monitoring treatment response. Three stages of pharmacotherapy are initial titration, maintenance, and termination.

Titration of medication is required to determine efficacy and optimal dosage with minimal side effects. The titration used most commonly is an open trial (nonblinded), although placebo-controlled trials can be useful in clinical practice, especially when strong biases exist either for or against medication use. The usual starting dose for school-age children is 5 mg/dose of methylphenidate (MPH) two to three times a day given at or just after meals. Dosage adjustments of 2.5 to 5 mg are made weekly until therapeutic effect or adverse effects occur. Dosage and schedules must be individualized.

Titration is best begun with short-acting medication. When optimal dosage is achieved, the comparable daily dose of long-acting (sustained release) medication can then be tried. Combined long- and short-acting stimulants may be useful. Some children require medication only on school days, but many benefit from daily medication when their symptoms impair functioning significantly at home or with peers.

Monitoring treatment response is critical. AD/HD specific rating scales, such as the *ADD-H Comprehensive Teacher's Rating Scale (ACTeRS)* or the revised *Conners Parent and Teacher Rating Scale*, short form can be completed by teachers and parents (see list of resources at the end of this chapter). It is important to obtain a baseline rating and at least weekly assessments during a trial. Comments from teachers often are very informative. In secondary school, it is useful to obtain feedback from two teachers because multiple factors influence behavior at that age. Children and adolescents should be involved in any discussion of a medication trial. Blood levels are not useful for monitoring stimulant therapy.

Nonstimulant medications. Nonstimulant medications have been used in the treatment of AD/HD, but controlled studies are limited. They may be beneficial in children who respond poorly to an adequate trial of stimulants, experience unacceptable side effects, or have significant comorbid conditions. Referral to a developmental-behavioral pediatrician or child psychiatrist should be considered if it is determined that stimulants are ineffective.

ANTIDEPRESSANTS. Antidepressants that have been studied in AD/HD include tricyclic antidepressants (TCAs) such as imipramine (Tofranil), desipramine (Norpramin), nortriptyline (Pamelor), and an atypical antidepressant, bupropion (Wellbutrin). Tricyclic antidepressants have shown clinical efficacy in children who have AD/HD and may be useful when comorbid anxiety, depression, or tic disorders are present. Improvement in cognitive symptoms (inattention) has not been documented objectively, and effects seem to be short lived for some children.

Anticholinergic side effects (dry mouth, constipation), and cardiovascular and neurological side effects limit the usefulness of TCAs further. Potentially serious cardiovascular side effects, especially induction of arrhythmias, are possible, and TCA use must be preceded by baseline ECG, which should be repeated when optimal dosage is reached. TCAs can lower the seizure threshold.

Bupropion is a heterocyclic antidepressant that has dopaminergic activity similar to that of stimulants. It shows modest efficacy in decreasing hyperactivity and aggressive behavior. Bupropion may increase tics and decrease seizure threshold. Selective serotonin reuptake inhibitors, such as fluoxetine (Prozac), have generated interest, but little evidence exists of efficacy on the core symptoms of AD/HD, although they may be useful for comorbid conditions. Venlafaxine (Effexor), a mixed serotonin/norepinephrine reuptake inhibitor, is being investigated for efficacy in AD/HD.

ANTIHYPERTENSIVES. Clonidine (Catapres), an alpha-2 adrenergic agonist, has been found, in the few controlled studies, to be effective for patients who have AD/HD, although not as effective as stimulants. Clonidine may be useful in overaroused, easily frustrated, extremely hyperactive or aggressive individuals. Clonidine has been used as a first-line treatment in children who have comorbid tics or Tourette's syndrome. It has been used clinically for AD/HD-related sleep problems and in combination with stimulants, although there are concerns about the safety of this practice. Side effects include sedation, depression, headache, and possible hypotension. Guanfacine (Tenex) is a more selective alpha-2a agonist. Preliminary studies indicate that it may have a longer half-life than clonidine, permitting once- or twice-daily dosing and less sedation.

Maintenance phase. Regular monitoring to review progress, assess current interventions, and prevent secondary complications is essential. Children taking medications are often seen every 3 to 4 months. Medication dosage should be reassessed and adjusted continually. It also is important to review the child's understanding of medication as he or she develops. Noncompliance during adolescence is greatly reduced when this step in management is followed.

Those who are not on medication should be seen twice yearly, especially around critical junctures, such as transitions to middle and high school. Functioning at school, at home, and with peers should be surveyed. Follow-up behavior ratings are useful. Medical evaluation should include height, weight, blood pressure, and pulse. Laboratory studies are obtained if indicated by symptoms or physical examination findings. Follow-up visits also function as "booster sessions," because dealing with a chronic condition can become discouraging for both parents and child. The goal is to instill a sense of competence and hope.

Termination of medication. The duration of treatment with medication is highly individualized and has lengthened as research has shown that stimulants continue to be effective in adolescence and adulthood. Noncompliance is a significant problem in adolescence. At times a placebo-controlled, cross-over trial of medication is an effective way to convince a reluctant adolescent of the continuing effectiveness of medication. Procedures for a trial off medication should be discussed routinely to prevent unsupervised termination. Trials off medication (2 to 4 weeks) should not be conducted at the beginning of a new school year or when other aspects of the child's life and treatment are unstable. Clear-cut benefits should be present to warrant continued use of psychotropic medication.

Management of Special Populations That Have AD/HD

Children who have pervasive developmental disorders or mental retardation who exhibit significant symptoms of inattention, impulsivity, and hyperactivity may benefit from stimulant medication. Response tends to be less predictable, and these children may manifest increased rates of tics, anxiety, and social withdrawal, even at fairly low doses.

Preschool children who are suspected of having AD/HD can be challenging to assess and manage. Developmentally appropriate behavior, temperament variations, and developmental problems, especially language delays, often imitate or compound AD/HD. Initial treatment should focus on parent counseling, behavior management, and placement in a structured preschool program. Stimulant medication usually is reserved for severe cases. Stimulants may reduce hyperactivity and oppositional behavior and improve mother-child interactions. Response to stimulants is more variable in preschool children; the behavioral half-life is shorter, and side effects are increased.

Controversial Interventions

Families frequently explore alternative treatments that lack scientific validation. Dietary treatments have been a source of controversy and extensive investigation. Methodically rigorous studies show that fewer than 5% of patients, primarily of preschool age, improve behaviorally on restrictive diets. EEG biofeedback training continues to be an unproven and expensive treatment. Other unproven treatments include herbal remedies, anti–motion sickness medication, anti–yeast treatments, sensory integrative training, and chiropractic manipulation. Megavitamin therapy is ineffective and potentially toxic.

OUTCOME

Outcome is affected significantly by persistence of AD/HD symptoms, comorbid conditions, and psychosocial factors. As many as 70% of children and adolescents continue to be symptomatic as adults. Only those who have the mildest degree of symptomatology are likely to outgrow their problems completely. Persistence of symptoms is associated with lower educational attainment, vocational instability, and problems with interpersonal relationships. Outcome is improved for those who have higher IQs, when the family is stable and supportive of the child, and treatment has been ongoing.

SUMMARY

AD/HD is a common neurobehavioral syndrome that has serious consequences for affected children and their families. The core symptoms of inattention and/or hyperactivity/impulsivity often impair social and academic functioning. Diagnostic criteria are well established, but a thoughtful differential diagnosis and careful assessment for possible comorbid conditions is essential. Management includes educating the child and family about AD/HD, behavior management, emotional support, academic interventions, and quite often, medication. Stimulant medication is highly effective and safe when titrated and monitored appropriately. Nonstimulant medications should be considered only after failure of adequate trials of more than one stimulant. AD/HD is a chronic disorder in the majority of cases, but successful adaption to persisting symptoms and positive outcome can be achieved with appropriate support and management.

SUGGESTED READINGS

American Academy of Pediatrics Committee on Children with Disabilities and Committee on Drugs: Medications for Children with Attention Disorders, *Pediatrics* 98:301, 1996.

Barkley RA: Attention deficit hyperactivity disorder, *Scientific American* Sept 1998, p 66.

Biederman J, et al: Pharmacotherapy of attention-deficit/hyperactivity disorder reduces risk for substance abuse disorder, *Pediatrics* 104:e20, 1999.

Cantwell DP: Attention deficit disorder: a review of the past 10 years, *J Am Acad Child Adolesc Psychiatry* 35:978, 1996.

Cassidy LJ, Jellinek MS: Approaches to recognition and management of childhood psychiatric disorders in pediatric primary care, *Pediatr Clin North Am* 45:1037, 1998.

Dulcan M: Practice parameters for the assessment and treatment of children, adolescents and adults with attention-deficit/hyperactivity disorder, *J Am Acad Child Adolesc Psychiatry* 36:85S, 1997.

Elia J, Ambrosini PJ, Rapoport JL: Treatment of attention-deficit/hyperactivity disorder, *N Engl J Med* 340:780, 1999.

Goldman LS, et al: Diagnosis and treatment of attention-deficit/hyperactivity disorder in children and adolescents: AMA council on scientific affairs report, *JAMA* 279:110, 1998.

Green WH: Treatment of attention-deficit/hyperactivity disorder with nonstimulant medications, *Child Adolesc Psych Clin North Am* 4:169, 1995.

Greenhill LL: Attention-deficit hyperactivity disorder: the stimulants, *Child Adolesc Psych Clin North Am* 4:123, 1995.

Miller KJ, Castellanos FX: Management of attention deficit hyperactivity disorders, *Pediatr Rev* 19:373,1998.

Pelham WE, Sams SE: Behavior modification, *Child Adolesc Psych Clin North Am* 1:505, 1992.

Safer D, Zito JM, Fine EM: Increased methylphenidate usage for attention deficit disorder in the 1990's, *Pediatrics* 98:1084, 1996.

Solanto MV: Neuropsychopharmacological mechanisms of stimulant drug action in attention-deficit hyperactivity disorder: a review and integration, *Behavioral Brain Research* 94:127, 1998.

Whalen CK, Henker B: Therapies for hyperactive children: comparisons, combinations and compromises, *J Consult Clin Psychol* 59:126, 1991.

Zametkin AJ, Ernst M: Problems in the management of attention-deficit-hyperactivity disorder, *N Engl J Med* 340:40, 1999.

RESOURCES

Books for Professionals

American Academy of Pediatrics: *Diagnostic and statistical manual for primary care: child and adolescent version*, Elk Grove Village, Ill, 1996, American Academy of Pediatrics.

American Psychiatric Association: *Diagnostic and statistical manual*, ed 4, (DSM-IV), Washington, DC, 1994, The Association.

Barkley R: *Attention deficit hyperactivity disorder*, ed 2, New York, NY, 1998, Guilford Publishing.

Pediatric Clinics of North America: *Attention deficit hyperactivity disorder*, vol 46, Philadelphia, 1999, WB Saunders.

Questionnaires and Rating Scales

Conners CK: *Conners rating scales—revised* (1997), North Tonawanda, NY, Multi-Health Systems (800) 456-3003.

Gadow KD, Sprafkin J: Child and adolescent symptom inventories: parent and teacher checklist, *Screening instruments for childhood emotional and behavioral disorders*, Stony Brook, NY, 1996, Checkmate Plus, Ltd. (516) 360-3432.

Levine MD, et al: *ANSER System—revised*, Cambridge, Mass, 1996, Educators Publishing Service (800) 225-5750. (Developmental questionnaires.)

Ullman RK, Sleator E, Sprague RL: *ACTeRs*. (ADD Comprehensive Teachers Rating Scale) Champaign, Ill, Metritech, Inc. (800) 747-4868. (Parent forms available.)

Books for Parents, Teachers and Children

American Academy of Pediatrics: *Understanding the AD/HD child: information for parents about attention deficit hyperactivity disorder*, Elk Grove Village, Ill, 1994, American Academy of Pediatrics. (800) 433-9016. Pamphlet for the office.

Barkley RA: *Taking charge of AD/HD: the complete, authoritative guide for parents*, New York, 1995, Guilford Publications (800) 365-7006.

Hallowell EM, Ratey JJ: *Driven to distraction: recognizing and coping with attention deficit disorder from childhood through adulthood*, Newark, NJ, 1994, Simon and Schuster (800) 223-2336.

National Institute of Mental Health: *Attention deficit hyperactivity disorder*, Bethesda, Md, 1994, National Institute of Mental Health (202) 783-3238. 42-page booklet, free single copy.

Quinn PO, Stern JM: *Putting on the brakes: young people's guide to understanding attention deficit hyperactivity disorder*, New York, 1991, Magination Press, Brunner/Mazel Inc. (212) 924-3344.

Parent Organization

Children and Adults with Attention Deficit Disorders (CHADD) National Office: 499 NW 70th Ave, Plantation, FL, 33317. (800) 233-4050. http://www.chadd.org/

74 School Behavioral Problems

Jack Kamins • William A. Shine

Classroom behavioral problems not only disrupt the learning process but may be precursors of more serious behavior disorders and even criminality. The primary care physician can play a major role in helping to ameliorate the effects of classroom behavior by the following:

1. Identifying potential difficulties as early as possible
2. Offering guidance to the parents
3. Monitoring the relationship between the school and the parents
4. Working in concert with school personnel to facilitate appropriate responses to a child's behavioral problems
5. Assessing behavior disorders
6. Making appropriate referrals

A child's classroom behavior is defined as a problem by either a teacher or a parent. The teacher's definition is based on internalized standards for this age group developed through his or her own experiences and conventional norms.[7] The parent's definition is concerned more with the effect of the behavior on the child's academic success and social viability. As defined by teachers, most classroom problems involve adjustment and relate either to disruptive or withdrawn behavior. This definition is situational; teachers', schools', and parents' interpretations of behavior and its consequences may differ. Most classroom behavioral problems are brought to the physician's attention by parents. The parents' perception of the problem, however, may not be sufficient for a full understanding of the situation. Contact with the child's teacher, school administrator, school psychologist, or guidance counselor may help in formulating a plan of action.

School stress often provokes behavior that elsewhere could go unattended. Usually, the school is the first setting outside the family in which children are evaluated. An undesirable consequence of schooling is the invidious comparisons that may occur among children, their parents, and teachers. A primary care physician who is knowledgeable about school organization and has a reliable medical history of the child can help the school and the parents protect the child from such comparisons by focusing on the child's individual needs. Early intervention offers the greatest chance for success in modifying reactive behavior that may become socially or academically dysfunctional.

By forming a close relationship with the local school system, a mutually beneficial alliance can be forged in which the physician increases his or her knowledge base on the working of schools and the functioning of the wide variety of school staff. In turn, the physician provides insight to school staff on the implications of childhood illness and child development on the educational process. This bond enables more effective and coordinated service provision for children and families.

EARLY CHILDHOOD

The primary care physician's role is unique in its potential to assist schools and families in the early identification of behavioral issues that can develop into school behavioral problems. Noncompliance, aggressive behavior, and pre–fire-setting behaviors, such as higher than expected interest in fires and fire play, including lighting matches (see Chapter 89, Fire-Setting), which are the precursors to oppositional-defiant disorder, conduct disorders, and more severe pathology, frequently are in evidence as early as 2 or 3 years of age.[2,11,15] This is prior to a child's entrance into school. By being the first provider working with a family, an unusual bond or trust is formed in the physician-family relationship. Using this bond to help families seek either private assistance or public-sponsored early intervention services (0 to 2 years), special education preschool services (3 to 5 years), or school-age interventions (5 to 21 years) is vital in addressing the child's needs. The physician is recognized by education law (Individuals with Disabilities Education Act of 1997, etc.) as a referring party for special services. Unfortunately, families do not always bring the same degree of trust to their relationship with the public schools. The physician, however, can serve as a liaison, preventing the development of an adversarial relationship.

In good school practice, the nursery school or kindergarten teacher informs the parents of problem behavior. A physician who has established a rapport with the family is often able to facilitate appropriate intervention. He or she may counsel a moderate "wait and see" approach or suggest a parent-teacher conference. Although the danger of diagnosing "false positives" is always a possibility, school psychologists have many instruments that can assist in making early assessments of potential behavioral problems, including aggression, hyperactivity, depression, and anxiety, even at the preschool level. These include, but are not limited to, the *Behavior Assessment System for Children, Children's Apperception Test, Social Skills Rating System, Children's Depression Inventory, Human Figure Drawings, Connors Parent and Teacher Rating Scales,* and *Reynold Depression and Suicide Inventories.* (Some of these are described in Appendix D, Table D-1.) At this point, the physician can assist the parents by delineating the problem and suggesting an approach to the family that will focus on resolving the problem rather than establishing causation or fixing blame. The most important point to emphasize is that the parents and school personnel respect each other. The physician who assumes professional competence on the part of the school will communicate that attitude to the parents.

If the parent-teacher conference fails to resolve the problem, the physician may choose to intervene directly. Otherwise, valuable time may be wasted in a clash of opinion between the school and the parents regarding the cause of the problem and, consequently, in reaching agreement on the best course of action to address it. It is here, as well as at any other point along the continuum of schooling, that the physician can provide trusted advice and counsel to prevent the development of an adversarial relationship between the home and the school.

It also is good practice for school personnel to view the physician as an ally in addressing the child's school-related problems. Good rapport between the school and the physician is vital to successful intervention. If the physician is not familiar with the school, he or she should arrange for a meeting to assess that climate. A visit to the child's classroom often provides valuable insight into the child and the environment.

Prekindergarten and kindergarten programs are characterized by their flexibility. When behavioral problems occur, they usually can be addressed by a change in the child's routine or in the quality of the teacher's interaction with the child. An accepting environment that reflects an understanding of the child's temperament and that reinforces behavior positively is often enough to resolve the immediate problem.[25] Unless the child presents serious behavioral problems such as bizarre, extremely withdrawn, or dangerous behavior, the natural maturation process should be allowed to occur. This process can be aided by good modeling by the parents and teacher and by using behavior modification techniques such as instant recognition of good behavior and time-out periods immediately after poor behavior. Because a temperamentally difficult child is vulnerable to developing a behavior disorder later in life, the length and severity of any school-related problem should be recorded by the parents and physician for future reference.[9]

ELEMENTARY SCHOOL

Elementary school places an increasingly heavier emphasis on academic skills. Throughout these grades, classroom behavioral problems are related closely to a lack of academic success, for a child's self-esteem is closely tied to his or her competence at the tasks imposed. Most students encounter few academic barriers during this period, but even these can result in school adjustment problems. Very active children may find the relative physical inactivity of the classroom oppressive, and their reaction to this inactivity often disrupts the class. If the child's behavior is not affecting his or her schoolwork but is disruptive to others, strategies to focus this excess energy should be developed.

Some children do not complete the demanding developmental tasks of early childhood. At critical points in their school career, they may refuse to go to school. Parents should try to identify any specific events, persons, or situations that may be the cause of the problem. If no school situation is identified as a cause, the child should be assessed or referred immediately (see Chapter 75, School Absenteeism and School Refusal).

In most situations a family-school conference can resolve the problem, whether it is related to academic frustration, physical inactivity, or undefined school refusal. These conferences should be planned carefully, with sufficient time and privacy provided. Because emotions tend to run high in these cases, hasty, episodic, or fragmentary encounters usually are counterproductive.[26]

Organic Bases for Behavioral Problems

In exceptional cases the classroom behavioral problem cannot be resolved solely through home and school collaboration. In such cases the child may have an organic problem that is unrecognized by either the parents or the teacher. Attention deficit/hyperactivity disorder (AD/HD) is receiving increasing attention as an organic disability that relates to school problems (see Chapter 73, Attention Deficit/Hyperactivity Disorder). An estimated 5% of school-age children are affected by this condition, which is considered a behavior disorder.[18] This condition should be diagnosed medically only after intensive cognitive and behavioral investigation has ruled out primary environmental causes. Behavior rating scales for children who have AD/HD can provide information important to proper diagnosis. Neuropsychological testing and psychiatric evaluation also may be required.[1]

AD/HD does not define the child; rather, it identifies a condition that probably will require some environmental modification to address associated problem behavior. Many children who have AD/HD have coexisting learning problems and anxiety disorders, oppositional-defiant disorder, or conduct disorder. School officials should be alert to the existence of these multiple educational disabilities.

Symptoms of a behavior disorder commonly first appear before age 7 years.[18] First noticed at home, these can become disruptive behaviors in school, generally manifested by physical aggression that discounts the rights of others. Identification of a child's disability is useful only to explain his or her behavioral reaction to situations at school; judgments about the inevitability of failure or "delinquency" should be avoided. These children deserve the presumption of achieving success.

Pharmacological therapy is considered the most effective management for AD/HD.[18] This therapy requires medical decisions and supervision.[19] Close monitoring of the child's progress is essential to help the physician determine the success of treatment. Because the problematic behavior associated with AD/HD is most prevalent in the school and seen rarely at home, parent feedback alone is insufficient to titrate medication dosages appropriately. Direct school feedback via the periodic completion of behavior rating scales and narratives, coordinated by the school psychologist, will better inform the physician's prescriptive decisions. This therapy is not a cure, but coupled with behavior modification techniques it is thought to offer the best hope for behavioral adjustment to academic and social norms.[1]

The most common cause of learning problems, some of which result in classroom behavioral problems, is a group of specific developmental disorders known as *learning disabilities* (LDs) (see Chapter 76, School Learning Problems and Developmental Differences). Frustration in coping with one or more of a plethora of cognitive, social, and motor skill deficiencies can cause the child to develop inappropriate strategies designed to obscure the problem and to protect him- or herself from failure. A teacher or school may focus on the inappropriate behavior and fail to address the causal academic frustration. A team of learning specialists, including a school psychologist, should identify the specific learning disability and develop a plan to address it.

Unfortunately, more research is directed to the diagnosis of academic problems than to remediation. A search of the literature indicates that few "proven" methods have been verified scientifically. Behavior modification and direct, intensive early intervention, peer tutoring, parent effectiveness training, and use of computers are considered to have the best nonpharmacological efficacy. To succeed, these approaches require extensive record keeping, perseverance, emotional control on the part of the parents and teacher, and a heavy time commitment.[5] However, such strategies are inconsistent with the "discovery method," favored by most teachers, involving higher-order thinking skills.[4,18] With the introduction of school practices such as curriculum-based assessment and functional behavioral analysis, these behavioral recording techniques are beginning to gain greater pedagogical acceptance.

For schools, categories of disabilities listed in Public Law 105-17 (Individuals With Disabilities Education Act [IDEA]) are as significant as those in the American Psychiatric Association's *Diagnostic and Statistical Manual of Mental Disorders, Fourth Edition*. Although IDEA categories are intended for funding rather than diagnosis, they direct resources to the school districts and as such are highly influential. Fifty percent of federal money spent under this law is for children classified as having LDs. AD/HD is not listed, but because it is a medical diagnosis, students who have AD/HD can be classified as LD or emotionally disturbed (ED) if the condition's primary symptoms or comorbid features are primarily in these areas. Some states administer the federal law to permit funding for AD/HD under the category "other health impaired."

IDEA addresses many of the problems antecedent to classroom behavioral problems. Its sufficiency, however, depends on its implementation by the state and by the local school district. The law is administered locally by an IEP (Individual Educational Program) team. Each school district has such a team, called by different names in various states, that is responsible for evaluating children identified by a teacher, parent, physician, or judicial officer as potentially disabled. A primary care physician may refer a child for an evaluation of special education needs with or without the parents' agreement. School districts vary in their application of this law; their attitude toward children and behavior greatly determines eligibility for treatment of behavior disorders.

Environmental Bases for Behavioral Problems

When classroom behavior is closely tied to an organic problem, it is more likely to be addressed because of the legal requirements of IDEA. However, some cases of poor classroom behavior are primarily the result of environmental factors. At times a classroom behavioral problem stems from family stress. In these cases, the physician plays a unique role by virtue of his or her intimate knowledge of family dynamics. He or she may either counsel the family or refer to an appropriate resource.

One often-overlooked resource is pastoral counseling. In many cases where a family may reject "psychological intervention," a rabbi, minister, or priest has access to that family's emotional core not available to others. Although it is not appropriate for the counselor to share the details of the family strife with all school personnel, it is helpful for a child's school to know that family problems might explain the child's behavior. Parental consent can be obtained to share information between the family counselor and the school psychologist or social worker, who will maintain appropriate confidentiality.

Many behavioral problems are cultural in origin. When the values of the parents and community are at odds with those of the school, the clash of values often manifests itself in the child's inability to control his or her anger through appropriate behavior. Some children and young people who are culturally alienated also have problems associated with AD/HD, LD, conduct disorder, and psychiatric illness. These conditions often are undiagnosed, and the child's behavior is interpreted as being merely a reaction to social circumstances.[20] School authorities tend to generalize disruptive behavior and adopt disciplinary practices that serve only to alienate these children further. There is evidence that bureaucratic use of suspension, although expedient, results in more disruptive behavior and a higher dropout rate.[4,6,24] Many of these children and young people do not have access to a primary care physician. Their plight could be addressed through establishment of a school-based primary health care program in any school that has students whose health care needs are unmet.

More boys than girls are identified as having behavior disorders; however, this does not necessarily mean that more boys than girls have such disorders. Some theorists hold that boys manifest their disorders by more disruptive behavior, whereas girls, more externally suppressed by powerful social controls, mask their disorders by withdrawn behavior. Gender bias in research and practice can blind schools and institutions to the social constraints that prevent girls from expressing their frustration as overtly as boys.[13] Teachers and physicians should be alert to these less overt classroom behavioral problems.

ADOLESCENCE

In early adolescence the entire school milieu becomes the arena in which problems occur. Middle schools have been created in response to the need for a school environment that provides the necessary freedom and control to meet the early adolescent's developmental needs.[17]

Children who adapted well to elementary school usually find this new environment stimulating and productive. One current theory of adolescent behavior holds that adolescent turmoil is not as pervasive as previously thought.[21,22] Although most adolescents have mood swings, only a small number experience serious emotional distress. The myth of adolescent turmoil could lead to a dangerous failure to identify serious behavior disorders.[17]

Symptoms of behavior disorders commonly appear between 2 and 3 years of age.[2,14] These symptoms may be suppressed by authoritarian punishment, only to appear overtly in adolescence when the child gains the physical strength and social mobility to resist authority. Low self-esteem, poor peer relationships, and increasingly poor school performance can deteriorate into physical aggression during later adolescence. A school that has many "at-risk" children and limited resources lacks the capacity to identify or address behavior disorders and tends to rely on punishment as a deterrent. Only a school that has sufficient resources and child-centered values can identify behavior disorders and implement individualized approaches to help children develop appropriate social skills. However, schools in poor areas typically do not have such resources, nor can families in such deprived neighborhoods find affordable mental health care.

Violence

In light of the 1990s school tragedies and their extensive media coverage, it is important to note that for most children school is not only a safe haven but also a place where they feel secure in a chaotic world.[12] Because of the complexity of the violence issue, the solutions also will be complex and require both a national and community response. Violence is not just a school problem; it is a societal problem.[14]

Although the fear of violence often is exaggerated, violence actually is a problem for many adolescents. Bullying has long been a fact of life for countless children who have suffered its physical and emotional effects; it is probably one of the most severely underrated educational problems.[3] The introduction of weapons into the schools has increased further the anxiety level of children who see themselves as potential victims. Some classroom behavior problems are the direct result of victims' efforts to mollify their tormentors by rejecting authority and adopting the oppositional style of their abusive peers. When a school climate is oppressive, this strategy often is all that remains for children who lack effective adult guidance and support.

The chronic bully requires early therapeutic intervention. Parents and teachers should not rationalize violent behavior.[16] Although anger can be useful, uncontrolled aggression cannot be tolerated. Controlling aggression can be one of an adolescent boy's most difficult developmental tasks.[21] Most learn to master their emotions through sublimation (e.g., athletics) and productive social activities. Schools must differentiate between violent behavior and other discipline problems. Recent federal legislation requires expulsion for any student determined to have brought a firearm to school (Title VIII, Gun-Free Schools Act of 1994). Treatment of the violent offender is a responsibility of the larger society (see Chapter 112, Violent and Aggressive Behavior).

Children killing children or multiple shootings at schools have created a new set of problems for behavioral theorists. Availability of weapons, media glorification of violence, poor schooling in social responsibility, absence of adult care and supervision, poverty, and inborn temperament are all factors in this relatively new phenomenon.[10,24] Although we need to learn much more about the profile of students who commit such acts, early identification and intervention of children who have violent, oppositional tendencies are the keys to preventing the development of the level of alienation and rage that characterizes these events. Once again, the primary care physician can play an important role in this identification process.

Academic Failure

Most school behavioral problems are associated with academic failure. This is even truer for adolescents than for elementary school children because this developmental period is characterized by heightened self-awareness and the need for peer group validation. For students who have poor impulse control, organizational deficiencies, or weak skills, productive classroom and school participation seems impossible. There is strong evidence that most children's perception of their own ability is set by the seventh grade.[23] Sometimes the disappointment felt by academically successful parents clouds their vision of the strengths of their mildly disabled child. These children often struggle to achieve a good self-image in the absence of authentic parental approval.[8]

A plan to address learning problems should be the focus of any attempt to deal with classroom behavioral problems for two reasons: (1) it addresses the probable cause and (2) it communicates to the adolescent a sense of his or her worth. Such a plan should demystify the learning problem and thus alleviate guilt. Educational methodology should include behavior modification, parent training, where appropriate, as well as strategies to bypass areas of vulnerability. The latter might include the use of assistive technology, such as having a student whose handwriting is poor use a computer for word processing or using audio books to supplement or even supplant reading. These strategies encourage participation in peer-related learning that might otherwise be foreclosed. A deficiency in mathematics, reading, or writing skill can be addressed better within the context of the adolescent's emerging social needs than in remedial isolation.

Opportunities should be provided for the student to develop and display nonacademic skills and abilities in or out of school. The school day can be modified to encourage community service or work. In some communities, for example, membership in the fire department provides a disciplined, prestigious outlet for adolescents who crave action and recognition. School activities also can provide important cocurricular experience. Therefore, it is of questionable value to deny students the opportunity to participate in athletics or other cocurricular activities as a punishment for improper behavior or academic failure. Although this practice is widely employed and often appears to be the only solution to an intractable problem, it takes away what often is the only opportunity for that student to experience the success necessary to maintain his or her self-esteem. A decision to remove a student from a valued activity should be subject to intensive review, which might well include the opinion of the child's physician.

For most young people in late adolescence, college life offers a healthy moratorium from the responsibility of choosing a lifetime companion and a vocation. Ironically and unfairly, lifetime choices are thrust upon those who drop out of high school or whose lives are filled with unresolved turbulence. For centuries, military service, the farm, or the factory provided a viable occupational goal for many adolescents. The current complexity of military and civilian vocational requirements forecloses these options for a large percentage of those who have not achieved a modicum of school success. This group often lacks the social skills necessary for these positions. Society cannot afford to discount this group. Alternative training opportunities and dignified entry-level employment, coordinated with adult counseling programs directed at life skills, should be available in each community.

SUMMARY

Occasional classroom misbehavior is common for many children and young people. For most middle-class children, their interaction with their environment is an exciting opportunity for growth. For the child who has a difficult temperament, a behavior or learning problem, or who is culturally deprived, the school often is a less than comfortable place. For this child to achieve a healthy future, the parents and school must, as early as possible, assess his or her ability and temperament accurately to develop a program that fits. However, this early identification sometimes is impeded because (1) some parents and teachers are reluctant to identify problems to avoid confrontation; (2) some parents resist special education classification for fear of stigmatizing their child; and (3) some school districts constrain special education expenditures.

Tragically for economically and culturally deprived children, it is doubtful that sufficient resources will be made available to address all of their behavioral problems and educational needs.

Physicians who lend their considerable prestige and expertise to creating an environment where the problems inherent in behavior disorders are identified early and receive long-term attention can have a positive effect on the lives of the children they serve. The primary care physician's potential role in addressing school behavioral problems is significant. The physician can:

- Help to identify potential behavioral issues in very young children to enable early intervention and the prevention of further exacerbation of behavioral difficulties
- Make parents aware of services available through the public schools, such as those provided through IDEA
- Provide trusted advice and counsel to break the logjam of inaction and prevent the development of an adversarial relationship between the home and the school

REFERENCES

1. Barkley RA: *Attention deficit hyperactivity disorder: a handbook for diagnosis and treatment,* New York, 1990, Guilford Press.
2. Barkley RA: *Defiant children: a clinician's manual for assessment and parent training, second edition,* New York, 1997, Guilford Press.
3. Batsche G: Bullying. In Bear GG, Minke KM, Thomas A, editors: *Children's needs II: development, problems and alternatives,* Silver Spring, Md, 1997, National Association of School Psychologists.
4. Bear GG: School discipline in the United States: prevention, correction, and long-term social development, *School Psychol Rev* 27:1, 1998.
5. Blechman EA: *Solving child behavior problems at home and at school,* Champaign, Ill, 1985, Research Press.
6. Bowditch C: Getting rid of troublemakers: high school disciplinary procedures and the production of dropouts, *Soc Probl* 40:493, 1993.
7. Brophy J, McCaslin M: Teacher's reports of how they perceive and cope with problem students, *Elem School J* 93:3, 1992.
8. Casey R, et al: Impaired emotional health in children with mild reading disability, *J Dev Behav Pediatr* 13:256, 1992.
9. Chess S, Alexander T: *Origins and evolution of behavior disorders from infancy to early adult life,* New York, 1984, Brunner/Mazel.
10. Dwyer KP: Children killing children: strategies to prevent youth violence. In Canter AS, Carroll SA, editors: *Crisis prevention & response: a collection of NASP resources,* Silver Spring, Md, 1999, National Association of School Psychologists.
11. Ehrhardt KE, et al: Fire setting. In Bear GG, Minke KM, Thomas A, editors: *Children's needs II: development, problems and alternatives,* Silver Spring, Md, 1997, National Association of School Psychologists.
12. Furlong M, et al: School violence in Canter AS, Carroll SA, editors: *Crisis prevention & response: a collection of NASP resources,* Silver Spring, Md, 1999, National Association of School Psychologists.
13. Gilligan C: *In a different voice: psychological theory and women's development,* Cambridge Mass, 1982, Harvard University Press.
14. Goldstein AP, Conoley JC: *School violence intervention: a practical handbook,* New York, 1997, The Guilford Press.
15. Goldstein AP, Glick B, Gibbs JC: *Aggression replacement training: a comprehensive intervention for aggressive youth,* Champaign, Ill, 1998, Research Press.
16. Greenbaum S, Turner, B, Stephens, RD: *Set straight on bullies,* Malibu, Calif, 1989, Pepperdine University Press.
17. Hamburg BA: Psychosocial development. In Friedman SB, Fisher M, Schonberg SK, editors: *Comprehensive adolescent health care,* St Louis, 1992, Quality Medical Publishing.
18. Ingersol BD, Goldstein S: *Attention deficit disorder and learning disabilities: realities, myths, and controversial treatments,* New York, 1993, Doubleday.
19. Klee B, Hack S: Child and adolescent psychopharmacology at a glance. In Koplewicz HS: *The NYU Child Study Center Letter* 3:4, 1999.
20. McIntyre T: Reflections on the new definition for emotional or behavioral disorders: who still falls through the cracks and why, *Behav Disorders* 18:148, 1993.
21. Offer D: *The psychological world of the teenager,* New York, 1969, Basic Books.
22. Offer D, Ostrov E, Howard KI: *The adolescent: a psychological self-portrait,* New York, 1981, Basic Books.
23. Sandler AD, Levine MD: Learning and attention deficit disorders. In Friedman SB, Fisher M, Schonberg SK, editors: *Comprehensive adolescent health care,* St Louis, 1992, Quality Medical Publishing.
24. Skiba RJ: Conduct Disorders. In Bear GG, Minke KM, Thomas A, editors: *Children's needs II: development, problems and alternatives,* Silver Spring, Md, 1997, National Association of School Psychologists.
25. Turecki S, Tonner L: *The difficult child,* New York, 1989, Bantam Books.
26. Turecki S, Wernick S: *The emotional problems of normal children: how parents can understand and help,* New York, 1994, Bantam Books.

75 School Absenteeism and School Refusal

Ronald V. Marino

A major developmental task of childhood is separating from one's family and accepting the functional demands of society. One of the most obvious indicators that this process may not be occurring normally is lack of attendance at school. It is the responsibility of child health professionals to assess the child's school attendance and functioning in the context of biopsychosocial health supervision.

Nonattendance may be due to a variety of underlying reasons. Absenteeism generally is considered to be parentally sanctioned nonattendance, most commonly attributed to medical illness. Truancy is nonattendance without parental consent, in which the time allegedly spent at school often is spent engaging in antisocial behaviors or rebelling against authority. School refusal is characterized by inappropriate fear about leaving home, inappropriate fear of school, or both.

ABSENTEEISM

Excessive absenteeism is important to health professionals because it is an excellent marker for both physical and mental health problems (Box 75-1). It also is negatively correlated with social adjustment and academic performance. In fact, excessive absenteeism and failure to read at grade level in third grade are the two strongest predictors of subsequent dropping out of school. National surveys indicate that healthy children average four or five absences a school year, whereas children who have a chronic disease typically are absent at least twice as often. Educators believe that missing more than 10 days in a 90-day semester results in difficulty staying at grade level.

Acute physical health problems are given as the reason for nonattendance 75% of the time. However, the variability in absenteeism among children who have the same medical condition suggests that in determining attendance, individual and family responses to the physical condition are more important than the actual condition. The decision not to attend school reflects subtle and complex relationships between the physical, social, and psychological states of the student, family, and community. Individual rates of absenteeism tend to be stable for a given child and also for a given school district.

The minor health complaints cited most commonly are upper respiratory tract infections, headaches, abdominal distress, and menstrual cramps. Parental characteristics associated with excessive absenteeism include lower socioeconomic class, cigarette smoking, chronic parental illness (including mental illness), lower educational expectations, and "vulnerable child syndrome." A plethora of nonmedical conditions, including transportation difficulties, illness of other family members, religious holidays, family vacations, inclement weather, and professional appointments, also are reasons children miss school.

Chronically ill children typically miss more school than their healthy peers. This may result from a wide variety of causes, including acute exacerbations of the underlying condition, health care visits, side effects of medications, and parental misconceptions about the child's ability to attend school. Healthy adjustment by the child and family to the chronic condition minimizes the potential impact of the increase in school days missed. A significant increase in absenteeism over baseline is always a "red flag." It is the clinician's responsibility to explore the reasons why a particular child seeks to avoid school. Sudden changes in school attendance may be the first concrete symptom of family dysfunction, mental illness, physical deterioration of the student or a family member, alcohol or drug abuse, or school refusal.

SCHOOL REFUSAL

Difficulties attending school despite caretakers' support for it have been a problem for clinicians for most of the twentieth century. Initial views of school refusal focused on truancy and its linkage to delinquency. In 1932, Broadwin focused attention to the frequent role of anxiety in attendance difficulties; in 1939, Partridge labeled this clinical condition "psycho-neurotic truancy." Johnson et al introduced the term school phobia in 1941, stressing that the child's anxiety about separating from mother was displaced to fear of attending school. This view was strengthened further in the 1950s when Estes, Haylett, and Johnson concluded that school phobia was a variant of separation anxiety.

This view and nomenclature persisted until the late 1970s when the term *school refusal* was introduced. The term has descriptive merits that recognize the heterogeneity of the underlying disorders. These disorders include but are not limited to major depression, simple and social phobia, or separation anxiety disorder. Criteria for making this diagnosis include (1) severe difficulty in attending school or refusal to attend school, (2) severe emotional upset when attempting to go to school, (3) absence of significant antisocial disorders, and (4) staying at home with the parent's knowledge.

A variety of vague physical symptoms frequently accompany the child's request to not attend school. Symptoms can

BOX 75-1

CHRONIC SCHOOL ABSENCE: DIFFERENTIAL DIAGNOSIS

School refusal
Overresponse to minor illnesses
Chronic physical disease with poor adaptation
Learning disability with poor adaptation
Truancy
Substance abuse
Psychosis
Teenage pregnancy
Family dysfunction

Modified from Nader P, editor: *School health: policy and practice,* Elk Grove Village, Ill, 1993, The American Academy of Pediatrics.

be quite impressive to parents and emulate organic medical problems.

Prevalence

The prevalence of school refusal has been estimated to be between 0.4% and 18%. There are two peaks in the incidence of school refusal. The first is associated with beginning school attendance (4 to 6 years) and the second is at the age of 11 to 12 years, a time of change from elementary to intermediate school as well as the onset of early adolescence. The AAP estimates that 5% of elementary school children and 2% of junior high students have this disorder.[6]

School refusal represents a symptom that has a variety of underlying dynamics. Attempts to classify it into acute versus chronic (or anxiety types) versus characterological (or secondary gain type) have little to offer the primary care physician in the development of therapeutic strategies. Clinicians should employ a sensitive, holistic approach to data gathering, because history-taking technique provides the first opportunity for creating a therapeutic alliance. Factors related to the child, parents, family, and school environment must be investigated when exploring school maladaptation. An open mind that recognizes the unique and complex interactions of temperament, stressful life events, family systems function, learning style, parental psychopathology, and school system variables will be helpful in solving this problem.

Child-Related Factors

Children who have "school refusal" usually have at least average intelligence and academic achievement. Numerous studies have shown that girls are more fearful than boys in relation to school-related activities. However, cultural norms encourage girls to admit fear and discourage boys from doing the same. The actual incidence of school refusal is nearly identical between the genders. Younger children report more fear of being scolded or performing before a group, whereas older children seem to be more intimidated by tests and the possibility of failure.

Vague somatic symptomatology, which typically is offered as a rationale for nonattendance, belies the underlying anxiety frequently present. Symptoms may amplify in response to parental pressure to attend and excel in school. Over dependency on a parent, usually the mother, also is common. Classic descriptions refer to passive, dependent, inhibited, timid, and willful children. Some children set unrealistic expectations of themselves, which contributes to the problem. Depression has been noted by numerous authors, as has panic disorder and agoraphobia. There have been some reports of suicide among school refusers. Thus, any reference to this possibility must be addressed seriously.

Parent-Related Factors

More attention has been paid to mothers of school refusers than fathers. There appears to be a higher incidence of neurosis associated with anxiety and depression in these women, and they have unresolved conflicts with their own mothers. Overindulgence and overprotection may reflect underlying maternal ambivalence or hostility toward the parental role. Other maternal characteristics include perfectionism, fear of illness, and an inability to set limits effectively.

Fathers commonly are professionals or skilled workers and good "material" providers. They frequently have been described as passive and ineffectual. They may be indifferent to or withdrawn from parental decision making. Conversely, some authors have described the father as firm, active, and overenmeshed. Both fathers and mothers tend to be older than average.

Family Factors

The family context always is a major factor in understanding the symptoms. Marital conflict or constricted communication patterns frequently are found in families who have school refusers. The child's presence at home due to physical illness may provide a cohesive force to an otherwise unstable marital relationship.

Nader has described three common patterns of communication in families in which school refusal occurs: (1) both parents are overly concerned and solicitous of the child's medical problem; (2) one parent, usually the mother, is overprotective and concerned, whereas the other overtly disagrees; and (3) one parent, typically the mother, is over involved in caring for the child's every need, whereas the other parent is absent emotionally.[7] Understanding and clarifying the family dynamics are important in developing an effective treatment plan.

School Environment Factors

The role of the school environment in school refusal has received little attention. Institutional factors such as changing classrooms or lack of privacy in the school bathroom have been associated with fear of school. Humiliation caused by an insensitive teacher also may be a precipitating stressor in the onset of clinical symptomatology. Temperamental mismatch between teacher, student, and parents may serve a maintaining role.

Recent developments in secondary school violence have provided children a seemingly appropriate reason for refusing to attend school. A survey of 12,000 students and school personnel conducted by the New York State Education Department during the 1992-1993 academic year revealed that 26% of junior and senior high school students had been assaulted on school grounds, 20% of students admitted bringing a knife or gun to school, and 10% admitted not going to school because of fear of violence.[8] Clearly, school-associated stressors are emerging as a concern in understanding and treating school refusal.

Associated Stressors

While exploring child, parent, family, and school environment factors, the clinician also must search for a precipitating event or stress that may have tipped the balance in causing a child to refuse to attend school. Illness or injury of a family member or of the child may be the initial reason for nonattendance. Likewise, the death of a relative or close friend may precipitate the refusal. Moving to a new home, community, or school also may contribute to refusal. The longer a child has been out of school, the more potentially stressful and difficult returning becomes.

Clinical Management

In 1958, Eisenberg stated, "it is essential that the paralyzing force of the school phobia on the child's whole life be recognized. The symptom itself serves to isolate him from normal experience and makes further psychological growth almost impossible. If we do no more than check this central symptom, we have nonetheless done a great deal."[2] The foundations of any clinical treatment plan are rapport, trust, and respect. The initial interview should serve not only as a means of gathering data but also as the start of a therapeutic alliance. The child must understand that the physician being involved in treatment begins a change in the existing behavior.

Organic disease should be ruled out through a careful history and physical examination, coupled with judicious laboratory evaluation. Time spent in conducting a thorough medical examination communicates the physician's sincere acceptance of the child's presenting symptom as being real. Parents are better able to confront the lack of organic disease when it is explained to them by a clinician who is completely familiar with the child's history and physical examination. The laboratory should be used in a symptom-specific, noninvasive, cost-effective manner consistent with ruling out possible organic disease. Additionally, addressing the potential contributions of parental psychopathology or specific environmental problems will be helpful in formulating a treatment plan.

The parents, physician, and school personnel all must agree that returning to school as quickly as possible is the immediate goal of treatment. Allowing the child to stay home while awaiting laboratory data results or using home tutors only makes the return to school more difficult. A specific plan must be developed to respond to clinical symptoms. Objective criteria such as a temperature elevation should be utilized consistently in modifying performance expectations both at home and in school. Parents in doubt should seek the guidance of the child's physician regarding the significance of acute symptoms before keeping the child home. Also, the patient must understand that the significant attachment figures in his or her life will adhere to the therapeutic program consistently and persistently.

In most cases of school refusal, especially in the elementary years, the above program, carried out by the primary care giver, is curative. Other treatment modalities, typically employed by a mental health professional, include desensitization, psychotherapy, hypnotherapy, cognitive restructuring, and behavior modification.[5] Numerous papers have been published about the use of various psychopharmacological agents as aids in the management of school refusal. Psychotropics are commonly used when depression or separation anxiety underlies the symptom. Scientific studies fail to demonstrate consistent reproducible positive effects of drug treatment.[1] However, in experienced hands, as part of a multimodal approach, medication may help a problematic child return to school sooner. Suggested criteria for mental health referral are listed in Box 75-2.

BOX 75-2

CRITERIA FOR MENTAL HEALTH REFERRAL

Unresponsive to pediatric management
Out of school for 2 months
Onset in adolescence
Psychosis
Depression
Panic reactions
Parental inability to cooperate with treatment plan

Prognosis

Pediatric experience suggests that the vast majority of children who refuse to attend school overcome the difficulty rapidly with appropriate clinical management. Intermittent relapses associated with stress or new separation experiences, such as camp or sleepovers, occur in approximately 5% of children. Children who require psychiatric management do not fare as well. Most published series in the psychiatric literature reveal significant cohorts of patients requiring ongoing therapy and having persistent difficulties in emancipating themselves from their family. Phobias, depression, and anxiety are more common in adults who have a history of childhood school refusal.[3]

Prevention

Anticipatory guidance is an excellent means of primary prevention, which allows the pediatrician to advise parents on developmentally appropriate "separation" guidelines. For example, by the time an infant is 6 months old, the parents should be able to spend some evenings out alone. By 1 year of age, peer contact should be encouraged. Toddlers should experience baby-sitters while awake. By age 3 the child should experience being away from home without a parent, such as in a play group or neighbor's home. Age 4 is a good time to consider preschool for the child. Such guidance can be shared in the context of routine health supervision. Parents also should be discouraged from keeping children home because of minor illness, and physicians must avoid unnecessary medical restrictions.

Preventing "vulnerable child syndrome" also is important when caring for ill children. This disorder arises when parents feel that their child's life has been threatened significantly, and it results in separation difficulties, overprotection, bodily concerns, and underachievement in school.[4] Parents need to be informed about the true significance and prognosis of any medical difficulty the child has experienced. Practitioners have a responsibility to avoid creating iatrogenic misconceptions about a child's health; they can do this by using everyday language as much as possible, rather than medical jargon, and by demystifying anxiety associated with insignificant findings such as a functional murmur. Parents need to be reassured that children who have recovered fully from an acute illness are at no increased risk for future illness. By inquiring about children's school attendance and promoting healthy parenting styles, pediatricians can help prevent school refusal.

TRUANCY AND DROPPING OUT

Truancy is a good predictor of dropping out later on. Many schools in inner cities report daily absence rates above 20%; an equal or greater percentage of these children never finish high school. Truancy is a serious social problem that has potentially lifelong consequences. Unemployment or underemployment, criminal behavior, marital problems, and chronic social maladjustment often are seen in both truants and dropouts. These same long-term outcomes have been identified in groups of children who have learning disabilities. Clearly, an unrecognized learning disability is a risk factor for school failure, with subsequent disengagement and truancy.

Truancy also has been noted among children who have a history of having been sexually abused. Other risk factors are low socioeconomic status, conduct disorder, gang membership, substance abuse, cigarette smoking, and family discord. Early recognition of children at risk should prompt immediate intervention to promote optimal adjustment. Mobilization of resources in the school, community, and family is critical to help prevent progression from truancy to dropping out. Creative programs to foster school attendance and success have been conducted with variable results. An emerging new truancy variant is the child who goes to school or its immediate environment but doesn't attend class. This "in-school truant" is participating in the social aspects of the school community but shuns the academics. Medical clinicians can assume an advocacy role in guiding and supporting therapeutic interventions in the educational and social welfare arenas.

CONCLUSION

Absenteeism is a simple symptom that has multiple causes. Because success in school often is the foundation for continuing success in life, health care professionals must devote thoughtful attention to understanding and treating absentees. Using a biopsychosocial model and mobilizing multidisciplinary resources are the keys to clinical success.

REFERENCES

1. Bernstein GA, Garfinkel BD, Borchardt CM: Comparative studies of pharmacotherapy for school refusal, *J Am Acad Child Adolesc Psychiatry* 2:772, 1990.
2. Eisenberg L: School phobia: a study on the communication of anxiety, *Am J Psychiatry* 114:712, 1958.
3. Flakierska-Praquin N, Lindstrom M, Gillberg C: School phobia with separation anxiety disorder and a comparative 20- to 29-year follow-up study of 35 school refusers, *Compr Psychiatry* 38:17, 1997.
4. Green M, Solnit AJ: Reactions to the threatened loss of a child: a vulnerable child syndrome, *Pediatrics* 34:58, 1964.
5. Last CG, Hansen C, Franco N: Cognitive behavioral treatment of school phobia, *J Am Acad Child Adolesc Psychiatry* 37:404, 1998.
6. Nader PR, editor: *School health: policy and practice*, Elk Grove Village, Ill, 1993, The American Academy of Pediatrics.
7. Nader PR, Bullock D, Caldwell B: School phobia, *Pediatr Clin North Am* 22:605, 1975.
8. New York State Education Department, Division of Criminal Justice Services, unpublished survey data, February 1994.

SUGGESTED READINGS

Berg I: Absence from school and mental health, *Br J Psychiatry* 161:154, 1992.

Dworkin PH: *Learning and behavior problems of school children*, Philadelphia, 1985, WB Saunders.

King NJ, Ollendick TH, Tonge BJ: *School refusal, assessment, and treatment,* Needham Heights, Mass, 1995, Allyn & Bacon.

Nader PR, editor: *School health: policy and practice*, Elk Grove Village, Ill, 1993, The American Academy of Pediatrics.

Weitzman M, et al: School absence: a problem for the pediatrician, *Pediatrics* 69:739, 1982.

76 School Learning Problems and Developmental Differences

Paul H. Dworkin

School learning problems are complex issues that defy traditional methods of pediatric assessment and management. Learning problems are not the exclusive responsibility of the pediatrician but rather are of multidisciplinary concern. Furthermore, pediatricians neither diagnose definitively nor treat learning disabilities independently. Nonetheless, pediatricians should assume critical roles when their patients manifest learning problems. Such roles include clarifying the reasons for poor school performance and facilitating appropriate intervention. The importance of such pediatric involvement has become evident; parents and educators regard such problems as learning disabilities to be within the pediatrician's area of responsibility and demand pediatric attention to the needs of children who perform poorly in school. Unfortunately, many pediatricians view themselves as inadequately prepared to deal with school learning problems.

REASONS FOR LEARNING PROBLEMS

The British pediatrician Martin Bax noted that a student's learning problems may result from a variety of causes, "from his school burning down to the lack of the appropriate textbook."[2] Causes of school failure may be classified somewhat simplistically into "intrinsic" and "extrinsic." Intrinsic causes comprise the inherent characteristics of the failing child, such as specific learning disabilities, mental retardation, and sensory impairment. Extrinsic causes are adverse external influences, such as family dysfunction and social stressors within the home or ineffective schooling.

Actually, however, learning problems typically are the consequence of a complex interaction of variables related to the child, the family, and the school (Fig. 76-1). For example, a subtle learning disability can be particularly devastating for a child reared in poverty who attends a school of inferior quality. Furthermore, learning problems often coexist with "clusters" of adverse influences. For example, a child with a learning disability may be at a particular disadvantage if he or she has a slow-to-warm-up temperament that precludes active classroom participation or if the child is confronted with the trauma of parental divorce. Thus, the pediatrician's assessment of school learning problems must include the child's capabilities and weaknesses within the context of social and environmental circumstances.

Specific Learning Disabilities

Of the many causes of school learning problems, specific learning disabilities are the most prevalent and perplexing. Learning disabilities are regarded as a heterogeneous group of disorders manifested by significant difficulties in the acquisition and use of listening, speaking, reading, writing, reasoning, or mathematical abilities. These disorders are presumed to be due to central nervous system (CNS) dysfunction and not directly to other handicapping conditions or environmental influences.[6] The hallmark of learning disabilities is a discrepancy between a student's potential for academic achievement, as suggested by cognitive abilities, and actual performance, as documented by achievement tests. The prevalence of learning disabilities is estimated to be 3% to 5% of students.

No single cause of learning disabilities has been identified. The search for biological, neurophysiological, and neuroanatomical correlates, in general, has been disappointing. Even the identification of a so-called "dyslexia gene" on chromosome 15 has limited implications for the large population of children with learning disabilities. Some researchers have suggested, based on longitudinal study, that learning disabilities are not discrete disorders but rather represent the extreme lower end of a continuum of learning abilities.[12]

Research has emphasized the critical importance of language development in learning. Many children with learning disabilities have experienced delayed or disordered language acquisition, supporting the belief that learning disabilities may be the expression of a more general linguistic disability. More recently, the importance of weaknesses in higher-order cognitive functions (i.e., thinking and reasoning processes and memory) has been emphasized. Deficits in so-called metacognitive skills, such as being able to access acquired knowledge when needed and knowing how to apply learned skills, may be the reason that children with learning disabilities are unable to focus attention on the salient features of tasks or effectively devise problem-solving strategies.[4] Such children have been described as passive learners because of their difficulty with strategy selection and problem solving.[13]

Children with learning disabilities typically display deficits in various areas of developmental functioning. When developmentally assessed, these children are more likely than their learning-normal peers to be confused by sequences and time relationships (temporal-sequential deficits), to have "right-left confusion" (directional disorientation), to fail to appreciate spatial relationships and visual detail (visuoper-

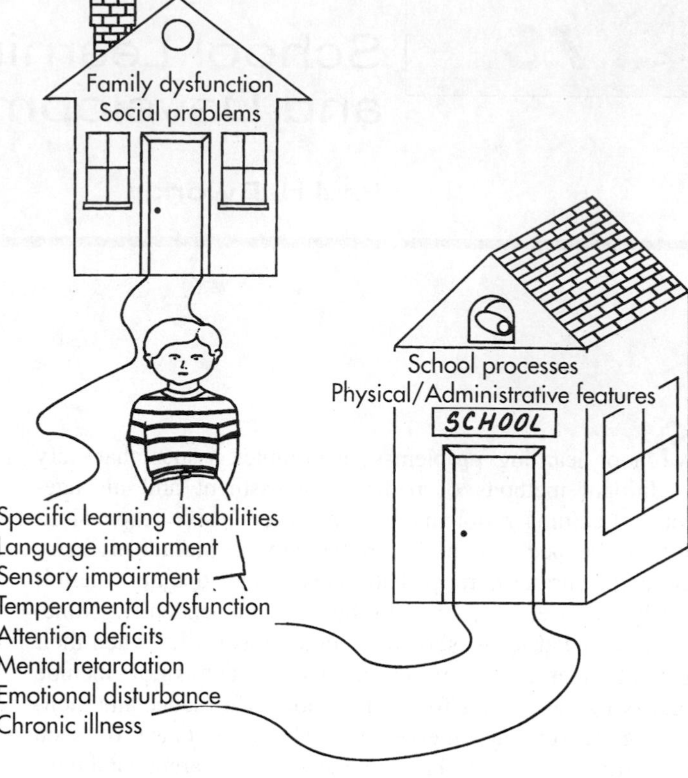

Fig. 76-1 Learning problems typically stem from a complex interaction of variables related to the child, family, and school.
(From Dworkin PH: *Pediatr Rev* 10:301, 1989.)

ceptual difficulties), and to have difficulty integrating auditory and visual stimuli, such as the sounds of words and the visual configurations of letters (deficits in intersensory integration). These children also are more likely to be clumsy and awkward (motor abnormalities) and neurologically immature (i.e., to exhibit neuromaturational delay or so-called soft neurological signs). In addition, behavioral or emotional problems, such as diminished self-esteem, are more common among such students.

Except for language and cognitive deficits, the extent to which these clinical correlates contribute to, result from, or merely coexist with learning disabilities is uncertain. For example, extensive research fails to substantiate a significant causal relationship between faulty visuoperceptual skills and academic deficits. The presence of such correlates should not form the basis of a diagnosis of learning disability. Rather, findings such as temporal-sequential deficits and directional disorientation should serve as "red flags" that increase the clinician's suspicion about the possibility of learning disabilities and prompt a referral for psychoeducational evaluation to document the potential-performance disparity required for diagnosis.

Children with learning disabilities most commonly have problems with the language arts (reading, spelling, and written expression). They also may have difficulties with arithmetic and handwriting skills, although isolated problems with arithmetic are less common. A child's pattern of academic performance may change over time. For example, some children with learning disabilities may cope satisfactorily during the first 3 years of school, only to experience increasing problems with academic achievement and organization of assignments by third or fourth grade, as classroom expectations increase and demands for the rapid retrieval of information and work productivity escalate.[9]

Other Reasons for Learning Problems

Whether attention deficit disorders represent a specific syndrome (attention deficit/hyperactivity disorder) or result from complex interactions between child-related and environmental factors is highly controversial. Regardless, for a group of children difficulties such as inattention, distractibility, lack of persistence, and impulsivity impair school functioning. These attention deficits often are associated with other causes of learning problems, such as specific learning disabilities.

Mild mental retardation usually is not identified until the child is confronted with the cognitive demands of school. The academic performance of such children is characterized by slow learning and acquisition of skills to at most the fifth or sixth grade level. Mental retardation and learning disabilities may coexist, and both contribute to a child's learning problems.

Sensory impairment may contribute to school learning problems. Of the five senses, hearing and vision are the most crucial for academic learning. Of these two, hearing loss results in the more profound educational handicap, primarily because of impaired language acquisition and communication skills. The learning problems of children with hearing impairments are characterized by difficulties in reading, mathematical reasoning, and problem solving. Deaf students also may struggle with classroom maladjustment, behavioral problems, and social immaturity. Children who have visual disturbances usually fare better than their peers with hearing impairments in the classroom. In general, such children tend to perform rather well; thus, their academic achievement has received only limited scrutiny.

Although 30% to 80% of emotionally disturbed students have problems with academic achievement and classroom behavior, emotional illness (e.g., depression or conduct disorders) is the primary cause of learning problems for only a small percentage of children facing school failure. Rather, emotional factors may be far more important in the exacerbation of academic difficulties caused by other problems. For example, the inevitable feelings of diminished self-esteem and frustration that accompany school failure because of learning disabilities may serve to impair classroom functioning even further.

One fourth to one third of children who have a chronic illness have problems achieving academically. Chronic illness may contribute to school learning problems as a consequence of limited alertness or stamina, chronic pain, side effects of medication, absenteeism, altered or inappropriate expectations of teachers or parents, maladjustment, or inappropriate placement in special classes. Low intelligence and learning disabilities may be problems for children who have certain neurological disorders.

A child's behavioral style, or temperament, may contribute to school learning problems. The temperamentally "difficult" child quickly may become frustrated and angry when confronted with material not easily mastered. Or the initial reluctance of the "slow to warm up" child to participate and his or her tendency to withdraw may be misinterpreted as anxiety or a limited capability for learning. Although the "easy" child usually fares well in the classroom, problems may arise when expectations for behavior differ markedly between home and school.

Social and environmental factors also can contribute to school learning problems. These include parental divorce or separation, child abuse or neglect, illness or death of immediate family members, parental emotional illness, early parenthood, substance abuse, and poverty. Ineffective schooling itself may contribute to learning problems. Some studies have revealed that school processes (e.g., academic emphasis, use of rewards and praise, teachers' actions during lessons) are more important than physical or administrative features.[11] Factors such as school climate and social environment may be particularly important for children from disadvantaged homes who attend schools that have limited resources.

For children of ethnocultural minorities, additional factors may influence school performance. Cultural factors include differences in concepts necessary to learn such subjects as math and science, teaching and learning styles, assumptions about interpersonal relations, and language. The influence of bilingual education is controversial. Select studies report that acquisition of English as a second language may interfere with school achievement, but other studies indicate that acquisition of a second language facilitates school achievement and cognitive development in the bilingual child.[1] A recent review from the National Research Council found effects favorable to bilingual education when such confounding factors as socioeconomic status are taken into account.[10]

PEDIATRIC EVALUATION OF LEARNING PROBLEMS

The goal of pediatric evaluation of school learning problems depends on the specific circumstances of a child's referral. When school-based assessment has already raised the possibility of a child being learning disabled, pediatric evaluation assumes a relatively limited role in excluding medical problems that may contribute to poor school functioning. Alternatively, pediatric evaluation is far more challenging when a child is experiencing unsuspected or unexplained learning problems. The goals of such evaluation are diagnosing "medical" conditions that may contribute to school problems (e.g., sensory impairment or a seizure disorder) and identifying clinical correlates (medical, neurophysiological, and psychological) of other causes of learning problems, such as specific learning disabilities.

The pediatrician should follow certain guidelines when evaluating school learning problems. For example, the numerous factors that can contribute to school failure must be considered. Communication with school personnel is invaluable in obtaining information about classroom functioning, past assessments, and school resources. The child must be evaluated within the context of the learning environment; for example, the expectations of a 5-year-old entering an academically oriented kindergarten class are quite different from those of a child entering a more developmentally and socially oriented program.

History

Important historical information should be sought from parents, teachers, and the child (Table 76-1); questionnaires may facilitate the gathering of necessary information.[7] Certain aspects of school functioning should be examined in detail, including the child's academic achievement, classroom behavior, school attendance, past psychoeducational testing, and special school services provided. Findings that suggest the possibility of specific learning disabilities may include the following:

1. Discrete delays in select subjects, such as the language arts, or an adequate early performance with later emergence of difficulties
2. Behavioral problems such as long-standing, pervasive problems with inattention, impulsivity, overactivity; acting out; disorganization and poor strategy formation; or depression, sadness, and moodiness resulting from frustration and diminished self-esteem
3. School avoidance because of frustration
4. Discrepancy between cognitive abilities and academic achievement on past psychoeducational testing
5. Poor response to special teaching techniques, which suggests special learning requirements

Other aspects of the traditional medical history also should be examined in detail. The perinatal history of children with learning disabilities is characterized by a somewhat increased incidence of "clusters" of adverse events, such as anoxic encephalopathy, prematurity, and bronchopulmonary dysplasia, as well as maternal alcohol and drug intake (e.g., substance abuse and anticonvulsants). The past medical history may be significant for recurrent or persistent otitis me-

Table 76-1 Role of the History in the Evaluation of School Learning Problems

Aspect	Findings Suggesting Specific Learning Disabilities
School functioning	
Academic achievement	Discrete delays in select subjects (e.g., language); adequate early performance with difficulties emerging later (e.g., mathematics, writing)
Classroom behavior	Long-standing, pervasive problems with inattention, impulsivity, overactivity; disorganization and poor strategy formation; depression, moodiness
Attendance	Excessive absenteeism; school avoidance
Past psychoeducational testing	Discrepancy between cognitive abilities and academic achievement
Special required school services	Response to "diagnostic teaching"
Perinatal history	"Clusters" of adverse events; maternal alcohol or drug intake
Medical history	Recurrent and/or persistent otitis media; iron-deficiency anemia; lead poisoning; seizures; frequent accidents; chronic use of medication
Development	Delayed or disordered language acquisition and communication skills; subtle delays in select milestones; "uneven" pattern of skills and interests
Behavioral history	Long-standing problems with attention span, impulsivity, overactivity; sadness; acting out; poor self-esteem
Family history	Learning problems, school failure among first-degree relatives
Social history	Child abuse or neglect; other stressors

dia, iron-deficiency anemia, lead poisoning, seizures, frequent injuries as a result of overactivity, or chronic use of medication (e.g., phenobarbital, theophylline, or antihistamines). The developmental history of children with learning disabilities may suggest delayed or disordered language acquisition and communication skills; subtle delays in select milestones, such as speaking, sitting, or walking; or an "uneven" pattern of skills and interests, with discrete areas of strength and weakness. The behavioral history may reveal long-standing problems with attention span, impulsivity, and overactivity; sadness; acting out; or poor self-esteem. The family history may corroborate the increased incidence of learning problems and school failure among first-degree relatives of children with learning disabilities. The social history may reveal such stressors as child abuse or neglect, known to be associated with specific learning disabilities.

Physical Examination

The physical examination has a limited but important role in the evaluation of children who have learning problems (Table 76-2). The physician's general observation of the youngster may note sadness, anxiety, a short attention span, impulsivity, or overactivity. Tics may indicate Tourette's syndrome, which is known to be associated in some cases with learning disabilities. Physical features may be observed that suggest syndromes associated with learning disabilities, such as fragile X syndrome, fetal alcohol effects, or Turner's syndrome. Alternatively, an increased incidence of so-called minor congenital anomalies (epicanthal folds, hypertelorism, low-set ears, high-arched palate, clinodactyly, and syndactyly of the toes) has been observed among some children who have specific learning disabilities and attention deficits.

Certain specific aspects of the physical examination deserve special emphasis. Examination of the skin should include a search for multiple café-au-lait spots (neurofibromatosis), as well as "ash leaf" spots and adenoma sebaceum (tuberous sclerosis), inasmuch as both conditions are associated with learning problems. Examination of the tympanic membranes may reveal signs suggesting recurrent or chronic otitis media. Among older boys, examination of the genitalia may reveal delayed sexual maturation, which has been correlated with learning problems. Growth measurements may indicate problems such as short stature, microcephaly, and macrocephaly, which also have been associated with learning disabilities. Sensory screening should exclude hearing impairment or vision defects.

Examination of Mental Status

Simple projective testing may identify emotional issues as either the cause or, more likely, the consequence of school learning problems. Techniques such as asking the child for three wishes, asking the child to draw a picture of his or her family, or playing the Winnicott Squiggle Game[3] may reveal the child's sadness, diminished self-esteem, or concerns regarding family functioning.

Neurodevelopmental Screening

Surveying the child's functioning in different areas of development may help identify factors that contribute to learning problems. As noted previously, children who have specific learning disabilities are more likely to have deficits in language functioning and cognitive abilities. Furthermore, the developmental profile of children with learning disabilities is characterized by an uneven pattern, with discrete areas of relative strength and weakness.

A few tools have been developed for assessing school-age children. One is the Pediatric Early Elementary Examination (PEEX),[8] which requires about 45 minutes to administer and surveys the following areas of development: temporal-sequential organization, visuospatial orientation, auditory-language function, memory, fine motor function, and gross motor function. The PEEX also includes a search for minor neurological indicators of dysfunction ("soft" neurological signs) such as dysdiadochokinesia (difficulty with rapid alternating movements), synkinesis (mirror movements), and dys-

Table 76-2 Role of the Physical Examination in Evaluation of School Learning Problems

Aspect	Findings Suggesting Specific Learning Disabilities
General observations	Sadness, anxiety, short attention span, impulsivity, overactivity; tics
Phenotypical features	Stigmata of genetic syndromes (e.g., sex chromosome abnormalities, fetal alcohol syndrome); minor congenital anomalies
Skin	Multiple café-au-lait spots; "ash leaf" spots, adenoma sebaceum
Tympanic membranes	Signs of recurrent or chronic otitis media
Genitalia	Delayed sexual maturation in boys
Growth measurements	Short stature; microcephaly and macrocephaly
Sensory screening	Poor hearing or vision

tonic posturing of the upper extremities, associated with heel walking. An increased incidence of such signs has been observed among boys who have attention deficits and, to a lesser extent, specific learning disabilities.

Laboratory Studies

Laboratory tests are of limited value in assessing school learning problems and should be used only in studies of children at specific risk for conditions known to be associated with learning disabilities. Examples include anemia screening for children at risk because of nutritional or socioeconomic factors; lead screening for those at risk because of their home environment or a history of pica; thyroid function studies if signs or symptoms of thyroid disease are noted or if the possibility is suggested by family history; and chromosome analysis (and molecular genetic testing for fragile X syndrome in all children who are mentally retarded) if the child has phenotypical features or multiple congenital anomalies that are associated with mental retardation. Drug screening is recommended for older children and adolescents who have shown a precipitous decline in school performance or erratic, unpredictable behavior.

Neuroanatomical and neurophysiological studies should be performed only for specific indications. For example, an electroencephalogram (EEG) should be reserved for children suspected of having a seizure disorder; computed tomography (CT) or magnetic resonance imaging (MRI) is indicated for suspected CNS malformations, microcephaly, or macrocephaly.

Further Investigations and Referrals

Referral for psychoeducational evaluation is indicated when the pediatric assessment suggests the possibility of learning disabilities as a cause of learning problems. For example, learning disabilities may be suspected if (1) the pediatric history reveals difficulties with discrete subjects such as reading and spelling, (2) developmental testing indicates an "uneven" profile, with areas of strength and weakness, and (3) a child demonstrates poor self-esteem and poor self-image. The goals of psychoeducational evaluation are to examine the child's academic strengths and weaknesses, to determine cognitive ability, to assess perceptual strengths and weaknesses, to examine communicative ability, and to assess social and emotional adaptation. Ideally, such evaluations are performed by the child's school system, although specific circumstances may dictate a private referral. School personnel participating in such evaluations may include psychologists, special educators and learning disability specialists, speech-language pathologists, and social workers. Tests typically administered include those for intelligence, general learning abilities, academic achievement in reading, mathematics and writing, perceptual and motor function, and speech and language skills. Diagnostic teaching also may be an effective test.

Pediatric assessment may indicate the need for referral to a variety of other professionals. For example, concern about language functioning may result in direct referral to a speech-language pathologist, and emotional disturbance or family dysfunction may suggest the need for referral to a mental health professional (e.g., psychologist, social worker, or psychiatrist). Concern about sensory impairment may suggest referral to an ophthalmologist, otolaryngologist, or audiologist.

PEDIATRIC INTERVENTION

A variety of actions may follow assessment of the child who has school learning problems. Although educational programming is the mainstay of treatment for specific learning disabilities, pediatric participation may involve a variety of traditional and nontraditional roles.

Examples of traditional roles include specific medical intervention for underlying conditions, such as treatment of a seizure disorder that may contribute to learning problems, as well as pharmacological management of attention deficits. Counseling is another traditional role, which may include clarifying a child's strengths and weaknesses, alleviating undue concern, guilt, and anxiety, explaining the legal rights of children and families under state and federal regulations (e.g., the Individuals with Disabilities Education Act), offering guidance on such alternative treatment strategies as diet, megavitamins, and optometric training, and depending on the pediatrician's expertise, giving advice about such specific behavioral management strategies as positive reinforcement and "time-out." Arranging for further investigations and referrals is yet another traditional role, and it may involve coordinating indicated laboratory studies and referring the child for psychoeducational testing and other evaluations.

With their access to young children and families and their responsibility for monitoring children's growth and development during the preschool years, pediatricians are well positioned to contribute to early detection of potential school dysfunction.[5] Developmental surveillance may be the most effective process for enabling the pediatrician to predict school readiness. Surveillance has four components: (1) eliciting and attending to parents' concerns and impressions, thereby acknowledging the importance of their opinions and descriptions of their child's development, (2) observing the child's development, which may be done longitudinally by using an informal collection of age-appropriate tasks or a developmental screening test, (3) obtaining the opinion of preschool teachers, which is important because such opinions are the single best predictor of kindergarten success, and (4) interpreting findings, including social and environmental circumstances, within the context of the child's overall well-being.

A less traditional but nonetheless important pediatric role is serving as ombudsman to help students and families use community services and resources effectively. Specific measures may include facilitating communication with school systems, introducing families to helpful parent and peer support groups, and initiating referrals to mental health and social service agencies. Although pediatricians are unlikely to have the expertise to suggest educational strategies for learning disabilities, participation as a member of a multidisciplinary planning team is both helpful and feasible. Such participation often is reassuring to the parents and children, who regard the pediatrician as an effective child advocate.

REFERENCES

1. Baca L, Amato C: Bilingual special education: training issues, *Except Child* 56:168, 1989.
2. Bax M: Looking at learning disorders, *Dev Med Child Neurol* 24:731, 1982 (editorial).
3. Berger LR: The Winnicott Squiggle Game: a vehicle for communication with the school-aged child, *Pediatrics* 66:921, 1980.
4. Denckla MB: Biological correlates of learning and attention: what is relevant to learning disability and attention-deficit hyperactivity disorder? *J Dev Behav Pediatr* 15:348, 1994.
5. Dworkin PH: Ready to learn: a mandate for pediatrics, *J Dev Behav Pediatr* 14:192, 1993.
6. Interagency Committee on Learning Disabilities: *Learning disabilities: a report to the US Congress,* Washington, DC, 1987, US Department of Education.
7. Levine MD: *The ANSER system,* Cambridge, Mass, 1981, Educators Publishing Service.
8. Levine MD, et al: The Pediatric Early Elementary Examination: studies of a neurodevelopmental examination for 7- to 9-year-old children, *Pediatrics* 71:894, 1983.
9. Levine MD, Oberklaid F, Meltzer L: Developmental output failure: a study of low productivity in school-aged children, *Pediatrics* 67:18, 1981.
10. National Research Council: *Improving schooling for language-minority children: a research agenda,* Washington, DC, 1997, National Academy Press.
11. Rutter M, et al: *Fifteen thousand hours: secondary schools and their effects on children,* Cambridge, Mass, 1979, Harvard University Press.
12. Shaywitz SE, et al: Evidence that dyslexia may represent the lower tail of a normal distribution of reading ability, *N Engl J Med* 326:145, 1992.
13. Torgesen JK: The learning-disabled child as an inactive learner, *Top Learn Disabil* 2:45, 1982.

SUGGESTED READINGS

Dworkin PH: *Learning and behavior problems of schoolchildren*, Philadelphia, 1985, WB Saunders.

Dworkin PH: School failure, *Pediatr Rev* 10:301, 1989.

Levine MD: *Educational care*, Cambridge, Mass, 1994, Educators Publishing Service, Inc.

Wender ED, editor: School dysfunction in children and youth: the role of the primary care provider for children who struggle in school, Report of the Twenty-Fourth Ross Roundtable on Critical Approaches to Common Pediatric Problems, Columbus, Ohio, September, 1993, Ross Products Division, Abbott Laboratories.

77 Nursing Roles in School Health

Patricia Chiverton • Bernadette Mazurek Melnyk

Nursing roles in schools today have changed significantly from 1902 when the first school nurse was employed by the New York City schools. School nursing developed from the public health movement in an effort to control communicable disease and ensure that children were healthy and attended school.[8] Today, the role of the school nurse remains one of the key elements for implementing a viable, effective school health service. This role is multifaceted and complex, and the work varies from one school to another depending on the nurse's educational preparation, priorities of the school board, funding sources, and the school's health program.

School systems are struggling with societal issues such as poverty, drug and alcohol abuse, and an altering of the family structure as a result of single parenting, divorce, and remarriage. In addition, sexually transmitted diseases, pregnancy, chronic illness, mental health and behavioral disorders, and violence in the school place increasing demands on the school nurse.

Responsibilities are diverse, and the school nurse must be able to work with a variety of individuals, including children and their families, school administrators, teachers, other school personnel, school physicians, primary care physicians, nurse practitioners, and community agencies. The school nurse, with direct access to children, families, and school personnel, is uniquely positioned to improve children's health and maximize their learning.

FUNCTIONS OF THE SCHOOL NURSE

The school nurse practice is a non–health care setting where the primary mission of the school system is education rather than health care. Often, the focus of school health has been on obtaining emergency care for children and adolescents rather than on preventing illness and injury.[4] With the current paradigm shift in health care delivery toward wellness and prevention, community- and population-based care, and health outcomes, the school nurse can integrate health education and promotion into the learning environment of the school and can measure outcomes.

Educational preparation of school nurses ranges from 1 year of study for licensed practical nurses to nurse practitioners with master's degrees. Opinions differ regarding the appropriate educational experience required for a school nurse, but most experts recommend, at minimum, a baccalaureate education with additional preparation in health education.[7,12] With the expansion of technology, increasingly complex health care problems in schools, and the need for outcomes research, some experts are recommending that school nurses be prepared nurse practitioners at the masters degree level.[9,12]

In most schools that have a well-established traditional school health program, school nurses provide primary, secondary, and tertiary prevention. School nurses are responsible for assessing, managing, and controlling any health problems they discover in students or in the environment. According to the American Nursing Association (ANA) Standards of School Nursing Practice,[2] school nurses implement programs that "enhance the educational process by the modification or removal of health-related behaviors detrimental to learning and by promotion of an optimal level of wellness."

The school nurse is responsible for planning a systematical health appraisal of all school children and often is the first professional to detect a child's health problem. Screening programs for vision and hearing problems are conducted routinely at specified grade levels. When health problems are identified, a referral process is initiated that involves counseling the student and family about the nature of the problem, the necessity of further treatment, and the health resources available in the community. After obtaining the family's consent, the school nurse speaks directly with the primary care practitioner about the problem and, after medical evaluation, discusses any educational implications and follow-up care indicated. The school nurse can provide the primary care practitioner with useful information about a child's response to the treatment and facilitate any temporary or long-term modification of the child's school milieu to meet health needs.

Virtually every contact with a student is an opportunity for health teaching or counseling. The nurse may develop special programs in the school for students who have similar health needs (e.g., teenagers who need to lose weight). Some nurses are involved in the health education curriculum, directly or indirectly as primary instructors or in collaboration with a teacher or health educator.

The school nurse works closely with parents and teachers of children who have a chronic illness. Increasing numbers of children who have major health problems are included in regular classrooms. Approximately 10% to 15% of school-age children have chronic health conditions,[11] whereas 12% to 22% of children suffer from a mental illness or a behavioral disorder.[1] The Individuals with Disabilities Act (IDEA), Section 504 of the Rehabilitation Act, the Americans with Disabilities Act (ADA), and state laws and regulations address education of the disabled and broaden the scope of

Public Law 94-142 broadly, which allowed many children to be enrolled in school for the first time. These students and their families often require physical and rehabilitative nursing care, as well as individual health teaching and counseling, to help them cope with chronic health problems. Comprehensive education of teachers by school nurses about childhood chronic illnesses can increase their comfort level with these children and enhance early detection of complications.

The school nurse coordinates emergency care for ill or injured pupils or staff members. First aid policies and procedures are developed by the school nurse, school administrators, and medical consultants. Although many school nurses are involved directly in providing some emergency care, teaching basic first aid procedures to all school personnel is a priority. Many emergencies can be prevented by analyzing previous injury data, checking for health and safety hazards in the school, and ensuring that appropriate protective equipment is available for students involved in laboratories, workshops, and athletic activities.

MODELS OF SCHOOL NURSE SERVICES

Although the approximate number of nurses who work in schools has remained relatively constant in recent years, the number of students served by one nurse generally has increased, often surpassing the recommended ratio of 1 nurse to 750 students.[2] A few schools have attempted to meet basic school health needs by employing paraprofessional aides in lieu of nurses or nurse practitioners. Although less costly to the school, these personnel require careful training and supervision by a registered professional nurse to provide safe and effective care.[6]

Other schools have used the nursing services provided by local public health departments. In this model of service, the nurse's school-related activities may constitute only a part of his or her total community nursing role, because the nurse provides care to all age groups within a geographical district and may be responsible for health department clinics and other activities. Assigning a high priority to school health activities within the context of community health needs has been a problem because children ordinarily are the healthiest segment of the community's population.

The role of the nurse practitioner in schools developed in response to the need for primary care services by school-age children.[13] It is a natural extension of the role of the pediatric nurse practitioner in other ambulatory child health care settings. Studies have documented the effectiveness of nurse practitioners in improving and maintaining the health of school-age children.[10,14] Working with a pediatrician colleague, the nurse practitioner may assume a primary care role that involves providing comprehensive well-child care, assessing and managing minor illnesses, and performing initial assessments of more serious acute and chronic conditions.

Diagnostic laboratory tests, as well as developmental and psychological screening procedures to identify behavioral and learning problems, are conducted as indicated. On the basis of the findings, appropriate health teaching and counseling are initiated with the student and family. If referral outside the school is indicated, a report of the nurse practitioner's findings assists in further management of the problem. Although hospital-based nursing certificate preparation was once common, nurse practitioners are now prepared in graduate programs that emphasize comprehensive education in all aspects of well-child care and the assessment and management of acute and chronic illnesses, as well as developmental, learning, and mental health disorders.

Some schools are trying to achieve an optimal mix of the services provided by the health aide, physician consultant, school nurse, and nurse practitioner to meet the health needs of a diverse school population. In times of rising educational costs and limited resources, many schools choose less expensive and, thus, less comprehensive health services. Studies of cost effectiveness and national trends in the financing of health care may well determine the composition of school nursing services in the future.[9]

NURSING INVOLVEMENT IN PRIMARY CARE

Changes are occurring in the health care delivery system due to health reform and market forces. School systems have begun to address these changes by altering the scope and nature of their school health services. New models of care are being utilized by school systems interested in illness prevention and health promotion. Many of these models utilize a diverse group of health professionals that provide comprehensive, integrative health services. Nurse practitioners play a key role in the provision of these health care services.

Edwards[3] describes four models of primary care services in schools. In the first model, the clinic is administered by the school system and the nurse is a school employee. Nurse practitioners are trained specifically to offer children comprehensive primary care and to assess factors affecting learning. This model allows the services of the nurse practitioner to be concentrated in areas underserved by community primary care resources.

In the second model, the local health department employs the nurse practitioner, and the clinic services provided are under the control of the health department. In some instances, personnel may be funded jointly by the school district.

The third model is a school-based or school-linked clinic that is designed to reduce health risks, identify problems, and provide primary health care. Nurse practitioners, part-time physicians, and mental health professionals usually staff school-based or school-linked clinics. The fiscal and administrative responsibility for the clinic is separate from that of the school system. According to a survey by *Making the Grade*,[5] a national grant program that provides funding for school-based health centers, 1154 school-based clinics are in operation around the country, up from 900 in 1996. School-based clinics do not substitute for school health services but function as complementary services to the school health program.[8]

The fourth model is a family health center located at or near the school. In this model, the clinic provides services to individuals or families both inside and outside the school and is fiscally operated as an ambulatory center. This type of clinic often is staffed with nurse practitioners, but these nurses do not participate in the school health program.

When a primary care clinic is present, activities of the school health program often are altered based on the type of primary care services provided. The scope of the school nurse's role is related to the organizational structure under which health services are provided. The school nurse may be fully integrated into the functioning of the clinic or remain separate from the clinic and serve as a liaison with the school health program. No matter which model is provided by a school health system, the role of the school nurse involves collaboration on interdisciplinary and intradisciplinary teams. An awareness of some of the variations in the school nurse's role can help the physician establish a collaborative relationship with the nurse and become familiar with the school health program.

PHYSICIAN AND SCHOOL NURSE COLLABORATION

Although communication between the physician and the school may occur in many contexts, most often it is the school nurse who interacts with the primary care physician. School and health care agencies have different "languages," priorities, and backgrounds. The school nurse can help the physician bridge the gap; at the same time, the nurse may gain valuable consultation and support for health-related activities in the school. Mutual respect, open communication, and some understanding of each other's view of the world can enhance cooperation between the physician and the school nurse. Collaboration in pursuit of common goals ultimately improves the health of school-age children.

REFERENCES

1. Adelman HS, et al: Mental health in schools: expanded opportunities for school nurses, *J Sch Nurs* 13:3, 1997.
2. American Nurses' Association: *Standards of school nursing practice*, Kansas City, Mo, 1993, American Nurses Publishing.
3. Edwards LH: The school nurse's role in school based clinics, *J Sch Health* 57:4, 1987.
4. Harvey GM: Making the transition from acute care to school nursing, *J Sch Nurs* 14:1, 1998.
5. Managed Care Interface: *Making the grade: national survey of state school-based health centers initiatives,* Washington, DC, 1998, Making the Grade National Program, George Washington University, p 38.
6. National Association of State School Nurse Consultants: Delegation of school health services to unlicensed personnel, *J Sch Nurs* 11:13, 1995.
7. National Association of School Nurses: *Resolution and policy statements*, Scarborough, Maine, 1990, The Association.
8. Passarelli C: School nursing: trends for the future, *J Sch Nurs* 10:2, 1994.
9. Proctor S, Lordi S, Zaiger D: *School nursing practice-roles and standards,* Scarborough, Maine, 1993, National Association of School Nurses.
10. Salmon ME: School nursing in the era of health care reform: what is the outlook? *J Sch Health* 64:4, 1994.
11. School health nursing services: exploring national issues and priorities, *J Sch Nurs*, 12:23, 1996.
12. Spanier AL: Development of a school nurse educational model, *J Sch Nurs* 13:1, 1997.
13. Urbinati D, et al: The evolution of the school nurse practitioner: past, present and future, *J Sch Nurs* 12:2, 1996.
14. Yates S: The practice of nursing: integration with new models of health service delivery, *J Sch Nurs* 10:1, 1994.

SUGGESTED READINGS

Bergren MD, Murphy EA: The best of the web for school health, *J Sch Nurs* 13:5, 1997.

Bradley BJ: Establishing a research agenda for school nursing, *J Sch Nurs* 14:1, 1998.

Brainerd E: School health nursing services progress review: report of 1996 National Meeting, *J Sch Health* 68:1, 1998.

Henry SB: A nursing informatics approach for addressing national issues and priorities for school nursing services, *J Sch Nurs* 13:4, 1997.

78 Developmental Approach to Behavioral Problems

T. Berry Brazelton • David M. Snyder • Michael W. Yogman

Every encounter between pediatrician and child is an opportunity for developmental assessment. The continuous, long-term relationship the pediatrician maintains with the child and family offers data about physiological and behavioral functioning under a variety of circumstances. When questions arise about the normality of a child's behavior, this data base gives the pediatrician a diagnostic and therapeutic edge, which a consultant can duplicate only with much time and effort.

The spectrum of behaviors about which parents become concerned is broad. Its range encompasses the following:

1. Nonproblems—concerns based on simple misinformation, which require support and corrective information only
2. "Problem behaviors," which are normal behaviors that often are difficult for the parents to deal with, such as negativism in the second year of life
3. Long-standing, relatively fixed "behavioral problems," such as continued, too-frequent night waking by 2-year-olds
4. Clearly pathological behavior based on psychopathology or organicity, such as that seen in an autistic child or a child who has lead encephalopathy or major psychiatric deviance that essentially is irreversible

This chapter takes a conceptual approach to the assessment of reversible behavioral problems as opposed to irreversible ones. The emphasis is on the center of the spectrum: problem behaviors and behavioral problems. These represent both the majority of parental concerns brought to pediatricians' attention and some of the most taxing diagnostic entities in behavioral pediatrics. This chapter shows how a conceptual approach based on normal development can be applied to these everyday problems in an office practice.

In pediatric practice it may not be possible to diagnose a behavioral problem in a single encounter; the rush to "make a diagnosis" on the first visit may well be inappropriate. It takes time to assess the dimensions of parental concern and the meaning of the behavior to the child. An early diagnosis may miss the appropriate dimensions of each of these factors. It can lead to extensive diagnostic studies or to referrals that not only may be unnecessary and costly but also actually may make diagnosis and treatment more elusive by reinforcing parental concerns.

This pursuit of a physical diagnosis often diverts the parents from approaching the child's problem. Frequently, the true nature and severity of the behavioral problem emerge only as we observe the parents' responsiveness to counseling or the child's reaction to altered parental approaches. This does not imply an interminable diagnostic phase. Rather, it reflects that in managing behavioral problems, diagnosis and treatment often proceed in parallel, the diagnostic hypotheses suggesting counseling approaches, the family's response to these generating more precise diagnostic formulations, and so forth.

ETIOLOGY

Behavioral problems arise in the course of growing up, as a consequence of the normal stresses of coping with new situations.[10] These problems must be viewed as part of the "coping process," the steps through which the child comes to terms with a challenge and successfully masters the difficulties inherent in learning about oneself and about the environment. The coping process may be modified by genetic, biological, and environmental factors, but it always is present and needs to be assessed even in those infrequent instances in which a severe, underlying pathological condition is present (e.g., brain damage, autism, or parental psychosis). The progression from a limited problem behavior to a more global behavioral problem and occasionally even to a severe psychopathological condition depends heavily on how effectively the parent-child unit supports this coping process.

In those few instances when problems are becoming more severe, the parents often show excessive concern about the child's symptoms rather than the underlying cause. The symptom may, in fact, be adaptive and represent a coping response to the stress of growing up or to illness or somatic defect. Most often the presenting symptom has had its beginning long before, and the parents' concerns have reinforced a chain of behavior-concern-problem behavior-increasing concern-increasing problem behavior. To understand the cause and to achieve any change in this ever-lengthening chain, a pediatrician must understand each link in its development.[10]

Evaluation

The most valuable clinical technique the pediatrician can use to assess developmental behavior in children is to observe the behavior of all participants as they interact. Clinical judgments about parents and children at every encounter are based on the physician's observational skills. Although formal tests of the child's intellectual and emotional functioning can structure these observations and articulate clinical judgments more clearly, tests can never entirely replace careful observation.

When parents make us, as pediatric observers, feel angry or depressed as they describe a problem, this becomes an important measure of the parents' own depth of reactions to the child and the behavioral problem. Do these feelings represent the parents' emotions about their conflicts with the child? Why are they generating parallel feelings in us as we observe them? Moments of intense emotion may provide the best clue to the depth of underlying issues. For example, when a mother brightens and becomes animated as she talks about her child's negativism, the pediatrician can be certain that she enjoys it and can identify with it; this will not create a serious problem for either mother or child. Similarly, when a young father begins to hold on grimly to his contention that his 5-year-old son's enuresis is punishable, the depth of tension and frustration created in us becomes our best measure of his inability to react appropriately to this symptom in the boy and indicates that a "fixed" problem area exists between them.

Mostly, pediatricians must begin by "listening with a third ear" or observing the behavior and documenting their own reactions to understand clearly what parents mean as they present their children's problem behaviors.[1] As the pediatrician attempts to gather the necessary information about a disturbing behavior (e.g., when it was first noted, the circumstances in which it occurs, how the parents react to it, and how the child responds to their reactions), he or she should be most alert to behavioral signs of deeper concerns.

These deeper, often unconsciously controlled concerns usually are the real reasons the parents seek help. Parents often are reluctant to begin discussing their fears about brain damage, mental retardation, or psychological disorder in the child; expressed concerns may not be expressed on the first visit. To the degree that they are, they signify that the parents feel the pediatrician is taking them seriously and can be trusted to accept their feelings without censure. Establishing this alliance with the pediatrician is the parents' first step toward solving the problem they are having with their child.

Evaluation of the Parents

In general, a child's behavior becomes problematic because it does not conform to the parents' expectations. Evaluation of the parents should start with the assumption that they are concerned about this dichotomy. It should proceed with specification of the worrisome behavior and how it deviates from their expectations. Regarding the parents, we are interested in the following:

1. How realistic their expectations are
2. How rigid they are in their expectations
3. Whether the child violates these expectations in a narrow or broad area of functioning
4. Whether the violation means abnormality or "badness" in the child or their own failure in parenting

It also is important to determine the origin of their expectations; for example, their own experiences in growing up, their experiences with their older children, the grandparents' comments, or their cultural expectations.[8] Parents come to the pediatrician feeling guilty, inadequate, often isolated from their children, and defensive about the difficulties they are having. These feelings, which invariably impede problem solving, may well be the tragic result of our cultural biases that blame parents for everything "wrong" with their children. These feelings commonly raise questions about the impact of medications taken during pregnancy, genetic factors, and their own child-rearing style as it affects the child's behavior.

In some cases these concerns are realistic; in others, the overconcern can be a symptom and measure of the severity of the problem. However, in all cases this concern and guilt interfere with the parents' relationship with their child and therefore need to be brought out and examined in a positive and supportive manner. This entails accepting the parents' concern, validating their right to get help, and above all, feeding back to them a perception of their own basic competence and of their child's strengths, along with an assessment of the child's problem.

Occasionally, signs of markedly unrealistic expectations, such as attributing adult goals to an infant or small child, may surface. Significant parental thought disorders may become apparent. A parent's own needs and concerns about his or her marriage or about another child may turn out to be the underlying motive for the visit. In any case, the degree to which the parents are conscious of their feelings about their child and his or her problematical behavior, and the ease with which they can express them, can tell us much about the kind of treatment most likely to work.

If the pediatrician's assessment of the child reveals that he or she is markedly different from the parents' description, or if their level of concern seems out of proportion to the problem they report, the physician should suspect an undiscovered parental concern. However, two alternative hypotheses also should be considered: (1) that the behavior observed is not typical of the child and (2) that the discrepancy represents an actual distortion of the child's behavior by the parents.

In the case of significant parental psychological disorder, pediatricians may first sense that their observations do not parallel the expressed complaints. Then they may realize that they cannot "reach" the parents to help them with their reaction to the child. This, then, may suggest that the primary problem is outside the realm of pediatrics altogether. Even in such situations, the manner in which the pediatrician talks with the parents about their feelings can influence significantly their acceptance of referral for psychiatric help. If they have learned that candidly expressing their concerns and feelings is met with acceptance and understanding rather than with censure or disinterest, it will be easier for them to make use of such psychiatric consultation.

Evaluation of the Child

In evaluating a child's behavior at any one time, pediatricians must keep in mind the following questions:

1. How is inborn individual temperament influencing

the child's behavior (either overreactivity or underreactivity)?[5,11]

2. Is the symptom appropriate to the child's age?[6,9]
3. How do the child's reactions to all stress reflect either adaptive strengths or inadequate coping mechanisms?[4,10]
4. To what degree has the symptom influenced broad areas of a child's functioning (e.g., with the family or peers or in school)?
5. What is the duration of the symptom as a sign of "fixation"?

Not changing over time should cause concern; if the symptom has increased in severity, the situation becomes even more ominous.[11]

In practice the pediatrician evaluates a problem on all five levels simultaneously, but separate discussion may clarify the importance of each level.

Temperament as a background for a symptom. An understanding of infant temperament is helpful in assessing the child's contribution to common problems such as crying, feeding, sleeping disorders, temper tantrums, and poor weight gain.[2] Children vary in the rhythmicity of repetitive biological functions. These include sleep-wake cycles, appetite, and elimination. Interviews with the parents enable a pediatrician to assess a child's temperament in vital areas of function (activity, intensity, mood, adaptability, rhythmicity, threshold, distractibility, persistence, and approach-withdrawal), as suggested by the longitudinal studies of Thomas, Chess, and Birch.[11] Knowing patterns of individual differences such as that of the temperamentally difficult child (high intensity, low adaptability, low threshold) helps a pediatrician understand the child's intrinsic contributions to a sleep problem, and this understanding in turn can help the parents manage this "difficult" yet still normal child.

Age appropriateness of behavior. A given behavior has different meanings in children of each age. Although this is obvious in the case of motor milestones, it is equally true for behavioral problems. Temper tantrums, nightmares, phobias, stuttering, and other types of behavior are seen regularly at certain ages and usually pass without consequence. For example, temper tantrums in an 18-month-old are an appropriate indicator of the child's growing sense of independence.[3] A tantrum of similar intensity at age 4 years deserves exploration for an answer to why the child's striving for autonomy does not take a more mature form. By being aware of the individual temperamental and maturational differences, a pediatrician not only can better evaluate problems when they arise but also can use this information preventively to understand the child as an individual. By sharing this information with the parents, the pediatrician establishes an alliance to optimize the child's development.[6]

Child's pattern for coping with stress. Because the pressures of growing up are a part of everyday life, children's behavioral problems must always be evaluated in the context of how they handle these stresses, as well as others that confront them. A pediatrician can note whether the behavioral symptoms in question provide a way for the child to cope better with the pressures of his or her environment. For example, thumb-sucking and holding onto a bottle, blanket, or beloved toy through the stressful second and third years of life seem to be healthy solutions to stress. Unless the parents' concern about such a "lovey" makes it nonadaptive, one should see such behavior as a source of strength for the child and help the parents to see it as such. Assessing a child by means of a "stress model" allows the practitioner to generalize and view the child's underlying resources for coping with any challenging situation.

A psychological testing instrument, such as the revised *Denver Developmental Screening Test,*[7] can be administered easily in the pediatrician's office, and it may be viewed as just such a stress. Such an assessment can become a way to evaluate the child's "level" of development, as well as his or her reaction to the stress of being tested. See Chapter 20 (Thirteen), Developmental Surveillance and Intervention. This, then, becomes a way to attend to the child's responses to the stress of testing and how the child is likely to cope with other stresses of life. In other words, we are given an opportunity to see how a child approaches any given problem or item rather than merely whether the test is passed or failed. When a 14-month-old boy turns to his mother to seek help when he is asked to stack blocks, this not only tells us about the child's response to the stress of the test but also tells us something about the strength of his attachment to his mother and something about his level of autonomy.[10]

The idea of identifying a child's mechanisms for coping is part of the broader principle of being able to list the child's individual strengths, as well as problems, in a "problem list." When asked to stack blocks, a 2-year-old may take great delight in knocking them over rather than stacking them. Negativism is a healthy sign of the toddler's growing independence and should not be overlooked.[3]

Influence of the symptom on other areas of function. In determining the significance of any problem to a child, it is crucial to determine how isolated and discrete the problem is. A 4-year-old's bed-wetting at night may represent a discrete delay in maturation, whereas the same symptom in a 6-year-old may interfere with peer relations (e.g., the child is unable to spend the night at a friend's house). As children grow and attempt to identify with their peers, such a symptom becomes a real source of anxiety about their own adequacy. This anxiety can begin to interfere with all areas of function. They may begin to show signs of deficit in school performance and in their self-esteem in general. In a small child and in the area of feeding, the problem may range from a discrete attempt to control choices, such as refusing vegetables (a transient, self-limited problem) to a more global feeding disturbance, such as a refusal to eat any solid food. When the problem no longer is confined to feeding and involves other areas of adjustment, such as sleep and toilet problems, it suggests an even more global impairment in the parent-child relationship. The degree to which a problem is clinically significant commonly is related to the number of functional areas affected in the child's life.

Determining the degree to which any symptom affects the child's overall level of function not only has diagnostic implications but also helps in the management of the problem. A therapeutic plan should account for and support the child's achievement and areas of success while attempting to improve any weaknesses.[8]

Chronicity of a symptom. Because development implies change over time, any symptom that becomes chronic is worrisome. Crying, for instance, reaches a developmental peak between 3 and 6 weeks of age and tapers off by 3 months of age.[3] A 6-month-old who shows a persistent problem of "colicky" crying requires evaluation and intervention. Thus, the degree of fixation in a behavior becomes a measure of the extent of the problem.

Finally, behavioral symptoms that become inflexible should arouse even more concern. If appropriate 2-year-old negativism is replaced by intense temper tantrums accompanied by persistent head-banging whenever the child does not get his or her way, this constrained, inflexible behavior pattern indicates a need for therapeutic to the child's relationship with the parents.

Delaying a diagnostic decision while collecting observations at several visits allows a pediatrician to assess the flexibility of any symptom by observing the parents' and child's responses to various therapeutic suggestions. Although an assessment of the parents' concerns, as well as the five areas of child behavior described, aids the pediatrician, no evaluation is complete without similarly observing the parent-child interaction.

Evaluation of Parent-Child Interaction

The pediatrician should evaluate not only the parents and the child separately but also the interaction of the parent and child over time. The essence of the parent-child interaction may be seen in the mutual request for attention and responses by parents with their children.

Pediatricians should record observations of these interactions. They can distinguish the mother who sensitively shapes and shows her child how to achieve a task from one who either angrily shoves the child to a task or is completely unavailable to the child. Similarly, pediatricians can distinguish between the child who explores the surrounding environment, using a parent as a secure base, and the child whose interactions with a parent are either minimal or provocative. Value judgments should never substitute for repeated careful observations that attempt to understand the interaction of parent and child on its own terms and in its own culture.

MANAGEMENT

The therapeutic first step may be for the physician to try a simple suggestion. If the parent cannot establish a working relationship with the pediatrician and misuses the suggestion so that the behavioral problem becomes worse or reinforced, it becomes a measure of the depth of the parent's inability to accept help and of the need for more intensive therapy if the problem is to be solved. Pediatricians tend to blame themselves when a helping relationship cannot be established, instead of recognizing the diagnostic implications of the parent's inability to let down their defenses and to join in a therapeutic effort to help the child.

Pediatric management of childhood behavioral problems usually requires seeing parent and child together. By using the child's behavior as a way of communication with parents and pointing out the child's behavior and their response to it, the pediatrician can help parents see their child as an individual who has strengths as well as weaknesses. For instance, when parents understand and accept their toddler's negativism as striving for independence, they can pursue the goal of allowing the child the opportunity to "work out" negative struggles and to define his or her own capacities and limits. In this way the pediatrician forms an alliance with the parents that supports them in their concern. However, it also gives them a goal that enables them to work together at finding adaptive parental responses to help the child.

A pediatrician who no longer feels able to understand or help a family should consider referral to a psychiatric or social worker who is trained to work with more difficult parents. Because of the nature of the problem and the nature of their relationships with families, pediatricians should approach such referrals even more sympathetically than they might a referral to another specialist. The parents' need for defenses against acknowledging that they have a family problem must be respected. The pediatrician may have to see a family several times to understand what kind of referral they will accept and to outline the questions that should be answered. The pediatrician must remain the primary health care provider for the family and must continue to support them after therapy is instituted by the consultant. The pediatrician not only should remain involved in the assessment but also must understand clearly the consultant's assessment of the problem, because the pediatrician most often will be left to carry out the consultant's treatment and management recommendations after the diagnostic or therapeutic interval has terminated.

Pediatric management of behavioral problems and the fostering of normal development can be among the most challenging and rewarding aspects of practice. They need not be especially time consuming. However, they do require a knowledge of normal development as a dynamic process, as well as concerned attention in understanding the parents' reports and in observing both the child's and the parent's behavior.

REFERENCES

1. Balint M: *The doctor, his patient and the illness*, New York, 1972, International Universities Press.
2. Brazelton TB: Crying in infancy, *Pediatrics* 29:579, 1962.
3. Brazelton TB: *Toddlers and parents*, New York, 1974, Delacorte Press.
4. Brazelton TB: *Touchpoints*, Reading, Mass, 1992, Addison-Wesley.
5. Carey WB: A simplified method for measuring infant temperament, *J Pediatr* 77:188, 1970.
6. Erikson E: *Childhood and society*, New York, 1950, WW Norton.
7. Frankenburg WK, Dodds JB, Fanato A: *Revised Denver Developmental Screening Test*, Denver, 1989, Denver Developmental Materials.
8. Lewis M: *Clinical aspects of child development*, Philadelphia, 1971, Lea & Febiger.
9. Murphy L: *The widening world of childhood*, New York, 1962, Basic Books.
10. Murphy L, Moriarty A: *Vulnerability, coping, and growth*, New Haven, Conn, 1976, Yale University Press.
11. Thomas A, Chess S, Birch H: *Temperament and behavior disorders in children*, New York, 1968, New York University Press.

79 Interviewing Children

David I. Bromberg

In assessing pediatric problems in which psychosocial and emotional factors are particularly important, the pediatrician must have a clear understanding of these children and their relationship to their world. For each child, this relationship has three interrelated parts: the relationship with the family, the relationship with the community (mainly school), and the relationship with peers. Diagnostic interviewing is the primary method of attaining this understanding. A great deal of information is available from the parents (see Chapter 7, The Pediatric History) and the school (see Chapter 70, Overview of School Health and School Health Program Goals). However, a wealth of qualitatively unique information and insight can be obtained through a careful interview with the child.

STRUCTURE OF THE INTERVIEW

The interview can be divided into three parts: (1) establishment of rapport, (2) the body of the interview (data collection), and (3) summation of the session (closure). The major goal is to collect data about the child, but other important functions also are served. For example, over the course of the interview, the pediatrician can establish him- or herself as a "helping" person by showing an understanding of the child's feelings and problems and a willingness to offer help rather than judgmental advice.

Establishment of Rapport

Attempting to teach a person how to establish rapport is somewhat akin to teaching someone how to ride a bike; you have to do it to learn it. Nevertheless, several concepts are useful. Rapport is built continually throughout the interview and the ongoing relationship and is not limited to introductory remarks. Showing a sincere interest in and empathy for what the youngster has to say is essential. Verbalizing the feelings represented by a child's story can be very helpful in this regard.

Patient (an 8-year-old boy being evaluated for school underachievement): I got sent to the principal's office yesterday.

Physician: Oh, really? What did you do?

Patient: We had a substitute, and everyone was throwing this eraser around the room.

Physician: Then what happened?

Patient: I guess I threw it last, and she yelled at me and sent me to the office.

Physician: Sometimes it doesn't seem fair to get into trouble for something the whole class is doing.

Patient: (brightening) Yeah, but I guess I shouldn't have thrown it.

Interpreting nonverbal behavior also can help by demonstrating that the pediatrician is "in tune" with the youngster. For example, 11- and 12-year-olds are seen routinely for physical examinations upon entering middle or junior high school. Sitting undressed and draped on an examining table, many of these youngsters appear angry or overly shy. They often avoid eye contact, scowl, and give brief answers. By saying, "I guess it's pretty embarrassing to have to undress and have a physical examination," the physician acknowledges the youngster's feelings, which can aid substantially in establishing rapport. Once rapport has been established, the examiner can watch the hostility wash away and the subsequent interview progress much more profitably.

"Reflecting" feelings generally is a useful way for the health care practitioner to display caring and a desire to communicate. This can involve responding to an "unspoken" message, for example, by commenting, "It sounds like you're pretty angry about that" or by summarizing the point of a story.

Patient (a 10-year-old boy being seen for behavioral problems after his parents' separation): It's just not the same since my dad left.

Physician: Really? What differences have you noticed?

Patient: Well, yesterday I had soccer practice, and my dad usually takes me, but he wasn't around to do it.

Physician: Didn't your mom take you?

Patient: Oh, yeah. She's really trying hard to do all the things. But Dad and I always talk about the practice, and Mom just doesn't know much about soccer.

Physician: So you've really missed your dad since he moved away but don't want to say so to your mom.

The same message can be communicated by "checking back" with the child, prefaced by saying something like, "Just to be sure we're understanding each other . . . "

When performing a behavioral assessment, it is important to remember that the consultation rarely is initiated by 8- or 10-year-olds. Such children often are brought to the office with little or no explanation. Exploring their fears and expectations, as well as the activities they may be missing by being there, can help "break the ice." For younger children this may involve clarifying that they will not be undergoing any blood tests or receiving immunizations. The physician should discuss the format of the evaluation and the demands that will be placed on the youngster. Explicitly stating the following clearly establishes the format of the sessions: "Mary, first I will be talking with you and your family about your school difficulty, and afterwards I will be meeting just with you so that we can get to know one another better; then next week I will give you a physical examination." For older children, recognizing how difficult it is to talk about oneself (or to be talked about) is worthwhile.

Physician: What concerns has the school expressed about John's behavior in the third grade?

Mother: The teacher is worried that he can't "stay on task" and is always out of his seat. He can be very disruptive in class.

Physician: How about at home?

Mother: Well, he leaves things all over the house, and he often annoys his younger sister and brother. He tends . . .

Patient: I do not. They always pick on me.

Physician: John, it can be pretty hard to have people talk about you, especially about things that are difficult for you. Remember, it's not that everyone is just angry at you, but rather that we're trying to understand a problem in order to make it better.

Third-person techniques can facilitate conversation with a child. Rather than attributing feelings or characteristics to the patient, the interviewer can talk about these feelings in other youngsters. The statement, "Many 9-year-olds who wet the bed are embarrassed and afraid of sleeping over at a friend's house" allows a youngster to claim these same feelings but does not confront him or her directly. It also shows that the physician will not be shocked or dismayed by this information.

As with all pediatrics, the interviewer must maintain a developmental perspective in relating to the patient. Complimenting a 3-year-old on climbing the steps to the examining table would be quite appropriate, whereas the same comment to an 8-year-old would be condescending.

In his book *Childhood and Society,*[2] Erikson describes the "eight ages of man," or critical periods of development. Each "age" is presented as a task in development of the ego. The eight ages are summarized as the accomplishment of the following characteristics: (1) basic trust versus basic mistrust, (2) autonomy versus shame and doubt, (3) initiative versus guilt, (4) industry versus inferiority, (5) identity versus role confusion, (6) intimacy versus isolation, (7) generativity versus stagnation, and (8) ego integrity versus despair. Erikson's tasks of development provide a useful framework for both evaluating and relating to children. Commenting on issues of autonomy in the 3- to 4-year-old, issues of initiative in the 5- to 6-year-old, and issues of industry in the 7- to 9-year-old often engages the child successfully.

Physician (to an 8-year-old who is being counseled for encopresis): To review, we've discussed why you soil your pants. We've also come up with a plan for helping you stop. Do you think you would be interested in this program?

Patient: Sure, it sounds easy.

Physician: Actually, it involves a lot of hard work. In talking with you today, I think that you are a pretty hard worker and I believe that you could do a very good job with this program. So, if you're willing, we could start this week.

Patient: Yeah, I think I'd like to do it.

It also is important to proceed from very concrete "here and now" discussions with the preschooler and early school-age child to more abstract explanations as the child gets older.

Data Collection

By the conclusion of the interview, the examiner ideally should have accumulated data covering three main areas: (1) the child's perceptions about the presenting problem, (2) information about the child's relationships with family, school, and peers, and (3) an assessment of the youngster's psychological and cognitive functioning.

Understanding the child's perception of the presenting problem usually is very difficult. Denial of emotional issues is common in school-age children. The 5- to 12-year-old frequently claims to be neither worried nor upset about the problem being evaluated. The physician must listen with his or her "third ear" and be sensitive to nonverbal cues to understand the youngster's relationship to the presenting complaint. Using third-person techniques may be helpful.

Physician: How has school been going?

Patient: Oh, I do OK. My grades are pretty good.

Physician: Your mother had mentioned that reading and phonics are sometimes difficult for you.

Patient: Well, maybe a little bit.

Physician: Many children have told me that they feel dumb when they have trouble with reading.

Patient: Yeah, I know I do. Sometimes I just get so mad.

When a child is reluctant to discuss problems, another useful approach is to ask him or her for "both sides of the coin"—for example, to state what he or she likes and dislikes about school. The same technique can be used to assess the child's feelings toward individuals or toward him- or herself. For example, "Can you brag about yourself and then run yourself down?" Social skills also can be evaluated in this manner: "What do your friends like about you? What things do you do that make them mad at you?"

Information about the child's relationships with family, school, and peers is obtained best by using open-ended questions, which leave the respondent a great deal of latitude in interpretation. This often is information that the pediatrician will obtain during routine health supervision visits. A multidisciplinary group under the auspices of the National Center for Education in Maternal and Child Health published *Bright Futures National Guidelines for Health Supervision of Infants, Children, and Adolescents,*[5] in which they outlined the preventive and health promotion needs of youngsters. For each health supervision visit, they suggested "trigger questions" the pediatrician should ask the parents and the child. These questions form a valuable foundation for a semistructured interview with children. Below is a sample interview using these "trigger questions" (in italics) during a checkup for a 10-year-old girl.

Physician: *How is school going?*

Patient: Fine.

Physician: *And how are your grades?*

Patient: They're OK, straight As.

Physician: That's terrific. You should be quite proud. *What do you do to have fun and with whom do you like to do it?*

Patient: I'm interested in acting and am rehearsing for a play. Some of my friends are in acting with me.

Physician: *Are you involved in any other after-school activities?*

Patient: I wanted to play indoor soccer, but my mother doesn't want me to do it.

Physician: Why is that?
Patient: She thinks that I'm involved in too many activities.

This interview could serve as the basis for discussion of a healthy lifestyle, overcommitment, and balancing of physical and sedentary activities. Other "trigger questions" explore safety, health risk behaviors, including drugs, alcohol, and cigarettes, sexual activity, pressures, and body image.

The physician should attempt to be nonjudgmental and allow the youngster maximum leeway in presenting his or her thoughts or feelings. Asking, for example, "You have lots of friends, don't you?" displays the examiner's preference for friendships and closes the subject to the child. A more effective question might be, "Do you have many friends or do you prefer doing things by yourself?" This allows the child to choose either option, without the physician prejudicing the choices.

Psychological functioning can be assessed by paying careful attention to both the content and the process of the interview. The assessment should include an estimate of intellectual functioning, an evaluation of the child's approach to problem solving (e.g., impulsivity, frustration), and the child's fears and fantasies, self-concept, and superego functioning (conscience). A useful framework for this analysis is the mental status examination. Because a complete discussion of this examination is beyond the scope of this textbook, the interested reader is referred to Simmons' *Psychiatric Examination of Children*.[6]

Numerous assessment techniques are available for gathering important data, ranging from the very unstructured "play" evaluation to the very structured questionnaire. The choice of particular tools depends on the patient's age and verbal abilities and the examiner's expertise and style. For school-age children, a semistructured interview probably is the most appropriate. This combines specific questions about the specific problem, peer relations, and related issues with the use of projective techniques. A discussion of several diagnostic techniques the pediatrician can use is included later in this chapter.

Closure

At the end of the interview, it is important to summarize for the child. A review of the session, highlighting the important points, is useful. An attempt should be made to offer the youngster honest, positive reinforcement and an optimistic outlook wherever possible. Plans for future meetings also should be discussed. A typical ending statement might be, "Bobby, I know you really worked very hard today, having to tell me all those things about yourself. It was especially hard to tell me how sad you were when your grandma died. But now I think we'll be able to make it easier for you to get back to school. I look forward to seeing you and your family next week."

The end of a session typically is the time that unanswered questions may be raised. The following excerpt is from an AD/HD summation conference with a patient and the parents:

Physician: I am glad we had the opportunity to review attention deficit/hyperactivity disorder today and to discuss James' medical treatment. I would like to see you again in 3 months.

Patient: (hesitatingly) Doctor, during the visit you told my mother that I was taking stimulants. Does that mean that I take drugs?

Physician: That must have been confusing. Let's review the differences between medications and drugs.

THE PARENTS' ROLE

The relationship binding physician, patient, and parents is complex. Children are brought to the physician to have a problem "fixed." As we have noted previously, the consultation rarely is initiated by the youngster. The pediatrician must define his or her relationship to the child and parents, paying careful attention to the issue of confidentiality and to the patient's therapeutic needs. What format the interview should take and in what order the practitioner will see the child and parents is the initial decision. Then the physician must decide how to share information among the parties.

Mature preadolescents and teenagers often are seen alone and first in the diagnostic process. The physician thereby demonstrates the primacy of the doctor-teenager relationship. Although establishing a similar relationship with a latency-age or preschool-age patient may be equally important, these youngsters may be frightened by an initial separation from their parents. It usually is better to see the child and parents together for the first diagnostic interview. This allows the youngster a chance to become more comfortable with the examiner in a less threatening setting. Parents occasionally are uncomfortable about discussing behavioral or emotional concerns with their children present. Children, however, usually are well aware of these concerns and find an honest discussion much less frightening than their fantasies about the process should they not be included. After an initial joint interview, both parents and child should be seen separately.

The issue of confidentiality is a difficult one to balance. On the one hand, the youngster has the right to tell the examiner specific things that should be held in confidence. On the other hand, the parents need information to play an effective role in the therapeutic process. It may be helpful to discuss treatment recommendations with the youngster before the final sum-up session with the family. The parents play a crucial role, both in the diagnostic process and in execution of the therapeutic program. The physician should plan the consultation process carefully so as to maximize an effective relationship with both patient and parents.

PEDIATRIC PSYCHODIAGNOSTICS

Many techniques and types of questions are available to help engage youngsters in an interview as well as to uncover "defended" emotional material. Projective techniques allow the youngster to respond to loosely structured stimuli, giving answers that reflect his or her personality. Examples include, "If a genie were to come and give you three wishes, what would you wish for?" or "If you were stranded on a desert island and could have only one person with you, who would it be?" Another area involves the child's happiest, saddest, and maddest times.

Physician: What is the happiest time that you remember?

Patient: Probably when the whole family took the vacation at the beach last summer.

Physician: How about the saddest time?
Patient: I really can't think of one.
Physician: Really, no sad times?
Patient: Well, I guess when my grandma had to go to the hospital last year.
Physician: That certainly can be frightening. Have you ever been so sad that you've thought of hurting yourself or wanting to die?
Patient: Oh, no, I've never considered that.
Physician: How about the maddest you've been? Does your temper ever get the better of you?

The responses to these questions must be evaluated in the context of what is known about the child. Other semistructured projective techniques are described below.

Sentence Completion

The physician should tell the child that they are going to play a sentence game. The physician gives the first part of a sentence, and the child has to finish it with the first thought that comes to mind. Short sentence fragments are used, such as "Boys are . . . ," "Girls are . . . ," "Mothers should . . . ," "I feel bad when I . . . " The answers may indicate areas of conflict or may introduce other topics of interest to the child.

Drawings

Many children find it easier to express themselves through drawings than through verbal communication. Several formats can be used. The pediatrician might ask a youngster to make the best drawing of a person that he or she can. Standards are available in using the "Draw-a-Person" test to assess an IQ.[4] Kinetic family drawings are obtained by asking the child to draw a picture of his or her family doing something.[1] Family relationships and activity can be discussed by using this stimulus. Figure placement, size relationships, and use of symbols all may be useful in interpreting the drawing. Allowing a child simply to draw a picture and tell you a story about it also can be very helpful.

Storytelling

Stories can be useful for talking about emotions or conflicts. A storytelling format that uses fables was developed by Despert and expanded by Fine.[3] With this technique, the physician tells the child that they are going to play a storytelling game in which the child must finish stories that the doctor begins. The child then is given a series of up to 20 fables that touch on many characteristic areas of conflict.

Physician: A boy and his mother go for a nice walk in the park all by themselves. They have a lot of fun together. When he comes home, the boy finds that his daddy is angry. Why is he angry?
Patient: Because the dinner wasn't ready.
Physician: What do you think the boy's father did when he got angry?
Patient: He yelled a lot at the mommy.
Physician: What does your father do when he gets angry?

The storytelling has offered several insights about this family that might have been difficult to obtain in other ways.

SUMMARY

Engaging children in a helping relationship is the core of pediatric practice. The formation of a close, empathic relationship with a patient begins with the diagnostic interview. It is important, therefore, to be alert to both the process and content of this interview and to select diagnostic tools that will foster development of the desired relationship between physician and child.

REFERENCES

1. Burns RC, Kaufman SH: *Actions, styles, and symbols in kinetic family drawings,* New York, 1972, Brunner/Mazel.
2. Erikson EH: *Childhood and society,* ed 2, New York, 1963, WW Norton.
3. Fine R: Use of Despert fables (revised form) in diagnostic work with children, *J Projective Techniques* 12:106, 1948.
4. Goodenough FL: *Measurement of intelligence by drawings,* New York, 1926, World.
5. Green M, editor: *Bright futures national guidelines for health supervision of infants, children, and adolescents,* Arlington, Va, 1994, National Center for Education in Maternal and Child Health.
6. Simmons JE: *Psychiatric examination of children,* ed 4, Philadelphia, 1987, Lea & Febiger.

80 Concepts of Psychosomatic Illness

Stanford B. Friedman

The notion that psychological and emotional factors influence a variety of disease states can be traced to antiquity. Only since the mid 1900s, however, have such relationships been exposed to systematic observation and scientific study. From his clinical observations of patients in the 1940s, Alexander[1] proposed that specific *psychological conflicts* could be identified in individuals suffering from seven disease entities: peptic ulcer, ulcerative colitis, regional enteritis, hyperthyroidism, rheumatoid arthritis, essential hypertension, and bronchial asthma. At about the same time, Dunbar[2] proposed specific *personality types,* rather than the nature of the existing conflicts, as being of etiological importance. Common to both theoretical formulations was a belief that specific psychological phenomena caused or predisposed to specific diseases, and thus evolved the "theory of specificity." This approach to the conceptualization of "psychosomatic medicine" has led to the common belief that some diseases are influenced significantly by psychological factors and others are "purely" physical. This "either-or" concept represents a simplistic attempt to relate a disease, as it exists in a particular individual, to a single cause.

In contrast, Engel, beginning in the 1950s, emphasized a "multifactorial" concept of etiology and, more recently, developed the "biopsychosocial model" of disease.[3,4] This model acknowledges that most diseases are the result of the complex interaction of multiple factors—biological, psychological, and sociocultural—converging at a particular point of time in the life of an individual. In addition, regardless of etiological considerations, disease obviously affects psychological and social functioning, which in turn influences the course of disease further. Thus, a cycle is established that is not captured fully by the term "psychosomatic"; indeed, in 1999, the American Psychosomatic Society was debating a change in name to acknowledge this fact.

BIOPSYCHOSOCIAL MODEL OF DISEASE

The degree to which any one etiological factor contributes to the development of disease depends on a number of considerations. First, some diseases appear to be influenced more than others by psychological and sociocultural factors. The clinical course of inflammatory bowel disease, for example, may be related to the psychological status of the patient. On the other hand, no evidence exists that brain tumors in children are affected by such factors. However, the lack of evidence of such a relationship may, in any given instance, be a result of insufficient study of this possibility. Second, just as the virulence and dose of a microorganism affect the development and severity of an infectious disease, so may the nature and intensity of a psychosocial stimulus influence its impact on a disease process. Third, individual biological differences attributable to genetic makeup, or previous experiences, modify the effect of psychological and sociocultural factors on the health status of the individual. Fourth, of special interest to those caring for children, temporal and developmental factors may alter the role of psychological and sociocultural stimuli in disease. Thus, an individual's vulnerability to develop the clinical manifestations of a particular disease may change with progression from infancy to late adulthood, with biological, psychological, and sociocultural factors all interacting within the context of age.

That psychosocial factors may influence diseases that traditionally are not considered "psychosomatic" in nature has been observed clinically and, as reviewed by Plaut and Friedman,[6] has been supported by experimental findings in infectious illnesses. Therefore, no specific number of diseases can be identified as psychosomatic, but rather a spectrum of illnesses exists with varying degrees of susceptibility to psychological and sociocultural stimuli. Diseases such as asthma and peptic ulcer, for example, traditionally have been viewed as influenced by psychological factors, but in managing these diseases the clinician should not necessarily assign etiological importance to psychological factors in every patient who has these illnesses. Extreme biological vulnerability in a given patient may result in disease symptoms without psychological distress or conflict beyond that normally experienced in everyday life. On the other hand, the presence or absence of psychosocial stressors may, in another individual, determine whether predisposition toward a disease will become a clinical problem later. Further, psychosocial factors may influence the response to drugs or other forms of therapy.

Understanding is beginning to emerge of the underlying physiological mechanisms that may link psychosocial stimuli to clinical symptomatology. For instance, numerous studies have demonstrated the influence of a wide range of stressors on immune function.[5]

ROLE OF THE PEDIATRICIAN

In the evaluation of symptoms and disease, the pediatrician always should consider psychosocial factors of possible etiologic importance.[7] In many instances, however, the benign and infrequent nature of the illness, such as occasional upper respiratory infection, does not warrant an extensive psychosocial assessment of the patient and family. In other instances, the pediatrician would be remiss not to evaluate the psychological status of the patient thoroughly; examples include severe headaches, hypertension, and chronic gastrointestinal symptoms.

In the medical evaluation, the physician should be aware of those diseases that frequently appear to be influenced by psychosocial stressors (e.g., asthma, inflammatory bowel disease). In addition, the interactions between disease and psychosocial factors that are characteristic of some diseases should be explored, such as exacerbation of asthmatic symptoms secondary to persistent family dysfunction.

The psychological environment of the child or adolescent also should be addressed. This evaluation may be divided into the three major spheres of a child's life: relationship to peers, functioning within the family, and successes and failures at school, work, or both. Basically, the psychological world of the child should be defined, including parental expectations and environmental pressures, as well as sources of psychological and social support. For example, within the context of the child's family, social, and community environments, is the child feeling excessive pressure to conform? Are expectations unreasonable? Are these expectations related more to parental needs than to those of the child? The answers to such questions should be accompanied by evaluation of the child's past and current coping abilities, psychological strengths, and the existence or lack of social support systems.

The child's physical, psychosocial, and cognitive development also should be assessed, with a focus on identifying biological or experiential factors that might predispose him or her to certain diseases or might make psychological adaptations more difficult. In terms of temperament, was this child's early behavior that of the "difficult child?" Is there a history of hyperactivity or learning problems in the family? Has the patient been abused or rejected by his or her parents? Counseling and/or referral to a mental health professional is then based on this overall assessment.

In the psychosocial evaluation of a child or adolescent, the developmental status is critical in interpreting the child's "psychological world" (see Chapter 52, Theories and Concepts of Development as They Relate to Pediatric Practice). Are the child's behaviors age appropriate? Of at least equal importance, are the expectations of parents (and grandparents) age appropriate for the child? The pediatrician should have an ongoing clinical impression of the "match" between the patient's chronological age and developmental status.

In conclusion, the concept of a defined number of "psychosomatic diseases" is overly limited. Rather, a spectrum of susceptibility to psychosocial factors exists that is related to the disease entity, the biological and psychological makeup of the patient, the psychological and sociocultural environment, and the developmental status of the child or adolescent. The clinical importance of these considerations must be individualized by the primary care practitioner. The clinical management, including the advisability of mental health consultation, must be planned accordingly.

REFERENCES

1. Alexander F: *Psychosomatic medicine,* New York, 1950, WW Norton.
2. Dunbar HF: *Psychosomatic diagnosis,* New York, 1943, Hoeber (Harper & Row).
3. Engel GL: The need for a new medical model: a challenge for biomedicine, *Science* 196:129, 1977.
4. Engel GL: Selection of clinical material in psychosomatic medicine, *Psychosom Med* 16:368, 1954.
5. Kiecolt-Glaser JK, Glaser R: Psychoneuroimmunology and health consequences: data and shared mechanisms, *Psychosom Med* 57:269, 1995.
6. Plaut SM, Friedman SB: Psychological factors in infectious disease. In Ader R, editor: *Psychoneuroimmunology,* New York, 1981, Academic Press.
7. Prazar G: Psychosomatic disorders and conversion reactions. In Friedman SB, et al, editors: *Comprehensive adolescent health care*, ed 2, St Louis, 1998, Mosby.

81 Prediction of Adult Behavior from Childhood

David S. Pellegrini

The common assumption is that adult psychopathology has its roots in childhood adjustment difficulties. By extension, earlier intervention in such difficulties generally is assumed better, because psychopathology is likely to crystallize over time, making subsequent remediation more difficult. Epidemiological studies suggest that a large proportion of children show some behavioral or emotional deviance at some stage of their development. However, according to Rutter et al,[9] such problems prove to be transitory in the majority of cases. Moreover, a number of well-intentioned early intervention programs have yielded adverse or mixed results.

Clearly, therapeutic efforts are not without risk. Unnecessary treatment might best be avoided if children otherwise would grow out of their difficulties through the natural process of development. Therefore, identifying those children prone to suffer serious lifetime maladjustment would be enormously advantageous.

Unfortunately, although childhood behavior and early life circumstances show some tendency to predict adult behavior, the correlations generally are too modest to allow useful prediction with regard to individuals.[8] For example, in a large-scale study published in 1973, West and Farrington[11] obtained a false-positive identification rate greater than 50% when predicting delinquency based on early family and child characteristics. Nevertheless, available findings offer some important and useful clues to guide the primary care physician in referring appropriate children for treatment.

Temperamental differences among infants and very young children frequently are noted by parents and hence are likely to be of interest to their pediatricians. Such temperamental qualities as irritability, low regularity, and low malleability are widely assumed to identify children who are likely to remain "difficult" throughout their life spans. However, most dimensions of temperament have proven to be elusive, and the characteristics ascribed to temperament generally appear to be unstable over time. Kagan and Snidman[4] have established "inhibition" as a relatively stable, potentially important temperamental contributor to social behavior. Inhibited children tend to be markedly quiet, fearful, and restrained in their approach to unfamiliar and risk-taking situations. (The physiological profile of such children is characterized by a low heart rate and a relatively low level of circulating cortisol.) Recent research suggests that temperamental inhibition may be an early marker of emotional dysregulation, of which anxiety disorder is one eventual consequence later in life.[6] Temperamental disinhibition, on the other hand, appears to be a possible risk factor in the subsequent development of conduct disorder and various forms of antisocial behavior, especially in children living under adverse social circumstances.[3]

Various symptoms of neurotic or emotional disorders also are readily observed and are very common in childhood. These include nail-biting, thumb-sucking, bed-wetting, eating and sleeping difficulties, and fears of animals, situations, and places. Such symptoms appear to be of little long-term significance when they are mildly intense and when they occur in isolation, rather than as part of a general pattern of multiple symptomatology. Isolated symptoms of this kind might best be thought of as exaggerations of normal developmental trends rather than as signs of a childhood disorder or as precursors of an adult disorder. On the other hand, the timing of such symptoms is interesting. Manifestations of emotional distress appear to be less benign when they are age inappropriate than when they occur at ages when the conditions are more common. For example, school refusal or phobia in an 11-year-old typically has a poorer long-term prognosis than the same clinical condition in a child just beginning school. See Chapter 75, School Absenteeism and School Refusal.

General emotional disorder, in contrast to isolated symptomatology, does appear to have some long-term risk. Rutter et al[9] observed that children who manifested emotional disorder at age 10 years were twice as likely as the general population to show such disorders at age 14 years. However, even those children who show severe and persistent disorders of this kind appear to have a relatively good adult prognosis, with or without treatment. Moreover, when emotional disorders do persist into adulthood, they tend to remain true to type, rather than evolving into more troubling conditions such as adult sociopathy or psychosis. Finally, emotionally troubled children seem to respond better to treatment than any other maladjusted group. Evidence suggests that appropriate and timely intervention can shorten the course of emotional disorders.

Childhood depression is one such condition for which the empirical picture is considerably less clear. Unlike most other symptoms of emotional maladjustment, depressive indicators such as sad mood, apathy, and self-deprecation become increasingly prevalent with age, especially among girls. It appears that isolated symptoms of depression are much more common among prepubertal children than was once thought.[10] Such symptoms have been recognized increasingly as common corollaries or consequences of physical illness and injury in childhood.

Less consensus exists regarding the prevalence of depression as a syndrome in childhood, although it probably is much less common before than after puberty. Most mood disturbances appear to be so short-lived before puberty that some have argued against clinical intervention in all but the most severe cases. However, adequate long-term data particularly are sparse in this area. Although depressive illness arising in adolescence has been shown to have a relatively poor long-term prognosis, possible links between untreated depressive symptomatology in childhood and chronic mood problems or other difficulties in adulthood have not been explored adequately.

In contrast to most indicators of neurosis or emotional disorder, certain indicators of social and behavioral maladjustment in childhood have demonstrated considerable predictive power with regard to adult psychopathology. However, few such predictors exhibit clear continuity with or a direct developmental path to specific and unique outcomes. Rather, they tend to predict a range of adverse outcomes. Moreover, predictive stability of this kind does not emerge until the early school years.

One such indicator pertains to the quality of peer relations. Recent research suggests that peers play a number of important roles in child development. For example, as agents of socialization, peers help to shape sexual and aggressive behavior. They also are a major source of emotional support, while providing instruction in a variety of social, cognitive, and motor skills. It should not be surprising, then, that poor peer relations in early childhood have been linked with later emotional difficulties, delinquency, substance abuse, suicide, and psychosis.

In one classic study, Cowen et al[2] attempted to uncover the early signs of persistent psychiatric disturbance. Of 537 schoolchildren, 33% (180) were identified as being at risk on the basis of ineffective school performance and behavior. By the time of follow-up 11 years later, 19% of this group, compared with only 5% of nondesignated children, had received some form of psychiatric care, as indexed by appearance on a cumulative county register. Negative peer evaluations in third grade exceeded a variety of other adjustment indicators (including teacher and school nurse judgments) in predicting later mental health difficulties.

Active rejection by peers seems to be more critical in the prediction and the development of later psychopathology than is social isolation resulting from shyness and social withdrawal. Indeed, shyness alone appears not to be as closely linked to adult disorders, such as schizophrenia, as once was thought. In a long-term epidemiological study undertaken in the Woodlawn area of Chicago, Kellam et al[5] found that shyness in first grade actually was correlated with reduced rates of delinquency and substance abuse in adolescent boys and with reduced intake of hard liquor in adolescent girls. However, shyness was related to higher levels of anxiety in adolescent boys (see Chapter 91, Peer Relationship Problems).

Early antisocial behavior and aggressiveness appear to be the sturdiest predictors of adult maladjustment. For example, in an exceptionally thorough and well-planned study, Robins[7] followed up with 500 individuals who had attended child psychiatry clinics 30 years earlier. Whereas most neurotic children went on to lead psychiatrically normal lives, children who engaged in early and repeated delinquent or aggressive acts grew up to be, with disturbing regularity, adult sociopaths. Looking backward, Robins noted that 95% of the adult sociopaths had been referred initially for antisocial and aggressive behavior.

In the Woodlawn study,[5] aggressiveness in first-grade boys clearly was linked to delinquency and heavy drug, alcohol, and cigarette use in adolescence. Although such associations were not apparent for girls, aggressiveness in conjunction with social isolation was associated with the poorest outcome for both genders. Aggressive behavior also has emerged as a primary prognostic component of hyperactivity.

Troublesome behavior patterns appear most likely to persist into adulthood when other social, psychological, and cognitive handicaps are present. According to Rutter et al,[9] parental antisocial behavior or alcoholism, chronic marital discord, and poor academic achievement tend to potentiate emerging behavioral difficulties for the child. Pervasive behavioral problems also tend to persist more than situation-specific problems. For example, those few youngsters who demonstrate hyperactivity, poor impulse control, and attentional problems in multiple settings (e.g., school, home, and the community at large) are more likely to show a variety of difficulties later in life (e.g., antisocial behavior, poor academic achievement, and depression) than are youngsters who are hyperactive in only one such setting (the majority of such cases). Similarly, children who engage in a variety of delinquent acts in multiple settings are at greater risk for adult criminality than are those who engage in isolated delinquent acts (see Chapter 106, Juvenile Delinquency).

Clearly, much more work is needed to determine the early precursors of, turning points in, and contextual (family, peer, and community) influences on psychopathology. In the interim we are left with only general guidelines regarding the appropriate timing of clinical intervention.[1] Available findings to date highlight the particular importance of early treatment for pervasive conduct and relational problems, especially because intervention efforts with antisocial adolescents and adults so far have proved to be singularly unsuccessful.

Early intervention also seems warranted whenever symptoms appear likely to interfere with the acquisition of social and academic skills, which could, in turn, lead to social rejection and school or work failure. Beyond that, intervention may be justified on the grounds of relieving or shortening the immediate distress caused by the symptoms themselves, even when they may bear little or no functional relationship to later difficulties.

REFERENCES

1. Coie JD, et al: The science of prevention: a conceptual framework and some directions for a national research program, *Am Psychol* 48:1013, 1993.
2. Cowen EL, et al: Long-term follow-up of early detected vulnerable children, *J Consult Clin Psychol* 41:438, 1973.
3. Earls F: Oppositional-defiant and conduct disorders. In Rutter M, Taylor E, Hersov L, editors: *Child and adolescent psychiatry: modern approaches*, ed 3, London, 1994, Blackwell.
4. Kagan J, Snidman N: Temperamental factors in human development, *Am Psychol* 46:856, 1991.
5. Kellam SG, et al: Paths leading to teenage psychiatric symptoms and substance use: developmental epidemiological studies in Woodlawn. In Guze SB, Earls FJ, Barrett JE, editors: *Childhood psychopathology and development*, New York, 1983, Raven Press.

6. Klein RG: Anxiety disorders. In Rutter M, Taylor E, Hersov L, editors: *Child and adolescent psychiatry: modern approaches*, ed 3, London, 1994, Blackwell.
7. Robins L: Sturdy childhood predictors of adult antisocial behavior: replications form longitudinal studies, *Psychol Med* 8:611, 1978.
8. Rutter M: Pathways from childhood to adult life, *J Child Psychol Psychiatry* 30:23, 1989.
9. Rutter M, et al: Isle of Wight studies, 1964-1974, *Psychol Med* 6:313, 1976.
10. Rutter M, Izard CE, Read PB, editors: *Depression in young people: developmental and clinical perspectives*, New York, 1986, Guilford Press.
11. West DJ, Farrington DG: *Who becomes delinquent?* London, 1973, Heinemann.

82 Options for Psychosocial Intervention with Children and Adolescents

Sheridan Phillips

Pediatricians may be unsure about what therapeutic options exist for children and adolescents who have psychosocial problems, as well as about what actually will transpire in the course of treatment. This hampers the effort to refer the patient appropriately and to prepare the child and parents for what to expect.

This chapter acquaints the pediatrician with the most common forms of therapeutic interventions available and provides a brief review of their efficacy. Discussion is focused on treatment rather than on assessment. Also, only "psychological" treatment is described (pharmacotherapy is not discussed), although it must be noted that a combination of psychotherapy and pharmacotherapy is indicated for some disorders.[12] The key aspects of major approaches to child therapy are highlighted. There are also a plethora of techniques: Kazdin,[13,14] in his review of the child psychotherapy literature, identified more than 230 therapy techniques from "activity-interview" therapy to "Z-process therapy."

Much of the confusion regarding psychotherapy is caused by two confounding variables: the therapist's theoretical orientation and the modality in which it is used. For example, one can take a behavioral approach with a child or with a family. Alternatively, family therapy can be conducted from a "systems" point of view. This chapter examines the five major schools of thought, or theoretical orientations, as well as the modalities in which they most commonly are applied (sometimes in adapted form), as shown in Table 82-1. Each school of thought listed at the left in the table is presented as a separate and distinct orientation. It is important, however, to emphasize that these are artificial divisions. Much more melding and blending occurs in the actual practice of child therapy, and combinations of approaches are both sensible and common. The modalities in which these theoretical orientations are typically applied are indicated under the appropriate column in the table.

Discussion of each therapeutic orientation includes the basic premises and goals of treatment, its typical course (e.g., length), examples of techniques or procedures used, most appropriate recipients, and a brief review of the efficacy of that approach. Evaluating the efficacy of treatment, however, is so important yet complex that a general discussion of psychotherapy research precedes the presentation of specific therapeutic orientations.

In an attempt to provide an overview, this review undoubtedly oversimplifies both theories and issues and omits much of the detail and nuance each orientation deserves. Specific discussion of when and how to refer children is not included, because this is provided throughout this section of the textbook for each specific clinical problem, as well as general indicators in Chapter 83, Consultation and Referral for Behavioral and Developmental Problems.

THERAPEUTIC EFFECTIVENESS: GENERAL CONSIDERATIONS

Physicians, consumers, and society at large have an abiding concern to document the usefulness of therapy. The "bottom line" questions are, "Does it work?" and "Is it cost effective?" These questions are easy to ask but extraordinarily difficult to answer. Conceptual, methodological, pragmatic, and ethical considerations appear to conspire against a clear-cut assessment of therapeutic efforts. Before discussing the effectiveness of specific orientations and modalities, this section reviews the general types of research strategies used to evaluate therapies and the complexity of and problems inherent in such research.

One form of psychotherapy research is focused on the *process* of treatment and examines aspects of therapy as it is unfolding (i.e., what transpires within a session). This large body of literature has yielded useful information about treatment[2] (e.g., see section on client-centered therapy in this chapter). However, for the sake of brevity this section reviews the other major type of research, *outcome* research, which investigates change that occurs from the beginning to the end of therapy and following the conclusion of treatment. Ideally such investigations document the nature and extent of change and demonstrate that such outcomes result directly from specific aspects of the intervention.

One approach is a *within-subject* design, whereby the experimental control is internal (i.e., no control groups are used). In this approach each subject or patient serves as his or her own control. Such an evaluation typically begins with a "baseline" period, during which the patient's behavior is recorded before any attempt at intervention. Recording continues during an intervention phase, when specific therapeutic procedures are in effect. One then may cease intervention and return to the baseline condition and subsequently reinstitute treatment. Repeated alternation accompanied by substantial changes in the observed behavior is an indication that the treatment is responsible for the behavior change. A variant of this design is to introduce one component of the treatment at a time (e.g., each might be targeted at a different type of behavior) to determine whether a behavior changes when—and only when—the relevant intervention is intro-

Table 82-1 Overview of Therapeutic Orientations and Therapeutic Modalities

	Therapeutic Modality					
Therapeutic Orientation	**Individual (Child Alone)**	**Parents Alone**	**Parents and Child**	**Family**	**Group (Children and/or Parents)**	**Residential**
Psychodynamic	X	Adapted		Adapted	Adapted	Adapted
Behavioral	X	X	X	X	X	X
Phenomenological						
Client-centered	X				X	
Gestalt	X				X	
Systems		X		X		
Eclectic	X	X	X	X	X	X

duced. The durability of change is assessed at various follow-up points.

The advantages of this design are the degree of experimental control and specificity it offers and its applicability with only a small number of patients or even with a single case (a "single-subject" design). Although internally valid, however, it is difficult to generalize from only one case; replications and extensions thus are required to increase confidence in the efficacy of treatment. Another difficulty is the "irreversibility" of some interventions, either for pragmatic or ethical reasons. It also has been argued that a therapeutic effect should be permanent and not so easily reversible.

A *within-group* design employs a homogeneous group of subjects (e.g., fourth- and fifth-grade children diagnosed with AD/HD) who receive several treatment phases in sequence, such as a baseline followed by methylphenidate treatment, then behavioral academic intervention, then social skills training, then methylphenidate plus behavioral academic contingencies. Such studies may include placebo phases and, ideally, variations in sequence so that not all children receive different treatments in the same order. Sophisticated studies employ several outcome measures, with hypothesized differences regarding how each will be affected by the various treatments.

In *between-subject* research, the nature of change is compared for a therapy group (or groups) versus a control group (or groups), typically before and after treatment and at various follow-up points (e.g., 6 months and 1 year after treatment). If done well, such research is costly and complex. For example, studies generally include several treatment groups. One group might receive a complete treatment "package" consisting of two components; a second group might receive one component only and a third group the second component only, with appropriate "fillers" to equate time spent in treatment. (Note how a three-component package would generate seven treatment groups.) Alternatively, or in addition, another group might receive a different type of treatment (e.g., behavior therapy versus client-centered therapy). With this approach the difficulty is in controlling for therapist characteristics: using a "switch-hitter" most likely would result in differential levels of skill confounded with therapeutic orientation, whereas using different individuals would confound personal characteristics and therapeutic orientation.

Devising appropriate control groups is no easier. One option is to use a "no treatment," or "waiting list," control group. This is accomplished by collecting a large group of comparable patients who have requested treatment and then randomly assigning them to therapy conditions: (1) immediate treatment or (2) treatment following a waiting period, with a delay at least as long as therapy for the treatment group (and longer if maintenance is to be assessed). It is common for at least some patients in the waiting-list group to improve over time. This is thought to occur because the individuals who have requested treatment have come to recognize that they have a problem and have made a commitment to change; deprived of access to professional therapists, they often turn to therapists in their environment (e.g., friends, pastor, self-help groups) or simply apply for treatment elsewhere. With children, one also must consider the effect of maturation during the waiting period.

Another important control is the "placebo," or "attention-control," group, in which the therapist is given the challenging task of conducting sessions with patients but not actually doing anything specific. This controls for the patient's expectation that he or she is being helped and for "nonspecific" effects of therapy. The "nonspecificity" hypothesis asserts that significant change in therapy can be attributed to four primary factors: (1) providing a trusting and caring relationship, (2) working within a "safe" atmosphere, (3) explaining confusing feelings and behaviors, and (4) implementing a set of procedures based on some conceptual scheme.[19] Such nonspecific factors are used to explain why placebo control groups typically display some improvement and why different forms of therapy can achieve equivalent results. To demonstrate its efficacy, then, a therapeutic intervention must demonstrate that it produced significantly greater change than could be accounted for by the nonspecific aspects of treatment.

A host of other difficulties besets research endeavors, such as the selection of appropriate dependent measures (behavior to be recorded) and the reliability and validity of the methods by which behaviors are assessed. Assuming that these challenges can be met and that a large enough pool of comparable patients and comparable therapists is available, the researcher still is confronted by major ethical concerns. Withholding treatment for an extended time and offering placebo intervention or a treatment hypothesized to be less than optimal all pose clear ethical obstacles.

It is understandable, therefore, to find that some investigators have chosen to conduct analog research, which attempts to simulate clinical conditions in the laboratory. In earlier analog research, participants typically were undergraduates who volunteered for course credit or monetary incentives or who had minor problems (e.g., mild fear of snakes or dogs or mild test-taking or speech-giving anxiety). More recent clinical research has recruited volunteers from the community who experienced more substantial problems but generally did not qualify for a diagnosis and had not been referred for treatment. Even when diagnosed patients are used, they typically are selected with stringent criteria, eliminating single-parent or foster-care children, and any children with comorbidity, to ensure "pure" instances of a disorder. The difficulty with this approach is the trade-off between internal and external validity: although greater experimental control is gained, the ability to generalize to real clinical situations is lessened.

Given the numerous and varied obstacles to be confronted, it is admirable to find investigators who remain undaunted and struggle valiantly to conduct the best possible evaluations of their therapeutic efforts. Accepting this challenge has continued to improve the level of sophistication evidenced in psychotherapy research. Even the questions asked have become more sophisticated and have moved well beyond the question of, "Does it work?" The ultimate outcome question posed by Paul is, "What treatment, by whom, is most effective for this individual, with this problem, under this set of circumstances, and how does it come about?"[2] Clearly this question cannot be answered by a single study but will represent the cumulative knowledge of multiple efforts to address the effectiveness of therapy.

THERAPEUTIC EFFICACY: EMPIRICALLY SUPPORTED TREATMENTS

Social pressure, particularly from managed health care and government agencies, has prompted professional organizations to develop guidelines for effective psychosocial intervention. The American Psychological Association (APA) convened a task force that published a report in 1995[23] delineating a number of empirically validated treatments that had demonstrated efficacy in psychotherapy outcome research. Because the original task force report focused largely on adult disorders, the APA's Division of Clinical Psychology subsequently commissioned a divisional task force to examine the evidence for psychosocial intervention with children. The first report was published in a special issue of the *Journal of Clinical Child Psychology*.[17] Criteria were established for determining adequate study design and empirical support, and several efficacious interventions were identified for children with anxiety disorders, conduct problems and AD/HD; "probably efficacious" treatments were identified for childhood depression, and interventions for autism came close to "probably efficacious." These findings confirm those of various meta-analyses that examined child outcome research published between 1952 and 1993:

1. The majority (75% or more) of empirically-supported treatments are behavioral or cognitive-behavioral in focus, followed by family therapy, with fewer than 10% involving psychoanalytic, psychodynamic, client-centered, or existential-humanistic models.
2. The average treatment effect is similar to that for adult psychotherapy.
3. Treatment effects are specific (i.e., stronger for targeted than for nontargeted problems).
4. Follow-up assessments (an average of 6 months posttreatment) show maintenance of treatment effects.[26]

The development of practice guidelines based on outcome research has significant limitations,[17] not the least of which is the difference between treatment *efficacy* demonstrated in controlled clinical research and clinical *effectiveness* in everyday clinical practice. When and how intervention must be adapted to the messier and more challenging realities of clinical service remains to be investigated. Nevertheless, the search for empirically supported treatments (EST) is a vital first step towards improving clinical practice. First, although most EST are behavioral or cognitive-behavioral, much of clinical practice involves other intervention approaches[14,17]; this suggests the need to scrutinize clinical practice with greater rigor. Second, the few studies that have investigated effectiveness of current practice in service settings have yielded generally negligible effects.[26] Although EST will undoubtedly need to be modified for practice, they at least provide a promising place to start. Treatments that are not efficacious in clinical trials are unlikely to be effective in clinical practice. Third, those EST that have been identified to date suggest that there are currently interventions of choice for some specific childhood disorders: depression, anxiety, conduct problems, and AD/HD.[15]

PSYCHODYNAMIC THERAPY

Basic Assumptions

Psychodynamic therapy covers a wide variety of approaches, from traditional analysis to neofreudian variants such as sociocultural, object relations, and ego psychology. The fundamental assumptions, however, were derived from Freud by his daughter, Anna Freud, by Melanie Klein, and by subsequent analytical theorists who specialized in work with children.[7] The concept of unconscious conflict is central: the child's disturbed or abnormal behavior is hypothesized to result from intrapsychic conflict in the same manner that an infection causes the overt manifestation of a fever.

Therefore, treatment is focused on identifying and resolving the underlying conflict among instinctual urges (id), conscious thoughtful regulation or reality orientation (ego), and self-evaluative thoughts, or "conscience" (superego). In contrast with other therapy approaches, psychodynamic therapists do not base decisions related to termination of therapy on whether presenting symptoms have improved. Instead, therapy continues until internal conflicts are brought to the surface and worked through. The belief is that, without resolution of underlying problems, other symptoms will develop to replace the original symptoms, what some dynamic therapists refer to as "old wine in new bottles."

Therapeutic Activities

The therapist first attempts to establish a relationship with the child that will enable the child to feel free to express any thoughts and feelings, such as anger and sadness. In fact this freedom of expression is seen by many theorists to be therapeutic in itself. With this relationship in place the therapist comments on the child's expressed feelings, generally interpreting the meaning of symbols revealed in the child's fantasies, dreams, or, most often, free play. Most of the therapeutic work is conducted in a playroom, using materials such as clay and sand, fingerpaints, games, and human figures and a dollhouse. The "depth" of interpretation provided varies among different theorists. For example, a doll thrown across the room might be seen by Anna Freud as anger toward the situation, whereas others might interpret it as hatred for the mother.

Although interpretation is an important therapeutic device, it is used parsimoniously, especially at the outset of treatment. Most therapists draw on additional devices, such as developing the transference reaction (or reaction to the therapist), "working through" past interpersonal conflicts, and gratifying dependency needs. The many different adaptations of psychodynamic treatment and variation among therapists make it difficult to provide a unitary picture of therapeutic activities. Many therapists vary the intensity of treatment and their approach, depending on the developmental stage of the child, the nature of the psychopathology, and the family situation.

Certain obvious adjustments have been made to apply psychodynamic treatment to children. Because children find it more difficult than adults to express their inner lives verbally, play is used more often than techniques based on free association (method of encouraging the patient to reveal anything that comes to mind, without censorship or guiding efforts by the therapist, in an effort to bring forth unconscious processes). Also, children generally do not seek therapy themselves; thus it is the therapist's responsibility to develop the child's insight so that he or she understands that a problem exists. Even with these modifications, however, analytical intervention generally is not attempted with children younger than 4 years of age. For the most part adolescents have not been considered to be appropriate candidates for such treatment because they are too old for play therapy and too young for the traditional analytical couch.

Less traditional forms of psychodynamic therapy increasingly have been used with children and adolescents.[6] Particularly when children and adolescents have experienced severe trauma such as sexual abuse, psychodynamic therapy techniques play a central role in treatment. In addition to education regarding common misperceptions of sexually abused children (e.g., feelings of self-blame, guilt, inferiority), these children are assisted in reporting on what happened to them and in expressing emotions associated with the abuse. Such processing and working through of abuse-related perceptions and emotions is viewed as central in removing threatening and disabling aspects of the abusive experience. The ultimate aim is for the child to achieve some perspective and self-acceptance such as, "Yes, that happened to me, and I can talk about it. But I know that I did nothing wrong and many other children have experienced what I have. I also know that I can cope with what happened and move on with my life."[11] Many therapists believe that for the abused child or adolescent to reach this perspective it is necessary to revisit and work through painful historical events and conflicts, the sine qua non of psychodynamic therapy.

As shown in Table 82-1 the traditional form of psychodynamic treatment has been conducted alone with the child. Whereas Anna Freud believed that it was the therapist's responsibility to educate parents about their child's problems, many psychodynamic therapists deliberately have little contact with the parents and other family members. Such therapists generally consider it inappropriate to work with both the child and any other family member; thus it is quite possible to find a family that uses three or more therapists: one for the child, another for a second child, and a third for the parents' marital problems. A major concern of psychodynamic therapists is that, when working with parents and the child together, the child will perceive an alliance between the adults and thus feel that his or her relationship with the therapist has been compromised. Additional rationales for this approach are the avoidance of "competition" for the therapist and "transference" problems that may arise when parents and children are seen together.

The disadvantage of separate therapists is the frequent lack of coordination among their efforts, so at times they may be working at cross purposes. The absence of contact between the therapist and the child's parents also often results in the parents' ignorance of the child's problems, of the goals and progress of therapy, and of what parents might do to assist the child's progress. Meeting only with the child may leave parents with the impression that they are expending significant money and effort, often over a period of several years, to enable the child to play with toys such as those he or she has at home. This obviously does a disservice to the therapist's efforts. Such problems have prompted adaptations of psychodynamic treatment, with some therapists seeing the entire family together or meeting with the parents separately.[6]

The psychodynamic approach also has been adapted for use with groups of children and adolescents (usually from five to eight children). Group therapy has two major assets: it makes more efficient use of professional time and provides therapy in a different setting, where children interact with and learn from each other as well as from the therapist. Groups of younger children typically play games or engage in activities such as arts and crafts, with the therapist guiding the group indirectly (i.e., by example). Psychodrama and more "talking" techniques generally are employed with older children and adolescents. The main goals of treatment continue to be achieving insight into and resolving unconscious conflict. Such groups may be homogeneous (e.g., victims of sexual abuse) or more heterogeneous (e.g., including both aggressive and withdrawn children). It also is possible to structure residential treatment with many psychodynamic features—combining individual and group treatment in an accepting, tolerant atmosphere that highlights the use of expressive materials such as paints and clay.

The course of traditional child psychoanalysis is lengthy, typically requiring two to four sessions per week for anywhere from 2 to 5 years. The obvious expense of such treatment and the limited number of children who can receive it have led to the development of less extensive psychotherapy that incorporates many aspects of analysis. Such intervention might involve one or two sessions a week for 1 to 3 years. The more limited goals of this shorter-term treatment have been described as (1) increasing capacity for reality testing, (2) strengthening object relations, and (3) loosening fixations. The appropriate adult candidate for psychodynamic treatment has been semijokingly referred to as a "YAVIS," young, attractive, verbal, intelligent, and salaried. The same general point can be applied to children because the typical patient is only mildly to moderately disturbed and has many assets. Aspects of the analytical approach, however, have been included in other interventions with more universal applicability (see section on eclectic therapy in this chapter).

Efficacy

Although a considerable amount of study has been devoted to child psychoanalysis and new adaptations of psychodynamic therapy, the majority of these investigations represent either uncontrolled case studies or investigations of the therapeutic process. Thus, some data are available regarding process questions, such as (1) who is an appropriate candidate for psychodynamic therapy, and (2) the effect of therapists' interpretations.

As with all forms of therapy, less research has been conducted with children than with adults. For both children and adults, psychodynamic therapists have paid the least amount of attention to outcome research, or controlled investigation of actual change or improvement produced by treatment.

Following Eysenck's devastating 1952 critique of the outcome of psychodynamic psychotherapy with adults, a similar analysis of traditional psychotherapy with children was conducted.[21] This work, published in 1957 and 1963, failed to find any sound support for the contention that traditional psychotherapy facilitates children's recovery from mental illness. These startling reports prompted attempts to broaden approaches to the treatment of children and to develop other alternatives, notably that of behavior therapy.

In recent years investigators have used "meta-analysis" in an attempt to evaluate the effectiveness of various therapies. Meta-analysis enables quantification of the results of studies so that they are comparable with other investigations. The most common meta-analytic technique is to compute "effect size," defined as the difference between the means of treatment and control groups divided by the standard deviation of the control group. A number of meta-analyses have been conducted on the adult psychotherapy literature, with findings generally indicating that treatment is better than no treatment and that alternative models of therapy typically have equivalent impacts; for specific problems such as fears, behavior therapy has been shown to be superior.

Very few meta-analyses have been conducted on child therapies. Casey and Berman[3] reviewed 75 psychotherapy interventions among children published between 1952 and 1983 and found that only 5 of the 75 studies (9%) used a psychodynamic approach. Effect size for these psychodynamic interventions was 0.21, the lowest effect size of any therapy (compared with effect sizes of 0.49 for client-centered therapy and 0.91 for behavior therapy). However, interpretation of this finding is constrained by the small number of psychodynamic studies reviewed. An additional consideration is that outcomes in psychodynamic interventions tend to be defined broadly (and subjectively), which decreases the likelihood of documenting significant change, particularly compared with behavioral studies, which generally use specific and discrete outcome criteria (e.g., the number of fears reported on a self-report measure). Other child therapy meta-analyses have since replicated Casey and Berman's findings, indicating the relative inferiority of psychodynamic techniques compared with behavioral techniques.[17,26] Studies of group psychotherapies similarly have shown relatively limited impacts of psychodynamic approaches, particularly compared with behavioral methods.[13]

Part of the difficulty in conducting scientific research of psychoanalysis lies in the very nature of the concepts used. For example, how can one gain access to an unconscious that by definition is inaccessible? However, the crux of the problem is determining acceptable criteria for measuring outcome: symptom relief is viewed as being too superficial an index of the change brought about in the child. Furthermore, many analysts maintain that each situation or case is unique; therefore, no situation can be replicated and no two patients adequately matched. They also argue that it is impossible to differentiate changes caused by maturation from those resulting from therapy. Finally, most analytically oriented therapists agree with Freud in insisting that psychoanalysis can be judged only by experienced analysts. However, Freud himself was not optimistic about a scientific study of psychoanalysis.

One must observe that these obstacles have not hindered therapists of other orientations from at least attempting to evaluate the effectiveness of their interventions in a controlled manner. Ultimately, then, the lack of scientific study of psychoanalysis probably reflects the values of its practitioners, who typically are uninterested in research.

BEHAVIOR THERAPY

A behavioral approach to treatment has grown with amazing rapidity. For example, the first report of a token-economy intervention was published in 1968; its use was widespread by the mid-1970s. Behavior therapists who were trained 15 years ago are surprised to find themselves no longer a rebellious, vocal minority but a part of the establishment. Surveys indicate that approximately 50% of all clinical psychologists in the United States and more than 60% of clinical child psychologists identify their orientation as behavioral or cognitive-behavioral. Behavior therapy associations now exist in more than 30 countries.

Basic Assumptions

Behavior therapy is not, as often is thought, a collection of techniques. Rather, it is an approach to conceptualizing and changing human behavior, an approach characterized by empirical methodology.[8,20] The key assumption of behavior therapists is that they must "anchor" their understanding by reference to observable behavior. An abstract concept, such as anxiety, thus is understood by asking questions such as how the patient experiences anxiety, when it is worse and when it is better, what the "trigger" events are, how the patient responds to these anxious situations, and what the consequences are for him or her and for others.

Each patient represents a "miniexperiment" in which the therapist examines the presenting problem and its development in the context of the patient's history. The therapist then searches for those variables that control the problem behavior. The resulting functional analysis represents a hypothesis that guides the therapist. This hypothesis is tested by the therapist and the patient as intervention proceeds. The therapist also typically relies heavily on data collection to assess the progress of treatment and the adequacy of his or her working hypothesis; thus the therapist often asks the patient to monitor and record specific behavior and will track its frequency over time.

A very early focus for behavioral analysis was a search for the stimuli that prompted the behavior and for the patient's response (hence S-R, or stimulus-response). This fairly rapidly evolved to SORC (stimulus-organism-response-consequence), which incorporates "organismic" factors such as the patient's perception of the stimulus and the consequences that the response engendered (e.g., the reaction of others). In the past 20 years growing numbers of behavior therapists have emphasized the importance of patients' thought processes or cognitions, as well as their overt behavior. This approach, referred to as cognitive-behavior therapy, has become the second most common therapy orientation after the "eclectic" orientation.[13] The cognitive-behavior therapist attends to factors such as the patients' expectations for themselves and others, how patients label an event, and what kinds of statements the patients make to themselves.[5] For example, in their work with impulsive children Kendall and Braswell have developed and evaluated interventions that focus on the use of behavioral principles to alter cognition (internal behavior) rather than overt behavior. These children are trained to use a series of self-statements (e.g., "What is my problem?" "What is a good plan?" "How is my plan working?" "How did I do?") in approaching, negotiating, and evaluating their performance in problematic situations.[16]

Increased understanding of such attitudinal and perceptual processes and deliberate attempts to modify them have brought behavior therapy much closer to other therapeutic approaches, such as ego psychology. In fact, the past few years have seen several laudable attempts to bring about a rapprochement between behavioral and psychodynamic formulations.[8]

Even though cognitive-behavioral approaches are gaining increasing prominence, more traditional approaches (manipulating antecedents and reward and punishment contingencies for target behaviors) continue to play a central role in child behavioral interventions, particularly those used with developmentally disabled children and conduct disorder.[18,20]

In designing therapeutic interventions, the behavior therapist draws on the principles and models of experimental psychology.[20] Many of these come from learning theory: classical and operant conditioning, observational-social learning (i.e., modeling), and the development of self-control. Other paradigms also are useful, such as research in social psychology regarding the process of attitude change and "commitment" to a specific course of action. Probably the broadest theory employed is social learning theory, which presumes a continuity between normal and abnormal behavior, implying that maladaptive behaviors are acquired through the same processes as normal behaviors.

Accordingly, specific efforts to learn and use more adaptive behavior are expected to bring about changes in the way patients view themselves and in how others see and react to them. Thus, intervention is a cyclical process involving change in behavior, attitudes, and cognitions. Bandura's more recent "self-efficacy" theory[1] attempts to synthesize a variety of therapeutic interventions as procedures that gradually convince the individual of his or her ability to cope with difficult and frightening situations.

Therapeutic Activities

It is difficult to state succinctly what a behavior therapist does with a patient, because the hallmark of the behavioral approach is to tailor intervention to the particular needs of a given patient. Therefore, therapy is very different for different problems. Although various treatment "packages" have been developed for specific problems, these are standardized largely for research and demonstration and subsequently are adapted for the individual patient. The key, as noted before, is the functional analysis or behavioral formulation of the problem. Treatment then is derived logically from assessment. For example, one important distinction is that of a behavioral *deficit* versus an *inhibition*. In the case of a deficit of the appropriate skills, the therapist would focus on acquiring skills (e.g., for social skills training: see Chapter 91, Peer Relationship Problems). Alternatively a patient might possess the appropriate skills but be inhibited in using them in certain situations because of excessive anxiety or fear of the consequences; therapy then would focus on reducing these inhibitions.

Regardless of the specific problem, some commonalties exist in behavioral and cognitive-behavioral approaches. The focus largely (although not exclusively) is on the present. A commitment to experimental evaluation is critical; the behavior therapist is likely to set concrete goals to be achieved within a relatively short time, with progress then being evaluated by both the therapist and the patient. Whenever possible, targets for intervention are selected based on empirical evidence that changes in such targets will result in enhanced clinical outcomes for the patient, rather than targets being selected by subjective judgment or clinical intuition.[25] Therapy is active and involves joint planning and homework assignments for the patient (and sometimes for the therapist). It is assumed that insight almost always is insufficient for satisfactory behavioral change and that it needs to be accompanied by gradual learning and implementation of new behavior in a concrete manner. Finally, therapy obviously takes place in an interpersonal context, and practitioner characteristics are an important aspect of therapeutic change. Goldfried and Davison[8] have pointed out that a tough-minded approach to conceptualizing human problems in no way precludes a warm, genuine, and empathic interaction with patients. In fact, patients of behavior therapists who were asked to describe their therapist identified the same personal qualities that have been found to be therapeutic in other orientations, such as client-centered therapy (discussed below).

Behavior therapy initially was applied with psychotic, retarded, and autistic populations and with patients who had severe phobias—that is, people who had intractable problems that no one else wanted to treat. This approach to therapy subsequently has been applied to an enormous array of problems and situations and is not restricted by the age of the patient or the type of problem. It may be applied in conjunction with pharmacotherapy (e.g., for treatment of AD/HD), although the goal sometimes is to withdraw medication when feasible (e.g., when treating anxiety or depression).

The same basic principles can be applied with a child who

has a conduct disorder and with a group of hospitalized patients who are not functioning optimally. In fact a behavioral approach has been applied to many nontherapeutic situations (e.g., examining the voting behavior of Congress and energy conservation behaviors of the public) and thus is used in businesses and other consultative settings. For example, one could analyze a pediatric clinic to determine whether the existing contingencies promote desired behavior of its users, such as keeping appointments. Other general education efforts include self-help books (e.g., on toilet training). This broader application of behavior principles generally is referred to as *behavior modification,* with *behavior therapy* referring specifically to clinical problems.

Behavior therapy appears deceptively simple to the neophyte therapist. In fact, the therapist is merely guided by general principles and must rely on considerable improvisation and inventiveness in the clinical situation. Many inexperienced practitioners (and teachers) have failed because of insufficient expertise both with clinical practice and with the theoretical principles on which therapy is based. Thus, it is not uncommon to be told before instituting a successful behavioral program, "Oh, we tried behavior modification and that didn't work."

When using behavior therapy with individual children, therapists typically employ a combination of sessions with the child and parents and, if indicated, the school or other extrafamilial agency. With infants and toddlers the therapist typically works almost exclusively through the parents, although the child may be present for sessions when the therapist "models" a type of interaction with the child or provides feedback to parents as they attempt to interact with the child in a different manner. With older children and adolescents, the extent to which the parents and other family members are involved depends on the analysis of the problem and the focus of treatment. Seeing all family members together for all sessions is indicated in some situations, whereas in others the therapist may choose to focus on the teenager and his or her parents. In cases of multiple problems the therapist may alternate family sessions (e.g., to work on communication and problem solving) with individual sessions (e.g., to address problems with peers). Sessions typically occur once or twice a week, and the length of treatment can be as short as four sessions or can continue for more than a year.

Behavior therapy can be employed also with groups of children or adolescents or with groups of children and their parents. This form of treatment, when appropriate, makes efficient use of professional time and provides an opportunity to interact therapeutically with peers (e.g., engage in role playing). Group therapy typically, although not necessarily, is employed with a relatively homogeneous group, such as shy and withdrawn boys, to enable treatment to focus on specific problems. A group approach also has been employed with parents; some parent-training groups are specifically therapeutic, and others are more educational and designed for a "normal" population.[20]

In any form groups generally are limited in time and rarely continue for longer than 6 months. It is not uncommon for two therapists to lead the group because they offer two models of behavior and also can model interaction with each other (e.g., a male and female therapist with a parent group). In addition, group interactions are so complex that having two therapists helps in tracking events in the group and ensuring that all patients receive therapeutic attention.

Behavioral group therapies often focus on training of skills in a sequential and cumulative fashion (i.e., skills taught earlier are reviewed as new skills are taught). As each skill is taught, group leaders use a format of instruction (on the skill and when and how to use it), demonstration (leaders model the skill), rehearsal (participants take turns practicing the behavior), feedback (leaders and participants provide feedback to each other), continued rehearsal (incorporating feedback), and reinforcement (praise and encouragement from the leaders and participants). In addition, considerable efforts ensure that the trained skills generalize to relevant settings in the child's natural environment (e.g., by incorporating realistic stimuli into training sessions, conducting training in natural environments) and are maintained over time (e.g., by thinning reinforcement schedules from frequent to random).

Behavioral interventions also have had widespread use in the classroom. These range from management tips developed for use in the normal classroom to special classroom programs for children who have attention deficit hyperactivity disorder (AD/HD) or conduct disorder.[7,21] Residential programs also have been developed for a variety of populations.[10,18,24] Two examples are Project Re-ED and Achievement Place, the first for emotionally disturbed children and the second for delinquent children and adolescents.[7] Children are placed in an intensive treatment environment that includes sessions with parents and then are returned gradually to the home. (Achievement Place, a community-based program, even enables children to continue attending their own school during treatment.)

Probably the most extensively evaluated out-of-home programs are those of the Oregon Social Learning Center, using intensified foster care.[4] In residential settings, usually some form of token economy or behavior management system acts as a framework, delineating behavioral expectations for residents and rewards and privileges that correspond to how well they meet these expectations. It is now difficult to find residential programs for emotionally disturbed and retarded children that do not make at least some use of behavioral principles. In fact, behavior therapy's greatest contribution may be the introduction of successful toilet training and management of children with mental retardation. This has released an enormous amount of staff time and reoriented such programs from being almost completely custodial to emphasizing self-care and education.

Efficacy

With the possible exception of client-centered therapy for adults, no other therapeutic approach has been subjected to as much systematic evaluation as has behavior therapy. Investigations of behavior therapy thus dominate most scientific journals that report on professional treatment outcomes. More than 70% of investigations of treatment efficacy funded by the National Institutes of Mental Health are conducted by behavior therapists. Although less research has been conducted on children than on adults, literally hundreds of outcome studies have been published in the past 20 years.

Notwithstanding the limitations of child therapy meta-analyses, evidence is strong for both the efficacy and the superiority of behavior therapy (1) for children who are retarded, autistic, conduct disordered, enuretic (especially those who have primary enuresis), anxious, depressed, engaging in self-injurious behavior, or have AD/HD, and (2) for classroom management.[7,18,21] This is based on reviews of treatment that sometimes combine behavior therapy with other forms of intervention (e.g., pharmacotherapy).

Early concern regarding "symptom substitution" has proved to be unfounded; given appropriate problem analysis and intervention, the substitution of a new symptom for the one that was treated has not been evident. Behavior therapy has had a more modest degree of success to date with problems such as obesity, addiction, and lack of assertion.[7,21,24] In addition, support is developing for the utility of behavioral treatment of headaches and other somatic disorders such as asthma, seizures, and persistent vomiting, as well as for helping children to cope with chronic illness and with medical and dental procedures, and for promoting compliance with medical regimens.[9,21]

Although its accomplishments to date have been gratifying, much remains to be learned about behavior therapy. One prominent criticism is that behavior therapists do not understand completely why successful procedures are successful. For example, relaxation training and desensitization, although clearly efficacious, have been variously explained as counterconditioning (using a classic conditioning model), as operant conditioning, and as a process of cognitive change.

Second, it is true that meta-analyses of child therapy efforts have shown larger-sized effects for behavioral compared with nonbehavioral (e.g., client-centered, psychodynamic) methods. However, considering the different types of outcome measures and clinical problems and considering the relatively smaller number of nonbehavioral interventions, definitive conclusions cannot be drawn regarding the relative efficacy of the different therapeutic approaches. "Dismantling treatment designs," wherein components of treatments are reduced systematically in an attempt to identify the core therapeutic factors, could be used to address this question, but such studies are sorely lacking.

An additional problem is that, whereas behavior therapists tend to be more concerned with the generalization and maintenance of treatment impacts than do nonbehavioral therapists, treatment effects that generalize across settings and maintain over time still are relatively rare.[13] This has led to attempts to identify and focus on classes of behavior that promote generalization and maintenance of more specific behaviors. For example, encouraging children to be energetic and attentive in social interaction often leads to concomitant improvement in behaviors such as smiling and initiating conversation. Other approaches to bolster and lengthen the impact of behavioral treatments include training patients to handle expected relapses (e.g., for problems such as enuresis and drug addiction) and using combined treatment approaches to address complex problems (e.g., desensitization for specific fears and relaxation training/cognitive restructuring to address generalized anxiety).

Finally, most evaluation of behavior therapy and cognitive-behavior therapy has employed controlled studies that demonstrate *efficacy* but not necessarily *effectiveness* in real-life clinical settings.[14,17] Although documentation of efficacy is a crucial first step, much study of clinical practice remains to be done.

PHENOMENOLOGICAL THERAPIES

Phenomenological (or humanistic) therapy is insight oriented, as is psychodynamic therapy, and assumes that disordered behavior can best be altered by increased awareness of one's own motivations and needs. The distinction of humanistic therapy, however, is its emphasis on free will, attributing considerable freedom of choice to the patient. Phenomenological therapies focus on promoting the patient's "growth as a person," the primary vehicle for doing so being the patient-therapist relationship.

Client-Centered Therapy

Basic assumptions. The major phenomenological model is Carl Rogers' client-centered therapy. (Rogerians refer to "clients" rather than "patients" because they maintain that these individuals are healthy and responsible, not "sick.") This approach assumes that patients can best be understood by the way in which they construe events subjectively (a phenomenological perspective) rather than by an objective view of the events themselves.[2] The focus of therapy, therefore, is to attend to the client's perceptions and feelings and to let the client take the lead in the therapeutic process. Rogers postulates an innate tendency to actualize, or to realize one's potential, which is as much a human drive as the reduction of biological tensions (e.g., hunger).

Because people are assumed to be innately striving for good, total and nonjudgmental acceptance by the therapist is the key to providing an atmosphere in which the client's natural growth may proceed unhindered. Rogers assumes that maximal development will take place when the client does not need to struggle for and be concerned about approval by others. This approach is thus believed to be the appropriate remedy when people have been thwarted in their growth by the evaluations and judgments imposed on them by others, creating "conditions of worth" that force individuals to distort or become unaware of their own real feelings.

Therapeutic activities. The key therapeutic relationship is based on three vital attitudes of the therapist: (1) unconditional positive regard (sometimes also referred to as "warmth"), (2) empathy, and (3) congruence (sometimes referred to as "genuineness"). To display unconditional positive regard, the therapist must convey the message that he or she cares about the client as a person, accepts the client, and trusts the client's ability to change. The therapist is willing to listen and avoid interpretation and value judgments. To display empathy, the therapist actively attempts to perceive the client's feelings and to communicate this understanding by "reflecting," or paraphrasing, what he or she believes to be the client's views. This is more than merely repeating what the client has said; it represents the distillation and "playback" of the client's feelings. Finally, in displaying congruence, the therapist establishes a real, human relationship by abandoning any facade and expressing himself or herself genuinely. In so doing, the therapist leaves the responsibility for the client's life with the client and indicates confidence in the client's ability to handle the therapist's feelings.

This individual, verbal form of client-centered therapy, although developed for adults, also is appropriate for many adolescents. Its course typically consists of one or two sessions weekly, for a period ranging from a few months to several years. Client-centered therapy generally is used for individuals who have a mild or moderate disturbance; Rogers himself has warned that it probably is not appropriate for those who have severe pathological conditions. The Rogerian approach also has been applied with groups, most notably with encounter groups. The goals of individual and group treatment are similar: increasing awareness, self-acceptance, interpersonal comfort, and self-reliance.

Client-centered therapy has been adapted by Virginia Axline and others for young children through the use of play therapy, using much the same setting and material as do psychodynamic therapists.[2,7] The key difference is that the Rogerian therapist does not use play to make symbolic interpretations. Analogous to treatment with adults, the therapist encourages the child to lead the session and displays unconditional positive regard by his or her words and actions.

Many aspects of client-centered therapy are used by therapists who represent other approaches. For example, behavior therapists often spend considerable time in developing a relationship with children and adolescents before specific interventions are implemented, and this relationship focus is no less important when clients are learning to modify maladaptive behaviors and cognitions and to develop skills. As such, Rogerian elements of interpersonal warmth, empathy, and genuineness toward the client commonly will be evidenced throughout therapy by the behavioral clinician. Although the therapist may express concern or unhappiness over a child's *behavior,* such a reaction would occur in the context of unconditional positive regard for the *child.* Psychodynamic therapists vary the presentation of these qualities more, as some adopt a passive posture with minimal talking to avoid disruption of the child's expressed feelings, memories, and symbolic play.

Gestalt Therapy

Basic assumptions. As with client-centered therapy, Fritz Perls' gestalt therapy promotes growth by increasing self-awareness and encouraging patients to assume responsibility for their actions and feelings.[2] Identifying theoretical differences between the two models is difficult, because the language used to describe gestalt therapy often is esoteric and unclear, and because it seems only to be loosely related, at best, to principles of gestalt psychology (a laboratory-based study of human perception). Gestalt therapy is discriminated from client-centered therapy most easily by the methods used in treatment, which involve an active, directive therapist and often dramatic techniques.

Therapeutic activities. A major focus of gestalt therapists is to emphasize the present; this therapy takes place in the "here and now." The therapist thus insists that the patient talk in the present tense and discuss current feelings. Use of language also is important in assisting the patient to assume direct responsibility for his or her feelings. For example, a patient who says, "It's really aggravating to hear that," might be asked to restate this as, "I am angry with you for saying that to me." Another technique is to ask the patient to project himself or herself into another person or object. For example, if a patient says she senses a wall between her and her parents, she may be asked to "become" that wall and talk about how it feels.

Possibly the most useful technique used by gestalt therapists is to externalize conflicts and feelings. For example, a patient may confront an empty chair, imagine that his father is there, and tell his father the things he has wanted to say but has been unable to say to him. Or if the patient is stuck in her decision making (e.g., whether to go to a local college and live at home or to go away to college), she may be asked to alternate sitting in two chairs. When she is in one, she takes the side of staying at home and tells why she wants to stay at home and how she feels about it; sitting in the other chair she fully experiences and relates to the therapist the part of herself that wants to go away to college. This enables the patient to sort out the emotional aspects of the conflict, and it is fascinating to observe how the balance gradually shifts as one side predominates and the decision begins to be made.

Gestalt therapy has not been adapted systematically for children and thus is used typically only with adolescents. As with client-centered treatment, it generally is appropriate only for mildly or moderately disturbed patients. Gestalt therapy is used both with individuals and with groups. Individual therapy generally consists of one or two sessions weekly for anywhere from a few months to several years. Groups often are begun with an intensive weekend experience and then typically meet for one evening a week for 6 months to a year, although some groups continue almost indefinitely.

Efficacy. Largely at Rogers' own insistence there have been numerous attempts to study and evaluate client-centered therapy.[2] In fact it has been suggested that Rogers can be credited with stimulating the whole field of psychotherapy research. Much of this has been a study of the process of therapy, and Rogerians have been responsive to the findings. For example, Rogers no longer calls his therapy "nondirective" (the original label); a careful analysis of his own therapy transcripts has shown that the therapist does "shape" or subtly guide the client's verbal statements.

Outcome studies of adults also have shown changes in clients' self-perceptions following treatment, in contrast to a normal control group (not in therapy) and a waiting-list control group. This research has been criticized, however, because it is based on clients' self-reports, with no external judgment of how clients actually behave after treatment. Also, it is not clear how much change is attributable to this form of therapy per se and how much to the nonspecific aspects of this and other forms of treatment.

As with all therapeutic modalities, less study of client-centered therapy has been directed to the treatment of children. Investigators have reported positive changes following child therapy, but some of these evaluations suffer from flaws, such as the selective assignment of children to treated and nontreated groups and the use of ratings by observers who were not "blind" to the therapeutic status of the children. The results of these evaluations currently are therefore suggestive rather than conclusive.

Gestalt therapy has been evaluated much less. Like psychodynamic therapists, many gestalt therapists are uninterested in or relatively inimical toward the collection of data. Those who have attempted to study therapeutic outcome have been hampered by the gap between Perls' concepts and his techniques. Gestalt therapy (and to some extent client-centered therapy) has been criticized for being incomplete: by deemphasizing clinical assessment and the patient's history, the therapist may miss diagnostic signs or background information that could be important in planning treatment. The danger of inadequate screening of group members, for example, can be seen in an estimated 8% "casualty" rate from phenomenological group experiences (e.g., sensitivity training, encounter groups).[2] Although these casualties are not all as dramatic as a psychotic episode, evidence suggests that these participants have been harmed in some way by the experience. This intervention thus may be beneficial for many but not all participants.

SYSTEMS THERAPY

Basic Assumptions

Systems therapy represents an approach to family therapy that views the family as a unit, a dynamic system, rather than a collection of individuals. The relationships among the family members are hypothesized to have developed in the specific manner in which they did so that the family could achieve homeostasis. This relatively stable state is disrupted periodically by external events (e.g., geographical relocation) or change within the family (e.g., birth of a child). This triggers changes in the family members' relationships and the subsequent reemergence of a homeostatic state, which may be different from the previous one, in much the same way that a mobile is affected by a gust of wind. Homeostasis sometimes may be achieved in ways that are not beneficial for all members, such as a "problem child" distracting attention from an unhappy marriage.[27]

Systems therapists therefore view the child who has behavior problems as merely the "identified patient" and believe that treatment is focused most appropriately on the entire family. This form of intervention, conjoint family therapy, treats the family as a group and includes all members who live together except for infants and toddlers. Treatment may focus initially on the "problem child," but the therapist often attempts to move fairly quickly to "reframe," or redefine, the problem as a disturbance in family process, faulty communication, or both. The therapist thus encourages all family members to see their own contribution to the problem and the positive changes that each can make.

The systems approach examines the roles played by family members and the function of the child's problem in maintaining the homeostasis of the family.[27] One goal of treatment is to identify covert family rules that produce the same maladaptive interactions consistently. For example, a stepfather believes that his marriage could be threatened by his stepdaughter, who dislikes him; he thus is overly critical of her and promotes conflict between her and her mother to diminish her influence on her mother. Another goal of treatment is to promote appropriate communication, such as providing direct messages, using noncoercive communication, and minimizing "scapegoating" of the identified patient. Note the similarity of the above to the functional analysis and skill training conducted by behavior therapists.

Therapeutic Activities

Therapeutic goals are achieved by analyzing and commenting on the verbal and nonverbal messages exchanged by family members. As the family becomes more aware of these maladaptive "rules" and messages, it is assumed that they are better able to change them. The therapist also may ask family members to relabel a behavior more positively (e.g., use the term "independent" rather than "selfish"). Another tactic might be to direct family members to exaggerate their customary style (be the ultimately critical father or ultimately martyred mother) to foster awareness and change.

Minuchin's structural family therapy is an adaptation that emphasizes family "sets" as the target for change.[2,27] These sets refer to the hierarchy, or structure, of family relations and the alliances between members. For example, an *enmeshed* family is one in which the members are overinvolved with one another. Here the therapist would attempt to strengthen the alliance between the parents and clearly designate their status as parents (e.g., he or she might even say, "You are a child; be quiet, this is a matter for your parents to settle"). The therapist would then encourage members to interact more with others of their own age and would promote more activities outside the family. With a *disengaged* family might be an uninvolved father, kept distant by a strong "coalition" between mother and son. The therapist again would attempt to reorder these alliances and reestablish the father in the family structure.

Systems therapy has been used for a variety of problems, both with children and adolescents (although typically not with very young children). Some therapists insist that all family members always attend; others may work with the parents alone for a part of the treatment (e.g., for marital problems). The course of therapy typically consists of one session a week (although this may be longer than the usual 50-minute session), with the active participation of the family between sessions by the use of assigned homework. (Again, note the similarity to behavior therapy.) Treatment may continue for several months or several years.

Efficacy

Evaluation of "pure" systems therapy to date is inconclusive because of the lack of appropriately controlled outcome studies. A combined behavioral-systems approach has demonstrated beneficial effects for both the identified patient and other family members (e.g., siblings).[7,22] A combined approach also has been shown to be as effective or more so than individual therapy and client-centered family therapy.[7,21]

Determining the key elements required for successful intervention can be complex. For example, Robin and Foster[22] developed an integrated approach to negotiating parent-adolescent conflict that combines aspects of behavior therapy, cognitive-behavior therapy, and systems therapy. Summarizing the results of their research and other outcome studies, they report that family intervention that consists of relationship enhancement, behavioral contracting or communication skill training will generally be effective only with mildly or moderately distressed families. Treatment necessitates both family system *and* communication skills when distress is severe, multiple problems are evidenced, and/or the adolescent is inappropriately involved with maladaptive interaction patterns or marital conflict.

In general, available data indicate that *conjoint* family therapy with all members present, regardless of theoretical orientation, appears superior to other methods, such as providing individual treatment for each family member. This particularly is true when the presenting problems relate to family crises and conflicts about values, lifestyles, or goals. Treatment outcomes have been found to be superior when fathers agree to participate in treatment. Interestingly, this has been shown to be the case when parents are separated as well as when they are together.[7]

ECLECTIC THERAPY

Basic Assumptions

Eclectic therapy is not so much a school of thought as the *absence* of an identified school. It has been included in this chapter because surveys of psychologists have indicated that eclecticism frequently is identified as a therapeutic orientation (eclectic, behavioral, and psychodynamic being the most common). As discussed previously, experienced therapists often employ procedures and techniques from a variety of therapies. Furthermore, they also may incorporate concepts from orientations other than that of their original training. With increasing borrowing and blending, a therapist may come to believe that his or her orientation no longer can be classified accurately as that of an identified school or theory; such therapists will label themselves "eclectic."

It is important to distinguish between *technical eclecticism* and *theoretical eclecticism.* The former refers to a therapist (1) who consistently is guided by a theoretical framework as he or she conceptualizes and understands a patient, the patient's problems, and his or her attempts to change, but (2) who employs techniques borrowed from other modalities when appropriate for a particular patient. For example, it is not uncommon for a behavior therapist to be guided by the principles of social learning theory and yet employ gestalt exercises to help an overly intellectual patient identify the emotional factors involved in his or her problem solving or decision making. Similarly a behavior therapist may use play materials when working with children. These techniques, however, are selected carefully to fulfill a specific purpose, which is part of an overall therapeutic strategy; in other words, the therapist uses them as a behavior therapist. In addition, as mentioned earlier, behavior and other therapists often use Rogerian methods to develop and maintain rapport throughout therapy. In contrast, theoretical eclecticism eschews the guidance of any theoretical system.

It is the author's bias that any theory is better than no theory, because successful therapy requires some purposive stance on the part of the therapist and an overall framework within which to interpret the patient's thoughts and actions. Victor Meyer has semi-jokingly said that a theoretical framework is therapeutic for the therapist, because the therapist at least thinks he or she understands what is going on.[8]

Eclecticism also may be an appropriate label for interventions that have been developed for very specific situations or populations, even though they may be associated loosely with some theoretical system. Probably one of the clearest examples of this is Synanon, an intensive, residential program developed to treat drug addiction. Although much of this program is translated readily into social learning (or behavioral) terms, it also makes extensive use of client-centered techniques and encounter group sessions. Other examples abound in community psychology, such as crisis intervention, suicide hotlines, and prevention efforts. Although some programs are explicitly behavioral, many community programs are atheoretical.

Efficacy

Given the plethora of programs and treatments that are essentially eclectic and the general absence of sound evaluative study, no pretense will be made here of discussing the efficacy of eclectic modalities.

SUMMARY

The goal of this chapter has been to increase the pediatrician's understanding of variants of psychotherapy that are available for use with children and to increase the practitioner's ability to effect an appropriate referral and prepare the patient and family for treatment. In becoming more familiar with the different therapeutic orientations described, it is hoped that the reader will appreciate the extent to which these are not completely separate and distinct.

With increasing clinical experience therapists become more similar to one another, and many combine elements from different schools of thought. Therapeutic orientation is only one of several factors important in the selection of a therapist; quality of training, personal characteristics, general reputation, responsiveness, and ability to work with the pediatrician clearly are vital considerations (see Chapter 83, Consultation and Referral for Behavioral and Developmental Problems).

Finally, it is hoped that the reader will appreciate the difficulty and complexity of psychotherapy research and thus be tolerant of the therapist's inability to make categorical and unqualified claims regarding the effectiveness of his or her intervention. In fact, some degree of humility should be evidenced by individual therapists and proponents of particular therapeutic approaches. Even those instances of "demonstrated efficacy" reviewed earlier represent a conclusion based on a number of studies, each of which is imperfect and rarely, if ever, reports unqualified, long-term success with all patients.

REFERENCES

1. Bandura A: *Self-efficacy: the exercise of control,* New York, 1997, WH Freeman.
2. Bernstein DA, Nietzel MT: *Introduction to clinical psychology,* New York, 1980, McGraw-Hill.

3. Casey RJ, Berman JS: The outcome of psychotherapy with children, *Psychol Bull* 98:388, 1985.
4. Chamberlain P: Intensified foster care: multi-level treatment for adolescents with conduct disorders in out-of-home care. In Hibbs ED, Jensen PJ, editors: *Psychosocial treatments for child & adolescent disorders: empirically based strategies for clinical practice,* Washington DC, 1996, American Psychological Association.
5. Finch Jr AJ, Nelson III WM, Ott ES: *Cognitive-behavioral procedures with children and adolescents: a practical guide,* Needham Heights, Mass, 1993, Allyn and Bacon.
6. Fonagy P, Target M: A contemporary psychoanalytical perspective: Psychodynamic developmental therapy. In Hibbs ED, Jensen PS, editors: *Psychosocial treatment for child and adolescent disorders: empirically based strategies for clinical practice*, Washington DC, 1996, American Psychological Association.
7. Gelfand DM, Jenson WR, Drew CJ: *Understanding child behavior disorders,* ed 3, New York, 1997, Holt, Rinehart & Winston.
8. Goldfried MR, Davison GC: *Clinical behavior therapy,* ed 2, New York, 1994, Wiley.
9. Hersen M, editor: *Innovations in child behavior therapy,* New York, 1989, Springer.
10. Hibbs ED, Jensen PJ: *Psychosocial treatments for child and adolescent disorders: empirically based strategies for clinical practice*, Washington, DC, 1996, American Psychological Association.
11. James B: *Treating traumatized children: new insights and creative interventions,* Lexington, Mass, 1989, Lexington Books.
12. Joshi PT: Pharmacotherapy in children and adolescents. In Ghuman HG, Sarles RM, editors: *Handbook of child and adolescent outpatient, day treatment and community psychiatry,* Philadelphia, 1998, Brunner/Mazel.
13. Kazdin AE: *Child psychotherapy: developing and identifying effective treatments*, New York, 1988, Pergamon Press.
14. Kazdin AE: Developing effective treatments for children and adolescents. In Hibbs ED, Jensen PS, editors: *Psychosocial treatments for child and adolescent disorders: empirically based strategies for clinical practice*, Washington DC, 1996, American Psychological Association.
15. Kazdin AE, Kendall PC: Current progress and future plans for developing effective treatments: comments and perspectives, *J Clin Child Psychol* 27: 217, 1998.
16. Kendall PC: *Child and adolescent therapy: cognitive-behavioral procedures,* New York, 1991, Guilford Press.
17. Lonigan CJ, Elbert JC, editors: Special issue on empirically supported psychosocial interventions for children, *J Clin Child Psychol* 27:138, 1998.
18. Mash EJ, Barkley RA, editors: *Childhood psychopathology,* New York, 1996, Guilford.
19. Parloff MB: Psychotherapy research and its incredible credibility crisis, *Clin Psychol Rev* 4:95, 1984.
20. Phillips S: Behavior therapy with children and adolescents. In Ghuman HG, Sarles RM, editors: *Handbook of child and adolescent outpatient, day treatment and community psychiatry,* Philadelphia, 1998, Brunner/Mazel.
21. Quay HC, Werry JS, editors: *Psychopathological disorders of childhood*, ed 3, New York, 1986, Wiley.
22. Robin A, Foster SL: *Negotiating parent-adolescent conflict: a behavioral-family systems approach,* New York, 1989, Guilford Press.
23. Task Force on Promotion and Dissemination of Psychological Procedures: Training in and dissemination of empirically-validated psychosocial treatments: report and recommendations, *Clin Psychol* 48:3, 1995.
24. Walker CE, Roberts MC: *Handbook of clinical child psychology,* ed 2, New York, 1992, Wiley.
25. Weist MD, Ollendick TH, Finney JW: Toward the empirical validation of treatment targets in children, *Clin Psychol Rev* 11:515, 1991.
26. Weisz JR, Hawley KM: Finding, evaluating, refining, and applying empirically supported treatments for children and adolescents, *J Clin Child Psychol* 27:206, 1998.
27. Zuk G: *Family therapy: a triadic-based approach,* New York, 1981, Behavioral Books.

83 Consultation and Referral for Behavioral and Developmental Problems

Sheridan Phillips • Richard M. Sarles • Stanford B. Friedman

INDICATORS FOR CONSULTATION OR REFERRAL

Certain types of behavior are such clear indicators of psychosocial problems that a single occurrence should signal the pediatrician to consider referral. For example, autism[1] usually is apparent before 30 months of age. These children generally show a lack of responsiveness to others, self-isolation, grossly deficient language development, and peculiar attachments to animate or inanimate objects. Autistic children do vary in symptomatology, and few are totally unresponsive to environmental stimuli, including people; however, their responses are characteristically unusual, variable, or inappropriate. Similarly, schizophrenic children typically display such bizarre behavior or preoccupations and such grossly impaired emotional relationships that they are readily identifiable. In fact, a major shortcoming of even relatively successful therapy is the inability to make the psychotic child socially inconspicuous.

Generally, it also is easy to identify certain acting out behaviors as clear signals for referral. These include behaviors that are dangerous to the child or others, vandalism, fire-setting, and cruelty to animals. Family intervention often is indicated, especially for problems such as child abuse and secondary enuresis. Also, a skilled therapist can help both patient and family deal with the aftermath of rape or exposure to violence.

Unfortunately, most problems cannot be readily identified by the occurrence of a single behavior. Probably the most difficult determination is whether certain behaviors, such as mood swings in adolescence, represent merely the normal developmental process or are manifestations of a more serious problem. This very dilemma prompted the development of the *Diagnostic and Statistical Manual for Primary Care (DSM-PC)*[7] sponsored by the American Academy of Pediatrics. A task force of behavioral specialists was convened to describe and distinguish normal developmental variation versus behavior problems versus psychiatric disorders. Clinical field trials for the *DSM-PC* currently are being conducted.

Signals for Concern

One indicator for concern is any sudden change in behavior, such as a significant drop in grades or withdrawal from peers or family. Such change may be related to a change in environment (e.g., moving to a new school or neighborhood) and may be transient, with the child's behavior returning to normal in a week or two. If the change persists for more than a month, however, the child probably needs special assistance to cope with the new environment or other stressor.

In general, the difference between "normal" and "problematic" behavior is not the actual behavior (or behaviors) but rather the quantity (frequency of occurrences), distribution (different manifestations), and duration (generally, at least 4 weeks).Two additional factors also determine when behavior warrants attention: if it is maladaptive, impairing social or cognitive functioning, or when the concomitant level of distress is inappropriate (either elevated distress or a total lack of distress when some would be anticipated). For example, many young boys occasionally dress as girls or prefer girls as playmates, or say things like "I wish boys could have babies." These behaviors should be distinguished from genuine cross-sex behavior, which is characterized by a variety of manifestations, by the frequency and duration of each behavior, by the degree to which these behaviors interfere with other socialization, and by the level of tension the behavior causes in the patient or family. See Chapter 86, Cross-Sex Behavior and Gender Identity Disorder.

Similarly, all five factors (quantity, distribution, duration, maladaptiveness, and level of distress) are relevant in discriminating between a very energetic child and one who is hyperactive. In other instances, the problem behavior may be more circumscribed but still of concern because of its frequency, duration, or maladaptiveness (e.g., drug abuse, sexual promiscuity, stealing, and poor academic performance). Children often have conduct problems at home but not at school or at school but not at home.[3] The maladaptiveness of the behavior, however, may signal a need for intervention, even though the behavior occurs in only one setting.

The problems most likely to be missed are the "quiet" ones that do not make life difficult for parents or teachers, such as poor peer relationships, emotional and social withdrawal, apathy, dysphoria, and poor self-esteem. Pediatricians also may not recognize "quiet" parenting problems. Some parents consistently express concern about their children's behavior or how they manage them. The specific behavior in question may be different at each visit, but the pediatrician may be providing brief reassurance continually, which often is ineffective. At such times the pediatrician should consider why these parents do not realize that their children's behavior is well within the norm. Are they isolated from other parents who have children the same age? Do they need education and anticipatory guidance? The parents' questions may indicate that they are excessively protective or concerned or that they have unrealistic expectations of their child. If so, this will continue to be a problem for the child and warrants intervention.

Determining the Need

A biopsychosocial model provides the framework for discriminating between problems that do and do not warrant referral. For example, in the case of a closed head injury, the pediatrician would assess for three things: (1) biological risk factors that might predispose the patient to a coexisting psychological (comorbid) disorder (e.g., Is there a significant family history of or genetic predisposition for depression?), (2) psychological risk factors that may affect the treatment course and outcome (e.g., Does this patient have previously documented cognitive deficits or behavior problems?), and (3) social stressors that may prevent the patient from achieving an optimal recovery (e.g., Will lack of financial resources or family support systems play a role?). Using this framework with every patient will not always generate referral to a behavioral specialist, but it will ensure that factors possibly inhibiting treatment will not be missed.

When deciding whether to refer patients, the pediatrician must consider not only the current maladaptiveness of the problem but also the potential benefit of early intervention, which may prevent severe problems or significantly improve the quality of life for a child or family. Despite the potential benefits, however, at least some children are not referred for consultation or treatment.

SOURCES OF RELUCTANCE TO EMPLOY BEHAVIORAL SPECIALISTS

For a variety of reasons, physicians often are reluctant to use behavioral consultation or referral. For example, the primary care practitioner may feel pressured to comply with the current medical trend to treat the "total" patient. However, any individual physician may not have the time, expertise, or interest to do so. In such cases only the insecure professional fears consultation with a colleague. Generally, parents acknowledge a physician's honesty in delineating his or her own area of expertise and concomitant limitations and appreciate the concern and interest evidenced by the physician suggesting appropriate consultation or referral.

Conversion disorder[1] illustrates the advisability of simultaneously exploring organic and psychosocial factors (see Chapter 100, Conversion Reactions in Adolescents). First, when a patient is admitted to the hospital for diagnostic evaluation, behavioral consultation should be requested at the outset of the hospitalization. Many behavioral specialists have been frustrated by the request to evaluate such a patient on the last day of the hospital stay after no significant physical reason for the patient's problem was identified.

Involvement of a specialist at the outset permits a more reasonable and thorough assessment. For example, it provides the opportunity to observe the child's behavior during the hospital stay, thus generating information difficult to obtain in any other way. Second, if the behavioral assessment is requested early, parents do not view it as a "last resort." Third, the specialist can consult with hospital staff and parents when gathering data about the patient's condition. This initial contact is crucial in establishing a relationship that allows the specialist to offer specific recommendations about the patient's condition. Last, should the patient begin exhibiting troublesome behavior while still hospitalized, the consultant may offer valuable recommendations to the hospital staff about treating these behaviors.

The tendency to request a behavioral consultation *only after* a variety of other subspecialty consultations have been conducted poses problems not only for the child and family but also for the consultation service per se. Many insurance and medical assistance plans limit the number of reimbursable consultations per hospital stay. Delaying the request for behavioral evaluation, therefore, is one of the reasons consultation/liaison services typically have trouble remaining solvent and viable.

Consequences for the Patient

Pediatricians may avoid referring a child who has a behavioral problem because they are reluctant to label a child or adolescent as having such a problem and fear that both parents and child will see the referral as an indication that the patient is "crazy" or seriously disturbed. Thus, many physicians tend to be excessively conservative and recommend referral only for a blatant and obviously severe problem or when all else has failed.

This implicit acceptance of the social stereotype of therapy is unfortunate, because early intervention can be extremely advantageous. For example, it is much easier for a child to catch up, whether with academic or social skills, when the performance gap is small. Similarly, intervening with a 16-year-old who truly is out of control is different from treating that same youngster at age 12.

Certainly, it is not always clear that the problem will become progressively more serious. Many parents and adolescents do survive several stormy years of teenage rebellion and ineffective parental efforts to exert control. However, family disruption and stress can be reduced by a brief series of sessions with a specialist who is skilled in teaching communication and problem-solving skills.[6] Many parents and teenagers would probably consider this a worthwhile investment of time and money. The same argument can be made for many other difficulties that are "problem behaviors" rather than "behavior problems" (see Chapter 78, Developmental Approach to Behavioral Problems).

Many behavioral problems reflect a child's lack of skills rather than deep-seated pathological conditions. However, it probably is the latter, psychodynamic view of behavioral problems that underlies current negative social prejudice toward psychosocial treatment. Thus, many individuals avoid using behavioral services, yet they readily turn to experts in virtually every other area of life—accountants, physicians, teachers, plumbers—as a natural and clever use of specialists. A pediatrician familiar with the nature and purpose of different treatments can encourage families to use behavioral resources effectively.

Obstacles to Accessing Mental Health Services

Pediatricians frequently have complaints about accessing mental health services promptly and effectively.[5] Most of these concerns are legitimate, reflecting the often incompatible structures of pediatric and mental health services as well as some attitudinal differences regarding what constitutes an emergency. These obstacles can be reduced, however, if pediatricians (1) become more familiar with behavioral services and how to access them[5] and (2) clearly communicate their expectations regarding referral questions, reports, and ongoing feedback. Good mutual communication of expectations and needs appears to be the key. For example, evaluation of suicidal risk (a crucial question for pediatricians) often is missing in psychiatric reports,[5] whereas the family's attitude and involvement of other agencies (important data for mental health specialists) often are missing in referrals from primary care practitioners.[5]

Usefulness of Mental Health Services

Pediatricians also may hesitate to refer patients if they are concerned about the efficacy of behavioral intervention—that is, how much good it will do. A related concern, which also is appropriate, is the effort involved for physicians, parents, and children in going to a different place and person for consultation, then possibly having to adapt to yet another professional. Financial considerations may present another difficulty. In general, the question is whether a referral involves much more effort and expense than it is worth.

Although no therapeutic approach or therapist can be totally effective, a skilled therapist generally is at least helpful, often very successful, and unlikely to be harmful. Many behavioral specialists now routinely generate a "treatment contract" with their patients, by which both parties agree to an initial series of sessions (usually between four and six), after which they jointly assess whether progress has been made. If the parents or patient believe that the initial experience has been productive, they may continue with the intervention plan; if not, there should be a change in either the plan or the therapist. This practice ensures that patients will not continue in a long and expensive course of treatment that is deemed unnecessary or unproductive by the therapist or the family. However, the length and intensity of appropriate intervention vary tremendously with the particular patient and problem. Even a highly effective and responsible therapist will have a range of cases, some requiring four sessions or fewer and others 100 sessions or more. The key is to select and use a behavioral specialist to provide optimum care while maintaining contact with the primary care physician.

GENERAL CONSIDERATIONS

The physician sometimes can select a consultant to reduce the chances of a "patient shunt," in which the child first must relate to a consultant and then adjust to another professional for intervention. When the primary care practitioner suspects that treatment is indicated, he or she should recommend a consultant who can both assess and intervene. In some cases this will not be possible, nor would it always represent optimum use of specialized skills. Knowledge of available behavioral resources, however, enables the physician to recommend appropriately.

Another consideration is how best to structure interaction with behavioral specialists. One possibility is to include behavioral specialists within general pediatric practices. Increasingly, pediatricians have invited mental health professionals to base their practices in adjacent offices. Even better, such professionals have become members of group practices. This approach has obvious advantages for providing many behavioral services to patients naturally and efficiently. This approach also allows the behavioral specialist the opportunity to provide a variety of other services. The specialist may offer suggestions to office staff concerning aspects of patient treatment (e.g., behavioral techniques or interventions for reducing anxiety during painful procedures). One or two brief sessions with this specialist before an inpatient hospitalization for treatments or procedures, such as chemotherapy, magnetic resonance imaging (MRI), and computed tomography (CT) scans, to familiarize the patient and family with these events also would be an excellent use of the specialist's consultation skills. Another example would be short-term group sessions for common problems of young mothers or diabetic teenagers. Although any particular professional cannot possess the entire range of skills required, he or she can enhance the effective use of other resources in the community.

Preparing the Parents

Preparation of the parents for behavioral consultation begins during the first discussion of the differential diagnosis, when both physical and emotional factors are included as potential causes of the symptoms. Even when the primary care physician has correctly introduced the possibility of emotional issues early in the diagnostic workup, parents may resist exploring emotional factors. Such resistance is most likely when the symptoms appear to have an organic origin or when no overt behavioral disruption has occurred.

In some instances, parents may not be aware that they foster their child's aberrant behavior; instead, they often blame the school or their child's peers. In other instances, parents may deny any problems with their child, partly to avoid revealing their own interpersonal or marital difficulties or a problem such as alcoholism. Nevertheless, the physician should present an honest appraisal of the situation (with appropriate recommendations for behavioral consultation) without trying to please or appease the parents by avoiding a discussion of his or her true assessment of the clinical situation.

If parents are reluctant to consider a behavioral consultation, it may help to address their concern for their child's health and welfare. In explaining the need for such consultation, the pediatrician should suggest that this is an important service for complete, comprehensive care of their child. The pediatrician should emphasize that behavioral consultation does not imply that the child is crazy; rather, it suggests that emotional factors may totally or partly account for their child's difficulty.

When the complaint is somatic, a useful example most parents can understand is the feeling of "butterflies in the stomach" or sweating before an examination, when speaking in public, during a marriage ceremony, or at other times of stress. A tension headache is another common symptom that can be used to demonstrate that a person can experience physical distress or pain without actual structural or physical disease being present.

The pediatrician can reduce the stigma of many emotional or behavioral problems by conceptualizing them as an absence of skills rather than deep-seated pathology. Further, treatment that improves a child's coping skills or social skills can have lifelong benefits, going well beyond resolution of the current problem. Finally, the good news is that behavioral problems generally are treatable; from this perspective, they are "better" problems to have than many organic disorders that are less responsive to intervention.

If the parents agree to the consultation, the pediatrician should give them the consultant's name and the reasons for this selection, the consultant's credentials, and how closely the consultant works with the primary care physician. It is the pediatrician's responsibility to contact the consultant initially and to discuss the reasons for consultation.

The parents also should be informed that the consultant probably will want to see both parents together to collect important data about the child's development and a detailed family history. The number of visits generally required for a consultation and its approximate cost also should be discussed with the parents. After the consultation, the primary care physician should meet with the parents to discuss the consultant's findings and recommendations. It often is useful to include the consultant and the child in this meeting, as well. If treatment is recommended, similar details should be provided regarding the nature of therapeutic activity and probable length of treatment (see Chapter 82, Options for Psychosocial Intervention with Children and Adolescents).

If the parents are reluctant to follow a consultant's recommendation for intervention, the primary care physician should be careful not to support the parents' hesitation. Such a stance engenders lack of faith in the consultant the physician has recommended. It also suggests expertise by the primary care physician in a field in which he or she has just recommended consultation. If, however, both parents and pediatrician drastically disagree with the findings and recommendations of the consultant, a second opinion is indicated.

Preparing the Child

The child should be told that his or her parents and the physician are concerned about aspects of the child's behavior, such as an inability to get along with friends, anger, nightmares, or difficulty coping with a physical illness. In the case of a psychosomatic symptom, the child needs to be told that pain or illness often is caused by emotional feelings or worries. The child should be informed that he or she will be seeing a professional known to the pediatrician who is an expert in helping with these kinds of problems; it should be emphasized that the consultant may help by playing with children and by talking with them about their thoughts and feelings.

With an older child or adolescent, the pediatrician begins to prepare the patient for consultation even while obtaining a physical and psychosocial history. As the physician concentrates on social and emotional aspects, the teenager may become indignant and confront the physician about the personal nature of the questions.

The physician should not retreat or become defensive but should emphasize the need for such probing personal questions to understand the symptoms or illness troubling the patient. As with parents, relating everyday examples can help the older child or adolescent understand the connection between emotions and physical well-being. Teenagers, because they are struggling with the developmental tasks of adolescence, may be concerned about confidentiality. Also, given the normal mood swings during this period, it is common for teenagers to wonder about their own mental health. Suggesting behavioral consultation can trigger a protest that may reflect their own worst fear: that they really are different or "crazy." In most cases the pediatrician can reassure teenage patients that they indeed are not.

However, the physician must convey concern if a significant psychopathological condition is suspected. Not to do so is frightening to the patient or parent, who may recognize that reassurance is premature and inappropriate. If severe problems are present, the pediatrician should explain that the teenager's behavior does signal a departure from normal and indicates some excessive stress, which may be interfering with optimum well-being. Also, it is extremely useful to identify some specific potential benefit of intervention that is likely to be meaningful to the patient (e.g., better relationships with peers) as well as the alleviation of a problem (e.g., reducing conflict with parents or feelings of anxiety).

It is essential that the physician be firm but not argumentative about the need for referral. While acknowledging the adolescent's anger or dismay, the physician needs to assert professional responsibility to render the best medical opinion, even if it is not to the patient's liking. It seems paradoxical that a sturdy posture in this regard often is reassuring, but it does convey the idea that someone is listening and hearing the patient's troubles and is concerned about his or her behavior.

In most instances, the child or adolescent should be informed of the approximate number of visits usually required and the type of interaction to expect. If the patient inquires about the cost of the consultation and evidences concern, the physician can assure the patient that only the parents can make this decision. In most situations, the physician can emphasize that the patient's parents are concerned enough and care enough to be willing to spend whatever it may take to obtain proper help.

In cases of overt psychosis, in which "reality testing" is seriously impaired, psychological preparation of the patient may be ineffective. However, the physician cannot assume that the patient is totally oblivious to the surroundings. In fact, the pediatrician can provide a stabilizing, reliable, and predictable influence for the patient. The physician can introduce the consultant as an expert in helping patients whose thoughts are confused or jumbled. It may even be helpful for the primary care physician to offer to be present during the first consultative session as a source of security for the patient.

Selecting a Consultant

Choosing the appropriate professional or agency probably is the most important service provided by the primary care physician to a patient who has psychosocial or learning problems. Although the common practice of suggesting a list of specialists protects the physician from any accusation of favoritism, it actually is not helpful to parents. A specific referral is preferable because it relieves the family of wondering if they made the best choice.

A common question is whether it is best to use a pediatrician interested and expert in behavioral disorders, a child psychiatrist, a clinical psychologist, a psychiatric nurse, or a social worker.[5] Although a thorough discussion of this issue is beyond the scope of this chapter, a brief review of relevant training and credentials may be helpful.

Pediatricians well versed in managing behavioral disorders generally have had training in behavioral or developmental pediatrics (or both) after their pediatric residency. Their specialized training typically consists of a 1- to 3-year fellowship in behavioral pediatrics and/or child development, including academic and clinical experience. Such fellowships vary greatly in their emphasis, some focusing almost exclusively on infants and young children, others covering a broad range of ages and problems. The behavioral pediatrician's area of expertise, theoretical orientation, and interests obviously reflect the specific training received.

Most physicians formally engaged in psychotherapy have been trained in psychiatry. The internship year can be the first year of a 4-year residency in psychiatry or it can consist of a year in internal medicine, pediatrics, or neurology. Three additional years of psychiatric residency are required for board eligibility in psychiatry. Two years of child and adolescent psychiatric training (1 year of which can constitute the fourth year of psychiatric residency) are needed for board eligibility in child and adolescent psychiatry. Certification in child and adolescent psychiatry is allowed only after an individual has been certified in general psychiatry.

Psychologists vary greatly in their educational background and may have a master's or doctoral degree. Those qualified to provide clinical service, both diagnostic assessment and therapy, have received a degree in clinical psychology (as opposed to developmental, experimental, physiological, or social psychology) or have completed a formal, accredited respecialization program in clinical psychology. Such training includes, in addition to a dissertation, 3 or 4 years of graduate coursework, with accompanying practicum experience, and a year of clinical internship. Graduate programs in clinical psychology and clinical internships are reviewed and accredited by the American Psychological Association (APA)[2]. Also, the referring physician may wish to determine whether the consultant is listed in the National Register of Health Service Providers, which is published biannually.[4] Finally, most states have licensing procedures for psychologists, and the physician should not use an individual who is unlicensed in those states. It should be noted, however, that such licensure often is generic—that is, it does not distinguish areas of training in psychology (e.g., clinical, developmental, experimental, industrial).

A clinical specialist in child and adolescent psychiatry and mental health nursing (psychiatric nurse) is required to have earned a 4-year bachelor's degree in nursing, to have obtained registered nursing licensure, and to have been involved in direct clinical nursing practice. Completion of an 18- to 24-month master's degree in psychiatric nursing is then necessary; this program consists of academic and clinical work focused on children, adolescents, and families. Upon providing evidence of post-master's degree, clinical experience and access to supervision, these clinicians must pass a national examination, which results in certification by the American Nurses Association. These clinicians must be recertified every 5 years.

Social workers may have a bachelor's degree (BSW), a master's degree (MSW), or a doctoral degree (DSW or PhD). Social workers are accredited nationally by the Academy of Certified Social Workers (ACSW), a component of the National Association of Social Workers (NASW), the primary professional association. The ACSW accreditation requirements include (1) a master's degree from a school of social work accredited by the Council of Social Work Education, (2) 2 years of supervised, post-master's degree social work practice, and (3) successful completion of a written examination. Many states now have licensing procedures for social workers, with requirements similar to those of the ACSW. The ACSW and most state licenses are generic, however, and do not distinguish among practitioners in clinical social work, administration, and community organization. The NASW maintains a national register of clinical social workers who have demonstrated clinical training and experience.

Accreditation and organizational affiliations indicate only minimum standards of professional competence. Even in their original training, behavioral specialists vary substantially with regard to orientation and areas of expertise (see Chapter 82, Options for Psychosocial Intervention with Children and Adolescents). For example, many child psychiatry programs have a largely organic focus and emphasize psychopharmacology, whereas others provide more training in psychotherapy. Similarly, some psychologists have more expertise in assessment, whereas others have focused on intervention; some are much better trained in behavioral or cognitive-behavioral intervention than others. Mental health specialists diverge even more after their training because their knowledge and skills are influenced by their professional activities and the continuing education experiences they select.

The lines between disciplines can become blurred, with individuals "crossing over" and developing expertise in other areas.[5] Such blurring is exacerbated by individual differences in dedication and talent[5]; it is clear that each mental health discipline has individuals who are inadequate and those who are superb. This unevenness of skill simply highlights the importance of the referring physician's systematic evaluation of consultative resources.

Knowing what behavioral resources are available in a particular community and arranging ongoing contact with appropriate individuals requires deliberate effort. Pediatricians should meet with an experienced and respected mental health professional to discuss appropriate referral resources within the community. Acquiring appropriate sophistication about available referral sources undoubtedly is time consuming, but it will ensure more meaningful referrals and, ultimately, save time.

The role of the primary care physician does not end once the referral has been made. The physician should contact the family to see that an appointment actually has been made. With the appropriate permission, he or she should provide a summary of the pertinent information to the professional or agency and, in turn, expect periodic reports. It is helpful if the primary care physician clearly states at the time of referral his or her expectations for feedback—how much detail is to be included and how often this feedback is to occur. Ongoing communication allows the pediatrician to maintain an integral role in providing total care to patients. Over time, it also allows evaluation of the quality of service available from a particular professional or agency.

REFERENCES

1. American Psychiatric Association: *Diagnostic and statistical manual of mental disorders,* ed 4, Washington, DC, 1994, The Association.
2. American Psychological Association: *General guidelines for providers of psychological services,* Washington, DC, 1987, The Association.
3. Ammerman RT, Hersen RT: *Handbook of child behavior therapy in the psychiatric setting,* New York, 1995, Wiley.
4. *National Register of Health Service Providers in Psychology*, Washington, DC, Council for the National Register of Health Service Providers in Psychology.
5. Phillips S, Clawson L, Osinski A: Pediatricians' pet peeves about mental health referrals. In Friedman SB, DeMaso D, editors: Adolescent psychiatric and behavioral disorders, *Adolescent medicine: state of the art reviews,* vol 9, Philadelphia, 1998, Hanley and Belfus.
6. Robin A, Foster SL: *Negotiating parent-adolescent conflict: a behavioral-family systems approach*, New York, 1989, Guilford Press.
7. Wolraich ML, Felice ME, Drotar D, editors: *The classification of child and adolescent mental diagnoses in primary care: diagnostic and statistical manual for primary care (DSM-PC) child and adolescent version*, Elk Grove Village, Ill, 1996, American Academy of Pediatrics.

84 Colic

David I. Bromberg

Certain problems in pediatrics demand a multifactorial approach to etiology to be understood well. The clinician must consider biological, developmental, psychosocial, and environmental causes to appreciate fully their contributions to the clinical problem. Only in understanding the interaction of these factors can the physician evaluate the problem accurately and offer a meaningful interpretation and effective treatment plan to the patient and family. Infantile colic is such a problem.

Colic is a poorly defined syndrome of paroxysmal infant crying. Illingworth[3] described the clinical picture of the infant "beginning with flushing of the face, a frown, drawing up of the legs, followed in a few seconds by high pitched screaming, suddenly ending in a few minutes, and followed in a few minutes by another paroxysm. The attacks recur for up to 2 or 3 hours . . . "

These symptoms, in affected babies, begin at several days to weeks of life, increase through the fourth to sixth weeks, and often are gone by 3 to 4 months of age. The research definition used by Wessel et al[7] in 1954 defines colic as occurring in an infant who in the first 3 months cries for greater than 3 hours in a day, 3 or more days a week. Other terms for this entity include "3-month colic," "evening colic," and "paroxysmal fussing." Studies suggest that colic occurs in an estimated 10% to 30% of infants and equally in males and females.

Two major issues emerge in understanding the definition and evaluation of colic. First, crying is a behavior in infants that spans a spectrum from normalcy to pathology both quantitatively and qualitatively. When Brazelton[1] had mothers keep a detailed diary of infant behaviors, he found that crying increased over the first 6 weeks of life, peaking at a median of 2¾ hours per day. Crying then gradually decreased over the remainder of the study through 3 months of age. The descriptions of crying infants also varied from those of a hungry baby, through the crying of a bored, fussy baby, to the above description of the colicky baby. The demarcation between normal and abnormal amounts of crying and normal cries and those of pain is not clear.

Second, Carey[2] raised the issue of primary versus secondary excessive crying. Crying is a behavioral final pathway for a multitude of reasons. The infant who has a urinary tract infection and cries because of bladder spasm or the child who is fussy because of a subdural bleed would cry because of these conditions. The otherwise healthy infant who exhibits paroxysmal crying over a protracted period of time would be the colicky infant whose excessive crying is primary. Again, the demarcation between these groups is not totally clear. To many researchers and clinicians, the healthy colicky infant appears to be in pain that often is thought to be gastrointestinal, albeit of undetermined origin.

Regardless of the cause, the effect on families of having a paroxysmally crying infant is dramatic. Families of colicky infants demonstrate negative alterations in family functioning up to 3 years after the infantile colic. Parents often describe feelings of guilt and inadequacy over their inability to soothe their babies. Families excited over the prospect of having a newborn at home begin to respond very dysfunctionally when colic occurs. One mother notes, "When I was pregnant, I had these romantic visions of having a sweet, cuddly, happy baby. The reality was quite different. I spent day after day walking this screaming baby from room to room, crying right along with her. I snapped at my husband so much that I'm amazed we're still together."[5]

Another mother remembers, "I used to walk up and down the hall with this screaming baby. I'd say, 'Stop it Emma,' and squeeze her leg real hard. Later I'd look at her, so innocent, and I'd cry that I could have done that. How could I want to hurt her when I love her so much?"[5]

ETIOLOGY

Infant Factors

Any condition causing pain in the infant may result in excessive crying. Consideration should be given to the possibility of gastroesophageal reflux (GER), incarcerated inguinal hernia, chronic subdural bleeds, corneal abrasion, renal disease or infection, or acute otitis media. Factors related to increased infant irritability, such as prenatal drug exposure, also must be considered.

Infant temperament has been shown to have a relationship to the development of symptoms of colic. Infants who have the temperamental cluster characterized as difficult and infants who have a low sensory threshold both are at greater risk for being colicky. These are infants who respond to environmental stimuli of a low level. At times, when they already may be "bored" or fussy—for example, during the evening, minor additional stimuli may "set them off."

The question remains open as to whether there is any gastrointestinal predisposition to the development of colic. A Swedish study demonstrated elevated levels of the gastrointestinal hormone, motilin, in the cord blood of infants who developed colic compared with noncolicky controls.[4] These differences are demonstrable on cord blood. Similarly, differences in the absorption of lactalbumin can be shown between colic and noncolic groups. The significance of these findings is unknown. Infants who have colic appear to many observers to be experiencing abdominal pain.

The final category of infant factors relates to feeding techniques and diet. No clear pattern of feeding technique, or alteration in technique, has been clearly demonstrated to relate to colic. An extensive amount of literature relates cow milk protein, both in formula and in the maternal diet for breast-feeding infants, to the course of colic. Although much of this literature is conflicting, it does suggest that the elimination of cow milk protein improves the course of colic in a small group of colicky infants.

Parents

Parental ability to cope with an inconsolable infant, as well as their ability to read and respond to infant cues, alters the course of colic. Parents develop "tunnel vision" in regard to their infant's crying. They feel unable to offer any comfort to their child and talk of the frustration of being out of control. This is not to say that parental anxiety or conflict is the cause of the problem; these feelings usually develop secondarily to the infant's crying pattern. They do, however, interfere with the parents interacting effectively with the child. Additional family stressors may exacerbate the situation. These might include such issues as poor maternal support, marital difficulties, criticism from the extended family, and maternal depression.

EVALUATION

A complete pediatric history and physical examination must precede any interventions for colic. The history should be obtained empathically and optimistically. Included should be a history of any physical signs of illness, an evaluation of the impact of the colic on the family, a detailed psychosocial history, and a complete feeding and sleeping history. As part of the assessment, the physician should evaluate the observed interaction between the mother and infant. Through the course of the evaluation the physician should attempt to identify temperamental factors that may have put this infant at greater risk for colic. This information is helpful in educating the parents about the dynamics of the problem. In most cases of colic, the physical examination will be normal; however, it is essential that this be done thoroughly and carefully. Parents enter this session angry and frightened. They are sure that something is seriously wrong with their child. Only with the reassurance of a careful normal examination can they be satisfied that the infant is healthy. Laboratory studies generally are not indicated.

MANAGEMENT

Management should be aimed at parental education, family support, and counseling about interventions for handling a crying infant. Parents come in mystified by their baby's crying. Explaining the multifactorial nature of colic, with specific reference to those features most applicable to this family, can be very helpful. Allowing parents to see the infant's contribution to the symptoms, which may include an explanation of normal crying patterns in infants or the temperamental characteristics of their child, can help alleviate their guilt. Knowing that the pediatric office will follow and share this problem with them also is very relieving. Frequent telephone and office follow-up are critical. A tone of reassurance and optimism, based on the good prognosis, should be maintained.

As noted previously, parents of colicky babies often see few options in trying to calm their crying infants. Counseling should be directed at problem solving with the parents and alternatives for handling a crying infant. Many of the studies of colic suggest that doing something unique with an infant will at least calm them temporarily. Strategies might include swaddling and holding in different positions, keeping the baby in a front carrier, or using an infant swing. Reviewing with the family the reasons that infants cry may give them a logical approach to handle the crying. A sequence of feeding, changing, holding, and resting can be agreed upon. Empowering parents with these strategies is a first step. Parents also must be reminded, however, that in spite of these efforts, the baby may continue crying. Under these circumstances parents must recognize that putting a crying infant down also is permissible and that no physical or psychological harm will result from the crying.

The clinician must always keep in mind the dictum of doing no harm. The parents' complaints must be taken seriously. Callous reassurance such as reminding the parents that "all babies cry" or advising them to just sit it out can be destructive. Pharmacological interventions should be considered only in very limited circumstances. Phenobarbital (4 to 6 mg/kg/day in 4 divided doses given orally 15 to 30 minutes before feedings) or elixir of meperidine (2 to 6 mg/kg/day given orally in divided doses every 4 to 6 hours) can be prescribed in intractable cases in an emotionally deteriorating household. Results with the former are variable, whereas those with the latter are almost always successful without adverse side effects. Enemas should be avoided. For infants on a cow milk formula, a 1-week trial on a hypoallergenic formula is indicated. Multiple formula changes can be discouraging to the family, may suggest medical problems that do not exist, and should be avoided. Studies have suggested that herbal teas prepared from chamomile, balm-mint, fennel, licorice, or vervain have been effective in reducing colic symptoms.[6] Lastly, most infants who have colic are free of symptoms by 3 to 4 months of age.

REFERENCES

1. Brazelton TB: Crying in infancy, *Pediatrics* 29:579, 1962.
2. Carey WB: "Colic": primary excessive crying as an infant-environment interaction, *Pediatr Clin North Am* 31:993, 1984.
3. Illingworth RS: Infantile colic revisited, *Arch Dis Child* 60:981, 1985.
4. Lothe L, et al: Motilin and infantile colic: a prospective study, *Acta Paediatr Scand* 79:410, 1990.
5. Waldman W: *Coping with infant colic: a guide for parents,* Columbus, Ohio, 1982, Ross Laboratories.
6. Weizman Z, et al: Efficacy of herbal tea preparation in infantile colic, *J Pediatr* 122:650, 1993.
7. Wessel MA, et al: Paroxysmal fussing in infancy, sometimes called "colic," *Pediatrics* 14:421, 1954.

SUGGESTED READINGS

Barr RG: Normality: a clinically useless concept: the case of infant crying and colic, *J Dev Behav Pediatr* 14:264, 1993.

Lehtonen LA, Rautava PT: Infantile colic: natural history and treatment, *Curr Prob Pediatr* 26:79, 1996.

Lucassen PL, et al: Effectiveness of treatments for infantile colic: systematic review, *BMJ* 316:1563, 1998.

Pinyerd BJ: Strategies for consoling the infant with colic: fact or fiction? *J Pediatr Nurs* 7:403, 1992.

Taubman B: Clinical trial of the treatment of colic by modification of parent-infant interaction, *Pediatrics* 74:998, 1984.

85 Conduct Disorders

Michael S. Jellinek • Asha Parekh • Linda M. Forsythe

All children and adolescents misbehave at one time or another. Epidemiological studies indicate that disruptive, oppositional, and problematical behaviors tend to cluster at certain developmental stages. Many such behavioral problems resolve in the process of development and do not predict future patterns; some of them reemerge in a more mature form at a later stage, and a few more indicate lifelong patterns. For example, infantile temper tantrums, a manifestation of aggression, remain common during the preschool years but decrease to less than 10% in 5-year-olds and occur rarely in 15-year-olds.[9] Through the school-age years, most children disobey their parents at one time or another, but few break the major rules of society. Although local police become familiar with nearly one third of adolescents, only a small percentage of these youths will continue to break the law beyond adolescence.[10]

A conduct disorder, defined as a persistent pattern of behavior in which a child or adolescent violates the basic rights of others or age-appropriate rules of society, does not emerge suddenly; it evolves slowly within a context. Children and adolescents do not come into the office with organized complaints that lead easily to the diagnosis of a conduct disorder. They, or their parents, present fragments of unexplained impairments in social and academic functioning, of altered attachments with vague explanations, and of violent or violating misconduct.

Pediatricians evaluate children daily who have a wide range of behaviors. Their clinical assessment includes attempts to recognize patterns and elicit relevant information. Throughout this process they consider whether instances of misconduct are due primarily to expectable temperamental or developmental variations or whether they are early manifestations of psychopathology. Routine assessment of the severity of the behavioral patterns helps predict both its trajectory and prognoses. Pediatricians search for the meaning and the quality of particular behaviors in an effort to answer parental questions such as "Why is this happening?" and "What have we done wrong?" The process of generating a differential diagnosis and of considering various managements flows naturally from a thorough clinical assessment.

CLINICAL ASSESSMENT

Statistically valid, reliable diagnostic measures of behavioral characteristics are being developed for research purposes but are impractical for the primary care setting. Clinicians rely on clinical judgment and experience when addressing parental concerns about disruptive behavior, asking themselves whether the child is behaving normally within his or her developmental stage, what the severity of the disruptive behavior is, and why it is happening now.

Is the Child Behaving Normally for His or Her Developmental Stage?

Some behaviors are normal for very young children but are less appropriate at later stages. Preschoolers do not understand distinctions among wanting, grabbing, and "stealing" because of their egocentric view of the world; they own everything they see or desire. The concept of "lying" is equally problematic in the young child, for he or she naturally mixes fantasy and reality in stories.

School-age children may tell lies to avoid doing something or to gain immediate favor. Older children, fearing harsh consequences, momentarily may prefer the risk of a lie to the certainty of punishment. Until a child's cognitive development reaches the abstract stage (usually not until the teen years), his and her moral reasoning remains organized around avoiding punishment and seeking rewards. Parents who witness their school-age children cheating on board games may worry that their child is obsessed with winning. Sometimes this cheating is an early sign of a child's neediness and insecurity and warrants concern. More often, however, it is an aspect of made-up rules and is a normal variant of play.

Adolescents may feel justified when a lie is used to avoid hurting the feelings of a friend or to maintain their privacy. These differences are key to the clinical assessment and crucial to diagnosis and management. Lying that seems to occur when a child is unable to deal with overwhelming demands may be an early sign of more severe difficulties. Whereas the threats of some adolescents to run away are early signs of a lifelong pattern of truancy, drug use, or prostitution, other threats are merely temporary, clumsy attempts to counteract strongly felt attachments.

Some parents, at the time of a first, even minor, legal infraction, may become paralyzed in their fear that their child will become a menace. Parents may be tempted to compensate for their child's lack of internal controls by imposing severe external controls on all independent and self-assertive behavior. Alternatively, they may threaten to sever all emotional or supportive ties. Efforts to counter the adolescent's developmental path to autonomy are unlikely to succeed. More often, they have the unintended consequence of inhibiting further development of the youngster's appropriate internal controls or of forcing the teenager prematurely to be independent. Minor violations are most likely to become important learning experiences when parents are able to initiate age-appropriate discussions, negotiations, and consequences thoughtfully (see Chapter 101, Counseling Parents of Adolescents).

As with all pediatric care, the clinician must listen carefully to the degree of parental anxiety about issues such as dependency and control. Are both parents in agreement, or is the youngster caught in parental discord? Are other adults in the child's life (e.g., teachers and coaches) equally concerned about the path the youngster is following? Are the parents seen as overly rigid and critical? Is the child having difficulties in other areas of functioning such as with peers, at school, or in after-school activities?

What is the Severity of the Disruptive Behavior?

Severity is a complex judgment that includes separate considerations of (1) the symptomatic behavior, including developmental considerations, intensity, frequency, duration, and context; (2) the impact of the behavior on family functioning, school performance, and peer relations; (3) the cumulative effect of psychosocial risk factors in the child's life, including neglect, abuse, poverty, violence, parental illness and strife, access to guns, and the influence of cultural norms; and (4) an appreciation of the child's or family's preoccupation with the behavior and an assessment of additional psychiatric or neurological illnesses (Box 85-1). See Chapter 23 (Four), Violence Prevention.

The assessment of severity is made even more complicated by severity factors themselves often being interrelated. For example, an 18-month-old child's difficult temperament, although often perceived as a sign of disobedience, is likely to be divided among the following factors: biological determination, emerging autonomy, degree of mother's tolerance, goodness of fit, and empathy, and deleterious factors such as poverty and frequent moving. Each of these factors affects the child-parent relationship directly and at the same time affects each of the other factors. Parental sociopathy and alcoholism may mask serious underlying parental psychopathology such as major depression, posttraumatic stress disorder, or psychosis. Similarly, parental pathology may contribute to parental denial, symptom dismissal, and the rejection of assistance.

As parental stresses increase and supportive resources decrease, children tend to adapt more slowly, function more poorly, and become more aggressive. Parental abuse toward each other and toward their children is known to promote, or may even cause, a child's or adolescent's violent behavior (see Chapter 61, Domestic Violence and the Family). Abuse incites intense levels of rage in the child, provides violent role models, and may cause neurological damage to impulse control. The histories of the most behaviorally disturbed children and violent adolescents typically reveal physical or sexual abuse—often by adults, including parents.

A direct interview with the child should be used to ascertain the degree of the youth's burden of suffering,[5] his or her mood state, (especially depression), and any related, coexisting psychiatric, neurological, or cognitive vulnerabilities. For example, when facing a substance-abusing adolescent, pediatricians should consider whether a given street drug is being used as a self-medication for a psychosis, depression, an attentional deficit, or an anxiety disorder. Depressed children may exhibit sad facies or a bored and irritable demeanor. Beneath the "coolest" or most obnoxious facades may lie severely psychotic, depressed, or aggressive states.

An organic basis of behavioral dyscontrol and limited affect tolerance should be considered and investigated. Perinatal difficulties, headaches, loss of consciousness, dizziness, accidents, seizures, and injuries may give subtle signs of central nervous system dysfunction with etiological clues. However, a neurological assessment usually is nondiagnostic.

Truancy and poor school performance may indicate cognitive difficulties such as below-average intelligence, poor judgment, or undeveloped abstract reasoning. Specific language disabilities may involve particular difficulties with verbal expression that lead to increased physical expression of mood states.

BOX 85-1

FACTORS THAT INFLUENCE SEVERITY OF MISCONDUCT

- Academic underachievement
- Access to weapons
- Age older than 13 years
- Associated psychiatric disorders
  - Attention deficit/hyperactivity disorder
  - Substance abuse
  - Depression
  - Posttraumatic stress syndrome
- Family history of violence
- History of having been physically or sexually abused
- Low intelligence
- Low socioeconomic status and neighborhood with a high crime rate
- Neurological disorders
  - Learning disabilities
  - Seizures
  - Head trauma
- Parental mental illness
  - Substance abuse
  - Depression
  - Antisocial/criminal behavior
- Past personal history of violence
- Poor parental supervision/neglect
- Poor peer relationships

Why Is the Disruptive Behavior Happening Now?

Specific information about the context in which the behavior surfaces may provide insights into its cause and development. Traditionally, socioeconomic pressures and peer influences were emphasized as causal factors of delinquency. More recent evidence suggests that individual characteristics, such as violent behavior before the joining of a gang, may be the most powerful predictor (see Chapter 112, Violent and Aggressive Behavior).[4]

An exploration of the child's character structure and internal motivations is critical, as is an understanding of the nature and context of the rules the child tends to break. For instance, are the broken rules those of his or her parents, of teachers, or of society as a whole? How violent is the behavior? Does it surface more when the child is alone or in a group? Does the child in question take on a leadership role or become a passive follower?

Inevitably, both the parents and pediatrician will wonder if the given severity and quality of the behavior are manifestations of a deeper flaw in the child's personality or character. The expression of anger and feelings of helplessness are major problems for youths who are verbally and physically aggressive with other children and with adults. Some of the most violent and aggressive youths have histories of severe neglect or serious emotional, physical, or sexual abuse. "Identification with the aggressor" may provide a temporary feeling of control and superiority in an otherwise distraught, empty, or wounded teenager.

The terms *character* and *personality* attempt to define a person and to predict an individual's reaction to given circumstances. It integrates genetics, temperament, child rearing, and critical life events with cognitive, affective, moral, language, and social development. As with all other behavior, most isolated or intermittent instances of misconduct (e.g., cheating, stealing, lying, or threats to run away from parents) have their roots in the child's or adolescent's developing personality. When this style is rigid and dysfunctional, a disorder of character or personality should be considered. A character disorder is a serious, often lifelong, distortion of an individual's approach to inner feelings and the feelings of others. Characterological defenses usually are unyielding, and reality tends to have little impact; therefore, dealings are likely to be taxing and irritating. Either as a result of character pathology of their own or in response to their child, parents may be anxious, demanding, and hostile.

Characterological behavioral disorders involve rigid and relentless patterns of cheating, stealing, lying, bullying, and running away. A character-disordered adolescent may engage in repetitive stealing and bullying as an unconscious solution to feeling unworthy (of friends, favors, kindness, or gifts), as well as to satisfying the need for immediate relief. Because the gain is superficial, the relief temporary, and the satisfaction limited, the behavioral pattern continues. As long as the reasons for the disturbance of behavior remain unconscious, these behavioral solutions for dealing with extremely painful feelings are likely to continue. Once the child or adolescent is able to face the anxiety, anger, and sadness connected to relationships or expectations, the reliance on behavioral solutions may diminish, and he or she may be free, psychologically, to love and to work.

Although most children outgrow developmental immaturities naturally and others do so with the aid of psychotherapeutic interventions, a small percentage persist with immature patterns as a defining aspect of their adult interactions and are diagnosed with adult personality disorders. At the extreme, pediatricians may be asked to assess adolescents who have long-standing criminal records who have committed serious acts of violence such as assault, arson, and rape. These severely disturbed youngsters should raise concerns about character structure, severe psychopathology, neurological injury, and histories of extreme deprivation or abuse.

DIAGNOSIS

The American Psychiatric Association's *Diagnostic and Statistic Manual of Mental Disorders (DSM-IV)* lists specific criteria for each diagnostic category. Rather than being fully based on new research findings, however, the *DSM-IV* has resolved some diagnostic debates by committee consensus. For example, the manual refers to age 18 as the age at which adolescents complete child development. By convention, then, adult character–disordered terms such as "antisocial personality" or "sociopathic character disorder" do not apply to persons younger than age 18. Minors who have behavioral disorders are diagnosed as having attention deficit/hyperactivity disorder, oppositional defiant disorder, or conduct disorder. The terms *delinquent, status offender, and criminal* are legal terms (Table 85-1).

According to the *DSM-IV* (Box 85-2), conduct disorder is a disturbance of behavior lasting at least 6 months, during which the basic rights of others or the major age-appropriate norms and rules of society are violated. To meet diagnostic criteria, a child or adolescent needs to demonstrate at least 3 of the 15 behaviors. The behavioral symptoms or individual acts of misconduct that make up the diagnosis have relatively low base rates and relatively high predictive value.[2,3] The *Diagnostic and Statistical Manual for Primary*

Table 85-1 Comparative Factors in Key Disruptive Behavioral Disorders

	Oppositional Defiant Disorder	Conduct Disorder	Antisocial Disorder
Age	Under 18	Under 18	18 and over
Whose rules broken?	Parents' and teachers' rules only	Society rules/laws violating the basic rights of others and/or age-appropriate norms	Society rules/laws violating the basic rights of others
Key diagnostic features	Angry, resentful, spiteful, and/or vindictive	Bullies, threatens, harms, and/or intimidates with or without breaking any one of a number of age-appropriate societal rules such as stealing, breaking and entering, arson, and assault	Law-breaking

From Frick P: *Conduct disorders and severe antisocial behavior,* New York and London, 1998, Plenum Press; and Frick P, et al: *J Am Acad Child Adolesc Psychiatry* 33:529, 1994.

Care (DSM-PC) is a modified version of the *DSM-IV* for clinicians not familiar with the diagnosis of psychiatric disorders. It is intended to help identify, treat, and refer patients who have psychiatric diagnoses.[11]

The causes of conduct disorders are multifactorial. The relative importance of genetics and environmental factors has been debated in various studies. Several reviews have shown a substantial genetic component to juvenile psychotherapy (aggressive behaviors). This is important when considering the comorbidity between attention deficit/hyperactivity disorder (AD/HD) and conduct disorder. AD/HD, which is highly heritable,[1] is the most common comorbid diagnosis in children who have conduct disorder (see Chapter 73, Attention Deficit/Hyperactivity Disorder).[11] The presence of this co-occurring comorbidity is strongly associated with more severe and aggressive behavioral problems, including substance abuse.[11]

BOX 85-2

DSM-IV DIAGNOSTIC CRITERIA FOR CONDUCT DISORDER

A. A repetitive and persistent pattern of behavior in which the basic rights of others or major age-appropriate societal norms or rules are violated, as manifested by the presence of three (or more) of the following criteria in the past 12 months, with at least one criterion present in the past 6 months:

Aggression to People and Animals

1. Often bullies, threatens, or intimidates others
2. Often initiates physical fights with others
3. Has used a weapon that can cause serious physical harm to others (e.g., bat, brick, broken bottle, knife, gun)
4. Has been physically cruel to people
5. Has been physically cruel to animals
6. Has stolen while confronting a victim (e.g., mugging, purse snatching, extorting, armed robbery)
7. Has forced someone into sexual activity

Destruction of Property

8. Has deliberately engaged in fire-setting with the intention of causing serious damage
9. Has deliberately destroyed others' property (other than by fire-setting)

Deceitfulness or Theft

10. Has broken into someone else's house, building, or car
11. Often lies to obtain goods or favors or to avoid obligations (i.e., "cons" others)
12. Has stolen items of nontrivial value without confronting a victim (i.e., shoplifting, but without breaking and entering, or forgery)

Serious Violations of Rules

13. Often stays out at night despite parental prohibitions, beginning before age 13 years
14. Has run away from home overnight at least twice while living in parental or parental-surrogate home (or once without returning for a lengthy period)
15. Often is truant from school, beginning before age 13 years

B. The disturbance in behavior causes clinically significant impairment in social, academic, or occupational functioning.

C. If the individual is age 18 years or older, criteria are not met for antisocial personality disorder.

MANAGEMENT

Management of children and adolescents who have conduct disorders is difficult and time consuming; the causes of the illness are complex, and each youngster's situation requires individual treatment. Treatment often requires the development of new attitudes and behavioral patterns. It is made more complicated by negative attitude toward and distrust of adults.

Research shows that the future of conduct-disordered youngsters is likely to be grim if they and their families do not receive early, ongoing, and comprehensive treatment. All management considerations need to include simultaneous efforts to treat existing disruptive behavioral problems and comorbid disorders while attempting to prevent future antisocial behavior. Attempts to prevent or treat disruptive behavior in the early years should focus on altering individual and family functioning, irrespective of differences in developmental stages. Prevention and treatment of later adolescent disruptive states require more attention to alterations in the peer culture, the school system, and larger social contexts.

Mild disturbances of behavior are not likely to cause serious developmental difficulties or dysfunction. As the behavioral disorder increases in severity, more intensive evaluation, treatment planning, and possibly, referral is indicated. In the most severe cases, in which behavioral disturbances are causing serious developmental difficulties and dysfunction in one or more key areas of the child's life, mental health referral and comprehensive treatment planning are indicated, possibly on an urgent basis (see Chapter 83, Consultation and Referral for Behavioral and Developmental Problems).

Research findings suggest that those adolescents who terminate treatment prematurely show greater impairment at home, at school, and in the community compared with children who complete treatment. Selection factors and severity of impairment before the initiation of psychotherapy are important predictors of both attrition rates and limited response rates among patients who continue in therapy.[6]

Clinical follow-up studies of formerly incarcerated male delinquents have found little psychiatric treatment for identified vulnerabilities, inadequate supports, and the perpetuation of risk factors for violence.[7] Without earlier interventions and longer-term tracking studies, the hope to target treatment and improve the prognoses of subsequent generations is poor.

Ever-increasing numbers of young people engage in violence and criminal acts. Unfortunately, it is not until tragic events such as the 1999 Columbine High School shootings in Colorado that the precariousness of this growing social concern is brought to light. Violence and criminal acts pose an enormous challenge to the family, school, justice, and health care systems and to society as a whole. Currently, we can categorize violent and criminal behavior and suggest the multiple biological, psychological, familial, and social forces that contribute to the rising trend. For an individual child or adolescent, pediatricians should work with a number of colleagues to design the best available treatment. Other steps can be taken, albeit challenging and costly in time and money, that would help many teenagers and likely decrease, though not eliminate, the number who are out of control and the extent of harm they cause; these include:

- Involving teenagers in organized after-school activities. Many teenagers live in single-parent households or in a home in which both parents work. Rather than eliminating junior high sports, arts, clubs, and other after-school activities from school budgets, increased opportunities for teenagers to feel connected and cared for are needed. School buildings, gyms, and playing fields are all potentially available after school, but actually are not because of no staff and program. Being alone at home or on the streets for 4 or more hours after school until a parent comes home is not reasonable.
- Increasing the number of school-based guidance counselors. We know that at least 20% of teenagers are impaired by psychiatric disorders (especially depression), learning difficulties, use of substances, or problems in the home. A single school-based guidance counselor cannot provide services for 20% of 300 to 500 students, even if the needs of the remaining hundreds of students are ignored.
- Providing guidance counselors with assistance. Guidance counselors need expert backup from school psychologists and administrators, as well as truancy officers, courts, and the medical care system, to be effective. Information needs to be shared among guidance counselors, teachers, school psychologists, administrators, and parents. Each junior high school and senior high school must develop a philosophy and set of values regarding teenager behavior, including how the school community will deal with typical teen-group rivalries, substance use, bullying, and other aberrant behaviors and then stick to these values fairly and consistently.
- Increasing access to mental health services. Schools and parents cannot do this alone. Our society spends approximately half of what it did 10 years ago for mental health services for children. In Massachusetts, for-profit managed care companies have been encouraged to compete, based on low cost. Winning bids based on low cost means that there will be fewer mental health services available. More children are being given psychiatric medications and limited comprehensive treatment. Reimbursement for services, even hospitalization, is so low that quality is suffering. We know that the use of alcohol and other substances adds to the risk of violence and accidents, yet very few programs treat teenagers who have drug addiction. If we want to identify and help teenagers in need, we cannot keep cutting mental health services.
- Coordinating care for the most troubled teenagers. Many severely disturbed children will be known to some agency, especially if adequate medical and school guidance services are in place. Some who have been abused or neglected or who have had psychiatric problems during childhood may not be known of for years. In Massachusetts, agencies such as departments of social services, mental health, public health, and the juvenile courts are underfunded and face administrative barriers that limit their effectiveness in tracking disturbed children into adolescence or in working together to provide comprehensive treatment for them; limiting teenager access to guns, including locking any guns that are accessible, will save lives.

These steps would help many teenagers feel connected and cared for, rather than feeling left alone or overcontrolled. Some disturbed youth can be prevented from creating a tragedy, but a few will always elude the best efforts of all involved. Money is required to take these steps. When we deal with repeat criminal offenders, we seem to have the money for more police and prisons. Money spent on the prevention of conduct disorders and their early management will eventually reduce that spent on criminal offenders and will improve the society in which we live and the lives of disturbed children and their families.

REFERENCES

1. Eaves LJ, et al: Genetics and developmental psychopathology. 2. The main effects of genes and environment on behavioral problems in the Virginia twin study of adolescent behavioral development, *J Child Psychiatry* 38:965, 1997.
2. Frick P: *Conduct disorders and severe antisocial behavior,* New York and London, 1998, Plenum Press.
3. Frick P, et al: DSM-IV field trials for the disruptive behavior disorders: symptom utility estimates, *J Am Acad Child Adolesc Psychiatry* 33:529, 1994.
4. Friedman C, Mann F, Friedman A: A profile of juvenile street gang members, *Adolescence* 40:563, 1975.
5. Green M: Personal communication, 1994.
6. Kazdin A, Mazurick J, Siegel T: Treatment outcome among children with externalizing disorder who terminate prematurely versus those who complete psychotherapy, *J Am Acad Child Adolesc Psychiatry* 33:549, 1994.
7. Lewis DO, et al: A clinical follow-up of delinquent males: ignored vulnerabilities, unmet needs, and the perpetuation of violence, *J Am Acad Child Adolesc Psychiatry* 33:518, 1994.
8. Scott CL: Juvenile violence, *Psychiatr Clin North Am* 22:71, 1999.
9. Shepherd M, Oppenheim B, Mitchell S, editors: *Childhood behaviour and mental health,* London, 1971, University of London Press.
10. Wolfgang ME, Figlio RM, Sellin T: *Delinquency in a birth cohort,* Chicago, 1972, University of Chicago Press.
11. Wolraich ML, Felice ME, Drotar D, editors: The classification of child and adolescent mental diagnoses in primary care. In *Diagnostic and statistical manual for primary care* (DSM-PC) *child and adolescent version,* Elk Grove, Ill, 1996, American Academy of Pediatrics.

SUGGESTED READINGS

Lewis DO: Conduct disorder. In Lewis M, editor: *Child and adolescent psychiatry: a comprehensive textbook,* Baltimore, 1991, Williams & Wilkins.

Robins L: *Deviant children grown up: a sociological and psychiatric study of sociopathic personality,* Baltimore, 1966, Williams & Wilkins.

Sanson A, et al: Precursors of hyperactivity and aggression, *J Am Acad Child Adolesc Psychiatry* 32:1207, 1992.

86 Cross-Sex Behavior and Gender Identity Disorder

George A. Rekers • Howard J. Heinze

In preschool and elementary school-age children, cross-sex behavior may represent either a normal episodic exploration of sex role behaviors or an emerging stereotyped pattern of persistent and compulsively performed behavior indicative of a "gender identity disorder of childhood."[1,13,20] In adolescent males, cross-dressing also can be associated with a gender identity disorder or may be part of the development of transvestism, in which female undergarments, stockings, or other women's clothing articles are used for sexual arousal.[20,24] Although many arbitrary sex-role stereotypes for males and females increasingly are being challenged in our culture, and although values regarding fathers sharing child-rearing and household duties are changing, a cultural consensus remains concerning certain sex role distinctions that children normally master in early development (e.g., females but not males normally are permitted to appear in public wearing lipstick or wearing a dress).

Cross-sex behavior in prepubertal boys includes the following:

- Dressing in feminine clothing
- Using cosmetics
- Avoiding male playmates and rough-and-tumble play
- Being rather rigidly and exclusively preoccupied with girls' activities
- Taking a predominantly female role in play
- Talking predominantly about stereotypical female activities
- Projecting the voice into a high, feminine voice inflection
- Displaying effeminate gait and body movements ("swishing hips") or feminine-appearing gestures such as "limp wrist" (flexing the wrist toward the palmar surface of the forearm), "arm flutters" (rapid up and down movements of the forearm or upper arm or both, while the wrist remains relaxed), or "palming" (touching the palm or palms to the back, front, or sides of the head above the ear level).[15,20,21,24]

Boys outnumber girls more than six to one in numbers of diagnosed cases of gender identity disorder.[25]

For girls, the clinician needs to differentiate the normal prepubertal "tomboy" phase of many girls from pathological cross-sex behavior, which typically includes some combination of the following behaviors:

- Chronic rejection of feminine clothing, cosmetics, and jewelry
- Regular avoidance of female playmates
- Stated desire to be "one of the boys"
- Frequent projection of the voice into a low, masculine voice inflection
- Predominant talk about male activities, and habitual attempts to stand, sit, or walk in a hypermasculine manner (e.g., sitting with legs crossed with the ankle of one leg resting on the other knee)[20,21,25]

If the cross-sex behavior described by a parent or child is an isolated occurrence, such episodic cross-sex behavior falls within the normal range of childhood exploration of sex-roles.[20] However, if the behavior has continued over a 6-month period, parents should not be counseled that the behavior is "just a passing phase." Many children subsequently diagnosed with a "gender identity disorder" were told erroneously by a doctor that the cross-sex behaviors were only a temporary phase that the child would outgrow. This served only to delay onset of psychotherapeutic intervention, and unfortunately, resulted in progressive worsening of the condition. Early detection and early intervention holds greater promise of normalizing gender identification in children developing a gender identity disorder.[15]

In 1980, "gender identity disorder of childhood" first became an official diagnosis in the third edition of *Diagnostic and Statistical Manual of Mental Disorders (DSM-III)* for prepubertal children who are persistently and intensely distressed about their gender role or anatomical sex. As of 1994, *DSM-IV* official criteria[1] for "gender identity disorder" included strong and persistent cross-gender identification (not merely a desire for any perceived cultural advantages of being the other sex) manifested by at least four of the following:

1. Repeatedly stated desire to be, or insistence that he or she is, a member of the opposite sex
2. In boys, preference for cross-dressing or simulating feminine attire; in girls, insistence of wearing only stereotypical masculine clothing
3. Strong and persistent preferences for cross-sex roles in make-believe play or persistent fantasies of being a member of the opposite sex
4. Intense desire to participate in the stereotypical games and activities of the opposite sex
5. Strong preference for playmates of the opposite sex

Among adolescents and adults, gender identity disorder is manifested by symptoms such as "a stated desire to be the opposite sex, frequent 'passing' as the other sex, desire to live or be treated as the other sex, or the conviction that one has the typical feelings and reactions of the other sex."[1] This condition must be differentiated diagnostically from pretransvestic behavior,[20,24] in which female garments are worn or used for masturbation by males who have a normal gender identity.

Another essential criterion for gender identity disorder is a persistent discomfort with one's sex or a sense of inappropriateness in assuming the gender role of one's anatomical sex.[1] This is manifested in children by any of the following:

1. A boy's assertion that his penis or testes are disgusting or will disappear or that it would be better not to have a penis
2. A boy's aversion toward rough-and-tumble play and rejection of male stereotypical toys, games, and activities
3. A girl's rejection of urinating in a sitting position
4. A girl's assertion that she does not want to grow breasts or menstruate
5. A girl's marked aversion toward normative feminine clothing[1]

Among adolescents and adults, manifested symptoms include preoccupation with getting rid of one's primary and secondary sex characteristics (e.g., request for hormones, surgery, or other procedures to alter sexual characteristics physically to simulate the other sex) or belief that one was born as a member of the wrong sex.[1]

"Gender identity disorder" may not be "concurrent with a physical intersex condition." In addition, gender identity disorder causes clinically significant distress or impairment in social, occupational, or other important areas of functioning.[1]

The formation of gender identity is related to the child's appropriate identification with his or her sexual anatomy and its reproductive function.[16,18,20] Normal child-rearing experiences contribute to identification with the parent figure and peers of the same sex and to development of complementary role behaviors toward members of the opposite sex. Some reports suggest that a mother's prenatal preference that the newborn child be a girl[24] and/or excessive and extremely prolonged physical and emotional closeness between mother and her male infant, coupled with physical or psychological absence of the father during early childhood years, contribute to gender identity disorders in boys.[13,15,20] Similarly, some young girls whose mothers are physically or emotionally "unavailable" may be at risk for a compensatory identification with the father, contributing to a male gender identity.[18,21] However, children reared in a single-parent home are not necessarily at risk for a gender identity disorder, especially when the child is afforded the opportunity to develop positive and enduring attachments with adults of both sexes to compensate for the missing parent.

Gender identity disorders infrequently are associated with a variety of endocrinological, genetic, and anatomical abnormalities. A study of women who had congenital adrenal hyperplasia (CAH) found only 50% to be heterosexually active and a higher rate of bi- and homosexuality, raising questions regarding the impact of pre- and perinatal androgen exposure on the developing brain.[12,14] In a similar manner, Berenbaum demonstrated sex-atypical play in young girls ages 9 to 19 years with CAH.[4] In only rare cases, transsexuals have been found to have an abnormal karyotype—for example, a fertile male having an extra Y chromosome.[23] However, the vast majority of those who have gender identity disorder have normal chromosome numbers, external genitals, and hormone levels, and only in extremely rare cases are gender identity disorders associated with any detectable abnormalities in genetic constitution, gonads, external sex organ anatomy, internal accessory genital structures, sex endocrinology, or maternal health during pregnancy.[7,20,21]

An anecdotal report of sex reassignment in two male infants during the first year of life following penile trauma demonstrated inconsistent gender identity patterns through adolescence and adulthood.[6] A recent study of 59 children born with genital ambiguity of various etiologies revealed psychopathology in 39% (despite intensive counseling of the parents and individual psychotherapy of the children), and 13% of children assigned as female developed a cross-gender identification.[22]

Male pseudohermaphroditism secondary to alpha$_5$-reductase deficiency and the adoption of the male gender identity at puberty despite a female sex assignment at birth suggest that a culturally recognized phenomenon may be a powerful influence beyond the imprinting effects of androgens on the brain.[11] Further, strong family support plays a vital role in the acceptance of sex reassignment.[9,10]

Guidelines regarding sex assignment at birth for those infants who have genital ambiguity are available.[8,9] Clearly, the majority of children develop without gender identity problems. We will continue to struggle with sex assignment in certain forms of hermaphroditism in addition to accidental genital trauma despite our best efforts to understand how best to proceed. The presence of a nurturing and supportive family cannot be overstated.

Gender identity disorder occurs infrequently, its onset is before puberty, and cross-sex behavior patterns often begin before 4 years of age.[13,20,24] In later grade school years, overt cross-sex behavior may lessen in public, even though a gender identity disorder is present. Both retrospective and prospective data indicate an unusually high incidence of depression and suicide attempts in the adult years for boys who are untreated and that 64% to 75% of boys whose gender identity disorders are untreated develop homosexual or bisexual orientation during their adolescence.[2,18] A small minority of girls who have a gender identity disorder retain a masculine identification, with some also developing a homosexual orientation.[18] These reports indicate further that 5% to 12% of untreated males develop adulthood transsexualism accompanied by severe depression and suicide attempts, whereas approximately 1% to 5% develop heterosexual transvestism.[18,20] The remaining 6% to 23% develop a heterosexual orientation in adulthood.

DIAGNOSTIC CONSIDERATIONS AND ISSUES

Clinicians have found it useful to assess a child who exhibits cross-sex behavior across the seven major psychosexual dimensions as outlined in Table 86-1, because a complete diagnosis must consider all these levels of assessment.[20] The evaluation of cross-sex behavior should involve notation of frequency and setting, as well as the social labeling attached to the behavior pattern.[15] The developmental context of the behavior and the child's overall emotional and psychosocial

Table 86-1 Dimensions for Psychosexual Assessment

Level of Assessment	Dimension	Major Categories
Sexual status	Physical sex	Male, female, or intersexed; Tanner's stages for prepubertal, pubertal, or postpubertal development
	Social assignment	Male, female, or intersexed; child, adolescent, or adult (boy, girl, man)
Intrapersonal behavior	Gender identity	Normal, undifferentiated, cross-gender, or conflicted
	Sexual role identity	Heterosexual, bisexual, homosexual, transsexual, transvestite, "queen," "fag," "drag queen," "gay," etc.
	Sexual arousal orientation	Human object choice (male, female, both); animal object choice; magnitude and frequency; fantasies
Interpersonal behavior	Gender role behavior	Masculine, feminine, undifferentiated, androgynous
	Sexual behavior	Human partner (male, female, both); animal partner; inanimate object; intrusive versus receptive roles; group versus individual partner, etc.

From Rekers GA, Kilgus MD: Differential diagnosis and rationale for treatment of gender identity disorders and transvestism. In Rekers GA, editor: *Handbook of child and adolescent sexual problems,* New York, 1995, Lexington Books/Macmillan/Jossey-Bass.

functioning also should be considered.[20] An inquiry should be made regarding the cultural context of the stereotypic behavior, the presence or absence of a compulsive cross-sex behavior pattern, and the significance of the behavior to the child or adolescent.[21] The cluster of behaviors should be considered, because it is the ratio of masculine to feminine behavior rather than the exact number of cross-sex behaviors that is diagnostically significant.[20,24] Parents can be asked specific questions:

1. How do you categorize masculine and feminine behaviors?
2. Does your child identify with and model after the parent and peers of the same sex?
3. In what ways does your child relate to boys and girls differently?
4. To what degree does your child identify with his or her sexual anatomy and understand its future reproductive function?
5. What is the history and frequency of the following behaviors in your child: cross-dressing, masculine and feminine gestures, play with cosmetics, avoidance of play with peers of the same sex, play with girls' toys and activities, play with boys' toys and activities, feminine and masculine voice inflection, desire to be called by a name of the opposite sex, "deviant" sexual behaviors, and masturbation in association with cross-dressing articles?
6. Does your child insist on being or pretend to be a member of the other sex?
7. Has your child expressed disgust or dislike for any body part, particularly a primary or secondary sex characteristic?
8. Has your child ever asked for a sex change (request for hormones or surgical change to the other sex), and if so, how often?

The parents can be asked to record the frequency of several key masculine and feminine behaviors daily for 1 or 2 weeks.[15,21] Parental inquiries with the school teacher on how the child relates to male and female classmates may be recommended.[15]

In interviewing the child, the pediatrician simply can ask the boy or girl to draw a person or a picture of himself or herself and talk about the drawing.[3,20] A significant number of boys who have gender identity disorder will draw a female figure, making this a quick diagnostic screening test that may provide clues to the child's gender identity.[3] After establishing rapport with the child, interview questions[20] similar to the ones that follow can help clarify progress in gender identity development.

1. What are the first names of your friends and playmates at home and school? (Note and compare the number of female and male friends.)
2. Are you more like your mom or your dad? How?
3. If you could have three wishes, what would you wish for?
4. What are your favorite subjects and activities at school?
5. How often do you feel like a boy? How often do you feel like a girl?
6. When you have free time, what are your favorite things to do?
7. Most kids are called names at some time or other; what names do the other kids call you?

Although children younger than 8 years of age often are open to disclosing truthful answers to such interview questions, older children and adolescents are more aware of the social significance of their gender role behavior and may have gone "underground" with their true interests at home, and they may conceal their cross-gender preferences from the physician, as well. In such cases, a more comprehensive evaluation with use of psychological testing by a clinical psychologist is recommended.[20,24]

If appropriate, parallel questions from the parent interview described previously should be asked. Even when the criteria for a gender identity disorder are not all present, a persisting "gender role behavior disturbance" (which can be diagnosed as an example of "gender identity disorder not otherwise specified," as defined earlier) can be detected in a child as young as 4 years of age.[20,21,24] In cases of chronic cross-sex behavior, evaluation should include medical and pregnancy history, physical examination (including external genitalia), chromosome analysis, and sex chromatin studies, even though these diagnostic procedures result in negative findings in the vast majority of cases.[7,20]

For adolescents, in addition to interviewing the parent and young person along the lines described above, the pediatrician also will find it necessary to assess sexual arousal patterns and frequency of specific sexual behaviors by interviewing the adolescent and/or by asking the patient to record the occurrence of sexual urges and sexual behaviors over a 2- to 4-week period.[15]

Many cross-dressing adolescents privately seek sexual information about their attraction to female garments from books, magazines, and/or the Internet. With the increasing availability of printed and Internet pornography, increasing numbers of adolescent males encounter information that depriving oneself of oxygen, and/or bondage, can heighten sexual sensations.[5,16,17] "Bondage" refers to tying together one's hands or feet with a rope or similar binder, or having another individual tie one's hands or feet together, so as to induce a deviant sexual arousal pattern. "Autoerotic asphyxia"[5,17] refers to unconsciousness resulting from oxygen deprivation and the systemic accumulation of carbon dioxide, which occurs accidentally as a result of the deviant (and potentially life-threatening) sexual practice in which an adolescent intends to induce temporary anoxia (oxygen deprivation) while masturbating. These practices include tightening a plastic bag over one's own head or tightening a rope around one's own neck to heighten sexual sensations during the sexual self-stimulation. Adolescents often do not realize that the deviant sexual practice of autoerotic asphyxia can lead to death.

Pediatricians also should tactfully inquire about the possible occurrence of bondage or attempted autoerotic asphyxia, which sometimes, although rarely, is associated with transvestic behavior among adolescents.[5] If interview information from the parent or adolescent confirms or hints at a masturbatory practice associated with intentional behavior to induce temporary anoxia, the adolescent urgently needs a specific warning from the pediatrician that such practices are life threatening. Immediate referral to a clinical psychologist or psychiatrist is indicated, together with the obtaining of parental permission to release patient information to that psychotherapist concerning the suspected or confirmed sexual practice.[17]

SUGGESTIONS FOR MANAGEMENT

If psychodiagnostic questions are raised regarding a potential gender identity disorder, the child should be refereed immediately to a clinical child psychologist for a psychological evaluation and recommendations regarding potential psychotherapeutic treatment.[15,20] Early detection accompanied by early intervention is the preferred clinical strategy.

Specific child behavioral therapy techniques have been demonstrated to be effective in the successful treatment of gender identity disorders and other cross-sex behavior problems in childhood.[15] Positive reinforcement for normal sex-type play, normal speech pattern, and sex-appropriate behavioral mannerisms as noted previously has been found to be effective in the clinic, home, and school in the successful treatment of deviant cross-sex behaviors in boys and girls, particularly when the parents are trained and supervised closely by a child psychologist or psychiatrist to carry out behavior-shaping programs in the child's environment.[15,21]

In cases of cross-sex behavior lacking conclusive evidence of gender identity disorder, the following management strategies are recommended:

1. Encourage the same-sex parent to invest time in positive play and interaction with the child, avoiding criticism of the child.[15,21]
2. Where a same-sex parent is unavailable, recommend finding a substitute same-sex adult (such as a grandparent) who can be a positive role model.
3. Recommend ignoring cross-sex behavior where possible.[15]
4. Advise parents to reward or praise appropriate "sex-typed" play and mannerisms.[15]
5. Provide appropriate sex education[19] where needed.
6. Inquire at regular office visits about the child's sex-typed behavior; if only limited improvement is apparent after several months, refer the child to a clinical child psychologist or child psychiatrist for behavioral therapy.

For emerging transvestic-like behavior in male adolescents (where female garments are used for sexual arousal), referral should be made to a clinical psychologist, behavioral pediatrician, or psychiatrist for specific psychotherapeutic and behavior therapy interventions.[15,24]

REFERENCES

1. American Psychiatric Association: *Diagnostic and statistical manual of mental disorders (DSM-IV),* Washington, DC, 1994, American Psychiatric Press.
2. Bailey JM, Zucker KJ: Childhood sex-typed behavior and sexual orientation: a conceptual analysis and quantitative review, *Dev Psychol* 31: 43, 1995.
3. Benziman H, Marodes S: Indicators of feminine gender identity in latency-aged boys in the Draw a Person and the Rorschach tests, *J Clin Psychol* 53:143, 1997.
4. Berenbaum SA: Effects of early androgens on sex-typed activities and interests in adolescents with congenital adrenal hyperplasia, *Horm Behav* 35:102, 1999.
5. Blanchard R, Hunker SJ: Age, transvestism, bondage, and concurrent paraphilic activities in 117 fatal cases of autoerotic asphyxia, *Br J Psychiatry* 159:371, 1991.
6. Bradley SJ, et al: Experiment of nature: ablatio penis at 2 months, sex assignment at 7 months, and a psychosexual follow-up in young adulthood, *Pediatrics* 102:132, 1998.
7. Byne W, Parsons B: Human sexual orientation: the biologic theories reappraised, *Arch Gen Psychiatry* 50:228, 1993.
8. Chase C: Long-term psychological evaluation of intersex children (commentary), *Arch Sex Behav* 28:103, 1999.
9. Diamond M: Intersexuality: recommendations for management, *Arch Sex Behav* 27:634, 1998.
10. Landen M, et al: Factors predictive of regret in sex reassignment, *Acta Psychiatr Scand* 97:254, 1998.
11. Mendonca BB, et al: Male pseudohermaphroditism due to steroid 5 alpha reductase 2 deficiency: diagnosis, psychological evaluation and management, *Medicine* 75:64, 1996.
12. Meyer-Bahlburg HFL: What causes low rates of child-bearing in congenital adrenal hyperplasia, *J Clin Endocrinol Metab* 84:1844, 1999.
13. Money J, Lehne GK: Gender identity disorders. In Ammerman RT, et al: *Handbook of prescriptive treatments for children and adolescents*, ed 2, Boston, 1999, Allyn & Bacon.
14. Mulaikal RM, Migeon CJ, Rock JA: Fertility rates in female patients with congenital adrenal hyperplasia due to 21-hydroxylase deficiency, *N Engl J Med* 316:178, 1987.
15. Rekers GA: Assessment and treatment methods for gender identity disorders and transvestism. In Rekers GA, editor: *Handbook of child and adolescent sexual problems*, New York, 1995, Lexington Books/Jossey-Bass.
16. Rekers GA: Development of problems in puberty and sex roles in adolescence. In Walker CE, Roberts MC, editors: *Handbook of clinical child psychology*, ed 3, New York, 1999, John Wiley & Sons.
17. Rekers GA, editor: *Handbook of child and adolescent sexual problems*, New York, 1995, Lexington Books/Macmillan/Jossey-Bass.

18. Rekers GA: The development of a homosexual orientation. In Wolfe C, editor: *Homosexuality and American public life*, Dallas, 1999, Spence Publishing.
19. Rekers GA, Hohn R: Sex education. In Sears J, Carper J, editors: *Curriculum, religion, and public education: conversations for enlarging the public square*, New York, 1998, Teachers College Press.
20. Rekers GA, Kilgus MD: Differential diagnosis and rationale for treatment of gender identity disorders and transvestism. In Rekers GA, editor: *Handbook of child and adolescent sexual problems*, New York, 1995, Lexington Books/Macmillan/Jossey-Bass.
21. Rekers GA, Kilgus MD: Practical issues in the diagnosis and treatment of gender identity disorders in children and adolescents. In VandeCreek L, et al: *Innovations in clinical practice: a sourcebook,* vol 16, Sarasota, Fla, 1998, Professional Resource Press.
22. Slijper FM, et al: Long term psychological evaluation of intersex children, *Arch Sex Behav* 27:125, 1998.
23. Taneja N, et al: A transsexual male with 47 XYY karyotype, *All India Inst Med Sci* 161:698, 1992.
24. Zucker KJ, Bradley SJ: Gender identity disorders and transvestic fetishism. In Netherton SD, et al, editors: *Child and adolescent psychological disorders: a comprehensive textbook*, New York, 1999, Oxford University Press.
25. Zucker KJ, Bradley SJ, Sanikhani M: Sex differences in referral rates of children with gender identity disorder, *J Abnormal Child Psychol* 25: 217, 1997.

87 Encopresis

Barton D. Schmitt

Encopresis (soiling) is the voluntary or involuntary passage of feces into the clothing. Some children who have encopresis leak fecal material involuntarily from an impaction (retentive encopresis). Others simply pass normal movements into their underwear rather than use the toilet (nonretentive encopresis). Retentive and nonretentive encopresis should be separated because the treatment for each type is radically different. The minor fecal staining that occurs when children do not wipe themselves adequately after using the toilet should not be mistaken for encopresis.

Encopresis affects approximately 2% of kindergarten and first-grade students. The *DSM-IV* inclusion criteria for encopresis require the child to be 4 years of age or older, although any child older than age 3 years who is not toilet-trained may be considered encopretic. Without professional advice for this age range, many parents mistreat encopresis with coercion or punishment, and the condition worsens.[9] Most children who have encopresis are brought in for examination by age 5 years, when their symptom interferes with school entry.[8] Affected boys outnumber affected girls by a ratio of 3:1.

ETIOLOGY

To understand retentive encopresis, one first must understand the pathophysiology of an impaction, which occurs when constipation has gone unrelieved for about a week. By then, the rectum is so distended with stool that the sacrospinal defecation reflex is no longer energized and the mass is so wide that voluntary effort alone cannot force it through the anal canal. Hence, an impaction is fairly irreversible by natural events. The pressure of the impaction dilates the internal anal sphincter and makes it incompetent. Small amounts of the impaction are extruded intermittently through the external sphincter as a result of gravity, exercise, and relaxation. A few children become impacted because of organic factors. Most children hold back stool in an attempt to avoid the pain associated with passage or because they are enmeshed in a control issue with a parent.

Approximately 10% to 20% of children who are encopretic are not constipated. Frequently, preschoolers who are of this type are resisting bowel training deliberately. Most school-age children who have this type are postponing bowel movements ("waiting too long") because they don't want to leave some enjoyable activity (e.g., video games) or they don't want to use public toilets (e.g., school bathrooms).

All encopretic children (of either type) eventually develop secondary emotional problems; this embarrassing symptom takes a great toll in shame. The unpredictable nature of the symptom in retentive children causes constant fear of exposure. Many of these children are "scapegoated" at home, teased by peers (e.g., called "stinky"), and ostracized at school.

EVALUATION

History

A careful history usually distinguishes between retentive and nonretentive encopresis (Table 87-1). The clinician asks about size and consistency of stools and soiling intervals. In the retentive form, leakage occurs many times a day or even continuously. Commonly, one elicits a history of periodic pain or crying with bowel movements, blood on the toilet tissue, passage of a huge bowel movement that clogs the toilet, or posturing that suggests deliberate holding back. By contrast, the child who has nonretentive soiling passes a bowel movement of normal size and consistency into the underwear once or twice a day; all symptoms of constipation are denied.

Other helpful parts of the history are diet and use of the toilet. The intake of milk products, fruit juice, and fiber should be recorded, as should information about sitting on the toilet: how many times per day and if sitting is spontaneous or prompted by parents or teachers. If the stool pattern is unknown, sending the parent home with an encopresis diary to complete for the child can be most illuminating.

Physical Examination

The physical examination provides definitive information. In retentive soiling, an abdominal mass usually is palpable. Sometimes the mass extends throughout the entire colon, but more commonly it involves only the rectosigmoid area. The mass is midline, suprapubic, irregular, and moveable. The mass can be missed if the rectus abdominis muscles are not relaxed. The back-up of gas and stool can cause a protuberant abdomen.

A rectal examination must be performed on every patient; it can be done without any pain or distress in most children. Overlooking this procedure can lead to an erroneous diagnosis. Inspection of the anal opening often reveals protruding fecal material in those children who are deliberate stool holders. The rectum in all impacted children is dilated and packed with wall-to-wall stool (often 6 to 10 cm across). The consis-

Table 87-1 Differentiation of Retentive Soiling from Nonretentive Soiling

	Retentive Soiling	Nonretentive Soiling
History		
Symptoms of constipation	Yes	No
Interval	Many times per day	Once per day
Size	Small	Normal
Consistency	Loose	Normal
Previous need for laxatives, suppositories, or enemas	Yes	No
Examination		
Abdominal mass	Yes	No
Abdominal distention	Often	No
Anal canal	Sometimes full	Empty
Rectum	Packed	Normal

Table 87-2 Organic Causes of Constipation and Retentive Soiling

Entity	Diagnostic Criteria
Constipating medication	History positive
Constipating diet	History positive
Chronic anal fissure	Examination positive
Perianal cellulitis	Examination positive
Hypothyroidism	Linear growth delayed
Anal or rectal stenosis	Finger cannot enter rectum
Pelvic mass	Mass found on rectal examination (usually posteriorly)
Hirschsprung's disease	Rectal ampulla repeatedly empty; rectum is tight

tency of the impaction more commonly is like wet clay, rather than hard. By contrast, the child who has nonretentive soiling has a normal abdominal examination, and the rectal vault contains either a stool of normal caliber or nothing if the child has evacuated recently.

Retentive encopresis has an organic basis in fewer than 5% of encopretic children. Organic causes of constipation and retentive soiling often are noted on physical examination (Table 87-2).

Laboratory Studies

Children who are encopretic generally need no routine laboratory confirmation of this diagnosis. Because an impaction can cause partial bladder emptying and urine retention, a urinalysis for nitrite and pyuria may be helpful to screen for urinary tract infection, especially if there is any associated enuresis. Suspicious perianal erythema should be cultured for group A *Streptococcus*. Occasionally, thyroid function tests are warranted.

Radiographic Findings

If the examiner cannot determine whether the patient is impacted (e.g., empty rectum), a plain post-voiding, supine abdominal radiograph can be helpful. Other indications include sexually abused children who might be emotionally traumatized by a rectal examination and those who refuse a rectal examination. A child who is impacted will demonstrate on roentgenogram a rectum grossly dilated with granular stool and increased stool in the transverse and descending colon, which normally is empty.[2] A normal child has granular stool in the ascending colon and formed stool of normal diameter in the rectosigmoid area. A barium enema or rectosigmoid manometric study is indicated only if Hirschsprung's disease is strongly suspected. Children who have retentive soiling and experience repeated treatment failures occasionally may warrant a barium enema to reassure the family (and physician) that some rare diagnosis has not been overlooked.

BOX 87-1

TREATMENT OF RETENTIVE ENCOPRESIS

- Hyperphosphate enemas (two or three) to remove impaction
- Mineral oil or lactulose for 3 months to keep the stools soft
- Laxatives if stool softeners are ineffective
- Sitting on the toilet for 10 minutes after meals
- Nonconstipating, high-fiber diet

MANAGEMENT OF RETENTIVE ENCOPRESIS

Most children older than age 5 years want to stay clean; they do not want the embarrassment of "messing" their underwear (Box 87-1). However, they may not understand how to become free of this symptom. Tell them they "need to have a BM every day." They need to keep their rectum empty. Help them understand that holding back BMs is the main cause of "leaking" or "messing" their pants.

Initial Disimpaction

Unless the impaction is removed, the child will be unable to maintain any bowel control. The traditional way to remove an impaction is to give two or three sodium phosphate enemas over 2 days. Warn the parents that phosphate enemas given in excessive dosage can cause tetany or dehydration. Gleghorn, Heyman, and Rudolph[3] showed that for children who refuse enemas, administering 1 oz of mineral oil per year of age (8 oz maximum) per day orally also can dislodge the impaction if the treatment is continued for approximately 4 days. A combination of these two approaches, starting with mineral oil orally and followed by enemas on day 3, may be useful. Occasionally, enemas have to be administered in the office or clinic. For severe impactions involving the entire colon, the child may need to be hospitalized for polyethylene glycol-electrolyte solution by nasogastric tube for 8 to 24 hours.[1]

Stool Softeners

As soon as the impaction is eliminated, the long-term treatment of constipation should be administered orally. Mineral oil or lactulose is prescribed (Table 87-3). The goal is the passage of one or two normal-size bowel movements per day. Stool softeners must be continued for 3 months, because bowel diameter and tone require this long to return to normal. If the child refuses to take straight mineral oil, consider a better-tasting (though more expensive) emulsified derivative of mineral oil.

Laxatives

Stool softeners are the first line of therapy for constipation. If stool softeners such as mineral oil or lactulose are not effective, recommend laxatives (bowel stimulants) to help the child keep the rectum empty. Laxatives usually are needed for children who deliberately hold back bowel movements or for those who have acquired megarectum and megacolon (for dosages, see Table 87-3).[7,10]

Undermedicating is the main cause of treatment failure and recurrences. If the child is not having a bowel movement daily, the dosage should be increased. Some children temporarily require dosages that exceed the "standard" dosage recommended by textbooks and the package insert. Many parents worry unnecessarily about laxative dependency. They

Table 87-3 Medications for Constipation and Impaction

Medication	Dosage	Comments
Stool Softeners		
Mineral oil	1-2 ml/kg/dose bid Adolescents: 60 ml/dose (max 8 oz/day)	Do not use in children who have GE reflux or vomiting or who are not yet walking Emulsified types (Petrogalar, plain Agoral, Kondremul) taste better
Lactulose	0.5-1.0 ml/kg/dose bid Adolescents: 15 ml bid (max 3 oz/day)	This is a prescription item
Polyethylene glucol (Miralox)	<5 yr: 5 g 6-12 yr: 8 g Adolescents: 17 g	This is a prescription item
Laxatives		
(Listed in order of increasing potency)		
Phillips' Milk of Magnesia or Haley's M-O (75% MOM, 25% mineral oil)	1 ml/kg/dose Adolescents: 30-60 ml	1 tablet MOM = 2.5 ml liquid
Senokot (senna)	<5 yr: 1-2 tsp syrup >5 yr: 2-3 tsp syrup Adolescents: 1 tbsp (max 2.5 tbsp or 8 tablets)	1 tablet = 3 ml granules = 5 ml syrup
Fletcher's Castoria	<5 yr: 1-2 tsp >5 yr: 2-3 tsp Adolescents: 2 tbsp max	
Ex-Lax (senna)	>5 years: 1 tablet Adolescents: 2 tablets	Chewable tablets
Dulcolax, 5-mg tablet	>5 yr: 5 mg >12 yr: 10 mg (2 tablets) Adolescents: 4 tablets max	No liquid form
Rectal Suppositories		
Glycerin suppository	1 or 2	
Dulcolax, 10 mg	>2 yr: 1 suppository	
Enemas		
Mineral oil enema	1-2 oz/20 lb of weight Adolescents: 4 oz	Squeeze-bottle size: 4.5 oz
Sodium phosphate enema (Fleet)	1 oz/20 lb of weight Adolescents: 4 oz (max 8 oz)	Squeeze-bottle size: 2.25 oz children, 4.5 oz adult

Modified from Schmitt BD, Mauro RD: *Contemp Pediatr* 9:47, 1992.

should be reassured that children can be tapered off laxatives successfully, even after 6 months of taking them.[6]

All affected children need stool softeners or laxatives for at least 3 months, and many for 6 months or longer. Many parents are in a hurry to stop the medications. They should be told on the first visit that to achieve a cure, medications need to be continued until the child has gone at least 1 month without any soiling. The medications then can be tapered gradually over 1 to 2 months.

Toilet Habits

The child must sit on the toilet for at least 10 minutes once a day with a timer. The gastrocolic reflex, which takes effect 20 to 30 minutes after a meal (especially breakfast), should be used to advantage. Any treatment that neglects this opportunistic timing will fail.

Children who have been impacted for many months have no urge to defecate. The defecation urge may not return until the rectum is kept empty for 2 to 4 weeks. Other important tips to impart to children are to flex the hips to open the rectum and to use a footstool for leverage and apply some pressure to the abdomen while pushing down. If they have no bowel movement for 24 hours, they need to sit on the toilet more often and longer each time. Soiling (leakage) also requires sitting on the toilet, as well as cleanup.

Some preschoolers and toddlers adamantly refuse to sit on the toilet, holding back their stools when they are forced to do so. The overriding goal is to produce a bowel movement daily. Passing it into the diaper is better than holding it in. This is a case where pediatricians and parents need to lower their expectations. The child can be told that the "poop wants to come out every day and it needs your help." Going in the diaper is fine.

Nonconstipating, High-Fiber Diet

All constipated children need more fiber in their diet, as is found in such foods as popcorn, grains, fruits, and vegetables. However, diet therapy alone will cure only those children who have mild constipation. The only foods that have been shown to be constipating are milk products. It is critical to identify the 10% or so of children who have impactions and who are drinking great amounts of milk (more than 32 oz per day). Milk intake can be limited to 16 oz per day in children older than 1 year of age. Fluid requirements for these children can be met with fruit juices, especially those that have a high sorbitol content such as pear, peach, or prune juice. This can increase the frequency of stools.

Follow-up Visits

All children who have impactions need follow-up about 1 week into treatment; over 30% still will be impacted.[10] Repeat the abdominal examination even if patients tells you that they are having normal bowel movements and no soiling. Children who have an impaction actually can keep themselves clean temporarily by making a superhuman effort at control and sitting on the toilet several times a day. If the history and abdominal examination leave you uncertain, repeat the rectal examination.

If a child still is impacted at the follow-up examination, a more detailed explanation of the disimpaction process is called for. Some children need enemas in the office at this point.

Back-up Plan for Recurrence of Constipation or Encopresis

Back-up plans are critical for preventing all-too-frequent relapses. If the child goes more than 48 hours without a bowel movement, the parents should be instructed to increase the dosage of stool softener or laxative.[1,10] This is critical to prevent impactions from recurring.

If soiling occurs more than twice over a few days, the child is becoming reimpacted. At this point, the parents should intervene vigorously by giving a double dose of laxative, a suppository, or an enema. Sometimes merely mentioning an enema results in the child sitting on the toilet and producing a bowel movement. For older children who are cooperative about sitting on the toilet, sitting there for 10 minutes out of every hour usually will relieve an early impaction. Again, the family should be made to realize that soiling always means that the rectum is full and the impaction is returning.

Biofeedback Treatment

Treatment failure has been attributed to rectal hyposensitivity and inability to relax the external anal sphincter.[5] Both of these pathophysiological conditions probably are acquired, the former caused by prolonged stretching of the rectum and the latter resulting from voluntary attempts to prevent stool leakage or pain. Both of these conditions usually revert to normal after a cure. No outcome study has shown the advantage of biofeedback training over using stool softeners, changing toileting habits, and instituting behavior modification.

MANAGEMENT OF NONRETENTIVE ENCOPRESIS

For those children who simply postpone BMs, a simple admonition "to find a toilet whenever you feel rectal pressure" or "don't make your body wait" usually removes the symptom (Box 87-2). Most of these children, however, are resistant to toilet training, and they need more intensive intervention.

BOX 87-2

TREATMENT OF NONRETENTIVE ENCOPRESIS

Do not give medications
Stop all reminders, lectures, or punishments
Give incentives for BMs into the toilet
For soiling, insist on immediate cleanup
Refer treatment failures

Medications

Stool softeners, laxatives, and enemas clearly are not needed in any of these cases.

Reminders and Lectures

The parents should be reassured that there is nothing more for them to teach their child. To eliminate the control issue, the parents should be told to stop all reminders about using the toilet and to let the child decide when he or she needs to go to the bathroom. Such children should neither be reminded to go to the bathroom nor be asked if they need to go. Reminders, inquiries, and lectures are a form of pressure, and pressure does not work. The parents should not threaten punishment. Many young children try to hold back all bowel movements to avoid punishment, such as being spanked or grounded for soiling. They are under the mistaken impression that not passing any bowel movements is the best way to avoid punishment. The parents should be told about the importance of not punishing their child for soiling. The child should be reassured that he or she will no longer be punished for soiling.

Incentives

Incentives for passing BMs into the toilet should be given and the parents reassured that this is how they can turn the tide. If the child passes a BM into the toilet, the parents should give immediate positive feedback such as praise, a hug, and a sticker. To achieve a breakthrough with some children who have never had a bowel movement into a potty chair or toilet, the parent should offer major incentives such as going out to their favorite fast-food restaurant, watching their favorite video, or giving them treats.[9] A "star" chart also helps many children stay focused on the goal of using the potty chair or toilet. Incentives also are helpful in younger children who deliberately hold back BMs and refuse to sit on the potty.

Changing Soiled Underwear

Soiling should not be ignored. The parents' only remaining assignment is to help the child change clothes when he or she is soiled. As soon as the parents notice that the child has messy pants, they should clean him or her up immediately. Changing should be made a neutral, timely interaction.

PROGNOSIS

Pediatric management can cure 99% of children who have mainly pain-related impaction. The physician will be successful with approximately 70% of children who have psychogenic impaction and will need to work in conjunction with a mental health professional for the others. Levine studied 127 encopretic children for more than 1 year.[4] At that time, 51% were cured and 27% had marked improvement.

Nonretentive encopresis is much easier to treat. These children have good results if the problem is recent and poor results if the problem is long-standing (more than 5 years). In mildly resistive children, primary care management can achieve a 90% to 95% cure rate. Those who have severe resistance need early referral. Box 87-3 lists the reasons for referral of encopretic children to a mental health professional.

BOX 87-3

WHEN TO REFER ENCOPRESIS TO A MENTAL HEALTH PROFESSIONAL

- Unresponsive to pediatric management
- Refuses to sit on the toilet and is older than 5 years of age
- Refuses to take medications
- Has nonretentive encopresis and is older than 8 years of age
- Has nonretentive encopresis and deliberately passes bowel movements on family possessions or at school (overt anger)
- Is depressed
- Parent-child relationship is severely disturbed

SUMMARY

The primary care pediatrician plays a critical role in the evaluation of children with encopresis. Most nonphysicians cannot distinguish between the retentive and nonretentive types. The physician also can treat many of these children successfully by using combined therapy (stool softeners, laxatives, diet, altered toilet habits, and positive reinforcement). If a child who has retentive soiling is referred to a mental health professional, the pediatrician should remain involved in titrating medications with the child's symptoms.

REFERENCES

1. Abi-Hanna A, Lake AM: Constipation and encopresis in childhood, *Pediatr Rev* 19:23, 1998.
2. Barr RG, et al: Chronic and occult stool retention: a clinical tool for its evaluation in school-aged children, *Clin Pediatr* 18:674, 1979.
3. Gleghorn EE, Heyman MB, Rudolph CD: No-enema therapy for idiopathic constipation and encopresis, *Clin Pediatr* 130:669, 1991.
4. Levine MD, Bakow H: Children with encopresis: a study of treatment outcome, *Pediatrics* 58:845, 1976.
5. Loening-Baucke V: Modulation of abnormal defecation dynamics by biofeedback treatment in chronically constipated children with encopresis, *J Pediatr* 116:214, 1990.
6. McClung HJ, et al: Is combination therapy for encopresis nutritionally safe? *Pediatrics* 91:591, 1993.
7. Nolan T, et al: Randomised trial of laxatives in treatment of childhood encopresis, *Lancet* 338:523, 1991.
8. Nolan T, Oberklaid F: New concepts in the management of encopresis, *Pediatr Rev* 14:447, 1993.
9. Schmitt BD: Toilet training refusal: avoid the battle and win the war, *Contemp Pediatr* 4:32, 1987.
10. Schmitt BD, Mauro RD: 20 common errors in treating encopresis, *Contemp Pediatr* 9:47, 1992.

88 Enuresis

Michael W. Cohen

Enuresis is defined as the involuntary discharge of urine, although it often is used to mean wetting during nighttime sleep *(nocturnal enuresis)*. Daytime wetting is termed *diurnal enuresis*. The diagnosis of enuresis should be reserved for girls wetting beyond the age of 5 years and for boys beyond 6 years; the gender-related age differences reflect developmental variations.

Nocturnal enuresis affects 5 to 7 million children in the United States and occurs in approximately 15% of all 5-year-olds, 7% of 8-year-olds, and 3% of 12-year-olds. Lower socioeconomic groups, families of lower educational levels, and institutionalized populations have a higher reported prevalence of enuresis. Males predominate at all ages, with the differential being greater in older children. Fewer than 10% of all children who have nocturnal enuresis wet in the daytime, and diurnal enuresis infrequently occurs without nocturnal enuresis.[1]

Primary enuresis exists when a child has never achieved consistent dryness. A child who has secondary enuresis generally is considered to have had a period of dryness of at least 3 to 5 months. As many as 25% of young children will have some minor relapse in bed-wetting after a period of initial dryness; this form of secondary enuresis usually is self-limiting and may occur only at times of illness or emotional stress.

ETIOLOGY

Enuresis is multifactorial in etiology, and a greatly increased prevalence of primary enuresis occurs in offspring of parents who themselves had been enuretic.[2,6] Developmental "delays," organic disorders, and psychological factors all have been emphasized as causes of enuresis. Although definitive proof is lacking, many believe that a delay in the enuretic child's adequate neuromuscular bladder control is the major cause, although this view is not universally held.[5]

Early studies suggested that enuresis occurs in lighter stages of sleep. Subsequent studies described nocturnal enuresis as a "disorder of arousal," with the voiding episodes beginning in the deepest stages of sleep. It currently is believed that nocturnal enuresis is independent of sleep stage and not specifically related to the depth of sleep, with enuretic episodes occurring randomly throughout the night.[3,4] Organic explanations have focused primarily on the genitourinary and nervous systems. Obstructive lesions of the distal outflow tract, such as posterior urethral valves, have received particular attention both as a cause of urinary tract infections and as an independent cause of enuresis. A current urinary tract infection or the history of previous infections may be causal factors in enuresis. However, in a primary care setting, only about 3% to 4% of youngsters who have enuresis demonstrate significant urological pathology.

Nervous system dysfunction may be associated with enuresis, either through lumbosacral disorders that affect bladder innervation or as a reflection of global mental retardation. Although true myelodysplastic disorders may affect bladder function, the radiological finding of spina bifida occulta has not been shown to be related causally to enuresis.[2]

In contrast to the normal nighttime increase in antidiuretic hormone (arginine vasopressin), some patients who have enuresis maintain constant serum levels of this hormone at night. Enuresis for these children appears to be a result of polyuria secondary to a lack of circadian rhythm in antidiuretic hormone secretion. This information is consistent with parental reports of multiple nighttime wetting episodes and an apparent excessive urinary output in their children.[5] Diabetes mellitus, sickle cell anemia, and sickle cell trait, and ingestion of foods or medications that have diuretic actions all have been implicated as infrequent causes of enuresis.

Psychological functioning may relate to enuresis at two levels. The enuresis may be only one aspect of a child's general difficulty in behavioral adaptation, or it may be an isolated symptom in a child whose behavioral functioning otherwise is normal. The prevalence of behavioral problems in children who have enuresis is somewhat increased, but most such children are not maladjusted or otherwise psychologically impaired.[3]

The evaluation should be considered the initial phase of therapy. The positive therapeutic value of a complete evaluation that satisfies the concerns and expectations of the child and family is well documented. Potential parental guilt associated with toilet-training approaches and management failures can be alleviated by a brief explanation of the multifactorial origin of the condition and the common difficulties in management.

HISTORY

The type of enuresis (primary versus secondary, nocturnal versus diurnal) should be established. The severity of the enuresis should be estimated and expressed as the number of wet nights per week or month (e.g., 4/7, 16/30). Quantification of the enuresis allows for a relatively accurate demonstration of a trend and the effect of intervention. The effect of environmental factors on the severity of the symptoms also should be explored. Parental management should be discussed, beginning with a history of initial toilet-training efforts. The age and response of the child, the attitudes and approach of the parents, and the results of such efforts are important. An interview with the child is quite important to elicit his perception of the problem, his feelings about enuresis and his sense of parental reactions. The presence of a significant negative emotional response by the child and whether the enuresis is limiting age-appropriate activities may influence decisions about intervention.

The medical history will reveal any perinatal difficulties that may have led to neurological trauma; the weight and gestation of the patient can alter developmental expectations. The review of systems should focus on the genitourinary and nervous systems. Delays in perceptual-motor or communication skills might coexist with a delay in bladder control. In addition to frequency and urgency of urination and symptoms of urinary tract infection, dysuria and dribbling after and between micturition have been found to be more common in enuretic children than in nonenuretic children. Approximately 1 in 10 children who have enuresis also will have encopresis (see Chapter 87). This association is firmly established and may reflect an underlying deficiency in toilet training or an organic pathology.

PHYSICAL EXAMINATION

A full examination is essential. Renal disease may be reflected in poor growth or elevated blood pressure. Examination of the genitalia should be complete and sensitive to the feelings of a developing youngster or teenager. A search for major and minor anomalies should be followed by an observation of micturition. Anomalies, including undescended testes, underdeveloped scrotum, epispadias, phimosis, and abnormalities in the urethral meatus in males, and location and characteristics of the urethral meatus in females should be observed because they may be associated with internal anomalies. Abnormalities or difficulties in voiding, such as changes in the quality (e.g., size and velocity) of the urinary stream, an inability to initiate or stop micturition voluntarily, and the presence of dysuria or dribbling, should be noted.

A neurological examination may reveal lower spinovertebral dysfunction that reflects abnormalities of bladder innervation. Gait, muscular strength and tone, deep tendon reflexes, sensory responses, and rectal sphincter tone, therefore, should be examined.

LABORATORY TESTS

A urinalysis provides valuable information about a wide range of organic disorders that may be associated with enuresis, including diabetes insipidus, psychogenic water drinking, diabetes mellitus, urinary tract infection, and various forms of renal pathology. Beyond the urinalysis and urine culture, the indication for further evaluation remains quite controversial.

Rushton[8] has divided nocturnal enuresis into uncomplicated and complicated, with the second category requiring additional diagnostic studies. Factors that dictate these studies include persistent secondary onset of bed-wetting, severe voiding dysfunction, associated encopresis, urinary tract infection, and abnormal findings on neurological examination. Further studies may include a renal or bladder sonogram, intravenous pyelogram (IVP), a voiding cystourethrogram (VCUG), or urodynamic measurements. If these procedures are indicated, the child must be prepared in a manner that will minimize the psychological trauma, with the nature of this preparation depending on the age, gender, and developmental maturity of the child. Functional bladder capacity should be measured if bladder training is the proposed form of treatment. Unless an undiagnosed seizure disorder is strongly suspected, the presence of enuresis does not warrant an electroencephalogram.

By the end of this type of evaluation, the majority of children who have enuresis who also have significant organic dysfunction or psychopathological dysfunction will have been discovered. When their needs exceed the expertise of the primary care physician, these patients should be referred to the appropriate specialist (urologist, neurologist, endocrinologist, nephrologist, or mental health or behavioral specialist). The remaining group, which constitutes the vast majority of children who have enuresis, will present a picture consistent with a basic developmental delay in bladder control with associated psychological factors. This population is managed best by the clinician who is most familiar with the child and the child's family and environment.

MANAGEMENT

An air of optimism is realistic and may be immeasurably therapeutic. Although a positive clinical response to the process of evaluation and intervention often has been labeled a placebo effect, the benefit of a carefully planned approach has been documented and should be considered therapeutic. An annual spontaneous remission rate of approximately 15% between ages 5 and 19 applies primarily to boys[9]; remission rates for girls are highest early in this age range. Optimism also may be bolstered by uncovering a history of parental enuresis.

The participation of the child enhances the efficacy of any specific mode of therapy and should be solicited. The child's involvement should begin with a demystification and an explanation of the probable cause of his or her enuresis at the child's level of understanding. A clarification of the involuntary nature of the symptoms usually removes any sense of guilt and allows the child to develop an optimistic perspective. Such involvement also decreases the chances of struggle between child and parents and promotes the child's responsibility for alleviating the symptoms.[6]

Reassurance may be the therapy of choice for younger children or for children developing transient secondary enuresis in response to an environmental stress. For parents who feel compelled to do something while awaiting a remission, various simple measures have been recommended, such as limiting the child's fluid intake, having the child empty his or her bladder at bedtime, or taking the child to the bathroom during the night. If these are suggested, it should be explained that although they may decrease the symptoms somewhat, they have not been shown to hasten a remission. These tactics also may initiate or aggravate a struggle between parent and child.

Supportive counseling may be required as the sole mode of therapy or as an adjunct to other specific regimens. The goals of counseling could include (1) parental understanding of the multifactorial nature of enuresis, (2) parental acceptance of the child and the symptoms in a manner that allows them to provide maximum emotional support, (3) acceptance by the child of the symptom and an appreciation of "individual differences" that many children demonstrate in other areas of functioning, and (4) appreciation by the patient that he or she can have some control over the enuresis. The requirement for counseling depends on the age of the child, the child's general developmental and behavioral pattern, the family's experience with enuresis, the coexistence of emotional problems, intrafamily communication patterns, and the response to the initial management.

If the enuresis is deterring the child's social, emotional, or cognitive development, therapy beyond reassurance and supportive counseling is indicated. Conditioning devices, bladder training, self-hypnosis, and drug therapy all have been shown to be effective. However, both parents and child should be alerted to the potential for relapse and, thus, the need for a "second dose" of treatment.

Enuresis-conditioning instruments involve a moisture-activated sensor, which is connected to an alarm that provides auditory or vibratory stimulation to wake the child or parent at the initiation of wetting.[6] Older devices involve a mattress pad; the new ones have portable sensors that attach to the child's underpants. The auditory alarms are contained in a wristwatch or small pin-on battery-powered alarm. Because the temporal relationship between the wetting episode and the alarm is critical for effective conditioning, a refined instrument of adequate sensitivity is required.

Cure rates have varied among studies, but several controlled studies have yielded rates between 60% and 85%. Personal resistance by the child may lead to as high as a 10% to 20% noncompliance rate. Permanent responders require an average of 60 days of therapy. A 20% to 40% relapse rate is reported in all studies, but dryness often is obtained more quickly and permanently with a second course of treatment. The technique of "overlearning" by increasing fluid intake before bedtime to stress the bladder and increase the waking episode decreases the relapse rate. An intermittent reinforcement program, with the alarm sounding during 70% of the wetting episodes, also may lead to a lower relapse rate. The safety and portable nature of the new devices and the reported successful results of such conditioning therapy make this an attractive therapeutic technique.

Self-hypnosis or self-conditioning has been effective in primary nocturnal enuresis.[7] The enuretic episode is viewed as a habit disorder that allows the wetting episode without the child awakening. The child is taught the technique of self-induced relaxation, to be practiced before sleep. During this "trance," children tell themselves that they will wake up when they experience the need to void, thus allowing a dry bed and very happy feelings on waking in the morning. This happiness can be associated with a visual image of some warm, tranquil, and enjoyable experience in the youngster's memory to enhance the desirability of the feeling upon waking in a dry bed. Significant improvement and cure rates (80%) have been reported after only a few training visits. This technique requires special therapy skills but appears to be a potent and safe alternative treatment with much promise.

Bladder-training therapy is based on the observation that functional bladder capacity in many children who have enuresis is decreased. The goal of this training is to transform a functionally infantile bladder into one of adult volume and coordination. The procedure involves the participation of the child in holding the urine as long as possible once a day for several months. Increasing urine volumes and number of dry nights are recorded on a calendar, which serves as a reinforcement for the child. The clinician must be cautious that the discomfort caused by urine retention does not discourage the participation of the youngster and create a struggle with the parents. In addition, measured increases in bladder volume do not generalize to nighttime dryness.

Several pharmacological agents have been used to treat enuresis. Sedatives, stimulants, and sympathomimetic agents are not beneficial. Oxybutynin, an anticholinergic agent, is not significantly better than a placebo in reducing the frequency of bed-wetting but may help some children who have diurnal enuresis. Tricyclic antidepressants, particularly imipramine, have been used extensively to treat enuresis, with total dryness being achieved in 10% to 20%, a "50% improvement" in 67% of children, and the remainder receiving less or no benefit. A very high relapse rate is noted when the medication is discontinued. Three proposed mechanisms of action are (1) a direct relaxation effect on the bladder detrusor muscle, (2) an alteration in the arousal state of the nervous system during sleep, or (3) an antidepressant effect. Because there is no evidence that children who have enuresis are depressed and because enuretic improvement can be immediate, whereas antidepressant benefits take more than 7 to 10 days, depression is unlikely to be the mechanism. The arousal proposal also is questionable because the relationship between depth of sleep and enuresis has been questioned.[8] Imipramine generally is given 30 minutes to 1 hour before bedtime, with no proven advantage to multiple daily doses. The initial dose of imipramine is 25 mg for children younger than age 12 years and 50 mg for older children. Although the maximum recommended dose has been 75 mg, studies measuring plasma levels at 12 hours after the bedtime dose suggest dramatic variations in levels and in the need for and safety of higher doses in some children. Measuring plasma levels routinely is not indicated but may be useful before concluding that imipramine is unhelpful.

The child should be asked to maintain a diary of success. At the first follow-up visit, the imipramine dosage can be altered and the youngster supplied positive feedback. Once the therapeutic response is successful, the child should be maintained on the medication for approximately 3 months. At the end of this period, a gradual discontinuation of the drug may decrease the likelihood of a relapse. The drug should be tapered to once every other night and then every third night over 4 to 6 weeks. The maximum psychological benefit of dryness on "nondrug" nights can be supplied by emphasizing and praising the child's newly developed bladder control, which it is hoped can be sustained without medication. The most common adverse effects are nervousness, insomnia, headaches, and anticholinergic symptoms.

Imipramine is well known for its toxicity and thin margin

of safety. The triad of coma, convulsions, and cardiac disturbances can occur at relatively low-dosage accidental ingestions in young children and may be fatal. School-age youngsters are vulnerable to overdosage because of magical thinking that leads them to believe that more medication might be more beneficial. A number of deaths have been reported under these circumstances. Caution must be used in prescribing this agent, and the parents and child must be well aware of the potential dangers involved in, and their control over, its administration.[5] Drug therapy with this agent should be reserved for the older child who has not responded successfully to other therapies.

The diuresis theory of causality has led to initial clinical trials with desmopressin (antidiuretic hormone). This agent was thought to serve as a substitute for endogenous nocturnal vasopressin, leading to a reduction in overnight urine volume. Increased dose and clinical benefit are correlated.

An initial dose of 20 μg can be increased gradually to 40 μg until dryness is achieved. Most studies have used intranasal administration, although the oral route appears to be just as effective and causes fewer electrolyte changes. Desmopressin has been used for 20 years in the treatment of central diabetes insipidus, with few adverse effects. Water intoxication and hyponatremia are a theoretical concern but have not occurred in otherwise healthy children given only a bedtime dose. Headaches, nausea, mild abdominal cramps, and vulvar pain have been reported but disappear when the dose is reduced. The drug neither suppresses endogenous production of vasopressin nor induces destructive antibodies.

A recent literature review indicated that desmopressin reduces the number of wet nights but that only about 25% of the subjects studied achieved complete dryness.[4] The best responses were in those who had a family history of enuresis and those who could achieve a urine osmolality greater than 1000 mmol/kg before or after the administration of desmopressin. A small proportion of responders remained dry after the medication was withdrawn, independent of how long they were treated. At this point, desmopressin should be viewed as a symptomatic treatment. Compared with conditioning devices, desmopressin had a more immediate benefit, but conditioning provided significantly more long-term results and less chance of relapse.[5] Long-term treatment is viewed as being well tolerated, safe, and appropriate for adults.

The specific indications for the use of desmopressin have not been defined. It may be most useful in patients older than 10 to 11 years of age who have not benefited from prior therapies. It also may help in conjunction with conditioning devices to achieve a rapid improvement while the conditioning response is developing, allowing eventual withdrawal of the medication. Intermittent use may be helpful in special situations in which children who have enuresis need to be dry to avoid embarrassment while awaiting results of other therapy or spontaneous resolution.

TREATMENT FAILURES AND RELAPSES

Relapses and treatment failures are relatively frequent for all methods of therapy. A particular therapy should not be considered a failure until it has been tried for at least 4 to 6 weeks. A failure of one type of therapy might dictate the addition of another. If combination therapy fails, the practitioner may have to tell the child and the family that the neuromuscular bladder control mechanisms still are too immature and that the symptoms must be tolerated for several more months, when the treatment can be reinstituted. Reassurance of physical and mental normality must accompany this message. However, if any new information concerning organic dysfunction or a psychopathological problem becomes apparent, further evaluation is indicated. For example, a treatment failure could result from noncompliance, which reflects either (1) an underlying family interactional pattern that precludes the necessary empathy and understanding or (2) emotional needs of family members that require persistence of the symptom. This aspect should be investigated appropriately by the primary care clinician or a mental health associate. Relapses may be handled by explaining to patients that the nervous system–bladder control mechanism is developing but is not yet fully mature and that a few more months of specific therapy will be required. The previously successful temporary mode of therapy then is reinstituted. This approach allows for maintenance of an optimistic posture and, if necessary, the use of several courses of therapy.

When to Refer

1. Significant history of recurrent urinary tract infections
2. Coexisting substantial constipation or encopresis
3. Concerns regarding a bladder innervation disorder
4. Evidence of vesicular outflow obstruction or reflux on pelvic sonogram
5. Urinalysis evidence of a metabolic or renal disorder
6. Inadequate therapeutic response to reasonably implemented, age-appropriate individual or combined treatment approaches
7. Major family dynamic or individual psychopathology causing, perpetuating, or escalating enuresis symptomatology

REFERENCES

1. Foxman B, Valdez RB, Brook RH: Childhood enuresis: prevalence, perceived impact and prescribed treatment, *Pediatrics* 77:482, 1986.
2. McLorie GA, Husmann DA: Incontinence and enuresis, *Pediatr Clin North Am* 4:1159, 1987.
3. Mikkelson EJ, Rapoport JL: Enuresis: psychopathology, sleep stage and drug response, *Urol Clin North Am* 7:361, 1980.
4. Moffatt MEK, Harlos S, Kirshen AJ: Desmopressin acetate and nocturnal enuresis: how much do we know? *Pediatrics* 94:420, 1993.
5. Norgaard JP: Pathopsychology of nocturnal enuresis, *Scand J Urol Nephrol Suppl* 140:1, 1991.
6. Novello AC, Novello JR: Enuresis, *Pediatr Clin North Am* 34:719, 1987.
7. Olness K, Gardner GG: *Hypnosis and hypnotherapy with children,* Philadelphia, 1988, Grune & Stratton.
8. Rushton HG: Nocturnal enuresis: epidemiology, evaluation and currently available treatment options, *J Pediatr Suppl* 114:691, 1989.
9. Schmitt BD: Nocturnal enuresis: an update on treatment, *Pediatr Clin North Am* 29:21, 1982.

89 Fire-Setting

Amy L. Suss

Childhood fire-setting is common and results in significant property damage, injury, loss of life, and other serious consequences for families and communities. Between 1983 and 1989, the United States averaged more than 2 million fire-settings and arson- and fire-setting-related fires annually, resulting in $8 billion in property loss, 28,500 injuries, and 5800 deaths.[5] Although the epidemiology of fire-setting is sketchy, studies suggest that children and adolescents represent a significant proportion of fire-setting– and arson-related behaviors. According to FBI statistics, in 1990 44% of all offenders who had committed arson were juveniles younger than 18 years of age.[16] Demographic information indicates that it is 10 times more common for adolescent boys to start fires than for girls.[6] The majority of these boys typically fall into the age group of 13 to 15 years.[2] Reported prevalence rates among both outpatient and inpatient psychiatric populations of children and adolescents range between 19% and 35%, respectively.[11] Younger children are more likely to set fires at home; older children are more likely to set fires outside their home and cause more overall damage.

ETIOLOGY

The development of fire behavior in children can be viewed as following a naturally occurring sequence of psychosocial phases.[3,4] Fire interest, fireplay, and fire-setting are three such phases, with progression toward increasing involvement with fire. Interest in fire is experienced by the majority of children between the ages of 3 and 5 years.[8] These children may express interest and/or curiosity in fire by playing with toy fire trucks and cooking food on their toy stoves. Fireplay usually occurs in boys between the ages of 5 and 9 years and involves experimenting with matches or other fire-starting materials.[9,17] Although all fireplay should be under the supervision of adults/parents in a controlled environment, studies indicate that the majority of these children engage in at least one unsupervised fireplay activity.[1,9] One study involving interviewing kindergartners, second-, and fourth-graders and their parents from three randomly selected schools found that 60% of children admitted to participating in unsupervised fireplay.[9] Fortunately, most unsupervised fireplay represents a single-episode firestart motivated by curiosity; the resulting fire is either accidental or unintentional. If the fire becomes uncontrolled, the children will make serious attempts to either extinguish the fire themselves or go for help.[1,4,9] By the age of 10 years, most children have learned the rules of fire safety and prevention. These children are capable of participating in age-appropriate fire-setting activities such as building a campfire or helping to light the family barbecue. However, for some children, what may begin as one or two unsupervised fireplay activities may lead to repeated, intentional fire-setting behavior.

Pathological fire-setting is characterized by a history of multiple firestarts taking place for at least a 6-month period.[4] Psychoanalytical theory has assigned unconscious meaning to fire as a symbol of sexuality. Fire-setting by children and adolescents is viewed as a substitute for masturbatory behavior in response to parental prohibitions. Although some instances of fire-setting may be a manifestation of sexual problems, subsequent study has revealed more complex and diverse etiological factors. Child and adolescent fire-setting involves the interaction of individual, social, and environmental factors. Researchers have examined the family background, the social and psychiatric history, and the stated reasons for engaging in fire-setting behavior. A high incidence of family dysfunction, including parental alcoholism, psychosis, and criminality is noted among pathological fire-setters.[5] Similarly, child and adolescent emotional disturbances, including hyperactivity, psychosis, rage reactions, and enuresis have been described.[5] Fire-setters exhibit higher levels of aggressive and antisocial behavior than their non–fire-setting peers. Characteristics consistently attributed to child fire-setters include male predominance (females constitute fewer than 10% of fire-setters), absence of a parent, a history of abuse or neglect, school problems, and either below-average intelligence or above-average incidence of learning disabilities.[13,14,17]

Although no typical profile of childhood fire-setters has been established, high risk for future fire-setting can be identified by several characteristics. Children at high risk for fire-setting generally are motivated by anger or revenge and often have a history of repeated fire-setting behaviors.[8] As previously noted, high-risk children tend to have individual or family-related psychopathology, including psychosis, alcoholism, abuse, and neglect. One- and 5-year prospective studies of childhood fire-setting describe recidivists as coming from less stable homes and tending to be more antisocial than children who no longer set fires.[10,12,18] Of particular note is the symptom triad of fire-setting, enuresis, and cruelty to animals. This syndrome has been suggested as a possible predictor of adult violent behavior.[7] Children at lower risk tend to have intact families and no history of abuse or neglect. Studies have described fire-setting adolescents as being restless, impulsive, and defiant.[3,4] These adolescents do not feel guilt or remorse for their actions.[3,4] Once they have set the fire they are not likely to call for help to extinguish the fire. Fire-setting adolescents have histories of academic and behavioral difficulties in school.[3,11,13] Statistical studies indicate that approximately 75% of middle school and high school fires are caused by adolescents.[15] Thus, not only do fire-setting adolescents fail to achieve or adjust to their school environment but also there is evidence that schools may be one of their primary targets.[15]

MANAGEMENT

Approaches to the management of fire-setting depend on recognition and assessment of the seriousness of the problem. Physicians can facilitate early recognition by screening routinely for fire-setting behaviors. Early detection of childhood fire-setting is critical to improving prognosis and reducing the potential for damage, injury, and death. The physician may assess the seriousness of the problem by differentiating low-risk from high-risk fire-setters based on the previously described characteristics.

Low-risk fire-setters are, in general, described as being "curious" and experimenting or playing with fire in an isolated incident. They tend to be younger, show remorse or guilt after the incident, express no other deviant behaviors, and reside in intact families.[5,10] These children are suitable for brief interventions that consist of education from parents or physicians about the dangers of fire and may benefit from training in fire safety. For example, parents can allow children to light the candles on their birthday cake; thus, they learn the conditions under which it is safe to strike a match and light candles. The physician, in discussing fire-setting behavior, should attempt to prevent inappropriate and extreme parental responses such as burning a child to teach him or her a lesson. Children have difficulty discriminating between permissive and nonpermissive opportunities to light fires. Parents should be provided with guidance about techniques to modify the behavior by communicating clearly the inappropriateness of the behavior, supervising the child (e.g., limiting access to matches), and reinforcing appropriate behavior positively (e.g., returning found matches without lighting them).

In contrast, high-risk fire-setters tend to be older, to use fire more deliberately as an expression of anger or revenge, to be emotionally disturbed, and to reside in dysfunctional families.[5,10] In this context, the physician should address the behavior as being representative of a broader pattern of disturbance that is in need of immediate attention. The possibility that the fire-setting is a response to environmental factors, including family dysfunction, needs to be explored. This exploration should be nonaccusatory, emphasizing action to help the child or adolescent. At this point, referral to a mental health professional for treatment may be appropriate. Owing to the potential dangers of continued fire-setting, the physician should make a routine call to the family to ensure compliance with any referrals. Although outpatient treatment is the method of choice, hospitalization may be necessary in cases of severe underlying psychiatric disturbances. A purpose of such hospitalization is to reestablish control if the child or adolescent represents an imminent danger and the parents are unable to ensure safety or supervision.

The goals of effective treatment are to abate fire-setting behavior and attain and sustain significant improvement in the underlying psychopathology. Thus, the treatment of pathological fire-setting is directed toward exploring the motivation, targeting therapeutic interventions toward individual/familial dysfunction, and teaching acceptable alternatives to fire-setting. Treatment must include close follow-up of the child or adolescent to prevent repeated episodes. The prognosis is guarded in children and adolescents who have high-risk behaviors such as repetitive fire-setting motivated by anger or revenge. To the contrary, the prognosis generally is good for children and adolescents who have low-risk fire-setting behaviors such as playing with matches out of curiosity or experimentation; complete remission in these children is realistic.

REFERENCES

1. Cole RE, Grolnick WS, Laurentis LL: *Children and fire: Rochester Fire-Related Youth Project (second report),* New York, 1986, Department of State Office of Fire Prevention and Control.
2. Federal Bureau of Investigation: *Uniform Crime Reports,* Washington, DC, 1978-1988, US Government Printing Office.
3. Gaynor J: Firesetting. In Lewis M, editor: *A comprehensive textbook of child and adolescent psychiatry,* Baltimore, 1991, Williams & Wilkins.
4. Gaynor J, Hatcher C: *The psychology of child firesetting: detection and intervention,* New York, 1987, Brunner/Mazel.
5. Geller JL: Arson in review: from profit to pathology, *Psychiatr Clin North Am* 15:623, 1992.
6. Heath GA, Hardesty VA, Goldfine PE: Diagnosis and childhood firesetting, *J Clin Psychol* 41:571, 1985.
7. Hellman DS, Blackman N: Enuresis, firesetting, and cruelty to animals: a triad predictive of adult crime, *Am J Psychiatry* 12:1431, 1966.
8. Jackson H, Glass C, Hope S: A functional analysis of recidivistic arson, *Br J Clin Psychol* 26:175, 1987.
9. Kafry D, Block JH, Block J: *Children's survival skills: a basis for functioning in society.* Final report prepared for the Maternal and Child Health and Crippled Services Research Program, Rockville, Md, 1980, Bureau of Community Health Services.
10. Kolko DJ, Kazdin AE: Motives of childhood firesetters: firesetting characteristics and psychological correlates, *J Child Psychol Psychiatry* 32: 535, 1991.
11. Kolko DJ, Kazdin AE: Prevalence of firesetting and related behaviors among child psychiatric patients, *J Consult Clin Psychol* 56:628, 1988.
12. Kolko DJ, Kazdin AE: The emergence and recurrence of child firesetting: a one-year prospective study, *J Abnorm Child Psychol* 20:17, 1992.
13. Kuhnley EJ, Hendren RL, Quinlan DM: Firesetting by children, *J Am Acad Child Adolesc Psychiatry* 21:560, 1982.
14. Moore JM, Thompson-Pope SK, Whited RM: MMPI-A profiles of adolescent boys with a history of firesetting, *J Pers Assess* 67:116, 1996.
15. National Fire Protection Agency: Fires and fire losses classified, *Fire J* Sept 1978-1988.
16. Rasanen P, Hakko H, Vaisanen E: Arson trend increasing: a real challenge to psychiatry, *J Forensic Sci* 40:976, 1995.
17. Showers J, Pickrell E: Child firesetters: a study of three populations, *Hosp Community Psychiatry* 38:495, 1987.
18. Stewart MA, Culver KW: Children who set fires: the clinical picture and a follow-up, *Br J Psychiatry* 140:357, 1982.

SUGGESTED READINGS

Fineman K: Firesetting in childhood and adolescence, *Psychiatr Clin North Am* 3:483, 1980.

Kaufman I, Henis LW: A reevaluation of the psychodynamics of firesetting, *Am J Orthopsychiatry* 31:123, 1961.

Yarnell H: Firesetting in children, *Am J Orthopsychiatry* 10:272, 1940.

90 Lying and Stealing

Gregory E. Prazar

Acts of lying and stealing by children often evoke strong emotional reactions from parents. Truthfulness and respect for property are two highly valued mores espoused by our society, even though adults frequently violate their own moral codes. Lying and stealing can represent a psychopathological spectrum from a common transient developmental phenomenon to an ominous indication of severe psychiatric disturbance. Frequently, both parents and professionals overreact to symptoms of lying and stealing before analyzing all the relevant information.

Prevalence figures for lying and stealing indicate that these behaviors occur more frequently in boys than in girls and achieve highest rates between 5 and 8 years of age. In one study by MacFarlane, Allen, and Honzik,[3] 49% of mothers of 5-year-old boys and 42% of mothers of 5-year-old girls reported that their children had lied; stealing among 5-year-old boys was reported for 10% and for 4% of 5-year-old girls. By age 8, 41% of the boys and 19% of the girls exhibited some lying, and 9% of the boys and 5% of the girls exhibited stealing behavior.

Given the prevalence of these behaviors, the responsibility of the primary care physician is to inquire about symptoms of lying and stealing during routine visits and to help families understand the nature of the problem and to respond appropriately. To identify and manage these problems adequately, a complete history should be obtained from parents and child, encompassing aspects of the home environment (patterns of child rearing, child's interaction with siblings and parents), peer relationships, and school performance.

LYING

When lying is presented as a problem to the pediatrician, either directly by the parents or indirectly from questions asked by the physician during a regular visit, several important aspects of the child's functioning should be considered before definitive action is taken: his or her maturational level; the influence of family, peers, and school; and, above all, the situation in which lying occurs.

The child's chronological age and developmental level greatly influence the extent to which lying should be evaluated. Children younger than 3 years are beginning to establish independence from their parents; for these children, the differentiation between what Stone and Church[5] refer to as "private self and public self" is tenuous. Children at this age have no concept of deception and, therefore, do not lie intentionally. Their experimentation with concepts of language often is interpreted by adults as lying. The toddler, attempting to understand presence and absence of individuals, may tell the father that "Mommy is not here," when she may indeed be in the next room.[4] Emotionally painful situations are avoided by all children, especially by toddlers younger than 3 years. The child, whose moral code is immature, thinks nothing of denying a misdeed, because admission might bring painful consequences.

The mental life of the preschool child (3 to 7 years) is one filled with fantasy. According to Stone and Church,[5] 20% to 50% of this age group create imaginary companions, pets, or situations. The imaginary companion usually is a helpful, empathic playmate, although he or she may function as a disciplinarian for the child. By serving as a surrogate friend, the imaginary companion helps the child adapt to new social situations. By serving as a disciplinarian, the imaginary companion helps the child to develop a sense of right and wrong. The imaginary companion usually has a very short life span, generally dying of "old age" by the time the child is 5 to 7 years old. For the preschooler, fantasy and reality frequently are not well delineated, as evidenced by the existence of imaginary companions and also by the child's love of fairy tales. A 4- to 5-year-old unabashedly tells tall tales, although he or she will, when encouraged, admit to creating a make-believe situation. By the age of 6 or 7 years, children are aware of the morality of lying. Although they are quick to accuse peers of cheating and lying, they often continue to cheat, seemingly guiltlessly, while playing.

Between the ages of 6 and 12 years, the child understands the concept of lying and its moral implications. However, lying may continue in an attempt to test adult-imposed moral codes. Children may admit to lying but have many rationalizations for their behavior. Rules are more important at this age than is winning, so cheating is less important and, therefore, less frequent. "Half-beliefs" become a part of the child's life; children become believers of superstitions, from the dangers of walking under a ladder to stepping on sidewalk cracks. Half-beliefs may extend into adulthood, and they are invested heavily with emotion. Their level of acceptance by the individual is inversely proportional to the individual's level of intellectual development.

Aside from developmental issues, external influences (family, school, and peers) affect the incidence of lying in children. Parents unconsciously may encourage their children to lie if expectations for the children exceed their ability to fulfill them and if truthfulness is not valued by the parents (i.e., if parents frequently lie). Parents who overestimate their child's academic capabilities frequently find that their child lies about grades received. Parents who tell "white lies" to protect the feelings of others, or for personal gain, fail to realize that young children cannot discern the moral issues involved in lying. Parents demanding to know why their son hit his younger sister or why the child broke the cookie jar are unaware that the child often cannot explain these behaviors to himself, much less to them. When interrogated, the confused child, in desperation, lies. According to Ginott,[2] "awkward lies" are told to avoid "embarrassing confessions"—confessions that the child knows from experience parents do not want to hear. For example, after hitting his younger sister, the son knows that his parents do not want to hear that he hit her because he does not like her. The parents want to believe that their children love each other, and they find it difficult to accept verbalizations to the contrary.

The child who is disciplined inconsistently but harshly who receives little positive reinforcement from parents, and who lives in an inflexible, demanding environment often is the child who lies. Physicians can help parents deal with childhood lying in several ways. First, by apprising parents of what behavior is normal during maturational stages, the physician helps the parents understand more easily why their 5-year-old makes up stories or why their 7-year-old cheats at games. Second, by helping parents become aware of their importance as role models for their child, the physician effectively guides the parents in explaining to their child the importance of truthfulness. Third, when specific problems arise, the physician, by counseling gently and nonpunitively, encourages parents to be as tactful and nonthreatening with the child as possible. For example, according to Spock,[4] the child who spends much time with imaginary companions may need more age-appropriate friends or may be asking indirectly for more parental involvement in play activities.

Children who cheat at games past age 7 years (when rules become more important and, therefore, cheating becomes a form of breaking the rules) need guidance from parents. If the parent is playing with a child who is cheating, the behavior should be identified calmly. The parent should tell the child that everyone likes to win and that losing is difficult to accept. Cheating among children, when identified, should best be settled among the players, without parental "judicial" intervention. Academic cheating is a more serious problem, frequently signaling that unrealistic expectations for performance have been placed on the child. Parents should be counseled to explore with school personnel possible academic problems.

Parents should be made cognizant of their importance as role models for their child and of the child's need for reasonable and clear expectations. Similarly, physicians must understand that they are role models for the parents whom they counsel. The physician who assumes a flexible, constructive, nonthreatening approach to problems raised by parents and who has been honest with the family in the past is more likely to be successful in counseling.

Lying becomes a symptom of more severe psychopathology under several circumstances. If other behaviors exist concomitantly (such as fire-setting, cruelty to animals, sleep disturbances, hyperactivity, phobias), there is a much greater likelihood of significant emotional disturbance. Similarly, if lying or fantasizing becomes a predominant behavior for children, more serious behavior disturbances must be suspected, such as chronically poor self-esteem, endogenous depression, and sociopathic behavior. Children who have few friends and limited interest in group activities often suffer from low self-esteem and depression. Children who lie for material gain and, apparently, guiltlessly may be displaying early signs of a conduct behavior. If these symptoms are present and if attempts at counseling fail to dissipate lying, referral to a mental health professional should be considered.

STEALING

Stealing often represents a much more worrisome symptom to parents than does lying because the former more often involves situations outside the home, represents a much more severe societal taboo, and affects other people more directly. Indeed, especially during school years, stealing can be an ominous sign of psychiatric disturbance. However, it may represent conformity to peer pressure and consequently is a transient phenomenon. Children younger than 3 years of age take things because they want them and have an immature sense of "mine" and "not mine," a concept related to their beginning struggle for independence from parents. Slowly they develop a conception of their own bodies (or property) and those of their parents. By age 3 years, children have a firmer sense of what belongs to them. They become possessive of their things and jealous of those of others, although they have only a tenuous grasp of others' property rights.

Between 3 and 7 years of age, as they begin to develop peer relationships, children become more respectful of property rights. However, they frequently give away their possessions and have not developed a concept of one thing being more valuable than many things (e.g., 25 hoarded pennies may be treasured much more than one piece of paper currency). The school-age child, though not yet completely mature, has a much more sophisticated sense of property rights. Consequently, an 8-year-old may pick up loose change from the table while unsupervised. However, after about age 9 years, respect for property should be well integrated in the child. Children who steal at this age or beyond are motivated by one or more factors. They may steal in a group, especially during adolescence, to conform to peer pressure. They may suffer from poor self-esteem because they feel unloved by parents or because they have difficulty making friends. They may steal to buy friendship, to achieve peer acceptance, or to display to themselves and their parents that they are worthwhile because they can succeed in at least one activity. Stealing as a mechanism to improve self-esteem especially is common with adolescents, who are concomitantly attempting to separate from parents and to establish satisfactory same-sex and heterosexual relationships. If adolescents feel that they have failed in both tasks, they frequently steal.

Families exert an important influence with respect to childhood stealing. If parents stole as children, they are more likely to assume a permissive role to intrafamilial stealing. Their reactions to extrafamilial stealing, however, may be extremely punitive, because their child's stealing will reflect unfavorably on them as parents. This value discrepancy between intrafamilial and extrafamilial acts is recognized easily by the child, whose resentment frequently precipitates intensified stealing. Parents giving little attention, affection, or approval to their child will potentiate poor self-esteem, which may result in stealing as the child attempts to attract attention and approval. Punishment may be ineffective, because the child may rationalize that, as Fraiberg[1] states, "Any ensuing punishment will cancel the crime."

Management of stealing, as in management of lying, requires an empathic but firm approach by both physician and parents. Parents should be advised to deal with the specific incident forthrightly. The child older than 3 years of age should be confronted with the evidence but should not suffer interrogative techniques (e.g., the parent should say, "I believe you took $5 from my wallet," rather than, "Why did you take $5 from my wallet?"). Immediate restitution of the stolen item is extremely important. If the article has been taken from a friend, the child should return it. If the article has been stolen from a store, the parent should accompany the child to the store and explain to the manager tactfully that the child took an item without paying for it and now wants to return it. The parents should voice their disapproval of stealing to the child but should also reinforce their belief in the child's basic integrity. A child who has stolen usually has poor self-esteem; punitive measures serve to damage self-concept further and imbue in the child the parent's mistrust.

Several specific questions should come to mind when the child steals, because the answers may aid in management. Is the child receiving a reasonable allowance? If not, the child may feel the need to resort to stealing to obtain spending money. Are there unrealistic academic pressures on the child? Children who feel that they cannot fulfill academic expectations of parents frequently steal to display at least transiently their success in one activity. Is the child having difficulty making friends? Stealing often occurs in situations in which the child feels that peer group acceptance can be achieved by offering peers stolen material goods. In cases of group stealing, are alternative community facilities available to occupy extracurricular hours? Although structured community activities may not obliterate all acts of group stealing, they may help to discourage such acts by offering alternative activities to occupy preadolescents' and adolescents' time.

Stealing assumes more ominous connotations in several situations. As in lying, if other behavioral disturbances coexist, a more psychiatrically sophisticated approach may be necessary. A child who steals without guilt, who compulsively steals (kleptomania), or who seemingly steals in a setting in which apprehension is inevitable may have serious emotional problems. Frequently, these are children who received little or inconsistent love and security as infants. Without psychiatric intervention, they will progress to delinquent and ultimately criminal lifestyles (see Chapter 106, Juvenile Delinquency). Unfortunately, psychic damage to these children often is severe by the time psychiatric referral finally is made.

REFERRAL CRITERIA

Effective referral to mental health specialists for problems of lying and stealing requires several things of referring physicians. The family should be informed of the possible need for referral when the physician first suspects a potential for significant psychopathology. As in managing less severe cases, the referring physician should be empathic and nonpunitive in the explanation given to parents. The physician should make sure that the parents do not think that their child is "crazy" because he or she is being referred. The parents also should know that the referral does not sever the physician's relationship with the family. Continued communication by the referring physician, both with the family and with the specialist, often solidifies recommendations made to parents by the therapist and encourages compliance with recommendations. If possible, the physician personally should introduce the family to the therapist. If this is not possible, the physician should call the counselor to ensure that the counselor can see the family. In general, a team approach between the referring doctor and specialist increases the treatment's efficacy.

SUMMARY

Lying and stealing in childhood usually cause both parents and physicians concern and also create anxiety for the involved child. The seriousness of these behaviors depends on many factors: the age of the child, the circumstances that precipitate the behavior, the psychosocial adjustment of the child (in school, with peers, and at home), and the reaction of parents. The physician's approach to the problem influences whether the behavior disappears or intensifies. In dealing with problems of lying and stealing, the physician should obtain a complete history, explain carefully to the parents and the patient the significance of the behavior, and ensure regular follow-up for the problem. If referral to psychologically trained professionals becomes necessary, the physician is obligated to prepare the family for the referral, to maintain communication with the consultant, and to offer the family emotional support before and after the consultation. In most cases, lying and stealing represent transient developmental behavioral problems that resolve if an empathic approach is used by parents and physician. However, the symptoms are not to be ignored in hopes that the child will "grow out of it" or because "all children lie and steal."

REFERENCES

1. Fraiberg S: *The magic years*, New York, 1996, Charles Scribner's Sons.
2. Ginott HG: *Between parent and child*, New York, 1985, Macmillan.
3. MacFarlane JW, Allen L, Honzik MP: *A developmental study of the behavior problems of normal children between twenty-one months and fourteen years*, Berkeley and Los Angeles, 1954, University of California Press.
4. Spock B: *Baby and child care*, New York, 1998, Pocket Books.
5. Stone LJ, Church JC: *Childhood and adolescence: a psychology of the growing person*, ed 5, New York, 1989, Random House.

91 Peer Relationship Problems

Sharon L. Foster • Nandita Chawla

Peer relations and positive social interaction are crucial to the normal development of children. A child's relations with peers serve important functions in his or her life, including promoting the development of social skills through interaction and feedback; providing emotional support and security; enhancing feelings of self-worth; providing guidance, assistance, and companionship; and offering validation through sharing information about common situations and events during childhood and adolescence. The importance of peer relations is highlighted by middle childhood children spending approximately 30% of their time with peers and 13% percent of their time with parents, a trend that continues through adolescence.[43]

EPIDEMIOLOGY

The major identifying characteristic of children who have peer relationship problems is being poorly accepted by one's peer group. This can be manifested in three ways: social withdrawal, peer rejection, and victimization by peers. Socially withdrawn children interact infrequently and isolate themselves from the peer group.[44] Socially rejected children are openly and actively rejected by peers. Victimized children are the targets of regular bullying by other children, which can take the form of physical intimidation, teasing, or severe social ostracism.

Epidemiological data from stratified national samples are not available to examine the incidence and prevalence of peer relationship difficulties. Rejection generally is defined statistically by selecting the 5% to 16% of children who are most disliked by their peers in a group,[49] rather than by formal diagnostic criteria. Although prevalence rates of social withdrawal depend on how "withdrawal" is defined, one reviewer estimated that as many as 33% of all children in regular classrooms have low levels of social interaction and that 3% are classified as being socially withdrawn.[15] Reports indicate that 10% of elementary school children are especially lonely.[30]

Victimization rates based on surveys in England, Australia, and Scandinavia indicate that between 3% (Norway) and 25% (Australia) of children report serious bullying, generally defined as being "picked on" once a week or more, although occasional teasing is much more common.[32,46,47] Rates are highest in elementary school and decline in adolescence.[32,47] Girls are more likely than boys to be victimized via social exclusion; boys are more likely than girls to be harassed via physical or verbal means.[10,11]

All three types of peer relationship problems are relatively stable, at least over relatively short intervals. Investigations found that 34% to 67% of rejected children assessed in elementary school still had peer problems 2 to 5 years later.[6,34] Social withdrawal also is stable: two thirds of children who are extremely withdrawn at age 5 years are still withdrawn six years later.[44] Indicators of victimization by peers correlated 0.69 over a 1-year period in one study[22] and 0.75 in the fall and spring of the school year in another.[16]

Considerable evidence indicates that children who are rejected by peers experience short- and long-term social and emotional problems. Chronically rejected children are at higher risk for concurrent and future difficulties than are children whose rejected status is more transient.[14,36] Being rejected in childhood predicts academic difficulties; truancy; dropping out of high school; delinquent and antisocial behavior such as aggression, criminality, and substance use; and higher use of mental health services.[1,14,34,43,50] Rejected children who are aggressive have elevated rates of externalizing disorders, such as aggression, attention deficit/hyperactive disorder (AD/HD), or conduct disorder (CD); rejected children who are submissive or withdrawn have higher than expected rates of internalizing disorders, such as depression or anxiety.[43] Relative to their peers, many poorly accepted children feel lonelier, are more depressed and anxious, and are less satisfied with both their peer relationships and with their friendships.[27,33]

Determining whether withdrawn children experience serious concurrent or future difficulties is complicated by social isolation taking many forms.[44] Children may choose not to interact with peers because they are shy and anxious, for example, or because they prefer solitary pastimes. The former appears to be associated with other difficulties, whereas the latter is not.[2] Furthermore, quiet, subdued behavior is valued more highly in Eastern than in Western societies, and has desirable correlates in those cultures.[44] Nonetheless, forms of social avoidance and withdrawal characterize many psychiatric diagnostic categories (e.g., separation anxiety disorder, reactive attachment disorder, social phobia, major depression). Many children who interact infrequently with familiar and unfamiliar peers also voice feelings of loneliness, both concurrently and in later childhood and adolescence. Withdrawal also is associated with peer rejection. In addition, the combination of social withdrawal, anxiety, and negative views of one's own social skills at age 7 years predicts later feelings of loneliness and depression at age 11 years.[44]

The long-term sequelae of victimization by peers have

received little attention, although victimization in elementary school is associated with concurrent reports of internalizing behavior problems, including loneliness and emotional distress; peer rejection; and—less consistently—with acting out and impulsive behavior problems.[10,11,23,25]

Unfortunately, causal relationships between early peer problems and later difficulties have not been established. Nonetheless, the substantial number of associations noted above strongly suggests that intervening early with children who have poor peer relationships may alleviate current dysfunction and prevent dysfunction later in life.

ETIOLOGICAL FACTORS

Understanding the etiology of peer relationship problems is complicated by findings that children may be rejected or victimized by peers for a variety of reasons. Many characteristics of the child, including physical attractiveness, race or minority status, gender, and academic competence, may affect his or her social status with peers. In addition, social isolation, peer rejection, and victimization have different developmental precursors, despite their overlap. Finally, most approaches to the etiology of peer relationship problems have focused on understanding social isolation and rejection rather than victimization.

One major hypothesis with respect to why children have difficulties in peer relationships is that children who have problems possess inadequate repertoires of social skills, which result in ineffective social interaction, causing them to be ignored or actively rejected by their peers. This negative experience may encourage further maladaptive responses such as increased social withdrawal or retaliatory verbal or physical aggression. These behaviors could, in turn, create a vicious circle by making children even less accepted by their peers and more prone to biased evaluations by peers, as they develop negative reputations.

Various theories of the development of socially skillful and socially maladaptive behavior have some empirical support, but none has unequivocal acceptance. Behavioral theories of etiology propose that early socialization by parents influences the acquisition of social repertoires through modeling, direct teaching, classical conditioning, and providing consequences for the child's social behavior.[39] Others hypothesize that poor social skills result from inadequate development of information-processing skills believed to be prerequisites for effective social intervention.[12] These include (1) perceiving and interpreting social situations correctly, (2) formulating appropriate social goals, (3) generating and evaluating possible ways of responding, (4) selecting and performing an appropriate response, (5) and monitoring the impact of that response. Related hypotheses emphasize the roles of social role-taking (the ability to view situations from others' perspectives) and empathy (actually experiencing another's feelings) in adaptive peer relationships and of managing disruptive emotional responses, particularly in upsetting situations. Most contemporary writers concur that all of these processes are likely to be involved and interact to influence the acquisition and performance of adaptive and maladaptive social behaviors.[34] In addition, the peer group can contribute to further growth of maladaptive behavior when rejected children form relationships with other deviant peers.

Research with preschool and elementary school children highlights the relationship between family experience and children's social competence. The parents of young children who have adaptive peer relations are more likely than parents of less well-accepted children to arrange play opportunities for their children, coach their children about peer problems, and supervise their play without excessive intrusion.[34] Negative family events and interactions, in contrast, characterize the lives of rejected children. Children who have had many parenting transitions, such as divorce or remarriage, and who experience excessive family conflict and stress are likely to experience peer adjustment problems.[24,37] Parent-reported spousal and parent-child aggressive conflict also relate negatively to peer acceptance,[48] as does sibling aggression.[29] Children who are poorly accepted and their mothers interact in more negative and demanding ways than do well-accepted children. Fathers of unpopular children issue more commands and engage less in their child's play.[28] Finally, deviant maternal values and expectations (e.g., positive endorsement of aggression as a solution to interpersonal problems and mothers' reports of more coercive discipline) are associated both with how children think about social problems and with peers' and teachers' views of children's social competence in the classroom.[21,37] Most of these correlates of peer rejection also are associated with disruptive and aggressive child behavior. Together, these findings suggest that early social experiences play an important role in children's development of socially competent behavior and social cognition, which then act as proximal causes for peer acceptance and rejection.[4]

Only a few studies have examined the family characteristics of children who are victimized by peers. One of these revealed that victimization in kindergarten children was associated with observations of low responsivity and high demandingness displayed by the primary caregiver. With boys only, intense closeness with the caregiver also predicted victimization.[26] A second study compared male aggressive and nonaggressive victims, finding that aggressive (but not passive) victims at ages 8 to 9 years came from families high in marital conflict, restrictive discipline, parental aggression, and maternal hostility assessed before the boys' entry into kindergarten.[45] These factors characterize the emergence of aggression in general, however, and are not unique to aggressive victimization.

Theories of withdrawal emphasize temperament to a greater extent than do theories of peer rejection. These perspectives draw from research on behavioral inhibition postulating that certain infants are physiologically predisposed to be aroused easily and to display high rates of negative affect, which lead to later caution and fearfulness in unfamiliar situations (see Rubin and Stewart[44] for a review). In the context of socialization patterns that exacerbate these tendencies, children can develop fearful and withdrawn ways of interacting with peers. Research indicates that behaviorally inhibited children are prone to develop insecure attachments to their primary caregivers and that these attachment styles are linked to later indicators of social withdrawal. In addition, compared with mothers of less anxious and more sociable children, mothers of anxious, withdrawn children report placing more importance on controlling and directive strategies for teaching the child social behaviors in general and for dealing with social problems in particular. Related literature links authoritarian, controlling parenting styles to anxiety and insecurity in children.[44]

CHARACTERISTICS AND DIAGNOSIS

Observations of socially withdrawn children reveal that children who spend little time interacting with familiar peers at school spend more time in solitary activities and play submissive or deferent roles when they do interact with more sociable partners.[42] They also are more unassertive and request help more often from adults than do their peers. In addition, peers comply less frequently with their requests than with those of children who interact more frequently.[44] These children may experience more anxiety, loneliness, negative views of themselves, and depression than their peers,[44] although for what percentage of children these reactions are outside the normal range is not yet clear.

Rejected children display a different constellation of behavior, particularly during preschool and early elementary school years (see Newcomb, Bukowski, and Pattee[31] for a review). Although rejected children form a heterogenous group, peer rejection in preschool and the primary grades generally has been associated with more actively negative behavior—higher rates of "off-task" behavior as well as solitary activity, greater dependence on adults, negative statements, interference with ongoing activities, and failure to conform to classroom rules. Poorly accepted children have difficulty joining ongoing play activities and are more likely than their peers to disengage from the group, to make weak demands, to engage in incoherent behavior (i.e., inaudible, ambiguous, or nonsensical), or to hover near the peer group. They interrupt the flow of social exchange by being disagreeable and demanding.[40] Rejected children also are consistently more physically and verbally aggressive than their better-accepted peers.[2]

Rejection also has been linked to *relational aggression* (behavior such as social ostracism or malicious gossip intended to harm another's social relationships) in both boys and girls. Researchers find girls to be equally or more relationally aggressive than boys; physical aggression is consistently more common among boys.[9,13,41] Although aggression is the most consistent correlate of peer rejection, only about 50% of rejected children are aggressive, and some aggressive children are not rejected.[2]

Children also treat rejected classmates differently than they treat their better-accepted peers. Peers initiate relatively few interactions with rejected children and may view their positive behavior less favorably than they do similar behavior by better-accepted peers. Nonetheless, most rejected children have one or more mutual friends. These friends, however, are likely to be similarly rejected.[19] This compounds the rejected child's difficulties because having antisocial and socially unskilled friends is a risk factor for the development of further antisocial and delinquent behavior.[5]

In addition, poorly accepted children differ from their better-accepted peers in how they think about and try to solve social dilemmas.[12] When questioned about handling interpersonal problems, rejected children's responses indicate that their knowledge of appropriate behavior may be deficient. Rejected children may be able to verbalize only one or two appropriate strategies to cope with a problem, and they voice unusual or inappropriate responses when pressed for other options. Furthermore, compared with average boys, aggressive boys are less accurate at detecting prosocial intentions but more accurate at detecting hostile intentions, generate a higher proportion of aggressive responses to hypothetical situations, and are less likely to choose appropriate responses when evaluating the possible ways of reacting to problems.

Although many studies treat rejected children as a homogenous group, findings suggest that there are at least two distinct subtypes of rejected boys: aggressive-rejected and nonaggressive-rejected, with different behavioral profiles.[17,38] Peers view aggressive-rejected boys as more aggressive and disruptive than accepted boys; teachers report that these children lack self-control and academic motivation and appear anxious. Peers view nonaggressive-rejected boys as more withdrawn, inattentive, and immature than others.

Subgroups seen by peers as aggressive and nonaggressive also emerge among girls.[18] Peers see both groups as withdrawn. Teachers view the nonaggressive subgroup of girls as more deviant than nonaggressive boys and as having particular difficulties with anxiety and academic performance.

In contrast with rejected children, most victims of peer aggression or bullying are submissive[10] and respond anxiously rather than assertively when provoked[32] (see Chapter 23 [Four], Violence Prevention, and Chapter 112, Violent and Aggressive Behavior). Male victims tend to be physically weak.[23,32] Nonetheless, some victims are also aggressive:[32,35] These victims often are impulsive and annoying to others. An estimated 48% to 64% of victims of peer maltreatment are also rejected.[5] As mentioned earlier, these children—particularly those who recognize their victimization and lack supportive friends—may express feelings of anxiety and loneliness.[20,22,25] In addition, they may indicate that they dislike and would prefer to avoid going to school.[25]

Detection of peer relationship problems by the physician is complicated by several factors. Most children's problems are first noted by teachers and peers and occur in the school. Parents may be unaware that the child has difficulties because they are uninformed, they ignore the teacher's feedback, or the child behaves differently at home. Although some rejected children recognize their difficulties and will admit to loneliness and low self-esteem, others view themselves no differently than their well-accepted peers and may deny that they have difficulties.[3] Victimized children may be keenly aware of their maltreatment, but be afraid to disclose it. Indications that peer relationship problems may be present include reports from the child's teacher, complaints by the child that he or she has few or no friends, evidence that the child frequently is used as a scapegoat by others, or reports of excessive shyness around other children, particularly at school. In addition, interpersonal difficulties have been associated with physical disabilities, learning disabilities, child abuse, obesity, conduct disorders, attention deficit problems, and delinquency; thus, assessment of the child's functioning with peers is warranted when any of these correlated problems is present.

MANAGEMENT AND INTERVENTION

The physician's direct intervention with a child having peer relationship problems is of questionable use unless the physician plans to meet frequently with the child, teachers, or parents, perhaps as often as every week. However, the physician who sees the child only occasionally can still help to educate parents and teachers about the importance of developing good peer relationship skills. Furthermore, he or she may be able to advise them of initial strategies to address the problem. The physician also may be able to identify the cases in which the child's rejection may be a result of poor physical appearance and instruct the parents and child in more appropriate dress or personal hygiene. Finally, the physician can encourage the parents to advocate for active school personnel involvement to reduce bullying when the child is victimized regularly by peers.

For the young child who has more minor or circumscribed peer relationship difficulties, advising the parents or teacher to provide the child with toys that require cooperation and sharing (e.g., seesaw, board games, flash cards) can lead to increased positive social interaction. Cooperative parents and teachers also can be advised to engineer opportunities for the child to interact positively with well-adjusted peers and then attend to and positively reinforce desirable social behaviors, such as cooperative play, while ignoring negative or nonsocial behaviors.

Children rejected because of off-task and disruptive behavior that results from academic problems may improve behaviorally when provided with effective tutoring so that they can keep up with their peers academically.

With children whose difficulties are pervasive or whose parents and teachers are uncooperative, more extensive intervention is advisable. Intervention methods that have documented effectiveness vary, depending on the age of the child and the nature of the child's difficulties with peers. With preschoolers and young primary grade-age withdrawn children, modeling can increase positive peer interactions. Modeling procedures typically include observation of other children (usually filmed) engaged in positive interaction, followed by opportunities for the child to engage in similar activities with peers. Modeling has been shown to be effective generally, although less so for children from families of lower socioeconomic status. Alternatively, reinforcement programs can be instituted in which the teacher or parent rewards positive social participation with praise, attention, or tokens that can be exchanged later for privileges or other rewards. A variant of this procedure appropriate for withdrawn children involves praising peers verbally for interacting with the withdrawn child, which presumably leads others to get to know the withdrawn child better and to begin to include him or her in their activities. This approach, however, is contraindicated for the child whose responses to peers often are negative, because the child's annoying behavior is likely to lead to increased exclusion in other situations. In addition, highly fearful avoidant children may need additional intervention targeted at managing and reducing anxiety.

Interventions with older children have focused primarily on those who are rejected. Intervention frequently consists of one-to-one or group training in specific social skills. Training may focus on teaching specific social interaction skills, such as helping others, conversing, and taking turns. "Coaching" procedures frequently are used to teach the child the skill to be mastered. Coaching includes providing a rationale for the target skill, having the child rehearse the skill in a "mock" situation with an adult or child partner, providing feedback on the child's performance, and sometimes reenacting the scene. In general, social skills training programs are most effective for children who lack positive behaviors and are less effective for children who drive others away with frequent negative behavior. The latter generally require interventions designed specifically to reduce aggressive, disruptive, or immature behavior, as well as approaches to build prosocial skills.

Coaching usually results in the child learning the trained skills, but generalizing the new skills to ongoing social interactions is a problem for some children and requires additional intervention. Peer-mediated interventions sometimes are used in an attempt to generalize trained skills. Typically, same-gender accepted peers are recruited as "co-therapists" and trained to initiate interactions, to respond to refusals, to maintain interactions, and to respond to the target child's negative behavior in order to engage that child in the activities of the larger peer group. Teachers also can provide rewards (e.g., classroom privileges, access to special activities) for a child's efforts to perform new skills, then gradually lengthen the period between performance and reward. These procedures need to be conducted and monitored carefully, however, to avoid even more stigmatization of the rejected child in the peer group.

Changing the child's school is another intervention sometimes considered by parents or teachers. However, research shows that rejected boys quickly reestablish their rejected status when placed in a group of children all unknown to one another.[7] These findings suggest that simply changing a child's school, without a concomitant change in a child's social behavior, will merely perpetuate a rejected child's negative peer relations. Changing the child's school may be indicated, however, if his or her previous negative reputation is making it difficult for the child to be accepted by peers even though the child is performing new socially appropriate behaviors.

Similar to social skills training are interventions that address general interpersonal problem-solving skills. In this approach the child is taught (usually by means of coaching) to handle interpersonal dilemmas by defining the problem, generating several alternatives that might resolve the situation, and selecting the solution most likely to produce desirable results. Although these programs are successful at improving children's social knowledge, their effects on actual social behavior (particularly negative behavior) are less clear. When combined with a comprehensive approach that involves parent training in managing child behavior, academic tutoring, and teacher involvement, results can be positive.[8]

Most interventions to date address social skills deficits and peer rejection rather than active victimization or bullying. The best-documented intervention for reducing bullying to date has used a multifaceted approach to reducing bullying in Norwegian schools.[32] Olweus (the developer of this intervention) emphasizes that adults must take whatever steps necessary to guarantee the victim protection from harassment from peers. Intervention strategies include having school-wide meetings to discuss the problem of bullying, improving adult monitoring of settings in which the bullying takes place, planning ways teachers can intervene swiftly and with appropriate sanctions when bullying occurs, encouraging contact between parents of victimized students and the students' teachers, and formulating classroom rules about bullying. Olweus also recommends that parents of victims help the victimized child to develop his or her talents and skills to build self-assurance and self-esteem and that parents encourage the child to build positive relationships with nonaggressive peers. Provocative victims also may need coaching in ways to reduce their impulsive acting-out behavior. When necessary, the provocateur and victim can be separated by changes in classrooms or schools, although this strategy alone does not change the interpersonal dynamics that promoted the bullying in the first place.

The health care worker who elects to work directly with the child is best advised to assess the effects of the intervention after approximately six sessions. If progress is not apparent, referral to a child psychiatrist, psychologist, social worker, or school counselor experienced with peer relationship problems is warranted. In addition, preschools and elementary schools (particularly in urban and academic communities) sometimes include curricula related to social development; such classrooms are referral possibilities if available in the local area.

REFERENCES

1. Bagwell CL, Newcomb AF, Bukowski WM: Preadolescent friendship and peer rejection as predictors of adult adjustment, *Child Dev* 69:140, 1998.
2. Bierman KL, Welsh JA: Social relationship deficits. In Mash EJ, Terdal LG, editors: *Assessment of childhood disorders,* ed 3, New York, 1997, Guilford Press.
3. Boivin M, Begin G: Peer status and self-perception among early elementary school children: the case of the rejected children, *Child Dev* 60:591, 1989.
4. Coie JD: Toward a theory of peer rejection. In Asher SR, Coie JD, editors: *Peer rejection in childhood*, New York, 1990, Cambridge University Press.
5. Coie JD, Dodge KA: Aggression and antisocial behavior. In Eisenberg N, editor; Damon W, series editor: *Handbook of child psychology, vol 3: social, emotional, and personality development*, New York, 1998, Wiley.
6. Coie JD, Dodge KA: Continuities and changes in children's social status: a five-year longitudinal study, *Merrill-Palmer Q* 29:261, 1983.
7. Coie JD, Kupersmidt JB: A behavioral analysis of emerging social status in boys' groups, *Child Dev* 54:1400, 1983.
8. Conduct Problems Prevention Research Group: Initial impact of the Fast Track prevention trial. I. The high-risk sample, *J Consult Clin Psychol* 67:631, 1999.
9. Crick NR: Engagement in gender nonnormative vs. normative forms of aggression: links to social-psychological adjustment, *Dev Psychol* 33: 610, 1997.
10. Crick NR, Bigbee MA: Relational and overt forms of peer victimization: a multiinformant approach, *J Consult Clin Psychol* 66:337, 1998.
11. Crick NR, Casas JF, Ku HC: Relational and physical forms of peer victimization in preschool, *Dev Psychol* 35:376, 1999.
12. Crick NR, Dodge KA: A review and reformulation of social-information-processing mechanisms in children's social adjustment, *Psychol Bull* 115:74, 1994.
13. Crick NR, Grotpeter JK: Relational aggression, gender, and social-psychological adjustment, *Child Dev* 66:710, 1995.
14. DeRoiser ME, Kupersmidt JB, Patterson CJ: Children's academic and behavioral adjustment as a function of the chronicity and proximity of peer rejection, *Child Dev* 65:1799, 1994.
15. Dodge KA: Problems in social relationships. In Mash EJ, Barkley RA, editors: *Treatment of childhood disorders*, New York, 1989, Guilford Press.
16. Egan SK, Perry DG: Does low self-regard invite victimization? *Dev Psychol* 34:299, 1998.
17. French DC: Heterogeneity of peer-rejected boys: aggressive and nonaggressive subtypes, *Child Dev* 59:976, 1988.
18. French DC: Heterogeneity of peer-rejected girls, *Child Dev* 61:2028, 1990.
19. George TP, Hartmann DP: Friendship networks of unpopular, average, and popular children, *Child Dev* 67:2301, 1996.
20. Graham S, Juvonen J: Self-blame and peer victimization in middle school: an attributional analysis, *Dev Psychol* 34:587, 1998.
21. Hart CH, Ladd GW, Burleson BR: Children's expectations of the outcomes of social strategies: relations with sociometric status and maternal disciplinary styles, *Child Dev* 61:127, 1990.
22. Hodges EV, et al: The power of friendship: protection against an escalating cycle of peer victimization, *Dev Psychol* 35:94, 1999.
23. Hodges EV, Malone MJ, Perry DG: Individual risk and social risk as interacting determinants of victimization in the peer group, *Dev Psychol* 33:1032, 1997.
24. Kurdek LA, Fine M, Sinclair RJ: School adjustment in sixth graders: parenting transitions, family climate, and peer norm effects, *Child Dev* 66:430, 1995.
25. Ladd GW, Kochendefer BJ, Coleman CC: Classroom peer acceptance, friendship, and victimization: distinct relational systems that contribute uniquely to children's social adjustment? *Child Dev* 68:1181, 1997.
26. Ladd GW, Ladd B: Parenting behaviors and parent-child relationship correlates of peer victimization in kindergarten, *Dev Psychol* 34:1450, 1998.
27. LaGreca AM, Lopez, N: Social anxiety among adolescents: linkages with peer relations and friendships, *J Abnorm Child Psychol* 26:83, 1998.
28. MacDonald K, Parke RD: Bridging the gap: parent-child play interaction and peer interactive competence, *Child Dev* 55:1265, 1984.
29. Mac-Kinnon-Lewis C, Starnes R, Vollig B: Perceptions of parenting as predictors of boy's sibling and peer relationships, *Dev Psychol* 33:1024, 1997.
30. McFaydn-Ketchum SA, Dodge KA: Problems in social relationships. In Mash EJ, Barkley RA, editors: *Treatment of childhood disorders,* ed 2, New York, 1998, Guilford Press.
31. Newcomb AF, Bukowski WM, Pattee L: Children's peer relations: a meta-analytic review of popular, rejected, controversial, and average sociometric status, *Psychol Bull* 113:91, 1993.
32. Olweus D: *Bullying at school: what we know and what we can do,* Oxford, 1993, Blackwell.
33. Parker JG, Asher SR: Friendship and friendship quality in middle childhood: links with peer group acceptance and feelings of loneliness and social dissatisfaction, *Dev Psychol* 29:611, 1994.
34. Parker JG, et al: Peer relationships, child development, and adjustment:a developmental psychopathology perspective. In Cichetti D, Cohen JD, editors: *Developmental psychopathology*, vol 2, New York, 1995, Wiley.
35. Perry DG, Kusel SJ, Perry LC: Victims of peer aggression, *Dev Psychol* 24:807, 1998.
36. Pettit GS, Clawson MA, Dodge KA: Stability and change in peer rejected status: the role of child behavior, parenting and family ecology, *Merrill-Palmer Q* 42:267, 1996.
37. Pettit GS, Dodge KA, Brown MM: Early family experience, social problem solving patterns, and children's social competence, *Child Dev* 59:107, 1988.
38. Pope AW, Bierman KL, Mumma GH: Aggression, hyperactivity, and inattention-immaturity: behavior dimensions associated with peer rejection in elementary school boys, *Dev Psychol* 27:663, 1991.

39. Putallaz M, Heflin AH: Parent-child interaction. In Asher SR, Coie JD, editors: *Peer rejection in childhood*, New York, 1990, Cambridge University Press.
40. Putallaz M, Wasserman A: Children's naturalistic entry behavior and sociometric status: a developmental perspective, *Dev Psychol* 25:297, 1989.
41. Rhys GS, Bear GG: Relational aggression and peer relations: gender and developmental issues, *Merrill-Palmer Q* 43:87, 1997.
42. Rubin KH: Social and social-cognitive developmental characteristics of young isolate, normal, and sociable children. In Rubin KH, Ross HS, editors: *Peer relationships and social skills in childhood*, New York, 1982, Springer-Verlag.
43. Rubin KH, Bukowski W, Parker J: Peer interactions, relationships and groups. In Eisenberg N, editor; Damon W, series editor: *Handook of child psychology, vol 3: social, emotional, and personality development*, New York, 1998, Wiley.
44. Rubin KH, Stewart SL: Social withdrawal. In Mash EJ, Barkley RA, editors: *Developmental psychopathology*, New York, 1996, Guilford Press.
45. Schwartz D, et al: The early socialization of aggressive victims of bullying, *Child Dev* 68:665, 1997.
46. Slee PT: Situational and interpersonal correlates of anxiety associated with peer victimization, *Child Psychiatry Hum Dev* 25:97, 1994.
47. Smith PK, Sharp S: *School bullying*, London and New York, 1994, Routledge.
48. Strassbourg Z, et al: The longitudinal relation between parental conflict strategies and children's sociometric standing in kindergarten, *Merrill-Palmer Q* 38:477, 1992.
49. Terry R, Coie JD: A comparison of methods for defining sociometric status among children, *Dev Psychol* 27:867, 1991.
50. Woodward LJ, Ferguson DM: Childhood peer relationship problems and psychosocial adjustment in late adolescence, *J Abnorm Child Psychol* 27: 87, 1999.

92 Phobias

Pieter le Roux • Christina M. McCann

A phobia is an extreme and persistent fear of an object, event, or situation that in reality is not dangerous to the individual and would not be of concern to most people. There are three categories of phobias: specific phobia, social phobia, and agoraphobia (often associated with panic disorder), all of which may occur in children and adolescents.

EPIDEMIOLOGY

In large-scale population studies of adults, phobias and other anxiety disorders are the most frequent psychiatric disorders occurring in the general population.[11] Although there are no comparable studies of the frequency of psychiatric disorders in childhood or adolescence, phobias clearly are common in these age groups.[6,10] In Rutter's Isle of Wight Study, about 2.5% of children had disabling specific fears or phobias.[13] A more recent community study found specific phobias in 2.6% of children.[6] In a study of children and adolescents who have anxiety disorders, except for separation anxiety disorders, specific phobias and social phobias were extremely common.[7]

The most common specific phobias occurring in children and adolescents involve animals, insects, and objects in the natural environment (e.g., storms, water) and are likely to begin before the age of 7 years. Other common phobias of closed spaces *(claustrophobia)* and heights *(acrophobia)* are much less frequent and tend to have their origins in adulthood.

Certain phobias associated with injury, blood, and health care (e.g., injections, other invasive medical procedures) also are common and should not be dismissed as trivial.[8] Extreme responses such as panic, fainting, or vomiting as a reaction to injury, venipuncture, or injection (even when such events happen to another person) may interfere with a phobic person seeking any health care.

DEVELOPMENTAL ISSUES

Some fears are common and expected at various developmental levels. For example, stranger anxiety is seen at roughly 8 months of age and usually decreases around the middle of the second year. It also is common for toddlers to be fearful of being left alone or with babysitters and for preschool children to be afraid of the dark. Because such fears are so common and so readily recognized as part of childhood, parents often do not consult physicians about them.

Many children have fears that technically might meet the criteria for a diagnosis of specific phobia but that disappear over time without specific intervention. However, the avoidance behavior associated with a phobia may interfere with usual activities and productive social relationships. Animal phobias may prevent a child from playing with neighbors or attending after-school activities because of a need to avoid the feared object. Even when a particular specific phobia disappears spontaneously, the consequences of the missed opportunities, embarrassment, or interference with social development may linger.

ETIOLOGY

The literature offers various theoretical speculations about the etiology of phobias.[9,14] Earlier theories postulated unconscious conflicts as the source. Others suggest that phobias are learned responses in the context of a child's experience. According to classical and operant conditioning theories, once a child experiences fear and physiological arousal in association with the stimulus (classical conditioning), the phobia is maintained and strengthened by avoiding the feared stimulus (negative reinforcement). Empirical research indicates that early correlates of anxiety disorders may be present. In very young children, behavioral inhibition, the tendency to exhibit withdrawal, and autonomic arousal to challenge or novelty is correlated with the later risk for anxiety and phobic disorders.[12]

SYMPTOMS

The key symptoms of phobias include a fear often associated with sweating, tachycardia, difficulty in breathing, and lightheadedness or dizziness and avoidance of the fear-provoking object or situation. According to the *Diagnostic and Statistical Manual of Mental Disorders, Fourth Edition (DSM-IV)*[3] and *DSM-PC*,[15] children may express anxiety by crying, tantrums, clinging, or freezing, and they typically do not realize that their fears are unreasonable. In extreme cases, panic may occur for adolescents. The degree to which avoidance or anticipatory anxiety occurs often is the critical factor in parents' seeking help.

Although specific phobias are defined as being related to

single feared objects, they may occur in multiples or at times in sequence (e.g., one phobia develops as another disappears). Such patterns, along with the lengthy persistence of a single phobia, suggest a more severe problem and the need for further evaluation.

Social phobia is more complex, potentially more disabling, and has a less optimistic prognosis. This disorder, which often begins in late childhood or early adolescence, is characterized by a child's fear that he may do or say something that will be socially inappropriate and thus humiliating. Because of the fear of social situations, such children limit contacts and become at risk for social immaturity and stigmatization by other children. Following are two examples of social phobia:

A 14-year-old girl, the daughter of a minister, developed a fear that she might vomit if she ate at church suppers. This progressed to the point where she could not attend such social functions or eat in public—at school, restaurants, or at friends' homes.

A 12-year-old boy had such a fear of "making a fool" of himself that he was unable to respond verbally in school or present oral reports.

In both these cases, even the thought of these social activities produced severe anxiety and led to avoidance behavior sufficient for the patient to appear "ill" enough to remain at home rather than face the social situations that were so feared.

Agoraphobia, the fear of being in places from which escape may not be possible or those where help might not be available, often begins in late adolescence. It may be associated with panic disorder or fears of panic or embarrassing happenings such as the loss of bowel or bladder control. Because of these fears, individuals often will progressively limit outside activities. This disorder usually is persistent and disabling if left untreated. Following is an example of agoraphobia:

At age 13, one girl began to be unable to go anywhere except school without her mother. Shortly, she was unable to go to school or anywhere else where there would be numbers of people (e.g., the grocery store or a shopping mall), even with her mother. Initially, she could take rides in the car with her mother, but by about 17, she was unable to leave her home unless heavily sedated.

DIAGNOSIS

A careful history usually will define the diagnosis. The report of fearful behavior, the symptoms of anxiety, or the development of avoidance behavior or compulsions (repetitive, purposeful, intentional behaviors in response to fears or obsessions) should prompt an evaluation. A detailed history of the symptoms and behaviors; the circumstances in which they occur; the responses of parents, teachers, peers, and others; and the general pattern of psychosocial development should be explored. Because children, and more commonly adolescents, may recognize that their fear is irrational, they may invent another reason for their avoidance behavior. The possibility of traumatic experience with the phobic object (such as having been frightened by even a playful dog, being lost, threatened, or abused) should be explored.

Although the history may seem to define the problem clearly, particularly if the patient can describe the object of the fear, a careful physical examination should be completed if physical problems are likely. Hypoglycemia, hyperthyroidism, and pheochromocytoma all can present with symptoms similar to anxiety. Withdrawal from some abused substances may be associated with episodes of severe anxiety, and some substances, particularly psychostimulants, may produce similar symptoms.

According to the *DSM-IV*,[3] the symptoms of specific phobia should persist for a minimum of 6 months for children and adolescents younger than age 18 years. The following subtypes should be considered when making a diagnosis of specific phobia: (1) animal (e.g., fear of animals or insects); (2) natural environment (e.g., fear is cued by natural occurrences such as storms, heights, or water); (3) blood-infection-injury (e.g., fear is cued by seeing blood or an injury or receiving an invasive medical procedure such as injections); (4) situational (e.g., fear is cued by specific situations such as tunnels or other closed spaces, public transportation, bridges, elevators, flying, or driving); and (5) other (e.g., fear cued by some other stimulus such as loud sounds or costumed characters).[3]

The differential diagnosis of specific phobia, social phobia, and agoraphobia includes:

1. *Separation anxiety disorder.* Children suffering from separation anxiety are afraid of leaving parents or others to whom they are attached and often fear that something may happen to parents when they are not present. Fear of the dark, animals, or objects may be present, but unlike a specific phobia, there is the added fear of separation from loved ones. So-called school phobia or school refusal is a specific manifestation of this disorder (see Chapter 75, School Absenteeism and School Refusal).
2. *Generalized anxiety disorder.* The essential feature of generalized anxiety disorder is excessive or unrealistic anxiety or worry for a period of 6 months or longer. Although phobias often are present, this disorder is more global and has less focused fears. Children may worry about the future, about past behavior, or about many other things.
3. *Obsessive-compulsive disorder.* When ruling out the presence of obsessive-compulsive disorder (OCD), avoidance behaviors associated with OCD are associated specifically with the content of the obsession, such as dirt and contamination, rather than a feared stimulus. Repetitive, purposeful, and intentional behavior also may develop to neutralize or prevent the occurrence of anxiety or worry, in addition to the development of anxiety and avoidance behaviors.[2]
4. *Posttraumatic stress disorder.* Posttraumatic stress disorder (PTSD) develops subsequent to experiencing a life-threatening stressor. In addition to avoidance behaviors that are typical for phobias, symptoms present with PTSD include reexperiencing the trauma (e.g., flashbacks, being retraumatized by witnessing a similar event, frightening dreams, or repetitive play in which the child expresses themes or aspects of the trauma), and restricted affect. **Note:** Acute stress disorder may be diagnosed if disturbances related to the trauma persist for a minimum of 2 days and a maximum of

4 weeks, and occur within 4 weeks of the traumatic event.

5. *Hypochondriasis*. Distinguishing between specific phobia, blood-infection-injury type, and hypochondriasis depends on the presence or absence of disease conviction. People with hypochondria are preoccupied with fears of having a disease, whereas individuals who have a specific phobia fear contracting disease but do not believe it already is present. A vasovagal fainting response also is typical for phobia of the blood-infection-injury type, whereas this is not common for hypochondriasis.

Avoidance behaviors or phobias themselves may be present with other anxiety disorders, depressive disorders, substance abuse, and psychotic disorders. However, the symptoms of these other disorders are typically the focus of treatment because they tend to produce more distress and impairment of daily functioning than symptoms of phobias.

TREATMENT

Treatment of phobias includes thorough assessment, initial intervention, and short-term follow-up. If the phobia persists, further assessment and potential consultation and referral may be necessary. It is important to inform the patient and his or her family of the diagnosis and treatment because the parents need to be partners in the treatment—their responses may be crucial to the outcome. For example, without intending to do so, parents can reinforce and perpetuate symptoms by allowing the child to avoid the feared stimulus.

When evaluating the patient, it is important to consider developmental issues. For example, children may exhibit "phobic" behaviors, such as a fear of the dark, that are common and likely to be self-limited. Providing a night light and using simple cognitive self-control strategies (e.g., relaxation, visualizing a pleasant scene, and teaching the child positive self-statements such as "I am brave; I can take care of myself in the dark.") may be all that is needed.[4] There is little point in attempting to insist that the child remain in the dark when such specific intervention is effective. More likely the "phobia" will abate spontaneously over time.

Patients who have specific phobias are treated typically with systematic desensitization that includes a combination of progressive exposure to the phobic stimulus and use of relaxation techniques. As anxiety occurs in response to the feared stimulus or imagined stimulus, the relaxation techniques are invoked and the stimuli or image removed. The feared stimulus gradually will become paired with a relaxed state instead of an anxious state, resulting in a decrease or absence of the fear response.[10]

Other behavioral approaches can enhance the effectiveness of systematic exposure, including the use of behavioral contracts and modeling procedures.[2] Contracts can increase the patient's compliance by using specific contingencies to reinforce, positively, the desired behavior toward the feared stimulus (e.g., the child earns stickers when she allows the dog she fears to come closer to her). Contracts also can ensure that treatment guidelines are followed consistently outside of the office by the patient and family. Modeling includes direct observation of the desired behavior (e.g., not avoiding the feared stimulus) demonstrated by the practitioner, family members, or peers, who initially show a comparable level of fear, which they are able to overcome.

Psychological consultation is indicated if the initial treatment does not result in symptom relief, which may result in referral for further assessment and cognitive-behavioral psychotherapy. Maintaining collaboration with referral sources helps coordinate treatment planning.[2]

Social phobia and agoraphobia are more difficult to treat and often require psychological treatment and pharmacotherapy. Systematic desensitization often is difficult to establish because of the complexity of the anxiety-provoking stimuli and social immaturity of the patient. A range of psychotherapeutic interventions, including cognitive-behavioral individual therapy, family therapy, and group therapy with age-appropriate peers, may be used to promote socialization and improve social skills. In vivo exposure with response prevention is the most effective treatment for agoraphobia with and without panic attacks, with effectiveness ranging from 60% to 70%. Booster sessions for symptoms of panic usually are necessary when panic and anxiety are still present once treatment has been completed.[4]

MEDICATIONS

Medications are most useful when used in combination with behavioral interventions. If medications are contemplated, anxiolytics or antidepressants are the medications of choice for the vast majority of children and adolescents.

In some cases, anxiolytics can help reduce anxiety for patients who find it difficult or even impossible to tolerate anxiety and to participate in treatment. Benzodiazepines are the anxiolytics used most commonly. These agents treat both acute anxiety and anticipatory anxiety. Common side effects include lethargy and sleepiness, which can interfere with academic performance. The most worrisome problem is dependency, which can develop with use for more than 3 to 6 weeks. A withdrawal syndrome including rebound anxiety, tremulousness, abdominal pain, and seizures has been described. Sudden discontinuation of medication, therefore, is not recommended. These agents are most useful for treating acute anxiety while other treatments are being put into place and in situations in which patients are not responsive to behavioral approaches. Newer anxiolytic agents have not yet been shown to have greater efficacy.[5]

Antidepressants are a better choice for long-term anxiolytic therapy because they do not carry the risk of dependency and because they are quite effective. Individuals who have comorbid depressive disorders are good candidates for antidepressants. Antidepressants will decrease or block panic attacks and other severe episodes of anxiety. Traditional tricyclics can be used, although they have anticholinergic and cardiac side effects. Selective serotonin reuptake inhibitors are equally efficacious in adults and have far fewer side effects, and probably are a better choice for children and adolescents, as well as adults. The most common side effects are sedation or sleeplessness, nausea, or diarrhea.

PROGNOSIS

Most phobias in children and adolescents seem to respond to treatment, at least in terms of relief of major symptoms, although the lack of controlled studies makes it difficult to attribute remission clearly to treatment. Follow-up studies are limited, but those that exist suggest a positive long-term outcome.[1,10] However, adults seeking treatment for phobias and other anxiety disorders often report a childhood onset of a phobia or similar symptoms during childhood or adolescence that diminished or disappeared for some time.

The prognosis for children and adolescents who have social phobia is less clear, but experience suggests that these disorders are less likely to remit spontaneously or as a consequence of treatment. Agoraphobia also has a more guarded prognosis, although outcome studies and long-term follow-up information are lacking.

Acknowledgments

The authors wish to acknowledge Norbert B. Enger, M.D., and Jed G. Magen, D.O., authors of this chapter in the third edition of *Primary Pediatric Care*. The chapter has been partially revised for this edition.

REFERENCES

1. Agres WS, Chapin HN, Oliveau DC: The natural history of phobia, *Arch Gen Psychiatry* 26:315, 1972.
2. Albano AM, Chorpita BF: Treatment of anxiety disorders of childhood, *Psych Clin North Am* 18:4, 1995.
3. American Psychological Association: *Diagnostic and statistical manual of mental disorders,* ed 4, Washington, DC, 1994.
4. Craske MG, Brown TA, Barlow DH: Behavioral treatment of panic disorder: a two-year follow-up, *Behav Therapy* 22:3, 1991.
5. Graae F, et al: Clonazepam in childhood anxiety disorder, *J Am Acad Child Adolesc Psychiatry* 33:373, 1994.
6. Kashani JH, Orvaschel H: A community study of anxiety in children and adolescents, *Am J Psychiatry* 147:313, 1990.
7. Last CG, et al: DSM-III-R anxiety disorders in children: sociodemographic and clinical characteristics, *J Am Acad Child Adolesc Psychiatry* 31:1071, 1992.
8. Marks I: Blood injury phobia: a review, *Am J Psychiatry* 145:1207, 1988.
9. Merckelback H, et al: The etiology of specific phobias: a review, *Clin Psychology Rev* 16:4, 1996.
10. Ollendick TH, King NJ, Yule W, editors: *International handbook of phobic and anxiety disorders in children and adolescents,* New York, 1994, Plenum Press.
11. Robius LN, et al: Lifetime prevalence of specific psychiatric disorders in three sites, *Arch Gen Psychiatry* 41:949, 1984.
12. Rosenbaum JF, et al: Further evidence of an association between behavioral inhibition and anxiety disorders: result from a family study of children from a non-clinical sample, *J Psychiatr Res* 25:49, 1991.
13. Rutter M, et al: Research report: Isle of Wight studies, 1964-1974, *Psychol Med* 6:313, 1976.
14. Schowalter JE: Fears and phobias, *Pediatr Rev* 15:10, 1994.
15. Wolraich ML, Marianne EF, Drotar D, editors: *The classification of child and adolescent mental diagnoses in primary care,* Elk Grove Village, Ill, 1996, American Academy of Pediatrics.

SUGGESTED READINGS

American Psychiatric Association: *Diagnostic and statistical manual of mental disorders,* ed 4, Washington, DC, 1994, American Psychiatric Association.

Baer L: *Getting control: overcoming your obsessions and compulsions,* Boston, 1991, Little, Brown.

Gitteman R, Koplewicz HS: Pharmacotherapy of childhood anxiety disorders. In Gittelman R, editor: *Anxiety disorders of childhood,* New York, 1986, Guilford Press.

Husain SA, Kushani JW: *Anxiety disorders in children and adolescents,* Washington, DC, 1992, American Psychiatric Press.

Klesges RC, Malott JM, Ugland M: The effects of graded exposure and parental modeling on the dental phobias of a four-year-old girl and her mother, *J Behav Ther Exp Psychiatry* 15:161, 1984.

Kohen DP, et al: The use of relaxation-mental imagery (self-hypnosis) in the management of 505 pediatric behavioral encounters, *J Dev Behav Pediatr* 5:21, 1984.

Leonard LL, Rapoport JL: Simple phobia, social phobia and panic disorders. In Wiener JL, editor: *Textbook of child and adolescent psychiatry,* Washington, DC, 1991, American Psychiatric Press.

Marks IM: *Fears, phobias, and rituals,* New York, 1987, Oxford University Press.

Morris RJ, Kratochwill TR: Behavioral treatment of children's fears and phobias, *School Psychol Rev* 14:84, 1985.

Parker S, Zuckerman B, editors: *A handbook for primary care: behavioral and developmental pediatrics,* Boston, 1995, Little, Brown.

93 Psychosis

Irving B. Weiner

The term *psychosis* refers to a serious degree of psychological disturbance in which an impaired grasp of reality prevents people from perceiving themselves and their experiences accurately. As a result of being out of touch with reality, psychotic individuals often misinterpret the meaning of events and misjudge the consequences of their own actions; thus, they are likely to behave strangely, inappropriately, unpredictably, and sometimes destructively. Other people frequently cannot comprehend why psychotic persons think, feel, and act as they do and are likely to regard them as being "crazy."

In young people, disorders of psychotic proportion appear mainly in three patterns, distinguishable by their typical age of onset: *infantile autism,* which is a form of pervasive developmental disorder that almost always begins before 3 years of age and interferes with the development of social interactions and communication skills from infancy on; *childhood onset schizophrenia,* which usually begins between 7 and 12 years of age and is continuous with adolescent and adult forms of schizophrenic disorder; and *adolescent onset schizophrenia,* which begins after puberty and, like schizophrenia in childhood, constitutes a breakdown or regression in psychological functioning following some years of more or less normal development.

INFANTILE AUTISM

The primary characteristic of infantile autism is a lack of relatedness to people. Autistic children are indifferent and unresponsive to social overtures. As infants they do not clamor for attention, they do not enjoy being picked up, and they do not cuddle or cling when someone holds them. They rarely look or smile directly at other people, and they seem happiest when left alone. For these reasons, parents of autistic children usually find little pleasure in nurturing them: "It was like taking care of an object; he never seemed to know or care whether I was around, and I never got any feeling of warmth from him." Nevertheless, because autistic infants tend to be healthy babies who develop normally physically, their serious deficits in social attachment often go unnoticed initially or are attributed to their being placid or reserved.

During the preschool years, however, the detachment and unresponsiveness of these children become noticeably persistent; they also begin to display a number of other unmistakable abnormalities. Most prominent in this regard are (1) a need to preserve sameness, which makes them intolerant of any change in their environment, such as moving their playpen or taking a piece of furniture out of their bedroom; (2) marked language abnormalities consisting of failing to develop any communicative speech or developing speech that is difficult to understand because of peculiar word usage, unusual grammatical constructions, and lack of relatedness to ongoing conversations; (3) repetitive and ritualistic behaviors, such as sitting for hours staring off into space or passing a toy back and forth from one hand to the other; and (4) other indices of developmental disorder that may include strange body movements or posturing, neuropsychological abnormalities, and "soft" signs of neurological impairment.

Infantile autism is a rare condition that is found in 4 to 5 live births per 10,000 and occurs three to four times more frequently in boys than in girls. Autism has a strong genetic base, however, and its frequency increases considerably in families that have an autistic member: An estimated 6% to 8% of subsequently born siblings of an autistic child are likely to exhibit the disorder, which is more than 200 times the rate in the general population. Monozygotic twins show an approximately 60% concordance for the condition, compared with 0% among dizygotic twins.[4,14]

However infrequently it may occur, autism is noteworthy for its devastating interference with psychological development virtually from birth and for its serious long-term consequences. Some autistic children improve spontaneously, especially if they are among the few who develop near-average intellectual and communication skills. Others respond favorably to specialized treatment programs that combine behavioral, educational, and pharmacological approaches. The general prognosis for the condition is poor, however. No more than 25% of autistic children make any substantial social or educational progress; of these, most achieve only fair academic and interpersonal functioning. As adults, only 10% of these children are likely to do well in work or family situations, and 60% will remain totally dependent on other adults for the rest of their lives.[5,8,10]

SCHIZOPHRENIA IN CHILDHOOD

Although schizophrenia can begin as early as the preschool years, children who are first identified as psychotic between ages 3 and 7 years very probably are youngsters who have autism or other pervasive developmental disorders whose problems previously have been overlooked. Children who become schizophrenic develop the same features of impaired personality functioning that characterize adult schizophrenia: disorganized and illogical thinking, distorted perception of reality, inappropriate ways of relating to people, and poor control of feelings and impulses. Schizophrenic children not infrequently exhibit many of the symptoms characteristic of infantile autism, including compulsive routines and self-preoccupied behavior; incoherent or incomprehensible speech patterns; excessive, diminished, or unpredictable responses to sensory stimulation; body rigidity and strange posturing; poor social skills; and periods of unaccountably severe anxiety or violent temper tantrums. Children whose schizophrenia is of early onset also are likely to develop delusions or hallucinations that detach them even further from reality and from appropriate relationships to people. Common in this regard are unrealistic fears about other children being "out to get me," bizarre fantasies about possessing special powers, and the conviction of being a machine or some kind of animal rather than a person. Schizophrenic youngsters are more likely than autistic children to have a history of poor physical health and development, but they are less likely to be intellectually or linguistically handicapped.[6,16,17]

The distinction between childhood onset schizophrenia and infantile autism is based not only on symptom patterns and age of onset but also on differences in etiology and course. Autism appears primarily to be a genetically transmitted disorder involving dysfunction in areas of the brain that are crucial to the development of language comprehension and social relationships. There is no convincing evidence that prenatal or perinatal factors contribute substantially to its etiology, and psychosocial factors have not been demonstrated to play any role in whether or when autism appears.[15] Schizophrenia, on the other hand, is understood best as a disorder of interactive origin in which biogenetic dispositions and psychosocial stressors combine to precipitate personality breakdown. Genetic transmission of some type of neurointegrative defect appears to be the most likely source of constitutional vulnerability to schizophrenia; pregnancy and birth complications may be implicated in this central nervous system (CNS) dysfunction; and patterns of family interaction, especially confusing and negatively toned parent-child communications, have considerable bearing on the severity and duration of schizophrenic breakdowns. For both biogenetic and psychosocial reasons, schizophrenia occurs in families, and the more closely two people are related, the more likely they are to be concordant for the disorder.[2,12,13]

Once begun, the symptoms of autism run a continuous, unrelenting course, whereas schizophrenia is an episodic disorder in which periods of severe symptomatology alternate with periods of reasonably adequate functioning. Autistic children who do not improve tend eventually to develop primary features of mental retardation, epilepsy, or aphasia. By contrast, the vast majority of schizophrenic children, perhaps as many as 90%, subsequently present evidence of schizophrenia as they progress through adolescence and into adulthood. Generally speaking, childhood onset schizophrenia (which also is referred to as *very early onset schizophrenia*) is a more serious disorder than schizophrenia beginning in adolescence (*early onset schizophrenia*). Adolescent onset schizophrenia is less likely than schizophrenia beginning in childhood to involve a discernable neurological substrate and a prominent family history of the disorder; it is more likely to show an acute rather than insidious onset; and it has a more favorable prognosis.[1,3,7,10]

SCHIZOPHRENIA IN ADOLESCENCE

Childhood onset schizophrenia occurs somewhat more frequently than infantile autism, but schizophrenia remains a rare condition until adolescence. Following puberty the incidence of the disorder increases sharply. The population prevalence of schizophrenia is approximately 1%, and most schizophrenic persons experience their first psychotic breakdown in late adolescence or early adulthood (15 to 25 years of age). Schizophrenia is diagnosed in 25% to 30% of 12- to 18-year-olds admitted to public psychiatric hospitals and in about 15% of those admitted to psychiatric units of general hospitals. Approximately 15% of schizophrenic patients being treated in private psychiatric hospitals are younger than age 18 years.[9]

In addition to these instances of overt schizophrenia, many adolescents who are destined to become schizophrenically disturbed as adults show prodromal signs of the disorder during their teenage years. This means that pediatricians who care for adolescents will see an appreciable number of young people in whom various kinds of apparently minor behavioral problems in fact constitute the early stages of a schizophrenic disorder.

The adolescent personality patterns from which schizophrenia emerges usually involve either *schizoid* or *stormy* behavior. Schizoid adolescents tend to withdraw into themselves, avoiding activities that would bring them into contact with people and sharing few interests in common with others. They express little or no emotion, and they may appear apathetic and unenthused about life, as if depressed. "Stormy" adolescents, by contrast, exercise little control over their emotions or actions. They consequently tend to be in constant conflict with their parents, peers, and teachers over such behavior as fighting, stealing, running away, being disobedient, being truant, and failing in school. Neither schizoid nor stormy personality patterns are by themselves diagnostic of schizophrenia, and both can occur in the context of numerous other behavior disorders. However, either pattern appearing in adolescence, especially if it represents a marked change from a youngster's childhood behavior, should alert the clinician to the possibility of incipient schizophrenia.[18]

Generally, the older people are when they develop serious psychological disorder, the less constitutionally disposed or vulnerable they are to psychotic breakdown and the better their prospects are for improvement and recovery. Accordingly, adolescent onset schizophrenia, as noted previously, offers a less guarded prognosis for improvement and at least marginal social adaptation than schizophrenia beginning in childhood. Schizophrenia beginning in adolescence, nevertheless, is in many cases a persistent and disabling disorder. As many as 90% of adolescents experiencing a first psychotic episode of schizophrenia are likely to have at least one further episode of breakdown. Among adolescents hospitalized for schizophrenia, about 25% recover and 25% improve substantially but suffer lingering symptoms or occasional relapses; the remaining 50% make little or no progress and are likely to require continuing residential care.[6,8,10]

TREATMENT

Contemporary treatment of infantile autism combines educational, psychosocial, and psychopharmacological approaches in a multimodal process involving considerable attention to family relationships. Educational methods are focused particularly on helping autistic children improve their language and communication skills; psychosocial approaches such as behavior modification, social skills training, individual psychotherapy, and vocational training are employed to promote socially adaptive and interpersonally rewarding behavior. A variety of psychotropic medications are used, as appropriate, to alleviate numerous specific symptoms that may accompany autistic disorder, including hyperactivity, aggressiveness, withdrawal, depression, and obsessive-compulsive behavior. Working with parents to help them understand their autistic child's behavior and participate in helping their child acquire coping skills is an important part of the treatment, and some type of residential placement, at least for brief periods, also may be necessary to implement a fully effective treatment program.[5]

The treatment of child and adolescent schizophrenia is, similarly, a multimodal process involving pharmacotherapy, social skills training, family treatment, and supportive psychotherapy. Antipsychotic medications may not be as effective with younger schizophrenic patients as with adults, but there is evidence to suggest that young people respond to them similarly. Whereas neuroleptic medications are employed primarily to alleviate the characteristic symptoms of schizophrenia, psychoeducational, family, and supportive psychotherapies are focused on helping the child or adolescent not only return to a premorbid level of functioning but also to promote the young person's progress through age-appropriate developmental tasks.[11] Because of the complexities of medication management in the pharmacological treatment of infantile autism and schizophrenia and the highly specialized nature of psychosocial interventions for these disorders, referral to a child psychiatrist for further evaluation and treatment is indicated when pediatricians suspect such severe psychopathology.

REFERENCES

1. Alaghband-Rad J, et al: Childhood-onset schizophrenia: the severity of premorbid course, *J Am Acad Child Adolesc Psychiatry* 34:1273, 1995.
2. Asarnow JR, Asarnow RF: Childhood schizophrenia. In Mash EJ, Barkley RA, editors: *Child psychopathology,* New York, 1996, Guilford.
3. Asarnow JR, Thompson MC, Goldstein MJ: Childhood-onset schizophrenia: a follow-up study, *Schiz Bull* 20:599, 1994.
4. Bailey A, et al: Autism as a strongly genetic disorder: evidence from a British twin study, *Psychol Med* 25:63, 1995.
5. Campbell M, et al: Treatment of autistic disorder, *J Am Acad Child Adolesc Psychiatry* 35:134, 1996.
6. Caplan R: Thought disorder in childhood, *J Am Acad Child Adolesc Psychiatry* 33:605, 1994.
7. Eggers C, Bunk D: The long-term course of childhood-onset schizophrenia, *Schiz Bull* 23:105, 1997.
8. Klinger LG, Dawson G: Autistic disorder. In Mash EG, Barkley RA, editors: *Child psychopathology,* New York, 1996, Guilford.
9. Krausz M, Müller-Thomsen T: Schizophrenia with onset in adolescence: an 11-year follow-up, *Schiz Bull* 19:831, 1993.
10. Kronenberger WG, Meyer RG: *The child clinician's handbook,* Boston, 1996, Alllyn & Bacon.
11. McClellan JM, Werry JS: Practice parameters for the assessment and treatment of children and adolescents with schizophrenia, *J Am Acad Child Adolesc Psychiatry* 33:616, 1994.
12. McKenna K, Gordon CT, Rapoport JL: Childhood-onset schizophrenia: timely neurobiological research, *J Am Acad Child Adolesc Psychiatry* 33:771, 1994.
13. Milkowitz DJ: Family risk indicators in schizophrenia, *Schiz Bull* 20: 137, 1994.
14. Piven J, Folstein S: The genetics of autism. In Bauman ML, Kemper TL, editors: *The neurobiology of autism,* Baltimore, 1994, Johns Hopkins University Press.
15. Piven J, et al: The etiology of autism: pre-, peri-, and neonatal factors, *J Am Acad Child Adolesc Psychiatry* 32:1256, 1993.
16. Russell AT: The clinical presentation of childhood-onset schizophrenia, *Schiz Bull* 20:631, 1994.
17. Volkmar FR: Childhood and adolescent psychosis: a review of the past 10 years, *J Am Acad Child Adolesc Psychiatry* 35:843, 1996.
18. Weiner IB: Early identification of schizophrenia, *Adolesc Med State Art Rev* 9:391, 1998.

94 Self-Stimulating Behaviors

Richard M. Sarles • Alice B. Heisler

Self-stimulating behaviors, such as head-banging, head-rolling, rocking, thumb-sucking and masturbation, and habits such as hair-pulling and nail-biting are of concern to both parents and primary care practitioners. It has been suggested that there are commonalties among such behaviors, sometimes classified as *stereotypies,* and that they represent an interaction of the stage of neuromotor development with environmental influences (e.g., restrictive car seats and cribs) and are a homeostatic mechanism that serves to regulate stimulation from the environment. Several of these behaviors, such as head-banging, head-rolling, and rocking, typically appear before 12 months of age, peak soon thereafter, and subsequently decline rapidly.[3] Thumb-sucking (25%) and nail biting (23%) are the most common behaviors described in preschool children, with only 4% manifesting motor stereotypies. In general, most of these behaviors are self-limited to the preschool period and usually are viewed as normal, common, and expected behaviors. As such, these habits generally do not signify psychological maladjustment; thus, they often require little intervention other than reassuring the parents and recommending adequate stimulation of their child.[8]

HEAD-BANGING AND ROCKING BEHAVIOR

Head-banging consists of rhythmic movements of the head against a solid object, such as the crib mattress or the headboard itself, and often is associated with rocking the head and the entire body. It is observed most commonly at bedtime or at times of fatigue or stress and may vary in duration from several minutes to hours. It has been noted that head-banging often continues even when the child is asleep. The age of onset shows wide variability, but the behavior is witnessed most commonly during the preschool years. The reported incidence of head-banging or rocking behavior varies between 3% and 20%, with a male-to-female ratio of approximately 3:1. There occasionally is a family history of such behavior, but only 20% of siblings of "rockers" exhibit similar or other rhythmic pattern disturbances.[7]

Various theories have been developed to understand these self-limited but often disturbing behaviors.[9] Rocking is thought to be a soothing, pleasurable experience every infant encounters in utero and most infants encounter from the neonatal period onward. The pleasure from movement is repeated throughout life, from early childhood rocking in the mother's arms, for example, to childhood jump rope games, the playground swing, and dancing in adulthood. Individual constitutional patterns in childhood account for a wide variability in the amount of stimulation any particular child may require. However, in certain children, such as those who are hearing impaired, sight impaired, emotionally disturbed, or severely mentally retarded, marked rhythmic movements are found commonly. In these cases the movements may represent a compensatory reaction for the lack of, or the inability to integrate, stimuli. In addition, the child who has no disability but who is inactive because of physical illness generally shows a need for motor release often manifested in bed rocking or other rhythmic body movements, which generally disappear once normal mobility is restored to the child.

Physical and neurological examinations show these children to be predominantly within normal limits, and electroencephalogram (EEG) studies are not indicated because they generally have been nonrevealing. It appears that these behaviors are linked to maturational patterns and correlate closely with teething and other transitions of growth and development, perhaps as a mechanism for increasing or reducing arousal and maintaining homeostasis. Even though psychosocial growth and development apparently are not disturbed in these children and studies indicate no connection between rocking behavior and parental divorce or separation, the question of inadequate stimulation for the child should be raised, or the presence of family turmoil and stress should be investigated.

Treatment generally is directed toward assuring the parents that head-banging cannot cause brain injury and that the child will show no adverse neurological residual in later life; in fact, "head-bangers" usually grow up to be coordinated and completely normal children. Padding the crib and securing the bed to prevent rolling may help during the limited rocking behavior. Sedation in the form of diphenhydramine may prove effective, but psychotropic medication generally is unnecessary and, thus, discouraged. Rarely, if ever, do fractures of the skull or cerebral hemorrhages result from head-banging, but soft-tissue swelling and scalp contusions have been reported. A protective helmet may be advised in severe cases. Consultation with a child psychiatrist or psychologist is indicated if the head-banging or rocking behavior persists beyond 3 years of age (see "When to Refer" on p. 857). For the child who shows a lack of social interaction or a preoccupation with himself or herself or with self-stimulatory behavior, such as overt, compulsive masturbation, consultation also is indicated.

THUMB-SUCKING AND NAIL-BITING

Thumb-sucking occurs almost universally in infancy but varies among cultures. Infants may place virtually every object in the mouth until parents restrict certain objects for reasons of safety.

The pleasurable sensations associated with the double tactile experience of sucking and being sucked and the feelings of security and comfort that these evoke tend to reinforce this type of behavior. Many families substitute artificial pacifiers as a more socially acceptable means of oral pleasure, and children themselves often suck a security blanket, a doll, or a stuffed animal spontaneously. Thumb-sucking usually occurs during times of stress or boredom and at bedtime. Social and family pressures generally limit thumb-sucking to the preschool years. However, the habit may persist into adolescence. It is estimated that approximately 25% to 40% of American children engage in finger-sucking during the preschool years, and 10% to 20% continue beyond 6 years of age.

Nail-biting is an extension or permutation of the habit of thumb-sucking. Some consider this behavior a form of more overt aggression directed toward one's self; others would define nail-biting simply as a variation of thumb-sucking because this behavior also is seen typically during times of stress. It is estimated that 25% of preschoolers and as many as 40% of all children older than 6 years of age bite their nails at some time or other, and 20% of college students continue to bite their nails. Thus, nail-biting, in contrast to thumb-sucking, often continues throughout childhood and into adulthood. There appears to be a family history in most cases, but this habit is so common that such an apparent association may be of no significance. There does not appear to be any correlation with the number of children in the family, the birth order, the type of feeding or type of feeding schedule, or the age or race of the parents. However, there is a significant association with the time of weaning, in that the later the weaning takes place, the less likely the chance of thumb-sucking.[2]

Thumb-sucking, nail-biting, and cuticle-biting or picking generate an increase in the probability of dental malocclusion and an increase in the incidence of digital cutaneous infections. The probability of malocclusion in the thumb-sucker appears directly related to the age at which the habit is discontinued. Thus, those children who cease the habit only after 6 years of age generally manifest malocclusion to some degree when seen at 12 years of age. In addition, thumb-sucking that persists into school age can bring on teasing from peers and criticism from teachers and family, leaving the child with decreased self-esteem and increased psychological distress. Excessive thumb-sucking, nail biting, and cuticle picking or biting should alert the clinician to investigate other possible obsessive-compulsive behaviors.[6]

Clarifying with parents the nature of these habits is important, as is encouraging them to avoid punishing or shaming the child for them. An underlying cause of tension always should be investigated, but often, simple behavioral therapy (based on positive reinforcement) is sufficient to alleviate this habit. The parents should be advised to avoid punishment, threats, or anger. Encouragement in the place of restrictions is helpful in engaging the child in his or her own program to decrease or eliminate this behavior.

Bitter-tasting commercial preparations applied to the fingers may be used as a reminder for the child but generally are inadequate unless supplemented by consistent positive reinforcement. This choice of reinforcement reward should be the child's and might represent a "Chinese menu" of extra television privileges, dessert, or other special treats. Friman and Leibowitz [4] found a combination of aversive taste treatment and a reward system to be effective in treating chronic thumb-sucking. Weekly visits to the physician for the first month of treatment are important to reinforce the change in behavior. Hypnosis is another treatment that often is quite successful and poses no dangers; psychotropic medications, on the other hand, are of little value. If these habits are linked to other signs of emotional distress, referral to a specialist in behavioral disorders is warranted.

MASTURBATION

Masturbatory activity in children is almost universal and often leads to great parental concern. Such activity may vary from direct manual genital stimulation to movements of the thighs against each other. Rhythmic swaying or thrusting motions of the child while straddling a hobby horse, pillow, stuffed animal, or other objects also are common methods of masturbation. Infants and children are capable of a physiological orgasmic response similar to that experienced by the adult, except for the absence of ejaculation in the male child. This was demonstrated by the common practice in Europe at about the turn of the century of masturbating an irritable child to induce relaxation and sleep. Occasionally, this orgasmic response has been thought incorrectly to represent a convulsive disorder in the preschool child. Masturbatory activity generally is initiated as a response to the learned pleasure associated with touching of the genitalia first experienced in infancy during normal body exploration. Masturbation will continue as a lifelong pleasurable experience unless suppressed by parents or other adults.

It is important for the practitioner to counsel parents about masturbatory practices and emphasize that masturbation is a normal, harmless, and healthy practice that helps the child to derive pleasure from his or her own body. Myths must be dispelled concerning the belief that masturbation may cause mental retardation, physical deformity, blindness, poor physical and mental health, facial pimples, hair on the palms of the hand, homosexuality, and sexual perversions. Parents should be aware that masturbation is normal and occurs almost universally in children, and should be encouraged not to punish or shame their child. If parents observe masturbatory activity in their child, they may want to suggest to the child the inappropriateness of manipulating their genitalia in public places or in front of others and inform the child that certain practices such as "toileting" and masturbation are best carried out in private.

Because local genital irritation, candidal infection, or pinworms in rare cases may cause one to masturbate, a physical examination helps to exclude such possibilities. Compulsive, overt masturbation among children and adolescents may lead to social ridicule and condemnation, or may signify a deeper emotional problem. Consultation with a specialist in behavioral disorders of children and adolescents is indicated if the practitioner suspects that the masturbatory activity is excessive, compulsive, or overt or may indicate the presence of a more complicated, troublesome emotional problem.

The practitioner should be aware that even with the current trend within our society of sexual openness and enlightenment, myths and feelings concerning masturbation often are deep-seated and persistent. Thus, counseling and advice given by the practitioner may be met with covert or overt resistance by parents or school authorities. The practitioner should be well prepared to educate those responsible for the growth and development of children.

HAIR-PULLING AND TWISTING

Hair-pulling and twisting *(trichotillomania)* is an uncommon form of self-stimulating behavior and often is indicative of psychological stress on the child. The scalp is the most common area affected; eyebrows and eyelashes are the next most likely sites. The obvious cosmetic damage often results in ridicule by peers and shame for the child. The possibility of a hair ball, or trichobezoar, forming in the stomach if the child ingests the hair is a serious problem that often results in hospitalization for surgical removal of the accumulated matted hair. This behavior, more frequent in females than males, has been reported in preschoolers, school-age children, adolescents, and adults. Classified as a disorder of impulse control *(DSM-IV),* some suggest that this disorder might best be grouped with the obsessive-compulsive disorder spectrum because of the common pathological compulsion of excessive grooming.[6] In general, the patient is totally unaware of the behavior during the hair pulling or twisting itself, and the patient often recognizes the action as senseless and undesirable.

Treatment usually is indicated and varies from initial behavior modification techniques, such as a positive reinforcement-reward system, to the wearing of a cap. Local irritation from a primary dermatological condition rarely is the cause of this disorder, but the possibility should be investigated. Referral to a mental health professional often is warranted to investigate possible underlying causes of tension, anxiety, depression, or obsessive-compulsive disorder. Hypnosis or psychotherapy may be required in many of these cases. Clomipramine, fluoxetine, and selective serotonin reuptake inhibitors, but not desipramine, have proven useful in cases that are unresponsive to nonmedication treatment.

SPECIAL PROBLEMS IN DISTURBED CHILDREN

A broad spectrum of self-stimulating behaviors may be seen in the severely retarded or the emotionally disturbed child. The behaviors, including body-twirling or spinning and hand- or arm-flapping, often are seen in cases of infantile autism or childhood schizophrenia.

Excessive rocking behavior is common in the severely retarded and emotionally disturbed child. In addition, severe self-mutilating behaviors such as compulsive self-biting, severe head-banging, and skin-gouging occasionally may be seen in these disorders but are more characteristic of certain metabolic/genetic disorders such as Lesch-Nyhan syndrome and Cornelia de Lange's syndrome.[5] Patients who have Prader-Willi syndrome frequently manifest severe skin picking.[1]

It is believed that these behaviors are part of a symptom complex in a severe disorder, in contrast to the generally isolated behavior discussed previously in normal children. The etiology generally is linked to the basic disorder and also may reflect the lack of, or disordered integration of sensory stimuli.

All these cases require treatment for the basic disorder and generally demand special treatment beyond the scope and expertise of the primary care physician. Institutionalization often is required, and methods of treatment include the application of aversive behavior modification techniques; the use of arm and neck restraints, head helmets, and psychotropic medications; and the institution of psychotherapeutic behavioral programs.

When to Refer

- Persistence of head-banging or rocking beyond the age of 3 years
- Preoccupation with self-stimulating behavior to the point that it interferes with healthy social and emotional interaction
- Presence of accompanying symptoms such as decreased socialization or other behavioral problems

REFERENCES

1. Donaldson MDC, et al: The Prader Willi syndrome, *Arch Dis Child* 70: 58, 1994.
2. Fletcher B: Etiology of fingersucking: review of literature, *J Dent Children* 42:293, 1975.
3. Foster LG: Nervous habits and stereotyped behaviors in preschool children, *J Am Acad Child Adolesc Psychiatry* 37:711, 1998.
4. Friman PC, Leibowitz JM: An effective and acceptable treatment alternative for chronic thumb- and finger-sucking, *J Pediatr Psychol* 15:1, 1990.
5. Harris JC: Destructive behavior: aggression and self injury. In Harris JC, editor: *Developmental neuropsychiatry: the fundamentals,* New York, 1995, Oxford University Press.
6. King RA, et al: Summary of practice parameters for the assessment and treatment of children and adolescents with obsessive compulsive disorder, *J Am Acad Child Adolesc Psychiatry* 37(10 Suppl):27S, 1998.
7. Kravitz H, et al: A study of head-banging in infants and children, *Dis Nerv Sys* 21:203, 1960.
8. Lourie R: The role of rhythmic patterns in childhood, *Am J Psychiatry* 105:653, 1949.
9. Werry JS, Carlielle J, Fitzpatrick J: Rhythmic motor activities (stereotypies) in children under five: etiology and prevalence, *J Am Acad Child Adolesc Psychiatry* 22:329, 1983.

95 Sleep Disturbances

Barbara J. Howard

Sleep problems are very common during childhood, occurring in 20% to 30% of healthy children younger than age 5 years and even more commonly in the presence of medical conditions. They are important for the pediatrician to ask about and recognize because parents may not realize that change is possible, even when the sleep problem is resulting in stress and sleeplessness for them and behavioral or learning difficulties for the child. Sleep problems often are a clue to underlying emotional, interactional, or family problems deserving attention and may be the aspect of the child's functioning that the family is most open to addressing initially. Sleep problems in children are associated with mothers who tend to be more irritable, be less in control, use more physical punishment, show less affection, and have more negative attitudes toward their children.[13] Treatment can improve the mother's emotional state and parenting confidence and improve mother-child interaction.[8] Sleep disturbances generally are resolved easily by the primary care physician in less than 3 weeks, using behavioral interventions based on a careful history about course, management, and family factors, yet persist more than 3 years when left untreated.

DEVELOPMENT OF SLEEP

The development of physiological sleep patterns starting in utero is predictable, which is important to understand when dealing with sleep problems. By 6 to 7 months gestational age, rapid eye movement (REM) sleep can be discerned via fetal ultrasound. Nonrapid eye movement (NREM) sleep develops around 7 to 8 months gestational age. At birth, infants have a basic pattern of alternating quiet and active sleep states, with waking every 2 to 6 hours. Quiet sleep is characterized by body stillness, regular respirations, and higher muscle tone. Active sleep has a pattern of body movements including eye movements, more irregular respirations, and lower muscle tone. The total amount of sleep at birth ranges from 11 to 23 hours, with an average of 16.5 hours, and cycles between active and quiet states every 50 to 60 minutes. By 6 weeks postterm, infants develop sleep spindles discernible on electroencephalogram (EEG). Paralleling changes in neurophysiological reorganization, the random distribution of sleep and wake periods gradually changes to cluster sleep and waking into longer bouts but without any significant change in total sleep. The timing of sleep and waking is determined by environmental influences, the so-called Zietgebers, the most powerful of which is light. Feeding and social interaction also affect sleep-wake cycles and need to be coordinated in any interventions. By 3 months of age, stages III and IV sleep can be seen on EEG, sleep begins with NREM, and babies begin the more mature pattern of sleeping longer periods at night. By 4 months, quiet sleep comprises more of total sleep than does active sleep. By 3 years of age, the child reaches an adult pattern of sleep, with cycles lasting 70 to 100 minutes and NREM occurring more in the first part of the night, with REM more toward the end of sleep. During each sleep cycle, the child progresses from light sleep stage I to deeper sleep stage II, then arouses through stages III and IV, called *slow wave sleep* because of its synchronous high-voltage slow waves on EEG, and then has a variable period of REM or dreaming sleep. Slow wave sleep is increased during adolescence, along with a slight increase in sleep requirement. The tendency to sleep is determined by the independent factors of circadian rhythm, set by the suprachiasmatic nucleus of the hypothalamus, and sleep debt. Different sleep states are associated with specific changes in endocrine release, seizure threshold, breathing, cardiovascular and gastrointestinal physiological changes, and differences in muscle tone. Genetic factors account for about half of the variability in sleep patterns. Sleep stages determine the timing of the different sleep disturbances.

SLEEP EVALUATION

In sorting out a sleep concern, the history is the major diagnostic tool. Questions should be open-ended to determine level of concern and detailed to elicit maladaptive patterns if no concern is expressed (Table 95-1). Having the family keep a sleep diary (Fig. 95-1) is helpful and often resolves the problem when distributed along with guidelines for sleep hygiene (Box 95-1). A general medical, developmental, and mental health history is needed, including any medications, substances, and/or tobacco the child is taking.

Eliciting parental perceptions and differences of opinion about sleep often is critical to any problem-solving efforts. Sleeping with the child is the norm internationally but not in North America except among blacks and Hispanics. When it is a planned arrangement agreed to by both spouses, not for anyone's sexual satisfaction, and is not occurring as a result of failure to manage the child's behavior, it is not associated with any greater than average behavioral or emotional problems in the child. When co-sleeping is planned, the desired duration should be discussed because it is easier to change this arrangement before 6 months of age if an end is intended during infancy. Purported cases of death by overlying almost

Table 95-1 Questions to Clarify Sleep Problems

Questions	To Clarify
To the Parents	
Do you have any concerns about his sleeping?	Problem versus disorder
How do you think he is sleeping compared with other children his age?	Traumas/stress
How did his sleep problems start?	Secondary gain
Were there other changes in his life happening around that time?	Traumas/stress
What have you tried to solve this problem?	
What ideas have you had about this problem?	
What have others told you about this problem?	
How has all this been for you?	
What is the room like where he sleeps? Temperature, darkness, noise, presence of siblings, type of bed	Sleep environment
When is the last time he eats before falling asleep?	Circadian disorders
	Sleep associations
Does he consume any caffeine/nicotine in the evening?	Pharmacological effects
What is he doing just before bedtime?	Bedtime resistance
What routines do you use to put him to bed?	Bedtime resistance
Tell me exactly what you do at bedtime.	Sleep associations
How does he act at bedtime?	Bedtime resistance
Where and with whom does he sleep?	Sleep associations
What does your spouse or partner think about this?	Family conflict
Who else has something to say about his sleeping?	Family conflict
Is he already asleep when you put him in the crib or bed?	Sleep associations
What time is he put in bed?	Circadian disorders
What time is he asleep?	Circadian disorders
Does he do anything in his sleep?	Restless legs
	Enuresis
	Disorders of arousal
What times does he wake up?	Trained night feeders
	Trained night wakers
	Disorders of arousal
What does he look like or do when he wakes up?	Disorders of arousal
What are you afraid of?	Developmental night waking
	Trained night feeders
	Trained night wakers
	Nightmare disorder
	Seizures
	REM behavior disorder
	Family conflict
	Overprotectiveness
What works to resettle him?	Sleep associations
	Trained night waking
	Trained night feeding
	Gastroesophageal reflux
How is that for you?	Secondary gain
Does he snore or seem to stop breathing during the night?	Breathing-related sleep disorders
What time is he up for the day?	Circadian disorders
Is the schedule the same on weekends, or does he sleep in?	Circadian disorders
How does he wake up in the morning?	Circadian disorders
When you wake him up, does he seem rested and cheerful?	Circadian disorders
	Sleep debt
What time does he eat in the morning?	Circadian disorders
Does he remember what happened during the night?	Disorders of arousal
Does he fall asleep during the day? When, where, for how long?	Circadian disorders
	Narcolepsy
How is he settled for naps?	Sleep associations
Does he sleep differently at other people's houses? How?	Bedtime resistance
Has he ever been given any medications for sleep?	
What? How did it work?	
Is there anyone in the family who ever had sleep problems?	Genetic factors

Continued

Table 95-1 Questions to Clarify Sleep Problems—cont'd

Questions	To Clarify
To the Child	
What do you think about before you go to sleep?	Bedtime fears
How do you feel when you wake up in the night?	Nightmares Disorders of arousal Anxiety/mood disorders
Do you still feel sleepy in the morning?	Circadian disorders
How do you feel about this sleeping problem?	Anxiety Secondary gain
What do you think your parents should do about this?	Secondary gain
How are your concentration and grades at school?	Breathing-related sleep disorder Narcolepsy

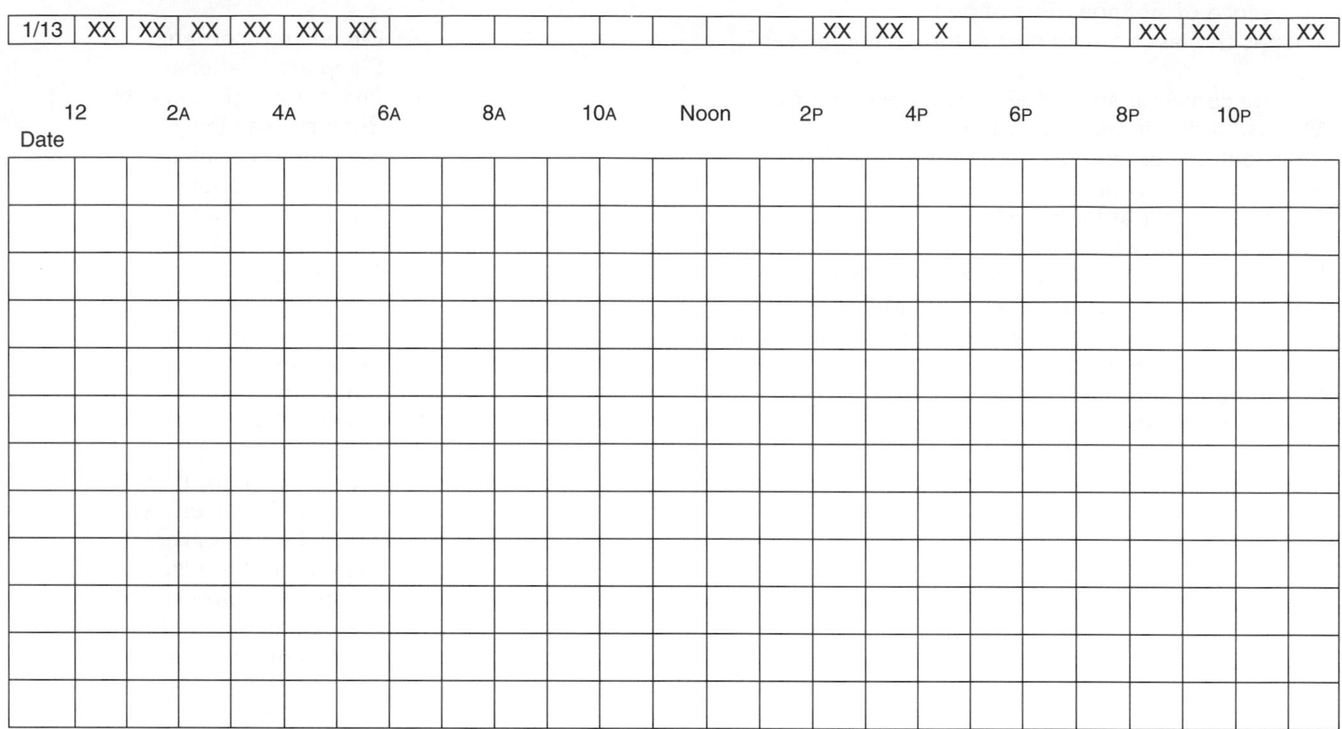

Fig. 95-1 Sleep diary. Shade in the times your child was asleep for each day. Bring this record to your next visit. Example: Child slept from 8 PM to 6 AM and napped from 2 PM to 4:30 PM.

BOX 95-1

SLEEP HYGIENE PRINCIPLES

1. Establish a good sleep environment that is dark, quiet, and comfortable, and has a steady, slightly cool temperature. Sleep should be in the same place for night and naps as much as possible.
2. Establish a soothing bedtime routine that involves friendly interaction between the parent and child. This may include a snack, then tooth brushing, use of the toilet, then several stories read to the child while in his or her own bed, presence of lovies or favorite toys, prayers or a song, and the parent leaving the room while the child is still awake.
3. Infants should be fed in your arms and placed in the crib without a bottle. Avoid excessive feeding close to bedtime to reduce the need to void during the night.
4. The child should be put to bed when tired to protect energy and yet avoid resistance.
5. Teach the child the skill of falling asleep on his or her own by avoiding pacifiers or body contact with the parent as the child drifts into sleep. This makes it possible for the child to go back to sleep on his or her own when he or she wakes up during the night.
6. Avoid changing the routine because of demands or tantrums at bedtime, or these can become habits.
7. Have no television in the child's room.
8. Try to keep bedtime, naps, and morning wake-up at the same times 7 days a week to avoid shifting the child's internal clock. Naps should not be too close to bedtime so the child will be sleepy.
9. Avoid caffeine beverages or cigarette smoke, very active play, television or movies, or arguments before bedtime. They stimulate the child and make falling asleep more difficult.

always have been due to adult intoxication or extremely deep sleeping, extreme obesity, or child abuse.

Parental mental health needs to be screened in sorting out sleep difficulties because it affects both the incidence of problems in children and adult motivation and ability to carry out treatment. Histories from babysitters or relatives who observe the child's sleep may be diagnostic, especially when there is no problem in those settings. If the history is not defining or further information is needed, the family can collect audiotapes of snoring or videotapes of night arousals. Rarely, other tests are needed, such as polysomnography, which can define sleep architecture, apnea/hypoxia, the relationship between episodic behavior and sleep stage, and sleep latency times needed to diagnose various sleep disorders. Video sleep EEGs may be needed to diagnose seizures during sleep. Haplotyping and karyotyping or fluorescent in situ hybridization (FISH) studies can be helpful for diagnosing some of the genetic conditions associated with sleep disorders.

Medication generally is not helpful more than briefly and may make childhood sleep disorders and behavior worse unless specifically indicated. Its use also can mislead families about the causes and the behavior management needed.

CLASSIFICATION OF SLEEP DISTURBANCES

Sleep disturbances can be characterized as (1) difficulty falling asleep (dyssomnias and protodyssomnias), (2) difficulties with arousals once asleep (parasomnias); and (3) excessive sleepiness (hypersomnia). These different kinds of sleep problems tend to occur in sequence because of developmental changes in sleep physiology. Infants spend a greater proportion of their sleep time in REM periods, resulting in more frequent arousals, which may present as sleep problems depending on how the family puts the infant to sleep and manages the wakings. In the preschool and school-age years, deeper NREM stages III and IV predominate, with greater risk for disorders of arousal such as confusional arousals or terrors. Adolescents have a greater need for sleep, yet more independence and demands on their time commonly result in circadian rhythm disturbances and excessive sleepiness. However, children of all ages can have the different kinds of sleep disturbances. The differential diagnosis and management strategies for a specific type of sleep problem and the general principles of sleep hygiene apply at any age (Table 95-2).

Table 95-2 Average Sleep by Age (Hours)

Age	Nighttime Sleep	Daytime Sleep
1 wk	8.25	8.25
1 mo	8.5	7.0
3 mo	9.5	5.5
6 mo	10.5	3.75
9 mo	11.0	3.0
12 mo	11.25	2.5
18 mo	11.5	2.0
2 yr	11.5	1.5
3	11.0	1.0
4	11.5	
5	11.0	
6	10.75	
7	10.5	
8	10.25	
9	10.0	
10	9.75	
11	9.5	
12	9.25	
13	9.25	
14	9.0	
15	8.75	
16	8.5	
17	8.25	
18	8.25	

DIFFICULTY FALLING ASLEEP

Difficulty falling asleep is very common in young children and the most common sleep complaint (27%) of parents of school-age children.[3] It usually is a problem of sleep routines for infants, limit setting with or without circadian rhythm problems in older children, and circadian problems created by lifestyle in adolescents. Difficulty falling asleep is termed *insomnia* or *sleeplessness*. It includes the dyssomnias and protodyssomnias (the less severe problems of young children that do not qualify as dyssomnias). The *Diagnostic and Statistical Manual for Classification of Mental Disorders in Children and Adolescents, Primary Care Version*[17] or *DSM-PC,* calls these Insomnia/Sleeplessness Variation V65.49 or Insomnia/Sleeplessness Problem V40.3, depending on their severity as judged by their duration and the extent to which they result in symptoms in the child or disrupt family life.

Day-Night Reversals

The earliest difficulty falling asleep is day-night reversal presenting around 2 weeks of age. This is predictable given the random sleep pattern described previously for this age. A concern at this time presents a valuable opportunity to assess parental coping versus maternal depression and to help first-time parents understand their important role in the child's physiological regulation. Day-night reversals can be shifted easily by establishing a general bedtime, keeping the lights off or low, and keeping handling and interaction to a minimum during nighttime feedings. In the morning, lights should be bright and social interaction encouraged. The bath may soothe some infants or arouse others and should be adjusted accordingly. If the infant sleeps more than 3 hours during the day, he or she can be awakened, ideally as one watches for active sleep and arouses the infant then, because this tends to be more effective.

Delayed Settling

The next chronologically occurring difficulty in falling asleep for infants is a delay in the much desired ability to sleep through the night. This so-called settling is defined as 5 hours of sleep after midnight for 4 weeks. Unrealistic parental expectations for settling are common and should be tempered by the statistics that 70% of infants have settled at 3 months of age, 83% at 6 months, 90% at 9 months, and

90% at 12 months. Delays in settling occur most commonly in breast-fed infants, perhaps because their mothers learn to be so responsive to them that they feed them at the slightest stirring. Other hypotheses for the prevalence of delayed settling in breast-fed infants include the habit of frequent daytime feedings, the high digestibility of human milk, and the common association of every nursing with defecation. It has been demonstrated, however, that breast-fed infants can begin to be helped to settle as early as 5 weeks postterm age if daytime feedings are spaced progressively farther apart and the longest nighttime sleep period is lengthened by delaying feeding a few minutes. Infants who have a low threshold of sensitivity by temperamental disposition also tend to settle later. Infants who have delays in central nervous system maturation often have delays in settling. Premature infants tend to settle around the time expected for their gestational age, although there is greater variability than in the full-term group. Infants who have frank neurological impairment may not only be delayed in settling but also have other severe sleep problems that can be difficult to treat.

Sleep Associations

Sleep associations, or habits of falling asleep with a person or object, may begin in the first 2 months and persist for years, leading to difficulties in falling asleep independently. This pattern develops when the child habitually falls asleep at the breast or with a bottle or simply in body contact with the parent. When placed in the crib, however, they reawaken and cry until the same circumstances are re-created for them. Repeated rearousals also can happen every 1½ to 2 hours at times of lighter sleep or when the pacifier falls out. A sleep association also may result in night waking, even if initially there is no difficulty falling asleep. The best treatment is avoidance through advising parents to place the infant in bed awake for both night and naps, even if it requires reawakening them, starting by 2 months after term. Placing in the crib a shirt that the mother has worn for several days without washing for the infant to smell also may be helpful, as long as it is not too near the face. If a sleep association has already developed, the infant or child may need the parent to sit beside him or her or sing as the infant learns to fall asleep on his or her own over several days.

Prolonged Routines and Curtain Calls

Taking longer than 30 minutes to be put to bed is considered a prolonged routine. This can be seen as a problem of falling asleep, even if the parent is complicit because of enjoying the time with the child, feeling guilty after being away all day, or avoiding being alone with his or her spouse. The child may plead charmingly for one more story, game, or glass of water or may be tearful. Toddlers and preschool children no longer sleeping in a crib may reappear after being put to bed, thus prolonging the routine. These "curtain calls" are unintentionally reinforced easily by the parental attention needed to return the child to bed, even if done with obvious displeasure. Some children pretend to be fearful at bedtime to gain extra time, although their affect exposes the act.

In assisting with a complaint of prolonged routine, the possibility of a phase-shift problem needs to be determined. In this case the child is not tired, usually because of excessive or late day napping. Total sleep time, including naps, is typically 11½ to 13 hours for the child between 2 and 4 years old (Table 95-2). A 3-year-old child given a 3-hour nap who wakes up at 7 AM may not be tired until 10:30 PM. The total sleep may be unknown to the parent if the nap is being allowed by a babysitter, which must be investigated. The best management of prolonged routines is prevention through reasonable daily routines and assurance of adequate "special" individual time with each parent every day.[11] This reduces child and parent urgency about being together, as well as parental guilt. The bedtime routine should be limited to a defined set of activities and/or length and ended on time. The parent may then either notify the child that they will not respond to further requests or to "only one more" and adhere to this. They should be warned not to respond to the excuses that will likely ensue. Having the parent promise to "check" the child in 5 minutes also can be reassuring. Bedtime in phase-shift situations should first be conducted at the time the child is tired rather than the desired bedtime to avoid struggles and then advanced by 10 minutes per night until it is an acceptable hour. Waking time must be adjusted either first or simultaneously and both times held constant 7 days per week. Curtain calls, in addition to the strategies just mentioned, require that the parent lead the child back to bed as many times as necessary without talking to him or her at all. Children succeeding in staying in bed without calling out may be rewarded with two stories at the next bedtime and/or a reward in the morning. If they come out or call out, they receive only one story. An alternative is for the parent to offer the choice of having the door open or closed, the light on or off. The child then is informed that the door will be closed and the light shut off if the child comes out or calls out. If the child starts to come out or calls out, the consequence is delayed for a few seconds before the door is opened to give the child a second chance. Toddlers who come out may need their doorway gated if they are not mature enough to respond to these other measures. A child who protests the parent leaving the room can have progressive weaning of this need by having the parent sit silently in the room as the child falls asleep, moving one foot closer to the door each night until he or she is out. Feigned fears should be verbally minimized with a brief response or turned into a joke. Real fears at bedtime are discussed below. Some children are noncompliant at bedtime similarly to their general noncompliance. Parents may need coaching on limit setting or referral if discipline is a major problem. Parents prolonging routines to avoid each other may need marital counseling. Domestic discord or violence should be considered as a potential reason for children avoiding bedtime, after which time they can hear parents fighting.

Bedtime Fears

Preschool and early school-age children are most susceptible to fears at bedtime because of their active fantasies yet limited abilities to distinguish reality. Exposure to violent or frightening media or videogames can be the major contributing factor and should be eliminated for their overall benefit as well. Fears also may be generated by the child's daily stresses such as problems with child care or after-school settings, aggressive peers, learning problems, pressure for the young child to be toilet trained, problems separating from parents, corporal punishment, witnessing or hearing about violence, moves, sibling birth, or experiencing a loss. Stresses should be reduced as much as possible and counseling provided when indicated. Sexual issues may result in fears if the child is overstimulated by home nudity, cobathing, or lack of limits on physical intimacy with adults, which should be discontinued. Sexual misuse also can result in bedtime fears, especially if the child was molested in his or her own bed. Some aggressive children have bedtime fears apparently in reaction to their own lack of control. These children need better limits and behavior management during the day. Fears deserve sympathy for the emotion but reassurance that the fear is unwarranted and the adult will keep the child safe. A ritual of the adult "spraying for monsters" may be helpful. Having the child help to buy a special flashlight to use to check out the room at night provides a sense of mastery. Older children benefit from relaxation exercises accompanied by empowerment stories. Any child may do better with a night-light as long as it does not interfere with sleep once achieved.

Circadian Rhythm Sleep Disorder

The most common difficulty with falling asleep is a sleep phase shift or circadian rhythm disturbance. Because the natural circadian cycle is about 25 hours, some individuals living a 24-hour day are vulnerable to shifting day-night cycles over time. This is especially likely when families do not adhere to routines by the clock but allow the child to set his or her own schedule. Children of any age may have a circadian disorder that is differentiated from an oppositional disorder by lack of resistance to going to bed but inability to fall asleep. In the morning the child is difficult to arouse and does not feel rested. Sometimes there is an early phase shift, usually in infants or toddlers who fall asleep early but then awaken early in the morning. Either type of circadian shift can be adjusted by simultaneously shifting naps, bedtime, waking time, and meals to a desired schedule that matches the child's sleep needs. Although puberty brings slightly increased sleep needs, adolescents almost universally are sleep deprived during weekdays because of school, work, and social activities. They become accustomed to a late bedtime and cannot readjust easily even though they are tired. Instead, they sleep late on weekends and often are irritable and hard to arouse in the morning. Adolescents must stick to a schedule of bedtime and waking matching their school needs and avoid napping 4 days per week to readjust. If this is insufficient, it is necessary either to advance the sleep phase 15 minutes every 2 to 3 days around the 24-hour day, using a set, reasonable amount of sleep, until reaching a bedtime more synchronous with the family then sticking to this schedule 7 days per week or delay sleep time by 1 to 2 hours more each day during a school break. Either treatment requires intense commitment by the teenager, who instead may be motivated to avoid family or school obligations by staying up late at night and getting up late in the morning.

Primary Insomnia

Primary insomnia is unusual in children, occurring only rarely in adolescents as a diagnosis of exclusion. It must last at least 1 month, interfere significantly with functioning or cause significant distress, and not be part of another sleep or mental disorder to be diagnosed. Impaired concentration, vigilance, or attention; low energy; increased fatigue; and bad mood may be associated symptoms.

Other Difficulties Falling Asleep

Dyssomnias can be used to describe other situations of insomnia that do not meet disorder criteria, mainly in preschool and older children. These include environmental factors interfering with sleep onset such as chaotic or noisy households, which often also are arousing because of tension and discord. Sleep deprivation may result in an overly tired child having difficulty falling asleep. Reestablishing a routine that includes adequate sleep is necessary to resolve this. Restless-legs syndrome has been noted in children old enough to report discomfort, usually at bedtime but also often awakening the child from sleep (see p. 866).

DIFFICULTIES WITH AROUSALS FROM SLEEP

Waking at night occurs in more than 80% of children and, of course, in infants who still need to feed at night. Night waking is only problematic when the child cannot return to sleep on her or his own. As many as 20% of 2-year-olds, 14% of 3-year-olds,[16] and 6.5% of 5- to 12-year-olds have problematic night wakings.[3] Difficulties caused by arousals from established sleep are called *parasomnias.* Difficulties less severe than disorder include nocturnal arousals variation and nocturnal arousals problem. During sleep cycles after III and IV, there often is a behaviorally inapparent arousal. When this arousal is disordered or results in awakening from which the child cannot return to sleep independently, it becomes an arousal problem. Because NREM III and IV are more predominant in the preschool and school-age child, arousal problems are more frequent then.

Sleep Associations

Just as sleep associations can cause difficulty falling asleep, they also can interfere with falling back to sleep. Management of any sleep association (see the preceding discussion) needs to be part of solving any kind of sleep difficulty. It is classified as sleep association resulting in nocturnal arousals problem.

Trained night feeding. Fifty percent of infants can go 8 hours without a feeding at 1.3 months of age, and 95% of full-term infants do not need a 2 AM feeding by 4 months of age. Despite this, many babies wake up in the night and are fed to return to sleep. Their sleep cycle is changed by the introduction of food to produce an arousal—basically, learned hunger—and they will consume a full feeding. Trained night feeding generally should not be diagnosed before 4 months postterm because of the frequent continued need for a feeding during the night earlier or in premature infants. Infants who were sleeping all night and begin waking inconsolable except by feeding are probably ready for solids or increased volumes of feeds during the day.

Trained night feeding can be prevented best through appropriate parent education to teach ways to recognize and console a fussy infant by other means than feeding during the day. Often it is the most responsive parents who continue to feed their infants at night by going to them when they stir, even though they may have been able to resettle given the chance. Expectations of the appropriate need for a late (e.g., a 10 PM) feeding should be clarified. Daytime feeding intervals can be lengthened gradually and any sleep associations retrained simultaneously. Then the infant can be allowed to cry at least 1 minute to try to resettle him- or herself before getting up for a feeding in the middle of the night. Each night the infant can be fed 1 oz less or spend 1 minute less at the breast. This will resolve trained night feeding in about 1 week.

Trained night waking. Waking at night without requiring a feeding in the infant between 4 and 8 months of age is called *trained night waking*. This often begins when the infant is ill or has been subjected to travel or some other change, but then persists when the child gets a secondary reward by the parent's attention. One parent may feel it necessary to quiet the infant quickly so as not to disturb other family members or neighbors, especially if this would evoke an angry response. Sometimes a parent working shifts or a mother busy during the day with other children looks forward to and reinforces night waking with play. Trained night waking also is more common in infants who have difficult temperament and twice as frequent in those who have depressed mothers. It is theorized that the latter infants are left to cry excessively during the day and therefore cannot self-console well at night. It also could be that depressed mothers feel guilty about deficient daytime interactions and try to make up for it at night, or they may have sleep disorders of their own that leave them awake and desiring company. Management of trained night waking requires management of the precipitant pain or stresses and, ideally, collaboration with spouse or neighbors to tolerate some crying during treatment and provide support for the parent. Bedtime routines need to be established, perhaps with a transitional object—that is, a lovie or smelly shirt from the mother, and the infant should be put in bed awake. Naps should be limited to 2 hours to consolidate the longest sleep period at night. When the infant awakens during the night, he or she should be allowed 5 minutes of crying before being checked, but not fed, then checked every 10 minutes. This may require the more involved parent to take a shower, turn up music, go out of the house, or otherwise distract themselves for this to be successful. Brief sedation should be needed only rarely to change this habit.

Developmental night waking. Although most infants are sleeping all night by 6 months of age, many begin awakening again starting around 8 to 10 months of age. This new behavior corresponds to several coincident developmental processes, including increased mobility, fear reactions to strangers, and object permanence or the ability to remember and seek something once it is out of sight and, therefore, is called *developmental night waking*. The arousal often begins suddenly after the infant awakens to a stranger, such as a babysitter, and becomes hysterical. It subsequently reoccurs nightly. Developmental night waking represents fear about separation and therefore is a common sleep problem whenever separation difficulties are present, generally only up to age 4 years, with the same solution applicable.

The best management is advising parents at the 6-month health supervision visit to expect a recurrence of night waking and to wait a few minutes before going in to the infant, but to avoid feeding or other reinforcement. If waking is already established, the parents should have the contributing developmental forces explained and be advised to create a bedtime routine, including a transitional object and a dim night-light. When the infant awakens, he or she should be allowed to cry at least 2 minutes to be given a chance to self-console. If crying continues, one parent can go to the child, reassure her or him briefly, without touching or feeding, and settle down within sight to sleep the rest of the night without talking to the child. The child often becomes enraged instead of fearful, which is more tolerable to the parent, who can see that the child is safe. Parents, therefore, are more likely to be able to carry out this plan than one that requires repeated separations. For children no longer constrained to a crib, the parent must require the child to stay out of body contact by giving them the alternative that the parent will leave the room to avoid establishing a sleep association. If vomiting occurs, cleanup should be postponed until morning to avoid reinforcement. In an average of four nights, the child no longer will awaken during the night, presumably because of increased trust in the availability of the parent.

Arousal disorders. Sleep terror disorder, sleepwalking disorder, and confusional arousals all are related episodic behaviors, often occurring in the same child and family because of genetic predisposition. In all of these conditions, children show automatic behaviors and lack of awareness of others. They are difficult to arouse and have little or no recall of dreams at the time. They are confused and have no recall of the arousal later. Sleep terrors may begin at 18 months, sleep walking during preschool or school age, and confusional arousals at any age, but all are diminished during adolescence. Because the deepest stage IV sleep is in the first cycles of the night, disorders of arousal are most likely to occur in the first 3 hours of sleep. Sleep talking and nocturnal leg cramps are part of normal developmental variation. Enuresis is a disorder of arousal discussed in Chapter 88.

CONFUSIONAL AROUSALS. Young children sleep so deeply that the transition from stage IV to REM sleep may result in progressively stronger thrashing and moaning lasting 5 to 15 minutes, usually in the first half of the night, and is difficult to interrupt. When multiple arousals occur, they also may extend into the second half of the night, although generally decreasing in intensity. These are most common when children are overtired, the schedule is altered, or the child is ill. If the child has behaviorally caused awakenings during the night, it can make partial arousals disturbing sleep more likely earlier in the same night. Management of the behavioral problem waking generally resolves the partial wakings also. Older children who have partial arousals may be responding to internal stresses. Most children who have partial arousals need adequate sleep and a routine schedule but minimal intervention at the time of the episode to avoid reinforcement or conveying a sense of concern. In severe cases, a few weeks of a benzodiazepine, such as clonazepam 0.125 to 0.5 mg at bedtime, may be needed to interrupt the sequence, avoiding prolonged use, which results in tolerance. A sleep study to confirm the diagnosis is needed only in these cases.

SLEEP TERRORS. Sleep terrors are disordered arousals from stage III or IV sleep characterized by physiological arousal including pallor, sweating, pupil dilation, piloerection, and tachycardia. The child may speak, but incoherently; is not responsive to others; and may even thrash violently, but with amnesia for any of this in the morning. Sleep terrors occur in 3% of children, mostly from 18 months to 6 years, and do not reflect mental health problems at these ages, although they may be increased by stress. There often is a family history of sleep terrors, enuresis, and sleep walking or talking—all disorders of arousal. Sleep terrors may be precipitated by fatigue, stress, a full bladder, or loud noises. They tend to occur in bouts up to 20 per night for several weeks and then disappear only to recur several weeks later. Parents deserve reassurance about the benign nature of sleep terrors and their tendency to resolve around age 6 to 8 years of age. The bladder should be emptied routinely, and the environment kept dark and quiet. The bouts may be interrupted by awakening the child a half hour before the expected episode, generally 1 hour into sleep each night for about a week. A 30- to 60-minute afternoon nap also can reduce stage IV sleep and decrease the number of episodes. Brief sedation with diazepam can reduce the frequency, but such terrors may recur when the child is weaned or tolerance occurs. Having a parent sleep in the child's room also may be helpful, presumably because it reassures the child and possibly alters sleep stages. Seizures should be ruled out in intractable cases or those that have their onset in adolescence.

SLEEPWALKING DISORDER. About 15% of children sleep walk at some time, 1% to 6% having one to four attacks per week, mostly between ages 4 and 12 years.[2] Sleep walking, like other disorders of arousal, occurs in stage IV sleep, generally 60 to 120 minutes into sleep. During sleep walking, children are difficult to arouse, are uncoordinated, and tend to wander in illogical places, often urinating outside the toilet. Chronic sleepwalkers need to be carefully safeguarded so that they do not injure themselves. Alarms and door or window locks may be necessary. There is amnesia for the event in the morning. Sleep walking usually can be differentiated by history or videotapes from dissociative states or seizures.

Sleep-Wake Transition Disorder

Disturbing behaviors while falling asleep are especially common in preschoolers because of their initial NREM states. Rhythmic movement disorders include head banging, sleep starts, and body rocking. Some rhythmic activity at bedtime occurs in 58% of 9-month-olds, decreasing to 33% at 18 months, and 22% at 2 years. Head banging is very common, occurring in 3% to 15% of children, often after an initial history of head rolling starting at 6 months. It typically is monotonous, occurring 60 to 80 times per minute for fewer than 15 minutes. Head banging may be due to CNS injury, headache, ear pathology, sensory deprivation (including visual or hearing impairment), neglect, or abuse. Children of intense temperament are especially likely to bang. Although head banging does not cause brain injury, it often can be reduced by kinesthetic stimulation during the evening and holding the child as part of the bedtime routine. Imipramine or hydroxyzine also are effective but rarely are needed. Parents may need reassurance that the child is not autistic or retarded because the prevalence in these conditions is well known.

Nightmare Disorder

Nightmares are extremely common parasomnias occurring during REM sleep, therefore, typically in the last one third of sleep. The dream content often is recalled as frightening and reflects daytime stresses. Although children clearly dream by 14 months of age, nightmares are most common between 3 and 6 years, occurring in 10% to 50% of children. During this stage, children have vivid imaginations, weak ability to differentiate fantasy from reality, and many drives that they are trying to master, such as aggression, sexuality, sibling rivalry, and toileting control. Severe traumas such as sexual abuse or the viewing of violence can produce nightmares. Nightmares are uniformly part of post-traumatic stress disorder. Nightmares may result after withdrawal of REM-suppressing medications such as alcohol, methylphenidate, benzodiazepines, or antidepressants. Nightmares deserve comforting but preferably in the child's bed, keeping intervention brief to avoid secondary gain by adult attention. The same concerns as listed under the discussion of "Bedtime Fears" should be addressed when nightmares are frequent. Children who have chronic nightmares have been shown to improve with targeted relaxation exercises and stories in which the child masters a situation. Children can prepare to have good dreams through rehearsal and imaging at bedtime. Severe nightmares may respond to bedtime diphenhydramine, trazodone, or cyproheptadine, although counseling is mandatory if the condition is of this severity.

Violent behavior during sleep

PARASOMNIA. A REM behavior disorder has been described during which, instead of hypotonia during REM, muscle activity is restored and dream content can be acted out, sometimes in violent ways. It is rare in children and is associated with neurological lesions, which must be sought through neuroimaging and sleep studies. Treatment with clonazepam has been beneficial in adults.[2]

Other parasomnias

Bruxism is the annoying habit of grinding the teeth during sleep. This occurs in 50% of normal infants at the time of tooth eruption but also occurs in those 10 to 20 years old, secondary to stress. Bruxism also can be caused by dental malocclusion and neurological conditions. Tooth guards can protect the teeth and reduce potential damage to the temporomandibular joint. Relaxation exercises at bedtime also can be helpful.

Sleep environment problems, such as a chaotic or excessively noisy home environment, can result in arousals.

Sleep association by falling asleep to music or television can result in awakenings and difficulty falling back to sleep at any age but is most common during adolescence.

Breathing-Related Sleep Disorder

Breathing-related sleep problems include central apnea, usually in infants born prematurely, and obstructive apnea or mixed forms. Central apnea in the premature infant rarely has any physical sequelae but may result in parental hypervigilance about the child. Breathing-related sleep disorder is defined as five 10-second apneas per hour or 10 apneic periods of oxygen saturations less than 50% of normal per hour of sleep. Episodes may occur 200 to 300 times per night, severely fragmenting sleep and resulting in sleep debt. In toddlers, this can even result in failure to thrive, possibly secondary to insufficient growth hormone secretion.[2] Obstructive sleep apnea occurs in 0.7% to 1.1% of children and consists of collapse of the upper airway, periodically obstructing breathing and disrupting sleep. Snoring occurs in about 75% of children who have obstructive sleep apnea. A sleep study often is needed to make the diagnosis if the history and/or audiotapes are not diagnostic of apnea, paradoxical abdominal breathing, grunting, choking, or gasping. Profuse sweating during sleep, hyperextension posturing, very restless sleep, and distress upon waking from obstructive episodes may all be clues. Because of the hypoxia, these episodes can result in concurrent negative mood, aggression, hyperactivity, poor attention, memory, visuomotor performance, and school success, and, long term, in high blood pressure, cor pulmonale, and increased risk of cardiovascular accidents, and death. All of these outcomes are reduced with relief of the obstruction.[1] There is evidence for genetic differences in the central control of breathing in some cases. Obesity, alcohol use, and differences in the soft tissue and bony structures also may contribute to airway obstruction. Children who have Prader-Willi syndrome, Down syndrome, mucopolysaccharidoses, craniofacial anomalies, and neuromuscular disorders are predisposed. In children, however, adenotonsilar hypertrophy is the major cause and removal the treatment. Severe cases may require other surgical procedures.

Restless-Leg Syndrome

Restless-leg syndrome is a common (2% to 5% of the population), highly familial condition, worsening with age and usually including periodic, brief, painful, or uncomfortable jerking leg movements during stage II sleep, which cause the individual to awake from sleep. They present as nocturnal arousals problem.

EXCESSIVE SLEEPINESS

Excessive daytime sleepiness can be due to a circadian or other dyssomnia. Less severe cases that do not affect daytime functioning constitute excessive sleepiness variation; mild difficulties constitute excessive sleepiness problem. Excessive sleepiness in children may present as hyperactivity, restlessness, poor concentration, impulsivity, aggressiveness, irritability, or sadness, rather than complaints of daytime sleepiness. It should be differentiated from fatigue and from sleepiness feigned to avoid something. The most common cause of daytime sleepiness is lack of adequate sleep, especially in adolescents who set their own schedules or children who are not maintained with a reasonable bedtime. However, multiple chronic sleep disruptions from any cause may result in daytime sleepiness. Primary hypersomnias (intrinsic dyssomnias) in children include breathing-related sleep disorder (described elsewhere on this page) and narcolepsy.

Narcolepsy

Narcolepsy is a potentially disabling syndrome of irresistible daytime sleep attacks that last 20 to 40 minutes, automatic behaviors, and abnormal REM transitions disrupting nighttime sleep occurring in 0.04% to 0.07% of the population. Cataplexy, sleep paralysis, and hypnagogic hallucinations are highly associated with narcolepsy. Ninety percent to 100% of patients who have narcolepsy have the HLA DQB1*0602 gene, a weakly penetrating factor, although other genetic factors also play a role. Narcolepsy rarely has onset before puberty, with peak onset of 15 to 25 years, but shortened REM onset has been noted in preadolescent offspring of narcoleptic adults.[2] Sleep paralysis or inability to move for a few seconds to minutes when awakening or falling asleep is commonly associated but not specific to narcolepsy. Sleep paralysis is highly familial. Cataplexy, in which the person has brief episodes of bilateral muscle weakness that may result in falling, head bobbing, or jaw sagging several times per day to several times per year during laughter or a period of elation, is specific to narcolepsy. Hypnagogic hallucinations or dream states at the time of falling asleep or during sleep attacks, along with sleep paralysis, are upsetting and can result in fear of falling asleep. Diagnosis can be aided by polysomnography showing sleep-onset REM and the Multiple Sleep Latency Test showing shortened sleep-onset times, as well as the absence of other diagnoses. Differential diagnosis includes hydrocephalus, postviral or trauma state, or the rare idiopathic CNS hypersomnia. Absence of HLA DQB1*0602 effectively excludes the diagnosis of narcolepsy. Treatment includes daytime stimulants such as methylphenidate, regular adequate sleep, two to three planned half-hour daytime naps, and timing activities at best hours. Support for the difficulties of this lifelong condition and any treatment needed for concomitant depression also are needed. Antidepressants, such as clomipramine 10 to 20 mg/day in divided doses, also can help eliminate cataplexy. Monoamine oxidase inhibitors can reduce sleep paralysis, hallucinations, and cataplexy.

Circadian Rhythm Sleep Disorder

Excessive sleepiness is most common in adolescence because of circadian rhythm disturbances caused by slightly increased sleep needs during puberty combined with demanding lifestyles that do not afford adequate sleep. This is exacerbated by make-up sleep on weekends and/or the use of stimulants or tobacco to stay up and alcohol or sedatives to fall asleep.

SLEEP DISORDERS ASSOCIATED WITH MENTAL DISORDER

Sleep problems may occur in association with any mental disorder, which becomes the primary diagnosis. Mood disorders are among the most common mental health disorders affecting sleep. Depression has been shown to include increased time to fall asleep, corresponding to neuroendocrine dysregulation at that time and reduced REM latency, even when the sleep schedule is controlled, although this is less common the younger the child. The early-morning waking of depressed adults is not seen prepubertally and rarely even in adolescents.[6] Hypersomnia predominates over insomnia in depression after puberty.[5] The problem with sleep intrinsic to depression is complicated by intrusive thoughts or worries that also may interfere with sleep. Bipolar disorder may include inadequate sleep during the manic phases because of agitation. Anxiety/panic disorders may result in difficulties falling asleep because of specific or nonspecific fears, as well as difficulties returning to sleep if aroused during the night. Children who have been abused, whether or not they have been diagnosed as having post traumatic stress disorder, have more sleep problems, including nightmares, increased activity during sleep, and troubles falling and staying asleep.[7] Personality disorders in adolescence have been associated with delays in falling asleep. Psychoses may include troubling intrusive thoughts, especially at night. Substance abuse disorders should be considered in sleep disorders in older children. Alcohol may induce sleep but also fragment it, and withdrawal from chronic use alters sleep. Stimulants can prevent falling asleep. Medications such as fluoxetine and tricyclics used to treat mental health disorders also may have adverse effects on sleep, including eliminating REM atonia, thus generating abnormal movements during sleep.

SLEEP DISORDERS ASSOCIATED WITH MEDICAL PROBLEMS

A variety of medical and behavioral problems can cause sleep difficulties, which then are classified as secondary. On the other hand, sleep disorders can result in behavioral and learning problems, so both etiologies must be considered, and both deserve treatment.

Neurological Disorders

Any CNS impairment can result in dysregulation of the sleep cycle. As many as 88% of children who have major developmental disabilities may experience chronic sleep problems, often of several types.[9] Even multiple behavioral sleep problems in these children can be improved by establishing a bedtime routine, delaying bedtime for a half hour and then removing the child from bed and keeping her or him awake and playing for 1 hour each time he or she does not go to sleep within 15 minutes. This procedure is repeated until the child falls asleep within 15 minutes of being put in bed. Wake-up time is kept constant. Each night the bedtime is made 30 minutes earlier than the prior effective bedtime, moving it 30 minutes later the next night if the child did not fall asleep within 15 minutes. Daytime naps are not allowed for children older than 4 years of age.[9] Children who are blind have special problems with circadian rhythm because of the lack of light stimulation in stabilizing the biological clock. Other factors, such as the timing of medications, difficulty repositioning during the night, pain, headache, and caregiver anxiety, can contribute to sleep problems in the neurologically impaired child. Melatonin at bedtime has been shown to be helpful in some children who have CNS problems or blindness as the cause of their sleep disturbance but also has been associated with reversible increased seizure activity.[12] The Kleine-Levin syndrome, comprising episodic severe daytime sleepiness, hyperphagia, and hypersexuality, is a cause of hypersomnia beginning in adolescence, with episodes lasting hours to weeks. Tumors of the third ventricle also may present as daytime sleepiness.

Sleep-related epilepsy. Seizures are more likely to occur during REM, perhaps because of the increase in metabolic rate then. Seizures occurring during the night affect sleep efficiency by causing multiple awakenings. The possibility of a seizure disorder should be considered in new-onset parasomnias in adolescents. Nonconvulsive epilepsy may present as excessive daytime sleepiness.

Sleep-related headaches. Cluster headaches occur 2.5 times more frequently at night and often disrupt sleep. Headaches causing night or early-morning awakening should be evaluated carefully for the presence of increased intracranial pressure as a cause.

Degenerative Disorders

Degenerative brain disorders result in frequent awakenings, difficulty falling asleep, early-morning waking, sleep deprivation, and daytime sleepiness.

Developmental disorders. Learning disabilities are associated with higher rates of sleep disturbance, including night waking and troubles falling asleep. Half of these sleep difficulties persist for more than 3 years.[16] Attention deficit/hyperactivity disorder (AD/HD) in particular has been studied, with mixed results, as to whether sleep problems are more common than in control children. Parent questionnaire studies show that 25% to 50% of children who have AD/HD have sleep problems of all types: troubles settling to sleep, waking from sleep, and morning difficulties, but no difference in total sleep time. In a review of multiple studies, 38% of studies reported lower sleep efficiency in those who had AD/HD[4]; 67% showed more movements during sleep, with medications used to treat AD/HD prolonging sleep latency in 75% of studies. Clonidine was shown to be effective; 85% improved in their sleeping when behavioral measures failed.[10] Children with autism have serious sleep problems more than 75% of the time, with onset before age 3 but resolving by age 5 years. They have difficulties with falling asleep, waking in the night, and early-morning waking.[15] Asperger syndrome has been associated with hypersomnia. Children who have Tourette's syndrome have increased parasomnias.

Other medical disorders. Any condition causing pain, including juvenile arthritis, can result in disrupted sleep.[18] Eczema with associated scratching results in more short and long awakenings. Menstruation can cause insomnia or hypersomnia. These symptoms are helped by oral contraceptives.

Sleep-related asthma. Asthma episodes are increased during sleep, presumably because the neuroendocrine regulators of respiration are sensitive to diurnal regulation. Children who have sleep-related asthma have fragmented sleep and may resist sleeping and develop sleep debt because of the anxiety associated with breathing discomfort. They may have impaired concentration abilities and more depressed mood and conduct problems. Of children who have asthma, 34% awaken at least once a week and 5% every night from asthma symptoms. They have more short and long awakenings, and 59% report daytime sleepiness, with 51% reporting difficulty with concentration. These all improve with successful asthma management.[14]

Gastroesophageal Reflux

Gastroesophageal reflux may produce sleep problems in a variety of ways. The reflux itself can be painful, resulting in night waking and crying. Reflux also can result in sleep apnea. Reflux may not always be an obvious diagnosis from daytime signs and symptoms, although excessive spitting up, reswallowing motions, increased fussiness, and even refusal of feedings and failure to thrive can be among them. Esophagoscopy, looking for erosions, may be needed to determine the cause of nighttime pain. Failure to be consoled while being held can be a clue that the child is suffering pain. Holding the child upright reduces the amount of acid in the esophagus and may comfort a child with reflux. See Chapter 180, Vomiting, for further discussion of gastroesophageal reflux.

When to Refer

If the clinician is unable to relieve a sleep disturbance after working with the family over the course of 4 to 6 weeks, assistance may be needed either from a sleep specialist or family therapist if the barrier is family dynamics. One should always consider, and generally respect, a family that really does not care to change what would seem to be a sleep disturbance to others. Children with chronic, physically based sleep disorders, such as narcolepsy and breathing-related sleep disorder, will benefit from referral to a sleep center for treatment and group support.

Use of Alternative Medicine

Alternative therapies have been devised by many cultures to restore the essential health-giving function of sleep. Chamomile and other soothing teas are the most common. Any treatment that requires scheduled rest and mental expectation of sleep would be expected to result in improvement.

When to Hospitalize

Primary sleep disturbances should never require hospitalization other than the overnight stay needed for a sleep study. Hospitalization may be needed for some of the underlying disorders, such as CNS tumors or serious depression, that can present as sleep disturbances.

REFERENCES

1. Ali NJ, Pitson D, Stradling JR: Sleep disordered breathing: effects of adenotonsillectomy on behavior and psychological functioning, *Eur J Pediatr* 155:56, 1996.
2. Anders TF, Eiben LA: Pediatric sleep disorders: a review of the past 10 years, *J Am Acad Child Adolesc Psychiatry* 36:9, 1997.
3. Blader JC, et al: Sleep problems of elementary school children, *Arch Pediatr Adolesc Med* 151:473, 1997.
4. Corkum P, Tannock R, Moldofsky H: Sleep disturbances in children with attention-deficit/hyperactivity disorder, *J Am Acad Child Adolesc Psychiatry* 37:637, 1998.
5. Dahl R: Sleep in behavioral and emotional problems. In Ferber R, Kryger M, editors: *Principles and practice of sleep medicine in the child*, Philadelphia, 1995, WB Saunders.
6. Dahl RE, et al: Sleep onset abnormalities in depressed adolescents, *Biol Psychiatry* 39:400, 1996.
7. Glod CA, et al: Increased nocturnal activity and impaired sleep maintenance in abused children, *J Am Acad Child Adolesc Psychiatry* 36:1236, 1997.
8. Minde K, Faucon A, Falkner S: Sleep problems in toddlers: effects of treatment on their daytime behavior, *J Am Acad Child Adolesc Psychiatry* 33:1114, 1994.
9. Piazza CC, Fisher WW, Sherer M: Treatment of multiple sleep problems in children with developmental disabilities: faded bedtime with response cost versus bedtime scheduling, *Dev Med Child Neurol* 39:414, 1997.
10. Prince JB, et al: Clonidine for sleep disturbances associated with attention-deficit disorder: a systematic chart review of 62 cases, *J Am Acad Child Adolesc Psychiatry* 35:599, 1996.
11. Sadeh A, Anders T: Infant sleep problems: origins, assessment, interventions, *Infant Mental Health J* 14:17, 1993.
12. Sheldon SH: Pro-convulsant effects of oral melatonin in neurologically disabled children, *Lancet* 351(9111):1254, 1998.
13. Stores G: Practitioner review: assessment and treatment of sleep disorders in children and adolescents, *J Child Psychol Psychiatry* 37:907, 1996.
14. Stores G, Ellis AJ, Wiggs L, et al: Sleep and psychological disturbance in nocturnal asthma, *Arch Dis Child* 78:413, 1998.
15. Taira M, Takase M, Sasaki H: Sleep disorder in children with autism, *Psychiatry Clin Neurosci* 52:182, 1998.
16. Wiggs L, Stores G: Severe sleep disturbances and daytime challenging behavior, *J Intell Dis Res* 40:518, 1996.
17. Wolraich M, editor: *Diagnostic and statistical manual for primary care* (DSM-PC), *child and adolescent version*, 1996, American Academy of Pediatrics.
18. Zamir G, et al: Sleep fragmentation in children with juvenile rheumatoid arthritis, *J Rheumatology* 25:1191, 1998.

96 Stuttering

Pearl A. Gordon

Stuttering is a disorder in the continuity or flow of speech characterized by repetitions, prolongations of speech sounds, and abnormal pauses. Typically, stuttering is observed first during the preschool years as children are progressing through various stages of language development. Onset is typically reported in the early preschool years (2 to 5 years of age) and rarely is observed after puberty.[3] The disorder is more prevalent in males than females. Among school-age children the male-to-female ratio is 3:1, is lower at preschool age, and increases to about 4 or 5:1 among adults.[1] Although all children are disfluent, only 4% to 5% demonstrate true stuttering at some point in their lives. Most children will be disfluent only for a few months and show no reaction to it. Unfortunately, about 20% to 30% of those who begin to stutter will have a lifelong problem.[1] In general, the longer the stuttering continues, the greater the likelihood that the disorder will become chronic and increase in complexity and severity. This complexity usually includes a very individualized pattern of reactions to the disorder, including fear and avoidance of speech. The pattern of stuttering described above sometimes is called *developmental stuttering* to distinguish it from the much rarer type, *acquired stuttering*. The latter usually appears suddenly, long after speech and language skills have been developed, and is associated with neurological or psychological trauma.

When developmental stuttering is treated appropriately, especially in its beginning stages, the prognosis for recovery generally is good. The types of behaviors typically seen in advanced stuttering (severe struggling and fear of talking) usually can be prevented. Even adults who have stuttered for years often can learn to decrease the severity of their stuttering and improve their attitudes about speaking.

The prognosis for acquired stuttering is much less certain. The small number of cases and the wide differences in type of cortical damage or psychogenic trauma make prediction of recovery much more tenuous.[4]

ETIOLOGY

Despite much research, the specific causes of developmental stuttering are unknown. Findings from several studies suggest a weak genetic inheritance pattern. Both physiological and environmental factors appear to play a role in the origin and progression of stuttering.[3]

Considerable evidence exists indicating that developmental stuttering is related to children's efforts to learn to talk. Most young children experience a period of normal disfluencies. Parents frequently observe their children having difficulty "getting started" or frequently repeating a word, especially at the beginning of a phrase or sentence.[3] This pattern is typically observed between the ages of 2 and 5 years, when children are mastering speech and language skills rapidly. This overlap between the occurrence of normal disfluencies and onset of early stuttering presents a problem for both parents and professionals in the diagnosis of stuttering. Disfluencies in both stuttering and nonstuttering children are more likely to occur when the child is using more complex speech or language.[2] It long has been observed that many children who stutter have a history of slow speech and language development.[1]

A current explanation of childhood stuttering, useful for counseling parents, explains etiology by a "demands and capacities" model,[5] which states that stuttering develops when either internal or external demands for fluency exceed the child's capacities for fluent speech. This model allows for the variability of environmental demands (e.g., parental or self-imposed pressures for speech performance) that might exceed the child's capacities for fluent speech—capacities such as motor speech skills and cognitive and language abilities.

In contrast to the lack of definitive known causes for developmental stuttering, acquired stuttering usually has a neurogenic or, more rarely, a psychogenic origin. Neurogenic stuttering usually is a sequela of brain damage. No consistent pattern in type of damage (e.g., stroke, tumor, or disease) or site of lesion (hemisphere or lobe) has been found.[4]

DIFFERENTIAL DIAGNOSIS

At its onset, stuttering is difficult to differentiate from normally disfluent speech. All speakers are disfluent, and young children are even more likely to have interruptions in their speech. To differentiate stuttering from normally disfluent speech, it is necessary to estimate the frequency, duration, and type of disfluencies in the child's speech; observe the child's reactions to his or her stuttering; and determine the presence of struggling as the child tries to speak. Because stuttering frequently varies among children who stutter, it may be necessary to obtain much of this information by questioning the parents or parent-surrogates. The Physician's Checklist for Referral presented in Table 96-1 summarizes key criteria for determining if a child normally is disfluent or is showing signs of early stuttering. These criteria are expanded on below.

Table 96-1 Physician's Checklist for Referral

	Normal Disfluencies Age of Onset: 1½ to 7 Years of Age	Mild Stuttering Age of Onset: 1½ to 7 Years of Age	Severe Stuttering Age of Onset: 1½ to 7 Years of Age
Speech behaviors you may see or hear	Occasional (not more than once in every 10 sentences), brief (typical ½ second or shorter) repetitions of sounds, syllables, or short words (e.g., "li-li-like this")	Frequent (3% or more of speech), long (½ to 1 second) repetitions of sounds, syllables, or short words (e.g., "li-li-li-like this"); occasional prolongations of sounds	Very frequent (10% or more of speech) and often very long (1 second or longer) repetitions of sounds, syllables, or short words; frequent sound prolongations and blockages
Other behaviors you may see or hear	Occasional pauses, hesitations in speech, or fillers such as "uh," "er," or "um"; changing of words or thoughts	Repetitions and prolongations begin to be associated with eyelid closing and blinking, looking to the side, and some physical tension in and around the lips	Similar to mild stutterers only more frequent and noticeable; some rise in pitch of voice during stuttering; extra sounds or words used as "starters"
When problem is most noticeable	Come and go when child is tired, excited, talking about complex/new topics, asking or answering questions, or talking to unresponsive listeners	Come and go in similar situations but more often present than absent	Tends to be present in most speaking; far more consistent and nonfluctuating
Child reaction	None apparent	Some show little concern, some will be frustrated and embarrassed	Most are embarrassed and some also fear speaking
Parent reaction	None to a great deal	Most concerned, but concern may be minimal	All have some degree of concern
Referral decision	Refer only if parents moderately to overly concerned	Refer if continues for 6 to 8 weeks or if parental concern justifies it	Refer as soon as possible

Modified for use by permission of the Stuttering Foundation of America, Memphis, Tenn, 1-800-992-9392, www.stutteringhelp.org.

Normally Disfluent Speech

The repetitions usually are brief (typically ½ second or less) and occur infrequently (only once in 10 sentences), and there are no signs of struggle in speaking. Repetitions of a word or a phrase (rather than of a sound or syllable) are considered normal and often are associated with the search for a word (e.g., "Mommy, where is my, where is my—you know, my uh, twicycle?"). Disfluencies often increase when a child is excited or tired.

Early stuttering often occurs on the initial sound or syllable of a word; excess tension may be visible around the lips or eyes. There usually is little concern on the part of the child other than occasional embarrassment or frustration.

Stuttering is considered severe when the following conditions are found: stuttering is very frequent (on 10% or more of the words spoken), the repetitions are very rapid and uneven, sound prolongations or blockings typically last 1 second or longer, the child appears to struggle in his or her attempts to say a word, and fear or avoidance of speaking is evident.

EFFECTS OF STUTTERING

A child's initial reactions to stuttering usually are surprise and frustration. If the stuttering continues, the frustration can change to a fear of "being stuck." Because severe stuttering occurs in only about 1% of the population, many young children have difficulty understanding why they are different from others. In the primary grades a stuttering problem can make reading aloud difficult and interfere with the acquisition of reading skills. Stuttering may interfere with a child's learning in other ways. Many stuttering children will not ask or answer questions of a teacher, even when they want information or know the answers. The psychosocial aspects of stuttering are particularly insidious. School-age stutterers are frequent targets of teasing.[3] The embarrassment about stuttering usually increases in adolescence, and teens may begin to avoid social situations. Even adults who formerly stuttered often report feeling embarrassed and guilty about their use of tactics to avoid or conceal a problem, such as pretending to not have heard a question or substituting a word for one on which stuttering is anticipated.

REFERRAL

There is no need to refer a child whose speech is considered normally disfluent. However, there are some suggestions that one can give to parents at this point. They should be advised to reduce communication time pressure. This includes pausing briefly before responding to the child; using a slower, less hurried model in their own speech; avoiding bringing attention to the disfluencies; giving the child their full attention; and allowing the child plenty of time to say what he or she wants to say.

Children who stutter mildly should be referred to a speech-language pathologist (SLP)* if they have stuttered for 3 months or more or if the stuttering continues for a few weeks after the parents have been trying to follow the suggestions mentioned on the facing page.

If a child's speech meets the criteria for severe stuttering, he or she should be referred to a qualified SLP as soon as possible. The course of treatment may well last a year or more. The pediatrician can assist teenagers who stutter by showing an understanding for the difficulty they encounter but urging them not to let the stuttering prevent them from engaging in activities they otherwise would attempt. In the case of the older child who stutters, a qualified SLP is essential in aiding the child and parents to identify an appropriate course of speech therapy.

In the past, parents concerned about their child's stuttering frequently were advised to ignore the problem and told that the child would outgrow it eventually. Although it is true that many young children who have incipient stuttering become fluent without treatment, children whose speech is diagnosed appropriately as stuttering usually require professional attention from an SLP to avoid the long-term embarrassment and frustration of a stuttering problem that gets worse rather than better as the child gets older. The pediatrician often is the first professional to recognize stuttering in a child. If a child (or his or her parents) can be seen for therapy when the problem consists primarily of easy, effortless repetitions, the chances for success are much higher than when the stuttering has become complicated by habitual struggle, fear of speaking, and avoidance behaviors. The key to success is early identification and intervention.

*The SLP should hold a Certificate of Clinical Competence from the American Speech-Language-Hearing Association and be experienced in working with childhood stuttering.

Acknowledgment

Acknowledgment is given to Harold L. Luper, Ph.D., friend and mentor, who died in 1994. His chapter in the third edition of this textbook provided the basis for this current version.

REFERENCES

1. Bloodstein O: *A handbook on stuttering*, Chicago, 1995, National Easter Seal Society.
2. Gordon PA, Luper HL: Speech disfluencies in nonstutterers: syntactic complexity and production task effects, *J Fluency Disorders* 14:429, 1989.
3. Guitar B: *Stuttering: an integrated approach to its nature and treatment,* Baltimore, 1998, Williams & Wilkins.
4. Helms-Estabrooks N: Stuttering associated with acquired neurological disorders. In Curlee RF, editor: *Stuttering and related disorders of fluency,* New York, 1999, Thieme Medical Publications.
5. Starkweather CW, Gottwald SR, Halfond MM: *Stuttering prevention: a clinical method,* Englewood Cliffs, NJ, 1990, Prentice-Hall.

SUGGESTED READINGS

Fraser J, Perkins WH, editors: *Do you stutter? A guide for teens,* Memphis, 1987, Stuttering Foundation of America.

Guitar B: Is it stuttering or just normal language development? *Contemp Pediatr* Feb 1988, p 109.

Guitar B, Conture EG: *The child who stutters: to the pediatrician,* Memphis, 1991, Stuttering Foundation of America.

Siegel GM, Gold C: Principles and practices of current stuttering therapy. In Curlee RF, editor: *Stuttering and related disorders of fluency,* New York, 1999, Thieme Medical Publications.

ADDITIONAL RESOURCES

Printed materials, videos, and referral services are available from the Stuttering Foundation of America, 3100 Walnut Grove Road, Suite 603, Memphis, TN 38111-0749, www.stutteringhelp.org, or call 1-800-992-9392.

97 Temper Tantrums and Breath-Holding Spells

Gregory E. Prazar

TEMPER TANTRUMS

Temper tantrums represent a behavior that children exhibit almost inevitably during the second through fourth years of life. Therefore, this generally is a "problem behavior" rather than a "behavioral problem." Displays of temper can run the gamut from a verbalized "no" to dramatic breath-holding spells, during which the child may lose consciousness. Helping parents cope with temper tantrums involves providing anticipatory guidance, sharing information on developmental psychology, and offering strategies to deal with tantrums.

Temper tantrums usually become part of the child's emotional repertoire during the second and third years of life. Early signs of the negativism that is part of tantrums can be appreciated as early as 12 months of age. Some children continue to display occasional tantrums until the age of 5 or 6 years. Tantrums typically then reappear in a slightly less intense form during adolescence, when independence once more becomes an issue for the developing child.

Several aspects of the toddler's development appear to make tantrums almost inevitable. First, because the 1-year-old can walk and climb, the child begins to achieve physical mastery over the environment. This increased physical independence and an insatiable curiosity frequently place the child in dangerous situations that require parental intervention. Imposition of adult safety limits thwarts and frustrates the child, often precipitating tantrums. Second, the child's increased exploration of the environment immediately creates a conflict because he or she must adapt to rules of an adult world. The child enters a hostile environment of adult social values, where people are expected to use the bathroom appropriately, verbalize their dissatisfactions rather than "act" them out physically, sit quietly while eating, and sometimes subjugate their own wants to those of others. This is too much for the egocentric toddler to bear, and frustration is inevitable.

Third, between the ages of 1 and 4 years the toddler begins to develop an increased awareness of how he or she is separate and different from his or her mother. The child experiences a conflict between desires for autonomy and desires to remain close to the mother. Frustration in dealing with these intense feelings frequently results in tantrums.

Tensions, therefore, are created in "establishing ego boundaries as separate from those of parents," as Brazelton[1] states, and in coping with physical limitations placed on exploring an adult world. Adults frequently deal with their own tensions and frustrations by verbalizing their feelings; the toddler, however, lacks a sophisticated ability to verbalize. A toddler's frustration with the adult world may be displayed in doing the exact opposite of what the adult requests, by saying "no, no" yet following through with the adult request (what Fraiberg[3] refers to as the "cheerful no"), by dawdling, or by displaying physical behavior outright (e.g., kicking, screaming, lying on the floor, hitting, throwing, biting).

Most parents probably would agree that intellectual appreciation of the cause of tantrums does not necessarily aid in coping with a screaming and inconsolable child. Reasons for parental frustration are understandable. Well-meaning relatives and friends (who likely have forgotten their experience as young parents) may propagate myths about tantrums, which intensify parental anxiety and confusion. Myths of causation suggest that children who display tantrums are underdisciplined or parented by inadequate adults. Myths of management suggest that tantrums be quelled by spanking, dousing with cold water, or threats.

Anticipatory Guidance for Tantrums

It is the responsibility of the primary care physician to provide anticipatory guidance about temper tantrums. Such guidance may forestall events that precipitate tantrums and prevent future parental confusion in dealing with negative behaviors. The physician has many opportunities during the child's first 2 years to provide behavioral counseling.

At the 6-month infant visit the importance of time away from the infant should be emphasized. Parents who occasionally leave their infants and toddlers with responsible babysitters provide their children with the security that adults can leave and *will* come back; they also provide themselves with important mental health holidays from the rigors of parenting.

At the 9- or 12-month infant visit, environmental engineering should be discussed. The importance of home safety (e.g., safety plugs in outlets, safety latches on drawers), the removal of valuables or breakables from the child's reach, and the availability of a safe place for the child to play (playpen or enclosed area) are examples of such engineering. Therefore, this visit not only may reduce chances for childhood accidents but also it may forestall potential adult-toddler power struggles over environmental dangers.

The 15- or 18-month visit provides the physician another opportunity to offer the parent alternatives to negative interactions with the toddler. Afternoon naps (to allow for renewal of toddler and parental energy), the importance of praising cooperative toddler efforts, and the concept of limited decision making for the toddler ("Do you want to wear the green or blue shirt today?" versus "Which shirt do you want to wear today?") represent issues that may help parents minimize hostile encounters with their toddler.

The approach here should be one that encourages parents to describe how they believe tantrums should be handled rather than one that displays the physician's personal biases about child rearing. Several excellent books describing turbulent toddlerhood can be suggested to parents, including Brazelton's *Toddlers and Parents,*[1] Ilg and Ames' *Child Behavior,*[4] and Schmitt's *Your Child's Health.*[8] Furthermore, general guidelines concerning tantrums can be given. Tantrums are best ignored unless, as Fraiberg[3] states, "they encroach on rights of others or potentially endanger." If safety is the issue, either environmental engineering should take place or the child should be restricted to his or her room for 2 to 3 minutes (a kitchen timer is helpful to remind both parent and toddler of the time). If the child hits, bites, or throws in anger, room restriction for 2 to 3 minutes once again should be suggested. Some behavioral psychologists suggest 1 minute of time out for each year of age (therefore, a 5-year-old child would have a 5-minute time-out). Other behaviorists recommend that time-out not be fixed. Because the goal is to help the child develop "self-regulation," the time-out should end when the tantrum subsides.[5] The child should receive a brief hug or be praised and then be allowed to resume his or her previous activity.

Parents may be reluctant to use bedroom restriction because they worry either that the child will associate the bedroom with unpleasant experiences or that the child will not feel adequately remorseful if placed in a room full of toys. Parents should be reassured that room restriction does not cause bedroom fears. Similarly, goals of discipline are to teach rules and to help the child understand which behaviors are acceptable. Discipline does not need to be severe to be effective.

Time-outs are an effective method of dealing with temper tantrums. Time-ins represent a method to reward acceptable behavior. Specifically, when a toddler is playing quietly, the parent should pat the child on the shoulder, give a brief hug, or otherwise offer some form of nonverbal affection. Such attention from the parent indicates simply but effectively approval of the current behavior. Some behavioral psychologists believe that time-ins are a more powerful method of encouraging acceptable behavior than are time-outs.

Temper tantrums occur much more frequently in the presence of parents; they are much less common in the presence of alternative care providers. Most experienced child care providers feel comfortable dealing with temper tantrums. If the child care provider expresses concern to a parent about a child's temper tantrums, several questions should be considered. Does the child care provider have adequate training to deal with such a common behavior? Is this child care setting the most appropriate for the child (in terms of adult-child ratio, philosophy of discipline used by the provider, and realistic developmental expectations for the child's behavior in the child care setting)? Are the child's temper tantrums much more severe or frequent than those of his or her peers? These questions should be addressed with the child care provider. Subsequently, parents and the child care provider should formulate a plan for dealing with the tantrums that is followed consistently at home *and* at the child care location. If the parent and the child care provider cannot agree on such a plan, the child's primary practitioner should be consulted.

More specific guidelines for managing tantrums may be necessary in other individual situations. Parents should be encouraged by the physician to ventilate their feelings (to the physician) about tantrums and reassured that they are doing the best job they can for their toddler.

Management of Problem Tantrums

Although tantrums represent a stage of the normal developing toddler personality, several factors suggest that further professional intervention is advisable. Toddlers who display persistent negativism or tantrums may suffer from too restrictive parenting, may receive too little positive reinforcement and affection, or may have parents who place unreasonable behavioral expectations on them. One study of 3-year-olds defined severe temper tantrums as "episodes of shouting, banging, kicking, or screaming occurring three or more times a day or lasting more than 15 minutes."[7] Approximately 50% of these children had behavior problems. Furthermore, such severe tantrums were associated with specific psychosocial issues, including maternal depression, use of corporal punishment, marital stress, and low maternal education.

Children who display tantrums regularly beyond 5 or 6 years of age may be displaying signs of depression or poor self-esteem, or they may be children who live in a family in which emotional problems exist. When temper tantrums regularly occur at school, academic problems should be suspected, because peer pressure usually inhibits displays of tantrums.

Children exhibiting persistent tantrums along with other associated behaviors (e.g., inability to concentrate, stereotypical behaviors, unrealistic fears, inability to display affection) may have underlying emotional problems. Similarly, parents who verbalize persistent frustration with tantrums or an inability to cope with age-appropriate tantrums may need more comprehensive counseling than the primary practitioner can provide.

Many parenting groups are available to help parents cope with negative behaviors. Programs such as Systematic Training for Effective Parenting (STEP) and Parent Effectiveness Training (PET) provide valuable community referral sources for families. If such services are not available or if it is obvious that more sophisticated professional counseling is warranted, the family should be referred to a psychiatrically trained counselor.

Referral should be discussed as soon as the physician anticipates its necessity and should stress the involvement of *both* parents. The physician should maintain contact with the family about the problem after the referral has been made. Such ongoing contact may solidify the family's commitment to obtain and comply with the counseling (see Chapter 83, Consultation and Referral for Behavioral and Developmental Problems).

BREATH-HOLDING SPELLS

Breath-holding spells represent a childhood behavior that causes particular anxiety for parents. Spells occur between ages 4 months and 5 years, with most occurring between 12 and 18 months of age. According to Menkes,[6] approximately 5% of all children display breath-holding spells. A positive family history of breath-holding spells occurs in approximately 25% of cases.

Such spells are precipitated by anger, frustration, fear, or minor injury (often a very minor head injury) and are categorized as cyanotic or pallid. Both types of spells are unlikely to occur more often than once a day and are not associated with an increased predisposition to epilepsy (although brief seizurelike activity can occur as a terminating event in either form of spell).

Cyanotic breath-holding spells are precipitated more often by anger or frustration than by fear or injury. The child emits a short, loud cry, takes a deep breath, and holds it. Cyanosis occurs after approximately 30 seconds. Either the episode terminates at this point or the child becomes rigid or limp and loses consciousness (loss of consciousness occurs in approximately 50% of all children who have breath-holding spells). In rare situations, mild clonic movements of the extremities follow.

Pallid breath-holding spells are similar to cyanotic spells in most respects but more often are precipitated by fear or minor injury. The initial cry is brief or silent. The spell then proceeds as with a cyanotic spell. Toddlers who suffer from pallid spells often are from families that have a history of syncope and, in fact, themselves have an increased chance of syncopal attacks as adults.

Both cyanotic and pallid breath-holding spells are caused by autonomic nervous system dysregulation. Cerebral anoxia is responsible for spells that terminate with loss of consciousness. Furthermore, both forms of spells are involuntary and reflexive, despite spells often being precipitated when the child is angry or frustrated.

Children who display pallid breath-holding spells may, as adults, suffer from neurocardiogenic syncope. Neurocardiogenic syncope is a form of vasovagal response to postural changes. Adults who suffer from neurocardiogenic syncope are more likely to faint at the sight of blood or when injured than are adults who do not have this disorder.

Because both forms of breath-holding spells potentially can terminate with seizurelike movements, differentiation between spells and epilepsy is important. Patients who have epilepsy, when they have seizures, display cyanosis during or after the seizures, not before seizure onset. Furthermore, electroencephalograms (EEGs) performed on patients who suffer from breath-holding spells are normal during non-breath-holding periods; patients who have epilepsy often have abnormal EEGs during seizure-free periods.

Management of Breath-Holding

No effective medical therapy exists for breath-holding spells, although some toddlers who experience seizurelike activity along with spells are prescribed anticonvulsant therapy. However, the decision to use medication remains controversial among pediatric neurologists.

Iron-deficiency anemia has been associated with breath-holding spells. A study involving 67 children who had breath-holding spells revealed that iron therapy reduced spells in the treatment group by 88%. These results suggest that iron may be important in the regulation of the autonomic nervous system.[2]

Coping with breath-holding spells can be extremely difficult for parents. Spells that terminate with loss of consciousness or with seizurelike movements obviously are frightening. Convincing parents that no harm will come to their child is important. Nevertheless, parents of a breath-holder frequently will not enforce limits for fear of precipitating the child's anger and a subsequent attack. Such parents need repeated reassurance and encouragement to continue age-appropriate limits on their child's behavior. To do otherwise will create an overindulged child who subsequently may fear loss of parental love because limits have been rescinded.

When to refer a breath-holding patient to a neurologist or a psychiatrically trained professional may not be an easy decision for the physician. If parents request further consultation, their wish certainly should be respected, even if the physician is confident that further evaluation is unnecessary. If parents indicate agreement with the physician that spells are of no consequence yet continue to withhold appropriate limit-setting, referral to a mental health professional should take place. The physician who is unsure of the diagnosis of breath-holding (especially in situations in which loss of consciousness or seizurelike activity occurs) always should refer the family to a pediatric neurologist. Referral must not end the physician-parent communication concerning the spells, however, because an ongoing dialogue may ensure compliance with the referral.

SUMMARY

Temper tantrums and breath-holding spells usually represent benign forms of childhood behavior, evolving from the child's preverbal attempts to express feelings of frustration and anger. Unfortunately, parents frequently find it difficult to appreciate the benign course of such behaviors when they daily must face a screaming, inconsolable toddler who may even lose consciousness and then display seizurelike movements. Parents can best deal with negative behaviors when they are adequately prepared by the physician before such behaviors occur and when they are offered empathic guidance and positive reinforcement during regular office visits.

REFERENCES

1. Brazelton TB: *Toddlers and parents,* New York, 1989, Dell.
2. Daoud AS, et al: Effectiveness of iron therapy on breath-holding spells, *J Pediatr* 130:547, 1997.
3. Fraiberg S: *The magic years,* New York, 1996, Charles Scribner's Sons.
4. Ilg FL, Ames LB: *Child behavior,* New York, 1992, Harper & Row.
5. Levine MD, Carey WB, Crocker AC: *Developmental and behavioral pediatrics,* Philadelphia, 1993, WB Saunders.
6. Menkes JH: *Textbook of child neurology,* ed 2, Philadelphia, 1995, Lea & Febiger.
7. Needlman R, Stevenson J, Zuckerman B: Psychosocial correlates of severe temper tantrums, *J Dev Behav Pediatr* 12:77, 1991.
8. Schmitt B: *Your child's health,* New York, 1991, Bantam Books.

98 Adolescence

W. Sam Yancy

Adolescence generally is defined as the period of psychological growth and development during the transition from childhood to adulthood. Physical growth and development, or pubescence, also occur during this period. Many of these changes can be confusing for both teenagers and the adults who care for them. "Rebellious" and "tumultuous" are negative adjectives often associated with this age group; "joyous" and "carefree" are more positive adjectives also used to describe adolescents. In 1989, the U.S. Public Health Service, having collaborated with a consortium of more than 300 national organizations and all 50 state departments of health, presented a broad-based plan to improve the health of all Americans. *Healthy People 2000: The National Health Promotion and Disease Prevention Objectives* outlines a 10-year course for individual, collective, and environmental change. From this work, numerous projects to promote the objectives for the improvement of adolescent health have been instigated by many groups and organizations, including the American Medical Association, the American Academy of Pediatrics, and the Society for Adolescent Medicine (Healthier Youth by 2000 Project, Guidelines for Adolescent Preventive Services,[4] Partners in Program Planning for Adolescent Health). It is discouraging to note that a mid-decade review reveals little change toward meeting objectives for physical activity and fitness, nutrition, smoking, alcohol and substance abuse, family planning, and suicide.[5] Recent information from the National Center for Health Statistics, however, does report that the birth rate among girls 15 to 19 years old dropped 16% from 1991 to 1997, most likely because of increased contraceptive use. Although it is unlikely that Healthy Youth 2000 objectives will be met, it is encouraging that there appears to be increased recognition of the needs of youth and a greater understanding of this age group.

Efforts on behalf of adolescents have come about not necessarily because of increasing problems in this age group and certainly not because of increasing demands by teenagers themselves, but because adolescents' unmet needs have been recognized. It was believed formerly that this was a carefree, healthy age, one that required no special interest from health care professionals. This is no longer true. Citing vital statistics data, Blum[1] reported in 1987 that violence has replaced communicable diseases as the chief cause of mortality among teenagers and that more than 75% of adolescent deaths are caused by accidents, suicide, and homicide. Subsequent reports from the Centers for Disease Control and Prevention have shown no improvement.[2] The prevalence of sexually transmitted disease, pregnancy, substance abuse, suicide, delinquency, chronic illness, mental illness, and school problems cannot be ignored.[7,8] The ability to provide preventive and therapeutic programs for the medical and psychological problems related to these high-risk behaviors requires practitioners who are knowledgeable about normal adolescent development and about adolescent behaviors that concern these patients and their parents. Diagnosis and treatment of the physical and psychosocial problems of adolescents, as well as early recognition of risk factors and appropriate anticipatory guidance, should be incorporated into the practice of all primary care physicians. A new site for the delivery of health care to adolescents, the school-based or school-linked clinic, may afford additional comprehensive care for this age group,[6] and a new format for diagnostic coding will be of much benefit to primary care and mental health practitioners who treat adolescents who have mental health problems.[9] *The Diagnostic and Statistical Manual for Primary Care (DSM-PC) Child and Adolescent Version* includes consideration of the different presentation of problems during the various developmental stages of childhood and adolescence and provides codes for a broader spectrum of problems than is included in previous classifications. This manual should assist practitioners in the early recognition of mental health problems and provide them with diagnostic descriptions and codes for common developmental and behavioral problems that require intervention but do not meet criteria for inclusion in *The Diagnostic and Statistical Manual, Fourth Edition (DSM-IV)*.

Although attention was focused on the health care needs of adolescents in England as early as the late 1800s, it was not until the 1930s that significant reports about this age group began to appear in the U.S. medical literature. And it was not until 1951 that the first separate hospital inpatient adolescent unit was established, at Boston Children's Hospital. Progress in the area of adolescent medicine is outlined in Box 98-1.

Pediatricians have led the way in providing health care for adolescents. In 1980, the report of the Task Force on Pediatric Education[3] called for more training in adolescent medi-

BOX 98-1

PROGRESS IN ADOLESCENT MEDICINE

1938: Publication of Greulich WW, et al: A handbook of methods for the study of adolescent children, *Monogr Soc Res Child Dev*, vol 3, no 2, serial no 13, Washington, DC.
1941: Publication of American Academy of Pediatrics: Symposium on adolescence, *J Pediatr* 19:289, 1941.
1951: Boston Children's Hospital establishes the first hospital adolescent unit.
1965: The *Journal of Pediatrics* lists four fellowship programs for adolescent medicine.
1968: The Society for Adolescent Medicine is founded. Also, federal funding of training programs in adolescent medicine is established through the Division of Maternal and Child Health of the Department of Health, Education, and Welfare.
1975: The First International Symposium on Adolescent Medicine is held in Helsinki.
1977: The American Medical Association (AMA) recognizes adolescent medicine as a specialty.
1978: The National Conference on Adolescent Behavior and Health is established as part of the National Academy of Sciences' Institute of Medicine.
1979: The American Academy of Pediatrics (AAP) creates its Section on Adolescent Health.
1980: The first volume of the *Journal of Adolescent Health Care* is published (the name is changed to the *Journal of Adolescent Health* in 1992).
1986: Health Futures of Youth, a national invitational conference, is held to develop an action plan for research, demonstration programming, and training.
1987: The International Association for Adolescent Health is founded.
1988: The AMA's First Annual National Congress on Adolescent Health is held in Chicago.
1994: The first certifying examination in adolescent medicine is administered by the American Board of Pediatrics and the American Board of Internal Medicine.
1998: *The Journal of Adolescent Health* lists 33 fellowship training programs in adolescent medicine.

cine. The Pediatric Residency Review Committee of the Accreditation Council for Graduate Medical Education requires all pediatric residency programs to include training in adolescent medicine. Also, 95% of all adolescent medicine fellowship training programs and divisions of adolescent medicine are based in pediatrics departments. Similar progress is now being made in departments of internal medicine and family practice.

Teenagers are cared for by professionals in many disciplines other than pediatrics (e.g., internists, obstetrician-gynecologists, psychiatrists, psychologists, family physicians, social workers, nurses, and educators). The new Subspecialty Board for Adolescent Medicine was developed by the American Board of Pediatrics and the American Board of Internal Medicine, and efforts are under way to include family physicians. The most effective health care programs for young people depend on collaboration among all interested disciplines to provide comprehensive care for these patients (see Chapter 99, Challenges of Health Care Delivery to Adolescents).

REFERENCES

1. Blum R: Contemporary threats to adolescent health in the United States, *JAMA* 257:3390, 1987.
2. Centers for Disease Control and Prevention: Mortality trends, causes of death, and related risk behaviors among US adolescents, CDC Pub No 099-4112, Atlanta, 1993, CDC.
3. Cohen MI: Importance, implementation, and impact of the adolescent medicine components of the report of the Task Force on Pediatric Education, *J Adolesc Health Care* 1:1, 1980.
4. Elster AB, Kuznets NJ: *AMA guidelines for adolescent preventive services (GAPS),* Chicago, 1992, American Medical Association.
5. Fleming M: *Healthy youth 2000: a mid-decade review,* Chicago, 1996, American Medical Association.
6. Fothergill K, Ballard E: The school-linked health center: a promising model of community-based care for adolescents, *J Adolesc Health* 23:29, 1998.
7. Hein K: *Issues in adolescent health: an overview,* Washington, DC, 1988, Carnegie Council on Adolescent Development.
8. Wilson MD, Joffe A: Adolescent medicine, *JAMA* 273:1657, 1995.
9. Wolraich ML, editor: *Diagnostic and statistical manual for primary care (DSM-PC) child and adolescent version,* Elk Grove Village, Ill, 1996, American Academy of Pediatrics.

SUGGESTED READINGS

Cromer BA, McLean CS, Heald FP: A critical review of comprehensive health screening in adolescents, *J Adolesc Health* (suppl)13:3S, 1992.

Marks A, Fisher M: Health assessment and screening during adolescence, *Pediatrics* (suppl)80:135, 1987.

Rosen DS, et al: Clinical preventive services for adolescents, *J Adolesc Health* 21:203, 1997.

99 Challenges of Health Care Delivery to Adolescents

Richard E. Kreipe

Several challenges threaten health care delivery to contemporary adolescents. First is the inherently unsteady nature of adolescence itself, the transitional stage between childhood and adulthood.[17] Developmentally, adolescents share characteristics of both children and adults, often vacillating from one extreme to the other, depending on circumstances. Therefore, they are not accommodated easily by health care designed for younger or for older individuals. Second is the nature of the problems threatening their health. The causes of mortality and morbidity for adolescents at this time are related largely to modifiable behaviors[15] rather than to diseases such as polio or congenital heart disease. Thus, health care should focus on prevention rather than on treatment. Our ability to treat most conditions generally exceeds our ability to prevent them, but a body of knowledge is emerging because of research focused on changing health-related behaviors in adolescents. Third is the highly variable contexts of health care delivery—the settings in which it occurs as well as the practitioners who render the care.[9] For example, ambulatory settings include private physician's offices, hospital clinics, school-based clinics, and private agencies. In addition, adolescents may receive care in free clinics that emphasize confidential services; homeless youth may receive care from a mobile van. Likewise, the clinician providing these services can range from a board-certified adolescent medicine physician to a youth worker. The wide variety of settings and providers, with little in the way of standardization or best-practice models, represents a major challenge to the delivery of consistently high-quality health care to adolescents. Fourth is the "system" in which health care is delivered.[1] Issues related to health insurance and other factors affecting the ability of adolescents to benefit from services are being addressed but continue to offer significant obstacles to improving the health of adolescents.

This chapter addresses each of these four factors, noting not only the challenges but also the opportunities in each of these areas for improving health care delivered to adolescents. The dedication to improving the health of infants and children must be carried forward for adolescents as well. Although many pediatricians prefer caring for prepubertal patients, it is important to note that the American Academy of Pediatrics (AAP) is dedicated to improving the health of infants, children, adolescents, and young adults. Improving the health of adolescents and young adults often requires strong advocacy and innovative methods. However, the challenges regarding health care delivery to adolescents are not insurmountable, if the emphasis is on the word "care." As Peabody noted more than 70 years ago, the secret of patient care is in caring for the patient.[14]

DEVELOPMENTAL ISSUES RELATED TO ADOLESCENCE

Tanner has observed that the only thing constant about adolescence is change.[16] Within the realm of pubertal changes, there is a well-recognized sequence of events of sexual maturation for boys and for girls, but the timing of the onset and the velocity of the tempo are highly variable from individual to individual. Thus, normal 12-year-olds can range from having no secondary sex characteristics to full sexual maturation. Recent evidence indicates that girls experience the onset of breast development up to 2 years earlier than they did a generation ago.[8] This is important because girls who develop earlier are at greater risk of engaging in high-risk health behaviors than are those who develop later and because girls who develop precociously sexually may not be mature cognitively. Likewise, androgen levels may account for some aggressive behaviors in males. None of the psychosocial aspects of adolescence necessarily is synchronous with each other or with sexual maturation. Those delivering health care need to be aware of these developmental issues; failure to appreciate the highly dynamic nature of adolescents' developmental experience will most likely hinder the provision of care to them.

The emergence of independence and autonomy—hallmarks of adolescence—also affects health care delivery.[4] Adolescents who have not yet reached the age of majority have legal rights to seek health care without parental consent, as determined by several factors, including (1) their status as an "emancipated" or as a "mature" minor, (2) the nature of the condition for which they are seeking confidential care, and (3) the laws governing their state of residence. Confidential health care tends to be sought most commonly for conditions that are highly charged emotionally, such as reproductive health care. To the degree that an adolescent's right to confidential health care is honored, his or her parents may feel excluded and argue that their parental rights and responsibilities are not being honored. Health care clinicians, especially family practitioners or others who provide care for both adolescents and adults in a family, may be caught in the middle of this conflict. It sometimes is difficult to determine the best interest of the adolescent in such situations. Nonadherence to treatment, especially for chronic illnesses such as diabetes, HIV, or cystic fibrosis, that requires a complex regimen often emerges during adolescence as a manifestation of autonomy—the adolescent not wanting to be told what to do or "using" the disease as a "weapon" in conflict with parents.

Alternatively, nonadherence to a treatment may be related to cognitive limitation imposed by an adolescent being "concrete operational" in his or her thinking. For example, a 15-year-old who has pelvic inflammatory disease might be encouraged by a physician to complete her 14-day course of antibiotics to prevent infertility. After taking the medication for 2 days, she might stop treatment because she feels well. However, she also might interpret the warning about infertility to mean that she no longer needs to use birth control, because she now is infertile. A better method to increase adherence would be to warn about the possibility of chronic pain or internal scarring if she does not complete treatment. The delivery of health care to adolescents should take into consideration the cognitive functioning (including the literacy) of each patient and adapt education and interventions accordingly.

Finally, identity development, sometimes characterized as the "essence of adolescence," can present a challenge to professionals delivering health care to individuals in this age group. As the major task of adolescence, identity development generally occurs in the context of a peer group, which can mean that it is attended by various high-risk behaviors. Not only can this predispose individuals to sexually transmitted diseases, unintended pregnancy, violence, substance abuse, and addiction, but also it can make obtaining the history extremely difficult. For example, if a girl has been forbidden by her parents to see her boyfriend, she may deny sexual activity with him; if a boy is a member of an athletic team that uses drugs, he may not be willing to admit to substance use. Likewise, a male who has an emerging homosexual sexual orientation may have numerous concerns related to health and be engaging in high-risk behaviors but not be able to bring these issues up spontaneously with a health care practitioner. Thus, the developmental aspects of adolescence themselves present significant challenges to the delivery of health care in several domains.

However, not all developmental challenges should be seen as barriers to the delivery of care. For example, adolescents focusing on their own identities are normally very self-centered or ego-centric. Instead of viewing this as a narcissistic shortcoming of the patient, the clinician can make use of it by offering authoritative advice to help the adolescent feel better about herself or himself, rather than an authoritarian prescription of what must be done. Alternatively, adolescents often modify their physical appearance as a personal statement. Multicolored hair, body piercings, tattoos, and kooky clothes all relate to the emerging individual's sense of self (even if he or she assumes an appearance that is remarkably similar to peers). For health care professionals, the challenge is to continue to respect the adolescent, regardless of how outlandish or unusual he or she may appear, and to seek the positive qualities and assets that each adolescent possesses. A patient recently came to clinic wearing a shirt displaying the message, "I dress this way to bother you." An appropriate response to this might be for clinicians to remind themselves, "Be not provoked."

CAUSES OF MORBIDITY AND MORTALITY AMONG ADOLESCENTS

More than 75% of the mortality among adolescents is caused by motor vehicle accidents, homicide, or suicide—most of which is preventable and generally related to behavior. The morbidity caused by violence; sexually transmitted diseases, including HIV; pregnancy; substance abuse; eating disorders; and obesity also is linked to modifiable behaviors. However, we have not yet discovered an effective way to prevent most of these health problems.[1] The "content" of adolescent health care must focus on their behaviors, knowledge, and attitudes rather than on their diseases, because adolescents generally are healthy and notably free of disease. However, the training of physicians often is focused on the diagnosis and treatment of "disease," with less attention to helping patients change behavior so as to prevent health problems. In addition, mental health concerns, such as depression, are important threats to the health of adolescents. Thus, many conditions affecting the health of adolescents are not easily preventable, may be resistant to treatment, or may require interventions that clinicians are unable to provide.

Moreover, health problems of adolescents may elicit from adults (e.g., parents, teachers, health care professionals, community leaders, elected officials) negative responses, labeling, and stereotyping. Because they are no longer children but not yet adults and because they may exercise their adult "rights" without displaying concomitant adult responsibilities when it comes to their health, adolescents do not create a cohesive constituency and have little advocacy on their behalf. As a result, they often are marginalized in society.

Given the nature of health problems facing contemporary adolescents, it is not unusual for health care practitioners to feel unprepared to address either the problems or the adolescents who must contend with them.[7] Thus, adolescent health care requires a high degree of self-awareness on the part of professionals providing care. Moreover, they need to have training and experience related specifically to the care of adolescents. This is available through publications, continuing education services, and programs by professional organizations, such as the American Academy of Pediatrics (http://www.aap.org) or the Society for Adolescent Medicine (http://www.adolescenthealth.org), as well as through numerous university medical centers that provide hands-on or distance-learning opportunities in adolescent health.

In response to the need for greater efforts at prevention of morbidity and mortality among adolescents, different comprehensive preventive strategies have been developed, most notably the American Medical Association's *Guidelines for Adolescent Preventive Services* (*GAPS*, http://www.ama-assn.org/adolhlth/adolhlth.htm) and the Maternal and Child Health Bureau's *Bright Futures Guidelines* (http://www.brightfutures.org/). These structure both initial and follow-up health supervision visits by providing paper forms that patients and parents complete, as well as specific questions that clinicians can use in assessment and management.

CONTEXTS (SETTINGS AND PROVIDERS) OF HEALTH SERVICE DELIVERY TO ADOLESCENTS

As the concept of health care expands to include services to adolescents that are more preventive and as the specific needs of various populations create a demand to develop "alternative" methods of providing services, the settings in which health services are delivered to adolescents can no longer be described in the simple dichotomy of "doctor's office" or "hospital bed." There is a wide variability of service settings and an even wider variability of service professionals. For example, within the category of private office, the physician might be a pediatrician, internist, or family practitioner, each of whom have different training in adolescent health. Even within the domain of pediatrics, the adolescent may be seen by a physician who has had no formal training and no interest in adolescent medicine or by a board-certified subspecialist in adolescent medicine. In addition, nurse practitioners and physician's assistants often provide health care to adolescents, depending on the type of setting (e.g., college health- or institution-based care) and geographical location.

School-based clinics offer many advantages over the other settings, most notably convenience, ready access, and the ability to minimize school absence.[11,13] Because schools represent a focal point of youth activity for many communities, some argue for "full-service schools," meaning that not only would education take place there but also health services could be rendered, after-school activities could be offered, and other family members would be welcomed.[2] This has special advantages for inner-city communities that offer little in the way of quality health care or safe out-of-school activities to their residents. Although there are many obstacles in the development of full-service schools, Dryfoos has highlighted examples of success in this regard.[2] The challenge is to get the community involved in the program, which generally requires a dedicated leader in the school.

Because of the public nature of schools, political controversy often surrounds school-based health services, especially related to reproductive health care. For example, the use of condoms is considered a central element in the reduction of unintended pregnancy and sexually transmitted diseases (STDs) for sexually active adolescents (recognizing that condoms are not 100% effective in preventing the transmission of human papillomavirus). On the other hand, abstinence-only proponents argue that providing condoms to adolescents encourages all adolescents to be sexually active; in response, proponents of condom use may let adolescents know where condoms are available, rather than distribute them in school.[6]

The variety of settings can be seen as a challenge or as an opportunity. For example, homeless "street" youth constitute an extremely high-risk, yet largely underserved, group with respect to health. Because the needs of these adolescents cannot be met in traditional medical settings, leaders in cities such as Seattle, Los Angeles, and New York have established programs that include free clinics that have late evening hours, links with community-based youth workers, mobile units that provide information and services, and telephone hotlines, as well as job-training, high school equivalency education, and referral to adolescent-friendly specialists. Likewise, obstetrical or gynecology services often are clustered in a clinic specifically for adolescents, but with adolescent obstetrical services provided at times different than adolescent gynecological services. This recognizes the differences between pregnant teens and adults (e.g., greater need for assistance with high school education, nutrition assistance, child care, and transportation), as well as the difference between the obstetrical and gynecological needs of teens.

Regardless of the outpatient setting, several considerations need to be given to the needs of adolescents.[12] In pediatrics, for example, it is optimal for them to have a waiting area that is adolescent oriented, with minimal evidence that they will be seeing a "baby doctor." Contemporary posters, magazines, and patient education materials should focus on adolescents in a positive light. The AAP has many adolescent health brochures and pamphlets available. Researchers are developing interactive computer-based programs that can obtain important aspects of medical history and provide immediate feedback to the adolescent while he or she is waiting for a scheduled appointment and then to the professional during the visit. Such innovative technology can serve several purposes simultaneously: entertaining, educating, and medical record keeping. With respect to appointments, it is optimal to arrange schedules at times when teens will not need to miss school (e.g., late afternoon and early evening) and when only other adolescents will be in the waiting room.

Perhaps the most important aspect of making an outpatient setting attractive to adolescents, however, is the attitude of the receptionist toward adolescents. The first impression that teenagers get from their reception, whether on the telephone or on being greeted in person, strongly influences their overall experience and may even determine whether the appointment is kept. When adolescents perceive that they are welcomed and respected, a positive tone is set for their visit. Feeling negatively regarded can be a barrier that may cause them to approach the visit negatively or to "blow off" the visit entirely. In such circumstances, the skills and training of the health care professional are irrelevant because the staff has made him or her "inaccessible" to the adolescent. Unfortunately, this often is most likely to occur for patients who are most in need of care.

INPATIENT HEALTH CARE DELIVERY

Most hospitals, even large, university-based facilities, do not have a distinct adolescent inpatient unit. Despite the advantages of being able to create a therapeutic adolescent-oriented milieu and to develop a professional staff that has expertise working with this challenging age group in an adolescent unit,[5] most institutions have neither the critical mass of specialists who have experience (or interest) in adolescent health care nor an average census of adolescent patients to sustain such a unit. Thus, adolescents tend to be admitted to hospital units based on their age (to pediatrics) or their admitting diagnosis (e.g., to orthopedics for a fractured femur or to psychiatry for depression). This can result in additional challenges in delivering appropriate inpatient services. For example, in some hospitals the age limit for pediatrics is 16 years old, resulting in middle adolescents being admitted to a unit in which the average patient is older than 50 years. This can be less than optimal for the adolescent, for the adult patients, and for the professional staff working there. This is especially true if the adolescent also has behavioral problems, which tend to become more prominent under the stress of hospitalization.

Hospitalizing adolescents on units based on the admitting diagnosis can present other challenges. For example, orthopedic units generally are unprepared to address the psychosocial needs of a 15-year-old boy who has attention deficit/hyperactivity disorder who breaks his femur driving a car while intoxicated and having no license. Without an understanding of his need for concrete, concise, and clear explanations of any treatment planned, for consistent and reasonable limits on behavior (his and his visitor friends), for a sense of control over his environment when he is rendered relatively vulnerable as a result of his injury, and for the need to express his feelings in socially acceptable and productive ways, the hospital unit staff may respond to expected behavior with escalating frustration or punitive restrictions. Even when adolescents are admitted to a pediatric unit—possibly even "cohorted" with other adolescents—they may not have their psychosocial needs met if they have chronic symptoms or undiagnosed conditions. If the staff is not aware of the mental health needs of these adolescents, especially those who have life-threatening conditions or somatic symptoms such as headache or abdominal pain, opportunities to help the patient may be missed. For example, the "rule-out" approach, in which an adolescent is admitted for a battery of tests or procedures but finally is judged to have a "psychosomatic" condition because of a "negative" work-up, rarely is of much benefit. The biopsychosocial model recognizes the complex interplay between biological, psychological, and social factors and includes mental health issues in considering the differential diagnosis and treatment for each patient.

Even if a hospital does not have a geographically distinct adolescent unit, several things can be done to improve adolescent inpatient services. First, it is advisable to have a recreation room in which adolescents can congregate for social interaction and leisure activity. It usually is best for this to be sufficiently far away from patient rooms that noise levels will not bother other patients. Second, having a "child life" professional on the unit staff will ensure that developmentally appropriate activities are available and that the psychosocial needs of hospitalized adolescents (such as keeping up with schoolwork) are identified. Third, the importance of developing a daily schedule for, and with, hospitalized adolescents cannot be overestimated, especially for anyone in the hospital for more than 3 days. This provides structure and predictability and also enhances the adolescent's sense of control. Fourth, regardless of the length of stay, a unit should have clear "rules" for adolescents regarding visitors, timing of various activities, leaving the unit, and doing schoolwork. It is better to emphasize what the adolescent is encouraged to do rather than to list a series of "don'ts." Fifth, in the absence of a geographically distinct unit, it is best to "cohort" adolescents together, rather than distribute them throughout a pediatric inpatient service. Sixth, a close working relationship with one or more physicians who have subspecialty training in adolescent medicine provides important support in staff development and consultation services. Now that the American Board of Pediatrics has required at least a 1-month elective in adolescent medicine for pediatric residents during their training, most institutions have such a specialist, albeit often as a part-time faculty member. Seventh, mental health consultation needs to be readily available. Such consultation may be patient- or staff-oriented. That is, the mental health services often are requested not only to address diagnosis and treatment for the adolescent but also to address staff concerns about their response to behavior and how an adolescent's behavior affects other patients and staff on the unit. Likewise, when a simple behavior modification program needs to be established for an adolescent inpatient, the hospital staff may need assistance in developing and implementing it.

THE HEALTH CARE SYSTEM AND THE DELIVERY OF SERVICES TO ADOLESCENTS

Relevant system elements include the *availability* of acute, as well as comprehensive, preventive health care (determined by the sites, the professionals at those sites, and the content of services provided); *access* to services (determined by details such as schedules, location and transportation, and adolescents' perceptions regarding the sites and services that are offered); and *appropriateness* (determined by items such as standards of care, cultural competence, and meeting the specific needs of adolescents). In addition, health care visits tend to take longer for adolescents than for older or younger individuals, yet adolescents are more likely than any age group to be uninsured. Even adolescents who have medical insurance may present a challenge because they request that their care be confidential and that no bill be sent to their parents.

The National Adolescent Health Information Center (NAHIC)[1] has proposed five recommendations to improve health care for adolescents: (1) ensure the delivery of high-quality services (by improving training in adolescent health, by improving workforce distribution for providing adolescent-related services, and by enhancing coordination and support for adolescent health services), (2) provide access to comprehensive health services[3] (by ensuring that appropriate services are readily available and by implementing strategies to overcome adolescents' barriers to access), (3) improve financial access to comprehensive health services (by improving existing health coverage and by expanding coverage for adolescents beyond existing parameters), (4) ensure the legal right to health care and confidentiality (by improving legal access to health services and by ensuring legal protection of confidential care), and (5) provide adolescent-focused, adolescent-acceptable health services (by providing services that focus on adolescents' needs and by involving adolescents directly in the planning and delivery of their health services). These recommendations must be considered as improvements in health care delivery are planned.

In addition, the NAHIC described five cross-cutting themes related to the adolescent health care systems. These themes include the need to (1) prioritize the health and well-being of adolescents on a national level; (2) coordinate, reduce fragmentation, and maximize existing resources at the local, state, and federal levels; (3) use resources effectively with joint collaborative efforts and sustainable funding to close major gaps in adolescent health services; (4) focus more on primary prevention and early intervention that is substantiated by rigorous research[10]; and (5) increase the role of families and other meaningful adults who play critical roles in the lives of adolescents.

PRACTICAL ISSUES IN PROVIDING ADOLESCENT HEALTH SERVICES

Much of the discussion about challenges to delivering health care to adolescents focuses on adolescents, rather than on health care professionals. Some specific suggestions have been made in each of the preceding sections of this chapter to enhance services. However, additional practical suggestions deserve consideration. These include altering the structure and format of adolescent visits, billings, and referrals of patients who have a chronic illness. Recognizing the multiplicity of service sites and professional training in adolescent medicine, this section will address these issues in the context of traditional office visits.

Ideally, patients enter adolescence having been in the care of a clinician who has provided continuity of care during the transition from childhood to adolescence. In anticipation of the inevitable emergence of puberty, clinicians often advise parents of patients around age 8 or 9 years of an office policy to begin to provide the patient some time alone with the professional at about the age of 10 years. This can be framed in the context of preparing the early adolescent to take increasing responsibility for his or her health (paralleling the increasing responsibility in other domains, such as school and work). Then, at the next visit, the parent can be reminded of the clinician's desire to talk to the emerging adolescent alone.

As adolescents progress developmentally, there is an increasing need for, and a right to, confidential care. This is best discussed with the adolescent and his or her parents at the outset of the visit and usually only needs to be addressed once. Two points need to be emphasized with respect to confidentiality. First, the principle underlying confidentiality is respect for the adolescent as a person, not keeping secrets from parents. Second, absolute confidentiality should never be offered. One might say: "It is important for my adolescent patients to have time alone with me, because by the time they are 18 years old, they legally can see me completely on their own. To help you prepare for that, you will have time at each visit when we can talk alone. What we talk about will be between us, unless I believe that you or others are in danger—such as if you were seriously thinking about hurting yourself. I would only do what I think is in your best interest, and I will not talk to your parents about my concerns without your knowledge. But most things we talk about will remain private." Parents usually are very comfortable with this policy. If they are not, there usually is a serious problem with trust in their relationship, which itself could be a focus for intervention.

A question commonly asked by clinicians is, "How do I get the parent to leave the room?" A useful technique is to get some background history from the accompanying parent, then give the patient an examination gown while saying, "Please put on this gown, so that I can do your physical. Your mom (or dad) and I will step out to give you some privacy." Then, after shepherding the parent or the parents out of the room, it is possible to ask if there are any concerns that either parent has. This gives parents an opportunity to mention their concerns privately. Parents then can be asked to have a seat in the waiting room while the adolescent is examined privately. Again, most parents accept this readily. Parents who refuse to leave the room generally have serious problems trusting their adolescent or the clinician.

Most clinicians allow at least 30 minutes for follow-up adolescent visits and more for an initial visit. Using structured survey forms, such as those of *GAPS* or *Bright Futures*, greatly facilitates data gathering, but the information contained in such formats needs to be reviewed before the patient leaves the office. It is essential that the adolescent know what is going to happen at the visit, how much time has been allotted, and that additional visits may be necessary if all concerns cannot be addressed initially. It is necessary to bill for services appropriately to avoid resenting the adolescent as a source of lost revenue.

Billing issues need to be discussed openly and early in the delivery of services to adolescents. Although many adolescents are without health care insurance, the new federal-supported State Child Health Improvement Program (SCHIP) promises to provide much-needed coverage for many uninsured teenagers. Some insurance companies or managed-care organizations allow confidential billing. Alternatively, services can be provided under a broad generic code (such as CPT No. 99215) when the medical decision making is of high complexity. For example, a pelvic examination could be recorded in the chart but might not be noted on the bill. The fees for counseling sessions should reflect the time spent. In addition, parents may be willing to pay bills that do not have a detailed list of the services rendered, reassured that their adolescent is acting responsibly toward health maintenance. Adolescents who prefer to pay for services with their own money generally need an installment plan. Finally, patients who cannot pay for services can be referred to free clinics, if they are available locally.

The referral of an adolescent to a subspecialist is most likely going to represent a challenge when the subspecialist is a mental health provider. Adolescents tend to interpret the referral to a psychiatrist, psychologist, social worker, or counselor as an indication that they are "crazy." To minimize resistance, it may be helpful to let the adolescent know the reason for the referral ("I am concerned that you seem to be feeling very sad, at times hopeless, and recently thinking that life's not worth living"), to frame the referral in terms of bringing the consultant onto the treatment team ("I need the help of Dr. Smith. He's a psychiatrist who helps me help my patients who are feeling the way you are"), and to plan a follow-up so that the referral does not evoke feelings of rejection or abandonment ("I want to meet with you 2 weeks after you have had a chance to talk to him. I want to make sure that things are improving. You also know that you can call me if you feel as if you're going to harm yourself in any way before you see him").

Patients who have chronic conditions that previously were fatal during childhood or adolescence are now living into adulthood. As a result, there is an increasing need for transition from pediatric to adult health care that should be anticipated and planned early on. Hearing from a pediatrician, "And when Jenny gets to be an older adolescent or young adult, we will need to make sure that the physician who will be assuming care for her knows about her cystic fibrosis," is interpreted by parents as positive, because it reflects an expectation that she will live to adulthood. Combined training in medicine and pediatrics prepares physicians especially well for the care of such patients, because there is no need for transfer of care as the patient grows out of the pediatric age group. Physicians who have such training are especially well prepared to address the needs of those adolescents who have complex medical and surgical problems as they enter adulthood.

REFERENCES

1. Brindis CD, et al: *Improving adolescent health: an analysis and synthesis of health policy recommendations,* San Francisco, University of California at San Francisco, 1998, National Adolescent Health Information Center.
2. Dryfoos JG: *Safe passage: making it through adolescence in a risky society,* New York, 1998, Oxford University Press.
3. Elster AB, Levenberg P: Integrating comprehensive adolescent preventive services into routine medicine care: rationale and approaches, *Pediatr Clin North Am* 44:1365, 1997.
4. English A, Simmons PS: Legal issues in reproductive health care for adolescents, *Adolesc Med: State of the Art Reviews* 10:181, 1999.
5. Fisher M: Adolescent inpatient units, *Arch Dis Child* 70:461, 1994.
6. Fortenberry JD: Condom availability in high schools, *Adolesc Med: State of the Art Reviews* 8:449, 1997.
7. Hedberg VA, Bracken AC, Stashwick CA: Long-term consequences of adolescent health behaviors: implications for adolescent health services, *Adolesc Med: State of the Art Reviews* 10:137, 1999.
8. Herman-Giddens ME, et al: Secondary sexual characteristics and menses in young girls seen in office practice: a study from the Pediatric Research in Office Settings network, *Pediatrics* 99:505, 1997.
9. Hofmann AD: Providing care to adolescents. In Hofmann AD, Greydanus DE, editors: *Adolescent medicine,* ed 3, Stamford, Connecticut, 1997, Appleton & Lange.
10. Millstein SG, Petersen AC, Nightingale EO, editors: *Promoting the health of adolescents: new directions for the twenty-first century,* New York, 1993, Oxford University Press.
11. Murray PJ: School-based health centers, *Adolesc Med: State of the Art Reviews* 8:433, 1997.
12. Neinstein LS: The office visit, interview techniques, and recommendations to parents. In Neinstein LS, editor: *Adolescent health care: a practical guide*, ed 3, Philadelphia, 1996, Williams & Wilkins.
13. Pastore DR, et al: School-based health center utilization: a survey of users and nonusers, *Arch Pediatr Adolesc Med* 152:763, 1998.
14. Peabody FW: The care of the patient (1927). Reprinted *JAMA* 252:813, 1984.
15. Rosen DS, Xiangdong M, Blum RW: Adolescent health: current trends and critical issues, *Adolesc Med: State of the Art Reviews* 1:15, 1990.
16. Tanner JM: Issues and advances in adolescent growth and development, *J Adolesc Health Care* 8:470, 1987.
17. Weiner IB: *Psychological disturbance in adolescence,* ed 2, New York, 1992, John Wiley & Sons.

100 Conversion Reactions in Adolescents

Gregory E. Prazar • Stanford B. Friedman

DEFINITION, INCIDENCE, AND ETIOLOGICAL FACTORS

The amalgamation of emotions and physical symptoms in patients challenges the primary care physician to formulate priorities in history-taking, diagnosis, and management. Some somatic complaints, such as headaches, nausea, and vomiting, can result directly from emotional upsets. Indeed, anxiety often is associated with palpitations, sweating, and tremulousness; depression often is manifested by symptoms of fatigue and weakness. Other somatic complaints reflect organic disorders, such as neuromuscular headaches, which may be associated with emotional turmoil. Still other physical problems are attributed to conversion symptoms.

Conversion reactions are a way of communicating the uncomfortable, or as Engel writes, "a psychic mechanism whereby an idea, fantasy, or wish is expressed in bodily rather than in verbal terms and is experienced by the patient as a physical symptom rather than as a mental symptom."[2] The idea or wish is psychologically threatening to the individual or is unacceptable for him or her to express directly. A conversion symptom serves as a form of decompression, whereby unpleasant affects associated with acknowledgment of the wish are dissipated through the use of a somatic symptom. Because the wish is completely unconscious, the patient in no way relates any psychological stigmata to the somatic complaint. As Hollender succinctly states, "The conversion symptom is a code that conceals the message from the sender as well as from the receiver."[6]

To understand why a wish or thought is represented by a bodily symptom, it is necessary to explore patterns of everyday behavior and infant development. Body activity (i.e., gestures) is used to express ideas during verbal interaction. Common conversational phrases frequently allude, metaphorically, to the intermixing of emotion and body functioning. "I'm fed up" and "He gives me a pain in the neck" are two such examples. Developmentally, infants express feelings and communicate through visible behavior long before spoken language becomes their dominant mode of communication. Furthermore, infants explore and learn about their environment, including the people in it, by using their bodies as investigative tools (e.g., placing new objects in the mouth) and as a means of making contact. Any bodily process that can be perceived by the individual can serve as the focus for conversion symptoms. Similarly, somatic symptoms of relatives or close friends also can serve as the source of a patient's complaint. It is the patient's *interpretation* of the other person's symptom that provides a model for the somatic complaint. When the symptom is adapted from one observed in the other person, that person frequently evokes strong feelings in the patient. Because the patient feels guilty about his or her feelings or impulses toward that person, he or she may take the other person's symptoms as a form of self-punishment, while at the same time psychologically expressing his or her own forbidden idea or wish.

All body systems may be invoked in a conversion reaction. The sensory system frequently is involved (e.g., paresthesia, anesthesia, or diffuse pain), although typically these symptoms are not distributed in the correct pattern of innervation of the implicated cutaneous nerves. Motor system involvement can be represented by paralysis, tremors, or weakness of an extremity. Hyperventilation and dizziness are other common conversion symptoms, as are nausea and vomiting and visual problems.

A common conversion symptom seen in children and young adolescents is abdominal pain. After an extensive investigation of 100 children who had abdominal pain, Apley[1] found an organic cause in only 8 cases. Another study, by Oster,[11] revealed abdominal pain in 14% of the children studied. The incidence was highest in those 9 years of age and lowest in those 16 to 17 years of age. Recurrent abdominal pain and its etiology remain controversial (see Chapter 114, Abdominal Pain). However, it is important to remember that many patients who have recurrent abdominal pain may have emotional concerns of which they are unaware. Many of these patients may be suffering from conversion symptoms.

Although the incidence of certain individual somatic complaints has been studied, the specific overall incidence of conversion symptoms in children and adolescents is not known. Available data suggest an incidence of 5% to 13%.[4] Lack of more definitive data reflects the difficulty in ascertaining whether a somatic complaint indeed represents a conversion symptom. Conversion symptoms may appear to be more common among adolescents than among children because the former more often have alarming somatic complaints, such as chest pains and fainting spells, whereas children frequently suffer from more indolent complaints, such as sporadic abdominal pains. Conversion symptoms are two to three times more common in girls than in boys and may appear as early as 7 or 8 years of age.[2] There appears to be no correlation between the occurrence of conversion symptoms and socioeconomic status; less sophisticated patients, however, tend to have bizarre and physiologically unexplained symptoms.

Conversion symptoms can appear as a group phenomenon. Such a situation often is referred to as *epidemic hysteria*. Adolescent girls swooning and fainting at rock concerts is an easily appreciated example. In this situation the unacceptable wish relates to sexualized thoughts involving rock stars. Other examples of epidemic hysteria are explained less easily. Episodes of epidemic hysteria appear to have several characteristics in common: (1) audiovisual cues (e.g., seeing ambulances arrive to care for accident victims) seem to be important as precipitators; (2) adolescent girls are involved more often than adolescent boys; (3) the reaction is more likely if it is initiated by a group member identified either as a leader (of a large subgroup) or as an outsider; and (4) episodes are likely to involve larger numbers of adolescents if the youngsters are allowed to confer among themselves without adults present. Entire school populations may be involved in mass conversion reactions.[7,10]

Although conversion symptoms have no organic basis by themselves, their perpetuation may result in biochemical or physiological body changes, known as *conversion complications*. These can include changes such as muscle atrophy secondary to long-standing paralysis and respiratory alkalosis secondary to acute hyperventilation. It is important to differentiate conversion complications from psychophysiologically mediated lesions, such as peptic ulcers, in which physiological processes concomitant with emotions contribute to altered activity of an involuntary body function.

INTERVIEW TECHNIQUES

Because symptoms caused by conversion and somatic processes can be easily confused, the practitioner evaluating any patient who has a somatic complaint always should consider the possibility of a conversion symptom. Attention to the personal history (family functioning, school performance, and peer relationships), as well as to physical functioning, demonstrates to the patient and family that the physician appreciates without prejudice the importance of all elements that may be contributing to ill health. Showing respect for the importance of emotional-physical interaction is thereby suggested so that this concept will not be foreign if it later is presented to the family in a diagnostic framework. Such an approach also contributes to the physician's understanding, as Engel[2] states, "of those personal, family, and social circumstances that are most relevant to the understanding of the illness and the care of the patient, whether or not the ultimate diagnosis is conversion."

Nondirective interviewing proves more rewarding than direct questioning. For example, asking the patient to describe the pain ("Tell me how it feels") almost always provides insight into the emotions the patient associates with the symptom. Suggesting how the symptom feels to the patient ("Is it dull or sharp pain?") limits his or her possible responses. If the patient spontaneously offers information about recent events, the interviewer should obtain further data related to such changes in the patient's life. However, care should be taken to avoid suggesting a cause-and-effect relationship between the patient's feelings and the symptoms. Because the patient who has conversion symptoms has no conscious knowledge of such an association, the suggestion of such a relationship may alienate him or her and prevent establishment of a trusting relationship.

DIAGNOSTIC CRITERIA FOR CONVERSION SYMPTOMS

The conversion symptom has a specific, but unconscious, symbolic meaning to the patient. In other words, the conversion symptom often is related to an unconscious wish, and the physical impairment serves to prevent acting out the wish. For example, the adolescent boy who has hand paralysis may have anxieties about masturbating. The physician treating children and adolescents may not always be aware of the symbolic meaning of the symptom. Indeed, the concept that conversion symptoms have a symbolic meaning to the patient was formulated only after a series of these patients had undergone extensive psychotherapy. Although it may be intellectually rewarding for the physician to be cognizant of the presence of the symbolic meaning, ignorance of the specific symbolism does not prevent adequate treatment of the patient. For example:

Jane, a 12-year-old, suddenly developed an inability to walk. Physical examination, including a neurological evaluation, revealed no abnormalities. Interviews by a psychiatrist and a pediatrician working as a team revealed no apparent symbolic etiological factor. The pediatrician formulated a system to reward Jane's progress in walking and implemented this approach; the psychiatrist was similarly supportive with the patient. Over a period of 3 weeks, the patient regained her ability to walk.

Adolescents who have conversion symptoms frequently display characteristic patterns of behavior, sometimes designated as traits of the "hysterical personality." Such characteristics include egocentricity; labile emotional states (quick shifts from sadness to elation and from anger to passivity); dramatic, attention-seeking behavior; and sexual provocativeness (displayed in gestures and in dress). Patients who have such characteristics also usually are demanding, display an air of pseudomaturity, and are dependent in personal interactions. Their personal relationships, however, rarely are intimate or satisfying. Although many aspects of the hysterical personality are seen in adolescent patients who have conversion symptoms, such characteristics also are demonstrable in adolescents who do not have such symptoms. Therefore, hysterical behavior traits in adolescents are not synonymous with conversion symptoms and, in isolation, are not indicative of a psychopathological condition.

The manner in which patients who have a conversion symptom describe their problem often is distinctive. The account frequently is dramatic. A pain may be described as "thousands of burning needles thrust into my leg" or as "a giant spike being driven into my chest." Because these patients are suggestible, any symptom description alluded to by the physician may be adopted readily and thereafter reported, which again emphasizes the importance of a nondirective approach in the interview.

As described previously, conversion symptoms are adopted unconsciously in an attempt to reduce unpleasant affects, especially anxiety, depression, and guilt. Therefore, although the patient may describe incapacitating pain, he or she often affects an air of unconcern. Psychiatrists refer to this as *la belle indifference*. The extent to which the conversion symptom diminishes the unpleasant affect and symbolically communicates the forbidden wish for the patient is referred to as the *primary gain*. Patients who have conversion reactions often are stubborn in their belief that the symptom is caused by organic problems. This reflects denial of the underlying emotional problem. Conversely, insistence (especially by an adolescent) that a symptom is psychological in origin may indicate denial of a physical problem. Therefore, differentiating between conversion symptoms and physical disease in adolescent patients cannot depend solely on the patient's emotional response.

Conversion symptoms not only effect a primary gain for the patient but also help him or her cope with the environment. In this respect the conversion symptom achieves a *secondary gain* for the patient. For example, the patient who has a conversion symptom defending against homosexual thoughts may be excused from attending school, where anxiety may have been intensified (e.g., in the locker room). Limitations imposed by the symptom may contradict the patient's verbalized wish to participate in activities but, nevertheless, remove him or her from potentially threatening social interactions. Interference with daily activities also provides a secondary gain for the patient in that attention and more frequent expressions of love are elicited from concerned parents and friends. This situation may be resistant to change, not only because the symptom is reinforced continually but also because the symptom meets the parents' psychological needs. In effect, the symptom may provide the parents with a reason for nurturing or infantilizing their child. Consequently, the patient and his or her entire family may fall into a vicious circle of dependence on the symptom.

Demonstration of a secondary gain does not ensure a diagnosis of conversion. To an extent, all illness is involved with some secondary gain. Bedridden patients must accept increased attention to cope with their physical confinement. Therefore, a degree of secondary gain is necessary for adequate adaptation to a physical disability. However, in the case of a conversion symptom, secondary gain not only intensifies symptoms but also may be associated with further occurrence of somatic complaints. Because perpetuation of secondary gain depends on concern from others, a conversion symptom is exhibited more readily in the presence of individuals meaningful to the patient.

Children and adolescents who develop conversion symptoms often are overprotected and become extremely dependent on their parents. Daily familial communication may have been invested heavily in somatic complaints, the child recognizing how often activities may have been canceled because of the father's headaches or the mother's cramps. Therefore, the patient's symptom may conform to the unspoken interactional rules of the family. The patient's problem is thereby reinforced indirectly by family members, who may even assume an air of indifference with respect to his or her symptoms. For example:

James was a 13-year-old who had severe abdominal pain and was referred to a pediatrician by his family practitioner. Physical examination revealed little objective evidence of abdominal pain in the physician's office. However, his return home quickly resulted in intensified pain. Abdominal pain appeared to be well controlled during a subsequent 4-day hospitalization (all organic tests were unremarkable). His return home again produced an immediate exacerbation of the abdominal discomfort. Furthermore, John, James' identical twin, began exhibiting signs of abdominal pain. The boys' mother admitted feeling trapped by the demands of her children and volunteered that in the past she had been treated for chronic abdominal pain. The appearance of abdominal pain in both twins reassured her that the pain was "probably a virus." She chose not to pursue further counseling for the boys.

Precipitation of a conversion symptom may be related to specific stressful events. A change of school, final examinations, new social experiences, and parental conflict are examples of events that may induce a conversion symptom. A study by Maloney[9] suggests that unresolved grief reactions may represent a source of stress that can precipitate a conversion symptom. Examples of grief reactions listed in the study include loss of a parent through death, divorce, or moving. Furthermore, a study by Griffith, Polles, and Griffith of adolescent and adult patients experiencing pseudoseizures revealed that this conversion symptom occurred more often in families in which there was "an unspeakable dilemma."[5] Specifically, the dilemma often was associated with a fear of physical or sexual assault. Even though other family members were aware of the specific dilemma, they often underestimated how severely the family member who experienced the pseudoseizures was affected by the dilemma. Because the patient's association between conflict and the conversion reaction is unconscious, a history is helpful only if the interviewer elicits details about daily activities. Often the stressful event precipitating a conversion symptom becomes apparent only after many visits. For example:

Chip, a 13-year-old, was brought by his mother to his pediatrician because of chronic abdominal pain, which appeared to be precipitated by his competing in horse-riding events. His history revealed the death of a grandparent 4 months previously, but his mother related that her son's pain preceded the onset of the fatal illness. Other family stresses were denied. The teenager did not appear for follow-up care but returned 6 months later, primarily because his mother wanted to discuss her son's reaction to her upcoming divorce. At this visit, the mother volunteered that marital stress had been ongoing for several years.

Symptom selection is based on the patient's unconscious remembrance of his or her own body function or on his or her understanding of symptoms in others. The patient's conversion symptom may appear quite dissimilar to that displayed by the other (often a parent or a close relative) because it is the patient's *perception* of disease that governs the display of symptoms. Parents and relatives often misinform children and adolescents about diseases, fearing that the truth would be too frightening. However, such misinformation actually may potentiate the adolescent's fantasies and result in the development of a symptom quite different from the one actually experienced by the individual serving as the model. For example:

During a routine physical examination, Jeff, a 14-year-old, mentioned that he experienced "migraine headaches," which appeared to be focused "behind my left eye" and occurred approximately once a month. Jeff's mother attached more importance to the symptoms than did Jeff. Initially, exploration of the family history proved unremarkable. Persistent questioning about stress led the mother to mention almost parenthetically that she had recently been diagnosed as having multiple sclerosis. She felt that the case was mild and therefore had not told Jeff and her other children directly about the diagnosis, although she sensed that the children knew. Her initial symptom that precipitated the diagnosis of multiple sclerosis was temporary loss of vision in her left eye.

The choice of a symptom also may be based on a physical illness the patient had suffered previously. Thus, patients who have a history of seizures may, after many years of adequate anticonvulsant control, have atypical and physiologically unexplainable seizures. Unfortunately, these patients often receive only a physiological workup for seizures. Despite the atypical history, the physician assumes that the diagnosis rests "where the money is, or was" in the past. For example:

Terry, a 15-year-old girl, recently had been treated for otitis media, which was characterized by pain and some dizziness. After the ear appeared adequately healed, her dizziness persisted. By encouraging Terry to discuss her daily schedule, it became apparent that she was under significant academic pressure, having recently transferred to an extremely competitive private school. In addition, extracurricular pressures were heavy, including her fervent commitment to gymnastics and her hope to achieve professional status. On further questioning, Terry related that she had had dizzy spells in past years just before competitions.

Because the somatic complaint expressed by the patient is based on a model symptom, a physical disease often is mimicked. Close scrutiny of the symptom's history and description often reveals anatomical and physiological discrepancies. The child or adolescent who has a *stocking anesthesia,* an anesthesia confined to a specific area of an extremity without any relationship to cutaneous nerve innervation, demonstrates an example of such symptom inaccuracy. It is based on the patient's concept of his or her body rather than on anatomical principles.

A thorough history may not only elicit symptom inconsistencies in the present illness but also may reveal a record of inexplicable or recurrent bouts of illness associated with life events. A history of chronic abdominal pain that occurs only on school days, a history of somatic complaints associated with stressful social events, or documentation of abdominal surgery with equivocal findings should raise suspicion that the patient's current problem represents conversion. A list of the diagnostic criteria for conversion symptoms appears in Box 100-1. No one criterion can be confirmatory, and each patient who has a conversion symptom may not display every criterion listed. However, a conversion symptom cannot be diagnosed solely based on negative physical and laboratory findings; it is not a diagnosis of exclusion.

BOX 100-1

CRITERIA FOR DIAGNOSIS OF CONVERSION SYMPTOMS

- The symptom has symbolic meaning to the patient.
- The patient frequently exhibits characteristic interpersonal behaviors.
- Conversion symptoms are more common in girls than boys.
- There is a characteristic style of reporting symptoms.
- The symptom helps the patient cope with his or her environment ("secondary gain").
- Health issues and symptoms frequently are used in family communication.
- Symptoms occur at times of stress.
- The symptom has a model.
- History and physical findings often are inconsistent with anatomical and physiological concepts.

From Prazar G: *Pediatr Rev* 8:279, 1987.

DIFFERENTIAL DIAGNOSIS OF OTHER PSYCHOSOMATIC DISORDERS

Other psychosomatic disorders at times may be confused with conversion symptoms. Patients exhibiting *hypochondriasis,* a common entity, especially in adolescents, view their symptoms with extreme concern. There is none of the apparent indifference seen in patients who have conversion symptoms. Patients who have conversion symptoms frequently seem relieved when an organic cause is considered; patients who have hypochondriasis become more concerned if an organic diagnosis is suggested because they suspect and fear a serious or fatal disease. However, neither type of patient is reassured more than transiently by being informed that he or she has no disease.

Malingering is an uncommon problem in adolescents, except in institutionalized adolescents or those who are in restrictive situations (e.g., military service). Malingering may even be regarded as an appropriate means of avoiding threatening or unpleasant circumstances. Attempts to feign illness often are naive, especially in younger patients. As Engel states, malingerers exhibit "an intense need to be nurtured or suffer."[2] Many appear to be accident prone, and many submit to painful procedures readily and without objection. Malingering adolescents are aloof and hostile to the physician; thus, discovery of their deception often is delayed. In contrast, patients who have conversion symptoms often are appropriately fearful of procedures and may appear charming and garrulous with the physician. Patients who have conversion symptoms and malingerers are similar in that their parents may have an unconscious psychological need to have their children be ill and therefore may reinforce their children's symptoms.

Somatic delusions are symptoms of psychosis and usually are not confused with conversion symptoms. Other signs of severe mental illness usually are present, such as an inability to relate to peers, visual or auditory hallucinations, and stereotypical behaviors. Furthermore, the symptoms described sometimes are intermittent and often are extremely bizarre. For example, a patient who has somatic delusions may express the conviction that his or her heart is shriveling or that something is wrong with the blood that is running from the head to the leg.

Psychophysiological symptoms may occur when conversion symptoms have failed to dissipate anxiety. Thus, continuing anxiety activates biological systems (especially the autonomic nervous system), resulting in physiological changes such as tachycardia, hyperperistalsis, and vasoconstriction. A patient's cognizance of these changes is manifested by palpitations, diarrhea, and sweating. In this situation the symptom itself has no organic symbolic meaning and results from a reaction to actual body changes. Therefore, psychophysiological symptoms can occur when conversion symptoms have failed. Similarly, conversion symptoms can replace psychophysiological symptoms.

CARE OF THE PATIENT WHO HAS CONVERSION SYMPTOMS

Adolescents who have conversion symptoms are seen most often initially, and eventually managed, by pediatricians or other primary care physicians. Families see this as appropriate because the obvious aspect of the problem is physical. They typically will accept a diagnosis of conversion only from a medical professional they consider an expert in physical disease. Nevertheless, when the physician undertakes a case of suspected conversion, his or her interviewing acumen and sensitivity to the patient's feelings are paramount. The initial interaction between the physician and the patient is crucial to the degree of success achieved in dealing with a conversion symptom. In essence, treatment of the patient begins before a definitive diagnosis is made. Some considerations involved in the initial evaluation of patients suspected of having conversion symptoms appear in Box 100-2.

The physician should advise the patient and family that the cause of any disorder involves both physical and emotional factors. As Schmitt[13] states, the family should be told that "everyone's body has a certain physical way of responding to emotional stress." Similarly, every individual has an emotional response to physical stress. Simple examples should be given (e.g., most people have learned that headaches often are intensified when they are upset). If the physician communicates an appreciation of the role of emotions in physical disease, the family may volunteer information more readily about psychosocial functioning. Furthermore, an eventual diagnosis involving emotional aspects may be more acceptable because the family has been prepared for the possibility. Focusing only on an organic diagnosis intimates to the parents that psychological involvement is unlikely, unimportant, and improbable. Turning to psychological issues after all physical tests prove unremarkable implies to parents that this tack was chosen as a last resort because the physician was unable to ascertain an organic cause. A concurrent physical-psychological diagnostic approach not only prepares the physician to consider the problem with some psychotherapeutic intent but also may save the family time and money because multiple laboratory tests often can be avoided.

After the evaluation has been completed, the physician must develop a treatment plan. Before embarking on this venture, the physician must be satisfied with the completeness of the medical evaluation. Common sense should dictate when he or she feels that further organic tests will be futile. The patient and family often can sense a physician's uncertainty, especially if the family is averse to accepting a psychological diagnosis. Therefore, it is prudent to ask the family what additional tests they might expect to have performed and what other diagnoses they may have considered. Involvement of the patient and family in this diagnostic process frequently dissipates anxiety and allows eventual psychological counseling.

Although patients who have conversion symptoms are suggestible, reassurance that the symptom will go away rarely is effective and also does not contribute to a psychological investigation of the symptom. On the contrary, suggesting that the symptom will persist allows time to work out a therapeutic relationship with the patient and sometimes has a paradoxical effect. Because the symptom is unlikely to disappear after two or three visits, the patient retrospectively will view the physician's suggestion as sound. Trust in the physician will be reinforced, and the patient may be more comfortable communicating information about his or her feelings. Placebo medication usually is ineffective and raises questions of medical ethics. Tranquilizers may reduce attendant anxiety transiently in some cases of conversion symptoms; however, using medication as the sole therapy rarely results in lasting improvement. Because medication does not relieve the underlying conflict responsible for the symptom, another symptom eventually may appear. Furthermore, there is risk that the medication's side effects may become the model for new conversion symptoms or that new symptoms may be confused with side effects.

At the conclusion of the evaluation, the number and type of counseling sessions the physician anticipates should be discussed. The number of sessions should be flexible so that it can be renegotiated if needed. Follow-up sessions with the teenager usually can be limited to 20 to 30 minutes every 2 to 4 weeks. More frequent visits may be necessary if the symptom interferes with school attendance, peer relationships, or family functioning. During follow-up sessions, the teenager should be encouraged to talk about his or her daily life (e.g.,

BOX 100-2

IMPORTANT CONSIDERATIONS IN THE INITIAL EVALUATION OF PATIENTS SUSPECTED OF HAVING CONVERSION SYMPTOMS

From the outset, parents and patient should be told that everyone's body has a certain physical way of responding to emotional stress.

Parents and patient should be encouraged to suggest diagnostic tests that they may want performed and to suggest possible diagnoses for consideration by the physician.

Parents and patient should understand that the symptom may persist but that the goal is to help maintain normal daily functioning in school and with peers.

Parents and patient should understand that referral to a psychiatrically trained professional may be necessary if progress is not made in coping with the symptom.

Modified from Prazar G: *Pediatr Rev* 8:279, 1987.

school, friends, family, dating). If the teenager volunteers information about recurrence of the somatic complaint, the physician should inquire about events that were transpiring concurrently when the symptom occurred and how the teenager felt about these events. In this way the physician can help the adolescent become reacquainted with how daily events and feelings are related. Suggesting that the adolescent keep a symptom diary may be helpful. The patient records when the symptom occurred, and what was happening at the time the symptom began. Such a record may illustrate to the patient the association of the symptom with feelings or emotionally charged life events.

Because the physician may serve both as therapist for the teenager and provider of acute medical care, there may be occasions when the teenager has a new physical symptom or complaint. If the physician suspects a physical illness unrelated to the conversion symptom, he or she must perform whatever evaluation is indicated, including a full or partial physical examination. However, an overzealous search for disease should be avoided. Treatment goals need to be realistic. Conversion symptoms seldom disappear completely. However, adolescents often acquire increased coping skills so that their daily functioning is unimpaired and dependence on secondary gain is minimized.

Follow-up visits with parents should take place every 4 to 6 weeks. Such meetings should serve to elicit persistent or new concerns that parents may have about their teenager's progress and should attempt to assess the parents' reaction to their teenager's continuing complaints. The practitioner should emphasize the validity of the teenager's concerns so that misconceptions about the symptom being "faked" are dispelled. Furthermore, positive reinforcement needs to be offered so that parents believe they are doing what is best for their child. Selected follow-up sessions with the parents should include the teenager. Not only do such family meetings demonstrate to the patient that confidentiality of individual sessions is not being violated but also they offer the physician an opportunity to observe parent-adolescent interaction. These observations may provide an important index to the effectiveness of ongoing therapy.

REFERRAL

Referral to mental health professionals is indicated if symptoms continue to interfere with the patient's daily activities or functioning or when the physician or school personnel feel that the teenager's symptoms have not diminished. School officials can provide valuable information about the effect of the conversion symptom on school functioning and peer interaction. Referral is dictated if the family feels that inadequate progress has been made after an agreed-upon duration of therapy.

Referral also is indicated if the patient's symptom creates uncomfortable feelings in the pediatrician. Situations involving seductive adolescent behavior in association with a conversion symptom may create feelings in the pediatrician that can prevent effective intervention. It is unrealistic to assume that a pediatrician can treat all psychological and medical problems adequately. Cognizance of one's own limitations is an important professional attribute. Another situation requiring referral involves the patient or family member who is a social acquaintance or a relative of the pediatrician. Dealing with the emotional problems of friends' or relatives' children is inappropriate. Obtaining personal details of family or sexual functioning often is indicated in the evaluation and may jeopardize the social relationship. Conversely, failure or hesitancy to obtain appropriate data may jeopardize subsequent resolution of the problem.

BOX 100-3

INDICATIONS FOR REFERRAL OF PATIENTS WHO HAVE CONVERSION SYMPTOMS

The symptom continues to interfere with daily functioning (school attendance, participation in extracurricular activities, involvement with peers).

Parents and patient believe that no progress is being made in dealing with the symptom.

The physician feels uncomfortable with the patient's symptom or behavior (e.g., patients exhibiting seductive behavior).

The patient's family includes a social friend or relative of the physician.

From Prazar G: *Pediatr Rev* 8:279, 1987.

In all cases, when referral is suggested, parental and patient compliance with the referral is improved if the possibility has been mentioned as a contingency early in the evaluation. The pediatrician should always help families understand that seeing a psychiatrically trained professional does *not* connote "craziness." Rather, the pediatrician may suggest that a psychiatrist could help because a physician trained in psychiatry can help teenagers understand feelings about unusual symptoms better than can most pediatricians. The physician should recommend a specific counselor rather than offering a list of suggested therapists. Before the name of the therapist is given to the family, the physician should verify that the counselor feels comfortable with the referral and has time available to see the patient.

After the referral is made, continued pediatrician contact with the family concerning the conversion symptom promotes compliance with the therapy. Indications for referring patients who have conversion symptoms are listed in Box 100-3.[12]

The prognosis for patients who have conversion reactions is unknown. In a report of 74 children who had psychogenic pain, Friedman[3] found many patients who were judged to be improved after several years regardless of whether professional intervention took place. In a 7-year follow-up of patients hospitalized with conversion, 23 of 41 patients no longer suffered from their presenting physical symptom, were free of underlying stress, and had experienced no symptom substitution or new associated complaint.[8] Patients who have conversion symptoms, indeed, may have an encouraging future. On the other hand, in some patients, adolescent conversion symptoms mark the beginning of a lifelong course of conversion illness.

SUMMARY

Conversion reactions represent an emotionally charged issue, not only literally for the adolescent but also figuratively for the physician, because patients displaying such symptoms often elicit a wide range of emotions from their physician. The physician's emotional response results from his or her frustration in dealing with such difficult patients. Every patient who has a somatic complaint has feelings about his or her symptoms. An evaluation of any somatic complaint should involve inquiry into aspects of the patient's family, school attendance and performance, and peer relationships. A better understanding of the patient's baseline emotional functioning can be achieved in this way. The physician must advise both parents and patient that it is acceptable to have feelings about somatic complaints. Both family and patient may be much more accepting of primary emotional involvement if permission for expressing feelings is given early in the physician-patient relationship. The diagnosis of a conversion reaction should never be one of exclusion and should follow specific diagnostic criteria.

Care of the adolescent patient who has a conversion reaction involves establishing a renegotiable number of regular visits, encouraging the patient to discuss daily activities and interrelated feelings, meeting with parents regularly to provide them with emotional support and counseling, and knowing that palliation rather than a cure may be the optimal goal. When the physician feels uncomfortable treating a patient who has a conversion reaction or when ongoing follow-up care appears to have made no progress in reducing the symptom, the patient should be referred to a mental health professional. However, referral should not end the pediatrician's contact with the patient, because ongoing physician interest may improve patient compliance with the referral source and may increase the physician's ability to resume responsibility later for the patient's care. The patient who has a conversion symptom usually will not outgrow it and will not respond permanently to placebo medication. Such patients severely tax the primary care physician's diagnostic and therapeutic acumen. However, the physician who respects the involvement of emotions with somatic complaints can help patients who have conversion symptoms cope with their disorders.

REFERENCES

1. Apley J: *The child with abdominal pains,* ed 2, Oxford, England, 1975, Blackwell Scientific.
2. Engel GL: Conversion symptoms. In MacBryde CM, Blacklow RS, editors: *Signs and symptoms: applied pathologic physiology and clinical interpretation,* ed 6, Philadelphia, 1983, JB Lippincott.
3. Friedman R: Some characteristics of children with "psychogenic" pain: observations on prognosis and management, *Clin Pediatr* 11:331, 1972.
4. Friedman SB: Conversion symptoms in adolescents, *Pediatr Clin North Am* 20:873, 1973.
5. Griffith JL, Polles A, Griffith ME: Pseudoseizures, families and unspeakable dilemmas, *Psychosomatics* 39:144, 1998.
6. Hollender MH: Conversion hysteria: a post-Freudian reinterpretation of nineteenth century psychosocial data, *Arch Gen Psychiatry* 26:31, 1972.
7. Levine RJ: Epidemic faintness and syncope in a school marching band, *JAMA* 238:2373, 1977.
8. Maisami M, Freeman JM: Conversion reactions in children as body language: a combined child psychiatry/neurology team approach to the management of functional neurologic disorders in children, *Pediatrics* 80:46, 1987.
9. Maloney MJ: Diagnosing hysterical conversion reactions in children, *J Pediatr* 97:1016, 1980.
10. Moffett MEK: Epidemic hysteria in a Montreal train station, *Pediatrics* 70:308, 1982.
11. Oster J: Recurrent abdominal pain, headache, and limb pains in children and adolescents, *Pediatrics* 50:429, 1972.
12. Prazar G: Conversion reactions in adolescents, *Pediatr Rev* 8:279, 1987.
13. Schmitt BD: School phobia—the great imitator: a pediatrician's viewpoint, *Pediatrics* 48:433, 1971.

101 Counseling Parents of Adolescents

Frances C. Paolini-Masucci

A pediatrician's relationship with the parents of adolescents has the benefit of time in which to develop a trusting partnership. Parents tend to see the pediatrician as a person from whom to seek advice, particularly with regard to physiological and behavioral issues and as less threatening than a mental health provider. The pediatrician's ongoing relationship with the family presents him or her with the opportunity to provide anticipatory guidance and to support the parents as their children enter and move through adolescence.

Adolescence is notable for the dramatic, uneven integration of development characterized by a changing body image, mood swings, burgeoning sexuality, intense need for peer acceptance, increasing independence from the family, expectations to achieve and "act one's age," and fragile egos. At the conclusion of this developmental phase the emergent young adult is expected to comprehend the nuances of complex issues and arrive at decisions, develop an ethical and moral value system, prepare for a chosen field of work, and be capable of intimacy. These daunting tasks are realized largely within a family unit (see Chapter 52, Theories and Concepts of Development as They Relate to Pediatric Practice).

It is crucial to note that adolescent autonomy or independence evolves from a *fluctuating process* that progresses within an environment of continuous connectedness to parents and family. Most adolescents do not achieve independence through a sudden break with their parents; rather, the process is one of gradual redefinition of the relationship. The adolescent years represent but one phase of a developmental continuum as the young person continues the process begun in childhood of broader boundaries with more latitude for the adolescent while continuing to use the family as a mainstay. It is well recognized that adolescents do not accept the presumed wisdom of their elders. They need to experience the tension created by going forth and experimenting with ideas and lifestyles that often are in marked contrast to those of the family. It is a time of "trying on" diverse personalities, like an actor in the center of an imaginary stage. At the same time, the adolescent needs to know that return to the refuge of the family is ensured.

A parent's greatest challenge is to maintain that delicate balance between enabling the adolescent's independent behavior and supporting his or her sense of trust and security in the family. Herein lies the principal source of conflicting emotional distress experienced simultaneously by parents and adolescents. The parents' pain is the result of feelings of loss of control provoked by the young person's independent behavior; the adolescent's discomfort is activated by feelings of loss of childhood security as he or she struggles to cope with greater freedom and responsibility. Unfortunately, all too often such emotional conflict and pain remain unrecognized and unarticulated and yet underlie many confrontations between parents and adolescents. Helping parents to understand the developmental basis for this inherent parent-adolescent conflict serves to reduce their frustration, as does acknowledging and empathizing with the parents' emotional separation, which may be as intensely painful for them as it is for the adolescent.

PARENTING GOALS

With the ever-widening array of diverse family systems and complex choices facing adolescents, what counsel can the pediatrician give parents to help them navigate the turbulent adolescent waters? Practitioners can begin by providing parents information about the physical, cognitive, and psychosocial developmental tasks of adolescence and by helping parents realize that adolescent development is a fluctuating process that occurs within the family system. Parents, as authoritative figures, should be encouraged to assume the role of facilitator and teacher for their adolescent, with two critical major goals. The first goal for parents is to promote expression and resolution of conflict between themselves and their teenager through *mutual respect*. Parents should maintain the adolescent's trust in the family by seeing to it that their child speaks respectfully to them and that they, in turn, speak respectfully to their child. The second goal for parents is to tolerate the adolescent's expression of differing views. This heightens the teenager's perception of parental support and nurtures the adolescent's ego. In this way, the parents become leaders in a process in which collaboration and mutuality are affirmed and the ultimate goal of a partnership can be achieved.

PARENT/ADOLESCENT COMMUNICATION

Open communication probably is the most important skill for parents to develop and maintain with their maturing child (Box 101-1). Adolescents need a trusted sounding board before venturing forth. As facilitators, parents need to *listen* more than speak. When parents start to lecture, the adolescent's attention automatically shuts down. The axiom "Actions speak louder than words" makes a useful parental

BOX 101-1

DO AND DON'T OF PARENT/ADOLESCENT COMMUNICATION

1. Listen more, speak less.
2. Respond empathetically rather than intellectually.
3. Resist saying "I told you so!"
4. Clarify expectations by allowing adolescents to participate in decision making.

motto, far better than "Do as I say, not as I do." This latter philosophy raises the question of hypocrisy, often diminishing the adolescent's respect for the parent. Such a situation can result in more angry confrontations and a weakening of the parent-teen collaborative relationship.

Adolescents' continuing need for parental affection and acceptance, plus a not yet fully developed sense of self, leaves them highly vulnerable to self-perceived injustices, put-downs, and negative innuendoes. Parents gain immeasurably when they respond to their adolescents' feelings with an empathetic rather than an intellectual response. For example, during the teen years, peer relationships are experienced with intense emotions characteristic of adolescent egocentricity. Should a break occur in a heretofore close friendship, it is a wise parent who demonstrates support by empathizing with their child's hurt feelings. Statements such as "I'm so sorry that you are in such pain," "I can imagine how bad you are feeling," or "It seems that your friend has really hurt you; do you want to talk about it?" are appropriate and allow room for continued discussion. Sometimes, in an attempt to "make it better," parents tend to minimize the adolescent's pain, perceiving it as "only" a short-lived adolescent drama. They respond with statements such as "You'll find other friends," or "Don't worry, you're young and have your whole life ahead of you." Rather than finding this helpful, the adolescent feels misunderstood and may cut off further communication by saying, "You just don't understand!"

If the parent did not approve of the friend, the end of the relationship may be a source of relief for the parent. Telling a teenager to "forget about it" may be more representative of the parent's wish than of the teen's. The ultimate negative scenario is a parent who adds, "I told you so!" Few, if any, adults respond kindly to such admonishment. The thoughtful parent refrains from statements that serve only to belittle the adolescent. In fact, adolescents feel devastated when berated by a parent, despite their attempts to defend against the hurt by false bravado or an "I don't care!" response. When parents appropriately empathize with their teenagers' emotional intensity and allow their youngsters to express their emotions without restraint or embarrassment, adolescents are comforted and feel supported. This reinforces open communication with parents and minimizes the need for adolescents to act out angry or hurt feelings maladaptively.

Parents also have an obligation to clarify expectations, responsibilities, and privileges; these decisions are not made in a vacuum. Just as a parent of a 2-year-old might give the toddler a choice between a red or a blue outfit, it is imperative for the parent of an adolescent to allow him or her to participate as a member of the contractual, decision-making team. It is well known that the success of any contract between two or more parties requires that each person be allowed to express, *without dissent,* what he or she wants. It also is important that both sides negotiating the contract *gain something* from the outcome. An "all-or-nothing" result breeds discontent and nonadherence by the person who perceives no gain. *Nothing less is required between parents and adolescents.* Open communication and decision making founded on mutual respect are skills best learned within a family and ensure a win-win outcome.

Another important aspect of the decision-making process concerns the consequences of breaking a contract. Here, too, the process of open discussion *by all family members* should apply—that is, the reason for the infraction should be discussed and renegotiated. Many parents have little difficulty "grounding" their adolescent for nonadherence to an agreement, but they have more difficulty acknowledging that they, themselves, have failed to abide by an agreement. An example of such a situation involved a family in which the parents conceded that they nagged their daughter about not spending enough time on school work, fearing her academic failure. The parents agreed with the physician's counsel that they respect the adolescent's privacy and give her the responsibility for her school work. A "contract" was signed by the pediatrician, as mediator, the parents, and the adolescent. The terms included the adolescent's decision about the time to set aside for study, and the parents agreed to permit her to experience her decision and not to nag. If the adolescent's grades declined, she would be grounded; if the parents continued to harangue, they would be grounded for that weekend!

ASSESSING THE PARENT/ ADOLESCENT RELATIONSHIP

One way pediatricians can assess how families are coping with adolescent development is to ask the parents how parent-teen decision making is progressing. Curfew, the generations-old source of conflict, especially when associated with social events, is a good issue to discuss with parents. There is an inherent conflict about curfew decisions. Curfew contains issues of the adolescent's safety, the purview of parental authority, as well as the adolescent's choice of friends and events to be attended, the domain of the adolescent's jurisdiction. Here the physician should explore whether the parents are able to have an open discussion with their adolescent about his or her plans. Do the parents routinely inquire about the location of the social function and the travel plans? Are they easily able to work out an agreed-upon curfew with which everyone is reasonably satisfied? In the event of a disagreement, how are compromises negotiated (Box 101-2)? Parents should be counseled to avoid making arbitrarily rigid time limits. An example of the type of statement best avoided is, "Your Dad and/or I have decided that you are to be home no later than midnight." Such unilateral decisions usually end in angry, unresolvable confrontations. Sometimes the rigidity of the curfew time is confounded by the parents' disapproval of the adolescent's choice of friends or lifestyle.

Not infrequently, parental disapproval of the adolescent's friends may be the *expressed* reason for parental inflexibility

BOX 101-2

GUIDELINES FOR PARENTS

*P*articipate as partners with the adolescent
*A*cknowledge your parental authority
*R*espect each other's differences
*E*ncourage open communication
*N*egotiate win-win agreements
*T*olerate the adolescent's separateness

about the young person's curfew. However, the *underlying* cause for concern may have more to do with the parents' fear of adolescent sexual activity. The pediatrician might ask the parents whether they and their adolescent have been able to share their views about adolescent sexual activity and sexual relationships. If so, did such a discussion result in a consensual understanding? If not, the pediatrician can suggest that such a meeting take place "to clear the air." Although the issue of sexuality may be unexpressed, it is never far from parents' thoughts.

Parents also may feel anxious because they fear adverse outcomes when they perceive their adolescent's behavior as "deviant." In particular, parents may be afraid that such behavior will be permanent and will destroy the teen's opportunity to mature into a responsible, productive adult. It may reassure the parents to know that extremes of adolescent behavior generally are transient and that most adolescents mature into adults who have lifestyles, values, and mores fairly similar to those of their families. Here, it might be pointed out that the more rigid the parents' control, the greater the adolescent's rebellion. The adolescent's perception of parental acceptance, interest, warmth, and respect is associated positively with the adolescent's self-esteem. Nevertheless, parents should be supported in their efforts to protect the adolescent from accidents and other dangerous behavior that might occur during these experimental ventures. Thus, flexibility and reasonableness are traits to strive for as parents negotiate behavioral limits with their teenagers.

Parents also are well advised not to abdicate their authority abruptly. Rather, they need to be encouraged to maintain confidence in their authority to negotiate limits, particularly where true issues of safety are involved. A striking example was presented by a mother and her 14-year-old son during a pediatric visit. In response to a question about how things were going, the mother angrily reported that her son thought he no longer needed a parent. The boy silently reacted by rolling his eyes upward. Each was given an opportunity to explain. The mother focused on her son's defiant behavior after the parents had denied his request for an extended curfew to join in a friend's birthday celebration at a downtown urban center. The pediatrician encouraged the mother to give her main objection. She cited their fear for their son's safety, given the lateness of return. At this the boy blurted, "Why didn't you just say that!" The parents' perceived loss of control undermined their authority; as a result, their son's "immaturity" became the focus of their confrontation. Here, the pediatrician facilitated a reframing of the problem to highlight the safety issues, on which both the parents and the son agreed.

MANAGEMENT OF PARENT/ ADOLESCENT CONFLICT

Some families are unable to make use of a pediatrician's counsel and require the intervention of a mental health practitioner. For example, some parents resist acknowledging the relevance of understanding adolescent development and the *mutuality* of the parent-adolescent interaction. Instead, they chronically respond to the adolescent's point of view with "Yes . . . but," followed by a litany of the adolescent's misdeeds. Other parents themselves are immature and needy and rely inappropriately on their adolescent for nurturance and support. The unmet needs of such adolescents generally are manifested in a chronic pattern of acting-out behaviors, such as poor school performance, loss of friends, somatic complaints, and in extreme situations, depression or suicide attempts. For the less serious behaviors, pediatricians might consider meeting with the parents to assess their willingness and capacity to understand the developmental and family communication issues. If parents are refractory to counseling after one or two meetings, the pediatrician will be in a better position to make an appropriate mental health referral than he or she would have been at the initial visit (see Chapter 83, Consultation and Referral for Behavioral and Developmental Problems).

Pediatricians who counsel parents in a mutually satisfying working relationship can make a significant difference. By enhancing the parents' knowledge, reducing their stress, and increasing their coping abilities, pediatricians can help provide a safe familial harbor for their adolescent patients.

SUGGESTED READINGS

McCurdy SJ, Scherman A: Effects of family structure on the adolescent separation-individuation process, *Adolescence* 31:122, 307, 1996.

Rueter MA, Conger RD: Interaction style, problem-solving behavior, and family problem-solving effectiveness, *Child Dev* 66:l, 1995.

Smetana JG, Asquith P: Adolescents' and parents' conceptions of parental authority and personal autonomy, *Child Dev* 65:1147, 1994.

102 Anorexia and Bulimia Nervosa

Marcie B. Schneider • Martin Mandell Fisher

The eating disorders, a group of conditions that affect adolescents and young adults primarily, have increased dramatically in prevalence during the past three decades. Marked by a combination of medical and psychological factors in their etiology and outcome, they predominantly include the well-known entities of anorexia and bulimia nervosa. Anorexia nervosa, viewed most simply as the *purposeful loss of weight beyond that which is healthy,* is said to affect 1 of every 200 adolescent girls in the United States and Great Britain. Bulimia, which is marked by *recurrent episodes of binge eating and/or vomiting,* has been estimated to affect 2% to 20% of young women of high school and college age in these same countries, depending on the criteria used. The diagnosis and prevalence of these disorders are much debated, and many questions remain about their etiology and outcome. Nevertheless, the growing prevalence of eating disorders has made it increasingly important for the primary care physician to have some knowledge of the principles involved in the evaluation and treatment of both anorexia and bulimia nervosa.

DIAGNOSIS AND PREVALENCE

Although individual cases suggestive of anorexia nervosa and cultural behaviors suggestive of bulimia have been described from antiquity, neither disorder was defined specifically as a medical condition until the 1880s. At that time, Charles Lasègue in France described a condition he called "anorexia hysterica"; William Gull in England referred to the same condition as "anorexia nervosa." Although the latter term is a misnomer, because patients who have eating disorders do not simply have a loss of appetite as the name implies, it has prevailed since that time.

Individual cases of "anorexia nervosa" appear in the medical literature from the 1880s through the 1950s. Beginning in the 1960s, more cases of anorexia nervosa began to be seen. At first considered only a component of anorexia nervosa, bulimia (now more formally called *bulimia nervosa*) was recognized as a separate entity in the 1970s. It now is well known that anorexia nervosa and bulimia may appear as separate syndromes, that they may occur concomitantly or sequentially in the same individual, and that both may be associated with several other entities, including laxative abuse or alternating with obesity.

The first officially published criteria for the diagnosis of anorexia nervosa were in 1972.[12] The original criteria stipulated that an individual considered as having anorexia nervosa must (1) be younger than 25 years of age; (2) have lost at least 25% of her initial body weight; (3) not have an alternative medical diagnosis to account for the weight loss; (4) not have an alternative psychiatric diagnosis to account for the weight loss; (5) display evidence of a distorted body image, desire for extreme thinness, and a preoccupation with food and weight; and (6) have at least two of the following signs or symptoms associated with anorexia nervosa: amenorrhea, lanugo hair, bradycardia, periods of hyperactivity, episodes of binge eating, and vomiting.

Changes in both the nature and our understanding of anorexia nervosa have occurred in the ensuing years. It now is acknowledged that some patients may develop the illness after age 25. A 25% weight loss may be the result of an appropriate diet for those who start out overweight, whereas a 15% to 20% weight loss may be extremely unhealthy for those already underweight. Patients who have anorexia nervosa may have other psychiatric diagnoses (e.g., depression),[23] and a few patients may manipulate the treatment of other medical conditions (e.g., diabetes mellitus or cystic fibrosis) to lose weight (i.e., a concomitant diagnosis of anorexia nervosa). Furthermore, the emergence of bulimia as a distinct entity required specific criteria for this disorder as well. The best current criteria for both disorders are those listed by the American Psychiatric Association in the fourth edition of the *Diagnostic and Statistical Manual of Mental Disorders (DSM-IV),*[2] as shown in Box 102-1. The *DSM-IV* acknowledges that some patients who have eating disorders do not meet the strict criteria for either anorexia or bulimia nervosa; therefore, an additional category, "eating disorders not otherwise specified," has been established.

It has become apparent in recent years that increasingly larger numbers of adolescents, and even children, are displaying abnormal attitudes toward weight and food, and many are showing evidence of subclinical eating disorders.[14] Included in this category are adolescents who lose enough weight to cause irregular periods but not enough to meet *DSM-IV* criteria for anorexia nervosa and those who use vomiting to control their weight but do not binge and, therefore, do not meet specific criteria for bulimia nervosa. These adolescents often have medical and psychological difficulties similar to those described in patients whose eating disorders are more overt and generally require similar treatment.[7]

Changes in diagnostic criteria are partly responsible for the debates about incidence that have taken place over the past several years. Most researchers in the field believe that eating disorders have increased in both incidence and prevalence during the past 30 years. One long-term study has dem-

BOX 102-1

CRITERIA FOR THE DIAGNOSIS OF EATING DISORDERS

Anorexia Nervosa

Refusal to maintain body weight at or above a minimally normal weight for age and height (e.g., weight loss leading to maintenance of body weight less than 85% of that expected; or failure to make expected weight gain during period of growth, leading to body weight less than 85% of that expected)

Intense fear of gaining weight or becoming fat, even though underweight

Disturbance in the way in which one's body weight or shape is experienced, undue influence of body weight or shape on self-evaluation, or denial of seriousness of the current low body weight

In postmenarchal females, amenorrhea—that is, the absence of at least three consecutive menstrual cycles. (A woman is considered to have amenorrhea if her periods occur only following hormone [e.g., estrogen] administration.)

Restricting type: during the current episode of anorexia nervosa, the person has not regularly engaged in binge-eating or purging behavior (i.e., self-induced vomiting or the misuse of laxatives, diuretics, or enemas)

Binge-eating/purging type: during the current episode of anorexia nervosa, the person has regularly engaged in binge-eating or purging behavior (i.e., self-induced vomiting or the misuse of laxatives, diuretics, or enemas)

Bulimia Nervosa

Recurrent episodes of binge eating. An episode of binge eating is characterized by both of the following:

- Eating, in a discrete period of time (e.g., within any 2-hour period), an amount of food that is definitely larger than most people would eat during a similar period and under similar circumstances
- A sense of lack of control over eating during the episode (e.g., a feeling that one cannot stop eating or control what or how much one is eating)
- Recurrent inappropriate compensatory behavior so as to prevent weight gain, such as self-induced vomiting; misuse of laxatives, diuretics, enemas, or other medications; fasting; or excessive exercise
- The binge eating and inappropriate compensatory behaviors both occur, on average, at least twice a week for 3 months
- Self-evaluation is unduly influenced by body shape and weight
- The disturbance does not occur exclusively during episodes of anorexia nervosa

Purging type: during the current episode of bulimia nervosa, the person has regularly engaged in self-induced vomiting or the misuse of laxatives, diuretics, or enemas

Nonpurging type: during the current episode of bulimia nervosa, the person has used other inappropriate compensatory behaviors, such as fasting or excessive exercise, but has not regularly engaged in self-induced vomiting or the misuse of laxatives, diuretics, or enemas

From The American Psychiatric Association: *Diagnostic and statistical manual of mental disorders,* ed 4, Washington, DC, 1994, The Association.

onstrated a steady rise in incidence and prevalence among adolescents but smaller increases in adults.[32] More than 90% of patients who have anorexia and bulimia nervosa are girls or young women; although most cases of anorexia nervosa begin in the teenage years, bulimia is more apt to begin in the late teens and early twenties. It generally is accepted that 0.5% of all adolescent girls meet strict criteria for anorexia nervosa. With the criteria for bulimia nervosa being somewhat more vague, some researchers have found prevalences of binge eating and vomiting in 20% to 30% of college-age women; others, using strict criteria, limit the diagnosis to only 2% to 3% of the same populations.[41] Both diagnoses are far less common in developing nations and among minorities and those of lower socioeconomic status in industrialized societies, although recent increases in these populations have been noted as well.

PRESENTATION AND ETIOLOGY

The patient who has an eating disorder may seek medical care in a variety of ways. Some visit their pediatrician or family physician because of concern about weight loss, vomiting, or abnormal eating attitudes noticed by family, friends, or school authorities. Others visit a gynecologist because of the menstrual irregularities that characteristically accompany the disorder. Many are seen first by a psychiatrist, psychologist, or social worker; others may be seen for the first time in an emergency department because of dehydration or other medical complications. Some patients may be seen within weeks of the disorder's onset; others avoid medical care for months or even years. It is common for many patients to be brought for their initial evaluation against their will, although some patients may seek help willingly. Large-scale questionnaire surveys have shown that many patients who have mild to moderate eating disorders, both anorexia nervosa and bulimia, avoid medical care altogether by hiding or denying their illness.

A considerable body of literature has explored the possible etiological factors in these disorders.[17] Several key questions are addressed: Why has there been an apparent increase in these disorders during the past three decades? Why are women affected predominantly? What factors cause any particular individual to develop the disorder? Cultural, psychological, and biochemical factors all have been invoked in responding to these questions.

Several cultural changes that have taken place during the past 30 years may bear directly on the increased incidence of eating disorders. Foremost among these is the strong emphasis our society places on the desirability of a thin appearance, especially for women. Certain vulnerable individuals may feel it necessary to choose an unhealthy means, whether it be excessive dieting, vomiting, laxative abuse, or a combination thereof, striving for a dangerously thin weight goal. Societal changes in sexual mores, which have lowered the mean age of initiating sexual intercourse from the late teens to the midteens, thereby putting increased pressure on adolescent and young adult women, also are hypothesized to play a role in furthering the psychological vulnerability of some individuals. The issue of career versus family may create another level of vulnerability for some individuals at risk for the development of psychological difficulties. Of further interest is issues of sexual identity having been noted in some young men who develop these disorders.

The psychological factors responsible for the development of an eating disorder in any given individual are numerous and complex.[26] When anorexia nervosa first came to prominence in the 1960s, it was found that most of the girls who had this disorder exhibited a set of similar characteristics, some of which were manifested openly; others emerged with intensive therapy. Specifically, these girls were described as having been excellent students, compulsive workers, and compliant daughters before the onset of their illness. These same girls then became hostile, withdrawn, and depressed after the illness began. In therapy they revealed exceedingly low self-esteem despite their apparent outward success. Their families, outwardly healthy and often so-called pillars of society, were found to have significant hidden psychopathological disorders.

Based on these early findings, three major lines of reasoning, often overlapping, have been proposed to explain the psychological basis of eating disorders. The first theory concentrates on the psychopathological condition of the individual, postulating that poor self-esteem in the face of outward success poses a major difficulty, which the vulnerable adolescent tries to alleviate by striving for one achievable goal—the thinnest possible body. The second focuses on the family, postulating that patients who have anorexia nervosa come from families in which the natural childhood processes of separation and individuation are not allowed to proceed normally. The refusal to eat represents the ultimate rebelliousness in a teenager who previously has done "everything you've asked of me." A third, older theory developed around a series of sexual themes, hypothesizing that the weight loss in anorexia nervosa serves to diminish the female figure of a young lady who is afraid of becoming a sexual adult. The basis of this fear may be sexual taboos in the family, in some cases, or sexual overstimulation in the family in other cases. In the extreme psychoanalytical interpretation of this theory, patients who have anorexia nervosa may even be refusing food intake for fear of "oral impregnation."

In many cases of anorexia nervosa, however, the patient does not fit the traditional "good girl" mold. Furthermore, the previous finding that most girls who have anorexia nervosa are excellent students from apparently healthy and intact families is no longer as true as in the past. In fact, increasing numbers of girls who have anorexia nervosa are noted to have learning disabilities or mental retardation or to live in difficult family situations. More recently, the role of sexual abuse as an etiological factor in the development of eating disorders, especially intractable bulimia, has been the focus of increased attention and debate.[8]

The possibility that a biological vulnerability may be present in the initiation and continuance of the eating disorders also has received much attention. Because cases of anorexia and bulimia have been associated in family studies with depression, addiction, or both, it is surmised that a biochemical predeterminant may be present in both disorders. Changes in either dopamine or serotonin metabolism may help bring on these disorders, and the cholecystokinin and endorphin systems have been implicated in maintaining them. It is very possible that the biochemical factors that may predispose an individual to begin losing weight or vomiting may be different from those that prevent reversal of these behaviors.

Most likely, several factors converge in the development of an eating disorder. The adolescent girl who is culturally primed, biologically at risk, and psychologically vulnerable may begin dieting or vomiting in response to a particular precipitant (often an insult by family or friends, exposure to another individual who has an eating disorder, or a stressful situation). The positive psychological feedback that initially accompanies an "improved" appearance and the biochemical changes that occur in response to decreased nutrition may serve to perpetuate the behavior. It is at this stage that family and friends become concerned and the individual patient seeks medical care.

EVALUATION

Initial evaluation of the patient includes a determination of the diagnosis and its severity, an evaluation of other possible causes of weight loss and effects of malnutrition, an analysis of the psychological context of the illness, and a decision about treatment.

As presented in Box 102-1, specific diagnostic criteria currently exist for the eating disorders. Evaluation of these criteria serves both to elucidate the diagnosis and determine the severity of the illness. Distortion of body image, a hallmark in the diagnosis of anorexia nervosa, may be evaluated by exploring the patient's views of her initial, current, and desired weight. A history of vomiting and binge eating is elicited in the patient who has bulimia. This information is used to gain insight into the severity of the disorder, but many patients who have eating disorders will not be completely truthful. Establishing the patient's eating and exercise patterns and use of vomiting or medications designed to promote weight loss (including diet pills, laxatives, diuretics, or ipecac) provides hints both to the diagnosis and the possibility of medical complications. Care must be taken to avoid being misled by the patient who is not completely forthright; often the physical examination and laboratory tests suggest the true extent of the patient's disorder.

The first steps in the physical examination of the patient who is thought to have an eating disorder are calculation of the percentage below ideal body weight (IBW) and determination of vital signs. The percentage below IBW, which may be calculated by comparing the patient's current weight with the average weight expected for height, age, and gender (as determined by standard growth charts), serves both as one of the diagnostic criteria and as a gross estimate of the degree of malnutrition. In general, body weight more than 30% below IBW represents severe malnutrition; 20% to 30% below IBW represents moderate malnutrition; and that not yet 20% below IBW represents mild malnutrition. For example, a 16-year-old girl who is 5 feet, 4 inches tall would be expected to have a body weight of 120 pounds, plus or minus 10%; she would be 20% below IBW at 96 pounds and 30% below IBW at 84 pounds. BMI, or body mass index, is being used increasingly to describe nutritional status. In addition, pediatric growth curves may be needed for premenarchal girls to determine previous height and weight curves and to establish appropriate weight goals for achievement of expected adult height.

Vital signs provide further evidence of the degree of malnutrition because chronic malnutrition is accompanied by declines in blood pressure, pulse, and electrocardiographic (ECG) voltage.[13] Other physical changes associated with malnutrition or its concomitant hormonal changes include the findings of scaphoid abdomen, muscle weakness, lanugo hair similar to that seen in newborns, diminished reflexes, and dry skin. Few physical findings are associated with the vomiting of bulimia, although telltale bite marks on the knuckles (used to induce gagging) may be evident in some patients.

Laboratory tests further elucidate the severity of the illness. Most patients who have anorexia and bulimia nervosa have normal laboratory results initially, although all organ systems probably are affected by the malnutrition. The laboratory abnormalities found on routine testing are related generally to the individual's particular nutritional pattern. Thus, the patient who is chronically malnourished usually has leukopenia; occasionally, thrombocytopenia; and in rare cases, severe anemia (being protected for some time from iron-deficiency anemia by the concomitant amenorrhea). The patient who restricts fluid intake may show evidence of dehydration on blood chemistry abnormalities (including an elevated sodium or blood urea nitrogen), whereas the patient who drinks excessive fluids to satisfy hunger or the physician's scale may show signs of hyponatremia and a dilute urine. Conversely, the patient who vomits or uses laxatives may show evidence of hypokalemia, which often is very severe in those who use both methods of weight control. Nutrient values, including levels of zinc, calcium, magnesium, copper, vitamin B_{12}, and folate, all may be altered in the malnourished patient; amylase levels and urinary pH may be elevated in some patients who have bulimia.[3]

Hormonal testing may produce evidence of dysfunction in endocrine systems.[36] The development of hypothyroidism, believed to be an adaptive response to inadequate nutrition, generally is evident in low-normal levels of triiodothyronine (T_3), thyroxine (T_4), and thyroid-stimulating hormone (TSH). Amenorrhea, a hallmark of the disorder, generally develops when the patient's weight reaches approximately 15% below IBW but may be seen earlier; it is accompanied by low levels of luteinizing hormone (LH) and follicle-stimulating hormone (FSH). Loss of the diurnal variation in cortisol production and abnormalities in antidiuretic hormone may be noted as well, although these tests need not be performed in most patients. Evidence of abnormalities may be found on computed tomography (CT) and magnetic resonance imaging (MRI) scans of the brain or echocardiograms of the heart, but these tests generally are reserved for evaluating other possible causes when the diagnosis is in question. It has been demonstrated recently that the MRI changes in the brain, including gray matter deficits and elevated cerebrospinal fluid volumes, may not be reversible.[27] In general, the initial laboratory workup of eating disorders may include a complete blood count, urinalysis, and ECG, as well as evaluation of serum electrolytes, liver function, thyroid function, and levels of LH, FSH, estradiol, and prolactin in patients who have amenorrhea. This battery of tests generally is sufficient to provide a barometer of current status, a baseline to follow further changes, and screening for other possible causes of weight loss.

Recent data have demonstrated that patients who have eating disorders, especially those whose amenorrhea is prolonged secondary to malnutrition, show evidence of osteopenia on bone density studies.[30] Initial studies have shown that this effect may not be preventable, even with calcium supplementation or hormonal replacement, or completely reversible, even after the patient regains her normal weight.[4] Concern is growing, therefore, that patients who have eating disorders may be at significant risk for developing osteoporosis and fractures later in life. Studies are under way to determine whether the osteopenia is due solely to low levels of estrogen or also to the effects of increased cortisol production and whether hormonal replacement, in fact, might be able to lessen the development of this complication.[1] Bone densitometry, using dual energy radiograph absorptiometry (DEXA), has become a routine test in the evaluation of patients who have eating disorders and amenorrhea of at least 6 to 12 months' duration.[10] The treatment of choice is weight gain and menstrual restoration, which generally occurs at an estradiol level of 30 μg/dl.[19] Estrogen replacement may be able to increase bone density in some or at least help maintain bone density in others.[24,29] Researchers are exploring other treatments such as recombinant human insulin growth factors (rhIGF)[2] and dehydroepiandrosterone (DHEA).[20]

DIFFERENTIAL DIAGNOSIS

The differential diagnosis of the eating disorders includes possible medical causes of weight loss or vomiting and other psychiatric causes of poor appetite. The history, physical examination, and baseline laboratory tests should help rule out infectious, inflammatory, neoplastic, or endocrine disease; further testing may be necessary if the weight loss or vomiting cannot be explained adequately. A brain MRI, gastrointestinal (GI) series, or other tests may be considered in rare cases for patients who claim to be eating well or not vomiting on purpose. Case reports abound with instances of hypothalamic tumors, inflammatory bowel disease, mesenteric artery syndrome, or GI tract tumors being diagnosed mistakenly as eating disorders in patients whose weight loss or vomiting was not understood adequately. Occasionally a patient may show obvious pleasure in the weight loss or vomiting brought on by another disorder, but this must not be confused with a positive diagnosis of anorexia or bulimia nervosa.

Psychiatric causes of weight loss can include depression and psychosis (especially schizophrenia). The patient who refuses to eat because of a desire to lose weight must be differentiated from the patient who cannot eat because of depression or the patient who will not eat because of delusional fears (e.g., that the food is poisoned). Although patients may have concomitant depression or psychosis with anorexia or bulimia nervosa, separate criteria must be used to establish each entity. A full psychosocial history must be obtained as part of the initial evaluation to establish both the diagnosis and the psychosocial severity of the disorder. The patient's functioning in the family, in school, and among peers must be determined, and possible psychiatric symptoms such as sleep disorders, hallucinations, delusions, or obsessions should be elicited. It is the rare patient who has an eating disorder who does not exhibit psychosocial changes with the onset of the illness. These generally include fighting with the family, withdrawing from friends, and performing less optimally in school, although some patients paradoxically report improved school performance as they withdraw from friends and family. If additional psychiatric symptoms are found, the possibility of an additional diagnosis should be pursued.

BOX 102-2

INDICATIONS FOR HOSPITALIZATION IN AN ADOLESCENT WITH AN EATING DISORDER

Any one or more of the following:
- Severe malnutrition (weight <75% ideal body weight)
- Dehydration
- Electrolyte disturbances
- Cardiac disturbances
- Physiological instability (bradycardia, hypotension, hypothermia, orthostatic changes)
- Arrested growth and development
- Failure of outpatient treatment
- Acute food refusal
- Uncontrollable bingeing and purging
- Acute medical complication of malnutrition (e.g., syncope, seizures, cardiac failure, pancreatitis)
- Acute psychiatric emergencies (e.g., suicidal ideation, acute psychosis)
- Comorbid diagnosis that interferes with the treatment of the eating disorder (e.g., severe depression, obsessive-compulsive disorder, severe family dysfunction)

From Fisher M, et al: Eating disorders in adolescence: a background paper, *J Adolesc Health* 16:420, 1995.

TREATMENT

The results of the initial medical and psychiatric evaluation play a major role in establishing a treatment protocol for the patient.[31] Although most patients who have an eating disorder may be treated as outpatients, those whose medical findings are significant (including severe malnutrition, electrolyte disturbance, or vital sign abnormalities) require hospitalization. Patients who fail to gain weight with outpatient treatment, whose vomiting is extreme, or whose psychiatric condition is out of control also may require hospitalization. Specific criteria for hospitalization are listed in Box 102-2.[15] Hospitalization may be shorter term in an adolescent medical unit or longer term in a psychiatric unit.[37] It has been shown that restoration to an appropriate "goal" weight is one way to prevent relapse and rehospitalization.[5,22] In this day of managed care, however, where every attempt is made to contain cost, hospitalizations often are for medical stabilization rather than weight restoration. In response to this, day treatment programs have been developed. These programs may be attempted in lieu of hospitalization or in transition from an inpatient program. Reviews of these programs have been favorable, although weight is more difficult to gain in this setting, and managed care remains an issue.[18,38] The struggle over managed care and the treatment for eating disorders remains powerful, with lawsuits being fought to allow patients the appropriate treatment for this chronic illness. Treatment approaches, whether in a hospital, a day program, or an outpatient setting, are aimed at restoring more normal physical and psychological functioning.

Most clinicians consider patients who have an eating disorder to be among the most difficult and frustrating patients to treat. Undoubtedly, several factors are responsible for this perception. The combination of medical and psychological care required makes it difficult for any single professional to be proficient in all aspects of a patient's care. If the patient is hostile to the physician (e.g., often chooses to ignore suggestions and tests how much she can "get away with"), the physician may find him- or herself in an uncomfortable and adversarial relationship with the patient. The difficult families within which many of these patients live often make it a challenge to establish the most rational treatment plans. For these reasons it is advisable that no single individual be responsible totally for any patient's care beyond the initial evaluation or for the most straightforward of cases.[46] Rather, a team approach should be used. The team may consist of a primary care physician, a psychiatrist, a psychologist, a social worker, and a nutritionist, with the exact combination determined by local availability and preference. Generally, each team member manages specific aspects of care, and team meetings and discussions are held frequently to avoid miscommunication that can sabotage the treatment. One team member serves as spokesperson to the patient and, especially, the family.

The treatment team may use several modalities, including nutritional rehabilitation, behavior therapy, individual psychotherapy, family and group therapy, and psychopharmacology. It generally is acknowledged that a "multimodality therapy" that includes aspects of each of these approaches holds the best promise for successful treatment.[47] The degree to which each of these approaches is incorporated into the treatment varies, both with the preferences of the treatment team and the requirements of the individual patient. Each of these approaches may be used for inpatients, day program patients, and outpatients.

NUTRITIONAL REHABILITATION

The malnutrition that accompanies anorexia nervosa is directly responsible for most, if not all, of the physical abnormalities noted in the disorder and also for some of the mental deterioration. Accordingly, nutritional rehabilitation is crucial in the treatment of the patient who has anorexia nervosa. Restoration of body weight, generally to an end point of within 10% of IBW, with restoration of menses, should be among the main goals of treatment. For many patients whose malnutrition is mild to moderate (15% to 25% below IBW), this may be accomplished on an outpatient basis; patients who have moderate to severe malnutrition (more than 25% below IBW) rarely can accomplish the required weight gain without hospitalization.

Nutritional rehabilitation generally can be achieved through oral feedings; a daily intake of three substantial meals and three to four snacks usually is sufficient to bring about the required weight gain. On inpatient units, meals generally are provided as part of a strict regimen, and snacks generally consist of high-calorie supplements, available as liquids or puddings in various brands and flavors. Care is taken not to overfeed patients whose malnutrition is severe because a too-rapid weight gain has been associated with severe metabolic abnormalities in some patients.[16] In the outpatient setting, an appropriate meal pattern may be developed based on the patient's and family's prior eating habits or on a specific dietary plan offered by the physician or a nutritionist. The dietary plan should be specific so that ambiguities that can lead to family fighting are avoided; it should provide approximately 2000 to 3000 calories a day, with up to 1000 calories supplied in the form of high-calorie supplements. The plan should be well balanced and include foods from each of the major food groups. Compliance with the dietary regimen may be evaluated by having the patient keep a diet diary; however, many patients do not always keep these accurately and honestly. Except for the high-calorie supplements, a similar dietary plan may be offered to the normal-weight patient who has bulimia because these patients generally require "nutritional adjustment" rather than nutritional rehabilitation.

BEHAVIORAL THERAPY

Merely offering a nutritious diet to a patient who has either anorexia or bulimia nervosa is unlikely to result in a drastic change in the patient's status. For this reason, behavioral therapy normally is a necessary component of treatment. The goal of behavioral therapy in the treatment of eating disorders is to offer a set of external positive and negative reinforcements to replace those internal sensors that usually control appetite and weight gain but that currently are missing. Behavioral therapy is not intended to be definitive but rather to accomplish specific goals in the areas of weight and diet stabilization, thus allowing the psychological modalities of treatment to proceed in a more "medically healthy" patient.

Various behavioral approaches may be used. The strict behavioral plans used on some psychiatric units involve removal of all "privileges," including use of the telephone, television, and regular clothing, if a particular weight goal is not achieved each day. A somewhat less strict plan the authors use on their adolescent unit involves four phases of treatment, with patients moving from one phase to another, based on achievement of progressively higher weight goals. Each phase incorporates additional privileges into the patient's daily activities (e.g., mobility on the unit, exercise, meals, snacks, and passes) in such a way that improved weight and eating patterns lead to additional privileges and responsibilities. For patients unable to respond to the positive reinforcements provided by such a phased system, an all-liquid diet, provided by mouth or, more rarely, nasogastric tube, may be substituted. Use of such methods ultimately achieves the necessary weight goals in almost all patients. However, behavioral therapy alone cannot be considered adequate treatment; controlled studies have been unable to distinguish between the effects of the various behavioral approaches.

Applying behavioral principles may be somewhat more difficult when treating anorexia nervosa patients or patients who have bulimia in the outpatient setting. For many patients who have anorexia nervosa, the usual approaches to behavioral therapy in outpatient settings (e.g., use of monetary or similar rewards) may not be strong enough to overcome the fear of eating. Fear of hospitalization itself may be the sole motivation. Similarly, classic approaches may not be effective for the patient who has bulimia because the symptom of vomiting cannot be measured readily. More sophisticated cognitive-behavioral approaches have been developed, therefore, so that the patient who has bulimia may understand and participate in her own behavioral therapy.[11] These approaches make use of diaries and changes in daily patterns to effect change in the bulimic patient.

INDIVIDUAL, FAMILY, AND GROUP THERAPY

Individual psychotherapy remains an essential part of the treatment for most patients who have an eating disorder. Although therapeutic styles differ based on the treatment team and the individual therapist, exploration of underlying psychological features and possible mechanisms for change is appropriate for most patients who have either anorexia or bulimia nervosa. Although several common themes have been noted in many of these patients, including poor self-esteem, family conflicts, difficulties with friends, and fear of sexuality, there is great individual variety in the way these themes are expressed and manifested. For many patients, it is apparent that the eating disorder serves as a defense against other difficult aspects of life; an important secondary gain also may be involved. It generally is acknowledged that psychological change is a necessary precursor to significant improvement in the disordered thinking and behavior exhibited by most patients who have an eating disorder.

Family therapy has become an increasingly popular treatment, especially for younger patients, as the major role that family conflicts and problems play in symptom continuation has become more apparent. Family sessions, arranged in varying combinations to include parents and siblings, generally focus on the disordered communication patterns that preceded and presumably contributed to the eating disorder. Resolving specific conflicts arising from the presence of the eating disorder itself also becomes an important area for discussion. It has been found that the course of the eating disorder is much more difficult for adolescent patients whose families are unable or unwilling to make necessary changes in their customary patterns of communication and parenting. It also has been demonstrated that family therapy is particularly important for adolescents who have eating disorders.[40]

Many patients who have eating disorders participate in group therapy during the course of their treatment. For some patients whose anorexia nervosa is mild and for college-age patients who have bulimia, this may be the only approach to therapy used. Groups may be organized in many different ways—some focusing on a psychotherapeutic approach, others concentrating more specifically on behavioral changes. Initial fears that patients who have eating disorders will "learn bad habits" from one another in the group have been outweighed by the apparent benefit most patients derive from group therapy. This is especially true for patients who have had social difficulties during their adolescence.

PSYCHOPHARMACOLOGY

The use of medication to treat eating disorders has a long history of decidedly mixed results. Numerous medications have been tried, from thyroid hormone and insulin in the 1940s and 1950s to phenytoin (Dilantin) and hydroxyzine (Atarax) in the 1960s and 1970s, as attempts were made to improve appetite, increase weight gain, and reverse physiological abnormalities. More recently, pharmacological treatment of the eating disorders has concentrated on psychoactive medications, including antidepressants, lithium, and antipsychotics. Two specific lines of reasoning have guided the use of these medications. In patients who are diagnosed as having an eating disorder along with, or as part of, another psychiatric diagnosis, medication for the associated diagnosis is offered with the expectation that the eating disorder will improve as other depressive or psychotic symptomatology is relieved. Alternately, more recent evidence has demonstrated that use of psychoactive drugs, especially the increasingly newer and safer serotonin reuptake inhibitors, diminish the urge to binge and vomit in patients who have bulimia and help treat obsessive-compulsive disorders in these patients as well.[45] Fluoxetine currently is the only drug approved by the Federal Drug Administration (FDA) for the treatment of bulimia.[6] Although earlier studies failed to show definitive benefits from the use of medication in the eating disorders, recent studies have delineated subgroups of patients most likely to improve with their use.[45] With antidepressants being used increasingly in the management of the eating disorders, it is important that only those familiar with their use prescribe these medications as part of the treatment.

OUTCOME AND PROGNOSIS

Eating disorders must be viewed as a chronic illness, similar to other medical or psychiatric chronic illnesses. A wide range of outcomes can be expected.[25] Recent reviews of follow-up studies of patients who have bulimia reveal that approximately 50% recover, 30% experience relapse, and 20% continue to meet the full criteria for bulimia nervosa 5 years after diagnosis.[28,42] A recent study on the long-term course of adolescents who have severe anorexia nervosa revealed a protracted course, yet 10 to 15 years later, almost 76% recovered fully.[44] Contradicting this, another study of severe anorexia nervosa revealed 24% full recovery at 10 years.[9] Although many different approaches are used to evaluate outcome, it is estimated that at least 25% of patients do well in the long term, 50% show varying degrees of improvement, and 25% do poorly despite adequate treatment. Patients who are younger, as well as those whose forms of the disease are milder, appear to have a better prognosis than these general numbers indicate.

Numerous personal, family, and treatment factors have been considered for their significance in predicting the outcome of an eating disorder. Several factors have been found to be associated with the prognosis, yet none of these may be predictive for an individual patient. For instance, a poorer outcome in anorexia nervosa has been associated with factors such as older age, vomiting, and premorbid personality problems, yet any particular patient who has this constellation of findings may do well with treatment. Furthermore, no specific treatment has been shown by controlled studies to be more effective than others, in general or for any particular type of patient. Thus, the eating disorders remain complicated and challenging for the patient, the family, and the treatment team.

PREVENTION

Although the focus on both primary and secondary prevention has increased, the best strategies for the prevention of eating disorders remain unclear.[39] To date, several programs geared toward both female and male adolescents, primarily in school settings, have been implemented. These programs generally provide factual information and are aimed at maintenance of a healthy body image, healthy eating, and promotion of self-esteem without relation to weight, and they appear to succeed in terms of increasing awareness and knowledge about eating disorders.[43] However, there are mixed results as to whether these programs prevent or actually promote eating-disordered behavior.[33,35] Although not documented in the literature, specific programs have aimed at populations at increased risk for the development of eating disorders, such as ballet dancers, which do not focus as much on eating, but rather on self-esteem, and seem to show promise. The concept of preventing eating disorders through more generic programs focused on building self-esteem is currently being explored. In keeping with this, the concept of a comprehensive school-based approach has been advocated.[34] This would include classroom interventions, staff training throughout the school, informal discussions between staff and students, integration of material about eating issues into the curriculum, more intensive work with those at high risk, changes within the school with respect to cafeteria food and physical education, and referrals and outreach, both within the school and to the community.

REFERENCES

1. Abrams SA, et al: Mineral balance and bone turnover in adolescents with anorexia nervosa, *J Pediatr* 123:326, 1993.
2. American Psychiatric Association: *Diagnostic and statistical manual of mental disorders* (DSM-IV), Washington, DC, 1994, APA Press.

3. Arden MR, Budow L, Bunnell DW: Alkaline urine is associated with eating disorders, *Am J Dis Child* 145:28, 1991 (letter).
4. Bachrach LK, et al: Recovery from osteopenia in adolescent girls with anorexia nervosa, *J Clin Endocrinol Metab* 72:602, 1991.
5. Baran SA, Weltzin TE, Kaye WH: Low discharge weight and outcome in anorexia nervosa, *Am J Psychiatry* 152:1070, 1995.
6. Becker AE, et al: Eating disorders, *N Engl J Med* 340:1092, 1999.
7. Bunnell DW, et al: Subclinical versus formal eating disorders: differentiating psychological features, *Int J Eat Disord* 9:357, 1990.
8. Connors ME, Morse W: Sexual abuse and eating disorders: a review, *Int J Eat Disord* 13:1, 1993.
9. Eckert ED, et al: Ten-year follow-up of anorexia nervosa: clinical course and outcome, *Psychol Med* 25:143, 1995.
10. Emans SJ, et al: Estrogen deficiency in adolescents and young adults: impact on bone mineral content and effects of estrogen replacement therapy, *Obstet Gynecol* 76:585, 1990.
11. Fairburn CG, et al: Psychotherapy and bulimia nervosa: longer-term effects of interpersonal psychotherapy, behavior therapy, and cognitive behavior therapy, *Arch Gen Psychiatry* 50:419, 1993.
12. Feighner JP, et al: Diagnostic criteria for use in psychiatric research, *Arch Gen Psychiatry* 26:57, 1972.
13. Fisher M: Medical complications of anorexia and bulimia nervosa, *Adolesc Med: State of the Art Reviews* 3:487, 1992.
14. Fisher M, et al: Eating attitudes, health-risk behaviors, self-esteem and anxiety among adolescent females in a suburban high school, *J Adolesc Health* 12:377, 1991.
15. Fisher M, et al: Eating disorders in adolescents: a background paper, *J Adolesc Health* 16:420, 1995.
16. Fisher M, Simpser E, Schneier M: Hypophosphatemia secondary to oral refeeding in anorexia nervosa, *Int J Eat Disord* (in press).
17. Garner DM: Pathogenesis of anorexia nervosa, *Lancet* 341:1631, 1993.
18. Gerlinghoff M, Backmund H, Franzen U: Evaluation of a day treatment programme for eating disorders, *Eur Eat Disord Rev* 6:96, 1998.
19. Golden N, et al: Resumption of menses in anorexia nervosa, *Arch Pediatr Adolesc Med* 151:16, 1997.
20. Gordon CM, et al: Use of DHEA to prevent osteoporosis in patients with anorexia nervosa, *J Adolesc Health* 22:176, 1998.
21. Grinspoon S, et al: Effects of short term recombinant human insulin-like growth factor I administration on bone turnover in osteopenic women with anorexia nervosa, *J Clin Endocrinol Metab* 81:3864, 1996.
22. Halmi KA, Licinio E: *Outcome: hospital program for eating disorders.* In Syllabus and Proceedings Summary, 142nd Annual Meeting of the American Psychiatric Association, Washington DC, 1989.
23. Halmi KA, et al: Comorbidity of psychiatric diagnoses in anorexia nervosa, *Arch Gen Psychiatry* 48:712, 1991.
24. Hergenroder AC, et al: Bone mineral changes in young women with hypothalamic amenorrhea treated with oral contraceptives, medroxyprogesterone, or placebo over 12 months, *Am J Obstet Gynecol* 176: 1017, 1997.
25. Herzog DB, Keller MB, Lavori PN: Outcome in anorexia nervosa and bulimia nervosa, *J Nerv Ment Dis* 176:131, 1988.
26. Johnson CL, Sansone RA, Chewning M: Good reasons why young women would develop anorexia nervosa: the adoptive context, *Pediatr Ann* 21:731, 1992.
27. Katzman DK, et al: A longitudinal magnetic resonance imaging study of brain changes in adolescents with anorexia nervosa, *Arch Pediatr Adolesc Med* 151:793, 1997.
28. Keel PK, Mitchell JE: Outcome in bulimia nervosa, *Am J Psychiatry* 154:313, 1997.
29. Klibanski A, et al: The effects of estrogen administration on trabecular bone loss in young women with anorexia nervosa, *J Clin Endocrinol Metab* 80:898, 1995.
30. Kreipe RE, Forbes GB: Osteoporosis: a "new morbidity" for dieting female adolescents? *Pediatrics* 86:478, 1990.
31. Kreipe RE, Uphoff M: Treatment and outcome of adolescents with anorexia nervosa, *Adolesc Med: State of the Art Reviews* 3:519, 1992.
32. Lucas AR, et al: Fifty-year trends in the incidence of anorexia nervosa in Rochester, Minnesota: a population-based study, *Am J Psychiatry* 148:917, 1991.
33. Mann T, et al: Are two interventions worse than none? Joint primary and secondary prevention of eating disorders in college females, *Health Psychol* 16:215,1997.
34. Neumark-Sztainer D: School-based programs for the prevention of eating disturbances, *J Sch Health* 66:64, 1996.
35. Neumark-Sztainer D, Butler R, Palti H: Eating disturbances among adolescent girls: evaluation of a school-based primary prevention program, *J Nutr Educ* 27:24, 1995.
36. Newman MW, Halmi KA: The endocrinology of anorexia nervosa and bulimia nervosa, *Neurol Clin* 6:195, 1988.
37. Nussbaum M, et al: Follow-up investigation in patients with anorexia nervosa, *J Pediatr* 106:835, 1985.
38. Piran N, et al: Evaluation of a day hospital programme for eating disorders, *Int J Eat Disord* 8:523, 1989.
39. Rosen DS, Neumark-Sztainer DN: Review of options for primary prevention of eating disturbances among adolescents, *J Adolesc Health* 23:354, 1998.
40. Russell GFM, et al: An evaluation of family therapy in anorexia nervosa and bulimia nervosa, *Arch Gen Psychiatry* 44:1047, 1987.
41. Stein DM: The prevalence of bulimia: a review of the empirical research, *J Nutr Educ* 23:205, 1991.
42. Steinhausen HC: Outcome of anorexia nervosa in the younger patient, *J Child Psychol Psychiatry* 38:271, 1997.
43. Story M, Neumark-Sztainer D: Promoting healthy eating and physical activity in adolescents, *Adolesc Med: State of the Art Reviews* 10:109, 1999.
44. Strober M, Freeman R, Morrell W: The long-term course of severe anorexia nervosa in adolescents: survival analysis of recovery, relapse and outcome predictors over 10-15 years in a prospective study, *Int J Eat Disord* 22:339, 1997.
45. Walsh BT, Devlin MJ: The pharmacologic treatment of eating disorders, *Psychiatr Clin North Am* 15:149, 1992.
46. Yager J, et al: American Psychiatric Association Practice Guidelines for Eating Disorders, *Am J Psychiatry* 150:207, 1993.
47. Yates A: Current perspectives on the eating disorders. II. Treatment, outcome, and research directions, *J Am Acad Child Adolesc Psychiatry* 29:1, 1990.

103 Drug, Alcohol, and Tobacco Abuse

Susan M. Coupey • S. Kenneth Schonberg

The use of drugs or, more precisely, the use of substances that alter the state of consciousness, has become nearly a universal rite of passage for American adolescents. Whereas the use of alcohol always has been widespread among youth, the past three decades have witnessed a dramatic rise in the amount and types of other substances abused by teenagers and young adults. Opiates, barbiturates, cocaine, hallucinogens, amphetamines, inhalants, anabolic steroids, and marijuana all have become familiar terms to those who provide care for youth.

The pattern of substance use by adolescents is continually evolving. New drugs, new fads, and new epidemics have been an invariable feature of substance abuse. The late 1960s and early 1970s were marked by a major concern with the abuse of opiates and barbiturates. Addiction, overdose, and medical sequelae from these drugs led to frequent hospitalizations, serious illnesses, and significant mortality. By the mid-1970s the use of these "hard" drugs had declined markedly. A variety of hallucinogens appeared, gained widespread popularity, and subsequently faded from the spotlight as their use lessened; however, hallucinogens remain readily available. Among these agents are peyote (which contains mescaline), lysergic acid diethylamide (LSD), and phencyclidine (PCP, angel dust).

During the 1980s, major attention focused on the use of milder intoxicants—alcohol and marijuana. Although these drugs are less likely to cause serious somatic illness during the teenage years, their widespread use and frequent association with both accidents and behavioral disruption are cause for significant health concern. In addition, in the latter part of the 1980s, cocaine use and abuse became quite common among both adolescents and adults. The emergence of "crack" (a smokable form of free-base cocaine) as a major public health problem, especially in inner cities, was accompanied by greater public awareness of the addictive and destructive properties of the drug.

As the decade of the 1990s began, cocaine use by adolescents declined. Many young people switched to amphetamines as their stimulant of choice; the use of this class of drug, including crystal methamphetamine ("ice"), rose among high school students in the mid- and late-1990s. At the same time, an increase in hallucinogens, including the designer hallucinogen "ecstasy" (3,4-methylenedioxymethamphetamine, or MDMA), and anabolic steroid use became apparent. In 1995, heroin use by high school seniors increased markedly, coinciding with a heroin epidemic among adults in the United States. This increase has continued through 1998. Most adolescents now use heroin by nasal inhalation (snorting, sniffing) rather than by injection. Because of the high purity of the heroin sold in the 1990s, nasal inhalation allows users to achieve the desired "rush" formerly achieved only by intravenous injection. Also during the early- to mid-1990s, an upsurge in marijuana use by high school students occurred, peaking in 1997 and beginning a slight downturn in 1998.

Traditionally, discussion of drug-related issues with teenagers has been approached either by outlining the physiological consequences associated with the abuse of a particular substance or by reviewing the effects of abuse on different organ systems. Such approaches, however, are at variance with the usual way most teenage drug abusers are seen for medical care. The substances now abused most commonly are not associated with frequent illness; therefore, teenagers using these agents most often are encountered when they seek routine health maintenance or care for an illness unrelated to drugs. Only through routine questioning is such drug use discovered.

Even the adolescent suffering from a drug-related illness seldom seeks care because of a particular drug habit or the impairment of a specific body organ, but rather because a symptom complex mandates medical attention. In this respect, teenage drug abusers are like other patients: Determining the etiological factors and the pathological conditions of their illnesses requires a comprehensive analysis of all possibilities. If drug abuse, of either one or several agents, is not considered along with other possible etiological factors to explain the symptoms, the physician may miss an opportunity for meaningful therapeutic intervention. Therefore, in keeping with the more usual method by which such adolescent patients come to medical attention, drug abuse-related illnesses are discussed as they initially appear to the primary care health professional.

THE MEDICAL HISTORY AND ANTICIPATORY GUIDANCE

His or her extent of drug involvement should be asked of every teenager during a periodic health examination. Such inquiries should be a natural adjunct to the assessment of other psychosocial indicators, including academic progress, sexual behavior, family and peer relationships, and recreation. An accurate drug history can be obtained only in an atmosphere of confidentiality and privacy, with parents excluded from the interview. In the proper setting, positive responses should be expected from the majority of teenagers when queried about current or past use of alcohol and cigarettes. Information should be obtained about not only the specific type of drug used, but about the frequency of use, the setting in which use occurs, and the degree of social, educational, and vocational disruption attributable to the drug use behavior. This information is necessary for a proper appraisal of the need for intervention. Obtaining such information depends largely on the physician's ability to listen to the adolescent without alarm or dismay, to establish an atmosphere of trust, and to direct the interview to obtain the specific information required.

Alcohol and marijuana are the substances used most commonly on a recreational basis by adolescents; frequently, they lead to problems in this age group. Although approximately 80% of adolescents will have tried alcohol and nearly 50% will have tried marijuana before graduating from high school (a significant percentage of whom report daily use), teenagers seldom volunteer information on the extent of their substance use unless questioned specifically. The medical complications of chronic alcoholism or marijuana abuse, although severe, usually do not appear until after adolescence. The physician's task is to identify those teenagers who are experiencing psychosocial disruption or who are at greatest risk of becoming alcoholic or chemically dependent adults. The youngster who is doing poorly in school, is having difficulty with family and peer relationships, or is engaging in delinquent behavior and who is drinking or smoking marijuana daily or weekly is not difficult to identify as one in need of special attention. In addition, a history of marijuana smoking, alcohol consumption, or the abuse of any drug by an adolescent indicates the need for further exploration into the possibility of underlying psychopathological conditions. Frequently the psychosocial problems that initiate drug-taking are as important as the specific complications of abuse.

The teenager who has not experienced academic or social failure but whose substance use goes beyond experimentation or occasional use represents a more difficult problem. Although no specific criteria determine who is at greatest risk of future difficulty, a history of parental alcoholism, drug abuse, or other serious family dysfunction or widespread alcohol or marijuana abuse within the teenager's peer group is associated with a poor prognosis. Even for youngsters in this high-risk but still high-functioning category, no specific therapy may be indicated beyond the need for periodic reevaluation of the situation. The history of substance use by most teenagers in this category should be noted, quantitated, and used as a reference point by which to evaluate information obtained during subsequent visits.

Counseling about Alcohol and Marijuana Intoxication

All teenagers, including the minority who do not drink or use drugs at all, need to be counseled about the relationship between intoxicants and accidents, the leading cause of death among adolescents. The majority of these fatal accidents are automotive; intoxicants are involved in many, if not most. A teenager who will not at some time drive while intoxicated or be a passenger in the automobile of an intoxicated driver is rare. Preventive health care for adolescents and their families must include a discussion of alternatives to such risk-taking behavior.

The prevalence of drinking among youth has not changed much during the 1990s. In 1998, just under 25% of eighth-graders, nearly 20% of tenth-graders, and just over 50% of twelfth-graders reported drinking alcohol in the past month, with 14%, 24%, and 32% of drinkers, respectively, consuming five or more drinks in a row in the past 2 weeks (binge drinkers). Teenage binge drinkers are at especially high risk for accidents and for significant developmental, educational, and emotional difficulties. These youth should be identified and counseled to reduce their health-risk behavior. A higher legal drinking age is associated with reduced deaths not only for motor vehicle drivers but also for pedestrians, unintentional injuries, and suicide in the adolescent and young adult age group, indicating that many categories of violent death in youth are associated with alcohol use. In addition, when counseling about alcohol use, it is important to note that women have higher blood alcohol concentrations than men after consuming comparable amounts of alcohol. Adolescent girls and young women thus are more vulnerable than men to acute complications of drinking and may have greater deterioration in their ability to drive and perform other psychomotor tasks.

Although the intoxicating effects of alcohol and the importance of its role in causing motor vehicle accidents are well known, the effects of marijuana (cannabis) are understood less widely. For appropriate counseling, the health care clinician should have an understanding of marijuana's physiological and behavioral effects. First, it is important to know that there have been exponential increases in the potency of marijuana over the past two decades: In the 1970s, the delta-9-tetrahydrocannabinol (THC) content of marijuana was between 0.5% and 2%; in the late 1990s, the average THC content was between 8% and 10%. The drug is a euphoriant and most often produces feelings of relaxation and well-being. The behavioral effects of marijuana are probably mediated by specific cannabinoid receptors (identified and cloned in 1990) and interaction with other neurochemical systems. Like other drugs that have addictive potential, such as heroin and nicotine, THC has been shown in experiments with rats to result in a release of dopamine in the brain's "reward" pathway in the nucleus accumbens, and long-term administration alters the limbic system in the brain similarly to other drugs of abuse.

As already mentioned, prevalence of marijuana use increased dramatically during the 1990s. In 1998, 10% of ninth-graders, 19% of tenth-graders, and 23% of twelfth-graders in the United States used marijuana within the past month; 1%, 3.6%, and 5.6%, respectively, were daily users of the drug. These represent the youth at high risk of addiction and significant health problems who should be identified and appropriately counseled and referred for treatment if necessary.

Although marijuana causes electroencephalographic changes and alterations in neurotransmitters, neither structural damage to the brain nor an increase in seizure potential has been demonstrated. In contrast, a number of acute behavioral changes are of clinical significance because of their potential to cause accidents. In addition to euphoria, the marijuana "high" causes a loss of critical judgment, distortions in time perception, impairment of tracking (the ability to follow a moving object accurately), and poor performance on "divided attention" tasks, such as driving. The infrequent correlation between marijuana intoxication and accidents probably is because the users show no specific signs of drug abuse and the authorities lack a quick, convenient method to detect marijuana. Other behavioral effects include impaired short-term memory, interference with learning, and difficulty with oral communication, all of which can affect school performance adversely. Occasionally a physician will encounter a patient who has an acute adverse reaction to marijuana manifested as a toxic psychosis with depression or panic. Both the symptoms and the treatment of these reactions are similar to those for hallucinogen abuse. Prolonged (and possibly permanent) personality changes have been reported in long-term marijuana users. This amotivational syndrome is marked by lethargy and a lack of goal-directed activity.

Physiological effects do occur with marijuana use but generally are less worrisome than the behavioral effects of the drug. Respiratory effects with more prolonged exposure include bronchodilation with acute inhalation and bronchoconstriction. Thus, adolescents who have asthma may experience either relief or exacerbation of symptoms. Allergic reactions to marijuana do occur and may cause asthmatic attacks. A potential long-term pulmonary consequence in the chronic marijuana abuser is lung cancer. Bronchial biopsies of marijuana smokers who have clinical diagnoses of chronic bronchitis have revealed precancerous epithelial lesions. Cardiovascular effects include both tachycardia and a transient low-grade elevation of systolic and diastolic blood pressure. Neither of these cardiac consequences is clinically significant. Marijuana has been reported to have numerous effects on the endocrine system in males who have histories of prolonged and frequent use, including depression of testosterone levels in the blood, diminished sperm counts, impaired sexual function, and gynecomastia. The associated clinical problems of impotence and infertility should respond to abstinence from marijuana. The long-term effects of these endocrine imbalances on the developing adolescent, however, as yet are unclear.

Counseling about Tobacco Use

Although fewer teenagers use tobacco than alcohol, 35% of high school seniors smoke cigarettes at least monthly, and 12.6% smoke half a pack or more per day. Nearly 9% use smokeless tobacco at least monthly. The active ingredient of cigarette smoke and chewed or snorted tobacco is nicotine. Nicotine plays a central role in the dependence-producing process of cigarette smoking and smokeless tobacco use. Tobacco use fits all the criteria of drug dependence or addiction, which is determined primarily by the effect of nicotine on the brain. The long-term cardiac, pulmonary, and carcinogenic consequences of cigarette smoking have been well publicized, and this information has not escaped the teenage population. Although the physician may have little to add in the way of warning to what already has been proffered by the schools and the media, it is negligent not to inquire about the adolescent's smoking habits and offer counsel on those health issues regarding tobacco use that are immediately relevant to the life of the teenager. The adverse effect of smoking on pulmonary function may affect the adolescent who has athletic aspirations. The pregnant teenager concerned with the welfare of her unborn baby may alter her smoking habits when informed of the possible association between tobacco and low birth weight and neonatal mortality. The adolescent girl who is starting to use oral contraceptives may be counseled that although "the pill" does not cause cancer, smoking certainly does, and she may be motivated to give up cigarettes. Adolescents who have a respiratory illness, particularly asthma, must be apprised of the immediate effects of smoking on their day-to-day health. All these issues lend themselves to discussion in the give-and-take atmosphere of the personal history interview.

The 1997 Youth Risk Behavior Survey conducted by the Centers for Disease Control and Prevention found that of U.S. high school students who had ever been daily smokers, 73% had tried to quit but only 13.5% were former smokers. These data underscore the prominent role of nicotine addiction in the maintenance of smoking behavior in adolescents. Thus, treatment should address pharmacological as well as behavioral factors. In addition to attempting to prevent the onset of smoking, health care practitioners should focus on preventing occasional smokers from progressing to daily smokers, thus preventing addiction. Nicotine patch therapy as an adjunct to smoking cessation treatment has been studied in adolescents and appears to be safe and well tolerated. The patch should be used for 8 weeks. There appears to be very little difference among the different brands. The use of sustained-release bupropion (Zyban) may be helpful, although no studies have been done in adolescents. New regulations restricting the sale, distribution, promotion, and advertising of nicotine-containing cigarettes and smokeless tobacco to minors were issued in 1996 by the Food and Drug Administration (FDA). These regulations are based on the emerging evidence of the addictive quality of nicotine and the vulnerability of youth to exploitation by the tobacco industry.

PHYSICAL EXAMINATION

The teenager who is heavily involved in the abuse of hard drugs is more likely to come to medical attention with a specific illness associated with drug abuse than through a routine physical examination. However, even those adolescents who use less dangerous drugs often have some concern about the potential somatic consequences of their behavior, and they may seek the reassurance of a check-up to prove to themselves that all is well. In such circumstances, the teenager may deny a history of drug abuse even when questioned directly so as not to prejudice the results of the examination. The physician must be alert to those physical findings that either are pathognomonic of or associated with illicit substance abuse.

The abuser of either marijuana or the stimulants cocaine and amphetamines may have an accelerated pulse rate. Stimulant abuse also is associated with weight loss and may mimic the symptoms of hyperthyroidism or eating disorders. In contrast, anabolic steroid use is associated with a marked weight gain, particularly in muscle mass. Pinpoint pupils unresponsive to light are characteristic of opiate abuse. Barbiturates usually produce sluggish pupillary responses. Conjunctivitis and irritation or ulceration of the nasal mucosa may be found in the teenager abusing drugs by inhalation. Glue "sniffers," marijuana smokers, and "snorters" of heroin or cocaine are likely to manifest these conditions.

Dermatological Manifestations

The majority of the specific physical signs of drug abuse are found on the skin and are associated with the subcutaneous or intravenous abuse of opiates, cocaine, anabolic steroids, and less commonly, barbiturates. Subcutaneous fat necrosis, similar to that experienced by persons who have diabetes and receive insulin injections, is common in teenagers who inject heroin under their skin ("skin popping"). Cutaneous scars ("tracks") following the course of superficial veins are found in teenagers who have a prolonged history of injecting drugs intravenously ("mainlining"). They are caused by chronic inflammation associated with repeated injections or by the deposition of carbonaceous material from needles that were "flamed" briefly in an attempt at sterilization. The teenager frequently disguises these tracks by covering them with a self-administered tattoo applied with a needle and India ink. Any tattoo placed by an amateur or professional and found in the antecubital fossa should be examined closely for tracks or needle marks. Plastic surgery for the removal of tracks and tattoos should be suggested to the patient because these stigmata often interfere with later employability and thereby compromise rehabilitative efforts.

Both the intravenous and subcutaneous routes of drug administration are characterized by a lack of sterile technique. Skin abscesses and cellulitis are common among teenage addicts. When these conditions come to medical attention, drug abuse should be considered a possible cause. The presence of needle marks confirms drug abuse as an etiological factor. Localized pain is the most frequent symptom of skin abscesses, with *Staphylococcus aureus* being the most common causative organism. Fever and leukocytosis are relatively uncommon, and regional adenopathy may be present. Treatment involves incision and drainage and the administration of an appropriate antibiotic as determined by isolation of the causative organism by culture. Skin abscesses and superficial skin ulcers are potential sites for the growth of *Clostridium* organisms, and tetanus has been reported in adult heroin addicts. A similar incidence of tetanus in teenagers has not been encountered, probably because of residual protection from childhood immunizations; nevertheless, the administration of a tetanus toxoid booster should be considered. Superficial thrombophlebitis, particularly of the upper extremities, is common among intravenous opiate-abusing teenagers and is a cause of both localized symptoms and systemic infection. Treatment includes local soaks and systemic antibiotic therapy. Anticoagulation is not a necessary part of the treatment for superficial thrombophlebitis.

Serious Systemic Infections and Opportunistic Infections

In the course of evaluating the teenager who has a systemic infection or a fever of unknown origin, the physician should remember that intravenous drug abuse may be an etiological factor in the development of the infectious process. The direct injection of bacteria or viruses into the bloodstream during intravenous drug administration or septic embolization from a site of superficial thrombophlebitis will give rise to the hematogenous dissemination of infectious agents to the heart, brain, osseous structures, and less commonly, other organs.

Human immunodeficiency virus (HIV) is the most serious of such infections transmitted by contaminated injection apparatus. Because of the prolonged asymptomatic period associated with this virus, clinical illness often is not expressed during the teenage years. However, an adolescent who has a history of injecting any illicit drug, including opiates, cocaine, amphetamines, or anabolic steroids, should be offered counseling and testing for HIV. Adolescents who have an unexplained weight loss, night sweats, generalized lymphadenopathy, oral thrush, recurrent bacterial infections, severe prolonged diarrhea, tuberculosis, or *Pneumocystis carinii* pneumonia should have HIV-related illness considered in the differential diagnosis. Teenagers who are HIV-positive and asymptomatic should have their immune function assessed initially and at least twice per year thereafter. Antiretroviral treatment and prophylaxis for opportunistic infections then can be instituted according to current guidelines based on significantly decreased immunocompetence. Because HIV is transmitted sexually as well as by contaminated needles, adolescent girls who are not drug users but whose sexual partners use drugs intravenously require counseling and testing for HIV infection.

Endocarditis in the intravenous drug abuser may affect either the right or left side of the heart. Beyond fever and occasional pulmonary symptoms, right-sided endocarditis is associated with few if any systemic signs and almost always affects a previously undamaged tricuspid valve. *S. aureus* frequently is the causative organism. Left-sided endocarditis may involve either normal or abnormal mitral or aortic valves and usually is associated with systemic evidence of infection. *S. aureus* and streptococcal species are the organisms encountered most frequently, and fungal infections with *Candida* organisms also have been reported. The teenager who has endocarditis must be hospitalized and treated with intravenous antibiotics as determined by the isolation of the causative organism.

Central nervous system (CNS) infection may be associated with endocarditis or may be a primary manifestation of drug abuse–related septicemia. Brain abscess is rare during adolescence; thus, when present, intravenous drug abuse should be suspected. Multiple microabscesses are found more frequently than a single large abscess; therefore, focal neurological signs may be absent. Because the only manifestation of multiple microabscesses of the brain may be fever or a personality change, lumbar puncture, electroencephalography, transaxial computed tomography, and magnetic resonance imaging may be required to reach the correct diagnosis. *S. aureus* is found most often to be the causative organism. The same organism has been associated with the increased frequency of osteomyelitis among intravenous drug abusers. The treatment and prognosis for CNS infection and osteomyelitis are the same for the user and the nonuser of drugs.

The intravenous injection of starch and talc, used as fillers for medicinal preparations designed solely for oral use, may lead to pulmonary angiothrombosis and granulomatosis. Although pulmonary hypertension and cor pulmonale eventually can result from this process, for these problems to become clinically apparent during adolescence is unusual. Nevertheless, the evaluation of teenagers manifesting unexplained compromise to respiratory function should include the consideration of intravenous drug abuse; thus, chest roentgenograms, blood cultures, and tuberculin skin testing should be performed.

Sexually Transmitted Diseases and Other Urological and Gynecological Manifestations

Because of the lifestyle often adopted by adolescents who use drugs frequently, sexually transmitted diseases (STDs) are common in this population and may be the reason for seeking medical care. Syphilis can be acquired both sexually and through contaminated needles; therefore, a serological test for syphilis always should be obtained, keeping in mind that false-positive results are common in heroin users. Gonococcal and nongonococcal urethritis, cervicitis, salpingitis, proctitis, and pharyngitis often are diagnosed in adolescents who abuse a variety of illicit substances. The signs, symptoms, and treatment of these conditions are the same as for patients who do not abuse drugs.

HIV infection transmitted sexually has been noted in adolescents who abuse drugs other than by the intravenous route. Both male and female adolescent "crack" abusers are at particular risk for sexually acquired HIV infection because of the practice of trading sex for drugs. The highly addictive nature and short duration of the crack "high" encourage drug binges that often include frequent acts of sexual intercourse with multiple partners. This has resulted in an increased prevalence among crack abusers of many sexually transmitted infections, including syphilis and HIV-related illness.

Amenorrhea occurs frequently in teenage girls who are opiate addicts. Because amenorrhea is associated with anovulation, these girls experience no increase in pregnancies despite their often increased sexual activity. Ovulation, menses, and fertility usually return to normal within a few months of cessation of opiate use; thus, contraceptive counseling and prescription must be part of rehabilitation.

Unfortunately, no such protection from pregnancy occurs in girls who abuse cocaine and crack. Cocaine use during pregnancy is associated with an increased incidence of spontaneous abortion, abruptio placentae, intrauterine growth retardation, premature delivery, and irritability in newborns. Contraceptive management is particularly important for these girls during the period of assessment and treatment for their drug abuse.

Anabolic steroid use is associated with testicular atrophy, lowered sperm count, gynecomastia, and accelerated male pattern baldness in males, and with menstrual irregularities, lowered voice pitch, clitoral hypertrophy, and hirsutism in females. Both sexes experience increased libido as a result of steroid abuse.

Flunitrazepam (Rohypnol), a benzodiazepine drug that is not licensed for sale in the United States but is sold legally in 64 other countries, including Mexico, is also known as the "date rape drug." The small white pills of flunitrazepam are 10 times more potent than diazepam, dissolve easily in liquid, and are odorless, colorless, and tasteless. They are used to spike the drinks of unsuspecting young women for the purpose of rape.

Abdominal Pain

Many physiological and psychosomatic illnesses produce abdominal pain in teenagers. Among them are a variety of illicit drug-related conditions. Severe abdominal pain, anorexia, vomiting, and gastrointestinal hemorrhage may accompany a large and acute ingestion of alcohol. Although the chronic medical complications of alcoholism, such as cirrhosis, are not found in teenagers, acute gastritis and acute pancreatitis may accompany the consumption of a large quantity of alcohol. The pain of acute gastritis usually will subside with the administration of antacids alone. However, persistent pain or bleeding requires therapy with medications that suppress acid secretion, such as ranitidine or omeprazole. Specific diagnostic studies to determine the origin of the hemorrhage may be indicated. In addition to severe abdominal pain and profuse vomiting, acute pancreatitis usually is accompanied by elevation of serum amylase and lipase levels. An increased incidence of peptic ulcer disease has been reported in adult opiate addicts, although no such increase has been noted in adolescents.

If ulcer disease or any other cause of acute abdominal pain does occur, the addict may attribute the discomfort falsely to withdrawal symptoms and quickly administer opiates as a form of self-treatment. Having thus masked the symptoms of possible intraabdominal pathological findings, the opiate-addicted teenager may not seek medical attention until gastric perforation has occurred. Similarly, the physician faced with a patient experiencing opiate withdrawal must be cautious not to overlook other serious illness by attributing all of the patient's symptoms to the abstinence syndrome.

Constipation almost is universal among opiate abusers and, at the extreme, causes symptoms of intestinal obstruction. Hemorrhoids, otherwise uncommon during adolescence, may result and cause rectal bleeding. Constipation responds rapidly to interruption of opiate abuse. Although constipation is one of the more benign complaints, it represents the most common complaint of the young methadone-maintained patient. In most instances the drug-abusing teenager who has abdominal pain should be hospitalized for evaluation because close observation and testing are required to reach a definitive diagnosis.

Jaundice

When evaluating the teenager who has jaundice, the physician must consider the possibility of drug abuse as an etiological factor. Acute viral hepatitis is common among intravenous drug abusers. Although primarily associated with the mainlining of heroin, hepatitis also has been reported in intravenous abusers of other substances, including cocaine, amphetamines, and anabolic steroids. In addition, hepatitis viruses can be transmitted by saliva and semen, and cases have been attributed to the sharing of marijuana joints. The inhalation of cleaning fluid fumes, an abuse practiced most often by younger adolescents and preadolescents, can cause acute toxic hepatitis. Anabolic steroid users can develop cholestatic hepatitis along with jaundice, hepatic cysts, and benign and malignant hepatic tumors. Recently, MDMA ("ecstasy") has been reported to have significant hepatotoxicity and has been associated with several cases of fulminant hepatic failure requiring intensive care or even liver transplantation.

The symptoms, signs, and serological abnormalities found in patients who use drugs do not differ from those of nondrug users who have acute hepatitis. The assessment of a jaundiced teenager who has acute hepatitis should include measurement of the prothrombin time because prolongation may indicate impending hepatic encephalopathy. Other indications of early hepatic encephalopathy are changes in sensorium and behavior. In the drug-using teenager, belligerence and lack of cooperation often are attributed incorrectly to drug withdrawal or an underlying personality disturbance rather than to hepatic encephalopathy. This error in judgment may lead to inappropriate treatment with sedatives; the administration of sedatives to patients in acute hepatic failure can precipitate coma. Dehydration or evidence of impending hepatic encephalopathy is an indication for hospitalization in any patient, but particularly for the drug-abusing teenager who has hepatitis, because noncompliance and lack of supportive care at home are more likely. Hepatitis B immunization should be offered to adolescent drug abusers who are antibody negative and who are at high risk for infection by either the intravenous or sexual route. All intravenous drug abusers should be tested for hepatitis C.

LABORATORY TESTING

The teenager who is well clinically occasionally will have abnormal findings on laboratory tests that raise suspicion of covert drug use. Although neither anemia nor total peripheral white blood cell count abnormalities are associated with substance abuse, peripheral eosinophilia may be found in up to one third of heroin users. The cause of eosinophilia in heroin users is unknown. Users of anabolic steroids often will show elevated serum concentrations of low-density lipoprotein cholesterol and reduced levels of high-density lipoprotein cholesterol. These adolescents are at increased risk for accelerated atherosclerosis. The routine urinalysis yields no findings specific to drug abuse, with the rare exception of mild proteinuria associated with serum glutamic-pyruvic transaminase elevations, which may be present in heroin-abusing adolescents. These patients show evidence of focal glomerulonephritis when their proteinuria is evaluated using renal biopsy. A false-positive serological test for syphilis may be found in approximately 10% of heroin abusers. Although these false-positive test results may occur for any teenager who has active liver disease, they have been observed for heroin abusers who have no evidence of hepatic dysfunction.

Liver function is not usually assessed as a part of the usual laboratory evaluation in teenagers; however, it represents the most fruitful method of screening for unsuspected opiate abuse because the liver is the best source for abnormal chemical findings in the known intravenous heroin abuser. Many clinically well adolescents who have a history of intravenous heroin abuse have serum elevations of glutamic-pyruvic transaminase and glutamic-oxaloacetic transaminase. Other indicators of hepatic function, including serum bilirubin and alkaline phosphatase levels, usually are normal. Adolescents who abuse heroin by nasal inhalation are less likely to have abnormal liver function tests.

Technological advances have made it possible to detect specific drugs of abuse in body fluids. However, the appropriate use of this testing ability has become an issue of some controversy, especially with regard to teenagers. Routine urine screening for drugs of abuse such as marijuana or cocaine of all adolescent patients without their knowledge and without clinical indicators of substance abuse is not advocated by most thoughtful authorities. Under such conditions, with an expected low prevalence of actual use, many false-positive tests would result, leading to accusations of and confrontations with adolescents who are not abusing drugs. In addition, only recent drug use would be detected, and no information about patterns and frequency of use or degrees of impairment would be obtained. However, urine drug testing may be a helpful adjunct to the treatment and rehabilitation of adolescents who are known to be drug abusers. Indeed, many drug treatment programs use random urine toxicological testing, with the knowledge and consent of the patient, as an early warning system for relapse and as an additional way of helping the adolescent to abstain from drugs. Blood and urine toxicological testing for illicit substances also can help in the assessment of an acutely ill adolescent whose mental status is altered and who is unable to give a history because of coma or psychotic behavior.

CHANGES IN SENSORIUM

The teenager who apparently is intoxicated or is disoriented, lethargic, or comatose represents a complex diagnostic and therapeutic problem. Even when head trauma, diabetic ketoacidosis, hypoglycemia, encephalitis, and other causes of coma and confusion can be excluded and the diagnosis of intoxication is clear, the specific causative drug must be determined. Information from the patient, the family, or friends may provide a ready answer, but such information may be unavailable or unreliable. Serum and urine toxicological screening can be extremely helpful in such a situation. An attempt must always be made to determine the reason for the intoxication. Was it accidental or deliberate? If the patient is suicidal, the physician must offer appropriate assessment, protection, and treatment.

Hospitalization for observation almost always is indicated for the teenager who has a drug intoxication, although emergency department treatment may negate all immediate medical risks. Even in those instances in which self-destruction was not a motivation, an overdose may signal the loss of the adolescent's ability to control his or her drug-abuse behavior. The teenager should not be released from care until a concerted effort has been made to minimize future risk.

Intoxication

Although the overwhelming majority of mild intoxications never come to medical attention, sometimes a youngster will be brought for care for being "high." A wide variety of substances are capable of producing a high, including inhaled fumes from airplane glue or cleaning fluid, marijuana, alcohol, and cocaine. Teenagers who exhibit euphoria or minimal disorientation require only protection against self-injury. At an appropriate time after the sensorium has cleared, inquiries should be made as to the nature, frequency, and pattern of episodes of intoxication to determine the need, if any, for further psychosocial intervention.

Teenagers who have severe alcohol intoxication usually can be distinguished by their ethanoic breath and, except in instances of extremely large or mixed ingestions, are not at serious physiological risk. Treatment need only be supportive, with protection provided against the aspiration of vomitus and observation for the development of respiratory depression, hypoglycemia, or the gastrointestinal complications of a large alcohol ingestion. Even when the teenager is not at risk, a brief hospitalization while sobriety is regained may be preferable to immediate discharge to the care of distraught parents.

Acute Psychosis

The adolescent who comes for medical attention as a result of an acute psychosis may be suffering from a hallucinogen ingestion or "bad trip." A wide variety of compounds are capable of producing hallucinations, including LSD, peyote, PCP, and occasionally, marijuana or hashish. Hallucinations may recur weeks or months after the ingestion of a hallucinogen as part of a "flashback" phenomenon. In addition, large doses of amphetamines or cocaine may precipitate a psychotic state marked by paranoia and aggression. A similar psychotic episode may follow abrupt cessation of amphetamine abuse. Along with the hallucinations that, in contrast to the auditory hallucinations of schizophrenia, almost always are visual, the teenager who has ingested one of the previously mentioned drugs often has dilated pupils, hyperreflexia, hyperthermia, and tachycardia. Identification of the specific abused hallucinogen is difficult. Even when the substance is known, the adolescent seldom has accurate knowledge of its exact composition because the compounds frequently are adulterated and misrepresented by the seller. Detection of the presence of PCP, tetrahydrocannabinol, amphetamines, or cocaine in the patient's blood or urine can help in determining the prognosis of acute psychosis.

Regardless of the hallucinogen abused, treatment is nonspecific and directed at allaying anxiety and protecting the patient from injury to self or others. The teenager should be placed in a quiet, nonthreatening environment. Verbal contact should be established and maintained, with frequent reassurance that the hallucinogenic experience is temporary and drug related. If at all possible, physical restraints should be avoided because they are certain to increase anxiety and panic in the already frightened adolescent.

Sedatives should be administered only if verbal contact does not control behavior successfully or cannot be maintained because of limitations of time and staff. Any sedation administered will compromise sensorium further and thereby may increase the severity of hallucinations. All the most commonly used sedative medications carry additional risks. The administration of phenothiazines is potentially dangerous because hallucinogens often are adulterated with anticholinergics, and this combination of drugs may precipitate circulatory collapse. However, small doses of benzodiazepine may help to allay anxiety. Haloperidol in a dose of 2 to 5 mg may be administered intramuscularly to control the agitation of an acute drug-related psychosis. This dose may be repeated as soon as 1 hour later if severe symptoms persist or recur.

PCP is among the most toxic of the hallucinogenic agents. Toxic reactions, which may be indistinguishable from schizophrenia and include elements of paranoia, agitation, or catatonia, may last for days and, in rare cases, weeks. With high-dose ingestions, convulsions, opisthotonos, coma, and very rarely, apnea may ensue. Treatment of overdose reactions includes (1) anticonvulsants for seizures, (2) support of respiration, and (3) enhancement of drug excretion by gastric lavage with half normal saline, the administration of furosemide, and the acidification of the urine by administering ammonium chloride or ascorbic acid.

In most instances, teenagers who have an acute drug-related psychosis should be hospitalized. These adolescents may have brief periods of lucidity and then relapse into hallucinations. It is difficult to determine with certainty if the teenager has recovered fully without having an opportunity to observe behavior over at least a few hours. In addition, there always is a question of whether the drug ingestion unmasked a preexistent psychosis or simply precipitated psychotic behavior in an otherwise healthy individual. The answer to that question is gained best through an opportunity to observe and evaluate the adolescent during hospitalization.

Lethargy and Coma

Acute methamphetamine toxicity can present with coma, shock, convulsions, oliguria, and hyperthermia. A common complication is rhabdomyolysis with acute renal failure. Intracerebral hemorrhage can occur even with small doses of amphetamines. Signs of MDMA ("ecstasy") toxicity include sympathetic overactivity, disturbed behavior, and increased temperature. Serious complications including delirium, seizures, and coma are more common when MDMA is used in combination with other substances, especially other stimulants. Rhabdomyolysis and acute renal failure have been reported with MDMA use by adolescents who use the drug at all-night dance parties called "raves."

The adolescent who has had an opiate or barbiturate overdose will have respiratory depression and constricted or sluggish pupils and be lethargic or comatose. For patients who have respiratory depression precipitated by an unknown agent, the use of naloxone has both diagnostic and therapeutic potential. Although it has no therapeutic benefit for the teenager who has had a sedative overdose, it is free of the effects of respiratory depression common to other narcotic antagonists and therefore can be used without fear of accentuating respiratory compromise in the nonopiate intoxication. Naloxone also is useful in treating propoxyphene ingestions. Failure of the teenager to respond to naloxone given intravenously indicates that the symptoms are not due to an opiate. Pupillary dilation, an improved level of consciousness, and an increase in the respiratory rate in response to the administration of naloxone strongly suggest that an opiate produced the syndrome. The presence of clinical signs of intravenous drug use supports the diagnosis of opiate overdose. Pulmonary edema and hypoxemia may occur in the teenager who has had an opiate overdose who then requires intubation, assisted ventilation, and administration of oxygen under positive pressure. Even the adolescent who responds dramatically to naloxone alone will require hospitalization for continued observation and continuous naloxone infusion. A relapse with respiratory depression may occur if the infusion is discontinued too early. This is a particular hazard in the patient who has had a methadone overdose because its duration of action is between 24 and 48 hours.

As noted previously, the teenager who has become intoxicated on a sedative displays clinical characteristics similar to those of one who has overdosed on an opiate. The patient who has overdosed on a barbiturate has pinpoint or slowly reactive pupils unresponsive to naloxone. Treatment is supportive. The respiratory rate and arterial blood gases must be monitored and mechanical ventilation instituted at the first sign of ventilatory failure. Intravenous fluids should be administered to ensure a high urine output. Analeptics have no role in the treatment of sedative overdose, and although hemodialysis may be effective, it seldom is necessary, because the supportive measures just described usually are adequate.

ABSTINENCE SYNDROMES

The addicted teenager who is hospitalized involuntarily requires treatment to prevent the discomfort and danger inherent in a withdrawal syndrome. At times, drug withdrawal is not imposed on the adolescent; rather, some life event, such as the death of a family member or a close friend, provides the motivation for voluntary detoxification. In either case, adolescents often are ambivalent regarding their abstinence and require careful, meticulous attention to their symptoms lest they become disruptive in the hospital or interrupt attempts to free them from addiction.

Opiate Withdrawal

A teenager must abuse opiates daily for weeks before the risk of suffering an opiate withdrawal syndrome develops. Within 12 hours after the last dose of heroin and 36 hours after the last dose of methadone, the addicted adolescent begins experiencing a progression of symptoms, including yawning, "gooseflesh," lacrimation, restlessness, dilated pupils, muscle cramps, diarrhea, and tachycardia. Insomnia may be severe during the first week of withdrawal and may persist to some degree for up to a month after abstinence from drugs.

Most teenagers who report less than daily heroin use are not physiologically addicted but rather are psychologically habituated. Nevertheless, they are quite fearful of becoming ill if their opiate supply is interrupted. Most often, these teenagers require no specific therapy beyond reassurance that relief for discomfort will be offered if symptoms appear. The adolescent who manifests symptoms and signs of opiate abstinence can be treated in a variety of ways. Methadone may be offered in a dosage of approximately 40 mg/day orally and then withdrawn slowly at a rate of 5 mg every 1 or 2 days over the course of 1 to 2 weeks. An alternative therapy is to administer 10 mg of diazepam every 4 to 6 hours. Diazepam relieves most symptoms, except diarrhea and insomnia. Persistent or severe diarrhea can be treated with diphenoxylate hydrochloride. Clonidine is a useful drug for opiate detoxification. It is an alpha-$_2$ agonist and reduces many of the autonomic signs and symptoms of opiate withdrawal, as well as produces mild sedation and a sense of well-being that facilitates withdrawal. Naltrexone, a specific μ opioid receptor antagonist, effectively blocks the cognitive and behavioral effects of opiates. It has a long half-life, permitting once-a-day dosing, and is useful in rapid detoxification regimens. The opiate abstinence syndrome can be managed on either an ambulatory or an inpatient basis. In general, greater success can be anticipated with hospitalization because this separates the addicted teenager physically from a supply of illicit opiates and provides him or her continual support and reassurance.

Methadone maintenance treatment programs may be appropriate for the older, opiate-addicted teenager. This treatment modality substitutes a synthetic opiate, methadone, for the abused opiate. A single daily oral dose of methadone can prevent both opiate craving and block the euphoric effect of subsequently self-administered heroin. With interruption of the need to obtain illegal opiates, the adolescent now is free to take advantage of support services and work toward restructuring his or her life. Therapy is aimed toward eventually withdrawing methadone treatment and preparing the patient for a drug-free existence. Unfortunately, although many adolescents do well while in treatment, evidence to date indicates a high incidence of subsequent drug abuse and significant morbidity and mortality after discharge from these programs.

Barbiturate Withdrawal

Unlike opiate-addicted adolescents, barbiturate addicts are at grave risk of a life-threatening withdrawal syndrome if their sedative dosage is discontinued abruptly. They become restless, develop postural hypotension, and have seizures in rapid succession, usually within 36 hours following their last dose. Occasionally a teenager may not come for medical attention until after a seizure has occurred and then may require large doses of anticonvulsants. The teenager who seeks medical attention for voluntary detoxification before seizures have occurred should be offered phenobarbital as a substitute for the abused sedative; an initial dose comparable to the barbiturate dose to which the patient is addicted should be used. This should be divided into four equal parts, with each given daily every 6 hours. The daily dosage then should be reduced slowly at a rate of 120 mg/day to zero. Because this method of detoxification relies on the accuracy of the original estimate by the addict of daily abuse, it is extremely difficult to judge the appropriate initial dose of phenobarbital to be given. If too much medication is offered, the teenager is at risk of iatrogenically induced barbiturate overdose and coma. If too little phenobarbital is given, convulsions may ensue. To be confident that an adequate dose has been administered, it often is necessary to induce mild barbiturate toxicity, which is accompanied by nystagmus, ataxia, and dysarthria, but which stops short of respiratory depression and coma. Treatment within this narrow therapeutic range requires careful observation of the adolescent, particularly during the first few days. Because an excessive initial dose of phenobarbital may cause the teenager to become somnolent during the initial stages of treatment, a concomitant interruption of oral intake may develop. Therefore, intravenous fluids should be administered routinely and the patient's fluid intake and output monitored carefully.

The high incidence of convulsions during barbiturate withdrawal and the need for frequent reevaluation and adjustment of therapy mandate in-hospital treatment of this abstinence syndrome. In many instances the guidance of a neurologist or a physician who has expertise in addictive illnesses may be necessary.

Stimulant Withdrawal

Stimulants such as cocaine and amphetamines are not associated with a dramatic or life-threatening withdrawal syndrome. Nevertheless, they are considered addictive because of the biochemical changes in the brain induced by these drugs that lead to the intense cravings and compulsive drug abuse behavior noted in both animal and human studies. A stimulant-abstinence syndrome has been described that follows a three-phase pattern. An initial crash after a drug-taking binge is characterized by a craving for sleep, often leading to the use of opiates, alcohol, or benzodiazepines. After 1 to 3 days of hypersomnolence, the stimulant abuser begins to experience an increasing intensity of withdrawal symptoms, including anergia, anhedonia (inability to feel pleasure or happiness), limited interest in the environment, and marked drug cravings. If abstinence is sustained for 6 to 18 weeks, the anhedonia, fatigue, and dysphoric mood usually improve. In the final extinction phase of abstinence, brief episodes of drug cravings recur with gradually diminishing frequency, often provoked by circumstances or objects that cue conditioned memories of drug euphoria. Treatment for adolescent stimulant abusers is conducted best within a highly structured chemical dependency program and often does not require hospitalization because the withdrawal syndrome does not necessitate intensive medical management. Inpatient treatment may be necessary, however, if outpatient treatment fails, if the adolescent exhibits suicidal or psychotic behavior, or if he or she is addicted to alcohol, sedatives, or opiates in addition to stimulants.

Cannabis Withdrawal

Marijuana produces pharmacological tolerance after several days of regular use and addiction after long-term daily use. A clinical withdrawal syndrome begins within 24 to 48 hours of discontinuing the drug. Withdrawal symptoms peak in intensity by the fourth day and gradually resolve by 10 to 14 days. The cannabis abstinence syndrome is characterized by a flu-like illness. Adolescents who are heavy cannabis users report withdrawal symptoms including malaise, irritability, agitation, insomnia, drug craving, shakiness, diaphoresis, night sweats, and gastrointestinal disturbance. The most persistent symptoms appear to be insomnia and irritable mood and, to a lesser extent, drug cravings. The insomnia is effectively treated with trazodone. It is important to appreciate that the magnitude of the cannabis withdrawal syndrome described by today's adolescents is much greater than that described in the 1970s because of the higher potency of the drug available today. Given the new understanding of the neurochemistry of cannabis addiction, it is not surprising that the withdrawal syndrome is similar to that seen with opiate dependence.

Alcohol Withdrawal

Frequent consumption of alcohol over prolonged periods produces physical dependence resulting in withdrawal syndromes of varying severity. The most common withdrawal symptoms include nausea, vomiting, insomnia, autonomic hyperactivity, and a mild confusional state. Symptoms begin within hours after drinking has stopped and peak at 24 to 36 hours. Benzodiazepines will suppress the symptoms as will resumption of drinking. Delirium tremens, the major alcohol withdrawal syndrome, is rarely if ever seen in adolescents. Teenagers whose drinking history suggests the possibility of withdrawal symptoms should be hospitalized for observation if they become abstinent.

SUMMARY

Whether the adolescent voluntarily comes for treatment for a drug abuse problem, is compelled to seek medical attention because of a drug- or alcohol-related illness, or is discovered to be using drugs or alcohol during a routine evaluation, the physician is in an advantageous position to intercede beyond the confines of treating somatic illness. The illegality and stigma attached to drug abuse often prevent the teenager from seeking help from clergy, educators, and particularly, family members. Protected by federal guidelines that ensure the confidentiality of the physician-patient relationship in drug abuse treatment, the physician who uses a nonjudgmental, sympathetic approach to these teenagers may be able to establish trust and thereby gather sufficient information to make a knowledgeable judgment as to the need for further intervention. Such information must include not only the history of past and present drug or alcohol abuse but also the nature of peer and family relationships, the extent of involvement with law enforcement authorities, the degree of educational or vocational disruption, and the adolescent's own interpretation of the need for therapy.

Often, the extent of substance abuse and related disruption is so minimal that no further action beyond the counsel of the physician is required. Such counsel should address the potential somatic effects of the teenager's current drug practices, the potential for escalation of drug-taking behavior, and the risks of accidents and death from even occasional intoxication. Alternatives to driving while intoxicated should be discussed with the adolescent and his or her family.

At the other extreme are teenagers who have severe psychopathological conditions and who are in obvious need of psychiatric care. A variety of other therapeutic modalities, not all of which may be present in a given community, are available for treatment of substance-abusing teenagers. Group or individual counseling may be indicated for the teenager who has less than severe drug involvement but has some evidence of psychosocial disruption. Group residences are available for adolescents from unsupportive homes. They usually offer counseling and a place to stay while teenagers continue their education or employment. Therapeutic communities are appropriate for those teenagers who are involved more deeply in drugs and are considered chemically dependent. These programs often are operated communally and staffed by former addicts, with or without professional support. The retention rate for teenagers within these programs is poor and may reflect the adolescents' inability to tolerate the rigors of relative incarceration and abrasive therapy.

Often, limitations of time for adequate psychosocial evaluation or lack of familiarity with available therapeutic resources prevent practitioners from reaching a meaningful long-term disposition for their patients. In these instances, referrals need to be made to other professionals or agencies that have expertise and interest in the field of teenage drug and alcohol abuse. In this regard, substance abuse does not differ from certain other behavioral problems for which specific therapeutic interventions are beyond the primary care physician's professional scope.

SUGGESTED READINGS

Alcohol, Drug Abuse, and Mental Health Administration: Cannabinoid receptor gene cloned, *JAMA* 264:1389, 1990.

American Academy of Pediatrics, Committee on Substance Abuse: Tobacco, alcohol, and other drugs: the role of the pediatrician in prevention and management of substance abuse, *Pediatrics* 101:125, 1998.

Andreu V, et al: Ecstasy: a common cause of severe acute hepatotoxicity, *J Hepatol* 29:394, 1998.

Barsky SH, et al: Histopathologic and molecular alterations in bronchial epithelium in habitual smokers of marijuana, cocaine, and/or tobacco, *J Natl Cancer Inst* 90:1198, 1998.

Brown RT, Coupey SM: Illicit drugs of abuse, *Adolescent medicine state of the art reviews* 4:321, 1993.

Bruner AB, Fishman M: Adolescents and illicit drug use, *JAMA* 280:597, 1998.

Canadian Center for Drug-free Sport: The use of anabolic-androgenic steroids by Canadian students, *Clin J Sport Med* 6:9, 1996.

Centers for Disease Control and Prevention: Selected cigarette smoking initiation and quitting behaviors among high school students—United States, 1997, *MMWR* 47:386, 1998.

Council on Scientific Affairs: Medical and nonmedical uses of anabolic-androgenic steroids, *JAMA* 264:2923, 1990.

Coupey SM: Barbiturates, *Pediatr Rev* 18:260, 1997.

DuRant RH, Escobedo LG, Heath GW: Anabolic steroid use, strength training, and multiple drug use among adolescents in the United States, *Pediatrics* 96:23, 1995.

Johnson LD, O'Malley PM, Bachman JG: *Monitoring the future study—1998*. US Department of Health and Human Services, 1998 (www.isr.umich.edu/src/mtf).

Jones NE, Pieper CF, Robertson LS: The effect of legal drinking age on fatal injuries of adolescents and young adults, *Am J Public Health* 82:112, 1992.

Kessler DA, et al: Nicotine addiction: a pediatric disease, *J Pediatr* 130:518, 1997.

Lan KC, et al: Clinical manifestations and prognostic features of acute methamphetamine intoxication, *J Formos Med Assoc* 97:528, 1998.

Markel H, et al: LSD flashback syndrome exacerbated by selective serotonin reuptake inhibitor antidepressants in adolescents, *J Pediatr* 125:817, 1994.

Mendelson JH, Mello NK: Management of cocaine abuse and dependence, *New Engl J Med* 334:965, 1996.

Middleman AB, et al: High-risk behaviors among high school students in Massachusetts who use anabolic steroids, *Pediatrics* 96:268, 1995.

National Consensus Development Panel on Effective Medical Treatment of Opiate Addiction: Effective medical treatment of opiate addiction, *JAMA* 280:1936, 1998.

Pope HG Jr, Gruber AJ, Yurgelun-Todd D: The residual neuropsychological effects of cannabis: the current status of research, *Drug Alcohol Depend* 38:25, 1995.

Pope HG Jr, Yurgelun-Todd D: The residual cognitive effects of heavy marijuana use in college students, *JAMA* 275:521, 1996.

Rickert VI, Wiemann CM, Berenson AB: Prevalence, patterns, and correlates of voluntary flunitrazepam use, *Pediatrics* 103:e6, 1999.

Schonberg SK, editor: *Substance abuse: a guide for health professionals*, ed 2, Elk Grove Village, Ill, 1999, American Academy of Pediatrics/Pacific Institute for Research and Evaluation.

Schwartz RH: LSD: its rise, fall, and renewed popularity among high school students, *Pediatr Clin North Am* 42:403, 1995.

Schwartz RH, Miller NS: MDMA (ecstasy) and the rave: a review, *Pediatrics* 100:705, 1997.

Smoking cessation: clinical practice guideline (No 18) US Department of Health and Human Services, 1997.

Weisbeck GA, et al: An evaluation of the history of a marijuana withdrawal syndrome in a large population, *Addiction* 91:1469, 1996.

Wickelgren I: Marijuana: harder than thought? *Science* 276:1967, 1997.

Williams H, et al: Saturday night fever: ecstasy related problems in a London accident and emergency department, *J Accid Emerg Med* 15:322, 1998.

Yesalis CE, et al: Trends in anabolic-androgenic steroid use among adolescents, *Arch Pediatr Adolesc Med* 151:1197, 1997.

104 Homosexuality: Challenges of Treating Lesbian and Gay Adolescents

Robert J. Bidwell

Lesbian and gay youths, although often unrecognized regarding their sexual orientation, make up a part of the practice of all physicians working with adolescents. In 1993, the American Academy of Pediatrics Committee on Adolescence[1] published its statement on "Homosexuality and Adolescence," which affirms the existence of lesbian and gay youth, acknowledges their special experience and needs, and provides physicians' guidelines for helping these adolescents reach a healthy, productive adulthood. Despite the greater recognition and acceptance of lesbian and gay youth, society still disagrees over homosexuality, especially as it relates to this age group. This controversy has presented obstacles to the development of strategies to meet the significant physical and mental health risks faced by these adolescents. This failure to address their experience and needs has led to many damaged and lost young lives over the past decades.

BACKGROUND

Human sexuality, its origins and manifestations, is an extremely complex phenomenon. Chromosomal sex, anatomical sex, gender identity, gender role behavior, sexual behavior, and sexual orientation all are interrelated aspects of an individual's sexuality. Sexual orientation generally refers to one's prevailing pattern(s) of erotic and affectional attraction to members of the same or opposite gender. Homosexuality refers to same-gender attraction, heterosexuality to opposite-gender attraction, and bisexuality to attraction to members of both genders. However, Kinsey's research in the 1930s and 1940s showed that these categories are not discrete; rather, human beings fall along a continuum of sexual orientation from same-sex to opposite-sex attraction. To add to the complexity, an individual's sexual orientation also is reflected in his or her fantasies, lifestyle, self-identification as gay or lesbian, and choice of friends for emotional and social, as well as erotic, fulfillment.

The origins of sexual orientation have been debated widely, often with limited scientific support for proposed theories. Some have suggested that sexual orientation is determined primarily by nature—that is, through genetic programming, brain anatomy, or prenatal hormonal influences on a developing central nervous system. Others have presented sociological or psychoanalytical theories suggesting that environment or "upbringing" are of primary importance. The preponderance of recent research, consisting primarily of anatomical studies and studies of twins, appears to support a biological explanation for sexual orientation. Whether the major determinants reflect "nature," "nurture," or a combination of the two, sexual orientation generally is believed not to be chosen and is established well before puberty; moreover, a gay or lesbian person's homosexuality is no less deeply rooted, and therefore no more amenable to change, than another person's heterosexuality. Furthermore, no scientific evidence exists that homosexuality is a matter of "something gone wrong." The lack of such evidence led the American Psychiatric Association in 1973 to accept homosexuality as simply a part of the spectrum of human sexuality.

The process of acquiring a gay or lesbian identity is long and often painful.[7] Troiden[8] has proposed a model describing a process that begins in childhood, continues through the confusion and first explorations of adolescence, and culminates in a healthy and open self-acceptance sometime during adulthood. Remafedi's study[5] of gay male youth has reconfirmed the adolescent years as particularly tumultuous and also has demonstrated that far from being "just a phase," homosexuality is a firmly established identity for a certain proportion of adolescents. They also found that for these adolescents, homosexuality was not simply sexual behaviors but involved a broader "attraction and affinity" to other men. A small subset of lesbian and gay individuals includes those who are "nontraditional" in their gender role behaviors as children. This is made up of very effeminate boys or very masculine girls. Green's[2] longitudinal study of boys having cross-gender behavior found that two thirds of prepubertal boys labeled as "sissies" because of their interest in stereotypical girls' games and activities or their displaying of feminine mannerisms were bisexually or homosexually oriented as adults.

The estimated percentage of Americans who are lesbian or gay is imprecise at best. Research techniques have been refined and sexual mores redefined since Kinsey's studies 50 years ago. Many studies have surveyed only sexual behaviors. These may be an imprecise measurement of sexual orientation, especially during adolescence. Some lesbian and gay teens have been active only heterosexually, and many have not yet become sexually active at all. Remafedi et al[6] found that among Minnesota adolescents, the prevalence of predominantly homosexual attractions increased generally with age (6.4% by age 18). Although only a small proportion (0.8%) of 18-year-old boys labeled themselves as homosexual, 8.9% report being "uncertain" about their sexual orientation. About 3% of 18-year-old boys acknowledged homosexual activity. Most studies conclude that somewhere between 3% and 10% of the population is lesbian or gay, and perhaps a larger percentage is bisexual in orientation.

GROWING UP LESBIAN OR GAY

Gay and lesbian adolescents are ordinary teenagers in every regard except that they grow up in an environment that often is unaccepting of a deepest part of who they are—their sexual orientation. Despite this, most of these youths grow up to be happy, healthy, and productive adults. Nevertheless, recent research has shown that for some adolescents the experience of growing up lesbian or gay can be difficult and even dangerous.[3,4]

Many gay and lesbian youths face an adolescence of profound isolation, believing that they are the only ones in their families or among their friends who have feelings of same-sex attraction. They have little access to objective information on sexual orientation, although their daily lives may be filled with antigay messages in school hallways and at home. They often have no access to informed and supportive counseling in schools or youth agencies. Accompanying this isolation is a fear of discovery; because most of these youths are "invisible," not fitting the gay or lesbian stereotypes, much of their energy is spent in "living a lie" that creates a wall between them and those they respect and love. It also prevents many of them from achieving the developmental tasks of adolescence related to self-esteem, identity, and intimacy. Harassment and violence are additional burdens faced by those gay and lesbian teenagers who identify themselves or are identified by others as homosexual. The results of isolation, fear, and violence are predictable, as they are for any group of alienated youth. Gay youth are at higher risk of dropping out of school, being kicked out of their homes, and turning to life on the streets for survival. There they often encounter violence and sexual exploitation with the attendant risks of pregnancy and sexually transmitted diseases, including HIV. Some gay and lesbian youth engage in substance use, and a significant number attempt suicide.

Many gay and lesbian youths have never had sex with another person. Some have been active heterosexually. Because of the social barriers to the exploration of their sexuality, those teenagers who are active homosexually often become so through anonymous sexual encounters, these sometimes facilitated through the Internet, in circumstances that engender feelings of guilt, self-loathing, and fear.

To date, more is known about the experience of urban white gay male youth than other groups of gay or of lesbian adolescents. Lesbian teens, gay and lesbian youth of color, and rural youths may be even more isolated and, therefore, at risk.

Unfortunately, society's response to the experience and needs of gay and lesbian youth has been one primarily of silence. Health practitioners, counselors, teachers, clergy, and other youth-serving professionals have failed to address these issues because of their own discomfort, disapproval, or fear. This failure has increased the alienation of gay and lesbian adolescents and has contributed, in part, to the significant morbidity and mortality among them.

WORKING WITH LESBIAN AND GAY YOUTH

Lesbian and gay youth come to the attention of health practitioners in a variety of ways. A small percentage will self-refer or self-identify themselves to receive appropriate medical services or counseling. More often they are brought in by concerned parents or referred by youth agencies. The stated concerns may not relate specifically to sexual orientation but rather represent "red flags," including substance use or depression. Most gay and lesbian teenagers, however, are "invisible" and will pass through clinics and counselors' offices without raising the issue of sexual orientation on their own, even if it has caused them distress and led to high-risk behaviors. Therefore, health practitioners must be able to address issues of sexual orientation with all adolescent patients. Only if these issues are addressed can specifically targeted medical screening, medical treatment, and anticipatory guidance be provided.

Health providers are not responsible for identifying each and every lesbian and gay teen. Instead, the provider should create a clinical environment in which clear messages are given that sensitive personal issues, including sexual orientation, can be discussed whenever the adolescent feels ready to do so. The provider should be ready to raise and discuss issues of sexual orientation with all teenagers, particularly any adolescent in distress or engaged in high-risk behaviors. If a youth acknowledges homosexual behavior or concerns about possibly being lesbian or gay, the practitioner should be able to explore the teenager's understanding and concerns about homosexuality, dispel any misconceptions, provide appropriate medical care and anticipatory guidance, and connect the teen to appropriate supportive community resources. One of the most important responsibilities of the practitioner is to facilitate every adolescent's growth toward a healthy homosexual, bisexual, or heterosexual adulthood.

HISTORY

Clinical settings and procedures must give clear, explicit messages that sexual orientation is among the personal issues that can be discussed with the practitioner. Otherwise, most gay and lesbian youth will believe that discussion of their possible homosexual orientation or behaviors is far beyond the limits of what health practitioners might be able to address supportively and knowledgeably. This message can be given through posters and brochures in the waiting area, a teen questionnaire that asks about sexual orientation concerns among other health issues, a clearly defined confidentiality policy, and by routinely seeing adolescent patients without their parents being present. The practitioner also must be careful not to presume heterosexual or homosexual orientation based on stereotypes. Any teenager should be considered as possibly dealing with issues of sexual orientation. Sexual orientation should be addressed in all "well-teen" visit interviews. To explore this area is especially important when "red flags" appear, including school problems, teen-parent conflicts, substance use, runaway behavior, depression, and self-destructive behaviors of any kind, including increased heterosexual or homosexual activity. How the issue is raised and explored depends on the individual teen and on the practitioner's interviewing style. Most gay and lesbian teenagers do not raise concerns about sexual orientation on their own. The practitioner, therefore, must open the door to discussion. If the adolescent has been referred by parents or the school, the practitioner's best policy usually is to let teenagers know what information has been given as a starting point for discussion. More commonly, the practitioner is alerted by "red flags" to the possibility of concerns regarding sexual orientation.

Sexual orientation can be explored in a number of ways. The practitioner might first ask if the adolescent has ever dated. Whether or not teenagers have dated, they also should be asked whether they have ever "had sex" with another person and whether their sexual partners have been males, females, or both males and females. Homosexually active youths, as well as heterosexual youths who engage only in oral or anal sex, may answer "no" to the question, "Have you ever had sexual intercourse?" Whether adolescents have been sexually active or not (and many gay and lesbian adolescents have not been so), all teenagers should be asked whether they have ever been concerned about feelings of sexual attraction to people of the same sex. Many teens who have same-sex attractions or activity have not labeled themselves as gay or lesbian, and so asking "Are you gay?" may be inappropriate. If a teenager acknowledges or hints at same-sex attractions, however, asking "Have you ever thought you might be gay?" may be appropriate.

If an adolescent denies homosexual feelings or behavior (sometimes with an expression of disgust), the practitioner can conclude by saying, "This may or may not ever be a part of your life. But if it ever is, I want you to know that I'm someone with whom you can come to talk about it."

It is necessary to ask any adolescent acknowledging same-sex activity about kinds of sexual behaviors, frequency, number of partners, consensual and nonconsensual sex, sex exchanged for money or drugs, the nature of partners (anonymous versus boyfriend or girlfriend), "safer sex" practices, and symptoms of sexually transmitted diseases. All teens acknowledging homosexual attractions or activity should be asked about substance use, depression, and other risky behaviors common to alienated youths.

If teenagers believe that they might be lesbian or gay, the origins of these concerns should be explored. Homosexual feelings and experiences do not necessarily mean that one is gay. Similarly, heterosexual feelings and experience do not necessarily represent a heterosexual orientation. Certainly, to tell a teenager that homosexual feelings are "just a phase" would be a mistake. For a significant percentage of adolescents, they do, in fact, represent an emerging lesbian or gay identity.

PHYSICAL EXAMINATION

Lesbian and gay adolescents face the same health risks as their heterosexual peers. Therefore, they should receive the same "well-teen" screening and acute-care examinations as any teenager. Because teenagers may fear disclosing homosexual, bisexual, or heterosexual activity, the physical examination should not be guided solely by the history given in the interview.

The incidence of sexually transmitted diseases (STDs) among lesbian adolescents who are exclusively homosexually active is low. These consist primarily of *Gardnerella vaginalis, Candida* organisms, and *Trichomonas* organisms. However, many lesbian teenagers occasionally may be active heterosexually, have female partners who are heterosexually active, or be the victims of heterosexual rape. Therefore, all lesbian adolescents should be considered at risk for STDs, including gonorrhea (pharyngeal, cervical, rectal), chlamydia (cervical, rectal), genital herpes, syphilis, genital warts, and HIV infection. Pregnancy, too, may be a possibility. Lesbian adolescents also should have regular Papanicolaou and breast examinations. All gay male youth, whether or not acknowledging sexual activity, should have a general screening examination with careful attention paid to the skin, lymph nodes, oropharynx, abdomen, genitals, and anorectal region. They should be considered for a complete STD evaluation. As with other adolescents, the content and frequency of screening examinations depends on the frequency and nature of the teenager's sexual activity. The evaluation and treatment of sexually transmitted diseases are discussed in Chapter 262, Sexually Transmitted Diseases.

LABORATORY EVALUATION

All sexually active gay male youths and lesbian adolescents should have serological studies performed to detect syphilis and be offered HIV testing. All adolescents, regardless of sexual orientation, should receive hepatitis B immunization.

ANTICIPATORY GUIDANCE

Because so little information is available to lesbian and gay youth about their sexual orientation, the health practitioner should address the following seven areas to ensure their safe passage into adulthood:

1. *Information about sexual orientation.* Although different segments of society and various religions may view homosexuality either positively or negatively, the field of pediatrics generally accepts that homosexuality is not a choice, that its origins appear to be established early in childhood, and that it appears to be a healthy or natural outcome for perhaps 3% to 10% of the population.
2. *Feelings about sexual orientation.* A teenager's feelings about the possibility of being lesbian or gay likely will come from a mixture of societal, religious, ethnic, and familial influences. The practitioner should not attempt to argue against any of these influences but rather allow teenagers the time to explore the effect of these in their lives and correct any misconceptions or matters of fact related to homosexuality or what it means to be lesbian or gay.
3. *Experience of lesbian and gay adolescents and adults.* Although lesbian and gay people historically have been subjected to ridicule, harassment, and discrimination, increased understanding and acceptance has been a definite trend in large segments of society, including some religious denominations. Teenagers should understand that they can aspire to rewarding careers;

long-term, loving relationships; and parenthood in their adult lives.

4. *Risk behaviors and safer-sex practices.* The practitioner should evaluate every adolescent's decision-making abilities related to risky behaviors and attempt to enhance negotiation skills related to sex and drugs. Helping the teen to postpone serious sexual involvement until older should be a goal in working with younger adolescents. All teenagers, sexually active or not, should understand in detail the rationale and techniques of safer sex, particularly the use of condoms.
5. *"Coming out" to parents and friends.* "Coming out" (revealing one's sexual orientation to others) is a strong urge some adolescents feel as they become more comfortable with their gay or lesbian identity. Many professionals who work with gay and lesbian youth suggest waiting until one is legally and financially independent before coming out to parents. Before coming out, a review of the range of possible responses from parents or friends and how the teenager will handle these is helpful.
6. *Resources for lesbian and gay teenagers.* Many larger towns have agencies that sponsor lesbian and gay teen support groups. Local gay and lesbian community organizations will know whether such groups exist in a particular area. Several excellent books have been written for lesbian and gay teenagers and their friends or parents. Teenagers in significant distress should be referred to experienced supportive counselors (social workers, psychologists, or psychiatrists). Care should be taken in making such referrals, because counselors who claim to be able to alter an adolescent's sexual orientation are engaging in an unethical and dangerous practice.
7. *Special experience of rural youth and youth of color.* Health practitioners should be sensitive to the possibility that rural youth and youth of color may be especially isolated and, therefore, have their own unique experience and needs.

PARENTS

Most lesbian and gay teenagers will decide to postpone telling their parents of their sexual orientation. This decision should be respected by the health practitioner. At times the practitioner, at the teen's request, might facilitate the coming-out process by meeting with both adolescent and parents to discuss these issues. Parents who become aware that their teenager is gay or lesbian often go through a very difficult period. Like their teen son or daughter, they may experience fear, anger, guilt, confusion, and a sense of isolation. Some may reject their child or seek out therapies to change their child's sexual orientation. The practitioner can ease parental distress by providing information and connecting them to community resources such as experienced counselors and local chapters of Parents/Friends of Lesbians and Gays. The practitioner also can acknowledge the pain and anger that parents may feel, but at the same time stress that what their sons or daughters need most is renewed assurance of their continuing love.

ADVOCACY

Although much is known about sexual orientation and the experience of lesbian and gay youth, a great deal of societal ignorance and fear still is related to working openly with them. Health practitioners are well situated to dispel the myths, initiate community dialogues, and create a network of supportive community service for these young people. These networks must include schools, churches, youth agencies, health centers, correctional facilities, and all other youth-serving institutions. These efforts are beginning in many communities throughout the country and enable these young people to become the happy, healthy, and productive gay and lesbian adults they are meant to be.

REFERENCES

1. Committee on Adolescence, American Academy of Pediatrics: Homosexuality and adolescence, *Pediatrics* 92:631, 1993.
2. Green R: *The "sissy boy syndrome" and the development of homosexuality,* New Haven, Conn, 1987, Yale University Press.
3. *Hawaii Gay and Lesbian Teen Task Force: A report on Hawaii's gay and lesbian youth,* Honolulu, Nov 1992.
4. Remafedi G: Adolescent homosexuality: psychosocial and medical implications, *Pediatrics* 79:331, 1987.
5. Remafedi G: Male homosexuality: the adolescents' perspective, *Pediatrics* 79:326, 1987.
6. Remafedi G, et al: Demography of sexual orientation in adolescents, *Pediatrics* 89:714, 1992.
7. Ryan CC, Futterman D: *Lesbian and gay youth: care and counseling,* New York, 1997, Columbia University Press.
8. Troiden RR: Homosexual identity development, *J Adolesc Health Care* 9:105, 1988.

SUGGESTED READINGS

Fairchild B, Hayward N: *Now that you know: a parents' guide to understanding their gay and lesbian children,* San Diego, 1998, Harcourt Brace.

Gold MA, et al: Children of gay or lesbian parents, *Pediatr Rev* 15:354, 1994.

Rench JE: *Understanding sexual identity: a book for gay teens and their friends,* Minneapolis, 1990, Lerner.

Ryan CC, Futterman D: *Lesbian and gay youth: care and counseling,* New York, 1997, Columbia University Press.

Whitlock K: *Bridges of respect: creating support for lesbian and gay youth,* Philadelphia, 1989, American Friends Service Committee.

RESOURCES

1. Lambert House: A Gay/Lesbian/Bisexual Youth Center, 1818 Fifteenth Avenue, Seattle, WA 98122. Provides a drop-in center, support groups, recreation, education, and health services.
2. Out Youth Austin Helpline: Provides a national toll-free helpline for sexual minority adolescents providing referrals to supportive gay/lesbian youth services nationwide. 1-800-96YOUTH.
3. Parents, Families and Friends of Lesbians and Gays, 1101 14th Street NW, Suite 1030, Washington, DC 20005. Web address: http://www.pflag.com/. Provides information on local chapters, written materials for parents, and advocacy on lesbian and gay issues.

105 Interviewing Adolescents

Esther H. Wender • Susan M. Coupey

The skill of interviewing is put to a strong test in the practice of adolescent medicine because the relationship between the adolescent patient and adults in positions of authority is changing rapidly and often is fragile. Yet, good interviewing requires establishing a relationship that enhances communication between the interacting parties. The information most relevant and useful to both people emerges if the relationship promotes communication. Conversely, the questions most skillfully formulated do not yield useful information if the interaction between the conversing parties is tense or hostile.

WHOM TO INTERVIEW

During adolescence, a transition from dependence to independence should be made by the teenager and should be facilitated by the parents. In early adolescence the parents still are largely responsible for their teen's health care, although by late adolescence these patients often are managing their own medical needs completely. These changes occur over a relatively brief period; therefore, the physician is faced with assessing the stage of transition toward independence each time the adolescent patient is seen. Whom to interview should be decided in the context of this transition, and several potential problems need to be considered.

The Adolescent's Developmental Level

Nothing is more upsetting to adolescents than feeling that they are being treated like younger children. This particularly is a problem in early adolescence when lack of sexual maturation on the part of teens causes insensitive adults to underestimate the patients' psychological age. Adolescent patients, when they feel free to comment, resent an office or hospital setting designed only for younger children. Even more upsetting, however, is the adult who talks to adolescents as though they are younger children. Therefore, to gain the respect of adolescent patients, the physician should take a genuine interest in them at the beginning of the interview.

It usually is best to greet the adolescent patient before greeting the parent. It also is helpful to chat with the patient briefly before the interview begins, being careful to gear the conversation to the appropriate level for that patient. To accomplish this, the physician should know enough about normal adolescent development to judge the appropriateness of this preinterview conversation (see Chapter 52, Theories and Concepts of Development as They Relate to Pediatric Practice).

The Parents' Role

Although it is essential to make the adolescent feel comfortable, the physician should not ignore the importance of the parents' role. In early and middle adolescence, the parents' input is critical for a thorough evaluation because adolescents still have only limited insight about themselves and have inadequate perspective on the timing and importance of symptoms. During late adolescence, seeing the adolescent without the parents' involvement may be appropriate, if that is the teenager's wish. When the parents are involved, the physician should allow them time to discuss their concerns without their child being present. Parents may be reluctant to discuss their concerns openly, particularly in the presence of their adolescent.

A younger (12- to 16-year-old) adolescent may request to be seen alone, particularly regarding sexual issues. The physician should be aware of the particular state's laws regarding the adolescent's rights to confidential evaluation, and these rights must be respected. However, because of adolescents' limited perspective and their need for emotional and financial support, the physician would be wise in most cases to encourage younger adolescents to involve their parents. Although the adolescent's independence should be encouraged and he or she should always have some time to see the physician alone, the appropriate role of the parents should not be ignored. In our culture parents still are responsible for their children through adolescence.

Adolescent Sensitivity to Parents-Only Interviews

Adolescent patients often are both upset and resentful when the parents and physician talk about them in their absence. This particularly is true if the adolescent disagrees with the parents' assessment of the problem or objects to consulting a physician. Therefore, the need to obtain information from the parents may be in direct conflict with consideration for the adolescent's feelings. One way to solve this problem is to see the patient and parents together for the initial portion of the interview. During this session the physician should tell both the adolescent and parents that each will be able to talk to the physician alone and that these conversations will be confidential. This approach, which allows disagreements between parents and patient to be aired openly, usually reduces the natural "paranoia" that the adolescent feels when in conflict with his or her parents' assessment of the problem.

Physician Neutrality

If a significant disagreement exists between the adolescent and parents, the physician must avoid seeming to take sides on these issues. Again, this can be accomplished best by interviewing the adolescent and parents together, concentrating on understanding and clarifying their disagreements, and thus conveying an appropriately neutral attitude about the conflict. The following vignette illustrates this technique. The evaluation has been initiated by parents, concerned that their 15-year-old son has behavioral problems.

Mr. Jones: We think his choice of friends leaves a lot to be desired.

Jim: What's the matter with my friends?

Mr. Jones: Most of them have no ambition. They don't care about school and spend their time just hanging around.

Jim: It's just that we're not like you. You don't care about anything except work. At least my friends know how to have fun.

Physician: Jim, you think your father devotes too much attention to work?

Jim: Yeah.

Physician: And, Mr. Jones, you wish Jim were more ambitious and also picked friends who were?

Mr. Jones: Yes. I worry that Jim isn't going to succeed.

Jim (to his father): I'll succeed in my own way.

Physician: What are your ideas about success, Jim?

In this interaction, the physician has facilitated communication between the father and son without stating an opinion that would appear to commit him to either's point of view.

A review of these issues before the interview helps the physician to make a reasonable decision about whom to interview first; no rigid rules apply. The choice depends on the age of the patient, the person who initiates the contact, and whether conflict exists between the adolescent and parents regarding the problem.

PHYSICAL SETTING

Adolescent patients often are sensitive to the atmosphere of the physician's office or hospital ward that emphasizes the interests of the young child. Therefore, the pediatrician should arrange the office waiting room with a section that contains reading material and decor appropriate for adolescent patients. At least one examining room should be equipped and decorated with the adolescent patient in mind. The hospital ward also should have a section furnished and decorated specifically for adolescent patients, and an interviewing room to be used exclusively for teens should be available. The need for privacy during the interview is never more important than in the practice of adolescent medicine. If the adolescent believes that the conversation will be interrupted or overheard, important information may not be revealed. Privacy may be particularly difficult to find on the hospital ward or in the emergency room, but every effort should be made to achieve it.

The interview room should be arranged with physician, patient, and parents seated at the same level, at a comfortable conversational distance, and without desks between the physician and the other person or persons to whom the physician is speaking. The few moments it takes to rearrange furniture to meet these requirements are well spent.

INTERVIEWING TECHNIQUE

The key to good interviewing is building a trusting relationship among the physician, patient, and parents. This goal can be accomplished if the physician makes an effort to understand how the adolescent patient perceives the problem and relationships with important people in his or her life. Most physicians would say that they do attempt to understand their patients. However, physicians often become involved in their own agenda of obtaining answers to specific medical questions and miss important clues about their patients' feelings.

The following vignette illustrates the insensitivity that results when medical issues are pursued vigorously and the physician becomes more interested in the answers than in the relationship. The patient is a 16-year-old girl who has diabetes.

Physician: How much insulin do you take?

Susan: Sixteen units of NPH and four units of regular each morning.

Physician: Do you test your urine?

Susan: Yeah.

Physician: How often?

Susan: Every morning and in the late afternoon, when my mother doesn't bug me.

Physician: Do you ever spill sugar?

Susan: Sometimes; not too often.

Physician: How much? One plus, two plus?

Susan: Just one plus a couple of times a week. Mom's always asking me that, but I tell her to leave me alone.

Physician: Do you ever have insulin reactions?

Susan: Not for a long time.

Physician: How's school?

One can sense the physician's need to fill in the blanks of the medical history. In the process, this physician has failed to pick up the clues of the daughter-mother conflict. The physician completed the agenda and then turned to a question about the adolescent's life that probably will be perceived by the patient as a "mechanical" question, because the physician did not "hear" previous comments.

Techniques that promote the acquisition of useful information fall into two main categories: listening skills and facilitative responses (see Interviewing Techniques in Chapter 7, The Pediatric History). Component aspects of these two techniques, discussed briefly in the next two sections, are outlined as follows:

1. Listening skills
    a. Clarification of meaning
    b. Verbal asides
    c. Nonverbal communication
2. Facilitative responses
    a. Repetition and review
    b. Acknowledgment of feelings
    c. Periods of silence

Listening Skills

Unless physicians pay attention to the meaning of words, they often will think that they understand when they really do not. Every time patients use words or phrases that are abstract or unclear, physicians should ask for clarification. Skilled interviewers continually ask themselves if they understand what has just been said. In the following vignette, the importance of this technique is illustrated. The patient is a 15-year-old boy who has school problems.

Physician: Your parents seem concerned about how you are doing in school. What do you think?

Gary: Sometimes I think I'm a wreck.

Physician: A wreck?

Gary: Yeah, you know, all washed up.

Physician: I don't know, Gary; what does that feel like?

Gary: Like I get these funny feelings, and I think I'm falling apart.

Physician: Tell me about one of these funny feelings.

Gary: Well . . . sometimes it's like my fingers are growing really big, or small. It's weird.

Physician: You mean like parts of your body are changing size?

Gary: Yeah.

Physician: Anything else?

Gary: Sometimes I feel like I'm walking just a little off the ground, like I was floating.

If the physician did not pursue the meaning of Gary's words, he or she might have been left with the vague statement that Gary feels he is a "wreck," which many people would assume means that he thinks he is a failure. Instead, the physician now has evidence that Gary is experiencing somatic symptoms of anxiety or psychotic thinking, and he or she can pursue the source of these feelings.

Verbal asides are parenthetical statements that often reveal the patient's true feelings, but that are stated as though they are unimportant. They usually reflect the adolescent's ambivalence about exposing his or her real feelings. The diabetic patient, described earlier, who said that she tested her urine twice a day "when my mother doesn't bug me" is giving a verbal aside. Statements about her mother constitute unsolicited information. Physicians often focus only on the solicited information and, therefore, fail to hear such asides. All that usually is required to facilitate further communication is to echo the phrase back to the patient in the form of a question.

Nonverbal communication consists of body movements and facial expressions that reveal a person's feelings. A physician who is preoccupied with asking the right questions and accumulating the answers will miss these important clues. The skilled interviewer learns to divide attention between the words that are being said and the body language of the person being interviewed. Because body language usually is outside the patient's awareness, it may be premature to comment immediately on such observations. Part of the art of interviewing is to sense when such comments may be useful.

A good rule to remember is that when body language reveals something the person seems to be trying to hide, it should be left alone. For example, a person's clenched fists may indicate tension, when his or her words suggest calm. However, when a facial expression suggests an inner thought or feeling, it often is useful to comment. The patient may say something funny, for example, and then appear sad. In this instance, it usually is helpful to say something like, "It looks as if that thought suddenly made you feel sad."

Facilitative Responses

The person who is talking usually feels good when the listener can synthesize what the speaker has just said into a summary that reflects the thoughts accurately. If, for example, the patient has had difficulty finding the right words to describe his or her symptoms and the physician then restates those symptoms briefly and accurately, the patient realizes that he or she has been heard. People like to be understood, and this type of *repetition and review* greatly facilitates further communication.

An important component of repetition and review is the *acknowledgment of feelings,* as well as the recognition of facts. Often, patients make a series of statements that really are meant to build a case for the underlying feelings they are experiencing. If the physician can hear and then acknowledge these feelings, the relationship may be significantly enhanced. The following segment of an interview illustrates this interaction. The patient is a 13-year-old girl brought in by parents because of acting-out behavior.

Physician: Your parents are upset over some of the things you have done. What do you think?

Judy: They really bug me. Last week, Mom wouldn't let me go to the roller rink with my friends. She said that we were too young to go by ourselves, but all my friends' parents let them go. Then, a couple of nights ago, I wanted to stay at Sally's house for dinner and Dad made me come home. He said that it's getting too dark at night. Geez, you'd think I was a baby.

Physician: It sounds like you don't feel that your parents trust you.

Judy: I *know* they don't trust me. It makes me feel like doing whatever I want, since they don't trust me anyway.

Another important facilitative response is the carefully timed use of *silences*. This is particularly important when the patient has difficulty expressing himself or herself. Physicians usually are highly verbal people and respond to such patients by asking more and more questions. When a question has been asked and the response is not immediate, the interviewer should look closely for cues that the patient is processing the question. If the patient appears to be thinking about the answer, the physician should learn to pause to allow a response. Further statements might include facilitative responses such as, "What thoughts are you having?" or "It's hard, sometimes, to find the right words." Such replies tend to encourage the response.

The periods of silence should not be so long that the patient is made to feel uncomfortable. Sometimes in psychiatric interviews, long silences are used purposefully, but this approach would be too threatening for most medical interviews. Instead, the recommended approach is to allow time for the person whose verbal responses are slow.

APPROACHING THE SENSITIVE ISSUES OF DRUGS, SEX, AND EMOTIONAL PROBLEMS

Vital issues in adolescent medicine include a healthy response to emerging sexuality and the avoidance of addiction to drugs or alcohol. Health care professionals should address these issues from the perspective of prevention. This approach requires inquiring about these topics throughout the period of adolescent development. However, both adolescents and physicians often feel uncomfortable with these issues. Questions about sexual activity, the use of drugs and alcohol, and the possibility of serious emotional problems often seem intrusive and embarrassing. One useful approach to these issues is to provide an anonymous questionnaire that the adolescent is instructed to complete while in the waiting room without "help" from the parents. Such questionnaires usually begin with questions that are medical, such as questions about the adolescent's perception of his or her weight, skin condition, and development of secondary sexual characteristics. This section also should include self-perceived bodily symptoms such as headache, stomach ache, heart palpitations, breathing problems and dizziness, or pain. Such a questionnaire may then move to more sensitive areas such as sexual activity and orientation, use of alcohol and drugs, and exposure to violence and abuse. Questions also should address mental health problems such as feelings of depression, suicidal thoughts, and symptoms of anxiety. The questionnaire also should ask about school performance, including possible problems with teachers or peers. The anonymity of the questionnaire is important. It should contain no identifying data, and the adolescent should be told that it will be reviewed only by the physician alone with the adolescent, and then be discarded—that is, not placed in the patient chart. The physician can then use the questionnaire to address issues that are pertinent to that adolescent at that point. If, for example, the adolescent indicates that he or she is sexually active, the physician can address issues of pregnancy prevention and the prevention of sexually transmitted diseases. If the patient is not sexually active, the physician can emphasize making informed choices about sexual activity in the future.

Another helpful approach, especially in addressing issues of drug and alcohol use, is to precede any direct questions about such use with indirect statements about the possible use of such substances by others. The following vignette illustrates this approach. The patient is a 15-year-old boy.

Physician: Sometimes kids your age try alcohol, like beer or hard drinks, when they're at parties or hanging out together. Has this ever happened to you?

Justin: Yeah. Like, you know, a couple of times.

Physician: Sometimes it can be a little scary. How was it for you?

Justin: Once I was with a friend who was driving and I thought he was, like, kind of crazy. I was really afraid he might get us in a wreck.

Physician: Was there anything you felt you could do? to protect yourself?

Justin: Well, no, but I sure wish there was.

Physician: How about yourself? Did you ever feel you drank too much?

Justin: Well, yeah, once I woke up the next day and I couldn't remember what happened for the life of me!

These responses probably would not have been forthcoming had the physician asked the questions directly—for example, "Do you drink or take drugs?" This indirect approach is face saving, and is likely, therefore, to yield more truthful information. The physician can now give much more targeted advice.

The importance of possible drug or alcohol abuse also has led to screening questionnaires that may be helpful in a population of adolescents at particularly high risk of abuse. Such questionnaires usually assume some alcohol or drug use and are designed to measure the severity of that use.

SUMMARY

The interviewing techniques described provide some suggestions for the practitioner who provides health care for adolescents. Effective interviewing requires practice. However, the skill is well worth learning, because it leads to the completion of better medical histories and improved patient compliance. The result is improved health care for adolescents and their families.

SUGGESTED READINGS

Coupey SM: Interviewing adolescents, *Pediatr Clin North Am* 44:1349, 1997.

Felice ME, Friedman SB: Behavioral considerations in the health care of adolescents, *Pediatr Clin North Am* 29:399, 1982.

Ginott HG: *Between parent and teenager,* New York, 1969, Macmillan.

Knight JR, et al: A new brief screen for adolescent substance abuse, *Arch Pediatr Adolesc Med* 153:591, 1999.

106 Juvenile Delinquency

Irving B. Weiner

Juvenile delinquency is the legal term for youthful behavior that violates the law. This broad legal definition embraces two specific questions pediatricians must address when dealing with delinquent behavior: Does the kind and extent of a patient's illegal activity call for clinical intervention? If so, what is the cause of the delinquent behavior in which he or she has been involved?

The first of these questions is important because delinquent acts, regardless of whether they have been detected by the police, can range widely in severity and frequency. Young people may have committed major felonies such as assault or armed robbery, which have serious implications for criminal tendencies, or they may be guilty only of misdemeanors such as running away or disturbing the peace, which have few such implications. Likewise, a particular kind of delinquent act may have occurred only once or may have become a repetitive pattern of illegal behavior. The point at which delinquent acts come to professional attention often is influenced by the tolerance level for such behavior in a particular child's family, neighborhood, or community. Generally, however, the more serious the delinquent acts and the more frequently they have been occurring, the more likely they are to require clinical evaluation and treatment.

Regarding the causes of delinquent behavior, juvenile delinquency does not constitute a unitary phenomenon that identifies universally applicable explanations of its etiology and uniformly appropriate ways of dealing with it. Instead, delinquent youngsters are a psychologically heterogeneous group. Some are socialized delinquents who are well-integrated members of a delinquent subculture and display few, if any, psychological problems; others are delinquent as a result of various psychological maladjustments, some of which are characterological in nature and some of which reflect neurotic tendencies.

Characterological maladjustments usually begin forming early in life and crystallize into various forms of personality disorder during adolescence. Individuals who have personality disorders are satisfied with their basic nature and have no wish to change it; they feel comfortable with themselves and attribute any difficulties they encounter to external events over which they have no control and for which they bear no responsibility. Neurotic maladjustments, by contrast, usually do not appear until the elementary school years and may emerge at any subsequent time of life with little previous warning. They constitute immature or unrealistic ways of attempting to solve problems or to reduce anxiety and are uncharacteristic of how the affected person usually behaves. Neurotic individuals usually are concerned about how they are feeling (e.g., phobic or depressed) or acting (e.g., being compulsive or having temper tantrums) and wish they could change themselves back to what they were like before these symptoms began.[15]

DIFFERENTIAL DIAGNOSIS OF DELINQUENT BEHAVIOR

The differential diagnosis of delinquent behavior in young people flows from the particular origin of their misconduct in socialized, characterological, or neurotic determinants.

Socialized Delinquency

In socialized delinquency, illegal activity emerges among members of a subculture who share antisocial standards of conduct. Whereas psychological forms of delinquency are maladaptive for the individual, socialized delinquency constitutes adaptive behavior in the sense that it earns delinquents praise and acceptance from their immediate social group and thereby provides them a sense of satisfaction and belonging. Socialized delinquency usually is a group or gang activity; it seldom accounts for delinquent acts that are committed alone or without the approval of neighborhood peer groups.[1]

Accordingly, the differential diagnosis of socialized delinquency is suggested by four findings in the clinical history: (1) the delinquent acts have been performed with valued companions rather than alone or with strangers; (2) the delinquent young people see themselves as accepted and integral members of their peer group and rarely exhibit feelings of personal alienation or social inadequacy; (3) unlike people who have psychological disorders, socialized delinquents evidence little in the way of neurotic symptom formation or basic character flaws; and (4) although socialized delinquency may result, in part, from inadequate parental supervision, socialized delinquents typically will have enjoyed close and supportive family relationships during their early years, which stands in contrast to the kinds of family tensions and disruption that contribute to psychological problems.

Characterological Delinquency

The illegal behavior of characterological delinquents reflects a basically asocial personality orientation. These young people manifest many features of what commonly is termed *psy-*

chopathy. Because of prominent guiltlessness (defective conscience) and lovelessness (incapacity for loyalty to others), they are highly prone to committing illegal acts against persons and property. Characterological delinquents tend to be loners who neither trust nor expect to be trusted by others. They break the law primarily as a result of disregard for the feelings and rights of others and an inability or unwillingness to control their own behavior. Such personality impairments derive from parental rejection early in life, which deprives children of an opportunity to learn to share mutual bonds of affection and attachment with other people, and parental neglect in middle childhood, which deprives young people of the discipline and guidance necessary to inculcate self-control and internal standards of moral conduct. Lacking such parenting, future psychopaths grow from childhood into adolescence loving no one and guided by an external morality in which acceptable behavior is whatever they can get away with.[5,9]

The differential diagnosis of characterological delinquency is based on adolescents' personality style, their behavioral history, and the nature of their past and current family relationships. The more patients appear basically to be aggressive, impulsive, and amoral, with little sympathy for others and little capacity to tolerate frustration of their own wishes, the more likely their delinquency will reflect a psychopathic personality disorder. Because the roots of psychopathy extend far back into childhood, characterological delinquents usually will have a long history of such problem behaviors as fighting, lying, stealing, being unruly in school, and being cruel to people and animals. The diagnosis of characterological delinquency rarely is justified in the absence of this kind of history, and it also should be avoided for children who appear to have enjoyed close and supportive care from reasonably well-adjusted parents. Evidence of early affective deprivation, on the other hand, especially when combined with a family history of irresponsible behavior, increases the probability considerably that delinquent activity is characterological in origin.

Occasionally, the long-term consequences of having had a childhood learning disability produce patterns of misconduct during adolescence that bear a superficial resemblance to characterological delinquency. The blows to self-esteem typically suffered by learning-disabled children at home, in the classroom, and on the playground can result in their becoming insecure and short-tempered teenagers who need to bolster their self-image and beat down unwanted criticism. Hence, like characterological delinquents, they tend at times to show the kinds of aggressive, self-centered behavior seen in psychopathic individuals. However, the basic nature of the difficulties of learning-disabled adolescents can be differentiated readily from psychopathy by a good clinical history. Instead of early affective deprivation or other family problems, these adolescents usually will have demonstrated evidence of an attention deficit/hyperactivity disorder in early childhood (including hyperactivity, delayed motor and language development, and impaired perceptual-motor coordination); in elementary school they will have been slow to learn (especially reading), despite having adequate intelligence, and will have had strained relationships with their teachers and classmates.

Neurotic Delinquency

Neurotic delinquents commit illegal acts neither as commonplace pursuits shared with their peer group nor as a reflection of a long-standing characterological disorder. Rather, their delinquency emerges without previous warning as a way of expressing needs for recognition or help. Young people who feel ignored or unappreciated by others may carry out daring or dramatic acts of delinquency to bask, even if only briefly, in the notoriety they achieve. Children and adolescents who cannot find direct ways of communicating a need for help in dealing with some problem may act delinquently as an indirect means of getting this message across. The kind of distress associated most frequently with such delinquency is underlying depression, and the onset of uncharacteristic misconduct commonly can be traced to feelings of loneliness or discouragement that a young person cannot express or get others to hear through more direct channels of communication.[7,14]

A key to identifying this particular pattern of delinquency is the regularity with which neurotic delinquents manage to get caught in the act or give themselves away. Because the symptomatic use of delinquency to express underlying concerns serves its purpose only if the misdeeds come to light, successful concealment of law-breaking usually contraindicates neurotic delinquency. The differential diagnosis of neurotic delinquency also is facilitated by certain elements of the history and family circumstances. Unlike psychopathic individuals, neurotic delinquents have little or no history of earlier behavioral problems. Their current misconduct deviates sharply from how they have acted before and how others have come to expect them to act.

Moreover, in their relationships with their parents, neurotic delinquents ordinarily have enjoyed both the close supervision denied socialized delinquents and the warmth and affection denied characterological delinquents. Nevertheless, specific problems in family communication often are the final factor in prompting otherwise law-abiding youngsters to resort to delinquent behavior as a means of getting their parents to recognize and respond to their needs. The more clearly these or other kinds of specific precipitating events (such as a painful rebuff from peers or loss of a parent through death or divorce) can be identified as occurring just before the onset of delinquent behavior, the more likely is the illegal activity to constitute neurotic symptom formation.

DIFFERENTIAL TREATMENT PLANNING IN DELINQUENCY

Differential treatment planning for delinquent youth depends on the type of delinquent behavior manifest. In socialized delinquency, antisocial actions are adaptive group behaviors that neither reflect nor lead to diagnosable psychological disturbance; hence, little is gained from efforts at psychological intervention in the practitioner's office. Socialized delinquents need (1) supervision and control, (2) guidance and models that can encourage them to exchange their antisocial values for more conventional standards of conduct, and (3) help in preparing themselves for an adult life in which they can find ways of enjoying and supporting themselves within rather than outside the law. Accordingly, the indicated treatment for adolescents displaying subcultural delinquency usually is referral to community-based activities or agencies that provide group-oriented programs for developing the talents and redirecting the energies of delinquent youth.[4,11,13]

Characterological delinquency, because of its integral relationship to psychopathic personality formation beginning early in life, constitutes a serious and usually chronic form of psychopathology. Successful intervention in characterological delinquency accordingly requires intensive, long-term psychotherapy, which even under the best circumstances offers much less hope for a favorable outcome than can be expected for most other child and adolescent behavioral problems. Pediatricians are unlikely to undertake the long and arduous treatment of characterological delinquents themselves, unless they have had extensive training in child and adolescent psychiatry or behavioral pediatrics and can commit large amounts of time to such work. Instead, their usual choice will be to refer these patients to mental health practitioners or agencies, many of whom, in turn, feel that only an extended period of residential treatment can affect these young people sufficiently to alter their chronic personality disorder.[2,10,12]

Recent advances in theory and practice have begun to improve this gloomy prognosis for psychopathy. The likelihood of psychopathic adolescents becoming seriously and persistently delinquent appears related to their lacking social skills that could help them find noncriminal ways of satisfying their needs. Attention, accordingly, is being directed to modifying the behavior of these delinquents, not by attempting to change their character style, but by enhancing their coping capacities through a variety of training exercises designed to increase their repertoire of interpersonal skills and their capacity for judgment and self-control. Adolescents' parents frequently are brought into this type of treatment program, not for traditional family therapy but to receive training themselves in interacting with their child in ways that encourage and reward prosocial behavior.[3,6,8]

Neurotic delinquency, because of its specific symptomatic meaning and relatively recent onset, frequently responds promptly to brief psychotherapy. Psychotherapy in correctly diagnosed instances of neurotic delinquency offers much greater promise of altering antisocial conduct than do any of the known ways of intervening in socialized or characterological delinquency, and pediatricians who conduct psychotherapy can provide the necessary treatment in the office. Because the deviant behavior of neurotic delinquents is motivated by needs for attention and help, the very act of hearing them out and offering to work with them can, in short order, result in their stopping delinquent activity.[7]

Beyond this immediate salutary impact, effective psychotherapy with neurotic delinquents consists mainly of (1) gaining the patient's trust and confidence and (2) adopting the stance of an interested and concerned listener who makes observations from time to time on the apparent significance of what is being said, rather than of someone who judges and advises. If these patients also can be helped to recognize connections between the onset of their delinquency and the onset of certain psychological problems they could not express in other ways, the likelihood of their resorting to such indirect channels of expression in the future will be diminished substantially.

REFERENCES

1. Dishion TJ, French DC, Patterson GR: The development and ecology of antisocial behavior. In Cicchetti D, Cohen DJ, editors: *Developmental psychopathology*, vol 2, New York, 1995, Wiley.
2. Glaser BA, Horne AM: A treatment program for children with conduct disorders. In LeCroy CW, editor: *Handbook of child and adolescent treatment manuals*, New York, 1994, Lexington Books.
3. Hengeller SW, et al: *Multisystemic treatment of antisocial behavior in children and adolescents*, New York, 1998, Guilford.
4. Johnson JH, Fennel EB: Aggressive, antisocial, and delinquent behavior in childhood and adolescence. In Walker CE, Roberts MC, editors: *Handbook of clinical child psychology*, New York, 1996, Wiley.
5. Kazdin AE: *Conduct disorders in childhood and adolescence*, ed 2, Thousand Oaks, Calif, 1995, Sage.
6. Kazdin AE, Siegel TC, Bass D: Cognitive problem-solving skills training and parent management training in the treatment of antisocial behavior in children, *J Consult Clin Psychol* 60:733, 1992.
7. Kimmel DC, Weiner IB: *Adolescence: a developmental transition*, ed 2, New York, 1995, Wiley.
8. Kirigin KA, Wolf MM: Application of the teaching-family model to children and adolescents with conduct disorder. In Van Hasselt VB, Hersen M, editors: *Handbook of psychological treatment protocols for children and adolescents*, Mahwah, NJ, 1998, Erlbaum.
9. Lykken DT: *The antisocial personalities*, Hillsdale, NJ, 1995, Erlbaum.
10. Marohn RC: Residential services. In Tolan PH, Cohler BJ, editors: *Handbook of clinical research and practice with adolescents*, New York, 1993, Wiley.
11. Mulvey EP, Arthur MW, Reppucci ND: The prevention and treatment of juvenile delinquency: a review of the research, *Clin Psychol Rev* 13:133, 1993.
12. Offord DR, Bennett KJ: Conduct disorder: long-term outcomes and intervention effectiveness, *J Am Acad Child Adolesc Psychiatry* 33:1069, 1994.
13. Patterson GR: Some characteristics of a developmental theory for early-onset delinquency. In Lenzenweger MF, Haugaard JJ, editors: *Frontiers of developmental psychopathology*, New York, 1996, Oxford.
14. Walker ML, Schmidt LM, Lunghofer LL: Youth gangs. In Singer MI, Singer LT, Angin TM, editors: *Handbook for screening adolescents at psychological risk*, New York, 1993, Lexington Books.
15. Weiner IB: *Psychological disturbance in adolescence*, ed 2, New York, 1992, Wiley.

107 Mood Disorders in Children and Adolescents

David A. Brent

Mood disorders are important contributors to the morbidity and mortality of children and adolescents. In fact, evidence shows that the prevalence of depression and bipolar disorder has increased within the past three decades and that their age of onset of has become younger. As the nature of pediatric practice shifts to accommodate an emphasis on psychosocial issues, it is important for the pediatrician to recognize and share in the management of these relatively common and serious problems of childhood and adolescence.

CLASSIFICATION

One of the advances in child and adolescent psychiatry has been the development of consistent nomenclature and criteria for various psychiatric disorders. Mood disorders are classified based on three factors: (1) severity, (2) course, and (3) presence or absence of mania. In terms of depressive symptomatology, the diagnosis of major depressive disorder requires at least 2 weeks of depressed mood more than half of the time and four additional depressive symptoms (Box 107-1). A more chronic, intermittent disorder such as dysthymic disorder may have periods of depression interspersed with normal mood (Box 107-2). Adjustment disorder is a still milder disturbance of affect that follows a serious life stressor (Box 107-3). A history of manic symptomatology in a person who has dysthymia or major depression confers a diagnosis of bipolar affective or cyclothymic disorder (Boxes 107-4 and 107-5).

DESCRIPTIVE EPIDEMIOLOGY

Mood disorders are relatively rare in prepubertal children, with estimates of point prevalences ranging from 1.8% to 2.9%. The incidence of mood disorder is estimated to be three to four times more common in adolescence (around 8.7%). Whereas the gender ratio for affectively ill prepubertal children approaches unity, depression among adolescents is approximately two to three times more common among females than males. Earlier onset of puberty may be associated with an increased risk of depression, especially in girls.

RISK FACTORS

The most potent risk factor for developing a depressive disorder in childhood is having at least one parent who has a history of depression. Anxiety disorders also may predispose to the development of depression. The risk of depression is greater and age of onset of depression younger with a greater familial "loading" for depression, an earlier age of onset of depression in parents, and a family history of either bipolarity or recurrent unipolar disorder. Physical or sexual abuse and exposure to family and community violence also may be associated with depressive symptoms. Certain medications may predispose to depression, namely, antihypertensive agents, steroids, and phenobarbital. The incidence of depression may be increased in patients who have some chronic illnesses, such as epilepsy, inflammatory bowel disease, and juvenile-onset diabetes. Although the etiology of depression is unknown, it is likely that genetic and biological factors play an important role in light of familial aggregation and neuroendocrine genetic and biological markers that have been described in early-onset depression. These neuroendocrine findings are most consistent with disordered noradrenergic and serotonergic neurotransmission and may be present before the onset of depressive illness.

CLINICAL PICTURE

The clinical picture of depressive disorders in children and adolescents is similar to that described in adults. It is important to remember that *depressed mood* can refer to sadness, irritability, or boredom. Depressed children, compared with depressed adolescents, present similarly, although depressed adolescents are more likely to have made a suicide attempt and to be using illicit drugs. However, suicidal thoughts are a very frequent symptom in both pre- and postpubertal depression. Patients who have either dysthymia or major depression frequently have other comorbid psychiatric disorders (anxiety disorders, attention deficit disorder, conduct disorder, and substance abuse) simultaneously. Prepubertal-onset depressive illness frequently is associated with psychotic features, specifically, mood-congruent delusions (e.g., "I am dead," "The world is coming to an end"), self-deprecatory auditory hallucinations, and paranoid ideation. The depressive picture for patients who have bipolar illness often includes psychotic features, along with hypersomnia, hyperphagia, and anergia.

Mood in the manic or hypomanic phase may be characterized by either expansive mood, euphoria, and grandiosity or by anger and irritability. Symptoms of mania and hypomania (a milder form of mania without functional impairment) may occur separately from depressive episodes or may co-occur with them. The simultaneous occurrence of manic and depressive symptoms is known as a *mixed state*. This combina-

BOX 107-1

CRITERIA FOR THE DIAGNOSIS OF A MAJOR DEPRESSIVE EPISODE

For at least 2 weeks for more than 50% of the time:

A. Depressed mood (sad, blue, "down in the dumps," angry, bored) or loss of interest and pleasure in almost all of the usual activities
B. Coincident with depressed mood, at least four of the following symptoms (three for children younger than age 6 years):
   1. Change in appetite or weight (either decreased or increased)
   2. Insomnia or hypersomnia
   3. Observable psychomotor agitation or retardation
   4. Loss of interest or pleasure; diminished libido
   5. Loss of energy; fatigue
   6. Feelings of worthlessness or inappropriate guilt
   7. Difficulty concentrating; indecision
   8. Recurrent thoughts of death; suicidal ideation or behavior
C. Not due to organic mental disorder (e.g., medical condition, drug treatment, or substance abuse) or uncomplicated bereavement

Modified from *Diagnostic and statistical manual of mental disorders,* ed 4, Washington, DC, 1994, American Psychiatric Association Press.

tion is a very common method of presentation in early-onset bipolar disorder, often is characterized by marked irritability and mood lability, comorbid-morbid substance abuse, and lack of clinical response to lithium. Mixed states pose a high risk for suicide attempt and completed suicide. Delusions associated with either grandiosity or paranoia often accompany severe mania, particularly if prolonged sleep deprivation has occurred.

DIFFERENTIAL DIAGNOSIS

Within depressive disorders, the main differential diagnosis is among the triad of dysthymia, depression, and adjustment disorder with depressed mood. Dysthymia is both a more chronic and intermittent depression than major depression, although the two disorders can coexist (major depression developing "on top" of dysthymia). Adjustment disorder with depressed mood has less severe mood disturbance and fewer symptoms and is self-limited in course compared with dysthymia or major depression. However, if a life stressor precedes a syndrome of depression, the presence of the stressor does *not* invalidate the diagnosis of major depressive disorder. The symptoms of bereavement may be indistinguishable from depressive symptoms. Depression in a bereaved patient is diagnosed if bereavement is associated with severe functional impairment, suicidal ideation, psychotic features, feelings of worthlessness, and prolonged course. A previous psychiatric disorder and a family history of depression predispose to depression following bereavement.

BOX 107-2

CRITERIA FOR THE DIAGNOSIS OF DYSTHYMIC DISORDER

A. During past year (2 years for adults), the patient has been bothered by symptoms of major depression, but of lesser severity
B. The periods of depressive symptoms may be separated by periods of normal mood of a few days or weeks
C. During the depressed periods, the patient has prominent depressed mood or loss of interest and pleasure
D. During depressed periods, the patient has at least three symptoms:
   1. Insomnia or hypersomnia
   2. Low energy level and fatigue
   3. Decreased productivity at school, work, or home
   4. Difficulty concentrating
   5. Feelings of inadequacy and poor self-esteem
   6. Social withdrawal
   7. Loss of interest and pleasure in usual activities
   8. Anhedonia (inability to experience pleasure)
   9. Tearfulness
   10. Suicidal thoughts
   11. Hopelessness and pessimism about the future, brooding about the past

Modified from American Psychiatric Association: *Diagnostic and statistical manual of mental disorders,* ed 4, Washington, DC, 1994, American Psychiatric Association Press.

BOX 107-3

CRITERIA FOR THE DIAGNOSIS OF ADJUSTMENT DISORDER WITH DEPRESSED MOOD

A. A reaction to an identified social stressor, characterized by depressed mood, tearfulness, and hopelessness
B. Occurrence within 3 months of the onset of the stressor
C. Syndrome characterized by symptoms in excess of "expectable reaction" to the stressor, the functional impairment, or both
D. Disorder is self-limited and should remit when the stress ceases
E. Disorder does not meet criteria for major depression or dysthymia

Modified from American Psychiatric Association: *Diagnostic and statistical manual of mental disorders,* ed 4, Washington, DC, 1994, American Psychiatric Association Press.

Various other psychiatric disorders also may have associated mood disturbances. Patients who have learning disabilities or attention deficit disorder may have poor self-esteem and feel demoralized but should not be diagnosed as being depressed unless they meet criteria for the syndrome. Chil-

BOX 107-4

CRITERIA FOR THE DIAGNOSIS OF BIPOLAR DISORDER

Past or current history of a manic episode, characterized by:

A. At least 1 week in which mood has been primarily elevated, expansive, or irritable
B. During this week, at least three of the following symptoms are experienced (four if mood is primarily irritable):
   1. Increase in activity (socially, at work, sexually) or physical restlessness
   2. Increased pressure of speech
   3. Flight of ideas or subjective sense of racing thoughts
   4. Inflated self-esteem (grandiosity)
   5. Diminished need for sleep
   6. Distractibility
   7. Poor judgment and impulsive, reckless action (e.g., being promiscuous, going on buying sprees, driving recklessly)
C. Episode not due to organic mental disorder (e.g., amphetamine intoxication)

BOX 107-5

CRITERIA FOR THE DIAGNOSIS OF CYCLOTHYMIC DISORDER

A. During the past year (2 years for adults), periods of depressive and manic symptoms of insufficient duration or severity to meet criteria for major depressive or manic disorders
B. The depressive and manic periods may be separated by periods of normal mood for a few days
C. During the depressive periods, there is a depressed mood and loss of interest and pleasure and at least three symptoms for dysthymic disorder (see Box 107-2)
D. During the hypomanic periods, there is an expansive, elevated, or irritable mood (but of less severity than for mania) and at least three manic symptoms
E. Psychotic features (which would suggest more severe depression or mania) are absent

Modified from American Psychiatric Association: *Diagnostic and statistical manual of mental disorders,* ed 3, Washington, DC, 1980, American Psychiatric Association Press.

dren who have separation anxiety disorder are often dysphoric when separated from their parents, but in the absence of premorbid depression, the dysphoria will be relieved by reunion with the parent. Anorectic patients, particularly if malnourished, may show a markedly depressed affect. However, depression should not be diagnosed until nutritional status has been normalized. Patients who abuse drugs and alcohol often show disturbances of mood. At times, the mood disorder may antedate and even predispose to substance abuse, but often the mood disorder is secondary to substance abuse and subsides within a month of detoxification. The differential diagnosis of depression and chronic medical illness can be difficult, given that the incidence of depression may be higher in certain illnesses and that chronic illness may affect sleep, appetite, and energy similarly to depression. Feelings of guilt, worthlessness, and hopelessness and suicidal thoughts are unlikely to be attributable to the illness itself and, if present, strongly suggest the presence of a depressive disorder.

Mania can be mimicked by stimulant abuse (e.g., cocaine, amphetamine). The irritability of mania also can be seen in depression, so that the differential diagnosis of depression and mania rests on whether the preponderance of associated symptoms is more consistent with mania or with depression. Euphoria, increased energy, and increase in sexuality are three symptoms that are seen much more commonly in bipolar than in unipolar (i.e., only experiencing depression and not mania) depressed patients. Irritability, anger, and poor judgment also may be prominent features of conduct disorder, but the lack of changes in energy, sleep, sexuality, and thought patterns in conduct disorder generally will exclude mania as a diagnosis. Similarly, the features of attention deficit disorder may suggest mania, but manic patients are more likely to have mood swings and neurovegetative changes and to show hypersexuality and inappropriate joking and punning. A severe clinical deterioration of an attention deficit-disordered patient after a trial of stimulants, particularly with some of the manic clinical features mentioned earlier or with a positive family history of mania, also suggests bipolar disorder. Sexually abused children may show sexually provocative behavior and depressed mood, but euphoria or increased energy in the absence of bipolar disorder is rarely seen. These guidelines for differential diagnosis notwithstanding, affective and non-affective disorders frequently co-occur.

CLINICAL COURSE

Naturalistic studies indicate that depressive disorders in children and adolescents run a chronic and recurrent course. According to one longitudinal study (see Kovacs et al, Depressive disorders in childhood. I. 1984, in Suggested Readings), untreated major depressive disorder lasts an average of 7.2 months and dysthymic disorder an average of 45.9 months. Those patients who have both major depressive disorder and nonaffective morbidity (e.g., additional diagnoses of conduct disorder, attention deficit disorder) may show a more prolonged course, as do those depressed youth whose parents also are depressed. On the average, 40% of depressed children experience a recurrence within 2 years, and nearly 75% have a recurrence within 5 years. Earlier age of onset and co-occurrence of an underlying dysthymic disorder increase the risk of depressive recurrences. Even after recovery from depression, prepubertal children show significant social impairment. The adult sequelae of adolescent depressive symptomatology include drug and alcohol use, development of antisocial behavior, and interference with interpersonal relationships. Moreover, depression confers a substantially increased risk for suicide in both male and female adolescents.

IDENTIFICATION OF DEPRESSED PATIENTS IN PEDIATRIC SETTINGS

Any disturbance in mood that is associated with functional impairment should be considered a psychiatric disorder until proved otherwise. Parents and children alike frequently have a tendency to mislabel *bona fide* depressive disorders as "the ups and downs" of childhood or adolescence. Mood disorder should be a strong consideration for any child who presents with unexplained somatic complaints, drop in school performance, apathy and loss of interest, social withdrawal, increased irritability or tearfulness, sleep and appetite changes, or suicidal ideation or behavior. Moreover, depressive illnesses frequently accompany tobacco, alcohol, and drug abuse; promiscuous sexual behavior; and risk-taking behavior. Depressive disorders may follow bereavement, particularly if the patient has a personal or family history of depression. Depression also may follow other severe stressors, such as physical or sexual assault. The pediatrician should be aware of a family history of depression, because such a history will increase the risk of depressive disorder at least threefold. A family history of bipolar disorder greatly increases the risk that other biological family members will develop this disorder.

Both the child and the parent usually will contribute important information to be used by the pediatrician in diagnosing depression. The child is likely to be the most accurate reporter of symptoms that refer to an internal state-depressed mood, anhedonia, guilt, worthlessness, and suicidal thoughts; the parent, by contrast, may be able to note such externally validated symptoms as irritability, decline in school performance, listlessness, withdrawal from social and other pleasurable activities, and weight loss. An important issue in the identification of mood disorder in children is to recognize that the depressed mood in children may be described as "grouchy," "mad," or "bored" rather than "sad."

MANAGEMENT

Children and adolescents who have mood disorders are best managed by a collaboration between pediatrician, mental health specialist, and child psychiatrist. Generally, psychiatric intervention has three components: (1) psychoeducation, (2) psychotherapy, and (3) pharmacotherapy. Most mood-disordered patients can be managed as outpatients. Inpatient referral should be reserved for those who are psychotic, acutely suicidal, acutely manic or in a mixed state, abusing substances, or unresponsive to outpatient intervention.

FAMILY PSYCHOEDUCATION

Family psychoeducation approaches depression as a chronic illness, with its aim to instruct family members about the nature and course of the illness. Such an approach is likely to improve compliance with treatment and reduce the rate of relapse. Psychoeducation also is aimed at reducing the tensions of living with a mood-disordered person by altering familial expectations. This alteration involves parents' accepting the illness and making appropriate expectations of the patient and themselves. Finally, psychoeducation should enable the child and family to identify early signs of recurrence of the disorder and to seek treatment before the recurrent mood disorder becomes severe and chronic. Identification and treatment of parental depression is critical because there is evidence that parental depression may prolong the child's depressive episodes and interfere with recovery.

PSYCHOTHERAPY

Individual, brief (3 months) cognitive behavior treatment (CBT) has been shown to be more efficacious than either family or supportive treatment for the relief of adolescent depression. Group CBT also has been shown to be helpful both in the treatment of depression and in the prevention of depression in at-risk youth.

PHARMACOTHERAPY

Fluoxetine and paroxetine, both selective serotonin reuptake inhibitors (SSRIs), have been shown to be more effective than placebo for child and adolescent depression. SSRIs have a more favorable side effect profile than do tricyclic antidepressants (TCAs), the most notable of which is their lack of fatality in overdose.

TCAs are no longer first-line agents for early-onset depression insofar as (1) no study having shown a difference between TCAs and placebo, and (2) their danger of fatality in overdose. In fact, one large multi-site study of adolescent depression found paroxetine superior to placebo, but imipramine no different from placebo. However, TCAs may be useful for the treatment of attention deficit/hyperactivity disorder (AD/HD) with comorbid anxiety or depression. Their use requires careful monitoring for cardiotoxicity, with a baseline electrocardiogram and rhythm strip.

For patients who present with a "bipolar-type" depression (anergia hypersomnia, hyperphagia, psychotic symptoms), particularly those who have a positive family history of mania, but who have never had a manic or hypomanic episode, one may use an SSRI, but it is necessary to monitor closely for the precipitation of mania. Studies in adults indicate that use of SSRIs results in a relatively low incidence of manic switch, but data are not yet available in younger populations.

For those adolescents who fail to respond to a first SSRI, standard practice is to try another SSRI at adequate dosage for 6 to 8 weeks. If the patient still fails to respond, the next choice is an agent out of the SSRI class such as bupropion, venlafaxine, or nefazodone.

COMBINATION OF CBT AND MEDICATION

Naturalistic and open treatment studies suggest that for patients who have chronic (2 years or longer) depression, a combination of medication and psychotherapy yields optimal results, and recovery may take close to 1 year.

CONTINUATION TREATMENT

After termination of either CBT or pharmacotherapy the risk of relapse is high; therefore, continued treatment is recommended at a lower frequency of contact for 6 months after recovery is achieved. For CBT, this consists of monthly visits or "booster sessions"; for pharmacotherapy, this involves continued treatment at the same dosage of medication for 6 months *after* recovery. This is a critical phase in the treatment of early-onset depression because it is not enough just to get depressed patients well; it also is critical to *keep* them well.

BIPOLAR DISORDER

Treatment of bipolar disorder consists of the use of mood stabilizers for prophylaxis, as well as for acute treatment of manic or depressive episodes. One of the most challenging aspects of the management of the disease is encouragement of continued treatment after normalization of mood. Therefore, psychoeducation for the patient and family are key.

Traditionally, lithium has been the mainstay of mood stabilization, but this agent may be less effective than valproate or carbamazepine for early-onset (e.g., prepubertal) bipolar disorder, those in mixed states, and those who present with rapid cycling, the latter two of which may be more common modes of presentation in juvenile populations. Neuroleptics may be important in the management of acute mania and of psychosis. However, there is a paucity of controlled studies in this population.

With regard to the use of lithium, blood levels for lithium should be monitored to check compliance and to avoid toxicity. Therapeutic levels are between 0.6 and 1.0 mEq/L. Renal effects of lithium are rare, but kidney function should be monitored by urinalyses and blood creatinine and blood urea nitrogen (BUN) levels. Hypothyroidism is a frequent complication of lithium treatment, so thyroid function tests should be performed at 4- to 6-month intervals on patients who receive maintenance lithium. For manic patients who do not respond to lithium alone, it may be necessary to add valproate or carbamazepine. Lithium is contraindicated in pregnancy because its use is associated with congenital malformations, namely Ebstein anomaly. Bipolar patients who experience a depressive episode should be continued on lithium, but an antidepressant should be added.

Valproate has become used more frequently for the management of juvenile bipolar disorder. The most significant side effect is that of hepatotoxicity, and the drug is contraindicated in those who have liver disease. Thrombocytopenia and other hematological abnormalities have been reported, necessitating monitoring of liver function tests and complete blood counts. Other significant side effects include sedation, weight gain, nausea, and vomiting, with the latter two generally transient. A serious problem in adolescent females is polycystic ovarian disease, which has been reported as a complication of valproate therapy, and may be secondary to weight gain. In adults, valproate was found to be superior to lithium in the treatment of mania complicated by depression, but comparable studies have not been conducted in younger populations. Plasma levels of 50 to 100 μg/ml are considered in the therapeutic range.

This chapter has been adapted with permission from Brent DA: Mood disorders and suicide. In Green M, Haggerty RJ, Weitzman M, editors: *Ambulatory pediatrics,* ed 5, Philadelphia, 1999, WB Saunders.

This work was supported by William T. Grant Foundation grant 1063-85 and NIMH grants MH43366, MH44711, and MH55123.

SUGGESTED READINGS

Birmaher B, Brent DA, Work Group on Quality Issues: Practice parameters for the assessment and treatment of children and adolescents with depressive disorders, *J Am Acad Child Adolesc Psychiatry* 37:63S, 1998.

Birmaher B, et al: Child and adolescent depression: a review of the past ten years. Part I. *J Am Acad Child Adolesc Psychiatry* 35:1427, 1996.

Birmaher B, et al: Childhood and adolescent depression: a review of the past ten years. Part II. *J Am Acad Child Adolesc Psychiatry* 35:1575, 1996.

Brent DA, et al: A clinical psychotherapy trial for adolescent depression comparing cognitive, family, and supportive treatments, *Arch Gen Psychiatry* 54:877, 1997.

Emslie GJ, et al: Recurrence of major depressive disorder in hospitalized children and adolescents, *J Am Acad Child Adolesc Psychiatry* 36:785, 1997.

Geller B, et al: Double-blind and placebo-controlled study of lithium for adolescent bipolar disorders with secondary substance dependency, *J Am Acad Child Adolesc Psychiatry* 37:171, 1998.

Kovacs M, Paulauskas SL: Developmental stage and the expression of depressive disorders in children: an empirical analysis. In Cicchetti D, Schneider-Rosen K, editors: *Childhood depression,* San Francisco, 1984, Jossey-Bass.

Kovacs M, et al: Depressive disorders in childhood. I. A longitudinal study of characteristics and recovery, *Arch Gen Psychiatry* 41:229, 1984.

Kovacs M, et al: Depressive disorders in childhood. II. A longitudinal study of the risk for a subsequent major depression, *Arch Gen Psychiatry* 41: 643, 1984.

Wood A, Harrington R, Moore A: Controlled trial of a brief cognitive-behavioural intervention in adolescent patients with depressive disorders, *J Am Acad Child Adolesc Psychiatry* 37:737, 1996.

108 Suicide and Suicidal Behavior in Children and Adolescents

David A. Brent

Suicide is the third-leading cause of death among adolescents and young adults ages 15 to 24 and accounts for 13% of the mortality in this age group. The rate of suicide among 15- to 19-year-olds has more than tripled, from 2.7 per 100,000 in 1950 to 11.1 per 100,000 in 1996. This may be related in part to increased use and availability of alcohol and firearms among youth, as well as to the increasing prevalence of depression. Suicidal behavior (i.e., attempts) also has become increasingly common, with recent surveys showing 4% of high school students having made an attempt within the previous 12 months and 8% having made a suicide attempt within their lifetime. However, only 12% of adolescent suicide attempts ever come to medical attention.

AGE

The increase in the suicide rate has been noted among 15- to 19-year-olds for the past three decades; only more recently has an increase been recorded for 10- to 14-year-olds. Among children and adolescents, the rate of attempted and completed suicide increases dramatically with age. Although prepubertal children do think about suicide, they may be protected against committing suicide by their cognitive immaturity, which prevents them from planning and attempting suicide despite suicidal thoughts. When suicidal behavior is observed in preschool children, it almost invariably is associated with physical or sexual abuse. Suicide in adolescents younger than 16 years of age is more difficult to predict, appears less often in the context of chronic and severe psychopathology, may be more impulsive than suicide in older adolescents, and may be influenced greatly by the presence of firearms in the home.

GENDER

The completed suicide rate is much higher among males, whereas the suicide attempt rate is much higher among females. This difference may be related to males' tendency to use more violent means of committing suicide and their higher rate of aggressive and antisocial behavior.

RACE AND SOCIOECONOMIC STATUS

The suicide rate is higher among whites than among blacks, although the rate among black males has increased dramatically in recent years and now is about 80% of the rate among whites. Young Native Americans have a particularly high suicide rate, especially those in tribes that have experienced erosion of traditional culture and high rates of delinquency, alcoholism, and family disorganization. Suicidal behavior may be more common among lower socioeconomic groups. Among young black males, higher socioeconomic status appears to be a risk factor for completed suicide. Hispanic youth have higher rates of suicidal ideation and attempts than either black or white youths.

PRECIPITANTS

The precipitants for suicidal behavior and suicide among children and adolescents are similar, most frequently involving problems such as interpersonal conflict or interpersonal loss, family discord, legal or disciplinary problems, physical or sexual abuse, or a failure or disappointment.

METHOD

In the United States, firearms are the most common method of suicide, followed by hanging, jumping, asphyxiation by carbon monoxide, and self-poisoning. Suicide by firearms may be related to their availability in the home and also to a state of intoxication in the victim. Several case-control studies show that (1) guns are much more common in the homes of suicide completers than suicide attempters or community controls, and (2) if a gun is in the home, it is very likely to be used as a method for suicide. Therefore, it is critical to secure and (ideally) remove firearms from the homes of suicidal individuals. Even in those who have no apparent psychopathology, a loaded gun in the home can pose a thirtyfold increased risk for successful suicide. By contrast, self-poisoning is the most common method of suicide attempt, followed by wrist cutting.

MOTIVATION AND INTENT

Youthful suicide victims frequently are intoxicated at the time of death. Nevertheless, many adolescent suicide victims show evidence of high intent (i.e., a strong wish to die), as manifested by timing the suicide so as not to be discovered, planning ahead, leaving a note, choosing an irreversible method, and verbalizing suicidal intent before the actual suicide. Older adolescent suicide victims show higher intent than younger ones. In contrast, only about one third of adolescents who attempt suicide actually wish to die. In fact, most adolescent suicide attempts are impulsive, with little threat to the patient's life. The motivation for most attempts appears to be the desire to influence others, gain attention, communicate love or anger, or escape a difficult or painful situation.

PSYCHIATRIC DISORDER AND PSYCHOLOGICAL TRAITS

The majority of adolescent suicide victims appear to have been suffering from at least one major debilitating psychiatric disorder, predominately mood disorder (depression or bipolar disorder), substance abuse, or conduct disorder. At least 50% had made suicide threats or attempted suicide in the past. The constellation of depression, conduct disorder, substance abuse, and past suicidal behavior also is characteristic of adolescents who attempt suicide, particularly older males. Among depressed patients, those who have a chronic course (duration of at least 2 years) and who have comorbid substance use are most likely to be suicidal. Suicidal patients also have been shown to feel more hopeless and to show poorer problem-solving and social skills than comparable patients who had not attempted suicide. Several community studies suggest that homosexual or bisexual orientation may increase the risk for suicide attempt and that the impact of homosexuality may be more pronounced in males. However, no empirical studies have examined the role of sexuality in completed suicide among adolescents because it is very difficult to ascertain sexual attitudes from secondary informants.

FAMILY HISTORY

The relatives of both adolescent suicide victims and suicide attempters have high prevalences of mood disorder, alcohol and drug abuse, suicide, and suicidal behavior. Suicidal behavior seems to be transmitted familially, independently of psychiatric illness per se.

FAMILY ENVIRONMENT

In the families of both suicide victims and suicide attempters, a high prevalence of divorce, parental absence, and abuse has been noted. Physical and sexual abuse convey substantial risks for completed suicide above and beyond psychopathology. The family environments of suicidal versus nonsuicidal patients have been characterized as less supportive, more conflicted, and more hostile. In community samples, suicide attempters have been exposed to family violence and have been victims of physical or sexual abuse more frequently than have psychiatric or community-control individuals.

EXPOSURE TO SUICIDE

Exposure to suicidal behavior via the suicide attempt of a schoolmate or the fictional or nonfictional representation of suicide on television may increase the risk for suicide and suicidal behavior, particularly among the psychiatrically vulnerable. The impact of exposure to suicide in the friends of suicide victims results in a markedly increased risk of depression and posttraumatic stress disorder, but does *not* result in an increased risk of suicide attempt. Although suicides in epidemiologically defined "clusters" do occur, they account for only 3% to 5% of all suicides.

MEDICAL ILLNESSES

Children who have epilepsy have been overrepresented in series of suicides and attempted suicides. Some of this increased risk in epilepsy may be related to the iatrogenic effects of phenobarbital. In a study of American adolescents attending inner city pediatric clinics, presenting complaints more prevalent among those who have a history of suicide attempts included any psychological concerns, having been a runaway, physical and sexual abuse, recent physical or sexual assault, problems with substance abuse, concerns about pregnancy, and presentation with a sexually transmitted disease. Suicide attempters seen in emergency rooms are more likely to use the emergency department as their source of primary care.

RISK OF REPETITION OF SUICIDAL BEHAVIOR

In follow-up studies of adolescent suicide attempters ranging from 1 to almost 3 years in length, the reattempt rate is between 6% and 15% per year. The risk for repetition is greatest within the first 3 months of the initial attempt. The risk is particularly high shortly after discharge from an inpatient psychiatric unit and may be related to poor coordination of subsequent outpatient care. Factors associated with reattempts are: previous suicidal behavior, high suicidal intent, serious psychopathology (either depression or substance abuse), hostility and aggression, hopelessness, noncompliance with treatment, social isolation, poor school performance, family discord, abuse and neglect, and parental psychiatric illness.

RISK FACTORS FOR COMPLETED SUICIDE AMONG SUICIDE ATTEMPTERS

Among males, the risk for suicide ranges from 0.7% among suicide attempters who present to an emergency room for a drug overdose to 10% among those who are psychiatrically hospitalized. Among females, the risk ranges from 0.1% of attempters seen in an emergency room to 2.9% on follow-up of those who are psychiatrically hospitalized. The risk factors for completed suicide are male gender, no apparent precipitant, high suicidal intent, "active" method, and bipolar or psychotic disorder. One cross-sectional case-control study suggests that in addition to bipolar disorder and high suicidal intent, risk for suicide is related to availability of firearms in the home.

SUICIDAL IDEATION

Suicidal ideation, or thoughts about suicide, is even more common than suicidal behavior. Suicidal ideation can be thought of as a continuum from nonspecific ideation (e.g., "Life is not worth living," "I wish I were dead"), to specific ideation (e.g., suicidal ideation with intent to die or with a suicidal plan), and finally, to actual suicidal behavior (Box

BOX 108-1

INTERVIEWING FOR SUICIDAL IDEATION

1. Have you ever thought that life was not worth living?
2. Have you ever wished that you were dead?
3. Have you ever tried to hurt yourself?
4. Do you intend to hurt yourself?
5. Do you have a plan to hurt yourself?
6. Have you ever attempted suicide?

From Brent DA: Suicide and suicidal behavior in children and adolescents, *Pediatr Rev* 10:269, 1989.

108-1). Community-based surveys indicate that between 12% and 25% of primary and high school children have some form of suicidal ideation. Specific suicidal ideation (e.g., ideation with a concrete suicidal plan), such as suicidal behavior, is much less common and associated most closely with depression, feelings of helplessness, substance abuse, and conduct disorder. Also, suicidal ideation (and behavior) frequently are associated with physical or sexual abuse. Given the clinical overlap between those who have specific suicidal ideation and those who actually attempt suicide, it follows that those patients who have specific suicidal ideation be considered to be at high risk of acting on their suicidal thoughts. In fact, as noted previously, youth who commit suicide frequently tell others (usually peers) about their suicidal thoughts.

IDENTIFYING YOUTH AT RISK FOR SUICIDE AND SUICIDAL BEHAVIOR

Box 108-2 outlines the three categories of personal problems that should induce the physician to probe further for suicidal risk: (1) psychiatric, (2) social adjustment, and (3) family or environmental. Any child who is suspected of being at risk should be questioned about suicidal ideation (see Box 108-1), by moving from nonspecific to more specific questions if the answers to the nonspecific queries are positive.

After the identification of someone at risk for suicide, it is important to listen to the patient nonjudgmentally. The pediatrician should avoid promising of confidentiality, which will have to be broken to protect and properly treat the child. The patient's parents should always be given some feedback about the assessment, because parental motivation is an important predictor of compliance with treatment recommendations. On discovering that a patient is suicidal, it is critical to obtain a no-suicide agreement, in which the patient promises to refrain from physically self-destructive behavior and to notify the physician or a caretaking adult if he or she does feel suicidal again (Box 108-3). In formulating the no-suicide agreement, the pediatrician should review with the patient those precipitants for the wish to commit suicide and rehearse alternative methods for coping with these stressors. It also is important to ensure that potential means of suicide, such as firearms, are removed from the home.

Whether the pediatrician elects to manage a suicidal child or to refer him or her to a specialist depends on the pediatrician's level of training and comfort with these types of patients. The ideal procedure is to obtain a specialist mental health consultation; then the pediatrician, specialist, and family can decide jointly about the next appropriate step. If psychiatric treatment is recommended, the pediatrician can play a critical role in monitoring compliance and satisfaction with treatment, because many suicidal patients and their families are noncompliant.

Referrals to a therapist are much more likely to go smoothly if (1) the patient and family are given a definite appointment; (2) the therapist meets the family before the first session and, preferably, is introduced to the family by

BOX 108-2

CIRC… ING SUICIDAL RISK

Psychiatric
Depression
Bipolar disorder
Substance abuse
Conduct problems
Psychosis
Past suicidal threats or at…

Psychological Factors
Hopelessness
Impulsivity

Poor Social Adjustment
School failure or dropout
Legal problems
Social isolation
Interpersonal conflict

Family or Environment
Interpersonal loss
Family problems
- Abuse or neglect
- Family history of psychiatric disorder or suicide

Exposure to suicide (in those already psychiatrically vulnerable)

Modified from Brent DA: Suicide and suicidal behavior in children and adolescents, *Pediatr Rev* 10:269, 1989.

BOX 108-3

STEPS IN A "NO-SUICIDE" CONTRACT

1. The child or adolescent agrees not to hurt him- or herself.
2. The child or adolescent, parents, and therapist rehearse strategies to cope with suicidal thoughts should similar precipitants recur.
3. The child or adolescent will tell parents or counselor if he or she is having suicidal thoughts.
4. The child or adolescent will present him- or herself at an emergency room if there is no one available to help.
5. The child or adolescent will structure his or her activities in a way that will reduce suicidal potential.

…atient and family are
the referring profe… e of the initial referral.
seen as soon as … with the mental health
The pediatrician… to be able to refer in the
resources in th… …rral to a psychiatrist, as op-
midst of a po… …al health professional, is indi-
posed to ano… …ient is psychotic, has a serious
cated speci… detoxification from drugs or alco-
affective d… medical condition that may be con-
hol, has … …atric presentation, or requires complex
tributing … …cal intervention.
psychor…

MA… …EMENT OF SU… ATTEMPTERS

Id… suicide attempter should ever by discharged di-
r… …om the emergency room, regardless of medical con-
…r Whereas a small number of highly suicidal and psy-
…rically disturbed patients should be admitted directly to
…psychiatric inpatient unit, most patients will not require such intensive or restrictive treatment. For this less-disturbed majority, a 48-hour admission to a pediatric ward is recommended to evaluate the patient and family. Even though the medical consequences alone might not warrant admission, the decision to admit to the hospital communicates to the family that the suicide attempt has been noticed and taken seriously. Many of the families of these attempters are chaotic, and a substantial minority are abusive or neglectful. In the emergency room, it is almost impossible to accurately determine the precipitants, motivation, mental status, and family environment of the attempter; hence, the recommendation to admit.

REFERRAL FOR INPATIENT PSYCHIATRIC TREATMENT

Suicidal children and adolescents who are judged to be at serious risk for committing or attempting suicide are most appropriate for inpatient hospitalization. The specific indications for psychiatric hospitalization are listed in Box 108-4.

THERAPEUTIC INTERVENTIONS

Treatment of suicidal youngsters should proceed on three levels: (1) treatment of the underlying psychiatric illness, (2) remediation of social and problem-solving deficits, and (3) family psychoeducation and conflict resolution. For example, a depressed, suicidal patient who is socially isolated and has a severely conflicted relationship with her alcoholic mother might require antidepressant treatment for her illness, augmentation of social skills to relieve her social isolation, referral of her mother for psychiatric treatment, and family sessions to relieve the family discord and provide psychoeducation about both the parent and child psychiatric illnesses.

BOX 108-4

INDICATIONS FOR PSYCHIATRIC INPATIENT HOSPITALIZATION

Characteristics of Suicidality
Inability to maintain a no-suicide contract
Active suicidal ideation (with plan and intent)
High intent or lethality of suicide attempt

Psychiatric Disorder
Psychosis
Severe depression
Substance abuse
Bipolar illness
Serious aggression
Previous attempts
Previous noncompliance or failure with outpatient treatment

Family Problems
Abuse
Severe parental psychiatric illness
Family unable or unwilling to monitor or protect patient

From Brent DA: Suicide and suicidal behavior in children and adolescents, *Pediatr Rev* 10:269, 1989.

This chapter has been adapted with permission from Brent DA: Mood disorders and suicide. In Green M, Haggerty RJ, Weitzman M, editors: *Ambulatory pediatrics,* ed 5, Philadelphia, 1999, WB Saunders.

This work was supported by William T. Grant Foundation grant 1063-85 and NIMH grants MH43366, MH44711, and MH55123.

SUGGESTED READINGS

Berman AL, Jobes DA: Suicide prevention in adolescents (age 12-18), *Suicide Life Threat Behav* 25:143, 1995.

Brent DA, Practioner review: the aftercare of adolescents with deliberate self-harm, *J Child Psychol Psychiatry* 38:277, 1997.

Brent DA, Perper JA: Risk factors for adolescent suicide and suicidal behavior: mental and substance abuse disorders, family environmental factors, and life stress, *Suicide Life Threat Behav* 25:52, 1995.

Brent DA, et al: Risk factors for adolescent suicide: a comparison of adolescent suicide victims with suicidal inpatients, *Arch Gen Psychiatry* 45:581, 1988.

Brent DA, et al: Psychiatric risk factors of adolescent suicide: a case control study, *J Am Acad Child Adolesc Psychiatry* 32:521, 1993.

Lewinsohn PM, Rohde P, Seeley JR: Adolescent suicidal ideation and attempts: prevalence, risk factors and clinical implications, *Clin Psychol: Science Practice* 3:25, 1996.

National Center for Health Statistics (NCHS): *Center for Disease Control WONDER*, 1998.

Shaffer D, et al: Psychiatric diagnosis in child and adolescent suicide, *Arch Gen Psychiatry* 53:339, 1996.

109 Runaway Youth

Gerald R. Adams

DEMOGRAPHIC ESTIMATES

In 1976, the National Opinion Research Corporation conducted the largest, most comprehensive study of the problem of runaway adolescents in the United States. This study, the National Statistical Survey on Runaway Youth,[19] was a nationwide probability study of nearly 14,000 households with teenagers. It found that 5.7% of the households surveyed had at least one runaway incident in 1976. When extrapolated to the general population, this statistic reflects an annual incidence of 985,000 to 1,134,200 episodes. The same numbers are estimated in the 1990s.[14]

During the 1980s, Cairns[9,10] tracked 695 children for 8 years. She reported that 22% of the children in her sample had run away from home; furthermore, 29% of the girls and 41% of the boys had considered running away. Reasons for running away range from an act of independence to escaping physical and sexual abuse.[10]

The federal General Accounting Office (GAO) analyzed data on runaways for the years 1985 to 1988 (the data were obtained from the Department of Health and Human Services). The GAO study found that only 35% of boys, but 65% of girls, who run away use federally funded shelters for youths. Recent evidence, from a study of 929 homeless and runaway youth (ages 12 to 23 years), indicates that the older youth are least likely to use services and may actually be the most vulnerable runaway youth because of it.[11]

From all these studies and statistics we can conclude that one in three children considers running away, one in five actually does so, and younger girls are more likely than boys of any age to use shelter services. However, older runaways of either gender are the least likely to turn to center services for assistance.

According to the National Statistical Survey on Runaway Youth, those most likely to run away are teenagers 15 through 17 years old (the median age was 16). Additional data from the GAO reveal that 71% of runaways fall in the 10- to 17-year age group.[32] Slightly more than 50% of all runaways were boys. Racial and socioeconomic differences were not apparent, but regional differences were observed. The incidence of runaway behavior tended to be higher in the Western and North Central states than in Northeastern or Southern states.

DISTINGUISHING RUNAWAYS FROM THROWAWAYS

In the early 1970s, runaways were considered a homogeneous group.[1] However, several subsequent investigations have established that runaway adolescents are divided into several subtypes.[23] In a study of Colorado youngsters, Brennan, Huizinga, and Elliott[8] identified two broad categories of runaways. One group (class 1) consisted of young people who were not delinquent or particularly alienated. In general, they appeared to be psychologically healthy and had nondelinquent or nondeviant friends. The second group (class 2), in contrast, were delinquent and manifested considerable alienation in their attitudes and behavior. These youngsters experienced considerable conflict with and rejection from their parents, had delinquent peers, manifested school alienation, reported low self-esteem, and behaved deviantly. The class 1 youngsters mostly were escaping temporarily from a conflict-laden home, had unrestrained peer activities without supervision, and tended to be lonely or isolated from their peers. The class 2 youngsters were rejected, rebellious, and unrestrained youths who were labeled negatively and were pushed away from their families. One recent finding from the National Incidence Study of Missing, Abducted, Runaway, and Throwaway Children indicates an intergenerational transmission of runaway behavior. That is, in families in which parents left home, there was a strong probability that these families would have children who run away.[24]

In 1985, Adams, Gullotta, and Clancy[2] substantiated the theory of multiple types of runaways. Runaways were interviewed while still away from home at a YMCA facility that had a shelter program. Three classes of runaways were identified. The first group consisted of runaways who were similar to Brennan's class 1 youths. These youths left home because of family conflict (hostile, confrontational, and unpleasant, but endurable); alienation from family, schools, and sometimes, peers; and poor social relationships with others.[see also 34] A second group consisted of "throwaways," children who had been encouraged or forced to leave home and were told not to return. A third group were societal rejects. These youngsters were rejected by their families, their neighborhood and school peers, their teachers, and even the justice and public social service systems. They lived independently, usually through criminal behavior, and were an integral part of street culture. The throwaways and societal rejects were similar to Brennan's class 2 runaways. Very little is documented empirically on class 2 throwaways and societal rejects. Further, these youth's behaviors are placing pressure on communities to endorse tough legal standards and the inclusion of incarceration for status offenses.[30] Because of the difficulty involved in identifying class 2 youths and obtaining their cooperation, our knowledge base about runaways is limited primarily to information obtained from class 1 youngsters. Allison[5] and Bass[6] have provided additional information on classification and easy-to-read, comprehensive review of much of the pertinent research on runaway adolescents.

UNDERSTANDING RUNAWAY BEHAVIOR

To speak authoritatively to parents and with adolescents about runaway behavior, medical professionals should be knowledgeable about the typical behaviors, psychological characteristics, social and familial circumstances, and documented negative consequences of running away.[16,27]

Typical Behavioral Patterns

Reviews by Nye,[20,21] Nye and Edelbrock,[22] Allison,[5] Adams and Munro,[3] and Gullotta, Adams, and Markstrom[14] describe the similarity of behavioral patterns of runaways. About 50% of the adolescents who run away do not run far and stay near home. Many stay with friends, relatives, or neighborhood families (sometimes with their parents' knowledge). Most stay away just briefly (overnight absences are most common). In fact, most runaways express the desire for reconciliation.[29] Gullotta, Adams, and Markstrom[14] estimate that approximately 40% of runaways return home in 1 day and 60% after 3 days. More than 80% return in 1 month or sooner. These researchers also reported that 52% of runaways stay within a 10-mile radius of home; only 18% travel more than 50 miles from home. Fewer than 5% of runaways run away more than three times, and most run away without companions. However, girls are slightly more likely than boys to run away with a partner. There is some evidence that older runaways are likely to travel greater distances and stay away longer. Cairns[9] reports that boys are more likely to run away only overnight or up to 1 week, whereas girls are more likely to run away for extended periods or permanently. Furthermore, although some runaways deliberate over their decision, most do not plan the episode substantially; usually the quick decision to leave is a result of emotional reactions.[12]

Nye and Edelbrock[22] found that more than 50% of runaways reported their experience neutrally and as relatively noneventful. About 25% reported a positive adventure resulting in a sense of independence and confidence in their ability to survive on their own. Approximately 20% reported negative consequences, with 3% reporting at least one violent experience. According to Nye,[20,21] approximately 40% of runaways returned willingly and on their own initiative. Approximately 20% were found by parents and brought home, and another 20% were returned by the police. The remaining 20% were returned by relatives and friends or by other individuals the family did not know personally. Among those adolescents who remain on the streets, survival is a daily, even hourly struggle.[18]

Psychological Characteristics

Adams and Munro[3] have reviewed the numerous investigations comparing youngsters who run away and those who do not. They concluded that runaways are more likely to have low self-esteem,[see also 31] to show more signs of depression, to feel that they had less control over their environment, and to use poor judgment. They also concluded that runaways are more impulsive, easily frustrated, and less tolerant or sustaining of close interpersonal relationships. Allison[5] came to similar conclusions. However, as Walker[33] correctly cautions, we are uncertain whether these psychological characteristics are antecedents or consequences of runaway behavior. However, growing evidence regarding a history of physical and sexual abuse suggests that a large portion of runaways are escaping some form of abuse in the family or kinship network.

Social and Familial Circumstances

Problems in social and family relationships are important factors in running away. Many forms of evidence indicate problems not only between parents and runaways but also between the parents themselves.[3] Family life generally is tense and conflict laden. Evidence summarized in the National Statistical Survey on Runaway Youth[19] clearly indicates that parents of runaways make few positive comments about their children, have more drinking problems, and physically abuse their children more than do parents of children who do not run away. These same parents are uninvolved in their child's community and school activities, and they show marked problems in communicating with their child. Roberts[26] reports that the severity of family conflict often is associated with an increased probability of physical or sexual abuse.

According to Wolk and Brandon,[35] parents of runaways commonly are unable to supervise effectively. Parents of runaway adolescent boys seem unable to control them, whereas parents of runaway adolescent girls tend to overcontrol and punish their daughters. According to Gottlieb and Chafetz,[13] this inability to supervise effectively tends to result in a long series of confrontations between parents and adolescent. These researchers also found that upon returning home, runaways were likely to face even worse communication problems, which are reflected in increased conflict and withdrawal.[13] According to GAO[32] data, approximately one third of runaways return home from shelters. Another third move into foster care, and the remaining third live in crisis houses, with friends, or in other unstable situations.

NEGATIVE CONSEQUENCES

Runaways leave home for several reasons; contributing factors include psychological characteristics, home environment, school and peer influence, abuse and neglect (particularly for throwaways), and delinquency. Throwaways are considerably more likely to leave for extended periods or even permanently, thus placing themselves at considerable risk; however, most runaways return home within 1 to

2 weeks and consider their experience as relatively benign. But the greater the distance from home and the longer the youngster is on the streets, the greater the risk of negative consequences. Longitudinal research shows that repeat runaways often have violent confrontations with family members and show extremely high levels of alcohol and drug abuse.[5,17] Young et al[36] have studied the evidence concerning the potential negative consequences for runaway youngsters. Clearly, the risk factors are substantial; they include confrontation with the legal system,[15] substance abuse, coercive sexual behavior, contraction of sexually transmitted diseases (including acquired immunodeficiency syndrome [AIDS]), nutritional and general health problems, loss of educational training opportunities, pregnancy, and early parenting. Furthermore, the negative conditions that may have motivated the adolescent to run away are only likely to be exacerbated because tension in the home is likely to increase when the adolescent returns.

Of particular concern to health care practitioners is the greater likelihood that the runaway will be abusing drugs or will have contracted a sexually transmitted disease.[28] Runaways are more likely to sell drugs to support their own habits, and their potential for addiction is extremely high. Furthermore, the risk of prostitution is evident. Boyer and James[7] estimate that there are 600,000 prostitutes between the ages of 6 and 16 years. Most emerge from runaway and abandonment backgrounds. Unplanned pregnancies commonly result from selling sex. Not only does an early pregnancy have negative health consequences for the teenage girl but also it places the newborn at risk for numerous medical problems. Indeed, Young et al[36] have summarized evidence indicating that children born to young adolescents are at risk of becoming socially maladjusted, commonly manifesting poor peer relationships and having a propensity for temper tantrums and impulsivity during their childhood.

A final cautionary note about negative consequences: According to Allison,[5] 61% of youths in shelters are depressed; 24% of shelter users indicate that they have made one or more serious suicide attempts, and 82% manifest serious psychiatric impairment in their responses on the Achenbach Child Behavior Checklist. Therefore, treating runaways must be seen as a potentially volatile and unpredictable situation requiring close observation and supervision during the initial period of crisis.

INTERVENTION SERVICES AND RECOMMENDATIONS

Services for runaway and throwaway youngsters are enmeshed in federal and state statutory definitions of emancipation. Running away is referred to as *functional emancipation* when the departure is undertaken without the benefit of legal maneuvering. In most states, *statutory emancipation* can occur if the minor comes under a judicial order, gets married, or joins the military. When a known runaway is treated medically, most states require either parental permission or contact with a parent after a designated period. Because the laws vary considerably, interested professionals must refer to their state's laws and requirements.

Adams and Adams[4] have suggested a three-phase method for intervening with and treating runaways. The first phase consists of *crisis intervention* and *stabilized placement,* the second involves *supportive counseling* and *assessment,* and the third includes *long-term therapy, education and training,* and *support services.* The agency (or physician, where appropriate) that first interacts with the youngster should assume responsibility for crisis intervention and the initiation of a stabilized placement. Assessment and supportive counseling should be undertaken by local mental health providers. Long-term therapy, education and training, and supportive services should be provided through family and social welfare assistance.

The purpose of crisis intervention is to defuse existing and looming physical, social, and mental crises. A recent report on a needs assessment of adolescent runaways indicates that runaways report the greatest immediate needs of reduced stress, better living situations, and better communication with parents (while viewing themselves as having disappointed their family).[25] The desired outcome is to resolve immediate crises sufficiently to make stable placement possible. The purpose of stabilization is to provide security, calm the runaway, and ensure assessment of the situation. The assessment should elicit the information necessary to enhance supportive counseling and to determine appropriate long-term treatment and placement. Long-term treatment, education and training, and supportive services should be undertaken to deal with the medical, social, and mental health issues of the youngster. The desired outcome is diminution of runaway reactions, increased skill and coping abilities, and reunion of the adolescent with the family and/or the establishment of alternative care.[6] The National Statistical Survey on Runaway Youth found that few runaways use hotlines to contact their parents; nevertheless, practitioners can encourage the youngster to make contact. The current National Runaway Switchboard number is 1-800-621-4000; the Youth Crisis Hotline is 1-800-448-4663. There also are several useful websites with a variety of links: http://www.child.net/runaway.htm and www.toronto.com/E/V/TORON/0011/86/85.

REFERENCES

1. Adams GR: Runaway youth projects: comments on care programs for runaways and throwaways, *J Adolesc* 3:321, 1980.
2. Adams GR, Gullotta T, Clancy M: Homeless adolescents: a descriptive study of similarities and differences between runaways and throwaways, *Adolescence* 20:715, 1985.
3. Adams GR, Munro G: Portrait of the North American runaway: a critical review, *J Youth Adolesc* 8:359, 1979.
4. Adams PR, Adams GR: Intervention with runaway youth and their families: theory and practice. In Coleman JC, editor: *Working with troubled adolescents,* London, 1987, Academic Press.
5. Allison KW: Adolescents living in "nonfamily" and alternative settings. In Lerner RM, editor: *Early adolescence: perspectives on research, policy, and intervention,* Hillsdale, NJ, 1993, Lawrence Erlbaum.
6. Bass DS: *Helping vulnerable youths: runaway and homeless adolescents in the United States,* Washington, DC, 1992, National Association of Social Workers.
7. Boyer D, James J: Easy money: adolescent involvement in prostitution. In Weisberg K, editor: *Women and the law,* Cambridge, Mass, 1981, Schuckman.
8. Brennan T, Huizinga D, Elliott DS: *The social psychology of runaways,* Lexington, Mass, 1978, DC Heath.
9. Cairns BD: Emancipation, abdication, and running away: a longitudinal perspective. Paper presented at the biennial meeting of the Society for Research in Child Development, Kansas City, Mo, April 1989.

10. Cairns RB, Cairns BD: *Lifelines and risks: pathways of youth in our time,* Cambridge, England, 1995, Cambridge University Press.
11. Clatts MC, et al: Correlates and distribution of HIV risk behaviors among homeless youths in New York City: implications for prevention and policy, *Child Welfare* 77:195, 1998.
12. de-Man A, et al: Adolescent runaways: familial and personal correlates, *Soc Behav Personality* 21:163, 1993.
13. Gottlieb D, Chafetz JS: Dynamics of familial generational conflict and reconciliation, *Youth Society* 9:213, 1977.
14. Gullotta TP, Adams GR, Markstrom C: *The adolescent experience,* ed 4, New York, 2000, Academic Press.
15. Hagan J, McCarthy B: *Mean streets: youth crime and homelessness,* New York, 1987, Cambridge University Press.
16. Janus M, et al: *Adolescent runaways: causes and consequences,* Lexington, Mass, 1989, Lexington Books.
17. Koopman C, Rosario M, Rotheram-Borus MJ: Alcohol and drug use and sexual behaviors placing runaways at risk for HIV infection, *Addict Behav* 19:95, 1994.
18. McCarthy B, Hagan J: Surviving on the street: the experiences of homeless youth, *J Adolesc Res* 7:412, 1992.
19. National Opinion Research Corporation: *National statistical survey on runaway youth,* Princeton, NJ, 1976, NORC.
20. Nye IF: *Runaways: a report for parents.* Extension Bulletin No 0743, Pullman, Wash, 1980, Washington State University.
21. Nye IF: *Runaways: some critical issues for professionals and society.* Extension Bulletin No 0744, Pullman, Wash, 1980, Washington State University.
22. Nye IF, Edelbrock C: Some social characteristics of runaways, *J Fam Issues* 1:147, 1980.
23. Payne M: Understanding "going missing": issues for social work and social services, *Br J Soc Work* 25:14, 1995.
24. Plass PS, Hotaling GT: The intergenerational transmission of running away: childhood experiences of the parents of runaways, *J Youth Adolesc* 24:335, 1995.
25. Post P, McCoard D: Needs and self-concept of runaway adolescents, *Sch Counselor* 41:212, 1994.
26. Roberts A: Adolescent runaways in suburbia: a new typology, *Adolescence* 17:387, 1982.
27. Rohr ME: Identifying adolescent runaways: the predictive validity of the Personality Inventory for Children, *Adolescence* 31:605, 1996.
28. Rotheram-Borus MJ, et al: Lifetime sexual behaviors among runaway males and females, *J Sex Research* 29:15, 1992.
29. Schaffner L: Searching for connection: a new look at teenage runaways, *Adolescence* 33:619, 1998.
30. Steinhart DJ: Status offenses, *Future Child* 6:86, 1996.
31. Swaim KF, Bracken BA: Global and domain-specific self-concepts of a matched sample of adolescent runaways and nonrunaways, *J Clin Child Psychol* 26:397, 1997.
32. US General Accounting Office: Homeless: homeless and runaway youth receiving services at federally funded shelters, Washington, DC, US General Accounting Office.
33. Walker D: Suburban runaway youth in the 1970s. Paper presented at the biennial meeting of the American Psychological Association, Washington, DC, September 1976.
34. Whitbeck L, Hoyt D, Ackley KA: Families of homeless and runaway adolescents, *Child Abuse Neglect* 21:517, 1997.
35. Wolk S, Brandon J: Runaway adolescents' perception of parents and self, *Adolescence* 12:175, 1977.
36. Young RL, et al: Runaways: a review of negative consequences, *Fam Relations* 32:275, 1983.

110 Adolescent Sexuality

Susan M. Coupey

All humans are born with the capacity for sexual response, but it is only during adolescence that we become conscious of certain thoughts and feelings as being sexual. It is then that we begin to integrate our sexuality as part of our self-concept. Gender identity as boy or girl develops much earlier in childhood; however, the sexual specifics of that gender identity, including sexual orientation and behaviors, become clear to the individual only during adolescence or young adulthood. Overt expression of sexuality depends on the biopsychosocial environment in which the individual exists. The biological changes of puberty prime the adolescent brain and body for reproduction; individual and family psychodynamics influence sexual behavior choices. The larger sociocultural environment sets the norms for sexual behaviors and controls them through its institutions (e.g., churches, schools, government, and the media). As adolescents experiment with sexual expression, they inevitably make errors of judgment. Most such errors are minor, but many have significant health consequences.

Pediatricians and other primary care providers have an essential role to play in helping adolescent patients maintain their biopsychosocial sexual health (Box 110-1). Monitoring pubertal changes and providing anticipatory guidance to adolescents and their parents regarding timing of the growth spurt or onset of menstruation traditionally have been viewed as appropriate tasks for pediatricians. However, with the trend toward initiation of sexual intercourse at younger ages, practitioners of adolescent health care now are being called on to deliver preventive care related to sexual behavior, including contraceptive counseling and prescription, screening for sexually transmitted diseases (STDs), and counseling on issues of gender orientation and abuse. Because of the high prevalence of health problems stemming from sexual behavior in the adolescent age group, practitioners must be able to diagnose and manage such conditions as pregnancy, STDs, sexual dysfunction, and sexual victimization. In addition, schools and other community organizations often can benefit from the expertise of health care practitioners who may help to design sexuality education classes, pregnancy prevention programs, or HIV/AIDS management. This expanded societal role gives clinicians a broader influence on the environment than is possible within just the patient-provider-family relationship.

HEALTH CONSEQUENCES

Sexually Transmitted Diseases

Sexually transmitted diseases (STDs) are common among sexually active adolescents. Young people who begin to have sexual intercourse in early or middle adolescence are much more likely to develop an STD than are those who postpone intercourse until later adolescence or adulthood. This is due both to anatomical and behavioral factors. Within the first few years after menarche, girls usually have cervical ectopy with immaturity of the epithelial lining of the cervix. Columnar epithelium, which is infected more readily by STD organisms than is stratified squamous epithelium, is exposed in the vagina. Thus, girls who initiate sexual activity before maturation of the cervical epithelium are at high risk of infection. In addition, asymptomatic STD infections are prevalent in both boys and girls. Because of the many barriers adolescents face in obtaining routine STD screening and gynecological care, asymptomatic infections are likely to go undetected unless some complication develops. For young adolescents, "love" relationships may last only for a few days or weeks, but if such relationships include sexual intercourse, younger teens may accumulate several different sexual partners before they are developmentally able to sustain a relationship that lasts months or years. Thus, they are more likely to be exposed to STDs than are their peers who wait until they are older to initiate sexual intercourse.

Some STDs are associated with a high rate of permanent damage to the reproductive tract, especially for girls. For example, salpingitis caused by *Chlamydia trachomatis* is the leading cause of acquired infertility in women. In a study of more than 3000 inner-city 12- to 19-year-old black females, 14-year-olds had the highest age-specific chlamydia prevalence rate, with more than one of every four girls (27.5%) infected.[2] Genital infection caused by the human papillomavirus (HPV) can cause cancer of the cervix, vulva, anus, and penis; studies of adolescents report that up to one third of sexually active girls are infected with this virus.[8] Infection with the human immunodeficiency virus (HIV), a potentially lethal condition, is becoming more prevalent among adolescents. Factors found to be associated significantly with HIV seropositivity in adolescents include having been sexually abused, engaging in survival sex, having sex under the influence of drugs, using multiple drugs, having sex with casual partners, having had an STD, and engaging in multiple problem behaviors.[9]

BOX 110-1

ADOLESCENT SEXUALITY: ROLE OF THE PRIMARY CARE PROVIDER

Anticipatory Guidance
Pubertal development
Postponing coitus
Family planning
Safer sex practices
Sexual victimization
Genetic counseling

Preventive Care
Screening for sexually transmitted diseases (STDs)
Prescribing contraceptives
Providing psychological support (sexual orientation and abuse)

Diagnosing, Treating, and Referring
STDs
Pregnancy
Sexual dysfunction
Sexual victimization

Unintended Pregnancy

Unintended pregnancy, with all of the accompanying physical and psychosocial costs of either early parenthood or therapeutic abortion, is endemic in the United States. Among all U.S. high school girls in 1997, a total of 8.5% have been pregnant: 5% of ninth-grade girls and 11% of twelfth-grade girls.[3] Pregnancy outcomes are comparable to those in older women if prenatal care and social supports are adequate, but the social consequences are considerable. Adolescent mothers are more likely than women whose first birth occurs in their twenties to live in poverty, and their children tend to have poorer health, lower IQs, and higher rates of adolescent incarceration and childbearing than children of older mothers.

Depression and Suicide

For some young people, the onset of adolescence stirs up feelings of uncertainty about sexual orientation or reminders of childhood sexual abuse. These psychosocial issues may be associated with significant depression and suicide attempts. For example, among 104 self-identified gay, lesbian, and bisexual high school students responding to a survey of more than 4000 students in Massachusetts, 35% had attempted suicide in the past 12 months compared with 10% of heterosexual youth.[7] In another school-based survey of a representative sample of nearly 8000 sexually active students in Vermont, 30% of the girls reported ever being forced or pressured to have sex, and they were twice as likely also to report seriously considering suicide than were girls who had not experienced forced sex.[17]

PUBERTAL DEVELOPMENT AND SEXUALITY

In the United States today, girls enter puberty on average at 9 or 10 years of age, reach menarche at age 12½, and achieve full fertility at age 15. Boys enter puberty somewhat later, at 11 or 12 years of age, begin to produce sperm (spermarche) and have their first ejaculation at age 13 or 14, and achieve full fertility at about age 15. Thus, by middle adolescence, most boys and girls have completed the biological developmental requirements for reproduction. How do these pubertal changes affect sexuality? Udry[21] and Udry and Billy[22] have conducted studies to elucidate the biosocial factors that contribute to sexual behavior in adolescence. Pubertal development can contribute in at least two ways: first, through hormonal effects on the brain that stimulate the adolescent's sexual interest and behaviors, and second, by changing the adolescent's outward appearance, thus signaling to others the individual's readiness for sexual intercourse (Fig. 110-1). Androgenic hormones primarily are responsible for sexual motivation (libido) in both boys and girls and for the visible pubertal increase in muscle mass in boys. Estrogenic hormones are important for skeletal growth in both sexes and for pubertal breast development and body fat redistribution in girls. Levels of these hormones increase dramatically during puberty. Udry's studies indicate that in developing adolescents, the subjective sexual state and noncoital sexual behavior (e.g., sexual fantasies and masturbation) depend on androgen levels in both boys and girls. Coital behaviors are more complex, however, and are subject to sociocultural influence.

Adolescents who undergo late pubertal development and those who have lower secretion levels of androgens when fully developed (and thus lower libido) would be expected to respond more readily to social controls aimed at their sexual behavior. Conversely, those who have developed earlier physically and/or have higher postpubertal androgen levels would require different or more intense social controls to influence coital behavior appreciably. Factors shown to be significantly associated with postponing initiation of coitus to later adolescence or adulthood in girls include later pubertal development (menarche after age 13), careful parental supervision, good communication with mother, and high educational aspirations. Few studies have looked at postponing coitus in boys, and sociocultural influences are less well understood for male coital behavior. A program devised by Howard and McCabe,[10] entitled "Postponing Sexual Involvement: Educational Series for Young Teens," was used with all eighth-grade students in 24 Atlanta city schools and was evaluated in the mid-1980s. The evaluation found that the program was helpful to both boys and girls. By the end of the ninth grade, boys who had not had sexual intercourse before they participated in the program were significantly more likely to postpone sexual involvement than were similar boys who had not participated. This result indicates that boys do respond to educational intervention aimed at helping them control their sexual behavior. However, in this study, 44% of the eighth-grade boys (ages 13 and 14) had already initiated sexual intercourse before the program was given, and they did not benefit from it.

ADOLESCENT SEXUAL BEHAVIOR

Historical Trends

Dramatic changes in the economic and sociocultural environment have taken place in most industrialized countries since the end of World War II. This period has seen the rise

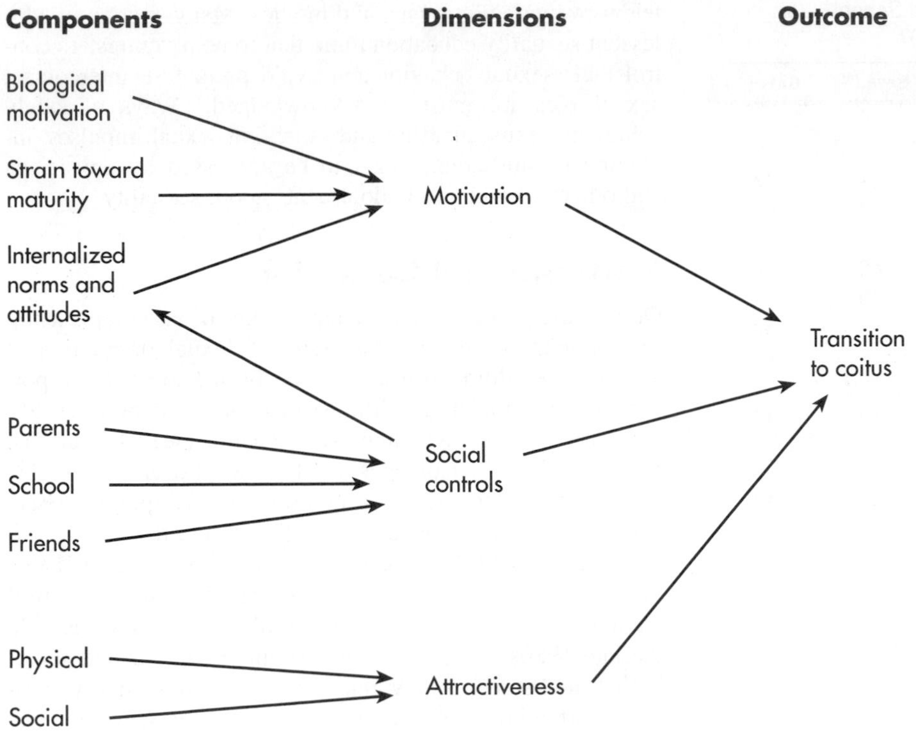

Components	Dimensions	Outcome
Biological motivation; Strain toward maturity; Internalized norms and attitudes	Motivation	Transition to coitus
Parents; School; Friends	Social controls	
Physical; Social	Attractiveness	

Fig. 110-1 Conceptual model of transition to coitus in adolescence. (Modified from Udry JR: Hormonal and social determinants of adolescent sexual initiation. In Bancroft J, Reinisch JM, editors: *Adolescence and puberty,* The Kinsey Institute Series, vol 3, 1990, Oxford University Press.)

of the middle class, support of the poor through the welfare state, the decline of both the extended family and the nuclear family, a reduction in the influence of religion, a vast increase in the influence of the media, and a huge "baby boom" generation whose members began to reach adolescence in the early 1960s. All these changes have had a profound influence on sexual mores in general and on adolescent sexual behavior in particular. The rising economic status of industrialized countries and improvements in medical science have allowed for better nutrition in pregnant women and children and fewer childhood infectious diseases. These, in turn, are the major causes of the downward trend in the age at which fertility is achieved in both boys and girls. At the turn of the twentieth century, the mean age at menarche in the United States was nearly 15 years, with significant socioeconomic differences in timing (wealthy adolescents matured earlier); by 1960 it had declined to about 13 years and now seems to have leveled off at 12½ years, with no significant socioeconomic differences. At the same time that puberty has been occurring at earlier ages, marriage and economic independence have been occurring at older ages. This is related partly to the need for young people to acquire more education to function adequately in an increasingly complex society. For young women, the interval between puberty and marriage rose from 7 years in 1890 to nearly 12 years in 1988. A similar phenomenon has occurred for young men. Earlier maturation of adolescents, in addition to looser legal and religious controls over marriage (as seen in the dramatically rising divorce rate), less supervision in the home (single-parent families, more women in the work force), and a barrage of sexual imagery in the media, have contributed to a declining mean age at first sexual intercourse and an increasing interval between first intercourse and marriage.

Prevalence of Sexual Intercourse

More than 50% of young people between the ages of 15 and 19 years have had sexual intercourse. However, nearly one in five wait until after their teenage years before beginning to have sex. More boys than girls report being sexually experienced at every age. Over the past three decades, the transition to coitus has become more common in the middle adolescent years. According to data collected by the Centers for Disease Control and Prevention (CDC), in 1970 only 4.6% of 15-year-old girls in the United States reported premarital sexual intercourse; by 1988, 25.6% had had premarital sexual intercourse, and in 1997, 34% of girls in grade 9 (age 14 to 15 years) reported that they were sexually active.[3,12] In 1988, 33% of 15-year-old boys had experienced sexual intercourse; in 1997, 42% of 14- to 15-year-old boys in grade 9 reported sexual intercourse.[3,19] Every 2 years the CDC collects data on a representative sample of U.S. high school students through the National Youth Risk Behavior Surveillance system. Data from the 1997 survey are summarized in Table 110-1.[3]

Details about the patterns of sexual behaviors among adolescents who have made the transition to sexual intercourse are only beginning to be studied, spurred on by the urgency to design effective AIDS prevention programs. Of adolescents who are sexually active, the overwhelming majority practice serial monogamy—that is, they have only one sexual partner at a time. Nevertheless, those boys and girls who begin having intercourse in early or middle adolescence often will accumulate three to five different sexual partners before they leave their teens (see Table 110-1). We do not know what percentage of young people have intercourse once or twice and then stop the behavior for months or years. Some studies indicate that younger adolescents who are unlikely to be living with a sexual partner have intercourse relatively

Table 110-1 Sexual Behavior among High School Students—United States, 1997

	All (%)	Boys (%)	Girls (%)
Students who have ever had sexual intercourse			
White	44	43	44
Black	73	80	66
Hispanic	52	58	46
Ninth grade	38	42	34
Twelfth grade	61	60	62
Students who have had sexual intercourse within the past 3 months	35	33	37
Students who have had four or more lifetime sexual partners	16	18	14
Students who used a condom at last intercourse	57	63	51
Students who used drugs or alcohol at last intercourse	25	31	19

Modified from *MMWR* 47(SS-3):1, 1998.

infrequently. For example, sexually active 15-year-old boys report spending an average of nearly 8 months of the year without a sexual partner.[19] Among U.S. high school students in 1997 who had had sex during their lifetime, 28% had been abstinent during the 3 months preceding the survey, with boys (32%) significantly more likely to be abstinent than girls (23%).[3] Intercourse behaviors other than penile-vaginal intercourse, such as anal or oral intercourse, are less well studied in the adolescent age group, but indications from studies of small nonrepresentative samples are that these behaviors are practiced with some frequency. A survey of more than 2000 high school students found that 47% were virgins. Of those who were virgins, about 30% had engaged in heterosexual masturbation with a partner, and 10% had participated in oral sex with a partner.[15]

Masturbation

Many adolescents learn about their sexuality and their bodily responses through masturbation. Masturbation is an activity associated primarily with male adolescent sexuality; there is less information concerning this behavior in girls.

Sarrel and Sarrel[14] have been gathering data from Yale undergraduates for many years. They noted that in the early 1970s, 33% of college women acknowledged masturbating. In the late 1980s, more than 80% reported this activity, a prevalence of masturbation very similar to that reported by young men at the same college. A report of masturbatory experiences of Australian high school students ages 15 to 18 found that boys were more likely than girls to report ever having masturbated (59% versus 43%) and to masturbate three or more times per week (38% versus 9%).[18] Despite the high prevalence of this sexual behavior, it still is not viewed as a normal, harmless part of sexuality by many adults. Our culture seems to have an official "erotophobia"; at the same time, our daily lives are permeated with erotica in the form of advertisements (e.g., Calvin Klein underwear, Guess jeans), television, popular music, and movies. Many experts in adolescent sexuality education think that to help youngsters control their sexual behavior and avoid premature intercourse, sexual pleasure must be acknowledged.[1] Ways of safely achieving sexual pleasure and satisfying sexual impulses, including masturbation, ought to be addressed by physicians and others who counsel adolescents about sexuality.

Homosexual Behavior

Only in the past decade have any studies of large representative populations tackled the issue of sexual orientation in adolescence, although it always has been known that a portion of the population, variously estimated at between 2% and 10%, grow up to be homosexual adults (see Chapter 104, Homosexuality: Challenges of Treating Lesbian and Gay Adolescents). A survey of a representative sample of Massachusetts high school students in 1995 found that 2.5% self-identified as gay, lesbian, or bisexual (67% male) and that these youth were at disproportionate risk for suicide, victimization, sexual risk behaviors, and multiple substance use.[7] In the late 1980s, a representative sample of junior and senior high school students in Minnesota responded to survey questions pertaining to sexual attraction, fantasy, behavior, and affiliation.[13] Overall, 1.1% of students described themselves as bisexual or homosexual, and 11% were unsure of their sexual orientation. Boys were significantly more likely than girls to label themselves as "mostly" or "100%" homosexual. As would be expected, uncertainty about sexual orientation gradually diminished with increasing age, from 26% of 12-year-olds to 5% of 18-year-olds, with corresponding increases in heterosexual and homosexual affiliation. Nearly 5% of students reported homosexual attractions, but only 1% reported such behavior. Boys were more likely than girls to report homosexual behavior (1.6% versus 0.9%), and the prevalence of homosexual behavior increased with increasing age in boys, from 0.4% at age 12 to 2.8% at age 18. These data do not support the widely held concept that homosexual behavior is common among early adolescent boys and gradually diminishes with age. Rather, the opposite may be true—that there is a gradual unfolding of sexual orientation during adolescence and that the behavior follows the awareness of homosexual attraction.

Much less is known about the adolescence of lesbian women. The pathways by which girls develop a same-sex sexual orientation are more diverse than those of boys. Girls tend to develop a homosexual identity at an older age than boys, often not until young adulthood or even later. Because of the severe social stigma associated with homosexuality, homosexual adolescents frequently are under considerable psychological stress, and as many as 30% of gay adolescent boys attempt suicide. Initial parental reaction to disclosure of a teenager's homosexuality usually is negative. Families often need help adjusting to the news and grieving for their lost "ideal" heterosexual child.

Sexual Victimization

Both adolescent boys and girls who have been victims of forced sex, either as young children by an adult perpetrator or as adolescents on a date or by a stranger, have higher rates of health risk behaviors and mental health problems. Large surveys of high school students regularly show 5% to 10% of students reporting sexual abuse. A prior history of sexual abuse in these nonclinical samples correlates significantly with young age at onset of voluntary sexual intercourse, unintended pregnancy, suicide attempts, drug and alcohol abuse, eating disorders, and violence.[11] The younger a sexually experienced girl, the more likely she is to have had forced sex. Seventy-four percent of girls who had intercourse before age 14 and 60% of those who had sex before age 15 report having had forced sex.[16] Data from a survey of high school girls in Washington State in 1992 found that girls who had been sexually abused were twice as likely as those not abused to have had intercourse by age 15 and three times more likely to have been pregnant.[20] Sexual abuse always should be considered a diagnostic possibility when an adolescent has very early onset of sexual intercourse and/or has multiple behavioral problems.

Sexual Dysfunction

Sexual dysfunction is an area not well studied in adolescence, although the prevalence in both boys and girls probably is quite high. Clinical reports indicate that many sexually active adolescent girls do not enjoy sexual intercourse and have never had an orgasm. Reasons for engaging in the behavior have more to do with intimacy and closeness to the partner than with personal sexual gratification.[4] Some girls who are anxious and unsure about sexual activity or who have previously been abused develop vaginismus. Large numbers of adolescent boys are thought to have premature ejaculation, but they rarely complain of the problem. Impotence does occur in adolescence, often as a result of "performance anxiety" and other psychogenic causes.[6] Heavy alcohol or marijuana use can be responsible for erectile dysfunction and should be explored in the medical history. Prescription medications often are implicated in erectile dysfunction in men and anorgasmia in women. Frequent offenders in this regard are antihypertensives, antipsychotics, and antidepressants. Other drugs that cause sexual dysfunction and that may be taken by adolescents are cimetidine, ranitidine, sulfasalazine, and some anticonvulsants.

ADOLESCENT SEXUALITY AND THE PATIENT-PRACTITIONER-PARENT RELATIONSHIP

Even though sexual feelings and behaviors are of great concern to adolescents and their families and adverse effects of sexual behavior are common in this age group, most patients and parents will not introduce the subject at the health care visit. Primary care clinicians must set the stage for frank, honest discussions of feelings and behaviors that often are embarrassing, shameful, and psychologically painful. Setting the stage requires that the provider pay particular attention to privacy for both adolescent patients and parents.[5] A seemingly innocuous question directed to the teenager when her mother is still in the room about whether she has had sex can significantly erode the patient's confidence that the practitioner understands the private nature of this subject. It would be equally inappropriate to ask the mother about her own sexual behavior in front of her daughter. Asking questions that do not make assumptions or presuppose certain behaviors is difficult but well worth the trouble, because adolescents are more likely to disclose closely guarded information when interviewed in this way. For example, if the physician assumes that everyone is heterosexual and asks girls if they have a boyfriend and boys if they have a girlfriend, adolescents who are questioning their sexual orientation or who know they are homosexual will be unlikely to offer this information. If, on the other hand, the question asks about sexual attraction to women, men, or both men and women or includes a gender-neutral term, such as "sexual partner," the patient is more likely to understand that the provider is ready to hear nontraditional information.

In interviewing adolescents about sexual issues, it is a mistake to assume that just because a question has been asked and answered, the full story has been told. Eliciting a history of sexual abuse is a case in point. As part of their screening sexual history, many physicians and nurses ask a question such as "Have you ever been sexually abused?" or "Has anyone ever done anything to you sexually that you didn't want them to do?" There is nothing wrong with these questions, but some adolescents who have been abused will answer them in the negative. They are afraid to disclose painful secrets because they have not yet developed a secure, trusting relationship with the health care practitioner. It is important to understand this, not to push too hard too soon for disclosure, and to explore the topic in more depth at a later visit when the relationship has had a chance to develop.

Negotiating confidentiality between adolescents and parents around sexual issues is another thorny area for the patient-practitioner-parent relationship. In general, the medical interview with the adolescent should take place in private. When a problem is diagnosed, the specifics of what will be disclosed to parents need to be negotiated with the patient. Providers should refuse to lie to parents; this sets a bad example and is unprofessional. However, it usually is not necessary to disclose all the details of the situation. For example, a 16-year-old girl is being seen for her annual checkup; the screening sexual history reveals that since the previous year's examination, she has become sexually active. She reports that she has had two partners in the past 8 months. She complains of a slight vaginal discharge. The clinician does a pelvic examination as part of the physical examination and discovers a mucopurulent cervicitis, most likely caused by a sexually transmitted infection. Appropriate antibiotics are prescribed. What should the mother be told? Most adolescents would agree to allow the physician to tell the mother that a pelvic examination was done because of a vaginal discharge and that he or she thinks that it is a minor infection that will clear up with antibiotics. The clinician can tell the adolescent beforehand that if the mother asks directly whether the infection is sexually transmitted, she will be told that information about her daughter's sexuality is kept in confidence. However, the adolescent patient should know that the physician will encourage a dialogue between mother and daughter about sexual behavior. The clinician must resist acting as a go-between in the mother-daughter relationship, and he or she should emphasize the necessity of direct communication between parent and child.

SUMMARY

Providing health care related to adolescent sexuality is one of the more difficult tasks of the primary care clinician. It demands in-depth knowledge of pubertal and psychosexual development, familiarity with the norms of adolescent sexual behavior, knowledge of pertinent gynecological and urological medicine, and superior communication skills. Adolescents are in great need of this type of care and are very appreciative when it is done well; the large majority want to be sexually healthy and eventually to have children and raise healthy families themselves.

REFERENCES

1. Brick P: Toward a positive approach to adolescent sexuality, *SIECUS Report* 17:1, 1989.
2. Burstein GR, et al: Incident *Chlamydia trachomatis* infections among inner-city adolescent females, *JAMA* 280:521, 1998.
3. Centers for Disease Control and Prevention: Youth risk behavior surveillance—United States, 1997, *MMWR* 47(SS-3):1, 1998.
4. Cohen MW: Adolescent sexual activity as expression of nonsexual needs, *Pediatr Ann* 24:324, 1995.
5. Coupey SM: Interviewing adolescents, *Pediatr Clin North Am* 44:1349, 1997.
6. Farrow JA: An approach to the management of sexual dysfunction in the adolescent male, *Sexually Active Teenagers* 2:39, 1988.
7. Garofalo R, et al: The association between health risk behaviors and sexual orientation among a school-based sample of adolescents, *Pediatrics* 101:895, 1998.
8. Gutman LT: Human papillomavirus infections of the genital tract in adolescents, *Adolesc Med* 6:115, 1995.
9. Hein K, et al: Comparison of HIV+ and HIV- adolescents: risk factors and psychosocial determinants, *Pediatrics* 95:96, 1995.
10. Howard M, McCabe JB: Helping teenagers postpone sexual involvement, *Fam Plann Perspect* 22:21, 1990.
11. Nagy S, Adock AG, Nagy CN: A comparison of risky health behaviors of sexually active, sexually abused, and abstaining adolescents, *Pediatrics* 93:570, 1994.
12. Premarital sexual experience among adolescent women: United States, 1970-1988, *MMWR* 39:929, 1991.
13. Remafedi G, et al: Demography of sexual orientation in adolescents, *Pediatrics* 89:714, 1992.
14. Sarrel LJ, Sarrel PM: Sexual unfolding, *J Adolesc Health Care* 2:93, 1981.
15. Schuster MA, Bell RM, Kanouse DE: The sexual practices of adolescent virgins: genital sexual activities of high school students who have never had vaginal intercourse, *Am J Public Health* 86:1570, 1996.
16. *Sex and America's teenagers,* New York, 1994, The Alan Guttmacher Institute.
17. Shrier LA, et al: Gender differences in risk behaviors associated with forced or pressured sex, *Arch Pediatr Adolesc Med* 152:57, 1998.
18. Smith AM, Rosenthal DA, Reichler H: High schoolers masturbatory practices: their relationship to sexual intercourse and personal characteristics, *Psychol Rep* 79:499, 1996.
19. Sonenstein FL, Pleck JH, Ku LC: Levels of sexual activity among adolescent males in the United States, *Fam Plann Perspect* 23:162, 1991.
20. Stock JL, et al: Adolescent pregnancy and sexual risk-taking among sexually abused girls, *Fam Plann Perspect* 29:200, 227, 1997.
21. Udry JR: Hormonal and social determinants of adolescent sexual initiation. In Bancroft J, Reinisch JM, editors: *Adolescence and puberty,* The Kinsey Institute Series, vol 3, New York, 1990, Oxford University Press.
22. Udry JR, Billy JO: Initiation of coitus in early adolescence, *Am Soc Rev* 52:841, 1987.

SUGGESTED READINGS

Bancroft J, Reinisch JM, editors: *Adolescence and puberty,* The Kinsey Institute Series, vol 3, New York, 1990, Oxford University Press.

Coupey SM, editor: *Primary care of adolescent girls,* Philadelphia, 1999, Hanley & Belfus.

Coupey SM, Klerman LV, editors: Adolescent sexuality: preventing unhealthy consequences, *Adolescent medicine: state of the art reviews,* vol 3, Philadelphia, 1992.

Drugs that cause sexual dysfunction: an update, *Med Lett Drugs Ther* 34:73, 1992.

111 Adolescent Pregnancy and Parenthood

Catherine Stevens-Simon • Elizabeth R. McAnarney

The true incidence of adolescent pregnancy in the United States is unknown, but it is estimated that each year more than 1 million adolescents, or approximately 1 of every 10 American teenage girls, are diagnosed as being pregnant. Studies suggest that approximately 50% of these young women give birth, 40% obtain abortions, and the remainder miscarry.[1] There is no way to determine the number of teenage pregnancies that terminate in spontaneous abortion without the teenager's knowledge. Thus, many more than a million teenage pregnancies occur each year.[1]

From the mid-1970s to the mid-1980s, births to women younger than age 20 years declined in number and rate, but the data presented in Fig. 111-1 show that, thereafter, the overall pregnancy rate among American teenagers rose, reaching an all-time high in 1991 and then declining again.[6] Of note, the data presented in Fig. 111-1 demonstrate that the convention of reporting on birth rates within the entire cohort of "15- to 19-year-old girls" has masked the steady decline in the pregnancy rate among sexually experienced teenagers in this country since the 1980s (a reflection of increased contraceptive use). Although it is encouraging that recent vital statistic data indicate that the teen birth rates in this country have reached an apex, the data presented in Fig. 111-1 give no reason for complacency or diminishing concern about the soaring number and the plummeting age of sexually experienced American teenagers. The teen pregnancy rate in this country is still higher than it was in the 1960s and remains one of the highest in the Western developed world.[1,16] Furthermore, although concerns about adolescent sexual experimentation traditionally have been focused almost exclusively on the risk of pregnancy, recent medical reports showing a dramatic increase in the prevalence of sexually transmitted diseases among American teenagers signal the need for broader concern. When one adds the millions of teenagers whose sexual lives are destroyed by the aftermaths of sexually transmitted diseases, including chronic pelvic pain, ectopic pregnancies, cervical cancer, and acquired immunodeficiency syndrome (AIDS), to the millions of teenagers whose futures are unnecessarily limited by pregnancy, it is easy to understand why curbing unprotected teenage sexual activity has become a national priority.

During the past three decades we have increased substantially our understanding of the risks associated with adolescent childbearing. Although vital statistical data still indicate that infants born to very young adolescent mothers (those younger than age 16 years at conception) are significantly more likely to be of low birth weight and to die during the first year of life than are infants born to older mothers, evidence is minimal that this is causally related to the physiological immaturity of the young adolescent mother.[1,16] Rather, most believe that the majority of the medical risks associated with adolescent childbearing reflect young adolescent mothers being significantly more likely to encounter adverse social environments than older mothers. Indeed, studies that control for potentially confounding psychosocial factors such as poor health habits (e.g., late prenatal care and substance abuse), poverty, and stress find no association between young maternal age and most of the obstetrical complications traditionally linked to adolescent childbearing.[16]

Nevertheless, adolescent pregnancy has become a source of increasing social, economic, and political concern in this country because of substantial evidence that early childbearing seriously jeopardizes the life chances of most young parents and their children.[1,8,16] The results of studies conducted over the past 30 years suggest that by limiting the educational achievements and vocational opportunities of successive generations, adolescent childbearing both contributes to the impoverishment of one of the most socioeconomically disadvantaged segments of American society and promotes intergenerational transmission of this socioeconomic disadvantage.[1,8,16]

It is not possible to prove that adolescent childbearing and poverty are causally related because studies of the sequelae of adolescent childbearing invariably are confounded by personal characteristics and environmental conditions known to predispose nulliparous adolescents to school failure and welfare dependency. However, current data suggest that few adolescent parents are prepared adequately to assume the economic, social, and psychological responsibility of child care and child rearing.[1,4,8,16] Many recent reports indicate that over the past two decades, the increased availability of alternative schools that have child care and flexible hours has enabled an increasingly large number of adolescent parents to obtain a high school education, to overcome economic and social barriers, and to become productive members of their communities. The numerous psychosocial problems still associated with youthful childbearing, however, challenge the concept that adolescent childbearing is a culturally adaptive response to socioeconomic and political disadvantage.[1,4,8,14,16]

Teenagers' ability to care for their offspring effectively has become the subject of investigation during recent years. Even though some professionals think that adolescents are

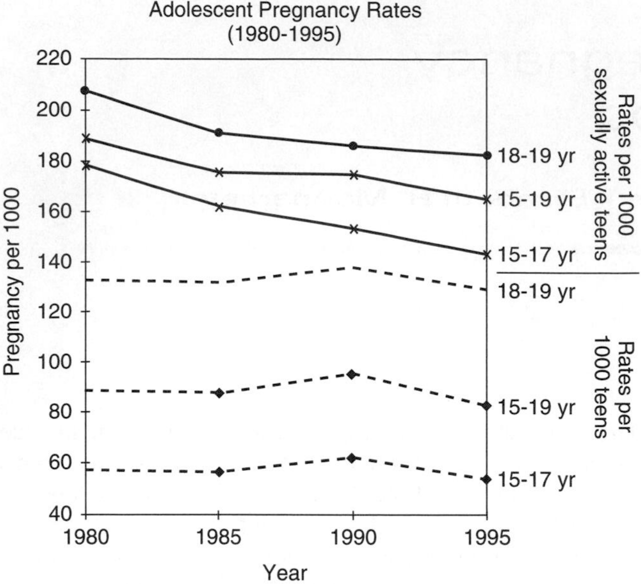

Fig. 111-1 Adolescent pregnancy rates (1980-1995).

(Data from Spitz AM, et al: Pregnancy, abortion, and birth rates among US adolescents—1980, 1985, and 1990, *JAMA* 275:989, 1996; *Mon Vital Stat Rep,* US Department of Health and Human Services, 46 No 1, 1997; and National Survey of Family Growth, 1995, US Department of Health and Human Services, series 23 No 19, 1998.)

more likely than adults to abuse their children, the data supporting this contention are far from conclusive. Some professionals are more concerned about adolescents' passive neglect of their children, a more benign neglect caused by their lack of child-rearing experience and ability to think causally, rather than by active, aggressive abuse.[15]

Current investigations of adolescents as parents are focusing on (1) adolescent mother-infant interaction during the neonatal period and subsequently during the first year of the child's life; (2) adolescent fathers—their strengths, needs, and behavior toward their children; (3) the intellectual, social, and emotional development of the children of adolescents; and (4) intervention programs for adolescent mothers and the effects of these programs on their offspring. These investigations will take time to complete because a methodology must be developed to study the many variables other than age that affect parenting, such as the adolescent's socioeconomic status, marital status, parity, educational level, and child-rearing experience.

PSYCHOSOCIAL REASONS THAT ADOLESCENTS BECOME PREGNANT

Teenagers become pregnant for many reasons, some conscious and some subconscious. The circumstances are unique for each individual and invariably color the nature and intensity of the conflicts that arise between the competing developmental needs of adolescence and parenthood. Although only a minority of young Americans actually state that they wish to become pregnant, many more clearly are ambivalent about postponing childbearing. The results of a study of 200 teenagers who had never been pregnant, conducted in Denver, revealed that even though only 10% of the young women seeking routine health care in the city's teen clinics openly admitted that they wanted to become pregnant, 40% said they "wouldn't mind being pregnant."[10] Other investigators have substantiated these findings among many American teenagers.[17] The results of these studies are a matter of concern because they have been consistent in showing that young women who have ambivalent feelings about postponing childbearing are significantly less likely than their peers to use contraceptives and therefore are at greater risk for conception. Indeed, one study reported that when adolescents in the third trimester of pregnancy were asked, "Why weren't you using birth control before you got pregnant?" the most frequent reply was, "I didn't mind getting pregnant."[12] Because teenage parents who express this sort of ambivalence about childbearing are significantly more likely to become pregnant again, it is imperative that we gain a better understanding of the reasons why so many American teenagers "don't mind" or want to get pregnant.[12]

An extensive body of literature exists concerning the antecedents of adolescent pregnancy. Some young people seek pregnancy to escape from intolerable home or living situations; others seek it as part of a complex pattern of "problem behaviors" to defy parental authority. Still others wish to become pregnant because their early sexual experiences have raised concern about their ability to conceive, and some adolescents seek pregnancy as a rite of passage, particularly if they are doing poorly in school or living in impoverished social environments in which adolescent pregnancy is rampant and adult roles, other than parenthood, are perceived to be inaccessible.[1,3,7,8,12]

Pregnancy may be the teenager's way of trying to resolve acute or chronic depression. Acute, reactive depression may result from the loss of a loved one (parent, grandparent, or caring relative) through death, separation, divorce, or a move. The teenager may conceive in an attempt to replace the individual who has been removed from her life.

Chronic, unresolved depression may precede the pregnancy by some years. A series of problems starting in childhood (e.g., poor school attendance, running away, suicidal behaviors, or drug overdoses) may precede pregnancy. Young women who report problem behaviors are more likely to have a child before age 19 years than are women who report no problem behaviors. Pregnancy, like the other behaviors, reflects the girl's chronic inability to resolve her depression. For example:

> Jeannie, a 13-year-old, was 6 months pregnant when she initially was seen in the clinic. Her widowed mother worked outside the home to keep Jeannie and her two older siblings together at home. Jeannie had a history of absenteeism and withdrawn behavior at school. When she was 12 years old, she had run away and was returned to her mother by the authorities. In the year before conception, she had gone to the emergency department of the local hospital twice, the first time with acute alcoholism, the second after a suicide gesture. Evaluation of Jeannie during the last emergency department visit revealed a depressed teenager who stated that she had been sad for as long as she could remember.

Jeannie's history indicates that she had been chronically depressed for several years and that her numerous attempts to gain attention had failed. Her history of school absenteeism, running away, alcohol ingestion, suicide-gestures, and finally, pregnancy suggested a long history of unresolved depression.

Peer pressure may be another important reason some teenagers become pregnant. Peer pressure for boys may come from friends of the same gender and for girls from friends of the opposite gender. For example:

Carrie, a 15-year-old, became pregnant during the same time period as three of her classmates. She was unable to say why she had become pregnant. The four girls often had talked about having babies. Carrie's boyfriend had not wanted her to use birth control pills, and he was pleased when she told him of the pregnancy.

Pregnancy and parenthood may represent positive accomplishments for teenagers who have experienced few. For example:

Beth, an 18-year-old school dropout, had a history of school problems and also had few friends. When she was told that she was pregnant, she was very happy. During the last trimester of pregnancy, she began to talk about her baby and all she expected it would be able to do. After the baby was born, she brought her proudly to the clinic to show her to the other pregnant girls. One year later, she still talked with great pride about the baby and was trying to become pregnant again. Beth saw her child as her first real achievement and was seeking greater achievement through a second pregnancy and child.

In some families an adolescent is encouraged to become pregnant either through overt approval of the young woman's sexual activity or through indirect encouragement. Still other teenagers become pregnant as a direct confrontation of parental authority or as a way of showing their growing independence. The need to show independence may be most particularly intense for middle adolescents (15 to 17 years old) because they normally are in the midst of struggling for their independence and, thus, may be most threatened if it is challenged. Adolescents' ignorance about their sexuality and their potential for becoming pregnant also are contributing factors for teenage conception. Although some adolescents are misinformed about the details of sexuality, contraception, and pregnancy, ignorance about coitus possibly resulting in pregnancy contributes to only a limited number of teenage pregnancies.

DIAGNOSIS OF PREGNANCY

The diagnosis of teenage pregnancy poses problems for both the adolescent and the practitioner that usually do not occur with adults. Teenagers concerned about being pregnant initially may hesitate to seek help from their primary care physician. The physician may find it difficult to talk with pregnant teenagers about confidentiality, sexuality, and pregnancy if he or she and the adolescent have not discussed these topics before the pregnancy. In pediatric settings in which these issues have been raised before the teenager seeks care for pregnancy, few problems arise between physician and adolescent.[11,16]

Pregnant girls raise their concerns to the physician in several ways. Some (often older adolescents) who have achieved formal operational thinking say that they think they may be pregnant. Others, particularly younger teenagers, may complain of vague, somatic symptoms, such as headaches, abdominal pain, or joint pains, when their real concern is pregnancy. Still others expect the physician to guess that they are pregnant and do not indicate that pregnancy even is a possibility. This belief in the physician guessing that they are pregnant may represent the magical thinking of some adolescents. If a reproductive history is included in the general medical history for all female teenagers, the physician will be able to move easily into the question of pregnancy in a situation such as the one just described. Questions about the menstrual cycle, including last menstrual period (LMP) and menstrual irregularities, should be incorporated into the reproductive history. Questions about previous pregnancies; contraceptive use; sexually transmitted diseases, particularly AIDS; and tampon use also should be included. If pregnancy is possible, the teenager should be asked whether she may be pregnant. Most teenagers are relieved to have the question of pregnancy raised. The physician then should decide how much of the pregnancy evaluation he or she will do and when the teenager will be referred for obstetrical care.

Confirmation of pregnancy clearly is within the role of the primary care physician. In addition to the medical and reproductive history, symptoms of pregnancy should be explored; a physical examination that includes a pelvic evaluation should be performed. Unless the pregnancy is well advanced, a pregnancy test is needed to confirm the diagnosis. Serum pregnancy testing may be necessary if there still is question after the urine screen. Urine tests for pregnancy are sensitive enough to give accurate results 10 to 14 days after conception. Laboratory screening is endorsed because many teenagers report their LMP inaccurately.

When pregnancy has been diagnosed, the teenager should be referred to a special program for pregnant adolescents, if one is available. If not, the teenager can be referred to a private obstetrical office or clinic. The primary care physician then may choose to continue seeing the teenager for counseling and education throughout her pregnancy. Practitioners who have good counseling skills and knowledge of pregnancy options also can be involved in abortion or adoption counseling. Referral to agencies providing these services also is appropriate.

COUNSELING PREGNANT TEENAGERS

Counseling in the practitioner's office might concentrate on the discussion of immediate considerations, such as the course of the pregnancy, labor, and childbirth, as well as on future considerations—the effects of the pregnancy on education, vocation, and finances. Every effort should be made to work with the adolescent father-to-be if he and his partner still are in contact.

Some discussion should be directed toward the circumstances under which the teenager became pregnant and how she and her partner feel about the pregnancy. Problems may include the academic future for both, as well as the possibility of finding child care and money for child care for their child. Finances are a major concern for most teenagers, and referral to the appropriate social service agency often is helpful.

Group counseling provides an effective method of communication with and education for teenagers. If there are two or more pregnant adolescents in one practice and the health professional is knowledgeable about group processes, group counseling can be provided.

An unstructured format for groups is optimal because it allows adolescents to choose the subjects to be discussed and to exert some control in that setting. Both tasks are consistent with the developmental tasks of adolescence. Significant others, such as parents, husbands, boyfriends, or labor coaches, also can attend, allowing the group leader to help these people reorder their relationships, a task similar to altering relationships when a new baby is added to the family.

Because some teenagers are not developmentally at the level of formal operational thinking, techniques traditionally used in adult groups need modification. For example, rather than presenting didactic information on a particular subject, role-playing provides an experience that teenagers enjoy. Although adolescents need to consider concrete, nonthreatening information at first, they soon become aware of their personal feelings about the meaning of pregnancy and are able to express these as the group process progresses. Although they may be unable to label their emotions abstractly, they can discuss their feelings by describing the thinking or behaviors of others. Written materials, videotapes, and movies at developmentally appropriate stages can be most helpful. Within groups, teenagers can learn to solve problems; resolve conflicts with their parents; clarify their independent, individual identities; and plan for their future.

POSTPARTUM CARE

Adolescents who become pregnant are at high risk for a repeat pregnancy during adolescence. Preventing repeat adolescent pregnancies is critical because current data indicate that the risk of adverse neonatal and maternal outcomes increases with subsequent pregnancies in this age group.[16] A major goal in providing care to teenagers during pregnancy is preparing both partners for responsible planning of their reproductive future. Ideally, responsibility for contraception after the first pregnancy is shared by both partners.

Adolescent contraception imposes many problems that do not diminish once the baby is born. Circumstances that were present before and that contributed to the initial conception may still exist, even though some teenagers are motivated to prevent a second pregnancy. Contraceptive failure caused by noncompliance in taking pills or sporadic or improper use of condoms or foam, as well as barriers to the use of these contraceptives that are inherent in the health care system, may continue to be particular problems for teenagers seeking effective contraception.

Norplant (a subdermal implant of levonorgestrel) and Depo-Provera (an injectable hormonal contraceptive agent) are particularly attractive to health care workers who provide contraceptive care to adolescents because they require less active patient participation to remain effective and, thus, bridge the gap in contraceptive vigilance that can be created by a painful break-up with an old boyfriend or the acquisition of a new boyfriend who wants a child.[12,16] Indeed, postpartum Norplant insertion is the only intervention that has been consistently associated with a significant reduction in the repeat pregnancy rate among American teenagers.[11,13]

For young people at risk for AIDS, special emphasis should be placed on counseling and education about condom use. The primary care practitioner may decide to assume the responsibility for contraceptive education and for prescribing birth control for adolescent parents.

TEENAGERS AS PARENTS

Teenage parents face numerous problems. Although often experienced in baby-sitting, teenagers are not prepared for the reality of round-the-clock child care. Adolescents may expect to have complacent babies who eat and sleep with regularity; they may become disillusioned easily when the child demands far more time and effort than they are able to give.

The attitudes of adolescent mothers suggest that they often use physical punishment for discipline and frequently have a minimal understanding of the need for stimulation. Although these attitudes may reflect sociocultural influences rather than the mother's age, professionals should be aware of this issue. Most teenagers are fond of children, want to be good parents, and are eager to learn about child rearing.

Adolescent parents frequently live with their own parents or other family members. Studies indicate that children who have the advantage of substantial daily input from grandmothers or other adults do not develop the same behavioral, academic, and health problems and are less likely to be maltreated than are children who are raised primarily by their adolescent mothers.[2] It is unclear if the presence of a more mature adult in the home has a direct, beneficial effect on the development of these children or if the same personal attributes and qualities that enable some adolescent mothers to elicit the daily support of adults in their environment may also make them more nurturing parents.[15] However, evidence that within multigenerational families the quality of both the mothering and the grandmothering behaviors is related inversely to the age of the adolescent mother favors the latter explanation.[2] Apparently the same factors that prevent some late adolescents from moving out of their parents' home and completing the normal process of emancipation also make them more dysfunctional parents and their mothers less helpful parenting partners. Although longitudinal studies are needed, available data suggest that those multigenerational families that are most likely to provide positive parenting are those in which young adolescent mothers cohabitate with their mothers and receive the support that they need to resolve the emancipation and identity struggles successfully. The tasks of emancipation and identity formation are characteristic of the early and middles stages of adolescence. If successfully achieved, they are prepared to establish independent households during late adolescence.[2] Unfortunately, observing the efficiency with which their relatives care for the child may add to the young mother's own lack of confidence. The adolescents' reaction may be to give up parenting and to relinquish this task to other caretakers in the home. The child, in turn, may become confused and have difficulty forming a bond with his or her own parents and may not even identify them as the actual parents. Simply teaching about child care and role modeling can help the adolescent parent. Home visits are an effective way to observe teenage parents with their baby and provide an excellent opportunity to help them learn to care for the infant.

Some teenagers expect their baby to fulfill their own

needs for love immediately and are disappointed when the infant does not respond as they had expected. Data indicate that younger adolescent mothers are less accepting of, cooperative with, and accessible and sensitive to their children during the first postnatal year than are older adolescent mothers. For example, a teenager may think her crying baby will be immediately comforted when picked up. If the infant does not respond as anticipated, the young mother may feel rejected and unloved by her child. However, with time and patience, teenagers can be taught about the needs of infants and the variety of responses that meet those needs.

Adolescent fathers who want to be actively involved with the rearing of their children should receive the same support as adolescent mothers.[9] Few adolescent boys are prepared for fatherhood and as a group tend to have more academic, drug, and conduct problems than do their nonparenting peers.[9] Teenage fathers may choose to relieve the mother of total responsibility for their child by being available to provide care when the mother needs time for her education, job, or other activities. Even if the adolescent father is not available personally, he may want to ask members of his extended family to provide direct help and support for the mother.

Mixed feelings about parenthood are appropriate for teenagers. They want to be good parents and to love their children, but they also want to engage in normal teenage activities.[4] It is important for the practitioner to remember that teenagers need to gain knowledge and expertise to fulfill their role as parents and also need to move through the adolescent period in concert with their peers. Often, families will need help in effecting an appropriate balance for the adolescent mother and father between their duties as parents and their peer, school, and social activities.

LONG-TERM FOLLOW-UP

Data from a long-term follow-up study in Baltimore indicate that many women who became mothers as adolescents actually finish their education and become independent of welfare assistance. In a 17-year follow-up of a group of poor, inner city adolescents, 67% of the group had obtained their high school diplomas and 35% had graduated from college or had taken some postsecondary courses. Only 12% of those who went on welfare assistance during the first 5 years of the study continued to be on assistance nearly two decades later.[5]

SUMMARY

Even though fewer adolescents than in the past are choosing to become pregnant or to continue their pregnancies (primarily because of the availability of contraception and abortion) the ability of teenagers to care for their children effectively still is an area in which intensive investigation is needed. Although adolescence and early parenthood can both be times of tremendous stress, professionals who have worked with teenage parents are often impressed by their strengths and their ability to learn how to be effective parents when they receive adequate instruction.

REFERENCES

1. Brown SS, Eisenberg L: *The best intentions: unintended pregnancy and the well-being of children and families,* Washington, DC, 1995, National Academy Press.
2. Chase-Lansdale PL, Brooks-Gunn J, Zamsky E: Young African-American multigenerational families in poverty: quality of mothering and grandmothering, *Child Dev* 65:373, 1994.
3. Dryfoos JG: A new strategy for preventing unintended teenage childbearing, *Fam Plann Perpect* 16:193, 1984.
4. Flanagan P, et al: Adolescent development and transitions to motherhood, *Pediatrics* 96:273, 1995.
5. Furstenberg FF, Brooks-Gunn J, Morgan SP: Adolescent mothers and their children in later life, *Fam Plann Perspect* 19:142, 1987.
6. Kaufmann R, et al: The decline in United States teen pregnancy rates. Teen pregnancy rates 1990-1995, *Pediatrics* 102:1141, 1998.
7. Klerman LV: Adolescent pregnancy and parenting: controversies of the past and lessons for the future, *J Adolesc Health* 14:553, 1993.
8. Luker K: *Dubious conceptions: the politics of teenage pregnancy,* Cambridge, Mass, 1996, Harvard University Press.
9. Marsiglio W: Adolescent males' orientation toward paternity and contraception, *Fam Plann Perspect* 25:22, 1993.
10. Rainey DY, Stevens-Simon C, Kaplan DW: Self-perception of infertility among female adolescents, *Am J Dis Child* 147:1053, 1993.
11. Stevens-Simon C: Providing effective reproductive health care and prescribing contraceptives for adolescents, *Pediatr Rev* 19:409, 1998.
12. Stevens-Simon C, et al: Reasons for first teen pregnancies predict the rate of subsequent teen conceptions, *Pediatrics* 101:e8, 1998.
13. Stevens-Simon C, Kelly LS: Effect of Norplant on repeat conceptions among adolescent mothers, *Fam Plann Perspect* 31:88, 1999.
14. Stevens-Simon C, Lowy R: Is teenage childbearing an adaptive strategy for the socioeconomically disadvantaged or a strategy for adapting to socioeconomic disadvantage? *Arch Pediatr Adolesc Med* 149:912, 1995.
15. Stevens-Simon C, Nelligan D: Identification and treatment of adolescent parents at risk for child abuse in a comprehensive adolescent-oriented maternity program, *Aggress Viol Behav* 3:197, 1998.
16. Stevens-Simon C, White M: Adolescent pregnancy, *Pediatr Ann* 20: 322, 1991.
17. Zabin LS, Astone NM, Emerson MR: Do adolescents want babies? The relationship between attitudes and behavior, *J Res Adolesc* 3:67, 1993.

SUGGESTED READINGS

Brooks-Gunn J, Chase-Lansdale L: Children having children: effects on the family system, *Pediatr Ann* 20:467, 1991.

Furstenberg FF: Teenage childbearing and cultural rationality: a thesis in search of evidence, *Fam Relations* 41:239, 1992.

Miller BC: Adolescent parenthood, economic issues, and social policies, *J Fam Econ Issues* 13:467, 1992.

112 Violent and Aggressive Behavior

Trina Menden Anglin

Adolescent violence is an important societal problem that has grave public health implications for the United States. The definition of interpersonal violence is based on the concept of intentional aggression. It is the threat to use or the actual use of physical force with the intent of intimidating or actually causing physical injury or harm to another person.[9] Two major categories of aggressive behavior have been described in psychophysiological terms. Instrumental, proactive, or predatory aggression, which is goal directed, is usually carried out with little emotional display and may be associated with psychophysiological underarousal. In contrast, hostile, or reactive, aggression is carried out in an emotionally charged, physically aroused state; is founded on anger in response to a perceived provocation; and frequently is impulsive and not well controlled. In practice, however, most aggressive adolescents exhibit both categories of behavior.[16,17] This chapter aims to increase clinicians' effectiveness in the area of adolescent interpersonal violence.[1,3] It provides clinical guidance for identifying adolescents involved in interpersonal violence, either as perpetrators or as victims, and explores health counseling and interventions for them.

CHANGING FREQUENCIES OF VIOLENT BEHAVIOR

Compared with all other age groups, adolescents and young adults have disproportionately high rates of involvement in interpersonal violence as perpetrators, victims, and witnesses.[7] In particular, adolescents living in urban areas grow up under the pervasive influence of violence, which affects both their social and cognitive development. Although they remain at unacceptably high levels, most indicators of violent behavior have demonstrated significant improvement during the latter part of the 1990s.[4,7,21]

Fighting and Weapons

Nationally, in 1997, 36.6% of adolescents reported having been in a physical fight within the preceding year, and 3.5% reported having received physical injuries from fighting. By carrying weapons, adolescents increase the risk of causing serious physical injury or death if they become involved in a fight; in a 1-year period, 18% carried a weapon, including 8.5% who carried a weapon to school. These 1997 data represent significant decreases compared with those in 1991.[4]

Delinquency

Delinquency rates are a second indicator of violent behavior. Between 1986 and 1996, the juvenile court delinquency case rate increased by 36%, from 45.5 to 61.8 per 1000 population. Juveniles represented 30% of arrests for all serious crimes and 14% of arrests for homicide in 1997. Violent offenses currently account for 7.8% of all juvenile court delinquency cases and have increased by 93% over the preceding decade. However, there has been a recent downward trend; the number of juvenile arrests for violent crime, including homicide, aggravated assault, and weapon law violations, decreased consistently between 1994 and 1997.[21]

Homicide

A third major indicator of violence is the homicide rate. In 1997, homicide remained the second leading cause of death among 15- to 24-year-olds in the United States (16.8 per 100,000 population).[11] Adolescents between 13 and 19 years of age represented 14% of all homicide victims, and young adults ages 20 to 24 years accounted for an additional 18%. The overall homicide rate in the United States has demonstrated an encouraging downward trend of 34% since 1993; it was 6.3 per 100,000 population in 1998. This rate is the lowest since 1967.[5]

During the past 3.5 decades, the homicide rates among male adolescents ages 15 to 19 years have paralleled the rates for young adults. The homicide rates for male adolescents gradually increased from 1963, when they were about 6 per 100,000 population, to 1974 and then remained at approximately the same level, between 12 and 15 per 100,000 population, until 1985. At this time, the homicide rate for male teenagers started a steep ascent to a peak of about 35 per 100,000 population in 1994. Since then, the rate has declined consistently.[7] However, the homicide rate remains unacceptably high among minority males between the ages of 15 and 24 years. In 1997, when the homicide rate was 6.5 per 100,000 population for white males in this age group, it was 117.4 for black and 42.7 for Hispanic adolescent and young adult males. Firearm injuries account for 84% of homicide deaths in this age group. The homicide rate is significantly lower for female adolescents and young adults; it was 4.7 per 100,000 population in 1997.[11]

THEORIES OF AGGRESSIVE BEHAVIOR

Contemporary explanations for aggressive and violent behavior are based on interactions among individuals' psychosocial development and cognitive processes, hormonal and neurological functioning, and surrounding social influences. Although information is available about the effects of each of these categories, we know little about how they interact.[7]

Psychosocial Development and Cognitive Processes

Aggressive adolescents and adults who commit acts of violence characteristically first demonstrate aggressive behaviors during early childhood. Their behavior patterns stabilize before adolescence; as these children mature, their aggressive behavior becomes more serious, violent, and harmful to others[9,10,16] (See Chapter 81, Prediction of Adult Behavior from Childhood). Some children do not display aggressive behaviors until early adolescence; the prognosis for positive change over time is relatively good for this group.[16]

Aggressive and violent behaviors appear to represent children's learned responses to solving problems of frustration; their learning is facilitated by observing successful outcomes to their own and others' aggressive behaviors. One example is the child who learns that a parent can be coerced into giving into a demand if the child behaves aggressively. Children subjected to harsh discipline or abuse by parents and children whose family dynamics reflect negativity and disapproval may be at heightened risk for long-term aggressive behavior. Children store such successful behavioral strategies or "scripts" in their memory and retrieve them for use in future similar situations. Once behavioral "scripts" are well encoded, they may be retrieved and acted on so quickly that the behavior appears impulsive rather than reflective.[9,16] In addition, based on numerous studies, there now is general agreement that intense, prolonged childhood exposure to violence portrayed on television also boosts the risk for long-term aggressive behavior (see Chapter 69, Children, Adolescents, and the Media). Children and young adolescents who display aggressive behavior usually have poor social problem-solving skills and are rejected by their conventional, nonaggressive peers.

Another psychological explanation for aggressive behavior is adapted by Kohlberg's theory of moral development. Aggressive adolescents who victimize others do not perceive predatory or aggressive behavior in moral terms but as a matter of personal choice. They believe that the "right" behavior is the one that serves their own interests. Their beliefs may bias them to disparage victims or to believe that they deserve to be attacked.[16]

Biological Explanations

Although multiple lines of research have demonstrated positive associations between biological differences and aggressive behavior, biological causality has not been determined and complex interactions are postulated among biological systems that are influenced by environmental conditions.

Genetic explanations. It currently is thought that genetic processes are an important influence on the biological potential for aggressive behavior, but that adverse environmental conditions must be present for aggressive behavior to become manifest. There is no clear evidence in humans that any simple chromosomal syndrome transmits the potential for violent behavior; multiple genetic loci must work synchronously.[6]

Hormonal explanations. Testosterone has been linked to adolescent aggressive behavior. Male adolescents who have relatively high testosterone levels are more likely to react physically when threatened or provoked. In addition, higher testosterone levels appear to lower tolerance for frustration among younger male adolescents, which in turn is associated with the likelihood of engaging in unprovoked aggressive behavior. Similarly, adult male violent offenders have higher testosterone levels than do nonviolent offenders.[12]

Neurotransmitters. Four neurotransmitters—dopamine, norepinephrine, serotonin, and gamma-aminobutyric acid (GABA)—have been studied to explore their relationships to aggressive and violent behavior. None can serve as a specific biological marker for aggression potential. However, the serotonin system appears to be linked consistently to human aggressive behaviors. An inverse correlation exists between the concentration of serotonin and its metabolites (e.g., 5-HIAA) in the cerebrospinal fluid and various measures of aggressive, impulsive, and suicidal behaviors. Serotonin is considered to inhibit impulsive aggression, but not premeditated aggression.[12] Both dopamine and norepinephrine also have been found to play roles in impulsive aggressive behavior.[12] Despite our inability to define specific roles for neurotransmitters in causing aggressive behavior, major classes of psychotropic drugs that are used to manage violent behavior and agitation (e.g., neuroleptics and anxiolytic agents) include inhibition of specific neurotransmitters as part of their spectrum of pharmacological action.

Neuroanatomical and neurophysiological abnormalities. Abnormalities of certain brain sites, such as structures in the limbic system, may be associated with violent behavior. For example, children who exhibit violent or aggressive behavior often have neuropsychological problems such as deficits in memory, attention, and language/verbal skills. These problems frequently follow damage to the limbic system from a head injury. About 70% of patients who have a history of blunt head trauma demonstrate aggressive behavior and irritability for varying periods thereafter. Hyperactivity at age 10 years and during the adolescent years is a strong predictor of future violent behavior.[10,16]

Social Influences

Several root community characteristics are associated with high epidemiological levels of interpersonal violence and crime. The most important are extreme poverty and its covariates, including the density of multiunit housing, residential mobility, disrupted family structures, low levels of participation in community social life and organization, and lack of legitimate employment opportunities. Other factors associated with risk for violent behavior among adolescents include positive parental attitudes toward violence, family conflict and poor family management, low academic performance, peer delinquency, criminal activity by neighborhood adults, and illicit substance use. The higher the number of risk factors identified for a child or young adolescent, the greater the likelihood for that young person's involvement in aggressive behavior and violence by age 18 years.[7,10,15,16] Community minority race and ethnicity status are not strongly associated with violence and crime rates once poverty and the other listed factors are controlled. The extremely high homicide rates of the past decade are attributed to the escalated rate of substance abuse and the acceptance of a violent lifestyle, especially the carrying and use of firearms.[19]

CLINICAL APPLICATIONS

There is a broad range of involvement in interpersonal violence among adolescents. Most commonly, teenagers occasionally become involved in physical fights but otherwise appear to demonstrate adequate psychosocial adjustment. A smaller proportion of youngsters demonstrates recurrent antisocial physical aggression. For these adolescents, physically aggressive behavior usually is part of a package of deviant problem behaviors. Common associated problems include conduct disorder (see Chapter 85, Conduct Disorders), adjudication for juvenile delinquency, commission of nonviolent felonies (see Chapter 106, Juvenile Delinquency), substance abuse (see Chapter 103, Drug, Alcohol, and Tobacco Abuse), the selling of drugs, bipolar disorder (see Chapter 107, Mood Disorders in Children and Adolescents) and other mental health problems, poor academic performance, and rejection by conventional peers.* The question of gang membership also must be raised. Although overlap clearly exists among adjudicated delinquents, adolescents who have conduct disorder, and adolescents who engage in physical aggression, the three groups are not synonymous.

Primary care clinicians are the professional group most likely to encounter adolescents individually from an evaluation perspective. Given the high rate of interpersonal violence and the substantial risk it carries for psychological trauma, serious injury, and death, all adolescents deserve to be screened clinically for involvement.[1,2] Adolescents should be assessed routinely as part of the following types of health care encounters and observations: visits for health maintenance and for care of acute injuries, findings of recent physical trauma and/or older scars, and symptoms of anxiety or depression. Adolescent engagement in violence does not occur as an isolated behavior; clinical screening for aggressive behavior and violence should be placed in the context of a comprehensive psychosocial history (see Chapter 105, Interviewing Adolescents). The triad of fighting, use of illicit drugs, and poor academic performance has successfully predicted the future occurrence of violence-related injuries among adolescents.[18] Adolescents who engage in violent behavior are likely to have symptoms of anger and to have been exposed to serious violence.[20]

Box 112-1 outlines a clinically useful sequence of questions to help identify and assess adolescents who are engaged in interpersonal violence. In addition, a short clinical screening instrument is based on the acronym FISTS. Its questions address *f*ighting, *i*njuries from fighting, *s*exual and dating violence, *t*hreats from weapons, and *s*elf-defense.[1] The screening and assessment interview should be interactive, use open-ended questions, and be low-keyed and conversational. The questions are phrased so that no assignment of blame is implied. It also is useful to ask the adolescent's parents about anger issues, trouble with fighting, problems with the law or police, and their own parenting styles and family safety policies.[15,16]

In addition to determining factual information, the primary care clinician should attempt to identify issues that may help motivate an adolescent to try to change his or her aggressive behavior (Box 112-2).

Counseling Strategies for Adolescents Who Fight

Useful counseling strategies are outlined in Box 112-3. Although adolescents who exhibit multiple, long-standing problem behaviors probably are not amenable to change through office-based counseling and may require referral for meaningful intervention, many other adolescents may benefit from interactive counseling discussions. First, the primary care clinician and adolescent must together define fighting or carrying weapons as a problem behavior. The clinician may need to indicate that such behavior is dangerous and express concern for the adolescent's well-being. The focus should be on helping the adolescent to explore nonviolent alternatives to fighting. The clinician may also point out that bystanders to fights frequently play active roles in either escalating or defusing the central aggressive behavior.

Aggressive adolescents frequently have different cognitions than nonaggressive adolescents. For example, they are more likely to perceive that other people have a hostile intent toward them. It is logical for them to adopt a physically aggressive solution to a problem. In addition, aggressive adolescents have a limited repertoire of means for solving social problems without resorting to physical violence.[10,16] The primary care clinician can help the adolescent correct these cognitive distortions and appreciate the potential effectiveness of prosocial, nonviolent solutions to interpersonal problems.

Referral for More Intensive Intervention

Office-based counseling by the primary care clinician usually is adequate for adolescents who demonstrate normal psychosocial functioning. The clinician probably will need to refer adolescents who exhibit recurrent significant antisocial behavior (see Chapter 83, Consultation and Referral for Behavioral and Developmental Problems). The following categories of programs may be effective[7,13]:

1. Parent management training, which is based on behavioral modification techniques of social learning theory.

*References 7, 8, 10, 14, 16, 20.

BOX 112-1

CLINICAL QUESTIONS TO HELP IDENTIFY ADOLESCENTS ENGAGED IN INTERPERSONAL VIOLENCE

1. How much of a problem is losing your temper or getting angry for you?
2. How much of a problem is fighting for you?
3. About how often do you get involved in fights? About how often do you watch other people fight?
4. What happened the last time you were part of a fight?
   - How did the fight get started?
   - Was the fight more name calling, pushing/shoving/wrestling, or hitting/punching/kicking?
   - Was the fight one on one, or were more people involved?
   - Had anyone used alcohol or drugs before the fight broke out?
   - Did anyone use weapons such as a bat, stick, knife, or gun?
   - Did anyone get hurt or injured because of the fight? What happened? Did anyone need to get medical care?
   - Did the police get involved? What happened?
5. Have you ever gotten hurt or injured from being part of a fight? What happened? Did you need to get medical care?
6. Have you ever hurt anyone else during a fight? What happened? Did that person need to get medical care?
7. Have you ever gotten into trouble for fighting?
   - Any problems at school? Have you ever been suspended for being part of a fight?
   - Any problems with the police or law? Did you need to go to court? Were you locked up (placed in detention)? What did the court say you needed to do? (Ask about probation, house arrest, community service time, reparation to the victim(s), and incarceration.)
   - When you were younger, did you ever get into trouble for fighting? What happened? About how old were you the first time you got into a fight with someone outside your family?
8. Has anyone ever threatened you with a gun? With a knife or some other weapon? Has anyone ever shot at you?
9. Have you ever needed to threaten someone or do something physical to get what you wanted or needed? What happened?
10. If you wanted a gun, how easy would it be for you to get it? How long would it take?
11. Have you ever carried a gun or knife? Where did you carry it? Was there any special reason for you to carry it? About how often do you carry it?
12. Have you ever shot at anyone? Have you ever shot at and hit a person? What happened?
13. Does anyone at home own a gun? Are you allowed to use it? How could you get it if you wanted to?
14. Do you own a gun? What kind is it? About how often do you use it?
15. Here are some reasons why people get into fights. What do you think about them?
   - Someone calls you a name, insults you, or says something untrue about you.
   - Someone insults a member of your family.
   - Someone wants to fight you or dares you to fight.
   - Someone hits you first.
   - Someone physically hurts or kills a friend or a member of your family.
   - You want to show how tough you are, to keep up your reputation.
16. What do you think about people who get picked on by other people or who get beaten up in a fight? Do you think it's their own fault? Does it matter if they get hurt?
17. How do you get along with your romantic partner (boyfriend/girlfriend)? When you are joking around or playing, does either of you ever slap, pinch, hit, punch, or kick the other one? When you argue, does one person always "win?" Does one person put the other one down with names or insults? During an argument, have you ever been slapped, pinched, hit, punched, or kicked by your boyfriend/girlfriend? Have you ever slapped, pinched, hit, punched, or kicked your boyfriend/girlfriend during an argument? Were either of you ever physically hurt from an argument and got a bruise, cut, or sprain?

This strategy may be effective for families that have young adolescents, have few dysfunctional factors, and are not socioeconomically disadvantaged (see Chapter 101, Counseling Parents of Adolescents).

2. Cognitive problem-solving skills training, which is a formal extension of the office-based strategy outlined in this chapter. It seeks to change how adolescents approach conflicts by teaching them a step-by-step approach to solving interpersonal problems. It also may include a sociomoral reasoning component.
3. Community-based interventions preventing adolescents' entry into violence by reducing children's and adolescents' exposure to antisocial peers, strengthening ties to their families, schools, and communities, and fostering connectedness among adult community residents to enhance the neighborhood's supervision of its

BOX 112-2

MOTIVATING INFLUENCES FOR AVERTING VIOLENT BEHAVIOR

1. Determine the adolescent's sense of future. Teenagers who expect to die violently at a young age may not be open to problem-solving strategies until this perception is addressed.
2. Determine the adolescent's connections to family members. Many teenagers have younger siblings, cousins, or their own children whom they wish to protect from their negative experiences. They may be persuaded that their own lives are important to members of their families and that their own behavior is a powerful model for the younger "generation."
3. Determine the adolescent's beliefs about familial attitudes toward fighting and the use of weapons. Many adolescents perceive that their parents would support their fighting and using a weapon in self-defense.
4. Determine the meanings that peer status and respect have for the adolescent. How important is "toughness?"
5. Determine the adolescent's concerns about ability to control anger and impulses. Many adolescents are worried about their emotional reactivity.
6. Determine the adolescent's emotional responses to fighting. Look for thrill seeking, need to retaliate, fear, and remorse.

BOX 112-3

COUNSELING APPROACHES FOR ANGRY, IMPULSIVE ADOLESCENTS

1. *Help the adolescent develop strategies to defuse anger and to lessen his or her emotional reactivity.* A combination of relaxation techniques and cognitive exercises appears to work most effectively. Teenagers can be taught that anger represents a highly charged physical state during which the body is prepared to react strongly in response to their feeling very upset. Together, these sensations lead to impulsive behavior (fast physical action without thinking). They can learn to control their bodies by using relaxation techniques. Cognitive exercises consist of rehearsing four steps that correspond to the stages of a provocation sequence. Teenagers can practice scenarios with the clinician and at home.
   - Prepare for a provocation. Rehearse self-efficacy statements, such as "I can manage this situation. I know how to control my anger. I know what to do if I get upset."
   - Confront the provocation. Rehearse self-instruction, such as "Stay calm. Keep cool. Relax." Recognize that "You don't need to prove yourself."
   - Cope with the psychological arousal and agitation. "My muscles are feeling tight. It's time to relax and slow things down."
   - Reflect on the provocation. These self-statements are meant to provide perspective if the situation was not resolved and to enhance self-efficacy for anger control if the adolescent was successful in controlling his or her anger.

   Other strategies include purposeful diversion—allowing the course of time to exert a cooling effect and confiding angry feelings to a trusted friend or adult. Teenagers who enjoy creating art may want to draw or paint their feelings. It is important not to brood about what occurred. In addition, it is not beneficial to recommend that angry feelings be released through imaginary acts of aggression, such as punching a pillow, which do not purge aggressive wishes and may even inflame aggressive fantasies.
2. *Work on effective problem-solving skills.* The primary care clinician can model effective prosocial problem solving by working through specific situations with the adolescent to seek alternative possible solutions, evaluating each possibility, and to examine the likely consequences of each alternative before deciding on a course of prosocial action. Role playing helps to engage the adolescent and promotes exploration of perspective taking (see approach 3).
3. *Help the adolescent develop sociomoral reasoning.* The goal is to promote an aggressive adolescent's belief that it is morally wrong to cause harm to others and that this belief is important to hold. The adolescent learns to respect others' humanity and rights and to become sensitive to and care about others' emotions (emotional empathy) rather than to focus on one's own immediate self-interests. The clinician can use the following probes when modeling problem-solving skills: Ask the adolescent to (a) summarize the problem from the perspectives of both players, (b) clarify the meaning of moral terms (e.g., what do you mean by fair when you say "it isn't fair"?), (c) explain why a certain alternative was decided on, (d) consider an issue from a universal perspective (e.g., what would happen if everyone stole from stores?), and (e) consider the issue's context (e.g., under what conditions would it be justifiable to break a promise?).

Modified from Berkowitz L: *Aggression: its causes, consequences and control,* New York, 1993, McGraw Hill; and from Pepler DJ, Rubin KH, editors: *The development and treatment of childhood aggression,* Hillsdale, NJ, 1991, Lawrence Erlbaum Associates.

young people. Community-based programs serve adolescents best who appear at risk for antisocial, aggressive behaviors but who do not exhibit severe problems. However, most community-level efforts have not been rigorously evaluated.

Primary care clinicians can successfully refer adolescents and their families for more intensive help when either adolescents or their parents are motivated. It is important, however, for the clinician to participate in the referral process. The clinician should explore the following types of community resources: school-based programs (programs for disruptive students and conflict mediation curricula that the guidance department or school social worker may offer), mental health agencies (group programs for troubled youngsters), a local university's department of psychology (experimental program if a faculty member has an interest in this area), juvenile court (court diversion programs), and a police department's juvenile or gang unit (officers may be charismatic and often have a broad knowledge of community resources for adolescents).

JUVENILE GANGS

Although juvenile gangs are a long-standing phenomenon in the United States, they are perceived as major threats to a community's well-being. A gang is a group of individuals that has an identifiable leadership, organizational structure, and a developed system of symbolic representation and that engages in antisocial and criminal behaviors. Many gangs also have territorial identification. Beyond this definition, gangs are heterogeneous in their membership and level of organization, degree of involvement in aggressive violence, and use and sale of drugs. Major gangs have extensive rules and codes of conduct, as well as specialized symbols and alphabets. Although there are no accurate national data on gang membership and gang activity distribution geographically, gangs, while present in suburban and rural areas, appear to be concentrated in impoverished urban neighborhoods.

Children and adolescents join gangs for a variety of reasons. Many drift into membership because gang activities dominate the social and economic structures of their neighborhoods and provide opportunities for recognition and status, money, physical protection and safety, and a social life. Gang membership, similar to membership in conventional prosocial youth organizations, is congruent with the developmental tasks of adolescence. It offers the peer associations that allow emancipation from the family unit, and it promotes a sense of belonging through group identity. Positive gang values include respect and the forging of intimate bonds among members. However, gang membership, especially as adolescents become more deeply involved, also promotes a corruptive power that stems from the ability to intimidate others through physical aggression. Many gang members relish the excitement brought by participation in antisocial activities and violence, as well as the quick affluence brought by selling drugs. Some gangs' formal rules and expectations have such strong and pervasive influences that they discourage independent thinking by individual members and make it virtually impossible to resign membership peacefully.

Violent behaviors by gang members occur in a variety of contexts. First, new gang members' initiations virtually always involve ritual violence and humiliation because they need to demonstrate courage, a willingness to fight, and an ability to carry out orders. (Examples include being "beaten in," participating in a drive-by shooting, assaulting an innocent victim, and for girls, being gang raped.) Second, internal violence occurs when members who disobey rules or leaders' orders are disciplined physically. Violence between members of rival gangs is founded on the needs for controlling territory and, very importantly, for maintaining or enhancing respect or honor.

Compared with other adolescents living in similar environments, youngsters who are gang members have significantly greater use of illicit drugs and engagement in a variety of violent and illegal activities. They also report higher rates of being victimized by others' physical aggression. Although gang members are less likely to be fully integrated with their families, they are as likely as non-gang youngsters to participate in conventional family, school, and neighborhood activities. It is probable that many gang members have some conventional values but that their behavior is shaped largely by gang membership.

Clinical Issues

Primary care clinicians may be able to identify individuals who belong to gangs by noting unusual tattoos, special clothing (with care taken not to confuse clothing identifiers with contemporary adolescent fashion), nicknames (monikers) that have violent or seemingly bizarre connotations, stylized verbal and body language, and the appearance and demeanor of accompanying friends. Many adolescents who belong to gangs are secretive about their involvement and may deny their membership.

It is not necessary to confirm gang membership to determine whether an adolescent is asking for help in solving a problem or to discuss issues of personal safety, substance abuse, and expectations for the future. Although physically aggressive adolescents are likely to report anger as an emotional issue, they are less likely to report depression and anxiety.[20] However, some gang members are dismayed about the violence to which they are exposed and demonstrate mental health symptoms or request help leaving a gang. The clinician should recognize the social complexity of these adolescents' lives and the ambivalence and disloyalty that they may experience in questioning their gang involvement. In addition, they may jeopardize their personal safety if they attempt to distance themselves from gang activities. A primary care clinician who has gained the adolescent's trust and respect may eventually be able to refer the teenager to the community's juvenile or gang control unit for assistance in leaving the gang.

DATING VIOLENCE

A significant proportion of teenaged couples involved in romantic relationships exhibit physically violent behavior. These patterns presage the domestic violence of adult relationships and are more common among couples who have relationship insecurities and who have experienced family maltreatment or instability. About 10% to 25% of high school couples have physical or sexual coercion in their relationships, and the chance for its occurring increases with the duration of the relationship. In contrast to the dominant pattern of male coercion in adult relationships, the physical and sexual coercion of adolescent relationships is more evenly divided between the male and female partners. However, given her smaller body mass and lesser strength, the female partner remains at significantly greater risk for sustaining physical injury. Many teenagers do not recognize violence in dating relationships as destructive but may interpret it as a sign of love, caring, and commitment. It is important to prevent and intervene with such violence before its behavioral patterns become ingrained and cause domestic violence in adult relationships. Many communities now offer programming for youthful romantic couples whose relationships contain elements of coercive and violent behavior.[23] Violence between romantic partners is not limited to heterosexual couples; it also is a major problem for gay couples, who may have even greater difficulty disclosing it because of the stigma attached to homosexual relationships.

VIOLENCE AT SCHOOL (See also Chapter 23 [Four], Violence Prevention)

Violent crimes are common occurrences at school or while going to or from school. Although there has been a 33% improvement since 1993, the overall school crime rate was 102 incidents per 1000 junior and high school students in 1997; about 10% were serious violent crimes.[22] That same year, about 7% of high school students reported being threatened or injured with a weapon on school property at least once during the preceding 12 months. In addition, about 20% of all middle and high schools reported serious violent incidents to the police during the 1996-97 school year.[21] Not surprisingly, many students feel vulnerable and are afraid to go to school. In 1997, about 4% of high school students felt too unsafe to attend school at least once during the preceding month.[4,22] Students attending schools serving lower income urban and suburban communities report the chronic effects of daily exposure to the tension of multiple acts of verbal and physical hostility and aggression between and among students, because provocation and confrontation are frequent occurrences. The emotional tension associated with vigilance for, avoidance of, and the need to respond accurately to provocation makes it difficult for students to attend to learning and for faculty to teach effectively.[9]

Bullying

Recurrent bullying of vulnerable children and young adolescents by aggressive agemates or older youngsters is a common phenomenon at school. About 15% of young adolescents report having been bullied because of their race or religion[22]; the proportion of youngsters who are bullied for other reasons is unknown. Teachers and classmates perceive bullied children as shy, passive or submissive, and insecure; they do not provoke attacks upon themselves. Bullied children report anxiety and also may be rejected socially. As young adults, they appear to function well and are not likely to be bullied at work, but are likely to be depressed and have low self-esteem. The primary care clinician can identify bullied adolescents by assessing the quality of their peer relationships. They may benefit from programs that teach assertive social skills. Whole-school intervention programs aimed at changing students' social norms appear to function effectively.[9]

Multiple-Victim Homicides

At least one nationally reported, tragic episode of student-perpetrated violence, in which multiple victims were shot and killed or severely wounded, has occurred on the campuses of United States public schools each school year since 1992-93 except 1993-94. Five such incidents occurred during school year 1997-98. That year a total of 46 deaths by homicide on public school campuses occurred, including the multiple homicide victims.[22] The incident that had the largest number of victims to date occurred in suburban Colorado during 1999. Each episode has taken its surrounding community by surprise and has left severely traumatized students, faculty, and families as an aftermath. Some of the lessons learned from these tragedies, which have taken place in suburban and rural settings, have been the realizations that the young students who committed such devastatingly horrifying acts have serious mental health problems that had not previously been recognized, identified, or addressed; that mental health problems among students are common; that our schools need assistance in identifying students in need and providing assistance to them and their families; that middle class communities are not immune to the consequences of the interaction between disturbed youth and firearms; and that the school social environment, climate, or milieu is very important to students' mental health, behavior, and ability to focus on academic work.

Schools are excellent sites for reducing violent behavior among young people. Four proactive strategies include developing students' social bonding to their school and commitment to academic success, promoting anti-violence attitudes among students, teaching conflict resolution skills, and minimizing the availability and acceptance of weapons.[9]

ADOLESCENTS VICTIMIZED BY AGGRESSION AND VIOLENCE

Adolescents have the highest rate of victimization by violent crime of any age group. In 1997, 88 per 1000 12- to 15-year-olds and 96 per 1000 16- to 19-year-olds were victimized.[21] Adolescents who themselves behave aggressively and engage in violent behavior are at heightened risk for victimization, including physical injury and death.

Adolescents who belong to minority groups may be at special risk for victimization by hate-motivated aggression. In addition to race, minority status may include sexual orientation, ethnicity/national origin, religion, social class, and disability.[22] However, victims of hate crimes frequently do not report them to the police because of stigma and fear. Victimized adolescents whose families compose a significant proportion of residents in the community may engage in reciprocal aggression against their attackers.

Adolescents who have been exposed to serious acts of

violence report a variety of mental health symptoms, including depression, anger, anxiety, and dissociation.[14] However, many teenagers who have witnessed violence or have been victimized may not volunteer such information spontaneously. It is important clinically, therefore, to ask adolescents who have mental health symptoms about acute or recurrent exposure to violence or whether such events have happened to friends or members of their families. In particular, adolescents may show depression or recurrent somatic symptoms linked to anxiety (see Chapters 100, Conversion Reactions in Adolescents, and 158, Nervousness). They may display features of posttraumatic stress disorder, which may function as a mediating factor for problems such as depression and suicidal ideation.[14] Adolescents exposed to violence may report fear of dying and may have difficulty sleeping and concentrating, with a concomitant deterioration in school performance, or may avoid situations that arouse recollection of the trauma. Many adolescents welcome insight into the etiology of their somatic symptoms and mental health problems. Adolescents who have significant psychological symptoms should be referred for mental health evaluation and treatment.

REFERENCES

1. Alpert EJ, et al: Interpersonal violence and the education of physicians, *Acad Med* 72(suppl):S41, 1997.
2. American Academy of Pediatrics, Task Force on Violence: The role of the pediatrician in youth violence prevention in clinical practice and at the community level, *Pediatrics* 103:173, 1999.
3. Borowsky IW, Ireland M: National survey of pediatricians' violence prevention counseling: *Arch Pediatr Adolesc Med* 153:1170, 1999.
4. Brener ND, et al: Recent trends in violence-related behaviors among high school students in the United States, *JAMA* 282:440, 1999.
5. Bureau of Justice Statistics, Office of Justice Programs, US Department of Justice: Homicide trends in the US, 1998. http://www.ojp.usdoj.gov/bjs/homicide
6. Cadoret RJ, et al: Genetics of aggressive and violent behavior, *Psychiatr Clin North Am* 20:301, 1997.
7. Dahlberg LL: Youth violence in the United States: major trends, risk factors, and prevention approaches, *Am J Prev Med* 14:259, 1998.
8. Ellickson P, et al: Profiles of violent youth: substance use and other concurrent problems, *Am J Public Health* 87:985, 1997.
9. Elliott DS, Hamburg BA, Williams KR, editors: *Violence in American schools,* New York, 1998, Cambridge University Press.
10. Herrenkohl TI, et al: Developmental risk factors for youth violence, *J Adolesc Health* 26:176, 2000.
11. Hoyert DL, et al: *Deaths: final data for 1997,* National Vital Statistics Reports, National Center for Health Statistics, Centers for Disease and Control and Prevention, USPHS, USDHHS, June 30, 1999.
12. Kavoussi R, et al: The neurobiology of impulsive aggression, *Psychiatr Clin North Am* 20:395, 1997.
13. Kellerman AK, et al: Preventing youth violence: what works? *Ann Rev Public Health* 19:271, 1998.
14. Mazza JJ, Reynolds WM: Exposure to violence in young inner-city adolescents: relationships with suicidal ideation, depression, and PTSD symptomatology, *J Abnorm Child Psychol* 27:203, 1999.
15. Orpinas P, et al: Parental influences on students' aggressive behaviors and weapon carrying, *Health Educ Behav* 26:774, 1999.
16. Pettit GS: The developmental course of violence and aggression, *Psychiatr Clin North Am* 20:283, 1997.
17. Scarpe A, Raine A: Psychophysiology of anger and violent behavior, *Psychiatr Clin North Am* 20:375, 1997.
18. Sege R, et al: Ten years after: examination of adolescent screening questions that predict future violence-related injury, *J Adolesc Health* 24:395, 1999.
19. Shahpar C, Li G: Homicide mortality in the United States: 1935-1994: age, period, cohort effects, *Am J Epidemiol* 150:1213, 1999.
20. Song LY, Singer MI, Anglin TM: Violence exposure and emotional trauma as contributors to adolescents' violent behaviors, *Arch Pediatr Adolesc Med* 152:531, 1998.
21. US Census Bureau: Statistical abstract of the United States: 1999 (ed 119), Washington, DC, 1999.
22. US Department of Education and US Department of Justice: 1999 Annual report on school safety.
23. Wekerle C, Wolfe DA: Dating violence in mid-adolescence: theory, significance, and emerging prevention initiatives, *Clin Psychol Rev* 19:435, 1999.

part seven

Presenting Signs and Symptoms

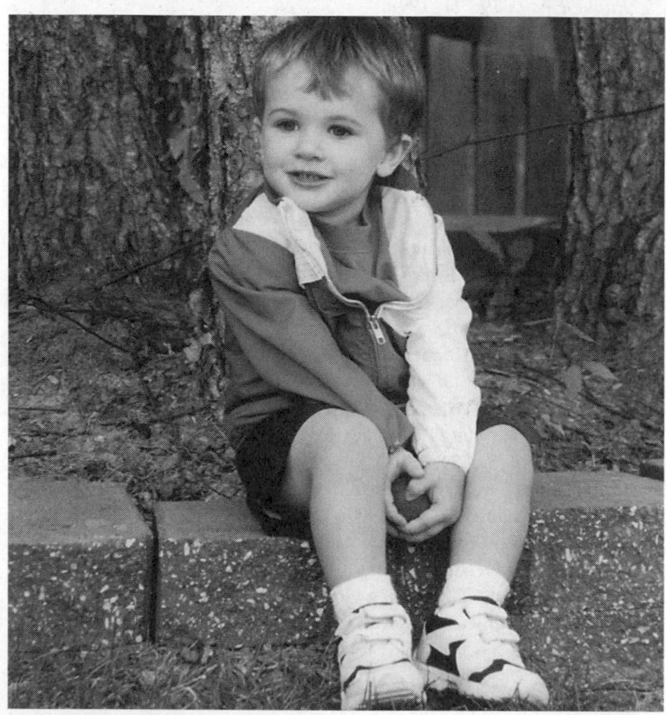

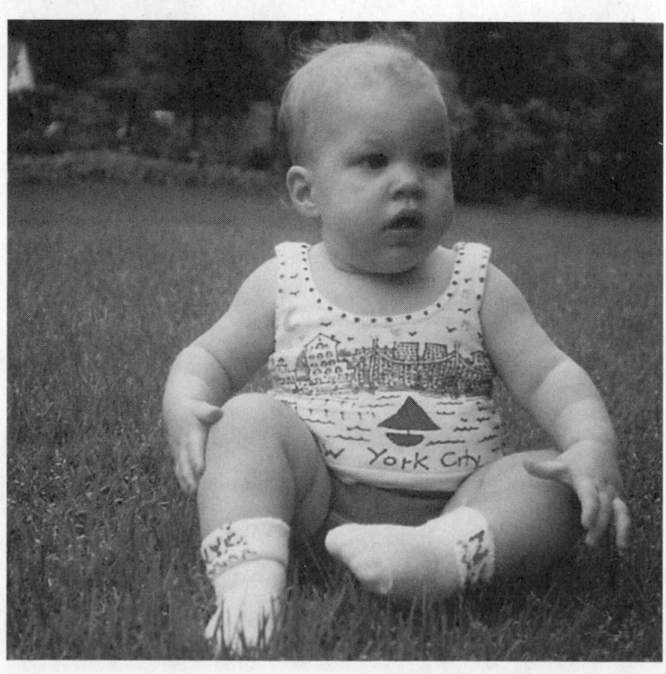

143 Hematuria

144 Hemoptysis

145 Hepatomegaly

146 High Blood Pressure in Infants, Children, and Adolescents

147 Hirsutism, Hypertrichosis, and Precocious Sexual Hair Development

148 Hoarseness

149 Hyperhidrosis

150 Hypotonia

151 Irritability

152 Jaundice

153 Joint Pian

154 Limp

155 Loss of Appetite

156 Lymphadenopathy

157 Malocclusion

158 Nervousness

159 Nonconvulsive Periodic Disorders

160 Odor (Unusual Urine and Body)

161 Petechiae and Purpura

162 Polyruia

163 Proteinuria

164 Pruritus

165 Puberty: Normal and Abnormal

166 Rash

167 Recurrent Infections

168 Red Eye

169 Scrotal Swelling

170 Splenomegaly

171 Strabismus

172 Strange Behavior

173 Stridor

174 Syncope

175 Tics

176 Torticollis

177 Vaginal Bleeding

178 Vaginal Discharge

179 Visual Disturbance

180 Vomiting

181 Weight Loss

182 Wheezing

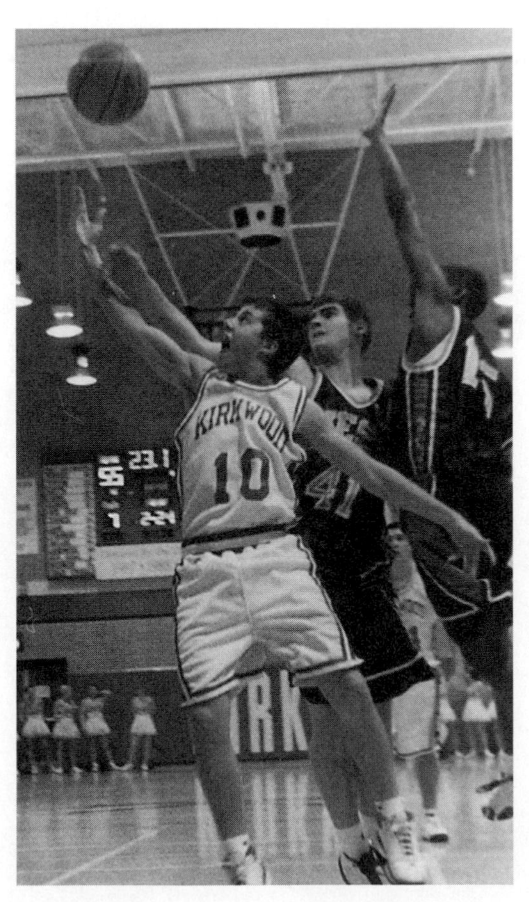

113 Abdominal Distention

Peter F. Belamarich

The child who has abdominal distention can be a formidable clinical challenge. The number of possible diagnoses is large, and the most likely diagnosis varies greatly with the child's age. Furthermore, not all distention is pathological. Healthy infants may have variable degrees of abdominal distention caused by aerophagia during feeding or crying or from transient constipation; healthy toddlers have a "pot belly" resulting from a combination of lumbar lordosis and hypotonia of the abdominal rectus muscles. This nonpathological distention often seen in infants and toddlers may exceed the mild distention seen with some intraabdominal malignancies. Thus, it is not surprising that numerous cautionary tales exist of parents being reassured by a physician that a child's mild and otherwise asymptomatic abdominal distention was "normal," only later to learn that in actuality it was a tumor. Therefore, a careful systematic approach should be employed whenever concerns about abdominal distention are raised.

APPROACH TO THE CHILD WHO HAS ABDOMINAL DISTENTION

History

Historical clues to the etiology of distention in newborns often are absent, although they may at times be found in the pregnancy history. Thus, a history of oligohydramnios suggests distal urinary obstruction, whereas polyhydramnios is seen with upper gastrointestinal obstruction. Although the burgeoning use of prenatal sonography has led to the increased antenatal recognition of numerous congenital conditions, particularly hydronephrosis, sonography is not as sensitive or diagnostically accurate prenatally as is sonography done on the newborn; therefore, a report of a "normal" prenatal sonogram does not rule out congenital causes of abdominal distention.

In older infants and children, the history should establish the duration and pattern of the child's distention. Whereas intermittent distention suggests intermittent gastrointestinal obstruction, progressive distention suggests an intraabdominal tumor. One must be careful to differentiate a parent's question about whether a toddler's pot-belly appearance is normal from more ominous reports of progressive or marked distention. When parents report that they have felt an abdominal mass, radiological evaluation is indicated even if the physician does not appreciate it. Constitutional symptoms such as fever, weight loss, failure to thrive, anorexia, fatigue, irritability, or bone pain also suggest a malignancy; however, their absence does not exclude one. Next, a systematic review of symptoms referable to the intraabdominal organs should be sought. Symptoms of gastrointestinal obstruction (vomiting, distention, pain, obstipation, delayed passage of meconium at birth) or malabsorption (diarrhea or greasy, bulky, malodorous stools) should be sought. The possibility of occult hydronephrosis should be considered. In the newborn, this may present initially as an asymptomatic flank mass. In older infants and children, recurrent fever from urinary tract infection (often misdiagnosed as viral illness or otitis media), gross hematuria following minor trauma, and voiding difficulty in boys who have posterior urethral valves are possible presentations.

A confidential history of sexual activity in all adolescent females who have abdominal distention should be obtained, as well as a history of the onset of puberty and menarche.

Preexisting conditions that should be reviewed include any prior intraabdominal surgery or a history of necrotizing enterocolitis. The family history should include questions about cystic fibrosis (meconium ileus), polycystic kidney disease, and whether there is any prior history of fetal demise or early neonatal deaths that could indicate an unrecognized metabolic disease, some of which produce hepatomegaly, splenomegaly, and/or congenital ascites.

Although rare, the presence of conditions that predispose a child to an intraabdominal malignancy should be remembered. In the case of Wilms' tumor, these include genitourinary anomalies, hemihypertrophy, aniridia, and Beckwith-Wiedemann syndrome (macrosomia, macroglossia, visceromegaly, and omphalocele). An increased incidence of neuroblastoma is observed in children who have Hirschsprung's disease, Beckwith-Wiedemann syndrome, and neurofibromatosis.[5]

Physical Examination

The profile of the abdomen with the child in a supine position should be inspected, noting whether the distention is generalized (maximal at the umbilicus) or localized. Box 113-1 presents commonly encountered etiologies for focal abdominal distention and common masses. The degree of lumbar lordosis should be noted in toddlers. The pattern and prominence of the abdominal veins should be noted. Prominent superficial veins on the abdomen may indicate portal hypertension or obstruction to the systemic venous return. The abdomen should be auscultated for hyperactive bowel sounds (malabsorption, acute obstruction), rushes (incomplete obstruction), and absence of sounds (paralytic ileus), as well as for bruits (vascular malformation).

Gentle palpation should begin from the lower quadrants and progress upward, so that the inferior edge of the liver and spleen are appreciated (massive hepatomegaly may be missed if the liver is compressible and the liver's edge is near the child's pelvis). The abdomen should be assessed for focal or generalized tenderness. Involuntary guarding noted on gentle palpation is a sensitive sign of peritoneal inflammation; assessment of rebound tenderness in young children is rife with false-positive results.

When an abdominal mass is appreciated, the examiner should note its location, whether it is painful, is mobile (intraabdominal) or nonmobile (retroperitoneal, malignant), moves with respiration (liver and spleen), is cystic or solid, is smooth or nodular, and whether it crosses the midline (often seen with neuroblastoma). Although rectal examination often is avoided as unduly invasive, properly done it can add considerable information to the evaluation of children who have constipation, anal stenosis, Hirschsprung's disease, and pelvic masses. Parents who are skeptical about the need for rectal examination are sometimes accepting when it is explained that intestinal bleeding can be excluded by the stool guaiac test.

Infants who have ascites will have bilateral bulging flanks in the supine position. In older children who have ascites, it may be possible to elicit shifting dullness and a fluid wave. An acquired umbilical hernia may indicate massive ascites.

In females, a genital examination is necessary to exclude imperforate hymen with hydrometrocolpos, or hematocolpos and pregnancy in adolescents. In both sexes, lower genitourinary tract malformation raises the question of upper genitourinary tract malformation.

BOX 113-1

CAUSES OF FOCAL ABDOMINAL DISTENTION OR MASS

Epigastrium
Duodenal atresia
Pyloric stenosis
Malrotation
Gastric duplication
Bezoar

Flank
Wilms' tumor
Hydronephrosis
Multicystic kidney
Polycystic kidney
Neuroblastoma
Renal vein thrombosis
Adrenal hemorrhage

Right Upper Quadrant
Choledochal cyst
Hepatomegaly
Hepatic tumors
Acute hydrops of the gallbladder

Left Upper Quadrant
Splenomegaly
Splenic cyst

Right Lower Quadrant
Intussusception
Appendiceal abscess
Crohn's disease
Fecal mass

Left Lower Quadrant
Ovarian mass
Fecal mass

Hypogastrium
Hydrometrocolpos
Hematocolpos
Presacral teratoma
Obstructed bladder
Urachal cyst

DIFFERENTIAL DIAGNOSIS

Table 113-1 narrows the differential diagnosis based on whether the child has a tympanitic abdomen, a palpable mass, ascites, or hypotonia of the abdominal wall. Hepatomegaly and splenomegaly are important causes of abdominal distention; these are reviewed in Chapter 145 and Chapter 170, respectively.

Tympanitic Abdomen

The newborn and neonate. Tympanitic abdominal distention may occur in healthy infants, in infants who have systemic conditions, and in newborns who have congenital causes of intestinal obstruction.

Some healthy infants experience mild distention because of air swallowing with crying and/or feeding. Their distention is variable, being greatest after feeding or "fussing" and being absent at other times. Vomiting is absent, and the stool-

Table 113-1 Differential Diagnosis of Abdominal Distention Based on Physical Examination Findings

Physical Sign	Possible Causes
Tympanitic abdomen	Gastrointestinal ileus Gastrointestinal obstruction Malabsorption Aerophagia Pneumoperitoneum
Palpable mass	Renal Adrenal/sympathetic Gastrointestinal Mesenteric/omentum Uterine/vaginal/ovarian Splenic/lymphatic
Ascites	Urinary Idiopathic Cardiac Hepatic Biliary/gastrointestinal Chylous
Abdominal wall hypotonia	Generalized hypotonia Rickets Hypothyroidism

ing pattern and physical examination are normal. This transient generalized distention responds to changes in feeding technique and burping and in consoling techniques for the crying infant.

In the ill newborn, many systemic conditions cause a paralytic intestinal ileus characterized by quiet, nontender abdominal distention. These conditions include sepsis, birth asphyxia, hypothyroidism, and electrolyte imbalance. Newborns who have pneumonia or respiratory distress may also develop distention from aerophagia.

The most common cause of acquired abdominal distention in premature infants is necrotizing enterocolitis (NEC), typically a disease of ill, very low–birth-weight infants. NEC affects 1 to 2/1000 live births and is characterized by focal areas of small intestinal or colonic ischemia, thrombosis, and bacterial invasion. Signs of NEC include generalized distention, vomiting, occult or frank gastrointestinal bleeding in association with temperature instability, and apnea. Transmural intestinal necrosis may ensue, causing perforation with peritonitis, or an ominous gray-blue discoloration of the affected bowel appreciable through the abdominal wall. Definitive radiographic evidence of NEC includes findings of (1) pneumatosis intestinalis and (2) gas visible in the portal venous system of the liver (Fig. 113-1). Shock, disseminated intravascular coagulation, and uncorrectable metabolic acidosis are complications of severe NEC that mandate emergent resection of the affected bowel.

Congenital causes of proximal gastrointestinal obstruction in the newborn include intestinal atresia, annular pancreas, abnormalities of intestinal rotation, and fixation (see Chapter 210, Gastrointestinal Obstruction). The most common proximal gastrointestinal obstruction is duodenal atresia,[1] characterized by polyhydramnios in 50% and the onset of bilious vomiting in the first hours of life in conjunction with focal epigastric distention (Fig. 113-2). At times, forceful gastroduodenal peristaltic waves are appreciable through the abdominal wall.

Upright plain radiographs are diagnostic of duodenal obstruction when they demonstrate the double bubble sign (see Fig. 210-1). Occasionally, it is necessary to evacuate the stomach of bile and amniotic fluid and instill air to appreciate this. Although intestinal atresias themselves are not operative emergencies, they are medical emergencies in so far as urgent decompression via nasogastric suction is indicated to diminish the risk of aspiration and gastrointestinal perforation while fluid and electrolyte abnormalities are corrected. However, because malrotation is seen in up to 19% of patients who have intrinsic duodenal obstruction, a barium enema should be obtained to establish normal placement of the cecum (which rules out malrotation) in those infants whose surgery is deferred.

Upper abdominal distention is a common, though not universal, finding in newborns and infants who have symptomatic intestinal malrotation (Fig. 113-3),[6] the majority of whom present in the first 4 weeks of life with bilious vomiting. It should be noted that 25% of infants who have malrotation may have nonbilious vomiting at presentation, and a high index of suspicion is warranted, given the severe morbidity of a delay in diagnosis. Plain radiographs may demonstrate a distended stomach or duodenal distention that has a paucity of gas distally (Fig. 113-4). Most significantly, plain radiographs may appear normal. Therefore, a stable infant suspected of having malrotation should undergo an upper gastrointestinal series, which is diagnostic when the duodenal-jejunal junction is seen on the right side of the midline or when there is a beak or corkscrew obstruction noted in the second or third part of the duodenum. Symptomatic malrotation is an operative emergency whether or not signs of intestinal ischemia (hematochezia, acidosis, shock, a blue-gray tinge to the abdomen, or peritonitis) have developed.

Congenital causes of lower intestinal obstruction include distal intestinal atresias, meconium ileus (Fig. 113-5), Hirschsprung's disease, small left colon syndrome, and anorectal malformations (see Chapter 210, Gastrointestinal Obstruction). Newborns who have lower intestinal obstruction typically develop generalized tympanitic distention over the

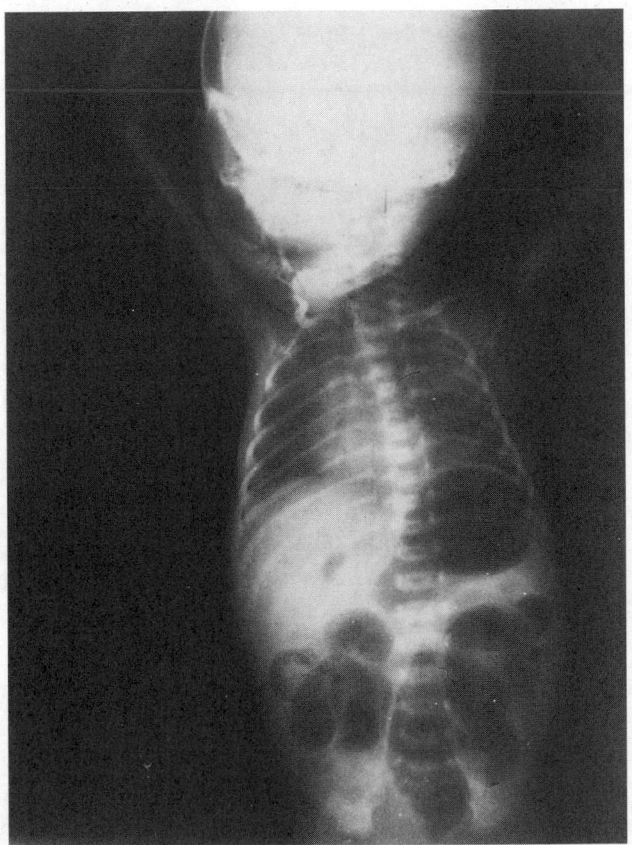

Fig. 113-1 Premature infant with necrotizing enterocolitis showing gas in the wall of the intestine and in the liver.

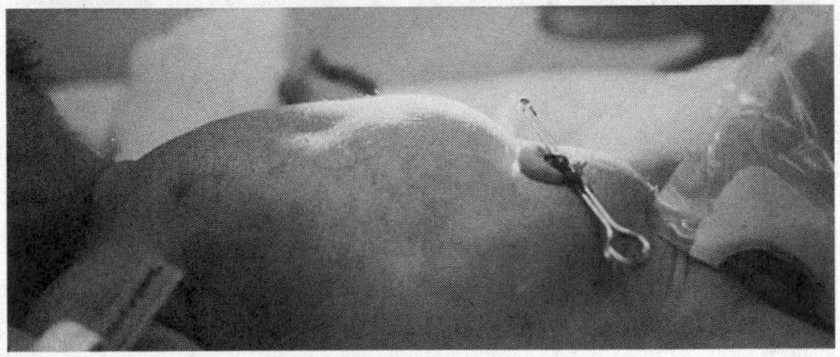

Fig. 113-2 Newborn infant with duodenal atresia and upper abdominal distention.

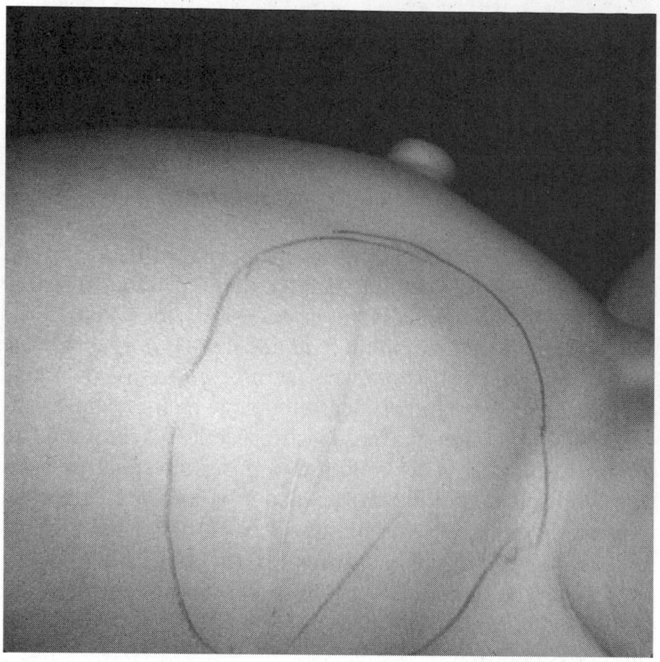

Fig. 113-3 Newborn with distention secondary to torsion.

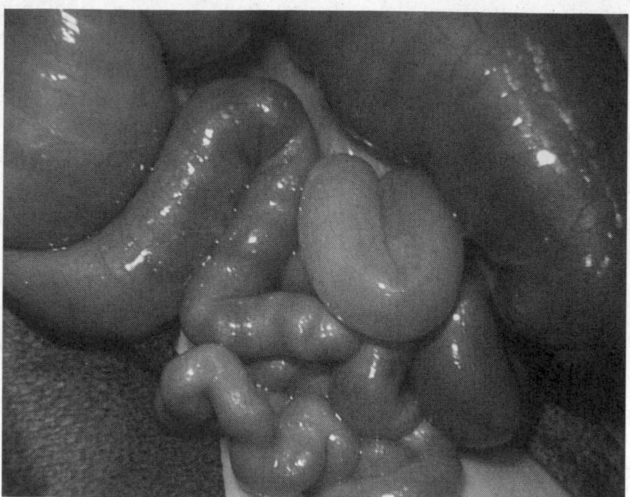

Fig. 113-5 Distal ileum segment with inspissated meconium secondary to meconium ileus surrounded by lilated proximal loops of bowel.

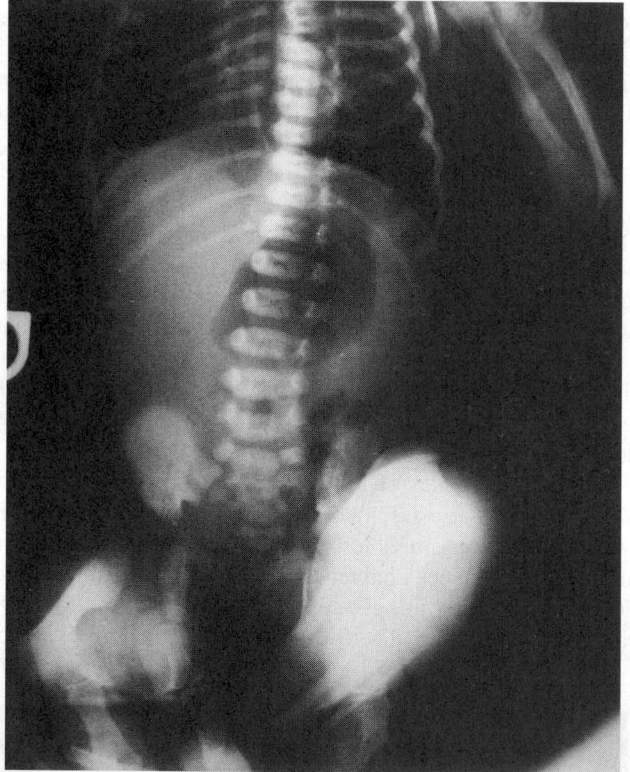

Fig. 113-4 Malrotation with distended stomach and paucity of distal gas.

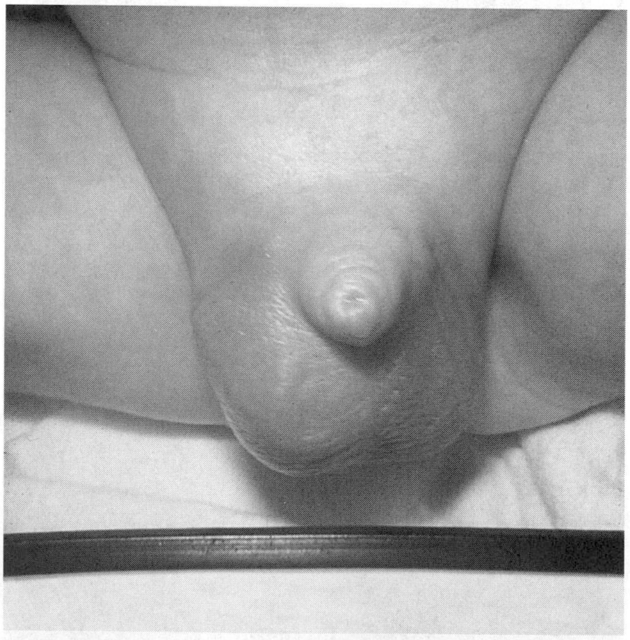

Fig. 113-6 Incarcerated right inguinal hernia in a newborn.

course of 24 to 48 hours, with bilious vomiting and failure to pass meconium. Although an imperforate anus or an incarcerated hernia (Fig. 113-6) will be apparent on physical examination, differentiation of the remaining causes of lower intestinal obstruction involves radiographic evaluation (outlined in Table 210-2).

Marked tympanitic abdominal distention can be a manifestation of pneumoperitoneum, which is demonstrated by upright and cross-table lateral abdominal radiographs revealing free air within the peritoneum. When this occurs as a complication of intestinal perforation, the associated peritonitis produces an ill newborn who has a tense, tender, and

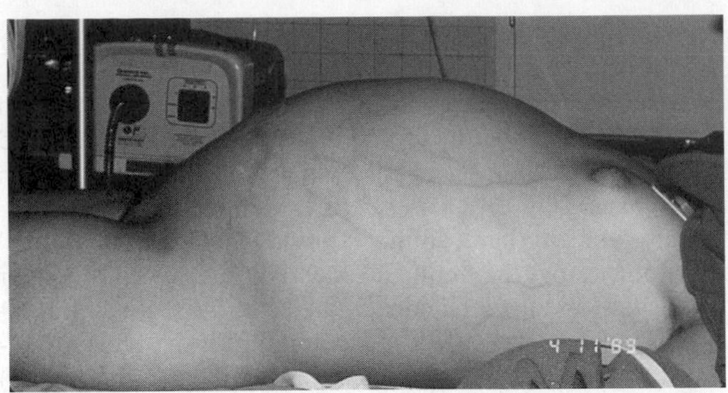

Fig. 113-7 Thirteen-year-old girl with stool withholding.

quiet abdomen. The most common cause of intestinal perforation is NEC; however, isolated spontaneous intestinal perforations affecting the stomach, duodenum, ileum, and colon do occur. Furthermore, intestinal perforation can complicate midgut volvulus, intestinal obstruction, and meconium ileus. In infants on a respirator, pneumoperitoneum may occur without peritonitis as a complication of pneumomediastinum when air tracts down through diaphragmatic fenestrations into the peritoneal cavity.

Postneonatal causes. Beyond the neonatal period, the etiology of a tympanitic abdomen includes constipation, mechanical obstruction, paralytic ileus, and malabsorption.

Idiopathic constipation is extremely common throughout childhood but is accompanied only infrequently by abdominal distention (Fig. 113-7). The diagnosis is supported by a history of hard or large, infrequent stools beginning after the neonatal period. Frequently, periumbilical pain is present. Rectal examination should reveal a hard, large fecal mass in a generous rectal vault. Occasionally a plain radiograph is necessary to establish the diagnosis when the rectal examination fails to reveal a fecal mass. The child's distention should be relieved completely by an enema or laxative therapy. Constipation associated with persistent distention that is refractory to therapy or that has its origins in the first month of life is suggestive of Hirschsprung's disease.

Gastrointestinal obstructions that cause a tympanitic abdomen beyond the neonatal period are discussed in Chapter 210, Gastrointestinal Obstruction. Some represent "late presentations" of congenital problems, rather than newly acquired obstructions. Thus, up to 20% of infants who have Hirschsprung's disease are diagnosed after the first year of life as having refractory constipation,[3] and one third of patients who have malrotation present beyond the neonatal period with episodes of intermittent obstruction.

Causes of acquired gastrointestinal obstruction beyond the neonatal period include pyloric stenosis, intussusception, postoperative adhesions, appendiceal abscesses, and intraluminal obstructions. In advanced cases of pyloric stenosis, forceful peristaltic waves moving from left to right in the epigastrium are visible through the abdominal wall. Vomiting relieves the distention, and the infant remains hungry. The diagnosis can be confirmed with palpation of an olive-sized mass in the right upper quadrant or sonographically by the demonstration of an elongated and thickened pyloric tumor (see Chapter 255, Pyloric Stenosis). Tympanitic distention may be seen in children who have intussusception; however, this is a late and relatively unusual sign preceded characteristically by intermittent pain, vomiting, rectal bleeding, or lethargy. Crampy abdominal pain progressing to bilious vomiting accompanied by generalized tympanitic distention and high-pitched bowel sounds is seen in children who have mechanical bowel obstruction from postoperative adhesions, of which 80% to 90% occur within 1 to 2 years of the initial operation. A similar picture may occur in the 10% to 30% of infants who develop obstructive intestinal stenoses following an episode of severe necrotizing enterocolitis. These stenoses typically involve the left colon and may remain asymptomatic for up to 1 year before presentation. Early in their clinical presentations, both adhesions and stenoses following NEC frequently are misdiagnosed as "gastroenteritis," despite the typical absence of fever. Many of the abdominal masses described later in this chapter may compress the bowel and present clinically as either complete or partial bowel obstruction; this also is true for inflammatory masses, such as appendiceal abscesses, which promote the formation of obstructive adhesions. In many areas of the developing world, the most common cause of acquired bowel obstruction is an obstructing mass of *Ascaris lumbricoides* worms. Other intraluminal obstructions include bezoars, meconium ileus equivalent, intestinal polyps, and intrinsic tumors.

Children who have paralytic ileus present with a clinical picture similar to that seen with distal mechanical bowel obstruction; however, bowel sounds are diminished or absent, and plain radiographs demonstrate air throughout the gastrointestinal tract. Common precipitants include abdominal surgery, peritonitis, trauma, shock, sepsis, hypokalemia, and numerous medications. Recurrent attacks of unexplained ileus characterize intestinal pseudoobstruction syndrome.

Lastly, tympanitic distention occurs in conjunction with the fat malabsorption syndromes, cystic fibrosis, and celiac disease. These conditions are characterized by steatorrhea and malnutrition with muscle wasting, creating the picture of a thin-limbed child who has a bloated abdomen.

Abdominal Masses

The newborn and neonate. Two thirds of abdominal masses in neonates originate from the kidney or the urinary tract.[4] Renal masses are retroperitoneal, nonmobile, and appreciated either in the flank or on deep abdominal palpation. Cystic masses predominate and have a slightly compressible quality. A multicystic kidney is the single most common neonatal flank mass. It is unilateral in 70% to 80% of cases. The affected kidney lacks parenchyma, is associated with ipsilateral ureteral atresia, and is composed of macroscopically visible, variably sized, fluid-filled cysts that may be appreciable on physical examination as a soft mass with a slightly irregular contour.

The next renal mass encountered most frequently is caused by hydronephrosis (see Chapter 240, Obstructive Uropathy and Vesicoureteral Reflux). A smooth flank mass in an otherwise well newborn is due usually to ureteral-pelvic junction obstruction. Posterior urethral valves, a common cause of bilateral hydronephrosis and hydroureters in male infants, may present with a low-pressure urinary stream and bilateral flank masses or a palpable bladder. Newborns who have autosomal recessive polycystic kidney disease may present with palpable bilateral firm flank masses, oliguria, hematuria, and hypertension. Ultrasonography reveals the kidneys to be enlarged. Renal vein thrombosis is a rare but important cause of a smooth flank mass and hematuria, which develop concurrently in an ill newborn following an episode of asphyxia, sepsis, or dehydration, or in an infant whose mother has diabetes.

Lastly, the most common renal tumor encountered in the newborn is not Wilms' tumor but mesoblastic nephroma, a surgically curable tumor that may cause massive unilateral nephromegaly.

The remaining one third of neonatal abdominal masses arise outside of the urinary tract. Of these, neuroblastoma, gastrointestinal duplications, hydrometrocolpos, and ovarian cysts account for a large proportion.[4] Neuroblastomas are discussed elsewhere on this page. Gastrointestinal duplications, which may be found as mobile asymptomatic abdominal masses in the newborn, arise most often from the jejunum, ileum, or cecum. Duplications may obstruct the gastrointestinal tract by direct compression or by acting as a lead point for an intussusception or for a volvulus, or they may contain heterotopic gastric mucosa that produces enough acid to cause an ulceration, resulting in lower gastrointestinal bleeding and sometimes perforation with peritonitis.

Female newborns may have a lower abdominal or pelvic mass from hydrometrocolpos, which develops as a result of an upper or lower vaginal obstruction in combination with a secretory response to a high level of maternal estrogens in utero. When this is caused by an imperforate hymen, it will be evident on the genital examination as a bulging round membrane within the introitus. Rectal examination confirms the presence of a dilated vagina. Maternal estrogens may also induce the development of a large functional or follicular ovarian cyst in newborns.

When a neonate has a palpable flank mass following a traumatic or breech delivery, the possibility of an adrenal hemorrhage should be considered, as should hepatic and splenic hematomas. Other hepatic masses and hepatomegaly are discussed in Chapter 145, Hepatomegaly. Although rare, a number of benign epithelial cysts may present in the neonatal period, including choledochal cysts (right upper quadrant), splenic cysts (left upper quadrant), mesenteric cysts (mid-abdominal, mobile in the transverse plane), and urachal cysts (hypogastrium). Retroperitoneal cysts include abdominal lymphangiomas and pancreatic cysts.

Postneonatal causes. The differential diagnosis of masses in infants and older children includes late presentations of congenital masses, malignancies, fecal masses, bezoars, and pancreatic pseudocysts. Of the congenital masses, gastrointestinal duplications, mesenteric cysts, and choledochal cysts may enlarge slowly and present in later infancy or childhood. Similarly, an adolescent who has an imperforate hymen or vaginal septum may not become symptomatic with a pelvic mass from hematocolpos until the onset of cyclical uterine bleeding.

The abdomen is the site of origin of Wilms' tumor, hepatic tumors, ovarian tumors, approximately 70% of neuroblastomas, and 30% of non-Hodgkin's lymphomas (see Chapter 193, Cancers in Childhood). Neuroblastoma, Wilms' tumor, and hepatoblastoma in particular have a propensity to produce asymptomatic abdominal distention that frequently is noted by the parent during bathing or dressing the child or by the physician on routine physical examination. Neuroblastoma is seen in newborns and also is the most common solid tumor in the first year of life. It arises from the adrenal gland or from the retroperitoneal paraspinal sympathetic ganglia in approximately 70% of cases. On examination, neuroblastomas are typically hard, immobile, and in contrast to Wilms' tumor, may cross the midline. They may be painful or tender to palpation and the incidence of metastatic disease at presentation is approximately 70%, accounting for the greater likelihood of constitutional symptoms (fever, anemia, bone pain) at presentation than with either Wilms' tumor or hepatoblastoma. Wilms' tumor tends to occur in older infants and toddlers, with a peak incidence in 2- to 5-year-old children. Hypertension is common, and macroscopic hematuria occurs in one third of cases (Fig. 113-8). Hepatoblastoma, the most common primary hepatic malignancy in childhood, is also overwhelmingly discovered as an asymptomatic abdominal mass, with a median age at diagnosis of 12 months. In the second decade, tumors presenting as an abdominal mass are predominantly ovarian (Fig. 113-9) or non-Hodgkin's lymphoma (see Chapter 193, Cancers in Childhood).

Fecal masses are extremely common in childhood and adolescence; they may be found either in the right lower quadrant (when a redundant sigmoid colon loops to the right) or in the left lower quadrant. These masses are mobile, nontender, and malleable. Questionable cases should have plain radiographs to confirm the diagnosis. In those children not needing radiographs, reexamination after laxative therapy is mandatory to confirm that the masses are no longer present.

Bezoars, intragastric concretions of indigestible material, cause upper abdominal discomfort and a large mass. Most bezoars are seen in mentally retarded girls, commonly resulting from the ingestion of hair (Fig. 113-10).

Ascites

The newborn and neonate. The newborn who has ascites has a distended, nontympanitic abdomen with bulging and dullness in the flanks. These findings may be mimicked by a massively dilated bladder, a severely hydronephrotic kidney, or a large ovarian cyst. In the newborn, ascites results most often from urine leaking from an obstructed urinary tract that has suffered a spontaneous perforation; posterior urethral valves are a common precipitant.[2] Idiopathic or benign ascites, a diagnosis of exclusion, is equally frequent and resolves without treatment. Ascites can occur as a complication of congestive heart failure or of liver disease caused by congenital infections, galactosemia, or a lysosomal storage disease. Chylous ascites is a rare condition that occurs when lymphatic fluid leaks directly into the peritoneum because of a malformation or perforation of the intestinal lymphatics occurring in utero. The diagnosis is made by paracentesis, when the characteristic milky-appearing ascitic fluid is found to have a high level of triglycerides. Massive neonatal ascites may occur as a complication of meconium peritonitis after intestinal rupture in utero. Usually, this is a manifestation of intestinal obstruction, with intestinal contents producing an intense chemical peritonitis. Typically, diffuse calcifications and signs of obstruction are seen on plain radiographs.

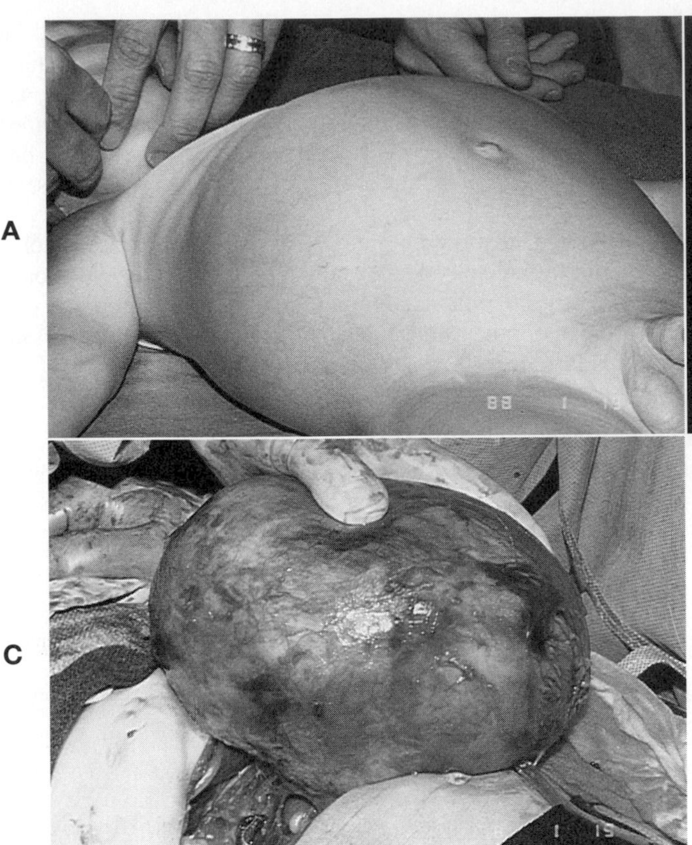

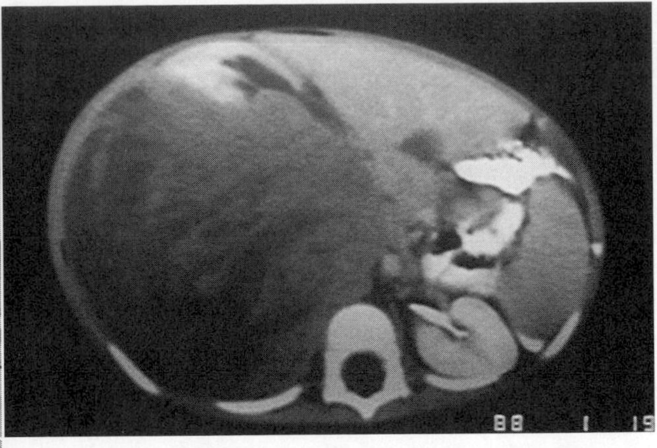

Fig. 113-8 **A,** Abdominal distention secondary to right Wilms' tumor. **B,** CT scan of tumor. **C,** Tumor exposed during surgery.

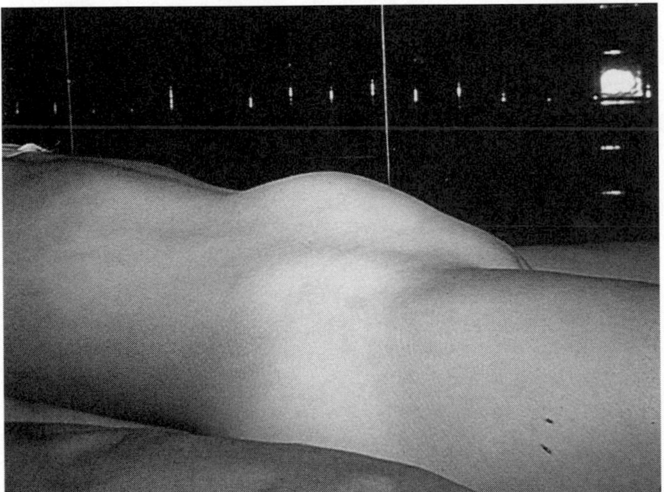

Fig. 113-9 Lower abdominal distention caused by ovarian teratoma.

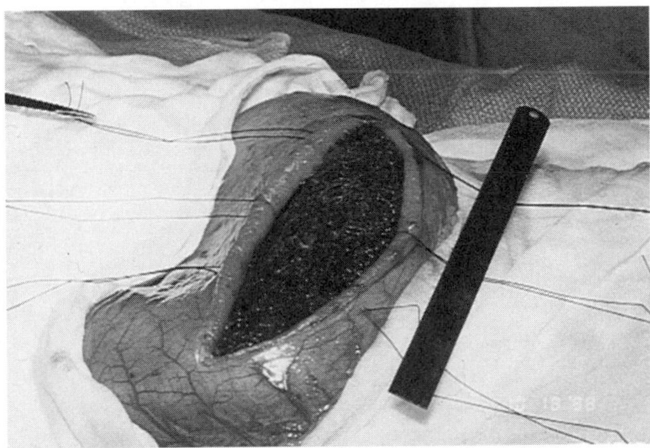

Fig. 113-10 Trichobezoar in the stomach.

Beyond the neonatal period, ascites occurs most commonly as a consequence of chronic liver disease with cirrhosis and portal hypertension.

Abdominal Wall Hypotonia

Abdominal distention frequently is encountered in healthy infants and also may be seen in infants who have varieties of neuromuscular conditions causing generalized hypotonia. In two treatable conditions, hypothyroidism and rickets, abdominal distention may be part of a subtle symptom complex that develops insidiously.

RADIOGRAPHIC APPROACH

Although the history and physical examination sometimes will provide a precise diagnosis, many children who have abdominal distention require radiographic imaging. The choice of initial imaging modality is dictated both by clinical suspicion and by locally available resources and expertise. Therefore, consulting with the radiologist is helpful.

The following general guidelines often apply. When the abdomen is tympanitic or gastrointestinal symptoms predominate, the initial study should be abdominal plain films obtained in the upright, supine, and prone positions. Used in conjunction with the clinical findings, plain films will differentiate mechanical gastrointestinal obstruction from paralytic ileus and constipation. The classic radiological signs of obstruction (distention and air-fluid levels proximally with collapse and a paucity of gas distally) may not be apparent early in an obstructive event. Further radiological investigation (unless urgent laparotomy is indicated) with serial plain films, GI contrast studies, or computed tomography (CT) scan may be used to localize and define the etiology more precisely. Pneumoperitoneum is diagnosed on upright or cross-table lateral radiographs; its presence warrants a chest radiograph to rule out pneumomediastinum, particularly in an infant on a respirator.

Sonography is invaluable in the initial assessment of palpable or suspected abdominal masses. It will definitively identify many pediatric masses (pyloric stenosis, pancreatic pseudocyst, choledochal cyst, ovarian cyst, multicystic kidney) and will differentiate effectively cystic from solid intraabdominal masses. When hydronephrosis is found on sonography, a staged evaluation is needed to differentiate from obstructive lesions; a combination of renal scintigraphy, excretory urography, and cystography usually is appropriate.[4]

When a solid mass is noted on sonography, CT and magnetic resonance imaging (MRI) are used to delineate its origin, size, and resectability.

If ascites is suspected, both plain radiography and sonography are useful. Both will differentiate centrally placed, large, fluid-filled cysts from true ascites. Plain films will be diagnostic when ascites accompanies meconium peritonitis because bowel obstruction, diffuse calcifications, and free air will be demonstrated. Sonography will detect small volumes of ascites and may reveal a dilated urinary tract that has ruptured, a large ruptured cyst, or the hepatomegaly seen with congestive heart failure or primary hepatic disease.

Lastly, distention reported or discovered in an asymptomatic child whose physical examination is inconclusive should be investigated with sonography because of the propensity of Wilms' tumor, neuroblastoma, and hepatoblastoma to present in this fashion.

Acknowledgement

The author wishes to thank Kenneth Kenigsberg, M.D., for providing the photographs used in this chapter.

REFERENCES

1. Fonkalsrud EW, et al: Congenital atresia and stenosis of the duodenum, *Pediatrics* 43:79, 1969.
2. Griscom NY, et al: Diagnostic aspects of neonatal ascites: report of 27 cases, *Am J Roentgenol* 128:961, 1977.
3. Kleinhaus S, et al: Hirschsprung's disease: a survey of the members of the surgical section of the American Academy of Pediatrics, *J Pediatr Surg* 14:588, 1979.
4. McVicar M, Margoulett D, Chandra M: Diagnosis and imaging of the fetal and neonatal abdominal mass: an integrated approach, *Adv Pediatr* 38:135, 1991.
5. Shapiro DN, et al: Molecular pathogenesis. In Behrman RE, Kliegman RM, Arvin AM, editors: *Nelson Textbook of pediatrics,* ed 15, Philadelphia, 1996, WB Saunders.
6. Torres MA, Ziegler MM: Malrotation of the intestine, *World J Surg* 17: 326, 1993.

114 Abdominal Pain

Jean C. Smith

Abdominal pain is one of the most common presenting symptoms of children and adolescents and is estimated to account for about 5% of pediatric office visits. Acute abdominal pain may require medical or surgical intervention to prevent disability or even death. The number of children who have had acute abdominal pain is unknown, but each year 4 in 1000 children have surgery for suspected appendicitis.[6] More often, abdominal pain is recurring and is not associated with physical disability or mortality. Yet recurring abdominal pain often results in serious dysfunction for both the child and the family. Apley[2] has estimated that 10% of school-age children are affected with recurring abdominal pain at some point in their development. In a community-based study of adolescents, 75% reported having had abdominal pain. Of the teens who had abdominal pain, 13% to 17% reported weekly pain, and about 21% had pain severe enough to interfere with their daily activities.[13]

CLINICAL CLASSIFICATION

Classification of abdominal pain as simply organic or nonorganic has ceased to be helpful. A more meaningful approach is to distinguish acute conditions that may require urgent or immediate intervention from the less life-threatening but nonetheless potentially disabling chronic or recurrent abdominal pains. Boxes 114-1 and 114-2 list some of the major diagnostic considerations for acute abdominal pain by pediatric age groups.[1,6,10,12-14] Although the diagnostic considerations clearly overlap for each age group, the child's age and physiological development can help the physician focus the differential diagnosis. For example, Hirschsprung's disease should be considered more likely in a young infant in the first weeks of life; pelvic inflammatory disease most certainly should be in the differential diagnosis for the adolescent female.

Acute Abdominal Pain

In the diagnosis of patients who have acute abdominal pain, it always is important to remember that many of the conditions that cause acute abdominal pain require immediate surgical or medical treatment. These conditions range from the infant who has intestinal malrotation or intussusception, who may develop bowel obstruction with bowel ischemia if appropriate surgical intervention is not performed, to the child or adolescent who has a urinary tract infection that requires appropriate antibiotic treatment to prevent progression of the infection. The possibility of drug reaction or overdose, or toxins, also should be considered as a cause of acute abdominal pain that requires immediate medical intervention. Eliminating further exposure to the offending agent is crucial, and specific detoxification or supportive care should be initiated promptly.

The concept of *referred pain* deserves special consideration when discussing acute abdominal pain in children. In these patients, a complete history may provide crucial information that suggests that the abdominal pain may originate outside the abdomen. Thus, a 3-year-old who has pneumonia may have inflammatory irritation of the diaphragm, resulting in acute abdominal pain as the presenting complaint. Also, testicular torsion can manifest as acute abdominal pain, and the physician should be sensitive to a teenager's possible reluctance to disclose a history of genital trauma or pain spontaneously.

Recurrent Abdominal Pain

Clinical studies have defined recurrent abdominal pain (RAP) as (1) occurring in children older than 3 years of age, (2) involving at least three episodes of pain over a period of more than 3 months, and (3) producing pain severe enough to limit the child's usual activities. Although this definition is useful for studying outcomes and the effect of treatment on the clinical course, it is less helpful for investigating the natural pattern of RAP in a particular patient. Researchers point out that in most studies, only the children are included who themselves or whose families express a concern about the pain. Other children may have similar painful experiences but because it either does not affect their usual activities or because they do not complain, they are not included in such studies.[17] The influence of age and developmental maturation, individual differences (e.g., temperament, coping patterns), family interactions, and the community and cultural contexts are hypothesized to influence the expression of RAP. Box 114-3 lists causes of recurrent RAP.

For RAP, the clinical categories "organic," "psychogenic," and "dysfunctional" can be helpful with the assessment and, more particularly, with the development of a treatment plan. The traditional model of RAP was modified by Barr[3] to include the larger category of "dysfunctional," in which no specific organic or psychological disease is identified. However, the category of dysfunctional pain includes conditions with identifiable primary physiological disorders of the abdomen such as chronic stool retention, lactose intol-

BOX 114-1

CAUSES OF ACUTE ABDOMINAL PAIN IN INFANCY AND EARLY CHILDHOOD

Gastrointestinal Causes
Meconium ileus
Hirschsprung's disease
Intestinal stenosis/atresia
Infectious enteritis/gastritis
Pyloric stenosis
Malrotation
Intestinal duplication
Inguinal hernia
Intussusception
Adhesions
Appendicitis

Genitourinary Causes
Testicular torsion
Urinary tract infection
Urinary obstruction (posterior urethral valves, tumors)

Trauma
Intraluminal hematoma
Pancreatic pseudocyst

Drugs/Toxins
Lead
Lactose intolerance
Salicylates
Erythromycin
Ibuprofen

Other
Sickle cell disease
Henoch-Schönlein purpura
Primary peritonitis
Pneumonia

BOX 114-2

CAUSES OF ACUTE ABDOMINAL PAIN IN LATE CHILDHOOD AND ADOLESCENCE

Gastrointestinal Causes
Appendicitis
Adhesions
Infectious enteritis/gastritis
Intussusception
Obstruction
Gastroesophageal reflux
Ulcer
Inguinal hernia

Genitourinary Causes
Pregnancy (tubular, incomplete/threatened abortion)
Pelvic inflammatory disease
Genital tract obstruction (imperforate hymen with menarche, bifid uterus)
Dysmenorrhea
Ovulation/ovarian cysts
Tuboovarian abscess
Ovarian or uterine tumors
Torsion of ovaries or testes
Undescended testicle
Urinary tract infection
Urinary calculi

Trauma
Intraluminal hematoma
Pancreatic pseudocyst

Drugs/Toxins
Lead and other heavy metals
Lactose intolerance
Alcohol
Salicylates
Erythromycin
Tetracycline
Ibuprofen

Other
Sickle cell disease
Henoch-Schönlein purpura
Primary peritonitis
Pneumonia
Muscle strain/sprain
Cholecystitis
Pancreatitis
Familial Mediterranean fever
Porphyrias

BOX 114-3

CAUSES OF RECURRENT ABDOMINAL PAIN

Organic (see acute causes in Boxes 114-1 and 114-2)
Infectious gastroenteritis (*Giardia lamblia, Salmonella, Shigella, Yersinia enterocolitica*, viral)
Peptic ulcer disease
Gastritis
Esophagitis
Hiatal hernia
Inflammatory bowel disease (Crohn's disease, regional enteritis)

Dysfunctional
Constipation/chronic stool retention
Lactose intolerance
Intestinal gas with heightened awareness of intestinal motility
Dysmenorrhea
Mittelschmerz
Sexual abuse
Overeating
Irritable colon

Psychogenic
Acute reactive anxiety
School phobia
Conversion reaction
Depression
Complaint modeling
Hypochondriasis
Factitious

erance, or dysmenorrhea. The degree to which these disorders lead to the expression of pain as a concern or interfere with the child's routine functioning varies among children.[4,9] Even within each child, expression of pain may vary. For example, the child who has chronic stool retention, who generally has few or no complaints, can have significant (and possibly even acute) pain when superimposed physiological (e.g., infectious gastroenteritis) or psychological problems (e.g., parental separation) are present. Psychogenic causes of abdominal pain generally are considered to have no primary physiological initiator of the painful expression. This includes entities such as school phobia, acute reactive anxiety, or conversion reaction. All of the RAP syndromes can lead to significant dysfunction and disability, with school absences, repeated visits to several health care professionals, and secondary psychological problems if assessment and initiation of treatment are either ignored or delayed inappropriately.[16]

ASSESSMENT

To identify the major diagnostic category to which further assessment and treatment recommendations can be directed, it is important to develop a systematic approach (Fig. 114-1) to the evaluation of the child or adolescent who has abdominal pain.[11,15] Because abdominal pain can be such a complex problem, systematic application of the cornerstones of medical care—history, physical examination, selected laboratory studies, and clear therapeutic recommendations based on the differential diagnosis—is essential. The history alone can account for about 80% to 90% of the data the physician uses in making a differential diagnosis. A systematic history should elicit information about the location, onset, severity, alleviating and precipitating factors, and associated symptoms. Timing of the onset of pain and the change in intensity, location, and quality of pain over time are essential factors in defining the etiology of the symptom. For children or adolescents who have recurring abdominal pain, information about the timing of the onset of the pain in relation to other events (e.g., mealtime or school days), as well as the duration of each episode and the frequency of recurrence, is helpful. Additional information about family (inherited disorders, concurrent illnesses, chronic pain disorders), medical history (prior surgery, chronic medication, faltering growth), and environmental/behavioral factors (recent changes in family or school, travel, unusual food intake) also should be obtained. In addition to the presence of specific symptoms and positive history, negative aspects of the history can provide important information to narrow the differential diagnosis. For example, the absence of dysuria in an older child or adolescent would make the diagnosis of urinary tract infection unlikely.

Laboratory and diagnostic studies that are done without any medical indications generally are unhelpful and actually may hinder the pediatrician's therapeutic recommendations. This common pitfall occurs when the pediatrician responds to the parents' initial requests to "rule everything out" by laboratory or radiographic studies.[7] The pediatrician needs to help the family understand how essential their history is in

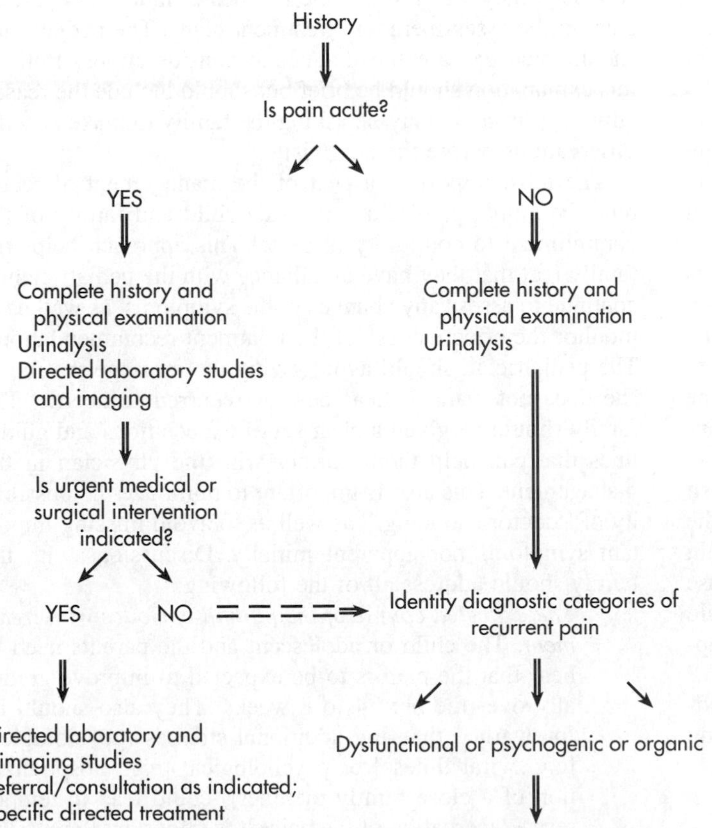

Fig. 114-1 Systematic approach to the evaluation of abdominal pain.

the assessment. The history from the child or adolescent himself or herself also is crucial and calls on the special skills of the pediatrician (see Chapter 79, Interviewing Children). The child or adolescent must feel comfortable in discussing his or her symptoms and concerns, even if these are different from those expressed by the parents. It is useful to obtain a history from the child or adolescent alone. Parents, too, may need to relate some of their concerns without the child present. In both instances, important diagnostic information can be missed if the pediatrician does not give the child and parents this opportunity to give separate histories.

The historical information should serve to focus the physical examination and specific diagnostic studies. A complete physical examination, including a careful external examination of the urethral orifice, vaginal orifice, and anus, always should be part of an initial assessment of abdominal pain. It is the history of the presenting symptoms, however, that will alert the pediatrician to more specific aspects of the physical examination (see Chapter 8, The Pediatric Physical Examination).

Laboratory and other diagnostic studies such as urine, stool, or genital tract cultures; serum chemistries (e.g., erythrocyte sedimentation rate); radiographic studies (e.g., barium swallow, upper or lower GI series, gallbladder series); and abdominal or pelvic ultrasound or computed tomography (CT) scans should be directed to clarification of a specific organic concern identified in the history and physical examination. When indicated, abdominal and pelvic ultrasound provide a safe, noninvasive way to assess bowel and pelvic organ structures and help clarify the need for urgent surgical intervention (e.g., intussusception, ovarian torsion, kidney abscess).[5] In general, the physician should consider the least invasive procedures first, while keeping in mind the cost of special studies in terms of pain, discomfort, and time.

In approaching recurrent abdominal pain, it is important to remember that dysfunctional and psychogenic causes account for most diagnoses, with organic causes identified in only about 5% to 8% of cases. When the history and physical examination indicate a dysfunctional or psychogenic cause, urinalysis should suffice as the initial laboratory study. It is wise to take a cautious approach when considering ordering laboratory studies to reassure the family and "rule out" disorders. These attempts to "test for everything" can lead to a series of tests that can distract both the family and the pediatrician from the differential diagnosis based on the clinical presentation.

Focusing on one particular diagnosis at the initial visit may be difficult if not impossible. At the same time, the parents want both to know what exactly is causing the pain and to obtain immediate relief for their child. Pressures to use the "shotgun" approach are great, but the pediatrician should consider the long-term therapeutic effects of such an approach. The costs of not using a systematic approach to RAP are great and include expensive, unnecessary laboratory studies, multiple acute emergency visits, and delay in beginning effective treatment.

MANAGEMENT

Treatment of abdominal pain that has a specific etiology obviously is directed to the indicated therapeutic interventions. For recurrent pain, continual review of the history is important to identify a change in symptoms, which could indicate that an acute process also is occurring, superimposed on the more chronic condition. For example, an adolescent girl who has recurring abdominal pain as a result of occult sexual abuse may present acutely with the pain now caused by a tubal pregnancy. Reviewing the symptoms will also facilitate the early recognition of chronic conditions such as inflammatory bowel disease.

Even though a specific cause may not be identified initially in the child who has RAP, this should not be viewed as a hindrance to developing a management plan. In the practice of medicine there are many instances of effective therapies available without complete understanding of the exact diagnosis or pathophysiology of the symptom. The pediatrician should be no less willing to offer such care to the child or adolescent who has recurrent abdominal pain.

The treatment of RAP begins at the first visit to the pediatrician for assessment. This initial interaction serves as the basis for establishing clear communication with the family. Effective communication is needed to facilitate the family's participation with and confidence in the treatment and management recommendations.

The next step is to provide the child and family with "informed reassurance." The therapeutic relationship is fostered when the physician explains the specific factors in the presenting history and physical examination that are not consistent with urgent intervention. Until the parents are reassured that acute or serious problems (e.g., appendicitis or tumors) and their particular concerns have been considered seriously, they will not be able to "hear," much less participate, in the assessment and treatment plans. The pediatrician should then explain the diagnostic considerations. Initially this explanation should be brief but should include the reason why the physician may be asking the family to make specific observations before the next visit.

The most important aspect of the management of recurrent abdominal pain is assuring the child and family of the commitment to continuity of care.[8] This approach helps the family feel that they have an alliance with the pediatrician to continue to assess any changes in the symptoms, as well as to monitor the effectiveness of the treatment recommendations. The pediatrician should avoid giving the message that he or she does not want to hear new or recurrent concerns. The family should be given a clear set of expectations and guidelines that can help them partner with the physician in the management. This also is important to minimize the possibility of "doctor shopping," as well as to avoid missing important symptoms not apparent initially. Discussions with the family should address all of the following:

1. *The expected course of the painful episodes with treatment.* The child or adolescent and the parents need to hear that the pain is to be expected to improve gradually over the next 4 to 8 weeks. They also should be forewarned that any additional stresses (physiological [e.g., viral illness] or psychological [e.g., hospitalization of a close family member]) could lead to temporary exacerbation of the pain. It is important to reassure the parents that this is a common and temporary problem rather than a worsening or more serious condition than originally explained to them. This helps avoid

a renewed search for a different diagnosis and redirects attention to the treatment plan and anticipated improvement.

2. *The frequency of follow-up visits to monitor progress and adjust treatment recommendations.* The first follow-up visit should take place within 1 to 2 weeks, depending on the degree of dysfunction caused by the pain. Thus a child who has not been in school for the past 2 weeks would need an early follow-up visit to reinforce a return to school. A common mistake is asking the family to call for an appointment only if there is no improvement. Generally the pediatrician does this to minimize any more school absences for visits to the doctor and may have the mistaken assumption that he or she will not really "do" anything at a visit so close to the initial one. Because symptoms often improve immediately after the first office visit, the pediatrician is wise to take the opportunity to reinforce this positive change. At this second visit the family and child also can be helped to recognize some of the control they have been able to have over the severity and frequency of the symptoms. The number of subsequent visits should be tailored to the individual case, but two to four follow-up visits spaced every 2 to 3 weeks apart generally is sufficient for treating uncomplicated recurrent abdominal pain.
3. *The modification of pain reinforcers.* Once recurrent abdominal pain has been diagnosed, neither the parents at home nor the pediatrician in follow-up should initiate discussion about the pain with the child. When children or adolescents feel the pain, they should be encouraged to identify any precipitating stresses, should be reassured that they can deal with the pain themselves, and, if needed, should rest for a short period before resuming activities. Likewise, when children report no painful episodes, they should be praised for how well they are doing. The obvious treatment goal is to alleviate pain. A less apparent, twofold goal is to reduce the number of reports of pain and to encourage children, when they do report it, to be able to describe how they coped with it and then returned to normal activities. Parents should plan rewards for improved school attendance and resumption of usual activities. The pediatrician can explain that he or she will be checking "how well" the child is doing in follow-up (by visits *or* phone calls) and focus attention on the child's positive coping strategies.
4. *The conditions and symptoms that need to be brought to the physician's attention and the degree of urgency for reporting them.* As previously mentioned, in children and adolescents acute abdominal pain can develop superimposed on recurrent abdominal pain; thus, the pediatrician should review with the family symptoms for which they should call immediately (e.g., localized pain, persistent vomiting, hematochezia) or urgently (e.g., fever, dysuria, decreased appetite). Parents should be instructed to note recurrent episodes and how their child dealt with the pain. This information is best reviewed without the child present to avoid reinforcing the reporting of pain. Parents should be encouraged to call and discuss any symptoms about which they are unsure. In this way the pediatrician can help alleviate the parents' guilt about minimizing their child's pain while making sure there are no new or changing symptoms.
5. *The pediatrician's willingness to discuss and assist in making appropriate referrals for second opinions and treatment recommendations.* The family will be more confident in the diagnosis if they know the pediatrician can initiate consultations readily should the need arise.

Longitudinal studies have shown that 30% to 60% of children continue to have pain for years because it can take some time to "grow out of it." The goal for pediatricians should be to help the child's or adolescent's abdominal pain from interfering with their functioning and well-being by a systematic approach to assessment and developing good communication and management strategies with the family.

REFERENCES

1. Ammerman S, Shafer MA, Snyder D: Ectopic pregnancy in adolescents: a clinical review for pediatricians, *J Pediatr* 117:677, 1990.
2. Apley J: Pathogenesis of recurrent abdominal pain. In Apley J: *The child with abdominal pains,* ed 2, London, 1975, Blackwell Scientific.
3. Barr RG: Abdominal pain in the female adolescent, *Pediatr Rev* 4:281, 1983.
4. Barr RG, Feuerstein M: Recurrent abdominal pain in children: how appropriate are our usual clinical assumptions? In Firestone P, McGrath P, editors: *Pediatric and adolescent behavioural medicine,* New York, 1983, Springer-Verlag.
5. Bhisitkul DM, et al: Clinical application of ultrasonography in the diagnosis of intussusception, *J Pediatr* 121:182, 1992.
6. Caty MG, Azizkhan RG: Acute surgical conditions of the abdomen, *Pediatr Ann* 23:192, 1994.
7. Coleman WL, Levine MD: Recurrent abdominal pain: the cost of the aches and the aches of the cost, *Pediatr Rev* 8:143, 1986.
8. Edwards MC, et al: Survey of pediatricians' management practices for recurrent abdominal pain, *J Pediatr Psychol* 19:241, 1994.
9. Feuerstein M, et al: Potential biobehavioral mechanisms of recurrent abdominal pain in children, *Pain* 13:287, 1982.
10. Fields KR, Neinstein LS: Uterine myomas in adolescents: case reports and a review of the literature, *J Pediatr Adolesc Gynecol* 9:195, 1996.
11. Green M: Diagnosis and treatment: psychogenic, recurrent, abdominal pain, *Pediatrics* 40:84, 1967.
12. Huang A, Jay MS, Uhler M: Tuboovarian abscess in the adolescent, *J Pediatr Adolesc Gynecol* 10:73, 1997.
13. Hyams JS, et al: Abdominal pain and irritable bowel syndrome in adolescents: a community-based study, *J Pediatr* 129:220, 1996.
14. Mollitt DL, Dokler ML: Acute abdomen: the teenage girl, *Semin Pediatr Surg* 6:100, 1997.
15. Poole SR, Schmitt BD, Mauro RD: Recurrent pain syndromes in children: a streamlined approach, *Contemp Pediatr* 12:47, 1995.
16. Stone RT, Barbero GJ: Recurrent abdominal pain in childhood, *Pediatrics* 45:732, 1970.
17. Zeltzer LK, et al: Pediatric pain: interacting behavioral and physical factors, *Pediatrics* 90:816, 1992.

115 Alopecia and Hair Shaft Anomalies

Nancy K. Barnett

Perhaps one of the lessons of the 1960s was that hair matters. It certainly does not serve an essential function, inasmuch as one can live without it. Nevertheless, the symbolism over the ages, from Samson to John Lennon, and the emotional investment everyone has in his or her hair make any of its abnormalities a matter of concern. This is particularly so with alopecia; loss of hair is a disturbing event.

A sequence of events makes up the life of a single hair, from active growth, a busy period known as the *anagen phase,* to passivity, a resting period known as the *telogen phase.* As many as 15% of scalp hairs may be in the telogen phase at any one time. These hairs soon are lost in the constant turnover of scalp hair, a continuous shedding that is hardly apparent to a casual observer. Surprisingly, about 50% of the hair must be shed for loss to be noticeable. Normally, up to 100 hairs are lost from the scalp daily.

Hair loss may increase to as much as 60% during a period known as a *telogen effluvium.* During such a period the situation is much like that of animals, which shed seasonally. In humans, this change in the normal anagen/telogen ratio may occur after a stress, such as high, relatively prolonged fever; a period of time after pregnancy; or after a severe illness. It may appear in either gender. The diagnosis of telogen effluvium can be confirmed simply by plucking a group of hairs and examining them microscopically. Note that plucking these hairs does not hurt because they are in the resting phase. The number of resting hairs is increased well beyond the usual 10% to 15%. This is a diffuse, nonpatterned, and nonscarring hair loss.

Obviously, then, hair loss is a matter deserving careful attention. A precise, pointed history and physical examination are necessary. The pediatrician must not limit the examination simply to the site of loss. The whole body and all hair-bearing parts of the body must be observed and the hairs themselves examined microscopically. There are unusual congenital alopecias, and under the light microscope the normality of the individual hair and the ratio of anagen to telogen hairs can be judged. The pediatrician may need to consult with a dermatologist.

The constant ebb and flow of growth and shedding and the extreme activity of the hair follicle—mitotic and metabolic—put the follicle at great risk when exposed to antimetabolites and mitotic inhibitors. If a child should lose scalp hair rather suddenly, the physician should be concerned with the possibility of a toxic event. This is most common in children who have a malignancy and have been treated with antimetabolites and therefore suffer loss because of the damage done by those drugs during the anagen phase, resulting in an anagen effluvium. Occasionally, sudden hair loss is caused by accidental poisoning, as with rat poison that contains thallium or coumarin. Children must be protected from toxins, and parents must be educated in this regard. In most instances, over a period of several months, new hairs will replace those lost, unless the exposure to the toxic element is repeated or becomes chronic.

The prognosis for the return of hair depends in large part on elimination of the toxic stimulus (when the practitioner is aware of what it might be) or on the hair loss not being accompanied by scarring. Loss with scarring (e.g., from iatrogenic scalp injury during delivery or from a burn) is permanent. In children, the various alopecias of both known and unknown causes usually occur without scarring. This is true of alopecia areata (spotty loss of scalp hair), alopecia totalis (loss of all scalp hair), and alopecia universalis (loss of all scalp and body hair); drug-induced, postfebrile, and postpartum alopecias; and alopecias associated with the endocrinopathies (hypothyroidism, hyperthyroidism, and hypoparathyroidism) or nutritional deficiency, particularly deficiencies of vitamins A, B, and C and the protein deficiency that causes kwashiorkor. Occasionally, some frontal hair can be lost in sickle cell anemia or some patchy, "moth-eaten" hair lost in secondary syphilis. In parathyroid insufficiency, the long-term calcium deficiency is associated with ectodermal abnormalities—not only alopecia and dental abnormalities but also cataracts and pitting and ridging of the fingernails. Also, hair will not grow at the site of most nevi and hemangiomas.

When there is scarring, as with the kerion associated with severe tinea capitis, keloid formation, or discoid lupus erythematosus, there is little hope for recovery. (Systemic lupus erythematosus may result in some hair loss, particularly frontally, but scarring does not necessarily occur.)

MICROSCOPIC EXAMINATION

Appropriate diagnosis requires microscopic differentiation of hair and its root in both the anagen and telogen stages. Deformities of the hair shaft can be seen, particularly with aminoacidopathy and in a variety of rare syndromes, including Menkes' kinky hair syndrome. One can differentiate monilethrix (usually an inherited, autosomal dominant disorder in which the diameter of the hair shaft varies) from pili torti (a disorder in which the hair is twisted on its long axis). However, the common causes of hair loss usually are innocuous, and the most common ones are distinctly age related.

PHYSIOLOGICAL LOSS OF HAIR

The first hair made by hair follicles in utero feels "silky," covers the entire body of the fetus, and is known as *lanugo*. It most often is shed in utero, to be replaced by hair that begins to grow on the scalp in the third trimester and continues to grow after birth. This is lost a few months after birth in a normal process that results in a temporary near-baldness. Often, parents are concerned with the thinning or with a more markedly localized area of loss, usually over the occiput, the result of the pressure of the head as the baby lies in the crib. Finally, however, this hair gradually is replaced by the new, which has more of a "feel" to it. It is thicker, usually darker, and more stable, growing longer before loss and shedding not quite so readily.

CAUSES OF ABNORMAL HAIR LOSS

A variety of congenital and hereditary disorders can be heralded by hair loss, either a total loss or a less obvious thinning. A true congenital alopecia may be inherited as an autosomal recessive trait. If the loss is not due to this genetic circumstance, it most often is evidence of an equally disturbing possibility of a significant hereditary disorder. The hair may not only be thin or possibly lost but also abnormal in a variety of ways. The pediatrician must look for signs of ectodermal dysplasia and consider radiographic exploration for skeletal defects (e.g., as with cartilage-hair hypoplasia, congenital ectodermal dysplasia, orofaciodigital syndrome), inherited metabolic disorders such as phenylketonuria or homocystinuria, or congenital problems such as hypothyroidism. These and other clinical pictures that result from serious chromosome defects (e.g., Cornelia de Lange's syndrome, Down syndrome) obviously provide a surfeit of signs and symptoms beyond the simple loss of hair. Acquired significant hair loss from telogen effluvium, occasionally even baldness, may follow intense and persistent fever, severe surgical insult, or precipitous weight loss, for any reason, with concomitant malnourishment and hypovitaminosis.

Hair Shaft Anomalies

Anomalies of the hair may result in a stubbly growth—a short, bumpy terrain most often of the scalp alone, the effect of broken hair and usually not true alopecia. There may be accompanying ectodermal defects, brittle fingernails, or perhaps cataracts and tooth anomalies. Actually, the fragility of hair and the resultant breakage (trichorrhexis) and stubble can be seen in a variety of conditions, all of which are rather rare. These may be familial or congenital, as in trichorrhexis nodosa, a familial circumstance in which the hair is fragile but in which there are no associated findings, or as with the stubbly hair associated with argininosuccinic aciduria, the stubbly hair being the least of the problems in a disease that, fortunately, is uncommon. Children who have argininosuccinic aciduria show evidence of severe mental retardation in the first year of life.

The feel of the hair may be helpful in finding the source of difficulty. In an infant who has hypothyroidism, the hair may be coarse, brittle, and without luster; in progeria and cartilage-hair hypoplasia syndrome, it may be fine and even silky. In all these circumstances the hair may break off and baldness increase. Whenever the hair is abnormal, it becomes weakened, fragile, and fractured, and it may be lost or unevenly shortened, often resulting in a stubbly, ragged alopecia. Various abnormalities—congenital, traumatic, or endocrine—all can lead to such fragility and loss. Referral to a dermatologist is appropriate so that, at the very least, a specific diagnosis can be made.

Loose anagen syndrome. Loose anagen syndrome is characterized by anagen hairs that are quite easily and painlessly pulled from the scalp.[3] Affected children are generally, but not always, blond and female preschoolers between 2 and 5 years of age.[5] Their hair appears sparse. The individual hairs are not fragile and on examination have misshapen bulbs with absent external root sheaths. Typically the child's hair is said to be slow growing, seldom requiring cutting. The hair over the occiput often is matted and sticky. The condition may wane with time, and adult onset cases have been reported.[5] The hair grows thicker and longer, and its pigmentation increases. Still, even in adulthood it may pull out easily and painlessly. A hereditary factor may be involved, but most cases are sporadic. The diagnosis can be made based on the history and examination, the painless "pull test" (when the hair is normal, it may hurt to pull), and light microscopy to view the recovered hairs. Management is limited to reassurance and allowance for the passage of time.

Trichorrhexis nodosa. Trichorrhexis nodosa is a common abnormality of the hair shaft that becomes obvious under the light microscope. The "nodes" seen resemble the effect one observes when the ends of two brushes are pushed together. This most often is congenital and results in breakage of hair and a short stubble over the scalp. It also is probably a genetic predisposition in black patients who experience hair breakage over large areas of the scalp and whose hair will not grow beyond a relatively short length. There usually is an accompanying history of hair straightening or repeated vigorous brushing and combing. Avoiding this kind of steady abuse and a more gentle cosmetic approach can result in some gradual improvement. White and Asian individuals can experience the same difficulty, probably without congenital or familial relationship, and the breakage occurs most often at the distal end of the hair. White specks may appear after some physical or chemical injury. Here again, the gentle approach and elimination of any noxious element are appropriate.

Monilethrix. Monilethrix (beaded hair syndrome) is a condition in which scalp hairs have regularly spaced differences in their circumference, suggesting a chain of beads. The cause is unknown, but probably genetic, and there is no known treatment; however, the outlook occasionally is promising in that a degree of recovery may occur spontaneously, particularly after puberty or during pregnancy. This is a long time to wait, inasmuch as hair breakage becomes obvious during infancy. Variable expressivity was noted in three kindreds in whom monilethrix was mapped to the type II keratin gene cluster at chromosome 12q13.[1] Occasionally, there are associated problems—cataracts, brittle nails, faulty teeth—suggestive of a more widespread ectodermal defect.

Pili torti. Pili torti simply means "twisted hair," and indeed, that is the way this type of hair looks under the microscope. The color is "off," and the hair is coarse and lusterless. It is as though straight and curly hair were competing for a place in the same strand. If one looks at a straight hair in cross section, it is round; a curly hair is oval. In pili torti, both configurations may be seen in a single strand. This abnormality can be an important clue to Menkes' kinky hair syndrome, an X-linked disease characterized by progressive cerebral degeneration, arterial degeneration, and the suggestion of scurvy in the bones. The serum copper level is low because of poor intestinal absorption of copper. This fatal disease has not yielded to administration of parenteral copper.

Alopecia Areata

Alopecia areata, most often seen as an acute problem, results in a rather sudden and total loss of hair in sharply circumscribed, round areas, often several centimeters in diameter, usually on the scalp but possibly anywhere on the body where there is hair. There is no evidence of inflammation except histologically. Hairs at the periphery of an area are plucked easily and may be particularly colorless and thin. "Exclamation point" hairs may appear throughout the patch, which sometimes is salmon colored. The fingernails may be pitted, as though nature were trying to tell us that the as yet undiscovered cause goes beyond the hair to another ectodermal expression. There may be just a few patches of loss or a total absence of body hair (alopecia universalis), including eyebrows and eyelashes. The more extensive the loss and the younger the child, the less likely a full recovery. The prognosis is best when the loss is less widespread, and only one or two patches are present. Although the cause is unknown, there has been some suggestion of an autoimmune process. Occasionally, autoimmune antibodies are identified in patients who have alopecia areata when there is no other clinical evidence of autoimmune disease. An increased incidence of alopecia areata also occurs in persons who have acute autoimmune thyroid disease and vitiligo. There may be a genetic predisposition to alopecia areata, for there is evidence that it is associated with certain class 2 genes in the HLA locus.

About one third of patients who have alopecia areata will regrow hair spontaneously in 6 months and about one third in 5 years, but for the remaining third, treatments must be tried to stimulate hair growth.

Cortisone creams applied topically have been used with some apparent success. It is possible in the older, more cooperative child to inject the hair follicles with corticosteroids, but the process is painful. It should be performed with a very small-gauge needle and topical anesthesia—for example, an ethyl chloride spray or EMLA cream. In any event, the primary care pediatrician should seriously question the need for this procedure, carefully assessing the impact of the disease and of the treatment on the patient, and should refer the patient to a dermatologist for further consideration of this form of treatment. Large areas that require infiltration present obvious difficulty. Oral steroid therapy can complicate the treatment further, but occasionally is tried.

There also has been some use of irritants (e.g., dinitrochlorobenzene and tars) and psoralen with ultraviolet light (PUVA therapy). These agents should be used only in children older than age 12 and only by a knowledgeable dermatologist in controlled circumstances. PUVA treatment possibly is justified in alopecia universalis, when all hair is lost. The poor prognosis, however, suggests that although a trial is appropriate, it should not be pushed to unreasonable lengths. It is odd that when hair does regrow after alopecia areata, it may be white. This, however, is temporary, and in the long run it will be impossible for casual observers to identify the formerly affected area.

It is difficult to assess the efficacy of various treatments because of the waxing and waning nature of this disorder.

Common Baldness

There is a genetically determined loss of hair that begins most often with a receding hairline and some thinning over the occiput. This androgenetic baldness occurs most often in men, but it can happen in women. Fortunately, its fullest expression is most common in the mature adult; the pediatrician rarely is confronted with the problem except in some older adolescents. There is no effective therapy, although topical minoxidil and hair transplant micrografts may help some individuals.

Trichotillomania

Some children have a considerable compulsive need to pull out their hair, even their eyebrows or eyelashes. Although this does not always have important emotional significance, it may provide a major clue to an underlying psychosocial problem when there are patchy, ill-defined bizarre patterns of hair loss. The pediatrician should begin with that assumption and follow this lead gently. The family structure and the interaction with siblings and parents and with friends at home and at school should be explored. Consulting a psychiatrist also should be considered. One can paint the attacked areas with petroleum jelly in an attempt to frustrate the habit; however, without attention to the possibility of a basic emotional problem, this approach quite obviously is temporary.

The hair that is lost is that which is most accessible to the probing hand. Sometimes enough is pulled to simulate alopecia areata, and the patient who eats hair may accumulate it in the stomach and create a trichobezoar (hairball), which ultimately may lead to acute intestinal obstruction or, most often, to the complaint of abdominal pain. It may be possible to palpate a mass and to demonstrate it on a roentgenogram; at this point, referral to a surgeon is mandatory. Both imipramine and fluoxetine have been used successfully to control trichotillomania in certain children.[4]

Traumatic Alopecia

Hair is a relatively fragile adornment. It does not respond positively to assault, and it should be handled gently and without physical or chemical importuning. It probably is best left alone, except for simple washing and, to suit the fashion, simple cutting.

For some, vanity can lead to alopecia. Constant teasing or straightening with heat or chemicals may seriously damage hair. Some hairstyles, particularly when one uses barrettes or has ponytails, braids, or corn-rows, cause traction that is constant and often tense and prolonged. The hair may then fall out, and there may be an accompanying redness and inflammation with some pustular involvement of the follicles. Generally, simply discontinuing the stress will help; the hair almost always will return. It should be remembered, however, that regrowth can be slow. The loss of any hair in this way, because of trichotillomania or a simple, excessively playful tug, will be slow to repair. Injured hair follicles do not heal quickly and often take 3 months or longer to return to an anagen phase.

Hypoparathyroidism

Sometimes, hypoparathyroidism is preceded by an acute bacterial infection and sometimes by candidiasis. The nature of the association between hypoparathyroidism and candidiasis is poorly understood. Chronic hypocalcemia and dental abnormalities can abound in this condition, along with other ectodermal defects such as pitted and ridged fingernails, cataracts, and a stringy, patchy loss of hair.

The candidiasis does not cause the hypoparathyroidism but, rather, follows the hormonal dysfunction; an immune mechanism possibly is common to both. The pediatrician should consult with an endocrinologist to develop a firm diagnostic and management plan.

Tinea Capitis

Whenever a child has patches of alopecia or stubbly hair growth, even in the absence of crusting, scaling, redness, or other inflammatory signs, the practitioner should consider the possibility of tinea capitis, seborrheic dermatitis, or psoriasis. Obviously, if there is crusting, scaling, or redness, the likelihood of alopecia areata is diminished because inflammation is not a symptom of that condition. In any event, the practitioner should perform a mycological examination, looking particularly for the usual *Trichophyton tonsurans,* in which case the lesions tend to be more elevated than in other forms of tinea and may be characterized by black dots. In rare cases, the fungi *Microsporum canis* and *M. audouinii* can invade the hair shaft and thereby cause breakage and stubbiness. *M. canis* tends to cause much more inflammation than does *M. audouinii*. The clinician can look for evidence of these fungal infections by shining the Wood's light on the affected area in a darkened room. There may well be a greenish fluorescence, although some chemical treatments in the hair also may simulate this fluorescence, making this test less worthwhile than years ago. In any event, the absence of this finding, while not precluding the diagnosis, may suggest a source other than *M. audouinii* or *M. canis*.

On occasion, particularly with *M. canis* or after treatment with an irritant, the area may become secondarily infected and seriously inflamed, requiring treatment with an antibiotic. Kerion, a delayed hypersensitivity reaction, may develop; the resultant scarring interferes with the regrowth of hair. Early diagnosis and treatment, therefore, are helpful. The long 10-to 12-week course of oral antifungal therapy may present difficulties with compliance in a young child. Topical antifungal agents, however, do not effect a cure. Several systemic fungistatic agents are effective for control of tinea capitis, although griseofulvin remains the most accepted. The fungicidal drug terbinafine is being investigated and appears effective for tinea capitis, but it currently is not approved for this use by the Federal Drug Administration. Liver function should be tested if antifungal medications are used for longer than 12 weeks. Oral prednisone tapered over 10 days may help to decrease the tenderness and inflammation of a kerion rapidly and help prevent a widespread "id" reaction.

Acrodermatitis Enteropathica

Acrodermatitis enteropathica, an autosomal recessive disorder characterized by abnormal zinc absorption, has several important cutaneous manifestations, simulating, at times, psoriasis, epidermolysis bullosa, pyoderma, or candidiasis. With zinc deficiency there is abdominal pain and diarrhea; there also can be an associated "wispy alopecia" and dystrophic development of the fingernails, suggesting widespread ectodermal involvement. Zinc sulfate given orally is the treatment of choice.

Discoid and Systemic Lupus Erythematosus

Discoid lupus erythematosus can be disfiguring to the scalp, and with scarring it can cause a permanent loss of hair. Therefore, early treatment is necessary. Scarring can be avoided with topical or intralesional steroids in most cases. Systemic lupus erythematosus also can cause alopecia, and the scalp itself can be erythematous; however, the loss of hair generally is temporary and does not involve the scarring characteristic of discoid lupus erythematosus.

GENERAL MANAGEMENT

Treatment for alopecia depends, of course, on the cause. Practitioners have become all too accustomed to seeing hospitalized children who have a malignancy being treated with antimetabolites and wearing baseball caps to hide their full or partial baldness. However, a noticeable loss of hair at any point may be disturbing to both patient and parent; therefore, the suggestion that the child wear a baseball cap or some other unobtrusive, concealing adornment may be appropriate. Even a hairpiece can be designed for a child. These steps serve only for the interim while practitioners attend to the discovery of a potentially helpful treatment or while they wait expectantly in those circumstances in which they do not have a specific treatment and in which their role is diagnostic and supportive. The possibility that hair will not regrow cannot be discarded when loss (1) follows high fever or chronic toxicity, (2) is accompanied by scarring, or (3) occurs in the areas of nevi, aplasia cutis, or persistent hemangiomas. Therefore, the supportive aspect should not be minimized because hair loss does matter. It is necessary to talk this through with the child who is old enough and also with the parents, exploring the source of emotional reaction and discomfort and, if recovery of hair is questionable, working with the patient to achieve an emotional balance consistent with reality and to adopt suitable coping mechanisms. Most often this is achievable, and the pediatrician should not back away from trying. The practitioner, sometimes frustrated by the lack of a practical, successful management regimen, should not forget the value of a willing, listening ear—in this, as in all things. Plastic surgery expertise should be sought for consideration of hair transplants and scalp reduction (for scarred areas) when possible.

When to Refer

Rapid, diffuse hair loss
Chronic, progressive, localized or diffuse hair loss without regrowth
Scarring alopecia
Inability to grow hair as a result of breakage, loss, abnormal texture of hair
Appearance of scalp mass or plaque affecting localized hair loss

REFERENCES

1. Birch-Machin MA, et al: Mapping of monilethrix to the type II keratin gene cluster at chromosome 12q13 in three new families, including one with variable expressivity, *Br J Dermatol* 137:339, 1997.
2. Gupta AK, Soloman RS, Adam P: Itraconazole oral solution for the treatment of tinea capitis, *Br J Dermatol* 139:104, 1998.
3. Price VH, Gummer CL: Loose anagen syndrome, *J Am Acad Dermatol* 20:249, 1989.
4. Sheika SH, Wagner KD, Wagner RF: Fluoxetine treatment of trichotillomania and depression in a prepubertal child, *Cutis* 51:50, 1993.
5. Tosti A, et al: Loose anagen hair, *Arch Dermatol* 133:1089, 1997.

SUGGESTED READINGS

Atton A, Tunnessen W: Alopecia in children: the most common causes, *Pediatr Rev* 12:25, 1990.

Datloff J, Esterly NB: A system for sorting out pediatric alopecia, *Contemp Pediatr* 3:53, 1986.

Price VH: Office diagnosis of structural hair anomalies, *Cutis* 15:231, 1975.

116 Amenorrhea

Alain Joffe

Amenorrhea is a symptom, not a disease, and has a variety of causes. Traditionally, amenorrhea has been classified as being either primary or secondary. *Primary amenorrhea* is defined as the failure to initiate menstruation; *secondary amenorrhea* refers to cessation of menses in an adolescent whose menstrual function previously was normal. In clinical situations, this distinction is of limited utility because many diseases can cause either primary or secondary amenorrhea. However, certain anatomical conditions (imperforate hymen, transverse vaginal septum, absent uterus [Mayer-Rokitansky-Küster-Hauser syndrome]), and endocrine disorders (androgen insensitivity syndrome) need be considered only in the evaluation of primary amenorrhea.

The mean age of menarche in the United States today is 12½ to 13 years; 95% of girls will have menstruated by age 16 years. Menstruation usually begins approximately 2 years after breast budding, the earliest sign of puberty in 85% of girls. However, the interval between the two can be as short as 6 months or as long as 5¾ years. Given this broad range of individual variation in the onset of puberty and menarche, the physician first must note whether breast budding or pubic hair is present. If no signs of secondary sexual development are present by age 14 years, the patient should be evaluated for delayed puberty (see Chapter 165, Puberty: Normal and Abnormal).[4]

If signs of puberty are present, the age at which they appeared must be determined. If progression through puberty appears normal, the findings of a thorough history and physical examination are unremarkable, and fewer than 4 years have elapsed since the onset of puberty at the time the patient seeks advice, the patient should be counseled about the variability of development and reassured that hers is normal, particularly if her mother indicates that she first menstruated at a relatively late age. A urine pregnancy test should first be done if there is any possibility that the patient is sexually active. Regularly scheduled follow-up visits until menarche occurs or the 4-year limit is reached are warranted. If more than 4 years have elapsed since the onset of puberty, the patient has true primary amenorrhea, and a more in-depth evaluation is indicated. In general, girls who have secondary sexual characteristics who have not menstruated by age 16 years require further evaluation.[6] The major causes of amenorrhea are listed in Box 116-1.

By definition, secondary amenorrhea implies some previous level of normal menstrual function. Thus, certain causes of primary amenorrhea, mainly abnormalities of the genitalia, are not in the differential diagnosis.

When evaluating an adolescent who appears to have secondary amenorrhea, it is important to consider her gynecological age (the number of months or years elapsed since menarche). After the onset of menarche, many teenagers will menstruate sporadically; regular monthly cycles often are not established until 1 to 2 years after menarche.[9]

Clearly, the abrupt cessation of menstruation in a teenager who has established regular cycles is of greater concern than the absence of menses for 3 to 4 months in a teenager who has a gynecological age of 6 months to 1 year. The point at which the clinician elects to pursue an evaluation depends on the anxiety of the patient and her family, the possibility of pregnancy, and the physician's assessment of the likelihood that a potentially serious disease is responsible for the amenorrhea. A teenager whose menses previously were regular should be evaluated if amenorrhea persists for three cycles or 6 months, whichever is the shorter period.[8] A general approach to the evaluation of amenorrhea is shown in Fig. 116-1.

History

The history and physical examination are essential in formulating a reasonable diagnostic approach. The hypothalamic-pituitary-ovarian axis of the adolescent is more sensitive to either physical or psychological stress than is that of the adult woman. Stress, emotional upset, fever accompanying viral illness, and changes in weight or environment (e.g., going away to college) all can induce amenorrhea. Casual comments about weight or body image may be a clue to anorexia nervosa. The history also should include questions about drug or medication use, particularly oral contraceptives, depot medroxyprogesterone acetate (Depo-Provera), or levonorgestrel implants (Norplant), all of which can cause amenorrhea. Most women who become amenorrheic while taking oral contraceptives resume menstruation within 6 months of stopping them. Whether the patient is sexually active also needs to be ascertained. If she is, pregnancy should be the primary consideration. Unfortunately, denial of sexual activity does not exclude pregnancy, inasmuch as many teenagers are reluctant to admit to something they feel will be met with condemnation from adults. Sudden cessation of menstruation is more likely to indicate pregnancy or stress as a cause, whereas a gradual cessation suggests polycystic ovarian disease or premature ovarian failure. A history of uterine surgery or abortion raises the possibility of uterine synechiae. With more and more women involved

BOX 116-1

CAUSES OF AMENORRHEA IN ADOLESCENTS IN WHOM SECONDARY SEXUAL CHARACTERISTICS ARE PRESENT

1. Familial (primary amenorrhea only)
2. Psychosocial stress
3. Obesity, severe weight loss (similarly, thin body habitus associated with strenuous exercise programs, as seen in ballet dancers and in patients who have anorexia nervosa), or failure to gain weight expected with pubertal development
4. Endocrine cause
   a. Hypopituitarism
   b. Adrenal disorders, including late-onset adrenal hyperplasia (21-OH deficiency) and adrenal tumors; hirsutism and/or virilization often present
   c. Gonadal dysgenesis (e.g., Turner's syndrome or Turner mosaic)
   d. Premature ovarian failure
   e. Androgen insensitivity syndrome (primary amenorrhea only)
   f. Thyroid disorders (hypothyroidism most common)
   g. Polycystic ovary disease
5. Chronic disease
6. Pregnancy
7. Anatomical anomalies (primary amenorrhea only)
   a. Vaginal, cervical and/or uterine agenesis
   b. Imperforate hymen or transverse vaginal septum
8. CNS tumor or lesions (e.g., prolactinoma) or CNS developmental defects (e.g., Kallman syndrome [primary amenorrhea only])
9. Drugs, including hormonal contraception

in sports, questions about exercise patterns or participation in athletics (frequency, duration, intensity) have become essential.[3] Clues to any of the endocrine abnormalities (e.g., galactorrhea), as well as a history of past central nervous system insults (e.g., meningitis) or symptoms of an intracranial tumor, need to be sought. The age at which the patient's mother and sisters first menstruated also is helpful information because such a pattern may be familial.[2] Finally, chronic diseases such as inflammatory bowel disease or renal failure may be subtle in their early presentation; hence, questions aimed at uncovering these illnesses must be included in the review of systems.

Physical Examination

Plotting of previous growth data (both height and weight) is essential. A short girl who has amenorrhea should prompt a search for the other physical characteristics of Turner's syndrome.[1] Diagnostic criteria for anorexia nervosa include loss of weight or *failure to gain the weight expected with pubertal development.* A complete physical examination, which in most cases will include a pelvic examination, should be performed. Obesity or excessive thinness can result in amenorrhea. Abnormalities of the visual field, smell or other cranial nerve function, papilledema, or disturbances of reflexes suggest a brain tumor. Hirsutism, a receding hairline, excessive acne, moon facies, striae, an enlarged thyroid, or buffalo hump suggests an endocrine disorder. A webbed neck, short stature, or widely spaced nipples suggest gonadal dysgenesis (e.g., Turner's syndrome). Physical signs and symptoms indicative of anorexia nervosa also should be sought (see Chapter 102, Anorexia and Bulimia Nervosa). Nipple discharge may be indicative of elevated prolactin levels, and lack of or scant pubic hair in a female who has Tanner stage 3 to 4 breast development suggests androgen insensitivity syndrome.

A pelvic examination is essential to ensure the presence of normal internal and external female genitalia. An imperforate hymen or transverse vaginal septum prevents menstrual blood from escaping. If the hymenal opening is patent, the examination should proceed to determine the presence of a normal vagina, cervix, and uterus. If the hymenal opening is very small, the cervix and uterus can be palpated by means of a bimanual rectoabdominal examination. The size of the clitoris should be noted because clitoromegaly indicates the presence of excess androgens (e.g., partial 21-hydroxylase deficiency). A pink vaginal mucosa indicates the presence of some degree of estrogenization. In those few cases in which a pelvic or rectoabdominal examination cannot be performed to determine the presence or absence of a uterus, an ultrasound may be necessary.

Laboratory Tests

For the girl who has primary amenorrhea who has an unremarkable history, review of systems, general physical examination, and no evidence of vaginal outlet obstruction, the next step is to determine, either by pelvic examination and/or ultrasound, whether a uterus is present. If not, karyotyping and serum testosterone levels should be determined to screen for Müllerian agenesis or androgen insensitivity syndrome. If a uterus is present, an evaluation comparable to that for secondary amenorrhea should be pursued.

The diagnostic algorithm recommended by Speroff, Glass, and Kase is very helpful.[8] The first step is to rule out pregnancy, thyroid disease, and hyperprolactinemia. If the pregnancy test is negative and thyroid stimulating hormone (TSH) and prolactin levels (prolactin levels must be obtained before any manipulation of the breast) are normal, the next step is to determine if anovulation accompanied by normal circulating estrogen levels is the cause of the amenorrhea. Progesterone 10 mg po for 5 to 10 days is administered; any spotting or bleeding in the week following is considered a positive test and evidence that anovulation is the cause. Some authors recommend measuring follicle-stimulating hormone (FSH) levels before administering progesterone because some women who have hypergonadotropic amenorrhea will have a withdrawal bleed.[7] Patients who have hypothalamic amenorrhea will need supplemental progesterone on a regular basis (or combination oral contraceptive pills if sexually active) to prevent unopposed estrogen stimulation of the uterus.

Absence of withdrawal bleeding requires further evalua-

Step 1: History to screen for pattern of familial delay, stress, chronic illness, other endocrine disorders, eating disorders, athletic competition, drugs, current or past CNS lesions, risk for pregnancy, past surgeries

↓

Step 2: Complete physical examination, including: plotting of past and current height and growth data; Tanner staging of breast and pubic hair: evidence of hirsutism or virilization; galactorrhea. (Primary amenorrhea: test for sense of smell and perform digital vaginal examination, if possible)

→ Examination normal

→ Specific cause identified: evaluate and treat as indicated

Step 3: Urine HCG

→ Negative (to evaluate for secondary amenorrhea, go to step 5)

→ Positive → Pregnancy

Step 4: Perform bimanual pelvic examination or if unable, rectoabdominal examination

→ Normal

→ Abnormal/equivocal/unable to complete → Ultrasound
 - → Normal: go to step 5
 - → Abnormal: further evaluation and treatment, as indicated

Step 5: TSH, prolactin levels

→ Normal

→ Abnormal: evaluate and treat, as indicated

Step 6: Progesterone challenge test

→ No withdrawal bleeding

→ Withdrawal bleeding → Treat with cyclic OCPs or progesterone; re-evaluate every 6 months

Step 7: Obtain FSH level. If high (hypergonadotropic hypogonadism), evaluate for ovarian failure. If low or normal, reassess for anorexia nervosa, intense exercise (low percent body fat), symptoms of CNS tumor, or chronic illness. MRI may be indicated. If all negative, follow closely or begin oral contraceptive (estrogen replacement) therapy. If no bleeding occurs on OCPs, refer to adolescent medicine specialist or gynecologist.

HCG, Human chronic gonadotropin; *OCPs*, oral contraceptive pills.

Fig. 116-1 Evaluation of patients who have amenorrhea in whom secondary sex characteristics are present.

tion, with measurement of FSH. If any signs of hirsutism or virilization are present (e.g., clitoromegaly), the evaluation is more complex. Useful laboratory tests include serum testosterone (total and free) and dehydroepiandrosterone and its sulfate, as well as measurement of 24-hour urinary excretion of 17-hydroxycorticosteroids and 17-ketosteroids. Individuals differ as to which of these tests or others are needed. High FSH/luteinizing hormone (LH) levels indicate ovarian failure and should prompt karyotyping; low or low-normal FSH/LH levels are consistent with either hypothalamic amenorrhea or a central nervous system lesion. The latter possibility can be evaluated with magnetic resonance imaging. An LH/FSH ratio greater than 3:1 strongly suggests polycystic ovary syndrome.[5] Definitive recommendations for treatment of secondary amenorrhea will depend on the underlying etiology.

When to Refer

1. If there is evidence of anatomical or chromosomal abnormality
2. If signs of virilization are present
3. If there is evidence of a CNS tumor
4. If the amenorrhea appears secondary to a chronic illness that the pediatrician is unable to manage
5. If the pediatrician feels uncomfortable performing a pelvic examination
6. If long-term hormonal therapy is required
7. If the patient has an eating disorder

REFERENCES

1. Emans SJ, Laufer MR, Goldstein DP: *Pediatric and adolescent gynecology,* ed 4, Philadelphia, 1998, Lippincott-Raven.
2. Ghai K, Rosenfield RL: Disorders of pubertal development: too early, too much, too late, or too little, *Adolesc Med* 5:19, 1994.
3. Gidwani GP: Amenorrhea in the athlete, *Adolesc Med* 10:275, 1999.
4. Iglesias EA, Coupey SM: Menstrual cycle abnormalities: diagnosis and management, *Adolesc Med* 10:255, 1999.
5. Neinstein LS: *Adolescent health care,* ed 3, Baltimore, 1996, Williams and Wilkins.
6. Polaneczky MM, Slap GB: Menstrual disorders in the adolescent: amenorrhea, *Pediatr Rev* 13:43, 1992.
7. Rebar RW, Connolly HV: Clinical features of young women with hypergonadotropic amenorrhea, *Fertil Steril* 53:804, 1990.
8. Speroff L, Glass RH, Kase NG: *Clinical gynecologic endocrinology and infertility,* ed 6, Baltimore, 1999, Lippincott Williams and Wilkins.
9. World Health Organization Task Force on Adolescent Reproductive Health: World Health Organization multicenter study on menstrual and ovulatory patterns in adolescent girls, *J Adolesc Health* 7:236, 1986.

117 Anemia and Pallor

David N. Korones • Harvey J. Cohen

Pallor and anemia are among the clinical problems encountered most frequently in pediatric practice. Pallor is a physical sign; anemia is a laboratory value. Neither is a diagnosis, and although both may be variations of normal, the pediatrician must investigate these findings thoroughly and determine their cause.

PALLOR

Pallor is pale complexion of the skin. Although it often may be a familial trait or a consequence of limited exposure to the sun, pallor also is observed in a variety of pathological conditions. Vasoconstriction of subcutaneous blood vessels causes the pallor associated with shock, exposure to cold, or syncope. Accumulation of fluid in the interstitium sometimes causes the pallor seen in edematous states such as myxedema, hypoproteinemia, and congestive heart failure. When the hemoglobin concentration is low, pallor may be due to anemia.

Assessment of skin color for pallor often is confounded by clinical and environmental factors. Fluorescent lighting, a common fixture in physicians' offices, distorts the true hue of the skin. It is particularly difficult to recognize pallor in dark-skinned patients. Assessment of pallor also may be complicated by coexistent disorders that cause changes in skin color; for example, jaundice and cyanosis may mask pallor entirely.

ANEMIA

Because most pediatricians screen children for anemia routinely in the first or second year of life and in adolescence, they frequently encounter children who have this problem. Like pallor, anemia is not a diagnosis; it is a laboratory finding that alerts the health provider to a reduction in red blood cell mass. The physician or nurse practitioner, therefore, must be familiar with anemia and prepared to evaluate it for a broad range of etiological possibilities. Armed with a thorough history and physical examination, as well as routine laboratory data that can be obtained in the office, the pediatric health care professional in most instances can determine the cause of anemia.

Definition

Anemia is a decrease in red blood cell mass as determined by a low hemoglobin or hematocrit value. Determining whether a child is anemic sometimes is problematic. Efforts to define a normal hemoglobin level have been hampered by sampling of small or nonrepresentative groups of infants and children, by differences in the normal range of hemoglobin in various ethnic groups, and by failure to exclude patients who have mild anemia from the sample populations. In one of the most thorough studies of normal hematological values of childhood,[6] large numbers of children from different ethnic groups, socioeconomic strata, and ages were sampled. Children who had findings suggestive of iron deficiency, thalassemia, or hemoglobinopathies were excluded. It was found that normal ranges varied depending on age and gender (Table 117-1). Normal hemoglobin levels in blacks are approximately 0.5 g/dl lower than those in whites and Asians.

Normal ranges for hematocrit and hemoglobin values usually are defined as the mean of these values ±2 standard deviations. This definition results in the arbitrary classification of 2.5% of children as anemic. Some of these children may not be anemic; others whose values fall within the normal range actually may be anemic relative to their usual value. For example, a 3-year-old whose hematocrit value has dropped from 40 to 34 still has a value that falls within the normal range, but this decrease merits further evaluation. A table of normal values serves only as a guideline for the pediatric health care practitioner. The hematological values of an individual child should be compared with any previous values obtained on that child and must be evaluated in the full context of the child's age, race, history and physical examination, and general state of health.

History

Because most anemic children are asymptomatic, a careful history may reveal clues to the existence of an anemia that otherwise would remain undetected. Demographic factors such as age, gender, and ethnic background define important risk groups for different types of anemias. Toddlers and adolescent girls are at highest risk for iron-deficiency anemia. Sickle cell disease is observed almost exclusively in blacks. Thalassemia occurs with increased frequency in blacks and people of Mediterranean and Southeast Asian descent. A dietary history should be elicited. A poor or unbalanced diet may result in a nutritional deficiency, and young children who demonstrate pica are at risk for lead toxicity. Certain drugs can cause anemia; sulfa drugs can precipitate hemolysis in children deficient in the red blood cell enzyme glucose-6-phosphate dehydrogenase (G6PD). Acute infections may

Table 117-1 Values (Mean and Lower Limit of Normal) for Hemoglobin, Hematocrit, and Mean Corpuscular Volume Determinations

	Hemoglobin (g/dl)		Hematocrit (%)		Mean Corpuscular Volume (fL)	
Age (Yr)	**Mean**	**Lower Limit**	**Mean**	**Lower Limit**	**Mean**	**Lower Limit**
0.5-1.9	12.5	11.0	37	33	77	70
2-4	12.5	11.0	38	34	79	73
5-7	13.0	11.5	39	35	81	75
8-11	13.5	12.0	40	36	83	76
12-14:						
Female	13.5	12.0	41	36	85	78
Male	14.0	12.5	43	37	84	77
15-17:						
Female	14.0	12.0	41	36	87	79
Male	15.0	13.0	46	38	86	78
18-49:						
Female	14.0	12.0	42	37	90	80
Male	16.0	14.0	47	40	90	80

From Nathan DG, Oski F: *Hematology of infancy and childhood,* ed 3, Philadelphia, 1987, WB Saunders.

suppress production or accelerate destruction of red blood cells. The patient should be screened for signs of acute or chronic bleeding in the most common sites for blood loss—the gastrointestinal tract and the female genitourinary tract. Anemia also may be part of an underlying systemic disorder such as juvenile rheumatoid arthritis or Crohn's disease. A family history should be taken; family members who have jaundice or a history of cholecystectomy or splenectomy at a young age may have a hereditary hemolytic anemia such as spherocytosis or hemoglobinopathy.

Signs and Symptoms

Children who have mild or moderate anemia show few signs or symptoms. Infants and toddlers may manifest irritability, longer periods of sleep, changes in behavior, or pallor. Older children may have similar signs or, like adults, may complain of a decrease in exercise tolerance, weakness or dizziness, fatigue, shortness of breath, or palpitations.

Signs of anemia often are subtle. It is not uncommon for a child to receive a clean bill of health at a routine health care visit, only to be called back for reevaluation because of a low hematocrit value on routine screening. Pallor may indicate anemia, but it is not appreciable in mild anemia and may not be detectable until the hemoglobin level is as low as 8 g/dl.[10] Careful examination of the conjunctivae, mucous membranes, palmar creases, and nail beds may reveal pallor when the skin does not. The presence of scleral icterus or jaundice suggests a hemolytic anemia. Frontal bossing and prominent maxillae may represent expansion of bone marrow red blood cell production caused by a chronic hemolytic anemia such as thalassemia major. Diffuse lymphadenopathy and organomegaly may indicate leukemia or lymphoma. Auscultation of the heart often reveals a pulmonary flow murmur with mild to moderate anemia, and a gallop rhythm may be heard when a profound anemia results in congestive heart failure. Splenomegaly is apparent in patients who have certain hemolytic anemias or infiltrative diseases.

Laboratory Data

In addition to the hemoglobin or hematocrit determinations, three other laboratory tests can be performed in most offices—the reticulocyte count, the peripheral blood film, and the mean corpuscular volume (MCV). These tests can provide the clinician with enough information to determine the cause of most anemias. The reticulocyte count is a measure of red blood cell production and thus provides valuable information about the bone marrow's ability to respond to an anemia. Reviewing the peripheral blood film allows the practitioner to assess the morphology and color of the erythrocytes. The MCV is an index of red cell size and serves as a starting point for morphological classification of anemia. Observation of the plasma in a centrifuged sample of blood is a simple test that may provide additional clues: (1) clear plasma suggests iron deficiency, (2) icteric plasma may occur secondary to extravascular hemolysis, and (3) pink plasma may develop secondary to intravascular hemolysis. Other laboratory tests may be indicated when particular causes of anemia are suspected; these are summarized in Tables 117-2 to 117-4.

CLASSIFICATION OF ANEMIA

Anemias often are classified based on decreased production or increased destruction of red blood cells. Another basis for classification is red cell morphology; the information gained from the peripheral blood film and the MCV enables the clinician to classify an anemia as microcytic, normocytic, or macrocytic. One then can follow an algorithm systematically to evaluate the subtype of anemia (Fig. 117-1) and minimize the number of laboratory tests done to arrive at a diagnosis.

Microcytic Anemias

In children, microcytic anemia has five causes: iron deficiency, thalassemia, lead poisoning, chronic inflammation, and sideroblastic anemia.

Table 117-2 Laboratory Evaluation of Hypochromic and Microcytic Anemias

Diagnosis	Laboratory Test	Expected Result
Iron deficiency	Serum ferritin	Low <25 μg/L
	Serum iron and total iron-binding capacity	Low/high
	% iron saturation	Low <15%
	Bone marrow iron stores	Absent
	Stool for occult blood	Positive (if gastrointestinal bleeding)
	Urine for blood, hemoglobin, or hemosiderin	Present (if renal loss)
	MCV/RBC ratio	>13
Beta-thalassemia trait	Blood film	Basophilic stippling
	Hemoglobin electrophoresis	Increased A_2 or F hemoglobin
	Biosynthetic beta/alpha-globin chain ratio	<1
	MCV/RBC ratio	<13
	Family studies	Hgb/Hct decreased
		Blood film
		Anisocysotis
		Poikilocytosis
		Basophilic stippling
		MCV <70 fL/cell
Alpha-thalassemia trait	No routine specific test	Normal A_2 hemoglobin
	Family studies	Hgb/Hct normal or slightly decreased
		Blood film
		Anisocytosis
		Poikilocytosis
		MCV <70 fL/cell
	Biosynthetic beta/alpha-globin chain ratio	>1
	Specific genetic probe analysis	Absent genes
Chronic inflammation	Nonspecific tests	
	Erythrocyte sedimentation rate	Increased
	Acute phase reactants	Increased
	C-reactive protein	
	Fibrinogen	
	Haptoglobin	
	Serum ferritin	Increased
	Serum iron + total iron-binding capacity	Low/low
	% iron saturation	Low
	Bone marrow iron stores	Increased
	Bone marrow sideroblasts	Decreased
Sideroblastic anemia	Serum ferritin	Increased
	Serum iron + total iron-binding capacity	Normal to increased/normal
	% iron saturation	High
	Bone marrow iron stores	Increased
	Bone marrow sideroblasts	Increased sideroblasts plus "ringed" sideroblasts
Lead poisoning	Blood film	Basophilic stippling
	Erythrocyte protoporphyrin	Increased
	Blood lead	Increased

From Segel GB: *Pediatr Rev* 10:77, 1988.
MCV, Mean corpuscular volume; *RBC,* red blood cell, *Hgb,* hemoglobin; *Hct,* hematocrit.

Iron deficiency. Iron deficiency is by far the most common cause of anemia in children.[7] The clinician must determine whether the deficiency is due to poor dietary intake of iron, blood loss, or other less common causes. Children between the ages of 12 and 24 months are at the highest risk of iron-deficiency anemia. Most of these children are no longer breast-feeding or taking iron-containing formula but are drinking cow milk instead, and their intake of solid foods is erratic. Adolescents also may develop an anemia as a result of poor dietary intake of iron; adolescent girls may have further loss of iron from blood loss with frequent or heavy menses. Iron-deficiency anemia is unusual in full-term infants in the first 6 months of life. These infants are born with sufficient iron stores to maintain a normal hematocrit level for 6 months, even if their mothers were anemic during pregnancy.

When children of any age have an iron-deficiency anemia, it is essential to consider the possibility of blood loss. Because the gastrointestinal (GI) tract is a common site of occult or chronic blood loss, patients and families should be queried about black or tarry stools, hematochezia, and bloody or coffee-ground emesis. Stool guaiac tests should

Table 117-3 Laboratory Evaluation of Normocytic Anemias

Diagnosis	Laboratory Test	Expected Result
Anemias with Low Reticulocyte Percentage		
Diamond-Blackfan anemia	Bone marrow examination	Decreased erythroid precursors
	Fetal hemoglobin and i antigen	± Increased
	Mean corpuscular volume	± Macrocytosis
Transient erythroblastopenia of childhood	Bone marrow examination	Decreased erythroid precursors
Aplastic crises	History	Underlying hemolytic disease
	Bone marrow examination	Decreased erythroid precursors
	Serology and/or viral culture	Parvovirus
Anemias with High Reticulocyte Percentage		
Extrinsic		
Autoimmune hemolysis	Blood film	Spherocytes
	Antiglobulin (Coombs) test	Positive
	Complement consumption assay	Positive (used if Coombs test is negative)
	Tests for underlying disease	
Fragmentation hemolytic anemia	Blood film	Fragmented RBC
	Tests for underlying disease	
Intrinsic		
Membrane disorders	Blood film	Characteristic RBC: spherocytes, stomatocytes, elliptocytes
	Incubated osmotic fragility	Increased fragility if spherocytes present
	Autohemolysis	Increased and corrected by glucose
	Membrane protein-structural analysis (investigational)	Abnormal (e.g., decreased spectrin in spherocytosis)
Hemoglobin disorders	Blood film	Irreversibly sickled cells in severe sickle syndromes: SS-, SC-, or S-thalassemia
		Targeting in CC, also in SS-, SC-, and S-thalassemia
	Hemoglobin electrophoresis	Abnormal hemoglobins
Enzyme disorders	Screening tests	Positive
G6PD	Enzyme assay	Low activity
Pyruvate kinase and other glycolytic defects	Enzyme assay	Low activity

From Segel GB: *Pediatr Rev* 10:77, 1988.

Table 117-4 Laboratory Evaluation of Macrocytic Anemias

Diagnosis	Laboratory Test	Expected Result
Vitamin B_{12} deficiency	Blood film	Macroovalocytes, Howell-Jolly bodies; nucleated RBC and hypersegmented granulocytes
	Serum vitamin B_{12}	Low <100 pg/ml
	Bone marrow examination	Megaloblastic erythroid and granulocyte precursors
Folic acid deficiency	Blood film	Same as above
	Serum folate	Low <3 ng/ml
	RBC folate	Low <160 ng/ml
	Bone marrow examination	Same as above

From Segel GB: *Pediatr Rev* 10:77, 1988.

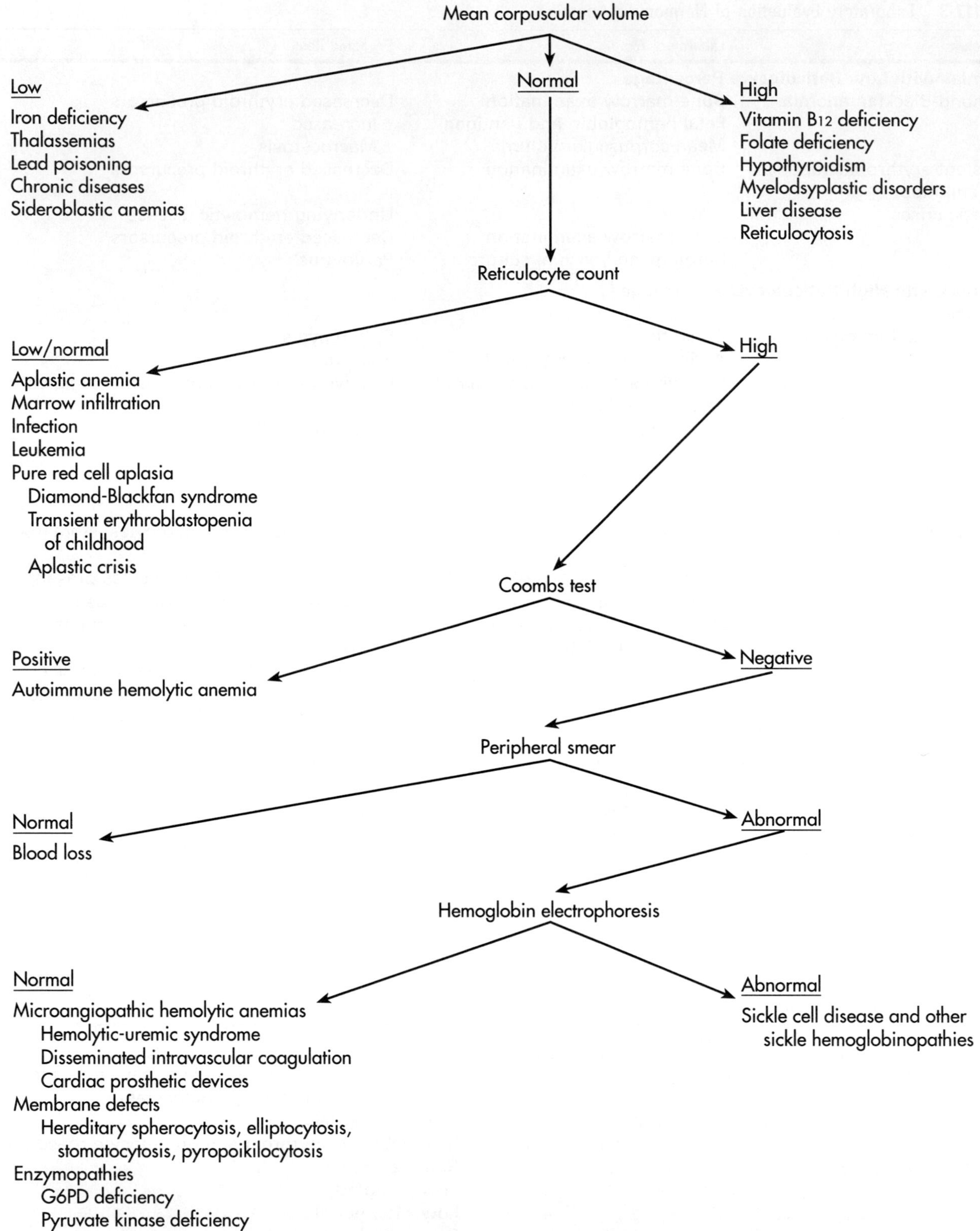

Fig. 117-1 Diagnostic approach to anemia in a child, based on the mean corpuscular volume.

be done at several different times because blood loss through the GI tract may be intermittent. Gastric or duodenal ulcers, Meckel's diverticula, polyps, hemorrhoids, and aspirin-induced bleeding should be considered. Other possibilities include epistaxis and inflammatory bowel disease. Cow milk may induce GI bleeding.[18] Iron deficiency itself, through damage to iron-dependent enzymes in the intestinal mucosa, may cause occult blood loss.[11] The signs and symptoms of iron-deficiency anemia do not differ significantly from those of any other slowly developing anemia. Irritability, pica, and craving for ice and unusual foods occasionally have been observed with anemia specifically caused by iron deficiency.[16]

If the iron deficiency is sufficient to cause anemia, changes in other laboratory parameters will be present. The MCV and the absolute reticulocyte count will be low, and the peripheral blood film will show a predominance of hypochromic and microcytic cells. Target cells and elliptocytes also may be observed. These data usually are sufficient to diagnose iron deficiency. When the diagnosis is not certain, confirmatory laboratory tests may include determining the serum ferritin and serum iron levels (both of which will be low) and the total iron-binding capacity (which will be elevated). The plasma of patients who have iron-deficiency anemia is clear rather than the normal straw color, and the anemia frequently is associated with thrombocytosis.

It is reasonable to give a patient a therapeutic trial of supplemental iron (6 mg/kg of iron per day) if the patient has laboratory evidence of iron-deficiency anemia and his or her age and history suggest poor dietary iron intake. For patients who do not fall into this category or who are compliant and yet do not respond (or respond only transiently) to supplemental iron, additional evaluations for blood loss are imperative. It must be remembered that iron-deficiency anemia is a pathophysiological state for which an etiology needs to be found. For individuals who have moderate to severe iron-deficiency anemia, the reticulocyte count should increase within 5 to 7 days after therapy is started. The therapy for iron deficiency requires continuous iron supplementation for approximately 2 to 3 months after the anemia is corrected. For a more complete discussion of iron-deficiency anemia, see Chapter 228.

Thalassemias. The thalassemias are a heterogeneous group of disorders of hemoglobin production. In alpha-thalassemia the synthesis of the alpha-chain is reduced; in beta-thalassemia, similar deficits occur in beta-chain production. A decrease in production of one leads to a surplus of the other. This imbalance results in precipitation of the surplus chains and destruction of the red blood cells. In general, the greater the imbalance in production of the two chains, the more severe the clinical syndrome.

BETA-THALASSEMIA. Two genes (one on each chromosome 11) direct the synthesis of the beta-chain of hemoglobin. An abnormality in one of these genes causes a mild decrease in beta-chain production. The associated clinical syndrome is called *beta-thalassemia trait* (or *thalassemia minor*) and commonly is observed in patients of African, Mediterranean, and Southeast Asian descent. These patients are completely asymptomatic and usually are diagnosed incidentally or when undergoing routine screening for anemia. The children are mildly anemic; they have a low MCV (usually 60 to 70 fL, a mild increase in the number of red cells (children who have iron-deficiency anemia have a decreased number of red cells), and a peripheral blood film showing microcytosis, hypochromia, and target cells. Iron deficiency may be confused with this entity because of the similarity of laboratory findings in these two disorders. A useful guideline for distinguishing between them is the Mentzer index,[15] which is based on the premise that numbers of red blood cells in beta-thalassemia trait are greater than in iron deficiency. Hemoglobin electrophoresis usually shows mild elevation of hemoglobin F or hemoglobin A_2. Genetic counseling is recommended for families of patients who have beta-thalassemia trait; individuals who inherit this defect from one parent and a similar or second defect from the other parent (e.g., sickle cell trait) may be afflicted with more severe hemoglobinopathies.

Severe beta-thalassemia (Cooley's anemia, thalassemia major) is the result of defects in both genes that direct synthesis of the beta-chain. The marked deficiency in beta-chain production that results is reflected in the more severe clinical syndromes. Patients are severely anemic; there is brisk hemolysis, and the compensatory erythropoiesis is responsible for the characteristic prominence of the cheeks and for the frontal bossing seen in these patients.

Extramedullary hematopoiesis and red blood cell destruction cause marked hepatosplenomegaly. Effective genetic counseling has led to a dramatic decrease in the incidence of this disorder in the United States. Treatment consists of repeated blood transfusions and administration of deferoxamine to minimize iron overload from the transfusions.

ALPHA-THALASSEMIA. Four identical genes (two on each chromosome 16) code for the synthesis of the alpha-chains. Abnormalities in these genes are encountered most often in blacks and Asians. The silent carrier has a mutation in one of the four genes and is asymptomatic and clinically undetectable. Abnormalities in two genes cause alpha-thalassemia trait. Patients who have this mutation also are asymptomatic; their laboratory findings are similar to those of patients who have beta-thalassemia trait. However, they are even less anemic (if at all), and their hemoglobin electrophoresis is normal. The diagnosis of alpha-thalassemia trait therefore must be based on a constellation of clinical findings—a patient who has the appropriate ethnic background and a mild anemia, microcytosis, normal hemoglobin electrophoresis, and normal iron status. Hemoglobin H disease is the result of abnormalities in three of the four alpha-chain genes. Patients usually are asymptomatic but have moderate anemia (hemoglobin 7 to 10 g/dl), microcytosis, hypochromia, and red cell fragments. The hemoglobin electrophoresis shows 5% to 30% hemoglobin H (four beta-chains). An abnormality in all four genes results in no production of alpha-chains and is not compatible with life except with extraordinary measures, such as intrauterine transfusions.

Other hemoglobinopathies associated with microcytosis and anemia include hemoglobin E syndromes (common in southeast Asians) and sickle thalassemia (a combination of beta-thalassemia trait and sickle trait).

Lead poisoning. Although lead has no known physiological role in humans, virtually everyone has measurable levels because of the widespread use of lead in industrial societies. Lead exerts its hematological effect at low plasma levels, inactivating heme synthesis by inhibiting the insertion of iron into the protoporphyrin ring. Thus, with lead poisoning, the hematological picture is similar to that of iron-deficiency anemia: microcytosis, hypochromia, and a low

MCV. In addition, target cells and intense basophilic stippling of red blood cells may be observed. Because iron cannot be inserted into the protoporphyrin ring, the latter compound builds up in the red cell, and levels of free erythrocyte protoporphyrin (FEP) rise.

Children are exposed to lead in the air (from combustion of lead-containing gasoline), in dust, and in lead-based paint found in old houses. With the elimination of lead-containing gasoline in the United States, the frequency of lead poisoning has dropped significantly. The number of children who have blood lead levels ≥20 μg/ml dropped from 3,335,000 during 1976 to 1980 to 206,000 during 1988 to 1991.[2] Although it is generally acknowledged that any measurable lead in plasma is abnormal, debate exists concerning the minimum level associated with clinically significant symptoms and concerning the level at which it is necessary to intervene. According to the 1991 Centers for Disease Control and Prevention guidelines, education and periodic monitoring are recommended for children who have lead levels of 10 to 20 μg/ml, and chelation therapy as well as home visits to remove potential sources of lead are to be considered for children who have lead levels ≥20 μg/ml.[5]

Because lead screening is routine, lead poisoning usually is detected before children are symptomatic or anemic. Symptoms of the anemia are nonspecific, but children who have associated lead encephalopathy may show malaise or behavioral changes. Some physicians use the FEP level to screen for lead poisoning because it is a very sensitive indicator of the pathophysiological effect of the heavy metal. Elevated FEP also is a marker of iron deficiency. Children who have an elevated FEP should have their blood lead level checked. The most important aspect of treatment is removal of any known sources of lead from the child's environment. Medical treatment consists of chelation therapy with dimercaprol or calcium EDTA, both of which chelate lead and subsequently are excreted with the lead into the urine. Lead poisoning is discussed in greater detail in Chapter 293, Poisoning, and in Chapter 20 (Six), Screening for Lead Poisoning.

Chronic inflammation. A wide variety of chronic illnesses may be associated with a mild microcytic anemia. This anemia can be seen in children who have cancer, collagen-vascular disease, chronic renal failure, and chronic infection. Although the red cells of these patients more often are normocytic and normochromic, they sometimes are microcytic and hypochromic. The anemia is moderate (hemoglobin 7 to 10 g/dl), and the reticulocyte count is normal or low. Plasma iron and total iron-binding capacity are low, and ferritin is high. This anemia is believed to be caused by a combination of decreased red blood cell survival, poor marrow response to anemia, and diminished flow of iron from the reticuloendothelial cells to the erythroblasts. The hypochromic microcytic anemia develops when the flow of iron is affected.

Sideroblastic anemias. These rare forms of anemia are a heterogenous group of disorders caused by retention of iron in the mitochondria of developing erythrocytes. Inherited forms are extremely rare but may be seen in children. Some may respond to pyridoxine. Acquired forms of the disease are encountered more often but almost exclusively in adults.

Normocytic Anemias

Normocytic anemias can be caused by increased destruction or decreased production of red blood cells. The reticulocyte count is a valuable test for distinguishing between these two processes. It generally is high in disorders of increased destruction and low in diseases of impaired red cell production.

Normocytic anemia with reticulocytopenia. A normocytic anemia with a low reticulocyte count is uncommon; it may be due to either an isolated problem in the erythroid line or to a disorder that affects all hematopoietic cell lines.

PURE RED CELL APLASIA. Diamond-Blackfan anemia and transient erythroblastopenia of childhood are the most common pure red cell aplasias in children. Diamond-Blackfan anemia is a rare congenital disorder. Children usually manifest the disease in the first year of life with profound anemia and reticulocytopenia. As many as 25% of affected children have physical abnormalities such as short stature or malformed thumbs.[1] Additional laboratory features may include slight macrocytosis, persistent fetal hemoglobin, and persistence of the fetal "little i" red blood cell surface antigen. The etiology is unknown. Patients usually respond to treatment with prednisone.

Transient erythroblastopenia of childhood is a recently recognized,[14] benign, transient hypoplastic anemia that occurs most often in children between the ages of 1 and 4 years. These otherwise healthy children have marked pallor and are severely anemic, with reticulocyte counts of less than 1%. They have normal-appearing erythrocytes that show none of the fetal characteristics of the red cells of Diamond-Blackfan anemia. Although the cause is unknown, several studies suggest that there is humoral suppression of erythropoiesis.[12] Recovery is spontaneous; treatment consists only of red cell transfusions when the anemia is profound. Patients sometimes present in the recovery phase with anemia and reticulocytosis. In these instances the diagnosis may be confused with a hemolytic anemia.

PANCYTOPENIAS. Because anemia may be but one manifestation of a more global disorder of the bone marrow, a white blood cell count and differential and platelet count always should be performed when the hematocrit is low. When these other cell lines are abnormal, serious disorders must be considered in the differential diagnosis. Such disorders include leukemia, primary bone marrow failure syndromes (e.g., aplastic anemia or myelodysplasia), and infiltration of the marrow, as is seen with bone marrow metastases or granulomatous diseases. Occasionally a viral illness will cause a transient suppression of all cell lines.

APLASTIC CRISES. Children who have chronic hemolytic anemia (e.g., sickle cell anemia or hereditary spherocytosis) compensate for increased hemolysis with an increase in the rate of red cell production. Occasionally, these children have transient suppression of red cell production, while the hemolysis continues at the same rate. The result is a precipitous drop in the hematocrit value, and patients may have a sudden onset of weakness, fatigue, pallor, and even shock.

Laboratory values include a low hematocrit and reticulocytopenia. A patient who has a known hemolytic anemia who manifests these findings must be treated immediately. The principal treatment is infusion of red blood cells. The aplasia is transient and in many instances is associated with acute parvovirus infection.[13]

OTHER. A normocytic, normochromic anemia often is seen with chronic illness, as noted previously. Acute blood loss may be mistaken for a hypoproductive anemia when the patient is seen shortly after the blood loss but before generating a reticulocyte response.

Normocytic anemia with elevated reticulocyte count. Normocytic anemias with reticulocytosis are characterized by accelerated destruction of red blood cells and a compensatory increase in erythropoiesis. These hemolytic anemias can be classified further by the nature of the red blood cell destruction: those secondary to destruction of normal red cells by extrinsic forces and those in which intrinsic abnormalities of the erythrocytes result in their premature destruction.

HEMOLYSIS CAUSED BY EXTRINSIC FACTORS. Disseminated intravascular coagulation (DIC), hemolytic-uremic syndrome (HUS), certain types of cardiac prosthetic devices, and immune-mediated hemolysis all cause destruction of otherwise normal red blood cells. In DIC and HUS, fibrin is deposited in the small vessels, and erythrocytes are torn apart as they attempt to flow through the maze of fibrin strands. The peripheral blood film shows red cell fragments (schistocytes). A similar morphological picture is seen when erythrocytes are destroyed by prosthetic devices such as artificial heart valves or foreign bodies such as arterial or central venous catheters.

Immune-mediated hemolysis is uncommon beyond the neonatal period; when it occurs, it usually is an autoimmune phenomenon. Autoimmune hemolytic anemia may be idiopathic or a feature of an underlying systemic disorder. Idiopathic autoimmune hemolytic anemia often is associated with an antecedent viral infection and occurs in children of all ages. In most instances the red cell destruction resolves over several months, although children younger than age 4 years or older than age 10 years are more likely to develop a chronic hemolytic anemia.[3]

Symptoms of autoimmune hemolytic anemia depend on the rapidity and degree of the drop in the hematocrit level. Patients usually are jaundiced secondary to the hemolysis and often have splenomegaly. Patients who have intravascular hemolysis may have pink or red urine as a result of excretion of free hemoglobin. The hematocrit may range from normal to profoundly low, reflecting the intensity of the hemolysis. The reticulocyte count usually is elevated but is normal or low in as many as one third to half of children,[8] presumably because autoantibodies are directed to reticulocytes as well as to the mature red blood cells. The peripheral blood film shows a preponderance of spherocytes. A positive Coombs test is diagnostic. It is imperative to evaluate the patient who has an autoimmune hemolytic anemia for an underlying systemic disorder. Autoimmune hemolysis is seen in association with malignancies, immune deficiencies, collagen vascular disease, certain drugs, and infections such as *Mycoplasma pneumoniae,* Epstein-Barr virus, and the human immunodeficiency virus (HIV). Treatment of autoimmune hemolytic anemia is directed at correcting the underlying disorder. In cases of idiopathic disease, treatment with prednisone is recommended. Patients should be maintained on a dose of 2 mg/kg/day until the hematocrit value is in the normal range and there is little or no evidence of red cell destruction. Patients who do not respond to steroids may respond to other immunosuppressives or to high doses of intravenous gamma globulin.[4]

Wilson's disease must always be considered in any patient who has a nonimmune hemolytic anemia. Hemolysis in Wilson's disease is due to elevated levels of serum copper. Early diagnosis leads to early treatment and prevention of severe liver disease and mental retardation associated with more advanced Wilson's disease. Vitamin E deficiency also causes hemolysis. It occurs in premature infants and patients who have fat malabsorption (e.g., children who have cystic fibrosis).

HEMOLYSIS CAUSED BY INTRINSIC ABNORMALITIES OF RED BLOOD CELLS. Three types of intrinsic abnormalities of red blood cells predispose them to premature destruction: a defective red cell membrane, deficiencies in red cell enzymes, and production of abnormal forms of hemoglobin.

Membrane defects. Hereditary spherocytosis is the most common of the membrane disorders. The membrane defect usually is due to a deficiency in spectrin, the main structural protein of the red cell membrane. This deficiency renders the red blood cell more fragile and, as a result, more susceptible to hemolysis.

Hereditary spherocytosis is transmitted as an autosomal dominant trait in 75% of cases and occurs in at least 1 in 5000 people of Northern European descent. The spectrum of disease is highly variable. Classically, patients who have hereditary spherocytosis have anemia, jaundice, and splenomegaly; in fact, many are identified incidentally on routine screening. Affected patients often report family members who have a history of anemia, jaundice, and splenectomy or cholecystectomy at an early age. Laboratory studies reveal anemia, reticulocytosis, and increased numbers of spherocytes on the peripheral blood film. The osmotic fragility of the red blood cells is increased. This test is not diagnostic, however, because spherocytes or red cells in any disorder characterized by unstable membranes show increased osmotic fragility. The hemolytic anemia resolves with splenectomy, because the spleen is the sole site of red cell destruction in this disease. Most patients eventually require a splenectomy to avoid complications of hereditary spherocytosis such as aplastic crises, gallstones, or splenic trauma.

Hereditary elliptocytosis and hereditary stomatocytosis and pyropoikilocytosis are less common congenital defects of red cell membranes and are encountered infrequently in children.

Enzyme deficiencies. Glucose-6-phosphate dehydrogenase (G6PD) deficiency is the most common enzymopathy affecting red blood cells. G6PD generates nicotinamide adenine dinucleotide phosphate (NADPH) by catalyzing the conversion of glucose-6-phosphate to 6-phosphogluconate. The NADPH is used by the red blood cell to reduce potentially toxic oxidizing agents that accumulate with exposure to certain drugs, chemicals, and infections.

Two of the most common types of G6PD deficiencies are a mild variant (Gd^{A}) that occurs in approximately 10% of black males and a more severe variant ($G^{Mediterranean}$) observed in people of Mediterranean descent. The disorder is transmitted as an X-linked trait; thus, males are affected more often than females. Most patients in the United States (those who have the Gd^{A} variant) are asymptomatic, and their deficiency is not apparent unless they are exposed to an oxidant stress such as an infection or a medication. Agents that precipitate hemolysis most often include sulfa drugs and chloramphenicol, antimalarial drugs, aspirin, ascorbic acid, chemicals such as benzene or naphthalene, infection (hepatitis), and diabetic ketoacidosis.

Patients manifest jaundice and symptoms of a rapidly falling hematocrit. Because the hemolysis is intravascular, patients may have hemoglobinuria. Laboratory findings include anemia and reticulocytosis. There may be pitted red blood cells on the blood film, but findings often are nonspecific. Special stains reveal the presence of precipitated hemoglobin aggregates, called *Heinz bodies.* A test for red cell G6PD often is normal or elevated at the time of a hemolytic episode because only the younger, more enzyme-replete cells remain. If G6PD deficiency is strongly suspected, the test should be repeated 1 to 2 months after the acute crisis or performed in the mother. Treatment is supportive and consists of eliminating exposure to the offending agent and, if necessary, giving the patient a transfusion.

Many other enzyme deficiencies predispose the red cell to hemolysis. Perhaps that occurring most frequently (excluding G6PD) is pyruvate kinase deficiency. Patients who have this rare enzymopathy suffer from a chronic hemolytic anemia. Routine laboratory studies are nondiagnostic; specific assays for pyruvate kinase must be ordered if the diagnosis is suspected.

Hemoglobinopathies. The hemoglobinopathies are a group of hemolytic disorders in which there are abnormalities in the amino acid composition of the alpha- or beta-chain of the hemoglobin molecule. Sickle cell anemia is the most prevalent disease in this group. The defect in sickle cell anemia is a single amino acid substitution of valine for glutamic acid in position 6 of the beta-chain of hemoglobin. This substitution renders hemoglobin susceptible to polymerization when it is exposed to low tensions of oxygen; as a result, the red cell "sickles" irreversibly.

Sickle cell anemia is transmitted as an autosomal recessive trait. Approximately 8% of blacks carry this trait. Although 30% to 45% of their hemoglobin is the sickle variant, this is not sufficient to cause their red cells to "sickle" under normal circumstances. These patients grow and develop normally and have normal hematocrit levels and reticulocyte counts. They occasionally may develop renal papillary necrosis, and when at high altitudes (over 10,000 feet) they are at risk of splenic infarction or other manifestations of vasoocclusive disease. For purposes of genetic counseling, it is important to identify patients who have the sickle hemoglobin trait.

Homozygous sickle cell anemia occurs in approximately 1 in 650 blacks. Although the vast majority of people afflicted with the disease in the United States are black, it occasionally has been reported in Greeks, Arabs, and natives of India.

Children who have sickle cell anemia usually do not have symptoms of the disease until they are approximately 6 months of age. From age 6 months to 3 years, however, most affected children have experienced the pain of vasoocclusive crises; by age 4 years many already show delayed growth and development along with maxillary hyperplasia. Typically, these children have hematocrit values ranging from the low to middle 20s, with reticulocyte counts of 5% to 15%. The MCV is normal. The peripheral blood film reveals some irreversibly sickled cells, but target cells, polychromasia, and Howell-Jolly bodies also are present. Hemoglobin electrophoresis is diagnostic; there usually is more than 90% hemoglobin S and less than 10% hemoglobin F and/or hemoglobin A_2.

Most of the signs and symptoms of sickle cell anemia are a consequence of intravascular sickling and occlusion of blood vessels by the sickled cells. This vasoocclusion (often referred to as a *vasoocclusive crisis*) occurs episodically, usually in association with infection, dehydration, acidosis, or exposure to cold. The most common type of vasoocclusive crisis is the "painful" crisis that results from widespread ischemia and infarction of bone marrow, bone cortex, or other organs. Infants and toddlers may have dactylitis; older patients complain of excruciating extremity, back, or chest pain and usually have a paucity of physical findings. Treatment consists of hydration, pain control, and careful monitoring for other complications of vasoocclusion. Patients may have focal rather than diffuse bone pain. When this occurs in association with a high fever, it often is difficult to distinguish whether the patient is experiencing a bone infarction or an osteomyelitis.

Patients also may have chest pain, respiratory distress, a high fever, and an infiltrate on the roentgenogram of the chest. This constellation of signs and symptoms is called the *acute chest syndrome* and may be caused by pneumonia, pulmonary infarction, or both. Patients who have acute chest syndrome are particularly vulnerable to severe, widespread vasoocclusive crises because the pulmonary involvement can cause hypoxia and exacerbate the sickling. Treatment should include vigorous hydration, supplemental oxygen, antibiotics to treat the presumed pneumonia and, if the patient is hypoxic, red blood cell transfusion or exchange transfusion to lower the amount of hemoglobin S and increase the oxygen-carrying capacity of red blood cells. Other complications of vasoocclusion include stroke, priapism, and splenic infarction.

Younger patients (ages 6 months to 3 years) are susceptible to splenic sequestration, a sudden accumulation of blood in the spleen. The result is rapid enlargement of the spleen and a precipitous drop in the hematocrit level. Treatment consists of blood transfusions and volume expanders. Patients who experience splenic sequestration are at increased risk of subsequent episodes. Some physicians advocate splenectomy for patients who have two or more episodes.

As noted previously, patients who have sickle cell anemia also are at risk for aplastic crises. The etiology, presentation, laboratory values, and treatment are similar to the aplastic crises of other chronic hemolytic anemias.

Perhaps the gravest threat to patients who have sickle cell anemia is their susceptibility to serious bacterial infection. This increased risk of infection is due largely to a hypofunctional spleen; defects in opsonization of bacteria also may play a role.[9] These children are at great risk of overwhelming sepsis, meningitis, and pneumonia secondary to infection with *Streptococcus pneumoniae* or *Haemophilus influenzae* type b. They also may experience severe *Mycoplasma* pneumonia and are unusually susceptible to osteomyelitis secondary to *Salmonella* organisms.

So great is the risk of serious bacterial infection in children who have sickle cell anemia that in most centers they are started on penicillin prophylaxis at age 2 to 3 months. It also is recommended that they receive the pneumococcal, *H. influenzae* type b, and influenza virus vaccines. Patients who have sickle cell anemia who develop a fever should be evaluated carefully; if no simple cause is found, they should be admitted to the hospital and treated empirically with intravenous antibiotics. Some investigators advocate initial treatment of well-appearing febrile children with ceftriaxone and subsequent management as outpatients.[17]

Several other hemoglobin defects can occur in combination with the sickle hemoglobin trait and cause a syndrome similar to sickle cell anemia. Patients heterozygous for both hemoglobin S and hemoglobin C may have signs and symptoms of sickle cell anemia, although generally they are less affected than children who have homozygous sickle cell disease. Patients who inherit both the sickle and beta-thalassemia traits may have signs and symptoms of mild or severe sickle cell disease. Patients who have any of these sickle syndromes (as well as those who have the more rare types such as hemoglobin SD or SO^{Arab}) should be managed similarly to patients who have homozygous sickle cell disease; they should receive penicillin prophylaxis and the appropriate vaccines and should be treated similarly for any clinical manifestations of sickling.

Macrocytic Anemias

Macrocytosis is very unusual in children. It can be seen with deficiencies in folic acid or vitamin B_{12}. Folate deficiency may occur secondary to inborn errors of metabolism, poor dietary intake, malabsorption, increased requirements for folate (as in chronic hemolytic anemias), and drugs that inhibit the metabolism of folate (e.g., methotrexate). Vitamin B_{12} deficiency also may be due to inborn errors of metabolism, poor dietary intake, or malabsorption.

The anemia associated with either of these vitamin deficiencies can be severe, and the MCV often is 100 to 140 fL. The peripheral blood film shows numerous normochromic macrocytes and hypersegmented neutrophils. The diagnosis can be confirmed with a serum folate or vitamin B_{12} level; as with iron deficiency, once the deficit is documented, the cause must be determined.

Macrocytosis also is observed in hypothyroidism, children who have Down syndrome, myelodysplastic disorders, dyserythropoietic disorders, and liver disease and in patients who have a significant reticulocytosis. It frequently is seen in patients taking valproic acid or zidovudine, and it is a normal finding in the red blood cells of newborns.

ANEMIA IN THE NEWBORN

The approach to anemia in the newborn must be considered apart from that of anemia in an older infant or child. Many of the etiologies of anemia in the newborn (e.g., isoimmune disease) are unique to this age group. Conversely, some common causes of anemia in older children, such as iron-deficiency anemia, are rare in infants. Furthermore, some of the etiologies of anemia common to both newborns and older children may manifest themselves quite differently in the newborn period than at an older age. A useful algorithm for evaluation of anemia in the newborn is illustrated in Fig. 117-2.

The normal hematological parameters of a newborn are markedly different from those of older children (Table 117-5). The mean hemoglobin level of term infants at birth is approximately 19 g/dl, but the level falls gradually over 8 to 12 weeks to a nadir of 10 to 11 g/dl. This phenomenon is known as the *physiological anemia of infancy*. The drop is even more pronounced in premature infants, in whom hemoglobin levels may fall to 7 to 8 g/dl. This "physiological anemia" is normal in premature and term infants, and despite the low hemoglobin levels, blood transfusion is not necessary in an asymptomatic, otherwise healthy infant.

There are three broad classifications for the etiology of anemia in the newborn: blood loss, hemolysis, and decreased red blood cell production. Blood loss may occur prenatally or perinatally. Common causes include fetomaternal or twin-to-twin transfusion, placenta previa, placental abruption, and internal hemorrhage caused by cephalohematoma, caput succedaneum, or intracranial hemorrhage. Fetomaternal hemorrhage can be confirmed by the Kleihauer-Betke test, which detects the presence of fetal red cells in maternal blood. (The test may result in a false negative if the mother has type O blood and the child does not.) The clinical presentation depends on the rapidity and degree of blood loss. Infants who have experienced chronic blood loss are hemodynamically stable but pale and have a microcytic, hypochromic anemia. Infants who have acute blood loss often are pale and floppy and have tachypnea, tachycardia, and hypotension. The initial hematocrit may be normal, but the infant soon develops a normocytic normochromic anemia with a reticulocytosis.

Isoimmune disease (erythroblastosis fetalis) is the most common cause of hemolytic anemia in newborns. It is caused by an incompatibility between fetal and maternal Rh, ABO, or minor blood group antigens. In Rh incompatibility, the mother's red blood cells are Rh negative, and those of the infant are Rh positive. If the Rh-negative mother previously was sensitized to Rh-positive blood (from a previous pregnancy), she may have developed antibodies to the Rh antigen; these antibodies cross the placenta and destroy the Rh-positive red cells of the infant. The result is a brisk hemolytic anemia, which occurs in utero and continues after the birth of the child. The hematocrit may fall quickly, and the associated hyperbilirubinemia can cause kernicterus. Rh disease can be prevented by prenatal administration of Rh immune globulin to Rh-negative mothers. Life-threatening Rh incompatibility is rare today, largely because of the routine use of Rh immune globulin. ABO incompatibility (a mother who has type O blood and her infant who has type A, B, or AB) is common, but the hemolysis is mild and infrequently causes hyperbilirubinemia or anemia. Hemolysis occasionally occurs when the mother has been sensitized to one of the minor blood groups, such as the Kell or Duffy antigen. An alloimmune hemolytic anemia or drug-induced hemolysis also may occur in the newborn secondary to passive transfer of maternal autoantibody or maternal drug.

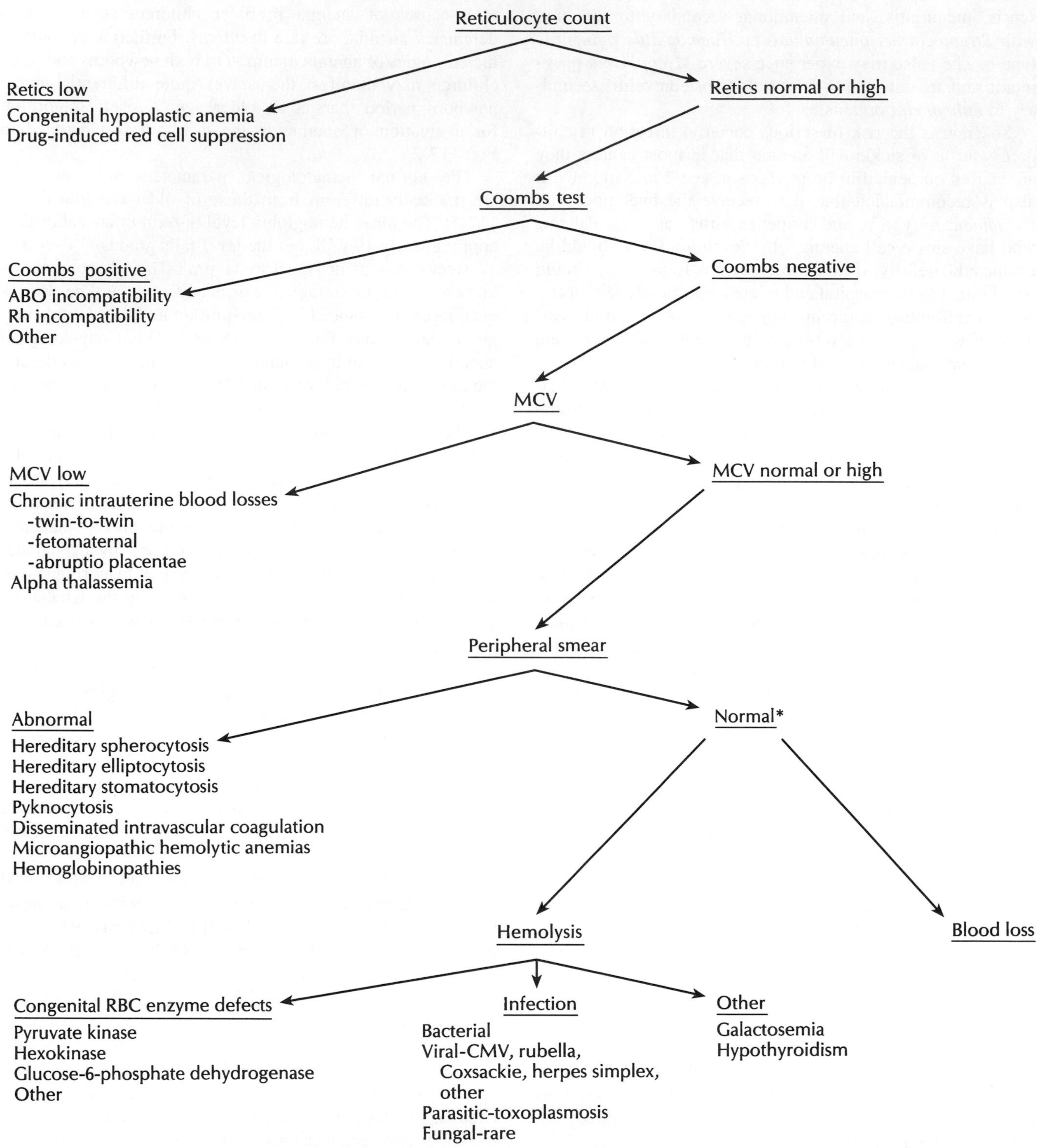

Fig. 117-2 Diagnostic approach to anemia in a newborn, based on the reticulocyte count. The asterisk indicates a peripheral blood smear that shows no specifically diagnostic abnormalities.

(From Nathan DC, Oski F: *Hematology of infancy and childhood,* ed 3, Philadelphia, 1987, WB Saunders.)

Table 117-5 Normal Hematological Values During First 2 Weeks of Life in Term Infant

	Cord Blood	Day 1	Day 3	Day 7	Day 14
Hemoglobin (g/dl)	16.8	18.4	17.8	17.0	16.8
Hematocrit (%)	53.0	58.0	55.0	54.0	52.0
Red cells ($mm^3 \times 10^6$)	5.25	5.8	5.6	5.2	5.1
MCV (fL)	107.0	108.0	99.0	98.0	96.0
MCH (pg/cell)	34.0	35.0	33.0	32.5	31.5
MCHC (g/dl RBCs)	31.7	32.5	33.0	33.0	33.0
Reticulocytes (%)	3-7	3-7	1-3	0-1	0-1
Nucleated RBC/(mm^3)	500	200	0-5	0	0
Platelets (1000/mm^3)	290	192	213	248	252

From Nathan DG, Oski F: *Hematology of infancy and childhood,* ed 3, Philadelphia, 1987, WB Saunders.
MCV, mean corpuscular volume; *MCH,* mean corpuscular hemoglobin; *MCHC,* mean corpuscular hemoglobin concentration; *RBC,* red blood cells.

Hemolytic anemia in the newborn is associated with many types of infection. Bacterial sepsis and cytomegalovirus, toxoplasmosis, herpes, and rubella infections all can cause hemolysis. A microangiopathic hemolytic anemia can occur secondary to DIC, cavernous hemangiomas (as in Kasabach-Merritt syndrome), and localized thrombi.

Hemoglobinopathies rarely cause symptoms in the neonatal period. Beta-chain defects, such as sickle cell syndromes, are not apparent until later in infancy, when appreciable concentrations of the beta-chain of hemoglobin have been produced. Similarly, beta-thalassemias are not detectable clinically at birth. Newborns who have alpha-thalassemia major present with erythroblastosis fetalis. Infants who have red blood cell membrane defects or enzymopathies occasionally are diagnosed in the newborn period but more often manifest symptoms at a later age.

Disorders of red cell production are rare in the newborn. Hypoproduction of red cells occurs most often secondary to drugs or infection. Diamond-Blackfan syndrome is a rare congenital pure red blood cell aplasia, but infants who have this disease are not anemic at birth. They usually are not diagnosed until the anemia is apparent clinically, sometime between the ages of 3 and 12 months; they may be diagnosed earlier if they have one of the characteristic physical anomalies. Congenital leukemia and osteopetrosis are other very rare causes of red cell aplasia and are associated with abnormalities in other cell lines.

When to Refer

Hematocrit <25%
Unexplained anemia
Bicytopenia or pancytopenia

When to Hospitalize

Profound anemia (i.e., hematocrit <15% to 20%)
Rapidly dropping hematocrit
Anemia in an ill child

REFERENCES

1. Alter BA, Young NS: The bone marrow failure syndromes. In Nathan DG, Orkin S, editors: *Nathan and Oski's hematology of infants and children,* ed 5, Philadelphia, 1998, WB Saunders.
2. Brody DJ, et al: Blood lead levels in the US population. Phase I of the Third National Health and Nutrition Examination Survey (NHANES III, 1988-1991), *JAMA* 272:277, 1994.
3. Buchanan GR, et al: The acute and transient nature of idiopathic immune hemolytic anemia in childhood, *J Pediatr* 88:780, 1976.
4. Bussel JB, Cunningham-Rundles C, Abraham C: Intravenous treatment of autoimmune hemolytic anemia with very-high-dose gammaglobulin, *Vox Sang* 51:264, 1986.
5. Centers for Disease Control: *Preventing lead poisoning in young children,* Atlanta, 1991, US Department of Health and Human Services.
6. Dallman PR, Siimes MA: Percentile curves for hemoglobin and red cell volume in infancy and childhood, *J Pediatr* 94:26, 1979.
7. Dallman PR, Yip R, Johnson C: Prevalence and causes of anemia in the United States, *Am J Clin Nutr* 39:437, 1984.
8. Habibi B, et al: Autoimmune hemolytic anemia in children: a review of 80 cases, *Am J Med* 56:61, 1974.
9. Johnston RB, Newman SL, Struth AG: Increased susceptibility to infection in sickle cell disease: defects of opsonization and of splenic function, *Birth Defects* 11:322, 1975.
10. Kay R, Oski FA, Barness LA: *Core textbook of pediatrics,* ed 3, Philadelphia, 1988, JB Lippincott.
11. Kimber C, Weintraub LR: Malabsorption of iron secondary to iron deficiency, *N Engl J Med* 279:453, 1968.
12. Koening HM, et al: Immune suppression of erythropoiesis in TEC, *Blood* 54:742, 1979.
13. Lefrere JJ, et al: Six cases of hereditary spherocytosis revealed by human parvovirus infection, *Br J Haematol* 62:653, 1986.
14. Lovric VA: Anemia and temporary erythroblastopenia in children, *Aust Ann Med* 1:34, 1970.
15. Mentzer WC: Differentiation of iron deficiency from thalassemia trait, *Lancet* 1:449, 1973.
16. Schorin MA: Pallor and anemia. In Ziai M, editor: *Bedside pediatrics,* Boston, 1983, Little, Brown.
17. Williams JA, et al: A randomized study of outpatient treatment with ceftriaxone for selected febrile children with sickle cell disease, *N Engl J Med* 329:472, 1993.
18. Wilson JF, et al: Studies on iron metabolism. V. Further observations on cow's milk-induced gastrointestinal bleeding in infants with iron deficiency anemia, *J Pediatr* 84:335, 1974.

SUGGESTED READINGS

Pearson HA: Sickle cell diseases: diagnosis and management in infancy and childhood, *Pediatr Rev* 9:121, 1987.

Segel GB: Anemia, *Pediatr Rev* 10:77, 1988.

118 Back Pain

Robert A. Pendergrast, Jr.

Back pain is an uncommon presenting symptom in pediatric practice. Population-based data on back pain in children are limited, and estimates of prevalence vary considerably depending on sample size and methodology. At the least, most authors have consistently shown that prevalence of back pain increases with age. In nonclinical populations, prevalence is less than 10% in preteens, progressing to nearly 50% of 18- to 20-year-olds reporting at least one episode of low back pain.[7] Clearly, most of those experiencing such pain do not seek medical care, and in preadolescent children back pain is not only unusual but also likely to indicate serious underlying illness when severe or persistent enough to prompt a medical visit.[5] One 6-year study in a tertiary orthopedic setting found that back pain constituted less than 2% of referrals in children age 15 years or younger, but that roughly 50% of these children had serious underlying disease.[12] From early adolescence onward, back pain not only becomes more common as a presenting complaint but also is more likely to be a benign condition related to acute injury or repetitive stress. The clinician presented with a child or adolescent complaining of back pain may use a careful history and physical examination to guide any further laboratory or radiological evaluation but should be aware of the relatively higher risk of serious underlying disease in younger children, even without specific physical findings.

DEFINITION AND CHARACTERISTICS

For purposes of this discussion, the back encompasses the region from the upper thoracic vertebra (T1) and shoulder girdle to the sacrum and surrounding musculature. The patient who complains of pain in this region may have a specific sense of localization to a muscle group or vertebral body, for example, or the pain may be more diffuse or sensed by the patient as "deep" and difficult to localize. Allowing the patient to define in his or her own words the nature, location, and duration of the pain is an important first step in arriving at a clinical diagnosis. Confirmation of the pain history should be obtained from parents, especially for young children but also for teens, who may minimize the pain out of imagined fears of diagnostic or therapeutic procedures. Pain that is acute, lasting fewer than 3 weeks, especially with a history of musculoskeletal injury, may be managed expectantly in many cases, whereas more chronic pain in a child or adolescent demands more immediate attention.[2,10] Any functional disability that accompanies pain (such as interference with sports or play) also lends urgency to the diagnostic evaluation, and the corroboration of other observers, such as parents, coaches, and school personnel, can assist the clinician at this point.

ASSOCIATED SIGNS AND SYMPTOMS

A variety of additional signs and symptoms may provide diagnostic clues to the etiology of back pain. Young children or adolescents who have fever and back pain must be considered to have an infectious, inflammatory, or neoplastic process until proven otherwise; examples include diskitis, vertebral osteomyelitis, ankylosing spondylitis, pyelonephritis, vasoocclusive crisis in a patient who has sickle cell anemia, acute lymphoblastic leukemia, Ewing's sarcoma, or Hodgkin's lymphoma.[2,8] Spinal tuberculosis (Pott's disease), fortunately is rare but should be considered when back pain is accompanied by low-grade fever.[10] Dysuria, urgency, or urinary frequency, especially if accompanied by fever, warrants consideration of pyelonephritis. Weight loss, bone pain in other locations, and adenopathy should prompt aggressive diagnostic evaluation for malignancies such as leukemia, lymphoma, or sarcomas. Accompanying neurological symptoms, including radicular pain down the leg, numbness or tingling, bowel or bladder problems, erectile dysfunction, or loss of sphincter tone on neurological examination,[2] may indicate disk herniation in adolescent athletes or other nerve compression and should prompt an urgent evaluation and referral.[8] Low-back pain associated with excessive lordotic curvature, especially in an athlete subjected to repetitive extension loading (e.g., gymnasts or football linemen) may indicate spondylolysis or spondylolisthesis. Idiopathic scoliosis usually would not be expected to cause back pain[10]; rather, the scoliosis and the pain may be secondary to a neoplasm in the region of the spine, such as a benign osteoid osteoma. A child who has nocturnal back pain, even if relieved by nonprescription analgesics, should be evaluated for osteoid osteoma or osteoblastoma with bone scans if plain films are normal.[5,8] Stigmata of Marfan syndrome found on physical examination usually include joint hyperextensibility, pectus excavation, pes planus, dislocated lenses, hernias, arachnodactyly, and scoliosis. Scoliosis may be due to a dural ectasia or widening of the subarachnoid space in the lumbar area, which has been associated with low-back pain in adolescents and young adults.[9] Patients who have Marfan syndrome are also at increased risk of spondylolysis.[10] Scheuermann's disease typically presents in an adolescent who has back pain after exercise or late in the day, thoracic kyphosis on examination, and pain worsened by forward flexion.[5,8]

CIRCUMSTANCES SURROUNDING PRESENTATION

The type of diagnostic evaluation and the therapeutic modalities chosen depend on several key factors at presentation. The age of the patient perhaps is the most critical of these, with the extent and urgency of evaluation usually being greater for preadolescent patients.[2,10] Another factor is the duration of symptoms; chronic pain, even in adolescent patients, is uncommon and may indicate structural or serious underlying disease. Chronic back pain in an adolescent should prompt a diagnostic evaluation to include rectal examination for sphincter tone loss, roentgenograms of the spine (anteroposterior, lateral, and oblique views), blood count and sedimentation rate, and urinalysis and culture. In the adolescent patient who can date the onset of pain to a specific event or injury, whose pain lasts fewer than 3 weeks, and whose pain clearly is exacerbated by mechanical factors such as lifting, stooping, or exercise, a diagnosis of mechanical low-back pain is most likely, and these symptoms in most cases will resolve in 2 to 3 weeks regardless of the therapeutic approach.[2] However, very localized tenderness in the spine following injury (e.g., motor vehicle accident or athletic trauma) warrants radiological evaluation for compression fracture.[8] Other presentations in adolescents often are sport specific: Gymnasts whose lumbar spines are subject to hyperextension and repetitive microtrauma should be highly suspect for spondylolysis or spondylolisthesis; ballet dancers as a group have great flexibility but may be predisposed to lumbar lordosis by postural demands and relatively weak abdominal musculature; they also are prone to spondylolysis as well as to disk disease.[1] Competitive swimmers can present with Scheuermann's disease, or "butterflyer's back." The classic presentation of Scheuermann's disease is thoracic kyphosis and wedging of three or more contiguous vertebrae shown on plain spine films.

DIFFERENTIAL DIAGNOSIS

Infants

From infancy through the second year of life, the patient will not be capable of localizing or complaining of pain in the back. Unexplained fever or toxicity along with refusal to walk or stand may be the presenting signs of diskitis in this age group.[8,11] Leukemia, lymphoma, vasoocclusive crisis, or vertebral osteomyelitis in a child who has sickle cell disease, or trauma (especially intentional injury) may present as disease localized to the back in this age group.

Children

As children mature and become more capable of localizing symptoms, a specific history of the duration, quality, associated symptoms, and radiation of back pain becomes possible to elicit. Back pain upon walking may be the only presenting sign of a tethered cord.[8] The differential diagnosis in this age group also includes diskitis, an inflammatory process presumed to be a bacterial infection in the intervertebral disk space, which typically is associated with an elevated erythrocyte sedimentation rate and a high white blood cell count. It is most common in children younger than 10 years of age (mean age about 6 years). A child who has diskitis is typically uncomfortable in an upright posture and may have pain when bending forward. A child who has fever who refuses to walk should be evaluated promptly for diskitis and treated with parenteral antibiotics pending diagnosis. Magnetic resonance imaging (MRI) generally is thought to be a sensitive test in evaluating for diskitis.[8,11] Vertebral osteomyelitis usually affects older children and teenagers and presents with severe back pain and systemic symptoms. Staphylococcal infection is most common and should be treated with antibiotics, rest, and a prompt orthopedic consult.[5] A family history of rheumatoid disease should prompt consideration of ankylosing spondylitis. In the presence of sickle hemoglobinopathy, a vasoocclusive crisis is a strong consideration. Especially in the presence of fever or other systemic signs and symptoms such as adenopathy, bruising, or organomegaly, acute leukemia must be ruled out by complete blood count and evaluation of the peripheral smear; the possibility of lymphoma must be evaluated further by lymph node biopsy, if available, or by MRI of the chest, abdomen, and spine. Primary vertebral tumors almost always will be visible on plain radiographs; these tumors include Ewing's sarcoma, aneurysmal bone cyst, benign osteoblastoma, and osteoid osteoma.[8] It is only after a thorough diagnostic evaluation that one should consider a diagnosis of idiopathic or mechanical back pain in younger children.

Adolescents

In adolescent patients, a diagnostic consideration of mechanical back pain without underlying cause becomes reasonable. The typical presentation for this diagnosis is an adolescent who has low-back pain of 3 weeks' or fewer duration, with or without recollection of an acute injury, and whose pain is exacerbated by postural changes or specific movements. Associated signs and symptoms such as neurological defects of the lower extremities; limited straight leg-raising; sciatic pain; bowel, bladder, or sexual dysfunction; fever; weight loss; adenopathy; urinary urgency or frequency; scoliosis; or Marfanoid habitus should be absent.[12] Fever accompanied by back pain in this age group should prompt an aggressive diagnostic evaluation and orthopedic consultation, because aspiration and culture to evaluate possible vertebral osteomyelitis should be considered.[5] The adolescent who has chronic pain (greater than 3 weeks) still may have idiopathic or mechanical low-back pain, but stronger consideration should be given at this point to plain films of the spine to rule out spondylolysis or spondylolisthesis, which are the most common identifiable causes of low-back pain in this age group.[5] Spondylolysis is a stress fracture of the pars interarticularis (posterior arch) of the spine, thought to be acquired through repetitive extension loading such as when a gymnast lands from a vault. It is visible on oblique lumbar spine films. Normal plain films alone do not rule out a healing spondylolysis completely, and a bone scan may be positive. Spondylolysis may be unilateral or bilateral and is most common at L5. Symptoms of spondylolysis are not usually acute; it more commonly presents as a gradual worsening of back pain in an athlete during his or her growth spurt. Pain can be reproduced reliably by having the patient hyperextend the back while standing on one leg.[5] Hamstring tightness is a common associated finding.[8] Spondylolisthesis is a forward slippage of one vertebral body on top of the other (usually L5 on S1), resulting from bilateral spondylolysis. Scheuermann's kyphosis predisposes to spondylolisthesis because of a compensatory lumbar lordosis.[8] Spondylolisthesis may be accompanied on physical examination not only by excess lumbar lordosis but also by the sensation of a shelf at the base of the lordotic curvature, where the lower of the two affected vertebrae has held its position while the upper vertebral body slipped forward. In rare cases, radiographs will reveal congenital absence of a lumbosacral articular process.[6]

Chronic low-back pain, especially in adolescent athletes or others who have cumulative trauma, may indicate lumbar disk disease. Symptoms typically are worsened by mechanical strain, as with lifting or coughing.[8] A positive straight leg-raising test is highly suggestive of a herniated disk. Using cervical flexion to accentuate the patient's symptoms during straight-leg raising may add to the test's sensitivity, and any reproduction of the patient's usual symptoms during testing, or marked asymmetry in symptoms, should be considered a positive test.[3] Chronic low-back pain without any of these signs may be a disorder of the soft tissues of the low back, perhaps secondary to repetitive strain coupled with genetic predisposition and environmental factors, such as prolonged seated posture or forward bending of the spine, as with studying or reading while sitting at a desk for long periods.

PSYCHOSOCIAL CONSIDERATIONS

Although malingering or the use of pain symptoms for secondary gain may be relatively common in adults, it should not be a strong consideration in the diagnosis of back pain in children or adolescents. However, whereas back pain is not as common a somatoform symptom among adolescents as is headache, abdominal pain, or chest pain, if a thorough diagnostic evaluation of chronic back pain in an adolescent is unrevealing and the usual management involving exercise and stretching is not beneficial, a psychosocial etiology should be considered. Referral to a mental health professional may not be necessary; if the physician has built a high degree of trust with the family, a sensitive evaluation of family and social factors may be an effective first step. In these cases, the pain should not be assumed to be feigned or "in the patient's head" but rather a very real physical symptom rooted in psychological or emotional distress. At the very least, chronic pain and its accompanying disability can, of itself, lead to psychological distress, and this should be addressed openly by the clinician.

MANAGEMENT

In cases in which back pain is secondary to an underlying disorder, treatment of the pain itself, though important, is secondary to treatment of its etiological condition. Specifically in spondylolysis, continued athletic activity while symptomatic (especially weight bearing in extension) should be discouraged and a program of physical therapy (abdominal and paraspinous muscle strengthening) prescribed. The following discussion focuses on treatment of pain and its associated weakness or disability in the adolescent patient who has acute mechanical back pain or whose chronic pain is idiopathic and thought to be a disorder of the soft tissues of the low back.

When the adolescent presents with back pain acutely after an injury and there is no indication of fracture or intraabdominal trauma, the RICE mnemonic (rest, ice, compression, elevation) is useful, as in other acute injuries, for the first 48 to 72 hours. Pain-free activity may be resumed gradually after this, and low-back and hamstring flexibility, as well as the strengthening of abdominal muscles and back extensors, should be emphasized.

The scientific evidence supporting these measures as effective rehabilitation is marginal, but experience strongly associates inflexibility of the hamstrings and the low back, as well as weakness of abdominal and back extensor muscles, with low-back pain, so the rationale for supporting such exercises seems sound.[4] Full sit-ups with the feet fixed and the knees bent should be discouraged, as this uses hip flexors rather than the abdominal muscles to complete the sit-up; evidence indicates that this type of sit-up is associated with higher intervertebral disk pressure. The goal of abdominal muscle strengthening is to reduce pelvic tilt and its accompanying tendency toward lordosis and low-back strain. It also has been shown that decreased strength and endurance of spinal extensor muscles is associated with low-back pain; thus, extensor exercises such as raising the torso and head off the floor while lying prone are recommended. These same exercises, and stretching after warming the muscles by gentle exercise or heat, are recommended for chronic low-back pain thought to be muscular in origin.

When to Refer

Fever
Abnormality of posture or gait
Neurological findings
Persistent pain in a preteen
Pain unrelated to activity or awakening from sleep
Functional disability (decreased play or sports activity)

When to Hospitalize

Whenever a prompt and thorough outpatient diagnostic assessment cannot be completed for a child who has back pain and associated fever or neurological findings

REFERENCES

1. Bryan N, Smith BM: Back school programs: the ballet dancer, *Occup Med* 7:67, 1992.
2. Dyment PG: Low back pain in adolescents, *Pediatr Ann* 20:170, 1991.
3. Farrell JP, Drye CD: Back school programs: the young patient, *Occup Med* 7:55, 1992.

4. Harvey J, Tanner S: Low back pain in young athletes, *Sports Med* 12:394, 1991.
5. Hollingworth P: Back pain in children, *Br J Rheumatol* 35:1022, 1996.
6. Ikeda K, Nakayama Y, Ishii S: Congenital absence of lumbosacral articular process: report of three cases, *J Spinal Disord* 5:232, 1992.
7. Leboeuf-Yde C, Kyvik KO: At what age does low back pain become a common problem? *Spine* 23:228, 1998.
8. Payne WK, Ogilvie JW: Back pain in children and adolescents, *Pediatr Clin North Am* 43:899, 1996.
9. Schlesinger EB: The significance of genetic contributions and markers in disorders of spinal structure, *Neurosurgery* 26:944, 1990.
10. Sponseller PD: Evaluating the child with back pain, *Am Fam Physician* 54: 1933, 1996.
11. Staheli LT: Pain of musculoskeletal origin in children, *Curr Opin Rheumatol* 4:748, 1992.
12. Turner PG, Green JH, Galasko CSB: Back pain in childhood, *Spine* 14:812, 1989.

119 Cardiac Arrhythmias

J. Peter Harris

Arrhythmias in the young are common and usually benign but may be life-altering and potentially lethal. Age at onset varies from in utero up to the later teenage years, with a higher incidence in early infancy and mid-adolescence. Newer investigative modalities such as event recorders to capture infrequent episodes have enhanced our ability to detect and treat arrhythmias properly. Empirical therapy without arrhythmia detection does not meet the current standard of practice. A 12-lead electrocardiogram (ECG) should always be obtained because rhythm alterations may be quite subtle and not always identified on a rhythm strip. In addition, a thorough family history is required, with particular emphasis on sudden and premature death, syncope, and recurrent arrhythmias.

APPROACH TO ARRHYTHMIAS

As a part of the systematic approach to ECG interpretation, the cardiac rhythm should be analyzed in an organized fashion. The answers to the following three questions will define the majority of arrhythmias:

1. Is the rhythm regular or irregular?
2. Are the QRS complexes narrow or wide?
3. What is the relationship between the P waves and the QRS complexes?

NORMAL RHYTHM VARIATIONS

Recognition of normal rhythm variations is important to allay patient and parental anxiety and to avoid unnecessary investigations and interventions. For instance, sinus arrhythmia and phasic respiratory variations of sinus rate with inspiratory slowing and expiratory acceleration are common throughout the pediatric age range. So too is wandering atrial pacemaker, usually noted with slower heart rates and characterized by different P wave morphologies. These rhythm variations are related to alterations in vagal tone.

A wide range of heart rates is present in the young. Sinus tachycardia has been documented at rates of 230 to 250 beats/min during infancy, but a rate in excess of 200 beats/min in a teenager not involved in maximum exertion would be abnormal. Greater consternation occurs with slow heart rates. Sinus bradycardia is a sinus rate below what is expected for a patient's age. A sinus rate below 100 beats/min in an awake neonate would be abnormal, but during sleep, rates down to 80 beats/min are commonly observed on ECG monitoring. Brief dips into the 60- to 80-beats/min range also are observed in sleeping neonates during normal, vagally induced episodes of junctional rhythm that arises from either the atrioventricular node or the bundle of His and which is characterized by a narrow QRS complex without a preceding P wave. A highly conditioned adolescent endurance athlete may have a resting heart rate of 40 beats/min or less. Table 119-1 provides guidelines for the diagnosis of sinus bradycardia on the surface electrocardiogram and during ambulatory monitoring.

PREMATURE BEATS

Premature beats are common but usually benign arrhythmias, which may arise in the atria, the atrioventricular junction, or the ventricles. By definition, premature beats are early and, thus, are distinguished from escape beats occurring when higher pacemaker cells fail to produce an impulse at the expected interval. Two premature beats in a row constitute a couplet; three or more premature contractions in a row define tachycardia. If every second or third beat is a premature impulse, a bigeminal or trigeminal rhythm is present.

Atrial premature contractions (APCs) are characterized by premature P waves with an axis and morphology different from the sinus P waves. If an APC occurs when one of the bundle branches is refractory, the premature beat will be conducted down the other bundle branch, resulting in an aberrated APC with a QRS morphology different from sinus QRS complexes (Fig. 119-1). If both bundle branches are refractory, the APC will not be conducted to the ventricles (blocked APC) but may reset the sinus node with a resultant pause greater than the previous RR intervals. If every other beat is a blocked APC (blocked atrial bigeminy) in a newborn infant, sufficient slowing of the heart rate to alter feeding and arousal time may be present. T waves usually are smoothly inscribed, and consistent sharp deflections in the T waves may represent P waves (Fig. 119-2). APCs usually occur with normally conducted QRS complexes, but if wide beats also are noted, the apparently prolonged QRS beats are likely to be aberrated APCs because premature atrial and ventricular contractions rarely occur together.

The incidence of APCs in pediatric patients is 50% to 75%. Although associated with myocarditis, atrial stretch, sympathomimetic or other stimulant drugs, intracardiac catheters, and electrolyte disturbances, the majority of patients do not have an obvious incitant, and these usually are not recognized by the child or adolescent. Therapy is not necessary unless the APCs initiate supraventricular tachycardia or result in blocked impulses in a newborn infant dependent, in part, on heart rate to maintain an adequate cardiac output. If suppressive therapy is required, either digoxin (7 to 10 µg/kg/day orally in two divided doses after an initial digitalizing dose of 25 µg/kg) or propranolol (beginning with 0.25 mg/kg every 6 hours orally) is suitable.

Premature ventricular contractions (PVCs) are less common than APCs but may affect up to 25% of healthy infants, children, and adolescents. PVCs are characterized by a QRS morphology different from sinus QRS beats, occur before the next expected sinus beat, and are not preceded by a premature P wave. The QRS duration may be only slightly prolonged. Uniform PVCs have a similar morphology in contrast to multiform beats. The designations "unifocal" and "multifocal" are no longer used because PVCs that have different origins may appear similar, and depending on the direction of exit from a particular spot in the myocardium, PVCs arising from the same focus may have different morphologies. If a PVC occurs late, just before the next expected sinus beat, it will produce a hybrid or fusion beat, in part derived from the normal conduction pathway and in part from the PVC. Fusion beats have a morphology intermediate between the sinus QRS and PVC.

Although seen most often in healthy children and adolescents, PVCs occur in patients who have underlying heart disease, especially cardiomyopathic processes such as myocarditis, hypertrophic and dilated cardiomyopathies, and ventricular dysfunction in congenital cardiac malformations. Other etiologies include sympathomimetic and street stimulant drugs, electrolyte imbalances, and intraventricular catheters. A 12-lead ECG always should be obtained to assess the premature beat morphology and to look for chamber enlargement but also to calculate the corrected QT (QTc) interval.

$$\text{QTc} = \frac{\text{QT interval (seconds)}}{\sqrt{\text{Preceding RR interval (seconds)}}}$$

PVCs are considered benign if there is no evidence for heart disease, the QTc is normal (≤0.44 seconds), the family history is not adverse (no sudden premature deaths or cardiac arrests, important arrhythmias, or cardiomyopathies), and the PVCs are uniform in appearance and are suppressed with exercise. On the other hand, the presence of any of these risk factors defines worrisome PVCs and the need for referral and further investigation. The new appearance of PVCs in the setting of a febrile illness should raise the question of myocarditis. Because underlying heart disease may be subtle, an echocardiogram to assess cardiac structure and function usually is obtained in referred patients. Benign PVCs do not require treatment or curtailment of exercise, even if a bigeminal rhythm is present. However, if very frequent PVCs persist, long-term yearly follow-up should be instituted to detect the unusual situation of arrhythmia-induced left ventricular dilation and/or dysfunction. If worrisome PVCs are present, the need for therapy should be determined by a pediatric cardiologist.

Ventricular couplets are assessed in the same manner, but triplets represent ventricular tachycardia and are discussed on p. 999.

Table 119-1 Age-Related Parameters for Sinus Bradycardia

Surface Electrocardiogram	Heart Rate
Neonates/infants	<100 beats/min awake, resting
Children to 3 yr	<100 beats/min
Children 3 to 9 yr	<60 beats/min
Adolescents 9 to 16 yr	<50 beats/min
Adolescents >16 yr	<40 beats/min
Ambulatory (Holter) Monitoring	**Heart Rate**
Neonates/infants	<60 beats/min sleeping, 80 beats/min awake, quiet
Children 2 to 6 yr	<60 beats/min
Children 7 to 11 yr	<45 beats/min
Adolescents >11 yr	<40 beats/min
Athletes	<30 beats/min

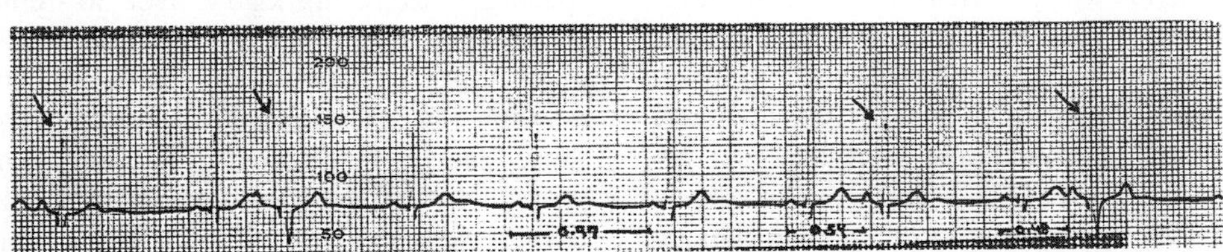

Fig. 119-1 Atrial premature contractions *(arrows)* with normal and aberrated conduction.

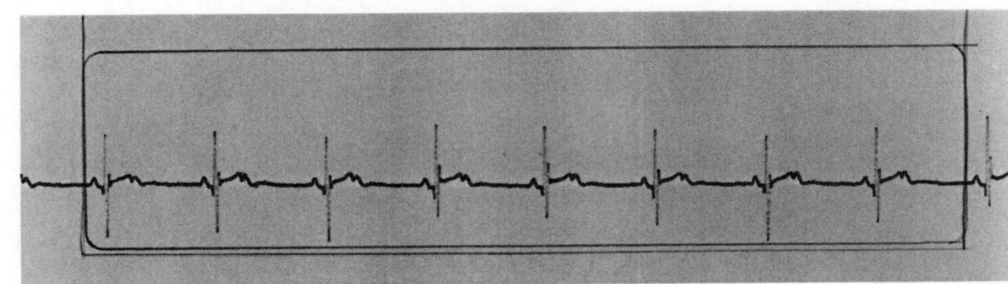

Fig. 119-2 Every other beat is a blocked atrial premature contraction (blocked atrial bigeminy) represented by a consistent sharp deflection in the T waves.

SUPRAVENTRICULAR TACHYCARDIA

Supraventricular tachycardia (SVT) is very common in the young, affecting as many as 1 of every 250 children. More than 90% of SVT is reentrant in nature, involving two distinct pathways that have different conduction characteristics and unidirectional block in one pathway. The impulse enters the second unblocked pathway and then reenters the blocked pathway from the opposite direction. Most of the reentrant SVTs encountered in children are due to an accessory pathway, but the incidence of atrioventricular (AV) nodal reentry increases during adolescence. Unlike reentrant SVT, automatic supraventricular tachycardias cannot be initiated or terminated by a premature beat or pacing and tend to be incessant. Automatic tachycardias account for fewer than 10% of SVT in children.

In decreasing order of frequency, the mechanisms underlying SVT in the young include atrioventricular reentry tachycardia through an accessory pathway (preexcitation), AV nodal reentry tachycardia using the fast and slow pathways in the AV nodal region, and primary atrial tachycardias such as automatic SVT, atrial flutter, and atrial fibrillation.

Approximately 50% of patients who have SVT will have the onset of tachycardia during the first 4 months of life. Although potentially still inducible during an electrophysiological study, more than 90% of these patients will be free of clinical episodes of tachycardia by 1 year of age. However, one third of those who have a history of SVT in early infancy and clinical resolution by 1 year of age will have a recurrence at a mean age of 8 years. The age range of 1 to 5 years is usually electrically quiescent. If SVT occurs for the first time in a child age 5 years or older, there is a 75% to 80% chance of persistent episodes of tachycardia. SVT usually is initiated by an APC or sinus tachycardia in early infancy, but in childhood and adolescence, PVCs and sinus pauses with junctional escape beats are additional initiators.

Most pediatric patients who have SVT have a structurally normal heart, but, if Wolff-Parkinson-White (WPW) syndrome is present (shortened PR interval, delta wave, and wide QRS on the ECG), an echocardiogram should be performed to look for subtle congenital cardiac defects such as Ebstein's malformation of the tricuspid valve or levo-transposition of the great vessels. If surgery for a cardiac defect is contemplated and episodes of SVT have occurred, preoperative assessment and ablation should be considered to reduce arrhythmia-related postoperative morbidity and potential mortality.

The incidence of WPW syndrome in the general population is 0.15%, but in many affected individuals, no SVT occurs. WPW syndrome may be inherited in an autosomal dominant fashion in which situation the risk of sudden death substantially increases (Fig. 119-3).

During infancy, SVT may be detected incidentally on a routine examination; more commonly, however, young infants present with varying degrees of congestive heart failure related to the rate and duration of tachycardia and the presence of associated heart disease. As a general rule, 25% of these infants are in congestive heart failure with a tachycardia duration of 24 hours, and 50% have heart failure after SVT for 48 hours. Frequently, there is a history of poor feeding and pallor over several days, culminating in respiratory distress. Children older than 5 years usually are able to communicate their distress soon after the onset of SVT, hence the relative paucity of congestive heart failure caused by SVT in older pediatric patients. The duration of SVT in childhood and adolescence ranges from a few seconds to several hours. Palpitations may be the only symptom in some; others have initial light-headedness as well as subsequent chest discomfort, pallor, diaphoresis, and nausea. In infancy, the rate of SVT may range from 230 to 300 beats/min but usually is between 260 and 280 beats/min, in contrast to older patients who typically have rates between 180 and 240 beats/min. The QRS complexes usually are narrow but may be wide, especially with a left bundle branch block in early infancy (Fig. 119-4). However, as a general rule, wide QRS tachycardias should be considered as ventricular in origin until proved otherwise. A 12-lead ECG should be obtained, with careful attention paid to the T waves for sharp deflections representing retrograde conduction from the ventricles to the atria via an accessory pathway (Fig. 119-5).

If cardiogenic shock is present with SVT, direct current synchronized cardioversion should be performed by using ½ to 2 watt-seconds or J/kg with the largest paddles allowing effective chest contact. Adenosine can be administered via intravenous bolus, if intravenous access is available, beginning with a dose of 100 μg/kg and increasing by 50 μg/kg per attempt up to a maximum of 350 μg/kg. Adenosine always should be administered with electrocardiographic monitoring to detect the rare conversion to a more malignant arrhythmia. Adenosine is effective in approximately 90% of episodes. If ineffective or if SVT quickly recurs, an infusion of intravenous procainamide at 40 to 50 μg/kg/min can be administered to infants and young children after appropriate loading (7 to 10 mg/kg IV over 30 minutes) with a subsequent repeat trial of adenosine. If conversion does not ensue, a procainamide level should be obtained 4 hours into the infusion (therapeutic range = 4 to 8 μg/ml). In general, in those younger than 1 year of age, intravenous verapamil and propranolol are contraindicated. Once conversion to a sinus rhythm is achieved, a 12-lead ECG should be repeated to look for evidence of preexcitation. If WPW syndrome is present, suppressive therapy with propranolol is appropriate. Digoxin and verapamil should be avoided because both medications may shorten the antegrade refractory period of the

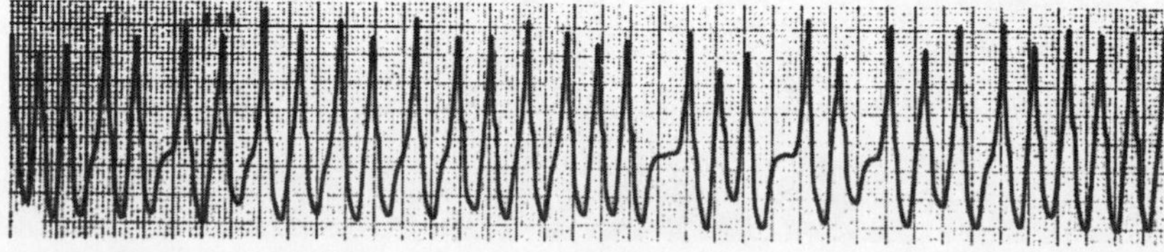

Fig. 119-3 Antegrade conduction over an accessory pathway during atrial fibrillation in a 15-year-old boy who presented with syncope. The short RR intervals represent rapid conduction over the accessory connection and a risk for ventricular fibrillation.

accessory pathway, allowing more rapid conduction to the ventricles, a potentially fatal scenario if atrial fibrillation develops. If preexcitation is not present, either digoxin or propranolol can be used to prevent recurrences. Beta-blockers should be avoided in the presence of congestive heart failure, sick sinus syndrome, or a history of bronchospasm. If these agents are ineffective, other medical therapies include flecainide, sotalol, or amiodarone, all of which require hospitalization for drug initiation.

Infants who have SVT usually are treated for 6 to 12 months and then observed in view of the risk of later recurrence. Ablations are not recommended during the first 2 years

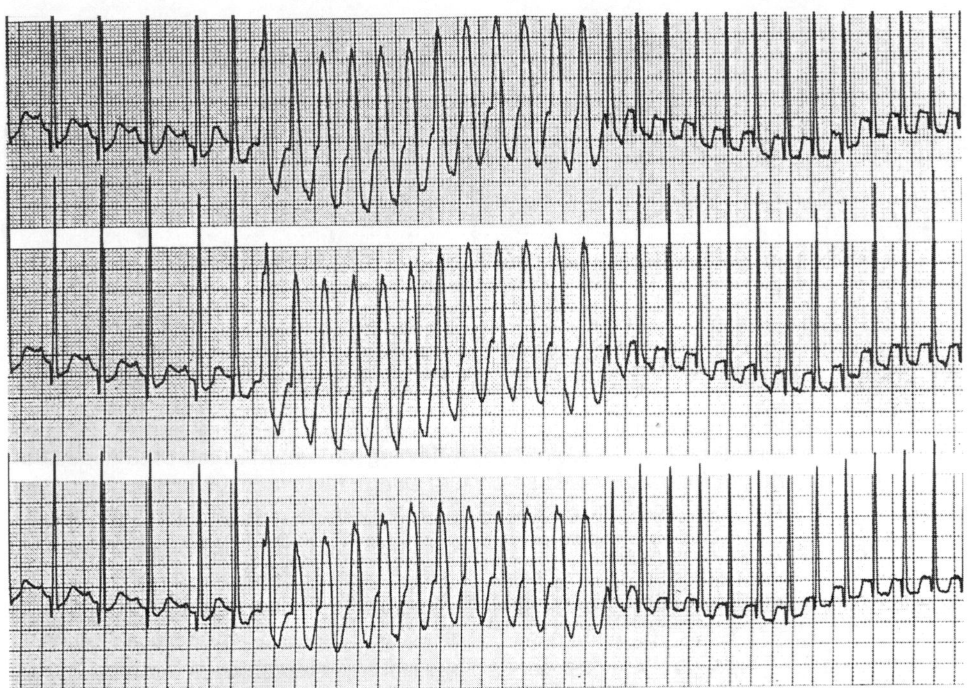

Fig. 119-4 Transient aberrant conduction at the onset of SVT during an exercise test in a 14-year-old male. The QRS duration then returns to normal.

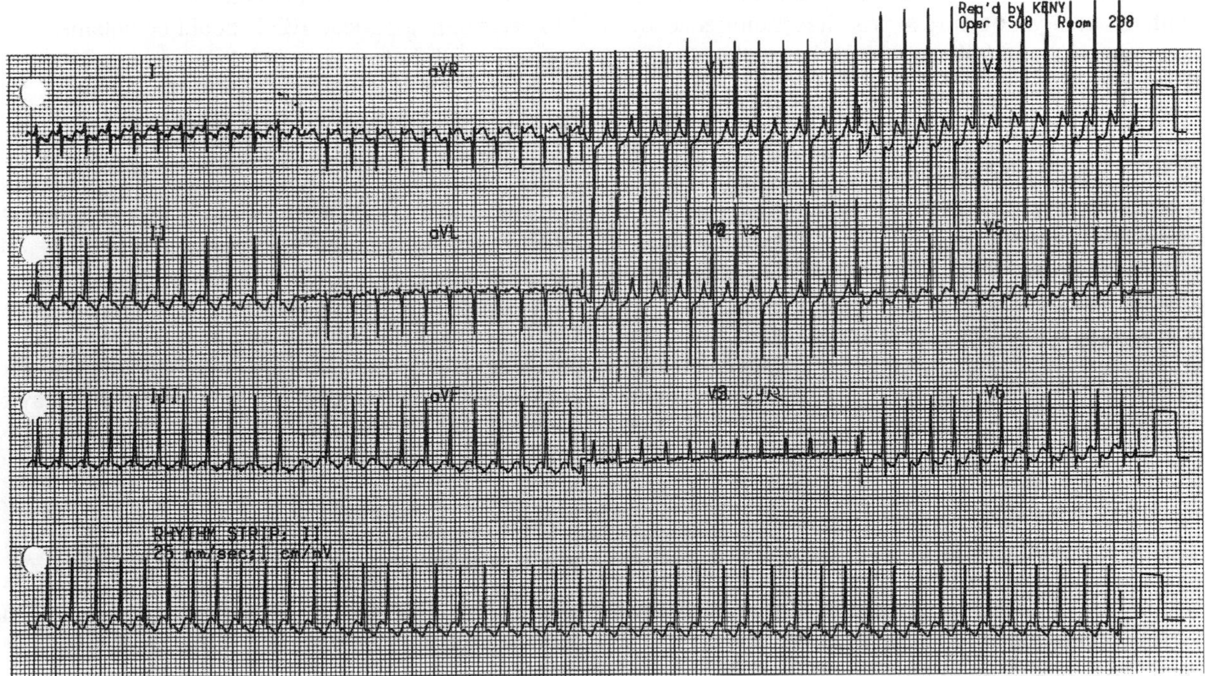

Fig. 119-5 Twelve-lead ECG of SVT in a 2-week-old infant. Consistent sharp deflections in the T waves are present in lead III, indicating retrograde atrial activation via an accessory pathway. A repeat ECG after conversion to sinus rhythm did not reveal any preexcitation, so a concealed accessory pathway is present.

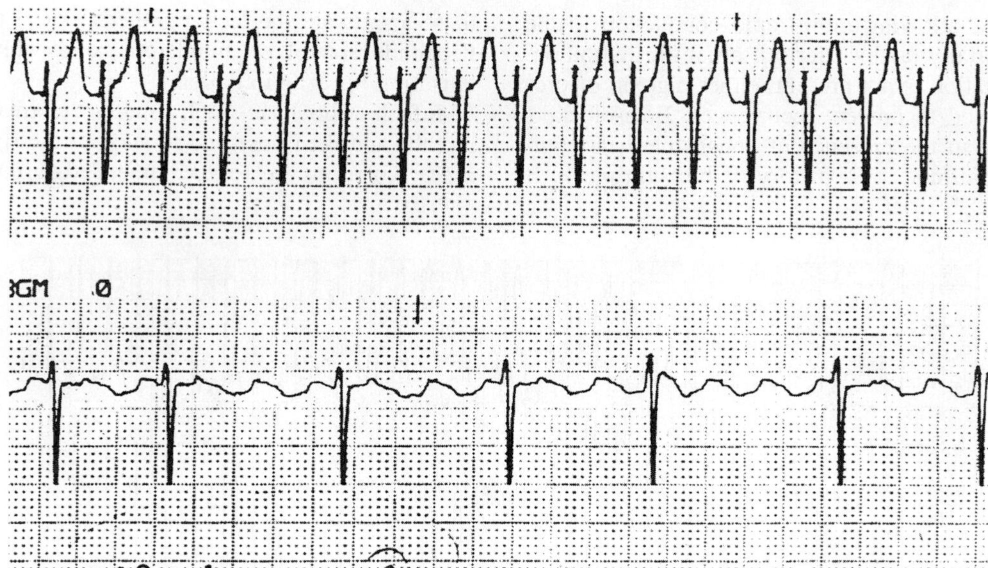

Fig. 119-6 Atypical atrial flutter or intraatrial reentry tachycardia before and immediately after adenosine treatment in a 12-year-old boy following a Mustard repair of transposition of the great arteries in infancy (see Chapter 198, Congenital Heart Disease). Adenosine produces high-grade AV block revealing, but not converting, the underlying atypical atrial flutter.

of life because the resultant myocardial scar may grow with the patient and become a subsequent nidus for malignant, often drug-refractory arrhythmias. Depending on the frequency and ease of conversion of episodes, older children and adolescents have three therapeutic choices. The first is no therapy other than self-conversion via a Valsalva maneuver or headstand. The second is drug therapy, but the duration, compliance issues, and cost of this approach need to be addressed with the family. The third approach is radiofrequency ablation, currently at least 90% successful but with a chance of a later recurrence.

ATRIAL FLUTTER

Atrial flutter, a primary atrial reentrant tachycardia, generally is seen in newborn infants and in older children, the latter usually with cardiomyopathies and after repair of congenital heart malformations.

In the newborn infant, the characteristic rapid sawtooth pattern is found with an atrial rate typically between 350 and 500 beats/min with 2:1 atrioventricular conduction and brief interruptions caused by higher degrees of AV block. If the onset is in utero, hydrops fetalis may develop. After birth, congestive heart failure may be seen but not as dramatically as in infants who have the usual variety of SVT. Structural cardiac problems are uncommon. One third of very young patients respond to in utero or postnatal digoxin. The remainder usually require electrical cardioversion. Chronic therapy usually is unnecessary because recurrences are rare.

Although the typical form of atrial flutter may be seen in older children and adolescents, more commonly an atypical variety called *intraatrial reentrant tachycardia* is found. The atypical form is characterized by a slower atrial rate and distinct P waves separated by isoelectric periods and usually is seen after repair of complex congenital cardiac lesions (Fig. 119-6). Management often is difficult, but if conversion to and maintenance in a sinus rhythm cannot be achieved, morbidity is substantial and a four- to fivefold increase in the risk of sudden death ensues. Commonly, after atrial repair of transposition of the great vessels or after a Fontan operation* for underlying single ventricular morphology and physiology, the patient's resting heart rate is in the 50 to 70 beats/min range. If such a patient is then seen with a rate of 100 to 140 beats/min, a 12-lead ECG should be obtained to look for atypical atrial flutter.

ATRIAL FIBRILLATION

Atrial fibrillation, an irregular tachycardia with variable atrioventricular conduction, is much less common than the other forms of SVT and is seen in older patients who have structural heart disease and cardiomyopathies. However, the incidence of lone (no underlying etiology) and paroxysmal atrial fibrillation in adolescence may be underestimated. If preexcitation is present and the accessory pathway is capable of rapid antegrade conduction, atrial fibrillation may conduct quickly to the ventricles, with a resultant decrease in cardiac output, syncope, and the potential for ventricular fibrillation (see Fig. 119-3).

VENTRICULAR TACHYCARDIA

Ventricular tachycardia (VT) is defined as three or more repetitive excitations arising from the ventricles with a rate

*The Fontan operation is a complex reconstruction of the heart in three stages such that upon completion, venous blood flows passively to the lungs and oxygenated blood is actively pumped by a single ventricular chamber into the aorta.

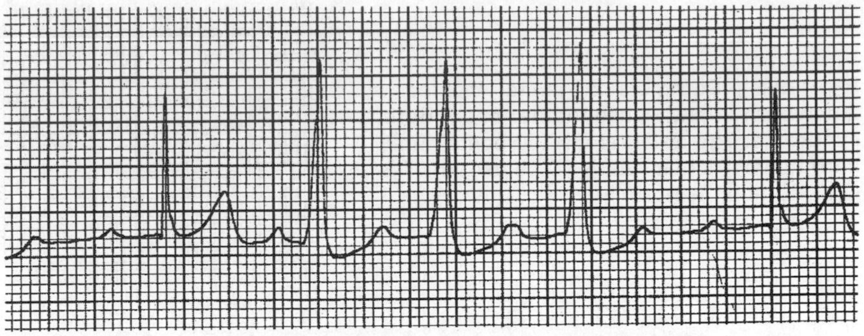

Fig. 119-7 Accelerated ventricular rhythm with a ventricular rate of 110 beats/min in a healthy 7-year-old girl. First-degree block is present in the sinus beats.

greater than 120 beats/min or 25% faster than the sinus rate. The QRS complexes are different from the sinus QRS complexes and typically are wide, except in young infants in whom minimal QRS prolongation (0.08 to 0.09 seconds) may be seen. VT may be extremely rapid, up to 500 beats/min, and slightly irregular because of intermittent sinus capture beats. The differential diagnosis includes SVT with persistent aberrancy (see Fig. 119-4) and SVT with antegrade conduction across an accessory pathway (see Fig. 119-3), both of which are uncommon. Safety dictates that all wide QRS tachycardias be considered VT until proved otherwise. The presence of similar but isolated PVCs and fusion beats in sinus rhythm assist in establishing the diagnosis, but VT is confirmed by the presence of atrioventricular dissociation.

VT in the newborn and young infant is rare, but if it is drug-resistant and incessant, a ventricular tumor may be present. Predisposing factors in older children and adolescents include myocarditis, repaired and unrepaired congenital cardiac lesions, cardiomyopathies, the long QT syndrome, catecholamine- or exercise-induced VT, marked electrolyte imbalances, and street drugs—for example, cocaine, amphetamines, and hallucinogens. In general, VT is a marker for myocardial disease.

Acute management depends on the patient's clinical status, which is determined by the rate and duration of VT and the presence of structural cardiac lesions or prior myocardial dysfunction. Hemodynamic compromise dictates electrical cardioversion with 1 to 2 watt-seconds/kg. If reasonable clinical stability is present, intravenous lidocaine, procainamide, magnesium, or amiodarone can be administered.

Chronic suppressive therapy is predicated on the risk of recurrence, the morbidity and mortality of the type of VT, and the risk-benefit ratio of treatment. Beta-blockers, sotalol, and amiodarone are commonly used antiarrhythmic agents to prevent VT recurrences. Other modalities include implantation of an automatic cardioverter-defibrillator and surgical VT ablation. One form of VT, accelerated ventricular rhythm, has a rate ≤120 beats/min or less than 25% faster than the basic sinus rate; it is benign, requiring observation only (Fig. 119-7).

CONDUCTION ABNORMALITIES

First-degree atrioventricular (AV) block is a prolongation of the PR interval beyond the upper limit of normal for age, with all impulses conducted. It may be seen in patients who have congenital cardiac malformations (especially AV septal defects), electrolyte disorders, rheumatic fever, myocarditis, and congenital muscular disorders. Patients on antiarrhythmic agents frequently exhibit first-degree AV block. This is a benign finding that does not require therapy.

Type I second-degree AV block (called *Wenckebach block* or *Mobitz type I block*) is a progressive prolongation of the PR interval until a dropped ventricular beat (nonconducted P wave) occurs. It is a normal finding in healthy children during sleep and in highly conditioned athletes at rest—circumstances associated with a predominance of vagal tone. In general, this is a benign entity; but if syncope occurs, especially with exertion, a cardiology referral is mandated.

On the other hand, type II second-degree AV block *(Mobitz type II block)* is characterized by intermittent loss of AV conduction without preceding lengthening of the PR interval. In contrast to type I, in which the site of block is in the AV node and little risk of progression to complete block is present, the site of block in Mobitz type II is more distally located in the bundle of His. Symptoms are more common, and progression to higher levels of AV block does occur. The presence of type II block implies an abnormal conduction system with a need for ongoing medical surveillance and a potential need for pacemaker implantation.

Complete AV block, in which no atrial impulses are conducted to the ventricles, may be acquired or congenital. Acquired block usually is a consequence of conduction system injury at the time of repair of congenital cardiac malformations but also can be seen in myocarditis. The need for pacemaker insertion in these situations depends on the presence of symptoms, the ventricular rate, and the stability of the ventricular escape rhythm. Approximately 50% of newborns who have complete congenital AV block (CCAVB) have underlying complex congenital heart malformations, particularly levo-transposition of the great vessels and AV septal defects. The other 50% of neonates who have CCAVB have immune-mediated block caused by the passage in utero of IgG SS-A/Ro and SS-B/La antibodies from a mother who has overt or occult collagen vascular disease. When the fetus is exposed to these maternal antibodies, especially between 15 and 24 weeks of gestation, the result may be fibrotic replacement of AV nodal tissue (Fig. 119-8). About 5% of infants born to mothers who have collagen vascular disease have CCAVB. If a mother bears one child who has CCAVB, the risk in future pregnancies is 20%. An immune-mediated myocarditis also may occur in fetuses exposed to maternal anti-Ro and anti-La antibodies, with possible development of a postnatal dilated cardiomyopathy.

Risk factors for fetal or neonatal death with CCAVB include fetal hydrops, the presence of complex structural heart disease, and a ventricular rate of ≤55 beats/min. In view of the 30% risk of mortality, early pacemaker implantation is

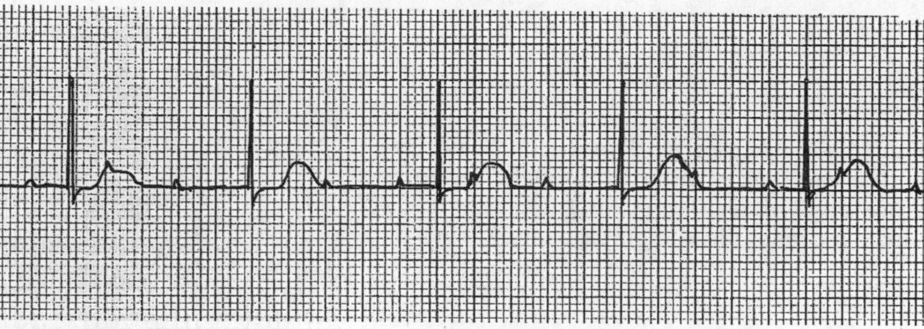

Fig. 119-8 Complete congenital AV block in a newborn infant whose mother has Sjögren's syndrome. The atrial rate is 150 beats/min, and the ventricular rate is 60 beats/min. The QRS duration is normal.

advised if any of these risk factors or symptoms of an inadequate cardiac output are present. An infusion of isoproterenol at 0.05 to 0.5 μg/kg/min can be administered, if necessary, to increase the heart rate while awaiting pacemaker therapy but should not delay implantation.

SUDDEN CARDIAC DEATH

Sudden cardiac death, a rare but obviously devastating event in the young, strikes approximately 1:100,000 children and teenagers, with the highest incidence in mid-adolescence. In decreasing order of frequency, predisposing factors include repaired complex congenital heart malformations, cardiomyopathies, myocarditis, congenital coronary artery anomalies (especially origin of the left main coronary artery from the right sinus of Valsalva), and primary arrhythmias such as the long QT syndrome (LQTS).

The LQTS is a familial, clinically and genetically heterogeneous ion channel cardiac disorder that may cause syncope, "seizures," and sudden death as a consequence of polymorphic ventricular tachycardia. The Romano-Ward subcategory is related to a heterozygotic mutation on chromosomes 11, 7, 3, or 5. Homozygotic mutations on chromosome 11 lead to the Jervell and Lange-Nielsen syndrome, which is characterized by prolongation of the corrected QT intervals and congenital deafness. Potassium channel function is affected by mutations on chromosomes 11 and 7, whereas the sodium channel is perturbed as a consequence of mutations on chromosome 3.

The incidence of LQTS is 1 in 10,000 individuals, with no gender preference. The annual mortality after onset of symptoms in untreated patients is 5% to 20%, with a nearly 10% risk of sudden death as the initial symptom. Syncope, atypical seizures, or cardiac arrest usually occur during exertion or emotional stress. Other than bradycardia, the physical examination is usually normal. The LQTS is defined by a corrected QT interval in excess of 460 ms, with a borderline QTc defined by an interval of 440 to 460 ms. In general, the longer the QTc, the greater the risk of polymorphic VT. The differential diagnosis includes electrolyte abnormalities such as hypokalemia, hypocalcemia, and hypomagnesemia. Myocardial ischemia or injury, acute central nervous system events, and cardiomyopathies may be associated with mild QTc prolongation. Cisapride, imipramine, pentamidine, and intravenous erythromycin may also prolong the QT interval. Therapy for the LQTS includes avoidance of competitive sports, beta-blocker therapy, avoidance of drugs capable of prolonging the QTc and sympathomimetics, and avoidance of and rapid correction of electrolyte abnormalities, followed by cardiac pacing, a left stellate ganglionectomy, and implantation of a cardioverter-defibrillator, if necessary. Insufficient evidence exists at present to incriminate QTc prolongation as an etiology of sudden infant death syndrome.

Twenty-five percent of sudden deaths in the young occur during exercise; the vast majority are electrical in nature, with ventricular fibrillation as the final common pathway. For any child or adolescent who collapses suddenly with no discernible cardiac output, rapid resuscitation including early defibrillation is mandated. This will become easier to accomplish in the future with greater public access to defibrillation equipment.

When to Refer

- Arrhythmias associated with:
- Presyncope, syncope, or chest pain
- Underlying heart disease
- Family history of premature (<35 years) sudden cardiac death
- Persistent or repetitive bradycardias or tachycardias
- Premature beats that increase with exercise

When to Hospitalize

- Arrhythmias associated with syncope or low cardiac output
- Symptomatic high-grade AV block
- Difficult-to-control SVT, atrial flutter
- VT
- LQTS with syncope, aborted sudden death

SUGGESTED READINGS

Carboni MP, Garson A Jr: Ventricular arrhythmias. In Garson A Jr, et al, editors: *The science and practice of pediatric cardiology,* ed 2, Baltimore, 1998, Williams and Wilkins.

Deal BJ, Wolff GS, Gelbard H, editors: *Current concepts in diagnosis and management of arrhythmias in infants and children,* Armonk, NY, 1998, Futura Publishing.

Gillette PC, Garson A Jr, editors: *Pediatric arrhythmias: electrophysiology and pacing,* Philadelphia, 1990, WB Saunders.

Perry JC: Supraventricular tachycardia. In Garson A Jr, et al, editors: *The science and practice of pediatric cardiology,* ed 2, Baltimore, 1998, Williams and Wilkins.

Wren C, Campbell RW, editors: *Pediatric cardiac arrhythmias,* Oxford, 1996, Oxford University Press.

120 Chest Pain

Scott A. Schroeder

No pain strikes more fear and anxiety in children and their parents than chest pain. In children and adolescents, chest pain rarely is caused by heart disease, but in a study of teenagers who had chest pain, 66% of them attributed their pain to heart disease and 44% thought that they were having a heart attack.[8] Where it has been studied, only a third of all parents seemed to have a clear understanding that children and adults have different types of heart disease.[12]

Despite chest pain being due to cardiac disease in only 1% to 3% of children, much of the evaluation and teaching is focused on convincing families that the heart is normal. Unfortunately, physicians often give wrong or confusing information to parents about their children's risk of heart disease.[2] If a child who has chest pain is managed inappropriately, there potentially can be unnecessary grief, anxiety, restriction of activities, and distrust by the family. However, a thorough history and physical examination usually will uncover the etiology for the chest pain in the majority of children and allow the clinician to state emphatically that chest pain in healthy children rarely is due to heart disease.

PATHOPHYSIOLOGY

Different diseases produce characteristic patterns of tissue damage. Because there are numerous organ systems within the thorax and because of the confusing overlap of sensory inputs from the various tissues in the chest, a systematic approach to the thorax is essential to determine the source of the child's pain. Pain from the chest wall and the supporting musculoskeletal structures is transmitted from these inflamed or irritated tissues to the central nervous system (CNS) via the primary sensory afferent nerves that terminate in the dorsal root ganglia. Spinal neurons then transmit the sensation to the brain where it is perceived as a sharp, localized pain. This is why chest wall pain is sharp, localized, and easily reproduced.

Spinal neurons that receive input from the organs within the thorax also receive sensory input from the thoracic dermatomes. This overlap of sensory input leads to the phenomenon of referred pain that often makes the evaluation of chest pain perplexing. Diffuse, poorly localized chest pain can originate from any of the organs within the thorax. Inflammation of the structures that pass through the mediastinum results in pain over dermatomes T1 to T4, from the retroclaviclular to the retrosternal regions. Pain over dermatomes T5 to T8, especially in the xiphoid area, suggests lower chest wall or diaphragmatic irritation or even intraabdominal pathology. Because both the intercostal nerves and the phrenic nerve innervate the diaphragm, peripheral diaphragmatic irritation causes pain in the lower anterior chest or epigastric regions. Central diaphragmatic inflammation results in ipsilateral shoulder pain because of its innervation by the phrenic nerve.

The pericardium, positioned on the central diaphragm, has pleural connections and is innervated by the phrenic, vagus, and recurrent laryngeal nerves. Therefore, when the pericardium is inflamed or infected, there can be sharp substernal pain. If there is pleural inflammation as a result of the pericardial inflammation, there will be pleural pain that will be aggravated by respiratory movements. If these patterns of pain are not confusing enough, the pain of pericarditis may be limited to the sternal and precordial areas; however, if the left lobe of the diaphragm is irritated, pain will be referred to the ipsilateral shoulder or neck.

Pleural pain results from distention or inflammation of the pleura that can occur during the course of a pneumonia, pneumothorax, or empyema. The pain is characterized as a well-localized, sharp pain that is exaggerated by coughing, laughing, or deep inspiration. The pain associated with a pneumothorax can be pleuritic in nature or it can be referred to the ipsilateral shoulder.

The pain associated with esophageal disorders can seem indistinguishable from that associated with myocardial ischemia, because the sensory afferents from the esophagus are through the cardiac and esophageal plexuses as well as the sympathetic trunk. Within the lungs, there is only sensory input from the larger airways and parietal pleura, so the pain arising from pulmonary parenchymal disease is due to inflammation of, or traction on, contiguous structures.

EVALUATION

Because there usually are no pathognomonic findings on physical examination, a detailed history will help focus the differential diagnosis, develop a logical intervention, and allow the child and family to voice their concerns. A meticulous history should address the nature of the pain as well as the child's response to the pain. If possible, children should describe the pain in their own words and should be asked what they think is causing the pain. Along with a description of the location, duration, radiation, and quality of the pain, it is important to elicit any associated signs and symptoms and aggravating and alleviating factors and to uncover the family history and dynamics. To many adolescents, chest pain is

Table 120-1 Indications that Chest Pain Warrants Referral or Hospitalization

History	Physical Examination
Syncope	Cyanosis, toxic appearance, or respiratory distress
Fevers, chills, weight loss, malaise, anorexia	Murmur that increases with Valsalva maneuver
History of Kawasaki disease, Turner's syndrome, Marfan syndrome, sickle cell disease, or cystic fibrosis	Pleural or pericardial friction rub
Recent elective abortion, pain in the calf, or oral contraceptive use	Pulsus paradoxus
Family history of hypertrophic obstructive cardiomyopathy or unexplained syncope	Cardiac clicks, thrills, gallop, or S_3
Pica	Chest pain with exercise
	Palpitation and/or tachycardia

synonymous with heart disease. Therefore, it is important to address this issue; if no cardiac etiology is discovered, it should be stated unequivocally to the child and family that the heart is normal.

Pain that occurs with exercise points toward either a cardiac or a respiratory cause. If the pain awakens the child from sleep, the etiology could be a respiratory, cardiac, musculoskeletal, or gastroesophageal problem but is never psychological.[16] When the pain is poorly localized, associated with recurrent somatic complaints or family or school stress, and there is a family history of chest pain, a psychogenic source of the pain is likely. On the other hand, deep, poorly localized pain that radiates to the neck or shoulders is characteristic of visceral pain. Superficial sharp pain that is exacerbated by lifting or movements of the torso suggests musculoskeletal pain. Peripheral pain that increases with inspiratory efforts originates from pleural inflammation. Questions regarding trauma to the chest wall should always be elicited, and even if the trauma occurred 1 to 3 months before the pain, it should not be discounted because the pain could represent a posttraumatic pericardial effusion. Sharp pain that decreases when the child leans forward is characteristic of pericardial inflammation. Children who have a family history of Marfan or Turner's syndrome, as well as those who have a history of Kawasaki disease or congenital heart disease, warrant referral to a pediatric cardiologist.

Even if the history is highly suggestive of the etiology for the chest pain, the clinician should be careful and thorough because there could be two different causes for the pain. Children who have asthma also not uncommonly have gastroesophageal reflux. Children who have acute chest syndrome may have chest pain secondary to medication-induced gastritis as well as vasoocclusive crisis.

After ascertaining that the child is in no distress, inspection of the thorax will determine whether bruising, swelling over joints, splinting, signs of trauma, or an abnormal breathing pattern is present. Palpation and percussion are extremely important to try to localize and reproduce the pain. Each rib cartilage should be palpated with only one finger or with the child's finger because palpation with two or more digits may cause splinting and not re-create the pain. Reproduction of point tenderness at the origin of the spontaneous pain is the strongest evidence favoring the diagnosis of chest wall disease.[5] Pain from the thoracic cage that can be elicited by movements of the torso or flexion of the arms is highly suggestive of a musculoskeletal chest wall injury. The pain of costochondritis causes tenderness over the affected costochondral or costosternal junctions and can occur at rest or with movement. Adolescents who have gynecomastia may present with chest pain that is easily discernible upon inspection and palpation of the developing breast tissue.

Findings on auscultation that point to a cardiac source of pain include clicks, rubs, and systolic murmurs. A murmur can be worrisome if it increases in intensity with the Valsalva maneuver or any other procedure that expands the degree of left ventricular outlet obstruction. A third heart sound or gallop is heard in myocarditis and congestive heart failure. Pleural friction rubs, wheezes, tachypnea, and crackles suggest a pulmonary etiology. On the other hand, hyperventilation associated with light-headedness, paresthesia, dizziness, and a high level of stress or anxiety suggests a hyperventilation syndrome.

Laboratory tests usually are not helpful in establishing a specific diagnosis. Therefore, a careful history and physical examination should guide the clinician in selecting laboratory investigations. In most cases, chest radiographs and electrocardiographs will confirm what is suspected clinically. If a child has a fever, acute onset of chest pain, and an abnormal cardiac examination suggestive of pericarditis, a chest radiograph and electrocardiogram are indicated. If a child has fever, tachypnea, chest pain, and decreased breath sounds over a segment of the lungs, a chest radiograph is appropriate to determine if there is a pneumonia or a pleural effusion. If the pain occurs with exercise, exercise testing or spirometry may help uncover underlying asthma or exercise-induced bronchospasm. Of adolescents who had idiopathic chest pain who were referred to a pediatric gastroenterologist, 63% had esophageal disorders diagnosed as the cause of their pain.[1] Signs and symptoms of children who have chest pain who would benefit from specialty evaluation or hospitalization are listed in Table 120-1.

ETIOLOGY

Of the 883 children and adolescents who had chest pain who were evaluated in four prospective studies, 25% had chest wall abnormalities identified as the source of their pain. Pulmonary diseases (pneumonia, asthma, and cough) accounted for 19%, 18% were idiopathic, 9% were secondary to trauma, 10% were due to hyperventilation or psychiatric causes, 2% were due to gastrointestinal disorders, 2% were due to cardiac disease, and 15% were due to a potpourri of etiolo-

Table 120-2 Common, Uncommon, and Rare Causes of Chest Pain and Associated Signs and Symptoms

Cause of Chest Pain	Signs and Symptoms
Musculoskeletal	
Costochondritis (common)	Localized, superficial, reproducible pain over rib cartilage
Protracted coughing or vomiting (common)	Intercostal muscle tenderness
Trauma	Localized pain; pain upon movement of involved areas
Stitch (common)	Sharp, crampy costal pain that occurs with running
Precordial catch (uncommon)	Transient, stabbing pain at left sternal border. Relieved by forced inspiration
Pulmonary	
Asthma (common)	Associated with cough, shortness of breath, wheezing, abnormal PFTs
Exercise-induced bronchospasm (common)	Abnormal exercise tests, improvement with bronchodilators or leukotriene receptor antagonists
Pneumonia (common)	Crackles, fever, cough
Pleural effusion (uncommon)	Pleural rub, fever, decreased breath sounds
Pneumothorax (uncommon)	Sudden pain, referred shoulder pain, dyspnea
Pulmonary embolus (rare)	Contraceptive use or recent abortion, pleuritic pain
Gastrointestinal	
Esophagitis (common)	Retrosternal pain; relief with antacids
Gastroesophageal reflux (common)	Retrosternal burning pain, worse after eating and upon reclining, relief with antacids
Cardiac	
Hypertrophic cardiomyopathy (rare)	Syncope, positive family history, systolic ejection murmur
Pericarditis (rare)	Associated fever with acute onset of pain, pain increases with movement, pain alleviated by leaning forward, narrow pulse pressure, distant heart sounds
Myocarditis (rare)	Precedent viral illness, anorexia, shortness of breath, S_3 or gallop, cardiomegaly
Nonorganic	
Pyschogenic (common)	Normal physical examination, trouble sleeping, family or school problems, life stresses, family history of chest pain, other somatic complaints
Hyperventilation (common)	Associated light-headedness, paresthesias, underlying anxiety

gies.[4,12,13,16] None of these studies rigorously assessed for the presence of esophageal disorders or reactive airway disease, and both of these have been shown to be common among children who have idiopathic chest pain.[7,17] Common and selected uncommon, but important causes of chest pain are listed in Table 120-2.

MUSCULOSKELETAL CAUSES

Musculoskeletal injuries to the thoracic cage are the etiologies of chest pain identified most commonly. They usually are suggested by a history of trauma and overuse or repetitive use of certain muscle groups of the anterior chest wall or shoulder girdle and are confirmed on palpation of the chest wall. On examination, maneuvers that stress specific chest wall muscle groups and palpation of the joints between the ribs and the sternum will elicit the pain easily. Costochondritis, an inflammation of the costochondral junctions, is characterized by sharp, localized tenderness elicited easily by palpation. This inflammatory process can be precipitated by direct trauma or an upper respiratory infection and can occur at rest or with exercise. The pain may be evanescent or last for minutes at a time and may persist for months. Tietze's syndrome, a rare form of costochondritis, differs from common costochondritis in that there is visible swelling at the costosternal junction. Another problem with the cartilage that can cause chest pain is the slipping rib syndrome, which probably occurs secondary to trauma to the floating ribs. Although annoying, all of the inflammatory conditions of the chest wall cartilage are benign and resolve without long-term sequelae. Treatment of the muscle strains and overuse syndromes include rest, change in weight-bearing behaviors, and local analgesia.

With excessive coughing or vomiting, the intercostal muscles can become tender and painful. The treatment of this type of pain should be directed at treating the underlying cause of the pain rather than suppressing the cough or the emesis.

PULMONARY CAUSES

A variety of diseases of the airways, pleurae, and parenchyma can cause substernal or pleuritic chest pain. Pneumonia, asthma, exercise-induced bronchospasm, pleural effusions, and air in the pleural space can cause pain, but the chest pain is never the sole presenting sign of the underlying disease process. A child who has a parapneumonic effusion will classically have fever, tachypnea, tachycardia, a pleural friction rub and/or crackles on auscultation, and dullness to percussion in addition to the pleuritic chest pain that heightens with inspiration. Exercise-induced chest pain or chest tightness that resolves with the cessation of the exercise or the administration of bronchodilators may be a manifestation of cardiac disease but more commonly is due to exercise-induced bronchospasm.[11,17] Exercise testing, cold air challenge, or a therapeutic trial of bronchodilators can confirm the diagnosis of exercise-induced bronchospasm. Treatment with bronchodilators or leukotriene modifiers will help these children participate in sports activities and allow them to lead normal, active lives.

Spontaneous pneumothorax can occur in teenagers who have a chronic illness such as cystic fibrosis, asthma, and Marfan syndrome but also can occur in unaffected teenagers.

A child who has cystic fibrosis who presents with chest pain should be assumed to have a pneumothorax until proved otherwise. Dyspnea, shoulder pain, and tachypnea often are observed in addition to the chest pain in children who have pneumothoraces.

PSYCHOGENIC CHEST PAIN

A child who has a long history of chest pain, other recurrent somatic problems, school or sleep problems, and/or a family history of chest pain may have a psychogenic etiology for the chest pain. If a psychogenic cause is entertained, the condition should not be diagnosed by exclusion of organic disease; rather, the diagnosis should be based on positive psychiatric evidence. As with any somatic illness, if the family or the child is able to articulate that the chest pain may be due to stress or emotional upheaval, the diagnosis will be easier for them to comprehend and accept.[9] Emotional causes for chest pain seem to be more common in adolescents than in children younger than 12 years of age.[16]

Hyperventilation can be associated with the chest wall syndrome but is seen more commonly in teenagers who have underlying anxiety.[12] The condition usually is diagnosed by history alone because the child may need to hyperventilate for 20 minutes to reproduce the pain. Almost all children who have hyperventilation syndrome have associated paresthesias, carpopedal spasm, and light-headedness.[18] If a child is in the midst of an acute episode of hyperventilation, the treatment is to breathe into a paper bag to relieve the hypocapnia. Resolution of the chronic problem is based on techniques to allow the child to understand the nature of the anxiety and to allow the child to regain control of his or her emotional state. The treatment of other forms of psychogenic chest pain should be focused on the family's comprehension of the etiology of the pain and reassurance that there are no long-term sequelae, all the while acknowledging that the pain is real to the child. For children who have severe psychiatric problems, referral to a psychiatrist may be necessary.

GASTROINTESTINAL CAUSES

Esophageal disorders have been shown to mimic the pain of angina and can cause acute as well as chronic chest pain.[7] Pain that originates from the esophagus or stomach is described as an uncomfortable, gnawing, substernal, burning sensation. The pain can last for hours and intensifies after meals and upon reclining. Any inflammation of the esophagus, abnormalities of peristalsis, or an esophageal foreign body or trauma can cause chest pain. Esophagitis is the most common gastrointestinal cause of chest pain, but the clinical presentation of esophagitis may not be specific. Children who have idiopathic chest pain may benefit from a trial of antacids or H_2 receptor antagonists before embarking on an exhaustive evaluation.[7]

CARDIAC CAUSES OF CHEST PAIN

The least likely but most worrisome causes of chest pain in children are those cardiac disorders that cause myocardial ischemia. Cardiac disease in children rarely presents with isolated chest pain and always is associated with other findings. Sudden death resulting from cardiac disease in children is caused by a small subgroup of disorders: abnormalities of the myocardium or coronary vessels, specific congenital heart lesions, and arrhythmia and conduction disorders.[10] Signs and symptoms that will identify children who have these disorders and warrant cardiology evaluation include exertional nonrespiratory dyspnea, syncope, and palpitations. A pediatric cardiologist also should see children who have chest pain and a family history of sudden death.

A child who has chest pain from myocarditis or pericarditis usually appears ill and has fever, dyspnea, changes in the pain associated with the respiratory cycle, and abnormal auscultatory findings. Usually the echoviruses, especially coxsackie B virus, are identified as the culprit responsible for myocarditis, whereas pericarditis can result from either an infectious agent or an autoimmune process.

Aortic stenosis and idiopathic hypertrophic cardiomyopathy, which are the most significant lesions that cause left ventricular outflow obstruction, can cause chest pain as a result of the heart's inability to increase cardiac output with exercise. These disorders cause syncope and chest pain with exertion. Mild aortic stenosis does not cause chest pain.[3]

Chest pain usually is not the primary complaint of children who have arrhythmias unless they perceive the palpitations as being painful. More commonly, older children complain of light-headedness or dizziness along with palpitations. The arrhythmia usually can be detected on auscultation and confirmed with a resting electrocardiogram. If the palpitations or chest pain occur infrequently or are not associated with exercise, referral to a pediatric cardiologist is indicated for Holter monitoring.

Although mitral valve prolapse (MVP) commonly is thought to cause chest pain in adolescents, most children who have MVP are asymptomatic. In the Framingham study, chest pain was no more common among teenagers who had MVP than it was in those who had no MVP.[15] In a study of adolescents who had MVP and chest pain, esophageal causes for the pain were demonstrated in 14 of 17 patients.[19]

IDIOPATHIC CAUSES OF CHEST PAIN

In two studies of adolescents who had chest pain, 39% of them were classified as having idiopathic chest pain.[4,12] Unfortunately, in neither of these studies were gastrointestinal or pulmonary causes of chest pain evaluated adequately. The clinician should feel confident that the child who has chronic chest pain, no history of respiratory or cardiac disease, and a normal physical examination is unlikely to have a serious cause for the pain. In teenagers, a careful, concrete explanation of the pathophysiology ultimately will be part of their therapeutic regimen. Long-term studies of children who have idiopathic chest pain showed that the vast majority of them had no further pain 1 to 2 years after their evaluation.[6,14]

HOSPITALIZATION FOR CHILDREN WHO HAVE CHEST PAIN

Rarely will a child who has chest pain need to be hospitalized because, for the most part, chest pain usually is benign, self-limited, and unassociated with severe intrathoracic illness. Children who have myocarditis, pericarditis, empyema, pneumothorax, significant thoracic trauma, acute chest syndrome, an esophageal foreign body, a coronary artery anomaly, or other cardiac lesions where it is thought that there might be myocardial ischemia should be hospitalized for stabilization and evaluation. Children who have chest pain and palpitations, cyanosis, or who are in distress also should be hospitalized.

REFERENCES

1. Berezin S, et al: Chest pain of gastrointestinal origin, *Arch Dis Child* 63:1457, 1988.
2. Bergman A, Stamm S: The morbidity of cardiac nondisease in school children, *N Engl J Med* 276:1008, 1967.
3. Brenner JI, et al: Cardiologic perspectives of chest pain in childhood: a referral problem? To whom? *Pediatr Clin North Am* 31:1241, 1984.
4. Driscoll DJ, et al: Chest pain in children: a prospective study, *Pediatrics* 57:648, 1976.
5. Epstein S, et al: Chest wall syndrome: a common cause of unexplained cardiac pain, *JAMA* 241:2793, 1979.
6. Fyfe DA, Moodie DS: Chest pain in pediatric patients presenting to a cardiac clinic, *Clin Pediatr* 23:3212, 1984.
7. Glassman MS, et al: Spectrum of esophageal disorders in children with chest pain, *Dig Dis Sci* 37:663, 1992.
8. Goodman BW, Pantell RH: Chest pain in adolescents: functional consequences, *West J Med* 141:342, 1984.
9. Green M: *Sources of pain,* Philadelphia, 1983, WB Saunders.
10. Liberthson RR: Sudden death from cardiac causes in children and young adults, *N Engl J Med* 334:1039, 1996.
11. Nudel D, et al: Chest pain: dyspnea on exertion, and exercise-induced asthma in children and adolescents, *Clin Pediatr* 26:388, 1987.
12. Pantell RH, Goodman JBW: Adolescent chest pain: a prospective study, *Pediatrics* 71:881, 1983.
13. Rowe BH, Dulberg CS, et al: Characteristics of children presenting with chest pain to a pediatric emergency department, *Can Med Assoc J* 143: 388, 1990.
14. Rowland TW, Richards MM: The natural history of idiopathic chest pain in children, *Clin Pediatr* 25:612, 1986.
15. Savage D, et al: Mitral valve prolapse in the general population. 2. Clinical features: the Framingham study, *Am Heart J* 106:577, 1980.
16. Selbst SM, et al: Pediatric chest pain: a prospective study, *Pediatrics* 82:319, 1988.
17. Weins L, et al: Chest pain in otherwise healthy children and adolescents is frequently caused by exercise-induced asthma, *Pediatrics* 90:350, 1992.
18. Wheatley C: Hyperventilation syndrome: a frequent cause of chest pain, *Chest* 68:195, 1975.
19. Woolf PK, et al: Noncardiac chest pain in adolescents and children with mitral valve prolapse, *J Adolesc Health* 12:247, 1991.

121 Constipation

Peter F. Belamarich

The term *constipation,* which is used to denote both a symptom and a chronic condition, refers to the infrequent elimination of large or hard stools that cause pain on defecation and other symptoms. In childhood, chronic constipation that is not caused by another condition is known by several different names, including functional constipation, dysfunctional stool retention, psychogenic constipation, and idiopathic constipation. The later term, which reflects our lack of understanding of the cause and is not pejorative, is used in this chapter. Numerous definitions of constipation exist. One useful definition of idiopathic constipation frequently used in pediatric clinical studies is stool frequency fewer than three times per week with the periodic passage of very large additional amounts of stool every 7 to 30 days. It also may be defined as the presence of a palpable fecal mass in the rectum or abdomen.

However defined and named, constipation is a common symptom among children in the industrialized world. In parental surveys, from 16% to 37% of toddlers are reported to suffer from it.[7] Most often, constipation is a self-limited symptom relieved by dietary changes or transient laxative use. Idiopathic constipation presents a challenge to the pediatrician, as suggested by the evaluation and treatment of constipation occupying a significant percentage of all referrals to pediatric gastroenterology services, even though these children rarely require an invasive procedure.[14] To pediatricians caring for chronically constipated children, treatment failure raises the question of Hirschsprung's disease. Among referral populations, more than 90% of childhood constipation is idiopathic; ultimately, 50% to 90% of these children are cured.[10]

The approach to chronically constipated children used in referral centers is well within the scope of the primary care pediatric practice and represents a therapeutic opportunity with a good cure rate.[5,10,12] The focus of this chapter is on the identification and treatment of children who have idiopathic constipation.

PATHOPHYSIOLOGY OF IDIOPATHIC CONSTIPATION

The role of the colon is the reclamation of water from the liquid ileal effluent. This is accomplished in part by a motility pattern that includes focal circular contractions, which impede the progress of the luminal contents while solutes and water are absorbed. Subsequently, forward progress of the relatively dehydrated fecal stream is achieved by coordinated contractile waves, which propel the bolus of stool to the next colonic segment and ultimately to the rectum. The final elimination of stool is controlled by defecation, a coordinated sequence of neuromuscular events with both reflexive and conscious components. Control of defecation, continence, is a critically important social achievement in early childhood. At rest, continence is maintained by the involuntary resting tonic contraction of the smooth muscle cuff of the internal anal sphincter and by the posterior turn of the anal canal in relation to the anterior angulation of the rectal vault. This angle is modulated by the puborectalis "sling" muscle, which loops posteriorly around the anorectal junction and is anchored anteriorly on the pubic bone. When stool arrives into the rectal ampulla, causing distention of the rectal walls, a reflexive relaxation of the internal anal sphincter occurs, which lowers the pressure of the anal canal and allows the stool bolus to descend to the anal canal. This phenomenon is known as the *rectoanal inhibitory reflex.* Control of defecation then occurs by the voluntary (and learned) deliberate contraction of the striated muscle of the external sphincter and puborectalis sling muscles, which increase the pressure in the anal canal and make the exiting angle more acute. Conversely, a Valsalva maneuver in combination with relaxation of the external anal sphincter and the puborectalis sling permit defecation to proceed.

The etiology of idiopathic constipation is not clear. Based on current knowledge, it is likely that idiopathic constipation may result from several distinct initiating pathophysiological events.[12] These include (1) a disorder of colonic transit leading to impacted, overly desiccated stool in the colon; (2) a disorder of the dynamics of defecation; and (3) a problem with rectal sensation. Stool withholding, the act of voluntarily deferring defection (as pain-avoidance behavior), significantly contributes to the chronicity of constipation in childhood.

Constipation from abnormally slow transit of the fecal stream through the colon occurs predominantly in young women but can occur in children.[4] Whether slowed colonic transit is the primary problem or an acquired epiphenomenon of more distal difficulties with defecation is unclear. Slow-transit constipation in children is not easily differentiated clinically from normal-transit constipation. A unique therapeutic approach to slow-transit constipation has not emerged.

Anorectal manometric studies have documented abnormalities in the dynamics of defecation in a large proportion of chronically constipated children. The most common abnormality noted in these studies is a paradoxical contraction of the external anal sphincter and the puborectalis sling in response to the rectoanal inhibitory reflex. This commonly identified abnormality is known variously as *rectoanal dyssynergia, abnormal defecation dynamics,* and *animus.*[9] Most experts consider dyssynergia a learned phenomenon. It has been observed that for a large proportion of chronically constipated children, painful defecation and withholding antedate the clinical presentation of constipation by 1 to 5 years.[13] In a significant subset of children who experience persistent constipation, withholding becomes entrenched and particularly difficult to unlearn. In fact, great initial enthusiasm over manometrically based biofeedback training was based on its potential to help patients identify and unlearn this withholding behavior. However, controlled studies have not documented greater improvements in the outcome for patients who have unlearned this behavior than for those given a standard treatment regimen.[9]

Another common described manometric abnormality found in chronically constipated children is known as *megarectum.* As the name implies, the rectum is dilated with a chronic impaction, a finding associated with an increase in the sensory threshold to minimal rectal distention as well as an increase in the minimum volume required to initiate the urge to defecate. These sensory abnormalities have been shown to persist for several years in some patients after successful treatment, suggesting that persistent sensory abnormalities contribute to relapses and perhaps to the initial pathogenesis of constipation in some children.

Despite experimental evidence in children who have established constipation that documents several varieties of abnormal anorectal physiology, no studies identify any of the abnormalities prospectively. Thus, it still is unclear what abnormality is primary and what abnormalities are secondary.

In practical terms, several commonly recognized clinical scenarios can result in constipation. These include painful anal fissures, perianal streptococcal cellulitis, traumatic toilet training experiences, anal sexual abuse, and transient periods of dehydration, illness, or immobility. It seems likely that stool withholding figures prominently in the perpetuation of constipation when these are the recognized precipitants. Withholding behavior in the toddler or child is strongly self-reinforcing. The child is avoiding painful bowel movements, which makes the stool harder and more painful to pass. Stool withholding also is reinforced unwittingly by parents who focus with great concern on the withholding crisis, often believing that the child is valiantly trying to defecate rather than to withhold. Toddlers love the worried attention of their parents! The lack of privacy commonly found in some school bathrooms can engender withholding by older children.

Interestingly, although an increase in dietary fiber intake is useful in the maintenance phase of the treatment of constipation, little prospective scientific data exist that implicate a fiber deficiency or the lack of a particular food or food group in the pathogenesis of constipation.[12] Nonetheless, many clinicians have remarked that periods of excess protein intake, such as occurs with excessive whole cow milk consumption, are associated with constipation. The tenacious and harmful myth that iron-containing formula causes constipation has been disproved a number of times.

Recently, one group of researchers reported that constipation is a manifestation of an atopic intolerance of cow milk protein. In a study of 65 children who have treatment-resistant chronic constipation, 44 had a positive therapeutic response to the substitution of soy milk for cow milk.[6] Questions remain, however, about the generalizability of these findings.

DIFFERENTIAL DIAGNOSIS

The differential diagnosis of chronic childhood constipation includes many conditions (Box 121-1). Despite the high number of possible diagnoses, studies of chronically constipated children have documented that at least 90% of individuals have idiopathic constipation.

Frequently, the foremost consideration in the differential diagnosis of chronic constipation is Hirschsprung's disease.[7] The most common basis for this concern is treatment failure, an appropriate concern in early infancy when idiopathic constipation is unusual and is easily treatable. However, treatment failure in the toddler and school-age child more often reflects the complexity and duration of interven-

BOX 121-1

DIFFERENTIAL DIAGNOSIS OF CONSTIPATION IN CHILDHOOD

Idiopathic Constipation

Disorders of Intestinal Neuromuscular Functions
Hirschsprung's disease
Pseudo-obstruction syndromes
Scleroderma
Systemic lupus erythematosus

Anal and Rectal Disorders
Anal fissure
Anterior ectopic anus
Anal stenosis
Rectal duplication
Anal trauma (abuse)
Pelvic tumor (presacral teratoma, ganglioneuroma)

Neurological
Spinal cord lesions
Cerebral palsy
Neuromuscular diseases with hypotonia

Metabolic/Endocrine
Hypothyroidism
Diabetes insipidus
Hypercalcemia
Hypokalemia

Medication- and Toxin-Related
Antihistamines
Anticholinergics
Anticonvulsants
Opioids
Bismuth, aluminum hydroxide
Tricyclic antidepressants
Iron preparations
Plumbism
Infant botulism

Table 121-1 Comparison of Hirschsprung's Disease to Idiopathic Constipation

Characteristic	Hirschsprung's Disease	Idiopathic Constipation
Prevalence	~ 1 in 6000 births	1.5% of 7-year-old boys
Failure to pass meconium <24 hr	58%-94%	~ 5%
Constipation in first 3 mo	90%	Rare
Obstruction	Common	Rare
Abdominal distention	Common	Mild or absent
Stool size	Narrow, ribbonlike	Intermittent large-caliber stools
General appearance	Chronically ill	Well
Stool-withholding behavior	Rare	Extremely common
Soiling	Unusual	Common
Stool in ampulla	Unusual	Common
Plain roentgenograms	Empty rectum	Dilated enlarged rectum
Rectal manometry	Recto-anal reflex absent	Recto-anal reflex present
Typical barium enema	Distal spasm, proximal dilation	Diffusely dilated colon and rectum

tion required to treat idiopathic constipation adequately than a missed diagnosis of Hirschsprung's disease. Fortunately, several findings in the history have an extremely high negative predictive value in ruling out Hirschsprung's disease (Table 121-1). Perhaps most useful is that almost all children who have idiopathic constipation withhold stool in response to the rectoanal inhibitory reflex, whereas this reflex is absent with Hirschsprung's disease. Simply put, "doodie dancing" is a historical finding that almost always rules out Hirschsprung's disease. Conversely, Hirschsprung's disease should be considered in any child who has refractory constipation who has had any of the following: (1) failure to pass meconium in the first 24 hours of life; (2) onset of constipation at less than 3 months of age; (3) symptoms of intestinal obstruction at any point (distention, emesis); (4) life-long dependence on laxatives, enemas, or mechanical manipulation to initiate defecation; and (5) a history of enterocolitis in early infancy (sometimes misdiagnosed as gastroenteritis). Intestinal neuronal dysplasia is a rare disorder, which may imitate or coexist with Hirschsprung's disease. Pathologically, it is distinct insofar as ganglia are present, although they may be poorly differentiated or inadequately innervated.

Other conditions that specifically affect the neuromuscular function of the colon include the pseudoobstruction syndromes, which are characterized by intermittent episodes of functional intestinal obstruction. Furthermore, a large percentage of children who have generalized neuromuscular disabilities (e.g., cerebral palsy, muscular dystrophy, generalized hypotonia) have refractory constipation that frequently is multifactorial and often difficult to treat.

Anorectal disorders producing constipation include anal fissures, anal stenosis, anterior ectopic anus, and extrinsic masses that partially obstruct the rectum. Fissures may induce a self-perpetuating cycle of withholding, worsening constipation, and reinjury. Congenital anal stenosis is characterized by straining during the production of small-caliber stools; it frequently is diagnosed during infancy. The anal canal is noted to be narrow and not distendible during digital examination. Occasionally, chronic constipation will be caused by a subtle anorectal malformation known as *anterior ectopic anus*.[8] In this condition the anal orifice is misplaced anteriorly[6]; consequently, the stool bolus must turn anteriorly at the perineum to exit. The parents may report seeing a perineal bulge when the baby attempts to defecate. Surgical reconstruction may be necessary in those who fail to improve with medical therapy. Rarely, constipation will be a manifestation of an intermittent or partial extrinsic obstruction of the rectum by a rectal duplication cyst, or by a pelvic mass such as a neuroblastoma, presacral teratoma, or ovarian tumor.

Spinal cord lesions affecting the second, third, and fourth sacral nerves are associated with both sensory and motor deficits affecting defecation. Examples of acquired lesions include trauma, intra- and extraspinal tumors, and a tethered spinal cord. These lesions commonly present with fecal incontinence rather than constipation and rarely affect defecation without accompanying abnormalities in bladder function and/or gait.

Metabolic and endocrine disorders associated with constipation include hypothyroidism, hypercalcemia, diabetes insipidus, hypokalemia, and plumbism. These conditions do not present with chronic constipation as a sole symptom. Finally, some medications and toxins are reported to cause constipation (see Box 121-1).

COMMON PRESENTATIONS OF IDIOPATHIC CONSTIPATION

Infancy

Particularly in the first 6 months of life, parental notions of what constitutes constipation may be mistaken. Breast-fed infants may have a mushy stool as infrequently as once a week. In the otherwise healthy infant, this does not deserve the label constipation and requires no intervention. For infants fed cow-milk formulas, infrequent stools are more likely to be a problem because fewer than 5% of these infants stool less than once a day. In general, stool consistency rather than frequency is the critical determinant of constipation in the infant.

Parents also worry about infants who strain or grunt excessively (often turning deep red) in the course of producing a soft stool of normal caliber. Manometric studies have documented the presence of a functioning rectoanal inhibitory reflex at birth, and it is likely that infants exhibiting this behavior are attempting, unsuccessfully, to coordinate the voluntary with the involuntary components of defecation. This problem does not predispose the child to future constipation.

The truly constipated infant typically presents with a pattern of straining and either the production of a desiccated plug of stool followed by loose stool or by the production of a consistently desiccated stool that has a pebbly consistency. These infants require treatment.

Toddlers

Although parents of toddlers usually are aware of when their child is constipated, they frequently do not recognize stool withholding. During the act of withholding, the child may hide quietly, clinging on to an inanimate object, while squeezing his buttocks together. Numerous variations of stool withholding behavior exist, including crouching, dancing or walking on tip-toes, and crying out in anticipation of the pain. Not infrequently, these episodes are misinterpreted by the parents as valiant attempts to defecate, and they generate great concern. Eliciting a history of stool withholding is critical for both diagnostic and therapeutic purposes.

Childhood

Once the child has attained privacy in the bathroom, parents are not likely to be involved in the toilet routine, and constipation becomes occult. The child often goes to the bathroom with a regular or increased frequency but during defecation passes only a small, hard piece of stool. Not infrequently, the child emerges from the bathroom not terribly bothered; the parent inquires, "Did you go?"; the child answers "yes"; and both parties are happy. This stooling pattern, known as *incomplete evacuation,* is extremely common in school-age children. It is punctuated episodically by the passage of massive bowel movements. Children do not seem terribly bothered by constipation; therefore, they often are brought in by their parents for the epiphenomena of constipation, which include: soiling, recurrent abdominal pain, blood streaks seen on the stool, excessive flatus, anorexia, or, occasionally, by urinary symptoms including those associated with urinary tract infection.

EVALUATION

Idiopathic constipation frequently can be diagnosed by history, physical examination, and therapeutic response to a comprehensive treatment regimen. The history should incorporate the frequency, consistency, and caliber of the stools that the child passes, as well as the age of the child at the onset of constipation. The newborn history should specifically establish whether the child passed meconium in the first day of life. A history of traumatic toileting experiences or periods of high protein intake (excessive whole cow milk consumption) should be sought. Common complications of constipation should be asked about: fissures, bleeding, abdominal pain, anorexia, and urinary tract infection. Significant distention and vomiting are not caused by idiopathic constipation. Eliciting a history suggesting stool withholding is critical.

Specific questions should address the differential diagnosis. Symptoms of Hirschsprung's, endocrine, metabolic, and neurological disease should be sought. The possibility of an occult spinal process affecting the sacral nerves can be addressed by inquiring about any changes in the urinary voiding pattern (urinary stream, or urinary continence) or in the child's gait.

On physical examination the child's growth parameters (including recent growth velocity) should be normal. The child should appear well and not wasted or malnourished. The abdomen should not be distended significantly. The external examination of the perineal area is performed to establish normal placement of the anal orifice and to look for evidence of soiling, fissures, skin tags, and a normal anal wink in response to touch.

In the majority of children who have idiopathic constipation, desiccated stool is found in the rectal vault on rectal examination. For older children who have long-standing constipation and a megarectum, chronic rectal distention may efface the internal sphincter along the rectal wall, making the anal canal feel foreshortened.

Children who soil from chronic constipation with a megarectum have only a sensory disorder; thus, the tone of the internal sphincter should be normal. The examiner should be alert during the digital examination for the rare situation in which an extrinsic mass is compressing the rectum. A patulous anus is indicative of a neurological lesion or of sexual abuse involving the anus. Especially in infants, an empty rectum on digital examination raises the possibility of Hirschsprung's disease, particularly in conjunction with a hard impaction mass palpated in the pelvis or lower abdomen. In the older child who has idiopathic constipation, an empty rectum may be found occasionally if the child has just stooled. Nonetheless, the possibility of Hirschsprung's disease should be considered carefully. The evaluation should continue with an examination of the spine, looking for a dimple, hair tuft, or palpable vertebral deformity (signs of spina bifida occulta), and from there to a thorough neurological examination that stresses the tone, strength, symmetry, and reflexes of the lower extremities, and an analysis of the patient's gait.

Routine laboratory tests are not indicted in the evaluation of idiopathic constipation, but plain radiographs of the abdomen can be used to assess the degree of impaction and colonic distention and to confirm that the patient has an enlarged stool-filled rectum, a finding consistent with idiopathic constipation.[2]

Children suspected of having Hirschsprung's disease should be discussed with a consulting surgeon and radiologist to decide on the choice of initial diagnostic testing. Typically, except in infants younger than 3 to 4 months of age, an unprepped barium enema is performed initially.

Treatment

Treatment of constipation involves parental education, pharmacotherapy, diet, and behavioral modification.[1,10,12] Consideration must be given to the age of the patient and the duration of symptoms. Whereas transient constipation of several days' duration typically can be managed with one to several days of laxative use and dietary change, the majority of patients who have idiopathic constipation require a phased approach and months of treatment. Successful treatment of idiopathic constipation in older children may even require 1 to 2 years of laxative therapy. Ultimately, the goals of treatment are to establish a pattern of soft bowel movements at a regular frequency (at least three per week), to wean the child from pharmacotherapy, and to have the child and family manage the problem on their own with diet and behavioral modification.

Infants are the easiest to treat. Before they are introduced to baby food, constipated infants can be treated by the addition to the diet of undigestible, osmotically active carbohydrates. This is accomplished by adding either dark corn syrup (Karo) or malt soup extract to the formula in a dose of 2 to 6 teaspoons divided in several bottles per day. Once juice and baby food are introduced, apple or prune juice and fruits can be added or substituted for the Karo. Barley cereal is substituted for rice cereal. Infant glycerine suppositories can be used at the beginning of therapy to remove a desiccated rectal plug but should not be the mainstay of therapy because infants can become behaviorally conditioned to depend on rectal stimulation to initiate stooling. Infants should not receive mineral oil because of the risk of pneumonia from aspiration. A small dose of Senna (¼ to ½ teaspoon) can be given at bedtime for a brief period until dietary changes take effect. Externally visible anal fissures should be treated with petroleum jelly. Infants whose constipation is refractory to these measures should be referred to a pediatric gastroenterologist.

A very successful treatment paradigm for toddlers and children who have long-standing idiopathic constipation was developed by Dr. Murray Davidson in the 1960s and was refined by Dr. Melvin Levine in the 1970s. This method divides the treatment of established constipation into three phases: (1) education and disimpaction, (2) maintenance, and (3) weaning. Its use has been adopted widely by pediatric gastroenterologists.

The treatment of constipation begins with parental education. Particular focus is given to the concept that, once established, constipation engenders withholding, which is self-perpetuating. Toddlers, in particular, require several months of laxative treatment that produces soft stools before they abandon this behavior. A corollary to this point is to address the widely held parental fear that long-term laxative use in childhood is not safe or engenders laxative dependence. This fear, compounded by a general reluctance to medicate children for what is widely perceived as a transient problem, almost always leads to premature discontinuation of therapy. In fact, innumerable studies have established that nonstimulant laxatives such as mineral oil, milk of magnesia, and lactulose do not result in dependence. Limited periods (weeks to months) of using Senna, an anthraquinone-stimulant laxative, also has a long history of safe use in childhood. Concerns that prolonged periods of mineral oil use may impair fat-soluble vitamin absorption have not been substantiated in a very carefully done study of this question.[11] Some time must be spent educating parents on the nearly universal behavioral phenomenon of stool withholding. As difficult as it may be, parents should be instructed to ignore these events, as they would a temper tantrum. Parents should talk directly to toddlers and engage them in the therapeutic program: "I want you to push the poo-poo out of your body; don't hold it in. That's how you will get better, and it will stop hurting!"

In the toddler or child who has had months to years of symptoms and/or an impaction on examination or on the abdominal flat plate, treatment begins with disimpaction. For older children, disimpaction treatment should be deferred until the weekend; in the interim, the child should be treated with mineral oil to lubricate the impacted stool (Table 121-2). Enemas once a day for 3 to 6 days are simple and effective and, with some important caveats, are safe. Dosage guidelines should be followed, and the child should be brought to medical attention in the rare event of failure to stool following an enema. Sodium phosphate enemas are contraindicated in children who weigh less than 10 kg, in those who have any cardiac or renal impairment or electrolyte disorders, and in children who may have any form of intestinal obstruction.[5]

The goal of disimpaction is to remove all the hard-formed stools throughout the colon. A follow-up telephone call after 2 days can ascertain whether the child is still passing hard stools. Following a series of three enemas, any questions about whether the disimpaction phase of treatment is complete should prompt a revisit for a rectal examination or an abdominal radiograph. Some children absolutely refuse to

Table 121-2 Regimens for Older Toddlers and Children Who Have Chronic Constipation

	Laxative Dosages
Disimpaction	
Enema	
Hypertonic sodium phosphate*	3 ml/kg/dose pr qd × 1-6 days
Mineral oil	30-60 ml pr qd × 1-6 days
Oral	
Mineral oil†	30 ml/year of age to maximum 8 oz bid × 3 days
Polyethylene glycol	10-40 ml/kg/hr per ng (maximum $2^{L}/_{h}$) until effluent clear
Maintenance	
Mineral oil†	1-3 ml/kg/day
Milk of magnesia	1-3 ml/kg/day
Lactulose 10 g/15 ml	1-2 ml/kg/day
Senna—syrup 218 mg/5 ml*	10-20 mg/kg/dose po qhs

*See maximum doses in the PDR.
†Not recommended for children ≤2 years of age.

cooperate with enemas; these patients may be disimpacted with a high-dose oral regimen of mineral oil. Lastly, children who have extremely hard or treatment-resistant impactions can be admitted for nasogastric administration of a polyethylene glycol solution. Failure to achieve a thorough disimpaction undermines successful treatment because laxatives given in maintenance doses do not penetrate or remove the impaction. For the same reason, fiber is withheld during the disimpaction phase of treatment.

The maintenance phase of treatment follows disimpaction and incorporates laxative use, dietary changes, and attention to the child's behavior. Maintenance doses of laxatives are listed in Table 121-2. Telephone follow-up within 2 to 3 days of starting therapy is essential so that the laxative can be titrated to a dose that induces a daily soft bowel movement. Choice of laxative is less important than close follow-up for dosage adjustment. Mineral oil should not be used in children younger than 2 years and in those who are at risk for pulmonary aspiration.[3] Parents should be counseled explicitly never to force the child to take it. At this point, dietary changes that increase the child's fiber intake also are made and include the introduction of whole-grain breads and of cereals and increasing the child's fruit and vegetable intake.

The maintenance phase of therapy incorporates behavioral modification as well. Behavioral modification for toddlers is focused on replacing stool withholding behavior with deliberate attempts to defecate. Frequently, toilet-training efforts are deferred until the child stops withholding. For older children, a behavioral modification program of sitting on the toilet for 5 to 10 minutes after meals is advocated and rewarded by the use of a star-chart system. The child should be rewarded for the targeted behavior (sitting). The physician is responsible for titrating the laxative dose to achieve the desired effect (a soft bowel movement every day). This requires an active partnership with the child and parents, who need to report back to the physician frequently. When parents' skills are limited, children can benefit greatly from referral to a child behavior specialist.

Weaning, as opposed to abrupt cessation, of laxative therapy is the next phase of treatment. Successful weaning can occur following 6 to 12 weeks of maintenance treatment in some toddlers but may not be possible for 6 to 12 months in older children. Typically, the daily laxative dose is decreased to 75%, 50%, and 25% of the initial dose over successive months, or the full dose is given every second day for 6 to 8 weeks and then every third day for another 6 to 8 weeks. Efforts to increase the child's fiber intake and comply with the behavioral program are redoubled during weaning. The older school-age child is encouraged to practice "self-monitoring" of the frequency and adequacy of his or her bowel movements, and a plan for an enema or suppository must be in place for a transient relapse (no stool for more than 3 days) that may occur during weaning. The inability to wean from laxatives following 12 months of therapy is not uncommon in idiopathic constipation but may reasonably justify referral to a pediatric gastroenterologist. It is important to remain optimistic and involved at this point because improvement beyond 12 months of therapy is well documented.[10,12]

REFERENCES

1. Abi-Hanna A, Lake AM: Constipation and encopresis in childhood, *Pediatr Rev* 19:23, 1998.
2. Barr RG, et al: Chronic and occult stool retention: a clinical tool for its evaluation in school aged children, *Clin Pediatr* 18:674, 1979.
3. Baudla HP, Davis SH, Hopkins NE: Lipoid pneumonia: a silent complication of mineral oil aspiration, *Pediatrics* 103:E19, 1999.
4. Benninga MA, et al: Colonic transit time in constipated children: does pediatric slow transit constipation exist? *J Pediatr Gastroenterol Nutr* 23:241, 1996.
5. Harrington L, Schuh S: Complication of Fleet enema administration and suggested guidelines for use in the pediatric emergency department, *Pediatr Emerg Care* 13:225, 1997.
6. Iocono G, et al: Intolerance of cow's milk and chronic constipation in children, *N Engl. J Med* 339:1100, 1998.
7. Issenman RM, et al: Are chronic digestive complaints the result of abnormal dietary patterns? Diet and digestive complaint in children at 22 and 40 months of age, *Am J Dis Child* 141:679, 1987.
8. Leape LL, Ramenofsky ML: Anterior ectopic anus: a common cause of constipation in children, *J Pediatr Surg* 13:627, 1978.
9. Loening-Baucke V: Biofeedback training in children with functional constipation: a critical review, *Dig Dis Sci* 41:65, 1996.
10. Loening-Baucke V: Chronic constipation in children, *Gastroenterology* 105:1557, 1993.
11. McClung HJ, et al: Is combination therapy to encopresis nutritionally safe? *Pediatrics* 91:591, 1993.
12. Murphy MS, Clauden G: Constipation. In Walker WA, et al, editors: *Pediatric gastroenterointestinal disease,* ed 2, St Louis, 1996, Mosby.
13. Partin JC, et al: Painful defecation and fecal soiling in children, *Pediatrics* 103:1007, 1992.
14. Taitz LS, et al: Factors associated with outcome in management of defecation disorders, *Arch Dis Child* 61:472, 1986.

122 Cough

William Jerry Durbin

Cough is one of the most common symptoms that pediatric practitioners are asked to evaluate and manage. Fortunately, as a symptom, cough generally is innocuous; furthermore, the underlying disease process that produces cough rarely is serious and usually is self-limited. Despite its generally benign nature, however, a cough may be disruptive to the child and annoying and anxiety-provoking for parents. In some instances, a cough may be a symptom of a chronic illness or of a worrisome acute process.

PATHOPHYSIOLOGY

From a pathophysiological point of view, cough is a forceful expiration. This "convulsion of the lungs," as Samuel Johnson put it, serves along with the mucociliary elevator to remove secretions and inhaled foreign material from the respiratory tract. The cough reflex can be triggered either voluntarily or by stimulation of cough receptors located throughout the respiratory tract—in the nose, sinuses, pharynx, larynx, trachea, large bronchi, and terminal bronchioles. Afferent impulses from these airway cough receptors travel through cranial nerve afferent pathways to the medullary cough center; from there, efferent stimuli activate coordinated closure of the glottis and contraction of diaphragmatic, chest wall, abdominal wall, and pelvic floor musculature.

The cough sequence is composed of three phases. In the *inspiratory* phase, there is an initial deep inspiration, followed by closure of the glottis. During the second, brief *compressive* phase, intrathoracic pressure increases following contraction of all the expiratory muscles. At the end of this phase, the glottis opens suddenly, leading to the cough, caused by a sudden, explosive release of intrathoracic air. It is during this *expiratory* phase that material from the respiratory tract is eliminated. Children often swallow rather than expectorate such secretions.

CLASSIFICATION

A number of classification schemes of cough have been developed. These focus on aspects such as the duration and descriptive qualities of the cough, the age of the child, and the various types of anatomical lesions and stimuli that can induce cough. The most basic classification is by duration, with cough being characterized as *acute* or *chronic* (3 weeks or longer). When evaluating acute coughs, the physician considers infection and foreign body inhalation; in chronic cough, structural, allergic, irritative, and habit causes become more important, as do chronic infections such as tuberculosis.

A second classification scheme is based on the characteristics of the cough. Thus, a staccato coughing paroxysm in an infant suggests pertussis or chlamydial infection; a barking or brassy cough and voice changes are associated with laryngotracheal infection; a "hawking," or throat-clearing, sound suggests postnasal drip; a ringing or grunting cough may be heard with asthma; and a "honking" or "foghorn" cough may suggest a psychogenic "habit" origin, especially if the cough disappears with sleep. Children who expectorate purulent sputum may have bacterial pneumonia, a lung abscess, bronchiectasis, or cystic fibrosis. Nighttime coughs suggest the possibility of postnasal drip related to sinus infection or allergy. Productive morning coughs suggest bronchiectasis; coughs that commence after feeding suggest aspiration; coughs induced by cold air or exercise may indicate reactive airway disease; and seasonal coughs suggest reactive disease or allergic rhinitis with postnasal drip. Hemoptysis raises concern about diseases such as tuberculosis, cystic fibrosis, bronchiectasis, and pulmonary hemosiderosis; it also occurs occasionally with foreign body aspiration or severe nasopharyngitis. In addition, blood arising from the gastrointestinal tract is often thought mistakenly to have been coughed from the respiratory tract.

A third approach to classifying cough is based on age. Infections are a prime concern in all age groups. In small infants, physiological or structural alterations should also be considered—for example, gastroesophageal reflux, tracheobronchomalacia, tracheoesophageal fistula, vascular ring, and other airway anomalies. In toddlers, foreign body aspiration, irritation of airways (e.g., from passive smoking), and reactive airway disease are important causes of cough. For school-age children who have asthma, sinusitis, and allergic rhinitis with postnasal drip assume greater importance, whereas in adolescents, smoking and psychogenic cough should be considered.

A fourth classification is strictly anatomical, in which the practitioner considers lesions at all levels of the respiratory tract that can stimulate cough. This includes diseases of the larynx, pharynx, nose, and sinuses (infections, irritations, allergies, foreign bodies, structural anomalies); the trachea and bronchi (infections, irritations, foreign bodies, structural anomalies, asthma, cystic fibrosis); the lung parenchyma (pneumonia, lung abscess, congenital malformations, pulmonary edema); the pleura (effusion, empyema); and the mediastinum (great-vessel malformations, adenopathy, tumors). In addition, nonrespiratory tract causes (external auditory canal irritation, diaphragmatic and subdiaphragmatic lesions, and cough tic) should be considered.

Perhaps the most satisfactory classification is one in which the types of stimuli that can produce cough are considered. *Mechanical* stimuli include intraluminal secretions and foreign bodies (e.g., dust, or gastric contents with gastroesophageal reflux or other causes of aspiration). In addition, extraluminal lesions that compress the airway must be considered—both extramural (e.g., vascular rings and other anomalies) and intramural (e.g., the contraction of bronchial smooth muscle, manifested by asthma). *Inflammatory* stimuli include all the infectious conditions of the respiratory tract in which edema or exudate involves either the airway or the alveoli. *Chemical* stimuli include irritative gases, such as cigarette or wood stove smoke or glue-sniffing allergens, which cause cough on inhalation. *Thermal* stimuli—that is, hot or cold air—also produce cough, as can *psychogenic* stimuli. Lastly, toxic reactions (e.g., to latex or drugs) should be considered.

These classification schemes provide the physician with a general framework with which to guide the evaluation of a coughing child. Implicit in the evaluation is the knowledge that most coughs of short duration are related to acute respiratory tract infections; the most common causes of chronic cough are reactive airway disease (classic or cough-variant asthma), postnasal drip (resulting from recurrent upper respiratory tract infections, sinusitis, allergic and vasomotor rhinitis), and airway irritants (e.g., smoke, dust, chemicals, and aspirated food or gastric contents).

HISTORY

The history should include a description of the cough, including its duration, frequency, quality, timing, and sputum productivity. A history of episodes of cough, respiratory infections, and allergies should be sought. The family history may be helpful in identifying children who have diseases such as asthma, cystic fibrosis, and tuberculosis. The environmental history will help identify those children whose symptoms are related to passive smoking or other chemical inhalation, to a respiratory virus that has affected a household, or to an exotic pathogen acquired while traveling. An awareness of family setting and home dynamics may aid in recognizing children at risk for foreign body aspiration or development of a cough tic. It also is important to elicit a history of associated clinical findings. Fever usually suggests an acute infectious process; rhinorrhea may indicate an upper respiratory tract infection, sinusitis, or allergy. Wheezing suggests that asthma or a foreign body is the cause of cough; a history of atopic dermatitis or allergic rhinitis provides evidence for the former. Shortness of breath is associated with asthma, upper airway obstruction, pleural effusions, pneumothorax, pneumonias, and congestive heart failure.

Timing of the cough is helpful—for example, the cough of asthma is often more notable at night, during sleep; nighttime cough also suggests postnasal drainage.

PHYSICAL EXAMINATION

When performing the physical examination, the clinician is looking for signs of an acute process (fever, tender adenopathy, pharyngitis, or a rash), as well as signs of a chronic or recurrent process (growth failure or clubbing, which may be seen in children who have severe asthma, cystic fibrosis, immunodeficiency, or congenital heart disease). It is important to define the level of involvement of the respiratory tract: crackles, wheezes, rhonchi, altered breath sounds, and changes in resonance signify lower respiratory tract involvement; stridor and dysphagia indicate laryngeal involvement; and changes in the mouth, nose, ears, and sinuses signify upper airway disease. Observation of color, state of hydration, respiratory rate, chest movement, retractions, flaring of the chest, and handling of oral secretions indicates the severity of the process. It also is useful to have the child demonstrate the cough. Last, inspection for stigmata of allergic disease (e.g., eczema; pale, boggy nasal mucosa; clear rhinorrhea; allergic shiners; a horizontal nasal crease) and for posterior pharyngeal wall cobblestoning (hypertrophic lymphoid follicles seen in chronic postnasal drainage) is important (see Chapter 184, Allergic Rhinitis). A foul breath may indicate sinusitis or an intranasal foreign body.

LABORATORY TESTS

Most children who have coughs do not require any laboratory testing. For those children in whom the cough is chronic or associated with respiratory distress, some investigations may be undertaken. A complete blood count may provide evidence of acute infection, atopy (eosinophilia), or polycythemia. Examination of the sputum, including its macroscopic appearance, cellular composition (polymorphonuclear leukocytes, eosinophils), and bacterial content (Gram stain, culture), may be useful in children who are able to expectorate. A similar examination of the nasal discharge also may help to distinguish allergic rhinitis from purulent rhinitis or sinusitis. Imaging studies of the neck or sinuses may yield useful information, as might a barium swallow test in an infant thought to be aspirating or having airway obstruction. Pulmonary function testing may be carried out in children who have suspected restrictive or obstructive airway disease; reversible reactive airway disease (asthma) is indicated either by improvement in an obstructive breathing pattern after bronchodilator administration or by the development of obstructive breathing after exposure to agents such as cold air, methacholine, histamine, or specific allergens. Pulmonary function testing may identify children who have cough-variant asthma, whose reactive airway disease is manifested clinically by coughing rather than by wheezing. The performance of pH probe monitoring, sweat testing, tuberculin skin testing, and immunoglobulin and alpha$_1$-antitrypsin measurements may be indicated in children who have chronic or recurrent cough and demonstrable pulmonary disease. Bronchoscopy is useful in searching for a foreign body, investigating persistent collapse, confirming anatomical malformations, or obtaining tissue from children who have undiagnosed infiltrates or suspected ciliary dyskinesia syndrome.

MANAGEMENT

Having completed the assessment of the coughing child, the clinician is faced with the problem of management. Several caveats are in order. First, the physician often needs to defuse parental anxiety about a cough, particularly when it is part of an acute respiratory infection. An explanation of the normalcy of a cough as part of the disease process, of the protective role that it may play, and of the usually self-limited nature of coughs may be necessary. The practitioner must acknowledge that the cough may be annoying and disruptive but also should reassure the child and parent that coughs in children in and of themselves rarely are harmful.

Second, treating the underlying disorder, thereby reducing the stimulation to cough, is more important than providing nonspecific cough medication. Thus, the child who has the productive cough caused by a postnasal drip may benefit from decongestants; the child who has the barking cough of croup should receive humidification; the child who has allergen- or irritant-induced cough may need environmental alteration, bronchodilators, or corticosteroids; the child who has gastroesophageal reflux may need thickened feedings, gastric motility agents, and upright positioning after feedings.

Third, the physician who prescribes cough medicines should explain their therapeutic purpose carefully—for example, expectorants to loosen (not diminish) the cough or antitussives to partially suppress (not eliminate) the cough. Such discussion helps avoid unrealistic expectations. Cough medicines generally are contraindicated in the first few months of life because of their potential toxicity. Antitussives generally are avoided in patients who have productive coughs.

There are several categories of potential cough medicines: expectorants, mucolytics, antitussives, antihistamines, and decongestants. *Expectorants* are drugs that increase sputum volume and, thus, promote removal of secretions from the airways. Water is the expectorant used most commonly, given both orally and by inhalation. It probably works because of its demulcent effect in the upper airway; whether administration of water actually affects lower airway secretions is unclear. Another expectorant, guaifenesin (glyceryl guaiacolate), is used commonly in cough preparations; however, although it may reduce sputum thickness, it has not been shown to reduce coughing in children. Ammonium chloride and potassium iodide rarely are prescribed for children, in part because of untoward side effects associated with effective dosages.

Mucolytic agents are drugs, such as acetylcysteine, that liquefy tenacious secretions. They occasionally are administered by inhalation for children who have bronchiectasis (e.g., cystic fibrosis). Poor taste, the potential for inducing airway reactivity, and uncertain clinical benefit severely limit their use.

Antitussives are drugs that suppress coughing; they are the most effective cough modifiers. Peripherally acting antitussives work by coating or by anesthetizing irritated oropharyngeal receptors. This group includes the demulcents (e.g., throat lozenges, cough drops, lollipops, honey), as well as topical anesthetics administered by swallowing or spraying. These local measures generally are safe and well tolerated and may be useful in a cough related to upper respiratory tract infections or other pharyngeal irritation. Their duration of benefit is limited, however, because they are washed away quickly. Centrally acting antitussives include both narcotic and nonnarcotic agents that suppress the cough reflex at the brainstem level. Narcotic agents are of proven efficacy in adults in suppressing cough; codeine and hydrocodone are those used most widely and in children have a low potential for abuse or for adverse effects. Among the nonnarcotic drugs, dextromethorphan is the most commonly prescribed. Unfortunately, objective clinical trials in children demonstrating a clinical benefit are lacking.

Antihistamines often are used in cough and cold medications. Although effective for allergy symptoms, these agents are not likely to help symptoms of an upper respiratory infection because histamines are not major mediators of cold symptoms. However, first generation H_1-receptor antihistamines exert an anticholinergic effect that results in drying of the nasal mucosa and a resultant decrease in postnasal drip and cough. Additionally, diphenhydramine may have a direct suppressive effect on the medullary cough center.

Decongestants such as pseudoephedrine hydrochloride may be given either topically or systemically and are used to relieve nasal congestion by shrinking nasal mucosa and increasing airway patency. They may promote sinus drainage by opening the ostia. Antihistamines and decongestants often are combined to treat allergy symptoms, balancing the sedative effects of the antihistamine with the stimulatory effects of the decongestant. By extension, such combinations often are used in treating cold symptoms, sometimes also in combination with antitussives or expectorants, although there are no studies to support the effectiveness of these combinations.

When to Refer

1. When the cough is persistent and disabling
2. When there is an associated undiagnosed pulmonary or systemic illness
3. When there is associated failure to thrive

When to Hospitalize

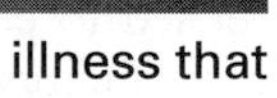

1. When the cough is part of a systemic illness that requires hospitalization for workup or treatment
2. When the child is having unrelieved respiratory distress

SUGGESTED READINGS

American Academy of Pediatrics: Use of codeine- and dextromethorphan-containing cough remedies in children, *Pediatrics* 99:918, 1997.

Brooke AM, et al: Recurrent cough: natural history and significance in infancy and early childhood, *Pulmonology* 26:256, 1998.

Callahan C: Etiology of chronic cough in a population of children referred to a pediatric pulmonologist, *J Am Board Fam Pract* 9:324, 1996.

Callahan CW: Primary tracheomalacia and gastroesophageal reflux in infants with cough, *Clin Pediatr* 37:725, 1998.

Chang AB, Phelan PD, Robertson CF: Cough receptor sensitivity in children with acute and non-acute asthma, *Thorax* 52:770, 1997.

Chang AB, Powell CV: Non-specific cough in children: diagnosis and treatment, *Hosp Med* 59:680, 1998.

Chang AB, et al: Airway hyper-responsiveness and cough-receptor sensitivity in children with recurrent cough, *Am J Respir Crit Care Med* 155:1935, 1997.

Chang AB, et al: A randomized, placebo-controlled trial of inhaled albuterol and beclomethasone for recurrent cough, *Arch Dis Child* 79:6, 1998.

Cochrane D: Diagnosing and treating chesty infants: a short trial of inhaled corticosteroids is probably the best approach, *BMJ* 316:1546, 1998.

Corrao WM: Chronic persistent cough: diagnosis and treatment update, *Pediatr Ann* 25:162, 1996.

Duull IJ: Descriptive study of cough, wheeze and school absence in childhood, *Thorax* 51:630, 1996.

Faniran AO, Peat TK, Woolrock AJ: Persistent cough: is it asthma? *Arch Dis Child* 79:411, 1998.

Guilbert TW, Tuussig LM: Chronic cough, *Contemp Pediatr* 15:155, 1998.

Irwin RJ: Silencing chronic cough, *Hosp Pract* 34:53, 1999.

Irwin RJ, et al: Managing cough as a defense mechanism and as a symptom: a consensus panel report of the American College of Chest Physicians, *Chest* 114(2 suppl):133S, 1998.

Kutcher ML: Cold, cough and allergy medications: uses and abuses, *Pediatr Rev* 17:12, 1996.

Munyam P, Bush A: How much coughing is normal? *Arch Dis Child* 74:531, 1996.

O'Brien KL, et al: Cough illness/bronchitis: principles of judicious use of antimicrobial agents, *Pediatrics* 101(suppl):178, 1998.

Rietveld S, et al: Diagnosis of spontaneous cough in childhood asthma: results of continuous tracheal sound recording in the homes of children, *Chest* 113:50, 1998.

Rose VL: American College of Chest Physicians issues consensus statements on the management of cough, *Am Fam Physician* 59:697, 1999.

Ruisler J, Alexander C, Campo P: Breast-feeding and illness: a dose-response relationship? *Am J Public Health* 89:25, 1999.

Schidlow DV: Cough in children, *J Asthma* 33:81, 1996.

Wright AL, et al: Recurrent cough in childhood and its relation to asthma, *Am J Respir Crit Care Med* 153:1259, 1996.

123 Dental Stains

Lindsey K. Grossman

Parental concerns about changes in tooth color, often the cause of much anxiety, frequently are brought to the pediatrician first. Normal tooth color varies greatly from one tooth to another, from one individual to another, and between the usual blue-white of the primary dentition and the yellowish ivory of the permanent teeth.

EXTRINSIC STAINS

Teeth often are discolored as a result of staining from external deposits on their surface layer. These extrinsic stains usually are removable by careful daily brushing and professional oral prophylaxis (scaling). Chromogenic bacteria in plaque can result in green, orange, or black stains along the gingival margins of the teeth. Although in most cases this is associated with poor oral hygiene, black stains may be seen with good hygiene and a low incidence of caries. Excessive use of certain foods or beverages and smoking can stain the teeth, but the discoloration usually disappears with oral prophylaxis and avoidance of the staining substance. Some liquid medications, especially iron preparations, may leave teeth with a dark stain that either resolves with professional scaling after the medication is discontinued or may be completely prevented if the medication is administered through a straw from the onset.

Recently a new dental calculus has been identified in children who are intensive swimmers.[1] Unusual in both appearance and location, the deposits often are yellow to dark brown and are most noticeable on the facial and lingual surfaces of the anterior teeth. These stains can be accompanied with gingivitis and are caused by the mixture of pool water (chemicals) with saliva.

INTRINSIC STAIN

When a staining substance is incorporated into the deep structures of the tooth (the enamel or dentin or both), it cannot be removed by scaling and is referred to as an intrinsic stain. Certain problems of the neonatal period, such as erythroblastosis fetalis, biliary atresia, neonatal hepatitis, or other conditions resulting in high serum concentrations of bilirubin pigments, can cause yellow-green or blue-green staining from pigment deposition in the structures of the primary teeth. As many as 50% of children who have cyanotic congenital heart disease may have dull, pale, bluish-white teeth, resembling skim milk in color, believed to be caused, at least in part, by prolonged hypoxemia.

Intrinsic stains may be associated with certain rare childhood conditions. The erythrodontia of porphyria, caused by deposition of red-brown porphyrin pigments into the tooth structure, is readily apparent in ultraviolet light if not in daylight. The inherited disorders amelogenesis imperfecta and dentinogenesis imperfecta are associated with hypoplastic enamel and a yellow, opalescent blue-gray or brown-violet tooth color. Major dental work is required to restore normal appearance in all of these disorders.

Common pedodontic problems often result in a change in tooth color. Tooth trauma and associated bleeding into dentin can cause a pink color that fades, first to gray as pulp degenerates, and eventually to yellow. In certain cases the dentin resorption results in a permanent pink hue. Active caries in teeth may appear chalky white or yellow but gradually change to shiny black as the caries convert to the arrested state. An unusual secondary complication of certain childhood infections is Turner tooth, a brown or yellow-brown discoloration associated with hypoplasia of the enamel in a tooth undergoing odontogenesis at the time of the illness.

Persons living in areas where the water contains fluoride have increased resistance to caries. However, as the fluoride content rises over 1.5 parts per million (ppm), many individuals begin to demonstrate hypoplastic enamel, with characteristic dull, opaque white mottled patches in the permanent teeth. If the amount of fluoride consumed is extremely high (more than 5 ppm), the teeth show a blotchy brown or black-brown color that is highly disfiguring and requires extensive restoration of the dental surfaces.

The routine use of fluoride toothpastes in young children who tend to swallow and not spit the dentifrice and the use of fluoride supplementation in breast-fed infants have caused fluorosis in young children in areas where the natural fluoride level in water is low. Parents should be counseled to give young children a very small amount of toothpaste on the brush and to supervise their tooth hygiene. Fluoride supplementation for breast-fed infants should not be recommended.

A similarly involved course of treatment often is required for the severe intrinsic staining problems caused by tetracycline, a dose-dependent and duration-linked problem caused by the incorporation of tetracycline itself into the mineral complex at the dentinoenamel junction during odontogenesis. If the tetracycline was ingested by the mother before birth or by the child in the first months after birth, the primary teeth will be affected. Permanent teeth will be stained if drug ingestion occurs between 3 months and 7 to 8 years of age. The result may be yellow, gray, or brown tooth discoloration in a linear pattern that, without restoration, may be quite disfiguring. For this reason tetracycline should be avoided by pregnant or lactating women and by young children.

MANAGEMENT

After allaying parental anxieties, the pediatrician should consider referring any child who has extrinsic or intrinsic stains. Simple office dental procedures and preventive education can resolve all extrinsic staining problems, and esthetic improvement is possible with the vast majority of intrinsic discoloration problems. Table 123-1

Table 123-1 Common Colorations of Primary and Permanent Teeth

Color	Distribution and Pattern	Causes	Treatment
Green	Several teeth; gingival third of crowns; extrinsic stain	Chromogenic bacteria in plaque, associated with poor oral hygiene	Oral prophylaxis; preventive education
Orange	Several teeth; gingival third of crowns; less common than green stain; extrinsic stain	Chromogenic bacteria in plaque, associated with poor oral hygiene	Oral prophylaxis; preventive education
Black	Several teeth; gingival third of crowns; less common than green and orange stains; extrinsic stain	Chromogenic bacteria in plaque, associated with poor oral hygiene	Oral prophylaxis; preventive education
	Several teeth; extrinsic stain	Oral medications, especially iron	Oral prophylaxis after discontinuing medication
	One or several teeth; occlusal or interproximal surfaces; hard, shiny	Arrested caries	Dental evaluation, observation, or restoration
Brown-black	Several teeth; occlusal pits and fissures or smooth surfaces	Accumulation of tin or staining of demineralized enamel after strontium fluoride (SrF_2) topical treatment	None or esthetic restoration
Pink	Single tooth; entire crown	Posttraumatic change	
		Within 1-2 days—bleeding into dentin; changes to gray in 1-3 wk	None or observation
		After several months—internal resorption of dentin	Minor resorption—endodontics; severe resorption—extraction
Gray	Several teeth; linear pattern or entire crown, depending on stage of tooth development	Tetracycline incorporation in tooth and subsequent oxidation by sunlight; exhibits other colors	Esthetic improvement—endodontic therapy and bleaching and/or esthetic restoration
	All primary and permanent teeth; entire crown	Dentinogenesis imperfecta (autosomal dominant)	Esthetic improvement and protection from wear—prosthetic coverage
	Single tooth; entire crown	Posttraumatic change	
		Within 1-3 wk—hemosiderin pigment in dentin	Observation
		After several months—pulpal necrosis	Endodontic treatment or extraction
Yellow	Several teeth; entire crown	Natural color of permanent compared with primary teeth	None necessary
	Several teeth; linear pattern or entire crown	Tetracyclines; systemic infections	Esthetic restoration
	All primary and permanent teeth; entire crown	Amelogenesis imperfecta (various inheritance patterns)	Esthetic restoration and protection from occlusal wear

Modified from Abrams RG, Josell SD: *Pediatr Clin North Am* 29:705, 1982.

Continued

Table 123-1 Common Colorations of Primary and Permanent Teeth—cont'd

Color	Distribution and Pattern	Causes	Treatment
Yellow—cont'd	Single tooth; entire crown	Posttraumatic change—pulpal obliteration by dentin	Observation or esthetic restoration
	Several teeth; gingival third of crown; extrinsic stain	Food debris and chromogenic bacteria in plaque, associated with poor oral hygiene	Oral prophylaxis; preventive education
	Several teeth; extrinsic stain; part of or entire crown	Tea, coffee, cola, tobacco	Oral prophylaxis; avoid excessive use of substance
Yellow-brown	Several teeth	Premature birth; enamel disturbance—hypoplasia and hypocalcification	None
	One or several teeth; one or more surfaces with cavitations	Advanced active caries	Restoration
Brown	Several teeth; entire crown	Amelogenesis imperfecta; dentinogenesis imperfecta; premature birth; jaundice	As suggested above under gray and yellow colorations
	Individual teeth; localized area	Turner hypoplasia secondary to infection	None or esthetic restoration
		Hypocalcified or hypoplastic area—traumatized primary tooth affecting permanent crown	None or esthetic restoration
	Several teeth; linear or generalized distribution; associated hypoplasia	Fluorosis; systemic infections, especially with high fever; nutritional deficiencies	None or esthetic restoration
	Several teeth; generalized or linear	Tetracycline	Esthetic restoration
	Several teeth; one or more surfaces; loss of tooth structure	Advanced active caries	Restoration
Red-brown	Several teeth; primary and permanent; generalized	Porphyria	None or esthetic restoration
Blue	Several teeth; extrinsic stain; part of or entire crown	Berries	Oral prophylaxis; avoid excessive use of substance
Blue-green or yellow-green	All primary teeth; entire crown	Bilirubin pigments incorporated into dentin—erythroblastosis fetalis, biliary atresia, neonatal hepatitis	None; generally fades; permanent teeth not affected if condition does not continue
White or cream	Several teeth; linear or entire crown	Fluorosis; systemic infections	None; generally fades; permanent teeth not affected if condition does not continue
	All primary and permanent teeth; entire crown	Amelogenesis imperfecta	None; generally fades; permanent teeth not affected if condition does not continue
	Individual teeth; localized area	Turner hypoplasia	None; generally fades; permanent teeth not affected if condition does not continue
	One or several teeth; occlusal or gingival third of smooth surface	Early active caries—demineralization of enamel	Preventive therapy
	Several teeth; any surface; extrinsic stain	Plaque and food debris (materia alba)—removed easily with gauze	Oral hygiene instruction

Modified from Abrams RG, Josell SD: *Pediatr Clin North Am* 29:705, 1982.

should be helpful in identifying the cause of any staining problem.

REFERENCE

1. Rose KJ, Carey CM: Intensive swimming: can it affect your patients' smiles? *JADA* 126:1402, 1995.

SUGGESTED READINGS

Acosta F, Carrel R, Binns WH: Dental stains and their relationship to periodontal diseases in children, *Acta Odontol Pediatr* 3:13, 1983.

Creightons PR: Common pediatric dental problems, *Pediatr Clin North Am* 45:1579, 1998.

Dayan D, et al: Tooth discoloration—extrinsic and intrinsic factors, *Quintessence Int* 14:195, 1983.

Faunce F: Management of discolored teeth, *Dent Clin North Am* 27:657, 1983.

Pindborg JJ: *Pathology of dental hard tissues,* Philadelphia, 1973, WB Saunders.

Sweeney EA: Pediatric dentistry, *Curr Probl Pediatr* 11:1, 1980.

Vogel RI: Intrinsic and extrinsic discoloration of the dentition, *J Oral Med* 30:99, 1975.

124 Diarrhea and Steatorrhea

Martin H. Ulshen

Diarrhea, like vomiting, is a common symptom in the young child, especially during infancy. Loosely defined, diarrhea is characterized by an increase in the frequency and water content of stools. The normal daily stool volume varies with the size of the child. Adults and older children have a normal daily stool weight in the range of 100 to 200 g (consisting of 60% to 85% water); infants weighing fewer than 10 kg can have approximately 5 g/kg/day of stool. An intermediate range of 50 to 75 g/day is an appropriate approximation for the preschool child. In infancy the frequency and quality of "normal" stools depend very much on diet.

During the first weeks of life, the breast-fed infant commonly has up to eight loose stools per day, which at times may contain mucus. These stools frequently follow feedings (as a result of the "gastrocolic reflex") and do not constitute diarrhea. Infants receiving cow milk or soy formula usually have firmer and somewhat less frequent stools. After the first few weeks of life, the normal breast-fed infant tends to have less frequent stools, which may become infrequent (i.e., less than once a week), although they remain soft. Commonly the stool of the nursing infant becomes firm when solids or cow milk are introduced into the diet.

Steatorrhea signifies an excess of fat in the stool and is a symptom of malabsorption. However, disorders associated with malabsorption (e.g., gluten-sensitive enteropathy) do not always produce steatorrhea. Stools that contain an increased quantity of fat can be greasy, bulky, and foul smelling; however, with mild steatorrhea, the stool may appear normal. The stool can be evaluated quickly for fat content by using light microscopy with Sudan staining. Fat excretion can be measured more precisely by quantitative chemical analysis of a 72-hour collection of stool. A record of the diet is kept during this period, and fat intake is calculated. The percentage of the ingested fat that is absorbed equals

$$\frac{(\text{Fat intake} - \text{Fat output})}{\text{Fat intake}} \times 100$$

This is called the *coefficient of absorption.*

Absorption of fat by young infants varies with the type of fat that is fed and with the maturity of the infant. A normal premature infant may absorb as little as 65% to 75% of dietary fat, but this improves to 90% in the full-term infant. Furthermore, the neonate absorbs vegetable fat much more efficiently than butterfat, but human milk fat best of all. Children and adults typically absorb at least 95% of the fat in a normal diet.

PATHOPHYSIOLOGY

Advances in the understanding of the pathophysiology of diarrhea allow a more rational approach to diagnosis and treatment. Normally, large volumes of fluid are processed by the gastrointestinal tract; data for adults are illustrated in Fig. 124-1. It is not difficult to see how an infant rapidly can become fluid depleted from diarrhea when such large gastrointestinal fluid shifts take place each day. Under normal circumstances, about 90% of fluid absorption takes place in the small bowel. However, the colon has a reserve capacity for fluid absorption that must be overcome before diarrhea will result. In adults, as much as 2 liters of ileal fluid can be reabsorbed by the colon daily without diarrhea occurring.

Movement of water across the gastrointestinal tract mucosa is passive, following osmotic gradients created by electrolytes and other osmotically active solutes (such as glucose and amino acids). Nutrients are absorbed by active transport or passive diffusion; some first require digestion to simpler compounds. The flux of electrolytes across the mucosa is bidirectional. The net result of absorption and secretion of these osmotically active solutes is net water retention or loss in the stool. In this sense, diarrhea can be thought of as the result of either malabsorption or net secretion of osmotically active substances.

Many nutrients (including glucose and most amino acids) are absorbed by active, carrier-mediated transport, which is coupled with sodium transport. The osmotic gradient created promotes the absorption of water. Movement of water, in turn, also carries small solutes such as sodium and chloride. This process is known as *solvent drag* and appears to be an important route for sodium absorption during normal digestion. As noted later in this chapter, these mechanisms of sodium movement associated with carrier-mediated nonelectrolyte transport are important to preserve normal fluid and electrolyte balance during some episodes of diarrhea.

Active absorption of chloride in exchange for bicarbonate (HCO_3^-) takes place in the ileum. Potassium moves passively along electrochemical gradients in the small intestine, but both active absorption and secretion of potassium occur in the colon and probably also in the small bowel. The permeability of the intestinal mucosa to passive fluid and electrolyte movement is high in the duodenum and proximal jejunum and decreases distally to the ileum and colon, which are poorly permeable. This feature allows the proximal intestinal contents to equilibrate rapidly with the isotonic extracel-

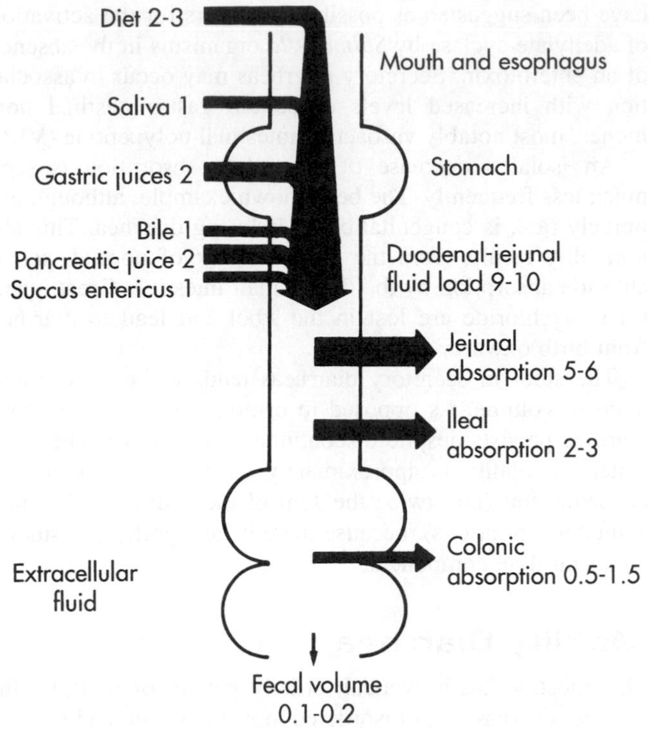

Diet 2-3
Mouth and esophagus
Saliva 1
Gastric juices 2
Stomach
Bile 1
Pancreatic juice 2
Succus entericus 1
Duodenal-jejunal fluid load 9-10
Jejunal absorption 5-6
Ileal absorption 2-3
Colonic absorption 0.5-1.5
Extracellular fluid
Fecal volume 0.1-0.2

Fig. 124-1 Ingestion, secretion, and absorption of water in the gastrointestinal tract of an adult. Numbers refer to liters of water.

lular fluid and facilitates the rapid absorption of water and small solutes by diffusion. Conversely, the ileum and colon are poorly permeable and are able to absorb water and sodium against high electrochemical gradients.

The pathophysiological mechanisms for diarrhea fall into three basic groups[49]: (1) osmotic diarrhea, (2) diarrhea resulting from secretion or altered absorption of electrolytes, and (3) diarrhea resulting from abnormal intestinal motility. Each mechanism has unique clinical characteristics and requires a different therapeutic approach. Therefore, for the physician considering an individual patient who has diarrhea, this framework provides a rational approach for both diagnosis and treatment. Frequently, more than one mechanism of diarrhea will be involved in an episode of diarrhea, but this will be apparent in the evaluation.

Osmotic Diarrhea

The ingestion of a poorly absorbable, osmotically active substance and its presence in the bowel lumen create an osmotic gradient that encourages movement of water into the lumen and subsequently into the stool. Electrolyte losses increase because electrolytes will follow water into the lumen through solvent drag and will tend not to be reabsorbed because of unfavorable electrochemical gradients.

Two main groups of poorly absorbed solutes exist, the ingestion of which results in osmotic diarrhea. The first group includes normal dietary components that may be malabsorbed either transiently or permanently. For example, disaccharides usually are hydrolyzed to monosaccharides before they are absorbed. If a mucosal disaccharidase (such as lactase) is deficient, the disaccharide (in this case lactose) will be malabsorbed and will represent an osmotic load that will produce diarrhea. Similarly, monosaccharides at times may be poorly absorbed. Medium-chain triglycerides (MCTs) also are osmotically active and may lead occasionally to diarrhea when ingested in high concentration, such as when infants who have compromised mucosal function are given an elemental formula containing MCTs. Malabsorption of long-chain triglycerides (LCTs) does not lead to osmotic diarrhea because LCTs are large hydrophobic molecules and, therefore, have little osmotic activity. Malabsorption of LCTs, however, may lead to diarrhea by mechanisms described later in this chapter. In addition, any osmotically active solute may produce diarrhea in normal persons if given in quantities great enough to surpass the intestinal capacity for absorption.

Thus, some infants whose bowel function is normal will not tolerate the high osmolality of an elemental formula, especially if it is undiluted. Similarly, older children may develop functional gastrointestinal symptoms, including diarrhea, from ingestion of large amounts of fructose in fruits and juices.[37] Patients who have decreased mucosal surface area may have decreased functional capacity and resultant osmotic diarrhea. This problem is seen in infants after small bowel resection. Protein malabsorption does not appear to be associated with diarrhea except in the rare instance of congenital trypsinogen or enterokinase deficiency. For example, Hartnup syndrome, with its malabsorption of primary amino acids, is not associated with diarrhea.

The second group of poorly absorbed solutes includes substances that are transported in limited amounts, even by normal individuals. This group includes magnesium, phosphates, and sulfates. Because these ions invariably lead to diarrhea when given in large enough quantities, they are used as cathartics. The introduction of lactulose in the treatment of hepatic encephalopathy takes advantage of its being a nondigestible disaccharide that leads to acidification of colonic contents by bacterial fermentation of nonabsorbed sugar. Its side effect is diarrhea. In fact, lactulose has become a popular alternative for the treatment of constipation, because it tastes better than many other stool softeners.

The key characteristic of an osmotic diarrhea is its association with the oral ingestion of the offending solute. When a patient who has an osmotic diarrhea is given nothing by mouth, the diarrhea will stop dramatically within 24 hours or less. If the agent is reintroduced (as in a lactose tolerance test), the diarrhea will reappear. The diarrhea is of a moderate volume compared with that in secretory diarrhea. The sodium and potassium ion concentrations in the stool fluid are very useful in establishing a diagnosis. As ileal and colonic sodium absorption continue to function against a concentration gradient, stool sodium concentration will be lower than in the plasma. Normally, the electrolyte concentration in the stool is roughly twice its combined sodium and potassium concentration, usually about 280 milliosmoles. When total stool osmolality is significantly greater than twice its sodium and potassium concentration, there must be osmotically active nonelectrolytes in the stool, and an osmotic diarrhea is present.[19] In some instances, one may be able to find the osmotic component in the stool (such as a reducing substance in lactose malabsorption).

Diarrhea Secondary to Secretion or Altered Electrolyte Absorption

Net movement of an electrolyte across the intestinal mucosa (i.e., into or out of the bowel lumen) is the sum of the simultaneous bidirectional electrolyte flux across the mucosal surface epithelium. Thus, under normal circumstances, opposing secretory and absorptive processes (both active and passive) take place, and the resulting balance is reflected in normal luminal electrolyte and water content. Secretory diarrhea occurs when a physiological electrolyte secretory process is pathologically stimulated. Under such circumstances, there is a net increase in luminal electrolytes and, subsequently, a secondary increase in water. In addition, an associated decrease in absorptive processes may occur. The electrolytes that have been implicated are sodium, chloride, and perhaps bicarbonate. Diarrhea also may result from a decrease in active electrolyte absorption in the absence of any change in secretory function.

It is very difficult clinically to distinguish increased electrolyte secretion from decreased absorption; the results are similar.

The prototype for a secretory diarrhea has been cholera. Cholera enterotoxin has been shown to lead to increased intestinal secretion of chloride and, possibly, bicarbonate, as well as to inhibition of the absorption of sodium. Cholera enterotoxin stimulates surface epithelial adenylate cyclase, leading to an increase in cellular levels of cyclic 3′5′-adenosine monophosphate (AMP). An important observation has been the normal histological appearance of the intestinal mucosa during cholera infection or in vitro exposure to cholera enterotoxin. Specifically, no evidence exists of cell necrosis, inflammation, or local bacterial invasion; other cell absorptive functions remain normal. The normal absorption of glucose provides a route for secondary sodium absorption; oral glucose- and electrolyte-containing solutions have gained wide use in the management of cholera.

A growing number of infectious agents may be associated with secretory diarrhea. Toxigenic *Escherichia coli* produces an enterotoxin antigenically distinct from cholera enterotoxin, which also activates adenylate cyclase. Infantile diarrhea resulting from this toxin is well known. Other bacteria that have been associated with stimulation of intestinal secretion are strains of *Shigella dysenteriae, Salmonella typhimurium, Klebsiella pneumoniae, Clostridium perfringens, Staphylococcus aureus,* and *Pseudomonas aeruginosa*. Experimental work with viral enteritis suggests that this diarrhea has a significant secretory component.[32] Secretion is the result of viral damage to villous epithelial cells in the small intestine and repopulation of the villi with immature crypt cells, rather than toxin production.

A number of noninfectious causes of secretory diarrhea exist as well. Malabsorbed bile acids and long-chain fats both have been shown to stimulate a colonic secretory diarrhea.[44] Certain prostaglandins have been shown to activate adenylate cyclase and produce intestinal secretion in experimental models. Because prostaglandins are released during inflammation, it has been hypothesized that diarrhea associated with certain inflammatory states may be caused by these hormones. This is a particularly appealing hypothesis to explain the small bowel secretion that may take place with chronic inflammatory bowel disease. Prostaglandins also have been suggested as possible mediators for the activation of adenylate cyclase by *Salmonella* organisms in the absence of an enterotoxin. Secretory diarrheas may occur in association with increased levels of certain gastrointestinal hormones, most notably vasoactive intestinal polypeptide (VIP).

An isolated decrease of electrolyte absorption is seen much less frequently. The best-known example, although extremely rare, is congenital chloride-losing diarrhea. This abnormality results from the apparent lack of normal, active chloride absorption by the distal small intestine. Great quantities of chloride are lost in the stool and lead to diarrhea from birth onward.

The stool in secretory diarrheas tends to be watery and large in volume. As opposed to osmotic diarrhea, secretory diarrhea persists despite discontinuing oral intake. The stool water osmolality is approximately equal to the electrolyte concentration (i.e., twice the sum of the sodium and potassium concentrations), because there is no significant osmotic nonelectrolyte component.[19]

Motility Diarrhea

The intestine has a cyclical, orderly pattern of motility. Increased, decreased, or disordered movement can lead to diarrhea. Rapid intestinal transit often occurs in association with osmotic and secretory diarrheas. Increased intraluminal volume has been implicated in stimulating increased peristaltic action. Increased motility may cause diarrhea by allowing less time for the contact of intraluminal contents with absorptive surfaces. When bowel function is compromised (as with the short bowel syndrome), the time of contact with the limited functioning surface may be a crucial factor. In irritable bowel syndrome, disordered motility also may play a role.[16]

Slowed transit and severely disordered motility lead to intraluminal stasis. In normal bowel, steady, progressive movement of chyme is one of the protective mechanisms that prevent the development of bacterial overgrowth, whereas stasis encourages overgrowth. Certain bacteria deconjugate bile acids when present in the upper small bowel and produce fat malabsorption secondarily. In addition, bacterial proteases may damage the small bowel surface. Stasis may result from an anatomical obstruction (e.g., blind loop or stricture), as well as from functional motor disorders. Motility disorder frequently is an associated factor in chronic inflammatory bowel disease. Stools associated with motility disorder, except those secondary to fatty acid malabsorption, tend to be small in volume. The response to feeding is variable, and the gastrocolic reflex may be heightened. Patients who have chronic inflammatory bowel disease may find that meals stimulate intestinal activity, resulting in postprandial abdominal cramps and bowel movements.

ACUTE DIARRHEA

Acute diarrhea is common in children, is transient and usually self-limited, and most often is caused by infection. In the United States, in the first few years of life, children average about one or two episodes per year.[21] The role of the physician is to rule out causes that require specific treatment, to advise the parents in supportive management, and to provide follow-up for possible complications. Box 124-1 lists some

BOX 124-1

CAUSES OF ACUTE DIARRHEA

Usually Without Blood in Stool

Viral enteritis—reovirus (rotavirus[5] and orbivirus), Norwalk agent, enteric adenovirus,[66] calicivirus, and astrovirus[40]

Enterotoxin—*Escherichia coli,*[26] *Klebsiella* organisms, cholera, *Clostridium perfringens, Staphylococcus* organisms, and *Vibrio* species

Parasitic—*Giardia, Cryptosporidium*[2,65] and *Cyclospora* organisms

Extraintestinal infection—otitis media and urinary tract infection

Antibiotic-induced and *Clostridium difficile* toxin (without pseudomembranous colitis)

Commonly Associated With Blood in Stool

Bacterial—*Shigella, Salmonella,* and *Campylobacter* organisms, *Yersinia enterocolitica,* invasive *E. coli,*[26] gonococcus (venereal spread), enteroadherent *E. coli,*[61] *Aeromonas hydrophilia,* and *Plesiomonas shigelloides*

Amebic dysentery

Hemolytic-uremic syndrome

Henoch-Schönlein purpura

Pseudomembranous enterocolitis *(C. difficile* toxin)[10,54]

Ulcerative or granulomatous colitis (acute presentation)

Necrotizing enterocolitis (neonates)

of the more frequent causes of acute diarrhea divided by the usual presentation with or without gross blood in the stool. Child care centers are likely sites for the spread of enteric pathogens. Pathogens that have been associated with epidemics include *Giardia lamblia,* rotavirus, *Shigella, Campylobacter, Cryptosporidium,* and *Clostridium difficile* organisms.[2,5,6] Asymptomatic fecal shedding of *Giardia* organisms is common in this setting.

The neonate who has acute diarrhea must be considered different from the older infant and child, both because of lower tolerance to the associated fluid shifts and because of the greater likelihood of severe infection or of a congenital anomaly. In addition, signs that suggest necrotizing enterocolitis must be sought, including gastric retention (frequently bilious), distention, and occult or bright red blood in the stool. Although this disease usually occurs in premature infants, it also has been reported in ill full-term infants. The presence of pneumatosis intestinalis, gas in the portal vein, or free intraperitoneal gas seen on abdominal roentgenograms supports this diagnosis. Epidemics of diarrhea associated with rotavirus, enteropathogenic *E. coli,* salmonellae, and other organisms, including klebsiellae, have been reported in nurseries. If the onset of diarrhea is associated with early feedings, one must consider congenital digestive defects, especially sugar intolerance. Hirschsprung's disease may manifest with acute diarrhea and enterocolitis in the neonatal period and should be suspected especially in the infant who has not passed meconium in the first 24 hours. Bloody diarrhea that results from cow milk or soy protein intolerance may develop in infants still in the nursery. Resolution and exacerbation on removal and reintroduction of cow milk or soy formula, as well as an atopic family history, are clues to this diagnosis.

In the older infant and child, the usual episode of acute diarrhea is transient and benign. On the initial visit the physician must evaluate the course in terms of both possible causes and the status of hydration. The diarrhea usually is the result of viral enteritis, typically occurring with low-grade fever, vomiting, and frequent watery stools. Generally, the stools are without blood or white blood cells. Enterotoxin-producing organisms (such as toxigenic *E. coli*) are associated with watery stools and are without evidence of mucosal invasion (no high fever or blood in the stool). *Giardia lamblia* produces watery diarrhea associated with intestinal gas and crampy abdominal pain. Diarrhea may be present in association with extraintestinal infections, most notably otitis media and pyelonephritis. This has been called *parenteral diarrhea,* and its mechanism is obscure. There may be an associated viral enteritis in some cases of otitis media. Certain antibiotics, especially ampicillin, have been associated with transient diarrhea. Less common but of greater danger is the association of pseudomembranous colitis with most antibiotics, most commonly clindamycin.[10] In childhood, pseudomembranous colitis may occur acutely or as a more chronic illness of 1 or 2 months' duration.[54] *C. difficile* toxin, which is considered the cause of most cases of pseudomembranous colitis, also may be associated with chronic childhood diarrhea in the absence of colitis.[56]

The presence of blood in the stool, especially with symptoms of colonic involvement (tenesmus, urgency, and crampy lower abdominal pain), should make one think of infection with *Campylobacter, Shigella,* or *Salmonella* organisms. The symptoms of dysentery may be less striking with *Salmonella.* When the *Shigella* is an enterotoxin-producing organism, watery diarrhea actually may precede the onset of dysentery.

Patients who have *Shigella* organisms tend to appear severely ill and may have meningismus or seizures. The stools tend to be foul smelling. Up to 40% of individuals who have Guillain-Barré syndrome have evidence of a *Campylobacter* infection occurring before the onset of neurological symptoms.[1] *Yersinia* enterocolitis also may be associated with blood in the stool, but *Yersinia* appears to be incriminated less commonly as an etiological agent in the United States. *E. coli* can produce diarrhea by a number of pathogenic mechanisms; the enteroadherent, enteroinvasive, and enterohemorrhagic forms all can be associated with blood in the stool.[26] Hemolytic-uremic syndrome is the result largely of enterohemorrhagic *E. coli* (especially serotype O157) and less commonly *Shigella* infections.

Amebiasis is unusual in the United States, but *Entamoeba histolytica* can produce a picture of acute colitis. Causes of bloody diarrhea that are not obviously infectious include intussusception, immune deficiencies, and chronic inflammatory bowel disease. The last may present with an initial episode of acute dysentery, although the history may reveal previous episodes; arthralgia or growth failure may have preceded the diarrhea. The history of recent similar diarrheal illness in family members or friends suggests an infectious diarrhea.

Foodborne spread of organisms or toxins is an important

cause of acute diarrheal illness[11] (Box 124-2). Improperly prepared poultry is the major source for both campylobacteriosis and salmonellosis. Explosive diarrhea after ingestion of seafood is likely to be due to infection with *Vibrio* species. Tetrodotoxin poisoning is caused by naturally occurring toxins in certain seafoods. Symptoms of the latter disorders usually are associated with neurological manifestations (e.g., headache, myalgia, paresthesia, or paralysis).

At the initial evaluation (Box 124-3), the physician should establish the quantity of the diarrhea, the child's ability to maintain oral intake, and the presence of associated vomiting. On physical examination the state of hydration should be estimated. The presence of tears and saliva usually is evidence of adequate hydration. A simple guideline to hydration is that the absence of tears and the presence of a dry mouth suggest 5% dehydration; the addition of sunken eyes, sunken fontanelle, and poor skin turgor suggests 10% dehydration. In the presence of hypernatremia, the state of dehydration typically is more severe than suggested on physical examination inasmuch as extracellular fluid volume tends to be preserved at the expense of intracellular volume (see Chapter 278, Dehydration). A recorded weight is essential; it can be compared with previous weights and also will be available to reevaluate the state of hydration during the illness. Information about the frequency and quantity of urination is important. A history of good urine output is reassuring. Parents may underestimate urinary frequency, especially when urine becomes mixed with liquid stool.

A stool culture should be obtained if blood or leukocytes are noted in the stool and the child is severely ill. Examination of the stool for leukocytes is helpful in establishing the presence of colitis. A small sample of stool is placed on a microscope slide and mixed with a drop of methylene blue. Multiple fields then are scanned. In the presence of both infectious and noninfectious colitis, white blood cells (WBCs) usually are found in high numbers—frequently in sheets. Polymorphonuclear leukocytes usually account for at least 60% to 80% of the cells; the presence of only occasional cells is considered a negative finding. The absence of WBCs in grossly bloody diarrheal stool occurs with enterohemorrhagic *E. coli* infection but also should direct attention to entities such as intussusception and Meckel diverticulum when these diagnoses seem clinically appropriate. Amebic colitis also may not be associated with WBCs in the stool, although the trophozoites and numerous RBCs may be visible on a saline wet mount preparation of the stool. Invasive bacterial diarrhea frequently is associated with a peripheral blood leukocytosis.

The cornerstone of treatment in acute gastroenteritis is good fluid and electrolyte management (Box 124-4). Commercial oral hydration solutions provide more sodium than traditional clear liquids. Human milk contains low concentrations of sodium (6 to 7 mEq/L); therefore, when diarrhea is persistent or severe, a supplemental rehydration solution should be used.

BOX 124-2

FOODBORNE DIARRHEA

Reportable Pathogens, Percentage of Reportable Cases (%)*	
Campylobacter	41
Salmonella	27
Shigella	15
Cryptosporidium	6
E. coli O157	5
Yersinia	2
Vibrio	0.5
Cyclospora	0.1

Nonreportable Pathogens

Clostridium perfringens
Bacillus cereus
Enterotoxigenic *E. coli*
Staphylococcus aureus
Tetrodotoxin poisoning (naturally occurring toxins in certain seafoods)

*Percent of 9787 laboratory-confirmed cases reported in 1998 among nine diseases under surveillance by the Foodborne Diseases Active Surveillance Network (includes *Listeria* 1%, a foodborne pathogen not producing diarrheal symptoms). CDC: Incidence of foodborne illnesses: preliminary data from the foodborne diseases active surveillance network (FoodNet)—United States 1998, *MMWR* 48:189, 1999.

BOX 124-3

EVALUATION OF ACUTE DIARRHEA

History

1. Length of illness
2. Stools: frequency, looseness (watery versus mushy), and presence of gross blood
3. Oral intake: diet, quantity of fluids and solids taken, and presence of vomiting
4. Associated symptoms: fever, rash, and arthralgia
5. Urine output
6. Contacts with diarrhea or other infectious illness (including child care exposure)

Physical Examination

1. Hydration status: weight (stable or loss), mucosa (moist or dry), saliva and tears (present or absent), skin turgor (normal or poor), eyeballs and fontanelle (normal or sunken), and vital signs
2. Alertness
3. Infant: vigor of suck

Laboratory

1. Stool culture, smear for white blood cells, and evaluation for occult blood
2. Stool ova and parasites and reducing substances
3. Complete blood count
4. If hydration status is in question: blood urea nitrogen (BUN) and serum electrolyte levels
5. Urinalysis
6. If child is lethargic or has had a seizure, culture for sepsis: measure the BUN and serum electrolyte and glucose levels and examine and culture the cerebrospinal fluid

BOX 124-4

FLUID AND ELECTROLYTE MANAGEMENT OF ACUTE DIARRHEA

A. General rules for management of acute diarrhea
   1. Age-appropriate feedings should be continued during acute diarrhea, except as noted below. Diet may be better tolerated if fatty foods and foods high in simple sugars (such as undiluted juices and soft drinks) are avoided.
   2. Breast-feeding should be continued when possible.
   3. Lactose-free diet generally is unnecessary. If stools worsen on reintroduction of lactose (human milk, cow milk, or lactose-containing formula), lactose intolerance should be considered. If stools become acid and contain reducing substances, lactose intolerance is likely.
   4. Oral rehydration therapy with glucose-electrolyte solution (oral rehydration solution [ORS]) is the preferred treatment of fluid and electrolyte loss except as noted below. These solutions generally contain 25 g/L glucose (or 30 g/L rice starch), 45 to 90 mEq/L sodium, 20 to 25 mEq/L potassium, and 30 mEq/L bicarbonate. The higher sodium concentration is appropriate for rehydration; the lower concentration is usually adequate for rehydration with mild diarrhea and is appropriate for maintenance.
   5. Moderate to large stool output should be replaced with ORS at 10 ml/kg/stool. Losses from emesis should be estimated for replacement with ORS.
   6. The use of ORS is labor intensive. If a caregiver is not available to give small amounts of fluid frequently, intravenous therapy is indicated. If the child is not severely dehydrated, oral rehydration may be completed at home with close follow-up. Otherwise, intravenous fluids should include replacement of deficit, ongoing losses, and maintenance fluids. Addition of intravenous potassium should wait until urine output is established
   7. ORS therapy is effective for hypernatremic as well as hyponatremic and isotonic dehydration.

B. No dehydration
   1. Continue age-appropriate feeding (see A.1, A.2).
   2. Use ORS only to replace excessive stool output (see A.5).

C. Mild dehydration (3% to 5%)
   1. Correct dehydration with 60 ml/kg ORS over 4 hours and replace continuing losses from stool and emesis with additional ORS (see A.5).
   2. Reevaluate hydration and replacement of losses at least every 2 hours.
   3. Once dehydration is corrected, begin feeding (see A.1, A.2).

D. Moderate dehydration (6% to 9%)
   1. Correct dehydration with 80 ml/kg ORS over 4 hours and replace continuing losses from stool and emesis with additional ORS (see A.5).
   2. Reevaluate hydration and replacement of losses at least every hour. Best accomplished under medical supervision (ER, hospital outpatient unit, or physician's office).
   3. Once dehydration is corrected, begin feeding (see A.1, A.2).

E. Severe dehydration (at least 10%)
   1. Resuscitate with intravenous or intraosseous normal saline or lactated Ringer's solution 20 ml/kg of body weight over 1 hour. Repeat until pulse and state of consciousness return to normal. Larger volumes and shorter periods of administration may be required. Delay giving intravenous potassium until urine output is established.
   2. Determine serum electrolyte levels.
   3. Lack of response to initial resuscitation suggests an underlying problem such as septic shock, toxic shock syndrome, myocarditis, myocardiopathy, or pericarditis. Persistently poor urine output may be seen with hemolytic-uremic syndrome.
   4. ORS may be initiated when the child's condition has stabilized and mental status is satisfactory. An intravenous line should be maintained until no longer needed.
   5. Feeding may be restarted when rehydration is complete (see A.1, A.2).

F. Special considerations
   1. Vomiting
      a. Vomiting occurs commonly during acute gastroenteritis.
      b. Children who are dehydrated and vomit usually tolerate ORS.
      c. Intractable, severe vomiting, unconsciousness and ileus are contraindications to ORS treatment.
      d. ORS should be started at 5 ml every 1 to 2 minutes.
      e. Vomiting usually decreases as dehydration improves, and larger amounts can be given at less frequent intervals.
      f. Nasogastric tube can be used for continuous ORS infusion (not in comatose child or one who has ileus or intestinal obstruction).
      g. Intravenous fluids should be used if ORS treatment is unsuccessful.
   2. Refusal to take ORS
      a. Children who are not dehydrated may not take ORS because of the salty taste. However, dehydrated children generally take it well.
      b. Giving ORS in small amounts at first allows child to become accustomed to the taste.
      c. ORS can be frozen in ice-pop form.

Modified from *Pediatrics* 97:424, 1996.

Electrolyte content in diarrheal stool varies widely, with the highest concentrations occurring in secretory diarrheas such as cholera. Fecal sodium levels may range from 40 to 100 mEq/L and occasionally may be as high as 150 mEq/L. In rotavirus diarrhea, fecal sodium concentration is typically 20 to 40 mEq/L.

At least 40% to 50% of epidemic diarrhea may be of viral origin (in winter this proportion probably is higher). Viral enteritis has been shown to result in a transient, patchy, mucosal lesion of the small intestine, which may be associated with temporary lactose and fat malabsorption. Decreased mucosal lactase levels may be seen. In experimental viral diarrhea in piglets (transmissible gastroenteritis), intestinal glucose-stimulated absorption of sodium (and therefore water) is impaired because of villus damage.[32,33] Abnormal glucose absorption also has been observed in infants who have rotavirus enteritis. Nevertheless, secretion can be converted to net absorption in most children by providing oral glucose electrolyte solution, because of the patchy nature of the lesion in viral gastroenteritis.

Oral rehydration solutions have been used safely and successfully to treat acute diarrhea with dehydration.[53,57] Infants who have diarrhea usually drink large volumes of salty tasting liquids ad libitum, appropriate for the stool output. Episodes of diarrhea in previously healthy, well-nourished children often are mild, and under these circumstances, the use of clear liquids is not of crucial importance. Liquids can be offered ad libitum, although smaller volumes per feeding may be tolerated better when diarrhea is associated with vomiting. If the episode is more severe, an oral rehydration solution as described in Box 124-4 should be used. Commercial rehydration solutions are available (e.g., Rehydralyte). The contents of these solutions have evolved in conjunction with advances in the understanding of optimal absorption during oral rehydration, so the clinician should consult current manufacturer specifications before choosing a product. Continuing regular feedings with supplemental oral rehydration solution generally is tolerated and thought to lead to quicker recovery.[17] Vomiting usually is not a contraindication for oral rehydration.

This treatment appears to be associated with shorter hospitalization and lower medical costs. Infants who have hypernatremic dehydration have fewer problems with seizures during oral, as compared with intravenous, rehydration.[53] Oral rehydration therapy, however, requires the constant presence of a caretaker, although this individual does not need to have previous medical experience. The use of starches in oral maintenance or rehydration solution may improve sodium and water absorption. For further discussion of oral rehydration, see Chapter 29, Fluid Therapy, and Chapter 278, Dehydration.

Indications for medications in the treatment of acute gastroenteritis in infants and children are limited. As already noted, the key mechanisms involved are intestinal secretion and transient malabsorption. Therefore, although medications sometimes are used, there is no apparent rationale regarding the pathophysiology of the disorder for medications that slow gut motility—diphenoxylate, loperamide, paregoric, and anticholinergics. In fact, pooling of fluid in the intestinal lumen after treatment may give a false impression that the diarrhea has improved. The limited reduction in stool output with these drugs is outweighed by the potential risk of lethargy, ileus, respiratory depression, coma, and death. Although Kaopectate does not carry the hazards of these drugs, it has not been shown to slow fluid output and also may lead to a false impression that the diarrhea has resolved. Slowing intestinal transit with drugs may allow greater mucosal contact with pathogens and thereby allow for local mucosal invasion. Bismuth subsalicylate, which may decrease the duration of diarrhea, has been shown to be a safe adjunct to oral rehydration, but is not used routinely.[20] Antibiotics are useful in specific situations: *Shigella* dysentery, *Yersinia* or *Campylobacter* gastroenteritis, pseudomembranous colitis, *Salmonella* infections in infants younger than 6 months of age, and *Salmonella* infections in older patients who have enteric fever, typhoid fever, or complications of bacteremia.[64] *Campylobacter* gastroenteritis must be identified very early for antibiotics to shorten the illness. For the individual patient, the presence of an *E. coli* serotype previously labeled enteropathogenic correlates poorly with the presence of diarrhea and alone is not an indication for antibiotic treatment.[26] Recent interest exists in the use of *Lactobacillus* or other probiotics to prevent or treat infectious diarrhea.[18]

Most episodes of gastroenteritis are self-limited and of short duration. Symptoms of rotavirus enteritis typically last 4 to 10 days. However, prolonged excretion of rotavirus in stool (up to 8 weeks) has been demonstrated in association with severe gastroenteritis in immunocompetent children.[51] The current approach to treatment is to restart the previous formula and solids early after the onset of diarrhea. If diarrhea recurs on the introduction of lactose-containing formula, the child may have a transient lactose intolerance. In this situation a lactose-free formula should be offered (the sugar in this formula can be either sucrose or a glucose polymer). As noted in the section on disaccharide intolerance, sugar malabsorption can be identified by the determination of reducing substance in the stool (sucrose must be hydrolyzed first with hydrochloric acid). A secondary lactose intolerance usually lasts only a week or less but at times can persist for months.

If the degree of dehydration is 5% or greater, use of oral rehydration solution should be instituted, if possible, in the manner presented in Box 124-4. For severe dehydration or shock, rapid intravenous administration of 10 to 20 ml/kg of isotonic fluid or colloid is required initially and may need to be repeated early. Hyponatremia and hypernatremia must be corrected slowly to prevent complications of the central nervous system (CNS). Oral solutions are better tolerated and result in fewer CNS complications than intravenous solutions in infants who have hypernatremia.[53] Potassium should not be added to intravenous fluids until adequate urine output is established. Urine specific gravity may be misleading inasmuch as kidney-concentrating ability may be poor as a result of reduced renal urea or whole body potassium. Inability to acidify the urine during acute diarrhea occurs commonly in infants despite the presence of metabolic acidosis.[27] This finding is thought to be secondary to sodium deficiency and the resulting inadequate delivery of sodium to the distal nephron. Complete discussion of intravenous treatment is presented in Chapter 29, Fluid Therapy.

CHRONIC DIARRHEA

Chronic diarrhea occurs in children of all ages; however, it is most frequent and often most challenging to diagnose in infants.[9] Both healthy and ill infants can develop diarrhea in response to a variety of stresses. The younger the infant, the more likely he or she is to enter the cycle of diarrhea and secondary malnutrition that leads to further diarrhea, malnutrition, and susceptibility to infection. Many of the causes of chronic diarrhea may appear at any time during childhood. Certain diseases, however, occur much more commonly in infancy; others are more likely to begin in later childhood. The division of etiologies of diarrhea in this section between infancy and older childhood is artificial because the groups overlap, but it is a helpful guide in initiating the evaluation of the child who has chronic diarrhea. All the causes discussed are listed in Box 124-5.

BOX 124-5

CAUSES OF CHRONIC DIARRHEA

Common Causes

Chronic enteric infection: *Salmonella* organisms, *Yersinia enterocolitica, Campylobacter, Giardia, Cryptosporidium,* and *Cyclospora* organisms, *Clostridium difficile* toxin,[54,56] enteroadherent *Escherichia coli,*[61] rotavirus (in immunodeficient patients), cytomegalovirus, and HIV
Food allergy
Chronic nonspecific diarrhea (toddler's diarrhea, irritable colon of childhood)[13]
Disaccharide intolerance[60]
Chronic constipation with overflow "diarrhea"
Cystic fibrosis
Gluten-sensitive enteropathy (celiac disease)
Inflammatory bowel disease: Crohn's disease and ulcerative colitis
Hirschsprung's disease
Immunodeficiency states
Monosaccharide intolerance
Eosinophilic (allergic) gastroenteritis
Short bowel syndrome
Urinary tract infection
Factitious causes

Less Common Causes

Autoimmune enteropathy[8]
Hormonal: adrenal insufficiency and hyperthyroidism
Vasoactive intestinal polypeptide-secreting tumor
Neural crest tumor and carcinoid
Intestinal lymphangiectasia
Acrodermatitis enteropathica
Intestinal stricture or blind loop
Pancreatic insufficiency with neutropenia
Trypsinogen or enterokinase deficiency
Congenital chloride-losing diarrhea
Abetalipoproteinemia
Microvillus inclusion disease[14]
Intestinal pseudoobstruction

Infants

The physician confronted with an infant who has a history of chronic diarrhea must decide first whether the stool pattern is abnormal. A nursing mother who has not been forewarned may become concerned about the appearance and frequency of her child's transitional stools. The infant's weight gain and healthy appearance, combined with an explanation about stools of breast-fed infants, should dispel these concerns.

In the latter half of the first year and in the second year, the most common cause for persistent diarrhea is chronic nonspecific diarrhea (also called *toddler's diarrhea*).[13,37] Affected infants and toddlers have intermittent loose stools for no apparent reason. Often the stools occur early in the day and typically not overnight. These children appear healthy and are thriving according to weight and length growth curves, unless the treatment has led to caloric deprivation. This condition represents a stool pattern rather than a pathological state and requires minimal or no laboratory evaluation. Symptoms may begin initially after an apparent acute enteritis (postenteritis irritable bowel).

Treatment may include (1) restricting the frequency of feedings, whether liquids or solids, in an effort to decrease stimulation of the gastrocolic reflex (in the toddler, three meals and a bedtime snack with nothing by mouth in between), (2) restricting the volumes of fluids ingested, which often are excessive, (3) avoiding excessive intake of juices,[37] and (4) reassuring the parents of the benign nature of this entity. A high-fat diet may be helpful in some children, although probably is of less importance.[13] Cholestyramine (2 g by mouth one to three times daily) also is effective at times; however, the duration of use should be restricted because of the potential for interference with fat-soluble vitamin absorption. In any event, this is a self-limited condition that typically resolves by 3½ years of age. The only danger is that well-intentioned parents may restrict oral intake to clear liquids repeatedly in an effort to treat the child; this may result in poor weight gain. Bile acid malabsorption is an occasional sequela of gastroenteritis that can produce persistent, watery diarrhea. This condition also will respond to cholestyramine therapy.

Protracted diarrhea of infancy. This syndrome of chronic diarrhea occurring during infancy is poorly understood.[36] It is defined somewhat arbitrarily as occurring in infants younger than 3 months of age and persisting for more than 2 weeks. Historically this syndrome, previously called intractable diarrhea of infancy, has been associated with a high mortality secondary to irreversible diarrhea and related malnutrition. However, the outcome has been improved markedly with the advent of oral elemental diets and total parenteral nutrition. Now intractable diarrhea is rare and related to more specific causes (e.g., microvillus inclusion disease).

Protracted diarrhea of infancy probably is the final pathway for multiple causes, including gastrointestinal infection and, perhaps, food intolerances. Generally, malnutrition develops and in concert with the persistent diarrhea leads to alteration of gastrointestinal flora sometimes associated with bacterial overgrowth of the small intestine. Altered mucosal function of the small intestine and pancreatic function may occur with malnutrition and protracted diarrhea. Bile salts may be deconjugated as a result of bacterial overgrowth. Commonly the initiating cause of protracted diarrhea is not found; it is likely that it may no longer be present when the diarrhea has become chronic. The small bowel biopsy specimen may show patchy villous shortening with a decreased villus/crypt ratio and marked inflammation, as well as a damaged surface epithelium. However, the results of the small bowel biopsy also may be normal. Likewise, a rectal biopsy specimen may show evidence of inflammation, including crypt abscesses, or may be normal. The presence or absence of these biopsy findings may not correlate with the severity of the clinical syndrome.[22] Affected infants are severely malnourished and have low serum protein and hemoglobin levels. Frequently they have had repeated treatment with oral clear liquids and peripheral intravenous fluids, all of which provide inadequate caloric intake.

When evaluating a young infant who has protracted diarrhea, the physician must rule out those causes that require urgent treatment while correcting hydration and nutrition. Rehydration is similar to the treatment of acute diarrhea, although it is more difficult to estimate the level of dehydration accurately in the presence of malnutrition, and initial oral therapy is less likely to be successful. Stool output should be measured. If the urine is collected in a urine bag, diapers can be weighed before and after stools to give an accurate measure of stool output. Urine specific gravity and volume may be deceptive because of poor concentration by the kidneys in the presence of malnutrition and total body hypokalemia. The infant should be weighed at least daily.

It is important to rule out infection as a cause early in the evaluation. Several stools for culture and examination for parasites, as well as blood and urine cultures, should be taken initially. The diagnosis of Hirschsprung's disease with enterocolitis should be considered early because infants who have this disorder are prone to perforation of the colon unless a decompression colostomy is performed. In such babies it usually is possible to elicit a history of the absence of stools in the first 24 hours of life and of early obstipation.

In Hirschsprung's disease a flat plate roentgenogram of the abdomen may show a dilated colon with absence of air in the rectum. Toxic megacolon also may be seen in infectious colitis or in chronic inflammatory bowel disease in infancy. Air-fluid levels throughout the bowel are common in infants who have gastroenteritis, and this sign is not helpful in defining a cause. A barium enema under low pressure in the unprepared patient may show the narrow distal segment of rectum; however, this finding may not be present in neonates, and evaluation for ganglion cells on rectal biopsy may be necessary. Hirschsprung's disease often is more obvious on a delayed roentgenogram (24 to 48 hours after the barium enema).

For a child who has chronic diarrhea and has been fed recently, the levels of stool pH and reducing substance should be determined to evaluate sugar malabsorption. The stool pH is not a good measure of the effect of diarrhea on total body acid-base balance. If stool concentration of sodium and potassium minus chloride is greater than the plasma bicarbonate, the infant is losing bicarbonate. An acid stool pH suggests carbohydrate malabsorption.[19] White blood cells or gross blood in the stool usually indicate colonic inflammation; occult blood in the stool suggests loss of blood across the mucosa anywhere in the gastrointestinal tract.

It is important to begin nutritional rehabilitation at once. Currently the best choices in treatment are either enteral alimentation with an elemental or modular formula[34] or total parenteral nutrition (TPN), peripheral or central (see Chapter 29, Fluid Therapy). Often, enteral nutrition is tolerated best by the continuous drip method, and recovery may be more rapid when enteral alimentation is used.[46] Nevertheless, unsuccessful attempts at enteral feeding necessitate initiation of TPN therapy in some infants. Initial treatment with TPN and a gradually increasing, continuous enteral drip is a good approach to patients who do not tolerate elemental diet alone. Elemental formulas are composed of predigested components in fixed proportions; modular formulas allow one to vary the components. Stool output and weight gain may be measured to assess the infant's response.

During the treatment, further workup, including an upper gastrointestinal series with small bowel roentgenogram, barium enema, small bowel biopsy, proctoscopy, the measurement of sweat electrolytes, and other specific tests to rule out the entities noted below, should be carried out as indicated. If disaccharidase levels are abnormal on small bowel biopsy, disaccharides should be avoided.

Malabsorption syndromes. Infants and children who have malabsorption syndromes typically have diarrhea, steatorrhea, growth failure, or a combination of these. Cystic fibrosis (see Chapter 36, Cystic Fibrosis) is the most common chronic disease that causes malabsorption in children in the United States. Steatorrhea results from pancreatic insufficiency and secondary maldigestion. Infants who have cystic fibrosis who nurse or are fed soy formula (but not cow milk formula) may present in the first months of life with protein malabsorption.

Although cystic fibrosis is thought of primarily as a respiratory disease, some infants and children have malabsorption and little history of respiratory symptoms; these patients typically have voracious appetites. The diagnosis must be confirmed by sweat electrolyte studies or genetic testing. Other diseases much less common than cystic fibrosis may be associated with prominent steatorrhea in early infancy, including congenital pancreatic insufficiency with cyclic neutropenia (Shwachman-Diamond syndrome),[38] intestinal lymphangiectasia, and abetalipoproteinemia. Transient steatorrhea may follow an acute enteritis.[29] Measurement of serum trypsinogen is a useful screening test for pancreatic insufficiency. Values are low in Shwachman-Diamond syndrome but may be high, normal, or low in cystic fibrosis, depending on the stage of the pancreatic disease.

In infancy, the age at which celiac disease (gluten-sensitive enteropathy) becomes apparent varies with the age of dietary introduction of gluten-containing products (wheat, rye, and barley). Usually the onset ranges from 1 month to several months later following their introduction (see Chapter 209, Gastrointestinal Allergy).[28,39] Infants who have celiac disease typically are irritable and have loose stools, a poor appetite, and poor weight gain. They also may have recurrent vomiting. The presentation, however, is quite variable. Steatorrhea often is not present, and results of absorptive studies such as the D-xylose tolerance test may be normal. Gluten-free dietary trials and antigliadin antibody studies may be misleading. The presence of endomysial IgA antibody in the serum is a much more reliable predictor of celiac disease and is useful in evaluating compliance with diet.[12,52] Tissue transglutaminase has been identified as the antigen recognized by endomysial antibody; assays for antibody recognizing this antigen are likely to replace the more cumbersome measurement of endomysial antibody.[15,55] In IgA-deficient individuals, the absence of these serum antibodies does not rule out celiac disease.

A diagnosis of celiac disease should be confirmed by small bowel biopsy. A later challenge with gluten and a repeat biopsy has been done in the past to confirm the diagnosis; however, with the advent of the current antibody studies, this may no longer be necessary. *Giardia* infection can produce small bowel malabsorption that mimics celiac disease.

Carbohydrate (monosaccharide or disaccharide) intolerance may be primary or more commonly secondary to other gastrointestinal disorders.[60] The congenital form of lactase deficiency is much less common than congenital sucrase-isomaltase deficiency.[59] The latter disorder typically appears after introduction of sucrose into the diet in solids. In carbohydrate intolerance the extent of symptoms varies directly with the quantity of the offending sugar in the diet. Similarly, the age at presentation varies with the age at which the sugar is introduced into the diet. Infants who have congenital sucrase-isomaltase deficiency may present with diarrhea when fed formula containing glucose polymers.[42] The diagnosis may be established by conducting standard sugar tolerance tests, measuring hydrogen excretion in the breath, or assaying the enzymes present in tissue obtained by a small bowel biopsy. Examination of the stool for reducing sugars is an imprecise screening test for stool carbohydrate content.[3] Sorbitol,[25] an artificial sweetener, as well as fructose,[50] may produce diarrhea when ingested in large amounts, and both are present in fruits.

The congenital deficiency of trypsinogen, the zymogen precursor of the pancreatic protease trypsin, has been reported to be a very rare cause of congenital diarrhea. The absence of trypsin in the stool suggests the diagnosis (in the absence of cystic fibrosis and congenital pancreatic insufficiency), but evaluation of the pancreatic proteases in the duodenal aspirate is necessary to confirm this impression. Congenital deficiency of enterokinase, the intestinal enzyme that activates trypsinogen to trypsin, appears in a similar fashion to that of congenital trypsinogen deficiency and is reversed with very small amounts of pancreatic replacement.

Infection. Acute bacterial or viral enteritis may be an important initiator of protracted diarrhea in infancy.[40,66] If the initial infection is no longer present at the time of evaluation for chronic diarrhea, this association will be difficult to prove. Infections at distant sites, especially urinary tract infections, also have been incriminated as a cause of chronic diarrhea in infancy. A urinalysis and urine culture should be obtained routinely in the evaluation of children who have chronic diarrhea. *Salmonella* enteritis commonly is associated with a chronic asymptomatic carrier state, especially in infancy. *Salmonella* infection, however, also may be associated with persistent diarrhea in infants. *Yersinia enterocolitica* enteritis has been associated with a chronic relapsing diarrhea. *Yersinia* organisms do not appear to be common pathogens in the United States; however, one must be sure that the microbiology laboratory specifically looks for this organism or it will be missed. *Campylobacter* enteritis also may have a protracted course. Persistence of rotavirus excretion has been identified in immunocompromised individuals but also rarely in immunocompetent children after severe gastroenteritis.[51] *Candida* has been described as a rare cause of persistent diarrhea in immunocompetent individuals.[30] However, the incidental finding of *Candida* is so common that one must be cautious before identifying it as the cause of diarrhea. A dramatic response to treatment for *Candida* would support this diagnosis.

Parasites. The principal parasite causing diarrhea in the United States is *Giardia lamblia*. It may be associated with watery diarrhea and crampy abdominal pain and may manifest in epidemic form. This protozoon may be difficult to detect in stools; the best yield of organisms comes from a duodenal fluid aspirate or a small bowel biopsy. Recent serological tests and stool antigen studies for *Giardia* appear to be very promising. Diarrhea secondary to *Cryptosporidium* occurs in immunocompetent individuals.[48,65] *Cyclospora* has been introduced into the United States on contaminated fruits. *Blastocystis hominis* and *Dientamoeba fragilis* may cause persistent diarrhea. Amebic dysentery may be indistinguishable from the colitis of inflammatory bowel disease and must be ruled out along with bacterial colitis before a diagnosis of inflammatory bowel disease can be made.

Hirschsprung's disease. This congenital abnormality involving the submucosal and myenteric plexuses of the colon (rarely involving the small intestine) accounts for about 25% of intestinal obstructions in newborns. Such neonates almost invariably fail to pass meconium early and have persistent obstipation and recurrent abdominal distention. These features may be overlooked, however, and the infants subsequently may have chronic diarrhea. The diarrhea is secondary to enterocolitis, which can be a surgical emergency that demands rapid diagnosis and treatment. A barium enema in the neonate may reveal false negative findings; anorectal manometric examination may be helpful, but an adequate rectal biopsy specimen showing absence of ganglion cells will confirm the diagnosis. Properly performed, suction biopsy of the rectum is highly reliable.[4]

Food intolerance. Dietary protein intolerance occurs in as many as 6% of children during the first 3 years of life and most commonly is a hypersensitivity to cow milk protein. In 85% of children who have dietary protein intolerance, the symptoms resolve by 3 years of age.[7] This entity should be considered when an infant who has chronic diarrhea has any of the following manifestations: occult or gross blood in the stool (colitis), protein-losing enteropathy, peripheral eosinophilia, or other extraintestinal manifestations of allergy such as eczema, hives, or asthma.[43] Continued manifestations when the infant is fed a soy formula diet (free of cow milk) do not rule out the diagnosis, inasmuch as more than 30% of children who have cow milk protein intolerance also will be intolerant to soy protein. Typically, symptoms improve when the feeding is changed to a protein hydrolysate formula, although the response to specific protein hydrolysate formulas may not be equivalent, and rarely an amino acid formula may be necessary.[62] Bloody diarrhea develops in some infants while nursing, which then resolves when they are given a protein hydrolysate formula, suggesting an allergic basis.[35] Some but not most infants respond to the reinstitution of nursing with the removal of dairy products from the mother's diet. Eosinophilic gastroenteritis may have an allergic component.

Short bowel syndrome. This syndrome of chronic malabsorption and diarrhea follows extensive resection of the small intestine.[23] Short bowel syndrome begins most commonly in the newborn period in association with necrotizing enterocolitis or a congenital anomaly of the small intestine (e.g., gastroschisis, intestinal atresia, or malrotation with secondary midgut volvulus). Recovery may be prolonged, requiring the use of TPN for the first several years of life. The factors that appear to contribute to persistence of symptoms include a decrease in intestinal absorptive surface, altered intestinal motility, intraluminal bacterial overgrowth[31] (with secondary deconjugation of bile salts and hydroxylation of fatty acids), malabsorption of bile salts secondary to terminal ileal resection, and disaccharidase deficiency. Symptoms of colitis often are noted during the initiation of enteral feedings.[58]

Intestinal lymphangiectasia. This syndrome of dilated intestinal lymphatic vessels is associated with protein-losing enteropathy, steatorrhea, lymphocytopenia, and chronic diarrhea. As a result of the bowel protein loss, affected children may have hypogammaglobulinemia and hypoalbuminemia, usually with peripheral edema. Primary intestinal lymphangiectasia appears to be a developmental anomaly of unknown origin and frequently is associated with lymphatic abnormalities of the extremities. Secondary lymphangiectasia may result from chronic volvulus secondary to malrotation with malfixation of the bowel, constrictive pericarditis, tumor, malformation, or any other factor that leads to obstruction of intestinal lymphatic flow. The diagnosis is suggested by a history of chronic diarrhea and poor growth and the presence of peripheral edema, hypoalbuminemia, hypogammaglobulinemia, and lymphocytopenia. The latter two abnormalities may lead to a decreased immune defense and an increased risk for infections.

A radiological small bowel follow-through study may show generalized thickening of the intestinal folds. The diagnosis is confirmed by the presence of characteristically dilated lymphatics on a small bowel biopsy specimen. The treatment includes the dietary use of medium-chain triglycerides and avoidance of long-chain fat. Protection from and early treatment of infection also are important.

Acrodermatitis enteropathica. This rare familial disease of poorly understood etiology often appears when breast-fed infants are weaned. Typically the infant has chronic diarrhea, intermittent vomiting, and an intractable erythematous, raw, crusty rash, which is most prominent in the perianal and perioral regions but may be seen on the extremities. Alopecia characteristically is present, and conjunctivitis and dystrophic changes of the nails may occur. Infants who have acrodermatitis enteropathica usually are irritable and unhappy. The disorder is associated with a zinc deficiency (perhaps secondary to malabsorption) and responds dramatically to zinc salts given orally.[41] Nutritional zinc deficiency (e.g., total parenteral nutrition without zinc supplementation or cystic fibrosis) may produce a syndrome similar to acrodermatitis enteropathica.

Factitious diarrhea. Factitious diarrhea undoubtedly is more common than pediatricians recognize. It is reasonable to screen a stool specimen for laxative abuse when an infant has persistent diarrhea that does not seem to fit any known pattern. Surreptitious administration of laxative to an infant is a symptom of the caretaker's psychosocial dysfunction; problems in other areas often become apparent during the social history. Frequently a parent is a medically knowledgeable person (e.g., nurse or laboratory technician) and often seems to prefer staying in the hospital to being at home. These parents usually are very helpful to the nursing staff, often to the degree of excessive involvement in the nursing care, and commonly are described by the nurses as caring and concerned parents. The pediatrician may note that the parent seems to encourage invasive diagnostic studies and treatment even beyond the medical plan and does not show an appropriate degree of hesitancy. Another form of factitious diarrhea occurs among teenage girls who take laxatives surreptitiously to lose weight.

Hormone-related diarrhea. Adrenal insufficiency secondary to either adrenogenital syndrome or adrenal hemorrhage may be associated with significant diarrhea, as may congenital thyrotoxicosis. Vasoactive intestinal polypeptide (VIP)–secreting tumors of the pancreas have been reported as a rare cause of diarrhea in adults and an even rarer cause in children.

Ganglioneuroma, as well as the more malignant ganglioneuroblastoma, has been associated with chronic secretory diarrhea. The tumors usually are abdominal but also have been reported in the mediastinum. Although these are catecholamine-secreting tumors, prostaglandins or VIP may be the mediator of the diarrhea. A workup of the infant who has persistent, undiagnosed, secretory diarrhea should include urinary catecholamine studies, prostaglandin and VIP levels, and CT scans of chest and abdomen. Even when the findings of these studies are negative, one must strongly consider arteriographic examination or surgical exploration if a severe secretory diarrhea persists. When a tumor is found and is completely excised, the diarrhea usually resolves abruptly.

Immune disorders. Immunodeficiency should be considered in any child who has chronic diarrhea. AIDS has become a major cause of immunodeficiency in childhood, and its first manifestation may be diarrhea. The two major inborn disorders associated with diarrhea in early infancy are severe combined immunodeficiency (SCID) and Wiskott-Aldrich syndrome. The most common primary disorder seen in later childhood is late-onset, variable hypogammaglobulinemia. Pure T-cell abnormalities (DiGeorge syndrome and other T-cell deficiencies) also are associated with diarrhea. The incidence of celiac disease is increased among persons who have selected IgA deficiency; therefore, measurement of immunoglobulin levels should be a routine part of the workup of any patient who has chronic diarrhea. If the diagnosis remains unclear, a T-cell evaluation should be carried out. Chronic parasitic or rotavirus infection can be seen with immunodeficiencies. Diarrhea in association with granulomas of the intestinal tract has been noted in chronic granulomatous disease of childhood. These children may have perianal fistulas or gastric outlet obstruction; the disorder initially may be mistaken for Crohn's disease.

A number of mechanisms of diarrhea have been described in infants and children who have AIDS.[63] In addition to the organisms one usually considers in individuals who have persistent diarrhea (especially *Giardia*), one must consider cytomegalovirus, *Mycobacterium avium-intracellulare, Cryptosporidium parvum, Isospora belli,* and *Enterocytozoon bieneusi.* Astrovirus, calicivirus, and adenovirus have been associated with diarrhea in HIV-infected individuals and may be more important than rotavirus as agents of AIDS diarrhea.[24] HIV may be a primary pathogen in the bowel of these patients as well. Lactose intolerance occurs commonly in individuals who have AIDS, presumably occurring secondary to injury to small bowel mucosa. Pancreatic insufficiency with steatorrhea also has been noted in these patients.

One must consider the full range of enteric infections associated with immunosuppression in children who have received organ transplants. Diarrhea also may be the presentation of tacrolimus toxicity or of lymphoproliferative disease.

Autoimmune enteropathy. Autoimmune enteropathy is a poorly understood disorder, with inflammatory small bowel mucosal damage leading to chronic diarrhea and failure to thrive. Serum antienterocyte antibodies are identified in at least 50% of these patients. Extraintestinal autoimmune disorders (e.g., diabetes mellitus, arthritis, thrombocytopenia, or hemolytic anemia) are common. Celiac disease, food allergy, and gastrointestinal infection must be ruled out. Treatment includes immunosuppressive therapy.[8]

Idiopathic intestinal pseudoobstruction. Idiopathic intestinal pseudoobstruction constitutes a group of rare disorders characterized by widespread gastrointestinal dysmotility. When this syndrome occurs in early infancy, vomiting and diarrhea often are major components. Diarrhea may alternate with constipation. In older children the presentation frequently is more insidious; a long history of constipation may precede the onset of diarrhea. Persons who have this syndrome usually have intermittent or constant abdominal distention. The syndrome is characterized by the roentgenographic findings of bowel dilation with disordered motility; urinary bladder dysfunction also often is present. These disorders can be sporadic or transmitted in an autosomal dominant fashion. They can result from a visceral myopathy or neuropathy or from a combination of both. Bacterial overgrowth is an important cause of diarrhea in this disorder.

Microvillus inclusion disease. Microvillus inclusion disease (familial enteropathy) is a disorder that occurs at birth and causes severe intractable secretory diarrhea with malabsorption.[14] These infants have small bowel villous atrophy and crypt hypoplasia. The villous surface epithelial cells lack a normal brush border, and on electron microscopic examination the microvilli are absent or severely abnormal. These defective cells contain intracytoplasmic inclusions, which in turn contain the components of the brush border, suggesting that the cells are either unable to assemble normal brush borders or that they rapidly dismantle them. A number of families reportedly have more than one child having this disorder. Microvillus inclusion disease, although rare, perhaps is the most common cause of intractable diarrhea in the newborn.

Tufting enteropathy. This disorder presents in the first few weeks of life with watery diarrhea. In contrast to microvillus inclusion disease, symptoms do not present at birth. The name derives from a typical light microscopic "tufted" configuration of the small bowel mucosal epithelium.[47]

Congenital disorders of electrolyte absorption. Congenital chloride-losing diarrhea is a very rare, familial disorder associated with maternal polyhydramnios. These infants have persistent diarrhea resulting from congenital absence of the normal ileal mechanism for active absorption of chloride in exchange for bicarbonate but histologically normal mucosa. They have a chronic metabolic alkalosis instead of the metabolic acidosis usually seen in chronic diarrhea. Stool chloride concentration is high, usually exceeding the sum of concentrations of Na and K. The stool chloride of children who have this disorder may be in the range of 100 to 150 mEq/L, although in infants it may be 30 to 100 mEq/L (normally adult stool chloride is less than 20 mEq/L). Although no satisfactory treatment exists, support with oral fluids and potassium chloride is recommended.

Congenital sodium diarrhea also is a rare cause of watery diarrhea from birth with histologically normal mucosa. However, these infants are acidotic, and stool chloride concentration is not excessive. The disorder is the result of defective mucosal Na^+/H^+ exchange in small and large bowel.

Infant of a drug-addicted mother. The syndrome of neonatal drug abstinence syndrome has become a more common problem, especially in urban areas. Diarrhea may be a prominent manifestation, and this diagnosis should be entertained in newborns who have persistent diarrhea, especially when other symptoms of neonatal drug withdrawal are present (see Chapter 50, Prenatal Drug Abuse and Neonatal Drug Withdrawal Syndrome).

Older Children

A pediatrician will see fewer older children who have chronic diarrhea than infants, but older children are more likely to have chronic diarrhea associated with significant underlying disease (compared with toddler's diarrhea in young children). As in infancy, the association of poor growth, weight loss, or other systemic manifestations suggests a serious organic cause. Older children commonly tend to deny symptoms, and the true impact of the disorder may not be apparent except in retrospect after initiation of appropriate treatment. Subtle changes in personality, sense of well-being, and appetite, as well as other systemic clues, should be sought. Children may hesitate to talk about their stooling pattern, and the degree of deviation from the norm may become apparent only after improvement occurs.

The etiological focus differs somewhat after infancy. Many of the causes seen in infancy, even congenital anomalies, may manifest first in childhood and therefore must still be considered. Factors that determine the age at diagnosis include (1) variability of presentation of signs and symptoms, (2) parental expectations of normality, and (3) the index of suspicion of the physician consulted. However, certain diseases, including inflammatory bowel disease and chronic constipation with encopresis, are much more likely to be seen in childhood than in infancy. Symptoms of celiac disease may begin at any age. Cystic fibrosis may be associated with only mild manifestations in infancy and may be overlooked until frequent, bulky, foul-smelling stools become intolerable at home. AIDS is seen in older children as well as in infants.

Irritable bowel. Irritable bowel similar to that occurring in adults may be seen in children and adolescents.[16] Stools may alternate from diarrhea to constipation. In addition, the patient may have recurrent, crampy, abdominal pain. It is important to rule out late-onset lactose intolerance and fructose or sorbitol ingestion as causes of symptoms that may mimic irritable bowel.[25,50]

Inflammatory bowel disease (IBD). The manifestations and presentation of both Crohn's disease and ulcerative colitis are so variable that this group of diseases must be thought of and ruled out whenever one sees an older child who has chronic diarrhea. Systemic evidence of inflammation (fever, weight loss, and leukocytosis), abdominal pain, blood in the stool (gross or occult), perianal disease, anemia, or extraintestinal manifestations (arthralgia, arthritis, or erythema nodosum) are helpful in making a diagnosis. Growth failure can occur with or precede other symptoms. An elevated sedimentation rate also is a clue; however, normal sedimentation rates may occur in as many as 50% of patients who have IBD. Thrombocytosis has been associated with IBD and may be present in the absence of an elevated sedimentation rate. Suggestive signs and symptoms require evaluation, including a complete blood count, platelet count, erythrocyte sedimentation rate, serum protein levels, roentgenographic contrast studies of the upper bowel (including good views of the terminal ileum), and colonoscopic examination with biopsy. Newer antibody screening studies may be helpful in confirming an uncertain diagnosis of Crohn's disease or ulcerative colitis. Management of inflammatory bowel disease includes an array of medical, nutritional, and surgical measures.[45]

Chronic constipation. Occasionally, chronic constipation with overflow incontinence is mistaken for diarrhea. A thorough history and physical examination, including a rectal examination, should make the diagnosis apparent. If one goes back in the history, it often is found that the problem began with constipation. A large amount of stool may be palpable in the abdomen, but a hard mass of stool usually is found in the rectal ampulla. This presentation is treated in the usual fashion of chronic constipation (as noted in Chapter 121, Constipation).

When to Refer

- Persistent diarrhea when the workup for routine infectious causes is negative
- Steatorrhea
- Diarrhea and/or steatorrhea causing failure to thrive

When to Hospitalize

- Acute or chronic diarrhea with mild dehydration that cannot be managed successfully with outpatient rehydration solution
- Dehydration of at least 10% of body weight
- Diarrhea with intractable vomiting
- Severe electrolyte imbalance, including hypernatremic dehydration or serum potassium level less than 3.0 mEq/L
- Laboratory evidence of hemolytic-uremic syndrome
- Chronic diarrhea and/or steatorrhea with persistent malnutrition

REFERENCES

1. Allos BM: Association between *Campylobacter* infection and Guillain-Barré syndrome, *J Infect Dis* 176:S125, 1997.
2. Alpert G, et al: Outbreak of cryptosporidiosis in a day-care center, *Pediatrics* 77:152, 1986.
3. Ameen VZ, Powell GK, Jones LA: Quantitation of fecal carbohydrate excretion in patients with short bowel syndrome, *Gastroenterology* 92:493, 1987.
4. Andrassy RJ, Isaacs H, Weitzman JJ: Rectal suction biopsy for the diagnosis of Hirschsprung disease, *Ann Surg* 193:419, 1981.
5. Bartlett AV, Reves RR, Pickering LK: Rotavirus in infant-toddler day care centers: epidemiology relevant to disease control strategies, *J Pediatr* 113:435, 1988.
6. Bartlett AV, et al: Diarrheal illness among infants and toddlers in day care centers. I. Epidemiology and pathogens, *J Pediatr* 107:495, 1985.
7. Bock SA: Prospective appraisal of complaints of adverse reactions to foods in children during the first 3 years of life, *Pediatrics* 79:683, 1987.
8. Bousvaros A, et al: Treatment of pediatric autoimmune enteropathy with tacrolimus (FK506), *Gastroenterology* 111:237, 1996.
9. Branski D, et al: Chronic diarrhea and malabsorption, *Pediatr Clin North Am* 43:307, 1996.
10. Buts JP, et al: Pseudomembranous enterocolitis in childhood, *Gastroenterology* 73:823, 1977.
11. CDC: Incidence of foodborne illnesses: preliminary data from the foodborne diseases active surveillance network (FoodNet)—United States 1998, *MMWR* 48:189, 1999.
12. Chan KN, et al: Endomysial antibody screening in children, *J Pediatr Gastroenterol Nutr* 18:316, 1994.
13. Cohen SA, et al: Chronic nonspecific diarrhea: dietary relationships, *Pediatrics* 64:402, 1979.
14. Cutz E, et al: Microvillus inclusion disease: an inherited defect of brush-border assembly and differentiation, *N Engl J Med* 320:646, 1989.
15. Dieterich W, et al: Autoantibodies to tissue transglutaminase as predictors of celiac disease, *Gastroenterology* 115:1317, 1998.
16. Drossman DA, Whitehead WE, Camilleri M: Irritable bowel syndrome: a technical review for practice guideline development, *Gastroenterology* 112:2120, 1997.
17. Duggan C, Nurko S: "Feeding the gut": the scientific basis for continued enteral nutrition during acute diarrhea, *J Pediatr* 131:801, 1997.

18. DuPont HL: Prevention of diarrhea by the probiotic, *Lactobacillus* GG, *J Pediatr* 134:1, 1999.
19. Eherer AJ, Fordtran JS: Fecal osmotic gap and pH in experimental diarrhea of various causes, *Gastroenterology* 103:545, 1992.
20. Figueroa-Quintanilla D, et al: A controlled trial of bismuth subsalicylate in infants with acute watery diarrheal disease, *N Engl J Med* 328:1653, 1993.
21. Glass RI, et al: Estimates of morbidity and mortality rates for diarrheal diseases in American children, *J Pediatr* 118:S27, 1991.
22. Goldgar CM, Vanderhoof JA: Lack of correlation of small bowel biopsy and clinical course of patients with intractable diarrhea of infancy, *Gastroenterology* 90:527, 1986.
23. Goulet OJ, et al: Neonatal short bowel syndrome, *J Pediatr* 119:18, 1991.
24. Grohmann GS, et al: Enteric viruses and diarrhea in HIV-infected patients, *N Engl J Med* 329:14, 1993.
25. Hyams JS: Sorbitol malabsorption: an unappreciated cause of functional gastrointestinal complaints, *Gastroenterology* 84:30, 1983.
26. Infectious Diseases Committee, Canadian Paediatric Society: *Escherichia coli* gastroenteritis: making sense of the new acronyms, *Can Med Assoc J* 136:241, 1987.
27. Izraeli S, et al: Transient renal acidification defect during acute infantile diarrhea: the role of urinary sodium, *J Pediatr* 117:711, 1990.
28. Janatuinen EK, Pikkarainen PH, Kemppainen TA: A comparison of diets with and without oats in adults with celiac disease, *N Engl J Med* 333:1033, 1995.
29. Jonas A, et al: Disturbed fat absorption following infectious gastroenteritis in children, *J Pediatr* 95:366, 1979.
30. Kane JG, Chretien JH, Garagusi VF: Diarrhea caused by *Candida, Lancet* 1:335, 1976.
31. Kaufman SS, et al: Influence of bacterial overgrowth and intestinal inflammation on duration of parenteral nutrition in children with short bowel syndrome, *J Pediatr* 131:356, 1997.
32. Kerzner B, et al: Transmissible gastroenteritis: sodium transport and the intestinal epithelium during the course of viral enteritis, *Gastroenterology* 72:457, 1977.
33. Kirschner BS: Inflammatory bowel disease in children, *Pediatr Clin North Am* 35:189, 1988.
34. Klish WJ, et al: Modular formula: an approach to management of infants with specific or complex food intolerances, *J Pediatr* 88:948, 1976.
35. Lake AM, Whitington PF, Hamilton SR: Dietary protein-induced colitis in breast-fed infants, *J Pediatr* 101:906, 1982.
36. Larcher VF, et al: Protracted diarrhea in infancy, *Arch Dis Child* 52:597, 1977.
37. Lifshitz F, et al: Role of juice carbohydrate malabsorption in chronic nonspecific diarrhea in children, *J Pediatr* 120:825, 1992.
38. Mack DR, et al: Shwachman syndrome: exocrine pancreatic dysfunction and variable phenotypic expression, *Gastroenterology* 111:1593, 1996.
39. Mäki M, Collin P: Coeliac disease, *Lancet* 349:1755, 1997.
40. Mitchel DK, et al: Outbreaks of astrovirus gastroenteritis in day care center, *J Pediatr* 123:725, 1993.
41. Neldner KH, Hambridge KM: Zinc therapy of acrodermatitis enteropathica, *N Engl J Med* 292:879, 1975.
42. Newton T, et al: Glucose polymer as a cause of protracted diarrhea in infants with unsuspected congenital sucrase-isomaltase deficiency, *J Pediatr* 128:753, 1996.
43. Odze RD, et al: Allergic colitis in infants, *J Pediatr* 126:163, 1995.
44. Oelkers P, et al: Primary bile acid malabsorption caused by mutations in the ileal sodium-dependent bile acid transporter gene (SLC10A2), *J Clin Invest* 99:1880, 1997.
45. Oliva MM, Lake AM: Nutritional considerations and management of the child with inflammatory bowel disease, *Nutrition* 12:151, 1996.
46. Orenstein SR: Enteral versus parenteral therapy for intractable diarrhea of infancy: prospective, randomized trial, *J Pediatr* 109:277, 1986.
47. Patey N, et al: Distribution of cell adhesion molecules in infants with intestinal epithelial dysplasia (tufting enteropathy), *Gastroenterology* 113:833, 1997.
48. Phillips AD, Thomas AG, Walker-Smith JA: Cryptosporidium, chronic diarrhoea and the proximal small intestinal mucosa, *Gut* 33:1057, 1992.
49. Phillips SF: Diarrhea: a current view of the pathophysiology, *Gastroenterology* 63:495, 1972.
50. Riby JE, Fujisawa T, Kretchmer N: Fructose absorption, *Am J Clin Nutr* 58:748S, 1993.
51. Richardson S, et al: Extended excretion of rotavirus after severe diarrhoea in young children, *Lancet* 351:1844, 1998.
52. Rossi TM, Albini CH, Kumar V: Incidence of celiac disease identified by the presence of serum endomysial antibodies in children with chronic diarrhea, short stature, or insulin-dependent diabetes mellitus, *J Pediatr* 123:262, 1993.
53. Santosham M, et al: Oral rehydration therapy of infantile diarrhea: a controlled study of well-nourished children hospitalized in the United States and Panama, *N Engl J Med* 306:1070, 1982.
54. Schwarz RP, Ulshen MH: Pseudomembranous colitis presenting as mild, chronic diarrhea in childhood, *J Pediatr Gastroenterol Nutr* 2:570, 1983.
55. Sulkanen S, et al: Tissue transglutaminase autoantibody enzyme-linked immunosorbent assay in detecting celiac disease, *Gastroenterology* 115: 1322, 1998.
56. Sutphen JL, et al: Chronic diarrhea associated with *Clostridium difficile* in children, *Am J Dis Child* 137:275, 1983.
57. Tamer AM, et al: Oral rehydration of infants in a large urban U.S. medical center, *J Pediatr* 107:14, 1985.
58. Taylor SF, et al: Noninfectious colitis associated with short gut syndrome in infants, *J Pediatr* 119:24, 1991.
59. Treem WR: Congenital sucrase-isomaltase deficiency, *J Pediatr Gastroenterol Nutr* 21:1, 1995.
60. Ulshen MH: Carbohydrate absorption and malabsorption. In Walker WA, Watkins JB, editors: *Nutrition in pediatrics: basic science and clinical applications,* Hamilton, 1997, BC Decker, Inc.
61. Ulshen MH, Rollo RL: Pathogenesis of *Escherichia coli* gastroenteritis in man—another mechanism, *N Engl J Med* 302:99, 1980.
62. Vanderhoof JA, et al: Intolerance to protein hydrolysate infant formulas: an underrecognized cause of gastrointestinal symptoms in infants, *J Pediatr* 131:741, 1997.
63. Winter H, Chang TI: Gastrointestinal and nutritional problems in children with immunodeficiency and AIDS, *Pediatr Clin North Am* 43:573, 1996.
64. Wolfe DC, Giannella RA: Antibiotic therapy for bacterial enterocolitis: a comprehensive review, *Am J Gastroenterol* 88:1667, 1993.
65. Wolfen JS, et al: Cryptosporidiosis in immuno-competent patients, *N Engl J Med* 312:1278, 1985.
66. Yolken RH, et al: Gastroenteritis associated with enteric type adenovirus in hospitalized infants, *J Pediatr* 101:21, 1982.

SUGGESTED READINGS

Bishop WP, Ulshen MH: Bacterial gastroenteritis, *Pediatr Clin North Am* 35:69, 1988.

Branski D, Lerner A, Lebenthal E: Chronic diarrhea and malabsorption, *Pediatr Clin of NA* 43:307, 1996.

CDC: Incidence of foodborne illnesses: preliminary data from the foodborne diseases active surveillance network (FoodNet)—United States 1998, *MMWR* 48:189, 1999.

Di Lorenzo, C: Pseudo-obstruction: current approaches, *Gastroenterology* 116:980, 1999.

Esteban MM: Adverse reactions to foods in infancy and childhood, *J Pediatr* 121:S1, 1992.

Lifshitz F: Management of acute diarrheal disease, *J Pediatr* 118:S25, 1991.

Practice parameter: the management of acute gastroenteritis in young children, *Pediatrics* 97:424, 1996.

Sampson HA: Food allergy, *JAMA* 278:1888, 1997.

Targan SR, Shanahan F, editors: *Inflammatory bowel disease: from bench to bedside,* Baltimore, 1994, Williams & Wilkins.

125 Dizziness and Vertigo

Jane A. Curtis

Dizziness and vertigo, although often confused and placed together, are very different symptoms that have very different clinical implications. It may be especially difficult to distinguish them in young children because much of the distinction depends on the patient's account of his or her history.

Dizziness is "an imprecise term commonly used by patients in an attempt to describe various peculiar subjective symptoms such as faintness, giddiness, light-headedness, or unsteadiness."[4] Patients who have simple dizziness do not describe the room spinning around them, and they do not have nystagmus. Dizziness is a relatively common symptom in childhood and in adolescents. One large cross-sectional study of adolescents found that 8% of girls and 5% of boys reported frequent or rather frequent occurrence of dizziness in the 6 months prior to the study.[3]

Dizziness commonly is seen as a symptom of presyncope in children or adolescents who have fever, dehydration, orthostatic hypotension, and vasovagal syncope. It can also be seen with anemia. Dizziness often is felt as a symptom of anxiety and as part of panic attacks. The diagnostic approach to dizziness takes these differential diagnoses into account. A clear history of when the dizziness occurred (on rising from bed, after vomiting, when stressed in class, in a hot, crowded place); an exploration of recent life stressors (parental discord, school problems, abuse problems with friends/romantic partners); and questioning about concurrent symptoms of panic attacks such as rapid heart rate, feelings of intense anxiety and impending doom, and trouble breathing should all be sought. On physical examination the physician should document orthostatic vital signs, look for evidence of anemia or dehydration, and pay particular attention to cardiac and neurological findings. Most episodes of dizziness can be diagnosed simply on history and physical examination. However, if actual fainting has occurred, an electrocardiogram (ECG) may be warranted (see Chapter 174, Syncope). In adolescent girls who have a suggestive history or physical examination, a hematocrit may be appropriate.

For patients who have presyncopal or orthostatic dizziness, reassurance and instructions about adequate hydration, care when arising suddenly, and the necessity of putting the head lower than the heart when symptoms occur generally suffice for patient management. For patients in whom dizziness is part of a panic attack or a marker of significant stress, further history should be obtained, including any suicidal ideation, and referral for counseling considered.

When young children cannot describe dizziness or vertigo, observers tend to apply these terms to a child who is unsteady on his or her feet. Disequilibrium in this age group may reflect acute cerebellar problems, such as postviral acute cerebellar ataxia and posterior fossa tumors, and referral for neurological evaluation and CNS imaging should be considered. Another common cause of disequilibrium in young children is middle ear disease. One study found that 60% of children who had chronic middle ear effusions had evidence of balance disturbance on a motor proficiency test.[2] These findings resolved after the placement of ventilating tubes. The clinical significance of these findings is unclear, because most patients can adapt to bilateral vestibular dysfunction quite quickly by using visual and other cues. Some experts suggest testing balance while the patient is blindfolded to unmask vestibular dysfunction.[1]

Vertigo is "a sensation of spinning or whirling motion. Vertigo implies a definite sensation of rotation of the subject or of objects about the subject in any plane."[4] True vertigo almost always is accompanied by nystagmus, at least at the time of the episode.[5] Thus, ask observers about the presence of nystagmus and ask them to watch for it in future episodes. The differential diagnosis of vertigo depends on three elements in the history: whether the vertigo is acute or chronic, whether episodes are recurrent, and whether it is accompanied by hearing loss. Acute episodic vertigo is the most common type encountered by pediatricians, usually not accompanied by hearing loss.

The most common causes of acute episodic vertigo are migraine headaches and related syndromes. In children younger than 4 years of age, this is manifested as benign paroxysmal vertigo of childhood. These children have the sudden onset of extreme unsteadiness and inability to stand, usually with nystagmus and sometimes with vomiting. The episodes last seconds to minutes. Often the family has a history of migraine headaches, and many of these patients develop migraine headaches in later life. Older children and adolescents may have episodic vertigo as a result of basilar artery migraines. These patients often have scintillating scotomas or visual obscuration, oral paresthesias, tinnitus, and occasionally "drop attacks" with or without loss of consciousness. This commonly but not always is followed by a pounding headache. Treatments are those used for migraines (see Chapter 140, Headache).

Vertigo associated with hearing loss in childhood is usually associated with severe otitis media leading to labyrinthitis. These patients are acutely uncomfortable, both from ear pain and from severe vertigo, usually with nausea, vomiting, and nystagmus. Treatment includes antibiotics for the infection and dimenhydrinate for vertigo and nausea. Less common in children is Meniere's syndrome, consisting of vertigo, fluctuating hearing loss, pressure in the ear, and tinnitus.

Chronic persistent vertigo, especially if accompanied by neurological signs, is usually indicative of CNS disease, including tumors, acoustic neurinomas (seen in neurofibromatosis type II), and demyelinating and degenerative diseases. These patients require referral for neurology consultation and neuroimaging.

In the evaluation of a first episode of acute vertigo, other etiologies include ingestions or overdoses of medication, trauma leading to perilymphatic fistula or labyrinthine concussion, and a postinfectious vestibular neuronitis. In the case of a history of significant head or ear trauma (including barotrauma), referral should be made to an ear, nose, and throat specialist because prompt surgical repair of a perilymphatic fistula may lead to some improvement in hearing loss.[1] Besides a thorough history and physical examination, formal audiometry and an electronystagmogram (ENG) usually are recommended for the initial evaluation of vertigo.

Thus, although dizziness frequently can be managed by the pediatrician alone, the description of true vertigo, especially if accompanied by nystagmus, usually requires consultation with either a neurologist or an otolaryngologist.

When to Refer

1. Patients who have acute ataxia
2. Patients who have a clear history of vertigo, especially with other neurological signs or after head or barotrauma

REFERENCES

1. Eviatar L: Dizziness in children, *Otolaryngol Clin North Am* 27:557, 1994.
2. Golz A, Angel-Yeger B, Parush S: Evaluation of balance disturbances in children with middle ear effusion, *Int J Pediatr Otorhinolaryngol* 43:21, 1998.
3. Poikolainen K, Kanerva R, Lonnqvist J: Life events and other risk factors for somatic symptoms in adolescents, *Pediatrics* 96:59, 1995.
4. *Stedman's Medical Dictionary*, ed 26, Baltimore, 1995, Williams & Wilkins.
5. Tusa RJ, Saada AA, Niparko JK: Dizziness in childhood, *J Child Neurol* 9:261, 1994.

126 Dysmenorrhea

Alain Joffe

Dysmenorrhea, generally meaning painful menstruation, is a syndrome associated with varying degrees of crampy lower abdominal pain and other symptoms such as nausea, vomiting, urinary frequency, low back pain, diarrhea, fatigue, and headache. The pain may radiate to the anterior thighs. Typically the pain begins just after menses and lasts for approximately 1 to 2 days, but it also can begin before menses starts and last up to 4 days.[4] Cramps may be more severe among teenagers who smoke.[6] The majority of surveys indicate that at least 40% to 60% of adolescent girls suffer some degree of discomfort during menstruation, and many miss school as a result.[6,7] Most affected teenage girls have primary dysmenorrhea—that is, a syndrome not associated with pelvic or other body system pathological conditions; however, causes of secondary dysmenorrhea always should be considered as the patient is evaluated.

PRIMARY DYSMENORRHEA

Although psychosocial and cultural factors may play some role in the pathogenesis of primary dysmenorrhea, the preponderance of current research indicates that this symptom complex results from increased amounts of prostaglandins E_2 and $F_{2\alpha}$ in the endometrium of women who have dysmenorrhea compared with women who do not have painful menses.[8,10] Such a biological explanation correlates with the clinical observation that women who have anovulatory cycles usually do not have dysmenorrhea.

The incidence of dysmenorrhea increases with chronological and gynecological age (as does the percentage of ovulatory cycles), and the increase in prostaglandin synthesis may be related to changes in serum progesterone levels not seen in anovulatory women. Additional confirmation comes from the dramatic response women experience with use of either prostaglandin synthetase inhibitors or oral contraceptives (which inhibit ovulation). Increased levels of prostaglandin activity are associated with increased uterine tone and high amplitude myometrial contractions, both of which result in reduced uterine blood flow and pain.

A careful history usually excludes most pathological causes of dysmenorrhea. Physicians differ in their opinions regarding what examination is necessary to evaluate the patient who has dysmenorrhea. In general, for a nonsexually active teenager who has mild to moderate menstrual cramps relieved by nonsteroidal antiinflammatory drugs (NSAIDs), only an external genital examination to rule out hymenal abnormalities is indicated. Some clinicians also would initiate oral contraceptive pills without first performing a pelvic examination for a few cycles if the dysmenorrhea is unresponsive to NSAIDs. For any sexually active teenager or, in the opinion of other clinicians, for one who is having significant pain unresponsive to NSAIDs,[2] a thorough pelvic examination is necessary. If a pelvic examination is not possible, a rectoabdominal examination will provide some useful information about the presence of masses or adnexal tenderness.

Although treatment of primary dysmenorrhea is likely to include drug therapy, the physician also should determine the mother's and daughter's understanding of menstruation.[1,2] Many teenagers do not understand the physiology of menstruation fully or may have inaccurate beliefs that have been passed on from mother to daughter. Evaluation and treatment of dysmenorrhea provide the clinician a valuable opportunity to teach the patient about her body.

Although teenagers who have very mild discomfort benefit from almost any analgesic, prostaglandin synthetase inhibitors in the form of nonsteroidal antiinflammatory drugs (NSAIDs) are the treatment of choice for most young women who have dysmenorrhea.[12] Dosage, both in terms of amount and timing, varies from patient to patient. Some need medication only for part or all of the first day; others require medication for 3 days or so. Ibuprofen (200 to 800 mg every 6 to 8 hours) is highly effective for dysmenorrhea, as is naproxen sodium (550 mg immediately and then 275 mg every 6 to 8 hours). Mefenamic acid, an NSAID that blocks the effect of prostaglandin at the end-organ level as well as inhibiting its production, can be used in a dose of 500 mg administered immediately, followed by 250 mg every 6 hours. In one study, 57% of adolescents used medications less often than the maximum daily frequency; thus, it is important to advise them of the range of correct dosages.[3] These medications are most effective if started at the first sign of menstrual bleeding; women who experience significant nausea with menses may benefit from starting treatment at the earliest symptom of menses, even before bleeding occurs. If the adolescent fails to respond to one type of NSAID (e.g., ibuprofen), another (e.g., naproxen sodium) should be tried.[9]

Some patients (perhaps as many as 30%) will not respond to these measures. In these young women, a trial of oral contraceptives used in the same way as for contraception usually provides relief. Patients should be told that 2 to 3 months may elapse before contraceptives exert their maximal effect. If the patient is sexually active, oral contraceptives are continued on a routine basis; for the non–sexually active teenager, therapy can be reassessed at 6-month intervals.

The efficacy of other treatments is still unproven. Some authors believe that pelvic exercise, general exercise, biofeedback, relaxation therapy, or various herbal remedies are effective; other authorities remain skeptical of these alternatives.[5] To the extent that smoking exacerbates dysmenorrhea, it provides yet another reason for clinicians to urge their patients to stop smoking.

Women who fail to respond to any of these measures should be referred to an adolescent medicine specialist or gynecologist for evaluation; they probably have secondary rather than primary dysmenorrhea.

SECONDARY DYSMENORRHEA

Causes of secondary dysmenorrhea, such as pelvic inflammatory disease (PID) or endometriosis, or conditions arising in a variety of other organ systems, usually can be excluded by a careful history and physical examination. Organic pathology should be suspected in a young woman whose pain begins after 20 years of age, who has a history of surgery related to the genitourinary or gastrointestinal tract, or whose pain begins before menses or is dull and constant rather than crampy.

Patients who have endometriosis will have failed therapy with NSAIDs and oral contraceptives, and their pain may be acyclic rather cyclic; a family history of endometriosis often is present. Endometriosis also may be associated with dyspareunia, tenesmus, and rectal pain. Pelvic inflammatory disease can cause dysmenorrhea acutely, and women often develop chronic pelvic pain as a consequence of PID. Even with assurances of confidentiality, some young women may still not admit to sexual activity. Hence, clinicians must maintain a high index of suspicion if other historical and physical examination findings suggest this diagnosis.

Teenagers who have a history of genital tract surgery (including abortions) may have outflow tract obstruction. A variety of Müllerian anomalies with incomplete obstruction of the outflow tract also produce dysmenorrhea.[4] Depending on the type of obstruction, a pelvic mass may be palpable. Endometrial polyps or fibroids are rare in women younger than 20 years of age but should be suspected if the menstrual bleeding is heavy, prolonged, or associated with the passage of clots. Whether these entities alone cause dysmenorrhea is unclear.

A pelvic examination that reveals cervical motion tenderness, adnexal masses, or fixation of the ovaries strongly suggests PID. If the cervical os is stenotic or the cervix or uterus feels atretic or abnormally shaped, outflow obstruction is possible (e.g., a uterus with a blind horn). Among adult women, physical finding such as small fixed nodules in the rectovaginal septum or cul de sac or fixation of the uterus indicated by the sensation of pain on stretching of the uterosacral ligaments suggests endometriosis. However, most adolescents generally have normal examinations; hence, endometriosis can be extremely difficult to detect on clinical grounds alone.[11] If a secondary cause of dysmenorrhea is suspected, consultation with an adolescent medicine specialist or gynecologist is warranted. Ultrasound examination of the uterus will rule out uterine anomalies but cannot exclude endometriosis.

Confirmation of endometriosis requires laparoscopy. Because the lesions of endometriosis in adolescent may differ from the "classic" lesions seen in adults, this procedure should be performed by a gynecologist experienced in evaluation of adolescents. Endometriosis may be difficult to manage, and women who have this condition are at increased risk for infertility.

Pelvic inflammatory disease should be treated according to standard antibiotic regimens (see Chapter 262, Sexually Transmitted Diseases). Follow-up is critical because these young women are at risk for further episodes of PID as well as for chronic pelvic pain, ectopic pregnancy, and infertility.

When to Refer

The point at which a clinician chooses to refer depends on his or her experience. For dysmenorrhea, referral might be appropriate

1. If the clinician feels uncomfortable prescribing oral contraceptive pills for the treatment of primary dysmenorrhea
2. If the patient fails to respond to NSAIDs and OCPs
3. If the clinical presentation/course suggests that the patient has secondary rather than primary dysmenorrhea
4. If the patient is sexually active and the clinician feels uncomfortable performing a pelvic examination

When to Hospitalize

If the cause of the dysmenorrhea is determined to be pelvic inflammatory disease, some clinicians would recommend hospitalization of all adolescents for treatment. Others recommend hospitalization under certain but not all circumstances (see Chapter 262, Sexually Transmitted Diseases).

REFERENCES

1. Beach R: Menstrual cramps need not be a curse, *Contemp Pediatr* 6:41, 1989.
2. Blythe M, Orr D: Common menstrual problems, Part 1. Management in the pediatric practice, *Adolesc Health Update* 3:3, 1991.
3. Campbell MA, McGrath PJ: Use of medication by adolescents for the management of menstrual discomfort, *Arch Pediatr Adolesc Med* 151: 905, 1997.
4. Emans SJ, Laufer MR, Goldstein DP: *Pediatric and adolescent gynecology*, ed 4, Philadelphia, 1998, Lippincott-Raven.
5. Golumb LM, Solidum AA, Warren MP: Primary dysmenorrhea and physical activity, *Med Sci Sports Exer* 30:906, 1998.

6. Harlow SD, Park M: A longitudinal study of risk factors for the occurrence, duration and severity of menstrual cramps in a cohort of college women, *Br J Obstet Gynaecol* 103:1134, 1996.
7. Klein JF, Litt IF: Epidemiology of adolescent dysmenorrhea, *Pediatrics* 68:661, 1981.
8. Neinstein LS: *Adolescent health care: a practical guide,* ed 3, Baltimore, 1996, Williams & Wilkins.
9. Osathanondh R: Dysmenorrhea, *Curr Ther Endocrinol Metab* 6:246, 1997.
10. Pickles VR, et al: Prostaglandins in endometrium and menstrual fluid from normal and dysmenorrheic subjects, *Br J Obstet Gynaecol* 72:185, 1965.
11. Schroeder B, Sanfilippo JS: Dysmenorrhea and pelvic pain in adolescents, *Pediatr Clin North Am* 46:555, 1999.
12. Zhang WY, Li WPA: Efficacy of minor analgesics in primary dysmenorrhea: a systematic review, *Br J Obstet Gynaecol* 105:780, 1998.

127 Dysphagia

Steven L. Werlin

Dysphagia refers to the sensation that something is wrong with the swallowing mechanism. True dysphagia is never psychogenic, and every patient who has this complaint requires a thorough evaluation. Globus, or "lump in the throat," is not related to swallowing and thus is not true dysphagia. Odynophagia, pain on swallowing, does not necessarily accompany dysphagia.

Preesophageal dysphagia almost always is accompanied by a more generalized neuromuscular disease such as cerebral palsy, muscular dystrophy, myasthenia gravis, or familial dysautonomia. In these conditions dysphagia is caused by primary or secondary involvement of skeletal muscles and difficulty in initiating or coordinating a swallow.

Symptoms associated with preesophageal dysphagia include cyanosis, coughing, choking, gagging during feeding, and nasal regurgitation. When these symptoms occur after a meal, they more commonly are due to gastroesophageal reflux than to a swallowing disorder. Refusal to feed leading to failure to thrive and aspiration pneumonia may occur when these symptoms are not addressed. In spite of multiple attempts, the child may be unable to initiate swallowing.

Esophageal dysphagia is the subjective sensation that a bolus of food cannot be transported normally down the esophagus. A barium swallow test can readily distinguish between motor and mechanical obstruction. Patients who have a motor disturbance usually have dysphagia for both solids and liquids; mechanical obstruction usually is accompanied by dysphagia for solids alone. This history may be difficult to elicit for the young child; such patients may be slow or "picky" eaters, may prefer liquids, or may refuse feedings.

NORMAL SWALLOWING

Swallowing is divided into oral, pharyngeal, and esophageal phases. In the mouth the food is chewed and lubricated, and a bolus is formed. The bolus then is presented to the pharynx, which must deliver it safely to the esophagus. Numerous protective reflexes are involved in keeping the food out of the airway, including elevation of the soft palate, closure of the glottis and epiglottis, relaxation and opening of the upper esophageal sphincter, and cessation of breathing. Failure of one or more of these reflexes may result in aspiration. Although the oral phase is voluntary and may take a variable amount of time, the pharyngeal phase of swallowing is brief, occurring in less than 1 second, and automatic.

Anatomically the esophagus is divided into the upper one third, composed of striated muscle, and the distal two thirds, composed of smooth muscle. Functionally the esophagus is composed of three zones: the upper esophageal sphincter (UES), the body, and the lower esophageal sphincter (LES). The UES is composed of the cricopharyngeus muscle and requires the participation of the inferior pharyngeal constrictors and the circular muscle of the proximal esophagus to function properly; it is contracted at rest. After pharyngeal contraction, but before esophageal peristalsis, the UES relaxes, contracting again when swallowing is completed. The cricopharyngeus is contracted at rest by constant discharge of motor nerves. Each swallow is followed by a monophasic pressure wave that traverses the esophagus aborally crossing the striated and smooth muscle.[6] Approximately 90% of swallows are followed by this "primary peristalsis." "Secondary peristalsis" is not preceded by a swallow but is induced by the failure of a bolus to pass into the stomach or by reflux of gastric contents into the esophagus. The velocity of a peristaltic wave is 2.5 to 6 cm/sec.

A zone of increased LES pressure is found on withdrawal of an intraluminal catheter from the stomach into the esophagus. The LES pressure drops promptly with a swallow and remains depressed until the peristaltic wave has passed. During this period of reduced LES pressure, the pressure gradient between the stomach and esophagus remains, preventing reflux of gastric contents. On the basis of studies of adults, it appears that the LES is the major barrier against reflux of acid gastric contents into the esophagus.[6,7] Resting LES tone is maintained by a combination of neural activity and intrinsic myogenic properties of the sphincter. Release of acetylcholine from excitatory neurons plays a major role in basal LES pressure. Nitric oxide mediates the final common pathway of LES relaxation. Anticholinergic drugs and theophylline-based compounds reduce LES pressure. Atropine decreases the incidence of transient LES relaxations, which are a major component of reflux.

METHODS OF STUDY

Radiology

The barium swallow examination is the most diagnostically useful method of evaluating oral, pharyngeal, and esophageal structure and function. The use of agents of a variety of textures, fluoroscopy, and videotape recording allow for accurate study of the transport function. Aspiration can be documented, the rate of propagation of the peristaltic wave can be measured, and mechanical and functional obstruction can be observed. The barium swallow is not a reliable method for diagnosing gastroesophageal reflux.[14]

Manometry

Intraluminal esophageal manometry has taken an important place alongside the roentgenographic study of the esophagus.[6,7,17,20] With perfused catheters or solid state catheters connected via transducers to a recording device, upper and lower esophageal sphincter pressures can be measured, relaxation of the sphincters can be documented, and the rate and strength of the peristaltic wave can be determined. Sedation usually is not required except in young children. Although clinically suspected, the diagnoses of achalasia and diffuse esophageal spasm can be confirmed only by manometric evaluation. At times, esophageal manometry is required to establish the diagnosis of scleroderma. It is important to note that gastroesophageal reflux cannot be diagnosed by manometry or by the measurement of LES pressure.

Esophagoscopy

Flexible fiberoptic esophagoscopy can be performed on children on an ambulatory basis. Inspection, biopsy, and photography of suspected lesions can be performed rapidly and safely.

CAUSES AND MANAGEMENT OF DYSPHAGIA

The many causes of dysphagia are listed in Box 127-1.

BOX 127-1

CAUSES OF DYSPHAGIA

Structural-Mechanical Disorders
Congenital stricture
Esophageal atresia
Esophageal web
Foreign bodies
Hiatal hernia
Paraesophageal hernia
Peptic stricture
Tumor
Vascular ring

Motor Disorders
Achalasia
Diffuse spasm
Scleroderma
Gastroesophageal reflux

Neuromuscular Disorders
Acquired central nervous system disease (tumor, infection, trauma)
Cerebral palsy
Dysautonomia
Muscular dystrophy
Myasthenia gravis

Inflammatory Disorders
Caustic ingestion
Epidermolysis bullosa
Esophagitis
- Gastroesophageal reflux
- *Candida albicans*
- Cytomegalovirus
- Herpes simplex

Oral-Pharyngeal Dysphagia

Dysphagia in children most commonly is secondary to central nervous system injury or disease. The primary disorder usually is brain injury, cerebral palsy, or a neurodegenerative disorder. The treatment, particularly when dysphagia is associated with aspiration, is insertion of a gastrostomy and avoidance of oral feeding. An accompanying antireflux procedure is needed only when pathological reflux is present.

Structural-Mechanical Disorders of the Esophagus

Congenital strictures and esophageal webs, usually located in the proximal esophagus, are uncommon and may be difficult to detect on a roentgenogram. Typically, the patient can point to the level of the obstruction. Esophageal foreign bodies frequently are seen in children and can be removed easily.[10] A hiatal hernia (Fig. 127-1) may be associated with gastroesophageal reflux and esophagitis, which are the true causes of the dysphagia and odynophagia.

Peptic strictures resulting from symptomatic or asymptomatic gastroesophageal reflux cause dysphagia by obstructing the esophageal lumen (Fig. 127-2). Dysphagia typically is greater for solids than for liquids. The diagnosis of peptic stricture is readily made roentgenographically. The stricture is treated with dilation, but the underlying reflux also must be treated. Even after successful repair of esophageal atresia, swallowing problems usually persist.[20,21] Peristalsis nearly always is abnormal, and symptomatic gastroesophageal reflux with or without esophagitis is found nearly universally. Anastomotic strictures may occur. Esophageal tumors are rare in children. Mediastinal tumors rarely cause esophageal obstruction. Although vascular rings are not rare, mechanical obstruction of the esophagus by an aberrant vessel is extremely rare.[8]

Motor Disorders of the Esophagus

Achalasia is a rare cause of functional obstruction of the distal esophagus caused by failure of the lower esophageal sphincter to relax and of the peristaltic wave to propagate.[3,9,12] Its prevalence is about 1:100,000; 10% of cases present in childhood. It is similar functionally and pathologically to Hirschsprung's disease. In both conditions the distal myenteric ganglion cells are absent, causing functional obstruction and proximal dilation. The onset of dysphagia usually is gradual but progressive, until weight loss and spiration occur in neglected cases. Symptoms often are surprisingly mild. Intermittent substernal pain also may be present.

A characteristic J-shaped megaesophagus, with a tapered distal beak, is seen on a barium swallow examination (Fig. 127-3). Peristalsis is absent, but sporadic aperistaltic contrac-

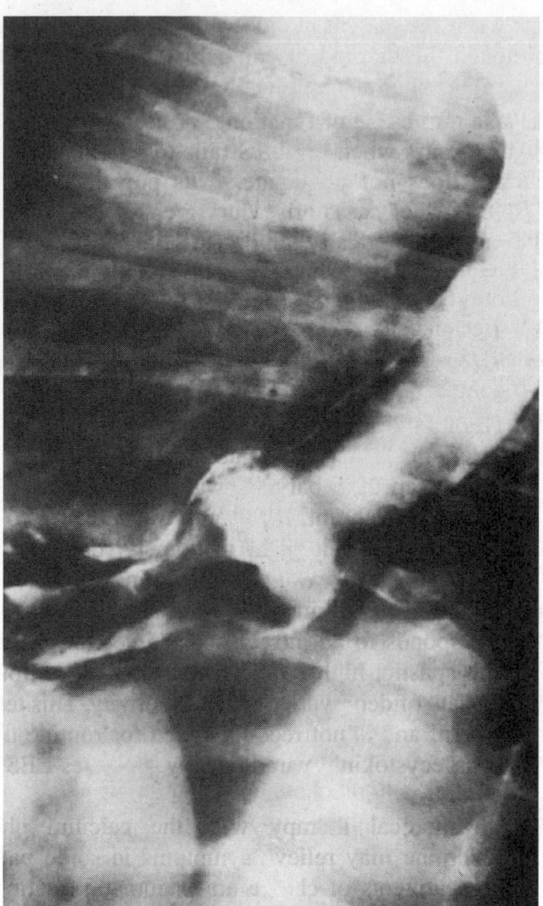

Fig. 127-1 A clearly defined, small hiatal hernia.

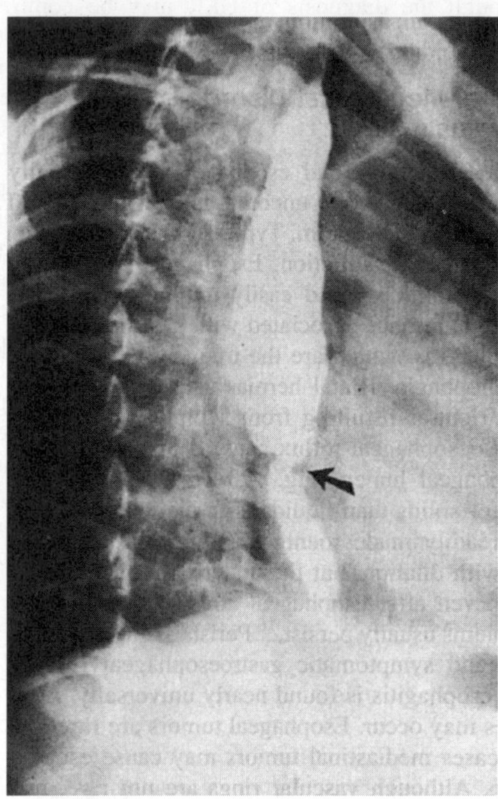

Fig. 127-2 Peptic esophagitis with stricture. Dilation is seen proximal to the tight stricture *(arrow)*. Note the irregularity of the distal esophageal mucosa.

tions may be seen. Intraluminal manometry documents the absence of peristalsis, as well as high resting pressure in the LES and failure of the sphincter to relax after a swallow. The esophagus responds to an intramuscular injection of methacholine with spastic, high-pressure contractions. This test can be quite painful and is not recommended for routine use. In achalasia, cholecystokinin paradoxically increases LES pressure.

Although medical therapy with the calcium channel blocker, nifedipine, may relieve symptoms in some patients, the current treatments of choice are pneumatic dilation and surgical myotomy, which successfully relieve the symptoms in nearly all patients.[3,9] Pneumatic dilation may need to be repeated. The long-term outlook is good, although there may be an increased risk of carcinoma of the esophagus in late adulthood.

Diffuse esophageal spasm is even less common than achalasia. Both dysphagia and pain are present. Symptoms typically wax and wane, often with long symptom-free intervals. Cold beverages frequently exacerbate symptoms. This is seen readily on manometry. The spastic contractions may be seen with a barium swallow. Medical therapy with nitroglycerin occasionally is successful. Otherwise, either pneumatic dilation or surgical myotomy is necessary. Neither approach is totally satisfactory.

Dysphagia may be the presenting symptom in a small but significant number of patients who have scleroderma. Roentgenographic or manometric examination may show aperistalsis in the distal esophagus, but a manometric study is required to confirm the diagnosis.

Gastroesophageal reflux may be associated with esophagitis, disordered peristalsis, and dysphagia. Dysphagia resolves when the esophagitis is treated successfully.

Inflammatory Disorders

It now is recognized that normal function of the LES is the critical factor in preventing reflux of gastric contents.[7] If the LES responds normally to swallowing and otherwise is intact, reflux esophagitis does not occur.

A hiatal hernia demonstrated by roentgenographic studies does not always need to be surgically repaired. A great deal of confusion has existed about which patients who have reflux should have surgery. Based on current knowledge, more than 85% of neurologically intact children referred for evaluation of reflux will respond to medical therapy. In the past, children who had neurological disorders required surgical therapy more frequently than neurologically intact children. This may change with the availability of proton pump inhibitors (omeprazole, lansoprazole) and the prokinetic agent, cisapride.[11]

Gastroesophageal reflux (GER) can be demonstrated in many normal infants. Usually reflux and benign regurgitation disappear by the age of 9 to 18 months. Infants who regurgitate chronically should be observed closely and, if symptomatic, evaluated for esophagitis. Esophageal inflammation and even stricture may occur in the absence of symptoms.

Although the diagnosis of GER may be confirmed by a barium swallow study, radiographic studies do not document reflux in as many as 40% of children who have it, even in patients who have known esophagitis. This is due to the intermittent nature of symptoms and the brief period of fluoroscopic observation. Esophagitis usually is not demonstrated roentgenographically. Although intraluminal esophageal pH recording and scintigraphic techniques can assist in diagnosing reflux, only esophagoscopy and biopsy can document the presence of esophagitis definitively.[19] A complete blood count, serum ferritin, and stool guaiac are useful determinations in documenting bleeding from an inflamed esophagus. A chest roentgenogram should be obtained because chronic GER has been incriminated as a cause of recurrent aspiration pneumonia and chronic obstructive pulmonary disease.

Although esophagitis has been considered uncommon in children, pediatricians are recognizing an increasing number of patients who have the classic symptoms of heartburn, foul taste in the mouth, bad breath, and vomiting.[19,21] Symptoms increase when the patient reclines. Infants may only regurgitate, although this finding, accompanied by failure to thrive and irritability, often is an indication of esophagitis.[4]

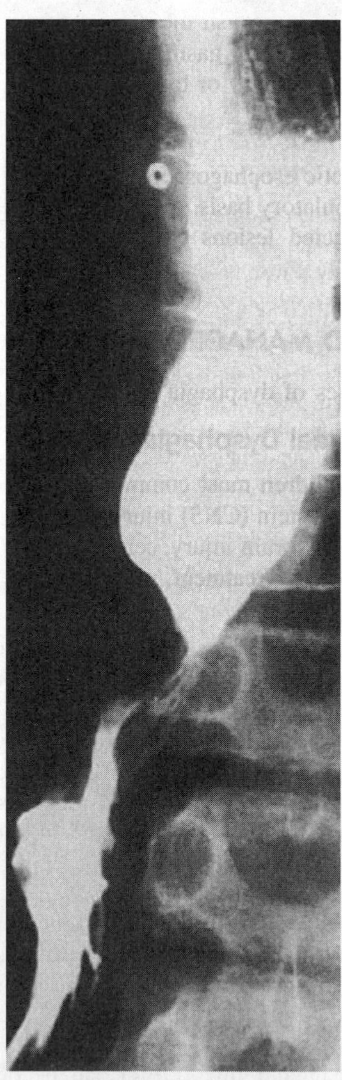

Fig. 127-3 Classic appearance of achalasia of the esophagus. The dilated esophagus ends in a narrow segment.

An important factor in the development of esophagitis is the rate at which refluxed material is cleared from the esophagus. In patients with esophagitis, the normal stripping action of the lower esophagus is impaired, and the distal esophagus remains acidic longer after reflux than in normal patients.

Traditional medical therapy consists of using the upright position during feedings and using feedings thickened with cereal.[15] Because the incidence of sudden infant death syndrome (SIDS) is more frequent in infants kept in the prone position compared with infants sleeping in the supine position, the prone position can no longer be recommended routinely for sleeping.[1]

Cisapride, the most effective prokinetic agent available,[5,18] has been withdrawn from the U.S. market because it can induce prolonged QTc and ventricular arrhythmias when given in excessive doses to premature infants and when given in combination with inhibitors of cytochrome P450 such as erythromycin, clarithromycin, azole antifungals (fluconazole, nitroconazole, miconazole, and itraconazole), and protease inhibitors. When a prokinetic agent is needed, bethanechol (0.1 to 0.2 mg/kg four times a day) may be used. Metoclopramide has not been shown to be an effective treatment for GER in children. H_2 blockers or proton pump inhibitors are administered when esophagitis is documented. In neurologically normal children, surgery rarely is needed for medical failure or stricture formation.

Inflammatory lesions of the esophagus are particularly common in association with infection by *Candida albicans*, cytomegalovirus, and herpes simplex virus. Although these agents may appear spontaneously, most pediatric patients who acquire infections by them are immunosuppressed. While the roentgenographic appearance of *C. albicans* and herpes may be suggestive in the appropriate clinical setting, the roentgenographic appearance may not be typical, and endoscopy and biopsy are usually required to confirm the diagnosis. The possibility of infection by these agents is not always considered in the uncompromised host.

Although not truly esophagitis, the esophageal lesions that occur in cases of epidermolysis bullosa may be recognized roentgenographically.

The most effective medical treatment for esophagitis consists of avoidance of foods such as coffee, alcohol, and fatty foods that reduce lower esophageal sphincter pressure, and elevation of the head of the bed at least 8 inches. Anticholinergic drugs, which decrease lower esophageal sphincter pressure, should be avoided. H_2 blockers may need to be given at higher doses than required for ulcer healing. Proton pump inhibitors (omeprazole, lansoprazole) are even more effective in healing esophagitis than are H_2 blockers and may be successful when H_2 blockers fail.[11] Surgery is indicated only for intractable symptoms and stricture development.

When *C. albicans* infection is documented, the therapy described above should be supplemented by the appropriate dosage of nystatin or ketoconazole. Amphotericin B frequently is required. Herpes esophagitis is treated with acyclovir. Cytomegalovirus esophagitis may be treated with ganciclovir.

Ingestion of caustic agents, especially liquid alkali, causes intense pain and dysphagia.[16] Symptoms commonly resolve after 3 or 4 days, but stricture formation associated with return of dysphagia may follow after 3 to 8 weeks. Early esophagoscopy, preferably 12 to 24 hours after the caustic ingestion, is essential to establish the extent and degree of the burn. If the burn is limited to the mouth, no therapy is necessary. The most recent reports in the literature suggest that steroids do not decrease stricture formation.[2] Strictures are treated by bougienage. Recurrent strictures may be treated with steroid injections. Esophagectomy and colon interposition rarely are necessary.[13]

REFERENCES

1. AAP Task Force on infant positioning and SIDS: Positioning and SIDS, *Pediatrics* 89:1120, 1992.
2. Anderson KD, Rouse TM, Randolph JG: A controlled trial of corticosteroids in children with corrosive injury of the esophagus, *N Engl J Med* 323:637, 1990.
3. Berquist WE, et al: Achalasia: diagnosis, management and clinical course in 16 children, *Pediatrics* 71:798, 1983.
4. Catto-Smith AG, et al: The role of gastroesophageal reflux in pediatric dysphagia, *J Pediatr Gastroenterol Nutr* 12:159, 1991.
5. Cucchiara A, et al: Cisapride for gastro-oesophageal reflux and peptic oesophagitis, *Arch Dis Child* 62:454, 1987.
6. Dodds WJ: Instrumentation and methods for intraluminal esophageal manometry, *Arch Intern Med* 136:515, 1976.
7. Dodds WJ, et al: Pathogenesis of reflux esophagitis, *Gastroenterology* 81:376, 1981.
8. Eklof O, et al: Arterial anomalies causing compression of the trachea and/or oesophagus, *Acta Paediatr Scand* 60:81, 1971.
9. Emblem R, et al: Current results of surgery for achalasia of the cardia, *Arch Dis Child* 68:749, 1993.
10. Ginsberg GG: Management of ingested foreign objects and food bolus impactions, *Gastrointest Endosc* 41:33, 1995.
11. Israel DM, Hassall E: Omeprazole and other proton pump inhibitors: pharmacology, efficacy, and safety, with special reference to use in children, *J Pediatr Gastroenterol Nutr* 27:568, 1998.
12. Khoshoo V, LaGarde DC, Udall JN: Intrasphincteric injection of botulinum toxin for treating achalasia in children, *J Pediatr Gastroenterol Nutr* 24:439, 1997.
13. Lee M, et al: Preliminary experience with endoscopic intralesional steroid injection therapy for refractory upper gastrointestinal strictures, *Gastrointest Endosc* 41:598, 1995.
14. Leonidas JC: Gastroesophageal reflux in infants: role of the upper gastrointestinal series, *AJR* 143:1350, 1984.
15. Orenstein SR, Whittington PF, Orenstein DM: The infant seat as treatment for gastroesophageal reflux, *N Engl J Med* 29:760, 1983.
16. Previtera C, Giusti F, Guglielmi: Predictive value of visible lesions (cheeks, lips, oropharynx) in suspected caustic ingestion: may endoscopy reasonably be omitted in completely negative pediatric patients? *Pediatr Emerg Care* 6:176, 1990.
17. Richter JE: Heartburn, dysphagia and other esophageal symptoms. In Sleisenger MH, Fordtran JS, editors: *Gastrointestinal disease*, ed 6, Philadelphia, 1998, WB Saunders.
18. Vandenplas Y: Clinical use of cisapride and its risk-benefit in pediatric patients, *Eur J Gastro Hepatol* 10:871, 1998.
19. Vandenplas Y, et al: A critical appraisal of current management practices for infant regurgitation: recommendations of a working party, *Eur J Pediatr* 156:343, 1997.
20. Werlin SL, et al: Esophageal function in esophageal atresia, *Dig Dis Sci* 26:796, 1981.
21. Werlin SL, et al: Mechanisms of gastroesophageal reflux in children, *J Pediatr* 97:244, 1980.

128 Dyspnea

Jay H. Mayefsky

Dyspnea is the uncomfortable feeling of not being able to satisfy "air hunger." Patients may complain of not being able to catch their breath or of a suffocating feeling. Dyspnea is a symptom, a subjective complaint by the patient, that describes the sensation caused by an underlying disorder. As with any subjective complaint, the diagnosis of dyspnea and its cause in an infant or young child can be problematic. Therefore, to evaluate fully a child in respiratory distress, the pediatric health care professional must be familiar with the pathophysiology, signs, and common causes of dyspnea. With the aid of the medical history, physical examination, and appropriate laboratory tests, the condition can be diagnosed and therapy initiated.

PATHOPHYSIOLOGY

Dyspnea is seen most commonly with exercise: The increased work of breathing necessary to keep up with the body's increased metabolic demands causes the dyspnea.[10] The sensation probably is transmitted from stretch receptors in the chest wall muscles to the central nervous system (CNS). Chemoreceptors, sensing changes in arterial pH, oxygen, and carbon dioxide concentrations, as well as chest wall proprioceptors, lung stretch receptors, and mechanoreceptors in the heart, skeletal muscles, and upper airway play a role.[2,12,16,29] The transmission is processed in the CNS, and the individual experiences the sensation of dyspnea. With exercise, the person who has dyspnea is aware of an increased ventilatory effort. A person who has obstructive or restrictive lung disease also experiences difficulty breathing, as will someone who has a neuromuscular disease who feels that he or she is not getting enough air.

To satisfy their oxygen needs, children who have dyspnea must increase their minute ventilation ($\dot{V}_E$) by working harder than normally to do so. In normal breathing, respiratory muscles work only during inspiration, and the diaphragm does most of the work. The work of inspiration is the sum of the work necessary to overcome the elastic forces of the lung, the tissue viscosity of the lung and chest wall, and airway resistance.[9] When any of these is increased (e.g., elastic force and tissue viscosity in restrictive pulmonary disease or resistance in obstructive airway disease), the work of inspiration must increase to maintain adequate $\dot{V}_E$. The accessory muscles of inspiration (the sternocleidomastoid, anterior serratus, and external intercostal muscles) are recruited to accomplish this. Contraction of these muscles causes forceful expansion of the thorax, resulting in an unusually large negative intrathoracic pressure. This negative pressure draws in the soft tissues of the chest wall and creates one of the classic signs of dyspnea—retractions. Retractions may be seen in the suprasternal, infrasternal, intercostal, subcostal, and supraclavicular areas. An alternative way to maintain an adequate $\dot{V}_E$ is to increase the rate of breathing—hence, the second classic sign of dyspnea—tachypnea. Nasal flaring and grunting are other signs seen and heard during respiration.

Little energy is expended during normal expiration. Relaxation of the diaphragm, elastic recoil of the lungs and chest wall, and compression of the lungs by the intraabdominal organs force air from the lungs. In obstructive airway disease the force generated by these processes may not be great enough to effect adequate expiration. In a child who has tachypnea the elastic recoil may not be fast enough to allow adequate exhalation between breaths.

In either instance the accessory muscles of expiration are used. The abdominal recti muscles contract and force the abdominal contents against the diaphragm to compress the lungs, and the internal intercostal muscles contract to pull the ribs downward and to create a positive intrathoracic pressure to force the air from the lungs. The contractions of these muscles provide the most important expiratory sign of dyspnea.

Although dyspnea is a respiratory symptom, it may be caused by primary disorders in other body systems. Cardiac, hematological, metabolic, circulatory, and psychogenic causes must be considered in the differential diagnosis of dyspnea. The child's age also is important, because various disorders occur with different frequency at different ages.

The history is essential. It starts with a complete description of the dyspnea. The patient or parent should be asked whether the onset was sudden (e.g., inhaled foreign body, lung collapse) or evolved over several hours (e.g., asthma, diabetic ketoacidosis). The patient also should be asked about the duration of the illness, the frequency of attacks of dyspnea, and whether there appears to be a trigger or temporally related event to the onset of dyspnea. An attempt should be made to quantify the severity of the dyspnea. This may be done by asking to what degree daily activities are restricted by shortness of breath.

An inquiry also should be made as to whether the dyspnea is affected by the patient's position. With unilateral lung disease, dyspnea may get worse when the patient lies with the affected lung down. Dyspnea that worsens with the recumbency often is due to left ventricular failure, obstructive airway disease, or muscle weakness. Dyspnea in the upright position relieved by lying down usually is due to intracardiac, vascular, or parenchymal lung shunts.

The patient also should be asked about associated symptoms such as cough, wheezing, sputum production, and pleuritic pain. In addition, a history of other known illnesses, allergies, illnesses in the family, medication, and environmental exposure must be obtained.

A thorough physical examination always is indicated, with special attention paid to the aforementioned systems. The most useful laboratory tests are the complete blood count (CBC) and peripheral blood smear, arterial blood gas measurement, and roentgenographic studies of the airways and lungs. Measurement of arterial oxygen saturation by pulse oximetry is invaluable for its ability to assess oxygenation status quickly and noninvasively. Pulmonary function tests are very helpful but may not be immediately available for evaluation of an acutely ill patient.

ETIOLOGY AND CLINICAL PRESENTATION

Pulmonary Disease

Pulmonary disease that causes dyspnea can be classified as obstructive, restrictive, or vascular.

Obstructive pulmonary disease. Obstructive disease is characterized by airway narrowing that can be caused by intraluminal objects (mucus, foreign bodies, or tumor), intramural factors (smooth muscle contraction, edema, or bronchomalacia), or extramural compression (tumor or lymph nodes). The narrowing increases both airway resistance and turbulent flow in the airways. If a fixed obstruction is present, affected areas of the lungs will become atelectatic. With a ball valve type of obstruction (i.e., air can get into the lungs but not out), air is trapped and affected areas become hyperinflated. In either case, an imbalance occurs between pulmonary ventilation and perfusion, and oxygen exchange is adversely affected.[27] All these processes force the patient to work harder to maintain adequate ventilation; hence, dyspnea ensues.

During normal respiration, inspiration and expiration are of equal length. With a fixed degree of obstruction, both are equally prolonged. If the obstruction varies and is extrathoracic (i.e., above the vocal cords), inspiration is affected more because the negative intraairway pressure during inspiration tends to collapse the extrathoracic airway. The characteristic sign of such an obstruction is inspiratory stridor.[11]

If the obstruction varies and affects the intrathoracic airways, expiration is prolonged, because the positive intrathoracic pressure tends to collapse these airways during expiration. If larger airways are involved, rhonchi are present. Airflow across an obstruction in smaller airways generates wheezing.

A paradoxical pulse and cyanosis are sensitive but nonspecific signs of severe obstruction. Patients who have chronic obstructive disease may be barrel chested and have signs of chronic hypoxia, such as clubbing. Children who have a systemic disease, such as cystic fibrosis, also will show the extrapulmonary manifestations of that disease. The common causes of obstructive airway disease in childhood are shown in Box 128-1. Obstruction in the nose or nasopharynx should not be overlooked, especially in infants, who are obligatory nasal breathers.

BOX 128-1

CAUSES OF OBSTRUCTIVE PULMONARY DISEASE

Newborns
- Choanal atresia or stenosis
- Dermoid cyst
- Encephalocele
- Nasolacrimal duct cyst
- Hemangioma
- Vocal cord paralysis
- Pierre Robin syndrome
- Ankyloglossia (tongue tie)[17]
- Pertussis

Infants
- Foreign body
- Vascular ring
- Tracheal web
- Bronchiolitis
- Asthma
- Cystic fibrosis
- Bronchomalacia
- Pyogenic thyroid[13]
- Accessory thyroid[13]

Children and Adolescents
- Foreign body (airway or esophagus)
- Asthma
- Adenopathy
  - Lymphoma
  - Systemic lupus erythematosus
  - Tuberculosis
  - Sarcoidosis
- Croup
- Epiglottitis
- Retropharyngeal abscess
- Enlarged tonsils or adenoids
- Cystic fibrosis
- Anaphylaxis
- Laryngeal tumor
- Vocal cord tumor
- Tracheal tumors
- Vocal cord polyp
- Laryngeal trauma
- Supraglottitis
- Diphtheria
- Bacterial tracheitis
- Ingestion of caustic substance
- Crack cocaine[20]
- Trauma

Blood gas values may be normal with mild obstructive disease. As the disease progresses, hypoxemia is the first abnormality seen. Hypocapnia, initially seen as a reflection of increased $\dot{V}_E$, is replaced by hypercapnia as the maldistribution of ventilation and perfusion increases. The patient then tires, and respiratory failure occurs.

The chest roentgenogram may reveal whether the cause of the obstruction is inside or outside the airway. Often hyperinflation with an increased anteroposterior chest diameter and flattened diaphragm are seen. Atelectasis may appear with a fixed obstruction. Fluoroscopic examination or inspiratory and expiratory roentgenograms may be useful in localizing a ball valve type obstruction.

Restrictive pulmonary disease. The cardinal features of restrictive pulmonary disease are a reduction in lung volume and pulmonary compliance secondary to pathological changes in the lung parenchyma or the pleura, deformities of the chest wall, or neuromuscular disease. Decreased volume necessitates an increase in respiratory rate to maintain a normal $\dot{V}_E$. The work of breathing must be increased to overcome the reduced compliance. Because it is more energy efficient to breathe rapidly with small tidal volumes than to breathe slowly and attempt to expand the chest against great restrictive forces, children who have restrictive diseases characteristically have rapid, shallow respirations.[27] The common pediatric causes of restrictive pulmonary disease are listed in Box 128-2.

Observation of the child often reveals skeletal and neuromuscular causes. Pleural and parenchymal diseases are detected best by palpation, percussion, and auscultation of the chest. Tactile fremitus can demonstrate pulmonary consolidation or pleural effusion. Careful percussion reveals effusions, consolidation, and abnormal diaphragmatic excursion. On auscultation, rales characteristic of alveolar disease may be heard, and changes in whispered pectoriloquy and egophony can be detected.

The CBC may be helpful in diagnosing an infectious cause. Arterial blood gases have a characteristic pattern of hypoxemia and hypocapnia. The chest roentgenogram is useful in that it can demonstrate decreased lung volume, pleural thickening and effusions, increased interstitial markings, parenchymal consolidation, skeletal deformities, and abnormal movement of the diaphragm.

Vascular pulmonary disease. Vascular lung disease is characterized by a decrease in the size of the pulmonary vascular bed. In the neonate, this is due often to "persistent pulmonary hypertension of the newborn."[7] Microemboli also have been reported in the lungs of infants

BOX 128-2

CAUSES OF RESTRICTIVE PULMONARY DISEASE

Newborns
- Hyaline membrane disease
- Hypoplastic lungs
- Eventration of the diaphragm
- Meconium aspiration
- Pneumonia (group B streptococci or gram-negative organisms)
- Diaphragmatic paralysis
- Osteogenesis imperfecta
- CNS depression
  - Hypoxia
  - Congenital
  - Maternal drugs
- Congenital myasthenia gravis
- Aspiration
- Pulmonary edema
  - Septicemia
  - Congenital heart disease

Infants
- Pneumonia
  - Bacterial
  - Viral
  - Aspiration
- Bronchopulmonary dysplasia
- Wilson-Mikity syndrome
- Hamman-Rich syndrome
- Pulmonary edema
- Infantile botulism
- Congenital lobar emphysema

Children and Adolescents
- Skeletal
  - Kyphoscoliosis
  - Ankylosing spondylitis
  - Pectus excavatum
  - Crush chest injury
- Parenchymal
  - Pneumonia
  - Hypersensitivity pneumonitis
  - Systemic lupus erythematosus
  - Scleroderma
  - Fibrosis
  - Toxin inhalation
  - Granulomatous disease
  - Drugs (e.g., antineoplastic agents and narcotics)[22]
  - Carcinoma
  - Fat embolus
  - Pneumothorax
- Smoke inhalation
- Pulmonary infarction
- Pulmonary edema
  - Congestive heart failure
  - Sepsis
  - Intracranial disease[6]
  - Croup[11]
  - Epiglottitis[11]
- Neuromuscular
  - Cord transection
  - Myasthenia gravis
  - Muscular dystrophy
  - Multiple sclerosis
  - Guillain-Barré syndrome
  - Pickwickian syndrome
  - Toxins
- Pleural effusion
  - Pneumonia
- Hypoproteinemia
- Renal failure
- Tumor
- Pulmonary infarction

who are in severe respiratory distress.[14] In older children, the most common cause of vascular pulmonary disease is intimal hyperplasia after persistent left-to-right shunting and resultant pulmonary hypertension. The size of the pulmonary vascular bed also can be reduced by obstruction caused by thromboembolic disease, obliteration (e.g., vasculitis),[8] or destruction, as in emphysema. The reduced blood flow through the lungs results in arterial hypoxemia and hypercapnia, which in turn lead to the symptoms and signs of dyspnea.

In addition to the common signs of dyspnea, the child who has vascular lung disease may have signs of pulmonary edema and pleural effusion. Systemic signs of right-sided heart failure secondary to pulmonary hypertension or left-sided failure that was the cause of the pulmonary hypertension may be present. The cardiac findings observed with pulmonary hypertension are an accentuated P_2, paradoxical splitting of S_2, an S_3, a pulmonary ejection click, and a right ventricular heave.

An electrocardiogram is helpful in the diagnosis of right ventricular hypertrophy. A chest roentgenogram may reveal increased right ventricular size, enlargement of the pulmonary artery silhouette, decreased pulmonary blood flow in advanced disease, or increased flow early in the course of disease, with a left-to-right shunt.

Cardiac Disease

Dyspnea occurs with cardiac disease when insufficient blood is being pumped to the lungs as a result of congenital structural anomalies in the heart, pump failure (myocarditis or cardiomyopathy), arrhythmia, or as already described, secondary pulmonary hypertension. Heart disease must be considered in all dyspneic newborns and older children who have a history of congenital heart disease. In the neonate, pulmonary disease often can be differentiated from cyanotic heart disease through a hyperoxia test. The nature of the cardiac defect can be delineated with the help of a thorough cardiac examination, an electrocardiogram, a chest roentgenogram, and an echocardiogram.

It must be remembered that what would be a trivial respiratory infection in a normal child may cause severe respiratory insufficiency in a child who has cardiopulmonary disease. Indeed, the mortality of infants who have respiratory syncytial viral pneumonia and congenital heart disease has been shown to exceed significantly the mortality of children who have normal hearts.[15]

Hematological Disease

If the oxygen-carrying capacity of the blood is reduced sufficiently, tissue hypoxia ensues. The resultant drop in arterial pH signals the CNS and stimulates the onset of dyspnea. Severe anemia, whether chronic or acute, congenital or acquired, can cause dyspnea. The oxygen-carrying capacity also can be lowered when the hemoglobin's ability to bind oxygen is reduced. This is seen most commonly with carbon monoxide poisoning, but it also occurs with cyanide poisoning and methemoglobinemia. In any of these cases the child will not be cyanotic. The blue color of cyanosis is caused by a level of at least 5 g/dl of reduced hemoglobin in the blood.[27] Such a concentration of reduced hemoglobin is not found in anemia uncomplicated by other diseases or in the other conditions cited. Conversely, a polycythemic infant whose blood is hyperviscous may have dyspnea because of poor perfusion. Because such an infant has an increased hemoglobin concentration and more oxygen is removed from the hemoglobin because his or her flow is decreased, this child may be cyanotic (having more than 5 g/dl unsaturated hemoglobin) and not hypoxic. An extreme elevation of leukocyte or platelet counts also can cause blood hyperviscosity and dyspnea.

Even though an anemic child may have tissue hypoxia and be dyspneic, he or she probably will not be hypoxemic; that is, the arterial oxygen tension (PaO_2) measured by blood gas analysis will be in the normal range.

Metabolic Disease

Disorders that increase the body's rate of metabolism and therefore oxygen consumption can cause dyspnea. Examples are hyperthyroidism[13] and fever. Metabolic disorders associated with an increased production of hydrogen ion and carbon dioxide cause a dyspnea-like breathing pattern to help rid the body of the carbon dioxide. The classic example is Kussmaul breathing with diabetic ketoacidosis. Aspirin poisoning can manifest similarly. In addition, children who have various muscle enzyme deficiencies, especially those affecting the mitochondria, may have dyspnea as part of their clinical presentation as a result of their increased acid production and decreased work tolerance.[21,23] In chronic renal failure the kidney's inability to remove acid from the blood adequately is the underlying cause of dyspnea. The history, physical examination, and appropriate laboratory tests should facilitate the proper diagnosis of these diseases.

If oxygen cannot reach the tissues, the body responds with dyspnea, cardiovascular collapse, and shock, a medical emergency that should not present a diagnostic problem.

Obesity

Dyspnea, especially with exertion, is a common complaint of obese children. An obese child is prone to dyspnea because his or her metabolic requirement for a given amount of work is increased.[30] In addition, the diaphragm of an obese child must move against increased abdominal pressure, and the chest wall is heavier; thus, more energy must be expended to maintain $\dot{V}_E$. Treatment should include dietary regulation and an exercise program graded to keep pace with the child's level of exercise tolerance.

Pregnancy

Dyspnea is normal during pregnancy.[32] The onset occurs during the first or second trimester, and 76% of women complain of dyspnea by the thirty-first week of gestation. The sensation is due to a subjective awareness of the hyperventilation normally present during pregnancy.

The normal dyspnea of pregnancy can be differentiated easily from dyspnea arising from heart or lung disease. First, the woman who has dyspnea of pregnancy has no other symptoms of cardiac or pulmonary disease. Second, dyspnea of pregnancy begins early and plateaus or improves as term approaches. Dyspnea resulting from heart disease begins during the second half of pregnancy and is worst during the seventh month. Finally, dyspnea of pregnancy rarely is severe, rarely occurs at rest, and does not interfere with the activities of daily life.

Intravenous Drug Use

Several causes of dyspnea must be considered with a history of intravenous drug use. Heroin can cause bronchospasm that responds to bronchodilator medications. In addition, heroin and other opioids may precipitate pulmonary edema.[22] Therapy consists of oxygen, diuretics, and naloxone.

Infections also may cause dyspnea in intravenous drug users. The most common infection is community-acquired pneumonia. However, opportunistic pulmonary infections, tuberculosis, and bacterial endocarditis with associated septic pulmonary emboli or heart failure must be considered.

Finally, talc granulomatosis must be considered. It is secondary to the intravenous injection of dissolved opioid tablets, with deposition of foreign bodies in the pulmonary vasculature and granuloma formation. It presents with chronic mild to moderate dyspnea.

Psychogenic Cause

Stress or hysteria may cause dyspnea.[28] A thorough history and physical examination are keys to the diagnosis. These patients are tachypneic and complain of air "hunger." When dyspnea is caused by pulmonary or cardiac conditions, the shortness of breath worsens with increasing activity and improves with rest. However, when dyspnea is due to hysteria, it does not improve with rest and may worsen. The patients also often complain of chest pain and sigh more often. Contrary to previous belief, tetany is an uncommon accompaniment of hysterical dyspnea.

The physical examination usually is normal. However, stress-induced paradoxical adduction of the vocal cords during inspiration has been reported.[18] Patients who have this disorder may have either stridor or wheezing. In this instance the diagnosis of hysterical dyspnea is one of exclusion, it can be made only after pathological lesions in the airways and lungs have been ruled out.

Normally the only laboratory abnormality found with hysteria-induced dyspnea is a diminished arterial carbon dioxide tension.

Treatment consists of calm reassurance and, occasionally, mild sedation. If the condition is chronic, psychotherapy may be required. When paradoxical vocal cord motion is the cause, the patient also should be taught laryngeal relaxation techniques.

MANAGEMENT

Severe dyspnea is a medical emergency. If not treated promptly, a child who has dyspnea may progress rapidly to respiratory failure and death. First the adequacy of the airway must be assessed. Foreign bodies must be removed and anatomical obstructions bypassed with endotracheal intubation or, in rare cases, tracheotomy. Bronchospasm, when present, should be treated with beta-agonistic drugs.

Subsequently, the efficacy of the child's ventilation must be evaluated. Normally, breathing uses 2% to 3% of the total body energy expenditure. When the work of breathing is increased during dyspnea, this amount may rise to 30% or more.[8] Such a degree of energy expenditure cannot be continued indefinitely, and the child tires. Even after an obstruction is removed, the child still may be unable to effect adequate ventilation. In this instance, or in the case of neuromuscular disease, the child requires mechanical ventilation.

Once ventilation is established, the cardiovascular system's ability to deliver oxygen to the tissues must be appraised. This involves evaluating the heart, peripheral circulation, intravascular volume status, and the blood's oxygen-carrying capacity. Therapy with vasopressors, fluids, blood transfusions, or diuretics should be initiated when indicated. Although not all children who have dyspnea require supplemental oxygen, every child should have oxygen administered until the cause of the dyspnea is known. Once the patient's condition has stabilized, the search for the underlying cause of the dyspnea should progress urgently, but calmly. At this point, a detailed history can be elicited, a full physical examination can be performed, and a chest roentgenogram and appropriate blood tests can be obtained. When the diagnosis is made, specific therapy can be initiated.

When dyspnea is caused by a chronic illness, no satisfactory therapy may be available to treat the underlying disease. However, simply relieving the dyspnea can improve the child's functional ability and quality of life significantly.[1] Several modalities can be used to treat the symptom of dyspnea in a chronically ill child.[3,26] Sedatives and narcotics reduce $\dot{V}_E$ and thereby diminish the intensity of the breathless feeling. Prostaglandin inhibitors and beta-agonists may blunt the perception of dyspnea without affecting ventilation.[25] Theophylline may improve diaphragmatic contractility. Continuous supplemental oxygen with or without continuous positive airway pressure reduces ventilatory drive.[31] Children who have chronic obstructive pulmonary disease may be taught to breathe through pursed lips. This reduces the respiratory rate, increases the tidal volume, and diminishes the sensation of dyspnea. Hypnosis has proved useful in treating the symptoms of dyspnea. Patients also have reported a decrease in dyspnea when seated next to an open window or a blowing fan.[24]

Exercise and proper nutrition are helpful in maintaining or increasing inspiratory muscle mass and thereby in reducing the perceived magnitude of dyspnea.[1,4,19] Finally, because dyspnea is a subjective complaint, there is a significant psychological contribution to its perceived severity.[5] Therefore, the child's emotional state, behavior, and personality must be monitored, because psychosocial intervention may be indicated.

When to Refer

- Chronic pulmonary disease
- Congenital or acquired heart disease
- Metabolic disease
- Conditions requiring surgical procedures

When to Hospitalize

Respiratory failure
Impending respiratory failure
Hypoxia while breathing room air

REFERENCES

1. Altose MD: Assessment and management of breathlessness, *Chest* 88(suppl 2):77, 1985.
2. Angelillo VA: Evaluation of dyspnea, *Postgrad Med* 73:336, 1983.
3. Belman MJ: Factors limiting exercise performance in lung disease: ventilatory insufficiency, *Chest* 101:253S, 1992.
4. Carter R, Coast JR, Idell S: Exercise training in patients with chronic obstructive pulmonary disease, *Med Sci Sports Exerc* 24:281, 1992.
5. Cherniak NS, Altose MD: Mechanisms of dyspnea, *Clin Chest Med* 8:207, 1978.
6. Drucker TB, Simmons RL, Martin AM: Pulmonary edema as a complication of intracranial disease, *Am J Dis Child* 118:638, 1969.
7. Fox WW, Duara S: Persistent pulmonary hypertension in the neonate: diagnosis and management, *J Pediatr* 103:505, 1983.
8. Goffman TE, Bloom RL, Dvorak VC: Acute dyspnea in a young woman taking birth control pills, *JAMA* 251:1465, 1984.
9. Guyton AC: *Textbook of medical physiology,* Philadelphia, 1981, WB Saunders.
10. Howell JB, Campbell EJM, editors: *Breathlessness,* Oxford, 1966, Blackwell Scientific.
11. Kanter RK, Watchko JF: Pulmonary edema associated with upper airway obstruction, *Am J Dis Child* 138:356, 1984.
12. Killian KJ, Campbell EJM: Dyspnea and exercise, *Annu Rev Physiol* 45:465, 1983.
13. Leigh M, Holman G, Rohn R: Dyspnea as the presenting symptom of thyroid disease, *Clin Pediatr* 19:773, 1980.
14. Levin DL, Weinberg AG, Perkin RM: Pulmonary microthrombi in newborn infants with unresponsive persistent pulmonary hypertension, *J Pediatr* 102:299, 1983.
15. Macdonald NE, et al: Respiratory syncytial virus infection in infants with congenital heart disease, *N Engl J Med* 307:397, 1982.
16. Manning HL, Schwartzstein RM: Pathophysiology of dyspnea, *N Engl J Med* 333:1547, 1995.
17. Mukai S, Mukai C, Asaoka K: Ankyloglossia with deviation of the epiglottis and larynx, *Ann Otol Rhinol Laryngol* 153:3, 1991.
18. O'Hollaren MT: Masqueraders in clinical allergy: laryngeal dysfunction causing dyspnea, *Ann Allergy* 65:351, 1990.
19. Olopade CO, et al: Exercise limitation and pulmonary rehabilitation in chronic obstructive pulmonary disease, *Mayo Clin Proc* 67:144, 1992.
20. Reino AJ, Lawson W: Upper airway distress in crack cocaine users, *Otolaryngol Head Neck Surg* 109:937, 1993.
21. Robinson BH, et al: Clinical presentation of mitochondrial respiratory chain defects in ADH-coenzyme Q reductase and cytochrome oxidase: clues to pathogenesis of Leigh disease, *J Pediatr* 110:216, 1987.
22. Rosenow EC: The spectrum of drug-induced pulmonary disease, *Ann Intern Med* 77:977, 1972.
23. Scholte HR et al: Defects in oxidative phosphorylation: biochemical investigations in skeletal muscle and expression of the lesion in other cells, *J Inherit Metab Dis* 10(suppl 1):81, 1987.
24. Schwartzstein RM, et al: Cold facial stimulation reduces breathlessness induced in normal individuals, *Am Rev Respir Dis* 136:58, 1987.
25. Stark RD: Dyspnoea: assessment and pharmacological manipulation, *Eur J Respir Dis* 1:280, 1988.
26. Sweer L, Zwillich CW: Dyspnea in the patient with chronic obstructive pulmonary disease: etiology and management, *Clin Chest Med* 11:417, 1990.
27. Tisi GM: *Pulmonary physiology in clinical medicine*, Baltimore, 1980, Williams & Wilkins.
28. Tobin MJ: Dyspnea: pathophysiologic basis, clinical presentation, and management, *Arch Intern Med* 150:1604, 1990.
29. Wasserman K, Casaburi R: Dyspnea: physiological and pathophysiological mechanisms, *Annu Rev Med* 39:503, 1988.
30. Wasserman K, et al: *Principles of exercise testing and interpretation,* Philadelphia, 1987, Lea & Febiger.
31. Younes M: Load responses, dyspnea, and respiratory failure, *Chest* 97: 59S, 1990.
32. Zeldis SM: Dyspnea during pregnancy: distinguishing cardiac from pulmonary causes, *Clin Chest Med* 13:567, 1992.

SUGGESTED READINGS

Burki NK: Dyspnea, *Lung* 165:269, 1987.

Cohen MH, et al: Treatment of intractable dyspnea: clinical and ethical issues, *Cancer Invest* 10:317, 1992.

Downes JJ, Fulgencio T, Raphaely RC: Acute respiratory failure in infants and children, *Pediatr Clin North Am* 19:423, 1972.

Gandevia SC: Neural mechanisms underlying the sensation of breathlessness: kinesthetic parallels between respiratory and limb muscles, *Aust N Z J Med* 18:83, 1988.

Harun MH, Yaacob I, Mohd Kassim Z: Spontaneous pneumothorax: a review of 29 admissions into Hospital Universiti Sains Malaysia 1984-90, *Singapore Med J* 34:150, 1993.

Heyse-Moore LH: Symptom control in palliative medicine: an update, *Br J Clin Pract* 43:273, 1989.

Huh J, et al: Management of tracheobronchial injuries following blunt and penetrating trauma, *Am Surg* 63:896, 1997.

Litam PP, Loughran TP Jr: Exertional dyspnea and headache in a 16-year-old girl, *Hosp Pract* 29:112, 1994.

Mahler DA: Dyspnea: diagnosis and management, *Clin Chest Med* 8:215, 1987.

Mahler DA, Horowitz MB: Clinical evaluation of exertional dyspnea, *Clin Chest Med* 15:259, 1994.

O'Connor PG, et al: Management of hospitalized intravenous drug users: role of the internist, *Am J Med* 96:551, 1994.

Poole-Wilson PA, Buller NP, Lindsay DC: Blood flow and skeletal muscle in patients with heart failure, *Chest* 101:330S, 1992.

Rebuck AS, Slutsky AS: Control of breathing in diseases of the respiratory tract and lungs. In Geiger SR, editor: *Handbook of physiology,* Bethesda, Md, 1986, American Physiological Society.

Schwartzstein RM, et al: Dyspnea: a sensory experience, *Lung* 168:185, 1990.

Seamens CM, Wrenn K: Breathlessness. Strategies aimed at identifying and treating the cause of dyspnea, *Postgrad Med* 98:215, 1995.

Shayevitz MB, Shayevitz BR: Athletic training in chronic obstructive pulmonary disease, *Clin Sports Med* 5:471, 1986.

van der Molen B: Dyspnoea: a study of measurement instruments for the assessment of dyspnoea and their application for patients with advanced cancer, *J Adv Nurs* 22:948, 1995.

129 Dysuria

Fred J. Heldrich

Dysuria is painful or difficult urination. Although this symptom occurs with some frequency in pediatric patients, it is interesting that the term rarely can be found in the index of standard pediatric texts and cannot be found in the *Cumulative Index Medicus*. The reason is that dysuria rarely occurs as an isolated symptom; far more often it occurs with other signs or symptoms of a pathological urinary tract condition and is discussed in concert with them. Although occasionally dysuria is the only complaint, it often is easier to identify the cause of the dysuria by considering the associated symptoms.

Identifying the cause of dysuria requires a thorough history, a careful physical examination, and a planned laboratory evaluation.[1] Failure to follow this routine usually leads to unnecessary expense, incorrect diagnosis, and improper management.

CLINICAL MANIFESTATIONS

Although older patients usually can tell the physician that urination is painful or difficult, infants and young children give other evidence of dysuria. Infants indicate pain on urination in a variety of ways (Box 129-1). Crying, the most typical sign, is associated with micturition. Just as voiding provokes crying, cessation of voiding provides relief, and the crying may stop. Characteristically, infants who cry because of discomfort associated with voiding flex their thighs. This combination of crying and drawing up of the legs frequently is described as colic. At times the association between crying and voiding is not appreciated, and the infant is thought merely to be hyperirritable. As a result of the frequent urination that usually accompanies painful urination in infants, these babies' diapers are seldom dry.

Young children unable to state accurately that urination is painful or difficult indicate dysuria by other signs (see Box 129-1). At this age the crying that occurs because of the pain experienced with urination is identified more readily. Because of the discomfort occasioned by voiding, the child may delay urination as long as possible. This can lead to bladder distention, suprapubic discomfort, and irritability or further crying. Difficulty in either initiating or continuing urination may produce a hesitant or an episodic urine stream, which may be seen or heard when the child is seated on a potty chair or commode. In an attempt to overcome resistance to urine flow, the child may assume a squatting position or sit with each voiding. Older children use terms such as "burn," "tingle," or "hurt" to express pain, and "strain," "bear down," or "it's hard to start" to indicate discomfort and difficulty in voiding.

Although dysuria may be the only symptom, other signs and symptoms that often occur concomitantly are extremely important and helpful in establishing the cause of dysuria. Regardless of the patient's age, the associated signs and symptoms are considerably similar, and they can be placed in one of two major categories: (1) other specific urinary symptoms (e.g., hematuria, malodorous urine, or frequency) or (2) nonspecific symptoms (e.g., fever, abdominal pain, diarrhea, or vomiting). Thus, dysuria may be either the primary complaint or simply an associated symptom that often occurs with other symptoms of greater significance.[3]

PHYSICAL FINDINGS

The physical examination often yields no positive findings. However, anomalies of the external genitalia may be seen. An obstructive uropathy may be discernible as an abdominal mass (enlarged bladder, ureters, or kidneys). Palpation may elicit pain at the costovertebral angles, above the symphysis pubis, or over the abdomen in general. In baby boys a small meatal opening, frequently ulcerated, may be seen. A rectal examination may identify a fecal mass or, in boys, a tender, swollen prostate. In girls, inspection of the perineum may reveal excoriation of the skin, labia, or meatal opening. Urethral prolapse is identified by a doughnut-shaped, red, swollen mucosa protruding from the urethral orifice. In addition to erythema, vesicles and a serous, serosanguineous, or purulent discharge may be found in the vagina.

DIFFERENTIAL DIAGNOSIS

Any condition that leads to inflammation or irritation of the urinary tract or obstructs the flow of urine may cause dysuria.[5] Dysuria as the dominant symptom suggests the diagnostic possibilities shown in Box 129-2.

Urinary Tract Infection

Urinary tract infection (UTI) is the most common cause of dysuria. Pain on urination also may lead to urgency, frequency, hesitancy, and enuresis. The urine may be clear, cloudy, bloody, or foul smelling. Dysuria typically is associated with infection of the lower urinary tract, but it also may

BOX 129-1

INDICATORS OF DYSURIA

Infants	Crying when voiding
Crying	Hesitancy in starting stream
Colic	Straining
Irritability	Squatting or sitting to void
Flexing of legs	Refusing to urinate
Diaper that is wet more often than usual	
Young children	

BOX 129-2

CAUSES OF DYSURIA

Urinary tract infection	Tumors
Urethritis	Drugs
Prostatitis	Trauma
Balanoposthitis	Sexual abuse
Meatal lesions	Hematological disorders
Vulvovaginitis	Perineal dermatitis (primary)
Kidney or bladder stones	Frequent masturbation
Obstruction	Psychogenic factors
Foreign bodies	

occur with upper tract disease. Although it is not always possible clinically to differentiate an upper urinary tract infection from a lower urinary tract infection, symptoms can be helpful. Systemic symptoms such as chills, fever, or abdominal or costovertebral angle pain usually indicate pyelonephritis. Suprapubic discomfort is more consistent with cystitis.

Indirect studies such as measurement of urinary leukocyte esterase and nitrites or by microscopic examination of the urine for leukocytes or bacteria may lead the physician to strongly suspect a diagnosis of UTI. However, urine culture is required to confirm the diagnosis. In infants and preschool children the specimen should be obtained by catheterization or suprapubic aspiration. Clean-caught specimens or bag urines are not reliable techniques and may result in contaminated specimens. It is advisable not to treat a suspected UTI before obtaining a urine sample for culture and sensitivity studies. However, should the severity of illness require antibiotics prior to knowing the result of the urine culture, one should obtain the specimen by catheterization or suprapubic aspiration, regardless of the patient's age.

Upper urinary tract infection could be identified by ureteral catheterization, collection of urine by use of the bladder washout technique, or renal biopsy; however, these are invasive techniques that require anesthesia. Nuclear imaging with technetium-labeled dimercaptosuccinic acid (DMSA) is a superior, noninvasive way of identifying upper tract infection.[2] A study performed initially will document pyelonephritis; one performed after therapy will allow evaluation of the effectiveness of therapy.[4]

Bacteria are the most common cause of both upper and lower urinary tract infections. Gram-negative organisms predominate, and *Escherichia coli* is found most frequently. A mixed bacterial flora, although unusual, is apt to exist if infection occurs in a urinary tract that has structural abnormalities or if the patient has had frequent reinfections.

In adolescent girls who have both frequency and dysuria, persistent recovery of a single organism at colony counts below 10^5/ml of a clean-caught, midstream specimen is consistent with the diagnosis of infection.[6]

Viruses, particularly coxsackieviruses A11 and A12, have been identified as a cause of hemorrhagic cystitis. Dysuria usually is pronounced, and blood clots pass frequently. *Ureaplasma urealyticum, Mycoplasma hominis,* and anaerobes are other potential pathogens.[6]

Tuberculosis is an uncommon cause of urinary tract infection today, but when it is the cause, it often is accompanied by dysuria and hematuria. Both the upper and lower urinary tracts may be affected. Fungi, especially *Candida albicans,* are an unusual cause of urinary tract infection, but they may occur, usually as a superimposed infection in a patient undergoing antibiotic therapy.

Pinworms *(Enterobius vermicularis)* may lead to perineal irritation and discomfort on urination.

Urethritis

Neisseria gonorrhoeae is a major cause of urethritis in sexually active adolescent boys. A profuse, creamy urethral discharge accompanies the dysuria. In prepubertal boys, urethritis often is nonspecific; that is, no etiological agent is recovered. *Chlamydia trachomatis,* yet another organism that has been identified as a cause of urethritis, frequently appears as a recurrent infection after the patient has been treated for gonorrhea. Burning on urination is a common symptom in nongonococcal forms of urethritis.

Prostatitis

Prostatitis is confined almost exclusively to sexually active patients. In addition to dysuria, the patient often has a sensation of deep, suprapubic discomfort, and he may urinate more frequently than usual. A rectal examination will reveal a tender prostate, which after massage yields a urethral discharge. The bacteria involved vary and are determined by culturing the discharge.

Balanoposthitis

Balanoposthitis, infection of the glans penis and prepuce, is an unusual infection that may occur in uncircumcised boys. The diagnosis is readily made by inspection, and the bacterium responsible is isolated by culturing the prepucal discharge.

Meatal Lesions

In a baby boy who is still in diapers (and most often circumcised), a meatal ulcer may develop as a result of irritation by the wet diaper. An ammoniacal diaper rash also is present in most instances. Bleeding at the site of the meatal ulceration may produce a spot of blood on the diaper covering the area.

A unique lesion of the female urethra is prolapse, which appears as a circumferential ring of red or bluish mucosa protruding from the urethral orifice.

Vulvovaginitis

Various organisms can cause vulvovaginitis; those encountered most often are *N. gonorrhoeae, Haemophilus vaginalis, C. trachomatis, Trichomonas vaginalis,* and herpes progenitalis. A discharge of varying degree is present in all instances. Herpes, an infection that is associated with severe dysuria, is characterized further by the presence of vesicles, or ulcerations after rupture of the vesicles, on the vulva and vagina. All these infections are sexually transmitted. In prepubertal girls, although any of the aforementioned agents may be identified, the infection usually is nonspecific. Gonococcal infection in a prepubertal girl should be considered as evidence of child abuse until proved otherwise.

Kidney Stones/Hypercalciuria

The pain caused by kidney stones usually is "colicky" and is associated with hematuria. The passage of the stone down the ureter or through the urethra is apt to produce pain that frequently radiates to the urethral meatus. Bladder stones typically produce pain at the end of micturition. Approximately 80% of kidney and bladder stones are radiopaque and contain calcium. The family history may be positive for nephrolithiasis. Hypercalciuria without stone formation may produce dysuria and hematuria.[7] Diseases associated with renal stones include hyperparathyroidism, gout, renal tubular acidosis, idiopathic hypercalciuria, cystinuria, inflammatory bowel disease, and immobilization hypercalcemia.

Obstruction

Lesions below the bladder (posterior urethral valves, urethral strictures, urethral diverticula, or meatal stenosis) almost always are found in boys and may cause difficulty with initiating urination. Obstruction in this area may produce bladder and bilateral ureteral dilation, which can lead to overflow incontinence and suprapubic discomfort. In mild forms of urethral obstruction, dysuria may be the most important symptom. Obstructive lesions of a ureter (ureteral stricture, ureteroceles, ectopic ureters, ureteropelvic obstruction) lead to unilateral hydronephrosis, which may remain silent or cause dysuria.

Either bilateral or unilateral hydronephrotic changes increase the probability of urinary tract infection, which can then produce dysuria. Hydronephrotic urinary tracts may also be traumatized, resulting in subsequent hematuria and dysuria.

Either infection or hematuria may lead to stone formation. Finally, hydronephrotic changes may produce ptosis of urinary tract structures and can be associated with pain that radiates toward the urethra and leads to an urge to urinate. In this instance the pain may be related to changes in body position.

Other Causes of Dysuria

Children may insert foreign bodies into their own urethras or those of their playmates. Evidence of trauma at the urethral orifice and discovery of a foreign body by roentgenography confirm the diagnosis. Bladder tumors are rare in children and usually are associated with bleeding. Wilms tumor, the most common renal tumor in children, may cause dysuria with hematuria, but this presentation is most unusual.

Use of the following drugs has been associated with dysuria: amitriptyline, chlordiazepoxide, imipramine, isoniazid, sulfonamides, cyclophosphamide, heparin, dicumarol, and antihistamines.

Trauma that produces hematuria may result in dysuria. Direct trauma to the perineum or external genitalia may be an obvious cause of dysuria. Irritation of the urethra by a catheter or a cystoscope is a self-limited cause.

A special form of trauma, sexual abuse, deserves consideration in all instances in which the history and physical findings are not compatible with the symptoms or when the accusation is made by the child or a person who brings the child for treatment.

Dysuria may occur in patients who have diaper rash as a result of pain caused by the flow of urine over an irritated perineum. Local lesions may be caused by soap or bubble bath, by local infections (e.g., varicella or candidiasis), or by masturbation. Wet diapers can cause perineal irritation if they are not changed frequently.

Cystoscopic examination, which may cause dysuria, should be avoided in the management of most urinary tract infections. It may be useful, however, in identifying bladder lesions, which often cause hematuria and dysuria. Other tests may be indicated to determine renal function and to rule out hematological disorders and rare forms of renal disease.

MANAGEMENT

The major cause of dysuria is a urinary tract infection, which the pediatrician usually can manage effectively. The principles of management are precise diagnosis, adequate evaluation of the genitourinary tract, appropriate antibiotic therapy, and long-term follow-up. Details are discussed in Chapter 273, Urinary Tract Infections. Sexually transmitted diseases should be treated as discussed in Chapter 262, Sexually Transmitted Diseases.

Drugs that cause dysuria should be discontinued. Patients who have idiopathic hypercalciuria may be managed with chlorothiazide. Offending irritants such as soaps, powders, or bubble bath should be removed. Tight-fitting diapers that restrict the entrance of air should be avoided. Local medications may be indicated for a candidal infection. If oxyuriasis (pinworm infestation) is present, mebendazole should be effective. (Other family members also must be treated.) After catheterization or cystoscopic examination, sitz baths in warm water may temporarily relieve acute symptoms of dysuria. If labial adhesions produce dysuria, they may be managed as discussed in Chapter 231, Labial Adhesions.

When evidence supports the diagnosis of functional dysuria, a positive approach to management begins with minimizing the laboratory workup. For example, imaging studies may not be required initially. Counseling to ensure understanding of the dynamics involved and methods to eliminate factors contributing to the symptom are of greatest importance. The patient, when old enough, should be reassured that organic disease does not exist but that the symptom of dysuria is real and steps will be taken to alleviate it. Pediatricians can manage functional dysuria effectively when they are willing and able to spend the time necessary and show appropriate concern for the problem. Suspicion of sexual abuse requires prompt protection of the child and warrants hospitalization pending adequate evaluation. Appropriate agencies should be notified.

Urological consultation occasionally is required, notably when the diagnosis of obstructive uropathy, renal calculi, foreign bodies, tumors, or urethral prolapse is suspected or confirmed.

REFERENCES

1. Carlton CE Jr: Initial evaluation: including history, physical examination, and urinalysis. In Harrison JL, et al, editors: *Campbell's urology,* ed 5, Philadelphia, 1986, WB Saunders.
2. Heldrich FJ: 99^{m} Technetium dimercaptosuccinic acid scan in evaluating patients with urinary tract infection, *Maryland Med J* 41:215, 1992.
3. Kaplan GW, Brock WA: Voiding dysfunction in children, *Curr Probl Pediatr* 10:41, 1980.
4. Merrich MV, et al: Long-term follow-up to determine the prognostic value of imaging after urinary tract infections. Part 2: scarring, *Arch Dis Child* 72:393, 1995.
5. Rubin MI, Barratt TM, editors: *Pediatric nephrology,* Baltimore, 1975, Williams & Wilkins.
6. Sobel J, Kaye D: Urinary tract infections. In Gillenwater JY, et al, editors: *Adult and pediatric urology,* Chicago, 1987, Mosby.
7. Stapleton FB, et al: Hypercalciuria in children with urolithiasis, *Am J Dis Child* 136:675, 1982.

130 Edema

Robert H. McLean

Recognizing edema can be a clinical challenge. Edema, the swelling of tissues caused by excessive fluid accumulation, often is labeled many other things before it is recognized as just what it is. Parents often notice weight gain, chubbiness, outgrown shoes, or irritability in their child, whereas the physician may diagnose allergic problems before the fundamental cause of swelling is determined.

Recognizing edema is important because any disturbance of salt and water homeostasis in the body is significant. Water makes up 65% of the adult's body weight and 75% of the newborn's. When edema is detected early, the clinical circumstances usually are dramatic enough to determine its cause. However, when it clinically is more subtle, the diagnosis can be delayed, often with serious consequences.

Edema reflects a profound abnormality in body fluid homeostasis because so much metabolic energy is spent regulating the body's water and sodium content. The patient's age and gender, as well as the organs involved and the duration of the edema, influence its ultimate importance. Edema usually is not idiopathic in children.

PATHOPHYSIOLOGY

Under normal circumstances the movement of water between the extracellular and the intracellular body compartments is regulated carefully, with the largest quantity of water located within the intracellular spaces. The appearance of edema results from disturbances in the distribution of fluid between the two extracellular space subcompartments—the intravascular and the interstitial spaces.

At the end of the nineteenth century, Starling[3] proposed the following hypothesis to explain the movement of water between the intravascular and the interstitial spaces: At the capillary and precapillary level, two types of forces cause water to leave the intravascular space (plasma)—hydrostatic pressure (blood pressure) and oncotic pressure within the interstitium. Opposing this movement of water out of plasma are two forces: the plasma oncotic pressure and tissue turgor. The forces that create egress of water from plasma slightly outweigh the opposing ingress forces at the arterial end of the capillary bed, but the reverse is true at the venule end of the capillary bed. The result is movement of water, nutrients, and electrolytes through the interstitium at both ends of the network, but no net change occurs in intravascular and interstitial fluid exchanges. Any slight accumulation of water in the interstitial spaces is carried away in the lymphatic system.

In quantitative terms, the most important force opposing movement of water into the interstitium is the oncotic pressure.[4] Plasma contains charged electrolytes (crystalloids such as sodium and chloride) and electrically charged proteins (colloids, such as albumin). The osmotic pressure is the function of the total number of such charged particles in any given fluid. A sodium molecule is osmotically as effective as an albumin molecule, even though the latter is much larger. The sum of the positive and negative particles in each compartment containing body fluid must balance, but the exact composition of these charges varies considerably. For example, because the capillary membrane is semipermeable rather than fully permeable, the protein content of plasma normally is much greater than that of the fluid in the interstitial spaces. Because of the high plasma protein concentration and the characteristics of the capillary membranes, the total number of osmotically active particles in plasma normally is higher than the number in the interstitium. This slight difference between the osmolarity of the plasma and the osmolarity of the interstitium creates the oncotic pressure. Because this difference is caused primarily (but not exclusively) by the protein content of plasma, determining the status of protein metabolism is important in evaluating edema. For example, mechanisms that reduce oncotic pressure, such as excessive loss of protein in the urine or gastrointestinal tract, may lead to edema.

Despite this, the role of body sodium in edema is paramount in most clinical situations. Several forces control sodium balance, including the rates of glomerular filtration and aldosterone production. Simply put, continued intake of the usual amount of sodium will lead to sodium retention if the sodium-controlling factors do not respond appropriately to maintain a proper balance between the intake and output of sodium.

Sodium moves freely throughout the plasma and extracellular water spaces. It constitutes the largest cationic (positively charged) crystalloid and thus exerts the greatest osmotic force for movement of water between these spaces. Therefore, it is not surprising that excessive accumulation of sodium in the body leads to accumulation of excessive body water.

The amount of sodium in the body is regulated primarily through the process of glomerular filtration, the renin-angiotensin-aldosterone hormonal axis, and atrial natriuretic factor (ANF).[2] Normally, most sodium filtered through the glomerulus is reabsorbed through the renal tubules before it reaches the pyelocaliceal system by a precisely controlled mechanism that responds to the amount of sodium consumed each day.

Total body sodium levels become abnormal when the glomerular filtration of sodium is so reduced that sodium balance no longer can be controlled through renal tubular resorption or nonresorption. Such is the case in renal failure, in which glomerular filtration is too low to excrete sodium to any significant degree. Aldosterone excess, which may occur in intravascular volume-depleted states (e.g., nephrotic syndrome), may be a primary cause of edema.

Edema confined to a single extremity or a well-circumscribed area of the body is a special situation. This can arise from obstruction of the vascular or lymphatic system of a limb through trauma, tumor, embolization, or thrombus formation. Local release of vasoactive substances that cause locally increased vascular permeability may occur in allergic individuals and in patients who lack a particular complement system inhibitor.

Edema formation in congestive heart failure develops secondary to stimulation of the kidneys to retain sodium. Many investigators previously attributed the cause of edema in cirrhosis and idiopathic nephrotic syndrome (INS) to hypoproteinemia, with the hypoproteinemia being a consequence of the formation of ascites in cirrhosis and of urinary loss in INS. In the presence of hypoproteinemia, the patient who has INS is predicted to have reduced renal cortical perfusion, which results in increased renin/aldosterone and catecholamine production. The result of increased aldosterone production is sodium resorption, which leads to edema formation (underfill theory; Fig. 130-1).

However, considerable evidence now suggests that as with congestive heart failure, edema formation in cirrhosis and INS is due primarily to augmented retention of sodium by the kidneys (overfill theory; see Fig. 130-1). When children who have INS have their blood volume measured, only about 50% have decreased values; the rest are normal or increased. In addition, plasma renin levels have been noted to increase rather than decrease with remission of nephrotic syndrome. The presence of pure hypoalbuminemia, such as with congenital analbuminemia, is not associated with edema. Experimental studies document a "blunted" response by the nephrotic kidney to atrial natriuretic factor.[2] Because of such observations, many investigators have concluded that the pathophysiology of edema in nephrotic syndrome may be due to a primary defect that results in increased sodium retention by the kidneys.

Recent studies confirm that children who have either minimal change nephrotic syndrome or secondary forms of nephrotic syndrome have episodes of hypovolemia.[5] During such episodes, salt retention is increased markedly, and vasoactive hormones (aldosterone, renin, and norepinephrine) are elevated. These metabolic abnormalities occur during episodes of rapid and severe loss of urinary protein and support the concept that hypovolemia mediates the development of edema.

Many edematous children who have nephrotic syndrome are stable and not hypovolemic. These children presumably have subtle abnormalities of salt retention that maintain the edematous state.

CAUSES

Various disorders can lead to edema (Box 130-1).[1] The history, physical examination, and some simple laboratory tests

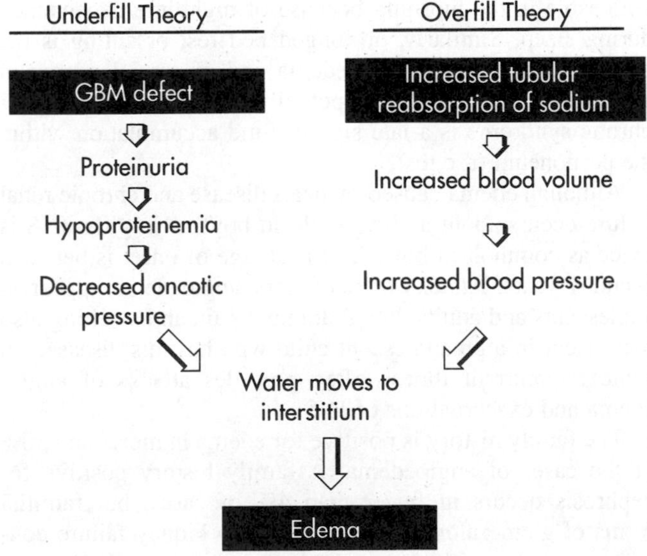

Fig. 130-1 Formation of edema in idiopathic nephrotic syndrome (INS) of childhood. Shown are the two current hypotheses for the formation of edema in INS. According to the underfill theory *(left),* fluid retention occurs secondary to the primary glomerular basement membrane (GBM) defect that produces proteinuria. According to the overfill theory *(right),* increased tubular resorption of sodium is the primary defect. Sodium retention leads to renal water resorption and the formation of edema.

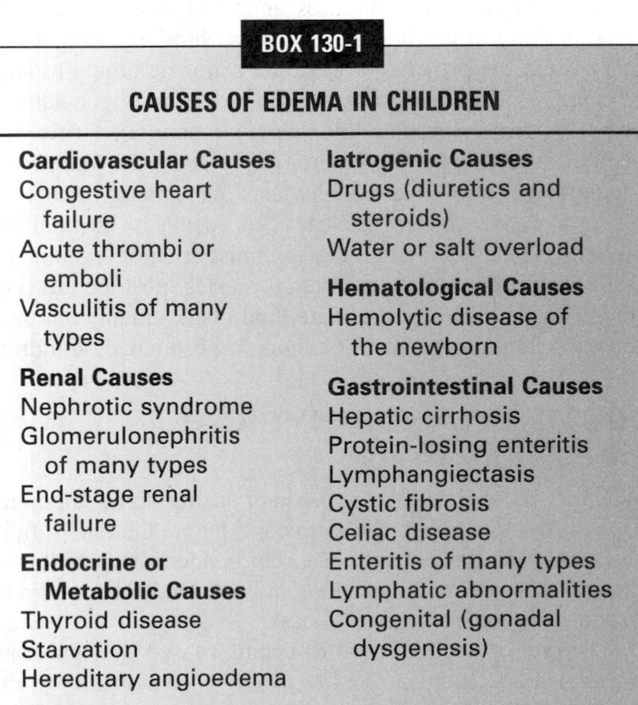
BOX 130-1

CAUSES OF EDEMA IN CHILDREN

Cardiovascular Causes
Congestive heart failure
Acute thrombi or emboli
Vasculitis of many types

Renal Causes
Nephrotic syndrome
Glomerulonephritis of many types
End-stage renal failure

Endocrine or Metabolic Causes
Thyroid disease
Starvation
Hereditary angioedema

Iatrogenic Causes
Drugs (diuretics and steroids)
Water or salt overload

Hematological Causes
Hemolytic disease of the newborn

Gastrointestinal Causes
Hepatic cirrhosis
Protein-losing enteritis
Lymphangiectasis
Cystic fibrosis
Celiac disease
Enteritis of many types
Lymphatic abnormalities
Congenital (gonadal dysgenesis)

Table 130-1 Causes of Edema and Age of Onset

Etiological Factor	Fetal or Neonatal	Infancy	Childhood	Adolescence
Hemolytic anemias	X			
Congenital heart disease	X	X	X	
Congenital kidney disease	X	X	X	X
Gastrointestinal disease	X	X	X	X
Vasculitis			X	X
Drug reactions				X
Infections	X	X		
Acute or chronic glomerulonephritis			X	X
Excessive salt and water administration	X	X	X	X
Hereditary angioedema			X	X

can point to the most likely cause, although more sophisticated procedures may be indicated.

It particularly is helpful to classify the cause of edema according to the usual age of onset (Table 130-1). In this regard the pediatrician has an advantage over the internist because this information often is less useful for diagnosis in adults.

The most common cause of chronic renal failure in children is either a congenital renal abnormality or glomerulonephritis. Signs of renal failure, such as edema, usually have their onset during infancy and childhood (unlike congenital heart disease, which so often causes edema and other symptoms at or soon after birth).

Certain forms of gastrointestinal disease cause edema early in life because of protein losses, but some congenital diseases (e.g., hepatic fibrosis associated with autosomal recessive diffuse cystic disease of the kidneys) cause signs of fluid retention only as the child grows older. Hepatic cirrhosis is an uncommon but important consideration in the evaluation of an edematous infant or child.

Vasculitis is a general term that includes anaphylactoid purpura, systemic lupus erythematosus, and a spectrum of inflammatory vascular diseases and syndromes. These diseases are rare in newborns and infants. Similarly, drug abuse and overuse of prescribed drugs are confined largely to adolescents. Abuse of narcotics can produce nephrotic syndrome and glomerulonephritis. Idiopathic glomerulonephritis and acute poststreptococcal glomerulonephritis are far more common among children and adolescents than among infants. At all ages the most common cause of edema in hospitalized patients is excessive parenteral administration of sodium and water. In the confusion of caring for a sick, postoperative, or traumatized child, inappropriate fluid management continues to be an important cause of edema in hospitalized children.

HISTORY AND PHYSICAL EXAMINATION

When trying to establish the cause of edema, some important aspects of the medical history to consider are the rate of fluid accumulation, the patient's age and gender, the location of the swelling, and the association of other medical conditions, including acute intercurrent illness.

The rate of accumulation of edema caused by significant organ damage may be so low as to go unnoticed by the parents or the child. The associated weight gain often is attributed to other causes. A change in shoe size or clothing size may be dismissed as compatible with changes that occur in a growing child.

Knowing the child's age when the edema first began is extremely helpful. The cause of edema in a newborn often can be clarified by weighing the placenta. With infants who have congenital nephrotic syndrome, the placenta is large and boggy and may weigh twice as much as normal. The appearance of edema in a newborn or infant is reason for concern because significant organ damage may be involved. Hematological and infectious disease in utero must be considered when evaluating an edematous newborn, whereas diseases of the heart, liver, and gastrointestinal tract are more common causes of edema in older infants or children.

Edema caused by nephrotic syndrome usually becomes noticeable early in the course of the disease (after a few weeks). Careful questioning can establish that subtle signs of fluid accumulation have been present for some time. Periorbital edema often is the first sign parents notice. This is more noticeable in the morning because of nighttime dependency during sleep. Similarly, prolonged bed rest or sitting is the primary cause of presacral edema and of scrotal edema in a nonambulatory child. The potbelly so characteristic of nephrotic syndrome is a late sign of fluid accumulation within the peritoneum (ascites).

Although edema caused by heart disease and chronic renal failure occurs about as frequently in boys as in girls, INS is twice as common in boys. The peak age of onset is between 3 and 4 years. Attacks of hereditary angioedema appear in adolescents and adults, but abdominal pain and swelling also may occur in a preadolescent child who has this disease. An acute intercurrent illness often precedes attacks of angioedema and exacerbations of INS.

The family history is positive for edema in more than 50% of the cases of angioedema. A family history positive for nephrosis occurs in fewer than 4% of cases, but familial forms of glomerulonephritis that lead to kidney failure constitute an identifiable cause of edema.

LABORATORY TESTS

The initial steps in the evaluation of edema must include a urinalysis. The presence of protein or abnormal cellular elements immediately focuses attention on a renal cause for the edema. The presence of large amounts of protein in a random urine specimen showing little or no blood strongly supports the diagnosis of nephrotic syndrome. The presence of red or white blood cells or casts suggests glomerulonephritis. Further evaluation of renal disease requires tests of renal function, including determining the serum urea nitrogen, creatinine, and total protein and albumin serum concentrations. If the results are abnormal, the (corrected) creatinine clearance and quantitative urine protein should be measured. Consultation with a pediatric nephrologist is appropriate at this point. Normal urinalysis and renal function tests associated with a low serum protein concentration should lead the physician to consider contrast studies of the gastrointestinal tract. Protein-losing enteropathies may be expected to be accompanied by significant symptoms of gastrointestinal aberrations (diarrhea and weight loss).

A complete blood count (CBC) and serological studies for red cell antibodies are emergency procedures in the evaluation of an edematous newborn. With chronic renal disease, anemia and an elevated sedimentation rate are expected findings; in acute infectious processes, the white blood cell (WBC) count should be elevated and the differential count should be shifted to the left.

Heart failure can be confirmed quickly with chest roentgenograms or through electrocardiography or echocardiography as the cause of edema. Unlike nephrotic syndrome or protein-losing enteropathy, congestive heart failure demands rapid corrective measures. The particular combination of abdominal cramps and localized edema (e.g., edema of the hands, feet, or larynx) should prompt the physician to consider measuring the concentration and function of the serum C_1 esterase inhibitor (C_1 INH). In 80% of individuals who have hereditary angioedema, the levels of C_1 INH are reduced; however, in the remaining 20% of cases, the levels are normal or elevated, but the functioning of the C_1 INH is reduced. Because of this, a special effort must be made to measure C_1 INH function. (Some commercial laboratories offer this test.)

MANAGEMENT

After the cause of the edema has been determined, treatment begins with managing the causative disorder. For example, if surgical correction of a cardiac lesion is possible, the appropriate corrective procedure becomes the primary therapeutic maneuver. Supportive care before specific therapy for a cardiac, renal, or other cause of edema is undertaken depends on the consequences of the edema collection. Generalized edema with dependency accumulation of fluid in the legs or abdominal or genital areas is not by itself reason for treatment. Slow accumulation of edema in nephrosis or cirrhosis generally is well tolerated. Treatment with diuretics or aldosterone inhibitors has only transient benefit in many of these chronic diseases, although such drugs may be tried if the situation demands such action. For example, if edema involves the lungs, as in heart failure, or if it may lead to a skin breakdown, as may occur in the scrotum in nephrotic syndrome, even the temporary relief provided by diuretics is indicated. In situations in which the "effective" vascular volume may be reduced, diminishing that volume further may produce acute renal failure. The use of plasma volume expanders with colloid, followed by diuretics, often is appropriate when the plasma volume is low, but this obviously should be avoided in cases involving heart failure.

Sodium requirements should be assessed carefully. Sodium and fluid restriction may be all that is required to correct the edema and is essential in iatrogenic cases. For chronic edema, patients and parents should be taught about the sodium content of foods so that the minimum sodium necessary for palatability of food is ingested. It is good practice to maintain this diet between episodes of edema, inasmuch as patients can adjust well to a low-sodium diet, but switching back and forth is difficult. Acute episodes of edema associated with nephrotic syndrome occasionally are accompanied by irritability and changes in behavior. The self-image of the child who has chronic edema can be affected seriously, either because the edema may be interpreted as obesity in an adolescent or because the underlying disease may require changes in the patient's activities and lifestyle. The physician and parents should be alert for such secondary effects of edema so that they can minimize the consequences for the child.

Several of the diseases that may cause significant edema require the assistance of a specialist. However, because these patients eventually return home, the primary care physician must be available for proper continuous care. The specialist should ensure that the patient and family are familiar with the early signs of recurrence or worsening of the process. The importance of keeping accurate records of weight, urine protein excretion, and blood pressure must be explained. Most parents and patients become more comfortable with a chronic disease when they acquire a working knowledge of the disorder and can participate in the required care. With such education, the primary physician can rely more fully on the parents' observations, which are of immeasurable help in managing edema at home.

REFERENCES

1. Fisher DA: Obscure and unusual edema, *Pediatrics* 37:506, 1966.
2. Perico N, Remuzzi G: Edema of the nephrotic syndrome: the role of the atrial peptide system, *Am J Kidney Dis* 22:355, 1993.
3. Starling EH: On the absorption of fluids from the connective tissue spaces, *J Physiol* 19:312, 1985.
4. Valtin H: *Renal function: mechanisms preserving fluid and solute balance in health*, ed 2, Boston, 1983, Little, Brown.
5. Vande Walle JGJ, Donckerwolcke RA, Koomans HA: Pathophysiology of edema formation in children with nephrotic syndrome not due to minimal change disease, *J Am Soc Nephrol* 10:2, 1999.

131 Epistaxis

David R. Edelstein • Nissim Khabie

Epistaxis, which occurs frequently in childhood, can be a frightening experience for a parent or child. Most nasal bleeding in childhood is minor and never comes to a physician's attention. Severe, prolonged, or recurrent bleeding, however, can indicate a more severe problem such as a bleeding disorder or nasal tumor. Epistaxis is rare in neonates and infants, increases in incidence in childhood, and again becomes less common after puberty until later in life.[12] It is more common in males than in females.[24]

The nose functions as an air filter, humidifier, and heater. It also serves as a buffer for central structures during trauma and acts as a resonance box for speech. To perform these functions, the nose is a highly vascular organ with a large surface area. Its high vascularity helps to warm the temperature of inspired air, deliver immunoglobulins and leukocytes to aid in immunity, and provide an expansile surface area that aids in filtration and cleaning. The most vascular areas are near the front of the nose in Little's area, which is the site of a plexus of vessels with branches from the internal and external carotid arteries (Table 131-1). Two other critical areas of the nose are the posterolateral portion, which contains large branches of the internal maxillary artery, and a portion high in the lateral nasal vault that contains other branches of the internal carotid artery.

There are many possible causes for nasal bleeding. Fortunately, most are benign. These include mucosal irritation from weather changes and allergies, trauma from nose picking, chronic rhinitis with nose blowing, chronic usage of nasal sprays or drying agents such as decongestants, and viral or bacterial infections. More serious epistaxis may occur as a result of blunt trauma from accidents or nasal surgery. In some cases, severe or recurrent bleeds may represent a bleeding diathesis such as von Willebrand's disease or a neoplasm such as nasopharyngeal angiofibroma. Distinguishing local from systemic causes is very important in order to institute early treatment and avoid the need for a blood transfusion. The correct diagnosis may have implications for the patient's family or community because many causes of epistaxis may be genetic or result from environmental problems.

CHARACTERISTICS

The type, location, and frequency of nasal bleeding may help the physician understand its cause and danger. In 1988, Katsanis et al[13] devised an epistaxis scoring system to help identify children who may need elaborate workups. This system is based on the frequency, duration, amount, and site of bleeding. Children who had high scores had a greater incidence of anemia and a family history of bleeding dyscrasias. Standard criteria are important in deciding whether to proceed with an elaborate evaluation for a bleeding disorder. Children who merit a high index of suspicion for a bleeding disorder need diagnostic tests beyond complete blood count (CBC), platelet count, prothrombin time (PT), and partial thromboplastin time (PTT) measurements.

In most instances, epistaxis is unilateral and is caused by local irritation or trauma. Bilateral epistaxis, in contrast, may be due to a bleeding disorder, a posterior source of bleeding, or severe craniofacial trauma. Gradual-onset bleeding often results from overuse of medications such as aspirin or ibuprofen in an older child[26] or from slowly growing tumors. In contrast, sudden-onset bleeding usually is due to trauma or nose picking. Intermittent bleeding may be caused by changes in the weather, allergies, or low humidification of inspired air. It also can be associated with menses.

The location of the bleeding may be useful in determining the cause and the treatment. An anterior bleed, which can be viewed with a nasal speculum, can be treated by simple compression. In contrast, a posterior bleed can be visualized only if the anatomy of the nose is normal and adequate premedication and special instruments are used. A high nasal bleed may represent a fracture involving the nasoethmoid complex and orbit. Recurrent epistaxis may occur in a patient who has a minor bleeding disorder or in one who suffers from chronic irritation of the nasal mucosa.

ASSOCIATED SIGNS AND SYMPTOMS

Although epistaxis is a dramatic symptom, it usually is not the only one related to the nose. Other symptoms and signs on physical examination can be useful in arriving at a diagnosis. For example, a child who has nasal obstruction and epistaxis may have a foreign body or a polyp in the nose. Anatomical causes of obstruction, such as a deviated septum or a unilateral choanal atresia, may present with bleeding from the affected side as a result of irritation or dryness.[10] Chronic nasal obstruction related to lower airway symptoms may indicate perennial allergic rhinitis associated with asthma.[19]

It is important to know if the patient has had facial pain or headaches. Facial pain may be present with sinusitis or an enlarging mucocele of one of the sinuses. It also can be caused by a tumor involving the nose, the sinuses, or the base of the skull, which may bleed intermittently. An encephalocele or meningocele can cause headaches associated with epistaxis in infants.

Children who have trauma-induced epistaxis should be tested for visual acuity because injury to the nose or ethmoid sinuses may disrupt the lamina papyracea and injure the eye, resulting in retroorbital bleeding, orbital fractures, and damage to the eye muscles. The cribriform plate also can be fractured, which can result in meningitis, anosmia (lack of smell), or chronic leakage of cerebrospinal fluid (CSF) through the nose.

Occasionally the only symptom noticed by the parents of a child who has chronic mild epistaxis is unexplained melena. This is due to the child swallowing blood from the posterior nares. Similarly, hematemesis can result from epistaxis when the child swallows blood.

All children who have epistaxis should have their vital signs monitored closely. Hypotension and syncope-like episodes can occur if the blood loss is significant. Some children who have had chronic nasal bleeding may tolerate a surprisingly low hematocrit. Younger children and infants tolerate blood loss less well than do older children; a blood transfusion may be required in severe cases.

One of the most useful observations the physician can make is whether other members of the family have bleeding disorders or problems with epistaxis. Although episodes of epistaxis are relatively rare in the general population, they are common in patients who have coagulation disorders. Inherited deficits such as factor V, VII, VIII, or X deficiencies can manifest as recurrent epistaxis.[17,22] Families of children who have chronic bleeding may have hereditary hemorrhagic telangiectasia syndrome (Osler-Weber-Rendu disease). This is an autosomal dominantly inherited disease associated with increased fragility of small blood vessels, with an incidence of only 1 to 2 per 100,000. Epistaxis is caused by defects in the walls of small mucosal vessels. Ninety percent of patients with this disorder present with epistaxis by age 12, and adults can average up to 18 episodes of epistaxis per month.[17]

Table 131-1 Blood Supply of the Nose

Vessel	Location
Internal Carotid Artery	
Ophthalmic artery	
Anterior ethmoid	Anterosuperior septum, anterior lateral wall
Posterior ethmoid	Posterior septum, posterior lateral wall
External Carotid Artery	
Internal maxillary artery	
Sphenopalatine branch	Posterior septum, posterior lateral wall
Nasopalatine branch	Posterior septum, floor of the nose
Descending palatine branch	Posterior lateral wall
Pharyngeal branch	Nasopharyngeal roof
Facial artery	
Superior labial branch	Tip of septum, nasal alar

DIFFERENTIAL DIAGNOSIS

The easiest way to conceptualize the many causes of epistaxis is to categorize them according to either local or systemic causes (Box 131-1). Local causes include trauma, surgery, infection, medications, or tumors. Systemic causes may be divided into bleeding disorders, other major diseases (e.g., leukemia, renal dysfunction, and hypertension), and cancer therapy (radiotherapy or chemotherapy).[7]

Most nasal injuries in children occur at home or during sporting events. Bleeding occurs because the nasal septum is abraded. Intranasal hematomas, abscesses, and lacerations can be overlooked unless the physician carefully inspects for

BOX 131-1

CAUSES OF EPISTAXIS IN CHILDREN

Local

1. *Trauma:* nose picking, surgery (septoplasty, turbinectomy), blunt impact (fist or instrument), foreign body, child abuse, sports, vehicular accident
2. *Infection:* viral, bacterial, fungal, and parasitic
3. *Chronic irritation:* allergies, recurrent colds, dry environment, chronic sniffers, smoking, cocaine abuse, ciliary dysfunction, chemicals, ingestion of a caustic substance
4. *Structural abnormality:* deviated septum, vomer spur, septal perforation
5. *Drugs:* topical sprays (phenylephrine, aerosol steroids), drying agents (decongestants, antihistamines)
6. *Neoplasms:* polyps, hemangiomas, rhabdomyosarcomas, and angiofibromas

Systemic

1. *Bleeding diseases:* von Willebrand's, coagulation factor deficiencies, vitamin deficiencies, Osler-Weber-Rendu, idiopathic thrombocytopenia, disseminated intravascular coagulation
2. *Infections:* rheumatic fever, diphtheria, malaria, and measles
3. *Neoplasms:* leukemia, lymphoma
4. *Granulomas:* Wegener, midline reticulosis, tuberculosis, and sarcoidosis
5. *Medications:* antiinflammatories (aspirin, ibuprofen), anticoagulants (warfarin), steroids
6. *Cancer treatment:* chemotherapy (methotrexate), radiotherapy
7. *Hormonal influences:* menses, birth control pills, and pregnancy
8. *Cardiovascular disease:* hypertension, arteriosclerosis
9. *Barometric pressure changes:* scuba diving, air flight, elevator rides
10. *Miscellaneous:* liver disease, renal dysfunction, aplastic anemia, and sepsis

them. Failure to recognize an infection or a blood clot lodged in this area may result in pressure necrosis of the nasal septum and eventual external and internal nasal deformities. Major facial fractures also can manifest in this way; thus a complete examination of the facial structures should be performed when this diagnosis is considered.

Occasionally, epistaxis may occur after surgery. Postoperative bleeding from the tonsils and adenoids can mimic epistaxis. Septal surgery, rhinoplasty, and turbinectomies also can lead to postoperative bleeding among adolescents. Whenever a child undergoes nasotracheal intubation, the nasal mucosa may be torn, which can lead to bleeding.

Chronic nasal irritation as a result of infection, allergies, or drugs can cause epistaxis. Local mucosal cellulitis and failure of the mucociliary lining of the nose to function properly after an infection may cause Little's area to become dry and cracked. Children who have chronic rhinorrhea may rub their noses frequently, thereby irritating the septum significantly. Chronic irritation also can occur from overuse of topical antiallergic sprays (e.g., cromolyn sulfate and dexamethasone). Cocaine use should be considered in adolescents with epistaxis. Cocaine causes local infection, chronic necrosis of the mucosa and septum, and foreign-body reactions and destroys nasal ciliary function.

A variety of nasal masses can cause bloody rhinorrhea in children. Hemangiomas, which are among the most common benign tumors of the nose during childhood, can cause epistaxis. Juvenile angiofibromas should be considered in adolescent boys who have unilateral spontaneous epistaxis and a nasopharyngeal mass or persistent unilateral serous otitis media.[14] Angiofibromas can be differentiated from benign choanoantral polyps by computed tomography (CT) scanning using a contrast medium.[20] Blind biopsies of the nasopharynx should be avoided because of the risk of life-threatening epistaxis.

Excessive nasal bleeding may be caused by a variety of acquired or inherited bleeding disorders. Aspirin and other nonsteroidal antiinflammatory drugs (NSAIDs) can cause a relative platelet dysfunction that results in a prolonged bleeding time.[26] Deficiencies of vitamins C and K also can predispose a child to epistaxis because of blood vessel changes and coagulopathies, respectively. Thrombocytopenia can occur after use of sulfisoxazole, chloroquine, carbamazepine, estrogens, and thiazide diuretics. Ingesting toxic substances and eating certain foods such as beans can lead to thrombocytopenia. Viral illnesses may cause idiopathic thrombocytopenic purpura. Inherited disorders such as Osler-Weber-Rendu disease, as well as coagulopathies, should be considered. The most common inherited bleeding disorders that cause epistaxis in children are von Willebrand's disease and factor XI deficiency (hemophilia C). Less common disorders are factor VIII deficiency (hemophilia A) and factor IX deficiency (hemophilia B, or Christmas disease).

Epistaxis may occur in immunocompromised children. Leukemia and lymphomas that involve the bone marrow can lead to thrombocytopenia and concomitant bleeding. In addition, the chemotherapeutic agents used to treat these malignant diseases (e.g., methotrexate and cyclophosphamide) can cause thrombocytopenia.[8] Radiotherapy often causes cracking, irritation in the nasal mucosa, and bleeding.

As noted, epistaxis has many causes. The patient's age and the circumstances that surround the onset of bleeding are important clues to the diagnosis. In neonates the most common cause is birth trauma, especially if forceps are used. Frequently the bleeding is caused by deflection of the nasal septum, which can be manipulated gently back into position or left as is if no deformity results. In childhood, simple nose picking and blunt trauma are the most common causes. In early adolescence, boys have a higher incidence of nasal tumors, such as angiofibromas,[20] than do girls. Pubescent girls may have occasional bleeding during their menses.

MANAGEMENT

The basic approach to treatment of children who have epistaxis should incorporate the "two Cs"—calmness and compression. The patient should be reassured during the history-taking and the assessment of his or her general condition and the amount of blood loss. Having the child sit upright and gently squeezing the anterior nose for 5 minutes can stop most bleeding. Blood pressure and other vital signs should be taken. Blood tests and roentgenograms should be performed only if the bleeding cannot be stopped with simple pressure or anterior or posterior nasal packing.[4] The first few minutes should be used to stem the bleeding while assessing its cause.

Once the initial bleeding has slowed, the nose should be examined more carefully with a nasal speculum and headlight. A simple solution of oxymetazoline (Afrin) can be sprayed into the nose for local vasoconstriction to control further bleeding and to help clear any clots that may have formed.[15] A 1% epinephrine solution with or without lidocaine can be used for the same purpose, if required.[2,9] Nose blowing should be avoided even though the nose will feel congested. Obvious bleeding sites in Little's area can be cauterized electrically or with silver nitrate sticks. If either form of cautery is used, the septum should be covered with a petroleum jelly-based antibiotic ointment to provide a moist environment for optimum healing. Care should be taken to clean any excess silver nitrate from the anterior nares because it will discolor the skin and may frighten the child and family.

If these simple measures fail to control the bleeding, the next step is to place bilateral anterior nasal packing, using a ½-inch gauze covered with petroleum jelly. Although this is not pleasant for the child, it is a highly effective way to stop anterior nasal bleeding. Bilateral packing is recommended to provide the greatest compression of the anterior septum. When packing is used, antibiotics should be given to prevent sinusitis. The packing usually is left in place for 3 days.

Another excellent choice for treatment of anterior epistaxis is the Merocel sponge. It is a compressed sponge that expands when wet, exerting pressure on the nasal lining.[23] This sponge comes in many sizes, can be cut down to fit a child's nose, and is easily placed, especially when the child is agitated. Its use is limited by its tendency to adhere to the nasal lining; it must be used with antibiotics to prevent staphylococcal toxic shock and should be removed within 48 hours. Additional agents include the use of oxidized cellulose (Surgicel) or Gelfoam, absorbable agents that also help provide hemostasis.[25] These agents may be the treatment of choice for patients in whom standard nasal packing might promote more bleeding by destroying the lining of the nose. This group of children includes those undergoing renal dialysis, those with coagulopathies, and those who are severely immunocompromised.

Refractory posterior bleeding can be controlled with placement of either posterior packs or nasopharyngeal balloons. Posterior packs are made from gauze pads inserted through the mouth into the nasopharynx and secured by ties through the nose.[3] Whenever they are used, an anterior pack also is placed. Easier to use, and often more effective, are balloon catheters. Some authors suggest the use of a single-balloon catheter, such as the Foley catheter, placed in the nasopharynx. Double-balloon catheters (Epistat) that have anterior (septal) and posterior (nasopharyngeal) balloons provide excellent hemostasis for difficult bleeding. When Foley catheters are used, they can be filled with methylene blue-stained saline to indicate if the Foley balloon has burst accidentally. All posterior packs cause significant discomfort for the patient. Furthermore, because of the possibility of hypoxia and pulmonary complications as a result of the "nasopulmonary reflex" (changes in pulmonary function induced by packing), most authors suggest patients with posterior packs should have supplemental oxygen and should be under close observation.[2,11,16]

Severe bleeding that does not respond to packing should prompt the physician to consider a different diagnosis and perhaps use more invasive therapeutic procedures. The use of tests for bleeding disorders, including determination of bleeding time, prothrombin time, partial thromboplastin time, and platelet count, as well as other hematological studies, should be based on the history. Roentgenographic studies should be reviewed for mass lesions, bone erosion, and other bony abnormalities. Angiographic examination of the internal and external carotid arteries should be considered for severe unremitting bleeding.

Nasal endoscopy enhances the physician's examination of the nose. Fiberoptic and rigid endoscopes are routine instruments in the office of most otolaryngologists. In experienced hands, endoscopic cauterization can stop posterior epistaxis in more than 90% of patients.[9,21] The advantage of this technique is that bleeding can be controlled under direct visualization. The limitations are absence of appropriate-size pediatric instruments in some otolaryngologists' offices and difficulty obtaining the patient's cooperation.

Persistent posterior nasal bleeding from the sphenopalatine artery sometimes requires ligation of the internal maxillary artery. This type of bleeding after trauma, which may be due to a tear of the anterior ethmoid artery, requires surgical ligation for control. Ligation of bleeding vessels can be performed either with open surgery or endoscopically.[5] Children may be more prone to traumatic tears of the anterior ethmoid artery because of immature bony development of the face and congenital dehiscences around the artery.

Embolization is a newly accepted method of controlling severe bleeding.[28] Recent articles have recorded success rates from 80% to 93%, compared with an average success rate of 88% in ligation.[6,18] Embolization is a useful procedure with hereditary hemorrhagic telangiectasia, juvenile angiofibromas, hemangiomas, vascular metastatic lesions, arteriovenous malformations, and traumatic arterial tears. The advantage of embolization is an overall lower rate of morbidity. However, most studies report a slightly increased rate of major complications, usually neurological.

When recurrent, moderate epistaxis fails to respond to conservative therapy, the underlying cause must be addressed. In some cases, this means medical correction of the bleeding diathesis. In others, surgical correction of anatomical defects must be performed. This includes septoplasty, laser photocoagulation of telangiectasias, or even skin grafts to cover diseased mucosal surfaces.[1] One study suggests that patients requiring multiple interventions, a 3-day hospital stay, or three or more units of blood should be considered for surgical intervention.[27]

Although the goals of epistaxis management are to stop the bleeding and determine its cause, the care of the patient often needs to be continued after the bleeding stops. Blood replacement or iron supplements may be required, and humidifying medications, such as saline nasal sprays, and petroleum jelly-based ointments often are needed to promote healing and adequate nasal mucociliary function. Children who have had severe epistaxis should be reexamined frequently to determine if further therapy is necessary. Recurrence of epistaxis can be prevented only if its many causes are considered and appropriate preventive measures are instituted.

REFERENCES

1. Bergler W, et al: Argon plasma coagulation for the treatment of hereditary hemorrhagic telangiectasias, *Laryngoscope* 109:15, 1999.
2. Bingham B, Dingle AF: Endoscopic management of severe epistaxis, *J Otolaryngol* 20:442, 1991.
3. Cannon CR: Effective treatment protocol for posterior epistaxis: a 10-year experience, *Otolaryngol Head Neck Surg* 109:722, 1993.
4. Cassisi NJ, Biller HF, Ogura JH: Changes in arterial oxygen tension and pulmonary mechanics with the use of posterior packing in epistaxis: a preliminary report, *Laryngoscope* 81:1261, 1971.
5. Christmas DA, Yanagisawa E, Pastrano JA: Transnasal endoscopic ligation of the sphenopalatine artery, *Ear Nose Throat J* 77:524, 1998.
6. Cullen MM, Tami TT: Comparison of internal maxillary artery ligation versus embolization for refractory posterior epistaxis, *Otolaryngol Head Neck Surg* 118:636, 1998.
7. della Faille D, et al: Posterior epistaxis: our experience with transantral ligation and embolisation, *Acta Otorhinolaryngol Belg* 51:167, 1997.
8. DiNardo LJ, Hendrix RA: The infectious and hematologic otolaryngologic complications of myelosuppressive cancer chemotherapy, *Otolaryngol Head Neck Surg* 105:101, 1991.
9. Frikart L, Agrifoglio A: Endoscopic treatment of posterior epistaxis, *Rhinology* 36:59, 1998.
10. Guarisco JL, Graham HD: Epistaxis in children: causes, diagnosis, and treatment, *Ear Nose Throat J* 68:522, 1989.
11. Jensen PF, et al: Episodic nocturnal hypoxia and nasal packs, *Clin Otolaryngol* 16:433, 1991.
12. Juselius H: Epistaxis: a clinical study of 1,724 patients, *J Laryngol Otol* 88:317, 1974.
13. Katsanis E, et al: Prevalence and significance of mild bleeding disorders in children with recurrent epistaxis, *J Pediatr* 113:73, 1988.
14. Komoroski EM: Nasopharyngeal carcinoma: early warning signs and symptoms, *Pediatr Emerg Care* 10:284, 1994.
15. Krempl GA, Noorily AD: Use of oxymetazoline in the management of epistaxis, *Ann Otol Rhinol Laryngol* 104:704, 1995.

16. Loftus BC, Blitzer A, Cozine K: Epistaxis, medical history, and the nasopulmonary reflex: what is clinically relevant? *Otolaryngol Head Neck Surg* 110:363, 1994.
17. Manning SC, Culbertson MC: Epistaxis. In Bluestone CD, Stool SE, Kenna MA, editors: *Pediatric otolaryngology,* ed 3, Philadelphia, 1996.
18. Moreau S, et al: Supraselective embolization in intractable epistaxis: review of 45 cases, *Laryngoscope* 108:887, 1998.
19. Murray AB, Milner RA: Allergic rhinitis and recurrent epistaxis in children, *Ann Allergy Asthma Immunol* 75:30, 1995.
20. Neel HB III, et al: Juvenile angiofibroma: review of 120 cases, *Am J Surg* 126:547, 1973.
21. O'Leary-Stickney K, Makielski K, Weymuller EA Jr: Rigid endoscopy for the control of epistaxis, *Arch Otolaryngol Head Neck Surg* 118:966, 1992.
22. Peyvandi F, et al: Bleeding symptoms in 27 Iranian patients with the combined deficiency of factor V and factor VIII, *Br J Haematol* 100: 773, 1998.
23. Pringle MB, Beasley P, Brightwell AP: The use of Merocel nasal packs in the treatment of epistaxis, *J Laryngol Otol* 110:543, 1996.
24. Sessions RB: Nasal hemorrhage, *Otolaryngol Clin North Am* 6:727, 1973.
25. Shaw CB, Wax MK, Wetmore SJ: Epistaxis: a comparison of treatment, *Otolaryngol Head Neck Surg* 109:60, 1993.
26. Tay HL, et al: Aspirin, nonsteroidal anti-inflammatory drugs, and epistaxis: a regional record linkage case control study, *Ann Otol Rhinol Laryngol* 107:671, 1998.
27. Tomkinson A, et al: Patterns of hospital attendance with epistaxis, *Rhinology* 35:129, 1997.
28. Welsh LW, et al: Role of angiography in the management of refractory epistaxis, *Ann Otol Rhinol Laryngol* 99:69, 1990.
29. Wurman LH, et al: The management of epistaxis, *Am J Otolaryngol* 13:193, 1992.

132 Extremity Pain

Michael G. Burke

Extremity pain is a common complaint in primary care pediatric practice. Up to 16% of school-age children report at least one episode of activity-limiting extremity pain annually.[1] Between 6% and 7% of pediatric office visits are related to extremity pain.[3,5] Fortunately, most of these visits involve pain secondary to only minor trauma. Occasionally, however, limb pain is the presenting complaint of a systemic illness, a neoplasm, an infectious process, a nutritional derangement, or a specific orthopedic disease. The challenge for the practitioner is to determine when the pain is significant without exposing the child to excessive diagnostic studies and without delaying treatment or referral. For the most part, this determination is based on the history and physical examination alone.

HISTORY

A careful history from patients and parents often reveals the etiology of extremity pain in children. Pain described as aching or cramping is likely to be muscular in origin. Bone pain often is described as deep, and nerve pain as burning, tingling, or numbness. Referred pain is common in children;thus, although usually helpful, the location of pain may be deceiving. Migrating extremity pain is less likely to occur secondary to trauma and is more typical of systemic illness such as leukemia, acute rheumatic fever, disseminated gonorrhea, and arthralgia or arthritis associated with inflammatory bowel disease. The mode of onset, variability, duration, and frequency of pain also help in determining its cause. Activities associated with worsening or relief of pain also can lead to a diagnosis. Likewise, color change associated with extremity pain may indicate inflammation (faint red), infection (intense red), or autonomic dysfunction (pallor, cyanosis, and erythema). Stiffness not associated with trauma should prompt concern about a rheumatological process.

A history specific to trauma associated with extremity pain can be helpful. Trauma accompanied by an audible "pop" or "snap" is more likely the result of a sprain or fracture. Mild trauma that leads to a fracture might indicate some previous defect in the bone, as with a pathological fracture. As always, if the physical findings of trauma are greater than would be expected from the history, physical abuse must be considered.

The child's general health history is needed to complete the picture of extremity pain. For example, the differential diagnosis changes with age. Toxic synovitis of the hip is a common diagnosis in a child younger than age 10 years; a slipped capital femoral epiphysis is more likely in an overweight adolescent.

As a screen for systemic disease, all systems should be reviewed briefly. Particular attention should be paid to a history of fever, recent weight loss, sweating, rashes, and gastrointestinal symptoms. A history of recent medications is important and might reveal a serum sickness–like illness (particularly associated with cefaclor). Even a short course of systemic steroids can cause aseptic necrosis of the hip or can result in demineralization of bone and the pain associated with osteoporosis. Immunizations, particularly for rubella, may cause joint or extremity pain, and a history of exposure to viral illness might explain myalgia or arthralgia. Specifically, the prodrome of hepatitis B can cause significant arthralgia.

The patient's family history may reveal a tendency toward autoimmune disease or recent exposure to infectious diseases. The family history particularly is helpful in identifying hemoglobinopathies. A family history of sickle cell anemia in a 6- to 24-month-old child whose hands and feet are painfully swollen may lead to the diagnosis of hand-foot syndrome and previously undiagnosed sickle cell disease. A sickle cell pain crisis always must be considered in a black child or one of Mediterranean origin who has a painful extremity. HLA-B27 is associated with Reiter's syndrome or ankylosing spondylitis and has been described in association with peripheral enthesitis (inflammation of tendons, ligaments, or fascia at their attachments to bone).[6] Joint hypermobility syndrome and fibromyalgia also can be familial.

Extremity pain may be a symptom of a functional disorder and can serve as an entry to the physician's office for the child or parent who has a hidden agenda. One large pediatric rheumatology group has estimated that 11% of their new patients suffer from psychosomatic musculoskeletal pain.[7] In cases of functional pain, the history may be either quite dramatic or highly understated. Pain in a nonanatomical distribution or that disturbs unpleasant but not pleasant activities (waxing on school days and waning on weekends) should raise suspicion of a functional disorder. Eliciting a history of recent events at home, recent school performance, and other social history can be essential to determining the diagnosis.

PHYSICAL EXAMINATION

It is worthwhile to do a brief general physical examination, even if the history points to extremity pain from minor local trauma. Abnormalities in blood pressure, heart rate, or growth pattern can reveal an endocrine cause. An elevated resting heart rate is associated with rheumatic fever. Pallor, fever, lymphadenopathy, or organomegaly may be clues to systemic disease. A rash, particularly, may be helpful. Dermatomyositis occurs with muscle pain and proximal weakness associated with a vasculitic rash on the extensor surfaces of knuckles, knees, and elbows (Gottron papules). Palpable purpura and extremity pain are associated with Schönlein-Henoch purpura. A photosensitive rash in a child who has limb pain might point to systemic lupus erythematosus (SLE), dermatomyositis, or parvovirus infection. Nail pitting is associated with psoriasis, a rare cause of extremity pain.

A thorough eye examination to detect the presence of various forms of uveitis can help diagnose juvenile rheumatoid arthritis (JRA), which may cause extremity pain. A complete physical examination can reveal generalized joint laxity and hyperextensibility, differentiating benign hypermobility syndrome from a focal ligament injury. In benign hypermobility syndrome, the joint laxity allows chronic hyperextension, which can cause pain, often located in the popliteal fossa. The pain often is worse in the evening and can be relieved by exercise that tightens the joint. This syndrome, particularly, is common in gymnasts and dancers.

Claudication is a rare cause of extremity pain in children. However, in popliteal artery entrapment syndrome, vascular calf pain that radiates to the foot is associated with an anomalous popliteal artery or anomalous placement of the gastrocnemius muscle.[2] The pain begins with activity, sometimes more with walking than with running. This syndrome is suggested if normal pedal pulses are lost with simultaneous knee extension and foot plantar flexion.

Because referred pain is common in children, the physical examination should include areas proximal and distal to the site of the complaint. A slipped capital femoral epiphysis and Legg-Calvé-Perthes disease, both of which affect the hip, can manifest as knee or thigh pain, whereas an abscess of the psoas muscle may cause hip pain. Some abdominal processes and diskitis also may cause extremity pain.

Examination of a painful extremity should include assessment of peripheral vascular status, muscle strength, soft-tissue swelling, and skeletal and joint integrity. Peripheral vascular status is assessed by palpating the pulses and determining the capillary refill time distal to the pain. Skin color and warmth, tenderness to palpation, and the extent of passive and active range of motion should all be assessed. Point tenderness over a bone raises suspicion of a fracture. Point tenderness in the absence of a clear history of trauma may indicate osteomyelitis. It is helpful to compare the opposite limb when assessing swelling, muscle wasting, or joint mobility. Observing the patient's gait or use of the painful limb when he or she is unaware of the observation helps in diagnosing a functional process. In evaluating strength, it is important to remember that isolated distal weakness is likely to be of neurological origin, whereas proximal weakness most likely is due to a muscular disease. Finally, with chronic extremity pain, serial examinations of the patient over the course of weeks can be the key to diagnosis.

LABORATORY AND ROENTGENOGRAPHIC EVALUATION

Laboratory studies are unnecessary for most extremity pain. However, if the history and physical examination do not lead to a definitive diagnosis, if they raise suspicion of a systemic or an infectious disease, or if the pain persists longer than anticipated, screening laboratory tests are in order. A basic evaluation should include a complete blood count (CBC), a sedimentation rate, a C-reactive protein, and a sickle cell preparation or hemoglobin electrophoresis when indicated. Rheumatological studies should be considered if the aforementioned diseases are suspected or if the pain becomes chronic. An elevated sedimentation rate raises suspicion of an infectious or inflammatory disorder, or occasionally of a neoplastic one. A CBC may reveal anemia or may suggest an infectious disease. With leukemia the white blood cell (WBC) count varies, but immature forms may be present in the differential WBC count or there may be thrombocytopenia. A creatine phosphokinase (CPK) determination occasionally is indicated if muscular pain is suspected.

Radiological studies often are unnecessary in evaluating limb pain. However, because of the plasticity of children's bones, traumatic injury that ordinarily would cause only a sprain in an adult is more likely to result in a greenstick or buckle fracture in a child. Therefore, a lower threshold for obtaining posttraumatic radiographs in children may be justified. The presence of point tenderness and/or gross deformity in an extremity or pain on motion of the involved limb increase the likelihood of fracture.

When there is no clear history of trauma, roentgenograms can help identify bony tumors, pathological fractures, some metabolic defects, and a number of orthopedic conditions.

A bone scan is a useful diagnostic tool in evaluating limb pain, and one should be considered when a stress fracture or osteomyelitis is suspected. Bone scans are more sensitive than plain roentgenograms for establishing these diagnoses.

DIFFERENTIAL DIAGNOSIS

The differential diagnosis of extremity pain is extremely broad (Box 132-1). However, most limb pain is benign, requires no intervention, and is self-limited. Characteristic patterns of pain and associated signs and symptoms signal the presence of certain diseases and conditions. A discussion of some of these disorders follows.

Growing Pains

"Growing pains" are a time-honored pediatric disorder. They are intermittent, deep extremity pains that affect the lower more often than the upper extremities. The pain nearly always is bilateral, rarely involves the joints, and almost universally is worse at night, resolving completely in the morning. Despite their name, growing pains do not occur most frequently during periods of rapid growth. Instead, their onset is described at 3 to 5 or 8 to 12 years of age. Most growing pains resolve in 12 to 24 months; however, they may persist into adolescence.

The cause of growing pains remains unclear. A previous

BOX 132-1

EXTREMITY PAIN IN CHILDHOOD: A DIFFERENTIAL DIAGNOSIS

Allergy/Collagen-Vascular Origin
Dermatomyositis
Familial Mediterranean fever
Henoch-Schönlein purpura
Inflammatory bowel disease
Juvenile rheumatoid arthritis
Mixed connective tissue disease
Polyarteritis nodosa
Rheumatic fever
Scleroderma
Serum sickness
Systemic lupus erythematosus

Congenital Origin
Caffey's disease
Hemophilia
Mucolipidosis
Mucopolysaccharidosis
Popliteal artery entrapment syndrome
Sickle cell anemia/thalassemia

Endocrine Origin
Hypercortisolism
Hyperparathyroidism
Hypothyroidism

Idiopathic Origin
Fibromyalgia
Growing pains
Guillain-Barré syndrome
Sarcoidosis

Infectious Origin
Bacterial
- Arthralgia/myalgia associated with streptococcal infection
- Diskitis/spinal epidural abscess
- Gonorrhea
- Osteomyelitis
- Pyogenic myositis
- Septic arthritis

Enteric disease
Histoplasmosis
Immunization reaction
Kawasaki disease
Lyme disease
Meningococcal disease
Syphilis: periostitis
Trichinosis
Tuberculosis
Viral
- Myalgia/arthralgia
- Myositis
- Toxic synovitis

Metabolic Origin
Carnitine palmityltransferase deficiency
Fabry's disease
McArdle syndrome
Phosphofructokinase deficiency

Neoplastic Origin
Histiocytosis X
Leukemia
Lymphoma
Neuroblastoma
Tumors of bone
- Chondrosarcoma
- Ewing's sarcoma
- Osteoblastoma (benign)
- Osteogenic sarcoma
- Osteoid osteoma (benign)

Tumors of soft tissue
- Fibrosarcoma
- Rhabdomyosarcoma
- Synovial cell sarcoma

Tumors of the spinal cord

Nutritional Origin
Gout
Hypercholesterolemia
Hypervitaminosis A
Osteoporosis
Rickets (vitamin D)
Scurvy (vitamin C)

Orthopedic Origin
Chondromalacia patellae
Freiberg's disease
Inflexible flat feet/tarsal coalition
Köhler's disease
Legg-Calvé-Perthes disease
Osgood-Schlatter disease
Osteochondritis dissecans
Osteogenesis imperfecta
Pathological fracture
Sever's disease
Slipped capital femoral epiphysis

Psychosocial Origin
Behavior disorders
Psychogenic pain
Reflex neurovascular dystrophy
School phobia

Trauma/Overuse
Compartment syndrome
Fracture
Hypermobility syndrome
Myohematoma
Myositis ossificans
Nerve compression syndrome
- Carpal tunnel syndrome
- Cervical nerve root entrapment
- Other peripheral nerve root compression

Physical abuse
Shin splint
Sprain
Stress fracture
Subluxed radial head
Thoracic outlet syndrome

Modified from Bowyer SL, Hollister JR: *Pediatr Clin North Am* 31:5, 1984.

emphasis on a psychological cause recently has given way to an emphasis on an overuse type of injury. Apparent worsening of the pain during times of increased activity and relief through use of heat and massage seem to support a physical cause. However, headache and abdominal pain—often associated with emotional illnesses—also have accompanied growing pains.

The diagnosis of growing pains is significant for its lack of associated physical signs. Thus, any abnormal finding on physical examination should provoke a search for another cause. Similarly, roentgenograms and the results of screening laboratory tests usually prove normal. Treatment involves heat, massage, and analgesics.

Sprains

A sprain is a physical disruption of a ligament. This occurs less commonly in children than in adults because a child's open epiphyseal plate or plastic bony cortex tends to give way more easily than does a ligament. Therefore, Salter-Harris fractures and buckle fractures should be considered when the history indicates a sprain and physical examination reveals tenderness on palpation or pain on stretching the ligament. Joint stability also should be assessed. Sprains can be graded according to the degree of associated ligament disruption. A mild, microscopic tear that results in no laxity of the involved joint is a grade I sprain. Grade II sprains involve macroscopic but incomplete ligament tears. Joint laxity is greater, but there is less than a 5-mm movement differential between the sprained and the contralateral joint. Grade III sprains result in more than 5 mm of increased mobility of the affected joint. Grade I sprains can be treated by the primary practitioner, icing and wrapping the involved joint to minimize swelling. Early range of motion exercises should be encouraged, with a gradual return to activity. The recurrence of pain indicates too rapid a return to a given level of activity. Grade II and grade III sprains generally should be referred to an orthopedist for immobilization and consideration of surgical repair of torn ligaments.

Overuse Syndromes

Overuse injuries have become more common as physical fitness has become popular nationwide. Localized, gradually increasing, persistent extremity pain that worsens with weight bearing, exercise, and activity but that diminishes with rest can indicate a stress fracture. Stress fractures are rare in children younger than age 12 years. They most commonly affect the second metatarsal, the proximal tibia, or the fibula. Although a roentgenogram may show normal findings, a bone scan can help establish the diagnosis. Treatment consists mostly of rest and treatment with nonsteroidal anti-inflammatory agents. Casting or splinting occasionally is necessary.

Little League elbow is an overuse injury caused by the repetitive motion of pitching a baseball; this motion compresses the radial aspect of the elbow and stretches the ulnar aspect. The result is painful inflammation of the epicondyles. The range of joint motion also may be diminished. Fragments of bone splintered into the joint may cause the joint to "catch" or "lock." Treatment consists of resting the arm by avoiding the repetitive movement. A change in pitching technique may reduce recurrences. To prevent this problem, some Little League systems limit the number of innings a youngster may pitch in one game.

Shin splints also are caused by overuse. The term originally referred to pain along the posteromedial aspect of the tibia as a result of irritation at the origin of the posterior tibial muscle. Shin splints now refer to any of a series of painful overuse syndromes of the lower portion of the leg, including irritation of the posterior or anterior tibial muscle, inflammation of the interosseous membrane located between the tibia and fibula, and both anterior and posterior compartment syndromes. All can cause pain in the lower legs. The condition, which is exacerbated by running and jumping, occurs most commonly at the beginning of a training season. Although the pain occurs initially after activity, it may occur during or before activity as the syndrome progresses. On examination, there may be tenderness over the posteromedial aspect of the tibia, over the proximal portion of the posterior tibia, or over the anterior tibia. Treatment involves rest, application of ice, and antiinflammatory drugs. For runners, training on a softer surface or with better quality running shoes may help.

Subluxation of the Radial Head

Nursemaids' elbow is a common injury in toddlers. The injury usually follows sudden, forceful traction of the hand or forearm, which pulls the immature radial head briefly from the cuff formed by the annular ligament. Release of the force allows the radius to trap the ligament against the capitellum. A verbal patient usually localizes the pain to the elbow or, occasionally, to the wrist. More often the child refuses to use the extremity and holds the arm with the elbow flexed, the forearm close to the chest, and the hand in pronation. The diagnosis usually is made by history alone. If the history is unclear or if attempts to reduce the subluxation are unsuccessful, radiographs may be obtained to rule out a fracture. Radiographic findings in subluxation of the radial head usually are negative. The practitioner can reduce the subluxation by using one hand to supinate the patient's forearm quickly while simultaneously exerting traction on the forearm and using the thumb of the other hand to create pressure over the patient's radial head. This maneuver is completed by placing the elbow through full extension and flexion while maintaining pressure over the radial head. Normal use of the extremity usually returns within 30 minutes. The rapid recovery is dramatic and rewarding to the parents and the physician. A prompt return to normal use of the affected arm may not occur if the subluxation has been present for some time because of swelling of the ligament. In such instances the affected arm should be placed in a simple sling and positioned across the upper portion of the abdomen for 12 to 24 hours. Referral to an orthopedist rarely is required.

Slipped Capital Femoral Epiphysis

A slipped capital femoral epiphysis is caused by a sudden or gradual dislocation of the head of the femur from its neck and shaft at the level of the upper epiphyseal plate. The characteristic pain occurs in the affected hip or the medial aspect of the ipsilateral knee. The displacement may be sudden, in which case the pain usually is severe and associated with the inability to bear weight. Gradual displacement is associated with slowly increasing, dull pain. This condition typically affects sedentary, obese adolescent boys. The physical examination may reveal diminished abduction and internal rotation of the hip. The diagnosis is made roentgenographically. Management involves surgical placement of a pin through the femoral head and the epiphysis to prevent further slippage. Avascular necrosis of the femoral head is a common complication, even with early recognition and treatment.

Toxic Synovitis

Toxic synovitis, a self-limited inflammation of the hip joint, commonly occurs in children younger than age 10 years. The cause is unknown, but because it often occurs within 2 weeks after an upper respiratory infection, a postviral inflammatory process is suspected. Typical presentation is that of a child who refuses to walk because of apparent pain in the hip. The hip is held in flexion, abduction, and external rotation. Findings may include a slight elevation in the WBC count and the sedimentation rate—a frustrating development for the practitioner, who hopes to rule out septic arthritis, a concern that may lead to consultation with an orthopedist. Treatment consists of bed rest, usually for fewer than 4 days. In rare instances, avascular necrosis of the femoral head may be a late complication.

Osteochondrosis

Osteochondrosis (see also Chapter 243) includes a group of disorders in which degeneration or aseptic necrosis of bone and overlying cartilage occurs at an ossification center and is followed by recalcification. The disorders vary in name and presentation according to their locations.

Legg-Calvé-Perthes disease, or osteochondrosis of the femoral head, results from compromise of the tenuous vascular supply to the area. The condition may be idiopathic or may result from a slipped capital femoral epiphysis, trauma, steroid use, sickle cell crisis, or congenital dislocation of the hip. Toxic synovitis also is associated with subsequent Legg-Calvé-Perthes disease, but again this is rare. After compromise of the vascular supply, the bone underlying the articular surface of the head of the femur becomes necrotic. Collapse of the necrotic bone flattens the femoral head and causes a poor fit with the acetabulum, even after new bone is formed. The pain associated with Legg-Calvé-Perthes disease, which results from necrosis of the involved bone, frequently is referred to the medial aspect of the ipsilateral knee. A limp may be the presenting complaint. Often, an early diagnosis eludes the practitioner because roentgenographic findings may be normal or show only swelling of the joint's capsule. A bone scan may demonstrate diminished blood flow to the femoral head compared with the contralateral hip. Later, radiographs may show areas of bone resorption, irregular widening of the epiphysis, or dense new bone formation. The goal of therapy is to prevent flattening of the femoral head as it undergoes new bone formation. This is accomplished by keeping the hip abducted so that the head of the femur is held well inside the rounded portion of the acetabulum. Either bracing or an osteotomy may accomplish this goal; both require referral to an orthopedic surgeon.

Two similar processes can affect the knee joint. Osteochondritis dissecans involves degeneration of bone and cartilage at the articular surface of the knee, particularly at the lateral aspect of the medial condyle of the femur. Knee pain and crepitus, caused by loose bone and cartilage fragments in the joint, can result. Chondromalacia patellae occurs because of a painful softening or breakdown of the inner surface of the patella. The pain is localized to the knee and increases with activities that require prolonged knee bending and even with prolonged sitting. The pain is described as grinding. It sometimes can be elicited by applying pressure over the patella. Crepitus may be felt by moving the patella from side to side over the knee joint. Treatment usually is limited to pain relief and reassurance that, in time, the condition will resolve. Exercise to strengthen the medial quadriceps muscles may promote better alignment of the patella with the knee and thereby diminish the pain. In severe cases, the patella may have to be realigned surgically. Osteochondrosis of the growth plate of the calcaneus, Sever's disease, can produce heel pain that worsens with activity. This usually mild process requires only padding of the heel to relieve the pain. Avascular necrosis and osteochondrosis of the tarsal navicular (Köhler's disease) and of the head of the second metatarsal (Freiberg's disease) can cause foot pain. Treatment usually requires only pain medication and rest.

Osgood-Schlatter disease is a painful degeneration of the tibial tubercle at the site of insertion of the quadriceps ligament. It is characterized by painful swelling of the anterior aspect of the tibial tubercle. Usually it occurs during adolescence. The degree of swelling may be alarming, and the area is tender to palpation. Pain is exacerbated by activity that involves increased use of the quadriceps muscles. The process is self-limited and resolves toward the end of adolescence when the epiphysis at the insertion site closes and the bone becomes stronger than the inserted ligament. Until it resolves, the condition is treated with rest and analgesics. In rare cases, casting or surgical attachment of the quadriceps ligament is required.

Osteomyelitis

Osteomyelitis (see also Chapter 244) is a local infection of bone, usually involving one of the long bones. The highest incidence is in children 3 to 12 years of age. Although infection often occurs by hematogenous seeding, it can be caused by direct entry after local trauma. In both children and adults, the most commonly isolated organism is *Staphylococcus aureus*. However, *Haemophilus influenzae* type b, *Salmonella* species, and group A streptococci all can infect the bone. Group B streptococcus is more likely the cause of infection in newborns. Osteomyelitis caused by *Salmonella* organisms tends to occur more often in children who have sickle cell anemia than in other children. In trauma from a puncture wound to the foot, especially through a sneaker, *Pseudomonas aeruginosa* must be considered. In addition, tuberculous osteomyelitis still occurs and may become more common with the resurgence of tuberculosis.

Osteomyelitis can manifest as extremity pain alone or extremity pain with signs of a systemic infectious disease (fever, irritability, septic appearance). In the absence of systemic signs, it often is difficult to distinguish between osteomyelitis and a traumatic cause of the pain. It may take 2 weeks or longer for roentgenographic evidence of osteomyelitis to develop. A bone scan usually, but not always, is diagnostic. In rare cases a reduction in perfusion caused by pressure from the exudative process may result in false-negative scans. In addition, the WBC count and sedimentation rate often are elevated in osteomyelitis. The effectiveness of treatment can be monitored by following the sedimentation rate or the C reactive protein.

Neoplasms

A neoplasm rarely is the cause of limb pain; however, the possibility of a tumor is a common concern for parents of children who have this complaint. And, although rare, benign and malignant bone tumors and systemic malignancies all can present in this fashion.

Osteoid osteoma is a benign bone tumor that occurs most often in adolescents. It usually involves the femur or tibia and occurs unilaterally. Pain, the presenting complaint, initially is dull and increases in intensity to deep and "boring." The pain is more intense at night and with weight bearing. Roentgenographic findings of sclerotic bone around a lucent center are diagnostic of this condition; sometimes tomograms are required for confirmation. Surgical excision is curative.

Systemic neoplasms in which extremity pain occurs include leukemia and metastatic neuroblastoma. One third of children who have acute lymphocytic leukemia have bone pain at the time of diagnosis, and in one fourth, joint or bone pain is a significant presenting complaint.[4] Unrelenting, increasing pain that worsens at night or with rest and that is not relieved by analgesics, heat, or massage may indicate the presence of a metastatic bone tumor. Systemic signs (weight loss, pallor, lymphadenopathy, hepatosplenomegaly, or fever) may accompany the pain. In leukemia, examination of the extremity may reveal strikingly little to account for the degree of pain. Radiographic studies of the extremities may show lucent "leukemic lines" in the subepiphyseal area.

Primary malignant tumors of bone may cause severe unilateral pain, with swelling and tenderness at the site. This supports the use of radiographic studies when unilateral limb pain is not explained adequately by a history of trauma and when pain from trauma does not resolve as expected. The peak incidence of both osteogenic sarcoma and the less common Ewing's sarcoma occurs in late childhood and during adolescence. The roentgenogram in osteogenic sarcoma may reveal a tumor in the metaphysis with the presence of both radiolucent and radiopaque areas. The characteristic "sunburst" results from extension of calcification into the overlying soft tissue. Although periosteal elevation may be present, it is not diagnostic of the disease.

REFERENCES

1. Abu-Arafeh I, Russell G: Recurrent limb pain in schoolchildren, *Arch Dis Child* 74:336, 1996.
2. Cummings JR, et al: The popliteal artery entrapment syndrome in children, *J Pediatr Orthop* 12:539, 1992.
3. de Inocencio J: Musculoskeletal pain in primary pediatric care: analysis of 1000 consecutive general pediatric clinic visits, *Pediatrics* 102:e63, 1998.
4. Leventhal BG: Neoplasms and neoplasm-like structures. In Behrman RE, Vaughan VC, editors: *Nelson's textbook of pediatrics,* ed 14, Philadelphia, 1992, WB Saunders.
5. National Center for Health Statistics: *Vital and health statistics: patient's reasons for visiting physicians—National Ambulatory Medical Care Survey, US, 1977-1978,* DHHS Pub No Pt82-1717, Hyattsville, Md, 1981.
6. Olivieri I, Pasero G: Long-standing isolated juvenile onset HLA-B27-associated peripheral enthesitis, *J Rheumatol* 19:164, 1992.
7. Sherry DD, et al: Psychosomatic musculoskeletal pain in childhood: clinical and psychological analyses of 100 children, *Pediatrics* 88:1093, 1991.

SUGGESTED READINGS

Cawkwell GD, Passo MH: Pursuing the source of musculoskeletal pain, *Contemp Pediatr* 11:72, 1994.

Sherry D: Limb pain in childhood, *Pediatr Rev* 12:39, 1990.

Szer IS: Musculoskeletal pain syndromes that affect adolescents, *Arch Pediatr Adolesc Med* 150:740, 1996.

Tunnessen WW Jr: *Signs and symptoms in pediatrics,* ed 2, Philadelphia, 1988, JB Lippincott.

133 Facial Dysmorphism

Marvin E. Miller

The face is the region of the body that reveals our identity to others. Although each person has two eyes, two ears, a nose, a mouth, a chin, and a head, it is the subtle uniqueness of these features in their form and their relationship to one another that marks each of us as a distinct and identifiable individual. Only monozygotic twins can have apparently identical faces, and even among them one finds facial differences that readily distinguish one from the other.

The face can appear dysmorphic or unusual if any facial part is abnormal in form or function or if a spatial relationship between or among these parts is abnormal.[1]

Physicians and other health care providers should be sensitive in the use of terminology to describe an individual who has a dysmorphic face. The terms "funny-looking kid," "FLK," or "funny-looking face" add little to the understanding of the situation and may arouse justified parental indignation. In discussing dysmorphic features with parents or describing them in written or verbal communication with colleagues, the physician should be objective in an evaluation that established a diagnosis and avoids an insensitive and derogatory approach to the patient. A dysmorphic face may be appropriate in relation to the family's physiognomy or it may indicate a particular syndrome. Thus, it is not surprising to find epicanthal folds and a flat nasal bridge in an Asian child; if these are found in a white child, however, the physician should be suspicious of Down syndrome and look for other features that suggest this diagnosis. The child who has a large head who also has a parent who has a large head does not prompt as much concern as the child who has a large head whose parents have normal-size heads. Thus, it is crucial to evaluate dysmorphic facial features in light of the child's genetic background.

If the child or baby looks like one of the parents or bears a strong resemblance to the baby pictures of one of the parents, the features obviously are familial. An autosomal dominant condition, such as Waardenburg's syndrome, could explain dysmorphism and parental similarity. However, if there is no parental or familial resemblance (especially with other problems in development or growth or other body symptoms), then the physician should consider further evaluation.

Facial morphogenesis is determined primarily by genetic information from multiple gene loci. Recently, the molecular characterization of several genetic disorders, each associated with characteristic facial dysmorphism, has provided some clues as to which specific genes are part of the process that determines the facial features of an individual.[5,6] These genetic loci include the PAX 3 gene (Waardenburg's syndrome type 1), the gene for fibroblast growth factor receptor 2 (several craniosynostosis syndromes, including Pfeiffer's syndrome, Crouzon's syndrome, Apert's syndrome, and Jackson-Weiss syndrome), the TWIST gene (Saethre-Chotzen syndrome), the sonic hedgehog gene (holoprosencephaly), and the Treacle gene (Treacher Collins syndrome). Other genes involved in facial morphogenesis will be characterized soon, when information from the Human Genome Project becomes available.

MECHANISMS OF DYSMORPHOGENESIS

Facial dysmorphogenesis has four general causes: deformation, disruption, primary malformation of the face, and central nervous system (CNS) malformations that cause secondary facial dysmorphism (anatomical and neuromuscular dysfunction).

Deformations

Deformations are structural abnormalities of newborns involving the musculoskeletal system that arise from intrauterine constraint.[2] Any situation that compromises the intrauterine space can cause a deformation, such as primigravida pregnancy, nonvertex presentation, multiple births, small mother, large baby, oligohydramnios, and structural uterine abnormality. Deformations are common and occur in 2% of all newborns. Common facial deformations include plagiocephaly (asymmetry of the head); asymmetry of the mandible, nose, ears, or chin; and micrognathia. The natural history of facial deformation almost always is benign, with restoration of the affected tissue to normal form and function within weeks after birth.

Disruptions

A disruption is the breakdown of previously normal fetal tissue.[3] The most common example is amniotic bands, which are estimated to occur in 1 in 2000 pregnancies. Although originally they were thought to affect limbs primarily, it now is clear that bands can attach to any part of the craniofacial region, causing a vast spectrum of structural defects of varying severity. This diagnosis should be considered in any newborn who has bizarre external craniofacial features. Evaluation of the placenta can be helpful in confirming this

Table 133-1 Examples of Causes of Facial Malformation

Cause	Example	Facial Dysmorphism
Genetic		
Chromosomal	Cri du chat syndrome (5p–)	Micrognathia, ocular hypertelorism
Autosomal dominant	Treacher Collins syndrome	Dysplastic ears, maxillary hypoplasia
Autosomal recessive	Hurler syndrome	Corneal clouding, coarse facies
Intrauterine infection	Congenital rubella	Cataracts
Drug induced	Fetal alcohol syndrome	Smooth philtrum, small eyes
Metabolic	Congenital hypothyroidism	Coarse facies; large, protruding tongue

diagnosis if strands of amnion can be demonstrated or if they are found attached to the affected tissues.

Malformations

Facial. A malformation is a structural defect resulting from an intrinsic abnormality in the cells of the affected tissue.[3] Malformations have a number of potential causes, including genetic disorders (chromosomes and single genes), drugs, intrauterine infections, metabolic derangements, and hyperthermia. Malformations can involve almost any part of the face; examples of these are given in Table 133-1.

Central nervous system. Malformations of the brain can cause facial dysmorphogenesis in two ways. First, the facial anatomy is directed partly by the growth of the forebrain. Any situation that grossly alters the normal development of the brain can alter facial development anatomically. An example of this is holoprosencephaly. When the forebrain fails to separate into the right and left ventricles, secondary midfacial abnormalities may occur. Another example is the upward slanting palpebral fissures in Down syndrome, which probably occurs secondary to forebrain underdevelopment. Second, neuromuscular dysfunction of the face resulting from a primary malformation of the brain can cause facial dysmorphism. Whenever a primary CNS malformation exists, neuromuscular control of a number of facial functions can be abnormal. These abnormal conditions include ptosis, nystagmus, strabismus, and lop ears. Prominent lateral palatal ridges that result from a deficit of tongue thrust into the palate are a sign of intrauterine CNS dysfunction.

BOX 133-1

EVALUATION OF THE INDIVIDUAL WHO HAS FACIAL DYSMORPHISM

1. Describe the dysmorphic facial features.
2. Describe any other dysmorphic somatic features.
3. Define the growth of the individual in weight, length, and head circumference.
4. Define the development of the individual.
5. Review the gestational and perinatal history.
6. Review the family history.
7. Consider laboratory tests.
8. Determine if the features fit a recognizable syndrome.
9. Discuss the findings with the family.

EVALUATION OF THE INDIVIDUAL WHO HAS FACIAL DYSMORPHISM

Evaluation of the baby or child who has a dysmorphic face is summarized in Box 133-1 and is aimed at establishing an etiological diagnosis. The physician should follow these steps:

1. *Describe the dysmorphic facial features.* The first task is to describe in objective terms why the face appears unusual. Rather than stating that the distance between the eyes appears increased or the ears appear small, the physician should measure these parameters and compare them with known standards.[2]
2. *Describe any other dysmorphic somatic features.* A thorough physical examination should be performed to determine if associated somatic abnormalities are present. Hearing and vision should be evaluated, and funduscopic examination should be performed. The cranial sutures should be palpated to evaluate for possible craniostenosis, which can cause facial dysmorphism.
3. *Define the growth of the individual in weight, length, and head circumference.* Data should be obtained and "plotted" to assess how the individual is growing in these parameters. The growth curves should be interpreted in light of the parental growth curves. Growth excess or, more often, growth deficiency can be seen as a part of malformation syndromes involving facial dysmorphism; for example, individuals who have cerebral gigantism (Sotos' syndrome), who have very characteristic facies, are macrocephalic and are very tall in childhood. Individuals who have any of the three common autosomal trisomies (trisomy 13, 18, or 21) all show postnatal growth deficiency.
4. *Define the development of the individual.* From the patient's history and the physician's examination and testing, the individual's development should be assessed. It is important to know of any developmental delay because it may indicate CNS dysfunction. However, psychosocial deprivation and chronic otitis media, two correctable situations, can cause developmental delay.
5. *Review the gestational and perinatal history.* The gestational history should be reviewed for maternal drug exposure, viral illness, fever, and alcohol consumption. Positive findings suggest an environmental cause of

a malformation. The history also should include factors that might predispose the patient to deformations, such as breech delivery, oligohydramnios, multiple births, or maternal structural uterine anomaly.

6. *Review the family history.* The importance of taking a good family history has already been mentioned; this information may suggest a genetic basis for the condition.[4] Some autosomal recessive disorders are found almost exclusively in certain ethnic groups. Ellis-van Creveld syndrome, a rare ectodermal dysplasia, has a high incidence in the Amish population. The offspring of parents who are related to each other, particularly if they are first-degree relatives (i.e., father-daughter, mother-son, brother-sister), are at greater risk for having autosomal recessive disorders. Incestuous matings probably are more common than thought, and the couple is at relatively high risk for dysmorphic offspring. An incestuous mating should be considered in any dysmorphic newborn of a very young mother and no reputed father. A dysmorphic individual born to an older mother suggests an autosomal trisomy and when born to an older father suggests an autosomal dominant disorder caused by a fresh mutation.
7. *Consider laboratory tests.* If the dysmorphic features and history suggest a primary CNS problem, brain imaging should be considered. If several systems are involved, chromosomes should be analyzed. Other laboratory tests and imaging studies of other organ systems should be performed when warranted. Magnetic resonance imaging (MRI), computed tomography (CT) scanning, and ultrasonography are extremely valuable imaging techniques that can be used selectively after consultation with a radiologist to evaluate internal structures.
8. *Determine if the features fit a known condition or syndrome* after all the information has been gathered.*
9. *Discuss the findings with the family.*

SUMMARY

The physician who is confronted with a patient who has dysmorphic facial features must decide whether the patient or family will benefit from a thorough evaluation or referral. The most important task initially is to determine whether the features are consistent with the individual's genetic background or whether they represent an abnormal phenotype. Through systematic gathering of information, the physician should attempt to establish an etiological diagnosis and then convey the implications (including genetic counseling) to the appropriate family members.

**Smith's Recognizable Patterns of Human Malformation* is the most valuable resource for this purpose. It also is helpful in determining if a particular condition is genetically based.

REFERENCES

1. Aase JM: *Diagnostic dysmorphology,* New York, 1990, Plenum.
2. Graham JM: *Smith's recognizable patterns of human deformation,* ed 2, Philadelphia, 1988, WB Saunders.
3. Jones KL: *Smith's recognizable patterns of human malformation,* ed 5, Philadelphia, 1997, WB Saunders.
4. McKusick VA: *Mendelian inheritance in man,* ed 12, Baltimore, 1998, Johns Hopkins University Press.
5. Nuckolls GH, Shum L, Slavkin HC: Progress toward understanding craniofacial malformations, *Cleft Palate Craniofac J* 36:12, 1999.
6. Winter RM: What's in a face, *Nat Genet* 12:124, 1996.

134 Failure to Thrive

Andrew D. Racine

The unfortunate term "failure to thrive" has served generations of practitioners and their patients poorly as an indecorous, unenlightening phrase that lumps together a heterogeneous group of infants and young children who have nothing more in common than a growth pattern irreconcilable with a predetermined standard for age. Perturbations in the homeostasis of a young infant or child that originate in abnormalities ranging from congestive heart failure to psychosocial deprivation can, like a series of convergent boulevards, eventually lead to the same common plaza we call "failure to thrive." To say that we have found a patient in such a location, however, tells us very little about the direction from which the child strayed to come to our attention.

Evaluation and management of a child who fails to gain weight adequately represents, therefore, a formidable challenge that requires of the physician:

- a determination to listen attentively and examine thoroughly, for no adequate substitute has yet been found for a complete history and physical examination
- a broad familiarity with the many pathophysiological sequences that can give rise to this condition
- an understanding of normal infant behavior and development requisite to identify aberrancies that may threaten weight gain at different ages
- a capacity to gather and synthesize information about the physical, psychological, emotional, familial, and social contexts of the patient's presentation
- a willingness to work with a team of other practitioners to evaluate and manage the infant
- the patience to persevere for as long as it may take to establish adequate weight gain

DEFINITION

In clinical medicine, the assignment of a diagnosis generally signals the culmination of a process of evaluation. By contrast, the diagnosis of failure to thrive merely serves to *initiate* the evaluation of a patient who has an abnormal pattern of weight gain. Deviation from normal weight gain has been defined conventionally by reference to age-adjusted nationally standardized norms of weight and rate of weight gain.[7] Infants or young children who either fall below a given percentile weight-for-age or weight-for-height or whose rate of weight gain has declined across two major percentiles (i.e., 90th, 75th, 50th, 25th, 10th, or 5th) invite close scrutiny.

Static measurements of a child's weight-for-age or weight-for-height that document a child's *size* should be distinguished from repeated measurements over time that record a child's *growth*. Deviations from the norm in the former measurements may or may not, depending on the clinical circumstances, indicate abnormalities in the latter.

A clinical entity defined by reference to statistical norms merits some additional comment. First, although an occasional child may present with obvious signs of severe malnutrition at the initial examination, a single observation of weight in a child generally is insufficient to make any diagnosis. We are concerned here, for the most part, with children who manifest abnormal *patterns* of weight gain.

Second, although we desire to identify children whose weight or weight gain is abnormal, some normal children will fall into the extreme tails of the standard distributions, be it 10%, 5%, or 3% of any cohort. The farther out on the curve we observe any individual child, however, the more likely the child is to be truly abnormal with respect to weight-for-age or weight-for-height.

Third, one must understand that the national standards are constructed by using serial cross sections of children, not longitudinal observations of cohorts as they grow. Therefore, the rate at which a child gains weight individually will differ from tracks across collections of different children at different ages that appear on these charts.

Finally, these statistical descriptions must not be allowed to obscure the salient feature common to most children who fail to gain weight adequately—they suffer from malnutrition and are, therefore, at risk for its attendant consequences. When acute malnutrition results in decreased weight-for-age, the condition is referred to as *wasting*. If caloric deprivation is prolonged, it eventually will affect the child's linear growth as well, at which point the child is said to be stunted. Abnormalities in linear growth not accompanied by wasting—the child who has short stature alone—is not the subject of failure to thrive.

One common set of criteria defines failure to thrive in children younger than 2 years of age:[33]

- weight consistently less than 80% of the median for age, or
- weight on more than one occasion falling below the third percentile for age, or
- weight that has fallen across two major percentiles on the National Center for Health Statistics (NCHS) standard growth charts[16]

One may anticipate that these criteria will identify as many as 10% of children seen in outpatient settings,[25] and 3% to 5% of hospital admissions.[2] Children who present with weights from 61% to 75% of the median for age are fewer but require intensive outpatient monitoring. When a child's weight falls below 60% of the median for age, the associated morbidity is severe and warrants inpatient hospitalization.[13] Children from lower socioeconomic backgrounds may be at heightened risk for malnutrition and consequent wasting.[15]

NORMAL WEIGHT GAIN IN INFANTS

The NCHS growth charts have received widespread application as tools for plotting the growth patterns of normal infants and children. (See Chapter 8, The Pediatric Physical Examination.) The ease of their use makes them an ideal screening instrument but, as with all "screens," their sensitivity and specificity are limited. They do not, for example, take into account parental size or the presence of preexisting chromosomal abnormalities, leading some to argue for the use of standards that control for mean parental height or the presence of certain genetic conditions such as trisomy 21.

Recent studies have examined the rate at which infants gain weight[14] and how regression to the mean accounts for the tendency of some heavier infants to lose weight and some lighter infants to gain weight over time.[31] The mean weight of a newborn infant is approximately 3.25 kg. (± 0.9 kg.). Many infants will lose between 6% and 10% of this weight in the first week as they undergo the normal diuresis associated with adaptation to the extrauterine environment. Birth weight usually is regained by the age of 10 days. Because an infant's weight at birth preferentially captures the influence of maternal characteristics and the intrauterine environment, it is an imperfect reflection of genetic growth potential. By 4 to 8 weeks of age, however, much catch-up growth in babies born light-for-dates has already occurred so that an infant's weight at this time appears to be a more reliable predictor of weight at 12 months than is birth weight.[8] In general, infants can be expected to gain a mean of 30 g (±15 g) a day during the first 3 months of life. Infants usually will triple their birth weight by 1 year of age, at which time the mean daily weight gain has declined to approximately 10 g (±3 g).

PATHOGENESIS

Infants and children grow in the presence of adequate amounts of four fundamental constituents: oxygen, substrate, hormones, and love. Deficient quantities of any one or a combination of these suffice to impede normal weight gain. Oxygen deprivation at the tissue level from causes as diverse as congestive heart failure, chronic lung disease, or anemia will result in poor weight gain. Inadequate quantities of calories, protein, or micronutrients either from environmental deprivation, malabsorption, or inability to metabolize them at the tissue level also will inhibit normal weight accumulation. Deficiencies in growth hormone, insulin-like growth factors, glucocorticoids, thyroid hormone, and other regulators of growth can result in failure to thrive. Finally, infants or children deprived of affection often will not grow despite what appears to be normal caloric intake. Chronic disease from many etiologies will interrupt normal weight gain through the induction of anorexia, malabsorption, increased metabolic needs, and the elaboration of inflammatory mediators, including tumor necrosis factor.

In the past, patients who had inadequate weight gain have been classified as a minority whose difficulty stems from a readily identifiable "organic" cause and a majority whose problem resides in a residual "nonorganic" category.[33] Others have emphasized the overlapping nature of these distinctions and have suggested a third, or "mixed," category of failure to thrive.[19] More recent approaches have tended to depart from the organic/nonorganic dichotomy in recognition of the somewhat arbitrary nature of this distinction.

A more useful categorization of infants and children who have inadequate weight gain acknowledges an imbalance between the energy needs of the organism that does not grow and the energy at its disposition. The largest share of energy consumed, approximately 55% to 60%, is devoted to maintain a basal metabolic rate. An additional 5% to 10% of energy is lost in urine and stool, 5% is accounted for by specific dynamic action, 15% is used for normal physical activity above basal metabolic functions, and 15% is directed toward growth. To provide for all these functions, infants need approximately 100 to 110 kcal/kg/day.

An imbalance between energy needs and energy supplies can arise either from increases in the former or deficiencies in the latter. Box 134-1 lists conditions that increase the energy needs of the organism. Energy needs increase either with increases in the intensity of energy expenditure or decreases in the efficiency of energy use. Conditions that increase the intensity of energy expenditure include chronic heart disease, chronic lung disease, chronic anemia, chronic

BOX 134-1

CONDITIONS THAT INCREASE ENERGY NEEDS

Increased Intensity of Energy Utilization:
Chronic heart disease (congenital or acquired)
Chronic lung disease (bronchopulmonary dysplasia, cystic fibrosis, pulmonary lymphangiectasis)
Chronic anemia (hemaglobinopathies, enzyme deficiencies, membrane abnormalities)
Chronic infection (urinary tract infections, respiratory infections, tuberculosis)
Endocrine abnormalities (hyperthyroidism)
Malignancy (neuroblastoma, ganglioneuroma)
Drugs or toxins

Decreased Efficiency of Energy Utilization:
Chronic infection
Chronic renal disease
Hepatic insufficiency (cirrhosis)
Metabolic disease (disorders of amino acid or carbohydrate metabolism, idiopathic hypercalcemia of infancy)
Hormonal disturbances (hypopituitarism, hypoparathyroidism, chronic adrenocortical insufficiency, diabetes insipidus, hypothyroidism)
Genetic conditions (Down syndrome, Cornelia de Lange's syndrome, cri du chat syndrome, Smith-Lemli-Opitz syndrome, familial dysautonomia)
Micronutrient deficiencies (iron, zinc, carnitine)

BOX 134-2

CONDITIONS THAT RESULT IN DEFICIENT ENERGY SUPPLY

- Calories withheld
  - In utero conditions
  - Formula preparation mistakes
  - Breast-feeding difficulties
  - Parent-child psychosocial dysfunction
  - Maternal depression
  - Intentional abuse or neglect
  - Poverty
  - Unsound parental beliefs regarding nutrition
  - Difficult feeders
- Calories not properly ingested or digested
  - Anorexia (reflux esophagitis, emotional deprivation, chronic infection, dysphagia)
  - Structural abnormalities of the oro- or nasopharynx (cleft palate, choanal atresia, Treacher Collins syndrome, Pierre Robin syndrome, laryngeal web)
  - Structural abnormalities of the gastrointestinal tract (stenosis or atresia of the esophagus or duodenum, tracheoesophageal fistula, vascular ring, strictures, achalasia, malrotation, antral web, pyloric stenosis)
  - Neuromuscular disorders (cerebral palsy, hydrocephalus, myopathies)
  - Conditions leading to excessive dyspnea (congestive heart failure, chronic lung disease)
- Vomiting and rumination
- Malabsorption
  - Small bowel (celiac disease, inflammatory bowel disease, disaccharide malabsorption, intestinal lymphagiectasia, jejunal atresia, duplication cysts, chronic parasitic infections)
  - Pancreas (cystic fibrosis, Schwachman-Diamond syndrome, chronic pancreatitis)
  - Liver (cirrhosis, intrahepatic cholestatic syndromes, biliary atresia)

infection, certain endocrine abnormalities, malignancy, and intoxications. The efficiency of energy utilization can be compromised by chronic infection, chronic renal disease, hepatic insufficiency, inborn errors of metabolism, hormonal abnormalities, certain genetic syndromes, and deficiencies of various micronutrients, including iron, zinc, and carnitine.

Conditions leading to deficiency in energy supply are listed in Box 134-2. These originate either because calories are withheld from or improperly presented to the child, because they are refused, not ingested, vomited, or not absorbed.

In the category of caloric deprivation, one must include nutritional deprivation in utero that may result in permanent growth retardation. After delivery an infant may not receive sufficient calories because of parenting difficulties ranging from unfamiliarity with proper preparation of infant formula[24] or appropriate breast-feeding techniques to psychosocial dysfunction, maternal depression, and even frank abuse or neglect.[10] Other conditions that fall into this category include economic deprivation, unsound parental beliefs regarding nutrition,[26] and subtle central nervous system (CNS) abnormalities in the child that make them difficult feeders.

Food refusal in children beginning even in infancy[30] can result from many causes, including pain (from reflux esophagitis), psychosocial adjustment disorders from emotional deprivation, anorexia from chronic infection or intoxication, and structural abnormalities resulting in dysphagia. Structural malformations of the nasal or oral pharynx such as cleft palate, choanal atresia, or Treacher Collins syndrome can lead to an inability to ingest nutrients properly, as can muscular weakness, cerebral palsy or other CNS abnormalities, and diseases that give rise to excessive dyspnea.

Vomiting of feeds secondary to structural abnormalities of the gastrointestinal tract, increased intracranial pressure from whatever source, chronic acidosis, rumination, and gastroesophageal reflux may all impede growth through caloric deprivation.

The principal organ of nutrient absorption is the small bowel. Malabsorption can occur from gross structural abnormalities, inflammatory conditions, infectious agents, or disorders of organs that elaborate enzymes essential for digestion.

In consideration of these potential etiologies for inadequate weight gain, two cardinal principles should be emphasized. First, the majority of cases encountered in ambulatory practice will result from inadequate caloric intake, with most of these originating in a disturbance in the parent-child feeding behavior.[3,17] At one time it was thought that maternal mental health disorders accounted for the majority of these cases; more recent analysis has dissected a more subtle web of causation.[21] What has been termed a transactional model allows for the complex interplay of social conditions,[11] family interactions,[22] and individual psychodynamics[27] in the creation of feeding abnormalities.

The second principle to be emphasized is that for the residual minority of cases not caused by caloric insufficiency, conducting a thorough history and physical examination is the surest route to diagnosis. If the etiology of the problem is not made clear by history and physical examination, laboratory investigation is unlikely to reveal it.

EVALUATION

Prompt evaluation of infants and children who do not gain weight as expected is important. The history and physical examination should be directed toward certain areas, and in cases in which psychosocial features predominate, most laboratory tests may be unnecessary.

HISTORY

Initial Approach

Every evaluation of an infant or child who is not gaining weight must begin with a thorough history. Although most often the history and physical examination will be conducted in the office, a home visit affords the pediatrician an opportunity to observe the family interaction around feeding in the context in which it normally occurs. A history of the present illness should assemble all data available from previous anthropometric measurements of the patient, including weight, height, and head circumference. Premature infants must have their measurements corrected for gestational age until 18 months of age for head circumference, 24 months of age for weight, and 40 months of age for height.[5] One should begin by asking the parent(s), guardian(s), or principal caregiver(s) how they feel the baby is doing and what they believe the problem to be. Knowledge of a parent's frame of mind may propel further evaluation toward or away from difficulty in parent-child interaction, including child neglect, as a potential explanation for a child's lack of weight gain.

Feeding

A careful feeding history is essential. Is the baby bottle-fed or breast-fed? How often does the child nurse if breast-fed and for how long? Does the mother feel as though the child is sucking well, and does the baby appear sated after he or she feeds? If bottle-fed, how is the formula prepared and by whom? How many ounces will the baby take in a 24-hour period? Does the infant wet six to eight diapers a day?

For older children, when were solids introduced? Does the parent find the child to be a "picky eater" or difficult to interest in food? Does she drink excessive amounts of juice during the day, substituting for more calorically rich nutrients? What are meal times like at home? Where does the child eat and with whom? Are distractions, such as television, game boys, or video games, present during meals? Is food being used for discipline or in battles over control? Often, a 24-hour dietary recall of a typical day can help to quantify the caloric intake of the patient. If this proves difficult to elicit, the parents can be sent home with a nutritional diary to fill out prospectively and bring in at the next visit.

Vomiting

One should inquire about any vomiting or spitting up, being sure to explore frequency, volume, and presence of blood or bile in the emesis. Gastric outlet obstructions (pyloric stenosis, antral web) often result in the generation of significant propulsive forces leading to projectile vomiting, whereas gastroesophageal reflux often results in less dramatic patterns of regurgitation. An obstruction distal to the ligament of Treitz generally will manifest bilious vomiting, a symptom that must be taken with utmost seriousness in infancy, as it may indicate the presence of a malrotation and midgut volvulus.

Stools

The pattern and frequency of stooling must not be overlooked in the history of present illness. The child who has liquid stools may have small-bowel pathology or bulky, foul-smelling stools from fat malabsorption. If mucus or blood is in the stools, an inflammatory condition may be present.

Past Medical History

Additional information should be obtained regarding past medical history, beginning with the parents' attitudes regarding their decision to have a baby and what their experience with the pregnancy was like. Did the mother gain a reasonable amount of weight? Did she experience any illnesses during her pregnancy? Hypertension or preeclampsia will result in an infant who is small for gestational age; gestational diabetes may produce a macrosomic infant who fails to gain weight because of postnatal cardiac complications.

One should ask about specific toxic exposures in utero, particularly to tobacco and alcohol. The former may result in a small baby who rapidly catches up in weight with her peers whereas the latter's influence on weight may be sustained throughout childhood. Recording the child's gestational age at birth, any unusual complications of the labor and delivery, and the presence of malformations or other obvious deformities will complete this portion of the history.

Family History

A family history should document the growth patterns of siblings, record the occurrence of fetal loss or infant deaths, review the presence in the family of immune deficiencies, neurological disorders, or metabolic derangements, and highlight any unexplained growth deficiencies in close relatives. These findings may provide clues to the etiology of the growth abnormality in the child.

Social History

The social history should focus on the availability of social supports for the parents, the existence of economic or legal circumstances that threaten the stability of the family, the nature of the relationship between the parents, and the presence of affective disorders in the primary caregiver. Any recent disruptive events in the family's life should be explored to determine what effect they may have had on the parents' ability to care for the patient. Finally, it is at this point that one often may uncover unrealistic expectations that parents may harbor regarding feeding patterns, dietary fads, or behavior in infancy that provide clues to why feeding this infant has developed into such a challenge.

Physical Examination

Repeated anthropometric measurements over time constitute the most important component of the physical evaluation of children who are not gaining weight. On the initial examination, one should begin with observing the child's general relatedness to the parent(s) and the examiner. Does she appear listless, easily distractible, or irritable? Can she be engaged to make eye contact or to play with an age-appropriate toy? After completely undressing the child, a notation should be made of any evidence of wasting, of the presence and distribution of normal subcutaneous body fat, of muscle mass and tone, and of the presence of dysmorphic features; these will serve to set the stage for more detailed examination.

Particular attention should be paid to those organ systems that may reflect evidence of malnutrition. The mucous membranes, hair, nails, and skin develop abnormalities in the presence of vitamin, protein, fat, and micronutrient deficiencies. The head, eyes, ears, nose, and throat may reveal conditions ranging from open fontanelles of hypothyroidism or craniotabes of nutritional rickets to the blurred disk margins of increased intracranial pressure in a child who has chronic emesis or a submucosal cleft of the hard palate in an infant who feeds poorly.

The thyroid should be palpated gently and then auscultated for evidence of hyperthyroidism before one moves to the lung and cardiac examination. Observation, palpation, and, particularly, auscultation of these organ systems may reveal wheezing, rales, or heart murmurs suggestive of the presence of chronic conditions. Often, these conditions result in substantial energy expenditures that outstrip the supply of nutrients available to the infant. Examination of the digits for clubbing in the older child should not be neglected. A careful abdominal examination will rule out organomegaly associated with tumor, infection, or storage disease. Intestinal distention can be associated with carbohydrate malabsorption from various causes. The neurological examination may suggest explanations for an infant's inability to ingest adequate calories. Disorders of mentation, cranial nerve abnormalities, generalized weakness, or spasticity should be carefully sought.

Laboratory Evaluation

In the absence of evidence from the history or physical examination indicating the need for specific laboratory testing, expectations of the yield of laboratory investigation should be modest. When charts of 185 patients hospitalized for failure to thrive at the Children's Hospital of Buffalo were reviewed, only 1.4% of the laboratory studies performed were found to be of diagnostic value.[29] A similar review of 122 infants hospitalized at the Boston Children's Hospital revealed that a mean of 40 laboratory tests were ordered, but only 0.8% revealed an abnormality that contributed to a diagnosis.[2]

Should the cause of a child's failure to gain weight adequately remain uncertain after careful history and physical examination, a limited number of screening studies might be considered, including a complete blood count, a blood pH, serum electrolytes, blood urea nitrogen and creatinine, a urinalysis and urine culture, and an examination of the stool for reducing substances, pH, occult blood, and ova and parasites.[28] More extensive testing for malabsorption, endocrine disorders, occult infection, malignancy, and cardiac, pulmonary, or renal abnormalities should be done only when there is historical or physical examination evidence of these diagnoses.

THERAPY AND FOLLOW-UP

The therapeutic approach to children failing to gain weight adequately must be tailored to the individual needs of the family and the child. For infants and children in whom a specific diagnosis has been identified, therapy should be directed toward the underlying disease or condition. More often, a disturbance in the parent-child interaction will be recognized as the cause of the patient's inability to gain weight. Regardless of the underlying etiology, the family should be approached nonjudgmentally and the severity of the child's condition should be allowed to dictate the initial approach to therapy.

Mild to Moderate Failure to Thrive

The primary care practitioner, with consultation from a nutritionist, can manage infants and children manifesting mild degrees of malnutrition (greater than 80% of ideal body weight for age) as outpatients, with occasional consultation from subspecialist colleagues. Patients who have evidence of more severe caloric deprivation will require the involvement of a multidisciplinary team including the primary care practitioner, nutritionist, mental health or behavioral therapist, and social worker.[18] Home visitation using either professionals[32] or lay personnel[4] has been demonstrated to be a useful intervention in select circumstances. Child protective services must be alerted regarding any child thought to be the victim of intentional neglect.

The goals of management must focus on nutritional rehabilitation, parental education, and behavioral intervention. Attempts to overfeed malnourished infants at the outset of therapy should be avoided because initially they may manifest some degree of anorexia, and refeeding that is too vigorous may induce malabsorption and diarrhea. The refeeding regimen should be calculated to provide approximately 10% to 15% of calories from protein, 50% to 60% from carbohydrate, and 30% to 40% from fat.[6]

A typical three-phase regimen[1] may begin with provision of 100% of daily energy and protein requirements based on the child's presenting weight on day 1. If well tolerated, this can be increased to the daily energy and protein requirements based on the 50th percentile weight for the child's age over the next 2 to 3 days.

In phase two, intake is increased to provide adequate nutrition to achieve catch-up growth. Multiplying the energy requirements (kcal/kg/day) of the 50th percentile weight for age by the ratio of the child's ideal body weight divided by the child's actual body weight at presentation will generate a reasonable estimate of the nutrition requirements for this stage. The same calculation can be made for protein requirements. Most often, the energy and protein requirements for these phases of infant refeeding can be accomplished with the use of a routine infant formula modified to increase its caloric density. Mixing 13 oz of concentrated formula with 10 oz of water rather than 13 oz of water will create a formula that is 24 cal/oz. Alternatively, the use of carbohydrate in the form of glucose polymers or fat in the form of medium-chain triglycerides will add calories while avoiding the complications of overhydration. For older children, the repertoire of caloric supplements will include a wide variety of solid foods as well.

In the third, or consolidation, phase of nutritional rehabilitation, a varied diet is offered ad libitum as the child gradually approaches ideal body weight. Multivitamin and iron supplementation should be part of every refeeding regimen for undernourished children.

Initiation of nutritional rehabilitation is an ideal time to engage the parents in an educational program that focuses on family interactions, psychological vulnerabilities, and social needs.[23] Emphasis should be placed on appropriate nutritional information, and concrete suggestions should be offered about how to structure mealtime at home to minimize distractions in a relaxed social environment that encourages good eating habits. For families in need, access to community resources such as WIC and food stamps must be facilitated.

Severe Failure to Thrive

Children who present at less than 60% of ideal body weight should be hospitalized and cared for by a multidisciplinary team of nutritionists, social workers, pediatricians, and pediatric subspecialists, when appropriate. The nutritional rehabilitation of these children will be more prolonged and may entail a period of tube feedings in addition to oral supplements. In cases in which the gastrointestinal tract is temporarily inaccessible, parenteral feedings with central venous access may be necessary.

Follow-up

Once identified, poor weight gain in infancy should be followed up assiduously. Initial weekly visits for infants may be necessary to reassure the parents and practitioner that the therapy undertaken is having the desired effects. Studies of hospitalized children have demonstrated that those younger than 6 months, when provided with adequate calories, begin to gain weight in a few days.[9] Older children may take longer before sustained weight gain is established. Ongoing developmental, behavioral, and social evaluations must be incorporated into any plan for follow-up. Abnormalities in these domains need to be monitored closely because frequently they are present in patients who gain weight poorly. Moreover, the lingering effects of calorie, protein, and micronutrient deprivation may manifest themselves in developmental and behavioral abnormalities,[12] particularly in families in which the mothers exhibit affective disorders.[20]

PROGNOSIS

Outcomes for children who have abnormal weight gain patterns in infancy and childhood should be predicted cautiously in view of the variety of conditions that may give rise to this clinical picture. Most children in the mild category will experience brisk nutritional rehabilitation and, with adequate follow-up, will do quite well. More severely affected children, depending on the etiology of their condition, may require more prolonged or repetitive interventions and may be left with residual cognitive, behavioral, and educational consequences of their malnutrition. It is imperative, therefore, that all children who manifest faltering weight gain during infancy and childhood receive early comprehensive evaluation and prompt treatment.

When to Refer

- If a diagnosis is made of a chronic disease pertaining to an organ subspecialty discipline such as cardiac, pulmonary, renal, gastrointestinal, or endocrine
- If the psychosocial family dynamic indicates a need for psychiatric intervention for either or both parents
- If nutritional rehabilitation warrants the attention of a nutritionist

When to Hospitalize

- Any child with a weight less than 60% of ideal body weight
- Any child who, despite aggressive outpatient management, continues to fail to gain weight at an acceptable rate
- Any child who presents with signs of marasmus or severe protein malnutrition (kwashiorkor)

REFERENCES

1. Adebonojo FO: Undernutrition. In Burg FD, et al, editors: *Gellis and Kagan's current pediatric therapy,* Philadelphia, 1996, WB Saunders.
2. Berwick DM, Levy JC, Kleinerman R: Failure to thrive: diagnostic yield of hospitalisation, *Arch Dis Child* 57:347, 1982.
3. Bithoney WG, Newberger EH: Child and family attributes of failure to thrive, *Dev Behav Pediatr* 8:32, 1987.
4. Black MM, et al: A randomized clinical trial of home intervention for children with failure to thrive, *Pediatrics* 95:807, 1995.
5. Brandt L: Growth dynamics of low birthweight infants with emphasis on the perinatal period. In Falkner F, Tanner J, editors: *Human growth: neurobiology and nutrition,* New York, 1979, Plenum Press.
6. Committee on Nutrition, American Academy of Pediatrics: *Pediatric nutrition handbook,* Elk Grove Village, Ill, 1993, American Academy of Pediatrics.
7. Drotar D, et al: Early preventive intervention in failure to thrive: methods and early outcome. In Drotar D, editor: *New directions in failure to thrive: implications for research and practice,* New York, 1985, Plenum Press.
8. Edwards AGK: Recognising failure to thrive in early childhood, *Arch Dis Child* 65:1263, 1990.
9. Ellerstein NS, Ostrov BE: Growth patterns in children hospitalized because of caloric-deprivation failure to thrive, *Am J Dis Child* 139:164, 1985.
10. Evans SL, Reinhart JB, Succop RA: Failure to thrive: a study of 45 children and their families, *J Am Acad Child Psychiatry* 2:440, 1972.
11. Frank DA, Allen D, Brown JL: Primary prevention of failure to thrive: social policy implications. In Drotar D, editor: *New directions in failure to thrive: implications for research and practice,* New York, 1985, Plenum Press.
12. Frank DA, Zeisel SH: Failure to thrive, *Pediatr Clin North Am* 35:1187, 1988.
13. Gomez F, et al: Mortality in second and third degree malnutrition, *J Trop Pediatr* 2:77, 1956.
14. Guo S, et al: Reference data on gains in weight and length during the first two years of life, *J Pediatr* 119:355, 1991.
15. Guyer B, et al: Anthropometric evidence of malnutrition among low income children in Massachusetts, *Massachusetts J Community Health* 1:3, 1986.
16. Hamill PVV, et al: *NCHS growth curves for children birth-18 years,* United States Vital and Health Statistics, Washington, DC, 1977, Government Printing Office, Department of Health, Education and Welfare Pub PHS 78-1650, series 11.
17. Hannaway PJ: Failure to thrive: a study of 100 infants and children, *Clin Pediatr* 9:96, 1970.
18. Hobbs C, Hanks HGI: A multidisciplinary approach for the treatment of children with failure to thrive, *Child Care Health Dev* 22:273, 1996.
19. Homer C, Ludwig S: Categorization of etiology of failure to thrive, *Am J Dis Child* 135:848, 1981.
20. Hutcheson JJ, et al: Risk status and home intervention among children with failure-to-thrive: follow-up at age 4, *J Pediatr Psychol* 22:651, 1997.
21. Kotelchuck M, Newberger EH: Failure to thrive: a controlled study of familial characteristics, *J Am Acad Child Psychiatry* 4:322, 1983.
22. Leonard MF, Rhymes JP, Solnit AJ: Failure to thrive in infants: a family problem, *Am J Dis Child* 111:600, 1966.

23. Maggioni A, Lifshitz F: Nutritional management of failure to thrive, *Pediatr Clin North Am* 42:791, 1995.
24. McJunkin JE, Bithoney WG, McCormick MC: Errors in formula concentration in an outpatient population, *J Pediatr* 111:848, 1987.
25. Mitchell WG, Gorrell RW, Greenberg RA: Failure-to-thrive: a study in a primary care setting epidemiology and follow-up, *Pediatrics* 65:971, 1980.
26. Pugliese MT, et al: Parental health beliefs as a cause of nonorganic failure to thrive, *Pediatrics* 65:971, 1987.
27. Rosenn DW, Loeb LS, Jura MB: Differentiation of organic from nonorganic failure to thrive syndrome in infancy, *Pediatrics* 66:698, 1980.
28. Schmitt BD, Mauro RD: Nonorganic failure to thrive: an outpatient approach, *Child Abuse Negl* 13:235, 1989.
29. Sills RJ: Failure to thrive: the role of clinical and laboratory evaluation, *Am J Dis Child* 132:967, 1978.
30. Tolia V: Very early onset nonorganic failure to thrive in infants, *J Pediatr Gastroenterol Nutr* 20:73, 1995.
31. Wright C, et al: New chart to evaluate weight faltering, *Arch Dis Child* 78: 40, 1998.
32. Wright CM, et al: Effect of community based management in failure to thrive: randomised controlled trial, *BMJ* 317:571, 1998.
33. Zenel JA Jr: Failure to thrive: a general pediatrician's perspective, *Pediatr Rev* 18:371, 1997.

SUGGESTED READINGS

Bithoney WG, Dubowitz H, Egan H: Failure to thrive/growth deficiency, *Pediatr Rev* 13: 453, 1992.

Drotar D, editor: *New directions in failure to thrive: implications for research and practice,* New York, 1985, Plenum Press.

Frank DA, Zeisel SH: Failure to thrive, *Pediatr Clin North Am* 35:1187, 1988.

Gahagan S, Holmes R: A stepwise approach to evaluation of undernutrition and failure to thrive, *Pediatr Clin North Am* 45:169, 1998.

Zenel JA Jr: Failure to thrive: a general pediatrician's perspective, *Pediatr Rev* 18:371, 1997.

135 Fatigue and Weakness

Philip O. Ozuah • Arnold T. Sigler

Fatigue and weakness are ubiquitous complaints that may or may not be related to medical diagnoses but are used commonly in medical and colloquial language. Both terms are difficult to define. To add to the confusion, the two concepts often are used interchangeably by both patients and physicians. Moreover, adolescents and children often use other terms to describe their perceptions of somatic weakness and fatigue. Fatigue, in fact, is very different from true body weakness. Therefore, it is important to define the two terms carefully, even though the definitions must be modified for each age group.

Fatigue involves extreme, unusual tiredness; decreased physical performance; and an excessive need for rest. It often is accompanied by feelings of sleepiness, weariness, irritability, lassitude, boredom, and decreased efficiency. *Weakness,* in contrast, refers to diminished body or muscle strength. True weakness can be identified only by demonstration of abnormal neurological or muscular function, either by history, by physical examination, or by laboratory techniques. Practically speaking, a history of weakness, on further questioning, will often suggest hypotonia in infants, and in older children will be expressed as trouble running or keeping up in gym class, clumsiness, or lack of agility.

FATIGUE

Fatigue may be a normal result of any physical or mental work in which energy expenditure exceeds the restorative processes. The temporary fatigue that follows intense exercise involves several complex mechanisms, including increased central inhibition mediated by group III and IV muscle afferents along with a decrease in muscle spindle facilitation and suboptimal cortical output.[6] At the level of the muscle cell, fatigue results from a reduction in adenosine triphosphate caused by high utilization rates, as well as a depletion of glycogen.[7] Normal fatigue also follows activities such as cramming for examinations and with food or sleep deprivation. In all of these instances, the degree of fatigue, even when prolonged, usually is appropriate for the amount of physical or mental exertion expended.

On the other hand, fatigue may be a pathological state with an organic or psychological foundation. The lassitude associated with somatic illness, often with definable physical or laboratory abnormalities, is well known. Fatigue also has been shown to have a strong correlation with the psychiatric diagnoses of depression and anxiety disorder.[4,5,8] Needless to say, any acute illness or trauma may be accompanied by fatigue but usually only prolonged fatigue is noteworthy. The differential diagnosis of prolonged fatigue is listed in Box 135-1.

FATIGUE IN INFANTS

The term *fatigue* rarely is pertinent for a very small child. Parents, however, report that the infant tires easily during feeds or seems droopy. Infants who are in heart failure often appear to tire easily and sweat excessively with feeds. Infants who have other serious conditions, including severe anemia and hypothyroidism, also may be described by their parents as being listless.

FATIGUE DURING CHILDHOOD

Children complain only infrequently of "feeling fatigued." Remarkably, even with chronic organic diseases, fatigue itself is not expressed verbally by the child. Rather, it is the concerned parent who usually reports that the child appears fatigued. Parents commonly say such things as "He has no energy," "She lies around all the time," "She seems bored and droopy," "He's sleeping a lot of the time," "She has no pep," "He drags around," or "I can't get her to do a thing." On questioning, younger children occasionally express a sense of lassitude and fatigue to a physician. Much of the difficulty in the middle years of childhood (before adolescence), however, is the child's inability to put into words what he or she feels. Fatigue, therefore, usually is exhibited in terms of a child's physical activity and performance in school, sports, and other organized activities. The younger the child the more likely that the expressed or observed fatigue has a pathological basis.

The most common problem associated with fatigue in children is recurrent or chronic infection. Otitis media, sinusitis, and tonsillitis of a recurrent and smoldering nature often are overlooked for their systemic effects, among which fatigue may be prominent. Often mistakenly considered insignificant, upper respiratory tract allergies may cause impressive fatigue, as well as irritability and mild depression, in children and adolescents.

Of the common endocrine disorders, only hypothyroidism is likely to be associated with fatigue. Certainly the hypothyroid child whose rate of growth has fallen off may manifest increasing fatigue and lassitude, at first subtle, as the only symptoms. Thyrotoxicosis, in contrast, is uncommon in young children but occasionally manifests with isolated fatigue in adolescents.

BOX 135-1

DISORDERS COMMONLY ASSOCIATED WITH PROLONGED FATIGUE IN DIFFERENT AGE GROUPS

Infancy
Cyanotic heart disease
Congestive heart disease
Severe anemia
Hypothyroidism

Childhood
Chronic upper respiratory tract infections
Otitis media and sinusitis
Tonsillitis
Chronic asthma
Chronic allergies
Hepatitis
Rheumatic fever
Disseminated malignancy
AIDS
Immunological disorders
Chronic renal disease

Adolescence
Mycoplasma and other viral pneumonias
Infectious mononucleosis
Hepatitis
Rheumatoid arthritis
Lupus erythematosus
Diabetes mellitus
Malignancy
Inflammatory bowel disease
AIDS
Drug abuse, including alcoholism
Chronic pulmonary disease
Depression
Severe obesity

Although any metabolic disorder can cause fatigue, only diabetes mellitus occurs with enough frequency to merit consideration here. Fatigue almost always accompanies the initial or uncontrolled diabetic state.

Inflammatory diseases, especially rheumatoid arthritis and other rheumatoid-like disorders, appear frequently in pediatric practice, and many children have significant fatigue, out of proportion to their musculoskeletal complaints. Lyme arthritis is a notable example. (See Chapter 233, Lyme Disease.)

Cyanotic heart disease and chronic advanced pulmonary disease, as seen with cystic fibrosis, commonly are associated with marked fatigue; in these cases, however, the underlying disease usually is readily evident before the fatigue becomes severe. The pediatrician occasionally may see an older child for the first time who has severe fatigue caused by a previously undiagnosed hypoxic disorder.

Overall, the condition suspected most often as a cause of fatigue in both children and adults is anemia—and, most often, incorrectly so. Although fatigue often is ascribed to mild or moderate anemia, from whatever source, symptoms usually are not seen in children until the hemoglobin level falls to 6 or 7 g/dl; if red cell levels fall gradually, even lower hemoglobin levels may ensue without clinically evident symptoms. Irritability and attention problems may be present with mild to moderate iron-deficiency anemia, but fatigue usually is not a common feature. Younger children, especially, seem to tolerate incredibly low hemoglobin levels with no symptoms at all.

Malignancy, particularly leukemia or lymphoma, occasionally develops insidiously, with fatigue as the major symptom. Although always feared, these diseases are seen infrequently in pediatric office practice.

Many children who come to the pediatrician with unexplained chronic fatigue are found to have an emotionally related disorder. Before adolescence, the complaint usually centers on the parents' concern about a child's reduced activity level. A younger child will be noted to prefer sedentary activities—to "lie around the house a lot," appear tired, lack energy, and shrink from social contacts. These traits may have been long standing, but a comment from grandparents or a teacher may arouse parental anxiety, precipitating the first visit to the pediatrician.

At this point the family often is convinced that the child has a serious organic disease. Further evaluation, however, usually reveals that the child is performing very satisfactorily, but not up to the family's excessive expectations. The child may be withdrawing because of failure to compete with an exceptional sibling or because of real or imagined failure in school. In other cases a child may feel a lack of well-being because of parental discord. Similarly, lack of parental involvement with a child may lead to lassitude and boredom. Stress and anxiety in children often result in either hyperactivity or withdrawal, and the more common withdrawal reaction may express itself as chronic fatigue.

Most children experience transient periods of lassitude or fatigue, but such instances are brief and usually self-limited. At the opposite extreme is the child whose chronic fatigue is a sign of true psychiatric depression. Here, as in the adolescent, the more protracted and severe the periods of withdrawal, the more likely that depression and fatigue are caused by a pathological process.

FATIGUE IN ADOLESCENTS

Complaints of chronic fatigue are encountered most often in adolescents. It is among the adolescent's most common presentations in pediatric practice and one that usually arouses excessive concern in parents. The normal swings in adolescent moods, from excessive exuberance to fatigue, usually are of more concern to parents and teachers than to the patient. Often, the adolescent may disagree vehemently with the parents' view and not share their concern. Adolescents, however, also initiate visits to the pediatrician because they themselves feel fatigue. Parents may be unable or may refuse to recognize the adolescent's symptoms.

Whereas a younger child who has a profound medical illness often does not present with fatigue, even minor illnesses often precipitate prolonged fatigue in adolescents.

Mycoplasma pneumonia, often low-grade and without fever, produces progressive fatigue. In addition, prolonged viral and parasitic illnesses (e.g., infectious mononucleosis, hepatitis, cytomegalovirus infection, and toxoplasmosis) commonly manifest with fatigue, especially in adolescents.

The terms *chronic infectious mononucleosis* and *chronic fatigue syndrome* have become popular with both physicians and the media. This attention has led to misuse of these terms and also, undoubtedly, to mild mass hysteria among young adults and adolescents who now are convinced they suffer from one of these disorders. Most adults and many infants and children have been infected with the Epstein-Barr (EB) virus. The clinical manifestations in proved cases are extremely variable: Some patients remain symptom free, whereas clinical, hematological, and serological findings support the diagnosis of infectious mononucleosis in others. The symptoms of infectious mononucleosis usually resolve in several weeks, but an occasional patient may have an atypical or a more prolonged course in which the initial clinical findings either persist or are intermittent over a period of months, or in rare cases, years. These unusual but documented cases of chronic infectious mononucleosis typically include complaints of chronic fatigue. Another much smaller group of patients has been described as having a serious, sometimes lethal, illness associated with EB virus infection. These patients usually do not manifest the classic findings of infectious mononucleosis; very often their conditions are proved to be either acquired or genetically determined immunological abnormalities.

Always unpredictable and often secretive, inflammatory bowel disease may arouse concern initially with unexplained fatigue and a loss of sense of well-being. Although eventually accompanied by fever, abdominal symptoms, or abnormal stools, this disorder can continue for months with fatigue as the only major symptom. Of more current importance in older children and adolescents are alcoholism and drug abuse—causes of chronic fatigue that easily are overlooked.

By far the most common and familiar patient complaining of protracted fatigue is the adolescent. The pediatrician can expect to see a generous number of adolescents who characteristically appear each spring complaining of fatigue or lassitude and lack of energy and seem mildly depressed. This disorder usually appears during periods of greatest school-related stress—before examinations. It is "spring fever." Although the patient may have a real fever, usually secondary to infection (e.g., infectious mononucleosis or influenza), the problem usually is emotionally based. All the uncertainties of late adolescence, including identity and sexual crises, may create a "spring fever" during *any* season, with fatigue often the dominant complaint.

Often, the adolescent collapses with fatigue after intense and exuberant activity involving schoolwork, extracurricular activity, sports, or social events. These individuals also may be short on sleep, may have "borderline" eating habits, and may complain of an additional variety of hypochondriacal symptoms. "Burnout" and fatigue are particularly common in overachieving high school and college students during late adolescence. The emotional reaction actually may be precipitated by a physical illness, particularly an infection. Most of these patients have normal findings on physical examinations and routine laboratory tests.

Since 1985, adolescents, adults, and occasionally, children have been described as having a disorder commonly referred to as *chronic fatigue syndrome* (CFS),[1-3,9-11] which most commonly involves persistent or relapsing severe fatigue, fever, headache, sore throat, tender lymphadenitis, nausea or vomiting, myalgia, arthralgia, and abdominal pain. Neurocognitive complaints, such as an inability to concentrate, sleep disturbances, episodic confusion and memory problems, depression, anxiety, and irritability, also are especially common in CFS.

The neurocognitive complaints are the most difficult to evaluate in CFS because of the extreme difference in emotional perception from person to person. Furthermore, careful physical examinations by experienced physicians often fail to document any physical abnormalities, and extensive laboratory evaluations usually produce normal results. In addition, much of the difficulty surrounding both the diagnosis and the search for a cause of CFS is attributable to confusion about the use of the terms *chronic fatigue* and *chronic fatigue syndrome*. Consequently, the Centers for Disease Control and Prevention (CDC) has formulated strict criteria for the case definition of CFS. Unfortunately, these criteria were based mainly on observations of adult populations and may not be completely pertinent to children and adolescents.

Nevertheless, the CDC criteria for CFS stipulate that the debilitating fatigue must last at least 6 months, and they exclude patients who have either a current or preexisting chronic psychiatric disorder such as depression. However, because depression and anxiety are so commonly reported in CFS, strict adherence to this definition may falsely exclude some patients who have CFS or may exclude some who have reactive depression secondary to their chronic physical fatigue.

CFS quickly became a popular diagnosis. Initially the syndrome was attributed to infection with the EB virus, although very few patients had documented physical findings or hematological abnormalities consistent with the diagnosis of infectious mononucleosis. In addition, most had no serological evidence of active EB virus infection. Recently, however, a better understanding of the natural course of EB virus antibody activity in healthy individuals months and years after an initial illness with infectious mononucleosis indicates that healthy patients who had mononucleosis years earlier could not be differentiated from fatigued patients who currently had the disease. See Chapter 195, Chronic Fatigue Syndrome, for further discussion of this syndrome.

WEAKNESS

True weakness in a pediatric patient should always be a cause of concern. Weakness is the result of a derangement of neuromuscular function at one of several levels, including the cerebral hemispheres, cerebellum, spinal cord, anterior horn cells, peripheral nerves, myeoneuronal junction, or the muscle. Box 135-2 lists some of the differential diagnoses for weakness in the pediatric age group.

Infants with weakness are often brought to the pediatrician with a complaint of being "floppy." It should be noted that a "floppy" infant is usually one who has hypotonia caused by a neuromuscular disorder. In the newborn period, some of these patients may assume a "frog-leg" position. Chromosomal anomalies such as Down syndrome, congenital hypothyroidism, and the infantile form of Werdnig-Hoffmann disease (spinal muscular atrophy) are some of the more common causes of hypotonia in infancy.

Older children and adolescents who have weakness pre-

BOX 135-2

DIFFERENTIAL DIAGNOSIS OF WEAKNESS AND HYPOTONIA

- Down syndrome
- Werdnig-Hoffmann disease
- Muscular dystrophies
- Congenital hypothyroidism
- Myasthenia gravis
- Guillain-Barré syndrome
- Dermatomyositis
- Polymyositis

sent with difficulty walking, running, and participating in athletic activities. Myasthenia gravis and Guillain-Barré syndrome (postinfectious polyneuropathy) are perhaps the two most common causes of weakness in this age group. A distinguishing clinical feature is that in myasthenia gravis, deep-tendon reflexes may be diminished but rarely are absent, whereas Guillain-Barré syndrome is remarkable for bilateral, symmetrically absent tendon stretch reflexes. Other causes of weakness in the older child include the muscular dystrophies, the juvenile form of Werdnig-Hoffmann disease, dermatomyositis, and polymyositis.

DIFFERENTIAL DIAGNOSIS AND EVALUATION

Although it may first appear that the patient who is chronically fatigued has an insignificant problem, great care must be taken to rule out underlying medical illness and also to return the child to a state of well-being and to relieve parental concerns. The physician must remember that either the child or the parents are worried about the child's fatigue. Because family members may disagree about the significance of the symptoms, adequate time and concern are needed to evaluate the history. The symptoms of chronic fatigue cannot be dismissed casually over the telephone or with a quick office visit.

Inasmuch as most patients who come to the physician complaining of fatigue have an emotionally based problem, a careful history, with information from both child and parents (taken separately when appropriate), often helps to narrow the differential diagnosis. Discrepancies between the child's and the parents' observations soon become evident, and the diagnosis of emotionally related fatigue emerges in most cases based on the history alone. Happily, the information derived from a long-standing physician-patient relationship contributes enormously to reducing tensions during the evaluation. Although fatigue may be the only presenting symptom, further questioning almost always uncovers other symptoms of somatic disease. Chronic fatigue, in the absence of other physical symptoms, usually is emotionally based. Other associated complaints are somnolence, depression, anxiety, boredom, decreased activity, and inappropriate affect. Often, emotional stress or some disruption in the patient's life is part of the history.

A physical examination, thoroughly performed, may be the only treatment necessary, working miracles to reassure the anxious child or parent. The child's affect and appearance are most revealing. The impression that the child "looks well" invariably proves to be an accurate measure of his or her health. The condition of the adolescent, in contrast, may be more difficult to interpret. Although the physical examination may be benign, the adolescent may be slovenly, uncommunicative, and depressed and be unable to express his or her feelings; thus, at first the adolescent sometimes appears to be physically ill.

In all age groups a search should be made for sites of chronic latent infection: adenopathy, enlargement or tenderness of the liver and spleen, and abdominal masses. Careful palpation for an enlarged or tender thyroid gland is essential. Mild scleral icterus and petechiae are easy to overlook. Similarly, a patient's pallor (a common finding, especially after long winters indoors) may evade even the most experienced pediatrician. On the other hand, the facies of the chronically allergic child, clubbing, and cyanosis are obvious.

A limited, well-selected group of laboratory tests should be performed on most patients who are chronically fatigued. These results will reassure the family, the patient, and the pediatrician and usually will erase any lingering doubt about the diagnosis.

The laboratory evaluation initially should include a complete blood count (CBC) with red cell indices, thyroid and liver function tests, a throat culture, and a stool examination for blood. The cold agglutinin test often is valuable, as is a simple initial screening test for a *Mycoplasma* infection. Roentgenograms rarely are necessary and should be discouraged. Critical evaluation of data collected from the history, physical examination, and laboratory tests should enable the pediatrician to detect quickly any organic causes of fatigue. Prolonged fever, however low grade, always must be viewed as significant and may suggest infection, inflammatory disease, or malignancy. Pallor points to the possibility of anemia or hypothyroidism.

Cervical adenopathy, even a single enlarged node, in the absence of other findings can be a clue to the diagnosis of infectious mononucleosis. In fact, in the autumn and early winter of each year every pediatrician begins to look for patients who have infectious mononucleosis. However, infectious mononucleosis is a protean illness, and the physical examination sometimes is normal. Children and adolescents who have infectious mononucleosis may have no fever or signs of toxicity but may manifest major fatigue. Furthermore, results of the heterophil antibody test for infectious mononucleosis may be negative in many young children and infants and in about 10% of older children and adolescents who have the disease. The reliability of EB virus antibody testing has improved to the point where the diagnosis of acute, active infectious mononucleosis can be confirmed. During the evaluation of chronic fatigue, EB virus antibody titers usually can differentiate long-past infection from recent and active infection, thus eliminating EB virus infection and infectious mononucleosis as causes for the fatigue and permitting a search for other likely neuropsychiatric causes. Toxoplasmosis and cytomegalovirus (CMV) infections may mimic mononucleosis closely and manifest with significant fatigue, but with only minimal cervical adenopathy and fever. Positive results of a fluorescent antibody test for toxoplasmosis or CMV with negative results of a heterophil antibody test will confirm the diagnosis. Similarly, fatigued children may have hepatitis and may be anicteric (or only slightly icteric), with little or no hepatic tenderness or enlargement. Other common viral infections, especially during convalescence, can cause a prolonged fatigue syndrome accompanied by depression.

The diagnosis of CFS should be restricted to patients who meet rigid criteria, including the new onset of persistent or relapsing fatigue with no prior history of such fatigue and the exclusion of other clinical conditions that might produce similar symptoms. In addition, two of the following three physical criteria should be documented on at least two occasions in a 1-month interval: (1) low-grade fever, (2) nonexudative pharyngitis, and (3) palpable or tender postcervical or axillary lymph nodes (less than 2 cm in diameter). Furthermore, symptoms must include several of the following: muscle weakness, muscle discomfort, headaches, migratory arthralgia, neuropsychological complaints, and sleep disturbances. After other medical conditions are excluded, some older children and adolescents may meet these criteria for diagnosis. Certainly these patients should not be labeled with a diagnosis of chronic infectious mononucleosis syndrome or chronic EB virus infection, which recently has become a "quick fix" diagnosis for patients who are chronically fatigued.

Children who have an autoimmune disease may have fatigue with little else at first. Mild articular or periarticular inflammation may be missed by the physician. The emphasis must be on a careful examination and the observation of subtle or minimal physical findings, inasmuch as children usually do not manifest fulminant findings initially. Children who have inflammatory bowel disease, arthritis, or an arthritis-like illness and some patients who have a malignancy (monocytic leukemia, in particular) may have especially prolonged symptoms, including fatigue, without any physical findings whatsoever.

An enlarged, tender thyroid gland and fatigue may indicate thyroiditis with emerging hypothyroidism. However, the thyroid often is palpable and full in healthy adolescents. In any event, chronic fatigue from thyroid disease usually can be ruled out quickly with a thyroxine (T_4) test. Some patients who have hypothyroidism also demonstrate mild to moderate anemia, and those who have active thyroiditis may have an elevated sedimentation rate. To be acceptable as an explanation for fatigue, the diagnosis of pure anemia requires marked reduction of hemoglobin. Red cell indices and a reticulocyte count will characterize the anemia and the probable cause. Anemia accompanied by thrombocytopenia, however, suggests leukemia or aplastic anemia. The white cell count may be normal in infectious mononucleosis or hepatitis, but lymphocytosis with atypical lymphocytes most likely will be present. The heterophil antibody screening test ("mono test") is diagnostic in most such circumstances.

The erythrocyte sedimentation rate is the most valuable screening test for inflammatory diseases of all varieties. A normal sedimentation rate almost always rules out autoimmune disease, inflammatory bowel disease, chronic smoldering infections, and disseminated malignancies. An elevated sedimentation rate requires further investigation. A routine urinalysis almost always reveals diabetes, and most patients who have chronic renal failure have abnormal urinalyses, as well as significant anemia. In these cases, the subsequent measurement of blood glucose in diabetes and of creatinine or blood urea nitrogen in renal disease can confirm these diagnoses.

The evaluation of a patient who has weakness may include chromosomal studies, muscle enzymes, nerve conduction studies, electromyography, edrophonium (Tensilon) challenge, muscle biopsy, and a lumbar puncture, depending on the suspected diagnosis. Consultation with a pediatric neurologist often is required.

MANAGEMENT

Inasmuch as significant organic disease is ruled out in most patients, further management requires meaningful communication between the pediatrician, the patient, and the parents. In younger children, one must put the variability in performance and behavior of normal children into perspective. Again, appropriate parental expectations must be emphasized. In addition, the child's and the family's daily schedule should be reviewed. A chaotic lifestyle that is frantic, with poorly structured activity and inadequate sleep patterns, often is revealed. Occasionally, true psychiatric depression is discovered, which calls for referral to a psychiatrist.

Older children and adolescents benefit from personal, warm attention. The value of a continuous relationship with one physician becomes self-evident. An understanding, thorough session with the patient's own pediatrician usually "streamlines" the evaluation and eliminates the need for excessive testing. Conversation after the physical examination should attempt to (1) reassure the child or adolescent about his or her basic health, (2) reiterate the common and "normal" occurrence of fatigue, (3) examine the daily routine and stresses on the patient, and (4) suggest modifications of the patient's lifestyle and approaches to life's situations. It is a time for respectful give-and-take. It is the pediatrician's responsibility to attempt to establish the probable cause of the fatigue before the patient is referred to a specialist. If emotional fatigue is suspected, the adolescent, in particular, must be comfortable with the conclusion that organic diseases have been ruled out. The patient then must be made aware of the emotional basis for the fatigue, and if psychiatric referral is needed, the reasons must be made clear. A knowledgeable pediatrician will be reassuring but firm in approaching the child or adolescent who needs referral. Fortunately, such a referral usually is not necessary.

When to Refer

1. Unexplained weight loss
2. Hypotonia in infants
3. Suspected major affective disorder
4. Suspected malignancy

When to Hospitalize

1. Severe depression and/or suicidal ideation
2. Need for evaluation of neuromuscular disorders such as Werdnig-Hoffmann disease, Guillain-Barré syndrome, and myasthenia gravis.

REFERENCES

1. Bou-Holaigah I, et al: The relationship between neurally mediated hypotension and the chronic fatigue syndrome, *JAMA* 274:961, 1995.
2. Carter BD, et al: Case control study of chronic fatigue in pediatric patients, *Pediatrics* 95:179, 1995.
3. Dale JK, Straus SE: The chronic fatigue syndrome: considerations relevant to children and adolescents, *Adv Pediatr Infect Dis* 7:63, 1992.
4. Epstein KR: The chronically fatigued patient, *Med Clin North Am* 79: 315, 1995.
5. Fuhrer R, Wessely S: The epidemiology of fatigue and depression: a French primary-care study, *Psychol Med* 25:895, 1995.
6. Gandevia SC, Allen GM, Mckenzie DK: Central fatigue: critical issues, quantification and practical implications, *Adv Exp Med Biol* 384:281, 1995.
7. Green HJ: Mechanisms of muscle fatigue in intense exercise, *J Sports Sci* 15:247, 1997.
8. Ridsdale L, et al: Patients with fatigue in general practice: a prospective study, *BMJ* 10:307(6896):103, 1993.
9. Sigler A: Chronic fatigue syndrome: fact or fiction, *Contemp Pediatr* 7:22, 1990.
10. Smith MS, et al: Chronic fatigue in adolescents, *Pediatrics* 88:195, 1991.
11. Wilson A, et al: The treatment of chronic fatigue syndrome: science and speculation, *Am J Med* 96:544, 1994.

136 Fever

Elise Willem van der Jagt

For centuries, fever has been associated with illness. Today, as many as 30% of all patients seen by pediatricians have fever as their principal complaint, making it one of the most common reasons children are taken to a physician. The multitude of telephone calls about fever received day and night by pediatricians makes it obvious that its proper evaluation and management is a basic and necessary skill for physicians and nurse practitioners.

Even though clinicians have dealt with this common clinical sign for decades, its mechanism, meaning, and management have remained sufficiently unclear and controversial that research on these matters continues. Although advances in neurochemistry and neurophysiology have improved our understanding of the pathophysiology of fever (see Chapter 25, Management of Fever), clinical investigators continue to search for practical knowledge that will enhance the care of the febrile patient. Availability of such information can simplify the challenging role of the physician, who must evaluate the patient quickly and effectively, arrive at a diagnosis, institute appropriate therapy, and both educate and support the parents and child during the entire process. The extent to which health care practitioners accomplish these goals depends on their knowledge of the mechanisms of disease, the various clinical manifestations of disease, and their awareness of the social context in which the disease occurs.

DEFINITION

The word *fever* is derived from the Latin *fovere* (to warm) and commonly means an elevation of body temperature. Although this general definition is acceptable in common parlance, fever is described more accurately as a disorder of thermoregulation. It must be differentiated from hyperthermia, an elevated body temperature resulting from conditions that overwhelm the normal process of thermoregulation. See Chapter 25, Management of Fever, for a full discussion of thermoregulation.

Excessive body heat generated during strenuous exercise, from excessive coverings, or from high environmental temperatures normally is dissipated by peripheral thermoregulation to maintain core body temperature at 37° C. If peripheral thermoregulation is unable to accomplish this task, heat will be retained and hyperthermia will occur. In the case of fever, however, the thermostat itself has been "reset" at a higher set point, causing core body temperature to be maintained at a higher level.

Ever since 1850, when the use of the thermometer first was recommended to measure body temperature,[38] normal core body temperature measured rectally ranges between 97° F and 100° F (36.1° C and 37.8° C), although on rare occasions it may be as low as 95.5° F (35.3° C) or as high as 101° F (38.3° C). The "normal temperature" of 98.6° F was derived from Wunderlich's study[38] of more than 1 million axillary temperatures taken in adults. This may have no relevance for children, not only because adults were studied but also because axillary and rectal (core) temperatures correlate poorly. Young children appear to have higher core body temperatures than do adults, with temperatures slightly higher than 37.8° C occurring frequently in those younger than 2 years of age. A study by Herzog and Coyne[16] suggested that the upper limits of normal for a rectal temperature is 38.0° C for infants younger than 1 month old, 38.1° C in 1-month-olds, and 38.2° C in 2-month-olds. In this study, 6.2% of infants (well babies) had a rectal temperature of 38.0° C. Lowest temperatures occur from 2 AM to 6 AM and highest ones from 5 PM to 7 PM, a diurnal variation that persists even during a febrile illness.

Because of the range of normal body temperatures, knowing a child's usual body temperature occasionally can be useful so that an abnormal elevation can be recognized more easily. The extent to which body temperature is elevated from normal may help determine the presence and significance of fever. This especially may be true in a young infant, in whom even a mild fever may be associated with serious disease. Although the variability and range of normal temperatures in children have made it difficult to define fever precisely and consistently, a recent consensus panel of experts[4] has recommended that the lower limit of fever be defined as a rectal temperature of 38° C (100.4° F).

MEASUREMENT

Inasmuch as accurate measurement of body temperature is relied on extensively to determine the presence of fever, every physician should ensure that patients and parents are knowledgeable about the techniques and rationale for temperature measurement. Ideally, this discussion should be held at the time of the child's birth, just before hospital discharge.

The traditional locations for measurement of temperature are the rectum, the mouth, and the axilla; the traditional devices are glass thermometers containing mercury or alcohol. However, concern about breakage and exposure to mercury has resulted in the increased use of electronic thermometers. These have digital readouts and disposable sheaths to reduce the spread of communicable disease. Attempts to measure temperature at home by use of a liquid crystal temperature strip applied to the forehead or sensor-containing pacifiers have neither been uniformly successful nor sufficiently reliable.

A recent advance in temperature measurement is the development of a device that is inserted into the outer part of the ear canal and measures thermal infrared energy emitted from the tympanic membrane. Because the tympanic membrane's blood supply is common with that going to the hypothalamus, the energy measured reflects core body temperature. This method is not uncomfortable, takes only 1 second, and has correlated well with pulmonary artery (r = 0.98) and rectal (r = 0.90) temperatures in both adults and children.[31] This "ear thermometer" is available for both home and health care provider use.

A number of studies have demonstrated that acceptable correlations of tympanic membrane temperatures with rectal temperatures exist in children.[8,36] However, in children who are very young (less than 3 months of age) or exceptionally active (toddlers), correlation with rectal temperatures is not as good, particularly if the child is febrile.[34] This may be due to the presence of wax in the ear canal and/or improper positioning of the instrument at the ear. Falsely low temperatures can result if the instrument is not aimed directly at the tympanic membrane. Caution is advised, therefore, in using this technique in the very young infant. In addition, environmental temperature (either hot or cold) has been shown to affect tympanic temperatures significantly,[39] something that is not true of rectal temperatures. Nevertheless, in the older infant or child and in the child for whom a rectal temperature is contraindicated (e.g., a neutropenic child), the advent of a tympanic thermometer has made the process of temperature-taking more pleasant, more reliable, more efficient, and more acceptable to parents.

Because the rectal temperature consistently reflects core body temperature best, this location (or a tympanic temperature) is preferred unless a specific contraindication to minor rectal trauma exists. After the procedure is explained to the parent and, as appropriate, to the child, a well-lubricated glass thermometer or a sheathed electronic thermometer should be inserted 3 to 7 cm into the anal canal. If care is taken that the thermometer stays in the anal canal, peak temperature will be reached in 2 to 3 minutes when a glass thermometer is used or in about 30 seconds when an electronic thermometer is used.

Taking temperatures orally should not be attempted until the child is older than 4 to 5 years and is cooperative. After the thermometer has been placed under the tongue for a minimum of 1 minute, a temperature reading will be obtained that is about 0.5° C less than the rectal temperature. Because hot and cold foods may alter the oral temperature by as much as 1° C to 2° C, they should be avoided for an hour before measurement.

Axillary temperature measurements have been recommended in the very young infant because of a concern that rectal temperature measurement in infants might result in rectal perforation. However, very few cases of rectal perforation have been reported (11 cases reported in the world literature over the past 30 years), and all have occurred in neonates, in the hospital, and in the first few days of life. Thus, there essentially are no risks in taking a rectal temperature after the first few days of life. Moreover, although axillary temperatures have been shown to correlate well with rectal temperatures in preterm infants under radiant warmers,[27] they correlate poorly in older infants and children.[28,29] Several recent studies have demonstrated that as much as 3° C difference can exist between the axillary and rectal temperature. In addition, although a mean difference of up to 1.8° C between axillary and rectal temperatures has been demonstrated in group studies, this cannot be used as a standard number to convert axillary to rectal temperatures, because of significant individual patient variability. For all these reasons, axillary temperature measurements should be avoided. If neither oral nor rectal temperatures can be measured, a tympanic temperature reading is preferable.

ASSOCIATED SIGNS AND SYMPTOMS

Donaldson[14] has noted the behavior of humans and animals to be remarkably similar when fever is present. When the set point in the hypothalamus is elevated, patients attempt to adjust the environment to keep their bodies at this higher temperature. Young children usually seek close contact with a warm person (generally a parent), wish to be covered by a blanket, sit near a warm stove or register, and refuse cold liquids or foods. Although children may be quite comfortable at this elevated body temperature, they interact less with others, have a decreased ability to concentrate, substitute quieter for energetic activities, and become less communicative except to indicate discomfort and distress. This "adaptive withdrawal" often is accompanied by loss of appetite and complaint of headache.

Such a combination of behavioral symptoms is a familiar indicator of illness to most parents and usually results in the "hand on the forehead" maneuver, followed by measurement of the temperature. Unfortunately, parents may not recognize the onset of fever in the younger child because the alterations in behavior are fewer and more subtle. In a small infant, irritability and anorexia may be the sole evidence of fever and disease. If a parent is not familiar with these subtle cues, recognition of serious illness may be significantly delayed.

In addition to the behavioral changes that may accompany fever, the general physical examination may reveal a pronounced hypermetabolic state. The child may have flushed cheeks, have an unusual glitter in the eyes, and be either sleepy and lethargic or exceptionally alert and excited (particularly 5- to 10-year-olds). With rare exception, the pulse is elevated by about 10 to 15 beats per degree centigrade of fever, and the respiratory rate is increased. (If the pulse rate is less than expected for the degree of fever, typhoid fever, tularemia, mycoplasma infection, or factitious fever should be considered.) The skin may feel very hot and dry ("burning up with fever"), although the distal extremities may be cold and pale (vasoconstricted), obscuring a very high core body temperature. Most children are not particularly uncomfortable, but some may shiver or sweat, mechanisms by which the body increases or decreases temperature. Sweating may be so excessive that significant dehydration may occur, particularly if the intake of fluids has been poor. Thus, a dry mouth and lips may result not only from rapid mouth breathing but also from dehydration. Finally, irritability of the central nervous system may increase, reflected in a febrile seizure.

The aforementioned signs and symptoms may be less obvious in a small infant. Shivering does not occur in the first few months of life, and diaphoresis is seen less frequently than in the older child. Because irritability and pallor may be the only suggestions of illness, a careful measurement of the temperature should be taken if the parent mentions these signs.

PRESENTATION

A febrile child may come to the attention of a physician or nurse practitioner in several ways. Probably the most dramatic and frightening manifestation of fever in a child is the sudden occurrence of a seizure. Usually lasting less than 15 minutes and occurring within 24 hours of the onset of fever, a generalized tonic or tonic-clonic seizure may begin without warning. Most parents are not aware that a fever was present and often feel guilty for not having noted it. The pediatrician may be called immediately after the seizure has occurred or after the child has been transported to the local emergency room. There the child is likely to be postictal and have a rectal temperature of 102° F to 104° F (39° C to 40° C). A careful assessment of the patient is indicated because a seizure may be the first sign of meningitis or encephalitis.

Although some have recommended that every patient who has a first febrile seizure should have a lumbar puncture routinely, most experts recommend that the diagnostic evaluation be individualized. Reexamination of the child after the convulsive episode may help determine whether an examination of the cerebrospinal fluid is needed. However, because the telltale signs of meningitis (meningismus, Kernig's sign, and Brudzinski's sign) may be absent in children younger than 24 months (especially under 18 months of age), it is prudent to perform a lumbar puncture in this age group.

More commonly, the patient is seen first when the fever has been present for longer than 24 hours and is associated either with nonspecific symptoms, such as those mentioned above, or with symptoms referable to a particular organ system. Inasmuch as many of the evaluations of the febrile child take place over the telephone (the first contact with the clinician), the physician must be able to take a pertinent history. Of particular significance are the age of the patient (the younger the child, the more careful the evaluation), any associated signs and symptoms, exposure to illness in the family or community, history of recent immunizations, and a history of any recurrent infections (e.g., urinary tract infections, streptococcal infections, or otitis media). The time of year should be considered, because certain viral illnesses are more prevalent at different times of the year. For example, respiratory syncytial and influenza virus infections are more common during the winter; parainfluenza virus infections (the most common cause of croup) are more common during the spring and especially in the fall; enterovirus infections occur primarily during the summer. In addition, questions should be asked about the duration and height of the fever. A low-grade fever that has been present for many days usually does not need to be evaluated as urgently as a temperature of 106° F (41° C) that has been present for a few hours. The former is likely to indicate a chronic or benign illness; the latter is more likely to be a potentially serious and rapidly progressive infectious disease.

A visit or telephone call for minimal fever and little evidence of disease should prompt a careful assessment of the psychosocial factors that may be contributing to parental concern. Is the main concern about something else—the "hidden agenda"? What knowledge about fever and disease does the caregiver have? Has there been a previous traumatic experience with disease? Could this be a "vulnerable child"? Is this a dysfunctional family in which minor illness either cannot be dealt with or is used as a means to meet other needs? These questions and others may clarify the situation.

DIFFERENTIAL DIAGNOSIS

Innumerable conditions may cause fever; an extensive discussion about each condition is beyond the scope of this chapter. However, it is useful to classify conditions associated with fever into broad categories: (1) infections, (2) autoimmune diseases, (3) neoplasias, (4) metabolic diseases (e.g., hyperthyroidism), (5) chronic inflammatory diseases, (6) hematological diseases (e.g., sickle cell disease, transfusion reaction), (7) drug fever and immunization reactions, (8) poisoning (e.g., aspirin, atropine), (9) central nervous system abnormalities, and (10) factitious fever. In addition, dehydration, excessive activity, and heat exposure all can cause hyperthermia.

Although any disease in these categories may cause fever at any age, some diseases are more likely to occur at some ages than at others. Autoimmune disease and inflammatory bowel disease, for example, are unusual in infants but become progressively more frequent with increasing age. Similarly, febrile immunization reactions are much more common during the first year of life, because this is when most immunizations are administered.

Infections affecting the respiratory and gastrointestinal tracts account for the majority of fevers in all age groups. Most of these infections have a viral origin (e.g., enterovirus, influenza virus, parainfluenza virus, respiratory syncytial virus, adenovirus, rhinovirus, rotavirus) and generally are self-limited. Knowledge of the seasonality of these viruses promotes correct and efficient diagnoses. In addition, knowledge of the typical physical findings in these infections and their course may help distinguish them from bacterial diseases. For example, high fever, irritability, posterior cervical adenopathy, and painful vesicles on the gums and tongue are characteristic of herpes gingivostomatitis. Failure to examine the tongue and gums may result in an unnecessary septic workup in search of a possible bacterial infection. On the other hand, assuming that a high fever in a 2-month-old child is due to roseola (exanthem subitum) would be erroneous because this infection (human herpesvirus-6) usually does not occur at such an early age.

Failure to evaluate the fever further might result in missing a serious bacterial infection. Although viral infections may cause significant morbidity and mortality, the more aggressive course and serious outcomes of bacterial infections make early diagnosis especially important, particularly because effective antibiotic treatment usually is available.

Bacterial infections may be especially devastating in younger children, who are relatively immunocompromised because of their immature immune system. An infection that remains localized in the older child may disseminate rapidly in the infant and toddler, particularly to the blood (bacteremia), the lungs (pneumonia), the meninges (meningitis), the bones (osteomyelitis), and the joints (arthritis). Because these infections may be fatal or seriously debilitating if not recognized, the physician must be able to differentiate bacterial infections from the more benign viral infections.

The younger the child, the more difficult it is to recognize bacterial infection. Complaints cannot be verbalized, and physical signs and symptoms are more subtle and easily missed unless a high index of suspicion is maintained. It is especially difficult to diagnose serious bacterial disease in children who have no obvious focus of infection. For this reason, many attempts have been made during the past 20 years to identify children in whom fever is a sign of a serious bacterial infection.[35] Children between birth and 36 months of age have been of special interest because fever is most common in this age group and may be difficult to assess, particularly during the first 6 months of life. Efforts have focused on three areas: (1) data from the history and physical examination,[17,26] (2) laboratory data,[24] and (3) response to antipyretics.[2] Of the three areas, the response to antipyretics has been shown most clearly not to be helpful in distinguishing between patients who have a serious bacterial infection and those who have a more benign viral infection.[2] Children who have a serious infection respond to antipyretics no differently than those whose illness is less significant. In fact, some children who have viral illnesses do not defervesce as well.

Many studies have attempted to delineate the precise combination of clinical or laboratory variables that might identify the febrile child at risk for serious disease. Clinical assessment using defined observational scales (e.g., Yale Observation Scale, Young Infant Observation Scale, Severity Scale) are not sufficiently discriminatory and predictive to be used alone.[7,23] Laboratory studies continue to be necessary as well.

During the early 1990s, Baraff et al[3] formulated and published specific practice guidelines to facilitate the initial management of febrile infants and children who do not have an obvious source of infection. Since these recommendations were published, as many as one third of pediatricians have found them to be helpful and have changed their management of fever.[11] However, although the recommendations are an excellent starting point, they remain controversial[3,5,15,21,33] and need to be applied in the individual context of each patient. Considerations of the inconvenience, discomfort, and cost of laboratory testing and the increasing resistance to antibiotics in the community must be weighed carefully against the risk of missing a serious bacterial infection, with its subsequent morbidity and mortality. Therefore, health care practitioners must make the best decisions possible in an environment of incomplete certainty about the presence of serious disease. Parents need to be part of these discussions, and adequate follow-up of all patients is crucial no matter what is decided in the initial visit.

Fever during the first 4 days of life has been associated with a high incidence of bacterial disease.[37] A temperature above 98.6° F (37° C) occurs in 1% of all newborns; of these children, 10% have a bacterial infection caused primarily by group B streptococcal or gram-negative enteric pathogens.

Although febrile (temperature of at least 100.4° F [38.0° C]) infants younger than 3 months of age previously were believed to have a higher incidence of bacteremia, more recent studies suggest that the incidence is similar to that in older infants and children. The presence of bacterial disease ranges between 8% and 15% and that of bacteremia between 3% and 4%.[4] In fact, neither age, gender, height of fever, nor apparent degree of toxicity has been a reliable predictor of bacteremia or serious bacterial infection.[6,25] Instead, several studies now have identified a combination of clinical and laboratory criteria that can be used to recognize infants who are at low risk for having a bacterial infection (low-risk criteria). The infants must satisfy all of the following conditions: previously healthy, no clinical signs of toxicity, no focal bacterial infection on physical examination (except otitis media), a WBC of 5000 to 15,000 with less than 1500 bands, a normal urinalysis (less than 5 WBC/hpf), and a Gram-stained smear of stool demonstrating less than 5 WBC/hpf if diarrhea is present.[13] Infants younger than 3 months old who satisfy these criteria have only a 1.4% probability of having a serious bacterial infection, a 1.1% probability of having bacteremia, and a 0.5% probability of having meningitis. Although there still is concern that infants younger than 28 days old should be evaluated and treated differently from those 2 to 3 months old, the "low-risk criteria" appear to be quite discriminatory in this group, as well. In fact, Chiu and Lin and Chiu, Lin, and Bullard have demonstrated only a 0.2% incidence of bacteremia/meningitis in neonates satisfying the low-risk criteria.[9,10]

Because it is so difficult to determine solely based on the degree of fever whether an infant younger than 3 months of age is at a low or high risk for bacterial disease (septicemia has occurred even in infants who have low-grade fevers[30]), evaluation should be prompt and thorough whenever a fever exists of at least 100.4° F (38° C), paying particular attention to obtaining the data necessary for classifying the child as low or high risk. Such a comprehensive evaluation generally should include a complete physical examination, total and differential white blood cell count, urinalysis[19] and urine culture, a Gram-stained smear of stool if diarrhea is present, blood culture, and examination/culture of the cerebrospinal fluid. A urine culture especially is important because a urinary tract infection is the most common bacterial infection observed in this age group, even in the absence of pyuria.[10,22] (Pyuria by itself has only a 40% positive predictive value, whereas a combination of pyuria and bacteriuria has a positive predictive value of 85%.[20]) At particular risk are girls who have a temperature of at least 102.2° F (39° C), because they have a 17% prevalence rate of urinary tract infection with temperatures this high or higher. Because urinary tract infections have been shown to occur more often in uncircumcised males, this physical characteristic should be noted.

However, if the infant appears nontoxic and meets the low risk criteria, examination/culture of the cerebrospinal fluid and blood cultures might reasonably be avoided as long as there is good observation (outpatient or inpatient), follow-up within 24 hours, and antibiotics are not administered. If antibiotics are to be administered, a full septic workup including blood and CSF cultures should be done.

For infants and children between 3 months and 3 years old who have a fever of at least 102.2° F (39° C) without an obvious source, the risk of bacteremia ranges from 3% to 11% (mean, 4.3%). Below this temperature, an associated bacteremia is much less common. *Streptococcus pneumoniae* (pneumococcus) and *Hemophilus influenzae* are the bacteria implicated most commonly in bacteremia and are associated with tissue invasion in 5% of cases of the former and in almost all cases of the latter. Fortunately, the advent of the *Hemophilus influenzae* type B vaccine (HIB) has diminished greatly the likelihood of developing a serious infection with this organism. In fact, *Hemophilus influenzae* meningitis and epiglottitis have become very uncommon since the vaccine has been used widely.

Based on many studies performed over the past decade, several recommendations can facilitate the identification of febrile children who have no obvious focus of infection but are most at risk for serious bacterial disease.[4] After a thorough history is obtained, including queries about illness of a similar nature in other family members, the child should be assessed for toxicity. If the child appears toxic (lethargic or very irritable, noninteractive, perfusion problems), hospitalization should be considered along with further diagnostic tests to assess for sepsis. If the child does not appear toxic, a white blood cell count should be considered; if this is greater than 15,000, a blood culture should be obtained. (Children who have a WBC greater than 15,000 are five times as likely to be bacteremic as those who have a WBC less than 15,000.[23] In addition, an absolute neutrophil count of at least 10,000 correlates with an increased [8.2%] risk of pneumococcal bacteremia.) Practically, obtaining the white cell count and blood culture at the same time is easiest, sending the blood for culture only if the white blood cell count warrants it.

A urine culture is recommended for male infants younger than 6 months of age and female infants younger than 2 years, because 5% to 8% of children in this age group who have an undifferentiated fever have a urinary tract infection.[18] A urinalysis is not adequate by itself as a screening tool to determine which child should have a urine culture, because 20% of children who have a urinary tract infection have a normal urinalysis, including a negative test for urinary nitrites or leukocyte esterase. A chest radiograph generally appears to be necessary only if clinical symptoms or signs suggest pneumonia (e.g., cough, tachypnea, dyspnea, rales, decreased breath sounds, dullness to percussion).[17] However, a recent study has suggested that up to 20% of children who have fever of at least 102.2° F (39° C) and a white blood cell count greater than 20,000 have pneumonia by chest radiograph, even in the absence of respiratory symptoms and signs.[1] Once the infant or child has been evaluated, a plan of management similar to the ones in Figs. 136-1 and 136-2 should be considered. (These plans were derived by Baraff et al from a meta-analysis of 85 published studies on undifferentiated febrile illness in young children.[4]) As discussed earlier in this chapter, the use of these protocols is controversial.

Children older than 3 years of age are more likely to have signs and symptoms consistent with a recognizable illness. If they have nonspecific symptoms, an urgent consultation with a physician probably is unnecessary; however, regardless of age, all febrile children who have localized signs and symptoms such as swollen joints, meningismus, labored respirations, chest pain, dysuria, petechiae, alteration of consciousness, and severe abdominal pain should be seen immediately.

Although many febrile children do not have signs and symptoms pointing to an obvious cause, a careful physical examination may reveal important clues to its origin. Because the majority of infections involve the respiratory tract, this area must be examined carefully. In all instances, the tympanic membranes should be examined for otitis media, the pharynx for pharyngitis, the nose for the nasal discharge of sinusitis or a viral upper respiratory tract infection, and the lungs for evidence of pneumonia or bronchiolitis. Conjunctivitis may be a clue to adenovirus infection, conjunctivitis-otitis syndrome, or Kawasaki disease.

The skin is no less important and may demonstrate typical viral exanthems, such as those associated with rubella, roseola, or chickenpox, or it may show the erythema marginatum of rheumatic fever or the rose spots of typhoid fever.

Generalized lymphadenopathy often occurs with viral illnesses, such as infectious mononucleosis, hepatitis, or cytomegalovirus infection, but it also may be a clue to the diagnosis of leukemia or lymphoma. Localized enlargement of lymph nodes should prompt a search for a skin infection or for a tumor. Isolated cervical lymphadenopathy may be associated with tuberculosis infection or cat-scratch disease.

The musculoskeletal system must be examined with care. Localized bone tenderness may suggest osteomyelitis, and a restricted range of motion in a warm joint may suggest arthritis. The latter finding may occur in many different diseases, but a careful examination of the heart always is indicated to detect the carditis of rheumatic fever or infective endocarditis. The spine should be palpated for any evidence of diskitis, and any costovertebral angle tenderness should prompt an examination of the urine for evidence of a urinary tract infection.

Although uncommon, factitious fever is a final consideration and a well-described entity, even in children. Children as young as 8 years of age have been known to increase the thermometer reading artificially by rubbing the mercury thermometer bulb on the sheets or by exposing it to warm liquids. Clues on physical examination include a pulse that is not correlated with the temperature elevation, inability to document fever when it is measured rectally, and an absence of sweating during defervescence. Investigation of psychosocial disturbances within the family usually is necessary.

MANAGEMENT

During the past decade, a large body of evidence has accumulated that appears to support the positive role fever and/or interleukin-1 plays as a part of the host defenses. Increased leukocyte mobility, increased leukocyte bactericidal activity, enhanced interferon effect, and decreased available trace metals (notably iron) for pathogenic bacteria are just a few of the ways in which fever improves the body's ability to fight

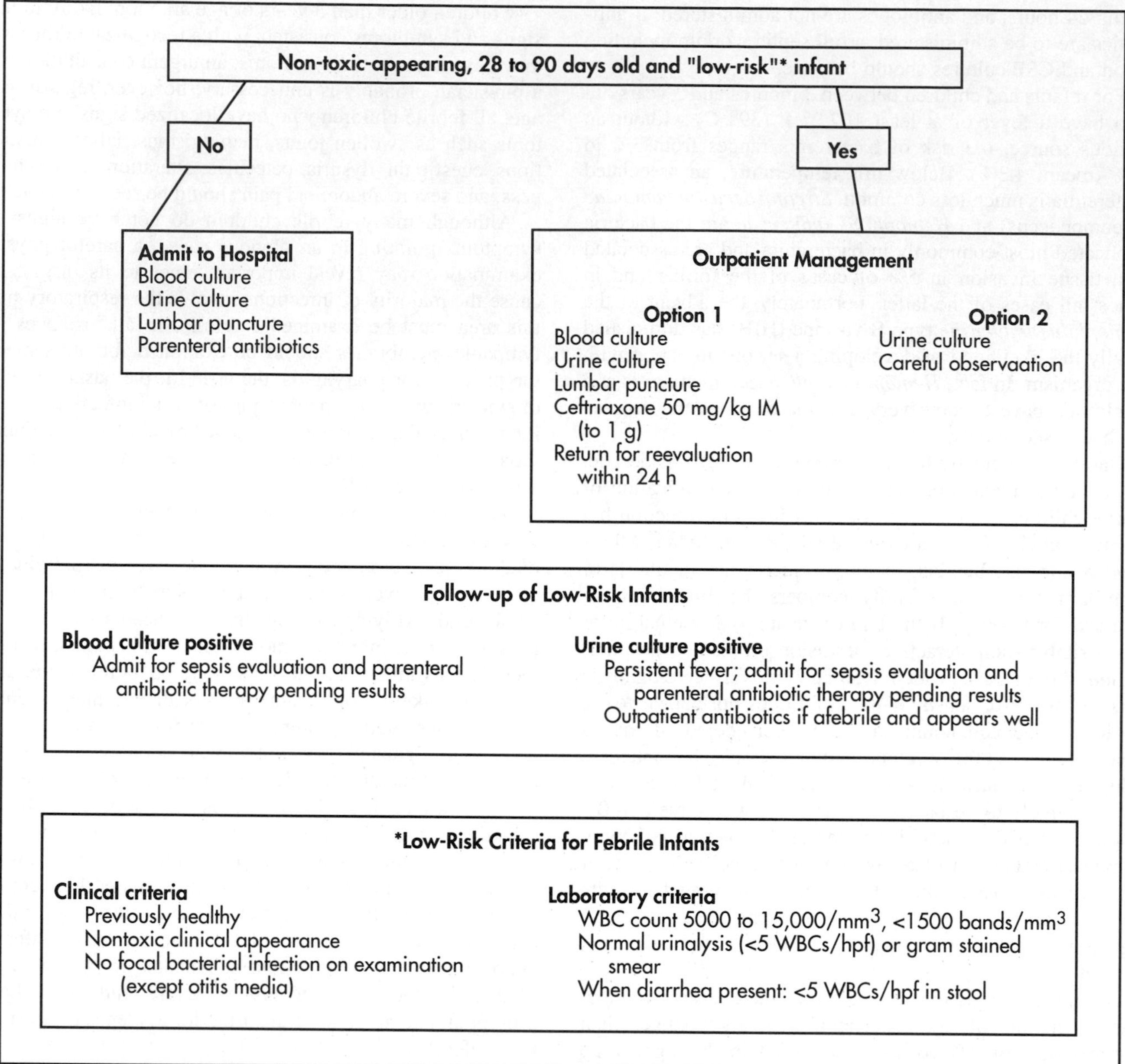

Fig. 136-1 Algorithm for the management of a previously healthy infant 0 to 90 days of age with fever without source at least 100.4° F (38° C).
(From Baraff LJ, et al: *Pediatrics* 92:1, 1993.)

infection. The inability of animals to mount a febrile response to infection has been demonstrated to be highly associated with increased mortality. Nevertheless, it still is not clear that fever has a beneficial effect independent of the release of interleukin-1.

As long as an appropriate evaluation has been undertaken and that specific therapy has been instituted for the underlying disease, the physician should question whether the best interest of the patient is served by eliminating fever through environmental and pharmacological manipulations. Three factors need to be considered in answering this question: (1) the complication rate associated with fever, (2) the ability of the patient to handle the increased metabolic demands of the fever, and (3) the comfort of the patient.

Complications in children who have a temperature below 105.8° F (41° C) are unusual unless the fever is associated with febrile status epilepticus or heatstroke. Of febrile seizures, 1% to 2% last longer than 15 minutes; if they continue beyond 60 minutes, they may be associated with severe brain injury (probably resulting from hypoxia). Heatstroke is uncommon in childhood and usually is associated with a temperature higher than 107.6° F (42° C), coma, and anhidrosis; it has a mortality rate of 80%. In both of these instances, body temperature obviously should be decreased. Children who have a seizure disorder may have an exacerbation of their seizures in the presence of fever and therefore may benefit from antipyretic management.

The child who has limited cardiopulmonary reserve, as might occur in congenital heart disease, cardiac infections, cystic fibrosis, or asthma, should be kept as normothermic as possible in spite of some of the benefits of fever in fighting disease. The high metabolic demand induced by fever other-

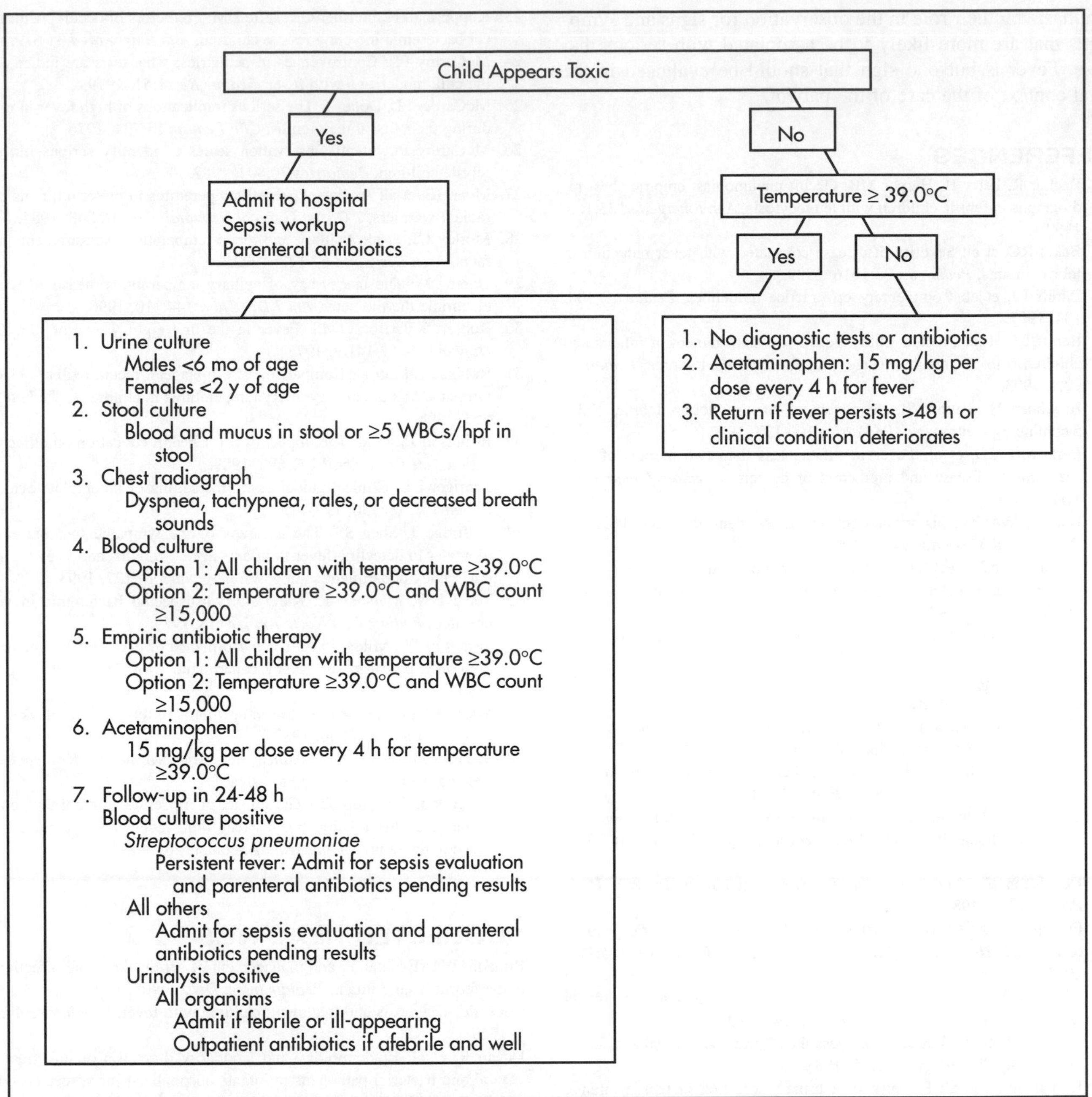

Fig. 136-2 Algorithm for the management of a previously healthy child 91 days to 36 months of age with fever without source.
(From Baraff LJ, et al: *Pediatrics* 92:1, 1993.)

wise may result in irreversible cardiopulmonary decompensation and death.

Although many children exhibit no discomfort until the temperature is higher than 102° F to 104° F (39° C to 40° C), discomfort at lower temperatures may be treated with antipyretic therapy. If the child is comfortable, no treatment is necessary up to a temperature of 105.8° F (41° C), except for the administration of additional fluids to prevent dehydration. A complete discussion of antipyretic therapy is provided in Chapter 25, Management of Fever.

Finally, the physician should provide sound education to parents about fever: its definition and meaning, its benefits and disadvantages, when to be concerned about it as an indicator of serious disease, its initial home management, including proper dosing with antipyretics, and when to contact the physician. Such education has been shown to improve home management and to enhance parental confidence in caring for their febrile child.[32]

SUMMARY

Although fever can be a frightening sign that may be associated with serious illness, its treatment is much less crucial than the evaluation and treatment of the illness causing the fever. Health care professionals are responsible for educating parents about the proper management of their febrile child, emphasizing their role in the observation for signs and symptoms that are more likely to be associated with serious disease. Fever is but one sign that should be evaluated in the total context of the care of the patient.

REFERENCES

1. Bachur R, Perry H, Harper MB: Occult pneumonias: empiric chest radiographs in febrile children with leukocytosis, *Ann Emerg Med* 33:166, 1999.
2. Baker RC, et al: Severity of disease correlated with fever reduction in febrile infants, *Pediatrics* 83:1016, 1989.
3. Baraff LJ, et al: Commentary on practice guidelines, *Pediatrics* 100: 134, 1997.
4. Baraff LJ, et al: Practice guideline for the management of infants and children 0 to 36 months of age with fever without source, *Pediatrics* 92:1, 1993.
5. Bauchner H, Pelton SI: Management of the young febrile child: a continuing controversy, *Pediatrics* 100:137, 1997.
6. Berkowitz CD, et al: Fever in infants less than two months of age: spectrum of disease and predictors of outcome, *Pediatr Emerg Care* 1:128, 1985.
7. Bonadio WA: The history and physical assessment of the febrile infant, *Pediatr Clin North Am* 45:65, 1998.
8. Chamberlain JM, et al: Comparison of a tympanic thermometer to rectal and oral thermometers in a pediatric emergency department, *Clin Pediatr* 30(suppl):24, 1991.
9. Chiu CH, Lin TY: Application of the Rochester criteria in febrile neonates, *Pediatr Infect Dis J* 17:267, 1998.
10. Chiu CH, Lin TY, Bullard MJ: Identification of febrile neonates unlikely to have bacterial infections, *Pediatr Infect Dis J* 16:59, 1997.
11. Christiakis DA, Rivara FP: Pediatrician awareness of and attitudes about four clinical practice guidelines, *Pediatrics* 101:825, 1998.
12. Crain EF, Gershel JC: Urinary tract infection in febrile infants younger than 8 weeks of age, *Pediatrics* 86:363, 1990.
13. Dagan R, et al: Identification of infants unlikely to have serious bacterial infection although hospitalized for suspected sepsis, *J Pediatr* 107:855, 1985.
14. Donaldson JF: Therapy of acute fever: a comparative approach, *Hosp Pract* 16:125, 1981.
15. Finkelstein JA, Christiansen CL, Platt R: Fever in pediatric primary care: occurrence, management, and outcomes, *Pediatrics* 105:260, 2000.
16. Herzog LW, Coyne JL: What is fever? Normal temperature in infants less than 3 months old, *Clin Pediatr* 32:142, 1993.
17. Heulitt MJ, et al: Febrile infants less than 3 months old: value of chest radiography, *Radiology* 167:135, 1988.
18. Hoberman A, et al: Prevalence of urinary infection in febrile infants, *J Pediatr* 123:17, 1993.
19. Hoberman A, et al: Pyuria and bacteriuria in urine specimens obtained by catheter from young children with fever, *J Pediatr* 124:513, 1994.
20. Hoberman A, Wald ER: Urinary tract infections in young febrile children, *Pediatr Infect Dis J* 16:11, 1997.
21. Kramer MS, Shapiro ED: Management of the young febrile child: a commentary on recent practice guidelines, *Pediatrics* 100:128, 1997.
22. Krober MS, et al: Bacterial and viral pathogens causing fever in infants less than 3 months old, *Am J Dis Child* 139:889, 1985.
23. Kupperman N, Fleisher GR, Jaffe DM: Predictors of occult pneumococcal bacteremia in young febrile children, *Ann Emerg Med* 31:679, 1998.
24. McCarthy PL: Controversies in pediatrics: what tests are indicated for the child under two with fever, *Pediatr Rev* 1:51, 1979.
25. McCarthy PL, Dolan T: The serious implications of high fever in infants during their first three months, *Clin Pediatr* 15:794, 1976.
26. McCarthy PL, et al: Observation scales to identify serious illness in febrile children, *Pediatrics* 70:802, 1982.
27. Moen JE, et al: Axillary vs rectal temperatures in preterm infants under radiant warmers, *J Obstet Gynecol Neonatal Nurs* 16:348, 1987.
28. Morley CJ, et al: Axillary and rectal temperature measurements in infants, *Arch Dis Child* 67:122, 1992.
29. Ogren JM: The inaccuracy of axillary temperatures measured with an electronic thermometer, *Am J Dis Child* 144:110, 1990.
30. Roberts KB, Borzy MS: Fever in the first eight weeks of life, *Johns Hopkins Med J* 141:9, 1977.
31. Robinson JL, et al: Comparison of esophageal, rectal, axillary, bladder, tympanic and pulmonary artery temperatures in children, *J Pediatr* 133: 553, 1998.
32. Robinson JS, et al: The impact of fever health education on clinic utilization, *Am J Dis Child* 143:698, 1989.
33. Schriger DL: Clinical guidelines in the setting of incomplete evidence, *Pediatrics* 100:136, 1997.
34. Selfridge J, Shea SS: The accuracy of the tympanic membrane thermometer in detecting fever in infants aged 3 months and younger in the emergency department setting, *J Emerg Nurs* 19:127, 1993.
35. Teele DW, Marshall R, Klein JO: Unsuspected bacteremia in young children, *Pediatr Clin North Am* 26:773, 1979.
36. Terndrup TE, Milewski A: The performance of two tympanic thermometers in a pediatric emergency department, *Clin Pediatr* 30(suppl):18, 1991.
37. Voora S, et al: Fever in full-term newborns in the first four days of life, *Pediatrics* 69(suppl):40, 1982.
38. Wunderlich C: *Das Verhalten der Eigenwarme in Krankenheiten*, Leipzig, Germany, 1868, Otto Wigard.
39. Zener WJ, Terndrup TE: The impact of moderate ambient temperature variance on the relationship between oral, rectal, and tympanic membrane temperatures, *Clin Pediatr* 30(suppl):61, 1991.

SUGGESTED READINGS

Bonadio WA: Evaluation and management of serious bacterial infections in the febrile young infant, *Pediatr Infect Dis J* 9:905, 1990.

Cone TE: Diagnosis and treatment: children with fevers, *Pediatrics* 43:290, 1969.

Dagan R, et al: Epidemiology and laboratory diagnosis of infection with viral and bacterial pathogens in infants hospitalized for suspected sepsis, *J Pediatr* 115:351, 1989.

Dinarello CA, Cannon JG, Wolff SM: New concepts on the pathogenesis of fever, *Rev Infect Dis* 10:168, 1988.

Jaffe DM, et al: Antibiotic administration to treat possible occult bacteremia in febrile children, *N Engl J Med* 317:1175, 1987.

Kluger MJ: Fever, *Pediatrics* 66:720, 1980.

Kramer MS, Naimark L, Leduc DG: Parental fever phobia and its correlates, *Pediatrics* 75:1110, 1985.

Schmitt BD: Fever phobia, *Am J Dis Child* 134:176, 1980.

137 Fever of Unknown Origin

Elise Willem van der Jagt

One of the more frustrating problems for the clinician to evaluate is that of a fever without a discernible cause. Because fever suggests disease, the inability to identify its cause strikes at one of the physician's raisons d'être and may undermine any credibility he or she previously had established with the patient and family. The longer the fever persists, the more concern is raised by the family and the more plentiful the demands made on the physician. A fever that is of only a few days' duration and not associated with any localizing signs or symptoms frequently does not even come to a physician's attention unless the child appears quite ill. Fever that continues beyond 5 to 7 days, however, usually alarms parents sufficiently to prompt a medical consultation. This discussion focuses on these more prolonged fevers and their evaluation.

DEFINITION

The classic definition for a fever of unknown origin (FUO) was proposed by Petersdorf and Beeson[8] in 1961 to be a fever (1) that is higher than 101° F (38.3° C) on several occasions, (2) that is present for more than 3 weeks, and (3) whose cause still is unexplained after 1 week of evaluation in the hospital. This definition, based on a study of adult patients, has not been accepted completely by most pediatricians, who would prefer not to delay evaluation for 3 weeks. More commonly, therefore, an FUO in children has been defined as a daily rectal temperature greater than 101° F (38.3° C), lasting for at least 2 weeks, whose cause has not been determined by simple diagnostic tests, including a thorough history and physical examination.[3] Some would add that 1 of the 2 weeks of fever should be documented in the hospital.

Careful documentation of fever is necessary before labeling a child with a diagnosis of FUO. A thorough explanation of the range of normal core body temperature for age, with its diurnal variation, may help in excluding patients who are not truly febrile but who instead have a high normal body temperature. The physician should instruct the parents in the technique of taking a rectal temperature and define a day of fever as a 24-hour period in which a temperature greater than 101° F (38.3° C) occurs at least once. All medications taken, the various activities in which the child has participated, and the environmental temperature during this time should be recorded, because each may affect body temperature. Although much importance has been attached to fever patterns in the past (i.e., remittent, intermittent, sustained), detailing them is not necessary because they rarely are diagnostic of a specific disease.[7]

Careful documentation of fever also should help exclude what Kleiman[6] has called a pseudo-FUO. Children who have a pseudo-FUO do not have a true fever if their body temperature is measured accurately and consistently (at times this needs to be done under hospital supervision), but do exhibit a definite constellation of findings that is recognizable and, many times, diagnostic (Box 137-1). In addition to the inability to corroborate fever and in the face of a completely normal physical examination, the parents may relate a previous serious illness and their concerns about its possible recurrence or lasting effect on the child ("vulnerable child syndrome"). Their child may have missed an excessive amount of school, given the general degree of illness described; school absence often is prompted by the presence of fatigue, abdominal pain, and headache in the morning—symptoms that are conspicuously absent during the rest of the day. Finally, a sequence of minor illnesses may have occurred, mimicking a single, continuous illness. Only careful questioning and record keeping will clarify this so that one can provide a reassuring explanation to the parents.

DIFFERENTIAL DIAGNOSIS

Box 137-2 lists the common causes of FUO in children. The causes are subdivided into four categories: infectious diseases, autoimmune diseases, malignancies, and miscellaneous. This list clearly shows that the majority of FUOs eventually are found to be caused by common pediatric illnesses that are either self-limited or treatable.

An infectious illness is the most common cause for an FUO in children, making up between 40% and 60%[3,5] of the reported cases; the second most common cause is autoimmune disease, making up between 7% and 20% of the cases. Children younger than 6 years of age are more likely to have an FUO resulting from an infection, whereas autoimmune diseases are found more frequently in children older than 6 years (Table 137-1).[9]

Although the majority of infections that manifest themselves as FUO are an atypical or incomplete manifestation of a common infectious disease, several types of infections recently have been added to the differential diagnosis. Jacobs'[5] prospective study of children who have fever of unknown origin (146 patients) in 1997 noted that Epstein-Barr virus was the most common of the infectious diseases, followed by osteomyelitis and bartonellosis. The advent of serologic test-

BOX 137-1

CHARACTERISTICS OF THE CHILD WHO HAS PSEUDO-FUO

1. Absence of documented, persistent fever
2. Lack of objective, abnormal physical findings
3. History of significant or near-fatal illness
4. Parental fear of malignant or crippling disease
5. Frequent environmental exposure to illness
6. Absence of persistent weight loss
7. Normal erythrocyte sedimentation rate and platelet count
8. Large number of missed school days because of subjective morning complaints
9. Discordance of fever and pulse rate
10. Medical or paramedical family background
11. Majority have, singly or in sequence, mild self-limited diseases, behavioral problems, parents who have misconceptions concerning health and disease, or families under stress

From Kleiman MB: *Pediatr Clin North Am* 29:201, 1982.

ing (indirect immunofluorescent antibodies) for Epstein-Barr virus and Bartonella infections has made these diagnoses easier to make. Although bartonellosis (caused by *Bartonella henselae*) usually presents as classic cat-scratch disease, it may present in an atypical, occult fashion such as hepatosplenic abscesses.[11] Thus, when there is a significant exposure to kittens and cats, serology for bartonella should be obtained; if positive, an abdominal ultrasound should be obtained.

Osteomyelitis, particularly of the axial skeleton (intervertebral diskspace/vertebral body infections) and the pelvis also should be strongly considered.

The appearance during the 1980s and subsequent increased incidence of human immunodeficiency virus (HIV) infection, with its associated acquired immunodeficiency syndrome (AIDS), should encourage the pediatrician to assess the child carefully for the presence of known risk factors (parental intravenous drug abuse, parental sexual contact with individuals who may be HIV positive, an HIV-positive mother, hemophilia requiring transfusion of blood products) and characteristic physical signs and symptoms. Fever usually is not the sole manifestation of HIV infection. However,

BOX 137-2

CAUSES OF FEVER OF UNKNOWN ORIGIN IN CHILDREN

Infectious Diseases
Bacterial
- Bacterial endocarditis
- Bartonellosis
- Brucellosis
- Leptospirosis
- Liver abscess
- Mastoiditis (chronic)
- Osteomyelitis
- Pelvic abscess
- Perinephric abscess
- Pyelonephritis
- Salmonellosis
- Sinusitis
- Subdiaphragmatic abscess
- Tuberculosis
- Tularemia

Viral
- Cytomegalovirus
- Epstein-Barr virus (infectious mononucleosis)
- Hepatitis viruses

Chlamydial
- Lymphogranuloma venereum
- Psittacosis

Rickettsial
- Q fever
- Rocky Mountain spotted fever

Fungal
- Blastomycosis (nonpulmonary)
- Histoplasmosis (disseminated)

Parasitic
- Malaria
- Toxoplasmosis
- Visceral larva migrans

Unclassified cause
- Sarcoidosis

Autoimmune Diseases
Juvenile rheumatoid arthritis
Polyarteritis nodosa
Systemic lupus erythematosus

Malignancies
Hodgkin's disease
Leukemia/lymphoma
Neuroblastoma

Miscellaneous Causes
Central diabetes insipidus
Drug fever
Ectodermal dysplasia
Factitious fever
Familial dysautonomia
Granulomatous colitis
Infantile cortical hyperostosis
Nephrogenic diabetes insipidus
Pancreatitis
Periodic fever
Serum sickness
Thyrotoxicosis
Ulcerative colitis

Modified from Feigin RD, Cherry JD: *Textbook of pediatric infectious diseases,* ed 4, Philadelphia, 1998, WB Saunders.

Table 137-1 Diagnosis of Prolonged Fever, Children's Hospital Medical Center, Boston[8]

	Infection						
Age	**"Viral"**	**Nonviral**	**Collagen**	**Malignancy**	**Miscellaneous**	**No Diagnosis**	**Totals**
<6 yr	14 (27%)	20 (38%)	4 (8%)	4 (8%)	7 (13%)	3 (6%)	52
>6 yr	7 (15%)	11 (23%)	16 (33%)	2 (4%)	3 (6%)	9 (19%)	49
TOTALS	21	31	20	6	10	12	100

HIV infection should be considered and the appropriate laboratory tests performed if the fever has been present for more than 2 months and is associated with one or more of the following: failure to thrive or a weight loss of more than 10% from baseline, hepatomegaly, splenomegaly, generalized lymphadenopathy (lymph nodes measuring at least 0.5 cm in two or more sites, with bilateral site involvement counting as one site), parotitis, and diarrhea that is either persistent or recurrent.[2]

Of the autoimmune diseases, juvenile rheumatoid arthritis is the most common. Fever is associated almost 100% of the time with systemic onset juvenile rheumatoid arthritis, frequently preceding the joint manifestations by weeks or months. The typical double quotidian fever (two fever spikes in 24 hours with a normal temperature in between) is a helpful clue to this diagnosis. Other autoimmune diseases that should be considered are lupus erythematosus and chronic regional enteritis. The latter is more common among children older than 6 years.

Malignancy, the most anxiety-producing diagnosis, is present in only a small percentage of patients in most studies (1.5% to 6%). This is in contrast to adults who have FUO, of whom as many as 31% may have a neoplastic process. Most common in children is leukemia, although solid tumors such as lymphoma, neuroblastoma, hypernephroma, and hepatoma all have been reported as presenting as FUO. The exact reason for fever in these diseases is unclear but may be related to endogenous pyrogen and other cytokines produced by the neoplastic cells.

As can be seen in Box 137-2, a large spectrum of miscellaneous diseases may cause prolonged fevers. In as many as 25% of patients who have persistent fevers, however, a true diagnosis never is obtained. (In one recent study,[10] no diagnosis was ever found in 67% of the children.) These are the genuine FUOs. The majority of these patients appear to do well, and the fever eventually disappears after months or even years.

EVALUATION

Whether the child has a true FUO or a pseudo-FUO cannot be determined without a thorough and precise history and physical examination, with the physician paying close attention to behavioral, social, and environmental factors. Information regarding travel, animal exposure, frequency of exposure to other persons who have common febrile illnesses, previous illness, hospitalizations, drug treatments, family history of disease, and the precise course of the manifested symptoms must be obtained methodically and efficiently. Meticulous documentation of dates is especially important.

For children older than 11 to 12 years of age, a separate interview is indicated to obtain the child's perspective on the illness and to elicit information that may be difficult to express in the presence of parents. School, peer relationships, family functioning, and sexual identity and activity all should be explored.

Once a complete history has been taken, a full physical examination must be performed. Rectal temperature, respiratory rate, heart rate, and blood pressure measurements should not be forgotten. Any discrepancy between heart rate and temperature should suggest factitious fever. A careful examination of the respiratory tract is indicated. Inspection of the pharynx for hyperemia and exudate, and the tympanic membranes for chronic otitis media, transillumination of the sinuses for sinusitis, a search for a purulent nasal discharge, and auscultation of the chest for localized wheezing all are important. In the older child, an examination of the teeth to exclude caries and periodontal disease must be included. A new cardiac murmur may be a clue to rheumatic fever or infective endocarditis. Lymphadenopathy, especially if generalized, may suggest a viral infection, such as infectious mononucleosis, cytomegalovirus infection, toxoplasmosis, or HIV infection. Joints must be examined meticulously for swelling, restricted range of motion, and tenderness. Skin rashes may suggest a viral disease or an autoimmune disease such as juvenile rheumatoid arthritis. The absence of sweating and the presence of a smooth tongue are consistent with familial dysautonomia, a rare genetic disorder of thermoregulation. Finally, a rectal examination with a sample of stool for a stool guaiac test is imperative, because pararectal lymphadenopathy suggests a pelvic infection, and a positive stool guaiac test can be consistent with inflammatory bowel disease.

If the history and physical examination disclose no specific findings, simple diagnostic tests are indicated. Routine blood counts and urinalysis have not been shown to be of major benefit, although no one advocates their elimination from the workup. A PPD (tuberculin skin test) with controls should be placed to detect tuberculosis, although anergy may occur in active tuberculosis infection. Negative blood, urine, and throat cultures exclude infections of these areas.

Probably the most useful laboratory tests are the erythrocyte sedimentation rate (ESR) and the albumin/globulin ratio. If the ESR is more than 30 or the albumin/globulin ratio is reversed, a high probability of serious disease exists—particularly an autoimmune vascular disease or a malignancy—and further evaluation should be pursued vigorously.

The remainder of the evaluation should individualized, based on historical and clinical findings. Because infectious causes are the most common, it is reasonable to pursue special serological tests for such diseases as hepatitis A and B, Epstein-Barr virus infection (infectious mononucleosis), bartonellosis, toxoplasmosis, and cytomegalovirus infection. Radioactive gallium scans may be useful in detecting occult abscesses and infections, although this scan has been found to be much less useful in children than in adults.[1] Total body computed tomography scans may help delineate tumors, although if the abdomen is of primary concern, an abdominal ultrasound will detect significant abnormalities, as well.[10] Radiological studies of the sinuses, the gastrointestinal tract, and the chest all may be appropriate in certain individuals but should not be routine. A bone marrow examination occasionally may help in the diagnosis of tuberculosis, leukemia, metastatic cancer, or fungal infections but should be considered only in those children who either have a clinical or laboratory suggestion of malignancy or are immunocompromised.[4] Finally, if the child is not deteriorating visibly, a period of observation may be necessary until new findings appear that can give more direction to the investigation.

If the ESR and the albumin/globulin ratio are normal and there are no signs and symptoms present that are specific to a particular disease, it is likely that little can be gained from any of the tests mentioned previously. Observation and periodic evaluation are all that are required while remaining alert for the occurrence of new symptoms or signs that might lead the investigation in a specific direction.

SUMMARY

The evaluation of the child who has FUO must be individualized to accommodate the history, the physical examination, and the particular social environment in which the child and family live. An intensive examination of all these factors is the physician's responsibility and is the first stage of managing the patient. Whether hospitalization is part of this approach depends ultimately on the amount of parental anxiety, the necessity to document fever, and the performance of diagnostic tests that cannot be done on an outpatient basis.

It is key that the health care professional continue to assess these children frequently to detect new findings early and to maintain the confidence of the family while the fever continues. Based on the existing literature, however, it is quite clear that children who have prolonged fever of unknown origin generally do well, even though the fever may last for weeks or months.

REFERENCES

1. Buonomo C, Treves ST: Gallium scanning in children with fever of unknown origin, *Pediatr Radiol* 23:307, 1993.
2. Centers for Disease Control: Classification system for human immunodeficiency virus (HIV) infection in children under 13 years of age, *MMWR* 36:225, 1987.
3. Feigin RD, Shearer WT: Fever of unknown origin in children, *Curr Probl Pediatr* 6:1, 1976.
4. Hayani A, Mahoney DH, Fernbach DJ: Role of bone marrow examination in the child with prolonged fever, *J Pediatr* 116:919, 1990.
5. Jacobs RF, Schutze GE: *Bartonella henselae* as a cause of prolonged fever and fever of unknown origin in children, *Clin Infect Dis* 26:80, 1998.
6. Kleiman MB: The complaint of persistent fever, *Pediatr Clin North Am* 29:201, 1982.
7. Musher DM, et al: Fever patterns: their lack of clinical significance, *Arch Intern Med* 139:1225, 1979.
8. Petersdorf RG, Beeson PB: Fever of unexplained origin: report on 100 cases, *Medicine* 40:1, 1961.
9. Pizzo PA, Lovejoy FH, Smith DH: Prolonged fever in children: review of 100 cases, *Pediatrics* 55:468, 1975.
10. Steele RW, et al: Usefulness of scanning procedures for diagnosis of fever of unknown origin in children, *J Pediatr* 119:526, 1991.
11. Ventura A, et al: Systemic *Bartonella henselae* infection with hepatosplenic involvement, *J Pediatr Gastroent Nutr* 29:52, 1999.

SUGGESTED READINGS

Lohr JA, Hendley JO: Prolonged fever of unknown origin: a record of experiences with 54 childhood patients, *Clin Pediatr* 16:768, 1977.

Miller LE, et al: Prolonged fevers of unknown origin in children: patterns of presentation and outcome, *J Pediatr* 12:419, 1996.

138 Foot and Leg Problems

Robert A. Hoekelman

Pediatricians and family practitioners often have to make judgments concerning actual or presumed problems of the feet and legs in infants and children. The frequency and natural history of these problems is such that referral to orthopedic consultants is not always appropriate. In most instances the problems presented require no treatment, others can be managed easily without consultations, and only a few require the services of an orthopedist.

The *ped* in pediatrics and orthopedics is derived from the Greek word *paidios,* meaning child, not from the Latin *pedalis* or French *ped,* meaning foot. Therefore, pediatrics is the medicine (Greek *iatrike*) of the child, and orthopedics is the straightening or correction (Greek *orthos*) of deformities in children. Orthopedics has expanded its scope well beyond this initial thrust; nevertheless, the orthopedist and the pediatrician are concerned with many problems involving the feet of children.

SHOES

Anatomy of the Shoe

Because some foot problems in childhood are treated with corrective shoes, understanding the anatomy of the shoe is necessary. The last is the wooden or metal form on which a shoe is constructed. Shoes for regular use are built on a straight last; shoes designed to deviate the forefoot outward are built on an out-flare last; those designed to deviate the forefoot inward are built on an in-flare last. Actually, most of the shoes sold for general use in the United States have an adducted forefoot last rather than a truly straight last.

The sole is that part of the shoe that covers the ventral surface of the foot. It consists of the outsole, usually made of firm leather or rubber that comes in contact with the surface on which the shoe is placed, and the insole, made of soft leather or synthetic material that comes in contact with the plantar surface of the foot. The heel, also made of leather, rubber, or synthetic material, elevates the rear portion of the shoe. It usually is absent in the shoes of infants and toddlers. It may be low and flat (common sense), somewhat higher (military), or more elevated and tapered (Cuban or high). The Thomas heel is of medium height and has a forward medial extension.

The shank of the shoe is that part of the sole between the forwardmost edge of the heel and ball of the foot. A narrow flat piece of steel sometimes is placed between the inner and outer soles to prevent flexion of the shank of the shoe. The counter of the shoe is placed above the heel between the outsole and insole and provides a shelf for the rear portion of the foot. It usually is made of firm leather and may be extended forward on the medial aspect of the shoe to provide added support to the instep. The upper or top of the shoe may be made of leather or a variety of other materials. The upper of low shoes (Oxfords) rises to a point below the malleoli; the upper of high shoes extends above the malleoli. The vamp is the part of the upper attached to the sole.

Functions of Shoes

Parents often ask the physician when their child should begin wearing shoes and what kind of shoe should be worn. In answering these questions, the reasons for wearing shoes must be borne in mind. The shoe has two functions, the most important of which is protection of the feet from trauma and extreme temperatures. Protection implies comfort; therefore, the shoe must fit properly to avoid discomfort to the foot. The second function of the shoe is to provide style. Older children often will sacrifice comfort for style despite parental or medical advice to the contrary.

Support to the foot and ankle is not a function of the shoe except when a pathological condition is present. Low shoes that have soft uppers are worn by athletes in all sports that place the feet and ankles under severe strain. Ski boots are worn not to support the foot and ankle but to make them "one with the ski," to ensure response to movements originating in the knee and lower leg. High shoes usually are worn by babies and toddlers not to provide support to the foot and ankle but to make it more difficult for the child to remove the shoes.

Style is the only reason for a baby to wear shoes at all until he or she begins walking outdoors or is taken out in cold weather. Some babies may gain a certain degree of stability from hard-sole shoes when beginning to stand, but this has not been shown to enhance learning to walk. Properly fitting shoes that have firm soles and soft uppers should be recommended initially and subsequently. They need not be expensive. Sneakers are perfectly adequate for summer wear and for winter indoor wear.

Fitting Shoes

Determining the proper fitting of shoes involves no great science. The counter should hug the heel snugly, the length should allow ¾ inch between the tip of the great toe and the front end of the upper, and the width should allow ¼ inch between the edge of the fifth toe and the lateral edge of the upper when the foot is pushed medially within the shoe. These measurements should be made with the child standing and should apply only to the time the shoes are newly acquired. Shoes in good condition can be handed down from one child to another.

The frequency with which shoes should be changed depends on the rate of growth of the feet, the quality of the shoes, and the degree of their use. Parents usually are able to tell when shoes become too small (or rather, feet become too large) without professional advice. The toes will be felt to press against the front end of the upper, and getting the shoes on or having the child keep them on will be increasingly difficult.

Lightweight cotton, nylon, or wool socks that adjust to the length and width of the foot present no problem in the attainment of maximal foot comfort for children of all ages.

ORTHOPEDIC TERMINOLOGY

Certain terms are used by practitioners to describe positional variations of the lower extremities and often are used in the nomenclature of specific orthopedic conditions.

In general, the joint that is primarily involved in the condition constitutes the first word; the subsequent word or words relate to the positioning of the extremity in relation to the midline of the body. For example, coxa vara is a condition of the hip (coxa) that results in a deviation of the leg toward the midline (varus position).

The following orthopedic terms have special reference to abnormalities of the feet (Fig. 138-1):

Talipes—congenital deformities of the foot that, if untreated, result in walking on the ankle (talus)
Pes—the foot
Inversion—foot twisted inward on its long axis
Eversion—foot twisted outward on its long axis
Adduction—deviation toward the midline of the body
Abduction—deviation away from the midline of the body
Varus—heel and forefoot inverted; forefoot adducted
Valgus—heel and forefoot everted; forefoot abducted
Equinus—foot plantar flexed, placing the toes below the level of the heel
Calcaneus—foot dorsiflexed, placing the heel below the level of the toes
Planus—medial longitudinal arch of the foot flattened
Cavus—medial longitudinal arch of the foot elevated

CLINICAL CONDITIONS

A variety of positional deformities of the legs and feet are encountered by physicians who provide primary care for children from birth through adolescence. The distinction between a pathological and functional cause must be made. The former should be referred to an orthopedist for treatment. When a pathological deformity of the legs or feet is diagnosed, the physician should look for other congenital anomalies, especially those involving the skeletal system. Most functional deformities of the legs and feet are self-correcting in time without treatment. This must be considered in weighing the results of any treatment prescribed. Unfortunately, studies of those conditions, analyzing treated versus untreated paired control patients, have not been performed, so clinicians are left to their own or others' anecdotal experiences in making therapeutic decisions.

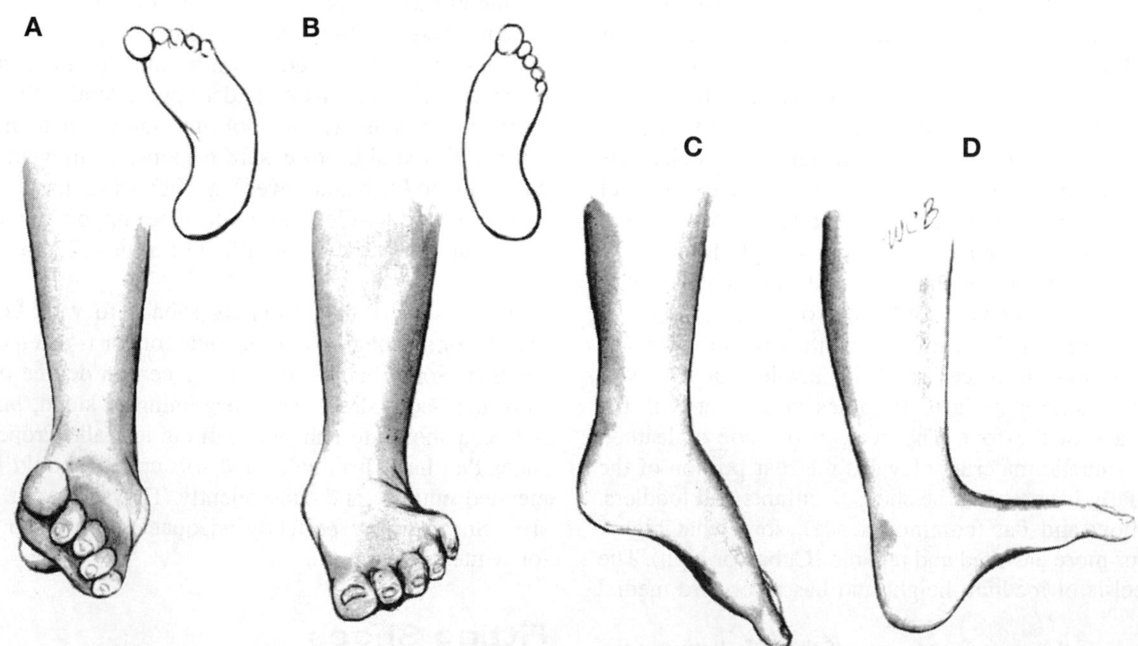

Fig. 138-1 Positional deformities of the foot and ankle. **A,** Varus. **B,** Valgus. **C,** Equinus. **D,** Calcaneus.

(From Tachdjian MO: *Pediatric orthopedics*, Philadelphia, 1977, WB Saunders.)

Clubfoot

The term *clubfoot* denotes a pathological deformity that causes the leg and its appended foot to resemble a clubbing instrument. Two varieties occur. The more severe is talipes equinovarus, in which the heel and forefoot are inverted, the forefoot is adducted, and the entire foot is plantar flexed. Fig. 138-2 shows bilateral clubfoot in a newborn; Fig. 138-3 shows an untreated right clubfoot. The other, talipes calcaneovalgus, is characterized by eversion of the heel and forefoot, abduction of the forefoot, and dorsiflexion of the entire foot (Fig. 138-4). Both forms occur in about 1 of every 200 live births, are bilateral in 50% of the cases, and affect boys almost twice as frequently as girls. When present, associated neurological, muscular, or other skeletal anomalies should be sought.

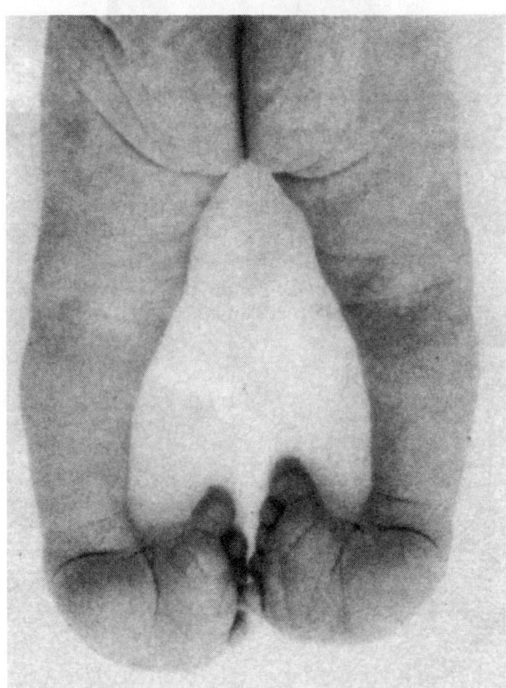

Fig. 138-2 Bilateral talipes equinovarus in a newborn infant.

(From Tachdjian MO: *Pediatric orthopedics,* ed 2, Philadelphia, 1990, WB Saunders.)

Often in the newborn period, functional deformities of the feet secondary to in utero positioning will mimic both varieties of clubfoot. These can be differentiated readily in that the functionally deformed foot can be brought easily to a neutral position and overcorrected. This is not possible when pathological deformities are present, and an orthopedic consultation should be sought immediately. Treatment with casting usually is required for initial correction. In severe cases, tenotomies, muscle transplants, and arthrodeses are necessary when the child is older. Functional deformities are self-correcting and require no treatment.

Metatarsus Varus

Much confusion surrounds the incidence and management of metatarsus varus, because three deformities are characterized by adduction of the forefoot: talipes varus (Fig. 138-5) in which the entire foot is inverted and the forefoot is adducted, metatarsus varus (Fig. 138-6) in which the forefoot is inverted and adducted while the hind foot and heel are in the normal position, and metatarsus adductus (Fig. 138-7) in which the only finding is adduction of the metatarsals at the tarsometatarsal joints. The combined incidence of these three forefoot adductive deformities is in the neighborhood of 1 per 100 live births (the most frequent musculoskeletal congenital malformation), with metatarsus adductus being the most common and talipes varus the least common.

Talipes varus and metatarsus varus have been considered lesser degrees of clubfoot and are fixed deformities of the

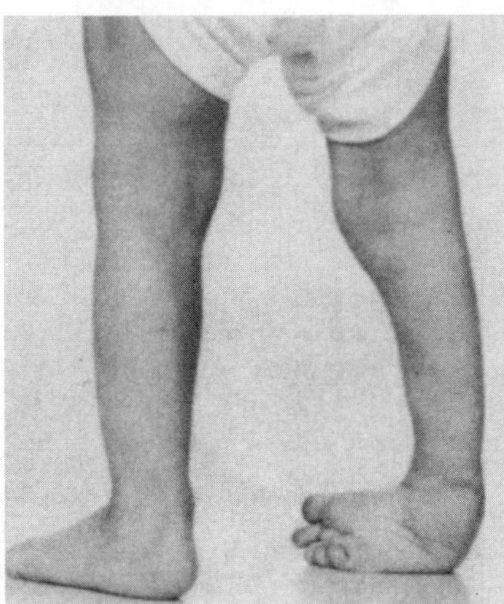

Fig. 138-3 Untreated talipes equinovarus in a 3-year-old child.

(From Tachdjian MO: *Pediatric orthopedics,* ed 2, Philadelphia, 1990, WB Saunders.)

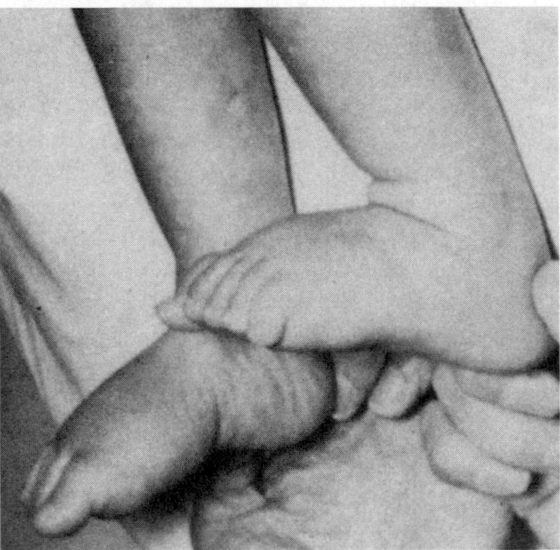

Fig. 138-4 Bilateral talipes calcaneovalgus. The left foot is held dorsiflexed and the right plantar flexed to show the range of ankle movement.

(From Sharrard WJW: *Paediatric orthopaedics and fractures,* ed 2, Oxford, 1979, Blackwell Scientific.)

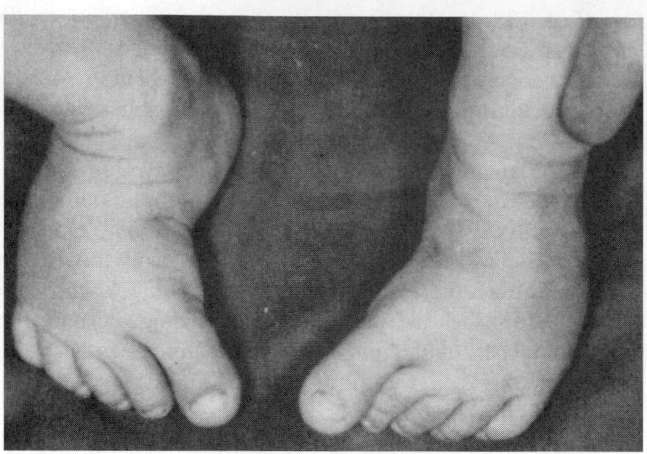

Fig. 138-5 Bilateral talipes varus. The entire foot is twisted inward on its longitudinal axis, and the forefoot is adducted.

(From Tachdjian MO: *Pediatric orthopedics*, ed 2, Philadelphia, 1990, WB Saunders.)

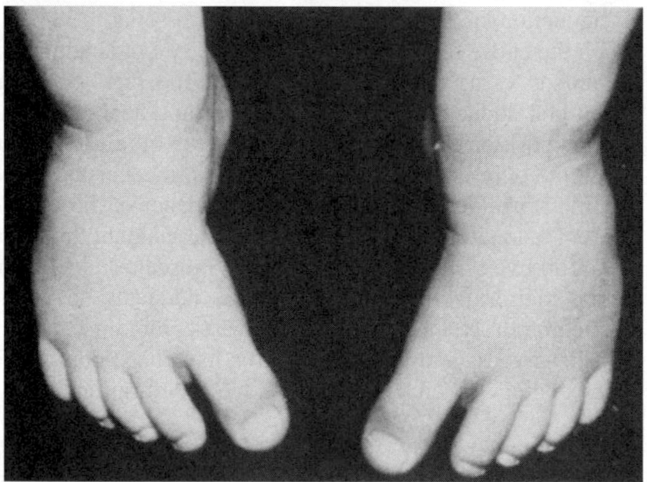

Fig. 138-6 Bilateral metatarsus varus. The forefoot is inverted and adducted, the great toe is widely separated from the second toe, and the lateral border of the foot is convex. The hindfoot is in a neutral position.

(From Sharrard WJW: *Paediatric orthopaedics and fractures,* ed 2, Oxford, 1979, Blackwell Scientific.)

foot that require early treatment. The medial border of the foot is concave with a widening of the space between the first and second toes and a high medial longitudinal arch. The lateral border of the foot is convex, and the base of the fifth metatarsal bone is prominent. Treatment consists of serial casting. Abduction stretching exercises and out-flare-last shoes may be used as an adjunct to cast treatment but should not be relied on as the only therapy.

Metatarsus adductus, a functional deformity, can be distinguished from the two fixed forefoot deformities by observing lateral movement of the infant's forefoot in response to stimulation of the sole. This condition requires no treatment because it corrects spontaneously, usually during the first year. Primary care physicians see metatarsus adductus frequently and observe its resolution without treatment, whereas orthopedists are more likely to see talipes varus and metatarsus through referrals, sometimes unfortunately in late infancy when treatment results are less satisfactory.

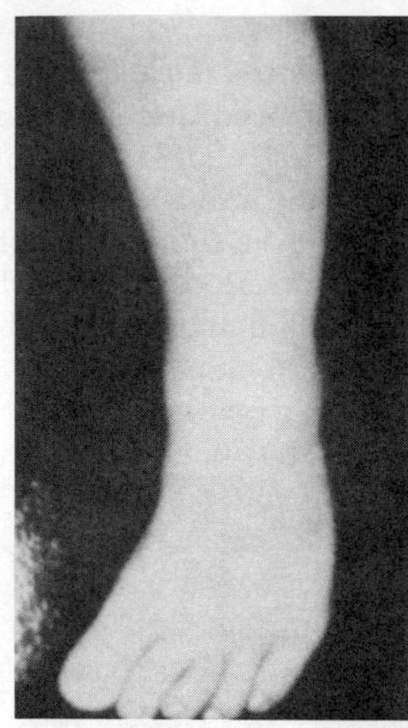

Fig. 138-7 Metatarsus adductus. The forefoot is adducted but not inverted.

(From Ferguson AB: *Orthopedic surgery in infancy and childhood,* ed 4, Baltimore, 1981, Williams & Wilkins.)

Pronation

Almost all children develop some degree of pronation during the early stages of weight-bearing. Pronation is characterized by an outward rolling of the foot with eversion of the heel and eversion and abduction of the forefoot. The Achilles tendon is seen to curve inward, and the medial longitudinal arch of the foot, observed without weight bearing, disappears on standing. These changes occur because a wide-based stance is assumed for balance (accentuated by bulky diapers), causing the weight to be borne on the medial aspect of the feet (Fig. 138-8). Laxity of the ligaments supporting the feet contributes to pronation. *Flexible foot, relaxed foot, fatfoot,* and *flatfoot* (pes planus) also are used to describe this condition, leading to considerable confusion in terminology.

Pronation is transient in most children, usually disappears before 2½ years of age and requires no treatment. In those in whom it persists, treatment is not necessary unless symptoms occur. These include aching of the feet and legs, muscle cramps in the calves at night, easy fatigability, and reluctance to participate in strenuous activity. Symptoms result from the strain caused by the child's continual attempt to shift weight bearing laterally toward the center of the foot, bringing about some degree of toeing-in. Persistent pronation without symptoms occurs in some children who may have a family history of pronation and often demonstrates hyperextensibility of other joints, including the knees, elbows, wrists, and thumbs.

When symptoms do occur, they may be alleviated by use of corrective shoes that have a long medial counter and a Thomas heel. Support to the medial longitudinal arch with a flexible felt, rubber, or leather pad placed beneath the inner sole may help. Wedges ⅛- to $\frac{3}{16}$-inch thick applied to the medial aspect of the heel and the lateral aspect of the sole of the shoe sometimes are helpful. Steel arch supports placed

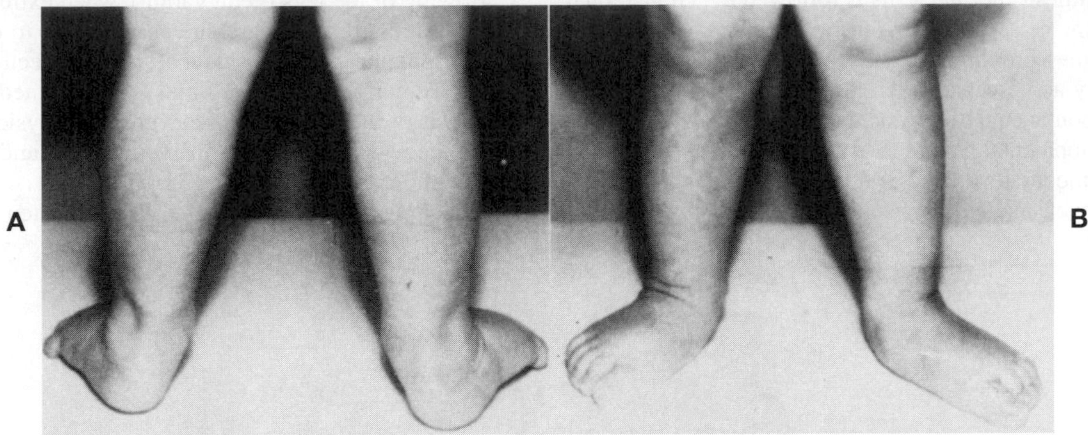

Fig. 138-8 Pronation. **A,** Viewed from behind, the hindfoot is everted. **B,** Viewed from in front, the forefoot is everted and abducted.
(From Sharrard WJW: *Paediatric orthopaedics and fractures,* ed 2, Oxford, 1979, Blackwell Scientific.)

within the shoe rarely are required, and foot exercises are of no value. Treatment with these simple measures usually brings relief of symptoms but may need to be continued for several years until the muscles and ligaments that support the foot mature sufficiently.

Planovalgus

Certain congenital anomalies involving the bones of the foot produce flattening of the medial longitudinal arch and eversion of the forefoot. These include vertical talus, accessory tarsonavicular, and fusion of one or more of the tarsal bones (tarsal coalition). The first two conditions usually can be detected in the newborn by the presence of a bony prominence on the medial and plantar aspects of the foot, with limitation of plantar flexion and inversion of the forefoot. Surgical correction should be accomplished early in infancy.

Tarsal conditions usually are not detected until late childhood or adolescence, when they produce pain with walking and inability to invert the foot. The foot is held in a pronated position with eversion of the forefoot. The peroneal tendons stand out prominently when attempts are made to invert the foot. This condition, commonly called *spastic flatfoot*, is not related etiologically to simple pronation. Treatment in most cases is symptomatic with orthopedic shoes. Surgical correction, usually performed in adulthood, is necessary in only about 10% of cases.

The incidence of pes planovalgus is unknown. Vertical talus and accessory tarsonavicular are very rare. Tarsal coalitions probably occur in 1% of the population and usually are hereditary.

Pes Cavus

Pes cavus is manifested by an equinus deformity of the forefoot in relation to the hindfoot, producing a high medial longitudinal arch (Fig. 138-9). It is referred to as *clawfoot* when associated with flexion deformities of the toes. The primary pathological condition is neuromuscular rather than bony, with weakness or paralysis of the intrinsic muscles of the foot and its dorsiflexors, leading to the deformity over time. It therefore is not seen at birth and usually does not manifest clinically until late childhood or adulthood, depending on the underlying neuromuscular disease.

Pes cavus is seen in muscular dystrophy, peripheral neuropathies, and disease of the spinal cord, brainstem, and cerebral cortex. Cerebral palsy, meningomyelocele, poliomyelitis, Charcot-Marie-Tooth disease, and Friedreich's ataxia are examples of conditions of neurological origin that produce pes cavus as a late manifestation. Because of the variety of conditions in which pes cavus is seen and its variability as a manifestation of some of these, its incidence in the general population is not known. A family history of pes cavus should be sought, because many of the conditions producing this deformity are inherited. Early treatment includes exercises designed to strengthen the affected muscles and application of metatarsal pads to the innersoles of the shoes or metatarsal bars to the outersoles. Surgical correction of the fixed deformities, including plantar fasciotomy, tendon transplants, osteotomies, and arthrodeses, may be required later.

Toe-Walking

Walking on the toes or the ball of the foot is a variation of normal gait for many children as they begin to walk. This usually progresses to a toe-heel gait and eventually to the normal heel-toe gait pattern within 3 to 6 months. Reassurance to parents is all that is required.

A congenitally short tendocalcaneus causes persistent toe-walking even though the child can toe-heel and heel-toe walk. These latter gaits are awkward and are less comfortable for the child until he or she is 6 to 8 years of age, when toe-walking disappears. No treatment is required.

As with pes cavus, certain rare muscular, peripheral, spinal, and central neurological diseases should be ruled out when toe-walking persists beyond 2 years of age.

Bowed Legs and Knocked Knees

From birth until 18 months of age a distinct bowing of the lower extremities is normal. This is followed by a transitional period over the next year or so, during which a knocked-knee pattern assumes prominence. This persists until later childhood or early adolescence when a balancing and straightening occur spontaneously. Physicians must be aware of this normal developmental pattern to avoid unnecessary treatment of mild to moderate degrees of bowed legs and knocked knees. However, marked degrees of these conditions require investigation to rule out underlying disease that can result in permanent deformity.

Bowing of the legs (genu varum), when extreme or unilateral, requires roentgenographic examination to exclude rickets, dyschondroplasia, osteogenesis imperfecta, osteochondritis (Blount disease), or injury to the medial proximal epiphysis of the tibia. Extreme degrees of physiological bowing of the legs may occur in the young child and resolve over time without treatment (Fig. 138-10).

Knocking of the knees (genu valgum) often is associated

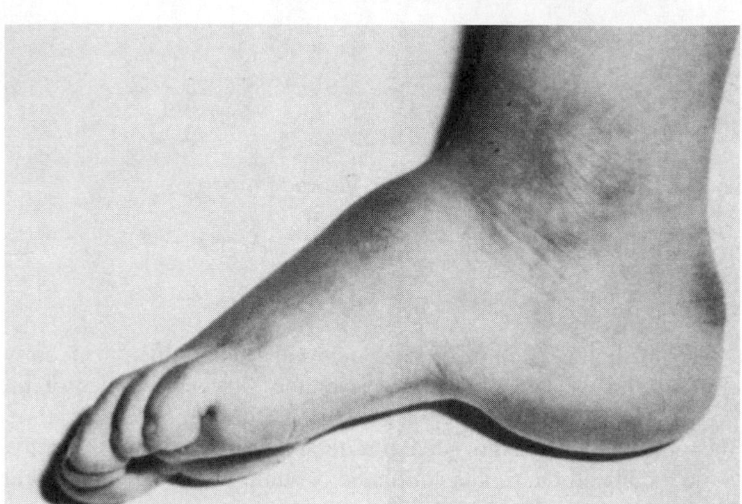

Fig. 138-9 Pes cavus, viewed from the outer side. There is abnormal height of the medial and lateral longitudinal arch.

(From Sharrard WJW: *Paediatric orthopaedics and fractures,* ed 2, Oxford, 1979, Blackwell Scientific.)

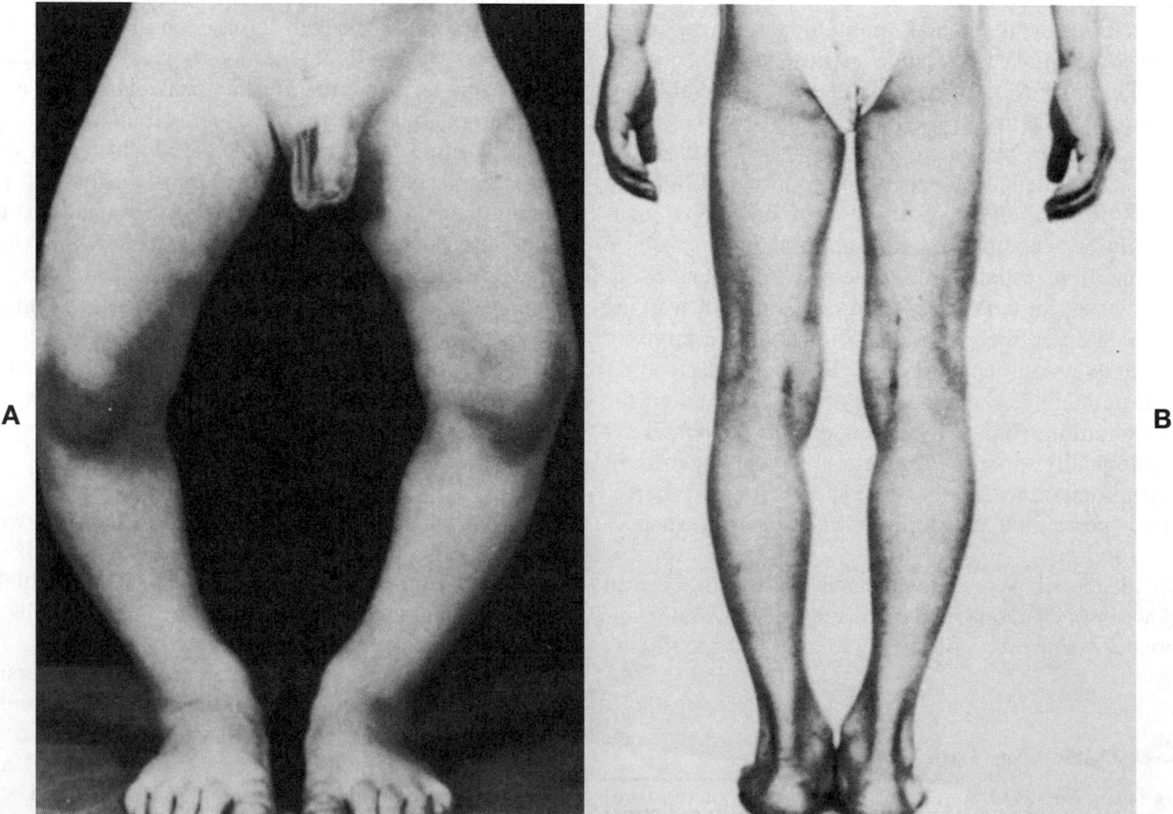

Fig. 138-10 **A,** Extreme physiological bowing of the legs at age 18 months. **B,** Spontaneous resolution over time (age 7 years).

(From Sharrard WJW: *Paediatric orthopaedics and fractures,* Oxford, 1971, Blackwell Scientific.)

with pronation and is more apt to be marked in the child who is overweight. The degrees of knocked knee can be gauged by measuring the distance between the medial malleoli when the child is standing with the knees approximated (Fig. 138-11). Injury to the lateral proximal tibial epiphysis can cause unilateral genu valgum (Fig. 138-12). As with extreme bowing, underlying generalized diseases of the bone can cause marked bilateral genu valgum.

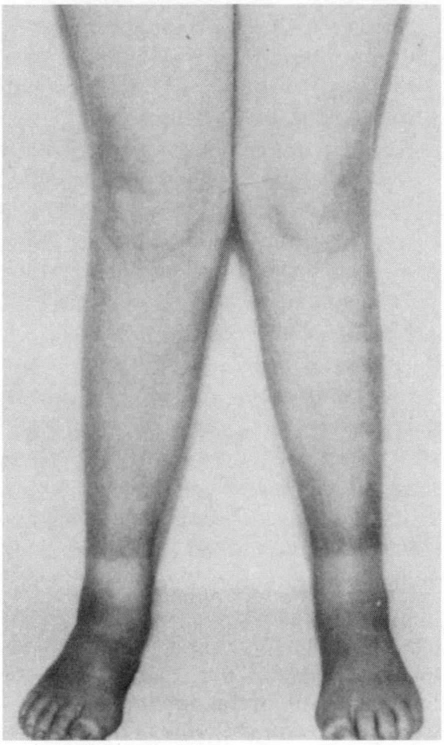

Fig. 138-11 Marked degree of physiological genu valgum. At age 11 years the distance between the medial malleoli measured 4 inches.

(From Sharrard WJW: *Paediatric orthopaedics and fractures,* ed 2, Oxford, 1979, Blackwell Scientific.)

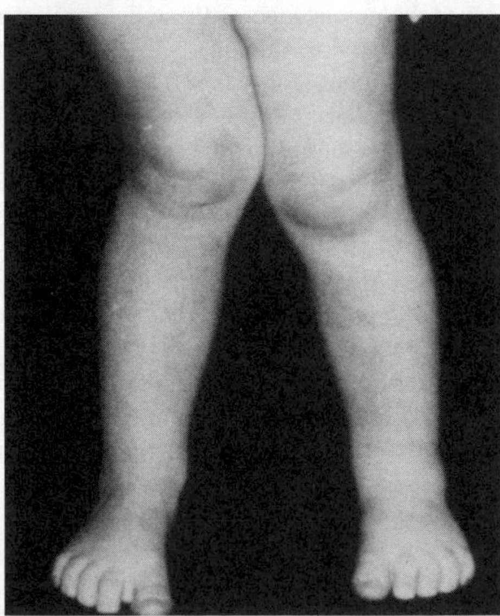

Fig. 138-12 Unilateral genu valgum caused by previous injury to the lateral aspect of the right proximal tibial epiphysis.

(From Sharrard WJW: *Paediatric orthopaedics and fractures,* ed 2, Oxford, 1979, Blackwell Scientific.)

Treatment of severe bowing or knocking of the knees caused by underlying disease is determined by the nature of the condition and may include wedge osteotomy or epiphyseal stapling.

Toeing-In and Toeing-Out

Toeing-in (pigeon toe) and toeing-out (slew foot) are frequently seen at all ages and are caused by a variety of conditions affecting the feet, ankles, legs, knees, and hips. Toeing-in is more common than toeing-out and is more likely to be caused by benign conditions. Protective or compensatory shifting of the body weight to the middle or outside of the foot in pronation and knocked knee, both normal developmental stages, is the most common cause of toeing-in and corrects itself in time. Developmental bowing of the legs, also self-correcting, may lead to temporary toeing-in. Talipes equinovarus and metatarsus varus are associated with toeing-in, whereas toeing-out is seen with calcaneovalgus and pes planovalgus. Spasticity of the internal rotator muscles of the hip, as seen in cerebral palsy, produces toeing-in; flaccid paralysis of these muscles results in toeing-out. Anterior and posterior maldirections of the acetabulum produce toeing-in and toeing-out, respectively. The remaining causes of both are related to internal or external torsion of the tibia and femur. In general, if in cases of toeing-in the child's patellae are noted to be rotated inward while walking, the underlying problem is above the knee; if they face straight forward, the underlying problem is below the knee.

Tibial torsion. During fetal life the tibia is rotated inward on its longitudinal axis relative to the transverse axes of the knee and ankle joints. At birth, it reaches a neutral position and thereafter gradually rotates outward, reaching 20 degrees of lateral torsion by the time walking is fully established and 23 degrees by adulthood. The degree of internal and external tibial torsion can be determined by observing the relative position of the medial and lateral malleoli while the child is sitting on the edge of a table or chair with legs dangling, the patellae facing forward, and the feet in their relaxed position (Fig. 138-13). The medial malleolus is placed posterior to the lateral malleolus in internal tibial torsion and anterior to it in external torsion.

The degree of torsion can be measured exactly either radiographically or with special instruments but is not required in most cases. The incidence of internal tibial torsion is 12% at birth. This gradually diminishes to near 0% at 2 years of age. External tibial torsion develops in most babies shortly after birth and is almost universal by age 2 years. Pathological degrees of internal and external tibial torsion are found only in association with deformities of the feet, ankles, knees, and hips or as a result of improperly applied casts, braces, or Denis Browne splints.

Treatment of primary internal tibial torsion is not required in most cases. Occasionally, if a child trips on his or her feet and falls frequently or if parents are unduly concerned over toeing-in, passive stretching exercises (externally rotating the foot at the ankle), corrective shoes (Thomas heel, longitudinal arch pad, inner-heel and outsole wedges), or application of torque heels may be prescribed. Denis Browne splints

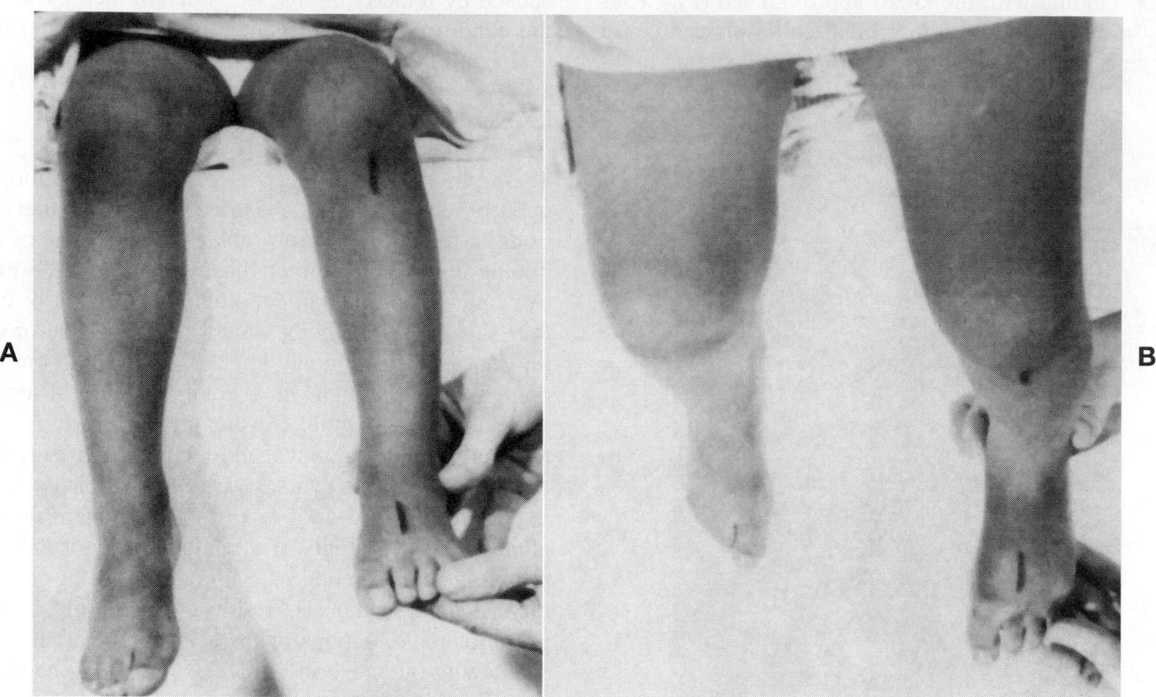

Fig. 138-13 Testing for tibial torsion. **A,** The patient is seated on the examining table with the knees flexed at 90 degrees and the legs hanging over the edge. A mark is drawn along the longitudinal axis of the tibia through the proximal tibial tubercle. Another mark is drawn over the second metatarsal bisecting the foot. The two marks are then aligned. **B,** With the left hand holding the foot in this neutral position, the thumb of the right hand is placed over the lateral malleolus and the forefinger over the medial malleolus. The angle at which an imaginary line joining the malleoli intersects the longitudinal axis will approximate the degree of internal or external tibial torsion.

(From Tachdjian MO: *Pediatric orthopedics,* ed 2, Philadelphia, 1990, WB Saunders.)

should not be used without orthopedic consultation because they may create abnormal stress on the hip joint. Derotation osteotomy of the tibia rarely is required and then almost always when tibial torsion is associated with other orthopedic anomalies of the lower extremity.

Femoral torsion. The proximal portion of the femur rotates on its longitudinal axis in relation to the transverse plane of the knee when the femoral neck is twisted anteriorly (anteversion) or posteriorly (retroversion) in relation to the femoral condyles. Anteversion produces "kissing knees," toeing-in, and a clumsy gait (Fig. 138-14). With the patella in neutral position, the greater trochanter of the femur lies posterior to the lateral, longitudinal midthigh line. External rotation is decreased and internal rotation of the hip in extension is increased (normally 35 to 45 degrees for both). External rotation of the hip in flexion is normal, however. The findings in retroversion are the opposite of those found in anteversion of the femoral neck.

In utero and postnatal positioning of the legs and hips produces stresses that bring about these rotational deformities of the femoral neck. The true incidence of anteversion and retroversion is not known, but the former is much more common and occurs twice as frequently in girls as in boys. Most femoral torsion deformities correct themselves by 7 years of age. If they do not, an orthopedist should be consulted, because the persistence of these deformities may lead to degenerative arthritis of the hip joint.

Orthopedic treatment consists of the use of a bivalve lower-trunk and leg cast during sleeping hours or in rare cases a derotation osteotomy of the middle or lower femoral shaft. A simple measure that can be employed by the primary care physician early on for parental concern over toeing-in is to have the child learn to sit in the tailor, modified lotus, or Indian-style sitting position. The use of Denis Browne splints is contraindicated, and corrective shoes are of no value.

Positions leading to toeing-in and toeing-out. Infants and children often assume certain positions during sleep or while sitting for long periods (watching television) that lead to positional deformities of the femur, tibia, or feet.

Sleeping in the prone, knee-chest position with the legs internally rotated may lead to anteversion of the femoral neck, internal tibial torsion, and varus of the forefoot; having the legs externally rotated may lead to valgus of the feet; and having the legs in a neutral position may lead to equinus of the feet and toe-walking. Sleeping in the prone position with

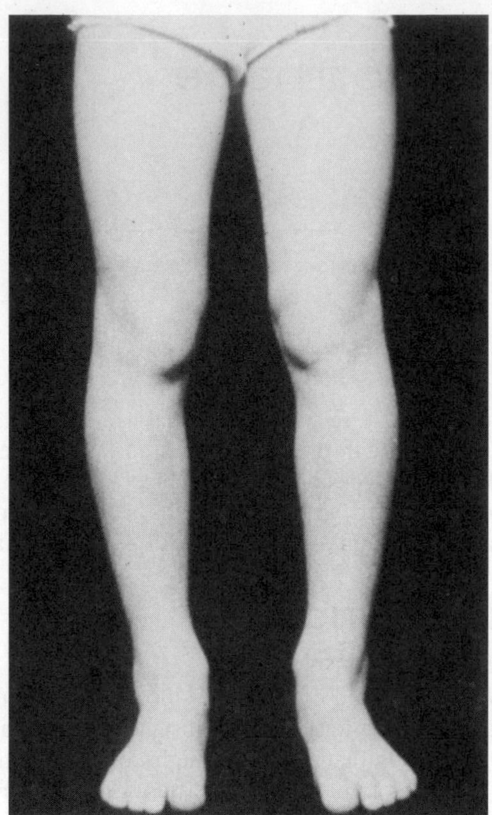

Fig. 138-14 Anteversion of the femoral neck or medial femoral torsion.

(From Sharrard WJW: *Paediatric orthopaedics and fractures,* ed 2, Oxford, 1979, Blackwell Scientific.)

the legs extended and rotated inward may lead to anteversion of the femoral neck, internal tibial torsion, and varus of the forefoot; having them rotated outward may lead to retroversion of the femoral neck and valgus of the feet. Sleeping in the frog-leg position prone or supine may lead to retroversion of the femoral neck and valgus and abduction of the feet.

Sitting in the reversed tailor position (on one's feet) with the feet internally rotated may produce anteversion of the femoral neck, internal tibial torsion, and varus of the forefoot; having the feet rotated externally may produce anteversion of the femoral neck and valgus of the feet.

When these sleeping or sitting positions are noted to occur in conjunction with the positional deformities listed, and when they raise concern, some effort can be made to change the positional sleeping or sitting habit. Success, however, is not often attained.

Although toeing-in or toeing-out may reflect a variety of underlying orthopedic diseases, no evidence suggests that toeing-in or toeing-out of developmental origin leads to any functional disabilities if left uncorrected.

SUGGESTED READINGS

Bleck EE: The shoeing of children: show or science? *Dev Med Child Neurol* 15:188, 1971.

Heinrich SD, Sharp CH: Lower extremity torsional deformities in children: a prospective comparison of two treatment modalities, *Orthopedics* 14:655, 1991.

Kling TF, Hensinger RN: Angular and torsional deformities of the lower limbs in children, *Clin Orthop* 176:136, 1983.

Staheli LT, et al: Lower-extremity rotational problems in children, *J Bone Joint Surg* 67:39, 1985.

Tachdjian MO: *Pediatric orthopedics*, ed 2, Philadelphia, 1990, WB Saunders.

139 Gastrointestinal Hemorrhage

Jeffrey R. Avner

A myriad of conditions can present with gastrointestinal (GI) bleeding in childhood. Most causes of GI bleeding in children, unlike in adults, are relatively benign and involve small amounts of blood loss. Although rare, some GI lesions may cause severe bleeding and lead to life-threatening conditions. In addition, GI bleeding may be a symptom of systemic illness or serious underlying chronic disease.

Evaluation of GI bleeding must center on a systematic approach. The age of the child, the history, the physical examination, and associated symptoms help focus the workup and allow the clinician to identify the source of the bleeding in the majority of cases. Endoscopy and new radiological techniques are particularly useful for both diagnosis and management of many conditions.

PATHOPHYSIOLOGY

Bleeding can occur at any point along the entire length of the GI tract, from the mouth to the anus. Multiple folds, coils, and villous borders of the GI mucosa provide a large surface area for secretion of enzymes and absorption of water and nutrients. In addition, there is a large vascular supply to the GI tract, which accounts for an appreciable fraction of the cardiac output, especially following meals. Bleeding may be arterial, venous, or both. Although most "bleeds" are slow and involve oozing from the mucosal surface, massive bleeding can result from lesions involving high-pressure arteries or large, engorged venous plexus.

Acute GI bleeding may occur with or without symptoms and can originate in either the upper or the lower GI tract. Chronic bleeding usually is slow and intermittent and may be identified only by occult blood in the stool. The slow nature of these bleeds allows the body ample time to compensate and preserve cardiac output. Chronic bleeding, therefore, presents with compensatory signs such as tachycardia, iron-deficiency anemia, fatigue, pallor, or change in stool color.

The nature, location, and duration of the bleeding lead to characteristic patterns of presentation. Hematemesis is bloody vomitus, which usually represents bleeding proximal to the ligament of Treitz. Blood, which is altered by gastric acid, becomes dark and coffee-ground in appearance. Bleeding that has little or no contact with gastric acid will be bright red. GI bleeding that occurs proximal to the ileocecal valve and is passed rectally usually will present with melena. Melena is black, tarry, sticky stools that results from the denaturing of hemoglobin by intestinal bacteria and enzymes. Hematochezia, bright red blood or maroon colored stools passed per rectum, usually results from distal GI bleeding. Blood usually is mixed with the stool or passed just before or just after defecation. Occasionally, rapid bleeding from an upper GI source combined with the cathartic action of blood can speed transit time and also present with hematochezia.

IDENTIFICATION OF TRUE BLEEDING

The appearance of red color in the stool is often assumed to be blood. However, many other substances cause change in stool color. Foods that contain a high concentration of red pigments such as tomatoes, cranberries, beets, and red fruit juices and gelatin (Jell-O) can cause red stools. Similarly, red-colored medications such as acetaminophen and amoxicillin can be passed in the stools, especially if there is diarrhea. Spinach, licorice, iron, and bismuth (Pepto-Bismol) often lead to dark, black stools, which can be confused with true melena. In infants, *Serratia marcescens* can cause "red diaper syndrome" as a result of the formation of red pigment in soiled diapers that were stored for more than 1 day.

Several biochemical tests are available to detect blood in the stool. The most common test, the stool guaiac, uses the peroxidase activity of hemoglobin to catalyze a color change on a test card or paper strip. The test is able to identify even trace amounts of blood and has a very high sensitivity. The following foods, which also have peroxidase activity, may cause false positive results if eaten within 3 days of testing: red meat, liver, processed meats, and raw fruits and vegetables, especially melon, turnip, radishes, and horseradish. High vitamin C intake interferes with the peroxidase reaction and can cause false negative results. Similarly, outdated guaiac cards and prolonged storage may affect the accuracy of the test. It is important to note that gastric acid can affect the reaction that causes the color change. Therefore, stool guaiac cards are not accurate for testing emesis for the presence of blood.

NONGASTROINTESTINAL SOURCE OF BLEEDING

Although blood is present in the GI tract, the bleeding may originate from a peripheral source. The most common example of this occurs in the newborn period. The infant may swallow maternal blood either during delivery or when breast-feeding if the mother has bleeding nipples. The Apt-Downey test is helpful in differentiating maternal blood from infant blood. One part of the bloody stool (or gastric aspirate) is mixed with five parts of water to lyse the red blood cells. After the mixture is centrifuged, 1 ml of 0.2N NaOH is added to the supernatant hemoglobin solution. After 2 minutes, fetal hemoglobin, which resists the alkaline reduction, remains pink, whereas maternal hemoglobin turns yellow-brown. Coffee-grounds or melena contains denatured hemoglobin and, therefore, cannot be used for the Apt-Downey test.

Swallowed blood by a child usually is the result of nosebleeds or bleeding mouth lesions. These nasopharyngeal bleeds can present as hematemesis or melena. Although rare in children, pulmonary hemorrhage may present acutely as hematemesis or more chronically with melena and anemia. Vaginal bleeding in the newborn who has estrogen withdrawal may be mistaken as rectal bleeding. In the menstruating teenager, vaginal blood may affect the accuracy of stool guaiac testing. The possibility of blood being added to the stool by a caretaker should arouse suspicion of Munchausen by proxy.

AGE AT PRESENTATION

Newborn

GI bleeding in newborns usually appears as rectal bleeding or blood suctioned from the stomach during routine postnatal care. Often, no lesion is readily discernible, and the bleeding resolves spontaneously and permanently. Common causes of GI bleeding in the first 24 hours of life include maternal blood swallowed during delivery and local trauma following nasogastric suctioning. Hemorrhagic disease of the newborn as a result of inherited deficits of coagulation factors or delay in administration of postnatal vitamin K occasionally presents as GI bleeding, although it is more common for these disorders to present as diffuse bleeding from venipuncture sites.

Premature infants and newborns who have low Apgar scores are at increased risk for having gastric ulcerations and erosions that can bleed. These lesions are rarely primary, usually resulting from asphyxia associated with a difficult delivery, a cardiac lesion, or sepsis. The diagnosis is made by radiograph or upper gastrointestinal endoscopy. Newborns who have persistent or severe gastroesophageal reflux can develop esophagitis. Although esophageal bleeding is upper GI bleeding, hematemesis is rare. Rather, the slow bleeding is occult and presents more commonly with signs of anemia or guaiac positive stools. Because a barium swallow has poor sensitivity, pH probe manometry and esophagoscopy are better tests for identifying gastroesophageal reflux. Treatment usually involves H_2-blockers.

Newborns who have necrotizing enterocolitis (NEC) usually present with the sudden onset of bilious vomiting, abdominal distention, lethargy, and lower GI bleeding. These symptoms usually follow the first feeding but may be delayed for a few weeks. NEC is most common in premature infants but occasionally can occur in stressed full-term infants. Up to 8% of neonates in intensive care units develop NEC, and the mortality may be as high as 40%. Complications of NEC include sepsis and shock. The diagnosis is confirmed by the presence of pneumatosis intestinalis on abdominal radiograph, but this finding is variable. These neonates remain hospitalized for bowel rest and intravenous antibiotics, and they occasionally need surgical intervention.

Intrinsic structural lesions of the GI tract also are a serious cause of lower GI bleeding in the newborn. Intestinal duplication, a tubular structure lined with normal GI mucosa adjacent to the true intestine, can be present anywhere along the GI tract. Duplication presents with lower GI bleeding, either acute or chronic, along with abdominal distention and vomiting. The diagnosis is confirmed by radiograph, CT scan, or ultrasound. Unrepaired duplications may lead to obstruction, volvulus, or perforation. A volvulus or malrotation of the GI tract should be suspected in any infant who has abdominal pain, bilious vomiting, and melena. However, because these symptoms and signs often are unreliable, the diagnosis should be considered in any newborn who vomits and has guaiac-positive stools. An abdominal radiograph may show loops of small bowel overriding the liver shadow with paucity of air in the GI tract distal to the volvulus. An upper GI series and/or barium enema sometimes is needed to confirm the diagnosis. Immediate surgical repair is necessary. Vascular malformations can occur anywhere along the GI tract and present with slow or diffuse lower GI bleeding. The bleeding usually is painless, and the color of the blood in the stool will vary depending on the level of the lesion. Vascular malformations may be associated with cutaneous hemangiomas or cardiac defects.

Milk or soy protein allergy can begin as early as the first week of life as severe diarrhea, gross blood in the stool, abdominal distention, and vomiting. Older infants may present with occult lower GI bleeding and mucus in the stool. The diagnosis is made by clinical response to withdrawal and rechallenge of the offending protein. Infectious enteritis, although rare in the newborn, may present later in the first month of life. In very young infants, bacterial gastroenteritis, especially that caused by *Salmonella,* can present with bloody diarrhea with or without fever, and 30% of infants may have associated bacteremia. Bright red blood streaks on the surface of the stool suggests an anal fissure. Often associated with hard stools, anal fissures are the most common cause of rectal bleeding. Visual inspection of the anus usually confirms the diagnosis. Medications, such as indomethacin and dexamethasone, can cause mucosal erosion and GI bleeding.

Infants and Young Children

Upper GI bleeding in the young child usually is secondary to mucosal lesions in the esophagus and the stomach. Esophagitis usually is of viral etiology, but fungal infections can be seen in the immunocompromised child. As infants become more mobile, with improved hand to mouth ability, they are at higher risk for foreign body and toxic ingestions. Foreign bodies such as coins and small toys, which lodge in the esophagus, can present with drooling, vomiting, and chest pain. Persistent or unrecognized esophageal foreign bodies lead to edema and erosion of the esophagus and may present with hematemesis. Caustic ingestion severe enough to burn the esophageal mucosa also can present with drooling and hematemesis. Children who have forceful or prolonged vomiting may develop a rent at the gastroesophageal junction known as a *Mallory-Weiss tear.* The emesis becomes streaked with bright red blood and may develop into coffee-ground emesis if the tear persists. Although the bleeding is minor and usually resolves spontaneously, an H_2-blocker may be needed to prevent continued irritation by stomach acid.

Gastroesophageal varices can occur at any age but usually present in children younger than 8 years of age. Variceal bleeding can range from slow, persistent oozing to acute massive hematemesis. Physical examination usually reveals signs of portal hypertension, such as enlarged liver and/or spleen. Most cases result from the cavernous transformation of the extrahepatic portion of the portal vein; this has been associated with umbilical vessel catheterization, omphalitis, or neonatal conditions associated with hypoxia, prolonged jaundice, or sepsis. Intrahepatic causes of cirrhosis, leading to portal hypertension that first may manifest during childhood, include Wilson's disease (after age 6 years), $alpha_1$-antitrypsin deficiency, biliary cirrhosis, and metabolic, infectious, or anatomical forms of chronic liver disease. These latter diseases also may be associated with coagulopathy and thrombocytopenia secondary to the hypersplenism that usually accompanies them. If the cause of the portal hypertension is extrahepatic, the bleeding may be tolerated remarkably well, in contrast to those patients who have cirrhotic liver disease in whom rapid hepatic decompensation may occur. Fortunately, most variceal bleeding stops spontaneously, but the incidence of rebleeding is high. The diagnosis is confirmed by endoscopy.

Juvenile polyps are the most common cause of lower GI bleeding, reaching a peak incidence in children ages 3 to 7 years old. Typically, they are located in the colon and are simple, solitary, benign hamartomatous lesions that may irritate the GI tract and cause intermittent, painless, bright red rectal bleeding. Many of these polyps will autoamputate if left alone and are passed with the stool. Because most polyps are located within 25 cm of the anus, they are easily identified by digital examination, air contrast barium enema, or sigmoidoscopy and can be removed with snare electrocautery.

Adenomatous polyps may present with rectal bleeding as early as infancy, but they are managed differently than juvenile polyps. Juvenile polyps are benign inflammatory lesions that do not cause later complications. Adenomatous polyps, on the other hand, are premalignant tumors, which may transform into a malignancy over an average period of 10 years.[2] Familial polyposis and Gardner's syndrome are associated with adenomatous polyps. Juvenile polyposis coli (JPC) is suggested by the presence of 5 to 10 juvenile polyps; 10 or more polyps is considered diagnostic. JPC, which occurs in about 10% of patients who have colonic polyps, is associated with anemia, right-colon polyps, and adenomas.[2]

Meckel's diverticulum, a remnant of the omphalomesenteric duct, is present in up to 2% of the population. The acid secreted by ectopic gastric mucosa, which usually is present in the diverticulum, causes peptic ulceration of the ileal mucosa. Presentation occurs typically in children younger than 3 years of age as painless, maroon or red-colored lower GI bleeding. Typically, the bleeding is severe enough to cause the hemoglobin level to fall to about 8 g%. Diagnosis is made by technetium-99 scan, which identifies the ectopic gastric mucosa. This test is fairly sensitive, but a repeat scan may be necessary. Treatment requires surgical excision.

Intussusception, the telescoping of an intestinal segment, is seen typically in children 6 to 24 months old. The occurrence often is idiopathic and usually involves invagination of the distal ileum through the ileocecal valve into the colon. Older children who have intussusception and those who have multiple recurrences may have pathological lesions that serve as lead points (Meckel's diverticulum, polyp, and tumor). The classic presentation begins as intermittent, severe, crampy abdominal pain, with vomiting following shortly thereafter. As the intussusception progresses, lethargy or paradoxical irritability develops. Guaiac-positive stools are seen as the bowel becomes ischemic and may develop into passage of red bloody mucus, classically referred to as "currant jelly stools." Hydrostatic reduction with barium enema, or more recently air enema, is successful in the majority of cases. Complications include intestinal perforation, peritonitis, and significant bleeding.

Symptoms associated with infectious enterocolitis range from mild diarrhea to fever, abdominal cramping, and watery and/or mucoid stools with or without blood. *Salmonella, Shigella, Yersinia,* and *Campylobacter* are the most common bacterial causes of bloody diarrhea. *Pseudomembranous colitis*, caused by *Clostridium difficile*, also presents with fever, diarrhea, abdominal cramping, and bloody stools. Often there is a history of recent hospitalization and antimicrobial therapy, but the presentation can be delayed for weeks. A variety of parasites, such as amoebae, can cause bloody diarrhea.

Systemic disease, in particular vasculitis, may present with or be accompanied by bloody stools. The constellation of arthritis, hematuria, purpura, intestinal cramping, and bloody stools suggests Henoch-Schönlein purpura (HSP). Children who have HSP are at increased risk of having an intussusception, or they may have severe GI bleeding. Hemolytic-uremic syndrome (HUS) often has a prodrome of hemorrhagic colitis recently shown to be caused by Shiga toxin-producing *E. coli* with a serotype O157:H7. The classic triad of HUS includes thrombocytopenia, hemolytic anemia, and renal disease.

Milk protein allergy, anal fissures, and congenital anatomic anomalies of the GI tract also can occur in this age group.

Older Children and Adolescents

Peptic ulcer disease can occur at any age but is more common in the older child and adolescent. Symptoms usually begin with epigastric or periumbilical pain accompanied by nausea. GI bleeding is evident in about 50% of children either as hematemesis or melena. *Helicobacter pylori*, a bacteria found in the gastric mucous layer or adherent to the epithelial lining of the stomach, has been implicated as the cause of more than 90% of duodenal ulcers and up to 80% of gastric ulcers.[1] Infection is uncommon in childhood but increases in adolescence and adulthood. *H. pylori* infection is diagnosed by culture of biopsy specimens from the stomach and duodenum. Serological tests, which measure specific *H. pylori* IgG antibodies, also are available. Treatment consists of a 10- to 14-day course of any of a variety of antibiotic regimens.

Hemangiomas and other vascular lesions, such as hereditary hemorrhagic telangiectasia (Rendu-Osler-Weber syndrome), must be considered in the evaluation of painless rectal bleeding. Its most common form is the larger cavernous hemangioma, either polypoid or diffuse, extending several centimeters through the submucosa of the small or large intestine. The large bowel, specifically the rectum, is the area usually involved in the diffuse type. Cutaneous vascular malformations often are present but may require scrupulous searching to detect. Selective arteriography or digital subtraction angiography may aid in demonstrating the abnormal vessels if they are not visible on direct inspection.

Inflammatory bowel disease may appear in the adolescent age group as episodes of bloody diarrhea, cramping, and tenesmus. The course may be atypical in children and, therefore, be difficult to diagnose. Growth failure, weight loss, or anemia with evidence of recurrent bouts of GI bleeding should alert the clinician to the diagnosis, which colonoscopy and biopsy usually confirm.

GENERAL APPROACH TO PATIENTS WHO HAVE GI BLEEDING

When evaluating a patient who has GI blood loss, the physician should keep two goals in mind. First, the severity of the blood loss must be assessed quickly in order to institute appropriate resuscitative measures. Second, the physician must consider the most likely causes so that problems requiring immediate surgery can be separated from those requiring medical evaluation and management. The workup is based on the patient's age and history, clinical appearance, and on the physician's familiarity with the patient. A list of lesions commonly associated with GI bleeding is provided in Box 139-1.

History

A detailed history may help the clinician determine the location and duration of the bleeding. Particular attention should be paid to the color of the stool and emesis and whether there has been a change in the preceding days or weeks. Massive red blood from the mouth or rectum is readily apparent to the parent and the patient. However, the importance of maroon or tarry stools may not be appreciated unless the clinician asks.

Antecedent symptoms also are a key to identification of many diseases. Vomiting that progresses from bile-stained to bloody is seen with intestinal obstruction (volvulus, intussusception, necrotizing enterocolitis) or with Mallory-Weiss tears. Bloody diarrhea may accompany infectious enteritis or precede the more serious hemolytic-uremic syndrome. Fever is common in infectious or inflammatory disorders. Arthritis and rash are seen with Henoch-Schönlein purpura. Abdominal pain, fever, and weight loss suggest the inflammatory bowel disease. Lower rectal disorders such as hemorrhoids or anal fissures present with blood-streaked stools and painful defecation. Young children who have upper GI bleeding should be questioned about foreign body or caustic ingestion. Medication use, especially of aspirin, nonsteroidal anti-inflammatory drugs, steroids, and tetracycline, is a frequent cause of gastritis. A family history of polyps, bleeding disorders, or GI diseases is important. Neonatal history should focus on risk factors for NEC or varices, including umbilical vein catheters, liver disease, and birth asphyxia. Sexual activ-

BOX 139-1

CAUSES OF GASTROINTESTINAL BLEEDING

Newborn

Upper GI bleeding

Hemorrhagic disease of the newborn
Gastritis
Stress ulcer
Esophagitis

Lower GI bleeding

Necrotizing enterocolitis (NEC)
Duplication
Volvulus/malrotation
Vascular malformations
Milk allergy
Infectious enteritis
Anal fissure

Infants and Young Children

Upper GI bleeding

Nasopharyngeal bleeding
Esophagitis
  Acid reflux
  Viral, fungal, caustic
Esophageal foreign body
Mallory-Weiss tear
Gastroesophageal varices
Gastritis

Lower GI bleeding

Juvenile polyps
Meckel's diverticulum
  Intussusception
Infectious enterocolitis
  Pseudomembranous colitis
Vasculitis (HSP, HUS)
  Milk allergy
Anal fissure/trauma (abuse)
  Duplication
Vascular malformation

Older Children and Adolescents

Upper GI bleeding

Nasopharyngeal bleeding
  Esophagitis
  Mallory-Weiss tear
Gastroesophageal varices
Gastritis
  Aspirin, NSAIDs
  Helicobacter pylori
Peptic ulcer disease

Lower GI bleeding

Polyps
  Infectious enterocolitis
Inflammatory bowel disease
  Vasculitis
Vascular malformation
Meckel's diverticulum
  Hemorrhoids
  Anal fissure

ity or abuse involving anal penetration should alert the clinician to anal and rectal trauma.

Physical Examination

The physical examination should be complete and systematic, because clues to the diagnosis may be present in any organ system. The general appearance and vital signs can be helpful in determining the duration of bleeding. Slow, chronic bleeding allows time for physiological changes such as tachycardia, orthostasis, and decreased pulse pressure. Children initially may appear comfortable but tired and have some degree of pallor. Patients who have acute, rapid bleeds present in various stages of shock depending on the amount of blood loss. The nose and mouth should be examined for bleeding lesions or burns. The abdominal examination should evaluate for tenderness, bowel sounds, masses, and hepatosplenomegaly. The physician also must look for signs of chronic liver disease, such as the presence of telangiectasias, jaundice, hepatosplenomegaly, and a prominent abdominal venous pattern. With lower GI bleeding, a careful rectal examination should be performed, with special attention paid to (1) the perianal region, observing for skin tags, abscesses, fissures, bleeding points, or much less commonly, hemorrhoids; (2) the character of the stool; and (3) the presence of occult blood. It also is necessary to palpate for polyps and pelvic masses during the rectal examination. Finally, skin lesions such as purpura and petechiae suggest a bleeding disorder, HSP, or HUS.

Management

For a child having acute massive GI bleeding, the approach must be the same as in any other emergency. The physician must approach the patient with an efficient, rational plan in mind that will allow him or her to obtain the pertinent historical information, perform a brief but adequate examination, stabilize the patient clinically, arrive at a working diagnosis, and institute appropriate therapy or consultations. Massive upper GI bleeding may lead to vomiting, aspiration, and airway obstruction that requires stabilization of the airway with endotracheal intubation. Administration of oxygen always is indicated. Evaluation of peripheral perfusion, quality of pulses, and capillary refill time assess the adequacy of circulation. In children, the initial response to hypovolemic shock is tachycardia. In acute bleeds, adequate blood pressure can be maintained with blood loss of up to 30% without replacement. Tachycardia and capillary refill time are essential criteria in determining the nature of the resuscitation required. Skin turgor and the color of the mucous membranes also should be noted.

If signs of shock are present (e.g., orthostasis or frank hypotension, tachycardia, poorly perfused extremities, pale mucous membranes, or altered mental status), a large-bore intravenous catheter should be placed. Initial laboratory studies include complete blood count, hematocrit, reticulocyte count, coagulation times, electrolytes, and blood typing and crossmatching. If percutaneous venous access is unobtainable within a few minutes, an intraosseous line should be placed, and 20 ml/kg of normal saline should be given rapidly to reexpand the vascular volume. This fluid bolus may need to be repeated several times. Additional fluid should be given as needed to allow equilibration of these solutions with the extravascular space. With greater than 30% to 40% acute blood loss, packed red blood cells should be given as soon as possible.

An appropriate size nasogastric (NG) tube, preferably of the vented sump type, helps determine the source of bleeding and estimate the volume of ongoing blood loss. This tube should be left in place and attached either to low-pressure continuous suction, if vented, or to intermittent suction, if nonvented. The only instance in which NG tube placement may aggravate bleeding is with a patient who has varices. Nonetheless, even in this case, an NG tube may be required to quantitate blood loss adequately.

Controlling the bleeding and determining the specific diagnosis are the next steps in management. If the nasogastric aspirate contains blood or if the patient has hematemesis, saline irrigation may be instituted in an attempt to decrease mucosal blood flow and thereby stop profuse bleeding. Although the efficacy of lavage in decreasing and controlling gastric bleeding has not been demonstrated conclusively, it allows easier assessment of the rate of bleeding and helps in removing clotted blood. Saline at room temperature should be used because irrigation with water can lead to hyponatremia, and iced or cold fluid may cause hypothermia. The saline is instilled through an NG tube and is withdrawn after 3 to 5 minutes. Aspirate returns that do not clear in 15 minutes suggest continued GI bleeding and should prompt additional evaluation.

If the bleeding ceases, gastroduodenoscopy should be performed to demonstrate the bleeding source and to determine the type of lesion present. Upper GI fiberoptic endoscopy can establish the diagnosis in 75% to 90% of patients. If the bleeding is massive and cannot be controlled with saline lavage, adequate visualization is not likely to be achieved with the fiberoptic endoscope. If the bleeding is not immediately life threatening, arteriography, which can demonstrate bleeding that occurs at a rate of 0.5 ml/minute or more, should be considered.

Of greater sensitivity and reduced invasiveness is the use of a sulfur-colloid isotopic study, which can demonstrate active bleeding at rates as low as 0.1 ml/minute. This method demonstrates active bleeding by using a tracer with a very short half-life. In small infants a large uptake of the isotope by the liver may mask the right upper quadrant. An additional isotopic method of determining the bleeding site consists of injecting the patient with technetium-99-pertechnetate-labeled red blood cells. These labeled cells may remain in the circulation for more than a day and allow repeated imaging to locate the site of intermittent bleeding.

If the lesion is one of mucosal erosion or inflammation, antacid therapy with or without the concomitant use of an H_2-blocker should be instituted. If the bleeding source is found to be variceal, the causes of these lesions must be considered, with appropriate treatment of the underlying disease. Liver or portal venous disease should be sought. Clotting factors and platelets should be replaced as indicated.

Variceal bleeding requires special mention because of the many settings in which varices may be seen. Although the treatment of variceal bleeding continues to evolve, it may be divided into those therapies that can be instituted in most emergency facilities and those that require a pediatric endoscopist skilled at sclerotherapy.

Of the former therapies, balloon tamponade and vasopressin therapy are the most commonly used. The Sengstaken-Blakemore tube is a nasogastric tube with additional lumina for a gastric balloon and an esophageal balloon. After placement, the gastric balloon is inflated and traction is applied so that the balloon abuts the gastroesophageal junction and tamponades the variceal bleeding. Inflation of the esophageal balloon is rarely needed in pediatric patients. Although Sengastaken-Blakemore tubes are available in pediatric sizes, their use has been associated with an unacceptably high incidence of airway problems and even esophageal rupture. Vasopressin may be used as a mesenteric vasoconstrictor to reduce portal blood flow and thus decrease variceal pressure. Initially, 0.1 unit/minute is infused, preferably through a central or intraosseous line. The infusion is increased by 0.05 unit/minute up to a continuous infusion of vasopressin 0.2 to 0.4 unit/minute, depending on the child's age. Infusion is continued for 12 to 24 hours after bleeding stops; the dose then is tapered gradually. Extreme care must be taken to avoid malignant hypertension in patients receiving vasopressin infusions, and arterial pressure and electrocardiograms must be monitored continuously.

Endoscopic sclerotherapy, which controls variceal bleeding caused by a variety of underlying diseases, has taken its place in recent years as a valuable treatment for children. The number and magnitude of complications are exceedingly small, with a low incidence of rebleeding. This technique is somewhat more effective when used for varices associated with extrahepatic portal hypertension rather than for those associated with primary liver disease. A major drawback to this technique is the frequent need for general anesthesia and endotracheal intubation when performed on small children and the need for a facility skilled at managing small children who are critically ill. For many patients, however, sclerotherapy offers a relatively less invasive means for controlling variceal bleeding than more risky portal shunting procedures.

Evaluation of lower GI bleeding differs in several aspects from that of upper GI bleeding. The abdomen, perineum, and rectum are carefully examined. Stool must be analyzed for the presence of blood, ova and parasites, and enteric pathogens. If diarrhea is present, the stool should be examined microscopically for polymorphonuclear leukocytes and mucus, both of which are evidence of bacterial infection. Digital rectal examination should follow in an attempt to discover the presence of anal fissures, rectal polyps, or hemorrhoids. Sigmoidoscopy may be necessary for children who have persistent rectal bleeding to identify polyps or mucosal lesions. The presence of blood coming from above the reach of the sigmoidoscope indicates the need to proceed with other diagnostic studies.

Persistent lower GI bleeding can be evaluated by several different imaging studies. An upright and supine view of the abdomen will reveal signs of obstruction or for calcifications. For severe, life-threatening bleeds, angiography can be both diagnostic and therapeutic, depending on the ability to embolize the bleeding vessels. Angiography must be performed during active bleeding, because the ability to detect slow or past bleeding is limited.

Children who have persistent, active bleeding who are clinically stable should have a radionuclide scan, which identifies accumulation of an isotope at the bleeding site. With a sulfur-colloid isotopic scan, the isotope is extracted rapidly so that there is low background radioactivity. Although there is high-contrast resolution around the bleeding site, it is effective only for identifying rapid bleeding. An isotope-labeled red blood cell infusion has a lower contrast ratio but is better at detecting slower or intermittent bleeds. A Meckel scan uses technetium-99 pertechnetate, which is secreted by ectopic gastric mucosa, to identify the diverticulum. If the rate of bleeding does not permit the time necessary to perform these studies, vasopressin may be administered parenterally in an attempt to control the bleeding and to stabilize the patient. Air contrast barium studies or endoscopy can identify sources of more chronic, low-grade bleeding. However, a barium enema or an upper GI series with small bowel follow-through should be the last studies performed because they make the further use of arteriography, isotope scans, and endoscopy impossible for several days thereafter.

In cases in which the intestine is compromised vascularly, or the rate of bleeding is excessive and uncontrollable by more conservative methods, prompt surgical intervention is required. Fortunately, however, conservative measures can control most acute episodes of GI bleeding relatively easily; those patients who eventually require surgical intervention usually can be handled electively at a later time.

When to Refer

Upper GI bleed
Lower GI bleed that is of moderate amount, persistent, or intermittent

When to Hospitalize

Any nontrivial upper GI bleeding (such as that associated with active bleeding, moderate amount of blood, anemia, abdominal pain)
Significant lower GI bleeding
Hemodynamic instability
Anemia (hematocrit <10%)
Severe abdominal pain
Associated systemic symptoms (e.g., HUS, IBD)
Altered mental status or lethargy
Suspicion of surgical etiology (e.g., Meckel's diverticulum, intussusception, volvulus)

REFERENCES

1. Centers for Disease Control and Prevention: *Helicobacter pylori,* fact sheet for health care providers, Centers for Disease Control and Prevention, July 1998.
2. Hoffenberg EF, et al: Symptomatic colonic polyps in childhood: not so benign, *J Pediatr Gastroenterol Nutr* 28:175, 1999.

SUGGESTED READINGS

Balkan E, et al: Sigmoidoscopy in minor lower gastrointestinal bleeding, *Arch Dis Child* 78:267, 1998.

Daneman A, et al: Recurrences of intussusception: barium vs air enema reduction, *Pediatr Radiol* 28:913,1988.

Goggin N, et al: Effect of *Helicobacter pylori* eradication on the natural history of duodenal ulcer disease, *Arch Dis Child* 79:502, 1998.

Pearl RH, et al: The approach to common abdominal diagnoses in infants and children. Part II. *Pediatr Clin North Am* 45:1287, 1998.

Proulx F, et al: Inflammatory mediators in *Escherichia coli* 0157:H7 hemorrhagic colitis and hemolytic-uremic syndrome, *Pediatr Clin North Am* 17:899, 1998.

Squires RH: Gastrointestinal bleeding, *Pediatr Rev* 20:95, 1999.

Stringer MD, McClean P: Treatment of oesophageal varices, *Arch Dis Child* 77:476, 1997.

140 Headache

Henry M. Seidel

Headache—literally, a pain in the head—is a common presenting complaint in childhood, increasing in frequency as the child becomes more verbal and better able to be explicit about aches and pains. We cannot, of course, accurately appreciate its frequency in the very young. Eventually, virtually everyone experiences a headache—probably humanity's most commonly experienced pain—usually, for the first time, at some point during childhood or adolescence. Becoming more frequent with age, chronic headaches may beset as many as 20% of adolescents at one time or another. It is a complaint that easily elicits empathy.

Occasionally, serious concern and frustration also accompany this complaint. The physician does not want to overlook the relatively infrequent causes that require lifesaving therapeutic interventions. Parents and many older children and adolescents who have headaches often worry about a major disease, particularly a brain tumor. Because of the several categories of headache (migraine, "abdominal" migraine, tension, and "cluster"), each with imprecise starting and end points, diagnosis and management can be difficult (Box 140-1).

Nonetheless, most headaches during childhood are transient, bearable, and associated with the general wear and tear of life, from the nonthreatening viral and upper respiratory tract infection to the results of stress-producing experiences of day-to-day living. The older the child, the more likely the latter. However, if an acute episode persists or the intensity of the complaint accelerates, one should be aware of the possibility of an organic cause for the complaint, particularly if any localizing findings are evident after the history has been taken and the physical examination performed.

MECHANISM OF HEADACHE

Headache may have both extracranial and intracranial origins. An extracranial cause is most common, not surprising in that almost all extracranial structures are pain sensitive. Thus, headache frequently is associated with dilation and distention of the extracranial vessels or with spasmodic contracture of the scalp and neck musculature. Infections or other diseases in any of the extracranial structures of the head—eyes, nose, teeth, sinuses, and ears—can cause headache and usually are identifiable readily with localized findings. However, this is not always so; extracranial causes may not be made immediately evident by localized signs.

Not all intracranial structures are pain sensitive. Those that are include cranial nerves V, VII, IX, and X; cervical nerves I through III; and the venous sinuses and some of their branches. Most of the rest of the intracranial structures—skull, substance of the brain, and most of the meninges—are not sensitive to pain. However, the "traction" produced by a mass of any sort, the pulls and displacements of the venous sinuses and their branches, and inflammation from any cause can and do influence those cranial and cervical nerves that respond to pain, although the exact mechanism by which pain results is not known, particularly when no identifiable anatomical displacements are evident.

CONCOMITANT SIGNS AND SYMPTOMS

Meningismus and fever, for example, may accompany headache and, when present, increase concern for an acute, treatable condition. Meningitis is an obvious first thought. However, other major conditions may produce a severe headache along with meningismus: retropharyngeal abscess, superior longitudinal sinus thrombosis, and subarachnoid hemorrhage, as well as typhoid fever and pneumonia. Of course, the common infecting bacteria and viruses may not always be the cause of meningitis or meningoencephalitis. Other agents (e.g., cryptococci) also must be considered.

HISTORY AND PHYSICAL EXAMINATION

The history and physical examination are, as usual, the bedrock of diagnosis. They often help to rule out many diagnoses quickly that require extensive investigation and therapeutic intervention. Actually, while taking the history, the pediatrician can begin to eliminate (or include) many concerns, for example, by an immediate look to observe the movement of the eyes (for evidence of cranial nerve VI palsy, frequently an early the first manifestation of increased intracranial pressure) or an initial question directed to the associated complaint of vomiting (whether it is accompanied by nausea, which usually is not the case with increased intracranial pressure).

Occasionally the acute circumstance for which treatment is sought requires great speed to reach even a tentative diagnosis. The patient's physical condition and level of consciousness may direct the diagnostic search. Certainly, the following accompanying complaints and findings suggest organic causes and, therefore, a less leisurely approach:

Fever
Meningismus

BOX 140-1

SOME CAUSES OF HEADACHES

Intracranial Masses (Sharply Localized or Diffuse)
Intracranial tumor, benign or malignant
Brain cyst
Subdural hematoma (and/or other hemorrhage localized or diffuse)
Central nervous system leukemia
Acute onset of hydrocephalus for any reason caused by obstruction within the ventricular system

Vascular Causes
Migraine
- Classic
- With ophthalmoplegia or hemiplegia
- Basilar artery
- Complicated by tension
- With ornithine transcarbamoylase deficiency

Cluster headache (histamine headaches)
Arteriovenous malformation
Venous sinus engorgement
Hypertension (pheochromocytoma)
Cranial arteritis (periarteritis nodosa)
Intracranial aneurysm
Subarachnoid hemorrhage
Vascular occlusion
- With congenital heart disease
- With sickle cell disease

Vascular dilation secondary to fever, hypoxia, hypercapnia, or severe anemia
Systemic lupus erythematosus

Specific Focal Disease
Inflammation, new growth, foreign body, or other injury of:
- Eye (glaucoma, orbital tumor)
- Ear
- Nose
- Throat
- Teeth
- Sinuses
- Cervical spine (osteoarthritis)
- Cranial bone

Emotional Causes
Conversion reactions
Daily stress, psychogenic causes, familial patterning
Depression
Possibility of secondary gain

Infections
Meningitis or encephalitis
- Bacterial cause
- Viral cause

Sinusitis (less frequent in the younger child, who has poorly developed sinuses)
Otitis media
Mastoiditis
Pharyngitis
Retropharyngeal abscess
Brain abscess
Cervical adenitis
Systemic infection
Subacute bacterial endocarditis

Neural Causes
Epileptic equivalent
Trigeminal neuralgia
Glossopharyngeal neuralgia
Excessive auditory, visual, or gustatory sensory stimuli
Seizures (postictal)

Trauma
Lumbar puncture (with subsequent decreased intracranial pressure)
Head injury
- Concussion
- Subdural hematoma
- Subarachnoid hemorrhage

Other posttraumatic events

Noxious Stimuli
"Gas leak" syndrome (carbon monoxide)
Alcohol
Lead
Oral contraceptives
Other drugs (e.g., steroid withdrawal)

Other Causes
Allergy
Hyperaldosteronism
Hypoglycemia
Hyponatremia
Hyperammonemia
Occipital neuralgia with malformation at C1 and C2
Pseudotumor cerebri (with otitis media, use of vitamin A, tetracyclines, steroids)
Renal disease
Temporomandibular joint disease
Unknown origin

Trauma (even if obscure or distant in time)
Seizures
Severe hypertension
Confusion
Diminished awareness
Petechiae and ecchymoses
Lethargy
Vomiting, with or without nausea
Intense irritability
Great specificity in description of headache
History of pica
Changes in gait, personality, behavior

Similarly, headaches characterized in the following manner suggest an organic cause:

Initial, dramatic episode
Sudden onset

Progressive severity and frequency over a short period (a history of several months tends to argue against the organic)
Intense pain upon awakening
A dramatic description (e.g., "jackhammer in the head")
Occurrence in the morning; subsidence after arising, particularly after vomiting
Precipitation by the Valsalva maneuver, cough, sneeze, strain (particularly if headache is of short duration, a few minutes to 30 minutes)

A sharply defined, acute onset is worrisome, and the age of the child is a prime consideration: the younger the child, the greater the risk. Also, the precision of the complaint suggests a more life-compromising diagnosis. Even the young child (usually by 3 to 4 years of age) can point a finger very accurately. A frontal location of the headache suggests frontal or ethmoid sinusitis, cerebral tumors, a migraine, and problems with the eyes; an occipital or suboccipital location suggests a cerebellar tumor, occipital neuralgia, sphenoid sinusitis, or tension. The more severe the complaint is, the more likely an organic cause. However, children younger than 8 to 10 years of age usually do not have recurrent headache as a result of sinusitis nor, in general, do those who have so-called eyestrain as a result of refractive errors or strabismus. Astigmatism may cause pain about the eyes and orbit, usually not severe, but may be confused with a frontal headache.

Some characteristics of headache particularly suggest increased intracranial pressure: those that wake the patient from sleep or occur in the morning and that are accompanied by vomiting free of nausea; those related to a change in position from prone to supine and from either of those to the sitting or standing positions; and those related to physical activity, coughing, sneezing, and straining. Increased intracranial pressure does not provide a warning, a prodrome like that of scotomata (visual "fireworks"), pallor, and abdominal pain that may precede a migraine headache. The headache that wakes the patient from sleep and that does not respond to aspirin, acetaminophen, or other over-the-counter drugs often may have a more serious cause; the simple, transient episode generally responds most readily. Pica, particularly in the younger child, suggests lead encephalopathy. The description of "throbbing" suggests hypertension. A clear history of trauma always requires particular attention.

These considerations underscore the need for a careful history and sharp dissection of the often intermingled psychosocial and organic variables. Clearly, the family history is important. Children who have migraine headaches tend to have parents who have them. Care should be taken, however: children under stress are apt to mimic their parents' behavior. Beyond that, the description of the headache, its frequency, duration, and location and the report of prodromata are all very important. Clues to stress and tension may reside in the events that precede the headache, such as the experience and thoughts of the patient, the time of day, and the day of the week. Understanding all the experiences of the child, both at home and at school, can help: the nature of relations with family, teachers, and friends, reading and television habits, eating patterns, environmental noise, sleep habits, and any recent change in bowel and urination patterns. Even the presence of a gas stove in the home is important, because it may be leaking. The search, then, must be for hints of organic cause and for evidence of emotional stress and tension.

A "concept" of the child emerges from this inquiry. The depiction of behavioral patterns, past coping mechanisms, any recent behavioral change, hints of any change in the flow of normal development, and diminished school performance all help characterize the child. Is the child shy or compulsive, too sensitive to the needs of others, obsessively neat—in all, a possible "worrywart"? These traits may facilitate a migraine or the so-called tension headache. Certainly, the physician should look for evidence of depression, because headache may be the prime complaint of a chronically depressed child.

The physical examination must be precise and include a careful neurological evaluation and a conscientious attempt at ophthalmoscopy, a visual field check, an evaluation of ocular muscle balance and convergence, palpation and auscultation of the skull and mastoid and of the optic globes, palpation and transillumination of the sinuses, a careful check of the teeth, ears, and throat, and a blood pressure reading. Eye drops may be used to improve the visualization of the fundus, but only after a description of the pupils and their reactions to light and accommodation are carefully recorded. Rarely, then, are laboratory and imaging examinations necessary.

INTERPRETING INFORMATION

Characterization of the headache is most important. Two major groups exist: those having an apparent first acute episode in the absence of a significant prior complaint and those suggesting chronicity and recurrence. This latter group bestows the advantage of hindsight in determining the patterns. However, the acute episode may be the first of many; the boundary can be obscure, at least at the start. A tendency to the diffuse and nondescript suggests tension or a more "distant" cause: an association, perhaps, with anemia, fever, some infectious process, or hypoglycemia. It is worth repeating that youth and specificity (the younger the child and/or the more specific the headache) increase the likelihood of an organic disorder. However, remember that time usually allows for a careful approach to differentiate the organic from the benign.

The trap to avoid is relying too greatly on a mechanical and unthinking use of the laboratory and other diagnostic aids—that is, the workup. Most headaches should be diagnosed and managed successfully without the skull roentgenographic series, computed tomography (CT) scan, magnetic resonance imaging (MRI), lumbar puncture, or arteriogram; most patients are helped by a conscientious history and physical examination, a meticulous explanation, and a ready and willing ear. It is the ability to listen wisely and to respond constructively that will do most for the patient who has a rather diffuse, chronic, or recurrent headache. Perhaps a little acetaminophen is helpful too.

Headache, more than most complaints, tends to force the physician's behavior to extremes: on the one hand, intervening forthrightly for major problems; on the other, responding gently in a conscientious attempt at understanding the patient's sometimes submerged feelings and needs. The physician must reject mechanistic diagnostic intervention unless the situation clearly calls for it.

DIFFERENTIAL DIAGNOSIS

Given a precise history and physical examination, resorting to the laboratory becomes necessary in cases of a genuine indication of CNS infection or increased intracranial pressure from whatever source. The choice of studies at the start is relatively simple. The suspicion of infection suggests the need for a complete blood count and, quite often, a lumbar puncture and blood culture. The lumbar puncture should be approached with care and only after verification that no papilledema or other evidence of increased intracranial pressure exists. A urinalysis is easy to obtain and certainly is indicated in the presence of hypertension. Auscultation for a cranial bruit may detect an aneurysm or other vascular deformity.

Although skull and sinus films can be helpful, a need for the CT scan, sonography, MRI, or radioactive isotope brain scans may arise, particularly if the history does not suggest a clearly definable diagnosis or when there are focal findings. If so, consultation is indicated with the neurologist and the "imagists," who can help decide on the most effective and least invasive of the various imaging techniques. Arteriography, still used occasionally, should be avoided if possible, because it increases morbidity and the risk of hemiplegia.

The electroencephalogram (EEG), of itself relatively benign (except for its cost and impressive, intimidating trappings), is of questionable help. Its findings, for example, often are abnormal in patients who have migraine and often normal in those who have epilepsy. It sometimes is helpful in localizing an intracranial lesion, but it is not nearly as specific as the imaging techniques, and it offers nothing in the way of establishing a prognosis. The EEG, therefore, is not the first line in the study of acute problems.

At this point, the individual problem often becomes sufficiently clear that an appropriate therapeutic intervention is evident. Infection can be defined further by appropriate cultures and treated with antibiotics, surgical drainage, or both; expanding lesions and any trauma and bleeding mandate neurosurgical consultation. Fortunately, pseudotumor cerebri sometimes can be diagnosed.

However, once the history and physical examination are complete, the pediatrician still may be confronted with a complaint that seems nonspecific and difficult to clarify. For example, some helpful information indicating a behavioral change may become evident, as well as information eliminating the possibility of organic disease; sometimes the organic and the functional components are concurrent. If migraine is present about 75% of the time in a family history, the physician should turn the evaluation in that direction. In this circumstance, other factors are helpful. Migraine, quite common in childhood, more so in boys than in girls, usually begins during the early school years, from 5 or 6 to about 9 years of age. However, it is not uncommon in the younger child. A history of cyclic vomiting or car sickness often is present. These headaches, usually unilateral, tend to predominate in females after puberty and sometimes are accompanied, particularly in "classic" migraine, by prodromal periods that may include sensory, motor, or visual auras, scotomas, abdominal pain, nausea and vomiting, irritability, or paresthesias; prodromes, however, are reported less commonly in children than in adults. At times, retroorbital pain occurs, usually on one side.

The physician should ask about odd visual phenomena, such as gaping "holes," dots, lines, and "stars." The older child should be asked to draw the scotoma. The often associated gastrointestinal complaint can be severe, and the occasional transient neurological finding of aphasia, hemiplegia, or ophthalmoplegia can be very disturbing. This complicates matters and leads to more extensive testing, particularly to the use of the CT scan or MRI and to the investigation of a urea-cycle abnormality (ornithine transcarbamoylase deficiency), believed by some to be a cause of migraine.

A migraine headache lacks consistency in that it may occur on either side of the head and may vary in frequency. It often may begin during periods of emotional stress, intense use of the eyes (reading, television), menstruation, use of oral contraceptives, or exposure to loud sound (rock music played at high volume); it may occur when menses have been missed or chocolate and cheeses have been eaten. A period of sleep following the headache often terminates the episode.

A variant of the "classic" migraine is "common" migraine, in which abdominal pain, nausea and vomiting, visual aura, and other prodromata are unusual; but family history of similar headaches and relief with sleep are typical. Notably, the headache accompanying "common" migraine tends to be somewhat less dramatic, and it is far more common, perhaps 9:1, than the classic form.

The presentation of migraine can be complicated by the absence of headache. A melange of visual auras, episodic abdominal pain, cyclic vomiting, periods of vertigo and confusion, and even torticollis represent migraine equivalents in infancy, childhood, and adolescence. These are very often self-limited. Many of these patients have a strong family history of migraine. Most often, however, there is recurrent headache even if but once a month in the beginning. The belly aches, nausea and vomiting, and the auras tend to be confirming of a diagnosis if there is a family history of migraine and a report of relief of pain with sleep.

Tension headaches, sometimes called muscle contraction headaches, usually follow periods of stress and may last for days or weeks; they are dull (not pulsating) and usually bilateral. They may be correlated with behavioral change and, particularly, with difficult relations with family, friends, or teachers. These undercurrents and any suspicion of them should have been explored during the history and should prompt the interviewer to go beyond initial denials. An effort must be made to gain a clear understanding of those feelings and attitudes that may provoke anger, hostility, or anxiety. The history also may reveal a disruption of sleep patterns, particularly difficulty in falling asleep.

Such headaches usually begin at about 8 to 12 or 13 years of age and usually in females, particularly those who are overweight. The description of a tension headache is more fuzzy than that of migraine (although it may be compulsively precise), and it often is said to involve the entire head or the occiput. No prodromal period akin to that of migraine occurs and, generally, no conclusion of the episode by a period of sleep takes place; neither are reports of aura, nausea and vomiting, or visual changes common. Finally, these headaches do not have associated objective findings, such as an abnormal EEG.

The depressed child often may have a severe headache that lasts for days or longer. Acute anger and subsequent guilt may underlie the depression. Although no particular behavioral pattern suggests either migraine or tension headache, these children frequently have a demeanor that sharpens the intensity of concerns common to all people, for example, sensitivity to criticism and meeting new people, worry about grades, and precision in doing homework. Such children may seem to be compulsive and to worry very much if they do not meet the personal demands they place on themselves.

Occipital neuralgia, often suggested by tenderness over the cervical spinous processes, usually occurs first during adolescence. A roentgenogram may reveal subluxation or narrowing at the level of the first and second cervical vertebrae. No prodrome occurs, nor does cessation of the pain with sleep.

Finally, vascular headaches, often called "cluster" headaches, begin to occur in older teenagers, predominantly in males. When they do occur in females, there is no association with menses. They usually are unilateral and accompanied by ipsilateral tearing of the eye. They are recurrent and tend to occur in clusters, often at night, each one lasting for perhaps an hour and then disappearing. Thus, cluster headaches are briefer and perhaps more frequent than migraine. They are not accompanied by vomiting or nausea.

Headache manifestations, then, are age related. The organic lesion is not confined to any age, yet headache in the very young suggests organicity. Thereafter, a sequence of diagnostic possibilities emerges: migraine during the early school years, tension headaches just before the onset of puberty, occipital neuralgia during adolescence, and finally, the vascular headache of the older teenager. It should be emphasized that the patient who has an already recognized headache disorder may, as time goes by, report a different sort of headache. Always respect the possibility of an evolving problem.

MANAGEMENT

The symptomatic management of headache is less difficult when there is a specific cause requiring a specific management. The therapeutic task is less certain in the circumstance when the headache is described less precisely and its true chronicity, severity, and recurrence often are obscured by fuzzy verbiage. The child most often involved is older than 6 or 7 years, and the presentation almost invariably suggests at least some emotional basis. The need, then, is to be more specific in getting at the cause, involving at times the psychologist or psychiatrist, and to use drugs sparingly. In fact, the very process of meticulous evaluation and sympathetic response sometimes is enough to break the cycle of complaint, particularly with the older child and adolescent.

Parents, properly advised, are central to the management. They can be effective in supervising the maintenance of the expected schedule (i.e., attendance at school) and helpful in arranging a compassionate yet disciplined approach when headaches occur at school. Depending on the age of the child, they can keep or help to keep a headache record, noting the time of occurrence, the characteristics, and the relationship to proximal events. The patient, of course, is central to all of this and should be expected to be a full participant in age-appropriate ways.

Although the cautious use of drugs has much to recommend it, do not be too cautious. A limited list of agents is helpful (Table 140-1). Headaches that are not severe, not particularly frequent, and not prolonged are managed best with acetaminophen rather than with aspirin or nonsteroidal antiinflammatory drugs, with their greater risk of side effects. Usually, the response is not dose related, and an increase in the amount or frequency of the dosage is *not* justified when the headache persists. In addition, a period of rest and sleep (if that is achievable) is synergistic. A migraine headache, particularly, responds to sleep. Although the chronic use of sedatives as an additional management "crutch" should be avoided, the use of short-term daily phenobarbital or phenytoin in anticonvulsant doses may help.

The next steps are guided by the diagnostic impression and the age of the child. Some children will persist in experiencing an intense and frequently recurrent headache (one or two times a month) and may, if they have migraine or cluster headaches, require ergot. The primary care pediatrician must then consider consulting with a neurologist or a physician whose expertise is the treatment of headache. The use of ergot derivatives to treat acute migraine is uncommon in pediatric practice, and they certainly should not be used in the prepubertal child or in any young person in whom gastrointestinal symptoms predominate. If they are used, they should be given in the prodromatal phase so that the subsequent headache might be prevented. In addition, the cluster headache often is managed more effectively by potentiating the effect of ergot with methysergide. However, the potential toxic effect of methysergide (retroperitoneal fibrosis and fibrotic syndromes) suggests the need for great caution.

Therefore, the pediatrician's usual unfamiliarity with these drugs and occasional inadequate understanding of their toxicity in the young (e.g., ergot will intensify an abdominal complaint) require the direction of a consultant more experienced in their use. If the clinical picture is suggestive of depression, an antidepressant can be prescribed. This, too, frequently requires the advice of a consultant, preferably a psychiatrist.

Eliminating certain foods thought to be associated with migraine, such as chocolate, citrus fruits, red wines, and some beans may be relatively easy, but one should first try to establish some association between the use of these foods and the occurrence of migrainous episodes. After all, abstinence from some foods can lead more often to problems than help and in any event can be difficult to enforce in children. In any event, it generally is acknowledged that special diets or other "allergic" interventions are not helpful. Suggested preventive or prophylactic medications for migraine (propranolol and cyproheptadine hydrochloride [Periactin]) should be used with caution. Propranolol is not to be used once an attack has begun, and its value compared with a placebo is not certain. Periactin's sedative and appetite-stimulant properties make it less desirable.

Tension headache is apt not to respond to acetaminophen, particularly if the underlying circumstances go beyond the usual wear and tear of living and involve a more deep-seated

Table 140-1 Drug Dosage for Relief of Headache

Drug	Dosage	Comments
Acetaminophen	<1 yr: 120 mg q4-6h PO 2-3 yr: 160 mg q4-6h PO 4-5 yr: 240 mg q4-6h PO 6-8 yr: 320 mg q4-6h PO 9-10 yr: 400 mg q4-6h PO 11-12 yr: 480 mg q4-6h PO Adult: 325-650 mg q4-6h PO Alternative: 5-10 mg/kg q4-6h Maximum adult dosage: 4 g/day	
Codeine phosphate	0.5-1 mg/kg PO, IM, or SC stat; repeat q4-6h Maximum dosage: 60 mg/kg/day	May be habit forming
Cyproheptadine	0.25-0.5 mg/kg/24h, divided, q8-12h PO Maximum total dose: 2-6 yr: 12 mg/24h 7-14 yr: 16 mg/24h Adults: 32 mg/24h	Use with caution in asthma because of atropine-like effects; contraindicated in neonates
Diazepam	0.2-0.8 mg/kg/day, divided, q6-8h PO	
Ergot	Older children and adolescents: no more than 3 mg per episode; may be used in tabs or sublingually; suggested approach: 1 mg to start and 1 mg q30 min prn to maximum dose	Prescribe only after consultation; caution with renal or hepatic disease
Phenobarbital	2-4 mg/kg/dose PO, IM, or PR; repeat prn q8h	
Propranolol (When used for migraine prophylaxis)	<35 kg: 10-20 mg PO tid >35 kg: 20-40 mg PO tid	May cause hypotension, nausea and vomiting, and bradycardia; contraindicated in asthma and heart block; caution advised in presence of obstructive pulmonary, renal, or liver disease; may interfere with thyroxine medication in patients who have hypothyroidism

problem, intense anxiety, or depression and especially if these contributors have been present for some time. In fact, the failure to respond to simple medication strongly suggests a tension headache. The temptation to intervene with a tranquilizer should be resisted despite an occasional reason to offer one. However, a frequent need for its use in a particular patient should suggest intense underlying factors that must, if possible, be discovered. Given this, sometimes with the help of a psychologist or psychiatrist, the pediatrician may be more secure in the use of diazepam or, in the instance of a child who is chronically depressed, amitriptyline. Such a serious and persistent problem usually requires psychiatric intervention. Biofeedback and relaxation techniques can help if supervised by an experienced person, but only when the child is old enough and motivated enough to use them consistently.

Occasionally, patients have a headache so severe and persistent that the physician is tempted to prescribe narcotics or an intramuscular sedative. In this event the diagnosis must be certain, because an unrecognized organic cause may exist, requiring a specific intervention. The primary care practitioner should seek consultation at this point. Severity, whether defined by intensity of the episodes, their frequency, or the persistence of an individual episode, often requires consultation. The failure of relatively simple medication to provide relief also suggests consultation before riskier drugs are tried. In any event, the long-term outlook for children who have nonorganic headaches generally is good, although adolescents who have tension headaches often may suffer them into and throughout adulthood.

Sumatriptan succinate, an agonist that causes vasoconstriction, has been approved for use in adults but not thus far in the young. Trials in adolescents have not demonstrated significant benefit. It appears to be useful in adults in an acute migrainous attack only. Sumatriptan succinate has no demonstrated prophylactic value for any type headache and no therapeutic relief in basilar or cluster headaches.

When to Refer

- When concern for an organic cause overpowers all other considerations; in such a circumstance, urgency may be dictated the younger the child and the more specific the headache
- For determination of the most effective and least invasive of the various imaging techniques
- When the severity overcomes good response to conventional treatment, and other efforts, e.g., ergot, may be needed
- For psychological or psychiatric counseling and for advice in the use of drugs in this regard

When to Hospitalize

Infection—meningitis or any other potentially invasive infection close to or inside the head
Any instance of increased intracranial pressure or neurologic aberration, particularly of the cranial nerves
Cranial bruits from an aneurysm or other vascular deformities
Any other organic cause that is not clearly understood and may have a life-threatening potential
Emotional/psychiatric issues may mandate at least a temporary change of place for the patient

SUGGESTED READINGS

Barlow CF: *Headaches and migraine in childhood,* Philadelphia, 1984, JB Lippincott.

Barone MA, editor: *The Harriett Lane Handbook*, ed 14, St Louis, 1996, Mosby.

Basbaum AI, Fields HL: Endogenous pain control mechanisms: review and hypothesis, *Ann Neurol* 4:451, 1979.

Cohen BH: Headaches as a symptom of neurologic disease, *Semin Pediatr Neurol* 2:144, 1995.

Elser JM: Easing the pain of childhood headaches, *Contemp Pediatr* 8:108, 1991.

O'Hara J, Koch TK: Heading off headaches, *Contemp Pediatr* 15:97, 1998.

Sargent J, et al: Oral sumatriptan is effective and well tolerated for the acute treatment of migraine: results of a multicenter study, *Neurology* 45(suppl 7):510, 1995.

Sheveli H: A guide to migraine equivalents, *Contemp Pediatr* 15:71, 1998.

Singer HS, Rowe S: Chronic recurrent headaches in children, *Pediatr Ann* 21:369, 1992.

Welch KMA: Drug therapy of migraine, *N Engl J Med* 329:1476, 1993.

141 Hearing Loss

Anne Marie Tharpe • Holly M. Huta

Throughout the course of their practice lifetime, pediatricians will encounter approximately a dozen children who have severe to profound hearing loss.[14] Pediatricians typically are the first health care practitioners approached by parents when they have concerns about their children's hearing. We know, however, that although parents become concerned about their children's hearing rather early (at approximately 6 months of age) when the hearing loss is severe, milder forms of hearing loss typically do not generate concern until children reach school age. As such, it is imperative that pediatricians learn to recognize the signs, symptoms, and risk factors for hearing loss in children and become aware of appropriate referral paths. Hearing loss secondary to otitis media is the most common type of loss encountered by pediatricians. That topic is discussed in Chapter 20 (Ten), Auditory Screening, and Chapter 245, Otitis Media and Otitis Externa. This chapter primarily addresses the identification of permanent hearing loss in children.

DEMOGRAPHICS

We have seen a dramatic change in the demographics of hearing loss over the past several decades. Although rubella and meningitis were once leading causes of severe to profound hearing loss in children, the advent of vaccines for these disorders has virtually eliminated hearing loss secondary to congenital rubella and has dramatically reduced hearing loss resulting from meningitis. Severe to profound hearing losses are not as common as they once were, and more cases now typically are the result of hereditary factors.

Although estimates of the prevalence of severe bilateral hearing loss in newborns are 1 per 1000, estimates for very mild or minimal losses approach 1 per 20.[3] Estimates of prevalence for hearing loss in the neonatal intensive care unit (NICU) are closer to 20 to 40 per 1000.[13] Two of the more typical patterns of hearing loss encountered today can be seen in Figs. 141-1 through 141-3. Note that the speech sounds represented on these audiograms demonstrate the audibility of normal conversational loudness levels. Fig. 141-1 represents the audiogram of a child who has normal hearing sensitivity in both ears; therefore, all the speech sounds fall within the range of audibility. Fig. 141-2 demonstrates a child who has normal hearing sensitivity for all pitches of sounds, or frequencies, through 1000 Hz, but exhibits a high-frequency hearing loss. This hearing loss is typical of that seen with ototoxic drug use or perinatal anoxia. Although this child would be expected to develop speech in a timely manner, distortions or omissions of the high-frequency consonant sounds of speech are expected. Parents may report that this child has difficulty hearing in the presence of background noise but appears to have little difficulty in quiet settings. The hearing loss depicted in Fig. 141-3 is a profound unilateral loss that typically is not identified until a child enters school. Similar to the child who has high-frequency hearing loss, a child who has unilateral hearing loss may reach age-appropriate speech and language milestones but experience difficulty hearing in the presence of background noise. In addition, children who have unilateral hearing loss often demonstrate difficulty localizing sound sources.

Although these patterns of hearing loss are termed mild or minimal, recent evidence suggests that their impact is far from benign. School-age children who have minimal and mild losses have been found to demonstrate greater academic, communicative, social, and emotional difficulty than normally hearing children. In fact, approximately 35% of children who have minimal hearing losses enrolled in two studies failed at least one grade in school compared with an overall failure rate of 3% in their district.[3,4] Therefore, a growing body of evidence suggests that such losses warrant the concern of pediatricians.

ASSOCIATED SIGNS AND SYMPTOMS

The Joint Committee on Infant Hearing[10] has outlined the high-risk indicators for hearing loss in infants: These are shown in Box 20-4 on p. 265.

Risk factors for infants ages 29 days through 3 years who require periodic rescreening to detect acquired hearing loss, either from other medical conditions or late-onset or progressive hereditary factors, are shown in Box 20-5 on p. 265.

The Joint Committee's list of risk factors provide an excellent starting place when attempting to identify hearing loss in children; however, approximately 35% to 50% of children who have hearing loss will not have any of those risk factors.[6,12] Therefore, a thorough history and keen observation accompanied by hearing screening is essential if hearing loss in children is to be identified. Although most congenital hearing loss is hereditary, one must not be misled by parental report of a negative family history: 80% of inherited hearing loss is the result of autosomal recessive transmission, 18% by autosomal dominant transmission, and about 2% by X-linked recessive transmission. Further, even those who have dominantly inherited hearing loss may have families who demonstrate incomplete penetrance. Evidence of the gene expression can be highly variable. Therefore, a negative family

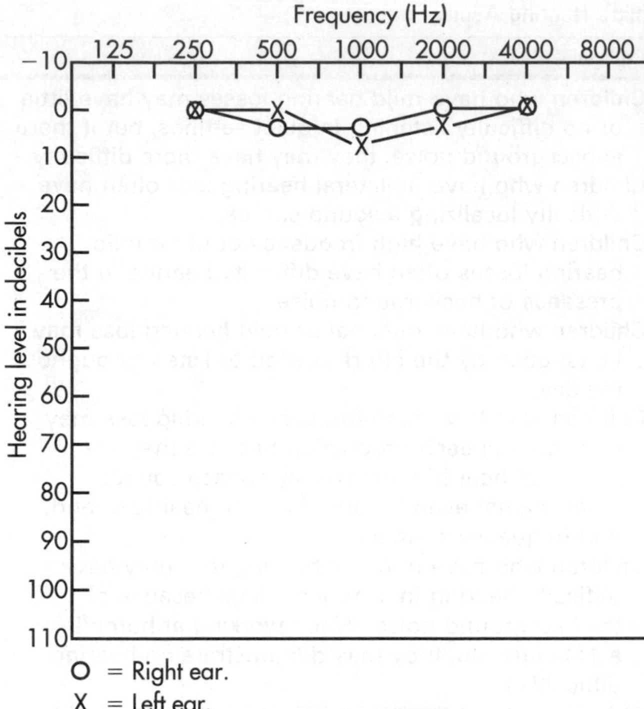

Fig. 141-1 An audiogram reflecting normal hearing sensitivity in both ears.

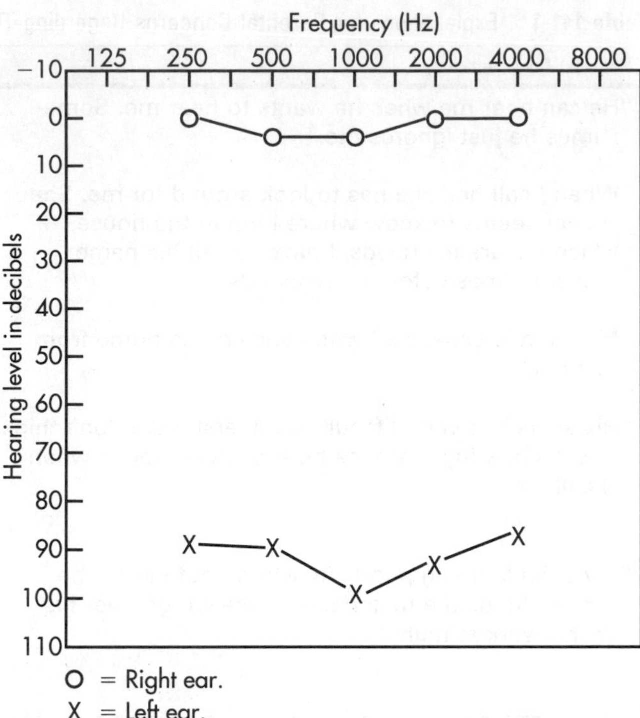

Fig. 141-3 An audiogram reflecting a profound hearing loss of the left ear.

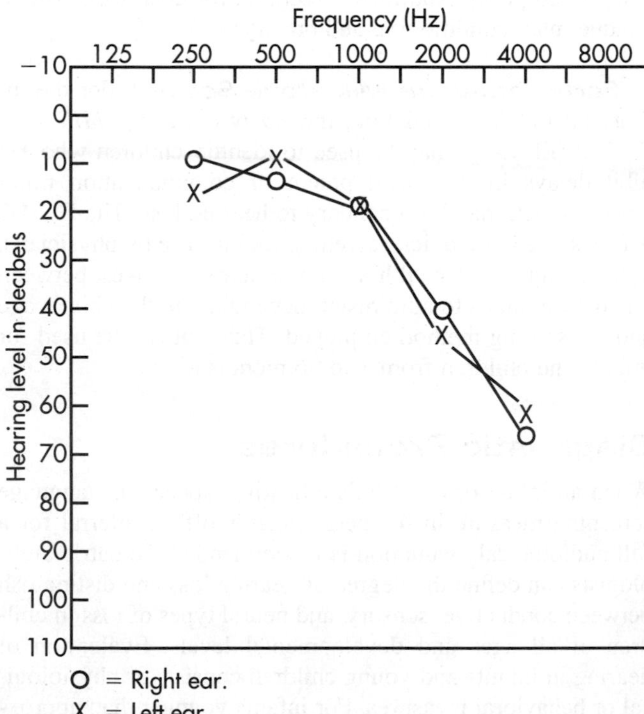

Fig. 141-2 An audiogram reflecting a high-frequency hearing loss bilaterally.

history of hearing loss should not lead one to conclude that a child is unlikely to have hearing loss, especially in today's society in which family members often live at some distance from their nuclear family and detailed knowledge of family members outside of the nuclear family may be limited. In addition, most children who have inherited hearing loss are nonsyndromic, therefore providing no additional clues and potentially limiting the pediatrician's level of suspicion.

The significant speech and language delays associated with severe to profound childhood hearing loss serve to provide a high level of suspicion to parents and physicians. The identification of milder degrees of hearing loss, however, may be more elusive. In addition to children who have speech and language delays or disorders, children who exhibit behavioral, social, or academic difficulties should be screened for hearing loss. Some of the concerns expressed commonly by parents of children who have milder forms of hearing loss are included in Table 141-1.

IDENTIFICATION

Office Tools

In 1994, the Joint Committee on Infant Hearing declared the goal of universal detection of hearing loss in children before 3 months and intervention by 6 months of age. To meet this goal, many hospitals have initiated universal hearing screening of all newborns before discharge. At this writing, 29 states have passed some form of newborn hearing screening legislation; several others are in the process of doing so. In 1999, the American Academy of Pediatrics convened a task force that issued a statement endorsing universal hearing screening of newborns.[1]

As hospitals begin to implement universal screening programs, there are two points to keep in mind. First, it is important to recognize that a large percentage of infants are not brought back to the screening hospital for follow-up, especially early in a screening program's development.[9] These non–follow-up rates have ranged from 32% to 52%.[9,11] It is reasonable to expect that many of these infants will be seen

Table 141-1 Explanations for Parental Concerns Regarding Their Child's Hearing Acuity

Parental Comments	Explanations
"He can hear me when he wants to hear me. Sometimes he just ignores me."	Children who have mild hearing losses may have little or no difficulty listening in quiet settings, but if there is background noise, they may have more difficulty.
"When I call her, she has to look around for me. She never seems to know where I am in the house."	Children who have unilateral hearing loss often have difficulty localizing a sound source.
"When we are in crowds, I have to call his name several times before he responds."	Children who have high-frequency or other mild hearing losses often have difficulty hearing in the presence of background noise.
"My child is exhausted when she comes home from school."	Children who have minimal or mild hearing loss may be fatigued by the effort exerted to listen throughout the day.
"His speech is very difficult to understand. I don't think it's his hearing, because he always responds when I call him."	Children who have high-frequency hearing loss may have poor speech production because they are unable to hear high-frequency speech sounds (consonants) even though they can hear low- and mid-frequency sounds.
"My child is doing poorly in school, but I know he understands the material because we go over his homework at night."	Children who have minimal hearing loss may have difficulty hearing in school settings because of the background noise. When working at home in a 1:1 situation, they may demonstrate no hearing difficulties.

in pediatricians' offices for well- or sick-baby visits. Second, even if an infant is screened for hearing loss at birth, many children ultimately diagnosed with hearing loss acquire their deficits after birth. Pediatricians should have a means of screening the hearing of these infants and young children within the confines of a busy practice. The following section discusses some options for hearing screening in such a setting.

Otoacoustic emissions. Evoked otoacoustic emissions (EOAEs) are low-intensity sounds, sometimes termed *echoes,* produced by healthy ears in response to auditory stimuli introduced into a sealed ear canal. These emissions are measured with the use of a sensitive microphone and provide evidence of cochlear function. Because EOAEs do not require any response by the patient, they provide objective information regarding cochlear integrity and make them ideal for screening infants and young children. EOAEs are believed to be present in all adults and children whose hearing thresholds are 20 dB or better but, if absent, do not provide information regarding the degree of hearing loss. Therefore, absence of EOAEs serves as an indication that further evaluation is needed. Handheld EOAE devices (similar in appearance to otoscopes) provide results in approximately 8 seconds per ear, making them an efficient way to screen hearing in pediatricians' offices.[8] Several manufacturers recently have introduced these devices; however, sensitivity and specificity data are not yet available.

Play audiometry. Children approximately 3 years of age and older can be efficiently and effectively screened in physicians' offices by the use of behavioral measures. Screening is recommended at 1000, 2000, and 4000 Hz in both ears at 20 dB.[2] If a child does not respond at least two of three times at any frequency in either ear, or if the child cannot be conditioned to the task, a referral to a pediatric audiologist is recommended. Handheld devices and more traditional audiometers are available for play audiometry (see Chapter 20 [Ten], Auditory Screening, for details on how to conduct play-conditioning audiometry).

Early Language Milestone Scale-2. For the infant and toddler population, the *Early Language Milestone Scale-2* (ELM-2)[5] may be used to identify children who exhibit delays in the development of communication milestones, which may be secondary to hearing loss. The ELM-2 was designed as a quick screening tool for use by physicians, nurses, and other health care providers; it takes between 1 and 10 minutes to administer, depending on the child's age and the scoring method employed. This tool can be used for infants and children from 1 to 36 months of age.

Diagnostic Procedures

When an infant or child fails a hearing, speech, or language screening measure in the pediatrician's office, referral for a full audiological evaluation is recommended. Pediatric audiologists can define the degree of hearing loss and distinguish between conductive, sensory, and neural types of loss in children of all ages and developmental levels. Evaluation of hearing in infants and young children consists of physiological or behavioral measures. For infants younger than approximately 6 months of age, testing typically is limited to physiological measures, because their behavioral responses are not yet reliable enough for defining the extent of hearing loss. A brief description of the diagnostic procedures of choice follows.

Auditory brainstem response. The auditory brainstem response (ABR) is an electrophysiological test that measures electrical potentials evoked from the brainstem by auditory stimuli. The beauty of this procedure for use with infants and young children is that it requires minimal cooperation from the patient. A sleeping state is ideal for reducing muscle artifact that could interfere with the electrical potentials. Occasionally a mild sedative is required but will not affect the ABR. Click-evoked ABRs can be elicited from infants as young as 27 weeks' gestation, making it a valuable predictor of auditory integrity from the external ear through the brainstem. Although not a true test of hearing, ABR results have been found to be strong predictors of hearing sensitivity. Absence of the ABR, however, may be the result of neural asynchrony rather than peripheral hearing loss in a child. Used in combination with EOAEs and other test procedures, the distinction between neural asynchrony and peripheral hearing loss can be made.

Behavioral assessment. Even with the widespread use of advanced technological evaluation tools, behavioral testing remains a valuable part of hearing assessment in children. Behavioral responses to sound are the only true tests of hearing incorporating all portions of the auditory system. Therefore, whenever possible, behavioral auditory thresholds should be obtained. Several techniques for obtaining behavioral responses can be used, depending on the age or developmental level of the child. Complete behavioral audiograms can be obtained easily for the majority of normally developing infants older than age 6 months if the proper procedures are followed. For children from approximately 6 to 30 months of age, visual reinforcement audiometry (VRA) is the behavioral procedure of choice. Using a conditioning paradigm, children are reinforced for their responses to controlled sound stimuli emitted from loudspeakers or earphones. The test/re-test reliability of the VRA procedure has been well supported in the literature.[7] For children older than approximately 2½ years of age, conditioned play audiometric techniques are used.

MANAGEMENT

The early identification of hearing loss in children is of little value if intervention is not initiated in a timely manner. Many children have conductive and sensorineural hearing losses that are not amenable to medical treatment. For these children, several options remain, the most familiar being the traditional hearing aid. These devices are designed to pick up sounds in the child's environment and convert them to electrical signals that are amplified, filtered, and converted back to acoustic signals by a receiver. For children in noisy settings (such as child care centers or classrooms), frequency-modulated (FM) systems usually are the devices of choice. These systems use a microphone worn by the teacher to amplify only the teacher's voice while minimizing the interfering background noise. The signal is transmitted to the child via an FM signal and is received by Walkman-type earphones, hearing aids, or speakers.

Most children who have hearing loss benefit from some form of amplification. In cases of profound hearing loss, however, conventional amplification may not be enough. An alternative to traditional hearing aids for these children is the cochlear implant, a surgically implanted device with electrodes that are coiled into the cochlea to stimulate the auditory nerve with electrical current. Although cochlear implants do not restore normal hearing and children vary markedly in terms of the benefits received from the implant, the vast majority experience at least an awareness of sound, and some reach a high level of speech recognition.

As the gatekeepers for children's health care, pediatricians are responsible for recognizing the signs and symptoms of hearing loss in their young patients. Only through the vigilance of pediatricians and other health care practitioners will the age of identification of hearing loss in children be lowered, thus avoiding delays in intervention.

REFERENCES

1. American Academy of Pediatrics, Task Force on Newborn Hearing: Newborn and infant hearing loss: detection and intervention, *Pediatrics* 103:527, 1999.
2. American Speech-Language-Hearing Association: *Guidelines for audiologic screening,* Rockville, MD, 1997.
3. Bess FH, Dodd-Murphy J, Parker R: Children with minimal sensorineural hearing loss: prevalence, educational performance and functional status, *Ear Hear* 19:339, 1998.
4. Bess FH, Tharpe AM: Unilateral hearing impairment in children, *Pediatrics* 74:206, 1984.
5. Coplan J: ELM Scale: the Early Language Milestone Scale, Austin, Texas, 1993, Pro-Ed.
6. Davis A, et al: Risk factors for hearing disorders: epidemiologic evidence of change over time in the UK, *J Am Acad Audiol* 6:365, 1995.
7. Diefendorf AO: Behavioral evaluation of hearing impaired children. In Bess FH, editor: *Hearing impairment in children,* Parkton, Md, 1988, York Press.
8. *ERO-SCAN DPOAE test instrument user manual,* rev 990315, Elk Grove Village, Ill, 1999, Etymotic Research.
9. Finitzo T, Albright K, Neal JO: The newborn with hearing loss: detection in the nursery, *Pediatrics* 102:1452, 1998.
10. Joint Committee on Infant Hearing: 1994 position statement, *Pediatrics* 95:152, 1995.
11. Mehl AL, Thomson V: Newborn hearing screening: the great omission, *Pediatrics* 101:4, 1998.
12. Pappas DB, Schaibly M: A two-year diagnostic report on bilateral sensorineural hearing loss in infants and children, *Am J Otol* 5:339, 1984.
13. Stein LK: Factors influencing the efficacy of universal newborn hearing screening, *Pediatr Clin North Am* 46:95, 1999.
14. Tomaski SM, Grundfast KM: A stepwise approach to the diagnosis and treatment of hereditary hearing loss, *Pediatr Clin North Am* 46:35, 1999.

142 Heart Murmurs

Chloe G. Alexson • James A. Manning • Joanne L. Fioravanti

Approximately 90% of infants, children, and adolescents will have heart murmurs at some time. Fewer than 5% of these murmurs will denote cardiac pathology. It is the practitioner's responsibility to distinguish between the common, innocent murmur and the murmurs denoting heart disease. Knowledge of the cardiac physical examination and the recognition of normal and abnormal findings will help in this differentiation.

CARDIOVASCULAR EXAMINATION

Adequate evaluation of the heart includes assessment of color, pulses, perfusion, respiratory effort and pattern, palpation of the chest, and auscultation of heart rate, rhythm, and sounds arising from the heart and great vessels. Many other physical findings are associated with significant heart disease, such as failure to thrive, clubbing of the fingers and toes, respiratory alteration, rales, hepatomegaly, and peripheral edema, usually seen in the periorbital area in infants, rather than in dependent areas. Congestive heart failure has the classic triad of tachycardia, tachypnea, and hepatomegaly, but these may be mimicked by severe respiratory distress, with tachycardia and tachypnea from increased physical effort and an apparent hepatomegaly because the diaphragms are flattened.

It is important for the practitioner to learn to recognize syndromes that may have congenital or acquired heart disease as one of their manifestations. Chromosomal defects such as trisomy 21, trisomy 13, and trisomy 18 have characteristic physical features and typical cardiac malformations. Many other conditions, including Marfan syndrome, Williams syndrome, and the mucopolysaccharidoses are clinically recognizable and should lead to a search for heart disease. Abnormal facial features or combinations of congenital defects also should lead to a search for cardiac disease.

Color

Assessment of color, particularly in a neonate, may be difficult. Cyanosis is not usually apparent until oxygen saturation drops below 85%. It is necessary to look at the nail beds, the palms and soles, the lips, and the conjunctivae to identify mild cyanosis or pallor. Comparison of an infant's color with your own nail beds may help. For black infants, an even more careful search is necessary, and it may be wise to ask a family member if the child looks blue. Sometimes, comparing color to strawberry ice cream for full saturation and raspberry sherbet for mild degrees of unsaturation is helpful. Cyanosis may not be general; therefore, the face and all the extremities should be examined. Extreme pallor also is an abnormal sign that may indicate anemia or poor perfusion and decreased cardiac output.

Pulses and Blood Pressure

The adequacy and symmetry of all the pulses must be evaluated. It is difficult to feel radial pulses in a neonate; therefore, comparing the brachial pulses with the femoral pulses is more reasonable. The brachial pulses are best felt in the antecubital area. The femoral pulse lies in the midline in the inguinal crease. In addition to pulses in the extremities, both temporal pulses should be felt, thus permitting evaluation of all the major branches of the aorta.

In older children, but not always in neonates, it may be possible to determine a lag between the brachial and femoral pulses in the presence of a coarctation; in the newborn or younger child, absent femoral pulses are a more common finding. Abnormally full or bounding pulses may be felt when there is a patent ductus arteriosus, aortic valve insufficiency, and occasionally in truncus arteriosus, all situations with aortic run-off to a lower-pressured area. The pulses also may be unusually full when there is a hyperdynamic state, as with fever, chronic anemia, or volume overload. Weak pulses may indicate ventricular dysfunction and/or heart failure.

In the evaluation of possible organic heart disease, accurate blood pressure measurements in both arms and at least one leg are important. In general, the pediatrician may rely on palpation of the pulses until the child reaches an age at which blood pressure measurement is less time-consuming than in infants. A convenient time to measure all blood pressures may be at age 3 years, when most children will be able to cooperate, or at the preschool examination. An appropriate-size cuff should be used, covering two thirds of the length of the upper arm or thigh. (See the section on measurement of blood pressure in Chapter 146, High Blood Pressure in Infants, Children, and Adolescents.) Leg blood pressure may be measured with the cuff around the thigh and the stethoscope in the popliteal fossa. This may be painful, and the child should be told what to expect. Care should be taken not to inflate the cuff excessively. The leg blood pressure should be at least 10 mm Hg higher than the arm pressure to rule out a coarctation of the aorta. Pulsus paradoxus, in which systolic pressure varies by more than 10 mm Hg between inspiration and expiration, is seen in pericardial effusion with tamponade and also in asthma.

Perfusion

In addition to evaluation of the pulses, it is important to evaluate perfusion. Well-perfused extremities are warm, with rapid capillary refill. Poor peripheral perfusion is accompanied by cool or cold extremities, which often are grayish-white, sometimes mottled, and have delayed capillary refill (>2 seconds).

Respiratory Effort and Pattern

Tachypnea is a common accompaniment of congestive heart failure. As opposed to respiratory disease producing tachypnea, infants who are tachypneic because of hypoxemia may have surprisingly rapid respiratory rates with no evidence of increased respiratory effort. This is because they have normal lungs and no need to use accessory muscles for inspiration or to grunt on expiration. Infants in respiratory distress who have lung disease rarely breathe more rapidly than 90 times per minute. Infants who have severe cyanotic heart disease, such as transposition of the great arteries, may have "peaceful tachypnea," with rates well above 100 breaths/min and no labored respirations.

Palpation

The precordium should be felt carefully. Normally, there is a soft impulse in the midclavicular line, most easily felt with the palm of the hand. A hyperdynamic precordium implies a large volume change within the heart, particularly the right ventricle, which lies directly beneath the chest wall. A vigorous heaving impulse suggests a ventricle generating a high pressure. A palpable thrill—a coarse tremor also felt best with the palm of the hand—reflects significant turbulence beneath the chest wall, helping to localize the abnormality.

Heart Rate and Rhythm

An assessment of rate, rhythm, and regularity of the heart beat is integral to the cardiac examination. This can be done by feeling the pulses but is done more easily by listening to the heart sounds. There are no absolute standards of heart rate for children as there are for adults, because infants' and children's rates vary widely with activity and normally are faster than those of adults. The rhythm should be regular, but many children demonstrate a normal sinus arrhythmia with changes in rate varying with respiration—increasing with inspiration, decreasing with expiration. Although sinus arrhythmia usually has smooth rate changes, some children who have sinus arrhythmia have fairly abrupt rate changes. Individual abnormal beats (heard as extra, premature beats or as skipped beats) in a healthy child usually are benign. This is true particularly if they can be suppressed by exercise, such as jumping in place. They may occur more frequently as the heart rate slows when exercise is discontinued.

Heart Sounds

Heart sounds should be clear and crisp; they are louder and more distinct in children than in adults. The heart sounds correspond to the hemodynamic events occurring during the cardiac cycle. The first sound, S_1, results from closure of the tricuspid and mitral valves. It usually is heard as a single sound but may be narrowly split, particularly in adolescence. The second heart sound (S_2) is produced by aortic and pulmonic valve closure. The first component of the second sound is produced by aortic valve closure and the second component by pulmonic valve closure. It should be possible to hear both components of the second sound at the upper left sternal border. The intensity of these sounds reflects the closing systolic pressure in the great vessels. The pulmonic component should be softer than the aortic component. If the second sound is as loud or louder than the first sound, pulmonary hypertension should be suspected.

In the normal child, the closure sounds at the base of the heart will vary in timing, with S_2 widely split during inspiration but coming together completely in deep expiration. Persistent splitting of the second sounds during all phases of respiration suggests right ventricular volume overload, which occurs in patients who have atrial septal defects, or with a delay in right ventricular depolarization, which occurs when a right bundle branch block is present.

Third and fourth heart sounds, "gallop sounds," may reflect ventricular failure, but an audible S_3 is relatively common in normal children.

Opening snaps, frequently heard in adults who have mitral valve stenosis, are not often heard in children. Early systolic clicks, known as *ejection clicks,* are common with pulmonic valve stenosis and somewhat less so with congenital aortic valve stenosis. Single or multiple mid- and late systolic clicks may be heard with mitral valve prolapse.

A pericardial friction rub (a multiphase, coarse, scratchy sound) may sometimes be heard with pericarditis. Usually, it is well localized to a small area of the precordium but may be widespread over the chest wall. The heart sounds may be distant and difficult to hear when a significant pericardial effusion is present.

Abnormal sounds also may arise entirely within the blood vessels and are heard in areas overlying an arteriovenous fistula. Listening over the head, the lung fields, the liver, and major muscles may reveal a hollow, continuous sound (a bruit), indicating a communication between artery and vein. A bruit also may be heard in the back left posterior thorax medial to the scapula over the site of a coarctation of the aorta.

Heart Murmurs

Heart murmurs are sounds in addition to the valve closure sounds and may reflect either normal flow or abnormal, turbulent flow in the heart or great vessels. They must be characterized by their location, timing, intensity, and quality.

Localizing heart murmurs exactly will help in identifying their cause, because turbulence is transmitted directly to the chest wall and, thus, represents blood flow through that part of the heart that lies beneath the thoracic surface. In some instances, the murmur arises from the great vessels and may reflect the location and direction of blood flow in those vessels. The pulmonic area lies high along the left sternal border above the pulmonary valve, whereas the midsternal border more accurately reflects sounds of the outflow tract of the right ventricle. The lower left sternal border overlies the ventricular septum and the tricuspid and mitral valves. Mitral valve murmurs may be heard most clearly at the apex, but when the anterior leaflet of the mitral valve is involved, those murmurs may be heard much closer to the left sternal border. Murmurs arising from the aortic valve should be heard well over the midsternum, with transmission to the upper right sternal border—the aortic area. It is important to remember that murmurs go where the blood goes, so murmurs of aortic and pulmonic insufficiency will be transmitted back to the areas of the ventricular chambers.

The timing of murmurs is important. They may be systolic, diastolic, systolic and diastolic, or continuous throughout systole and diastole without interruption by the S_1 and S_2 heart sounds. Systolic murmurs that begin with the first sound and end with the second sound are called *holosystolic, pansystolic,* or *regurgitant murmurs.* They imply an abnormal way out of the ventricle immediately after ventricular pressure rises with the onset of systole. Examples are ventricular septal defects or atrioventricular valve regurgitation. In contrast, systolic murmurs that begin after the first sound are crescendo-decrescendo in nature and end before the second sound are caused by ventricular outflow obstruction, when the ventricle has to build up sufficient pressure to overcome the obstruction. These ejection murmurs may be quite short, with an early peak of the crescendo-decrescendo quality, when there is little obstruction. As the degree of obstruction increases, so does the time necessary for the ventricle to overcome it, and the peak sound will be heard later.

The intensity of murmurs is reasonably well correlated with their significance. Standard grading of murmurs is from I to VI: Grade I is heard with difficulty; grade II is heard immediately; grade III is louder than grade II but does not have a thrill; grade IV is loud enough to have a palpable thrill; grade V has a thrill and can be heard with the stethoscope only partly on the chest; grade VI, the loudest of the heart murmurs, can be heard with the stethoscope held slightly off the chest.

FUNCTIONAL HEART MURMURS

Nearly all children will at some time have an innocent, or functional, murmur, which is not caused by any abnormal cardiac structures, representing, instead, normal flow patterns. The murmur will have recognizable characteristics, and cardiac evaluation will be normal.

Neonates and Young Infants

In the neonate, the most common of these innocent murmurs is a soft, short, transient grade I to II ejection murmur in the pulmonic area, representing the ductus arteriosis as it begins to close. It may be heard very briefly in the first few days of life. At 2 to 3 weeks of age there may be a soft grade I to II systolic murmur heard slightly at the upper left sternal border but more clearly over the lung fields and in the axillae. This is a peripheral pulmonary flow murmur caused by turbulence at the bifurcation of the branch pulmonary arteries; it usually disappears by 6 or 8 months of age. There are, however, syndromes in which anatomical branch pulmonary artery stenosis occurs, such as Williams syndrome or congenital rubella syndrome, that must be considered in the differential diagnosis.

Toddlers and Early School-Age Children

At age 2 or 3 years, many children will have other functional murmurs. One of the more common is the venous hum, a hollow, continuous sound heard under the right clavicle and, less commonly, under the left clavicle. This represents venous flow back to the heart and is loudest where the main venous channels come together. The venous hum is louder in diastole and can be eliminated completely by alterations in venous flow. Maneuvers such as having the child turn his or her head sharply to the right, left, or upward will eradicate the venous hum. Having the child lie supine or compressing the jugular vein also will eradicate the hum. This sound should not be considered functional if it cannot be completely eradicated.

Another common functional murmur of the middle-age child is the Still's, or vibratory, murmur. This is located at the mid- and/or lower left sternal border, is early and midsystolic in timing, and is grade I or II in intensity. It usually is decrescendo and frequently has musical overtones or a vibratory, grunting, or groaning quality. An ejection quality to a vibratory murmur should raise the question of subaortic obstruction. Carotid bruits, heard over the base of the neck, are early and midsystolic murmurs that have many of the characteristics of vibratory murmurs. They are common in children and adolescents and, unless the neck is auscultated carefully, may be confused with aortic or pulmonic valve stenosis. The sound of a carotid bruit sometimes may be heard over the midprecordium and is similar to the Still's murmur. It may be eradicated by carotid artery compression.

Adolescence

As adolescence begins, many teenagers will have the appearance of a pulmonary flow functional murmur. This is a systolic murmur, best heard at the upper left sternal border, and although it has the timing of an ejection murmur, it is no louder than grade II and does not have the harshness of a murmur caused by valvular obstruction. The pulmonary closure sound should be of normal intensity and have a normal, physiological split. This murmur may persist into adulthood and also may be heard in situations of a volume overload, such as pregnancy or chronic anemia. Carotid bruits are common in adolescents as well.

Functional murmurs are quite variable on a day-to-day basis, are occasionally absent, and are affected by increased cardiac output as with exercise or fever. They vary widely with position and with phases of respiration. No structural cause for these murmurs is found on routine evaluation.

Murmurs caused by organic or structural disease have characteristic sounds and may be associated with abnormal radiographic and echocardiographic findings, depending on the physiological effects of the cardiac disease.

ORGANIC HEART MURMURS

Ventricular septal defects (VSD) produce systolic murmurs at the lower left sternal border. Only very small VSDs are heard at birth. Larger defects are heard first as pulmonary vascular resistance decreases at 7 to 10 days of age. Occasionally a VSD is not heard until systemic vascular resistance rises considerably. The murmur is pansystolic and may be as soft as grade I in intensity but also may be increasingly loud, frequently grade IV with a palpable thrill. Small VSDs that have relatively small left-to-right shunts and normal pulmonary artery pressure will generate a pulmonary closure sound of normal intensity. However, as the pulmonary artery pressure rises, the pulmonary closure sound will be louder. Most small VSDs have murmurs of grade I to III intensity; high-flow VSDs that have a large left-to-right shunt will have a grade IV murmur. Some VSDs that have maximal pulmonary vascular resistance will have no murmur but will have a very loud pulmonary component of the second heart sound. In infants and small children who have small VSDs, the murmur may be eradicated completely by a spontaneous or induced Valsalva maneuver. Steady, firm compression of the child's abdomen with the examiner's hand will force the child to hold his or her breath and push back against the examiner's hand, suppressing the murmur as intrathoracic pressure raises right-heart pressure to equal left-heart pressure. This same maneuver will accentuate the murmur of tricuspid valve regurgitation. In children who have a high-flow VSD and a pulmonary-to-systemic flow ratio of 2 to 1 or greater, there may be a low-pitched mid-diastolic murmur of relative mitral stenosis heard at the apex. This reflects a large amount of blood flow across a normal mitral valve.

Tricuspid valve regurgitation is heard at the lower left sternal border and may sound very much like the murmur of a VSD. The murmur often is higher pitched and will be accentuated, rather than diminished, by a Valsalva maneuver. Tricuspid regurgitation is commonly heard in the neonate, particularly in situations of stress, such as aspiration, low Apgar scores, and acute illness. It is one of the sounds heard with Ebstein malformation of the tricuspid valve and may be part of the atrioventricular canal defect complex. It may, however, be of no clinical significance. Anatomical tricuspid stenosis produces a low-pitched diastolic murmur at the lower left sternal border.

Mitral valve regurgitation may be heard close to or at the apex, at the point of maximal apical impulse. It is a pansystolic, somewhat high, unvarying-pitched systolic murmur. The exception is mitral valve prolapse, in which the murmur is more likely to be heard in mid- to late systole, with late systolic accentuation and with single or multiple clicks. Either the posterior or the anterior mitral valve leaflet may be involved in mitral valve regurgitation, and it usually is possible to distinguish between the two on examination. Posterior leaflet mitral valve regurgitation is the classic murmur of rheumatic heart disease and may be transmitted to the axilla. In an atrioventricular canal defect, however, it is the anterior leaflet of the mitral valve that is involved, and the murmur may be closer to, or at, the lower left sternal border. Murmurs of mitral valve regurgitation are accentuated by maneuvers that increase systemic vascular resistance, such as hand gripping or squatting. Anatomical mitral valve stenosis, often heard later after acute rheumatic carditis, produces a low-pitched mid- and late diastolic murmur just within the area of the apex. It may well have presystolic accentuation.

The murmur of an atrial level shunt is not the sound of flow through the defect but rather the sound of increased blood flow through a normal pulmonary valve. It rarely is heard before 1 year of age because time is needed for pulmonary vascular resistance to drop after birth and for right ventricular compliance to increase, resulting in a greater shunt. In an atrial septal defect, chest development may be somewhat asymmetrical, with the left side more prominent because the heart has enlarged gradually over time. A hyperdynamic precordium reflects an increased volume change within the right ventricle. The heart sounds are of normal intensity, but the second sounds at the base of the heart are persistently split through all phases of respiration. There is a flow murmur in the pulmonic area, a soft grade I to II (occasionally III) murmur with the timing of an ejection murmur but without its harshness. In the presence of a large left-to-right atrial shunt with a pulmonary-to-systemic flow ratio of 2 to 1 or greater, a low-pitched, mid-diastolic murmur of relative tricuspid stenosis may be heard at the lower left sternal border.

Murmurs heard with aortic-pulmonary artery communications, such as a patent ductus arteriosus, have characteristics dependent on the systemic and pulmonary vascular resistance. The typical murmur of a patent ductus is a hollow, continuous sound, uninterrupted by the heart sounds, heard best at or just to the left of the upper left sternal border. It is louder in systole and, unlike the venous hum, cannot be eradicated by position change or compression of the jugular vein. As pulmonary artery pressure increases in the presence of a large, hypertensive ductus, the murmur will lose its continuous characteristics, become shorter and systolic only, or will disappear completely, and the pulmonary component of the closure sound will be louder. The murmur of an aortic-pulmonary window may be the same but located closer to the sternal border and a bit lower down. It also may be confined to systole. Murmurs heard with truncus arteriosus are quite variable, usually reflecting truncal valve stenosis and insufficiency or narrowing of the pulmonary arteries as they leave the truncus, thus having an ejection quality transmitted to the lung fields. Continuous murmurs also may be heard over arteriovenous fistulas; carefully listening over the head, liver, and major muscles may lead to this diagnosis.

The ejection murmur of pulmonic valve stenosis is heard at the upper left sternal border. It is a crescendo-decrescendo murmur, increasing in intensity as the degree of obstruction increases. As obstruction increases, the peak of the murmur occurs later in systole and the pulmonic component of the closure sounds is delayed and diminished, eventually becoming inaudible. In the presence of a relatively mobile valve, there is a prominent ejection click—a short, snapping sound heard immediately after the first sound. Thick, dysplastic pulmonary valves are less likely to produce a click. If the murmur reflects significant turbulence across the valve, there will be a palpable thrill in the same area. Pulmonary valve insufficiency or regurgitation causes a low-pitched, somewhat rumbling sound, beginning just after the second heart sound. The murmurs of pulmonary stenosis and insufficiency are to and fro rather than continuous. The ejection murmur of tetralogy of Fallot is mid-peaking and heard just below the pulmonic area because it arises from the right ventricular outflow tract rather than exclusively from the pulmonic valve. Following repair for tetralogy of Fallot, a soft, short grade I to II ejection murmur and an early diastolic murmur commonly are heard.

The murmur of aortic valve stenosis is heard over the midsternum and is transmitted to the upper right sternal border. Its intensity increases with the degree of obstruction and may be accentuated by exercise. The aortic closure sound may be accentuated, and there may be a prominent ejection click. Aortic regurgitation or insufficiency is a high-pitched, tambour, metallic sound and is heard best over the midsternum to the apex, where the cavity of the left ventricle is located. Murmurs of aortic stenosis and insufficiency are to-and-fro, not continuous. Subaortic stenosis produces an ejection murmur heard best at the lower left sternal border or over the lower sternum.

There are many complex cardiac defects that have combinations of two or more of the basic abnormalities noted herein. Their physical findings will be related to the intracardiac abnormality, the relative systemic and pulmonary vascular resistances, the presence of left-to-right or right-to-left shunting, and the adequacy of cardiac function. An understanding of the complex defects is necessary to evaluate the findings.

SUGGESTED READINGS

Allen HD, et al: *Moss and Adams' heart disease in infants, children and adolescents,* ed 6, Philadelphia, 2000, Lippincott Williams and Wilkins.

McCrindle BW, et al: Cardinal clinical signs in the differentiation of heart murmurs in children, *Arch Pediatr Adolesc Med* 150:169, 1996.

Park MK: *Pediatric cardiology for practitioners,* ed 3, St Louis, 1996, Mosby.

143 Hematuria

Edward J. Ruley

The diagnostic approach to hematuria in pediatric patients is quite different from the strategy employed for adults. Having an organized plan of investigation is important if one is to determine the diagnosis most cost effectively while subjecting the child to the fewest invasive and uncomfortable procedures.

It is helpful to consider the occurrence of hematuria in several clinical presentations: (1) macroscopic or gross hematuria; (2) spots of blood found on the underclothing or diapers, with an otherwise clear urine; and (3) microhematuria found by chemical or direct microscopy in an otherwise grossly normal-appearing urine. The presence of symptoms, either localized to the urinary tract or more generalized, is variable in each of these circumstances. The most likely causes of the hematuria in these clinical scenarios are different; therefore, the clinical approach to the diagnosis of each also differs.

GROSS HEMATURIA

Incidence

Gross hematuria is a relatively uncommon urinary symptom, the occurrence of which varies according to the population being studied. In a report of more than 128,000 consecutive patients visiting an emergency clinic in a large city in the northeastern United States, the incidence of "red urine" as the chief complaint was 1.4 per 1000 visits. When other causes of a red urine were eliminated, the incidence of true gross hematuria was 1.3 per 1000 visits.[3]

Etiology

Urinary tract infection (either bacterial or viral) is the most common cause of gross hematuria in children, accounting for approximately half the cases. Irritation or ulceration of the perineum or urethral meatus is the next most common cause, constituting about 20% of the cases. Trauma is the third most common etiology. When relatively minor trauma results in gross hematuria, the clinician should be alerted to the possibility of an undiagnosed dilated urinary system. Such dilated structures may be fluid-filled cysts associated with various types of congenital cystic kidney diseases or a urine-filled renal pelvis and ureter caused by obstructive uropathy. These dilated systems are much more susceptible to gross bleeding after minor direct or indirect trauma than is the normal urinary system. Urinary stones, as well as hypercalciuria without lithiasis, have been recognized as important causes of gross hematuria in children. In one study, significant hypercalciuria was found in 64% of the children who had gross hematuria.[2] Although coagulopathy has always been included among causes of gross hematuria, it is very uncommon. In contrast, gross hematuria is not uncommon in patients who have sickle cell trait or sickle cell disease. Glomerulonephritis usually accounts for fewer than 10% of patients who have gross hematuria, although the incidence varies considerably. Even with a complete and thoughtful approach, a specific cause will not be obvious in 10% to 20% of children.

History

It is important to ascertain a description of the color, clarity, and pattern of the gross hematuria. Pink or red urine most often indicates bladder or urethral bleeding; greenish or brown urine is seen most commonly in upper tract or renal parenchymal bleeding. An opaque or cloudy specimen usually results from the presence of blood cells in the urine, whether they originate from the upper or lower urinary tract. In contrast, a urine that is discolored but clear in character usually indicates the presence of pigmenturia (hemoglobinuria or myoglobinuria). Gross hematuria that occurs sequentially in each voiding, even though it may differ in the degree of discoloration, usually is consistent with infection or the presence of upper tract (parenchymal) disease. Gross hematuria that occurs interspersed with normal-appearing urine is most consistent with hypercalciuria and lithiasis.

The presence of symptoms, either generalized or localized to the urinary tract, is important in determining the most likely cause. Generalized symptoms such as fever, abdominal pain, arthralgia, arthritis, edema, and rash imply that the gross hematuria is part of a more extensive illness. In contrast, urinary frequency, urgency, and dysuria would lead one to consider the lower urinary system and the bladder outlet as the site of the pathology. The past medical history, in particular previous diagnoses, prior episodes of gross hematuria, recent or concurrent illness, as well as the events surrounding the onset of gross hematuria, are important. Certain diagnoses such as sickle cell disease, hypercalciuria, or IgA nephropathy are characterized by recurrent episodes of gross hematuria. The occurrence of antecedent or concurrent upper respiratory tract infections may favor a particular type of glomerulonephritis as the etiology (see Chapter 237, Nephritis). A history of vigorous exercise, such as riding a mountain bike or jogging, may be associated with transient gross or microscopic hematuria. Prior voiding habits such as the frequency and style of voiding can be important clues to the

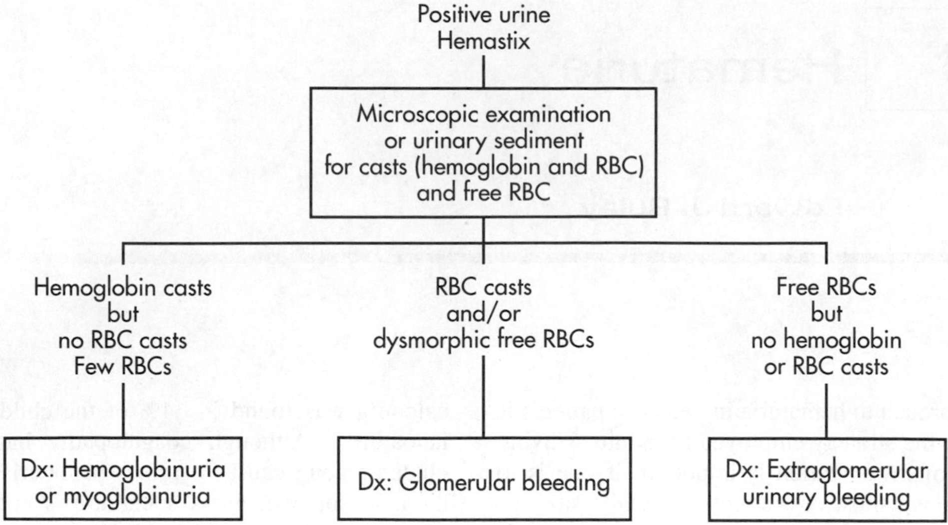

Fig. 143-1 A clinical algorithm for hematuria in children.

etiology. It has been noted that young boys may squeeze or compress their penis in an attempt to thwart an urge to micturate when it is experienced at a time when they do not want to interrupt their play or activities. Other boys may have the habit of bending their penis over the elastic in their underpants when voiding, causing a sharp bend in the urethra. Both of these practices may lead to urethral irritation and produce gross or microscopic bleeding. In girls, it is important to consider menarche as being misinterpreted as an episode of gross hematuria. Finally, a history of other family members who have gross hematuria, urinary stones, hearing loss, sickle cell disease, or coagulopathies can be pertinent.

Physical Findings

A comprehensive general physical examination is appropriate for children who have gross hematuria. Specifically, blood pressure measurement, abdominal examination, and direct visualization of the penile meatus or the female introitus, including the urethral meatus, is important.

BOX 143-1

CAUSES OF HEMOGLOBINURIA AND MYOGLOBINURIA

Hemoglobinuria

Hemolytic anemia (e.g., glucose-6-phosphate dehydrogenase [G6PD] deficiency, Coombs'-positive hemolytic anemia)
Mismatched blood transfusions
Intravascular coagulation (e.g., disseminated intravascular coagulation [DIC], hemolytic-uremic syndrome)
Infections (e.g., sepsis, malaria)
Freshwater near-drowning
Mechanical erythrocyte damage (e.g., artificial heart valves, cardiopulmonary bypass)

Myoglobinuria

Muscle injury (e.g., crush injuries, electrical burns)
Myositis
Rhabdomyolysis

Laboratory Findings

Obviously, the most important laboratory test is the urinalysis. The centrifuged sediment of a freshly voided urine specimen should be examined very carefully under the microscope, giving attention to the presence and morphology of any erythrocytes, as well as to the presence of any cellular casts (Fig. 143-1). Should there be only relatively homogeneous pigmented casts without significant numbers of erythrocytes, one should suspect hemoglobinuria or myoglobinuria as the cause of the discolored urine. The dip-and-read strips for blood react to both hemoglobin and myoglobin. Some causes of hemoglobinuria and myoglobinuria are given in Box 143-1. These situations are relatively uncommon in pediatric patients.

When erythrocytes are present, scrutiny of their appearance helps to determine their origin.[1] Red blood cells that originate from the urinary structures outside the nephrons look like normal peripheral-circulating erythrocytes on a blood smear. They will be eumorphic—that is, of uniform size and shape. Also, no casts will be seen. In contrast, erythrocytes originating from the kidney parenchyma are dysmorphic—that is, they vary in size and have irregular outlines, with blebs of cytoplasm appearing to bud from the cell surface (Fig. 143-2). The dysmorphic appearance of the erythrocytes may be the result of their damage during extrusion through the glomerular basement membrane, the effect of osmotic forces during the cell's passage down the tubule, or some other as yet undefined factor. In addition to dysmorphic erythrocytes, a variety of casts containing erythrocytes, leukocytes, or tubular cells, as well as casts that appear coarsely and finely granular or hyaline, may be present. Although up to 10% of erythrocytes may be dysmorphic in nonglomerular bleeding, nearly all the erythrocytes will be dysmorphic in glomerular bleeding.[5] Regardless, erythrocyte casts originate only from diseases in the kidney parenchyma,

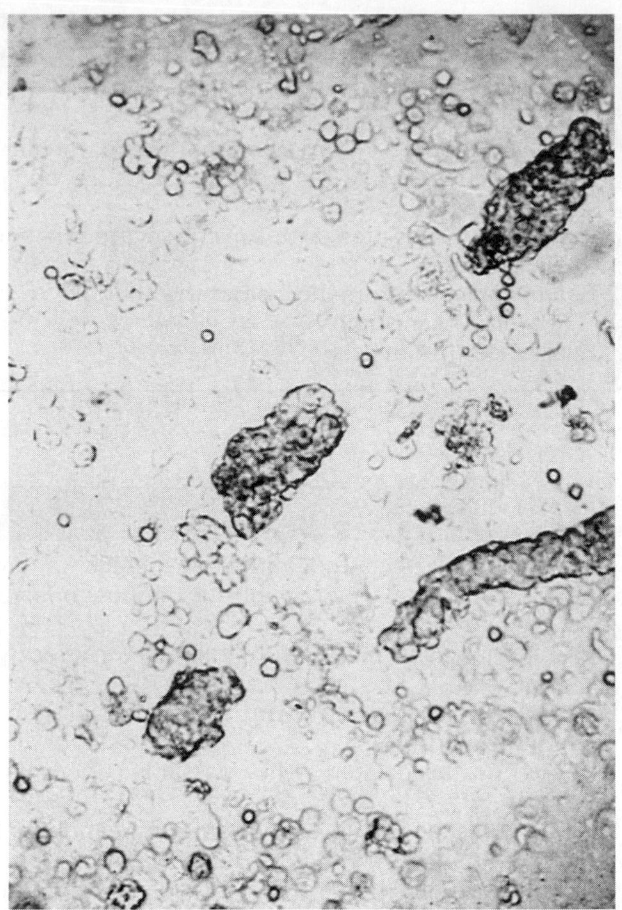

Fig. 143-2 Unstained urine sediment showing a red blood cell cast and dysmorphic red blood cells (×100).

making their presence an important clue to a glomerular origin for the hematuria. However, there are certain situations in which kidney insult can cause some overlap. One of the most obvious is trauma, in which bleeding can come from the kidney parenchyma and the urinary system at the same time. In this circumstance, both dysmorphic and eumorphic erythrocytes, as well as erythrocyte casts, may be present in the same specimen.

Proteinuria also can be found in urine specimens in which there is gross hematuria. However, the dip-and-read test for protein is inaccurate in the presence of gross hematuria because of the effect on interpretation of color change. Therefore, another method of protein quantitation, such as sulfosalicylic acid precipitation, must be used to assess proteinuria when gross hematuria is present. In urine specimens that are isotonic or hypertonic, gross hematuria can result in modest amounts of protein being detectable. In urine specimens that are hypotonic, the degree of proteinuria can be marked. Studies have shown that the protein in this latter circumstance originates from the hemoglobin released from the lysed erythrocytes. Microhematuria does not result in any significant proteinuria;[7] therefore, proteinuria in the presence of microhematuria needs to be investigated as an additional harbinger of significant renal disease.

Because urinary tract infection is so common, a urine culture is indicated in all instances of gross hematuria. The presence of pyuria or bacteruria and a positive urinary leukocyte esterase test support an infectious origin. To investigate hypercalciuria, a 24-hour specimen should be obtained for measuring urinary creatinine and calcium. The calculation of creatinine excretion (mg/kg/day) can be used to determine the adequacy of collection. Children of normal habitus excrete about 18 mg of creatinine per kilogram each day, although there is individual variation that is determined partly by age and gender.[4] Once the adequacy of collection is known, the calcium excretion (mg/kg/day) can be evaluated. A normal child should excrete fewer than 4 mg of calcium per kilogram of body weight each day.[2,6] Ultrasound of the kidneys and the urinary system also is indicated to investigate kidney size and the character of the kidney parenchyma and to screen for dilated collecting systems. Gross hematuria is one instance in which cystoscopy may be indicated to look for sites of bleeding within the bladder or to determine from which kidney the blood is originating. Obviously, such direct visualization is indicated for selected cases only and must be done when the patient is bleeding to be of value. Further investigation and the institution of treatment depend on the working diagnosis as suggested by recent, past, and family histories and the results of the preliminary tests. In contrast to adults, tumors of the urinary system are very uncommon causes of gross hematuria in children.

Blood on Underclothing

The discovery of dried spots of blood on diapers or underclothing can be very distressing for parents. The urine usually is normal in appearance and actually may dilute the appearance of the blood spots. This is seen most often in male infants who otherwise are well. The most common cause of this finding is irritation of the urethra, particularly at the meatus. These infants usually pass a normal urine, but at the end of urination a drop or two of blood seeps out of the meatus, creating a discolored spot in a wet diaper. This can be diagnosed by direct observation of the penile urethral meatus. If urethral meatal erosion is evident and the rest of the physical examination is normal, more invasive tests are not indicated. Applying petroleum jelly to the meatus and leaving the infant undiapered for a short period is all that is needed to resolve the problem.

MICROHEMATURIA

Incidence

Microhematuria occurs much more frequently than gross hematuria in the pediatric population, with a prevalence of 0.05% to 2.0%, depending on the definition of significant hematuria (see Chapter 20 [Eight], Use of Urinalysis and the Urine Culture in Screening). Although the definition of significant microhematuria differs among studies, many investigators consider more than 10 erythrocytes per high-power field in the sediment of a centrifuged aliquot of freshly voided urine to be significant.

Etiology

Many of the causes of gross hematuria also may cause isolated microhematuria (i.e., microhematuria in the absence of proteinuria). Microscopic hematuria in the asymptomatic

BOX 143-2

CAUSES OF EXTRAGLOMERULAR HEMATURIA

Infection (e.g., cystitis, urethritis, balinitis)
Hypercalciuria (e.g., absorptive hypercalcinuria, renal tubular hypercalciuria)
Trauma (e.g., vehicular accidents, falls, child abuse)
Urinary lithiasis (e.g., hypercalcinuria, cysteinuria)
Malformations (e.g., cystic kidney diseases, posterior urethral valves, ureteropelvic junction obstruction)
Hemoglobinopathy (e.g., sickle cell disease, thalassemia)
Drugs (e.g., antibiotics, cytoxan)
Bleeding diathesis (e.g., von Willebrand's disease, hemophilia)
Instrumentation (e.g., suprapubic aspiration, urinary catheterization, cystoscopy, self-stimulation)
Tumors (e.g., Wilms' tumor, rhabdomyosarcoma, bladder papilloma)

child usually is discovered during a routine well-child examination. This frequent clinical problem requires a thoughtful, systematic approach. The same algorithm given for macroscopic hematuria (see Fig. 143-1) can be applied to the child who has microhematuria.

History and Physical Findings

The same questions should be asked and a similar physical examination performed in the child who has microhematuria as that outlined for the child who has gross hematuria. Not uncommonly, the history is noncontributory, and the physical examination is unrevealing.

Laboratory Findings

As with gross hematuria, the carefully done urinalysis becomes the crucial first test for the child who has microhematuria. Pigmenturia should be considered, although significant hemoglobin or myoglobin filtration more often causes macroscopic urine discoloration rather than microhematuria. When true hematuria exists, the morphology of the erythrocytes and the presence of casts assume the same significance as in gross hematuria. Differentiation of the causes of glomerular bleeding often requires hospitalization and more extensive testing (see Chapter 237, Nephritis). Should the urine contain mainly eumorphic erythrocytes and be free of casts, extraglomerular bleeding is most likely. Some causes are listed in Box 143-2. Twenty-four-hour urine specimens should be collected for calcium excretion determination. Specific treatment regimens depend on the cause of the microhematuria.

When to Refer

Hematuria associated with recurrent urinary tract infections and pyelonephritis
Suspected acute glomerulonephritis, particularly if associated with high blood pressure and/or azotemia
Hematuria associated with thrombocytopenia and/or azotemia
Recurrent asymptomatic hematuria thought to be of glomerular origin
Suspected urolithiasis

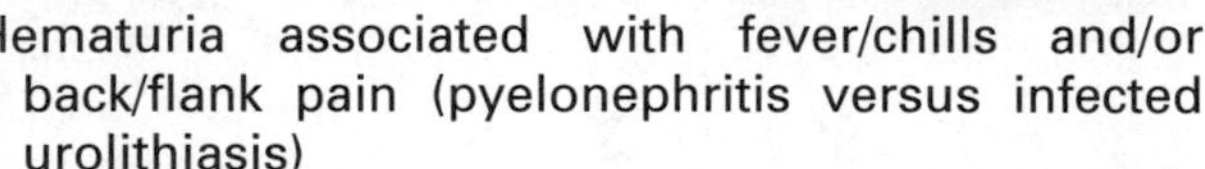

When to Hospitalize

Hematuria associated with fever/chills and/or back/flank pain (pyelonephritis versus infected urolithiasis)
Hematuria associated with rapidly progressive azotemia
Hematuria associated with hemoptysis (lung-kidney syndrome)
Hematuria associated with palpable abdominal mass
Stone passage symptoms (hematuria and flank/abdominal pain) with intractable vomiting
Stone passage symptoms with documented urinary obstruction

REFERENCES

1. Birch DF, et al: Urinary erythrocyte morphology in the diagnosis of glomerular hematuria, *Clin Nephrol* 20:78, 1983.
2. Garcia CD, Miller MLT, Stapleton FB: Natural history of hematuria associated with hypercalciuria in children, *Am J Dis Child* 145:1204, 1991.
3. Ingelfinger JR, Davis AE, Grupe WE: Frequency and etiology of gross hematuria in a general pediatric setting, *Pediatrics* 59:557, 1977.
4. Meites S: *Pediatric clinical chemistry,* ed 3, Washington, DC, 1989, AACC press.
5. Stapleton FB: Morphology of urinary red blood cells: a simple guide in localizing the site of hematuria, *Pediatr Clin North Am* 34:561, 1987.
6. Stapleton FB, et al: Hypercalciuria in children with hematuria, *N Engl J Med* 310:1345, 1984.
7. Tapp DC, Copley JB: Effect of red blood cell lysis on protein quantitation in hematuric states, *Am J Nephrol* 8:190, 1988.

SUGGESTED READINGS

Feld LG, et al: Hematuria: an integrated medical and surgical approach, *Pediatr Clin North Am* 44:1191, 1997.

Lieu TA, Grasmeder HM, Kaplan BS: An approach to the evaluation and treatment of microscopic hematuria, *Pediatr Clin North Am* 38:579, 1991.

Mahan JD, Turman MA, Mentser MI: Evaluation of hematuria, proteinuria and hypertension in adolescents, *Pediatr Clin North Am* 44:1573, 1997.

144 Hemoptysis

Scott A. Schroeder

Hemoptysis, the spitting or coughing of blood that originates within the thorax, can vary from flecks of blood in the sputum to massive, potentially life-threatening bleeding that can lead to severe respiratory distress or death. Unlike adults, for whom more than 100 different causes of hemoptysis are described, hemoptysis is a rare occurrence in children. At our large, inner-city general hospital, over a 3-year period, 23 children, none of whom had cystic fibrosis, were hospitalized for the evaluation of hemoptysis. The causes for their hemoptysis are listed in Table 144-1. Six of these patients developed respiratory distress and required mechanical ventilation. During the evaluation, seven of the children were found to have a nonpulmonary source for their bleeding. Three of the children had diffuse alveolar hemorrhage rather than bleeding from a localized site.

Our experience illustrates four important considerations in the evaluation of children who have hemoptysis. First, it is essential to determine if the bleeding requires an emergency resuscitative effort. Second, what appears to be hemoptysis may actually be bleeding from the upper airway or gastrointestinal tract. Third, those children who have no chronic diseases who develop hemoptysis with associated symptoms of a lower respiratory tract infection usually have mild, self-limited bleeding that requires no specific treatment other than management of the pneumonia. Fourth, the management of hemoptysis that arises from a localized site differs from that which is due to diffuse alveolar hemorrhage, because the latter may be the presenting sign of an underlying collagen-vascular or immunological disorder.

IS THE HEMOPTYSIS LIFE-THREATENING?

As with any potential emergency, the first question to be answered is, "Is the hemoptysis life-threatening?" Because the expectoration of blood understandably arouses anxiety and fear, and the blood can be mixed with saliva or phlegm, swallowed or aspirated, it often is difficult for children and their parents to determine accurately the amount of blood coughed up from the lower respiratory tract. In children, the gravity of the hemoptysis is determined more by their clinical status and their ability to keep their airways clear rather than the amount of blood expectorated. The greatest danger to a child who has hemoptysis is not exsanguination but rather asphyxiation from aspirated blood. The management of the child who has life-threatening hemoptysis is beyond the scope of this chapter, but if the child has evidence of cardiorespiratory distress, hypotension, orthostatic changes, poor perfusion, pallor, tachypnea, tachycardia, mental status changes, arterial hypoxemia, or hypercapnia, stabilization and evaluation should occur simultaneously in a pediatric intensive care unit.

EVALUATION

Before summoning the bronchoscopist, echocardiographer, and interventional radiologist and before scheduling pulmonary arteriography and radionuclide scanning, it is essential to ascertain if the source of bleeding is, indeed, from within the thorax. Careful inspection of the oropharynx and nasal passages may identify an upper airway source of bleeding. Infants and young children who have hemoptysis may cough up and swallow the blood and vomit it later, rather than expectorating it immediately. Therefore, in infants, one often has to distinguish hematemesis from hemoptysis. Examination of the blood-stained vomitus may help to determine if the bleeding site is from the respiratory tract or the gastrointestinal tract (Table 144-2).

PATHOGENESIS

Hemoptysis can result from the disruption of either arm of the dual pulmonary vascular system or from damage to the alveolar endothelial junction. The low-pressure, high-capacity pulmonary arterial system accepts the entire cardiac output from the right ventricle and carries blood to be oxygenated in the alveolar capillaries before returning the oxygenated blood to the left atrium via the pulmonary veins. Although the pulmonary arteries travel alongside the bronchial tree, they interact with the airways only at the level of the terminal bronchiole.[5] The second arm of the blood supply within the lungs is the high-pressure bronchial system. The bronchial arteries originate from the aorta or, less commonly, the intercostal arteries, and they receive 1% to 2% of the cardiac output. The bronchial arteries enter the lungs at the hili and branch with the bronchi. As they branch, they anastomose and penetrate the bronchial mucosa, forming an extensive submucosal plexus. The high flow, low-pressure pulmonary capillary bed allows for the exchange of gases between the alveoli and the capillaries to occur with little risk of hemorrhage in the normal state. When hemoptysis is localized, it usually is the result of bleeding from the high-pressure bronchial circulation in inflamed airways. The pulmonary circulation is rarely to blame for hemoptysis except with necrotic infarcts and from pulmonary arterial aneurysms in tuberculous cavities. Both of these conditions are extremely rare in children.

Table 144-1 Etiologies of Children Who Have Hemoptysis Who Presented to Montefiore Medical Center Over a 3-Year Period*

Discharge Diagnosis	Number of Children
Hematemesis or upper airway hemorrhage	7
Congenital heart disease	5
Pneumonia	4
Acute chest syndrome	2
Pulmonary hypertension	1
Idiopathic pulmonary hemosiderosis	1
Goodpasture's syndrome	1
Tracheostomy-related tracheitis	1
Sarcoma	1

*Thirteen of the children had no previous illnesses and 10 children had an underlying medical condition that is associated with hemoptysis. Six of the children needed to be placed on mechanical ventilation. Children who had cystic fibrosis were excluded from this analysis.

Table 144-2 Differentiation of Hemoptysis from Hematemesis and Upper Airway Hemorrhage

	Hemoptysis	Hematemesis/Upper Airway Hemorrhage
pH	Alkaline	Acidic
Color	Bright red	Dark red or brown
Consistency	Clotted, liquid, or frothy	Coffee ground
Symptoms	Cough	Nausea and vomiting
Gram stain	Macrophages	Food particles and epithelial cells

Younger children and infants may swallow blood that originates from the lungs, appearing to have a nonpulmonary source of bleeding.

Inflammation within the lungs, pulmonary vascular obstruction, and neoplasia can all cause an increase in the bronchial circulation. In chronic inflammatory conditions, such as bronchiectasis, the cardiac output to the bronchial circulation can triple, and bronchopulmonary anastomoses also increase. Therefore, with chronic inflammatory lung diseases, vessels can erode into the airways with superimposed infection.

The pathogenesis of disease states in which there is diffuse pulmonary hemorrhage (e.g., Wegener's granulomatosis or hemosiderosis) is not entirely understood, but the bleeding into the alveoli appears to be due to neutrophil-mediated injury to pulmonary capillaries, with interstitial and airspace fibrosis as a result of the chronic hemorrhage.[18]

HISTORY

As is the case for any sign or symptom that has many possible etiologies, a detailed history of both pulmonary and nonpulmonary symptoms often will allow a tentative diagnosis to be made. The presumptive diagnosis can then be proved or not by the use of specific laboratory tests and procedures. For a child or adolescent who has no preexisting medical condition who presents with a first episode of hemoptysis, the most common causes are acute infections of the tracheobronchial tree, pneumonia, and foreign-body aspiration.[7,16,17] Although rare, hemoptysis can be the presenting symptom for a connective tissue disorder or immunological abnormality. Travel to or from developing countries and sheep-raising areas may necessitate evaluation for mycobacterial, mycotic, or parasitic lung infections. Recurrent pneumonitis, sinus infections, and chronic sputum production may indicate bronchiectasis caused by cystic fibrosis, foreign-body aspiration, ciliary dyskinesias, or other chronic lung diseases. Other aspects of the history that will help focus the evaluation include recent trauma, easy bruising, changes in urine color, weight loss, arthralgias, previous heart disease or cardiac surgery, medication use, substance abuse, family history of bleeding disorders, surgical procedures, pica, fever, pleuritic chest pain, menstrual irregularities, and asthma not responsive to appropriate medical therapy.

PHYSICAL EXAMINATION

Physical examination begins with a determination of the vital signs to decide the urgency with which the examination should be conducted. A thorough inspection of the nasal passages and oropharynx is conducted to rule out a nonpulmonary cause of the hemoptysis. As the examination proceeds caudally, certain findings on inspection and auscultation may suggest a specific diagnosis. Cutaneous telangiectasias with a murmur or bruit over the lung fields suggests hereditary hemorrhagic telangiectasia. Clubbing of the fingers and toes, with or without pulmonary crackles, suggests bronchiectasis. A saddle nose and stridor suggestive of subglottic stenosis are often seen in persons who have Wegener's granulomatosis.[14] A pleuritic rub, acute pleuritic chest pain, and a history of oral contraceptive use or recent abortion raises the specter of a pulmonary embolic event or other pleural lesions. Localized homophonous wheezing over a major airway and decreased breath sounds, with or without a cough, suggest an intraluminal obstruction such as an aspirated foreign body. Evidence of trauma to the thorax may not always be obvious; 30% of children who sustain major trauma to other organ systems will be found to have thoracic trauma as well.[15] Examination of the heart may provide evidence of pulmonary hypertension or a new murmur. Lymphadenopathy and hepatosplenomegaly should raise the possibility of a bleeding diathesis or other hematological abnormality.

IMAGING STUDIES

The history and physical examination should allow a tentative diagnosis and help direct the imaging studies or procedures that are required to make a definitive diagnosis. If the child is stable, a chest radiograph should be obtained. Any abnormality on a chest radiograph should be considered a potential source for the hemoptysis, but a normal radiograph does not exclude the thorax as the source of bleeding. In about one third of children and up to half of adults who have hemoptysis, the initial chest radiograph will be normal.[17] Findings on the chest film that help focus the evaluation include hilar adenopathy, an air-fluid level in an abscess, a mass, a cavitary lesion, mediastinal widening, and alveolar infiltrates. Finding alveolar infiltrates in a child who has hemoptysis is common with autoimmune and collagen-vascular diseases that involve the lungs.[4] Thickening of the bronchial walls with ring shadows and tramlines suggest bronchiectasis. If a foreign body is suspected of being the cause, inspiratory and expiratory films or left and right lateral decubitus films may help localize the aspirated object. If a foreign body causes obstruction of an airway, the side that does not deflate normally on expiration or when dependent is the side that contains the foreign body. If the foreign body is embedded within the mucosa of the airway, or if obstruction is only partial, the chest radiographs may be normal.

The next imaging studies depend on the presumptive diagnosis because not every child who has hemoptysis needs special radiographic evaluation. If a chest radiograph is normal or does not add any information to that obtained from the history and physical examination, computerized tomography (CT) or high-resolution computerized tomography (HRCT) may be helpful. CT is good for the detection of parenchymal disease and has replaced bronchography to diagnosis bronchiectasis.[1] CT can identify airway abnormalities, elucidate abnormalities seen on chest radiographs, define mediastinal structures, and help categorize congenital pulmonary malformations and pulmonary vasculitis syndromes. CT also may serve as a road map for subsequent bronchoscopy.

Magnetic resonance imaging (MRI) is useful for the evaluation of congenital vascular malformations and for the differentiation of structures within the mediastinum and hilum. Perhaps in the future, MRI will supplant CT in the evaluation of hemoptysis, but for now the advantages of MRI do not outweigh its disadvantages, especially if there is excessive respiratory motion or the child's condition is unstable.

BRONCHOSCOPY

The timing and need for bronchoscopy, either rigid or flexible, depends on the stability of the child and the suspected etiology of the hemoptysis. Not every child who has hemoptysis needs bronchoscopy. If the child's hemoptysis has resolved rapidly following medical therapy, then there is no reason to perform bronchoscopy. Bronchoscopy should be performed if the diagnosis is in question, if there is massive hemoptysis, or if the response to therapy is incomplete.

No studies exist that compare the use of fiberoptic and rigid bronchoscopy for the evaluation of hemoptysis in either adults or children. Both instruments can be used to sample bronchial fluids, obtain biopsy samples, and administer therapeutic agents to the airways. With the rigid bronchoscope, the bronchoscopist has complete airway control, can suction through a larger channel, can obtain samples of suspicious lesions for biopsy, and can insert packing material to control the bleeding. The rigid bronchoscope is the instrument of choice for removal of foreign bodies in the airways. On the other hand, fiberoptic bronchoscopy (FOB) does not require the use of general anesthesia and is usually performed transnasally, so the upper airways can be examined as well. Further, in FOB the bronchoscope can be maneuvered into the upper lobes and more distal airways with greater ease. If a child who has hemoptysis needs bronchoscopy, FOB should be used for the initial evaluation. If an anatomical lesion or foreign body is discovered, rigid bronchoscopy will be needed.

LABORATORY EVALUATION

Numerous laboratory tests may be helpful, but they should be selected based on the history and physical examination. If the patient has a compromised airway, arterial blood gas measurement may help to determine how quickly the intensive care unit needs to be alerted. Urinalysis and specific serological markers will help determine if the child has an immunological disease that involves the basement membranes of both the kidneys and the lungs. A complete blood count with an eosinophil count may help differentiate a bacterial from a parasitic pneumonia. Although clotting studies are ordered routinely, they usually are normal, because bleeding disorders generally do not cause spontaneous hemoptysis. Skin tests for mycobacteria should always be placed, but additional skin tests for fungi or other infectious agents should be guided by clinical indications. If sputum is produced or bronchoscopy is performed, pulmonary fluids should be cultured for bacteria, fungi, ova, parasites, and mycobacteria. The fluid also should be examined microscopically for the presence of hemosiderin-laden macrophages. If a skilled bronchoscopist is not available, early-morning gastric aspirates can be cultured and viewed microscopically for microorganisms and macrophages.

ETIOLOGY

Hemoptysis in Children Who Have No Preexisitng Medical Condition

In children who do not have a preexisting medical condition and present with acute hemoptysis, the most common causes are acute infectious pneumonias and the aspiration of a foreign body (Table 144-3). A child who has a pneumococcal pneumonia who is old enough to expectorate, classically is ill appearing with fever and has a cough that is productive of rusty sputum. Certain other bacterial and viral lower respiratory tract infections can cause hemoptysis, but the hemoptysis occurs early in the course of the illness, is self-limited, and consists of only blood-tinged sputum. Worldwide, tuberculosis, echinococcus, and paragonimiasis probably are the most common causes of hemoptysis in children.

After acute infectious processes, the most common cause of hemoptysis in a previously healthy child is the aspiration of a foreign body. For many children who aspirate foreign bodies, the initial choking episode is not observed or not remembered.[12] There may be a bout of paroxysmal coughing after the initial event, but as the cough receptors in the bronchi or trachea adapt, the coughing will subside. Over time, and depending on the location and composition of the foreign object, there will be airway inflammation. If the inflammation results in airway obstruction, there will be wheezing, or recurrent pneumonitis. If there is neovascularization of granulation tissue in the airways or if bronchiectasis develops, there can be hemoptysis weeks to months after the initial event. Only 40% of children who have foreign body aspiration will present with the classic triad of wheezing, cough, and decreased breath sounds distal to the site of obstruction. The chest roentgenogram will be normal in 25% of children who have bronchial foreign bodies and in more than 50% of children who have tracheal foreign bodies.[12]

Because only 10% of aspirated foreign bodies are radiopaque, a normal chest radiograph does not preclude aspiration. Inspiratory and expiratory films, decubitus films, and fluoroscopy may be necessary to confirm the diagnosis. If the evidence for aspiration is definitive, then referral for rigid bronchoscopy to a pediatric surgeon or oto-

Table 144-3 Common, Less Common, and Rare Causes of Hemoptysis

Common Causes in Children Who Have No Preexisting Medical Problems	Diagnostic Clues
Pneumonia	Usually rusty-colored sputum early in the course of the illness
Foreign-body aspiration	Needs a high index of suspicion; may have a normal chest radiograph; localized wheezing that does not respond to medical therapy
Less Common Causes in Children Who Have No Preexisting Medical Problems	**Diagnostic Clues**
Pulmonary tuberculosis	Usually with systemic manifestations, such as anorexia and weight loss; may have negative PPD
Autoimmune disorders	Diffuse pulmonary hemorrhage, often with weight loss or other systems involved, including the kidneys and joints
Congenital malformations	Symptoms depend on the nature of the lesion; may be associated with massive hemoptysis or respiratory distress in newborns
Rare Causes in Children Who Have a Preexisting Medical Problem	**Diagnostic Clues**
Primary pulmonary neoplasms	Primary pulmonary cancers reported in fewer than 400 children; usually present with cough and recurrent pneumonitis
Pulmonary embolism	Associated with pleuritic pain, cough, and dyspnea; oral contraceptive use; recent abortion; or trauma to lower extremities
Parasitic lung infections	Travel to endemic areas or sheep-raising areas; peripheral eosinophilia
Arteriovenous malformations	Recurrent epistaxis, a positive family history for Osler-Weber-Rendu syndrome, or cutaneous telangiectasia
Idiopathic pulmonary hemosiderosis	Cough, wheezing, iron-deficiency anemia, and diffuse pulmonary hemorrhage on chest radiograph
Catamenial hemoptysis	Hemoptysis occurs with onset of menses
Factitious hemoptysis	A form of Munchausen syndrome
Common Causes in Children Who Have a Preexisting Medical Problem	**Diagnostic Clues**
Bronchiectasis	Blood-tinged sputum; clubbing; signs of increasing airway inflammation
Congenital heart lesions	Seen with Eisenmenger's complex and pulmonary venous congestion
Less Common Causes in Children Who Have a Preexisting Medical Problem	**Diagnostic Clues**
Sickle cell anemia	Hemoptysis associated with acute chest syndrome or pulmonary infarction
Aspergillosis	Seen in association with cystic fibrosis or asthma; peripheral eosinophilia and fungi seen on Gram stain of sputum

laryngologist experienced in retrieving foreign bodies is indicated. If the diagnosis is uncertain, referral to a pediatric pulmonologist or other clinician skilled in the use of the fiberoptic bronchoscope is appropriate to determine if a foreign body is present.

Diffuse pulmonary hemorrhage. Children who have acute hemoptysis, cough, wheezing, or pulmonary crackles, diffuse patchy infiltrates on chest roentgenogram, and bronchoscopic evidence of blood or hemosiderin-laden macrophages in all lobes should be assumed to have diffuse pulmonary hemorrhage or hemosiderosis. The four categories of diffuse hemorrhagic syndromes that occur in children are: (1) those associated with antiglomerular basement membrane antibodies in serum or tissue (e.g., Goodpasture's syndrome), (2) those associated with an immune-mediated collagen vascular disease (e.g., systemic lupus erythematosus), (3) those associated without any immunological abnormalities but with antibodies to cow milk, and (4) idiopathic pulmonary hemosiderosis.[2]

Goodpasture's syndrome, which occurs most commonly in males in their second and third decades of life, is characterized by diffuse pulmonary hemorrhage, antiglomerular basement membrane antibodies in serum or tissue, and glomerulonephritis. The collagen vascular diseases, which are more common in females, rarely present with hemoptysis; more common are systemic manifestations of fever, weight loss, malaise, anorexia, amenorrhea, rashes, or hypertension. Treatment for the pulmonary hemorrhage in these disorders should be directed to the underlying disease process.

With Heiner syndrome (pulmonary hemosiderosis associated with cow milk allergy), infants and children present with failure to thrive, vomiting, gastrointestinal bleeding, and upper respiratory tract congestion in addition to hemoptysis.[10] Although the mechanism whereby the milk causes the multisystem damage is unclear, elimination of milk from the diet results in a dramatic improvement in the child.

In idiopathic pulmonary hemosiderosis (IPH), no evidence exists for an immune-mediated mechanism. The majority of children who have IPH are diagnosed before 7 or after 16 years of age. They usually present with respiratory distress, bilateral alveolar infiltrates, and iron-deficiency anemia. The treatment of acute exacerbations of IPH includes the use of high-dose oral or intravenous corticosteroids, as well as supportive care for the acute bleeding into the lungs. The need for chronic immunosuppressive therapy is controversial, but most clinicians caring for children who have IPH use azathioprine, chloroquine, or Cytoxan to help maintain normal lung function.

Primary pulmonary neoplasms. Unlike adults, primary pulmonary neoplasms are extremely rare in the pediatric age group: Only 383 primary pulmonary neoplasms have been reported in the English medical literature to 1993, and only 8% of these tumors were associated with hemoptysis. The most frequent presentations of primary pulmonary neoplasms in children are fever, cough, and pneumonitis.[8]

Hemoptysis in Children Who Have a Preexisting Medical Condition

The most common chronic disease associated with hemoptysis is cystic fibrosis (CF). Hemoptysis in CF, which usually begins in the second or third decade of life, can range from the production of blood-tinged sputum with excessive coughing to massive bleeding. Mild hemoptysis can be treated with conservative medical therapy, which includes bed rest, intravenous or oral antibiotics, withholding of chest physiotherapy, and administration of vitamin K.[11] Massive hemoptysis has an annual incidence of 1% among CF patients and carries a high mortality.[3] Massive or recurrent hemoptysis in CF and other diseases is now treated with bronchial artery embolization. Despite a moderately high rate of recurrent bleeding, embolization can relieve symptoms for a significant period. A team comprised of a pulmonologist, thoracic surgeon, and interventional radiologist should evaluate these patients before bronchial artery embolization.

Although the number of children who have bronchiectasis has declined because of the decline of tuberculosis and the use of effective vaccines against measles and pertussis, children who have primary immunodeficiencies, recurrent aspiration, and ciliary dyskinesias may develop bronchiectasis and have episodes of hemoptysis. In most cases, a history of a chronic productive cough with purulent sputum and changes on the lung examination precede the hemoptysis. The diagnosis is made by high-resolution chest tomography, and management is similar to that for cystic fibrosis.

Hemoptysis is a well-recognized complication of congenital heart disease but is becoming an uncommon problem because of advances in corrective cardiac surgery.[9] Hemoptysis in primary or secondary pulmonary hypertension occurs because of thromboembolic events. In right ventricular outflow obstruction with increased bronchial arterial circulation, hemoptysis is due to hemorrhage from enlarged and tortuous bronchial arteries. Hemoptysis is seen in pulmonary vascular obstructive disease because of pulmonary hypertension, as well as thrombosis. These vascular changes take years to develop and usually are observed first in adolescents.

Hemoptysis in the Newborn Period

Infants who have a variety of congenital defects can develop localized hemoptysis and diffuse pulmonary hemorrhage in the newborn period. Arteriovenous malformations, extralobar sequestration, or Osler-Weber-Rendu syndrome (hereditary hemorrhagic telangiectasia) can present in the nursery with respiratory distress or mild to massive hemoptysis. All of these vascular malformations have abnormal connections between the bronchial and pulmonary circulations. The diagnosis of these lesions is made by angiography, and children who have these defects need to be hospitalized in a center that has a pediatric surgeon and an interventional radiologist.

Diffuse pulmonary hemorrhage is not an uncommon occurrence in very low-birth-weight infants. The more premature the infant, the higher the likelihood of hemorrhage. The pathogenesis of the diffuse bleeding is thought to be due to effects of barotrauma on an immature pulmonary capillary endothelium. The risk of pulmonary hemorrhage increases slightly with the administration of exogenous surfactant therapy.[13] Numerous nonpulmonary conditions also have been associated with diffuse hemorrhage in premature newborns, including central nervous system insults and coagulation and metabolic defects.

Ten infants between the ages of 6 weeks to 6 months in the Cleveland area have been described with acute hemoptysis, respiratory failure, and cyanosis following exposure to mold growing in water-damaged homes and to environmental tobacco smoke.[6] Similar cases have been reported from Chicago, and in both cohorts, all of these children needed to be hospitalized and placed on mechanical ventilation.

REFERENCES

1. Ablin DS, Newell JD II: Diagnostic imaging for evaluation of the pediatric chest, *Clin Chest Med* 8:641, 1987.
2. Albelda SM, et al: Diffuse pulmonary hemorrhage: a review and classification, *Radiology* 154:289, 1985.
3. Brinson GM, et al: Bronchial artery embolization for the treatment of hemoptysis in patients with cystic fibrosis, *Am J Resp Crit Care Med* 157:1951, 1998.
4. Connolly B, et al: CT appearance of pulmonary vasculitis in children, *AJR* 167:901, 1996.
5. Deffebach ME, et al: The bronchial circulation: small, but a vital attribute of the lung, *Am Rev Resp Dis* 135:463, 1987.
6. Etzel RA, et al: Acute pulmonary hemorrhage in infants associated with exposure to *Stachybotrys atra* and other fungi, *Arch Pediatr Adolesc Med* 152:757, 1998.
7. Fabian MC, Smitheringale A: Hemoptysis in children: the Hospital for Sick Children Experience, *J Otolaryngol* 25:44, 1996.
8. Hancock BJ, et al: Childhood primary pulmonary neoplasms, *J Pediatr Surg* 28:1133, 1993.
9. Haroutunian L, Neill CA: Pulmonary complications of congenital heart disease: hemoptysis, *Am Heart J* 84:540, 1972.
10. Heiner DC, Kniker WT: Multiple precipitins to cow's milk in chronic respiratory disease, *Am J Dis Child* 103:634, 1962.
11. Holsclaw DS, Grand RJ, Shwachmann H: Massive hemoptysis in cystic fibrosis, *J Pediatr* 76:829, 1970.

12. Pyman C: Inhaled foreign bodies in childhood: a review of 230 cases, *Med J Aust* 1:62, 1971.
13. Raju TN, Langenberg P: Pulmonary hemorrhage and exogenous surfactant therapy: a metaanalysis, *J Pediatr* 123:603, 1993.
14. Rottem M, et al: Wegener granulomatosis in children and adolescents: clinical presentation and outcome, *J Pediatr* 122:26, 1993.
15. Sinclair M, Moore T: Major surgery for abdominal and thoracic trauma in childhood and adolescence, *J Pediatr Surg* 9:155, 1974.
16. Thompson JW, et al: Evaluation and management of hemoptysis in infants and children: a report of nine cases, *Ann Otol Rhinol Laryngol* 105:516, 1996.
17. Tom LW, Weisman RA, Handler SD: Hemoptysis in children, *Ann Otolaryngol* 89:419, 1980.
18. Travis WD, et al: A clinicopathologic study of 34 cases of diffuse pulmonary hemorrhage with lung biopsy confirmation, *Am J Surg Pathol* 14:1112, 1990.

145 Hepatomegaly

Philip O. Ozuah

Hepatomegaly is defined as an enlargement of the liver resulting from an increase in the number or size of cells and structures within the liver. Although hepatomegaly usually presents clinically as a palpable liver, not all palpable livers result from hepatomegaly. In normal children, the liver edge may be palpable up to 2 cm below the right coastal margin at the midclavicular line. Clinical estimation of the liver span has a much stronger correlation with hepatomegaly than does reporting the liver projection below the costal margin as a single indicator of liver size.[16] The liver span is the distance between the upper and lower margins of the liver at the right mid clavicular line. The upper margin should be determined by percussion and the lower edge by either percussion or palpation. Liver span is related curvilinearly to age, height, weight, and body surface area.[4,8] Recent studies have demonstrated no consistent gender differences in liver size.[5,7] A normal liver span ranges from 5.9 cm (±0.8 cm) in the first week of life to 6.5 to 8 cm by 15 years of age.[4,8,16] The upper edge of liver dullness is usually at the level of the fifth rib in the right midclavicular line. Radiographic assessment of liver size can be a helpful adjunct to the clinical examination. Ultrasonography, computed tomography (CT) scan, and sulfur colloid scintigraphy have all been demonstrated to measure liver size reliably.[5-7,9-11] The differential diagnosis of a palpable liver and hepatomegaly is presented in Box 145-1.

PALPABLE LIVER WITHOUT HEPATOMEGALY

Several intrathoracic conditions may push the right hemidiaphragm down and thereby result in a palpable liver. For example, asthma, bronchiolitis, and pneumonitis may produce a palpable liver through hyperinflation of the lungs. Tension pneumothorax usually has other accompanying clinical features, including dyspnea, tachycardia, tracheal deviation, and hypotension. Congenital diaphragmatic hernias often present in the neonatal period with a scaphoid abdomen and the presence of bowel sounds in the chest. Other thoracic space-occupying lesions also can displace the diaphragm.

Abdominal sepsis with a subdiaphragmatic abscess may push the liver caudally. Riedel's lobe is an occasional tongue-like process extending downward from the right lobe of the liver lateral to the gall bladder. A palpable liver without hepatomegaly also may be a normal variant.

INFLAMMATORY DISORDERS

Inflammatory liver disorders frequently present clinically with jaundice and a liver that is firm and tender to palpation. Viral hepatitis (including A, B, C, D, and E) may be fulminant or insidious in onset. Hepatitis A may be anicteric in 50% of infected children younger than 4 years of age and in more than 80% of children younger than 2 years. Bacterial sepsis may result in hepatomegaly as part of a generalized process or a localized liver abscess.[3] Toxic hepatitis may result from exposure to several agents, including isoniazid. Idiopathic neonatal hepatitis presents with direct hyperbilirubinemia and may be difficult to distinguish clinically from congenital biliary atresia. Liver biopsy in idiopathic neonatal hepatitis reveals marked infiltration with inflammatory cells in contrast to bile duct proliferation found in biliary atresia. Giant-cell transformation is found in both conditions. Rarely, autoimmune diseases such as systemic lupus erythematosus and sarcoidosis may involve the liver, leading to a hepatitis with hepatomegaly.

INFILTRATIVE DISORDERS

Primary or metastatic neoplasia may infiltrate the liver and often are associated with other clinical findings. Malignant hepatic tumors present clinically with a hard, palpable liver. Benign tumors include large hemangiomas, which occasionally lead to a platelet consumption coagulopathy (Kasabach-Merritt syndrome), as a result of excessive trapping and destruction of platelets within the vascular bed. Clinically, a bruit may be heard over the liver in patients who have hemangiomas and arteriovenous shunts.

STORAGE DISORDERS

Several genetic and enzyme defects result in excessive accumulation of metabolites in the liver. These conditions produce a smooth, distended liver. Many of these syndromes also are associated with other clinical features besides hepatomegaly. Fat and glycogen accumulation are well known causes of hepatomegaly. Less frequently, copper accumulation results in Indian childhood cirrhosis or Wilson's disease.[1,12,13,15,17] Indian childhood cirrhosis presents as jaundice and hepatomegaly predominantly in middle-income, rural Hindu children, but it also has been described in other parts of the world. Its onset is at about 1 to 3 years of age, usually with rapid evolution to cirrhosis and hepatic failure if

BOX 145-1

DIFFERENTIAL DIAGNOSIS OF A PALPABLE LIVER AND HEPATOMEGALY

- A. Palpable liver without hepatomegaly
  1. Downward displacement of right hemidiaphragm
     - Hyperinflated lung (e.g., asthma, bronchiolitis, pneumonitis)
     - Tension pneumothorax
     - Congenital diaphragmatic hernia
     - Thoracic tumors
  2. Subdiaphragmatic lesions (e.g., abscess)
  3. Normal variant
  4. Aberrant lobe of liver (Riedel's lobe)
- B. Hepatomegaly
  1. Inflammatory disorders
     - Viral hepatitis
     - Bacterial hepatitis (e.g., abscess, sepsis)
     - Toxic hepatitis (e.g., drugs)
     - Neonatal hepatitis
     - Autoimmune hepatitis (e.g., systemic lupus erythematosus, sarcoidosis)
  2. Infiltrative disorders
     - Primary tumors
       - Hepatoblastoma
       - Hepatocellular carcinoma
       - Hemangioma
       - Focal nodular hyperplasia
     - Metastatic tumors
       - Lymphoma
       - Leukemia
       - Neuroblastoma
       - Wilms' tumor
       - Histiocytosis
  3. Storage disorders
     - Fat accumulation
       - Obesity
       - Malnutrition
       - Reye's syndrome
       - Cystic fibrosis
       - Diabetes mellitus
       - Lipid infusion
       - Metabolic liver disease
       - Lipidoses (e.g., Niemann-Pick, Gaucher's, Wolman's diseases)
     - Glycogen excess
       - Glycogen storage diseases
       - Infant of mother who has diabetes
       - Beckwith-Wiedemann syndrome
       - Total parenteral nutrition
     - Copper accumulation
       - Indian childhood cirrhosis
       - Wilson's disease
     - Miscellaneous
       - Alpha$_1$-antitrypsin deficiency
       - Hypervitaminosis A
  4. Vascular congestion
     - Suprahepatic
       - Congestive heart failure
       - Cardiac tamponade
       - Constrictive pericarditis
     - Intrahepatic
       - Hepatic vein thrombosis (Budd-Chiari syndrome)
       - Hepatic vein web
       - Vascular malformations
         - Cavernous hemangioma
         - Capillary hemangioma
         - Hemangio-endothelioma
  5. Biliary obstruction
     - Congenital biliary atresia
     - Congenital hepatic fibrosis
     - Caroli's disease

left untreated. Until recently, this familial disorder was thought to be uniformly fatal, but chelation therapy has shown very promising results. Wilson's disease, an autosomal recessively inherited disorder of copper metabolism, presents with hepatomegaly in young children but generally is not manifested clinically until after 5 years of age. Children older than age 10 years often present with neuropsychiatric symptoms; they also may have hemolytic anemia. Alpha$_1$-antitrypsin deficiency may present with hepatomegaly, icterus, and acholic stools in the first week of life. Signs of chronic liver disease and portal hypertension are seen in older children. Excessive ingestion and accumulation of vitamin A can also result in hepatomegaly.

VASCULAR CONGESTION

Congestive heart failure, cardiac tamponade, and constrictive pericarditis all lead to impaired cardiac filling and pressure back-up into the inferior vena cava and portal vein, all of which produce a smooth, distended, and tender liver. Other signs of cardiac decompensation, including dyspnea, cough, chest pain, and tachycardia, usually are present.

Budd-Chiari syndrome may be caused by a thrombus, mass, or web occluding the inferior vena cava or the hepatic veins and tributaries, resulting in an enlarged liver.

Vascular malformations produce hepatomegaly via several mechanisms, including hemorrhage into the liver or high-output cardiac failure with secondary vascular congestion or by the size of the malformation itself.

BILIARY OBSTRUCTION

Biliary atresia occurs in approximately 1 of 8000 births and is the most frequent reason for liver transplantation in pediatric patients. The bile duct atresia may be extrahepatic, intrahepatic, or a combination thereof. The presence of jaundice, hepatomegaly, and acholic stools beginning during the first months of life in otherwise healthy appearing infants is characteristic. Extrahepatic atresia can be corrected surgically, and intrahepatic atresia can be treated using the hepatoportoenterostomy procedure of Kasai. Nevertheless, many patients will develop cirrhosis and portal hypertension.

Congenital hepatic fibrosis is an autosomal recessive disorder that presents in childhood with hepatosplenomegaly, portal hypertension, and bleeding esophageal varices. Up to 75% of affected children have associated renal disease. Histology reveals diffuse periportal and perilobular fibrosis. Caroli's disease is a congenital saccular dilation of intrahepatic bile ducts that is inherited in an autosomal recessive fashion. Presenting symptoms usually are those of acute cholangitis manifesting in late childhood or young adulthood, with fever, icterus, abdominal pain, and a large, tender liver.

DIAGNOSIS

History and physical examination remain the cornerstone of establishing a prompt diagnosis in patients who have hepatomegaly. A careful history that explores not only gastrointestinal symptoms but also pulmonary and cardiac manifestations will often point in the right diagnostic direction. Physical examination of the liver should include an assessment of its size, consistency, texture, and tenderness. In addition, the liver should be auscultated with a stethoscope.

A firm and tender liver suggests an acute inflammatory disorder; a hard liver often is neoplastic. A smooth and exquisitely tender liver is found in conditions that cause vascular distention. Bruits are heard in arteriovenous malformations. It should be noted that although a palpable liver may be a normal variant, the concomitant physical finding of an enlarged spleen usually suggests significant pathology.

Laboratory investigations should be directed at the suspected diagnosis. Liver function studies usually are necessary. The imaging study used most widely is ultrasonography, which is cheap, portable, reliable, and quickly obtainable in most settings. Liver masses detected on ultrasonography may be defined further by CT scan or sulfur colloid scintigraphy. Hepatic angiography may be indicated in the evaluation of suspected vascular tumors. In patients who have probable metabolic or genetic disorders, a percutaneous liver biopsy may be necessary to establish a diagnosis. Also, the definitive diagnosis of a liver abscess can be made by percutaneous liver aspiration.

TREATMENT

Treatment should be aimed at the underlying disease entity. Patients who have inflammatory hepatitis require supportive care; those who have bacterial infections should receive appropriate antimicrobials. Surgical excision is the definitive treatment for liver tumors. Chemotherapy may be a helpful adjunct in reducing tumor size either pre- or postoperatively.

The treatment of metabolic-genetic disorders includes dietary modifications and chelation therapy. Frequent small feedings of a high-protein, complex-carbohydrate diet, including continuous nighttime feeding via gastrostomy tubes, have been used successfully to manage glycogen storage disorders. Early treatment with D-penicillamine can prevent the progression of Wilson's disease.

Exciting new developments have provided optimism for some disease entities for which there were no treatments formerly. For example, a synthetic enzyme, Ceredase, has been promising in the experimental treatment of Gaucher's disease. Until recently, Indian childhood cirrhosis was thought to be uniformly fatal, but chelation therapy with penicillamine has now been shown to reduce mortality significantly if administered early in the course of the disease.[2,14]

When to Refer

1. Hepatomegaly with concomitant splenomegaly
2. Palpation of a hard liver
3. Hepatomegaly with distended abdominal veins
4. Audible bruit over the liver
5. Suspicion of malignancy

When to Hospitalize

Liver failure
Impending liver failure

REFERENCES

1. Baker A, et al: Copper-associated liver disease in childhood, *J Hepatol* 23:538, 1995.
2. Bavdekar AR, et al: Long term survival in Indian childhood cirrhosis treated with D-penicillamine, *Arch Dis Child* 74:32, 1996.
3. Brook I, Frazier EH: Microbiology of liver and spleen abscesses, *J Med Microbiol* 47:1075, 1998.
4. Carpentieri U, et al: Liver size in normal infants and children, *South Med J* 70:1096, 1977.
5. Friis H, et al: Ultrasonographic organometry: liver and spleen dimensions among children in Zimbabwe, *Trop Med Int Health* 1:183, 1996.
6. Holmes JH, et al: A simple ultrasonic method for evaluating liver size, *J Clin Ultrasound* 5:89, 1977.
7. Konus OL, et al: Normal liver, spleen, and kidney dimensions in neonates, infants, and children: evaluation with sonography, *Am J Roentgenol* 171:1693, 1998.
8. Lawson EE, et al: Clinical estimation of liver span in infants and children, *Am J Dis Child* 132:474, 1978.
9. Markisz JA, Treves ST, Davis RT: Normal hepatic and splenic size in children: scintigraphic determination, *Pediatr Radiol* 17:273, 1987.
10. Niederau C, et al: Sonographic measurements of the normal liver, spleen, pancreas, and portal vein, *Radiology* 149:537, 1983.
11. Noda T, et al: Liver volume in children measured by computed tomography, *Pediatr Radiol* 27:250, 1997.
12. Pandit A, Bhave S: Present interpretation of the role of copper in Indian childhood cirrhosis, *Am J Clin Nutr* 63:830S, 1996.
13. Petrukhin K, Gilliam TC: Genetic disorders of copper metabolism, *Curr Opin Pediatr* 6:698, 1994.
14. Pradhan AM, et al: Reversal of Indian childhood cirrhosis by D-penicillamine therapy, *J Pediatr Gastroenterol Nutr* 20:28, 1995.
15. Prasad R, et al: Molecular basis of pathophysiology of Indian childhood cirrhosis: role of copper accumulation in liver, *Mol Cell Biochem* 156:25, 1996.
16. Reiff MI, Osborn LM: Clinical estimation of liver size in newborn infants, *Pediatrics* 71:46, 1983.
17. Tanner MS: Role of copper in Indian childhood cirrhosis, *Am J Clin Nutr* 67(5 suppl):1074S, 1998.

146 High Blood Pressure in Infants, Children, and Adolescents

Carol J. Buzzard • Steven E. Lipshultz

Hypertension long has been recognized as the cause of significant morbidity and mortality in adults.[9,25] Although the data available are based primarily on studies of adult males, many physicians have been increasingly concerned that there may be a causal link between blood pressure (BP) elevations in children and primary hypertension in adults. Many long-term tracking studies document the familial nature of essential hypertension,[29] and others support the theory that elevated BP in children correlates with hypertension in early adulthood.[14] Most pediatricians feel that even mild to moderate elevations of BP in children warrant close watching and possible therapy. Mild and moderate hypertension in childhood generally is not associated with significant symptoms; therefore, routine screening can identify a fair number of children who have either primary or secondary hypertension. Definitive therapy can decrease later morbidity. All pediatricians should be familiar with the basic aspects of hypertension in children, including the diagnosis of normal and abnormal BP, the etiology of high BP, and possible therapeutic options.[27]

DEFINITION

In children, BP normally will vary considerably throughout the day. Evaluation of patients who have 24-hour BP monitoring devices has shown that diastolic and systolic BPs appear to be lower in the morning and reach a peak in the afternoon.[7,19] BP measurements also change with posture, emotional state, and exercise.[11,16] This variability can make the diagnosis of true hypertension in the infant, child, or adolescent difficult. The second National Heart, Lung, and Blood Institute Task Force on Blood Pressure Control in Children developed definitions based on the distribution of BP in healthy children as well as on clinical experience and consensus.[18,28] The report and subsequent updates[28] define normal systolic and diastolic BPs as less than the 90th percentile for age and gender. High-normal BP is defined as that greater than or equal to the 90th but less than the 95th percentile. Hypertension is defined as an average systolic or diastolic BP greater than or equal to the 95th percentile for age and gender measured on at least three separate occasions. Physicians should use three distribution patterns provided by the task force to evaluate their individual patients. Tables 146-1 and 146-2 represent 90th and 95th percentiles in girls and boys ages 1 to 17 years by percentiles of height. Because body size is the most important determining factor of BP in children and adolescents, using height as a variable should help eliminate falsely classifying extremely tall or short individuals. Fig. 146-1 shows age- and gender-specific distribution curves for infants during their first year of life.

Normotensive children are those in whom the average systolic and diastolic BP is less than the 90th percentile for age and gender. Those whose BP falls between the 90th and 95th percentile are considered to be at risk for developing hypertension and, although they do not require intervention, should have their BP monitored yearly. Hypertension is defined as a BP greater than the 95th percentile on three consecutive measurements, and severe hypertension (with the risk of end-organ injury) as BP greater than the 99th percentile.[21]

MEASUREMENT OF BLOOD PRESSURE

Appropriate BP measurement techniques are important to review because of the risk of false-positive readings when proper care is not taken.[18] The normal data were obtained in seated children and adolescents and in supine infants. The child should be at rest. It is very important that an appropriately sized BP cuff be used to take the measurement. The inner bladder should go more than halfway around the arm and extend from the antecubital fossa to two thirds of the distance to the shoulder. The cuff should be inflated to at least 30 mm Hg above the expected systolic BP, although if inflated too high in young children or infants, it may cause them to become agitated. The stethoscope or Doppler crystal should be placed lightly over the antecubital fossa, with the arm at the level of the heart. The heart sounds (or Korotkoff sounds) are used to determine the systolic and diastolic BPs. The systolic BP is defined as the onset of the first Korotkoff sound, and the diastolic as the fifth Korotkoff (K5) sound or the disappearance or muffling of the Korotkoff sounds. In some children, Korotkoff sounds can continue to be heard until 0 mm Hg. This generally excludes diastolic hypertension.

Automated BP devices can be very helpful in providing serial noninvasive BP measurements in the intensive care unit; BP measurements taken this way appear to correlate well with intraarterial readings.[4] However, the reliability of these instruments in the physician's office is less clear because they require frequent calibration and suffer from a lack of established reference standards. In general, the recommended method of measuring BP in children is auscultation. There recently has been an interest in using ambulatory monitoring devices to help establish the diagnosis of hypertension as well as to track the diurnal variations of BP

Table 146-1 Blood Pressure Levels for the 90th and 95th Percentiles of Blood Pressure for Girls Aged 1 to 17 Years by Percentiles of Height

Age (yr)	Blood Pressure Percentile*	Systolic Blood Pressure by Percentile of Height, mm Hg†							Diastolic Blood Pressure by Percentile of Height, mm Hg†						
		5%	10%	25%	50%	75%	90%	95%	5%	10%	25%	50%	75%	90%	95%
1	90th	97	98	99	100	102	103	104	53	53	53	54	55	56	56
	95th	101	102	103	104	105	107	107	57	57	57	58	59	60	60
2	90th	99	99	100	102	103	104	105	57	57	58	58	59	60	61
	95th	102	103	104	105	107	108	109	61	61	62	62	63	64	65
3	90th	100	100	102	103	104	105	106	61	61	61	62	63	63	64
	95th	104	104	105	107	108	109	110	65	65	65	66	67	67	68
4	90th	101	102	103	104	106	107	108	63	63	64	65	65	66	67
	95th	105	106	107	108	109	111	111	67	67	68	69	69	70	71
5	90th	103	103	104	106	107	108	109	65	66	66	67	68	68	69
	95th	107	107	108	110	111	112	113	69	70	70	71	72	72	73
6	90th	104	105	106	107	109	110	111	67	67	68	69	69	70	71
	95th	108	109	110	111	112	114	114	71	71	72	73	73	74	75
7	90th	106	107	108	109	110	112	112	69	69	69	70	71	72	72
	95th	110	110	112	113	114	115	116	73	73	73	74	75	76	76
8	90th	108	109	110	111	112	113	114	70	70	71	71	72	73	74
	95th	112	112	113	115	116	117	118	74	74	75	75	76	77	78
9	90th	110	110	112	113	114	115	116	71	72	72	73	74	74	75
	95th	114	114	115	117	118	119	120	75	76	76	77	78	78	79
10	90th	112	112	114	115	116	117	118	73	73	73	74	75	76	76
	95th	116	116	117	119	120	121	122	77	77	77	78	79	80	80
11	90th	114	114	116	117	118	119	120	74	74	75	75	76	77	77
	95th	118	118	119	121	122	123	124	78	78	79	79	80	81	81
12	90th	116	116	118	119	120	121	122	75	75	76	76	77	78	78
	95th	120	120	121	123	124	125	126	79	79	80	80	81	82	82
13	90th	118	118	119	121	122	123	124	76	76	77	78	78	79	80
	95th	121	122	123	125	126	127	128	80	80	81	82	82	83	84
14	90th	119	120	121	122	124	125	126	77	77	78	79	79	80	81
	95th	123	124	125	126	128	129	130	81	81	82	83	83	84	85
15	90th	121	121	122	124	125	126	127	78	78	79	79	80	81	82
	95th	124	125	126	128	129	130	131	82	82	83	83	84	85	86
16	90th	122	122	123	125	126	127	128	79	79	79	80	81	82	82
	95th	125	126	127	128	130	131	132	83	83	83	84	85	86	86
17	90th	122	123	124	125	126	128	128	79	79	79	80	81	82	82
	95th	126	126	127	129	130	131	132	83	83	83	84	85	86	86

From Update on the 1987 Task Force Report on High Blood Pressure in Children and Adolescents: *Pediatrics* 98:654, 1996; with permission.
*Blood pressure percentile was determined by a single measurement.
†Height percentile was determined by standard growth curves.

in the older child. The devices are worn on the arm for 24 hours, and BP levels are measured periodically and stored for later analysis.

REGULATION OF BLOOD PRESSURE

A complete discussion of the complex and intricately balanced hormonal and physical factors that influence BP regulation is beyond the scope of this chapter. A summary of the more important concepts is presented here. BP is the product of cardiac output and systemic resistance; therefore, anything that affects the heart rate, stroke volume, blood volume, or peripheral resistance will alter the BP. Resistance is affected not only by physical changes but also by the effect of various hormones on a given vascular bed. Angiotensin II is the major end-product of the renin-angiotensin system, which exerts the major hormonal control of BP. Angiotensin II is a potent vasoconstrictor and is closely related to renal blood flow. Renin release is stimulated by volume depletion, hypotension, and salt depletion, and is inhibited by volume expansion, salt loading, and elevated electrolyte levels. Several other hormonal systems also affect renin release.[13] Circulating catecholamines and glucagon stimulate renin release, as do adrenocorticotropic and parathyroid hormones. Angiotensin II itself acts as a feedback to inhibit renin release, and both mineralocorticoids and antidiuretic hormone do the same.

Drugs also can affect renin release. Both vasodilators and diuretics stimulate renin; mineralocorticoids and beta-blockers inhibit it. Other hormonal systems also play a role in BP regulation.[10,12] Catecholamine secretion increases

Table 146-2 Blood Pressure Levels for the 90th and 95th Percentiles of Blood Pressure for Boys Aged 1 to 17 Years by Percentiles of Height

Age (yr)	Blood Pressure Percentile*	Systolic Blood Pressure by Percentile of Height, mm Hg†							Diastolic Blood Pressure by Percentile of Height, mm Hg†						
		5%	10%	25%	50%	75%	90%	95%	5%	10%	25%	50%	75%	90%	95%
1	90th	94	95	97	98	100	102	102	50	51	52	53	54	54	55
	95th	98	99	101	102	104	106	106	55	55	56	57	58	59	59
2	90th	98	99	100	102	104	105	106	55	55	56	57	58	59	59
	95th	101	102	104	106	108	109	110	59	59	60	61	62	63	63
3	90th	100	101	103	105	107	108	109	59	59	60	61	62	63	63
	95th	104	105	107	109	111	112	113	63	63	64	65	66	67	67
4	90th	102	103	105	107	109	110	111	62	62	63	64	65	66	66
	95th	106	107	109	111	113	114	115	66	67	67	68	69	70	71
5	90th	104	105	106	108	110	112	112	65	65	66	67	68	69	69
	95th	108	109	110	112	114	115	116	69	70	70	71	72	73	74
6	90th	105	106	108	110	111	113	114	67	68	69	70	70	71	72
	95th	109	110	112	114	115	117	117	72	72	73	74	75	76	76
7	90th	106	107	109	111	113	114	115	69	70	71	72	72	73	74
	95th	110	111	113	115	116	118	119	74	74	75	76	77	78	78
8	90th	107	108	110	112	114	115	116	71	71	72	73	74	75	75
	95th	111	112	114	116	118	119	120	75	76	76	77	78	79	80
9	90th	109	110	112	113	115	117	117	72	73	73	74	75	76	77
	95th	113	114	116	117	119	121	121	76	77	78	79	80	80	81
10	90th	110	112	113	115	117	118	119	73	74	74	75	76	77	78
	95th	114	115	117	119	121	122	123	77	78	79	80	80	81	82
11	90th	112	113	115	117	119	120	121	74	74	75	76	77	78	78
	95th	116	117	119	121	123	124	125	78	79	79	80	81	82	83
12	90th	115	116	117	119	121	123	123	75	75	76	77	78	78	79
	95th	119	120	121	123	125	126	127	79	79	80	81	82	83	83
13	90th	117	118	120	122	124	125	126	75	76	76	77	78	79	80
	95th	121	122	124	126	128	129	130	79	80	81	82	83	83	84
14	90th	120	121	123	125	126	128	128	76	76	77	78	79	80	80
	95th	124	125	127	128	130	132	132	80	81	81	82	83	84	85
15	90th	123	124	125	127	129	131	131	77	77	78	79	80	81	81
	95th	127	128	129	131	133	134	135	81	82	83	83	84	85	86
16	90th	125	126	128	130	132	133	134	79	79	80	81	82	82	83
	95th	129	130	132	134	136	137	138	83	83	84	85	86	87	87
17	90th	128	129	131	133	134	136	136	81	81	82	83	84	85	85
	95th	132	133	135	136	138	140	140	85	85	86	87	88	89	89

From Update on the 1987 Task Force Report on High Blood Pressure in Children and Adolescents: *Pediatrics* 98:653, 1996; with permission.
*Blood pressure percentile was determined by a single measurement.
†Height percentile was determined by standard growth curves.

BP, and in the presence of a pheochromocytoma or neuroblastoma, it can cause severe hypertension. Both mineralocorticoids and glucocorticoids affect BP, and adrenal hypertrophy and tumors may lead to severe hypertension. Other, less well known, hormonal systems also may play a role in BP regulation.

FACTORS INFLUENCING BLOOD PRESSURE IN CHILDREN

BP tends to increase with age throughout the first two decades of life.[26] The average systolic BP on the first day of life is 70 mm Hg, and it increases steadily for the first 2 months of age.[29] It tends to remain stable until 1 year of age, when it increases until adulthood. Diastolic BP increases slowly for the first week and then declines until age 3 months. It then increases gradually until 1 year of age, when it reaches the level found in the first week. Diastolic BP remains steady for the first 5 to 6 years, after which it begins to increase along with the systolic BP.[23] Children tend to maintain the same BP percentile rank relative to their peers as they grow up, a pattern that continues through adolescence, supporting the idea that essential hypertension begins in childhood.

Body size is a major factor that influences BP in children. As in adults, there is a particularly prominent relationship between BP and weight in the teenage years.[14,23,26] Height also is related independently to BP at all ages.[18] (See Tables 146-1 and 146-2.)

BP is not significantly affected by racial or ethnic origin, and differences between the genders do not become important until later in adolescence. Children from families that have a history of hypertension tend to have higher blood

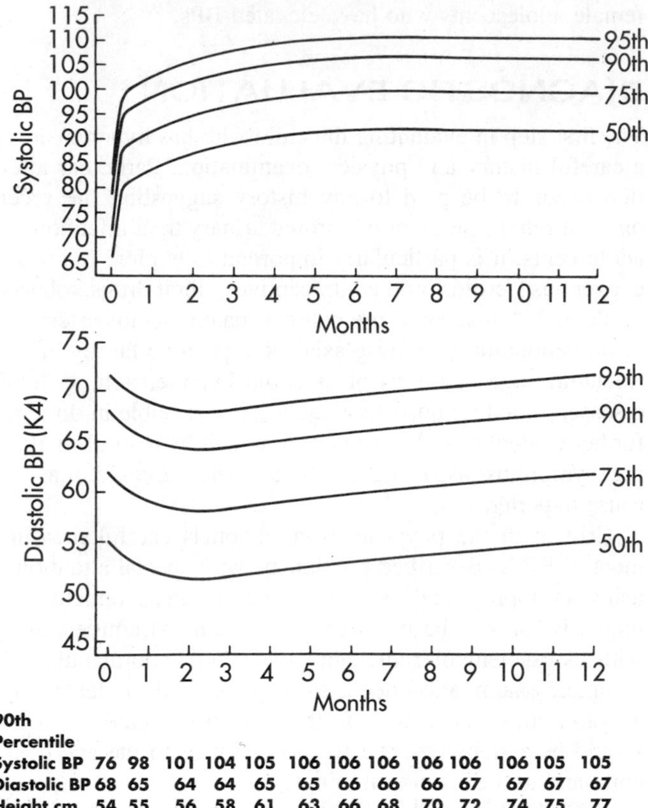

90th Percentile													
Systolic BP	76	98	101	104	105	106	106	106	106	106	106	105	105
Diastolic BP	68	65	64	64	65	65	66	66	66	67	67	67	67
Height cm	54	55	56	58	61	63	66	68	70	72	74	75	77
Weight kg	4	4	4	5	5	6	7	8	9	9	10	10	11

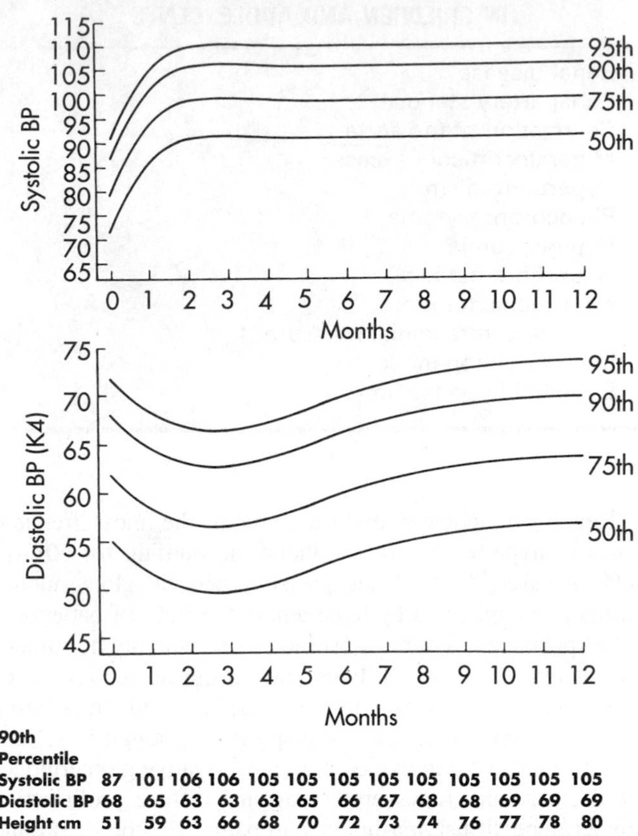

90th Percentile													
Systolic BP	87	101	106	106	105	105	105	105	105	105	105	105	105
Diastolic BP	68	65	63	63	63	65	66	67	68	68	69	69	69
Height cm	51	59	63	66	68	70	72	73	74	76	77	78	80
Weight kg	4	4	5	5	6	7	8	9	9	10	10	11	11

Fig. 146-1 Age-, gender-, height-, and weight-specific percentiles of systolic and diastolic blood pressure from birth to 12 months of age.

(From *Pediatrics* 79:1, 1987; courtesy Dr. Michael J. Horan.)

pressures than do children from normotensive families, supporting the generally accepted conclusion that there is a genetic influence on blood pressure levels.[17,24] There also are significant correlations between parents' and their children's other cardiovascular risk factors.[26]

ETIOLOGY

Primary, or essential, hypertension is a diagnosis of exclusion. It is increasingly obvious that this syndrome is yet to be completely defined. It appears to be associated with family history, sensitivity to high salt intake, and failure to regulate angiotensin II and renal blood flow properly.[12] Although children, and particularly adolescents, who have mild to moderate elevations in BP will have no identifiable underlying disease process, a diagnosis of essential hypertension should not be made until treatable causes have been excluded. Boxes 146-1 and 146-2 list the most common (but not all) causes of hypertension in infants, children, and adolescents.

Severe hypertension can be seen in the neonatal intensive care unit and has been reported in 2% to 3% of former premature infants.[1] Hypertensive neonates often present with evidence of congestive heart failure, respiratory distress, feeding difficulties, irritability, lethargy, coma, or seizures. In almost all cases the hypertension is renal or renovascular in origin, most commonly from renal artery thrombi related to umbilical vessel catheterization. Medical therapy usually is effective in these infants, and the long-term prognosis is surprisingly good.[1,2] High blood pressure also can occur in infants who have bronchopulmonary dysplasia, commonly from the use of glucocorticoids or theophylline in its treatment.[23] Hypertension also has been described in neonates undergoing extracorporeal membrane oxygenation, possibly secondary to volume overload.[3]

BOX 146-1

CAUSES OF HIGH BLOOD PRESSURE IN NEONATES AND INFANTS

- Renal artery thrombosis after umbilical artery catheterization
- Coarctation of the aorta
- Congenital renal parenchymal or structural disease
- Renal artery stenosis
- Bronchopulmonary dysplasia
- Extracorporeal membrane oxygenation

BOX 146-2

CAUSES OF HIGH BLOOD PRESSURE IN CHILDREN AND ADOLESCENTS

Renal disease
Renal artery stenosis
Coarctation of the aorta
Mineralocorticoid excess
Hyperthyroidism
Pheochromocytoma
Hypercalcemia
Neurofibromatosis
Neurogenic tumors
Increased intracranial pressure
Immobilization-induced
Essential hypertension

Renal parenchymal disease remains the most frequent cause of hypertension in childhood, accounting for 60% to 80% of cases.[10,23,26] Acute poststreptococcal glomerulonephritis is complicated by hypertension in 80% of patients at initial presentation; almost 50% of those who are normotensive at first will develop hypertension during the course of their illness. Hypertension also is associated with other forms of immune complex glomerulonephritis, although less commonly. It can be seen in membranoproliferative glomerulonephritis, systemic lupus erythematosus, diffuse proliferative glomerulonephritis, and IgA nephropathy. Hemolytic uremic syndrome also is associated with hypertension, in proportion to the degree of arteriolar thrombosis. Nephrotic syndrome rarely leads to severe hypertension in childhood, unless it is a manifestation of more serious renal disease. Reflux nephropathy is an important cause of hypertension in children, with a reported prevalence of 5% to 38%. Hypertension also is seen with polycystic kidney disease and Wilms' tumor but is less common with other renal structural malformations.[12,23]

Coarctation of the aorta is the most common nonrenal cause of hypertension in childhood, accounting for 5% to 15% of cases.[6,23] Hypertension also can occur immediately following repair of coarctation of the aorta and for years thereafter.[20,22] The risk for postoperative hypertension appears to be lower if the lesion is repaired before 5 years of age.[15,23]

Renal artery stenosis, caused by fibromuscular dysplasia, Takayasu's arteritis, Williams syndrome, or neurofibromatosis, is an uncommon cause of hypertension in childhood. Patients who have renal artery stenosis may present with significant symptoms, caused by end-organ damage (congestive heart failure, left ventricular hypertrophy, retinal changes, and renal impairment).[5,10] Endocrinological causes of hypertension may be exogenous (from administration of glucocorticoid or anabolic steroids) or primary. Overall, they are relatively rare. Hyperthyroidism can cause high BP and always should be considered in the evaluation of isolated hypertension. Increased catecholamines, as with pheochromocytoma, adrenal cortical hyperplasia, and hypercalcemia, all may result in hypertension.

Increased intracranial pressure can cause hypertension, often episodic in nature. Various drugs also can be associated with hypertension, particularly sympathomimetics (cocaine, amphetamines, phenylephrine, and pseudoephedrine). A history of oral contraceptive use should always be sought in female adolescents who have elevated BPs.[10,23]

DIAGNOSTIC EVALUATION

The first step in evaluating the child who has hypertension is a careful history and physical examination. Particular attention needs to be paid to any history suggesting the recent onset of renal disease or of chronic urinary tract infections. In adolescents, it is particularly important to explore the use of exogenous steroids, oral contraceptives, illicit drugs, tobacco, or alcohol. A history of prematurity, patent ductus arteriosus, or bronchopulmonary dysplasia and a positive family history (including age of onset) of essential hypertension, systemic disease, or endocrinopathy may be very valuable in directing further evaluations. A system review will be helpful in eliciting symptoms associated with specific diseases that can cause hypertension.

Critical in the physical examination is careful measurement of BP, as described previously, with special attention to using an appropriately sized cuff and to measurement technique. BP should be measured in all four extremities, along with assessment of radial, brachial, and femoral pulses. A complete examination needs to be performed to identify any abnormalities. This will further direct evaluation, which should be a stepwise investigation tailored to the age of the child and to the specific findings.

Fig. 146-2 is an algorithm for the diagnosis and management of patients who have hypertension. BP should be an average of at least two separate measurements or, better, measurements obtained during several visits. All patients should have a general laboratory screening for possible renal etiologies, including urinalysis, complete blood count, serum urea nitrogen and creatinine, and serum electrolytes. A urine culture and a renal ultrasound usually are necessary. If there is a positive family history for essential hypertension, a lipid profile will help to assess cardiovascular risk factors.

If the BP remains elevated, further, more intensive investigation should proceed, based on the results of the initial history, physical examination, and laboratory findings. If a renal etiology is suspected, further imaging of the genitourinary system may be necessary. A renal ultrasound will identify most causes of renovascular hypertension; however, a diagnosis of renal artery stenosis will often require renal arteriography. Captopril-challenged renal scans also may have some utility in diagnosing renal artery stenosis. Studies of plasma renin activity can be helpful, and if low, suggest the presence of excess mineralocorticoids. Elevated renin levels are less helpful because of the overlap between normal and affected patients. Thyroid function tests or serum catecholamines may be necessary if hyperthyroidism or pheochromocytoma is suspected.

Cardiac evaluation is important.[8] In addition to a careful physical examination, an electrocardiogram and echocardiogram provide information about left ventricular size and function. Formal stress testing can help assess normal and abnormal BP responses to exercise. Ambulatory BP measurements can help establish the presence of hypertension

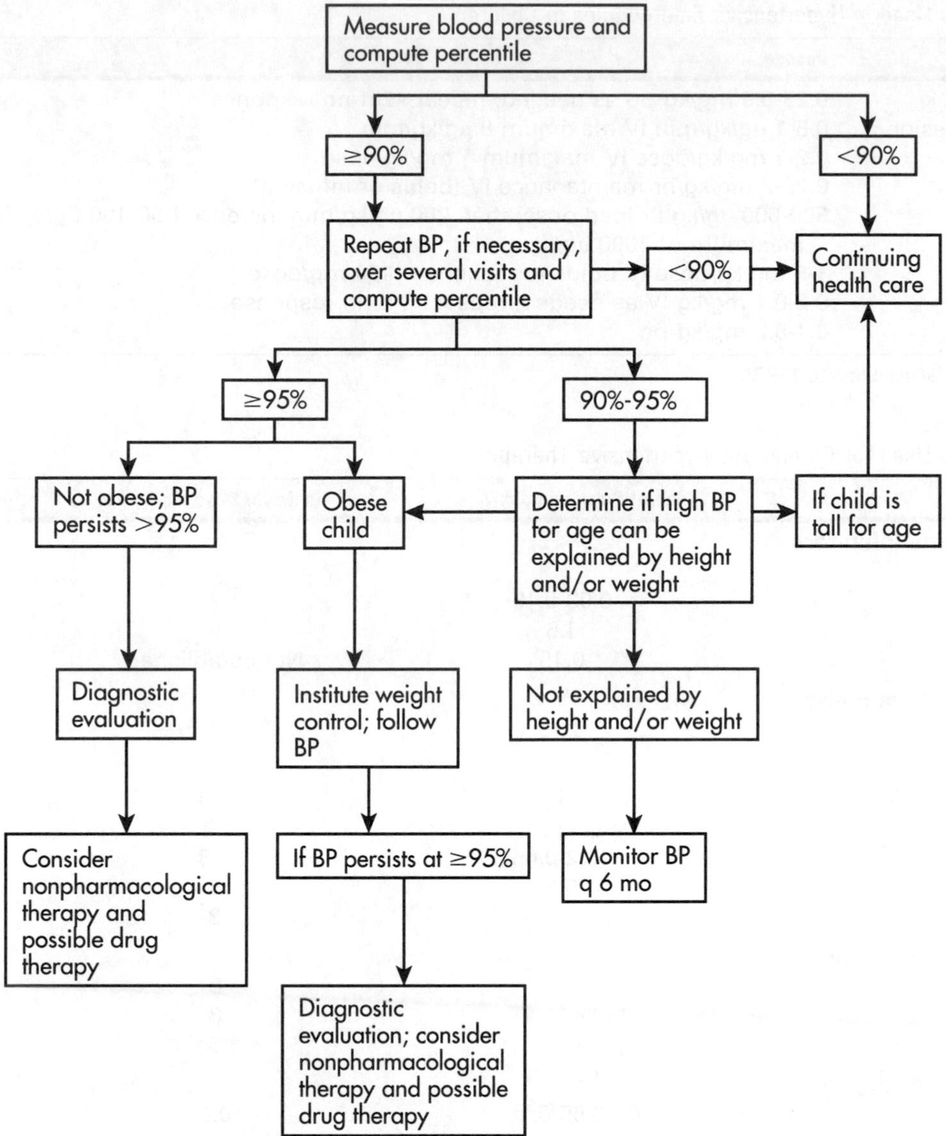

Fig. 146-2 Algorithm for the diagnosis of children with high blood pressure. (Modified from *Pediatrics* 79:8, 1987, with permission.)

and determine the amount of time each day the BP is above the norm.

It also is important to determine if the BP will respond to salt restriction, and if it is sensitive to stress. Isometric hand grip exercises and serial subtractions from 100 are easy to perform; if the diastolic BP increases by 20 mm Hg or more and the systolic by 30 mm Hg or more, the patient is a stress reactor and may respond to behavioral modification techniques, as well as to diet and exercise.

THERAPY FOR HIGH BLOOD PRESSURE

The justification for treating children who have significant hypertension is an extension of adult trials showing that a reduction in BP reduces the risk of target organ damage. Nonpharmacological therapy generally is recommended for mild or moderate hypertension. The initiation of a low-salt or no-added-salt diet is reasonable because many patients will be salt-sensitive. Body size is a major determinant of BP, and weight loss often is associated with reduction in both systolic and diastolic pressures. Exercise as an adjunct to weight loss often provides an even greater degree of BP reduction.

Table 146-3 reviews treatments for hypertensive emergencies. Treatment should be directed at reducing the BP enough to alleviate acute symptoms, not necessarily to make the patient normotensive. Table 146-4 reviews the drugs used most commonly for the treatment of chronic hypertension. The basic strategy of pharmacological therapy is to start with a single drug and assess the response. Additional agents should be added one at a time, always attempting to target a different organ system. The drug of first choice is usually an ACE inhibitor or a calcium channel blocker. Beta-blocking agents can be used also but tend to have more side effects and can be troublesome for patients who have reactive airway disease. The alpha agonists generally are considered to be second-line drugs, and recently diuretics are being used less often for initial therapy of chronic hypertension.

Table 146-3 Drugs Used in Hypertensive Emergencies in Children

Drug	Dosage
Nifedipine	0.25-0.5 mg/kg po as needed; repeat ×2 if no response
Sodium nitroprusside	0.5-1 μg/kg/min IV maximum 8 μg/kg/min
Labetalol	0.2-1 mg/kg/dose IV maximum 1 mg/kg/dose 0.25-2 mg/kg/hr maintenance IV (bolus or infusion)
Esmolol	500-600 μg/kg IV load dose; then 200 μg/kg/min increased 50-100 μg/kg every 5-10 min to maximum of 1000 μg/kg
Diazoxide	1-5 mg/kg/dose IV bolus to maximum 150 mg/dose
Hydralazine	0.2-0.4 mg/kg IV as needed; repeat ×2 if no response
Minoxidil	0.1-0.2 mg/kg po

Modified from *Pediatrics* 98:649, 1996.

Table 146-4 Drugs Used for Chronic Antihypertensive Therapy

	Initial Dose mg/kg/day	Maximum Dose mg/kg/day	Interval (q = every)
Converting Enzyme Inhibitors			
Captopril			
Neonates	0.03-0.15	2	q 8-24h
Children	1.5	6	q 8h
Enalapril	0.15	Not established	q 12-24h
Calcium Channel Antagonist			
Nifedipine	0.25	3	q 4-6h
Diuretics			
Hydrochlorothiazide	1	2-3	q 12h
Furosemide	1	12	q 4-12h
Bumetanide	0.02-0.05	0.3	q 4-12h
Metolazone	0.1	3	q 12-24h
Spironolactone	1	3	q 6-12h
Beta-Adrenergic Antagonist			
Propranolol	1	8	q 6-12h
Atenolol	1	8	q 12-24h
Metoprolol	1	8	q 12-24h
Alpha-Adrenergic Antagonist			
Prazosin	0.05-0.1	0.5	q 6-8h
Alpha-Adrenergic Agonist			
Clonidine	0.05-0.1 (dose in mg)	0.5-0.6 (dose in mg)	q 6h
Vasodilators			
Hydralazine	0.75	7.5	q 6h
Minoxidil	0.1-0.2	1	q 12h

Modified from *Pediatrics* 98:649, 1996.

CONCLUSION

Evidence of a link between the onset of hypertension in childhood and adult morbidity and mortality from end-organ damage is increasing. As pediatricians become more aware of the importance of monitoring blood pressure in childhood, the opportunity exists for decreasing long-term adverse cardiovascular effects. Of equal importance are the continuing efforts to identify the underlying genetic and environmental causes of this potentially devastating condition.

REFERENCES

1. Adelman R: Neonatal hypertension, *Pediatr Clin North Am* 25:99, 1978.
2. Adelman RD: Long-term follow-up of neonatal renovascular hypertension, *Pediatr Nephrol* 1:35, 1987.
3. Bowdy RF, et al: Incidence of hypertension in infants on extracorporeal membrane oxygenation, *J Pediatr Surg* 25:258, 1990.
4. Colan S, et al: Noninvasive determination of systolic, diastolic and end-systolic blood pressure in neonates, infants and young children: comparison with central aortic pressure measurements, *Am J Cardiol* 52:867, 1983.
5. Deal JE, et al: Renovascular disease in childhood, *J Pediatr* 121:378, 1992.
6. DeSwiet M: The epidemiology of hypertension in children, *Br Med Bull* 42:34, 1986.
7. Fixler DE, et al: Ambulatory blood pressure monitoring in hypertensive adolescents, *Am J Hypertens* 3:289, 1990.
8. Frohlich ED, et al: The heart in hypertension, *New Engl J Med* 327:998, 1992.
9. Gordon T, Kannel WB, editors: *An epidemiological investigation of cardiovascular disease: the Framingham Study,* US DHEW, Sec 1-27, 1968-1971.

10. Hackman AM, Bricker JT: Preventive cardiology, hypertension and dyslipedemia. In Garson A Jr, editor: *The science and practice of pediatric cardiology,* ed 2, Baltimore, 1998, Williams and Wilkins.
11. Hagberg JM, et al: Effect of weight training on blood pressure and hemodynamics in hypertensive adolescents, *J Pediatr* 104:147, 1984.
12. Ingelfinger JR: Endocrine causes of hypertension. In Ingelfinger JR: *Pediatric hypertension,* Philadelphia, 1982, WB Saunders.
13. Ingelfinger JR: The renin-angiotensin system and other hormonal systems in the control of blood pressure. In Ingelfinger JR: *Pediatric hypertension,* Philadelphia, 1982, WB Saunders.
14. Lauer RM, Clarke WR: Childhood risk factors for high adult blood pressure: the Muscatine Study, *Pediatrics* 84:633, 1984.
15. Liberthson RR, et al: Coarctation of the aorta: review of 234 patients and clarification of management problems, *Am J Cardiol* 43:835, 1979.
16. McGrory WW, Klein AA, Rosenthal RA: Blood pressure, heart rate and plasma catecholamines in normal and hypertensive children and their siblings at rest and after standing, *Hypertension* 4:507, 1982.
17. Munger RG, Prineas RJ, Gomez-Marin O: Persistent elevation of blood pressure among children with a family history of hypertension: the Minneapolis Children's Blood Pressure Study, *J Hypertens* 6:647, 1988.
18. National Heart, Lung, and Blood Institute: Report of Second Task Force on Blood Pressure Control in Children—1987, *Pediatrics* 79:1, 1987.
19. Portman RJ, Yetman RJ, West MS: Efficacy of 24-hour ambulatory blood pressure monitoring in children, *J Pediatr* 118:842, 1991.
20. Rocchini AP, et al: Pathogenesis of paradoxical hypertension after coarctation repair, *Circulation* 54:382, 1976.
21. Sadowski RH, Falkner B: Hypertension in pediatric patients, *Am J Kid Dis* 3:305, 1996.
22. Sealey WC: Paradoxical hypertension after repair of coarctation of the aorta: a review of its causes, *Ann Thorac Surg* 50:323, 1990.
23. Sharma A, Sinaiko AR: Systemic hypertension. In Emmanouilides GC, editor: *Moss and Adams heart disease in infants, children and adolescents,* ed 5, Baltimore, 1995, Williams and Wilkins.
24. Shear CL, et al: Values of childhood blood pressure measurements and family history in predicting future blood pressure status: results from eight years of follow-up in the Bogalusa Heart Study, *Pediatrics* 77:862, 1986.
25. Shurtleff D: *Some characteristics related to the incidence of cardiovascular disease and death: the Framingham Study, 18-year follow-up,* US DHEW, Pub No (NIH) 74-599, Sept 30, 1974.
26. Sinaiko AR: Hypertension in children, *N Engl J Med* 335:1968, 1996.
27. Sinaiko AR: Treatment of hypertension in children (review), *Pediatr Nephrol* 8:603, 1994.
28. Update on the 1987 Task Force Report on High Blood Pressure in Children and Adolescents: a working group report from the National High Blood Pressure Education Program, *Pediatrics* 98:649, 1996.
29. Zinner SH, et al: Significance of blood pressure in infancy: familial aggregation and predictive effect on later blood pressure, *Hypertension* 7:411, 1985.

147 Hirsutism, Hypertrichosis, and Precocious Sexual Hair Development

Joan DiMartino-Nardi

The growth and distribution of body hair depends on the subject's ethnic background, age, and sex. Body hair generally is classified as either vellus or terminal.[9] Vellus hair is soft, short, fine, and less pigmented; terminal hair is coarse, long, and more pigmented. The term *sexual hair growth* refers to the presence of terminal hair on the face, chin, neck, midline chest, abdomen, upper and lower back, buttocks, axilla, pubic area, and inner aspect of the thigh. The transformation of vellus hair into terminal sexual hair is androgen dependent. Normal androgen production, in turn, depends on the gender and age of the patient. In girls, androgens normally are produced after the age of 8 years and in boys after the age of 9 years. Hence, pathological hair growth refers to the timing, as well as to the amount, of sexual hair growth.

Hirsutism refers to excessive body hair growth involving the sex hormone-dependent areas already described. The presence of hirsutism represents either androgen overproduction or enhanced androgen metabolism in the skin tissue. Androgen production and metabolism affect hair follicles and the sebaceous glands of the skin. Hence, hirsutism may be associated with acne vulgaris, although the degree of hirsutism and acne in patients varies tremendously.

Hypertrichosis refers to the generalized increase in fine body hair with no special preferential sites, most often not associated with pathological sex hormone production. Its presence usually is determined by genetic or ethnic background, but it may be induced by chronic ingestion of certain drugs such as oral diazoxide used for the treatment of islet cell dysmaturation syndrome. Hypertrichosis can be a feature of several congenital syndromes, including congenital hypertrichosis lanuginosa, generalized lipodystrophy, fetal hydantoin syndrome, mucopolysaccharidoses, trisomy 18, leprechaunism, and Cornelia de Lange's syndrome. In some cases, hypertrichosis may be an early manifestation of mild androgen excess and should be monitored closely.

Virilization, or *masculinization,* refers to the following symptoms of androgen excess: phallic or clitoral enlargement, masculine body habitus, temporal hair loss, voice changes, breast atrophy, and menstrual disorders. These symptoms are manifestations of significant pathological conditions causing androgen overproduction. These conditions are presented in this chapter and are discussed further in Chapter 165, Puberty: Normal and Abnormal.

Excessive androgen exposure can occur either prenatally or postnatally. As the development of the external genitalia occurs in the first trimester, exposure of the female infant to significant androgens during this time (as in the congenital adrenal hyperplasia syndromes) will cause genital ambiguity, including varying degrees of clitoral enlargement and labial fusion. The exposure of the female infant to excessive androgens after the first trimester does not result in labial fusion. The male infant exposed to excessive androgens in utero is not born with abnormal genitalia. If the condition causing androgen overproduction is left either undiagnosed or inadequately treated, the child will develop early sexual hair growth and will continue to virilize. In the growing child, excessive androgens contribute to an increased growth velocity, rapid epiphyseal maturation, excessive bone age advancement, and short adult stature.

HYPERANDROGENISM

Hirsutism in women and early sexual hair growth in girls and boys may represent either excessive or early hyperandrogenism from either gonadal or adrenal pathology.

Gonadal Androgen Production

Ovarian androgen production. *Gondarche* refers to the maturation of the hypothalamic/pituitary/gonadal axis.[16] The maturation of the pulsatile release of gonadotropin releasing hormone (GnRH) from the hypothalamus causes an increase in the amplitude and frequency of pituitary gonadotropin secretion and resultant gonadal maturation. Pituitary luteinizing hormone (LH) stimulates ovarian androgen synthesis occurring mainly in the theca cells, stroma cells, and the corpus luteum. The major androgens secreted by the ovaries include Δ-4-androstenedione and testosterone, and their levels gradually increase during gonadarche. These androgens contribute to the development of pubic hair, axillary hair and odor, and acne. The ovary converts androgens to estrogen in the granulosa cell layer via stimulation from pituitary follicle-stimulating hormone (FSH). Estrogens contribute to breast development, uterine enlargement, vaginal discharge, and menarche. Recently, insulin and insulin-like growth factor (IGF-1) have been shown to have a role in normal ovarian steroidogenesis.[10] The presence of true puberty can be confirmed by detecting a rise in gonadotropins in response to a bolus dose of GnRH in the GnRH stimulation test.[24] In addition, puberty is characterized by an increase in growth velocity (pubertal growth spurt) that results from an increase in growth hormone secretion.

TRUE PRECOCIOUS PUBERTY. The early maturation of the hypothalamic/pituitary/gonadal axis in girls before the age of 8 years is termed *true precocious puberty.* Clinically, girls present with the early development of pubic hair, axillary hair and odor, acne, and breast development. Most commonly, breast development occurs initially, but sexual hair growth actually may precede breast development. The suspicion of true precocious puberty can be confirmed by finding a pubertal gonadotropin response to a GnRH stimulation test. In most cases, early puberty is not caused by a specific identifiable lesion. However, in some cases, especially in the very young child (younger than 6 years of age), a hypothalamic or pituitary lesion may be the cause of early puberty. Hence, the evaluation of the precocious child should include magnetic resonance imaging (MRI) with gadolinium of the hypothalamic/pituitary area.

Precocious puberty can be associated with astrocytomas, craniopharyngiomas, ependymomas, germinomas, and gliomas. A hypothalamic hamartoma is a congenital malformation consisting of benign neurovascular tissue containing its own GnRH pulse generator.[29] Identification of a hamartoma is important because these lesions are amenable to medical therapy with GnRH analogs (see below). Precocious puberty also can be associated with virtually any CNS insult, such as trauma, surgery, inflammation, and neurological-mental deficits. Prolonged exposure to sex steroids also can precipitate precocious puberty. For example, in children who have poorly controlled adrenal hyperplasia or who have ovarian cysts, the chronic exposure to hyperandrogenism and estrogen can cause early maturation of the hypothalamic/pituitary/gonadal axis.[4]

Pubertal progression can be vary considerably in the child who is precocious. There are many children in whom puberty is slowly progressive and, hence, may not be of major concern to the patients or their families. However, some children can have rapid pubertal progression. In the latter group, psychosocial issues surrounding early puberty may be of particular concern. In general, a child's social maturity reflects chronological age rather than pubertal status. Furthermore, the early production of sex steroids can cause rapid epiphyseal maturation and resultant short stature. Obtaining a bone-age radiograph can help identify the child who is at risk for short stature.[2] Treatment with long-acting preparations of GnRH (GnRH analog) is available for those children whose families are particularly concerned about the psychosocial issues surrounding their child's early sexual development or the risk for short adult stature.[20] The GnRH analogs are effective in halting pubertal progression and preventing menses. In addition, via a reduction in growth hormone secretion, the child's growth velocity declines.[7] The reduction in sex steroids either halts or reduces the rate of bone-age maturation. The net result is an improvement in height prediction and, ultimately, adult stature.

OVARIAN ANDROGEN-PRODUCING TUMORS. Ovarian tumors producing androgens can present with either early sexual hair growth, hirsutism, or virilization. The concurrent secretion of estrogen can result in premature breast development, vaginal discharge, or irregular uterine bleeding. Patients may have excessive weight gain, acceleration of linear growth, and an advanced bone age. Abdominal symptoms (cramps, pain, mass, distention) also may occur. In the young child, these symptoms can mimic true precocious puberty. Rapid pubertal progression suggests the presence of a tumor. However, pubertal progression can appear to be normal. Virilization is never normal. Finding markedly elevated estradiol, androstenedione, or testosterone is consistent with an ovarian lesion. In contrast to true precocious puberty, the pseudo-precocious puberty resulting from an ovarian tumor occurs independently of the hypothalamic/pituitary axis. A GnRH stimulation test can distinguish between the two conditions, because the gonadotropin response is suppressed in pseudo-precocious puberty. Pelvic ultrasound can be useful in identifying ovarian lesions that may be cystic, solid, or both. The tumorous androgen-producing cells can occur in association with embryonal carcinomas, dysgerminomas, choriocarcinomas, gonadoblastomas, granulosa-thecal cell tumors, Sertoli-Leydig cell tumors, and arrhenoblastomas.[26,31] These tumors can occur in phenotypic females having an abnormal karyotype containing components of the Y chromosome. These dysgenetic gonads, in which differentiation into testis or ovary is either absent or incomplete, are at risk for malignant deterioration. Hence, prophylactic gonadectomy is recommended in these girls.

POLYCYSTIC OVARY SYNDROME. Polycystic ovary syndrome (PCOS) is a disorder that has a wide spectrum of hyperandrogenic signs and symptoms, including hirsutism, acne, and chronic anovulation with resultant irregular menses, amenorrhea, dysfunctional uterine bleeding, or infertility.[8] Virilization is not common with this condition. The precise etiology of chronic ovarian hyperandrogenism is not known, but several factors have been implicated, including altered gonadotropin secretion, hyperinsulinism, IGF-1 and alterations of IGF-1 binding proteins, hyperprolactinemia, thyroid disease, and adrenal hyperandrogenism. Hyperinsulinism stemming from insulin resistance is a frequent component of this condition. Ovarian hyperandrogenism also can occur in certain insulin-resistant syndromes such as leprechaunism (associated with severe congenital growth retardation) and the Kahn type B insulin resistance syndrome caused by the presence of circulating antibodies for the insulin receptor.[13,14] Women who have insulin resistance are at risk of developing the complications of chronic hyperinsulinism, including hyperpigmentation in the intertriginal skin sites known as *acanthosis nigricans,* impaired glucose tolerance, type 2 diabetes mellitus, lipid abnormalities (low HDL-cholesterol and high LDL-cholesterol), atherosclerosis, and cardiovascular disease.

The hormonal findings in PCOS can include an increased LH/FSH ratio greater than 2, generous levels of Δ-4-androstenedione, increased total and free testosterone with a reduced level of sex hormone–binding globulin and variable levels of estradiol. The presence of a total testosterone level greater than 150 ng/dl suggests the presence of a tumor. Insulin resistance can be confirmed by fasting hyperinsulinism and a reduced fasting glucose/insulin ratio.

Grossly, the ovaries in PCOS have subcapsular cysts that may be detected by ultrasound, but the absence of cysts on ultrasound does not exclude the diagnosis of PCOS. Hormonal evidence of PCOS can be discerned before the morphological changes can be appreciated by ultrasound. However, an ultrasound should be performed if an ovarian lesion is suspected.

Although PCOS has been studied extensively in adolescents and adult women, the developmental aspects of PCOS are yet to be elucidated. Recently, premature adrenarche has been identified as a possible risk factor for PCOS (see the section on premature adrenarche on this page).

Testicular androgen production

TRUE CENTRAL PRECOCIOUS PUBERTY. True central precocious puberty in boys refers to the activation of the hypothalamic/pituitary/gonadal axis before the age of 9 years. Levels of testosterone rise and a pubertal pattern of gonadotropin release can be detected with a GnRH stimulation test. The rise of gonadotropins causes testicular growth and full physical pubertal development. As in girls, an MRI of the pituitary gland should be performed to identify a hypothalamic or pituitary lesion. Although idiopathic central precocious puberty is more frequent in girls, boys more commonly have CNS pathology. Rarely, severe chronic hypothyroidism can be associated with true precocious puberty.[23] True precocious puberty in boys can be suppressed with GnRH analogs as outlined previously for girls.

PERIPHERAL OR PSEUDO-PRECOCIOUS PUBERTY. The production of sex steroids from either the testes or the adrenals independent of an activated hypothalamic/pituitary/gonadal axis is referred to as *peripheral* or *pseudo-precocious puberty*. The evaluation entails identifying the source of hyperandrogenism. The presence of enlarged testes suggests a gonadal source of hyperandrogenism; the presence of small (1 to 2 ml) testes is consistent with adrenal pathology (see the section on adrenal hyperandrogenism below).

TESTICULAR TUMORS. Leydig cell tumors and seminomas can produce testosterone. However, many testicular tumors can cause testicular enlargement without symptoms of hyperandrogenism. These can include germ cell tumors (embryonal carcinoma, endodermal sinus tumor, and teratoma). Boys who have cryptorchidism and delayed orchidopexy after the age of 6 years are at increased risk.[3,18] Dysgenetic gonads associated with androgen insensitivity, persistent Müllerian syndrome, true hermaphroditism, and Klinefelter's syndrome have a higher incidence of germ cell tumors as well.[5,6]

FAMILIAL GONADOTROPIN-INDEPENDENT PUBERTY. Familial gonadotropin-independent puberty is a condition in which an autosomal dominant, male-limited mutation of the LH receptor results in autonomous Leydig cell activity with resultant gonadotropin-independent precocity including gonadal steroidogenesis and spermatogenesis.[27] In these boys, who clinically present with precocious puberty, testosterone levels are high and GnRH-stimulated gonadotropins are low. If left undiagnosed, the chronic hyperandrogenism will eventually precipitate true precocious puberty.

CHORIONIC GONADOTROPIN-SECRETING TUMORS. Teratomas, embryonal tumors, hepatoblastomas, and CNS germinomas can produce human chorionic gonadotropin, which has been implicated in peripheral precocious puberty among males.

Adrenal hyperandrogenism. The adrenal glands produce three groups of steroids: glucocorticoids (cortisol), mineralocorticoids (aldosterone and desoxycorticosterone), and androgens (dehydroepiandrosterone, Δ-4-androstenedione, and testosterone). Glucocorticoid and androgen production are stimulated primarily by pituitary adrenocorticotropic hormone (ACTH). Exogenous glucocorticoids, such as dexamethasone, by suppressing ACTH, suppress glucocorticoid and androgen production. The mineralocorticoids are regulated primarily by the renin-angiotensin enzyme system, which is stimulated and suppressed by low and high salt diets, respectively. Disorders of adrenal hyperandrogenism caused by enzymatic defects of steroidogenesis (congenital adrenal hyperplasia) respond to stimulation and suppression tests. On the other hand, the functional adrenal tumors are characterized by their autonomous ability to produce any of the mentioned steroids independent of pituitary ACTH or the renin-angiotensin enzyme system. Hence, by and large, they do not respond to the dynamic tests known to effect adrenal steroidogenesis.

PREMATURE ADRENARCHE. Normal puberty is characterized by two generally simultaneous processes after the age of 8 years in girls and 9 years in boys: gonadarche and adrenarche. As outlined previously, gonadarche refers to the activation of the hypothalamic/pituitary/gonadal axis, and adrenarche refers to the activation of the hypothalamic/pituitary/adrenal axis, although the precise trigger for adrenarche is not known. Normal adrenarche results from the gradual increase in androgen biosynthesis that occurs as the innermost zona reticularis of the adrenal cortex matures. As puberty progresses, one can detect the gradual rise in androgen levels in response to a standard test of adrenal steroidogenesis known as the ACTH Stimulation test.[15] The adrenal androgen response depends on the age, gender, and pubertal status of the child. When adrenarche occurs in girls before the age of 8 years, and in boys before the age of 9 years, the condition is referred to as *premature adrenarche*. Clinically, these children present with the development of early sexual hair growth usually limited to the axilla and pubic area (i.e., the presence of facial, abdominal, or back hair is not consistent with this syndrome). These children may develop mild oily skin and minimal acne (especially on the nose and forehead). Axillary odor is a frequent occurrence and generally requires deodorant. These children are never virilized. In fact, the presence of virilization suggests either a tumor or an enzymatic defect of steroidogenesis. The child's growth velocity may increase slightly, and the bone-age maturation also may advance (but generally within 2 years of the chronological age). Androgen levels are in the range one usually sees during the early Tanner II-III stages of puberty.

In the past, pubertal progression was considered to be normal in children who had premature adrenarche. However, recent data indicate that the pubertal outcome may not always be benign. Of 35 adolescent girls from Italy and Spain who had functional ovarian hyperandrogenism, 45% had a history of premature adrenarche.[11] In a recent study of a large cohort of black and Caribbean Hispanic girls who had premature adrenarche, approximately one third of the 72 girls who underwent ACTH testing had ACTH-stimulated androgens more than two standard deviations above the mean for normal Tanner II-III pubertal girls.[1] In another study, the same group noted that approximately 50% of the black and Hispanic girls who had premature adrenarche had mild acanthosis nigricans.[21] Knowing the association between acanthosis nigricans, hyperinsulinism stemming from insulin resistance, and hyperandrogenism in adolescent and adult women who have polycystic ovarian disease, the authors assessed insulin sensitivity in 35 minority youths who had premature adrenarche.[30] Essentially, those girls who were markedly insulin resistant had the more severe hyperandrogenism. These insulin-resistant girls were heavier than those girls whose insulin sensitivity was normal. This suggests that hyperinsulinism in these patients, possibly exacerbated by their obesity, has a role in the hyperandrogenism of these girls who have premature adrenarche just as it does in the more severe hyperandrogenism of women who have PCOS. This is of particular concern because these minority children are known to be at increased risk for the complications of hyperinsulinism (including noninsulin-dependent diabetes mellitus, lipid abnormalities, PCOS, and cardiovascular disease). Long-term studies are necessary to determine which of these girls are truly at risk for these complications. Perhaps early identification will permit early intervention.

Obesity is not the sole factor causing insulin resistance. Children born with intrauterine growth retardation have been noted to develop insulin resistance, short stature, and premature adrenarche. In addition, in a recent study, girls who had premature adrenarche, functional ovarian hyperandrogenism, and hyperinsulinism had the lowest birth weights of the entire group of girls who had premature adrenarche.[12] Perhaps the stress of intrauterine growth retardation induces insulin resistance and alterations in adrenal physiology.

ENZYMATIC DEFECTS OF STEROIDOGENESIS. The term *adrenal hyperplasia* refers to the histological change that occurs in the adrenal glands as a result of a deficiency of one of the several enzymes necessary for normal steroid biosynthesis.[19] Cortisol is the most important of the glucocorticoids made by the adrenal gland, and its synthesis is regulated primarily by a sensitive negative feedback system with pituitary ACTH. Any condition that causes a decrease in cortisol biosynthesis results in a compensatory rise in ACTH. In the enzymatic defects of cortisol biosynthesis, cortisol levels fall. The compensatory rise in ACTH stimulates adrenal steroidogenesis, with the resultant accumulation of steroids proximal to the enzymatic defect. These precursor steroids then are shunted to the androgen pathways, with resultant hyperandrogenism. Three autosomal recessive disorders of adrenal steroidogenesis cause cortisol deficiency and hyperandrogenism: 21-hydroxylase deficiency, 11-beta-hydroxylase deficiency, and 3-beta-hydroxysteroid dehydrogenase deficiency. Diagnosis is confirmed by finding elevated precursor steroids either in the basal state or in response to a bolus dose of ACTH.

The specific symptoms of the disorder depend on which class of steroids is deficient and which is overproduced. In the severe salt-wasting form of 21-hydroxylase deficiency, both cortisol and mineralocorticoid synthesis are interrupted and androgens are overproduced. The prenatal exposure of the genetic female external genitalia to the high androgens in the first trimester will cause genital ambiguity. Males do not present with genital abnormalities. Children of either gender will develop salt-wasting symptoms generally within the first 3 months of life. In the simple virilizing form of 21-hydroxylase deficiency, the genetic female will be born with genital ambiguity; the genetic male will appear normal. In either form of 21-hydroxylase deficiency, delay in diagnosis or inadequate treatment will result in postnatal virilization, with progressive clitoral and phallic enlargement, early development of axillary and pubic hair, axillary odor and acne, increased growth velocity with crossing of percentile growth channels, advanced bone age, precocious puberty, and ultimately, short stature. Young women inadequately treated will develop PCOS, with its associated menstrual irregularities and infertility. The diagnosis is confirmed by finding an elevated 17-hydroxyprogesterone level either basally or in response to a bolus dose of ACTH.

The 21-hydroxylase gene is situated in the HLA major histocompatibility complex on the short arm of the sixth chromosome. Molecular genetic studies have identified the precise location of the gene. Currently, an affected fetus can be identified by chorionic villus sampling (CVS) between the eighth and eleventh week of gestation.[28] This permits early diagnosis and treatment by administration of dexamethasone to the mother. The goal is to prevent genital ambiguity in the affected female fetus. The effectiveness of therapy depends on the early initiation of suppressive glucocorticoid therapy to the mother by 6 to 7 weeks of gestation before onset of adrenal androgen secretion. Hence, effective treatment must be initiated before the diagnosis of 21-hydroxylase deficiency can be made by CVS. This form of preventive therapy has resulted in considerable controversy because, by the nature of the treatment protocols, many unaffected fetuses would be treated.

The nonclassic late-onset form of 21-hydroxylase deficiency has clinical variability and can present at any age with symptoms of hyperandrogenism. However, affected girls do not have genital ambiguity. The spectrum of symptoms include premature pubic and axillary hair growth, premature axillary odor, acne, increased growth velocity and advanced bone age, hirsutism, male-pattern baldness in young women, and PCOS. Because the hyperandrogenism in this form of 21-hydroxylase deficiency is not as severe as the congenital classic form, the basal unstimulated 17-hydroxyprogesterone may not be elevated. Hence, the diagnosis is confirmed by detecting an exaggerated 17-hydroxyprogesterone response to ACTH stimulation.

Treatment of 21-hydroxylase deficiency includes glucocorticoid replacement therapy as hydrocortisone at a dose of 10 to 25 mg/m^2/day to maintain normal growth and development and a normal rate of bone-age advancement. The salt-retaining steroid 9-alpha fludrocortisone acetate is used to treat those children who have the salt-wasting variant and sometimes is useful for those simple virilizers who tend to have elevated plasma renin activity. Although the introduction of steroid radioimmunoassay methods has facilitated management of these children, growth and development are not always optimal. Studies are under way to determine if the addition of androgen-receptor blockers will improve growth.

Deficiency of the 11-beta-hydroxylase enzyme can also present with the more severe congenital syndrome characterized by sexual ambiguity in affected females. Like 21-hydroxylase deficiency, inadequate therapy can result in early virilization. The accumulation of desoxy-corticosterone, a weak mineralocorticoid, will eventually lead to low renin hypertension. Milder forms of 11-beta-hydroxylase deficiency have been described and present very similarly to the late-onset form of 21-hydroxylase deficiency. The diagnosis is made by finding an elevated 11-deoxycortisol that is stimulated by ACTH and is suppressed by dexamethasone.

Complete 3-beta-hydroxysteroid deficiency presents with ambiguity in both sexes, as well as a salt-wasting crisis. Milder forms have been described and present similarly to late-onset 21-hydroxylase deficiency.[17,25] Treatment is similar to that already described for 21-hydroxylase deficiency.

IDIOPATHIC HIRSUTISM/ACNE

The term *idiopathic hirsutism/acne* refers to females who present with these signs without any other signs of androgen excess and who have normal circulating androgen concentrations. Menses and reproductive function also should be normal. The hirsutism and acne in these women have been attributed to "increased peripheral metabolism" of androgens.[22]

EVALUATION

The evaluation of the child or adolescent who has either early sexual hair development or hirsutism begins with the history. The rapid development of sexual hair associated with symptoms of virilization (e.g., severe acne, voice changes, change in body habitus, clitoral or phallic enlargement, rapid growth) suggests the presence of marked hyperandrogenism as would occur in the severe adrenal enzyme deficiencies or with either an adrenal or ovarian tumor. The presence of sexual hair growth with early breast development is consistent with either true or pseudo-precocious puberty. The family history should include information regarding cardiovascular disease, atherosclerosis, obesity, and diabetes, which can be seen in the families of patients who have premature adrenarche and PCOS. A family history of early fetal demise suggests the presence of adrenal hyperplasia. Hypertension on physical examination can occur with either 11-hydroxylase deficiency, an adrenal tumor, or obesity. The presence of virilization should be noted carefully because this indicates severe hyperandrogenism. An increase in growth velocity with "crossing percentile channels" suggests precocious puberty, tumor, or adrenal hyperplasia. Labial fusion indicates exposure to hyperandrogenism during fetal life, as occurs in the congenital adrenal hyperplasia syndromes.

The hormonal evaluation should include the GnRH Stimulation test if precocious puberty is identified to distinguish true from pseudo-sexual precocity. The evaluation of early sexual hair growth or hirsutism without virilization should include an ACTH stimulation test to identify an enzymatic defect of adrenal hormone biosynthesis. The presence of virilization and high levels of testosterone (>150 ng/dl) or of dehydroepiandrosterone sulfate (>750 μg/dl) suggests an ovarian or adrenal tumor; appropriate imaging should be done with ultrasound, computed tomography (CT) scan, or MRI. A karyotype should be obtained if an ovarian tumor is suspected, because dysgenetic gonads may deteriorate to malignancy. If the ACTH testing is consistent with an enzymatic defect in the virilized patient, the benign nature of the condition should be confirmed by suppression of hyperandrogenism with dexamethasone. Imaging studies always should be done in equivocal cases.

SUMMARY

Fortunately, our knowledge of androgen physiology and metabolism has made us more aware of the pathophysiology of hirsutism and early sexual hair growth. Historically, children and adolescents who presented with these signs were neglected and not evaluated because their abnormal hair growth was often minimized or was attributed to a familial tendency without underlying pathology. Although our tools for evaluation and treatment have improved during the past 20 years, much needs to be learned about the natural history of PCOS and of idiopathic hirsutism so that prevention and treatment can be improved. Furthermore, improvement in therapy is needed.

REFERENCES

1. Banerjee S, et al: Hormonal findings in African-American and Caribbean Hispanic girls with premature adrenarche: implications for polycystic ovarian syndrome, *Pediatrics* 102, e36, 1998.
2. Bar A, et al: Bayley-Pinneau method of height prediction in girls with central precocious puberty: correlation with adult height, *J Pediatr* 126: 955, 1995.
3. Batata MA, Whitmore WFJ, Chu FCH: Cryptorchidism and testicular cancer, *J Urol* 124:382, 1980.
4. Boepple PA, et al: The natural history of autonomous gonadal function, adrenarche, and central puberty in gonadotropin-independent precocious puberty, *J Clin Endocrinol Metab* 75:1550, 1992.
5. Cassio A, et al: Incidence of intratubular germ cell neoplasia in androgen insensitivity syndrome, *Acta Endocrinol (Copenh)* 123:416, 1990.
6. Dexeus FH, et al: Genetic abnormalities in men with germ cell tumors, *J Urol* 140:80, 1988.
7. DiMartino-Nardi J: The effect of luteinizing hormone-releasing hormone analog for central precocious puberty on growth hormone (GH) and GH binding protein, *J Clin Endocrinol Metab* 78:664, 1994.
8. Dunaif A: Insulin resistance and the polycystic ovary syndrome: mechanism and implications for pathogenesis, *Endocr Rev* 18:774, 1997.
9. Ebling FJG: Hair follicles and associated glands as androgen targets in androgen metabolism in hirsute and normal females. In Horton R, Lobo RA, editors: *Clinics in endocrinology and metabolism,* Philadelphia, 1986, WB Saunders.
10. Giudice L: The insulin and insulin-like growth factor system in normal and abnormal ovarian follicle development, *Am J Med* (suppl 1A):485, 1995.
11. Ibanez L, et al: Postpubertal outcome in girls diagnosed of premature pubarche during childhood: increased frequency of functional ovarian hyperandrogenism, *J Clin Endocrinol Metab* 76:1599, 1993.
12. Ibanez L, et al: Precocious pubarche, hyperinsulinism and ovarian hyperandrogenism in girls: relation to reduced fetal growth, *J Clin Edocrinol Metab* 83:3558, 1998.
13. Kadawaki T, et al: Two mutant alleles of the insulin receptor gene in a patient with extreme insulin resistance, *Science* 240:787, 1998.
14. Kahn CR, White MF: The insulin receptor and the molecular mechanism of insulin action, *J Clin Invest* 82:1151, 1988.
15. Lashansky G, et al: Normative data for adrenal steroidogenesis in a healthy pediatric population age and sex related changes after adrenocorticotropin stimulation, *J Clin Endocrinol Metab* 73:674, 1991.
16. Lee PA: Disorders of puberty. In Lifshitz F, editor: *Pediatric endocrinology,* New York, 1996, Marcel Dekker.
17. Lobo RA, Goebelsmann U, Horton R: Evidence for the importance of peripheral tissue events in the development of hirsutism in polycystic ovary syndrome, *J Clin Endocrinol Metab* 57:393, 1983.
18. Martin DC: Germinal cell tumors of the testis after orchiopexy, *J Urol* 121:422, 1979.
19. New MI, Ghizzoni L, Speiser PW: Update on congenital adrenal hyperplasia. In Lifshitz F, editor: *Pediatric endocrinology,* New York, 1996, Marcel Dekker.
20. Oerter KE, et al: Adult height in precocious puberty after long-term treatment with deslorelin, *J Clin Endocrinol Metab* 73:1235, 1991.
21. Oppenheimer E, Linder B, DiMartino-Nardi J: Decreased insulin sensitivity in prepubertal girls with premature adrenarche and acanthosis nigricans, *J Clin Endocrinol Metab* 80:614, 1995.
22. Pang S: Hirsutism and polycystic ovary syndrome. In Lifshitz F, editor: *Pediatric endocrinology,* New York, 1996, Marcel Dekker.
23. Pringle PJ, et al: Abnormal pubertal development in primary hypothyroidism, *Clin Endocrinol (Oxf)* 28:479, 1988.

24. Reiter EO, Kaplan SL, Conte FA: Responsitivity of pituitary gonadotropes to luteinizing hormone-releasing factor in idiopathic precocious puberty, precocious thelarche, precocious adrenarche and in patients treated with medroxy-progesterone acetate, *Pediatr Res* 9:111, 1975.
25. Rosenfield RL, et al: Pubertal presentation of congenital Δ-5-3β-hydroxysteroid dehydrogenase deficiency, *J Clin Endocrinol Metab* 51:345, 1980.
26. Roth LM, et al: Sertoli-Leydig cell tumors: a clinicopathological study of 34 cases, *Cancer* 48:187, 1981.
27. Shenker A, et al: A constitutively activating mutation of the luteinizing hormone receptor in familial male precocious puberty, *Nature* 365:652, 1993.
28. Speiser PW, et al: First trimester prenatal treatment and molecular genetic diagnosis of congenital adrenal hyperplasia (21-hydroxylase deficiency), *J Clin Endocrinol Metab* 70:838, 1990.
29. Starceski PJ, et al: Hypothalamic hamartomas and sexual precocity: evaluation of treatment options, *Am J Dis Child* 144:225, 1990.
30. Vuguin P, et al: The role of insulin sensitivity, insulin-like growth factor and insulin-like growth factor binding proteins 1 and 3 in the hyperandrogenism of African-American and Caribbean Hispanic girls with premature adrenarche, *J Clin Endocrinol Metab* 84:2037, 1999.
31. Young RH, Dickerson RG, Scully RE: Juvenile granulosa cell tumor of the ovary: a clinicopathological analysis of 125 cases, *Am J Surg Pathol* 8:575, 1984.

148 Hoarseness

Susan E. Levitzky

Hoarseness, a symptom of voice dysfunction, is a change in voice quality often described as harsh, grating, rough, noisy, or raspy. Hoarseness should not be confused with (1) stridor, which is a high-pitched whistling sound; (2) the muffled "hot potato mouth" speech of persons who have supraglottic lesions; or (3) the weak, "breathy" speech of persons who have neuromuscular disorders. The main significance of hoarseness is that some process has affected the structure or function of the vocal cords. This may be an early sign of local disease or a manifestation of a systemic illness. This chapter highlights the common causes of hoarseness in newborns, infants, children, and adolescents.

According to voice surveys conducted among elementary school children, the prevalence of chronic hoarseness ranges from 5% to more than 20%.[25,37,58] Statistics reflecting the incidence of acute hoarseness are not available.

HISTORY

When evaluating a child who is hoarse, it is essential to obtain a thorough history from the parents. In hoarseness of sudden onset, an inflammatory process should be considered. In acute laryngitis, symptoms of rhinorrhea, cough, and sore throat often precede the hoarseness. Occasionally a history of foreign-body aspiration or direct laryngeal trauma may explain acute hoarseness. Gradually progressive or persistent hoarseness implies a more insidious and chronic disease process. Information should be gleaned regarding age of onset, excessive use of the voice, associated allergies, chronic chest congestion with recurrent wheezing or pneumonia (gastroesophageal reflux), sluggishness associated with any decrease in the yearly rate of height increase (hypothyroidism), chronic postnasal drip, recent tuberculosis intradermal test conversion, underlying systemic disease, and change of hoarseness with change in position (mobile lesion). Thus, a thorough review of systems is indicated to uncover any conditions that may be responsible for or associated with persistent hoarseness.

PHYSICAL EXAMINATION

A complete physical examination should be performed to detect any unsuspected disease. One especially should observe for any signs of increased respiratory effort (stridor, drooling, nasal flaring, retractions, tachypnea, or use of accessory muscles). If any of these is present, the child should be evaluated promptly by a qualified, experienced physician for potentially life-threatening airway obstruction (see Chapters 173, Stridor, and 275, Airway Obstruction). If stridor is not present, the physician may proceed with the examination, noting any of the following: neck masses (hemangiomas, lymphangiomas); local adenopathy; tracheal shift; thyromegaly or thyroid nodules; pale, boggy nasal mucosa (allergies); chest congestion (gastroesophageal reflux); cardiac murmurs or enlargement; cutaneous hemangiomas; café-au-lait spots; pallor; rash; joint swelling; or splenomegaly. With clues from the history and physical examination, the physician must decide what further investigation is indicated.

FURTHER INVESTIGATION

Direct laryngoscopy by a skilled endoscopist has become the mainstay in diagnosing laryngeal disease.[29,43,61] Categories of hoarseness meriting direct laryngoscopy include (1) congenital hoarseness; (2) possible foreign body in the larynx; (3) progressive, unremitting hoarseness of unknown cause; (4) hoarseness of unknown cause with stridor; and (5) acquired hoarseness persisting for longer than 2 to 3 weeks.[24] Other diagnostic modalities complement but do not replace laryngoscopy. True lateral and anteroposterior roentgenographic views of the soft tissues of the neck, computed tomography (CT) scans, and magnetic resonance imaging (MRI) studies may reveal vocal cord immobility, cysts, foreign bodies, or masses.[33] A chest roentgenogram may demonstrate a mediastinal mass. Fiberscopic stroboscopic videolaryngoscopy, a procedure described recently for documenting laryngeal images and voice simultaneously, can be very useful for clinical diagnosis.[57,63] Oscilloscopic readings of both pitch and intensity using equipment such as the Visi-Pitch (Kay Elemetrics) serve as valuable adjuncts in following perturbation (the degree of hoarseness of the voice). This procedure is simple, brief, highly accurate, and cost effective.[21]

CAUSES OF HOARSENESS

Newborns

Lifesaving measures increasingly are successful in treating premature and newborn infants who are in respiratory distress, but reports on resultant laryngeal injuries also have increased. Following intubation, an infant may sustain arytenoid cartilage dislocation, or ulceration or edema of the vocal cords. Unilateral or bilateral vocal cord palsy may result from birth trauma, with stretching of the neck and with it the recurrent laryngeal nerve during a breech delivery. The prognosis is good for unilateral laryngeal paralysis and poor for bilateral paralysis.[17]

Congenital anomalies causing hoarseness include the following[4]:

1. *Laryngeal web.* This is a persistent membrane of tissue usually located at the anterior commissure between the true vocal cords. The thickness and extent of the web are variable and determine the mode of therapy. Webs have been associated with cardiac defects, most often with ventricular septal defects.
2. *Laryngeal cysts and laryngoceles.* Cysts arise from the mucus glands of the laryngeal ventricle and contain fluid, causing stridorous symptoms soon after birth. The endoscopist must be prepared to deal with complete airway obstruction because laryngeal edema or hemorrhage into the cyst may occur during endoscopy. Laryngoceles are dilations of the laryngeal saccule that contain air and communicate with the lumen of the larynx. Symptoms are typically intermittent, especially during acute respiratory infections. Lateral neck roentgenograms show a supraglottic mass that may disappear when the child is quiet. Endoscopic deroofing of symptomatic laryngoceles may be advised.[21]
3. *Laryngeal fissure or cleft.* This is a rare anomaly characterized by an incomplete closure of the posterior larynx. This vertical slit often extends below the vocal cords, causing a tracheoesophageal fistula in 20% of cases. Feeding-associated respiratory distress usually overshadows the voice disorder.
4. *Laryngeal hemangiomas.* These rarely cause hoarseness in newborns. In 50% of cases, skin hemangiomas also are present. Symptoms worsen with crying or with an intercurrent upper respiratory tract infection. Most of these hemangiomas regress spontaneously, but if airway compromise develops, steroid and/or surgical laser therapy may avert the need for a tracheostomy.

Infants who have Down syndrome have a harsh, flat, low-pitched cry. Infants who have de Lange's syndrome have a coarse, growling cry. The cry of babies who have untreated hypothyroidism has a hoarse, "gravelly" quality resulting from myxedematous infiltration of the vocal cords. Rarer causes of hoarseness with onset in the newborn period include Farber's lipogranulomatosis,[38] lipoid proteinosis of Urbach and Wiethe,[8,16] pachyonychia congenita,[62] and laryngoonychocutaneous syndrome.[31] Hypocalcemic tetany may cause laryngospasm with accompanying hoarseness and stridor.

Infants, Children, and Adolescents

Infectious inflammatory causes. By far the majority of cases of acute hoarseness in childhood are related to respiratory tract infections, especially those caused by adenoviruses 4 and 7, influenza A, and parainfluenza I. Acute laryngitis and acute laryngotracheobronchitis (infectious croup) result in vocal cord inflammation.[49] Impaired nasal respiration during a cold leads to mouth-breathing and drying of the vocal cord mucosa, with resultant hoarseness on arising in the morning. Children who have spasmodic croup have recurrent episodes of laryngeal obstruction and wake up at night with a hoarse voice, a croupy cough, and inspiratory stridor (see Chapter 277, Croup [Acute Laryngotracheobronchitis]). Children who have epiglottitis are not hoarse, and cough is not a prominent symptom, but inspiratory and expiratory stridor are (see Chapter 284, Epiglottitis). As the epiglottis swells, the voice becomes muffled and drooling sets in. Laryngeal diphtheria should be considered in the differential diagnosis of progressive hoarseness. With lapses in immunization practices and the ongoing influx of refugees into the United States, sporadic outbreaks of diphtheria still occur. Laryngeal diphtheria usually develops as a downward extension of the tonsillar-pharyngeal membrane. Sudden death from laryngeal obstruction also may occur. Membranous laryngitis after infectious mononucleosis also has been reported.[18] Other causes of hoarseness in this age group are laryngeal candidiasis and tuberculosis, especially in the immunocompromised host, either following immunosuppressive treatment in a transplant patient or complicating combined steroid and antibiotic usage in croup[10,42] Febrile, immunocompromised or neutropenic children who are hoarse should have laryngoscopy promptly so that fungal involvement can be ruled out.[23,54] Cytomegalovirus (CMV) infection of the laryngeal nerve has resulted in hoarseness in adults who have acquired immunodeficiency syndrome (AIDS)[56] and should be considered in immunocompromised children who have CMV infection who also develop vocal cord paralysis. Rarely, cryptococcal laryngitis may occur in patients who have AIDS.[13] Hoarseness secondary to left recurrent laryngeal nerve palsy can develop during the healing stage of fibrosing tuberculous mediastinitis and may be permanent.[41,55] The recent upsurge in maternal and congenital syphilis requires physicians to consider this infection in the evaluation of a hoarse infant.[48]

Noninfectious inflammatory disease. Gastroesophageal reflux may result in hoarseness secondary to acid or chemical laryngitis.* Thickened feedings; 30-degree prone, upright positioning; antacids; and histamine H_2 receptor antagonists usually control the reflux, and eventually a normal voice returns. In allergic laryngeal disease, children who have respiratory allergies and rhinosinusitis may develop vocal cord edema and inflammation and the hoarseness that accompanies these changes.[30] Occasionally, patients using inhaled steroids for asthma control may develop secondary dysphonia. Discontinuation of treatment or the addition of a volumetric spacer device for administration leads to resolution.[10]

Inhalation of a caustic or hot gas or ingestion of salicylic acid may lead to vocal cord edema and hoarseness in susceptible individuals. Cricoarytenoid arthritis, sometimes associated with juvenile rheumatoid arthritis, can cause painful hoarseness.

Traumatic causes. The most common cause of chronic hoarseness in school-age children is the development of vocal cord nodules. The nodules usually occur bilaterally and are whitish protuberances on the free margin of the true vocal cords, located at the junction of their anterior and middle thirds, which is the area of maximum vibration. Nodule

*References 7, 15, 22, 26, 36, 53, 60.

formation is attributed to submucosal hemorrhages caused by screaming or shouting. The hemorrhages then are organized into fibrous nodules or polyps. Speech therapy may resolve the nodules and alleviate the hoarseness. Personality and emotional factors have been implicated in the abnormal vocal outbursts of these children, more often boys. Surgical removal of the nodules usually is not indicated, but in specific situations, such as when the hoarseness has lasted for several years without improvement, with worsening, or with psychological sequelae, vocal nodule microsurgical removal should be considered.[28,40,52]

Acute hoarseness may follow endotracheal intubation, aspiration of a foreign body, fracture of the larynx, or cardiac surgery.[5,34] Laryngoscopic investigation and laryngeal electromyography of postoperative hoarseness can be helpful in clarifying the type of laryngeal injury.[43,64]

Tumors. Juvenile laryngeal papillomatosis is the most common benign laryngeal tumor that occurs during childhood. Such papillomas usually present with hoarseness in children between 2 and 7 years of age, but they may occur in newborns. The tumor consists of wartlike proliferations of stratified squamous epithelium arising in the glottic region, but occasionally it spreads to involve the trachea, the bronchi, and rarely, the lung parenchyma. Caused by human papillomaviruses, this tumor may involute spontaneously during puberty.[3,19,20,27] Rarely, lethal asphyxiation can occur.[2,59] Carbon dioxide laser excision has been very successful in maintaining a patent airway and preserving vocal cord function.[39,50] Leukocyte interferon administration and ribavirin treatment have shown promise in inducing remission.[12,46] A mediastinal cystic hygroma has been reported in a patient who has AIDS whose only symptom was hoarseness.[1] Laryngeal granular cell tumor is an uncommon benign tumor usually seen in adults. However, this tumor should be considered in a hoarse child who has a vocal cord tumor or a subglottic mass. Local excision performed endoscopically usually is curative.[14,32]

Rhabdomyosarcoma of the larynx is a rare but highly malignant tumor that presents with painful hoarseness. Combined partial laryngectomy, radiotherapy, and chemotherapy have effected high cure rates.[35,44,47]

Miscellaneous causes. Miscellaneous causes of hoarseness during childhood and adolescence include sarcoidosis,[6] which may cause supraglottic granulomas and compression of the left recurrent laryngeal nerve by enlarged lymph nodes; laryngeal neurofibromatosis, amyloidosis, or lipoid proteinosis; and vocal cord paralysis secondary to central nervous system malfunction, such as the Arnold-Chiari malformation. In cardiovocal syndrome, vocal cord paralysis results from impingement on the left recurrent laryngeal nerve by an enlarged pulmonary artery or an enlarged left atrium.[11]

Relapsing polychondritis is a rare autoimmune-related disorder that has an insidious onset of hoarseness, airway narrowing, and nonspecific systemic complaints. Its management includes steroids and immunosuppressive agents; tracheostomy to maintain an airway is required in some patients.[51]

Other causes of hoarseness that occur during adolescence include abusive, vigorous, loud singing and yelling (without vocal cord nodule formation)[52]; pubertal voice changes,[9] laryngeal trauma sustained during automobile and motorcycle accidents,[45] smoking, myasthenia gravis, multiple sclerosis, and functional dysphonia (whispering syndrome in girls and falsetto voice use in boys).[14]

RESTORING AND PRESERVING NORMAL PHONATION

Speaking in a pleasant-sounding voice is especially important for older children and adolescents because peers are very cognizant and often intolerant of deviations from the norm. Once the cause of a child's or adolescent's hoarseness is determined, every attempt should be made to restore and preserve vocal function. Voice therapy with a speech pathologist is useful for children who have functional hoarseness as well as for those who have organic hoarseness.

REFERENCES

1. Agartan C, et al: A case of mediastinal cystic hygroma whose only symptom was hoarseness, *J Pediatr Surg* 33:642, 1998.
2. Balazic J, Masera A, Poljak M: Sudden death caused by laryngeal papillomatosis, *Acta Otolaryngol Suppl* 517:111, 1997.
3. Bauman NM, Smith RJH: Recurrent respiratory papillomatosis, *Pediatr Clin North Am* 43:1385, 1996.
4. Benjamin B: Congenital disorders of the larynx. In Cummings CW, editor: *Otolaryngology, head and neck surgery,* ed 2, St Louis, 1993, Mosby.
5. Benjamin B: Prolonged intubation injuries of the larynx: endoscopic diagnosis, classification and treatment, *Ann Otol Rhinol Laryngol* 160 (suppl):1, 1993.
6. Benjamin B, Dalton C, Croxson G: Laryngoscopic diagnosis of laryngeal sarcoid, *Ann Otol, Rhinol Laryngol* 104:529, 1995.
7. Bobin S, Attal P: Laryngotracheal manifestations of gastrointestinal esophageal reflux in children, *Pediatr Pulmonol* 18 (suppl):73, 1999.
8. Bohme M, Wahlgren CF: Lipoid proteinosis in three children, *Acta Paediatr* 85:1003, 1996.
9. Boltezar IH, Burger ZR, Zargi M: Instability of voice in adolescence: pathologic condition or normal developmental variation? *Pediatrics* 130:185, 1997.
10. Burton DM, et al: Candida laryngotracheitis: a complication of combined steroid and antibiotic usage in croup, *Int J Pediatr Otolaryngol* 23:171, 1992.
11. Chan P, et al: Cardiovocal (Ortner's) syndrome: left recurrent laryngeal nerve palsy, *Eur J Med* 1:492, 1992.
12. Chireshkin DG, et al: Effectiveness of human leukocytic interferon in children with papillomatosis of the larynx, trachea and bronchi, *Vestn Otol Rhinol Laryngol* 5:19, 1991.
13. Chongkolwatana C, et al: Primary cryptococcal infection of the larynx in a patient with AIDS: a case report, *J Med Assoc Thailand* 81:462, 1998.
14. Conley SF, Milbrath MM, Beste DJ: Pediatric laryngeal granular cell tumor, *J Otolaryngol* 21:450, 1992.
15. Contencin P, et al: Gastroesophageal reflux and dysphonia in children, *Rev Laryngol Otol Rhinol* 118(4):253, 1997.
16. Cote DN: Head and neck manifestation of lipoid proteinosis, *Otolaryngol Head Neck Surg* 119:144, 1998.
17. de Gaudemar I, et al: Outcome of laryngeal paralysis in neonates: a long-term retrospective study of 113 cases, *Int J Pediatr Otorhinolaryngol* 34:101, 1996.
18. Di Giorolamo S, et al: A specific membranous laryngitis after infectious mononucleosis, *Int J Pediatr Otorhinolaryngol* 34:171, 1996.

19. Doyle DJ, et al: Recurrent respiratory papillomatosis: juvenile vs adult forms, *Laryngoscope* 104:524, 1994.
20. Doyle-Lloyd DJ, Gianoli GJ: Laryngeal papillomatosis, *J La State Med Soc* 144:551, 1992.
21. Drake MK, Zubick HH: Evaluation of vocal function. In Fried MP, editor: *The larynx: a multidisciplinary approach,* St Louis, 1996, Mosby.
22. Euler AR: Upper respiratory complications of gastroesophageal reflux in adult and pediatric age patients, *Digest Dis* 16:111, 1998.
23. Forest LA, Weed H: Candida laryngitis appearing as leukoplakia and gastroesophageal reflux disease, *J Voice* 12:91, 1998.
24. Garrett CG, Ossoff RH: Hoarseness: contemporary diagnosis and management *Compr Ther* 21:705, 1995.
25. Gray SD, Smith MC, Schneider H: Voice disorders in children, *Pediatr Clin North Am* 43:1357, 1996.
26. Gumpert L, et al: Hoarseness and gastroesophageal reflux in children, *J Laryngol Otol* 112:49, 1998.
27. Hartley C, et al: Recurrent respiratory papillomatosis: the Manchester experience, 1974-1992, *J Laryngol Otol* 108:226, 1994.
28. Hirschberg J, et al: Voice disorders in children, *Int J Pediatr Otorhinolaryngol* 32(suppl):S109, 1995.
29. Hocevar-Boltezar I, et al: Neonatal and pediatric micro subglottiscope set, *Ann Otol Rhinol Laryngol* 100(4 Pt I):325, 1991.
30. Hocevar-Boltezar I, Radsel Z, Zargi M: The role of allergy in the etiopathogens of laryngeal mucosal lesions, *Acta Laryngologica* 527(suppl): 134, 1997.
31. Hodges UM, Lloyd-Thomas A: Anaesthesia for airway obstruction in laryngo-onycho-cutaneous syndrome, *Anaesth* 48:503, 1993.
32. Holland RS: Granular cell tumor of the larynx in a six-year-old child: case report and review of the literature, *Ear Nose Throat* 77:652, 1998.
33. Hudgins PA, et al: The normal pediatric larynx on CT and MR, *Am J Neuroradiol* 18:239, 1997.
34. Inada T, Fujise K, Shingu K: Hoarseness after cardiac surgery, *J Cardiovasc Surg* 39:455, 1998.
35. Kato MA, et al: Rhabdomyosarcoma of the larynx in children: a series of five patients treated in the Institute Gustave, *Med Pediatr Oncol* 19:110, 1991.
36. Katz P: Ambulatory esophageal and hypopharyngeal pH monitoring in patients with hoarseness, *Am J Gastroenterol* 85:38, 1990.
37. Kauffmann I, et al: Chronic hoarseness in children: evaluation based on personal series of 64 cases, *Pediatrics* 47:319, 1992.
38. Kim YJ, et al: A case of Farber lipogranulomatosis, *J Korean Med Sci* 13:95, 1998.
39. Kolomenskii EE, et al: Use of transcatheter high-frequency artificial ventilation of the lungs in surgical treatment of obliterating papillomatosis of the larynx and trachea in children, *Vestn Otorhinolaryngol* 4:34, 1996.
40. Koufman JA, Blalock PD: Functional voice disorders, *Otolaryngol Clin North Am* 24:1059, 1991.
41. Leek KC, Schecter G: Tuberculous infections of the head and neck, *Ear Nose Throat J* 74:395, 1995.
42. Lopez-Amado M, Yebra-Pimentel MT, Garcia-Sarandeses A: Cytomegalovirus causing necrotizing laryngitis in a renal and cardiac transplant recipient, *Head Neck* 18:455, 1996.
43. Lotz WK, et al: Successful nasoendoscopic and aerodynamic examination of children with speech and voice disorders, *Int J Pediatr Otolaryngol* 26:165, 1993.
44. McGuirt WF Jr, Little JP: Laryngeal cancer in children and adolescents, *Otol Clin North Am* 30:207, 1997.
45. Merritt RM, Bent JP, Porubsky ES: Acute laryngeal trauma in the pediatric patient, *Ann Otol Rhinol Laryngol* 107:104, 1998.
46. Morrison GAJ, Kotecha S, Evans JNG: Ribavirin treatment for juvenile respiratory papillomatosis, *J Laryngol Otol* 105:423, 1993.
47. Mortele K, et al: Laryngeal embryonal rhabdomyosis coma in a child: MRI appearance, *Eur Radiol* 8:1251, 1998.
48. Murphy FK, Patamasuon P: Congenital syphilis. In Holmes KK, et al, editors: *Sexually transmitted diseases*, New York, 1990, McGraw-Hill.
49. Ng ML, Gilbert HR, Lerman JW: Some aerodynamic and acoustic characteristics of acute laryngitis, *J Voice* 11:356, 1997.
50. Ossoff RH, et al: The clinical application of lasers in otolaryngology, head and neck surgery, *Laser Surg Med* 15:217, 1994.
51. Prasid S: Airway obstruction in an adolescent with relapsing polychondritis, *Otolaryngol Head Neck Surg* 103:113, 1990.
52. Reilly JS: The "singing-acting" child: the laryngologist's perspective, 1995. *J Voice* 11:126, 1997.
53. Richter JE: Hoarseness and gastroesophageal reflux: what is the relationship? *Gastroenterol* 98:1717, 1990.
54. Roig P, et al: Candida laryngitis and HIV infection: description of four cases, *Revista Clin Esp* 19:261, 1992.
55. Shah P, Ramakantan R: Hoarseness of the voice due to recurrent laryngeal nerve palsy in tuberculosis mediastinitis, *Arch Otol Laryngol Head Neck Surg* 116:108, 1990.
56. Siegel RJ, et al: Cytomegalovirus laryngitis and probable malignant lymphoma of the larynx in a patient with AIDS, *Arch Pathol Lab Med* 116:539, 1992.
57. Smith ME, et al: Voice problems after pediatric laryngotracheal reconstruction: videolaryngostrobosopic, acoustic and perceptual assessment, *Int J Pediatr Otolaryngol* 25:173, 1993.
58. Soderholm E, et al: Aetiologic factors associated with hoarseness in ten-year-old children, *Folia Phoniatr Logop* 47J:262, 1995.
59. Sperry K: Lethal asphyxiation in juvenile laryngeal papillomatosis, *Am J Forens Pathol* 15:146, 1994.
60. Sutphen JL: Pediatric gastroesophageal reflux disease, *Gastroenterol Clin North Am* 19:617, 1990.
61. Wed DT, Courey MS, Ossoff RH: Microlaryngoscopy in the difficult surgical exposure: a new microlaryngoscopy, *Otorhinolaryngol Head Neck Surg* 110:247, 1994.
62. Wudy SA, et al: Diagnosis and management of laryngeal obstruction in childhood pachyonychia congenita, *Int J Pediatr Otorhinolaryngol* 31: 109, 1995.
63. Yanagisawa E, Yanagisawa K: Stroboscopic videolaryngoscopy: a comparison of fiberscopic and telescopic documentation, *Ann Otol Rhinol Laryngol* 102:255, 1993.
64. Yin SS, Qiu WW, Stucker FJ: Value of electromyography in differential diagnosis of laryngeal joint injuries after intubation, *Ann Otol Rhinol Laryngol* 105:446, 1996.

SUGGESTED READINGS

Aronson A: *Clinical voice disorders: an interdisciplinary approach,* New York, 1980, Thieme-Stratton.

Bluestone CD, Stool SE, Kenna M: *Pediatric otolaryngology,* Philadelphia, 1990, WB Saunders.

Colton RH, Casper JK, Hirano M: *Understanding voice problems: a physiological perspective for diagnosis and treatment,* Baltimore, 1996, Williams and Wilkins.

Cotton RT, Myer CM, editors: *Practical pediatric otolaryngology,* Philadelphia, 1999, Lippincott-Raven.

Hirano M, Bless DM: *Videostroboscopic examination of the larynx,* San Diego, 1993, Singular Publishing.

Holinger LD, Lusk RP, Green CG, editors: *Pediatric laryngology and bronchoesophagology,* Philadelphia, 1997, Lippincott-Raven.

Tewfik TL, Der Kaloustian VM, editors: *Congenital anomalies of the ear, nose and throat,* New York, 1997, Oxford University Press.

Tucker HM: *The larynx,* New York, 1993, Thieme.

149 Hyperhidrosis

Nancy K. Barnett

Hyperhidrosis, or sweating more than is normal, occurs commonly in childhood. The child or the family usually expresses concern because the sweating is either odiferous or so intense that it interferes with hand or foot functions (e.g., holding a pencil). Axillary hyperhidrosis usually becomes more of a problem in adolescence because of the odor associated with bacterial degradation of apocrine sweat, the apocrine glands being stimulated at puberty by androgenic hormones. However, palmar and plantar hyperhidrosis secondary to eccrine sweat production may occur at any age.

Palmoplantar hyperhidrosis is thought to be stimulated by anxiety, whereas axillary hyperhidrosis probably is stimulated by both heat and emotion. It is postulated that emotions and the temperature of the blood perfusing the hypothalamus stimulate the secretion of the hormones that regulate the autonomic nervous system's control of perspiration.[1]

Excessive sweating that is not chronic or limited to the palms, soles, and axillae may indicate a systemic disorder, such as infection, lymphoma, thyrotoxicosis, Riley-Day syndrome, hypoglycemia, drug withdrawal, or pheochromocytoma. These disorders should be evaluated only in the face of generalized increased perspiring.

Systemic anticholinergic agents will control hyperhidrosis, but the side effects of cholinergic blockage preclude their long-term use. The application of aluminum salts (e.g., Drysol) every other day had been the most effective treatment for palmar sweating. Plantar hyperhidrosis also responds to aluminum salts, and absorbent powders (e.g., Zeasorb) are used more easily here than on the palms. However, palmar and plantar hyperhidrosis can be controlled by inhibiting sweat production with subepidermal injections of botulinum A toxin. The toxin purportedly blocks the presynaptic acetylcholine release and is effective for as long as 12 months. Patients as young as 14 years of age have been treated in this manner.[6] For bromhidrosis (malodorous hyperhidrosis) of the soles, cleansing frequently with drying deodorant soaps and applying topical antibiotics (erythromycin, tetracycline, or clindamycin) may help. The patient should go barefoot whenever possible.

Axillary hyperhidrosis is troublesome because in the face of continual sweating it is difficult to maintain an effective antiperspirant in contact with the axillary skin. One approach consists of applying a saturated solution of aluminum chloride in absolute ethanol or isopropyl alcohol to the axillary vault. For individuals who have axillary hyperhidrosis and bromhidrosis, frequent clothing changes may be necessary, as well as the use of topical antibiotics and deodorant powders. Successful chemodenervation with intracutaneous botulinum toxin injections is being reported increasingly.[3,4] In extreme cases, when these measures fail and the patient is desperate for relief, local axillary skin can be excised with reasonable expectation of success. Because of its attendant complications, ganglion sympathectomy cannot be recommended for most patients who have axillary hyperhidrosis.[2,5]

When to Refer

- Hyperhidrosis that interferes with the function of a body part (e.g., hand so slippery wet that the child cannot hold a pencil)
- Generalized excessive sweating
- Socially isolating hyperhidrosis as a result of odor or excessive drenching of clothing

REFERENCES

1. Cage GW, Shwachman H, Sato K: Hyperhidrosis. In Fitzpatrick TB, et al, editors: *Dermatology in general medicine,* New York, 1979, McGraw-Hill.
2. Hurwitz S: *Clinical pediatric dermatology,* Philadelphia, 1981, WB Saunders.
3. Naumann M, et al: Focal hyperhidrosis, *Arch Dermatol* 134:301, 1998.
4. Odderson IR: Axillary hyperhidrosis: treatment with botulinum toxin A, *Arch Phys Med Rehabil* 79:350, 1998.
5. Shelley WB, Hurley HJ: Studies on topical antiperspirant control of axillary hyperhidrosis, *Acta Derm Venereol (Stockh)* 55:241, 1975.
6. Shelley WB, Talanin NY, Shelley ED: Botulinum toxin therapy for palmar hyperhidrosis, *J Am Acad Dermatol* 38:227, 1998.

150 Hypotonia

Alfred J. Spiro

Hypotonia is a term used to indicate diminished resistance to passive movement around the range of motion of a joint. The commonly used term "floppy" refers to hypotonia and/or weakness. There is no accurate test to enable a clinician to quantitate hypotonicity, and it must be remembered that tone, especially in a young infant, may vary greatly during the day. Hypotonia is not in itself a diagnosis, but the origin of a neonate's floppiness may be obvious in, for example, overwhelming sepsis, meningitis, or marked hyperbilirubinemia. Central nervous system (CNS) abnormalities are commonly associated with hypotonia; generally, "central" hypotonia just involves diminished tone but not appreciably diminished strength, coupled with preserved or hyperactive deep tendon reflexes. In disorders of the motor unit—namely, lesions of the anterior horn cell, peripheral nerve, myoneural junction, and muscle—strength usually is diminished, and tone, as a result, may be reduced. Testing of strength in infants and young children is very difficult, even for experienced examiners; it usually can be done by observation of how strong a baby's kicking and pushing are, for example, or by functional testing. Hypotonia caused by an underlying motor unit disorder is much less common than hypotonia not the result of a motor unit disorder.

HYPOTONIA NOT CAUSED BY MOTOR UNIT DISORDERS

Disorders virtually anywhere in the brain may be associated with hypotonia; global developmental delay is a common, but not universal, accompanying feature, as is microcephaly. Magnetic resonance imaging (MRI) of the brain may be helpful in documenting the lesion in some cases but is not always helpful; in many instances, a specific diagnosis cannot be made. As infants who have hypotonicity get older, the abnormal tone may evolve into spasticity, and the diagnosis of spastic quadriplegia, spastic diplegia, or other form of cerebral palsy (a static disorder of the CNS beginning in the first few months of life resulting in motor dysfunction) becomes evident. It is a common misconception that cerebral palsy is caused by obstetrical trauma; the cause of most instances of cerebral palsy is unknown.[6,11] Despite this, a review of birth records, drug administration, and factors surrounding prematurity is indicated. On examination, deep tendon reflexes usually, but not always, are hyperactive. Abnormalities of tone usually are global—that is, both proximal and distal. Treatment of various types of cerebral palsy is supportive and symptomatic and usually requires a multidisciplinary team effort.

Several genetic syndromes, Down syndrome being the most common, are associated with hypotonia; the diagnosis can be made on clinical grounds and with appropriate genetic studies. Newborns and young infants who have Prader-Willi syndrome may be extremely hypotonic and obtunded. As these babies get older, tone may improve and they may become obese. They have characteristic almond-shaped eyes, short stature, and some degree of mental retardation and hypogonadism; some have a severe eating disorder and scoliosis, but these are not usually present until school age. The clinical features coupled with a deletion in the chromosome 15q11-13 region can establish the diagnosis.

Several of the Ehlers-Danlos syndromes[4] may simulate hypotonicity, but the major feature of this group of connective tissue disorders is hyperlaxity of joints. Weakness is not a prominent feature.

Hypothyroidism and other metabolic disorders may be accompanied by hypotonia. Neonatal "screens" generally include a test for hypothyroidism; if the diagnosis is not obvious on physical examination, appropriate other studies can be done.

HYPOTONIA CAUSED BY MOTOR UNIT DISORDERS

History

In taking the history, it should be ascertained when the floppiness was first noted—that is, whether it was present at birth or was recognized later. Parents of first children may have no basis for comparison and may not recognize an abnormality. Occasionally, photographs or family videotapes can be extremely useful in revealing abnormalities denied or not noted by parents. Breech presentation is a common mode of delivery in babies subsequently diagnosed as having a motor unit disorder, but the reason for this has not been established. Congenital hip dislocation may be present in children who have central core disease, a congenital myopathy.

Careful questioning usually can determine if the floppiness is getting better or worse or if weakness is periodic, as observed in hyperkalemic periodic paralysis, the onset of which often is in infancy or early childhood. The distribution of weakness, namely whether it is more proximal, distal, or global, also can be identified with questions such as whether the baby or child moves the fingers and toes better than the large muscles of the pelvic and shoulder girdles. Details of the baby's or child's developmental milestones also can provide a clue to the nature of the lesion. For example, language development is normal in infantile progressive spinal muscular atrophy and impaired in myotonic dystrophy.

Facial muscle weakness, as observed in some congenital myopathies, can be diagnosed if the parents state that the child sleeps with the eyelids partially open. Extraocular muscles, in addition to facial muscles, are abnormal in myotubular myopathy. Acquired autoimmune myasthenia gravis can occur in young children and may present with ptosis, extraocular muscle weakness, and in some cases, with generalized weakness and respiratory distress. Less severely affected patients may have only very limited abnormal findings at the time of examination; reassessment or inspection of family videotapes can be very useful. Practitioners should inquire about swallowing and sucking difficulties, since these are not always recognized by parents.

Details of the family history can be very helpful, because many of the motor unit disorders are genetic. Inquiries should be made concerning consanguinity, the presence of which suggests an autosomal recessive entity. Examination of parents and siblings can sometimes be very revealing, because some genetic disorders may be expressed quite subtly in family members and frequently are overlooked. Facial muscle weakness is one common example; patients do not seek medical attention if they cannot puff up their cheeks, whistle, or squeeze their eyelids closed completely, all features seen in certain congenital myopathies or facioscapulohumeral muscular dystrophy. If early-onset myotonic dystrophy is suspected, other family members should be examined for myotonia, because neither percussion nor electrical myotonia is observed in very young children.

Physical Examination

A careful search for systemic disorders should be carried out. Dysmorphic features, such as high-arched palate and dental malocclusion, are observed in some congenital myopathies, such as nemaline myopathy. An enlarged heart and congestive heart failure are observed in glycogen storage disease caused by acid maltase deficiency. Club feet deformity is seen in the infantile form of myotonic dystrophy. Joint abnormalities and scoliosis are encountered frequently in several motor unit disorders.

A striking paucity of spontaneous movement is observed in infantile progressive spinal muscular atrophy; paradoxical respiration, in which the chest wall moves inward during inspiration instead of expanding, also is observed frequently.

In infants and in children younger than 5 years of age, manual muscle testing generally cannot be accomplished reliably, making observation of spontaneous movement and functional testing, such as the ability to hold the head erect, sit, roll over, and stand, mandatory. Assessment of cranial nerve function should emphasize the searching for weakness of facial and extraocular muscles, as well as for fasciculation and atrophy of the tongue. Fasciculation of the tongue, observed in infantile progressive spinal muscular atrophy, should be assessed with the tongue not protruded and with the child not crying. Tremulousness of the outstretched fingers (minipolymyoclonus) is seen almost exclusively in spinal muscular atrophy with a protracted course. Generally, deep tendon reflexes are reduced or absent in motor unit disorders. However, in most cases of myasthenia gravis, they are preserved. With hypotonia of "central" origin, reflexes are preserved or hyperactive; however, there are many exceptions to this rule. The presence or absence of extensor plantar responses is also frequently difficult to assess in young children; these responses may be present variably up to a year or more of age.

Laboratory Studies

Laboratory studies can be categorized into blood testing, neurophysiological evaluation, and histological examination of muscle. Laboratory studies should be goal-directed. Serum muscle enzyme levels, particularly creatine kinase, are always markedly elevated in Duchenne's and Becker's muscular dystrophy, but are not always increased in congenital myopathies. They generally are normal or minimally increased in spinal muscular atrophy. DNA studies for diagnostic purposes are readily available in many commercial and research laboratories (see Helix or OMIM on the Internet) for several motor unit disorders, including infantile progressive spinal muscular atrophy, myotonic dystrophy, various hereditary sensorimotor neuropathies, selected mitochondrial myopathies, and Duchenne's and Becker's muscular dystrophy. When these disorders are suspected on clinical grounds, appropriate DNA studies may be all that is needed to substantiate the diagnosis. Thus, a child who has classic infantile progressive spinal muscular atrophy can be spared many painful studies when the DNA studies are conclusive.[7] Other noninvasive studies, such as CT, MRI, or sonographic imaging of muscles, can assess muscle mass accurately; in the presence of very small muscles, imaging is indicated if a muscle biopsy is contemplated.

Electromyographic studies can be very useful in the diagnosis of motor unit disorders,[12] but because of the pain involved and the need for sedation in some cases, they should be used with discretion when DNA studies are not helpful. Nerve conduction studies can be extremely useful in distinguishing the various types of peripheral neuropathies seen in infants and children. Repetitive stimulation studies are very helpful in diagnosing infantile botulism, but these are quite painful. An edrophonium test can be diagnostic when myasthenia gravis is suspected. All electrodiagnostic studies done in young children should be performed by a clinician experienced in the particular technical and other problems encountered in this age group.

Muscle biopsies, performed either with a special needle or surgically, are most useful in myopathies such as congenital myopathies, congenital muscular dystrophy, metabolic myopathies, and mitochondrial disorders. Many specialized analytical studies are available when needed. In virtually all instances, when a biopsy is performed, sections should be taken for histochemical, biochemical, ultrastructural, and genetic studies, although all of these studies are not always needed.

Selected Motor Unit Disorders

Anterior horn cell disease. Since the disappearance of paralytic poliomyelitis in the United States, the various types of infantile progressive spinal muscular atrophy

Table 150-1 Infantile Progressive Spinal Muscular Atrophy

Type	Age of Onset	Course
I	Birth to 6 mo	Never sits independently, even when placed; progressive; demise <2 years of age
II	6-18 mo	Sits independently when placed; life expectancy into the twenties or later
III	>18 mo	Weakness after having learned to walk; normal life expectancy

constitute the major disease in this category. Eponyms have been applied to these disorders, including the term *Werdnig-Hoffmann disease,* but these terms may be misleading and confusing. A much more useful operational classification of infantile progressive spinal muscular atrophy, as shown in Table 150-1, is now commonly used.[13]

In all types of infantile progressive spinal muscular atrophy, cognition is normal, as are extraocular muscles. Weakness and muscle wasting are proximal more than distal and are more pronounced in the legs than in the arms. Fasciculation of the tongue and minipolymyoclonus (in types I and II) are observed frequently, and areflexia and normal sensation are the rule. Joint contractures and scoliosis may develop, especially in type II. All forms are autosomal recessive, with the responsible gene having been located at 5q11-q13. A deletion of the survival motor neuron gene has been identified in the vast majority of patients, making this useful for diagnostic purposes and for prenatal diagnosis.[1] Recent evidence suggests that phenotype-genotype correlation will be available soon. Treatment generally is supportive and includes physical therapy and, when needed, respiratory and nutritional support and genetic counseling. Scoliosis is common in type II and must be addressed appropriately with a body jacket, molded back support, or surgery. Most children who have type II can use a motorized wheelchair at about 2 to 3 years of age. Life expectancy in type II, contrary to outdated reports, can be well into adult life.

Peripheral nerve disorders. Peripheral nerve disorders are rare in infancy and early childhood. Hypomyelinating neuropathy[8] can present with severe weakness, hypotonia, and areflexia in a neonate or young infant. The diagnosis can be suspected when extremely abnormal nerve conduction studies are encountered and can be confirmed with a nerve biopsy. Hereditary sensorimotor neuropathies (Charcot-Marie-Tooth disease), the most common cause of childhood peripheral nerve disorders, may present with gait abnormalities resulting from weakness of the anterior tibialis muscles or foot deformities.[9,17] Ankle jerks frequently are diminished or absent, but all reflexes may be preserved in the early phases of peripheral neuropathies. Nerve conduction studies can be extremely useful in separating axonal from demyelination neuropathies. DNA studies can be diagnostic in selected hereditary neuropathies, especially the autosomal dominant demyelinating and the X-linked varieties. Treatment is symptomatic; some children who have foot drop may require bracing.

Several CNS disorders may have peripheral nerve involvement; these include metachromatic leukodystrophy, Krabbe's disease, and adrenoleukodystrophy, among others.

Myoneural junction disorders.[15] Several disorders of the myoneural junction affect children and infants: (1) passively acquired autoimmune myasthenia gravis, also known as transient neonatal myasthenia; (2) acquired autoimmune myasthenia gravis, also known as juvenile myasthenia; (3) nonautoimmune myasthenic syndromes, also known as congenital myasthenia gravis; and (4) infantile botulism.

Passively acquired autoimmune myasthenia gravis is seen in approximately 20% of infants born to mothers who have myasthenia gravis. All newborns of seropositive mothers have acetylcholine receptor antibodies, but only a small portion are symptomatic—most mildly, but some more severely—with hypotonia, a weak cry, swallowing and sucking difficulty, facial diapiresis, respiratory distress, external ophthalmoparesis, and ptosis. The diagnosis can be made quickly by using intravenous edrophonium; when the newborns are symptomatic, pyridostigmine can be given therapeutically until symptoms no longer are present. The dose then is tapered, usually over a period of a week or two after the treatment has commenced. These infants do not have myasthenia gravis after the initial involvement. If the weakness does not occur by 1 week of age, it is highly unlikely to develop.

Major features of acquired autoimmune myasthenia include fatigability and fluctuating weakness of extraocular, facial, and lingual muscles, and in some instances, mild or severe generalized weakness and hypotonicity of the limbs. An acute fulminating onset may be encountered in young children. The diagnosis can be made by using the edrophonium test and confirmed with the acetylcholine receptor antibody test, although the latter is not necessarily positive in milder cases and is less useful in children than in older individuals. Electrodiagnostic studies can be used in selected instances in children but generally are less useful than in adults. The mediastinum should be radiographed to assess thymic size. Treatment includes judicious use of anticholinesterase drugs, and, when needed, immunosuppressive treatment, intravenous gamma globulin, corticosteroids, and thymectomy.

Nonautoimmune myasthenic syndromes may be associated with ocular, bulbar, or respiratory involvement, and in some instances, with progressive weakness and hypotonicity. Some disorders may be genetic; patients are seronegative. Specialized electrodiagnostic and ultrastructural studies are required to establish an exact diagnosis.

Infantile botulism is characterized by onset (at an average age of a little more than 3 months) of weakness and hypotonia, poor feeding, constipation, and diminished activity. The onset may be rapid, developing over 2 to 3 days. The diagnosis is confirmed when the toxin is documented in the stool or when the organism is isolated from culture, but repetitive stimulation studies can by extremely useful in establishing the diagnosis quickly. Treatment is supportive.

Myopathies

Myopathies constitute a diverse group of genetic, inflammatory, and metabolic disorders that involve muscle, and in many cases, other organ systems, including the brain and heart. Inflammatory myopathies (dermatomyositis) are seen rarely in very young children and generally present with subacute weakness.

In the infantile form of myotonic dystrophy,[5] hypotonia can be severe at birth. Obtundation, difficulty with sucking and swallowing, weakness of facial muscles, club feet, and areflexia may be present. Myotonia (spasmodic increased muscular contractility with decreased relaxation) will not be present either clinically or electrically until after age 5 years. A patient who survives the neonatal period will gain strength and tone and eventually will walk. Until strength and tone improve, assisted ventilation and gastrostomy tube feedings often are needed. Myotonic dystrophy is an autosomal dominant disorder; however, when it is manifest in the neonatal period, it virtually is always the mother who transmitted the gene. She should be examined for the characteristic features of the disease, which include reflex and percussion myotonia, weakness of the neck flexor muscles, smallness of the sternocleidomastoid muscles, weakness of the wrist extensors and anterior tibialis muscles and facial muscles, and often, mental retardation. For children who first manifest myotonic dystrophy beyond infancy, either parent may have transmitted the gene, which is located on 19q13. DNA studies can be done to document the diagnosis. Family members should be provided with genetic counseling if they so desire, since prenatal diagnosis is available. Treatment is supportive.

There are several congenital myopathies,[3] generally diagnosed by their characteristic morphology on muscle biopsy. These myopathies, typified by nemaline myopathy, frequently are hereditary and are associated with varying degrees of floppiness and weakness and sometimes with respiratory and sucking problems early in life. Some have rather characteristic clinical features. For example, in myotubular myopathy of very early onset, an X-linked disorder, the extraocular and facial muscles are weak, in addition to generalized hypotonia and weakness. Central core disease is associated with congenital hip dislocation and a propensity for malignant hyperpyrexia. In some congenital myopathies, the gene location has been identified, but DNA testing is not yet available for establishing the diagnosis.

The congenital muscular dystrophies comprise a diverse group of diseases in which varying degrees of weakness and hypotonia are present early in life (see Chapter 37, Muscular Dystrophy). Muscle biopsy shows characteristic pathological findings. The serum muscle enzymes (creatine phosphokinase) generally are elevated and, in some forms of this disorder, merosin is absent on the biopsy specimen.[16] The merosin-deficient type of congenital muscular dystrophy seen in the United States has been localized to chromosome 6q2. In Japan, the Fukuyama type of muscular dystrophy, which is associated with severe central nervous system abnormalities, is common.

Facioscapulohumeral muscular dystrophy[10] usually becomes symptomatic in older children but, at times, will present with severe facial weakness in early childhood. This is an autosomal dominant disorder, although there are sporadic cases, and parents of suspected children should be examined for involvement that may be very mild and go unnoticed, such as facial muscular weakness, scapular winging, and a round-shouldered stance. This disease is linked to high-frequency hearing deficits. Treatment is symptomatic. DNA studies are available to document the diagnosis when this disorder is suspected.

Glycogen storage disease caused by deficient acid maltase, in addition to its neuromuscular manifestations (hypotonia and weakness), is associated with a markedly enlarged heart and congestive heart failure. The diagnosis can be made readily by muscle biopsy. Treatment is directed toward the cardiac manifestations, but prognosis for life is poor. This is an autosomal recessive disorder; the responsible gene has been located at 17q23.

An increasing number of mitochondrial encephalomyopathies[2,14] are being reported that have varying CNS and muscle involvement. Lacticacidemia is common, but specialized genetic and other studies on muscle mitochondria are needed to provide a specific diagnosis if DNA studies are unrevealing. Treatment generally is symptomatic.

When to Refer

- Persistent lack of normal motor development
- Regression of motor development
- Sudden or precipitous worsening of tone or strength
- Swallowing dysfunction
- New onset of neurological signs

REFERENCES

1. DiDonato CJ, et al: Deletion and conversion in spinal muscular atrophy patients: is there a relationship to severity? *Ann Neurol* 41:230, 1997.
2. DiMauro S, et al: Mitochondria in neuromuscular disorders, *Biochim Biophys Acta* 1366:199, 1998.
3. Goebel JJ: Congenital myopathies: the current status, *J Child Neurol* 14:30, 1999.
4. Grahame R: Joint hypermobility and genetic collagen disorders: are they related? *Arch Dis Child* 80:188, 1999.
5. Keller C, et al: Congenital myotonic dystrophy requiring prolonged endotracheal and noninvasive assisted ventilation: not a uniformly fatal condition, *Pediatrics* 101:704, 1998.
6. Kuban KCK, Leviton A: Cerebral palsy, *N Engl J Med* 330:188, 1994.
7. Lefebvre S, et al: Identification and characterization of a spinal muscular atrophy-determining gene, *Cell* 80:155, 1995.
8. Mandich P, et al: Congenital hypomyelination due to myelin protein zero Q215X mutation, *Ann Neurol* 45:676, 1999.
9. Mouton P, et al: Spectrum of clinical and electrophysiologic features in HNPP patients with the 17p11.2 deletion, *Neurology* 52:1440, 1999.
10. Okinaga A, et al: Early-onset facioscapulohumeral muscular dystrophy: two case reports, *Brain Dev* 19:563, 1997.
11. Perlman JM: Intrapartum hypoxic-ischemic cerebral injury and subsequent cerebral palsy: medicolegal issues, *Pediatrics* 99:851, 1997.
12. Russell JW, Afifi AK, Ross MA: Predictive value of electromyography in diagnosis and prognosis of the hypotonic infant, *J Child Neurol* 7:387, 1992.
13. Russman BS, et al: Function changes in spinal muscular atrophy II & III, *Neurology* 47:973, 1996.
14. Shoubridge BA: Mitochondrial encephalomyelopathies, *Curr Opin Neurol* 11:491, 1998.
15. Spiro AJ: Disorders of the myoneural junction. In Berg BO, editor: *Principles of child neurology,* New York, 1996, McGraw-Hill.
16. Tome FMS, et al: Congenital muscular dystrophy with merosin deficiency, *C R Acad Sci Paris* 317:351, 1994.
17. Warner LE, Garcia CA, Lupski JR: Hereditary peripheral neuropathies: clinical forms, genetics, and molecular mechanisms, *Ann Rev Med* 50: 263, 1999.

151 Irritability

C. Jean Ogborn

Irritability is a common and vexing presenting complaint in the pediatric age group. Although experienced clinicians can recognize irritability in a child, agreeing on a concise definition is difficult. *Webster's Ninth New Collegiate Dictionary* defines irritability as "abnormal or excessive excitability of an organ or body part." In the context of pediatrics, irritability is an alteration in sensorium that evokes negative behaviors outside the range of normal for the child, including overreaction or inappropriate reaction to normal stimuli.

At the root of the symptom of irritability is the lack of something vital (e.g., oxygen, glucose), the presence of something noxious (e.g., pain, toxins), or an emotion (e.g., anger, frustration). Irritability may have different causes and manifestations in infants, children, and adolescents. An infant or preverbal child will be unable to offer information about his or her complaint, whereas some older children and adolescents may offer verbal clues to the disease process. In addition, an infant or child who is irritable and has other symptoms generally will have a different underlying disorder than one who has irritability as a sole presenting complaint. An organized approach to the differential diagnosis is essential to minimizing unnecessary testing while making the correct diagnosis.

ACUTE IRRITABILITY

Categories of conditions that can cause acute irritability include infections, trauma, toxins or drugs, metabolic derangements, hypoxic/ischemic events, allergies, inflammatory processes, and emotional disturbances, among others. Acute irritability may be associated with life-threatening illnesses and physical findings, requiring urgent intervention. A parent who seeks care for an infant who is "fussier than usual" may present with a child who is in shock, in respiratory distress, or having a seizure. The child must be stabilized before a search for the cause begins. Some life-threatening conditions that may cause acute irritability are listed in Box 151-1.

If the child does not have an immediately life-threatening condition, a careful history and physical examination are the first steps in the evaluation of irritability and, in many cases, will reveal the cause of the symptom. Many common infectious, traumatic, toxic, allergic, and inflammatory conditions can be diagnosed by history and physical examination alone. Laboratory or radiological procedures may confirm a clinical suspicion. Some conditions associated with acute irritability but generally without life-threatening presentations are listed in Box 151-2. Common and some unusual causes of acute irritability are discussed below.

Infections

Meningitis often is suspected when the complaint is irritability in the presence of fever. Lumbar puncture followed by spinal fluid analysis often settles the issue quickly. Encephalitis also must be considered when the infant or child is irritable and has fever without another apparent focus or fever associated with hallucinations, seizures, or rash. Spinal fluid pleocytosis and focal findings on magnetic resonance imaging (MRI) or electroencephalogram (EEG) may be suggestive, and viral cultures may yield a pathogen. Treatment mostly is supportive, with parenteral acyclovir for proven or suspected herpes simplex encephalitis.

Urosepsis, *Escherichia coli* sepsis, or group B streptococcal sepsis in a neonate or young infant may present with irritability, fever, and a toxic or "shocky" appearance. Urinary tract infections in preverbal or nonverbal children may cause fever and irritability without the expressed specific complaints of dysuria or flank pain. Examination of the urine for blood, leukocytes, nitrites, and bacteria is necessary to establish the diagnosis.

Myocarditis and pericarditis with poor cardiac output can present with fever and irritability as the most prominent signs. The presence of tachypnea, tachycardia, and cough may mislead the examiner toward a diagnosis of pneumonia. Chest radiography may show cardiomegaly or pulmonary edema in early stages of these disorders. The findings of hepatomegaly, poor capillary refill, or tachycardia out of proportion to the fever may be clues to the presence of these underrecognized and sometimes deadly causes of heart failure. An echocardiogram and electrocardiogram (ECG) are useful in making the diagnosis.

Kawasaki disease (see Chapter 230) is thought to result from an infectious process leading to a toxin-mediated generalized vasculitis.[16] Early in its course, fever and extreme irritability may be the most pronounced signs. Conjunctival, dermal, and mucosal vasculitis are responsible for the red eyes, rash, and stomatitis that occur in typical cases. No definitive diagnostic tests exist, but an elevated erythrocyte sedimentation rate (ESR), sterile pyuria, toxic granulations of the neutrophils, and uveitis on slit lamp examination, in conjunction with fever, rash, and lymphadenitis, all combine to make the diagnosis. Although not immediately life threatening, recognition of this disorder and treatment with intrave-

BOX 151-1

SOME LIFE-THREATENING CAUSES OF ACUTE IRRITABILITY

Infections
Meningitis
Encephalitis
Myocarditis
Pericarditis
Kawasaki disease*

Trauma
Shaken-baby syndrome
Child abuse
Cerebral edema
Acute blood loss

Hypoxia/Ischemia
Stroke
Myocardial infarction
Respiratory failure
Carbon monoxide poisoning
Methemoglobinemia
Pulmonary embolism

Metabolic Causes
Hypoglycemia
Hyponatremia
Hypernatremia
Hypocalcemia
Hypercalcemia
Acidosis
Hyperammonemia
Pheochromocytoma
Thyrotoxicosis

Toxins/Drugs
Heavy-metal intoxication
Chemical exposure
Medication toxicity
Drugs of abuse

Miscellaneous
Heat illness
Malignancy*

*May be life threatening but may not present with emergent symptoms.

BOX 151-2

SOME CAUSES OF ACUTE IRRITABILITY

Infections
Otitis media and externa
Urinary tract infection
Stomatitis
Dental caries and abscess
Balanitis
Gastroenteritis
Sinusitis
Measles
Osteomyelitis
Septic hip

Trauma
Fractures and dislocations
Corneal abrasions
Anal fissures
Foreign body (eye, ear, nose, skin)
Sunburn
Bites and stings

Toxins/Drugs
Medication toxicity and side effects
Substance abuse or withdrawal
Chemical or drug exposure

Allergies
Food and environment
Contact dermatitis
Eczema

Inflammations
Juvenile rheumatoid arthritis
Toxic synovitis
Inflammatory bowel disease

Miscellaneous
Teething
Colic
Constipation
Hunger
Hyperthermia or hypothermia
Dactylitis and vaso-occlusive crisis
Hernia
Diaper rash
Constrictive or abrasive clothing and shoes
Altitude sickness
Phimosis
Torsion of the testis or the ovary
Insect bites or stings

nous immunoglobulin within the first 10 days of illness are critical to decreasing the likelihood of coronary artery vasculitis and the formation of an aneurysm.[17,22]

Musculoskeletal infections such as osteomyelitis, diskitis, and septic arthritis may cause fever with pain and irritability. A careful history and physical examination may yield these diagnoses, or the suspicion of them, but skeletal infectious processes may be nearly indistinguishable from inflammatory or malignant processes or even behavioral reactions in young infants. Diagnosis may require serial examinations and tests. Plain films of bones and joints may be unrevealing, and further evaluations including ESR, C-reactive protein, complete blood count, blood cultures, bone scan, bone biopsy, and joint aspiration may be necessary.

Trauma

In general, irritability will not be the most salient finding in a child who has sustained life-threatening trauma. Important exceptions to this generalization are the shaken-baby syndrome, the battered child syndrome (see Chapter 57, Child Abuse and Neglect), and massive occult blood loss. Infants and very young children who have been shaken may suffer retinal hemorrhages and detachment, subdural or subarachnoid hemorrhages, and cerebral edema.[5] Irritability without an obvious source may be the only external sign of these life-threatening situations and may be erroneously attributed to other causes, even by experienced clinicians.[11] An infant or young child who is battered (and ultimately at high risk for death) may have occult fractures, intracranial bleeding, and/or intraabdominal contusions and yet evidence very few outward findings except irritability. The clinician should consider carefully the issue of child abuse or neglect in the case of unexplained irritability or irritability resulting from fracture or dislocation, especially in very young or nonambulatory children.[1,5,13]

The pressure of the lap belt of a restraint system in a motor vehicle crash or other blunt abdominal trauma can lead to intraabdominal bleeding from a laceration of the liver, spleen, or bowel wall and the resultant irritability that occurs from hypoperfusion and pain.

Many traumatic causes of irritability that are not life threatening may be apparent on initial physical examination and include fractures or dislocations, anal fissures, corneal abrasions, sunburn, and foreign bodies (including insects) in the eye, nose, and ear or under the skin.

Hypoxic/Ischemic Events

Carbon monoxide poisoning and methemoglobinemia cause irritability by producing hypoxia. The history and arterial measurement of carboxyhemoglobin or methemoglobin are diagnostic. A cherry red (carboxyhemoglobin) or chocolate brown (methemoglobin) appearance of arterial blood is an immediate clue. Pulmonary embolism can cause irritability by inducing sudden hypoxia, and respiratory failure from any cause may be associated with irritability progressing to lethargy.

Altitude sickness from relative hypoxia may cause acute irritability in infants and children, as it may in adults.[2] Reactions to changes in altitude vary among individuals and are difficult to predict. Altitude sickness must be considered in a child from a lower altitude who recently has arrived in the mountains.

Cerebral ischemia from thrombosis or a hemorrhagic stroke may produce irritability. Myocardial ischemia is not common in children but can present with irritability. Children who have had Kawasaki disease or have certain congenital heart defects are at risk for thrombosis, arrhythmia, ischemia, and infarction. Vasoocclusive crisis in a child who has sickle cell anemia is an ischemic cause of pain and irritability. With any ischemic insult, older children and adolescents may be able to describe pain, but younger children and infants simply may be irritable.

Metabolic Derangements

Hypoglycemia, hyponatremia or hypernatremia, hypocalcemia or hypercalcemia, hyperammonemia, and acidosis can cause irritability. In a child who appears toxic and irritable, a quick check of electrolytes may indicate sodium, glucose, calcium, and acid-base abnormalities. Dehydration, hyponatremia, hypernatremia, and acidosis can result from common gastrointestinal illnesses in infants and young children. Hypoglycemia can result from many causes, including starvation. Infants who are underfed acutely or chronically (e.g., have marasmus or kwashiorkor) may be quite irritable. Older children and adolescents also may exhibit an irritable response to the relative hypoglycemia that occurs if regular meals are delayed. Obtaining ammonia levels is not often part of initial screening in a child, but the clinician should consider checking in children who have encephalopathy or evidence of liver disease along with their irritability, all of which could indicate Reye's syndrome or congenital enzyme deficiencies.[24] Detection of a metabolic derangement is far simpler than determining the precise cause; see Chapter 20 (Three), Recognition of Genetic-Metabolic Diseases by Clinical Diagnosis and Screening.

Toxins and Drugs

Life-threatening intoxications may result from heavy metals such as lead and mercury,[9] drugs of abuse such as cocaine and alcohol, envenomations by scorpions and snakes, overdoses of or idiosyncratic reactions to medications, and contact with agricultural, industrial, or household chemicals. Careful questioning about recent use of lawn chemicals, pesticides, and cleaning products may be the only clues to these as a cause of irritability because many of these chemicals will not be detected by standard toxicology screenings of blood and urine. Prescribed or over-the-counter medications such as theophylline, beta-agonists, antiepileptics, decongestants, antihistamines, antitussives, and various "cold preparations" may cause irritability even when used as directed, and certainly when overused. Cocaine,[21] alcohol, phencyclidine hydrochloride (PCP),[25] inhalants, and other drugs of abuse are known to cause irritability. Infants and children may be exposed to these substances by passive means transplacentally,[18] by ingestion of breast milk,[6] or by inhalation. They may accidentally ingest alcohol or cigarettes and other substances left within reach. A positive history may be difficult to elicit, and a toxicology screen may be helpful. Substance use or withdrawal should be considered in the differential diagnosis when any adolescent presents with irritability. Rarely, intentional poisoning may be the cause of a child's distress.[26]

Allergies

Allergies are a controversial cause of irritability, but one that more and more parents and clinicians recognize. Food allergies, environmental allergies, contact allergies, and severe eczema may result in irritability. Bizarre behavior, temper tantrums, and outbursts of rage reportedly have been caused in some children by allergic responses to foods and environmental allergens.[14,23]

Miscellaneous

Increased intracranial pressure from a brain tumor may present with acute irritability and altered behavior without preceding symptoms such as headache or loss of coordination. Many clinicians remember at least one child who presented with complaints of irritability and intermittent fever in whom leukemia with bone pain was diagnosed. Malignancies of all sorts may have a component of irritability among their symptoms and must be considered carefully when no other diagnosis is forthcoming.

Heat illness, heat stroke, and malignant hyperthermia are life-threatening alterations in the body's homeostatic mechanism that may present with irritability. Thyrotoxicosis and pheochromocytoma also may have irritability as a symptom.

Irritability in infants has been attributed to a variety of causes of pain or discomfort that may become obvious during the evaluation, including teething, colic, constipation, diaper rash, hernia, hair wrapped around a digit or penis, prolapsed rectum or urethra, phimosis, testicular torsion, dactylitis, insect and spider bites or stings, constrictive clothing, and inappropriate clothing leading to hyperthermia or hypothermia. Ovarian torsion is fairly uncommon but can cause pain and irritability and can be difficult to diagnose. An ultrasound examination can be helpful in this regard.

CHRONIC OR RECURRENT IRRITABILITY

Chronic or recurrent irritability in a child challenges both the parents'[12] and the clinician's skills. Psychosocial causes may head the list, but toxic, neurological, metabolic, and miscellaneous causes must be considered and are shown in Box 151-3.

Psychosocial/Psychiatric Disorders

Irritability as a chronic feature of a child's behavior may indicate significant problems with his or her familial relationships and ability to master the environment. Infants may be irritable because of maternal/infant temperament mismatches, maternal depression,[27] or stress within the family surrounding the addition of a new child. Abuse and neglect of a child may provoke irritable behavior or outbursts. An older child or adolescent who has a psychiatric problem such as depression, psychosis, autism, or posttraumatic stress

BOX 151-3

SOME CAUSES OF CHRONIC/ RECURRENT IRRITABILITY

Psychosocial/Psychiatric
Abuse and neglect*
Temperament mismatch
Family discord
Maternal depression
Substance abuse or withdrawal*
Depression*
Psychosis*
Autism

Toxins/Drugs
Lead poisoning*
Mercury poisoning*
Hypervitaminosis A
Medications

Neurological Causes
Seizures
Migraine
Tumors*
Degenerative diseases*
Postconcussion syndrome

Metabolic/Genetic Causes
Urea cycle defects*
Storage diseases*
Fetal alcohol syndrome
Phenylketonuria
Acute intermittent porphyria
Dietary deficit

Miscellaneous
Colic
Vision or hearing impairment
Glaucoma
Reflux esophagitis
Kwashiorkor/ marasmus*
Idiopathic hypercalciuria
Pseudotumor cerebri
Hormones

*Potentially life threatening.

disorder may be described as irritable by parents and others. The investigation and treatment of irritability in these situations may require a multidisciplinary and long-term approach.

Toxins and Drugs

As discussed earlier, any medication or drug of abuse may cause irritable behavior in some individuals in some circumstances. Hypervitaminosis A, pseudotumor cerebri,[15] and transient intracranial hypertension of infancy[19] can cause chronic recurrent irritability resulting from elevations in intracranial pressure. The use of steroids among adolescents who are trying to "bulk up" for sports is known to cause irritability and aggression.[3]

Neurological Disorders

Degenerative diseases, brain tumors, migraine headaches, seizures, and postconcussion syndrome are neurological causes for cyclical, chronic, or recurrent irritability among older children and adolescents. Postconcussion or post-head trauma syndrome is particularly distressing to families because the head injury may have occurred months or years before and even might have been minor, yet the irritability and behavior changes may be major and persistent.[7,10]

Metabolic/Genetic Diseases

Urea cycle defects,[24] storage diseases, congenital drug or alcohol syndromes, phenylketonuria, vitamin B_{12} deficit, and acute intermittent porphyria are a few significant disorders that must be considered in the recurrently irritable child.

Miscellaneous

A wide variety of chronic disorders have irritability as a prominent or sole component. Colic is one well-known but little understood disorder that is characterized by recurrent bouts of irritability and crying. Other causes in infants or young children include vision or hearing impairment, glaucoma, reflux esophagitis, and idiopathic hypercalciuria.[8] Hormonal effects associated with adolescence in both males and females can cause moodiness and irritability.[4,20]

SUMMARY

Irritability has a variety of causes and can be indicative of life-threatening or relatively trivial or transient disorders. A careful history and physical examination most often can determine the cause. In puzzling cases, serial examinations and staged laboratory investigations may be necessary. Treatment of irritability depends on its cause.

REFERENCES

1. AAP Committee on Child Abuse and Neglect: Shaken baby syndrome: inflicted cerebral trauma, *Pediatrics* 92:872, 1993.
2. Bahrke MS, Shukitt-Hale B: Effects of altitude on mood, behavior and cognitive functioning: a review, *Sports Med* 16:97, 1993.
3. Bahrke MS, et al: Psychological moods and subjectively perceived behavioral and somatic changes accompanying anabolic-androgenic steroid use, *Am J Sports Med* 20:717, 1992.
4. Buchanan CM, Eccles JS, Becker JB: Are adolescents the victims of raging hormones: evidence for activational effects of hormones on moods and behavior at adolescence, *Psychol Bull* 111:62, 1992.
5. Caffey J: On the theory and practice of shaking infants, *Am J Dis Child* 124:161, 1972.
6. Chasnoff IJ, Lewis DE, Squires L: Cocaine intoxication in a breast-fed infant, *Pediatrics* 80:836, 1987.
7. Evans RW: The postconcussion syndrome and the sequelae of mild head injury, *Neurol Clin* 10:815, 1992.
8. Fivush B: Irritability and dysuria in infants with idiopathic hypercalciuria, *Pediatr Nephrol* 4:262, 1990.
9. Florentine MJ, Sanfilippo DJ: Elemental mercury poisoning (clinical conference), *Clin Pharmacol* 10:213, 1991.
10. Goldstein J: Posttraumatic headache and the postconcussion syndrome, *Med Clin North Am* 75:641, 1991.
11. Jenny C, et al: Analysis of missed cases of abusive head trauma, *JAMA* 281:621, 1999.
12. Keefe MR, Froese-Fretz A: Living with an irritable infant: maternal perspectives, *Am J Child Nurs* 16:255, 1991.
13. Kempe CH, et al: The battered-child syndrome, *JAMA* 181:17, 1962.
14. Klein GL, et al: The allergic irritability syndrome: four case reports and a position statement from the Neuroallergy Committee of the American College of Allergy, *Ann Allerg* 55:22, 1985.
15. Lessell S: Pediatric pseudotumor cerebri (idiopathic intracranial hypertension), *Surv Ophthalmol* 37:155, 1992.
16. Leung DYM, et al: Toxic shock syndrome toxin-secreting *Staphylococcus aureus* in Kawasaki syndrome, *Lancet* 342:1385, 1993.
17. Levy M, Koren G: Atypical Kawasaki disease: analysis of clinical presentation and diagnostic clues, *Pediatr Infect Dis J* 9:122, 1990.
18. Levy M, Spino M: Neonatal withdrawal syndrome: associated drugs and pharmacologic management, *Pharmacotherapy* 13:202, 1993.
19. Mann NP, McLellan NJ, Cartlidge PH: Transient intracranial hypertension of infancy, *Arch Dis Child* 63:966, 1988.

20. Mortola JF: Issues in the diagnosis and research of premenstrual syndrome, *Clin Obstet Gynecol* 35:587, 1992.
21. Mott SH, Packer RJ, Soldin SJ: Neurologic manifestations of cocaine exposure in childhood, *Pediatrics* 93:557, 1994.
22. Nadel S, Levin M: Kawasaki disease, *Curr Sci* 5:29, 1993.
23. Price CE, Rona RJ, Chinn S: Associations of excessive irritability with common illnesses and food intolerance, *Paediatr Perinat Epidemiol* 4:156, 1990.
24. Rowe PC, Newman SL, Brusilow SW: Natural history of symptomatic partial ornithine transcarbamylase deficiency, *N Engl J Med* 314:541, 1986.
25. Schwartz RH, Einhorn A: PCP intoxication in seven young children, *Pediatr Emerg Care* 2:238, 1986.
26. Woolf AD, et al: Intentional infantile ethylene glycol poisoning presenting as an inherited metabolic disorder, *J Pediatr* 120:421, 1992.
27. Zuckerman B, et al: Maternal depressive symptoms during pregnancy, and newborn irritability, *J Dev Behav Pediatr* 11:190, 1990.

152 Jaundice

Joel M. Andres • Mary Pat Francisco

Jaundice, a yellow discoloration of skin and mucous membranes, is the most common presenting manifestation of liver dysfunction in infants and children. This important physical finding is a direct indicator of hyperbilirubinemia, or excessive unconjugated and/or conjugated bilirubin in blood and tissues. Jaundice becomes clinically apparent in infants, children, and adults when the serum bilirubin approaches a concentration of 3 mg/dl. In neonates, these serum levels are usually in the 6- to 8-mg/dl range before jaundice is observed. The spectrum of conditions associated with jaundice ranges from physiological immaturity of bilirubin metabolism in the neonate to life-threatening disruption of liver function in the adolescent who is using illicit drugs. Jaundice always prompts concern and anxiety in the physician, parents, and older child; it is a clinical sign that demands evaluation.

EVALUATION

History

The history is important in determining the patient's age at the onset of the illness, in defining the chronicity of the hepatic dysfunction, and in understanding the clinical manifestations, especially jaundice and hepatomegaly. Inquiry may point to prolonged abdominal distention suggestive of longstanding hepatomegaly, splenomegaly, or ascites, or combinations of these. Other manifestations of chronic liver disease are easy bleeding or bruising and peripheral edema. The occurrence of jaundice, dark urine, and acholic stools may help date the onset of illness; also, jaundice usually appears in a cephalad to caudad progression. Pruritus and skin excoriations suggest prolonged cholestasis. The historical assessment also should include questions about maternal illness during pregnancy, exposure to sick individuals, blood products, or hepatotoxins, or recent surgery involving anesthesia. Because inheritable metabolic disease is a more common cause of liver dysfunction in the infant than in the older child or adult, a careful family history is essential and should include information about early-childhood deaths, pulmonary problems, neurological or liver disease, pregnancy loss, oligohydramnios, or hydrops fetalis.

Clinical Assessment

The infant liver, a large organ relative to body size during the first 2 years of life, normally is palpable about 2 cm below the right costal margin[106] and should not be felt to the left of the midline. Knowledge of vertical liver span for normal children may provide a guideline for estimating liver size in children younger than age 2 years: A liver span greater than 7 cm, usually determined by percussion, should be considered an indication for further evaluation.[110] Changes in structures adjacent to the liver can influence apparent liver size; for example, gas in the hepatic flexure of the colon may obscure hepatic dullness, and hyperinflation of the lungs, with subsequent depression of the diaphragm, may displace the liver downward, making it easier to palpate and appear to be enlarged.

The consistency and character of the liver's surface may help determine the nature of the underlying liver disorder. The liver's edge normally is sharp, but soft and nontender. A large liver that develops secondary to congestive heart failure has a rounded, smooth edge and a firm consistency; a cirrhotic liver is hard and has an irregular surface and edge. Auscultation over the liver area is valuable for detecting increased hepatic arterial blood flow (bruit) caused by primary liver tumors, metastatic disease of the liver, hepatic hemangiomas, or arteriovenous fistulas. (See Chapter 145, Hepatomegaly.) A complete abdominal evaluation of an infant who has jaundice or is suspected of having hepatomegaly should include palpation of the spleen. In normal infants younger than age 2 years, the spleen can be palpated 1 to 2 cm below the left costal margin; under most circumstances this organ should not be felt in normal children older than age 2. Splenomegaly suggests portal hypertension, especially in a child who has a prominent abdominal venous pattern, peripheral edema, and ascites. Splenic enlargement may be the first manifestation of previously undiagnosed progressive liver disease because it may precede the onset of jaundice. (See Chapter 170, Splenomegaly.)

JAUNDICE IN THE NEONATE AND YOUNG INFANT

In this chapter, jaundice in the neonate and young infant (Box 152-1) is considered separately from jaundice in the older infant and child (Box 152-2) for two reasons: (1) the young infant liver mounts a unique response to injury (i.e., active fibroblastic proliferation, Kupffer cell hyperplasia, and formation of multinucleated giant cells), and (2) unconjugated hyperbilirubinemia is common in early life and relatively uncommon after the neonatal period.

BOX 152-1

DIFFERENTIAL DIAGNOSIS OF JAUNDICE IN THE NEONATE AND YOUNG INFANT

Unconjugated Hyperbilirubinemia* (Nonconjugated Jaundice)

Overproduction of bilirubin
- Sepsis
- Rh/ABO incompatibility
- Hematoma (birth trauma)
- Drugs (e.g., vitamin K)
- Polycythemia
  - Maternal-fetal or twin-to-twin transfusion
  - Delayed clamping of umbilical cord
- Erythrocyte defects (e.g., congenital spherocytosis)
- Erythrocyte enzyme defects (e.g., glucose-6-phosphate dehydrogenase)
- Hemoglobinopathies
- Physiological jaundice

Impaired transport of bilirubin
- Hypoxia, acidosis
- Drugs (e.g., sulfonamides, aminosalicylic acid [ASA])
- Serum free fatty acids
  - Breast milk
  - Fat emulsions
- Hypoalbuminemia of prematurity

Impaired hepatic uptake of bilirubin
- Decreased sinusoidal perfusion (e.g., diminished venous flow after birth)
- Gilbert syndrome
- Physiological jaundice

Impaired conjugation of bilirubin
- Breast milk jaundice
- Drugs (e.g., chloramphenicol)
- Hypoglycemia
- Hypothyroidism
- High intestinal obstruction
- Glucuronyl transferase deficiency (types I and II)
- Physiological jaundice
- Gilbert syndrome

Enterohepatic circulation of bilirubin
- Delayed passage of meconium
  - Low intestinal obstruction (e.g., ileal atresia)
  - Cystic fibrosis
- Diminished intestinal motility
- Physiological jaundice
  - Negligible intestinal bacterial flora
  - Presence of intestinal beta-glucuronidase

Conjugated Hyperbilirubinemia* (Cholestatic Jaundice)

Acquired cholestatic jaundice
- Sepsis
- Other infections
  - Bacterial
  - Congenital (TORCH)
  - Viral (e.g., hepatitis A, B, C, or D)
  - Other viruses
    - Echovirus
    - Adenovirus
    - Parvovirus B-19
    - Paramyxovirus
    - HIV
  - Parasitic (e.g., toxoplasmosis)
- Chemical liver injury (e.g., drugs)
- Total parenteral nutrition (TPN)

Idiopathic cholestatic jaundice
- Hepatocellular cholestatic jaundice
  - Neonatal hepatitis
- Ductal cholestatic jaundice
  - Biliary atresia
  - Biliary hypoplasia
  - Paucity of intrahepatic bile ducts
  - Choledochal cyst

Inherited cholestatic jaundice
- Familial cholestatic syndromes (e.g., benign recurrent cholestasis)
- Metabolic cholestasis
  - Galactosemia
  - Hereditary fructose intolerance
  - Hereditary tyrosinemia
  - Neonatal iron storage disease
  - Cystic fibrosis
  - $Alpha_1$-antitrypsin deficiency
  - Glycogen storage disease
  - Inborn errors of bile acid metabolism
- Other storage disease
  - Niemann-Pick disease
  - Gaucher's disease
- "Noncholestatic" syndromes
  - Dubin-Johnson syndrome
  - Rotor's syndrome

*When this is the predominant form of bilirubin, the following diagnoses should be considered.

Unconjugated Hyperbilirubinemia

Unconjugated bilirubin in neonates is hazardous because of the potential for deposition of free bilirubin in neuronal tissues, with associated brain damage (kernicterus), especially in premature infants. Also, more subtle central nervous system (CNS) abnormalities can occur in infants, although a critical level of serum unconjugated bilirubin (at which only physiological changes rather than brain cell injury occur) has not yet been identified clearly. A total bilirubin of 14 mg/dl or higher may be associated with a significant risk of deafness in high-risk preterm infants whose birth weight is 1500 g or less.[21] Others have suggested that moderate hyperbilirubinemia (10 to 20 mg/dl) in full-term infants affects adjoining areas of the brainstem, including both the auditory pathway and the cry production pathways.[105]

A persistent unconjugated hyperbilirubinemia suggests excessive production of bilirubin, an inherited or acquired block in bilirubin transport, uptake, or conjugation, or abnormal enterohepatic circulation of bilirubin. More than one mechanism may be involved at any time during the course of

BOX 152-2

DIFFERENTIAL DIAGNOSIS OF JAUNDICE IN THE OLDER INFANT AND CHILD

Unconjugated Hyperbilirubinemia* (Noncholestatic Jaundice)

Overproduction of bilirubin

Hemoglobinopathies (e.g., sickle cell disease)
Erythrocyte defects (e.g., congenital spherocytosis)

Impaired uptake of bilirubin

Gilbert syndrome

Impaired conjugation of bilirubin

Glucuronyl transferase deficiency (types I and II)

Conjugated Hyperbilirubinemia* (Cholestatic Jaundice)

Acquired cholestatic jaundice

Sepsis
Other infections
- Bacterial (e.g., syphilis, leptospirosis)
- Viral (e.g., hepatitis A, B, C, D, and E; HIV, Epstein-Barr virus)
- Parasitic (e.g., toxoplasmosis)

Chemical liver injury
- Drugs (e.g., valproic acid, erythromycin, sulfonamides, isoniazid, methyldopa)
- Total parenteral nutrition (TPN)

Idiopathic cholestatic jaundice

Autoimmune hepatitis
Sclerosing cholangitis

Inherited cholestatic jaundice

Wilson's disease
Cystic fibrosis
$Alpha_1$-antitrypsin deficiency

*When this is the predominant form of bilirubin, the following diagnoses should be considered.

an illness. Normally, bilirubin metabolism commences with the breakdown of hemoglobin and subsequent conversion of heme (by the enzyme heme oxygenase) to biliverdin, which then is reduced to bilirubin. Unconjugated bilirubin binds to albumin, is transported to the hepatocyte, and then is taken up across the hepatocyte-sinusoidal membrane. Cytoplasmic proteins help transport bilirubin to the smooth endoplasmic reticulum for conjugation. Only bilirubin glucuronide conjugates are secreted at the bile canaliculus into bile and subsequently to the small intestine. Because unconjugated bilirubin is not secreted into bile, urobilinogen does not appear in the intestine or subsequently in the urine.

Sepsis, one of the important treatable problems associated with bilirubin overproduction, causes a hyperbilirubinemia that is a consequence of rapid hemolysis. Severe infection eventually causes a more prominent conjugated hyperbilirubinemia because of the bacterial or viral hepatocellular damage. The jaundice associated with hemolytic states such as erythroblastosis occurs during the first 36 hours of life; the risk of kernicterus is high if the infant develops early severe anemia and splenomegaly. Blood group typing and a direct Coombs test will establish the diagnosis of Rh incompatibility. Late hyporegenerative anemia occurs in some of these infants.[43] In a patient who has ABO incompatibility, numerous spherocytes may be noted in the blood smear, which can be obtained in addition to the appropriate blood group typing of infant and mother. A hematoma or polycythemia can lead to hemolysis because of the increased red blood cell (RBC) mass. Certain drugs administered during pregnancy or to the infant after birth may increase the risk of significant unconjugated hyperbilirubinemia. Vitamin K, for example, may cause hemolysis by acting as an oxidizing agent. Congenital erythrocyte defects such as spherocytosis cause chronic hyperbilirubinemia in infancy. The diagnosis is suspected when maternal agglutination antibodies are not demonstrated, especially if there is a family history of splenomegaly or hemolysis.

Most cases of neonatal unconjugated hyperbilirubinemia occur secondary to physiological jaundice, a transient, benign condition. This common form of jaundice has no single cause; it results from the interaction of many complex factors and is noted in approximately 15% of normal newborn infants. Overproduction of bilirubin occurs in these children because catabolism of fetal hemoglobin is increased and RBC survival is shortened.

Other newborn developmental factors include delayed conjugation of bilirubin that occurs secondary to immaturity of the glucuronyl transferase enzyme, poor hepatocellular transport of bilirubin because of a decrease in cytoplasmic transport proteins, and increased intestinal reabsorption of unconjugated bilirubin. For a full-term infant the serum bilirubin concentration rarely exceeds 10 mg/dl; jaundice occurs on the second or third day after birth and usually disappears by the fifth to eighth day of life. Bilirubin levels may increase to 12 mg/dl by the fifth to seventh day of life in a premature infant, returning to normal by the fourteenth day. Physiological jaundice is of no clinical significance unless additional factors such as prematurity, acidosis, or hemolysis also are present. Odell[66] has identified four criteria to help distinguish physiological jaundice from pathological jaundice; the presence of any of these criteria should prompt careful diagnostic evaluation: (1) jaundice before 36 hours of age, (2) jaundice that persists beyond the eighth day of life, (3) serum total bilirubin concentration above 12 mg/dl, and (4) a conjugated bilirubin level above 1.5 mg/dl.

Numerous other conditions can cause unconjugated hyperbilirubinemia in the neonate. Drugs such as aspirin and sulfonamides can lead to impaired transport of bilirubin as a result of displacement of the bilirubin molecule from albumin-binding sites. Other albumin-binding sites also can be blocked by free fatty acids, known to be in high concentration in breast milk and the main metabolic product of intravenous lipid (e.g., Intralipid or Liposyn).[3,68] Various cephalosporins[77] and sodium fusidate[10] also increase the risk of bilirubin encephalopathy by altering bilirubin-albumin binding. Although the precise mechanism of action is not known, benzyl alcohol, a bacteriostatic agent used to flush intravascular catheters, has been associated with the development of kernicterus in infants.[39] Other changes in care may have contributed to the findings in this latter group of patients (many also had intraventricular hemorrhages), but drug interference with bilirubin-albumin binding was suspected. Bilirubin displacement from albumin is amplified in the neonate who is hypoxic and acidotic, especially in a premature infant who has hypoalbuminemia.

Impaired hepatic uptake of bilirubin occurs in Gilbert syndrome, a common familial condition that usually is diagnosed in the second decade of life and in sick neonates who have diminished hepatic sinusoidal blood flow or persistent patency of the ductus venosus. Although alteration of bilirubin-albumin binding probably is the main defect, breast milk jaundice may occur because of the hormone pregnanediol in the mother's milk.[27] This hormone is capable of inhibiting glucuronyl transferase activity, which leads to impaired conjugation of bilirubin. Clinical jaundice occurs in about 1% of breast-fed infants, usually between the sixth and eighth days of life in a normal-appearing, thriving child. The serum concentration of unconjugated bilirubin rarely exceeds 20 mg/dl; this level recedes after breast-feeding is discontinued, and the jaundice usually does not recur if breast-feeding is reinstituted after 2 or 3 days.[46] Even if breast-feeding is continued, the serum bilirubin usually declines over a period of 2 to 3 months. Kernicterus has never been reported with this common form of jaundice; however, a brief discontinuance of breast milk always should be considered because of the small potential for subtle neurological dysfunction after prolonged exposure to unconjugated bilirubin. This should be done before the child is subjected to a detailed diagnostic evaluation.

The possibility of drug-induced jaundice again should be emphasized. For example, chloramphenicol and novobiocin can diminish bilirubin conjugation by competing for glucuronyl transferase. Hypoglycemia also may exacerbate jaundice in young infants because glucose is a required substrate for synthesis of the bilirubin-glucuronide conjugate. Prolonged elevation of unconjugated bilirubin is seen in congenital hypothyroidism, presumably because of delay in maturation of the bilirubin-conjugating enzyme.[50] Because this is a treatable disease, it is critical to obtain thyroid function studies in all children who have indirect hyperbilirubinemia. Some infants who have intestinal obstruction (e.g., pyloric stenosis or duodenal atresia) develop unconjugated hyperbilirubinemia. The mechanism for jaundice in this circumstance is not known, but some evidence suggests diminished glucuronyl transferase activity in these infants, who improve rapidly after the anatomical problem is corrected surgically.

A rare familial cause of unconjugated hyperbilirubinemia is glucuronyl transferase deficiency.[5] Two forms have been described, depending on the patient's clinical response to phenobarbital. Type I, Crigler-Najjar syndrome, is a severe, rare autosomal recessive disease in which no glucuronyl transferase enzyme can be demonstrated. Nonhemolytic jaundice develops in the first hours of life, and early signs of kernicterus often are present. Phototherapy is required, and exchange transfusion often is necessary. As the child becomes older, phototherapy is less effective. Plasmapheresis can then be tried, but patients usually require liver transplantation; phenobarbital therapy is ineffective. The type II deficiency is autosomal dominant. These infants have reduced levels of glucuronyl transferase enzyme, and the action of the enzyme is enhanced by phenobarbital. Serum bilirubin levels may decline dramatically with the use of phenobarbital, which is required for the individual's entire life. Lower intestinal obstruction syndromes and clinical conditions that lead to decreased intestinal motility promote increased enterohepatic circulation of unconjugated bilirubin. Elevated serum bilirubin can occur, especially in the early days of life when the intestinal lumen sequesters bilirubin-rich meconium together with deconjugating glucuronidase enzyme.

Conjugated Hyperbilirubinemia

Immature secretory mechanisms, damage to the hepatocyte canalicular membrane, or an anatomical abnormality of bile ducts can cause conjugated hyperbilirubinemia. This always is a pathological condition, and it usually is associated with hepatocellular disease. The conjugated molecule is not known to be harmful to body tissues, including the central nervous system, but a serum conjugated bilirubin level above 1.5 mg/dl always should be considered abnormal and a development that occurs secondary to hepatic injury.

Hepatic excretion of organic anions such as bilirubin depends in part on the movement of bile acid and water across the canalicular membrane. Jaundice usually is associated closely with a reduction in bile flow, or cholestasis—hence the term *cholestatic jaundice*. Various acquired, idiopathic, and inherited conditions that cause neonatal cholestatic jaundice are discussed briefly in this section (see Box 152-1).[56]

Hepatocellular cholestatic jaundice includes neonatal hepatitis and is the diagnosis given for most infants who have conjugated hyperbilirubinemia in the early months of life. Symptoms usually occur in the first 2 weeks after birth, and the typical presentation is that of an unwell, jaundiced infant who has hepatomegaly. The main differential diagnostic consideration is ductal cholestatic jaundice, especially biliary atresia—that is, determining whether the jaundice occurs secondary to a surgical or a nonsurgical problem. An evaluation to determine the type of hyperbilirubinemia and to establish an early diagnosis of a treatable disease always should be considered immediately. Studies that should be done include total and direct serum bilirubin determinations, a hemoglobin level, Coombs test, blood glucose test, serum amino acid determinations, and serological tests for toxoplasmosis, syphilis, hepatitis B virus (HBV) (especially anti-HBc), and human immunodeficiency virus (HIV). HIV infection is slowly beginning to emerge as an important problem affecting the liver in neonates and young infants. Clinical symptoms of HIV perinatal infection can develop as early as 1 month of age; however, the median interval from birth to the emergence of symptoms is 8 months. The commonest early manifestations of HIV infection in infants are poor growth, interstitial pneumonitis, and hepatosplenomegaly. However, the overall spectrum of liver disease and pathological features among neonates and young infants is unknown, and jaundice is not common. Cholestatic jaundice and hepatitis occurred in a study of seven infants as the first manifestation of their perinatally acquired disease.[70] No specific etiological agent was identified as the cause of the cholestasis. Six of the seven infants died within 12 weeks of the onset of hepatitis, mainly because of complications of *Pneumocystis carinii* pneumonia and cytomegalovirus infection. Only one infant died as a consequence of liver failure. Other uncommon, but important viral infections of the liver not associated with HIV infection include parvovirus B-19 and paramyxovirus (rubeola and parainfluenza 4).[71] Cell fusion is part of the basic pathobiology of the paramyxoviruses, including fusion with cell membranes to form syncytial giant cells.

Other important tests include urine testing for nonglucose-reducing substances and organic acids, blood cultures, and urine cultures. The syndrome of cholestatic jaundice in association with urinary tract infection is not uncommon, especially among neonates and infants younger than 2 months of age. The liver histology may suggest the cause of the infant's problem, but failure to diagnose hepatocellular cholestasis specifically necessitates studies to determine patency of the biliary tree such as hepatobiliary scintigraphy (e.g., diisopropyl iminodiacetic acid [DISIDA]), duodenal intubation for bile, and percutaneous liver biopsy. Intraoperative laparoscopic cholangiography or magnetic resonance cholangiography also may emerge as important diagnostic procedures for evaluation of cholestatic jaundice in neonates and young infants. Factors related to an unfavorable prognosis are prolonged jaundice and cholestasis, early appearance of portal fibrosis, and coexistence of systemic disease.[17] Approximately 30% of infants who have hepatocellular cholestatic jaundice develop progressive liver failure, another 10% survive the early months of illness but have chronic disease (including cirrhosis), and the remainder recover completely. The overall outlook for these patients has improved because of the success of liver transplantation. The major challenge is to identify the infant who has biliary atresia before the age of 8 to 10 weeks and avoid unnecessary surgery in infants who have hepatocellular forms of cholestasis.

Children who have cholestatic jaundice who die have significantly more liver histological abnormalities, including prominent periportal inflammation and fibrosis and diffuse giant cell transformation.[93] Ductal cholestatic jaundice includes diagnoses such as biliary atresia, sclerosing cholangitis, biliary hypoplasia, and choledochal cyst. Infants who have biliary atresia usually appear well until jaundice persists beyond the first week after birth. About 20% of infants who have biliary atresia have other congenital anomalies, mainly cardiovascular, gastrointestinal, or splenic malformations.[87] Although the theory is controversial, *Reovirus* (type 3) has been implicated as an important etiological agent for hepatobiliary disease in infants.[61] This virus has been localized in biliary remnants in the inflamed porta hepatis.[62] Jaundice increases with time, and the liver becomes hard and firm as cirrhosis progresses over the first months of life.

In the past, the prognosis for infants who had biliary atresia correlated best for those who had expert surgical treatment performed by operating teams skilled in biliary microsurgery[16]; however, the long-term outcome for these children now is related more strongly to the skills of the liver transplantation surgeon. In some Japanese surgery units, bile drainage is reported in almost 90% of patients who undergo portoenterostomy (the Kasai procedure); in North America, the overall success rate of Kasai portoenterostomy is less satisfactory,[73] but this procedure always should be done before transplantation is considered except for infants seen after 120 days of life, in whom liver transplantation may be considered primary therapy.[22] The Kasai operation restores bile flow in about 80% of children operated on before 60 days of life. Despite this success, fewer than 20% of patients who have biliary atresia survive for long periods.[60] Most of these patients have portal hypertension and abnormal liver function. Postoperative cholangitis often leads to deteriorating liver function; it occurs in more than half of successful portoenterostomies before the age of 1 year, but is unusual after age 2.[29] Predictors of poor outcome after portoenterostomy include age greater than 2 months, presence of cirrhosis at initial biopsy, total nonpatency of extrahepatic ducts, absence of bile ducts at transected liver hilus, and subsequent development of varices or ascites. Liver transplantation is the only chance of survival for many patients who have this form of end-stage liver disease.[101] Transplantation is a curative procedure; portoenterostomy is primarily palliative. The long-term outcome of liver transplantation for children who have biliary atresia is excellent. Factors that enhance survival include surgical technical precision, aggressive retransplantation, antifungal chemoprophylaxis and therapy, and judicious immunosuppression.[12]

Sclerosing cholangitis of neonatal onset may be confused with biliary atresia. The former is a cholestatic syndrome associated with abnormal intrahepatic bile ducts and increased serum levels of gamma-glutamyl transpeptidase (an index of bile duct damage). Infants who have hypoplasia of bile ducts and antitrypsin deficiency also have high serum levels of this transpeptidase enzyme.[51]

Biliary hypoplasia is noted in infants who have acute infections of the liver, various familial cholestatic syndromes such as arteriohepatic dysplasia (Alagille syndrome),[1,20] and the more common metabolic cholestatic syndrome, alpha$_1$-antitrypsin deficiency.[83] The clinical course of infants who have biliary hypoplasia varies; overall survival is much longer than for children who have biliary atresia, but some patients require liver transplantation.[100] Patients who have Alagille syndrome often have a significant heart murmur and characteristic facies. The presence of congenital heart disease is the main feature associated with increased mortality. Butterfly vertebrae and posterior corneal embryotoxons (opaque rings) occur in more than 50% of these patients.[24] Less common ocular abnormalities include diffuse fundus hypopigmentation, iris changes, and optic disc anomalies.[33] Ophthalmological examination of children who have cholestatic jaundice should allow early diagnosis of Alagille syndrome.

Clinical recognition of a jaundiced child who has a choledochal cyst depends on the size of the cyst and whether biliary obstruction occurs.[84] Ultrasonographic scans can improve the preoperative diagnosis of this problem, which can be resolved surgically before progressive biliary obstruction and cirrhosis occur. Identifying the gallbladder by using ultrasound and noting a change in its size after oral feeding aids in the differential diagnosis of ductal versus hepatocellular problems.[38] For example, infants who have biliary atresia may have a small gallbladder that is not affected by oral feeding. Further, ultrasound-guided percutaneous cholecystocholangiography may help differentiate extrahepatic from intrahepatic causes of cholestatic jaundice in infancy.[98]

Just as rare as the familial cholestasis syndromes are the metabolic hepatocellular problems (except for cystic fibrosis and $alpha_1$-antitrypsin deficiency); nevertheless, they are important to diagnose because of the potential for effective treatment. Specifically, infants who have galactosemia, fructose intolerance, and tyrosinemia have similar clinical manifestations, usually within days to weeks after birth. Marked jaundice, hepatosplenomegaly, bleeding, and failure to thrive usually are prominent. However, infants who have galactosemia may have less apparent findings; after several months they may develop cataracts, cirrhosis, and psychomotor retardation. Similarly, the tyrosinemic infant may escape the acute phase of illness and be discovered months later to have cirrhosis, rickets, and renal disease; these patients have a high incidence of hepatoma in later childhood.[107] Hereditary tyrosinemia (type I) is caused by a deficiency of fumarylacetoacetate hydrolase (FAH), the last enzyme in the catabolic pathway of tyrosine. It is a disease reported most commonly in infants from French Canada. Most patients are homozygous for a splice mutation.[31] A variety of other mutations have been described; therefore, there is heterogeneity in the expression of this rare, but interesting, inborn error of metabolism. Tyrosinemia occurs in chronic and acute forms. Patients who have the chronic form have immunoreactive FAH at a level of about 20% of normal enzymatic activity. The prognosis is poor, and survival after the onset of symptoms varies with the age of onset[102]—the earlier the symptoms, the poorer the outlook. Besides hepatoma, the most common causes of death are liver failure and a porphyria-like syndrome with respiratory failure (secondary to a block of porphyrin biosynthesis by succinylacetone, a metabolic byproduct of abnormal tyrosine metabolism). The acute form of tyrosinemia, when FAH is at undetectable levels, can cause a neurological crisis presenting as a peripheral neuropathy with pain and extensor hypertonia, vomiting and paralytic ileus, muscle weakness, and self-mutilation.[59] Between crises, most children regain normal function. Serum levels of tyrosine usually are elevated, and markedly increased urinary succinylacetone is diagnostic of this inborn error. It has been suggested that succinylacetone might have neurotoxic effects, in addition to delta-aminolevulinic acid, an intermediate metabolite of porphyrin metabolism. A jaundiced child who has cataracts and psychomotor retardation might very well have galactosemia, whereas jaundice associated with a history of vomiting, distaste for sweet foods, and fructosuria more likely would result from fructose intolerance. Each of these metabolic disorders also may cause renal dysfunction manifested by aminoaciduria, glycosuria, and phosphaturia (Fanconi's syndrome). Their definitive diagnosis depends on specific tolerance tests and the measurement of enzyme activity in the red blood cells (galactosemia), liver, or kidney (fructose intolerance). Analyzing the urine for non-glucose-reducing sugars, organic acids, and amino acids is appropriate for initial screening. The long-term prognosis for all of these metabolic diseases depends on early introduction of dietary restrictions and possible pharmacological therapy for tyrosinemia.

Neonatal iron storage disease (NISD) is a poorly understood, uncommon, inherited disorder of iron metabolism characterized by severe hepatic insufficiency of intrauterine onset.[42] This problem is referred to inappropriately as neonatal hemochromatosis because of its association with extrahepatic siderosis and sparing of the reticuloendothelial system. The precise cause of NISD and nature of the basic defect remain unknown. Although patients who have NISD and adult-onset hereditary hemochromatosis have similar patterns of iron loading, all studies have failed to demonstrate a familial linkage between NISD and iron storage disease in later life. Infants who have NISD usually have a normal serum iron and transferrin levels, markedly elevated serum ferritin, and prominent siderosis of the liver, pancreas, kidneys, and adrenal glands. Abnormal iron levels also are detected in minor salivary glands, a fact that allows for confirmation of the diagnosis of iron overload because of easy accessibility of the salivary glands to buccal mucosal biopsy. If antenatal death does not occur, infants who have NISD are almost always severely ill at birth with jaundice, hypoglycemia, coagulopathy, and ascites secondary to perinatal cirrhosis. The diagnosis can be associated with fetal nonimmune hydrops.[109] It is not known whether intrauterine infection can lead to NISD, but the differential diagnosis of neonatal intra- and extrahepatic siderosis is important and includes cytomegalovirus liver disease,[41] neonatal echovirus 9 disease,[9] tyrosinemia, and disorders of bile acid synthesis.[86] Deferoxamine has not proved to be effective in infants who have NISD.

Jaundice is unusual in children who have glycogen storage disease,[58] except for types III and IV. Hepatocellular dysfunction is more prominent in infants who have type IV glycogenosis; jaundice occurs in the first months of life and usually is followed by cirrhosis and death before age 2 years. Persistent jaundice is unusual in infants who have cystic fibrosis, but it may occur when the disease is associated with increased enterohepatic circulation of bilirubin (meconium ileus), drug hypersensitivity, parenteral alimentation, or common bile duct inflammation secondary to inspissation of biliary secretions. $Alpha_1$-antitrypsin (AAT) deficiency,[83] a genetic defect of glycoprotein metabolism, is the most common metabolic disorder associated with liver disease among infants. The AAT gene is a single copy gene on chromosome 14 and is known to have numerous variants, including the deficiency "Z" type AAT gene, which is associated with reduced serum antitrypsin.[13] Abnormal Z-AAT is retained in the endoplasmic reticulum, with consequent intrahepatocellular accumulation as insoluble inclusions that may be associated with liver damage. The usual presentation is that of cholestasis with associated jaundice and hepatomegaly. The diagnosis is confirmed by a low serum $alpha_1$-antitrypsin level and protease inhibitor (Pi) typing. There is an estimated 80% to 85% decrease in serum ATT levels. No specific treatment is available, but infants at risk must be identified and proper genetic counseling provided to the family. Liver transplantation has been performed in older children who have end-stage liver disease caused by antitrypsin deficiency.[34] The prognosis varies considerably. Despite the persistence of mild hepatocellular dysfunction, clinical improvement may occur a few months after birth. Biliary cirrhosis and portal hypertension eventually develop in about 15% of patients who have homozygous Z antitrypsin deficiency.

In rare cases, an infant who has cholestatic jaundice will be discovered to have a primary metabolic defect in bile acid synthesis,[11,81] a disorder that affects transformations in the bile acid steroid nucleus. This rare but important inborn error of metabolism has the potential for successful diagnosis (urine and serum analysis for the presence of bile acids and bile precursors). Neonates who have bile acid metabolism defects may present with liver failure and appear, at least initially, to have giant-cell hepatitis.[11,15,81] Detection is difficult because the bile acid analysis requires fast atom bombardment ionization-mass spectrometry and gas chromatography-mass spectrometry. Although these inborn errors probably are rare, their true incidence is not known. More importantly, bile acid therapy has been successful in many of these infants, with normalization of liver function abnormalities and liver histology.

Inherited storage diseases (e.g., Niemann-Pick and Gaucher's disease) usually cause hepatosplenomegaly in infants, but jaundice is unusual. These diseases are exceedingly rare and should not be considered in the initial evaluation of children who have cholestatic jaundice.

Dubin-Johnson syndrome[4] is another type of familial jaundice that probably has an autosomal recessive mode of inheritance. It is considered a benign condition, but the child has a reduced capacity to secrete several organic anions, especially conjugated bilirubin, sulfobromophthalein, rose bengal, and cholecystographic dye. Interestingly, excretion of bile acids is normal; therefore, the term *noncholestatic jaundice* is applicable and the extrahepatic biliary tree always is patent. Recurrent episodes of jaundice, which can be precipitated by infection, may begin in infancy and can be misdiagnosed as acute hepatitis because of the abrupt onset of illness. There often is a family history of jaundice and vague upper abdominal pain in older children. Routine tests of liver function produce normal results except for an increase in total bilirubin (usually below 15 mg/dl) with predominance of conjugated bilirubin. Grossly, the liver appears black, owing to accumulation of melanin-like pigment in lysosomes. Rotor's syndrome is similar to (or may be a variant of) Dubin-Johnson syndrome except that pigmentation of hepatocytes has not been demonstrated and secretion of cholecystographic dye is normal. Recognition of these benign noncholestatic jaundice syndromes may obviate the need for extensive diagnostic tests.

JAUNDICE IN THE OLDER INFANT AND CHILD

Unconjugated Hyperbilirubinemia

Unconjugated hyperbilirubinemia in 1- to 2-year-old infants (after maturation of the blood-brain barrier) and in older children usually is of no pathological significance. It is uncommon in an older child who does not have an underlying hemolytic disease such as sickle cell disease or spherocytosis. Gilbert syndrome[72] is a common familial syndrome of autosomal dominant inheritance that may occur secondary to an abnormality of bilirubin uptake at the hepatocyte sinusoidal membrane. Mild fluctuating jaundice can be noted during early infancy, but the syndrome usually is not diagnosed until the second decade of life. Fatigue and caloric deprivation accentuate the jaundice. The mechanism is not understood, but it may be related to increased production of bilirubin after fasting. Abdominal pain, malaise, and other vague symptoms usually accompany the jaundice. The criteria for diagnosing Gilbert syndrome are a serum unconjugated bilirubin level above 1.5 mg/dl but below 6 mg/dl, lack of other demonstrable abnormalities of liver function, absence of overt hemolysis, and no evidence of liver disease on examination except for jaundice. The main differential diagnostic considerations are glucuronyl transferase deficiency (type II) and mild hemolytic syndromes. No treatment is necessary for Gilbert syndrome except resumption of an adequate caloric intake. This is a benign condition but one important to recognize so that unnecessary diagnostic investigations are avoided.

Conjugated Hyperbilirubinemia

Acute viral hepatitis is the most common cause of jaundice in older infants and children. Hepatitis A virus (HAV) often is the etiological agent, but most of these children do not have jaundice or significant liver dysfunction. Fulminant hepatitis may occur, however, and is associated with a high mortality.[26] The newly developed HAV vaccine is recommended before travel and for patients who have chronic liver disease, especially hepatitis C infection. Hepatitis B virus (HBV) produces a similar symptom complex of nausea, vomiting, and anorexia that often precedes the jaundice. In children, liver disease that occurs secondary to HBV may be mild, but persistent jaundice and hepatocellular dysfunction with eventual occurrence of chronic hepatitis can occur. Antigenemia and clinical disease occur often in infants born to mothers who have acute hepatitis during the latter part of pregnancy or early in the postpartum period.[80] Although HBV infection was once considered a contraindication to breast-feeding, the availability of HBIG and HBV vaccine for infants has made breast milk safe.[2] From a worldwide perspective, perinatal and postnatal transmission of HBV is an extremely important public health problem. For example, before an extensive, controlled HBV vaccine trial in Senegal, striking evidence of the endemicity of HBV infection was found: 12% of blood donors were HBsAg positive, and 80% of 6- and 7-year-olds had at least one serum marker of past or present HBV infection.[57] In areas where HBV is endemic, the relative risk of hepatocellular carcinoma is much higher in carriers than in noncarriers.

Routine HBV screening of all pregnant women is essential. If the woman proves to be positive, the newborn should receive hepatitis B immunoglobulin (HBIG) for passive immunity and begin the recombinant vaccine series immediately at birth. In the United States and other developed countries, adolescent users of parenterally administered illicit drugs may develop acute HBV liver disease. The HBV vaccine needs to be given to patients at risk of developing this serious infection.[91,95]

Interferon is the only agent known to have a lasting beneficial effect in the treatment of hepatitis B. The results of large, multicenter adult trials[35] are encouraging, but further studies are necessary to evaluate the degree and duration of resolution of HBV infections after use of interferon. Therapy with interferon is now for a duration of 4 months, with subcutaneous injections given every other day or three times a week. Lamivudine, a nucleoside that suppresses HBV replication, may produce higher response rates when used in combination with interferon.[45]

Hepatitis C virus (HCV), formerly known as non-A, non-B hepatitis virus, recently was discovered to be an important pathogen in children.[7,8] The significance of this virus in infant cholestatic jaundice is not clear, but it is known that HCV probably transmits vertically[49] and that the risk of HCV transmission to the infant is directly related to the level of viremia in the mother.[67] Similar to the low transmission rate of HCV at birth, breast milk does not appear to contribute to the spread of this important virus.[44] Further, infants born to HCV-positive mothers coinfected with HIV have a higher vertical transmission rate.[97] It also is known that anti-HCV antibodies can be detected, although infrequently, in infants who have jaundice, abnormal liver function, and biopsy-proven hepatitis. HCV is transmitted to older infants and children through transfusion of infected blood; this virus probably is responsible for most cases identified as posttransfusion hepatitis. Acute and chronic infection with HCV usually is milder and anicteric compared with HBV infections; however, persistent HCV infection leads to chronic liver disease in 25% to 50% of patients. For example, 24% of multiply transfused leukemic children in long-term remission were discovered by anti-HCV reactivity to have a persistently polyphasic pattern of elevated serum transaminase and abnormal liver histology, such as chronic active hepatitis.[49] In general, anti-HCV antibodies persist in patients who have chronic disease. The mean interval from onset of hepatitis to detection of anti-HCV antibodies may be 15 weeks but can be much longer. HCV is detected much more rapidly by polymerase chain reaction (PCR) technology.[65] Detection of HCV-RNA by reverse transcription PCR is the best means of confirming the diagnosis,[47] although recombinant immunoblot assay (RIBA) now is readily available and also confirms the presence of infection. Treatment of HCV is problematical, and clinical trials using alpha-interferon and ribavirin have just commenced in children at this writing. In adults, 50% of patients who have persistent HCV infection respond to interferon with normalization of serum alanine aminotransferase (ALT) and improvement in liver histology.[18] Unfortunately, 50% of these patients relapse after therapy is discontinued. Prolonged therapy is becoming the rule, with interferon being administered three times a week for up to 12 months. Combination therapy with ribavirin, a nucleoside analogue, is now being evaluated for patients who have hepatitis C infection.[14]

Hepatitis D virus (HDV) is diagnosed as a concurrent infection in patients who have acute and chronic HBV hepatitis. Transmission of HDV (delta agent) from mother to infant has been reported.[111] This RNA virus requires HBV for replication. The severity of HBV infection is greatly increased by the presence of HDV. Testing for anti-HDV antibodies is recommended for any patient who is HBV positive. No therapy is available to treat this viral infection, which is not common in the United States.

Hepatitis E virus (HEV) may be the most common cause of acute sporadic hepatitis among children living in some developing countries.[36,37] Its fecal-oral or waterborne transmission is similar to that of HAV infection. Hepatitis E infection has not been documented to occur in Western countries; it is endemic to Southeast Asia and India and should be suspected in travelers returning from these areas of the world. Clinical manifestations of HEV resemble those of HAV except that the attack rates are highest among adolescents and young adults. Fulminant hepatitis may occur in outbreaks of HEV disease, especially in young pregnant women. This infection is confirmed by a Western blot assay for anti-HEV IgM.[37]

Chronic active hepatitis was discovered in older infants and children who had clinical and immunological characteristics of acquired immunodeficiency syndrome (AIDS).[23] Epstein-Barr virus (EBV) infection may have been the cause of the hepatic inflammation in these AIDS patients as a consequence of a generalized immune disturbance. Another report documented hepatic opportunistic infections caused by *Cryptosporidium* organisms and *Mycobacterium avium-intracellulare,* as well as small epithelioid granulomas on liver histology.[69] In general, liver histopathology in pediatric patients shares some features with that in adults. However, granulomas are less common in children, whereas young patients who have interstitial pneumonitis are more likely to have evidence of hepatic lymphoplasmacytic infiltrates.[40] In adults who have AIDS, macrocytosis and nonspecific portal inflammation are the most common histological abnormalities. See Chapter 216 for further discussion of hepatitis.

Sporadic cases of jaundice in childhood may be noted with other infections, such as infectious mononucleosis. Jaundice occurs in only a small percentage of children infected with EBV, despite hepatic involvement in most patients. This diagnosis should be suspected in an adolescent who has acute pharyngitis and splenomegaly with or without hepatomegaly. A large number of children younger than age 4 years also acquire this disease and are prone to develop pneumonia during their acute course.[94]

Cholecystitis is a rare problem in children. Acute disease usually develops among adolescent girls, who often experience jaundice, right upper quadrant pain, vomiting, and fever. Gallbladder ultrasonography will suggest the correct diagnosis and identify the presence of gallstones, which are discovered most often in children who have hemolysis. Gallstones also are seen in pregnant adolescents, in patients receiving parenteral nutrition or ceftriaxone therapy, in patients who have cystic fibrosis, and in some children who have cirrhosis.[75,76] Laparoscopic cholecystectomy is the treatment of choice for most children who have cholelithiasis.[103] Cholangiography may be important to exclude the presence of stones in the common bile duct, especially in a patient who has hemolytic disease who is acutely ill with fever and abdominal pain. For children who have evidence of common duct stones, especially those who have undergone cholecystectomy previously, endoscopic sphincterotomy is the treatment of choice.[32] Hemolytic anemia may be the mode of presentation for Wilson's disease in children older than age 5 years. Individuals who have this important, rare, treatable disease have jaundice during the early hepatic stage of illness, when the liver is becoming saturated with copper. A careful evaluation should be made to detect Kayser-Fleischer rings and subtle neurological dysfunction.

Chronic active hepatitis probably is rare in infants younger than age 2 years. In more than 25% of these children, the illness begins as acute hepatitis with jaundice, and the severity, course, and prognosis vary considerably. An immunological form of chronic active liver disease (autoimmune hepatitis) occurs primarily in young girls. The extrahepatic autoimmune manifestations they develop are skin rash, arthritis, and hemolytic anemia. This inflammatory liver disease often is associated with high serum titers of anti-liver-kidney-microsomal (anti-LKM) antibody, and it is a potentially fatal disease for which immunosuppressive treatment must be started early.[52]

Exposure to drugs such as isoniazid and methyldopa occasionally leads to liver dysfunction and a histological abnormality indistinguishable from chronic active hepatitis. The appearance of jaundice may be delayed for months after institution of isoniazid therapy, and the severity of the liver dysfunction correlates with continued use of the drug.[90]

The anticonvulsant agent valproic acid also causes cholestatic jaundice with diffuse hepatocellular injury.[92] The mechanism for hepatic damage is uncertain; concurrent administration of valproic acid with other anticonvulsants should be monitored carefully. Other common drugs (e.g., erythromycin estolate and sulfonamides) can cause jaundice with either a hepatitis-like or a cholestatic pattern. Hepatotoxic reactions occur in children who have tuberculosis and are treated with isoniazid combined with rifampin; jaundice occurs more rapidly if the dose of isoniazid exceeds 10 mg/kg/day.[99]

Jaundice occurs in children, especially infants, who are receiving total parenteral nutrition (TPN). The precise mechanism is unknown, but the problem may be related to amino acid imbalance and a subsequent decrease in bile acid synthesis or to inadequate secretin stimulation of bile flow in a child who has minimal oral alimentation. Clinical characteristics associated with the development of TPN-associated jaundice include low birth weight, duration of TPN administration, interval before enteral feeding is initiated, sepsis, central venous catheter infection, and the number of surgical procedures performed.[28,63]

Children who have immunodeficiency syndromes and increased serum gamma-glutamyl transferase activity may have sclerosing cholangitis.[19] This chronic cholestatic disease also is associated with chronic inflammatory bowel disease, histiocytosis X, congenital psoriasis, and cholestatic jaundice of the neonate. Cholangiography reveals abnormal intrahepatic bile ducts in all these children. The prognosis is poor, but liver transplantation should be considered except in those who have severe immunodeficiency disorders.

MANAGEMENT

Unconjugated Hyperbilirubinemia

Excellent general reviews are available in the literature on the treatment of newborns who have unconjugated hyperbilirubinemia.[53] An extensive discussion of such treatment can be found in Chapter 48, Common Neonatal Illnesses. Intravenous infusion of albumin, especially before exchange transfusion, increases the potential binding sites for unconjugated molecules. A double-volume exchange transfusion is indicated infrequently except for hemolytic disease when the serum indirect bilirubin concentration exceeds 20 mg/dl in full-term neonates or 10 mg/dl in ill premature infants or in any child who experiences a rapid rise (more than 0.5 mg/dl/hour) in serum bilirubin. Phototherapy is more efficacious than exchange transfusion for nonhemolytic jaundice and may help prevent a rapid increase in serum bilirubin. However, its effectiveness in terms of preventing brain injury is unknown, and as noted earlier, it should not be instituted before any underlying pathological condition is excluded. This form of therapy never is considered routine and should be reserved for premature infants or term infants who have high serum bilirubin concentrations, as well as for the rare patient who has type I glucuronyl transferase deficiency who requires continuous therapy. Specific guidelines for initiating phototherapy include treatment if the bilirubin level exceeds 15 mg/dl at any time of life in the full-term infant, at 12 hours of age in neonates weighing less than 1500 g at birth, and when the serum bilirubin rises to 10 mg/dl in infants weighing 1500 to 2000 g at birth. Phototherapy probably induces increased biliary excretion of photoisomers of bilirubin after the molecule in exposed skin reacts photochemically.[25] Potential side effects are well recognized, including an increase in insensible water loss, retinal damage, unusual bronzing of the skin,[25] and even alteration of intracellular deoxyribonucleic acid. When the hyperbilirubinemia is refractory to conventional phototherapy, treatment with high-dose intravenous gamma globulin may be useful in some patients who have isoimmune hemolytic disease.[78]

The effectiveness of oral agar in treating neonates who have jaundice is uncertain, but it may be associated with reduced peak serum bilirubin levels by binding bilirubin in the gut. Recently, a new treatment with tin (Sn)-mesoporphyrin has been proposed for infants who have unconjugated hyperbilirubinemia.[55] This synthetic metalloporphyrin is a competitive enzyme inhibitor (of heme oxygenase) that blocks the degradation of heme to the bile pigment, biliverdin. The excess heme is not converted to bilirubin; instead, it is excreted in bile. This synthetic compound may prove useful, especially if it helps lessen dependence on phototherapy and exchange transfusion.

Phenobarbital is used to treat unconjugated hyperbilirubinemia in older infants who have type II glucuronyl transferase deficiency. In this situation, continuous use of phenobarbital is necessary in the early weeks of life when the risk of kernicterus is greatest. Children who have Crigler-Najjar syndrome do not respond to phenobarbital. An exchange transfusion is the only effective early therapy to reduce toxic serum bilirubin levels in these patients, but curative treatment has been reported with home phototherapy, followed by orthotopic liver transplantation at an early age.[85]

Collaborative perinatal projects have examined the association between neonatal bilirubin levels and subsequent neurodevelopmental outcome in terms of intelligence quotient (IQ), neurological examination, and sensorineural hearing loss. In general, there is little evidence to suggest that a level of indirect bilirubin of less than 25 mg/dl affects the neurodevelopment of healthy, full-term infants who do not have hemolytic disease. However, infants born prematurely have a greater susceptibility to kernicterus. The percentage of children born prematurely who had minor and major disabilities increased consistently as the bilirubin concentration increased.[64,79,104] Finally, because newborn infants are now being discharged earlier from the hospital, there is a higher risk of morbidity from hyperbilirubinemia. Guidelines from the American Academy of Pediatrics recommend that infants discharged less than 48 hours after birth should be evaluated by a health care professional within 2 to 3 days of discharge.[54] Discharge of many newborns before 36 hours is common.[108] Recently, the accuracy of predischarge total serum bilirubin (TSB) values as a predictor of subsequent degree of hyperbilirubinemia was measured in direct Coombs negative, healthy term, and near-term newborns.[6] It was determined that an hour-specific TSB before discharge can predict which newborn is at high, intermediate, or low risk for developing clinically significant hyperbilirubinemia. This was easily monitored on an hour-specific, percentile-based, predictive bilirubin nomogram, which should help identify those infants who require more careful follow-up surveillance. These data are a reminder of the importance of relating the serum bilirubin level to the infant's age in hours and not days, and emphasize the important fact that if newborns are discharged at less than 36 hours, their bilirubin levels can only be increasing.[54] Repeated transcutaneous measurements of bilirubin, using a computer-driven, handheld device (Chromatics Colormate III) may eventually make hour-specific TSB predictions even more valuable by obviating the need for serum bilirubin determinations.[96]

Conjugated Hyperbilirubinemia

In general, it is not necessary to treat the jaundice of patients who have conjugated hyperbilirubinemia, because the conjugated molecule is nontoxic. Therapy is aimed at optimizing nutrition and controlling pruritus. Using choleretic agents (e.g., phenobarbital [3 to 4 mg/kg/day], cholestyramine [250 to 500 mg/kg/day], and ursodeoxycholic acid [10 to 15 mg/kg/day]) may increase bile flow effectively, which, in turn, lowers the level of total serum bilirubin. Fat-soluble vitamins also are essential in children who have cholestatic liver disease. Rifampin (5 to 10 mg/kg/day), which inhibits hepatocyte uptake of bile acids, has been used to treat pruritus, especially refractory pruritus.[30]

Vitamin K is given at a starting dose of 2.5 to 5 mg every day or every other day. The dose is monitored by following coagulation studies, especially prothrombin time. Excessive vitamin K can cause hemolysis. Vitamin D is administered as 25-hydroxy vitamin D (3 to 5 μg/kg/day). Serum calcium levels are monitored carefully because vitamin D intoxication leads to hypercalcemia, which is responsible for CNS depression, ectopic calcification, and nephrolithiasis.

A water-miscible preparation of vitamin A is given in a dose of 5000 to 25,000 IU/day. Vitamin A deficiency can cause xerophthalmia, keratomalacia, night blindness, and pigmentary retinopathy. Manifestations of vitamin A toxicity include hepatotoxicity and pseudotumor cerebri. Serum vitamin A and retinol ester levels should be followed.

Vitamin E supplementation is indicated in all infants and young children who have cholestatic jaundice. For vitamin E-deficient patients (who have hyperreflexia, areflexia, ptosis, mild truncal ataxia, or hypotonia),[88] 50 IU/kg/day of vitamin E or standard alpha-tocopherol acetate suspension should be administered. Tocopherol polyethylene glycol-1000 succinate (TPGS) is a water-soluble ester of vitamin E (e.g., Liqui-E) that is more effective in maintaining vitamin E sufficiency.[89] The dose of vitamin E is modified according to serum concentrations and the ratio of serum vitamin E to total serum lipid concentration (normally above 0.8 mg : 1 g).

Liver transplantation or more specific therapy is available for some of the metabolic diseases. Currently, liver transplantation is the only therapy available for children who have severe liver disease caused by alpha$_1$-antitrypsin (AAT) deficiency. The future treatment of patients who have AAT may involve therapy using recombinant retroviruses to transduce normal genes (via genetically corrected cells) into the child's own hepatoyctes.[74]

Until recently, there was no treatment for infants who had tyrosinemia (type I) except for early institution of tyrosine-restricted diets and liver transplantation. Cloning of cDNA-encoding FAH via recombinant retroviral vectors may lead to consideration of gene therapy in the future. For now, pharmacological therapy for tyrosinemia is recommended.[48] A pesticide derivative, nitro-trifluoromethylbenzoyl-cyclohexane (NTBC) perturbs tyrosine metabolism via inhibition of hydroxyphenylpyruvate dioxygenase, preventing the formation and accumulation of succinylacetone and succinylacetoacetate (clinical trial doses of 0.1 to 0.6 mg/kg/day). Improvement in liver function occurs as well as a decrease in serum fetoprotein. It is not known if NTBC will influence the development of hepatoma. Consequently, liver transplantation is still the accepted treatment of choice for tyrosinemia.

As previously noted, deferoxamine has not proved to be effective in infants who have neonatal iron storage disease (NISD), and liver transplantation is usually not possible, because of the delayed liver procurement in these very sick infants. Recently, infants who have NISD have been treated with a combination of antioxidants, cryoprotective agents, and chelation. Three antioxidants are used: *N*-acetylcysteine (200 mg/kg/day), tocopherol polyethylene glycol succinate (TPGS, 20 to 25 IU/kg/day), and selenium (2 to 3 mg/kg/day) for the entire course of therapy.[82] Prostaglandin E (0.5 mg/kg/hr for 4 weeks) and deferoxamine (30 mg/kg intravenously until serum ferritin is less than 500 mg/L) are used for the cryoprotective effect and iron chelation, respectively.[82]

REFERENCES

1. Alagille D, Odievre M, Gautier M: Hepatic ductular hypoplasia associated with characteristic facies, vertebral malformations, retarded physical, mental, sexual development, and cardiac murmur, *J Pediatr* 86:63, 1975.
2. American Academy of Pediatrics: Recommendations for care of children in special circumstances. In Peter G, editor: *1997 Redbook: Report of the Committee on Infectious Diseases*, ed 24, Elk Grove Village, Ill, 1997, American Academy of Pediatrics.
3. Andrew G, Chan G, Schiff D: Lipid metabolism in the neonate. II. The effect of Intralipid on bilirubin binding in vitro and in vivo, *J Pediatr* 88:279, 1976.
4. Arias IM: Inheritable and congenital hyperbilirubinemia: models for the study of drug metabolism, *N Engl J Med* 285:1416, 1971.
5. Arias IM, et al: Chronic nonhemolytic unconjugated hyperbilirubinemia with glucuronyl transferase deficiency: clinical, biochemical, pharmacologic, and genetic evidence for heterogeneity, *Am J Med* 47:395, 1969.
6. Bhutani VK, Johnson L, Sivieri EM: Predictive ability of a predischarge hour-specific serum bilirubin for subsequent significant hyperbilirubinemia in healthy term and near-term infants, *Pediatrics* 103:6, 1999.

7. Blanchett VS, et al: Hepatitis C virus infection in children with hemophilia A and B, *Blood* 78:285, 1991.
8. Bortolotti F, et al: Cryptogenic chronic liver disease and hepatitis C virus infection in children, *J Hepatol* 15:73, 1992.
9. Bove KE, et al: Exogenous iron overload in perinatal hemochromatosis, *Pediatr Pathol* 11:389, 1991.
10. Brodersen R: Fusidic acid binding to serum albumin and interaction with binding of bilirubin, *Acta Paediatr Scand* 78:874, 1985.
11. Buchmann MS, et al: Lack of 3B-hydroxy-C27-steroid dehydrogenase/isomerase in fibroblasts from a child with urinary excretion of 3B-hydroxy bile acids, *J Clin Invest* 12:2034, 1990.
12. Busuttil RW, et al: Liver transplantation in children, *Ann Surg* 213:48, 1991.
13. Byth BC, et al: Physical and genetic mapping of the serpin gene cluster at 14q32.1: allelic association and unique haplotype associated with alpha-1-antitrypsin deficiency, *Am J Hum Genet* 55:126, 1994.
14. Chemello L, et al: The effect of interferon alfa and ribavirin combination therapy in naïve patients with chronic hepatitis C, *J Hepatol* 23:8, 1995.
15. Clayton PT, et al: Familial giant cell hepatitis with low bile acid concentration and increased urinary excretion of specific bile alcohols: a new inborn error of bile acid synthesis, *Pediatr Res* 37:424, 1995.
16. Danks DM: Biliary atresia: lessons from Japan, *Lancet* 1:219, 1981.
17. Danks DM, et al: Prognosis of babies with neonatal hepatitis, *Arch Dis Child* 52:368, 1977.
18. Davis GL, et al: Treatment of chronic hepatitis C with recombinant interferon-alpha: a multicenter randomized controlled trial, *N Engl J Med* 321:1501, 1989.
19. Debray D, et al: Sclerosing cholangitis in children, *J Pediatr* 124:49, 1994.
20. Deprettere A, Portmann B, Mowat AP: Syndromatic paucity of the intrahepatic bile ducts: diagnostic difficulty: severe morbidity throughout early childhood, *J Pediatr Gastroenterol Nutr* 6:865, 1987.
21. DeVries LS, Lary S, Dubowitz LMS: Relationship of serum bilirubin levels to ototoxicity and deafness in high-risk low-birth-weight infants, *Pediatrics* 76:351, 1985.
22. Dorney SF, et al: Outcome of surgery for biliary atresia, *Aust N Z J Surg* 59:855, 1989.
23. Duffy LF, et al: Hepatitis in children with acquired immune deficiency syndrome: histopathologic and immunocytologic features, *Gastroenterology* 90:173, 1986.
24. Emerick KM, et al: Features of Alagille syndrome in 92 patients: frequency and relation to prognosis, *Hepatology* 29:822, 1999.
25. Ennever JF, Knox I, Speck WT: Differences in bilirubin isomer composition in infants treated with green and white light phototherapy, *J Pediatr* 109:119, 1986.
26. Friedland IR, et al: Fulminant hepatitis in children: report of 12 cases, *Ann Trop Paediatr* 11:207, 1991.
27. Gartner LM, Arias IM: Studies of prolonged neonatal jaundice in the breast-fed infant, *J Pediatr* 68:54, 1966.
28. Ginn-Pease ME, Pantolos D, King DR: TPN-associated hyperbilirubinemia: a common problem in newborn surgical patients, *J Pediatr Surg* 20:436, 1985.
29. Gottrand F, et al: Late cholangitis after successful surgical repair of biliary atresia, *Am J Dis Child* 145:213, 1991.
30. Gregorio GV, et al: Effect of rifampicin in the treatment of pruritus in hepatic cholestasis, *Arch Dis Child* 69:141, 1993.
31. Grompe M, et al: A single mutation of the fumarylacetoacetate hydrolase gene in French Canadians with hereditary tyrosinemia type I, *N Engl J Med* 331:353, 1994.
32. Guelrud M, et al: ERCP and endoscopic sphincterotomy in infants and children with jaundice due to common bile duct stones, *Gastrointest Endosc* 38:450, 1992.
33. Hingorani M, et al: Ocular abnormalities in Alagille syndrome, *Ophthalmology* 106:330, 1999.
34. Hood JM, et al: Liver transplantation for advanced liver disease with alpha-1-antitrypsin deficiency, *N Engl J Med* 302:272, 1980.
35. Hoofnagle JH, diBisceglie AM: The treatment of chronic viral hepatitis, *N Engl J Med* 336:347, 1997.
36. Hyams KC, et al: Acute sporadic hepatitis E in children living in Cairo, Egypt, *J Med Virol* 37:274, 1992.
37. Hyams KC, et al: Acute sporadic hepatitis E in Sudanese children: analysis based on a new Western blot assay, *J Infect Dis* 165:1001, 1992.
38. Ikeda S, Sera Y, Akagi M: Serial ultrasonic examination to differentiate biliary atresia from neonatal hepatitis: special reference to changes in size of the gallbladder, *Eur J Pediatr* 148:396, 1989.
39. Jardine DS, Rogers K: Relationship of benzyl alcohol to kernicterus, intraventricular hemorrhage, and mortality in preterm infants, *Pediatrics* 83:153, 1989.
40. Jonas MM, et al: Histopathologic features of the liver in pediatric acquired immune deficiency syndrome, *J Pediatr Gastroenterol Nutr* 9:73, 1989.
41. Kershisnik MM, et al: Cytomegalovirus infection, fetal liver disease, and neonatal hemochromatosis, *Hum Pathol* 23:1075, 1992.
42. Knisely AS, et al: Neonatal hemochromatosis, *Birth Defects* 23:75, 1987.
43. Koenig JM, et al: Late hyporegenerative anemia in Rh hemolytic disease, *J Pediatr* 115:315, 1989.
44. Kurauchi O, et al: Studies on transmission of hepatitis C virus from mother to child in the perinatal period, *Arch Gyn Obstet* 253:121, 1993.
45. Lai CL, et al: Lamivudine is effective in suppressing hepatitis B virus DNA in Chinese hepatitis B surface antigen carriers: a placebo controlled trial, *Hepatology* 25:241, 1997.
46. Lascari AD: Early breast-feeding jaundice: clinical significance, *J Pediatr* 108:156, 1986.
47. Lau JYN, et al: Significance of antibody to the host cellular gene-derived epitope GOR in chronic hepatitis C virus infection, *J Hepatol* 17:253, 1993.
48. Lindstedt S, et al: Treatment of hereditary tyrosinemia type I by inhibition of 4-hydroxyphenylpyruvate dioxygenase, *Lancet* 340:813, 1992.
49. Locasciulli A, et al: Hepatitis C virus infection and chronic liver disease in children with leukemia in long-term remission, *Blood* 78:1619, 1991.
50. MacGillivray MH, Crawford JD, Robey JS: Congenital hypothyroidism and prolonged neonatal hyperbilirubinemia, *Pediatrics* 40:283, 1967.
51. Maggiore G, et al: Diagnostic value of serum gamma-glutamyl transpeptidase activity in liver disease in children, *J Pediatr Gastroenterol Nutr* 12:21, 1991.
52. Maggiore G, et al: Liver disease associated with anti-liver-kidney microsome antibody in children, *J Pediatr* 108:399, 1986.
53. Maisels MJ: Jaundice in the newborn, *Pediatr Rev* 3:305, 1982.
54. Maisels MJ, Kring E: Length of stay, jaundice, and hospital readmission, *Pediatrics* 101:995, 1998.
55. Martinez JC, et al: Control of severe hyperbilirubinemia in full-term newborns with the inhibitor of bilirubin production Sn-mesoporphyrin, *Pediatrics* 103:1, 1999.
56. Mathis RK, Andres JM, Walker WA: Liver disease in infants. II. Hepatic disease states, *J Pediatr* 90:864, 1977.
57. Maupas P, et al: Efficacy of hepatitis B vaccine in prevention of early HBsAg carrier state in children: controlled trial in an endemic area (Senegal), *Lancet* 1:289, 1981.
58. McAdams AJ, Hug G, Bove BE: Glycogen storage disease, types I to X: criteria for morphologic diagnosis, *Hum Pathol* 5:463, 1974.
59. Mitchell G, et al: Neurologic crises in hereditary tyrosinemia, *N Engl J Med* 332:432, 1990.
60. Miyano T, et al: Current concept of the treatment of biliary atresia, *World J Surg* 17:332, 1993.
61. Morecki R, et al: Biliary atresia and *Reovirus* type 3 infection, *N Engl J Med* 307:481, 1982.
62. Morecki R, et al: Detection of *Reovirus* type 3 in the porta hepatis of an infant with extrahepatic biliary atresia: ultrastructural and immunocytochemical study, *Hepatology* 4:1137, 1984.
63. Moss RL, Das JB, Raffensperger JG: Total parenteral nutrition-associated cholestasis: clinical and histopathologic correlation, *J Pediatr Surg* 28:1270, 1993.

64. Newman TB, Klebanoff MD: Neonatal hyperbilirubinemia and long-term outcome: another look at the Collaborative Perinatal Project, *Pediatrics* 92:651, 1993.
65. Novati R, et al: Mother-to-child transmission of hepatitis C virus detected by polymerase chain reaction, *J Infect Dis* 165:720, 1992.
66. Odell GB: Neonatal jaundice. In Popper H, Schaffner F, editors: *Progress in liver disease,* New York, 1976, Grune & Stratton.
67. Ohto H, et al: Vertical Transmission of Hepatitis C Virus Collaborative Study Group: transmission of hepatitis C virus from mothers to their infants, *N Engl J Med* 330:744, 1994.
68. Ostrea EM, et al: Influence of free fatty acids and glucose infusion on serum bilirubin and bilirubin binding to albumin: clinical implications, *J Pediatr* 102:426, 1983.
69. Patrick CC, et al: A patient with leukemia in remission and acute abdominal pain, *J Pediatr* 111:624, 1987.
70. Persaud D, et al: Cholestatic hepatitis in children infected with the human immunodeficiency virus, *Pediatr Infect Dis J* 12:492, 1993.
71. Phillips MJ, et al: Sporadic hepatitis with distinctive pathologic features, a severe clinical course, and paramyxoviral features, *N Engl J Med* 324:455, 1991.
72. Powell LW: Clinical aspects of unconjugated hyperbilirubinemia, *Semin Hematol* 9:91, 1972.
73. Psacharapoulos HT, et al: Extrahepatic biliary atresia: preoperative assessment and surgical results in 47 consecutive cases, *Arch Dis Child* 55:351, 1980.
74. Raper SI, Wilson JM: Cell transplantation in liver directed gene therapy, *Cell Transplant* 2:381, 1993.
75. Reif S, Sloven DG, Lebenthal E: Gallstones in children: characterization by age, etiology, and outcome, *Am J Dis Child* 145:105, 1991.
76. Riccabona M, et al: Ceftriaxone-induced cholelithiasis: a harmless side-effect? *Klin Padiatr* 205:421, 1993.
77. Robertson A, Fink S, Karp W: Effect of cephalosporins on bilirubin-albumin binding, *J Pediatr* 114:291, 1988.
78. Sato K, et al: High-dose intravenous gamma globulin therapy for neonatal immune hemolytic jaundice due to blood group incompatibility, *Acta Paediatr Scand* 80:163, 1991.
79. Scheidt PC, et al: Intelligence at six years in relation to neonatal bilirubin levels: follow-up of the National Institute of Child Health and Human Development Clinical Trial of Phototherapy, *Pediatrics* 87:797, 1991.
80. Schweitzer IL: Vertical transmission of the hepatitis B surface antigen, *Am J Med Sci* 270:287, 1975.
81. Setchel KDR, et al: 3-Oxosteroid 5B-reductase deficiency described in identical twins with neonatal hepatitis: a new inborn error in bile acid synthesis, *J Clin Invest* 82:2135, 1988.
82. Shamieh I, et al: Antioxidant therapy for neonatal iron storage disease, *Pediatr Res* 33:109A, 1993.
83. Sharp HL: The current status of alpha-1-antitrypsin, a protease inhibitor, in gastrointestinal disease, *Gastroenterology* 70:621, 1976.
84. Sherman P, et al: Choledochal cysts: heterogeneity of clinical presentation, *J Pediatr Gastroenterol Nutr* 5:867, 1986.
85. Shevell MI, et al: Crigler-Najjar syndrome type I: treatment by home phototherapy followed by orthotopic hepatic transplantation, *J Pediatr* 110:429, 1987.
86. Shneider BL, et al: Delta 4-3 oxosteroid 5-beta reductase deficiency causing neonatal liver failure and hemochromatosis, *J Pediatr* 124:234, 1994.
87. Silveira TR, et al: Congenital structural abnormalities in biliary atresia: evidence for etiopathogenic heterogeneity and therapeutic implications, *Acta Paediatr Scand* 80:1192, 1991.
88. Sokol RJ, et al: Frequency and clinical progression of the vitamin E deficiency neurologic disorder in children with prolonged neonatal cholestasis, *Am J Dis Child* 139:1211, 1985.
89. Sokol RJ, et al: Treatment of vitamin E deficiency during chronic childhood cholestasis with oral d-alpha-tocopheryl polyethylene glycol 1000 succinate (TPGS), *Gastroenterology* 93:975, 1987.
90. Stein MT, Liang D: Clinical hepatotoxicity of isoniazid in children, *Pediatrics* 64:499, 1979.
91. Stevens CE, et al: Yeast-recombinant hepatitis B vaccine: efficacy with hepatitis B immune globulin in prevention of perinatal hepatitis B virus transmission, *JAMA* 257:2612, 1987.
92. Suchy FJ, et al: Acute hepatic failure associated with the use of sodium valproate, *N Engl J Med* 300:962, 1979.
93. Suita S, et al: Fate of infants with neonatal hepatitis: pediatric surgeons' dilemma, *J Pediatr Surg* 27:696, 1992.
94. Sumaya CV, Ench Y: Epstein-Barr virus infectious mononucleosis in children. I. Clinical and general laboratory findings, *Pediatrics* 75:1003, 1985.
95. Szmuness W, et al: Hepatitis B vaccine: demonstrations of efficacy in a controlled clinical trial in a high-risk population in the United States, *N Engl J Med* 303:833, 1980.
96. Tayaba R, et al: Noninvasive estimation of serum bilirubin, *Pediatrics* 102:E28, 1998.
97. Thaler MM, et al: Vertical transmission of hepatitis C virus, *Lancet* 338:17, 1991.
98. Treem WR, et al: Ultrasound-guided percutaneous cholecystocholangiography for early differentiation of cholestatic liver disease in infants, *J Pediatr Gastroenterol Nutr* 7:347, 1988.
99. Tsagaropoulou-Stinga H, et al: Hepatotoxic reactions in children with severe tuberculosis treated with isoniazid-rifampin, *Pediatr Infect Dis J* 4:270, 1985.
100. Tzakis AG, et al: Liver transplantation for Alagille's syndrome, *Arch Surg* 128:337, 1993.
101. Vacanti JP, et al: The therapy of biliary atresia combining the Kasai portoenterostomy with liver transplantation: a single center experience, *J Pediatr Surg* 25:149, 1990.
102. Van Spronsen FJ, et al: Hereditary tyrosinemia type I: a new clinical classification with difference in prognosis on dietary treatment, *Hepatology* 20:1187, 1994.
103. Vinograd I, et al: Laparoscopic cholecystectomy: treatment of choice for cholelithiasis in children, *World J Surg* 17:263, 1993.
104. Vohr BR, et al: Abnormal brainstem function (brainstem auditory evoked response) correlates with acoustic cry features in term infants with hyperbilirubinemia, *J Pediatr* 115:303, 1989.
105. Vohr BR: New approaches to assessing the risks of hyperbilirubinemia, *Clin Perinatol* 17:293, 1990.
106. Walker WA, Mathis RK: Hepatomegaly: an approach to the differential diagnosis, *Pediatr Clin North Am* 22:929, 1975.
107. Weinberg AG, Mize CE, Worthan HG: The occurrence of hepatoma in the chronic form of hereditary tyrosinemia, *J Pediatr* 88:434, 1976.
108. Wiley CC, et al: Nursery practices and detection of jaundice after newborn discharge, *Arch Pediatr Adolesc Med* 152:972, 1998.
109. Wisser J, et al: Neonatal hemochromatosis: a rare cause of nonimmune hydrops fetalis and fetal anemia, *Fetal Diagn Ther* 8:273, 1993.
110. Younoszai MK, Mueller S: Clinical assessment of liver size in normal children, *Clin Pediatr* 14:378, 1975.
111. Zanetti AR, Ferroni P, Magliano EM: Perinatal transmission of the hepatitis B virus and the HBV-associated delta agent from mothers to offspring in northern Italy, *J Med Virol* 9:139, 1982.

SUGGESTED READINGS

Barrera JM, et al: Incidence of non-A, non-B hepatitis after screening blood donors for antibodies to hepatitis C virus and surrogate markers, *Ann Intern Med* 115:596, 1991.

Krugman S: Viral hepatitis: A, B, C, D and E infection, *Pediatr Rev* 13:204, 1992.

Newman TB, Maisels MJ: Evaluation and treatment of jaundice in the term newborn: a kinder, gentler approach, *Pediatrics* 89:809, 1992.

Nowicki MJ, Balisteri WF: Hepatitis A to E: building up the alphabet, *Contemp Pediatr* 9:23, 1992.

Ramirez RO, Sokol RJ: Medical management of cholestasis. In Suchy FJ, editor: *Liver disease in children,* St Louis, 1994, Mosby.

Suchy FJ: Approach to the infant with cholestasis. In Suchy FJ, editor: *Liver disease in children,* St Louis, 1994, Mosby.

153 Joint Pain

David M. Siegel • John Baum

Pediatricians and others who provide primary health care to children often are faced with clinical situations involving musculoskeletal aches and pains; within this group of symptoms is the subset of joint pain. In fact, 1 of every 6 to 10 pediatric outpatient visits includes a musculoskeletal complaint.[1] Discomfort in a joint can result from a wide variety of diagnoses that must be sorted out to allow appropriate evaluation and management. Using a systematic approach to patients who have pain and swelling in one or more joints helps the clinician arrive at an accurate diagnosis and course of therapy.

ARTHRALGIA VERSUS ARTHRITIS

As always, a careful, thorough history is indispensable in initially approaching a child who has joint pain; the physical examination then can substantiate or alleviate suspicions raised during the interview. It is essential to distinguish between arthralgia and arthritis. Joint pain, or arthralgia, is the subjective experience of pain referable to a bony articulation. In a young child, this sensation of pain might be inferred from the patient's refusal to move a particular extremity or joint, but the term *arthralgia* refers only to discomfort in a joint. On the other hand, the term *arthritis* (as indicated by the *-itis* suffix) should be used only when the joint can be shown to be inflamed, as evidenced by the classic signs of inflammation: redness, warmth, swelling, tenderness, plus pain with motion. In the joint, this kind of inflammation can be accompanied by loss of motion. Thus, all that is arthralgia is not arthritis—a critical distinction in the differential diagnosis of joint pain.

With these definitions in mind, what are the characteristics of children who have joint pain, and what information must be elicited through the interview and physical examination? Before enumerating specific entities, it is helpful to review the general characteristics of clinical presentations.

The onset of joint pain can be rather sudden or quite indolent (over days or weeks). In cases of sudden onset, an associated history of a fall or direct blow to the joint immediately suggests a traumatic etiology, whereas the presence of fever points to an infectious process such as septic arthritis or a systemic inflammatory disease such as juvenile arthritis. Often, the complaint expressed to the physician is loss of motion in a joint, with or without obvious swelling. Further clues are provided by the time of day the stiffness occurs and its duration. A child who has juvenile arthritis typically complains of joint stiffness on arising in the morning. The stiffness may last from half an hour to several hours and may be relieved by gradual exercise. On the other hand, a patient who has hypermobility syndrome or some other mechanical, noninflammatory condition associated with joint pain usually gives a history of pain and stiffness occurring at the end of a vigorous day. Besides fever, other distinguishing signs can include rash, mucous membrane involvement, lymph node inflammation or enlargement, or the presence of some recognizable chronic disease that can involve the joints.

DIFFERENTIAL DIAGNOSIS AND MANAGEMENT

A useful format for beginning a discussion of the differential diagnosis of joint pain is the division between rheumatic and nonrheumatic diseases. Juvenile arthritis, sometimes called *Still disease,*[9] is a classic rheumatic disease of childhood involving the joints. It typically peaks in children 1½ to 2 years of age, although onset can occur through late adolescence. The clinical presentation can be limited to four or fewer, usually large joints (pauciarticular disease), or a greater number of joints, both large and small, might be involved (polyarticular disease). There also is a systemic and at times initially fulminant form of juvenile arthritis known as *systemic-onset disease* that is marked by high, spiking fevers; a typical salmon-pink, maculopapular, evanescent rash; lymph node, spleen, and liver enlargement; subcutaneous nodules; anemia; and general malaise. These more systemic findings often precede the onset of any joint involvement, although arthritis must be present for at least 6 consecutive weeks to establish the diagnosis of the other two subgroups of juvenile arthritis (pauciarticular and polyarticular). The clinician may glean only a history of ill-defined arthralgias and stiffness, whereas on physical examination he or she may find contractures of the elbows, knees, and wrists or limitation of cervical motion (ankylosing spondylitis), all of which provide evidence of previous episodes of active inflammation in these joints. Iridocyclitis and keratopathy also may be present. Although not a common disease, juvenile arthritis has a prevalence of 0.1 to 1 child per 1000 children worldwide.[2,14]

The diagnosis can be reinforced by laboratory studies, including the erythrocyte sedimentation rate (ESR), the C-reactive protein (CRP), and a complete blood count (CBC), as well as by more specialized studies such as (1) the antinuclear antibody (ANA) test (among patients who have juvenile arthritis, the most common result is positive in those who have pauciarticular disease), (2) rheumatoid factor titer (RF factor is present in only a small subset of children who have polyarticular juvenile arthritis), and (3) serum immunoglobulin levels.

Management focuses on subduing inflammation and preserving the normal range of joint motion. In the past, salicylate therapy was a mainstay of treatment, but other nonsteroidal antiinflammatory drugs (NSAIDs) now are used as initial therapy. The long-acting agents of gold and D-penicillamine are rarely used any more in patients who have juvenile arthritis; instead, methotrexate has come to play a central role in medical management of children who require therapy beyond NSAIDs. Other long-acting agents also are prescribed, as well as the judicious (and infrequent) use of systemic corticosteroids. For the patient who has a single persistently active joint, intraarticular corticosteroids (e.g., triamcinolone hexacetonide) can be effective. The most recent developments in drug treatment of arthritis include a new class of selective cyclooxygenase-2 inhibitor NSAID and biological preparations that interfere with specific cytokines, such as tumor necrosis factor alpha (TNF-α).[8] Surgery is used mostly in joint reconstruction or prosthetic replacement as a means of dealing with sequelae of synovial inflammation and destruction (see Chapter 229, Juvenile Arthritis).

Acute rheumatic fever (ARF) is another classic rheumatic disease of childhood. Although not the scourge that it once was, the incidence of ARF is increasing, and its inclusion in the differential diagnosis of arthritis and arthralgia remains important. The characteristics of the disease are described at length in Chapter 257, Rheumatic Fever; suffice it to say that the arthritis usually involves large joints, such as the knees, and typically is migratory, with the joints being quite tender to palpation. Although signs of marked inflammation commonly are present, arthralgia alone can be seen.

Ankylosing spondylitis, or spondyloarthropathy, which can involve large joints of the lower extremities during childhood and early adolescence, is typified in late adolescence by involvement of the sacroiliac joint (which can be seen on roentgenograms) and by pain elicited on palpation over the joint. In adulthood, further axial involvement can occur; the classic "bamboo spine" develops, with its diffuse paravertebral fusions and often severe limitation of back motion. The HLA-B27 transplantation antigen is seen in 90% of patients who have ankylosing spondylitis, although the converse is not true (only 20% of those born with HLA-B27 develop arthritis). Treatment begins with NSAIDs and progresses to more aggressive medication as needed.

Reiter's syndrome, a triad of urethritis, conjunctivitis, and arthritis, can be seen in adolescents and children. In children, it often starts with enteritis. It is more common in boys, and making the diagnosis depends on ruling out infectious causes of the inflammation. The arthritis occurs predominantly in large joints; again, there is a strong association with the HLA-B27 locus in these patients (about 60%). The disorder is treated with antiinflammatory drugs. Most children recover within a few months, although some follow a more chronic and relapsing course, occasionally progressing to ankylosing spondylitis.

Also showing a predisposition for larger joints is an arthritis sometimes seen with psoriasis: either the characteristic involvement of the skin is present or there is at least a history of psoriatic skin disease.

Systemic lupus erythematosus (SLE) can cause chronic joint pain. Seen most commonly in girls, SLE is a true multisystem disease that can involve almost every organ in the body; the joints, however, may merely be stiff and painful, or they may show frank signs of inflammation. This disorder, then, would be within the differential diagnosis of joint pain or arthritis in an adolescent girl. Dermatomyositis and polymyositis also can cause inflamed joints in addition to muscle and skin involvement. Other rheumatic diseases that can affect children and cause joint involvement are scleroderma, mixed connective tissue disease, and mucocutaneous lymph node syndrome (Kawasaki disease; see Chapter 230). Each of these entities has its own distinguishing features, as seen on physical examination and found in laboratory tests.

Unlike most of the rheumatic diseases that cause joint pain and tend to be chronic (having waxing and waning courses), many of the nonrheumatic diseases are acute in onset and short in duration, given appropriate therapy. Foremost among this group, and representing something of a medical emergency, is acute bacterial infection of the joint, or septic arthritis (see Chapter 261). The usual presentation is one of a child complaining of a painful joint (rapid onset), usually accompanied by fever. The joint itself is red, warm, swollen, and exquisitely tender to palpation or with movement. This clinical situation demands immediate arthrocentesis for diagnosis and therapy. Analysis of the fluid for appearance (opaque), viscosity (usually low), mucin clot (friable), cell count (more than 100,000 WBC/mm^3 with at least 80% polymorphonuclear cells), glucose (usually low, much less than serum), and protein (high) helps to establish the diagnosis. Most important, a portion of the fluid must be Gram-stained to check for bacterial organisms. Cultures can direct definitive antimicrobial therapy. In the past, for a child younger than age 4 years, *Haemophilus influenzae* infection (seeding from a bacteremia) was the most commonly responsible organism, but with institution of regular immunization this bacterium is no longer a major consideration in septic arthritis. *Staphylococcus aureus* and *Streptococcus* organisms now are more likely to be the offending organisms. In addition to joint fluid cultures, blood cultures also may yield growth of the organism, occasionally in the absence of a positive joint fluid culture.

Systemic bacterial infections, notably those caused by *Neisseria gonorrhoeae* and *Neisseria meningitidis,* also can produce arthritis, although the organism usually is not isolated from the joint in these cases. After joint aspiration and establishment of at least a strong suspicion of a purulent arthritis, the child should be hospitalized and appropriate intravenous antibiotic therapy started. Prompt, aggressive therapy usually effects recovery without sequelae, although some foci, such as the hip joint, can remain persistent problems. Because of the tenuous blood supply to the femoral capital epiphysis (as it courses intracapsularly via the ligamentum teres), purulent arthritis of the hip can lead to chronic problems despite timely intervention.[5]

In addition to bacteria, other infectious organisms can cause joint disease. Viruses, including rubella, mumps, chickenpox, and adenovirus, as well as the Epstein-Barr virus (in infectious mononucleosis), all can affect synovial tissue. Manifestations of the viral syndrome (rash, fever, mucous membrane involvement) usually precede joint involvement.

Infectious hepatitis, on the other hand, can cause arthritis before overt hepatic involvement. Rubella immunization is associated with arthralgia and arthritis in as many as 3% of children who receive the vaccine—rarely, if ever, with any sequelae.[6] Other infections that can involve the joints include brucellosis, leptospirosis, tularemia, Rocky Mountain spotted fever, and rat-bite fever. Mycobacteria can cause arthritis, as can various fungal agents, particularly in immunocompromised individuals.

Ixodes scapularis (previously referred to as *I. dammini*) is a tick that harbors the spirochete *Borrelia burgdorferi* and is carried by numerous mammals. The infection and arthritis produce the syndrome of Lyme disease.[11] First described in Old Lyme, Connecticut, the syndrome is characterized by an initial tick bite that often (but not always) causes a large, circular, spreading, erythematous lesion known as *erythema migrans*. Meningoencephalitis, neuritis, and carditis also may occur. The arthritis manifests later in the course as recurrent attacks of inflammation of the large joints (85% of cases involve the knee), with each recurrence usually lasting no more than a week or two. Occasionally, symptoms may persist for several months, and chronic, persistent arthritis of the knee has been reported. A short course of high-dose penicillin therapy seems to shorten the course of the rash and perhaps attenuate the arthritis, and NSAID therapy relieves the symptoms. Specific antibiotic regimens are recommended for different stages of disease and age of patient.[13] Vaccination against *B. burgdorferi* now is available and appropriate for those in endemic areas(see Chapter 233, Lyme Disease).[10,12]

Congenital syphilis (see Chapter 262, Sexually Transmitted Diseases) can be seen in the infant as painful bony lesions and refusal to move the involved limb (Parrot pseudoparalysis), along with other associated stigmata. In adolescence, an individual who was born with this disease can develop bilateral knee effusions known as *Clutton joints*.

Osteomyelitis is an acute infection of the bone (see Chapter 244, Osteomyelitis). However, when one of the long bones is infected adjacent to a joint (such as the distal femur and knee), the patient may describe pain in the joint, and a sterile effusion may even be present.[5] In some rare instances, particularly in younger patients, the bacterial infection directly invades the joint space from the bone.

Diskitis, a disorder manifested by low-grade fever, back pain, and tenderness over the spinous process contiguous to the involved disk space, causes joint pain. *S. aureus* has been isolated from the blood and disk space in some instances, but often there is no culture-proven cause. The presentation can involve sensory and motor complications that occur secondary to nerve root impingement, and an epidural abscess must be considered in the differential diagnosis.

Noninfectious origins of arthralgia and arthritis abound. Large joint involvement is the most common extraintestinal manifestation of inflammatory bowel disease. This can manifest as pain alone or inflammation as well; the joint complaints may precede the appearance of bowel disease. The activity of the bowel disease may or may not correlate with joint flare-ups. Sarcoidosis can include arthritis, as can the unrelated diseases of polyarteritis nodosa and Marfan syndrome, although arthralgia is more likely than arthritis in the latter. In the group of vasculitic disorders, Henoch-Schönlein purpura is a disease of childhood evidenced by fever, abdominal pain (with or without melena), purpuric lesions of the buttocks and lower extremities, and warm, swollen, painful, tender joints (usually large joints such as the knees and ankles). Hematological diseases that have articular manifestations include hemophilia and sickle cell disease. In the latter disorder, the physician must consider the hand-foot syndrome type of vasoocclusive crisis in a child between 1 and 4 years of age. Although primary gout is exceedingly rare in children, hyperuricemia and subsequent joint disease can be seen in those who have leukemia (with chemotherapy producing sudden lysis of cells), hemolytic anemia, glycogen storage disease, and Lesch-Nyhan syndrome. In Lesch-Nyhan syndrome, a sex-linked, recessive, genetic, inborn metabolic error results in overproduction of uric acid. Polyarthritis and limb pains can be seen in children following traumatic pancreatitis. Infantile cortical hyperostosis (Caffey's disease), which occurs in infants younger than 6 months of age, involves fever, irritability, an increased ESR, and tender swellings of facial, trunk, and limb bones, with associated arthralgia. Toxic synovitis of the hip also can cause arthralgia and/or arthritis (see Chapter 132, Extremity Pain).

A fascinating condition seen primarily in children and adolescents that can induce arthralgia without arthritis is hypermobility syndrome. Children who have this disorder have increased joint laxity, and with vigorous activity, especially those requiring extremes of joint flexion and extension, they can experience significant arthralgia. The diagnosis is made by physical examination and observation of at least three of the following five signs: (1) hyperflexion of the wrist, bringing the thumb in contact with the volar surface of the forearm; (2) hyperextension of the fingers to parallel with the forearm; (3) hyperextension of the elbow to at least -10 degrees; (4) hyperextension of the knee to at least -10 degrees; and (5) hyperflexion of the spine such that with forward flexion the palms can be placed flat on the ground with the feet together and without flexing the knees. The arthralgia can be seen in only one or two of these sites, with examination showing hypermobility in only the joints that are the source of the complaints. All laboratory and radiological studies are normal. The syndrome is treated with NSAIDs and reassurance.

In chondromalacia patellae, or patellofemoral pain syndrome, the child has knee pain that usually is related to activity. The problem is a roughening of the cartilage on the underside of the patella, with resultant pain as the patella moves in the patellofemoral groove. Exercises directed toward strengthening the quadriceps femoris and adductor muscles can produce marked improvement. NSAID and/or analgesic medication can be used as an adjunct to the physical therapy.

"Growing pains" are an actual discomfort in the lower limbs and joints (often worse at night) that children experience during a phase of rapid linear growth. A bedtime dose of NSAID can help alleviate this pain until it resolves spontaneously with the slowing of growth. Adolescent females who have fibromyalgia syndrome can experience diffuse arthralgia but, more typically, their pain is muscular and/or periarticular.

Physical abuse must be strongly considered whenever signs of trauma are evident, and accidents that represent neglect on the part of parents or guardians need to be recognized and pursued. Any suspicious history or circumstance demands complete investigation.

There are other orthopedic reasons for joint pain. See Chapter 208, Fractures and Dislocations.

Management of Psychological Aspects

Having arrived at a diagnosis and plan of therapy, the practitioner also must offer management for the psychological aspects of joint disease. In children afflicted with an ongoing joint problem, all the issues of chronic pediatric disease also must be addressed. The child may not be able to keep up with his or her peers in physical activity and also may be faced with making numerous health care visits and, thus, a substantial number of school absences. Many clinicians feel that in addition to the stress caused by the disease in these patients, stress in their environment can exacerbate the disease, as may occur in children who have juvenile arthritis. A child faced with hospitalization for an acute problem, such as septic arthritis, is exposed to all the complications of being taken out of his or her family and school environment, as well as those dealing with an institutional setting. Any child who has ongoing joint disease, even those who have a mild disability, should be provided with the expertise and services of a social worker, counselor, or psychologist experienced with this population of patients. Family resources (both emotional and financial) need to be assessed, and support provided when needed. Discussion groups composed of these children and their families can be very beneficial because they offer an opportunity to compare experiences and coping mechanisms. Attention to the physical dimension alone does not provide adequate care in these diseases. A functionally minor disability can cause major problems of body image and feelings of lack of independence that must be dealt with appropriately.[3,4] As with other chronic physical disorders of childhood and adolescence, long-term psychosocial sequelae also may develop.[7]

REFERENCES

1. Cassidy JT, Petty RE: An introduction to the study of the rheumatic diseases of children. In Cassidy JT, Petty RE, editors: *Textbook of pediatric rheumatology*, ed 3, Philadelphia, 1995, WB Saunders.
2. Gewanter HL, Roghmann KJ, Baum J: The prevalence of juvenile arthritis, *Arthritis Rheum* 26:599, 1983.
3. Lowit IM: Social and psychological consequences of chronic illness in children, *Dev Med Child Neurol* 15:75, 1973.
4. McAnarney ER, et al: Psychological problems of children with chronic juvenile arthritis, *Pediatrics* 53:523, 1974.
5. Petty RE: Septic arthritis and osteomyelitis in children, *Curr Opin Rheumatol* 2:616, 1990.
6. Phillips P: Viral arthritis in children, *Arthritis Rheum* 20(suppl 2):584, 1977.
7. Pless IB, et al: Long-term psychosocial sequelae of chronic physical disorders in childhood, *Pediatrics* 91:1131, 1993.
8. Siegel DM: Drug treatment of juvenile arthritis: accepted therapeutic options, *Drug Today* 34:377, 1998.
9. Siegel DM, Baum J: Juvenile arthritis, *Prim Care* 20:883, 1993.
10. Sigal LH, et al: A vaccine consisting of recombinant *Borrelia burgdorferi* outer surface protein A to prevent Lyme disease, *N Engl J Med* 339:216, 1998.
11. Steere AC, et al: The spirochetal etiology of Lyme disease, *N Engl J Med* 308:733, 1983.
12. Steere AC, et al: Vaccination against Lyme disease with recombinant *Borrelia burgdorferi* outer-surface lipoprotein A with adjuvant, *N Engl J Med* 339:209, 1998.
13. The Medical Letter: *Treatment of Lyme disease*, 39:47, 1997.
14. Towner SR, et al: The epidemiology of juvenile rheumatoid arthritis in Rochester, Minnesota, *Arthritis Rheum* 26:1208, 1983.

154 Limp

Erica M.S. Sibinga • Alain Joffe

Limp, defined as an abnormality in a child's pattern of walking, is a common presenting complaint in pediatric primary care. It usually is unilateral, thereby creating an asymmetrical gait, and may be painful (antalgic) or not (Trendelenburg). Limp has many causes, ranging from a stone between the toes to leukemia. Distinguishing among the potential etiologies requires a careful history and physical examination, with special attention given to the age- and activity-related aspects of possible diagnoses.

CAUSES AND CHARACTERISTICS

Table 154-1 lists possible causes of limp in children and adolescents. Certain causes of limp may be characterized by their association with systemic signs and symptoms, specific ages, and varying degrees of pain. (See Chapter 132, Extremity Pain.)

Systemic signs and symptoms, such as fever, malaise, anorexia, weight loss, and ill appearance, usually accompany limp when the etiology is infectious or neoplastic. The onset and duration of these symptoms may be useful in understanding the cause.

The child's age can help determine the cause of a limp. As an infant begins to bear weight and walk, congenital coxa vara or developmental dysplasia of the hip may become evident as an asymmetrical gait. Legg-Calvé-Perthes disease (LCPD) occurs most frequently from ages 4 to 10 years. Osgood-Schlatter and slipped capital femoral epiphysis (SCFE) are more common in adolescents.

The degree to which a limp is painful also assists in determining its etiology. An antalgic gait may result from infection, fracture, trauma, repetitive microtrauma, synovitis, or neoplasia. Severe pain is associated with fractures, dislocations, and joint or bone infections. SCFE, LCPD, synovitis, and trauma without fracture generally cause mild to moderate pain. Limp caused by muscle weakness (as in muscular dystrophy) or leg length discrepancy is unlikely to be painful. The practitioner should keep in mind that pain may be referred distally: Pain in the knee or thigh may be caused by a pathological process in the hip; pain in the hip may indicate pelvic, vertebral, or spinal cord problems.

HISTORY

A thoughtful history and physical examination are the cornerstones of diagnosis. Important historical points include the duration of limp; trauma; antecedent symptoms including fever, viral illness, rash, and weight loss; and changes in exercise patterns. The most common cause of limp is trauma,[2] resulting in soft-tissue or musculoskeletal injury. It is essential to consider whether the history and the physical examination findings correlate. If the nature or degree of the child's injury does not fit the history given, child abuse should be considered and evaluated further. As the child's advocate, the pediatrician is in a unique position to intervene if there is concern about intentional injury.

Other historical points of relevance may fall into specific diagnostic patterns. Recurrent fevers, rash, and joint pain suggest juvenile rheumatoid arthritis. Adolescent girls who receive a rubella vaccination often develop a transient but painful arthritis 1 to 2 weeks after vaccination. Hemarthrosis from hemophilia should be considered as a cause of limp in a boy who has a swollen, painful knee and a family history of bleeding problems. Lyme arthritis should be added to the differential diagnosis if there is a history of flu-like illness and erythematous rash with central clearing.[9]

Also important to explore are the child's or adolescent's physical activities. Stress fractures, patellofemoral arthralgia syndrome, and Osgood-Schlatter disease are more common among runners.[5,7] Overuse syndromes may be the result of repetitive microtrauma of the tibia (Osgood-Schlatter disease), the calcaneus (Sever's disease), or patella (patellofemoral arthralgia syndrome).[8] A sudden increase in the amount or duration of exercise frequently is associated with injury.[3]

PHYSICAL EXAMINATION

The extent and focus of the physical examination should be tailored to the individual, based on the history obtained. If there is any indication that a systemic illness is causing the limp, a complete examination should be conducted, including measurement of height, weight, and temperature. In the absence of systemic signs, most of the examination can be directed toward the back and lower extremities.

Observation of the patient's gait can yield important diagnostic clues. Close attention should be paid to signs of pain, pattern of weight bearing, and suggestion of muscle weakness. These observations can direct the physical examination further and should correlate with the pathophysiology of the diagnosis.

Inspection of the affected side for erythema, warmth, bruising, swelling, muscle atrophy, and asymmetry (compared with the unaffected limb) may localize the etiology of the limp. Erythema, warmth, and swelling suggest an infectious or inflammatory process of the underlying subcutane-

Table 154-1 Possible Causes of Limp in Children and Adolescents

Causes	Infants and Toddlers (0-3 yrs)	Children (4-10 yrs)	Adolescents (11 yrs and older)
Trauma			
Fracture, sprain, contusion	++	++	++
Infection			
Septic arthritis (hip, knee)	++	++	+
Osteomyelitis	++	++	+
Myositis	−	+	+
Transient Synovitis of the Hip Developmental Causes			
Developmental dysplasia of the hip	++	−	−
Leg length discrepancy	++	+	+
Acquired Causes			
Legg-Calvé-Perthes disease	−	++	−
Slipped capital femoral epiphysis	−	+	++
Systemic Disease			
Juvenile rheumatoid arthritis	+	++	+
Rheumatic fever	−	+	+
Autoimmune disease	+	+	+
Lyme arthritis	+	++	++
Activity-Related Causes			
Osgood-Schlatter disease	−	−	++
Overuse syndromes (knee, heel, foot)	−	+	++
Neoplastic Disease			
Leukemia	−	++	+
Bone tumors (e.g., Ewing's sarcoma, osteogenic sarcoma)	−	+	+
Metastatic neoplasia	−	+	+
Hematological Disease			
Sickle cell anemia	+	+	+
Hemophilia	+	+	+
Neuromuscular Disorder			
Muscle weakness/dystrophy	−	+	+
Spinal cord compression	−	+	+
Other			
Foreign body in foot	++	++	++
Appendicitis	+	+	+
Rubella vaccination	−	+	++

Modified from Green M: *Pediatric diagnosis,* ed 3, Philadelphia, 1980, WB Saunders.
−; uncommon cause of limp in this age group.
+; causes limp in this age group.
++; common cause of limp in this age group.

ous tissue, muscle, bone, or joint. If there is a question of swelling or asymmetry, the examiner should measure both limbs at the same level, comparing the affected with the unaffected side.

Palpation along the limb from the lower spine to the toes may localize any area of pain. Pinpoint tenderness suggests a process involving structures at that point and is found most often with fractures or focal infection. If the hip or upper thigh appears to be involved, the lower spine, paraspinal areas, abdomen, and inguinal areas also should be examined. A rectal examination may help confirm a diagnosis of appendicitis or a pathological pelvic condition.

Each joint of the limb should be examined systematically for erythema, warmth, swelling, pain, and range of motion (both active and passive). Again, infection and/or inflammation are suggested by erythema, warmth, and swelling. Significant limitation in range of motion is a concern because it may represent an intraarticular process. Pain with active but not passive range of motion suggests a muscle or tendon problem. Examination of the knee joint should include attention to the patella, evaluating for pain by applying pressure, and the ligaments, assessing the stability of the joint. The ankle and foot should be assessed for range of motion and flexibility.

If the limp's etiology remains unclear or another process is suspected, other physical findings should be evaluated. Discrepancy in leg length can be detected by measuring both legs from the anterior superior spine of the ilium to the distal end of the ipsilateral medial malleolus. Performing the Ortolani maneuver to check for hip dislocation may be useful in an ambulatory toddler but a negative test is not necessarily reassuring. Asymmetry in deep tendon reflexes or altered sensation suggests a pathological condition of the spinal cord. Difficulty raising the leg against mild resistance indicates muscle weakness.

DIFFERENTIAL DIAGNOSIS AND MANAGEMENT

Trauma

Most cases of limp in primary care are due to trauma, and unless the mechanism of injury or the physical examination suggests fracture or ligament damage, rest, elevation, the application of ice, and mild analgesics are the mainstays of therapy. Other causes require further evaluation.

Plain radiographs remain an important tool in the evaluation of limp,[6] particularly in diagnosing fractures, hip pathology, spinal abnormalities, and foot pathology (e.g., tarsal coalition). Obtaining at least two views of the affected area is essential, with suspected hip pathology usually requiring anteroposterior (AP) and frog-leg lateral (Lauenstein) views of the pelvis. Laboratory evaluations also are useful in the further evaluation of limp: Most commonly, the complete blood count (CBC) and erythrocyte sedimentation rate (ESR) or C-reactive protein (CRP) are obtained. In the evaluation of limp, an ESR less than 20 mm/hr is unlikely to be associated with a serious infectious, inflammatory, or neoplastic etiology.[4]

Infection

If an infectious etiology of limp is suggested, such as a septic arthritis or osteomyelitis, a low threshold for further evaluation is appropriate, because of the high morbidity of these conditions. Septic arthritis is more likely to be found in infants or young children who exhibit a painful limp. They often are febrile, ill-appearing, have joint pain and guarding, and may have "pseudoparalysis" (the affected leg held in flexion, abduction, and external rotation to decrease the pressure in the hip joint).[8] An elevated white blood cell (WBC) count, ESR, or CRP is consistent with an infectious or inflammatory process. Early in the course, a radiograph is not diagnostic in septic arthritis; bone scintigraphy is the most sensitive modality.[6] Ultrasound may show a joint effusion, but aspiration of the fluid is required for diagnosis. Septic arthritis is a surgical emergency and necessitates emergent orthopedic involvement for diagnosis and treatment.

Osteomyelitis has a broad range of clinical presentation. A child may be afebrile and mildly uncomfortable or toxic in appearance. A specific area of tenderness on physical examination is found, and the WBC, ESR, and CRP are usually elevated. Radiographs may be normal early in the process, because periosteal elevation and osteolysis are not visible until 7 to 14 days after the onset of infection. Radionuclide bone scintigraphy is positive earlier in the disease process.[6] An effort also should be made to obtain a bacterial culture of the infected area by using needle aspiration before initiating antibiotic treatment.

Transient Synovitis

Transient synovitis of the hip is a common cause of limp in children, especially in those who are 3 to 10 years of age. The etiology is unknown, but many affected children have had a viral infection before the onset of symptoms. Limp results from acute unilateral hip pain and mild limitation in the range of motion. Pain may be referred to the groin, thigh, or knee and the patient may preferentially hold the leg in flexion, abduction, and external rotation (usually less so than with a septic arthritis). A child who has transient synovitis is typically not ill-appearing or febrile, has mild pain in the hip joint, and slight limitation of adduction and internal rotation. Often the diagnosis can be made by history and physical examination alone, but severe transient synovitis is difficult to distinguish from septic arthritis of the hip, and further evaluation may be necessary. In transient synovitis, laboratory values usually are normal, although the ESR may be slightly elevated, and hip radiographs typically are normal. Ultrasound may show fluid in the joint space, and aspiration may be necessary to distinguish synovitis from septic arthritis. The treatment of transient synovitis of the hip is symptomatic, usually requiring some limitation of activity. It is a self-limited process, and full recovery should be anticipated, usually in a matter of weeks.[11]

Developmental/Acquired Etiology

Unilateral developmental dysplasia of the hip (DDH) may present as a limp in an infant beginning to walk; bilateral DDH causes a "waddling" gait. Otherwise, the patient is asymptomatic. Examination reveals an apparent leg length discrepancy and/or asymmetrical skin folds in unilateral DDH. Because bilateral DDH affects both hips, it typically is very difficult to detect by physical examination alone. In the toddler or childhood years, AP and frog-leg radiographs of the pelvis are necessary, and referral to an orthopedist is needed for treatment. Prognosis depends on the age of the child at diagnosis and on the extent of dysplasia. Careful physical examinations during infancy will detect DDH as unilateral or bilateral congenital dislocation of the hip(s). (See Chapter 208, Fractures and Dislocations.)

Legg-Calvé-Perthes disease (avascular necrosis of the femoral head) is a common cause of limp in children 2 to 10 years of age. It is fivefold more likely in boys than in girls. The typical presentation is limp, usually accompanied by mild pain in the thigh or knee, with mild weakness or atrophy of the hip abductor, thigh, and buttock muscles. Approximately 5 months after the initial ischemia, AP radiographs of the pelvis show a dense femoral epiphysis and apparent widening of the medial joint space. Earlier diagnosis may require magnetic resonance imaging (MRI) or a bone scan.[6] LCPD is self-limited, with resolution in 18 to 24 months, although there may be intermittent synovitis with discomfort, requiring limitation of normal activity.

Slipped capital femoral epiphysis (SCFE) occurs most commonly among adolescents, often during or just before the pubertal growth spurt (ages 10 to 15 years). Boys are affected more than girls (3:2), with obesity and tall stature being risk factors. There usually is acute onset of limp, a painful hip, and limitation of internal rotation. However, some patients present subtly, with dull aching in the hip or leg and pain occurring only with exercise, which may result in a delayed diagnosis.[1] AP radiographs may show asymmetry and widening of the growth plate, but SCFE is seen best on frog-leg films, where the displaced femoral head is more apparent. Because further displacement of the epiphysis is a risk, this diagnosis and an orthopedic referral should be made quickly. Treatment consists of pinning the femoral epiphysis for stabilization. Many patients who have SCFE eventually will have bilateral involvement.

Systemic Disease

Arthritis caused by a systemic process also may cause limp. Juvenile rheumatoid arthritis, acute rheumatic fever, Lyme arthritis, and lupus erythematosus are likely to be suggested by a history of fever, rashes, migrating arthralgias, recent pharyngitis, or tick exposure. Further evaluation should include a CBC, ESR, and specific antibody titers, as indicated by clinical suspicion. Consultation with a rheumatologist may be beneficial. (See Chapter 229, Juvenile Arthritis.)

Activity-Related Etiology

Activity-related causes of limp also should be considered. Overuse, as with excessive training or participation in athletics, can result in repetitive microtrauma and specific pain syndromes. Osgood-Schlatter disease is commonly seen in active adolescents, the result of repetitive microtrauma to the tibial tubercle. Tenderness is localized over the tibial tubercle; treatment requires some limitation of activity. Patients who have patellofemoral arthralgia syndrome present with knee pain, made worse by activity, particularly stair climbing. On physical examination, compression of the patella on the femur causes pain. Rest and limited activity is the treatment of choice. Overuse syndromes also can affect the heel and foot.[8] Intense or excessive exercise (such as occurs with young women who have eating disorders) may cause stress fractures of the lower extremities.

Neoplastic Disease

Limp may be the presenting symptom of a benign tumor or malignant neoplasm. Malignant conditions include leukemia, Ewing's sarcoma, and osteosarcoma; plain radiographs are helpful in leading to the diagnosis. Multiple lesions on radiograph should raise concern of a metastatic process. An MRI or a bone scan may be used to better define the extent of involvement. Osteoid osteoma is a benign lesion that presents with pain that is worse at night and is relieved by aspirin.[10] It may be identified on computed tomography (CT) scan, but a bone scan is most sensitive for detection of this lesion.[6]

Spine and Abdomen

It also is important to recognize that limp may be caused by a process of the spine or abdomen. Vertebral body pathology or infection, intervertebral disc herniation, and spinal neoplasms can cause limp. Plain radiographs typically are helpful in these diagnoses. Intraabdominal processes, including appendicitis or psoas muscle abscess, may cause limp.

If, despite a thorough history and physical examination, a diagnosis is unclear and a condition associated with high morbidity is not a concern, a short period of observation (perhaps 1 to 2 weeks) may be appropriate. If the limp persists, the history and physical examination should be repeated. A repeat ESR or CRP and radiological examination likely will establish the diagnosis. If the diagnosis remains confusing, consultation with an orthopedist or neurologist is warranted.

When to Refer

Fracture
Clinical, radiographic, or laboratory concern for:
- Septic arthritis
- Osteomyelitis
- Developmental dysplasia of the hip
- Slipped capital femoral epiphysis
- Neoplastic disease
- Appendicitis/psoas abscess
- Persistent limp of unclear etiology

REFERENCES

1. Causey AL, et al: Missed slipped capital femoral epiphysis: illustrative cases and a review, *J Emerg Med* 13:175, 1995.
2. Doughty RA, Rose C: Limp. In Fleischer GR, editor: *Textbook of pediatric emergency medicine*, ed 3, Baltimore, 1993, Williams & Wilkins.
3. Garrick JG: Knee problems in adolescents, *Pediatr Rev* 4:235, 1983.
4. Huttenlocher A, Newman TB: Evaluation of the erythrocyte sedimentation rate in children presenting with limp, fever, or abdominal pain, *Clin Pediatr* 36:339, 1997.
5. Keller EK: Patellar management syndrome in runners, *Nurs Pract* 8:27, 1983.
6. Myers MT, Thompson GH: Imaging the child with a limp, *Pediatr Clin North Am* 44:637, 1997.
7. Newell SG, Bramwell ST: Overuse injuries to the knee in runners, *Physician Sports Med* 12:81, 1984.
8. Renshaw TS: The child who has a limp, *Pediatr Rev* 16:458, 1995.
9. Steere AC, Schoen RT, Taylor, E: The clinical evolution of Lyme arthritis, *Ann Intern Med* 107:725, 1987.
10. Thompson GT: Gait disturbances. In Kliegman RM, editor: *Practical strategies in pediatric diagnosis and therapy*, Philadelphia, 1996, WB Saunders.
11. Waters E: Toxic synovitis of the hip in children, *Nurse Pract* 20:44-51, 1995.

155 Loss of Appetite

Martin H. Ulshen

Loss of appetite (anorexia) is a common symptom in pediatric practice. Acute illness in childhood often is associated with transient loss of appetite. Prolonged loss of appetite associated with poor weight gain or loss of weight usually signifies a serious chronic illness, either organic or psychogenic.

The mechanisms that regulate hunger and satiety are complex and redundant, remaining incompletely understood.[5,8,12] Appetite is regulated by the hypothalamus, which includes the "satiety center" in the ventromedial hypothalamus and the "feeding center" in the lateral hypothalamus. Central control of appetite is influenced by anticipation of a pleasurable meal, visual and taste sensations, ambient temperature, and changes in blood levels of glucose or other nutrients, as well as by limbic signals from higher central nervous system (CNS) regions. Initiators of satiety include vagal input from gastric distention, cholecystokinin from the intestine and CNS, and other humoral factors, including insulin, glucagon, and endorphins. Each individual may have a set point for body fat content, and deviations may cause alterations in diet intake. This process appears to be mediated by the interaction of the hormone leptin, produced in adipose cells, with receptors in the hypothalamus.[1] The CNS hormones neuropeptide Y and melanocyte-stimulating hormone, respectively, stimulate and suppress appetite.[12] Changes in leptin levels influence release of these hormones. A newly characterized family of neuropeptides, the orexins, act on the lateral hypothalamus and, thus, stimulate appetite as well.

Cytokines are key mediators of the appetite suppression that occurs with acute and chronic illnesses.[6] Beta-interleukin-1 and tumor necrosis factor-α, for example, both have been shown to induce anorexia by acting directly on the hypothalamus. Effects on the peripheral nervous system and on hormone levels occur as well.

When considering anorexia, the physician first must separate complaints based on unrealistic parental dietary expectations from justified parental concern over a child's diminished nutritional intake. This usually is not difficult because children in the former situation thrive and gain weight appropriately. Although significant gastrointestinal disease commonly leads to poor appetite, anorexia may be the result of disease distant from the bowel. In the newborn period, poor oral intake by an infant developmentally capable of feeding may be the first indication of a major disorder, such as sepsis, meningitis, urinary tract infection, congenital viral infection, a gastrointestinal anomaly, CNS disease, renal failure, or a metabolic disorder.

During infancy, a wide spectrum of causes can account for inadequate caloric intake. An acute infectious disease is a common cause of transient anorexia in infants. If there is no obvious explanation for poor feeding, the practitioner always should consider the possibility of an oral disease (such as thrush), gastroesophageal reflux, renal tubular acidosis, dietary protein intolerance, or a neurological disease. Emotional deprivation is a common cause of failure to thrive; a careful social history is essential to the evaluation. Early observation of parent-infant interaction in the hospital, including feeding techniques, may be appropriate. An infant who has not received oral feedings for a prolonged period because of medical problems (e.g., esophageal disease or short-bowel syndrome) may not be interested when feedings are introduced by mouth. The mother and infant may require training (typically provided by a physical therapist or speech pathologist) and gradual advancement of an oral diet.

A state of chronically inadequate caloric intake can be established objectively by computing the total calories ingested (most of which come from formula) and comparing this with the estimated caloric requirements for weight. This is more difficult with breast-fed infants, although intake may be established by weighing the infant before and after feedings. If the nursing infant has a reduced intake, the physician must establish whether maternal milk production is inadequate or the infant is too weak or disinterested to nurse.

In older children and adolescents, an adequate evaluation of nutritional intake requires careful calorie counts. If the possibility of malabsorption is a concern, calories may be counted in conjunction with a 72-hour stool fat collection. It is important at the outset to separate children who have poor appetites from children who do not eat for fear of worsening their symptoms. Children who have abdominal pain resulting from chronic inflammatory bowel disease or chronic constipation may not eat because this increases their pain. Similarly, children who have chronic diarrhea may eat less if doing so seems to lead to less stool. These individuals actually may not have anorexia, and treatment aimed at improving the other symptoms may result in a rapid improvement in appetite.

Box 155-1 presents a list of causes of loss of appetite applicable to both infants and children. Generally, the best approach to anorexia is to treat the underlying condition.

Enlisting the help of a dietitian to plan diets can be useful for maximizing nutritional intake in older children. Nutritional supplements may be indicated (e.g., high-calorie milk shakes or commercial high-calorie supplements). Several medications, including cyproheptadine and megestrol acetate, have been shown to stimulate appetite. Although cyproheptadine does not seem to affect appetite in all children treated, when successful the response is dramatic. Megestrol

BOX 155-1

CAUSES OF DECREASED APPETITE IN INFANTS AND CHILDREN

Organic Disease
- Infectious (acute or chronic)[6]
- Neurological
  - Cerebral palsy
  - Congenital degenerative disease (e.g., spinomuscular atrophy, muscular dystrophy)
  - Hypothalamic lesion
  - Increased intracranial pressure (including a brain tumor)
- Gastrointestinal
  - Oral or esophageal lesions (e.g., thrush or herpes simplex)
  - Gastroesophageal reflux[3]
  - Dietary protein intolerance (including eosinophilic esophagitis)[4]
  - Obstruction (especially with gastric or intestinal distention)
  - Inflammatory bowel disease
  - Celiac disease
  - Constipation
  - Esophageal motility disorder (e.g., cricopharyngeal dysfunction, achalasia, connective tissue disorder)
- Cardiac
  - Congestive heart failure or cyanotic heart disease
- Metabolic
  - Renal failure and/or renal tubular acidosis
  - Liver failure
  - Congenital metabolic disease
  - Lead poisoning
- Nutritional
  - Marasmus
  - Iron deficiency
  - Zinc deficiency
- Drugs
  - Morphine
  - Digitalis
  - Antimetabolites
  - Methylphenidate
  - Amphetamines
- Miscellaneous
  - Prolonged restriction of oral feedings, beginning in the neonatal period
  - Tumor[2,6]
  - Chronic febrile conditions (e.g., rheumatoid arthritis, rheumatic fever)[6]

Psychological Factors
- Anxiety, fear, depression, mania (limbic influence on the hypothalamus)[7]
- Avoidance of symptoms associated with meals (abdominal pain, diarrhea, bloating, urgency, dumping syndrome)
- Anorexia nervosa (see Chapter 102)
- Excessive weight loss and food aversion in athletes, simulating anorexia nervosa[9,13]

acetate, a progesterone derivative, has been administered for cancer-related anorexia, primarily in adults.[6] Potential side effects of this medication include effects on the endocrine system, including adrenal insufficiency. The weight gain of treatment with megestrol acetate may be associated to a large extent with increased fat mass. In some disorders (e.g., congenital heart disease), initial nasogastric or nasoduodenal infusion of nutrients may be necessary to promote growth.[11] Parenteral nutrition may be indicated in very specific situations; however, both expertise with this modality and close supervision are required. Caretakers need special training if parenteral nutrition is to be provided at home. Refeeding after severe malnutrition requires careful consideration of potential cardiac and metabolic complications.[10]

When to Refer

1. Loss of appetite without an obvious explanation
2. Anorexia nervosa

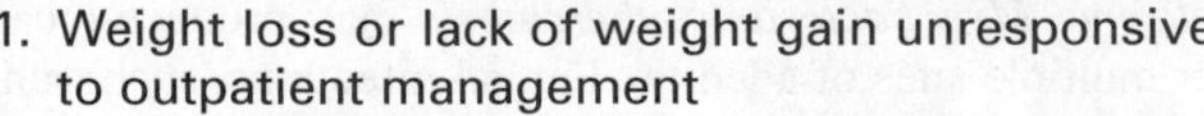

When to Hospitalize

1. Weight loss or lack of weight gain unresponsive to outpatient management
2. Need to initiate enteral or parenteral feeding because of inadequate oral intake

REFERENCES

1. Auwerx J, Staels B: Leptin, *Lancet* 351:737, 1998.
2. Bernstein IL, Sigmundi RA: Tumor anorexia: a learned food aversion? *Science* 209:416, 1980.
3. Dellert SF, et al: Feeding resistance and gastroesophageal reflux in infancy, *J Pediatr Gastroenterol Nutr* 17:66, 1993.
4. Liacouras CA, et al: Primary eosinophilic esophagitis in children: successful treatment with oral corticosteroids, *J Pediatr Gastroenterol Nutr* 26:380, 1998.
5. Plata-Salaman CR: Regulation of hunger and satiety in man, *Dig Dis Sci* 9:253, 1991.
6. Plata-Salaman CR: Cytokines and anorexia: a brief overview, *Semin Oncol* 25(suppl 1):66, 1998.
7. Pugliese MT, et al: Fear of obesity: a cause of short stature and delayed puberty, *N Engl J Med* 309:513, 1983.
8. Robinson PH, et al: Gastric control of food intake, *J Psychosom Res* 32:593, 1988.
9. Smith NJ: Excessive weight loss and food aversion in athletes simulating anorexia nervosa, *Pediatrics* 66:139, 1980.
10. Solomon SM, Kirby DF: The refeeding syndrome: a review, *J Parenter Enteral Nutr* 14:90, 1990.
11. Vanderhoff JA, et al: Continuous enteral feedings: an important adjunct to the management of complex congenital heart disease, *Am J Dis Child* 136:825, 1982.
12. Woods SC, et al: Signals that regulate food intake and energy homeostasis, *Science* 280:1378, 1998.
13. Yates A, Leehey K, Shisslak CM: Running: an analogue of anorexia? *N Engl J Med* 308:251, 1983.

156 Lymphadenopathy

George B. Segel • Caroline Breese Hall

Lymphadenopathy, or enlargement of the lymph nodes, is a common problem in childhood. Lymphadenopathy may be defined as any lymph node enlargement; all lymph nodes that are palpable are technically considered to be enlarged. However, nodes in the cervical, occipital, and inguinal areas drain regions commonly infected in childhood and often are mildly enlarged (less than 1 cm in diameter) in children who otherwise are normal.

The clinically relevant problems in assessing lymphadenopathy are (1) whether any lymph node or lymph node aggregate or chain is abnormal and requires further assessment; (2) if abnormal, whether the nodes are benign, primarily inflammatory, or malignant; and (3) what is the appropriate evaluation, diagnosis, and management.

CHARACTERISTICS OF LYMPH NODE ENLARGEMENT

Components of the Lymphatic System

The lymphatic system includes not only lymph nodes but also the spleen, thymus, tonsils, Waldeyer ring, and Peyer's patches in the intestine, as well as the appendix. Potentially palpable lymph node groups and their drainage areas are shown in Table 156-1, which may serve as a guide to palpation of these superficial nodes.

Lymph Node Features

Abnormalities of the palpable lymph nodes are assessed by noting the node's size, location, mobility, inflammatory reaction, and consistency. Nodes less than 1 cm often are found in the cervical chain and in the femoral and inguinal areas. Likewise, nodes less than 0.5 cm may be palpated in the occipital, postauricular (mastoid), and axillary chains (see Table 156-1). Small occipital and postauricular nodes are common in infants but not older children; cervical and inguinal nodes are common after age 2 years. The distribution by age is shown in Table 156-2. In the submental or submaxillary regions, intraoral or facial infections may enlarge the nodes to more than 1 cm. It is unusual, however, to find lymph nodes of any size in the supraclavicular or epitrochlear areas. Thus, the same size lymph node observed in two different regions may have markedly different implications. For example, a 1-cm node in the cervical region of a 5-year-old child is very likely to be benign, whereas a 1-cm supraclavicular node requires a biopsy because it is unlikely to result from superficial inflammatory disease and may reflect intrathoracic or intraabdominal malignancy.

Table 156-3 shows the correlation between lymph node location and disease origin. These associations help narrow the differential diagnosis. Fluctuance and signs of inflammation surrounding a group of enlarged lymph nodes are helpful in reaching a diagnosis, particularly if an infectious source is present distal to the node area. These findings strongly suggest an infectious etiology (Table 156-4), usually requiring systemic antibiotic therapy. If no inflammation is found, the consistency and mobility of the nodes may heighten suspicion of underlying malignancy. Hard, fixed nodes are seen more often in adults who have metastatic carcinoma. The nodes of Hodgkin's disease and lymphoma are more matted than hard, although nodes associated with neuroblastoma, rhabdomyosarcoma, and other childhood malignancies may mimic the findings in adults.

DIFFERENTIAL DIAGNOSIS

The major differential diagnostic categories for enlarged lymph nodes include infectious (inflammatory) and neoplastic diseases. Table 156-4 provides a summary of the common and uncommon conditions associated with lymphadenopathy for newborns, infants, children, and adolescents (the relative occurrence varies with age). The classification of these conditions is somewhat arbitrary and not all-inclusive but does reflect the diagnostic likelihood within a given age group.

Infections

Infectious problems may be localized or systemic. If localized, the primary site of infection draining to the involved lymph node area should be identified. Most often, lymph nodes enlarge in reaction to a localized or generalized infection, but a node can, itself, become intrinsically infected, resulting in lymphadenitis.

The common pyogenic bacteria, atypical mycobacteria, and anaerobic bacteria are most likely to cause localized adenopathy. Generalized adenopathy and regional adenopathy associated with adenopathy elsewhere are more likely caused by infections from viruses, spirochetes, or sometimes, *Toxoplasma. Mycobacterium tuberculosis* may produce localized or multiple sites of adenitis. Fungal infections, such as histoplasmosis, occasionally may cause generalized lymphadenopathy, but most fungal infections, if associated with adenopathy at all, produce regional enlargement.

Table 156-1 Palpable Lymph Nodes and Lymphatic Drainage

Lymph Node Area	Area of Drainage
Occipital	Posterior scalp, neck
Mastoid	Mastoid area
Submental	Apex of tongue and lower lip
Submaxillary	Tongue, buccal cavity, lips, and cheek
Cervical	Cranium, neck, and oropharynx
Axillary	Greater part of arm, shoulder, superficial anterior and lateral thoracic and upper abdominal wall
Supraclavicular	Right: Inferior neck and mediastinum Left: Inferior neck, mediastinum, and upper abdomen
Epitrochlear	Hand, forearm, and elbow
Inguinal	Leg and genitalia
Femoral	Leg
Popliteal	Posterior leg and knee

Table 156-2 Prevalence of Lymphadenopathy by Age

		Palpable Lymph Nodes									
	Number of	Occipital		Postauricular		Submandibular		Cervical		No Palpable Nodes	
Age	Patients	No.	(%)	No.	(%)	No.	(%)	No.	(%)	No.	(%)
0-6 mo	52	17	(32)	7	(13)	1	(2)	1	(2)	32	(62)
7-12 mo	31	8	(26)	4	(13)	1	(3)	8	(26)	16	(52)
13-23 mo	39	4	(10)	3	(7)	7	(18)	11	(28)	20	(52)
2 yr	35	3	(8)	2	(6)	7	(20)	16	(45)	11	(32)
3 yr	27	2	(7)	0	(0)	7	(26)	9	(33)	11	(41)
4 yr	20	0	(0)	0	(0)	5	(25)	11	(55)	7	(35)
5 yr	19	0	(0)	1	(5)	4	(21)	12	(63)	5	(26)
TOTAL	223	34	(15)	17	(8)	32	(14)	68	(30)	102	(45)

Reproduced from Herzog LW: *Clin Pediatr* 22:485, 1983 with permission.

Table 156-3 Correlations Between Lymph Node Locations and Disease Origin

Lymph Node Groups	Associated Cause
Occipital	Scalp infections, insect bites, ringworm
Posterior auricular	Rubella
Anterior auricular	Eye or conjunctival infections
Posterior cervical	Toxoplasmosis
Submental	Tongue, gum, buccal mucosal, and dental infections
Anterior cervical	Infections of pharynx and oral cavity, tuberculosis, Epstein-Barr virus
Supraclavicular	Malignancy—lymphomas, metastatic disease
Mediastinal	Sarcoidosis, histoplasmosis, coccidiomycosis, tuberculosis, lymphoma, metastatic disease
Axillary	Cat-scratch disease, pyogenic infections of upper arms, brucellosis, dermatopathic lymphadenopathy, lymphoma
Epitrochlear	Viral diseases, sarcoidosis, tularemia, infections of hands
Abdominal/retroperitoneal	Tuberculosis, lymphoma, metastatic disease
Inguinal	Herpes, lymphogranuloma venereum, syphillis, gonococcal infection, lymphoma

Reproduced from Perkins SL, et al: *Semin Diagn Pathol* 12:284, 1995 with permission.

Table 156-4 Etiology of Lymphadenopathy

Differential Diagnosis	Newborn	Infant	Child	Adolescent
Infections				
Bacterial				
Pyogenic	Group B streptococci			
		Streptococci/staphylococci and other gram-positive and gram-negative organisms		
			Cat-scratch fever →	→
			Typhoid fever →	→
			Tularemia →	→
Spirochetal	Syphilis →	→		Syphilis
Anaerobes				Acute necrotizing, ulcerating gingivitis
Granulomatous		Mycobacteria →	→	→
		Atypical mycobacteria →	→	→
Viral			Rubella →	→
			Rubeola →	→
			Varicella →	→
		HHV-6 syndrome →		
		Adenovirus →	→	→
		Enterovirus →	→	→
			Epstein-Barr virus (EBV) →	→
			Cytomegalovirus (CMV) →	→
			Herpes simplex virus (HSV) (stomatitis, pharyngitis, or skin infection) →	→
		Human immunodeficiency virus (HIV) →	→	→
Protozoan	Toxoplasmosis →	→	→	→
Fungal		Histoplasmosis →	→	→
		Other fungi (rare cases) →	→	→
Rickettsial			Rocky Mountain spotted fever →	→
Chlamydial				Lymphogranuloma →
Parasitic			Toxocara →	→
			Myiasis →	→
Neoplastic				
Endogenous		Leukemia →	→	→
		Lymphoma →	→	→
		Langerhans histiocytosis →	→	→
			Hodgkin's disease →	→
Exogenous (Metastatic)		Neuroblastoma →	→	→
		Wilms' tumor →	→	→
			Ewing's sarcoma →	→
			Rhabdomyosarcoma	
Immunological		Juvenile rheumatoid arthritis (JRA) →	→	→
			Systemic lupus erythematosus (SLE) →	→
		Serum sickness →	→	→
			Sarcoidosis →	→
Other				
(Reactive)		Kawasaki disease →	→	→
			Hemoglobinopathies →	→
			Hemophilia →	→
			Phenytoin →	→
			Addison's disease →	→
			Hyperthyroidism →	→
				Sinus histiocytosis →
				Histiocytic necrotizing lymphadenitis
	Chronic granulomatous disease (CGD) →	→	→	→
	Agammaglobulinemia →	→	→	→

Neoplastic Diseases

Primary neoplastic diseases are the other major consideration in both localized and generalized adenopathy. Included in this category are lymphomas, leukemia, histiocytosis, and metastases from solid tumors such as neuroblastoma, Wilms' tumor, Ewing's sarcoma, and rhabdomyosarcoma.

Immunological and Inflammatory Diseases

Generalized lymphadenopathy also may be associated with chronic inflammatory conditions, such as collagen-vascular diseases and sarcoidosis, and with reactions to certain drugs, such as phenytoin and isoniazid, or serum sickness. Such divergent causes as hyperthyroidism and Addison's disease also must be included in the differential diagnosis of generalized adenopathy.

ASSESSMENT

History, Physical Examination, and Chest Roentgenogram

The history and physical examination may reveal a source of a localized infection, such as a dental abscess, mastoiditis, scalp infection, insect bite, or cat scratch. Alternatively, systemic diseases, such as infectious mononucleosis, juvenile rheumatoid arthritis (JRA), and infection with the human immunodeficiency virus (HIV), may be suggested by other characteristic historical and physical findings. The physical examination should include all the palpable nodes listed in Table 156-1. Furthermore, assessment of enlarged lymph nodes that have no obvious inflammatory explanation requires a chest roentgenogram to determine whether enlarged mediastinal or hilar nodes are present. Mediastinal or hilar adenopathy would preclude "trials of antibiotics," with the attendant delay in performing a diagnostic biopsy.

Imaging

The abdominal lymph nodes, including retroperitoneal, periportal, and celiac nodes, as well as the nodes of the splenic hilum, are more difficult to evaluate without more sophisticated imaging techniques. The spleen, which is primarily lymphoid tissue, may be enlarged in infectious, immunological, collagen-vascular, and neoplastic disorders and may be delineated by ultrasound or computed tomography (CT) examination. Abdominal and pelvic lymph nodes may be visualized by ultrasonography or may require techniques such as CT and magnetic resonance imaging (MRI). Newer techniques, including positron emission tomography and scintigraphy, are being evaluated.

Complete Blood Count

Numerous other studies may be useful in the assessment of lymphadenopathy. The complete blood count (CBC) may reveal the reactive lymphocytes of infectious mononucleosis or a granulocytosis with a "shift to the left," suggesting systemic bacterial infection. Any cytopenia (e.g., anemia, granulocytopenia, or thrombocytopenia) would be a "red flag" that a hematological malignancy, such as leukemia or lymphoma, or metastatic disease invading the bone marrow, such as neuroblastoma, may underlie the lymphadenopathy. The finding of nucleated erythrocytes and immature granulocytes ("leukoerythroblastic blood picture") on the blood film is ominous, suggesting bone marrow "irritation" with premature release of cell precursors. This may be seen in metastatic diseases such as neuroblastoma and rhabdomyosarcoma, with immunological vasculitis, and with granulomas (mycobacteria) in the marrow.

Infectious Evaluation

The diagnostic workup of potential infectious lymphadenopathy is diverse and depends on the history, the patient's age, the location of the nodes, and the signs of inflammation accompanying the adenopathy, as noted previously. For acute, inflamed, and localized adenopathy, an infectious etiological diagnosis is achieved most frequently by obtaining material for culture and histological or pathological examination. In children who have acute cervical adenitis, needle aspiration of an acutely inflamed, sometimes fluctuant node demonstrates the infecting organism in two thirds or more of cases. The aspirated material should be cultured aerobically and anaerobically and for fungi and mycobacteria. Histochemical evaluation should include Gram and acid-fast stains. In certain cases, a biopsy may be required, and this may be evaluated by additional special stains, such as the Warthin-Starry silver stain for cat-scratch disease. Intradermal skin tests should be applied when mycobacterial infection is suspected. Although a skin test exists for cat-scratch disease, the antigen is neither standardized nor available commercially. However, serological tests for *Bartonella henselae*, the major agent of cat-scratch disease, have been developed and are available commercially. Specific serological or antigen detection tests also are available for syphilis, toxoplasmosis, brucellosis, tularemia, fungi, and some viral infections such as Epstein-Barr virus, HIV, cytomegalovirus, and herpes simplex virus (HSV). Viral cultures are appropriate for the last two and for the common respiratory viruses, such as the adenoviruses and enteroviruses. The erythrocyte sedimentation rate may be useful in assessing underlying inflammation, but it is not unique to infectious diseases because it also may be elevated in immunological and neoplastic diseases.

After initial evaluation by history, physical examination, chest roentgenogram, and preliminary laboratory studies, the clinician may not yet have an obvious explanation for the node enlargement. If a bacterial source for localized adenopathy (e.g., pharyngitis and cervical nodes) is suggested, a limited course of 7 to 10 days of antibiotic therapy may be tried. However, if the nodes have not regressed significantly, prompt further evaluation is necessary. At this time, a chest roentgenogram should be obtained, if it has not already been done; even in the absence of mediastinal or hilar adenopathy, significantly enlarged, unexplained lymph nodes should be biopsied promptly to establish the diagnosis and permit institution of appropriate therapy.

Biopsy

Biopsy of significant adenopathy should be performed early if there is no evidence to suggest an infection or other etiology, and particularly if mediastinal or hilar nodes are enlarged. The biopsy should encompass the central mass of the enlarged nodes so that a misdiagnosis of reactive inflammation in adjacent nodes can be avoided. This is particularly common in Hodgkin's disease, in which an adjacent smaller lymph node may be more accessible and technically easier to biopsy but may not demonstrate the presence of Reed-Sternberg cells. Fine-needle aspiration is not recommended for biopsy of superficial, accessible nodes, although it is useful for intrathoracic nodes to avoid thoracotomy. Appropriate expertise is required for interpretation, and negative findings are not definitive.

It is critical that any biopsy be performed at a medical center specializing in the care of children so that all of the appropriate touch preparations, cultures, special cytochemical or immunological stains, and biochemical or cytogenetic studies are obtained. The pathology of Hodgkin's disease, lymphoma, and other similar round-cell tumors may be difficult to establish and requires the expertise of a pediatric pathologist who has experience in assessing these diseases. Immunophenotyping, cytogenetic analysis, molecular studies of gene rearrangement, and electron microscopy may be required for precise diagnosis. These studies, in conjunction with the histopathology, are central to the assessment and subsequent management, which may involve treatment with radiation, chemotherapy, or both.

TREATMENT

Infectious Diseases

Therapy of lymphadenitis depends on its etiology or the most likely cause. Acute adenitis, particularly of the cervical area in young children, frequently is associated with infection from group A beta-hemolytic streptococci or *Staphylococcus aureus* organisms. The latter are particularly likely in adenitis that progresses to fluctuance. In the neonate and rarely in older children, group B streptococci may cause localized adenitis with or without cellulitis. In children beyond the neonatal period who have acute localized adenitis, particularly cervical adenitis, antibiotic therapy should be directed at group A streptococci with an antibiotic that also covers penicillinase-producing strains of *S. aureus*. For most patients, oral therapy is adequate.

The usual course of therapy is 10 to 14 days, but therapy should be continued for at least 5 days after the signs of acute inflammation have subsided. For patients who have suppurative adenitis from these organisms, drainage is not only diagnostic (by culturing the exudate obtained) but also therapeutic. A few patients may not respond to oral therapy, even with a drug to which the organism is sensitive. Parenteral antibiotic therapy then is required.

If an anaerobic infection is suspected, therapy depends in part on the location of the adenitis and the type of organism. Most anaerobic infections of the cervical and submental areas are associated with mouth flora, most of which are sensitive to penicillin. Occasionally, however, such infections require alternative therapy such as clindamycin, metronidazole, or a cephalosporin.

Both *M. tuberculosis* and atypical mycobacteria can cause adenitis, with the latter being more frequent in children. Differentiating the two may be difficult but is important because many strains of atypical mycobacteria are resistant to the usual antitubercular chemotherapy, and excisional biopsy may be required. If tubercular infection is suspected, appropriate therapy for *M. tuberculosis* should be initiated while awaiting identification and sensitivities of the organism. Adenitis suspected to be tubercular should not be incised for biopsy or drainage.

Cat-scratch adenitis usually is self-limited. The recent discovery of *Bartonella* spp., especially *B. henselae* as the prime cause of cat-scratch disease, has raised the potential for specific antibiotic therapy. A recent study has shown clinical benefit with azithromycin treatment.[1] If nodes become markedly enlarged, tender, and fluctuant, aspiration may help relieve symptoms; incision and drainage, however, should be avoided.

For the unusual case of severe primary HSV infection with localized adenitis, treatment with oral acyclovir in some studies has shortened the clinical course.

Neoplastic Disease

The treatment of neoplastic diseases today is oriented in most instances toward cure. The effectiveness of treatment for lymphocytic and myelocytic leukemia, lymphomas, and Wilms' and other tumors has improved markedly in the past two decades. The specific treatment of childhood cancer often involves combinations of chemotherapy, radiation therapy, and surgery, which depend on the individual diagnosis and are beyond the scope of this presentation (see Chapter 193, Cancers in Childhood). However, prompt, accurate diagnosis is essential for institution of specific treatment and optimum care of these patients.

When to Refer

1. When history and physical examination do not suggest an infectious etiology.
2. When apparently infected nodes have not responded to a course of antibiotics.
3. When there is mediastinal or hilar adenopathy
4. When a biopsy is considered. Biopsies should be performed only at a center specializing in the care of children.

When to Hospitalize

1. When biopsy requires hospitalization (e.g., mediastinal or hilar biopsy)
2. When biopsy results require inpatient treatment or further evaluation
3. When an infection requires intravenous antibiotic therapy

REFERENCE

1. Bass JW, et al: Prospective randomized double-blind placebo-controlled evaluation of azithromycin for treatment of cat scratch disease, *Pediatr Infect Dis* 17:4, 1998.

SUGGESTED READINGS

Ferrer R: Lymphadenopathy: differential diagnosis and evaluation, *Am Fam Physician* 58:1313, 1998.

Filston HC: Common lumps and bumps of the head and neck in infants and children, *Peditatr Ann* 18:180, 1989.

Freidig EE, et al: Clinical-histologic-microbiologic analysis of 419 lymph node biopsy specimens, *Rev Infect Dis* 8:322, 1986.

Kaji AV, Mohuchy T, Swartz JD: Imaging of cervical lymphadenopathy, *Semin Ultrasound* 18:220, 1997.

Knight PJ, Mulne AF, Vassy LE: When is lymph node biopsy indicated in children with enlarged peripheral nodes? *Pediatrics* 69:391, 1982.

Lake AM, Oski FA: Peripheral lymphadenopathy in childhood, *Am J Dis Child* 132:357, 1978.

Morland B: Lymphadenopathy, *Arch Dis Child* 73:476, 1995.

Starke JR: Nontuberculous mycobacterial infections in children, *Adv Pediatr Infect Dis* 7:123, 1992.

157 Malocclusion

Lindsey K. Grossman

The incidence of malocclusion in school-age children and adolescents may be as high as 90% or more, according to some reports. In evaluating such statistics, however, one first must consider the definition involved, because in the field of orthodontics any deviation from absolutely ideal tooth alignment is considered malocclusion, although probably only 10% to 15% of these can be viewed as disabling.[11] The 1963 to 1965 National Health Survey, which examined 7400 children 6 to 11 years of age, found 14.2% to have severe or very severe malocclusion.[5] This national survey of malocclusion has not been repeated to date; however, there is no reason to believe that the incidence has changed since then.

A major problem hindering objective evaluation of orthodontic treatment is the lack of a universally acceptable classification system. The Treatment Priority Index, which was used in the National Health Survey, is a quantitative measure of severity, but because of its complexity has not been adopted widely. The commonly used Angle classification system effectively expresses qualitative but not quantitative differences in dental occlusion; hence, it is not helpful in determining the need for referral or in evaluating treatment outcome.[4] It, therefore, is difficult to determine objectively which patients require orthodontic correction or to compare the results of various treatments.

It is not always easy to determine the etiology of malocclusion, which involves both genetic and environmental factors. Only in about 5% of cases is a cause clearly identifiable.[13] Significant evidence links nasal obstruction, especially when caused by enlarged tonsils or adenoids, with the development of a high arched palate and posterior crossbite.[9,13]

Significantly abnormal dental occlusion has been said to predispose individuals to many risks.[9] Caries, periodontal disease, increased susceptibility to trauma or root resorption, and disturbances of physiological functioning, including muscular dysfunction, speech defects, and masticatory disturbances, have been linked to malocclusion, although the data supporting such outcomes are either scanty or conflicting.[6] Temporomandibular joint (TMJ) dysfunction increasingly has been cited as a possible cause of headache and other symptoms in adolescents and school-age children. Some studies show an amazingly high incidence of signs referable to the temporomandibular joint but usually without symptoms of TMJ dysfunction. Signs such as joint sounds with movement or condyle position do not correlate well with symptomatic TMJ dysfunction requiring treatment, especially in children. Furthermore, there is no convincing evidence that malocclusion or orthodontic therapy has a relationship to the development of temporomandibular symptoms.[7,12]

Most patients seek orthodontic treatment because of malocclusion's effect on their appearance. In our society, the individual's own sense of attractiveness can influence behavior and success in life. However, there is no direct evidence that treating dental irregularities affects these outcomes positively.

Pacifiers, as well as thumb- and finger-sucking habits,[8] play a role in malocclusion problems. Most children develop such habits during infancy, and by 4 or 5 years of age most have stopped the practice; however, as many as 5.9% of children may continue into school age.[3] If sucking continues into the periods of mixed and permanent dentition, the potential for developing malocclusion is greater, although a specific causal relationship may not always hold. Often, abnormal bites revert to normal after the habit is stopped. Anterior open bite, overjet, crossbites, and other malocclusions have been reported in association with sucking habits, although other children who have such habits may show no abnormalities.[14] Thumb-sucking may be preferable to finger-sucking because fewer physical stresses are exerted on the teeth. A pacifier probably has the least deleterious effect. Most studies show that use of a pacifier stops earlier than thumb- or finger-sucking.

In the assessment of occlusion, both the maxillary and mandibular arches should be observed with the mouth open to determine if the teeth are crowded or have excess space between them.[11] Crowding almost always increases over time, whereas excess space may either improve or worsen. Excess space, especially between the upper lateral incisors and canines and the lower canines and first deciduous molars, is the norm in young children who have primary dentition and allows room for the eruption of the larger, permanent teeth.

Occlusion of the posterior teeth is assessed with the teeth set in the biting position. The tongue should not be visible between the upper and lower teeth; the presence of such a space, albeit very small, or the contrasting problem of a deep bite (lower incisors biting on palatal gingiva) nearly always requires treatment. The maxillary teeth should overlap their mandibular partners slightly in the lateral plane and be placed slightly anterior (approximately half a tooth width) to them. Posterior crossbites are common discrepancies that rarely self-correct. Timely treatment of such problems, during the primary or early mixed stages of dentition, is recommended for establishing optimal function to normalize dental, skeletal, and neuromuscular growth during these times of active change.[15]

Anterior dentition problems, readily apparent when the patient smiles, are the source of many orthodontic referrals. An open bite with space visible between the upper and lower arches, and underbite, are difficult to treat, whereas overbite ("buck teeth") or anterior crossbite often can be corrected easily. Occasionally, one or more of the permanent teeth, often incisors, may erupt before the corresponding primary teeth have been shed, giving the child a double row of teeth and causing much parental concern. Extraction rarely is necessary because the primary teeth almost always are shed by age 8 years. Normal tongue movements usually ensure correct final placement of the permanent teeth.

Few data link maloccluded primary dentition with maloccluded permanent teeth. However, the presence of anterior crossbite, wherein the upper lateral incisors erupt behind the lower ones or the upper posterior teeth erupt medial to the lower ones, may interfere with ultimate maxillary growth and tooth position. The absence of normal spacing in primary dentition almost always leads to severe crowding of the permanent teeth. Children who have such conditions should be referred to an orthodontist early.[1] Probably the most important influence pediatricians can have in promoting good dental occlusion is their advice concerning primary dentition. Congenital absence or loss of one or more of the primary teeth to decay or trauma can seriously affect the spacing required for normal occlusion of the permanent teeth. Thus, a dental referral is advisable if any primary tooth fails to erupt or is prematurely lost.[10]

In general, however, the decision to refer a child or young adolescent for orthodontic treatment may be difficult; there are few objective referral guidelines.[2] Treatment nearly always results in an improved, although not necessarily a flawless, appearance. The pediatrician should assess the patient's and family's expectations, as well as their willingness to comply with the discomfort and cost of treatment, before arranging for referral.

When to Refer

Posterior crossbites rarely self-correct, and treatment during the stage of primary or mixed dentition may be optimal to promote normal development of the teeth, bones, and muscular structures.

The absence of normal dental spacing in the primary dentition requires early referral. This is especially important if any primary tooth is lost or fails to erupt.

REFERENCES

1. Agapas TR: Early orthodontic treatment, *Ont Dent* 71:26, 1994.
2. Currier GF: Fundamentals of orthodontics with criteria for referral, *Pediatr Ann* 14:117, 1985.
3. Gellin ME: Digital sucking and tongue thrusting in children, *Dent Clin North Am* 22:603, 1978.
4. Jago JD: The epidemiology of dental occlusion: a critical appraisal, *J Public Health Dent* 34:80, 1974.
5. Kelly JE, Sanchez M, VanKirk LE: *An assessment of the occlusion of teeth of children 6-11 years,* NHS Series 11, No 130, US Department of Health, Education and Welfare Publications (PHS) 74-1612, 1973.
6. McLain JB, Profitt WR: Oral health status in the United States: prevalence of malocclusion, *J Dent Educ* 49:386, 1985.
7. McNamara JA, Seligman DA, Okeson JP: Occlusion, orthodontic treatment and temporomandibular disorders: a review, *J Orofac Pain* 9:73, 1995.
8. Moore MB: Digits, dummies and malocclusions, *Dent Update* 23:415, 1996.
9. Richter HJ: Obstruction of the pediatric upper airway, *Ear Nose Throat J* 66:209, 1987.
10. Schneider PE, Peterson J: Oral habits: considerations in management, *Pediatr Clin North Am* 29:523, 1982.
11. Smith RJ: Development of occlusion and malocclusion, *Pediatr Clin North Am* 29:475, 1982.
12. Tallents RN, Catania J, Dommers E: Temporomandibular joint findings in pediatric populations and young adults: a critical review, *Angle Orthod* 61:7, 1991.
13. Turner S, Nattrass C, Sandy JR: The role of soft tissue in the etiology of malocclusion, *Dent Update* 24:209, 1997.
14. Vanderas AP, Manetas KJ: Relationship between malocclusion and bruxism in children and adolescents: a review, *Pediatr Dent* 17:7, 1995.
15. Zhu JF, et al: Posterior crossbites in children, *Compend Contin Educ Dent* 17:1051, 1996.

SUGGESTED READINGS

Sadowsky PL: Craniofacial growth and the timing of treatment, *Am J Orthod Dentofacial Orthop* 113:19, 1998.

Turgeon-O'Brien H, et al: Nutritive and nonnutritive sucking habits: a review, *ASDC J Dent Child* 63:321, 1996.

158 Nervousness

Richard M. Sarles

Some chief complaints occasion a sinking feeling in a busy physician, especially when he or she first hears them in the middle of a busy afternoon in the office. The nature of such complaints implies that the physician and patient are about to embark on an often murky and abstract search for the root of an evanescent symptom or problem. One such complaint is nervousness, whether it is voiced by an older child or an adolescent or by a parent about a child: for example, the mother who describes her 12-year-old as "nervous all the time," to which the patient responds vaguely, "I don't know, maybe, I just feel funny."

Such moments call for discipline on the part of the physician. They remind us that this may be a circumstance in which an inarticulate patient literally is shouting for help. It is the kind of complaint with which patients may signal that they are among those most in need of attention. The physician must look beyond the chief complaint to the "doctor-seeking" stimulus: Why does this patient have this complaint? What does it mean?

Finding the answer will take time, perhaps a great deal of time. The approach, however, is clear. A good history and physical examination are needed. The circumstance is not life threatening; everything does not have to be done immediately. Indeed, some of the effort may be delayed until a time when the physician can schedule more time and is more at ease and less stressed. Certainly the abstraction of the term *nervousness* and the difficulty in defining it more precisely underscore the need to devote adequate time to take a complete history, conduct a thorough physical examination, and discuss the problem in depth.

What accompanies the nervousness: anorexia, restlessness at night, sluggishness, overactivity? A physical problem is implied but quite often is not at the root. Nervousness, for example, often is part of the constellation of complaints in a variety of endocrine disorders (hyperthyroidism, hypoglycemia, Addison's disease) and in dermatitis, pinworm infestation, and allergy. Caffeine ingestion (colas and coffee) and abuse of a variety of drugs also can cause "nervousness." Mitral valve prolapse and paroxysmal tachycardia are cardiac diseases that can create symptoms of nervousness. Clearly, a careful history and thorough physical examination can be productive.

The physician also should consider the possibility of an attention deficit disorder with or without hyperactivity, as well as an anxiety disorder, such as separation anxiety or school phobia, and somatization of depression. Many more serious problems, such as autism, childhood psychoses, obsessive-compulsive and manic-depressive disorders, panic attacks, and Tourette's syndrome, all can present with a complaint of nervousness as the parents or patient try to define perceptions and feelings. However, such problems rarely are defined as nervousness alone; the history and physical examination quickly can uncover a host of concomitant findings.

It is after a conscientious biopsychosocial search has been made, and when little if anything more has been discovered, that the chief complaint of nervousness becomes even more difficult to approach. Time, caring, and sensitive understanding of the patient's needs are required. Unfortunately, little help is available in the literature. Nervousness usually is not defined or described in textbooks and is not listed in the American Psychiatric Association's *Diagnostic and Statistical Manual of Mental Disorders, Fourth Edition (DSM-IV)* or in any standard psychiatric textbook, and a discussion of its implications generally is not included in most medical school curricula.

How, then, is the practitioner to conceptualize, diagnose, and treat nervousness, nervous stomach, or other disorders that occur as symptoms without any readily discernible underlying pathophysiology? First, of course, comes the careful search; then come the devotion of time, the "listening ear," the sensitive exploration, and if necessary, referral to a colleague who has expertise in emotional disorders of childhood and adolescence to attempt to unravel the sometimes intricate psychosocial puzzle.

Even when the physician knows the patient has no physical disorder, emotional tension, restlessness, agitation, fearful apprehension, acute uneasiness, undue excitability, or excessive irritability may be evident. These manifestations, quite real and requiring care, call for individual attention to the child or for work with the family collectively. Indeed, the approach needed may vary as widely as the range of complaints. A physician who is unprepared to provide the necessary time and effort should refer the patient to ease the morbidity inevitably associated with these complaints.

159 Nonconvulsive Periodic Disorders

Sarah M. Roddy

A variety of paroxysmal nonepileptic disorders occur in children. These disorders have a wide range of clinical features that mimic seizures, and it is important to distinguish them from seizures so that the child is not treated with anticonvulsants inappropriately. A careful history often is all that is needed to make the diagnosis, although a few patients may require a more extensive evaluation. Some of the more common paroxysmal nonepileptic disorders are reviewed here.

BREATH-HOLDING SPELLS

Breath-holding spells, or infantile syncope, occur in approximately 5% of children.[18] Most children who have breath-holding spells begin having episodes between 6 and 18 months of age, although some may begin in the first few weeks of life. The frequency of episodes ranges from once a year to several times daily. The history of the episode and of the surrounding events is the most important part of the evaluation of a child who has such spells. Because the familial incidence of breath-holding spells is high, the parents should be questioned about episodes in other family members.

Two types of breath-holding spells occur—cyanotic and pallid. The cyanotic type is more common and usually is precipitated by frustration or anger. The child cries vigorously and then holds his or her breath in expiration. This apnea is followed by cyanosis with opisthotonic posturing and loss of consciousness. Recovery usually is quick, with return of respiration and consciousness within 1 minute. Evaluation of children who have severe cyanotic breath-holding spells has shown an underlying autonomic system dysregulation that may contribute to the pathophysiology of the episodes.[8] Pallid breath-holding episodes usually are provoked by sudden fright or minor injuries, especially falling and hitting the occiput. The child gasps or cries briefly and then abruptly becomes quiet, loses consciousness, has pallor, and becomes limp. The child then may develop clonic jerks. Pallid breath-holding spells are a vasovagal phenomenon. The precipitating event induces a vagally mediated asystole, leading to cerebral ischemia. Ocular compression during simultaneous electroencephalographic and electrocardiographic tracing in children who have pallid breath-holding spells has shown asystole with flattening of the electroencephalogram without electrical seizure activity.[18] The clonic jerks are caused by cerebral hypoxia rather than by epileptiform discharges from the brain.

The prognosis for children who have either type of breath holding is excellent; most outgrow the episodes by school age. Children who have pallid breath-holding spells later may develop syncope.[18] Treatment is directed mainly at reassuring the family of the benign nature of the episodes. It is important to emphasize that the episodes are not seizures and that they do not lead to mental retardation or epilepsy. Because cyanotic episodes often are precipitated by temper tantrums, anger, and frustration, advice about behavior management may be helpful. Anemia has been described as a contributing factor in breath-holding spells, and treating it may reduce the incidence of the episodes.[5,6] Atropine is effective for pallid breath-holding episodes, but its use rarely is warranted. Anticonvulsants should not be used because they are not effective in the treatment of either type of breath-holding spell. (See Chapter 97, Temper Tantrums and Breath-Holding Spells.)

SYNCOPE

Syncope, or fainting, is an acute and transient loss of consciousness caused by reduced cerebral perfusion. These episodes are relatively common among teenagers.[10] Postural hypotension, which may occur after a sudden change from a sitting or reclining position to a standing position, can precipitate an episode. Emotional upset, fright, or overheating also are common provoking stimuli. Cardiac disorders, including arrhythmias, aortic stenosis, and severe cyanotic heart disease, may cause syncope by reducing cardiac output and causing cerebral hypoxia. In rare cases, episodes of syncope have been reported with swallowing, coughing, urinating, and defecating.[14]

Patients have presyncopal symptoms that may include light-headedness, anxiety, sweating, nausea, generalized numbness, and visual changes described as constriction or darkening of vision. Observers notice marked pallor and clammy skin. These symptoms are followed by loss of consciousness and slumping to the floor. Once the patient is recumbent and cerebral perfusion is restored, consciousness returns within a few seconds. If the patient is held with his or her head above the body and cerebral perfusion is not restored, clonic movements may occur. As with the pallid breath-holding spells, these movements occur secondary to cerebral ischemia rather than to epileptiform discharges from the brain. Patients are not disoriented or confused after an episode of syncope, although they may be tired.

The history is very important in diagnosing syncope, and it should include a description of the event by the patient and an observer. Laboratory evaluation seldom is needed, but if atypical features are involved, such as absence of a precipitating factor or confusion after the episode, an electroencephalogram or a cardiac evaluation, including Holter monitoring, may be appropriate. Evaluation with tilt table testing has been recommended for children who have unexplained syncope.[20] Treatment consists of teaching the patient and family about managing an episode. Because patients have presyncopal symptoms, they should be instructed to sit or lie down as soon as the symptoms begin, thereby preventing progression to loss of consciousness. If the patient does lose consciousness, the family should place him or her in a recumbent position with the head lower than the body. Parents often pick up a child who has fainted; they should be cautioned against doing this because they may prolong the period of unconsciousness (see Chapter 174, Syncope, for a more detailed discussion of syncope and its causes.)

BENIGN PAROXYSMAL VERTIGO

Benign paroxysmal vertigo of childhood is a disorder characterized by brief attacks of vertigo. Symptoms usually appear within the first 3 or 4 years of life, although they may begin later. Episodes are characterized by abrupt onset, with the child appearing fearful and unable to maintain normal posture and gait. The child may seek support and clutch the parent or abruptly sit down or fall. In severe cases the child may be limp and incapable of using his or her extremities. Pallor and diaphoresis usually are apparent, and vomiting and nystagmus sometimes occur. Typically an episode lasts less than 30 seconds, and in rare cases, a few minutes. A brief period of postural instability may follow the episode, but within a few minutes the child is back to normal and playing. Consciousness is not altered during the episode, nor does the child feel sleepy after it. The frequency of episodes varies from as many as several weekly to as few as one every 4 months. Audiograms are normal. Oculovestibular testing with cold water calorics is difficult to perform in young children, and results vary. When properly done, no abnormalities in vestibular function have been found.[12] Radiographic studies of the temporal bone and electroencephalographic recordings also are normal. Included in the differential diagnosis of vertigo in childhood are brainstem lesions, posterior fossa tumors, and epilepsy. Usually the history and physical examination differentiate benign paroxysmal vertigo from these more serious disorders. In most cases no treatment is necessary, and anticonvulsants are not effective. Antihistamines such as dimenhydrinate have been used in some patients who have frequent episodes, with an apparent reduction in the number of episodes. Because the frequency of attacks varies, it is difficult to assess the effect of therapy accurately. Attacks of vertigo usually stop spontaneously over a period of a few years. Some children who had had benign paroxysmal vertigo have later developed migraine headaches[17] (see Chapter 125, Dizziness and Vertigo).

SHUDDERING ATTACKS

Shuddering or shivering episodes are a benign movement disorder that probably occurs in many children at one time or another. The episodes are brief and characterized by paroxysmal rapid tremors involving primarily the head and arms. Some episodes may involve flexion of the head, elbow, trunk, and knees, with adduction of the elbows and knees.[21] Consciousness is not altered during the episodes. The frequency varies, with some children having more than 100 episodes daily. Emotional factors, including excitement, fear, anger, and frustration, may precipitate episodes. Shuddering episodes may start as early as a few months of age or not until later in childhood. Usually the number of episodes declines gradually. The pathophysiology of the episodes is unclear, although it has been postulated that the attacks are an expression of an essential tremor.[21] Electroencephalographic monitoring has shown that the episodes are not epileptiform in nature.[15] Usually, no treatment is necessary. If episodes are severe and interfere with activities, treatment with propranolol may be helpful;[2] anticonvulsants are ineffective and should not be used.

BENIGN NEONATAL SLEEP MYOCLONUS

Sudden brief jerks of the extremities are normal in children and adults when falling asleep. Sleep-related myoclonus in neonates is called *benign neonatal sleep myoclonus*. The myoclonic jerks begin in the first month of life, often within the first day, and are present only during quiet sleep, disappearing when the baby awakens.[7] The jerking movements may start in one extremity and then progress to involve the other extremities, or they may begin bilaterally. The upper extremities are involved more often than the lower extremities. Jerks occur every 2 to 3 seconds for several minutes, although they have been reported to last up to 90 minutes.[4] Rocking the crib has been described as a maneuver to provoke the myoclonus.[1] Development is normal, and there are no neurological deficits. Electroencephalographic results are normal, with no epileptiform discharges associated with the myoclonus.[1,11] The major differential diagnosis of neonatal sleep myoclonus is a seizure disorder. A history of episodes only during sleep and a normal electroencephalogram help to differentiate this benign disorder from seizures. The myoclonus usually diminishes gradually during the first 6 months of life. No treatment is necessary.

NIGHT TERRORS

Night terrors are a sleep disorder that has some features that mimic partial complex seizures. They occur in up to 6% of children, with a peak incidence in late preschool and early school-age children.[9] There often is a family history of either night terrors or another sleep disorder. The episodes usually occur during the first 2 hours after falling asleep. The child sits up in bed abruptly and screams or talks unintelligibly. If the child's eyes are open, they have a glazed look. During the episode, the child appears to be hallucinating and does not respond to the parents. Tachycardia and diaphoresis result from the response of the sympathetic nervous system. In some cases the child may sleepwalk. A night terror usually lasts about 10 minutes, with the child then relaxing and abruptly falling back to sleep. Upon awakening, the child does not remember the episode. Night terrors are caused by a rapid partial arousal from deep, slow-wave sleep.

Electroencephalography does not show seizure activity during the episodes. It is important to differentiate night terrors from nightmares, which occur during rapid eye movement (REM) sleep and are associated with easy arousal and recall of the content, or at least the occurrence, of the nightmare. Night terrors usually occur less often as the child gets older, although episodes may continue into adolescence and adulthood. The nature of the episodes should be explained to the parents. Although parents tend to try to wake and reassure the child, they should be told that the child is not aware of their presence, and attempts to awaken him or her are not helpful. Usually, no medication is indicated, but if episodes are frequent or severe, diazepam is the drug of choice.[13]

NARCOLEPSY

Narcolepsy is a sleep-wake disorder characterized by excessive and inappropriate periods of sleep during the day. The daytime sleepiness interrupts activities and does not diminish in response to adequate amounts of sleep at night. Naps may last from a few minutes to longer than an hour. In addition to the excessive daytime sleep, patients often have cataplexy, sleep paralysis, and hypnagogic hallucinations. Cataplexy is a transient partial or complete loss of tone, often triggered by an emotional reaction such as laughter or fright. The individual does not lose consciousness. Sleep paralysis occurs as the patient falls asleep or awakens and is characterized by the inability to move or speak. Hypnagogic hallucinations occur while falling asleep, can be auditory or visual, and may be very frightening to a child.

The estimated prevalence of narcolepsy is 0.02% to 0.05%.[16] Onset usually occurs in the second decade, although it has been reported in children as young as age 3 years. Sleep studies in patients who have narcolepsy show that REM sleep occurs within 15 minutes of sleep onset; in normal subjects, 90 minutes of non-REM sleep precede the first REM period. In whites and Japanese, there is a strong association between narcolepsy and the haplotype DR15, which is a subtype of the HLA-DR2 antigen. In blacks, there is an association with the haplotype DQ6, which is a subtype of HLA-DQ1.[3,19] HLA typing may be helpful but is not diagnostic. Sleep studies are important in diagnosing narcolepsy. Included in the differential diagnosis of excessive daytime sleepiness are chronic illness, sleep apnea, hypothyroidism, depression, and seizures.

Narcolepsy is a lifelong condition, but central nervous system stimulants such as methylphenidate help reduce the frequency of naps. Tricyclic medications such as imipramine are used to treat cataplexy and the other associated symptoms.[3]

When to Refer

- If a diagnosis cannot be made by history and physical examination
- Need for subspecialty expertise

When to Hospitalize

- If the child needs video electroencephalographic monitoring to evaluate an episode

REFERENCES

1. Alfonso Y, et al: Simple maneuver to provoke benign neonatal sleep myoclonus, *Pediatrics* 96:1161, 1995.
2. Barron TF, Younkin DP: Propranolol therapy for shuddering attacks, *Neurology* 42:258, 1992.
3. Bassetti C, Aldrich MS: Narcolepsy, *Neurol Clin* 14:545, 1996.
4. Blennow G: Benign infantile nocturnal myoclonus, *Acta Paediatr Scand* 74:505, 1985.
5. Colina KF, Abelson HT: Resolution of breath-holding spells with treatment of concomitant anemia, *J Pediatr* 126:395, 1995.
6. Daoud AS, et al: Effectiveness of iron therapy on breath-holding spells, *J Pediatr* 130:547, 1997.
7. Di Capua M, et al: Benign neonatal sleep myoclonus: clinical features and video-polygraphic recordings, *Mov Disord* 8:191, 1993.
8. DiMario FJ Jr, Burleson JA: Autonomic nervous system function in severe breath holding spells, *Pediatr Neurol* 9:268, 1993.
9. DiMario FJ Jr, Emery S III: The natural history of night terrors, *Clin Pediatr* 26:505, 1987.
10. Driscoll DJ, et al: Syncope in children and adolescents, *J Am Coll Cardiol* 29:1030, 1997.
11. Fejerman N: Nonepileptic neurologic paroxysmal disorders and episodic symptoms in infancy and early childhood, *Int Pediatr* 11:364, 1996.
12. Finkelhor BK, Harker LA: Benign paroxysmal vertigo of childhood, *Laryngoscope* 97:1161, 1987.
13. Golden GS: Nonepileptic paroxysmal events in childhood, *Pediatr Clin North Am* 39:715, 1992.
14. Hannon DW, Knilas TK: Syncope in children and adolescents, *Curr Probl Pediatr* 23:358, 1993.
15. Holmes GL, Russman BS: Shuddering attacks: evaluation using electroencephalographic frequency modulation radiotelemetry and videotape monitoring, *Am J Dis Child* 140:72, 1985.
16. Hublin C, et al: The prevalence of narcolepsy: an epidemiological study of a Finnish twin cohort, *Ann Neurol* 35:709, 1994.
17. Lanzi D, et al: Benign paroxysmal vertigo of childhood: a long-term follow-up, *Cephalagia* 14:458, 1994.
18. Lombroso CT, Lerman P: Breathholding spells (cyanotic and pallid infantile syncope), *Pediatrics* 39:563, 1967.
19. Matsuki K, et al: DQ (rather than DR) marks susceptibility for narcolepsy, *Lancet* 339:1052, 1992.
20. Samoil D, et al: Head-upright tilt table testing in children with unexplained syncope, *Pediatrics* 92:426, 1993.
21. Vanasse M, Bedard P, Andermann F: Shuddering attacks in children: an early clinical manifestation of essential tremor, *Neurology* 26:1027, 1976.

160 Odor (Unusual Urine and Body)

Modena Hoover Wilson

An unusual or offensive odor associated with the body may be the presenting complaint or be noted incidentally by the examiner. Odor may provide a diagnostic clue when other symptoms have prompted a visit to the pediatrician, or it may confirm a suspected diagnosis.

UNUSUAL ODOR AS THE CHIEF COMPLAINT

When an unusual body odor is the chief complaint, relevant questions include: When was the odor first noticed? What does it smell like to the patient or parents? Does it seem to come from any particular part of the body or piece of clothing? Does bathing modify it, and if so, for how long? What other symptoms have been noted? Is there any reason to suspect that the child might have an object lodged in a body orifice? Is there drainage from any orifice or skin lesion? Is the child using any medications, either taken by mouth or applied topically? How has the odor affected the child and family?

ODOR AS A CLUE TO DIAGNOSIS

When a particular infection, metabolic defect, or ingestion is suspected for reasons other than odor, the practitioner may inquire about or note the presence or absence of an odor that often is associated with that condition to clarify the clinical situation.[14,17,26]

Any unexpected odor the physician detects while taking a history or examining a child requires explanation. For example, the lingering odor of feces or urine on a child who should have attained continence may prompt consideration of encopresis or enuresis.

If a patient reports an unusual odor (especially intermittently) but it is never detected by others, the possibility of temporal lobe epilepsy should be entertained. On the other hand, if the practitioner notices a clearly offensive body odor but the patient or parent does not, anosmia in either the child or the parent should be considered.

ODOR AND THE PHYSICAL EXAMINATION

In assessing an odor, the examiner should (1) note the character of the odor, (2) determine the patient's age (and stage of pubertal development), (3) check for any other signs or symptoms during a complete examination with the child unclothed, and (4) localize the odor, if possible, to a particular body site.

In a routine medical examination, the sense the physician uses least is smell. Satisfactory methods of classifying, quantifying, or even describing odors have been lacking. Gas-liquid chromatography now allows more precise identification of odors. Historically and practically, odors have been compared with others for which we have common experience, and their strength is characterized either by the distance from which the odor is obvious or by such adjectives as "strong" or "faint." Also, individuals differ in their ability to detect at least some odors and in their assessments of whether certain odors are offensive. Artificial nose technology, which can sense a wide range of volatile chemicals and be trained in pattern recognition, may soon become a tool to supplement the clinician's own nose. Bioelectronic noses are already being tested in the diagnosis of conditions such as bacterial vaginosis[5] and diabetes.[22]

CAUSES OF UNUSUAL ODOR

An array of odors can be associated with the human body and with personal effects, such as clothing, and subtle differences in odor can be found among people as well. Therefore, the first task may be to decide whether a particular odor truly is peculiar and whether it emanates from the body. The odor may be simply a normal body odor that drew attention because of its intensity or because the complainant is unusually sensitive to or concerned about it.

Normal Body Odor

Normal body odors derive from secretions of the sweat and apocrine glands, vagina, cervix, and respiratory tract and from urine, feces, breath, and flatus.[14] Odor may be produced or modified by the action of normal or abnormal microbial flora. Halitosis is offensive breath, and bromhidrosis is fetid perspiration.

In Western culture, people often minimize body odors by frequently changing their clothing, bathing, and using deodorants or antiperspirants, mouthwashes, douches, or scents applied to the skin. If one of these artificial odors is too strong, the practitioner may wonder what the patient is trying to hide. On the other hand, if a patient does not practice these customs, the physician may detect an odor that he or she finds offensive and then must decide whether the patient's noncompliance with social expectations is either precipitating or precipitated by stress.

Body odor changes with puberty, and a characteristic adult odor may prompt a child (or the child's parents) to seek medical attention.

Axillary Odor

Axillary odor, which varies in intensity from person to person, often is the strongest odor associated with adolescents and adults.[14] Its pungency long has been attributed to the action of aerobic diphtheroids on apocrine secretions. Recent work has identified odor-binding proteins that originate in the apocrine glands. The most abundant of the smelly compounds may be (E)-3-methyl-2-hexenoic acid.[27] Bacterial decomposition of androsterone is another possible etiology of axillary odor.[8] Axillary hair appears to retain or spread odor.[13]

Some adolescents and adults, both male and female, have axillary odor that is unusually strong, a condition called *osmidrosis axillae,* or as previously noted, *bromhidrosis.* The odor emanates from the apocrine glands. Possible explanations have included specific features of apocrine androgen metabolism,[23] bacterial alteration of sweat,[30] and abnormally large and numerous apocrine glands.[1] A variety of topical interventions, as well as surgical excisions, have been tried.

Vaginal Odor

The odor of postpubertal vaginal secretions varies among individuals and with the menstrual cycle. Vulvar secretions, vaginal wall transudates, exfoliated cells, cervical mucus, fluids from the endometrium and uterine tubes, and metabolic products of the vaginal microflora all contribute.[11] Some characterize the resulting odor as unpleasant, even in the absence of vaginitis. Odor during menses usually is rated as the most offensive.[11] Some individuals may be concerned about these normal odors. The "rotten fish" smell of the vaginal discharge associated with bacterial vaginosis is caused by trimethylamine.[3,18]

Mouth Odor

The odor of a healthy mouth is assumed to be inoffensive in childhood; however, "bad breath" is not uncommon, even in an otherwise well child. Halitosis in the absence of disease is thought to be caused at least partly by volatile sulfur compounds, which are formed when the oral flora metabolize compounds containing amino acids that are found in the saliva or adhering to the teeth, tongue, or gums. Halitosis is exacerbated by infrequent eating and drinking, which ordinarily have a flushing action. Halitosis also accompanies a variety of childhood respiratory tract and gastrointestinal infections. Persistent halitosis should prompt a search for dental or gingival disease or a nasal foreign body. In some cases, halitosis may reflect lung disease or gastroesophageal reflux.

Simple oral hygiene can modify mouth odor for about 3 hours. Brushing the teeth and the dorsoposterior surface of the tongue and then rinsing with water or a mouthwash supposedly reduces both the concentrations of volatile sulfur compounds and the offensive odor.[25,29]

Foot Odor

Several types of localized dermatitis, including eczema, tinea pedis infection (athlete's foot), and pitted keratolysis, have been associated with increased foot odor. Occlusive footwear (e.g., boots) and a hot, humid climate provide the most common setting for the development of pitted keratolysis. White plaques appear on the plantar surface of the feet and are interrupted by shallow pits that may coalesce. Various gram-positive bacteria and dermatophytes have been cultured from the lesions, and the condition responds to a combination of moisture control, topical antibiotics, and antifungal agents. The overpowering rotten odor is believed to derive from thiols, thioesters, and sulfides that are released when microbial proteolytic enzymes attack the stratum corneum.[24] Little is known about the causes of excessive foot odor that occurs despite the seeming absence of skin lesions. One group of investigators found that cultures of particularly smelly feet, compared with those from other feet, had higher bacterial counts, especially of organisms that produce lipid- and protein-degrading exoenzymes.[16] Moisture may promote the growth of such bacteria.

Metabolic Abnormalities

Certain metabolic defects are associated with an unusual odor of the urine,[4] sweat, and other body fluids because of accumulation of odoriferous metabolic precursors or byproducts. These disorders (listed in Table 160-1), although infrequently the cause of odor, are the pediatric conditions most commonly linked to diagnosis by odor.[6,15] They should be suspected if an infant has an unusual body odor, especially if he or she is doing poorly or is ketotic. Recognizing the odor in a compatible clinical situation may lead to early diagnosis and therapy, which may prevent progressive brain damage or death. A specialist in metabolic disease should be consulted and an appropriate diet instituted while blood and urine amino acid analyses are completed. The odor itself may lead to embarrassment, low self- esteem, and psychosocial problems. In some conditions, dietary manipulation may reduce the malodor as well as other symptoms.[2]

Foreign Bodies

Retention of a foreign body in an orifice may lead to a fetid or foul smell with or without drainage or to generalized body odor, apparently because odoriferous substances are absorbed and secreted in sweat.[7] Nasal foreign bodies are the most common.[12,20] Vaginal tampons or diaphragms that have not been removed also may promote odor. All orifices must be inspected.

Inhalation, Poisoning, and Ingestion

When inhalation or ingestion of a toxic substance is suspected, odor may provide a clue to the substance involved. Table 160-2 lists some common associations. When puzzled, the practitioner should consult a poison control center.

Penicillin and cephalosporins give the urine a "medicinal" or musty smell. Topical benzoyl peroxide has been implicated in at least one case of persistent body odor.[19] Thiourea compounds give the breath a sweet smell, resembling

Table 160-1 Abnormalities of Metabolism Associated with Unusual Odor

Disease	Description of Odor	Clinical Features	Metabolic Defect
Phenylketonuria	Musty, like a mouse, horse, wolf, or barn	Vomiting, progressive mental retardation and microcephaly, eczema, decreasing pigmentation, seizures, spasticity	Phenylalanine hydroxylase
Maple syrup urine disease	Maple syrup, burnt sugar, curry, malt, caramel, fenugreek beans	Feeding difficulty, irregular respiration beginning in first week, marked acidosis, seizures, coma leading to death in first 1-2 years of life Intermittent form without mental retardation but with episodes of ataxia and lethargy that may progress to coma Other variants, including thiamine, respond to treatment	Branched chain decarboxylase
Oasthouse urine disease (methionine malabsorption syndrome)	Yeast, dried celery, malt, hops, beer	Diarrhea, mental retardation, spasticity, attacks of hyperpnea, fever, edema	Kidney and intestinal transport of methionine, branched chain amino acids, tyrosine, and phenylalanine
Odor of sweaty feet syndrome 1 (isovalericacidemia)	Sweaty feet, cheese	Recurrent bouts of acidosis, vomiting, dehydration, coma, mild to moderate mental retardation, aversion to protein foods	Isovaleryl CoA dehydrogenase
Odor of sweaty feet syndrome 2 (*N*-butyric and *N*-hexanoic acidemia; may be same as odor of sweaty feet syndrome 1)	Sweaty feet	Poor feeding, weakness and lethargy developing in first week of life with acidosis, dehydration, seizures, and death in early months of life from bone marrow depression	Green acyldehydrogenase
Odor of cat urine syndrome (beta-methylcrotonylglycinuria)	Cat urine	Neurological symptoms resembling Werdnig-Hoffmann disease, failure to thrive, ketoacidosis Biotin-responsive form	Multiple carboxylase deficiency
Fish odor syndrome (trimethylaminuria)	Dead or rotting fish, rancid butter, boiled cabbage	Fish odor of urine; breath and sweat not associated necessarily with other problems	*N*-oxidation enzyme deficiencies
Rancid butter syndrome	Rancid butter, boiled cabbage, decaying fish	Poor feeding, irritability, progressive neurological deterioration with coma and seizures, death caused by infection in first 3 months	Unknown; hypermethioninemia, hypertyrosinemia, and generalized aminoaciduria present; may be a form of acute tyrosinosis

Data from Mace JW, et al: *Clin Pediatr* 15:57, 1976; Hayden GF: *Postgrad Med* 67:110, 1980; Monastiri K, et al: Fenugreek odour in maple syrup urine disease, *J Inherit Metab Dis* 20:614, 1997.

Table 160-2 Inhalations, Poisonings, and Ingestions Associated with Recognizable Odors

Odor	Site	Substance Implicated
Fruity, like acetone or decomposing apples	Breath	Lacquer, chloroform, salicylates
Fruity, alcohol	Breath	Alcohol, phenol
Fruity, pearlike, acrid	Breath	Chloral hydrate, paraldehyde
Wintergreen	Breath	Methyl salicylate
Severe bad breath	Breath	Amphetamines
Bitter almond	Breath	Cyanide (chokecherry, apricot pits), jetberry bush
Burned rope	Breath	Marijuana
Camphor	Breath	Naphthalene (mothballs)
Coal gas	Breath	Coal gas (associated with odorless but toxic carbon monoxide)
Disinfectant	Breath	Phenol, creosote
Garlic	Breath	Phosphorus, arsenic, tellurium, parathion, malathion
Metallic	Breath	Iodine
	Stool	Arsenic
	Vomitus	Arsenic, phosphorus
Shoe polish	Breath	Nitrobenzene
Stale tobacco	Breath	Nicotine
Hydrocarbon	Breath, vomitus	Hydrocarbons
Violets	Urine, vomitus	Turpentine
Medicinal	Urine	Penicillins
Sulfides or amines	Skin	War gases

Data from Hayden GF: *Postgrad Med* 67:110, 1980; McMillan JA, Nieburg PI, Oski FA: Diseases and poisonings associated with unusual breath odor. In *The whole pediatrician catalog,* Philadelphia, 1977, WB Saunders; Goldfrank L, Kirstein R: *Hosp Phys* 3:12, 1976; Smith M, Smith LG, Levinson B: *Lancet* 2:1452, 1982.

Table 160-3 Odor As a Clue to Infection

Odor	Infection
Foul, putrid breath or sputum	Lung abscess, empyema (especially anaerobic), bronchiectasis, fetid bronchitis
Severe halitosis	Trench mouth, tonsillitis, gingivitis
Ammoniacal urine	Urinary tract infection with urea-splitting bacteria
Musty, fruity, grapelike, like wet corn tortillas, especially in a patient who has burns or wounds	*Pseudomonas* skin infection
Fetid sweat	Intranasal foreign body
Rancid stool	Shigellosis
Fishy vaginal discharge	Bacterial vaginosis
Foul vaginal discharge	Vaginal foreign body
Pus that smells like feces or overripe cheese	Proteolytic bacteria
Foul cerumen	*Pseudomonas* infection
Putrid smell from skin	Scurvy
Sweetish odor from mouth	Diphtheria
Butcher shop	Yellow fever
Beer odor in peritoneal dialysate	*Candida* infection[31]
Mousy	*Proteus* infection
Rotten apples	*Clostridium* gas gangrene
Stale beer	Scrofula
Fresh-baked brown bread	Typhoid fever
Alcohol smell to cerebrospinal fluid	*Cryptococcus* meningitis
Malodorous newborn	Amnionitis
Rotten-potato odor of culture specimen	*Pseudomonas aeruginosa*
Foul-smelling wound	Anaerobic bacteria
Rotten smell from feet	Gram-positive bacteria and dermatophytes (pitted keratolysis)

Data from Hayden GF: *Postgrad Med J* 67:110, 1980; Smith M, Smith LG, Levinson B: *Lancet* 2:1452, 1982; Schiffman SS: *N Engl J Med* 308:1337, 1983; Labaren JA, et al: *Clin Infect Dis* 26:1440, 1998; Kavic SM, Cohn SM: *J Trauma* 41:1077, 1996.

Table 160-4 Some Other Diseases Associated with Specific Odors

Disease	Odor
Diabetic ketoacidosis, starvation	Ketones are present in the breath and smell fruity, like acetone or decomposing apples
Uremia	Fishy smell to urine caused by dimethylamine and trimethylamine Ammoniacal smell to the breath caused by ammonia
Acute tubular necrosis	Urine smells like stale water[21]
Hepatic failure	Breath smells like musty fish, raw liver, feces, or newly mown clover; caused by mercaptans and/or dimethyl sulfide
Intestinal obstruction, esophageal diverticulum	Breath smells feculent, foul
Schizophrenia	Sweat smells unpleasant, pungent, heavy; caused by trans-3-methyl-2-hexanoic acid
Skin diseases with protein breakdown	Skin smells foul, unpleasant
Intestinal obstruction, peritonitis	Vomitus smells like feces
Malabsorption	Stool smells foul
Portacaval shunt, portal vein thrombosis	Breath smells sweet

Data from Hayden GF: *Postgrad Med J* 67:110, 1980; McMillan JA, Nieburg PI, Oski FA: Diseases and poisonings associated with unusual breath odor. In *The whole pediatrician catalog,* Philadelphia, 1977, WB Saunders; Smith M, Smith LG, Levinson B: *Lancet* 2:1452, 1982.

that of decaying vegetables.[28] Newborns have smelled spicy when their mothers ate particular curries before labor.[9]

Other Diseases

Odor may suggest either the presence of an infection or the type of infection (Table 160-3), or it may confirm an acquired but noninfectious medical condition (Table 160-4).[10]

SUMMARY

Odor is imprecise. It is not surprising that, with many other diagnostic aids at hand, today's practitioners have minimized olfactory cues.[7] However, odor should not be neglected; it may be the patient's chief concern, can cause severe psychosocial distress, and, more important to the clinician, it may be the most specific early indication of a diagnosis, thereby guiding the choice of diagnostic tools and prompt initiation of therapy.

REFERENCES

1. Bang YH, et al: Histopathology of apocrine bromhidrosis, *Plast Reconstr Surg* 98:288, 1996.
2. Boustead C: Fish-odour syndrome: dealing with offensive body odor, *Nurs Times* 92:30, 1996.
3. Brand JM, Galask RP: Trimethylamine: the substance mainly responsible for the fishy odor often associated with bacterial vaginosis, *Obstet Gynecol* 68:682, 1986.
4. Burke DG, et al: Profiles of urinary volatiles from metabolic disorders characterized by unusual odors, *Clin Chem* 29:1834, 1983.
5. Chandoik S, et al: Screening for bacterial vaginosis: a novel application of artificial nose technology, *J Clin Pathol* 50:790, 1997.
6. Cone TE: Diagnosis and treatment: some diseases, syndromes, and conditions associated with an unusual odor, *Pediatrics* 41:993, 1968.
7. Feinstein RJ: Nasal foreign bodies and bromhidrosis (comment), *JAMA* 242:1031, 1979.
8. Gower DB, et al: Transformations of steroid sulphates by human axillary bacteria: a mechanism for human odour formation? *Biochem Soc Trans* 25:16S, 1997.
9. Hauser GJ, et al: Peculiar odors in newborns and maternal prenatal ingestion of spicy food, *Eur J Pediatr* 144:403, 1985.
10. Hayden GF: Olfactory diagnosis in medicine, *Postgrad Med J* 67:110, 1980.
11. Huggins GR, Preti G: Vaginal odors and secretions, *Clin Obstet Gynecol* 24:355, 1981.
12. Katz HP, et al: Unusual presentation of nasal foreign bodies in children, *JAMA* 241:1496, 1979.
13. Leyden JJ, et al: The microbiology of the human axilla and its relationships to axillary odor, *J Invest Dermatol* 77:413, 1981.
14. Liddell K: Smell as a diagnostic marker, *Postgrad Med J* 52:136, 1976.
15. Mace JW, et al: The child with an unusual odor, *Clin Pediatr* 15:57, 1976.
16. Marshall J, Holland KT, Gribbon EM: A comparative study of the cutaneous microflora of normal feet with low and high levels of odor, *J Appl Bacteriol* 65:61, 1988.
17. McMillan JA, Neiburg PI, Oski FA: Diseases and poisonings associated with unusual breath odor. In *The whole pediatrician catalog,* Philadelphia, 1977, WB Saunders.
18. Mitchell SC, Zhang A, Smith RL: Fish-odour syndrome and impaired *N*-oxidation, *Biochem Soc Trans* 24:96S, 1996.
19. Molberg P: Body odor from topical benzoyl peroxide, *N Engl J Med* 304:1366, 1981 (letter).
20. Moriarty RA: Nasal foreign body presenting as an unusual odor, *Am J Dis Child* 132:97, 1978.
21. Najarian JS: The diagnostic importance of the odor of urine, *N Engl J Med* 303:1128, 1980 (letter).
22. Ping W, et al: A novel method for diabetes diagnosis based on electronic nose, *Biosens Bioelectron* 12:1031, 1997.
23. Sato T, et al: Predominance of type I 5 alpha-reductase in apocrine sweat glands of patients with excessive or abnormal odour derived from apocrine sweat (osmidrosis), *Br J Dermatol* 139:806, 1998.
24. Schissel DJ, Aydelotte J: Case report: road rash with a rotten odor, *Milit Med* 164:65, 1999.
25. Schmidt NF, Tarbet WJ: The effect of oral rinses on organoleptic mouth odor ratings and levels of volatile sulfur compounds, *Oral Surg* 45:876, 1978.
26. Smith M, Smith LG, Levinson B: The use of smell in differential diagnosis, *Lancet* 2:1452, 1982.
27. Spielman AI, et al: Identification and immunohistochemical localization of protein precursors to human axillary odors in apocrine glands and secretions, *Arch Dermatol* 134:813, 1998.
28. Stewart WK, Fleming LW: Use your nose, *Lancet* 1:426, 1983 (letter).
29. Tonzetich J, Ng SK: Reduction of malodor by oral cleansing procedures, *J Oral Surg* 42:172, 1976.
30. Tung TC, Wei FC: Excision of subcutaneous tissue for treatment of axillary osmidrosis, *Br J Plast Surg* 50:61, 1997.
31. Turney JH: Use your nose, *Lancet* 1:426, 1983 (letter).

161 Petechiae and Purpura

Reggie E. Duerst

Although patency of the body's vascular system is required to ensure continued delivery of nutrients and oxygen to the tissues, immediate steps must be taken to limit any blood loss if the integrity of a blood vessel is disrupted. In primary hemostasis, platelets adhere to the injured endothelium or subendothelium, and a thrombus begins to form. Defects in primary hemostasis are manifested after capillary injury by minute, 1- to 2-mm hemorrhagic spots called *petechiae*. Purpuric lesions represent a confluence of petechiae or extravasated blood from a larger vessel; ecchymoses result if the extravasated blood extends along a fascial plane.

Many disorders cause the formation of petechiae or purpura or both. Although the underlying etiology may be benign, serious life-threatening illnesses also must be considered such as meningococcemia, disseminated intravascular coagulopathy (DIC), and purpura fulminans. Immediate action must be taken to halt progression of these life-threatening diseases. Also, intracranial hemorrhage must be considered in any child being evaluated for changes in consciousness who also has petechiae or purpuric lesions. Hemolytic-uremic syndrome (HUS) and thrombotic thrombocytopenic purpura (TTP) are clinical syndromes considered to represent a continuum of a process manifesting thrombocytopenia, hemolysis, and microvascular occlusion. Organ system dysfunction secondary to ischemic injury from microvascular occlusion can be minimized by prompt recognition of these syndromes and appropriate intervention.

The differential diagnosis of disorders leading to development of petechiae or purpura includes many other serious, potentially life-threatening syndromes or diseases. The pathophysiology of these disorders, although varied, ultimately leads to defective primary hemostasis. These disorders can be manifestations of (1) a decrease in the number of platelets, (2) platelet dysfunction, or (3) defective vessels. Alternatively, deficiency of anticoagulant proteins (C or S) can result in neonatal purpura secondary to microvascular thrombosis. An approach for evaluating a patient who has petechiae or purpura (or both) is presented in Box 161-1.

The child's age, family history of bleeding disorders, rapidity of onset of the purpura, and associated signs of systemic illness provide clues that help the physician initially assess the gravity of the illness. A well-appearing child who has petechiae isolated to a well-circumscribed location may have self-inflicted them by suction (factitious petechiae). A lethargic, febrile patient who has had a rapid onset of diffuse petechiae needs immediate management of sepsis and DIC. As noted previously, the distribution of purpuric lesions also may help the examiner make a diagnosis. Involvement of the buttocks and lower extremities is classic for Henoch-Schönlein purpura; prominence of purpura around hair follicles is characteristic of scurvy. Localization of petechiae to the head and neck may result from increased transmural pressure transmitted to vessels after a prolonged Valsalva maneuver (e.g., cough, weight lifting). Well-circumscribed lesions also may result from trauma, and child abuse must be considered.

NORMAL HEMOSTASIS

The pathophysiological mechanisms underlying formation of petechiae are associated with different steps in primary hemostasis. Following vascular injury, the subendothelium is exposed, and the blood elements are no longer confined within the vessel. Primary hemostasis (Fig. 161-1) is initiated when von Willebrand factor is released from endothelial cells and adheres to the exposed collagen matrix; von Willebrand factor, in turn, binds to platelets via the platelet surface glycoprotein Ib (gpIb-IX). Next, the platelets that have adhered to the subendothelium release their granule contents. Additional platelets aggregate in response to adenosine diphosphate (ADP) released from the granules. Synthesis and release of thromboxane A_2 (TxA_2) by the platelets result in vasoconstriction and further enhancement of platelet plug formation.

Secondary hemostatic mechanisms include activation of factor X at the platelet membrane surface, prothrombin conversion to thrombin, and thrombin-catalyzed polymerization of fibrin. Thrombin also provides positive feedback for primary hemostasis by stimulating platelets to release ADP and synthesize TxA_2. Finally, the clot is stabilized by cross-linking of fibrin strands, a reaction catalyzed by activated factor XIII.

After the damaged endothelium has been repaired, the clot that was formed needs to be degraded so that normal blood flow may resume. Plasminogen (which is incorporated into the fibrin clot as it is produced) is converted to the proteolytic enzyme plasmin by the action of plasminogen activators (e.g., tissue plasminogen activator and urokinase). Plasmin cleaves fibrin, forming fibrin degradation products (or fibrin split products) and causing clot dissolution. Thus, hemostasis—formation and degradation of a clot—is an ongoing "homeostatic" process designed to maintain vascular integrity and thereby blood flow.

BOX 161-1

EVALUATION OF PETECHIAE AND PURPURA

1. **History and Physical Examination**
   Age/family history
   Duration/speed of onset
   "Sick versus well"
   Distribution of lesions
2. **Low Platelet Count (<150,000/mm^3)**
   a. ***Blood smear***
   Verify low platelet count
   Look for microangiopathic changes
   - Kasabach-Merritt syndrome
   - Disseminated intravascular coagulation (DIC)/purpura fulminans
   - Hemolytic-uremic syndrome (HUS)
   - Thrombotic thrombocytopenic purpura (TTP)
   - Liver disease

   b. ***PT, aPTT (±FDP, fibrinogen)***
   ABNORMAL
   As above plus:
   Langerhans' cell histiocytosis
   Familial erythrophagocytic lymphohistiocytosis (FEL)
   NORMAL
   See below

   c. ***Bone marrow examination***
   DECREASED MEGAKARYOCYTES
   Aplasia, congenital
   - Thrombocytopenia with absent radii (TAR) syndrome
   - Fanconi anemia
   - Bernard-Soulier syndrome
   - Wiskott-Aldrich syndrome
   - Metabolic disorders

   Aplasia, acquired
   - Idiopathic
   - Nutritional (iron, vitamin B_{12}, folate)
   - Drug, chemical, toxin, radiation
   - Rubella, other "TORCH," hepatitis B

   Infiltration
   - Leukemia, lymphoma
   - Neuroblastoma or other metastatic solid tumor
   - Storage disease

   NORMAL OR INCREASED MEGAKARYOCYTES
   Immune destruction
   - Immune thrombocytopenic purpura (ITP) (acute and chronic)
   - Evan's syndrome
   - Alloimmune thrombocytopenia
   - Posttransfusion purpura
   - Drugs
   - HIV/AIDS

   Other
   - Langerhans' cell histiocytosis
   - Virally associated hematophagocytic syndrome (VAHS)
   - Familial erythrophagocytic lymphohistiocytosis (FEL)
   - Intravascular prosthesis
   - May-Hegglin anomaly
   - Hypersplenism with sequestration
   - Protein C or S deficiency
3. **Normal Platelet Count (>150,000/mm^3)**
   Platelet dysfunction, congenital
   Glanzmann thrombasthenia
   Bernard-Soulier syndrome
   Wiskott-Aldrich syndrome
   Storage pool defect

   Platelet dysfunction, acquired
   Aspirin or aspirin-like drugs
   Liver disease
   Uremia
   Paraproteinemia (dysgammaglobulinemia, cystic fibrosis)

   Von Willebrand's disease
   Vascular defect, congenital
   Ehlers-Danlos syndrome
   Osler-Weber-Rendu syndrome

   Vascular defect, acquired
   Trauma
   - Lacerations
   - Abuse
   - Factitious

   Vasculitis
   - Drugs
   - Infection (bacterial, viral, rickettsial)
   - Henoch-Schönlein purpura

   Senile purpura
   Steroid purpura
   Scurvy

THROMBOCYTOPENIA

Thrombocytopenia is the most common cause of bleeding. Regulation of platelet production and maintenance of the normal platelet count (150,000 to 400,000/mm^3) is poorly understood. The megakaryocyte growth factor, thrombopoietin, has been identified and cloned; its receptor, c-mpl, also has been characterized. Thus, further insight regarding regulation of platelet production should ensue. If platelet function is normal, abnormal bleeding usually will not occur unless the platelet count is below 100,000/mm^3. Declines in the platelet count may result from inadequate production, enhanced destruction, maldistribution, or dilution (e.g., a patient who is hemorrhaging and receiving insufficient platelet replacement). If the decrease in the platelet count is caused by excessive platelet destruction despite greatly increased production, symptomatic bleeding often does not develop until the platelet count falls below 20,000/mm^3. This clinical observation has implied that the newly produced platelets may have enhanced coagulant function. Similar to erythrocytes, the youngest platelets contain relatively higher

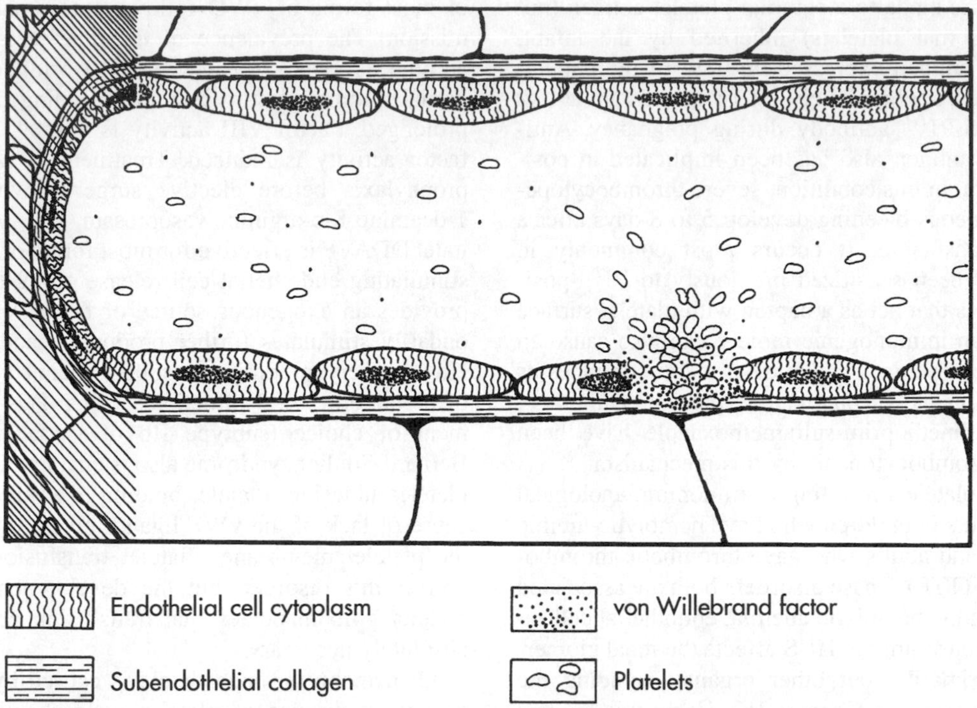

Fig. 161-1 In primary hemostasis, platelets adhere to subendothelial collagen coated with von Willebrand factor. Platelet aggregation ensues, and a platelet "plug" forms.

amounts of RNA and, thus, are "reticulated." The amount of hemostatic proteins released from the α-granules of reticulated platelets appears to be greater than from "older" platelets. Thus, patients who have destructive thrombocytopenia have platelets that have enhanced hemostatic function.

Thrombocytopenia from Inadequate Production

Inadequate production of platelets can be divided into congenital and acquired conditions. One such congenital disorder is thrombocytopenia with absent radii (TAR) syndrome. Infants who have TAR syndrome are recognized readily by their upper extremity deformities. The platelet count is in the 15,000 to 30,000/mm^3 range, and megakaryocytes are reduced or absent in the bone marrow. Platelet production improves gradually after the first year of life. Congenital amegakaryocytic thrombocytopenia also is present in Fanconi anemia. Patients who have Bernard-Soulier syndrome also may be mildly thrombocytopenic secondary to inadequate production. The functional defect—reduced to absent surface glycoproteins Ib, V, and IX, in the platelets of these individuals—is the more significant cause of bleeding. May-Hegglin anomaly (giant platelets and Döhle bodies in the leukocytes) rarely is associated with thrombocytopenia and bleeding. Wiskott-Aldrich syndrome (WAS) is an X-linked recessive disorder characterized by eczema, immunodeficiency, and thrombocytopenia with platelet dysfunction; the combination of thrombocytopenia and platelet dysfunction places the patient at great risk for hemorrhage. Treatment of these disorders is supportive—avoiding aspirin or aspirin-like drugs and using protective head gear, plus administering of the antifibrinolytic agent ϵ-aminocaproic acid (EACA) and, if necessary, platelet transfusions.

Marrow aplasia also results in underproduction of platelets. When caused by exposure to drugs or other toxic chemicals, marrow aplasia and its resultant thrombocytopenia may be temporary and may resolve when the causative agent is withdrawn. Immunosuppressive therapy, bone marrow transplantation, or both may be required for patients who have severe aplastic anemia. Extensive infiltration of bone marrow in patients who have leukemia, lymphoma, or a metastatic solid tumor prevents normal platelet production. Infectious agents (e.g., congenital CMV or rubella) also may cause ineffective thrombocytopoiesis and thrombocytopenia.

Destructive Thrombocytopenia

Acute idiopathic thrombocytopenic purpura (ITP) is the most frequent cause of severe thrombocytopenia and bleeding in childhood. ITP usually is a temporary disorder, and 80% to 90% of children recover completely within 1 year of diagnosis. The incidence of life-threatening hemorrhage or intracranial bleeding is less than 0.1% to 1%. Intracranial hemorrhage and other significant bleeding events have been reported most often when the platelet count is less than 20,000/mm^3. Furthermore, the risk appears to be greatest at the onset (initial 48 hours) of the disease. Chronic ITP or other diseases associated with immune dysfunction (e.g., lupus erythematosus, Evan's syndrome) develop in 10% to 20% of patients who manifest acute ITP. Thrombocytopenia is a result of increased removal of platelets from the circulation by monocyte-macrophage cells of the reticuloendothelial (RE) cell system. Adherence to the platelet surface of specific antiplatelet autoantibody or immune complexes leads to phagocytosis of the platelets by the RE cells. See Chapter 225 for a more complete discussion of ITP.

Neonatal alloimmune thrombocytopenia develops when

maternal antibody is made to a paternal platelet antigen (not expressed on maternal platelets) inherited by the infant. $P1^{A1}$ is a platelet antigen expressed on 98% of the population's platelets; thus, approximately 1% of women are at risk of developing anti-$P1^{A1}$ antibody during pregnancy. Antibody to the $P1^{A1}$ antigen also has been implicated in posttransfusion purpura. In this condition, severe thrombocytopenia and mucocutaneous bleeding develop 5 to 8 days after a blood product transfusion. It occurs most commonly in women who have been sensitized previously to $P1^{A1}$-positive platelets. Drugs that act as a hapten with platelet surface antigens to form an immunogenic moiety can also cause an immune thrombocytopenia. Platelet destruction continues as long as the drug-platelet neoantigen is present. Quinidine, cimetidine, and trimethoprim-sulfamethoxazole have been shown to cause thrombocytopenia by this mechanism.

Destruction of platelets resulting from nonimmunological platelet injury occurs in children who have hemolytic-uremic syndrome (HUS) and adults who have thrombotic thrombocytopenic purpura (TTP). These disorders both are associated with microangiopathic hemolytic anemia, endothelial cell injury, and platelet consumption. HUS affects the renal glomerular capillaries primarily, but other organs, including the brain, may be involved. See Chapter 213, Hemolytic-Uremic Syndrome.

The thrombocytopenia of Kasabach-Merritt syndrome results from platelet consumption in a giant hemangioma. Intravascular prostheses also may cause significant platelet destruction.

Several disorders associated with reticuloendothelial cell proliferation also result in platelet consumption that is not antibody mediated. Patients who have histiocytosis X, virally associated hematophagocytic syndrome (VAHS), and familial erythrophagocytic lymphohistiocytosis (FEL) can develop thrombocytopenia as a result of excessive phagocytosis of platelets by abnormal histiocytic cells. If these disease processes are active, splenomegaly often is present, and the spleen is a major site of platelet destruction. Sequestration of platelets in an enlarged spleen (regardless of cause) also causes a reduction in measured circulating platelet concentration. However, bleeding symptoms are uncommon because the platelet count is not reduced severely.

DEFECTIVE PLATELET FUNCTION

Defects in platelet function can be subdivided by the step in primary hemostasis (platelet adhesion, release, and aggregation) at which the defect is expressed. Adherence of platelets to the exposed subendothelium is mediated primarily by the collagen receptor glycoprotein Ia/IIa and von Willebrand factor. Von Willebrand factor (vWF) is a glycoprotein of 240,000 molecular weight subunits synthesized primarily by endothelial cells. It is "complexed" with factor VIII and circulates as multimers of the basic subunit. Larger multimers are more active in promoting coagulation than are monomers or small oligomers. Von Willebrand's disease (vWD) is a heterogeneous disorder involving vWF. It has three major subtypes: patients may have (1) reduced synthesis of vWF, (2) synthesis of defective vWF, or (3) disordered assembly of the vWF complexes. Type I accounts for 75% of patients who have the disease. The inheritance of most forms of vWD follows autosomal dominant transmission. The prevalence of the disease is estimated to be as high as 1 per 100 individuals worldwide. The activated partial thromboplastin time and bleeding time generally are prolonged. Factor VIII activity is normal, but ristocetin cofactor activity is reduced. Treatment of active bleeding or prophylaxis before elective surgery involves infusion of 1-deamino-8-D-arginine vasopressin (DDAVP) or cryoprecipitate. DDAVP is effective for most forms of vWD and acts by stimulating endothelial cell release of vWF. Cryoprecipitate provides an exogenous source of factor VIII-vWF and secondarily stimulates further production and release of vWF. However, cryoprecipitate can be associated with transmission of bloodborne viral infections. DDAVP is the current treatment of choice (subtype IIb of vWD is the exception). Bernard-Soulier syndrome also is characterized by a defect in platelet adhesion. Platelet binding to vWF is diminished because of lack of the vWF ligand, glycoprotein Ib (gpIb), on the platelet membrane. Platelet transfusion is necessary to correct this disorder, but the development of antibody to platelet gpIb mandates that transfusion be withheld unless absolutely necessary.

Glanzmann thrombasthenia is caused by congenital deficiency or absence of platelet surface antigen glycoprotein IIb/IIIa. This deficiency results in defective binding of platelets to fibrinogen and a decrease in platelet aggregation after activation. Platelet transfusion can be lifesaving, but its use should be minimized to prevent antibody formation. Deficiency of α-granules in the platelets of patients who have gray platelet syndrome (named for the platelet appearance on routine blood smears) results in a decrease of coagulation factors available for release after aggregation. Several heterogeneous deficiencies in dense granules, collectively called *storage pool defects,* result in defective platelet release of ADP and serotonin. This defect also is associated with Wiskott-Aldrich syndrome, Chédiak-Steinbrinck-Higashi syndrome, and Hermansky-Pudlak syndrome. Other diseases associated with defects in platelet granule release include disorders of platelet arachidonic acid metabolism and type 1 glycogen storage disease (glucose-6-phosphatase deficiency). The latter disorder is associated with decreased ADP release during episodes of hypoglycemia.

Acquired platelet dysfunction is characteristic of uremia. Retention of metabolites otherwise cleared by the kidneys appears to be causative, and significant bleeding may occur as a result. DDAVP is very useful for prophylaxis against bleeding if a uremic patient requires a surgical procedure. Liver disease and myeloproliferative and lymphoproliferative disorders also have been associated with acquired platelet dysfunction.

VASCULAR DEFECTS

Congenital Defects

Predisposition to the development of purpuric lesions is a consequence of several congenital vascular disorders. The telangiectasias of Osler-Weber-Rendu disease result from vascular anomalies that include a thin endothelial lining. The thrombocytopenia of Kasabach-Merritt syndrome is a result of consumption within the cavernous arteriovenous malformation. Patients who have congenital connective tissue disorders that result in defective collagen or elastin can exhibit "vascular purpura." These disorders include osteogenesis imperfecta, Ehlers-Danlos syndrome, Marfan syndrome, and pseudoxanthoma elasticum.

Acquired Defects

Acquired vascular conditions can be manifested by petechiae or purpura. Vasculitis develops in response to drugs, toxins, or a host of infectious organisms (e.g., meningococcus, yellow fever virus, and rickettsiae). In response to endotoxin (or other mediators of inflammation), interleukin-1 and tumor necrosis factor are produced by endothelial cells. These cytokines, in turn, bring about endothelial cell changes that impair primary hemostasis, and petechiae or purpura result. Similarly, systemic lupus erythematosus, rheumatoid arthritis, and other collagen-vascular diseases can produce purpura resulting from vasculitis.

Henoch-Schönlein purpura (see Chapter 215) is a syndrome of widespread acute vasculitis that may cause a rash (vasculitis in the skin) and arthralgia (vasculitis in the joints). Vasculitis in the gastrointestinal tract may cause abdominal pain, bowel wall edema, partial obstruction, and intussusception. Renal complications (proteinuria, hypertension, renal failure) are possible. Late renal sequelae are confined to patients who have renal involvement during the acute illness.

Vitamin C is required for normal collagen synthesis. Patients who have scurvy may develop purpuric lesions as a result of the abnormal collagen in the subendothelium. Prominence of bleeding at the base of hair follicles is characteristic of scurvy. Senile purpura (purpura of the elderly) is another manifestation of abnormal collagen in the subendothelium. Dysproteinemias and conditions that result in elevated gamma globulinemia (including cystic fibrosis) have been shown to promote development of petechiae or purpura.

SUGGESTED READINGS

Beardsley DS, Nathan DG: Platelet abnormalities in infancy and childhood. In Nathan DG, Orkin SH, editors: *Hematology of infancy and childhood,* Philadelphia, 1998, WB Saunders.

Handin RI: Blood platelets and the vessel wall. In Nathan DG, Orkin SH, editors: *Hematology of infancy and childhood,* Philadelphia, 1998, WB Saunders.

Medeiros D, Buchanan GR: Major hemorrhage in children with idiopathic thrombocytopenic purpura: immediate response to therapy and long-term outcome, *J Pediatr* 133:334, 1998.

Moake JL, Chow TW: Thrombotic thrombocytopenic purpura: understanding a disease no longer rare, *Am J Med Sci* 316:105, 1998.

Rinder HM, et al: Differences in platelet alpha-granule release between normals and immune thrombocytopenic patients and between young and old platelets, *Thromb Haemost* 80:457, 1998.

162 Polyuria

Samuel M. Libber • Leslie P. Plotnick

Polyuria, or excessive urinary volume, is a symptom common to many pediatric disorders. It may be defined clinically as urine production of more than 900 ml/m^2/day or functionally as an inappropriately high urine output relative to circulating volume and osmolarity.[13] It often is associated with frequent urination, nocturia, or enuresis. Sometimes the pediatrician is called on to evaluate this symptom without knowing the exact daily urinary volume; in such situations a detailed history of fluid intake and urinary habits may help delineate the primary symptom.

A normal homeostatic response to polyuria is increased thirst; with subsequent liquid intake, water balance remains intact. In an older child the parent may perceive this symptom to be more prominent than the polyuria. However, in infants who have polyuria and are unable to maintain free access to fluids, negative water balance results, and weight loss, dehydration, and electrolyte disturbances often occur. When chronic or recurrent electrolyte disturbances plague the infant, growth failure and central nervous system (CNS) injury may result.

DIFFERENTIAL DIAGNOSIS

In reaching a diagnosis in a patient who has polyuria, the clinician must bear in mind a general overview of the systems that may cause this symptom, as indicated in Box 162-1. A CNS or pituitary lesion may reduce vasopressin secretion; a renal defect may limit the kidney's ability to respond to vasopressin; an excessive fluid intake may be the primary cause of polyuria; or excretion of an osmotically active urine may effect a large volume loss.

Central or neurogenic diabetes insipidus is a condition in which secretion of vasopressin by the posterior lobe of the pituitary gland is limited. Consequently, a dilute urine of large volume is passed, and the crucial function of water conservation in times of volume depletion is lost. In rare cases there may be a familial idiopathic vasopressin deficiency, inherited generally as an autosomal dominant trait but occasionally in an X-linked recessive pattern. More commonly, however, cases are sporadic; although many of these are idiopathic, a search for a specific underlying organic lesion and concomitant anterior pituitary dysfunction is necessary. Injury to the CNS, whether traumatic or surgical, may be associated with a decline in the production or release of vasopressin. Likewise, thrombosis or hemorrhage involving the hypothalamus or pituitary gland may result in vasopressin deficiency. Abnormalities in vasopressin secretion may accompany CNS infections. Just as the syndrome of inappropriate antidiuretic hormone (SIADH) may accompany meningitis in the acute state, clinical diabetes insipidus may supervene as a chronic sequela to CNS infections. Recently, central diabetes insipidus has been described in an infant who has congenital toxoplasmosis.[17]

Congenital intracranial defects (such as septooptic dysplasia, holoprosencephaly, and encephalocele) also have been associated with diabetes insipidus. Brain tumors (craniopharyngioma, glioma, dysgerminoma, and metastatic tumor) are the most common causes of central diabetes insipidus. In addition, patients who have any of a variety of systemic illnesses (histiocytosis, syphilis, tuberculosis, sarcoidosis, and Guillain-Barré syndrome) have developed vasopressin deficiency.

An unusual association between diabetes mellitus, diabetes insipidus, optic atrophy, and hearing loss (Wolfram syndrome) has been described.[7] A review by Greger et al[6] suggests that in recent years, fewer cases of diabetes insipidus have been diagnosed as idiopathic and that a higher proportion has been diagnosed as occurring secondary to CNS infection or intracranial birth defects. Also, autoantibodies to hypothalamic vasopressin cells have been detected in some children previously thought to have idiopathic diabetes insipidus. Interestingly, about 50% of the patients who have histiocytosis also have vasopressin cell antibodies.[20] Adolescents who have acquired lymphocytic or granulomatous hypophysitis recently have been described. In these individuals, hyperprolactinemia and other anterior pituitary dysfunction may accompany the diabetes insipidus.[8] The practitioner must search diligently for an organic lesion because an underlying lesion may not be evident at the initial evaluation.

Polyuria sometimes is a consequence rather than a cause of excessive fluid intake. Primary polydipsia, or compulsive water drinking, is a rare cause of polyuria in childhood.[12] It occurs most often in older children or adults who have emotional disturbances; about 80% of cases are believed to occur in girls and women. The ailment has a gradual onset, unlike the more abrupt onset typical of central diabetes insipidus. Although some believe this disorder to be caused by a primary psychiatric disturbance, a study of adult psychiatric patients who have polydipsia and hyponatremia showed evidence of a defect in water excretion, osmoregulation of water intake, and vasopressin secretion.[5]

Water intoxication is another cause of polyuria, seen in increasing numbers over the past 20 years.[10] It is particularly common among infants living in impoverished circumstances

BOX 162-1

DIFFERENTIAL DIAGNOSIS OF POLYURIA IN CHILDHOOD

I. Neurogenic vasopressin deficiency
   A. Idiopathic
      1. Familial
      2. Sporadic
   B. Organic
      1. Posttraumatic
      2. Vascular event
      3. After infection
      4. CNS tumor
      5. Systemic infiltrative diseases (histiocytosis, syphilis, tuberculosis, sarcoidosis)
      6. Guillain-Barré syndrome
      7. Congenital intracranial defect
      8. Autoimmune disorders
II. Excessive fluid intake
   A. Primary polydipsia
   B. Water intoxication
III. Renal vasopressin insensitivity
   A. Congenital
      1. Hereditary nephrogenic diabetes insipidus
      2. Other renal tubular defects (cystinosis, distal renal tubular acidosis, Bartter's syndrome, renal Fanconi syndrome, ARC syndrome)
      3. Structural defect
   B. Acquired
      1. Postinfectious
      2. Postobstructive
      3. Drug induced
      4. Associated with systemic disease (sickle cell disease, sarcoidosis, amyloidosis)
      5. Metabolic (hypercalcemia, hypokalemia)
IV. Osmotic diuresis
   A. Diet induced
   B. Drug induced
   C. Type I diabetes mellitus
   D. Type II diabetes mellitus
   E. Renal glycosuria

in which caretakers feed diluted formula or water when formula supplies are exhausted. Life-threatening hyponatremia may ensue unless such infants are treated promptly.

Renal disorders may be associated with polyuria because of an inability of the renal tubule to concentrate urine despite normal circulating levels of vasopressin. This may be a congenital or an acquired abnormality. In hereditary nephrogenic diabetes insipidus, renal tubular cells lack the ability to respond to vasopressin because of a defect in vasopressin V_2 receptors in the distal convoluted tubule and collecting duct.[16] This is an X-linked recessive disorder in which polyuria, fever, failure to thrive, and hypernatremic dehydration occur in early infancy. Older children and adults may be able to adjust their oral fluid intake to maintain constant serum osmolality, but infants do not have this ability. The condition can be associated with damage to the CNS or even death if the infant develops recurrent hypernatremic dehydration. A recent follow-up study of such patients suggested an increased risk of attention deficit/hyperactivity disorder and impaired short-term memory. Two of 17 patients had cognitive abilities greater than 2 standard deviations (SDs) below the mean.[9] Thus, prompt recognition and treatment are needed to prevent such sequelae.

Besides the hereditary form of nephrogenic diabetes insipidus, the clinician must consider other renal tubular defects in which vasopressin resistance has been observed. Patients who have cystinosis, distal renal tubular acidosis, renal Fanconi syndrome, and Bartter's syndrome may have polyuria. An association between nephrogenic diabetes insipidus and the ARC syndrome (arthrogryposis, renal tubular dysfunction, and cholestasis) recently has been recognized; such children also are prone to severe growth impairment as well as to mental retardation and deafness.[2]

In addition to functional tubular impairment, congenital structural abnormalities also can cause polyuria. In medullary cystic disease and oligomeganephronia, a condition in which the renal tubules are abnormally large and reduced in number, the architecture of the kidney is distorted, resulting in an abnormality in the regulation of renal output. In chronic pyelonephritis or obstructive uropathy, damage to the tubules or a disturbance in the medullary osmotic gradient may result in nephrogenic diabetes insipidus. A child who has a lipoma of the cauda equina and subsequent tethered cord syndrome and neurogenic bladder may develop nephrogenic diabetes insipidus as a result of hydronephrosis.[4] Drugs such as lithium, demeclocycline, and amphotericin have been known to result in functional vasopressin insensitivity. Likewise, hypercalcemia and hypokalemia each may be associated with a nephropathy in which tubular ability to conserve water is lost. Certain systemic disorders such as sickle cell disease, sarcoidosis, and amyloidosis also may cause renal tubular dysfunction and result in polyuria.

Finally, polyuria may accompany any disorder in which renal water loss results from an osmotic diuresis. In rare cases this may be diet induced, as in individuals who are tube fed a diet high in protein and sodium. Drugs such as mannitol, urea, and glycerol, as well as radiological contrast agents, may be responsible for this situation. Glycosuria is one of the most frequent findings in children who have acquired polyuria; in these patients, type I diabetes mellitus is the most likely explanation (see Chapter 202, Diabetes Mellitus). Polyuria, polydipsia, polyphagia, and weight loss compose the symptom complex seen most commonly in diabetic patients. Type II diabetes mellitus is less common in childhood but is being recognized increasingly in obese children and adolescents. In both situations, glycosuria results from diminished carbohydrate utilization, and loss of water and electrolytes ensues. In renal glycosuria, insulin secretion and activity are entirely normal, but the maximum glucose reabsorption rate of renal tubular cells is diminished. As a result, glycosuria occurs without hyperglycemia. When present in the urine in large amounts, glucose acts as an osmotic diuretic and causes polyuria.

EVALUATION

The initial laboratory procedure of highest yield is a urinalysis performed on a first-voided morning specimen. A high

Table 162-1 Interpretation of Vasopressin Test

	Intake	Output	Urine Specific Gravity
Normal	↓	↓	↑
Psychogenic polydipsia	Unchanged	↓	↑
Central diabetes insipidus	↓	↓	↑
Nephrogenic diabetes insipidus	Unchanged	Unchanged	Unchanged

specific gravity (1.020 or higher) generally is found in patients who have osmotic diuresis or in normal individuals; a specific gravity of 1.008 or lower is found in patients who have nephrogenic or central diabetes insipidus. Patients whose renal tubular epithelium has been damaged (e.g., individuals who have sickle cell disease) are more likely to have isosthenuria with specific gravities in the neighborhood of 1.010. Protein, casts, or formed blood elements in the urine likewise would suggest a renal disorder. In patients who have glycosuria, ketonuria would strongly suggest type I diabetes mellitus; if glycosuria without ketonuria is present, one must distinguish further between diabetes mellitus and renal glycosuria.

A normal serum glucose concentration would be more suggestive of a diagnosis of renal glycosuria.

Examination of serum electrolytes, glucose, urea nitrogen, phosphate, creatinine, calcium, and osmolality also is indicated, as is evaluation of urinary amino acid excretion. A hyperosmolar state would suggest vasopressin deficiency or insensitivity, provided the serum glucose concentration is normal. A low serum osmolality would suggest either primary polydipsia or water intoxication as the most likely diagnosis. A careful feeding history can help identify infants who have water intoxication. Evidence of renal impairment, hypercalcemia, and hypokalemia also will be uncovered in such an examination.

In polyuric individuals who have a low urine specific gravity and no glycosuria, the next step in evaluation is a water deprivation test to determine the child's ability to conserve water at times when antidiuresis is necessary for homeostasis. After a 24-hour period of adequate hydration, blood is drawn to determine sodium, osmolality, and urea nitrogen levels and to perform a hematocrit; the urine osmolality and specific gravity are measured, the child is weighed, and his or her intake and output are recorded. The child then is restricted from any food or fluid intake for 6 to 8 hours, during which the child's weight, urine output, urine specific gravity, and serum sodium are determined periodically. After the study period, the initial blood tests are repeated, urine osmolality is measured again, and the final weight is recorded. If at any point the child has lost 5% or more of his or her body weight, the test is stopped, once final blood studies are obtained. Because of the possibility of volume depletion, it is recommended that the study be carried out during the day when supervision is optimal. In normal children and in most children who have psychogenic polydipsia, the weight remains constant, the urine specific gravity increases to at least 1.010, the urine volume decreases, and the ratio of urine to plasma osmolality rises to at least 2:1. However, if diuresis continues in the absence of oral intake and if weight loss and hyperosmolarity ensue, one should suspect a diagnosis of diabetes insipidus, either central or nephrogenic.

The vasopressin test is the next step in the evaluation of a polyuric patient when the water deprivation test shows a specific gravity of less than 1.015 (Table 162-1). The purpose of this test is to determine whether the excessive urine flow responds to exogenous vasopressin. This test is done best immediately after the water deprivation test. Aqueous vasopressin in a dose of 6 U/m^2 is administered subcutaneously, and the patient is allowed free access to water. Subsequently, intake, output, and urine specific gravity are recorded every 30 to 60 minutes. Normal subjects and patients who have vasopressin deficiency evidence a reduced fluid intake and output and a rise in urine specific gravity to at least 1.015. Urine osmolality, likewise, increases significantly. Individuals who have partial diabetes insipidus demonstrate a modest rise in urine concentration on water deprivation testing (urine osmolality less than 400 mOsm/kg), but the urine becomes concentrated after administration of vasopressin. Patients who have primary polydipsia maintain a constant intake but generally have a reduced urine output and increased urine specific gravity. If no response to vasopressin occurs after 6 hours, the test should be repeated by using a dose of 12 U/m^2 subcutaneously. If the patient shows no effect after this double dose, nephrogenic diabetes insipidus probably is the diagnosis.

MANAGEMENT

Patients who show evidence of vasopressin deficiency are best referred to an endocrinologist or neurologist so that the cause of the diabetes insipidus can be determined. A full investigation of other pituitary functions, visual field examination, and either magnetic resonance imaging (MRI) or computed tomography (CT) scans of the head likely will be the next steps in evaluation. Patients should be allowed free access to fluids, and their serum and urine osmolality should be monitored closely. In a severely ill patient, aqueous vasopressin (0.1 to 0.2 U/kg) may be given subcutaneously every 4 to 6 hours.

Aqueous vasopressin also may be given by constant intravenous infusion. Reported starting dosages vary from 0.5 to 4.6 mU/kg/hour; these should be increased or decreased as needed.[15,19] The clinician is reminded that vasopressin is a potent vasoconstrictor and that tissue ischemia, skin infarction, and severe lactic acidosis may develop, particularly at high infusion rates. Once the child's condition has stabilized, management consists of desmopressin acetate (DDAVP), a synthetic derivative of vasopressin, instilled or sprayed intranasally at a dosage of 5 to 20 μg twice daily. Infants and children receiving dose multiples of 10 μg may use the nasal spray; those on smaller or intermediate doses must use the rhinal tube. Recent studies have shown that DDAVP may be administered effectively and safely either orally[1,3] or sublingually, although therapeutic doses are larger and more variable than those administered intranasally. Use of thiazide diuretics, chlorpropamide, and clofibrate has met with some success in the management of diabetes insipidus but generally lacks the efficacy of vasopressin derivatives. There is some evidence that patients who have central diabetes insipidus have decreased bone mineral density and should be closely followed for this over time.[18]

In patients who have primary polydipsia, once a neurogenic lesion has been ruled out, medical therapy is not indicated. Psychotherapy, however, may be useful in addressing the emotional problem causing the polydipsia.

Water-intoxicated infants require prompt attention to fluid and electrolyte balance, and some whose hyponatremia is severe have required treatment with either isotonic or hypertonic (3%) saline solution. Once the acute sequelae have been treated, preventive efforts should focus on educating caretakers so that feeding techniques may be corrected.

Patients who have structural renal diseases leading to polyuria can be referred to a nephrologist; patients who have nephrogenic diabetes insipidus commonly are seen by an endocrinologist or a nephrologist. They should be allowed free access to fluids; parents of infants who have this disorder need to offer frequent water feedings to allow their infants to maintain osmotic homeostasis. A low-salt diet has been helpful in reducing urine output; thiazide diuretics can reduce polyuria further by reducing the amount of urine delivered to the distal tubule. Indomethacin[14] and amiloride,[11] when given concurrently with a thiazide, have each been found effective at reducing urine output.

Osmotic diuresis induced by drugs or diet generally is self-limited. Although renal glycosuria requires no specific therapy, such a diagnosis can be made only when other renal tubular functions are normal. In overweight patients who have type II diabetes mellitus, weight reduction is paramount. This measure alone often is sufficient to reverse the carbohydrate intolerance. If hyperglycemia persists, an endocrinologist may prescribe an oral hypoglycemic agent or insulin. In type I diabetes mellitus, patients who have polydipsia and polyuria may be hospitalized to stabilize the abnormal carbohydrate metabolism with exogenous insulin, to correct the electrolyte disturbance, and to educate the patient and family about home management (see Chapter 202, Diabetes Mellitus).

Management of polyuria, therefore, depends largely on the underlying diagnosis and must be individualized carefully. In most cases the results are gratifying, but patients often are found to have a chronic disease that requires close, long-term surveillance.

REFERENCES

1. Boulgourdjian EM, et al: Oral desmopressin treatment of central diabetes insipidus in children, *Acta Paeditr* 86:1261, 1997.
2. Coleman RA, et al: Cerebral defects and nephrogenic diabetes insipidus with the ARC syndrome: additional findings or a new syndrome (ARCC-NDI)? *Am J Med Genet* 72:335, 1997.
3. Fjellestad-Paulsen A, et al: Central diabetes insipidus: oral treatment with dDAVP, *Regul Pept* 45:303, 1993.
4. Fujii T, et al: Nephrogenic diabetes insipidus and tethered cord syndrome with a lipoma of the cauda equina, *Brain Dev* 20:47, 1998.
5. Goldman M, Luchins D, Robertson G: Mechanisms of altered water metabolism in psychotic patients with polydipsia and hyponatremia, *N Engl J Med* 318:397, 1988.
6. Greger N, et al: Central diabetes insipidus: 22 years' experience, *Am J Dis Child* 140:551, 1986.
7. Grosse Aldenhovel H, Gallenkamp U, Sulemana C: Juvenile onset diabetes mellitus, central diabetes insipidus, and optic atrophy (Wolfram syndrome): neurological findings and prognostic implications, *Neuropediatrics* 22:103, 1991.
8. Heinz HJ, Bercu BB: Acquired hypophysitis in adolescence, *J Pediatr Endocrinol Metab* 10:315, 1997.
9. Hoekstra JA, et al: Cognitive and psychosocial functioning of patients with congenital nephrogenic diabetes insipidus, *Am J Med Genet* 61:81, 1996.
10. Keating J, Schears G, Dodge P: Oral water intoxication in infants: an American epidemic, *Am J Dis Child* 145:985, 1991.
11. Knoers N, Monnens L: Amiloride-hydrochlorothiazide versus indomethacin-hydrochlorothiazide in the treatment of nephrogenic diabetes insipidus, *J Pediatr* 117:499, 1990.
12. Kohn B, et al: Hysterical polydipsia (compulsive water drinking) in children, *Am J Dis Child* 130:210, 1976.
13. Leung A, Robson W, Halperin M: Polyuria in childhood, *Clin Pediatr* 30:634, 1991.
14. Libber S, Harrison H, Spector D: Treatment of nephrogenic diabetes insipidus with prostaglandin synthesis inhibitors, *J Pediatr* 108:305, 1986.
15. McDonald J, et al: Treatment of the young child with postoperative central diabetes insipidus, *Am J Dis Child* 143:201, 1989.
16. Merendino J, et al: A mutation in the vasopressin V_2-receptor gene in a kindred with X-linked nephrogenic diabetes insipidus, *N Engl J Med* 328:1538, 1993.
17. Oygur N, et al: Central diabetes insipidus in a patient with congenital toxoplasmosis, *Am J Perinatol* 15:191, 1998.
18. Pivonello R, et al: Impairment of bone status in patients with central diabetes insipidus, *J Clin Endocrinol Metab* 83:2275, 1998.
19. Rogers MC, Helfaer MA: *Handbook of pediatric intensive care,* ed 2, Baltimore, 1995, Williams and Wilkins.
20. Scherbaum W: Autoimmune hypothalamic diabetes insipidus ("autoimmune hypothalamitis"), *Prog Brain Res* 93:283, 1992.

163 Proteinuria

Edward J. Ruley

The presence of abnormal amounts of protein in the urine may be asymptomatic or, if severe enough to cause hypoproteinemia, associated with varying degrees of edema. The techniques and pitfalls of detecting proteinuria and determining its prevalence are discussed in Chapter 20 (Eight), Use of Urinalysis and the Urine Culture in Screening.

The crucial factors in the consideration of proteinuria are (1) its constancy, (2) its quantitation, and (3) its concurrence with other urinary or systemic abnormalities. The first two factors can be determined simultaneously by having the patient collect a 24-hour urine specimen following the instructions shown in Box 163-1.

The constancy of proteinuria in relation to posture and activity can be determined if the amount of protein in each voiding during the 24-hour collection is measured by the patient or parent by using dip-and-read strips. Because the collection begins and ends with the first void after waking on consecutive days, two urine protein determinations after the patient has been supine overnight will be available. More information on the effect of activity on proteinuria can be obtained if the patient is instructed to have periods of both vigorous and quiet activity during the waking hours of the 24-hour collection.

The total collection should be assayed for volume, creatinine, and protein content. One can determine whether the 24-hour urine was collected properly by calculating the urinary creatinine excretion (mg/kg/day). Children of normal habitus excrete about 18 mg/kg/day of creatinine, although there is individual variation that is determined partly by age and gender.[1] If the creatinine excretion is near this amount, one can presume that the 24-hour urine specimen was obtained correctly and that the urinary protein quantitation is a good reflection of the degree of proteinuria. Although creatinine excretion may vary among individuals, each person is very consistent in his or her creatinine excretion. Thus, if the urinary creatinine excretion varies in serial collections, one must suspect that the collection methodology has been inconsistent, and the protein quantitations cannot be compared in terms of trends. If the creatinine excretion is not near normal or varies greatly, the urine collection should be repeated after the technique of urine collection has been reviewed with the patient and parents. Normally, children excrete fewer than 200 mg of protein per square meter (95th percentile), although quantity may very among diagnostic laboratories because of different methods of measurement.

The third crucial factor is the concurrence of other urinary abnormalities or the presence of signs of systemic disease. The presence of hematuria or cylindruria should alert the clinician to the possibility of significant renal disease. Furthermore, clinical abnormalities such as hypertension or edema suggest that the proteinuria may be part of a more systemic illness. An algorithm for the investigation of proteinuria using the 24-hour urine collection in which each individual specimen has been tested is shown in Fig. 163-1. If all specimens are negative and the total 24-hour protein excretion is normal for the child's size, the previous finding of proteinuria in random urine samples probably was an artifact. Such an occurrence is not unusual in pediatric practice. The two most common causes of artifactual proteinuria are (1) improper urine collection, in that the cleansing solution or an extraneous source of protein (e.g., vaginal discharge) contaminates the specimen, and (2) collection of a specimen from a person who has had a poor fluid intake. In this latter circumstance, the normal amount of excreted protein that usually is below the range of detection by the dip-and-read strips is concentrated to a detectable level. Usually a history of poor fluid ingestion and infrequent voiding can be obtained. Despite the positive result on the dip-and-read test, the quantitative protein will be normal. High positive dip-and-read results (3+ and 4+) usually are not caused by poor fluid intake.

If the patient has negative urine protein results after he or she has been supine or inactive but has positive results following upright posture or physical activity, a clinical diagnosis of postural, or orthostatic, proteinuria is justified, providing that such a postural effect occurs (1) as an isolated urine abnormality, (2) with a quantitative protein excretion that is less than five times the 95th percentile for surface area, (3) in the absence of symptoms and of a personal or family history of renal disease, and (4) with a normal physical examination and laboratory tests of renal function. Orthostatic proteinuria usually is discovered on routine urinalysis in an asymptomatic adolescent or young adult. The diagnosis of orthostatic proteinuria is a clinical one; therefore, renal biopsy and an extensive radiographic investigation are not indicated. When renal biopsies have been performed, they have been normal or have shown only nonspecific changes.[4] Orthostatic proteinuria resolves in early adulthood in 50% of these patients. Follow-up studies of patients (for as long as 50 years after diagnosis) have revealed no tendency for the urinary abnormality to progress to serious renal disease.[2,3] Even so, the child should have a semiannual reexamination and a repeat 24-hour urine collection with individual specimen testing. Such a follow-up can detect any change in the pattern of

BOX 163-1

PATIENT INSTRUCTIONS FOR SIMULTANEOUS COLLECTION OF 24-HOUR URINE SPECIMEN AND POSTURAL PROTEIN TEST

This test involves the simultaneous collection of a 24-hour urine specimen (for quantitation of total urinary protein) and the testing of each individual urine specimen for protein. The amount of protein in each urination should be recorded along with the date, time of day, and the activities of the patient since the previous urination. The specific instructions for the patient are as follows:

1. On the day the test begins, urinate immediately after rising (________ AM), test for protein, record the results, and then *discard* the urine.
2. Test each subsequent urination, record the result, and add the entire specimen to the 24-hour collection, which should be kept refrigerated. A good intake of fluid is helpful throughout this test.
3. Sometime during the day, exercise (e.g., bike riding, playing ball) so that there is a urine specimen to test after a period of vigorous activity. Test it, record the results, and add it to the collection as you did with the others.
4. During another time of day (evening is best), remain relatively quiet (e.g., doing homework, watching television) so that there is urine to test after a period of rest. Test it and add it to the collection.
5. On the next day, rise at the same time, urinate immediately, test for protein, record the results, and add to the 24-hour collection.
6. Bring this paper with the written urine tests results, the unused protein test strips, and the 24-hour specimen to the office. The patient need not come to the office unless an appointment has been scheduled.

Results

Date	Time	Activity	Urine Protein

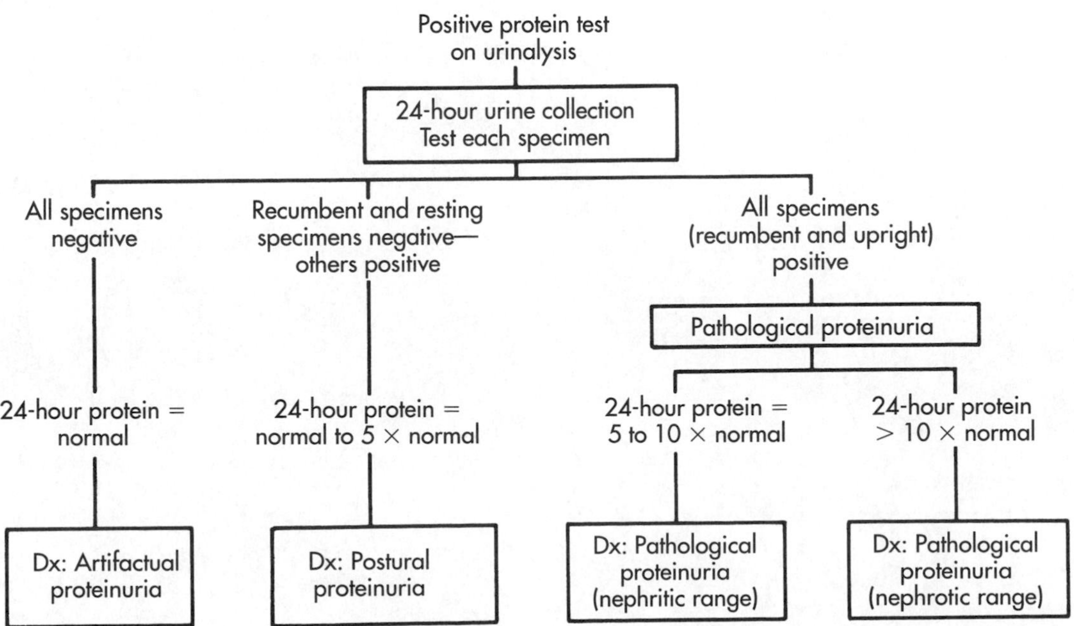

Fig. 163-1 A clinical algorithm for proteinuria in children.

proteinuria, which may be a harbinger of an underlying serious renal problem.

If all urinary specimens test positive for protein regardless of position or activity, a significant renal pathological condition is likely. Such pathological proteinuria also is associated more frequently with hematuria or other abnormalities of the urinary sediment. The nephritic range for total 24-hour proteinuria usually is 5 to 10 times the 95th percentile for surface area and may be associated with hypertension, mild edema, and nonspecific generalized symptoms, such as malaise and fatigue. In such patients a complete renal functional examination and imaging of the kidneys are important. Most of these children should be referred to a pediatric nephrologist for more complete evaluation, which usually includes a renal biopsy[5] (see Chapter 237, Nephritis).

Pathological total 24-hour proteinuria greater than 10 times the 95th percentile for surface area can be labeled as being in the nephrotic range. Hypoproteinemia and hypercholesterolemia often are found concomitantly. These patients usually have edema or other obvious signs and symptoms that bring them to medical attention. A complete evaluation is indicated in these circumstances (see Chapter 238, Nephrotic Syndrome).

When to Refer

- Urinary protein excretion greater than 1 g/m^2/day
- Proteinuria associated with hypertension and/or hematuria
- Proteinuria associated with azotemia
- Repeated measurements show an increasing amount of proteinuria

When to Hospitalize

- Anasarca
- Proteinuria associated with significant hypertension
- Proteinuria associated with significant azotemia

REFERENCES

1. Meites S: *Pediatric clinical chemistry*, ed 3, Washington, DC, 1989, AACC Press.
2. Robinson RR: Isolated proteinuria in asymptomatic patients, *Kidney Int* 18:395, 1980.
3. Rytand DA, Spreiter S: Prognosis in postural (orthostatic) proteinuria: forty- to fifty-year follow-up of six patients after diagnosis by Thomas Addis, *N Engl J Med* 305:618, 1981.
4. Sinniah R, Law CH, Pwee HS: Glomerular lesions in patients with asymptomatic persistent and orthostatic proteinuria discovered on routine medical examination, *Clin Nephrol* 7:1, 1977.
5. Trachtman H, Bergwerk A, Gauthier B: Isolated proteinuria in children: natural history and indications for renal biopsy, *Clin Pediatr* 33:468, 1994.

SUGGESTED READINGS

Ettenger RB: The evaluation of the child with proteinuria, *Pediatr Ann* 23:486, 1994.

Mahan JD, Turman MA, Mentser MI: Evaluation of hematuria, proteinuria, and hypertension in adolescents, *Pediatr Clin North Am* 44:1573, 1997.

164 Pruritus

Nancy K. Barnett

Pruritus, or itch, is the subjective perception of a cutaneous disturbance that is relieved by scratching or rubbing. It usually is not brought to the pediatrician's attention unless it is generalized, chronic, or associated with an eruption. In such instances, however, it must be treated with great respect because severe itching can be physically incapacitating. In addition, scratching or rubbing the itch can produce extensive disfigurement in the form of linear excoriations or lichenified plaques and can set up cutaneous infections. Constant scratching can even cause social isolation, for at times the pruritic child is viewed by others as contagious or unclean.

PATHOPHYSIOLOGY

Because itch is a subjective sensation, objective evaluation to delineate its pathophysiology has been difficult. However, current thinking implicates a local production of chemomediators that stimulate "itch receptors," thought to be free, fine nerve endings at the dermoepidermal junction.[6] The exact mediators and their release triggers are unknown. Histamine and endopeptidases have elicited itch fairly consistently in experimental settings and may be active in human disease. Experimental triggers that have produced itch are physical pressure, heat, and electric shock.

It is believed that the nerve impulses travel along the anterolateral spinothalamic tract to the thalamus, where they are transferred to the sensory cortex via the internal capsule, where they are interpreted as itch.[4,7] This is the same pathway for pain, and some contend that itch is a mild degree of "pain"; however, aspirin alone does not relieve itch.

Certain circumstances alter the interpretation of the degree of pruritus. For example, the itch threshold in and around areas of active dermatitis can be lowered by psychic stress, decreased skin hydration, or increased skin temperature, and during the night.[2,3]

CLINICAL MANIFESTATIONS

In children, local cutaneous rather than systemic disease is by far the most common cause of generalized pruritus. The major differential diagnoses of generalized pruritus with skin lesions in children are infestation (scabies, pediculosis, insect bites, and papular urticaria), atopic dermatitis, miliaria, contact dermatitis, and acute or chronic urticaria.[7]

Children may itch with cutaneous diseases such as psoriasis, lichen planus, and bullous disease of childhood. These children should be referred to a dermatologist for evaluation and management, as should a pruritic child who otherwise is healthy and does not have bites, eczema, "heat rash," contact dermatitis, or hives. The child who has pruritus, from whatever cause, is at risk for psychological damage, infection secondary to impetiginization, and scarification.

Systemic causes of pruritus in childhood that should be sought in the occasional child who has pruritus but no evident skin lesions are hyperthyroidism, leukemia or lymphoma, chronic renal failure, obstructive biliary disease, and xerosis (generalized dry skin).

EVALUATION AND TREATMENT

All of the common cutaneous diseases associated with generalized pruritus can be diagnosed based on a good history and physical examination. The answers to the following questions may help in diagnosing infestation of one sort or another and direct therapy toward topical steroids, long clothes, and repellents: Are there individual pruritic papules with a central punctum? If so, are they on exposed or nonexposed areas? Does anyone else in the family have similar lesions?

A family history of allergy, asthma, or eczema in a child who has a chronic eczematous dermatitis over extensor surfaces in infancy and flexural areas in childhood suggests atopic dermatitis. Hydration and emollients will reduce the pruritus and should be the mainstay of therapy, although topical steroids, antibiotics, and cool compresses may be required to bring the scratch-itch cycle under control. A tolerable (nonsoporific) dose of an antihistamine may relieve itch, especially if it is given about 1 hour before bedtime, because the itch threshold is lower at night. Hydroxyzine seems to be the most effective agent.[5] Data conflict about the use of nonsedating antihistamines for controlling itch.[1]

Pinpoint crystalline or erythematous papules in areas of occlusion and sweating—that is, miliaria crystallina and miliaria rubra (heat rash)—can be controlled by simple measures such as applying dusting powders, avoiding tight clothing, and reducing exposure to high ambient temperatures.

Contact dermatitis usually is readily recognizable because of the linear array of papulovesicular, erythematous lesions and sharp borders that conform to the shape of the contactant. The use of antihistamines, topical steroids, and compresses is discussed in detail in Chapter 199, Contact Dermatitis.

Acute urticaria that occurs secondary to a drug or other ingestant is indicated by intensely pruritic, erythematous, and edematous plaques and papules. Careful historical and environmental sleuthing may reveal the cause of contact allergic or contact irritant dermatitis, but the cause of 90% of acute urticaria cases remains a mystery. If the patient has not used any new drug or food and if the hives persist despite regular use of antihistamines for several days, it is reasonable to obtain a throat culture and a complete blood count with differential and to screen for mycoplasmal disease and infectious mononucleosis to rule out occult streptococcal, mycoplasmal, and viral infections. Rarely, a skin biopsy may be helpful.[8]

To relieve itching and prevent scarring (both mental and physical), the scratch-itch cycle must be broken. Scratching relieves itching only temporarily, perhaps by substituting the perception of pain for that of itch. Itching provokes scratching, and when the scratching stops, the itching returns. To control itching, the following steps can be helpful: keep the patient's fingernails short (to prevent damage from scratching); keep the patient fully clothed except when applying medications; apply bland emollient creams frequently, especially after bathing; apply cool compresses to relieve intense pruritus and to remove crusts and debris; apply topical steroids for short periods (fewer than 10 days) to control inflammation; increase the dosage of antihistamine until the scratching stops or marked drowsiness occurs, and then reduce the dosage to a level that controls the scratching but does not cause drowsiness; have the patient avoid stress, heat, and irritants; and see the patient frequently to provide support. If the child is old enough to understand, explain why these methods are being used. Topical capsaicin and pramoxine may be indicated in some cases. Referral to the dermatologist generally is indicated in such a circumstance. Ultraviolet B (UVB) light therapy may be very helpful for generalized pruritus such as occurs in biliary cirrhosis or severe chronic atopic dermatitis.

When to Refer

- Pruritus with uncommon disease (e.g., psoriasis or bullae)
- Chronic pruritus without cutaneous disease to evaluate for systemic cause
- Pruritus uncontrolled by usual topical steroids and antihistamines

REFERENCES

1. Bernhard JD: Itching: some answers but no panacea, *Dermatol Perspect* 5:1, 1989.
2. Cormia FE: Experimental histamine pruritus, *J Invest Dermatol* 19:21, 1952.
3. Edwards AE, et al: Pruritic skin disease, psychological stress, and the itch sensation, *Arch Dermatol* 112:339, 1976.
4. Gilchrest BA: Pruritus: pathogenesis, therapy, and significance in systemic disease states, *Arch Intern Med* 142:101, 1982.
5. Rhoades RB, et al: Suppression of histamine-induced pruritus by three antihistamine drugs, *J Allergy Clin Immunol* 55:180, 1975.
6. Shelly WB, Arthur RP: The neurohistology and neurophysiology of the itch sensation in man, *Arch Dermatol* 76:296, 1957.
7. Tonnesen MG: Pruritus. In Fitzpatrick TB, et al, editors: *Dermatology in general medicine,* ed 3, New York, 1987, McGraw-Hill.
8. Toppe E, et al: Neutrophilic urticaria: clinical features, histological changes and possible mechanisms, *Br J Dermatol* 138:248, 1998.

165 Puberty: Normal and Abnormal

Leslie P. Plotnick • Robert K. Kritzler

Disorders of pubertal development constitute one of the most frequent referrals to pediatric endocrinology clinics. In many cases, no endocrine problem is found. Frequently, a costly referral can be avoided by a careful evaluation, including family history, and a few simple laboratory procedures.

NORMAL PUBERTY

At puberty, a series of complex hormonal changes takes place. The hypothalamus secretes pulses of gonadotropin-releasing hormone (GnRH), which stimulates pituitary gonadotropin production of luteinizing hormone (LH) and follicle-stimulating hormone (FSH). Concomitantly, the previously very sensitive hypothalamic-pituitary-gonadal feedback loop becomes less sensitive to the negative effect of gonadal steroids; thus, gonadotropin levels rise. This results in the secretion of greater amounts of androgens or estrogens, depending on the gender of the child, leading to the physical changes of puberty. Secretion of adrenal androgens also are increased. The mechanism that triggers the maturation of the adrenal cortex at puberty remains poorly understood.

In girls, breast development usually is the first sign of puberty, with the mean age of onset at about 10½ years and a standard deviation of 2½ years. This is followed in about 6 months by the appearance of pubic hair. Menarche follows the onset of breast development by about 2 years. A growth spurt accompanies the changes, usually peaking before menarche. The range of normal variation, however, is quite wide. In boys, testicular enlargement and scrotal thinning are the first signs of puberty, with a mean age of onset at about 11½ years and a standard deviation of 2 years; this is followed in about 6 months by pubic hair growth and some penile enlargement. Approximately 2 years after the first changes, axillary hair and then facial hair appear. The male growth spurt peaks about 2 years after that of the female. As with girls, the normal range is wide.

The time of puberty is one of profound change, both physical and psychological. Problems of sexual identity, body image, adolescent independence, and peer acceptance are frequent. Because the ranges of age of normal puberty are wide, children of similar chronological age may have markedly different physical maturity. When pubertal development is precocious or delayed, many of these problems are compounded.

DELAYED PUBERTY

Few matters are of greater concern to the adolescent than remaining short in stature or sexually underdeveloped. Delayed development demands the immediate attention of the practitioner.

Puberty is considered delayed in girls who have no breast development by 13 years of age or in boys who have no testicular enlargement at 14 years of age. In girls a delay of more than 4 to 5 years from onset of puberty to menarche also is cause for concern. Similarly, maturation arrest in boys warrants evaluation. Delayed puberty is more common in boys than in girls.

Constitutional delay, a slow maturation with appropriate hormonal levels and delayed bone age, accounts for the majority of all cases of delayed pubertal development. This problem is identified much more frequently in boys, perhaps because of general societal and peer group reaction to short and sexually underdeveloped boys. It frequently is familial. Often, early signs of puberty are found on careful examination, which permits the physician to reassure the child and the parents. These children should be followed closely. Chronic systemic diseases that can lead to delayed puberty may be difficult to differentiate from constitutional delay as a cause for the difficulty; these diseases are listed in Box 165-1.

The remainder of the differential diagnosis of delayed development relates to failure at either the hypothalamic-pituitary level, shown by low serum gonadotropins (hypogonadotropic hypogonadism), or at the gonadal level, shown by elevated gonadotropins (hypergonadotropic hypogonadism). Either of these conditions may result from genetic disorders or acquired illnesses (see Box 165-1). The workup of the patient is directed toward identifying the specific cause.

Treatment should be directed, when possible, toward the cause of the delayed development. If sex steroid secretion is deficient, because of either gonadal failure or gonadotropin deficiency, treatment focuses on replacing the appropriate sex steroid. In constitutional delay, waiting is the best course. In males, however, a short course of injectable testosterone may be indicated if the delayed development is affecting the boy's psychological well-being. In girls, cosmetic treatment, such as the use of a padded bra, is very helpful. Estrogen therapy is necessary only occasionally. In patients who have GnRH or gonadotropin deficiency, fertility may be induced with GnRH or gonadotropin therapy. In any case, strong psychological support must be provided to the adolescent and sometimes to the family. If the problem is difficult diagnostically

BOX 165-1

CAUSES OF DELAYED PUBERTY

I. Constitutional delay
II. Deficiency of GnRH secretion by the hypothalamus
    A. Genetic and molecular causes
        1. Isolated deficiency
        2. Kallmann's syndrome
        3. Laurence-Moon-Bardet-Biedl syndrome
        4. Prader-Willi syndrome
    B. Acquired causes
        1. Infection
        2. Neoplasm
        3. Infiltrative disease
        4. Trauma
III. Deficiency of gonadotropin secretion by the pituitary
    A. Genetic
        1. Panhypopituitarism
        2. Isolated deficiency
        3. Fertile eunuch (normal FSH, low LH)
    B. Acquired
        1. Infection
        2. Tumor
        3. Excess prolactin secretion
        4. Trauma
IV. Gonadal disorders
    A. Genetic and molecular
        1. Turner's syndrome (45, X or structural X abnormalities or mosaicism)
        2. Klinefelter's syndrome (47, XXY abnormality)
        3. Noonan's syndrome
        4. Syndromes of complete androgen insensitivity (no sexual hair)
        5. del Castillo's syndrome (Sertoli cells only)
        6. Pure gonadal dysgenesis
        7. Myotonic dystrophy
        8. Receptor mutations
    B. Acquired
        1. Infections
            a. Gonorrhea (male)
            b. Virus (usually mumps)
            c. Tuberculosis (male)
        2. Postradiation or chemotherapy
        3. Mechanical causes
            a. Torsion
            b. Surgery
            c. Congenital anorchia ("vanishing testes" syndrome)
        4. Autoimmune
V. Adrenal and gonadal steroid enzyme deficiencies
VI. Excessive exercise
VII. Chronic systemic diseases
    A. Congenital heart disease
    B. Chronic pulmonary disease
    C. Inflammatory bowel disease
    D. Chronic renal failure and renal tubular acidosis
    E. Hypothyroidism
    F. Poorly controlled diabetes mellitus
    G. Sickle cell anemia
    H. Collagen-vascular disease
    I. Anorexia nervosa

or if hormonal therapy is desired, referral should be made to a pediatric endocrinologist.

PRECOCIOUS PUBERTY

Precocious puberty is the appearance of secondary sexual characteristics classically before 8 years of age in girls and 9 years in boys. Recent data, however, show that 5.0% of white and 15.4% of black girls begin breast development by 7 to 7.99 years of age and 2.8% and 17.7%, respectively, begin pubic hair development by this age.[1] These data suggest that more appropriate ages for concern may be 7 years for white and 6 years for black girls. Precocity may be isosexual (appropriate for phenotype) or heterosexual (appropriate for opposite sex phenotype) and is much more common in girls than in boys. In girls, idiopathic precocious puberty is the single most common diagnosis; precocious puberty in boys is more likely to be secondary to organic causes. Girls adopted from developing countries may be at particular risk for precocious puberty.[2]

Isosexual Precocious Puberty

Early stimulation of the hypothalamic-pituitary axis, with resultant gonadotropin secretion and sex steroid secretion, is termed *central precocious puberty.* Sex steroid secretion independent of pituitary gonadotropin secretion may be termed *peripheral* or *pseudoprecocious puberty.* Box 165-2 lists the causes of these two conditions.

The diagnosis of precocious puberty is based on the physical examination and laboratory evidence of sex steroid secretion. Measurement of serum gonadotropin levels before and after an injection of GnRH usually allows classification of the condition as either central or peripheral precocious puberty. In central precocious puberty, further workup focuses on a search for the cause of the gonadotropin secretion. The diagnosis of idiopathic central precocious puberty can be made only after a search for a pathological cause is negative. Although onset is at an early age, tempo and pattern of pubertal progression are normal in idiopathic central precocity. In peripheral precocious puberty, one must search for the source of sex steroid, remembering that exogenous sources (e.g., contraceptive pills in girls) are easily available. In males, physical examination of the testes is particularly useful in the differential diagnosis. If both testes are of pubertal size, then the patient has gonadotropin-stimulated precocious puberty; if one testis is enlarged, a testicular tumor may be present; if both testes are small, the androgens are either exogenous or of adrenal origin.

Treatment of the isosexual precocity centers on removal

BOX 165-2

CAUSES OF ISOSEXUAL PRECOCIOUS PUBERTY

I. Central (with pituitary gonadotropin secretion)
  A. Idiopathic
  B. Central nervous system abnormalities
    1. Congenital anomalies (hydrocephalus)
    2. Tumors (hypothalamic, pineal, other)
    3. Hamartoma
    4. Postinflammatory condition
    5. Trauma
    6. Syndromes
      a. Neurofibromatosis
      b. Tuberous sclerosis
  C. Hypothyroidism (severe)
II. Peripheral
  A. Exogenous sex steroids
  B. Gonadal tumors or cysts
  C. Adrenal hyperplasia or tumor
  D. Ectopic gonadotropin-secreting tumors (chorioepithelioma, hepatoblastoma, teratoma)
  E. Familial Leydig cell hyperplasia/receptor mutation
  F. McCune-Albright syndrome/G-protein mutation

of the underlying cause. The treatment of idiopathic central precocious puberty is with GnRH analogs, which lead to pituitary desensitization and a reduction in gonadotropin secretion to prepubertal levels. Several GnRH analogs are available in intramuscular (depot), subcutaneous, and intranasal forms. This treatment has been used for years and is effective and generally safe. For gonadotropin-independent precocious puberty, testolactone, spironolactone, and ketoconazole may be used. In all cases, psychological support is important. Evaluation and treatment of precocious puberty is a matter for a pediatric endocrinologist.

Variations of Puberty

Two entities not requiring treatment are isolated premature breast development (thelarche) and isolated premature development of sexual hair (adrenarche). Premature thelarche typically occurs in girls between 6 months and 2 years of age. Breast development usually is moderate, often regresses, and is seen without other signs of precocious puberty. Specifically, estrogen or gonadotropic levels do not increase significantly, and statural and skeletal maturation accelerate only mildly, if at all. Premature thelarche does not progress to complete precocious puberty.

Premature adrenarche usually occurs between 5 and 7 to 8 years of age. The development of sexual hair frequently is accompanied by a mild growth spurt (with slight bone age advancement) and signs of increased adrenal androgen (slightly elevated urinary 17-ketosteroids and increased levels of plasma dehydroepiandrosterone and its sulfate); in girls there are no signs of increased estrogen secretion. An abnormal androgen source such as a tumor or adrenal hyperplasia must be excluded.

BOX 165-3

CAUSES OF HETEROSEXUAL PRECOCIOUS PUBERTY

I. Female
  A. Congenital adrenal hyperplasia
  B. Androgen-secreting tumors
    1. Adrenal
    2. Ovarian
    3. Teratoma
  C. Exogenous androgens
II. Male
  A. Estrogen-producing tumors
    1. Adrenal
    2. Teratoma
    3. Hepatoma
    4. Testicular
  B. Exogenous estrogens
  C. Increased peripheral conversion of androgens to estrogens

In both premature thelarche and premature adrenarche, careful follow-up is necessary to be sure they do not actually represent the early stages of complete sexual precocity.

Heterosexual Precocious Puberty

Heterosexual precocious puberty is uncommon. Box 165-3 lists its causes. Exogenous sex steroids (including creams) must be considered. The diagnostic workup must center on the search for a sex steroid-producing tumor. These patients should be referred to a pediatric endocrinologist. Treatment is aimed at removal of the sex hormone source (exogenous or tumor) or suppression with glucocorticoid replacement therapy (congenital adrenal hyperplasia).

SUMMARY

In most cases of delayed or precocious sexual development, a careful history and physical examination and a few basic laboratory tests identify those patients likely to have a pathological cause requiring referral to a pediatric endocrinologist. See Chapter 147, Hirsutism, Hypertrichosis, and Precocious Sexual Hair Development, for further discussion of various forms of precocious sexual development.

In all cases, along with physical care, psychological care and support are extremely important, particularly when medical therapy is only partially satisfactory.

REFERENCES

1. Herman-Giddens ME, et al: Secondary sexual characteristics and menses in young girls seen in office practice: a study from the Pediatric Research in Office Settings network, *Pediatrics* 99:505, 1997.
2. Virdis R, et al: Precocious puberty in girls adopted from developing countries, *Arch Dis Child* 78:152, 1998.

SUGGESTED READINGS

Blizzard PM, Rogol AD: Variations and disorders of pubertal development. In Kappy MS, et al, editors: *Wilkins diagnosis and treatment of endocrine disorders in childhood and adolescence,* ed 4, Springfield, Ill, 1994, Charles C Thomas.

Clemons RD, Kappy MS, et al: Long-term effectiveness of depot GnRH analogue in the treatment of children with central precocious puberty, *Am J Dis Child* 147:653, 1993.

DiMeglio LA, Pescovitz OH: Disorders of puberty: inactivating and activating molecular mutation, *J Pediatr* 131: S8, 1997.

Kelch RP, Beitins IZ: Adolescent sexual development. In Kappy MS et al, editors: *Wilkins the diagnosis and treatment of endocrine disorders in childhood and adolescence,* ed 4, Springfield, Ill, 1994, Charles C Thomas.

Kulin HE: Delayed puberty in boys, *Curr Ther Endocrinol Metab* 6:346, 1997.

Rosenfield RL: Selection of children with precocious puberty for treatment with GnRH analogs, *J Pediatr* 124:989, 1994.

Rosenfield RL: The ovary and female sexual maturation. In Kaplan SA, editor: *Clinical pediatric endocrinology,* Philadelphia, 1990, WB Saunders.

Saenger P, Reiter EO: Premature adrenarche: a normal variant of puberty? *J Clin Endocrinol Metab* 74:236, 1992.

Styne D: New aspects in the diagnosis and treatment of pubertal disorders, *Pediatr Clin North Am* 44: 505, 1997.

Styne D: The testes: disorders of sexual differentiation and puberty. In Kaplan SA, editor: *Clinical pediatric endocrinology,* Philadelphia, 1990, WB Saunders.

Tanner JM: Growth and endocrinology of the adolescent. In Gardner LI, editor: *Endocrine and genetic diseases of childhood and adolescence,* Philadelphia, 1975, WB Saunders.

Thomas MA, Rebar RW: Delayed puberty in girls and primary amenorrhea, *Curr Ther Endocrinol Metab* 6:223, 1997.

166 Rash

Michael Fisher • Judith L. Fisher • Nancy K. Barnett

Rash is an ambiguous term used to describe an acute skin eruption that usually is temporary. It does not define any specific lesion. The term also does not convey information about the evolution or progression of a disorder, which are data needed to arrive at a logical differential diagnosis.

Tables 166-1 and 166-2 list descriptions of lesions and contain historical or characteristic information for particular diagnoses. The tables are not valid for "rashes" that have been altered by therapy. They are not all-inclusive but cover the major acute eruptions that the pediatric practitioner will encounter.

To put the tables in context, a few points are worth making. As usual in medicine, a careful history is always helpful. We too often are prone to look at a rash before exploring its past, and by doing so we lose all that a history can contribute. We must know when it arose, how it progressed, and whether there were accompanying symptoms or signs—for example, an itch or a fever. A sound history includes that of the family. It is easy to ask if someone else in the family is scratching or similarly beset now or was so in the past.

The most important lesson one pediatrician learned early in his career about evaluating a rash involved light: The rash of scarlet fever became evident when he raised the window shade. The light should be adequate when performing a physical examination; natural lighting is preferred. Be sure your view of the field is unobstructed. Clothing must be shed. Do not limit your look to a rolled-up sleeve or a lifted shirttail. Feel the rash—is it smooth or rough? Once the site has been inspected and palpated, the rash must be described as accurately as possible. What does it look like? (Use a magnifier to discern, for example, a burrow or a pinpoint puncture.) Where is it? Are the lesions discrete or confluent, large or small? Use a tape measure to define the lesions accurately by size. Is it oozing or dry, excoriated or relatively untouched in appearance? Describe carefully in writing what you see.

A *macule* is a spot that is set apart from its immediate surroundings by a difference in color. It is a discoloration of the skin that is not elevated above the surface and may be of any color or of many colors. It is small, generally less than 1 cm. Larger areas may be described as patches. *Papules* are small (less than 5 mm in diameter), well-circumscribed, solid elevations of the skin. A *nodule,* too, is solid and usually elevated or palpable in the subcutaneous area, but it is larger than a papule. Its solidity, like the papule, enables it to be detected by touch, although its borders are indistinct. A *vesicle* is a small sac that contains liquid. With respect to the skin, it may be described as a circumscribed elevation of the epidermis containing a serous liquid. As the diameter approaches 1 cm, it is called more appropriately a bulla, bleb, or blister. A *bulla* is an elevation above the level of the skin that is filled with fluid, usually serous. It may have either a quite delicate or tough "roof," depending on the level of the skin in which it appears.

Once one has become familiar with Tables 166-1 and 166-2 and their precepts, it becomes evident that many dermatological diagnoses are not particularly difficult to make. On the other hand, problems of either diagnosis or treatment are sure to arise. Children and adolescents who have eczema, acne, and psoriasis, for example, often will benefit from consultation with a dermatologist.

Regardless, for pediatrician and dermatologist alike, *primum non nocere* (i.e., above all, do no harm) should be the rule. Iatrogenic difficulties from the overuse of drugs such as topical corticosteroids and antibiotics must be avoided. Seldom should adrenal suppression be risked because of continuous steroid use, and we already are too far along in encouraging bacterial readaptations to the environment. Fortunately, some principles of therapy help guide the pediatrician. First, the least amount necessary of the most effective medication should be given by mouth or applied locally. Second, the use of household aids can be convenient and inexpensive. For example, oatmeal can serve as a colloid compress or bath for itching; an emery board will keep the fingernails smooth and short to reduce excoriations from scratching; and tea bags can be used as compresses for odd places (weeping behind the ears). Third, a moistened gauze wrapped twice around atopic areas helps to reduce oozing, to relieve itching, and to potentiate the effect of topical steroids. Fourth, children whose itching is generalized, as in atopic dermatitis, should always be kept fully clothed, using long-sleeved shirts and leotards during the day and pajamas with feet at night. Fifth, emollients, such as Eucerin or Aquaphor, lubricate and smooth dry skin and diminish itching, whereas powder or cornstarch, dusted on lightly, is useful on moist or oozing surfaces (particularly between the toes and other intertriginous areas) to prevent maceration. And last, precise instruction is essential; the patient or parent should be asked to repeat the plan for treatment and the steps for its implementation to ensure complete understanding of what is to be done, and written instructions should be given to the patient or the parents.

Text continued on p. 1234

Table 166-1 Descriptions of Lesions

Diagnosis or Differential Diagnosis	Number			Pattern						Distribution									Size			Spread			Other Characteristics				
	Few	Many	TNTC*	Discrete	Confluent	Annular†	Localized	Generalized	Symmetrical	Face/scalp	Palmoplantar	Truncal	Intertriginous	Extremities	Acral	Extensor	Flexor	Mucosae	<1 mm	1-5 mm	>5 mm	Centripetal	Centrifugal	Caudal	Sun exposed	Fever/illness	Pruritus	Scale	Crust
Macule																													
Erythematous																													
Dermatomyositis‡					X					X						X									X			X	
Drug reaction‡			X	X	X			X		X	X	X	X	X	X				X	X	X						X		
Erythema infectiosum					X		X			X		X		X						X	X			X					
Erythema marginatum‡		X				X						X		X							X		X			X			
Erythema multiforme, Stevens-Johnson syndrome	X	X	X	X			X	X	X	X	X	X			X	X		X		X	X	X				X			
Infectious mononucleosis‡					X			X				X		X												X			
Juvenile rheumatoid arthritis‡		X		X	X			X				X		X						X	X					X			
Kawasaki disease‡					X			X		X	X	X		X				X								X			
Lupus erythematosus	X	X		X	X		X		X	X				X					X	X	X				X	X		X	
Lyme disease	X	X		X		X	X	X				X									X					X			
Roseola infantum (exanthem subitum)			X	X	X			X				X								X						X			
Rubella			X	X	X			X		X		X		X				X		X						X			
Rubeola			X	X	X			X		X		X		X				X		X				X		X			
Scarlet fever			X	X	X				X				X	X	X			X		X	X			X			X		
Staphylococcal scalded skin syndrome					X		X	X		X		X	X	X												X			X
Sunburn, phototoxic reaction	X				X		X	X													X				X				
Toxic epidermal necrolysis					X			X		X		X	X	X				X								X			
Toxic shock syndrome					X			X				X						X								X			
Viral exanthem‡			X	X	X			X		X	X	X		X				X		X						X			
Hypopigmented																													
Pityriasis alba	X	X	X	X	X		X	X		X		X		X						X	X						X		
Tinea versicolor‡	X	X	X	X	X		X	X		X		X		X						X	X			X		X	X		
Vitiligo in evolution	X	X		X	X		X	X	X	X	X	X		X	X	X				X	X								
Hyperpigmented																													
Tinea versicolor‡	X	X	X	X	X		X	X		X		X		X						X	X			X			X	X	
Transient neonatal pustular melanosis	X	X	X	X	X			X		X		X	X							X									
Nonblanching (petechiae, purpura)																													
Atypical measles		X	X	X	X			X		X		X		X	X			X	X	X					X	X			
Battered child syndrome‡	X	X		X			X			X		X		X							X								
Leukemia, coagulation defect, ITP	X	X	X	X	X			X		X		X		X				X	X	X									

Rocky Mountain spotted fever‡	X	X	X	X	X			X		X	X	X		X	X		X		X	X		X				X			
Viral exanthem, TORCH infection, drug, hepatitis‡		X	X	X	X			X		X		X		X				X	X	X					X	X			
Papules, Nodules																													
Erythematous																													
Atopic dermatitis	X	X	X	X	X		X	X		X		X		X		X	X		X	X	X						X		X
Gianotti-Crosti	X	X	X				X		X	X				X	X					X	X								
Granuloma annulare	X	X		X		X						X		X	X					X	X								
Insect bites	X	X	X	X			X			X		X	X	X	X					X					X				
Mastocytosis (urticaria pigmentosa)§	X	X	X	X	X		X	X		X		X		X						X	X						X		
Miliaria rubra (heat rash)	X	X	X	X			X			X		X	X						X							X	X		
Seborrheic dermatitis	X	X	X	X	X		X	X		X		X	X							X	X							X	
Tinea corporis	X	X		X		X	X			X		X		X					X	X	X			X					
Hypopigmented																													
Lichen nitidus		X	X	X			X					X		X					X	X									
Lichen striatus, linear lichen planus, epidermal nevus		X	X	X	X		X				X			X							X								
Molluscum contagiosum	X	X	X		X		X			X		X		X					X	X	X								
Violaceous																													
Lichen planus	X	X	X	X	X			X	X			X		X	X			X	X	X	X						X		
Nonblanching																													
Gonococcemia, SBE	X			X			X				X	X		X						X						X			
Henoch-Schönlein purpura§	X	X	X	X	X			X	X					X		X				X	X	X				X			
Letterer-Siwe disease	X	X	X	X	X		X	X		X	X	X	X	X						X	X					X		X	X
Leukemia cutis/lymphoma	X	X	X	X	X			X				X		X					X	X	X					X			
Meningococcemia, sepsis	X	X	X	X	X			X		X	X	X		X				X	X	X						X			
Neuroblastoma, TORCH infection, leukemia	X	X		X				X		X		X		X						X	X					X			
Pseudomonas sepsis	X	X		X			X					X		X	X					X	X					X			X
Staphylococcal sepsis	X	X		X			X					X		X	X					X	X					X			X
Vesicles																													
Congenital syphilis	X	X	X	X		X	X	X	X	X	X	X	X		X			X	X	X	X					X		X	X
Contact dermatitis	X	X	X	X	X		X	X		X		X	X	X	X				X	X						X	X		X
Coxsackievirus hand, foot, and mouth disease	X	X		X			X			X					X			X		X						X			
Dyshidrotic eczema (pompholyx)	X	X	X	X	X		X				X				X				X	X						X			
Flea bites	X	X	X	X			X							X	X					X							X		X
Herpes simplex; herpex zoster	X			X	X		X			X		X		X				X	X	X						X	X		X

*Too numerous to count.
†Raised border.
‡May be papular in parts.
§May be edematous.

Continued

Table 166-1 Descriptions of Lesions—cont'd

Diagnosis or Differential Diagnosis	Number			Pattern						Distribution								Size			Spread			Other Characteristics				
	Few	Many	TNTC*	Discrete	Confluent	Annular†	Localized	Generalized	Symmetrical	Face/scalp	Palmoplantar	Truncal	Intertriginous	Extremities	Acral	Extensor	Flexor	Mucosae	<1 mm	1-5 mm	>5 mm	Centripetal	Centrifugal	Caudal	Sun exposed	Fever/illness	Pruritus	Scale	Crust
Vesicles—cont'd																													
Kaposi's varicelliform eruption	X	X	X				X	X	X	X		X		X			X		X	X						X	X		X
Miliaria crystallina	X	X	X	X			X	X		X		X	X	X					X						X	X	X		
Rickettsial pox	X	X						X				X		X					X	X						X			X
Tinea pedis	X	X	X	X	X		X				X								X	X							X		X
Varicella		X	X	X				X	X	X	X	X	X	X				X	X	X		X				X	X		X
Bullae																													
Blistering distal dactylitis	X						X								X						X								
Bullous disease of childhood	X	X	X	X	X	X		X		X		X	X	X	X						X						X		X
Bullous impetigo	X	X		X	X		X			X		X	X	X							X						X		X
Pustules																													
Acne neonatorum	X	X		X			X		X	X									X	X									
Acral pustulosis	X	X					X		X		X				X				X	X							X		
Candidiasis	X	X	X	X	X		X	X		X	X	X	X	X				X		X						X		X	
Erythema toxicum neonatorum	X	X	X	X	X		X	X		X	X	X		X						X									
Folliculitis	X	X	X	X			X	X				X		X					X	X									
Transient neonatal pustular melanosis	X	X	X	X	X		X			X		X	X							X									
Plaques																													
Acute urticaria	X	X	X	X	X		X	X		X		X		X				X	X	X	X						X		
Erysipelas	X						X			X		X									X					X			
Hematogenous cellulitis	X						X			X		X									X					X			
Nummular eczema	X	X	X	X			X					X		X		X					X						X	X	X
Perianal streptococcal cellulitis	X						X						X								X						X		
Psoriasis	X	X	X	X	X		X	X	X	X	X	X		X		X				X	X				X		X	X	

Table 166-2 Laboratory Studies and Characteristics of Lesions

Diagnosis or Differential Diagnosis	Laboratory Studies	Comments
Macule		
Erythematous		
Dermatomyositis*	Electromyography, creatinine phosphokinase, aldolase	Muscle weakness; periungual telangiectasia; heliotrope eyelid edema; Gottron's papule
Drug reaction*	Leukocytosis with eosinophilia	History of drug ingestion
Erythema infectiosum	Lymphocytosis, eosinophilia	Reticulated pattern may appear for months with stress; arthritis; slapped-cheek appearance
Erythema marginatum*		Acute rheumatic fever with active carditis; fleeting
Erythema multiforme, Stevens-Johnson syndrome	Skin biopsy may aid diagnosis	Central papule or vesicle, iris lesions; may be bullous
Infectious mononucleosis*	Heterophil antibody; atypical lymphocytes on smear	Generalized adenopathy, splenomegaly; ampicillin use
Juvenile rheumatoid arthritis*	Rheumatoid factor may be positive	Arthritis; lesions may be papular
Kawasaki disease*	Thrombocytosis beginning second to third wk after onset	Conjunctival injection, cervical adenopathy
Lupus erythematous	Positive ANA, skin biopsy	Periungual telangiectasia
Lyme disease	Most nonspecific; may look for antibodies to *Borrelia burgdorferi* (see Chapter 233 on Lyme disease)	Erythema migrans appearing as enlargening rings after tick bite
Roseola infantum (exanthem subitum)	Leukopenia may be present	Eruption appears with resolution of fever; periorbital edema
Rubella	Fourfold rise in antibody titer	Postauricular lymphadenopathy; monarticular arthritis; palatal petechiae
Rubeola		Koplik spots, preauricular lymph nodes
Scarlet fever	Throat culture, ASO titer	Malar flush, circumoral pallor, Pastia lines, desquamation
Staphylococcal scalded skin syndrome	*S. aureus* cultured from focus	Tender erythema, positive Nikolsky's sign, bullae
Sunburn, phototoxic reaction		Look for patterns and sharp edges (e.g., clothing lines after exposure to sun)
Toxic epidermal necrolysis	*S. aureus* cultures negative	Search for new drug use
Toxic shock syndrome	Blood, throat, urine, stool, vaginal cultures for *Staphylococcus aureus* or *Streptococcus pyogenes*	Shock, tampon use
Viral exanthem*	Leukocytosis with lymphocytosis	
Hypopigmented		
Pityriasis alba	Wood light—hypopigmented	
Tinea versicolor*	Potassium hydroxide (KOH) smear—short, branched hyphae and spores	Chronic, prevalent if immunosuppressed
Vitiligo in evolution	Wood light—depigmented if vitiliginous, T_4, TSH to rule out thyroid disorder	Observe for scleroderma, melanoma
Hyperpigmented		
Tinea versicolor*	See above	See above
Transient neonatal pustular melanosis	Pustule Gram stain—sterile with polymorphonuclear neutrophils (PMNs)	Pustules; superficial desquamation
Nonblanching (petechiae, purpura)		
Atypical measles		History of killed measles vaccine; pneumonitis: acral petechiae, purpura, vesiculobullous lesions

*May be papular in parts.

Continued

Table 166-2 Laboratory Studies and Characteristics of Lesions—cont'd

Diagnosis or Differential Diagnosis	Laboratory Studies	Comments
Nonblanching (petechiae, purpura)—cont'd		
Battered child syndrome*		History incongruous with pattern and/or degree of lesions
Leukemia, coagulation defect, ITP	CBC, PT, PTT, platelet count, bone marrow aspirate and biopsy	
Rocky Mountain spotted fever*	Fluorescent antibody screen: OX-19. OX-2: skin biopsy of fluorescent stain	History of tick bite
Viral exanthem, TORCH infection, drug, hepatitis*	Complete blood count (CBC) liver enzymes, viral titers	Drug history
Papules, Nodules		
Erythematous		
Atopic dermatitis	IgE level	Family or personal history of allergies, asthma, eczema; flexural in infancy and extensor in childhood
Gianotti-Crosti	Hepatitis B surface antigen, EBV	May koebnerize
Granuloma annulare		Lack of scale distinguishes from tinea corporis; no epidermal component
Insect bites		Check for central punctae
Mastocytosis (urticaria pigmentosa)†	Skin biopsy—mast cells	Wheal and flare on stroking
Miliaria rubra (heat rash)		Prominent in occluded areas
Seborrheic dermatitis		Intertriginous with yellow, greasy scale; cradle cap
Tinea corporis	KOH smear—long, thin-branched hyphae	
Hypopigmented		
Lichen nitidus		Check penis for grouped lichenoid papules
Lichen striatus, linear lichen planus, epidermal nevus		Linear
Molluscum contagiosum		Pearly papule with central umbilication containing easily expressed, white, cheesy core
Violaceous		
Lichen planus		Purple, pruritic, polygonal papules
Nonblanching		
Gonococcemia, SBE	Blood, throat, cervical, rectal cultures	Check for heart murmur, arthritis, tenosynovitis; distal asymmetrical palpable purpura
Henoch-Schönlein purpura†	Stool guaiac, urinalysis, skin biopsy	Abdominal pain, arthritis; crops of lesions: palpable purpura—symmetrical
Letterer-Siwe disease	Skin biopsy—histiocytes	Distinguish from seborrheic dermatitis
Leukemia cutis/lymphoma	Skin biopsy—atypical leukemic infiltrate	Lymphoma, especially Hodgkin's disease, may be pruritic
Meningococcemia, sepsis	Blood cerebrospinal fluid (CSF) culture, Gram-stain lesion	Check conjunctivae for hemorrhage, palpable purpura
Neuroblastoma, TORCH infection, leukemia	Skin biopsy	"Blueberry muffin" baby
Pseudomonas sepsis	Gram stain	Palpable purpura, ecthyma gangrenosum
Staphylococcal sepsis	Gram stain	Palpable purpura

†May be edematous.

Table 166-2 Laboratory Studies and Characteristics of Lesions—cont'd

Diagnosis or Differential Diagnosis	Laboratory Studies	Comments
Vesicles		
Congenital syphilis	+ Dark-field examination +IgM FTA-ABS test	"Snuffles"
Contact dermatitis	Patch testing	Sharp borders, linear arrays, bizarre patterns, asymmetrical
Coxsackievirus hand foot, and mouth disease	Throat culture—coxsackievirus A16,5, and 10	May be recurrent
Flea bites		Treat pet
Herpes simplex; herpes zoster	Tzanck preparation—multinucleated giant cells, viral culture to distinguish simplex from zoster	Grouped vesicles on an erythematous base; simplex labialis, progenitalis, whitlow-zoster usually linear and dermatomal
Kaposi's varicelliform eruption	Tzanck preparation	
Miliaria crystallina		Superficial
Rickettsial pox		Eschar at site of house mouse, mite bite; vesicle on top of papule
Tinea pedis	KOH scraping of vesicle roof—hyphae	
Varicella		Crops in various stages—macule, papule, vesicle, pustule and crust
Bullae		
Blistering distal dactylitis	Gram stain—gram-positive cocci in chains, culture—*Streptococcus pyogenes*	
Bullous disease of childhood	Skin biopsy for hematoxylin and eosin (H&E) stain and immunofluorescence	Refer to dermatologist to rule out bullous pemphigoid and dermatitis herpetiformis
Bullous impetigo	Culture blister fluid for phage group II *S. aureus*	
Pustules		
Acral pustulosis	Gram stain—sterile with PMNs	
Candidiasis	KOH smear of scale or pustule budding yeast and pseudohyphae	
Erythema toxicum neonatorum	Wright stain of pustule—eosinophils	Pustule in center on erythematous macule
Folliculitis	Gram stain—staphylococcal or sterile	Follicular (i.e., hair shaft) central in pustule; *pseudomonas* causes hot-tub follicuitus
Transient neonatal pustular melanosis	Gram stain of pustule—sterile with PMNs	Hyperpigmented macules; superficial desquamation
Plaques		
Acute urticaria	Eosinophil count, throat culture for streptococci, HB_sAG	Erythematous, edematous plaque, drug history, food history (shellfish)
Erysipelas/cellulitis	Culture—*Streptococcus pyogenes;* may be *S. aureus*	
Haemophilus cellulitis		Face, upper torso—associated with otitis, pneumonitis
Nummular eczema		Papules and vesicles grouped into plaques
Perianal streptococcal cellulitis	Culture—*Streptococcus pyogenes*	
Psoriasis		Well-demarcated erythematous plaque with adherent scale; check family history, arthritis

SUGGESTED READINGS

Cohen BA: *Atlas of pediatric dermatology,* London, 1993, Wolfe.

Hurwitz S: *Clinical pediatric dermatology,* ed 2, Philadelphia, 1993, WB Saunders.

Rasmussen JE: Principles of diagnosis. In Schachner LA, Hansen RC, editors: *Pediatric dermatology,* New York, 1988, Churchill Livingstone.

167 Recurrent Infections

David L. Goldman

Pediatricians as part of their daily practice frequently encounter children who have recurrent infections. The vast majority of these children are healthy. For the parents of these children, reassurance that their child is normal and that no underlying abnormality exists is particularly important. Much less commonly, recurrent infections can be a sign of an underlying disorder that may be either immunological or nonimmunological in origin. Early identification of these children is critical because prompt intervention can lead to decreased morbidity and mortality. For some of these disorders, prenatal detection is now possible and can allow for disease prevention in subsequent siblings.

NORMAL PATTERN OF INFECTIONS IN CHILDHOOD

It is crucial that pediatricians be aware of the normal pattern of infections in childhood and the signs suggestive of an underlying disorder. On average, healthy children can experience six to eight upper respiratory tract infections per year in the first few years of life. However, up to 15 infections per year can still be considered within the normal range. The high frequency of infections in the first years of life results from the relative immunological immaturity of this age group and to their frequent exposure to respiratory pathogens. Certain factors, such as attendance in child care and exposure to second-hand smoke, may increase the anticipated number of infections. In the normal host, these infections are self-limited, occur more frequently in the winter, and are associated with periods of wellness in between illnesses. Considering that the average duration of a viral illness is 7 to 10 days, a normal toddler may be sick for up to 100 days or almost one third of the year.

NONIMMUNOLOGICAL DISORDERS ASSOCIATED WITH ENHANCED SUSCEPTIBILITY TO INFECTIONS

Defense of the human body against microbial pathogens involves anatomical, physiological, and inflammatory barriers. Defects in any of these systems can lead to recurrent infections. Noninflammatory (nonimmunological) causes of recurrent infection often involve defects in the functioning or integrity of an anatomical barrier. Recurrent or unusual infections also can occur as a result of alteration in the normal microbial flora associated with antibiotic use and circulatory disorders such as venostasis. In general, recurrent bacterial infections at the same anatomical site that are not associated with other infections or other signs of an underlying syndrome should suggest the possibility of an anatomical defect that may be either congenital or acquired. This is true especially of children who have urinary tract infections and otitis media, but also may be true for other organ systems. Recurrent meningitis may occur as the result of an occult cerebral spinal fluid (CSF) leak. Recurrent pneumonia also may occur as a result of various nonimmunological causes. Repeated infection within the same region of the lung may result from alteration of the normal barrier as a result of foreign body aspiration, tracheoesophageal fistula, and gastroesophageal reflux. Recurrent pneumonia may also occur as a result of impaired function of the normal mucociliary transport as seen in cystic fibrosis and immotile cilia syndrome. When repeated episodes of pneumonia are the sole presentation of recurrent infection, the clinician also must consider the possibility of reactive airway disease, which can produce recurrent respiratory symptoms in association with pulmonary infiltrates. Reactive airway disease can be distinguished from recurrent pneumonia by a careful history and physical examination.

CLINICAL FEATURES SUGGESTIVE OF AN UNDERLYING IMMUNE DISORDER

Infrequently, pediatricians encounter a child who appears to have a history of infections that is outside the range of normal. One pattern of presentation is an increased frequency of common infections. Although an immunocompetent child can experience a single serious bacterial infection such as pneumonia, meningitis, or osteomyelitis, repeated serious bacterial infections should alert the pediatrician to the possibility of an underlying disorder. For example, a child who has recurrent meningococcal infections may have a deficiency in one of the terminal components of the complement system. Immunodeficiency syndromes also may manifest as a common infection presenting uncommonly, either with increased severity, prolonged duration, or failure to respond to appropriate treatment. Varicella, a typically benign infection in healthy, immunocompetent children, can cause overwhelming infection in children who have leukemia and prolonged illness in children who have acquired immunodeficiency syndrome (AIDS). Immunodeficiency also may be suggested by a common infection presenting at an uncommon age. Thrush or candidal diaper dermatitis presenting after 1 year of age suggests a defect in

T-cell immunity, such as that associated with human immunodeficiency virus (HIV) infection. Alternatively, immunodeficiency may present as an uncommon or opportunistic infection or as an unusual reaction to a live, attenuated vaccine. A child who develops *Pneumocystis carinii* pneumonia or cryptococcal meningitis is likely to have an underlying defect in T-cell immunity. Finally, a child who develops polio infection after oral polio virus immunization may have X-linked agammaglobulinemia.

SECONDARY IMMUNODEFICIENCY

Abnormalities of the immune system may be categorized as either primary or secondary. Primary immunodeficiencies are due to intrinsic defects in the immune system that are genetically determined. Secondary immunodeficiencies are those that are either acquired or a consequence of a nonimmunological primary syndrome. Secondary immunodeficiencies are much more common than primary immunodeficiencies and may be acquired as a result of many factors, including infection, malignancy, medication, malnutrition, splenic dysfunction, and metabolic disorders. HIV infection, which produces a combined deficiency in both humoral and cellular immunity, has become an important cause of secondary immunodeficiency over the past two decades. Infection may be acquired congenitally or horizontally. Recent advances in HIV therapy have helped decrease the morbidity and mortality associated with this disease, making early recognition and prompt intervention essential for optimal management. Secondary immunodeficiencies also may occur in the context of a nonimmunological primary disorder, including chromosomal, metabolic, and hematological diseases. Examples of some secondary immunodeficiencies are listed in Table 167-1.

PRIMARY IMMUNODEFICIENCY

Overall, primary immunodeficiency syndromes are far less common than secondary immunodeficiencies. Excluding selective IgA deficiency, primary immunodeficiencies occur at an incidence of 1 : 10,000. Because many of these syndromes are X-linked, boys are affected more commonly than girls. Most children who have primary immunodeficiencies are symptomatic within the first few years of life, with several exceptions including common variable immunodeficiency and deficiencies of the terminal complement components (see p. 1238). Primary immunodeficiencies are classified by the component of the immune system that is affected: humoral, cellular, complement, and phagocytic. Defects in various arms of the immune system are associated with enhanced susceptibility to infections by particular types of pathogens. Hence, the type of infecting pathogen may be useful in guiding the evaluation of a child who has a suspected immunodeficiency.

Associated clinical findings also may suggest a primary immunodeficiency. These findings can be nonspecific or syndrome specific. A child who has serious recurrent infections will often experience growth failure. Some of the other physical, historical, and laboratory findings that can be found in association with primary immunodeficiency syndromes are listed in Table 167-2.

Defects in Humoral Immunity

The humoral arm of the immune system refers to antibody-mediated immunity. Defects in the humoral immune system comprise 50% to 70% of symptomatic primary immunodeficiencies and can occur at various stages of B-cell development, resulting in a wide variety of clinical presentations. Syndromes range in severity from a total absence of antibody production to a selective isotype defi-

Table 167-1 Secondary Immunodeficiencies

Causes	Diseases
Infection	HIV, congenital rubella
Malignancy	Leukemia, lymphoma
Metabolic	Uremia, malnutrition, protein-losing enteropathy, diabetes, galactosemia
Chromosomal	Down syndrome, Bloom syndrome
Medications	Corticosteroids, chemotherapy, anti-rejection medication
Splenic dysfunction	Splenectomy, sickle cell disease, congenital asplenia

Table 167-2 Findings Associated with Primary Immunodeficiencies

Findings	Associated Syndromes
Intractable diarrhea and malabsorption	Severe combined immunodeficiency (SCID), X-linked agammaglobulinemia (XLA), common variable immunodeficiency (CVID)
Rheumatological conditions	CVID, IgA deficiency, XLA
Hepatosplenomegaly, lymphadenopathy	Hyper IgM syndrome
Absence of lymph tissue	XLA
Thrombocytopenia	Wiskott-Aldrich syndrome
Eczema	Wiskott-Aldrich syndrome, Chronic granulomatous disease, Job's syndrome
Oculocutaneous albinism	Chédiak-Higashi syndrome

ciency. Given the protective effects of maternally acquired antibody, even the most severely affected children (i.e., those who have a total absence of antibody production) do not become symptomatic until after the first few months of life. Humoral immunity plays an important role in host response against a variety of pathogens and is recognized especially for its primary role in the immune response against encapsulated pathogens. Children who have defects in the humoral immune system are characteristically susceptible to recurrent infections with encapsulated bacteria, including *Streptococcus pneumonia* and *Haemophilus influenzae.* These children generally are not more susceptible to viral infections but may experience severe or persistent enterovirus and rotavirus infections. Persistent campylobacter infections also may occur. Children who have defects in humoral immunity also are predisposed to autoimmune disorders, such as dermatomyositis and asymmetric arthritis. Table 167-3 lists some of the more common humoral immunodeficiency syndromes.

Defects in Cellular Immunity

Cellular immunity refers to immune responses mediated primarily by T lymphocytes. Children who have defects in cellular immunity are characteristically more susceptible to fungal, mycobacterial, and viral infections. These children may present with recurrent and/or persistent candidiasis in the form of thrush and diaper candidiasis. Failure to thrive and *Pneumocystis carinii* pneumonia often are observed in association with T-cell defects. T cells play an important role in B-cell development and function; hence, children who have defects in T-cell immunity usually have associated defects in humoral immunity and can be susceptible to pyogenic bacterial infections. Severe combined immunodeficiency (SCID), which represents a collection of disorders, is characterized by combined deficiencies in both humoral and cellular immunity. Children who have SCID typically present in the first few months of life with intractable diarrhea, failure to thrive, recurrent candidiasis, and pneumonia, which often is due to *Pneumocystis carinii* infection. Table 167-4

Table 167-3 Humoral Immunodeficiencies

Syndrome	Clinical Features	Associated Features
X-linked agammaglobulinemia	Susceptibility to encapsulated bacterial pathogens. Sinopulmonary and gastrointestinal infections, sepsis, meningitis. Enhanced susceptibility to enterovirus and rotavirus. Symptomatic polio infection following live polio vaccination.	Asymmetric arthritis, dermatomyositis, malabsorption, absence of tonsils, adenoids, and lymph nodes
Transient hypogammaglobulinemia of infancy	Recurrent sinopulmonary infections; generally improves by 3-4 yr of age	May develop IgA deficiency
Hyper-IgM syndrome	X-linked. Recurrent bacterial infections including encapsulated pathogens. Infections associated with T-cell defects (e.g., *Pneumocystis carinii*) also seen.	Low levels of IgG, IgA, and IgE. Neutropenia, thrombocytopenia, T-cell defects
Common variable immunodeficiency	Sinopulmonary infections Bronchiectasis Giardiasis	Most common in second and third decade. Noncaseating granulomas, malabsorption, autoimmune disease
IgA deficiency	Very common (1 in 400 individuals) but usually asymptomatic. Recurrent pulmonary infections leading to bronchiectasis.	Systemic lupus erythematosus, rheumatoid arthritis, chronic diarrhea. Allergic reactions to gamma globulin preparations. IgG subclass deficiency in some
IgG subclass deficiency	Clinical significance not well delineated	

Table 167-4 Cellular Immunodeficiencies

Syndrome	Clinical Features	Associated Features
DiGeorge	Clinically variable. Increased viral and fungal infections	Hypocalcemia, hypoparathyroidism, congenital heart disease, abnormal facies
Severe combined immunodeficiency (SCID)	Both B-cell and T-cell deficiencies present. Includes a variety of disorders that have multiple modes of inheritance. Presents early in life (before 6 mo of age) with recurrent/severe infections with all types of pathogens.	Failure to thrive, diarrhea
Chronic mucocutaneous candidiasis	Chronic candidal infections affecting skin, mucous membranes, and nail beds	Hypoparathyroidism and other endocrinopathies

Table 167-5 Phagocytic Immunodeficiencies

Syndromes	Clinical Features	Associated Features
Chronic granulomatous disease (CGD)	Often X-linked. Recurrent infection of skin, lungs, liver, lymph nodes, and bone. Infections with catalase-positive organisms (staphylococci, *Escherichia coli,* and *Candida albicans*).	Eczema, lymphadenopathy, hepatosplenomegaly
Chédiak-Higashi syndrome	Autosomal recessive. Recurrent pyogenic infections with organisms similar to those seen in CGD.	Ocular albinism, lymphoreticular malignancies. Neutrophils have abnormally large granules.
Job's syndrome	Recurrent sinopulmonary infections and skin abscesses	Eczema, red hair, coarse facies, high IgE levels
Leukocyte adhesion defect	Autosomal recessive. Recurrent bacterial infections and necrotic skin lesions.	Leukocytosis with absence of neutrophils at infection site. Severe gingivitis, early loss of teeth. Delayed separation of umbilical cord.

lists some of the more common primary cellular immunodeficiency syndromes.

Defects in Phagocytic Immunity

Phagocytes form the first line of defense against a number of pathogens and are considered part of the nonspecific immune response. Children who have defects in phagocytic immunity are particularly predisposed to infections with staphylococci, nocardia, and fungal and gram-negative organisms. Recurrent skin infections and abscesses often are observed in affected children. A wide variety of defects in the phagocytic system exists, ranging from the absence of a particular phagocyte type (cyclical neutropenia) to defects in chemotaxis (leukocyte adhesion defect) and defects in effector function (chronic granulomatous disease). A description of some of the more common syndromes associated with defects in phagocytic immunity is given in Table 167-5.

Defects in the Complement System

Complement acts to lyse target cells and, as an opsonin, promotes the phagocytosis of microbial pathogens. Defects in the complement system are the least common among the primary immunodeficiencies. Congenital deficiencies in the late or terminal components of the complement system (C5, C6, C7, C8, and C9) are inherited as autosomal recessive traits and result in recurrent neisserial infections. In contrast to many of the primary immunodeficiencies, terminal complement deficiencies tend to present in older children and in adolescents. Those affected develop recurrent meningococcal infection (meningitis or meningococcemia) or gonococcal arthritis. Deficiencies in the C3 component result in an increased susceptibility to encapsulated bacterial pathogens. This disorder may present similarly to antibody deficiencies but tends to occur at an earlier age, within the first few months of life.

OTHER PRIMARY IMMUNODEFICIENCY DISORDERS

Some primary immunodeficiency disorders cannot be classified in any of the above categories. Wiskott-Aldrich is an X-linked disorder associated with the triad of thrombocytopenia, eczema, and recurrent infections. Affected infants often present with bleeding in the first few years of life. The basis for this disorder is not well understood. Ataxia-telangiectasia is an autosomal recessive disorder producing progressive ataxia and conjunctival telangiectasias. Affected children have decreased IgA levels and altered T-cell function; they experience an increased frequency of sinopulmonary infections and are at risk for malignancy.

EVALUATION OF THE CHILD WHO IS SUSPECTED OF HAVING PRIMARY IMMUNODEFICIENCY

History

An evaluation for a primary immunodeficiency should be performed after nonimmunological and secondary immunodeficiency syndromes have been considered. A complete history should be obtained for all children being evaluated for recurrent infections, including a history of risk factors for HIV infection: parental drug use, prostitution, blood-product transfusion, multiple sexual partners, or history of sexually transmitted disease and homosexual behavior. Particular attention should be paid to documenting the characteristics of previous infections: types of pathogens and infections, duration of illnesses, and need for hospitalizations. Because many of the primary immunodeficiencies are hereditary, a detailed family history is important. A complete review of systems should be obtained, with attention paid to known associated features of immunodeficiency syndromes, including failure to thrive. The immunization history is important, because failure to make protective antibodies in response to immunizations can be indicative of immunodeficiency.

Table 167-6 Laboratory Examination

Immunodeficiency	Screening Tests	General Comments
Humoral (B cell)	Serum immunoglobulin levels (IgG, IgM, IgA). Antibody titers against protein (diphtheria, tetanus toxoid) and polysaccharide *(Haemophilus)* antigens.	Antibody levels must be interpreted with respect to age-appropriate values. High or low levels can be significant.
Cellular (T cell)	Lymphocyte count Anergy testing	Total lymphocyte count obtained by multiplying total white blood cell count by the percent of lymphocytes. Value <1500/μl is considered lymphopenia. Anergy testing not reliable for children younger than 1 yr.
Phagocytic (macrophage/ neutrophil)	CBC IgE level NBT (Nitroblue tetrazolium test)/Flow cytometric respiratory burst assay	Abnormal neutrophil morphology may be present. IgE level elevated in Job's syndrome.
Complement	CH_{50}	Screening assay for components of classic complement pathway. May not be sensitive for limited deficiencies in individual complement components.

Physical Examination

A complete physical examination should be performed. Many children who have immunodeficiency appear chronically ill. Growth parameters (height, weight, and head circumference percentiles) should be obtained to determine the presence of failure to thrive. Physical findings that may indicate underlying immunodeficiency include absence of tonsils and generalized lymphadenopathy and hepatosplenomegaly. Skin lesions (eczema, abscesses, seborrhea) and mucous membrane involvement (telangiectasias, mucositis) are observed with some immunological disorders. Other findings of immunodeficiency may include signs of recurrent infection (e.g., dull, retracted tympanic membranes) and evidence of ongoing infection (e.g., thrush). Specific findings associated with a particular immunodeficiency syndrome, such as oculocutaneous albinism in Chédiak-Higashi syndrome, also may be present.

Laboratory Evaluation and Referral

Laboratory evaluation for a child who is suspected of having an immunodeficiency should be guided by the type of infections the child is experiencing. Initial screening tests usually include complete blood count and differential, serum immunoglobulin levels (IgG, IgA, IgM), and lymphocyte count. Most primary immunodeficiency syndromes will be associated with abnormal serum immunoglobulin levels. HIV testing should be strongly considered, as indicated by the history and physical findings. In an area that has a high prevalence of HIV infection, testing should be considered even if no obvious risk factor can be identified. Table 167-6 lists the initial screening tests to be considered for each component of the immune system. Regardless of the results of initial screening tests, referral to a specialist, either immunologist or infectious disease expert, should be considered for those children who have signs and symptoms suggestive of immunodeficiency. Pending a complete immunological evaluation, children who are suspected of having immunodeficiency syndromes should not receive live attenuated vaccines, such as OPV and measles, to avoid the possibility of vaccination-induced infection. Needed blood transfusions should be performed with cytomegalovirus (CMV)-negative, irradiated cells to prevent the possibility of transfusion-related CMV infection and graft-versus-host disease.

SUGGESTED READINGS

Dizon JG, Goldberg BJ, Kaplan MS: How to evaluate suspected immunodeficiency, *Pediatr Ann* 27 742, 1998.

Puck J: Primary immunodeficiency diseases, *JAMA* 278, 1835, 1997.

Stiehm ER: *Immunologic disorders in infants and children,* ed 4, Philadelphia, 1996, WB Saunders.

Ten RM: Primary immunodeficiencies, *Mayo Clin Proc* 73:865, 1998.

168 Red Eye

James W. McManaway III • Carl A. Frankel

Red eye is hyperemia of the bulbar conjunctiva, which occurs with inflammation of the conjunctiva, cornea, episclera, sclera, or anterior uvea. The differential diagnosis of red eye in childhood includes (1) conjunctivitis, (2) nasolacrimal duct obstruction, (3) keratitis, (4) iritis, and (5) glaucoma. "Pink eye" is a lay term that refers to conjunctivitis.

CONJUNCTIVITIS

Conjunctivitis means inflammation of the conjunctiva, which is characterized by conjunctival hyperemia and discharge that varies from clear to purulent. Because of the close association of the conjunctiva with them, many forms of conjunctivitis involve the eyelid and cornea as well. The causes of conjunctivitis in children include (1) allergens, (2) bacteria, (3) viruses, (4) chlamydia, (5) toxins, (6) immunological reactions, and (7) ophthalmia neonatorum. Although most types of conjunctivitis do not present an acute risk to the eye, conjunctivitis should be evaluated promptly so that appropriate intervention can be instituted.

Allergic Conjunctivitis

Allergic conjunctivitis is a noninfectious disorder characterized by itching, conjunctival chemosis (edema), and conjunctival hyperemia. Frequently, tearing also is present. The condition may be unilateral or bilateral and may be asymptomatic. The six types of allergic conjunctivitis are (1) seasonal allergic rhinoconjunctivitis, (2) vernal keratoconjunctivitis, (3) giant papillary conjunctivitis, (4) contact allergic dermatoconjunctivitis, (5) atopic keratoconjunctivitis, and (6) phlyctenular keratoconjunctivitis.[3]

Seasonal allergic rhinoconjunctivitis. Seasonal allergic rhinoconjunctivitis, also called hay fever conjunctivitis, is the most common form of allergic conjunctivitis. It is an IgE-mediated immediate hypersensitivity reaction to airborne allergens. During times of high pollen counts, patients have red, itchy, tearing eyes. Minimal ocular signs are present besides conjunctival redness, although patients occasionally may show eyelid edema or increased skin pigmentation called "allergic shiners." Treatment includes avoidance of known allergens and use of artificial tears as necessary. Children who have more severe symptoms can be treated with topical mast cell stabilizers, such as lodoxamide tromethamine (Alomide) or cromolyn sodium (Crolom). Olopatadine hydrochloride (Patanol) is a combination mast cell stabilizer and antihistamine. Children 12 years of age and older can be treated with the topical antihistamine levocabastine hydrochloride (Livostin) or the topical nonsteroidal anti-inflammatory agent ketorolac tromethamine (Acular); the safety and efficacy of these two drugs have not yet been established in younger children.

Vernal keratoconjunctivitis. Vernal keratoconjunctivitis is a rare form of allergic conjunctivitis characterized by severe ocular itching, ropy mucus discharge that can be pulled like a string from the conjunctival surface, and giant papillae on the upper tarsal conjunctiva (Fig. 168-1). Gelatinous nodules at the corneoscleral limbus are more common in dark-skinned children. Corneal complications such as limbal neovascularization, central epithelial keratitis, and corneal "shield" ulcer may occur. As the name implies, the allergy is much worse in the spring and early summer. Patients often develop symptoms first between age 10 and 13 years and may be symptomatic each spring for the next 10 or so years. Because of the severity of the symptoms, the frequent need for topical corticosteroids to control symptoms, and the risks of cataracts, glaucoma, and herpes simplex keratitis associated with long-term topical steroid use, these patients should be referred to an ophthalmologist for management. Typical management includes topical corticosteroids, topical mast cell stabilizers, and topical and systemic antihistamines.

Giant papillary conjunctivitis. Giant papillary conjunctivitis (GPC) nearly always is associated with contact lens wear and has been reported among patients wearing hard, rigid, gas-permeable, and soft contact lenses. Patients initially have conjunctival hyperemia, mucus accumulation, increased awareness of the contact lens, and itching on removal of the lens. End-stage GPC is characterized by the presence of giant papillae on the upper tarsal conjunctiva, copious mucus production, and contact lens intolerance. GPC is thought to be an allergic reaction to antigen (degraded mucus) coating the contact lens as well as a reaction to mechanical trauma caused by the lens. These patients should be referred for treatment to the eye care professional who dispensed the contact lenses. Treatment options include no contact lens wear, better contact lens hygiene, use of a different contact lens type, and topical cromolyn sodium.

Contact allergic conjunctivitis. Contact allergic conjunctivitis is characterized by itching, watery discharge; conjunctival edema; and hyperemia associated with redness and edema of the periorbital skin. Possible sources include

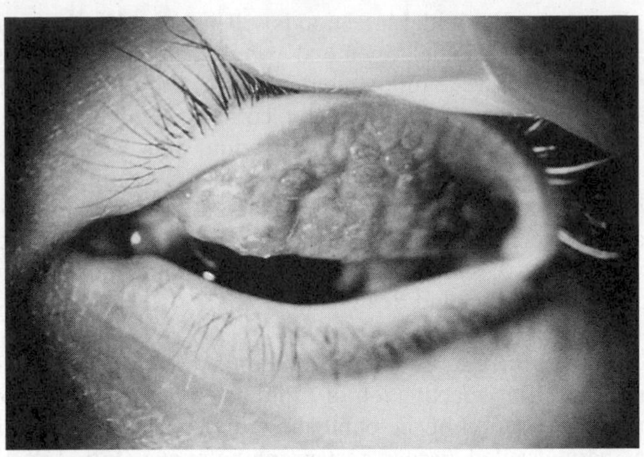

Fig. 168-1 Vernal conjunctivitis with giant papillae on the upper tarsal conjunctiva.

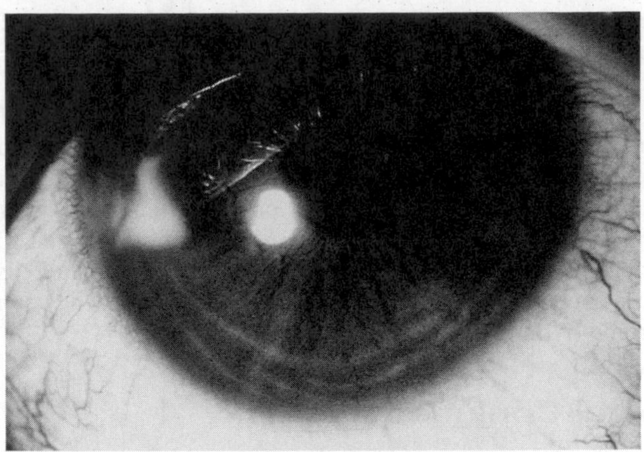

Fig. 168-2 Phlyctenular keratoconjunctivitis with corneal scarring and trailing "leash" of conjunctival vessels.

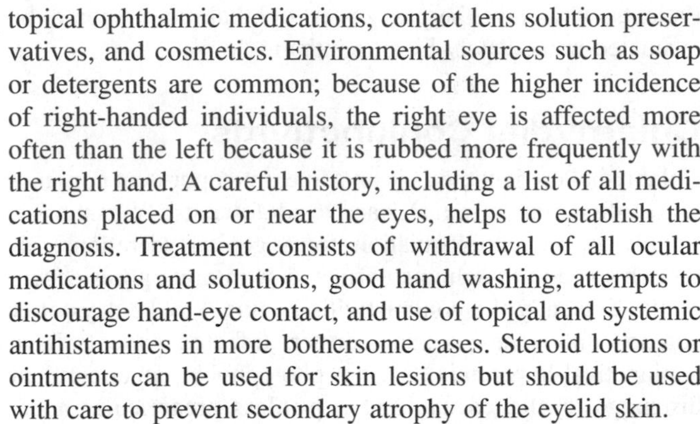

topical ophthalmic medications, contact lens solution preservatives, and cosmetics. Environmental sources such as soap or detergents are common; because of the higher incidence of right-handed individuals, the right eye is affected more often than the left because it is rubbed more frequently with the right hand. A careful history, including a list of all medications placed on or near the eyes, helps to establish the diagnosis. Treatment consists of withdrawal of all ocular medications and solutions, good hand washing, attempts to discourage hand-eye contact, and use of topical and systemic antihistamines in more bothersome cases. Steroid lotions or ointments can be used for skin lesions but should be used with care to prevent secondary atrophy of the eyelid skin.

Atopic keratoconjunctivitis. Atopic keratoconjunctivitis is a vision-threatening disease that occurs in 25% to 40% of atopic individuals. It occurs most frequently in males around 20 years of age. Patients have extreme itching, copious discharge of mucus, conjunctival hyperemia, and redness, scaling, and maceration of the eyelids and periorbital skin. Conjunctival papillae develop on the upper and lower tarsal conjunctiva; the location of the papillae and the older age of these patients differentiate atopic from vernal keratoconjunctivitis. The eyelid appearance and discharge of mucus distinguish atopic keratoconjunctivitis from seasonal allergic rhinoconjunctivitis. Corneal complications include epithelial keratitis, a chronic defect that can become infected secondarily, and corneal scarring and vascularization. Teenagers who have atopic keratoconjunctivitis are at risk of developing cataracts. Patients who have atopic keratoconjunctivitis should be referred to an ophthalmologist. Management includes short courses of topical corticosteroids, topical cromolyn sodium, oral antihistamines, eyelid hygiene to treat associated blepharitis, and steroid ointments to the eyelid skin.

Phlyctenular keratoconjunctivitis. Phlyctenular keratoconjunctivitis is characterized by a heavily vascularized, whitish yellow, elevated lesion, usually located near the limbus. Left untreated, the conjunctival phlyctenule advances into the cornea with a trailing leash of vessels (Fig. 168-2). In developing nations, tuberculosis is the most common association; however, in industrialized nations an allergic reaction to the *Staphylococcus* exotoxin is the suspected cause. Treatment with topical steroids is extremely effective but should be performed under the care of an ophthalmologist.

Bacterial Conjunctivitis

Patients who have bacterial conjunctivitis often experience tearing, photophobia, and a foreign-body sensation. The conjunctiva has moderate to severe hyperemia; the conjunctival discharge may be watery to serous initially, but becomes mucopurulent with a green to yellow color. The discharge may be mild or so copious that the eyelids become pasted shut. Eyelid edema and erythema may be worrisome. Typical causative agents include strains of *Staphylococcus, Streptococcus, Pneumococcus,* and *Haemophilus influenzae*; strains of *Pseudomonas, Klebsiella,* and *Neisseria* are encountered less frequently.

Neisseria gonorrhoeae causes a hyperacute conjunctivitis with copious purulent discharge and severe eyelid edema. The examiner should wear eye protection because infected secretions can be expelled forcibly upon attempts to open the swollen eyelids. Gonococcal conjunctivitis is a medical emergency: The organism can invade intact corneal epithelium, resulting in corneal ulceration or perforation with resultant bacterial endophthalmitis. An ophthalmologist should be consulted immediately.

Bacterial conjunctivitis generally is diagnosed on clinical grounds alone. Because most bacterial conjunctivitis responds readily to topical antibiotics, cultures and sensitivity determinations usually are not necessary unless *Pseudomonas, Neisseria,* or another particularly virulent organism is suspected. Treatment with ophthalmic solutions is easier than with ophthalmic ointments, and the response frequently is dramatic. Sodium sulfacetamide (10% solution) is useful in most cases, although polymyxin B sulfate-trimethoprim sulfate solution (Polytrim) has a broader spectrum and is well tolerated. Because of the small volume of the conjunctival cul-de-sac, only one drop is needed in each eye every 3 hours up to six times daily. Gentamicin and tobramycin should be reserved for suspected gram-negative bacterial conjunctivitis and for cases in which culture and sensitivity results justify their use. Treatment should be continued for 24 to 48 hours after the conjunctival hyperemia and purulence have subsided.

Gonococcal conjunctivitis should be treated with a single intramuscular dose of ceftriaxone (1 g or 50 mg/kg in patients weighing less than 20 kg).[2] If keratitis is present, saline lavage and topical erythromycin ointment four times daily should be added. The patients also should be evaluated for chlamydial conjunctivitis and other sexually transmitted diseases such as syphilis and acquired immunodeficiency syndrome (AIDS).

Viral Conjunctivitis

The three major causes of viral conjunctivitis are adenovirus, herpes simplex virus, and varicella-zoster virus. Adenoviral infections are the most common and have two types: epidemic keratoconjunctivitis and pharyngoconjunctival fever. Epidemic keratoconjunctivitis (EKC) is caused by adenovirus types 8, 19A, and 37. Transmission occurs through respiratory tract-to-eye and finger-to-eye pathways, as well as by contaminated swimming pools. Affected patients have moderate conjunctival hyperemia, watery discharge, photophobia, and a tender preauricular node. Treatment consists of artificial tears to lubricate the eyes and isolation of the patient to prevent further outbreaks. Some patients develop inflammatory membranes and keratitis; they should be treated with topical steroid drops by an ophthalmologist. Pharyngoconjunctival fever is caused by adenovirus types 3, 4, and 7. These patients have similar ocular signs but also have pharyngitis, fever, and malaise.

Herpes simplex virus. Herpes simplex virus can cause a host of ocular problems and is associated with disseminated encephalitis in infants. A primary herpetic ocular infection typically manifests as a unilateral conjunctivitis with watery discharge and photophobia several days to 2 weeks following close personal contact. Patients frequently have eyelid vesicles and a tender preauricular node. Some patients have an epithelial keratitis, which may be punctate or show a classical dendrite (Fig. 168-3) after application of fluorescein dye when the eye is viewed with a cobalt blue light source. The initial infection is self-limited, but the virus remains latent in the trigeminal ganglion and, with stress, fever, or exposure to ultraviolet light, infection can recur. The recurrences are characterized by corneal involvement and lead to corneal scarring, vascularization, and decreased vision. Amblyopia is a common problem in young children who have recurrent herpes simplex keratitis. Children who have conjunctivitis and lid vesicles or corneal staining with fluorescein dye should be referred to an ophthalmologist for further evaluation and treatment.

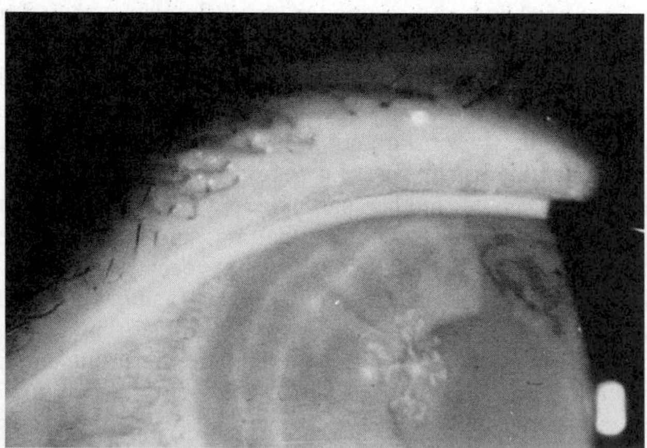

Fig. 168-3 Typical herpes simplex virus dendrites stained with fluorescein and viewed with a cobalt blue light.

Varicella-zoster virus. Immunocompromised children may have reactivation of a previous varicella infection in the distribution of the ophthalmic division of the trigeminal nerve, called *herpes zoster ophthalmicus* (Fig. 168-4). Affected patients can have conjunctivitis, keratitis, uveitis, glaucoma, optic neuritis, and other cranial nerve palsies. The diagnosis is easy when the characteristic skin changes are present, but these do not always precede the ocular signs. Patients who have herpes zoster ophthalmicus should be evaluated immediately by an ophthalmologist.

Chlamydial Conjunctivitis

Chlamydial conjunctivitis is an acute, mucopurulent conjunctivitis often seen in sexually active adolescents. Transmission usually is by autoinoculation from genital secretions, although spread through unchlorinated swimming pools occurs rarely. Typically the conjunctivitis begins 4 to 12 days after contact with a new sexual partner. Infected patients have conjunctival hyperemia, tearing, photophobia, mucopurulent discharge, eyelid edema, and a painless preauricular node.

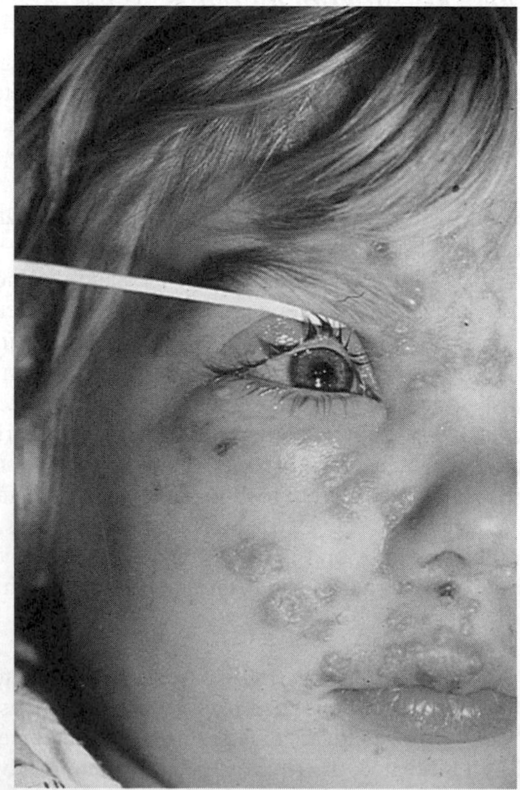

Fig. 168-4 Herpes zoster ophthalmicus in a child.

The diagnosis is made most readily by using direct immunofluorescent antibody testing of conjunctival scrapings. Topical therapy alone is ineffective; it must be combined with systemic antibiotics such as erythromycin (250 mg orally four times daily for 3 weeks). Untreated patients may have a chronic conjunctivitis for up to 18 months. Sexual contacts also must be treated to prevent spread to or reinfection from them.

Toxic Conjunctivitis

Toxic conjunctivitis occurs as a direct (not allergic) effect of some ocular medications and a host of foreign substances that can be splashed, sprayed, aerosolized, or rubbed into the eye. Toxic conjunctivitis occurs immediately to several hours after contact by the offending substance, whereas contact allergy generally requires about 2 days for symptoms to develop. Treatment of toxic conjunctivitis includes ocular irrigation and care to avoid future exposure. Ocular chemical injuries are discussed in Chapter 242, Ocular Trauma.

Immunological Conjunctivitis

Erythema multiforme is an acute systemic disorder thought to be an acute hypersensitivity reaction that occurs after exposure to infectious agents, drugs, or certain foods. Some patients develop a skin rash that resolves after several days. Other patients have severe skin and mucous membrane disease with conjunctival involvement, known as *Stevens-Johnson syndrome*. Patients who have Stevens-Johnson syndrome develop a mucopurulent conjunctivitis that may progress to conjunctival necrosis. The conjunctival damage leads to complications, including adhesions between the tarsal and bulbar conjunctiva (symblepharon), eyelid margin changes with inturned lashes (entropion with trichiasis), and a chronic dry eye syndrome caused by loss of normal conjunctival function. These problems can lead to corneal scarring and permanent visual loss.

Patients who have Stevens-Johnson syndrome require admission to the hospital. The use of systemic steroids to control the immune complex-mediated vasculitis is controversial. Ocular management includes topical ocular steroids and antibiotics to reduce conjunctival inflammation and prevent secondary infection. Conjunctival adhesions must be lysed daily with a glass rod under topical anesthesia. After the acute conjunctivitis resolves, these patients require artificial tears and careful observation for the development of vision-threatening corneal complications.

Ophthalmia Neonatorum

Ophthalmia neonatorum is defined as conjunctivitis occurring in the first month of life. The causes can be (1) chemical, (2) chlamydial, (3) bacterial, and (4) viral. The most common cause of ophthalmia neonatorum is a chemical conjunctivitis from the 1% silver nitrate drops given as prophylaxis for gonococcal or chlamydial conjunctivitis. This conjunctivitis usually is characterized by conjunctival hyperemia, mild lid edema, and scanty discharge. Chemical conjunctivitis usually resolves over 24 to 48 hours without sequelae. Because of the chemical conjunctivitis caused by silver nitrate drops, most hospitals use erythromycin ophthalmic ointment, which also prevents most cases of chlamydial and other bacterial ophthalmia neonatorum.

The most common infectious cause of ophthalmia neonatorum is inclusion conjunctivitis from *Chlamydia trachomatis*, characterized by a mucoid or mucopurulent discharge and mild lid edema with conjunctival hyperemia. Bacterial ophthalmia neonatorum usually is caused by *Neisseria, Staphylococcus, Pneumococcus,* or *H. influenzae* organisms. Bacterial conjunctivitis is characterized by a moderate or profuse purulent discharge with significant conjunctival hyperemia (Fig. 168-5); eyelid edema also may be severe. Viral ophthalmia neonatorum, caused by herpes simplex virus (see Fig. 168-3), has mild conjunctival hyperemia with a serous discharge, although the cornea may be hazy if a simultaneous keratitis is present.

The diagnosis is determined by direct immunofluorescent antibody testing for *Chlamydia* organisms and by culture for bacteria and herpes simplex virus. Conjunctival scraping and plating at the bedside recovers the organism more often than the use of a cotton applicator sent to the microbiology laboratory. Treatment is organism specific, with systemic therapy reserved for herpes simplex virus, *Chlamydia,* or *Neisseria* infections.

As a guide, gram-positive organisms usually are well treated with sodium sulfacetamide 10% solution every 4 hours. *Haemophilus* species should be treated with topical polymyxin B sulfate-trimethoprim sulfate solution (Polytrim). Gentamycin or tobramycin should be reserved for gram-negative organisms. Inclusion conjunctivitis should be treated with topical and systemic erythromycin (10 mg/kg four times a day) for at least 3 weeks. Herpes simplex keratoconjunctivitis is treated best with idoxuridine (Herplex) or trifluridine (Viroptic) solution topically, under the direction of an ophthalmologist, with appropriate systemic antiviral agents. *Neisseria gonorrhoeae* ophthalmia neonatorum is treated with a single dose of intramuscular ceftriaxone (50 mg/kg).[2] The parents and any sexual partners of either also need to be treated in cases of gonococcal and chlamydial ophthalmia neonatorum.

In the past, the causative agent of ophthalmia neonatorum was predicted based on the time of onset of the conjunctivi-

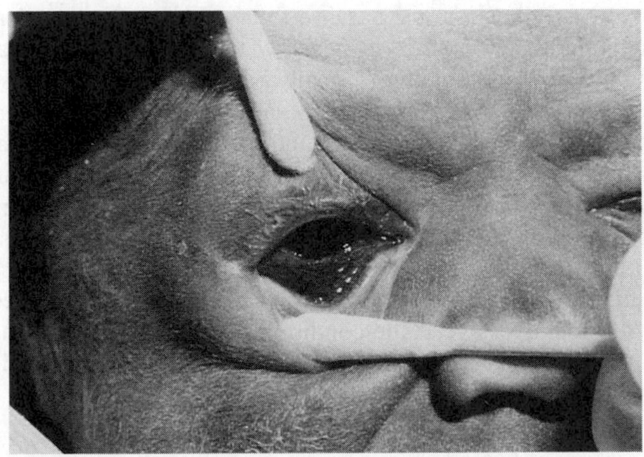

Fig. 168-5 Early bacterial ophthalmia neonatorum treated successfully with topical antibiotics.

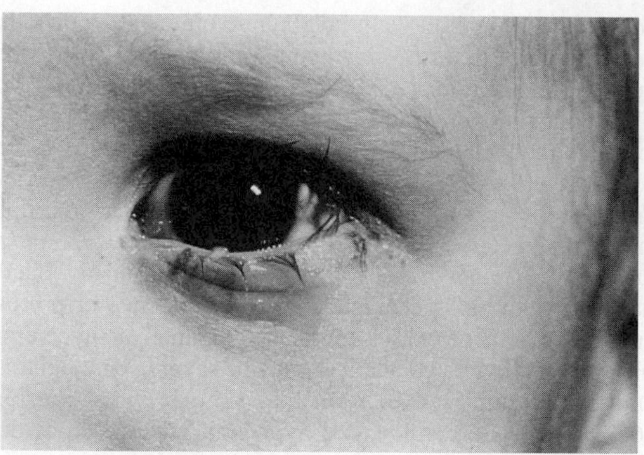

Fig. 168-6 Congenital nasolacrimal duct obstruction. Note the significant discharge, usually accompanied by epiphora. In the absence of conjunctival hyperemia, antibiotic therapy is not indicated and treatment is with nasolacrimal sac massage.

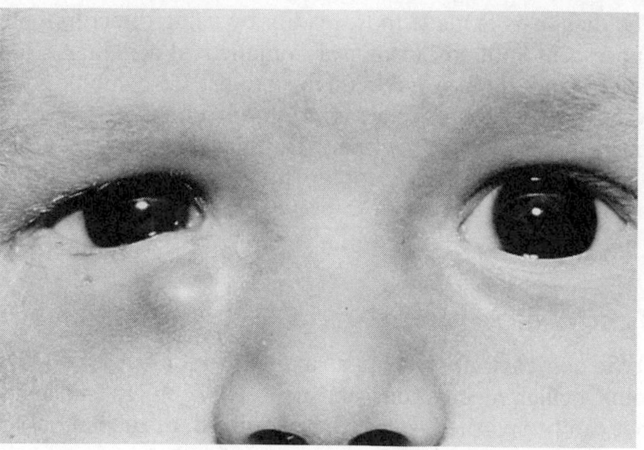

Fig. 168-7 Acute dacryocystitis secondary to nasolacrimal duct obstruction where massage was not performed. Pressure on the tear sac led to mucopurulent reflux from the superior and inferior puncta. Resolution of the dacryocystitis was complete with topical and systemic antibiotics, and nasolacrimal sac massage was successful in overcoming the obstruction.

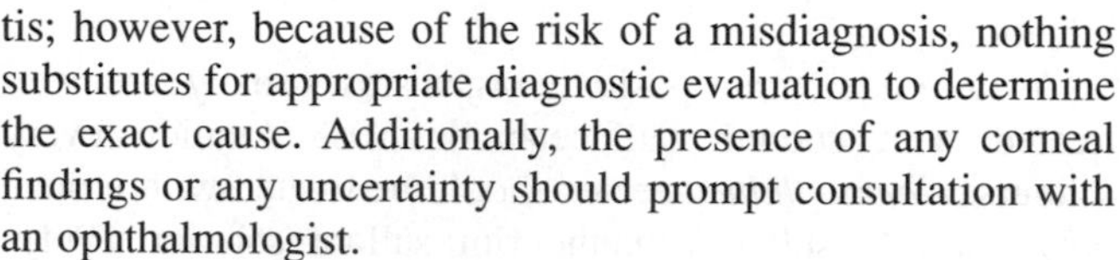

tis; however, because of the risk of a misdiagnosis, nothing substitutes for appropriate diagnostic evaluation to determine the exact cause. Additionally, the presence of any corneal findings or any uncertainty should prompt consultation with an ophthalmologist.

NASOLACRIMAL DUCT OBSTRUCTION

Nasolacrimal duct obstruction may be present in as many as 6% to 7% of healthy full-term infants (Fig. 168-6). Fortunately, this common condition resolves spontaneously in about 90% of infants by 12 months of age. Occasionally, dacryocystitis (infection in the nasolacrimal sac) (Fig. 168-7) may occur and can progress to preseptal or orbital cellulitis. Treatment of nasolacrimal duct obstruction is varied; ophthalmological opinion is split between early nasolacrimal duct probing and conservative management via nasolacrimal sac massage and topical antibiotics when purulence is present. Nasolacrimal sac massage is performed with five strokes from just beneath the medial aspect of the brow in a downward direction just nasal to the medial canthus and terminating about ¼ to ½ inch below the level of the medial canthus. The use solely of downward strokes serves to raise the pressure in the nasolacrimal sac in an attempt to overcome the obstruction usually found at the distal nasolacrimal duct. The success rate with conservative treatment is about 90% by 1 year of age, although nasolacrimal duct probing often is performed early to deal with parental unhappiness with the chronic tearing and accumulation of mucus in the conjunctival sac.[4] Referral to an ophthalmologist is indicated by 6 months of age if the condition persists or earlier if the purulent discharge cannot be controlled by topical antibiotic eye drops.

KERATITIS

Inflammation of the cornea (keratitis) indicates significant ocular disease that needs urgent attention from an ophthalmologist. Because the cornea is relatively avascular, keratitis usually is associated with perilimbal conjunctival hyperemia (ciliary flush), which may simulate conjunctivitis. If the corneal epithelium is damaged, the pain can be quite intense. Otherwise, a mild to moderate foreign-body sensation, blepharospasm, and significant tearing are present. Under normal conditions the cornea has a bright luster; however, when keratitis is present, the cornea often is hazy, with a dull corneal light reflex on direct illumination with a penlight. Important forms of keratitis include (1) trauma, such as a corneal abrasion or chemical injury; (2) exposure, such as in patients who have decreased corneal sensation (Fig. 168-8) or a facial nerve palsy; (3) infectious, such as in patients who have bacterial, viral, fungal, or parasitic infections of the cornea; and (4) interstitial, such as in patients who have congenital syphilis who develop eye symptoms between 5 and 15 years of age. Fluorescein staining can help distinguish herpes simplex virus keratitis from other forms by the characteristic dendrites associated with it.

IRITIS

Iritis is an inflammation of the anterior uvea (iris or ciliary body) and can indicate a severe, vision-threatening condition or even the initial manifestation of systemic disease. As in keratitis, the primary symptom frequently is a ciliary flush or generalized conjunctival hyperemia. Blepharospasm, reactive ptosis, photophobia, epiphora, and pupillary miosis (secondary to spasm of the constrictor muscle) are common. Iritis may be either unilateral or bilateral, and the more posterior layers of the uvea also may be involved. Untreated iritis can result in glaucoma, cataracts, posterior synechiae (adhesions between the iris and the lens), and blindness. Because of the conjunctival hyperemia and epiphora, a diagnosis of conjunctivitis often is entertained first, and treatment with a topical antibiotic is instituted; however, the lack of a rapid clinical response soon should prompt suspicion. Chronic treatment with an antibiotic may allow the posterior synechiae to become quite advanced (Fig. 168-9); thus, any patient who has

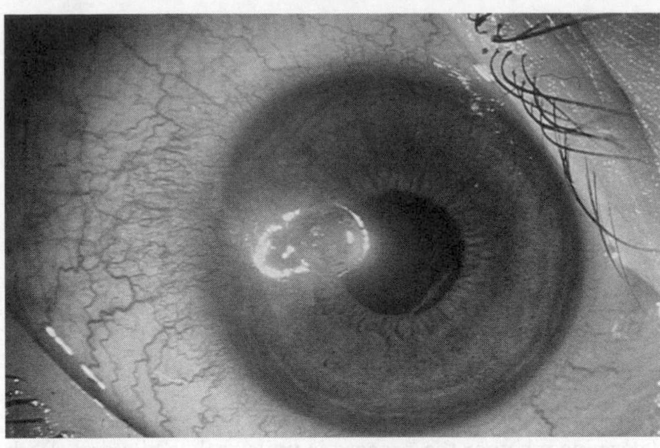

Fig. 168-8 Neurotrophic keratitis in a child who has neurofibromatosis and decreased corneal sensation of the right eye.

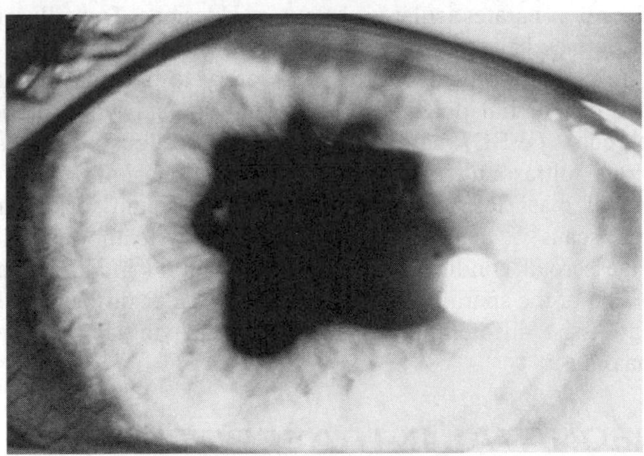

Fig. 168-9 Chronic anterior uveitis treated for 5 months as a chronic "conjunctivitis." Note the irregular pupil caused by posterior synechiae.

presumed conjunctivitis that does not respond readily should be referred to an ophthalmologist to rule out iritis. If iritis is diagnosed, systemic disease should be considered. Patients who have pauciarticular, antinuclear antibody–positive juvenile rheumatoid arthritis can have significant iridocyclitis without the typical conjunctival hyperemia; these patients must be examined by an ophthalmologist via a slit-lamp biomicroscope at the time of diagnosis and every 3 months thereafter for several years.[1] Iritis is treated with mydriatic and cycloplegic agents to reduce the ciliary spasm and topical steroid agents (under the care of an ophthalmologist) to reduce inflammation and lessen the risk of posterior synechiae.

GLAUCOMA

Infantile or congenital glaucoma usually is diagnosed readily by the presence of corneal enlargement. However, this rare condition sometimes is mistaken for conjunctivitis or nasolacrimal duct obstruction. The symptomatic constellation of tearing, photophobia, fussiness, and failure to thrive with signs of corneal enlargement (buphthalmos) and cloudiness should prompt urgent referral to an ophthalmologist so that the intraocular pressure can be managed (usually by surgery) to minimize loss of vision.

REFERENCES

1. American Academy of Pediatrics Section on Rheumatology and Section on Ophthalmology: Guidelines for ophthalmologic examinations in children with juvenile rheumatoid arthritis, *Pediatrics* 92:295, 1993.
2. Haimovici R, Roussel TJ: Treatment of gonococcal conjunctivitis with single-dose intramuscular ceftriaxone, *Am J Ophthalmol* 107:511, 1989.
3. Jackson WB: Differentiating conjunctivitis of diverse origins, *Surv Ophthalmol* 38(suppl):91, 1993.
4. Kushner BJ: Congenital nasolacrimal system obstruction, *Arch Ophthalmol* 100:597, 1982.

SUGGESTED READINGS

Beauchamp GR, Meisler DM: Disorders of the conjunctiva. In Nelson LB, Calhoun JH, Harley RD, editors: *Pediatric ophthalmology,* ed 3, Philadelphia, 1991, WB Saunders.

Calhoun JH: Disorders of the lacrimal apparatus in infancy and childhood. In Nelson LB, Calhoun JH, Harley RD, editors: *Pediatric ophthalmology,* ed 3, Philadelphia, 1991, WB Saunders.

Day S: Lacrimal system. In Taylor D, editor: *Pediatric ophthalmology,* Boston, 1990, Blackwell Scientific.

Day S: Uveal tract. In Taylor D, editor: *Pediatric ophthalmology,* Boston, 1990, Blackwell Scientific.

Friedlaender MH: Conjunctivitis of allergic origin: clinical presentation and differential diagnosis, *Surv Ophthalmol* 38(suppl):105, 1993.

Giles CL: Uveitis in children. In Nelson LB, Calhoun JH, Harley RD, editors: *Pediatric ophthalmology,* ed 3, Philadelphia, 1991, WB Saunders.

Good W, Hoyt C: Corneal abnormalities in childhood. In Taylor D, editor: *Pediatric ophthalmology,* Boston, 1990, Blackwell Scientific.

Hoyt C, Lambert S: Childhood glaucoma. In Taylor D, editor: *Pediatric ophthalmology,* Boston, 1990, Blackwell Scientific.

Jackson WB: Differentiating conjunctivitis of diverse origins, *Surv Ophthalmol* 38(suppl):91, 1993.

Laibson PR, Waring GO: Diseases of the cornea. In Nelson LB, Calhoun JH, Harley RD, editors: *Pediatric ophthalmology,* ed 3, Philadelphia, 1991, WB Saunders.

Lambert S, Hoyt C: Ophthalmia neonatorum. In Taylor D, editor: *Pediatric ophthalmology,* Boston, 1990, Blackwell Scientific.

Taylor D: External eye diseases. In Taylor D, editor: *Pediatric ophthalmology,* Boston, 1990, Blackwell Scientific.

Walton DS: Glaucoma in infants and children. In Nelson LB, Calhoun JH, Harley RD, editors: *Pediatric ophthalmology,* ed 3, Philadelphia, 1991, WB Saunders.

169 Scrotal Swelling

Mark F. Bellinger

The nature of the scrotal contents makes the differential diagnosis of scrotal swelling challenging. Swelling may be acute or chronic, congenital or infectious, traumatic or neoplastic. The source of the swelling may be the scrotal wall, the testis, its adnexa, or the cord structures (Box 169-1). Differential diagnosis requires an appreciation of both the embryology and anatomy of the scrotal contents.

The testis develops in the retroperitoneal space at the level of the internal inguinal ring. Descent through the inguinal canal occurs late in the third trimester of gestation and is complete within the first year of life.[1] As the testis descends, the spermatic cord becomes elongated so that the testis hangs on a pedicle containing its neurovascular supply and the vas deferens (Fig. 169-1). The tongue of peritoneum, which elongates to follow the testis into the scrotum (the processus vaginalis), forms a serous lubricating surface over most of the testis. The neck of the processus vaginalis normally pinches off during development, isolating the tunica vaginalis from the peritoneal cavity (Figs. 169-2, *A* and 169-3). The posterior testis and epididymis, excluded from the processus vaginalis, normally are attached to the scrotal wall, making torsion of the cord impossible. The testis and epididymis frequently exhibit small appendages (appendix testis and appendix epididymis) that are developmental remnants of embryonic ductal systems (Fig. 169-4). The testis and its adnexal structures are contained within the scrotum, a sac of smooth muscle capable of considerable contraction, whose rugated skin bears hair and sebaceous glands.

EVALUATION OF THE CHILD WHO HAS SCROTAL SWELLING

Determining both the circumstances of onset and the duration of scrotal swelling is important. A history of urinary symptoms, urethral instrumentation, urological anomalies, or urological surgery can indicate a predisposition to urinary infection and epididymitis. Because of the embryonic origin of the testis, pain from scrotal disease may be referred to the lower abdomen; conversely, pain of renal origin may be referred to the scrotal skin. Therefore, all children who have abdominal or scrotal complaints must have a complete abdominal and genital examination. Genital examination may be anxiety provoking and embarrassing, especially for teenagers. Younger boys generally are more comfortable having their parents present; teenage boys may prefer to be alone with a male physician. Examining the patient in both the upright and supine positions may facilitate differential diagnosis.

Inspection of the scrotum is important and may help to determine whether the process is unilateral or bilateral. With painful unilateral lesions, the patient may be put at ease by examination of the normal hemiscrotum first. Palpation may distinguish lesions of the scrotal wall from those of the spermatic cord. Testicular masses must be differentiated from adnexal or paratesticular spermatic cord lesions. Transillumination may help to differentiate cystic from solid lesions.

In certain clinical settings, laboratory testing may influence differential diagnosis. The urinalysis and white blood cell count (WBC) may be abnormal in infectious processes. Scrotal ultrasound may provide information about the nature of mass lesions. Color Doppler ultrasound[15] and nuclear scans[8,14] aid in evaluating blood flow to the testis in acute scrotal conditions and are most helpful in ruling out torsion of the spermatic cord. In addition, color flow Doppler may assist differential diagnosis by displaying intrascrotal anatomy.

NEONATAL INTRASCROTAL MASSES

In the newborn infant, a firm upper scrotal mass most likely is the result of torsion of the spermatic cord that has occurred before birth. Salvage of these testes is almost unheard of, and surgery is not indicated in most cases.[4] However, if a mass develops acutely after birth, prompt surgical exploration is appropriate. The role of prophylactic contralateral testicular fixation remains the subject of debate.[3] Testicular tumors in neonates are rare. Hydroceles are common, frequently imparting a bluish translucency to the scrotal skin; moreover, hydroceles transilluminate easily. The testis is normal but may be difficult to palpate if the hydrocele is tense. Infantile hydroceles usually resolve spontaneously over a period of months.

ACUTE, PAINFUL SCROTAL SWELLING

The acute onset of scrotal pain is a pediatric urological emergency. Any process causing acute inflammation may produce massive scrotal swelling and exquisite pain rapidly, making differential diagnosis difficult.

Torsion of the Spermatic Cord

Torsion of the spermatic cord is the most important diagnosis to exclude when acute scrotal swelling occurs. Be-

BOX 169-1

CAUSES OF SCROTAL SWELLING

Acute, Painful Scrotal Swelling
Torsion of spermatic cord
Torsion of appendix, testis, epididymis
Acute epididymitis, orchitis
Mumps orchitis
Henoch-Schönlein purpura
Trauma
Insect bite
Thrombosis of spermatic vein
Fat necrosis
Hernia
Folliculitis
Dermatitis

Acute, Painless Scrotal Swelling
Tumor
Idiopathic scrotal edema
Hydrocele
Henoch-Schönlein purpura
Hernia

Chronic Scrotal Swelling
Hydrocele
Hernia
Varicocele
Spermatocele
Sebaceous cyst
Tumor

cause the testis hangs at the end of a narrow vascular pedicle, ischemic necrosis occurs quickly in the absence of collateral blood supply. Salvage of endocrine function requires detorsion within 4 to 8 hours, and oligospermia or aspermia may result after only short periods of ischemia.[2] Torsion may occur at any age but is most common between 6 and 12 years. Severe unilateral scrotal pain of sudden onset is most commonly encountered. Frequently, a history of episodes of acute scrotal pain can be elicited (intermittent torsion with spontaneous detorsion). Vomiting is common, but fever is unusual. Although torsion may be triggered by trauma or athletic activity, many boys are awakened from sleep by pain. Inspection of the scrotum may reveal an immobile testis located high in the scrotum. This is the result of shortening of the cord as it twists (up to 720 degrees). The contralateral testis should be examined for a transverse axis, presumptive evidence of abnormal fixation—bell-clapper deformity (see Fig. 169-2, *B*). The cremasteric reflex may be absent in the presence of cord torsion but can be elicited in all other causes of acute scrotal swelling.[18] Scrotal skin over the involved testis may be reddened and taut, with loss of normal rugations. Transillumination usually is negative, although an acute, tense hydrocele may form. The scrotum is acutely tender, often making adequate examination difficult. Laboratory examination may reveal a slightly elevated white blood cell count and normal urinalysis.

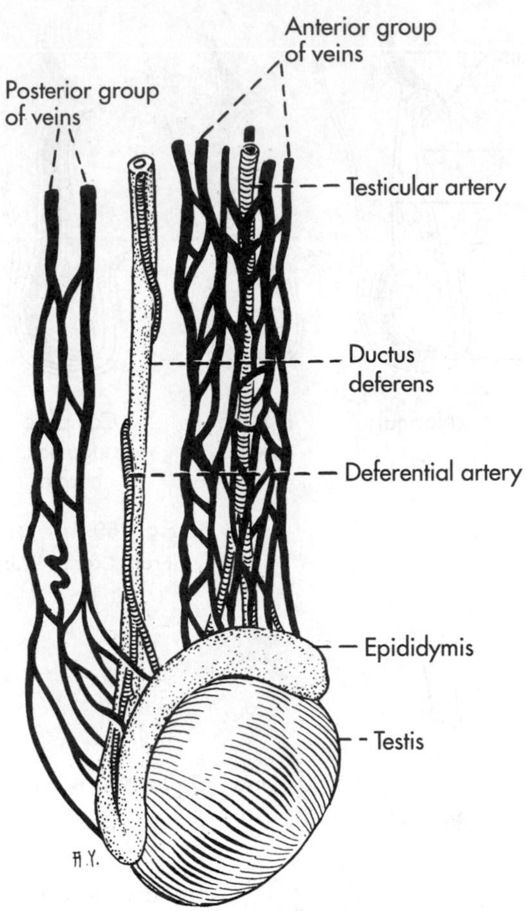

Fig. 169-1 Structure of the spermatic cord.
(From Rosse C, Gaddum-Rosse P: *Hollinshead's textbook of anatomy,* ed 5, Philadelphia, 1997, Lippincott-Raven.)

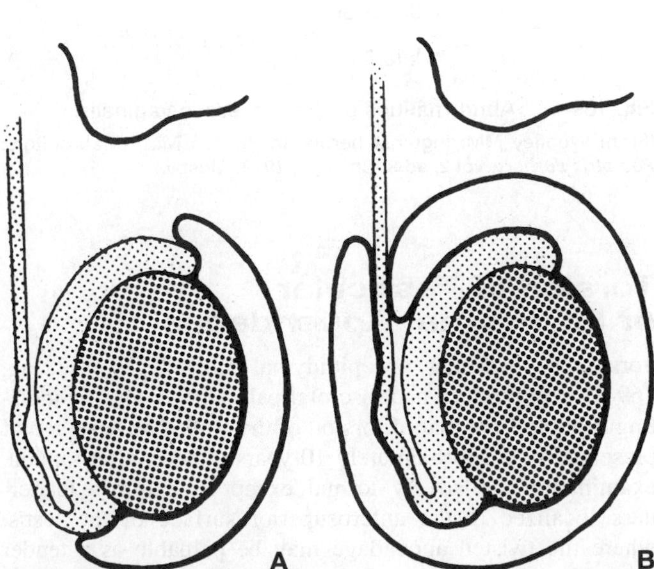

Fig. 169-2 **A,** Normal configuration of the tunica vaginalis. **B,** Bell-clapper configuration of the tunica vaginalis.
(From Gonzalez R: *J Urol* 116:673, 1976.)

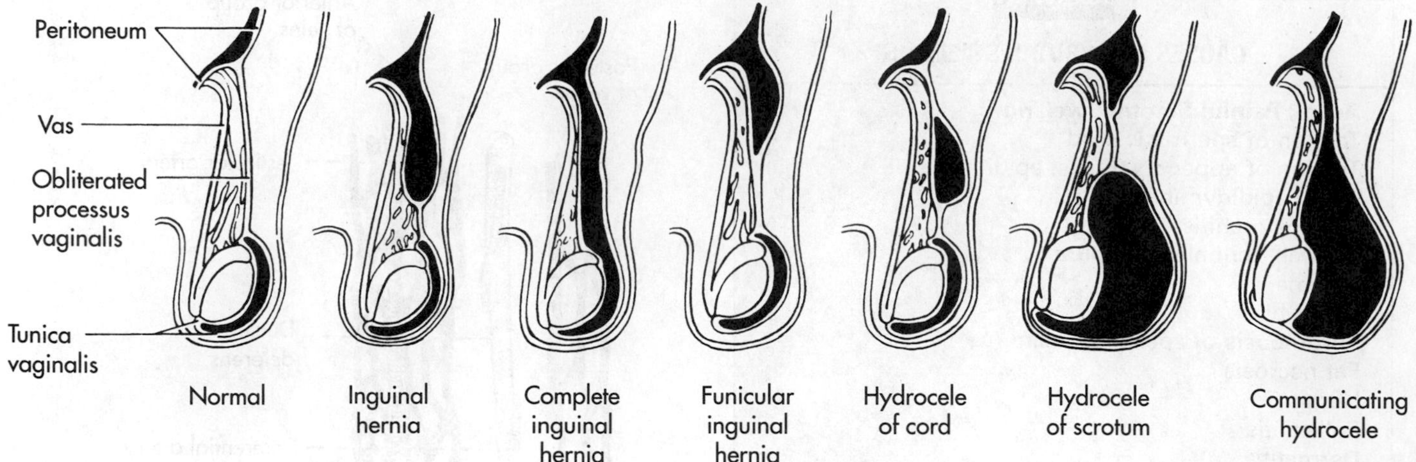

Fig. 169-3 Testicular appendages.
(From Cromie WJ: *Urol Clin North Am* 5:237, 1978.)

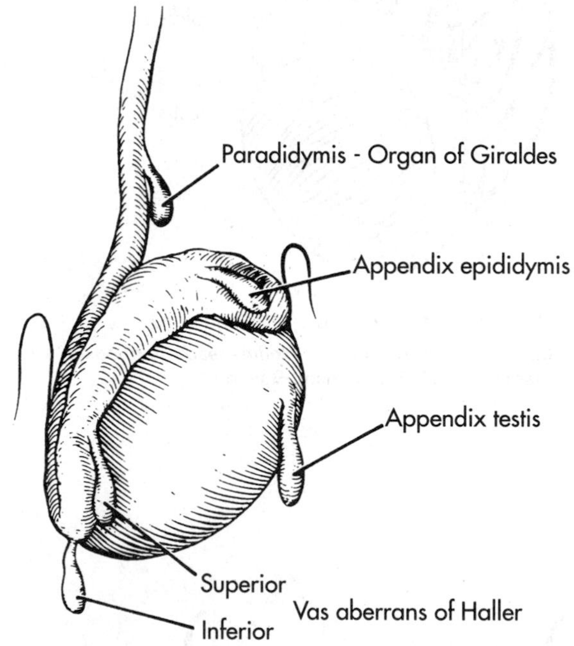

Fig. 169-4 Abnormalities of the processus vaginalis.
(From Woolley MM: Inguinal hernia. In Ravitch MM, et al, editors: *Pediatric surgery,* vol 2, ed 3, Chicago, 1979, Mosby.)

Torsion of Testicular or Epididymal Appendages

Torsion of testicular or epididymal appendages (see Fig. 169-4) may produce acute scrotal pain whose onset is indistinguishable from that of torsion of the cord. The peak age of presentation is approximately 10 years.[22] Soon after torsion, examination is relatively normal, except for exquisite tenderness localized at the anterosuperior surface of the testis, where the twisted appendage may be palpable as a tender mass. The black, necrotic appendage may be visible through the skin of light-skinned children, appearing as a "blue dot."[7] Testicular mobility is normal. When this entity is encountered at a later age, skin fixation, reactive hydrocele, and massive scrotal edema make it indistinguishable from torsion of the spermatic cord. Radionuclide scan or color flow Doppler examination will reveal normal or increased blood flow to the testis.[8,14,15]

Acute Epididymitis

Acute epididymitis is relatively uncommon in younger children and may indicate the presence of congenital or acquired lower urinary tract anomalies (ectopic ureter, urethral valves, urethral stricture). Although it has been recommended that all young boys have radiological investigation, including renal ultrasound and contrast voiding cystourethrography after the acute episode has resolved,[21] recent clinical experience-has called this practice into question. In the face of sterile urine, a normal ultrasound study of the upper urinary tract and bladder, and the absence of a fever, voiding cystourethrography will have a low yield. A history of sexual activity, dysuria, or urethral discharge should be sought in the older child and adolescent. The onset of pain and swelling usually is less acute than seen with torsion, but the two may be difficult to distinguish based on history alone. Pain and swelling usually are accompanied by fever, commonly 102° F (38.9° C) or greater. Dysuria may be present and may antedate other symptoms. Early examination may reveal a normal testis with posterior epididymal tenderness. Later, the epididymis and testis swell into a globular mass as scrotal swelling obliterates all landmarks. The cremasteric reflex usually is present.[18] Passive elevation of the testis may relieve pain (Prehn sign). Rectal examination may indicate prostatic tenderness or result in the expression of a urethral discharge, which should be examined microscopically and cultured for gonorrheal and other organisms. Urinalysis may suggest infection, but results of the microscopic examination and culture are frequently normal in adolescents who have epididymitis. The white blood cell count usually is elevated.

MANAGEMENT OF ACUTE CONDITIONS OF THE SCROTUM

Management of acute conditions of the scrotum should be based on the concept that all cases represent torsion of the spermatic cord until proved otherwise. Hence, urological consultation should be obtained while the patient is prepared for immediate surgery. If torsion of the cord cannot be ruled out definitively, scrotal exploration must be undertaken immediately.[5] Manual detorsion of the testis frequently is possible, resulting in immediate relief of pain and resolution of physical findings as blood flow is restored to the testis.[11] Manual detorsion may be simple or difficult to accomplish, and success will be due in part to the ability of the patient to cooperate while a painful testis is manipulated. The technique of manual detorsion involves a quick attempt at twisting the testis in a coronal plane. Because it is impossible to determine in which direction the cord rotated during spontaneous torsion, the examiner must use his or her best guess and rotate in the opposite direction. If this maneuver is not successful, detorsion in the opposite direction should be attempted. When manual detorsion has been successful and blood flow returned to the testis, an abrupt clinical improvement will be seen, with rapid diminution of pain and return of scrotal contents to more normal consistency and configuration. Although manual detorsion can provide evidence of blood flow to the testis, surgical exploration is mandatory to confirm complete detorsion of the cord, to fixate the testis, and to perform contralateral testicular fixation, because the opposite testis invariably has the same abnormal anatomy and thus is at risk for asynchronous torsion. If a testis is found to be even marginally viable, it usually is left in situ. Although laboratory evidence of possible immunological damage to the contralateral testis has rendered this practice controversial,[17] most urologists continue to be conservative if testicular viability is even marginally suspected. When torsion of the spermatic cord seems to be an unlikely diagnosis but confirmation of the clinical diagnosis is sought, either nuclear scan[8,14] or color flow Doppler ultrasound[15] is appropriate. Bedside Doppler examination, originally considered to be a reliable indicator of testicular blood flow, has proved to be unreliable and should no longer be employed. Torsion of a testicular or epididymal appendage may be treated conservatively when the diagnosis is certain, but many children undergo excision of the infarcted appendix because the diagnosis is uncertain or pain is severe or persistent. If epididymitis is diagnosed, cultures should be taken, scrotal elevation instituted, and antibiotic therapy begun. Severe cases may require hospitalization and parenteral antibiotics. Follow-up radiological examination should be performed.[21]

Rare Causes of Acute, Painful Scrotal Swelling

Acute, painful scrotal swelling may be caused by mumps orchitis,[19] Henoch-Schönlein purpura,[23] insect bites, or scrotal trauma. Mumps orchitis occurs commonly in adolescence but is rare in younger boys.[19] Acute orchitis or epididymitis usually occurs within a week after parotitis and rarely occurs in isolation. Clinical findings are typical of orchitis, and treatment is symptomatic. Infertility following bilateral disease may occur secondary to testicular atrophy, but this is quite unusual.

Henoch-Schönlein purpura may involve the scrotal wall, producing various degrees of erythema and edema, and may involve the testis and epididymis, producing acute pain of sufficient intensity to mimic testicular torsion.[23] Although some form of scrotal involvement may be seen in as many as 15% to 38% of cases, severe acute scrotal disease is uncommon. Testicular torsion coincident with purpura has been reported, so surgical exploration is warranted if the diagnosis is in doubt. Nuclear or color flow Doppler scans may be extremely valuable in determining the presence of testicular torsion.[8,14,15]

Insect bites and allergic dermatitis may cause edema of the scrotal wall; examination should reveal a normal spermatic cord and testis. Scrotal trauma may result in hematoma of the scrotal wall, a hematocele, or testicular rupture. Scrotal ultrasound may provide valuable information. If massive swelling makes diagnosis impossible, exploration is necessary.

Painless Scrotal Swelling

Painless scrotal swelling may be acute or chronic. Scrotal masses discovered on routine examination may have been present for an unknown period. Painless swelling may originate in the scrotal wall, testis, adnexal, or cord structures.

Idiopathic scrotal edema is a self-limited process of unknown origin that causes acute erythema, edema, and perhaps, mild tenderness of the scrotal wall.[9] The process usually involves the entire scrotum, although the testis and cord are normal. It may occur at any age from 18 months to 14 years. The process resolves spontaneously, although diphenhydramine has appeared to hasten resolution. Edema or lymphedema from any origin also may cause scrotal wall swelling, as may various other soft tissue processes.[6,12]

Painless swelling of the testis should be regarded as a tumor until proved otherwise. Most tumors occur after age 15 years, but a small peak in incidence occurs at 2 years.[13] Tumors are firm, painless masses that may give a sensation of heaviness in the testis; they do not transilluminate. The mass cannot be delineated from the substance of the testis. Because solid lesions of the epididymis are rare and invariably benign, firm lesions in the sulcus between the testis and the epididymis should be considered testicular in origin until proved otherwise. Testicular tumors require prompt inguinal exploration and orchiectomy. Preoperatively a chest roentgenogram and serum markers (alpha-fetoprotein, beta-human chorionic gonadotropin) should be obtained.

The most common cause of painless scrotal swelling in infants is a hydrocele, a collection of serous fluid within the tunica vaginalis surrounding the testis (see Fig. 169-3). These cystic swellings may impart a bluish tinge to the scrotum, especially when tense. They exhibit transillumination, and it usually is possible to palpate a normal testis within the hydrocele. Infantile hydroceles resolve spontaneously within several months. Communicating hydroceles vacillate in size. A reliable history of a flat scrotum in the morning with a gradual increase in fluid during the day is diagnostic because a hydrocele may not be grossly apparent at the time of office examination.

Examination may reveal a variable amount of fluid or a "silk glove" sign in the groin, as the surfaces of the tunica vaginalis glide over each other. Communicating hydroceles rarely resolve, and because of the potential for herniation of abdominal structures, elective repair is indicated.[20] Boys younger than 2 years of age should have a bilateral exploration because of the high incidence of a contralateral patent processus vaginalis. Adolescents who have communicating hydroceles frequently are found to have omental hernias. A hydrocele associated with an inguinal mass is likely a hernia. If the mass cannot be reduced or if vomiting or signs of intestinal obstruction occur, emergency surgery is indicated.

Painless masses of the epididymis occur with some frequency. Epididymal solid tumors are very rare and invariably are benign.[16] Cystic lesions of the epididymis (spermatocele, epididymal cyst) often are found in teenagers. These transilluminate, are nontender, and can be separated from the testis by examination. No surgical intervention is indicated unless discomfort arises, because postoperative epididymal scarring may obstruct ductal structures and result in infertility. Swellings of the spermatic cord are not uncommon in childhood. Solid, painless lesions should be pursued aggressively because spermatic cord and paratesticular sarcomas are not rare. Cystic lesions that transilluminate may represent encysted hydroceles of the cord, many of which are associated with a patent processus vaginalis (see Fig. 169-3).

Varicoceles are found in older boys and adolescents. These dilated veins of the pampiniform plexus commonly are asymptomatic and usually occur on the left side. The veins may collapse when the patient is sitting or supine. The left-sided predominance suggests origin from increased pressure in the left gonadal vein, which has no valves and enters the renal vein at a right angle. Acute onset of a varicocele, or a right-sided varicocele in a younger child, may represent acute venous obstruction from a retroperitoneal tumor. Abdominal sonography is indicated in these cases. Recent data indicate that diminished testicular volume may result from noxious effects of a varicocele, thought perhaps to be due to increased scrotal temperature. Although a subject of some debate and much uncertainty, indications for varicocele ablation include pain, ipsilateral testicular growth failure, and abnormal semen analysis. Varicocele ablation can be achieved by surgical, laparoscopic, or radiological means.[10]

Physical examination of a boy who has acute scrotal swelling should be sufficient to rule out folliculitis, sebaceous cyst, local trauma (e.g., zipper injury), and other miscellaneous local scrotal wall processes.

REFERENCES

1. Arey LB: *Developmental anatomy,* ed 7, Philadelphia, 1965, WB Saunders.
2. Bartsch G, et al: Testicular torsion: late results with special regard to fertility and endocrine function, *J Urol* 124:375, 1980.
3. Blyth B, editor: Neonatal testicular torsion, *Dialogues Pediatr Urol* 14:1, 1991.
4. Brandt MT, et al: Prenatal testicular torsion: principles of management, *J Urol* 147:670, 1992.
5. Cass AS, Cass BP, Veeraraghhavan K: Immediate exploration of the unilateral acute scrotum in young male subjects, *J Urol* 124:829, 1980.
6. Coolsaet B, Weinberg R: Thrombosis of the spermatic vein in children, *J Urol* 124:290, 1980.
7. Dresner ML: Torsed appendage: diagnosis and management—blue dot sign, *Urology* 1:63, 1973.
8. Falkowski WS, Firlit CF: Testicular torsion: the role of radioisotopic scanning, *J Urol* 124:886, 1980.
9. Kaplan GW: Acute idiopathic scrotal edema, *J Pediatr Surg* 12:647, 1977.
10. Kass EJ, editor: Options for adolescent varicocele, *Dialogues Pediatr Urol* 13:1, 1990.
11. Kiesling VJ, et al: Spermatic cord block and manual reduction: primary treatment for spermatic cord torsion, *J Urol* 132:921, 1984.
12. Koster LH, Antoon SH: Fat necrosis in the scrotum, *J Urol* 123:599, 1980.
13. Kramer SA, Kelalis PP: Pediatric surgical oncology. In Gillenwater JA, et al, editors: *Adult and pediatric urology,* ed 2, St Louis, 1991, Mosby.
14. Mendel JB, et al: Testicular torsion in children: scintigraphic assessment, *Pediatr Radiol* 15:110, 1985.
15. Meza MP, et al: Color flow imaging in children with clinically suspected testicular torsion, *Pediatr Radiol* 22:370, 1992.
16. Mostofi FK, Price EB: Tumors of the male genital system. In *Atlas of tumor pathology,* Series 2, Fasc 8, Washington, DC, 1973, Armed Forces Institute of Pathology.
17. Nagler HM, White RD: The effect of testicular torsion on the contralateral testis, *J Urol* 128:1343, 1982.
18. Rabinowitz R: The importance of the cremasteric reflex in acute scrotal swelling in children, *J Urol* 132:89, 1984.
19. Riggs S, Sandford JP: Viral orchitis, *N Engl J Med* 266:990, 1962.
20. Rowe MI, Lloyd DA: Inguinal hernia. In Welch KJ, et al, editors: *Pediatric surgery,* ed 4, Chicago, 1986, Mosby.
21. Siegel A, Snyder H, Duckett JW: Epididymitis in infants and boys: underlying urogenital anomalies and efficacy of imaging modalities, *J Urol* 138:1100, 1987.
22. Skoglund RW, McRoberts JW, Ragde H: Torsion of the testicular appendages: presentation of 43 new cases and a collective review, *J Urol* 104:598, 1970.
23. Turkish VJ, et al: Scrotal swelling in the Schönlein-Henoch syndrome, *J Urol* 115:317, 1976.

170 Splenomegaly

Allen E. Eskenazi

The spleen has intrigued physicians for centuries. Pliny the Elder associated it with mirth and laughter, and Galen described it as an organ full of mystery. Over the years the immunological and hematological roles of the spleen have been defined more precisely. Understanding the role of the spleen in health and disease permits the clinician to evaluate rationally the child or adolescent who has an enlarged spleen.

The spleen is fixed in the left upper quadrant of the abdomen by the splenorenal and phrenosplenic ligaments. Congenital or acquired abnormalities of the support structure can result in splenic ptosis and thus allow palpation of a spleen that actually is normal in size. An estimated 5% to 10% of normal infants have a palpable spleen tip, whereas a palpable spleen in an older child or adult almost always is pathological.

A useful framework for evaluating the child who has splenomegaly is to consider the four major physiological functions of the spleen: immunological, phagocytic, hemodynamic, and hematopoietic. First, the spleen is the major lymphoid organ in the body. It is the primary site of B-lymphocyte activity related to antibody production, and it is an important reservoir of T lymphocytes and natural killer cells, the mediators of cellular immune responses. Second, the spleen serves a major role in the removal of abnormal and senescent blood cells, as well as of circulating particulates. Third, the vasculature of the spleen plays an important role in the regulation of portal blood flow. Finally, the spleen is an important site of extramedullary hematopoiesis in the fetus, and in children and adults who have pathological conditions affecting the bone marrow.

Splenomegaly is a prominent or associated feature in numerous disease states (Box 170-1). Splenomegaly caused by recurrent viral infections often is seen in young infants. The degree of splenic enlargement is relatively small and should resolve within a short period. A greater degree of splenic enlargement occurs specifically in infectious mononucleosis (Epstein-Barr virus), cytomegalovirus, and human immunodeficiency virus (HIV) infections. Chronic bacterial infections (such as subacute bacterial endocarditis, syphilis, and tuberculosis) may be associated with splenomegaly. Acute overwhelming bacterial infections with pneumococcus or meningococcus also may result in splenic enlargement. In many areas of the world the spleen may harbor a large burden of protozoan-infected cells.

Inherited and acquired hemolytic anemias generally result in splenomegaly because of either increased phagocytic activity by the reticuloendothelial network (membranopathies, hemoglobinopathies, autoimmune hemolysis) or the development of extramedullary hematopoiesis (thalassemia major). Splenic sequestration of blood is a common, acute event in children who have sickle cell anemia, resulting in pallor, irritability, tachypnea, tachycardia, and variable degrees of splenic enlargement. Recognition of splenic sequestration is imperative because hypotension and shock can develop rapidly as a result of accumulation of blood in the spleen.

Infiltrative diseases of the spleen require prompt evaluation. The spleen rarely is the site of metastatic solid tumors but often is infiltrated by leukemias and lymphomas. Nonmalignant infiltration is seen in lipidosis and mucopolysaccharidosis, as well as in histiocytosis X. Autoimmune disorders (e.g., systemic lupus erythematosus and rheumatoid arthritis) and alloimmune disorders (serum sickness) may lead to expansion within the spleen of its lymphoid elements, as well as the phagocytic elements that remove antibody-coated cells and proteins. These conditions often mimic other infiltrative processes and may result in hypersplenism.

HYPERSPLENISM

Hypersplenism is not a specific disease entity. The term refers to the condition in which the spleen removes excessive numbers of normal circulating blood cells, resulting in one or more cytopenias. The affected blood element(s) are formed in the bone marrow to compensate for their accelerated destruction in the spleen. Splenectomy will correct the cytopenia(s). Establishing the cause of the hypersplenism is vital, however, inasmuch as other therapeutic modalities may correct the hypersplenism and thus obviate the need for splenectomy.

EVALUATION

Splenomegaly is diagnosed by physical examination and only rarely requires confirmation by radiographic, ultrasonographic, or radionuclide imaging. These studies, which may be useful in the evaluation of the child who has lymphoma, are not indicated in the routine evaluation of splenomegaly. A careful history, including family history, and physical examination permit the clinician to narrow the differential diagnosis to a few entities. A complete blood cell count, a reticulocyte count, and careful evaluation of the peripheral blood smear are extremely useful studies in the majority of patients who have splenomegaly. The results of these simple diagnostic procedures help dictate further diagnostic procedures such as hemoglobin electrophoresis, bone marrow aspiration, or lymph node biopsy.

BOX 170-1

SOME CAUSES OF SPLENOMEGALY

Infections
Viral: Epstein-Barr, cytomegalovirus, human immunodeficiency virus
Bacterial: acute bacterial infections, subacute bacterial endocarditis, congenital syphilis, tuberculosis
Protozoal: malaria, toxoplasmosis
Fungal: candidiasis, histoplasmosis, coccidioidomycosis

Hematological Disorders
Hemolytic anemias—congenital and acquired
Red cell membrane defects: hereditary spherocytosis, hereditary elliptocytosis
Red cell hemoglobin defects: sickle cell disease and related syndromes, thalassemia
Red cell enzyme defects: pyruvate kinase deficiency and others
Autoimmune hemolytic anemia
Extramedullary hematopoiesis
Thalassemia major, osteopetrosis, myelofibrosis

Infiltrative Disorders
Leukemias
Lymphomas
Lipidoses
Mucopolysaccharidosis
Histiocytosis X

Congestive Splenomegaly
Chronic congestive heart failure
Portal hypertension secondary to hepatic cirrhosis

Inflammatory Diseases
Systemic lupus erythematosus (SLE)
Rheumatoid arthritis (Still's disease)
Serum sickness
Sarcoidosis
Immune thrombocytopenias and neutropenias

Primary Splenic Disorders
Cysts
Hemangiomas and lymphangiomas
Subcapsular hemorrhage

SUGGESTED READINGS

Crosby WH: The spleen. In Wintrobe MM, editor: *Blood, pure and eloquent,* New York, 1980, McGraw-Hill.

Pearson H: The spleen and disturbances of splenic function. In Nathan D, Orkin S, editors: *Nathan and Oski's hematology of infancy and childhood,* Philadelphia, 1998, WB Saunders.

171 Strabismus

James W. McManaway III • Carl A. Frankel

Strabismus is the general term for any misalignment of the eye. The misalignment can be present under binocular conditions, in which case it is a manifest strabismus (tropia), or under monocular conditions, in which case it is a latent strabismus (phoria). Many persons have a small phoria, which is of no clinical significance; these latent deviations usually are found on routine ophthalmological examination. Tropias (manifest deviations) are present under binocular conditions, either intermittently or constantly, and may be alternating or unilateral. Alternating tropias imply equal or near-equal visual acuities; monocular tropias may indicate reduced vision (amblyopia) in the deviant eye (Fig. 171-1).

Strabismus occurs in approximately 3% of the population; although familial tendencies have been well documented, no clear-cut genetic mode of inheritance has been demonstrated. The direction of deviation of one eye with respect to the fixating eye names the deviation. An inward deviation is called an *esotropia,* an outward deviation an *exotropia.* A vertical deviation is referred to as a *hypertropia* or *hypotropia,* depending on whether the deviating (nonfixating) eye is higher or lower than the fixating eye. Torsional deviations are named for incyclotorsion or excyclotorsion of the 12 o'clock position of the eye and usually are associated with an abnormality in superior oblique muscle or inferior oblique muscle function with a secondary vertical strabismus; these conditions usually are referred to as *cyclovertical strabismus.*

Congenital or infantile strabismus deviations acquired before full maturation of the visual system (between the ages of 7 and 9 years for most children) are not associated with diplopia caused by suppression. Suppression is the adaptation to strabismus that inhibits the image at the deviating eye from reaching consciousness. In an alternating strabismus, alternating suppression is evidence for normal monocular visual development in both eyes and abnormal binocular visual development. However, in a youngster who has monocular strabismus, visual development in the fixating eye is expected to proceed normally, whereas binocular visual development and monocular visual development in the nonfixating eye can be expected to be impaired. This impairment in monocular visual development leads to amblyopia (poor vision, or "lazy eye"), which requires patching of the fixating eye to restore normal vision in the nonfixating eye. After the visual acuity of the amblyopic eye has been improved, surgery may be indicated to correct the ocular misalignment.

Because one eye is the fixating eye, bilateral strabismus is a misnomer. If both eyes appear deviated when the patient is facing an examiner, visual inattention or visual impairment is suggested and further evaluation is indicated to assess the function of the visual system. This assessment can be in the form of the visual evoked potential (VEP) or visual evoked response (VER), electroretinogram (ERG), or forced preferential looking (FPL). The first three are electrophysiological tests that require surface electrodes; the latter requires a visual stimulus that interests the child.

Because of the long-term implications for the patient, acquired strabismus, whether esotropia, exotropia, or a cyclovertical deviation, should prompt concern as to the exact cause. After leukocoria, strabismus is the second most common presenting sign of retinoblastoma, the most frequent intraocular tumor of children, with an incidence of 1 : 12,000 to 1 : 14,000 live births. Head trauma, either accidental or deliberate, can cause third, fourth, or sixth cranial nerve palsies that may result in an acute acquired strabismus. Any patient who has an acquired strabismus should be referred to an ophthalmologist for evaluation and intervention as needed, including that necessary to restore the integrity of binocular vision.

In a newborn infant, ocular alignment is variable, reflecting central nervous system (CNS) immaturity. About 70% of newborns show a variable, small exotropia; about 30% have straight eyes; and esotropia is very rare. By 2 months of age, most normally developing infants will have straight eyes. Any infant in whom strabismus persists beyond 10 to 12 weeks of age should be evaluated by an ophthalmologist. This should be done earlier if other signs of developmental delay are present or if the strabismus is constant.

DETECTION OF STRABISMUS

The Corneal Light Reflection Test

The simplest method to determine the presence of strabismus is the corneal light reflection test (Hirschberg method): A penlight is directed at the cornea, and the observer notes the position of the corneal reflection with respect to the center of the pupil (Fig. 171-2). If the light reflex is deviated toward the nose, an exotropia may be present; an esotropia should be suspected when the light reflex is deviated toward the lateral side of the visual axis. Although this method is used as a rapid screening test, the high incidence of false-positive findings results in unneeded referrals. On the other hand, the presence of a false-negative result may give an unwarranted sense of security.

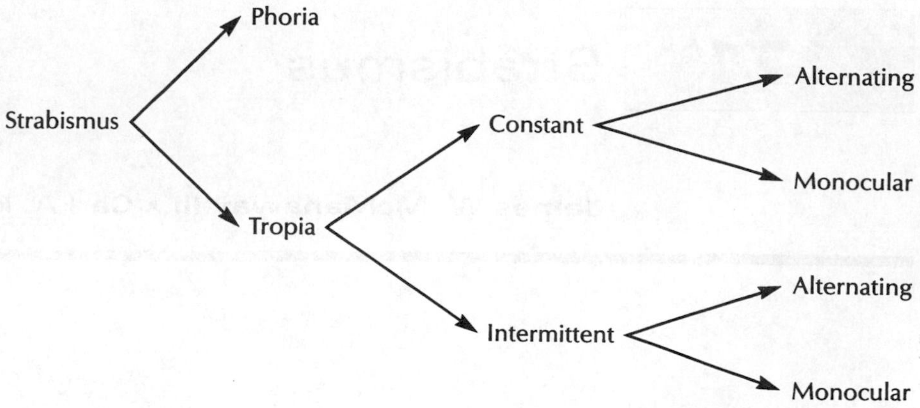

Strabismus → Phoria
Strabismus → Tropia
Tropia → Constant → Alternating / Monocular
Tropia → Intermittent → Alternating / Monocular

Fig. 171-1 Classification of strabismus.

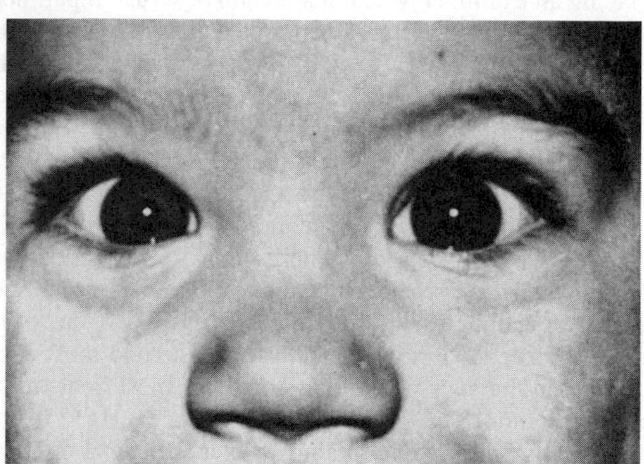

Fig. 171-2 Pseudostrabismus. This child's eyes, in fact, are aligned perfectly, even though the right eye appears "crossed" (esotropic). Epicanthal skin folds produce this illusion, which here is enhanced by the face being turned slightly toward the side. Notice that the corneal light reflections are quite symmetrical.

The Cover-Uncover Test

A more sensitive test for the presence of a strabismus is the cover-uncover test: The examiner uses some bright, pleasant object to attract the youngster's attention and then covers one eye with a hand, finger, or occluder. The examiner should watch the other eye carefully for a refixation movement, which indicates the presence of a tropia. The examiner then removes the cover and covers the other eye after 1 to 2 seconds, again watching for a refixation movement. Each eye must be tested several times, and the cover should be removed briefly before the next eye is covered. The presence of a shift of one eye while the fellow eye is covered is evidence of a strabismus (see Fig. 179-6) and should prompt referral for further evaluation and intervention, as indicated.

PSEUDOESOTROPIA

A common misconception among the lay public is that children may outgrow "crossed" eyes by the time they are 2 to 3 years of age. Unfortunately, this is not so. What children do tend to outgrow is the pseudoesotropia that is caused by the prominent epicanthal folds and broad, flat nasal bridge present in most infants. This condition creates an illusion of esotropia because of the decrease in the width of nasal conjunctiva visible to the observer (see Fig. 171-2). Because the nasal cornea tends to "dip" under the epicanthal fold on adduction, the parent frequently reports that the eyes are crossed more with right or left gaze and with near viewing (where convergence accentuates the illusion).

ESOTROPIA

The most common type of strabismus is esotropia, which is characterized by a nasal deviation of the nonfixating eye (Fig. 171-3). In patients in whom visual function is equal, alternate fixation may be present, giving rise to an alternating (not bilateral) deviation, whereas a monocular deviation is present in those in whom visual function is better in one eye. The corneal light reflection test will show the light to be centered in the pupil of the fixating eye, with the deviating eye showing the light reflection to be toward the temporal side of the center of the pupil. Because of variation in the location of the visual axis with respect to the center of the pupil, a small deviation may be either accentuated or, of greater concern, minimized. In fact, deviations of up to 7 degrees (15 prism diopters) may be missed. Thus the cover-uncover test is more reliable in the detection of a deviation.

Congenital Esotropia

Congenital esotropia is defined as having its onset within the first 6 months of life. Because the deviation may not be present at birth, a more accurate term is *infantile esotropia,* which is characterized by a large angle of deviation and, at least initially, by equal visual function and cross fixation. Cross fixation is that condition in which a patient prefers to look to the left with the already deviating right eye and to the right with the already deviating left eye. Because of cross fixation, a unilateral or even bilateral sixth cranial nerve palsy may be diagnosed. Normal abduction of each eye may be demonstrated by occluding one eye and using rotational testing or observing the following eye movements of the unpatched eye.

To normalize ocular alignment, early surgical intervention is indicated in youngsters who have congenital esotropia. Current medical opinion recommends surgical intervention

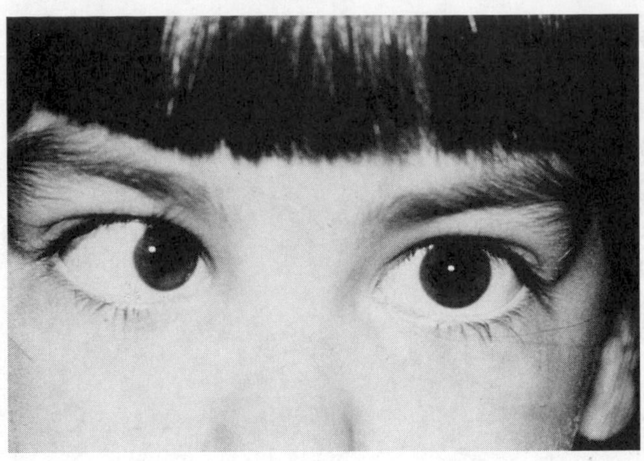

Fig. 171-3 Note the nasal deviation of the right eye with the corneal light reflection temporally displaced on the right eye and centered in the left pupil, indicating an esotropia.

between 6 and 18 months (possibly up to 24 months) to obtain more stable binocular vision than might be possible if the surgery were performed later. Prerequisites for early surgical intervention include stable ocular deviation, treatment of amblyopia (poor vision), and minimal risk for undergoing general anesthesia.

Less common conditions in which an esotropia is present include the congenital abducens nerve palsy (very rare) and Duane's syndrome, which typically affects the left eye. Duane's syndrome is distinguished from a true sixth nerve palsy by narrowing of the palpebral fissure with retraction of the globe on adduction as a result of contraction of the medial rectus muscle and inappropriate simultaneous contraction of the lateral rectus muscle of the same eye.

Acquired Esotropia

Any esotropia first detected beyond 6 months of age is classified as acquired; although it may represent a late-onset form of infantile esotropia, it requires careful diagnostic evaluation. Visual function needs to be assessed because unilateral visual loss in the first several years of life typically results in an acquired esotropia.

Accommodative esotropia. This type of acquired esotropia typically has its onset in patients between 2 and 3 years of age. The history is that of an intermittent esotropia that becomes more frequent in its occurrence and is of increasing duration. The condition is based on the accommodation reflex. For an emmetrope (person who has no refractive error) to focus at near objects, a synkinetic near reflex must occur. The three components of this synkinetic near reflex include accommodation (the alteration in the shape of the lens to make it a more powerful refracting element), accommodative convergence (nasal movement of the eyes so that the visual axes may be directed to the near object of regard), and pupillary miosis (irrelevant to this discussion). In accommodative esotropia, one of two scenarios typically is encountered and depends on the relationship between accommodation (A) and accommodative convergence (AC)—the AC/A ratio.

NORMAL AC/A RATIO. When the deviation (esotropia) of a patient who has a normal AC/A ratio is measured and found to be the same for both near and distant targets, a normal relationship between accommodation and accommodative convergence is defined. A hyperopic (farsighted) patient is not able to view distant objects clearly when the lens is in its normal, relaxed state (the usual state for distant viewing). To focus, the patient increases the refractive power of the eye by forced accommodation for distant viewing. Accommodative convergence ensues because of the synkinetic near reflex, and esotropia results (Fig. 171-4, *A*). Spectacle correction of the refractive error obviates the need for the accommodation reflex during distant viewing (with its secondary accommodative convergence) and promotes normal ocular alignment while spectacles are worn (Fig. 171-4, *B*).

HIGH AC/A RATIO. Patients who have a high AC/A ratio have excessive convergence for each unit of accommodation generated and have an esotropia that is more marked during near focusing then during distance focusing. Those patients who have no refractive error may have nearly straight eyes during distance focusing but develop an esotropia during near focusing because their normal accommodative effort results in excessive convergence. Hyperopic patients will have an esotropia during distance focusing that becomes larger during near focusing because of the additional accommodation required during near focusing.

These patients are treated with bifocal spectacles containing their distance refractive correction in the upper segment and a stronger correction for near focusing in the lower segment to relieve the need for accommodation during both distance and near focusing. An alternative treatment is the use of topical ophthalmic anticholinesterase agents such as isoflurophate or echothiophate iodide to facilitate accommodation (less effort needed) and thus reduce the excessive convergence. Unfortunately, these agents have ocular and systemic side effects, so they are used most commonly for short periods in the summer so that the child will not have esotropia at the swimming pool when glasses are not worn. Patients who have esotropia at distance looking through the upper segment of the glasses or esotropia at near looking through the lower segment of the glasses often are candidates for surgical correction of their strabismus. Fortunately, many children have their esotropia controlled with bifocal glasses. Because the AC/A ratio typically begins to normalize by about 8 years of age, the bifocals eventually can be discontinued.

Paralytic esotropia. An esotropia secondary to paralytic causes (abducens nerve palsy) is characterized by a deviation that varies with the direction of gaze and depends on whether the patient is fixating with the affected or the unaffected eye. When the patient looks in the direction of the affected side, the deviation is increased (horizontal incomitance). For example, in a patient who has left abducens nerve palsy, the esotropia will increase during left gaze and decrease during right gaze in relation to the primary (straight ahead) gaze position. Additionally, the deviation accompanying fixation by the unaffected eye (primary deviation) is less than the deviation with fixation by the affected eye (secondary deviation). If the paralytic strabismus is long-standing, the secondary deviation may approximate the primary deviation. An acquired abducens palsy is a nonlocalizing sign; it

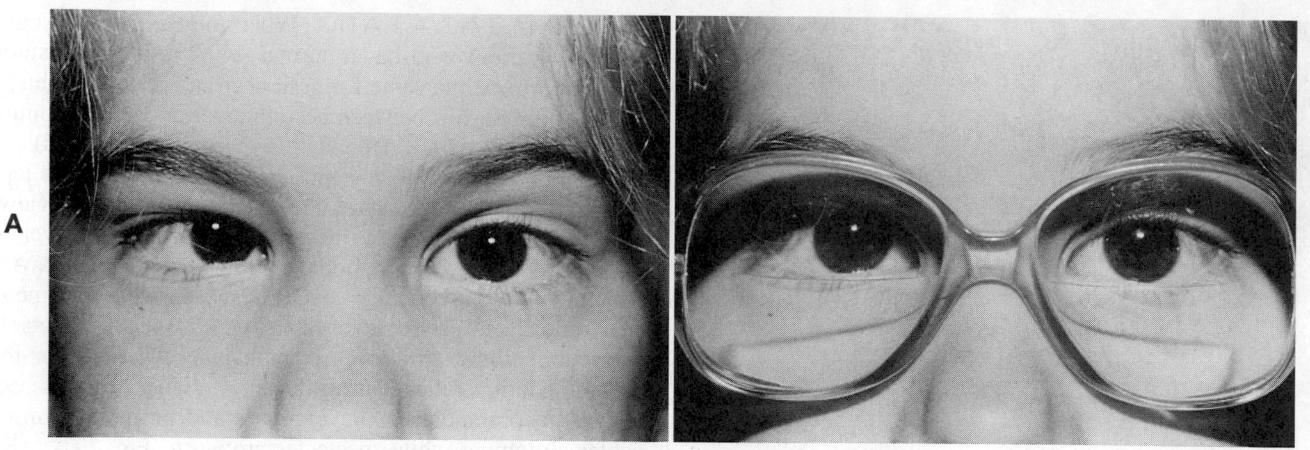

Fig. 171-4 **A,** Esotropia in a patient who has accommodative esotropia. **B,** Same patient, now having straight eyes upon refractive correction. Note the small increase in pupil size because of the reversal of accommodative miosis upon correction.

may reflect any cause of increased intracranial pressure or may be the benign sixth nerve palsy of childhood.[1,2] An appropriate evaluation to rule out the causes of increased intracranial pressure should be undertaken.

PSEUDOEXOTROPIA

Illusory exotropia occurs much less frequently than illusory esotropia. Because of the strikingly prominent appearance of pseudoexotropia, referral is made much more frequently and at a much earlier age, but the cover-uncover test reveals no refixation movement on covering either eye.

EXOTROPIA

Exotropia, or divergent strabismus (Fig. 171-5), occurs less frequently than does esotropia. As with esotropia, the deviation may be congenital or acquired and alternating or monocular. In addition, the exotropia may be constant or intermittent. Careful analysis of all these factors determines the treatment selected by the ophthalmologist.

Congenital Exotropia

Congenital exotropia is defined as having its onset in the first 6 months of life and is called, more appropriately, *infantile exotropia*. Infantile exotropia occurs much less frequently than infantile esotropia but similarly is characterized by a large angle of deviation and normal refractive error (mild hyperopia). Pseudoadduction deficit may be present, but full adduction usually is demonstrable on occlusion of one eye and then the other. As with infantile esotropia, early surgery is indicated.

Acquired Exotropia

Any exotropia that has its onset after 6 months of age is an acquired exotropia. Visual function must be assessed because the strabismus secondary to a retinoblastoma is more likely to be an exotropia than an esotropia.

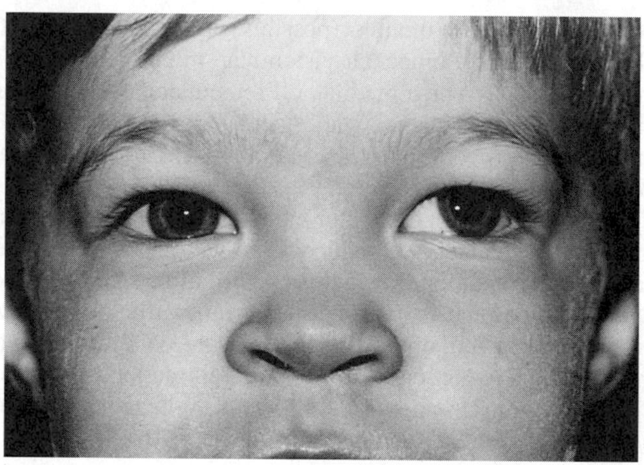

Fig. 171-5 Divergent strabismus of the left eye, defining an exotropia.

Intermittent exotropia. This is the most common type of exotropia seen in children and typically has its initial onset at about 2 to 3 years of age. Late-onset intermittent exotropias typically are diagnosed beyond 3 years of age, although these are perhaps atypical only in the age at which they are first noted. During periods when the eyes are well aligned, binocular vision may be developing normally, and the presence of binocular vision can help determine when, or if, surgical intervention is indicated. If binocular vision is deteriorating or if the frequency and duration of the deviation are increasing, surgical intervention is justified.

Convergence insufficiency. A subset of intermittent exotropia, convergence insufficiency is characterized by complaints of eyestrain, fatigue, blurred vision, diplopia, and headache. Orthoptic exercises for symptomatic convergence insufficiency have a high rate of success, as measured by relief of symptoms. Orthoptic exercises should not be confused with "vision training," which is of dubious value.

Divergence excess. Divergence excess is characterized by an exotropia that is larger at distant fixation than at near. The exotropia sometimes is noted only when a distant object is viewed. Surgical intervention is directed at the distance deviation, and a postoperative overcorrection (esotropia) for near fixation may occur.

Consecutive exotropia. This deviation may occur spontaneously in previously esotropic patients who have poor vision of one eye but generally follows surgical correction of an esotropia in patients who have poor fusional ability or unrecognized accommodative esotropia. Surgical intervention frequently is indicated in an attempt to obtain normal ocular alignment.

Paralytic exotropia. Paralytic exodeviations, which usually are seen with acute third cranial nerve palsies, are characterized by pupillary mydriasis, ptosis, an exotropia, and a hypotropia. Head trauma is the most frequent cause, and neuroradiological imaging (computed tomography or magnetic resonance imaging) usually is indicated. Because of the ptosis, diplopia is not a complaint. Special care should be taken in young children because of the possibility of deprivation amblyopia resulting from the ptotic lid.

VERTICAL AND CYCLOVERTICAL DEVIATIONS

Four muscles in each eye contribute to vertical and torsional eye movements: the superior and inferior rectus muscles and the superior and inferior oblique muscles. The two rectus muscles are concerned primarily with vertical eye movement, with secondary actions of incyclotorsion for the superior rectus muscle, and with excyclotorsion for the inferior rectus muscle. Conversely, the two oblique muscles are concerned primarily with torsional movements: the superior oblique for incyclotorsion and the inferior oblique for excyclotorsion. Secondary actions of the oblique muscles are depression and elevation for the superior and inferior oblique muscles, respectively. As a result of this arrangement, the two elevators (superior rectus and inferior oblique) have opposite torsional actions (incyclotorsion and excyclotorsion, respectively), whereas the two depressors (inferior rectus and superior oblique) also have opposite torsional actions (excyclotorsion and incyclotorsion, respectively). Thus, an imbalance in any one of the four muscles of either eye can result in a significant cyclovertical strabismus.

Superior Oblique Muscle Palsy

The superior oblique muscle is innervated by the trochlear nerve (fourth cranial nerve), and superior oblique muscle palsies are forms of strabismus undiagnosed the most commonly. Although head trauma is a frequent cause, most of these palsies are congenital and bilateral. In a youngster who has bilateral superior oblique muscle palsy, fusion is not possible (because of the bilateral excyclotorsion), and the head position typically is normal, giving no clue to the existence of a problem. On right gaze, however, a left hypertropia typically is present because of the relatively unopposed action of the left inferior oblique muscle (Fig. 171-6, *A*). Similarly, on left gaze a right hypertropia usually occurs as a result of the action of the right inferior oblique muscle (Fig. 171-6, *B*). In addition, in down gaze a large esotropia is typical, resulting from an absence of the abduction function of both superior oblique muscles.

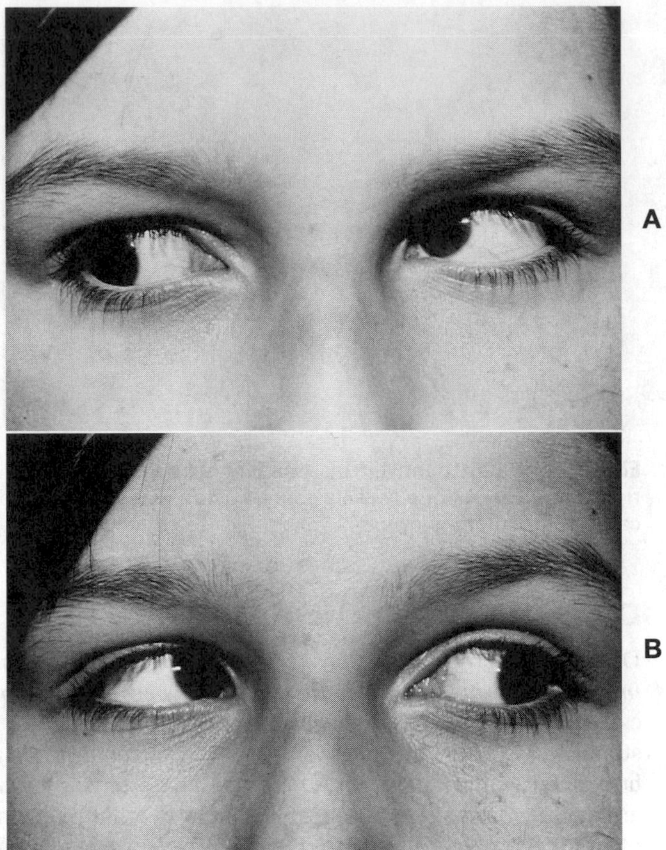

Fig. 171-6 **A,** Left hypertropia on right gaze characteristic of a left superior oblique muscle palsy. **B,** Right hypertropia on left gaze characteristic of a right superior oblique muscle palsy. This is the same patient shown in **A,** implying bilateral superior oblique muscle palsies.

In unilateral superior oblique muscle palsies, the unopposed excyclotorsion action of the inferior oblique muscle causes the affected eye to rotate outward. In an attempt to obtain and maintain fusion, a head tilt toward the opposite side from the palsied muscle results in normal ocular alignment, and fusion may be normal (Fig. 171-7). When the patient's head is straightened, the torsional action of the synergistic incycloductor (superior rectus muscle) results in an upward drift (hypertropia) of the affected eye, which is exaggerated by tilting of the head to the side opposite the naturally occurring head tilt. For example, a patient who has a right superior oblique muscle palsy usually will have a left head tilt to overcome the excyclotorsion of the right eye. On forced right head tilt, a large right hypertropia typically becomes obvious. Any patient who has torticollis should be evaluated for the presence of ocular torticollis, inasmuch as patients unwittingly may be subjected to unnecessary treatments such as physical therapy and braces for presumed nonocular torticollis. If any doubt exists about a possible superior oblique muscle palsy, the patient should be referred to a pediatric ophthalmologist for further evaluation.

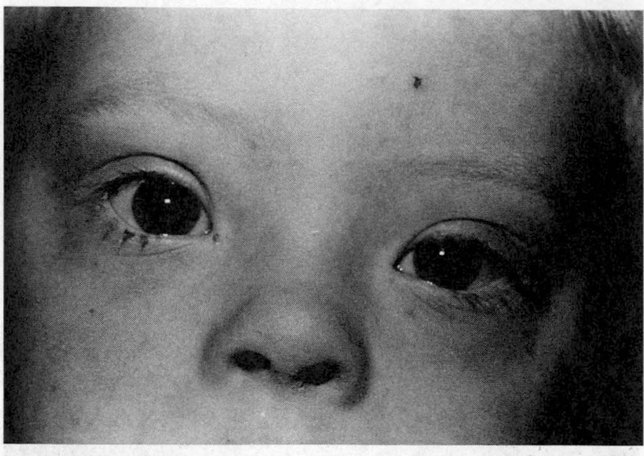

Fig. 171-7 Left head tilt in a patient who has a unilateral right superior oblique muscle palsy. Fusion was present, indicating binocular vision.

Dissociated Vertical Deviations

Dissociated vertical deviations (DVDs), also termed *alternating hyperphorias* or *double dissociated hyperphorias,* typically are seen in patients who have infantile esotropia, even if strabismus surgery has been successful in obtaining normal horizontal ocular alignment. DVDs are characterized by an alternating upward deviation of first one eye and then the other on alternate cover testing. Occasionally, excycloduction may be noted with a lateral deviation of the eye on its upward movement. The exact cause of DVD is unknown, but both superior rectus and inferior oblique muscle dysfunctions have been implicated. If the DVD is infrequent and asymptomatic, no treatment is indicated. If the DVD is frequently manifest or if it is associated with eye strain from the effort to keep the eyes aligned, surgery is appropriate.

REFERENCES

1. Knox RL, Clark DB, Schuster FF: Benign VI nerve palsies in children, *Pediatrics* 40:560, 1967.
2. Werner DB, Savino PJ, Schatz NJ: Benign recurrent 6th nerve palsies in children, *Arch Ophthalmol* 101:607, 1983.

SUGGESTED READINGS

Ernest JT, Costenbader FD: Lateral rectus muscle palsy, *Am J Ophthalmol* 65:721, 1968.

Harley RD: Paralytic strabismus in children, *Ophthalmol* 87:24, 1980.

Khawam E, Scott AB, Jampolsky A: Acquired superior oblique palsy, *Arch Ophthalmol* 88:761, 1967.

Kodsi SR, Younge BR: Acquired oculomotor, trochlear, and abducent cranial nerve palsies in pediatric patients, *Am J Ophthalmol* 114:568, 1992.

Nelson LB, et al: Congenital esotropia, *Surv Ophthalmol* 31:363, 1987.

Nelson LB: Strabismus disorders. In: Nelson LB, Calhoun JH, Harley RD, editors: *Pediatric ophthalmology,* ed 3, Philadelphia, 1991, WB Saunders.

Rubin SE, Wagner RS: Ocular torticollis, *Surv Ophthalmol* 30:366, 1986.

von Noorden GK: Cyclovertical deviations. In von Noorden GK, editor: *Binocular vision and ocular motility: theory and management of strabismus,* ed 5, St Louis, 1995, Mosby.

von Noorden GK: Esodeviations. In von Noorden GK, editor: *Binocular vision and ocular motility: theory and management of strabismus,* ed 5, St Louis, 1995, Mosby.

von Noorden GK: Exodeviations. In von Noorden GK, editor: *Binocular vision and ocular motility: theory and management of strabismus,* ed 5, St Louis, 1995, Mosby.

von Noorden GK: Paralytic strabismus. In von Noorden GK, editor: *Binocular vision and ocular motility: theory and management of strabismus,* ed 5, St Louis, 1995, Mosby.

von Noorden GK: Special forms of strabismus. In von Noorden GK, editor: *Binocular vision and ocular motility: theory and management of strabismus,* ed 5, St Louis, 1995, Mosby.

172 Strange Behavior

Audrey Walker

In the first two decades of life, the links between mind, body, and development are at their most complex and dynamic. Behaviors or thought processes, which at one phase are entirely normal, can, when they emerge in a different stage of development and with subtle differences in presentation, be a harbinger of serious psychopathy. To complicate this picture, the introduction of a medical illness during childhood or adolescence may cause temporary or permanent regressions or deviances in thinking and behavior, which may further blur the clinician's understanding of the patient. In a multicultural society, the nuances of different cultural and belief systems can, at times, masquerade as pathological thinking and behavior to the culturally naïve observer. For all these reasons, the successful collaboration between child psychiatry and pediatrics is crucial in the diagnostic understanding and treatment of the pediatric patient. Unfortunately, this collaboration has a disappointing history. In the past, the assessment of the child who has "organic illness" has not been adequately informed by a sophisticated approach to the psychological issues of the patient, even though this set of diagnostic skills has been shown to improve the quality of care and decrease the pain and suffering of the child. Conversely, an adequate knowledge of normal development solidified by the exposure to a large volume of normal children, which is so fundamental to pediatric training and practice, has not been a part of the clinical exposure of the child psychiatry trainee, resulting in a deficient understanding of the normal child in health and disease.[11] This chapter approaches the assessment of strange thinking and behavior in childhood and adolescence, focusing on four areas: normal development, development of abnormal thinking and behavior in the context of medical illness, psychopathology, and cultural beliefs and behaviors that can confuse the assessment of children.

INFANCY AND EARLY CHILDHOOD (BIRTH TO 5 YEARS)

Assessment in child psychiatry is unique in that the accurate evaluation of psychopathology requires a firm grasp of the vagaries of normal development. A behavior or thinking pattern, which may be completely normal in one developmental phase (for example, repetitive lining up of favorite objects in early childhood or masturbation in adolescence), may be a sign of trouble if observed in a phase in which these behaviors should not be found. Nowhere is this diagnostic endeavor more challenging than in the first 5 years of life, when keen observation must be combined with skilled and informed probing and the acquisition of supporting history to identify abnormalities. In the assessment of infants and preschoolers, it is most useful to break down observations into the four categories identified by Gesell:[10] motor skills, language abilities, personal-social abilities, and adaptive functioning, which includes manipulation of objects, alertness, and hand-eye coordination. The Bayley Scale,[3] which is a direct descendent of the work of Gesell, also breaks infant assessment into useful subdivisions focusing on social communication, object constancy, and capacity for discrimination. Abnormalities in any of these areas can direct the clinician to more serious consideration of the major types of psychopathology found in infancy and early childhood.

Pervasive Developmental Disorder

Pervasive developmental disorder (PDD) is a neuropsychiatric disorder that usually is identified, when present, in the first 5 years of life. Specific deviances are noted in the language/communication and personal-social domains, with related abnormalities in stereotypic and repetitive behaviors. Approximately two thirds of children who have PDD are mentally retarded, but cognitive delay is not intrinsic to the diagnosis. The social abnormalities seen in PDD are present in the first year of life.

Children who have PDD have little interest in the human face or interactions with others. In many cases, this deficit in social interaction can be identified in the first year of life by the astute and experienced observer. The communication impairments seen in children who have PDD include abnormalities in verbal and nonverbal communication, such as delay in spoken and gestural language, and the use of echolalia. Bizarre, restricted, and repetitive stereotypic behaviors such as flapping, spinning, and head banging frequently are seen. A subcategory of PDD, Asperger's disorder, differs from the classical presentation of PDD in that language and cognitive functioning are preserved, while social abnormalities and stereotypic behaviors are present.

Reactive Attachment Disorder of Infancy or Early Childhood

Abnormalities in the area of social relatedness are the hallmark of the child who has reactive attachment disorder (RAD); these abnormalities are rooted in grossly pathological care of the child in the earliest years of life. Social-relatedness abnormalities fall into two diametrically opposed categories. On the one hand, these children can display the "inhibited type" of RAD in which they appear withdrawn, hypervigilant, and resistant to all attempts at establishment of relatedness or comforting. On the other hand, in the "disinhibited type," children show indiscriminate, excessive, and superficial sociability. In both cases, the failure to develop developmental appropriate attachment behaviors is obvious. In extreme cases, these children also may fail to thrive, with severe growth and cognitive delays, or developmental deviances, related to failure of caretaking and attachment.

Separation Anxiety Disorder

In separation anxiety disorder (SAD), the child experiences excessive anxiety when separated from home or from those to whom he is attached. This anxiety is of a magnitude that leads to disruptions in social or academic function. Often the child refuses to go to school and is unwilling to travel independently or even to be separated from the parent for brief, developmentally appropriate activities such as play dates, sleepovers, or camp. The child who has SAD will often shadow the parent and refuse to be on a different floor of the house or to sleep alone. Excessive worries, including the generation of frightening fantasies about misfortune occurring to the parent, are common. SAD must be distinguished from the developmentally appropriate anxiety of early childhood during the "rapprochement phase," when the child, in the second year of life, shows normal separation and stranger anxiety. In addition, the cultural variations on acceptable child-from-parent separation must always be considered, as in traditional cultures where great emphasis is placed on family interdependence.

Posttraumatic Stress Disorder

Posttraumatic stress disorder (PTSD) is one of the few entities in psychiatry in which a specific etiology, the exposure to an extreme traumatic stressor involving direct personal experience of an event that involved actual or threatened death or serious injury, is necessary to diagnose PTSD. PTSD is well established in adults, adolescents, and children. However, it is a formidable challenge to diagnose PTSD in children younger than 5 years because the *Diagnostic and Statistical Manual of Mental Disorders, Fourth Edition (DSM-IV)*[1] criteria require verbal descriptions of thoughts and experiences that are difficult to obtain from young children whose language skills are limited. Terr[20] has made extensive clinical observations of the posttraumatic symptoms of early childhood and identified strongly visualized or repetitively perceived memories of the traumatic event, which can either take the form of the well known "flashback" or can be less intrusive in quality. Posttraumatic play, which is compulsive, repetitive, and grim and often incorporates a portion of the trauma known as "play reenactment," differs from normal play in being much less imaginative and more rigid; it does not relieve anxiety or trauma-specific fears or change attitudes about people and life, manifested by excessive pessimism and hopelessness about the future.[4] Scheeringa et al[16] did a preliminary investigation to explore whether *DSM-IV* PTSD criteria accurately describe the symptomology of young, traumatized children and found that it did not. The authors suggested more objective, behaviorally anchored and developmentally sensitive criteria, including assessment of posttraumatic play and sleep disturbances and emergence of new aggressive and separation anxiety symptoms.

Feeding and Eating Disorders of Infancy and Early Childhood

DSM-IV recognizes three feeding disorders in early childhood: pica, rumination disorder, and feeding disorder of infancy or early childhood. Pica is the persistent eating of nonnutritive substances. This is an activity that frequently is seen in association with mental retardation and developmental disorders. It is important to recognize that this practice is sanctioned in certain cultures and in this context would not be appropriately viewed as a pathological behavior. Rumination disorder is seen frequently in mentally retarded infants and children and is characterized by repeated regurgitation and rechewing of food. Feeding disorder of infancy or early childhood involves a persistent failure to eat adequately, judged by a failure to gain weight or significant weight loss over 1 month or more. Known in the pediatric literature as *failure to thrive,* this disorder must not be due to a medical condition and often is associated with parental psychopathology, child neglect, or abuse. Developmental disorders and extreme difficulties in temperament also may lead to feeding difficulties and must be distinguished from feeding disorders for proper management to occur.

Cross-Gender Behavior and Gender Identity Disorder

A child's sense of gender identity, that is, the sense of being male or female, emerges in early childhood and usually is consolidated by age 3 or 4 years. Children who suffer from clinically significant gender identity disorder (GID) commonly manifest a persistent, pervasive desire to be of the opposite gender.[6] In *DSM-IV,* this disorder is defined as having two important components. The child who has GID has a strong, persistent cross-gender identification as well as a persistent discomfort with his or her sex and a sense of inappropriateness in the assigned gender role. Boys who have GID will assert that their genitalia are disgusting or that they wish it to disappear. Rejection of male stereotypical toys, games, and activities is common. This entity must be distinguished from developmentally normal, nonconforming to stereotypical gender role behavior, such as the tomboyism of some latency age girls or cultural variants such as the effeminate style of the bohemian artist or dandy. These normal variants usually are distinguished easily from true GID by the lack of severe disgust with the individual's anatomy and assigned gender role and the absence of a strong identification with the other sex. See Chapter 86, Cross-Sex Behavior and Gender Identity Disorder, for further discussion of this entity.

Transitional Objects and Imaginary Companions

The existence of transitional objects and imaginary companions is a common experience of early childhood. In one study,[18] 65% of children between the ages of 3 and 5 years were found to have imaginary playmates, and 75% of children had transitional objects. Winnicott[22] first recognized and named the transitional object and defined it as a first possession that is used by the child as a defense against anxiety, which arises in the course of separation and individuation from the mother or primary caretaker. A soft object or stuffed animal, the transitional object will emerge at age 4 to 12 months and persist well into early childhood. This normal developmental element of early childhood is to be distinguished from the transitional phenomena and imaginary companions of the severely disturbed child. Children who have a history of severe physical or sexual abuse may develop symptoms of pathological dissociation or psychosis, which can include auditory hallucinations or imaginary companions. Unlike the more benign imaginary companion of the normal child, the hallucinatory experiences of the dissociative or psychotic child are threatening, frightening, and often express aggression toward others. The child feels little control over the experience and often is unable to distinguish between reality and this frightening product of the imagination. These experiences are not always easy to distinguish in early childhood and require assessment by an experienced child psychiatrist if there is doubt.

THE MIDDLE CHILDHOOD YEARS (5 YEARS TO PUBERTY)

The phase of middle childhood begins when the child enters elementary school and begins the stage of formal learning and participation in a structured peer group. In this developmental stage, the child emerges into the world beyond the family. Industriousness is called for in the acquisition of academic skills, social competence with peers, and a successful relationship with authority figures outside the family. One-to-one supervision by an adult gives way to the structured classroom setting, where formal rules of behavior within a distracting group of peers is the predominant experience of daily life. A number of psychiatric disorders emerge or are more readily identifiable in this developmental stage and social setting. When assessing the school-age child, the combination of a skilled interview and supporting information from parents, teachers, and other relevant reporters is necessary for an accurate understanding of symptomatology. Middle childhood ushers in the period during which the disruptive behavior disorders emerge and gain clinical attention.

Attention Deficit/ Hyperactivity Disorder

Attention deficit/hyperactivity disorder (AD/HD) is one of the most prevalent and important psychiatric disorders of the middle childhood years. Current prevalence estimates for AD/HD in the school-age population are between 3% and 5%.[4] The core symptoms of AD/HD according to *DSM-IV* require the onset of inattention and hyperactivity-impulsivity by age 7 years manifested in at least two settings. The symptoms must be more severe and frequent than those seen in a normal child at a comparable development level. Symptoms of AD/HD tend to emerge once the child enters school, in part because the highly structured setting, significant demands, and lack of one-to-one adult-to-child supervision all conspire to tax the limited attention and impulse control available to the child who has AD/HD. The most common entity that leads to a misdiagnosis of AD/HD in children is the normal exuberance of early childhood. See Chapter 73 for further discussion of AD/HD.

Oppositional Defiant Disorder

Oppositional defiant disorder (ODD) is a diagnosis that occurs frequently in children who have AD/HD. The core features of this disorder are a recurrent, severe pattern of negativistic, defiant, disobedient, and hostile behaviors toward authority figures, lasting more than 6 months. The symptoms of ODD are seen invariably in the home and frequently are focused on one particular authority figure. The behaviors must be particularly frequent, severe, and persistent to prevent the inappropriate labeling of children exhibiting developmentally normal oppositionalism as being ODD.

Conduct Disorder

Conduct disorder is characterized by a repetitive and persistent pattern of behavior in which the basic rights of others, as well as social rules and norms, are violated.[1] Although mild antisocial behaviors can be developmentally normal in certain settings, such as the preschooler who is unable to "play by the rules" in structured games, in the school-age child and adolescent, conduct disorder symptoms are grossly developmentally deviant and include aggressivity, deceitfulness, theft, serious rule violations, and property destruction. Children and adolescents who have conduct disorder are at high risk for the development of antisocial personality disorder in adulthood. See Chapter 85 for further discussion of conduct disorders.

Dissociative Disorders

The *DSM-IV* includes four diagnoses within the category of dissociative disorders, the most familiar to the nonpsychiatric clinician being dissociative identity disorder, also known as multiple personality disorder. The core of these disorders is the presence of pathological dissociation, which is defined as a disruption of the integrated functions of consciousness, memory, identity, or perception of the environment. Pathological dissociation can be transient or chronic, and its onset can be acute or gradual. The capacity for dissociation develops in childhood and is a normal process used in imaginative play. This normal process declines markedly by late adolescence. The key differences between the normal dissociation of a daydreaming child or a child in the throes of fantasy play and the pathological dissociation seen in the dissociative disorders are (1) amnesia for complex behaviors and (2) extreme forms of depersonalization, which is a subjective sense of being unreal, strange, or unfamiliar to oneself.[12] These symptoms rarely occur in normal children or even in children who have psychiatric disorders other than the dissociative disorders. Although the prevalence of dissociative disorders in children and adolescents is unknown, it is clear that childhood trauma, especially early sexual abuse, is the major risk factor for the development of pathological dissociation. Dissociation is a defensive coping mechanism that functions to protect the child against the extreme pain and vulnerability of severe childhood abuse; 85% to 100% of adults who have dissociative identity disorder have documented histories of severe childhood abuse.[14]

ADOLESCENCE

Adolescence is a developmental phase unique to human beings. In the human, hormonal and neurological changes develop slowly over many years and culminate during puberty.[7] Adolescence is the psychological, social, and maturational process initiated by the biological event of puberty. During puberty, marked and rapid changes in primary and secondary sexual characteristics occur. In girls, menstruation and breast development are the major physical events; for boys they are rapid enlargement of the external genitalia and attainment of adult height and muscle mass. With these biological changes come several psychological and social changes, including preoccupation with the body, development of sexuality, social anxiety and increased importance of the peer group over parents and other adult figures, and the development of more abstract cognitive abilities.[2] All these developments result in changes in thinking and behavior, which are unfamiliar and at times may be mistaken for psychopathology. Several major psychiatric disorders also present typically in adolescence.

Major Depressive Disorder and Bipolar Disorder

Major depressive disorder (MDD) is defined in the *DSM-IV* as the presence of a single major depressive episode, with five or more of the following symptoms lasting for at least 2 weeks and manifested daily: depressed mood for most of the day, markedly diminished interest or pleasure in almost all activities, significant weight loss or gain caused by a decrease or increase in appetite, insomnia or hypersomnia, psychomotor agitation or retardation, fatigue or loss of energy, feelings of excessive worthlessness or guilt, diminished ability to concentrate, and recurrent thoughts of death or suicide. Adolescents who have bipolar disorder (BPD) characteristically have the occurrence of a major depressive episode before a first manic episode. A manic episode is a distinct period of abnormally and persistently elevated, expansive, or irritable mood lasting for at least 1 week. A manic episode is characterized by symptoms that may include grandiosity, decreased sleep requirement, pressured speech, racing thoughts, agitation, and high-risk behaviors, including spending sprees, sexual promiscuity, and gambling. Although both MDD and BPD typically present in adolescence, prepubertal manic and depressive disorders have been diagnosed more frequently in recent years and are associated with a more severe course.[9] In addition, milder forms of depressive and manic disorders exist and can be seen in adolescence. Finally, aspects of normal adolescent development in the psychological and cognitive area can gain clinical attention and be mistaken for pathology. The tendency toward egocentric, grandiose thinking and abstract theorizing is pronounced during adolescence. Obsessive, ruminative focus on the body or on one's thinking process can be mistaken for anxiety disorders, a hypomanic episode, or oppositional behavior. See also Chapter 107, Mood Disorders in Children and Adolescents.

Schizophrenia and Other Psychotic Disorders (see also Chapter 93, Psychosis)

Before the *DSM-III*, published in 1980, all serious forms of childhood psychiatric disturbance were labeled schizophrenia. Over the past 20 years the label of psychosis has been significantly narrowed. The term *psychosis* currently implies a serious disturbance in an individual's reality testing, as evidenced by hallucinations, delusions, and disturbances in the form of thinking.[21] The narrowing of this diagnostic category has occurred in a climate of growing understanding that perception of reality differs in various developmental phases and, more broadly, in diverse cultural contexts. Psychotic disorders are very uncommon in prepubertal children and, when present, are harbingers of a poor prognosis.

In adolescence, the frequency of schizophrenia increases dramatically, and the symptomatology closely parallels that seen in adult-onset schizophrenia. *DSM-IV* identifies the characteristic symptoms of schizophrenia as being delusions, hallucinations, disorganized speech, grossly disorganized behavior, and the so-called negative symptoms, which include avolition, alogia, and affective flattening.[1] These symptoms are accompanied by significant occupational and social dysfunction. This severe picture is to be contrasted with the disturbances in reality testing seen in various phases of normal development. Transient hallucinatory experiences, often tactile or visual in nature, are seen commonly in early childhood and, in times of stress, in older children, as well.[15] Magical, animistic thinking is common and developmentally normal in the preschool and early school-age child. Imaginary companions and transitional objects imbued with lifelike qualities by the child are normal in early childhood. All such normal phenomena should gradually disappear by the end of mid-childhood.

Eating Disorders

The two classic eating disorders, anorexia nervosa (AN) and bulimia nervosa (BN), are common psychiatric disorders of childhood that commonly present in adolescence. The prevalence of eating disorders in adolescence has increased markedly over the past 50 years, and their signs and symptoms typically come to the attention of the pediatrician before any mental health intervention is sought.

In the eating disorders, both thinking and behavior are disturbed. In AN, there is an intense fear of gaining weight or becoming fat, even when the patient is underweight, and a disturbance in the way in which body weight is experienced. The patient refuses to maintain body weight above a minimally normal level, defined in *DSM-IV* as 85% of expected body weight. Restricting food intake and a cycle of binge eating followed by purging are two forms of behavior employed by patients who have AN to inhibit weight gain. Methods of purging may include self-induced vomiting, excessive use of laxatives, excessive exercise, and use of diuretic medications and enemas. Patients who have bulimia nervosa are typically within the normal weight range, but often have had a prior period of AN. BN is characterized by recurrent episodes of binge eating in which, during a discrete period of time, an excessive amount of food intake occurs accompanied by a feeling of total lack of control. The binge is then followed by purging behavior. Eating disorders are much more common in females, with onset typically in later adolescence. They are seen mostly in Western industrialized nations and more typically in white, upper middle class females.[19] It is clear that in puberty the need for the young girl to integrate the realities of menstruation, breast development, and the broadening of the hips can be a challenge that results in transient perturbations of body image and abnormal eating behaviors.[7] The distinguishing factors that identify eating disorders from the transient, developmentally normal process is the severity of the weight loss, the persistence of a disturbed body image, and in the case of AN, the loss of menses, which is necessary to make the diagnosis in females. See Chapter 102 for further discussion of anorexia nervosa and bulimia nervosa.

SPECIAL CONSIDERATIONS

Extreme Temperament in Childhood

In the 1940s and early 1950s, Chess and Thomas[5] did their renowned work in identifying and describing the importance of temperament, or behavioral style, in the functioning of children. They identified nine categories that defined temperament: activity level, rhythmicity or regularity, approach/withdrawal behavior, adaptability to new situations, threshold of responsiveness, intensity of reaction, quality of mood, distractibility, and attention span. Analyzing these categories, they identified three distinct temperamental styles: (1) the easy temperament, which encompasses a regular, easily adaptable child who displays a predominantly positive mood and only mild intensity; (2) the child who has the difficult temperament, behaviorally opposite of easy temperament and characterized by biological irregularity, withdrawal in reaction to novel stimuli, slow adaptability to change, predominantly negative mood, and high intensity (this group comprised 10% of Chess & Thomas's study group); and (3) the slow-to-warm-up temperament, also known as "shy," which comprised 15% of the group; they were described as slow adapters who had significant withdrawal responses, low intensity, and frequent negative mood. The difficult child and the slow-to-warm-up child are developmentally and psychologically normal and yet, because of their being difficult to manage, often can be labeled as behaviorally disordered by caretakers and brought to pediatric attention. Although extreme negative temperamental features have not been found to be equivalent to psychiatric disorders in childhood,[13] they can predict poor psychiatric functioning in adolescence, particularly in the context of poor caretaker-child interaction or dysfunctional behavioral control among adult family members.

The Medically Ill Child

"Where the defense mechanisms available at the time are strong enough to master the anxieties, all is well; where they have to be overstrained to integrate the experience, the child reacts to the operation with neurotic outbreaks; where the ego is unable to cope with the anxiety released, the operation becomes a trauma to the child."[8]

The pediatrician is a primary observer of the child in the sick role and therefore is in great need of an understanding of the emotional and developmental reactions to pain and illness that children manifest. Studies and clinical observations in both the areas of psychodynamic and cognitive development in children have been applied to the thinking and behavior of the medically ill child. This work has been helpful in the understanding of behavior of the child who has a medical illness and in the successful management of noncompliance in the pediatric setting.

Cognitive-developmental theory based on the work of Piaget and Inhelder defined a predictable sequence of stages by which cognitive concepts are acquired throughout childhood.[17] The sensorimotor stage of infancy through roughly the age of 2 years is when things exist only insofar as one can act on them, and the ultimate cognitive outcomes is the achievement of object permanence. From ages 2 through 7 years, the child is in the preoperational stage, in which symbolic thought and representations, including language, develop. During this stage, thinking is not logical but rather egocentric and animistic. Only when the child moves into the third, concrete operational stage, from ages 7 until the onset of puberty, does logical thinking take hold. Finally, in the formal operational stage, which begins at puberty, formal abstract thinking is the predominant mode of thought. It is important to note that not all individuals reach the formal operational stage, even in adulthood.

In cognitive-developmental theory there is a systematic and predictable sequence by which concepts of illness are acquired; this process is comparable to the acquisition of casual understanding described by Piaget for normal development.[17] An appreciation of the cognitive level of a child, as well as an understanding that children often regress to an earlier level of cognitive functioning under the stress of an illness, can be very helpful to the clinician's understanding of what may appear to be very strange behavior in children who are ill. Symptoms such as enuresis, soiling, sleep difficulties, and separation anxiety, which existed previously and were overcome by the child, may recur and persist during the course of the illness. An example can be seen in the preoperational child who becomes ill with diabetes, for instance. Unable to embrace the causes of his illness cognitively, his egocentric and magical thought processes lead him to believe that his disease has come upon him as a punishment for previous "bad behavior." The resulting feelings of guilt, shame, and anxiety pose major stumbling blocks to his care, including exaggerated pain behavior and poor compliance with his medical regimen. In adolescence, when abstract thought first emerges, the reaction to illness may have a much different quality. For example, placed in a life-threatening medical situation, the adolescent may take on an obsessive, ruminative, darkly philosophical caste that may resemble clinical depression.

Other elements specific to the plight of the child who has a medical illness also may predispose the child to unusual thinking and behavior. The experience of being nursed and a change in parental emotional climate, often with an uncharacteristic exclusive focus by the parents on the child, can cause great anxiety and may even be traumatic. Being forced into a passive role during hospitalization and medical procedures and being handled by the parent and medical/nursing staff like a much younger child can be very upsetting to the child who only recently has acquired independent functioning and detachment of his body from the parents. The resulting anxiety can create a difficult, even intractable, patient.

CONCLUSION

In the assessment of strange thinking and behavior in childhood, a number of important considerations must be kept in mind. First and foremost is that thinking or behavior in childhood can be categorized as normal or pathological based in large part on when in development it presents. An adequate understanding of the details of normal development is rooted best in the wide clinical exposure available to the pediatric practitioner. Phenomena such as dissociation and antisocial behavior, even unusual perceptual phenomena, can represent aspects of normal development or warning signs of serious psychopathology, depending on the developmental phase in which they occur and the severity and persistence of the symptoms over time. Cultural influences can at times confuse the diagnostic picture, either by widening the gap in belief systems between a child and his family or between a child of a culturally unfamiliar family and the assessing practitioner. Extremes of temperament that are in the normal range can also be confusing diagnostically, especially if the child and his parents interact negatively, leading to presenting complaints, which appear pathological. Finally, the child who is suffering from a major medical illness can "regress" to an earlier level of functioning, which can masquerade as psychopathology. In all these cases, the close collaboration between the pediatric practitioner and the child and adolescent psychiatrist is essential to assess the child or adolescent accurately who presents with strange thinking or behavior.

REFERENCES

1. American Psychiatric Association: *Diagnostic and statistical manual of mental disorders,* ed 4, Washington, DC, 1994, the Association.
2. Anthony EJ: Normal adolescent development from a cognitive viewpoint, *J Am Acad Child Psychiatry* 21:318, 1982.
3. Bayley N: *Bayley scales of infant development,* New York, 1969, Psychological Corporation.
4. Cantwell D: Attention deficit disorder: a review of the past 10 years, *J Am Acad Child Adolesc Psychiatry* 35:978, 1996.
5. Chess S, Thomas A: Temperament. In Lewis M, editor: *Child and adolescent psychiatry,* Philadelphia, 1991, Williams and Wilkins.
6. Coates S: Ontogenesis of boyhood gender identity disorder, *J Am Acad Psychoanalysis* 18:414, 1990.
7. Committee on Adolescence, Group for the Advancement of Psychiatry: *Normal adolescence,* New York, 1968, Charles Scribner's Sons.
8. Freud A: The role of bodily illness in the mental life of children. In Eissler R, et al, editors: *Physical illness and handicap in childhood,* New Haven, Conn, 1977, Yale University Press.
9. Geller B, Luby J: Child and adolescent bipolar disorder: a review of the past 10 years, *J Am Acad Child Adolesc Psychiatry* 36:1168, 1997.
10. Gesell A: *Mental growth in the preschool child,* New York, 1925, Macmillan.
11. Kaplan H, Sadoc B, Grebb J, editors: *Synopsis of psychiatry,* Baltimore, 1994, Williams and Wilkins.
12. Lewis DO: Diagnostic evaluation of the child with dissociative identity disorder/multiple personality disorder, *Child Adolesc Psychiatr Clin North Am* 5:285, 1996.
13. Maziade M, et al: Psychiatric status of adolescents who had extreme temperaments at age 7, *Am J Psychiatry* 147:1531, 1990.
14. Ross C: Epidemiology of dissociation in children and adolescents, *Child Adolescent Psychiatr Clin North Am* 5:273, 1996.
15. Rothstein A: Hallucinatory phenomena in childhood: a critique of the literature, *J Am Acad Child Psychiatry* 20:623, 1981.
16. Scheeringa MS, et al: Two approaches to the diagnosis of posttraumatic stress disorder in infancy and early childhood, *J Am Acad Child Adolesc Psychiatry* 34:191, 1995.
17. Schonfeld D: The child's cognitive understanding of illness. In Lewis M, editor: *Child and adolescent psychiatry,* Philadelphia, 1991, Williams and Wilkins.
18. Singer JL, Singer DG: Imaginative play and pretending in early childhood: some experimental approaches. In Davids A, editor: *Child personality and psychopathy, current topics,* New York, 1976, John Wiley and Sons.
19. Steiner H, Lock J: Anorexia nervosa and bulimia nervosa in children and adolescents: a review of the past 10 years, *J Am Acad Child Adolesc Psychiatry*, 37:1352, 1998.
20. Terr L: Childhood traumas: an outline and overview, *Am J Psychiatry* 148:10, 1991.
21. Volkmar F: Childhood and adolescent psychosis: a review of the past 10 years, *J Am Acad Child Adolesc Psychiatry* 35:843, 1996.
22. Winnicott D: Transitional objects and transitional phenomenon, *Int J Psychoanal* 34:89, 1953.

173 Stridor

Morton E. Salomon

Stridor is a high-pitched, crowing respiratory noise caused by partial obstruction of the large airways at the level of the pharynx, larynx, or trachea. Stridor commonly is heard on inspiration but may be heard on expiration or on both inspiration and expiration (biphasic stridor) if the obstructive lesion is more distal.[10,12,15]

Stridor must be differentiated from stertor, a noisy, heavy, snoring-type breathing heard during inspiration as a result of obstruction at the level of the nose, nasopharynx, or oropharynx. One also must distinguish stridor and stertor from wheezing. Wheezing is a high-pitched, musical whistling sound generally associated with prolongation of exhalation.[15]

Although stridor can be a manifestation of a benign, static, and self-limited condition, it also can herald a rapidly progressive deterioration in ventilation leading to complete airway obstruction. Therefore, a patient who has stridor requires prompt attention so that the degree of airway compromise can be assessed and its etiology determined.

PATHOPHYSIOLOGY

Stridor is produced by turbulence of air flow in the large airways. During inspiration, pressure gradients in the extrathoracic airway favor narrowing of the lumen because intraluminal pressure becomes slightly lower than atmospheric (extraluminal) pressure. During expiration, intraluminal pressure is greater than extraluminal pressure and the airway dilates. More distally, within the intrathoracic airway, the situation reverses itself and the airway tends to narrow during exhalation.[12]

These transmural gradients normally are not significant clinically. However, the airways of infants and young children are narrow in diameter and have a soft, cartilaginous superstructure. Therefore, the pediatric airway can experience air flow turbulence even with small degrees of edema, inflammation, mucus accumulation, or anatomical protuberances; for this reason, stridor is a common pediatric phenomenon.

APPROACH TO DIAGNOSIS

Stridor, of course, is a symptom and not a disease. As Boxes 173-1 and 173-2 demonstrate, numerous diagnostic entities cause stertor and stridor. How one approaches the diagnostic evaluation depends on the condition of the child at presentation. With the patient who has severe airway compromise, characterized by retractions, nasal flaring, diminished air entry, pallor or cyanosis, and change of mental status, airway maintenance takes precedence over diagnostic evaluation. Attention is directed toward controlling the airway, ventilating the patient, and relieving obstruction. Under these circumstances, most diagnostic maneuvers, including blood drawing, could compromise the integrity of the airway even further and should be postponed. On the other hand, in the uncompromised child whose obstruction does not seem life threatening, one can proceed with an orderly, thorough diagnostic investigation on an outpatient basis. But even in this situation, diagnosis must be prompt, because some pathological entities—for example, hemangiomas or papillomas—can progress to obstruction rapidly. (For detailed discussion of the management of acute airway obstruction, see Chapter 275, Airway Obstruction.)

For the child who has a single episode of acute stridor, the diagnosis might be obvious, and evaluation can stop with a history and physical examination. But for the patient who has congenital or continuous or frequently recurrent stridor, a more thorough investigation is warranted. In these situations, one follows the history and physical examination by radiographic studies—both plain films and specialized procedures—fiberoptic laryngoscopy, and possibly, bronchoscopy.

History

In evaluating stridor, two aspects of the patient's history are key to the diagnosis: age at onset and chronicity. Stridor, as well as other manifestations of airway problems that present soon after birth, usually indicates the presence of a congenital anatomical abnormality of the upper airway. Symptomatology within hours of birth most likely is caused by choanal atresia, bilateral vocal cord paralysis, or a large laryngeal web or cyst. On the other hand, stridor that presents at several days to weeks of life usually is caused by laryngomalacia, an external vascular compression of the trachea (a ring or sling), or a subglottic hemangioma. Subglottic stenosis—either congenital or acquired—often will not be evident until the infant develops his or her first respiratory illness, and thus usually is diagnosed initially as viral croup.

Acute stridor. Stridor that has been present for only a few hours to a few days is significantly more common than chronic stridor in the pediatric practice, and the cause often is readily apparent. A single episode of acute stridor usually is caused by an infectious process. It is estimated that 80% of all cases of stridor are caused by an airway infection. When one looks at these infectious episodes, laryngotracheobron-

BOX 173-1

CAUSES OF ACUTE STRIDOR IN PEDIATRIC PATIENTS

Infection
Laryngotracheobronchitis (croup)
Epiglottitis
Bacterial tracheitis
Retropharyngeal abscess
Peritonsillar abscess
Severe adenotonsillitis (infectious mononucleosis)
Ludwig's angina
Diphtheria
Membranous croup

Immune-Mediated Cause
Anaphylaxis
Angioneurotic edema

Trauma
Foreign body (in larynx, trachea, or esophagus)
Laryngeal fracture
Cricoarytenoid dislocation
Hematoma
Caustic ingestion
Thermal/inhalation injury

Metabolic Cause
Hypocalcemia (vocal cord tetany)
Biotinidase deficiency

chitis (viral croup) accounts for approximately 90% of all large-airway infections in the infant and child.[12] In addition to laryngotracheobronchitis (LTB), one also must consider supraglottitis (epiglottitis), bacterial tracheitis, and retropharyngeal abscess. The only fairly common noninfectious cause of acute stridor is foreign body of the airway or the esophagus. Of course, the practitioner must be aware that repeated episodes of crouplike illnesses might mean that the child has an underlying anatomical abnormality of the airway such as subglottic stenosis or hemangioma.[15]

Chronic stridor. Stridor present for weeks to months or frequently recurrent episodes of stridor are less common problems in pediatric practice and present a diagnostic challenge because the possibilities are much more numerous and less obvious (see Box 173-2). Chronic or recurrent stridor generally indicates a fixed anatomical obstruction and is significantly more common in males (about 70%).[5] In the young child, the lesion usually is congenital; in the older child, one must also consider acquired conditions.

The perinatal history is also useful in the evaluation of stridor. Children who have congenital airway problems frequently will have a perinatal history of polyhydramnios. A history of birth trauma or difficult delivery might suggest vocal cord paralysis; a history of neonatal intubation and ventilation raises the possibility of acquired subglottic stenosis.[8]

BOX 173-2

CAUSES OF CHRONIC/FREQUENTLY RECURRENT STRIDOR IN PEDIATRIC PATIENTS

Nasal Cavity
Bilateral choanal atresia
Anterior encephalocele
Polyps
Neoplasms
Dermoid cysts

Oropharynx/Nasopharynx
Craniofacial dysmorphia (micrognathia and glossoptosis; e.g., Pierre Robin and Treacher Collins syndromes)
Macroglossia (e.g., Beckwith's syndrome, congenital hypothyroidism, glycogen storage disease, lingual thyroid)
Hyperplasia of the tonsils and adenoids
Thyroglossal duct cyst
Cystic hygroma

Supraglottic Area
Laryngomalacia
Cysts of vallecular, epiglottis, arytenoids
Laryngeal web
Papillomatosis

Glottic and Subglottic Area
Vocal cord paralysis
Cricoarytenoid arthritis (manifestation of juvenile rheumatoid arthritis)
Psychogenic stridor (paradoxical vocal cord motion)
Glottic and subglottic webs
Subglottic stenosis (congenital and acquired)
Subglottic hemangioma

Trachea
Tracheal stenosis
Tracheomalacia
Vascular rings and slings
Enlarged thyroid
Spasmodic croup

Esophagus
Esophageal atresia
Tracheal-esophageal fistula
Laryngotracheal-esophageal cleft
Gastroesophageal reflux
Achalasia

Mediastinal Masses
Bronchogenic cysts
Ectopic or enlarged thymus
Neoplasm
Enlarged lymph nodes

Physical Examination

Once the degree of respiratory distress has been assessed and the airway stabilized (if necessary), the physical examination should focus on the quality of the stridorous sound. Low-pitched snoring sounds on inspiration (stertor) generally denote obstruction in the nose or nasopharynx. A harsh, high-pitched stridor generally will point to a lesion in the supraglottic area. Inspiratory stridor is produced mostly by obstruction above the level of the glottis. Biphasic stridor usually connotes obstruction at the glottic or subglottic level. Exclusively expiratory stridor generally points to a lesion in the intrathoracic trachea.

When examining the patient, it also is important to note the quality of the voice and cry. Hoarseness, aphonia, or a weak cry generally indicates a problem at the glottic level, either a glottic web or vocal cord paralysis.[1] Progressive hoarseness suggests an expanding lesion in the larynx such as a laryngeal papillomatosis or another form of neoplasm. A barking cough generally points to pathology in the subglottic and tracheal area. Pronounced drooling associated with stridor characteristically is associated with obstruction and inflammation in the oropharyngeal area and suggests epiglottitis or retropharyngeal abscess. Stridor that increases with agitation or crying probably stems from floppy airway structures and classically is associated with laryngomalacia. The position of the patient also should be noted. An infant whose stridor diminishes while in the prone position is likely to have laryngomalacia. In contrast, the child who holds his or her neck in the hyperextended position might have a mass in the retropharyngeal region or an aberrant artery in the mediastinum.[1,15] Finally, stridor that increases with drinking and eating suggests a tracheoesophageal connection such as a laryngotracheal-esophageal cleft or a tracheoesophageal fistula.

The practitioner should look for evidence of trauma to the body that would suggest an injury to the larynx or neck. Cutaneous hemangiomas should raise a suspicion of a hemangioma in the larynx. Craniofacial dysmorphia should prompt the examiner to look for micrognathia and glossoptosis. Tongue size should be noted and the oropharynx gently examined for enlarged tonsils, a retropharyngeal bulge, and an enlarged epiglottis. Any child who has both stridor and concomitant meningomyelocele or hydrocephalus should be assumed to have bilateral vocal cord paralysis unless proved otherwise.[10]

Associated Signs

The simultaneous occurrence of acute stridor and wheezing in a patient presents a diagnostic challenge frequently encountered by the clinician. Undoubtedly, any patient who has stridor and wheezes may have two pathological processes occurring together, such as croup and bronchiolitis or croup and asthma. But in one unscientifically sampled hospital-based series of 25 patients presenting with both symptoms, fewer than one third of the patients fit into this dual-diagnosis category. The other two thirds had a single problem accounting for both symptoms. The two largest groups were infants who had congenital lesions of the trachea (e.g., vascular ring) and children who had foreign bodies in the esophagus or airway.[14] The authors suggest that the history was not always reliable in these cases and that a physical examination could not distinguish between patients who had single lesions and those who had dual pathology. They do point out, however, that a thorough history and physical examination supplemented by plain radiography of neck and chest established the correct diagnosis in more than 75% of the patients.[14]

Radiography

Although the patient's history, physical examination, and associated findings may suggest the location of the obstruction and even the specific anatomical diagnosis, radiographic, and sometimes even endoscopic studies, generally are necessary for confirmation. A plain radiograph of the chest and the neck, coupled with fluoroscopy or a barium esophagram, can pinpoint the cause of chronic stridor in more than half of cases.[7]

A chest radiograph should be taken in all newborns who have stridor and in all older children in whom the cause of stridor is not evident immediately. Plain radiographs of the chest can reveal a mediastinal mass, external tracheal compression, or a right-sided aorta, which suggests the presence of a vascular ring.[10] One also might visualize a foreign body or infer its presence because of asymmetrical air trapping.

Anterior-posterior (AP) and lateral views of the neck can elucidate anatomical obstruction when done with the correct technique and when the clinical situation is not critical. The films should be taken with high-energy (high KV) exposure to emphasize soft-tissue detail. The lateral view is performed best with the head slightly extended in order to view the retropharyngeal space more accurately.[10,16] The AP view allows assessment of the subglottic and tracheal area and is particularly helpful in diagnosing subglottic stenosis, subglottic hemangioma, and tracheal stenosis. The lateral view allows assessment of the adenoids and tonsils, the epiglottis, and the retropharyngeal profile. However, it should be noted that radiographs are not always indicated in cases of acute stridor. An AP view of the neck is unnecessary to confirm the diagnosis of croup (see Chapter 277, Croup [Acute Laryngotracheobronchitis]). And for the patient who has epiglottitis (see Chapter 284), roentgenographic studies can be dangerous and generally are contraindicated when the diagnosis seems fairly certain.[10]

The diagnosis of a foreign body in the airway or esophagus is easily confirmed when the object is radiopaque. However, in the majority of cases one must look for more subtle findings. In addition to the unilateral air trapping that may be seen on a regular chest radiograph, forced expiratory films may be needed to establish the diagnosis. Because young children cannot perform this maneuver, one of the best approaches to the diagnosis of nonopaque foreign bodies is bilateral cross-table decubitus films of the chest. In this examination, one would expect, under normal circumstances, the dependent side to have increased vascular markings. However, when the side containing a foreign body is placed in the dependent position, vascular markings are not enhanced because of hyperinflation on that side.

Fluoroscopic evaluation of the airway also plays a role in diagnosis by providing a dynamic view of the airway during both phases of respiration. Thus, fluoroscopy can be used to confirm the diagnosis of subglottic stenosis (when suggested by an AP view of the neck) and can reveal other fixed lesions. It is particularly useful in diagnosing tracheomalacia. Fluoroscopy of the chest might reveal air trapping during exhalation, further confirming the diagnosis of bronchial foreign body.

Another radiographic study that is useful in the evaluation of airway obstruction is the barium esophagram. Although this study would not be done routinely, it is indicated if one suspects a nonradiopaque foreign body in the esophagus, a tracheoesophageal fistula, or a laryngotracheal-esophageal cleft. In the latter two instances, barium can be seen as it is aspirated into the trachea from the esophagus. Vascular compressions also are revealed by the esophagram because they are likely to indent the esophagus as well as the trachea.[10] Computerized tomography (CT) and magnetic resonance imaging (MRI) are not routinely used in the evaluation of stridor and airway obstruction; however, they have their place in specific instances. Computerized tomography is useful for defining masses in the neck and mediastinum, whereas MRI is particularly useful in delineating vascular anomalies. In some instances, MRI has obviated the need for angiography before surgical repair of aberrant vascular structures.[10,16]

Endoscopy

Whereas history, physical examination, plain radiographs of the chest and neck, and barium esophagram will define the cause of stridor in many cases—especially cases of acute stridor—endoscopy with a flexible fiberoptic laryngoscope or a rigid bronchoscope is required to reach a definitive diagnosis in most patients who have chronic or recurrent stridor.

Flexible fiberoptic laryngoscopy is a simple, safe, and well-tolerated procedure. Although some older children, especially those who are cooperative, can be examined by the heated mirror technique of indirect visualization, most are examined best by using a fiberoptic scope. This scope can visualize the airway anatomy from the nasal vestibule to the glottic opening. It can be done with the patient—even an infant—in a sitting position, awake, with local topical anesthesia and little or no sedation. The technique is enhanced by a video display and recording of the examination. The flexible endoscope is introduced through both nostrils so that the nasal cavities can be examined for atresia, masses, polyps, and foreign bodies. The scope then is advanced to the nasopharynx where the adenoids, tonsils, and base of the tongue are visualized. The supraglottic area is examined next, looking for hemangiomas and other masses, webs, and evidence of laryngomalacia. Finally, the examiner assesses vocal cord dynamics, noting abnormal movement or anatomical irregularities. On occasion the flexible endoscope reveals significant lesions below the vocal cords, in the subglottic area, although this area is better examined with roentgenograms and a rigid bronchoscope.[10,16]

More often than not, flexible laryngoscopy establishes the diagnosis in the evaluation of chronic stridor. However, in select cases a diagnosis cannot be determined definitively without rigid endoscopy of the esophagus and the airway below the glottis. Rigid endoscopy is the definitive procedure in airway evaluation. Not only does it allow for visualization but also it can be applied therapeutically. With a rigid endoscope one can biopsy lesions, drain abscesses and cysts, remove polyps, remove foreign bodies, and perform laser surgery.[16] In one study of chronic stridor, 12% of patients had two or more airway lesions. Of those patients who had two lesions, the majority of the lesions were below the vocal cords. Therefore, one can argue that patients who have severe airway symptomatology or cyanosis should be evaluated for multiple lesions, even if one diagnosis is made by laryngoscopy.[3,5] The practitioner should be aware that rigid endoscopy involves general anesthesia and must be done in the operating room.

SPECIFIC DIAGNOSTIC ENTITIES

A discussion of each of the stridor-producing diagnostic entities listed in Boxes 173-1 and 173-2 and their management is beyond the scope of this chapter. For an in-depth discussion of the management of severe acute airway obstruction, the reader is referred to Chapter 275, Airway Obstruction. The most important causes of acute airway obstruction are described in Chapters 277, Croup (Acute Laryngotracheobronchitis); 284, Epiglottitis; and 207, Foreign Bodies of the Ear, Nose, Airway, and Esophagus. Craniofacial abnormalities are discussed in Chapter 196, Cleft Lip and Cleft Palate, and other airway-obstructing abnormalities in Chapters 201, Cystic and Solid Masses of the Face and Neck, and 221, Hyperthyroidism.

One hospital-based series retrospectively reviewed 60 cases of children admitted for chronic stridor; the most common etiologies in this series are listed in Table 173-1.[3] As this table indicates, laryngomalacia is far and away the most common cause of congenital stridor in children and, along with tracheomalacia, makes up almost half of all cases of chronic stridor. Acquired and congenital subglottic stenosis occur with almost equal frequency and constitute another 30% of cases. Other common causes of chronic or recurrent stridor include subglottic hemangiomas, external vascular rings and slings, and vocal cord paralysis. The anatomy and physiology of each of these entities, as well as their diagnosis and management, are discussed briefly below. Some attention also will be directed to psychogenic stridor. Although this condition is not nearly as common as other causes of stridor, the practitioner caring for adolescent patients should be aware of it.

Laryngomalacia and Tracheomalacia

Laryngomalacia, also known as *congenital laryngeal stridor,* is the most common cause of chronic stridor in children and the most common congenital anomaly of the lar-

Table 173-1 Etiology of Chronic Stridor in Children*

Diagnosis	Frequency (%)
Laryngomalacia	45
Acquired subglottic stenosis	17
Congenital subglottic stenosis	13
Subglottic hemangioma	10
External vascular compression of trachea	6
Tracheomalacia	5
Vocal cord paralysis	3
All other diagnoses	1

*Based on retrospective review of 60 hospitalized patients.

ynx.[10,12,16] The problem arises from a weakness in the cartilaginous support of the laryngeal structures. As a result of this anatomical immaturity the epiglottis, aryepiglottic folds, and arytenoid cartilage collapse over the glottic opening, causing inspiratory stridor. Sixty percent of patients who have laryngomalacia demonstrate symptoms within the first week of life; almost all cases are apparent by the fifth week of life. However, most authors have described "outlying" cases that are not diagnosed in infancy and do not come to recognition until childhood or adolescence.[3,13] These late-presenting cases often are associated with additional abnormalities of the respiratory tract and, in some cases, probably are acquired rather than congenital.[13] In the typical congenital case, the infant's stridor is exacerbated by upper respiratory tract infection and by agitation and crying, but is relieved by prone positioning.

The prevailing understanding of laryngomalacia is that it is a benign, self-limited entity that requires no intervention, generally resolves by the time the infant is 18 months old, and has no long-term sequelae.[3] Although this is true in the majority of cases, 10% to 22% of infants who have laryngomalacia will develop life-threatening respiratory compromise that requires some sort of airway intervention.[3,6,12] These patients also will have feeding difficulties and failure to thrive secondary to their airway problems. This "sicker" subset of patients will go on to require intubation during respiratory tract infections and, in many cases, tracheostomy. With or without airway intervention the laryngomalacia ultimately will resolve when the larynx matures and the cartilaginous structures become firmer. In 17% of cases, symptomology will persist beyond 18 months of age. In some, the stridor will persist up to the fifth birthday.[3]

The simplest and most direct way to diagnose laryngomalacia is by flexible fiberoptic laryngoscopy. It also can be diagnosed by fluoroscopy, where the examiner notes inspiratory collapse of the laryngeal structure. However, many patients—up to 46% in one series and 68% in another—who have laryngomalacia will have additional abnormalities of their respiratory tract. The two most common anatomical defects associated with laryngomalacia are subglottic stenosis and tracheal compression by an anomalous innominate artery.[5,12,13] Patients who have additional airway lesions are the ones most likely to have severe airway obstruction and to require medical or surgical intervention. Therefore, it sometimes is necessary to go beyond flexible laryngoscopy in the evaluation of laryngomalacia and undertake bronchoscopy of the airway, especially for patients who have significant obstruction.

Most patients who have laryngomalacia will not require medical intervention. For those patients who have severe airway collapse, a tracheostomy is performed. More recently, a procedure in which the aryepiglottic folds are trimmed down endoscopically has been described; this allows some patients to have their symptoms relieved without a tracheostomy.[6]

Tracheomalacia similarly is caused by floppy cartilaginous support of the trachea. Patients who have tracheomalacia typically have biphasic stridor caused by inspiratory collapse of the extrathoracic trachea and expiratory collapse of the intrathoracic trachea. Although the pathophysiology of tracheomalacia is similar to that of laryngomalacia, the two entities usually occur independently and only rarely coexist in the same patient.[1] Like laryngomalacia, tracheomalacia often can be a benign, self-resolving condition that disappears in a child between 12 and 18 months of age as the cartilage becomes firmer. However, some patients who have this entity also have severe airway compromise and require surgical intervention. Although the diagnosis can be suggested by the disappearance of the tracheal air column above the carina on plain radiograph, it is confirmed by fluoroscopy or more definitively by flexible or rigid endoscopy of the trachea. Those patients who have severe and unremitting airway obstruction require continuous positive airway pressure, tracheostomy, or placement of a tracheal stent to prevent collapse.[1] Aortopexy, a surgical procedure in which the anterior surface of the ascending aorta is affixed to the sternum to stabilize the wall of the trachea, also has been used, with mixed results.[11]

Subglottic Stenosis

Subglottic stenosis is a narrowing of the larynx at the level of the cricoid cartilage, usually 2 to 3 mm below the glottic opening.[3] It can be caused by a congenital malformation or it can be acquired as a result of prolonged or especially traumatic neonatal intubation. Acquired subglottic stenosis is slightly more common than the congenital variety, but congenital stenosis often is more severe.[1]

Subglottic stenosis usually is not diagnosed until the patient is several months old. Frequently the patient will be asymptomatic until the airway is challenged by a respiratory tract infection. At this time the patient will develop respiratory distress, barking cough, and biphasic stridor and will be diagnosed as having croup. Subglottic stenosis is suspected when the croup fails to resolve with treatment or the patient develops recurrent episodes of stridor.

Subglottic stenosis is diagnosed initially by a high KV AP view of the neck that shows the characteristic "steeple" sign of subglottic narrowing. However, this is the same radiological finding seen in croup (see Fig. 277-3). If the clinical course of the patient suggests a fixed lesion, the diagnosis is made definitively by bronchoscopy.

If the patient does not develop critical airway obstruction during any bout of inflammation, the child eventually will outgrow the condition as the larynx enlarges and the obstruction becomes relatively less consequential. However, some patients who have subglottic stenosis will require an emergency tracheostomy during an acute episode of inflammation and obstruction. For patients who have severe obstruction and can escape emergency tracheostomy, an anterior cricoid split can be done to widen the airway diameter. This procedure, which usually requires 10 to 14 days in the hospital, is performed so that a tracheostomy can be avoided.[16]

Subglottic Hemangioma

Congenital cavernous hemangiomas of the airway are always located in the subglottic area. Like other congenital hemangiomas, airway hemangiomas grow rapidly in the first several months of life, and the patient generally becomes symptomatic at the age of 3 to 6 months. Symptoms include biphasic stridor, respiratory distress, and in more severe cases, feeding difficulties. Fifty percent of patients who have subglottic hemangiomas also have cutaneous hemangiomas, which provides a valuable clue to the diagnosis.[1,12]

The diagnosis is suggested by a lateral roentgenogram of the neck. One often can visualize larger hemangiomas by direct laryngoscopy, as they can be seen protruding below the glottic opening. However, a definitive diagnosis is made by rigid bronchoscopy, where a compressible lesion, located asymmetrically on one side of the subglottic area and covered by normal mucosa, is visualized. Biopsy is not necessary for confirmation.[1,12]

Like other hemangiomas, subglottic hemangiomas begin to regress spontaneously after the first year of life. For the patient who does not develop life-threatening airway obstruction, it therefore is possible to wait for remission; a tracheostomy is necessary in more severe cases.[16]

Vascular Rings and Slings

The trachea and/or esophagus can be compressed externally by persistent aberrant segments of the embryonic aortic arch. Although many individuals have anomalous vessels in their mediastinum and are asymptomatic, vascular anomalies account for 1% to 6% of all cases of congenital stridor.[3,12]

A vascular ring is created when the trachea and/or esophagus is encircled tightly by aberrant vascular structures. The most common vascular ring is created by a double aortic arch (approximately 50% of cases), encircling the trachea and esophagus.[9] Rings also can arise from a right-sided aortic arch and retroesophageal left subclavian artery with a left-sided ductus arteriosus or from an anomalous right subclavian artery arising from a left aortic arch.[1,9,12] A vascular sling is created by the anterior compression of the trachea by a nonencircling anomalous vessel. Slings generally are created by anomalous innominate or pulmonary arteries.[9,12]

The superior mediastinum of the infant is more crowded than that of a larger person, and the trachea is softer. Therefore, the infant is most prone to respiratory symptoms from anomalous vessels. Symptoms, when present, usually begin in the neonatal period. Biphasic stridor is common and is present in 95% of symptomatic patients. Other symptoms might include feeding problems secondary to esophageal compression, expiratory wheezing, cyanotic spells, and opisthotonic posturing to relieve the tracheal compression. If left untreated, these patients are prone to recurrent episodes of croup and recurrent lung infections.[1,9]

When suspected, diagnostic workup of a vascular compression starts with a chest radiograph to detect a right-sided aorta. A barium esophagram will reveal external compression of the esophagus and is diagnostic in 95% of cases.[2] The diagnosis is confirmed by rigid bronchoscopy, where one sees a pulsatile external indentation on the trachea. If surgery is contemplated, precise mapping of the vascular anatomy is required. Vascular anatomy is defined best by an arteriogram. However, this invasive procedure ultimately might be replaced by MRI. Echocardiography is not helpful in the diagnosis of thoracic vascular anomalies but should still be considered because about 25% of these children also will have significant congenital heart lesions.[9]

As the trachea firms and the mediastinum enlarges, becoming less crowded, the patient who has a vascular anomaly will become less symptomatic. Tracheostomy is contraindicated in patients who have vascular anomalies. Therefore, intubation is used to secure the airway. However, cardiovascular surgery is indicated for patients who have severe airway obstruction, recurrent pneumonia, or recurrent lung atelectasis. If surgical repair is undertaken early, one can expect the trachea to achieve normal configuration with growth. Because most vascular rings are associated with some degree of tracheomalacia, stridor does not always disappear immediately after vascular repair.[9]

Vocal Cord Paralysis

Vocal cord paralysis (VCP) can be congenital or acquired, unilateral or bilateral, benign or urgently life threatening. The paralyzed cord generally is frozen in adduction owing to paralysis of the vocal cord abductors. Unilateral VCP generally is caused by a peripheral injury to the recurrent laryngeal nerve (RLN). The RLN injury usually is caused by a cardiovascular impingement such as an enlarged left atrium or a dilated pulmonary artery. However, RLN dysfunction also can be caused by masses in the neck or mediastinum, traction on the neck at time of delivery, or surgery on the neck, chest, or mediastinum.[1,12]

Bilateral vocal cord paralysis sometimes can be caused by bilateral RLN impingement, but more likely is due to CNS pathology. Bilateral VCP occurs most frequently in patients who have Arnold-Chiari type II malformations. Patients who have this neural tube defect will manifest stridor alone or in association with dysphagia and apnea. In this setting, VCP heralds the onset of brainstem compression, which must be alleviated neurosurgically or death is certain. Brain tumors, and any other cause of increased intracranial pressure, can cause caudad displacement of the brainstem and traction on the vagal nerve before it exits the skull. Vocal cord paralysis and its associated symptoms can be the first manifestation of this intracranial pathology.[15]

The patient who has VCP generally will have stridor, continuous respiratory distress, difficulty with feeding, and a weak or absent cry. Patients who have unilateral VCP, however, often have minimal respiratory distress and normal phonation.[10,12,16]

VCP is diagnosed by direct fiberoptic laryngoscopy with the patient unanesthetized. The endoscopist will observe the absence of vocal cord motion during inspiration and phonation. Once vocal cord paralysis is diagnosed, it is necessary to do a chest roentgenogram and barium swallow to rule out mediastinal and cardiovascular anomalies. If the paralysis is bilateral, a head CT or MRI must be performed urgently to rule out intracranial pathology. Management of the patient who has vocal cord paralysis depends on the etiology and severity. Patients who have bilateral VCP need a tracheostomy to preserve their airway unless they have intracranial pathology that can be immediately addressed. If the vocal cord paralysis is not reversed within 24 hours, it generally becomes irreversible.[12] Unilateral VCP rarely requires tracheostomy and can be treated more temperately.

Psychogenic Stridor

The practitioner treating adolescent patients should be aware of the rare but instructive condition known as *psychogenic,* or *"functional," stridor.* This condition can be seen in adolescents and adults, males and females, but occurs most often among adolescent females. In most cases it represents a true conversion reaction (see Chapter 100, Conversion Reactions in Adolescents).

A person whose stridor is psychogenic often will present having intermittent and recurrent bouts of stridor. They typically show little anxiety about their symptoms and maintain normal oxygen saturation levels. However, sometimes their stridor is so convincing that they will be intubated repeatedly.

The diagnosis generally is made at laryngoscopy. With the patient awake, the vocal cords are noted to have normal anatomy and mobility. However, there is paradoxical adduction of the false and true cords during inspiration, with normal motion or abduction on expiration.[4] These laryngoscopy findings have led some to call this condition *paradoxical vocal cord motion.*[14]

Psychogenic stridor must be diagnosed by laryngoscopy. If suspected and confirmed early, it can save the patient many unnecessary diagnostic procedures and interventions. Effective treatment can be provided by psychotherapy, which allows patients to recognize their underlying depression and the symbolic import of their stridor.[4,14]

REFERENCES

1. Bellet PS: Stertor and stridor. In Bellet PS, editor: *The diagnostic approach to common symptoms and signs in infants, children and adolescents,* Philadelphia, 1989, Lea & Febiger.
2. Chun K, et al: Diagnosis and management of congenital vascular rings: a 22-year experience, *Ann Thoracic Surg* 53:597, 1992.
3. Friedman EM, et al: Chronic pediatric stridor: etiology and outcome, *Laryngoscope* 100:277, 1990.
4. Geist R: Diagnosis and management of psychogenic stridor caused by a conversion reaction, *Pediatrics* 86:315, 1990.
5. Holinger LD: Etiology of stridor in the neonate, infant and child, *Ann Otol* 89:397, 1980.
6. Jani P, et al: Surgical treatment of laryngomalacia, *J Laryngol Otol* 105:1040, 1991.
7. John SD, Swischuk LE: Stridor and upper airway obstruction in infants and children, *Radiographics* 12:625, 1992.
8. Kilham H, et al: Severe upper airway obstruction, *Pediatr Clin North Am* 34:1, 1987.
9. Ledwith MV, Duff DF: A review of vascular rings 1980-1992, *Irish Med J* 87:178, 1994.
10. Letourneau MA, et al: Respiratory disorders. In Barkin RM, editor: *Pediatric emergency medicine,* St Louis, 1992, Mosby.
11. Malone PS, Kiely EM: Role of aortopexy in the management of primary tracheomalacia and tracheobronchomalacia, *Arch Dis Child* 65:438, 1990.
12. Maze A, Bloch E: Stridor in pediatric patients, *Anesthesiology* 50:132, 1979.
13. Nussbaum E, Maggi JC: Laryngomalacia in children, *Chest* 98:942, 1990.
14. Poole SR, et al: The child with simultaneous stridor and wheezing, *Pediatr Emerg Care* 6:33, 1990.
15. Ross DA, Ward PH: Central vocal cord paralysis and paresis presenting as laryngeal stridor in children, *Laryngoscope* 100:10, 1990.
16. Tunkel DE, Zalzal GH: Stridor in infants and children: ambulatory evaluation and operative diagnosis, *Clin Pediatr* 31:48, 1992.

174 Syncope

Diane L. McDonald

Syncope (fainting) is defined as a rapid, transient, complete loss of consciousness and postural tone as a result of cerebral ischemia, hypoxia, or hypoglycemia. In the pediatric population, it usually occurs among older children and adolescents. In a study by Pratt and Fleisher,[3] 50% of the patients examined in the pediatric emergency room for fainting were diagnosed as having vasovagal syncope. Other diagnoses included orthostatic hypotension (20%), atypical seizure (7.5%), migraine (5%), and minor head trauma (5%). McHarg et al[2] looked at children referred to a subspecialty clinic for the evaluation of syncope and found that although most children had a vasovagal etiology, a significant percentage (25%) had a serious but treatable cardiac or neurological disorder.

Although syncope most often is benign, a thorough history and physical examination must be performed, with added attention to the patient's cardiac and neurological status. If the cause of the syncopal event is cardiac, the child may be at risk for an arrhythmia or even sudden death. In addition, a child who is lethargic or unconscious is not one who has simple syncope and needs to be evaluated for an underlying disorder of the central nervous system. A child in whom cardiac disease is suspected or one who manifests impairment of consciousness after the initial event requires immediate attention and intervention.

The history of the event usually will lead to the likely cause. Any available witness should be interviewed to obtain a full description of the event. Issues to be noted include the premorbid state of the child, circumstances surrounding the episode, the onset and duration of the loss of consciousness, any associated body movements, and the quality of the recovery period. Inquiry should include the circumstances precipitating the event. For example, with vasovagal syncope the child often is standing in a warm, stuffy room and is hungry, tired, or frightened. The prodrome of a seizure may consist of an aura, whereas a cardiac event often occurs without warning or is induced by exercise.

It is helpful to attempt to determine if the child was completely unconscious or if there was some degree of responsiveness, suggesting hysteria or malingering. A truly unconscious person will not respond if the eyelashes are lightly brushed; a hysterical person will respond, albeit often with just a mild flickering of the lids. Seizurelike movements are important; however, generalized tonic-clonic movements may be seen in all forms of syncope because of cerebral anoxia or hypoglycemia.

The duration of the episode should be estimated. In general, the conscious state is regained quickly in the case of vasovagal syncope (a few seconds to 1 or 2 minutes), whereas a seizure may last longer and the postictal state may be characterized by prolonged confusion and fatigue.

The past medical history is very important. A history of congenital heart disease, seizure disorder, or endocrine abnormalities such as diabetes may be important. Recurrent syncopal episodes are unusual and may require more extensive testing—for example, Holter (cardiac) monitoring, echocardiographic examination, electrophysiological studies, or an electroencephalogram to uncover occult cardiac or neurological disease.

The family history may be helpful. Seizure disorders and cardiac disease leading to syncope, such as Marfan syndrome, idiopathic hypertrophic subaortic stenosis, and prolonged QT syndrome, may be inherited. Breath-holding spells also have been noted to occur more frequently in those who have such a family history.

As can be inferred from the disorder-specific descriptions that follow, particular importance should be paid during the physical examination to the cardiorespiratory systems. Murmurs, gallops, and irregular rhythms suggest that the syncopal event is of cardiac origin. Wheezing, rales, and evidence of hypoxia suggest cardiac or respiratory disease. Attention also should be directed to the gastrointestinal tract for signs of hemorrhage or hypovolemia.

DIFFERENTIAL DIAGNOSIS

Syncope can be categorized by its various causes (Box 174-1).

Neurocardiogenic Syncope

A fainting episode in which the child has been standing or sitting for a prolonged period in an uncomfortable environment suggests neurocardiogenic syncope (also known as *vasovagal* or *vasodepressor syncope*). A noxious event that causes fear, pain, or anxiety also may precipitate the faint. The child may feel dizzy, weak, or nauseated and appear cold and clammy. A rapid drop in blood pressure associated with vagally stimulated bradycardia may lead to the loss of consciousness. The exact mechanism is not completely understood; however, it is known that the normal response to standing is a decrease in venous return to the heart. The ensuing message of hypotension to the brain results in an increase in sympathetic outflow and a consequent increase in heart rate and an increase in blood pressure. It is believed that patients who have vasodepressor syncope lack this adaptive

BOX 174-1

DIFFERENTIAL DIAGNOSIS OF SYNCOPE

Neurocardiogenic
Vasovagal/vasodepressor episodes
Breath-holding spells
  Cyanotic
  Pallid infantile syncope

Psychophysiological
Hyperventilation
Hysteria/conversion reaction

Neurological
Generalized tonic-clonic seizure
Atonic seizures
Complex partial seizures
Migraine
Trauma/concussion
Narcolepsy

Cardiac
Structural abnormalities
  Aortic stenosis
  Idiopathic hypertrophic subaortic stenosis
  Left atrial myxoma
  Tetralogy of Fallot
  Pulmonic stenosis
  Primary pulmonary hypertension
Arrhythmia
  Bradycardia
    Sick sinus syndrome
    Atrioventricular block
  Ventricular tachycardia/fibrillation
    Myocarditis/pericarditis
    Intoxication/medication
    Congenital heart disease
    Postoperative cardiac surgery
    Prolonged QT syndrome
    Ischemic heart disease
  Supraventricular tachycardia
    Wolff-Parkinson-White syndrome
    Caffeine/stress

Orthostatic
Hypovolemia
Postural hypotension
Medications

Metabolic
Hypoglycemia
Anemia

Miscellaneous
Cough
Swallowing
Micturition
Pregnancy

mechanism. Instead, a sudden decrease in venous return to the heart causes a forceful ventricular contraction, resulting in stretching of the mechanoreceptors. This sends a paradoxical message of hypertension to the brain, causing decreased sympathetic output and increased parasympathetic activity.[6] The resulting bradycardia and hypotension usually is short-lived and, depending on the degree of cerebral hypoperfusion, may end with tonic-clonic movements. The patient usually awakens to full consciousness within a short time.

Cyanotic breath-holding spells usually begin around the age of 6 months and end by age 6 years. Clinically the child is upset, frightened, or hurt, begins to cry, gasps, and then becomes apneic and cyanotic. Stiffening of the body and a loss of consciousness soon may follow. The pathophysiological basis is unclear, but it may be that crying during expiration causes increased intrathoracic pressure, which in turn leads to low cardiac output. Hypoxia combined with decreased cerebral blood flow leads to the loss of consciousness. The event is brief, and afterward the child becomes fully conscious. A pallid type of breath-holding spell (pallid infantile syncope) is less common, although it can occur in the same age range as does the cyanotic spell and likewise may begin with pain or crying. The mechanism differs: The child suddenly becomes pale and limp and loses consciousness. The pathophysiological basis is increased vagal tone, which causes an apparent asystole. The event ordinarily lasts only seconds to minutes, and the child awakens to full consciousness.[1] (See Chapter 159, Nonconvulsive Periodic Disorders).

Psychophysiological Syncope

Hyperventilation may occur as a response to anxiety or pain. For instance, the child may hyperventilate in anticipation of venipuncture or as a reaction to fright. Rapid, short breaths cause hypocapnia and a resultant cerebral vasoconstriction and hypoperfusion. The individual experiences a feeling of lightheadedness along with numbness and tingling of the hands and feet; loss of consciousness is brief and recovery rapid.

A conversion reaction transforms an unacceptable unconscious desire into a physical complaint. In the older child or adolescent the conversion reaction may take the form of hysterical fainting. The child often is sitting or recumbent or may exaggerate a fall from a standing position to avoid injury. The child usually responds quickly to a mildly painful stimulus, and the physical examination reveals nothing extraordinary.

Neurological Syncope

Generalized tonic-clonic movements can occur with all forms of syncope, so the diagnosis of seizure disorder as a specific underlying cause for syncope may be difficult. Intercurrent fever or a history of seizures, head trauma, or adverse perinatal events may be helpful leads; frequently, there is a family history of epilepsy.

The generalized tonic-clonic or grand mal seizure is characterized by a rather sudden onset of complete unconsciousness with stiffening of the body and rolling back of the eyes. After a tonic phase, clonic movements of the extremities may occur. Although the duration is variable, it usually lasts longer than a simple fainting spell. Incontinence is common, and the postictal recovery period is characterized by prolonged confusion and weakness.

Some complex partial seizures can resemble fainting episodes. Partial seizures may begin with an aura, which the child may describe as an uncomfortable feeling or an unusual visual or olfactory sensation. During the seizure the child may be unresponsive and lose postural tone. The complex partial seizure is characterized by semipurposeful yet involuntary action—for example, picking at clothing. In the postictal period the child is tired and returns to full consciousness slowly.

A basilar artery migraine may manifest as a syncopal event believed to result from impaired blood flow to the brainstem during the vasoconstrictive phase of migraine. After the initial spasm, the affected artery dilates and a classic or common migraine headache occurs. A family history of migraine may help in making this diagnosis.

It is not uncommon to lose consciousness after relatively minor head trauma (concussion). Other symptoms such as vomiting, headache, and amnesia also may occur. A significant episode of unconsciousness warrants a computed tomography (CT) scan followed by an observation period in the emergency department. Abnormal findings on neurological examination, clear drainage from the nose or ears, bleeding from the ears, a Battle sign, or a prolonged period of altered consciousness should alert the physician to the possibility of serious injury such as a subdural hematoma, basilar skull fracture, or cerebral contusion. If intracranial injuries are suspected, an immediate CT scan and neurosurgical consultation are required.

Cardiac Syncope

Cardiac syncope is rare in childhood; however, when it occurs, it may be life threatening. Cardiac disease can cause syncope in a number of ways. Structural heart disease may obstruct blood flow from the left ventricle, with consequent hypoperfusion, or may shunt blood flow from right to left, leading to hypoxia. A person who has a diseased or stressed myocardium from hypoxia, myocarditis, toxic drug ingestion, or a congenital heart lesion is at risk for a sudden arrhythmia. Arrhythmias, by decreasing either the cardiac stroke volume or the heart rate, can lead to a reduced cardiac output and cerebral hypoperfusion.

Structural lesions such as aortic stenosis and idiopathic hypertrophic subaortic stenosis (IHSS) can cause dizziness or fainting after exercise. On auscultation, a systolic murmur may be heard at the right sternal border. The murmur of IHSS is accentuated by a Valsalva maneuver, and the electrocardiogram shows signs of left ventricular enlargement. Children who have cyanotic congenital heart disease, in particular tetralogy of Fallot, may have spells of cyanosis that occasionally lead to unconsciousness. These episodes, called "tet spells," are caused by a sudden decrease in pulmonary blood flow and the shunting of deoxygenated blood from right to left through the ventricular septal defect and thence the aorta.

Bradycardia, as seen with sick sinus syndrome, is associated with periods of extreme sinus slowing or arrest and may require a pacemaker. Tachycardia, as with ventricular tachycardia and ventricular fibrillation, is most serious and usually is the result of severe underlying cardiac disease. Ventricular fibrillation and episodes of torsade de pointes can be seen with the prolonged QT syndrome. Two autosomal dominant inherited diseases characterized by a prolonged QT interval are notable. The Jervell and Lange-Nielsen syndrome is associated with deafness; the Romano-Ward syndrome occurs with normal hearing. Both are caused by mutations in genes encoding cardiac ion channels. This produces a prolonged action potential that can lead to arrhythmias and sudden death.[7] Sinus rates of 200 to 300 beats/min are possible with supraventricular tachycardia (SVT), which can be associated with Wolff-Parkinson-White syndrome. In this circumstance an accessory pathway, the bundle of Kent, bypasses the atrioventricular node and speeds conduction from the atria to the ventricles. Stress, coffee, and drugs (e.g., amphetamines) also can cause an attack.[4]

Orthostatic Syncope

Hypovolemia from dehydration or acute blood loss can lead to orthostatic hypotension and syncope. Medications (e.g., diuretics, antihypertensives, and antidepressants) also can cause orthostatic blood pressure changes. In addition, postural hypotension can occur from rising quickly, prolonged standing, or prolonged bed rest.

Metabolic Syncope

Syncope caused by hypoglycemia is encountered most frequently in the young patient who has insulin-dependent diabetes. Better control, with appropriate insulin dosing and an understanding of the warning signs of hypoglycemia, may prevent further episodes. Chronic anemia can lead to fatigue, weakness, or a syncopal attack. A thorough search for the source of decreased erythropoiesis or of blood loss is required, and a blood transfusion may be necessary.

Miscellaneous Causes of Syncope

Cough-induced syncope has been described in patients who have the paroxysms of pertussis, laryngeal spasm, laryngeal nerve irritation, and asthma. Rarely in childhood, syncope is associated with micturition or strenuous swallowing.

Pregnancy always should be considered when a female of childbearing age faints. Pregnancy-associated fainting results from increased estrogen and progesterone levels that cause decreased peripheral vascular resistance and hypotension.

PSYCHOSOCIAL CONSIDERATIONS

The majority of benign vasovagal fainting episodes occurs in places outside the home. Perhaps at school or church, for example, the child is forced to sit or stand for long periods but at home is more free to move about and alter body position. Thus, a "faint" at home or while exercising may suggest a more serious cause, including cardiac syncope.

Atypical syncopal episodes, hysteria, or pseudoseizures may reflect "acting-out" behavior and should prompt evaluation for evidence of physical, verbal, or sexual abuse. Efforts should be made to determine whether the family is subject to unusual stress—for example, marital conflict, divorce, or recent death.

MANAGEMENT

A simple workup for a first fainting episode should include an electrocardiogram. The electrocardiogram should be evalu-

BOX 174-2

WORKUP FOR THE FIRST EPISODE OF SYNCOPE

History
Physical examination
Vital signs, including orthostatic blood pressure and pulse
Electrocardiogram
Consider:
- Glucose level
- Electrolyte levels
- Hematocrit measurement
- Pregnancy test
- Toxicology screen
- CT scan
- EEG

Table 174-1 Relating History to Etiological Factors

History	Possible Causes
Prolonged seizure activity or postictal state	Seizure disorder
Precipitation by crying	Breath-holding spell
Precipitation by cough, swallow, or urination	Cough, swallow, micturition syncope
Precipitation by exercise or a sudden onset of syncope	Cardiac syncope
Head trauma	Concussion
Precipitation by noxious event or environmental stress	Vasovagal syncope
Inconsistent findings or incomplete unconsciousness	Hysteria or malingering

ated for rhythm disturbances, chamber hypertrophy, abnormal voltage, and a prolonged QT segment. Also, vital signs should be taken while the patient is upright and supine (Box 174-2). Further laboratory tests should be guided by the physical examination and the current and past medical history. The physical examination of the syncopal patient begins with assessment of neurological status. A child who arrives unconscious or with depressed consciousness has not had a simple fainting episode and requires immediate care. This may include a CT scan, toxicology screen, hematocrit, and electrolyte and glucose levels. If the child is alert, a careful physical examination should be performed with special attention to the cardiovascular system. The examiner should listen for murmurs, extra heart sounds, and an unusual rhythm or rate. If an abnormality is found on cardiac examination or electrocardiogram, monitoring and cardiology consultation most often are mandated. A patient who has recurrent syncopal episodes should be evaluated for occult cardiac disease. A referral to a cardiologist for Holter monitoring, an echocardiogram, stress testing, or an electrophysiological study is indicated. Abnormalities such as a low hematocrit or blood glucose level are rare but, if present, require a vigorous search for the cause. If postprandial hypoglycemia is suspected, a glucose tolerance test may help in making the diagnosis. Children who have symptoms of obvious dehydration or abnormal orthostatic vital signs require rehydration therapy.

Frequently the results of the physical examination are normal and no abnormality is found in the initial laboratory workup. As is so often the case, the history becomes most important in establishing a cause (Table 174-1). A seizure disorder can be particularly difficult to diagnose because seizurelike activity can occur with all forms of syncope, and the electroencephalogram often does not reveal significant findings. Therefore, a high index of suspicion and consultation with a neurologist may be needed.

Most other causes of syncope are benign. Reassurance and common-sense management are required. A child who has vasovagal syncope should be placed supine before venipuncture. Children who hyperventilate need to learn its relationship to fainting; attention should be paid to the reasons for hyperventilation. Breath-holding spells are best treated by educating the parents and by emphasizing the harmless nature of the spells. In severe instances a neurology consultation is warranted.

Hysteria or malingering may be difficult to diagnose. Hospitalization for observation and a psychiatric referral may be indicated. Finally, pregnancy always should be considered in the evaluation of postpubertal female who has syncope. If there is any possibility of pregnancy or if the date of the last menstrual period is unknown, a urine or serum pregnancy test should be done.

Recurrent Syncope

In the past, recurrent idiopathic syncope has been a diagnosis of exclusion. Although its utility in children is still controversial, head-upright tilt-table testing has become a means of provoking vasodepressor syncope in susceptible individuals, after other more serious causes have been ruled out. Patients are placed supine on a table that has a footboard. The table then is tilted up between 60 to 80 degrees for 30 to 60 minutes. Patients are monitored closely for a syncopal episode. Some centers use low-dose intravenous isoproterenol infusions to increase the sensitivity of the test, which ranges from 30% to 80% depending on the laboratory.

Therapy includes avoiding precipitating factors, educating the patient to lie down when symptoms occur, and treating pharmacologically. Fludrocortisone, beta-adrenergic-blocking agents, and transdermal scopolamine have been effective in some individuals.[5]

REFERENCES

1. Holmes GL: Breath-holding attacks in children, *Postgrad Med* 84:191, 1988.
2. McHarg ML, et al: Syncope in children, *Pediatr Cardiol* 18:367, 1997.
3. Pratt JL, Fleisher GR: Syncope in children and adolescents, *Pediatr Emerg Care* B5:80, 1989.
4. Ruckman RN: Cardiac causes of syncope, *Pediatr Rev* 9:101, 1987.
5. Samiol D, et al: Head-upright tilt-table testing in children with unexplained syncope, *Pediatrics* 92:426, 1993.
6. Tanel RE, Walsh RP: Syncope in the pediatric patient, *Cardiol Clin* 15: 277, 1997.
7. Vincent GM: The molecular genetics of the long QT syndrome: genes causing fainting and sudden death, *Annu Rev Med* 49:263, 1998.

SUGGESTED READINGS

Anderson RH, et al: *Pediatric cardiology*, Edinburgh, 1986, Churchill Livingstone.

Braden DS, Gaymes CH: The diagnosis and management of syncope in children and adolescents, *Pediatr Ann* 26:422, 1997.

Castor W, Skarin R, Roscelli JD: Orthostatic heart rate and arterial blood pressure changes in normovolemic children, *Pediatr Emerg Care* 1:123, 1985.

DiMario F, et al: Pallid breath-holding spells, *Clin Pediatr* 29:17, 1990.

Driscoll DJ, Edwards WD: Sudden unexpected death in children and adolescents, *Am Coll Cardiol* 5(6 suppl):118B, 1985.

Farmer TW: *Pediatric neurology*, Philadelphia, 1983, Harper & Row.

Katz RM: Cough syncope in children with asthma, *Pediatrics* 77:48, 1970.

Naschitz JE, et al: The role of the capnography head-up tilt test in the diagnosis of syncope in children and adolescents, *Pediatrics* 101:2, 1997.

Prodinger RJ, Reisdorff EJ: Syncope in children, *Emerg Med Clin North Am* 16:3, 1998.

Salim MA, et al: Syncope recurrence in children: relation to tilt-test results, *Pediatrics* 102:4, 1998.

Sugarman JM, Rodgers GC, Paul RI: Utility of toxicology screening in a pediatric emergency department, *Pediatr Emerg Care* 13:1, 1997.

Woody RC, Kiel EA: Swallowing syncope in a child, *Pediatrics* 78:507, 1986.

175 Tics

John S. Werry

DEFINITION AND CLASSIFICATION

Tics are recurring, nonrhythmic, sudden, rapid, stereotyped, involuntary movements or vocalizations.[2] The muscles affected mostly are those of the head, neck, and respiratory system. Tics may be motor or vocal and simple or complex in form. The commonest simple motor tics are eye-blinking, neck-twisting, shoulder-shrugging, and grimacing; coughing, throat-clearing, sniffing, grunting, and hiccuping are the usual simple vocal tics. Complex motor tics include facial gestures; grooming of the head or hair; touching, jumping, stomping on, or sniffing objects; and echokinesis (automatic imitation of another person's movements). Complex vocal tics include palilalia (repeating one's own words), echolalia (repeating the words of others), and coprolalia (uttering obscenities). Tics are exacerbated by emotion, disappear in sleep, and can be controlled to some degree, though not completely, with treatment. These characteristics are not as helpful in differential diagnosis as might be supposed because they also characterize many neurological movement disorders. Although children generally report that they are unaware of their tics, premonitory urges occur, especially in severe cases, and are reported more often as the child gets older.[8,10]

Motor tics are distinguishable easily from chorea (with which they often are confused) by their centripetal location, fixed repetitive form, and normal muscle tone and from most other neurologically based abnormal movements by their rapidity, fixity, and normal muscle tone. They are distinguished from self-stimulating behaviors, such as rocking or head-banging, by their later onset, more restricted localization and lower complexity, involuntary nature, and lack of apparent pleasure associated with the movement (see Chapter 94, Self-Stimulating Behaviors). Nevertheless, distinguishing these from complex motor tics can sometimes be difficult. Vocal tics often are mistaken for otolaryngological or respiratory symptoms, but other essential diagnostic characteristics of such disorders are absent.

The study of tics over the past 50 years is a fascinating microcosm of the history of psychiatry in that period. At first, lacking any definitive etiology or treatment, medicine confined tics to the psychiatric waste basket. However, psychiatrists proceeded to show that tics are actually a neurobiological disorder and like most medical disorders, not caused but only made worse by psychological factors.

The fourth edition of the American Psychiatric Association's *Diagnostic and Statistical Manual of Mental Disorders (DSM-IV)* describes four rather arbitrary subtypes of tic disorder: transient (duration longer than 4 weeks but less than 1 year), chronic (longer than 1 year), Tourette's disorder (at least 1 year duration with less than a 3-month remission; severe, multiple tics including vocal tics but not necessarily occurring contemporaneously), and tic disorder not otherwise specified (NOS), in which criteria of minimum duration of 4 weeks or frequency of many times a day and most every day are not met.[2] It is not known whether these four disorders simply are more or less severe instances of the same disorder;[22] most recent research has been restricted to Tourette's disorder. However, pedigree studies regarding Tourette's disorder suggest that they probably are related somewhat.[8] Tourette's disorder attracts a variety of sobriquets (e.g., Gilles de la Tourette syndrome, and combined vocal and motor tic disorder). The *DSM-IV* term used here is simpler, is in more general use, and should become standard.

FREQUENCY

Tics can begin as early as age 2 years. Peak prevalence is between 10 and 12 years (2 to 3 years earlier for Tourette's disorder), after which tics decline rapidly.[2,22] At peak they may affect from 5% to 24% of children, depending on the criteria used for diagnosis. Higher figures probably include many cases of tic disorder NOS that are short-lived and inconspicuous, because this is the commonest kind of tic disorder. However, recent epidemiological studies suggest that even Tourette's disorder is much more common than previously thought and in most cases is quite mild and not seen in clinical settings.[12] Boys are affected more often than girls, especially in severe cases; the ratio is as high as 3 to 1.[2]

ETIOLOGY

The cause of tics is unknown, but it is the focus of intensive and fascinating biobehavioral research[8-11] that shows the boundaries between psychiatry and neurology to be ill defined and increasingly obsolete. Not surprisingly, in view of its greater severity, most of this research is on Tourette's disorder, which may distort results. It reflects the increasing sophistication of neuropsychiatric and medical research. Notable in this research is its focus on the basal ganglia, genetics, and immunology,[11,14] though none of this yet has much clinical application. In a small number of cases, tics reflect or portend a neurological disorder.[22] Such tics are likely to be much more persistent and to be accompanied by signs of the causative disorder.

Some of the factors that have been shown to be associated with tics and thus may give clues to the cause are:[2,8,22]

1. *Developmental stage*. That tics are common in middle childhood and disappear soon after points to maturational factors in the neuromuscular apparatus mirrored in the high frequency of all spontaneous movements (such as choreiform movements) at this age.
2. *Gender*. The preponderance of boys affected also supports the motor developmental view because boys are more active motorically than girls at all ages, but especially in middle childhood.[22] There is evidence that androgens may mediate this vulnerability because postnatal exposure to such hormones may elicit Tourette's syndrome,[8] and anti-androgens may improve tics.[15]
3. *Prenatal, perinatal, and postnatal factors*. There is some association between tics and the same group of factors that has been proposed repeatedly for hyperactivity; as in that condition, however, this association is weak, because it has appeared only in epidemiological studies.[8,22] Nevertheless, recent studies suggest that prenatal and perinatal factors (including maternal vomiting and stress during pregnancy, poor fetal nutrition, and exposure to androgens) may be of more significance in Tourette's syndrome.[8] Apart from drugs (see item 7) and a few neurological disorders, thermal stress is the only other established physical insult.[8] One exception is streptococcal infection, which it is posited, may cause an autoimmune reaction attacking basal ganglia. Although this may be consequent on Syndenham's chorea, more often tics may be an alternative autoimmune outcome (along with obsessive-compulsive disorder with which Tourette's disorder shares some clinical and genetic features).[21]
4. *Psychological factors*. Anxiety is associated with tics, in that it makes existing tics worse and may precipitate them in some cases; furthermore, children who have anxiety disorders or overanxious personalities are overrepresented in clinical cases.[22] Little is known, however, about the psychological status of most children who have tics, for they rarely are seen in clinics.
5. *Psychiatric disorders*. Psychiatric disorders should be separated from psychological factors because some psychiatric disorders, especially those more severe, are biogenic or require a biological vulnerability to develop. Family pedigree and clinical studies of tics and occurrence of stimulant-induced tics in hyperactivity show that there is a strong relationship, most marked in Tourette's syndrome, between tics and attention deficit/hyperactivity disorder (AD/HD).[2,8,9] Although much has been made of these overlapping similarities, recent work has emphasized the differences, suggesting that much of the behavioral and neuropsychological disability ascribed to Tourette's disorder is actually a contaminant form of comorbid AD/HD (or other psychiatric disorder).[19] Similar problems of diagnostic promiscuity are widespread in pediatric psychiatry, for example, in ascribing to AD/HD characteristics that properly belong with comorbid but ignored oppositional or conduct disorder (see Chapter 73, Attention Deficit/Hyperactivity Disorder). Community studies show that most of those who have (mild) tics and Tourette's disorder probably have no comorbid psychiatric problems.[12] Nevertheless, there is some relationship between tics and obsessive-compulsive disorder because symptomatology (e.g., premonitory urges, intrusive thoughts, and compulsive actions), putative anatomical locus (cortico/striato/thalamic circuits), hypothesized pathophysiology (rogue reverberating microcircuits), and family pedigrees all show elements in common.[8,11]
6. *Genetic factors*. There is evidence to suggest that tics are, in some cases, a genetic disorder.[8,11,24] This is most true of Tourette's disorder, in which the gene seems to act as an autosomal dominant one. However, the gene seems to be of variable expression in that most relatives have much more mild and transient forms of tic disorder. This suggests that in addition to genes, protective and risk factors must also exist. Penetrance increases if obsessive-compulsive disorder is accepted as an alternative expression of the gene; indeed, a majority of patients who have Tourette's disorder develop obsessive-compulsive symptoms if the disorder persists into adulthood.[8] Although there is an association between tics and AD/HD, it is by no means clear that this is another expression of the tic/Tourette gene.[8] As previously noted, some of the supposed overlap may be due to confusion with unrecognized comorbid conditions.[19]
7. *Drugs*. Amphetamine and other dopaminergic drugs induce stereotypies in rats and occasionally can produce tics and other abnormal movements in children. Stimulants given for hyperactivity may precipitate tics or Tourette's disorder in vulnerable children,[9] though some believe that this merely reflects the common association of the two disorders.[23] However, it now is disputed whether it is prudent *not* to give stimulants to hyperactive children if there is any history or signs of tics or Tourette's disorder.[9] Stimulants certainly can aggravate tics, but this may fade after a few days and may be less with methylphenidate than with dextroamphetamine.[7,23] If tics emerge subsequently, the stimulants can be stopped and other medications such as antidepressants substituted.[9,23] However, current thinking is probably more in favor of titrating the effects of the tics, which are often mild and short-lived, against the benefit produced by stimulants.[7] Drugs of abuse, especially cocaine and other stimulants, are capable of producing tics. Neuroleptic drugs also can produce tics/Tourette's disorder as an analog of tardive dyskinesia[3] presumptively caused by hypersensitivity of dopamine receptors following chronic blockade. This is yet one more reason for caution in using these drugs, including in tic disorders.

It seems reasonable to posit that in most cases, tics appear spontaneously during middle childhood as exaggerations of spontaneous movements, normal at that stage of development, and as manifestations of normal maturation in dopaminergic or other systems. In others, they are catalyzed by states of increased motor activity or excitability such as in AD/HD or in anxiety disorders or the use or abuse of dopaminergic drugs interacting with neuromuscular developmental status. In some cases, notably Tourette's disorder, tics probably are the result of an as yet unestablished abnormality of the neuromotor system of genetic origin or rarely, some other neurological disorder. As with any other motor behavior, however, tics may be influenced by learning or conditioning, which may serve to prolong or shorten their course.

Tics should never be assumed to indicate a psychiatric disorder unless they are associated with other signs or symptoms of such a disorder that affect other areas of function beyond the motor system. Also, although tics can be controlled to some degree for variable periods in public situations (e.g., a pediatrician's office), this does not mean that the child can or should be expected to control them most of the time. Such control requires considerable emotional energy from the child[10] and can be sustained only for limited periods. As soon as the child relaxes, is distracted, or lets up concentration in the least, the tics will reappear.

Even if most tics do not represent disease, referral is likely to be influenced as much by associated problems as by the tics themselves.[12,19] This being so, the key to treatment may sometimes lie less in tics than in mapping other areas of disability and in the treatment of the whole child.[16]

TREATMENT

The vast majority of tics in children will be mild, be short-lived, and flit from one muscle group to another. As in so much of medicine, the best treatment for most tics is masterly inactivity coupled with authoritative information about the condition to child and parents.[22] Clearly, any unreasonable and avoidable stress on the child should be reduced; however, tics should not be a sign to treat the child as though she or he is necessarily overstressed or anxious. First, that presumes a cause that may not be present; second, if it is so, moderate stress is not only an inexorable part of life but also is one of the ways children learn how to cope. AD/HD, obsessive-compulsive disorder, or drug abuse also may be present and require attention. Other kinds of medication, such as stimulants, neuroleptics, androgenic steroids, or any drug that interferes with dopamine, such as metoclopramide or antiemetics, should be borne in mind because their removal may be the required treatment.

Once a tic has been present and unchanged in form or site for more than a year, treatment may be considered—but only if the tic is conspicuous, disabling, or distressing to the child. No treatment for tics can be said to be simple or entirely or even often effective or free from side effects. Treatments shown to have some limited efficacy include the following:

1. *Behavioral methods.*[4,13,22] These are the only methods that are potentially curative and then only in a minority of cases. More often, only variable improvement can be expected.There are various such techniques (e.g., massed practice, habit reversal, and avoidance learning); all, however, are specialized and best carried out by a psychologist who is used to working with children because the procedures are difficult and children are usually disinterested and passively resistant.
2. *Anxiety-reducing procedures.*[22] These include relaxation training, biofeedback, psychotherapy, and where possible, general adjustment of the child's lifestyle. Unlike behavioral methods, however, none of these is of proven value in tics. Neither should these procedures be considered specific; rather, they are ancillary and holistic in meeting therapeutic objectives.
3. *Acceptance.* In the overwhelming majority of cases, the best management is explaining to parents, teachers, and peers that the tics are a physical disability, that the child cannot help them, and that acceptance of both child and tics is the kindest, safest, and simplest way to deal with them. Criticizing and belittling the child are likely to make tics worse and prolong their course.[8] Peer problems can be a major difficulty for those who have tics and Tourette's syndrome.[5] Getting peer (and adult) acceptance, therefore, can be a major therapeutic task.
4. *Pharmacotherapy.* Only physicians thoroughly familiar with the drugs indicated and experienced in their use should undertake pharmacotherapy, and only after reading one of the specialized publications on the topic.[9,23] Because of the risks involved and the lack of any truly curative value, drugs should be used only when tics are seriously disabling. This is most likely to be in Tourette's disorder or in chronic severe tics. Medication should not be given simply for superficial reasons except for brief periods during special, socially embarrassing circumstances. Even then it is important to ensure that dramatic and distressing side effects such as dystonic reactions will not ensue or that the embarrassment will be far greater than that from the tics.

The mainstays of pharmacotherapy are the dopamine-blocking neuroleptic now renamed "antipsychotic" drugs. Their utility stems from tics, whatever their cause, being executed through the basal ganglia and appears to reflect a relative overactivity in the dopaminergic nigrostriatal systems that inhibit cholinergic basal ganglion systems. These latter regulate movement through the twin mechanisms of increased tone and synchronization seen in exaggeration in parkinsonian states. Dopamine has the opposite effect—that is, it produces unregulated or spontaneous movements seen in chorea or occasionally, with dopamine agonists such as dextroamphetamine or L-dopa.

Any one of the so-called high-potency (i.e., nonatropinic) neuroleptics may be used,[23] although haloperidol and pimozide in doses starting at 0.5 mg and increasing slowly up to 3 mg/day seem to be preferred.[9,17,23] Controlled trials are rare, but clinical experience and the occasional study seem to prefer pimozide;[17] however, it has a reputation for cardiotoxicity in doses in excess of 0.2 mg/kg.[9,23] Even these relatively low doses of neuroleptics may produce acute dystonic reactions, sedation, parkinsonism, the highly uncomfortable and usually overlooked akathisia (restless legs), and in the longer term, withdrawal or tardive dyskinesias, one type of which may be a worsening of tics caused by presumed dopamine-2 receptor hypersensitivity.[3] In some cases, initial effects wear off, subsequent doses needed may be quite high, and the risk of side effects rises accordingly. Although neuroleptics often are effective to some degree, their action is symptomatic rather than curative. A number of lawsuits in the United States have been successful against physicians for tardive dyskinesias, and it is necessary that this and other risks involved be discussed fully and that informed consent be obtained. A second opinion, by a specialist who has knowledge of tics/Tourette's disorder, before neuroleptic pharmacotherapy is undertaken, offers the physician added protection.

Increasingly, the traditional neuroleptics, renamed "typical antipsychotics," are being replaced in psychiatry by newer drugs called "atypical antipsychotics."[23] These have less effect on dopamine receptors and, as a result, have fewer extrapyramidal side effects and, it is hoped, less risk of tardive dyskinesia. A few case studies[6,18,20] suggest that risperidone, olanzapine, and even the potentially dangerous clozapine may be effective in Tourette's disorder, but this remains to be proved. If these newer drugs are preferred in psychiatry because they have less effect on dopamine receptors (which predominate in the basal ganglia), it needs to be asked how they could be effective in Tourette's syndrome without having to be used in high dosages, which would eliminate their superiority over typical antipsychotics. This may explain the mixed results so far and underlines the need for properly controlled trials.

If neuroleptics are unsuccessful or, more commonly, create unacceptable side effects, clonidine may be tried in doses of 50 μg/day and slowly raised, if needed, over several weeks to 150 to 300 μg/day after preliminary EKG and blood work has been done.[9,23] However, clonidine is not particularly successful in most cases.[23]

Although it may seem logical to use anxiolytic drugs in the management of tic disorders, these thoroughly undesirable drugs[23] should be used only in unusual instances in children. They affect the highest functions of the brain, including learning; can make children irritable and lead to dependence, and withdrawal symptoms[1] may make children more irritable.[23] The muscle relaxant properties of the benzodiazepines are insignificant clinically, so they cannot be defended on that basis either.[1,23]

In summary, tics should be treated pharmacotherapeutically only as a last resort and by a physician (ordinarily a child or adolescent psychiatrist) skilled in the use of the drugs concerned. Such treatment should be considered and discussed carefully, closely monitored, and undertaken only with knowledge and consideration of the risks and disadvantages involved.

REFERRAL TO MENTAL HEALTH SPECIALISTS

Criteria for referring children who have tics to a mental health specialist are: (1) tics associated with additional evidence of psychiatric disorder, such as AD/HD, generalized anxiety, or obsessive-compulsive disorder; (2) chronic or recurrent tics that seem to have a clear relationship to stress, particularly if there is reason to believe that mental health procedures may be helpful; (3) chronic, disabling, or discomforting tics for which differential diagnosis or treatment is indicated; (4) when the primary physician knows little about tics and feels the need of expert opinion; or (5) when psychoactive drugs such as antipsychotics (neuroleptics) or clonidine may be indicated, because psychiatrists use these medications routinely and are generally better informed about risks, side effects, doses, and newer drugs.

Of course, such referral may be only for consultation, not necessarily for continued management. In general, the preferred mental health specialist is a well-trained child or adolescent psychiatrist—one who has a broad biopsychosocial perspective, including a good grasp of neuropsychiatry and pharmacotherapy but a "light" prescribing hand and a capacity to work closely with behavioral psychologists. This kind of child psychiatrist most likely will also be alert to the possibilities of the rare neurologically induced tics and will order any appropriate neuroimaging studies and neurological consultations. Where the tic is disabling and no further diagnostic workup is required, or where pharmacotherapy is not an option or is already in place but some relief is necessary, an experienced psychologist is the best person. Care must be taken, however, that the psychologist is competent in behavioral types of treatment.[13]

PROGNOSIS

Most tics last only a few weeks, although they may flit from one muscle group to another or change their form at irregular intervals.[23] Even chronic tics are likely to disappear in adolescence, although the longer a tic has been present and unchanged in form or site, the less likely it will be to disappear. Because the prevalence drops sharply after age 13 years, a tic that persists after that age is more likely to become chronic. Tourette's disorder may be a lifelong condition, but better recognition of the disorder shows that most cases generally will improve somewhat and even abate in late adolescence or adulthood.[2,8,12] Behavioral methods of treatment can sometimes influence the course of tics,[13] but there is no evidence that any other treatment affects prognosis as opposed to suppressing symptoms.

Children who have tics and especially Tourette's disorder can suffer secondary problems of self-image when adult criticism and peer rejection ensue.[5,8] Occasionally, severe complex motor tics result in injury or self-mutilation.[2] Finally, obsessive-compulsive disorder may develop during adolescence or late in Tourette's disorder.[8]

When to Refer

If psychiatric disorder is present or a possibility
If psychiatric drugs or treatments are needed
For expert opinion

Use of Alternative Medicine

Masterly inactivity
Adjusting of world to child; not child to world
Behavior therapies

When to Hospitalize

Never in the first instance (for tics alone)
Occasionally, for complex assessments or to initiate treatments

REFERENCES

1. American Psychiatric Association: Benzodiazepine dependence, toxicity and abuse, Washington, DC, 1990, The Association.
2. American Psychiatric Association: *Diagnostic and statistical manual of mental disorders (DSM-IV),* ed 4, Washington, DC, 1994, American Psychiatric Press.
3. American Psychiatric Association: Tardive dyskinesia: a task force report, Washington, DC, 1992, The Association.
4. Azrin NH, Peterson AL: Behavior therapy for Tourette's syndrome and tic disorders. In Cohen DJ, Leckman JF, Bruun RD, editors: *Tourette's syndrome: clinical understanding and treatment,* New York, 1988, John Wiley & Sons.
5. Bawdin HN, et al: Peer relationship problems in children with Tourette's disorder or diabetes mellitus, *J Child Psychol Psychiatry* 39:663, 1998.
6. Bhadrinath BR: Olanzapine in Tourette syndrome, *Br J Psychiatry* 172: 366, 1998.
7. Castellanos FX, et al: Controlled stimulant treatment of ADHD and comorbid Tourette's syndrome: effects of stimulant and dose, *J Am Acad Child Adolesc Psychiatry* 36:589, 1997.
8. Cohen DJ, Leckman JF: Developmental psychopathology and neurobiology of Tourette's syndrome: advances in treatment and research, *J Am Acad Child Adolesc Psychiatry* 33:2, 1994.
9. Cohen DJ, et al: Pharmacotherapy of Tourette's syndrome and associated disorders, *Psychiatr Clin North Am* 15:109, 1992.
10. Leckman JF, et al: Premonitory urges in Tourette's syndrome, *Am J Psychiatry* 150:98, 1993.
11. Leckman JF, et al: Tic disorders, *Psychiatr Clin North Am* 20:839, 1997.
12. Mason A, et al: The prevalence of Tourette syndrome in a mainstream school population, *Develop Med Child Neurol* 40:292, 1998.
13. Miltenberger RG, et al: Applying behavior analysis to clinical problems: review and analysis of habit reversal, *J Appl Behav Analysis* 31:447, 1998.
14. Neurologic Clinics: Tourette syndrome, *Neurol Clin* 15:291, 1997.
15. Peterson BS, et al: A double-blind placebo-controlled trial of an antiandrogen in the treatment of Tourette's syndrome, *J Clin Psychopharmacol* 18:324, 1998.
16. Peterson BS, et al: The treatment of Tourette's syndrome: multimodal developmental intervention, *J Clin Psychiatry* 59(suppl 1):62 1998.
17. Sallee FR, et al: Relative efficacy of haloperidol and pimozide in children and adolescents with Tourette's disorder, *Am J Psychiatry* 154: 1057, 1997.
18. Schmider J, Hoff P: Clozapine in Tourette's syndrome, *J Clin Psychopharmacol* 18:88, 1998.
19. Schuerholz LJ, et al: Gender study of neuropsychological and neuromotor function in children with Tourette syndrome with and without attention-deficit hyperactivity disorder, *J Child Neurol* 13:277, 1998.
20. Stein DJ, et al: Risperidone augmentation of serotonin reuptake inhibitors in obsessive-compulsive and related disorders, *J Clin Psychiatry* 58:119, 1997.
21. Swedo SE, et al: Identification of children with pediatric autoimmune neuropsychiatric disorders associated with streptococcal infections by a marker associated with rheumatic fever, *Am J Psychiatry* 154:110, 1997.
22. Werry JS: Physical illness, symptoms and allied disorders. In Quay HC, Werry JS, editors: *Psychopathological disorders of childhood,* ed 3, New York, 1986, John Wiley & Sons.
23. Werry JS, Aman MG: *A practitioner's guide to psychoactive drugs for children and adolescents,* ed 2, New York, 1998, Plenum Press.
24. Zausmer DM, Dewey ME: Tics and heredity: a study of the relatives of child tiqueurs, *Br J Psychiatry* 150:628, 1987.

SUGGESTED READINGS

Cohen DJ, Leckman JF, Bruun RD, editors: *Tourette's syndrome: clinical understanding and treatment,* New York, 1988, John Wiley & Sons.

Leckman JF, et al: Tic disorders, *Psychiatr Clin North Am* 20:839, 1997.

Neurologic Clinics: Tourette syndrome, *Neurol Clin* 15:291, 1997.

176 Torticollis

Philip O. Ozuah

The word *torticollis* originates from two Latin words, *tortus* (twisted) and *collum* (neck). Hence, torticollis literally means *twisted neck* or *"wry" neck*. It often arises from a spasmodic contraction of the sternocleidomastoid (SCM) muscles of the neck, which are enervated by the spinal accessory nerve. The classic clinical picture of torticollis is that of the head tilted to one side and rotated in such a way that the chin and face point to the contralateral side. Torticollis can be broadly classified into congenital and acquired forms. Facial asymmetry often is encountered in congenital torticollis but not in acquired torticollis. This finding, therefore, can be useful in distinguishing clinically between the two forms. The differential diagnosis of torticollis is listed in Box 176-1.

CONGENITAL TORTICOLLIS

Congenital muscular torticollis is by far the most common form of congenital torticollis and presents clinically in the first 8 weeks of life. It frequently is not obvious at birth but manifests at about 2 weeks of age. Several theories have been proposed to explain the etiology of this disorder. One theory suggests that stretching of the neck during a difficult delivery results in rupture and hemorrhage within the sternocleidomastoid muscle. Subsequent muscle ischemia results from increased pressure arising from the blood, which is trapped within the fascial compartment. The culmination and resolution of these events is believed to produce progressive muscle fibrosis and contracture, hence, torticollis. This theory is supported by approximately 40% of patients who have congenital torticollis having had a difficult birth, including forceps delivery and breech presentation. However, congenital torticollis has been reported in children who have uncomplicated births; in addition, specimens of sternocleidomastoid muscles in patients who have torticollis sometimes have shown no evidence of trauma or hemorrhage. Another theory, therefore, is that the torticollis is a result of an intrauterine position that occludes the venous drainage from the sternocleidomastoid, leading to vascular congestion, ischemia, muscle damage, and fibrosis. This theory is supported in that 75% of congenital muscular torticollis cases are right-sided because of intrauterine, left-occiput-anterior positioning and about 20% of patients who have congenital torticollis also have other musculoskeletal anomalies, including congenital hip dysplasias, talipes equinovarus, and metatarsus adductus.[3]

The clinical picture of congenital muscular torticollis often includes a "tumor." This is characteristically a nontender, soft, and mobile mass in the inferior aspect of the sternocleidomastoid muscle. The mass enlarges in the first few weeks of life, reaching its maximum size at 1 month of age. Thereafter, it begins to shrink in size until it disappears by 4 to 6 months; at this point the mass is replaced by a contracture, which prevents normal growth and normal range of motion of the neck. Facial asymmetry results from the uneven growth forces that are present in this situation. Congenital postural torticollis presents similarly to congenital muscular torticollis, but without the presence of a palpable mass or "tumor."

Several congenital cervical spine anomalies can present with torticollis. Most of these can be diagnosed by radiographic studies of the cervical spine. Pterygium coli is a congenital web of the skin of the neck extending from the acromial process to the mastoid. This web can be restrictive and result in torticollis. Congenital remnant cysts within the body of the sternocleidomastoid are a less common cause of torticollis. Unilateral absence of one sternocleidomastoid muscle results in unopposed action of the other muscle and produces a contralateral torticollis.

ACQUIRED TORTICOLLIS

As with congenital torticollis, most cases of torticollis encountered in older children are primarily muscular in origin. Cervical muscle or ligament injury arising from trauma can present with a head-tilt and unilateral neck tenderness. This condition also may occur upon awakening, presumably as a result of awkward positioning of the neck during sleep. Benign paroxysmal torticollis is a disease of infancy that has an unknown etiology, although a familial pattern has been described. Manifestations of the condition begin in the first year of life with recurrent episodes of head-tilt that may be associated with emesis, pallor, agitation, ataxia, malaise, and other behavioral changes. Attacks may last from several hours to several days. Spontaneous and complete remission usually occurs by 5 years of age. Some patients, however, go on to develop migraines or benign paroxysmal vertigo.

Other conditions that need to be considered in the differential diagnosis of acquired torticollis include cervical spine subluxations, infections of the head and neck, neurological disorders, and neoplasia. Laxity of the transverse cervical ligaments results in atlanto-axial instability in up to 15% of patients who have Down syndrome.[5] Most of these children are asymptomatic, but subluxation of the cervical spine, most commonly a rotational atlanto-axial subluxation, may occur following trauma.[4] Nontraumatic subluxations of the atlanto-axial spine may arise secondary to head and neck

BOX 176-1

DIFFERENTIAL DIAGNOSIS OF TORTICOLLIS

Congenital
- Muscular torticollis
- Postural torticollis
- Cervical spine anomalies
  - Hemivertebra
  - Atlanto-occipital fusion
  - Klippel-Feil syndrome
  - Sprengel deformity
- Pterygium colli
- Sternocleidomastoid cysts
  - Cystic hygroma
  - Bronchial cleft cyst
  - Unilateral absence of sternocleidomastoid

Acquired
- Muscular
  - Cervical muscle injury
  - Psychogenic torticollis
  - Benign paroxysmal torticollis
- Vertebral
  - Atlanto-axial subluxation
  - Atlanto-occipital subluxation
  - C2-C3 subluxation
  - Rotary subluxation
  - Cervical fractures
  - Cervical vertebral osteomyelitis
  - Rheumatoid arthritis
  - Acute cervical disk calcification
  - Eosinophilic granuloma
- Infectious
  - Upper respiratory infection
  - Cervical vertebral osteomyelitis
  - Dental infections
- Neurological
  - Ocular torticollis
  - Spasmus nutans
  - Dystonic torticollis
  - Wilson's disease
  - Syringomyelia
  - Labyrinthine torticollis
  - Accessory nerve palsy
- Neoplastic
  - Cervical cord tumor
  - Posterior fossa tumor
  - Soft-tissue tumor
  - Histiocytosis X
- Other
  - Sandifer's syndrome
  - Dermatogenic torticollis
  - Spurious torticollis

infections or rheumatoid arthritis. The current theory is that inflammatory reactions around the spine produce hyperemia and edema, which in turn lead to laxity of the supporting ligaments and hence a predisposition to spontaneous subluxations and secondary torticollis.

Torticollis also may arise from acute cervical disk calcification secondary to trauma or an upper respiratory infection. Ocular torticollis may be secondary to paralysis of the extraocular muscles, strabismus, nystagmus, and refractive errors. Spasmus nutans, which also is known as *nodding spasms* or *salaam spasms,* includes a triad of acquired nystagmus, head nodding, and torticollis. The etiology is unknown. Signs and symptoms usually develop within the first 2 years of life and may persist for several months to years. However, the clinical course often is benign and self-limited. A dystonic torticollis may follow the administration of several drugs, including phenothiazines, carbamazepine, and phenytoin. The presence of other extrapyramidal signs often can be used to differentiate patients who have dystonic reactions.

Neoplasms associated with torticollis include cervical cord tumors and cerebellar tumors. Posterior fossa masses may present similarly to spasmus nutans with nystagmus, head nodding, and torticollis. For patients who have cerebellar tumors, however, ataxia often is a cardinal feature. Sandifer's syndrome is an abnormal posturing that includes torticollis and opisthotonos. It is believed to be a protective mechanism adopted by some patients who have one of several conditions, including gastroesophageal reflux, esophagitis, or hiatal hernia. Dermatogenic torticollis is a painful stiff neck that results from extensive local skin lesions. Stiffness of the neck resulting from dental malformations and caries is termed *spurious torticollis.*

DIAGNOSIS

The first step in determining the etiology of torticollis should be to obtain a careful and detailed history. Particular attention should be given to duration of symptoms, prior trauma, presence of fever, and other systemic manifestations. In younger patients, the birth history is essential.

Physical examination should not be limited to the head and neck areas but should include all organ systems. Findings such as craniofacial asymmetry suggest a congenital torticollis of long duration. The presence of webs or cysts in the neck should raise the suspicion of pterygium colli or remnant cysts. Patients who have acquired torticollis secondary to trauma often have a tender sternocleidomastoid muscle. Point tenderness over the cervical spine may suggest an underlying fracture or subluxation. Cervical vertebral osteomyelitis should be suspected in patients who have point tenderness in association with an unexplained fever.

Cervical spine radiography should be obtained in all neonates who have torticollis and in older children who have findings suggestive of vertebral involvement or who have persistent torticollis. Patients who have neurological deficits should undergo prompt computed tomography (CT) scanning or magnetic resonance imaging (MRI) of the head and neck. The presence of a peripheral leukocytosis and an elevated sedimentation rate can be helpful adjuncts in diagnosing infectious and inflammatory etiologies.

MANAGEMENT

Congenital muscular torticollis responds extremely well to early conservative treatment during the first year of life.[2] Medical management includes passive and active stretching of the neck. Gentle passive stretching can be performed daily by the parents of the child or by a physical therapist. Active stretching is achieved by manipulating the infant's environment in such a way that objects of interest are located on the opposite side of the room from the torticollis, inducing the infant to turn the neck in the desired direction. Surgical correction is essential if deformity persists beyond the first year of life, if there is greater than a 30% restriction in range of motion, or if there is a residual craniofacial deformity.[6,7] Craniofacial asymmetry is best reversed at an early age when growth potential is maximum. The surgical procedure that has the best results involves a bipolar tenotomy of the affected sternocleidomastoid muscle, followed by casting or bracing to maintain the corrected posture.[1]

Acquired muscular or ligamentous torticollis is managed with local heat, massage, analgesics, and a soft cervical collar. Symptoms usually resolve in 7 to 10 days. It should be noted, however, that patients who have acquired muscular or ligamentous torticollis experience only mild discomfort. All patients who have severe neck pain or tenderness over the vertebra require immediate cervical immobilization until a vertebral fracture or subluxation is excluded radiographically.

Drug-induced dystonic reactions are reversed by discontinuation of the offending agent and administration of intravenous diphenhydramine. The treatment of torticollis arising from other specific diseases should be directed at the cause.

When to Refer

1. Presence of craniofacial asymmetry
2. Radiographic evidence of cervical spine abnormality
3. Greater than 30% restriction in range of motion
4. Persistence beyond the first year of life

When to Hospitalize

1. Presence of neurological deficits
2. Severe neck pain
3. Point tenderness over the vertebrae

REFERENCES

1. Bharadwaj VK: Sternomastoid myoplasty: surgical correction of congenital torticollis, *J Otolaryngol* 26:44, 1997.
2. Binder H, et al: Congenital muscular torticollis: results of conservative management with long-term follow-up in 85 cases, *Arch Phys Med Rehabil* 68:222, 1987.
3. Davids JR, et al: Congenital muscular torticollis: sequela of intrauterine or perinatal compartment syndrome, *J Pediatr Orthop* 13:141, 1993.
4. Msall ME, et al: Symptomatic atlantoaxial instability associated with medical and rehabilitative procedures in children with Down syndrome, *Pediatrics* 85:447, 1990.
5. Peuschel SM, Scola FH, Pezzullo C: A longitudinal study of atlanto-dens relationships in asymptomatic individuals with Down syndrome, *Pediatrics* 89:1194, 1992.
6. Slate RK, et al: Cervical spine subluxation associated with congenital muscular torticollis and craniofacial asymmetry, *Plast Reconstr Surg* 91:1187, 1993.
7. Wolfort FG, Kanter MA, Miller LB: Torticollis, *Plast Reconstr Surg* 84:682, 1989.

177 Vaginal Bleeding

Alain Joffe

As with other symptoms referable to the female genital tract, physician assessment of vaginal bleeding depends largely on the pubertal status of the patient. In prepubertal girls, vaginal bleeding probably reflects a localized problem in the vagina or uterus; in pubertal females, the differential diagnosis includes disorders affecting the hypothalamic-pituitary-ovarian axis and complications of pregnancy, as well as local causes. In both cases, however, a careful history and physical examination will provide important clues to the diagnosis.

PREPUBERTAL GIRLS

In utero, maternal estrogen diffuses across the placenta into the fetal circulation. After birth, estrogen levels fall, resulting in a physiological discharge that can be either blood-tinged or frankly bloody. No treatment, except reassurance, is necessary, and the discharge usually disappears within 10 days.

A number of conditions can result in vaginal bleeding in the prepubertal child, including vulvovaginal infections, excoriations secondary to pruritus, foreign bodies, sexual abuse, trauma (such as that involving a straddle injury during bike riding), tumors, condyloma, hemangiomas, polyps, and coagulopathies.[1] If there is any suggestion of sexual abuse, such as bruises, hymenal tears, or other signs of trauma, careful, nonthreatening questioning of the child or caretaker may reveal whether further referral to child protective services is necessary.

Nighttime pruritus may indicate a pinworm infestation. The Scotch tape slide test, to look for pinworm eggs, can help to establish *Enterobius vermicularis* infestation. If the presence of petechiae or numerous bruises is noted on physical examination, platelet counts and clotting studies are indicated to screen for a coagulopathy. A foreign body in the vagina should always be considered, even if there is no history of such. Contrary to popular belief, most girls who have bleeding from a foreign body do not have an associated foul-smelling discharge. The physician also should make sure that the bleeding is vaginal in origin, because a prolapsed urethra can mimic vaginal bleeding.

If excoriation, erythema, or a rash in the perineal area is noted, vaginitis is a distinct possibility. If there is vaginal discharge and microscopic examination demonstrates large numbers of white blood cells, vaginitis is highly likely. Concern about sexual abuse should prompt cultures for *Neisseria gonorrhoeae* and *Chlamydia trachomatis*. Other bacterial cultures may be necessary; for example, a history of diarrhea in the weeks preceding onset of the bleeding suggests vaginitis caused by *Shigella* organisms. Group A beta-hemolytic streptococcus also can cause vaginitis.

Vaginal bleeding caused by vulvitis or foreign bodies will respond to removal of the foreign body and proper perineal hygiene. Occasionally, systemic antibiotics may be necessary. Foreign bodies often can be washed out with a soft, flexible catheter; sharp objects should be removed carefully, under direct visualization. Referral to a gynecologist may be required if the patient is uncooperative. Following removal of a foreign body, bleeding should subside within 10 days. If it does not, referral to a gynecologist is indicated. The entire foreign body may not have been removed, or a tumor, not readily visualized by the primary care clinician, may be the actual cause of the bleeding. Similarly, if treatment of the presumed cause does not end the bleeding, referral for a more thorough examination is indicated.

PUBERTAL FEMALES

Evaluation

Abnormal vaginal bleeding in pubertal females can indicate a variety of disorders. Evaluation of this symptom depends on the nature of the problem: Is she bleeding between normal periods, or have her previously regular menses become more frequent or heavier? It also is possible that a teenager whose prior menses have been regular will begin to have infrequent but heavy menstrual bleeding. In general, normal periods are 28 days apart (measured from the first day of one period to the first day of the next), with a range of 21 to 35 days, and should not last more than 5 days.[1,4] Thus, some teenagers will have only 2 weeks without bleeding between menses. How much bleeding is too much is difficult to quantify by history alone; normal blood loss during menses is 30 to 40 ml, with an upper limit of 80 ml.

The causes of abnormal bleeding in this age group are summarized in Box 177-1. Although dysfunctional uterine bleeding (DUB) secondary to an immaturity of the hypothalamic-pituitary-ovarian (HPO) axis with resultant anovulatory cycles is the most common etiology,[3] this diagnosis requires a careful search for and exclusion of many other causes. Nonetheless, it is worth noting that menstrual irregularity is frequent in the year following menarche: In one study of 5000 adolescents, 43% had irregular menses in the first year, and 20% still had irregular periods 5 years after menarche.

Normal menstrual function requires that the HPO axis function properly. When this occurs, the following sequence of events transpires: Follicle-stimulating hormone (FSH)

BOX 177-1

POSSIBLE CAUSES OF ABNORMAL UTERINE BLEEDING

Pregnancy Complications
Spontaneous abortion
Ectopic pregnancy
Retained gestational products
Trophoblastic disease

Coagulation Disorders
von Willebrand's disease
Idiopathic thrombocytopenia
Other causes of thrombocytopenia
Glanzmann's disease
Leukemia

Systemic Disease
Renal failure
Hepatic failure
Malignancy

Pathology of the Reproductive Tract
Vagina
Vaginitis
Trauma
Foreign body
Congenital anomaly (septum)
Neoplasia

Cervix
Cervicitis, erosion
Cervical polyp
Neoplasia

Uterus
Endometritis
Endometrial polyp
Submucosal leiomyoma
Arteriovenous malformation
Congenital anomaly
Neoplasia

Pelvis
Endometriosis

Endocrine Disorders
Hypothalamus/pituitary
Immature hypothalamic-pituitary-ovarian axis
Hyperprolactinemia
Anorexia nervosa, malnutrition
Excessive exercise

Ovary
Polycystic ovary syndrome
Luteal phase abnormality
Premature ovarian failure
Neoplasia (hormone secreting)

Adrenal
Congenital adrenal hyperplasia
Cushing's disease
Adrenal insufficiency
Neoplasm

Thyroid
Hypothyroidism
Hyperthyroidism

Iatrogenic
Hormonal medications
Anticoagulants
Neuroleptics
Intrauterine contraceptive device

From Namnoun AB, Carpenter SEK: *Adolescent Medicine: State of the Art Reviews* 5:162, 1994.

causes maturation of ovarian follicles, which produce estrogen. Rising levels of estrogen stimulate the endometrial lining of the uterus to proliferate and, at the same time, induce a midcycle surge of luteinizing hormone (LH) that causes the primary follicle to release an ovum, after which LH and FSH levels fall. The remnants of the follicle (termed *corpus luteum*) now produce progesterone, which converts the proliferative endometrium to a secretory phase. At the end of a normal cycle, the corpus luteum involutes, and both estrogen and progesterone levels fall. The endometrial lining is now shed, and bleeding occurs.

In adolescents, especially young adolescents, the HPO axis is relatively immature and highly sensitive to disturbance by a number of endogenous and exogenous factors; this perturbation leads to irregular bleeding. Among young adolescents (but in some older ones as well), the axis has not yet matured, and most cycles are anovulatory. Thus, the endometrium proliferates under estrogen stimulation from the maturing follicle, but the midcycle LH surge is absent, ovulation does not occur, and the progesterone-secreting corpus luteum never forms. Toward the end of the cycle, the follicle involutes, estrogen levels fall, and bleeding occurs. Influenced by estrogen only, endometrial shedding is incomplete and irregular, accounting for the excessive bleeding of anovulatory cycles. Alternatively, fluctuating estrogen levels during an anovulatory cycle result in estrogen withdrawal bleeding.[5] The occasional ovulatory cycle helps to stabilize endometrial growth, and because the corpeus luteum produces progesterone, a more organized withdrawal bleed occurs. Hence, any condition that increases the frequency of anovulatory cycles is more likely to produce the kind of uterine bleeding that prompts the teenager to seek medical care.

Most teenagers who seek evaluation for genital bleeding will have DUB; in one series, 74% did so.[6] Nonetheless, it is important to search for other causes that affect the integrity of the HPO axis and therefore can mimic DUB. Heavy bleeding at menarche, significant anemia, or the need to be hospitalized to control the bleeding increases the likelihood that a coagulopathy or another pathological condition is the cause of the bleeding.[4] Because any significant stress in a teenager's life can affect the HPO axis, a general assessment of her well-being is valuable. Fluctuations in weight, particularly if rapid and significant, also can affect menstrual function. The adolescent's dietary habits (including fad or crash diets), concerns about body image, and exercise patterns should be assessed as part of the physician's evaluation. Symptoms of the other endocrine disorders listed in Box 177-1 (e.g., cold intolerance, polyuria, nipple discharge, headache, and increased facial hair) also should be sought.

Most of the causes indicated in Box 177-1 can be ruled out by history and physical examination. Certain key aspects of the history may be difficult to obtain: A young woman may hesitate to reveal that she has engaged in sexual intercourse or that she has been sexually abused. If a discharge is foul smelling and bloody, a foreign body or retained tampon is likely; however, necrotic tumors can result in similar bleeding patterns. Pruritus or dysuria suggests vaginitis or cervicitis as the cause of the bleeding. Bleeding between periods is common during the first two or three cycles of oral contraceptive use and generally does not require any additional therapy; however, cervicitis secondary to *N. gonorrhoeae* or *C. trachomatis* infection also may result in intermenstrual spotting. Young women who have levonorgestrel implants (Norplant) or who receive depot medroxyprogesterone acetate (Depo-Provera) injections often have frequent and irregular periods of excess bleeding, particularly in the first months after beginning use of these contraceptive methods. Teenagers who forget to take one or two oral contraceptive pills may also have some bleeding.[2] Occasionally, women may have a small amount of bleeding or spotting after sexual intercourse, and some will have spotting around the time they ovulate. A careful family history is important to determine if other family members have any kind of bleeding problem. Complications of pregnancy (e.g., ectopic pregnancy or incomplete abortion) are more likely if there is a history of one or two missed periods, if the prior menstrual period was lighter than normal, if other symptoms of pregnancy are present (breast tenderness or nausea), or if the bleeding is accompanied by crampy lower abdominal pain. A history of passing tissue or tissue present in the vaginal canal also is suggestive. Blood dyscrasias, such as thrombocytopenia or von Willebrand's disease, can cause heavy vaginal bleeding without other cutaneous manifestations of bleeding.

The physical examination should include measurement of height, weight, and blood pressure, as well as careful palpation of the thyroid gland. Visual field and funduscopic examinations are necessary to help rule out a prolactinoma. Increased facial hair is consistent with polycystic ovaries or an adrenal tumor. Striae suggest Cushing's disease; enlargement of the clitoris is consistent with an androgen-secreting tumor or late-onset 21-hydoxylase deficiency. Normal findings on physical examination, including pelvic examination, help to rule out many of the causes listed in Box 177-1. Vulvar or vaginal bruising or lacerations suggest the probability of sexual abuse. Lack of adnexal or cervical motion tenderness excludes pelvic inflammatory disease. If the ovaries are of normal size, ovarian tumors or cysts are unlikely sources of the bleeding. A minimally enlarged uterus, consistent with early pregnancy, may not be noted by an inexperienced examiner. Endometrial polyps or submucous leiomyomas are distinctly unusual in women younger than 20 years of age. They cannot be felt by the examiner on the usual pelvic examination. If the patient has an intractably heavy flow, the presence of one of these entitles should be considered.

For most cases, relatively few laboratory tests are needed. A complete blood count with indices and a reticulocyte count provides some objective measurement of the amount and duration of bleeding. A urinalysis and urine pregnancy test also should be obtained; if an ectopic pregnancy is possible (bleeding associated with crampy lower abdominal pain), a serum pregnancy test is preferred. If suggested by the history or physical examination or if hormonal therapy is contemplated, thyroid function tests (TSH), prolactin, LH and FSH levels, and coagulation tests should be done. An LH:FSH ratio greater than 3:1 is highly suggestive of polycystic ovary syndrome but is not a sensitive indicator. Any evidence of hyperandrogenism necessitates measurement of testosterone, dehydroepiandrosterone and its sulfate, and 17-OH progesterone levels. Endometrial biopsy or dilation and curettage rarely are indicated in the evaluation or treatment of vaginal bleeding in adolescents.[6]

Management

If a specific cause for the bleeding is discovered, treatment should be directed at ameliorating this condition. As the aforementioned study[6] indicates, a specific cause is not found in most instances, and the clinician must manage the bleeding without knowing the etiology. Whether and how to treat is a matter of judgment: Some physicians may feel comfortable using hormonal therapy; others may prefer the guidance of a more experienced clinician.

Mild cases of bleeding that do not result in anemia and that do not upset the patient and her parents greatly can be managed expectantly with no immediate, specific therapy. Those who have mild anemia (hemoglobin value 11 to 12 g/dl) should receive iron supplementation. Some will have the problem resolved within three or four cycles. If the patient is sexually active, oral contraceptive pills can be prescribed to treat the bleeding as well as to provide contraception.

Hormonal therapy is indicated in those teenagers who have moderate bleeding—that is, enough to cause a small decrease in the hemoglobin level or to cause bleeding for 7 to 10 days per cycle.[1,3,4] Teenagers who have menses every 1 to 3 weeks also need treatment. Treatment includes combined estrogen-progestin oral contraceptive pills or progestin alone. Birth control pills are easier to use (one pill is taken daily every day of the month), but some patients or their parents may object to this approach. If this is the case, medroxyprogesterone 10 mg orally can be given daily for 10 to 14 days, beginning on the first of each month (calendar method) or on the fourteenth day of the menstrual cycle (day 1 being the first day of bleeding).[1] The patient should be reassessed after 3 to 6 months.

Heavier bleeding, accompanied by a drop in hemoglobin of 2 or 3 g/dl, needs to be treated more aggressively. Lo/Ovral or similar birth control pills (one tablet taken twice daily for 3 to 4 days) generally will stop the bleeding. However, it may be necessary to prescribe three or four doses daily. Emans, Laufer, and Goldstein[1] suggest a regimen such as Lo/Ovral four times daily for 4 days, then three times daily for 3 days and two times daily for 2 days. At these doses, use of antiemetics may be required.[1]

Should these methods fail or the hemoglobin level fall below 10 g/dl, gynecological or adolescent medicine consultation should be sought; clotting studies should be obtained and hospitalization strongly considered.[1,3] The need for blood transfusion will depend on the hemodynamic stability of the patient. Although some clinicians prefer to use conjugated estrogens, (25 mg intravenously every 4 hours) to stop the bleeding, use of Lo/Ovral or a similar contraceptive given six times a day and then gradually tapered to once a day over the next 7 to 10 days will usually stop the bleeding. Failure to stop the bleeding with this regimen should prompt referral to an adolescent medicine specialist or gynecologist. Even if these measures succeed in controlling the vaginal bleeding, these adolescents require long-term follow-up because an appreciable number of them will continue to have menstrual abnormalities.[5]

REFERENCES

1. Emans SJ, Laufer MR, Goldstein DP: *Pediatric and adolescent gynecology,* ed 4, Boston, 1998, Lippincott-Raven.
2. Hilliard PA: Abnormal uterine bleeding in adolescents, *Contemp Pediatr* 12:79, 1995.
3. Hilliard PA: Diagnosing and controlling abnormal uterine bleeding, *Contemp Adolesc Gynecol* 4:3, 1999.
4. Iglesias EA, Coupey SM: Menstrual cycle abnormalities: diagnosis and management, *Adolesc Med* 10:255, 1999.
5. Namnoun AB, Carpenter SEK: Abnormal uterine bleeding in the adolescent, *Adolesc Med* 5:157, 1994.
6. Polaneczky MM, Slap GB: Menstrual disorders in the adolescent: dysmenorrhea and dysfunctional uterine bleeding, *Pediatr Rev* 13:83, 1992.

178 Vaginal Discharge

Alain Joffe

Vaginal discharge is a common complaint that confronts the pediatrician. However, the presence of discharge is not necessarily abnormal; this symptom may represent the vagina's adaptation to changes in estrogen levels, and the pediatrician need only reassure the patient and her parents. In most circumstances, the age of the patient, her pubertal status, and whether she has ever had sexual intercourse are key elements in sorting out the etiology of the discharge.

NEWBORN PERIOD

In utero the vaginal epithelium of the neonate is stimulated by maternal hormones that cross the placenta into the fetal circulation. After delivery these hormone levels fall rapidly, and the parents may note a thick, grayish-white, mucoid discharge from the neonate's vagina. Often the discharge is blood tinged or even grossly bloody. No treatment is needed, and the discharge usually resolves by 10 days of age.

PREPUBERTAL GIRLS

The genital area of prepubertal girls is more susceptible to infection than that of older, pubertal girls. The labial folds are smaller and lack pubic hair, and there is a relatively short distance between the vagina and the rectum compared with adolescents and adults.[1,5] Low levels of circulating estrogen render the vaginal mucosa relatively thin and more susceptible to irritation or infection. The alkaline pH (approximately 7.0) of the vaginal secretions affords a hospitable environment to bacteria. In this environment, together with poor perineal hygiene, fecal flora can establish themselves more easily in the genital area. Box 178-1 lists causes of vaginal discharge in prepubertal girls.

Evaluation

When evaluating a premenarchal girl who has vaginal discharge, the physician should inquire about her hygiene. Wiping from the rectum toward the vagina brings intestinal flora to the vaginal introitus. Use of chemicals such as bubble baths or deodorants or of strong detergents to launder underwear can irritate the vulva and vagina. Occlusive nylon or rayon underwear provides a moist environment for potential pathogens, and the material itself can be an irritant. Although accounting for less than 5% of cases of vaginal discharge, the possibility that the child placed a foreign body, such as toilet paper, a coin, or a small toy, in her vagina should be considered.

The parents should be asked about recent or concomitant illness. For example, vaginal discharge is associated with *Streptococcus pyogenes* infection (with or without scarlet fever) and with *Shigella flexneri* infection, occurring coincident with or after an episode of diarrhea. Systemic illnesses such as varicella also may be associated with vaginal discharge. Rectal infestations with *Enterobius vermicularis* (pinworms) can lead to vaginitis if the eggs are deposited around or in the vagina. A history of nocturnal itching accompanying vaginal discharge suggests this diagnosis.

Sexually transmitted organisms, such as *Neisseria gonorrhoeae* or *Trichomonas vaginalis,* are known to cause vaginal infections in prepubertal girls; thus, the possibility of sexual abuse always should be considered in the evaluation.[3] Whether *C. trachomatis* alone can cause discharge is uncertain.[2]

Although these other entities should be carefully considered as the pediatrician evaluates the young patient, nonspecific vaginitis, in which no clear etiological agent for the discharge can be established, accounts for 25% or more of vaginal symptoms in prepubertal girls.[2] Rarer causes of discharge include polyps or tumors, ectopic ureters (which drain urine into the vagina, resulting in a wetness that is mistaken for discharge), or prolapsed urethra (often associated with a bloody discharge).

The physical examination should include the entire genital and rectal area. The condition of the vulva, urethral meatus, and vaginal introitus should be noted. Infections in prepubertal girls usually involve the vulva as opposed to only the vagina. Bruises, lacerations, or scrapes in the genital area should raise suspicion of sexual abuse. Excoriations around the rectum or vagina suggest itching caused by pinworms. A rash that spares skin folds is consistent with an irritative cause; one that is predominantly within the skin folds suggests candidiasis.

The use of a veterinary otoscope and speculum allows for examination of the outer portions of the vagina without causing undue discomfort to the girl. Having the girl sit on her mother's lap with her legs spread so that they dangle outside her mother's will often afford the examiner a clear view of the vulva and vaginal introitus. Alternatively, she may lie face down on the examining table in the knee-chest position. If a foreign body is suspected (because of a thick, yellowish discharge that is often bloody and sometimes foul-smelling) but not visualized, irrigating the vagina with a soft, flexible catheter and tepid saline solution often will flush out bits of toilet paper or small objects.

If sufficient vaginal discharge is present, several drops of

BOX 178-1

CAUSES OF VAGINAL DISCHARGE IN PREPUBERTAL GIRLS

"Nonspecific vaginitis" (the most common cause)
Irritative (bubble baths, sand); the vulva often is involved as well. Nonabsorbent, occlusive clothing such as nylon undergarments, tights, bathing suits, etc., also irritate the vulva, leading to skin breakdown and infection. *Candida* infections often arise under these circumstances
Poor perineal hygiene
Foreign body
Associated systemic illness (group A streptococci, chickenpox)
Other respiratory pathogens (e.g., *Haemophilus influenzae*) also may cause discharge
Enteric infections
- *Escherichia coli* with foreign body
- *Shigella* organisms
- *Yersinia* organisms
- *Enterobius vermicularis*

Infections (strong presumption of sexual abuse)
- *Neisseria gonorrhoeae*
- *Trichomonas vaginalis*
- *Chlamydia trachomatis* (it is unclear whether this organism alone can cause discharge.

C. trachomatis often is isolated in conjunction with *N. gonorrhoeae*)
Primary vulvar skin disease
Tumor, polyps (rare)

the secretion should be placed on three glass slides. If the discharge is scant, a saline-moistened cotton swab can be introduced into the vagina and the material obtained placed on the glass slides. Several drops of normal saline solution should be added to one slide to create a wet preparation. Several drops of 10% potassium hydroxide should be added to the second slide and the slide then gently heated to dissolve epithelial cells, which allows visualization of hyphae. A Gram stain of the material on the third slide also should be made. All slides should be examined as indicated in Table 178-1. A piece of Scotch tape with its sticky side applied to the rectal area and then on a glass slide for microscopic examination may reveal the typical eggs of *E. vermicularis*.

Management

If the history or physical examination suggests an irritative origin, parents should discontinue the offending agent and have the patient wear cotton underpants. Sitz baths will provide temporary relief until natural healing takes place. Removal of a foreign body will result in rapid improvement and cessation of the discharge. Pinworm infestations should be treated in the usual manner (see Chapter 246, Parasitic Infections). Infections caused by poor personal hygiene will respond to the general measures just listed, coupled with instructions about proper perineal hygiene. If the discharge is associated with another infection (such as *Streptococcus pyogenes* or *Shigella* organisms), it will disappear as the underlying infection is treated.

When the organism causing the vaginal discharge is found to be sexually transmitted, more comprehensive evaluation and treatment are required (see Chapters 68, Sexual Abuse of Children, and 262, Sexually Transmitted Diseases).[3] Appropriate antibiotic treatment should be prescribed and a report to child protective services made.

Nonspecific vaginitis usually will respond to careful perineal hygiene, Sitz baths, and mild soaps. For persistent cases, Emans, Laufer, and Goldstein[2] recommend treatment with amoxicillin, amoxicillin clavulanate, or a cephalosporin in standard childhood doses for 10 to 14 days.[2] If this approach is unsuccessful, estrogen creams or other antibiotic regimens may be used or a referral to a pediatric gynecologist made.

PUBERTAL AND POSTPUBERTAL ADOLESCENTS

With the onset of puberty, circulating estrogen and progesterone levels rise, stimulating vaginal mucus production and an increase in the turnover of vaginal epithelial cells. Bartholin and sebaceous glands also are stimulated. Generally, the clear mucoid discharge that results will not cause problems. The amount of secretion, however, can increase with sexual excitement, as well as midway through a normal menstrual cycle. This discharge is particularly prominent at the onset of puberty (physiological leukorrhea). Examination of a wet preparation will reveal vaginal epithelial cells only. The high protein content of this discharge, absorbed onto underwear, causes yellow staining. Traditionally, occlusive nylon or rayon underpants have been alleged to cause a nonspecific vaginal discharge; however, that association may be spurious.

A wide variety of organisms normally are found in the vagina. These organisms, especially the lactobacilli, help maintain the normal acidic pH of the vagina, which resists infection. Some of the organisms that cause vaginitis and vaginal discharge in this age group are sexually transmitted or associated with sexual activity.[6] Because many teenagers fear admitting to sexual intercourse, a negative response to queries about sexual activity should not rule out consideration of a sexually transmitted organism as the cause of the discharge. Sexual abuse and the presence of a foreign body (e.g., a retained tampon or condom) also should be considered. If the discharge is caused by a sexually transmitted organism, the patient's sexual partner should be notified and treated. The patient should refrain from sexual intercourse until she completes treatment. Otherwise, infection of her partner may occur. The use of spermicides or douching can cause vaginitis.[4]

Table 178-1 lists the organisms and conditions commonly responsible for vaginal infections or vaginal discharge in pubertal young women. Although the characteristics of each type of infection are said to be typical, the discharge observed on examination does not always fit these classic presentations.[7] The laboratory methods outlined in Table 178-1, therefore, are of considerable diagnostic utility. However, they are not 100% sensitive: *T. vaginalis* may not be noted during microscopic examination even if the vaginal fluid is

Table 178-1 Major Causes of Vaginal Discharge in Pubertal Girls

Agent	Discharge	Odor; pH	Dysuria; Pruritus	Other Clues	Diagnosis	Treatment*
Candida albicans	Thick, white, curdlike, "cheesy"	None usually; pH 4.5 (obtained from midvagina with nitrazine paper)	Dysuria frequent; pruritus (4+)	Vulva affected; association with use of some oral contraceptives and, in some women, with antibiotic use	Hyphae on potassium hydroxide examination	A variety of effective treatments are available for vaginal candidiasis, including creams, ointments, suppositories, and intravaginal tablets. Three-, 5-, and 7-day therapies offer no advantage over single-day treatments. Fluconazole 150 mg PO as a single dose is as effective as other regimens; however, there may be more systemic side effects. Ultimately, the "best" treatment is a combination of patient preference, what treatments are covered by her insurance, and whether it is cheaper and/or more convenient for the patient to obtain a prescription medication or purchase an over-the-counter treatment.
Trichomonas vaginalis	Frothy; yellow green or gray	Foul-smelling; pH 5.2-5.5	Dysuria frequent; pruritus	Low abdominal pain; "strawberry" cervix; punctate vaginal hemorrhages	Motile trichomonads on wet preparation; avoid drying specimen	Metronidazole 2 g orally in a single dose. Alternatively, this medication can be given as 500 mg bid for 7 days. Partners of the patient must be treated. Some strains of *T. vaginalis* have diminished susceptibility to metronidazole. If failure occurs with either of the indicated regimens (and reinfection is not a possibility), the patient should be treated with 500 mg bid for 7 days. Repeated failures should be treated with 2 g qd for 3 to 5 days. The patient should be told to avoid alcohol until 24 hours after completion of therapy.
Bacterial vaginosis (formerly *Gardnerella vaginalis*)	Gray or white, not curdlike†	Fishlike and foul; increased when mixed with potassium hydroxide†; pH 5.0-5.5†	No dysuria; slight pruritus	Occurs in association with anaerobes and *G. vaginalis*	Clue cells on wet preparation (bacteria-coated epithelial cells)†	Metronidazole 500 mg orally bid for 7 days or clindamycin cream 2%, one full applicator (5 g) intravaginally q hs for 7 days, or metronidazole gel 0.75% one full applicator (5 g) intravaginally bid for 5 days

Data from Amsel R, et al: *Am J Med* 74:14, 1983; Brunham RC, et al: *N Eng J Med* 311:1, 1984; Rein MF, Chapel TA: *Clin Obstet Gynecol* 18:73, 1975; and Sobel J: *N Engl J Med* 337:1896, 1997.

*See reference no. 1.

†Must have three of these four criteria to make diagnosis.

examined immediately under the microscope to avoid drying of the organisms. Microscopy is 60% to 90% sensitive compared with culture, depending on the experience of the microscopist. The role of *N. gonorrhoeae* and *C. trachomatis* in causing vaginal discharge has been reassessed recently. The presence of yellow vaginal discharge on speculum examination has been associated with infection by either organism; in contrast, neither profuse vaginal discharge nor a foul or "fishy odor" predicted infection with either.[4] Nonetheless, because sexually transmitted infections often co-occur, appropriate screening tests for *N. gonorrhoeae* and *C. trachomatis* should be part of the evaluation of vaginitis if *T. vaginalis* is found or if the patient reports a new sexual partner.

Bacterial vaginosis is a syndrome resulting from replacement of lactobacilli by high concentrations of a variety of anaerobic organisms.[9] There is mounting evidence that this infection is sexually transmitted, although treatment of sexual partners does not appear to reduce the risk of recurrence.[4] Current evidence indicates that women who have bacterial vaginosis are at increased risk for developing pelvic inflammatory disease, and if pregnant, are more likely to deliver a premature infant or experience postpartum complications. Therefore, prompt treatment of this cause of symptomatic vaginal discharge is essential. Treatment of sexual partners is not currently recommended.

Occasionally, herpesvirus infections of the vulvovaginal area and/or cervix are associated with vaginal discharge. Typically there is pain or a burning sensation in the genital area. The vulva is reddened, and groups of small vesicles are noted on the vulva, in the vagina, or on the cervix. If the vesicles have ruptured, the examiner sees only small ulcerations. Inguinal adenopathy, fever, and malaise usually are present if this is a first attack (see Chapter 217, Herpes Infections).

A teenager who has a persistent discharge unresponsive to therapy may not be complying with treatment or may have become reinfected by an untreated partner. If this not the case, if *N. gonorrhoeae*, *C. trachomatis,* and *T. vaginalis* are shown not to be present, and the discharge does not appear to fit any of the causes described earlier, a trial of Sitz baths, use of cotton as opposed to nylon underwear, and careful attention to perineal hygiene is warranted. If symptoms persist, the patient should be referred to an adolescent medicine specialist or a gynecologist.

Candidal infections can be especially difficult to treat and may recur. Factors that predispose to candidiasis include oral contraceptive or broad-spectrum antibiotic use[8] and diabetes mellitus. A variety of month-long antifungal treatments have been successful; male sexual partners also should be treated if they have any signs or symptoms of candidal penile involvement.

When to Refer

1. If the clinician is uncomfortable with evaluating genital complaints in prepubertal girls
2. If the clinician lacks experience in performing pelvic examinations
3. If the evaluation yields evidence of sexual abuse
4. If the discharge persists despite seemingly appropriate therapy

REFERENCES

1. Centers for Disease Control and Prevention: 1998 Guidelines for treatment of sexually transmitted diseases, *MMWR* 47 (No RR-1), 1998.
2. Emans SJ, Laufer MR, Goldstein DP: *Pediatric and adolescent gynecology,* ed 4, Boston, 1998, Lippincott-Raven.
3. Gardner JJ: Comparison of the vaginal flora in sexually abused and nonabused girls, *J Pediatr* 120:870, 1992.
4. Holmes KK, Stamm WE: Lower genital tract infection syndromes in women. In Holmes KK, et al, editors: *Sexually transmitted diseases,* ed 3, New York, 1999, McGraw-Hill.
5. Preminger MK, Pokorny SF: Vaginal discharge: a common pediatric complaint, *Contemp Pediatr* 15:115, 1998.
6. Shafer MB: Sexually transmitted diseases in adolescents: prevention, diagnosis, and treatment in pediatric practice, *Adolescent Health Update* 6:2, 1994.
7. Sobel J: Vaginitis, *N Engl J Med* 337:1896, 1997.
8. Spinillo A, et al: Effect of antibiotic use on the prevalence of symptomatic vulvovaginal candidiasis, *Am J Obstet Gynecol* 180:14, 1999.
9. Thomason JL, Gelbart SM, Scaglione NJ: Bacterial vaginosis: current review with indications for asymptomatic therapy, *Am J Obstet Gynecol* 165:1210, 1991.

179 Visual Problems

James W. McManaway III

Detection of visual problems in children may be difficult for several reasons: (1) children usually do not complain of monocular or mild bilateral visual loss, and even those who have significant bilateral visual loss may navigate familiar surroundings without notable difficulty; (2) vision-threatening ocular disease may have subtle ocular signs; (3) measurement of visual acuity in preverbal children requires special techniques; and (4) children who have monocular visual loss tend to peek around the occluder to escape detection (Fig. 179-1). Nonetheless, the primary care pediatrician must use accurate screening techniques to ensure the ocular health of children.

THE VISION SCREENING EXAMINATION

A basic but effective pediatric vision screening examination consists of three steps: (1) measurement of visual acuity in each eye, (2) assessment of ocular alignment, and (3) assessment of the fundus red reflex. All newborns' red reflex should be assessed in the nursery, and children should have this vision screening examination at 2, 4, and 6 years of age. Children passing all three steps are unlikely to have vision-threatening ocular problems.

Measurement of Visual Acuity

The method of visual acuity measurement (Table 179-1) depends largely on the age and level of cooperation of the child. The simplest of these tests is to look for a fixation preference by alternately covering one eye. The normal response is to maintain fixation with the uncovered eye. A child who consistently objects to covering one eye and has no objection to covering the other eye is said to have a fixation preference for one eye (Fig. 179-2). The methods used to measure visual acuity in young children do not yield a numerical measurement; what is important is that both eyes show the same response. Children often perform better if the test is practiced close up, using both eyes, before one eye is completely covered with an eye patch or an occluder. When performing a "fixes and follows" acuity test, be sure not to provide audible clues—a blind child can track with eye movements a subtle sound all over the examination room!

Children older than 2 to 3 months of age should be able to follow the examiner's face for several seconds with each eye. Children 6 to 12 months of age should be able to follow a brightly colored toy (Fig. 179-3). A very useful and well-accepted method is the localization of small candy beads in the examiner's hand; children 12 to 30 months of age should be able to sweep at or grasp a 1-mm bead at 13 inches using each eye. The examiner should extend both hands to force the child to choose the hand holding the candy (Fig. 179-4). Older children can be tested by use of the picture chart, E game, or letters in the usual fashion at a 20-foot testing distance. Children who have significant differences in visual acuity between their two eyes (two Snellen lines difference) or who have abnormal acuity in both eyes (20/50 or worse for a 3-year-old, 20/40 or worse for a 5-year-old) should be referred to an ophthalmologist.

Assessment of Ocular Alignment

Strabismus in children may be associated with amblyopia caused by suppression of the deviating eye or with vision- or life-threatening ocular disease such as cataracts, retinoblastoma, or congenital ocular malformations. Thus, detection of strabismus is a key part of the vision-screening examination. Two major methods to detect strabismus exist—the corneal light reflex test and the alternate cover test.

The corneal light reflex test shows centering of the corneal reflection of a penlight in both pupils of a child who has normal ocular alignment. Temporal displacement of the reflex occurs in esotropia (Fig. 179-5; also see Fig. 171-3), and nasal displacement occurs in exotropia. Any deviation of the reflection from the center is abnormal, but this test yields both false-positive and false-negative results because the visual axis may not coincide with the center of the pupil. A much superior test is the cover-uncover test. The examiner covers one of the child's eyes with a finger or occluder and looks for a refixation movement by the other eye. Both eyes must be tested, but the cover should not be moved from eye to eye; instead, the cover is used to cover one eye and then is removed. A few seconds later, the other eye is tested similarly. A refixation demonstrates the presence of strabismus (Fig. 179-6); an outward refixation means esotropia, and an inward refixation means exotropia. Further details of the testing methods can be found in Chapter 171, Strabismus. Any refixation is abnormal and should be referred for further evaluation.

Assessment of the Fundus Red Reflex

A normal fundus red reflex rules out any opacity of the ocular tissues that could cause amblyopia; it also rules out an intraocular tumor or coloboma involving the posterior retina. This

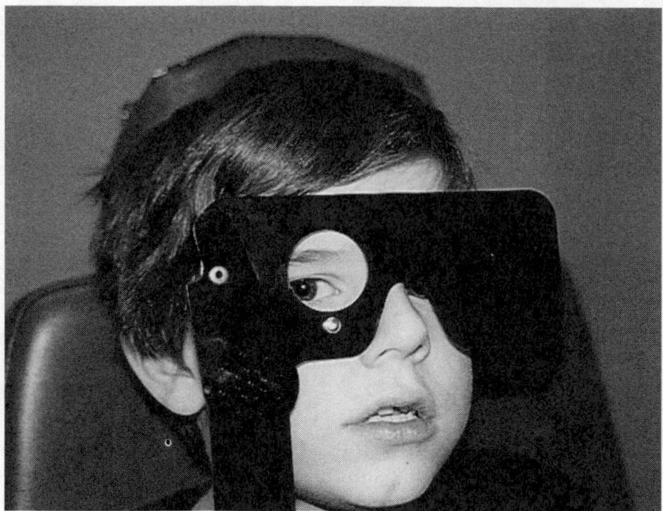

Fig. 179-1 This child is peeking around the occluder to use his left eye instead of the amblyopic right eye to see the visual acuity chart. This subtle behavior results in false-negative visual acuity testing and a delay in the diagnosis and treatment of his amblyopia.

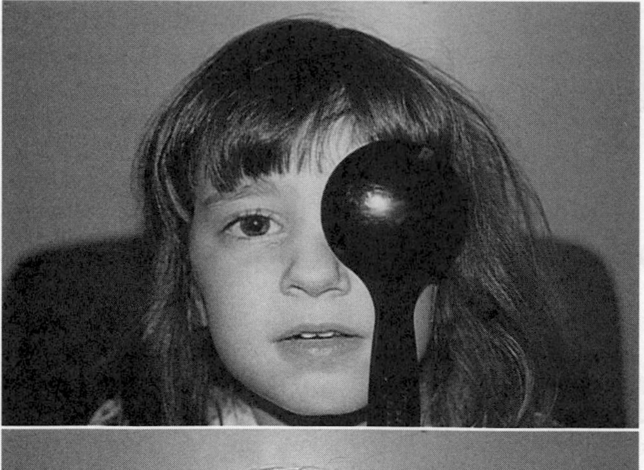

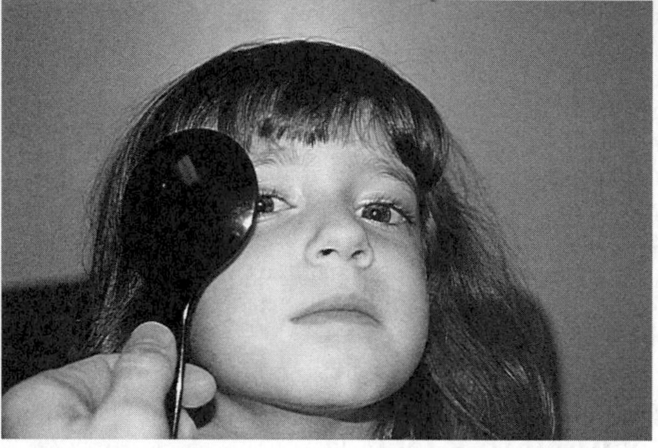

Fig. 179-2 **A,** This child happily fixes with her right eye and does not object if the left eye is covered. **B,** When the right eye is covered, she moves her head away and tries to remove the cover, demonstrating a fixation preference for the right eye and amblyopia of the left eye.

Table 179-1 Visual Acuity Measurement in Children

Method	Age of Child
Fixes and follows examiner's face	3-6 mo
Fixes and follows toy	6-12 mo
Localizes candy beads	12-30 mo
Picture chart	30-60 mo
E game	5-6 yr
Snellen letter chart	6+ yr

test is performed with a direct ophthalmoscope in a semidark room (Fig. 179-7). With the ophthalmoscope on the zero power setting, the examiner should sit 3 to 5 feet from the child and direct the ophthalmoscope beam on the child's face. When looking through the ophthalmoscope, the examiner immediately will see a bright orange-red reflection from the fundus through the patient's pupils. Asymmetry, dimness, or whiteness of the reflex (leukocoria) is abnormal and should be evaluated immediately by an ophthalmologist.

REFRACTIVE ERRORS

Refractive errors are the most common cause of decreased visual acuity in children. Four major types of refractive errors exist: (1) myopia, (2) hyperopia, (3) astigmatism, and (4) anisometropia. A detailed discussion of ophthalmic optics is beyond the scope of this chapter, but a few basic points will be set forth.

Myopia

Myopia (nearsightedness) exists when the refractive power of the eye is too strong for the length of the eye. Images from distant objects are focused in front of the retina and are blurred, but images from near objects are seen clearly. Myopia is the most common cause of decreased distance acuity in children. Mild myopia does not have to be corrected until the child reaches school age, but high myopia, as seen in many infants born prematurely, should be corrected by 9 to 12 months of age.

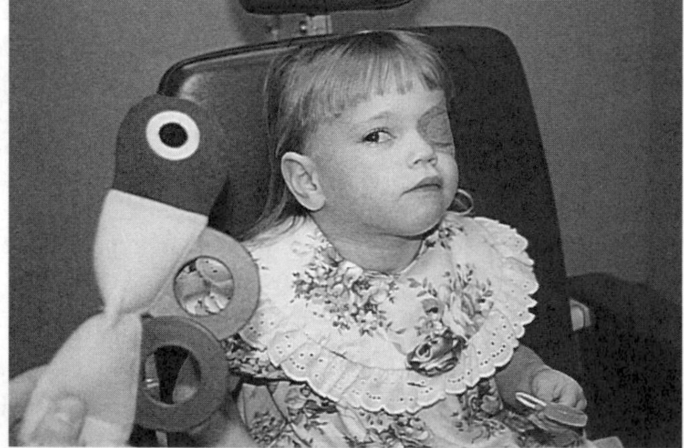

Fig. 179-3 This child follows the brightly colored toy easily with each eye.

Hyperopia

Hyperopia (farsightedness) exists when the refractive power of the eye is too weak for the length of the eye. Without

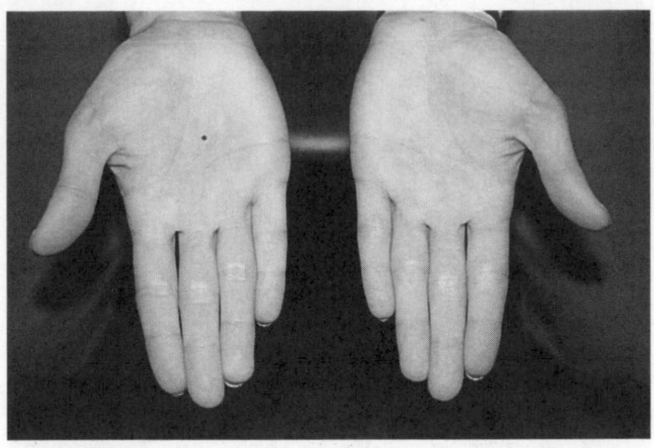

Fig. 179-4 Technique of visual acuity testing using a 1-mm candy bead in one hand while presenting both hands.

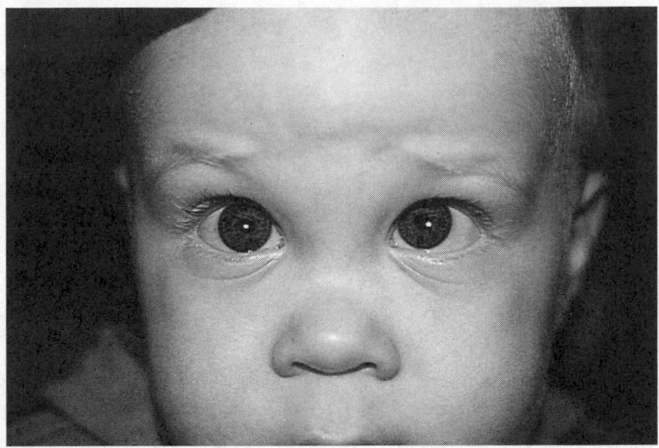

Fig. 179-5 The corneal light reflex test in a child who has esotropia.

accommodation (focusing of the crystalline lens of the eye for near vision), images from distant objects are focused "behind" the retina and are somewhat blurred, and images from near objects are focused farther "behind" the retina and are more blurred. Children have a tremendous amplitude of accommodation, and hyperopic children can easily accommodate somewhat to see distant objects clearly and can accommodate more to see near objects clearly. Some children who have uncorrected hyperopia have eyestrain from constant accommodation; others develop accommodative esotropia because excessive accommodation is linked to excessive convergence.

Astigmatism

Astigmatism occurs when the refractive power of the eye is different in the horizontal than in the vertical meridian of the eye. This generally occurs when the corneal curvature is steeper in one meridian than in the other. A descriptive exaggeration is that the cornea is shaped more like a football than a basketball. This causes a point object to be focused into a vertical line image in front of the retina and into a horizontal line image behind the retina. This lack of a point focus earns this condition the name *astigmatism* (without a point). Astigmatism causes both distant and near objects to be blurred.

Anisometropia

Anisometropia occurs when the refractive power between the two eyes is significantly different. One eye could be hyperopic and the other myopic, or one eye could have more hyperopia, myopia, or astigmatism than the other. Anisometropia is a common cause of amblyopia because the eye that has the larger refractive error has a constantly blurred image and does not have normal visual development.

FUNCTIONAL VISUAL LOSS

Functional (psychogenic) visual loss is a common cause of unilaterally or bilaterally decreased visual acuity. This occurs most commonly in the pediatric clinic because the child is fearful of upcoming injections or painful procedures. Another common cause is the desire to obtain glasses because a classmate or sibling has them. A pair of medium-size spectacle frames that have plano (no power) lenses can be made by a local optician and will establish the diagnosis quickly in the child who wants to obtain glasses. Some children will continue to show abnormal visual acuity despite encouragement and retesting with plano lenses; these children should be referred to an ophthalmologist to rule out amblyopia, refractive errors, or ocular disease.

AMBLYOPIA

Amblyopia is a decrease in visual acuity in one or both eyes, with no apparent abnormality on physical examination. It is a very important cause of permanent visual loss and affects 5% of the United States population; the incidence of amblyopia may be much higher in economically deprived children or in those who were born prematurely. Detection of amblyopia in young children is important for two reasons: (1) amblyopia can be treated successfully only in young children, and (2) life-threatening disorders (retinoblastoma) may present as amblyopia. Because the results of amblyopia treatment are much better in young children, the National Children's Eye Care Foundation aims to eliminate permanent visual loss caused by amblyopia through effective vision screening of all children before they reach 3 years of age.

Five types of amblyopia exist: (1) deprivation, (2) strabismic, (3) anisometropic, (4) occlusion, and (5) bilateral ametropic. Deprivation amblyopia occurs when the visual axis is blocked and a clear image cannot reach the retina. Typical causes include severe congenital or acquired ptosis, congenital cataract, and opacities of the vitreous body. Amblyopia often adds to the visual loss already caused by cataracts or other opacities of the ocular media. Bilateral deprivation amblyopia is possible in children who have bilateral occlusion of the visual axis. Strabismic amblyopia occurs when the same eye constantly is deviated; the brain ignores the image from the deviating eye, and amblyopia results. Anisometropic amblyopia occurs when a significant difference in refractive power exists between the two eyes. The brain ignores the blurred image from the eye that has the larger refractive error, and amblyopia results. Occlusion amblyopia is a subtype

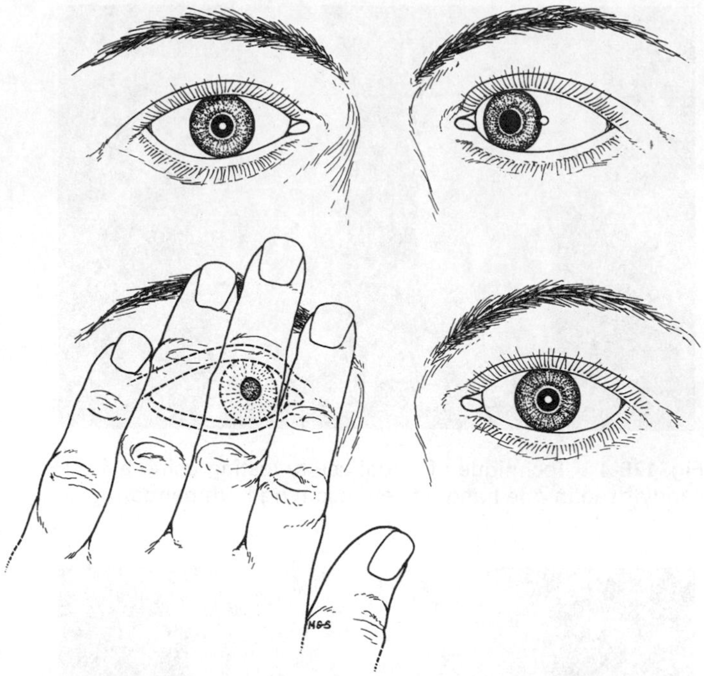

Fig. 179-6 The cover-uncover test demonstrating a temporal ocular refixation in a child who has esotropia.

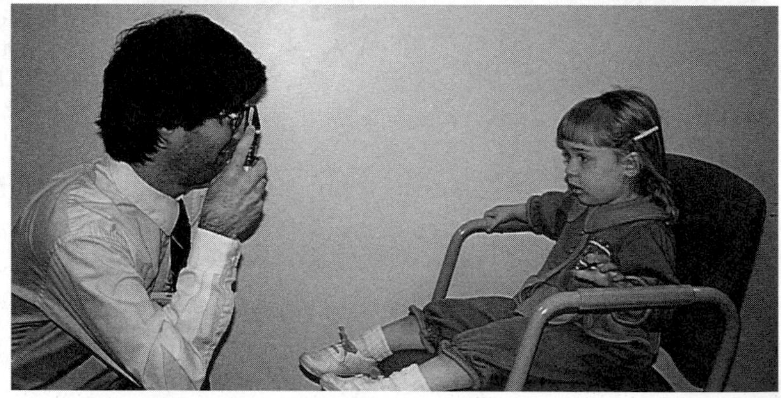

Fig. 179-7 The technique of assessing the fundus red reflex.

of deprivation amblyopia that occurs when the better-seeing eye is patched excessively in an attempt to improve the visual acuity of the amblyopic eye. The poorer-seeing eye becomes the better-seeing eye, and vice versa. Frequent follow-up visits during patching therapy prevent this complication. Bilateral ametropic amblyopia occurs when both eyes have a large and equal refractive error, typically hyperopic astigmatism. Neither eye sees well at a distance or close up, and bilateral amblyopia occurs.

OCULAR AND NEUROLOGICAL DISORDERS CAUSING VISUAL LOSS

Disorders causing visual loss can be categorized into (1) opacities of the optical media, (2) retinal disease and detachment, (3) optic nerve disorders, and (4) disorders of the visual pathways and the cerebral cortex. Common examples of each category will be provided, but summarizing the field of pediatric ophthalmology is beyond the scope of this chapter.

Opacities of the optical media can occur in the cornea, lens, and vitreous body. Corneal opacities can be caused by congenital anomalies, glaucoma, herpetic or bacterial keratitis, metabolic disease, corneal dystrophies, and trauma. Any opacity of the crystalline lens is called a *cataract,* which can be congenital, traumatic, or caused by other ocular or metabolic disorders. Common examples of vitreous opacities include persistent hyperplastic primary vitreous, a congenital anomaly, and vitreous hemorrhage caused by child abuse or bleeding abnormalities.

Many retinal diseases can cause visual loss in children. Common examples include cicatricial changes from retinopathy of prematurity, congenital retinal infections (TORCH*), metabolic storage diseases, and retinal dystrophies. Retinal detachment in children is rare but can occur congenitally or in association with retinopathy of prematurity (retrolental fibroplasia) or trauma to the eye. Optic nerve disorders include congenital anomalies of the optic disk, optic nerve hypoplasia, optic atrophy, and optic neuritis. Optic nerve hypoplasia is a very important cause of visual loss because of a common

*Toxoplasmosis, other, rubella, cytomegalovirus, herpes simplex

association with midline central nervous system (CNS) defects and a pituitary insufficiency (de Morsier's syndrome).

Disorders of the visual pathways posterior to the optic chiasm usually cause loss of visual field instead of an overall loss of visual acuity. Patients who have infarcts of both occipital lobes following prolonged hypotension or anoxia will have severe loss of overall visual acuity and of visual fields (cortical blindness). Some infants will have delayed myelination of the visual pathways or the visual cortex, and will demonstrate profound visual inattention during the first several months of life (delayed visual maturation). This usually resolves by 6 months of age in otherwise healthy infants but may take longer in infants who have other developmental delays caused by delay of myelination throughout the CNS.

Migraine is a disorder of the visual pathways that may cause transient visual loss in children as the scintillating scotoma expands from a small spot near the fixation point to a large area covering nearly half of the visual field of each eye. This scintillating scotoma may not be associated with a headache, and the child may not be able to explain the visual phenomenon sufficiently for the examiner to consider migraine as the diagnosis. A carefully directed history may allow the child to explain the visual symptoms.

SUGGESTED READINGS

Berson FG: *Basic ophthalmology for medical students and primary care residents,* San Francisco, 1993, American Academy of Ophthalmology.

Nelson LB, Calhoun JH, Harley RD: *Pediatric ophthalmology*, ed 3, Philadelphia, 1991, WB Saunders.

Taylor D: *Pediatric ophthalmology*, Boston, 1990, Blackwell Scientific.

180 Vomiting

Martin H. Ulshen

Vomiting is a common symptom of acute and chronic illness in childhood. This highly coordinated, active process must be distinguished from regurgitation, which is passive reflux of gastric contents into the esophagus and mouth through a relaxed lower esophageal sphincter. Vomiting is a coordinated event usually preceded by nausea in association with increased salivation, gastric atony, and reflux of duodenal contents into the stomach (resulting from nonperistaltic contractions of the small bowel). This phase may not be apparent in infants. Retching (coordinated contraction of abdominal and intercostal muscles as well as the diaphragm, with simultaneous closure of the glottis) immediately precedes the actual vomiting. Increased intragastric pressure from contraction of the abdominal wall musculature, lowering of the diaphragm, and pyloric contraction are associated with elevation and relaxation of the cardia, and vomiting occurs.

The total process of vomiting is coordinated in the medullary vomiting center. This center may be influenced directly by visceral afferent stimuli or indirectly through the chemoreceptor trigger zone. The latter region is the site of action of many of the drugs that cause nausea and vomiting, including apomorphine and digitalis. During motion sickness, stimulation of the vestibular system activates the vomiting center and perhaps the chemoreceptor trigger zone as well. Higher central nervous system (CNS) centers may also influence the medullary vomiting center.

Understanding the role of neurotransmitters as mediators of the initiation of vomiting has led to a range of new antiemetics. The area postrema, which is a major lower brainstem center for coordination of drug-induced vomiting, is rich in enkephalins, 5-hydroxytryptamine (HT) receptors, and dopamine receptors. Enkephalins and 5-HT both stimulate release of dopamine. Dopamine and 5-HT antagonists have been successful in the treatment of chemotherapy-induced nausea and vomiting. Antihistamines and anticholinergics prevent motion sickness by acting at H_1 and muscarinic cholinergic receptors, respectively, in the nucleus ambiguus in the lower brainstem and in the lateral vestibular nucleus in the midpons.[1]

CAUSES AND DIFFERENTIAL DIAGNOSIS

Box 180-1 lists the most frequent causes of emesis in infants and children. In infancy, regurgitation, or spitting up, is very common and most often a developmental event, which has no sequelae and gradually resolves. Pathological gastroesophageal reflux is defined by the association of regurgitation with severe complications (including esophagitis with or without anemia secondary to blood loss or stricture, recurrent apnea, aspiration pneumonia, or failure to thrive). Bilious vomiting (especially when associated with the first vomitus) usually occurs only with ileus or intestinal tract obstruction below the ampulla of Vater (in the second portion of the duodenum). In newborns, bilious vomiting can be associated with necrotizing enterocolitis. In older children who vomit persistently, reflux of bile from the duodenum into the stomach may lead to bilious vomiting without gastrointestinal tract obstruction. Projectile vomiting commonly occurs with pyloric stenosis. When this condition persists, however, gastric atony may eliminate the projectile character. A succussion splash (the splashing sound present when a patient who has fluid in a hollow organ [e.g., stomach] is shaken on physical examination) may be present, as in other causes of gastric outlet obstruction. Vomiting associated with increased intracranial pressure may be projectile and may take place in the absence of nausea or retching.

Persistent vomiting in a newborn or young infant who has no evidence of infection usually suggests a congenital gastrointestinal anomaly, inborn error of metabolism, or CNS abnormality such as hydrocephalus or subdural effusion. If the history and physical examination results do not suggest a cause, it is best to evaluate all three possibilities simultaneously. When the sudden onset of bilious vomiting, especially within the first few days of life, develops in a previously well newborn, one must consider a malrotation with secondary midgut volvulus. A plain film of the abdomen may show a paucity of gas distal to the upper small intestine; however, the plain film may not be helpful. If a midgut volvulus is suspected, an upper gastrointestinal roentgenographic series should be done at once, with the controlled introduction of barium through a nasogastric tube after gastric aspiration. A barium enema investigation of cecal position is a less reliable study when evaluating a patient for malrotation because of the lack of complete correlation of developmental rotation of the cecum with that of the duodenum. Midgut volvulus is a surgical emergency requiring early diagnosis and surgical intervention. In a sick newborn the diagnosis of necrotizing enterocolitis must be considered in the event of bilious vomiting, especially with blood in the stool. Beyond the first week of life, but within the first 2 months, pyloric stenosis is the most common cause of persistent vomiting. In the older infant or child, the entire spectrum of causes of vomiting listed in Box 180-1 should be considered. It is interesting that patients who have celiac

BOX 180-1

CAUSES OF EMESIS (ARRANGED BY USUAL AGE OF EARLIEST OCCURRENCE)

Infancy
Gastrointestinal
Congenital
- Regurgitation—gastroesophageal reflux (developmental or pathological)
- Atresia—stenosis (tracheoesophageal fistula, antral web, intestinal atresia, annular pancreas)
- Duplication
- Volvulus (secondary to an error in rotation and fixation or to Meckel's diverticulum)
- Congenital bands
- Meconium ileus (cystic fibrosis), meconium plug
- Hirschsprung's disease

Acquired
- Acute infectious gastroenteritis
- Pyloric stenosis
- Intussusception
- Incarcerated hernia—inguinal, internal secondary to old adhesions
- Food allergy, cow milk protein intolerance, eosinophilic gastroenteritis
- Disaccharidase deficiency
- Celiac disease—risk is inherited but presents after introduction of gluten in diet
- Postviral gastroparesis[8]
- Adynamic ileus—the mediator for many nongastrointestinal causes of vomiting
- Neonatal necrotizing enterocolitis
- Chronic granulomatous disease with gastric outlet obstruction

Nongastrointestinal
- Infectious—otitis, urinary tract infection, pneumonia, upper respiratory tract infection, sepsis, meningitis
- Metabolic—aminoaciduria and organic aciduria, galactosemia, fructosemia, adrenogenital syndrome, renal tubular acidosis, hyperammonemia, disorders of fatty acid oxidation, Reye's syndrome
- Central nervous system—trauma, tumor, infection, diencephalic syndrome, rumination, autonomic responses (pain, shock)
- Medications—anticholinergics, aspirin, alcohol, idiosyncratic reaction (e.g., codeine)

Childhood (Additional Causes)
Gastrointestinal
- Appendicitis
- Food poisoning (staphylococcal, clostridial)
- Peptic disease: ulcer, gastritis, duodenitis
- Trauma—duodenal hematoma, traumatic pancreatitis, perforated bowel
- Pancreatitis—mumps, trauma, cystic fibrosis, hyperparathyroidism, hyperlipidemia, organic acidemias
- Gallbladder—cholelithiasis, choledochal cyst
- Crohn's disease
- Adhesions—congenital or secondary to abdominal surgery
- Idiopathic intestinal pseudo-obstruction
- Superior mesenteric artery syndrome[7]

Nongastrointestinal
- Central nervous system—cyclic vomiting, migraine, anorexia nervosa, bulimia
- Motion sickness
- Metabolic—diabetic ketoacidosis, acute intermittent porphyria
- Pregnancy

disease occasionally may have minimal or no diarrhea but prominent vomiting. When an older child manifests acute vomiting and somnolence, one always should consider drug overdose (especially aspirin toxicity), meningoencephalitis, and Reye's syndrome in the differential diagnosis. Persistent or recurrent vomiting without other symptoms may be the major manifestation of an emotional disorder in childhood. Therefore, a careful psychosocial history is an important part of the evaluation.

Cyclic Vomiting

Cyclic vomiting is characterized by repeated episodes of vomiting (peak intensity at least four emeses/hour and frequency no more than two episodes/week), sometimes occurring in clusters and sometimes associated with abdominal pain.[4,6] Uncontrollable vomiting and retching are typical of an attack, but between episodes patients are well. About 10% of these children have an identifiable gastrointestinal or extraintestinal (e.g., renal, metabolic, or neurological) disorder as the probable cause.

Abdominal migraine is a common cause of cyclic vomiting and is characterized by the paroxysmal onset of repetitious attacks often relieved with sleep. A strong family history of migraine commonly is present. Headache typical of migraine may occur with episodes. Cyproheptadine, amitriptyline, and propranolol are highly effective as prophylactic treatment for abdominal migraine; treatment success helps to confirm the diagnosis.[2,11] Abdominal epilepsy is a much less common cause of cyclic vomiting. A careful history of the sequence of events and electroencephalographic evaluation are useful in the evaluation, and anticonvulsants can be tried when this condition is suspected. Low-dose erythromycin has been used successfully to treat some children who have idiopathic cyclic vomiting.[10]

EVALUATION

Evaluation of the gastrointestinal tract usually includes an upper gastrointestinal contrast roentgenographic study. However, in an infant between 2 and 12 weeks of age, the first study is often an ultrasound of the abdomen for pyloric stenosis. Endoscopy is feasible in all children, even newborns, if performed by an experienced examiner using a pediatric instrument.[9] Esophageal pH monitoring, esophageal biopsies, and gastroesophageal scintiscan all are useful in establishing a diagnosis of gastroesophageal reflux. If brain tumor is a consideration in an infant, magnetic resonance imaging (MRI) is more sensitive than a computed tomography (CT) scan of the head. Further workup for metabolic or neurological disease should be considered, as appropriate. With persistent vomiting, one expects to see a metabolic alkalosis; metabolic acidosis raises concerns about an underlying metabolic disorder or drug intoxication. In a postpubertal girl, pregnancy must always be considered in the differential diagnosis of vomiting.

COMPLICATIONS

The most significant complications of vomiting include aspiration pneumonia, hemorrhage from prolapse gastropathy (a hemorrhagic area on the posterior wall of the proximal stomach) or less commonly a tear at the gastroesophageal junction (Mallory-Weiss syndrome), rupture of the esophagus (very uncommon in children), and dehydration and electrolyte imbalance associated with persistent vomiting.

TREATMENT

Acute intercurrent vomiting without serious underlying disease or significant dehydration should be treated by administering clear liquids by mouth (e.g., in acute gastroenteritis or otitis media). It usually is advisable to start with a period of 4 to 6 hours without oral intake and then begin with frequent small quantities of clear liquids (1 teaspoonful every few minutes for infants) and gradually increase the volume and extension of the period between oral fluids. If vomiting is associated with diarrhea and dehydration, oral rehydration solution is indicated (see Chapter 278, Dehydration). Carbonated beverages may increase vomiting. Fluids of high osmolality, long-chain triglycerides, and anticholinergic drugs all tend to slow gastric emptying and should be avoided.

Antiemetic drugs should be avoided in infants, although they may at times be useful in older children.[1] The drug used most commonly for acute symptoms is promethazine (Phenergan). Trimethobenzamide (Tigan) may be less effective but also is used. Rectal suppositories are preferable to oral drugs because nausea is associated with gastric atony and unpredictable absorption. Dopamine-receptor antagonists (such as metoclopramide) are effective for chemotherapy-induced vomiting, although 5-HT_3 receptor antagonists (ondansetron) appear to have even greater efficacy without the risks of dystonic reactions associated with metoclopramide.[1] Histamine (H_1) receptor antagonists (including diphenhydramine, dimenhydrinate, meclizine, and promethazine) and muscarinic cholinergic receptor antagonists (e.g., scopolamine) prevent motion sickness.[1] Metoclopramide, cisapride, and erythromycin can help to treat poor gastric emptying without mechanical obstruction. Use of cisapride has been severely limited by concerns about increased risk of arrhythmias.[3] It can be used more safely if a normal QT interval is documented by ECG before and several days into use of cisapride. A number of antibiotics should not be administered with cisapride, including erythromycin and clarithromycin.

Patients should be monitored for signs of dehydration. For certain patients (e.g., those who have severe psychomotor retardation), a nasoduodenal infusion may be useful. Significant vomiting that requires intravenous fluid therapy usually is associated with hypochloremic alkalosis with secondary hypokalemia. Intravenous fluids should repair the deficits (see Chapter 29, Fluid Therapy).

Management of gastroesophageal reflux must be individualized. The extent of treatment depends on the volume of emesis and the presence of any of the complications of reflux (esophagitis with or without esophageal stricture or intractable anemia, failure to thrive, or respiratory manifestations). Medical management includes thickening feedings with cereal (a standard concentration is 1 tablespoonful of cereal for each 1 to 2 ounces of formula). The efficacy of placing an infant in a supine or lateral, head-elevated position for sleep is questionable, although elevating the head of the bed remains standard therapy for older children and adults.[5] Older children also should avoid snacks or liquids after dinner and agents that exacerbate esophagitis (alcohol, caffeine, and smoking). Medications can be used in an attempt to improve lower esophageal function and gastric emptying (e.g., metoclopramide) and to decrease exposure of the esophageal mucosa to acid (antacids, histamine receptor blockers, or proton pump inhibitors). A slurry of sucralfate (a cytoprotective agent) is used occasionally. When a child has severe gastroesophageal reflux, medical management may be unsatisfactory. In this case, antireflux surgery (fundoplication) should be considered. In this group of children the results of surgery generally are good when performed by an experienced surgeon, and the benefits can be long lasting. In children who have psychomotor retardation and gastroesophageal reflux, antireflux surgery may not eliminate respiratory symptoms inasmuch as other factors such as swallowing dysfunction may contribute to these findings. Among all children undergoing a Nissen fundoplication, the risk of a postoperative complication that requires further surgery may be as high as 10% and underscores the need for careful patient selection for this operation.

When to Refer

1. Persistent vomiting
2. Recurrent episodes of vomiting
3. Vomiting associated with a significant underlying process (e.g., surgical abdomen, neurological problem)

When to Hospitalize

1. Intractable vomiting with dehydration
2. Vomiting in association with symptoms or signs of an acute abdominal process (e.g., acute appendicitis, pancreatitis, cholecystitis)

REFERENCES

1. Allan SG: Antiemetics, *Gastroenterol Clin North Am* 21:597, 1992.
2. Andersen JM, et al: Effective prophylactic therapy for cyclic vomiting syndrome in children using amitriptyline or cyproheptadine, *Pediatrics* 100:977, 1997.

3. Hill SL, et al: Proarrhythmia associated with cisapride in children, *Pediatrics* 101:1053, 1998.
4. Li BUK, et al: Heterogeneity of diagnoses presenting as cyclic vomiting, *Pediatrics* 102:583, 1998.
5. Orenstein SR: Prone positioning in infant gastroesophageal reflux: is elevation of the head worth the trouble? *J Pediatr* 117:184, 1990.
6. Pfau BT, et al: Differentiating cyclic from chronic vomiting patterns in children: quantitative criteria and diagnostic implications, *Pediatrics* 97: 364, 1996.
7. Shandling B: The so-called superior mesenteric artery syndrome, *Am J Dis Child* 130:1371, 1976.
8. Sigurdsson L, et al: Postviral gastroparesis: presentation, treatment, and outcome, *J Pediatr* 130:751, 1997.
9. Ulshen MH: Unique aspects of gastrointestinal procedures for pediatric patients. In Drossman DA, editor: *Manual of gastroenterologic procedures,* ed 3, New York, 1993, Raven Press.
10. Vanderhoof JA, et al: Treatment of cyclic vomiting in childhood with erythromycin, *J Pediatr Gastroenterol Nutr* 17:387, 1993.
11. Worawattanakul M, et al: Abdominal migraine: prophylactic treatment and follow-up, *J Pediatr Gastroenterol Nutr* 28:37, 1999.

181 Weight Loss

Carole A. Stashwick

The documentation of weight loss in an infant, child, or adolescent is an uncommon but highly significant event. A child's weight should be measured at each visit and plotted on standard growth charts in the medical record. Weight loss, as the chief complaint or as an incidental finding, should be evaluated and followed carefully. Illingworth[8] ranked the symptom "loss of weight" as 1 of 13 that may signal a serious problem in the child.

Parents may have the impression that a child has lost weight based on a decrease in appetite or a change in the fit of clothing. Subjective impressions of weight loss always should be verified objectively before an evaluation is undertaken. True weight loss, however, sometimes may be difficult to differentiate from factitious weight loss, even when weights are documented in the medical record. It is estimated that specific errors in weighing children occur at frequencies ranging from 5% to 20% of all children weighed. Errors are caused by faulty equipment and by poor technique—for example, weighing with the clothes on.

NEWBORNS AND YOUNG INFANTS

The normal full-term newborn who is breast-fed is likely to lose about 6% (±3%) of weight during the first 3 days of life, and at least 7% of infants will lose more than 10% of their birth weight.[10,11] A loss of more than 10% to 12% of birth weight in the few days after birth is uncommon and is cause for an investigation to ensure that the infant is well, that adequate intake is being provided, and that fluid losses from vomitus, urine, or stool are not excessive.[10] It generally is believed that the infant who is breast-fed should have regained the lost weight and thus be at or above birth weight by 2 weeks of age.[11]

The most common reason for the breast-fed infant to have lost more weight than expected or to have failed to regain the lost weight by age 2 weeks is inadequate intake at the breast, not because of "insufficient milk" or milk that is not sufficiently "rich." Inadequate weight gain occurs because of infrequent or short feedings, failure of the let-down reflex, or improper positioning of the infant for an effective suck.[14] The infant will appear well, although perhaps slim, and may or may not act hungry. A number of reports have documented passivity and infrequent demands to be fed in some infants who are starving at the breast.[6,14]

The breast-feeding mother should be observed during a feeding, if possible, and specific evidence of a let-down or oxytocin reflex should be sought (uterine cramps, milk dripping or spraying from the opposite breast, a pins-and-needles sensation in the breast at the beginning of each nursing, and loud swallowing or occasional choking by the baby at the beginning of the feeding). The mother's motivation to breastfeed and her positive or negative feelings about the experience should be discussed; encouragement and support should be given for continuation of the nursing; and specific suggestions should be made for the mother to rest, to nurse frequently (every 2 to 3 hours in the day) to build up the milk supply, and to arrange relaxed, pleasant, and unhurried nursings. Formula or other fluids should not be recommended unless there are serious concerns about the infant's well-being. It is inappropriate for the physician to recommend discontinuing the nursing prematurely.[14] Demonstration of an appropriate weight gain in the following few days (120 to 200 g or more each week) is evidence that the infant is well and confirms the diagnosis of initial underfeeding. Infants who demonstrate failure to thrive while breast-feeding require more intensive nutritional rehabilitation while still preserving breast-feeding.[14]

The formula-fed infant rarely loses more than 5% of birth weight in the first few days, inasmuch as complete nutrition is available beginning a few hours after birth.[10] Because it is unusual for a bottle-fed infant to weigh less than birth weight at the age of 2 weeks, such an infant should be evaluated carefully. An error in feeding caused by maternal inexperience or ignorance is the usual explanation, but a careful search for an organic problem, as well as an evaluation of the family's functioning, support mechanisms, and adjustment to the new infant, are indicated. Rarely, the newborn will lose weight as a result of (1) inadequate intake for other reasons, such as infection, congenital heart disease, metabolic abnormality, somnolence from maternal medications or substance abuse, or poor suck resulting from a craniofacial or central nervous system (CNS) abnormality, or (2) excessive fluid loss, such as vomiting associated with congenital gastrointestinal malformations (duodenal atresia, annular pancreas, volvulus), diarrhea, or polyuria (diabetes insipidus, renal disease) (Box 181-1).

OLDER INFANTS, PRESCHOOLERS, AND SCHOOLCHILDREN

The infant may lose weight because of excessive vomiting, as in pyloric stenosis or severe gastroesophageal reflux. Tumors of the CNS in infancy may manifest with vomiting, anorexia, and cachexia.

BOX 181-1

DIFFERENTIAL DIAGNOSIS OF WEIGHT LOSS BY AGE GROUP

Newborns and Young Infants
- Difficulties in establishing breast-feeding
- Inappropriate dilution or choice of formula
- Inadequate intake
  - Infection
  - Metabolic abnormality
  - Craniofacial abnormalities
  - CNS dysfunction
  - Somnolence from maternal medications/substance abuse
  - Congenital heart disease
  - Maternal depression/inexperience/lack of knowledge
- Excessive losses
  - Vomiting because of gastrointestinal malformations (duodenal atresia, others)
  - Polyuria (diabetes insipidus, renal disease)
  - Diarrhea

Older Infants, Preschoolers, and Schoolchildren
- Excessive losses
  - Pyloric stenosis
  - Gastroesophageal reflux
  - CNS tumors
  - Vomiting
  - Diarrhea
  - Fever and infection
  - Diabetes mellitus
  - Excessive activity
- Inadequate intake
  - Fever and infection
  - Tuberculosis
  - Surgery
  - Medication effect (loss of appetite)
  - Malignancy
  - Congenital heart disease
- Poor utilization
  - Malabsorption syndromes
  - Inflammatory bowel disease
- Immunodeficiency disorders, especially HIV infection
- Psychosocial dysfunction
  - Neglect; nonorganic failure to thrive
  - Parental depression
  - Childhood depression
  - Rumination
  - Childhood eating disorder

Adolescents
- "Dieting" behavior
- Adolescent eating disorders
  - Anorexia nervosa
  - Bulimia nervosa
  - Other eating disorders
- Psychiatric affective disorders, especially depression
- Malignancy
- Inflammatory bowel disease
- Diabetes mellitus
- Hyperthyroidism
- Tuberculosis

The most common reason for weight loss in older infants and toddlers is fluid loss as a result of fever, vomiting, and diarrhea. The loss of weight may amount to 5% or more of premorbid body weight and usually is reversed with a few hours of oral or intravenous fluid replacement.

Weight loss also is a frequent concomitant of any severe febrile illness, such as pneumonia, pyelonephritis, septic arthritis, osteomyelitis, or meningitis, as well as less severe illnesses such as stomatitis and pharyngitis. Resolution of the infection often is followed by a period of "catch-up" growth and weight gain. Surgical procedures commonly result in a temporary loss of weight.

Weight loss also may be caused by poor utilization of ingested foodstuffs. Cystic fibrosis, the most common disease in which malabsorption occurs in childhood, may appear in infancy as poor weight gain or actual weight loss. Malabsorption, weight loss, and constipation may occur in the child who has Hirschsprung's disease. Children who have chronic diarrhea or severe immunodeficiency also may have weight loss. An infant or child who loses weight should be evaluated carefully for infection caused by the human immunodeficiency virus (HIV).[13]

Although emotional reasons often are the basis for an infant's or child's failure to thrive, actual weight loss is much less common than a slowdown or cessation of weight gain and linear growth. Psychosocial dysfunction (poor parent-child interaction, depression, rumination) that results in a child's weight loss requires a prompt and thorough evaluation.[5] Eating disorders have been described in prepubertal children as young as 7 years.[4]

The young child who has new-onset insulin-dependent diabetes mellitus commonly loses weight (often 10% or more of body weight) despite polyphagia and polydipsia. Hyperthyroidism in childhood may manifest as weight loss. Children who have inflammatory bowel disease usually demonstrate poor weight gain or actual weight loss.

A diagnosis of tuberculosis should be considered in every child who has lost weight, particularly in those who have night sweats or cough. Malignancies, such as lymphoma, also may cause loss of weight with few other symptoms initially.

ADOLESCENTS

Planned dieting is widespread among adolescent girls and is the most common cause of weight loss in adolescents. Dieting must be distinguished carefully from an eating disorder, such as anorexia nervosa, which may affect as many as 1% to 2% of adolescent women in the United States, or bulimia nervosa, which may affect 1% to 5% or more.[7] Anorexia nervosa should be suspected when the adolescent is unwill-

Table 181-1 Laboratory Studies Helpful in Weight Loss

Suggested Studies	Suggested Diagnoses
Complete blood count, smear	Anemia Infection Nutritional deficiencies Malabsorptive syndromes Malignancy
Erythrocyte sedimentation rate (ESR)	Collagen-vascular disease Infection Inflammatory bowel disease Malignancy Anorexia nervosa (very low ESR)
Serum electrolytes, kidney function tests	Dehydration Vomiting, self-induced or pernicious Renal dysfunction Adrenal disorders Metabolic disorder (with acidosis) Collagen-vascular disease
Serum protein and albumin levels	Liver dysfunction Malignancy Malnutrition Protein malabsorption Protein-losing enteropathy
Tuberculosis skin test	Tuberculosis
Stool for occult blood	Gastroenteritis Inflammatory bowel disease Enteropathies
Serum carotene; specific tests of malabsorption	Malabsorption syndromes Cystic fibrosis Anorexia nervosa (high carotene)
Urinalysis, including specific gravity; urine culture	Diabetes mellitus Diabetes insipidus Dehydration Urinary tract infection Renal disease Adolescent eating disorder (high pH)

ing or unable to maintain body weight over a minimally normal weight for age and height and when attitudes and behaviors about eating or body image are distorted.[1] The anorectic adolescent may experience amenorrhea associated with emaciation and overactivity and may demonstrate clinical signs of malnutrition (hypothyroidism, bradycardia, hypothermia, growth of lanugolike hair on the body and extremities).[7,9] Nutritional rehabilitation and psychiatric treatment are indicated (see Chapter 102, Anorexia and Bulimia Nervosa).

Bulimia is an eating disorder that to some degree overlaps anorexia nervosa. Adolescents who have bulimia indulge in binge eating, followed by self-induced vomiting, self-starvation, overactivity, or the use of cathartics or diuretics to reduce weight.[1] These behaviors are practiced in secret, and the adolescent often denies them. An elevated serum bicarbonate level, hypokalemia, or high urine pH may provide evidence of chronic vomiting.[3] The patient often is depressed and self-deprecating and may seek medical aid when the eating-vomiting pattern becomes compulsive and out of the patient's control. Psychiatric evaluation and intervention are indicated.[7,9]

Although severe degrees of weight loss during adolescence often can be ascribed to eating disorders, weight loss in adolescence also may result from other psychiatric disturbances, especially affective disorders; CNS tumors, particularly those of the hypothalamus, sella turcica, or other midline areas; or gastrointestinal problems, such as undiagnosed inflammatory bowel disease or other syndromes of malabsorption. Diabetes mellitus may manifest during adolescence with significant weight loss. Tuberculosis always should be considered and ruled out when an adolescent patient reports weight loss. Malignancies, particularly lymphoma, may present as weight loss.

INITIAL EVALUATION OF A COMPLAINT OF WEIGHT LOSS

The following should be included in the initial evaluation (Table 181-1):

1. A careful history and physical examination, with special attention to dietary intake, family functioning, and the patient's emotional well-being. The growth chart should be reviewed and updated..

2. A complete blood cell count (CBC) and erythrocyte sedimentation rate (ESR). The CBC screens for oncological factors and provides an overview of the nutritional state. The ESR may be elevated in collagen-vascular diseases, chronic infections, certain malignancies, and inflammatory bowel disease; it may be abnormally low in anorexia nervosa.[2]
3. Serum electrolyte and kidney function tests to evaluate dehydration, to reveal evidence of pernicious or self-induced vomiting, and to rule out renal or adrenal disease.
4. Serum protein and albumin levels to assess liver function, to determine whether the weight loss represents malnutrition, and to rule out protein malabsorption. Reversal of the albumin/globulin ratio is seen often in collagen-vascular diseases and malignancies.[12]
5. Tuberculosis skin test.
6. Stool for occult blood and tests of malabsorption to diagnose gastroenteritis, inflammatory bowel disease, and the various causes of malabsorption. The serum carotene level may be low in infancy and in malabsorptive conditions but often is elevated in anorexia nervosa.[2]
7. Urinalysis and urine culture to rule out diabetes mellitus, diabetes insipidus, dehydration, urinary tract infection, and renal disease. The urine pH may be high (>8) in adolescents who have eating disorders, particularly when vomiting occurs.[3]

When to Refer

Evidence or suspicion of:
- Malignancy
- Endocrinopathy (thyroid, adrenal, pituitary)
- Gastrointestinal disorder (e.g., gastroesophageal reflux; malabsorption, including cystic fibrosis; inflammatory bowel disease)
- Pancreatitis
- Heart disease
- Renal disease
- Pulmonary disease
- Rheumatological condition
- Central nervous system abnormality
- Metabolic disorder
- Surgical abdominal problem (e.g., pyloric stenosis, Hirschsprung's disease, volvulus)
- Immunodeficiency
- Unusual infection
- Psychiatric diagnosis in child or caretaker
- Anorexia nervosa or bulimia nervosa in child or adolescent

When to Hospitalize

In newborn, when weight loss cannot be managed as outpatient
- Weight loss of more than 12% to 15% of birth weight
- Excessive fluid loss (vomiting, diarrhea, polyuria)
- Evidence of infant hypernatremic dehydration
- Suspicion of infection, metabolic abnormality, congenital heart disease, other conditions requiring evaluation
- Extreme passivity of infant, which may require tube feeding
- Need for intensive maternal education and support

At any age, when:
- Weight loss is excessive (more than 5% to 10% of previous weight)
- Excessive fluid loss from vomiting or diarrhea
- New-onset diabetes mellitus (usually)
- Evidence of severe febrile illness (pneumonia, pyelonephritis, osteomyelitis, meningitis, septic arthritis, others)
- Evidence of dehydration
- Physiological instability
  - Severe bradycardia
  - Hypotension
  - Hypothermia
  - Orthostatic changes
- Electrolyte abnormalities (e.g., hypernatremia, hypokalemia)
- Evidence of significant psychosocial dysfunction

In adolescent, when eating disorder cannot be managed as outpatient
- Severe malnutrition, with weight <75% of ideal body weight
- Evidence of dehydration or electrolyte abnormalities
- Physiological instability
- Acute food refusal
- Uncontrollable binge eating and purging
- Acute medical complication of malnutrition (syncope, seizures, cardiac failure, pancreatitis)
- Suicidal intent or ideation, or psychosis

REFERENCES

1. American Psychiatric Association: *Diagnostic and statistical manual of mental disorders,* ed 4, Washington, DC, 1994, The Association.
2. Anyan WR: Changes in erythrocyte sedimentation rate and fibrinogen during anorexia nervosa, *J Pediatr* 85:525, 1974.
3. Arden MR, et al: Alkaline urine is associated with eating disorders, *Am J Dis Child* 145:28, 1991.
4. Atkins DM, Silber TJ: Clinical spectrum of anorexia nervosa in children, *J Dev Behav Pediatr* 14:211, 1993.
5. Bithoney WG, et al: Failure to thrive/growth deficiency, *Pediatr Rev* 13:453, 1992.
6. Cooper WO, et al: Increased incidence of severe breastfeeding malnutrition and hypernatremia in a metropolitan area, *Pediatrics* 96: 957, 1995.
7. Fisher M, et al: Eating disorders in adolescents: a background paper, *J Adolesc Health* 16:420, 1995.
8. Illingworth RS: *Common symptoms of disease in children,* ed 9, Oxford, 1988, Blackwell Scientific.

9. Kreipe RE: Eating disorders among children and adolescents, *Pediatr Rev* 16:370, 1995.
10. Lawrence RA, Lawrence RM: *Breastfeeding: a guide for the medical profession,* ed 5, St Louis, 1999, Mosby.
11. Maisels MJ, Gifford K: Breast-feeding, weight loss and jaundice, *J Pediatr* 102:117, 1983.
12. Pizzo PA, Lovejoy FH, Smith DH: Prolonged fever in children: review of 100 cases, *Pediatrics* 55:468, 1975.
13. Rand TH, Meyers A: Role of the general pediatrician in the management of human immunodeficiency virus infection in children, *Pediatr Rev* 14:371, 1994.
14. Stashwick CA: When a breastfed infant isn't gaining weight, *Contemp Pediatr* 10:116, 1993.

182 Wheezing

Thomas A. Hazinski

The term *wheezing* often is used by parents and children to refer to any noise made during breathing; to avoid ambiguity, however, the term should be used more precisely to describe a high-pitched sound heard with a stethoscope during the terminal phases of exhalation. Wheezes also may be heard without the use of a stethoscope, usually in patients who have chronic asthma, acute foreign-body inhalation, or psychogenic asthma.

Wheezing usually implies obstruction of the distal airway, but a wheezelike sound also can be produced by patients who have peribronchial edema (e.g., congestive heart failure) and disorders of the proximal or middle airway. The presence or absence of wheezing correlates poorly with the degree of impairment in pulmonary function. As shown in Tables 182-1 and 182-2, the differential diagnosis of wheezing is extensive, so if one approaches the wheezing patient with only asthma in mind, life-threatening but correctable disorders may be missed. Finally, it is important to remember that patients who have normal lungs can generate a wheeze sound during a rapid, forced exhalation maneuver; such a sound probably is produced in the larynx and disappears during a slow exhalation.

Lower airway obstruction usually causes wheezing only during exhalation, because of dynamic changes in airway caliber during spontaneous breathing. During inhalation, normal airways (or even narrowed or unstable airways) inside the thorax are expanded by the inspiratory decrease in pleural pressure (as the pressure in the airway becomes positive with respect to pleural pressure). During exhalation, narrowed or poorly supported intrathoracic airways will narrow further when intrathoracic pressure begins to exceed the pressure inside the airway lumen. Although small-airway closure thus can occur at the end of exhalation, in the normal lung this is counterbalanced by elastic elements in the alveolar walls, which act as springs to hold the small airways open at low lung volumes. In addition, at low flow rates (e.g., as respiratory muscle fatigue in the wheezing child develops), a wheeze may not be generated, despite the presence of severe obstruction. In these patients the appearance of wheezes actually may indicate a beneficial response to therapy as flow rates improve and airways open.

In addition to wheezing, another useful sign of airway obstruction is a prolongation of the expiratory time. During a normal breath the ratio of inspiratory time to expiratory time is approximately 1:1. During airway obstruction, however, expiratory airflow resistance increases, and this ratio approaches 1:2. Indeed, in some wheezing patients who have acute tachypnea, the next inhalation actually may occur before complete exhalation has occurred, thus eliminating the pause between breaths and producing a progressive increase in end-expiratory lung volume, termed *dynamic hyperinflation.* As airway obstruction worsens, accessory respiratory muscles are recruited. This is manifested as nasal flaring and intercostal retractions.

DIFFERENTIAL DIAGNOSIS

Among the anatomical causes of wheezing, large-airway instability is common in infancy and is termed *tracheomalacia.* Most of these infants have had intermittent inspiratory stridor as a major sign since birth, but wheezing only may occur if the lack of airway rigidity is limited to the bronchi. Wheezing develops as the abnormal airway is opened on inspiration but dynamically narrows on expiration, with airflow occurring through the unstable airways. A coarse, low-pitched expiratory sound is generated.

Fixed lesions of the trachea or bronchi may not cause wheezing, inasmuch as the degree of obstruction is not influenced by the respiratory cycle. These lesions, however, may cause or be associated with softening of the adjacent airway wall sufficient to cause wheezing occasionally. Two examples are a completely circular tracheal stenosis or a constricting vascular ring; these lesions encircle the airway and essentially are unyielding. Many of these patients have residual tracheomalacia after surgical correction.

In patients who have acute infections and asthma, wheezing is bilateral and diffuse on auscultation, whereas focal wheezing may indicate the presence of a discrete obstruction (mucus, foreign body, or tumor). Tumors or granulomas may be found in the lumen of the airway, but most lung tumors in children occur outside the lumen and compress the airway to produce obstruction with focal hyperinflation or atelectasis.

Patients who have emphysema or interstitial inflammation may wheeze because damaged alveolar walls cannot act as springs to hold the small airways open. The wheezing of patients who have bronchopulmonary dysplasia, bronchiectasis, or cystic fibrosis may be intermittent and asymmetrical because the wheezing is caused by a combination of mucous obstruction, inflammation, loss of airway tone, and bronchial hyperreactivity.

Most of the causes of wheezing in the lower airway are acquired. Viral infections are the most common cause of acute wheezing. The smaller airways are affected most often by respiratory syncytial virus (RSV) or parainfluenza virus,

Table 182-1 Causes of Diffuse Wheezing

Location	Pathological or Anatomical Cause	Clinical Diagnosis	Type of Wheeze Generated
Trachea	Loss of airway wall rigidity	Laryngotracheomalacia	Generalized, coarse
	Airway inflammation	Tracheobronchitis, bacterial tracheitis	Generalized, coarse to fine
Bronchi	Less airway wall rigidity	Bronchomalacia	Localized, fine
	Foreign body	Aspirated foreign body	Localized, fine
	Inflammation and mucous obstruction	Bronchiectasis	Localized, fine, bubbly
	Extrinsic compression	Mediastinal tumor or nodes	Localized, coarse
	Airway and elastic tissue destruction	Emphysema	Generalized, fine
	Inflammation	Bronchitis	Generalized, fine
Bronchioles	Inflammation and mucous obstruction	Bronchiolitis	Unusual—generalized, fine, but occasionally localized with mucous obstruction
	Airway wall edema, smooth-muscle hypertrophy	Asthma	Same as for bronchiolitis
	Peribronchial edema	Congestive heart failure	Diffuse, fine
	Peribronchial hemorrhage	Hemosiderosis	Focal or diffuse, fine

Table 182-2 Differential Diagnosis of Diffuse Wheezing as a Function of Age

Age Group	Acute	Chronic or Recurrent
Infants	Infection (bronchiolitis), including tuberculosis and opportunistic infection in immunosuppressed patients Congestive heart failure Asthma	Tracheomalacia Cystic fibrosis Tracheoesophageal malformations Vascular ring Tracheal stenosis Congenital lobar emphysema Diaphragmatic hernia Bronchopulmonary dysplasia Gastroesophageal reflux Aspiration pneumonitis Extrinsic compression of airway by tumors (e.g., neuroblastoma) Visceral larva migrans Histiocytosis Hemosiderosis Asthma
Children and adolescents	Infection Foreign body Asthma	Foreign body Asthma Allergic bronchopulmonary aspergillosis Cystic fibrosis Ciliary dysmotility syndromes Tumors, lymph nodes Alpha$_1$-antitrypsin deficiency Sarcoidosis Vocal cord dysfunction Psychogenic causes

but tracheal involvement, as in viral tracheobronchitis (croup) and bacterial tracheitis, may occur. Bacterial infections of the lower airway rarely are associated with wheezing. However, bacterial tracheitis can involve the large airway, creating such limited airflow that fine wheezing develops, which leads to its confusion with severe asthma.

Tables 182-1 and 182-2 summarize the causes of wheezing.

EVALUATION OF THE WHEEZING CHILD

Physical signs to be recorded are the expiratory time, respiration rate, and the degree to which accessory respiratory muscles are used. Anteroposterior and lateral chest radiographs provide the key laboratory procedure for diagnosis of the wheezing patient, because they allow identification of focal lesions. The clinician should remember that 50% of patients ultimately found to have a foreign body have no history of choking or cough and that a foreign body should be considered when the onset of wheezing is abrupt and unassociated with other respiratory symptoms. When a foreign body is suspected, additional radiographs (either decubiti or inspiratory/expiratory) should be obtained to demonstrate asymmetrical and sustained hyperinflation.

Asthma should not be diagnosed in an infant or child during the first episode of wheezing until a pattern of recurrent wheezing responsive to bronchodilator therapy is documented. In infants, the differential diagnosis of acute wheezing should include usual or unusual infections, a foreign body, and congenital malformations. Viral and bacterial infections may cause transient bronchial hyperreactivity, and wheezing with respiratory infections can develop in patients who have bronchial hyperreactivity. For this reason, patients who have respiratory infections often may respond to bronchodilator therapy. The differential diagnosis of recurrent or sustained wheezing includes asthma, reflux, aspiration, foreign body, cystic fibrosis, or congenital malformations.

SUGGESTED READINGS

Benjamin B: Tracheomalacia in infants and children, *Ann Otol Rhinol Laryngol* 93:438, 1984.

Gilbert EF, Opitz JM: Malformations and genetic disorders of the respiratory tract. In Stocker JT, editor: *Pediatric pulmonary disease,* New York, 1989, Hemisphere.

Michelson PH, McColley SA: Wheezing or stridor: intrinsic and extrinsic lesions causing noisy breathing, *Allergy Asthma Proc* 19:81, 1998.

Pasterkamp H, Kraman SS, Wodicka GR: Respiratory sounds: advances beyond the stethoscope, *Am J Respir Crit Care Med* 156(3 Pt 1):974, 1997.

Poirier MP, Pancioli AM, DiGiulio GA: Vocal cord dysfunction presenting as acute asthma in a pediatric patient, *Pediatr Emerg Care* 12:213, 1996.

Sporik R: Early childhood wheezing, *Curr Opin Pediatr* 6:650, 1994.

Valletta EA, et al: Tracheoesophageal compression due to congenital vascular anomalies (vascular rings), *Pediatr Pulmonol* 24:93, 1997.

part eight

Specific Clinical Problems

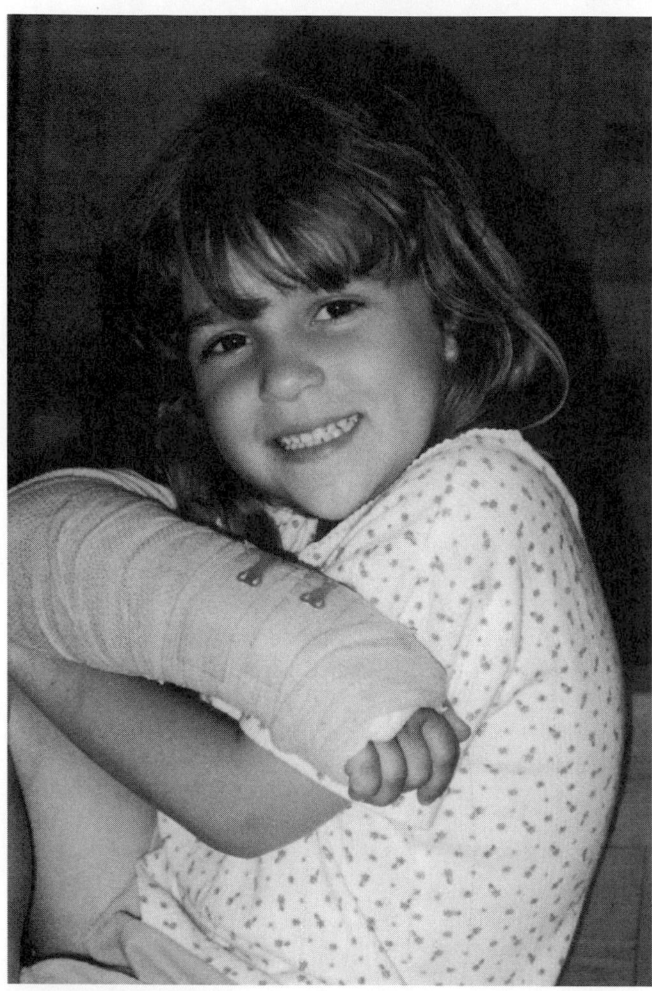

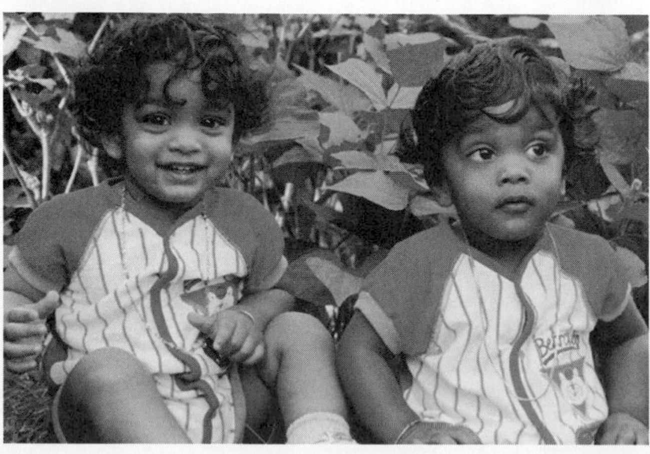

183 Acne

Judith V. Williams • Donald P. Lookingbill

Acne is so prevalent in adolescents and young adults that some consider it a physiological event. However, this perspective does not take into account the impact of acne on the patient, and it may preclude therapeutic intervention. This chapter addresses acne as a treatable disease that deserves medical attention.

ETIOLOGY

Hormones

Acne is a disease of the pilosebaceous unit.[1,14,18] Androgens stimulate the sebaceous glands, which enlarge and increase their production of sebum. Before puberty, the responsible androgens are of adrenal origin.[11] With puberty, gonadal androgens further stimulate the sebaceous glands. In most studies to date, patients who have acne have not had abnormal levels of circulating testosterone; therefore, tissue androgen metabolism may be the more important factor in the pathogenesis of acne.[9] One of the major organs for androgen metabolism is the skin, where the enzyme 5-alpha-reductase metabolizes testosterone to dihydrotestosterone, which has much more potent activity at the tissue level. Some evidence suggests that 5-alpha-reductase is more active in the skin of acne patients. This would be expected to increase androgenic stimulation of the sebaceous glands, ultimately causing acne. Increased sebaceous gland activity is necessary for acne to develop, yet alone it is insufficient to cause disease. Additional factors are needed.

Follicular Obstruction

If sebum is allowed to drain freely to the surface, the surface skin becomes oily, but acne does not develop. Acne can develop only if the outlet of the follicular canal is obstructed, which occurs when adherent, keratinized cells within the canal accumulate and form an impaction that blocks the flow of sebum (Fig. 183-1). Production of keratinized cells within the lining of the follicular canal is normal, but accumulation and subsequent impaction are not. This follicular obstruction, which also may be influenced by androgens, is a prerequisite for the development of acne.

Bacteria

Sebum and keratinous debris accumulate proximal to the follicular outlet obstruction. This provides an attractive environment for the growth of anaerobic bacteria, particularly *Propionibacterium acnes,* which plays a role in the pathogenesis of inflammatory acne.[17] Several factors may be involved in causing the inflammation. One theory suggests that the lipase enzymes elaborated by *P. acnes* hydrolyze sebaceous lipids, releasing free fatty acids, which then cause irritation when the follicle ruptures. *P. acnes* also produces chemotactic factors that may attract inflammatory cells directly to a sebaceous follicle. Some evidence indicates that complement-mediated inflammation is directed against *P. acnes* itself. Whatever the mechanism of inflammation, there is little question of the therapeutic benefit of antibiotics.

The pathogenic events involved in the development of acne, then, include (1) androgenic stimulation of sebaceous glands, which increases sebum production; (2) keratinous impaction in the pilosebaceous canal, causing outlet obstruction; (3) accumulation of sebaceous and keratinous debris behind the obstruction' and (4) proliferation of *P. acnes*, which alters this milieu in such a way as to contribute to the rupture of the dilated pilosebaceous unit, resulting in extravasation of its contents into the surrounding dermis and inflammatory acne lesions.

CLINICAL FINDINGS

The disease process may begin at a surprisingly young age. In a recent study of premenarchal girls, 78% were found to have some acne.[10] The same investigators found acne to be present in 100% of adolescent boys.[11] Although the severity of the disease increases during adolescence, acne by no means is confined to these years. It is not uncommon for acne activity to continue into the third and fourth decades of life, much to the consternation of the afflicted patient.

The pathogenic mechanisms described previously result in the following types of clinical lesions: noninflamed open and closed comedones and inflammatory papules, pustules, nodules, and cysts.

The acne found in prepubertal children is predominantly noninflammatory and so may easily be overlooked. The open comedo (blackhead) and closed comedo (whitehead) are lesions caused purely by obstruction of the pilosebaceous canal; there is no accompanying inflammation.

Inflammatory acne is rare in young children and should raise the suspicion of a possible hyperandrogenic condition, such as that associated with congenital adrenal hyperplasia or even a rare androgen-secreting tumor. Girls should be examined for virilization, and boys and girls should be checked for precocious puberty. Screening blood studies should include serum levels of testosterone, dehydroepiandrosterone sulfate (DHEA-S), and 17-hydroxyprogesterone.

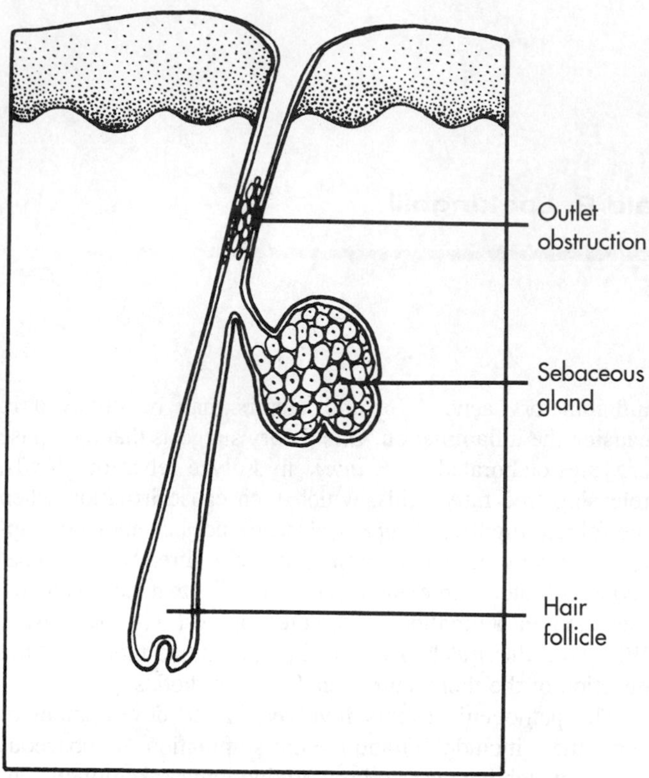

Fig. 183-1 Obstruction of the pilosebaceous unit in acne.

Not surprisingly, acne lesions have a predilection for skin rich in sebaceous glands. Accordingly, the face is the prevailing site, although acne also is found often on the chest and back. The lower portions of the trunk, buttocks, and thighs are involved much less commonly, and the distal extremities are always spared.

DIFFERENTIAL DIAGNOSIS

It rarely is difficult to diagnose acne; usually the condition can be diagnosed from "across the room," although, as mentioned, the comedonal lesions may require closer inspection (Fig. 183-2). Occasionally, acne may be confused with flat warts, milia, or adenoma sebaceum, and acne variants may occur.

Flat Warts

Small, flesh-colored warts may be confused clinically with closed comedones. The question usually can be resolved with very close inspection—a flat wart has a sharp, right-angled edge and a finely roughened surface; a closed comedo has a dome shape and a smooth surface. Flat warts also vary in size; closed comedones are uniformly small.

Milia

Milia are small epidermal inclusion cysts that sometimes are confused with comedones and occasionally with inflammatory pustules, especially in infants who have neonatal acne.

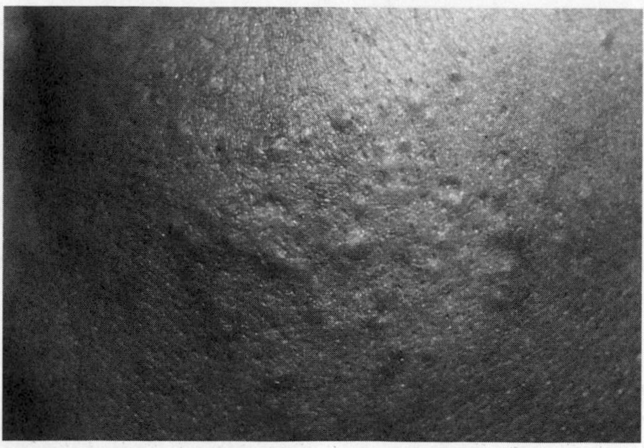

Fig. 183-2 Closed comedones (whiteheads) appear as dome-shaped, flesh-colored papules that often are overlooked.

Adenoma Sebaceum

A misnamed disorder (the lesions actually are angiofibromas), adenoma sebaceum is one of the skin manifestations in tuberous sclerosis. Clinically the lesions appear as pink papules, which occasionally are confused with the lesions of acne. Adenoma sebaceum should be suspected if the papules are (1) clustered primarily in the center of the face, (2) persistent, and (3) resistant to acne therapy.

Acne Rosacea[14]

Acne rosacea is an acneiform eruption that can be distinguished from acne by a background blush of erythema and telangiectasia and by the absence of comedones. Also, rosacea occurs most often in middle-age adults.

Steroid Acne[4]

Both systemic and topical steroids can induce acne. Acne from systemic steroids usually appears as numerous small, uniform-size papules and pustules that have a predilection for the upper trunk. The condition involutes slowly and spontaneously after the steroids are discontinued.

Gram-Negative Folliculitis

Gram-negative organisms occasionally can produce a pustular folliculitis in patients being treated for acne with systemic antibiotics. This condition should be suspected in any patient whose disease flares up during therapy, especially if the flare is manifested by numerous pustules. A bacterial culture with antibiotic sensitivity studies should be done so that the diagnosis can be confirmed and the antibiotic therapy changed.

PSYCHOSOCIAL CONSIDERATIONS

Acne can be a devastating disease. In an ironic quirk, it occurs at a time of life when personal appearance is of prime concern and self-consciousness is at its peak. Some young

Table 183-1 Retin-A Preparations

	Mildest	Mild	Moderate	Strongest
Cream	0.025%	0.05%	0.1%	
Gel		0.01%	0.025%	
Solution				0.05%

people appear to be more affected psychologically by acne than others, but no one is comfortable with it.[5,6] Patients who have severe cystic acne may even be socially ostracized. Regardless of the acne's severity, the condition is important to the patient seeking help and deserves serious attention. Patients are not impressed with soothing advice that trivializes their disease and reassures them that they eventually will "outgrow it." Fortunately, an alternative to this advice is possible—medical therapy is available that can produce effective, gratifying results.

MANAGEMENT

Three methods of treatment have proved effective for acne: topical comedolytic agents,[12] topical and systemic antibiotics,[3] and systemic retinoids.[8,13] The most traditional, yet still effective, treatment regimen comprises comedolytics and antibiotics.

Comedolytics

Topical retinoids (Retin-A, Differin, Avita, Tazarac) and benzoyl peroxide both help disimpact the keratinous plug in the follicular canal. They are most helpful in treating superficial acne lesions—that is, comedones and superficial papules and pustules.[14] Of the two agents, retinoic acid has a somewhat more active effect on comedones,[16] but benzoyl peroxide preparations also exert an antibacterial effect. When both agents are used, the patient should be instructed to apply the retinoic acid at bedtime and the benzoyl peroxide each morning. Both Retin-A and benzoyl peroxide are available in a variety of preparations. The "strength" of a given preparation reflects its irritancy and probably also its efficacy. Benzoyl peroxide gels are marketed in concentrations of 2.5%, 5%, and 10%. For Retin-A, the strength of the preparation depends both on the concentration of the drug and the nature of the vehicle in which it is contained (Table 183-1). Patients initially are prescribed the mildest preparations, and the potency is increased at subsequent visits if necessary.

Skin irritation, which usually becomes less of a problem with continued use, is the major side effect of the comedolytics. Also, about 1% of patients develop a true allergic contact dermatitis to benzoyl peroxide, in which case permanent discontinuation of this agent is required. Because topical retinoic acid may make the skin more susceptible to the effects of sunlight, patients should be instructed to avoid excessive exposure to the sun and to use sunscreens if they need to be exposed to the sun for prolonged periods. Patients should also be told that benzoyl peroxide can bleach clothing and bedlinens.

Antibiotics

Antibiotics are indicated for patients who have inflammatory acne lesions. Topical agents such as tetracycline, erythromycin, and clindamycin have been formulated for commercial use. However, if a patient already is using the two topical comedolytics mentioned earlier, the addition of a third topical agent becomes confusing. Therefore systemic antibiotics are preferred for most patients. Tetracycline is the drug of choice because of its proved efficacy, its relatively low cost, and its low incidence of side effects, even when given over a long period. However, because of dental staining, tetracycline should not be used in patients younger than age 9 years. Food, particularly dairy products, interferes with the absorption of tetracycline, and so it needs to be taken on an empty stomach. The most convenient times are on awakening in the morning and on retiring at night. Tetracycline usually is started at a dose of 500 mg orally twice daily. Once a sustained response is achieved, the dose can be decreased to 500 mg orally per day. For the occasional patient who does not respond adequately to tetracycline, erythromycin may be used as an alternative. Doxycycline and minocycline also may be substituted, but doxycycline is more likely to cause photosensitivity, and minocycline is very expensive. Topical combinations of benzoyl peroxide and erythromycin are often tried before an oral antibiotic is started. Benzamycin gel contains 5% benzoyl peroxide and 3% erythromycin base and can be applied twice daily.

Systemic Retinoids

The systemic retinoid 13-cis-retinoic acid (isotretinoin, or Accutane) became commercially available in September 1982 for use in the treatment of severe cystic acne.[8] This drug reduces follicular keratinization, sebum production, and intrafollicular bacterial counts. The result of these (and possibly other) effects is a dramatic improvement in acne. The therapeutic effect usually takes several months to begin and often is sustained long after the recommended 20-week course of therapy is discontinued. Unfortunately, side effects are common. Almost all patients experience mucocutaneous reactions (cheilitis, conjunctivitis, and dry mucous membranes of the mouth and nose), and extracutaneous complications also occur. For example, systemic retinoids can elevate plasma lipid levels, cause asymptomatic vertebral hyperostoses and, rarely, depression and pseudotumor cerebri.[2,8] Most important is the drug's teratogenicity. Exposure to isotretinoin in pregnancy has been associated with a twenty-fivefold increased risk of major fetal malformations.[7] Thus, it is mandatory that female patients exercise strict birth control while taking this drug. Isotretinoin is recommended only for those who have severe cystic and/or scarring acne, and a minority of patients who have severe noncystic acne who have not responded to standard therapy with topical comedolytics and oral antibiotics.

Patient Compliance

Patient compliance is the single most important aspect of successful acne treatment. Without patient compliance, even the most effective medications are doomed to failure.

To maximize compliance, the physician must take time at the initial visit to explain in detail the use of each medication, as well as the effects and side effects to be expected. To reinforce these instructions, it is helpful to give the patient printed instructions, an example of which is shown in Box 183-1. Medications are used only twice daily. If this activity is linked to an established daily routine, such as brushing the teeth, it, too, can become habitual. Given careful, specific instructions, most patients who have acne are exceptionally compliant and, given time, obtain good results for their efforts. In this regard, the "it takes time" concept needs to be emphasized to all patients; otherwise, they may become prematurely, and inappropriately, discouraged. The acne instruction sheet also can be used to answer several other questions, often unasked, that acne patients or their parents frequently have. The most common of these pertain to diet, cleanliness, cosmetics, and picking at the lesions.

Diet. Although some evidence indicates that the usual American diet may have adverse effects on acne,[15] specific foods have not been implicated. For the vast majority of patients, it is useful to remember Dr. A.M. Kligman's admonition,[14] "The disease is enough of a curse without gustatory deprivations." For most, a sensible diet is all that is suggested.

Cleanliness. The question of cleanliness is pondered more by parents than by patients. To help maintain peace at home, it is useful to dispel the notion that acne is a function of poor hygiene. It is not. In general, acne cleaning agents need not be recommended, because most irritate the skin, unnecessarily compounding the irritation caused by the recommended topical comedolytics. The use of mild non-soap cleanser is often suggested.

Cosmetics. Because cosmetics have been implicated as possibly contributing to the acne process, it is preferable not to use them. If cosmetics are used, they should be water based and used sparingly.

Picking. For many patients who have acne, much of the skin damage is self-inflicted. Although the temptation to squeeze a fresh pustule can be overwhelming, the practice must be discouraged. Picking, probing, and squeezing cause more tissue damage and sometimes produce scars. For some acne patients, picking may become so obsessive that excoriations are the only lesions seen.

COMPLICATIONS

The major complications of acne are its psychosocial ramifications.[5,6] In addition to the cosmetic liability of active

BOX 183-1

ACNE INSTRUCTION SHEET

Topical Medications: Benzoyl Peroxide and Retinoic Acid

A. Action
   1. Both help open up clogged pores.
   2. Benzoyl peroxide also helps kill bacteria in the pores.
B. Method of use (apply to *all* affected areas)
   1. Apply retinoic acid at bedtime.
   2. *Do not* use acne scrub cleaners.
   3. Apply benzoyl peroxide in the morning.
C. Possible problems
   1. May make the condition look worse rather than better after several weeks ("bringing acne to surface").
   2. May cause irritation (e.g., redness, dryness, and tenderness). If too much irritation occurs, use every other night until the skin becomes accustomed to it. If irritation is severe, medication should be stopped and a return visit scheduled.

Tetracycline

A. Action—helps kill bacteria; particularly useful for deep and inflamed lesions.
B. Method of use—needs to be taken on an *empty* stomach. Therefore, take it as soon as you get out of bed in the morning (wait ½ hour before eating breakfast) and at bedtime, at least 1 hour after taking any evening snack.
C. Potential side effects
   1. Uncommon; most patients have no trouble.
   2. May upset stomach and cause nausea and/or diarrhea.
   3. Occasionally causes a yeast vaginitis, particularly if you are taking birth control pills.
   4. Should not be taken if you are pregnant or trying to get pregnant.

General

A. Diet—for most patients, foods have no effect on acne. If you notice that a certain food aggravates the condition, simply avoid that food. Otherwise, no restrictions are necessary.
B. Washing—acne cannot be washed off. Wash your face with a mild cleanser two to three times and bathe or shower daily.
C. Results from medicines—*it takes time,* usually several months, to begin to see benefits. At a return visit in 2 months, some improvement should be present, but it is unlikely that the acne will be cleared. The medications and their dosage will be altered at that time, depending on the response.
D. Conscientious and *regular* use of the medications is essential. They will not do any good if not used regularly.
E. Cosmetics—they may aggravate your acne. If you must use them, do so sparingly and use only those that are water based.
F. No picking!

lesions, permanent scars compound and perpetuate the problem in some patients, mainly those who have inflammatory lesions. Established scars are difficult to treat. Many patients have been disappointed with the results of dermabrasion. It is recommended that patients who have been treated with isotretinoin wait a minimum of 1 year before having dermabrasion performed. Bovine collagen injections have been used in some patients, producing short-term improvement, but repeated injections often are necessary, and the long-term results are not yet known. Laser resurfacing by experienced operators has produced some promising results. Acne scars are best treated when inflammatory lesions are quiescent. Because scars are prevented more easily than treated, the emphasis in acne is on early, aggressive medical therapy such as that outlined earlier in this chapter.

PROGNOSIS

With proper treatment, the prognosis for acne is good, if not excellent. Patients should understand that most therapies control rather than cure the disease and that improvement does not occur overnight. However, improvement does occur, usually within 2 months of starting therapy, and it is at this time that the first revisit is best scheduled. At that visit the acne regimen can be adjusted as necessary. For example, the potency of the comedolytics can be increased (or reduced) and the dosage of the antibiotic altered, depending on the initial response. Continued improvement is to be expected with continuation of therapy. For many patients, the dose of systemic antibiotics can be reduced gradually and eliminated after 6 to 12 months, but most patients require prolonged maintenance therapy (often over years) with topical agents and, in some cases, continued antibiotic therapy.[3]

Historically, cystic acne has been the most difficult to treat, but isotretinoin has become a powerful tool for dealing with this disastrous disease. This drug has the potential to effect prolonged remissions, sometimes lasting for years after a single course of therapy. However, as was discussed previously, isotretinoin has serious side effects, and its use usually is reserved for patients who have severe cystic and/or scarring acne that does not respond to standard treatment.

When to Refer

- Patient unresponsive to oral antibiotics, topical retinoid, and benzoyl peroxide
- Cystic or scarring acne
- Young female with acne or female with acne and irregular menses
- Acne fulminans (abrupt onset of cystic acne, fever, arthralgias)

REFERENCES

1. Cunliffe WF: *Acne,* Chicago, 1989, Mosby.
2. Ellis CN, et al: Long-term radiographic follow-up after isotretinoin therapy, *J Am Acad Dermatol* 18:1252, 1988.
3. Hughes BR, et al: Strategy of acne therapy with long-term antibiotics, *Br J Dermatol* 121:623, 1989.
4. Hurwitz RM: Steroid acne, *J Am Acad Dermatol* 21:1179, 1989.
5. Koo JYM, Smith LL: Psychologic aspects of acne, *Pediatr Dermatol* 8:185, 1991.
6. Krowchuk DP, et al: The psychosocial effects of acne on adolescents, *Pediatr Dermatol* 8:332, 1991.
7. Lammer EJ, et al: Retinoic acid embryopathy, *N Engl J Med* 313:837, 1985.
8. Layton AM, Cunliffe WJ: Guidelines for optimal use of isotretinoin in acne, *J Am Acad Dermatol* 27:S2, 1992.
9. Lookingbill DP, et al: Tissue production of androgens in women with acne, *J Am Acad Dermatol* 12:481, 1985.
10. Lucky AW, et al: Acne vulgaris in early adolescent boys, *Arch Dermatol* 127:210, 1991.
11. Lucky AW, et al: Acne vulgaris in premenarchal girls: an early sign of puberty associated with rising levels of dehydroepiandrosterone, *Arch Dermatol* 130:308, 1994.
12. Melski JW, Arndt KA: Topical therapy for acne, *N Engl J Med* 302:503, 1980.
13. Peck GL, et al: Prolonged remissions of cystic and conglobate acne with 13-cis-retinoic acid, *N Engl J Med* 300:329, 1979.
14. Plewig G, Kligman AM: *Acne and rosacea,* ed 2, New York, 1993, Springer-Verlag.
15. Rosenberg EW: Acne diet reconsidered, *Arch Dermatol* 117:193, 1981.
16. Thomas JR, Doyle AR: The therapeutic uses of topical vitamin A acid, *J Am Acad Dermatol* 4:505, 1981.
17. Webster GF: Inflammatory acne, *Int J Dermatol* 29:313, 1990.
18. Winston MH, Shalita AR: Acne vulgaris: pathogenesis and treatment, *Pediatr Clin North Am* 38:889, 1991.

184 Allergic Rhinitis

Robert A. Wood

Allergic rhinitis is the most common of the atopic diseases. It occurs in as much as 15% of the general population and may exist alone or in combination with asthma or atopic dermatitis.[11] In children, its occurrence is unusual before the age of three years but increases in frequency thereafter, reaching a peak prevalence in adolescence. The most easily recognized form of allergic rhinitis occurs in a typical seasonal pattern, referred to as seasonal allergic rhinitis or hay fever. Year-round, or perennial, allergic rhinitis, which is triggered by indoor allergens such as dust mites or animal danders, is more common but often less dramatic and, therefore, more difficult to diagnose.

ETIOLOGY

As with all atopic disease, the tendency to develop allergic rhinitis is inherited. When a child who has a genetic predisposition to atopy is exposed to an allergen, antigen-specific IgE molecules are produced, which bind to mast cells in the respiratory tract. Once the child has been sensitized in this way, re-exposure to the same allergen causes an immediate, type I hypersensitivity reaction, in which cross-linking of cell surface IgE molecules triggers the rapid release of mast cell mediators (e.g., histamine, prostaglandins, and leukotrienes), as well as the synthesis of cell interactive compounds called cytokines.[7,9] Histamine causes immediate local vasodilation, mucosal edema, and increased mucus production. Cytokines summon inflammatory cells, especially eosinophils, to the site of the allergic reaction, which leads to the slower "late-phase reaction," characterized by inflammation and damage to the mucosal surface that progresses to chronic nasal obstruction. The severity of the symptoms varies tremendously and depends both on the individual's level of sensitivity and the intensity of the antigen exposure.

The allergens involved most commonly in allergic rhinitis include the following[10]:

1. *Pollens.* Wind-borne pollens from trees and grasses in the spring and from weeds (especially ragweed) in the fall cause well-defined seasonal symptoms, but variation is tremendous according to location. Most flower pollens are insect borne and, therefore, rarely cause allergic problems.
2. *Molds.* In colder climates, outdoor molds produce spores beginning in the early spring and peaking in the late fall. In warmer climates, outdoor molds can grow year-round. Molds may grow indoors year-round in most climates, with the highest levels occurring in warmer, more humid months.
3. *Animal danders.* Allergens from the skin and saliva of household pets such as dogs and cats can produce severe intermittent as well as perennial symptoms.
4. *Dust mites.* These ubiquitous, microscopic arthropods are the major allergen in house dust. Mites prosper in warm, moist, indoor environments and colonize pillows, mattresses, and carpets. They are the major cause of perennial allergic rhinitis.
5. *Cockroaches.* Cockroach allergens now are recognized as another common cause of perennial allergic rhinitis, especially in urban areas.

CLINICAL FEATURES

Allergic rhinitis is characterized clinically by a combination of nasal congestion, sneezing, rhinorrhea, and pruritus. Younger children usually have perennial symptoms, whereas pollen sensitivity becomes more common after the age of three or four years. In the acute, seasonal variety, the symptoms may be quite intense and often include severe congestion and rhinorrhea, as well as associated allergic conjunctivitis. The diagnosis usually is very clear based on the patient's history, and the specific allergens responsible for these seasonal exacerbations usually can be identified based on knowledge of the local pollen seasons. Perennial sufferers typically have less dramatic or fewer specific symptoms. Although nasal congestion is still the most prominent symptom, patients often display symptoms such as frequent colds, recurrent otitis media, nasal speech, mouth breathing, snoring, and fatigue; epistaxis also is common. The nasal discharge usually is clear unless the child has a superimposed infection. Many children perform the allergic salute, a maneuver in which they sniff and sweep the palm of their hand upward across the tip of the nose in an attempt to open their nasal passages, remove secretions, or relieve nasal itching. Facial grimacing also is used to relieve nasal itching.

Although the physical examination can be very striking, especially during periods of seasonal rhinitis, it also can be quite unremarkable when symptoms are quiescent. The nasal mucosa is pale, bluish, and boggy, with a clear serous discharge. The nasal turbinates are enlarged, sometimes enough to obstruct the airway almost completely. Children who have perennial problems often have the typical allergic facies, consisting of allergic shiners (a dark discoloration beneath both eyes), Dennie lines (extra folds below the lower eyelids), and an elongated facies due to chronic mouth breathing. The tonsils and adenoids often are enlarged, and there may be evidence of middle ear effusion.

Nasal polyps occur but are uncommon in childhood allergic rhinitis.

COMPLICATIONS

Early in life, children who have allergic rhinitis may suffer from an increased incidence of respiratory infections, acute otitis media, and eustachian tube dysfunction, leading to serous otitis media. Several studies have suggested an association between allergy and chronic serous otitis media, although this is only one of many risk factors. Abnormal facial development, a high arched palate, and orthodontic problems from chronic mouth breathing occasionally develop, especially if there is associated adenoid hypertrophy. Acute and chronic sinusitis are common, probably the result of reduced ciliary clearance and obstruction of sinus ostia. Asthma often is seen in combination with allergic rhinitis but is not viewed typically as a complication of untreated allergic rhinitis.

LABORATORY FINDINGS

The nasal smear for eosinophils is a simple office procedure that can help confirm the clinical diagnosis of allergic rhinitis. The patient blows his or her nose into plastic wrap or wax paper (a cotton swab may be used to obtain secretions if the patient cannot blow), and the secretions are spread onto a glass slide and left to dry. The slide then is prepared with Hansel or Wright stain. If more than 10% of the cells seen on the smear are eosinophils, an ongoing allergic process is probable. Strongly positive results are most likely during heavy exposure to the allergen. Concurrent nasal infection may obscure the results, and eosinophils may be absent during the off season.

Blood eosinophilia occasionally is found (more than 5% eosinophils on the differential white blood cell count or more than 250/mm^3 eosinophils in total). An elevated total serum IgE suggests atopy, but many patients who have allergic rhinitis have a normal serum IgE. Eosinophil counts and total serum IgE levels, therefore, are not recommended as screening tests for allergic rhinitis.

Skin tests and radioallergosorbent tests (RASTs) can detect antigen-specific IgE and identify specific allergic sensitivities in patients in whom the diagnosis is in question or who are in need of more aggressive management.[5] Skin tests should be performed by a physician trained in their use, and they should be interpreted in the context of the clinical history. Compared with skin testing, RASTs have the disadvantages of higher cost and slightly lower sensitivity. However, they are accurate overall and can be used very efficiently in the primary care physician's office as a limited screening test for allergy that also will identify specific allergens to be targeted for environmental control. When more extensive testing is needed, it usually will be more cost-effective to refer the patient to an allergist.

DIFFERENTIAL DIAGNOSIS

Usually there is very little difficulty diagnosing seasonal allergic rhinitis on the basis of the clinical presentation, physical examination, and a knowledge of local pollens. On the other hand, children who have nonspecific perennial symptoms often pose a more difficult diagnostic challenge. Three other conditions that often are confused with allergic rhinitis are recurrent upper respiratory tract infections, vasomotor rhinitis, and adenoid hypertrophy.

Recurrent viral and bacterial upper respiratory tract infections can be differentiated from allergies by their intermittent course; a history of contagion; and by the presence of fever, purulent nasal discharge, and/or erythematous, inflamed nasal mucosa. In addition, eosinophils will not be prominent on a nasal smear, and the family history for allergy is more likely to be negative.

Vasomotor rhinitis is an ill-defined condition that may begin at any age.[1] It is characterized by hyperreactivity of the nasal mucous membranes to a wide variety of irritant stimuli. The most prominent symptom usually is perennial nasal obstruction that responds poorly to environmental controls and/or medications. There is usually no family history of allergy, although other family members may report chronic nasal congestion as well. The nasal smear and skin test results are negative, the serum IgE is normal, and no eye signs or other atopic manifestations are present.

Another variant of perennial rhinitis, called nonallergic rhinitis with eosinophilia, also has been described. In this disorder, which affects adolescents and adults, the nasal smear results are positive for eosinophils, but the serum IgE is normal and skin test results are negative.

Anatomical abnormalities represent the last major cause of chronic nasal symptoms in children. By far the most common of these is adenoid hypertrophy, which typically will manifest as nasal obstruction with little or no rhinorrhea. Many of these children also will experience recurrent middle ear or nasal/sinus infections. In more severe cases the obstruction will lead to obvious changes in the structure of the face and palate due to chronic mouth breathing. Snoring is common, and often there is a typical nasal quality to the voice.

Other less common conditions that may mimic allergic rhinitis are the presence of a nasal foreign body, choanal atresia, congenital syphilis, rhinitis medicamentosa, cystic fibrosis, and nasopharyngeal tumors.

TREATMENT

Management of allergic rhinitis incorporates the information from a careful history and physical examination into a stepwise program that typically consists of allergen avoidance measures and pharmacotherapy.[5] It is critical that time be taken to individualize each child's treatment, taking into account the patient's age, the severity of the symptoms, specific environmental issues, the presence or absence of complications, and any other medical conditions that may be present. If the symptoms are perennial, do not respond to appropriate medications, or worsen each year, an allergist should be consulted. The allergist can confirm the diagnosis, identify specific allergens, fine tune environmental controls and pharmacotherapy, and possibly prescribe immunotherapy.

Environmental control for both allergens and nonspecific irritants should be the first line of therapy at all ages.[10] Particular attention should be directed to the child's bedroom and other settings where substantial amounts of time are spent. If an allergy to dust mites is suspected or has been confirmed by testing, the first steps to reduce exposure should include dust mite-proof encasements for mattresses, box springs, and pillows; removal of stuffed animals and similar items; and hot washing of bed linens every one to two weeks. Ideally, pets should be removed if they are the cause of allergic symptoms, although some relief may be obtained by keeping the pet out of the child's bedroom, using mattress and pillow encasements, removing carpets, and using an air cleaner in the bedroom. Children allergic to pollens can be helped dramatically by closing windows and using an air conditioner. Forced air heating and cooling systems can be improved by adding humidifiers and air filters, although it is very important that the relative humidity be kept below 50% so that dust mite and mold growth is not encouraged.

Oral antihistamines, which inhibit histamine-mediated symptoms by blocking histamine H_1-receptors on mast cells, should be the first line pharmacological treatment of childhood allergic rhinitis.[8] They are most effective in controlling rhinorrhea, sneezing, and pruritus, but are less effective in relieving symptoms of nasal congestion. The first-generation antihistamines, including diphenhydramine, chlorpheniramine, and hydroxyzine, are very effective, but their use may be limited in many children by their sedative side effects. They can impair school performance significantly and therefore should be used with caution in that age group.[6] Fortunately, several second-generation antihistamines, including loratadine, cetirizine, and fexofenadine, have now been approved for use in children. Although not necessarily more potent, their lack of sedation is an important advantage. Alternatively, many children can be treated effectively by use of a first-generation antihistamine as a single bedtime dose, especially if their symptoms are worse at night.

Oral decongestants, such as pseudoephedrine and phenylephrine, may have value in treating some children, especially when nasal congestion is a major symptom. They can be used either alone or in combination with an antihistamine. They should be used with some caution, however, because some children experience significant stimulatory effects, which may manifest as hyperactivity, irritability, and/or sleep disturbance. Topical decongestant nasal sprays may provide transient relief that often is followed after several days by rebound congestion. Because prolonged use of nasal sprays often leads to a worsening of symptoms (a condition known as rhinitis medicamentosa), their use should be discouraged.

Antiinflammatory nasal sprays also can be very helpful. Nasal cromolyn sodium (Nasalcrom) is an extremely safe drug, similar in potency to oral antihistamines without the side effects. It must be used preventively before and during seasons or before periodic exposure, and its usefulness is significantly limited by the need to use it four to six times a day.

Topical nasal corticosteroids are the most effective pharmacological agents for allergic rhinitis, and some agents now have been approved for use by patients 3 years of age and older.[3] Available preparations include beclomethasone, budesonide, flunisolide, fluticasone, mometasone, and triamcinolone. Nasal steroids do have the potential for adverse effects on growth in children; therefore, although their risk/benefit ratio generally is excellent, they should always be used at the lowest possible dose. In addition, short courses of oral steroids (e.g., prednisone) may be needed for severe cases that do not respond to other therapies.

Finally, ipratropium nasal spray is approved for children 6 years of age and older and may be very helpful in the control of rhinorrhea. It may have a particular advantage in cases of nonallergic rhinitis in which excessive rhinorrhea is a major complaint.

If the patient's symptoms do not respond to avoidance measures and reasonable doses of medication, he or she should be referred to an allergist for skin testing to identify specific allergens. If the clinical history and skin test results correlate, immunotherapy becomes a logical part of treatment.[2] Usually a 3- to 5-year course of regular injections is necessary. This regimen is most effective in the treatment of seasonal allergic rhinitis, but it also is beneficial for most cases of perennial disease. As treatment progresses, patients can expect a gradual decline in symptoms and reduced reliance on medication. Because of the risk of local and generalized reactions to the material injected and because of the inconvenience and expense associated with regular injections, it is essential that immunotherapy be used selectively.

PROGNOSIS

Allergic rhinitis, like other allergic disorders, is an illness that waxes and wanes over time. Most children tend to improve with time, although very few (probably fewer than 10%) lose their symptoms completely.[4] Remission of symptoms may result from changes in environment, avoidance programs, and immunotherapy. It is important to counsel patients that allergic symptoms can be controlled but not eliminated entirely and that the success of any treatment depends on the patient's understanding of the causes of symptoms and compliance with the prescribed regimen.

REFERENCES

1. Druce HM: Allergic and nonallergic rhinitis. In Middleton EJ, et al, editors. *Allergy principles and practice*, ed 5, St Louis, 1998, Mosby-Year Book.
2. Greenberger PA, editor: Immunotherapy of IgE-mediated disorders, *Immunol Allergy Clin North Am* 12:1, 1992.
3. Laforce C: Use of nasal steroids in managing allergic rhinitis, *J Allergy Clin Immunol* 103:S388, 1999.
4. Linna O, Kokkonen J, Lukin M: A 10-year prognosis for childhood allergic rhinitis, *Acta Pediatr* 81:100, 1992.
5. Lund VJ, et al: International consensus report on the diagnosis and management of rhinitis, *Allergy* 49(suppl 19):1, 1994.
6. Meltzer EO: Comparative safety of H_1 antihistamines, *Ann Allergy* 67: 625, 1991.
7. Naclerio RM: Allergic rhinitis, *N Engl J Med* 325:860, 1991.
8. Simons FER: H_1-receptor antagonists: clinical pharmacology and therapeutics, *J Allergy Clin Immunol* 84:845, 1989.
9. White MV, Kaliner MA: Mediators of allergic rhinitis, *J Allergy Clin Immunol* 90:699, 1992.
10. Wood RA: Allergens. In Mygind N, Naclerio RM, editors: *Allergic and non-allergic rhinitis: clinical aspects*, Copenhagen, 1993, Munksgaard.
11. Wright AL, et al: Epidemiology of physician-diagnosed allergic rhinitis in childhood, *Pediatrics* 94:895, 1994.

185 Animal Bites

Neil E. Herendeen • Peter G. Szilagyi

It is estimated that more than 2 million people across the United States are bitten by animals annually.[9,12] Dog bites account for more than 90% of these injuries, and cat bites account for most of the remainder. Although wild animal bites are rare, they potentially are more serious, given their risk of rabies and other infections. Half of all animal bites are trivial, requiring no medical treatment; only 10% are severe enough to require suturing, and only 2% result in hospitalization. Bite wounds account for an estimated 1% of pediatric visits to an emergency department. Children sustain the greatest number of animal bites (the peak age group is 5 to 14 years), with 50% of all school-age children reporting an animal bite at some point in their life. With dog bites, adults are bitten on an extremity; children, however, are bitten primarily on the head or neck 75% of the time.[4] Boys are twice as likely to be bitten by a dog, whereas girls receive twice as many cat bites.[9] Not surprisingly, the vast majority of the animals live in the victim's neighborhood (75%) or home (15%); in most instances the bites are provoked by humans. With the recent trend among many urban families of buying guard dogs, including pit bulls, the incidence of dog bites is likely to rise, and pediatricians should be familiar with preventive strategies and management of these injuries.[9]

The major morbidity from animal bites results from direct trauma and infection. Although dog bites are more likely to cause lacerations or avulsions, these open wounds can be debrided and cleaned to prevent infection. Puncture wounds, however, which usually do not require suturing, can result in deep-tissue infections.[2,3,5,6]

MICROBIOLOGY

As shown in Table 185-1, the risk of infection varies according to several factors. Hand wounds are most likely to become infected, partly because of the type of wound (most frequently a puncture wound), the relatively poor vascular supply, and the vulnerability of the closed spaces of the hand. If more than 24 hours has elapsed before medical attention is sought, the risk of infection is increased substantially. Cat and human bites pose a greater risk of infection than dog bites, partly because these bites more often cause puncture wounds, whereas dog bites frequently cause open lacerations.

Most bacteria associated with bite wounds are common organisms that reside in the animal's oral cavity. In addition, bacteria on the victim's skin may contribute to infection. Most infections involve several pathogens,[5] often both aerobes and anaerobes. *Pasteurella multocida,* a gram-negative, facultative anaerobe found in the mouths of most dogs and cats, is highly associated with cat bite infections (up to 80%) and to a lesser extent with dog bite infections (12% to 50%). Although the exact prevalence of other pathogenic bacteria isolated from infected animal bites varies across studies, gram-negative aerobes (e.g., *Pseudomonas, Klebsiella,* and *Enterobacter* spp.) are found more often than gram-positive aerobes (e.g., staphylococci and streptococci) or anaerobes (e.g., *Bacteroides, Fusobacterium,* and *Peptococcus* spp.).[1-7,11]

Another group of gram-negative bacteria, classified by the Centers for Disease Control and Prevention (CDC) as alphanumeric organisms, frequently has been isolated from dog bite wounds. Interestingly, human bites rarely are infected by *P. multocida* but often are associated with gram-positive organisms, gram-negative anaerobes, or *Eikenella corrodens,* a genus almost unique to human bites that in rare cases is found in cat bites. *Human bites have the potential to transmit the human immunodeficiency virus (HIV) and hepatitis B virus and should be evaluated in persons who are bitten by those at high risk for infection.*

CLINICAL DIAGNOSIS

Important historical points include the length of time since injury, the type of animal (including domestic or wild), the animal's present location and health, and the prior wound management. The physical examination entails a careful musculoskeletal and neurological examination to determine if underlying structures were damaged and a thorough inspection of the wound for signs of infection. Special attention must be given to bites on the hand because, particularly in deep puncture wounds, superficial signs of infection (redness, swelling, purulent drainage) may be absent. Finally, the clinician should be aware that deep infections of tendons or bones and systemic infections can occur if animal bites go untreated. The time of the infection's onset may be a clue to *P. multocida* infection. Cellulitis from this organism generally develops rapidly, within hours of the animal bite, whereas systemic signs (fever, lymphangitis) usually are absent.[11] A cellulitis that develops gradually, over days, is due more likely to gram-positive cocci or other pathogenic bacteria.

A Gram stain of a wound specimen is not useful, because findings do not correlate with culture results. Cultures of clinically infected animal bite wounds are reported to have "no growth" in as many as one third of cases; conversely, cultures of clinically noninfected bite wounds grow a wide spectrum of oral flora bacteria in the same proportion of

Table 185-1 Risk Factors for Infection in Animal Bites

Risk Factor	Infection Rates
Location of bite[6]	Hand (18%-36%) >arm or leg (12%-16%) >face (5%-11%)
Type of wound[2,6,10]	Puncture with laceration (17%-26%) >laceration alone (9%-12%)
Interval between bite and medical care	If >24 hr, risk of infection is higher
Type of animal	Cat bites (40%-50%) Dog bites (10%-30%) Human bites (13%-40%)[8]

cases.[7] Moreover, such cultures do not predict the likelihood of subsequent infection, nor do results correlate with culture findings when clinical infection becomes apparent. However, cultures of clinically infected wounds may help to ensure that the causative bacteria are sensitive to the antibiotic used.

The clinician should remember that cat-scratch disease is a relatively common complication of cat bites and, less commonly, of bites by other animals. This disease often begins with the development of a red, painless papule at the site of a recent scratch or bite; within weeks, a tender, enlarged, regional lymph node appears, usually associated with fever, malaise, and other systemic symptoms. This self-limited illness, caused by a gram-negative bacillus, is diagnosed clinically because the cat-scratch skin test reagent used to substantiate the clinical diagnosis is not licensed and therefore not available for use in most clinical settings. The role of antibiotics in the treatment of this disease is not clear; however, because the disease is self-limited, their use seldom is indicated. Large, tender, fluctuant lymph nodes may require aspiration or incision and drainage.

Animal bites from nondomestic animals require careful attention. Although most pediatricians will never treat a child who has rabies, they will evaluate children who may have been exposed to it. With the increasing spread of rabies among nondomestic animals, the number of people exposed to rabies and requiring vaccination is increasing dramatically. A full postexposure vaccination series can cost $2000 or more and requires five visits to the doctor in a single month. Knowing whom and when to treat requires an understanding of rabies transmission and epidemiology. Rabies is an RNA virus present in saliva and transmitted by bites or by licking of mucosa or open wounds. In the United States, in all cases of rabies resulting from a dog or cat bite, the infected animal has been noted to become ill during the standard 10-day confinement and observation period; thus, location, confinement, and observation of the animal are important.

In cases involving wild animal bites, consultation with the local health department is helpful in determining the risk of rabies in a specific animal for a particular geographical region. In general, bats, skunks, foxes, raccoons, and other carnivores are considered rabid until proved otherwise by laboratory tests;[8] in the interim, or if the animal cannot be found, treatment with human rabies immunoglobulin (HRIG) and human diploid cell vaccine (HDCV) is recommended.

A variety of rare diseases have been described after wild animal bites; consultation with the local health department may help in establishing the diagnosis and managing treatment. Rat bite fever, a systemic illness caused by *Streptobacillus moniliformis* or *Spirillum minus,* is one such example. The *Red Book* (published by the American Academy of Pediatrics' Committee on Infectious Diseases) contains comprehensive, up-to-date descriptions of unusual diseases transmitted by various domestic and wild animals.[8]

MANAGEMENT

The initial step in treating animal bites is meticulous wound care. This involves gently cleaning the wound with soap and water and vigorously irrigating with saline solution. Saline irrigation of the wound with a syringe and a 19-gauge needle generates increased pressure on the tissues that facilitates cleansing of the wound and reduces the risk of infection.[2] Devitalized tissue should be debrided. Puncture wounds should be cleaned, but irrigation is ineffective and may result in further damage to underlying structures. Elevation and immobilization are important for significant extremity injuries. The child's immunization status should be assessed and tetanus prophylaxis given if indicated. Primary closure of lacerations caused by animal (or human) bites is controversial.[2,4,13] Clearly, infected wounds should not be closed. The consensus is that most noninfected lacerations can be sutured, after meticulous cleansing and irrigation, for cosmetic purposes or for hemostasis, without increasing the risk of infection. Hand wounds may be an exception[2,6] because of the great likelihood of infection and the risk of serious complications from deep, closed-space infections; in these cases, suturing is recommended only for large wounds.

Radiological studies may be necessary for deep puncture wounds to determine if the periosteum has been penetrated. These include studies of the calvaria of small children who sustain bites to the head. The use of prophylactic antibiotics in noninfected animal bite wounds is controversial.[1-6] It is prudent to treat, prophylactically (for 5 to 7 days), bites that have a high likelihood of infection, including (1) puncture wounds (particularly from cat bites), (2) human bites, and (3) bites of the hands and face. If infected, bite wounds brought to medical attention after 24 hours should be treated with antibiotics. The choice of antibiotics depends on culture results or, if cultures are not available, on the likely pathogens. Although penicillin is active against *P. multocida* and many oral flora, the addition of a penicillinase-resistant antibiotic provides more effective coverage. Amoxicillin/clavulanic acid (Augmentin) is an excellent choice for empirical treatment of bites from all animals. As mentioned, administration of rabies prophylaxis depends on the type of animal and the prevalence of rabies in the community (Table 185-2). Current recommendations call for most, if not all, of the HRIG dose (20 IU/kg of body weight) to be infiltrated in and around the site of the bite. Rabies prophylaxis now also is recommended after exposure to bats in a confined setting, even when no bites are visible.[8,10]

ANTICIPATORY GUIDANCE

Although pets provide hours of delight and companionship for children, education about responsible care of a pet is important. Preschool-age children should not be left alone

Table 185-2 Rabies Vaccination Guidelines

Animal	Management
Wild carnivores	Begin HRIG and HDCV. Submit animal's head for testing.
Healthy domestic dogs and cats	Quarantine animal; treat only if animal develops symptoms.
Stray or sick dogs and cats	Submit animal's head for testing. Delay treatment until test results are known unless clinical likelihood of rabies is high. If animal is unavailable, complete full series of HRIG and HDCV.
Rodents, rabbits	Unlikely to be rabid (except woodchucks). Treat only if animal acted strangely and cannot be tested.

Data from Schmidt MJ, Olson JG, Krebs JW: *Contemp Pediatr* 10:36, 1993.

with a pet, and they should be advised never to tease animals, approach strange animals, or play with pets that are eating.[6,9] Families who have children should be advised not to buy wild animals or dogs bred for aggressiveness. Finally, vaccinations for pets and routine visits to a veterinarian should be encouraged (see Chapter 23 [Two], Injury Control for a more detailed discussion of animal safety rules for children).

REFERENCES

1. Boenning DA, Fleisher GR, Campos JM: Dog bites in children: epidemiology, microbiology, and penicillin prophylactic therapy, *Am J Emerg Med* 1:17, 1983.
2. Callaham M: Prophylactic antibiotics in common dog bite wounds: a controlled study, *Ann Emerg Med* 9:410, 1980.
3. Cummings P: Antibiotics to prevent infection in patients with dog bite wounds: a meta-analysis of randomized trials, *Ann Emerg Med* 23:535, 1994.
4. Kountakis SE, et al: Animal bites to the head and neck, *Ear Nose Throat J* 77:216, 1998.
5. Lindsey D, et al: Natural course of the human bite wound: incidence of infection and complications in 434 bites and 803 lacerations in the same group of patients, *J Trauma* 27:45, 1987.
6. Marcy SM: Management of pediatric infectious diseases in office practice: infections due to dog and cat bites (special series), *Pediatr Infect Dis J* 1:351, 1982.
7. Ordog GJ: The bacteriology of dog bite wounds on initial presentation, *Ann Emerg Med* 15:1324, 1986.
8. Pickering LK, et al: *Report of the Committee on Infectious Diseases (Red Book),* ed 25, Elk Grove, Ill, 2000, American Academy of Pediatrics.
9. Rosekrans JA: Animal bites: a summertime hazard, *Contemp Pediatr* 10:23, 1993.
10. Schmidt MJ, Olson JG, Krebs JW: Rabies goes wild, *Contemp Pediatr* 10:36, 1993.
11. Talan DA, et al: Bacteriologic analysis of infected dog and cat bites, *N Engl J Med* 340:85, 1999.
12. Weiss HB, Friedman DI, Coben JH: Incidence of dog bite injuries treated in emergency departments, *JAMA* 279:51, 1998.
13. Wolff KD: Management of animal bite injuries of the face: experience with 94 patients, *J Oral Maxillofac Surg* 56:838, 1998.

186 Anuria/Oliguria

Melissa J. Gregory

Decreased urine output, termed *oliguria* if less than 500ml/ 1.73 m^2/day in children and less than 0.5 ml/kg/hr in infants, and *anuria* if completely absent, can be either an appropriate physiological response or an indication of primary renal or urological pathology. In a volume-depleted child, the kidney tubules act to maintain body water by reabsorbing most of the glomerular filtrate, leading to diminished urine output. Bladder outlet obstruction can present with either anuria or oliguria, depending on the grade of obstruction. Alternatively, a large number of acute renal insults or chronic kidney diseases can reduce glomerular filtration by damaging the kidney parenchyma, with ensuing oliguria or anuria. Oliguria occurs more often than anuria.

EVALUATION

An organized approach to the child who has anuria or oliguria begins with a careful history and physical examination. A history of recent urological surgery or trauma to the lower abdomen or pelvis suggests a bladder outlet obstruction. Intrinsic renal pathology is suggested by a history of a recent pharyngitis or systemic symptoms such as malaise, anorexia, arthralgia, or rash. Vomiting, diarrhea, or diminished fluid intake are symptoms suggestive of dehydration. Hypertension can be associated with intrinsic renal disease. If the urinary bladder or one or both kidneys are palpable and enlarged, urine is being formed but for some reason is not being emptied from the urinary tract. In obese patients, it may not be possible to detect an enlarged bladder or kidney. In contrast, if the urinary bladder and kidneys are not palpable, the patient's state of hydration must be considered in assessing why urine apparently is not being formed. Tachycardia, orthostatic changes in pulse or blood pressure, dry mucous membranes, sunken eyes, and decreased skin turgor are all findings suggestive of dehydration. It should be remembered that hypotension is a late sign of dehydration in children, and its presence indicates impending vascular collapse. Associated findings such as petechiae or purpura, malar rash, joint effusions, or evidence of pneumonia can be seen with primary renal disease. A systematic approach to the evaluation and management of anuria/oliguria follows the algorithm shown in Fig. 186-1.

DIFFERENTIAL DIAGNOSIS

Dehydration

Dehydration is the most common cause of oliguria and anuria in children. Decreased intravascular volume leads to decreased renal perfusion, which initiates a cascade of events resulting in increased renal reabsorption of glomerular filtrate and decreased urine output. A history of vomiting and/or diarrhea and the physical findings described above are all consistent with dehydration. However, patients who have primary renal failure also can present with dehydration; thus, the clinical findings of dehydration do not rule out a primary renal process. Differentiation of the two etiologies depends on the assessment of urine quality and the patient's response to rehydration. In children who are not toilet trained or who are noncooperative, bladder catheterization may be necessary to permit adequate evaluation of these two parameters. If the initial urine shows a specific gravity greater than 1.020, intrinsic renal disease is unlikely because kidney function must be intact to allow this degree of concentration. Other laboratory findings such as elevated urine osmolarity and low urine sodium concentration also are indicative of dehydration and are discussed in more detail in Chapter 295, Renal Failure. If, following fluid resuscitation a child's urine production normalizes promptly, it can be presumed that that the patient's oliguria or anuria was a physiological response to dehydration. The condition should not recur, provided that hydration is maintained.

If urine production does not increase on rehydration or if oliguria or anuria has occurred with near-normal hydration, the patient most likely has severe intrinsic renal failure. This usually is the result of an extensive parenchymal disease, such as acute glomerulonephritis (in the outpatient setting) or acute tubular necrosis (in hospitalized patients).

A third possibility is a partial response to rehydration, in which urine output increases but remains suboptimal. Such a patient most likely has oliguria from partial intrinsic renal failure.

Prompt differentiation of functional (prerenal) failure from parenchymal renal failure is extremely important. Significant parenchymal renal failure may result if functional renal failure goes untreated, as in a dehydrated patient who does not undergo prompt rehydration. Diagnostic evaluation and management of a child who is in severe renal failure are discussed in Chapter 295, Renal Failure.

Acute Urinary Retention

Acute urinary retention is a relatively uncommon occurrence in children, compared to its incidence in adults. Urine production is normal, but the volume of retained urine is greater than expected for a patient's age (normal bladder capacity in ounces is approximated by the patient's age in years plus 2). When present, a distended, often painful urinary bladder can be palpated or percussed just above the symphysis pubis,

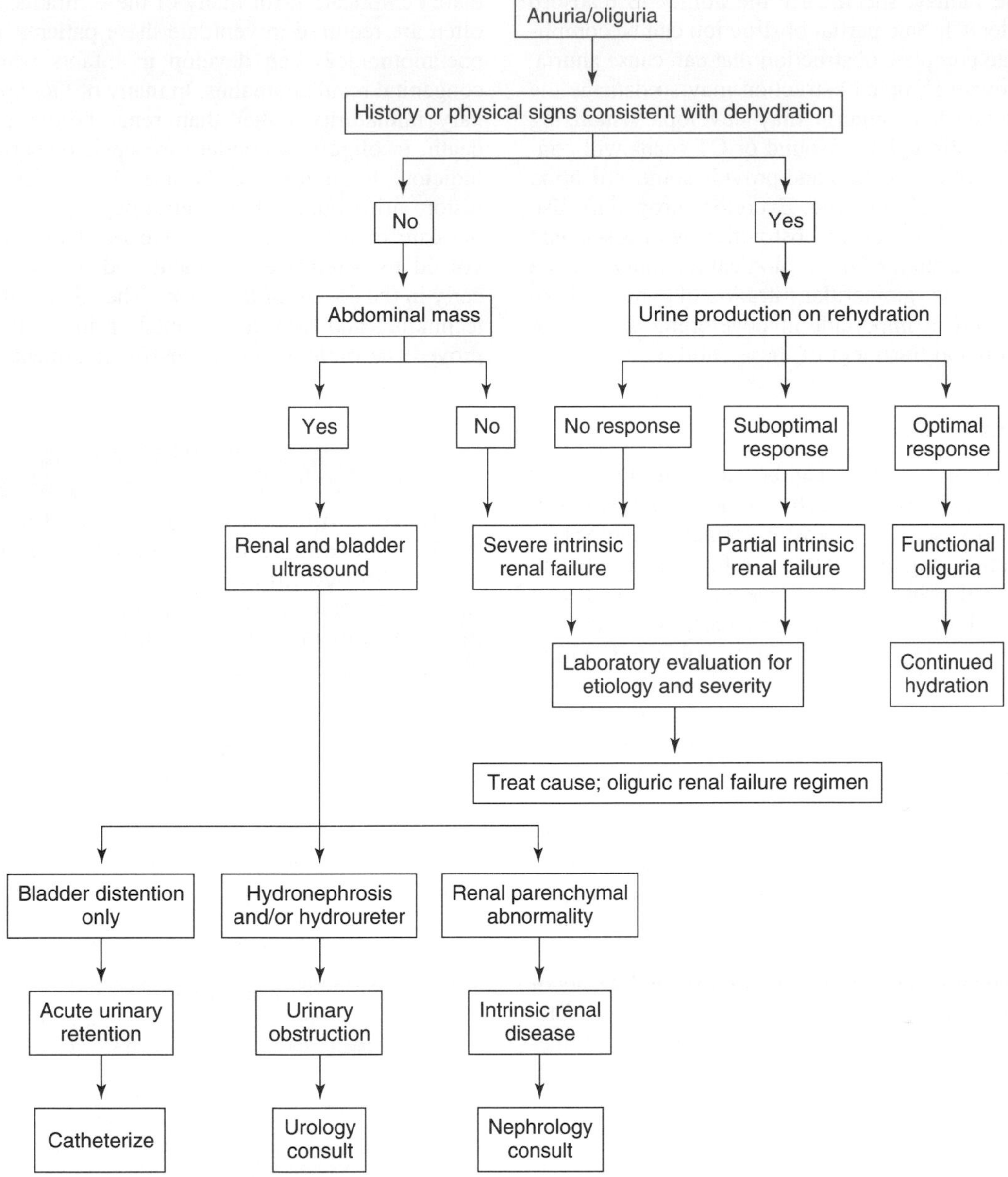

Fig. 186-1 Algorithm of the evaluation and management of a child who has anuria/oliguria.

sometimes extending as high as the umbilicus. Etiological factors can include cystitis, posterior urethral valves, severe constipation, hematocolpometra, appendiceal abscess, neurogenic bladder, reaction to anticholinergic drugs, and psychological causes. It can occur in otherwise normal children when the child consciously overrides the urge to micturate because the circumstances are not convenient for voiding, and the urinary bladder therefore becomes progressively more distended. Eventually, voluntary voiding is not possible because overdistention has exceeded the muscular compliance of the bladder, and an organized contraction coordinated with relaxation of the internal sphincter cannot be achieved. Simple catheterization to empty the bladder usually relieves the symptoms and restores the compliance of the bladder musculature. Urinary retention from this latter cause is unlikely to recur, and indwelling bladder catheterization is not indicated. However, in the majority of pediatric patients with acute urinary retention, the cause is pathological. Evaluation of these patients should include a urinalysis, urine culture, serum BUN and creatinine, an abdominal flatplate, and a renal ultrasound.

Urinary Obstruction

Urinary obstruction rarely causes anuria or oliguria in children. For anuria to occur secondary to obstruction, the obstruction must include the bladder outlet. Potential etiological factors include posterior urethral valves, urethral stones, and extrinsic compression. Evaluation should include visualization of the urinary system through ultrasound or computed tomography (CT) scans and urological consultation. Congenital and chronic urinary obstruction usually causes polyuria rather than anuria or oliguria. Polyuria occurs in these circumstances because obstruction first affects the medullary functions of the kidney, specifically the ability to reabsorb sodium and water. Chronic partial obstruction can be complicated by an acute complete obstruction that can cause anuria. Occasionally, severe chronic obstruction may so damage the kidney parenchyma that oliguria may develop. Visualizing the urinary system through ultrasound or CT scans will confirm the diagnosis of obstruction and provide some indication of the site and degree of blockage. Excretory urography also can be used, although in severe obstruction with associated renal failure, visualization of the urological anatomy may be limited because of poor glomerular filtration of contrast. Urological consultation is important in developing a plan for further evaluation and treatment of these children.

Newborns

Anuria or oliguria in a newborn can be secondary to a major congenital urological anomaly such as renal agenesis, posterior urethral valves, sepsis, or severe perinatal asphyxia. A history of maternal oligohydramnios, reflecting a deficient production of fetal urine, often is seen in newborns who have severe renal or urological anomalies. Maternal use of angiotensin-converting enzyme (ACE) inhibitors during pregnancy is associated with neonatal anuria and renal agenesis. Other clues to a major urinary anomaly include a maternal history of small uterine size for gestational age, scanty passage of amniotic fluid at delivery, and positional somatic abnormalities discovered on examination of the newborn. With the common use of prenatal sonography, many of these infants are identified prior to delivery. At birth the results of the newborn's blood chemistry tests are normal because the mother maintains the neonate's biochemical status in utero. Biochemical abnormalities attributable to renal failure usually become evident gradually over the first several weeks of life. Because adequate amniotic fluid is important to fetal lung development, pulmonary problems are the most immediate complication for many of these infants. High pressures often are required to ventilate these patients adequately, and pneumothoraces can develop in infants who have serious congenital renal anomalies. In many of these patients, pulmonary immaturity rather than renal failure is the cause of death. In oliguria secondary to sepsis or perinatal asphyxia, judicious hydration and the use of diuretics can sometimes restore urine output. A pediatric nephrologist experienced in the care of newborns who have renal failure should be involved to determine treatment and to counsel the parents early in the course of treatment. The advent of newer dialysis techniques and renal transplantation in small infants has improved the outlook for successful treatment of these cases.

When to Refer

1. No or minimal response to hydration
2. Abnormal renal function that does not correct with hydration
3. Associated hypertension
4. Abnormal renal or bladder ultrasound

SUGGESTED READINGS

Airede A, Bello M, Weerasinghe HD: Acute renal failure in the newborn: incidence and outcome, *J Pediatr Child Health* 33:246, 1997.

Kitapci F, Avsar AF, Senses DA: A girl with constipation and acute urinary retention, *Eur J Pediatr* 158:3337, 1999.

Peter JR, Stenhardt GF: Acute urinary retention in children, *Pediatr Emerg Care* 9:205, 1993.

Sehic A, Chesney RW: Acute renal failure: diagnosis, *Pediatr Rev* 16:101, 1995.

Shotan A, et al: Risks of angiotensin-converting enzyme inhibition during pregnancy: experimental and clinical evidence, potential mechanisms, and recommendations for use, *Am J Med* 96:451, 1994.

187 Appendicitis

R. Scott Strahlman

Although appendicitis is a surgical emergency, the pediatrician has a crucial role in its initial diagnosis and management and often is the first to suspect appendicitis and to contact the surgical team. The pediatrician's high index of suspicion can be the driving force that leads to an appropriate, timely appendectomy. Prompt diagnosis and preoperative management help to reduce the high morbidity associated with a perforated appendix.

Appendicitis is the most common cause of an acute surgical condition of the abdomen in childhood. The exact incidence is unknown, but appendicitis is rare in early childhood and becomes more common after age 10. Boys and girls are affected equally before puberty, but after age 15, twice as many boys are affected as girls. An increased incidence in the spring and autumn months also has been observed. In addition, appendicitis is more common in children who have a family history of appendicitis.[3] Whether this tendency is genetic or diet related is unclear, because the risk of appendicitis may be reduced with a high-fiber diet.[2]

ETIOLOGY AND PATHOPHYSIOLOGY

Appendicitis always is initiated by obstruction of the appendiceal lumen, usually by a fecalith or by lymphoid hyperplasia. In rare cases, a parasite, tumor, or foreign body may obstruct the lumen. Inspissated secretions of cystic fibrosis also may obstruct the appendiceal lumen (thus, although rarely, cystic fibrosis may manifest as appendicitis).[13] As secretions accumulate within the obstructed appendix, the walls become distended. Continued distention causes ischemia and necrosis of the appendix, leading to irritation of the surrounding peritoneum.

Clinically, the initial distention of the appendiceal wall is manifested by a dull, steady periumbilical pain. After 4 to 6 hours this pain often shifts to the right lower quadrant as local peritoneal inflammation develops. Without surgical intervention the appendix eventually may rupture, causing peritonitis. The incidence of rupture increases dramatically 24 to 36 hours after the onset of abdominal pain. Delaying surgery more than 36 hours results in at least a 65% incidence of perforation.[1] Organisms cultured from the peritoneal cavity after perforation have included both aerobic and anaerobic bacteria.[15] The most common aerobic bacteria are *Escherichia coli* and *Klebsiella* and *Proteus* organisms. Common anaerobes include *Bacteroides* and *Clostridium* species.

INITIAL ASSESSMENT

History

A thorough history is invaluable in differentiating appendicitis from other disorders; an important component of that history is pain. The onset of symptoms often is heralded by a dull, steady periumbilical pain. The pain more often is thought to be caused by acute appendicitis if it awakens the patient from sleep. Anorexia is a consistent finding. One or two episodes of vomiting may follow, but essentially never precede, the pain. After 4 to 6 hours the pain commonly migrates to the right lower quadrant. Given the many variations in the location of the appendix, however, the location of abdominal pain may vary. Usually, bowel habits do not change. The child may have a low-grade fever, but the temperature rarely is above 100.3° F (37.9° C). If the clinical picture suggests but does not convince the physician that appendicitis is the problem, it is best to watch the progression of signs and symptoms carefully over several hours. Because an appendix rarely perforates within 24 hours of the onset of pain, a period of observation can safely differentiate a potential surgical condition from a nonsurgical one.

Physical Examination

As always, a gentle, nonthreatening approach is most effective during the physical examination. The physician should look for peritoneal signs such as pain upon walking or coughing. If the patient can jump up on the examining table, he or she usually does not have appendicitis. Patients may be most comfortable lying supine with their legs flexed. Abdominal tenderness always is present and often is greatest at the McBurney point (two thirds of the distance on a direct line from the umbilicus to the anterosuperior iliac spine). Rebound tenderness of the abdomen (particularly that which is referred to the right lower quadrant) is common, as is hyperesthesia of the skin overlying the painful area. Pain in the right lower quadrant may be accentuated when the inflamed appendix is located rectrorecally by (1) placing the patient in the left decubitus position and extending the right leg at the hip, thereby placing tension on the right psoas muscle, the origins of which underlie the appendix (psoas sign), and (2) placing the patient supine and internally rotating the flexed right hip, thereby extending the right internal obturator muscle, the origins of which also underlie the appendix (obturator sign). When the inflamed appendix is located anteriorly, pain in the right lower quadrant may be accentuated when the child is asked to sit up from the supine position while pressure is placed against the forehead. Bowel sounds may be diminished or hyperactive. A rectal examination often will facilitate making the diagnosis, by revealing right-sided tenderness. Examination of the lungs is important to rule out a right lower lobe pneumonia that may generate referred pain to the right lower quadrant of the abdomen. A pelvic examination is indicated for any adolescent girl who has abdominal pain, to rule out gynecological conditions.

Laboratory Tests

The only essential laboratory studies are a blood count and urinalysis. Appendicitis has a characteristic blood count: The white blood cell count most often is in the range of 10,000 to 20,000/mm^3, with a slight increase in the number of neutrophils, particularly younger forms. The blood count helps to rule out viral and other processes that do not increase the white cell count. The erythrocyte sedimentation rate usually is normal. Urinalysis is performed to rule out urinary tract infection or diabetic ketoacidosis as causes of the abdominal pain.

If the diagnosis is in doubt, abdominal roentgenograms occasionally are helpful. Radiographic features that suggest appendicitis include a calcified appendicolith or an air-filled appendix, although the absence of abnormalities does not rule out the diagnosis. Ultrasonography, computerized tomography (CT), and even magnetic resonance image (MRI) scanning have helped to delineate appendicitis in cases that are not clear-cut.[8]

The typical progression of signs and symptoms in appendicitis may be summarized as follows: periumbilical abdominal pain, followed by nausea, vomiting, and localization of the pain to the right lower quadrant. Low-grade fever, direct tenderness to palpation in the right lower quadrant and indirect tenderness referred to the right lower quadrant, right-sided tenderness on rectal examination, and a mild leukocytosis often accompany these symptoms.

DIFFERENTIAL DIAGNOSIS

The differential diagnosis of appendicitis, which is the same as the differential diagnosis of acute abdominal pain, is extensive (Box 187-1). Gastroenteritis can be differentiated from appendicitis on the basis of a benign abdominal examination in the former condition. Vomiting and diarrhea usually occur before the onset of pain, not afterward as in appendicitis. Constipation often can appear to be appendicitis; however, this pain usually is diffuse, not localized to the right lower quadrant, and the patient often has a history of constipation. An abdominal flat plate roentgenogram can help in the diagnosis, and a small Fleet enema often is both diagnostic and therapeutic.

An appropriate initial evaluation can rule out the following nonsurgical conditions in a patient who has abdominal pain: urinary tract infection, diabetic ketoacidosis, sickle cell crisis, right lower lobe pneumonia with referred pain, nephrotic syndrome with primary peritonitis, and inflammatory bowel disease. Gynecological disorders can be ruled out based on the history and a pelvic examination; pelvic inflammatory disease, ovarian torsion, ectopic pregnancy, dysmenorrhea, and mittelschmerz all can mimic appendicitis.

BOX 187-1

DIFFERENTIAL DIAGNOSIS OF APPENDICITIS

- Common conditions
  - Gastroenteritis
  - Constipation
- Medical problems
  - Urinary tract infection
  - Diabetic ketoacidosis
  - Sickle cell crisis
  - Right lower lobe pneumonia
  - Primary peritonitis
  - Inflammatory bowel disease
- Gynecological problems
  - Pelvic inflammatory disease
  - Ovarian torsion
  - Ruptured ectopic pregnancy
  - Dysmenorrhea
  - Mittelschmerz
- Unusual conditions
  - Henoch-Schönlein purpura
  - Hemolytic-uremic syndrome
  - Rocky Mountain spotted fever
- Surgical emergencies
  - Meckel's diverticulitis
  - Intestinal adhesions
  - Intussusception
  - Necrotizing enterocolitis

Unusual conditions such as Henoch-Schönlein purpura and hemolytic-uremic syndrome may be indistinguishable from appendicitis.[6] Even Rocky Mountain spotted fever can mimic appendicitis.[5] Surgical emergencies that mimic appendicitis (see Box 187-1) can be ruled out only in the operating room.

NEONATAL APPENDICITIS

Appendicitis in the first 2 years of life is rare, accounting for fewer than 2% of all childhood cases.[7] The mortality is high, however, and approaches 100% in cases with perforation.[10] Therefore, appendicitis must be considered in any infant suspected of having abdominal pain. The presenting symptoms consist of vomiting and fever, and the baby may appear to be colicky. Physical examination shows abdominal distention with diffuse tenderness. Abdominal roentgenograms can be diagnostically helpful in a neonate by showing an appendicolith, free peritoneal fluid, bowel wall edema, or free air. With a high index of suspicion, surgery must be performed immediately to prevent or manage perforation, with its high mortality.

MANAGEMENT

Once the diagnosis is made, the patient must be prepared for immediate surgery. Nothing is given by mouth, and a nasogastric tube is inserted and placed on low suction. Intravenous hydration is started (e.g., 10 ml/kg/hr of lactated Ringer's solution), and fever may be controlled with acetaminophen given by rectum. Broad-spectrum antibiotics (e.g., ampicillin, gentamicin, and clindamycin, or a cephalosporin) are administered intravenously before surgery. Antibiotics have been shown to reduce morbidity even in nonperforated cases.[4] An appendectomy is performed as soon as the patient's condition has been stabilized. Many institutions are gaining experience with laparoscopic appendectomy[11] (see Chapter 32, Minimally Invasive Surgery).

For patients who have symptoms for 5 days or longer and a palpable mass consistent with an appendiceal abscess, many surgeons prefer nonsurgical management initially.[14] The patient is treated with broad-spectrum antibiotics and, barring interim complications, returns in 4 to 6 weeks for an elective appendectomy. This approach lowers the incidence of peritonitis and the associated complications precipitated by surgical manipulation during the acute inflammatory stages of the disease.

PROGNOSIS

For uncomplicated appendicitis treated with prompt surgical repair, the mortality is much less that 1%, and there essentially is no long-term morbidity. The average hospital stay is about 4 days.[9] A ruptured appendix increases the risk of mortality only slightly (with most of the increase occurring in the neonatal age group) but extends the average hospital stay to about 7 days. Complications that increase morbidity include peritonitis, postoperative abscesses, and prolonged ileus. In women, infertility is a possible long-term complication of a ruptured appendix due to intraabdominal adhesions affecting the fallopian tubes.[12]

The incidence of perforated appendicitis exceeds 20%, a disconcertingly high figure.[9] A higher index of suspicion on the part of pediatricians and the general public may lead to earlier diagnosis of the condition and reduce the incidence of appendiceal perforation and its morbid complications.

When to Refer

Refer to surgery immediately whenever appendicitis is suspected.

When to Hospitalize

Hospitalize for inpatient observation if the diagnosis is in doubt and for appendectomy when it is not.

REFERENCES

1. Brender JD, et al: Childhood appendicitis: factors associated with perforation, *Pediatrics* 76:2, 1985.
2. Brender JD, et al: Fiber intake and childhood appendicitis, *Am J Public Health* 75:399, 1985.
3. Brender JD, et al: Is childhood appendicitis familial? *Am J Dis Child* 139:338, 1985.
4. Busuttil RW, et al: Effect of prophylactic antibiotics in acute nonperforated appendicitis, *Ann Surg* 194:502, 1981.
5. Davis AE, Bradford WD: Abdominal pain resembling acute appendicitis in Rocky Mountain spotted fever, *JAMA* 247:2811, 1982.
6. Edmonson MB, Chesney RW: Hemolytic-uremic syndrome confused with acute appendicitis, *Arch Surg* 113:754, 1978.
7. Grosfeld JL, Weinberger M, Clatworthy HW: Acute appendicitis in the first two years of life, *J Pediatr Surg* 8:285, 1973.
8. Gupta H, Dupuy DE: Advances in imaging of the acute abdomen, *Surg Clin North Am* 77:1245, 1997.
9. Hale DA, et al: A contemporary appraisal of appendectomies, *Ann Surg* 225:252, 1997.
10. Kwong MS, Dinner M: Neonatal appendicitis masquerading as necrotizing enterocolitis, *J Pediatr* 96:917, 1980.
11. Miller JP: Laparoscopic appendectomy, *Pediatr Ann* 22:664, 1993.
12. Mueller BA, et al: Appendectomy and the risk of tubal infertility, *N Engl J Med* 315:1506, 1986.
13. Oestreich AE, Adelstein EH: Appendicitis as the presenting complaint in cystic fibrosis, *J Pediatr Surg* 17:191, 1982.
14. Powers RJ, et al: Alternate approach to the management of acute perforating appendicitis in children, *Surg Gynecol Obstet* 152:473, 1981.
15. Stone HH: Bacterial flora of appendicitis in children, *J Pediatr Surg* 11:37, 1976.

SUGGESTED READINGS

Ravitch MM: Appendicitis (review), *Pediatrics* 70:414, 1982.

Shaul WL: Clues to the early diagnosis of neonatal appendicitis, *J Pediatr* 98:473, 1981.

Silen ML: The right lower quadrant "revisited," *Pediatr Clin North Am* 40:1201, 1993.

Siler W, editor: *Cope's early diagnosis of the acute abdomen,* New York, 1983, Oxford University Press.

188 Asthma

Philip Fireman

Asthma is the most common chronic illness in childhood.[2] Unfortunately, no specific biological, genetic, physiological, or immunological marker defines the disease. Asthma can best be described as a chronic inflammatory obstructive lung disease associated with hyperreactive airways. The obstruction of the hyperreactive airways results from bronchial inflammation with smooth-muscle contraction, increased mucus secretion, and edema. Both large and small airways can be involved to a variable degree and are hyperresponsive to a variety of environmental stimuli. The typical symptoms of wheezing, cough, and shortness of breath usually are episodical because of reversible airway obstruction that can improve either spontaneously or as the result of therapy. Although it can occur at any age, asthma usually has its onset within the first 5 years of life.[7] U.S. Public Health questionnaire surveys estimate that 5% to 10% of children have asthma at some time during childhood.[4] However, its prevalence may be greater in certain communities. For example, a recent prospective study of asthma of more than 2000 children from birth to 6 years of age in a managed care organization in Tucson, Arizona, showed that 51% never wheezed, 20% had at least one transient episode of wheezing during the first 3 years of life but none at 6 years of age, 15% had no wheezing before 3 years of age but developed wheezing by 6 years of age, and 14% had persistent childhood wheezing.[8] Therefore, of those children who wheezed during infancy, the majority subsided by 6 years of age, but 40% had persistence of symptoms by 6 years. A survey conducted at Children's Hospital of Pittsburgh showed that asthma accounted for 10% of medical emergency room visits and 10% of medical hospitalizations. According to a U.S. Public Health Service survey, asthma is the most common cause of school absenteeism in children younger than age 17.[13] Before adolescence, boys are affected more often that girls (3:1), but the male preponderance does not persist past adolescence. The clinical spectrum of asthma is that of an illness that begins early in life, tends to improve in some, but continues on into adulthood in others. A matter of great concern is the increase in prevalence, hospital admissions, and mortality in recent years.[3] Asthma, therefore, is particularly important to pediatricians and to all physicians interested in the care of childhood respiratory illnesses.

ETIOLOGY AND PATHOGENESIS

The pathogenesis of asthma is only partly understood. Risk factors for persistent asthma include a family history of asthma, maternal cigarette smoking, and exposure to household pets.[8] It is a familial, multifactorial respiratory illness that involves allergic and other immunological, infectious, biochemical, autonomic nervous system, and psychological factors to a varying degree in different individuals. The pathology of the bronchial inflammation involves mast cells, eosinophils, and T and B lymphocytes. Thus, an affected individual may develop respiratory symptoms after exposure to a variety of environmental stimuli, such as specific inhalant allergens, infectious agents, cold air, tobacco smoke, aerosolized chemicals, inert dusts, strong aromas, and the hyperventilation that can be associated with exercise, laughing, or crying. These environmental factors trigger the release or generation of certain mediators of inflammation, such as histamine, leukotrienes, prostaglandins, and other cytokines, that can induce smooth-muscle contractions, mucus gland secretion, and inflammatory edema to provoke symptoms and, if persistent, lead to remodeling of the airway.[6]

Atopy, the genetic predisposition to develop an allergic immunoglobulin E (IgE)-mediated response to allergens and the genetically influenced hyperreactivity of the airway are two familial risk factors. Epidemiological linkage studies have proposed several candidate genetic loci: These include chromosome 5q with bronchial hyperresponsiveness, chromosome 5q with the IL4 cytokine gene cluster, chromosome 11q13 with the high-affinity IgE receptor, and chromosome 14q with the T-cell antigen receptor.[12] These data of different patient populations reflect the heterogenicity of the clinical spectrum of asthma and ultimately may lead to better definition of the disease. The airway hyperactivity may be manifest as enhanced airway responsiveness to provocative challenge with inhalation of cholinergic agents, cold air, or exercise. Inhalation challenge with methacholine or histamine to provoke airway obstruction has been developed as a diagnostic provocative test in individuals who have asthma, but it is not suitable as a test for children younger than age 6 years. Studies have confirmed the impression of many pediatricians that a history of respiratory syncytial virus (RSV) bronchiolitis or croup is a risk factor for the development of asthma; approximately 33% to 50% of children who have had more than one episode of bronchiolitis or croup during early life subsequently demonstrate bronchial hyperreactivity.[5] It is interesting that one third of these patients' first-degree relatives also had airway hyperreactivity, which suggests a genetic predisposition. A relation between allergy and asthma also exists whenever specific antigen (allergen) inhalation challenge is documented as provoking signs and symptoms of asthma in the hypersensitive (allergic) host. An increase in serum IgE has been documented in both familial and epidemiological studies of asthma patients.[1] In fact, specific allergen sensitization has been reported in 70% to 80% of children who have asthma.[8]

CLINICAL MANIFESTATIONS

Asthma in infants and children varies markedly among patients and sometimes even in the same patient. The illness may manifest in several clinical patterns. The National Institutes of Health (NIH) has set guidelines for asthma management; these classify the disease as intermittent or persistent mild, moderate, or severe (Table 188-1).[10] Patients may have occasional acute episodes of symptoms that can vary from mild (requiring only minimal medication) to severe, life-threatening attacks of status asthmaticus, which demands hospitalization and treatment in an intensive care unit. Other children may have episodes every several months, yet appear to be well and symptom free between episodes. Still others may have chronic or daily symptoms that interfere in some way with their lifestyle and have superimposed on this a number of acute episodes that can be severe but may vary in duration from several hours to days. Finally, a small number of patients (probably fewer than 2% of all asthmatic individuals) have severe daily symptoms that require several medications and careful clinical monitoring. Studies indicate that the most severely affected children experience the onset of wheezing during the first year of life and have a family history of asthma or other allergic disease, especially atopic dermatitis (infantile eczema).

Many pediatricians hesitate to diagnose asthma in infants because the illness may be transient or of the difficulty involved in documenting the signs and symptoms of reversible obstructive airway disease. Yet in most children who subsequently are diagnosed as having persistent asthma, suggestive signs appear during the first year or two of life, usually associated with a viral respiratory infection that induces cough and "wheezy," labored respirations. The mechanism of this virus-induced wheezing has been shown to involve virus-specific IgE antibody and increased release of histamine into the secretions of young children infected with RSV.[14] The infectious agents involved during the preschool years are primarily RSV, with fewer episodes associated with parainfluenza virus; rhinovirus and influenza viruses are more significant among older children and adults.[9] Mycoplasma infections can promote asthma symptoms in children of school age, especially adolescents. Bacterial infections rarely are associated with acute exacerbations of asthma except as secondary invaders or as a cause of an associated sinusitis. There is no correlation between the severity of allergic rhinitis or atopic dermatitis and the severity of asthma.

An acute episode of asthma may begin with rhinorrhea and fever, then rapidly progress to cough, audible wheeze, and dyspnea. Many pediatricians label these viral respiratory illnesses ("asthmatic bronchitis," "wheezy bronchitis," or "wheezy cold"), but this reluctance or actual failure to recognize the underlying reactive airway disease may delay institution of appropriate management. Between infections, an infant may be relatively free of respiratory symptoms, but cough can persist for longer than the usual 7 to 10 days.

Between the ages of 3 and 5 years, the typical persistent asthmatic child begins to have some episodes without apparent infection. Acute symptoms may commence abruptly and range from paroxysms of cough to severe dyspnea. Symptoms may be seasonal or perennial and can be precipitated by exercise, infection, allergens (e.g., pollens, dust mites, animal products, and organic dusts), tobacco smoke, fumes, odors, laughter, or other stimuli. In rare instances, foods can provoke an asthma attack. Allergic rhinitis, seasonal or perennial, often is evident in children whose asthma has an allergic basis. Between episodes the patient may be free of symptoms or may have latent reactive airway obstruction provoked by forced expiration (elicited by the astute clinician as compression expiratory rhonchi during chest auscultation). A chronic cough in children or adults may be the only manifestation of airway hyperreactivity. Sputum production is minimal in children, who usually swallow excess bronchial secretions.

During an acute episode of asthma, the patient appears anxious and dyspneic. The pediatrician will recognize the characteristic prolonged expiratory phase of respiration, the raised clavicles, and subcostal retractions. If the asthma has been long-standing, the child may have a distended or barrel-chest appearance caused by air-trapping. Auscultation of the chest may reveal the characteristic high-pitched musical expiratory rhonchi (wheeze), but both inspiratory and expiratory coarse rhonchi also can be heard. Lack of breath sounds or rhonchi in a dyspneic, asthmatic child should suggest poor air exchange and potential respiratory failure, requiring immediate therapy and close observation in the office, emergency room, or hospital.

Table 188-1 Classification of Asthma Severity

	Mild Intermittent	Mild Persistent	Moderate Persistent	Severe Persistent
Frequency of Symptoms	**<1 × week**	**>1 × week <1 × day**	**Daily**	**Continual**
Exacerbation	Brief/mild	May affect acuity	Affect acuity	Frequent/severe
Night-time symptoms	<2 × month	>2 × month	>1 × week	Frequent
Lung function*				
FEV_1 or FEF	≥80%	≥80%	>60% <80%	≤60%
% PEF validity	<20%	20% to 30%	>30%	>30%

Modified from National Heart, Lung, and Blood Institute: National Asthma Education Program: *Guidelines for the diagnosis and management of asthma,* Expert Panel Report 2 No 97-405, National Institutes of Health, Bethesda, Md, 1997.
**FEV_1* = Forced expiratory volume in 1 second; *FEF,* Forced expiratory flow; *PEF,* Peak expiratory flow.

LABORATORY FINDINGS

Laboratory studies of pulmonary function in mild cases of asthma during remission may well show no abnormalities. A chest roentgenogram shows hyperinflation during acute attacks, with persistent hyperinflation changes in the more severe and chronic states. Atelectasis, particularly in the right middle lobe, is a common finding on chest radiography during acute episodes and should not be misconstrued as pneumonia. Pulmonary function testing may be a valuable adjunct in assessing the degree of pulmonary impairment in children older than age 6, especially when performed both before and after treatment with an aerosolized sympathomimetic bronchodilator. Long-term management of the chronic asthmatic child may include home monitoring of pulmonary function (e.g., with the mini-Wright peak flow meter). Pulmonary testing after exercise can be helpful in assessing an asthmatic child who is involved in athletic activities. Monitoring patients by means of pulse oximetry during an acute asthma attack is a valuable adjunct, as is determining arterial blood gas and pH values in the intensive management of a child who has severe acute asthma or status asthmaticus.

All children suspected of allergic (immune-mediated) asthma should be evaluated for allergy. Skin testing usually is preferred over serological IgE antibody testing because of its greater sensitivity and lower cost. Serum immunoglobulins, especially total serum IgE, often are elevated but nonspecifically. Unconventional allergy tests, including the controversial cytotoxic, sublingual neutralization, and titration techniques, should be avoided until their sensitivity and specificity have been established in controlled studies. Eosinophilia in sputum and blood is a common finding in asthmatic individuals, but sputum bacterial cultures generally are not helpful.

DIFFERENTIAL DIAGNOSIS

During the first few years of life, other conditions that can partially obstruct the airway and provoke recurrent cough and wheezing must be considered. As already indicated, bronchiolitis and asthma often are difficult to differentiate in infants younger than 1 year of age. Cystic fibrosis may cause symptoms that mimic asthma, even in the absence of growth failure. Thus, a sweat test is warranted for children who have recurrent wheezing. Congenital anomalies of the respiratory, cardiovascular, and gastrointestinal tracts may obstruct the airway and produce symptoms that warrant appropriate radiological studies, especially during the first 2 years of life. Aspiration of a foreign body usually causes a sudden onset of symptoms, but if the acute event is not appreciated at the time of aspiration, it may result in chronic or recurrent wheezing. Gastroesophageal reflux may be associated with subtle aspiration that causes respiratory symptoms, including wheezing, during infancy and childhood. On occasion, an immunodeficiency may be associated with repeated respiratory infections accompanied by wheezing. IgG antibody deficiency should be considered in children who have recurrent infections and asthma.[11] Yet the child who has recurrent episodes of coughing and wheezing, after appropriate study, most often is shown to have asthma.

TREATMENT

The goals of therapy for asthma are to reverse symptoms and, of course, to prevent their development. To achieve both these goals, the clinician must classify the asthma as intermittent or persistent mild, moderate, or severe and, following NIH guidelines (see Table 188-1), institute appropriate incremental pharmacological therapy along with suitable measures of environmental control to reduce or eliminate specific and nonspecific factors that provoke symptoms.[10] The pharmacotherapy of children who have asthma comprises two classes of medication—bronchodilators and antiinflammatory agents (Table 188-2). The sympathomimetics, theophyllines, and anticholinergics are bronchodilators; antiinflammatory cromolyn, nedocromil, leukotriene modifiers, and steroids do not act promptly on the airway and provide clinical improvement only over hours or days. The efficacy of these medications can be additive, and they may be used simultaneously. Unfortunately, multiple-drug treatment regimens are potentially confusing, not only to the patient but also to the pediatrician.

To simplify the use of appropriate pharmacotherapy, Table 188-3 presents a step-up or step-down flowchart of drug treatment based on the clinical patterns of asthma described above.[10] Efficient reversal of symptoms requires a prompt-acting bronchodilator; thus, the β_2 agonists are the drugs of choice for the acute, occasional asthma attack. Theophylline does not appear to be effective during acute attacks. Several of these agents, along with their formulations and appropriate dosages, are listed in Table 188-2. Severe acute symptoms may require administration of subcutaneous epinephrine or a β_2 agonist aerosol; the latter is preferred as a faster and safer treatment route. Home use of metered-dose inhalers demands proper instruction and has the potential for overuse and abuse by some children, particularly adolescents. A sympathomimetic aerosol generated by an air compressor can be used for the child younger than age 6 who cannot use the metered-dose inhalers properly, and spacers and holding chambers have been devised that may facilitate metered-dose inhaler therapy. Mild occasional symptoms may be controlled with oral sympathomimetic agents. If symptoms are persistent, an antiinflammatory drug should be added to the regimen. If symptoms are severe or unresponsive, hospitalization is indicated. As an alternative to hospitalization for a known asthmatic child, administration of a short course of oral steroids may be warranted. Prednisone in a dosage of 2 mg/kg/24 hr (up to a maximum daily dose of 60 mg) can be given in several divided doses for 3 to 5 days; it then can be stopped or tapered over several days as clinically indicated.

Cromolyn can be effective for preventing asthma attacks in a patient who has recurrent or daily wheezing. It should be used as a prophylactic agent, however, and not as an acute bronchodilator for ongoing established episodes of asthma. Cromolyn and nedocromil are available as a metered dose that is used four times a day. For children younger than age 6, a liquid form of cromolyn is available for inhalation via a nebulizer with compressed air. If cromolyn therapy proves beneficial, certain children may be maintained on as few as two or three inhalations per day; it may even be possible, then, to reduce or stop administration of bronchodilators.

Table 188-2 Medications Used to Treat Children Who Have Asthma

Drug	Formulation/Administration	Dose/Duration*
Bronchodilators		
Sympathomimetics		
β_1-agonists		
Epinephrine	1:1000 solution, SQ	0.01 ml/kg up to 0.3 ml
Sus-Phrine†	1:200 suspension, SQ	0.005 ml/kg up to 0.25 ml
β_2-agonists		
Albuterol		
Proventil†	Metered aerosol	90 μg/puff qid
Ventolin†	Tablet: 2, 4 mg	0.1 mg/kg tid
	Syrup: 2 mg/5 ml	0.1 mg/kg tid
	Aerosol solution 1% (racemic formulation)	0.5 ml/2.5 ml saline qid
Levalbuterol		
Xopenex†	Aerosol solution: 0.63- and 1.25-mg, 3-ml unit-dose vials	0.63 mg tid
Metaproterenol		
Alupent†	Aerosol solution: 5%	0.25 ml/2.5 ml saline
	Metered aerosol	650 μg/puff qid
	Syrup: 10 mg/5 ml	
	Tablet: 10, 20 mg	0.5 mg/kg tid
Terbutaline		
Brethine†	1:1000 solution SQ	0.25 ml/dose qid
Bricanyl†	Tablet: 2.5, 5 mg	0.075 mg/kg tid
Anticholinergic		
Ipratropium	Metered aerosol	3-14 yr 1-2 puffs tid >14 yr 2 puffs qid
Atrovent†	Aerosol solution	3-14 yr 0.125-0.25 mg tid >14 yr 0.5 mg tid or qid
Salmeterol (long acting)		
Serevent†	Metered aerosol	2 puffs bid
Theophyllines (the normal dosage [12-16 mg/kg/24 hr] must be individualized)		
Theo-Dur Sprinkle†	Capsule: 50, 75, 125 mg	q8-12h (long duration)
Theo-Dur†	Tablet: 100, 200, 300 mg	q8-12h (long duration)
Slo-Phyllin†	Gyrocap: 60, 125, 200 mg	q8-12h (long duration)
Slo-Bid†	Gyrocap: 100, 200, 300 mg	q8-12h (long duration)
Antiinflammatory Drugs		
Cromolyn	Aerosol solution 20 mg/2 ml	20 mg qid
	Metered aerosol	2 puffs qid
Nedocromil	Metered aerosol	2 puffs qid
Leukotriene modifiers		
Montelukast (Singulair†)	Tablet: 5 mg (chewable), 10 mg	5 or 10 mg daily
Zafirlukast (Accolade†)	Tablet: 20 mg	20 mg bid
Zileuton (Zyflo†)	Tablet: 600 mg	600 mg q6-8h
Inhaled corticosteroids (dosage and frequency need to be individualized)		
Beclomethasone (Vanceril, Beclovent†)	Metered aerosol	44 mg/puff, 88 mg/puff
Fluticasone (Flovent† 44, 110, 220)	Metered aerosol	44 mg, 110 mg, 220 mg/puff
Triamcinolone (Azmacort†)	Metered aerosol	100 mg/puff
Flunisolide (AcroBid,† Acrobid-M†)	Metered aerosol	250 mg/puff
Budesonide (Pulmicort†)	Dry powder inhaler	200 mg/puff

*These dosages/frequency need to be individualized based on the patient's age or body surface area.
†Trade names.

Intermittent corticosteroid therapy with prednisone may be necessary in certain children who have chronic or severe asthma that has failed to respond to the other drugs. Judicious use of prednisone in dosages of 1 to 2 mg/kg/24 hr for several days, followed by rapid tapering of the dose over 1 week, may prevent frequent hospitalization of a child who has severe chronic asthma. The recommended alternative to oral corticosteroids is prophylactic use of a topical metered-dose inhaled steroid (beclomethasone, triamcinolone, flunisolide, fluticasone, or budesonide). The usual pediatric dose (two inhalations several times daily) produces minimal side effects, other than a rare instance of oral candi-

Table 188-3 Pharmacotherapy of Asthma: Stepwise Approach*

Controller	Reliever
Step 4: Severe Persistent Asthma	
Daily medications Inhaled corticosteroid (high dose), and Long-acting β_2 agonist, and Sustained-release theophylline, and Leukotriene modifiers, and Oral steroid (alternate day)	Short-acting β_2 agonist prn for symptoms
Step 3: Moderate Persistent Asthma	
Daily medications Inhaled corticosteroid (moderate dose), and Long-acting inhaled β_2 agonist, and Sustained release Theophylline	Short-acting β_2 agonist prn; not to exceed 3-4 times a day for symptoms
Step 2: Mild Persistent Asthma	
Daily medications Inhaled corticosteroid (low dose) or Inhaled cromolyn or nedocromil, or Leukotriene modifiers	Short-acting β_2 agonist prn; not to exceed 3-4 times a day for symptoms
Step 1: Intermittent Asthma	
Daily medications None needed	Short-acting β_2 agonist prn for symptoms Short-acting inhaled β_2 agonist or cromolyn before exercise or allergen exposure

*Step-up therapy progressively from step 1 to step 4: When asthma control is not achieved.
Step-down therapy progressively from step 4 to step 1: When asthma control is sustained.

diasis. Metered-dose fluticasone, flunisolide, triamcinolone, or beclomethasone also can be delivered via a spacer or holding chamber to children younger than age 6. At this writing, a corticosteroid solution of budesonide available in Canada and Europe is not yet available in the United States for aerosol use via an air compressor.

Severely affected children may require alternate-day steroids, which should be tapered to the smallest dose (given as a single morning dose) that controls symptoms. Long-term daily use of oral corticosteroid should be avoided in children at all costs because of the potential for development of Cushingoid changes and severe impairment of growth and development.

Leukotriene modifiers are a recent addition to the antiinflammation medications, especially for the patient who has mild persistent asthma, as an alternative to inhaled steroids or cromolyn. In addition, leukotriene modifiers may be useful in moderate or severe persistent asthma to reduce the dosage of inhaled steroids. Like steroids and cromolyn, leukotriene modifiers are not bronchodilators and are not indicated for therapy of acute asthma exacerbations. Montelukast is prescribed orally once daily as a 5-mg chewable tablet for children 6 to 13 years of age and a 10-mg tablet for those older than age 14. Zafirlukast is given orally as a 20-mg tablet twice daily for children 12 years and older. Zileuton is given three or four times a day as a 600-mg tablet by mouth, but liver function needs to be monitored several times a year.

The child who has persistent, moderate to severe recurrent asthma may benefit by the addition of regular maintenance therapy with a sustained-release theophylline, as may the child who has chronic daily wheezing. It must be remembered, however, that there is substantial intersubject variation in theophylline metabolism. The preschool and primary school-age child, for instance, metabolizes theophylline faster than does the adolescent or infant. Other factors that can alter theophylline metabolism include liver disease, viral infection, nicotine (from cigarette smoking), and other drugs. Ingestion of sustained-release theophylline with meals can alter its pharmacokinetics and should be avoided. It usually is best to begin with a moderate dose (12 to 16 mg/kg/24 hr) and then cautiously increase it weekly if wheezing persists. Chronically ill children who are to be treated with daily maintenance theophylline probably should have their serum theophylline concentration measured a week after therapy is begun and thereafter at approximately 6- to 12-month intervals. Still, it may be sufficient to monitor the serum theophylline level only in children who do not respond to the usual recommended dose or who have adverse symptoms while receiving the usual dosage. Although the therapeutic range for serum theophylline is 10 to 20 mg/ml, it probably is best not to exceed 16 mg/ml in most children. Several reliable sustained-release theophylline products are available. The bead-filled capsules may be particularly useful for a young child who is unable to swallow a capsule or tablet but who can swallow the beads mixed into or sprinkled on food. Another adjunct therapy for chronic asthma is the anticholinergic ipratropium (Atrovent), which is available as a metered-dose inhaler and a solution for nebulization.

Other aspects of therapy should not be overlooked in planning comprehensive treatment. Passive inhalation of cigarette smoke or other respiratory irritants can provoke hyperreactivity in the airways of an asthmatic person. Thus, appropriate environmental control should be pursued to prevent exposure to known irritants. Appropriate play and exercise are necessary for all children. Should exercise provoke asthma, prophylactic inhalation of an aerosolized bronchodilator 15 to 30 minutes before exertion may allow active play and can be especially useful for children engaged in competitive sports.

In many children, allergic asthma is associated with allergic rhinitis, and aggressive therapy of the allergic rhinitis will benefit asthma management and should not be ignored. If the offending allergens (which are not easily avoided) are identified, a trial of hyposensitization immunotherapy by injection, with the specific allergen, may be considered. The stresses, both emotional and financial, on the family of a child who has chronic asthma create an environment conducive to psychological problems. Attention to these potential behavioral problems should lessen the anxiety associated with asthma and improve compliance with the total therapeutic program.

PROGNOSIS

In general, the prognosis for a child who has asthma is good. Yet long-term studies of asthmatic patients show abnormal airway hyperreactivity, even among those who have been symptom free for years. Many children whose asthma is intermittent tend to improve during adolescence, with symptoms developing only during viral respiratory infections or strenuous exercise. Of those who have persistent daily wheezing during childhood, however, fewer than 20% become asthma free during adolescence. Thus, persistent daily bronchospasm may indicate an unfavorable prognosis; appropriate therapy should be pursued aggressively so that the child who has asthma can have a normal lifestyle, including regular school attendance, uninterrupted rest at night, appropriate recreation, and enjoyment of participation in sports.

When to Refer

1. Children older than 6 years of age who have persistent asthma should have pulmonary function tests (spirometry) every 1 to 2 years
2. Children who have persistent asthma who require frequent medications should have an allergic evaluation

When to Hospitalize

1. Children who have status asthmaticus who are not responsive to appropriate β antagonists and antiinflammation therapies
2. Children who have asthma who are in impending respiratory failure

REFERENCES

1. Burrows B, et al: Association of asthma with serum IgE levels and skin-test reactivity to allergens, *N Engl J Med* 320:271, 1989.
2. deBenedictis FM, Canny GJ, Levinson H: Progressive nature of childhood asthma, *Lung* 1:278S, 1990.
3. Evans R, et al: National trends in the morbidity and mortality of asthma in the United States, *Chest* 91:655, 1987.
4. Gergen PV, Mulladly DI, Evans R: National survey of prevalence of asthma among children in US: 1976-1980, *Pediatrics* 81:11, 1988.
5. Gurwitz D, Mindorff C, Levinson H: Increased incidence of bronchial reactivity in children with a history of bronchiolitis, *J Pediatr* 98:551, 1981.
6. Jeffrey RK, et al: Bronchial biopsies in asthma, *Am Rev Respir Dis* 140:1745, 1989.
7. Martin AJ, et al: Natural history of asthma from childhood to adult, *Br Med J* 280:1397, 1980.
8. Martinez FD, et al: Asthma and wheezing during the first six years of life, *N Engl J Med* 332:133, 1995.
9. McIntosh K, et al: The association of viral respiratory infections with wheezing in young asthmatic patients, *J Pediatr* 82:578, 1973.
10. National Heart, Lung, and Blood Institute: National Asthma Education Program: *Guidelines for the diagnosis and management of asthma,* Expert Panel Report 2 No 97-405, National Institutes of Health, Bethesda, Md, 1997.
11. Page R, et al: Asthma and selective IgG subclass deficiency: improvement of asthma following IgG replacement therapy, *J Pediatr* 112:127, 1988.
12. Sandford A, et al: The genetics of asthma, *Am J Respir Crit Care Med* 153:1749, 1996.
13. Schiffer CG, Hunt EP: Illness among children: data from the National Health Survey, US Public Health Service Pub No 2074, Washington, DC, 1970, US Government Printing Office.
14. Welliver RC, et al: The development of respiratory syncytial virus-specific IgE and release of histamine in nasopharyngeal secretion after infection, *N Engl J Med* 305:841, 1981.

189 Atopic Dermatitis

Ana M. Duarte • Lawrence A. Schachner

Atopic dermatitis (AD) is a multifactorial, chronic skin disorder that is common in children. It sometimes is referred to as *eczema,* which is a general term used to describe a condition of redness, scaling, vesicles, and crusting. Eczematous eruptions include AD, seborrheic dermatitis, contact dermatitis, and dermatophyte infection.

EPIDEMIOLOGY

AD is predominantly a disease of infancy and childhood. In 60% of affected individuals, the onset occurs in the first year of life; 85% have symptoms by age 5.[16] Studies indicate an increasing prevalence in developed countries, with as much as 10% to 20% of the general population having atopic disease. In the United States the prevalence of AD increased from 3% in the 1960s to 10% in the 1980s.[10,19] AD affects all races, but it is particularly common among whites and Asians.[17] Males and females are affected equally.[18] As many as 50% of children who have acquired immunodeficiency syndrome (AIDS) also have AD.

GENETICS

AD appears to be inherited in a polygenic pattern. When one parent is affected, there is a 60% chance the child will have AD; if both parents are affected, the likelihood increases to 80%.[9,12]

CLINICAL FEATURES

AD is characterized by three distinct stages—infantile, childhood, and adult. The patient may manifest acute dermatitis (Fig. 189-1), which is characterized by severe pruritus, redness, vesicles, and exudation, or may have a subacute pattern (Fig. 189-2), with pruritus, redness, and scaling. Over time, the lesions show the changes of chronic dermatitis, marked by excoriations, lichenification (thickened skin and deeper skin lines), and postinflammatory hypopigmentation or hyperpigmentation (Fig. 189-3).

The infantile stage begins at about 3 months of age and lasts through the first 2 years of life. The eruption begins on the cheeks and extensor surfaces of the arms and legs. The hair is dry, and the scalp often is scaly. The dermatitis usually is a more acute form.

The childhood stage begins at about age 3 years and lasts through puberty. The areas affected most often are the antecubital and popliteal areas, the neck, and the flexor surfaces of the wrists and ankles (Fig. 189-4). Clinically, the patients in this stage display a more subacute and chronic dermatitis.

The adult stage, which lasts from puberty onward, is an extension of the childhood stage. Additional clinical signs include diffuse involvement of the body, with xerosis, lichenification, and central facial pallor.

Associated Clinical Manifestations

Dennie-Morgan folds (infraorbital folds) and allergic shiners (infraorbital darkening), as well as hyperlinear palms and soles, frequently are seen in patients who have AD.

Twenty percent of patients who have AD have ichthyosis vulgaris, marked by areas of scaling, on the lower extremities. Keratosis pilaris, characterized by follicular keratotic papules, affects the lateral surfaces of the upper or lower extremities predominantly, although the face also may be involved.

Lichen spinulosus, marked by annular, grouped follicular keratotic papules, may occur on the trunk and extremities (Fig. 189-5). Pityriasis alba, a condition of ill-defined, mildly scaling hypopigmented patches, occurs primarily on the face, although other areas often are involved (Fig. 189-6).

Cataracts (anterior or posterior subcapsular form), keratoconjunctivitis, and keratoconus also are seen in AD patients. Periodic ophthalmological examinations are recommended.

Juvenile plantar dermatosis (Fig. 189-7), which manifests as redness, scaling, and painful fissuring of the plantar surfaces of the feet, often is worse in atopic individuals. Treatment involves applying a moderate-potency topical corticosteroid to the fissured areas for 7 days, followed by a low-potency corticosteroid in combination with a topical antibiotic. If the condition fails to improve, a dermatologist should be consulted.

Nummular eczema, a condition marked by coin-shaped, scaling, red lesions, also is seen in association with AD (Fig. 189-8). The treatment is the same as that for AD (see the section on management later in this chapter).

DIAGNOSIS

The criteria for diagnosing AD were defined by Hanifin and Lobitz.[7] These criteria are presented in Box 189-1.

PATHOGENESIS

AD is characterized by two basic immune abnormalities: an increase in immunoglobulin E (IgE) and a decrease in

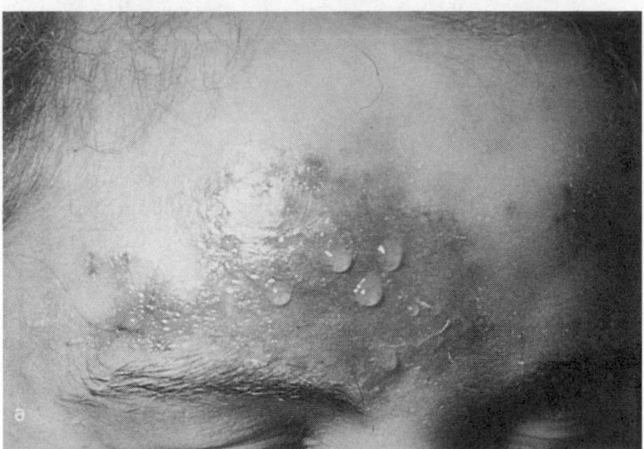

Fig. 189-1 Acute dermatitis characterized by redness and vesiculation.

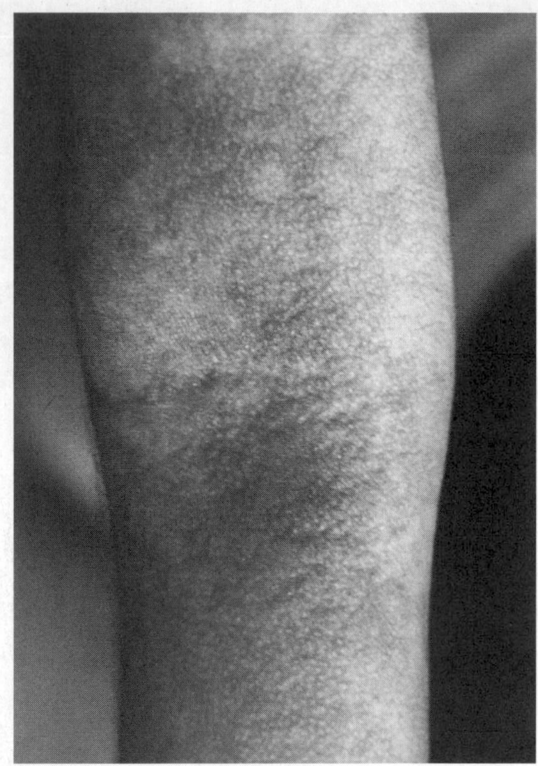

Fig. 189-2 Subactute dermatitis of the antecubital region. The skin is pink and dry and shows mild scaling.

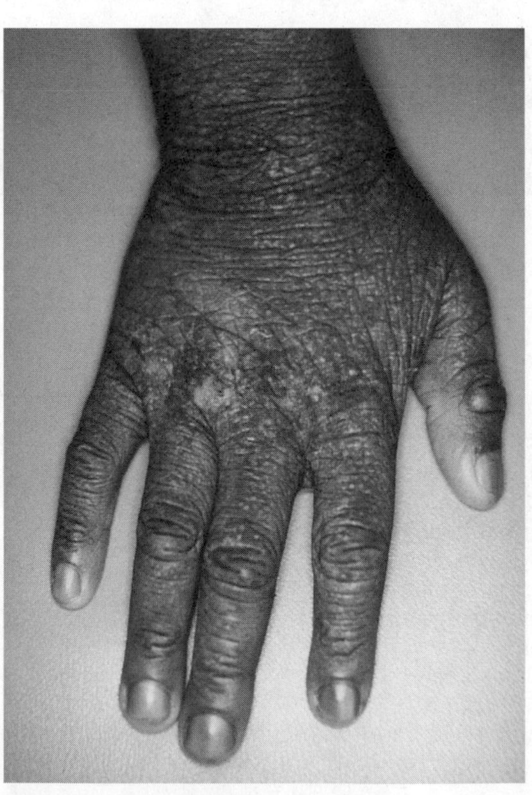

Fig. 189-3 Chronic dermatitis. The skin is dry and hyperpigmented, and the skin markings are accentuated.

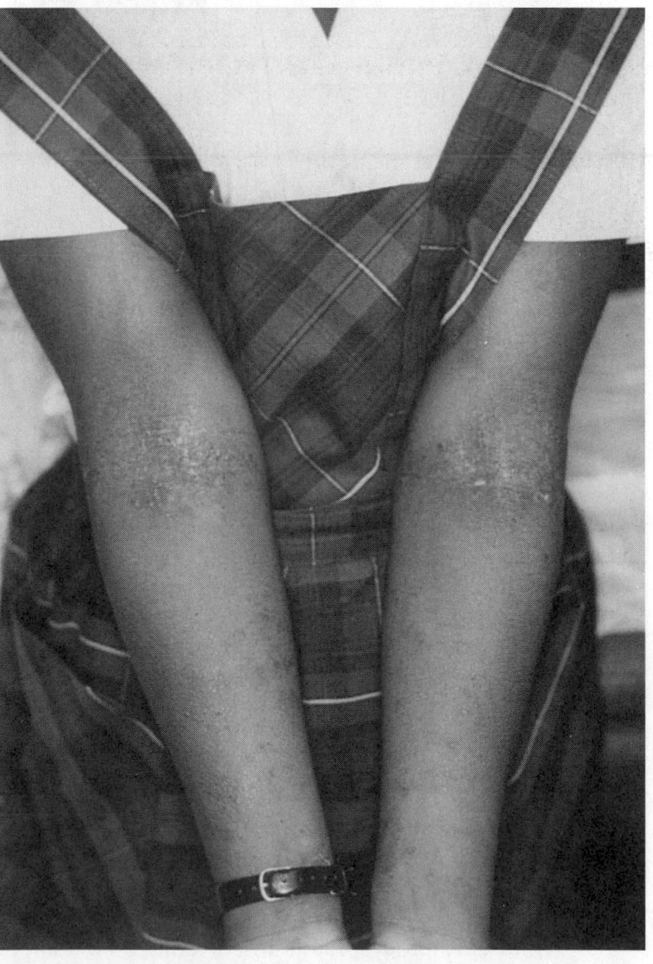

Fig. 189-4 Atopic dermatitis, childhood stage. Note the flexural distribution of the eruption.

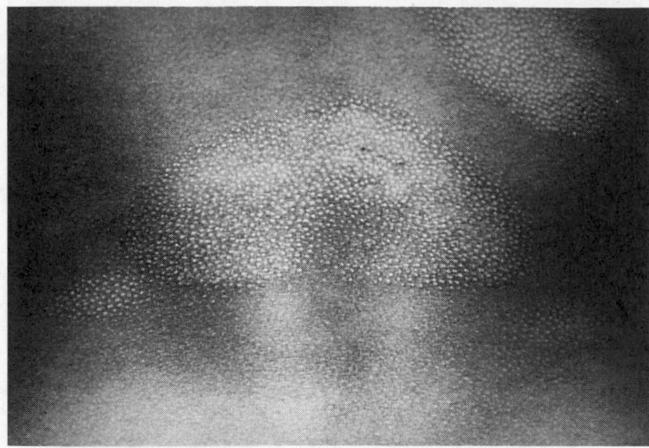

Fig. 189-5 Lichen spinulosus.

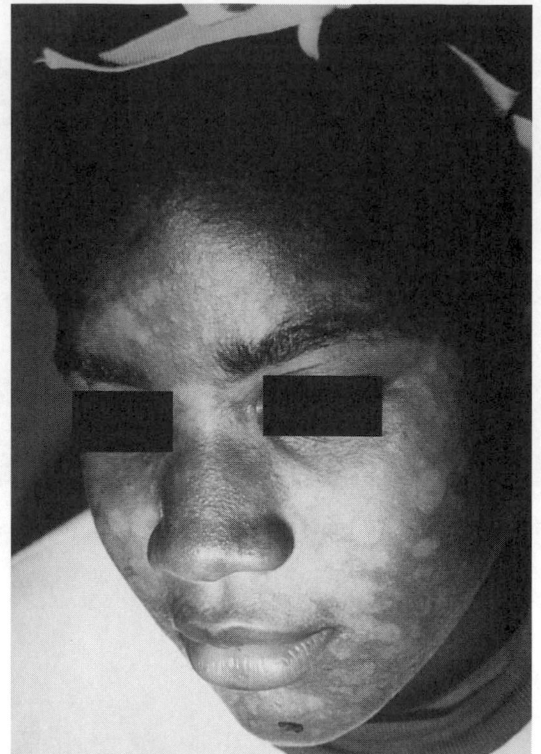

Fig. 189-6 Pityriasis alba.

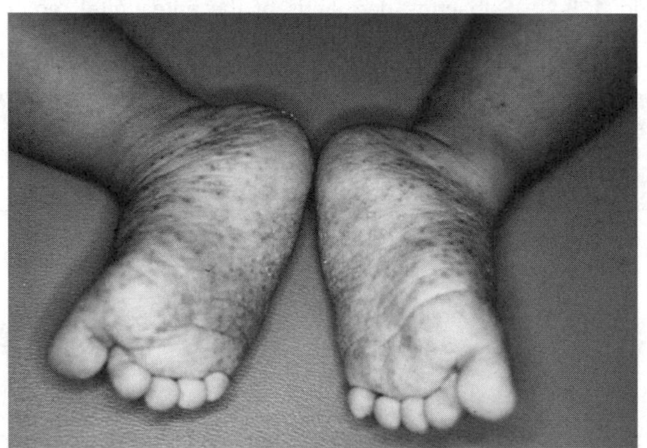

Fig. 189-7 Juvenile plantar dermatosis.

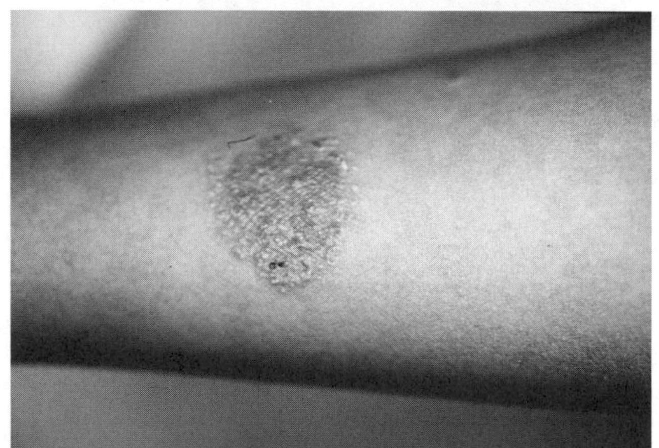

Fig. 189-8 Nummular eczema.

BOX 189-1

CRITERIA FOR THE DIAGNOSIS OF ATOPIC DERMATITIS

Major Criteria (All Three Must Be Present)

1. Pruritus
2. Typical morphology and distribution
   a. Facial and extensor involvement during infancy and early childhood
   b. Flexural lichenification and linearity by adolescence
3. Chronic or recurring dermatitis

Minor Criteria (Two or More Must Be Present)

1. Personal or family history of atopy (e.g., asthma, allergic rhinoconjunctivitis, atopic dermatitis)
2. Immediate skin test reactivity
3. White dermatographism and/or delayed blanch to cholinergic agents
4. Anterior subcapsular cataracts

Associated Conditions (Four or More Must Be Present)

1. Xerosis/ichthyosis/hyperlinear palms
2. Pityriasis alba
3. Keratosis pilaris
4. Facial pallor/infraorbital darkening
5. Dennie-Morgan fold
6. Elevated serum IgE
7. Keratoconus
8. Nonspecific hand dermatitis
9. Recurring cutaneous infections

T-suppressor cells. Also, production of gamma-interferon (INF-gamma) and interleukin-4 (IL-4), which play reciprocal roles in regulating IgE production, is abnormal. Production of INF-gamma is inadequate, and production of IL-4 is excessive.[21] These disturbances affect IgE-mediated activation of mast cells and mononuclear cells, which includes the release of histamine and other pharmacologically active mediators, resulting in the clinical manifestations of AD.

DIFFERENTIAL DIAGNOSIS

The differential diagnosis of AD includes disorders characterized by an eczematous eruption. These include seborrheic dermatitis, contact dermatitis (allergic and irritant forms), and dermatophyte infection, as well as other immunological and metabolic disorders.

Seborrheic dermatitis is a disease of unknown cause that affects infants and some adolescents. It usually manifests in the neonatal period and consists of asymptomatic, greasy, yellow, scaling plaques. When these occur on the scalp, the condition is called *cradle cap*. Areas typically affected include the flexural creases, the axillae, the retroauricular area, and the neck. Seborrheic dermatitis may occur with AD (see Chapter 259, Seborrheic Dermatitis).

Contact dermatitis may be a primary irritant reaction, resulting from application of an irritating substance, or the result of true allergic sensitization (a type 4 delayed hypersensitivity reaction). The most common causes of allergic contact dermatitis are poison ivy, nickel, and rubber. The lesions, which may be acute, subacute, or chronic, occur on exposed sites in the distribution of the contactant (Fig. 189-9). A careful history and patch testing can help determine the cause (see Chapter 199, Contact Dermatitis).

Dermatophyte infection (Fig. 189-10), which is characterized by red, scaling, annular plaques on the trunk and interdigital maceration and scaling of the feet, may be confused with nummular eczema and juvenile plantar dermatosis. A potassium hydroxide preparation will identify the septate hyphae.

A detailed discussion of other disorders that may produce eczematous lesions is beyond the scope of this chapter. Some of these diseases are Wiskott-Aldrich syndrome, Leiner's disease, histiocytosis X, ataxia telangiectasia, ahistidinemia, agammaglobulinemia, Hartnup disease, Hurler's syndrome, and phenylketonuria.

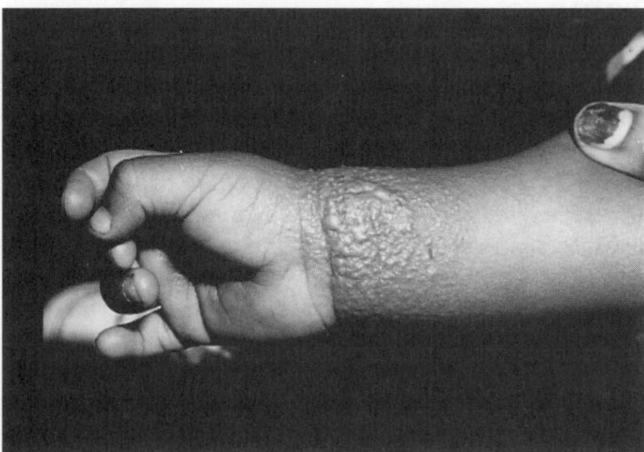

Fig. 189-9 Contact dermatitis caused by poison ivy. (Courtesy Dr. Harvey Blank.)

COMPLICATIONS OF ATOPIC DERMATITIS

Cutaneous Infection

Staphylococcal infections (impetigo). Many patients who have AD have significant colonization with *Staphylococcus aureus* and may easily develop a secondary infection, known as *impetigo* (Fig. 189-11), in areas of dermatitis. This infection usually responds well to topical or oral antibiotics. However, an *S. aureus* superinfection may be widespread and serious. Such patients may have generalized exfoliative erythroderma, which requires hospitalization for aggressive skin care and systemic antibiotics.

Herpes simplex infections. Eczema herpeticum (Fig. 189-12), also known as *Kaposi varicelliform eruption,* is a widespread herpes simplex virus or varicella virus infection of the skin that occurs in patients who have AD. The eruption may be serious, especially in very young or immunodeficient patients. The morbidity and mortality rates are greater than those for superinfection with *S. aureus*. Patients who have eczema herpeticum may require treatment with acyclovir.

Human papillomavirus. Verruca vulgaris (warts) also may occur more commonly in AD patients. Various types of treatment can be used, including topical vesicants (e.g., Duofilm or Cantharone). Some cases may require more

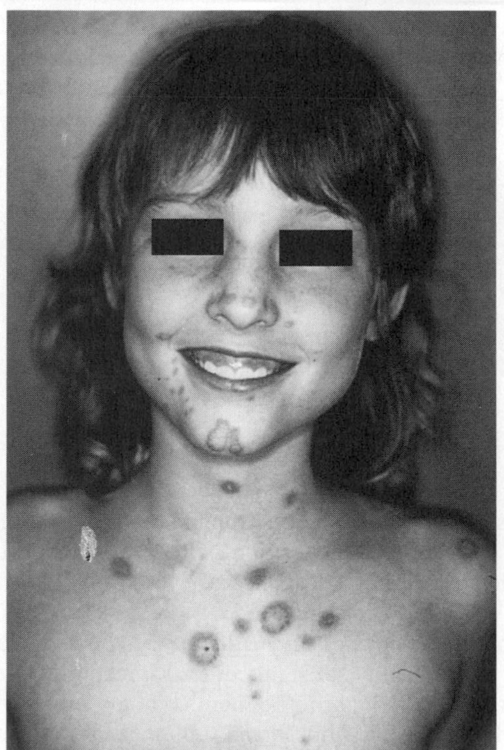

Fig. 189-10 Dermatophyte infection.

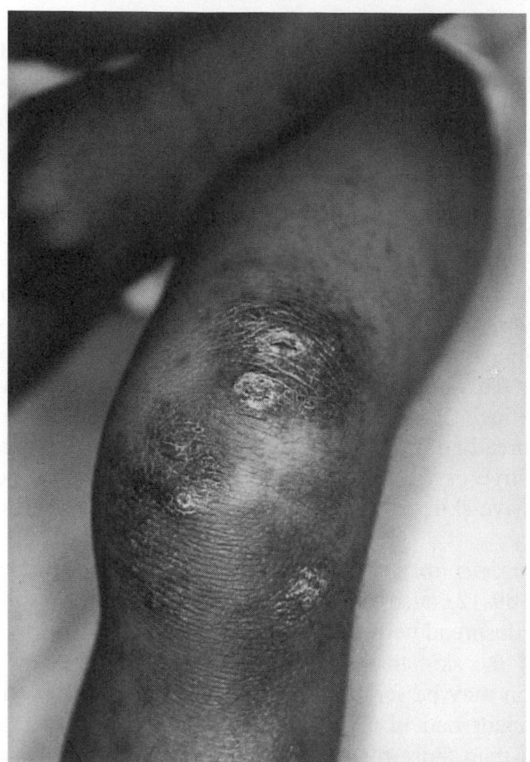

Fig. 189-11 Impetigo.

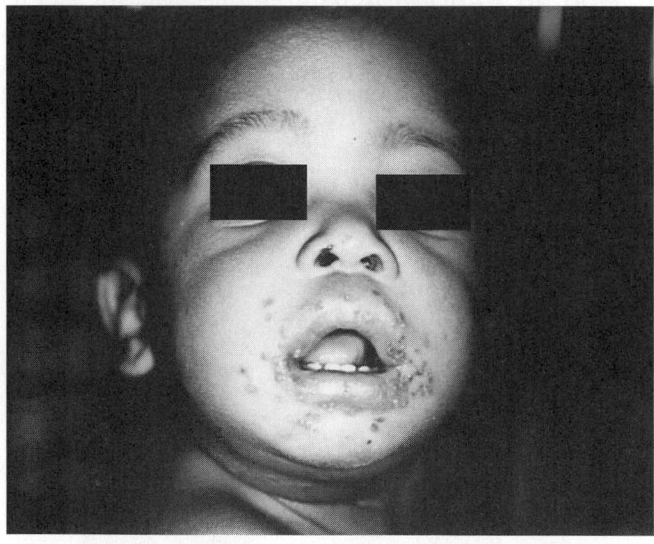

Fig. 189-12 Eczema herpeticum.

aggressive treatment, such as immunomodulaters (e.g., interferon), cryotherapy, or ablation with a carbon dioxide laser (see Chapter 274, Verrucae [Warts]).

Molluscum contagiosum. Molluscum contagiosum is a cutaneous, self-limited viral infection caused by a pox virus. It is thought to be more common in patients with AD, who may have widespread eruptions. Treatment is optional. In extensive cases, manual expression, cryotherapy, or topical applications of cantharidin (Cantharone) may be helpful.

Short Stature

In children who have severe AD (i.e., involvement of more than half of the body surface area), linear growth may be diminished.[13] Also, elimination diets and long-term treatment with corticosteroids may further retard growth.[13] The release of growth hormone may be diminished in some children who have AD who show growth retardation.[4]

MANAGEMENT

Treatment of AD is directed primarily at relieving inflammation, dryness, and pruritus, treating superinfection by *S. aureus,* and managing other associated conditions.

Inflammation

Inflammation is treated best with corticosteroids. A cream should be used for acute dermatitis (weeping, red lesions). For chronic dermatitis, in which dryness and lichenification predominate, an ointment base is more therapeutic.

Low-potency steroids (e.g., 1% hydrocortisone ointment or cream) can be used on the face and groin twice a day as needed. *Strong, halogenated steroids should not be used for the face, axillae, or groin.* A midpotency corticosteroid (e.g., 0.1% triamcinolone acetonide cream or ointment) may be applied to lesions on the extremities or trunk, as needed twice a day. Systemic corticosteroids are used only in rare cases because of the many undesirable side effects and the rebound flares that occur when the drug is discontinued. As a last resort, prednisone may be given at 1 mg/kg daily for 5 days and then tapered slowly over the next 2 weeks.

Some patients may respond to a modified Goeckerman regimen, which involves applying tar to the affected area and then exposing it to ultraviolet light (using sunlight or a light box). Narrowband UVB (311 nm) has proven to be superior to conventional ultraviolet therapy. This treatment is used in addition to the course of topical corticosteroids described in the paragraph above.

Newer treatments include immunosuppressive agents such as (1) topical tacrolimus (FK506)[14] in concentrations ranging from 0.1 to 0.3% twice a day, (2) oral cyclosporine (Neoral),[2] (3) interferon gamma,[5] and (4) thymopentin.[11]

Dryness

Dryness can be alleviated by having the patient take lukewarm baths instead of showers, which are more drying. The bath should last only about 5 minutes, and a mild soap, such as unscented Dove, Cetaphil, or Lowila, should be used. The patient should be patted dry (not rubbed) with a towel, and an oil-based emollient (e.g., Vaseline) should be applied immediately to unaffected skin and the prescribed corticosteroid to areas of dermatitis. This effectively seals in moisture.

Pruritus

Pruritus can be relieved with newer nonsedating antihistamines such as Loratadine and Stelazine alone and in combination with hydroxyzine or diphenhydramine, which are more likely to induce drowsiness. The latter is especially useful at bedtime, so that the child sleeps more peacefully.

Behavior modification, such as teaching the child to rub rather than scratch and having him or her wear mittens to bed, will lessen the itch-scratch cycle. Keeping the child's nails cut short is essential to help reduce skin damage and superinfection.

Staphylococcal Superinfection

A staphylococcal superinfection may manifest as a flare in the patient's dermatitis. Local infections are treated with topical antibiotics, and oral medications are used for more extensive involvement. Cultures of skin and nares may help identify appropriate antibiotic sensitivities, as well as a nasal carrier state, in which case Bactroban applied twice a day to the nares for 5 days may eradicate the bacteria.

Associated Manifestations

Ichthyosis vulgaris can be treated with keratolytics in combination with emollients. Treatment for keratosis pilaris and lichen spinulosus involves the use of topical isotretinoin, keratolytics, and emollients. Pityriasis alba may improve if treated with low-potency topical steroids, emollients, and sunscreen. As mentioned previously, juvenile plantar dermatosis may respond to a short course of a moderate-potency corticosteroid followed by a low-potency corticosteroid in combination with a topical antibiotic.

Chinese plant extracts have been found to be of therapeutic value compared with a placebo in many patients who have AD.[20] However, long-term, well-controlled studies are needed to evaluate hepatotoxicity further. The medications are available in pill, tablet, or liquid form.

Dietary Management

Dietary management of patients who have AD remains controversial. However, for patients whose food allergy has been identified (peanuts, milk, and eggs account for 80% of adverse reactions in patients who have AD), eliminating these allergens has been shown to improve the dermatitis. Prophylactic avoidance of food allergens, both for infants (i.e., breast-feeding exclusively for the first 6 months) and for lactating mothers who have a strong family history of atopy, may be helpful in some cases of AD.[8,22] Measuring the level of beta-lactoglobulin and soya protein antibody in affected children may help predict the response to an exclusionary diet.[3]

Oral sodium cromoglycate is useful in treating children who have AD that is aggravated by food hypersensitivities when the food or foods have high nutritional value or are very common in the diet and therefore cannot be eliminated easily.[1]

Environmental Control

Measures to control house dust mites may improve AD in patients who have this allergy. Such measures include encasing pillows and mattresses in plastic liners; eliminating plants, stuffed animals, drapes, and carpeting from the home; dusting frequently; and using acaricides (mite killers). Determining IgG antibody titers against Der P1 Ag (the major allergenic component of house dust mite extract) may predict which children will benefit from these control measures.[3]

The patient's environment should be kept cool, and 100% cotton clothing is recommended; wool should be avoided.

PSYCHOSOCIAL CONSIDERATIONS

AD is a chronic condition that very often is physically and psychologically distressing to both the patient and the family. Children who have a moderate to severe form of the disease often are irritable, restless, aggressive, and manipulative. Stress reduction and relaxation in the form of massage therapy may be an important therapeutic adjunct. Behavior modification directed to teaching the child not to scratch is important to relieving the itch-scratch cycle. In some cases, referral for professional family and individual counseling may be appropriate.

The child's activities, including sports, should be as "mainstream" as possible. If the child enjoys swimming, a thin barrier of petroleum jelly should be applied to the skin before the child enters the pool. He or she should shower quickly upon getting out and then reapply the petroleum to counteract the drying, irritating effects of chlorine.

PROGNOSIS

AD tends to resolve with age. Studies have shown clearing rates up to 40% of patients.[15] Those who have the most severe AD, as well as those who have food allergies, are more likely to have persistent cutaneous disease and respiratory involvement.[6,15] Hyperactive airway disease, or asthma, is found in up to 30% of cases. (See Chapter 188, Asthma.)

REFERENCES

1. Businco L, Cantani A: Oral sodium cromoglycate in the management of atopic dermatitis in children, *Allergy Proc* 12:333, 1991.
2. Camp RDR, et al: Cyclosporin A in severe, therapy-resistant atopic dermatitis: report of an international workshop, April 1993. *Br J Dermatol* 129:217, 1993.
3. Casimir GJ, et al: Atopic dermatitis: role of food and house dust mite allergens, *Pediatrics* 92:252, 1993.
4. David TJ, Ferguson AP, Newton RW: Nocturnal growth hormone release in children with short stature and atopic dermatitis, *Acta Derm Venereol* 71:229, 1991.
5. Friedman RM: Interferons. In Oppenheim JJ, Shevach EM, editors: *Immunophysiology: the role of cells and cytokines in immunity and inflammation,* New York, 1990, Oxford University Press.
6. Guillet G, Guillet MH: Natural history of sensitization in atopic dermatitis: a 3-year follow-up in 250 children: food allergy and high risk of respiratory symptoms, *Arch Dermatol* 128:187, 1992.
7. Hanifin JM, Lobitz WC: Newer concepts of atopic dermatology, *Arch Dermatol* 113:663, 1977.
8. Kajosaari M, Saarinen UM: Prophylaxis of atopic disease by six months total solid food elimination, *Acta Paediatr Scand* 27:411, 1983.
9. Kaufman HS, Frick OL: The development of allergy in infants of allergic parents: a prospective study concerning the role of heredity, *Ann Allergy* 38:339, 1983.
10. Larsson PA, Liden S: Prevalence of skin diseases among adolescents 12-16 years of age, *Acta Derm Venereol* 160:415, 1980.
11. Leung DY, et al: Thymopentin therapy reduces the clinical severity of atopic dermatitis, *J Allergy Clin Immunol* 85:927, 1990.
12. Luoma R, Koivikko A, Viander M: Development of asthma, allergic rhinitis, and atopic dermatitis by age five years, *Allergy* 38:339, 1983.

13. Massarano AA, et al: Growth in atopic eczema, *Arch Dis Child* 68:677, 1993.
14. Meigassner JG, Stutz A: Immunosuppressive macrolides of the type FK506: a novel class of topical agents for treatment of skin diseases? *J Invest Dermatol* 98:851, 1992.
15. Musgrive K, Morgan JK: Infantile eczema, *Br J Dermatol* 95:365, 1976.
16. Rajka G: Some aetiological data on atopic dermatitis. Paper presented at the Second International Symposium on Atopic Dermatitis, Norway, 1984.
17. Rajka G: Clinical aspects. In Rajka G, editor: *Essential aspects of atopic dermatitis*, Berlin, 1989, Springer-Verlag.
18. Schachner L, Ling NS, Press S: A statistical analysis of a pediatric dermatology clinic, *Pediatr Dermatol* 2:157, 1983.
19. Schultz-Larsen F: Atopic dermatitis: etiological studies based on a twin population, thesis, Copenhagen, 1985, Legeforeningens.
20. Sheehan MP, Atherton DJ: A controlled trial of traditional Chinese medicinal plants in widespread nonexudative atopic dermatitis, *Br J Dermatol* 126:179, 1992.
21. Tang M, Kemp A, Varigos G: IL-4 and interferon-gamma production in children with atopic disease, *Clin Exp Immunol* 92:120, 1993.
22. Zeiger RS, et al: Effect of combined maternal and infant food allergen avoidance on development of atopy in early infancy: a randomized study, *J Allergy Clin Immunol* 84:72, 1989.

190 Bacterial Skin Infections

Judith V. Williams • Donald P. Lookingbill

Bacterial infections of the skin are common.[10] Most often they are caused by gram-positive bacteria, specifically *Staphylococcus aureus* and group A streptococci.[1,18] The clinical disease that results depends on the infection's location within the skin. For example, staphylococcal impetigo involves only the most superficial layer of the epidermis; streptococcal cellulitis is an infection deep in the dermis, even involving subcutaneous fat.

STAPHYLOCOCCAL IMPETIGO

Etiology

The answer to which bacteria most commonly cause impetigo—*S. aureus* or group A beta-hemolytic streptococci—has changed over time.[2,12] Initially, impetigo was thought to be caused primarily by *S. aureus*, but studies of children living on the Red Lake Indian Reservation in Minnesota provided evidence that impetigo was caused primarily by group A streptococci.[5,8] Dillon's work[7] supported this thesis. The exception was staphylococcal bullous impetigo, which was not encountered often in these surveys. More recent studies, however, have shown that most cases of impetigo are caused by *S. aureus*.[2]

In nonbullous staphylococcal impetigo, the skin lesions may start with small vesicles or pustules, but these often are not evident by the time the physician sees the patient. Crusts, usually honey colored, are seen instead. Removing these crusts exposes a moist, glistening base, which is a very superficial erosion of the epidermis; culturing usually reveals *S. aureus*.

The differences between staphylococcal and streptococcal impetigo are summarized in Table 190-1. For the purposes of this chapter, the staphylococcus-induced lesion is designated staphylococcal impetigo. Although staphylococcal impetigo may be bullous, it most often is not. The streptococcus-induced lesion, which is designated streptococcal pyoderma, is a more inflammatory process and is discussed later.

History

With staphylococcal impetigo, the patient usually has no history of preceding trauma to the skin. Mild to moderate itching may be associated with the lesions. Other family members also may be affected.

Physical Findings

Staphylococcal impetigo is found most commonly on the face and may appear as single or multiple lesions. Lesions may be scattered elsewhere on the body, as well. As mentioned previously, the usual findings are yellow- or honey-colored crusts, which when removed reveal a pink, superficially eroded, glistening base (Fig. 190-1). The culture sample should be obtained from this base. With bullous impetigo, intact bullae, if present, contain deceptively clear fluid. These blisters break easily, leaving behind a superficially denuded skin surface covered with a thin brown varnish-like crust that is marginated by a thin rim of loose, ragged epidermis that represents the remnants of the blister roof (Fig. 190-2). With staphylococcal impetigo, surrounding erythema is minimal and regional lymphadenopathy is rare.

Laboratory Studies

A Gram stain of either the clear blister fluid or the serum underlying the crusts shows gram-positive cocci. Cultures grow *S. aureus,* usually resistant to penicillin.

Differential Diagnosis

Herpes simplex virus (HSV) infection is the condition most often confused with impetigo. Clinical clues that suggest herpes rather than impetigo are as follows:

1. Intact vesicles are more likely to be appreciated by both the patient and the physician in recurrent HSV than in impetigo. In herpes simplex, as the vesicles age they become cloudy and ultimately result in crusts that also may be honey colored. This crusted phase most often causes the diagnostic confusion.
2. Herpes simplex tends to be a recurrent condition, with the recurrences usually occurring in the same location (usually oral and perioral lesions). This is not the case with impetigo.
3. In impetigo, Gram staining shows numerous gram-positive cocci. In herpes simplex, Wright staining of a scraping from the base of a crust (or preferably a vesicle) reveals multinucleated giant cells.

Psychosocial Considerations

Given the potential infectious nature of both staphylococcal and streptococcal skin infections, school nurses are appropriately concerned with this disease, and a child may be asked to leave school until it is treated. Once treatment is begun, it probably is safe for the child to return to school, even though it will take at least several days for the lesions to heal.

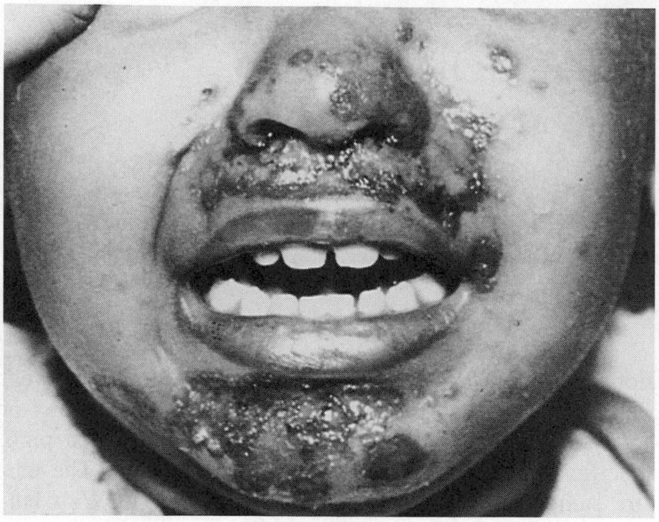

Fig. 190-1 Classic impetigo marked by superficial oozing and crusted ulcers. Note involvement of nares—the nose is the likely source of the infective organism.

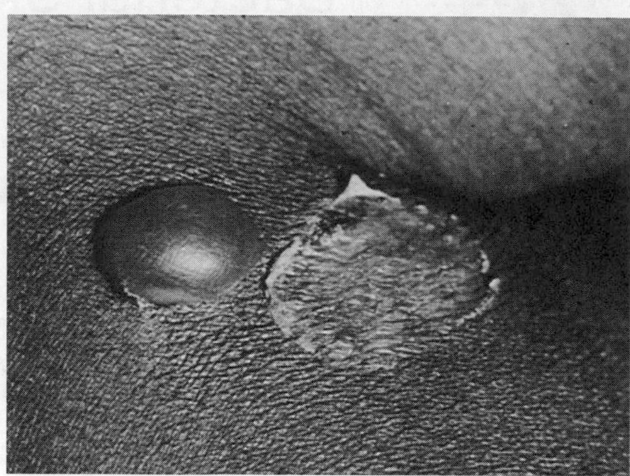

Fig. 190-2 Bullous impetigo. The roof of the bulla is thin and delicate; the contents consist of some leukocytes that have settled at the inferior pole and some slightly turbid supernatant fluid. The larger adjacent bulla already has ruptured and discharged its contents. The delicate roof has collapsed onto the base. Lesions of this type may be caused by exfoliatin-producing organisms.

Table 190-1 Features of Staphylococcal Impetigo Versus Streptococcal Pyoderma

	Staphylococcal Impetigo		
Feature	**Honey Crusted**	**Bullous**	**Streptococcal Pyoderma**
Most common location	Face	Trunk	Extremities (usually lower)
Nature of early lesion	Vesicle	Bulla	Pustule
Appearance of crust	Honey colored	Thin, brown, varnishlike	Thick, usually brown
Depth of lesion	Superficial	Superficial	Deep
Appearance when crust is removed	Shallow, glistening erosion	Shallow, glistening erosion	Ulcer
Surrounding erythema	None to minimal	None to minimal	Moderate to marked
History of preceding trauma	No	No	Yes
Other nomenclature	Impetigo	Bullous impetigo	Impetigo, nonbullous impetigo, ecthyma

Management

Both topical and systemic antibiotics have been advocated for treating staphylococcal impetigo. Traditional topical preparations that contain bacitracin or neomycin, either alone or in combination, have been used, especially for small lesions of staphylococcal origin. The infected area should be washed carefully and the crusts gently removed, if possible, three times daily before the antibiotic cream or ointment is applied. For more extensive lesions—and, in the opinion of some physicians, for all impetiginous lesions—systemic antibiotics should be used. Currently, most strains of *S. aureus,* including those encountered in outpatients, are penicillinase producing; thus, penicillin is *not* appropriate for treating this disease. Appropriate oral antibiotics include erythromycin, a penicillinase-resistant penicillin (e.g., dicloxacillin), or cephalexin.[6] The treatment course should be 7 to 10 days.

Mupirocin topical antibiotic ointment has been reported to equal or exceed the efficacy of oral erythromycin in the treatment of bacterial impetigo.[15] A cream form also is available.

Complications and Prognosis

With appropriate antibiotic therapy, prompt healing is expected; most patients show marked improvement within several days. Bacteriological cures occur within 7 to 10 days in nearly all cases. If the condition does not respond rapidly to therapy, the infection may be caused by an antibiotic-resistant strain. In such cases, the result of the initial culture and sensitivities serves as a guide in selecting an alternative antibiotic.

Inasmuch as acute glomerulonephritis is not a sequel of staphylococcal infection and streptococcal infection may be, the importance of discriminating between staphylococcal impetigo and streptococcal pyoderma assumes even greater importance. In this regard, the features of streptococcal pyoderma should be compared with those of staphylococcal impetigo (see Table 190-1).

STREPTOCOCCAL PYODERMA

Etiology

In contrast to the superficial nature of staphylococcal impetigo, which involves mainly the top layers of the epidermis, streptococcal pyoderma frequently extends through the epidermal layer into the underlying dermis. The process may start with small erythematous papules and rapidly proceed through vesicular, pustular, and crusted stages, during which it could be clinically confused with staphylococcal impetigo. *Ecthyma* is a term used for the more fully developed streptococcal lesion.

Streptococcal skin disease is more common in warm, humid environments; higher humidity favors the survival of group A streptococci on normal skin. Presumably, trauma to the skin results in inoculation, followed by infection.

History

Streptococcal pyoderma may occur in epidemics among children of lower socioeconomic status who live in crowded conditions in warm, humid environments. In contrast to staphylococcal impetigo, the streptococcal skin lesions occur most commonly on the lower extremities, where they usually are preceded by trauma such as a scratch or insect bite. Family members also may be affected.

Physical Findings

The early lesion is a pustule (hence the term *pyo*derma) with surrounding erythema, but the more advanced lesion of ecthyma is seen more often. At first glance, this looks like a thick, usually brown crust surrounded by erythema. When the crust is removed, an actual ulcer is revealed (Fig. 190-3) (in contrast to the superficial erosion underlying the crust of a staphylococcal lesion). Also in contrast to staphylococcal impetigo, regional adenopathy often is present with streptococcal pyoderma.

Laboratory Studies

A culture sample taken from the base of the denuded ulcer grows group A beta-hemolytic streptococci. *S. aureus* occasionally is recovered concomitantly, in which case it is thought to be a secondary invader. Because some strains of group A streptococci are nephritogenic, screening for renal complications may be done by obtaining a urinalysis 2 to 3 weeks after the onset of infection.

Differential Diagnosis

Ecthyma gangrenosa is an uncommon but serious manifestation of *Pseudomonas* septicemia. Clinical features that help differentiate this lesion from streptococcal ecthyma are (1) the location (usually inguinal or axillary folds), (2) the lesion's appearance (a deeper ulcer covered with a tightly adherent, black [gangrenous] crust), and (3) the host (a seriously ill, usually immunocompromised patient who manifests other signs of sepsis).

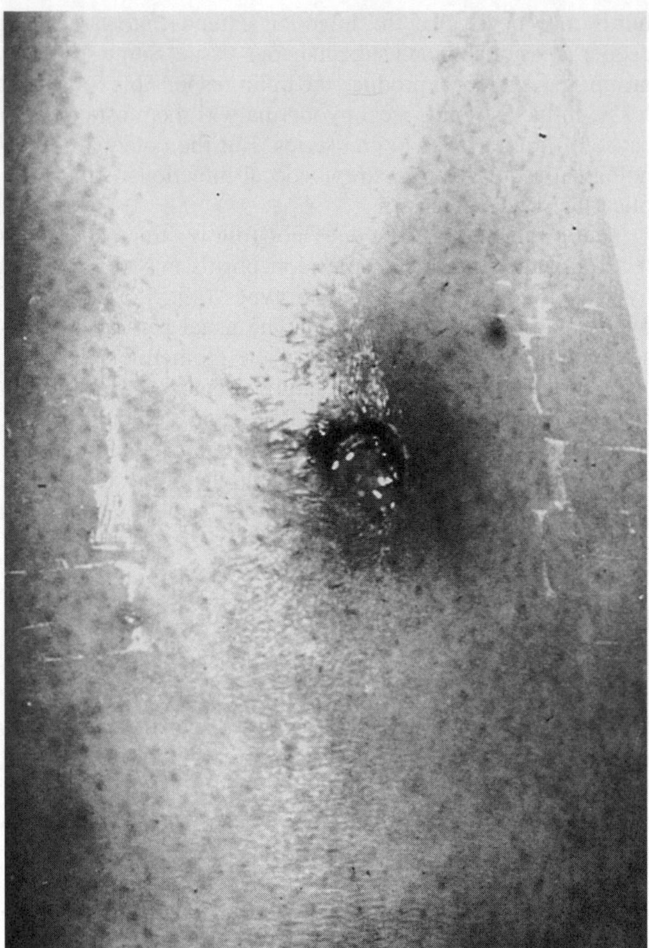

Fig. 190-3 Streptococcal pyoderma (ecthyma). After the crust is removed, the depth of this ulcerative lesion can be appreciated. The surrounding erythema and the location on the lower leg also are typical of this streptococcal lesion.

Management

Streptococcal pyoderma is treated with antibiotics, although the most appropriate route of administration is still a matter of debate. Some evidence indicates that applying topical antibiotics to scratches and insect bites reduces the incidence of subsequent pyoderma;[4] thus, topical antibiotics may be advocated prophylactically for traumatic skin lesions.[13] Although topical mupirocin has proven effective for impetigo caused by group A streptococci, systemic antibiotics still are recommended for streptococcal infections, particularly if the infection is extensive. Injectable benzathine penicillin G is effective, but a 7- to 10-day course of oral penicillin or erythromycin often is used with compliant patients. Penicillin treatment occasionally fails, presumably because of the persistence of coexisting penicillinase-producing *S. aureus* organisms.

Complications

Complications are uncommon, although both local and systemic problems can result from streptococcal pyoderma. Cellulitis may develop if the infection extends into larger and deeper areas of skin and subcutaneous tissue. Some strains of group A streptococci produce the toxin responsible for scarlet fever; in fact, streptococcal pyoderma was the most common cause of scarlet fever in one series. But the potential immunological sequelae from streptococcal infections is the complication of most concern.

Acute rheumatic fever does not follow streptococcal infection of the skin, but glomerulonephritis may. It is caused by only a few nephritogenic serotypes (49, 55, and 57) of pyoderma-inducing streptococci. The usual period from onset of infection to development of the glomerulonephritis is 18 to 21 days. Even though treating streptococcal pyoderma has not been proven to prevent this nephritic complication, treatment nonetheless is recommended. Systemic antibiotic therapy clears the skin infection and helps to reduce the spread of streptococcal infection to the patient's playmates and family.

Prognosis

The aforementioned complications are uncommon, and in most patients the lesions heal uneventfully. Because they are deeper, streptococcal lesions often take longer than staphylococcal lesions to heal; however, bacteriological cures usually are accomplished within a week. If a prompt response is not achieved, a secondary infection from a penicillinase-producing staphylococcal strain should be considered, particularly if penicillin was used for treatment. Erythromycin-resistant strains of group A streptococci also may be encountered.

FOLLICULITIS

Etiology

Bacterial folliculitis is a moderately common disorder that primarily affects older children and young adults. It is an infection of the hair follicles, caused almost exclusively by *S. aureus*. In rare cases the infection is caused by gram-negative organisms; this occurs occasionally in patients whose acne is being treated with antibiotics.[11] Also, with the recent popularity of hot tubs and whirlpools, some of which become contaminated, *Pseudomonas aeruginosa* has been identified as the cause of an uncommon and unusual type of folliculitis (hot tub dermatitis), which causes pruritic papules and pustules on the trunk and proximal extremities. The lesions usually clear without treatment, although antipruritics should be used. In the usual case, however, *S. aureus* is the responsible pathogen, and it is this type of infection that is the subject of discussion here.

History

Staphylococcal folliculitis appears most commonly as a chronic, smoldering eruption unaccompanied by symptoms, although occasionally a patient has mild discomfort or pruritus.

Physical Findings

The lesions in staphylococcal folliculitis usually are located on the buttocks and upper portion of the thighs, over which individual small papules and pustules are scattered. The key to the diagnosis is that on close inspection, hairs can be seen growing out of the very center of many of the lesions.

Laboratory Studies

In the typical case, culturing usually is not necessary. If, however, the presentation is atypical and laboratory confirmation is desired, the contents of a fresh pustule should be cultured.

Differential Diagnosis

Clinically, folliculitis caused by gram-negative organisms differs from staphylococcal folliculitis in its distribution, with lesions occurring primarily on the face and shoulders. Hot tub folliculitis usually appears on the lower trunk.

Keratosis pilaris is another common follicular disorder that manifests as tiny, rough, scaling papules on the back of the upper parts of the arms, the buttocks, and the thighs. Although the distribution may be similar to that of staphylococcal folliculitis, the appearance of the lesions is not. In keratosis pilaris the lesions are smaller, more numerous, and scaling, but not pustular.

Management

The usual mild case of staphylococcal folliculitis can be managed by having the patient use an antiseptic cleanser (e.g., chlorhexidine) or antibacterial soap containing triclosan or triclocarban daily or every other day for at least several weeks. For more extensive involvement, a 7- to 10-day course of systemic antibiotics (e.g., erythromycin or dicloxacillin) is suggested in addition to the topical regimen.

Complications and Prognosis

In rare cases the follicular infection extends more deeply, producing a furuncle. Most patients respond to the treatment outlined in the paragraph above; if not, a bacterial culture should be done to rule out infection by gram-negative organisms. Some patients are plagued with recurrences, for which a more prolonged course of antibiotic therapy is recommended.

FURUNCLES AND ABSCESSES

Etiology

Furuncles and abscesses are forms of skin infection (pus-filled nodules or boils) that usually follow folliculitis. *S. aureus* almost always is the responsible organism. Bacteria also may be inoculated into the skin and underlying soft tissue by traumatic injury, including surgery. Gram-negative and anaerobic organisms also can be causes.[3,14] In children, anaerobic organisms commonly are isolated from abscesses in the perirectal area, hand, fingers, and nail beds.

History

A history of trauma may be elicited but often is not, especially with furuncles. Immunodeficiency states and diabetes may predispose certain patients to bacterial skin infections, but the typical patient who has a furuncle or abscess has no underlying medical disease.

Physical Findings

Furuncles and abscesses are fluctuant masses filled with pus. They often begin as hard, tender, red nodules and become more fluctuant and painful with time. Abscesses tend to be larger and deeper than furuncles, but sometimes the two lesions may be difficult to differentiate clinically.

Laboratory Studies

A Gram stain of the pustular material may provide a clue to the bacterial cause, but for precise identification, cultures are required. If anaerobic cultures are desired, material ideally is collected by aspirating the pus, sealing the syringe, and promptly delivering it to the laboratory. If insufficient material is available to aspirate, a swab Culturette can be used for anaerobic as well as aerobic cultures. Blood culture results rarely are positive and are not indicated unless the patient shows signs of sepsis.

Management

Incision and drainage remains the mainstay of therapy. This results in complete healing in most cases, even in patients not treated with systemic antibiotics.[14] Systemic antibiotics may result in involution of early lesions, thereby halting their progression and averting the need for incision and drainage. Erythromycin or dicloxacillin is the antibiotic of choice. Culture results from abscesses may help in the ultimate selection of the appropriate antibiotic.

Complications

Recurrent furunculosis sometimes prompts a search for an underlying immunodeficiency—a search that almost always goes unrewarded. However, many such patients harbor *S. aureus* in a sequestered mucocutaneous site, the most common of which is the nose. The application of an antibiotic ointment (e.g., mupirocin) to the external nares twice daily for 1 week and then monthly may decrease this bacterial colonization and thereby prevent furuncles from recurring. This should be accompanied by an every-other-day total body scrub with an antiseptic cleansing agent, such as chlorhexidine, or antibacterial soap containing triclosan or triclocarban.

In rare cases a staphylococcal abscess may be the focus of toxin production, resulting in staphylococcal scalded skin syndrome (most commonly seen in infants and neonates), toxic shock syndrome, or staphylococcal scarlet fever.

Prognosis

Untreated lesions often rupture and drain spontaneously. After either surgical or spontaneous drainage, uneventful healing is the rule. Larger lesions may leave scars.

CELLULITIS

Etiology

Cellulitis is a deep, locally diffuse infection of the skin that has systemic manifestations and life-threatening potential.[9] It usually involves the face, an extremity, or the perianal area.[16] On an extremity the bacteria presumably have been externally inoculated into the deep dermal tissue, although the portal of entry often is not detectable clinically. A hematogenous or lymphangitic source also is possible and may explain the development of cellulitis in some cases in which the underlying skin is unbroken. Before the introduction of Hib conjugate vaccines in 1988, *Haemophilus influenzae* type b was a frequent cause of facial cellulitis in children. The incidence of invasive infections from this organism in the United States has declined by 95%, and now occurs primarily in undervaccinated children or young infants who have not completed the primary vaccination series.[1] Preseptal (periorbital) cellulitis is now likely to be caused by *Streptococcus pneumoniae* in younger children and by group A streptococci in older children.[17] *S. aureus* and group A streptococci more commonly are responsible for cellulitis of the extremities. Group A streptococci are the most common cause of perianal cellulitis. Two thirds of these patients also will have positive pharyngeal cultures. In rare cases other aerobic and anaerobic bacterial organisms, as well as deep fungal agents such as *Cryptococcus neoformans,* can cause cellulitis. These infections usually occur in immunosuppressed individuals.

History

Children who have cellulitis often feel and look ill. Fever frequently is present and may precede the clinical skin signs. Patients may complain of pain in the affected area. There may be symptoms of an accompanying otitis media in buccal cellulitis. Patients who have perianal cellulitis often have pain on defecation. However, patients who have this disorder usually are not systemically ill; thus, the disease may persist for weeks or months before it is correctly diagnosed.

Physical Findings

Fever at the time of presentation is common. The area of involved skin shows the classic signs of inflammation: redness, swelling, heat, and tenderness.

Laboratory Studies

Leukocytosis is a common finding. Cultures are required to identify the responsible pathogen, and samples should be obtained from the skin, the blood, and, with facial cellulitis, the cerebrospinal fluid (CSF). Middle ear aspirates also may reveal significant findings in patients who have otitis media. Skin aspirates from the leading edge of the lesion sometimes help in isolating pathogens when other cultures are negative.[9,19] This procedure is performed by preparing the skin with an antiseptic, introducing an 18- or 21-gauge needle into the deep dermis, and aspirating material. If no material is obtained (which usually is the case), 0.5 to 1 ml of nonbacteriostatic saline is injected and then aspirated. All aspirates should be Gram stained as well as cultured.

Differential Diagnosis

Erysipelas sometimes is considered separately from cellulitis. Classic erysipelas has more sharply demarcated borders than does cellulitis and may be caused more commonly by group A streptococci. However, the distinction between these two entities often is more semantic than real, inasmuch as the diagnosis and therapeutic considerations are the same.

A severe, local, confluent contact dermatitis sometimes may be confused with cellulitis in that both may show marked erythema of the skin. The important differences are that with contact dermatitis, the patient complains of itch rather than pain, the skin usually is not tender, and the patient is not febrile. The presence of vesicles also favors contact dermatitis, although vesicles and bullae sometimes may occur in erysipelas as the condition evolves.

Perianal cellulitis may be misdiagnosed as candidiasis or a diaper dermatitis. Pain and tenderness of the involved skin suggests bacterial infection, and a swab culture often confirms it.

Erythema of the cheeks occurs characteristically in erythema infectiosum (fifth disease, caused by parvovirus B19), in which a "slapped cheek" appearance is noted. Important diagnostic differences between erythema infectiosum and cellulitis are that in the former, the involvement is bilateral, the site usually is not very tender, and the patient does not appear toxic, although he or she may be mildly febrile.

Management

Systemic antibiotics are the mainstay of cellulitis therapy. Mild cases of cellulitis on an extremity may be treated with an oral antibiotic, warm soaks, and outpatient follow-up in several days. Inasmuch as cellulitis of the extremity most often is caused by gram-positive organisms, erythromycin, dicloxacillin, or cephalexin are appropriate drugs to use. More seriously ill patients in whom sepsis is suspected should be hospitalized for parenteral antibiotic therapy.

Complications

Bacterial sepsis often accompanies cellulitis and was present in 86% of one series of pediatric cases. Local abscesses and osteomyelitis are rare sequelae. Although cellulitis once was a serious, life-threatening disease, antibiotics have reduced the fatality rate to nearly zero in otherwise healthy patients.

Prognosis

With appropriate antibiotic therapy, fever usually resolves within 24 hours. If it does not, a change in antibiotic therapy should be considered, optimally guided by early culture and bacterial sensitivity results. The skin reaction resolves more slowly than does the fever, sometimes taking a week or longer to subside completely—the outcome to be expected in most patients.

When to Refer

Preseptal cellulitis

When to Hospitalize

Cellulitis with suspected sepsis
Invasive infections (necrotizing fasciitis)
Staphylococcal scalded skin syndrome
Toxic shock syndrome

REFERENCES

1. American Academy of Pediatrics: *Hemophilus influenza* infections. In Peter G, editor: *1997 Red Book: report of the committee on infectious diseases,* ed 24, Elk Grove Village, Ill, 1997, American Academy of Pediatrics.
2. Barton LL, Friedman AD: Impetigo: a reassessment of etiology and therapy, *Pediatr Dermatol* 4:185, 1987.
3. Brook I, Finegold SM: Aerobic and anaerobic bacteriology of cutaneous abscesses in children, *Pediatrics* 67:891, 1981.
4. Coskey RJ, Coskey LA: Diagnosis and treatment of impetigo, *J Am Acad Dermatol* 17:62, 1987.
5. Dajani AS, Ferrieri P, Wannamaker LW: Natural history of impetigo. II. Etiologic agents and bacterial interactions, *J Clin Invest* 51:2863, 1972.
6. Demidovich CW, et al: Impetigo: current etiology and comparison of penicillin, erythromycin, and cephalexin therapies, *Am J Dis Child* 144: 1313, 1990.
7. Dillon HC: Impetigo contagiosa: suppurative and nonsuppurative complications. I. Clinical, bacteriologic, and epidemiologic characteristics of impetigo, *Am J Dis Child* 115:530, 1968.
8. Ferrieri P, et al: Natural history of impetigo. I. Site sequence of acquisition and familial patterns of spread of cutaneous streptococci, *J Clin Invest* 51:2851, 1972.
9. Fleisher G, Ludwig S, Campos J: Cellulitis: bacterial etiology, clinical features, and laboratory findings, *J Pediatr* 97:591, 1980.
10. Hayden GF: Skin diseases encountered in a pediatric clinic, *Am J Dis Child* 139:36, 1985.
11. Leyden JJ, et al: *Pseudomonas aeruginosa* gram-negative folliculitis, *Arch Dermatol* 115:1203, 1979.
12. Lookingbill DP: Impetigo, *Pediatr Rev* 7:177, 1985.
13. Maddox JS, Dillon HC: The natural history of streptococcal skin infection: prevention with topical antibiotics, *J Am Acad Dermatol* 13:207, 1985.
14. Meislin HW, et al: Cutaneous abscesses: anaerobic and aerobic bacteriology and outpatient management, *Ann Intern Med* 87:145, 1977.
15. Mertz PM, et al: Topical mupirocin treatment of impetigo is equal to oral erythromycin therapy, *Arch Dermatol* 125:1069, 1989.
16. Rehder PA, Eliezer ET, Lane AT: Perianal cellulitis: cutaneous group A streptococcal disease, *Arch Dermatol* 124:702, 1988.
17. Schwartz GR, Wright SW. Changing bacteriology of periorbital cellulitis, *Ann Emerg Med* 28:617, 1996.
18. Tunnessen WW: Practical aspects of bacterial skin infections in children, *Pediatr Dermatol* 2:255, 1985.
19. Uman SJ, Kunin CM: Needle aspiration in the diagnosis of soft tissue infections, *Arch Intern Med* 135:959, 1975.

191 Brain Tumors

Jerome Y. Yager • Juliette Hukin

Primary brain tumors, the most common type of solid tumor in childhood,[8,32] are surpassing the incidence of leukemia in the United States. However, brain tumors have a threefold greater mortality rate than acute lymphocytic leukemia.[1] Advances in the fields of neuroradiology, neurosurgery, and cancer chemotherapy have improved the identification, management, and survival of affected children. Accordingly, pediatricians and other primary care physicians have become involved in the long-term management of children who have central nervous system (CNS) tumors, thereby increasing their own need to keep abreast of current trends in cancer diagnosis and treatment.

EPIDEMIOLOGY

The incidence of primary childhood brain tumors is 2.2 to 2.4 per 100,000 population at risk per year.[29,33] This figure equates to between 1200 and 1500 new cases a year. No significant gender or ethnic differences in incidence are evident.[33]

Both the incidence and histopathological typing of brain tumors in children vary with age. In the first year, supratentorial tumors—those of the cerebral hemispheres and the diencephalon—predominate. Thereafter, infratentorial tumors—those involving the brainstem and the cerebellum—are more prevalent. The highest incidence of tumors occurs between 5 and 9 years of age; these predominantly are astrocytic, with a smaller proportion being medulloblastomas. A slightly lower number of tumors occurs between birth and 4 years of age; these, unfortunately, tend to be both clinically and histologically more malignant than those that occur at an older age. Histopathological types and their respective locations are shown in Box 191-1. Astrocytomas (both in the cerebral hemisphere and the cerebellum) represent 48% of all CNS tumors of childhood, medulloblastomas 23%, brainstem gliomas 9%, ependymomas 8% (both supratentorial and infratentorial), and craniopharyngiomas between 6% and 10%. Oligodendrogliomas, optic nerve gliomas, choroid plexus papillomas, and pineal gland tumors each make up 2% or less.

PATHOGENESIS

The cause of the majority of primary brain tumors in childhood remains unknown. Recent work in the field of molecular biology, however, has brought us closer to an understanding of tumor pathogenesis in general.

Chromosomal abnormalities, manifested as deletions, translocations, and duplications, have long been known to exist in a variety of tumors, including brain tumors.[3,28,29] Highly malignant tumors appear to show extensive heterogeneity in DNA content. Benign tumors, on the other hand, display a more homogeneous cellular karyotype. Extensive evidence also exists, at least in laboratory animals, for a role of both RNA and DNA viruses in the induction of primary intracranial neoplasms.

The mechanism by which either viruses or chromosomal aberrations lead to tumor induction and propagation probably involves oncogenes, a group of genes involved in cell growth and differentiation.[30] Activation of these oncogenes releases the cell from its normal growth constraints and allows malignant transformation to occur. One theory proposes that viral genes integrate into host DNA and allow expression of the cellular oncogene; a second proposes that structural chromosomal abnormalities predispose a cell to oncogene enhancement.[28]

Several genetic syndromes are associated with an increased risk of CNS tumors; two of the most common are neurofibromatosis (NF) and tuberous sclerosis (TS). Both syndromes exhibit autosomal dominant modes of inheritance, with approximately 50% secondary to a spontaneous new gene mutation. Peripheral neurofibromatosis (NF-I) and central neurofibromatosis (NF-II) have been linked to loci on chromosomes 17 and 22, respectively.[31] The relative risk of benign or malignant CNS neoplasms in NF-I is four times that in the general population,[32] and optic gliomas occur in as many as 15% of affected individuals.[9] The same rate has been quoted for the occurrence of giant cell astrocytomas in patients who have TS.[17] The vast majority of these tumors are supratentorial gliomas. Whether an association exists between malignant transformation and the genetic abnormalities of these conditions is as yet unknown. Several investigators have suggested a role for neuronal growth factors as a possible cause of oncogenesis in patients who have NF-I.[27]

Other mechanisms that likely play a role in the development of childhood CNS tumors include prior radiation[18] and exposure to environmental toxins.[34] The incidence of brain tumors is decreased in the offspring of mothers who took multivitamins during pregnancy.[25] Some tumors, often appearing in the first year of life, are congenital in the sense that they arise from embryonic rests (e.g., craniopharyngioma) or result from errors in development (e.g., epidermal and dermoid cysts, hamartomas, and colloid cysts). A strong association exists between primary CNS lymphoma and acquired immunodeficiency syndrome.[19]

BOX 191-1

PRIMARY BRAIN TUMORS OF CHILDHOOD

Supratentorial (Cerebral Hemispheres)
Astrocytoma
Choroid plexus papilloma
Ependymoma
Meningioma
Oligodendroglioma

Midline (Diencephalon)
Craniopharyngioma
Pinealoma
Optic nerve glioma

Infratentorial (Brainstem and Cerebellum)
Astrocytoma
Medulloblastoma
Glioma
Ependymoma

Other
Primitive neuroectodermal tumors

CLINICAL MANIFESTATIONS

The diagnosis of brain tumor in a child is based on clinical suspicion, a thorough history, and a detailed neurological examination. Signs and symptoms may be subtle and depend on the age of the child and the location and biological aggressiveness of the tumor.

Although brain tumors lack pathognomonic features, several general concepts should be kept in mind. Intracranial mass lesions produce symptoms as a result of indirect effects caused by an increase in intracranial pressure (ICP) or of direct effects arising from the displacement or invasion of surrounding tissue. The duration of symptoms before diagnosis is affected by tumor site and growth characteristics. Symptoms typically are progressive rather than intermittent. Malignant, rapidly growing lesions have more explosive manifestations than do benign and slow-growing lesions.

In addition to tissue displacement within a fixed cranial volume, elevated ICP is caused by obstruction of cerebrospinal fluid (CSF) flow and secondary hydrocephalus or, more rarely, by increased CSF production. Symptoms appear insidiously; a change in personality, deterioration in school performance, headache, nausea, vomiting, and lethargy are the most common presenting complaints. In rare cases, acute ventricular obstruction leads rapidly to coma.

The signs of increased ICP may be subtle. Young infants and children, whose cranial sutures have not yet fused, are able to tolerate a relatively greater expansion of the intracranial contents than are older children and adults. Compensatory head growth and ultimate macrocephaly are presenting features and may be accompanied by (1) failure to thrive from anorexia, (2) lethargy, or (3) irritability. Funduscopic examination may reveal papilledema. If increased ICP is long-standing, optic atrophy can occur with associated visual loss and nystagmus. Pressure on the sensitive abducens cranial nerve VI causes lateral gaze impairment, resulting in diplopia.

Signs and symptoms of intracranial hypertension are common among children who have brain tumors, inasmuch as the majority of such mass lesions lie in the midline of the posterior fossa and cause ventricular obstruction. Such neoplasms include cerebellar astrocytomas, medulloblastomas, ependymomas, and pineal gland tumors. Choroid plexus papillomas, although rare, cause increased ICP by excessive production of CSF.

Direct symptom-producing effects of a brain tumor vary according to their site or origin. Supratentorial lesions within a cerebral hemisphere lead to headache, unilateral muscle weakness (hemiparesis), visual disturbance, or unilateral sensory loss. Headaches may not be localized, but their presence should arouse suspicion, particularly if they worsen while lying down or coughing, sneezing, or straining. Headaches that awaken a child in the early morning hours also are of concern.

Seizures occur rarely as an initial manifestation of brain tumors in children. When present, they typically are focal and tend to be refractory to anticonvulsant medication before definitive therapy for the tumor itself. The electroencephalogram shows persistent focal slowing. The tumors usually are benign and slow growing.[2]

Craniopharyngiomas and hypothalamic gliomas, both midline diencephalic tumors, manifest with headache, endocrine dysfunction (growth failure, precocious puberty, diabetes insipidus, hypothyroidism), and visual disturbance. The accompanying symptoms of abnormal visual fields and hormonal imbalance strongly suggest the presence of a midline supratentorial mass. Infratentorial tumors are associated with increased ICP, usually secondary to hydrocephalus, and brainstem or cerebellar dysfunction, including truncal and limb ataxia, long-tract signs (spasticity and hyperreflexia), and cranial nerve deficits.

The differential diagnosis of intracranial tumors includes less common space-occupying lesions and other causes of increased ICP, such as (1) arteriovenous malformation, (2) subdural hematoma, effusion, or empyema, (3) abscess, (4) infarction, (5) hemorrhage, and (6) demyelination. Pseudotumor cerebri, especially in the adolescent, is a common cause of increased ICP without clinical evidence of a mass lesion. Classic hemiplegic migraine or Todd's paralysis after a focal seizure may mimic the signs of an intracerebral mass lesion. The residual signs for migraine or a prior seizure, however, are transient and usually resolve within 24 hours. Occasionally, venous sinus thrombosis manifests with signs of increased ICP.

DIAGNOSIS

The advent of computed tomography (CT) and magnetic resonance imaging (MRI) has revolutionized the diagnosis and subsequent management of CNS tumors. Initial evaluation should include both an unenhanced and enhanced CT and an MRI scan. A noncontrast CT scan affords the opportunity to determine (1) tumor density compared with surrounding tissue, (2) the existence of hydrocephalus, and (3) the presence of calcifications or hemorrhage, which may suggest certain tumor types or their aggressiveness. Contrast enhancement delineates tumor margins from surrounding edema and differentiates neoplasms from suspected vascular malformations. Although CT scanning has shown a greater than 90%

sensitivity, relevant limitations exist in the assessment of pediatric tumors. In particular, poor resolution of posterior fossa structures (brainstem and cerebellum) hinders the evaluation of more than 55% of childhood tumors.[13]

Where available, MRI is now supplanting CT as the imaging procedure of choice.[35] Greater resolution, the ability to image in more than one plane, and the lack of artifact produced by the surrounding skull make MRI particularly suitable for assessment of posterior fossa structures. MRI has been reported to provide more information than does the CT scan in up to 50% of patients and has proved its superiority for the early detection of neoplasms and for determining the limits of their extension.[21] MRI is essential in the planning of the surgical approach. It also allows better visualization of the spinal cord without the need for a myelogram. Disadvantages of MRI include the inability to detect calcification and to distinguish tumor from surrounding edema, although contrast enhancement with gadolinium (a paramagnetic contrast agent) can obviate this limitation.[4] MRI requires a much longer scanning time—thus the need for prolonged sedation or even anesthesia, which potentially is hazardous in children who have increased ICP. MRI and CT scans currently are complementary; both provide important information regarding tumor location, type, and extent of invasion.

Once the diagnosis of an intracranial mass is confirmed, further imaging and CSF evaluation should be considered to delineate the presence of dissemination within the nervous system. In addition, histological typing is required to determine further management.

Approximately 30% of medulloblastomas have developed seeding along the subarachnoid pathways by the time of diagnosis.[13] MRI examination detects CSF dissemination most accurately and generally is performed as part of the initial assessment of posterior fossa tumors prior to surgery. Caution must be exercised in performing lumbar punctures in patients who have brain tumors, particularly of the posterior fossa, because of the risk of brainstem herniation. For the most part, lumbar punctures are performed postoperatively after decompression of the intracranial contents.

Determination of CSF cytology, although historically of interest in early tissue diagnosis, is of little value in the initial diagnosis of brain tumors. Although cells frequently are present initially in the CSF postoperatively, whether they are the result of preoperative seeding or intraoperative shedding is uncertain. Therefore, cytological examination of CSF for tumor staging usually is postponed until 2 weeks after surgery to determine the extent of disease. Several biochemical tumor markers are of assistance in the early diagnosis and progression of CNS tumor recurrences. The polyamines, specifically putrescine, are accurate markers for the recurrence of medulloblastomas, whereas CSF alpha-fetoprotein and beta-human chorionic gonadotropin are good indicators of germ cell tumor activity.[10,13]

MANAGEMENT

Substantial gains have accrued in the management of childhood brain tumors through microsurgical techniques, refined modes of radiation therapy, and chemotherapeutic agents that cross the blood-brain barrier.

Stabilization of the child's neurological condition through the use of osmotic agents and corticosteroids to reduce surrounding brain edema and early CSF shunting for hydrocephalus are the first steps toward comprehensive treatment. Histological diagnosis has been aided by the advent of stereotaxic biopsy for most tumors regardless of location, including certain brainstem gliomas.[11,35] Complete excision and cure are possible for several localized CNS tumors, including choroid plexus papilloma, craniopharyngioma, and cystic cerebellar astrocytoma. Operative mortality has been reduced in most centers to less than 5%. Refinement in the use of micro-operative techniques, laser surgery, and intraoperative monitoring has improved outcome further, with diminished morbidity.[15]

Survival generally is aided by a "debulking" procedure, followed by radiation or chemotherapy, or both, in those patients in whom the tumor cannot be safely resected completely. Substantial evidence now exists that chemotherapy plays a vital role in the treatment of primary childhood CNS tumors. The rationale for combination chemotherapy regimens relates to CNS malignant tumors displaying histological heterogeneity. This cellular diversification enables a greater degree of drug resistance to single-drug therapy, whereas multiple drugs attack a tumor by a variety of mechanisms, thereby increasing the likelihood of sensitivity.

The Children's Cancer Study Group (CCSG) has reported an improved 5-year survival rate of 42% among patients who have high-grade astrocytomas treated with combined radiation/chemotherapy compared with survival rates of only 10% among patients treated with radiation alone.[14] Low-grade gliomas that have residual tumor bulk that progresses and that are not surgically resectable are considered for chemotherapy if the patient is younger than 10 years of age so as to avoid, or at least defer, radiation.[23,24] Medulloblastoma is a radiosensitive tumor; therefore, the mainstay of therapy is involved field and craniospinal radiation. Improved survival and decreased morbidity have been achieved with the addition of chemotherapy to the therapy of medulloblastoma.[22] Adding chemotherapy has allowed a decrease in the dosage of craniospinal radiation in standard-risk patients. Germ cell tumors also are chemosensitive. The main thrust of therapy for ependymoma is radical resection. In the presence of possible residual disease, adjuvant radiation is used either early or when progression occurs.[16] The reports of the efficacy of chemotherapy in ependymoma are anecdotal only. It is not uncommon for diffuse pontine gliomas to show at least some transient radiographic[26] or clinical response to involved field radiation. To date, no chemotherapy regimens have been shown to be of value in this disease.

Children younger than 3 years of age who have malignant brain tumors tend to present with large tumors that seem to behave more aggressively than their histological counterparts in older children. Also, therapy is limited by reluctance to administer radiation to these children due to unacceptable long-term intellectual morbidity. Various intensive chemotherapy regimens, with and without stem cell support, have been used with some success to avoid, delay, or possibly decrease the dose of radiation.[7,20]

PROGNOSIS

Prognosis for brain tumors depends on tumor type, size, and location. Overall, 5-year survival rates approach or exceed 50% for all age groups and tumor types.[8] Low-grade cerebellar and supratentorial astrocytomas have excellent long-term survival rates of 70% to 80%. Survival of patients who have standard-risk medulloblastoma is 85%, and those who have high-risk medulloblastoma is 20% to 65%. The poorest prognosis occurs in children who have diffuse pontine gliomas; their 2-year survival rate is less than 20%. For all tumor types, the survival rate generally is poorest in children younger than 2 years of age.

The treatment of brain tumors carries with it significant morbidity. Acute effects of radiation and chemotherapy are well known. Bone marrow suppression brings the risks of infection and bleeding. Cranial radiation is accompanied by hair loss, emesis, headache, and sometimes, excessive somnolence.

As improvements in therapy lengthen survival, long-term adverse effects of treatment increase. Delayed effects of radiation include progressive demyelination, radiation necrosis, and a second malignancy, which can be misdiagnosed as tumor recurrence. Recent studies have documented a slow decline over years in intelligence quotients among children receiving radiation and chemotherapy.[5] The higher the dose of radiation (particularly to the supratentorium) and the younger the patient, the greater the deficits.

Growth hormone deficiency and subsequent growth deceleration occur frequently among children who receive cranial radiation. Replacement of multiple hormones is required for patients who have been treated for craniopharyngiomas by surgery, with or without radiation therapy.[6,26]

FUTURE PROSPECTS

Prospects for improved treatment modalities for childhood brain tumors continue with advances in our understanding of the molecular biology of tumors, better diagnostic techniques, microsurgical procedures, improved chemotherapeutic programs, and more sophisticated radiotherapy techniques. New approaches that may play a greater role in the future include gene therapy, antiangiogenesis agents, and immunotherapy. The care of children who have brain tumors involves a greater number of physicians as long-term survival and the rate of neurological morbidity continue to improve. Management requires an ongoing, multidisciplinary approach with participation by specialists in oncology, neurosurgery, neurology, primary care, social work, psychology, and rehabilitative services.

REFERENCES

1. Bleyer A, Sposto R, Sather H: In the United States, pediatric brain tumors and other nervous system tumors (NST) are now more common than childhood acute lymphoblastic leukemia (ALL) and have a 3-fold greater national mortality rate. Proceedings of the annual meeting of the American Society of Clinical Oncology, October 17, 1998.
2. Blume WT, Girvin JP, Kaufman JCE: Childhood brain tumors presenting as chronic uncontrolled focal seizure disorders, *Ann Neurol* 12:538, 1982.
3. Cusimano MD: An update on the cellular and molecular biology of brain tumors, *Can J Neurol Sci* 16:22, 1989.
4. Dickman CP, et al: Unenhanced and gadolinium-DTPA-enhanced MR imaging in postoperative evaluation in pediatric brain tumors, *J Neurosurg* 71:49, 1989.
5. Duffner PK, Cohen MR, Parker MS: Prospective intellectual testing in children with brain tumors, *Ann Neurol* 23:575, 1988.
6. Duffner PK, et al: Long-term effects of cranial irradiation on endocrine function in children with brain tumors: a prospective study, *Cancer* 56:2189, 1985.
7. Duffner PK, et al: Postoperative chemotherapy and delayed radiation in children less than three years of age with malignant brain tumors, *N Engl J Med* 328:24, 1993.
8. Duffner PK, et al: Survival of children with brain tumors: SEER program 1973-1980, *Neurology* 36:597, 1986.
9. Dunn DW: Neurofibromatosis in childhood. In Lockhart JD, editor: *Current problems in pediatrics*, vol 17, Chicago, 1987, Mosby-Year Book.
10. Edwards MSB, Davis RL, Laurent JP: Tumor markers and cytologic features of cerebrospinal fluid, *Cancer* 56:1773, 1985.
11. Edwards MSB, Prados M: Current management of brain stem glioma, *Pediatr Neurosci* 13:309, 1987.
12. Epstein F, McClearly EL: Intrinsic brain stem tumors of childhood: surgical indications, *J Neurosurg* 64:11, 1986.
13. Finlay JL, Goins SC: Brain tumors in children. I. Advances in diagnosis, *Am J Pediatr Hematol Oncol* 9:246, 1987.
14. Finlay JL, Goins SC: Brain tumors in children. III. Advances in chemotherapy, *Am J Pediatr Hematol Oncol* 9:264, 1987.
15. Finlay JL, Uteg R, Giese WL: Brain tumors in children. II. Advances in neurosurgery and radiation oncology, *Am J Pediatr Hematol Oncol* 9:256, 1987.
16. Hukin J, et al: Treatment of intracranial ependymoma by surgery alone, *Pediatr Neurosurg* 29:40, 1998.
17. Kingsley DPE, Kendall BE, Fitz CR: Tuberous sclerosis: a clinicoradiological evaluation of 110 cases with particular reference to atypical presentation, *Neuroradiology* 28:38, 1986.
18. Leviton A: Principles of epidemiology. In Cohen ME, Duffner PL, editors: *Brain tumors in children: principles of diagnosis and treatment*, New York, 1984, Raven Press.
19. List AF, Greco A, Vogler LB: Lymphoproliferative disease in immunocompromised hosts: the role of Epstein-Barr viruses, *J Clin Oncol* 5:1673, 1987.
20. Mason WP, et al: Intensive chemotherapy and bone marrow rescue for young children with newly diagnosed malignant brain tumors, *J Clin Oncol* 16:1, 1998.
21. Packer RJ, Batnitzky S, Cohen ME: Magnetic resonance imaging in the evaluation of intracranial tumors of childhood, *Cancer* 56:1767, 1985.
22. Packer RJ, et al: Outcome for children with medulloblastoma treated with radiation and cisplatin, CCNU and vincristine chemotherapy, *J Neurosurg* 81:690, 1994.
23. Packer RJ, et al: Carboplatin and vincristine chemotherapy for children with newly diagnosed progressive low-grade gliomas, *J Neurosurg* 86: 747, 1997.
24. Prados MD, et al: Treatment of pediatric low-grade gliomas with a nitrosourea-based multiagent chemotherapy regimen, *J Neurooncol* 32: 235, 1997.
25. Preston-Mann S, Pogoda JM: Prenatal vitamin supplementation and pediatric brain tumor: significant reduction in risk and high variation in use. Eighth International Symposium on Pediatric Neuro-Oncology Program and Proceedings, May, 1998.
26. Rappaport R, Brauner R: Growth and endocrine disorders secondary to cranial irradiation, *Pediatr Res* 25:561, 1989.
27. Riopelle RJ, Riccardi VM: Neuronal growth factors from tumors of von Recklinghausen neurofibromatosis, *Can J Neurol Sci* 14:141, 1987.
28. Schmidek HH: The molecular genetics of nervous system tumors, *J Neurosurg* 16:1, 1987.
29. Schoenberg BS, et al: The epidemiology of primary intracranial neoplasms of childhood: a population study, *Mayo Clin Proc* 51:51, 1976.
30. Shapiro JR: Biology of gliomas: heterogeneity, oncogenes, growth factors, *Semin Oncol* 13:4, 1986.
31. Sorensen SA, Mulvihill JJ, Nielsen A: Long-term follow-up of von Recklinghausen neurofibromatosis survival and malignant neoplasms, *N Engl J Med* 314:1010, 1986.
32. Tomita T, Mclone DG: Brain tumor during the first twenty-four months of life, *Neurosurgery* 17:913, 1985.
33. Young JL, et al: Cancer incidence, survival and mortality for children younger than age 15 years, *Cancer* 58:598, 1986.

34. Zeller WJ, et al: Experimental chemical production of brain tumors, *Ann N Y Acad Sci* 281:250, 1982.
35. Zimmerman RA: Neuroimaging of primary brainstem gliomas: diagnosis and course, *Pediatr Neurosurg* 25:45, 1996.

SUGGESTED READINGS

Cohen ME, Duffner PK: *Brain tumors in children: principles of diagnosis and treatment*, ed 2, New York, 1994, International Review of Child Neurology Series, Raven Press.

Cohen ME, Duffner PK: Tumors of the brain and spinal cord including leukemic involvement. In Swaiman KF, editor: *Pediatric neurology: principles and practices,* ed 2, St Louis, 1994, Mosby-Year Book.

Kadota RP, et al: Brain tumors in children, *J Pediatr* 114:511, 1989.

192 Bronchiolitis

Caroline Breese Hall • William J. Hall

Bronchiolitis is a common, acute infectious respiratory illness of children that usually occurs in the first 2 years of life. According to recent data from the Centers for Disease Control and Prevention,[46] bronchiolitis, primarily caused by respiratory syncytial virus (RSV), is an increasing cause of hospitalization among infants. The hallmarks of the clinical picture are wheezing and hyperaeration, commonly associated with tachypnea, respiratory distress, and retractions of the chest.

Although the clinical picture of bronchiolitis has been described since the beginning of the twentieth century, bronchiolitis was not recognized as a separate entity until Engle and Newns[10] gave it its sovereignty by designating the distinctive infantile disease as bronchiolitis.

ETIOLOGY

Viruses and occasionally, *Mycoplasma pneumoniae,* are now recognized as the causes of bronchiolitis.* As shown as Fig. 192-1, RSV is by far the most frequently isolated agent, with the parainfluenza viruses being the next most common agents.[11,23] In the study by Henderson et al[23] of bronchiolitis occurring among children in a private pediatric practice, RSV, parainfluenza viruses types 1 and 3, adenoviruses, rhinoviruses, and *M. pneumoniae* accounted for 87% of the isolates from children of all ages. Respiratory syncytial virus accounted for 44% of the isolates from children in the first 2 years of life, with parainfluenza type 1, parainfluenza type 3, and adenoviruses each accounting for about 13%. In two group practices in Monroe County, New York, RSV was isolated from 55% and parainfluenza type 3 from 11% of cases of bronchiolitis. If only hospitalized cases of bronchiolitis are examined, the contribution of RSV is much higher.[15,55] In the Newcastle-upon-Tyne studies, RSV was isolated from 74% of hospitalized bronchiolitis patients.[15]

EPIDEMIOLOGY

The seasonal pattern of bronchiolitis reflects the activities of its viral agents, particularly RSV.[4,13,18,19] Because RSV is causative in the majority of cases, bronchiolitis peaks during the winter to spring when RSV is epidemic in the community. As shown in Fig. 192-2 in Monroe County, New York, the greatest number of cases are reported during the yearly January to February peak of RSV activity. Lesser peaks are seen during the fall when parainfluenza virus type 1 has been present in the community and during the spring period of parainfluenza virus type 3 major activity. Cases of bronchiolitis commonly are designated as epidemic or sporadic bronchiolitis, which essentially means cases that are or are not associated with RSV.

The incidence of bronchiolitis varies according to the age and definition of the syndrome. More than 80% of bronchiolitis cases occur during the first year of life.* The peak attack rate occurs between 2 and 10 months of age, and bronchiolitis is relatively uncommon during the first weeks of life. The highest reported incidence is from Denny et al's long-term studies[8] in Chapel Hill, North Carolina, in which 115 cases per 100 children up to 6 months of age were detected per year. Because these children in a child care center were examined at regular intervals, and the diagnosis of bronchiolitis did not have to include tachypnea or air-trapping, the mildest cases were included. In subsequent Chapel Hill studies of ambulatory children, the incidence was 11 cases per 100 children per year for both the first and second 6 months of life.[7,23] In both of these studies, the incidence fell rapidly during the second year of life to 32 cases per 100 children per year in the child care center and to 6 cases per 100 children per year in the private practice. In hospitalized cases the incidence is highest during the first 6 months of life and in the study by Foy et al[13] was found to be 6 per 1000 children per year. The attack rate in boys generally is 1½ times greater than that in girls among both outpatients and hospitalized patients.[4,7,18]

PATHOPHYSIOLOGY

Host, environmental, and immunological factors appear to play a role in the development and severity of bronchiolitis. The risk of bronchiolitis appears to be increased in children who come from poorer socioeconomic areas and from crowded and polluted surroundings, who have more siblings attending child care, and who have not been breast fed.[5,29,55,56] Children who have a genetic predisposition to hyperreactive airways appear more likely to manifest their initial respiratory viral infections as bronchiolitis, especially if caused by RSV or the parainfluenza viruses, although the role of atopy, genetics, and an allergic family background is unclear.[5,29,35,47,56] Immunological mechanisms, however, have been suggested in the pathogenesis of bronchiol-

*References 4, 7, 8, 11, 13, 18, 23.

*References 4, 7, 8, 11, 18, 23, 55.

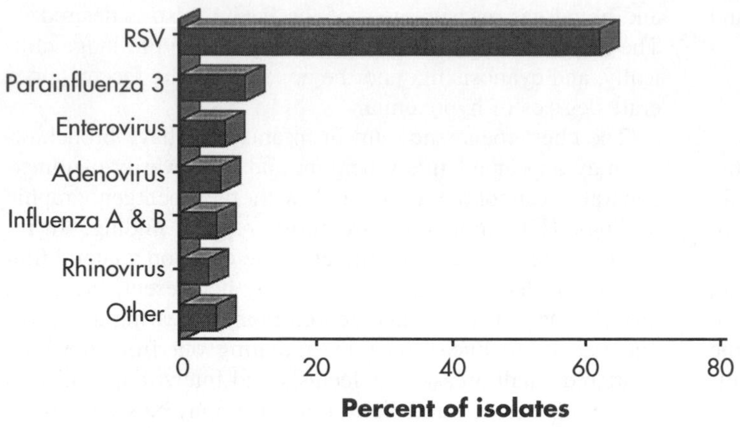

Fig. 192-1 Viral origin of bronchiolitis from patients in pediatric practices participating in a community surveillance program in Monroe County, New York, ongoing since 1976.

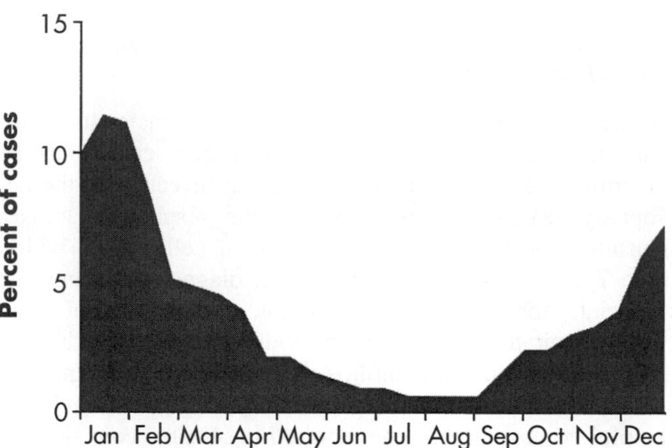

Fig. 192-2 Seasonal occurrence of bronchiolitis cases obtained over a 20-year period from a community surveillance program in Monroe County, New York.

itis.[29,42,52,53] An enhanced responsiveness to viral antigens and allergens in infants who have bronchiolitis has been suggested to result in release of lymphokines, inflammation, and hyperreactivity of the airways. Increased production of specific IgE antibody and histamine released in the secretions of infected infants, as well as leukotriene C4 and eosinophilic cationic protein (ECP), have been associated with the development and severity of bronchiolitis.[17,40,51-53] Additional cell-specific mediators, including the production of some chemokines (chemotactic cytokines), and neutrophilic chemotactic factors (IL-6 and IL-8), have been detected in the secretions of children who have RSV infection and bronchiolitis.[2,3] This suggests that RSV and other respiratory viruses may engender an inflammatory response by initiating local migration and activation of eosinophils, basophils, and neutrophils.

Paramount in the pathogenesis of bronchiolitis are the age of the child and the specific viral agents, particularly RSV and parainfluenza virus type 3, which infect children early in life and are capable of infecting the lower respiratory tract in a high proportion of young infants. As important as gender in this young age group are anatomical and physiological factors, such as the small diameter of the peripheral airways, the poor collateral ventilation, and the relatively increased number of mucus-secreting glands. Furthermore, males appear to have greater muscle tone of the airways and increased risk of hyperresponsiveness.[29,30,34]

Initially the viral agent infects the upper respiratory tract and subsequently spreads to affect the medium and small bronchi and bronchioles. The virus characteristically causes inflammation and necrosis of the respiratory epithelium.[55] Histologically, peribronchiolar infiltration and proliferation, mostly of mononuclear cells, are observed. The bronchiolar epithelium subsequently becomes necrotic and sloughs. In most cases of bronchiolitis, spread of the inflammation beyond the peribronchiolar area is slight, with little involvement of the surrounding alveoli. The inflammation of the small bronchi and bronchioles, nevertheless, is generalized, but with areas varying in severity. Because resistance to the flow of air is related inversely to the cube of the radius, the small diameter of the lumen makes the infant particularly vulnerable to obstruction caused by the developing edema and exudate. Peripheral to the sites of partial obstruction, air becomes trapped by a process similar to a "ball valve" mechanism. During inspiration, the negative intrapleural pressure allows air to flow past the site of partial obstruction. On expiration, however, the positive pressure decreases the lumen's size, causing an increase in the degree of obstruction. The lung becomes hyperinflated. Expiration, in particular, becomes difficult and prolonged. If the inflammation progresses, complete obstruction occurs. When the trapped air is absorbed, multiple areas of focal atelectasis result.

Two important physiological sequelae occur from these pathological processes. First, the resistance to airflow increases markedly.[55] This leads to dyspnea, an increased respiratory rate, and lower tidal volume. Thus, the volume of air reaching the gas-exchanging alveoli diminishes with each breath, and proportionately more air ventilates only "dead space." This eventually may elevate the $PaCO_2$. The second sequela resulting from small-airway obstruction is the marked change in the distribution of ventilation within the lung. This ventilation-perfusion mismatch is engendered by the characteristic distribution of infection of these respiratory viruses, which in young children is widespread rather than localized to a lobe or segment of the lung. The low ratio of ventilation compared with perfusion of the lung results in arterial hypoxemia. Almost all infants hospitalized with bronchiolitis have some degree of hypoxemia, which commonly is appreciable and protracted.[20,55] Despite clinical improvement, the hypoxemia may persist for weeks, reflecting the relatively slow resolution of the inflammation and atelectasis.

CLINICAL FEATURES

Bronchiolitis usually is heralded by the signs compatible with a common cold. Rhinorrhea, nasal congestion, a slight fever, and cough may develop over a prodromal period of 1 to 7 days. As bronchiolitis develops, the cough may become more prominent and an increased respiratory rate, pulse rate, and tachypnea appear. Fever commonly is present during the prodromal period but usually is not high; by the time bronchiolitis has developed, fewer than 50% of the children are febrile.

Physical examination of the infant who has bronchiolitis often is striking. Tachypnea is a constant finding, often accompanied by tachycardia; the respiratory rate usually is 45 to 80 breaths/min. The infant may appear lethargic and distressed, with circumoral cyanosis. The increased work of breathing is evidenced by flaring of the nasal alae and expiratory grunting. Retractions of the chest wall in the subcostal, intercostal, and suprasternal areas and use of the accessory muscles of respiration are notable.

Physical examination of the baby's chest verifies the hyperinflation resulting from the trapping of air peripheral to the small-airway obstruction. The diameter of the chest appears increased, and the percussion note is hyperresonant. The liver and spleen may become easily palpable from the downward placement of the overinflated lungs. Expiration usually, but not always, is prolonged and may be difficult to detect in a small baby who has a rapid respiratory rate. The flow of air also is obstructed on inspiration but to a lesser extent. Auscultation usually reveals the diagnostic hallmark of wheezing. The degree of wheezing and the fine, moist rales commonly heard on inspiration may vary from hour to hour. A decrease in the auscultatory findings with increasing respiratory distress may indicate progressive obstruction to the flow of air in the small airways and impending respiratory failure. As this stage of respiratory acidosis becomes manifest, the respirations become shallow and ineffective, as if the effort to breathe becomes too great for the infant.

Associated findings that may complicate the infant's course include otitis media and dehydration. Otitis media caused by RSV infection is observed most frequently in infants who have bronchiolitis. Babies who have bronchiolitis are prone to dehydration because of paroxysms of coughing that trigger vomiting and because of a decreased fluid intake resulting from their respiratory distress and lethargy. In addition, tachypnea and fever may increase fluid requirements.

Most infants who have bronchiolitis improve appreciably within several days, and the cough and other signs resolve gradually thereafter over 1 to 2 weeks. For some infants, the entire course is one of slow, gradual improvement. Most children who worsen and require hospitalization will do so within the first 3 or 4 days.

For most infants, the white blood cell count and differential count are within normal limits. However, in the more severely affected and hypoxemic infant, the white blood cell count may be elevated, and the differential count may demonstrate a shift to the left. For those more distressed infants, hypoxemia needs to be assessed by the use of pulse oximetry, and blood gas measurement of the $PaCO_2$ also is desired.[20] The degree of hypoxemia is extremely difficult to judge clinically, and cyanosis may not be apparent in the face of moderate degrees of hypoxemia.

The chest roentgenogram in infants who have bronchiolitis may appear relatively benign, and the severity of illness generally cannot be correlated with the roentgenographic findings. Hyperinflation is the most frequent finding. An increased anteroposterior diameter of the chest on a lateral film and flat or depressed diaphragms may be present. Increased bronchovascular markings are common, appearing as abnormal streaks or linear densities radiating out from the hila. Scattered small areas of atelectasis and interstitial infiltrates of varying intensity and distribution also may be seen. Differentiation of these areas of atelectasis from those of pneumonic infiltration often is not possible.

DIAGNOSIS

Bronchiolitis usually is diagnosed on the characteristic clinical and epidemiological features; a specific cause may be determined by viral isolation or antigen detection in the nasopharyngeal secretions. Most of the respiratory viruses causing bronchiolitis are identifiable in cell culture within 3 to 7 days. A variety of rapid viral diagnostic techniques, especially for RSV, are now available to detect within hours in the respiratory secretions those viruses that cause the majority of cases of bronchiolitis.[26,39] Antibody determinations on acute and convalescent sera in the young infant rarely are helpful because of the time required to obtain a convalescent serum, the presence of passive maternal antibody, and the diminished antibody response of young infants to RSV and other viral respiratory agents.

DIFFERENTIAL DIAGNOSIS

Asthma is the major consideration in the differential diagnosis of bronchiolitis.[32] Often in a single episode, it is not possible to differentiate these two entities; indeed, the two may be combined.[29] A great proportion of wheezing episodes occurring in an atopic child may arise from viral infections. In asthmatic children 1 to 5 years of age, McIntosh et al[36] found 42% of the episodes of wheezing to be associated with a viral infection and respiratory syncytial virus to be the agent isolated most frequently.

Respiratory syncytial virus has an unexplained propensity for producing wheezing in infants. Therefore, children who first wheeze during an epidemic of respiratory syncytial viral infections may be less likely to have an atopic predisposition than do children who develop sporadic bronchiolitis at other times of the year. The role of atopy also is apt to be greater in a child older than 18 months and in one who has a family history of allergy and previous episodes of wheezing.

Another diagnostic consideration is gastroesophageal reflux, which in the infant may produce a picture clinically identical to that of bronchiolitis. The differential diagnosis also should include a number of other entities that may result in wheezing and respiratory distress in the bronchiolitic age group, including obstruction from an aspirated foreign body, a vascular ring, retropharyngeal abscess, and rarely, significantly enlarged adenoids. Wheezing also may occur in congestive heart failure and in cystic fibrosis.

TREATMENT

Management of most infants who have bronchiolitis consists mainly of supportive care, including adequate hydration and antipyretics, if necessary. For the hospitalized child, the mainstay of care is supportive—that is, ensuring adequate oxygenation and hydration. For infants who have RSV bronchiolitis with more severe disease and for those who have underlying conditions predisposing them to more complicated disease, aerosolized ribavirin may be considered for use.[1,21,41] The duration of treatment should be guided by the infant's clinical improvement rather than by a set number of days. Infants in controlled studies treated with ribavirin have been shown to have diminished production in their secretions of specific IgE antibody and of leukotrienes associated with inflammation and wheezing.[16,44]

The use of bronchodilators in bronchiolitis remains controversial. Although bronchodilators appear to be the most commonly used therapy for bronchiolitis, evidence supporting their efficacy for most children who have bronchiolitis is lacking.[12,14,25,27] In young infants, inflammation from the viral infection often is the prime cause of the impedance to air flow, rather than airway hyperresponsiveness, although the latter may aggravate the obstruction. Studies evaluating bronchodilators in bronchiolitis have produced conflicting results. No significant clinical benefit or improvement in pulmonary function has been documented in the majority of studies.[12,14,25,31] Some modest degree of clinical benefit has been noted in a few studies, particularly those using epinephrine aerosols rather than albuterol.[24,37,45] Corticosteroid therapy also is used commonly in children who have bronchiolitis,[27] despite the lack of any significant benefits demonstrated in most controlled studies.[28,38,43,48,50]

Antibiotics should not be used to treat bronchiolitis because bacteria have no role in its origin. Secondary bacterial infection rarely is observed after bronchiolitis; unless such is documented, antibiotics should not be used.

COMPLICATIONS AND PROGNOSIS

The prognosis for normal infants who have bronchiolitis is good; mortality is less than 1%. In certain children who have underlying diseases such as cardiopulmonary disease, bronchiolitis may be accompanied by increased morbidity and mortality.

Viral pneumonia so commonly coexists with the clinical manifestations of bronchiolitis that the diseases may be considered a continuum, particularly in RSV infection. Bacterial pneumonia is an uncommon complication.

Apnea may complicate the course of approximately 20% of infants hospitalized with RSV infection.[6] Apnea is most likely to occur in the youngest infants and in premature infants. Occasionally, bronchiolitis, especially from RSV, may produce significant cardiovascular abnormalities, even in infants who have no underlying cardiac or lung disease.[49]

It has long been noted that infants who have had bronchiolitis, whether mild or severe, appear to be at risk for recurrent episodes of lower respiratory tract disease during their early years.[29,38,47,55]

These episodes tend to diminish with age in most children.[20,22] Studies recently have indicated that such children who have recurrent wheezing generally may be divided into two groups.[9,31,33,34,54] The larger of these two groups is composed of children who have no known predisposition for atopy and who at birth are clinically normal but are believed to have diminished lung function. The much smaller group consists of those who have an atopic predisposition. At the time of the initial episode of bronchiolitis, differentiation of these groups and, more importantly, even whether a child will become a "recurrent wheezer" usually is not possible.

When to Refer

When episodes of bronchiolitis or wheezing are recurrent
When wheezing continues despite clinical improvement

When to Hospitalize

When oral intake is inadequate
When toxic appearing; marked tachypnea, lethargy
When hypoxemic by pulse oximetry

REFERENCES

1. American Academy of Pediatrics: Respiratory syncytial virus. In Pickering LK, editor: *Red book 2000: report of the Committee on Infectious Diseases,* ed 25, Elk Grove Village, Ill, 2000, American Academy of Pediatrics.
2. Becker S, et al: RSV infection of human airway epithelial cells causes production of the β-chemokine RANTES, *Am J Physiol* 272 *(Lung Cell Mol Physiol 16)*:L512, 1997.
3. Berkman NA, et al: Expression of RANTES in human airway epithelial cells: effect of corticosteroids and interleukin -4, -10, and -13, *Immunology* 87:599, 1996.
4. Brandt CD, et al: Epidemiology of respiratory syncytial virus infection in Washington, DC. III. Composite analysis of eleven consecutive yearly outbreaks, *Am J Epidemiol* 98:355, 1973.
5. Carlsen KH, et al: Acute bronchiolitis: predisposing factors and characterization of infants at risk, *Pediatr Pulmonol* 3:153, 1987.
6. Church NR, et al: Respiratory syncytial virus related apnea in infants: demographics and outcome, *Am J Dis Child* 138:247, 1984.
7. Denny FW, Clyde WA: Acute lower respiratory tract infections in nonhospitalized children, *J Pediatr* 108:635, 1986.
8. Denny FW, et al: The epidemiology of bronchiolitis, *Pediatr Res* 11: 234, 1977.
9. Dodge R, et al: Early childhood respiratory symptoms and the subsequent diagnosis of asthma, *J Allergy Clin Immunol* 98:48, 1996.
10. Engle S, Newns GH: Proliferative mural bronchiolitis, *Arch Dis Child* 15:219, 1940.
11. Everard ML, Milner AD: The respiratory syncytial virus and its role in acute bronchiolitis, *Eur J Pediatr* 151:638, 1992.
12. Flores G, Horwitz RI: Efficacy of β_2-agonists in bronchiolitis: a reappraisal and meta-analysis, *Pediatrics* 100:233, 1997.
13. Foy HM, et al: Incidence and etiology of pneumonia, croup and bronchiolitis in preschool children belonging to a prepaid medical care group over a four year period, *Am J Epidemiol* 97:80, 1973.

14. Gadomski AM, et al: Oral virus nebulized albuterol in management of bronchiolitis in Egypt, *Pediatrics* 24:131, 1994.
15. Gardner PS: How etiologic, pathologic, and clinical diagnoses can be made in a correlated fashion, *Pediatr Res* 11:254, 1977.
16. Garofalo R, Welliver RC, Ogra PL: Modulation of leukotriene (LT) release with ribavirin during infection with respiratory syncytial virus (RSV), *Pediatr Res* 25:163A, 1989.
17. Garofalo R, et al: Peripheral blood eosinophil counts and eosinophil cationic protein content of respiratory secretions in bronchiolitis: relationship to severity of disease, *Pediatr Allergy Immunol* 5:111, 1994.
18. Glezen WP, Denny FW: Epidemiology of acute lower respiratory disease in children, *N Engl J Med* 288:498, 1973.
19. Hall CB, Douglas RG Jr: Respiratory syncytial virus and influenza: practical community surveillance, *Am J Dis Child* 130:615, 1976.
20. Hall CB, Hall WJ, Speers DM: Clinical and physiologic manifestations of bronchiolitis and pneumonia, *Am J Dis Child* 133:798, 1979.
21. Hall CB, et al: Aerosolized ribavirin treatment of infants with respiratory syncytial viral infection: a randomized double blind study, *N Engl J Med* 308:1443, 1983.
22. Hall CB, et al: A long term prospective study of children following respiratory syncytial virus infection, *J Pediatr* 105:358, 1984.
23. Henderson FW, et al: The etiologic and epidemiologic spectrum of bronchiolitis in pediatric practice, *J Pediatr* 95:183, 1979.
24. Hickey RW, et al: Albuterol delivered via metered-dose inhaler with spacer for outpatient treatment of young children with wheezing, *Arch Pediatr Adolesc Med* 148:189, 1994.
25. Kellner JD, et al: Efficacy of bronchodilator therapy in bronchiolitis, *Arch Pediatr Adolesc Med* 150:1166, 1996.
26. Kellogg JA: Culture vs. direct antigen assays for detection of microbial pathogens from lower respiratory tract specimens suspected of containing the respiratory syncytial virus, *Arch Pathol Lab Med* 115:451, 1991.
27. Kimpen JL, Schaad UB: Treatment of respiratory syncytial virus bronchiolitis: 1995 poll of members of the European Society for Paediatric Infectious Diseases, *Pediatr Infect Dis J* 16:479, 1997.
28. Klassen TP: Recent advances in the treatment of bronchiolitis and laryngitis, *Pediatr Clin North Am* 44:249, 1997.
29. Landau LI: Bronchiolitis and asthma: are they related? *Thorax* 49:293, 1994.
30. Landau LI, et al: Gender related differences in airway tone in children, *Pediatr Pulmonol* 16:31, 1993.
31. Mahesh VK, Taussig LM: The wheezing infant: acute and long-term management, *J Respir Dis* 11:799, 1990.
32. Mahesh VK, Taussig LM: When an infant wheezes: clues to the differential, *J Respir Dis* 11:739, 1990.
33. Martinez FD, et al: Asthma and wheezing in the first six years of life, *N Engl J Med* 332:133, 1995.
34. Martinez FD, et al: Diminished lung function as a predisposing factor for wheezing respiratory illness in infants, *N Engl J Med* 319:1112, 1988.
35. Martinez FD, et al: Initial airway function is a risk factor for recurrent wheezing respiratory illnesses during the first three years of life, *Am Rev Respir Dis* 143:312, 1991.
36. McIntosh K, et al: The association of viral and bacterial respiratory infections with exacerbations of wheezing in young asthmatic children, *J Pediatr* 82:578, 1973.
37. Menon K, et al: A randomized trial comparing the efficacy of epinephrine with salbutamol in the treatment of acute bronchiolitis, *J Pediatr* 126:1004, 1995.
38. Morgan WJ: Viral respiratory infection in infancy: provocation or propagation? *Semin Respir Med* 11:306, 1990.
39. Peter JB: *Use and interpretation of laboratory tests in infectious disease,* ed 5, Specialty Laboratories, Santa Monica, Calif, 1998.
40. Reijonen TM, et al: Serum eosinophil cationic protein as a predictor of wheezing after bronchiolitis, *Pediatr Pulmonol* 23:397, 1997.
41. Rodriguez WJ, et al: Aerosolized ribavirin in the treatment of patients with respiratory syncytial virus disease, *Pediatr Infect Dis J* 6:159, 1987.
42. Ronchetti R, et al: Enhanced allergic sensitization related to parental smoking, *Arch Dis Child* 67:496, 1992.
43. Roosevelt G, et al: Dexamethasone in bronchiolitis: a radomized controlled trial, *Lancet* 348:292, 1996.
44. Rosner IK, et al: Effect of ribavirin therapy on respiratory syncytial virus-specific IgE and IgA responses after infection, *J Infect Dis* 155: 1043, 1987.
45. Sanchez I, et al: Effect of racemic epinephrine and salbutamol on clinical score and pulmonary mechanics in infants with bronchiolitis, *J Pediatr* 122:145, 1993.
46. Shay DK, Holman RC, Anderson LJ: *Bronchiolitis-associated hospitalizations among United States children from 1980 through 1995,* IDSA Thirty-sixth Annual Meeting, Denver, Colo, November 12-15, 1998 (abstract 44).
47. Sims DG, et al: Atopy does not predispose to RSV bronchiolitis or postbronchiolitic wheezing, *Br Med J* 282:2086, 1981.
48. Springer C, et al: Corticosteroids do not affect the clinical or physiological status of infants with bronchiolitis, *Pediatr Pulmonol* 9:181, 1990.
49. Sreeram N, Watson JG, Hunter S: Cardiovascular effects of acute bronchiolitis, *Acta Paediatr* Scand 80:133, 1991.
50. Van Woensel JBM, et al: Randomized double blind placebo controlled trial of prednisolone in children admitted to hospital with respiratory syncytial virus bronchiolitis, *Thorax* 52:634, 1997.
51. Volovitz B, et al: The release of leukotrienes in the respiratory tract during infection with respiratory syncytial virus: role in obstructive airway disease, *Pediatr Res* 24:504, 1988.
52. Welliver RC, et al: The development of respiratory syncytial virus-specific IgE and the release of histamine in nasopharyngeal secretions after infection, *N Engl J Med* 305:841, 1981.
53. Welliver RC, et al: Parainfluenza virus bronchiolitis: epidemiology and pathogenesis, *Am J Dis Child* 140:34, 1986.
54. Wilson N: The significance of early wheezing, *Clin Exper Allergy* 24: 522, 1994.
55. Wohl MEB: Bronchiolitis. In Chernick V, Kendig EL Jr, editors: *Kendig's disorders of the respiratory tract in children,* ed 5, Philadelphia, 1990, WB Saunders.
56. Young S, et al: The influence of a family history of asthma and parental smoking on airway responsiveness in early infancy, *N Engl J Med* 324: 1168, 1991.

193 Cancers in Childhood

Andrea S. Hinkle • Cindy L. Schwartz

Advances in the treatment of solid tumors of childhood during the past 20 years have ensured the long-term survival of at least two thirds of children who have these diagnoses. The pediatrician who initially discovers a solid tumor may not, and need not, know the best treatment available. However, early referral of such a child to the appropriate specialist, a pediatric oncologist, significantly affects the likelihood and the quality of survival. Many common childhood tumors are unique in the pediatric age range. For all solid tumors in children, therapies must be designed to minimize effects on growth and development. Appropriate use of the therapeutic modalities—surgery, chemotherapy, and radiation—provides maximum efficacy and minimal toxicity of therapy.

The child and his or her family should be encouraged to plan for the future. Educational and developmental needs must be addressed by the pediatric team—generalist and specialist together. Such a team also is best able to address the needs of the child, the parents, and the siblings if treatment is not successful. Fortunately, most children are cured and return to the pediatrician for many years of general pediatric care.

The following solid tumors seen in the pediatric population are described herein: Wilms' tumor, neuroblastoma, retinoblastoma, rhabdomyosarcoma, germ cell tumors and teratomas, Ewing's sarcoma, osteogenic sarcoma, non-Hodgkin's lymphomas, and Hodgkin's disease. The role of the pediatrician in the care of these children also is examined.

WILMS' TUMOR

Wilms' tumor, or nephroblastoma, is a malignant renal tumor of childhood that occurs at an annual rate of approximately 8 per 1 million children in the United States. It is the second most common abdominal tumor of childhood. Wilms' tumor comprises 5% to 6% of pediatric cancers. This translates to approximately 600 to 700 new cases diagnosed each year in the United States.[73] Patients usually are between 2 and 5 years of age. Only rarely does the tumor occur in teenagers and adults. The incidence of bilateral disease is increased in younger patients and female patients. It is one of the few pediatric malignancies that has a higher incidence in blacks than in whites.

The chemosensitivity and radiosensitivity of this tumor, in conjunction with the ability to resect most nonmetastatic tumors, have allowed a multidisciplinary approach to be highly successful. Wilms' tumor has become the model for treatment of childhood cancer. The National Wilms' Tumor Study (NWTS) has evaluated over the past three decades successive therapeutic regimens with the goal of increasing the cure rate and decreasing the duration and toxicity of therapy. The cooperative group approach has made possible the gathering of more data than could have been obtained at single institutions. The findings, such as the superiority of multiagent chemotherapy and the importance of tumor histology, are relevant for many tumors.

Etiology

Wilms' tumor has occurred in siblings, cousins, and parent-child pairs, particularly in association with specific congenital anomalies and bilateral disease.[126] Although it has been proposed that 15% to 20% of patients who have Wilms' tumor have a genetic predisposition to the disease, a much lower incidence of Wilms' tumor in patients who have affected relatives has been reported (approximately 1% to 2%).[18,97]

Anomalies are commonly reported in patients who have Wilms' tumor, although present in only a minority of patients who have the disease.[18,97] Most of the reported anomalies involve the genitourinary tract. Hemihypertrophy is second in frequency, sometimes noted as a component of the Beckwith-Wiedemann syndrome (excessive growth of many body organs). Of children who have the sporadic form of congenital aniridia, 33% have Wilms' tumor. WAGR syndrome is the association of Wilms' tumor, aniridia, genitourinary abnormalities, and mental retardation. Denys-Drash syndrome represents the association of Wilms' tumor with ambiguous genitalia and diffuse glomerular disease.[29,47] These syndromes are associated with germline mutations of the WT1 gene, located at 11p13.[72] WT1 abnormalities have been identified in a small subset of patients who have apparently sporadic Wilms' tumor, usually in association with genitourinary anomalies.[43] A second Wilms' tumor suppressor locus may be at 11p15, also the locus for the familial form of Beckwith-Wiedemann. Loss of heterozygosity at 1p and 16q also has been identified in Wilms' tumors and may confer a worse prognosis.[72] Further investigation of chromosomal abnormalities in Wilms' tumor and other malignancies will provide insight into tumorigenesis and potential new directions for therapy.

Screening by ultrasound and urinalysis for Wilms' tumor in patients who have aniridia, WAGR syndrome, Denys-Drash syndrome, and hemihypertrophy/Beckwith-Wiedemann syndrome is recommended every 3 months until

Table 193-1 Differential Diagnosis of Abdominal and Pelvic Tumors in Infants and Children

Tumor*	Age	Clinical Signs	Laboratory Findings
Wilms'	Preschool	Unilateral flank mass, aniridia, hemihypertrophy	Hematuria
Neuroblastoma	Preschool	GI/GU obstruction, raccoon eyes, myoclonus-opsoclonus, diarrhea, skin nodules (infants)	Increased VMA; increased HVA; increased ferritin; stippled calcification in mass
Non-Hodgkin's lymphoma	>1 yr	Intussusception in >2-year-old	Increased urate
Rhabdomyosarcoma	All	GI/GU obstruction, sarcoma botryoides, vaginal bleeding, paratesticular mass	
Germ cell/teratoma	Preschool, teens	Girls: abdominal pain, vaginal bleeding Boys: testicular mass, new onset "hydrocele" Sacrococcygeal mass/dimple	Increased HCG; increased AFP
Hepatoblastoma	Birth-3 yr	Large, firm liver	Increased AFP
Hepatoma	School age, teens	Large, firm liver; hepatitis B, cirrhosis	Increased AFP

*Other causes: constipation, splenomegaly, hydronephrosis, kidney cyst, and full bladder.
AFP, Alpha-fetoprotein; *GI,* gastrointestinal; *GU,* genitourinary; *HCG,* human chorionic gonadotropin; *HVA,* homovanillic acid; *VMA,* vanillylmandelic acid.

age 7 years. Screening also may be appropriate for patients who have unexplained nephropathy and who have multiple other congenital anomaly syndromes.[29]

Clinical Manifestations[97]

Wilms' tumor in children usually manifests as a painless mass discovered by a relative, often during bathing. The mass usually is firm, occasionally lobulated, and confined to one side of the abdomen. Rapid abdominal enlargement, anemia, and hypertension (perhaps because of a sudden subcapsular hemorrhage) occasionally occur at the time of presentation. Hypertension, malaise, abdominal pain, hematuria, and fever each occur in 20% to 30% of patients. Hypertension has been attributed to hyperreninemia.

Table 193-1 presents the differential diagnosis of abdominal and pelvic tumors of childhood that may mimic Wilms' tumor.

Evaluation

The evaluation of a patient who presumably has Wilms' tumor begins with a history and physical examination. Particular attention should be paid to the associated congenital anomalies and the family history. Laboratory studies should include a complete blood cell count, urinalysis, and renal and liver function testing. Bleeding within the tumor may cause anemia.[143] An erythropoietin-secreting Wilms' tumor may cause polycythemia. Hypercalcemia may occur in patients who have congenital mesoblastic nephroma or a rhabdoid tumor.

A plain radiograph of the abdomen should be obtained. Calcification, if noted in a Wilms' tumor, usually is quite coarse, unlike the fine, stippled pattern commonly seen in neuroblastoma. Mass effect may be noted on the film. An abdominal computed tomography (CT) scan with contrast may reveal an intrarenal mass displacing and distorting the collecting system of the involved kidney. The tumors may be very large, and minimal kidney parenchyma may be identified. Ultrasonographic examination is often the initial study obtained, and this modality is particularly helpful in evaluating the renal vein, vena cava, and the right side of the heart for tumor spread.[7] Liver metastases may be diagnosed either by ultrasound or by CT scan. Although intravenous pyelography may demonstrate the tumor, with currently available imaging techniques it generally is not indicated. Magnetic resonance imaging (MRI) occasionally may be indicated to define tumor extent. A chest radiograph (CXR) should be obtained and may demonstrate pulmonary nodules. A CT scan of the chest to detect small pulmonary metastases should be performed before surgery, inasmuch as postoperative atelectasis can obscure the presence of metastatic nodules. Bone scans are indicated in patients who have clear-cell sarcoma of the kidney, which often spreads to bone.

At the time of surgery, the tumor is staged as follows:[54]

1. Stage I: Tumor is limited to the kidney and is completely resected.
2. Stage II: Tumor extends beyond the kidney but is completely resected.
3. Stage III: Residual, nonhematogenously spread tumor is confined to the abdomen, such as lymph node involvement, peritoneal contamination before or during surgery, peritoneal implants, residual tumor postoperatively, or incomplete resection caused by local infiltration. Unresectable tumors are also stage III.
4. Stage IV: Hematogenous metastases are present. Sites include lung (only site in 80% of patients who have metastases), liver, lymph node, and less commonly, bone, brain, and other sites.
5. Stage V: Bilateral renal involvement is present.

Wilms' tumors are pathologically designated as being of either favorable histology (FH) or unfavorable histology (UH). Favorable histology indicates the absence of unfavorable features. Unfavorable histology involves the presence of anaplasia, defined by the presence of gigantic polypoid nuclei within the tumor sample. Anaplasia may be focal or diffuse. Diffuse anaplasia conveys a worse prognosis, which appears to be due to resistance to chemotherapy and radiation therapy and not to biologically more aggressive disease.[11] Two other renal tumors, clear-cell sarcoma of the kidney and rhabdoid tumor of the kidney, previously were considered Wilms' tumor variants, but now are considered separate entities. Only clear-cell sarcoma continues to be studied as part of National Wilms' Tumor Study protocols.

Management

In the United States, the initial therapeutic approach is a complete resection by nephrectomy. This requires careful and gentle surgical techniques to prevent tumor spillage. The large transabdominal incision facilitates full exploration and excision. The entire ureter is removed, lymph nodes are sampled, and the contralateral kidney and abdominal cavity are examined for evidence of disease. For bilateral disease, chemotherapy is recommended after bilateral biopsy. "Second-look" excision of residual disease may be accomplished by partial nephrectomies, when possible.[93] Tumors deemed unresectable by clinical and radiological evaluation also are biopsied initially, then second-look resection is performed after adequate chemotherapy-induced shrinkage is achieved.

Actinomycin D and vincristine were noted to be effective agents in the mid-1960s. The initial NWTS-I study revealed that radiation therapy in combination with a single agent (actinomycin D or vincristine) provided approximately 55% relapse-free survival in patients whose disease was localized. An 81% relapse-free survival was found when both agents were administered in conjunction with radiation.[34] The two drugs have since been the mainstay of chemotherapy for Wilms' tumor. Subsequent studies demonstrated that radiation therapy was not necessary for stage I-II FH tumors and stage I UH, and that the addition of doxorubicin and 10 Gy of radiation to vincristine and actinomycin D improved the prognosis for patients who had stage III- IV FH tumors, as well as for those who had stage II-IV with focal anaplasia.[34,66] The addition of cyclophosphamide as a fourth agent is of benefit for patients who have stage II-IV tumors with diffuse anaplasia. The NWTS-IV evaluated shorter-duration and dose-intensified regimens. This study demonstrated that shorter-duration therapy (6 months versus 15 months) and fewer higher doses of chemotherapeutic agents versus multiple smaller doses (pulse-intensive therapy) resulted in the same outcome, with less toxicity and less cost.[67] The use of lower-dose radiation (10 Gy) and irradiation of the entire width of the vertebrae adjacent to the renal bed have decreased the severity—but not entirely prevented the development—of scoliosis.[172] Peritoneal seeding or a major tumor rupture necessitates radiation of the entire abdomen. Thoracic radiation is used for pulmonary metastasis visible on CXR or those seen on chest CT only, which do not resolve with chemotherapy.[68]

Prognosis

The prognosis of patients who have Wilms' tumor is determined by the histopathology of the tumor. In the NWTS-I, 50% of 26 patients who had UH findings died, compared with 6.9% of 376 patients who had FH findings.[12] The survival of both groups of patients has improved, but UH, particularly diffuse anaplasia, continues to confer a worse prognosis. More intensive regimens continue to be studied for those patients who have stage II-IV disease with UH features.

Prognosis also depends on the stage of disease at diagnosis. Most relapses occur within 2 years of diagnosis. Two-year relapse-free survival for stages I-III disease that has FH findings is approximately 91%. The 2-year relapse-free survival rate is 84% for patients who have stage IV disease and FH features.[67] Patients who have diffuse anaplasia have a poor prognosis, with only 59% of stage II patients, 45% of stage III patients, and 7% of stage IV patients surviving at 4 years following diagnosis.[11] Patients who relapse have a better prognosis if their initial management did not include radiation therapy or doxorubicin. Autologous transplant procedures are being investigated in patients who have high-risk, relapsed disease.

Follow-up

While patients are receiving therapy, they are monitored for disease recurrence at the primary site, usually with abdominal ultrasound, and in the lungs, usually with CXR. Some patients may be followed with CT of the chest and abdomen. Such monitoring continues at increasing intervals until approximately 5 years after diagnosis.

Long-term survival is likely in patients who have Wilms' tumor. Virtually all have had a nephrectomy and should be discouraged from engaging in contact sports. A kidney guard can be recommended for particularly active children, if only to serve as a reminder of the need for caution. In addition, patients should have their renal function monitored.

Scoliosis was a major problem for early survivors treated with moderate-dose radiation (30 to 40 Gy), particularly if the entire vertebrae were not included in the field, because of impaired growth of the irradiated portion of the vertebrae. The scoliosis is less severe in patients treated more recently. Close observation of patients who received irradiation, particularly during the pubertal growth spurt, remains necessary. Prevention of obesity will minimize the asymmetry associated with a decreased quantity of adipose tissue in the radiation field. Hypoplasia with a decrease in adipose tissue occurs in the radiation field and is accentuated by obesity. Therefore, prevention of obesity minimizes this asymmetry.

Fertility is preserved in most patients who have Wilms' tumor, although there is a risk of ovarian failure with whole-abdomen radiation therapy. The average size of infants born to female survivors of irradiation is smaller than that of non-irradiated women,[105] and increased pregnancy losses and premature births in female survivors of Wilms' tumor who received radiation therapy have been reported.[21] In addition, some of these females may have underlying uterine anomalies.[134] Continued follow-up of these offspring is necessary to evaluate the genetic factors involved in the occurrence of Wilms' tumor.

NEUROBLASTOMA

Neuroblastoma arises from the fetal neural cells that normally develop into the sympathetic nervous system. It is a tumor that provides insight into the biological processes of malignancy. Tumors in infants may regress spontaneously or mature to benign ganglioneuromas, whereas patients older than 1 year who have disseminated disease remain difficult to cure despite aggressive use of multimodal therapy.

Neuroblastoma is the most common extracranial solid tumor in children and is the most common malignancy of infants, accounting for more than half of infantile cancers. Neuroblastoma accounts for 7% of all children diagnosed as having cancer and 15% of childhood cancer mortality. Approximately 9.7 white children and 7.4 black children per million in the United States are afflicted with neuroblastoma each year. This equals approximately 800 to 900 new cases diagnosed each year in the United States.[73] Ninety percent of patients who have neuroblastoma are younger than 5 years of age, and 97% of patients will be diagnosed before the age of 10 years.

Etiology

The high incidence of neuroblastoma in early infancy suggests that its development may be related to abnormal maturation of fetal neural crest cells. The finding of microscopic nodules of adrenal neuroblastoma in infants younger than 3 months of age who have died of unrelated causes suggests that spontaneous maturation or regression occurs in many children.[13]

Families have been reported in which neuroblastoma occurred in multiple siblings or occasionally in multiple generations.[27,137] Some have proposed that 20% to 25% of neuroblastomas occur in patients who have a prezygotic germinal mutation.[96] Neuroblastoma has been reported to occur with an increased incidence in patients who have Hirschsprung's disease, which may be related to maldevelopment of the neural crest. The reported incidence in neurofibromatosis type I may be coincidence. Although reported in other syndromes, no clear increased frequency has been determined.

Clinical Manifestations

Neuroblastoma may arise anywhere along the sympathetic nervous system chain, including the adrenal gland (40%), the paraspinal regions of the abdomen (25%), the thorax (15%), the neck (5%), and the pelvis at the organ of Zuckerkandl (5%). The incidence of primary site varies by age, with thoracic and cervical tumors more common in infants. The presenting features depend to a large extent on the location of the tumor. A large, firm, irregular abdominal mass that may cross the midline often is the first sign of disease. Disturbances of bowel or bladder function may be due to compression by a pelvic mass. Thoracic masses may cause a persistent cough or respiratory distress and are detected by a CXR. Cervical masses often are diagnosed initially as lymphadenitis, but they do not respond to antibiotic therapy. Horner's syndromeor heterochromia iridis suggests the possibility of neuroblastoma.

Neuroblastomas that arise in the paravertebral ganglia tend to grow into the intervertebral foramina, forming a dumbbell-shaped mass. Pain, weakness of an extremity, paralysis, or incontinence may result from spinal cord compression by the intraspinal component. Incontinence may be difficult to assess, however, as many patients will still be in diapers. Cord compression is an oncological emergency that requires surgical decompression, radiation, or chemotherapy to prevent permanent paraplegia.

The majority of children who have neuroblastoma have metastatic disease at the time of diagnosis. The symptoms then usually are related to the metastatic tumor rather than to the primary tumor. Infants may have metastatic hepatic involvement. Rapid liver enlargement can cause marked abdominal distention followed by respiratory compromise. Bluish skin nodules, which may release catecholamines if palpated, sometimes are noted in infants who have neuroblastoma. Palpation causes an erythematous cutaneous flush, lasting for 2 to 3 minutes, and is followed by blanching because of vasoconstriction.[77]

The most common site for metastases is the bone marrow, reported in 70.5% of patients who have metastatic disease. The next most common site is bone in 55.7% of patients, followed by lymph nodes, liver, and intracranial and orbital sites. Lung and CNS disease was seen in only 3.3% and 0.6% of patients, respectively.[48] Infiltration of the bone marrow may cause pancytopenia. Bone involvement may produce pain, with or without palpable bone masses. Lytic bone lesions are found most often in the skull, orbit, or proximal long bones. A raccoonlike appearance caused by proptosis and eyelid ecchymosis has been described in those who have orbital involvement. Intracranial disease usually is due to meningeal metastases.[98] In infants, this may manifest as separation of cranial sutures caused by increased intracranial pressure. Infants and children who have neuroblastoma also may present with fever, malaise, and failure to thrive.

Secretory products of the tumor may be the cause of the presenting features. Vasoactive intestinal polypeptide (VIP) has been found in 7% to 9% of children who have neural crest tumors, most frequently ganglioneuromas or ganglioneuroblastomas.[156] Intractable diarrhea is caused by this hormone.

An unusual symptom of neuroblastoma is the syndrome of opsoclonus-myoclonus.[152] These patients have acute cerebellar ataxia and rapid, dancing-eye movements. Although these patients often have localized disease and usually are cured, residual neurological dysfunction, including residual ataxia and mental retardation, is common. The etiology of this syndrome is unclear. An autoimmune factor, perhaps an antibody directed against neuroblastoma that cross-reacts with the cerebellar cell antigen, may be causative.

Tables 193-1 to 193-3 present the differential diagnosis of abdominal, pelvic, head, neck, and mediastinal tumors that may mimic neuroblastoma.

Evaluation

After the initial physical examination, evaluation of a patient who has neuroblastoma requires radiological examination of the area of primary disease, as well as of areas to which neuroblastoma metastasizes. In addition to the CXR, a CT scan of the abdomen, pelvis, and chest should be performed. For those patients who have cervical masses, the CT scan should include this area. Because paravertebral lesions may extend into the intervertebral foramina, any patient who has such a lesion should be evaluated by MRI. A skeletal survey and a bone scan should be performed to detect bony lesions.[91] Radiographs are useful for the detection of small lytic lesions at the end of bones; the bone scan helps find

Table 193-2 Differential Diagnosis of Head and Neck Tumors in Infants and Children

Tumor*	Age	Clinical Signs	Laboratory Findings
Non-Hodgkin's lymphoma	>1 yr	Lymphadenopathy—NR to antibiotics; immunodeficiency; EBV (in Africa)	Increased urate
Hodgkin's disease	>10 yr	Lymphadenopathy—NR to antibiotics; weight loss, night sweats, fever, pruritus	Increased ESR
Rhabdomyosarcoma	All	Orbital mass; hoarseness; persistent otitis, sinusitis	
Neuroblastoma	Preschool	Heterochromia iridis, Horner's syndrome, myoclonus-opsoclonus, raccoon eyes, skin nodules (infants)	Increased HVA in urine; increased VMA in urine; calcification
Retinoblastoma	Preschool	Cat's eye reflex, strabismus, family history	Calcification

*Other causes: infectious lymphadenopathy, histiocytosis, Caffey's disease, acquired immunodeficiency syndrome.
EBV, Epstein-Barr virus; *ESR,* erythrocyte sedimentation rate; *HVA,* homovanillic acid; *NR,* no response; *VMA,* vanillylmandelic acid.

Table 193-3 Differential Diagnosis of Mediastinal Tumors in Infants and Children

Tumor*	Age	Clinical Signs	Laboratory Findings
Non-Hodgkin's lymphoma	All	Cough, respiratory distress, anterior mediastinal mass, immunodeficiency syndrome	Increased urate; malignant effusion
Hodgkin's disease	>10 yr	Middle mediastinum lymphadenopathy—NR to antibiotics; weight loss, night sweats, fever, pruritus	Increased ESR; increased copper
Neuroblastoma	Preschool	Posterior mediastinum; heterochromia iridis, myoclonus-opsoclonus, raccoon eyes, skin nodules (infants)	Increased HVA; increased VMA; calcification
Thymoma	>10 yr	Anterior mediastinum, myasthenia gravis, red cell aplasia, hypogammaglobulinemia	
Germ cell/teratoma	All	Anterior mediastinum (rarely, posterior mediastinum), cough, wheeze, dyspnea	Increased AFP; increased HCG

*Other causes: infection, bronchogenic cysts, aneurysms, lipoid tumors, thoracic meningocele.
AFP, Alpha-fetoprotein; *ESR,* erythrocyte sedimentation rate; *HCG,* human chorionic gonadotropin; *HVA,* homovanillic acid; *VMA,* vanillylmandelic acid.

lesions of the skull and tubular bones. Because of the frequency of metastatic involvement, bone marrow biopsy specimens should be obtained in all patients; bilateral specimens should be obtained to increase the probability of detecting metastases. The liver should be examined by contrast CT scan in all patients and by biopsy in those who have abdominal disease. Meta-iodobenzylguanidine (mIBG) is taken up by neuroblastomas and may be utilized for imaging but is not universally employed because of the difficulties in administering mIBG and in interpreting results.

The previously used Evans and St. Judes staging systems have been synthesized into an International Neuroblastoma Staging System (INSS). Stage 1 includes tumors with complete gross resection and microscopically negative ipsilateral and contralateral lymph nodes. Stage 2 tumors are unilateral tumors with complete or incomplete gross resections but, at the most, only ipsilateral microscopically positive lymph nodes. Stage 3 includes tumors that cross the midline or unilateral tumors that have contralateral lymph node involvement, and stage 4 designates metastatic disease. Stage 4S (for special) tumors occur in infants younger than 1 year of age who have stage 1 or 2 primary tumors with dissemination limited to liver, skin, or bone marrow.[19]

Neuroblastoma must be diagnosed by histological examination after biopsy. In patients who have localized disease, the biopsy specimen must be obtained from the primary tumor. For those who have metastatic disease, neuroblastoma cells can be identified in the primary tumor or in areas of metastases, including the bone, bone marrow, or liver. Neuroblastoma comprises small round cells with scant cytoplasm that must be differentiated from other small cell tumors of childhood, including lymphoma, leukemia, Ewing's sarcoma, and retinoblastoma. Neuroblastoma cells often are densely packed and separated by thin fibrils or bundles. Necrosis and calcification may be seen. The small round cells often form clusters (called Homer-Wright pseudorosettes) surrounded by pink neurofibrillary material. With increasing maturation, more fibrillary material is present, and ganglionic differentiation may be seen. Cytoplasmic structures consisting of neurofibrils, neurotubules, and neurosecretory granules that contain catecholamines may be noted.[111] Secretion of catecholamines from the granules results in elevated levels of vanillylmandelic acid (VMA) and homovanillic acid (HVA) in 24-hour urine samples or in elevated VMA:creatinine or HVA:creatinine ratios in "spot" urine samples.[62,99] These findings can be used to confirm the diagnosis of neuroblastoma in patients who have a small round-cell infiltrate in the bone marrow. In addition, elevated urinary catecholamine levels can be used to monitor the response to therapy. Ferritin and lactic dehydrogenase (LDH) levels may be obtained and have prognostic significance in that elevated levels predict a poor prognosis.[121]

Amplification of the N-*myc* oncogene is an intrinsic biological property of some neuroblastomas and has been associated with poor prognosis regardless of clinical stage (although most commonly it is seen in patients who have advanced disease).[151,157] Conversely, tumors that have hyperdiploid neuroblastoma (DNA index >1) are sensitive to chemotherapy, resulting in a good prognosis.[109] Specimens should be analyzed for both of these biological features, which are used to determine "risk groups" for treatment purposes. Newer findings, such as the association of the tyrosine kinase receptor *TRK A* with good risk and the association of deletion of chromosome 1p with poor risk, suggest that continued study of the molecular biology of neuroblastoma may lead to additional prognostic factors as well as to new therapeutic approaches.[118] Areas of interest include nerve growth factor receptors, multidrug resistance genes, and telomerase activity.

Management

Neuroblastoma is sensitive to both chemotherapy and radiation therapy. Surgical therapy alone may suffice for localized disease. Minimal residual disease may regress spontaneously in patients whose disease is localized. Although complete removal of the tumor offers the best chance of cure in higher-risk patients, often only a diagnostic biopsy is feasible. Tumor recurrence in such patients often is at the site of the primary tumor. Surgical reduction after initial cytoreductive therapy may enhance the likelihood of cure.

Chemotherapy is the major modality of therapy in neuroblastoma. Complete and partial responses have been found with multiple agents, including cyclophosphamide, doxorubicin, cisplatin, epipodophyllotoxin, and vincristine.[23] Ifosfamide, carboplatin, and topotecan also are effective agents. Combination therapy is used, most intensively in the more advanced stages of disease. Survival with conventional therapy remains inadequate for patients older than 1 year of age who have stage 4 disease or stage 3 disease with unfavorable biological features (e.g., N-*myc* amplification).

Intensive regimens are at the limits of bone marrow tolerance. Myeloablative therapy followed by purged autologous bone marrow transplantation to restore hematopoiesis has been shown in a randomized trial to improve event-free survival.[123] A second randomization performed after high-dose therapy showed that the differentiating agent, cis-retinoic acid, improved survival for high-risk patients, regardless of whether stem cell transplantation was used.[123] Peripheral blood stem cells (PBSC) also can be used for marrow rescue after myeloablative therapy. Stem cell preparations often are either purged of tumor cells[65] or the stem cells are preferentially selected. Consecutive PBSC transplant procedures to increase the dose intensity further and, it is hoped, the response in patients who have high-risk disease are being investigated.

Neuroblastoma is a radiation-sensitive tumor. Although rarely needed in early-stage disease, radiation therapy may facilitate surgical resection of residual disease or may reduce the risk of recurrence in surgically unresectable disease. Emergent situations, such as a large mediastinal mass resulting in respiratory compromise or a dumbbell lesion protruding into the intervertebral foramen that causes cord compression, may be treated with radiation. Total-body irradiation also may be a component of the preparative regimen used before bone marrow or PBSC transplantation. In the terminal stage of neuroblastoma, bone pain or compression of organs such as the trachea, bowel, or urinary tract may require palliative radiation therapy.

Investigations continue into other treatments to improve the outcome and potentially reduce the toxicities of therapy for children who have high-risk neuroblastoma. These include the use of desferrioxamine, radiolabeled mIBG, and targeted immunotherapy employing anti-GD_2 ganglioside antibodies.[28,57,59]

Prognosis

Age and stage of disease appear to be the most important predictors of survival. Patients who are younger than 1 year of age do markedly better than those who are older than 2 years. Patients who have stage 1, 2, or 4S neuroblastoma with favorable biological features have survival rates higher than 90%. Although some studies dispute the poor prognosis of N-*myc*-amplified tumors in infants, other studies report a significantly lower survival rate for those patients.[17,90] Long-term survival for patients who have stage III neuroblastoma has improved in recent years, with patients younger than 1 year of age and with those who have favorable biology having, respectively, survival rates of 100% and 90% at 4 years.[122] Thus, intensive multiagent chemotherapy appears to result in improved cure rates for these patients. In studies of stage 4 patients treated with bone marrow or stem cell transplants, event-free survival is 23% to 46 % at 3 to 6 years.[92,101] Skeletal disease and persisting bone marrow involvement were predictive of a poorer outcome, and patients who have complete response to chemotherapy benefit most from transplant procedures.

Follow-up

Although late recurrences have been reported, most tumors recur while patients are receiving therapy or shortly afterward. Close follow-up with physical examination and radiological studies should continue for 2 years after completion of therapy. Urinary catecholamine levels may be useful in the surveillance of those who had elevated values at diagnosis. Relapses may occur later after transplant procedures, and radiological evaluation and urinary catecholamine monitoring should continue for 5 years from diagnosis. Patients should be monitored for late toxicities (e.g., of cyclophosphamide, doxorubicin, and cisplatin). High-dose therapy associated with autologous BMT or PBSC procedures may result in significant late effects, including hearing loss, renal insufficiency, growth impairment, and gonadal failure.

RETINOBLASTOMA

Retinoblastoma is a congenital malignant tumor of the retina that occurs once in 18,000 live births.[41] Retinoblastoma develops in approximately 350 children in the United States annually, 20% to 30% of whom have bilateral disease. The disorder is diagnosed in 95% before age 4 years, with the median age of diagnosis being 2 years.[73] Patients who have bilateral disease appear to have an inherited form of this tumor that manifests at an earlier age. Most patients who have unilateral disease have a sporadic form of the tumor.

This tumor is the model for understanding the role of genetics in the development of malignancy. The pediatrician plays an important role in detecting this disorder initially and in providing support to the family, who may carry a genetic predisposition to this malignancy.

Etiology

Knudson[95] has proposed that two independent mutations must occur in a single retinal cell for retinoblastoma to develop. The initial mutation may occur in a germinal cell (inheritable form) or in the somatic retinal cell itself (sporadic form). Those patients who have an abnormality in the germinal cell have one mutation in each retinal cell. A second mutation is relatively likely to occur, causing retinoblastoma (often multiple, bilateral tumors). If the initial mutation arises in a retinal cell, it must be followed by a second mutation in the same cell for the sporadic form of retinoblastoma to arise. The likelihood of two such events is low; hence single, unilateral tumors develop. Because the germinal cell is not involved, the mutation is not inherited.

Clearly, a patient who has a family history of retinoblastoma or bilateral retinoblastoma has a germinal mutation and therefore the hereditary form of the disease. These patients have a 50% chance of transmitting retinoblastoma to their children. The germinal mutation also may have arisen in an affected parent or in one who had an undiagnosed retinal lesion. Parents are recommended to have an ophthalmological examination. If the first child of "normal" parents has unilateral retinoblastoma, their second child has a 1% risk of being affected. In some families, recombinant DNA techniques may aid in determining which relatives are predisposed to retinoblastoma.[178] All families should be referred for genetic counseling. Deletions of chromosome 13q14 have been detected in some patients who have retinoblastoma. This retinoblastoma gene (Rb) has been cloned, and the Rb gene product may play a role in the regulation of cell growth. Deletion or dysfunction of the gene also has been found in nonretinal tumors such as osteosarcomas, soft-tissue sarcomas, and breast carcinomas.

Clinical Manifestations[24]

Patients who have a family history of retinoblastoma currently are screened by examination under anesthesia every 2 to 3 months during early childhood, starting at birth. These patients therefore are diagnosed before the occurrence of any clinical symptoms. Pediatricians and parents usually detect the abnormality in children who have the sporadic form of disease, because young children rarely complain of unilaterally decreased vision. Leukocoria, or cat's eye reflex, describes a whiteness detected in the pupillary area caused by a large retrolental mass. It is the most commonly encountered sign of retinoblastoma. If a normal red reflex is not present in a young child, it should be investigated. The second most common presenting feature is strabismus. Although this is common in childhood because of abnormalities of ocular muscle strength, it rarely arises suddenly in a child who has had normal extraocular movements. Rarely, pain in the eye may occur as a result of glaucoma. New-onset strabismus or an abnormal red reflex (leukocoria) requires prompt ophthalmological evaluation.

The differential diagnosis of retinoblastoma includes Coats' disease, retrolental fibroplasia, persistent hyperplastic primary vitreous, toxoplasmosis, *Toxocara canis*, and other causes of severe uveitis. In one review, 25% of patients had nonneoplastic disorders at the time of enucleation,[116,163] but this is an uncommon occurrence with newer methodologies, including ultrasonic examinations and MRI. Patients in whom retinoblastoma is a possibility should be referred to an ophthalmologist who has a working relationship with radiation and pediatric oncologists and is experienced in the diagnosis and initial evaluation of these patients.

Evaluation

Examination under anesthesia, after pupillary dilation, is necessary to evaluate fully the retina in a young child. Ultrasonographic examination is useful to evaluate the mass, particularly if the fundal examination is obscured by hemorrhage or retinal detachment.[165] Calcification in retinoblastoma may be apparent on roentgenogram, ultrasound examination, or CT scanning. The CT scan is useful to demonstrate the extent of intraocular disease and to detect possible extraocular extension. MRI can help to evaluate the tumor's involvement with the optic nerve, the subarachnoid, and the brain.

Retinoblastoma is not a tumor for which biopsy is a feasible method of diagnosis. Patients who have a family history or bilateral disease do not need a tissue diagnosis. In many, but not all cases of unilateral disease, enucleation is necessary to establish the diagnosis and to treat the tumor. For high-risk patients, bone marrow and cerebrospinal fluid specimens are obtained for evidence of dissemination. The extent of local disease (extension beyond the globe or optic nerve infiltration) is assessed at the time of enucleation.

Management

Treatment for retinoblastoma is individualized based on the extent of disease and the possibility for the preservation of vision.[25,158] Treatments available include enucleation, cryotherapy, photocoagulation, radiotherapy, and chemotherapy. Most patients who have unilateral sporadic disease have large lesions and visual compromise. Enucleation is usually required, with removal of as long a segment of the optic nerve as possible. Chemotherapy is rarely used in this population. Photocoagulation and cryotherapy are used for small lesions, most commonly in those who have hereditary bilateral disease. Until recently, radiation therapy was the standard of care for those who had massive bilateral disease. Chemotherapy for bilateral disease is increasingly used to allow local therapy and to preserve vision.[140] The most commonly employed agent is carboplatin, often in association with etoposide. The number of children who ultimately will need enucleation or radiation and the long-term outcome is being studied. Emerging therapy also includes the use of thermotherapy (diode laser hyperthermia) with or without adjuvant chemotherapy.[104,160]

Cyclophosphamide, doxorubicin, vincristine, cisplatin, carboplatin, and epipodophyllotoxins have been used with some evidence of success in patients who have advanced or recurrent disease.[159] Cyclosporin has been used with chemotherapy to overcome multidrug resistance and has been shown in one study to improve the long-term response to chemotherapy, although definite benefit remains to be proved.[26] Bone marrow transplantation or peripheral blood stem cell support after high-dose therapy for the treatment of recurrent disease has been reported.[133]

Prognosis

Survival of patients who have retinoblastoma is excellent; more than 85% have no recurrence of their tumor. Unfortunately, those who have hereditary retinoblastoma have a high incidence of second malignancy. Approximately 50% occur within the radiation field; osteogenic sarcoma or other sarcomas particularly are common. Approximately one third of such patients have a second malignancy within 15 years. By 30 years, two thirds will have a second malignancy.[3,64] Avoidance of radiation therapy may reduce this risk.

Follow-up

Patients who have been treated for retinoblastoma will need close follow-up for evidence of recurrence and for second malignancies. Most recurrences manifest within 3 years of diagnosis. Examinations under anesthesia should be performed every 2 to 3 months during the first year, every 3 to 4 months during the second year, and every 6 months thereafter until age 6 years. Long-term risk depends on treatment. After enucleation, a prosthesis is necessary. Radiation impairs orbital growth and increases the risk for cataract development and retinal vascular injury. Growth and pubertal development usually are unaffected by orbital radiation, but monitoring of hypothalamic-pituitary axis function is warranted. The risk of second malignancy is high in those who have bilateral or familial disease, particularly in the radiation field. Medical care should be sought promptly for unexplained masses, pain, or other symptoms.

RHABDOMYOSARCOMA

Rhabdomyosarcoma is considered to be one of the small, round, blue cell tumors of childhood (along with neuroblastomas, Ewing's sarcoma, and lymphoma). It arises from embryonal mesenchyme that can differentiate into skeletal muscle. Rhabdomyosarcoma can occur almost anywhere in the body, even in sites that do not normally contain skeletal muscle. It is an aggressive tumor that disseminates early in the course of disease. Before the advent of chemotherapy, cure required extirpative surgery of localized disease and then radiotherapy. The rapid progress, with survival rates increasing from less than 20% in the 1960s to approximately 70% in the late 1990s, has been due to the multidisciplinary cooperative group approach of the Intergroup Rhabdomyosarcoma Study (IRS).[124]

Rhabdomyosarcoma is the most common pediatric soft-tissue sarcoma, accounting for 2% to 4% of childhood malignancies and 5% to 15% of childhood solid tumors. Its annual incidence among children through 18 years of age in the United States is 4.5 per million. Thus, there are approximately 400 new cases diagnosed each year. The incidence in males is greater than in females, and in whites is greater than in blacks.[73] Forty percent of affected children are younger than 5 years of age, 47% are 5 to 14 years of age, and the rest are older than 15 years.

Etiology

The cause of this tumor is unknown. It has occurred in association with neurofibromatosis, in families who have a history of multiple tumors, and in patients who have congenital abnormalities of the central nervous system, the heart, the gastrointestinal tract, and the urinary tract.[154]

There are two major histopathological subtypes: embryonal and alveolar. Embryonal rhabdomyosarcoma may have loss of heterozygosity at 11p15; the alveolar subtype is associated with a characteristic chromosomal translocation, t(2:13).[5,10] The latter is more common in extremity and trunk sites and older children. Younger children who have alveolar rhabdomyosarcoma may have t(1:13), which is associated with a somewhat better prognosis than t(2:13). Further investigation of the cytogenetic alterations identified in the histopathological subtypes will provide insight into tumorigenesis. Undifferentiated sarcomas do not express lineage markers but have been traditionally treated on rhabdomyosarcoma regimens.

Clinical Manifestations

Rhabdomyosarcoma manifests as a painless mass that has poorly defined margins.[44] No mass may be palpable, but patients may present with disturbance of a normal body function resulting from the presence of tumor. Pain may also be a presenting symptom. Thirty-five to forty percent of rhabdomyosarcomas arise in the head and neck region, 25% in the genitourinary region, 20% in the extremities, and the remainder from truncal and other sites. One common site of involvement is the orbit, in which swelling, proptosis, discoloration, and limitation of extraocular motion occur. Patients who have a tumor of the head and neck may have hoarseness, difficulty swallowing, nasopharyngeal polyps, nasopharyngeal obstruction, decreased hearing acuity, persistent otitis, sinusitis, bloody nasal discharge, parotitis, or cranial nerve palsies. In parameningeal sites, penetration to the brain may cause headache, vomiting, or diplopia. Retroperitoneal tumor may manifest as a mass or partial or complete bowel obstruction. Vaginal bleeding, pelvic or perineal masses, hematuria, urinary frequency, and urinary retention suggest genitourinary tract involvement. Tumor may even be extruded from the bladder or female genital tract. A hydrocele, incarcerated hernia, testicular torsion, or testicular mass may be an indication of paratesticular rhabdomyosarcoma. Symptoms may be related to metastatic disease, such as pain or difficulty or refusal to ambulate resulting from bone metastases. Patients may also have systemic symptoms, such as fever, fatigue, or weight loss.

Evaluation

Initial evaluation should include a complete history and physical examination. Roentgenograms, CT scans or MRIs, and in some instances (e.g., genitourinary tract) ultrasound examination of the involved and adjacent areas should be performed. For genitourinary disease, a cystourethrogram, barium enema, and cystoscopic and pelvic examinations may also be needed. Bone surveys, bone scans, a bone marrow biopsy, and liver CT scan are necessary to assess for metastatic disease. Basal skull erosion may be seen by CT scan, and spinal fluid may reveal meningeal disease in those who have parameningeal tumors. Dental films may be helpful. If spinal cord symptoms are present, a spinal MRI is necessary. Biopsy of the lesion establishes the diagnosis and should be performed before extensive resection. The current Intergroup Rhabdomyosarcoma Study (IRS) determines chemotherapy by preoperative extent and site of disease (stage). Radiotherapy is determined by residual disease postoperatively (clinical group).

Management

Rhabdomyosarcoma is a tumor that requires a multitherapeutic approach, including chemotherapy, surgery, and radiation. Aggressive surgical approaches have become less essential as chemotherapy and radiation therapy have become more efficacious.

The initial surgical procedure should be a diagnostic biopsy. A wide resection of the primary tumor, including surrounding normal tissue, is preferable if excessive functional and cosmetic morbidity can be avoided.[125] Extensive en bloc lymph node dissection is no longer indicated; however, large regional nodes should be biopsied. After chemotherapy or radiotherapy, second-look surgery provides assessment of therapeutic response by determining the presence of viable tumor and reduces the extent of residual disease by resecting the involved lymph nodes.

Chemotherapy regimens for rhabdomyosarcoma include vincristine, actinomycin D, and cyclophosphamide (VAC). Ifosfamide, doxorubicin, etoposide, and topotecan also are active agents. The benefit of adding any of these agents to VAC has not been demonstrated.

Rhabdomyosarcoma is an infiltrative disease, and radiation portals should include the entire extent of tumor volume. Although high doses of radiation (60 to 65 Gy) control local residual disease excellently, substantial late morbidity results.[169] Unfortunately, lower doses of radiation result in an increased recurrence rate. New methodologies using lower total doses of radiation administered twice preserve efficacy while minimizing late toxicities.[114] Brachytherapy is another investigational approach that may limit toxicity by using sealed radioisotopes placed inside or close to the tumor, thereby treating only tissues within a short distance and minimizing damage to the surrounding normal tissues.[132]

Prognosis

The likelihood of survival for patients who have rhabdomyosarcoma is determined by the site and the stage of disease.[102] Overall survival is 65% at 5 years from diagnosis. The prognosis is particularly good for patients who have orbital tumors; nonbladder and nonprostate genitourinary-tract tumors, and localized tumors that can be resected fully (90% to 95% long-term survivors). Group IV patients (those who have metastatic disease) younger than age 10 years who have embryonal histology have recently been noted to have a better prognosis than older patients who have group IV disease. The results of IRS I-III demonstrate that in group I patients (those who have completely resected disease) radiation therapy was not necessary for patients who had embryonal histology. Patients who had alveolar histology had a 10-year failure-free survival of 95% if treated with radiation therapy, but only 69% if they received chemotherapy only after resection.[180] Extremity lesions are particularly difficult to treat, perhaps because many present with metastatic disease. Treatment of genitourinary primary tumors has improved markedly in recent years with the use of extensive chemotherapy. Pelvic exenteration and other morbid surgeries now can be avoided in most patients, and radiation therapy may be avoided in some patients.[119] Cranial radiation and intrathecal chemotherapy were once used in all patients who had parameningeal lesions,[145] but such treatment now is reserved for those who have basal skull lesions or CNS involvement.

Eighty percent of recurrences occur within 2 years of treatment. Local relapse is most common, although distant spread to the lungs, central nervous system, lymph nodes, bone, liver, bone marrow, and soft tissues does occur. Twenty percent of patients have metastatic disease at diagnosis; these patients continue to have a low likelihood of survival.[153] Current studies indicate that 25% to 30% of these patients will survive 5 years from diagnosis. Bone marrow transplantation, autologous PBSC procedures, or the use of new agents may offer hope to these patients. For patients who relapse, survival depends on histology, initial grouping, and staging. Twenty percent of relapsed patients have favorable features, with 50% 5-year survival; the other 80% of patients have only 10% 5-year survival.[5]

Follow-up

Patients who have rhabdomyosarcoma should receive close follow-up for evidence of recurrent disease for approximately 3 years from the time of diagnosis. Later recurrences may occur thereafter. Most of these patients have been treated with high-dose radiotherapy; thus, bone films of the area should be obtained periodically. Patients who have orbital tumors often have significant cosmetic effects as a result of the radiation therapy. Those who have orbital parameningeal lesions have received radiation to the sinuses, hypothalamus, and pituitary gland. Sinusitis is a common complaint. Hormonal levels (e.g., growth hormone and gonadotrophins) may need monitoring. The patient also should be monitored for any potential late effects of chemotherapeutic agents (e.g., cyclophosphamide and doxorubicin) (Table 193-4).

GERM CELL TUMORS AND TERATOMAS

Germ cell tumors are growths arising from primordial germ cells. They account for 3% of tumors in children, with an annual incidence of approximately 4 cases per million children younger than 15 years of age.[73] Incidence is greatest in adolescents and very young children, as reflected in the three major categories of germ cell tumors: adolescent tes-

Table 193-4 Long-Term Side Effects of Chemotherapy

Drug	Potential Organ Damage	Evaluation
Anthracyclines, (e.g., doxorubicin)	Cardiac: myocardial damage, congestive failure, arrhythmias	*Cardiac* History: Exercise intolerance, palpitations; ECG (QTc interval); echocardiogram (shortening fraction q3-5 yr); Holter monitor; exercise ECG; exercise nuclear angiography
Bleomycin	Lungs: fibrosis, impaired diffusion capacity, exacerbated by increased oxygen (e.g., anesthesia)	*Pulmonary* History: Shortness of breath, dyspnea on exertion, cough. Chest film and pulmonary function tests (with diffusion capacity) q3-5 yr
Cyclophosphamide, ifosfamide	Gonadal damage: infertility, sterility, early menopause	*Gonadal* History: Menses, question of fertility; LH/FSH/ testosterone or estradiol during pubertal development, or if a problem with fertility/ amenorrhea exists; semen analysis (prn childbearing)
	Bladder: hemorrhagic cystitis	Urinalysis—annually
	Marrow: secondary AML	CBC—annually
Lomustine (CCNU) Carmustine (BCNU)	Gonadal, lungs	Pulmonary, gonadal evaluation (as above)
Cisplatin	Kidney: decreased glomerular filtration rate	Serum creatinine q1-3 yr Creatinine clearance q3-5 yr
	Ears: hearing loss (high frequency)	Audiogram q3-5 yr
Methotrexate	Liver dysfunction	Liver function tests q1-3 yr
	CNS: learning impairment (high intravenous dose)	
6-Mercaptopurine (6-MP), 6-thioguanine, actinomycin D	Liver dysfunction	Liver function tests q1-3 yr

AML, Acute myeloblastic leukemia; *CBC,* complete blood cell count; *ECG,* electrocardiogram; *FSH,* follicle-stimulating hormone; *LH,* luteinizing hormone; *prn,* as required.

tes and ovaries, extragonadal tumors of older children, and tumors of infants and young children. The sacrococcygeal teratoma (named from the Greek *teras,* or monster) is the most common germ cell tumor of childhood and is benign in 80% of patients. It occurs in 1 per 35,000 live births and is more common in girls than in boys (2 to 4 : 1). Sixty percent of childhood germ cell tumors originate in other sites, including the gonads, mediastinum, intracranial region, and retroperitoneum.

Etiology

Germ cells appear in the yolk sac endoderm, migrate around the hind gut to the genital ridge on the posterior abdominal wall of the embryo, and congregate, becoming part of the developing gonad. A slightly aberrant path of migration may account for the occurrence of extragonadal germ cell tumors along the dorsal wall of the embryo in midline sites (sacrococcygeal, retroperitoneal, mediastinal, and pineal regions).[6] Children who have sacrococcygeal teratomas have an approximately 15% incidence of associated anomalies (e.g., imperforate anus and rectal stenosis).[70] An association with a family history of twinning resulted in early theories suggesting that teratomas were abortive attempts at the development of twins. Of interest, the common sites of teratomas—the brain, mediastinum, abdomen, and sacrococcygeal region—are all sites of twin attachment. Although most germ cell tumors arise in "normal" individuals, a genetic tendency for abnormal germ cell development may exist in some families. These tumors have been reported to develop in siblings, twins, and subsequent generations. Gonadal dysgenesis has been associated with dysgerminoma or gonadoblastoma.[76]

The type of germ cell tumor that forms is determined by the subsequent development of the germ cell.[170] Those that maintain their total potentiality become embryonal sarcomas. The development of extraembryonic structures results in the formation of choriocarcinomas (placental tumors) or endodermal sinus tumors (yolk sac tumors). Seminomas or dysgerminomas arise when the gonads differentiate. Teratomas form as a result of embryonal differentiation into ectoderm, mesoderm, and endoderm.

Clinical Manifestations

The clinical manifestations of a germ cell tumor depend on the tumor's location. Sacrococcygeal tumors occur as a mass between the anus and the coccyx.[177] An abnormality of the overlying skin may be noted. An intrapelvic tumor may be associated with an external tumor or may be the only evidence of disease, noted by the onset of urinary or rectal obstruction. The incidence of intradural tumor extension is 3% to 5%. Maternal polyhydramnios may be associated with infantile sacrococcygeal teratomas.

Ovarian tumors[113] in infants manifest as abdominal masses. Older girls have symptoms of abdominal pain, nausea, vomiting, constipation, or urinary tract obstruction, with palpable masses noted in 50%. Torsion or hemorrhage within the tumor may be responsible for acute abdominal pain; 5% of such children have bilateral tumors. Vaginal germ cell tumors in preschool girls (younger than 3 years old) may cause bloody vaginal discharge.

Testicular tumors[52] most often manifest as symptom-free scrotal masses, sometimes with a coexisting hydrocele. Torsion of the tumor in an undescended testis may result in acute abdominal pain. Testicular malignancy is 20 to 40 times more common in boys who have undescended testes. Because the ipsilateral or contralateral testis may be affected, an intrinsic testicular defect is likely.

Retroperitoneal teratomas that occur in children younger than age 2 years usually are symptom-free abdominal masses. In older children, anorexia, vomiting, or abdominal pain may be noted. Intradural extensions also may occur, and gastric and hepatic tumors have been reported.

The symptoms of patients who have germ cell tumors of the anterior mediastinum include coughing, wheezing, dyspnea, and chest pain.[100] Newborns may require immediate intubation for respiratory distress caused by mediastinal, cervical, or oropharyngeal germ cell tumors. Intrapericardial tumors can cause heart failure and cardiac tamponade. In the fetus that has an oropharyngeal mass, the inability to swallow can cause maternal polyhydramnios. Cranial tumors (80% in the pineal region) cause hydrocephalus and increased intercranial pressure in infants. Teenagers have headaches, lethargy, vomiting, diabetes insipidus, seizures, and visual disturbance, especially loss of upward gaze.

The differential diagnosis of children who have germ cell tumors depends on the location of the primary tumor. For those who have sacrococcygeal masses, meningocele is the most frequent alternative diagnosis. Abdominal or pelvic masses may be due to neuroblastoma, Wilms' tumor, rhabdomyosarcoma, or lymphomas. Nonmalignant disorders such as hydronephrosis, benign ovarian cysts, constipation, and splenomegaly must be considered. Anterior mediastinal tumors include T cell lymphoma, leukemia, or thymoma. The differential diagnosis for an intrascrotal mass includes testicular torsion, epididymitis, and testicular infarction. (See Tables 193-1 and 193-3 for details of the differential diagnosis of germ cell tumors.)

Evaluation

As in any ill child, evaluation includes a careful physical examination. For those patients who have a sacrococcygeal mass or abdominal pain, particular attention should be given to the abdominal and rectal examination. A pelvic examination (performed under anesthesia in young girls) will be necessary if an ovarian or a vaginal tumor is suspected.

Careful evaluation by CT or ultrasound examination, or both, is essential. A CT scan of benign germ cell tumors often will reveal calcifications. A teratoma frequently shows cystic and solid components on ultrasound examination. A chest CT scan and bone scan should be performed to detect pulmonary and bony metastases.

Malignant germ cell tumors that have evidence of extraembryonic differentiation often produce proteins elaborated by the corresponding normal embryonic structure. Serum levels of these markers, alpha-fetoprotein (AFP) and beta-human chorionic gonadotropin (B-HCG), should be assayed before surgery. AFP is found in germ cell tumors that have endodermal sinus tumor histology. The evaluation of AFP levels must account for their elevation during fetal development; they do not fall to normal levels until the child is approximately 9 months old.[173] B-HCG, a glycoprotein normally produced by specialized placental cells, is present in increased quantity in patients who have choriocarcinomas and hydatidiform moles and during pregnancy. In adolescent females who have an abdominal mass and elevated B-HCG, pregnancy should not be assumed, especially if the patient denies sexual activity or symptoms are atypical. Detection of AFP or B-HCG improves the ability to follow the disease status. The rate of disappearance after resection reflects the adequacy of the tumor removal. With response to chemotherapy, the levels of these proteins fall. A significant rise in these levels suggests disease recurrence.

Management

Germ cell tumors may have components of teratoma, endodermal sinus tumor, embryonal carcinoma, choriocarcinoma, seminoma, or dysgerminoma. Teratomas are classified as mature, immature, or teratoma with malignant components. Mature teratomas (well-differentiated tissues) and immature teratomas (embryonic-appearing neuroglial elements and mature elements) most commonly are found in infants. A review of germ cell tumors that had a major component of immature teratoma revealed 55% to be mixed tumors, all of which at least contained elements of yolk sac tumor.[79] Malignant evolution may occur years after removal of an apparently benign tumor, particularly in the sacrococcygeal area. For this reason, complete excision of the coccyx often is recommended, and careful follow-up is necessary.

In the past, malignant teratomas, embryonal carcinomas, endodermal sinus tumors, and choriocarcinomas were almost uniformly fatal. Complete surgical resection rarely was attained and only infrequently was curative. Only embryonal carcinoma of the infant testis could be cured by radical orchiectomy. In the 1960s, however, the efficacy of methotrexate chemotherapy for gestational choriocarcinomas and testicular germ cell tumors was demonstrated.[106] Ovarian tumors responded to vincristine, actinomycin D, and cyclophosphamide. In the 1970s, additional agents such as vinblastine and cisplatin were found to have significant single-agent response in testicular germ cell tumors of young men. The combination of these two agents with bleomycin produced a 70% complete remission rate and a 55% long-term disease-free survival for patients who have advanced testicular carcinoma.[49]

The regimens initially studied in adults also were effective in children; in one early study, 79 children who had malignant germ cell tumors, 39% of whom had widely disseminated metastases at diagnosis, were treated with these agents.[1] Of these, 45% remained free of disease 4 years after diagnosis. Newer agents such as ifosfamide and etoposide, as well as higher doses of cisplatin, also are being studied in an effort to continue to increase the percentage of cured patients.

Prognosis

The French Society for Pediatric Oncology's analysis of treatment for germ cell tumors identified three prognostic groups for patients older than 1 year who had localized disease. The group with a poor prognosis included patients who had stage III disease (more than microscopic residual disease), sacrococcygeal or mediastinal primaries, and AFP greater than 10,000 ng/ml. This group had a 43% 3-year disease-free survival. Patients who had a good prognosis had stage I disease (complete resection) or stage II disease (microscopic residual); testicular, ovarian, perineal, or retroperitoneal primaries; and AFP less than 10,000 ng/ml. These patients had 100% 3-year disease-free survival. The remaining patients were in an intermediate prognosis group and had an 81% disease-free survival.[9] This study also detected improved prognosis for patients treated with cisplatin versus carboplatin.

The prognosis for a teratoma depends on its degree of maturity. Patients who have a mature teratoma do best. Age also is important: Sacrococcygeal teratomas usually are benign in children younger than 2 months of age; thereafter the likelihood of malignant evolution increases rapidly. This may be the reason that intrapelvic teratomas that are not detected early often are found to be malignant. Mediastinal teratomas behave benignly in children and young teenagers; in older patients they are more aggressive. Cervical and intracranial teratomas in infants usually are benign; those in adolescents and adults often are malignant.

Immature teratomas can be treated with surgery alone, with event-free survival of 97.8%, 100%, and 80% for patients who have ovarian, testicular, and extragonadal tumors, respectively. For patients who did relapse, cisplatin-based chemotherapy offered an excellent chance of cure.[117]

Follow-up

The response of malignant germ cell tumors to chemotherapy is very encouraging. These patients, however, may relapse late in the course of the disease, as many as 10 years from the time of diagnosis.[60] Late-brain metastases also have been described. For this reason, close follow-up care is essential, including frequent physical examinations, radiological evaluations, and monitoring of AFP and B-HCG if elevated at diagnosis. Salvage therapy may prolong survival or even provide a cure. Late effects of the chemotherapeutic agent administered (e.g., bleomycin, cisplatin, doxorubicin) should be monitored (see Table 193-4).

EWING'S SARCOMA

Ewing's sarcoma is a malignant nonosseous tumor that usually arises in bone but also may occur in soft tissues. The Ewing family of tumors includes Ewing's sarcoma of bone, extraosseous Ewing's and peripheral primitive neuroectodermal tumors (PNET). A PNET of the chest wall is referred to as *Askin's tumor.*

The Ewing family of tumors accounts for 3% of childhood cancers and is the most common bone tumor in children younger than 10 years of age. In the second decade of life it is second in incidence to osteogenic sarcoma. The peak incidence is between the ages of 11 and 17 years, when the annual incidence is approximately 7 per million.[73] Ewing's sarcoma is extremely rare in patients younger than 5 years or older than 30 years of age, as well as in blacks and Asians.

Etiology

The Ewing family of tumors is a primitive small round cell tumor. These tumors share a neural origin, with variable degrees of differentiation and a common chromosomal translocation, t(11:22).[39] The resulting gene fusion rearrangements provide insight into tumorigenesis of these malignancies and may have prognostic significance.[37,40] No evidence suggests hereditary transmission of Ewing's sarcoma, nor has it been associated with known congenital syndromes or constitutional karyotypic abnormalities. No specific environmental risk factors have been identified.[20]

Clinical Manifestations

Patients who have Ewing's sarcoma most commonly consult the clinician for pain.[51] Swelling also may be seen. Symptoms often begin insidiously, several months before diagnosis, and may initially be attributed to trauma. At the time of diagnosis a mass is palpable in 60% of patients, resulting from the propensity of this tumor to break through the bony cortex and involve the surrounding tissue.[127] This disruption of the cortex may also result in a pathological fracture. The primary tumor site is evenly distributed between central and extremity lesions. The primary lesion most often is found in the femur (22%), the fibula or tibula (21%), or the pelvis (22%). The ribs and vertebrae are other common sites of origin. Demonstrable metastatic lesions are present in 14% to 35% of patients, occurring in the lungs, bones, lymph nodes, and bone marrow.[175] Central nervous system involvement is uncommon.

The differential diagnosis includes osteogenic sarcoma, osteomyelitis, benign bone tumors, and bone cysts. Other tumors that occasionally involve the bone and have a similar histological pattern of small round cells include lymphoma, leukemia, neuroblastoma, and rhabdomyosarcoma (Table 193-5).

Evaluation

A roentgenogram should be obtained in a patient who has a mass overlying bone or bone pain that is not characteristic of trauma (by lack of history or duration of symptoms). Radiographs of a bone that has Ewing's sarcoma often show a destructive lesion in the diaphysis. An onion-skin appearance arises from periosteal elevation and subperiosteal new bone formation associated with tumor extension through the cortex. A mottled pattern may be seen as a result of bone destruction, sclerosis, and cystic formation. An associated soft-tissue mass occurs in more than 50% of patients who have primary tumors of long bones. In addition to a plain roentgenogram of the involved bone, a CT scan and espe-

Table 193-5 Differential Diagnosis of Malignant Tumors Involving the Extremities

Tumor*	Age	Clinical Signs	Laboratory Findings
Ewing's sarcoma	≥5 yr	Pain, swelling; GU/skeletal anomaly; weight loss, fever; malaise (metabolic)	"Onion skin" on roentgenogram
Osteogenic sarcoma	Teens	Pain, swelling; familial retinoblastoma; prior radiation to bone; Paget's disease	Codman triangle (cortical elevation, new bone formation); "sunburst" ossification of soft tissue; soft-tissue mass; elevated alkaline phosphatase level
Lymphoma	All	Pain	
Fibrosarcoma	Infants, teens	Painless mass; prior radiation; plastic implant	
Rhabdomyosarcoma	All	Mass	
Synovial sarcoma	Teens	Mass	Calcification (40%)

*Other causes: trauma, bone cysts, osteomyelitis.

cially an MRI may help to determine the extent of the primary lesion.

Radionuclide bone scanning detects primary and metastatic lesions, but it is not particularly useful in determining the extent of the primary disease. However, it may aid in following the response to therapy. A chest film and a CT scan of the chest are necessary to determine whether pulmonary lesions are present. The possibility of bone marrow involvement should be evaluated by bilateral bone marrow aspirates and biopsies. Cerebrospinal fluid should be examined in patients who have parameningeal tumors.

A biopsy of the lesion is necessary to establish the diagnosis. If possible, diagnostic tissue should be obtained from soft tissue rather than from cortical bone to reduce the potential for pathological fracture. Ewing's sarcoma is characterized by a pattern of monomorphic sheets of small tumors made up of round cells with hyperchromatic nuclei and relatively little cytoplasm.[51] Schiff stains of the cells show positivity, but this finding is not specific for Ewing's sarcoma.

Ewing's sarcoma has no staging system; tumors are classified and treated as being either localized or metastatic.

Management

Approximately 75% of patients who have Ewing's sarcoma apparently have localized disease. Localized therapies alone, however, are unlikely to be curative because of the presence of micrometastases. Chemotherapy has made it possible to cure the majority of patients who have Ewing's sarcoma, and it assists in the treatment of local disease by reducing the need for radical surgery or high-dose, large-volume irradiation.

The choice of radiation or surgery for local control is based on the likelihood of preserving function. Functionally expendable bones should be removed. Aggressive surgical procedures (amputation or radical limb-sparing excisions) are being used more commonly now than in the past decade. There is some evidence that complete surgical resection may improve prognosis. However, radiotherapy is often required for local control. Local control is attained after radiotherapy in 90% of patients who have distal-extremity lesions, 75% who have proximal-extremity lesions, and 65% who have central lesions.[171] Radiation therapy also may be helpful after subtotal resection of the primary tumor or for treatment of pulmonary or osseous metastases.

Ewing's sarcoma is extremely chemosensitive. Active agents, including regimens of vincristine, doxorubicin, cyclophosphamide, and actinomycin D, have been used successfully in the treatment of patients who have Ewing's sarcoma. Etoposide and ifosfamide, in combination, elicit good therapeutic responses in many patients whose disease has relapsed. Recent studies have shown improved survival for patients treated with etoposide and ifosfamide, alternating with vincristine, doxorubicin, and cyclophosphamide.[33,69,150] Studies have demonstrated the effectiveness of these regimens for extraosseous Ewing's and also peripheral PNETs.[4,74]

Dose intensity of the more active agents (cyclophosphamide and doxorubicin) has played a major role in improving disease-free survival.[147] However, the outcome remains extremely poor for patients who have bone metastases or bone marrow involvement. Further dose intensification is being investigated in new studies. Pulmonary metastases often can be treated effectively with intensive chemotherapy regimens and radiation therapy, but patients who have pulmonary metastases do not fare as well as patients who have other sites of metastatic disease.[136]

Prognosis

Before the use of multiagent chemotherapy, 85% of children who had Ewing's sarcoma died within 2 years of diagnosis.[53] Five-year, disease-free survival is now 55% to 70%, influenced by the extent and location of disease.[88,139] Approximately 80% of patients who have small, distal-extremity Ewing's sarcoma tumors survive, compared with only 30% of those who have large, proximal-extremity lesions, perhaps because of the difficulties in achieving surgical resection or delivering adequate amounts of radiation therapy. The most significant prognostic factor remains the presence of metastases. Other factors associated with worse prognosis include poor response to chemotherapy, extensive soft-tissue masses, large primary tumors, high serum levels of lactate dehydrogenase, and older age.[33,50,127] Histological response also affects prognosis in that patients who have significant tissue necrosis following chemotherapy have a better prognosis.

Follow-up

Patients who have Ewing's sarcoma require close follow-up for evidence of recurrent disease for approximately 5 years from the time of diagnosis, although recurrences may occur later. Particular attention should be paid to the irradiated field of long-term survivors, because second malignancies may arise (Table 193-6). Bone films should be obtained periodically. Patients who have lower-extremity lesions whose growth is incomplete should be monitored for evidence of leg length discrepancies, which may need to be treated by arresting the growth in the opposite limb. Monitoring for potential late effects of specific chemotherapeutic agents administered (e.g., cyclophosphamide and doxorubicin) is important (see Table 193-4).

OSTEOGENIC SARCOMA

Osteogenic sarcoma is the most common bone tumor encountered in the first three decades of life; approximately 300 patients are diagnosed per year in the United States. Osteogenic sarcoma comprises 60% of malignant bone tumors. Seven teenagers per million are diagnosed annually with osteogenic sarcoma, with a male to female ratio of approximately 1.5:1.[73] The peak incidence occurs at age 14.5 for boys and 13.5 for girls, corresponding to the age

Table 193-6 Long-Term Side Effects of Radiation

Irradiated Area*	Risks	Monitoring
Cranium and nasopharynx	Cataracts	Physical examination
	Growth: impaired	Growth charts (bone age, growth hormone)
	Central nervous system: learning impairment	Monitoring of school function; neuropsychological evaluation
	Dentition: abnormal formation	Dental evaluation
	Thyroid: overt or compensated hypothyroidism	Free T4, TSH levels
	High dose (>2500 Gy)	
	Hypothalamic dysfunction (decreased growth hormone; decreased gonadotropin, hyperprolactinemia)	Growth; pubertal, menstrual, and fertility history (growth hormone, LH, testosterone, estrogen, prolactin levels)
	Hearing (especially with cisplatin)	Audiogram
Neck and mandible	Hypoplasia of bone/soft tissues	Examination of area
	Dentition: abnormal formation, abnormal salivary function	Dental evaluation
	Thyroid: hypothyroidism	Free T_4, TSH
Thorax	Hypoplasia (includes impaired chest wall growth)	Examination of area
	Thyroid: hypothyroidism	Free T_4, TSH levels
	Lungs: fibrosis, decreased capacity	History, pulmonary function tests, chest film q3-5 yr
	Cardiac: pericardial and valvular thickening; possibility of early myocardial infarction	History, ECG, echocardiogram q3-5 yr
	Breasts: impaired growth, possibility of increased malignancy	Breast self-examination, early mammograms
Abdomen/pelvis	Hypoplasia (including scoliosis)	Examination of area, x-ray film of spine during puberty
	Liver (if in field)	Liver function tests
	Kidneys (if in field)	Serum creatinine, urinalysis protein, (24-hour collection for creatinine, protein)
	Gonads (if in field)	Pubertal, menstrual, and fertility history, LH, FSH, estradiol or testosterone levels during puberty and if fertility is doubtful, semen analysis
	Gastrointestinal tract	Nutritional history
Extremities	Hypoplasia	Examination of area

*All: Consider roentgenograms of bones every 5 to 10 years after ≥35 Gy radiation (risk of secondary malignancy). Examine skin for abnormal pigmented nevi (risk of second malignancy).

ECG, Electrocardiogram; *FSH,* follicle-stimulating hormone; *LH,* luteinizing hormone; *T_4,* thyroxine; *TSH,* thyroid-stimulating hormone.

of their growth spurts. Taller children appear to be at increased risk.[56]

Etiology

The hallmark of osteogenic sarcoma is the production of osteoid or mature bone by proliferating malignant spindle cell sarcoma. The high incidence of this tumor in adolescents who are undergoing rapid skeletal growth, as well as individuals who have Paget's disease of the bone, suggests that increased bone growth may play a role in the induction of the malignancy.[80] Although patients often report a history of trauma before the diagnosis, injuries most likely allow the recognition of an already proliferating tumor.

Patients at increased risk of osteogenic sarcoma include those who have received irradiation to the bone, usually for the treatment of malignancy.[161] Radiation itself can be causative, but patients who have one tumor may be at increased genetic risk for a second primary malignancy. Patients who have hereditary retinoblastoma and thus a constitutive deletion at Rb, the retinoblastoma tumor suppressor gene, have an increased incidence of osteogenic sarcoma, half of which occur within the retinoblastoma's radiation field.[2] However, the risk of sarcoma is significantly elevated, regardless of whether they receive radiation. Thus, the abnormality at Rb itself predisposes to osteogenic sarcoma. It is not surprising, then, that osteogenic sarcoma in otherwise normal hosts often is found to have mutation or loss of the RB1 gene.[61] Another tumor suppressor gene noted in osteogenic sarcoma tumors is p53, the gene associated with Li-Fraumeni syndrome (an autosomal dominant predisposition to multiple malignancies). P53 is present constitutively in 3% to 4% of children who have osteogenic sarcoma. No environmental risk factors have been identified.[20]

Clinical Manifestations

The presenting symptom of virtually all patients is pain. Palpable masses, swelling, and limited motion are common signs. Weight loss and other systemic effects such as anorexia are seen rarely; if these are present, overt metastatic disease is likely. A few patients have fractures. Cough, chest pain, or dyspnea may be seen in those who have extensive pulmonary metastases at the time of diagnosis, although most patients who have pulmonary metastases are symptom free. Ninety percent of tumors occur in the extremities; the metaphyses of bones are common sites of osteogenic sarcoma origin. The lower extremities are involved most frequently, with 60% of tumors occurring around the knee, 40% in the distal femur, and 20% in the proximal tibia.[174] The sacrum, jaw, and phalanges are involved less commonly. Patients who have Paget's disease of the bone or those who have had radiation therapy in the area of the orbit may have osteogenic sarcoma of the cranial bones.

The presenting symptom, bone pain, is ubiquitous. It commonly is associated with trauma. Prolonged symptoms, or a history inconsistent with trauma, suggest the need for further diagnostic consideration. Bone abnormalities that may be confused with osteogenic sarcoma include benign cysts, Ewing's sarcoma, lymphoma, or tumor metastases. Table 193-5 provides the differential diagnosis of osteogenic sarcoma involving the extremities.

Evaluation

Roentgenograms of the involved bone show bony destruction with periosteal new bone formation. A "sunburst" appearance is characteristic, a result of the eruption of tumor through the cortex with subsequent formation of new bone. Soft-tissue swelling often is noted. Adequate biopsy and histological examination are necessary to establish the diagnosis of osteogenic sarcoma.

Osteoid found within a sarcomatous tumor is the characteristic histological pattern. Osteogenic sarcoma in the child or adolescent usually is a high-grade tumor characterized by osteoblasts that demonstrate pleomorphism and bizarre mitoses. Necrosis, fibrosis, and calcification may be noted. This classic form usually arises from the medullary cavity. A less aggressive form of osteogenic sarcoma arises in the parosteal area of the bone and tends to spread along the shaft of the bone without invading the cortex. Periosteal, intracortical, and extraskeletal osteogenic sarcomas also have been described.

Baseline lactic dehydrogenase and alkaline phosphatase levels should be obtained. The extent of the primary lesion is defined further by the use of CT or more frequently by MRI scanning. Before MRI, arteriographic examination often was necessary in patients considered for limb salvage procedures, in which the vascular and neurological integrity of the limb must be ensured. Metastatic disease in the lung should be sought by the use of CT scanning. Bone scans can be helpful both for outlining the primary tumor and for detecting multiple primary lesions and metastasis.

Management

The traditional therapy of osteogenic sarcoma has been amputation of the affected limb. The natural history of disease in such patients is notable for the rapid appearance of pulmonary metastases 6 to 12 months after diagnosis.[35] Five years following the diagnosis, only 10% to 20% of patients treated with amputation alone are alive. High-dose radiotherapy is even less effective than amputation.[167] In the early 1970s, favorable responses to high-dose methotrexate with leucovorin and to doxorubicin were noted.[32,84,85] Patients treated with these agents had markedly improved survival rates (40% to 50%) compared with historical control subjects (treated with amputation alone). Unfortunately, a report of 50% survival after surgery alone suggested that the improved outcome was a result of improved surgical techniques rather than the chemotherapy.[168] Adjuvant chemotherapy, therefore, was not recommended by many physicians until the 1980s, when a controlled randomized study confirmed that adjuvant chemotherapy improves disease-free survival of patients who have osteogenic sarcoma.[107] Adjuvant chemotherapy regimens now being recommended use high doses of methotrexate, doxorubicin, and cisplatin. The role of ifosfamide in osteosarcoma is being investigated.

The availability of effective chemotherapy and improved surgical technique has made limb-sparing or subamputative therapies possible for many patients who have osteogenic sarcoma.[115] Survival after limb salvage is comparable to survival after amputation. Although the complication rate is higher, function is improved. The portion of bone involved with tumor is removed and replaced by an artificial prosthesis or a bone graft. This procedure can be performed only if the vascular and neurological integrity of the limb is not compromised. Preoperative chemotherapy may reduce the size of the mass so as to make such surgery possible. For those who have lower-extremity tumors, limb-salvage procedures are limited to patients who have achieved most of their growth potential. For patients who have lesions of the humerus, any preservation of hand function will improve the patient's lifestyle significantly.

For patients in whom pulmonary metastases develop, surgical resection of these nodules may result in long-term survival.[120,128] A similar approach has been used in patients who have metastatic pulmonary disease at the time of diagnosis, with long-term survivals of 20% to 40%.

Prognosis

Two randomized studies have confirmed the role of adjuvant chemotherapy in improving the long-term disease-free survival of patients who have nonmetastatic osteosarcoma. Approximately 65% to 75% overall disease-free survival can be achieved.[107,148] The initial histological response to chemotherapy appears to have prognostic significance, although it is unclear whether subsequent tailoring of therapy achieves a better result than aggressive, early chemotherapy for all patients.[8,142] The outcome after preoperative chemotherapy is similar to that of immediate surgical excision. Preoperative chemotherapy, however, allows for the possibility of limb-salvage procedures by decreasing tumor size, and allows early treatment of potential or demonstrated metastases.

The most significant prognostic variable is the presence of metastatic disease. The presence solely of pulmonary metastases is associated with a better prognosis than bone metastases. Among patients who have pulmonary disease, unilateral disease or fewer than eight nodules may carry a better prognosis.[75] Other prognostic factors in this disorder are related to the site of the tumor (patients who have distal tumors do better than those who have proximal or central-axis tumors) and the patient's age (prognosis improves with increased age).

Follow-up

Adjuvant chemotherapy has resulted in an increased number of long-term survivors of osteogenic sarcoma. Virtually all will have had either amputation or limb-salvage procedures. It is hoped that less disabling therapies will someday be feasible. Most of these patients maintain a relatively normal lifestyle, including participation in various sports. Long-term follow-up care includes imaging of the primary tumor site, bone scans, and chest CTs performed semiannually for 5 years and annually until 10 years from the time of diagnosis to monitor for recurrent disease. Orthopedic evaluations and monitoring for late effects of the chemotherapeutic agents used (e.g., doxorubicin, cisplatin, methotrexate, bleomycin, ifosfamide, and cyclophosphamide) also are necessary.

NON-HODGKIN'S LYMPHOMAS

Non-Hodgkin's lymphoma (NHL) of childhood comprises a heterogeneous group of malignancies arising from lymphocytes and lymphoid precursors. The migratory nature of these cells is reflected by the variable sites at which the tumors occur and to which they spread. Recognition of the systemic nature of the disease, even in those patients who have only locally detectable disease, has resulted in a marked improvement in survival rates in recent years. Childhood NHL is markedly different from adult NHL both in the immunohistopathological types that occur and in the better survival rates noted in children. Non-Hodgkin's lymphomas in children are generally of three types: lymphoblastic (30%); small noncleaved, including Burkitt's (50%); and large cell (15%).[103]

Lymphomas account for 10% of childhood cancer; 60% are NHLs. The incidence of NHL is low in children younger than 5 years and then increases steadily throughout life.[73] It occurs more commonly in males than in females (2 to 3:1). NHLs of childhood have a rapid growth rate, with the percentage of actively dividing tumor approaching 100% in some cases, and short doubling-in-size times as few as 12 hours. They have a high frequency of dissemination, particularly to the bone marrow and central nervous system. Although the distinction between lymphoma and lymphocytic leukemia is defined by less than 25% versus more than 25% bone marrow lymphoblasts, respectively, the distinguishing biological parameters are not clear.

Etiology

Childhood NHL arises from lymphoid precursors in the marrow and thymus. Burkitt's and non-Burkitt's small, noncleaved-cell lymphomas and most large-cell lymphomas are B-cell phenotypes, usually manifesting surface immunoglobulin and B-cell–specific antigens. Lymphoblastic lymphomas almost invariably express the enzyme terminal deoxynucleotidyl transferase (TdT), as well as T-cell markers. Anaplastic large-cell lymphomas generally have T-cell receptor gene rearrangements.[103]

Different breakpoints of chromosomal translocations may be seen in the Burkitt's lymphoma of equatorial Africa, which usually harbors Epstein-Barr virus (EBV), compared with the North American variety, which does so only occasionally.[138] The presence of EBV in lymphoma specimens suggests that viral infection may play a role in the development of NHL. Immunodeficiency states also are associated with the development of lymphomas, usually of the B-cell immunoblastic or large-cell variety.[55] A defect of T-cell regulation that permits the expansion of EBV-affected clones of B cells has been hypothesized to result in lymphomas, particularly in immunologically abnormal hosts. Lymphomas occur with increased frequency in children receiving immunosuppressive therapy for renal, cardiac, or bone marrow allografts.

Specific chromosomal aberrations have been described in Burkitt's lymphoma, which place the c-myc oncogene adjacent to immunoglobulin heavy or light chain constant region genes.[14,182] A number of specific, nonrandom chromosomal abnormalities have been reported in lymphoblastic lymphoma and large-cell lymphomas. The variation in subtypes described suggests that these tumors may be more heterogeneous than Burkitt's lymphoma.

Clinical Manifestations

Localized lymphadenopathy is a common presentation of NHL. Common areas of involvement are supradiaphragmatic, particularly the cervical, axillary, and mediastinal areas, or the Waldeyer ring.[130] The histological pattern of supradiaphragmatic disease often is lymphoblastic. Dissemination to the bone marrow, the central nervous system, or the gonads is common. Patients may also have skin or soft-tissue involvement, particularly patients who have B-lineage lymphoblastic lymphoma.[181] Patients who have mediastinal masses frequently have a history of cough and, occasionally, acute respiratory distress. Unless careful attention is paid to the state of the airway, obstruction can occur during evaluation, even in patients who have minimal symptoms, particularly with the administration of sedation. The obstruction may involve the lower airway, beyond the reach of an endotracheal tube, resulting in an inability to ventilate the lungs effectively.

An abdominal mass that may involve the ileocecal region, mesentery, ovaries, or retroperitoneum is seen in 30% to 40% of patients.[130,181] Such tumors often are of B-cell origin. Large-cell lymphomas may present with peripheral adenopathy, although potential primary sites include the mediastinum and extranodal sites including the tonsils, lungs, bone, testicles, and soft tissue.

Patients whose disease is localized often feel well. Those who have disseminated disease experience weight loss and malaise, as well as symptoms referable to the primary site of the disease.

The differential diagnosis of cervical adenopathy includes a variety of infectious and inflammatory processes. Malignant processes that cause enlarged cervical nodes include Hodgkin's disease, neuroblastoma, leukemia, nasopharyngeal carcinoma, rhabdomyosarcoma, and thyroid carcinoma. Anterior mediastinal masses may be due to T-cell leukemia or thymoma. Abdominal masses may be due to constipation, splenomegaly, Wilms' tumor, rhabdomyosarcoma, or neuroblastoma. Lymphoma is a rare type of bone tumor. (Tables 193-1 to 193-3 provide differential diagnostic aids in evaluating patients who have NHL.)

Evaluation

The diagnosis of NHL should be established by surgical biopsy; if adenopathy is present, removal of the most suspicious node is recommended. Complete resection of the diseased area(s) is not necessary. Frozen section and needle biopsies are to be discouraged to ensure proper diagnosis. Although the primary diagnosis is based on histological findings, for proper determination of subtype immunophenotyping, enzyme studies (TdT), or gene rearrangement studies may be helpful. If possible, cytogenetic studies should be performed. A sufficient number of malignant cells may be present in patients who have bone marrow involvement or pleural effusions to establish the diagnosis. In this instance, a lymph node biopsy may not be necessary. Biopsy may be contraindicated for patients who have large mediastinal masses with imminent airway obstruction unless endotracheal intubation will ensure airway patency. If the distal end of the endotracheal tube lies proximal to the mass, localized radiation to the mediastinum may be necessary before the diagnostic specimen is obtained. Alternative sites for obtaining diagnostic specimens then must be considered.

A lumbar puncture should be obtained with cytocentrifugation of cerebral spinal fluid to detect meningeal involvement. Imaging studies should include a CXR and a CT scan of the chest and abdomen in all patients. Bone scans and gallium scans can be helpful in selected patients.

A variety of staging systems are used for lymphomas. The most common, the Ann Arbor system used for Hodgkin's disease, is not of prognostic significance in pediatric NHL because of noncontinuous patterns of spread. The Murphy staging system is the most widely applied for pediatric NHL.[130] Stage I disease indicates a single tumor, nodal or extranodal. Stage II indicates the involvement of two or more nodal or extranodal sites, both on the same side of the diaphragm. Gastrointestinal tumors with only mesenteric nodes involved are also stage II. Stage III tumors involve both sides of the diaphragm, extensive abdominal disease, paraspinal or epidural tumors, or any primary intrathoracic tumors. Stage IV designates CNS or bone marrow involvement.

Management

The majority of patients who have NHL have disseminated disease at the time of diagnosis. Even those who have clinically localized disease rarely are curable with localized surgical or irradiation therapy alone. The choice of chemotherapeutic regimens is based on the clinical stage and the immunohistological tumor subtype.

Lymph node biopsy usually is required for diagnosis and characterization of NHL. Removal of the tumor may be indicated only for those patients who have Burkitt's lymphoma whose tumor can be removed en masse (90%) with minimal morbidity.[112] In general, major surgical procedures should be avoided because the healing time may delay initiation of chemotherapy, the most essential component of treatment.

The high incidence of micrometastatic disease at the time of diagnosis necessitates that all children who have NHL receive chemotherapy. Many agents are active in lymphomas. Optimal treatment regimens differ for patients who have lymphoblastic lymphoma compared with those who have nonlymphoblastic lymphoma. A study comparing two lymphoma regimens showed that the histological class of lymphoma predicted the efficacy of the regimens. Effective agents include cyclophosphamide, vincristine, prednisone, methotrexate, doxorubicin,[87] cytosine arabinoside, etoposide, and ifosfamide. Patients who have localized nonlymphoblastic lymphoma can be treated with short-course, low-intensity chemotherapy. Patients who have localized lymphoblastic lymphoma require continuation therapy.[108] High-risk patients who have lymphoblastic lymphoma are treated on acute lymphoblastic leukemia–like protocols.

Local measures of control rarely are essential in the treatment of childhood NHL. Although lymphomas are radiosensitive, the use of radiation therapy does not improve survival in chemotherapy-responsive patients and unnecessary morbidity may be added. Radiotherapy is helpful in the treatment of emergent situations such as airway compromise or spinal cord compression and for treating overt meningeal involvement. Radiation therapy also plays a role in the treatment of patients who do not achieve a complete remission after standard chemotherapy or for those patients who require bone marrow transplantation or palliative therapy.

Prognosis

The prognosis is excellent for most children who have NHL, approaching 90% event-free survival for patients who have localized disease and 60% to 80% for patients who have advanced disease. Although histological findings are not of great prognostic significance for outcome, they provide the basis for the choice of therapeutic regimen. Clinical staging is of particular relevance because it is determined by a combination of the tumor burden, disease extent, and primary location. New intensive chemotherapy or bone marrow transplantation regimens should improve the likelihood of survival in patients whose prognosis is poor or who relapse.

Follow-up

Patients who have NHL and are disease free 2 years from the time of diagnosis usually are cured. During this initial period they should be monitored based on complete blood cell counts, CXR, and evaluation of the primary site of disease. The follow-up of long-term survivors of childhood lymphomas should reflect the types of therapy (e.g., cyclophosphamide, doxorubicin, methotrexate) administered (see Table 193-4).

HODGKIN'S DISEASE

Hodgkin's disease, or Hodgkin's lymphoma, is a malignancy of the lymphoreticular system characterized by multinucleated giant cells, known as *Reed-Sternberg cells,* interspersed in an infiltration of normal-appearing cellular elements (lymphocytes, macrophages, histiocytes, plasma cells, and eosinophils).[146] The Reed-Sternberg cells appear to be the mitotically active malignant cell of Hodgkin's disease.[94] Controversy exists as to the normal counterpart from which these cells derive, although recent evidence supports a B-lymphocyte origin with a cytokine-induced cellular infiltrate.[164]

Hodgkin's disease comprises approximately 6% of pediatric malignancies; approximately 600 cases are diagnosed in the pediatric population of the United States each year.[73] In the more developed nations, the incidence of Hodgkin's disease exhibits two age peaks, one in young adults (15 to 30 years of age) and one in late adulthood.[71,162] In developing nations, the early peak occurs in preadolescence. Ten percent to 15% of the total incidence of Hodgkin's disease occurs in children younger than 16 years of age. Hodgkin's disease is extremely rare before the age of 5 years. A male predominance is present throughout the preadolescent age range; thereafter, the incidence is approximately equal in males and females. Hodgkin's disease in older teenagers and young adults is most common among whites.

Etiology

The role of environment or genetics in the acquisition of Hodgkin's disease is suggested by national and racial differences in the epidemiological features of the disease. First-degree relatives of patients who have Hodgkin's disease have an increased risk of acquiring the disease,[71] possibly because of genetic susceptibility or similar exposures (viral, environmental). Monozygotic twins have a much higher concordance for disease development than dizygotic twins.

High serum titers to EBV and EBV-associated antigens are identified in some patients who have Hodgkin's disease and may reflect a causative role for the virus.[135] Alternatively, patients may have an inappropriate immune response to this virus. Evidence of EBV infection is greater in certain subtypes of Hodgkin's disease. In addition, EBV may influence response to chemotherapy and prognosis.[131,144] The incidence of Hodgkin's disease is known to be increased in patients who have certain underlying immunodeficiency diseases (e.g., ataxia-telangiectasia and acquired immunodeficiency syndrome [AIDS]).[58,83]

Clinical Manifestations

The most common presenting feature of Hodgkin's disease is painless enlargement of the lower cervical lymph nodes. Approximately 50% of the patients who have this manifestation also have mediastinal disease. The classic pattern of spread is from the cervical lymph nodes to the mediastinum and then into the spleen and abdominal lymph nodes. Spread via the thoracic duct may result in disease of the right side of the neck and of the abdomen, without mediastinal involvement. Axillary or inguinal adenopathy or extranodal primary sites (e.g., bone) are seen occasionally. Mediastinal disease is present in 76% of adolescents and 33% of 1- to 10-year-olds who have Hodgkin's lymphoma. Pleural involvement occurs in approximately 10% of patients. Renal, skin, or nervous system involvement is less common. Constitutional symptoms related to Hodgkin's disease occur in approximately one third of patients at the time of diagnosis. The symptoms that predict a poor prognosis ("B" disease) are fever (oral temperature greater than 38° C), weight loss (more than 10% of body weight within 6 months), and drenching night sweats. Absence of these symptoms provides a better prognosis ("A" disease).[144]

Hematological abnormalities may be present in Hodgkin's disease (usually in advanced stages), even in the absence of bone marrow involvement. Hemolytic disease or the anemia of chronic disease associated with impaired mobilization of iron storage may occur. Neutrophilia in the absence of infection occurs in approximately 50% of patients. Thrombocytopenia caused by immunologically mediated platelet destruction also is seen.

Lymphadenopathy occurs in children for various reasons, including infection (with bacteria, viruses, tuberculosis, atypical mycobacteria, and toxoplasmosis), malignancies (non-Hodgkin's lymphoma, nasopharyngeal carcinoma, soft-tissue sarcoma, neuroblastoma), histiocytosis, and other inflammatory processes. A CXR, a complete blood cell count, and a sedimentation rate should be obtained in any patient who has lymphadenopathy that is atypical for infection. Persistent lymphadenopathy, even after a transient "response" to antibiotic therapy, requires biopsy. (Tables 193-2 and 193-3 provide differential diagnostic aids in evaluating patients who have Hodgkin's disease.)

Evaluation

Evaluation of the child who has Hodgkin's disease should begin with a careful history and physical examination. Particular attention should be paid to "B" disease symptoms. Lymphatic areas to be evaluated include Waldeyer ring and the cervical, supraclavicular, axillary, and inguinal lymph nodes. The sizes of the nodes found should be recorded carefully, and it should be noted whether they are tender. In addition, a careful abdominal examination should be performed, particularly to evaluate liver and splenic size. Retroperitoneal lymph nodes are not palpable. The blood cell counts may show anemia (caused by hemolysis or chronic disease), neutropenia, or thrombocytopenia. Elevation of the sedimentation rate and the serum copper level resulting from activation of the reticuloendothelial system occurs in some patients and may be useful for following response to therapy. Serum hepatic alkaline phosphatase isoenzyme levels also may be elevated.

Radiographic evaluation of a patient who has a possible diagnosis of Hodgkin's disease includes a CXR and CT scans of the chest and abdomen. Bipedal lymphangiography can be used to detect pelvic and paraaortic lymph nodes. However, this rarely is performed in pediatrics. Gallium scanning also detects Hodgkin's disease and can be particularly useful in detecting disease in obscure sites. Although bone involvement is rare, a bone scan should be considered in patients who have advanced disease, particularly those who have bone pain or an elevated serum alkaline phosphatase level.

Laparotomy with splenectomy is the only precise way to define the subdiaphragmatic extent of Hodgkin's disease.[63] Nonetheless, it is performed less commonly in children and adolescents, since chemotherapy is used in most. If performed, biopsy specimens of even normal-appearing lymph nodes should be obtained in each of the following areas: splenic hilar, celiac portal hepatic, mesenteric, paraaortic, and iliac regions. Any suspicious lesions should be removed. A careful examination of the spleen, sectioned at 1- to 3-mm intervals, detects small nodules. Wedge biopsies (rather than needle biopsies) of the liver are necessary to detect focal lesions. A bone marrow biopsy must be obtained either before or coincidentally with laparotomy. The finding of Hodgkin's disease in the bone marrow documents stage IV disease (see below), obviating the need for a staging laparotomy.

The importance of defining subdiaphragmatic involvement is most clear when radiation therapy is the primary therapeutic modality. A staging laparotomy with splenectomy allows limited fields to be irradiated, thus preventing the morbidity associated with total nodal irradiation. When chemotherapy is used, the benefits of staging laparotomy with splenectomy are lower. The current trend is to perform laparotomies in those situations in which exact staging of disease extent would facilitate reduction of radiotherapy or chemotherapy.[81,144]

Unfortunately, overwhelming bacteremia with polysaccharide-encapsulated organisms occurs in up to 10% of patients after splenectomy, with a mortality of 50%.[149] The risk is greatest for young children who previously have not been exposed to these pathogens. All patients who have undergone splenectomy will require presurgical vaccination against pneumococci, *Haemophilus influenzae* type b, and *Neisseria meningitidis*. Prophylactic antibiotics also are recommended throughout their lives. With these interventions, the risk of sepsis is lower than noted above.

The extent of disease spread usually is classified by the Ann Arbor staging system by means of either the clinical stage (CS) or the pathological stage (PS).[22] PS implies that the most extensive degree of involvement has been confirmed pathologically. The stages are as follows:

Stage I—involvement of one lymphatic region only

Stage II—involvement of two or more lymphatic regions on the same side of the diaphragm

Stage III—involvement on both sides of the diaphragm, including nodal regions and/or the spleen

Stage IV—involvement of extranodal organs such as lungs, liver, bone marrow, kidneys, bone, or skin, in addition to lymph nodes

Direct extranodal extension to adjacent tissue is denoted by the staging subscript E. Stage III disease is subdivided by the degree of abdominal involvement. Stage III1 involves nodes of the upper portion of the abdomen alone (celiac portal nodes and/or spleen). Stage III2 involves paraaortic nodes as well; stage III3 additionally involves iliac nodes.

Four subtypes of Hodgkin's disease are described by review of pathological specimens.[110] The nodular sclerosing subtype (NS) is distinctive because of collagenous bands that divide the lymphoid tissues into nodules and the presence of a "lacunar variant" of the Reed-Sternberg cell. It is the most common subtype in children, occurring in approximately 75% of adolescents and 40% of children younger than 10 years. The lymphocyte-predominant Hodgkin's disease subtype is characterized by destruction of the lymph node architecture, with the cellular proliferation of benign-appearing lymphocytes. Reed-Sternberg cells rarely are found in the absence of fibrosis. It is more common in young children; 33% of cases are in children younger than 15 years of age. Disease is usually localized. In the mixed-cellularity Hodgkin's disease subtype, lymph node architecture is not preserved. Approximately 10 Reed-Sternberg cells are seen per high-power field, often with interstitial fibrosis; necrosis is not pronounced. It is more common in children younger than 10 years than in adolescents and is associated with high-risk disease. The lymphocyte-depleted Hodgkin's disease subtype is characterized by the presence of fibrosis, necrosis, and abnormal cells (but only a rare lymphocyte). It is rare in children.

Management

Hodgkin's disease responds to radiation or chemotherapy. Protocols using radiation therapy alone, chemotherapy alone, or both forms of therapy all have been successful, at least in some groups of patients. Choosing an appropriate therapeutic plan necessitates assessing the risk of disease recurrence and the potential risk for long-term ill effects in a particular patient.

Contiguous spread of Hodgkin's disease via lymphoid organs allows for success with radiation therapy alone.[89] Full-dose radiation therapy (35 to 45 Gy) is used most frequently in the treatment of patients who have stages I, II, and III1 disease. The involved fields, and one field beyond the area of proved disease, are treated. Those patients who have large mediastinal masses (more than one third the thoracic diameter) also require chemotherapy for optimal results. Skeletal and soft-tissue growth, particularly in the neck and clavicular areas, are severely compromised when these doses of radiation are used. Cardiac and pulmonary complications, such as coronary artery disease, valvular disease, pneumonitis, or pulmonary fibrosis, occur as well. Children who have not achieved full adult size at the time of diagnosis will have significant skeletal deformity if full-dose irradiation is used to the neck and mediastinum. Low-dose radiation (20 to 25 Gy) to involved fields, in conjunction with chemotherapy, is being used for most younger children.[46]

Hodgkin's disease responds to numerous single chemotherapeutic agents but rarely are lasting, complete remissions achieved in this manner. Combination chemotherapy, with active agents that have differing mechanisms of action and nonoverlapping toxicities, is used. The original combination that proved to be successful in the treatment of Hodgkin's disease was MOPP (mechlorethamine, Oncovin [vincristine], procarbazine, and prednisone).[42] Cyclophosphamide or a nitrosurea may be substituted for mechlorethamine, or vinblastine for vincristine. In 1974, 10 years after the initial discovery of MOPP, another combination regimen ABVD (Adriamycin [doxorubicin], bleomycin, vinblastine, and dacarbazine) was devised for the treatment of patients whose disease had relapsed.[16] The efficacy of this combination resulted in combined ABVD/MOPP regimens. Currently, MOPP is used less often because of significant long-term toxicity, including infertility and risk of secondary leukemia.[82] Second-generation treatment protocols are being studied to decrease the number of courses and to eliminate particularly toxic components of therapy and substitute less toxic agents.

Combined therapies (chemotherapy and radiation together) are used (1) to improve cure rates in patients whose prognosis is poor and (2) to reduce the dose of radiotherapy administered to children so that skeletal development will proceed more normally. Chemotherapy has side effects as well, including infertility after MOPP chemotherapy, cardiotoxic effects of the doxorubicin of ABVD, and pulmonary toxicity caused by bleomycin.[36,155] Secondary leukemias have been described, particularly after the combination of MOPP and radiation.[30] In choosing an appropriate regimen for a given patient, the following must be considered: (1) the age and skeletal maturity of the patient (likely effects on the developing child), (2) the extent of disease present (how much therapy is necessary), and (3) symptoms that might predict a poor prognosis. Because so many regimens currently appear equivalent in terms of outcome, an investigational protocol should be used (if one is available) to help delineate the best treatment for patients in the future, while ensuring appropriate treatment for those under study.

Prognosis

Radiation therapy alone may cure up to 70% of patients who have stage I or IIA Hodgkin's disease and 50% of patients who have IIB or IIIA disease. The subsequent use of chemotherapy will enable half of those who relapse after radiation therapy to be cured of the disease.[166,176] The success of this approach varies significantly among institutions. In the 1980s, combined-modality therapy became the standard recommendation for younger patients who had not completed their growth and for those who have advanced-stage disease. Recent recognition of the toxicities of full-dose radiation have made combined modality therapy the standard of care for virtually all patients cared for by pediatric oncologists.

High-risk features include advanced-stage disease, a large mediastinal mass, more than four sites of involvement, and B symptoms.[81,144] Results of recent studies demonstrate 5-year, disease-free survivals of approximately 70% to 90% for patients who have advanced-stage disease and 85% to 100% for patients who have localized disease. In some patients who experience relapse, improvement can be effected with bone marrow transplantation.

Follow-up

Patients who have Hodgkin's disease should be monitored for evidence of recurrent disease for as long as 10 to 15 years after the original diagnosis. In addition to a careful physical examination, useful tests for prolonged follow-up include a complete blood cell count, a sedimentation rate, and a CXR.

Following high-dose radiotherapy to the neck and mediastinum, soft-tissue and bone growth abnormalities include shortening of clavicles and underdevelopment of the soft tissues of the neck. Sitting height decreases after radiation to the axial skeleton in proportion to the growth potential remaining at the time of radiation.[141] In prepubertal girls, breast development may be impaired. The incidence of breast cancer may be increased after irradiation,[15,86] particularly for girls who received radiation therapy during early adolescence during breast tissue proliferation. Annual mammography examinations beginning at an early age (approximately 25 years) are recommended.

Overt hypothyroidism (low thyroxine and elevated thyroid-stimulating hormone [TSH]) occurs in approximately 5% to 10% of patients who have undergone irradiation, whereas compensated hypothyroidism (elevated TSH and normal thyroxine) occurs in 50% to 90% of such patients.[31] Thyroid function should be assessed for at least 15 years. Thyroid replacement therapy is recommended when the TSH level is elevated.

Patients who receive mediastinal irradiation may have pulmonary fibrosis with variable abnormalities detected by pulmonary function testing.[46] Late cardiac abnormalities include pericardial thickening and, occasionally, valvular dysfunction. Early myocardial infarctions have been reported. These toxicities may be exacerbated by the use of bleomycin and anthracyclines.

Fertility in women is affected by the use of radiation

and chemotherapy. Pelvic irradiation of a woman causes infertility unless oophoropexy (moving ovaries to the midline) is performed. Following oophoropexy, all teenage girls treated with radiation alone and 88% of those treated with combined-modality therapy maintained normal menses.[45] Women older than 30 years of age experience ovarian failure after treatment with MOPP more frequently than do younger women. All should be advised of the possibility of early menopause. A menstrual history should be elicited at each visit.

Testes are more severely affected by cytotoxic therapies than are ovaries. Fortunately, the radiation fields used in Hodgkin's disease spare the gonads in male patients. Six courses of MOPP chemotherapy, however, result in universal male sterility. Approximately 50% of patients treated with three courses of MOPP are sterile.[38] ABVD causes less impairment of spermatogenesis. Men interested in fathering a child may benefit from sperm banking and posttherapy monitoring of gonadotropin levels and semen analysis. Recovery has been documented in previously sterile men.

Acute nonlymphocytic leukemia occurs in patients who have Hodgkin's disease at the rate of approximately 1% per year for the first 10 years after treatment with MOPP and radiotherapy.[30] Thereafter, the risk appears to decrease. The incidence is lower with single-modality therapy or after ABVD and radiation. Solid tumors, particularly breast cancer, thyroid cancer, bone tumors, and NHL, also may occur after Hodgkin's disease.

Patients who have had a splenectomy are at risk for overwhelming infection, particularly by polysaccharide-encapsulated organisms. Empirical treatment with intravenous antibiotics is recommended for fever (>101° F) in these patients.

GENERAL ONCOLOGICAL CARE

Referral to a Pediatric Oncologist

Fortunately, children who have malignancies represent a very small proportion of patients in a general pediatrics practice. The treatment of such patients is specialized and changes rapidly each year. Proper care of such patients begins with referral to a pediatric oncologist, even if the initial procedure indicated is surgical. Recognition of potential malignancy in the differential of a patient's presentation is essential to ensure inappropriate therapy will not be administered—for example, corticosteroids to a patient whose symptoms mimic EBV infection or reactive airway disease. For many tumors, appropriate baseline studies must be obtained before surgical procedures are instituted. For example, AFP and B-HCG levels fall rapidly after removal of the germ cell tumor, as do catecholamine levels after removal of a neuroblastoma. Delayed assays for such markers may result in an inability to recognize an important indicator of recurrent disease in a given patient. The chest CT scan should be performed before surgical procedures because perioperative atelectasis may interfere with the detection of metastatic disease in the pulmonary parenchyma.

The tumors of childhood behave differently from those of adults, even when histologically identical. In addition, children tolerate radiation and chemotherapy differently than do adults. Therefore, all children should benefit from the care of a pediatric oncologist. Services available for children and their families at pediatric referral hospitals often ease the pain of being diagnosed with a life-threatening disease. Pediatric social workers, child life workers, and nurses experienced in dealing with children and adolescents who have cancer are available. For patients living at a distance from a center, it often is possible to initiate therapy at a referral medical center and administer most of the subsequent treatments and evaluations closer to the patient's home. At times, a local oncologist can assist in administering chemotherapy to children living at a distance from a center, but such oncologists should not choose a therapeutic regimen or evaluate major problems that may arise without corroboration with the pediatric oncologists at the referral medical center.

A number of oncological emergencies exist that general pediatricians must recognize. Cord compression may result from neuroblastoma, Ewing's sarcoma, lymphoma, or any other tumor that invades the spinal canal. Such patients experience incontinence, loss of reflexes in the lower extremities, or decreased ability to use the lower extremities. Rectal sphincter tone may be decreased. Rapid institution of therapy may reverse such findings, markedly changing the long-term functioning of the patient. Thus, recognition of such findings should prompt immediate referral to a pediatric oncologist who, in conjunction with a neurosurgeon or radiation therapist, will be able to deliver emergent therapy.

Patients whose bone marrow has been infiltrated by leukemia, Ewing's sarcoma, neuroblastoma, or lymphoma may have pancytopenia and thus be at risk of infection as a result of neutropenia, bleeding caused by thrombocytopenia, and congestive heart failure as a result of anemia. Rapid lysis of cells (tumor lysis syndrome) because of the high cell turnover rate of the tumor itself (as is seen in Burkitt's lymphoma) or to cytotoxic therapy is characterized by elevated uric acid (risk of urate nephropathy), hyperkalemia, hypocalcemia, and hyperphosphatemia. Medical management includes allopurinol, urinary alkalinization, and binders of potassium and phosphate. Dialysis may be necessary. If delayed arrival to the medical center is anticipated, allopurinol should be started by the referring physician when a tumor that has a large cell burden (e.g., leukemia, Burkitt's lymphoma, and bone marrow involvement with either neuroblastoma, Ewing's sarcoma, or rhabdomyosarcoma) is suspected.

Pediatricians should recognize the signs and symptoms of superior vena cava (SVC) syndrome, which may include swelling, plethora, and cyanosis of the face, neck, and upper extremities; engorged vessels; cough and wheezing; chest pain; headache; diaphoresis; and visual changes. Lymphomas and other malignancies are the leading causes of SVC syndrome, which may progress rapidly to be life threatening. Therefore, prompt recognition of the potential for mediastinal mass as the etiology of the symptoms and appropriate referral is essential.

Role of the Pediatrician During Therapy

The most prominent toxicity that results from chemotherapy is myelosuppression. Infections in neutropenic patients can rapidly result in septic shock, particularly if gram-negative organisms are involved. Primary physicians who monitor these children can help by recognizing the risk of fever and referring the patient immediately to the pediatric oncologist when the patient becomes febrile. If the center is at a distance, the pediatrician becomes the frontline caretaker, obtaining proper culture specimens and initiating antibiotics (usually an aminoglycoside and semisynthetic penicillin or a fourth-generation cephalosporin). In such circumstances, the primary pediatrician should discuss aspects of care with the pediatric oncologist to ensure that all appropriate measures are taken. Many patients receiving intensive chemotherapy have indwelling central venous catheters that increase the risk for septicemia with gram-positive organisms. These patients, even in the absence of neutropenia, should have blood cultures taken and the administration of antibiotics considered if fever develops. Any person who is febrile and who has undergone a splenectomy should be given antibiotics empirically to treat potential infections with polysaccharide-encapsulated organisms.

In the absence of splenectomy and a central line, pediatric treatment of patients whose blood cell counts are normal usually is similar to that of the typical child. The primary pediatrician can see such children for common pediatric complaints, including skin rashes, earaches, and respiratory and gastrointestinal infections, inasmuch as these children appear to handle such infections without undue difficulty. Varicella, however, is a major threat to all immunocompromised patients (because dissemination of disease is likely even in the absence of neutropenia). Before the availability of acyclovir, significant morbidity and mortality occurred in such patients. Immunocompromised children who are exposed to varicella by a sibling or a close playmate should receive varicella-zoster immunoglobulin within 4 days of the exposure. Should chickenpox occur, the patient should be treated with acyclovir or related new-generation antivirals, often as an inpatient. Chemotherapy usually is withheld during the treatment of varicella.

Children who are receiving treatment for a malignancy should continue to see their primary pediatrician for well-child visits. This is in anticipation of their ultimate successful treatment and cure. Immunizations are delayed until 1 year after therapy is terminated, because live vaccines may cause disease, and inactivated vaccines rarely result in a normal immune response. The pediatrician should remain involved in continuing developmental issues that at times are exacerbated by the treatment of a malignancy. With the current success rates in treating children who have cancer, pediatricians should anticipate the return of these children to their practice for most of their care. Maintenance of a relationship with the patient and family, therefore, is essential.

Care of Long-Term Survivors

Patients treated for childhood malignancy have, for the most part, received a number of extremely toxic agents, the long-term implications of which are not known in their entirety. Studies of a new treatment regimen's late toxicities are often in their early stages, and as therapy evolves, so do the potential late side effects. Children should continue to return at least annually to the treating institution or to a similar institution elsewhere to be monitored for potential side effects and to be informed of problems occurring in patients treated similarly. Toxicities of radiation to particular areas and of currently used chemotherapeutic agents are listed in Tables 193-6 and 193-4, respectively, and recommended follow-up studies are described. The pediatrician should ensure that his or her patients are being screened appropriately.

Multidisciplinary clinics, which evaluate all survivors for potential late effects, are being formed in some hospitals. Subclinical evidence of cardiac damage after anthracycline administration and of pulmonary toxicity (decreased diffusing capacity) after bleomycin administration is found in some survivors, but whether the damage will be progressive is not clear. The long-term effects on renal function and hearing are not yet known. Fertility has been impaired in some adolescent patients who received alkylating therapies, but the incidence of this dysfunction is lower than in adults treated similarly. Radiation to the gonads also causes infertility. Affected women need hormone replacement for feminization and to prevent the osteoporosis associated with estrogen depletion. Testosterone levels in treated males usually remain in the normal range, but they should be monitored. Endocrine dysfunction after radiation may involve the thyroid, hypothalamus, and pituitary. Studies of the mechanism of impairment may help in treating other affected patients more effectively. Thyroid radiation often causes compensated (increased TSH, normal T_4) or overt (increased TSH, decreased T_4) hypothyroidism and should be treated with thyroid hormone.

Secondary malignancies are reported in long-term survivors. Mutagenic agents such as mechlorethamine, cyclophosphamide, etoposide, and radiation therapy play a role. A genetic predisposition to malignancy exists for those who have certain disorders (e.g., bilateral retinoblastoma).

Neurocognitive function and school performance will be affected in many children who are going through or have undergone treatment for childhood cancer. Education specialists and/or pediatric oncological nurse practitioners can be extremely helpful to the child and his or her teachers by (1) explaining the child's diagnosis and treatment to school administrators and teachers, and when appropriate, to classmates; (2) defining the problems and limitations the child will have in keeping up with school work during periods of intensive treatment; and (3) providing or arranging (through the school system) for lessons and special tutoring during prolonged hospitalizations and recovery periods at home.[179]

The psychosocial effects of childhood cancer also differ from patient to patient. Some were so young when they received treatment that they do not remember the ordeal; others had to forsake normal childhood experiences because of their illness. Some have no physical deficits; others have permanent deformities (amputations, scoliosis, hair loss, scars). Although memories and physical disabilities may linger, survivors usually are cured of their cancer. They are emotionally intact people who are able to live and work normally within the mainstream of society. Unfortunately, certain workplaces and insurance companies continue to discriminate based on a history of cancer. Because each tumor and treatment regimen is different, businesses and agencies must be taught to accept those who are cured and are likely to have a normal future. Legal protection is available to survivors via the Americans with Disabilities Act, and advocacy resources that exist within communities and at the national level.[78,129]

Pediatricians must be advocates for these successfully

treated persons. Past medical conditions that will not interfere with future health should not be a barrier to success; however, we must remain aware of potential late effects of therapy. Screening for toxicities will allow for interventions that can maintain health.

REFERENCES

1. Ablin AR, et al: Malignant germ cell tumors in childhood: an outcome analysis, *Proc Am Soc Clin Oncol* 5:213, 1986.
2. Abramson DH, Ellsworth R, Zimmerman L: Nonocular cancer in retinoblastoma survivors, *Trans Am Acad Ophthalmol Otolaryngol* 81: 454, 1976.
3. Abramson DH, et al: Retinoblastoma: survival, age at detection and comparison 1914-1958, 1958-1983, *J Pediatr Ophthalmol Strabismus* 22:246, 1985.
4. Ahmad R, et al: Extraskeletal Ewing's sarcoma, *Cancer* 85:725, 1999.
5. Arndt CAS, Crist WM: Medical progress: common musculoskeletal tumors of childhood and adolescence, *N Engl J Med* 341:342, 1999.
6. Ashley DJB, Path FRC: Origin of teratomas, *Cancer* 32:390, 1973.
7. Babyn P, et al: Imaging patients with Wilms tumor, *Hematol Oncol Clin North Am* 9:1217, 1995.
8. Bacci G, et al: Predictive factors of histologic response to primary chemotherapy in osteosarcoma of the extremity: study of 272 patients preoperatively treated with high-dose methotrexate, doxorubicin, and cisplatin, *J Clin Oncol* 16:658, 1998.
9. Baranzelli MC, et al: Prognostic factors in children with localized malignant nonseminomatous germ cell tumors, *J Clin Oncol* 17:1212, 1999.
10. Barr FG: Molecular genetics and pathogenesis of rhabdomyosarcoma, *J Pediatr Hematol Oncol* 19:483, 1997.
11. Beckwith JB: New developments in the pathology of Wilms tumor, *Cancer Invest* 15:153, 1997.
12. Beckwith JB, Palmer NF: Histopathology and prognosis of Wilms' tumor, *Cancer* 41:1937, 1978.
13. Beckwith JB, Perrin EV: In situ neuroblastoma: a contribution to the natural history of neural crest tumors, *Am J Pathol* 43:1089, 1963.
14. Bernheim A, Berger R, Lenoir G: Cytogenetic studies on African Burkitt's lymphoma cell lines: t(8,14), t(2,8) and t(8,22) translocation, *Cancer Genet Cytogenet* 3:307, 1981.
15. Bhatia S, et al: Breast cancer and other second neoplasms after childhood Hodgkin's disease, *N Engl J Med* 334:745, 1996.
16. Bonadonna G, et al: Combination chemotherapy of Hodgkin's disease with adriamycin, bleomycin, vinblastine, and imidazole carboxamide versus MOPP, *Cancer* 36:252, 1975.
17. Bordow S, et al: Prognostic significance of MYCN oncogene expression in childhood neuroblastoma, *J Clin Oncol* 16:3286, 1998.
18. Breslow NE, Beckwith JB: Epidemiological features of Wilms' tumor: results of the national Wilms' tumor study, *J Natl Cancer Inst* 68:429, 1982.
19. Brodeur G, et al: Revisions of the international criteria for neuroblastoma diagnosis, staging, and response to treatment, *J Clin Oncol* 11: 1466, 1993.
20. Buckley JD, et al: Epidemiology of osteosarcoma and Ewing's sarcoma in childhood, *Cancer* 83:1440, 1998.
21. Byrne J, et al: Reproductive problems and birth defects in survivors of Wilms' tumor and their relatives, *Med Pediatr Oncol* 16:233, 1988.
22. Carbone PP, et al: Report of the Committee on Hodgkin's Disease Staging Classification, *Cancer Res* 31:1860, 1971.
23. Carli M, et al: Therapeutic efficacy of single drugs for childhood neuroblastoma: a review. In Raybaud C, et al, editors: *Pediatric oncology,* Amsterdam, 1982, Excerpta Medica.
24. Cassady JR: Retinoblastoma: managing a childhood malignancy, *Contemp Oncol* April, p 29, 1994.
25. Cassady JR, et al: Radiation therapy in retinoblastoma, *Radiology* 93: 405, 1969.
26. Chan HSL, et al: Combining cyclosporin with chemotherapy controls intraocular retinoblastoma without requiring radiation, *Clin Cancer Res* 2:1499, 1996.
27. Chatten J, Voorhees ML: Familial neuroblastoma, *N Engl J Med* 277: 1230, 1967.
28. Cheung NKV, et al: Anti-GD2 antibody treatment of minimal residual stage 4 neuroblastoma diagnosed at more than 1 year of age, *J Clin Oncol* 16:3053, 1998.
29. Clericuzio CL, Johnson C: Screening for Wilms tumor in high risk individuals, *Hematol Oncol Clin North Am* 9:1253, 1995.
30. Coleman CN: Secondary malignancy after treatment of Hodgkin's disease: an evolving picture, *J Clin Oncol* 4:821, 1986.
31. Constine LS, et al: Thyroid dysfunction after radiotherapy in children with Hodgkin's disease, *Cancer* 53:878, 1984.
32. Cortes EP, et al: Amputation and adriamycin in primary osteosarcoma, *N Engl J Med* 291:998, 1974.
33. Craft A, et al: Ifosfamide-containing chemotherapy in Ewing's sarcoma: the second United Kingdom Children's Cancer Study Group and the Medical Research Council Ewing's Tumor Study, *J Clin Oncol* 16:3628, 1998.
34. D'Angio GJ, et al: The treatment of Wilms' tumor: results of national Wilms' tumor study, *Cancer* 38:633, 1976.
35. Dahlin CD, Coventry MB: Osteosarcoma: a study of 600 cases, *J Bone Joint Surg (Am)* 49:101, 1967.
36. Damewood MD, Grochow LB: Prospects for fertility after chemotherapy or radiation for neoplastic disease, *Fertil Steril* 45:443, 1986.
37. de Alava E, et al: EWS-FLII fusion transcript structure is an independent determinant of prognosis in Ewing's sarcoma, *J Clin Oncol* 16: 1248, 1998.
38. deCunha MF, et al: Recovery of spermatogenesis after treatment for Hodgkin's disease: limiting dose of MOPP chemotherapy, *J Clin Oncol* 2:571, 1984.
39. Delattre O, et al: The Ewing family of tumors: a subgroup of small round-cell tumors defined by specific chimeric transcripts, *N Engl J Med* 331:294, 1994.
40. Denny CT: Ewing's sarcoma: a clinical enigma coming into focus, *J Pediatr Hematol Oncol* 20:421, 1998.
41. Devesa SS: The incidence of retinoblastoma, *Am J Ophthalmol* 80:263, 1975.
42. DeVita VT Jr, Serpick A, Carbone PP: Combination chemotherapy in the treatment of advanced Hodgkin's disease, *Ann Intern Med* 73:881, 1970.
43. Diller L, et al: Constitutional WT 1 mutations in Wilms tumor patients, *J Clin Oncol* 16:3634, 1998.
44. Donaldson SS: Rhabdomyosarcoma. In Carter S, Glatstein E, Livingston RB, editors: *Principles of cancer treatment,* New York, 1982, McGraw-Hill.
45. Donaldson SS, Kaplan HS: Complications of treatment of Hodgkin's disease in children, *Cancer Treat Rep* 66:977, 1982.
46. Donaldson SS, Link MP: Combined modality treatment with low-dose radiation and MOPP chemotherapy for children with Hodgkin's disease, *J Clin Oncol* 5:742, 1987.
47. Drash A, et al: A syndrome of pseudohermaphrodism, Wilms' tumor, hypertension, and degenerative renal disease, *J Pediatr* 76:585, 1970.
48. DuBois S, et al: Metastatic sites in stage IV and IVS neuroblastoma correlate with age, tumor biology, and survival, *J Pediatr Hematol Oncol* 21:181, 1999.
49. Einhorn LG, Donahue JP: Combination chemotherapy in disseminated testicular cancer, *Semin Oncol* 6:87, 1979.
50. Evans R, et al: Local recurrence, rate and sites of metastases, and time to relapse as a function of treatment regimen, size of primary and surgical history in 62 patients presenting with non-metastatic Ewing's sarcoma of the pelvic bones, *Int J Radiat Oncol Biol Phys* 11:129, 1885.
51. Ewing J: Diffuse endothelioma of bone, *Proc N Y Pathol Soc* 21:17, 1921.
52. Exelby PR: Testicular cancer in children, *Cancer* 45:1803, 1980.
53. Falk S, Albert M: The clinical and roentgen aspects of Ewing's sarcoma, *Am J Med Sci* 54:44, 1965.
54. Farewell VT, et al: Retrospective validation of a new staging system for Wilms' tumor, *Cancer Clin Trials* 4:167, 1981.

55. Filipovitch A, et al: Lymphomas in persons with naturally occurring immunodeficiency disorders. In Magrath I, O'Connor G, Ramot B, editors: *Pathogenesis of leukemias and lymphomas: environmental influences,* New York, 1984, Raven Press.
56. Frauman JF: Stature and malignant tumors of bone in childhood and adolescence, *Cancer* 20:967, 1967.
57. Frost J, et al: A phase I/IB trial of murine monoclonal anti-GD2 antibody 14.G2a plus interleukin-2 in children with refractory neuroblastoma, *Cancer* 80:317, 1997.
58. Gatti RA, Good RA: Occurrence of malignancy in immunodeficiency disease: a literature review, *Cancer* 28:89, 1971.
59. Gaze MN, Wheldon TE: Radiolabeled mIBG in the treatment of neuroblastoma, *Eur J Cancer* 32:93, 1996.
60. Gerl A, et al: Late relapse of germ cell tumors after cisplatin-based chemotherapy, *Ann Oncol* 8:41, 1997.
61. Gilman PA, et al: Familial osteosarcoma associated with 13;14 chromosomal rearrangement, *Cancer Genet Cytogenet* 17:123, 1985.
62. Gitlow SE, et al: Diagnosis of neuroblastoma by qualitative and quantitative determination of catecholamine metabolites in urine, *Cancer* 25:1377, 1970.
63. Glatstein E, et al: The value of laparotomy and splenectomy in the staging of Hodgkin's disease, *Cancer* 24:709, 1969.
64. Grabowski EF, Abramson DH: Intraocular and extraocular retinoblastoma, *Hematol Oncol Clin North Am* 1:721, 1987.
65. Graham-Pole J, et al: High dose chemotherapy supported by marrow infusion for advanced neuroblastoma: a Pediatric Oncology Group study, *J Clin Oncol* 9:152, 1991.
66. Green D, Thomas PRM, Shochat S: The treatment of Wilms tumor, *Hematol Oncol Clin North Am* 9:1267, 1995.
67. Green DM, et al: Effect of duration of treatment on outcome and cost of treatment for Wilms' tumor: a report from the National Wilms' Tumor Study Group, *J Clin Oncol* 16:3744, 1998.
68. Green DM, et al: The treatment of Wilms tumor patients with pulmonary metastases detected only with computed tomography: a report from the National Wilms' Tumor Study Group, *J Clin Oncol* 9:1776, 1991.
69. Grier H, et al: Improved outcome in non-metastatic Ewing's sarcoma (EWS) and PNET of bone with the addition of ifosfamide (I) and etoposide (E) to vincristine (V), Adriamycin (Ad) and Actinomycin (A), *Proc ASCO* 13:421, 1994.
70. Grosfeld JL, et al: Benign and malignant teratomas in children: analysis of 85 patients, *Surgery* 80:297, 1976.
71. Grufferman SL, Delzell E: Epidemiology of Hodgkin's disease, *Epidemiol Rev* 6:76, 1984.
72. Grundy P, et al: Molecular genetics of Wilms tumor, *Hematol Oncol Clin North Am* 9:1201, 1995.
73. Gurney JG, et al: Trends in cancer incidence among children in the US, *Cancer* 78:532, 1996.
74. Gururangan S, et al: Treatment of children with peripheral primitive neuroectodermal tumor or extraosseous Ewing's tumor with Ewing's directed therapy, *J Pediatr Hematol Oncol* 20:55, 1998.
75. Harris MB, et al: Treatment of metastatic osteosarcoma at diagnosis: a Pediatric Oncology Group study, *J Clin Oncol* 16:3641, 1998.
76. Hart WR, Burkons DM: Germ cell neoplasms arising in gonadoblastomas, *Cancer* 43:669, 1979.
77. Hawthorne HC, et al: Blanching subcutaneous nodules in neonatal neuroblastoma, *J Pediatr* 77:297, 1970.
78. Hays D, et al: Educational achievement, employment and workplace experience of adult survivors of childhood cancer, *Int J Pediatr Hematol Oncol* 44:327, 1997.
79. Heifetz SA, et al: Immature teratomas in children: pathologic considerations: a report from the combined Pediatric Oncology Group/ Children's Cancer Group, *Am J Surg Pathol* 22:1115, 1998.
80. Hems G: An etiology of bone cancer, and some other cancers, in the young, *Br J Cancer* 24:208, 1970.
81. Hudson MM, Donaldson SS: Treatment of pediatric Hodgkin's lymphoma, *Semin Hematol* 36:313, 1999.
82. Hutchinson RJ, et al: MOPP or radiation in addition to ABVD in the treatment of pathologically staged advanced Hodgkin's disease in children: results of the Children's Cancer Group Phase III Trial, *J Clin Oncol* 16:897, 1998.
83. Ioachim HL, Cooper MC, Hellman GC: Lymphomas in men at high risk for acquired immune deficiency syndrome (AIDS): a study of 21 cases, *Cancer* 56:2831, 1985.
84. Jaffe N: Recent advance in the chemotherapy of metastatic osteogenic sarcoma, *Cancer* 30:1627, 1972.
85. Jaffe N, et al: Adjuvant methotrexate and citrovorum-factor treatment of osteogenic sarcoma, *N Engl J Med* 291:994, 1974.
86. Janjan NA, et al: Mammary carcinoma developing after radiotherapy and chemotherapy for Hodgkin's disease, *Cancer* 61:252, 1988.
87. Jenkin R, et al: The treatment of localized non-Hodgkin's lymphoma in children: a report from the Children's Cancer Study Group, *J Clin Oncol* 2:88, 1984.
88. Jurgens H, et al: Multidisciplinary treatment of primary Ewing's sarcoma of bone: a 6-year experience of a European Cooperative Trial, *Cancer* 61:23, 1988.
89. Kaplan HS: *Hodgkin's disease,* ed 2, Cambridge, 1980, Harvard University Press.
90. Katzenstein H, et al: Prognostic significance of age, MYCN oncogene amplification, tumor cell ploidy, and histology in 110 infants with stage D(S) neuroblastoma: the Pediatric Oncology Group experience—a Pediatric Oncology Group study, *J Clin Oncol* 16:2007, 1998.
91. Kauffman RA, et al: False negative bone scans in neuroblastoma metastatic to the ends of long bones, *Am J Roentgenol* 130:131, 1978.
92. Kawa K, et al: Long-term survivors of advanced neuroblastoma with MYCN amplification: a report of 19 patients surviving disease-free for more than 66 months, *J Clin Oncol* 17:3216, 1999.
93. Kay R, Tank E: The current management of bilateral Wilms' tumor, *J Urol* 135:983, 1986.
94. Keinzler H, et al: Hodgkin's and Reed Sternberg cells in Hodgkin's disease represent the outgrowth of a dominant tumor clone derived from germinal center B cells, *J Exp Med* 184:1495, 1996.
95. Knudson AG: Mutation and cancer: statistical study of retinoblastoma, *Proc Natl Acad Sci U S A* 68:820, 1971.
96. Knudson AG, Strong LC: Mutation and cancer: neuroblastoma and pheochromocytoma, *Am J Hum Genet* 24:514, 1972.
97. Kobrinsky NL, et al: Wilms' tumor, *Hematol Oncol Ann* 1:173, 1993.
98. Koizumi JH, Dal Canto MC: Retroperitoneal neuroblastoma metastatic to brain: report of a case and review of the literature, *Child Brain* 7:267, 1980.
99. LaBrosse EH: Biochemical diagnosis of neuroblastoma: use of a urine spot test, *Proc Am Assoc Cancer Res* 9:39, 1968.
100. Lack EE, Weinstein HJ, Welch KJ: Mediastinal germ cell tumors in childhood: a clinical and pathologic study of 21 cases, *J Thorac Cardiovasc Surg* 89:826, 1985.
101. Ladenstein R, et al: Multivariate analysis of risk factors in stage 4 neuroblastoma patients over the age of one year treated with megatherapy and stem-cell transplantation: a report from the European Bone Marrow Transplantation Solid Tumor Registry, *J Clin Oncol* 16:953, 1998.
102. Lawrence W, et al: Prognostic significance of staging factors of the UICC staging system in childhood RMS: a report from the Intergroup Rhabdomyosarcoma Study (IRS-II), *J Clin Oncol* 5:46, 1987.
103. Leventhal BG, Kato GJ: Childhood Hodgkin's and non-Hodgkin's lymphomas, *Pediatr Rev* 12:171, 1990.
104. Levy C, et al: Role of chemotherapy alone or in combination with hyperthermia in the primary treatment of intraocular retinoblastoma: preliminary results, *Br J Ophthalmol* 82:1154, 1998.
105. Li FP, et al: Adverse pregnancy outcome after radiotherapy for childhood Wilms' tumor, *Proc ASCO* 5:202, 1986.
106. Li MC, Hertz R, Spencer DB: Effect of methotrexate on choriocarcinoma and chorioadenoma, *Proc Soc Exp Biol Med* 96:361, 1956.
107. Link MP, et al: The effect of adjuvant chemotherapy on release-free survival in patients with osteosarcoma of the extremity, *N Engl J Med* 314:1600, 1986.
108. Link MP, et al: Treatment of children and young adults with early stage non-Hodgkin's lymphoma, *N Engl J Med* 337:1259, 1997.
109. Look AT, et al: Cellular DNA content as a predictor of response to chemotherapy in infants with unresectable neuroblastoma, *N Engl J Med* 311:231, 1984.

110. Lukes RJ, Butler JJ: The pathology and nomenclature of Hodgkin's disease, *Cancer Res* 26:1063, 1966.
111. Mackay B, et al: Diagnosis of neuroblastoma by electron microscopy of bone marrow aspirates, *Pediatrics* 56:1045, 1975.
112. Magrath IT, et al: Surgical reduction of tumor bulk in management of abdominal Burkitt's lymphoma, *BMJ* 2:308, 1974.
113. Mahour GH, Woolley GH, Landing BH: Ovarian tumors in children: a 33-year experience, *Am J Surg* 63:367, 1976.
114. Mandell L, et al: Preliminary results of alternating combination chemotherapy (CT) and hyperfractionated radiotherapy (HART) in advanced rhabdomyosarcoma (RMS), *Int J Radiat Oncol Biol Phys* 15:197, 1988.
115. Marcove RC, Rosen G: En bloc resections for osteogenic sarcoma, *Cancer* 45:3040, 1980.
116. Margo CE, Zimmerman LE: Retinoblastoma: the accuracy of clinical diagnosis in children treated by enucleation, *J Pediatr Ophthalmol Strabismus* 20:227, 1983.
117. Marina NM, et al: Complete surgical excision is effective treatment for children with immature teratomas with or without malignant elements: a Pediatric Oncology Group/Children's Cancer Group Intergroup study, *J Clin Oncol* 17:2157, 1999.
118. Maris J, Matthay KK: Molecular biology of neuroblastoma, *J Clin Oncol* 17: 2264, 1999.
119. Martelli H, et al: Conservative treatment for girls with nonmetastatic rhabdomyosarcoma of the genital tract: a report from the Study Committee of the International Society of Pediatric Oncology, *J Clin Oncol* 17:2117, 1999.
120. Martini N, et al: Multiple pulmonary resections in the treatment of osteogenic sarcoma, *Ann Thorac Surg* 12:271, 1971.
121. Matthay K: Neuroblastoma: biology and therapy, *Oncol* 11:1857, 1997.
122. Matthay K, et al: Successful treatment of stage III neuroblastoma based on prospective biologic staging: a Children's Cancer Group study, *J Clin Oncol* 16:1256, 1998.
123. Matthay KK, et al: Treatment of high-risk neuroblastoma with intensive chemotherapy, radiotherapy, autologous bone marrow transplantation, and 13-cis-retinoic acid, *N Engl J Med* 341:1165, 1999.
124. Maurer H, Beltangody M, Gehan E: The Intergroup Rhabdomyosarcoma study-1: a final report, *Cancer* 611:209, 1988.
125. Maurer H, et al: Rhabdomyosarcoma in childhood and adolescence, *Curr Probl Cancer* 2:3, 1977.
126. Meadows AT, Lichtenfield JL, Koop CE: Wilms' tumor in three children of a woman with congenital hemihypertrophy, *N Engl J Med* 291:23, 1974.
127. Mendenhall C, et al: The prognostic significance of soft tissue extension in Ewing's sarcoma, *Cancer* 51:913, 1983.
128. Meyer WH, et al: Thoracotomy for pulmonary metastatic osteosarcoma, *Cancer* 59:374, 1987.
129. Monaco GP, et al: Legal and societal issues facing survivors of childhood cancer, *Pediatr Clin North Am* 44:1043, 1997.
130. Murphy SB: Classification, staging, and end results of treatment of childhood non-Hodgkin's lymphomas: dissimilarities from lymphomas in adults, *Semin Oncol* 1:332, 1980.
131. Murray PG, et al: Effect of Epstein-Barr virus infection on response to chemotherapy and survival in Hodgkin's disease, *Blood* 94:442, 1999.
132. Nag S, et al: Use of brachytherapy to preserve function in children with soft tissue sarcomas, *Oncology* 13:361, 1999.
133. Namouni F, et al: High dose chemotherapy with carboplatin, etoposide, and cyclophosphamide followed by a hematopoietic stem cell rescue in patients with high risk retinoblastoma: a SFOP and SFGM study, *Eur J Cancer* 33:2368, 1997.
134. Nicholson HS, et al: Uterine anomalies in Wilms tumor survivors, *Cancer* 78:887, 1996.
135. Nonoyama M, et al: Epstein-Barr virus DNA in Hodgkin's disease, American Burkitt's lymphoma and other human tumors, *Cancer Res* 34:1228, 1974.
136. Paulussen M, et al: Ewing's tumors with primary lung metastases: survival analysis of 114 (European Intergroup) cooperative Ewing's sarcoma studies patients, *J Clin Oncol* 16:3044, 1998.
137. Pegelow GH, et al: Familial neuroblastoma, *J Pediatr* 87:763, 1975.
138. Pellici PG, et al: Chromosomal breakpoints and structural alterations of the c-myc locus differ in endemic sporadic forms of Burkitt lymphoma, *Proc Natl Acad Sci U S A* 83:2984, 1986.
139. Perez CA, et al: Radiation therapy in the multimodal management of Ewing's sarcoma of bone: report of the Intergroup Ewing's Study, *Natl Cancer Inst Monogr* 56:262, 1981.
140. Pratt CB: Use of chemotherapy for retinoblastoma, *Med Pediatr Oncol* 31:531, 1998.
141. Probert JC, Parker BR, Kaplan HS: Growth retardation in children after megavoltage irradiation of the spine, *Cancer* 32:634, 1973.
142. Provisor AJ, et al: Treatment of nonmetastatic osteosarcoma of the extremity with preoperative and postoperative chemotherapy: a report from the CCG, *J Clin Oncol* 15:76, 1997.
143. Ramsey NKC, et al: Acute hemorrhage into Wilms' tumor, *J Pediatr* 91:763, 1977.
144. Raney RB: Hodgkin's disease in childhood: a review, *J Pediatr Hematol Oncol* 19:502, 1997.
145. Raney R, et al: Improved prognosis with intensive treatment of children with cranial soft tissue sarcomas arising in nonorbital parameningeal sites: a report from the Intergroup Rhabdomyosarcoma Study, *Cancer* 59:147, 1987.
146. Reed DM: On the pathological changes in Hodgkin's disease, with especial reference to its relation to tuberculosis, *Johns Hopkins Hosp Rep* 10:133, 1902.
147. Rosen G, et al: Ewing's sarcoma: ten-year experience with adjuvant chemotherapy, *Cancer* 47:2204, 1981.
148. Rosen G, et al: Preoperative chemotherapy for osteogenic sarcoma, *Cancer* 49:1221, 1982.
149. Rosenstock JG, D'Angio GJ, Kiesewetter WB: The incidence of complications following staging laparotomy for Hodgkin's disease in children, *Am J Roentgenol* 120:531, 1974.
150. Rosito P, et al: Italian Cooperative Study for the treatment of children and young adults with localized Ewing sarcoma of bone, *Cancer* 86: 421, 1999.
151. Rubie H, et al: N-Myc gene amplification is a major prognostic factor in localized neuroblastoma: results of the French NBL 90 Study, *J Clin Oncol* 15:1171, 1997.
152. Russo C, et al: Long-term neurologic outcome in children with opsoclonus-myoclonus associated with neuroblastoma: a report from the Pediatric Oncology Group, *Med Pediatr Oncol* 29:284, 1997.
153. Ruymann F, et al: Bone marrow metastases at diagnosis in children and adolescents with RMS: a report from the Intergroup Rhabdomyosarcoma Study, *Cancer* 53:368, 1984.
154. Ruymann F, et al: Congenital anomalies associated with RMS: an autopsy study of 115 cases—a report from the Intergroup Rhabdomyosarcoma Study Committee, *Med Pediatr Oncol* 16:33, 1988.
155. Santoro A, et al: Long-term results of combined chemotherapy-radiotherapy approach in Hodgkin's disease: superiority of ABVD plus radiotherapy versus MOPP plus radiotherapy, *J Clin Oncol* 5:27, 1987.
156. Scheibel E, et al: Vasoactive intestinal polypeptide (VIP) in children with neural crest tumors, *Acta Paediatr Scand* 71:721, 1982.
157. Seeger RC, et al: Association of multiple copies of the N-myc oncogene with rapid progression of neuroblastomas, *N Engl J Med* 313:111, 1985.
158. Shields CL, Shields JA: Recent developments in the management of retinoblastoma, *J Pediatr Ophthalmol Strabismus* 36:8, 1999.
159. Shields CL, et al: Chemoreduction in the initial management of intraocular retinoblastoma, *Arch Ophthalmol* 114:1330, 1996.
160. Shields CL, et al. Thermotherapy for retinoblastoma, *Arch Ophthalmol* 117:885, 1999.
161. Sim F, et al: Postradiation sarcoma of bone, *J Bone Joint Surg* 54A: 1479, 1972.
162. Spitz MR, et al: Ethnic patterns of Hodgkin's disease incidence among children and adolescents in the United States, 1973-1982, *J Natl Cancer Inst* 76:235, 1986.
163. Stafford WR, Yanoff M, Parnell B: Retinoblastoma initially misdiagnosed as primary ocular inflammations, *Arch Ophthalmol* 82:771, 1969.

164. Stein H, et al: Cellular origin and clonality of classic Hodgkin's lymphoma: immunophenotypic and molecular studies, *Semin Hematol* 36: 233, 1999.
165. Sterns JK, Coleman DJ, Ellsworth RM: The ultrasonographic characteristics of retinoblastoma, *Am J Ophthalmol* 78:606, 1974.
166. Sullivan MP, et al: Intergroup Hodgkin's disease in children study of stages I and II: a preliminary report, *Cancer Treat Rep* 66:937, 1982.
167. Sweetnam R, Knowelden J, Jedden H: Bone sarcoma: treatment by irradiation, amputation, or a combination of the two, *BMJ* 2:363, 1971.
168. Taylor WF, et al: Trends and variability in survival from osteosarcoma, *Mayo Clin Proc* 53:695, 1978.
169. Tefft M, et al: Acute and late effects on normal tissues following chemo- and radiotherapy for childhood RMS and Ewing's sarcoma, *Cancer* 37:1201, 1986.
170. Teilum G: Special tumors of ovary and testis and related neoplasms. In Levine AS, editor: *Cancer in the young,* New York, 1982, Masson Publishing USA.
171. Tepper J, et al: Local control of Ewing's sarcoma of bone with radiotherapy and combination chemotherapy, *Cancer* 46:1969, 1983.
172. Thomas PRM, et al: Late effects of treatment for Wilms' tumor, *Int J Radiat Oncol Biol Phys* 9:651, 1983.
173. Tsuchida Y, et al: Evaluation of alpha-fetoprotein in early infancy, *Pediatr Surg* 13:155, 1978.
174. Uribe-Botero G, et al: Primary osteosarcoma of bone: a clinicopathologic investigation of 243 cases with necropsy studies in 54, *Am J Clin Pathol* 67:427, 1977.
175. Vietti TJ, et al: Multimodal therapy in metastatic Ewing's sarcoma: an intergroup study, *Natl Cancer Inst Monogr* 56:279, 1981.
176. Vinciguerra V, et al: Alternating cycles of combination chemotherapy for patients with recurrent Hodgkin's disease following radiotherapy: a prospectively randomized study by the Cancer and Leukemia Group B, *J Clin Oncol* 4:838, 1986.
177. Whalen T, et al: Sacrococcygeal teratomas in infants and children, *Am J Surg* 150:373, 1985.
178. Wiggs J, et al: Prediction of the risk of hereditary retinoblastoma using DNA polymorphisms within the retinoblastoma gene, *N Engl J Med* 318:151, 1988.
179. Wissler KH, Proukou C: Navigating the educational system: a practical guide for nurse practitioners, *J Pediatr Oncol Nurs* 16:145, 1999.
180. Wolden SL, et al: Indications for radiotherapy and chemotherapy after complete resection in rhabdomyosarcoma: a report from the Intergroup Rhabdomyosarcoma Studies I and II, *J Clin Oncol* 17:3468, 1999.
181. Wright D, McKeever P, Carter R: Childhood non-Hodgkin's lymphomas in the United Kingdom: findings from the UK Children's Cancer Study Group, *J Clin Pathol* 50:709, 1997.
182. Zech L, et al: Characteristic chromosomal abnormalities in biopsies and lymphoid-cell lines from patients with Burkitt and non-Burkitt lymphomas, *Int J Cancer* 17:47, 1976.

194 Chickenpox

George K. Siberry

Chickenpox (varicella) is a common childhood viral disease characterized by a pruritic vesicular rash that appears in crops. It is highly contagious and has been regarded as a relatively benign disease, inasmuch as complications are rare in healthy children. However, because of the increasing population of patients who are at risk for severe diseases because they are immunosuppressed or receiving therapy for malignancies, the educational impact of the disease through days lost from school, and the financial impact of days lost from the work force by parents,[61] interest in this disease and in its prevention though immunization has grown.

The *chicken* in *chickenpox* is believed to derive from its likeness to the chickpea *Cicer areitinum,* or from the French for chickpea, *pois chiche*.[26,35] Others postulate it may come from the Old English word for itch, *gican*.[56] The word *varicella* is derived from a disease that is similar in appearance but is much more severe: variola (smallpox).

ETIOLOGY

Chickenpox is caused by the varicella-zoster virus, a DNA virus and member of the herpesvirus family, along with the herpes simplex viruses, cytomegalovirus, and Epstein-Barr virus and others. It has been established that the same virus causes both chickenpox and herpes zoster, the latter being a reactivation (after a latent phase) of the initial varicella infection.[26] Varicella-zoster virus can be isolated from the vesicles of both chickenpox and herpes zoster. It also has been isolated from blood and tissue during an infection but has proved more difficult to isolate from respiratory secretions. The virus is highly labile, losing its infectivity quickly in the external environment. Inactivation also can be accomplished by heat and trypsin. There is only one serotype of varicella-zoster virus, but different virus strains have been identified by means of restriction endonuclease patterns of DNA.[39]

TRANSMISSION

Chickenpox is one of the most contagious viral infections to cause disease in humans and is only slightly less contagious than measles and smallpox. Infection is thought to be spread by respiratory secretions, because airborne particles from patients can transmit infection before onset of the rash.[24] Virus has not been cultured from these secretions, although its presence can be detected by PCR.[68] Contact with the vesicular fluid of chickenpox or herpes zoster also may result in the transmission of chickenpox infection. Indirect contact (fomite transmission) probably is rare because of the lability of the varicella-zoster virus.

Varicella-zoster virus can cross the placenta during the first and early second trimester of pregnancy to produce a congenital varicella syndrome.[2,22,27,45] Maternal infection during the late third trimester of pregnancy similarly may result in transplacentally acquired varicella in the newborn.[41,54] Transplacentally acquired antibody to varicella-zoster virus is partially protective to the newborn, but chickenpox can occur in young infants born to immune mothers.

EPIDEMIOLOGY

Humans are the only known reservoir, or natural host, of the varicella-zoster virus. The communicability period is considered to last from 1 or 2 days before the onset of the rash until 5 days after the onset or until all vesicles have crusted. Most vesicles have lost virus particles after 5 days. The incubation period is between 10 and 21 days, with an average of 14 to 15 days. With household exposure, clinical disease will develop in approximately 90% of susceptible contacts after one incubation period,[53] and secondary household cases are often more severe.

In temperate climates, chickenpox is mainly a disease of childhood, with 80% to 90% of children having historically been infected by 9 to 10 years of age.[26,40,50] Currently, the highest incidence of varicella in the United States is among children ages 1 to 6 years.[51] Recent data from the United Kingdom also reveal a shift in age distribution to a greater proportion of cases occurring in children of preschool ages.[20,69,71] This shift has been attributed, in part, to the increased use of out-of-home care for infants and children. Data from the United Kingdom also indicated an unexplained increase in the proportion of varicella cases occurring among teenagers.[20] The impact of increasing use of the varicella vaccine on chickenpox incidence and age distribution of cases remains to be seen.

Until 1995 (prevaccine era), approximately 4 million chickenpox cases occurred yearly in the United States, with 90% of cases occurring in children.[64] The disease occurs throughout the year, but most cases occur during the winter and spring months. There are epidemic occurrences every 2 to 3 years, distributed worldwide. Children in tropical climates have a lower rate of infection. Up to 40% to 90% enter adulthood without having had chickenpox, creating a much larger pool of susceptible persons among older age groups in the tropics than in temperate climates.[68]

Subclinical infections with serological conversion rarely occur. However, because varicella infects most people in temperate climates as children, most adults who report a negative or equivocal history of chickenpox are immune.[3] Infection generally confers lifelong immunity in normal hosts, but second clinical infections can occur.[24] Many such "second cases" may represent situations in which a prior non–varicella exanthematous illness was erroneously labeled as chickenpox.[66]

Death rates from chickenpox are estimated to be 2 per 100,000 for children, 50 per 100,000 for adults, 7000 per 100,000 for immunocompromised patients, and 31,000 per 100,000 for neonates. Prior to introduction of the vaccine, varicella caused 10,000 hospitalizations and 43 deaths annually among children in the United States. More than 90% of the childhood deaths occurred in children who had no risk factors for severe varicella.[63]

PATHOGENESIS

Varicella virus gains entry by droplet or airborne spread into the susceptible individual through the respiratory tract. It migrates to the regional lymph nodes, where primary replication occurs. Approximately 4 to 6 days later a primary viremia spreads the virus to internal organs, where secondary replication occurs. This is followed by a secondary viremia, which spreads the organism to the skin and is followed by clinical chickenpox. Viremia has been documented in blood-borne monocytes 9 to 12 days after exposure but 1 to 5 days before onset of the rash.[72] The appearance of the rash in crops may be the result of an intermittent secondary viremia.[28]

The rash at first is macular and then progresses to a papular lesion that contains a minute vacuole. Fluid accumulates in the vacuole, causing a vesicle to appear on a reddened base to produce the classic "dewdrop on a rose petal" lesion. Multinucleated giant cells and intranuclear inclusions can be identified microscopically in the base and on the edges of the vesicle. As the rash resolves, the vesicle becomes cloudy and fills with fibrinous fluid and leukocytes. A crust develops that may remain attached for 1 to 2 weeks. When a vesicle occurs on mucous membranes, its roof sloughs to leave a shallow ulcer. There is evidence that interferon, produced by the polymorphonuclear cells in the lesion, may contribute to resolution of the disease.[67]

CLINICAL MANIFESTATIONS

Normal Children

Chickenpox usually begins with no noticeable prodrome or with mild malaise and low-grade fever. This is followed in a few hours to days by a macular rash, usually beginning on the scalp, neck, or upper portion of the trunk. The macules progress to a papular, vesicular, pruritic rash usually within 12 to 24 hours. Vesicles appear in crops, with a new crop occurring every 1 to 2 days over the next 2 to 5 days, resulting in two to four crops during the illness. Typical childhood cases produce a total of 250 to 500 lesions.[51] The vesicles turn to pustules and then crust over. The illness usually runs its course in 5 to 10 days. At the height of the disease, lesions in all phases from early vesicles to crusts can be seen. Fever varies from none to 102° F (38.9° C) at the onset of the disease and may continue until vesicles cease to appear. The rash spreads centrifugally and involves all areas of the skin in severe cases. Vesicles are pruritic, and excoriations frequently are seen. Lesions occur more frequently in areas of irritation or dermatitis or in skinfolds. Occasionally the rash appears as a macular rash in the diaper area or on the trunk and remain for a day or two before becoming vesicular, making early diagnosis more difficult. Vesicles may occur on the mucous membranes of the mouth, conjunctiva, esophagus, trachea, rectum, or vagina. Generally, little scarring occurs, unless the lesions become superinfected or are continually traumatized. Areas where pox have occurred may, however, remain hypopigmented or hyperpigmented months after the rash has resolved. Occasionally, lesions are bullous, as a variant of the disease itself, but these more often are caused by staphylococcal superinfection. White blood cell counts and other laboratory test results usually are normal.

Older Children and Adults

Chickenpox in older children and adults usually is more severe than in younger age groups, with a prodrome that may include irritability, listlessness, headaches, chills, anorexia, and myalgias. Fever usually is present and is higher and more prolonged than in the young child. The rash, too, tends to be more severe. The risk of complications is 9 to 25 times greater; for example, varicella pneumonia occurs in 15% to 50% of older patients.[21]

Immunocompromised Children

Immunocompromised children usually have the most severe symptoms; they, along with neonates, are at greatest risk of death from chickenpox infection. "Progressive varicella" can be seen in children who have an immunocompromising condition or who are being treated with immunosuppressive therapy for leukemia or another malignancy.[67] Following a more severe prodrome, up to 30% of such immunocompromised children develop progressive varicella with spread of the varicella-zoster virus to the lungs, liver, pancreas, or CNS. Vesicles may be larger and hemorrhagic. All complications of chickenpox are increased in this population, with varicella pneumonia being the most common cause of death. Even if progressive varicella does not develop, these patients still have higher fevers and more prolonged vesicular eruption than do nonimmunocompromised children.

Although severe varicella can occur in HIV-infected children, especially those who have very low CD4 percentages, most HIV-infected children, including those who have low CD4 percentages, do not develop severe acute varicella.[25] Nevertheless, most experts still manage HIV-infected children as being at increased risk of severe disease.[3]

Children receiving systemic steroid therapy for disease other than cancer also are at risk for more severe involvement and complications.[14] Some of this increased risk may be attributable to the potentially immunocompromising effect of nononcological conditions for which steroids are prescribed.[46] Children receiving greater than 2 mg/kg or 20 mg prednisone (or equivalent) for more than 2 weeks should be considered at increased risk of severe varicella.[3] Inhaled corticosteroids are not thought to increase risk of severe varicella, but no studies have been done in children.

Congenital and Neonatal Varicella

Infants born to mothers who contract chickenpox during the first 20 weeks of pregnancy have a 2% to 17% risk of having congenital varicella syndrome. This syndrome includes one or more of the following defects: low birth weight, cicatricial skin lesions or scars, a hypotrophic limb, eye abnormalities, brain damage, and mental retardation.[2,16,22,29,45] In one series of 366 women who had herpes zoster in pregnancy, none of the infants had evidence of intrauterine infection.[16]

When mothers have clinical chickenpox in the 2 weeks before delivery, 24% of their infants will develop neonatal varicella. If the onset of maternal rash occurs more than 5 days before delivery or if the onset of rash in the infant occurs at fewer than 4 days of age, there seems to be little risk of death. This reprieve probably is attributable at least in part to maternally transferred immunity. If, on the other hand, the *maternal* rash emerges between 4 days before and 2 days after delivery or if the *newborn* rash begins at 5 to 10 days of age, there is an associated 21% to 31% neonatal mortality.[41,45,54] The risk is uncertain for infants who are nursing when the mother contracts chickenpox.

COMPLICATIONS

Secondary Bacterial Infection

Secondary bacterial infection is the most common complication of chickenpox. Children younger than 5 years of age appear to be at increased risk.[1,29,47] Symptoms of secondary bacterial infection begin, on average, 4 days after the appearance of the varicella rash, often with a secondary fever. Infections usually are by group A streptococci or *Staphylococcus aureus* and include impetigo, cellulitis, abscess, necrotizing fasciitis, myositis, gangrene, arthritis, osteomyelitis, pneumonia, empyema, conjunctivitis, toxic shock syndrome (usually streptococcal), sepsis, and erysipelas. Bullous lesions caused by *S. aureus* may begin on the second or third day of the rash and manifest as bullous impetigo. Although superficial bacterial skin infections remain most common, invasive Group A streptococcal infections have increased in recent years.[1]

Reye's Syndrome

Reye's syndrome (see also Chapter 256) is an acute illness occurring almost exclusively in children and characterized by encephalopathy and fatty degeneration of the liver. Reye's syndrome carries a high case fatality rate of 30% overall, reaching rates of 43% for children younger than 5 years old. In 1980, the association between Reye's syndrome and use of aspirin during varicella or influenza illnesses was first reported. This led to a CDC advisory in 1980, a Surgeon General advisory in 1982, and mandatory warning labels of all aspirin-containing medications in 1986 cautioning physicians and parents not to use salicylates in children who have varicella or influenza-like illnesses.The annual number of reported cases of Reye's syndrome in the United States fell from a high of 555 cases in 1980 to no more than 36 cases per year from 1987 to 1993 and no more than 2 cases per year from 1994 to 1997.[9] Given the rare occurrence of Reye's syndrome, any child suspected of Reye's syndrome should be evaluated thoroughly for the presence of another metabolic disorder.

Aspirin should be avoided in any child who has chickenpox.

Neurological Complications

Nervous system complications are the second most common complication of varicella and include acute cerebellar ataxia, encephalitis, seizures, aseptic meningitis, myelitis, and peripheral neuropathy. Many of the seizures occurring with chickenpox may simply be febrile seizures; in one series, 12 of 23 patients who had varicella and seizures had concomitant fever.[47] In older series, the mortality from neurological complications reached about 10% overall, but most of the deaths occurred among cases of encephalitis, some of which may have represented unrecognized Reye's syndrome.[57]

Acute cerebellar ataxia (ACA) is the most common neurological complication of varicella, occurring in 1 in 4000 cases of chickenpox.[29] The average age is 4 years old with the great majority of ACA cases occurring among children younger than 5 years old.[13] The onset of symptoms usually occurs 1 to 2 weeks following onset of varicella, but ranges from 2 to 21 days after the appearance of the rash, and, uncommonly, may even precede the rash.[57] The usual clinical features of varicella-related ACA are acute onset of vomiting and ataxic gait disturbance without major disturbance in mental status. Dysmetria (68%) and trunk ataxia (74%) also occur frequently; fever and nystagmus are much less common (5% to 10%). Laboratory studies usually reveal a normal peripheral white blood cell count, normal to mildly elevated CSF protein, and, in 50% of patients, a CSF pleocytosis. Between 95% and 100% of normal children who have varicella-related ACA recover completely with only supportive care.[13,57] Many cases are mild enough that hospitalization is not necessary. Recovery usually takes place within the first 3 months, although it may take longer for some children. There is some concern for longer-lasting subtle behavioral and learning difficulties, but these need further study with controlled comparisons.

Varicella Pneumonia

Varicella pneumonia occurs most often among adults, adolescents, and immunocompromised children.[21] It is one of the more common causes of death resulting from varicella. In children it occurs in fewer than 1 per 10,000 cases of chickenpox.[29] In adults it may be present in 30% to 50% of cases of varicella, although more recent studies estimate a lower incidence of 5% to 10%. Manifestations range from abnormal chest radiograph findings only to cough, rales, tachypnea, hemoptysis, chest pain, cyanosis, and respiratory failure. Onset of pneumonia typically occurs 5 to 6 days after onset of rash in immunodeficient children and adults, but occurs within the first 3 days of rash onset in immunocompetent hosts (adults). Chest radiographs typically show diffuse, reticulonodular densities of various sizes, best viewed in the lung periphery. As the disease progresses, nodules may enlarge and coalesce into extensive infiltrates. Treatment of varicella pneumonia with intravenous acyclovir is recommended; however, mortality is still 10% to 20%, reaching higher rates among severely immunodeficient patients.[21]

Hematological Complications

Thrombocytopenia is the most common hematological abnormality seen with varicella. Thrombocytopenia may occur with an invasive secondary bacterial infection or sepsis, in which case it is associated with more severe illness and worse outcome.[1] In the absence of secondary bacterial infections, however, varicella may produce thrombocytopenia (or even pancytopenia), attributed to infection-related suppression or antibody-mediated destruction (ITP) of platelets.[17,47,69] Onset occurs from 3 days to 3 weeks after the chickenpox rash appears. Febrile purpura, malignant chickenpox with purpura, postinfectious purpura, purpura fulminans, and Henoch-Schönlein purpura all have been described as occurring with varicella infection.[11]

Hepatitis

Hepatitis has been reported during chickenpox infections and is marked by the onset of abdominal pain, vomiting, and continued fever on the second to fourth day after the rash appears.[19] Liver function tests become abnormal but return to normal with resolution of the abdominal symptoms. No progression to classic Reye's syndrome occurs, and the blood ammonia level is normal. However, some experts believe that some of these cases may represent low-grade Reye's syndrome.[36] One study of 39 children who had uncomplicated chickenpox found 47% to have a mildly increased level of AST (SGOT) and 29% to have markedly increased AST levels.[48]

Zoster

Zoster, or shingles, is the reactivation of the varicella-zoster virus that has remained dormant after clinical chickenpox.[26] The virus resides in the dorsal nerve ganglia and is reactivated by periods of decreased host immunity or other unknown stimuli. During reactivation, the rash covers the dermatome that corresponds to the infected nerve root. Disseminated zoster, however, also can occur, involving multiple dermatomes. Zoster has been described in all age groups, including in infancy after prenatal exposure to varicella virus resulting from maternal chickenpox.

Children who have varicella infections at younger ages, especially when the infection occurs before the child is 1 year of age, have an increased incidence of zoster later in life.[6] Leukemic children who experience varicella develop zoster at an increased incidence of 25 cases per 1000 person-years,[30] a significantly lower rate than that for HIV-infected children. Twenty-seven percent of HIV-infected children who had primary varicella after 1 year of age developed zoster 2 years (on average) after primary varicella; among those children whose CD4 percentage was greater than 15% at the time of varicella infection, 70% developed zoster in the same time period.[25]

Other Complications

Appendicitis, myocarditis, arthritis (viral), nephritis, orchitis, splenic hemorrhage and rupture, pancreatitis, pericarditis, and parotitis have been reported, although rarely.[10,26,60] The most common ophthalmological complication is papillary conjunctivitis, but keratitis, uveitis, optic neuritis, and chorioretinitis also can occur.[32]

DIAGNOSIS

Chickenpox usually is diagnosed clinically. There may be a history of exposure in the previous 10 to 21 days. White blood cell counts usually are normal. A Tzanck smear (scraping of the base of a vesicle and staining with Giemsa or Wright stain) will be positive for multinucleated giant cells in varicella-zoster virus infections.[58,59] Herpes simplex types 1 and 2 also produce a positive Tzanck smear.[44] Electron microscopy and viral cultures can be used to demonstrate virus in the vesicular fluid. Viral antigen has been identified in vesicular fluid by countercurrent immunoelectrophoresis. Polymerase chain reaction (PCR) tests have been demonstrated to be superior to viral culture in identification of varicella virus from vesicles.[42] Viral titers during acute and convalescent stages can document a recent infection if acute titers are obtained early in the illness (preferably day 1 or 2), and higher titers are noted during convalescence 2 to 6 weeks later.

DIFFERENTIAL DIAGNOSIS

Smallpox (variola) historically was the most important disease to be differentiated from chickenpox. This can be done easily with a Tzanck smear or other of the aforementioned laboratory tests, but it has not been necessary since the eradication of smallpox.

Vaccinia (cowpox) produces a vesicular rash resulting from exposure to infected livestock or, in former years, from direct contact with a smallpox vaccination.

Disseminated herpes simplex can resemble the chickenpox rash, but the history and progression of the disease usually differentiate these two entities. Confusion ordinarily arises only in newborns, because disseminated herpes is rare in normal children; a Tzanck smear will be positive in both diseases.[44,58,59] Rickettsial pox can resemble chickenpox, but its vesicles are deeper and are at a uniform stage of development, and there is a more severe prodrome.

Other viruses, especially coxsackievirus and echovirus, can produce vesicular exanthema that usually do not crust and that follow a distinctly different course. The Tzanck smear is negative in these infections. Lesions of Stevens-Johnson syndrome can resemble chickenpox, but the two diseases follow different clinical courses and the rashes develop differently. A Tzanck smear will be negative. Contact dermatitis may produce a rash similar to that of chickenpox (including pruritus) but has a different distribution and evolution.

Insect bites and scabies occasionally cause confusion if they are vesicular. Bullous impetigo (especially staphylococcal skin infection) may produce bullae that resemble chickenpox.

TREATMENT

Treatment with acetaminophen for control of fever and relief of prodromal symptoms, along with measures to control pruritus, usually are sufficient. There is concern that use of ibuprofen during varicella may increase the risk of necrotizing fasciitis and other secondary bacterial (streptococcal) infections, but an association has not been firmly established, and its causal relationship may be confounded by the use of ibuprofen for the signs (e.g., secondary fever) of incipient bacterial complications.[12,52,73] Pruritus can be controlled with oral antihistamine (e.g., diphenhydramine), calamine lotion, Cetaphil lotion, or 0.25% menthol lotion. Uncommon but reported encephalopathic side effects of diphenhydramine may mimic neurological complications of varicella.[55,62]

Patients should be encouraged to take daily baths to help prevent bacterial superinfection. Adding baking soda or oatmeal preparations (Aveeno) to a warm bath helps to relieve the pruritus. Children's nails should be kept clean and trimmed to help discourage scratching. Occasionally, gloves or socks on the hands are required to prevent opening of lesions by scratching. If superinfection is present, it usually is a result of group A streptococci or *S. aureus*. Superinfection of a few lesions can be treated topically with bacitracin or mupirocin ointment; superinfection of many lesions or of lesions in difficult areas (e.g., around nares or the mouth) can be treated systemically with a first-generation cephalosporin (e.g., cephalexin, cefadroxil) or other antibiotics active against streptococci and staphylococci.

The Centers for Disease Control and Prevention recommend avoiding aspirin in the treatment of chickenpox because of its association with Reye's syndrome (see section on Reye's syndrome, p. 1387). Physicians caring for patients who are taking aspirin chronically for juvenile rheumatoid arthritis or other diseases need to consider the risks versus the benefits of this therapy on an individual basis if such a patient develops chickenpox.

Acyclovir has been shown to be effective in the treatment of varicella infections in healthy children and adolescents. When instituted within 24 hours of the onset of rash, treatment has resulted in modest reductions in duration of illness, number of cutaneous lesions, fever, and systemic symptoms.[7,8,15] Antibody titers 1 year later were equal in treated and untreated patients. In one study, treatment of the index case with acyclovir did not change the transmission rate to other susceptible household contacts.[7] Use of acyclovir for varicella infection in adolescents should be considered, because they are at greater risk for more severe disease[3]; however, routine use of acyclovir in healthy preadolescent children continues to be controversial in the pediatric literature. Valacyclovir and famciclovir have been licensed for treatment of zoster in adults, but there are no studies and no pediatric formulations upon which to base recommendations for their use in children.[3]

Acyclovir, generally by the intravenous route, has been recommended for the treatment of immunocompromised children who develop varicella infection.[3] Increasingly, children infected with HIV, particularly those who have higher CD4 percentages, have been treated successfully for primary varicella with oral acyclovir.[4,25]

Hospitalization should be avoided whenever possible because hospital epidemics can occur even when the strictest isolation procedures are followed. Generally, spread is by infection of staff members who were thought to be immune or by airborne spread of the virus through ventilation systems. When unavoidable, hospitalization requires strict isolation. Hospitalization on an adult ward that has no immunosuppressed patients may lessen the chances of spread in hospitals where effective strict isolation is not available.[23]

PREVENTION

Isolation or exclusion of the child who has chickenpox to prevent subsequent exposure of those susceptible is the easiest strategy of prevention in institutional settings such as hospitals, schools, or child care facilities. This is not always effective, however, inasmuch as the disease is contagious 1 to 2 days before the appearance of the rash. It also is generally not feasible for prevention of household exposures.

Passive prevention may be attempted by administering varicella-zoster immunoglobulin (VZIG) to susceptible persons within 72 to 96 hours of a known or suspected exposure.[27,38,70] VZIG administration usually prevents disease in normal children and modifies it in adults and immunocompromised patients. Varicella occurring despite VZIG prophylaxis may occur up to 28 days after exposure, instead of the usual incubation period limit of 21 days.

Prophylaxis with VZIG after exposure to varicella is recommended for *susceptible* individuals at high risk of severe varicella, including susceptible HIV-infected and other immunocompromised children, susceptible pregnant women, newborn infants whose mothers develop varicella eruption from 5 days before until 2 days after delivery, hospitalized premature infants older than 28 weeks' gestation whose mothers are susceptible, and hospitalized premature infants younger than 28 weeks or less than 1000 g, regardless of maternal susceptibility status.[3] VZIG may be repeated in individuals who are reexposed to varicella more than 3 weeks after an initial VZIG dose and have not developed varicella.VZIG also may be considered for susceptible adolescents and adults exposed to varicella, although acyclovir may be used instead to treat such patients if varicella develops. Alternatively, susceptible adults and children (older than 1 year old) who are exposed to chickenpox may be given varicella vaccine within 3 days and perhaps up to 5 days after exposure for prevention of disease.[51] Prophylactic use of acyclovir for prevention of varicella in exposed, susceptible children is not recommended based on inadequate data and concern about alteration by acyclovir of immune response to varicella.[3]

Varicella Vaccine

A live-attenuated varicella virus vaccine was licensed by the FDA in 1995. This vaccine has been shown to be effective in preventing varicella infection in most recipients.[33] A single dose is recommended for routine administration to normal children 1 year and older who are susceptible; two doses of the vaccine at least 1 month apart are recommended for susceptible adolescents, 13 years old or older. Susceptible is defined as a lack of reliable history of chickenpox. Routine serological confirmation of susceptibility in adolescence is not likely to be cost effective, but a positive serological result does exclude the need for vaccination.[3] Modified chickenpox (shorter duration, fewer lesions, less fever) occurs at a rate of about 2% to 3% per year among vaccinees and is associated with low 6-week postvaccination VZV antibody titers.[31] Limited data demonstrate persistence of humoral and cell-mediated immunity following vaccination for up to 20 years in Japan, but the contribution of boosting by continued circulation of wild-type varicella to maintenance of immunity is unknown.[5]

The adverse event attributed most commonly to the vaccine is a mild (two to five lesions on average) maculopapular or varicelliform rash at the injection site or other sites in the month following varicella vaccination.[3] Such lesions appear in 7% to 8% of vaccinated normal children; when tested by PCR, however, the majority of these rashes are determined to be due to natural infection. Other more serious but much less common adverse events—encephalitis, ataxia, erythema multiforme, pneumonia, thrombocytopenia, seizures, herpes zoster—occur at lower frequencies than would be expected following natural infection.[49,51]

Because immune globulin or other blood products may interfere with the immune response to varicella vaccination, vaccine should be deferred for 5 months (9 months for RSV-IVIG) after receipt of blood products other than washed RBCs. Salicylates should not be given for 6 weeks following vaccination because of the theoretical risk of Reye's syndrome.

Because the varicella vaccine is an attenuated-live virus vaccine, it generally is not recommended for use in pregnancy or in immunocompromised children, including those who have congenital immunodeficiencies, moderately to severely symptomatic HIV infection or HIV infection with age-specific CD4 percentages less than 25%, blood dyscrasias, leukemia, lymphoma, immunosuppressive therapy for malignancy, or high-dose steroid therapy (equivalent of prednisone 2 mg/kg/day or 20 mg per day).[3,51]

Clinical trials have demonstrated that for children whose leukemia is in remission, and with a break in chemotherapy before and after vaccination, two-dose varicella vaccine was safe, immunogenic, and completely effective in preventing severe varicella; 50% of these children developed a mild rash in the month following vaccination. They were less likely to develop zoster than were comparable leukemic children who had natural varicella infection.[34] The vaccine is not licensed or routinely recommended for susceptible children who have leukemia at this time, but these children may be eligible to receive the vaccine through a research protocol. (See *Red Book 2000* for details.[3])

Based on data from a recent clinical trial, varicella vaccine should be considered for children who have asymptomatic (CDC class N) or mildly symptomatic (CDC class A) HIV infection whose age-specific CD4 percentages are at least 25%.[51]

Transmission of vaccine virus to susceptible contacts has been extremely rare and has occurred only in the presence of a vaccine-associated rash; therefore, vaccinees who develop a rash should avoid direct contact with susceptible, immunocompromised individuals until the rash has resolved. Presence of an immunocompromised or pregnant contact does not preclude vaccination of an otherwise eligible child.

Acceptance by parents and pediatricians of routine use of varicella vaccine in children has not been universal. In 1997, coverage among U.S. children ages 19 to 35 months old was 26%.[18] In one study, the majority of pediatricians reported that they did not recommend routine varicella vaccination for their patients.[43] Perception that varicella had potentially serious complications was the strongest measured correlate with the recommendation for routine vaccination. Reasons commonly cited for reluctance to use varicella vaccine routinely are belief that varicella is not a serious illness, concern that immunity will not be long lasting, concern that disease might be delayed by the vaccine until adulthood, and cost.[49] When many factors are taken into account, including costs of health care visits and parental lost time from work, routine use of vaccine appears to be cost effective.[37] The Centers for Disease Control and Prevention's Advisory Committee on Immunization Practices has recommended that all states require varicella vaccination for susceptible children entering child care and school.[63]

Acknowledgment

The author gratefully acknowledges the past contributions of the previous author, Evan G. Pattishall III.

When to Refer

Chickenpox in immunodeficient child
Chickenpox in pregnant woman

When to Hospitalize

Varicella pneumonia
Moderately to severely immunosuppressed host
Moderate to severe bacterial complications
Chickenpox in neonate
Encephalopathy

REFERENCES

1. Aebi C, Ahmed A, Ramillo O: Bacterial complications of primary varicella in children, *Clin Infect Dis* 23:698, 1996.
2. Alkalay A, Pomerance JJ, Rimoin DL: Fetal varicella syndrome, *J Pediatr* 111:320, 1987.
3. American Academy of Pediatrics: Varicella-zoster infections. In Pickering LK, editor: *Red book 2000: report of the Committee on Infectious Diseases*, ed 25, Elk Grove Village, Ill, 2000, American Academy of Pediatrics.
4. Arvin AM: Oral therapy with acyclovir in infants and children, *Pediatr Infect Dis J* 6:56, 1987.
5. Asano Y: Varicella vaccine: the Japanese experience, *J Infect Dis* 174(suppl 3):310, 1996.
6. Baba K, et al: Increased incidence of herpes zoster in normal children infected with varicella zoster virus during infancy: community-based follow-up study, *J Pediatr* 108:372, 1986.
7. Balfour HH Jr, et al: Acyclovir treatment of varicella in otherwise healthy adolescents, *J Pediatr* 120:627, 1992.
8. Balfour HH Jr, et al: Acyclovir treatment of varicella in otherwise healthy children, *J Pediatr* 116:633, 1990.

9. Belay ED, et al: Reye's syndrome in the United States from 1981 through 1997, *New Engl J Med* 340:1377, 1997.
10. Bullowa J, Wishile SM: Complications of varicella, *Am J Dis Child* 49:923, 1935.
11. Charkes ND: Purpuric chickenpox: report of a case, review of the literature and classification by clinical features, *Ann Intern Med* 54:745, 1961.
12. Choo PW, et al: Ibuprofen and skin and soft tissue superinfections in children with varicella, *Ann Epidemiol* 7:440, 1997.
13. Connolly AM, et al: Course and outcome of acute cerebellar ataxia, *Ann Neurol* 35:673, 1994.
14. Dowell SF, Bresee JS: Severe varicella associated with steroid use, *Pediatrics* 92:223, 1993.
15. Dunkle LM, et al: A controlled trial of acyclovir for chickenpox in normal children, *N Engl J Med* 325:1539, 1991.
16. Enders G, et al: Consequences of varicella and herpes zoster in pregnancy: prospective study of 1739 cases, *Lancet* 343:1548, 1994.
17. Espinoza C, Kuhn C: Viral infection of megakaryocytes in varicella with purpura, *Am J Clin Pathol* 61:203, 1974.
18. Evaluation of varicella reporting to the national notifiable disease surveillance system—United States, 1972-1997, *MMWR* 48:55, 1999.
19. Ey J, Smith S, Fulginiti V: Varicella hepatitis without neurologic symptoms or findings, *Pediatrics* 67:285, 1981.
20. Farley CK, Miller E: Varicella-zoster virus epidemiology: a changing scene*?* *J Infect Dis* 174:S314, 1996.
21. Feldman S: Varicella-zoster virus pneumonitis, *Chest* 106:22S, 1994.
22. Fuccillo D: Congenital varicella, *Teratology* 15:329, 1977.
23. Gardner P, Breton S, Charles D: Hospital isolation and precaution guidelines, *Pediatrics* 53:663, 1974.
24. Gershon AA, et al: Clinical reinfection with varicella-zoster virus, *J Infect Dis* 149:137, 1984.
25. Gershon AA, et al: Varicella-zoster virus infections in children with underlying human immunodeficiency virus infection, *J Infect Dis* 176: 1496, 1997.
26. Gordon JE: Chickenpox: an epidemiological review, *Am J Med Sci* 244:362, 1962.
27. Greenspoon J: Fetal varicella syndrome, *J Pediatr* 223:505, 1988 (letter).
28. Grose C: Variation on a theme by Fenner: the pathogenesis of chickenpox, *Pediatrics* 68:735, 1981.
29. Guess HA, et al: Population-based studies of varicella complications, *Pediatrics* 78:723, 1986.
30. Hardy IB, et al: The incidence of zoster after immunization with live attenuated varicella vaccine: a study of children with leukemia, *N Engl J Med* 325:1545, 1991.
31. Johnson CE, et al: A long-term prospective study of varicella vaccine in healthy children, *Pediatrics* 100:761, 1997.
32. Kertes PJ, Baker JD, Noel LP: Neuro-ophthalmic complications of acute varicella, *Can J Ophthalmol* 33:324, 1998.
33. Krause PR, Klinman DM: Efficacy, immunogenicity, safety, and use of live attenuated chickenpox vaccine, *J Pediatr* 127:518, 1995.
34. LaRussa P, Steinberg S, Gershon AA: Varicella vaccine for immunocompromised children: results of collaborative studies in the United States and Canada, *J Infect Dis* 174:S320, 1996.
35. Lerman SC: Why is chickenpox called chickenpox? *Clin Pediatr* 20: 111, 1981.
36. Lichtenstein PK, et al: Grade I Reye syndrome: a frequent cause of vomiting and liver dysfunction after varicella and upper respiratory-tract infection, *N Engl J Med* 309:133, 1983.
37. Lieu TA, et al: Cost-effectiveness of a routine varicella vaccination program for US children, *JAMA* 27:375, 1994.
38. Lipton SV, Brunell PA: Management of varicella exposure in a neonatal intensive care unit, *JAMA* 26:1782, 1989.
39. Martin JH: Restriction endonuclease analysis of varicella-zoster vaccine virus and wild-type DNAs, *J Med Virol* 9:69, 1982.
40. Muench R, et al: Seroepidemiology of varicella, *J Infect Dis* 153:153, 1986.
41. Myers J: Congenital varicella in term infants: risks reconsidered, *J Infect Dis* 129:215, 1974.
42. Nahass GT, et al: Comparison of Tzanck smear, viral culture, and DNA diagnostic methods in detection of herpes simplex and varicella-zoster infections, *JAMA* 268:2541, 1992.
43. Newman RD, Taylor JA: Reactions of pediatricians to the recommendation for universal varicella vaccination, *Arch Pediatr Adolesc Med* 152: 792, 1998.
44. Oranje AP, et al: Diagnostic value of Tzanck smear in herpetic and non-herpetic vesicular and bullous skin disorders in pediatric practice, *Acta Derm Venereol (Stockh)* 66:127, 1986.
45. Paryani SG, Arvin AM: Intrauterine infection with varicella-zoster virus after maternal varicella, *N Engl J Med* 314:1542, 1986.
46. Patel H, Macarthur C, Johnson D: Recent corticosteroid use and the risk of complicated varicella in otherwise immunocompetent children, *Arch Pediatr Adolesc Med* 150:409, 1996.
47. Peterson CL, et al: Children hospitalized for varicella: a prevaccine review, *J Pediatr* 129:529, 1996.
48. Pitel PA, et al: Subclinical hepatic changes in varicella infection, *Pediatrics* 65:631, 1980.
49. Plotkin SA: Varicella vaccine, *Pediatrics* 97:251, 1996 (commentary).
50. Preblud S, D'Angelo L: Chickenpox in the United States 1972-1977, *J Infect Dis* 140:257, 1979.
51. Prevention of varicella: updated recommendations of the Advisory Committee on Immunization Practices (ACIP), *MMWR* 48(RR-6):1, 1999.
52. Rosefsky JB: Varicella and necrotizing fascitis, *Pediatr Infect Dis J* 15:556, 1996.
53. Ross AH: Modification of chickenpox in family contacts by administration of gamma globulin, *N Engl J Med* 267:369, 1962.
54. Rubin L, et al: Disseminated varicella in a neonate: implications for immunoprophylaxis of neonates postnatally exposed to varicella, *Pediatr Infect Dis* 5:100, 1986.
55. Schunk JE, Svendsen D: Diphenhydramine toxicity from combined oral and topical use, *Am J Dis Child* 142:1020, 1988 (letter).
56. Scott-Wilson JH: Why "chicken" pox? *Lancet* 1:1152, 1978.
57. Snodgrass SR: Syndromic diagnosis in para-infectious neurologic disease: varicella ataxic syndrome, *J Child Neurol* 13:83, 1998.
58. Solomon AR: The Tzanck smear: viable and valuable in the diagnosis of herpes simplex, zoster and varicella, *Int J Dermatol* 25:169, 1986.
59. Solomon AR, Rasmussen JE, Weiss JS: A comparison of the Tzanck smear and viral isolation in varicella and herpes zoster, *Arch Dermatol* 122:282, 1986.
60. Stebbings S, et al: Chickenpox monoarthritis: demonstration of varicella-zoster virus in joint fluid by polymerase chain reaction, *Br J Rheumatol* 37:311, 1998.
61. Sullivan-Bolyai JZ, et al: Impact of chickenpox on households of healthy children, *Pediatr Infect Dis J* 6:33, 1987.
62. Tomlinson G, Helfaer M, Wiedermann BL: Diphenhydramine toxicity mimicking varicella encephalitis, *Pediatr Infect Dis J* 6:220, 1987.
63. Tucker ME: Get varicella vaccine before school, ACIP says, *Pediatr News*, March 1999, p 12.
64. Varicella-related deaths among adults—United States, *MMWR* 46:409, 1997.
65. Varicella-related deaths among children—United States, 1997. *MMWR* 47:365, 1998.
66. Wallace MR, et al: Reliability of a history of previous varicella infection in adults, *JAMA* 278:1520, 1997.
67. Weller TH: Varicella and herpes zoster, *N Engl J Med* 309:1362, 1984.
68. Weller TH: Varicella: historical perspective and clinical overview, *J Infect Dis* 174:S306, 1996.
69. Winiarski J: Platelet antigens in varicella associated thrombocytopenia, *Arch Dis Child* 65:137, 1990.
70. Wurzel CL, Rubin LG, Krilov LR: Varicella zoster immunoglobulin after postnatal exposure to varicella: survey of experts, *Pediatr Infect Dis J* 6:466, 1987.
71. Yawn BP, Yawn RA, Lydick E: Community impact of childhood varicella infections, *J Pediatr* 130:759, 1997.
72. Yoshizo A, et al: Viremia is present in incubation period in nonimmunocompromised children with varicella, *J Pediatr* 106:69, 1985.

73. Zerr DM, et al: A case-control study of necrotizing fasciitis during primary varicella, *Pediatrics* 103:783, 1999.

SUGGESTED READINGS

Johnson CE, et al: A long-term prospective study of varicella vaccine in healthy children, *Pediatrics* 100:761, 1997.

Krause PR, Klinman DM: Efficacy, immunogenicity, safety and use of attenuated chickenpox vaccine, *J Pediatr* 127:518, 1995.

Prevention of varicella: updated recommendations of the Advisory Committee on Immunization Practices (ACIP), *MMWR* 48(RR-6):1, 1999.

Weller TH: Varicella: historical perspective and clinical overview, *J Infect Dis* 174:S306, 1996.

195 Chronic Fatigue Syndrome

Leonard R. Krilov • Stanford B. Friedman

Chronic fatigue syndrome (CFS) has been used to describe an illness characterized by prolonged periods of debilitating fatigue for which no definitive cause has been determined. Although the U.S. Centers for Disease Control and Prevention has created a working definition of CFS for study purposes,[2] CFS nevertheless is not a well-defined clinical entity. No specific etiological agent(s) and no characteristic pathophysiological model have been identified for CFS. Debate centers on the contributions of infectious and other medical conditions and immunological and psychological factors to the clinical manifestations of CFS. It is likely that all these factors interact to produce CFS, albeit to differing degrees in each individual.

Historically, a variety of syndromes that appear similar to CFS have been described.[11] These include chronic infectious mononucleosis, total allergy syndrome, chronic candidiasis, hypoglycemia, neurasthenia, myalgic encephalomyelitis, postviral syndrome, and fibromyalgia. All these diagnoses are characterized by signs and symptoms similar to those of CFS, as well as the inability to develop a definitive diagnostic test or confirm a definitive causative agent. Cases of CFS have been reported to occur both sporadically and epidemically.

More recently, an association between low blood pressure (neurally mediated hypotension [NMH]) and CFS has been suggested.[10] Other investigators have proposed hormonal factors, such as depressed cortisol responses, as contributing to the signs and symptoms of CFS.

The majority of reported cases of CFS have occurred in white women—a median age of 35 to 40 years and from upper socioeconomic groups, although adolescents who have the diagnosis also have been described.[4,6,9] Minorities, the indigent, and those living in developing countries are strikingly underrepresented in reports of CFS. Whether this observation reflects a bias in patient selection or predisposing factors for development of CFS remains to be determined.

CLINICAL MANIFESTATIONS

The primary manifestation of CFS is severe fatigue greater than 6 months in duration that limits the individual to activity less than 50% of the premorbid level of function. Associated symptoms frequently include sore throat, low-grade fever (oral temperatures of 37.5° to 38.6° C), painful lymph nodes, unexplained generalized weakness, myalgias and/or arthralgias, prolonged fatigue after exercise, headaches, difficulty concentrating or memory loss, and sleep disturbances (hypersomnia or insomnia). The majority of patients describe a sudden onset of the syndrome with an initial mononucleosis or flu-like illness, although in some cases a more gradual onset is related. Many patients also describe a history of atopy and/or multiple allergies.

The initial history should include questions about the nature and duration of symptoms, as well as possible exposures to or contacts with ill persons that might suggest an alternative diagnosis. Personal and social history to assess family dynamics, prior level of functioning, response to illness, family history of psychiatric illness, and psychological or marital problems may be helpful.

The physical examination may reveal abnormalities, including (1) mild inflammation of the pharynx, (2) cervical or axillary lymphadenopathy, or (3) low-grade temperature elevation in up to 50% of cases. However, the primary goal of the physical examination is to eliminate other causes for the patient's symptoms. Significantly elevated temperatures, enlarged lymph nodes (>2 cm), weight loss of more than 10% of body mass without dieting, or focal neurological abnormalities should suggest an alternative diagnosis. The differential diagnoses of illnesses associated with extensive fatigue are listed in Box 195-1.

PSYCHOLOGICAL FACTORS

Clinicians and investigators have noted a relationship of CFS to depressive symptoms, frank depression, and a family history of depression.[3] Conceptually, depression may be both part of the etiology of CFS and a reaction to having CFS. We have been impressed with the family dynamics of adolescents who have CFS.[4,7] School avoidance behaviors related to expectations for high academic performance, compared with the teenager's abilities, have been noted frequently. In many families we also have noted overprotection and overindulgence of the child, often associated with difficulty in mother-teen separation. A recent analysis of adolescents who have CFS compared with age-matched adolescent survivors of childhood cancer and a healthy control group showed that the CFS group had higher scores on measures of somatic complaints, depression, internalizing symptoms, and feeling different from others.[7]

The manifestations of CFS can be considered in this framework as a conversion reaction in which an infection or other stressor serves as a model for persistent symptoms that offer the individual a mechanism by which to maintain an overprotective environment or to avoid going to school (see Chapter 100, Conversion Reactions in Adolescents).

BOX 195-1

DIFFERENTIAL DIAGNOSIS OF A PATIENT WHO IS CHRONICALLY FATIGUED

- Malignancy
- Autoimmune disease
- Localized infection (e.g., sinusitis, occult abscess)
- Chronic or subacute infection (e.g., Lyme disease, endocarditis, tuberculosis)
- HIV infection
- Fungal disease (e.g., candidiasis, histoplasmosis, coccidioidomycosis, blastomycosis)
- Parasitic disease (e.g., toxoplasmosis, giardiasis)
- Chronic inflammatory disease (e.g., sarcoidosis, Wegener's granulomatosis)
- Endocrine disease (e.g., hypothyroidism, Addison's disease, diabetes)
- Neuromuscular disease (e.g., myasthenia gravis, multiple sclerosis)
- Drug dependency
- Side effects of chronic medications or other toxic agents (e.g., chemical solvent, heavy metal, pesticide)
- Psychiatric disorder

LABORATORY DIAGNOSIS

There are no specific laboratory tests by which to diagnose CFS. As with the physical examination, the primary aim of laboratory evaluations is to eliminate other conditions that may be responsible for the patient's symptoms. A suggested battery of screening tests might include a complete blood count and differential; measurement of the erythrocyte sedimentation rate (ESR), serum electrolytes, creatinine, BUN, and glucose; liver function tests; thyroid function tests; tuberculin skin test with controls; measurement of alkaline phosphatase, antinuclear antibodies (ANA), rheumatoid factor, and HIV antibody; and chest and sinus radiographs. Additional tests (e.g., Lyme disease and viral serologies) may be indicated based on history and physical examination findings. Although potential immunological abnormalities, including altered lymphocyte subsets, qualitative defects in natural killer cell activity, hypo- or hypergammaglobulinemia, elevated titers to herpes viruses (e.g., EBV, HHV-6), abnormal lymphokine levels, and decreased lymphocyte proliferation responses, have been described in patients who have CFS, they have not been observed consistently in different groups of patients.[1] Additionally, the magnitude of immunological abnormalities detected in patients who have CFS has been small compared with those who have classic immunodeficiencies; the degree of immune aberrations does not correlate with the severity of symptoms, and opportunistic infections do not occur in CFS.

The role of NMH, as discussed on p. 1393, in CFS is intriguing. Head-upright or tilt-table testing is the modality by which this abnormality is assessed. Such testing should be for a subset of patients in whom dizziness is a significant part of their symptom complex. Whether all CFS patients might benefit from such evaluation is currently unknown.

Although of uncertain significance, increased white matter on T2 magnetic resonance imaging (MRI) scans suggestive of possible infiltration of the perivascular spaces, focal demyelination, or disease of the small blood vessels of the cerebral white matter has been reported in a number of CFS patients.[8]

PROPOSED MODEL OF PATHOGENESIS

Exact definition of a case of CFS is difficult in that there are few objective findings in these individuals, and their most severe symptoms are difficult to quantify. To date, no specific infectious cause for CFS has been defined, and it is unlikely that a single infectious agent is responsible. It seems reasonable to suggest that it is the interaction of multiple factors, as depicted in Fig. 195-1, that results in the development of CFS. The relative importance of each of the factors probably varies from individual to individual.

THERAPY

No specific therapy for CFS has been proven to be effective. However, management aimed at alleviating the patient's symptoms may help. If NMH is documented, dietary (e.g., increased salt intake) and/or pharmacological management with drugs such as fludrocortisone, propranolol, or midodrine may be beneficial. In our experience, therapy of NMH has been only of partial benefit, even in those adolescents whose tilt-table tests are abnormal. An approach to the management of CFS is outlined in Box 195-2. The primary goals of this treatment are to provide symptomatic relief for depression, sleep disorders, and musculoskeletal pains; offer emotional support with involvement of a social worker, psychologist, or psychiatrist, as needed; identify and eliminate "secondary gain" from continuing to contribute to the illness; and devise programs with the patient to increase school (or work) attendance and exercise capability gradually. Periodic physical examinations for possible other conditions also are important. Family therapy often helps the parents manage these issues and addresses the role of family dynamics in the evolution of a patient's symptoms. A team approach with coordination of services to avoid "doctor shopping" and fad therapy is critical to the successful management of the patient who has CFS.

Some of the unproved fad therapies described are megavitamin treatment, immune modifiers (e.g., Ampligen, thymic extract, interleukin-2), magnesium sulfate, liver extract injections, anti-*Candida* diets, colonic irrigation, and removal of dental fillings. Immunoglobulin injections have been reported to be beneficial in one study of CFS patients,[5] although two subsequent studies failed to confirm this observation.

PROGNOSIS AND FUTURE PROSPECTS

Despite the vagaries associated with the diagnosis of CFS and differences in each case, long-term follow-up suggests that most individuals report improvement or resolution of symptoms over a 2- to 3-year period.[4] Few patients report

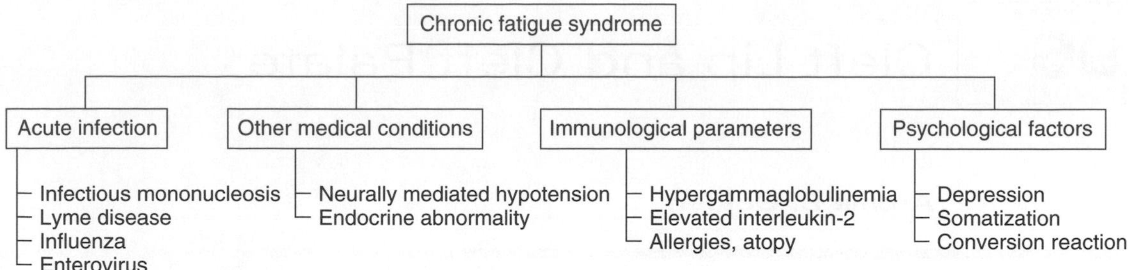

Fig. 195-1 Pathogenesis of chronic fatigue syndrome.

BOX 195-2

MANAGEMENT OF PEDIATRIC PATIENTS WHO ARE CHRONICALLY FATIGUED

Confirm the diagnosis of CFS and acknowledge the symptoms as real
Explain and explore the potential relationship to psychological symptoms
Stress a coordinated approach; minimize doctor shopping, unnecessary testing, and unconventional therapies
Consider tilt-table testing and/or cardiology evaluation if dizziness is a prominent complaint
Use stress-coping skills: modify lifestyles, decrease stress, develop a realistic schedule including working with school (gradual return to classes, home tutoring, neuropsychometric testing), and develop a graduated exercise program
Use cognitive-behavioral approaches: pay attention to sleep patterns and nutrition; increase activity gradually
Provide psychological support: individual therapy, family therapy, decrease secondary gain
Maintain follow-up: monitor physical symptoms and psychological issues; provide ongoing guidance and continued reassurance

progressive symptoms, although symptoms may wax and wane in severity. With better definition of the nature of the neurological, cardiovascular, endocrinological, and immunological alterations in CFS, additional therapeutic approaches may become available.

REFERENCES

1. Barker E, et al: Immunologic abnormalities associated with chronic fatigue syndrome, *Clin Infect Dis* 18(suppl 1):136, 1994.
2. Fukuda K, et al: The chronic fatigue syndrome: a comprehensive approach to its definition and study, *Ann Intern Med* 121:953, 1994.
3. Katon WJ, et al: Psychiatric assessment of patients with chronic fatigue and those with rheumatoid arthritis, *J Gen Intern Med* 6:278, 1991.
4. Krilov LR, et al: Course and outcome of chronic fatigue in children and adolescents, *Pediatrics* 102:360, 1998.
5. Lloyd A, et al: A double-blind, placebo-controlled trial of intravenous immunoglobulin therapy in patients with chronic fatigue syndrome, *Am J Med* 89:561, 1990.
6. Marshall GS, et al: Chronic fatigue in children: clinical features of Epstein-Barr virus and human herpes virus 6 serology and long-term follow-up, *Pediatr Infect Dis J* 10:287, 1991.
7. Pelcoviz D, et al: Psychosocial correlates of chronic fatigue syndrome in adolescence, *J Dev Behav Pediatr* 16:333, 1995.
8. Schwartz RB: Neuroradiologic features. In Dawson DM, Sabin TD, editors: *Chronic fatigue syndrome,* Boston, 1993, Little, Brown.
9. Smith MS, et al: Chronic fatigue in adolescents, *Pediatrics* 88:195, 1991.
10. Stewart JM, et al: Orthostatic intolerance in adolescent chronic fatigue syndrome, *Pediatrics* 103:116, 1999.
11. Straus SE: History of chronic fatigue syndrome, *Rev Infect Dis* 13 (suppl 1):2, 1991.

SUGGESTED READINGS

Dawson DM, Sabin TD, editors: *Chronic fatigue syndrome,* Boston, 1993, Little, Brown.
Klonoff DC: Chronic fatigue syndrome, *Clin Infect Dis* 15:812, 1992.
Marshall GS: Report of a workshop on the epidemiology, natural history, and pathogenesis of chronic fatigue syndrome in adolescents, *J Pediatr* 134:395, 1999.

196 Cleft Lip and Cleft Palate

Archie S. Golden

The complex problems associated with cleft lip and cleft palate require that the primary care pediatrician coordinate management, family support, and a variety of medical needs over the years. The goal is a good psychosocial outcome, as well as a satisfactory anatomical result. Cleft lip or cleft palate, or both, occurs in approximately 1 in 900 births. Cleft lip with or without cleft palate is most frequent in Native Americans and least so in blacks. Cleft palate alone has similar frequency in all groups. Isolated cleft lip is more common in girls, cleft lip and cleft palate more so in boys.

ETIOLOGY AND PATHOGENESIS

The pathogenesis of this malformation is related to hereditary and environmental factors and their interactions. Clefts of the face have been described as a component of more than 250 syndromes. Cleft palate, in particular, occurs more frequently as a constituent of certain syndromes (e.g., trisomy 13). Because many of these syndromes exhibit single-gene inheritance, their recognition is important so that genetic counseling can be provided. Although a specific environmental cause rarely is identified, several substances are known to increase the risk of this birth defect. Among these are alcohol, some tranquilizers, and a few anticonvulsant medications; retinoids and folate antagonists also have been implicated. One third of all infants who have fetal alcohol syndrome have a cleft. Amniotic bands and maternal phenylketonuria also may play a role. Because these deformities may have ramifications far beyond the oral cavity, affected children often present a continuing, complex diagnostic and treatment challenge to a wide range of professionals.

CLINICAL EVALUATION

History

A full family and gestational history is necessary, with particular attention to the maternal use of alcohol, medications, and drugs. A family tree is helpful in identifying those family members who have had clefts, other congenital anomalies and syndromes, mental retardation, odd speech and dental problems, and parental consanguinity. A physical examination of parents and other relatives can confirm the clues provided in the history.

Physical Examination

All infants must have visual inspection of their gums, the hard and soft palates, the uvula, and the throat, as well as palpation of the palate and gums. The degree of clefting will vary. A cleft lip may manifest as a small notch in the vermilion border or a complete separation extending into the nose. Clefts may be unilateral or bilateral. Isolated cleft palate occurs in the midline and can vary from minimal involvement of the uvula to extension through the soft and hard palates. Associated lip and palatal clefts can involve the soft or hard palate on one or both sides, thereby exposing one side of the nasal cavity, or both. A complete examination is necessary to uncover the existence of possible associated anomalies in a variety of described syndromes. Prognosis varies with the particular constellation of findings.

COMPLICATIONS AND THEIR MANAGEMENT

Family Reactions

Giving birth to a baby who has a facial defect can be emotionally traumatic for parents. The emotions experienced are varied and may include shock, anger, confusion, guilt, anxiety, and sadness. Because most parents are unprepared for the birth of a child who has a cleft and are not familiar with the defect, the manner in which the physician first presents the infant and the defect to the parents is of utmost importance. The knowledge, reassurance, and counseling that the primary physician can provide at such a critical time may do much to alleviate the uncertainties and anxieties of the parents. Parents should be encouraged to express their feelings openly and should be reassured that these feelings are normal. The physician should listen attentively and help the parents to understand the importance of their role in the baby's habilitation. Also, the physician should emphasize his or her intent to support the family after the infant is discharged from the hospital. The parents also should be advised that the treatment may take several years and include many types of management. Of paramount importance to the parents is knowing the degree of risk that the cleft will recur in subsequent children. Predictions can be made for individual families by using tables that provide risk data for almost every pedigree; consultation with a geneticist is essential.

Feeding

The most immediate need in the newborn period and during early infancy is adequate nutrition.[1] The infant born having a cleft lip only usually has little or no difficulty feeding; however, those who have a cleft palate with or without a cleft lip may have some difficulty. One of the major causes of difficulty in feeding is the inability to generate effective oral suction.

Breast-feeding should be encouraged and can be accomplished with most infants who have a cleft lip. If not possible directly, breasts can be pumped and the milk bottle-fed. When breast-feeding the infant is not possible or not desired, a variety of feeding techniques can be effective. The position of the infant while feeding is important. Holding the infant in an upright or semi-upright position generally works best and keeps food from coming out through the nose. This also decreases the probability of formula entering the eustachian tubes and causing ear problems. Because these babies often swallow an excessive amount of air, the feeding period may be prolonged and a great deal of energy used in obtaining a marginal amount of nourishment. The use of a squeezable bottle with a soft, enlarged cross-cut nipple often works well. Alternatively, a Haberman nipple or a Brecht feeder is used. Milk should be directed to the inside of the cheek, rather than into the throat. If choking on liquids is a problem, rice cereal may be used as a thickener.

The most important factor in feeding an infant who has a cleft lip or palate is patience. Smaller but more frequent feedings may help to avoid tiring the infant and frustrating the parents. Parents should be encouraged to be creative, determining what works best for their particular infant. Gavage feedings or gastrostomy rarely is needed. It is important that another person (or persons) knows how to feed the infant to enable the mother or other primary caretaker to obtain some respite.

Speech and Language

A hypernasal tone to the voice is the most common speech defect associated with clefts, particularly of the palate. Functioning of the palatal and pharyngeal muscles is impaired. The development of expressive language and speech may be retarded in children who have a cleft palate, and their articulation is less advanced than that of children who do not have such a defect. An associated hearing defect may play an important role in delayed or abnormal speech development. Because problems may persist even after successful anatomical closure, early referral to a speech therapist is important.

Dental and Orthodontic Problems

Irregularities in the upper anterior dental arch associated with cleft lip may result in supernumerary incisors, rotation and malformation of the lateral incisors, or malocclusions. When there is a cleft of both lip and palate, the dental deformities may be greater, involving the canine teeth and the molars. Children who have these problems tend to have more cavities, thus requiring meticulous oral hygiene and constant dental care. Orthodontic treatment usually is necessary.

Middle Ear Disease and Hearing Loss

Recurrent otitis media and hearing loss are almost universal complications of cleft palate. A key factor in the cause of secretory otitis in patients who have a cleft palate is eustachian tube dysfunction. Although middle ear disease is almost universal in these patients, the hearing loss that often accompanies recurrent disease usually can be avoided by close supervision that results in early recognition and treatment of middle ear infections. Educating the parents to recognize the signs of middle ear disease is important and can aid the physician tremendously. The likelihood of otitis media decreases after palate repair, but an increased incidence may continue, compared with unaffected children. Antibiotic prophylaxis should be prescribed readily for these infants and children; referral to the otolaryngologist member of the cleft palate team may be necessary for tympanostomy tubes or adenoidectomy. Careful audiological follow-up clearly is necessary.

Upper Airway Problems

Occasional apneic episodes have been described in children who have a cleft palate, especially in those who have the Pierre Robin malformation, which includes micrognathia and other craniofacial anomalies in addition to cleft lip and cleft palate.

Psychological Problems

Without question, the presence of such a visible defect adds to the challenges of child rearing and increases the stress experienced by the child and the parents. However, specific psychological disorders common to these children have not been found. It is most important that the primary physician, as well as others involved in the medical management, remain sensitive to the emotional needs of these children throughout the total process of rehabilitation. The stability of the family, available support, existing emotional problems and those arising from the condition, the possibility of the child being unwanted, and ethnic and cultural beliefs that might affect parental attitudes toward the baby should be explored. Economic status is important because children who have clefts require long-term medical care and rehabilitation, which is very expensive.

Because of our mobile society and changes in health care coverage, pediatricians may "inherit" children who have clefts at varying states of repair and rehabilitation. The practical matters of anatomical revisions must be addressed, as well as the psychosocial needs of older children and adolescents and peer and family relationships.

SURGICAL CORRECTION

A cleft lip usually is repaired in early infancy. Most surgeons prefer to wait until the child reaches a body weight of 10 to 12 pounds. In an otherwise healthy infant in whom no complications of general anesthesia are expected, the cleft lip is repaired at about 3 months of age, as an ambulatory procedure.

Speech development is of primary consideration in palate repair. The purpose of the operation is to close the palate anatomically and to minimize maxillary growth retardation accompanied by associated dental alveolar deformities. Eighteen months generally is accepted as the latest age for surgical repair of a cleft palate, because speech usually develops rapidly from that age on; 6 to 10 months of age is preferable. If the operation is delayed until 2 years of age or older, the child is more likely to have longstanding speech problems. Revisions of the primary procedure may be necessary by 5 or 6 years of age with further plastic surgery and rhinoplasty at 11 to 14 years.

LONG-TERM CARE: THE CLEFT LIP AND PALATE TEAM

Although the pediatrician must assume the responsibility for the child's overall health management and for parental counseling and guidance, immediate referral to an interdisciplinary cleft lip and cleft palate team is essential. There are at least 215 such groups in the United States today, varying in size from some 20 members in major academic centers to 3 in community-based programs; a plastic surgeon, a dentist or pedodontist, and a speech pathologist are the core members of the team. In addition, university-based teams often include an otolaryngologist, a geneticist, a psychologist, a public health nurse, a social worker, a vocational and rehabilitation counselor, an orthodontist, and a prosthodontist. A well-functioning team is cost effective in that it allows a comprehensive group of specialists to evaluate and manage a patient through a minimum of closely coordinated visits over time, thus limiting time lost from school by the patients and from work by the parents.

Clearly the specialization of team members mandates the pediatrician's coordinating effort. This need may continue for decades. Anatomical problems associated with clefts may emerge any time in a patient's life, and the rehabilitative process may be prolonged.

When to Refer

A call to the cleft lip/palate team should be made immediately after the cleft is noted.

REFERENCE

1. Clarren S, Anderson B, Wolf L: Feeding infants with cleft lip, cleft palate, or cleft lip and palate, *Cleft Palate J* 24:244, 1987.

SUGGESTED READINGS

The American Cleft Palate-Craniofacial Association: http//www.cleft.com.

Balasubrahmanyam G, Scherer NJ, Martin JA, Michal ML: Cleft lip and palate: keys to successful management, *Contemp Pediatr* 15:133, 1998.

Kaufman FL: Managing the cleft lip and palate patient, *Pediatr Clin North Am* 38:1127, 1991.

Moller KT, Starr CD, Johnson SA: *A parent's guide to cleft lip and palate*, Minneapolis, 1989, University of Minnesota Press.

Suslak L, Desposito F: Infants with cleft lip/cleft palate, *Pediatr Rev* 9:331, 1988.

197 Common Cold

Philip E. Thuma

Colds are viral infections of the upper respiratory tract, with involvement of the mucosal surfaces that are lined with respiratory epithelium. Thus, nasal passages, sinuses, eustachian tubes, middle ears, conjunctiva, and the nasopharynx potentially are affected with the symptoms of the common cold. The distribution of this illness is worldwide: adults and children of all ethnic and geographical groups may become afflicted. Colds are most common in children during the preschool years, who average three to eight colds per year, which is about half the number expected in adults. Those attending child care centers or exposed to other school-age children tend to have more colds than children spending most of their time at home.

Colds always have tended to occur more frequently during the cooler months in temperate climates, probably leading to the popular myth that exposure to cold weather leads to a cold. Fortunately the common cold has been researched extensively in the last 3 to four decades, allowing us to have a more scientific understanding of this age-old malady. In fact, in the northern hemisphere the incidence of colds peaks in early fall, followed by a peak in late January and another in early April. Studies have shown that exposure to a cold environment neither causes a cold nor decreases immunity that potentially may allow a viral infection to begin. It does appear clear, however, that colds are more frequent in crowded situations, and evidence suggests that the infection begins most commonly after self-inoculation of a virus onto one's own nasal or conjunctival mucosa.[11]

Because the viruses of infected individuals are shed in large numbers in nasal secretions, they can be spread easily by way of fingers and hands to objects such as clothing or environmental surfaces, where fingers of other children can acquire them and then self-inoculate their respiratory tracts by picking their noses or rubbing their eyes. Other epidemiological data suggest that colds and other respiratory tract infections may be more common in those exposed to passive tobacco smoke or other indoor air pollution. Studies in adult populations have shown that colds are more likely to develop after inoculation by rhinovirus in those who are under chronic stress; whether this is the case in children is not known.[3]

ETIOLOGY

More than 100 different infectious agents can cause cold symptoms, with rhinoviruses and small RNA viruses of the picornavirus family implicated most frequently. In addition to many rhinovirus serotypes, other viruses and a few nonviral organisms are associated with the common cold (Table 197-1). Although respiratory syncytial virus and parainfluenza viruses most commonly cause a croupy cough and bronchiolitis in infants, they may cause a cold in older children and adults. Adenoviruses and enteroviruses tend to cause other symptoms in addition to those of a common cold, including pharyngitis and gastrointestinal problems.

CLINICAL PRESENTATION

Once a cold-causing virus is introduced into the host's respiratory tract, assuming there is no immunity to that particular serotype, a local infection usually begins after an incubation period, the length of which depends on the specific virus. However, not all people who have a viral respiratory tract infection (defined as evidence of viral shedding and an increase in antibody titers) develop symptoms of a cold. In one study, only 75% of experimentally infected adults who shed rhinovirus type 2 and developed a greater than fourfold rise in antibody titers actually developed symptoms.[7] It has been shown that the symptoms of a cold are related primarily to the host's production of interleukin-8 and other vasoactive peptides in response to the viral infection,[17] resulting in increased vascular permeability and mucus hypersecretion.[19]

Younger infants may begin their illnesses with fever; an older child, however, is usually afebrile, with the earliest symptoms being a stuffy nose and watery nasal discharge, followed in a few days by sneezing. Generalized symptoms such as headache and malaise are uncommon with a rhinovirus infection, although they are seen in adenoviral and other viral infections. Infants tend to be irritable, have changes in feeding and sleep patterns, and sometimes develop mild diarrhea. By the third or fourth day of the illness, a dry cough may be present, and the nasal discharge usually becomes more purulent. Although such purulence has been interpreted in the past as indicating a secondary bacterial infection (such as sinusitis), little evidence is available to support that impression. Of adults who had colds and had sinus abnormalities on CT scan, only 2% developed bacterial sinusitis.[8] Furthermore, examination of purulent secretions has not shown increased aerobic bacterial growth or sloughing of nasal epithelial cells,[18] and biopsies in volunteers demonstrate only loss of cilia and ciliated cells.[15] Although viral sinusitis is a common finding during a cold, progression to bacterial sinusitis probably is quite rare in children.[14]

The symptoms of a cold generally last about a week, with

Table 197-1 Causative Agents of Colds

Agent	Relative Importance	Peak Season
Rhinovirus	++++	All seasons
Influenza virus	+++	Winter
Coronavirus	++	Winter
Respiratory syncytial virus	++	Winter
Parainfluenza virus	++	Autumn and spring
Enterovirus	+	All seasons
Mycoplasma pneumoniae	+	All seasons

From Welliver RC: The common cold. In Long SS, Pickering LK, Prober CG, editors: *Principles and practice of pediatric infectious diseases,* New York, 1997, Churchill Livingstone.
++++, most frequent cause; +++, frequent cause; ++, less frequent cause; +, occasional cause.

an occasional child having mild rhinorrhea and a dry cough for 2 to 3 weeks. The cilia necessary for proper function of the respiratory epithelium may take as many as 3 weeks to return to their normal state,[15] thus delaying the return to an absence of respiratory tract symptoms.

DIFFERENTIAL DIAGNOSIS

There are no routine confirmatory tests to diagnose the common cold. Viral cultures are expensive and generally unnecessary, so the diagnosis should be made on clinical grounds. The most common concern is that an underlying bacterial infection (such as a sinus or ear infection) is being missed or treated improperly. If a cold follows its expected course of causing usual symptoms for 5 to 7 days, a concurrent bacterial sinus or ear infection is unlikely. When the symptoms of a cold are prolonged, a secondary infection may be present, especially if fever persists or is prominent, or if ear pain or a productive cough develops. Thus, ear and lung examinations are essential for a child whose cold has persisted longer than expected. The routine use of radiographs or CT scans to diagnose sinusitis is not necessary, because when studied (albeit in older individuals) the radiological finding of opacification of the sinuses has not correlated with the clinical indications of sinusitis.[4]

Persistent nasal symptoms also can be caused by allergy. It is not uncommon for allergies to be diagnosed initially as colds and only later to be recognized as being seasonal or associated with nasal eosinophilia.[12] Cold symptoms associated with significant pharyngitis, rashes, or other systemic symptoms usually are caused by viruses other than those causing the common cold.

Occasionally a persistent purulent nasal discharge in children younger than 2 years of age results from beta-hemolytic streptococcal infection, although this usually is associated with mild excoriations around the nares. Unilateral nasal discharge also must be evaluated carefully to rule out a foreign body in the nose. Finally, irritation and swelling of the nasal passages from inhalation of drugs such as cocaine or the chronic use of medicated nasal sprays should be considered in the older child who has persistent cold symptoms.

MANAGEMENT

Although the various remedies available for the common cold take up a significant portion of any pharmacy's shelf space, all of them constitute symptomatic rather than curative treatment. In the pediatric population, most of the remedies give only marginal symptomatic relief, if any; in many cases, they are potentially harmful. Most pediatricians advise against using any of these cold remedies for infants and, at most, suggest saline nose drops with the use of a bulb syringe to aspirate secretions and a cool-mist vaporizer to humidify room air.[6] The malaise and fever sometimes associated with a cold can be treated with acetaminophen or ibuprofen; aspirin should be avoided because of its association with Reye syndrome. Some studies suggest that ibuprofen may be more beneficial during a cold than acetaminophen, because it leads to a shorter period of viral shedding and a better neutralizing antibody response.[7]

Studies conducted on preschoolers have not demonstrated a beneficial effect with decongestants, antihistamines, or their combinations that are readily available in multiple colors and flavors.[13,16] In older children and adolescents, an oral decongestant such as pseudoephedrine hydrochloride, either alone or with an antihistamine such as chlorpheniramine maleate, provides symptomatic relief with a low possibility of side effects. The use of nasal spray or drops containing vasoconstrictors such as oxymetazoline hydrochloride should be discouraged because of the high incidence of rebound nasal congestion after only a few days of use. Although recent studies in adults indicate some decrease in symptomatology when steroid or atropine-like nasal sprays are used, their use in children has not been evaluated and is not recommended.[9,14] The use of mast-cell stabilizers such as nedocromil and sodium cromoglycate given intranasally or by inhalation has shown some promise in adult studies. Their place in pediatric care is not clear, and they are not recommended currently.[1]

The use of zinc lozenges to reduce the duration of cold symptoms has been studied extensively in adults in recent years with conflicting results. Despite at least eight placebo-controlled trials and a number of reviews of these studies, the efficacy of zinc lozenges remains controversial. Studies of potential anti-rhinoviral drugs such as enviroxime[10] and pirodavir[9] are still too preliminary to gauge their therapeutic potential. Many parents will ask about the advisability of giving vitamin C during a cold, as well as request that the physician prescribe antibiotics. Neither has been proven efficacious, and both should be discouraged.[5] It is particularly important to discourage antibiotic use when bacterial infection is unlikely, given current evidence of increasing drug resistance among bacterial pathogens.

COMPLICATIONS

The vast majority of colds resolve without the help of the doctor or any medication. When a secondary fever occurs or symptoms continue longer than expected, a complication such as otitis media or pneumonia should be suspected. It appears that a cold can contribute to eustachian tube dysfunction, especially in younger children, resulting in an otitis media. A fever, headache, and unilateral purulent nasal discharge may herald a secondary bacterial sinusitis, although this is probably diagnosed much more frequently than it really occurs. On rare occasions a lower respiratory tract infection develops and can progress into pneumonia manifested by cough, tachypnea, and usually fever. It can be confirmed by chest radiograph.

The role of rhinovirus infection as a trigger for exacerbation of reactive airway disease now has been well documented;[2] thus, the development of wheezing or a prolonged cough after a cold should alert the clinician to that possibility.

REFERENCES

1. Aberg N, Aberg B, Alestig K: The effect of inhaled and intranasal sodium cromoglycate on symptoms of upper respiratory tract infections, *Clin Exp Allergy* 26:1045, 1996.
2. Busse WW: The role of the common cold in asthma, *J Clin Pharmacol* 39:241, 1999.
3. Cohen S, et al: Types of stressors that increase susceptibility to the common cold in healthy adults, *Health Psychol* 17:214, 1998.
4. Cooke LD, Hadley DM: MRI of the paranasal sinuses: incidental abnormalities and their relationship to symptoms, *J Laryngol Otol* 105:278, 1991.
5. Dowell SF, Schwartz B, Phillips WR: Appropriate use of antibiotics for URIs in children: part II, *Am Fam Physician* 58:1335, 1998.
6. Gadomski A, Horton L: The need for rational therapeutics in the use of cough and cold medicine in infants, *Pediatrics* 89:774, 1992.
7. Graham NM, et al: Adverse effects of aspirin, acetaminophen, and ibuprofen on immune function, viral shedding, and clinical status in rhinovirus-infected volunteers, *J Infect Dis* 162:1277, 1990.
8. Gwaltney JM Jr: Acute community acquired bacterial sinusitis: to treat or not to treat, *Can Respir J* 6:46A, 1999.
9. Hayden FG, et al: Intranasal pirodavir (R77,975) treatment of rhinovirus colds, *Antimicrob Agents Chemother* 39:290, 1995.
10. Heinz BA, Vance LM: The antiviral compound enviroxime targets the 3A coding region of rhinovirus and poliovirus, *J Virol* 69:4189, 1995.
11. Hendley JO, Wenzel RP, Gwaltney JM: Transmission of rhinovirus colds by self-inoculation, *N Engl J Med* 288:1361, 1973.
12. Huang SW, Kimbrough JW: Mold allergy is a risk factor for persistent cold-like symptoms in children, *Clin Pediatr* 36:695, 1997.
13. Hutton N, et al: Effectiveness of an antihistamine-decongestant combination for young children with the common cold: a randomized, controlled clinical trial, *J Pediatr* 118:125, 1991.
14. Puhakka T, et al: Sinusitis in the common cold, *J Allergy Clin Immunol* 102:403, 1998.
15. Rautiainen M, et al: Ultrastructural changes in human nasal cilia caused by the common cold and recovery of ciliated epithelium, *Ann Otol Rhinol Laryngol* 101:982, 1992.
16. Smith MB, Feldman W: Over-the-counter cold medications: a critical review of clinical trials between 1950 and 1991, *JAMA* 269:2258, 1993.
17. Turner RB, et al: Association between interleukin-8 concentration in nasal secretions and severity of symptoms of experimental rhinovirus colds, *Clin Infect Dis* 26:840, 1998.
18. Winther B, Kawana R, Saito H: Fireside conference 11: common cold, *Rhinol Suppl* 14:228, 1992.
19. Yuta A, et al: Rhinovirus infection induces mucus hypersecretion, *Am J Physiol* 274:L1017, 1998.

SUGGESTED READINGS

Hilding DA: Literature review: the common cold, *Ear Nose Throat J* 73:639, 1994.

Mossad SB: Treatment of the common cold, *BMJ* 317:33, 1998.

Turner RB: The common cold, *Pediatr Ann* 27:790, 1998.

198 Congenital Heart Disease

Alan M. Mendelsohn • Roger P. Vermilion • Lucian A. Durham III

Defects of the cardiovascular system are among the most common congenital lesions, with an incidence of 8 to 12 per 1000 live births.[22] Such defects are of an even higher incidence in the premature and stillborn infant. The fetal heart develops between weeks 3 and 8 of gestation. Incomplete septal formation leads to the varieties of atrial septal defects (ASDs) and ventricular septal defects (VSDs). Abnormalities in septation of the primitive bulbus cordis lead to truncus arteriosus and other anomalies. Of the six branchial aortic arches, only the left fourth and sixth remain. They become the aortic arch and ductus arteriosus, respectively. Remnants of the remaining branchial arches lead to vascular ring malformations.

Elevated vascular resistance and little pulmonary blood flow characterize the fetal circulation. Most of the blood entering the right atrium is shunted to the left atrium via the foramen ovale; blood reaching the pulmonary artery is shunted into the aorta via the ductus arteriosus. With expansion of the lungs and decreased pulmonary vascular resistance, the flap valve of the foramen ovale is closed (as left atrial [LA] pressure exceeds right atrial [RA] pressure); and then, within the first few days of life, the ductus closes. The most common congenital heart lesions and their incidences are outlined in Table 198-1.

ETIOLOGY

The etiology of congenital heart defects is incompletely understood. Causes are multiple, including multifactorial genetic and environmental interactions, in as many as 90% of patients who have these lesions. Significant chromosomal abnormalities occur in approximately 5% of patients who have congenital heart disease (e.g., trisomy 21, trisomy 18). Many single-mutant gene syndromes (both autosomal recessive and autosomal dominant) can have cardiovascular manifestations as a feature that has incomplete penetrance (Tables 198-2 and 198-3). For the majority of lesions, recurrence risk given one sibling who has a cardiovascular abnormality is 1% to 4%. If two siblings have similar congenital anomalies, the chance of a third sibling having a comparable lesion increases markedly to 25% to 50%. In cases of parental congenital heart disease (particularly maternal lesions), the incidence in the fetus may rise to 4 to 18 times the incidence in the general population. Paternal congenital cardiovascular disease raises risk only minimally (1.5 to 3 times). Except for the 45X Turner syndrome and the XXXY syndrome, the most common congenital heart lesions in the general population are also the most common ones seen in patients who have various chromosomal syndromes (Table 198-4). Other factors that influence the occurrence of congenital heart lesions are maternal infections, diabetes mellitus, systemic lupus erythematosus, and drug use during the pregnancy (Table 198-5).

LEFT-TO-RIGHT SHUNTS

Intra- and extracardiac flow from the systemic circulation to the pulmonary circulation is described as a left-to-right shunt. From a physiological standpoint, this allows oxygenated blood to recirculate through the pulmonary circulation without first entering the peripheral arterial circulation.

Four important and interrelated physiological factors influence the volume of blood shunting from left to right in the postnatal period and thus affect symptomatology significantly. These include the absolute diameter of the defect, the location of the defect within the cardiovascular system, the differences in pressures between the two "connected" chambers or vessels, and the portion of the cardiac cycle in which the majority of shunting occurs.

Physiological Correlates

Defect size. The absolute diameter of a VSD, for example, determines the physiological state of the patient's defect. For patients who have small to medium defects, the defect size itself may offer sufficient resistance to limit the magnitude of the left-to-right shunt; however, with large defects, there is almost no resistance to flow.

Pressure differences. For example, the child who has a VSD—in the early neonatal period when the child may have elevated pulmonary vascular resistance—flow is limited from the left ventricle to the right ventricle. As pulmonary vascular resistance falls with lung expansion and improved oxygenation occurs with pulmonary vasodilation following oxygen therapy, increasing flow across the defect may occur. In cases such as these, the classic "VSD murmur" may not be heard until a specific pressure gradient between the peripheral and pulmonary vascular beds occurs.

Cardiac cycle/location of defect. Some cardiac lesions that have left-to-right shunts may cause significant pulmonary overcirculation more rapidly than other lesions of similar diameter, mainly because of the portion of the cardiac cycle in which the shunt occurs. For example, in the case of

VSDs, the majority of the left-to-right shunt is ejected directly from the left ventricle through the VSD into the right ventricle, pulmonary valve, and pulmonary artery during systole. Because the excessive blood volume is ejected directly into the pulmonary vascular bed, patients tend to experience pulmonary vascular overcirculation and subsequent symptoms of congestive heart failure rapidly. Similarly, patients who have a large patent ductus arteriosus (PDA [a direct connection between the aorta and the pulmonary artery]) will tend to manifest symptoms of pulmonary overcirculation and congestive heart failure rapidly. On the other hand, patients who have large atrial septal defects may not be as likely to experience symptoms of pulmonary overcirculation. In these patients, the left-to-right shunt occurs predominantly during diastole and may lead to right atrial and right ventricular dilation (from volume overload) rather than to pulmonary overcirculation.

Table 198-1 Incidence* of Congenital Heart Disease

Lesion	Incidence†
Ventricular septal defect	30-50
Patent ductus arteriosus‡	10
Atrial septal defect (secundum)	7
Endocardial cushion defects	3
Coarctation of aorta	6
Aortic stenosis	5
Pulmonic stenosis	7
Tetralogy of fallot	5
Transposition of great arteries	5
Pulmonary atresia	1-2
Tricuspid atresia	1-2
Truncus arteriosus	1
Total anomalous pulmonary venous connection	1
Aortic atresia	1

Modified from Hoffman JIE: Congenital heart diseases. In Rudolph AM, Hoffman JIE, editors: *Pediatrics,* ed 18, Norwalk, Connecticut, 1987, Appleton & Lange.
*Does not include bicuspid aortic valves, which occur in about 2% to 3% of live-born children.
†Incidence per 100 children who have congenital heart disease.
‡Does not include preterm infants.

Ventricular Septal Defect

Deficiencies in formation of the ventricular septum occur in 30% to 50% of patients who have congenital heart lesions, making them the most common defect. Embryologically, septae of the heart develop between the twenty-seventh and thirty-seventh day of gestation by fusion of actively growing tissue within the lumen of the primitive cardiac tube. Continued growth of connective tissue upward from the ventricular apex forms the "muscular" septum; downward growth from the division of the conus and truncus arteriosus forms the "outlet" portion of the septum; and protuberances of the endocardial cushions form the atrioventricular canal, destined to be mitral and tricuspid valves, form the "inlet" portion of the septum. As a separate event, a new component of the ventricular septum (i.e., the perimembranous region) forms to unify at the meeting point of the other three components of the ventricular septum into an impervious structure. Errors in any one of these four elements may lead to developmental defects, which may explain the comparatively high incidence of congenital VSDs compared with other cardiac lesions.

Table 198-2 Autosomal Dominant Syndromes with Associated Cardiovascular Abnormalities

Syndrome	Abnormality
Apert's	VSD, TF
Crouzon	PDA, CA
Ehlers-Danlos	Rupture of large blood vessels (e.g., carotids, dissecting aneurysm of the aorta)
Familial periodic paralysis	Hypokalemia, supraventricular tachycardia
Forney	MI
Holt-Oram	ASD, VSD
Idiopathic hypertrophic subaortic stenosis (IHSS)	Subaortic muscular hypertrophy
Leopard	PS, prolonged P-R interval, abnormal p waves
Lymphedema (Milroy and Meige)	Lymphedema
Marfan	Great artery aneurysms, AI, MI
Myotonic-dystrophy (Steinert)	Myocardiopathy
Neurofibromatosis	PS, pheochromocytoma with hypertension, CA
Noonan	PS, ASD, IHSS
Osler-Weber-Rendu	Multiple telangiectasias, pulmonary arteriovenous fistulas
Osteogenesis imperfecta	AI
Romano-Ward	Prolonged Q-T, sudden death
Treacher Collins	VSD, PDA, ASD
Tuberous sclerosis	Myocardial rhabdomyoma
Von Hippel-Lindau	Hemangiomas, pheochromocytoma with hypertension

Modified from Nora JJ: Etiologic aspects of heart diseases. In Adams FH, Emmanouilides GC, Riemenschneider TA, editors: *Moss' heart disease in infants, children, and adolescents,* ed 4, Baltimore, 1989, Williams & Wilkins.
AI, Aortic insufficiency, *ASD,* atrial septal defect; *CA,* coarctation of the aorta; *IHSS,* idiopathic hypertrophic subaortic stenosis; *MI,* mitral insufficiency; *PDA,* patent ductus arteriosus; *PS,* pulmonary stenosis; *TF,* tetralogy of Fallot; *VSD,* ventricular septal defect.

Table 198-3 Autosomal Recessive Syndromes with Associated Cardiovascular Abnormalities

Syndrome	Abnormality
Adrenogenital (21 and 3)	Hyperkalemia, broad QRS, arrhythmias
Alkaptonuria	Atherosclerosis, valve disease
Carpenter's	PDA
Cockayne's	Accelerated atherosclerosis
Conradi's	VSD, PDA
Cutis laxa	Pulmonary hypertension, peripheral pulmonary artery stenosis
Cystic fibrosis	Cor pulmonale
Ellis-van Creveld	ASD, most commonly single atrium, and other CHD
Friedreich ataxia	Myocardiopathy
Glycogenosis IIa, IIIa, and IV	Myocardiopathy
Homocystinuria	Coronary and other vascular thromboses
Jervell-Lange-Nielsen	Prolonged Q-T, sudden death
Laurence-Moon-Biedl	VSD and other CHD
Mucolipidosis III	Aortic valve disease
Mucopolysaccharidosis (MPS) I-H (Hurler's)	Coronary artery disease, AI and MI
MPS I-S (Scheie's), MPS IV (Morquio's), MPS VI (Maroteaux-Larry)	Aortic valve disease, coronary artery disease
Osteogenesis imperfecta	Aortic valve disease
Progeria	Accelerated atherosclerosis
Pseudo-xanthoma elasticum	Coronary insufficiency, MI, hypertension
Refsum's	Atrioventricular (AV) conduction defects
Riley-Day	Episodic hypertension, postural hypotension
Seckel's	VSD, PDA
Sickle cell disease	Myocardiopathy, MI
Smith-Lemli-Opitz	VSD, PDA, and other CHD
Thalassemia major	Myocardiopathy
Thrombocytopenia and absent radius (TAR)	ASD, TF, dextrocardia
Weill-Marchesani	PDA
Werner's	Vascular sclerosis

Modified from Nora JJ: Etiologic aspects of heart diseases. In Adams FH, Emmanouilides GC, Riemenschneider TA, editors: *Moss' heart disease in infants, children, and adolescents,* ed 4, Baltimore, 1989, Williams & Wilkins.
AI, Aortic insufficiency; *ASD,* atrial septal defect; *CHD,* congenital heart disease; *MI,* mitral insufficiency; *PDA,* patent ductus arteriosus; *TF,* tetralogy of Fallot; *VSD,* ventricular septal defect.

Table 198-4 Congenital Heart Disease in Selected Chromosomal Aberrations

		Most Common Lesions		
Population Studied	Incidence of CHD (%)	1	2	3
General Population	1	VSD	PDA	ASD
4p–	40	VSD	ASD	PDA
5p– (cri du chat)	25	VSD	PDA	ASD
C group anomalies	25-50	VSD	PDA	
13 trisomy	90	VSD	PDA	Dext
13q–	50	VSD		
18 trisomy	99+	VSD	PDA	PS
18q–	50	VSD		
21 trisomy	50	ECD	VSD	ASD
45,X Turner	35	CA	AS	ASD
XXXXY	14	PDA	ASD	

Modified from Nora JJ: Etiologic aspects of heart diseases. In Adams FH, Emmanouilides GC, Riemenschneider TA, editors: *Moss' heart disease in infants, children, and adolescents,* ed 4, Baltimore, 1989, Williams & Wilkins.
AS, Aortic stenosis; *ASD,* atrial septal defect; *CA,* coarctation of aorta; *CHD,* congenital heart disease; *Dext,* dextroversion; *ECD,* endocardial cushion defect; *PDA,* patent ductus arteriosus; *PS,* pulmonary stenosis; *VSD,* ventricular septal defect.

Table 198-5 Selection of Potential Cardiovascular Teratogens

Potential Teratogens	Frequency of Cardiovascular Disease (%)	Most Common Malformations
Drugs		
Alcohol	25-30	VSD, PDA, ASD
Amphetamines	?5	VSD, PDA, ASD, TGA
Anticonvulsants		
Hydantoin	2-3	PS, AS, CA, PDA
Trimethadione	15-30	TGA, TF, HLHS
Chemotherapy	?5	PS, AS, VSD, ASD
Lithium	10	Ebstein, TA, ASD
Sex hormones	2-4	VSD, TGA, TF
Thalidomide	5-10	TF, VSD, ASD, truncus arteriosus
Retinoic acid	10	VSD
Infections		
Rubella	35	Peripheral pulmonary artery stenosis, PDA, VSD, ASD
Maternal conditions		
Diabetes	3-5	TGA, VSD, CA
	30-50	Cardiomegaly and cardiomyopathy
Lupus	40	Heart block
Phenylketonuria	10	TF, VSD, ASD

Modified from Nora JJ: Etiologic aspects of heart diseases. In Adams FH, Emmanouilides GC, Riemenschneider TA, editors: *Moss' heart disease in infants, children, and adolescents,* ed 4, Baltimore, 1989, Williams & Wilkins.

AS, Aortic stenosis; *ASD,* atrial septal defect; *CA,* coarctation of aorta; *HLHS,* hypoplastic left heart syndrome; *PDA,* patent ductus arteriosus; *PS,* pulmonary stenosis; *TA,* tricuspid atresia; *TF,* tetralogy of Fallot; *TGA,* transposition of the great arteries; *VSD,* ventricular septal defect.

Four different types of VSDs are important to identify to assess (1) the need for intervention better, (2) the possibility of spontaneous closure, and (3) the frequency of follow-up evaluations. The most common VSD (75% to 80%) occurs in the perimembranous region, which lies in the outflow tract of the left ventricle immediately beneath the aortic valve (Fig. 198-1). Physiological closure of this portion of the ventricular septum requires involution from the endocardial cushions, downgrowth from the conus, and ingrowth from the muscular septum. The defect may extend into the inlet, muscular, or even outlet portion of the ventricular septum. Many defects have associated minor abnormalities of the tricuspid valve, which may either be intrinsic or acquired, secondary to the intracardiac shunt. It is this abnormality of the tricuspid valve that aids in eventual postnatal spontaneous closure of these defects in many patients. A "windsock" of tissue grows to occlude the defect in an aneurysmal fashion, with 75% to 90% of small perimembranous VSDs undergoing spontaneous closure or diminution in size within the first 2 years of life. Surgical closure is indicated for perimembranous VSD patients who become symptomatic or have a defect that fails to regress spontaneously. The conduction system courses along the posterior-superior border of the defect and is at risk during repair.

Muscular VSDs are the second most common type (approximately 20% [see Fig. 198-1]). They can occur in any segment of the muscular ventricular septum from the anterior portion to the mid-muscular septum or the apex of the ventricle. Because these defects tend to be completely surrounded by muscle (except for the large apical defect or multiple "Swiss cheese" types), the defects tend to "open" and "close" with each cardiac cycle as the ventricular septum itself contracts in systole. It is this contraction of the septum that presumably leads to a high incidence (90% to 95%) of complete spontaneous closure of small muscular VSDs within the first 6 to 12 months of life. Small thrombi are trapped within the interstices of the muscular ventricular septum and the defect itself, leading to endothelialization of the defect and complete closure.

The management of patients who have multiple VSDs remains controversial. Primary closure, interventional catheter techniques, and palliative surgery all may have a role. Despite advances in diagnosis and surgical treatment, morbidity and mortality remain high. For all VSDs, banding of the pulmonary artery to protect the pulmonary vascular bed and relieve symptoms of congestive failure traditionally have been employed in an effort to delay definitive repair. This procedure may allow time for, or even promote, spontaneous closure, or possibly increase the likelihood of a successful surgical outcome. The location of the defects, symptoms, and presence of associated cardiovascular conditions influence the timing of corrective surgery. Associated major cardiac lesions and the complexity of the underlying malformation are significant factors in mortality associated with complete repair of muscular VSDs.

Inlet VSDs are referred to more commonly as *VSDs of the atrioventricular (AV) canal.* Anatomically, they are found posterior and inferior to the membranous defect and lie beneath the septal cusp of the tricuspid valve and septal papillary muscle. Approximately 5% of VSDs are of this type. Unlike muscular or perimembranous VSDs, spontaneous closure of these defects is exceedingly rare; thus, many patients who have even small to moderate defects may eventually require surgical repair. Large, nonrestrictive inlet VSDs that have shunts greater than 2:1 and/or congestive heart failure (CHF) will require earlier intervention to prevent early onset of pulmonary arteriolar disease secondary to pulmonary hypertension.

Outlet VSDs occur in all population groups but have a higher incidence in patients originally from the Pacific Rim

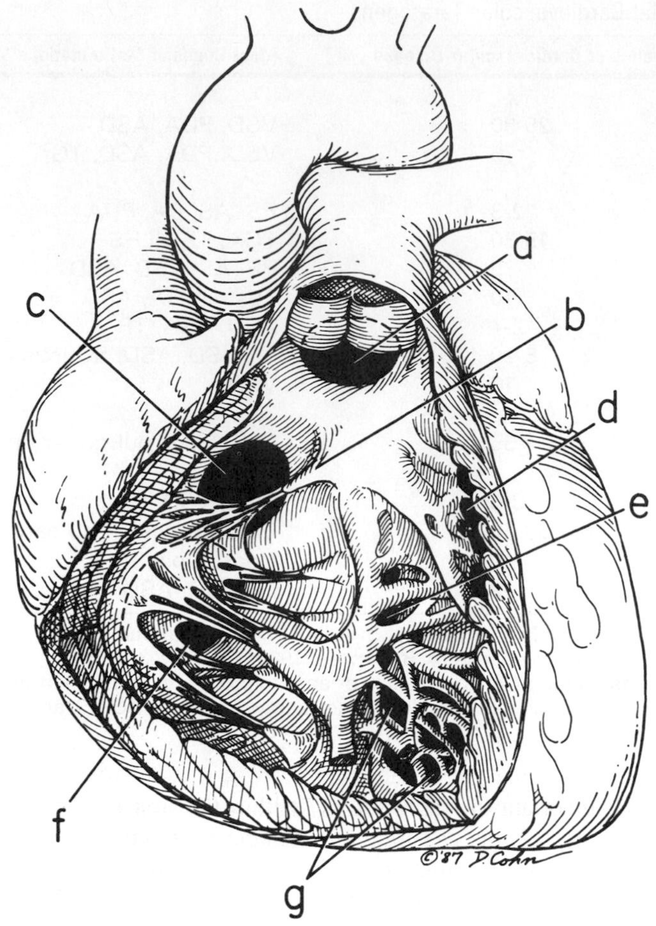

Fig. 198-1 Schematic drawing of locations of ventricular septal defects. *a,* Outlet defect; *b,* papillary muscle; *c,* perimembranous defect; *d,* muscular defect; *e,* muscular defect; *f,* inlet defect; *g,* apical muscular defect.

(From Graham TP, Bender HW, Spach MS: Ventricular septal defect. In Adams FH, Emmanouilides GC, Riemenschneider TA: *Moss' heart disease in infants, children and adolescents,* ed 4, Baltimore, 1989, Williams & Wilkins.)

(i.e., Japan, Korea, and Asia). Also referred to as *infundibular* or *supracristal VSDs,* these defects are located anterior to the crista supraventricularis, just beneath the pulmonary valve in the right ventricular outflow tract (RVOT) and away from the conduction system. In many cases, these defects extend into the perimembranous region. Early identification of these defects is important because of associated aortic valve prolapse and aortic insufficiency if the defect is located in close proximity to the aortic valve. These defects also tend to have low rates of spontaneous closure. Unlike the other types of VSDs, early surgical intervention may be indicated in cases in which aortic valve prolapse has occurred, even if the septal defect is small and of little hemodynamic consequence.

Clinical presentation. In patients who have small VSDs regardless of location, few symptoms are identified. In this group of patients, onset of a new murmur may be the only sign of any cardiac abnormality. Patients tend to have normal growth and development and otherwise normal physical examinations. Patients who have moderate to large VSDs may present both with new onset of a murmur and the primary signs and symptoms of CHF (i.e., poor weight gain, tachypnea, and tachycardia) caused primarily by pulmonary overcirculation. In some neonates or infants, no symptoms of pulmonary overcirculation are identified; poor weight gain or development may be the sole manifestation of small VSDs.

Physical examination. In the majority of neonates and children who have small ventricular level shunts, adequate growth and development are noted, and there are no significant vital sign abnormalities. The pulmonary examination usually reveals no rales or rhonchi. The heart sounds are normal, with normal splitting of the first and second sounds. In most children who have small defects, I-III/VI systolic regurgitant murmurs are heard on auscultation. In many, the murmur is well localized to the region of the defect (left lower sternal border for muscular or inlet defects, mid to upper sternal borders for perimembranous defects). The murmurs tend to be of mid to high frequency, reflecting the significant difference in pressures between the left and right ventricles. Patients who have small defects tend not to have the classic "diastolic rumble" evident in patients who have large defects, in whom increased left atrial filling yields a relative "mitral stenosis" murmur on physical examination. Paradoxically, children who have small septal defects may have loud IV-V/VI harsh systolic regurgitant murmurs. This depends on the location of the defect within the ventricular septum. Muscular or perimembranous defects that are parallel in the ventricular septum to the chest wall may yield a thrill as the high-resistance, low-flow jet strikes the anterior wall of the right ventricle, transmitting the energy of the jet to the chest wall. Such loud systolic murmurs in a child who has a small VSD can be differentiated from similar murmurs in the child who has a large VSD by the:

1. Lack of symptomatology in the child who has a small defect
2. Absence of a diastolic component in the patient who has the small defect
3. Absence of pulmonary hypertensive changes on physical examination (normal frequency and splitting of the second heart sound)
4. Absence of a gallop rhythm or rumble (i.e., S_3 or S_4)
5. Differences in murmur frequency. Because small VSDs tend to be restrictive to interventricular flow (manifesting a higher-resistance circuit between the high-pressure left ventricle and lower-pressure right ventricle), murmurs from smaller VSDs tend to be of higher frequency than those of larger defects.

Children who have hemodynamically significant VSDs tend to be smaller and more ill appearing secondary to CHF. Mild decreases in cardiac output, identified by thready pulses and prolonged capillary refill time, also may be noted. Respiratory discomfort presents with tachypnea and suprasternal retractions.

Infrequently, rales secondary to pulmonary edema may be auscultated. Patients also tend to be tachycardic for age but usually maintain normal blood pressures. Palpation of the precordium reveals hyperdynamic activity. Depending on the physiological status, such patients may have increases in their first and second heart sounds and/or a gallop rhythm. These children tend to have loud systolic regurgitant murmurs of mid to low frequency. Murmur frequency and intensity depend on equalization of pressures within the two ventricles. A "mid diastolic rumble" may occur secondary to increased filling of the left atrium and relative mitral stenosis (increased blood flow across a fixed mitral orifice).

Electrocardiogram. In patients who have small, hemodynamically insignificant VSDs, the electrocardiogram (ECG) tends to remain normal. Some patients demonstrate an RSR′ in lead V_1, indicating mild right ventricular volume overload. In some children who have inlet VSDs, a leftward and superior QRS axis (0 degrees to -90 degrees) may be identified, similar to that seen in children who have complete AV canal defects.

In patients whose defects are of moderate size, the ECG may still be normal, although in some patients who have elevated right ventricular pressures, right ventricular hypertrophy (particularly in leads V_{4R} or V_1) may be identified. These patients concomitantly have evidence of mild left atrial and left ventricular hypertrophy by voltage criteria. In patients who have large defects and normal pulmonary artery resistances, further increases in ventricular and atrial voltages may be seen. Once symptoms of fixed pulmonary hypertension are noted, the ECG may normalize (reduction in left ventricular and left atrial voltages) and/or switch to more prominent right ventricular voltages. Following either spontaneous or surgical closure of the VSD, many of the ECG changes may take months to years to resolve fully, even if the ventricular level shunt is obliterated.

Chest radiograph. Chest radiography in children who have VSDs may help define cardiac size and pulmonary vascular changes. Findings will vary depending on the physiological impact of the left-to-right shunt. In the majority of children who have small, hemodynamically insignificant defects, chest radiography will demonstrate a normal cardiac silhouette and normal pulmonary vascular markings. With increasing left-to-right shunting across the defect, increases in atrial and ventricular dimensions and increases in pulmonary vascular markings usually occur. As with the ECG, increases in pulmonary vascular resistance resulting in pulmonary hypertension may cause the chest radiograph to normalize. Additionally, as with the ECG, even in the acute postoperative or post-spontaneous-closure period, significant changes in cardiac silhouette may not resolve until remodeling of the atrial and ventricular muscle occurs.

Echocardiogram. Although not imperative for diagnosing a VSD, acquisition of two-dimensional echocardiographic images and Doppler flow studies can be helpful. In some neonates who have non-"classic" systolic regurgitant murmurs, the diagnosis may be difficult to make if based solely on physical examination, chest radiograph, and ECG. Second, localization of the defect may assist the physician in discussions with parents concerning the need for surgical closure versus observation. Third, the echocardiogram allows definition of subclinical abnormalities associated with VSDs (atrioventricular or semilunar valvar insufficiency, aortic valve prolapse, and formation of ventricular aneurysms from the tricuspid valve pouch).

Standard two-dimensional echocardiographic images and Doppler studies readily identify both the location, number (single versus multiple defects), and dimensions of the lesion; determine chamber sizes and cardiac function; define gradients and pressures across the ventricular septum; and determine the presence and degree of pulmonary hypertension.

Cardiac catheterization. Given the significant advances in two-dimensional echocardiography and magnetic resonance imaging (MRI), there usually is little need for angiographic definition of VSDs. The indications for cardiac catheterization are to determine the size of the physiological shunt, give additional definition of contiguous structures (i.e., aorta, pulmonary artery), or reveal the presence of multiple defects that may not be visualized completely by other imaging modalities. Physiological studies directly measure right ventricular and pulmonary artery pressures and, in cases of pulmonary hypertension, define the reactivity of the pulmonary vascular bed to vasodilator agents (i.e., oxygen, nitric oxide). Such studies also may suggest, in cases of large defects requiring surgery, whether significant postoperative complications can be anticipated.

Treatment. For patients who have small to moderate defects, the natural history studies of the 1970s and 1990s have demonstrated that many will close within the first 2 years of life.[27,57] In cases in which the defect does not close completely, the shunt may remain small and the patient asymptomatic. Follow-up is indicated routinely to detect continuing spontaneous closure and to reinforce the importance of prophylactic antibiotics to prevent endocarditis.

In most centers, treatment of VSDs is limited to those patients who have hemodynamically significant left-to-right shunts. Diuretic agents (i.e., furosemide and thiazide agents) are the initial treatment of choice in the face of pulmonary overcirculation by clinical history, physical examination, or imaging studies. Evidence is growing that inotropic support with digoxin is of little utility because the major symptomatology is related to pulmonary edema and not to ventricular systolic dysfunction.[28] Second-line agents may include afterload reduction with angiotensin-converting enzyme (ACE) inhibitors such as captopril.

When medical management has been exhausted with little improvement in symptomatology or somatic growth, surgical intervention is indicated. DuShane et al[9] showed that development of irreversible pulmonary vascular obstructive disease did not occur in patients who have moderate to large defects operated on when younger than 2 years of age, but occurred in 14 of 50 patients whose operation was performed later. Some recent data suggest that surgical closure of large VSDs within the first year of life may be associated with better long-term left ventricular function and regression of ventricular and atrial hypertrophy compared with surgical repair performed later.[8] Standard surgery utilizing cardiopulmonary bypass and patch closure of the VSD is highly effective in shunt obliteration, with success rates approaching 99% and significant morbidity and mortality of less than 5%. Postoperative complications include arrhythmias, particularly right bundle branch block or AV block; small residual VSDs or patch leaks; and progressive pulmonary hypertension.

Atrial Septal Defects

Atrial septation begins within the embryological common atrium within the first 5 weeks of gestation, with growth and proliferation of the septum primum and formation of the septum secundum. The point at which the two septae coapt forms the patent foramen ovale crucial for interatrial flow during the fetal period. Soon after birth, with the neonate's first breath and increases in pulmonary flow and left atrial filling, the flap valve of the septum secundum fuses with the septum primum, and anatomical closure of the interatrial communication occurs. When malalignment of the two septa or incomplete formation of the septum secundum occurs, atrial septal defects (ASDs) may form. They constitute 7% to 10% of all congenital heart lesions.

Similar to VSDs, there are four types of ASDs defined by location within the atrial septum. Ostium primum and ostium secundum ASDs are by far the most common, constituting 75% to 80% of atrial lesions.

AV canal defects constitute 20% of interatrial communications. AV canal defects represent various anomalies that may occur either as isolated lesions or as components of more complex cardiac lesions in conditions such as Down syndrome. Such defects are not defects of fusion of the two embryological septae but rather are defects in the endocardial cushion.

Defects in formation of the embryological sinus venosus (precursor of the superior vena cava and the atrial wall) or the coronary sinus may lead to ASDs as well, together accounting for 5% of cases. Sinus venosus defects often are associated with partial anomalous pulmonary venous return, particularly of the right upper pulmonary veins.

Clinical presentation. The majority of patients who have ASDs present with a heart murmur, with or without a history of pulmonary disease. Early signs and symptoms of excessive pulmonary blood flow are rare in patients who have ASDs. This is because the flow of blood across the ASD occurs both in atrial systole and diastole. The right ventricle thus has sufficient time within the cardiac cycle to accept the abnormal flow of blood from the left to the right atrium, which leads to progressive right atrial and right ventricular dilation. However, this also allows for near normal pulmonary artery pressures, even in patients who have moderate to large ASDs, so that symptoms may be few. When present, however, symptoms tend to be nondescript but do involve some changes in pulmonary function. In patients who have "recurrent asthma" only mildly responsive to standard medical therapy or multiple upper respiratory infections and/or pneumonias, suspicion of an interatrial communication should be raised. In adolescents and young adults, the initial manifesting symptoms may be a history of palpitations, sensed extra beats, or "chest pain."

Physical examination. The tell-tale signs on physical examination of an ASD are abnormalities of the second heart sound. In many patients, there is widening and fixed splitting of the second heart sound. Fixed splitting of the second heart sound also can occur in patients who have complete right bundle branch block. Most patients will have a II-III/VI systolic flow murmur heard best along the left upper sternal border. Interestingly, this murmur is not from blood rushing through the ASD but rather from increased flow across the pulmonary valve. In severe right ventricular volume overload, a right ventricular heave may be palpated. There appears to be no diminution in pulses or capillary refill, and the remainder of the examination tends to be within normal limits. However, in many patients who have ASDs, no significant abnormalities, except for the systolic flow murmur, may be noted on physical examination.

Electrocardiogram. Classically, patients who have significant ASDs will have right atrial and right ventricular abnormalities. The patients may meet voltage criteria for a volume-overloaded right ventricle with an RSR′ pattern (the R′ larger than the R) in leads V_1, V_2, and V_{3R}. Patients also may have mild to moderate right QRS axis deviation for age (95 to 170 degrees). Other abnormalities include mild first-degree AV block (PR interval 160 to 200 msec) secondary to right atrial dilation and lengthening of the conduction time from the sinoatrial (SA) node to the AV node.

Chest radiograph. In the majority of patients who have hemodynamically significant ASDs, there is moderate cardiomegaly (particularly the right atrium and ventricle) and a mild increase in pulmonary vascular markings. Some patients, however, may have a normal cardiac silhouette and pulmonary vascularity, even in the face of a hemodynamically significant shunt.

Echocardiography. When physical examination, history, or other noninvasive studies suggest the diagnosis of ASD, echocardiography is extremely valuable in determining the location and size of the ASD and associated anomalies of the pulmonary veins, as well as a general evaluation of cardiac function and anatomy. Classically, there is evidence of right atrial and right ventricular dilation with normal or minimally elevated right ventricular and pulmonary artery pressures. Echocardiography also can differentiate between a true ostium secundum ASD (i.e., absence of a component of the septum primum) and a patent foramen ovale with a residual flap valve and small leak between the collapsed portions of the septum primum and secundum. The majority of patients will demonstrate left-to-right shunting by color flow Doppler.

Cardiac catheterization. There is little role for diagnostic cardiac catheterization or angiography for the patient who has an uncomplicated ASD. Adequate information for decision-making can be gained through the noninvasive studies already discussed.

Treatment. For the asymptomatic patient who has a large ASD, elective surgery is usually performed after the age of 4 or 5 years. There is no significant disadvantage to waiting until that age to allow for possible spontaneous closure.[1] The symptomatic infant or small child who evidences CHF or pulmonary hypertension can undergo surgical repair sooner. Repair of the ASD (the first congenital intracardiac lesion ever repaired [1953]) involves cardiopulmonary bypass and either direct suture closure of the defect or patch repair with synthetic material (e.g., Dacron, Gore-Tex) or autologous pericardium. Complications may include atrial dysrhythmias, residual septal leaks, and postpericardiotomy syndrome (fever, pericardial effusion, and respiratory distress 1 to 4 weeks following surgical repair). Over the past 30 years, interventional cardiologists have shown that small, uncomplicated central ostium secundum defects can be closed via the transcatheter route.[34]

Typically, patients who have smaller, nonrepaired ASDs remain active and asymptomatic or may only have symptoms of pulmonary hypertension or dysrhythmias in late adulthood. Pulmonary hypertension occurs in only a small proportion of older adult patients, although there have been anecdotal reports of significant, irreversible pulmonary hypertension in patients younger than 12 years of age.

ENDOCARDIAL CUSHION DEFECTS

Embryologically, abnormalities of the endocardial cushion can cause defects of the atrial septum, the ventricular septum, or combined atrial and ventricular lesions (AVSD), with concomitant abnormalities of the atrioventricular valves. This type of lesion often is seen in children who have Down syndrome, who have an increased incidence of atrioventricular defects over the general population.

Ostium Primum Defects

Clinical presentation. The majority of patients who have ostium primum defects will have clinical histories similar to those of patients who have ostium secundum defects. There is no significant difference in physical examination or chest radiography in such patients except for those patients who have ostium primum defects and associated abnormalities of the mitral valve.

Physical examination. In many patients, significant mitral insufficiency (caused by a cleft of the anterior mitral valve leaflet) may lead to symptoms of CHF and may produce the dominant murmur on physical examination—a regurgitant murmur at the apex of the heart consistent with mitral insufficiency. Abnormalities of the second heart sound and a nonspecific systolic ejection murmur similar to that of an ostium secundum defect may lead the examiner to the diagnosis.

Electrocardiography. On ECG, patients who have ostium primum defects may be differentiated from those who have other ASDs by the presence of a leftward and superior QRS axis (between 0 degrees and -90 degrees). However, as with other ASDs, right atrial and right ventricular dilation and changes in the PR interval and right ventricular hypertrophy may be present. In the presence of significant mitral insufficiency, increased left ventricular and left atrial voltages may be detected.

Chest radiograph. Without significant mitral insufficiency, chest radiography will appear to be similar to that of those patients who have ostium secundum defects (i.e., variable from normal to significant cardiomegaly and increased pulmonary vascularity).

Echocardiography. Echocardiography can confirm the presence of an ostium primum versus an ostium secundum defect, as well as reveal any other associated valvar defects, particularly clefts of the mitral valve.

Treatment. Ostium primum defects currently are not amenable to transcatheter device closure, because of the lack of tissue rims inferior to the defect to which the device can appose. The surgical repair of such lesions is similar to that already described except for the use of pericardial patch material in these repairs (to reduce hemolysis by blood striking the patch). The mitral valve also can be repaired at the same time, usually by suture closure of the leaflet cleft through the ASD before its repair.

Complete Atrioventricular Canal Defects (Fig. 198-2)

Clinical presentation. The clinician's suspicion of partial or complete AV canal defects should be heightened when physical examination or genetic studies are consistent with Down syndrome. However, among patients who have normal chromosomes, patients who have AV canal defects tend to have clinical histories similar to those of patients who have other large intracardiac shunts, such as large VSDs, or extracardiac shunts. Congestive heart failure is common in the neonate and young infant, because of significant pulmonary overcirculation. Patients may present clinically with symptoms of poor feeding, poor weight gain, poor activity, and diaphoresis and/or shortness of breath on feeding. Significant mixing of oxygenated and deoxygenated blood may produce mild cyanosis (oxygen saturations of 85% to 95%).

Physical examination. Similar to the patient who has a large VSD early in the clinical course, loud systolic regurgitant murmurs may be auscultated, along with mid-diastolic rumbles. However, as ventricular pressures equilibrate across the ventricular septal component, murmurs may, in fact, be soft or absent. Development of increasing frequency and amplitude of the second heart sound, lack of splitting of the second heart sound, and/or disappearance of the murmurs may signify early onset of pulmonary hypertension. In the face of pulmonary hypertension, increases in the second heart sound, appearance of a third or fourth heart sound, and prominent right and left ventricular impulses may be present, consistent with combined CHF and increased pulmonary artery pressures. Hepatosplenomegaly also may be present.

Electrocardiography. Electrocardiography may show biventricular or biatrial hypertrophy and a leftward and superior QRS axis, as described for ostium primum defects.

Chest radiograph. Chest radiography routinely reveals evidence of pulmonary overcirculation and cardiomegaly resulting from the large left-to-right shunt. As pulmonary hypertension increases, decreasing left-to-right shunting may lead to normalization of the cardiac silhouette and pulmonary vascular markings.

Echocardiography. Echocardiography is important both for delineating the sizes of the atrial and ventricular components as well as for defining abnormalities of the right or left atrioventricular valves. Complete atrioventricular septal defects (AVSDs) are classified by the nature of the common AV valve, according to the Rastelli classification. The classification of the AVSD determines the method of repair. Serial measurements of pulmonary artery pressure by Doppler study are advantageous.

Cardiac catheterization. Cardiac catheterization may be indicated in some patients in whom insufficient echocardiographic images make it difficult to construct a surgical road map or in whom irreversible pulmonary hypertensive change is suspected.

Treatment. Standard diuretic therapy and/or afterload reduction (using ACE inhibitors) usually is the treatment of choice early in the patient's course, even before symptoms of CHF develop. In the face of poor ventricular function, positive inotropes such as digoxin may be added. Spontaneous closure of these defects is exceedingly rare; because of the large size of the intracardiac shunts, diligence toward prevention of pulmonary hypertension is important. Because of the size of this defect, transcatheter closure cannot be accomplished. Surgical repair usually is mandated within the first 2 to 6 months of life both to reduce pulmonary overflow and CHF and to prevent irreversible pulmonary vascular obstructive disease. Surgical repair is accomplished by either a one- or two-patch repair. The single-patch method uses a single piece of synthetic material both to divide the common five-leaflet AV valve and to repair the mitral valve. Because of the increased incidence of late mitral regurgitation, many surgeons have come to prefer the two-patch method. This repair utilizes a synthetic patch (for its rigid quality) to close the ventricular component of the defect along the midpoint of apposition of the common AV valve and an autologous pericardial patch to separately close the atrial component of the

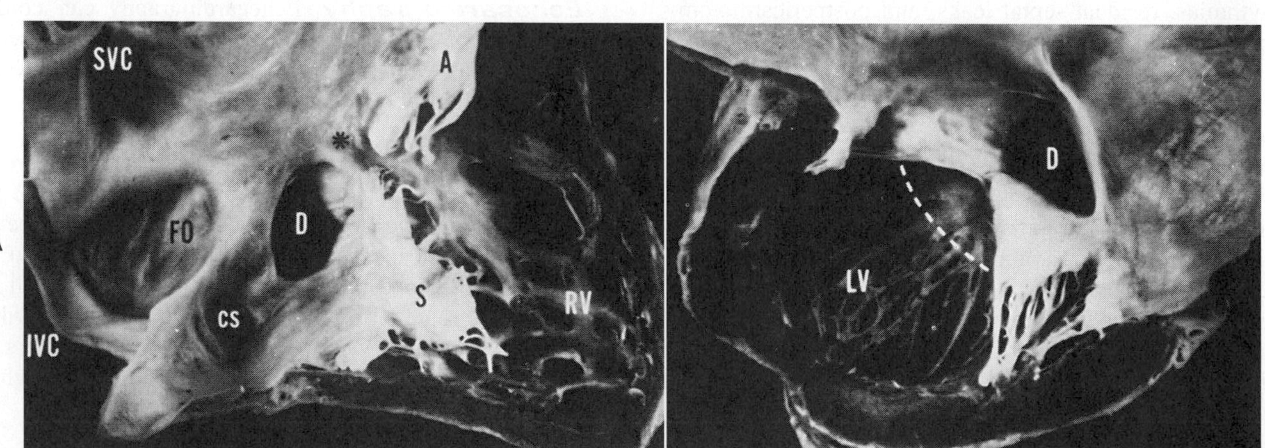

Fig. 198-2 **A,** Right ventricle and **B,** left ventricular views of a necropsy specimen demonstrating large atrial and ventricular septal components of endocardial cushion defect. *CS,* Coronary sinus; *D,* defect; *FO,* foramen ovale; *IVC,* inferior vena cava; *LV,* left ventricle; *RV,* right ventricle; *S,* septal leaflet of tricuspid valve; *SVC,* superior vena cava.

(From Feldt RH, et al: Defects of the atrial septum and atrioventricular canal. In Adams FH, Emmanouilides GC, Riemenschneider TA: *Moss' heart disease in infants, children and adolescents,* ed 4, Baltimore, 1989, Williams & Wilkins.)

AVSD. The anterior leaflet of the mitral valve must be evaluated for a cleft before closure of the atrial component.

Patent Ductus Arteriosus (Fig. 198-3)

The ductus arteriosus is a vessel found in all mammalian fetuses as an extension of the sixth aortic arch, which connects the main pulmonary artery with the descending aorta distal to the left subclavian artery. Its presence is imperative for decompression of the right ventricle. In utero, it directs more than 60% of systemic blood flow ejected from the right ventricle to the descending aorta. In 82% to 96% of full-term neonates, complete physiological closure of the ductus arteriosus occurs within the first 48 hours of life secondary to smooth-muscle constriction within the ductus on initial inspiration of oxygen. Full anatomical closure with scar formation usually occurs within the first 2 to 3 weeks; final closure is uncommon after 6 months of age. The overall incidence of failure of closure of the ductus arteriosus, resulting in a patent ductus arteriosus (PDA), is 1 in 5000 live births and is more common in premature infants, affecting at least 80% of neonates who weigh less than 1000 g at birth. There is a 2 to 3:1 female-to-male ratio, and PDA may be associated with first-trimester rubella infection. The incidence of PDA at higher altitudes both in full-term and premature infants is increased.

Clinical presentation. The majority of patients are asymptomatic and come to medical attention because of a continuous murmur along the upper sternal border. Patients who have large ductal diameters may present with classic signs and symptoms of CHF, as with any large left-to-right shunt. This occurs more commonly in children younger than 2 years of age and particularly in the neonatal population. In a rare patient, the initial presentation may be that of acute bacterial endocarditis. In cases in which the PDA is a component of a vascular ring, patients may present with stridor secondary to tracheal compression. Although exceedingly rare, a patient 6 to 24 months of age who has an undiagnosed large PDA may present with Eisenmenger's syndrome and irreversible pulmonary artery hypertension. In older adolescent and adult patients who have asymptomatic ductuses, a ductal aneurysm on imaging studies may be detected. Treatment of such ductal aneurysms becomes complicated because the tissue is friable and may rupture on surgical intervention. A small number of patients who have murmurs thought to be "benign" or "innocent" are found to have small-caliber PDA on echocardiography. The importance of this finding is discussed on the following page.

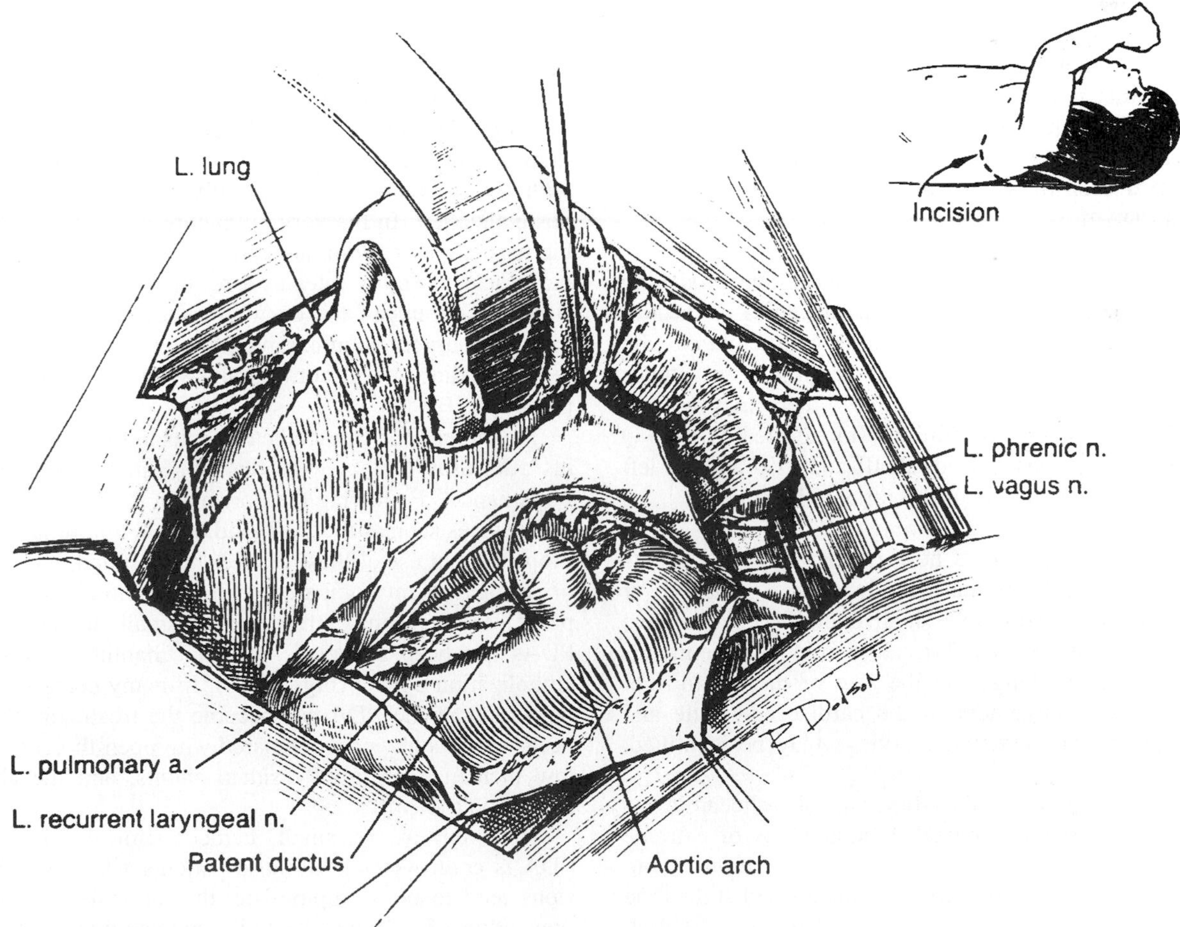

Fig. 198-3 Schematic drawing of surgical exposure of patent ductus arteriosus. Note proximity of all contiguous structures.

(From Castenda AR, Jonas RA, Mayer JE: *Cardiac surgery of the neonate and infant,* Philadelphia, 1994, WB Saunders.)

Physical examination. Patients who have a small PDA present with mildly increased palpable pulses and a widened pulse pressure by sphygmomanometry. Heart sounds tend to be normal, and a continuous murmur of variable intensity is heard usually just below the left clavicle (below the right clavicle in patients who have a right arch and a right PDA). Except in cases of CHF, no other systolic or diastolic components are heard on auscultation. Patients in whom the PDA is of hemodynamic significance may present with the full spectrum of CHF on physical examination—mid-diastolic rumble, loud continuous murmur, hyperdynamic precordium, and clinical manifestations of pulmonary overflow.

In patients who have continuous murmurs, the differential diagnosis should include arteriovenous or other forms of atriopulmonary fistulae and benign continuous murmurs such as carotid artery bruits, venous hums, or (in pregnant females) mammary souffles. These benign murmurs can be differentiated from the PDA by either direct compression over the jugular veins or breast or their disappearance when the patient assumes a supine position.

Because of their relative pulmonary hypertension, neonates who have a PDA may present with a short systolic ejection murmur along the left upper sternal border rather than a continuous murmur. Consequently, the differential diagnosis will include valvar aortic or vascular pulmonary stenosis, coarctation of the aorta, and benign peripheral pulmonary artery stenosis. Radiation of the murmur to the back (as in aortic coarctation or peripheral pulmonary artery stenosis) or to both axillae (as in peripheral pulmonary artery stenosis) may help distinguish these defects from the PDA. The presence of full pulses is a "soft sign" in the neonate population and has never been fully correlated with the presence or absence of a PDA.

Electrocardiogram. As with other lesions producing left-to-right shunts, ECG findings vary, depending on the size and hemodynamic significance of the PDA. In children who have a small PDA, the ECG tends to be normal; in patients who have moderate and large ductuses, there may be evidence of left ventricular hypertrophy (manifested by deep Q waves and tall R waves in leads II, III and aV_F, and the left lateral precordial leads) and/or left atrial enlargement.

Chest radiograph. Chest radiography in patients who have a PDA reflects the hemodynamic significance of the defect. Patients who have small ductuses tend to have normal cardiac silhouettes and trivial to mild increase in pulmonary vascular markings. As the size of the left-to-right shunt increases, enlargement of the cardiac silhouette and excessive pulmonary vascular markings may be identified.

Echocardiogram. Two-dimensional echocardiography, particularly in the neonatal population, is of extreme value not only in documenting the PDA but also in ruling out any ductal-dependent lesions not fully manifested at the time of the examination. These would include tetralogy of Fallot, pulmonary atresia with a VSD, or significant outflow-tract obstruction (valvar pulmonary stenosis, valvar aortic stenosis, coarctation of the aorta, hypoplastic left heart syndrome). In the vast majority of patients who have an uncomplicated PDA, adequate visualization of the PDA with directional shunt flow by color Doppler examination provides further substantiation of this diagnosis. Particularly in patients who have large PDA, echocardiography assists in determining cardiac function and chamber sizes, which may aid in assessing the need for transcatheter or surgical intervention.

Treatment. Medical therapy for the patient who has a hemodynamically significant PDA is similar to that for other left-to-right shunt lesions. In the neonatal population, diuretic therapy may be indicated, but other treatments include vascular-volume restriction and the use of prostaglandin inhibitors such as indomethacin. Inhibitors act antagonistically against intrinsic prostaglandin (which is a smooth-muscle relaxant) to induce vasoconstriction of smooth muscle within the PDA. A treatment course of three doses of 0.1 mg/kg of indomethacin daily has been shown to have good results (greater than 70% complete closure rate) in the small premature infant.[17] In the very small premature infant, some have advocated a 7-day course of treatment because of the dearth of smooth muscle at this age. In one such study,[19] rates of recurrence in patients treated with the 7-day course were 7% in contrast to 40% with a standard three-dose regimen.

Beyond the neonatal period or in the neonate not responsive to indomethacin (e.g., the usual full-term infant), the treatment of choice is complete occlusion of the PDA. Established in the late 1930s, surgical closure for patent ductus was, in fact, the first extracardiac surgery for congenital heart disease.[10] Surgical approaches to the ductus arteriosus may be through standard thoracotomy or developed more recently, via thoracoscopy. Simple ligation or ligation with division of the PDA may be accomplished by either approach with similar outcome and usually requires only overnight hospitalization. In the very premature neonate who has friable tissue, either technique carries an increased risk of morbidity and mortality rates as a result of ductal tears, so that surgical clipping of the ductus may be preferred. Mortality from this surgery is quite rare, although significant morbidity (e.g., bleeding, vocal cord paralysis) even in the 1990s approached 5%.[33]

Techniques for transcatheter occlusion of the patent ductus arteriosus in fact were described in the late 1960s by Portsmann.[46] Following the Portsmann Plug, other transcatheter devices such as the Rashkind double umbrella have been proposed, but use of these devices has resulted in higher rates of residual shunt compared with open-thoracic surgical repair.[23] More recently, treatment of small- to moderate-size PDAs has been achieved by using Gianturco transcatheter embolization coils[30] (Fig. 198-4). In many centers, coil embolization of the PDA has become the treatment of choice, because of its low cost compared with open-thoracic surgery, low incidence of small residual shunts, and the ability to reposition the coils.

Treatment of the small, hemodynamically insignificant PDA is controversial. Because patients who have these lesions tend to be asymptomatic, the rationale for closure is prevention of subacute bacterial endocarditis (SBE). When surgery was the only option, cardiologists were hesitant to recommend closure. Because coil embolization techniques have lower morbidity and require little or no hospital stay, more cardiologists have advocated closure using this method.

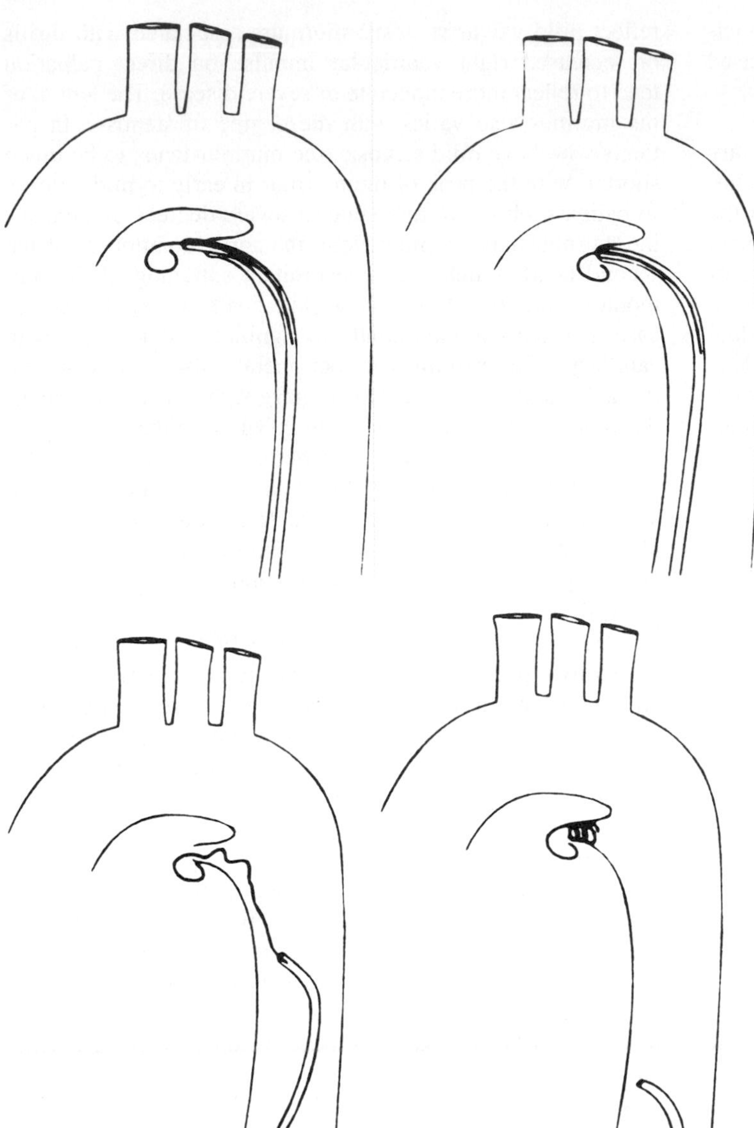

Fig. 198-4 Schematic drawing of retrograde (from aorta to pulmonary artery) coil embolization of patent ductus arteriosus. The embolization coil is implanted to allow for complete occlusion of patent ductus arteriosus.

(From Lloyd TR, Fedderly R, Mendelsohn AM: *Circulation* 88:1412, 1993.)

The "silent" PDA raises an even more interesting issue, because these defects, by definition, are not audible and usually are identified by echocardiography. Most cardiologists would not advocate either surgical or transcatheter closure of such lesions, and the literature does not support any significant increase in the incidence of SBE in patients in whom the PDA cannot be heard on auscultation.[29] Once discovered, however, most would recommend SBE prophylaxis, but even this approach is considered somewhat controversial.

OBSTRUCTIVE LESIONS

As a group, obstructive lesions of either the right ventricular or left ventricular outflow tract constitute the second largest group of congenital heart lesions (30% of all patients who have congenital heart disease). Obstruction to flow can occur in any part of the pulmonary or systemic vascular systems, although certain sites are more commonly affected than others. Lesions may be categorized from very mild and asymptomatic to severe, causing total obstruction to flow and hemodynamic instability.

Generally, severe stenoses in the neonatal period are associated with significant CHF symptoms and/or cyanosis, depending on the location of the lesion within the cardiopulmonary circulation systems. For example, neonates who have critical aortic stenosis or coarctation of the aorta tend to present with significant respiratory distress associated with pulmonary edema, ventricular failure secondary to the severe pressure overload caused by the obstruction, and poor weight gain due to poor feeding. In utero, most of these lesions are well tolerated, because multiple bypass tracks within the neonatal circulation (patent foramen ovale, patent ductus arteriosus) allow shunting of the blood flow away from the obstruction and into a patent circulation. These neonates, therefore, tend to be of normal weight and gestational age and develop symptoms only upon either ductal or patent foramen ovale closure.

Right Ventricular Outflow Tract Obstruction

Right ventricular tract obstruction may occur anatomically below, at, or above the pulmonary valve. Overall, about 8% to 10% of patients who have congenital heart disease have isolated stenosis. As with other congenital lesions, the incidence of pulmonary stenosis might be mildly increased among family members.

Valvar pulmonary stenosis. Valvar pulmonary stenosis is categorized from trivial to severe, based on echocardiographic measurements as defined on this page. In the majority of cases, a tricuspid pulmonic valve is identified, and the stenosis is due to partially fused raphae (commissures between leaflets) restricting leaflet movement. With increasing severity of the stenosis, clear definition of individual cusps becomes difficult. In addition, the cusps themselves become thickened and dysplastic. As valvar stenosis worsens, the infundibular (muscular) component of the right ventricular outflow tract may hypertrophy and the valve leaflets thicken, causing combined muscular/infundibular and valvar stenosis. The association between valvar pulmonary stenosis and Noonan's syndrome is high, with a greater incidence in this group of patients of myxomatous and dysplastic cusps.

Development of the right heart in neonates and the degree of right ventricular hypoplasia with valvar pulmonary stenosis depends on the stage at which the stenosis occurs. The earlier in gestation stenoses develop, the more diminutive will be the right ventricle and tricuspid valve.

CLINICAL PRESENTATION. In the neonatal period, patients who have "critical pulmonary valve stenosis" may present with symptomatology of right heart failure but more commonly present with cyanosis caused by the combination of diminished pulmonary blood flow and right-to-left shunting at the patent foramen ovale level. These infants are more likely to have a higher incidence of valve leaflet dysplasia and annular hypoplasia than are older children who present with heart murmurs.

In the majority of older patients, pulmonary stenosis will be diagnosed on routine murmur evaluation. With this defect, associated symptoms are notoriously unreliable in reflecting hemodynamic severity. The few patients who present with symptoms beyond the neonatal period have evidence of mild right heart failure (jugular venous distention and mild hepatosplenomegaly) or cyanosis, although this is exceedingly rare. In the vast majority of children, moderate to even severe valvar or subvalvar pulmonary stenosis is tolerated well.

PHYSICAL EXAMINATION. In patients who have mild valvar stenosis, there are usually no abnormalities of the heart sounds, and in some patients, no systolic ejection click may be auscultated. More commonly, however, a variable systolic ejection click (decreasing during inspiration and increasing during expiration) will be heard. Such variation in these findings has been related to the position of the stenotic valve at the onset of ventricular contraction. The presence of a click helps to differentiate valvar pulmonary stenosis from either subvalvar (infundibular) or supravalvar pulmonary stenosis, in which a click is absent. The presence of a third or fourth heart sound may reflect an associated atrial septal defect or abnormalities of the pulmonary veins. The systolic murmur of valvar pulmonary stenosis is ejection in quality with maximal intensity at the left upper sternal border. It may radiate widely through the precordium, neck, and back. The loudness of the murmur may not necessarily correlate with the severity of the stenosis, particularly in the face of poor cardiac output. Murmurs that are grade III/VI or less tend to reflect mild valvar stenosis; murmurs associated with thrills or increased right ventricular impulse on direct palpation tend to reflect more moderate or severe disease. The length of the murmur also varies with the degree of stenosis. In patients who have mild stenosis, the murmur tends to be much shorter, with the peak of the murmur in early to mid systole. In patients who have moderate to severe degrees of stenosis, the murmur may extend beyond the aortic component of the second heart sound, with concomitant softening of the pulmonary component of the second heart sound. Except in cases of poor cardiac output, no significant abnormalities in capillary refill or diminished peripheral pulses are identified. A small number of patients who have significant dysplasia of the pulmonary valve or patients in whom either surgery or balloon valvuloplasty has been performed may have a "to-fro" murmur reflecting residual pulmonary stenosis as well as insufficiency. In addition, particularly in the neonatal population, a second apical systolic murmur may be present, reflecting tricuspid insufficiency secondary to right ventricular dysfunction.

ELECTROCARDIOGRAM. The ECG in patients who have valvar pulmonary stenosis tends to be extremely helpful particularly because it defines the degree of right ventricular hypertrophy, which correlates with the degree of stenosis. In mild valvar obstruction, the ECG is normal in 40% to 50% of patients. In others, there may only be a mild abnormality reflected in a rightward QRS axis shift. Inversion of the T waves to the upright position in either V_1 or V_{3R} also may be present and reflect significant ventricular pressure overload. With increasing severity of valvular obstruction, a more rightward axis (up to 130 degrees) is found and there is an increase in right ventricular voltages reflected in an RSR′ pattern (R′ larger than R) in leads V_1 to V_{3R}. The following formula has been used by some to estimate valve gradients based on the size of the R wave in lead V_1:

Pressure gradient (in mm Hg) = height of R wave (in mm) × 5.[42] In some patients there also is right atrial hypertrophy with peaked P waves.

CHEST RADIOGRAPH. In most patients, chest radiography is not revealing. Beyond the neonatal period, when the hypertrophied right ventricle maintains adequate pulmonary blood flow, pulmonary vascular markings may be normal, and the cardiac silhouette may be within normal limits. Paradoxically, the less severe the stenosis, the greater the degree of "poststenotic dilation" reflected as enlargement of the main pulmonary artery segment on chest radiograph. This is because the wider jet in patients who have mild valvar stenosis causes greater dilation of the main pulmonary artery than the smaller jet delivered through a more restrictive orifice. In some patients, a prominent right atrial segment can be seen in the chest radiograph; in others, right ventricular hypertrophy may be identified in the lateral examination.

ECHOCARDIOGRAPHY. Echocardiography is the primary tool in defining the presence and severity of stenosis as well as the degree of compensatory right ventricular hypertrophy or dilation. Right ventricular pressures can be estimated in cases in which a tricuspid insufficiency jet is noted by color Doppler flow study. Estimated transvalvar gradients have been shown to correlate well with those directly measured during cardiac catheterization.[37] The severity of stenosis is categorized by the gradient across the pulmonary valve.

Stenosis may be considered trivial when the peak instantaneous gradient is less than 25 mm Hg, mild when it is between 25 and 50 mm Hg, moderate when it is between 50 and 75 mm Hg, and severe when it is greater than 75 mm Hg. In some cases, the echocardiogram can define the degree of leaflet dysplasia, any annular hypoplasia, and the presence of infundibular or supravalvar stenosis. Poststenotic dilation of the main pulmonary artery or inherent stenoses of the proximal branch pulmonary arteries also may be visualized.

CARDIAC CATHETERIZATION. Currently, cardiac catheterization and concomitant balloon valvuloplasty is considered the treatment of choice for most cases of valvar pulmonary stenosis. Both the timing and degree of stenosis at which to intervene is still controversial. In the asymptomatic patient who has moderate to severe valvar pulmonary stenosis, elective therapy should be performed somewhere between 2 and 4 years of age, although the procedure can be performed much sooner if the degree of stenosis is severe (right ventricular systolic pressure at or above the systemic systolic pressure). In contrast, other investigators have shown that long-term ECG changes and symptomatic improvement have occurred following intervention for gradients between 40 and 50 mm Hg.[37] Most recent studies have demonstrated that successful balloon valvuloplasty results in significant reduction of the systolic gradient (residual gradient less than 25 mm Hg) in 70% to 85% of patients, with no recurrent stenosis for up to 10 years of follow-up. Factors that negatively influence success include significant annular hypoplasia and severe leaflet dysplasia. Whether younger patients (<2 years) have poorer procedural success is controversial. Studies comparing long-term outcomes following surgical (mean 11.7 years postoperatively) and balloon valvuloplasty (mean 5.3 years after the procedure) have revealed similar residual gradients (16 ± 2 versus 24 ± 3 mm Hg; p = ns).[44]

TREATMENT. Interventional therapy in the symptomatic neonate (right ventricular failure, cyanosis) usually follows stabilization with prostaglandin E_1. Pulmonary balloon valvuloplasty in the neonate is technically more challenging, and results are less favorable. There is a much higher incidence of significant residual stenosis that may be secondary to residual infundibular obstruction or inadequate tearing of the fused commissures. Some have shown that neonates who have a tricuspid valve diameter less than 12 mm and a pulmonary valve diameter less than 7 mm tend to have a higher incidence of restenosis requiring treatment, the need for surgical augmentation of the right ventricular outflow tract, or an aortopulmonary shunt shortly after balloon valvuloplasty.[12] In cases in which significant infundibular or supravalvar stenosis is present, surgical valvulotomy with patch angioplasty of the supravalvar stenosis or infundibular muscle resection may be indicated. Such issues can be predicted either by echocardiography or by standard right ventricular angiography.

Most cardiologists believe that mild valvar pulmonary stenosis has a benign course and does not require treatment except for antibiotic prophylaxis for bacterial endocarditis. This view has been borne out by long-term studies in more than 400 patients.[42] On the other hand, most centers have shown that infants and children who have moderate to severe valvar stenosis develop increasing degrees of outflow tract obstruction, particularly during the periods of rapid somatic growth (i.e., infancy and adolescence). For this reason, observation and repeat echocardiograms are indicated throughout childhood.

Subvalvar pulmonic stenosis. Infundibular pulmonary stenosis with a normal pulmonary valve is exceedingly rare and may either be associated with a small VSD, or more commonly, is seen with cyanotic heart lesions such as tetralogy of Fallot. Mechanical obstruction may be attributable to a discrete fibrous or fibromuscular ring. Significant functional infundibular obstruction may occur from intracavitary muscular bands that form, dividing the right ventricle into low- and high-pressure chambers. Clinical features, ECG, and chest radiography findings are similar to those in patients who have valvar pulmonary stenosis. The physical examination differs from valvar disease by the absence of a systolic ejection click. Therapy for this lesion tends to be surgical. Balloon valvuloplasty has not proven to be effective in resolving gradients in these patients. The patient who has mechanical right ventricular outflow tract obstruction (RVOTO) secondary to infundibular hypertrophy generally is amenable to infundibular resection through the pulmonary valve; a right atrial approach is preferred for functional obstruction caused by trabeculations or septal bands, as is often the case with tetralogy of Fallot.

Supravalvar pulmonic stenosis. Stenosis of the main pulmonary arteries is rarely an isolated lesion. More often it occurs in conjunction with hypoplasia of the branch pulmonary arteries in such conditions as Alagille syndrome, Williams syndrome, and congenital rubella syndrome. The clinical presentation and laboratory examination in these patients is similar to those of the other two forms of RVOTO. Some investigators have shown that balloon angioplasty is effective, but it is not as successful as in patients who have valvar disease.[40] In addition, in many cases the extensive stenoses require patch angioplasty alone or in combination with endovascular stent therapy.

Peripheral pulmonary artery stenosis (Fig. 198-5). Significant stenoses of the branch pulmonary arteries are fairly rare pathological lesions. Many neonates, particularly those born prematurely, will have the murmur of benign peripheral pulmonary artery stenosis. This murmur results from flow disturbance rather than anatomical stenosis at the bifurcation of the branch pulmonary arteries from the main pulmonary artery. Usually, these benign murmurs resolve by 6 months of age, as the pulmonary artery contour at the bifurcation changes with growth.

As characterized by Gay et al,[15] two thirds of patients who have peripheral pulmonary artery stenosis have involvement of the main pulmonary trunk and its bifurcation to branch pulmonary arteries. In the remaining one third of patients, stenoses within the parenchymal vessels of the lung are identified. Pathological branch pulmonary artery stenosis occurs in 3% to 6% of patients who have congenital heart lesions, and its etiology may be secondary either to hypoplasia of the pulmonary arteries or maternal conditions (i.e., rubella, cocaine use). It also has been associated with Williams, Noonan's, Alagille, cutis laxa, and Ehlers-Danlos syndromes. Most commonly, however, it is diagnosed in patients following

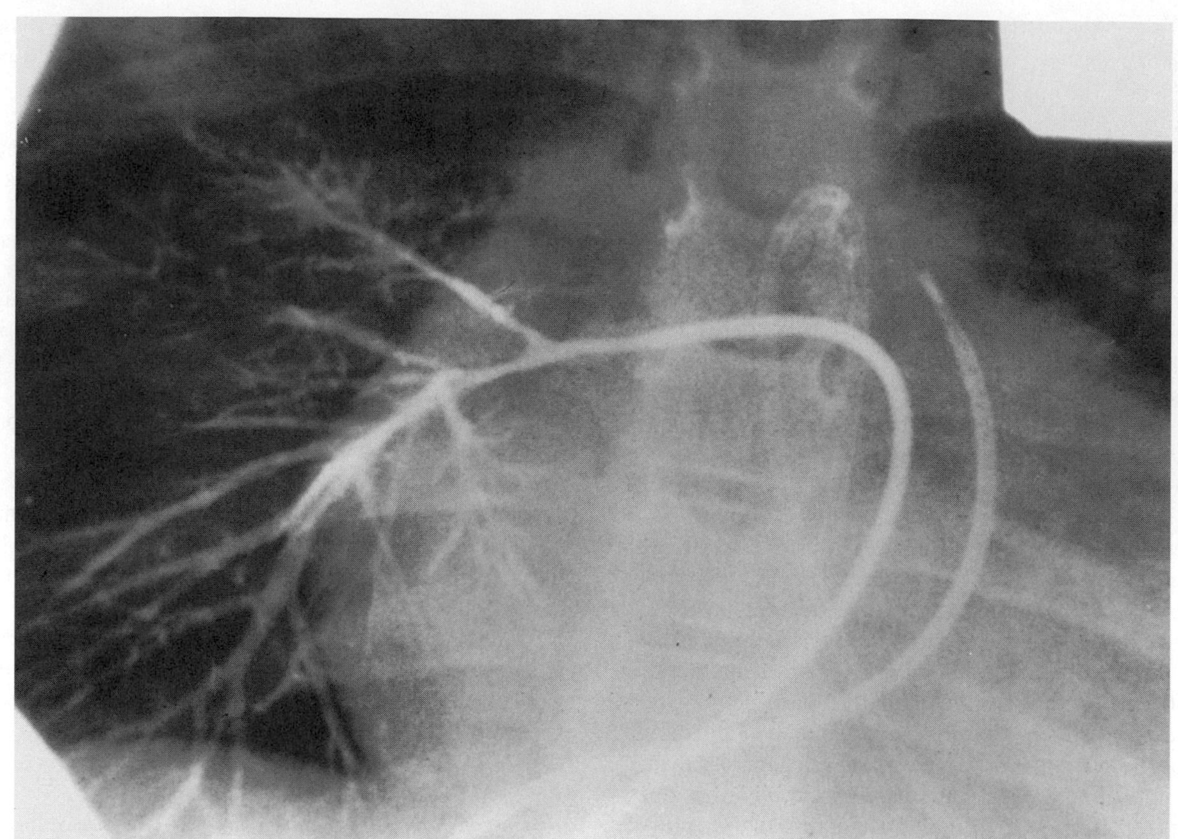

Fig. 198-5 Spot cineangiogram of isolated right pulmonary artery hypoplasia in a 16-year-old female. Note small parenchymal vessels within the lungs in addition to a hypoplastic main right pulmonary artery.

surgical repair of outflow tract lesions (i.e., tetralogy of Fallot, transposition of the great arteries).

CLINICAL PRESENTATION. Patients who have mild or moderate bilateral pulmonary artery stenoses, as well as those who have unilateral stenosis, usually are asymptomatic and a murmur may be the only physical sign. In those patients whose obstruction is severe, symptoms of dyspnea on exertion, easy fatigability, and signs of right heart failure may be seen as a result of severe pressure overload of the right ventricle. In patients who have previous cardiac surgery and new onset of a murmur, further workup to search for such stenoses is mandated.

PHYSICAL EXAMINATION. As with other forms of right ventricular outflow tract disease, the major presenting sign may be a harsh systolic ejection murmur. Localization of the murmur may aid in differentiating this diagnosis from that of valvar pulmonary stenosis. In the majority of patients who have significant branch pulmonary artery stenosis, the murmur, although heard well in the precordium, is heard better in the axilla and back; the murmurs of valvar disease usually are best auscultated in the precordium. The first heart sound usually is normal in patients who have peripheral pulmonary artery stenosis. It is not followed by a systolic ejection click as in patients who have valvar pulmonary stenosis. The second heart sound in patients who have peripheral pulmonary stenoses usually is split normally and is of normal intensity, again differentiating it from valvar pulmonary stenosis. With multiple peripheral artery stenoses, particularly with increasing severity, the murmurs become more continuous over the posterior lung fields. Other disease processes in the differential diagnosis include aortic coarctation, valvar aortic or pulmonary stenosis, and in the neonate, a PDA.

ELECTROCARDIOGRAM. Except in instances of severe stenosis causing right ventricular hypertrophy, the majority of patients who have peripheral pulmonary artery stenosis present with a normal electrocardiogram.

CHEST RADIOGRAPHY. Similarly, unless the stenosis is severe enough to diminish pulmonary vascular flow markedly, cardiac silhouette and pulmonary vascular markings appear to be normal on chest radiography. Unlike valvar pulmonary stenosis in which the main pulmonary artery may show evidence of poststenotic dilation, the main pulmonary artery in patients who have branch pulmonary artery stenosis appears to be normal. When stenoses are severe, however, varying degrees of right atrial and right ventricular enlargement may be seen. Certainly, if the patient has progressed to right heart failure, concomitant findings on chest radiography may be identified.

ECHOCARDIOGRAPHY. Standard two-dimensional and Doppler echocardiography usually can confirm this diagnosis. In addition to defining the size of and relative flow pattern to each pulmonary artery, echocardiography also can demonstrate degrees of right ventricular or right atrial hypertrophy. Associated lesions such as atrial or ventricular septal defects, valvar aortic or pulmonary stenosis, and tetralogy of Fallot can be detected by these methods, as well. At present, two-dimensional echocardiographic imaging is limited to definition of the main branch pulmonary arteries to the level of the hilum. Stenoses within the parenchymal vessels may be delineated better by other noninvasive testing such as MRI.

CARDIAC CATHETERIZATION. Cardiac catheterization is used to confirm and define the clinical diagnosis of significant peripheral pulmonary artery stenoses, particularly within the parenchymal vasculature. Hemodynamic tracings define the precise location of stenoses within the larger vessel and angiography further defines the vessels in particular. Basic hemodynamic tracings can differentiate patients who have significant branch pulmonary artery stenosis—those who have wide pulse pressure within the pulmonary artery from those who have pulmonary artery hypertension secondary to other etiologies resulting in narrow pulse pressure.

TREATMENT. In the majority of patients who have mild to moderate, isolated unilateral or bilateral peripheral artery stenosis, no therapy is indicated. The need for intervention is based on symptoms of right ventricular hypertension or hypertrophy, diminished pulmonary blood flow resulting in poor exercise tolerance or inactivity, and overall clinical status. From a hemodynamic standpoint, treatment usually is reserved for gradients of more than 40 to 60 mm Hg. In most centers, initial treatment tends to be transcatheter balloon angioplasty of the branch pulmonary artery stenoses. Past studies have demonstrated, however, that balloon angioplasty alone is successful in only about 50% of patients.[49] The more recent use of high-pressure balloons has increased success to about 70%,[16] but the greatest increase in success has followed the use of endovascular stent therapy,[35,45] with success rates of balloon angioplasty exceeding 85%, accompanied by a low rate of restenosis in short- and medium-term follow-up studies.

When peripheral pulmonary artery stenoses are identified as components of other surgical lesions (i.e., tetralogy of Fallot), full repair including patch angioplasty of the pulmonary arteries in the operating room can be performed. In cases in which the patch collapses as a result of low flow or pressure in the pulmonary arteries immediately following repair or patch angioplasty proves technically difficult, intraoperative stent implantation can be performed.[35]

In patients in whom peripheral pulmonary artery stenosis is associated with underlying complex abnormalities (i.e., congenital rubella syndrome, Williams syndrome, Alagille syndrome), both surgery and balloon angioplasty have been of limited utility.[49] Angioplasty and stent procedures are applicable only to stenoses within the main branches of the pulmonary artery. Significant stenoses within the parenchyma of the lungs are almost impossible to treat by any conventional therapy. Untreated or incompletely treated pulmonary artery stenoses may lead to significant right heart failure in adolescence and young adulthood.

Left Ventricular Outflow Tract Obstruction

Aortic stenosis. Lesions affecting the left ventricular outflow tract constitute 10% to 15% of congenital heart defects. Isolated aortic valve stenosis occurs in 3% to 6% of patients who have congenital cardiovascular defects. The incidence of mild abnormalities of the aortic valve is higher, with a bicuspid valve, occurring in 1% to 2% of the entire population. Among patients who have aortic valve disease, the male-to-female ratio is approximately 4 to 1. Associated cardiac lesions may occur in up to 20% of patients and include PDA or coarctation of the aorta. Aortic valve anomalies often are undetected in early life and may only come to evaluation with detection of an increasing murmur. Murmurs associated with valvar stenosis do not differ whether the abnormality is congenital or acquired, as may occur with advancing age.

Because normal valves are composed of three leaflets, the stenotic aortic valve is usually described as "unicuspid," in which two of the three leaflets are fused and an eccentrically formed orifice is identified; "bicuspid," which is the most common form of congenital aortic valve stenosis; or "tricuspid." Most commonly, unicuspid aortic valves present earlier and may be the principal abnormality in the neonate who has critical aortic valve stenosis. Abnormalities of the valve leaflets and hypoplasia of the valve annulus may combine as components of the outflow tract disease. As higher-velocity flow is ejected through the stenotic valve, increased thickening and deformity of the valve cusps may occur with time, potentially leading to valve calcification in the adult. Such secondary calcification is rare in childhood. The rate of progression of stenosis is variable, but congenital aortic stenosis frequently progresses, even early in life.

CLINICAL PRESENTATION. Clinical presentation in patients who have aortic stenosis is determined mainly by the degree of obstruction to left ventricular outflow. As noted, neonates who have significant left ventricular outflow tract obstruction (LVOTO) may present within the first few hours to days of life in severe CHF following closure of the PDA. Conversely, patients who have mild or moderate valvar disease may simply present in infancy or later with a systolic ejection murmur. Most children who have aortic valve stenosis are asymptomatic and grow and develop normally; however, symptoms of ventricular pressure overload may develop disease including fatigue, exertional dyspnea, angina pectoris, and syncope. Less commonly, patients may present with diaphoresis and abdominal pain. If symptoms develop, one can assume that the degree of stenosis is at least moderate. Syncope may be related to the inability of the left ventricle to increase cardiac output to maintain cerebral flow during exercise. Disparities between oxygen supply to the left ventricle and myocardial oxygen demands lead to angina pectoris. In a small number of patients, the diagnosis may not be confirmed until other illnesses arise (e.g., endocarditis). Rarely, sudden death has been reported, although usually such patients have had severe, long-standing obstruction and/or significant symptomatology beforehand. Patients who have a significant stenosis may present with ventricular dysrhythmias secondary to combined myocardial ischemia and a hypertrophic left ventricle. Rapid changes in severity of aortic stenosis may occur with rapid growth spurts in puberty or young adulthood as the effective valve orifice is insufficient to permit the needed increase in cardiac output.

PHYSICAL EXAMINATION. The systolic murmur characteristic of aortic stenosis begins soon after left ventricular contraction, is harsh in quality and loud, and has been described as "crescendo/decrescendo." The murmur is heard best at the base of the heart, although it does radiate well to the left lower sternal border and apex. In approximately 25%

of patients who have aortic stenosis, an early diastolic murmur of aortic insufficiency may be present. Such regurgitation usually is trivial to mild, and the murmur may be faint and the pulse pressure normal.

Paradoxically, the cardiac examination may or may not correlate with the degree of obstruction to ventricular outflow. For example, in the neonate who has critical aortic stenosis, only a soft systolic ejection murmur may be heard. Complete clinical examination, however, would reveal diminished pulses and capillary refill, systemic hypotension with narrow pulse pressures and clinical symptomatology of CHF—tachypnea, tachycardia, and diaphoresis.

When the degree of aortic stenosis is significant, a left ventricular heave or thrill usually is palpable. Gradients greater than 25 mm Hg usually result in a precordial systolic thrill, which radiates to the jugular notch and along the carotid arteries. When neither of these findings is present, the obstruction tends to be mild. On cardiac examination, the first and second heart sounds tend to be within normal limits. A systolic ejection click may be heard at the cardiac apex, with radiation to the right upper sternal border when the valve is fairly mobile. This click may be differentiated from a similar ejection sound in patients who have pulmonary valve disease because the ejection click in aortic disease is more constant and tends not to be influenced by the respiratory cycle. Ejection sounds are heard more often in patients who have mild to moderate disease, as those who have severe stenosis tend to have poorer mobility of their valve. The disappearance of such an ejection sound may suggest progression of stenosis. Prolongation of left ventricular emptying may lead to delayed valve closure and a single or closely split second heart sound. A third heart sound is common in normal children younger than 12 years of age and is even more common in children who have aortic valve stenosis and diastolic dysfunction. The presence of a fourth heart sound also may support the clinical impression of diastolic dysfunction in patients who have severe obstruction and concomitant left ventricular hypertrophy.

ELECTROCARDIOGRAM. Although absence of ECG findings does not preclude the presence of significant stenosis, the majority of patients who have significant stenosis do have left ventricular and/or left atrial hypertrophy by voltage criteria. Although better in younger patients, the correlation between ECG findings and transvalvar pressure gradients generally is poor.[14] Other findings consistent with significant ventricular pressure overload include T-wave inversion or flattening in the left precordial leads and/or ST depressions consistent with myocardial ischemia or diastolic dysfunction. In some patients, these abnormalities may not be present at rest but are exacerbated by graded exercise testing.

CHEST RADIOGRAPH. Chest radiography usually is inconclusive in defining the significance of valvar stenosis. The cardiac silhouette and size of the ventricle do not correlate closely with the size of the aortic orifice, systolic blood pressure, or transvalvar peak gradient. In some patients who have mild to moderate disease, poststenotic dilation of the ascending aorta may be noted. With severe stenosis, rounding of the left ventricular apex in the frontal plane may indicate concentric left ventricular hypertrophy. Evidence of left atrial dilation by chest radiography correlates better with significant aortic stenosis and left ventricular diastolic dysfunction. In patients who have significant stenosis and symptoms, radiographic findings of CHF (i.e., pulmonary edema) may be present.

ECHOCARDIOGRAPHY. The echocardiogram is valuable for distinguishing valvar from subvalvar or supravalvar aortic stenosis, for defining associated lesions (i.e., aortic insufficiency, VSD, aortic coarctation), and for gauging ventricular chamber sizes and thickness of the ventricular wall and septum. The presence of subclinical aortic insufficiency can be detected with echocardiography. Echocardiography also may be useful in determining aortic root measurements and valve morphology, which helps determine treatment.

EXERCISE TESTING. Bicycle or treadmill exercise testing is used frequently in the evaluation of patients who have aortic disease. Increasing severity of obstruction correlates well with worsening systolic blood pressure response, decreases in R-wave amplitude, and significant ST segment depression or inversion during maximal exercise. Several laboratories have reported that ST depressions of greater than 1 mm may indicate transvalvar pressure gradients in excess of 50 mm Hg. This sign, however, is inconsistent, as other reports have shown similar depression with gradients of less than 30 mm Hg.[25] The appearance of symptoms (i.e., dyspnea, chest pain, dizziness, or palpitations) during exercise does correlate well with the degree of stenosis. Similarly, an inadequate increase or even a decrease in systolic blood pressure suggests severe obstruction, and an inverse relationship does exist between severity of obstruction and time spent working or exercising. Cardiac function during exercise testing, even in patients who have severe obstruction, tends to remain normal. In contrast to adult patients, few children show reduction in stroke volume even with increasing ventricular end diastolic pressure.

TREATMENT. Cardiac catheterization is important for establishing the site and severity of obstruction to left ventricular outflow. In addition, cardiac catheterization in such patients can be therapeutic. Although the original criteria for intervention included a gradient of at least 60 mm Hg between the left ventricle and the ascending aorta, interventional catheterization now is performed when gradients are lower (i.e., 40 mm Hg) if there are symptoms (i.e., exercise intolerance) or significant ventricular dysfunction. Standard right and left heart catheterizations are performed, and either an antegrade (through the atrial septum into the left ventricle) or a retrograde (from the femoral artery to the left ventricle) approach may be used to cross the stenotic aortic valve. In most patients, technically adequate balloon valvulotomy results in reduction of the systolic gradient to 25 to 35 mm Hg. Patients who have significant concomitant aortic insufficiency, calcific aortic stenosis, or hypoplasia of the aortic annulus (less than 5 mm) usually are not good candidates for transcatheter aortic balloon valvulotomy. The procedure can be performed in the neonate who has "critical" aortic stenosis or low cardiac output, but the patient's size and tenuous clinical status increases procedural morbidity and mortality rates.

Successful balloon valvulotomy may be accomplished in 70% to 80% of carefully selected patients. In most patients, it does not worsen aortic insufficiency.[43] Unfortunately, the incidence of restenosis approaches 30% to 40% within 7 to 10 years. Restenosis rates are even higher when balloon valvulotomy is performed in the neonatal period. Repeat valvulotomy within 4 years of the initial procedure was required in 36% of one group of children who underwent balloon valvulotomy in the neonatal period.[11] Immediate postprocedural complications include arterial injury, hemorrhage, ventricular arrhythmias, endocarditis, leaflet tears or perforations, and aortic insufficiency. However, recent studies have demonstrated aortic insufficiency of equivalent degree following either balloon or surgical valvulotomy.[26] Beyond the neonatal period, postprocedural mortality or leaflet avulsion is rare. Repeat balloon dilations in the face of restenosis may provide further palliation.[53] Recent studies[20] have shown that each year following a balloon valvulotomy, 5% to 7% of patients will require aortic valve surgery, most for increasing severity of the aortic insufficiency. In many of these cases, however, valve repair rather than replacement may be accomplished.

Family choice, significant dysplasia of the valve leaflets, hypoplasia of the aortic annulus, or concomitant lesions (i.e., severe aortic insufficiency) may mandate surgical intervention. Long-term follow-up studies indicate that surgical valvulotomy is safe and effective, with excellent symptomatic relief. If aortic insufficiency progresses or valve morphology is inadequate for simple repair, valve replacement may be necessary. Mechanical valve replacement requires life-long anticoagulation with its inherent risks, yet requires replacement only if the child outgrows it or a complication such as bacterial endocarditis develops. Homograft or bioprosthetic replacement does not require anticoagulation, but the valves have a finite service lifetime of 10 to 15 years, after which they need replacement. The Ross procedure, originally performed in the late 1960s, has gained popularity as the procedure of choice in the pediatric population. The procedure consists of pulmonary autograft replacement of the aortic valve along with pulmonary allograft replacement of the right ventricular outflow tract (RVOT). The key benefit is that the autograft replacement of the aortic valve may last a lifetime, with only the homograft in the RVOT requiring replacement. Recent statistics have shown that 35% of patients will require prosthetic valve replacement within 15 to 20 years of the initial surgery.[7]

Subaortic stenosis. Subvalvar aortic stenosis accounts for 8% to 10% of all cases of congenital aortic stenosis and occurs more frequently in males than in females. It may be either a membranous diaphragm or fibrous ring encircling the left ventricular outflow tract just at the base of the aortic valve. The aortic valve itself may become dysplastic, thickened, and distorted. Occasionally, both valvar and subvalvar aortic stenosis occur in the same patient. In these cases, there may be diminution in the diameter of the ascending aorta, hypoplasia of the aortic valve annulus, and thickened valve leaflets. A combination of lesions makes surgical intervention more difficult. Obstructions beneath the aortic valve may occur not only from discrete membranes or muscular ridges but from impingement of the mitral valve leaflet into the left ventricular outflow tract (LVOT). This is observed in some patients, for example, who have an atrioventricular septal defect.

CLINICAL PRESENTATION. The clinical history of patients who have subvalvar aortic stenosis is similar to that of those who have valvar aortic stenosis. Until obstruction is severe, symptomatology usually is quite limited.

PHYSICAL EXAMINATION. Differentiating valvar from subvalvar aortic stenosis by physical examination can be difficult. Overall, the incidence of systolic ejection clicks is much higher in patients who have true valvar aortic disease than in patients who have subvalvar disease. The incidence of diastolic murmurs secondary to aortic insufficiency is higher in patients who have subvalvar disease.

ELECTROCARDIOGRAM. The ECG in patients who have subvalvar stenosis is similar to that of patients who have valvar aortic stenosis of a similar degree.

CHEST RADIOGRAPH. Chest radiography shows variable dilation of the ascending aorta with an otherwise normal cardiac silhouette. Pulmonary vascular markings are normal except in cases of severe outflow tract obstruction with which signs of CHF and pulmonary edema are seen.

ECHOCARDIOGRAPHY. Echocardiography is extremely valuable in confirming the clinical diagnosis and in defining the degree of subvalvar stenosis and its etiology. Subclinical degrees of aortic insufficiency may also be defined by color flow Doppler studies. Chamber sizes and ventricular function can be evaluated by these studies, as well.

CARDIAC CATHETERIZATION. Cardiac catheterization is valuable for further definition of the degree and etiology of the subvalvar stenosis and aids in planning of potential intervention. Aortography can help to define aortic insufficiency.

TREATMENT. Intervention for subvalvar aortic stenosis depends not only on the measured gradient but also on the overall clinical impression of the examiner concerning ventricular and valvar function. In most patients, a gradient greater than 40 mm Hg between the left ventricle and the ascending aorta is an indication for intervention, but intervention may be indicated for a lower gradient in the face of advancing aortic insufficiency. Resection of the membranous or the fibrous muscular ridge and resuspension of a prolapsing aortic valve to reduce aortic insufficiency is the primary therapy. In cases of long-segment, muscular-outflow-tract obstruction, further excision of muscle and, in some cases, valve replacement with enlargement of the subvalvar area (Konno operation) may be indicated.

In a small number of patients, secondary muscular hypertrophy of the outflow tract and pressure gradients may persist following operative relief of discrete subvalvar aortic stenoses. In 20% to 40% of patients, stenosis may recur within 7 to 10 years.

Supravalvar aortic stenosis. Supravalvar aortic stenosis can present either as a localized or diffuse narrowing of the aorta above the level of the coronary arteries and the superior annular margin of the sinus of Valsalva. Although it does occur in isolation, one significant associated abnormality is idiopathic infantile hypercalcemia, or Williams syndrome. Such patients have characteristic "elfin faces," mild mental retardation, and a friendly demeanor ("cocktail personality"). From a cardiovascular standpoint, such patients may have significant combined stenosis of both the peripheral systemic arteries and peripheral pulmonary arteries. Abnormalities of calcium metabolism are identified routinely. From a physiological and anatomical standpoint, prolonged supravalvar stenosis occurring distal to the origins of the coronary arteries may lead to thickened coronary artery media and intima. In some cases, premature coronary arteriosclerosis has been observed. Associated abnormalities of the aortic cusps themselves may cause further interference with coronary artery flow.

CLINICAL PRESENTATION. When a patient presents with the stigmata of Williams syndrome, supravalvar aortic or peripheral pulmonary arterial disease should be suspected. In other patients, discovery of a systolic murmur on physical examination and findings on echocardiography may lead to the diagnosis. Symptomatology consistent with other forms of LVOTO may be present.

PHYSICAL EXAMINATION. Physical examination in patients who have isolated supravalvar aortic stenosis differs little from that of those who have subvalvar aortic stenosis. Patients tend to have harsh systolic ejection murmurs with normal heart sounds and without systolic ejection clicks. In patients who have Williams syndrome and concomitant peripheral pulmonary artery stenosis, systolic ejection murmurs also may be heard over the axilla and back. Depending on the physiological state and degree of cardiac compromise, diminished pulses, tachycardia, and tachypnea may be present.

CARDIAC CATHETERIZATION. Cardiac catheterization defines the significant anatomy of the ascending aorta and provides evidence of coronary occlusion or medial thickening. Balloon angioplasty of the supravalvar region has had limited success.[24]

TREATMENT. Supravalvar aortic stenosis is often more difficult to treat than other forms of aortic stenosis. Surgical intervention involves patch angioplasty of the ascending aorta, creating an enlarged aortic root. If the aorta is markedly hypoplastic, further patch angioplasty or an interposition graft from ascending to descending aorta may be necessary. Intervention should be performed for gradients greater than 60 to 70 mm Hg, particularly in the face of hypoplasia of the ascending aorta. In patients who have little hypoplasia or a discrete narrowing, intervention may be performed for gradients greater than 50 mm Hg.

Coarctation of the aorta. Constriction of the aorta causing a coarctation may be either a discrete membranous narrowing or a long, hypoplastic segment. Invariably, the narrowing is located at the insertion point of the ductus arteriosus and the aorta. Embryologically, coarctation of the aorta usually is due to abnormal intrauterine aortic flow dynamics. In fetal life, the aortic isthmus (the region of the aorta between the subclavian artery and the ductus arteriosus) conducts only 10% to 12% of normal cardiac output. The majority of forward flow from the left ventricle is destined for bilateral carotid and right subclavian arterial filling, and ductal flow from the right ventricle perfuses the majority of the descending aorta. Thus, the "watershed" between these two regions is most prone to limited arterial flow and decreased growth.

Isolated coarctation of the aorta is among the most common congenital heart lesions; in the New England Regional Study of Congenital Heart Defects it constituted 7.5% of congenital heart defects in infants younger than 1 year of age. This may be an underestimate of the true incidence of this defect, because evolution of this lesion may be progressive in some children and may not appear until late infancy or young childhood. There is a male predominance of this lesion in older patients, but in infancy the gender ratio is approximately 1 : 1. There is a high association between coarctation and other congenital cardiac abnormalities, particularly PDA (67% of patients), VSD (30% to 35%), aortic stenosis and insufficiency, and mitral valve abnormalities. A bicuspid aortic valve is encountered most frequently and is found in upward of 85% of patients who have aortic coarctation. In addition, some patients will present with associated cerebral aneurysms, predisposing them to cerebrovascular accidents in the presence of severe systolic hypertension. A few patients (about 7%) may have noncardiac malformations, including clubbed foot, hypospadias, and ocular defects. Coarctation is the most common congenital cardiovascular abnormality found in patients who have Turner's syndrome.

CLINICAL PRESENTATION. Even with significant coarctation, neonates may have minimal differences in blood pressures or pulses between upper and lower extremities on physical examination until the ductus arteriosus closes (within the first 3 to 7 days). In a small number of neonates, there may be differential oxygen saturations between the upper and lower extremities (upper extremities filled by the left ventricle, descending aorta filled by the ductus arteriosus). At the time of ductal closure, infants who have severe aortic coarctation (nearly complete interruption of the aortic arch) may have differential oxygen saturations, blood pressure and pulses between upper and lower extremities, and cyanosis of the feet. Associated metabolic acidosis, oliguria and anuria, and potential right heart failure may ensue. Unless the coarctation is severe, it may not be discovered until a murmur or systemic systolic hypertension is investigated in childhood or adolescence. In some children in whom the coarctation is more severe, decreased lower extremity flow may lead to lower extremity claudication and diminished exercise tolerance. In infants who have aortic coarctation, associated anomalies occur quite frequently.

PHYSICAL EXAMINATION. The diagnosis of coarctation of the aorta, particularly in the infant beyond 3 to 7 days of age, is made principally by noting differential blood pressures between upper and lower extremities and diminished pulses in the lower extremities. In the older child, particularly those who have abnormalities of the brachiocephalic vessels (e.g., aberrant right subclavian artery arising below the coarctation) or development of aorto-aortic collaterals, differential blood pressures may not be present. Except for the neonate who evidences left or right ventricular failure, most infants and children will have normal growth and development.

Most often the first and second heart sounds are normal. If an associated bicuspid aortic valve is present, a systolic ejection click may be heard. The systolic ejection murmur of aortic coarctation usually is heard in the left hemithorax but can best be localized to the left axilla and the infrascapular areas. Unless there is clinical evidence of CHF, the third and fourth heart sounds are usually absent.

The differential diagnosis of the systolic ejection murmur in the neonate includes peripheral pulmonary artery stenosis, pulmonary valvar stenosis, and PDA. Soft, high-frequency, continuous murmurs, possibly emanating from aorto-aortic collaterals, may be heard throughout the chest, neck, and back.

ELECTROCARDIOGRAM. In the neonate and young infant who have aortic coarctation, the ECG may indicate right ventricular hypertrophy with or without strain and a right axis deviation pattern. The pattern derives from pressure overload secondary to the right ventricle supplying blood to the lower extremities. With ductal closure and worsening stenosis within the aorta, the right ventricular hypertrophy pattern may regress and convert to the more commonly seen left ventricular hypertrophy pattern. In cases of CHF, left atrial enlargement may also be indicated. Rarely, in some older patients in whom collateral vasculature has developed to bypass the aortic coarctation, the ECG may be normal.

CHEST RADIOGRAPH. In patients who have significant symptomatology, chest radiography may demonstrate both mild cardiomegaly and prominent pulmonary vascular markings consistent with CHF. A characteristic "3 sign" may be noted caused by the shelflike narrowing of the aorta (Fig. 198-6). In patients who have severe aortic coarctation and significant aorto-aortic collaterals, rib notching secondary to enlarged intercostal vasculature may lend supporting evidence for this diagnosis. Such notching occurs mainly in children older than 5 years of age. Prominence of the ascending and descending aorta may be identified, as well.

ECHOCARDIOGRAPHY. The echocardiogram is useful in confirming the diagnosis and determining associated abnormalities such as aortic valve lesions or a VSD. Two-dimensional echocardiography usually also will demonstrate the location of a discrete versus long-segment coarctation, which has important implications for treatment. In some older and larger patients, MRI may be necessary to delineate aortic anatomy fully.

CARDIAC CATHETERIZATION. Cardiac catheterization and angiography are useful in defining aorto-aortic collaterals that may not be visualized well on other studies and to define the nature of any obstruction further. Hemodynamic measurements of left ventricular function and coronary artery anatomy also can be defined. Transcatheter interventions for coarctation of the aorta can be performed in the cardiac catheterization laboratory by isolated balloon angioplasty and, more recently, by balloon angioplasty with associated endovascular stent implantation. Overall, the procedure successfully reduces systolic gradients in 65% to 75% of patients.[36] In patients who have gradients between the ascending and the descending aorta of greater than 50 mm Hg, success rates drop to below 50%.

TREATMENT. In the neonate who has severe left and/or right ventricular failure, attempts to reopen the ductus arteriosus (using standard infusions of prostaglandin E_1) are necessary to increase descending aortic flow and to reverse the metabolic acidosis and anuria seen in these patients. Stabilization of the patients by using either intravenous or oral inotropic support has improved survival and outcomes. In the neonate or infant who demonstrates clear evidence of CHF, intervention becomes more critical. Indications for intervention in the older child include systemic systolic hypertension unmanageable by medical therapy, systolic gradients be-

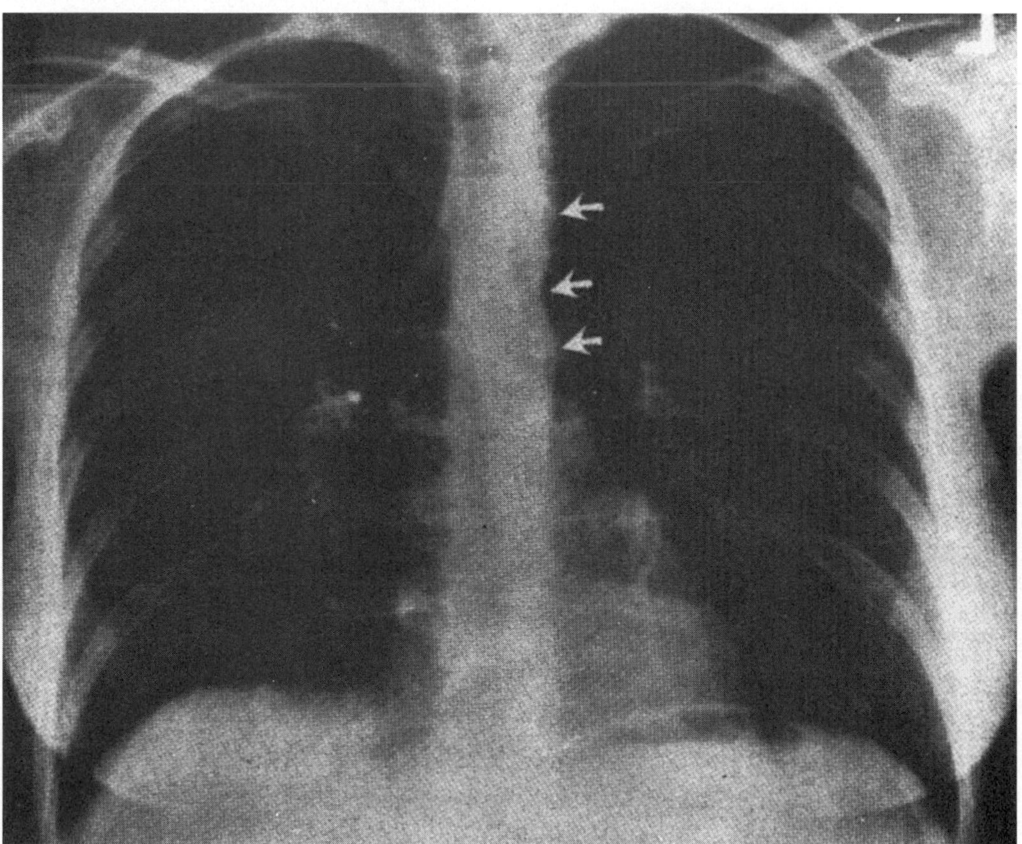

Fig. 198-6 Anteroposterior chest radiograph demonstrating characteristic "3 sign" (defined by arrows) in patient who has aortic coarctation.

tween upper and lower extremities of at least 25 mm Hg, or significant ventricular dysfunction.

Surgical repair of coarctation was first reported in the late 1930s and early 1940s and has undergone multiple transitions. Initial repair involved excision of the coarcted segment and reanastomosis of the two ends (end-to-end anastomosis).[18] Modifications of this operation have included resection of the discrete shelf and enlargement of the isthmus and descending aorta with a patch (patch aortoplasty) or bypass of the coarcted segment by turn-down of the ipsilateral subclavian artery (subclavian flap angioplasty).[55,56] Surgical repairs of these lesions have been somewhat complicated by restenosis after end-to-end anastomosis (as high as 40% in younger children), and by aneurysm formation at the site of repair following patch aortoplasty or subclavian flap angioplasty repair in upward of 30% of patients. Postoperative complications include postcoarctectomy syndrome, which manifests with acute onset of severe systolic and diastolic hypertension. The etiology of this complication may be transsection of sympathetic and parasympathetic nerves during surgery. Control of blood pressure by using various agents (i.e., beta-blockers, methyldopa) has proved effective. The incidence of postcoarctectomy syndrome in patients undergoing balloon angioplasty of the coarctation is low. Indications for balloon angioplasty are similar to those for surgery, except that patients who have long-segment coarctations (greater than 3 mm in length) are better served by surgical intervention. In a small number of patients who have berry aneurysms of the cerebral vasculature in whom the coarctation is not treated, rupture of aneurysms occurs.

LONG-TERM OUTCOME. A small number of patients developed subvalvar aortic stenosis years following repair of coarctation. Late recoarctation of the aorta may occur in 5% to 10% of patients, requiring a second surgical procedure or transcatheter balloon dilation. Evidence does exist for rebound hypertension during adolescence or young adult life, even with excellent surgical or interventional repairs. Whether the frequency of such hypertension in these patients is greater than would be expected in the general population is unclear. Long-standing hypertension can be managed medically, as with any other patient who has systolic hypertension.

CYANOTIC HEART DISEASE

Approximately 15% to 20% of infants and children who have congenital heart disease will present with cyanosis. This excludes patients in whom cyanosis is secondary to poor cardiac output or left ventricular disease. Most cyanotic congenital heart disease is associated with right-to-left shunts (i.e., systemic venous blood bypasses the lungs and mixes with the systemic arterial circulation.) From an anatomical standpoint, these shunts can occur with normally related great vessels, as in patients who have obstruction to inflow to the right ventricle (i.e., tricuspid atresia) or severe right ventricular outflow tract obstruction (i.e., tetralogy of Fallot, pulmonary atresia). Mixing may occur at the atrial level when obstruction to inflow to the right ventricle is present or at the ventricular septal or ductal level in patients who have true pulmonary outflow tract obstruction. Similarly, in the most extreme form of left heart obstruction, hypoplastic left heart syndrome, inability to generate significant forward flow from the diminutive left ventricle, may cause obligatory right-to-left shunting at the ductal level. In a second large group of patients, the right-to-left shunts may occur when the great vessels are abnormally configured. The most common form of cyanotic heart disease in a neonate is d-transposition of the great arteries, in which the aorta arises from the right ventricle and the pulmonary artery from the left ventricle. In such cases, systemic venous return to the right atrium and right ventricle is then ejected into the aorta without first being oxygenated normally within the lungs. Similarly, fully oxygenated blood returning from the lungs to the left atrium and left ventricle is then ejected back into the pulmonary circulation. In such cases, obligatory right-to-left shunts occur either at the atrial, ventricular, or ductal levels. In the case of double outlet right ventricle, both the pulmonary artery and the aorta arise from the right ventricle and the sole outflow from the left ventricle is through an obligatory VSD. Patients born with truncus arteriosus, in which a single great vessel gives rise to both the aorta and the pulmonary artery, have similar degrees of ventricular shunting. Because significant mixing occurs both through the VSD and within the truncus itself, both pulmonary arterial and aortic oxygen saturations tend to be decreased only minimally.

How cyanotic the child becomes is determined by multiple factors. For example, patients who have severe anemia may have less apparent clinical cyanosis because the absolute amount of reduced, deoxygenated hemoglobin in the capillary bed is limited by the anemia. In patients who have low cardiac output or polycythemia, cyanosis may appear worse because of increased concentrations of reduced hemoglobin in the distal capillary beds. Rarely, in neonates, placental transfusion of blood to the infant will result in polycythemia with transient cyanosis. Brain abscesses occur in up to 2% of patients who have cyanotic heart disease. These are potentially lethal complications and should always be suspected in any cyanotic patient older than 2 years of age who has unremitting headaches, focal neurological signs, or seizures. Treatment is with antibiotics and surgical aspiration of the abscess; even in the 1990s, however, mortality has been nearly 40%.[13]

Evaluation of Cyanosis in the Newborn

In the infant who has no pulmonary or cardiovascular disease, the arterial oxygen level (PaO_2) should be greater than 60 mm Hg after 2 hours of life. In the majority of neonates who have cyanotic heart disease, the PaO_2 is less than 50 mm Hg in room air and responds little to supplemental oxygen (PaO_2 < 150 mm Hg). Usually, carbon dioxide levels are normal or decreased. Conversely, the oxygen level of patients who are cyanotic because of lung disease is quite variable, but such patients usually do respond to supplemental oxygen (PaO_2 > 200 mm Hg). Because of intrinsic problems with gas exchange, carbon dioxide levels in patients who have pulmonary disease tend to be higher than those who have cyanotic heart disease. Other syndromes must be included in the differential diagnosis of cyanosis in the neonate. Mechanical interference with lung function (e.g., meconium aspiration) or persistent fetal circulation may lead to peripheral cyanosis. Polycythemia and methemoglobinemia may give the appearance of cyanosis. Patients in whom hypoglycemia, shock, and/or sepsis are present may appear gray, lethargic, and somewhat cyanotic. Primary central nervous system disease with hypoventilation may lead to cyanosis.

In evaluating the cyanotic neonate, noting the distribution of cyanosis is crucial. Peripheral cyanosis ("acrocyanosis"), involving only the hands and feet, is quite common in the neonate and is usually benign. True central cyanosis involves superficial capillary-rich beds, such as those of the lips, mucous membranes, and nail beds, and is more indicative of cyanotic heart disease. Full assessment of all of the vital signs, including respiratory status, capillary refill, and blood pressures, may assist in directing the examiner to the diagnosis. Assisting in the evaluation is the remainder of the physical examination, focusing on the presence or absence of murmurs, abnormalities of heart sounds, presence of systolic clicks, and hyperactivity of the precordium. Imperative to differentiating cardiac versus pulmonary etiologies of cyanosis is evaluation of the arterial blood gas sample. Ideally, samples should be obtained from a preductal position (either an umbilical arterial catheter placed in the transverse aortic arch or from the right arm) and a postductal position (left arm, low-lying umbilical artery catheter), looking for differential saturations reflecting right-to-left shunting at the ductal level. Testing should be performed both in room air and in 100% oxygen. Routine blood tests (complete blood count, glucose levels, and blood cultures) should be obtained, with more extensive testing when indicated either by history or physical examination. Chest radiography can be extremely helpful in the neonate in defining the size of the cardiac silhouette and the pulmonary vascular markings. In some cases, the chest radiograph may demonstrate an unanticipated etiology for the cyanosis, such as inadvertent selective intubation of a single bronchus, a congenital diaphragmatic hernia, or an umbilical arterial catheter inadvertently placed in the ductus arteriosus. In some patients who have cyanotic heart disease, characteristic ECG changes of the specific anomaly may be noted. The ultimate test in most cases will be either two-dimensional or Doppler echocardiography or cardiac catheterization.

Initial management of the cyanotic newborn should include oxygen supplementation and, if indicated, stabilization of the airway with endotracheal intubation. Acidosis, hypoglycemia, anemia, or sepsis should be treated aggressively. When suspicion of congenital cyanotic heart disease is high, prostaglandin E_1 therapy should be initiated.

Classification of Cyanotic Heart Disease

Once initial blood gas sampling has increased suspicion of cyanotic heart disease, results of noninvasive testing may allow for broad groupings of cyanotic lesions. Chest radiography becomes valuable in defining degrees of pulmonary over- or undercirculation. Cyanosis with increased pulmonary blood flow by chest radiography increases suspicion for lesions such as:

1. Complete transposition (d-transposition) of the great arteries
2. Total anomalous pulmonary venous return (with potential obstruction to pulmonary venous flow)
3. Truncus arteriosus (with significant pulmonary overcirculation)
4. Some forms of tricuspid atresia (associated with concomitant transposition of the great arteries)
5. Some forms of single ventricular anatomy

On the other hand, chest radiography demonstrating decreased pulmonary blood flow raises suspicion for right ventricular inflow or right ventricular outflow tract disease such as:

1. Critical pulmonary valve stenosis
2. Tetralogy of Fallot (with significant infundibular, valvar, and supravalvar pulmonary stenosis)
3. Pulmonary atresia (with or without a ventricular septal defect)
4. Most forms of tricuspid atresia.
5. Single-ventricle anatomy and severe pulmonary stenosis
6. Ebstein's anomaly

The ECG may be helpful. For example, in most patients who have tricuspid atresia, the diagnosis can be made simply by the degree of cyanosis and the ECG because of a characteristic leftward and superior QRS axis (0 degrees to -90 degrees), and associated ECG indicators of right atrial enlargement and left ventricular hypertrophy. Similarly, lesions that have significant RVOTO may present with more apparent and significant right ventricular hypertrophy on electrocardiography than is present in the average neonate. However, in many other cardiac lesions, the ECG may not be diagnostic.

Specific Lesions

Tetralogy of Fallot (Fig. 198-7). Beyond the neonatal period, tetralogy of Fallot is the most common form of cyanotic congenital heart disease (approximately 5% of patients). Anatomically, tetralogy of Fallot encompasses four components, primary among which is a large VSD with malaligned borders. Because of this malalignment, upward compression of the infundibulum and the RVOT occurs, leading to pulmonary outflow tract obstruction and concomitant right ventricular hypertrophy. Aortic attachments to the perimembranous septum lead to an overriding aorta. In many patients, a right aortic arch is identified. In addition, in approximately 5% to 15% of patients, the left anterior descending artery arises directly from the right coronary artery, which may have significant technical implications at the time of surgical repair.

The etiology of this lesion is unknown. Although it has been reported to follow maternal rubella during the first trimester of pregnancy, it is not closely associated. Tetralogy of Fallot occurs in 8% of patients who have Down syndrome and about 1% of patients who have Noonan's syndrome. There is a slight predominance among males.

CLINICAL PRESENTATION. Many patients who have tetralogy of Fallot present in the neonatal period for murmur evaluation. Because the VSD is large and nonrestrictive, the murmur that is auscultated usually is not caused by the VSD but rather by the RVOT obstruction. The differential diagnosis of such systolic ejection murmurs in the relatively "acya-

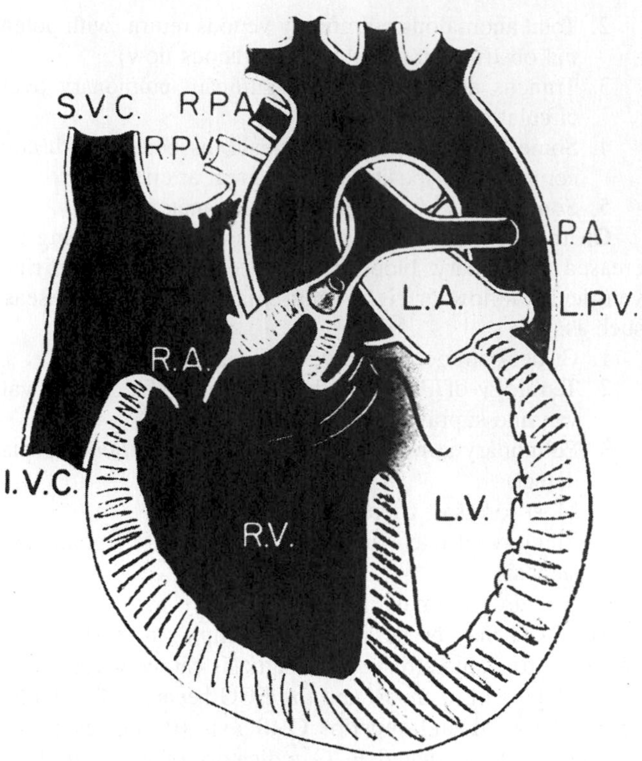

Fig. 198-7 Schematic drawing of major lesions in tetralogy of Fallot. Note significant aortic override, infundibular pulmonary stenosis, and hypoplasia of main and branch pulmonary arteries. *IVC,* Inferior vena cava; *LA,* left atrium; *LPA,* left pulmonary artery; *LPV,* left pulmonary vein; *LV,* left ventricle; *RA,* right atrium; *RPA,* right pulmonary artery; *RPV,* right pulmonary vein; *RV,* right ventricle; *SVC,* superior vena cava.

notic" newborn includes valvar pulmonary stenosis, peripheral pulmonary artery stenosis, PDA, and ASD. In many patients, RVOTO is progressive and may not be complete in the early neonatal period so that the neonate rarely is significantly cyanotic. Similarly, beyond the neonatal period, children who do not appear clinically cyanotic may present with a murmur. Pulse oximetry documentation of mild cyanosis along with a characteristic murmur should raise suspicion for this diagnosis.

A classic presentation in the infant is with a "hyperpneic spell," or tetralogy spell. These spells are postulated to occur secondary to infundibular spasm, causing decreased pulmonary blood flow. Precipitating mechanisms are multiple, although more commonly they occur on awakening in the morning and may be related to mild dehydration from limited oral intake during the night. Episodes also can occur when the infant performs a Valsalva maneuver during bowel movements or when crying. Right-to-left shunting at the ventricular level increases cyanosis. Systemic blood pressure usually is maintained. However, diminished systemic oxygenation leads to rapid initiation of metabolic acidosis, further worsening the infundibular spasm and branch pulmonary artery constriction. Such spells may, in fact, lead to a syncopal episode. At this point, however, autonomic mechanisms may cause the child to breathe more calmly and the infundibular spasm to abate. The appearance of such cyanotic spells is a semi-emergent indication for intervention with an aortopulmonary shunt or a complete surgical repair.

Exercise tolerance is related directly to the severity of the RVOTO. In patients who have relatively mild obstruction and normal oxygen saturations, exercise tolerance is not decreased. However, in more severe cases, excessive cyanosis (resulting in polycythemia) and diminished oxygenation may lead to diminished exercise activity.

Patients whose palliative surgery is delayed until 3 or 4 years of age may assume a "squatting" position frequently. Physiologically, bending the knees increases systemic vascular resistance and decreases systemic venous return, leading to increased left-to-right shunting and improved oxygenation. Patients rarely present with evidence of CHF, because the inherent pulmonary stenosis prevents pulmonary overcirculation. In patients who have an absent pulmonary valve or significant aortopulmonary collaterals, however, pulmonary overcirculation may be present and CHF may develop.

PHYSICAL EXAMINATION. In the most severe cases, the physical examination is dominated by significant cyanosis. The cyanosis may be generalized or limited to the lips, mucous membranes, or nail beds. With persistent cyanosis in the young child or adolescent, clubbing of the nail beds also may be seen. Palpation of the chest often reveals a quiet precordium and limited apical impulse. Usually, patients who have tetralogy of Fallot have normal blood pressures and heart rates. The first heart sound is normal, but consistent with severe pulmonary stenosis; the second sound may be either narrowly split or single. The second heart sound usually is of normal intensity or loudest at the upper left sternal border but may only reflect aortic valve closure. In the presence of significant pulmonary valvar disease, there may be a soft systolic ejection click. The ejection sound also may arise from the aortic valve because of increased transvalvar blood flow. The third and fourth heart sounds are not auscultated routinely in this disorder. Most patients present with systolic ejection murmurs along the left upper sternal borders with radiation to the axilla and the back, reflecting the RVOT disease. Because the VSD is large and nonrestrictive (i.e., no pressure gradient between ventricles), little if any murmur is generated there. The systolic ejection murmur may be either crescendo/decrescendo or holosystolic. Presence of the murmur is important when trying to differentiate between true hypercyanotic spells and other causes of distress. During a hypercyanotic spell, the loud systolic ejection murmur present previously usually decreases both in intensity and frequency as flow across the RVOT decreases. In contrast, in cases of apparent "cyanosis" not related to tetralogy of Fallot, the intensity and loudness of any murmur remains unchanged during these spells. Diastolic murmurs are rare but if present may represent aortic insufficiency. In a patient who has tetralogy of Fallot and no pulmonary valve, a "to-fro" murmur (secondary to combined pulmonary stenosis and insufficiency) may be heard. If aortopulmonary collaterals are present, continuous murmurs may be heard in the axilla and back.

ELECTROCARDIOGRAM. Common findings on the ECG include right axis deviation of the QRS complexes and right ventricular hypertrophy (dominant R wave in the right precordial leads, S wave in the left precordial leads). Because the right ventricular pressure does not exceed systemic pressure, severe right ventricular hypertrophy is rare. There may be T-wave inversion in the right precordial leads. Right atrial

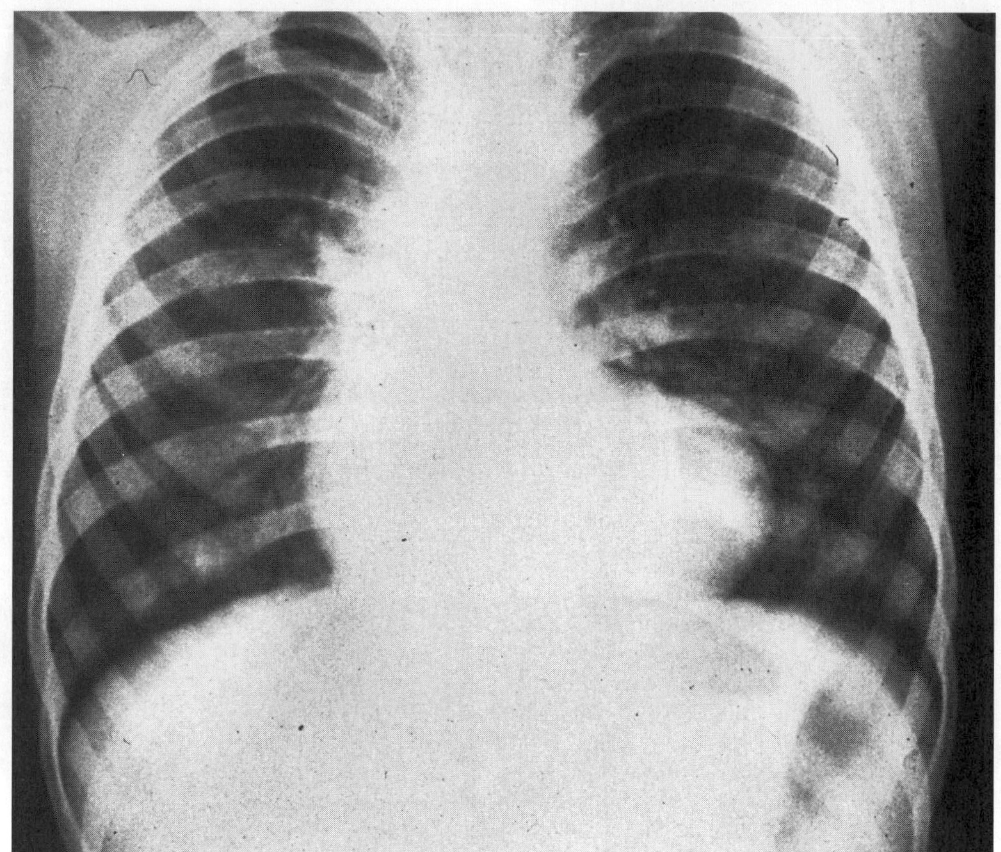

Fig. 198-8 Chest radiograph in a patient who has tetralogy of Fallot, demonstrating the "coeur de sabot" (boot-shaped heart) secondary to hypoplasia of main pulmonary artery.

enlargement is uncommon in infants and children but may be seen in adults. Conduction abnormalities are rare; in older patients, particularly following surgical repair of this lesion, premature ventricular contractions and varying degrees of heart block may be identified. Varying degrees of right bundle branch block also can be seen before and following surgical repair.

CHEST RADIOGRAPH. The classic chest radiograph in patients who have tetralogy of Fallot is a "coeur de sabot" (boot-shaped heart) cardiac silhouette reflective of the hypoplastic main pulmonary segment and upturned hypertrophied right ventricular apex (Fig. 198-8). It is important to determine the sidedness of the aortic arch, because approximately 20% of patients who have tetralogy of Fallot will have a right aortic arch, which becomes important from a surgical standpoint. Pulmonary vascular markings usually are normal or decreased, although in cases of tetralogy of Fallot and absent pulmonary valve, the pulmonary arteries and vascular markings may, in fact, appear full.

ECHOCARDIOGRAPHY. Echocardiography is valuable for confirming the diagnosis, identifying the level of RVOTO, defining the location and number of VSD(s), gauging the degree of right ventricular hypertrophy, delineating coronary and pulmonary artery anatomy, and revealing associated anomalies such as an absent pulmonary valve or pulmonary artery, ASDs, or abnormal origin of the left anterior descending coronary artery.

CARDIAC CATHETERIZATION. Angiography further defines the branch and hilar/parenchymal pulmonary arteries (which may not be fully visualized by echocardiography), and defects in the ventricular septum (Fig. 198-9). In some patients, aortography also reveals the presence of aortopulmonary collaterals. Coronary angiography confirms the location of the left anterior descending artery. In a small number of neonates, balloon valvuloplasty of the stenotic pulmonary valve has been performed as a temporizing procedure before full surgical repair. In many centers, diagnostic cardiac catheterization has been replaced by noninvasive imaging modalities.

TREATMENT. Medical management is important both before and after surgical repair. In the presence of increasing cyanosis, hemoglobin levels must be monitored carefully to avoid polycythemia and resultant complications (stroke, embolic phenomenon, brain abscess).

Hypercyanotic spells are a cardiovascular emergency. The majority of such spells respond to conservative measures such as calming of the child, administration of fluid boluses (10 ml/kg), and knee-to-chest maneuvers. If available, oxygen should be administered. In more severe spells, sodium bicarbonate boluses (1 to 2 mEq/kg) and intravenous sedation (morphine sulfate, lorazepam) can be valuable. Intravenous administration of beta-blocking agents (e.g., propranolol) may reduce infundibular spasm and improve cyanosis. If these standard measures do not resolve the spell, intravenous or intramuscular ketamine (1 to 2 mg/kg) or general anesthesia followed by emergency surgical intervention may be necessary. Oral beta-blockers have been administered prophylactically to prevent such spells.

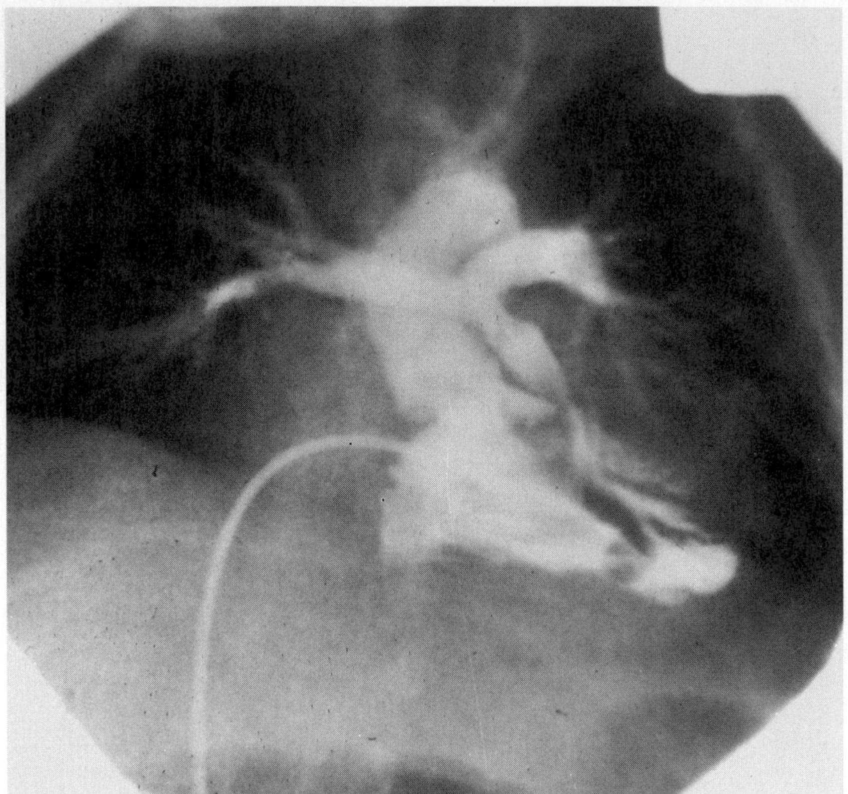

Fig. 198-9 Spot left ventricular cineangiogram in a patient who has tetralogy of Fallot. Aortic root dilation, severe infundibular muscular stenosis, and hypoplasia of the branch pulmonary arteries are shown.

Surgical intervention can be either palliative (Blalock-Taussig aortopulmonary shunt to increase pulmonary blood flow) or complete intracardiac repair. Most centers prefer to delay a complete repair until the child reaches 6 to 12 months of age, unless the child demonstrates increasing cyanosis. In cases in which the pulmonary arteries are small, a shunt may be performed in an attempt to increase their size by increasing pulmonary blood flow. Complete repair of the lesion involves closure of the VSD and varying approaches to enlargement of RVOT. In cases of significant infundibular stenosis, surgical myomectomy is indicated.

Surgical mortality is low, ranging in most centers from 2% to 4%. Residual hemodynamic abnormalities, however, are common and may include RVOTO or a VSD. More data are accumulating about long-term consequences of tetralogy of Fallot repair pertaining to significant ventricular dysrhythmias and sudden unexpected death.[58] Investigators have described a possible association between either right bundle branch block or left anterior hemiblock and sudden cardiac events, but no significant correlation has been proven. Twenty-four-hour Holter monitoring is necessary every 2 to 5 years because evidence of subclinical paroxysmal ventricular tachycardia is a potential harbinger for fatal ventricular dysrhythmias of other types.

Pulmonary valve atresia/ventricular septal defect. Pulmonary valve atresia and ventricular septal defect (PA/VSD) is considered to be the most extreme form of tetralogy of Fallot. These lesions are not rare, accounting for approximately 2% of patients in the New England Regional Heart Program. This diagnosis must be considered in the neonate who has significant cyanosis unresponsive to prostaglandin therapy.

Embryologically, PA/VSD occurs early in gestation before significant development of the pulmonary arteries. Consequently, management is more complicated than for most patients who have tetralogy of Fallot. Although deformities of the pulmonary arteries may accompany tetralogy of Fallot, they remain in continuity with the right ventricle. By definition, patients who have PA/VSD lack such continuity and are prone to severe hypoplasia of the pulmonary arteries or even discontinuity of the right and left branch vessels. Patients may depend on aortopulmonary collateral flow to supply their parenchymal pulmonary arteries. In some patients, either aortopulmonary collateral flow and/or flow from the PDA may supply all of the lung tissue, but only rarely do both sources of pulmonary blood flow coexist in the same lung. The aortopulmonary collaterals in the majority of cases arise from the descending thoracic aorta, although they also can arise from the subclavian arteries, abdominal aorta, or even the coronary arteries themselves. They are variable in number and diameter. In many patients, stenoses occur somewhere within this system.

PA/VSD is associated with a right aortic arch in up to 50% of cases, and a secundum ASD is present in approximately 50% of patients. Other associated anomalies include a persistent left superior vena cava connecting to the coronary sinus, abnormalities of the coronary sinus itself, abnormalities of pulmonary venous return, tricuspid valve abnormalities, complete atrioventricular canal, and transposition of the great arteries. Usually, the origin and distribution of the coronary arteries are normal.

CLINICAL PRESENTATION. The majority of patients present during the neonatal period, with the levels of hypoxemia and cyanosis depending on the volume of aortopulmonary collateral flow. While the ductus arteriosus is still patent, patients may be asymptomatic and only minimally cyanotic; however, with natural closure of the ductus, they become more hypoxemic. Because many who have this lesion have significant aortopulmonary collaterals, cyanosis may not be severe because of adequate pulmonary blood flow. In the face of inadequate aortopulmonary collateral vessels, however, hypoxemia may be severe, and prostaglandin E_1 therapy should be initiated to maintain ductal patency until surgery can be performed. The natural history of collaterals is for them to become more stenotic with advancing age, leading to worsening cyanosis. Although rare, patients who have extensive collateral flow may present with pulmonary overcirculation and CHF after 4 to 6 weeks of age. In such patients, standard medical therapy for CHF is indicated. The major presenting signs beyond the neonatal period are mild cyanosis and/or the presence of multiple continuous murmurs heard throughout the chest, back, and axillae consistent with the presence of aortopulmonary collaterals.

PHYSICAL EXAMINATION. Cyanosis usually is present in the early neonatal period except in the presence of a large PDA or significant aortopulmonary collaterals. In general, growth and development are delayed, although if pulmonary flow is adequate and cyanosis minimal, they may be normal. Early on, peripheral pulses and blood pressure are normal, even in patients who have large aortopulmonary collaterals. Beyond the neonatal period, however, large runoff lesions, either from the collaterals or the ductus arteriosus, may lead to widened pulse pressures and fuller pulses. Other signs and symptoms of CHF, such as hepatosplenomegaly and venous distention, are rare but can occur. The cardiac impulse usually is prominent at the left lower sternal border, and some patients may have a systolic thrill. Patients usually demonstrate normal first heart sounds and single second heart sounds, because of the absence of the pulmonary valve. Systolic murmurs do not represent the outflow tract obstruction, but rather the VSD or concomitant atrioventricular valve insufficiency. In older patients, as noted, continuous murmurs may be heard throughout the chest, back, and axillae.

ELECTROCARDIOGRAM. The ECG pattern is consistent with significant RVOTO. Right ventricular and right atrial hypertrophy and also right axis deviation of the QRS complex are most common. In patients who have CHF caused by pulmonary overcirculation from aortopulmonary collaterals, similar changes in left-sided voltages may be seen.

CHEST RADIOGRAPH. The "boot-shaped heart" is the most classic radiographic presentation in this lesion, similar to patients who have tetralogy of Fallot. Likewise, chest radiography is valuable in identifying sidedness of the aortic arch. Pulmonary vascular markings may be heterogeneous, not conforming to the usual pattern present with normal, pulmonary vessels.

ECHOCARDIOGRAPHY. The value of echocardiography is in confirming the diagnosis and clarifying other issue such as abnormalities of the atrioventricular connections, the number and location of atrial and/or ventricular septal defects, and anomalies of the systemic venous circulations and the aortic arch. However, echocardiography may not fully delineate aortopulmonary collaterals.

CARDIAC CATHETERIZATION. The principal indication for cardiac catheterization in this condition is an angiographic study of the aortopulmonary collaterals (Fig. 198-10). It defines the number of collaterals, the location of their origin from the aorta, and the segments of lung supplied. The hypoplastic native pulmonary arteries can be identified by retrograde filling from the aortopulmonary collaterals or by a pulmonary vein contrast injection and backfilling of the native pulmonary arteries. In addition, confluence of the proximal native pulmonary arteries is defined, which becomes important in eventual surgical repair.

TREATMENT. Therapy is primarily surgical. In the face of significant hypoxemia caused by spontaneous closure of the PDA and/or progressive stenosis of the aortopulmonary collaterals, a systemic to pulmonary shunt (i.e., Blalock-Taussig shunt) may be indicated either in the immediate neonatal period or in infancy. This shunt also may aid in increasing the size of the native pulmonary arteries. The goal of surgical intervention is to reconstitute normal continuity between the right ventricle and the pulmonary vasculature, which at times can be performed in one stage or may need to be performed in multiple stages, depending on the location of collaterals and severity of collateral stenoses. Such repairs always include creation of a right ventricle to pulmonary artery conduit. When pulmonary blood flow from the right ventricle to the lungs is sufficient, the VSD can be closed surgically. In patients who have less complex forms of this condition, minimally hypoplastic pulmonary arteries, and mild main pulmonary artery hypoplasia, the prognosis and late issues of concern are identical to those of patients who have true tetralogy of Fallot. A significant proportion of patients eventually will require replacement of their conduits as they either outgrow them or they develop stenosis and insufficiency. Patients who have residual pulmonary artery disease, right ventricular hypertension, or severe pulmonary artery abnormalities in whom only palliation can be performed may have less positive long-term outcomes.

Pulmonary atresia with intact ventricular septum (Fig. 198-11). Pulmonary atresia with intact ventricular septum (PA/IVS) is, in fact, a complex of significant right heart abnormalities that in many cases has poor long-term outcomes. Although uncommon overall (3% of all congenital defects), about 25% of cyanotic newborns have such lesions. In contrast to PA/VSD, PA/IVS occurs late in development; therefore, the pulmonary arteries of patients who have PA/IVS tend to be of normal size and distribution. Right ventricular and tricuspid anomalies are common. Many patients develop moderate to severe tricuspid insufficiency and significant right atrial dilatation. In other patients who have no tricuspid insufficiency, the right ventricle drains by fistulous connections between it and the coronary artery system. This anatomical problem alone is one of the most significant predictors of short- and long-term survival.

Patients who have PA/IVS have variable right ventricular dimensions, depending on the point in fetal life at which atresia of the pulmonary valve occurred. Earlier valvar atresia is associated with smaller ventricular chamber size. If atresia develops relatively late in gestation following full development of the tricuspid valve and right ventricle, patients may present with severe RVOTO but an otherwise normal right heart. In some patients, an imperforate diaphragm-like membrane beneath a well-formed pulmonary valve may

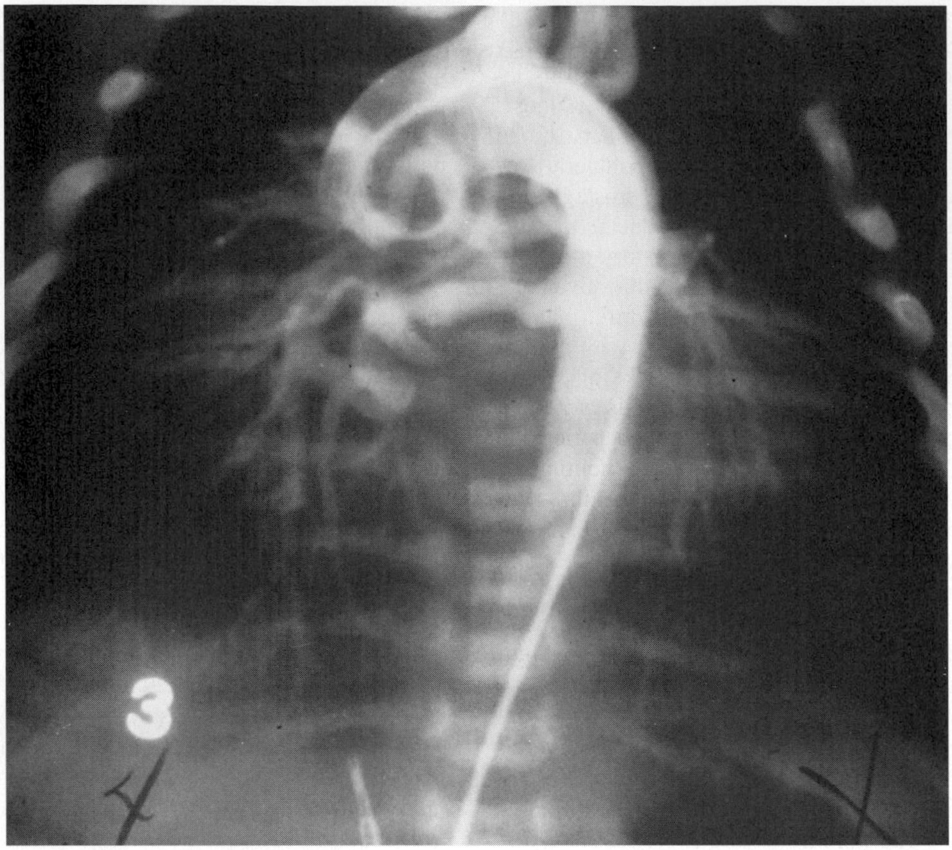

Fig. 198-10 Spot ascending aortic cineangiogram in a patient who has pulmonary atresia and ventricular septal defect. Note the aortic collateral flow into both the right and left pulmonary arteries.

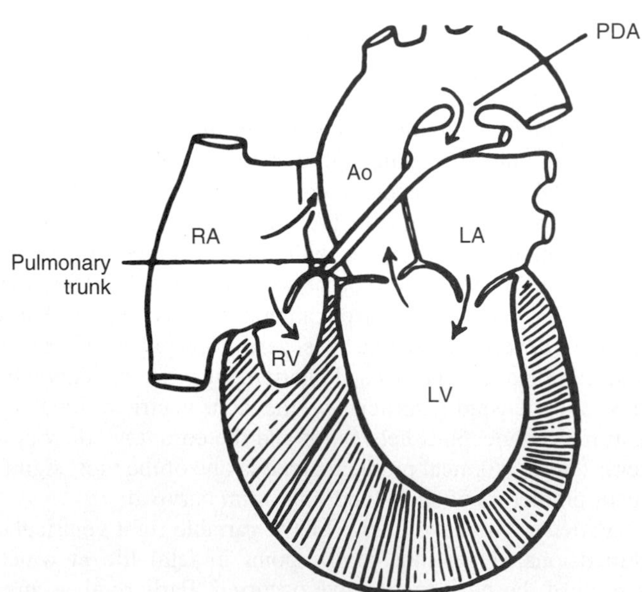

Fig. 198-11 Schematic drawing of patient who has pulmonary atresia and intact ventricular septum. Note hypoplasia of right ventricular mass and ductal filling of pulmonary arteries from aorta. *Ao,* Aorta; *LA,* left atrium; *LV,* left ventricle; *PDA,* patent ductus arteriosus; *RA,* right atrium; *RV,* right ventricle.

cause the "atresia." Significant aortopulmonary collateral vessels rarely are present at birth.

CLINICAL PRESENTATION. As with the other forms of severe RVOTO, the initial clinical symptom is significant cyanosis within hours or days after birth in conjunction with ductal involution and closure. Because these patients lack significant aortopulmonary collaterals, development of severe cyanosis usually is rapid and may be accompanied by progressive hypoxemia and metabolic acidosis with increasing evidence of right ventricular failure. Some neonates present with severe intrauterine tricuspid valve insufficiency and the classic signs and symptoms of CHF.

PHYSICAL EXAMINATION. General physical examination usually is unremarkable except for cyanosis. Vital signs tend to be normal except for some mild tachypnea. Palpation of the precordium usually is unremarkable. The first and second heart sounds are normal in intensity, but the second heart sound is single. No systolic ejection clicks are identified, and in many patients no murmurs are heard. If a systolic ejection murmur is identified, it may be due to the PDA. In patients who have severe tricuspid insufficiency, loud holosystolic murmurs may be heard at the right or left lower sternal borders. The regurgitant murmur must be differentiated from the similar sound of a VSD.

ELECTROCARDIOGRAM. The most striking findings on ECG are severe right ventricular hypertrophy with strain, right atrial enlargement, and a somewhat leftward axis (between 0 degrees and 90 degrees). The latter finding may be due to a paucity of right ventricular muscle mass to create sufficient right-sided voltages.

CHEST RADIOGRAPH. The majority of patients who have PA/IVS present with a normal to small cardiac silhouette and diminished pulmonary vascular markings. Patients who have associated severe tricuspid insufficiency may manifest severe cardiomegaly and right atrial enlargement. In contrast to patients who have pulmonary valve atresia and VSD, a right aortic arch is rare.

ECHOCARDIOGRAPHY. Two-dimensional echocardiography is diagnostic by demonstrating an intact ventricular septum and the absence of antegrade flow from the right ventricle to the pulmonary arteries. Early in the neonatal period when the patient has a PDA, there may be retrograde filling of the pulmonary arteries from the aorta. Determining the size of the tricuspid valve and the dimensions of the right ventricular mass and infundibulum are important in deciding which surgical procedure(s) are necessary. Color Doppler flow studies are invaluable in determining presence and degree of coronary sinusoidal flow.

CARDIAC CATHETERIZATION. In many patients, cardiac catheterization and angiography become crucial in defining the presence of coronary artery fistulae and sinusoids. In many patients who have sinusoidal connections between the apex of the right ventricle and the left anterior descending coronary artery, significant coronary stenoses may be found where the abnormal sinusoid meets with the normal coronary artery. In patients who have "membranous" pulmonary atresia, either standard balloon valvuloplasty or catheter perforation of the membrane may be performed.[47]

TREATMENT. Initial therapy should address maintaining ductal patency, particularly with worsening cyanosis and/or right heart failure. This usually can be achieved by initiation of a prostaglandin E_1 infusion. Supportive measures correcting hypoxemia and acidosis and improving the oxygen-carrying capacity of the blood (if necessary, with blood transfusions) should be performed. In the face of significant CHF, afterload reduction and/or inotropic support can be utilized. Following stabilization, if patients do not have lesions thought to be amenable to transcatheter therapy, surgical intervention becomes mandatory. Systemic to pulmonary arterial shunts, pulmonary valvulotomy, or combinations of these interventions have all been proposed as initial palliations, depending on the degree of right heart hypoplasia. Each case mandates its own surgical approach. A significant factor in long-term survival is the presence or absence of the coronary sinusoidal connections with coronary artery stenosis. Any operation or procedure that lowers systemic vascular resistance or arterial blood flow will have a direct influence on coronary filling and potential myocardial ischemia. In many centers, in patients who have severe coronary artery fistulae, primary orthotopic cardiac transplantation becomes the treatment option of choice, because of fears regarding precarious coronary supply to the ventricular mass.

Tricuspid atresia. Tricuspid atresia is a fairly uncommon form of congenital heart disease occurring in approximately 2.7% of patients in the New England Regional Infant Cardiac Program. There is complete agenesis of the tricuspid valve, and depending on associated anomalies, there may be hypoplasia of the remainder of the right heart. There is a slight male predominance of this lesion, and 20% of patients may have extracardiac abnormalities involving the musculoskeletal or gastrointestinal tracts.

Three different types of tricuspid atresia with associated anomalies have been broadly categorized. In approximately 70% of patients, tricuspid atresia exists in the face of normally related great vessels. In approximately 20% to 30% of patients, tricuspid atresia exists with d-transposition of the great arteries (aorta arising from right ventricle, pulmonary artery arising from left ventricle). Physiologically, such patients will behave as if they have mitral valve atresia and/or hypoplastic left heart syndrome. In 3% to 7% of patients, l-transposition of the great arteries (both ventricular and arterial inversion) is found. Such patients will be similar physiologically to those patients who have d-transposition of the great arteries. The presence of varying degrees of pulmonary stenosis and atresia and the presence and size of VSDs will subcategorize patients further. More than 80% have an ASD.[51]

Additionally, patients can have varying degrees of pulmonary obstruction, subaortic stenosis, or even coarctations of the aorta. Other anomalies include a persistent left superior vena cava, a PDA, and aortic arch abnormalities.

CLINICAL PRESENTATION. More than 50% of patients who have tricuspid atresia present with cyanosis within the first day of life; the remainder present within 1 month. Depending on the arrangement of the great vessels, patients can either present with low cardiac output and with diminished pulmonary blood flow (patients who have an intact ventricular septum and pulmonary atresia) or in CHF, secondary to excessive pulmonary blood flow (d-transposition of the great arteries with a large VSD and no pulmonary stenosis). This latter configuration is relatively uncommon. Patients have obligatory right-to-left shunts at the atrial septal level and may have left-to-right shunts at the ventricular level, as well. Infants may present with sudden-onset hypoxic spells related to spontaneous closure of the VSD or worsening infundibular stenosis. Some patients who have severe cyanosis and concomitant polycythemia may present with cerebrovascular accidents or brain abscesses, particularly following acute febrile illnesses. In subgroups of patients who have tricuspid atresia and diminished pulmonary blood flow, marked cyanosis and poor growth may occur. Clubbing may be identified on physical examination, occurring in more than 70%.

PHYSICAL EXAMINATION. In general, patients tend to have cyanosis, delayed growth, and clubbing. Other findings on physical examination in patients who have tricuspid atresia depend on associated anomalies. For example, in patients who have moderate-size VSDs and pulmonary valve stenosis, regurgitant and ejection murmurs may be heard, respectively. A dominant left ventricular impulse may be palpated. The first heart sound tends to be single (because of the absence of the tricuspid valve) and may be accentuated. The second heart sound in patients who have diminished pulmonary flow may be single or may be normally split. Patients who have a restrictive ASD may have a prominent fourth heart sound.

ELECTROCARDIOGRAM. In many cases, the ECG is diagnostic. In more than 95% of patients, the ECG demonstrates a leftward and superior axis (0 degrees to -90 degrees). Other lesions that have a similar QRS axis deviation include inlet VSDs or atrioventricular canal defects. In many cases, evidence of right atrial hypertrophy, decreased right ventricular forces, and increased left ventricular forces confirms the diagnosis. In patients who have a normal right ventricular mass, normal right-sided voltages may be noted. First-degree AV block is rare, even though the right atrium is dilated. Ischemic ST depressions and T-wave changes are common, particularly in patients who have increased pulmonary flow and ventricular volume overload.

CHEST RADIOGRAPH. Chest radiography varies depending on the constellation of anatomical abnormalities. Patients who have pulmonary atresia may have diminished pulmonary blood flow or, where pulmonary stenosis is minimal, markedly increased pulmonary blood flow. Similarly, normal, increased, or decreased cardiac silhouette dimensions may be seen, depending on the anatomy.

ECHOCARDIOGRAPHY. Echocardiograms provide data concerning the size of the right ventricle, the relationship of the great vessels, the presence and size of atrial and ventricular septal defects, and ventricular systolic function. They also are useful for assessing the sizes of the pulmonary arteries, particularly in patients who have undergone palliative procedures such as Blalock-Taussig shunts. Doppler flow studies are valuable in revealing mitral valve abnormalities, gradients across the VSDs, or other aortopulmonary collateral shunts.

CARDIAC CATHETERIZATION. Cardiac catheterization and angiography are valuable in further defining the relationship of the great vessels, the degree of left-to-right shunting at the ventricular level, and the degree of right-to-left shunting at the atrial level. The distal pulmonary arteries and their possible stenoses can be demonstrated. Also, coronary artery abnormalities may be noted. In patients who have restrictive ASDs, either balloon or blade atrial septostomies can be performed at the time of angiography. Cardiac catheterization is invaluable in documenting pulmonary artery blood flow, pulmonary artery pressures, ventricular systolic and diastolic function, restriction of the atrial septum, aortic valve disease, and distal pulmonary artery anatomy.

TREATMENT. Initial management of the cyanotic neonate with decreased pulmonary blood flow includes maintaining ductal patency by prostaglandin E_1 infusion. In patients presenting with CHF resulting from abnormalities of the great vessels, standard medical management (diuretic therapy, afterload reduction, inotropic support) can be used. In the face of diminished pulmonary blood flow, many patients undergo palliative procedures, including aortopulmonary shunts. Anastomosis of the superior vena cava to the pulmonary artery (Glenn shunt) can be performed between 3 and 6 months of age, and patients undergo the Fontan operation (connection of the inferior vena cava to the pulmonary artery) between 12 and 36 months, although these timeframes vary by patient and surgical center.

Survival into the second decade of life following full surgical intervention is greater than 60%, compared with less than 10% without any form of surgical therapy. Long-term complications following surgery include obstruction to right-sided flow, either within conduits or from thrombosis of vessels. Intracardiac leaks or intrapulmonary shunts may persist, and VSDs or aortopulmonary collaterals that have not been addressed surgically can cause ventricular volume overload and potential ventricular failure. Patients need to be observed for significant atrial dysrhythmias and particularly for complications of systemic venous hypertension, including liver dysfunction and protein-losing enteropathy.

Complete transposition of the great arteries (Fig. 198-12). Complete transposition (d-transposition) of the great arteries, occurring in 5% to 7% of all children who have congenital cardiac malformations, is the most common form of cyanotic heart disease presenting in the neonatal period. The term *transposition* implies that the great vessels arise from the opposite ventricle. Morphologically, the aorta arises from the right ventricle, the pulmonary artery from the left. In cases in which the right atrium and ventricle are in atrioventricular continuity (so that systemic venous blood returns to the right atrium and right ventricle), poorly oxygenated blood is returned to the aorta before passing through the oxygenation cycle in the lungs. Concurrently, fully oxygenated blood returning to the left atrium and left ventricle is ejected to the lungs to become further oxygenated. Thus, instead of normal circulation that is composed of two circulations in series, patients who have transposition of the great arteries have two circulations in parallel and little mixing of oxygenated and deoxygenated blood. Without any form of treatment, approximately 30% of the neonates die within the first week of life, 50% within the first month, and 90% within the first year. There is a strong male preponderance (up to 70%). Commonly, these children are born at full term of multiparous mothers, particularly with insulin-dependent diabetes during pregnancy. Compared with other outflow-tract lesions, such as tetralogy of Fallot and truncus arteriosus, the incidence of extracardiac anomalies is low; however, many of these neonates have other intracardiac lesions.

In most neonates who have transposition, the atria are normally formed. The majority have a patent foramen ovale, and about 5% have a true ASD. About 30% to 35% have a VSD, although in some it is of little hemodynamic consequence. Significant subvalvar LVOTO occurs in approximately 5% of children; true valvar stenosis is rare. Five percent of patients present with a concomitant aortic coarctation, and approximately 60% will have their coronary arteries arise from the appropriate aortic sinuses. However, in approximately 30% of patients, either a single coronary orifice or other permutations of coronary artery anatomy are seen. Usually, this has no clinical implications but is important in complete surgical repair.

CLINICAL PRESENTATION. Neonates who have transposition of the great arteries are usually full term and well-developed. They present with significant cyanosis unresponsive to supplemental oxygen therapy. The degree of cyanosis depends on the number and size of intra- and extracardiac shunts (i.e., PDA, interatrial communication, VSD). In some patients, upper-extremity saturations are lower than lower-extremity saturations because of reversed pulmonary to systemic blood flow through the large PDA. In the neonate, such effects may be transient, but in the older patient

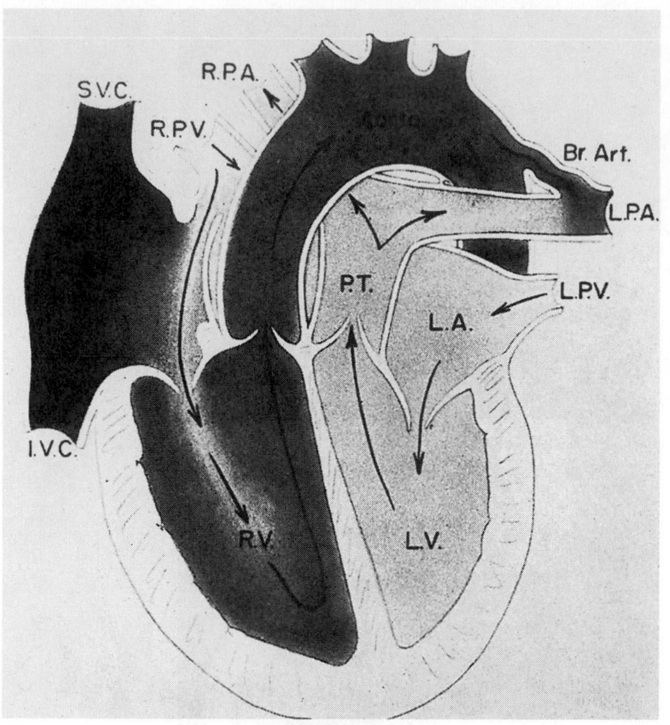

Fig. 198-12 Schematic drawing of complete transposition of the great arteries. The aorta arises directly from the right ventricle and the pulmonary trunk from the left ventricle. There is no significant interatrial or interventricular shunting. *Br Art,* Brachial artery; *IVC,* inferior vena cava; *LA,* left atrium; *LPA,* left pulmonary artery; *LPV,* left pulmonary vein; *LV,* left ventricle; *PT,* pulmonary trunk; *RA,* right atrium; *RPA,* right pulmonary artery; *RPV,* right pulmonary vein; *RV,* right ventricle; *SVC,* superior vena cava.

this may indicate more extensive aortic arch abnormalities. Unlike patients who have significant lung disease, patients who have transposition of the great arteries do not usually present with respiratory distress; however, it is not uncommon for them to develop signs and symptoms of pulmonary overcirculation with advancing age. Therefore, they may develop irreversible pulmonary vascular obstructive disease if left untreated. Whether this is due to an accelerated rate of pulmonary vessel development, the influence of systemic hypoxemia on pulmonary vasoconstriction, or inherent increases in pulmonary vascular muscularity and intimal hyperplasia is unknown. Significant changes in the pulmonary vascular bed (intimal fibrosis, vascular dilation) have developed in the majority of untreated infants older than 1 year of age, particularly if an associated VSD is present.

Hematological abnormalities associated with the cyanotic state, including polycythemia, thrombocytopenia, and coagulopathies, are fairly common and may result in pre- and perioperative complications in patients older than 6 to 9 months of age. Polycythemia may lead to thrombotic lesions within the lungs, kidneys, and central nervous system. Cerebrovascular accidents (more common in those younger than 2 years of age) and brain abscesses (more common in those older than 2 years of age) can occur.

PHYSICAL EXAMINATION. The neonate who has transposition of the great arteries, but no CHF, is usually well appearing except for significant cyanosis and has normal vital signs. Auscultation reveals a normal or loud first heart sound and, in the majority of patients, a single, or loud second heart sound. A second heart sound of normal intensity and normal splitting of the second heart sound may alternatively be heard. No murmur is heard in about 40% of patients, although the majority have a soft ejection murmur, which is nondescript in quality. Murmurs from a VSD or inflow abnormality are rarely heard. When there is significant right or left ventricular outflow tract obstruction, murmurs appropriate for those conditions will be heard.

In patients who have large VSDs who do not appear cyanotic at birth and are diagnosed later in infancy, signs and symptoms of left heart failure may develop within the first 2 to 6 weeks of life. Development of a loud III to IV/VI holosystolic murmur, a third heart sound, and a diastolic rumble are indicators of such a large intracardiac shunt.

ELECTROCARDIOGRAM. The ECG changes are variable. For example, the QRS axis in the neonate with transposition of the great arteries and a VSD may be normal. On the other hand, right QRS axis deviation with right ventricular hypertrophy may be noted. Increasing right ventricular hypertrophy may appear beyond 3 to 5 days of age. Other ECG findings may be present when there are associated lesions (i.e., subpulmonary stenosis, PDA).

CHEST RADIOGRAPH. The classic cardiac silhouette in patients who have transposition of the great arteries is described as an "egg on a string" (Fig. 198-13). This is due to mild ventricular rotation and narrowing of the mediastinum, with the great vessels being aligned in an anteroposterior position, yielding the "string." In the first few days of life, the cardiac silhouette is normal in size or slightly enlarged, and the pulmonary vascular markings are normal or mildly increased. A right aortic arch is relatively uncommon (4% to 11%). Beyond the first few weeks of life, increases in cardiomegaly and pulmonary vascular markings become evident as pulmonary vascular resistance drops. In patients who have residual pulmonary vasoconstriction, vascular markings may be somewhat reduced.

ECHOCARDIOGRAPHY. Echocardiography plays an important diagnostic role. With marked improvement in noninvasive imaging, many patients can undergo complete repair of d-transposition of the great arteries based solely on echocardiographic anatomical evaluation. Besides confirming the

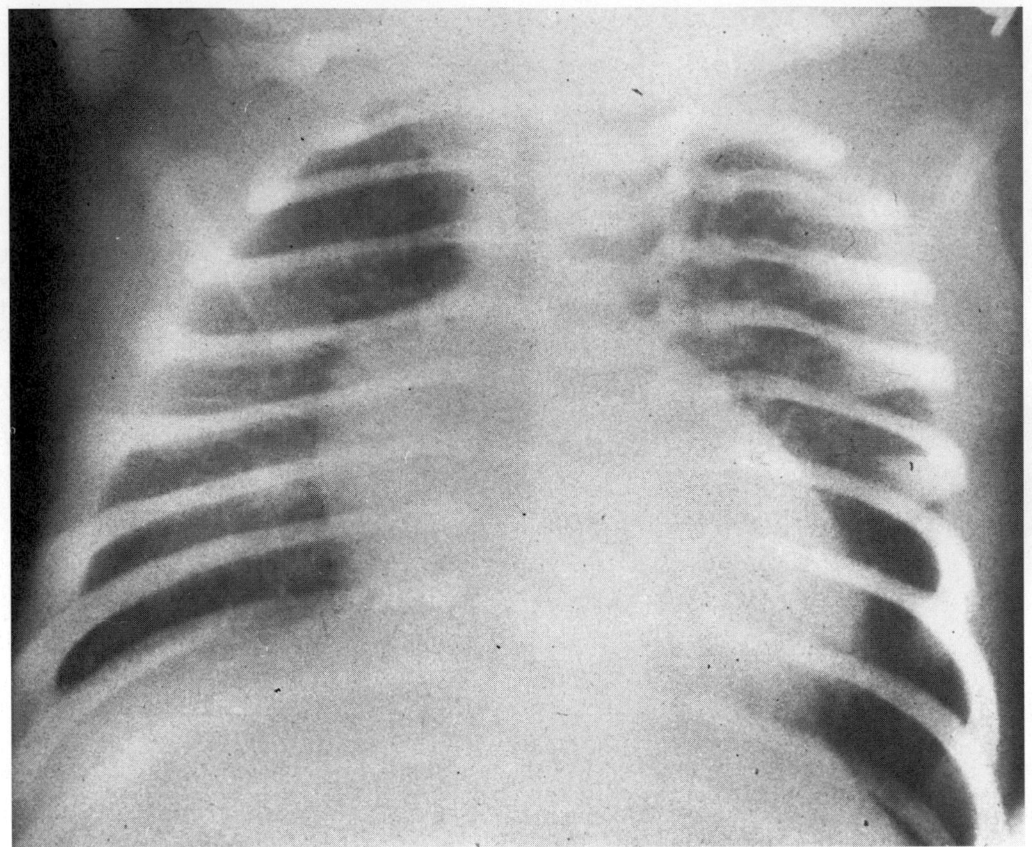

Fig. 198-13 Classic chest radiograph in patients who have d-transposition demonstrating "egg-on-a-string" configuration of cardiac silhouette. The narrow mediastinum is secondary to superimposition of the aorta and pulmonary artery in the anteroposterior plane.

diagnosis, echocardiography is crucial for defining ventricular and atrial septal anatomy and patency of the ductus arteriosus. In the majority of cases, the proximal coronary anatomy can be fully delineated by two-dimensional imaging. Definition of the aortic and pulmonary valves and subvalvar disease is important, as is definition of ventricular size and function. From a treatment standpoint, two-dimensional echocardiography can be invaluable in assisting in the performance of transcatheter balloon atrial septostomy (see below).

CARDIAC CATHETERIZATION. Currently, cardiac catheterization is indicated for better definition of coronary artery anatomy and, in most cases, for emergent transcatheter intervention (e.g., balloon atrial septostomy). Patients who have more complex forms of transposition of the great arteries may undergo full hemodynamic studies to define the anatomy and pulmonary artery pressures, flows, and vascular resistances.

In the late 1960s, Rashkind and Miller[48] noted that enhancement of intracardiac shunting in patients who have d-transposition of the great vessels would improve oxygenation and cardiac output, thus permitting atrial switch surgery at an older age. The procedural details are straightforward (Fig. 198-14). Either femoral venous or umbilical venous access is gained, and a balloon septostomy is performed by pull-through of either the ASD or the patent foramen ovale. Rapid improvement in oxygen saturation follows. Complications of balloon septostomy are rare but can sometimes be life threatening. These include significant atrioventricular valve or pulmonary vein damage or avulsion of the pulmonary veins from the posterior wall of the left atrium. Damage to the inferior vena cava also can occur. Balloon atrial septostomy has improved 1-month survival from 20% to more than 95%.

TREATMENT. Initial management of the neonate depends on presentation. In the face of severe cyanosis, initiation of prostaglandin E_1 therapy to preserve patency of the ductus arteriosus is indicated. Acidosis, hypoglycemia, pulmonary overcirculation, and CHF should be managed with standard medical therapy. The diagnosis should then be confirmed by noninvasive imaging studies. If there is evidence of restriction to atrial blood flow, patients should undergo balloon atrial septostomy.

SURGICAL REPAIR. Blalock and Hanlon first proposed surgical atrial septectomy[5] for this lesion in the early 1950s. In the late 1950s and early 1960s, Senning[52] and Mustard[39] developed the atrial switch operation. In this procedure, either the atrial septum or surgical material is used to channel inferior and superior vena caval flow to the left ventricle so that systemic venous return is then ejected through the transpositioned pulmonary artery to the lungs. Pulmonary venous return similarly is baffled to the right ventricle so that pulmonary venous return then is ejected into the transposed aorta. This surgical approach has been problematic long-term, because the right ventricle is ex-

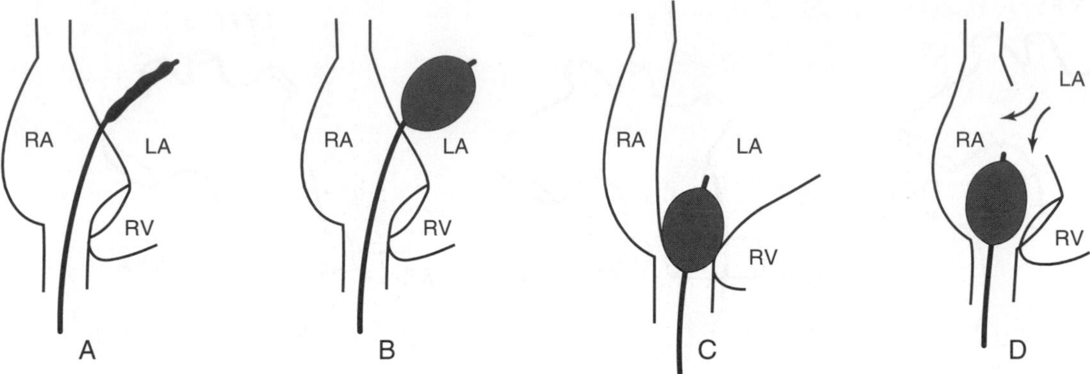

Fig. 198-14 Schematic drawing of balloon atrial septostomy procedure. Balloon catheter is passed across atrial septum into left atrium *(A)*. A balloon is inflated *(B)* and pulled back to cause tear in atrial septum (*C* and *D*). *LA,* Left atrium; *RA,* right atrium; *RV,* right ventricle.

pected to perform systemic work. Although 10-year survival rates of 85% to 90% are reported following surgery, longer follow-up has indicated worsening right ventricular failure and the eventual need for cardiac transplantation.[2] In addition, sinus and AV nodal disease have developed in a large minority of patients, eventually requiring pacemaker implantation.[4] Patients also are at risk for significant atrial and ventricular dysrhythmias.

In contrast, since the late 1970s and early 1980s, the surgical preference in most centers has been an arterial switch operation. In this procedure the pulmonary artery and aorta are transected and then reanastomosed to their appropriate ventricles. The coronary arteries are removed from their original position on the aorta and reimplanted in the new aortic anastomosis. This operation needs to be performed within the first 1 to 3 weeks of life before the left ventricle becomes conditioned to its low-pressure state within the pulmonary circulation. With improving techniques, significant operative morbidity and mortality is 5% or less. The major complication following arterial switch surgery involves coronary kinking or tension on the anastomotic line of the coronary vessels, which may lead to acute myocardial ischemia in the immediate postoperative period. Recent studies of radionucleotide coronary injections have revealed mild diminution of flow in the watershed areas of the distal coronary arteries following arterial switch operation.[21] In addition, concern has been voiced over coronary constriction with growth. Scarring at the anastomotic line, particularly in the suprapulmonary region, has been widely reported.[32] Because the neoaortic valve originally was the pulmonary valve, some patients develop valvar insufficiency.

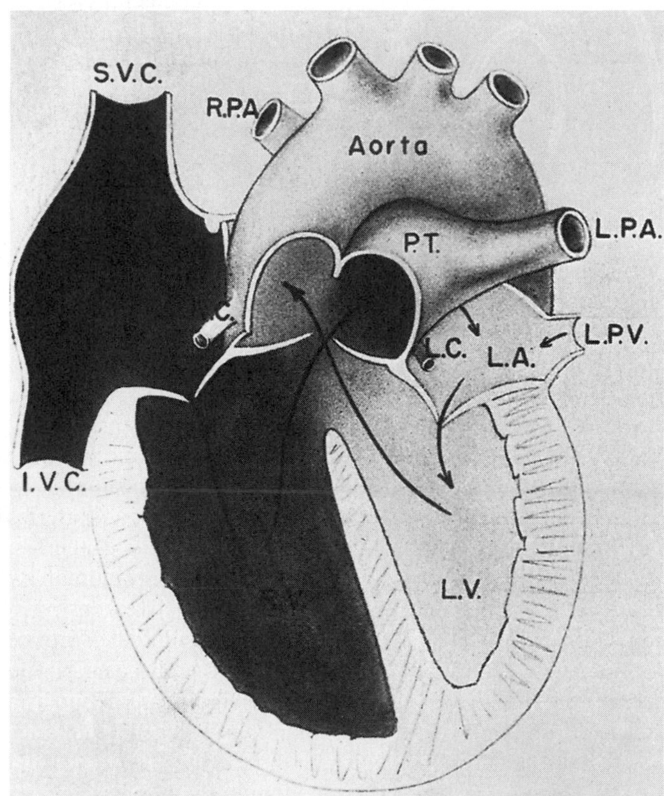

Fig. 198-15 Schematic drawing of truncus arteriosus. There is a large outlet ventricular septal defect and a common pulmonary and aortic trunk. *IVC,* inferior vena cava; *LA,* left atrium; *LC,* left coronary artery; *LPA,* left pulmonary artery; *LPV,* left pulmonary vein; *LV,* left ventricle; *PT,* pulmonary trunk; *RPA,* right pulmonary artery; *SVC,* superior vena cava.

Truncus arteriosus (Figs. 198-15 and 198-16). Persistence of the truncus arteriosus, the progenitor of the aorta and pulmonary artery, is an uncommon cardiac malformation (1% to 4% of cardiac deformities). There is no significant gender difference in incidence. The lesion usually is isolated, although it has been found with abnormalities of other systems, such as in patients who have DiGeorge syndrome. Incomplete division of the single truncus arteriosus into two separate components yields a single great vessel from which cardiac output from both ventricles is ejected. Because the portion of the conal septum that divides the truncus arteriosus into the two great vessels also is intimately involved in the formation of the ventricular septum, most patients who have truncus arteriosus have outlet ventricular septal defects. The single truncal valve may be deformed or functionally insufficient and may vary in number of cusps from two to six. It usually overrides the VSD in up to 80% of patients but may arise predominantly from one ventricle or the other. Truncal valve insufficiency is common. Because this portion of the conal septum contributes to the formation

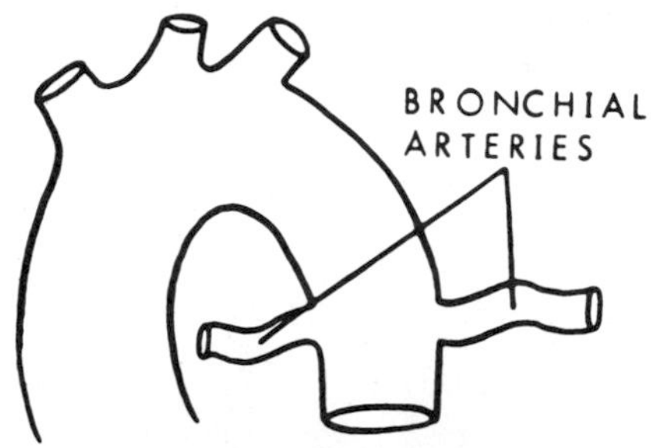

Fig. 198-16 Types of truncus arteriosus defined by the presence of a main pulmonary artery and arrangement of the branch pulmonary arteries from the main truncus.

(Modified from Mair DD, et al: Truncus arteriosus. In Adams FH, Emmanoulides GC, Moss AJ, Riemenschneider TA, editors: *Moss' heart disease in infants, children and adolescents,* ed 4, Baltimore, 1989, Williams & Wilkins.)

of the tricuspid valve leaflets and papillary muscles, abnormalities of these may be seen as well.

Collett and Edwards[6] subdivided patients who had truncus arteriosus into four categories based on the origin and anatomy of the main and branch pulmonary arteries. In type 1 (48% to 68% of patients), a well-formed, main pulmonary artery gives rise to normal branch pulmonary arteries. In type 2 (29% to 48% of patients), no significant main pulmonary artery is identified; however, both branch pulmonary arteries arise from the truncus in close proximity to each other. In type 3 (6% to 10% of patients), the two branch pulmonary arteries arise from the truncus separately in divergent positions. Type 4 truncus arteriosus now is considered a form of pulmonary atresia with VSD. Right aortic arch occurs in up to 35% of patients. A few patients have significant hypoplasia of the aortic arch; aortic coarctation may be seen; true interruption of the aortic arch occurs in up to 19% of patients and may be accompanied by ductal continuity with the ascending aorta. The ductus arteriosus remains patent in up to 70% of patients. Variations in coronary arterial origin are common. Secundum ASDs have been noted in up to 20% of patients, aberrant subclavian arteries in up to 10%, and persistent left superior vena cavae in up to 9%. Because of the significant pulmonary artery overcirculation in this condition, patients are prone to early pulmonary vascular obstructive disease.

Patients who have truncus arteriosus have an increased number of extracardiac anomalies, including skeletal abnormalities, genitourinary and gastrointestinal abnormalities, and other multisystem complex anomalies.

CLINICAL PRESENTATION. Because of the significant mixing both at the ventricular septal level and at the truncal level, patients present with mild cyanosis (oxygen saturations at 80% to 85%). Because pulmonary vascular resistance is high early in neonatal life, there may be little evidence for CHF unless there is severe truncal valve insufficiency. However, as pulmonary vascular resistance falls over the first 4 to 6 weeks and pulmonary flow increases, cyanosis may disappear and be replaced by the signs and symptoms of pulmonary overcirculation and CHF.

PHYSICAL EXAMINATION. Physical findings relate to the degree of pulmonary overcirculation and the presence or absence of truncal valve abnormalities. Patients who have significantly increased pulmonary blood flow may have minimal cyanosis. Depending on the degree of pulmonary blood flow, patients may be asymptomatic or present with signs or symptoms of CHF (tachypnea, tachycardia, and poor growth). Peripheral pulses usually are accentuated, and the pulse pressure is increased. There may be an increased left precordial impulse, and a systolic thrill usually is palpable over the left sternal border. The first heart sound is normal and frequently is followed by a loud ejection click from the single, redundant truncal valve. The second heart sound usually is single and loud because of the absence of a second semilunar valve. An apical third heart sound often is present in patients who have CHF. A loud holosystolic murmur often is heard along the left lower sternal border with radiation throughout the precordium, along with a low-pitched apical diastolic murmur of increased flow across the mitral valve. Patients who have truncal valve insufficiency may present with a high-pitched diastolic murmur heard along the left sternal border. Continuous murmurs rarely are heard in this condition, differentiating it from patients who have pulmonary atresia/VSD and significant aortopulmonary collaterals.

ELECTROCARDIOGRAM. The ECG demonstrates a normal QRS axis and/or minimal right axis deviation. Most patients who have increased pulmonary blood flow have biventricular hypertrophy with prominent left ventricular forces. In patients who have diminished pulmonary blood flow, isolated right ventricular hypertrophy may be seen.

CHEST RADIOGRAPH. Typically, the chest radiograph demonstrates moderate cardiomegaly. Pulmonary vascular markings depend on flow patterns. A right aortic arch may be present, and a dilated truncal root may be noted.

ECHOCARDIOGRAPHY. Echocardiography defines the cardiac anatomy and great vessel abnormalities in truncus arteriosis. In many patients, two-dimensional echocardiography demonstrates the posterolateral origin of the pulmonary arteries arising from the truncal root (types 2 and 3). Doppler techniques are useful in assessing pressure gradients and degrees of truncal valve stenosis and insufficiency.

CARDIAC CATHETERIZATION. The value of angiography in patients who have truncus arteriosus is in delineating coronary artery anatomy and pulmonary artery anatomy not well visualized by noninvasive imaging. The definition of truncal valve abnormalities (i.e., stenosis and/or insufficiency) is important. Angiography also is valuable in the definition of aortic arch abnormalities. Hemodynamic studies define degrees of pulmonary artery hypertension and its reversibility. Trials of inhaled, pharmacological pulmonary vasodilators can be valuable if the pulmonary vascular resistance is high, because such patients have an increased risk (39%) of operative mortality.[31]

TREATMENT. Without surgical intervention, the outcome for patients who have truncus arteriosus is poor. In one report, the mean age of death was 5 weeks.[54] Other studies have shown survival of only 15% to 30% beyond 1 year of age. Early mortality most commonly is secondary to heart failure, but later deaths may be secondary to severe pulmonary vascular obstructive disease. Because of these poor outcomes, surgical intervention is performed as early as possible, usually no later than 6 months of age.

Initial therapy for pulmonary overcirculation and ventricular dysfunction includes standard anticongestive medications (diuretic therapy, afterload reduction, positive inotropes). Once the patient is stabilized, the type of surgical approach can vary. In some centers, patients are palliated early in infancy by pulmonary artery banding, the placement of a tight "band" around the pulmonary artery to reduce pulmonary flow. Because of the significantly increased pulmonary artery flow in this condition, pulmonary artery bands have limited success and may produce severe distortion of the pulmonary arteries at the band site that will complicate future repair. Most centers, therefore, have advocated for complete repair in early infancy. The VSD is closed by standard patch technique and, after the pulmonary arteries are removed from the truncus, a right ventricle conduit to them is constructed. The site of the pulmonary arterial connections to the truncus is sewn closed, and the patient is left with a two-ventricle repair. Additional operations become necessary over the course of the patient's life to replace these conduits as they either fail or are outgrown. Significant truncal valve stenosis or insufficiency usually is treated at the same operation and may require valve replacement.

Early operative mortality in single center reports was 25% but has now fallen to below 10%. Severe incompetence of the truncal valve adds significantly to the risk. Long-term outcome depends on the severity of truncal valve abnormalities, ventricular dysfunction, and pulmonary vascular disease.

Hypoplastic left heart syndrome. Hypoplastic left heart syndrome constitutes a continuum of left ventricular hypoplasia, which may involve all levels (aorta, aortic valve, left ventricle, mitral valve, and left atrium). This malformation occurs in 7% to 9% of patients who have congenital heart disease, with a 2:1 male predominance. There has been some suggestion of autosomal recessive transmission of this lesion, but inheritance probably is multifactorial. The etiology is unclear, although it is suspected that underdevelopment of the left side of the heart may be related to diminution in size of the fetal interatrial communication. The atrial septum is intact in 10% of patients who have this syndrome. Only 20% of patients who have hypoplastic left heart syndrome have a true secundum ASD, and in most patients the ASD is restrictive. Because of this atrial septal abnormality, some patients present with anomalous pulmonary venous return and pulmonary lymphangiectasia. In most patients who have hypoplastic left heart syndrome, the mitral valve is stenotic or atretic. Varying degrees of aortic stenosis, atresia, and/or coarctation may be present. The vast majority of patients have a left-sided aortic arch. The coronary arteries are normal. In a small number of patients, left ventricular myocardial sinusoids, analogous to those seen in patients who have pulmonary atresia with an intact ventricular septum, may be identified. Other associated anomalies include atrioventricular septal defects and physiologically corrected and uncorrected transposition of the great arteries.

CLINICAL PRESENTATION. Nearly 40% of babies who have hypoplastic left heart syndrome present within the first 2 days of life and an additional 35% within the first week of life. Before ductal closure, patients are noncyanotic and hemodynamically stable. With ductal involution, cyanosis may be the initial presenting symptom, although patients also may present in shock with respiratory distress, hypotension, and hypothermia caused by decreased cardiac output. Without treatment, nearly 95% of all infants will die by the first month.

PHYSICAL EXAMINATION. With the development of low output cardiogenic shock, the physical examination will reveal tachycardia, tachypnea, and hepatosplenomegaly. The femoral pulses may vary in volume depending on the hemodynamic status. The first and second heart sounds tend to be single; third and fourth heart sounds may be present. Some patients have a pulmonary ejection click reflecting pulmonary hypertension and a dilated pulmonary artery. Patients may have soft systolic ejection murmurs and apical mid diastolic murmurs corresponding to increased flow across the tricuspid valve.

ELECTROCARDIOGRAM. Electrocardiograms may demonstrate decreased left-sided forces or apparent "increased" left-sided forces, generated by right ventricular rotation toward the apex of the heart. Large P waves, indicative of right atrial enlargement, also may be noted. Coronary insufficiency from ductal restriction and inadequate aortic flow may yield ST- and T-wave segment abnormalities.

CHEST RADIOGRAPH. There is no diagnostic pattern for this syndrome. Most patients do have mild cardiomegaly, and in some cases there is moderate to severe cardiac enlargement. The right heart border usually is conspicuous, consistent with right atrial enlargement. In some patients, absence of the ascending aortic shadow may be detected. Pulmonary vascular markings vary from normal to significant congestion.

ECHOCARDIOGRAPHY. Echocardiography fully delineates the anatomy, which can be quite variable in this syndrome. Diminutive mitral and aortic valves, left ventricular hypoplasia, and aortic arch abnormalities may be documented. Aortic root dimensions of less than 5 mm are consistent with aortic hypoplasia/atresia. The atrial septum should be examined for restriction to atrial level flow. Pulmonary venous drainage should also be studied.

CARDIAC CATHETERIZATION. Cardiac catheterization and angiography to establish this diagnosis are becoming less common as noninvasive imaging studies allow for its confirmation. When interatrial flow is restricted causing increasing pulmonary edema, balloon atrial septostomy, blade septostomy, or static balloon dilation of the interatrial communication have proved valuable. Angiocardiography also can be valuable in defining the entire aortic root in cases of suspected interruption of the aortic arch not fully documented by other studies. Clear definition of subaortic stenosis and VSDs can be valuable in planning surgical intervention. In some centers, ductal patency is maintained by transcatheter placement of an endovascular stent.[50]

TREATMENT. Initial therapy is supportive, once the diagnosis is suspected. Institution of prostaglandin E_1 therapy is mandatory to maintain systemic cardiac output through the ductus arteriosus. Reversal of metabolic acidosis, hypoxemia, and hypoglycemia is indicated by using glucose and sodium bicarbonate infusions and ventilation with supplemental oxygen. Intravenous inotropic support is indicated in the face of poor cardiac output.

Over the past 15 years, surgical management of hypoplastic left heart syndrome has increased dramatically. The two major surgical approaches at present are single-ventricle palliative therapy (Norwood operation[41]) and orthotopic heart transplantation. In the three-stage surgical palliation approach, patients undergo reconstruction of the aortic arch, combining the pulmonary artery and the aorta into a single great vessel. Care must be taken to maintain adequate coronary perfusion to prevent early morbidity and mortality. Pulmonary blood flow then is supplied by a small aortopulmonary shunt. This initial surgery is performed in the early neonatal period. At approximately age 3 to 6 months, a second stage, consisting of a bidirectional Glenn shunt (anastomosis of the superior vena cava to the pulmonary arteries), is performed to increase systemic arterial oxygen saturations, improve effective pulmonary blood flow, and decrease volume overload of the single ventricle. At 18 to 24 months of age, surgical intervention is completed by creating the Fontan circuit (connection of inferior and superior vena caval flow to the pulmonary arteries). Survival following the first stage repair varies between 65% and 90%; survival through the second stage drops to 60% to 85%, and following the third stage, varies from 50% to 75%. Multiple anatomical and physiological factors are related to outcome.[38] Long-term follow-up issues include possible ventricular dysfunction, dysrhythmias, and systemic venous hypertension, which may lead to liver dysfunction, varicosities, or protein-losing enteropathy.

With improvement in both the surgical and postoperative management of patients who have orthotopic heart transplantation and with rejection management, initial survival following transplantation is more than 90%.[3] Issues of acute rejection and the increased incidence of leukemias, lymphomas, and infections still limit 5-year survival to 75%. Patients also tend to have an increased incidence of premature atherosclerotic disease, which in some cases is severe enough to cause myocardial ischemia and necessitate a second transplant.

Anomalous pulmonary venous return. The frequency of abnormalities of pulmonary venous drainage from the lung at present is probably underestimated because it may be detected only at autopsy. Although these anomalies are quite variable in appearance, they usually have a common embryological origin. Almost any connection between the embryological pulmonary veins, common pulmonary vein, and the other neonatal systemic venous circuits can occur. In patients who have total anomalous pulmonary venous return, the pulmonary veins may drain into the superior vena cava, into the inferior vena cava, through the innominate vein via an embryological remnant (vertical vein), or to the coronary sinus. Patients are subgrouped into four major categories depending on the sites of venous drainage. These include the following:

1. Supracardiac (connections to the superior vena cava either directly or via the innominate vein)
2. Cardiac (directly to the right atrium or the coronary sinus)
3. Infracardiac (via a connecting vein to the inferior vena cava)
4. Mixed (a combination of two or more of the other categories).

The incidence of total anomalous pulmonary venous return is approximately 2% of patients who have congenital heart disease. Of patients who have infracardiac anomalous pulmonary venous return, there is a male preponderance; in the other forms, gender distribution is equal.

CLINICAL PRESENTATION. Patients who have partial anomalous pulmonary venous return may present similarly to that of patients who have ASDs (i.e., who have recurrent pulmonary infections, cardiomegaly found serendipitously on chest radiography, or with a murmur). No symptomatology may be present if the size of the anomalous left-to-right shunt is fairly small, as is particularly the case when only one pulmonary vein drains anomalously. Symptomatology increases if more than one pulmonary vein develops abnormally. Early cyanosis is unusual, although it may occur during the third and fourth decades of life as pulmonary vascular resistance increases or pulmonary hypertension develops.

Patients who have total anomalous pulmonary venous return usually present in the neonatal period. Associated anomalies are found in approximately 30% of patients, including a single ventricle, truncus arteriosus, transposition of the great arteries, pulmonary atresia, coarctation of the aorta, and anomalies of the superior and inferior venae cavae. The clinical presentation depends on the degree of pulmonary venous obstruction. Obstruction can occur at the atrial septal level or by stenosis of the connecting vein as it passes from the thorax through the diaphragm and into the inferior vena cava in patients who have infracardiac drainage. In the newborn who has no pulmonary venous obstruction and a large interatrial communication, the only symptom may be mild cyanosis, which can be so mild as to be inapparent. However, symptoms of CHF may develop in the first month of life. Pulmonary overcirculation may lead to frequent respiratory infections and cardiac failure within the first 6 months of life.

By 12 months, significant, irreversible pulmonary vascular change may occur if the condition is left untreated. With significant obstruction to pulmonary venous return, the clinical presentation will be striking. Patients demonstrate decreased cardiac output, shock with associated tachypnea and tachycardia, and significant cyanosis.

The prognosis of patients who have total anomalous pulmonary venous return depends on the size of the interatrial communication and the presence of obstruction to pulmonary venous return. Without intervention, mortality is approximately 50% by 3 months and 80% by 1 year. Mortality is even higher in patients who have inadequate interatrial communications.

PHYSICAL EXAMINATION. Cardiac examination findings depend on the degree of obstruction to pulmonary venous return. Usually, the first heart sound is increased and distinct, followed by a systolic ejection click caused by increased pulmonary flow. The second heart sound is widely split and does not vary with respiration, consistent with an ASD or other forms of right ventricular volume overload. The pulmonary component of the second heart sound may be accentuated from pulmonary hypertension. Many patients will have a third heart sound, and some will have a gallop rhythm. Occasionally, cardiac murmurs are absent, but a thrill is palpated. More characteristically, a soft, blowing systolic ejection murmur may be heard over the pulmonary area. Some patients may have diastolic murmurs at the left lower sternal border. Loud "venous hums," particularly in patients who have supracardiac pulmonary venous drainage, may be noted. This type of murmur, unlike the classic venous hum, will not change with variation in position.

ELECTROCARDIOGRAM. In patients who have anomalous pulmonary venous return, some degree of right atrial enlargement, reflected in enlarged P waves, is identified on ECG. Many patients will have right axis deviation of the QRS complexes, with right ventricular hypertrophy reflected in a right bundle branch block pattern.

CHEST RADIOGRAPH. Chest radiography reflects the degree of pulmonary venous obstruction. Patients who have partial anomalous pulmonary venous return will have a chest radiograph consistent with an ASD or right ventricular volume overload (i.e., enlarged right atrium and right ventricle with pulmonary overcirculation). Patients who have total anomalous pulmonary venous return without obstruction will have a similar picture. Patients who have significant pulmonary venous obstruction will present with marked pulmonary venous congestion and edema. Cardiac size tends to be within normal limits, particularly in the neonatal period. In patients who have supracardiac pulmonary venous drainage, a prominent innominate vein may yield what classically is referred to as the "snowman sign," with the shadow of innominate vein forming the head and the cardiac silhouette the body.

ECHOCARDIOGRAPHY. The echocardiogram is invaluable in defining the drainage patterns of the pulmonary veins. Evidence of obstruction either within the orifice of the pulmonary vein or at the atrial septal level also can be detected. Definition of left atrial anatomy, particularly ruling out interatrial membranes, is important. All patients who have any form of anomalous pulmonary venous return need full studies to define the exact drainage pattern of all four pulmonary veins and to confirm patency of the atrial septum. Definition of ventricular function and cardiac chamber sizes is important, as well. A search is made for coexisting lesions as previously described.

CARDIAC CATHETERIZATION. Selective pulmonary arteriography is undertaken when questions arise from noninvasive studies. It helps to define the exact location of the pulmonary venous drainage and can define better any intrapulmonary venous stenosis or stenosis at the orifices of the pulmonary veins. Careful hemodynamic measurements can confirm the diagnosis, particularly demonstrating increased oxygen saturations either in the superior vena cava, right atrium, or inferior vena cava.

TREATMENT. In patients who have partial anomalous pulmonary venous return or total anomalous pulmonary venous return without obstruction, intervention depends on the degree of symptomatology. In patients who have symptoms of CHF, standard medical management may be indicated, although it may provide only temporary benefit. Surgical intervention depends on the entry location of the anomalous veins and the presence or absence of an ASD. In most cases, the ASD can be baffled to include the anomalous pulmonary vein without causing obstruction to the right atrium or to the superior or inferior venae cavae.

In patients who have total anomalous pulmonary venous return and pulmonary venous obstruction, emergent surgical intervention is required. Surgery should be delayed only long enough to optimize the patient's clinical condition. In the majority of cases, the anatomy can be delineated solely by echocardiography and the stress of cardiac catheterization can be avoided.

Before surgery, balloon or blade atrial septostomy may be used to palliate patients and allow for improved venous mixing. However, because surgery is the definitive procedure, any delay in getting the patient to the operating room may increase the surgical risk. Depending on the location of drainage, the pulmonary veins are anastomosed in some fashion to the posterior wall of the left atrium, thus disconnecting the pulmonary veins from their systemic venous drainage. Postoperative mortality in the 1970s was as high as 50%; subsequently, mortality has dropped to 27%.

The long-term prognosis depends on the amount of preoperative damage that has occurred to the pulmonary vascular bed and the resultant pulmonary vascular obstructive disease. Stenosis at the anastomosis site to the left atrium requiring further intervention occurs in 5% to 10% of patients.

REFERENCES

1. Andersen M, et al: The natural history of small atrial septal defects, long-term follow-up with serial heart catheterizations, *Am Heart J* 92: 302, 1976.
2. Ashrof MH, et al: Fate of long-term survivors of Mustard procedure for simple and complex transposition of the great arteries, *Ann Thorac Surg* 42:385, 1986.
3. Bailey LL, et al: Cardiac allotransplantation as therapy for hypoplastic left heart syndrome, *N Engl J Med* 315:949, 1986.
4. Beerman LB, et al: Arrhythmias in transposition of the great arteries after the Mustard operation, *Am J Cardiol* 51:1530, 1983.
5. Blalock A, Hanlon CR: The surgical treatment of complete transposition of the aorta and the pulmonary artery, *Surg Gynecol Obstet* 90:1, 1950.
6. Collett RW, Edwards JE: Persistent truncus arteriosus: a classification according to anatomic types, *Surg Clin North Am* 1245, 1949.

7. Conkle DM, Jones M, Morrow AG: Treatment of congenital aortic stenosis: an evaluation of the late results of aortic valvotomy, *Am J Cardiol* 58:338, 1986.
8. Cordell D, et al: Left heart volume characteristics following ventricular septal defect closure in infancy, *Circulation* 54:294, 1976.
9. DuShane JW, et al: The fate of raised pulmonary vascular resistance after surgery in ventricular septal defect. In Rowe RD, Kidd BSL, editors: *The child with congenital heart disease after surgery,* Mt Kisco, NY, 1976, Futura.
10. Edmunds LH Jr, et al: Surgical closure of patent ductus arteriosus in premature infants, *Circulation* 48:856, 1973.
11. Egito ES, et al: Transvascular balloon dilatation for neonatal critical aortic stenosis: early and mid-term results, *J Am Coll Cardiol* 29:442, 1997.
12. Fedderly RT, et al: Determinants of successful balloon valvotomy in infants with critical pulmonary stenosis or membranous pulmonary atresia with intact ventricular septum, *J Am Coll Cardiol* 25:460, 1995.
13. Fischbein CA, et al: Risk factors for brain abscess in patients with congenital heart disease, *Am J Cardiol* 34:97, 1974.
14. Friedman WF, Pappelbaum SJ: Indications for hemodynamic evaluation and surgery in congenital aortic stenosis, *Pediatr Clin North Am* 18: 1207, 1971.
15. Gay BB, et al: Roentgenologic features of simple and multiple coarctations of the pulmonary artery and branches, *AJR* 90:599, 1963.
16. Gentles TL, Lock JE, Perry SB: High pressure balloon angioplasty for branch pulmonary artery stenosis: early experience, *J Am Coll Cardiol* 22:867, 1993.
17. Gersony WM, et al: Effects of indomethacin in premature infants with patent ductus arteriosus: results of a national collaborative study, *J Pediatr* 102:895, 1983.
18. Gross RE, Hufnagel CA: Coarctation of the aorta: experimental studies regarding its surgical correction, *N Engl J Med* 233:287, 1945.
19. Hammerman C, Aramburo MJ: Prolonged indomethacin therapy for the prevention of recurrences of patent ductus arteriosus, *J Pediatr* 117:771, 1990.
20. Hawkins JA, et al: Aortic valve repair and replacement after balloon aortic valvuloplasty in children, *Ann Thorac Surg* 61:1355, 1996.
21. Hayes AM, et al: Influence of anatomic correction for transposition of the great arteries on myocardial perfusion: radionuclide imaging with technetium-99m 2-methoxy isobutyl isonitrile, *J Am Coll Cardiol* 24: 769, 1994.
22. Hoffman JIE: Congenital heart diseases. In Rudolph AM, Hoffman JIE, editors: *Pediatrics,* ed 18, Norwalk, Conn, 1987, Appleton & Lange.
23. Hosking MCK, et al: Transcatheter occlusion of the persistently patent ductus arteriosus: forty-month follow-up and prevalence of residual shunts, *Circulation* 84:2313, 1991.
24. Jacob DL, et al: Initial experience with balloon dilatation of supravalvar aortic stenosis, *Br Heart J* 70:476, 1993.
25. James FW: Exercise testing in normal individuals and patients with cardiovascular disease, *Cardiovasc Clin* 11:227, 1981.
26. Justo RN, et al: Aortic valve regurgitation after surgical versus percutaneous balloon valvotomy for congenital aortic valve stenosis, *Am J Cardiol* 77:1332, 1996.
27. Kidd L, et al: Second natural history study of congenital heart defects: results of treatment of patients with ventricular septal defects, *Circulation* 87:1, 1993.
28. Kimball TR, et al: Effect of digoxin on contractility and symptoms in infants with a large ventricular septal defect, *Am J Cardiol* 68:1377, 1991.
29. Lloyd TR, Beekman RH III: Clinically silent patent ductus arteriosus, *Am Heart J* 127:1664, 1994.
30. Lloyd TR, et al: Transcatheter occlusion of patent ductus arteriosus with Gianturco coils, *Circulation* 88:1412, 1993.
31. Mair DD, et al: Selection of patients with truncus arteriosus for surgical correction: anatomic and hemodynamic considerations, *Circulation* 49: 144, 1974.
32. Martin RP, et al: Incidence and site of pulmonary stenosis after anatomical correction of TGA, *Br Heart J* 59:122, 1988.
33. Mavroudis C, Backer CL, Gevitz M: Forty-six years of patent ductus arteriosus division at Children's Memorial Hospital of Chicago, *Ann Surg* 220:402, 1994.
34. Mendelsohn AM, Shim D: Inroads in transcatheter therapy for congenital heart disease, *J Pediatr* 133:324, 1998.
35. Mendelsohn AM, et al: Intra-operative and percutaneous stenting of congenital pulmonary artery and vein stenosis, *Circulation* 88:11210, 1993.
36. Mendelsohn AM, et al: Late follow-up of balloon angioplasty in children with a native coarctation of the aorta, *Am J Cardiol* 74:696, 1994.
37. Mendelsohn AM, et al: Predictors of successful pulmonary balloon valvuloplasty: 10-year experience, *Cathet Cardiovasc Diagn* 38:236, 1996.
38. Moodie DS, et al: The hypoplastic left heart syndrome: evidence of preoperative myocardial and hepatic infarction in spite of prostaglandin therapy, *Ann Thorac Surg* 43:307, 1986.
39. Mustard WT: Successful two-stage correction of transposition of the great arteries, *Surgery* 55:469, 1964.
40. Nakanishi T, et al: Balloon angioplasty for postoperative pulmonary artery stenosis in transposition of the great arteries, *J Am Coll Cardiol* 22:859, 1993.
41. Norwood WI, Kirklin JK, Sanders SP: Hypoplastic left heart syndrome: experience with palliative surgery, *Am J Cardiol* 45:87, 1980.
42. Nugent EW, et al: Clinical course in pulmonary stenosis, *Circulation* 6:1, 1977.
43. O'Connor BK, et al: Intermediate-term effectiveness of balloon valvuloplasty for congenital aortic stenosis: a prospective follow-up study, *Circulation* 84:732, 1991.
44. O'Connor BK, et al: Intermediate-term outcome after pulmonary balloon valvuloplasty: comparison with a matched surgical control group, *J Am Coll Cardiol* 20:169, 1992.
45. O'Laughlin MP, et al: Implantation and intermediate-term follow-up of stents in congenital heart disease, *Circulation* 88:605, 1993.
46. Portsmann W, et al: Catheter closure of patent ductus arteriosus: 62 cases treated without thoracotomy, *Radiol Clin North Am* 9:203, 1971.
47. Qureshi SA, et al: Transcatheter laser-assisted balloon pulmonary valve dilation in pulmonic valve atresia, *Am J Cardiol* 64:428, 1991.
48. Rashkind WJ, Miller WW: Transposition of the great arteries: results of palliation by balloon atrioseptostomy in thirty-one infants, *Circulation* 38:453, 1968.
49. Rothman A, et al: Early results and follow-up of balloon angioplasty for branch pulmonary artery stenoses, *J Am Coll Cardiol* 15:1109, 1990.
50. Ruiz CE, et al: Stenting of the ductus arteriosus as a bridge to cardiac transplantation in infants with the hypoplastic left heart syndrome, *N Engl J Med* 328:1605, 1993.
51. Rumisek JD, et al: Coronary sinus septal defect associated with tricuspid atresia, *J Thorac Cardiovasc Surg* 92:142, 1986.
52. Senning A: Surgical correction of transposition of the great vessels, *Surgery* 45:966, 1959.
53. Shim D, Lloyd TR, Beekman RH: Usefulness of repeat balloon aortic valvuloplasty in children, *Am J Cardiol* 79:1141, 1997.
54. VanPraagh R, VanPraagh S: The anatomy of common aorticopulmonary trunk (truncus arteriosus communis) and its embryological implications: a study of 57 necropsy cases, *Am J Cardiol* 16:406, 1965.
55. Vosschulte K: Isthmusplastik zor behandlung der aortem isthmusstenose, *Thoraxchirugie* 4:443, 1957.
56. Waidhausen JA, Nahrwold DL: Repair of coarctation of the aorta with a subclavian flap, *J Thorac Cardiovasc Surg* 51:532, 1966.
57. Weidman WH, et al: Clinical course in ventricular septal defect, *Circulation* 56(1 suppl): I56, 1977.
58. Zimmerman M, et al: Ventricular late potentials and induced ventricular arrhythmias after surgical repair of tetralogy of Fallot, *Am J Cardiol* 67:873, 1991.

199 Contact Dermatitis

David H. Stein • Nancy K. Barnett

Contact dermatitis is eczematous dermatitis caused by external chemical substances. The basic types are irritant contact dermatitis and allergic contact dermatitis. Contact dermatitis caused by irritants (often referred to as *irritant contact* or *irritant dermatitis*) is toxicity to the skin from directly applied irritants, which can occur in any individual who has had adequate exposure. It is not immune or hypersensitivity mediated; therefore, no sensitization or prior exposure is needed. In contrast, allergic contact dermatitis develops only in individuals who manifest immune reactivity to a contact allergen through cell-mediated (delayed) hypersensitivity.[1,2]

Contact dermatitis is more common when the barrier function of the skin is weakened, as when the skin is thin, occluded, or excessively moist; it also depends on the toxicity of a substance. The onset of allergic contact dermatitis also depends on the immune competence of a child as well as adequate, usually repeated, exposure to substances that are sufficiently antigenic. Allergic contact dermatitis is uncommon in infancy, is more common in childhood, and, with maturity of immune function and repeated exposure to allergens, approaches adult incidence about the end of the first decade of life.[1] A diagnosis of either type of contact dermatitis should be considered when an eruption is most pronounced on skin surfaces in direct contact with a possible external triggering agent and/or shows obvious delineation of borders, linear arrays, or unusual asymmetrical patterns and distributions that suggest exposure to external surfaces or substances. In contrast, most systemic or idiopathic rashes are bilateral, often symmetrical, and lack the distinct borders seen with contact dermatitis. A good history should provide clues to the inciting agent, and an accurate diary often is extremely helpful.[3,4]

IRRITANT DERMATITIS

Various common childhood irritants, including soaps, detergents (especially bubble bath products[5]), lotions, oils, saliva, or foods cause eruptions; these vary in severity according to the duration of contact, the strength of the irritant, and the age of the patient. Dermatitis can occur in minutes to hours following exposure and often is associated initially with burning or discomfort other than itching; subsequently, itching can increase. Confluent papules and plaques of erythema and epidermal change, manifesting as eczematous dermatitis confined to the area of contact, is the most common presentation. It should respond to the application of a mild- to medium-strength topical steroid over approximately a week, but whenever possible only low-potency steroids should be used on the face. With more potent irritants, a more acute dermatitis with erythema, vesicles, weeping, and crusting may occur. Cool compresses (water, saline, or Burow's solution) applied approximately four times daily to the weeping areas for 10 minutes before applying the steroid will dry the involved areas and enhance steroid effectiveness.

Diaper Dermatitis

Diaper dermatitis is the most frequent contact irritant dermatitis during infancy (see Chapter 203, Diaper Rash). The usual irritant is urine or stool in prolonged direct contact with the skin, especially with occlusion. Diaper dermatitis appears as confluent erythematous papules or plaques confined to areas of direct contact, with sparing of inguinal folds. Irritants in oils or lotions applied to the diaper area can involve the skin folds. With severe irritation, the skin may macerate and erode, and crusts can form.

Involved areas should be kept dry, with gentle blotting or wiping and free air flow; further irritant contact can be prevented with the use of protective barriers such as ointments. A low-potency topical steroid can be applied up to three times a day. If the dermatitis persists, the area often becomes colonized and sometimes infected with *Candida albicans*. Candida infection causes beefy red plaques with frequent satellite papules and/or pustules. Potassium hydroxide (KOH) preparation of skin scrapings may reveal pseudohyphae or budding yeasts. An antifungal/antiyeast cream, such as clotrimazole or miconazole, applied twice daily, is alternated with a mild topical steroid or barrier cream.

Other Irritants

Soaps and detergents, and especially their additives such as perfumes, can be irritants when applied directly to the skin. Soaps tend to cause the most severe eruptions on the face and hands with repeated exposure. Bubble bath solutions often cause perivaginal dermatitis and vaginitis in young girls.[5] Flame retardants, formaldehyde resins, or other clothing treatments can cause irritant or allergic dermatitis; therefore, new clothes should be washed and rinsed before the first wearing.

ALLERGIC CONTACT DERMATITIS[6]

In allergic contact dermatitis,[1-6] contact allergens penetrate the epidermis and are bound by dendritic cells (Langerhans' cells) within the epidermal basal layer before T-cell processing. T lymphocytes that have specific antigen recognition properties then proliferate and return to the skin, where they are available for rapid (24 to 72 hours) antigen recognition and reactivity on subsequent contact with that antigen. The time required for initial sensitization varies with the allergen and can take more than a month for minimally antigenic substances, but a week or less for potent ones. On recognition of and reaction to a contact allergen, T lymphocytes release inflammatory mediators, causing acute eczematous dermatitis.[6]

On examination, erythematous papules, plaques, and often, vesicles or blisters are found in areas of allergen contact. In contrast to irritant contact, substantial itching is present from the onset. Gradual worsening and some extension beyond the original area of actual contact and involvement is expected, even after the allergen is removed.

Compared with treatment for irritant dermatitis, longer treatment times and higher-potency topical steroids often are necessary; this is because allergic contact dermatitis, especially when acute, tends to be less responsive than most dermatitis to topical treatment. Liberal use of oral antihistamines, cool compresses, cool baths, and soothing lotions (e.g., calamine) may be helpful. If the area involved is more than 10% to 15% of body surface or includes the face or genitals, oral prednisone can speed resolution; in healthy children, this usually begins with 1 mg/kg as a single morning dose, with tapering over 2 to 3 weeks to avoid a rebound of the dermatitis, as the oral steroid is discontinued. Simultaneous use of topical steroids also may lessen the likelihood of rebound.

Rhus Dermatitis

The most frequent allergic contact dermatitis in children is rhus (Toxicodendron) dermatitis from poison ivy, oak, or sumac. The contact allergen is urushiol, the plant's oleoresin. A very pruritic, vesicular, red, eczematous dermatitis is found on exposed surfaces, often in linear patterns where leaves and branches rub against the skin. The sensitizing oleoresin can persist on fur, clothing, or furniture for months until it is removed or discarded. The burning of rhus leaves or airborne carriage of other antigens, such as ragweed pollen, can create an airborne contact dermatitis that can be confluent and extensive over exposed sites, including the upper airway.

All skin surfaces and garments, as well as items such as shoes and backpacks, should be cleaned after possible oleoresin exposure to decrease potential ongoing contact exposure. Vesicle fluid does not spread the dermatitis, but resin trapped on clothing or under fingernails can be spread by scratching or rubbing. Education about toxic plants and exposure avoidance is essential.

Other Common Allergens

Nickel sensitivity, the second most frequent cause of allergic contact dermatitis, often is seen following ear piercing or other exposure of inflamed or damaged skin to metals. Most metal alloy contains some nickel; for example, nickel is found in zippers, watch bands, toys, coins, and metal snaps. Allergic contact dermatitis also can result from allergens such as parabens, lanolin, ethylenediamine, and paraphenylenediamine contained in nail polish, hair dyes, perfumes, deodorants, and other cosmetics. Sunscreen preparations can cause allergic contact dermatitis.[3] Latex allergy is increasingly a problem and can be serious or even life threatening.[4,7]

Shoe Contact Dermatitis

Contact dermatitis from shoes can be either irritant or allergic in nature. Usually a bilateral symmetrical dermatitis involves the dorsum of the toes and feet, with relative sparing of the web spaces and dorsal foot. Various shoe compounds are irritants or sensitizers; the most common of these compounds is rubber, but dyes and adhesives also can be causative. Patients who have shoe contact dermatitis should wear loose-fitting, open shoes. Plantar hyperhidrosis (see Chapter 149, Hyperhidrosis), frequently accompanies shoe contact dermatitis and should be managed with frequent sock changes and the application of absorbent powder and aluminum chloride (e.g., Xerac AC, Drysol). As mentioned previously, acute dermatitis will respond to topical steroids, oral antipruritic agents, and compresses. Patch (epicutaneous) testing, outlined in the following section, can determine if the patient is allergic to a shoe component. Patch testing can be done with a standard shoe patch test tray or parts of the suspected offending shoes. If problems persist, allergen-free footwear purchased according to patch test results is recommended.

PATCH TESTING

Patch testing to diagnose specific contact allergy involves applying suspected allergens at critically exact dilutions directly to the skin and serially inspecting the ensuing reaction; patch tests should not be performed while active dermatitis is present. Because specific patch tests are difficult to administer and interpret, tests should be performed by trained personnel. Positive results are only significant if there has been exposure to that allergen or a similar compound and if exposure to the identified allergen causes dermatitis. Results are questionable for young children.

REFERENCES

1. Kwangsukstith C, Maibach HI: Effect of age and sex on the induction and elicitation of allergic contact dermatitis, *Contact Dermatitis* 33:289, 1995.
2. Mortz CG, Andersen KE: Allergic contact dermatitis in children and adolescents, *Contact Dermatitis* 41:121, 1999.
3. Schauder S, Ippen H: Contact and photocontact sensitivity to sunscreens: review of a 15-year experience and of the literature, *Contact Dermatitis* 37:221, 1997.
4. Shaer C, Slater JE: Latex allergy in children, *Curr Opin Pediatr* 5:700, 1993.
5. West NY, Fitzpatrick JE, Jackson EM: Comparison testing of the irritancy of children's liquid bubble bath using a modified human repeat insult patch test, *Am J Contact Dermatitis* 9:212, 1998.
6. Weston WL: Contact dermatitis in children, *Curr Opin Pediatr* 9:372, 1997.
7. Ylitalo L, et al: Natural rubber latex allergy in children who had not undergone surgery and children who had undergone multiple operations, *J Allergy Clin Immunol* 100:606, 1997.

200 Contagious Exanthematous Diseases

Robert Iannone

The literal translation of *exanthem* is *to bloom* or *to break out*. It is commonly used to refer to an eruption or rash that usually is associated with fever and generally implies that the eruption is infectious in origin. These eruptions are extremely common in children and present the clinician with a major challenge in differential diagnosis, inasmuch as many manifest contagious exanthems have similar appearances. Consequently, the clinical manifestations other than the rash itself often must be explored to distinguish one disease from another. These would include the incubation period, prodromal signs, the age of the patient, immunization history, contact history, distribution and progression of the rash, evidence of other organ involvement, and pathognomonic signs, such as peeling, or Koplik spots.

Exanthems may be caused by viruses, bacteria, rickettsia, mycoplasma, and fungi. Moreover, certain allergic and immune-complex diseases such as childhood arthritis can mimic the infectious exanthems.

Some exanthems herald diseases for which treatment is necessary; others signal the need for quarantine or further evaluation. For example, if rubella or erythema infectiosum (human parvovirus) is included in the differential diagnoses, one needs to investigate recent and potential exposures of the sick child to pregnant women, because fetal infection with these viruses may be devastating. Diseases that might respond to specific therapy require special consideration. These include the exanthem of *Mycoplasma pneumoniae* infection, which will respond to erythromycin, or the exanthem of *Rickettsia rickettsii* (Rocky Mountain spotted fever), which requires early treatment with tetracycline or chloramphenicol. The rash of streptococcal or staphylococcal scarlet fever (scarlatina) needs specific identification so that it can be treated appropriately, and scarlatina must be differentiated from Kawasaki disease so that the latter receives careful monitoring and specific treatment. Some of the differentiating characteristics of these eruptions are found in Table 200-1 and in Tables 166-1 and 166-2 (see also Chapter 194 for a discussion of chickenpox).

ENTEROVIRAL EXANTHEMS

Inasmuch as rubeola (measles) and rubella have been controlled largely by the administration of effective vaccines, enteroviral infections are now the most common cause of exanthems in children. Many serotypes of echoviruses and coxsackieviruses are associated with rashes; often these are generalized maculopapular rashes that have discrete lesions much like those of rubella. They may appear very much like roseola, with an initial 2 to 3 days of fever followed by the eruption. Generally, though, the prodromal fever is much lower than that of roseola. Transmission is fecal-oral.

Although maculopapular rashes predominate, vesicular lesions have been observed in coxsackievirus A5, A9, and A16 infections. Hand-foot-mouth disease commonly is seen with coxsackievirus A16 infection and is manifested by vesicles on the palms and soles and ulcers in the mouth. The oral ulcerations of enteroviral herpangina typically occur in the back of the mouth, which can distinguish it from the more diffuse lesions of primary herpes stomatitis.

Enteroviral exanthems typically occur in the late summer and early fall and are associated with epidemics of aseptic meningitis. A more detailed discussion of enteroviral infections and aseptic meningitis can be found in Chapters 206 and 235, respectively.

EXANTHEM SUBITUM (ROSEOLA)

Based on its clinical course and epidemiology, roseola long has been presumed to be an infectious illness. In 1988, a newly discovered virus called *human herpesvirus-6* (HHV-6) was shown to be the infectious agent.[1] Transmission is via secretions from an asymptomatic contact. Roseola is characterized by 3 or 4 days of high fever (104° to 105° F [40° to 40.6° C]), followed by abrupt resolution of the fever and the eruption of a pink maculopapular rash that begins on the neck and then spreads to the trunk and extremities, usually sparing the face. The lesions are discrete and last only for 1 or 2 days.

The child usually has no other manifestation of illness and does not appear as ill as the severity of the fever might imply.

Roseola occurs year round and is limited to children between the ages of 6 months and 3 years.

Complications are limited to febrile seizures, which may be precipitated by the rapid rise in body temperature. Most children who have seizures associated with roseola show normal findings on spinal tap and have an excellent prognosis. See Chapter 218, Human Herpesvirus-6 and Human Herpesvirus-7 Infections, for a more complete discussion of this disease.

ERYTHEMA INFECTIOSUM (FIFTH DISEASE)

Erythema infectiosum is caused by infection with human parvovirus B19. Susceptible persons are infected by respiratory tract droplets.

Table 200-1 Differentiating Common Childhood Exanthems

Disease	Character of Rash	Prodrome	Pathognomonic Signs	Helpful Signs
Enterovirus infection	Maculopapular; generalized to most of body; discrete	May have 3-4 days of mild fever before rash, or rash may appear with constitutional signs	Herpangina, hand-foot-mouth syndrome	Aseptic meningitis, pharyngitis, petechiae with some coxsackievirus strains; occurs in summer and early fall
Exanthem subitum (roseola)	Maculopapular and discrete; begins on trunk and spreads to face and usually spares the limbs	3-4 days of high fever and irritability with no other signs	None	Dramatic drop in fever simultaneous with onset of rash
Erythema infectiosum (fifth disease)	Red and flushed cheeks with circumoral pallor; subsequent proximal maculopapular rash on extremities (lacelike)	None	Slapped-cheek appearance in otherwise healthy child	Possible recurrence of eruption with irritation of skin by heat, cold, or pressure
Rubella (German measles)	Pink, maculopapular, discrete; begins on face and spreads to trunk and extremities	Commonly none; adolescents may have 1-3 days of low-grade fever and malaise	None	Tender postauricular and suboccipital lymph nodes; possibly arthralgia in adolescents
Mumps	Maculopapular, discrete, concentrated on trunk; may have urticaria; may be first sign of illness	1-2 days of fever, headache, and malaise	None	Diffuse swelling of parotid glands, with pain and tenderness; aseptic meningitis; orchitis or pancreatitis; erythema of the Stensen duct
Infectious mononucleosis	Macular or maculopapular and discrete; when associated with ampicillin administration, is confluent (morbilliform) and more intense	2-4 days of fever, pharyngitis, malaise	None	Exudative pharyngitis, lymphadenopathy, splenomegaly, atypical lymphocytes on peripheral smear

The typical clinical presentation is one of rash without fever or other systemic signs, though fever can occur in 15% to 30% of patients. The rash first erupts as a bright red erythema of the cheeks and forehead, with circumoral pallor, 7 to 10 days after nonspecific symptoms of malaise, myalgias, and headache. This "slapped-cheek" appearance is the result of many large maculopapular lesions that coalesce to form a confluent red rash. These confluent lesions are hot to the touch and commonly palpable but are nontender.

After a single day, a maculopapular rash next appears on the proximal extremities. This then spreads gradually to the trunk and distal extremities, leaving a lacelike appearance as it clears. This second stage lasts 2 to 4 days. In a third stage the rash may reappear transiently when the skin is traumatized by pressure, sunlight, or extremes of hot and cold. Arthritis and arthralgia, which often occur in adults, are infrequent findings in children. Mild myelosuppression typically goes unnoticed in normal individuals, whereas a life-threatening aplastic crisis may occur in patients with shortened red cell survival, such as occurs in sickle cell disease or hereditary spherocytosis.

Clinical suspicion may be confirmed, when necessary, by testing for anti-parvovirus B19 IgM or through polymerase chain reaction testing.

RUBELLA

Rubella is also known as "German measles" or "3-day measles." These names served to distinguish the disease from rubeola ("hard measles" or "10-day measles"). The virus was cultivated first in 1962; its clinical spectrum was documented thoroughly in the 1965 epidemic. Transmission is through direct or droplet contact from nasopharyngeal secretions. The period of maximal communicability is just before and up to a week after onset of the rash.

The typical clinical illness is mild and brief. In most children the rash itself is the first sign of infection. It typically is a pink, maculopapular eruption beginning on the face and spreading downward to the trunk and extremities. The lesions

Table 200-1 Differentiating Common Childhood Exanthems—cont'd

Disease	Character of Rash	Prodrome	Pathognomonic Signs	Helpful Signs
Mycoplasma pneumonia	Maculopapular on trunk and extremities in 10% of cases; common spectrum of urticaria, erythema multiforme, and vesicular/bullous lesions	3-5 days of progressive fever, headache, malaise, and cough	None	Pneumonia, cold agglutinins may be elevated
Rubeola (measles)	Red to brown macular rash that spreads from face and neck to trunk and extremities; confluent (morbilliform), particularly on face; begins afer onset of fever and fades after 6-7 days with temporary staining of skin	3-4 days of high fever, conjunctivitis, cough, and coryza	Koplik spots	Always an associated conjunctivitis and cough
Atypical measles	Rash may be maculopapular, purpuric, petechial, or vesicular; prominent at wrists and ankles	2-3 days of fever, headache, and cough	None	History of killed measles vaccine, myalgia, pneumonia
Scarlet fever	Erythematous papular eruption sometimes associated with generalized erythema; concentrated on trunk and proximal extremities; feels like fine sandpaper	Occurs within 1-4 days of onset of focal infection	None	Focal infections such as pharyngitis, vaginitis, cellulitis, erythema of palms and soles; strawberry tongue; desquamation in recovery phase; Pastia lines
Kawasaki disease	Rash ranges from maculopapular to scarlatina form to urticaria; marked erythema of palms and soles	At least 5 days of fever and irritability is common	None	Conjunctivitis, tender lymphadenopathy, strawberry tongue, meatitis, diarrhea, prolonged fever, late desquamation, arthritis in recovery phase

remain discrete and pink, the appearance of which contrasts with the raised, confluent, and deep red lesions of rubeola. The facial rash clears as the extremity rash erupts, and all are cleared by the third to the fifth day.

Fever is very mild, ranging between 99° and 101° F (37.2° and 38.3° C). Lymphadenopathy frequently is impressive; the posterior auricular and suboccipital chains are most commonly involved. They usually are tender at the onset of rash, but the tenderness resolves rapidly over 2 to 3 days. Although lymphadenopathy is an important sign of rubella infection, it is not specific. Tiny reddish spots may occur on the soft palate, which are indistinguishable from those of scarlet fever or rubeola. The incubation period is 2 to 3 weeks, with a peak at 16 to 18 days.

The rubella virus usually can be grown from the pharynx within 5 days of the onset of the rash. Serological diagnosis is made by demonstrating an antibody titer rise between acute and convalescent sera. Hemagglutination-inhibition (HI) antibody titers are readily available, and a fourfold rise after 2 weeks indicates recent infection.

Complications of rubella are rare in children, but a transient arthritis develops in approximately 15% of adolescents and young adults. The arthritis rarely becomes chronic.

The major serious complications of rubella virus result from fetal infection. If a pregnant woman is infected in the first trimester of gestation, there is a very high probability that the fetus will become infected, with multi-organ involvement. See Chapter 42, The Fetus at Risk, for details on congenital rubella syndrome. For this reason, one might need to pursue objective confirmation of infection with the rubella virus by determining maternal antibody titers.

INFECTIOUS MONONUCLEOSIS

The exanthem of Epstein-Barr virus (EBV) occurs in approximately 15% of children who have infectious mononucleosis who are not treated with ampicillin. The rash is pink to red and macular or maculopapular. The lesions are discrete and have no specific distinguishing characteristic; therefore, the disease most often is diagnosed based on other signs of infectious mononucleosis and confirmed by the peripheral blood smear and serological tests.

The administration of ampicillin to persons who have infectious mononucleosis results in approximately 50% of them developing a much more intense rash, which also may occur with other penicillins. This ampicillin-associated rash is deep red and confluent, giving it a morbilliform appearance. This iatrogenic exanthem resolves spontaneously within a week. The appearance of such a rash in a patient treated for presumptive group A streptococcal pharyngitis is cause to reconsider the diagnosis. It also is important to reassure parents that this rash does not represent penicillin hypersensitivity. The full spectrum of EBV infection is discussed in Chapter 226, Infectious Mononucleosis and Other Epstein-Barr Virus Infections.

MEASLES (RUBEOLA)

Measles is the most serious of the childhood exanthems because of the morbidity of the acute infection and its potential for producing permanent sequelae. The virus is highly contagious and is transmitted via respiratory droplets. Typical clinical disease begins after an incubation period of 10 to 11 days. The prodromal illness is manifested by increasing fever, cough, conjunctivitis, and coryza. By the fourth day the fever commonly is high (104° F [40° C]) and the rash erupts. Typically, a deep red macular rash begins on the face and neck and spreads down the trunk and extremities, as in rubella. The lesions on the face and upper portion of the trunk soon become confluent to produce the characteristic morbilliform rash, whereas the rash of rubella tends to remain discrete. By the sixth day the fever subsides and the rash begins to fade; as it fades, it leaves a faint brown stain in the skin, and a fine desquamation ensues.

The enanthem of measles is pathognomonic. Koplik spots begin approximately 2 days before the rash erupts and increase in number until the first or second day of the exanthem. They are tiny bluish white spots on an erythematous base and cluster adjacent to the molars on the buccal mucosa.

The combination of Koplik spots, fever, cough, conjunctivitis, and morbilliform rash is sufficient to make a firm clinical diagnosis of measles. Although the children usually are very ill, they recover rapidly after the eighth or ninth day and most often are back to normal in a few days, hence, the moniker "10-day measles."

Measles virus induces inflammation throughout the respiratory tract; respiratory complications are common, including otitis media, pneumonia, and croup. The otitis media is treated as any acute otitis media. The pneumonia may be either a primary measles pneumonia or a superimposed bacterial pneumonia. All children who have measles should have careful follow-up, and the examiner should have a high degree of suspicion for secondary bacterial pneumonia.

Subacute sclerosing panencephalitis (SSPE), also known as *Dawson's encephalitis,* is the major complication of persistent measles virus infection. It occurs in approximately 1 per 1000 cases and commonly results in death or permanent neurological sequelae. It manifests by headache, vomiting, drowsiness, personality changes, seizures, and coma. In most cases the cerebrospinal fluid reveals pleocytosis and elevated protein levels. Some of these children have only a mild disease and recover in a few days; others have a fulminant course.

Prevention of measles is discussed in Chapter 18, Immunizations.

Atypical Measles

In recent years, some children who had been immunized with inactivated measles vaccine have had an atypical presentation of wild measles virus infection. Such children may have 2 to 3 days of fever and headache, followed by a rash erupting on the wrists and ankles. The rash may be maculopapular, purpuric, petechial, or vesicular. There also may be marked myalgia, with swelling of the hands and feet; pneumonia is common.

The constitutional symptoms and the distribution of the rash are similar to that of Rocky Mountain spotted fever. Elicitation of a history of having received killed measles vaccine assists in making the diagnosis.

MYCOPLASMA PNEUMONIA

Cutaneous signs are a minor manifestation of mycoplasmal infections. A maculopapular eruption may appear on the trunk and extremities of 10% to 15% of persons infected with *Mycoplasma pneumoniae*. It is even more common for these infections to be associated with allergic-type eruptions that display a spectrum of cutaneous lesions ranging from urticaria and erythema multiforme to vesicles or bullae. Such patients frequently have had a prodromal illness of fever, headache, malaise, and cough. The pneumonia may escape physical diagnosis, only to crop up on the chest radiograph as an "incidental" finding. Macrolide antibiotics may be used to treat mycoplasma pneumoniae infections. See Chapter 252, Pneumonia.

MUMPS

An exanthem will develop in fewer than 10% of persons infected with the mumps virus. The lesions are maculopapular, pale pink, discrete, and concentrated on the trunk. The virus more typically involves the salivary glands, the testicles (after puberty), the pancreas, and the meninges. After an incubation period of 16 to 18 days, clinical mumps develops in approximately 60% of infected persons. The remaining 40% have inapparent infections, without salivary gland swelling. Transmission is through direct contact via the respiratory route.

The typical illness begins with 1 or 2 days of anorexia, headache, and mild to moderate fever. This is followed by complaints of discomfort when chewing and of pain around the ear. There usually is a diffuse but noticeable enlargement and tenderness of the parotid gland, which can be distinguished from lymph node enlargement in that it extends anterior to the ear and below the ramus of the mandible posteriorly to the mastoid bone, usually obliterating the angle of the jaw. Lymph nodes are more discrete and generally submandibular in location. Accompanying the parotitis, one commonly sees erythema around the opening of the Stensen duct. The fever usually lasts 2 to 5 days. Rarely, only one parotid gland is involved, or the submandibular salivary glands rather than the parotids will be swollen.

Meningoencephalitis is estimated to occur in 10% of all cases of mumps and is characterized by headache, nausea, vomiting, and mild nuchal rigidity. It may occur before, during, or after the parotitis phase of the disease. It follows a course similar to the aseptic meningitis that is caused by other viruses, and it usually has no sequelae. Some cerebrospinal fluid pleocytosis is present in most cases of mumps without clinical evidence of meningeal irritation.

Orchitis is uncommon in children, but unilateral involvement of the testes and epididymis is observed in approximately 25% of males who are infected with mumps virus after puberty. Patients who have orchitis usually are quite ill; however, the incidence of sterility in males who experience mumps orchitis is no greater than in those who do not.

The pancreas and other exocrine glands rarely are involved.

Late neurological complications include nerve deafness and a very rare postinfectious encephalitis.

SCARLET FEVER

The rash of scarlet fever (scarlatina) is caused by a circulating erythrotoxin that is produced by certain strains of streptococci and staphylococci. This rash is characterized by a fine papular eruption on an erythematous base. Often there is a generalized erythema of the skin, including even those areas that are not yet involved with the papular rash. The eruption of scarlet fever is concentrated on the trunk and proximal extremities. It feels rough to the touch like fine sandpaper. The rash commonly is associated with prominent erythema of the lips, soles, and palms. Transverse red streaks (Pastia lines) sometimes are present, usually in the antecubital spaces. Desquamation of involved skin typically occurs in the recovery phase. On the tongue one can observe prominent papillae on a very red base, giving a "strawberry tongue" appearance.

If streptococci are the source of the erythrogenic toxin, the pharynx is the usual site of focal infection. Other focal infections, however (such as vaginitis or cellulitis), also may be found. When staphylococci are the source of erythrogenic toxin, the infective focus usually is some site other than the pharynx; infected surgical or traumatic wounds have been common sites.

The treatment of scarlet fever is directed toward eradication of the focal infection. Streptococcal infections are treated with penicillin or erythromycin, whereas staphylococcal infections are treated with parenteral cephalexin, amoxicillin-clavulanate, dicloxacillin, or oxacillin.

Kawasaki disease must be carefully differentiated from scarlet fever because coronary artery disease may complicate untreated Kawasaki disease. Its cutaneous manifestations overlap remarkably with those of scarlet fever, but it usually can be distinguished by the additional signs of discrete bulbar conjunctivitis without exudate, cracking of the lips, very tender lymphadenopathy (usually solitary, unilateral and more than 1.5 cm in diameter), changes in the extremities including induration with erythema of palms and soles, meatitis, and diarrhea. These children are profoundly irritable, and their fever persists for more than a week in most cases (5 days of fever is necessary for diagnosis). Just as in scarlet fever, however, they have erythema of the palms and soles, with striking desquamation during the second and third weeks of the disease. Kawasaki disease is presented in more detail in Chapter 230.

OTHER

Many other respiratory viral illnesses may result in nondescript "morbilliform" rashes, including respiratory syncytial virus, influenza A and B, adenovirus, and parainfluenza virus.

Acknowledgment

The author gratefully acknowledges the contribution of the previous author, John H. Dossett.

REFERENCE

1. Yamaniski K, et al: Identification of human herpesvirus-6 as a causal agent for exanthem subitum, *Lancet* 1:1065, 1988.

SUGGESTED READINGS

American Academy of Pediatrics: Pickering LK, editor, *Red book 2000, report of the Committee on Infectious Diseases,* ed 25, Elk Grove Village, Ill, 2000, American Academy of Pediatrics.

Feigin RD, Cherry JD: Viral infections. In Feigin RD, Cherry JD, editors: *Textbook of pediatric infectious diseases,* ed 4, Philadelphia, 1998, WB Saunders.

201 Cystic and Solid Masses of the Face and Neck

Neil E. Herendeen • Peter G. Szilagyi

The differential diagnosis of a neck mass is broad, ranging from common inflammatory lymph nodes and cysts to rare neoplasms. Therefore, an orderly approach to the workup and management of a neck mass is needed. The most practical approach involves differentiating the anatomical location of the mass into lateral neck masses versus midline neck masses and determining the exact anatomical position of the mass.[6] It is helpful to localize a lateral neck mass further into either the anterior cervical triangle (anterior to the sternocleidomastoid muscle) or the posterior cervical triangle.

ETIOLOGY

Masses in the neck can be classified into two broad categories: cystic lesions and solid masses.[3] Cystic lesions are either congenital cysts or vascular malformations; however, traumatic hematomas and abscesses may appear to be cystic. Solid neck masses usually are inflammatory lymph nodes or, rarely, neoplastic lesions. In general, a careful history and physical examination will lead the clinician to the correct diagnosis. Carefully chosen laboratory tests or radiological studies then may confirm the diagnosis.

When evaluating neck masses, it is important to be familiar with key anatomical structures of the neck. Because most neck masses encountered by pediatricians are lymph nodes and not cysts, it is crucial to understand the location of the different groups of lymph nodes within the anterior and posterior anatomical triangles of the neck. Fig. 201-1 shows the location of the major groups of lymph nodes, the sternocleidomastoid muscle, and the typical locations of the congenital cysts encountered most frequently.

HISTORY

It is important to determine whether the neck mass was observed at birth, whether it has increased or decreased in size, whether it has changed color, and whether the lesion has drained or opened. Knowing the age of onset may help, because lymph nodes rarely appear at birth, whereas many congenital cysts are noted in the newborn period. Some congenital cysts, however, may not be noted until childhood or beyond and are detected only when they become infected.

The history of pain or tenderness is important. Congenital cysts are nontender unless they become infected. Inflamed lymph nodes are quite tender and painful. Pain during eating suggests parotid gland involvement.

PHYSICAL EXAMINATION

The first step in the physical examination is to determine whether abnormalities exist in other parts of the body, such as other cysts, lymphadenopathy, hepatosplenomegaly, skin lesions, or signs of infection. The exact anatomical location of the neck mass must be determined, and the clinician should note whether the mass is in the typical location of a lymph node (see Fig. 201-1). The consistency, color, and firmness of the mass should be noted, as well as the presence of tenderness. The size of the mass also should be measured.

Midline masses usually are related to a thyroid abnormality. Those that move with swallowing or with tongue protrusion suggest a thyroglossal duct cyst, inasmuch as these lesions may be tethered to the foramen cecum by the thyroglossal duct remnant. A mass along the anterior edge of the sternocleidomastoid muscle that moves with swallowing or that has a sinus opening to the surface of the overlying skin is likely to be a branchial cleft cyst. Both cysts and benign lymph nodes are freely mobile; malignant lesions are more likely to be fixed to underlying structures.

Rapidly growing, painless neck masses are worrisome because they might be neoplastic. Additional signs associated with a neoplastic process include fixation of the mass to subcutaneous tissue, firm consistency, size of greater than 3 cm, and presence of constitutional symptoms. Neck masses in the posterior cervical triangle are more likely to be malignant than are masses anterior to the sternocleidomastoid muscle.

TYPES OF CONGENITAL CYSTS

Thyroglossal duct cysts account for more than 70% of congenital cysts of the neck, branchial cleft cysts for more than 20%, and vascular malformations and other lesions for 4% to 5%.[6]

Thyroglossal duct cysts result from failure of the embryological thyroglossal duct to degenerate during the fifth week of gestation, leaving a fistula, sinus tract, or cyst at the midline of the neck just below the hyoid bone.[3] Thyroglossal duct cysts often are not detected at birth but usually are noted first after the age of 2 years; initially, they may manifest as an inflamed, tender mass. When not infected, they are smooth, firm, mobile, and nontender and move upward with tongue protrusion or with swallowing. The differential diagnosis includes sebaceous cysts, epidermal cysts, submandibular lymph nodes, and lipomas. Unless normal thyroid tissue is palpable, it is important to confirm the presence of the thyroid gland by ultrasonography or technetium scan, because

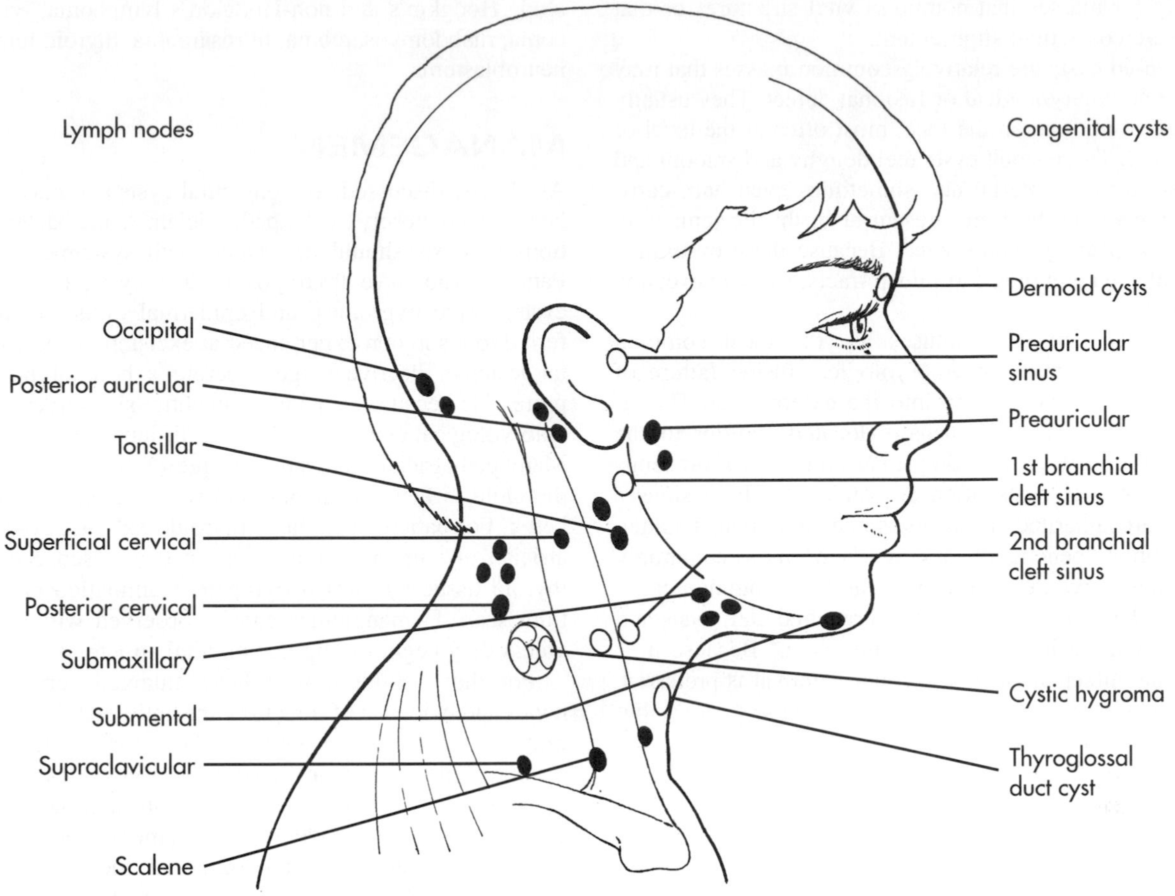

Fig. 201-1 Common locations for cystic *(open circles)* and lymph nodes *(solid circles)* of the face and neck.

what may appear to be a thyroglossal duct cyst actually may be an ectopic thyroid gland, and its removal would leave the child dependent on thyroid hormone supplementation throughout life.[5] Because the likelihood of infection is high, thyroglossal duct cysts should be removed surgically.

Branchial cleft cysts are congenital remnants of the lateral four branchial pouches and clefts, which, interestingly, correspond to embryological gill slits in fish.[2] The vast majority of branchial cleft cysts arise from the second cleft or pharyngeal pouch. They appear as a small dimple or opening anterior to the middle portion of the sternocleidomastoid muscle. The cyst is nontender, firm, and mobile and is located just under the skin. A small sinus, which occasionally drains fluid to the surface of the overlying skin, may be present, and a long fistulous tract may extend from it to the tonsil bed.[3] Branchial cleft cysts without sinuses often are unnoticed until later childhood when they become infected. Infected cysts can easily be confused with lymphadenitis. Other lesions included in the differential diagnosis are sternocleidomastoid muscle masses associated with torticollis, small cystic hygromas, epidermoid cysts, neurofibromas, lipomas, and an ectopic thyroid gland. Treatment involves surgical removal of the cyst and fistula.

Cystic hygromas are congenital, avascular masses derived from congenital obstruction of lymphatic vessels. They generally are multilocular, fluid-filled, soft, compressible, painless masses located in the posterior triangle just behind the sternocleidomastoid muscle and in the supraclavicular fossa. They usually can be transilluminated. These masses may grow rapidly because of accumulation of lymph and can reach an enormous size, compressing important structures and obstructing the airway.[1] Although the diagnosis usually is obvious on physical examination, smaller cystic hygromas may resemble hemangiomas or other cysts. Ultrasonographic examination will reveal fluid and multiple cystic components, confirming the diagnosis. Because spontaneous regression is rare and the risk of compression of vital upper airway structures is high, surgical removal is indicated. Often, multiple procedures are necessary to remove large lesions in their entirety. Cystic hygromas occur infrequently in the axilla, on the trunk, or on the extremities; in older children, when they occur within the subcutaneous tissues, they may be mistaken for a lipoma or a hemangioma.[2]

Cavernous hemangiomas are vascular lesions within the subcutaneous tissues that may appear in any part of the body and may be difficult to differentiate from congenital cysts. They often are noted in the newborn period and enlarge (sometimes very rapidly) during the first year of life. Cavernous hemangiomas are less firm, more diffuse, and more easily compressible than are cystic masses (except for cystic hygromas). Unlike cystic hygromas, cavernous hemangiomas do not transilluminate, and their size may increase with crying or straining. Often the skin overlying these vascular lesions is bluish; cavernous hemangiomas frequently begin to increase in size during the first few months of life but usually regress spontaneously by school age.[6] Thus, surgery is indicated only for masses that compress vital structures or that cause severe cosmetic disfigurement.

Epidermoid cysts are relatively common masses that may arise from an embryological or fusional defect. They usually are located at midline on the face, most often at the level of the eyebrows. These small cysts feel doughy and smooth and contain sebaceous material and sometimes even hair, cartilage, or bone. One third are present at birth; the remaining two thirds appear by school age.[4] Because these cysts may become infected and may form deep tracts, surgical excision is indicated.

Preauricular cysts and sinuses are the most common anomalies arising from an embryological fusion failure of precursor tissues that develop into the external ear. The sinuses are pinhole-size pits usually located anterior to the helix (see Fig. 201-1), and they may contain a short sinus tract.[3] Preauricular cysts often are bilateral. These sinuses and cysts are inherited in an autosomal dominant manner, with incomplete penetrance, and are found more commonly in blacks than in whites. They are a far more common cause of preauricular lesions than are first branchial cleft cysts and sinuses, which are located in the same area.[4] Because they may become infected, elective surgical removal is preferred. Hearing deficits may be associated with these lesions, but their prevalence is unknown.

Other congenital masses occur rarely in the head and neck; the aforementioned lesions account for the vast majority of congenital masses. The major challenge in the differential diagnosis involves (1) differentiating congenital masses from lymph nodes and (2) determining the type of congenital lesion.

SOLID NECK MASSES

Cervical lymph nodes frequently are palpable in normal children and can be distinguished by their location (see Fig. 201-1), size, shape, consistency, and mobility. Enlarged cervical lymph nodes (>1 cm) should be defined further by their association with surrounding nodes or generalized adenopathy, the presence of an infection of the head or pharynx, and localized signs of inflammation and erythema. Cervical adenitis typically presents in a child who has a fever as a swollen, tender, erythematous mass. *Staphylococcus aureus* and *Streptococcus pyogenes* account for 80% of acute unilateral cervical adenitis and usually respond to oral antibiotics such as a penicillin or cephalosporin. Lymph node aspiration usually is reserved for those patients who do not respond to the initial course of therapy. Incision and drainage is an option for those masses that become fluctuant. Some of the various causes of cervical lymphadenopathy include viral infections of the upper respiratory tract, bacterial infections, HIV infection, Kawasaki disease, and certain systemic disorders (lupus, juvenile rheumatoid arthritis, sarcoidosis, histoplasmosis). Chronic inflammation of the lymph nodes can be seen with infections such as cat-scratch disease (see Chapter 185, Animal Bites), atypical mycobacterium, and toxoplasmosis.

Malignant tumors often are found as a single mass in the posterior triangle or as multiple or matted masses crossing into both the anterior and posterior triangles. More than 25% of children who have malignancies have a tumor of the head or neck.[6] The most common neck malignancies include Hodgkin's and non-Hodgkin's lymphoma, lymphosarcoma, rhabdomyosarcoma, fibrosarcoma, thyroid tumors, and neuroblastoma.

MANAGEMENT

As already discussed, all congenital cysts and masses should be followed closely by the pediatrician. Acute bacterial infections of cysts should be treated with systemic antibiotics. Patients who have thyroglossal duct cysts, branchial cleft cysts, cystic hygromas, and epidermal cysts should be referred to a surgeon experienced at excision of these congenital lesions. Elective surgery before a bout of infection is preferable because excision of an entire sinus tract, fistula, or embryological connection is more difficult after an infection. Many pediatricians and surgeons prefer to delay surgery until the child is beyond infancy and will tolerate the procedure better. For patients who have thyroglossal duct cysts, a pediatrician or surgeon should confirm the presence of normal thyroid tissue by ultrasonographic examination or a technetium scan. Hemangiomas can be observed without referral unless they begin to impinge on vital structures.

For those children who have enlarged cervical lymph nodes and evidence of infection, the antibiotic therapy should improve the condition within 7 days; the condition should resolve completely over the next few weeks. If the adenopathy is persistent, with no inflammation, and has any worrisome characteristics (size >3 cm, not mobile, associated with systemic symptoms, in an abnormal location), the child should be evaluated further and followed closely until the enlarged node has resolved.[6]

When to Refer

- All congenital cysts/tracts should be removed
- Mass that does not resolve on antibiotics (≥2 weeks)
- Mass in thyroid gland
- Mass in parotid gland
- Rapidly enlarging mass (>3 cm)
- Mass is fixed or lymph nodes are matted
- Mass in a concerning area (posterior triangle, supraclavicular)
- Systemic signs and symptoms (e.g., fever, weight loss, easy fatigability) are present

REFERENCES

1. Armstrong WB, Giglio MF: Is this lump in the neck anything to worry about? *Postgrad Med* 104:63, 1998.
2. Feins NR, Raffensperger JG: Cystic hygromas, lymphangioma and lymphedema. In Raffensperger JG, editor: *Swenson's pediatric surgery,* ed 5, Norwalk, Conn, 1990, Appleton & Lange.
3. Friedberg J: Pharyngeal cleft sinuses and cysts, and other benign neck lesions, *Pediatr Clin North Am* 36:1451, 1989.
4. Hogan D, Wilkinson RD, Williams A: Congenital anomalies of the head and neck, *Int J Dermatol* 19:479, 1980.
5. Raffensperger JG: Congenital cysts and sinuses of the neck. In Raffensperger JG, editor: *Swenson's pediatric surgery,* ed 5, Norwalk, Conn, 1990, Appleton & Lange.
6. Zitelli BJ: Evaluating the child with a neck mass, *Contemp Pediatr* 7:90, 1990.

202 Diabetes Mellitus

Robert E. Greenberg

DEFINITIONS AND FREQUENCY

Diabetes mellitus refers to a number of related disorders, all characterized by impaired glucose tolerance associated with either a deficiency in insulin secretion or abnormalities of its metabolic effects. Although disordered glucose homeostasis is the most striking and well-recognized characteristic of diabetes, many other metabolic abnormalities occur, affecting amino acid, protein, and lipid metabolism. A new classification of diabetes in children reflects both the diversity and changing clinical picture of diabetes (Table 202-1).[15] Type I diabetes primarily reflects insulin deficiency, whereas type II diabetes results from resistance to the action of insulin. Over recent decades, there has been a striking increase in the number of children and youth who present with type II diabetes; this immense change in the clinical picture of diabetes correlates with the increasing prevalence of obesity.[9] Further, type II diabetes occurs more commonly in children and youth from minority groups (black, Native American, Hispanic). In atypical diabetes (ADM), hyperglycemia presents acutely, with or without ketoacidosis, but is then followed by a clinical pattern commonly seen in type II diabetes. Maturity-onset diabetes in the young (MODY) is a rare form of diabetes, genetically determined, associated with abnormalities in pancreatic recognition of glucose as a signal for insulin secretion.

The prevalence of type I diabetes varies strikingly among various populations, with the highest rate in Northern Europeans (1 in 300 to 500 18-year-olds) and much lower rates in African and Asian children. The incidence in Northern Europeans approximates 10 per 100,000, with the peak incidence between 11 and 14 years of age. There is some suggestion that type I diabetes is less common in those population groups in which the prevalence of type II diabetes appears to be increasing markedly, and can affect adults at any age.

HETEROGENEITY

Recognition of the heterogeneity within diabetes was a critical step in understanding the separate nature of type I and type II diabetes. This demonstration of heterogeneity has been based on family, twin, hormonal, immunological, and genetic studies. Family studies indicate that type I and type II diabetes segregate in an unrelated fashion. Studies of twins have set forth the difference between the two clinical syndromes: Only 50% or fewer of monozygotic twins demonstrate concordance for type I diabetes; 100% of twins show concordance for type II diabetes. Hormonal studies have demonstrated deficient insulin secretion as the primary event in type I diabetes. In type II diabetes, both insulin deficiency and resistance to the action of insulin are demonstrable, with the latter considered to be the primary event.[5] An altered immune response is associated with type I diabetes in that most type I diabetic patients have autoantibodies against several pancreatic antigens demonstrable in their sera at the time of clinical diagnosis. Finally, HLA association studies have continued to reveal the striking association between specific alleles in the major histocompatibility locus with type I but not type II diabetes; the HLA-DQB1 gene is the principal genetic susceptibility locus in humans.[13] More than 90% of white patients bear the serologically defined tissue specifications HLA-DR1, HLA-DR3, or HLA-DR4.[16] If the fifty-seventh amino acid on the DQB chain is aspartic acid, occurrence of diabetes is low; a noncharged amino acid at the same site raises the risk.[13] Distinguishing between type I and type II diabetes mellitus in those in the middle years of life may be difficult, requiring use of hormonal and immunological data in addition to demonstrating alterations in carbohydrate metabolism. Further, both forms of diabetes may exhibit common aspects of their natural history, especially because the vascular and neuropathic complications partly are a consequence of similar disturbances in metabolic regulation.[1,10]

ETIOLOGICAL MECHANISMS IN TYPE I INSULIN-DEPENDENT DIABETES MELLITUS (IDDM)

Genetic and Environmental Interplay

The striking fact that fewer than 50% of identical twins show concordance for type I diabetes strongly suggests that an interplay between genetic and other biological mechanisms occurs to produce disease.[13] Specific genes (primarily HLA-DQ) create genetic susceptibility to type I diabetes by regulating or influencing immune selection and activation in a process leading to autoimmune destruction of insulin-producing cells. Evidence supporting the role of immune mechanisms in the development of type I diabetes includes (1) the presence of infiltration of the pancreatic islets by lymphocytes and macrophages in newly diagnosed patients, (2) islet cell-reactive antibodies and T-cell clones in the sera of patients at the time of clinical onset, and (3) an increased frequency of non-islet cell specific autoimmunity in affected individuals or their family members. Of importance is the

Table 202-1 Classification of Diabetes in Children and Youth

	Type I Diabetes	Type II Diabetes	ADM	MODY
Age of onset	All of childhood	Often around puberty or later	Puberty	Puberty
Clinical onset	Acute	Mild, often insidious	Acute	Mild, insidious
Insulin secretion	Very low	Usually high	Low	Variable
Insulin sensitivity	Normal	Decreased	Normal	Normal
Genetics	Polygenic	Polygenic	Autosomal dominant	
Frequency (of all childhood diabetes)	~80%	10%-20%	5%-10%	Rare
Associated conditions				
Obesity	No	Strong	Variable	No
Acanthosis nigricans	No	Often	No	No
Autoimmunity	Yes	No	No	No

Modified from Rosenbloom AL, et al: *Diabetes Care* 22:345, 1999.
ADM, Atypical diabetes mellitus; *MODY*, maturity-onset diabetes in the young.

observation that autoantibodies may be demonstrated long before aberrant carbohydrate tolerance can be detected in both humans and experimental animal models. Further, a marked increase in the incidence of autoantibodies is seen in genetically predisposed, but healthy first-degree relatives of persons who have type I diabetes. There is, most likely, a significant environmental component to enhance susceptibility to type I diabetes. The mechanism(s) underlying the effect of environment remain conjectural; however, it is likely that infectious processes (primarily viral) or antigens that cross-react with islet cell autoantigens (e.g., bovine serum albumin or coxsackie virus) amplify parts of the immune mechanism.[7]

History

The classic presentation is that of a child who demonstrates the clinical consequences of reduced glucose utilization (polyphagia, weight loss) and hyperglycemia (polyuria, polydipsia). It still is common for the physician to be confronted with a child in whom the early clinical signs were unappreciated, leading to the classic clinical picture of diabetic ketoacidosis (vomiting, Kussmaul respirations, altered state of consciousness). Diabetic ketoacidosis is discussed in detail in Chapter 279. The coexistence of abdominal pain in a child who has diabetic ketoacidosis is extremely common and remains the leading cause of confusion in making the initial diagnosis. Although preexisting infections may be present (as in any child), no convincing evidence exists that newly diagnosed patients who have type I diabetes are more susceptible to significant infections. Although the majority of affected children have type I diabetes, the prevalence of type II diabetes is appreciable and increasing. In this circumstance, the clinical signs of diabetes usually are more subtle, although ketoacidosis may occur initially.

Decreased glucose utilization (leading to hyperglycemia) may be found in any severely ill young child, especially in those who have reduced blood volume and peripheral hypoperfusion. Hyperglycemia in these circumstances is neither diagnostic nor predictive of type I diabetes.

Physical Examination

The findings on physical examination are determined by the duration and severity of insulin deficiency (or resistance). If decreased glucose utilization has been present for weeks or months, poor weight gain will be an almost universal finding. If glucose utilization has been severely impaired, dehydration, respiratory compensation for metabolic acidosis, and altered consciousness will be the primary findings.

Laboratory Findings

Laboratory confirmation of carbohydrate intolerance requires the demonstration of hyperglycemia either when fasting or after food intake. Because of significant individual variations in the renal threshold for glucose reabsorption, *glucosuria alone is not diagnostic*. Elevation in the amount of glycosylated hemoglobin confirms persistent or chronic hyperglycemia. Depending on the severity and duration of insulin deficiency, the laboratory findings of diabetic ketoacidosis—reduced plasma bicarbonate, reduced blood pH, increased anion gap, and hyperlipemia (increased cholesterol and/or triglycerides)—may be present. Hyperkalemia often accompanies significant metabolic acidosis; hypokalemia in untreated diabetic ketoacidosis usually signifies a massive depletion of total body potassium. Hyponatremia may be partly artifactual because of the altered water distribution produced either by hyperglycemia or by the water displacement in plasma produced by severe hyperlipemia.

Rapid bedside diagnosis and management of diabetes are facilitated by use of glucometers for the determination of blood glucose and serial dilution of plasma for determination of ketone bodies (Acetest).

Differential Diagnosis

Glucose intolerance can result from a number of different conditions: (1) decreased insulin secretion (type I diabetes); (2) defects in the binding of insulin to receptors (altered affinity or numbers of receptors, antireceptor blocking antibodies); (3) defects in the glucose transport system, such as a reduced affinity and number or mobility of glucose transport proteins; (4) increased secretion of counterregulatory hormones (catecholamines, corticosteroids, growth hormones); and (5) postreceptor defects in insulin action (genetic or nongenetic).[8] A useful path through such confusion is to determine whether the glucose intolerance coexists with a reduced or an increased level of insulin secretion (plasma insulin or

C-peptide, determined by radioimmunoassay), as measured during a standard oral glucose tolerance test. If insulin levels are increased, the differential diagnosis of insulin-resistant states may be considered more confidently.

Management

Natural history. When diabetes mellitus is first diagnosed, insulin requirements may be high (>1 unit of insulin/kg/day). It should be noted, however, that the young child may be exquisitely sensitive to exogenous insulin, especially when the diabetes is diagnosed before the onset of ketoacidosis. Soon after initial stabilization, a respite may occur wherein requirements for exogenous insulin may fall or even vanish as endogenous insulin secretion resumes (documented by increased plasma C-peptide levels). This "honeymoon" period may last for weeks or even months, with longer periods following intensive intravenous insulin therapy at initial diagnosis; after this phase, insulin requirements are determined primarily by body weight, hormonal changes during puberty, and psychological factors.

The clinical course of the child who has diabetes is determined primarily by levels of understanding and the acceptance of the disease by the child/youth and family, psychological adjustment, family interactions, and stability of lifestyle. These factors are more significant determinants of metabolic control and frequency of illness and hospitalization than are the strictly biological factors affecting the action of insulin.

The progression of the natural history of type I diabetes depends on the attack rate and severity of occurrence of the vascular and neuropathic complications. The significance of these long-term complications is made dramatically evident by renal failure caused by diabetes being the most prevalent diagnosis among adults beginning hemodialysis or undergoing renal transplantation and by blindness being 25 times more common in individuals who have type I diabetes than in the nondiabetic population.

Critical significance of chronic hyperglycemia. The approach to the management of diabetes mellitus is directed and targeted by recent population studies regarding the effect of intensive metabolic control on the natural history of the disease. The Diabetes Control and Complications Trial (DCCT) was a multicenter randomized clinical trial designed to compare intensive with conventional diabetes therapy with regard to the development and progression of the early vascular and neurological complications of type I diabetes mellitus. This study demonstrated conclusively that the risk of microvascular complications in diabetes was reduced by improving glucose control.[17] Further confirmation of this relationship was found in the Stockholm Diabetes Intervention Study; in addition, no discernible threshold could be found below which hyperglycemia had no untoward effect.[1] The interpretation that hyperglycemia is a toxic state was also demonstrated in type II diabetes;[18] in addition, careful attention to blood pressure monitoring and control emerged as an important part of chronic diabetic management, especially because the relationship between hyperglycemia and coronary heart disease is not firmly established.[2]

These observations have markedly heightened the mandate to assist children and youth who have diabetes of any type in establishing glucoregulation as close to the normal range as possible. This mandate represents a significant departure from previous pediatric practice, wherein adequate control was defined simply as normal physical and emotional growth and development in the absence of significant hypoglycemia or ketoacidosis. The practical questions now focus on the best methods to effect such a demanding level of metabolic control.

The duration of prepubertal diabetes has, in previous years, been considered to exert much less impact on the development of microvascular and/or neuropathic complications compared with postpubertal duration. However, recent studies do not support the lack of significance of prepubertal years for the development of complications.[6]

Intensive management and hypoglycemia. Hypoglycemia, both severe and moderate, occurs in a significant percentage of diabetic children.[4] In all studies involving the attempt to provide intensive management to bring blood glucose as close to normal as possible, the incidence of significant hypoglycemia increases, with greater risks for younger children.

The response to hypoglycemia involves counterregulation, mediated principally by adrenal medullary and cortical hormones, and glucagon. Hypoglycemia unawareness refers to reduced adrenomedullary and sympathetic responses to falling blood glucose levels, resulting in reduced symptoms associated with both rapidly falling and low blood glucose. Hypoglycemia unawareness develops as a function of duration of diabetes and is accentuated by recurrent episodes of hypoglycemia.[14] If hypoglycemia is avoided, hypoglycemia unawareness often is reversible. Thus, the therapeutic challenge is to provide insulin replacement therapy in as physiological a manner as possible, in a child whose life has structure and consistency.

Monitoring

SHORT-TERM GLYCEMIA. Glucosuria will occur only when the concentration of glucose in blood exceeds the renal threshold for glucose reabsorption (the tubular maximum [Tm] for glucose). Inasmuch as the Tm for glucose normally approximates 180 mg/dl (with wide variations), glucosuria usually cannot occur without significant preceding hyperglycemia, nor does the absence of glucosuria ensure the absence of moderate hyperglycemia or distinguish normoglycemia from hypoglycemia. If metabolic balance is to be brought under more rigorous control, the glucose concentration of blood, rather than of urine, must be measured precisely. Hence, monitoring the blood glucose level is the modern cornerstone of diabetes management. Assuming use of proper technique, the self-monitoring of blood glucose has many potential positive consequences for the patient: (1) It can stimulate interest and motivation in self-control of the disease, (2) it documents the precise nature of metabolic problems, (3) it reinforces learning by demonstrating that metabolic control is possible, (4) it reinforces the acceptance of personal responsibility, and (5) it teaches through personal experience. Lack of compliance, however, may be associated with inaccurate and invalid blood glucose data, as has been recognized previously to be the case in home monitoring of urinary glucose levels.

Daily monitoring can easily become an unthinking routine, especially if the data are not used to alter management. When daily monitoring at multiple times is beyond the current capability of a child or family, the following approach has been shown to lead to improved control:

1. Determine the blood glucose level before each meal and before bedtime during 3 days of every week (Monday, Wednesday, Saturday or Tuesday, Thursday, Sunday).
2. Determine the blood glucose level whenever symptoms suggest hypoglycemia or hyperglycemia.
3. Determine the blood glucose level whenever clinical situations arise that often are associated with hyperglycemia (infections, injuries, emotional distress).
4. Analyze available data weekly in terms of average blood glucose at each time of sampling.
5. Determine urine ketone levels whenever the blood glucose level is elevated markedly or the patient is symptomatic.

By using the weekly blood glucose record to adjust insulin dosage, exercise pattern, or dietary intake systematically, diabetic control not only may be improved but also patients may be convinced that blood glucose measurements are used to make their lives better, rather than being just a mandate from either parents or physicians. Further, this approach provides an incentive for regularity and places responsibility for documenting and interpreting metabolic control with the patient and/or parent, depending on the age of the child.

LONG-TERM GLYCEMIA. When foods are heated or stored in the presence of reducing sugars for long periods, a brown color results, produced by a direct reaction between the free amino groups of proteins and the reducing sugars (this is the Schiff reaction of nonenzymatic glycosylation). Because some minor hemoglobin electrophoretic variants were found to be glycosylated, such variants might be a consequence of nonenzymatic glycosylation, just as in the browning of foods. The detection of elevated levels of the principal glycosylated hemoglobin variant Hb A_{1c} among diabetic patients supported this proposal. The rate and extent of nonenzymatic glycosylation of any protein in vivo depend in part on the concentration of protein and sugar, on the turnover rate of the protein, and on accessibility of sugar to the protein. Thus, if a protein has a rapid turnover rate, it cannot become significantly glycosylated, regardless of the concentration of blood glucose. Similarly, if the concentration of blood glucose is significantly elevated only for a small portion of time, the extent of protein glycosylation will be minimal, even if the specific protein has a very slow rate of turnover. The measurement of glycosylated hemoglobin (Hb A_{1c}) provides a sort of integrated assessment of the mean blood glucose concentration over the preceding 2 to 3 months. Measurement of glycosylated albumin or fructosamine reflects the mean blood glucose concentration over a much shorter period. However, many different methods of glycosylated protein assays are available, differing regarding glycated components, measured interferences, and nondiabetic ranges; thus, it is important that the clinician be aware of the method(s) used and their limitations.

More than simply providing a handy index of long-term glycemia, nonenzymatic glycosylation may have far greater implications in diabetes. Many proteins may exhibit significant changes in their functional properties after glycosylation and thus be responsible for some of the tissue-specific consequences of the diabetic state.[3]

MONITORING COMPLICATIONS. Careful monitoring of blood pressures is an important part of monitoring procedures. Monitoring quantitative urinary albumin excretion also appears to be significant because microalbuminuria exhibits a relationship to the development of significant nephropathy. Yearly monitoring of thyroid function and blood cholesterol/triglyceride levels is recommended. Complete ophthalmological examination and urinalysis must become regular components of ongoing management, beginning approximately 5 years after the clinical onset of type I or type II diabetes.

Patient and family education. Critical to the successful management of insulin-dependent diabetes is the extent to which the patient and family are engaged in and informed about the disease and its management. Living a life that is less restricted or affected by diabetes can only be achieved if the patient and parents fully understand the practical and theoretical aspects of the disease and its management. An outline of topics that must eventually be discussed fully with the patient and family is presented in Box 202-1. Several principles underlie the education of the diabetic family:

1. A natural period of shock and grieving accompanies a new diagnosis of diabetes, during which the family is not capable of easily assimilating extensive information.
2. Education about diabetes must be organized into discrete modules (digestible bites) of information.
3. Opportunity for self-study, using instructional aids, must be provided.
4. Educational outcome criteria need to be developed and incorporated into the patient's ongoing record; it is essential to know how much the patient and family actually comprehend.
5. Education must be directed initially toward the more practical procedures of blood glucose monitoring and insulin administration.
6. Education must be an ongoing, continuous part of patient-physician interaction and management.
7. Problem-solving situations to enhance education are most effective when two approaches are used: (a) analyzing and interpreting the data derived from the patient's own monitoring program, and (b) creating fictional "problem cases" that require the child/youth and the parent(s) both to understand the issues and to formulate approaches to management. Analysis of a patient's own blood glucose data may be facilitated by using computer-based systems for taking data stored in glucometers and displaying the data in a variety of ways.

Diet. Of overriding importance to helping children and their families manage diabetes is the concept of diet regularity. When an individual has lost the capacity to modulate the amount of insulin secreted from moment to moment in re-

BOX 202-1

TOPICS FOR PATIENT AND FAMILY EDUCATION

1. Nature of diabetes
   a. Blood glucose regulation in normal individuals
   b. Role of insulin
   c. Significance of hyperglycemia and ketoacidosis
   d. Significance of hypoglycemia
2. Monitoring
   a. Short term
      (1) Home blood glucose monitoring: technique and methods of analysis and interpretation
      (2) Urine testing
   b. Long term
      (1) Glycosylated protein levels
      (2) Clinical complications
3. Insulin therapy
   a. Types of insulin
   b. Methods of injection
4. Dietary management
   a. Importance of regularity
   b. Nutrient equivalents (exchange lists)
5. Effect of environment
   a. Emotional factors
   b. Exercise
6. Special problems and emergencies
   a. Ketoacidosis
   b. Insulin reactions (hypoglycemia)
   c. Illness
7. Informing family, friends, and school personnel about diabetes
8. Resources for diabetics
   a. Peer or family groups
   b. Organizations
   c. Camps

sponse to varying stimuli (glucose or amino acids), it becomes essential to keep constant from day to day the magnitude of the substrate load to be metabolized. Fortunately, the average child in a stable family usually has a uniform pattern of nutrient intake, but when that nutrient intake becomes the prime focus of parental attentions, mealtime can generate family anxiety. Soon, regularity in intake is replaced by marked irregularity and variation. In that situation, one asks the same dose of insulin to accomplish very different tasks from day to day—an impossible request. In addition to regularity in the timing and quantity of food intake, several other principles are important:

1. The diet should be adequate nutritionally, just as for a nondiabetic person.
2. The diet prescribed should be within the bounds of cultural patterns and individual preferences and also should be based, whenever possible, on the family's usual pattern of food served.
3. Caloric and protein intake should be sufficient for optimal growth without causing obesity.
4. Caloric intake in the morning should be proportionally less than at other meals. The "dawn phenomenon" refers to that period between approximately 5 AM and 9 AM when insulin requirements increase in the absence of antecedent hypoglycemia for both diabetic and nondiabetic individuals. Thus, the pancreas in a nondiabetic person secretes more insulin in the early morning to keep blood glucose normal. In the diabetic individual, blood glucose in the morning can be kept stable by reducing caloric intake at breakfast, compared with other meals.
5. Exchange diets, based on individual dietary assessment, may be used as an educational tool for establishing and maintaining a pattern of regularity in nutrient intake. However, the blood glucose response to various foods that contain isocaloric amounts of total carbohydrate varies widely; thus, the basic premise that underlies the older "exchange lists" actually may not be valid.
6. Readily available pure carbohydrate (e.g., candy) makes interpretation of blood glucose patterns difficult and thereby reduces the effectiveness of a self-monitoring program.

Insulin administration. All mammalian insulin is of a similar structure and contains 51 amino acids in two polypeptide chains (A and B). Human insulin (Humulin) made by use of recombinant DNA technology has largely replaced insulin isolated from animals.

The proper use of insulin in the management of diabetes is restricted by the following considerations:

1. The normal pattern of insulin secretion is one of rapid changes (pulses, almost) in response to substrate stimuli, with a subsequent rapid decline in insulin levels. No current system of insulin administration, including the newer extracorporeal and implanted pumps, can mimic the rapidly changing secretory patterns found in the nondiabetic individual.
2. Fifty percent of endogenous insulin, secreted into the portal vein, is extracted by the liver in a single passage, but when insulin is given parenterally (except by intraperitoneal administration), the liver is bypassed. Thus, the hepatic extraction rate for exogenously administered insulin theoretically can be only half the physiological secretory rate without producing peripheral hyperinsulinemia; at physiological peripheral blood insulin levels, the portal vein concentration remains only half that seen in the nondiabetic person.

Practical aspects of insulin administration include the following:

1. Insulin absorption from sites of injection is highly variable from site to site and from one individual to another. Insulin absorption is enhanced from sites in which vasodilation has been produced by exercise. Insulin should be injected in a rotating fashion, preferably within one area, for example, the abdominal wall or the upper, lateral thigh.
2. After administration of either intermediate- or long-acting forms of insulin, a relationship between the dose administered and the blood insulin level observed can be demonstrated *only* by measuring the total area under

the curve of blood insulin concentrations obtained over a period of 24 to 36 hours—that is, no single time after injection can be selected to measure "peak" levels. Thus, intermediate- and long-acting insulins cannot be used effectively where changing levels in circulating insulin are needed to handle sudden changes in substrate load (e.g., after meals).

3. For all type I and many type II patients, at least two or more injections of insulin are required per day, with each injection being a mixture of both rapid- or short- and longer-acting insulins. In the patient who can only tolerate two injections per day, the following guidelines are helpful: (a) in the "established" diabetic (i.e., beyond the honeymoon period), less than 1 U/kg/day of insulin should be given; (b) the usual division of insulin should approximate two thirds of the total dose before breakfast and one third before the evening meal; and (c) approximately one third to half of the morning insulin should be given as short-acting insulin, whereas increasing ratios of intermediate-acting insulin to regular insulin are given before the evening meal. The intermediate insulin in the evening may be given separately before bedtime to reduce the likelihood of hypoglycemia during sleep.
4. In those patients who choose to control their diabetes as precisely as possible, the short-acting insulin analog lispro (Lys[B28], Pro [B29]) offers some advantages. When given together with small doses of intermediate insulin (NPH) 15 to 30 minutes before mealtimes, diabetic control can be improved with a reduction in the frequency of hypoglycemia.[11]

Physical activity. Regular physical activity is an important part of diabetic management, not only as an effective means to facilitate glucose utilization but also as an integral component of a lifestyle designed to minimize the risk of large-vessel disease. Because the physical activity of children often is sporadic and unpredictable, it is wiser to ask the child to take extra calories than to attempt to alter insulin administration in anticipation of exercise, which can increase glucose utilization sufficiently to produce a relative insulin overdose and lead to hypoglycemia.

Psychological considerations. Like any chronic illness, diabetes presents new problems that may affect the child who has diabetes and his or her family. Many normal developmental tasks such as mealtime choices and acquiring independence during play. may be more difficult and less spontaneous for both child and parents. The family's ability to lead a normal life may be compromised by ignorance of the principles of good control or by unnecessary rigidities that impose excessive restrictions on lifestyle. An adolescent who has diabetes may use the disease and the quality control it requires as a weapon against his or her parents; the parents, in turn, may use the disease as a mechanism to restrain the adolescent's establishment of appropriate independence from them.

The intimate relation that exists between the emotional state and the metabolic control of diabetes is well recognized. Numerous studies have demonstrated that emotional disturbances lead to compromised rates of glucose utilization, presumably through increased secretion of counterregulatory hormones such as adrenal corticosteroids and catecholamines. Conversely, emotional well-being of a patient who has diabetes can be affected by disturbances in metabolic control.

Uninformed responses to the child's disease by the extended family, friends, and school personnel can magnify his or her emotional distress. Careful attention, therefore, must be paid to informing and educating such well-meaning contacts so that the child's living experiences are not restricted unnecessarily.

With careful attention to family dynamics, effort should be focused on improving the family's interactions, facilitating the communication of individual and group needs, and allowing both the child and family the opportunity to express the fears, concerns, and frustrations generated by the predictable problems every family with a child who has diabetes faces.

As the child grows older, the effect of microangiopathic and neuropathic complications on the emotional state becomes pronounced. Yet many patients remain able to maintain the balance necessary between the demands and excitement of their normal lives and the insistent constraints imposed by their disease.

FUTURE DEVELOPMENTS

Attempts to reduce the impact of type I diabetes reflect three primary approaches: (1) preventing the development of diabetes, (2) improving the physiological delivery of insulin, and (3) understanding the biological basis for the complications of diabetes, with the assumption that pharmacological tools will become available to impede the development of complications.

Prevention

The demonstration that therapy directed toward inhibiting an immune-mediated process at the time of clinical onset can delay the rate of beta-cell destruction has set the stage for multiple approaches toward either primary prevention or treatment of subclinical disease in high-risk individuals. Primary prevention would be feasible if it can be demonstrated that certain defined antigens such as cow milk proteins participate in "molecular mimicry." Clinical protocols are addressing several approaches to early treatment of islet-cell, antibody-positive relatives of persons who have type I diabetes. These include the use of: (1) nicotinamide; (2) parenteral insulin in autoantibody-positive family members who already have exhibited loss of the first phase of insulin secretion response to an intravenous glucose challenge; (3) oral insulin in a larger population; and (4) different immunotherapy programs directed toward minimizing side effects.[12]

Improving the Physiological Delivery of Insulin

Insulin delivery systems. "Open-loop" devices for long-term subcutaneous insulin infusions can provide normal metabolic control in certain patients, but they require a higher order of individual responsibility and compliance;

such devices also are associated with complications (infection, erratic absorption, ketoacidosis). The "brittle" and often unmotivated child who has diabetes usually is not a good candidate for use of these open-loop devices. "Closed-loop" infusion devices (where insulin is delivered in response to the blood glucose level) must await the development of a reliable and implantable or attachable glucose sensor. The recent developments of optical glucose sensing, radiotelemetry systems to link pump and sensor, and miniaturization and refinement of insulin pumps create the promise of a clinically useful "artificial pancreas."

Differing insulin forms. Compounds that mimic the action of insulin when given orally are being tested for their efficacy. These oral forms of insulin or insulin-like compounds, however, are of short duration in their action and cannot be used alone, without concomitant insulin injections, to provide necessary insulin levels during the overnight period.

Beta-cell transplantation. Islet-cell or intact-pancreas transplantation has been successful; however, ongoing immunosuppression is required to maintain graft acceptance. Attempts to alter the antigenicity of donor cells before transplantation so far have been only partially successful. Further, transplanted cells or tissue often become subject to the same autoimmune phenomena that led to islet-cell destruction in the patient initially. Development of immunobarrier devices, immunosuppression, improvements in the development of tolerance, and genetic manipulation represent approaches to preventing the transplant from being destroyed by either initial immune rejection or subsequent autoimmunity.

Understanding the Biological Bases of Diabetic Complications

If the biochemical mechanisms that underlie diabetic complications were completely understood, specific therapies might be formulated that could forestall or prevent pathophysiological sequelae. For instance, nonenzymatic glycosylation of proteins leads to increased protein cross-linking, a process that can be impeded chemically. In chronic hyperglycemia, shunting of glucose through the sorbitol or polyol pathway increases (leading to increased tissue concentrations of sorbitol), and this process can be impeded by inhibitors of the enzyme aldose reductase. Impaired synthesis of heparin proteoglycan may cause increased permeability of the vascular endothelium to macromolecules, a mechanism that also may be subject to chemical modification. These putative mechanisms exemplify exciting possibilities concerning chemical prevention of the pathological consequences of diabetes.

COMPLICATIONS

Insulin Resistance

The most common form of insulin resistance occurs as a normal phenomenon—that is, during puberty, when insulin requirements in diabetic patients may increase to 2 U/kg/day. Another common form of insulin resistance is that produced by excessive insulin administration (e.g., the Somogyi phenomenon). When poor metabolic control of the disease is attended by insulin dosages significantly exceeding 1 U/kg/day, concern should be raised about invoking the Somogyi phenomenon; a stepwise reduction in insulin dose eventually will lead to improved control. Insulin resistance also may accompany use of the same site for repetitive injections (leading to reduced insulin absorption). Further understanding of rare instances of insulin resistance requires sophisticated studies of insulin binding and postreceptor phenomena.[8] The child who has so-called brittle type I diabetes in reality most often is the child for whom family disruption and emotional factors lead to irregularity in diet, activity, and insulin administration, along with the metabolic consequences of emotional distress.

Organ-Specific Complications

The major goals in diabetic management are the facilitation of normal physical and emotional growth and development, as well as postponement or actual prevention of the microangiopathic and neuropathic complications of the disease. Signs of microangiopathy are observed readily in many (but not all) children within 5 to 10 years after the clinical onset of diabetes, although the actual clinical consequences are seen only rarely in childhood or adolescence. Individuals caring for children who have diabetes, therefore, constantly must recall the consequences of the disease in later life and, thus, the overriding importance of establishing and maintaining optimal metabolic control.

When to Refer

Inability to establish mechanism of hyperglycemia during and/or following initial presentation
Diabetic education and support program not available
Family desires access to specialized information and methodology

REFERENCES

1. American Diabetes Association: Implications of the United Kingdom Prospective Diabetes Study, *Diabetes Care* 22:S27, 1999.
2. Barrett-Connor E: Does hyperglycemia really cause coronary heart disease? *Diabetes Care* 20:1620, 1997.
3. Brownlee M: Glycation products and the pathogenesis of diabetic complications, *Diabetes Care* 15:1835, 1992.
4. Davis EA, et al: Hypoglycemia: incidence and clinical predictors in a large population-based sample of children and adolescents with IDDM, *Diabetes Care* 20:22, 1997.
5. DeFronzo RA, Bonadonna RC, Ferrannini E: Pathogenesis of NIDDM: a balanced overview, *Diabetes Care* 15:318, 1992.
6. Donaghue KC, et al: The effect of prepubertal diabetes duration on diabetes, *Diabetes Care* 20:77, 1997.
7. Dryberg T: Molecular mimicry between virus proteins and autoantigens in autoimmunity. In Demaine AG, Banga J-P, McGregor AM, editors: *The molecular biology of autoimmune disease,* Berlin, 1990, Springer-Verlag.
8. Flier JS: Syndromes of insulin resistance: from patient to gene and back again, *Diabetes* 41:1207, 1992.
9. Glaser NS: Non-insulin-dependent diabetes mellitus in childhood and adolescence, *Pediatr Clin North Am* 44:307, 1997.

10. Klein R: Hyperglycemia and microvascular and macrovascular disease in diabetes, *Diabetes Care* 18:258, 1995.
11. Lalli C, et al: Long-term intensive treatment of type 1 diabetes with the short-acting insulin analog lispro in variable combination with NPH insulin at mealtime, *Diabetes Care* 22:468, 1999.
12. Mahon JL, Dupre J: The limitations of clinical trials for prevention of IDDM, *Diabetes Care* 20:1027, 1997.
13. Nepom GT, Kwok WW: Molecular basis for HLA-DQ associations with IDDM, *Diabetes* 47:1177, 1998.
14. Ovalle F, et al: Brief twice-weekly episodes of hypoglycemia reduce detection of clinical hypoglycemia in type I diabetes mellitus, *Diabetes* 47:1472, 1998.
15. Rosenbloom AL, et al: Emerging epidemic of type 2 diabetes in youth, *Diabetes Care* 22:345, 1999.
16. Tait BD, et al: HLA antigens and age at diagnosis of insulin-dependent diabetes mellitus, *Hum Immunol* 42:116, 1995.
17. The Diabetes Control and Complications Trial Research Group: The effect of intensive treatment of diabetes on the development and progression of long-term complications in insulin-dependent diabetes mellitus, *N Engl J Med* 329:977, 1993.
18. UK Prospective Diabetes Study Group: Intensive blood-glucose control with sulphonylureas or insulin compared with conventional treatment and risk of complications in patients with type 2 diabetes (UKPDS 33), *Lancet* 352:837, 1998.

203 Diaper Rash

Gregory S. Liptak

Diaper rash is the most common skin disorder of infants and toddlers. For example, a survey of suburban infants revealed that 25% had some diaper dermatitis; 4% of the sample had a rash that was classified as severe.[10] The greatest frequency occurs in infants between 9 and 12 months of age.[1] Diaper rash is not a single disorder but represents the reaction of the skin to a host of factors, both local and systemic, and on occasion may result from serious illness.

ETIOLOGY

Four factors have been associated with the occurrence of diaper rash: (1) wetness of the skin, (2) elevated pH level of the skin, (3) fecal enzymes, and (4) microorganisms.[2,21] Wet skin has been shown experimentally to have greater friction and higher permeability. In one study, infants whose diapers had been changed eight or more times during the day (and presumably were drier) had less rash than those whose diapers were changed less often.[7] Diapers made with water-absorbent gel material (usually cross-linked sodium polyacrylates) have been shown to keep skin drier and decrease the occurrence of diaper rash.[4,13,19]

The normal pH concentration of the skin is between 4.5 and 5.5. Elevated pH levels increase irritation and have been associated with more severe diaper rash. When urine and stool mix on an infant's skin, urease from the stool breaks down urea in the urine, increasing the pH. Although ammonia, which once was believed to be the primary irritant causing diaper rash,[15] may play a role in increasing the pH level, it no longer is considered to be the major factor.

Normal stool contains enzymes such as proteases and lipases that inflame skin and increase permeability to substances such as bile salts, which worsen the inflammation. Infants who have more frequent bowel movements, such as those who have gastroenteritis or who are taking antibiotics, have a higher prevalence of diaper dermatitis.[4] Infants who are breast-fed have lower levels of enzymes in their stools, lower urinary pH, and a lower occurrence of diaper rash.

The most important microorganism found on the skin of infants who have diaper rash is *Candida albicans*. This yeast, which produces a protease that penetrates the skin, can (1) cause a primary infection, (2) be a secondary invader in systemic conditions such as seborrheic dermatitis, and (3) be found in many infants who have nonspecific diaper rash. Even a small number of *Candida* organisms can cause significant infection. In one survey, candidal species were isolated from half the mouths cultured in healthy infants.[5] Infants who routinely sucked a pacifier had a higher rate of oral candidal carriage. The use of oral or parenteral antibiotics can increase the number of *Candida* organisms on the skin (as well as the frequency of stools) and contribute to the occurrence of diaper rash.[8] *Staphylococcus aureus* also has been isolated as a secondary invader of systemic illness, such as atopic dermatitis; however, although present on the skin, it does not appear to be a common primary pathogen in other forms of diaper rash.[14]

PATHOLOGY

A few histopathological studies of diaper rash have been described; however, most of these have dealt with unusual or chronic cases. The more common diaper rashes are believed to manifest nonspecific inflammatory changes.

HISTORY

Historical factors that may help determine the factors contributing to diaper rash include duration of the rash; associated symptoms (e.g., diarrhea); type of diaper; frequency of changing; method of laundering (if cloth diapers are used); use of watertight coverings, such as plastic (rubber) pants; past illness (especially dermatological, allergic, infectious); medication use (e.g., antibiotics), including the therapy for the rash; exposure to contagious disease (e.g., scabies, varicella); the presence of systemic symptoms; and a family history of illness (e.g., psoriasis, allergy).

PHYSICAL EXAMINATION

Although diaper rashes can be classified by presentation (appearance and location), this approach should be viewed with caution because one agent (e.g., *C. albicans*) can lead to different presentations, and a single presentation may be caused by many agents (acting either alone or in concert).

Three common distribution patterns for diaper rash occur. Chafing (irritative or ammoniacal) dermatitis (Fig. 203-1) is an erythematous desquamative rash involving the convex surfaces that touch the diaper and spare the inguinal folds. There is mild erythema with or without papules. The skin has a shiny, glazed appearance. This rash is associated with the irritants mentioned previously. Prolonged contact with water (uncontaminated urine) probably facilitates the production of all diaper rashes, especially those in this category. Meatitis (urethritis) may be seen in boys who have this type of diaper rash. Diaper rashes that have persisted for more than 72

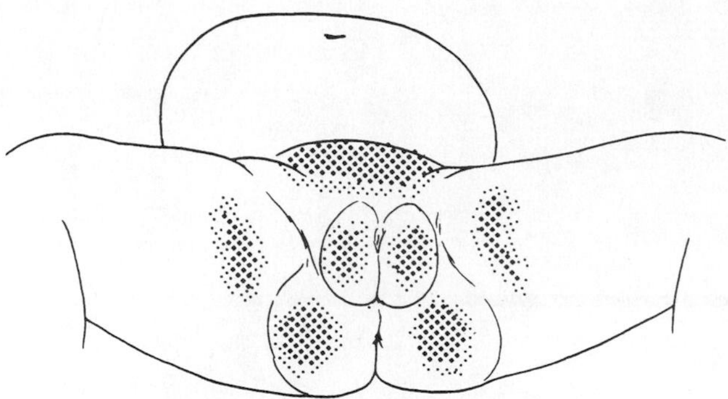

Fig. 203-1 Irritative pattern of diaper dermatitis.

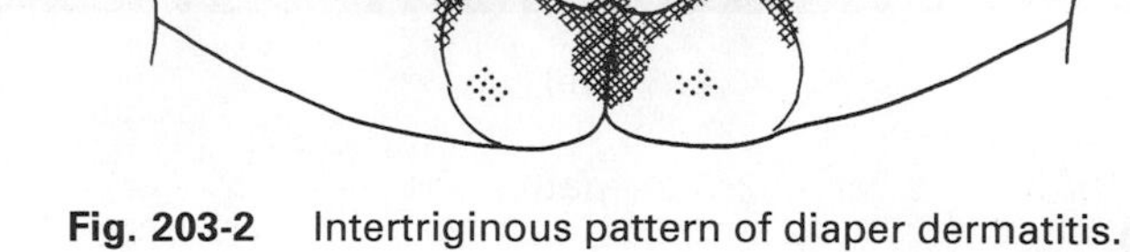

Fig. 203-2 Intertriginous pattern of diaper dermatitis.

hours usually are found to have significant *Candida* involvement.

Atopic dermatitis may have the same distribution as chafing, as do zinc deficiency, Kawasaki disease, and Wiskott-Aldrich syndrome. The eczematoid appearance with lichenification (thickening), pruritus, and the occurrence of the atopic dermatitis elsewhere on the child should help substantiate this diagnosis. Diaper rash caused by atopic dermatitis is uncommon in children younger than 6 months.

The second pattern of diaper dermatitis involves skinfolds and spares convex surfaces (Fig. 203-2). Rashes involving the perianal area only are common in the neonatal period and may be the result of irritation from diarrhea (and are especially common in children whose diarrhea is secondary to disaccharidase deficiency). They also may be caused by infection with *C. albicans.*

Moist, macerated symmetrical eruptions in the skinfolds and creases (see Fig. 203-2) may result from seborrhea or intertrigo, an ill-defined entity. Both commonly are infected secondarily by *C. albicans,* especially when satellite lesions are present. The classic primary candidal (monilial) diaper rash has this pattern, with bright red confluent lesions, often with raised borders, and occasionally with pustular-vesicular satellite lesions on the trunk and legs. Other areas, such as the folds of the neck, the postauricular area, and the oral mucosa (thrush), may be involved. Dermatitis caused by *Candida* organisms usually is painful and tender. Letterer-Siwe disease (histiocytosis) may have the same skin rash distribution as seborrhea or *Candida* infections but is more papular and more likely to be ulcerated. It also fails to respond to conventional therapy; the child may have constitutional symptoms such as malaise and abnormal physical findings such as hepatosplenomegaly. Seborrheic dermatitis, which also has been termed *psoriasiform napkin dermatitis,* is characterized by beefy red confluent erythema with scaling involving the entire diaper area; however, the intertriginous areas are involved more prominently. The rash looks worse than it appears to feel to the child. Some of these infants have a family history of psoriasis; true psoriasis will develop in approximately 3% as they get older.

The third major distribution pattern of diaper dermatitis is shown in Fig. 203-3. Erythema in this distribution has been termed *tide mark dermatitis* and is believed to be related to frequent cycles of wetting and drying. Irritation from diapers

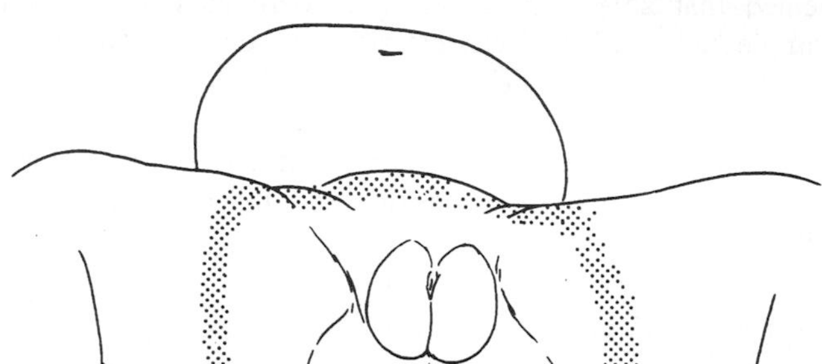

Fig. 203-3 Constrictive pattern of diaper dermatitis.

that are too tight (constrictive) and that may have an elastic band also can lead to a similar rash.

Diaper rashes that do not fit any of these patterns—for example, from herpes simplex virus infection, also occur. In one study, the less a rash looked like the one shown in Fig. 203-1, the more likely it was to be associated with *Candida* organisms.[4] Diaper dermatitis from any cause can become secondarily infected with *Staphylococcus* or *Streptococcus* organisms, leading to impetigo or bullous impetigo.

DIFFERENTIAL DIAGNOSIS

Systemic conditions such as seborrhea, atopic dermatitis, hand-foot-and-mouth disease, primary herpes simplex infection, psoriasis, varicella, miliaria, and scabies may begin or occur with greater intensity in the diaper area,[11] and may be altered morphologically.[16] Such predilections for the diaper area probably represents the Koebner (isomorphic) response in which the skin lesions of a systemic illness concentrate on areas previously inflamed by other factors—for example, friction.[10] Table 203-1 lists some of the less common causes of diaper rash.

In addition to the aforementioned conditions, histiocytosis (Letterer-Siwe disease), acrodermatitis enteropathica,[17] congenital syphilis, granuloma gluteale infantum,[3] and Wiskott-Aldrich syndrome may lead to rashes that are prominent in the diaper area. Kawasaki disease may manifest as a red, desquamating perineal eruption, often during the first week after onset of the syndrome[6] (see Chapter 230, Kawasaki

Table 203-1 Less Common Conditions Associated with Diaper Rash

Conditions	Comments
Infectious or presumed infectious	
Herpes simplex virus	Vesicular; may be associated with immunosuppression
Cytomegalovirus	Usually associated with immunosuppression
Kawasaki disease	Desquamating rash associated with fever
Syphilis	May have other manifestations of secondary syphilis
Trichophyton	Extremely uncommon; annular scaly patches
Neoplastic	
Histiocytosis (Letterer-Siwe)	Resembles seborrhea plus reddish brown papules
Nutritional and metabolic	
Zinc deficiency (acrodermatitis enteropathica)	Mimics monilial rash; vesicular eruptions elsewhere
Presumed iatrogenic	
Granuloma gluteale infantum	May be secondary to use of halogenated steroid creams
Genetic	
Wiskott-Aldrich	Thrombocytopenia and recurrent infections in boys

Disease). Serious illness always must be considered in the child who has an atypical or a severe rash, as well as in the child who fails to respond to customary therapy. For instance, the child who has severe "seborrhea" may have histiocytosis; fulminant atopic dermatitis may be the result of Wiskott-Aldrich syndrome; and severe, persistent, and recurrent infections with *Candida* organisms may (albeit rarely) result from immunodeficiency, including infection with human immunodeficiency virus (HIV) or diabetes mellitus. Children who are immunosuppressed from HIV infection or neoplasia (or its treatment) may have diaper rash from organisms such as herpes simplex or cytomegalovirus. If an immunosuppressed child has a serious or unresponsive diaper rash, aggressive pursuit of an etiological agent, including skin biopsy, should be considered.[20] The physician should suspect child (including sexual) abuse or neglect in the child who has lesions in the diaper area (especially burns) that are inconsistent with the history provided.

LABORATORY FINDINGS

Laboratory tests generally are not indicated for most diaper rashes. Those that may be helpful in identifying the cause of a diaper rash include a potassium hydroxide preparation and a fungal culture of skin scrapings for *Candida* organisms, a bacterial culture for *Staphylococcus* organisms, a mineral oil slide preparation for scabies, a serum zinc level (to rule out acrodermatitis enteropathica), serological tests for syphilis, and radiograms of the skull and long bones for evidence of child abuse. Rarely, a skin biopsy may be useful in cases in which the diaper rash is atypical or unresponsive to therapy.

MANAGEMENT

Because most diaper rashes, whatever the cause, are worsened by prolonged contact with wet or soiled diapers, the initial step in their management should be to keep the skin free of such diapers as much as possible. However, because total abstinence from diapers is impractical, most clinicians recommend that during therapy the diapers be changed frequently (at least eight times a day, using diapers with absorbent gel material) and kept off as much as possible and that plastic pants that retain water not be used.

Most systemic conditions such as scabies, atopic dermatitis, and varicella can be managed for the diaper area as they are for other parts of the skin. Seborrheic dermatitis, however, is an exception. Because it so often is infected secondarily with *Candida* organisms, measures to treat the yeast must be undertaken as well. For this and other diaper rashes in which *Candida* organisms are present, topical miconazole, clotrimazole, haloprogin, nystatin, or ketoconazole should be applied. Miconazole has the advantage of requiring only twice-daily applications, is less irritating than nystatin, and probably is more effective. It also is more expensive. Gentian violet also is effective but is extremely messy. The simultaneous use of 1% hydrocortisone usually hastens healing. Steroids more potent than 1% hydrocortisone should never be used in the diaper area because diapers form an occlusive dressing. Their chronic use may lead to granuloma gluteale infantum (a rash characterized by purple granulomatous nodules),[3] skin atrophy, telangiectasis, striae, irritation, and systemically, Cushing's syndrome. The effectiveness of oral nystatin in the therapy of candidal diaper rash is uncertain. In a controlled study, Hoppe et al found that oral nystatin did not decrease the recurrence of candidal diaper rash significantly.[9] In another controlled trial, oral miconazole was more effective than nystatin in eliminating oral *Candida* in infants who had oral thrush.[9]

For irritative diaper rashes, changing diapers frequently and washing the skin with plain water and allowing it to dry between diaper changes usually are the only interventions needed. The use of diapers with absorbent gel materials has been shown to decrease wetness in the diaper area and may hasten the disappearance of a diaper dermatitis.[13] Scrubbing the rash or diaper area should be discouraged; a soft cloth with water should provide sufficient cleansing in most cases. A barrier ointment that contains zinc oxide or vitamins A and D may help to protect the skin from further irritation. Rinsing cloth diapers in methylbenzethonium chloride (Diaperene), a bacteriostatic agent, or in a vinegar solution (1 ounce in a gallon of water) has been shown to reduce recurrences.[7] Agents to acidify the urine (cranberry juice, vitamin C), cornstarch, and ointments that contain vitamins A and D are widely used; however, there is no experimental evidence that they are effective. Eliminating fabric softeners and changing detergents may be effective in some cases, but this approach also is undocumented scientifically. In cases of significant inflammation, 1% hydrocortisone may promote healing. The meatitis that occurs in this form of rash may be treated with topical antibiotics to prevent stricture by use of an ophthalmic solution applied by partially inserting the tip of the dispensing bottle into the urethra every 4 to 6 hours.

Many more children have been harmed by well-intended diaper rash therapies than have ever been harmed by the rash itself. Boric acid, mercury compounds, and pentachlorophenol used in the treatment and prevention of irritative diaper rash have led to illness and death in infants.[10] Talcum powder never should be used because inhalation of a large quantity can produce serious, even fatal, pulmonary damage. The dangers of topical steroids already have been mentioned. Hair dryers should never be recommended as a means to dry the skin in the diaper area; perineal burns may result. Products containing iodochlorhydroxyquin, such as Vioform, should never be used because they may lead to optic atrophy and neuropathy. Prudent use of therapeutic agents is necessary to avoid harm. The use of commercial diaper wipes, which contain an emollient and cleansing agent, is on the increase. In one controlled study, no clinically detectable differences in erythema, frequency of rashes, edema, and desquamation were found in the perineal regions of infants compared with those times when soap and water were used. However, the wipes led to a lower pH. The significance of this is uncertain.[18]

PREVENTION

If there were no diapers, there would be no diaper rashes. Because the complete elimination of diapers is unacceptable, alternatives to keep the skin dry, such as changing as soon as the diaper becomes wet or soiled and avoiding plastic pants, have been recommended.

Most recent studies have shown that diapers that contain absorbent gel are associated with the lowest incidence of diaper rash in otherwise healthy children and those who have atopic dermatitis.[12,13,19] Although plastic diapers that contain absorbent gel material have been shown to decrease the occurrence of diaper rash and to contain stool and urine better, an important factor for decreasing the spread of disease in sites such as child care centers, attention also should be paid to the effect of plastic diapers on the environment. It is estimated that commercial nonbiodegradable diapers make up 1% to 2% of landfills. The cost of their disposal, which is borne by all citizens, should be considered when recommending their use. On the other hand, washing cloth diapers (and soiled clothes and bed linens) requires water and energy, as well as human labor.[22] Parents who usually use cloth diapers may consider using commercial diapers that contain absorbent gel materials when their children are at increased risk for developing diaper rash, such as when they are taking antibiotics or have gastroenteritis. Commercial diapers also are convenient during travel away from home.

Breast-feeding and frequent diaper changes have been associated with a lower occurrence of diaper rash; both should be recommended. Airing the diaper area, using barrier creams and ointments, cleansing the diaper area promptly, selecting the diaper, and educating caregivers should prevent much diaper rash. The physician should be certain that other recommendations do not harm the child.

When to Refer

If the rash has not responded to conventional treatment in several weeks or is worsening
If the rash is nodular
If abuse is suspected

Use of Alternative Medicine

May be used to treat or prevent rashes, as long as they are known not to be toxic or harmful

When to Hospitalize

If the child is systemically ill and cannot be treated safely at home

REFERENCES

1. Benjamin L: Clinical correlates with diaper dermatitis, *Pediatrician* 14:21, 1987.
2. Berg RW, Buckingham KW, Stewart RL: Etiologic factors in diaper dermatitis: the role of urine, *Pediatr Dermatol* 3:102, 1986.
3. Bluestein J, Furner BB, Phillips SD: Granuloma gluteale infantum: case report and review of the literature, *Pediatr Dermatol* 7:196, 1990.
4. Campbell RL, et al: Effects of diaper types on diaper dermatitis associated with diarrhea and antibiotic use of children in day-care centers, *Pediatr Dermatol* 5:83, 1988.
5. Darwazeh AM, al-Bashir A J: Oral candidal flora in healthy infants, *Oral Pathol Med* 24:361, 1995.
6. Friter BS, Lucky AW: The perineal eruption of Kawasaki syndrome, *Arch Dermatol* 124:1805, 1988.
7. Grant WW, Street L, Fearnow RG: Diaper rashes in infancy: studies on the effects of various methods of laundering, *Clin Pediatr* 12:714, 1973.
8. Honig PJ, et al: Amoxicillin and diaper dermatitis, *J Am Acad Dermatol* 19:275, 1988.
9. Hoppe JE, Hahn H: Randomized comparison of two nystatin oral gels with miconazole oral gel for treatment of oral thrush in infants, *Infection* 24:136, 1996.
10. Jacobs AH: Eruptions in the diaper area, *Pediatr Clin North Am* 25:209, 1978.
11. Jenson HB, Shapiro ED: Primary herpes simplex virus infection of a diaper rash, *Pediatr Infect Dis J* 6:1136, 1987.
12. Jordan WE, et al: Diaper dermatitis: frequency and severity among a general infant population, *Pediatr Dermatol* 3:198, 1986.
13. Lane AT, Rehder PA, Helm K: Evaluations of diapers containing absorbing gelling material with conventional diapers in newborn infants, *Am J Dis Child* 144:315, 1990.
14. Leyden JJ, Klingman AM: The role of microorganisms in diaper dermatitis, *Arch Dermatol* 114:56, 1978.
15. Leyden JJ, et al: Urinary ammonia and ammonia-producing microorganisms in infants with and without diaper dermatitis, *Arch Dermatol* 113:1678, 1977.

16. Messner J, et al: Accentuated viral exanthems in areas of inflammation, *J Am Acad Dermatol* 40:345, 1999.
17. Munro CS, Lazaro C, Lawrence CM: Symptomatic zinc deficiency in breast-fed premature infants, *Br J Dermatol* 121:773, 1989.
18. Priestley GC, McVittie E, Aldridge RD: Changes in skin pH after the use of baby wipes, *Pediatr Dermatol* 13:14, 1996.
19. Seymour JL, et al: Clinical effects of diaper types on the skin of normal infants and infants with ectopic dermatitis, *J Am Acad Dermatol* 17:988, 1987.
20. Thiboutot DM, et al: Cytomegalovirus diaper dermatitis, *Arch Dermatol* 127:396, 398, 1991.
21. Weston WL, Lane AT, Weston JA: Diaper dermatitis: current concepts, *Pediatrics* 66:532, 1980.
22. Wong DL, et al: Diapering choices: a critical review of the issues, *Pediatr Nurs* 18:41, 1992.

204 Down Syndrome: Managing the Child and Family

Paul T. Rogers

The pediatrician provides education and support for the family of a child born having Down syndrome (DS). The physician plays a critical role in helping the family adapt to their child's special needs. However, it may be frustrating at times to meet this responsibility. Often it is difficult to locate current information about the special health problems of a child who has DS. In addition, coordinating care with medical subspecialists and early child education specialists often can be time consuming. This chapter provides the pediatrician with a guide to the special needs of these families and children. It also discusses interventions that can identify and remediate many disorders that prevent a DS child from reaching his or her full potential.

DS occurs in about 1 in every 1250 births,[8] a decline from the incidence of 1 in 700 births just a decade ago.[34] Although the specific reason for this decline is not clear, termination of pregnancy may play a role.[7] The incidence of DS is closely related to advanced age of the mother, and the likelihood of bearing an infant who has DS increases dramatically when maternal age is greater than 35.[20]

Recent advances have improved noninvasive techniques for identifying fetuses that have DS. Previously, measurement of the maternal serum alpha-fetoprotein (AFP) level was offered to pregnant women younger than age 35 because low levels of AFP are associated with DS.[1] Diminished levels of other maternal serum factors, unconjugated estriol, and human chorionic gonadotropin (hCG) also are associated with DS.[1] Currently, for pregnant women younger than age 35, serum screening usually includes a combination of AFP, estriol, and hCG. For pregnant women older than age 35, amniocentesis or chorionic villous sampling (CVS) is offered instead of serum screening. In the future, prenatal testing almost entirely through noninvasive methods will be available to high-risk women.[24]

ETIOLOGY

An abnormality in chromosome replication leads to DS. The abnormality, known as *nondisjunction,* occurs during meiosis. During normal replication, the process of disjunction reduces the number of chromosomes in the sperm and ova from 46 to 23. At fertilization, the egg and sperm unite, giving the developing fetus the full number of 46 chromosomes in 23 pairs. Nondisjunction is the improper division of the 46 chromosomes in the cell, resulting in 24 chromosomes in the sperm or egg. At fertilization, 24 chromosome pairs, usually in the egg, unite with 23 pairs of chromosomes in the sperm, resulting in a total of 47 chromosomes. Recent DNA testing has shown that nondisjunction takes place in the egg 91.6% of the time.[4] In 90% of individuals who have DS, there is an extra chromosome in the 21 group (the extra chromosome plus the normal pair), which is designated *trisomy.*[24] A small group of DS patients have a mixture of cell types (mosaicism), some cells with 46 chromosomes and some with 47. *Translocation* refers to a chromosome rearrangement in which the extra chromosome attaches to yet another chromosome. In the case of DS, one of the chromosomes from the 21 group often attaches to one in the 14 group. This results in the normal number of 46 chromosomes in 23 pairs, but the karyotype shows the abnormally attached additional chromosomal material. Both translocation and mosaicism produce the clinical picture of DS. Translocation is especially significant because it can be inherited.

Every newborn who has DS requires chromosome testing. This information forms the basis of genetic counseling for the parents regarding the risk of recurrence. Chromosomal analysis complements a detailed family history. With this information, the family can better make decisions about future pregnancies.

Down syndrome, in effect, is a gene overdosage disease.[2] A DS-specific segment on a normal 21 chromosome produces excess proteins. The overproduction results in an imbalance of the biochemical pathways, which causes the physical characteristics of DS. Chromosome mapping shows that the DS-specific region is located around D21S55 in 21q22.2-22.3.[10]

Preventive management refers to early detection and correction of medical problems seen in children who have DS. Children who have this disorder require the usual preventive interventions and anticipatory guidance given to other children and families, but the special problems of children who have DS require additional evaluation and close monitoring. The most common types of problems include the following:

1. Ophthalmological: strabismus, myopia, and cataracts
2. Otological: chronic otitis media, conductive hearing loss
3. Cardiac: congenital heart disease (CHD)
4. Endocrine: hypothyroidism
5. Gastrointestinal: constipation, failure to thrive
6. Neurological: congenital malformation, seizures

Careful examination and testing should be done at critical ages to detect these common problems and correct them, if possible.

Occasionally a woman who has learned that she is carrying a fetus that has DS will contact a pediatrician with questions about the challenges of raising a child who has this

BOX 204-1

COMMON FEATURES OF DOWN SYNDROME

May or May not Be Present:

Head
Brachycephaly (flat occiput)

Dermatoglyphics
Increased ulnar loops
Single-flexion crease on fifth finger
Four-finger sign (simian crease): transverse palmar lines

Eyes
Brushfield spots (speckling of the iris)
Inner epicanthal folds
Upward slanting palpebral fissures (mongolian characteristic)

Face
Flat appearing
Low nasal bridge
Small shell-like ears with small or no earlobes

Fingers and toes
Brachydactyly (short hands and fingers)
Wide-spaced first and second toes

Heart (commonly, congenital defects)
Endocardial cushion defects
Ventricular septal defects

Hips and pelvis
Dysplasia

Neck
Short
Superabundant skin at nape

Neuromuscular system
Absent or diminished Moro reflex
Muscular hypotonia
Joint hyperflexibility

Tongue
Macroglossia
Excessive protrusion

Potential for:
Increased incidence of leukemia
Increased susceptibility to infection
Increased incidence of duodenal atresia

disorder. A good additional source of information is the National Down Syndrome Congress (1-800-232-6372). This organization can provide the names of parents in the caller's community who have a DS child, as well as information about DS, per se.

DIAGNOSIS

The birth of a child who has DS presents an abundance of clinical and family management issues. The first critical task is making an accurate diagnosis. This often can be done at the bedside by means of a careful examination. When eight of the many characteristics commonly associated with DS are present (Box 204-1), the diagnosis is relatively simple.[17]

BOX 204-2

SUGGESTIONS FOR INFORMING THE PARENTS

1. Talk to both parents in a quiet place.
2. Report the diagnostic information; be hopeful.
3. Allow time for the parents to respond.
4. Give the parents current information to read.
5. Give the parents the telephone number of the local Down syndrome support group.
6. Discuss future expectations briefly.
7. Allow the parents time to express their feelings and to ask questions.

BOX 204-3

MANAGING THE NEWBORN

History
1. Evaluate the feeding pattern
2. Evaluate the stooling pattern

Physical Examination
1. Perform a general physical examination and a neurological examination
2. Check for signs of CHD
3. Examine the eyes for congenital cataracts

Laboratory Tests
1. Chromosomal karyotyping
2. Thyroid screening

Consultation
1. Cardiological examination
2. Genetic counseling

However, when the diagnosis is based on one or two findings, errors can occur. For example, 50% of children who have DS have the four-finger sign (formerly called a *simian crease*), but so do 15% of normal children. Small ears also are characteristic, but not diagnostic, of DS.

Many pediatricians are reluctant to share the diagnosis of DS with the parents unless it is confirmed in the laboratory by chromosomal karyotyping. Physicians delay the diagnosis until it is definitive so as to avoid giving the family the wrong diagnosis. However, most families would like the physician to share the information with them as soon as the diagnosis of DS is suspected (Box 204-2). The pediatrician must decide which approach is best for the individual situation.

MANAGEMENT

Newborn to 2 Months of Age (Box 204-3)

After the diagnosis is made, the child is observed for signs of gastrointestinal malformations (vomiting, weight loss, and absence of stools), cardiac malformations (cyanosis, murmur, and irregular heart rate), and cataracts (absent red reflex). Laboratory testing includes karyotyping, thyroid screening, and a complete blood count (CBC). Thyroid screening is particularly important because children who have DS have a higher incidence of congenital hypothyroidism (see Chapter 223).[14] Occasionally a DS child has leukocytosis, suggesting congenital leukemia. This usually benign condition is called *leukemoid reaction* (transient myeloproliferative disease), but careful follow-up is needed.[12,36] Hearing screening is suggested because 15% of children who have DS may have congenital hearing loss. In addition, an ophthalmological consultation should be arranged for any abnormalities (e.g., lens opacities) seen on the eye examination. A pediatric cardiologist should evaluate the baby for cardiac disease. A genetic consultant can help educate the family about prenatal detection and the risk of recurrence.

Once the diagnosis is made, the physician must inform the family fully; the approach must be gentle and hopeful. Some suggestions in this regard include the following:

1. Inform both parents together. Do this in a quiet place where the physician and parents will not be interrupted.
2. Provide current information to the family; be hopeful. Provide the name and number of a local DS support group. The National Down Syndrome Congress (1-800-232-6372) will provide the names of local support groups, as well as educational information for the physician and family.
3. Discuss future expectations briefly. Also discuss the potential medical problems, but point out that many children who have DS are healthy and participate in most of the usual childhood activities. Point out that the average life span of those who have DS now is 55 years. Discuss the plan to identify and manage medical problems.
4. Allow time for the parents to respond, to voice concerns, and to raise questions. Parents need the opportunity to express feelings of anger, guilt, or depression.
5. Provide written information about DS. Parents find it useful to have something to read after their discussion with the physician. Most information more than 5 years old should be considered outdated.
6. Arrange for a follow-up meeting with the family to give them time to begin adjusting to the new information and to formulate questions. Offer to meet extended family members, as well as the parents, to answer questions.

Most families accept a child born having DS. Some have greater initial difficulty and require more extended counseling. In rare cases, a family will not be able to accept a child who has DS. In this event, adoption should be discussed. There often are families waiting to adopt children who have DS. The Down Syndrome Adoption Exchange (914-428-1236) can be called for more information.

In this time of abbreviated hospital stays, the physician should arrange a visit with the parents and child 1 to 2 weeks after discharge. This provides time for further discussion with the family as well as for a follow-up medical assessment.

In the first few weeks of the infant's life, the physician may be asked questions about the following:

1. *Oral motor problems.* Anatomical and neuromotor problems often result in a poor suck and frequent spitting. Mild feeding problems usually resolve in 2 to 3 weeks. However, some measures can help to simplify feeding. The parents should be instructed to (1) make sure the child is fully awake when fed at night, (2) clear mucus from the baby's nose and mouth before feeding so that breathing will be easier, and (3) support the infant's chin during feeding. The pediatrician should follow the baby's weight and caloric intake carefully. If feeding problems are particularly severe or do not resolve with these interventions, referral to an oral motor (swallowing) specialist should be considered.
2. *Breast-feeding problems.* Most babies who have DS can breast-feed successfully. If breast-feeding appears to be going poorly, the pediatrician should arrange a visit to review the baby's weight gain and the mother's breast-feeding technique. After a medical examination, particularly severe problems should be referred to a lactation specialist.
3. *Constipation.* If an infant has constipation that does not respond to dietary changes and stool softeners, evaluation for Hirschsprung's disease should be considered (see Chapter 121, Constipation).

Infants 2 to 12 Months of Age (Box 204-4)

In many cases, families who have a child who has DS need to see the pediatrician frequently for medical care and education. Often it is difficult to find the extra time in a busy office,

BOX 204-4

MANAGING THE INFANT: AGES 2 TO 12 MONTHS

Health Concerns

History

1. Evaluate the parents' concerns
2. Determine the incidence of otitis media and upper respiratory tract infection
3. Assess the infant's nutritional intake

Perform or refer the patient for the following tests and examinations:

Physical Examination

1. Plot growth on a DS Growth Chart
2. Conduct a general physical examination and neurological examination

Laboratory Tests

1. Thyroid screening

Consultation

1. Cardiological examination
2. Ophthalmological examination
3. Audiological screening

Psychosocial Concerns

Habilitation

1. Refer the parents to an infant education program
2. Continue educating the family about Down syndrome

where most visits may be for routine checkups or acute care. The following are a few suggestions on how the physician can find time for extended discussion:

1. Set aside a period each week, perhaps half a day, for consultation and family education. Keep this time free of acute care office visits.
2. Consider the contribution of a nurse practitioner (e.g., to help meet the extra educational and health care needs of the child and family).
3. Use a problem-oriented approach to the office chart. At the start, set up the medical record with special sections for:
   a. Problems
   b. Procedures (date, site, and result of all special medical procedures completed)
   c. Consultants involved in the child's care (with emergency numbers)
   d. An updated, one-page medical summary to be used for emergency admissions and consultations
   e. A flow chart of significant laboratory data and medications
4. Provide special check-out instructions for "covering" or "on-call" physicians, especially if they are outside the office and not familiar with the patient.

Medical care for infants in this age group who have DS involves particular diagnostic and consultative procedures, because more than 50% have serious or fatal medical disorders.[35] It is important to remember that the first year of life holds the highest probability of death for children who have DS.[3] Cardiac malformations cause 60% of the deaths that occur during the first 12 months.[5] Cancers also are more frequent because of a twentyfold increase of leukemias.[31]

During office visits for periodic health assessments, the physician should ask about the baby's feeding and discuss enrollment in an early education program.

On physical examination, the pediatrician should check carefully for signs of cardiac and neurological disorders. Because frequent episodes of otitis media and upper respiratory tract infection are common in this age group, the tympanic membranes should be inspected with particular care. Hearing screening should be repeated if the newborn testing was equivocal or if signs of recurrent middle ear effusion are seen. The ophthalmological examination needs to be repeated at 9 months of age. A repeat cardiac consultation is indicated even in the absence of a murmur. Occasionally a congenital heart lesion is missed in the newborn period and manifests without typical cardiac findings at 6 to 9 months of age. Children who have DS and CHD have a greater tendency to develop early pulmonary hypertension compared with other children who have the same heart lesions.[9]

The pediatrician can identify failure to thrive by plotting and following the infant's weight and height on the DS growth chart.[11] Further evaluation may be indicated for pulmonary, cardiac, and gastrointestinal malformations. Celiac disease is one of the disorders that must be considered when infants who have DS present with failure to thrive.[19]

Thyroid screening should be repeated at the end of the first year. Because clinical signs of hypothyroidism often are subtle, routine screening is suggested. Hypothyroidism occurs 28 times more often in infants who have DS than in the general population.[14]

Extra time should be arranged at office visits to allow families to talk about how they are adjusting. The practitioner should review with them information about DS provided earlier. The family also should be informed about Supplemental Security Income (SSI) and other government programs that help families financially with the extra costs of raising a child who has special needs.

Parents of infants who have DS often ask questions about the following issues:

1. *Tongue protrusion.* The factors that produce tongue protrusion include macroglossia, a small oral cavity, and mouth breathing.[2] Behavior management techniques can be used to manage tongue protrusion. Partial glossectomy should be considered when the macroglossia obstructs the airway.[30]
2. *Controversial therapies.* Some families contemplate controversial therapies as a means of obtaining a magical cure for their child—for example, tongue resection to improve speech and silicone implants to correct micrognathia. Experts still are not sure if tongue resection does improve speech,[25,26] and complications have been reported from facial surgery.[27,28] The pediatrician should try to inform families about the risks and benefits of any surgical procedures. Preparations high in vitamins and minerals initially seemed to result in increased intelligence scores.[18] However, because no studies to date have replicated these results and because side effects from megavitamin regimens have been reported,[6] unproved megavitamin and mineral therapies should be avoided. Routine nutritional screening should be done at health assessment visits and vitamins prescribed when warranted by standard criteria.

Child 1 to 12 Years of Age (Box 204-5)

Children who have DS need an annual health assessment. At these office visits, the pediatrician should ask about respiratory infections, constipation, hearing problems, and symptoms of sleep apnea (e.g., snoring, difficulty breathing during sleep, excessive drowsiness during the day).

The physician also should ask about behavior problems. The personalities of many children who have DS do not fit the stereotype of being placid or compliant, and parents may not volunteer information about obstinance or noncompliance. When there seems to be a behavior disorder, a careful history should be obtained, and the parents should be asked about changes in the environment or their expectations. A complete physical examination should be done, as well as laboratory tests, if warranted, to identify medical problems that may lead to behavior disorders. A trial of behavior management should be initiated for mild problems, and the diagnoses of pervasive developmental disability or physical abuse should be considered for serious behavior disorders. For severe behavior problems or persistent mild to moderate problems that have no medical cause, the child should be referred to a behavior specialist.

The pediatrician needs to review the current individual educational plan (IEP) to ensure that appropriate developmental testing has been completed and that the parents have

BOX 204-5

MANAGING THE CHILD: AGES 1 TO 12 YEARS

Health Concerns

History

1. Assess any parental concerns about the child's behavior and school program
2. Ask if the child has shown any symptoms of a vision or hearing disorder

Perform or refer the patient for the following tests and examinations:

Physical Examination

1. General physical examination plus a careful neurological examination
2. Height and weight plotted on a DS growth chart

Laboratory Tests

1. Thyroid screening each year
2. Hearing screening
3. Consider a cervical spine roentgenogram

Consultation

1. Eye examination every 2 years
2. Hearing test every 2 years
3. Roentgenogram of the cervical spine
4. Dental examination twice a year

Psychosocial Concerns

Habilitation

1. Discuss respite and long-term care plans with family
2. Review the child's education program

had an opportunity to provide information in the IEP process. School problems may come to the physician's attention more often as children who have DS are placed in mainstreamed or regular classes. School learning problems require further evaluation. The history should be reviewed carefully to ensure that the parents' and teachers' expectations are appropriate for the child's developmental age. Medical problems that can affect learning and behavior should be identified. For example, the ears should be examined for impacted cerumen that can cause a moderate hearing loss. An eye examination should be done to detect cataracts.[15] Vision screening should be done yearly or more often, if indicated.

The physical examination must include plotting of appropriate measurements on the DS growth chart. It also should include a careful neurological search, because atlantoaxial subluxation presents special problems for children who have DS. Atlantoaxial instability, which occurs in about 15% of children who have DS, refers to excess mobility of the atlantoaxial joint without neurological complications.[29] A roentgenogram of the cervical spine in flexion reveals an atlantoodontoid interval greater than 5 mm. Atlantoaxial subluxation, however, refers to backward movement of the odontoid process of the axis compressing the spinal cord, resulting in the signs and symptoms of cord compression, which may include neck pain, head tilt, progressive weakness, and loss of bladder or bowel control. Neurological examination reveals long-tract signs such as increased deep-tendon reflexes in the lower extremities, a positive Babinski sign, and ankle clonus. This is a neurosurgical emergency and requires immediate referral and treatment. Although atlantoaxial subluxation occurs in only 1.5% of children who have DS, it is life-threatening.

Unfortunately, the natural history of atlantoaxial instability and subluxation still is understood poorly. It is not clear if only one set of cervical spine roentgenograms is necessary or if these films need to be repeated. In addition, cervical spine roentgenograms may be unreliable in identifying all children at risk.[32] Until further information is available about the natural history of atlantoaxial subluxation, the diagnosis depends on a neurological examination plus neurophysiological and imaging studies.[28] Given incomplete understanding, the following are some general guidelines for the pediatrician:

1. Cervical roentgenograms should be taken at 3 and 12 years of age to identify atlantoaxial instability. The child also should have a yearly neurological examination to identify long-tract signs and a careful examination before participating in school sports or Special Olympics. Roentgenograms should be read by an experienced radiologist. If the child has a normal neurological examination and the roentgenograms are normal, he or she may participate in all sports. Roentgenograms should be repeated in adolescence.
2. If the roentgenograms are read as being abnormal (the atlantoodontoid distance is greater than 5 mm) and the neurological examination is normal, the child should be followed yearly with repeated neurological examinations. It also is prudent for the child to avoid certain sports that place the neck in extreme extension (e.g., tumbling, gymnastics, and diving). Careful monitoring during intubation for induction of anesthesia would be needed if surgery is necessary.
3. If the roentgenograms are normal but the neurological examination is abnormal, the child should be referred to a neurosurgeon or orthopedic physician experienced with DS. Further diagnostic testing may be suggested, such as a computed tomography (CT) scan of the cervical spine.

The studies suggested for DS children 1 to 12 years of age include annual thyroid, vision, and hearing screening.

General habilitation includes monitoring of exercise and recreational activities, good daily care of the teeth, and a dental examination twice a year beginning at the first birthday. Obesity often becomes a problem at about age 2 years. The pediatrician should ask about the child's snacks and the amount of time he or she spends watching television. The family should be asked again if they have checked into eligibility for SSI and Medicaid benefits. Parents also should investigate trust and guardian arrangements. The Association for Retarded Citizens (ARC) helps guide parents through these financial and custody arrangements. The local ARC chapter or the national office can be contacted for further information.

Parents of school-age children who have DS ask about the following issues most frequently:

1. *Obesity.* The cause of obesity in DS is multifactorial. Children who have greater hypotonia and shorter stature and those at preschool age and in adolescence are at greater risk. A preventive approach includes monitoring the child's diet, promoting regular exercise, and screening yearly for hypothyroidism.

BOX 204-6

MANAGING THE ADOLESCENT

Health Concerns

History

1. Answer the parents' questions
2. Ask about any education or behavioral problems
3. Make sure the patient is up to date on his or her immunizations

Perform or refer the patient for the following tests and examinations:

Physical examination

1. General physical examination
2. Obesity
3. Gynecological examination
4. Neurological examination

Laboratory tests

1. Thyroid screening

Consultation

1. Eye examination every 2 years
2. Hearing test every 2 years
3. Roentgenogram of the cervical spine
4. Dental examination twice a year

Psychosocial Concerns

Habilitation

1. Check to see whether the patient is obtaining vocational training
2. Have the patient continue speech therapy

Family Concerns

1. Ask about community living plans for the patient
2. Discuss enrolling the patient in Medicaid and Supplemental Security Income (SSI) if he or she is eligible
3. Discuss the issue of sexuality, including preventing pregnancy
4. Help the parents teach their child to avoid smoking and abusing drugs

2. *Hyperactivity.* Because children who have DS often attend regular schools for their education, hyperactivity frequently comes to the physician's attention. The child should be carefully assessed to identify medical problems associated with inattention. After obtaining a careful history that includes information from the child's teacher, the physician should perform a complete physical and neurological examination and evaluate the child's vision and hearing. Thyroid testing should be considered when clinically suggested to rule out hyperthyroidism.[22] Behavior management techniques and classroom adaptations should be tried before resorting to medications.

Adolescence (Box 204-6)

Adolescence is a special challenge for any family. The physical, emotional, and educational needs in adolescents who have DS, however, require a special approach. During the annual health assessment visit, the pediatrician should discuss with the family their child's infections, educational program, behavior problems, and prevocational experience and training.

The general physical examination should include plotting the child's height and weight to monitor for obesity. The need for a careful neurological examination for long-tract signs persists.

A gynecological examination of females should be done by at least 17 years of age. Because the examination often is not tolerated well by the adolescent, the pediatrician should consider referral to a specialist who has had experience evaluating women who have developmental disabilities. Often the examination can be done less invasively with pelvic ultrasound, which requires an examiner who has appropriate experience with the procedure.

Routine studies include thyroid screening, a cervical spine roentgenogram at 12 and 18 years of age, and vision and hearing screening. The higher risk for periodontal disease among children who have DS adds importance to the recommendation of a dental examination twice a year.

Although many adolescents who have DS receive some formal education about sexuality in school, it is important to make sure that it is complete and to discuss this with the family. Although young men who have DS usually are sterile, a small number of girls and women have given birth to children. When a young woman who has DS does become pregnant, the father usually is a close relative.[33] Families need to know about birth control options and routine procedures for safeguarding their adolescent. If the primary care physician is not experienced in answering these questions, referral to a specialist who is should be considered.

Adolescents who have DS also need education about smoking and drug abuse. If at all possible, they should have well-balanced diets, continue regular exercise, and be involved in appropriate social activities. When possible, they also should have opportunities for prevocational experiences such as doing volunteer work at a library or other facility that can provide adequate supervision. The school curriculum should make the transition to planning for a life vocation. Psychoeducational testing often is helpful in this regard to determine the individual's aptitudes, as well as his or her job interests.

Disruptive behavior, as well as anxiety disorders, may arise in adolescence.[23] A good mental status examination is helpful as part of the routine health assessment. When completing a mental status examination on an individual whose verbal skills are limited, it is necessary to talk with the family and teachers about any changes or regression in self-care skills. Often the family will report important information about withdrawal or loss of interest in recreational activities. Some emotional disorders manifest with excessive anger, frustration, or aggressive behaviors. Other signs of a possible disorder include self-injurious behavior (hitting or biting oneself), crying spells, or refusal to participate in self-care activities.

When the physician is evaluating a patient who has a sudden increase in behavior problems, it is important to look for underlying medical problems. For example, changes in vision or hearing may result in withdrawal or temper tantrums. Hypothyroidism can cause lethargy and lack of interest in activities. In rare cases, Alzheimer's disease may appear in adolescence. When skills have been lost, it is important to document this with psychological testing that includes an assessment of self-care skills. Referral to a neurologist is suggested if loss of skills is documented and initial assessment shows no signs of a correctable problem.

The pediatrician needs to discuss with the family a long-term plan for the adolescent's living arrangements. Most communities have a spectrum of community living facilities that range from small, heavily supervised group homes to apartments that have minimal supervision. Families need to arrange this 2 or 3 years before they anticipate need because often there is a waiting list for placement in a community facility.

Most families have questions about their adolescents and the following issues:

1. *Sexuality.* Families usually have many questions about a teenager's sexuality but often do not ask the pediatrician about them. For example, many parents wonder about the sexual interests of their children and the level at which they experience sexual feelings. They do not know how to deal with masturbation or questions about wanting to have a baby. Management of menstrual hygiene also presents problems. Referral to community resources should be considered if the pediatrician's expertise or the school curriculum needs to be complemented.
2. There may be inquiries about sterilization procedures for both young men and young women. In most states it is difficult to perform sterilization procedures because of the difficulty in obtaining consent. The pediatrician should counsel the family as well as the adolescent about preventing conception. Additional sources of counseling are available for families and professionals.[13]

Young Adult (Box 204-7)

Often, pediatricians continue to follow adolescents into the early adult years to maintain continuity of care. Families often are attached to the physician and ask about continuing care; this discussion can center on aspects of preventive medical care for the young adult.

Adults who have DS require an annual health assessment. The general physical examination includes a gynecological and breast examination in women and testicular examination in men. The neurological assessment must include testing for long-tract signs. Thyroid, vision, and hearing screening should continue, and the patient should be referred to a neurologist and/or a psychiatrist if symptoms of dementia, behavior problems, or depression arise. The dental examination continues at twice a year. Because about 50% of adults who have DS develop mitral valve prolapse, an echocardiogram needs to be done when clinical findings are suggestive.[16] A Pap smear is necessary annually for sexually active women; in addition, a baseline mammogram is appropriate at age 35, with follow-up based on the physical examination and family history. Immunizations should be reviewed and kept current. Hepatitis B and pneumococcal vaccines should be considered for adults at special risk.

BOX 204-7

MANAGING THE YOUNG ADULT

Health Concerns

History

1. Evaluate the family's concerns
2. Ask about symptoms of dementia and mental disorders

Perform or refer the patient for the following tests and examinations:

Physical examination

1. Gynecological examination and Pap smear
2. Testicular and breast examination
3. Neurological examination

Laboratory tests

1. Thyroid screening

Consultation

1. Cardiological examination and echocardiogram to check for mitral valve prolapse
2. Eye examination every 2 years
3. Hearing test every 2 years
4. Dental examination twice a year
5. Cervical spine examination at age 30 years

Psychosocial Concerns

Habilitation

1. Inquire about the patient's exercise and recreational activities
2. Urge the patient and family to continue with vocational and adult education programs to allow better job placement
3. When appropriate, check to see whether the patient has registered to vote and (for young men) has registered with the Selective Service Commission

Family Issues

1. Remind the family to update their estate planning and wills
2. Evaluate the patient for community living if he or she is not already in this type of setting
3. Check on patient's eligibility for Medicaid and Supplemental Security Income (SSI)

The young adult should be enrolled in a vocational training program to enhance his or her skills for either a community job or workshop placement. The program also should include some basic educational activities for continued improvement in skills.

The parents and patient should be asked about family or community living arrangements. Again, the physician should discuss with the family future living arrangements if the DS adult continues to live at home. Plans for guardianship and wills and trusts should be reviewed. The young adult also should be referred for voter registration and males with the Selective Service Commission. Health education, especially about drug and alcohol abuse, smoking, and sex, should continue.

A parent of an adult who have DS usually has a compelling question: What will happen to my child after I die? Most

BOX 204-8

ORGANIZATIONS PROVIDING PARENT EDUCATION AND SUPPORT

United States

National Down Syndrome Society
666 Broadway
New York, NY 10012
Telephone: 1-212-460-9330 or 1-800-221-4602
Net: www.ncdss.org

National Down Syndrome Congress
7000 Peachtree Dunwoody Road N.E.
Lake Ridge 400 Office Park
Building J, Suite 100
Atlanta, GA 30327
Telephone: 1-800-232-6372
Net: www.downsyndrome.com

Down Syndrome Adoption Exchange
56 Midchester Ave.
White Plains, NY 10606
Telephone: 1-914-428-1236

Association for Retarded Citizens
500 East Border Street, Suite 300
Arlington, TX 76010
Telephone: 1-817-261-6003
Net: www.the arc.org

Canada

The Canadian Down Syndrome Society
811-14 Street NW
Calgary, Alberta
Canada T2T 2AY
Telephone: 1-403-270-8500

adults who have DS will need supervision because they are not independent economically. The family should be counseled to seek community resources for information about community living options. The state office of disabilities can provide information about social insurance and medical benefits available for adults who have DS. A booklet published by ARC provides further information for the family.[21] The names and addresses of organizations providing parent education and support in the United States, Canada, and Mexico are listed in Box 204-8.

When to Refer a Newborn

1. All infants require cardiology and genetics consultation.
2. Infants who have leukocoria require ophthalmology assessment.
3. Families who have serious difficulty adapting to their new baby may need a family counselor.

When to Refer Infants 2 Months to 12 Months of Age

1. Infants who have severe constipation not responding to dietary control need a pediatric gastroenterology evaluation.
2. Infants who have chronic middle ear effusions need a consultation with an ear, nose, and throat specialist.
3. All infants to an infant therapy.

When to Refer Children 1 Year to 12 Years

1. Children who have infantile spasms need immediate referral to a pediatric neurologist.
2. Children who have neck pain, loss of bladder and bowel control, and gait disturbance need immediate pediatric neurosurgery consultation.
3. Children who have disruptive behavior or excessive sort attention span need an evaluation by developmental or behavioral specialists.

When to Refer Adolescents and Young Adults

1. All females to gynecologists by 17 years for pelvic examination and birth control options.
2. Neurologist for all teenagers who have lost skills with no obvious medical explanation.
3. All families to the Association For Retarded Citizens for guidance on financial and custody issues.
4. Psychiatrist for all adolescents who have severe behavior disturbances.

REFERENCES

1. American Academy of Pediatrics, Committee on Genetics: Prenatal genetic diagnosis for pediatricians, *Pediatrics* 93:1010, 1994.
2. Anneren G, Edman B: Down syndrome: a gene dosage disease caused by trisomy of genes within a small segment of the long arm of chromosome 21, exemplified by the study of effects from the superoxide-dismutase type 1 (SOD-1) gene, *APMIS* 40:71, 1993.
3. Baird P, Sadovnick A: Life expectancy in Down syndrome, *J Pediatr* 110:849, 1987.
4. Ballesta F, et al: Parental origin and meiotic stage of non-disjunction in 139 cases of trisomy, *Ann Genet* 42:11, 1999.
5. Bell JA, Pearn JH, Firman D: Childhood deaths in Down syndrome: survival curves and causes of death from a total population study in Queensland, Australia, 1976 to 1985, *J Med Genet* 26:764, 1989.
6. Bidder RT, et al: The effects of multivitamins and minerals on children with Down syndrome, *Dev Med Child Neurol* 31:532, 1989.
7. Carothers AD, et al: Trends in prenatal diagnosis of Down syndrome and other autosomal trisomies in Scotland 1990 to 1994, with associated cytogenetic and epidemiological findings, *Genet Epidemiol* 16:179, 1999.

8. Centers for Disease Control: Congenital malformation surveillance report: January 1981-December 1983, September 1985, US Department of Health and Human Services.
9. Chi TPL, Krovetz LJ: The pulmonary vascular bed in children with Down syndrome, *J Pediatr* 86:533, 1975.
10. Crete N, et al: Mapping the Down syndrome chromosomal abnormality, *Clin Pediatr* 5:4, 1966.
11. Cronk C, et al: Growth charts for children with Down syndrome: 1 month to 18 years of age, *Pediatrics* 18:102, 1988.
12. Duflos-Delaplace D, et al: Transient leukemoid disorder in a newborn with Down syndrome followed 19 months later by an acute myeloid leukemia: demonstration of the same structural change in both instances with clonal evolution, *Cancer Genet Cytogenet Hearing* 113:166, 1999.
13. Edwards JP, Elkins TE: *Just between us: a social sexual training guide for parents and professionals who have concerns for persons with retardation,* Portland, Ore, 1988, Ednick Communications.
14. Fort P, et al: Abnormalities of thyroid function in infants with Down syndrome, *J Pediatr* 104:545, 1984.
15. Gaynon MW, Schimek RA: Down's syndrome: a ten-year study, *Ann Ophthalmol* 9:1493, 1977.
16. Goldhar S, Brown WD, St John M: High frequency of mitral valve prolapse and aortic regurgitation among asymptomatic adults with Down syndrome, *JAMA* 258:1793, 1987.
17. Hall B: Mongolism in newborn infants: an examination of the criteria for recognition and some speculation on the pathogenic activity of the chromosomal abnormality, *Clin Pediatr* 5:4, 1966.
18. Harrell RR, et al: Can nutritional supplements help mentally retarded children? An exploratory study, *Proc Natl Acad Sci U S A* 78:574, 1981.
19. Hilhorst MI, et al: Down syndrome and coeliac disease: five new cases with a review of the literature, *Eur J Pediatr* 152:884, 1993.
20. Hook EB, Fabia JJ: Frequency of Down syndrome by single-year maternal age interval: results of a Massachusetts study, *Teratology* 17:223, 1978.
21. *How to provide for their future,* Association for Retarded Citizens, National Headquarters, PO Box 6109, Arlington, TX 76011.
22. Lambyah PA, Cheah JS: Hyperthyroidism and Down syndrome, *Ann Acad Med Singapore* 22:603, 1993.
23. Myers BA, Pueschel SM: Psychiatric disorders in persons with Down syndrome, *J Nerv Ment Dis* 179:609, 1991.
24. Nicolini U: Prenatal diagnosis and fetal therapy, *Curr Opin Obstet Gynecol* 5:50, 1993.
25. Olbrisch RR: Plastic surgical management of children with Down's syndrome: indications and results, *Br J Plast Surg* 35:195, 1982.
26. Parson CL, Lacono TA, Rozner L: Effect of tongue reduction on articulation in children with Down syndrome, *Am J Ment Deficiency* 91:328, 1987.
27. Peled IJ, et al: Mandibular resorption from silicone chin implants in children, *J Oral Maxillofac Surg* 44:346, 1986.
28. Pueschel SM, et al: Atlantoaxial instability in Down syndrome: roentgenographics, neurologic, and somatosensory evoked potential studies, *J Pediatr* 110:515, 1987.
29. Pueschel SM, Scola FH: Epidemiologic, radiographic and clinical studies of atlantoaxial instability in individuals with Down syndrome, *Pediatrics* 80:555, 1987.
30. Purdy AH, Deitz JC, Harris SR: Efficacy of two treatment approaches to reduce the tongue protrusion of children with Down syndrome, *Dev Med Child Neurol* 29:469, 1987.
31. Satge D, et al: A tumor profile in Down syndrome, *Am J Med Genet* 78:207, 1998.
32. Selby KA, et al: Clinical predictions and radiological reliability in atlantoaxial subluxation in Down's syndrome, *Arch Dis Child* 66:876, 1991.
33. Sheridan R, et al: Fertility in a male with trisomy, *J Med Genet* 26:294, 1989.
34. Smith GF, Berg JM: *Down's anomaly,* Edinburgh, 1976, Churchill Livingstone.
35. Torfs CP, Christianson RE: Maternal risk factors and major associated defects in infants with Down syndrome, *Epidemiology* 10:264, 1999.
36. Wong KY, et al: Transient myeloproliferative disease disorder and acute nonlymphoblastic leukemia in Down syndrome, *J Pediatr* 112:18, 1988.

SUGGESTED READINGS

Lou IT, McCoy EE: *Down syndrome: advances in medical care,* New York, 1992, Wiley-Liss.

Rogers RT, Coleman M: *Medical care in Down syndrome,* New York, 1992, Marcel Dekker.

205 Drug Eruptions

Judith V. Williams • Donald P. Lookingbill

The clinical expression of drug eruptions varies considerably. Because systemically administered drugs can cause almost any kind of rash, the practitioner should remember a general principle of dermatological diagnosis: "For any rash, think of drugs." The types of skin reactions caused by drugs include morbilliform eruptions, urticaria, erythema multiforme, erythema nodosum, vasculitis, photosensitivity reactions, acneform eruptions, alopecia, blistering disorders, fixed drug eruptions, lichenoid reactions, and drug-induced lupus erythematosus.[2,3] Tables in the general dermatology text by Fitzpatrick et al[2] conveniently list the drugs most commonly responsible for each of these different types of eruptions. This chapter deals only with the three types of eruptions seen most commonly in children; in order of decreasing incidence they are morbilliform eruptions, urticaria, and erythema multiforme.

MORBILLIFORM ERUPTIONS

Etiology

Morbilliform eruptions, also known as *exanthematous* or *maculopapular* eruptions, are the most common cutaneous expression of a drug reaction. Although a variety of drugs can cause this reaction, the drugs that cause morbilliform or urticarial eruptions most often are listed in Table 205-1.

History

A drug-induced morbilliform eruption usually does not have an immediate onset; rather, it begins within several days of initiation of the drug. The onset sometimes is delayed up to a week but seldom longer. Because no laboratory test can identify the responsible drug, heavy reliance is placed on the history. Patients receiving more than one drug obviously present a problem. In trying to select a single drug from a list of many, the two variables to consider are (1) the temporal relationship between the administration of the drug and the onset of the rash and (2) the likelihood that a given drug can cause a drug eruption. For the latter, incidence data such as those in Table 205-1 are used.[1] Itching usually is present but is not helpful as a diagnostic marker.

Physical Findings

The eruption is generalized and consists of brightly erythematous macules and papules that tend to be confluent in large areas. It usually starts proximally and proceeds distally, with the legs the last to be involved and also the last to clear. Palms and soles also are affected. Drug fever has been well described, but most drug eruptions are not accompanied by an elevation in body temperature.

Laboratory Studies

Laboratory tests usually are not helpful. A peripheral blood eosinophilia sometimes is present and may heighten the suspicion for a drug reaction, but no laboratory tests can incriminate a specific drug.

Differential Diagnosis

For a generalized erythematous, "maculopapular" eruption, the major differential diagnosis is (1) a drug reaction, (2) a viral exanthem, or (3) a toxic erythema.

As the name *morbilliform* (measleslike) suggests, a viral exanthem and a drug eruption can be indistinguishable clinically. Often a drug eruption is much more erythematous and more confluent, but not always. Other clinical information can help, including a drug history and the presence or absence of other signs and symptoms of a viral infection. Eosinophilia favors a drug etiology. Acute and convalescent serological tests can be obtained for some viral infections to provide a retrospective diagnosis. In most cases, however, a presumptive diagnosis is made based on the combined clinical data.

Examples of toxic erythema are scarlet fever, staphylococcal-induced scarlatiniform eruptions, and, possibly, Kawasaki disease. Features that help to distinguish these toxic erythemas from drug eruptions include a sandpaper-like roughened texture of the rash, mucous membrane involvement (scarlet fever and Kawasaki disease), fever, a focus of infection, and lymphadenopathy. Postinflammatory desquamation from the skin of the hands and feet often follows the rash of toxic erythema, but this is not specific. Drug eruptions and even viral exanthems also can involve the hands and feet, particularly the palms and soles in drug eruptions; if the inflammation has been sufficiently intense, desquamation follows.

Management

When an offending agent is identified, it should be discontinued. If a patient is taking several drugs and it is not possible to be certain of the culprit, the number of drugs administered should be reduced to an absolute minimum, and whenever possible, any remaining possible offenders should be changed to alternative agents.

Table 205-1 Allergic Skin Reactions to Drugs

Drug	Reaction Rate (Reactions per 100 Recipients)
Amoxicillin	5.1
Trimethoprim-sulfamethoxazole	3.4
Ampicillin	3.3
Blood	2.2
Cephalosporins	2.1
Semisynthetic penicillins	2.1
Erythromycin	2.0
Penicillin G	1.9
Allopurinol	0.8
Barbiturates	0.4
Diazepam	0.04

Data from Bigby M, et al: *JAMA* 256:3358, 1986.

Therapy, otherwise, is directed toward the symptoms, with antihistamines used most commonly for the pruritus. Topical agents usually are confined to moisturizing lotions, which are most helpful during the later, desquamative phase of the reaction. Topical steroids are of little value, and systemic steroids rarely are required.

Complications

The complications primarily are cutaneous. When large areas of skin are inflamed, body heat increases and water is lost. If the patient already is seriously ill, this could be a problem; for most patients, however, it is not.

Guessing wrong and continuing an offending agent in the face of a drug eruption can result in two main consequences: cutaneous and renal. The cutaneous risk is that of progressive worsening of the rash, possibly resulting in toxic epidermal necrolysis, a serious problem. Fortunately, this is rare. In fact, in some cases a drug eruption clears even when the offending agent is continued. Of course, it is not desirable to continue the drug if an alternative is available. The renal risk is that of allergic interstitial nephritis, an uncommon development that usually is associated with penicillins and cephalosporins and only rarely with other drugs.

Course

Drug eruptions clear with time after the responsible agent is discontinued. It is important to realize that it usually takes 1 to 2 weeks for the condition to clear completely and that the eruption actually may worsen for several days after the offending drug has been stopped. If a responsible drug has been identified, the patient should be advised about the allergy, and the medical record should be clearly labeled to that effect.

URTICARIA (HIVES)[5,6,8]

Etiology

Drug-induced hives can be mediated immunologically by either (1) immediate IgE reactions, usually within hours, or (2) delayed immune complexes that result in serum sickness–like reactions after 7 to 10 days. The immediate reactions are more common.

History

A precise cause usually is not found among patients who have hives. When it is, it is determined from the history. The drug history is the most important but the most difficult to obtain, at least among outpatients. Because many patients and their parents tend to consider over-the-counter (OTC) medications unimportant, it often is helpful to ask about specific medications to help jog their memories. Aspirin is particularly important, inasmuch as salicylates cause hives in some patients and aggravate them in as many as one third of all patients who have urticaria, regardless of its cause. Whenever a drug is suspected, the physician must be aggressive and persistent in eliciting a medication history. Otherwise, some drugs invariably are overlooked.

A history of associated symptoms also may be important. Itching nearly always is present. A history of an obstructed airway or other anaphylactic symptoms suggests a more serious problem. Fever and arthralgia often accompany hives in serum sickness reactions, for which the two most common causes are drugs and viral hepatitis.

Physical Findings

Hives are skin lesions that are recognized more easily than described. They appear as edematous plaques, often with pale centers and red borders. They frequently assume geographical shapes and sometimes are confluent. The lesions may be scattered but usually are generalized. By definition an individual hive is transient, lasting less than 24 hours, although new hives may develop continuously. In serum sickness reactions, lymphadenopathy, in addition to fever and arthralgia, may be present.

Laboratory Studies

Drug-induced hives may be accompanied by an eosinophilia. To evaluate for hepatitis, it is appropriate to obtain liver function tests in patients who have hives and fever. In patients who have no fever, however, laboratory tests rarely are helpful in eliciting a cause, and they are of no help in implicating a specific drug.

Differential Diagnosis

The differential diagnosis of urticaria may be approached in two ways: (1) from the causes of hives per se and (2) from consideration of the cause of lesions sometimes mistaken as hives. As already mentioned, the cause of hives most often cannot be determined. When a cause is found, it usually is drug related. Other causes include infection, physical modalities (e.g., cold, pressure, or sunlight), emotions and, albeit rarely, foods.

Lesions sometimes mistaken for hives include those seen in erythema multiforme and juvenile rheumatoid arthritis (JRA). The lesions in erythema multiforme are discussed later in this chapter. The individual lesions in JRA behave like hives in that they are transient but differ in size (only 2 to

3 mm), color (typically salmon), and timing (usually appearing with fever spikes).

Management

Any suspected medication, including aspirin, should be discontinued. Symptomatic therapy usually is achieved with antihistamines given on a regular, rather than an as-needed, schedule. Hydroxyzine is the preferred agent, administered in a dosage of 2 mg/kg/day divided so as to be given every 6 or 8 hours, with a maximum of 50 to 100 mg daily in children older than 6 years.

Complications

In rare cases, acute urticaria can be accompanied by anaphylactic reactions that require more immediate therapy; usually, however, hives are more of a nuisance than a morbid threat.

Course

Drug-induced hives usually clear within several days after the responsible medication is discontinued. As with any drug reaction, if a specific agent has been identified, the patient must be alerted to avoid that drug in the future. Because most hives are IgE mediated, rechallenge with the responsible drug is more likely to result in an anaphylactic response than is rechallenge in a patient who had a previous morbilliform eruption.

ERYTHEMA MULTIFORME[4,7]

Etiology

Erythema multiforme has been ascribed to innumerable causes, which are poorly substantiated except for two: (1) drugs and (2) infection, the latter primarily from *Mycoplasma pneumoniae* and recurrent herpes simplex. Circulating immune complexes have been detected in patients who have erythema multiforme, a finding consistent with the concept that this distinctive cutaneous disorder is an immunological reaction.

History

Sulfonamides, penicillins, barbiturates, and hydantoin have been the drugs implicated most commonly in erythema multiforme; however, a history for all drugs should be elicited. Recurrent herpes simplex infection is the most common cause of recurrent erythema multiforme. The herpetic lesion usually precedes the erythema multiforme by a few days to a week or more. Because, for the more extended intervals, the herpetic lesions may have healed by the time the patient comes for treatment, the history is important. In about half of all cases, a cause cannot be identified. In some patients a febrile prodrome precedes the cutaneous eruption by 1 to 14 days.

Physical Findings

As the name suggests, erythema multiforme is characterized by a variety of lesions, including erythematous plaques, blisters, and iris, or target, lesions. Hives sometimes are confused with target lesions. The difference is that a hive has only two zones of color: a central pale area surrounded by an erythematous halo. The criteria for a target lesion require three zones: a central dark area or blister, surrounded by a pale zone, surrounded by a peripheral rim of erythema. True target lesions are diagnostic for erythema multiforme. They are seen more often on the palms and soles but may occur anywhere. Typically, erythema multiforme is a strikingly symmetrical eruption that favors the extremities. The disorder can range from mild to severe. In the severe form (Stevens-Johnson syndrome), the skin lesions are more extensive, and mucous membrane involvement usually is severe as well.

Laboratory Studies

A chest roentgenogram is appropriate to screen for pulmonary involvement, including that caused by *Mycoplasma* infection, which can be confirmed further by acute and convalescent cold agglutinin titers. For herpes simplex disease, if the responsible vesicular lesion is still present, its fluid can be examined for multinucleated giant cells (Tzanck preparation) or cultured for herpesvirus. Laboratory evaluation usually is not helpful in drug-induced cases of erythema multiforme.

A complete blood cell count (CBC) and urinalysis are recommended because erythema multiforme occasionally is accompanied by leukocytosis and (although rarely) by renal involvement.

When the diagnosis is in doubt, a skin biopsy can be helpful. Erythema multiforme blisters are subepidermal.

Differential Diagnosis

The skin reactions most commonly considered in the differential diagnosis are urticaria, viral exanthems, vasculitis, staphylococcal scalded skin syndrome, and other blistering eruptions. The difference in appearance between a target lesion and a hive already has been discussed. In addition, individual hives last less than 24 hours; the lesions in erythema multiforme persist much longer. Viral exanthems usually are monomorphous and tend to be less red, more confluent, and more centrally distributed than the lesions of erythema multiforme. Purpura is the distinguishing feature of vasculitic lesions. The skin in scalded skin syndrome is diffusely red and strips off easily (Nikolsky sign). In the rare case when erythema multiforme involves the whole skin surface (toxic epidermal necrolysis), a skin biopsy helps distinguish it from staphylococcal scalded skin syndrome. In erythema multiforme, the split in the skin is subepidermal; in scalded skin syndrome, it is intraepidermal. Other blistering disorders that might be confused with erythema multiforme are rare in children.

Management

There is no convincing evidence that medical therapy favorably alters the course of erythema multiforme. Treating a precipitating infection seems appropriate, and erythromycin is recommended for *M. pneumoniae* infections, even though there is no proof that this alters the course of the skin reaction.

The use of systemic steroids is more controversial. They have been used frequently in Stevens-Johnson syndrome, but without documented benefit. In fact, Rasmussen's retrospective study[7] found that children who had Stevens-Johnson syndrome treated with systemic steroids required a longer hospital stay and had more complications (e.g., infection and gastrointestinal bleeding) than did untreated patients. Nevertheless, prednisone given systemically in doses ranging from 1 to 2 mg/kg/day sometimes is used early in the course of patients who have severe erythema multiforme. Intravenous gamma globulin (IVGG) may prove to be beneficial; however, more prospective studies are needed to determine optimal treatment. Supportive measures are vitally important. These are aimed mainly at (1) restoring and maintaining hydration, (2) preventing secondary infection, and (3) relieving pain. Patients who have severe oral involvement may be unable to drink and thus may require intravenous fluids. When skin involvement is extensive, transcutaneous fluid loss increases and replacement volumes must be adjusted accordingly. Local therapy with antiseptics and dressings may help to prevent secondary infection, and patients who have severe involvement may require treatments similar to those for burn patients. Systemic analgesics are used for pain. Topical anesthetics may be used intraorally to provide temporary relief for patients who have painful mouth lesions. "Magic swizzle," containing one part each of diphenhydramine HCl elixir, Maalox, and viscous lidocaine 2%, is one such agent. One must be aware of the potential for systemic effects from lidocaine when ordering this agent for young children.

Complications

The major complication of erythema multiforme, which occasionally results in death, is worsening of the mucocutaneous involvement. The entire skin surface can become involved with the blistering process, a condition often called *toxic epidermal necrolysis*. Mucous membrane involvement can restrict oral intake, resulting in dehydration. Conjunctivitis can produce residual ophthalmic complications, of which keratitis sicca is the most common, occurring in about 15% of patients who have Stevens-Johnson syndrome. Internal organs are affected less often; pulmonary involvement is reported occasionally and renal involvement in rare cases.

Course

Patients who have mild forms of erythema multiforme usually recover uneventfully within 2 to 3 weeks. The course of the disease is longer (4 to 6 weeks) in patients who have severe involvement, and death occasionally occurs from Stevens-Johnson syndrome, with reported rates ranging up to 15%. Erythema multiforme recurs in 10% to 20% of patients and is particularly common in those in whom the disease is precipitated by recurrent herpes simplex infection.

When to Refer

Recurrent erythema multiforme
Drug hypersensitivity reactions with multiorgan involvement

When to Hospitalize

Stevens-Johnson syndrome
Toxic epidermal necrolysis

REFERENCES

1. Bigby M, et al: Drug-induced cutaneous reactions: a report from the Boston Collaborative Drug Surveillance Program on 15,438 consecutive inpatients, 1975 to 1982, *JAMA* 256:3358, 1986.
2. Blacker KL, Stern RS, Wintroub BU: Cutaneous reactions to drugs. In Fitzpatrick TB, et al, editors: *Dermatology in general medicine,* ed 4, New York, 1993, McGraw-Hill.
3. Dunagin WG, Millikan LE: Drug eruptions, *Med Clin North Am* 64:983, 1982.
4. Huff JC, Weston WL, Tonnessen MG: Erythema multiforme: a critical review of characteristics, diagnostic criteria, and causes, *J Am Acad Dermatol* 8:767, 1983.
5. Jorizzo JL, editor: Symposium on urticaria and the reactive inflammatory vascular dermatoses, *Dermatol Clin* 3:1, 1985.
6. Monroe EW: Urticaria: an updated review, *Int J Dermatol* 20:32, 1981.
7. Rasmussen JE: Erythema multiforme in children: response to treatment with systemic corticosteroids, *Br J Dermatol* 95:181, 1976.
8. Wintroub BU, Stern RS: Cutaneous drug eruptions: pathogenesis and clinical classification, *J Am Acad Dermatol* 13:167, 1985.

206 Enterovirus Infections

Jerri Ann Jenista

Enteroviruses affect the practice of every pediatrician. The best known serotypes are the polioviruses, but the other enterovirus serotypes also cause widespread disease. A knowledge of these viruses can save both the practitioner and the patient considerable anxiety and can reduce diagnostic and therapeutic expenses.

CLASSIFICATION

Enteroviruses are *Picornaviridae,* small ribonucleic acid (RNA) viruses. They are classified into three groups: polioviruses, coxsackieviruses, and enteric cytopathogenic human orphan viruses (echoviruses).

The paralytic disease of poliovirus was known in ancient Egypt and was described clinically in 1789 in England. There are three polio serotypes.

Coxsackieviruses, named for the town in New York state where the first recognized patients lived, are divided into groups A and B, depending on the characteristic pathological changes induced in suckling mice; 23 and 6 serotypes, respectively, have been described.

Echoviruses initially were thought not to cause disease but now have been associated with nearly all the enterovirus syndromes. More than 30 types are known.

All newly identified enterovirus serotypes are designated simply as "enterovirus" followed by a number, beginning with 68. Recent dramatic gains in our understanding of enterovirus genetics have resulted in the reclassification of several echoviruses and the hepatitis A virus (formerly enterovirus 72) into nonenteroviral categories.[11]

EPIDEMIOLOGY

The epidemiology of enterovirus infection is complicated by host, virus, and environmental factors. In the United States alone, approximately 15 million cases of symptomatic enterovirus infection occur every year. Since up to 90% of infections are silent clinically and reinfection is common, clearly a large percentage of the population must encounter enteroviruses each year.

Environment

In temperate climates, enterovirus infections show a distinct seasonality, occurring from June through October in the Northern Hemisphere, although sporadic cases are noted in all seasons. In tropical regions, however, infection is noted throughout the year, with an increased incidence during rainy periods. Crowding, poor sanitation, and lower socioeconomic conditions also contribute to a higher incidence of infection.

Host

Age correlates inversely with the severity of clinical disease, probably because an individual becomes immune to an increasing number of serotypes over several seasons. With certain enteroviral serotypes, neonates may develop fatal sepsis rapidly, whereas most older children and adults have mild or no symptoms. Some enteroviral syndromes (e.g., poliomyelitis, acute hemorrhagic conjunctivitis, or myocarditis) may be severe at any age. Males seem to suffer both more infections and more disease than do females.

Individuals who have humoral immunodeficiencies may suffer chronic, debilitating infection with enteroviruses.[6] Except for poliovirus, enteroviral infection does not seem to pose a particular threat to individuals who have malignancy or acquired immunodeficiency syndrome (AIDS), although there are occasional reports of severe or fatal disease in these groups. Recipients of bone marrow transplants may experience severe or prolonged infection.

Virus

Most enteroviral syndromes are not serotype specific—that is, several different types may produce the same clinical disease. For example, the coxsackieviruses first were recognized in children who had classic paralytic disease without evidence of poliovirus infection. Conversely, a single serotype may produce varying clinical syndromes in different seasons and communities and even in different individuals infected at the same time and place.

Although outbreaks of illness associated with a single serotype often are reported, the far more common pattern is endemic infection caused by several enterovirus types. The predominant circulating serotypes may vary yearly, by locality, and even within the same year. The pattern of clinical syndromes seen also tends to change over the enterovirus season. A typical sequence for one serotype might be herpangina in June, nonspecific febrile exanthem in midsummer, and aseptic meningitis by early fall. Pandemic illness is unusual but not unknown. A modern example is the worldwide spread of acute hemorrhagic conjunctivitis caused by coxsackievirus A24 and enterovirus 70, which started in 1969 and affected millions of people.

Transmission and Incubation

Human beings are the only known reservoir for enteroviruses in nature. These viruses nearly always are transmitted by the fecal-oral route, although infections transmitted by food, water, blood, and perinatally occasionally have been reported. Nosocomial transmission has resulted in a number of severe nursery epidemics. In the special case of acute hemorrhagic conjunctivitis, the disease is spread by hand-to-eye contact.

The incubation period for enterovirus infection ordinarily is 3 to 5 days but may range from 2 to 20 days. The period of contagion probably is greatest several days before and immediately after the onset of symptoms; however, it may be prolonged. Because infection is so commonly asymptomatic and because virus excretion in the feces can persist for weeks after a person has recovered from the illness, it often is impossible to identify a patient's contact by history alone. Scrupulous hand washing may reduce the spread of enterovirus infection but is unlikely to control it completely, given the large pool of asymptomatic "shedders" usually present. Reinfection is common and usually clinically inapparent.

PATHOGENESIS

Over the past decade, the technological advances in molecular biology have produced a wealth of new information and have confirmed many long-held theories about the pathogenesis of enterovirus infection. For example, the development of monoclonal antibody systems has allowed researchers to isolate and clone poliovirus receptor sites on human cells.[11] As long suspected, these receptors are different from those for echoviruses. Antibodies directed against the poliovirus receptors block infection by any of the three serotypes of poliovirus but not infection by echoviruses or closely related nonenteroviruses. These and many other data constitute the first steps toward understanding the specificity of enteroviruses for primates and the tissue tropism of certain serotypes. The ultimate result of these studies may be an all-enterovirus vaccine.

Enterovirus infection is initiated by viral replication in the lymphoid tissues of the oropharynx and intestines. This phase occurs over 1 to 3 days and is symptom free. A *minor viremia* follows, with spread of virions to the reticuloendothelial system at 3 to 5 days. At this point, the patient is contagious, although symptoms of disease are not yet apparent. In a subclinical infection, the process is halted at this point by host defenses. A subsequent *major viremia* results in viral dissemination to secondary organs such as the skin, heart, liver, pancreas, adrenal glands, and central nervous system (CNS). This phase most often is recognized clinically as a nonspecific febrile illness, or the "minor illness" of poliomyelitis. In a very small percentage of cases, viral replication continues, producing the various clinical syndromes of enterovirus infection such as poliomyelitis, herpangina, or pleurodynia. We do not know why serotypes have a tropism for certain tissues, such as poliovirus for the neurons of the brain and spinal cord.

Antibody production may be detectable as early as 1 day after exposure to an enterovirus; both serum and secretory antibody forms are induced. Although some cross-reaction occurs among antibodies to different serotypes, protection against disease is not complete. Thus, a person who has suffered paralytic disease with one serotype of poliovirus may still be susceptible to a second episode with another serotype. Enterovirus antibody also is found in human milk; it may prevent enterovirus infection or may interfere with successful immunization with oral (live) poliovirus vaccine in the newborn period.

CLINICAL SYNDROMES

Large-scale epidemiological studies of poliovirus infection indicate that probably more than 90% of enterovirus infections are inapparent. When symptoms do occur, a variety of host factors (e.g., age, genetic background, and antibody status) and viral factors (e.g., strain virulence and inoculating dose of virions) determines the clinical disease present. Although nearly all the protean syndromes associated with enteroviruses have been noted with serotypes from each group, certain diseases are associated more frequently with specific groups (Table 206-1). For example, coxsackievirus A is the likely etiological agent of an outbreak of herpangina.

Nonspecific Febrile Illness

Any of the enteroviruses may cause a mild nonspecific febrile illness that lasts up to 7 or more days. Such seasonal infections account for the late summer and early fall peak of office visits noted in community surveillance studies of pediatric febrile illnesses. Because there are usually several serotypes circulating within a community during any particular year, a child may suffer several episodes of enterovirus-induced febrile illness within the same season.

Nonpolio enteroviruses are the major cause of hospitalization in febrile infants under 3 months of age. In prospective studies in Rochester, New York, enterovirus infection resulted in hospitalization in 2% of infants in the first month of life and accounted for 82% of admissions for "suspected sepsis." In other studies, enterovirus infection accounted for 33% of year-round admissions and 65% of summer-fall admissions for acute febrile illness in young infants.[7]

Enterovirus-associated symptoms serious enough to warrant laboratory evaluation in the emergency room are not uncommon in young children during the summer. Of 173 children requiring blood culture and/or lumbar puncture in four teaching hospitals over one summer season, 46% were ultimately diagnosed with enterovirus infection. Compared with enterovirus-negative children, those with enterovirus infection were hospitalized more often (82%) and had a higher risk of another hospitalization during the same illness (13%).[22]

Summer febrile illness associated with enterovirus infection probably is more common than recognized in older children also. In a prospective study of summer febrile illness in children 4 to 18 years of age presenting to private pediatric practices, at least 33% were confirmed to have enterovirus infection. Illness lasted 7 to 9 days; caused the children to miss 2 to 3 days of summer camp, work, or school; and spread to 50% of siblings and 25% of parents.[18]

The most frequent presenting symptoms of nonspecific

Table 206-1 Etiological Groups Most Often Implicated in Clinical Diseases Associated with Enteroviruses

	Poliovirus	Coxsackievirus A	Coxsackievirus B	Echovirus	Enterovirus
Asymptomatic infection	X	X	X	X	X
Nonspecific febrile illness	X	X	X	X	X
Common cold		X	X	X	X
Pharyngitis	X	X	X	X	X
Herpangina		X	X		X
Parotitis			X		
Croup		X	X		
Bronchitis, bronchiolitis			X	X	X
Pneumonia		X	X	X	X
Pleurodynia		X	X	X	
Myocarditis, pericarditis	X		X		
Gastrointestinal symptoms	X	X	X	X	
Hepatitis			X	X	
Pancreatitis			X		
Diabetes mellitus			X		
Orchitis			X		
Hand-foot-mouth disease		X			X
Exanthem		X	X	X	X
Conjunctivitis		X			X
Aseptic meningitis	X	X	X	X	X
Paralysis, encephalitis	X	X	X	X	X
Chronic meningoencephalitis	X			X	
Generalized neonatal disease		X	X	X	

Modified from Amstey MS, editor: *Virus infections in pregnancy,* New York, 1984, Grune & Stratton.

enteroviral illness are fever, irritability, lethargy, myalgia, malaise, and poor feeding. Diarrhea, vomiting, sore throat, or upper respiratory tract symptoms may be present but are not severe enough to be the cause of the admission. Concomitant aseptic meningitis in infants is common and is not predicted by clinical symptoms.[22] The illness occasionally takes a biphasic course. A relapse of fever associated with irritability within a day or two sometimes results in a second hospital admission for the same illness.

Respiratory Tract Disease

Nonexudative pharyngitis with or without lymphadenopathy is common and probably is the major cause of summertime sore throat. In a few cases, this illness may be the first manifestation of more severe disease that appears after an apparent recovery period of 1 to 3 days. Other respiratory syndromes (e.g., bronchitis, croup, or pneumonia) listed in Table 206-1 are less common and generally are mild.

Herpangina is a disease commonly diagnosed in a young child who has fever and sore throat or pain on swallowing. An enanthem may be noted early, but it soon is succeeded by small vesicles or tiny white papules and then by ulcers on the tonsils, pharynx, and soft palate. Herpangina is differentiated from herpes simplex stomatitis by the former's milder fever, primarily posterior oropharyngeal involvement, and epidemic seasonal occurrence.

The coxsackievirus B serotypes often are implicated in epidemic pleurodynia, or Bornholm disease.[14] Fever with severe pain in the intercostal and abdominal muscles occurring in spasms lasting minutes to hours is characteristic. The succeeding episodes are milder than the first but may occur days and sometimes even months later. In rare cases the symptoms are severe enough to prompt an exploratory laparotomy.

Enanthem and Exanthem Diseases

Hand-foot-mouth syndrome occurs in toddlers and school-age children. The hallmark signs are relatively painless vesicles on a red base, occasionally grouped, that appear on the buccal mucosa, tongue, hands, and feet. Rarely, the rash may spread to the extremities and buttocks. Patients usually have a low-grade fever and a sore throat and recover within a week.

A variety of exanthems may be the sole or major manifestation of enterovirus infection. Epidemics are reported with the classic macular blanching, rubella-like rash, the so-called Boston exanthem, which begins on the face and trunk and spreads to the extremities. It is distinguished from rubella by the lack of posterior auricular and suboccipital adenopathy. Unusual enterovirus rashes may be maculopapular, vesicular, roseola-like, urticarial, or petechial. When such exanthems occur in conjunction with other enterovirus syndromes, such as aseptic meningitis, the illness may be mistaken for a more serious disease, such as meningococcal meningitis.

Gastrointestinal Diseases

Despite the virus group name and the fecal-oral transmission of enteroviruses, enteric disease is not a prominent clinical syndrome. Gastrointestinal symptoms of nausea, vomiting, abdominal pain, constipation, diarrhea, or peritonitis occasionally are seen but almost always with other signs of systemic enterovirus infection, such as aseptic meningitis. Hepatitis or pancreatitis usually is part of a generalized enterovirus syndrome.

Anecdotal cases of juvenile diabetes mellitus have been related to coxsackievirus B infection.

Acute Hemorrhagic Conjunctivitis

Acute hemorrhagic conjunctivitis is an epidemic disease marked by the sudden onset of severe eye pain, photophobia, tearing, and dramatic subconjunctival hemorrhage and swelling. Recovery occurs in a week to 10 days. The illness most often is observed in middle-age individuals, but epidemics in schools have been noted. Neurological sequelae may be seen in adults; clinical improvement may take several months. A worldwide pandemic of this disease began in 1969 with waves of disease in Asia and Africa. The disease reached the continental United States only in the early 1980s and was confined mostly to the southeastern states.

Aseptic Meningitis

Enterovirus infection is the major cause of aseptic meningitis in countries that immunize against mumps. Most cases are sporadic although epidemic aseptic meningitis does occur, usually associated with person-to-person spread typically at summer camps or playgrounds and in day care centers.[5,15,19]

The classic disease manifests in a school-age child who has a headache, nuchal rigidity, fever, and often photophobia, pharyngitis, and/or a rash. Cerebrospinal fluid (CSF) analysis shows a moderate pleocytosis with a predominance of lymphocytes, normal glucose levels, and slightly increased protein levels. Occasionally, meningitis (as documented by isolation of the virus) is present with minimal or no pleocytosis, especially in a very young infant.[8]

Diagnostic dilemmas are not uncommon when such an illness occurs in an infant under 1 year of age, in sporadic cases, during a course of antibiotic therapy, or with atypical associated findings such as a petechial rash or encephalitis. Lyme meningitis occurs in a similar age group and during the same season as enteroviral meningitis but can usually be distinguished by the presence of cranial neuropathy, papilledema, or erythema migrans—clinical findings not noted in enteroviral disease.[9] See Chapter 233, Lyme Disease.

Spinal fluid obtained early in the course of enteroviral aseptic meningitis most often has a predominant polymorphonuclear (PMN) cell type; cell counts greater than 1000/mm^3 have been reported. A second spinal tap after a 12- to 24-hour observation period may clarify the diagnosis,[10] although in some children the PMN predominance persists for several days.[16] Other laboratory studies on CSF, such as C-reactive protein level or leukocyte aggregation, show too broad an overlap to distinguish it reliably from bacterial meningitis. The results of rapid virus identification techniques may reduce the empirical use of antibiotics and the length of hospitalization significantly.[23]

The course of enterovirus-associated meningitis usually is mild, although complications (e.g., the syndrome of inappropriate secretion of antidiuretic hormone [SIADH]) are seen occasionally. Adults and older children may complain of headache severe enough to require narcotic analgesia. Most patients recover within 2 weeks; in rare cases, relapses occur. Early information suggested that as many as 10% of survivors of aseptic meningitis that occurred before 3 months of age suffered long-term neurological sequelae, especially speech and language delays.[24,26] Recent prospective outcome studies are conflicting with reports of subtle receptive language problems in one series but no detectable neurodevelopmental disability in others.[3,20] Older children apparently recover completely.

Paralytic Disease

Paralytic disease with wild-type poliovirus has been eradicated in the Western Hemisphere. Virtually all cases of poliomyelitis acquired in the United States during the 1990s were associated with vaccine virus strains and occurred in young adults or in immunodeficient individuals. This should not occur any more because live polio vaccine is no longer used in the United States. (See Chapter 18, Immunizations.) Cases of wild-type disease are encountered in unimmunized individuals who travel to endemic regions of the world (i.e., Africa, the Middle East, and Asia). Infection with other enterovirus serotypes may also result in paralysis. Nonpolio enterovirus paralysis actually has been more common in the United States in recent years than has classic poliovirus-associated disease.[10]

Asymmetrical weakness and/or paralysis without sensory loss differentiates this illness from Guillain-Barré syndrome. Life-threatening disease usually involves paralysis of the primary and accessory respiratory muscles or bulbar poliomyelitis of the respiratory center. Recovery of muscle function may continue for several months.

In the 1980s, a new syndrome of progressive weakness and fatigue was recognized in long-term survivors of paralytic poliomyelitis. This "postpolio syndrome" is seen decades after the initial infection. Apparently, the previously affected muscles suffer denervation as overburdened motor neurons eventually "wear out." The long-term outcome of this syndrome is unknown.

Perinatal Infection

Enterovirus infection in neonates may occur as any of the syndromes seen in older children.[1] However, premature infants and newborns born without specific passively acquired maternal antibody may suffer a fulminant, rapidly fatal disease. Generalized neonatal infection begins as a syndrome of fever, lethargy, and poor feeding indistinguishable from early bacterial sepsis. Progression is swift, with multiorgan involvement, including hepatitis, pancreatitis, myocarditis, and encephalitis. Mortality is high in the disseminated forms of infection. The virus in neonates most often is transmitted from mother to infant at or near the time of delivery; however, nursery outbreaks with fatal cases have been reported.

There is some evidence that maternal enterovirus infection may affect the fetus, but no consistent teratogenic pattern has been recognized. Epidemiological evidence suggests that maternal exposure to certain enteroviruses during pregnancy may increase the risk of subsequent juvenile diabetes mellitus in the offspring.

Other Diseases

Unusual enterovirus syndromes include encephalitis (often occurring in severely ill neonates), the chronic meningoencephalitis of patients who have hypogammaglobulinemia, and the "dancing eyes-dancing feet" (opsoclonus-myoclonus) syndrome. In 1998, there was a dramatic outbreak of enteroviral disease in Taiwan. It is estimated that more than 1 million infections with coxsackievirus A16 and enterovirus 71 occurred. In particular, infection with enterovirus 71 was associated with an unusually high rate of severe disease including aseptic meningitis, acute flaccid paralysis, encephalomyelitis, and death, probably caused by neurogenic pulmonary edema.[12,13] Similar but less widespread outbreaks of enterovirus 71–associated neurological disease were noted in 1997 in Malaysia and in 1999 in Australia. Studies to determine if the virus strains are related are under way.

Myocarditis and pericarditis occur with a high mortality as part of the generalized disease of newborns. Fewer than 50% of older children and adults who have myocarditis die; recovery may be complete, but severe sequelae have been reported. Orchitis occasionally occurs in postpubertal patients in association with coxsackievirus B infection.

LABORATORY DIAGNOSIS

Interpretation of Laboratory Results

When obtaining specimens for enterovirus identification, the clinician must keep in mind the concept of "permissive" versus "nonpermissive" sites. Permissive sites (e.g., the nasopharynx and feces) are those in which enteroviruses may persist for weeks to months after infection. Identification of an enterovirus from a permissive site may be completely unrelated to the illness under investigation.

Nonpermissive sites are those from which virus is identified only during periods of disease. Shedding of virus in these sites usually is brief. Thus, finding an enterovirus in blood, spinal fluid, or a skin vesicle is strong evidence that the virus is related to the concurrent clinical illness.

Because almost all enterovirus serotypes can produce any enterovirus syndrome and because no disease is associated uniquely with any enterovirus serotype, an enterovirus usually need not be identified beyond its actual presence. Enterovirus presence from a nonpermissive site is sufficient to diagnose the etiology of the illness in question. In rare cases, both enteroviral and bacterial pathogens may be present in blood or spinal fluid. Invariably, the symptoms associated with the bacterial agent are more severe and dictate the clinical management.

Identification of an enterovirus from a permissive site specimen, especially feces, is more problematic. Vague, nonspecific symptoms or highly unusual or rare syndromes may be completely unrelated to the finding of an enterovirus shed in the gastrointestinal tract. Many disease associations with enteroviruses probably are explained by such incidental enterovirus identification. Classic enterovirus disease during a known epidemic season is interpreted more easily; isolating an enterovirus from the stool of an infant who has fever and CSF pleocytosis in the summer, without any other pathogen isolated, is presumptive evidence of enteroviral meningitis.

Virus Isolation

Except for most of the coxsackievirus A group, enteroviruses are isolated readily in cell cultures. A presumptive positive culture can be noted as early as 18 hours but more typically requires 2 to 5 days. Specific identification of an individual serotype takes somewhat longer. Suckling mouse inoculation, an expensive and difficult procedure, is the only available method of isolating most of the coxsackievirus A group serotypes.

Viruses may be isolated from throat swabs, feces, CSF, blood or serum, skin vesicles, and tissues obtained at autopsy. Specimens from several sites increase the diagnostic yield because it is not always possible to predict the pathological stage of infection and thus the most likely source of the virus.

Virus isolation by culture is time and labor intensive, requiring special expertise. In clinical laboratories, it may soon be supplanted by more rapid diagnostic tests such as polymerase chain reaction. These newer tests, however, do not detect all enterovirus serotypes and cannot differentiate among serotypes. When a specific diagnosis is required, as in the tracing of epidemic enterovirus 71 infection, virus isolation by culture remains the technique of choice.

Rapid Virus Identification

Currently, the only rapid diagnostic technique with clinical promise is the polymerase chain reaction (PCR). In areas in which the test is available, an enterovirus can be identified from a specimen such as CSF in as short a time as 5 hours.[2]

Numerous studies of the use of CSF enterovirus PCR tests in clinical settings indicate that PCR is more sensitive than viral culture in identifying aseptic meningitis.[4,23,25] The time needed to identify a positive specimen by using PCR is considerably shorter, typically 1 day versus 3 to 4 days for viral culture, and results in briefer hospitalizations and shorter courses of empirical antibiotic therapy. Experience with non-CSF specimens is limited. Although PCR assays are expensive, the cost is balanced by the savings in therapeutic expenses. As specific antiviral therapy directed against enteroviruses becomes available, PCR will be essential in the early identification of patients most likely to benefit from treatment.

Molecular Genetic Analysis

The genomes of the polioviruses and several of the echoviruses have been sequenced and cloned. These and other advances in genetic analysis have allowed researchers to examine viral strains isolated during epidemics precisely. Thus, the epidemic of paralytic poliomyelitis in Finland in 1984 and 1985 was discovered to be caused by a typical wild-type poliovirus strain, not a new mutant, as had been suspected.[11] Ten cases of paralysis and widespread minor infection occurred in this highly immunized population because of an inadequate response to one of the inactivated vaccine components. The epidemic was terminated quickly by mass administration of a live oral polio vaccine.

Investigations such as these may allow better vaccines to be engineered to accomplish the World Health Organization's goal of eradicating polio worldwide soon after the beginning of the twenty-first century.

Serological Diagnosis

It is not practical to obtain serum for analysis of enterovirus antibody titers because of the numerous serotypes and the complexity of the procedure. When the clinical or pathological picture strongly suggests one enterovirus group or a limited number of serotypes (i.e., myocarditis probably related to coxsackievirus B), measuring neutralizing antibody titers may be feasible.

In situations in which it might be desirable to prove the cause of an epidemic or a particularly unusual case, serum-neutralizing antibody titers in acute and convalescent samples may be useful. Unfortunately, because antibody production occurs early, titers already may be high during the acute phase of clinical illness, thus obscuring the diagnosis. Assays to detect enterovirus serotype-specific IgM in serum are not available commercially.

PREVENTION

Attenuated live or killed poliovirus vaccines are the only preventive enterovirus preparations currently available. Enhanced-potency inactivated poliovirus vaccine is now the recommended choice for routine immunization in the United States.

In the prevaccine years, 0.2 ml/kg of pooled immune serum globulin given intramuscularly prevented or ameliorated poliovirus infection. In view of the severity of the disease in neonates, such injections might be indicated in nursery epidemics and for infants of mothers who develop a probable enterovirus disease within a few days of delivery. Trials of intravenous immune globulin in neonates who have clinical disease or who have been exposed to enterovirus during a known nosocomial outbreak have not shown clear benefit.[17]

TREATMENT

Pleconaril, a novel oral anti-viral drug activity against picornaviruses, including enteroviruses, is now entering into clinical trials. Infants, older children, and adults who have enterovirus-associated aseptic meningitis treated with pleconaril suffered a shorter illness and returned to normal activity sooner. In particular, older children reported a marked decrease in headache that was apparent as early as 24 hours after the initiation of treatment.[21]

Pleconaril has been widely used in compassionate trials. It is effective in stopping the replication of virus in immunodeficient individuals. Clear benefit in neonates who had disseminated disease or in other enteroviral syndromes has not been demonstrated. Pleconaril is well tolerated, with few or no side effects attributed to the drug. Clinical enterovirus isolates resistant to plenconaril have not been detected.

When to Refer

- Neonates who have any evidence of disseminated or rapidly progressive enterovirus-like infection
- Immunocompromised individuals who have chronic enterovirus-like syndromes
- Normal hosts who have atypical progression of enteroviral disease, especially those who have neurological or cardiac involvement

When to Hospitalize

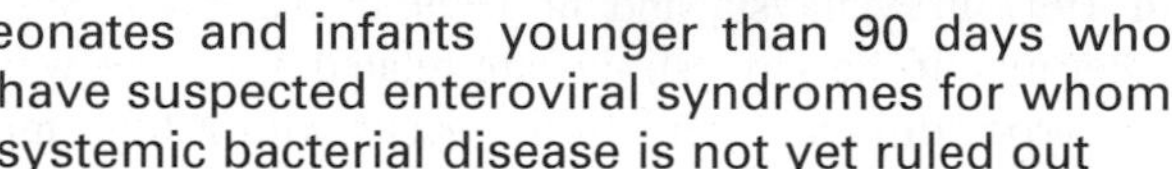

- Neonates and infants younger than 90 days who have suspected enteroviral syndromes for whom systemic bacterial disease is not yet ruled out
- Disease significant enough to require subspecialty expertise, especially cardiac, immunological and neurological disease
- Any enteroviral syndrome that has a rapidly progressive or atypical course
- Older children who have aseptic meningitis who require symptomatic treatment for severe headache or dehydration

REFERENCES

1. Abzug MJ: Perinatal enterovirus infections. In Rotbart HA, editor: *Human enterovirus infections,* Washington, DC, 1995, American Society for Microbiology.
2. Abzug MJ, et al: Diagnosis of neonatal enterovirus infection by polymerase chain reaction, *J Pediatr* 126:447, 1995.
3. Baker RC, et al.: Neurodevelopmental outcome of infants with viral meningitis in the first three months of life, *Clin Pediatr* (Phila) 35:295, 1996.
4. Byington CL, et al.: A polymerase chain reaction-based epidemiologic investigation of the incidence of non-polio enteroviral infections in febrile and afebrile infants 90 days and younger, *Pediatrics* 103:656, 1999, e27. (URL: http:\www.pediatrics.org/cgi/content//full/103/3/e27)
5. Centers for Disease Control and Prevention: Outbreak of aseptic meningitis, Whiteside County, Illinois, 1995, *MMWR* 46:221, 1997.
6. Centers for Disease Control and Prevention: Prolonged poliovirus excretion in an immunodeficient person with vaccine-associated paralytic poliomyelitis, *MMWR* 46:641, 1997.
7. Dagan R: Nonpolio enteroviruses and the febrile young infant: epidemiologic, clinical and diagnostic aspects. *Pediatr Infect Dis J* 15:67, 1996.
8. Dagan R, Jenista JA, Menegus MA: Association of clinical presentation, laboratory findings, and virus serotypes with the presence of meningitis in hospitalized infants with enterovirus infection, *J Pediatr* 113:975, 1988.
9. Eppes SC, et al: Characterization of Lyme meningitis and comparison with viral meningitis in children, *Pediatrics* 103:957, 1999.
10. Harrison SA, Risser WL: Repeat lumbar puncture in the differential diagnosis of meningitis, *Pediatr Infect Dis J* 7:143, 1988.
11. Hellen CUT, et al: Enterovirus genetics. In Rotbart HA, editor: *Human enterovirus infections,* Washington, DC, 1995, American Society for Microbiology.
12. Ho M, et al: An epidemic of enterovirus 71 infection in Taiwan, *N Engl J Med* 341:929, 1999.

13. Huang CC, et al: Neurologic complications in children with enterovirus 71 infection, *N Engl J Med* 341:939, 1999.
14. Ikeda RM, et al: Pleurodynia among football players at a high school: an outbreak associated with coxsackievirus B1, *JAMA* 270:2205, 1993.
15. Mohle-Doetani JC, et al: Viral meningitis in child care center staff and parents: an outbreak of echovirus 30 infections, *Public Health Reports* 114:249, 1999.
16. Negrini B, et al: Cerebrospinal fluid findings in aseptic versus bacterial meningitis, *Pediatrics* 105:316, 2000.
17. Pasic S, et al: Intravenous immunoglobulin prophylaxis in an echovirus 6 and echovirus 4 nursery outbreak, *Pediatr Infect Dis J* 16:718, 1997.
18. Pichichiero ME, et al: Clinical and economic impact of enterovirus illness in private pediatric practice, *Pediatrics* 102:1126, 1998.
19. Reintjes R, et al: Community-wide outbreak of enteroviral illness caused by echovirus 30: a cross-sectional survey and case-control study, *Pediatr Infect Dis J* 18:104, 1999.
20. Rorabaugh ML, et al: Aseptic meningitis in infants younger than 2 years of age: acute illness and neurologic complications, *Pediatrics* 92:206, 1993.
21. Rotbart HA: Antiviral therapy for enteroviral infections, *Pediatr Infect Dis J* 18:631, 1999.
22. Rotbart HA, et al: Clinical significance of enteroviruses in serious summer febrile illnesses of children, *Pediatr Infect Dis J* 18:869, 1999.
23. Sawyer MH: Enterovirus infections: diagnosis and treatment, *Pediatr Infect Dis J* 18:1033, 1999.
24. Sells CJ, Carpenter RL, Ray CG: Sequelae of central nervous system enterovirus infections, *N Engl J Med* 293:1, 1975.
25. Van Vliet K, et al.: Multicenter evaluation of the Amplicor enterovirus PCR test with cerebrospinal fluid from patients with aseptic meningitis, *J Clin Microbiol* 36:2652, 1998.
26. Wilfert CM, et al: Longitudinal assessment of children with enteroviral meningitis during the first three months of life, *Pediatrics* 67:811, 1981.

SUGGESTED READING

Rotbart HA, editor: *Human enterovirus infections,* Washington, DC, 1995, American Society for Microbiology.

207 Foreign Bodies of the Ear, Nose, Airway, and Esophagus

Jay N. Dolitsky • Robert F. Ward

Foreign bodies of the ear, nose, and upper aerodigestive tract are a common problem among children, particularly those younger than age 5 years. The scope of the problem was underscored first by National Safety Council statistics in 1969, which showed that more children died at home from accidental foreign body ingestion or aspiration than from any other cause.[1] By 1998, foreign body aspiration and asphyxiation was but the fourth leading cause of accidental death in the home among children younger than age 5 years; it is still a major problem.[15] The severity of the problem depends on several factors, including the site, composition, and duration of residence of the foreign body. Similarly, the clinical presentation and management of these objects are related to those factors.

Removal of a foreign body usually is not an emergency, unless the airway is compromised; it should be attempted only after the physician has as many factors as possible under control, including appropriate sedation or anesthesia, proper instrumentation and illumination, and most important, ability. If these elements are lacking, the problem probably will be aggravated by attempts to remove the foreign body, and the child's well-being may be jeopardized.

FOREIGN BODIES OF THE EAR

Earrings can become embedded in the auricle when a chronic infection of the pierced site is followed by overgrowth of granulation tissue. The use of the spring-loaded gun to pierce ears has resulted in numerous cases of embedded earrings as well.[6] Foreign bodies of the external auditory canal are found most commonly among children between 2 and 4 years of age. Curiosity, boredom, and imitation of others often are predisposing factors. Accidental entry of a foreign object through placement in the external auditory canal, either by the child or a companion, can occur during play. Insects also can find their way into the ear canal without any assistance. Das[7] reviewed 233 cases of foreign bodies in the ear and nose and found that the most consistent etiological factor was chronic irritation or inflammation of these orifices. Thus, children who have chronic external otitis or itching are more likely to place objects in their ear canals.

Clinical Presentation

Depending on the depth of the foreign object within the external auditory canal, the nature and composition of the object, and its duration in the canal, a wide spectrum of findings can be seen. Usually, there is no history of placing an object in the ear canal because most children are reluctant to admit to this activity for fear of punishment. If insertion is not witnessed, some foreign bodies may go undetected for extended periods.

Nonreactive substances, such as plastic, that are not obstructing the canal completely and are not abutting the tympanic membrane may not cause symptoms. Insects tend to incite local irritation, causing discomfort, erythema, and occasionally, drainage. Vegetable matter also may cause local inflammation, which often leads to local pain and itching. Objects that touch the tympanic membrane cause pain, particularly with movement of the drum, as when swallowing. If the entire canal is obstructed, hearing most likely will be decreased.

There have been several reports concerning button-size alkaline batteries as foreign bodies of the ear canal.[5,23,26] These objects may leak battery acid, causing a severe local tissue reaction or destruction with pain, swelling, and discharge. This relatively new type of foreign body should be handled expeditiously to prevent serious injury to the canal, tympanic membrane, or middle ear.

When a small foreign body is suspected from the history but cannot be visualized on examination, it may be lodged anteriorly in the tympanic sulcus. Instillation of water to fill the medial half of the external canal may act as a concave lens, thereby allowing visualization of the tympanic sulcus.[22] In a patient who has a small, narrow or swollen external ear canal, microscopic evaluation will aid in visualization.

Management

Nonreactive foreign bodies that do not occlude the external canal completely or impinge on the tympanic membrane do not present an emergency. These can be removed with a various instruments; the most useful will depend on the shape and composition of the object. Often a 5- or 7-mm Frazier tip suction, an alligator forceps, or a right-angle hook can be used to retrieve the object. The hook is used by passing it beyond the object, hooking it from behind, and pulling it out gently. Gentle irrigation also may be used on nonvegetable substances, provided the tympanic membrane can be visualized and is intact and there is no evidence of inflammation of the external canal; vegetable matter tends to swell when water is applied, making it more difficult to remove.

When the tympanic membrane cannot be visualized or if there is evidence of inflammation or injury to the external canal, the foreign body should be removed immediately. This is particularly important with an alkaline battery, because tympanic membrane perforations have been reported within only 8 hours of entry.[5] Magnets may be helpful for removing metallic objects such as batteries or metal beads.[17]

Insects should be killed before removal by instilling either mineral oil or 4% Xylocaine into the external canal. Extraction with suction or alligator forceps then may be undertaken.

After any foreign body is removed, the external canal and tympanic membrane should be inspected carefully and thoroughly. Aqueous-based acidic ear drops or ophthalmic drops should be used for 5 to 7 days if the external canal appears injured or inflamed. The affected ear should be protected from water until it has healed completely.

In older children who are cooperative, a local anesthetic injected with a small-gauge needle into the skin lining the external canal may allow complete removal of the foreign body and subsequent examination. For younger children or for those who are uncooperative, general anesthesia may be necessary and certainly is preferable to traumatic removal if a child is unable to cooperate or cannot be restrained adequately.

Complications

Complications can be caused by the foreign body itself or by traumatic removal. Laceration or inflammation of the external canal usually is not serious and resolves with instillation of liquid analgesics and antibiotics. Perforations of the tympanic membrane require careful inspection to ensure that a flap of the membrane has not folded into the middle ear, which can lead to a permanent perforation or the development of a cholesteatoma. Likewise, when the tympanic membrane is not intact, the middle ear space can become contaminated, and otitis media can develop. Balbani et al reviewed 93 cases of ear foreign bodies and found that all 12 complications (11 canal lacerations, 1 tympanic membrane perforation) occurred in patients who had undergone previous attempts at removal.[4] Engelsma reported one case of impacted foreign body following two attempts at removal that required surgical widening of the canal before extraction.[10]

If it is not possible to remove a foreign object from the ear canal safely or if the tympanic membrane may have been injured by either the foreign body or its removal, the patient must be seen by an otolaryngologist.

FOREIGN BODIES IN THE NOSE

The predicaments that lead to foreign objects in the nasal cavity are quite similar to those of the ear. Boredom, curiosity, and acts of imitation may lead a child to place an object in his or her nose. These objects typically are soft, such as tissues, erasers, clay, or pieces of a toy. Occasionally a foreign object enters the nose accidentally while the child is attempting to sniff or smell it. In Das' study, chronic rhinitis was found to be the most common underlying factor in children placing objects in the nose.[7] The frequency has been noted to increase during the summer and Christmas, when toy sales increase.[27]

Clinical Presentation

Children usually will not confess to having placed something in the nose. The most common finding with this problem is unilateral nasal discharge, which usually is foul smelling. In fact, a unilateral nasal discharge in a young child should be considered evidence of a foreign body until proved otherwise. Occasionally, epistaxis is the presenting symptom.[31] When an alkaline disk battery is lodged in the nose, the symptoms may be more acute. Tissue damage can occur through three mechanisms: electrical burn, liquefaction necrosis (from sodium hydroxide), and pressure necrosis.[2] If possible, the anterior nasal cavities should be examined with a nasal speculum and suction. The key to any evaluation is powerful illumination. Roentgenograms may be helpful if the object is radiopaque or has become calcified. An incidental finding of a nasal foreign body on a routine dental roentgenogram has been reported.[16] U.S. toy manufacturers are required by law to make toy parts radiopaque, a regulation that proves quite valuable when a physician is looking for foreign objects in the nasal cavity or in any part of the upper aerodigestive tract. However, toys and toy parts manufactured outside the United States do not have to conform to this regulation. In their review of children who had nasal foreign bodies, Tong et al reported that 28 of 71 (39%) radiographs demonstrated a foreign body.[27]

Management

Nasal foreign bodies should be removed as quickly as possible, particularly in the case of an alkaline battery, which can cause severe local inflammation with tissue damage occurring within 1 hour of placement.[5,13] When an alkaline disk battery is in the nasal cavity, saline irrigation should be avoided because it can cause further tissue damage.[2] Young children tend to detest any nasal instrumentation, and removal of a nasal foreign body requires some degree of cooperation or restraint. Thus, sedation or general anesthesia may be advised. Topical application of an epinephrine-like decongestant, (e.g., Neo-Synephrine, Afrin) in conjunction with removal of secretions by a small suction tip helps in visualizing the foreign object, particularly one lodged in the middle or posterior nasal cavity. Use of an endoscope is recommended to visualize this region.[31] A foreign body that has been allowed to remain in the nose for a long time may become calcified and form what is known as a rhinolith. Removing rhinoliths often is difficult and bloody. Various methods of foreign body removal have been described that can be attempted in the office, including using pepper to induce a sneeze while the uninvolved nostril is occluded or blowing in the child's mouth while the contralateral nostril is held shut. We do not recommend these methods. In a more controlled fashion, nebulized adrenaline together with nose blowing has been reported to expel nasal foreign bodies successfully.[9] Ambu-bag insufflation of the mouth with the patient in Trendelenburg position has also been described.[11] Another method of removal involves using a Fogarty or a small Foley catheter.[14,21] The catheter is placed beyond the foreign body into the posterior portion of the nasal cavity or nasopharynx and then inflated with 2 to 3 ml of saline solution. The catheter then is drawn gently forward and out of the nose, expelling the object. The danger with this technique is that the foreign object may be dislodged by pushing it posteriorly into the nasopharynx, which may lead to aspiration of the object.

Soft, friable objects usually can be removed with a Frazier tip suction. If the foreign body is firm and is flat or has an edge, it may be removed by using a nasal bayonet or Hartmann or alligator forceps. A wire loop may be placed beyond the foreign body that is spherical and removed by pulling it forward. After removal, local inflammation manifested by bloody or purulent oozing may be controlled with saline nose drops and an antibacterial ointment such as bacitracin or mupirocin (Bactroban). Sterile water should be used in place of saline if the foreign object removed was an alkaline battery.[2]

Complications

Complications of nasal foreign bodies include epistaxis, local infection, inflammation, and irritation. Occasionally a scar band, or synechia, may form between the turbinate and septum. These can be prevented by placing a splint made of Gelfilm or Silastic over the raw, exposed area. Nasal septal perforation has been reported.[27] Obstruction of a sinus ostium by a foreign object may lead to the development of sinusitis. This typically manifests as pain and tenderness over the affected sinus, or clouding and an air-fluid level on radiograph. Treatment includes oral antibiotics and nasal decongestant drops. The dreaded complication of aspiration of a nasal foreign body can be avoided in most cases by prompt and skilled removal.

The differential diagnosis of foreign bodies in the nose includes suppurative rhinitis, adenoiditis, sinusitis, and nasal or nasopharyngeal tumors. Nasal polyps also may manifest as a unilateral nasal discharge, and in a young child, the diagnosis of cystic fibrosis must be ruled out.

FOREIGN BODIES OF THE AIRWAY

A statistic mentioned earlier bears repeating: Only a few years ago, foreign body aspiration and asphyxiation was the fourth-leading cause of accidental death in the home among children younger than age 5 years. It accounts for approximately 9% of all home accidental deaths of children in this age group.[15] The incidence declines rapidly among those older than age 5, until age 65, when it increases again to an even higher percentage. Overall, the incidence of death from foreign body aspiration has declined significantly during the past two decades.[15] This probably is the result of increased parental awareness of the risks of leaving small objects within the reach of young children. Consumer education and awareness have been important in diminishing this potential hazard. Also, the development of lifesaving techniques, such as the Heimlich maneuver, that can be performed by people who are not medical personnel accounts for a higher survival rate.

With regard to foreign body impaction, the airway can be divided into three segments: the larynx, the trachea, and the bronchial tree. Lima[19] reviewed all airway foreign body admissions to his pediatric hospital from 1980 through 1987. Of the 91 cases, 11 involved a foreign body lodged in the larynx. Of these 11 patients, 5 died and 3 suffered anoxic encephalopathy. It is apparent that although most foreign bodies pass through the larynx, the outcome is grave when one does not.

Etiology

The causes of foreign body impaction in the airway are many. As with foreign bodies of the ears and nose, curiosity or boredom may lead a young child to put foreign objects in his or her mouth. Infants in particular will attempt to place almost anything they can handle into their mouths. A startle may cause inadvertent ingestion or aspiration. Lack of complete dentition, as well as lack of attention to chewing, allows large food particles to enter the posterior pharynx. Incomplete development of mouth and tongue coordination and the neuromuscular mechanism for swallowing in young children also may account for a greater incidence of foreign body ingestion or aspiration.[18] Reichert[24] reports that a positive association has been noted between the occurrence of upper respiratory tract infections and foreign body aspiration. He postulates that the need for continuous mouth breathing when a child suffers a cold interrupts a smooth breathing-swallowing pattern, leading to an increase in aspiration. Although this typically occurs in the younger child, Lemberg found, in a review of 105 patients who had foreign bodies of the airway, that 23% occurred in children older than 5 years of age.[18]

Clinical Presentation

A history of foreign body ingestion or aspiration may be obtained, depending on the patient's age or condition and whether the suspected incident was witnessed. Classically, when a foreign object is aspirated into the respiratory tract, initially it produces a choking, gagging, coughing, or wheezing episode. This may be followed by an asymptomatic interval during which there is little to suggest the presence of a foreign body. At this point the parents and physician often are lulled into a false sense of security.

Depending on the site of the foreign body in the airway, a patient may manifest a spectrum of findings, ranging from an almost complete lack of symptoms to signs of complete airway obstruction.

Laryngeal foreign bodies are likely to produce the most acute and dramatic presentation. Large objects that completely obstruct the airway may result in stridor, high-pitched wheezing, cough, dysphonia, or worse—aphonia and cyanosis. Children who have smaller, partly obstructing objects that allow adequate air exchange have cough, stridor, hoarseness, and pain or discomfort.

Tracheal foreign bodies usually are associated with cough and some degree of stridor or wheezing and may produce an audible "slap" as the object moves from the carina to the glottis with respiration. Bronchial foreign bodies usually cause wheezing or coughing if they are partly obstructing; this often is misdiagnosed as asthma. With complete obstruction of a bronchus, an initial asymptomatic period is followed by a postobstructive pneumonitis or bronchiectasis.[20] Sharp objects such as pins or tacks may cause pain or hemoptysis.

If aspiration of a foreign body into the upper airway is suspected, plain roentgenography may help. For objects suspected to be lodged in the laryngeal inlet, high-kilovolt, anteroposterior (AP) and lateral roentgenograms of the upper trachea or esophageal inlet should be obtained if the patient's condition permits. Bronchial foreign bodies may be suggested by some form of dynamic roentgen ray study, such as inspiratory-expiratory roentgenograms, lateral decubitus films, or videofluoroscopy. These studies can demonstrate air-trapping in the affected lung.

Management

Foreign bodies that completely obstruct the laryngeal inlet create a life-threatening emergency and should be expelled immediately by using the Heimlich maneuver (abdominal thrusts). For infants younger than 1 year of age, the American Academy of Pediatrics recommends five back blows in the head-down position followed by five chest thrusts in the supine position, in place of the Heimlich maneuver[3] (see Appendix A, Pediatric Basic and Advanced Life Support). Blind finger sweeps are dangerous and should be avoided.[3] If the foreign body cannot be expelled, a large-bore needle or angiocatheter (14 gauge) should be inserted into the cricothyroid space to allow some degree of ventilation until the patient can be taken to the operating room for removal of the object. Alternatively, if skilled personnel are present, an emergency tracheotomy may be necessary. Partly obstructing laryngeal foreign bodies should be treated in a way that prevents total obstruction of the airway; therefore, back blows and abdominal thrusts should not be used in these cases.

Tracheal and bronchial foreign bodies should be removed by a physician specifically trained for the task, which usually requires controlled endoscopic removal in the operating room. This usually is not an emergency; therefore, adequate preparations can be made.

Complications

Abdominal and chest thrusts may damage intraabdominal contents (e.g., liver, spleen) and ribs, respectively. Therefore, these techniques should be used only in cases of complete airway obstruction that otherwise would cause certain death. Conversion of a partial airway obstruction to a complete obstruction can best be avoided by having skilled personnel retrieve the foreign body. According to Wolach et al,[30] pneumonia was the most common complication in 127 cases of foreign body aspiration.

A bronchial foreign body that remains in place for an extended period may cause air-trapping and irreversible bronchiectatic changes distal to the obstruction.

Prolonged or difficult instrumentation of the airway during removal of a foreign body can lead to laryngeal edema or injury, with obstructive symptoms. This may require a period of intubation after surgery. As an alternative, postoperative edema sometimes can be avoided by using steroids during and after surgery.

FOREIGN BODIES INVOLVING THE ESOPHAGUS

More than half of the foreign bodies in children involve the esophagus, with the highest incidence in children 14 months to 6 years of age.[29] Younger children are inquisitive and tend to explore objects orally. The objects then are intentionally swallowed or accidentally ingested as the result of a startle. In the United States, coins are the most common foreign body to lodge in the esophagus.[28] In a recent review, coins were the most frequent esophageal foreign body in children younger than 10 years old, and fish bones were the most common in children older than 10 years.[25]

The esophagus has four physiological areas of narrowing: the cricopharyngeal sphincter, the aortic arch, the region of the left main bronchus, and the gastroesophageal sphincter. These correspond to the four most common sites of foreign body obstruction. The cricopharyngeus is the most common, the arch of the aortic region the most dangerous.

Clinical Presentation

The history of foreign body ingestion often is not obtained, and most foreign bodies pass through the normal esophagus undetected. Those that do not pass freely initially stimulate the larynx and cause gagging and coughing. Subsequent symptoms depend on the size, composition, and nature of the foreign body. With young children, poor feeding or refusal to eat or drink, as well as increased salivation, are typical. When the esophagus is completely or almost completely obstructed, choking and vomiting occur. The duration of obstruction can affect the clinical presentation: The longer a foreign object is present, the greater the tissue reaction and local inflammation. Thus, in the later stages, patients can have pain on swallowing, fever, and leukocytosis.

When a foreign body is suspected, posteroanterior (PA) and lateral chest roentgenograms, in addition to neck films, are diagnostic if the object is radiopaque, such as a coin. Contrast studies can be used when an esophageal foreign body that does not show on routine roentgenograms is strongly suspected.

Management

An esophageal foreign body does not usually require emergency measures, but it should be removed as soon as possible after proper evaluation and preparation.[12] Often, children will have eaten recently, and generally it is recommended that an appropriate period pass before they are given general anesthesia. If the foreign body is corrosive, such as an alkaline button battery, it should be removed as soon as possible to prevent severe inflammation and potential perforation of the esophageal wall.[8]

Endoscopic removal under anesthesia by a trained expert remains the method of choice because of the safety provided. This technique allows for direct visualization of the esophagus, its mucosa, and the foreign body. Removal with a flexible endoscope also is possible without general anesthesia.

Nonendoscopic techniques for removing an esophageal foreign body (i.e., with a Foley or Fogarty catheter) have been described.[14] The child is sedated and brought to the fluoroscopy suite. While the child is in a steep Trendelenburg position, the catheter is placed beyond the foreign object, and the balloon on the catheter is inflated and withdrawn. This technique can lead to aspiration and airway obstruction and generally is not recommended.

Complications

Perforation of the esophagus can result from the endoscopic procedure or may be caused by the foreign body itself, especially if it is sharp or caustic. Endoscopic removal is particularly dangerous with objects lodged at the level of the aortic arch. If an esophageal tear is suspected, contrast roentgenography usually will confirm or negate the suspicion.

Retropharyngeal abscess has been reported as the most frequent complication of a sharp esophageal foreign body, such as a fish bone.[25] Foreign bodies that have been in the esophagus for long periods also can cause a stricture to develop. In these cases, a contrast study, computed tomography scan, or esophagoscopy also should be performed to aid in the diagnosis.

REFERENCES

1. *Accident facts,* National Safety Council, Chicago, 1969.
2. Alvi A, et al: Miniature disc battery in the nose: a dangerous foreign body, *Clin Pediatr* 36: 427, 1997.
3. American Academy of Pediatrics Committee on Pediatric Emergency Medicine: First aid for the choking child, *Pediatrics* 92:477, 1993.
4. Balbani AP, et al: Ear and nose foreign body removal in children, *Int J Pediatr Otorhinolaryngol* 46:37, 1998.
5. Capo JM, Lucente FE: Alkaline battery foreign bodies of the ear and nose, *Arch Otolaryngol Head Neck Surg* 112:562, 1986.
6. Cohen HA, et al: Embedded earrings, *Cutis* 53:82, 1994.
7. Das SK: Etiological evaluation of foreign bodies in the ear and nose, *J Laryngol Otol* 98:989, 1984.
8. Derkay CS, et al: Retrieving foreign bodies from upper aerodigestive tracts of children, *AORN J* 60:53, 1994.
9. Douglas AR: Use of nebulized adrenaline to aid expulsion of intra-nasal foreign bodies in children, *J Laryngol Otol* 110:559, 1996.
10. Engelsma RA, Lee WC: Impacted aural foreign body requiring endaural incision and canal widening for removal, *Int J Pediatr Otorhinolaryngol* 44:169, 1998.
11. Finkelstein JA: Oral Ambu-bag insufflation to remove unilateral nasal foreign bodies, *Am J Emerg Med* 14:57, 1996.
12. Giordano A, et al: Current management of esophageal foreign bodies, *Arch Otol* 107:249, 1981.
13. Gomes CC, et al: Button battery as a foreign body in the nasal cavities: special aspects, *Rhinology* 32:98, 1994.
14. Henry LN, Chamberlain JW: Removal of foreign bodies from the esophagus and nose with the use of a Foley catheter, *Surgery* 71:918, 1972.
15. *Injury facts,* National Safety Council, Chicago, 1999.
16. Kittle PE, et al: Incidental finding of an intranasal foreign body discovered on routine dental examination, *Pediatr Dent* 13:49, 1991.
17. Landry GL, Edmanson MB: Attractive method for battery removal, *JAMA* 256:3351, 1986 (letter).
18. Lemberg PS, et al: Aerodigestive tract foreign bodies in the older child and adolescent, *Ann Otol Rhinol Laryngol* 105:267, 1996.
19. Lima JA: Laryngeal foreign bodies in children: a persistent life-threatening problem, *Laryngoscope* 99:415, 1989.
20. Mears AJ, England RM: Dissolving foreign bodies in the trachea and bronchus, *Thorax* 30:461, 1975.
21. Nandapalan V, McIlwain JC: Removal of nasal foreign bodies with a Fogarty biliary balloon catheter, *J Laryngol Otol* 108:758, 1994.
22. Peltola TJ, Scarento R: Water used to visualize and remove hidden foreign bodies from the external ear canal, *J Laryngol Otol* 106:157, 1992.
23. Rachlin LS: Assault with battery, *N Engl J Med* 311:921, 1984 (letter).
24. Reichert TJ: Foreign bodies of the larynx, trachea, and bronchi. In Bluestone CD, Stool SE, editors: *Pediatric otolaryngology*, ed 2, Philadelphia, 1990, WB Saunders.
25. Singh B, et al: Complications associated with 327 foreign bodies of the pharynx, larynx, and esophagus, *Ann Otol Rhinol Laryngol* 106:301, 1997.
26. Skinner DW, Chiu P: The hazards of "button-sized" batteries as foreign bodies in the nose and ear, *J Laryngol Otol* 100:1315, 1986.
27. Tong MC, et al: Nasal foreign bodies in children, *Int J Otorhinolaryngol* 35: 207, 1996.
28. Turtz MG, Stool SE: Foreign bodies of the pharynx and esophagus. In Bluestone CD, Stool SE, editors: *Pediatric otolaryngology*, ed 2, Philadelphia, 1990, WB Saunders.
29. Witt WJ: The role of rigid endoscopy in foreign body management, *Ear Nose Throat J* 64:70, 1985.
30. Wolach B, et al: Aspirated foreign bodies in the respiratory tract of children: eleven years experience with 127 patients, *Int J Pediatr Otorhinolaryngol* 30:1, 1994.
31. Yanagisawa E, Citardi MJ: Endoscopic view of a foreign body in the nose, *Ear Nose Throat J* 74:8, 1995.

208 Fractures and Dislocations

R. Scott Strahlman

At first glance the reader may feel that this chapter is unnecessary—that fractures and dislocations are a topic more appropriately discussed by orthopedic surgeons in an orthopedic textbook. The truth, however, is that pediatricians see scores of fractures and dislocations each year. Whether a particular injury is managed conservatively by the pediatrician or referred to an orthopedic specialist is up to the individual primary care practitioner; regardless, a familiarity with proper management and triage is essential. This chapter covers the pathophysiology, clinical assessment, and classification of fractures and dislocations, as well as some of the more common conditions encountered in primary care.

ETIOLOGY AND PATHOPHYSIOLOGY

A *fracture* is defined as a break or crack in a bone. The fracture may occur directly at the site of injury or indirectly when the break occurs at a site different from the applied force. Stress fractures result from recurrent trauma to a bone and often occur in athletes (e.g., long-bone fractures in distance runners). Pathological fractures can occur without trauma or with minor trauma when a bone is weakened, as with osteogenesis imperfecta or a tumor.

A *dislocation* is defined as a malposition of bone ends that normally appose each other within a joint. Dislocations are far less common in children than are fractures, because a child's ligaments are quite strong; with an injury, it is more likely that a bone will break or a growth plate will separate than that a ligament will tear.

Certain broad generalizations can be made about the pathophysiology of childhood fractures. First, fractures in children heal more quickly than in adults. For example, a fractured clavicle in a 4-year-old may heal in as few as 3 weeks! Second, the remodeling that occurs in the healing of pediatric fractures often corrects residual bony deformities. Third, children's bones are resilient; they bend instead of break, or they break on one side only (a greenstick fracture). Fourth, a phenomenon called *overgrowth* occurs in pediatric long-bone fractures. Overgrowth is an accelerated growth rate of bony fragments during healing. Long-bone fractures, therefore, must be corrected with overriding of the broken ends to prevent length discrepancies with the uninjured side. Finally, the growth plate must be protected when treating children's fractures because a growth plate injury can result in the loss of growth potential.

INITIAL ASSESSMENT

Whenever a fracture or dislocation is suspected, an accurate history is essential. Historical details may provide clues about the mechanism of injury. The practitioner should find out how, where, and when the injury occurred and where any pain is located. Does the parent or child report any loss of function in the affected limb? Is there a history of acute or recurrent trauma?

A complete physical examination, including vital signs, should be performed; a neurovascular assessment also is important. The relevance of a thorough examination is to reveal signs of serious trauma and to identify secondary sites of injury that otherwise might be overlooked. The examiner should look carefully for any unnatural or deformed position of joints or limbs. Pain on palpation or attempted movement may be a clue. Swelling and discoloration may be seen. Crepitus sometimes can be elicited at a fracture site.

Radiography is a mainstay in the diagnosis of fractures and dislocations. Roentgenograms from two angles are indicated to delineate subtle fractures. It sometimes is helpful to include the joint above and below the injury to rule out a dislocation; often it is necessary to get a film of the unaffected side for a comparison view. Stress fractures often are not seen on roentgenograms. If a stress fracture is suspected, a radionuclide bone scan may be indicated.[1] Occasionally, when injury to the growth plate is a concern, newer imaging techniques such as computed tomography (CT) or magnetic resonance image (MRI) scanning can be useful.[5]

CLASSIFICATION

Fractures are characterized in various ways to give the orthopedic surgeon information. This information, in turn, aids in the formulation of a management plan and prognosis for the fracture. Fractures may be classified according to the clinical appearance. A closed fracture has no break in the skin. With an open, or compound, fracture, a bone fragment is exposed to the air, increasing the risk of infection and injury to adjacent nerves and blood vessels. A hidden fracture causes slight pain and swelling but no obvious bone deformity. Roentgenograms are necessary to confirm the diagnosis. An obvious fracture or dislocation is an easily seen injury, even with a cursory examination. Immediate medical attention is necessary.

Fractures also are classified by their anatomical location and according to their radiographic appearance. Breaks in the

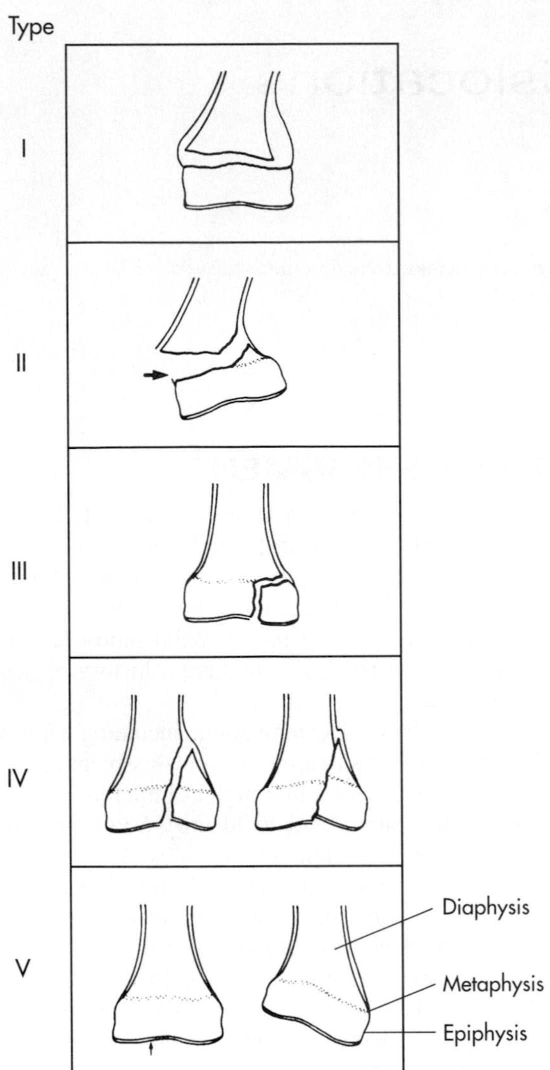

Fig. 208-1 Salter-Harris classification of growth plate injuries. (See text for explanation.)

(Modified from Canale ST, Beaty JH: *Operative pediatric orthopaedics,* St Louis, 1995, Mosby.)

bone may be described as transverse, oblique, torus, or spiral. A fracture is comminuted when the bone has three or more fragments. With an impacted fracture, the bone ends are compressed into each other.

Probably the most important classification system for fractures is the Salter-Harris system of describing injury to the growth plate (Fig. 208-1). Growth or epiphyseal plate injuries occur only in childhood. They must be treated with care to protect a bone's growth potential. Approximately 15% of all childhood fractures involve the growth plate.[6] In a Salter-Harris I fracture, the epiphysis is separated from the metaphysis without a true break in the bone. Roentgenograms often are normal, and the diagnosis is made based on the clinical picture: tenderness over the area of the growth plate. Growth usually is not disturbed. The treatment is immobilization by cast for approximately 3 weeks. The most common growth plate fracture is the type II fracture, in which a fragment of metaphyseal bone separates from the epiphysis. Closed reduction of the fracture usually is possible; with proper casting, growth is not disturbed. A Salter-Harris III fracture involves a partial growth plate injury through the epiphysis. Open repair of the fracture in the operating room is indicated to align articular surfaces and preserve joint function. A Salter-Harris IV fracture extends across the growth plate, injuring both the epiphysis and the metaphysis. The fracture must be perfectly realigned to protect growth potential. In a Salter-Harris V fracture, the growth plate is compressed. The prognosis for preserving growth is poor in this case because of a crush injury to the growth plate.

Chip fractures that do not cause any direct injury to the growth plate usually are not included in the Salter-Harris classification system.

MANAGEMENT

Fractures and dislocations should be splinted and immobilized immediately. For most, consultation with an orthopedic specialist is then necessary. Most pediatric fractures respond to closed reduction by the orthopedist. If the growth plate is affected, however, open reduction is performed. Close pediatric and orthopedic follow-up always are important. A child in a cast should be comfortable; if pain is persistent, the child needs reevaluation and possibly recasting.

COMMONLY ENCOUNTERED FRACTURES AND DISLOCATIONS

Fractured Clavicle

A broken collarbone is the most common fracture in children. It can occur at any time during childhood as a result of trauma. This fracture often occurs at birth when there is a difficult vaginal delivery. The incidence can be as high as 3.5% in babies delivered vaginally.[3] Physical findings include decreased arm motion on the affected side, crepitus, and swelling at the fracture site. A roentgenogram or ultrasound study may be needed to confirm the diagnosis.[4] If the condition is asymptomatic, no treatment is needed; indeed, the diagnosis often is made after the fact when a callus at the fracture site is noted at a well-baby visit. If the fracture causes pain or reduced arm movement, immobilization of the arm on the affected side for 2 to 3 weeks is indicated. In older children, treatment requires splinting for 3 to 4 weeks in a figure-of-8 bandage or a shoulder extension harness. Most of the fracture's healing and realignment are spontaneous.

Developmental Dysplasia of the Hip

The femoral head has a tendency to dislocate in as many as 5 of every 1000 infants.[2] This condition, formerly known as congenital hip dislocation, is termed *developmental dysplasia of the hip*. The condition is 6 to 8 times more common in girls than in boys. Because hip dysplasia is not always detected in the newborn period, children younger than 1 year of age should be examined for hip dislocation at every routine visit. Although the exact etiology is unknown, the disorder may be related to abnormal intrauterine positioning and, therefore, is more common in breech deliveries and in infants delivered by cesarean section.

Roentgenograms are of limited value during the neonatal

period in the diagnosis of developmental dysplasia of the hip. Therefore, the physical examination is of utmost importance. The Ortolani test is used to detect a dislocated hip. With the baby on his or her back, the hips and knees are flexed and the knees brought together. The examiner then places a hand on each of the baby's knees, with each middle finger over the greater trochanter and each thumb over the medial thigh. With gentle abduction of the knees, the dislocated femoral head will slip back into the acetabulum; an audible or palpable "clunk" results. Notably, a hip "click" (without a "clunk" and without any movement of the femoral head) does not indicate a hip dislocation. The Barlow test, essentially, is the reverse of the Ortolani test; the femoral head can be felt slipping out of the acetabulum when the knees are brought back together. An examiner may feel unusual laxity of the hip by pushing up and down on the thigh when the hips are flexed and adducted. Older infants should be examined for asymmetry of the thigh skin folds, a limp when cruising or walking, and leg length discrepancy. If the diagnosis is in doubt, an ultrasound study, and in older infants a roentgenogram, will confirm or rule out a dysplastic hip. Treatment requires referral to an orthopedist for a harness or casting. If the diagnosis is not made until later in infancy, surgery often is required.

Nursemaid Elbow

"Nursemaid elbow" is a common dislocation in pediatrics. A transient subluxation of the proximal radial head, it is caused by pulling or "yanking," sometimes inadvertent, of a child's arm, often by a parent or caretaker. The condition usually occurs in children between 1 and 4 years of age. The child refuses to move the arm and keeps it flexed and pronated. Roentgenograms rarely are necessary; the history and characteristic posture of the child's arm confirm the diagnosis. The treatment, easily performed by the pediatrician, requires rapid, forceful supination of the forearm while pressure is placed over the proximal radial head. Symptoms usually resolve within 30 minutes. The condition sometimes is recurrent, in which case great care must be taken when holding hands with the affected child, lest he or she suddenly tries to pull away.

Child Abuse

Unfortunately, fractures and dislocations are all too commonly suggestive of child abuse (see Chapter 57, Child Abuse and Neglect). Child abuse may be suspected when there is an unexplained injury or an inconsistency between the history and the physical findings in a childhood injury. There may be an unusually long delay between the time of injury and the time that medical attention is sought. Multiple bruises may be noted on physical examination. If abuse is suspected, a radiographic bone survey should be done in younger children. Silent fractures, or multiple fractures in varying stages of healing, may be seen.

When child abuse is suspected, the child should be hospitalized for protection as well as appropriate orthopedic care. Child protective services and social services should be involved. Pediatric care practitioners are morally and legally responsible for detecting child abuse and reporting all suspected cases.

TODDLER'S FRACTURE

Radiologists refer to a spiral fracture of the tibia as a *toddler's fracture* when the fracture occurs in a child younger than age 6 years. Torsion of the foot creates a spiral break in the tibia. The trauma to the leg often is minor or unwitnessed, so frequently there is no history of trauma. Symptoms can be minimal; the child may be brought for medical attention only because of reluctance to bear weight on the affected leg. The physical examination is significant for tenderness over the affected area of the tibia. A diagnosis can be made with anteroposterior and lateral roentgenograms of the tibia-fibula, but the fracture sometimes is not evident on a roentgenogram for a few days. The physician, therefore, should not hesitate to repeat films on a child who has an unexplained limp that is not resolving spontaneously. Treatment requires immobilization in a cast for 3 to 4 weeks.

Because the signs and symptoms of a toddler's fracture can be subtle, the examiner should have a high index of suspicion in a child who has a limp or fails to bear weight. Because the cause of the fracture often is unexplained, child abuse sometimes is a consideration. However, an isolated spiral fracture of the tibia usually does not imply child abuse in a young child.

When to Refer

All fractures and dislocations not easily managed in a primary care setting

When to Hospitalize

Whenever child abuse is suspected, or if the patient is not medically stable (i.e., multiple injuries)

REFERENCES

1. Anderson MW, Greenspan A: Stress fractures, *Radiology* 199:1, 1996.
2. Bialik V, et al: Developmental dysplasia of the hip: a new approach to incidence, *Pediatrics* 103:93, 1999.
3. Joseph PR, Rosenfeld W: Clavicular fractures in neonates, *Am J Dis Child* 144:165, 1990.
4. Katz R, et al: Fracture of the clavicle in the newborn: an ultrasound diagnosis, *J Ultrasound Med* 7:21, 1988.
5. Rogers LF, Poznanski AK: Imaging of epiphyseal injuries, *Radiology* 191:297, 1994.
6. Salter RB, Harris WR: Injuries involving the epiphyseal plate, *J Bone Joint Surg* 45a:591, 1963.

SUGGESTED READINGS

Beaty JH: Orthopedic aspects of child abuse, *Curr Opin Pediatr* 9:100, 1997.

England SP, Sundberg S: Management of common pediatric fractures, *Pediatr Clin North Am* 43:991, 1996.

Novachik TF: Developmental dysplasia of the hip, *Pediatr Clin North Am* 43:829, 1996.

Tachdjian MO: *Clinical pediatric orthopedics,* Stanford, Conn, 1997, Appleton and Lange.

209 Gastrointestinal Allergy

Aubrey J. Katz

Food allergy is a common but often unsubstantiated diagnosis in pediatric practice. Adverse reactions to foods are a feature of many gastrointestinal (GI) diseases; however, although food intolerance is caused by allergy in some patients, many other causes should be considered, such as malabsorption, lactose intolerance, toxic effects of contaminants and additives, and psychological factors.

The GI tract contains lymphoid tissue capable of mounting an immunological response to protect against the penetration of antigens across the epithelium. Lymphocytes and plasma cells are present in Peyer's patches and the lamina propria of the small and large intestine; IgA-containing plasma cells account for only 2%. The aberrations in immunological mechanisms that trigger GI allergic reactions are unknown.

Allergic disorders of the GI tract can be subdivided into two general groups: specific allergens and eosinophilic (allergic) gastroenteritis.[4] Removing specific allergens from the diet ameliorates symptoms, which are exacerbated with reintroduction of the allergen. These allergies are much more common in infants. Cow milk protein allergy and soy protein allergy are defined the best. Eosinophilic (allergic) gastroenteritis is a much rarer condition in which multiple food sensitivities are identified, also usually associated with other systemic allergies. Eosinophilic gastritis may occur at any age.

COW MILK PROTEIN ALLERGY

The incidence of cow milk allergy is estimated to vary between 0.5% and 7% of all infants under the age of 6 months.[2] Beta-lactoglobulin appears to be the most antigenic component of cow milk, but some babies also may be sensitive to casein or whey protein. The symptoms and signs are listed in Box 209-1. GI symptoms predominate in many patients. In other patients, anaphylaxis or pulmonary symptoms occur.[4] The GI manifestations depend on the site of predominant inflammation in the GI tract. Esophagitis manifests as recurrent vomiting; gastritis manifests as vomiting, irritability or pain, and occult GI bleeding; enteritis manifests as diarrhea, malabsorption, or protein-losing enteropathy[5]; and colitis manifests as rectal bleeding, with blood or mucus in the stool.

Allergic esophagitis is now well described. Patients who have allergic esophagitis have significant eosinophilic infiltration of the esophagus and improve when the specific allergen is removed. Many of these patients have concomitant gastroesophageal reflux disease. Food allergy or formula sensitivity should always be considered in patients with refractory esophagitis.

Antral gastritis is a common finding in these patients, with increased eosinophils and inflammatory cells in the antrum. Duodenal biopsy reveals patchy changes ranging from normal mucosa to "flat gut" lesions (see Chapter 212, Gluten-Sensitive Enteropathy [Celiac Sprue]). Colitis is common in these patients who have blood or mucus in the stool. Allergy is the most common cause of rectal bleeding among infants under 6 months of age. Rectal bleeding or guaiac-positive stools are probably the most common presenting symptoms in infants with formula sensitivity. A significant number of these infants present with straining or discomfort with stools.

SOY PROTEIN ALLERGY OR SENSITIVITY

Thirty percent to 50% of infants are allergic to milk protein or allergic to soy protein[1]; however, soy protein allergy may occur without a concomitant sensitivity to milk protein. The clinical features of soy protein allergy are similar to those of milk protein allergy, including esophagitis, gastritis, enteritis, and colitis.

ALLERGY VIA BREAST MILK

The term *breast milk colitis* is a misnomer. It is apparent that infants who are breast-fed may develop the same symptoms as patients who are formula-fed, manifesting either colitis or evidence of esophagitis, gastritis, or enteritis—the most common appears to be colitis.[8] These patients are commonly asymptomatic or may show significant irritability as a manifestation of their disease, with either occult blood or obvious rectal bleeding.

Treatment in this instance involves persuading the mothers to avoid dairy products, but only about 20% of infants respond to this measure alone. It then becomes extremely difficult, sometimes, to prevent many of the breast-feeding mothers from starting to eliminate many other foods from their diet, resulting in significant maternal weight loss. It is important to emphasize to mothers that, by far, most infants who show sensitivity to foods the mother is eating do not have severe disease. Therefore, breast-feeding can be continued unless the symptoms are significant. Sometimes using a hypoallergenic formula may be worth a trial to see if the baby's symptoms disappear.

BOX 209-1

COW MILK ALLERGY

Systemic Signs
Anaphylaxis
Iron-deficiency anemia (secondary to GI blood loss)
Rhinitis
Wheezing
Pulmonary hemosiderosis
Nasopharyngeal obstruction leading to cor pulmonale
Peripheral eosinophilia

Gastrointestinal Manifestations
Vomiting
Diarrhea/malabsorption/protein-losing enteropathy
Colic
Gastrointestinal bleeding
Failure to thrive

CLINICAL FEATURES OF A SPECIFIC FOOD SENSITIVITY

In most cases of formula sensitivity, the infant may have peripheral eosinophilia initially or, interestingly enough, the eosinophilia may occur once the allergen has been removed from the diet.

IgE determinations and radioallergosorbent tests (RASTs) to detect these specific milk and soy proteins usually are negative, suggesting that the immunological mechanism occurs by means of an IgG rather than an IgE mechanism. A significant number of these patients also appear to have a concomitant transient hypogammaglobulinemia; the sensitivity to either milk or soy or other specific allergens disappears once the immunoglobulin levels, particularly IgG, return to normal. The findings of an elevated IgE or positive RAST result with these foods at this age in most cases would suggest, perhaps, long-term, rather than self-limited, sensitivity.

The hallmark of GI biopsies in these patients is the increased number of eosinophils. It has been reported that more than 20 eosinophils per high-power field on rectal biopsy is indicative enough of an allergic etiology for colitis.[10] It must be remembered, however, that any inflammatory lesions of the GI tract appear to attract eosinophils.

TREATMENT

There are many formula choices today (see Chapter 17 [Two], Feeding of Infants and Children). It is important for the primary care pediatrician to be very familiar with the different protein bases.

Once the infant either is suspected of having or has been diagnosed with a specific formula sensitivity, he or she initially should be placed on a hypoallergenic formula. The choice of formula will depend on which formula the patient is on at the time of diagnosis. If the patient is on a milk-based or soy-based formula, it is appropriate to start with a casein hydrolysate formula such as Alimentum, Nutramigen, or Pregestimil. In view of their expense, however, many practitioners place their patients on a trial of a whey formula (GoodStart), because a fair number of patients appear to tolerate whey.

It appears most practical to choose a casein hydrolysate formula first (see Table C-14, Analysis of Human Milk and Fortifiers [Per Liter]), then to try to switch to the whey formula perhaps 4 to 6 months later. The sensitivity usually lasts from about 3 to 12 months, so this usually is a period of trial and error.

About 10% to 15% of infants placed on casein hydrolysate formula still have a persistent sensitivity as evidenced by continual guaiac-positive stools or overt GI bleeding. Many of these patients respond to the new amino acid formulas such as Neocate and Elecare.[6,11] These formulas are very expensive and should only be used when persistent sensitivity to all other formulas is well documented.

EOSINOPHILIC (ALLERGIC) GASTROENTERITIS

Eosinophilic (or allergic) gastroenteritis is a condition characterized by peripheral eosinophilia and infiltration of the GI tract with eosinophils.[12] Hypereosinophilic syndromes, which are characterized by infiltration of many organs with eosinophils, are not included in this category. Three types of disease manifestation are described, depending on the site of GI involvement: (1) mucosal disease manifests as protein-losing enteropathy, malabsorption, and GI blood loss; (2) submucosal disease usually manifests with pyloric obstruction; and (3) serosal disease manifests with eosinophilic ascites. The latter two types are less common in children.

Etiology

The presence of peripheral eosinophilia, systemic allergy, and elevated IgE levels, plus a therapeutic response to steroids, indicates an allergic basis for this disease in some patients.

Pathology

The small intestine reveals lesions, patchy in distribution, ranging from areas of normal mucosa to a flat villus lesion.[9] Eosinophilic infiltration may be mild or marked. Gastric abnormalities, found more commonly in the antrum, have been described as being consistent in the mucosal form of the disease. The stomach shows evidence of gastritis, with destruction and regeneration of gastric glands and surface epithelium. Eosinophilic infiltration usually is marked. Esophagitis with significant eosinophilic infiltration is a common finding in these patients. Preliminary data indicate that biopsies in these cases are identical to those for patients who have reflux esophagitis.

Clinical Features

Peripheral eosinophilia is common to all three types of disease. The mucosal form has many of the features listed in Box 209-2, whereas pyloric obstructive disease, especially serosal inflammation, commonly does not have all these features. Whether these are variants of a similar disease process or distinctly different conditions remains to be solved. Pylo-

BOX 209-2

EOSINOPHILIC (ALLERGIC) GASTROENTERITIS

Peripheral eosinophilia (common to all three types of disease)
Mucosal disease
  Protein-losing enteropathy leading to hypoalbuminemia and hypogammaglobulinemia
  Growth failure
  Iron-deficiency anemia secondary to occult gastrointestinal blood loss
  Systemic allergy
Submucosal disease
  May have features of mucosal disease
  Pyloric obstruction
Serosal disease: eosinophilic ascites

ric obstructive disease manifests with vomiting and serosal disease with ascites. Numerous eosinophils are present in the ascitic fluid. Growth failure is a prominent feature of mucosal disease in childhood; diarrhea often is not a feature. These patients usually have evidence of systemic allergy, especially asthma. Thus, this syndrome often is missed at initial presentation. Iron-deficiency anemia that occurs secondary to GI blood loss is another consistent feature, together with protein-losing enteropathy.

Diagnosis

The diagnosis of eosinophilic gastroenteritis is based on the clinical features and laboratory findings previously described. A biopsy of the small intestine reveals both normal mucosa (with or without eosinophilic infiltration) and a flat villus lesion. A gastric antral biopsy is of diagnostic value in the mucosal form of the disease and usually is positive, revealing evidence of gastritis with marked eosinophilic infiltration.[3,7]

Treatment

Dietary elimination of these allergens, which are found to be highly positive in affected patients, may alleviate most of the symptoms.[9] In many cases, corticosteroid therapy may be required intermittently. Pyloric obstructive disease may require surgery.

Prognosis

Extensive follow-up studies are lacking, but the evidence indicates that eosinophilic gastroenteritis is a lifelong condition with remissions and exacerbations, often requiring careful dietary manipulation and intermittent steroid therapy. Preliminary data also suggest that younger adolescents go through a phase in which they are much better able to tolerate foods to which they previously were sensitive.

CONCLUSION

GI food sensitivity can be divided into two types: that involving a specific allergen (a self-limited condition usually found in patients under 1 year of age) and that characterized by eosinophilic or allergic gastroenteritis with multiple food sensitivities (a more permanent condition usually associated with a positive RAST result and elevated IgE). However, the biopsy findings in both types are similar.

REFERENCES

1. Ament ME, Rubin CF: Soy protein: another cause of the flat intestinal lesion, *Gastroenterology* 62:227, 1972.
2. Gryboski JD: Gastrointestinal milk allergy in infants, *Pediatrics* 40:354, 1967.
3. Katz AJ, Goldman H, Grand RJ: Gastric mucosal biopsy in eosinophilic (allergic) gastroenteritis, *Gastroenterology* 73:705, 1977.
4. Katz AJ, et al: Milk-sensitive and eosinophilic gastroenteropathy: similar clinical features with contrasting mechanisms and clinical course, *J Allergy Clin Immunol* 74:72, 1984.
5. Kuitenen P, et al: Malabsorption syndrome with cow's milk intolerance, *Arch Dis Child* 50:351, 1975.
6. Lake AM: Beyond hydrolysates: use of l amino acid formula in resistant dietary protein-induced intestinal disease in infants, *J Pediatr* 131:658, 1997.
7. Lake AM: The polymorph in red is no lady, *J Pediatr Gastroenterol Nutr* 19:4, 1994.
8. Lake AM, Whittington PF, Hamilton SR: Dietary protein-induced colitis in breast-fed infants, *J Pediatr* 101:96, 1982.
9. Leinbach GE, Rubin CE: Eosinophilic gastroenteritis: a simple reaction to food allergens? *Gastroenterology* 59:874, 1970.
10. Machida HM, et al: Allergic colitis in infancy: clinical and pathologic aspects, *J Pediatr Gastroenterol Nutr* 19:22, 1994.
11. Vanderhoof JA, et al: Intolerance to protein hydrolysate infant formulas: an underrecognized cause of gastrointestinal symptoms in infants, *J Pediatr* 131:741, 1997.
12. Waldmann TA, et al: Allergic gastroenteropathy, *N Engl J Med* 276:761, 1967.

210 Gastrointestinal Obstruction

Anthony Stallion • David L. Dudgeon

Gastrointestinal obstruction (GIO) during infancy, childhood, and adolescence is relatively uncommon but always is a diagnostic challenge. Obstructions that occur distal to the pylorus are surgical emergencies, and the younger the patient, the more ominous the probable cause and the more urgent the required therapy.[35] Therefore, the pediatrician continually must be alert for a GIO to facilitate early diagnosis and thus prevent tragedy.

HISTORY

The symptoms and signs of a GIO (Table 210-1) vary considerably but involve the following, either singly or in combination: vomiting (often bilious), abdominal pain, abdominal distention (see Chapter 113), a change in bowel habits, fever, abdominal tenderness, or a palpable abdominal mass. The presence or absence of each of the key symptoms and signs, along with patient age, are important clues to etiology.

Vomiting

Vomiting is a ubiquitous symptom, the cause of which most often is not GIO. However, vomiting can be a sign of obstruction, particularly when marked by certain characteristics.

A small amount of nonbilious, nonprojectile vomitus by an infant is unlikely to indicate a GIO; it commonly denotes a benign, self-limited form of regurgitation or gastroesophageal reflux (chalazia). However, this picture in the newborn can be associated with an esophageal obstruction (atresia).[14] An esophageal block encountered during attempts to pass a transoral soft catheter into the stomach denotes esophageal atresia. Respiratory distress can be associated with this anomaly, caused by tracheal aspiration of saliva retained in the upper esophagus or aspiration via the commonly associated tracheoesophageal fistula proximal or distal to the atresia.[14] Esophageal atresia and the rare entity of pediatric gastric volvulus are the only two neonatal conditions in which a congenital or early acquired esophageal obstruction is likely to be encountered. Acute gastric volvulus, unlike esophageal atresia, often is accompanied by severe pain and can be associated with signs of shock. Nonbilious vomiting also can be produced by the rare anomaly of a complete or incomplete gastric antral web.[36] Frequently, this is a delayed diagnosis presenting in late infancy and associated with failure to thrive.

The more dramatic, projectile, nonbilious vomiting of early infancy is associated with the semiurgent medical condition of dehydration and electrolyte disturbances as a result of congenital hypertrophic pyloric stenosis.[38]

Bilious vomiting, usually nonprojectile, is a more ominous problem and denotes GIO below the level of the ampulla of Vater. Concern arises because of the possibility of intestinal nonrotation with a complicating volvulus, which can produce GIO with ischemia and subsequent bowel necrosis.[25,43,45] Although a premature infant who has an immature pyloric sphincter can have bilious regurgitation without obstruction, especially when associated with an ileus related to an underlying septic process, the threat of intestinal vascular compromise caused by an underlying volvulus mandates immediate radiological examination for diagnosis. Clinical signs of peritonitis preclude radiological study for diagnosis, and an immediate exploratory laparotomy is necessary. Usually an upper GI radiography series is the diagnostic study of choice in less ill neonates, although the diagnosis also may be made by ultrasound.[40] Other causes of bilious vomiting in the neonate and infant include duodenal, jejunal, and ileal atresias; duodenal stenosis secondary to an annular pancreas or Ladd bands (colonic peritoneal bands crossing the duodenum); meconium ileus; colonic atresia; congenital aganglionosis of the colon (Hirschsprung's disease); and imperforate anus.[20,22,26,48]

An infant or older toddler who has bilious vomiting can have a GIO produced by an incarcerated hernia, intussusception, or previously unrecognized malrotation with associated volvulus.[37] The etiology of bilious vomiting in an adolescent can include incarcerated hernias, postoperative adhesions, meconium ileus equivalent associated with cystic fibrosis, acute inflammation (appendicitis and pelvic inflammatory disease), and chronic inflammation (regional ileitis or ulcerative colitis).[16,21,31] At this age, malrotation is less likely. A significant number of all patients who have persistent bilious emesis will have underlying pathology requiring early diagnosis and definitive surgical treatment.

Vomitus containing minimal amounts of blood can be seen in infants who have congenital hypertrophic pyloric stenosis; it is secondary to gastric irritation as a result of repeated emesis.[38] In rare cases, hematemesis with larger amounts of blood is associated with GIO, as in the uncommon occurrence of an acute peptic ulcer resulting in obstruction in a newborn or, more frequently, in an older, chronically stressed infant or child.

Table 210-1 Pediatric Gastrointestinal Obstruction: Clinical Findings

	Findings						
Etiology	**Vomiting**	**Pain**	**Stool Pattern**	**Distention**	**Bowel Sounds**	**Tenderness**	**Masses**
Esophageal atresia	Nonbilious (saliva)	No	Normal meconium	No	Absent to normal	No	No
Gastric obstruction	Nonbilious (curdled formula)	Severe with gastric volvulus; none with antral web	Normal meconium	Epigastric	Absent to normal	Severe with volvulus	No
Hypertrophic pyloric stenosis	Nonbilious, projectile	No	Constipation (dehydration)	Epigastric	Hyperactive (epigastric)	No	Yes ("olive")
Duodenal obstruction	Bilious	Minimal	Small meconium stool	Epigastric	Absent to normal	No	No
Volvulus	Bilious	Severe	Hematochezia	Epigastric to generalized	Hyperactive	Yes (severe)	No
Jejunoileal atresia	Bilious	No	Small, hard, light-colored meconium stool	Generalized	Variable	No	No
Intussusception	Bilious	Yes (crampy)	Currant jelly stool	Generalized	Hyperactive	Yes	Yes ("sausage shaped")
Meconium ileus	Bilious	No	Obstipation	Generalized	Variable	No	Yes ("doughy beads")
Meconium plug	Bilious	No	Obstipation	Generalized	Variable	No	No
Congenital aganglionosis	Bilious	No	Obstipation, constipation, and intermittent diarrhea	Generalized	Hyperactive	No	Palpable stool
Obstipation of prematurity	Bilious	No	Obstipation	Generalized	Hyperactive	No	No
Incarcerated inguinal hernia	Bilious	Yes	Diarrhea or constipation	Generalized	Hyperactive	Yes	Inguinal or scrotal
Imperforate anus	Bilious	No	Obstipation	Generalized	Hyperactive	No	No

Abdominal Pain

Abdominal pain, presenting as inconsolable crying or irritability in an infant, usually accompanies GIO. It is likely to be "crampy" or intermittent and results in crying and flexion of the legs to the abdomen interspersed with periods of decreased levels or absence of distress. This is exemplified best by the toddler who has an intussusception.[37] However, approximately 10% of children who have intussusception will have lethargy as their only presenting symptom.[13] A complete or partial obstruction of the intestine produces acute intermittent abdominal pain, which in a matter of hours becomes constant and is caused by intestinal distention, or peritoneal inflammation, or both. Bowel wall edema ensues, increasing the degree of obstruction, causing a progression of changes that place the intussuscepted intestine at further risk for ischemic damage.

Stools

Obstipation in a newborn is a significant finding. Full-term, otherwise healthy infants spontaneously pass normal meconium within the first 24 hours of life. With premature infants, those who are small for gestational age, and infants of diabetic mothers, there may be a delay of up to 72 hours before the initial stool is passed.[24,32] The initial bowel movement also may be delayed if pregnancy is complicated by maternal drug abuse (narcotics such as morphine), drug therapy (e.g., magnesium sulfate for toxemia), or neonatal stress (hypoxemia or sepsis).[41]

Atresias of the upper GI portion of the tract do not cause obstipation routinely except for those involving the most distal terminal ileum; however, the meconium passed by these infants usually is sparse and lighter in color and may be hard and dry. The differential diagnosis of newborn obstipation includes congenital aganglionosis of the colon, meconium ileus (with underlying cystic fibrosis), meconium plug syndrome (30% of these are associated with congenital aganglionosis of the colon or cystic fibrosis), colonic atresia, imperforate anus, and in rare cases, rectal atresia.[30]

Strictures that occur secondary to episodes of neonatal necrotizing enterocolitis or intestinal surgery, as well as extrinsic compression of the GI tract caused by congenital cysts, intestinal duplication, inflammatory masses, and/or malignancies, produce obstipation or constipation in an older infant or child.[3,15,33]

Particularly in neonates and infants, diarrhea or alternating diarrhea and constipation can occur as a sign of functional GIO or as a partial or intermittent GIO. Congenital colonic aganglionosis, intussusception, or intermittent volvulus can produce this picture also. The latter two conditions frequently manifested with hematochezia or melena.

Hematochezia, or grossly bloody stools, in association with GIO symptoms, indicates intestinal vascular compromise. It occurs most commonly in patients who have an intussusception or volvulus.[37,43] The so-called currant jelly stools result from the admixture of blood and mucus and are a sign of superficial mucosal sloughing, but they also can accompany a full-thickness necrosis of the bowel wall. Occasionally, darker (mahogany to black), melena-type stools resulting from a more proximal intestinal bleeding site are noted, with the same potentially dire etiologies.

PHYSICAL EXAMINATION

When GIO is suspected, the physical examination of the abdomen includes evaluation for distention, which is likely to be prominent if the obstruction is distal to the duodenum (see Table 210-1). Gastric obstruction caused by a congenital antral web, hypertrophic pyloric stenosis, or duodenal atresia produces only mild to moderate epigastric distention; distal intestinal atresias or other forms of lower GIO produce generalized distention. The presence or absence of abdominal distention does not aid in the diagnosis of a potential underlying midgut volvulus because the obstruction may be at the level of the duodenum, with few air- and fluid-distended bowel loops present.

Abdominal auscultation should be performed before any other aspect of abdominal examination. An effort should be made to listen to all the abdominal quadrants. High-pitched, "tinkling" bowel sounds heard in "rushes" are diagnostic of a complete GIO. However, bowel sounds often are normal early in obstruction, becoming diminished to absent late in obstruction and in GIO produced by an inflammatory process.

If the abdomen is moderately to grossly distended, a mild amount of tenderness or discomfort with palpitation is to be expected because pressure applied to gas- or fluid-filled loops of bowel causes pain. However, marked tenderness clearly indicates an accompanying peritoneal inflammation. This inflammation (or peritonitis) in the face of GIO indicates ischemia of the bowel wall with possible necrosis and demands immediate surgical evaluation and treatment. In this situation, diagnostic radiological studies using contrast material are contraindicated.

The presence of multiple, "doughy," compressible, mobile, nontender abdominal masses in a newborn who has GIO is associated with meconium ileus.[27] A tender, palpable, immobile mass most likely is an area of cellulitis or abscess related to visceral perforation, secondary to necrotizing enterocolitis in infants or appendicitis or inflammatory bowel disease in children and adolescents. A nontender, extremely mobile mass that produces GIO symptoms is found with congenital intestinal duplication cysts or mesenteric cysts. Often there is a palpable mass associated with intussusception. Malignancies in the intestinal tract are rare and usually do not produce intestinal obstruction, but lymphomas may do so in older patients. When they cause GIO, intestinal or mesenteric lymphomas in patients older than age 4 years commonly are manifested as an intussusception. An immunocompromised host who has a malignancy or AIDS may develop primary or secondary inflammatory lesions that lead to obstruction.[18]

An incarcerated inguinal hernia is an important cause of GIO in children and adolescents. Detecting an inguinal hernia in an uncooperative, chubby infant is difficult and requires considerable patience and effort. Sedation with a tranquilizer, with or without an added narcotic analgesic, while keeping the patient supine in mild Trendelenburg position and applying an ice pack to the inguinal region may be helpful in the reduction of an incarcerated hernia. Medications must be used very cautiously to avoid excessive sedation, because vomiting and aspiration can occur. If possible, the hernia should be reduced gently and then repaired later when the effects of the GIO and local edema have subsided. If the hernia is reduced but left unrepaired, recurrent incarcerations are likely, with the potential consequences of strangulation and necrosis of the bowel.

Often a rectal examination can clarify the cause of GIO. In an infant who is suspected of having an incarcerated inguinal hernia, the clinician often can palpate the peritoneal side of the internal inguinal ring transanally and identify an exiting intraperitoneal structure. The rectal examination can be equally important in the diagnosis of any suspected colonic or distal GIO. Previously unsuspected perirectal or presacral pelvic masses (e.g., hydrometrocolpos, appendicial inflammatory mass, or a presacral teratoma) can be identified in this manner. Abnormal stool (as in the patient who has meconium plug syndrome) or blood (associated with intussusception or inflammatory bowel disease) can be detected during a rectal examination. In rare cases, an intraluminal rectal mass can be palpated, such as with a low-lying intussusception.

Accidental and inflicted blunt injury to the abdomen can result in early obstruction both from bowel wall edema and a hematoma.[23] A hematoma can also produce late sequelae such as an intestinal leak or stricture. The diagnosis of acute bowel wall trauma requires a high index of suspicion and often thorough and repeated radiological evaluations.

TREATMENT

Medical Management

A pediatric patient who has GIO requires gastric decompression to avoid continued bowel distention, vomiting, and possibly, aspiration. Intravenous fluid therapy is required immediately to replace the "third space" (i.e., intraluminal and intraperitoneal) fluid loss. When replacing the fluid deficit, it must be remembered that luminal GIO losses are high in electrolyte content, requiring administration of higher-than-maintenance concentrations of sodium, chloride, and potassium; therefore, solutions such as lactated Ringer's solution are needed to provide appropriate replacement. A urinalysis, with catheterization if necessary, as well as a complete blood count (CBC) and blood chemistry studies, are mandatory. Because almost all pediatric patients who have GIO require emergency or semi-emergency surgery, they must be well prepared for anesthesia and the surgical procedure. This requires correcting fluid and electrolyte, hematological, and metabolic imbalances preoperatively. Such corrective measures should begin before extensive diagnostic radiological studies are undertaken.

Diagnosis

With the widespread use of prenatal ultrasound, GIO may be diagnosed before the birth of the child. In up to 40% of cases, findings such as polyhydramnios, an inability to identify the stomach, cystic abdominal lesions, and dilated loops of bowel strongly suggest the presence of an obstructive intestinal lesion.[5] The prenatal diagnosis of GIO (i.e., atresia, volvulus) alleviates the need for emergent postnatal workup.

Table 210-2 lists roentgenographic diagnostic studies required for a patient who has GIO and their expected findings; these studies are dictated by the results of the history and physical examination. A plain roentgenogram of the abdomen should be obtained for all patients suspected of having GIO. In a newborn infant, air localized to the stomach and duodenum (double-bubble sign) is diagnostic of a duodenal obstruction[48] (Fig. 210-1). If no distal intestinal intraluminal air is seen, the GIO usually is caused by an atresia; however, if even a small amount of air is found distally, the diagnosis of a malrotation with possible volvulus must be suspected. Use of an upper GI series to determine the relationship between the duodenum, the jejunum, and the ligament of Treitz, or a barium enema to ascertain cecal position is necessary to rule out a malrotation or nonrotation of the intestine.[43] The presence of even a large number of air-filled loops on the plain roentgenographic study of the abdomen does not eliminate the need for a contrast study, because a volvulus still is possible. Visualization by barium enema of an "unused," small-caliber distal colon (microcolon) in a normal position makes the diagnosis of intestinal atresia or meconium ileus more likely than acute volvulus.

Calcifications visualized by an abdominal roentgenogram in a neonate who has suspected GIO are evidence of an intrauterine intestinal perforation (meconium peritonitis), which often is associated with intestinal atresia. The calcifications may be small, single, or multiple and scattered throughout the entire peritoneal cavity or may outline the peritoneal cavity (Fig. 210-2). Cystic fibrosis may be the underlying disease producing such a presentation.

Infants suspected of having hypertrophic pyloric stenosis usually do not require an upper GI series to confirm the diagnosis. The classic presentation of the characteristic upper abdominal peristaltic waves and a palpable, olive-size mass in the mid to right upper quadrant is diagnostic. An experienced pediatrician or surgeon will be successful in palpating the olive in approximately 80% to 90% of affected patients. An abdominal ultrasound scan can aid diagnosis in cases in which the diagnosis is suspected but there is no palpable mass.[44,47] Roentgenographic confirmation is needless, costly, and potentially hazardous because residual barium may remain in the dilated, obstructed stomach at the time of induction of anesthesia (see Chapter 255, Pyloric Stenosis).

An unusual presentation of nonbilious vomiting with no clinically palpable olive, a normal abdominal ultrasound examination, and a "normal" upper GI contrast study is possible. This sequence of events may lead to prolonged delay in diagnosing an underlying partial gastric antral web. This can be clarified by using esophageal gastric duodenoscopy to identify and potentially divide the web. If the web cannot be treated safely during endoscopy, open gastric antroplasty is effective.[36]

Often an abdominal roentgenogram of GIO in association with suspected cystic fibrosis (meconium ileus) has a peculiar hazy pattern described as a "ground-glass" or "soap bubble" appearance (Fig. 210-3). This is caused by the abnormal meconium mixed with air that is inspissated in the bowel lumen. Occasionally, this hard, dense stool, palpable as multiple abdominal masses, appears on the roentgenogram as a chain of radiolucencies, or a "string of beads" sign.[27,30] Meconium ileus, like ileal atresia, is associated with a complete GIO; however, air-fluid levels are rare in meconium ileus. Meconium ileus and meconium plug syndrome are two neonatal GIO conditions that can be diagnosed and frequently can be treated with a contrast enema.

Table 210-2 Common Causes of Pediatric Gastrointestinal Obstruction: Roentgenographic Findings

	Findings				
Etiology	**Dilated Area**	**Air or Fluid Levels**	**Calcium Deposits**	**Noncalcium Opacities**	**Further Studies That May Be Indicated**
Esophageal atresia	Esophagus and stomach	Yes (gastric)	No	No	Esophageal air instillation
Gastric obstruction	Stomach	Yes	No	No	Gastric barium instillation*
Hypertrophic pyloric stenosis	Stomach	Yes	No	No	Ultrasonography
Duodenal obstruction	Stomach, duodenum (double bubble)	Yes	No	No	None
Volvulus	Variable	Variable	No	No	Upper GI series or barium enema
Jejunoileal atresia	Stomach and small intestine	Yes	Yes (with prenatal perforation)	No	Barium enema to rule out nonrotation
Intussusception	Stomach and small intestine	Variable	No	Yes (soft tissue densities)	Ultrasonography and/or barium enema†
Meconium ileus	Stomach and small intestine	No	Yes (meconium peritonitis)	Yes (ground-glass appearance)	Water-soluble contrast enema†
Meconium plug	Stomach to colon	Yes	No	No	Barium enema‡
Congenital aganglionosis	Stomach to colon	Yes	No	No	Barium enema
Obstipation of prematurity (short left colon syndrome)	Stomach to colon	Yes	No	No	Barium enema‡
Incarcerated inguinal hernia	Stomach and small intestine	Yes	No	No	None
Imperforate anus	Stomach to colon	Yes	No	No	Complete evaluation of genitourinary tract

*Should be performed cautiously to avoid aspiration.
†Should be performed cautiously to avoid bowel perforation.
‡May be therapeutic and diagnostic.

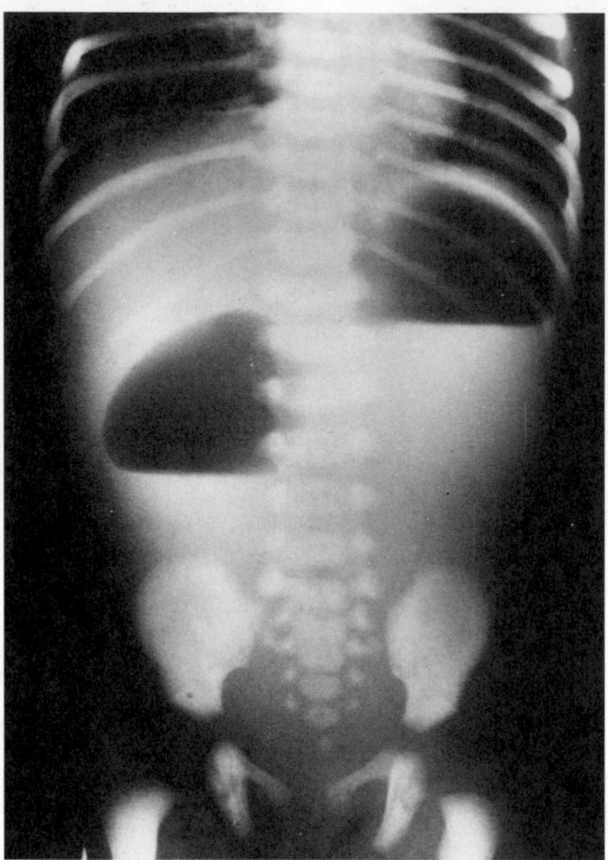

Fig. 210-1 Duodenal atresia. An upright roentgenogram of a 4-day-old girl who has had persistent vomiting since birth. The double-bubble sign is classic, showing the large gastric fluid-filled air bubble on the right and the similar duodenal bubble on the left.

(From Micro X-ray Recorder, Inc, Chicago.)

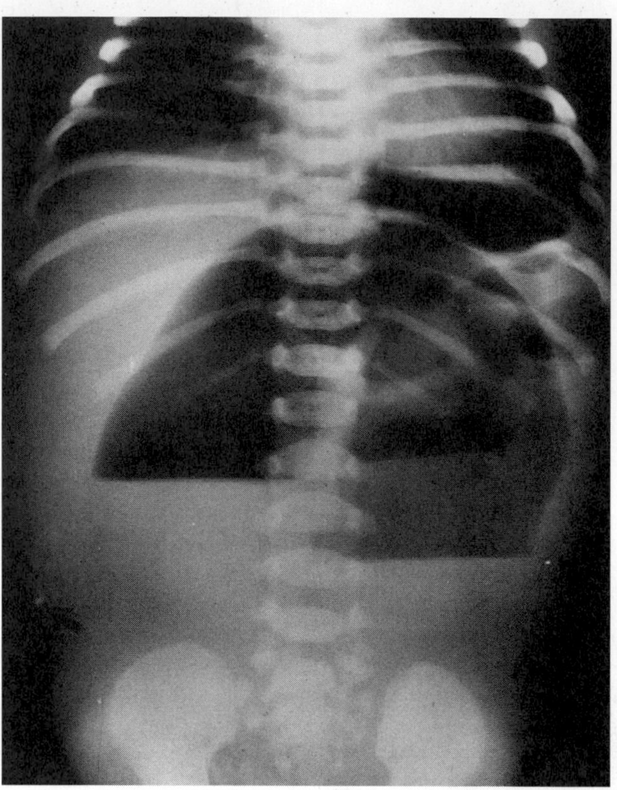

Fig. 210-2 Ileal atresia with meconium peritonitis. An upright roentgenogram of a 36-hour-old girl who has had persistent vomiting since birth. The numerous dilated loops of small bowel with fluid levels indicate atresia of the ileum; the calcification *(arrow)* is diagnostic of meconium peritonitis caused by prenatal rupture of the small bowel.

(From Micro X-ray Recorder, Inc, Chicago.)

A neonate who is suspected of having meconium ileus, who has no evidence of perforation, and who is well hydrated can be given a water-soluble contrast enema cautiously by an experienced radiologist. This identifies the inspissated meconium, localized to the distal ileum, and may free it from the bowel wall for spontaneous expulsion. This technique is somewhat limited in application and duration, with subsequent surgical therapy required in as many as 50% of patients treated in this way. Uncomplicated meconium plug syndrome, a lower GIO lesion infrequently associated with cystic fibrosis but occasionally associated with congenital aganglionosis, also is diagnosed and treated successfully with a barium enema.[6,30] Unlike meconium ileus, the abnormal meconium in meconium plug syndrome is localized to the distal colon. Contrast enemas in either syndrome are contraindicated when there is intestinal vascular compromise or perforation—that is, peritonitis, free intraperitoneal air, or intraperitoneal calcification.

Older infants and toddlers suspected of having GIO produced by intussusception can be diagnosed and often treated successfully with a barium enema.[37] The importance of an experienced radiologist for this maneuver cannot be overemphasized. The study is performed with a limited pressure (3-foot) barium column. The intussusception is slowly reduced by the hydrostatic pressure generated. Because of the potential hazard of a barium perforation, the study should never be performed without a surgical team standing by. The procedure, which can be used in about 75% of patients, successfully reduces the intussusception in 85% to 90% of those cases.[37,49] Surgical reduction is required in those that are unable to be reduced radiologically. Some have advocated the use of laparoscopy to aid in this hydrostatic reduction.[12,34] The diagnosis also can be made effectively by ultrasound or computed tomography (CT) scan.[4,11,39] Both are useful in a patient whose examination is unremarkable and whose history is equivocal. More recently, the use of air enema reduction of the intussusception has become available. This technique consists of air insufflation of the rectum and colon by using an in-line pressure-limiting valve while maintaining fluoroscopic or sonographic observation to ensure that the reduction is under control. The advantages of this technique are (1) elimination of barium, with the threat of severe chemical peritonitis if a perforation inadvertently occurs, and (2) possibly an improved mechanical advantage by using air reduction.[17,19,28] It has been stated that repeated attempts at pneumatic reduction improve the success rate

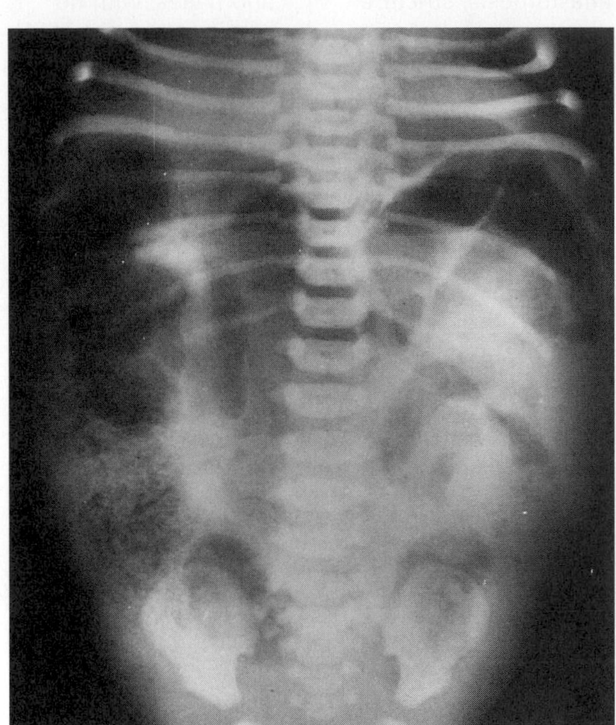

Fig. 210-3 Meconium ileus. An upright roentgenogram of a 2-day-old boy who has had abdominal distention since birth. The loops of distended bowel of varying size without fluid levels are filled with meconium shadows (radiolucent soap bubbles).

(From Micro X-ray Recorder, Inc, Chicago.)

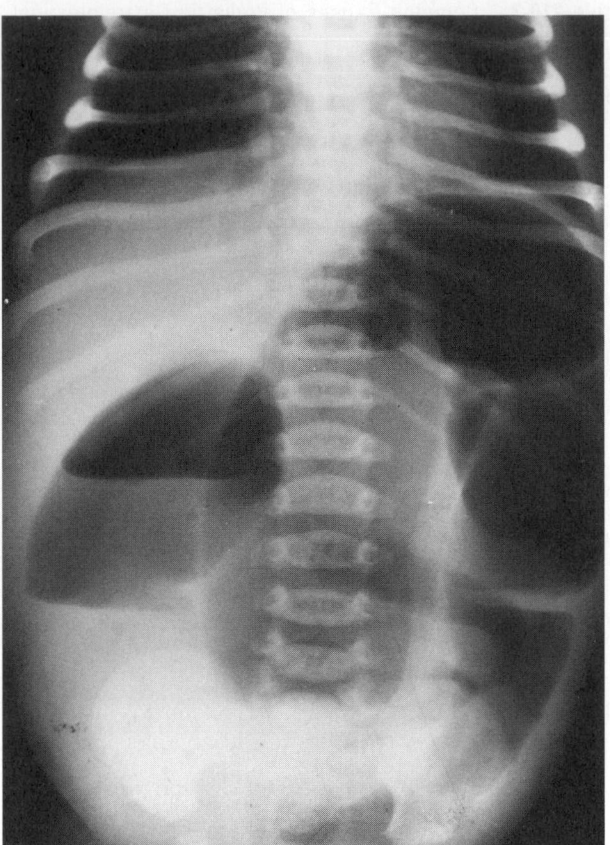

Fig. 210-4 Aganglionic megacolon (Hirschsprung's disease). An upright roentgenogram of a 2-day-old boy who has a distended abdomen and has failed to pass anything by rectum shows extreme distention of the colon with several fluid levels.

(From Micro X-ray Recorder, Inc, Chicago.)

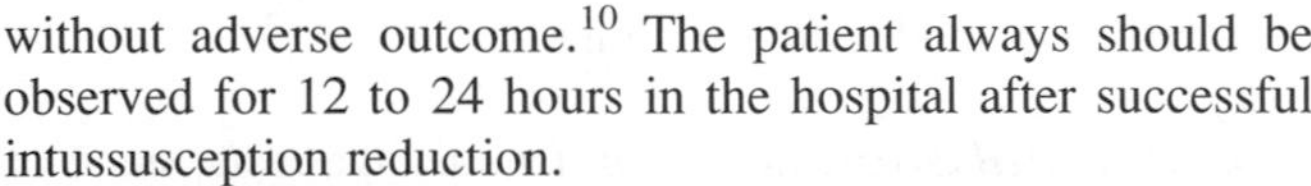

without adverse outcome.[10] The patient always should be observed for 12 to 24 hours in the hospital after successful intussusception reduction.

Congenital aganglionosis of the colon (Fig. 210-4), or Hirschsprung's disease, in infancy can be lethal if complicated by enterocolitis. Hirschsprung's disease seldom produces total GIO, which, when present, must be treated as an emergency. The initial diagnosis is made based on clinical suspicion because it cannot be verified by noninvasive diagnostic procedures. A barium enema often is helpful in diagnosing Hirschsprung's disease in older children, but either a rectal mucosal or full-thickness rectal wall biopsy specimen is required to confirm the diagnosis in infants.

Colonic dysfunction of prematurity, or small left colon syndrome (SLCS), produces a functional mechanical obstruction that mimics Hirschsprung's disease. SLCS can be related to extreme prematurity, maternal diabetes, prenatal maternal medications for eclampsia (magnesium sulfate), hyperthyroidism, or maternal narcotic use. SLCS is a diagnosis of exclusion because its barium contrast appearance resembles Hirschsprung's disease. Surgically, a temporary colostomy is indicated only for failure to respond to careful, small-volume, saline enema therapy or in the presence of signs of peritonitis or intestinal perforation.[32] The prognosis for uncomplicated cases is excellent.

Surgical Management

The type of surgical procedure performed and the patient's postoperative course and prognosis (Table 210-3) depend on the type of lesion causing the GIO.[2]

Esophageal obstruction. Esophageal atresia with associated tracheoesophageal fistula (TEF) constitutes a relative emergency requiring either primary repair or a staged procedure using an initial gastrostomy for gastric decompression and prevention of aspiration. Subsequent definitive repair, including a division of the fistula and anastomosis of the esophageal ends, is carried out after treatment of any existing underlying pneumonic process. Occasionally the gastrostomy and definitive repair are performed simultaneously, and in selected patients the esophageal repair is performed without gastrostomy. Complications of the definitive procedure include esophageal leaks, infection, and strictures. Anomalies, particularly of the cardiovascular system, are associated problems in as many as 50% of cases.[14] Patients who have

Table 210-3 Common Causes of Pediatric Gastrointestinal Obstruction: Surgery and Prognosis

Etiology	Surgical Procedure	Complications	Prognosis
Esophageal atresia	Divide tracheoesophageal fistula, perform primary esophageal anastomosis, with or without gastrostomy	Aspiration, leaking anastomosis, stricture	Depends on associated anomalies; with no cardiac anomaly, ≥95% survival
Gastric volvulus	Gastropexy, gastrostomy, with or without resection	Sepsis, leaking anastomosis	With no necrosis, very good; with necrosis, high mortality
Antral web	Gastrotomy, divide web, modified pyloroplasty	Leaking gastrotomy or pyloroplasty	Good
Hypertrophic pyloric stenosis	Pyloromyotomy	Incomplete procedure, mucosal leak	Good
Volvulus	Detorsion of mesentery, divide Ladd bands, and intestinal resection (if necrosis is present)	Leaking anastomosis, sepsis, short-gut syndrome	With no necrosis, good; with necrosis, guarded
Jejunal atresia	Resection and anastomosis	Strictures, leaking anastomosis, poor gut motility	Isolated anomaly, good; associated with cystic fibrosis, poor
Intussusception	Reduction with or without resection	Ischemic bowel, leaking anastomosis, recurrence	With no necrosis, good; with necrosis, potential short-gut syndrome
Meconium ileus	Intestinal cleansing through enterotomy, possible resection	Sepsis, malnutrition	Immediately after surgery, good; long term, poor
Obstipation of prematurity	Colostomy only for severe cases	Sepsis	Good
Congenital aganglionosis	Colostomy, delayed pull-through procedure	Sepsis, incontinence	Good
Incarcerated inguinal hernia	Reduction, possible intestinal resection	Sepsis	Good to guarded
Imperforate anus	Colostomy, delayed pull-through procedure	Sepsis, incontinence	High defects, guarded; low defects, good

uncomplicated atresia and TEF have a low morbidity and negligible mortality. However, associated cardiovascular anomalies and low birth weight lead to a mortality as high as 70%. Late complications of atresia and TEF include congenital hypertrophic pyloric stenosis and chronic gastroesophageal reflux with reactive airway symptoms.

Gastric obstructions. Gastric volvulus usually is an acute problem that requires an immediate surgical gastropexy to prevent ischemia and necrosis. If no gastric necrosis is found, recovery usually is uneventful. Gastric necrosis with secondary peritonitis results in high morbidity and mortality. A gastric antral web is difficult to diagnose and often requires repeated diagnostic studies, but it is not a critical problem. Surgical therapy consists of simple incision of the web and performance of a modified pyloroplasty, resulting in few postoperative complications.[46]

Hypertrophic pyloric stenosis requires surgical therapy following adequate correction of the associated, potentially life-threatening dehydration and hypochloremic alkalosis. The procedure is a muscle-splitting pyloromyotomy, leaving the mucosa intact. Acute complications are unusual, with the patient resuming postoperative feedings without sequelae within 8 to 24 hours, sometimes as early as in the immediate postoperative period in the recovery room. Chronic complications such as stricture related to intraoperative mucosal perforations and adhesions are rare.

Duodenal obstructions. Duodenal atresia, stenosis, and annular pancreas constitute semiurgent problems, as long as they are not accompanied by an associated volvulus, which demands immediate abdominal exploration. Surgical therapy consists of bypassing the obstructed area by means of a duodenoduodenostomy, a duodenojejunostomy, or a gastrojejunostomy.[48] Moderate feeding problems necessitating a longer hospitalization may be encountered, particularly when a gastrojejunostomy is performed. The prognosis is good; however, with associated congenital cardiac problems, mortality can be as high as 50%. Duodenal atresia is associated with Down syndrome (trisomy 21) in as many as 10% of cases. The growth and development of patients who have uncomplicated and isolated duodenal obstructions are normal.

Jejunal and ileal obstructions. Jejunal and ileal atresia also are semiurgent conditions unless they are associated with a volvulus. Surgical treatment involves excision of the atretic bowel and primary anastomosis of the dilated proximal and the narrowed distal segments.[26] When multiple atretic segments of bowel, or small-bowel atresias associated with the absence of the superior mesenteric artery are present, the overall intestinal length and therefore the absorptive surface may be reduced significantly. Total parenteral nutrition commonly is required after surgery. Overall survival and prognosis are good unless the atresia is complicated by cystic fibrosis or the remaining small intestine is too short for adequate absorption.

Nonrotation with a complicating volvulus is the most critical diagnosis in any pediatric patient suspected of having GIO. The twisted bowel mesentery may lead to ischemia and bowel necrosis within 4 to 6 hours after the onset of symptoms. Untreated volvulus has a high acute mortality rate because of associated metabolic imbalance and sepsis. Even after successful surgical resection of the involved necrotic bowel, high long-term morbidity can be expected. The entire embryonically derived midgut may have to be resected, leading to reduced intestinal absorption of nutrients and the so-called short-gut syndrome. Thus, early diagnosis, rapid correction of fluid and electrolyte imbalances, and surgical reduction of the mesenteric torsion with or without resection of potentially necrotic bowel are imperative.[43] Proximal and distal segments of involved intestine that appear ischemic but may be viable should be retained and abdominal enterostomas created in lieu of extensive initial intestinal resection and a second-look operation performed in 24 hours. Postoperative complications include marked fluid and electrolyte disturbances, local and systemic infections, and malnutrition. Long-term parenteral nutrition, dietary adjustments, and repeated surgical procedures should be expected. Survival with reasonable quality of life can be expected if the remaining viable small bowel is 30 cm or longer. Morbidity is lessened when the ileocecal valve remains intact. Long-term hospitalization and prolonged nutritional support through total parenteral nutrition usually are required.

As noted previously, meconium ileus may respond to water-soluble contrast enemas; however, evidence of an accompanying intestinal perforation or failure of a carefully managed water-soluble contrast enema necessitates surgical therapy.[27] Cystic fibrosis, which almost always is present as an underlying disease, complicates the patient's postoperative respiratory and nutritional status. Administration of cleansing solutions by means of an enterotomy usually frees the intestinal lumen of the inspissated material. Associated atretic or necrotic intestinal segments are excised, and primary anastomoses are performed. Enterostomas are created for postoperative lavage of massively impacted meconium or in instances in which the viability of the remaining bowel segments is in question. A stoma also may be needed to protect an anastomosis and so that postoperative intestinal irrigation may be performed. A T-tube may be left intraluminally to allow decompression and irrigation, and the appendix may be used as a conduit.[8,42] The surgical survival is good; however, the morbidity is high, and the ultimate prognosis is related to the severity of the other manifestations of cystic fibrosis.

Colonic and rectal obstruction. An intussusception uncomplicated by a lead point (i.e., a Meckel's diverticulum, a polyp, or a malignancy) can be successfully reduced hydrostatically or by air in up to 90% of appropriately selected patients.[37] Recurrences after air/hydrostatic reduction range from 5% to 7%. Surgical intervention is required if there is evidence of compromised bowel, such as a free perforation or peritoneal irritation, and in failures of air/hydrostatic reduction. Successful reduction requires retrograde reflux of contrast media or air into the terminal ileum. Most patients who have intussusceptions that are reduced intraoperatively do well postoperatively, with a low 2% to 5% recurrence rate. Bowel resection is required when an intraoperatively diagnosed pathological lead point is present or an ischemic complication is found. Early diagnosis and treatment of intussusception reduces morbidity and mortality.

Rectal atresia and imperforate anus require diagnosis and initial therapy (a colostomy) within 24 hours. Definitive therapy, which includes a pull-through procedure and anoplasty, is performed when the infant is 2 to 3 months of age.[20] If the lesion is not associated with any other congenital anomalies, survival is good. Other anomalies should be looked for, particularly those of the genitourinary tract (rectovaginal and rectovesicular fistulas, lower urinary tract obstructions with megacystis, hydroureter, and hydronephrosis). Future stool continence is related directly to the severity of the deformity, which is determined by the degree of normal embryological descent of the colon through the levator muscle. Definitive surgery for high lesions, in which colon descent is limited to a position above the levator muscle, results in daytime stool continence in approximately 60% of patients. The overall continence rate for high lesions is 10% to 20%. Repair of low lesions, in which the colon has descended below the levator muscle, results in an overall stool continence rate of at least 80% to 90%.

Surgical therapy for congenital aganglionosis of the colon (Hirschsprung's disease) can include creating a colostomy by using a segment of proximal ganglionic colon, followed in 6 months to 1 year by excision of the affected aganglionic segment and anastomosis of the normally innervated (ganglionic) bowel to the anus (pull-through procedure).[22] Many patients respond preoperatively to regular rectal stimulation and irrigations to evacuate the colon. This allows performance of a primary pull-through procedure during the immediate newborn period and up to several months of age and the avoidance of a colostomy. Infant morbidity and mortality rates are high when the disease is complicated by enterocolitis; however, patients who have no such complications usually do well, with good anal continence, growth, and development.

The availability of minimally invasive techniques and instruments for infants and toddlers has allowed many procedures such as pyloromyotomy and endorectal pull-throughs to be performed laparoscopically (see Chapter 32, Minimally Invasive Surgery). Obstructions from adhesions, inflammation (inflammatory bowel disease, appendicitis, and Meckel diverticulitis), and intussusception can be treated successfully with minimally invasive techniques by the skilled laparoscopist. However, procedures such as pyloromyotomy may be performed with a modified open technique in a less expensive, faster fashion that has equally acceptable cosmetic results.

Fetal surgery is the new frontier in the treatment of many congenital anomalies. Given the risk to the mother from invasive prenatal procedures, the demise of the unborn child without in utero treatment has to be almost certain for fetal surgery to warrant consideration. This also applies to the newly developed endoscopic fetal procedures ("fetendo"). None of the prenatal GIO diagnoses or their etiologies pose an immediate threat to the fetus or the mother, with overall combined mortality rates of less than 5%. The benefits to the baby do not, at the time, outweigh the risk to the mother; therefore, these lesions are not appropriate for prenatal interventional therapy.[1,7,9,29]

REFERENCES

1. Albanese CT, et al: Surgical treatment of fetal disease: the state of the art, *Ann N Y Acad Sci* 847:74, 1998.
2. Bagolan P, et al: Neonatal intestinal obstruction: reducing short-term complications by surgical refinements, *Eur J Pediatr Surg* 6:354, 1996.
3. Cirino E, et al: Intestinal obstruction and incomplete obstruction from mesenteric cyst formation, *Chir Ital* 31:543, 1979.
4. Cox TD, et al: CT of intussusception in the pediatric patient: diagnosis and pitfalls, *Pediatr Radiol* 26:26, 1996.
5. Dell'Agnola CA, et al: Prenatal diagnosis of gastrointestinal obstruction: a correlation between prenatal ultrasonic findings and postnatal operative findings, *Prenat Diagn* 13:629, 1993.
6. Ellis DG, Clatworthy WH Jr: The meconium plug syndrome revisited, *J Pediatr Surg* 1:54, 1966.
7. Farmer DL: Fetal surgery: a brief review, *Pediatr Radiol* 28:409, 1998.
8. Fitzgerald R, Conlon K: Use of the appendix stump in the treatment of meconium ileus, *J Pediatr Surg* 24:899, 1989.
9. Flake AW, et al: Fetal surgery, *Annu Rev Med* 46:67, 1995.
10. Gorenstein A, et al: Intussusception in children: reduction with repeated, delayed air enema, *Radiology* 206:721, 1998.
11. Harrington L, et al: Ultrasonographic and clinical predictors of intussusception, *J Pediatr* 132:836, 1998.
12. Hay SA, et al: Idiopathic intussusception: the role of laparoscopy, *J Pediatr Surg* 34:577, 1999.
13. Heldrich FJ: Lethargy as a presenting symptom in patients with intussusception, *Clin Pediatr* (Phila) 25:363, 1986.
14. Holder TM, Ashcraft KW: Esophageal atresia and tracheoesophageal fistula: collective review, *Ann Thorac Surg* 9:445, 1970.
15. Iyer CP, Mahour GH: Duplications of the alimentary tract in infants and children, *J Pediatr Surg* 30:1267, 1995.
16. Janik JS, Firor HV: Pediatric appendicitis: a 20-year study of 1640 children at Cook County (Illinois) Hospital, *Arch Surg* 114:717, 1979.
17. Jinzhe Z, Yenxia W, Linchi W: Rectal inflation reduction of intussusception in infants, *J Pediatr Surg* 21:30, 1986.
18. Kahn E: Gastrointestinal manifestations in pediatric AIDS, *Pediatr Pathol Lab Med* 17:171, 1997.
19. Katz M, et al: Gas enema for the reduction of intussusception: relationship between clinical signs and symptoms and outcome, *Am J Roentgenol* 160:363, 1993.
20. Kiesewetter WB, et al: Imperforate anus, *Arch Surg* 111:518, 1976.
21. Kirchmann HM, Bender SW: Intestinal obstruction in Crohn's disease in childhood, *J Pediatr Gastroenterol Nutr* 6:79, 1987.
22. Kleinhaus S, et al: Hirschsprung's disease: a survey of the members of the surgical section of the American Academy of Pediatrics, *J Pediatr Surg* 14:588, 1979.
23. Kurkchubasche AG, et al: Blunt intestinal injury in children: diagnostic and therapeutic considerations, *Arch Surg* 132:652, 1997.
24. LeQuesne GW, Reilly BJ: Functional immaturity of the large bowel in the newborn infant, *Radiol Clin North Am* 13:331, 1975.
25. Lilien LD, et al: Green vomiting in the first 72 hours in normal infants, *Am J Dis Child* 140:662, 1986.
26. Louw JH: Resection and end to end anastomosis in the management of atresia and stenosis of the small bowel, *Surgery* 62:940, 1967.
27. Mabogunjc OA, Wang CI, Mahour GH: Improved survival of neonates with meconium ileus, *Arch Surg* 117:37, 1982.
28. Menor F, et al: Effectiveness of pneumatic reduction of ileocolic intussusception in children, *Gastrointest Radiol* 17:339, 1992.
29. Milner, R, Adzick NS: Perinatal management of fetal malformations amenable to surgical correction, *Curr Opin Obstet Gynecol* 11:177, 1999.
30. Olsen MM, et al: The spectrum of meconium disease in infancy, *J Pediatr Surg* 17:479, 1982.
31. Penketh AR, et al: Cystic fibrosis in adolescents and adults, *Thorax* 42:526, 1987.
32. Philippart AI, Reed JO, Georgeson KE: Neonatal small left colon syndrome: intramural, not intraluminal obstruction, *J Pediatr Surg* 10:733, 1975.
33. Pinter AB, et al: Alimentary tract duplications in infants and children, *Eur J Pediatr Surg* 2:8, 1992.
34. Poddoubnyi IV, et al: Laparoscopy in the treatment of intussusception in children, *J Pediatr Surg* 33:1194, 1998.
35. Reyes HM, et al: Neonatal intestinal obstruction, *Chir Ital* 31:543, 1997.
36. Rodin D, Schwartz S, Dudgeon DL: Antral mucosal diaphragm, *Gastrointest Endosc* 24:33, 1977.
37. Rosenkrantz JG, et al: Intussusception in the 1970s: indications for operation, *J Pediatr Surg* 12:367, 1977.
38. Scharli A, Sieber WK, Kiesewetter WB: Hypertrophic pyloric stenosis at the Children's Hospital of Pittsburgh from 1912 to 1967: a critical review of current problems, *J Pediatr Surg* 40:108, 1969.
39. Shanbhogue RL, et al: Ultrasonography is accurate enough for the diagnosis of intussusception, *J Pediatr Surg* 29:324, 1994.
40. Shimanuki Y, et al: Clockwise whirlpool sign at color Doppler US: an objective and definite sign of midgut volvulus, *Radiology* 199:261, 1996.
41. Sokal MM, et al: Neonatal hypermagnesemia and the meconium plug syndrome, *N Engl J Med* 286:733, 1975.
42. Steiner Z, et al: T-tubes in the management of meconium ileus, *Pediatr Surg Int* 12:140, 1997.
43. Steward DR, Colodny AL, Daggett WC: Malrotation of the bowel in infants and children: a 15-year review, *Surgery* 79:716, 1976.
44. Studen RJ, LeQuesne GW, Little KE: The improved ultrasound diagnosis of hypertrophic pyloric stenosis, *Pediatr Radiol* 16:200, 1986.
45. Torres AM, Ziegler MM: Malrotation of the intestine, *World J Surg* 17:326, 1993.
46. Tunell WP, Smith EI: Antral web in infancy, *J Pediatr Surg* 15:152, 1980.
47. Weiskittel DA, Leary DL, Blane CE: Ultrasound diagnosis of evolving pyloric stenosis, *Gastrointest Radiol* 14:22, 1989.
48. Wesley JR, Majour GH: Congenital intrinsic duodenal obstruction: a 25-year review, *Surgery* 82:716, 1977.
49. West KW, et al: Intussusception: current management in infants and children, *Surgery* 102:704, 1987.

211 Giardiasis

Craig M. Wilson

ETIOLOGY

A *Giardia*-like organism was described and associated with gastrointestinal symptoms by Dutch microscopist Anton van Leeuwenhoek in 1681,[7] but only in the past 30 years has the true pathogenicity of this flagellate protozoan been recognized. It now is clear that *Giardia lamblia* is one of the most common intestinal parasites in the United States and the world,[1,20] and it has attained a certain notoriety as a result of diarrhea epidemics at fashionable ski resorts, in child care centers, in major metropolitan areas, among campers, and among international tourists. The prevalence of giardiasis in children is becoming more widely appreciated, particularly in the child care setting.[28]

G. lamblia is an extracellular parasite that has no intermediate development outside of the intestinal lumen. This unicellular protozoan exists in two forms: a motile, flagellated trophozoite that causes disease and a dormant cyst that transmits infection. The trophozoite is 12 to 15 μm long and has four pairs of flagella and two prominent nuclei (Fig. 211-1). It lacks many eukaryotic subcellular structures, including (1) mitochondria, (2) Golgi apparatus, and (3) a well-developed endoplasmic reticulum; it also has a ribosomal RNA structure suggestive of a very primitive organism.[10,27] A large sucking disk, which the parasite uses to attach to the intestinal mucosa, occupies most of the flat ventral surface. Attachment is regulated by contractile proteins, including actin and myosin, which alter the structure of the disk. It is not clear how the organism evades degradation in the intestinal lumen. The motile trophozoites divide by longitudinal binary fission in the upper small bowel and then encyst as they pass into the colon. Trophozoites usually are seen only in the stool when diarrhea is present. Cysts, the more common form seen in stool specimens, are 9 to 12 μm long. Recently formed cysts have two nuclei; mature cysts have four.

EPIDEMIOLOGY

Studies in human volunteers have demonstrated the high infectivity of *G. lamblia* cysts. Although one cyst rarely was infectious, infection occurred in virtually all volunteers receiving 100 to 1 million cysts orally and in 36% of those exposed to 10 to 25 cysts.[21]

G. lamblia is one of the most commonly identified pathogens in waterborne diarrheal disease in the United States, where the organism is holoendemic.[3,20] A number of large common-source outbreaks have been traced to contaminated drinking water. Epidemiological studies have attributed these epidemics to cross-contamination of municipal drinking water supplies that have sewage, defective or deficient filtration facilities, and reliance on chlorination as the principal method of water disinfection.[10,25] In mountainous regions, where the prevalence of disease appears to be higher,[4] use of surface water for drinking is the principal problem. It has been suggested that indigenous animal hosts, especially beavers, are responsible for contaminating mountain streams and reservoirs.[9] True zoonotic infection has been demonstrated.[11] As suggested by the occurrence of epidemic giardiasis despite chlorination of municipal water supplies, routine chlorination may not be adequate for killing *G. lamblia*.[21] The level of chlorine necessary to kill cysts depends on many other factors, including pH, contact time, turbidity, and temperature.[16] Thus, an adequate water purification system for clearing *G. lamblia* should include filtration, sedimentation, and flocculation systems. Halogen-based, small-quantity disinfection methods also are affected by water clarity and temperature.[17]

Because cysts may be shed in abundance in the stool, it is not surprising that *G. lamblia* may be transmitted by the fecal-oral route. This undoubtedly is the main route of spread in families, in institutions, in child care centers, and among homosexuals. With intensive exposure to stool, as in child care centers caring for infants in diapers, giardiasis quickly may become hyperendemic.[2,23,28] Although food-borne giardiasis is a theoretical hazard, only four such outbreaks have been reported; in all four, the implicated food probably was contaminated during preparation.

PATHOGENESIS

Although many mechanisms have been postulated for the diarrhea and malabsorption caused by *G. lamblia,* how this parasite causes disease remains a mystery. It seems likely that the process is multifactorial, with the severity of symptoms depending on the degree of focal small bowel injury. Infection is associated with injury to the mucosal brush border, with disruption of disaccharidase activity and transport mechanisms.[14] There is a basal membrane and intraepithelial inflammatory cell infiltrate[29] and evidence of an increased enterocyte turnover in the murine model.[12] In either case, less efficient villus function would be expected. In the extreme, the microvilli atrophy, results in the severe malabsorptive diarrhea that is a major complication of giardiasis.[14] Recent studies suggest that parasite-induced prostaglandin E_2 production plays a role in the pathophysiology of

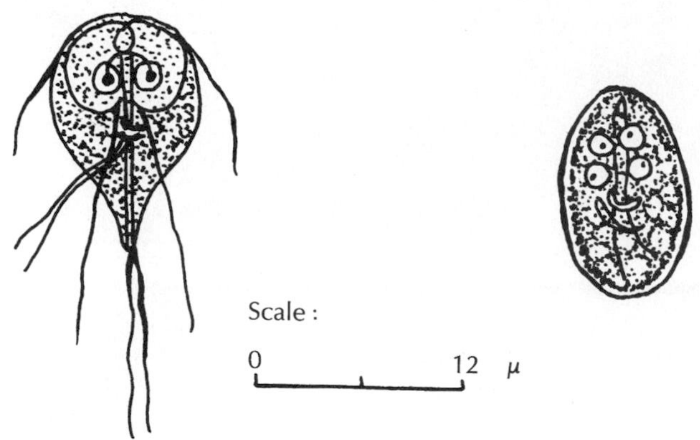

Fig. 211-1 *Giardia* organisms. The trophozoite *(left)* is 12 to 15 μm long and has four pairs of flagella and two prominent nuclei. This form is not commonly seen in stools. Cysts *(right)* are 9 to 12 μm long and may have two to four nuclei.

this infection.[26] Also, there is evidence that some *Giardia* strains produce more severe symptoms in humans than in other species,[19] and differences in phenotype and genotype have been correlated with virulence in experimental models of infection.

Host defense mechanisms appear to be relatively inefficient, given the small number of organisms required to initiate infection and the frequency of relapse and reinfection. However, intraluminal secretory antibody response, nonspecific inflammatory responses at the level of the mucosa, and antibody-dependent cell-mediated cytotoxicity (ADCC) appear to be important in limiting the severity of disease.[26] The role of antibody and ADCC in containing giardiasis is supported by the increased incidence and severity of disease in patients who have immunoglobulin deficiencies. Underlying IgA deficiency and both X-linked and common variable hypogammaglobulinemia have been associated with more severe or prolonged infection.

G. lamblia should be considered in the workup of diarrhea or malabsorption in patients who have human immunodeficiency (HIV) infection. The role and extent of *G. lamblia* infections in children who have HIV infection have not been established. Of course, diarrhea in patients who have acquired immunodeficiency syndrome (AIDS) often is multifactorial, and treatment of documented giardiasis may not result in clinical improvement if other pathogens still are present (see Chapter 219, Human Immunodeficiency Virus Infection and Acquired Immunodeficiency Syndrome).

CLINICAL MANIFESTATIONS

Based on experimental studies and point-source outbreak observational data, the incubation period of giardiasis is 7 to 14 days.[21] Most patients infected by *G. lamblia* probably remain asymptomatic, although they do shed cysts in their feces and are infectious.[13,21] Children are more likely than adults to have symptomatic disease.

The principal symptoms of giardiasis are gastrointestinal. Diarrhea, abdominal cramps, and nausea are reported most often.[24] Vomiting, malodorous stools, flatulence, bloating, anorexia, and even constipation are noted less frequently. Because the colon and rectum are not involved, tenesmus should suggest another diagnosis. Blood almost never is found in the stool, and the presence of mucus is unusual. Gastrointestinal symptoms generally last 7 to 10 days, although a more protracted course is common. Because of the disaccharidase deficiency that accompanies severe infections, some patients complain of milk intolerance, which may last for weeks.

Constitutional symptoms are not prominent in giardiasis, but up to 25% of patients experience fatigue, headache, or a low-grade fever.[24] Extraintestinal syndromes, such as urticaria, erythema multiforme, and arthralgia, have occurred, but very rarely, in association with giardiasis.

Some patients, particularly children, develop chronic diarrhea, frank malabsorption, weight loss, malnutrition, and growth retardation. Thus giardiasis must be considered in the differential diagnosis of failure to thrive. Occasionally, giardiasis may be misdiagnosed as sprue, food allergy, or psychogenic abdominal pain, and its protean clinical manifestations may mimic a wide variety of gastrointestinal disturbances. Malabsorption leading to an iron deficiency anemia also has been reported with *G. lamblia*.[6]

The physical examination generally is unremarkable unless secondary malnutrition has developed.

LABORATORY EVALUATION

The diagnosis often escapes a physician who performs a casual laboratory evaluation.[15] Unfortunately, eosinophilia, one of the hallmarks of parasitic helminth infections, generally is absent in giardiasis, supporting the observation that *G. lamblia* rarely is invasive beyond the intestinal mucosa.

Careful examination of the stool is of paramount importance in diagnosing giardiasis. Initially, fresh stool suspended in saline or 1% potassium iodide should be examined microscopically. Trophozoites are detected more readily in fresh diarrheal specimens. The yield of cyst detection can be increased if the stool is concentrated by either the formylether or zinc sulfate methods. Trichrome-stained, polyvinyl alcohol-fixed specimens also are useful for detecting trophozoites or cysts. At least three stool specimens obtained on separate days should be examined, particularly if diarrhea is not present, because cysts can be passed intermittently.

Traditional diagnostic techniques are relatively labor intensive, cumbersome, and slow. Recently the focus has been directed toward developing techniques for detecting *Giardia* antigens directly in stool specimens by a variety of technologies.[18] Overall, these tests compare well with standard microscopic procedures and in some cases are more sensitive. In some clinical centers, this methodology has replaced microscopic stool examination. The disadvantage is that the tests are singularly specific for *Giardia* and do not rule out other parasitic infestations that often are in the same diagnostic differential as giardiasis.

A few patients require additional measures to have the pathogen detected. Examining the duodenal contents provides the optimum yield in these patients. This can be done either by direct duodenal aspiration or by using the Entero-Test.[22] In rare patients who have chronic symptoms in whom the diagnosis must be excluded, the small bowel should be biopsied. Several sections of the biopsy specimen stained with Giemsa may have to be examined to find the parasite;

Giardia organisms are detected more easily in Giemsa-stained mucosal impression smears.

Serological tests are valuable in epidemiological studies but are of little use diagnostically. Upper gastrointestinal roentgenograms may reveal mild dilation of the small bowel, edema of the mucosa, segmentation of barium, and either increased or decreased transit times; however, these changes are nonspecific. The sedimentation rate is normal, and as noted above, there is no eosinophilia. There may be biochemical evidence of malabsorption, including disaccharidase deficiency, abnormal absorption of D-xylose and fat, and a deficiency of folic acid.

THERAPY

Most authorities agree that giardiasis should be treated when recognized, even if the patient is asymptomatic, because carriers of the parasite are potential transmitters of disease and may have subclinical malabsorption.[8] However, physicians may elect not to treat some patients, particularly if reexposure to *G. lamblia* seems unavoidable.

Furazolidone (Furoxone) has the distinct advantages of having a pleasant taste and being available in a pediatric suspension. Side effects, which have been minimal in children, include mild GI distress, hypersensitivity reactions, hemolysis in individuals who have glucose-6-phosphate dehydrogenase (G6PD) deficiency, brown discoloration of the urine, and disulfiram-like reactions (optic neuritis, peripheral neuritis, and/or polyneuritis). The efficacy in children has been as high as 92%, which is comparable if not superior to cure rates seen with alternative agents.[5] The dosage is 6 mg/kg/day (maximum dosage, 400 mg/day) given orally in four divided doses for 7 to 10 days.

Metronidazole (Flagyl) has been used widely to treat giardiasis in adults because it is well tolerated (except for the mild metallic aftertaste), has a very low incidence of serious side effects, and has an acceptable cure rate. However, the U.S. Food and Drug Administration (FDA) has not approved metronidazole for treating giardiasis in children. This agent has received considerable adverse publicity because studies have shown that it is carcinogenic in laboratory animals and mutagenic in bacteria. The relevance of these studies to humans has been questioned; no data suggest carcinogenicity in humans. The dosage of metronidazole is 250 mg three times a day for 5 days for children weighing more than 27 kg and 15 mg/kg/day for smaller children. The drug is not available as a suspension. Tinidazole, a nitroimidazole similar to metronidazole, is used extensively in a single-dose regimen outside the United States to treat giardiasis.

Relapse is possible after using any of these regimens. If this occurs, retreatment with the same agent or an alternative drug often is successful. There is no well-documented evidence for actual drug resistance in *Giardia*. Quinacrine, a previously recommended therapy for giardiasis, no longer is manufactured. Albendazole (400 mg/day for 5 days) has been reported to be as effective as metronidazole in a study of children 5 to 10 years of age.[13] This drug is not marketed in the United States but may be an alternative therapy when it becomes more widely available. Paromomycin, a nonabsorbable aminoglycoside, has been used to treat giardiasis in pregnancy, but data regarding its efficacy are limited.

PREVENTION

Because giardiasis is so prevalent, total prevention of transmission is virtually impossible. When the disease is known to be present in a household, institution, or child care center, good hand washing is essential to limit spread by the fecal-oral route. Personal hygiene is especially important when infants in diapers are affected. In child care centers that have infants in diapers, eradication is difficult unless all *Giardia* excretors are treated, whether or not symptomatic. Because parasitological examinations of the stool are expensive and diagnosis often is delayed because cysts are not always found in a single specimen, all infants in the center may need to be treated to terminate the outbreak.

As already noted, prevention of waterborne giardiasis is contingent on adequate water purification, including filtration, sedimentation, and flocculation in addition to chlorination. Tourists in endemic areas should avoid drinking tap water. Campers should not rely on chlorination tablets, which are ineffective against *Giardia* cysts. Iodination, boiling for at least 2 minutes, even at high altitudes, or filtration (pore size under 3 μm) are satisfactory means for preparing drinking water free of *G. lamblia*.

REFERENCES

1. Beaver PC, Jung RF, Cupp EW: *Clinical parasitology*, ed 9, Philadelphia, 1984, Lea & Febiger.
2. Black RE, et al: Giardiasis in day care centers: evidence of person-to-person transmission, *Pediatrics* 60:468, 1977.
3. Centers for Disease Control: Intestinal surveillance: United States, 1976, *MMWR* 27:167, 1978.
4. Centers for Disease Control: Waterborne giardiasis: California, Colorado, Oregon, and Pennsylvania, *MMWR* 29:121, 1980.
5. Craft JC, Murphy T, Nelson JD: Furazolidone and quinacrine: a comparative study of therapy for giardiasis in children, *Am J Dis Child* 135: 164, 1981.
6. DeVizia B, et al: Iron malabsorption in giardiasis, *J Pediatr* 107:75, 1985.
7. Dobell C: The discovery of the intestinal protozoa of man, *Proc R Soc Med Section Hist Med* 13:1, 1920.
8. Drugs for parasitic infections, *Med Lett Drugs Ther* 35:111, 1993.
9. Dykes AC, et al: Municipal waterborne giardiasis: an epidemiologic investigation: beavers implicated as a possible reservoir, *Ann Intern Med* 87:426, 1980.
10. Erlandsen SL, Meyer EA, editors: *Giardia and giardiasis: biology, pathogenesis, and epidemiology,* New York, 1984, Plenum.
11. Fathering MJG: Giardiasis, *Gastroenterol Clin North Am* 25:493, 1996.
12. Gillon J, Thamery AL, Ferguson A: Features of small intestine pathology (epithelial cell kinetics, intraepithelial lymphocytes, disaccharidases) in primary *Giardia muris* infection, *Gut* 23:498, 1982.
13. Hall A, Nahar Q: Albendazole as a treatment for infections with Giardia duodenalis in children in Bangladesh, *Trans R Soc Trop Med Hyg* 87:84, 1993.
14. Hartong WA, Gourley WK, Arvanitakas C: Giardiasis: clinical spectrum and functional structural abnormalities of the small intestinal mucosa, *Gastroenterology* 77:61, 1979.
15. Isaac-Renton JL: Laboratory diagnosis of giardiasis, *Clin Lab Med* 11: 811, 1991.
16. Jarroll EL, Bingham AK, Meyer EA: Effect of chlorine on *Giardia lamblia* cyst viability, *Appl Environ Microbiol* 41:483, 1981.
17. Jarroll EL, Bingham AK, Meyer EA: Cyst destruction: effectiveness of six small-quantity water disinfection methods, *Am J Trop Med Hyg* 29:8, 1980.
18. Marshall M, et al: Waterborne protozoan pathogens, *Clin Microbiol Rev* 10:67, 1997.

19. Nash TE, et al: Experimental infections with Giardia lamblia, *J Infect Dis* 156:974, 1987.
20. Nelson JD: Etiology and epidemiology of diarrheal disease in the United States, *Am J Med* 78:76, 1985.
21. Rendtorff RC: The experimental transmission of human intestinal protozoan parasites. II. Giardia lamblia cysts given in capsules, *Am J Trop Med Hyg* 59:209, 1954.
22. Rosenthal P, Liebman WM: Comparative study of stool examinations, duodenal aspiration, and pediatric Entero-Test for giardiasis in children, *J Pediatr* 96:278, 1980.
23. Sealy DP, Schuman SH: Endemic giardiasis and day care, *Pediatrics* 72:154, 1983.
24. Shaw PK, et al: A community outbreak of giardiasis with evidence of transmission by a municipal water supply, *Ann Intern Med* 87:426, 1977.
25. Smith PD: Giardia lamblia. In Walzer PD, Genta RM, editors: *Parasitic infections in the compromised host,* New York, 1989, Marcel Dekker.
26. Smith PD: Pathophysiology and immunology of giardiasis, *Annu Rev Med* 36:295, 1985.
27. Sogin ML, et al: Phylogenetic meaning of the kingdom concept: an unusual ribosomal RNA from *G. lamblia, Science* 243:75, 1989.
28. Thompson SC: Giardia lamblia in children and the child care setting: A review of the literature, *J Paediatr Child Health* 30:202, 1994.
29. Wright SG, Tomkins AM: Quantitative histology in giardiasis, *J Clin Pathol* 31:712, 1978.

212 Gluten-Sensitive Enteropathy (Celiac Sprue)

Aubrey J. Katz

Gluten-sensitive enteropathy (GSE), also called celiac sprue, is a condition characterized by clinical features of malabsorption and pathological changes in the jejunal mucosa, both of which improve when gluten is removed from the diet and recur when it is reintroduced. After cystic fibrosis, celiac sprue is the second most common cause of malabsorption in childhood.

HISTORY

The classic clinical description of celiac disease was given by Samuel Gee in 1888. In 1950, Dicke noted the association between the ingestion of gluten and celiac disease. During World War II, when grain products in Holland were in short supply, the incidence of gluten-sensitive enteropathy was reduced markedly, and children who had the disease improved. After the war, when cereal grain became plentiful, the incidence of GSE rapidly returned to the prewar level. In 1954, Paulley, studying surgical biopsy material, provided the first accurate description of the intestinal lesion in patients who have gluten-sensitive enteropathy. It was not until 1968 that Rubin and colleagues discovered that adult nontropical sprue and celiac disease in childhood were the same disease.

PATHOLOGY

Gluten-sensitive enteropathy primarily affects the mucosa of the small intestine.[6] The submucosa, muscularis, and serosa are not involved. The mucosal lesion of the small intestine in GSE varies in both severity and extent, the lesion in the jejunum being generally more severe than that in the ileum. This variability may explain the differences in the degree of malabsorption seen in some patients. Those in whom more intestinal area is involved presumably have a greater degree of malabsorption. This difference in the distribution of the lesion suggests that the proximal intestine has greater exposure to undigested gluten than the distal intestine because there is no greater sensitivity to gluten in the proximal than in the distal mucosa. Among patients who have active GSE, surface epithelial cell damage occurs, and the migration of cells from the crypt to the villus region is increased. Compensatory crypt hypertrophy occurs, with a marked increase in mitotic activity, and gradual villus flattening develops (Figs. 212-1 and 212-2). The surface epithelial cells demonstrate a loss of the basal nuclei polarity and become more cuboidal. Numerous intraepithelial lymphocytes are noted, and the lamina propria shows a marked increase in plasma cells (T cells) and lymphocytes. It should be emphasized at this stage that this flat villus lesion is not pathognomonic of GSE, because it may be seen in many other diseases. With the introduction of the flexible endoscope for focused biopsying rather than blind suction biopsying, investigators have found nonspecific antral gastritis in 10% of patients who have celiac disease, suggesting there may be some gastric sensitivity.

PATHOGENESIS

GSE is a genetic disease; the exact mode of inheritance, however, remains unknown. In 1972, Falchuk and colleagues observed the association between histocompatibility antigen HLA-B8 and GSE: 80% of patients had HLA-B8, whereas only 22% of the unaffected population carried this antigen. A similar incidence of HLA-B8 is observed in patients with dermatitis herpetiformis, a skin disorder characterized by vesicular eruptions and a gluten-sensitive intestinal lesion.[2]

The exact mechanism by which gluten damages the mucosa of the small intestine remains unknown. Two contrasting mechanisms have been proposed: (1) GSE results from the lack of a specific enzyme, perhaps a dipeptidase, which results in accumulation of toxic gluten peptides (evidence for this hypothesis is lacking); and (2) gluten toxicity is mediated through immunology aberrations associated with the genetically determined cell-surface markers discussed above.[8,9] Various immunological abnormalities have been described in GSE: (1) elevated levels of serum IgA and diminished levels of serum IgM are abnormalities that are reversed by a gluten-free diet; (2) intestinal mucosal immunoglobulin synthesis, notably IgA and IgM, is increased markedly in patients who have active GSE and returns to normal when remission occurs, and 50% of the elevated IgA is associated with specific antigluten antibody; (3) patients who have active GSE respond to treatment with corticosteroids; and (4) in vitro peripheral lymphocyte transformation in response to gluten has been described in GSE patients.

INCIDENCE AND AGE OF ONSET

The precise incidence of gluten-sensitive enteropathy is unknown because a large number of patients have asymptomatic disease. The disorder is more common in certain European countries than in the United States. This may relate to a larger intake of gluten by people in Europe or to the way in which wheat is refined in the United States. The incidence of GSE in the United States is estimated to be 1 case per 3000 people. In certain parts of Ireland, it is as high as 1 in 300.

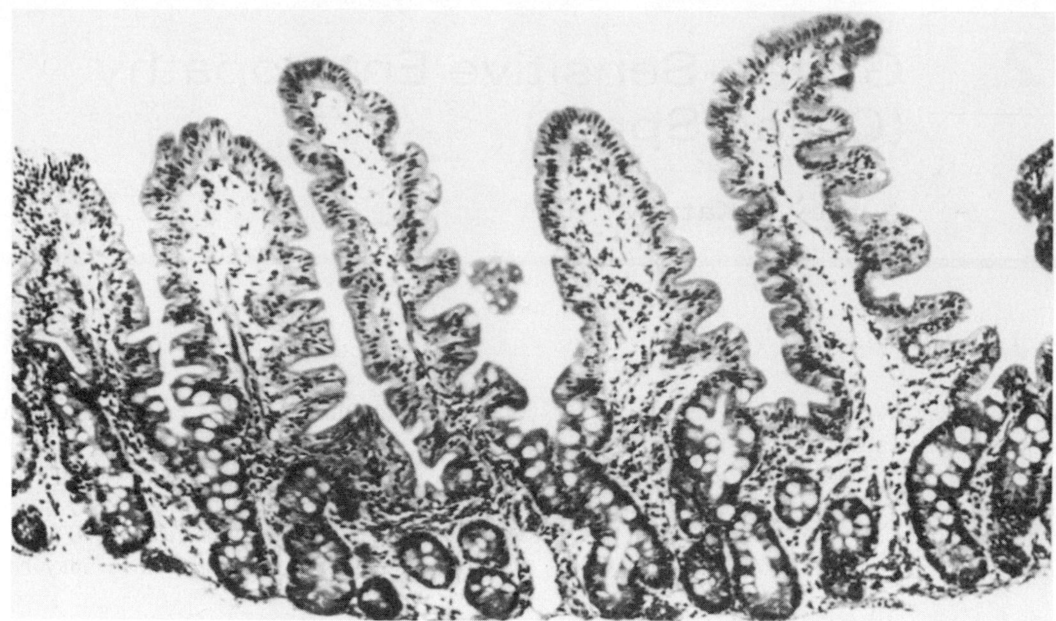

Fig. 212-1 Normal jejunal mucosa. Villi are tall, crypts are relatively short, and the crypt: villus ratio is approximately 1:4. Epithelial cells are columnar, and their nuclei are basally oriented. Some lymphocytes and plasma cells are found in the lamina propria (×160).

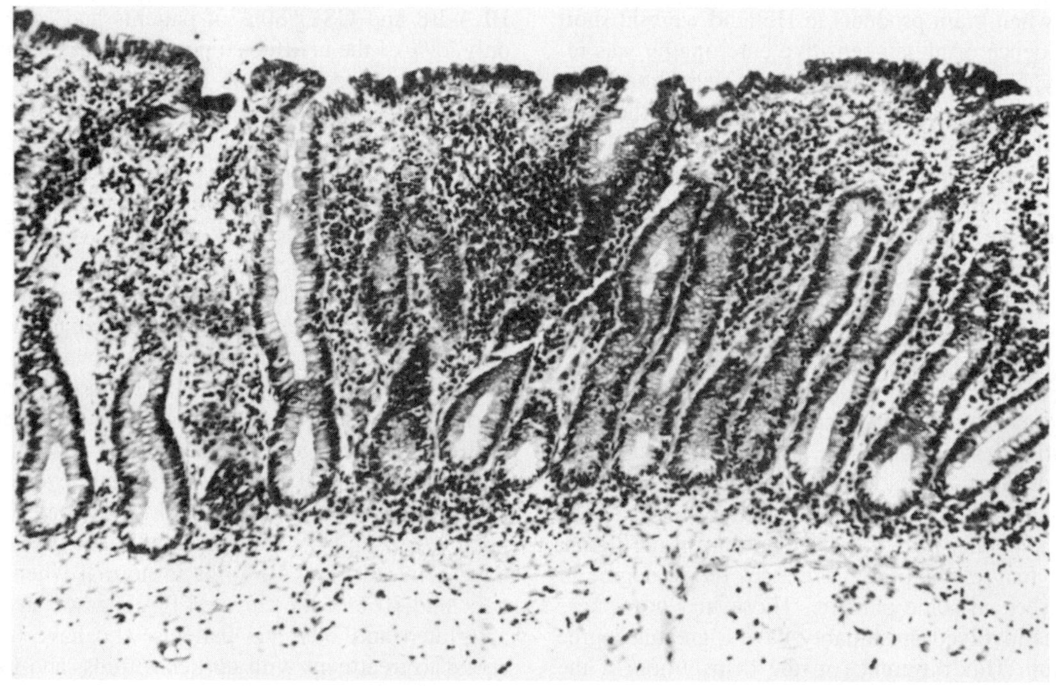

Fig. 212-2 Jejunal mucosa in gluten-sensitive enteropathy (celiac sprue). The mucosa is flat, villi are absent, and crypts are deep. Epithelial cells are cuboidal, and nuclei are not basally oriented. There are increased numbers of mitoses in the crypts. Inflammatory cells, especially plasma cells and lymphocytes, are markedly increased (×160).

Recent studies have estimated an incidence of 1 in 284 in Italy.

For pediatric patients, the average age at the time of diagnosis appears to be between 9 and 18 months, occurring earlier in infants who are fed cereal at an earlier age. The clinical incidence declines markedly after age 2 years, and it is less common to have a newly clinically diagnosed case of GSE in a teenager. There is a resurgence of clinically manifest disease in adult life, when GSE may be precipitated by infectious diarrhea, other illnesses, or surgical procedures such as gastrectomy.

It has become evident in the last few years that the clini-

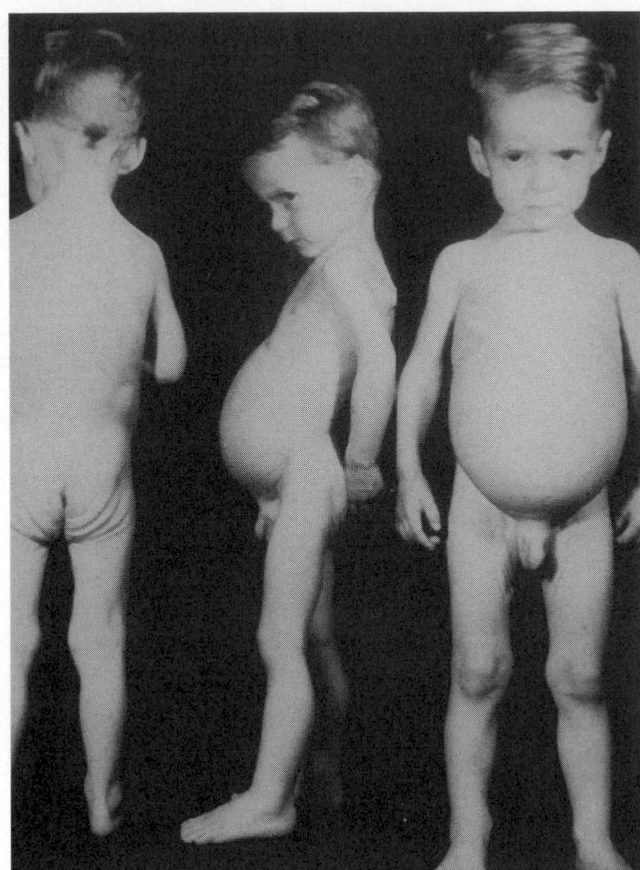

Fig. 212-3 Classic "celiac" profile. Note potbelly, thin buttocks, and proximal muscle wasting.

cal diagnosis of celiac disease or GSE is much more common. This increase in incidence is due to the advent of routine upper endoscopy in evaluation of patients with abdominal pain and the finding of a flat villus lesion on routine small bowel biopsy. In addition as is mentioned below the routine screening of family members has yielded many more patients.

CLINICAL FEATURES

A patient who has an advanced case of GSE typically is an irritable, anorectic child who has chronic diarrhea, failure to thrive, a potbelly, and muscle wasting, especially of the buttocks and proximal limbs.[5] These children usually are easy to diagnose (Fig. 212-3). It is extremely important to realize, however, that many patients manifest the disorder atypically (e.g., steatorrhea may be absent). Atypical features of patients who have GSE are listed in Box 212-1. These presentations usually are related to selective malabsorption of various nutrients. Thus it is not unusual for some patients to have rickets, osteoporosis with bone pain, or pathological fractures. Also seen are bleeding disorders secondary to vitamin K deficiency, iron-deficiency anemia, and megaloblastic anemia usually secondary to folate deficiency; deficiency of vitamin B_{12} is rare and usually indicates severe disease that extends to the terminal ileum. Constipation, rectal prolapse, clubbing of the fingernails, edema, and vomiting also have been described as presenting features. Gluten-sensitive enteropathy should always be considered in patients with specific nutritional defects who fail to respond to appropriate replacement therapy.

BOX 212-1

ATYPICAL PRESENTATIONS OF GLUTEN-SENSITIVE ENTEROPATHY

Growth failure (without GI symptoms)
Anemia
Iron deficiency
Folate deficiency
Vitamin B_{12} deficiency (rare)
Rickets, osteoporosis, pathological features
Bleeding disorders
Edema
Constipation
Vomiting
Recurrent abdominal pain

DIAGNOSIS

Laboratory Findings

Before GSE is diagnosed in childhood, a sweat test should be performed to exclude cystic fibrosis, the most common cause of malabsorption in childhood. A number of reports have described the coexistence of these two disorders. Tests are discussed in detail in Chapter 124, Diarrhea and Steatorrhea.

Anemia is common in gluten-sensitive enteropathy and usually occurs secondary to iron, folate, or vitamin B_{12} malabsorption. Hypoprothrombinemia may occur secondary to vitamin K malabsorption. Because protein-losing enteropathy may occur in GSE, serum albumin and globulins should be measured. Electrolyte disturbances, especially hypokalemia, are common; calcium, phosphorus, and alkaline phosphatase levels may be abnormal in patients who have rickets. The radiographic findings in gluten-sensitive enteropathy, which are nonspecific (Fig. 212-4), include distention of the small intestine and segmentation of barium as a result of hypersecretion of intestinal fluid.

Intestinal Biopsy

Biopsy of the small intestine is the definitive method of establishing the diagnosis of GSE. Previously, blind biopsies were performed with either the Crosby capsule or the Quinton-Rubin pediatric suction tube; currently, fiberoptic endoscopy is used routinely to obtain biopsy specimens to establish this diagnosis. Various studies have indicated that adequate tissue can be obtained with this technique. In addition, endoscopy allows visualization of the duodenum. Scalloping of the small intestinal valvulae of Kerckring[1] has been described as pathognomonic for GSE on endoscopy (Fig. 212-5). In young infants this appearance may not be visualized as easily, but edema of the duodenal mucosa appears to be more common.

Differential Diagnosis of Flat Villus Lesion

In children under 18 months of age, flat villus lesions can have many causes besides GSE. Many GI insults can damage surface epithelial cells, resulting in increased epithelial cell turnover, crypt hypertrophy, abnormal surface epithelial cells, and eventual villus flattening. Other causes of the flat villus lesion are listed in Box 212-2. Thus, for a definitive diagnosis of gluten-sensitive enteropathy, the following criteria must be met: (1) demonstration of clinical malabsorption and abnormal intestinal lesions, (2) clinical and histological response to gluten withdrawal, and (3) subsequent gluten challenge that may exacerbate clinical symptoms but always produces abnormal intestinal histology. Because the diagnosis of gluten-sensitive enteropathy means lifelong gluten restriction and, in an untreated patient, perhaps an increased risk for development of GI cancer in late adulthood, it is essential that this diagnosis be made with assurance.

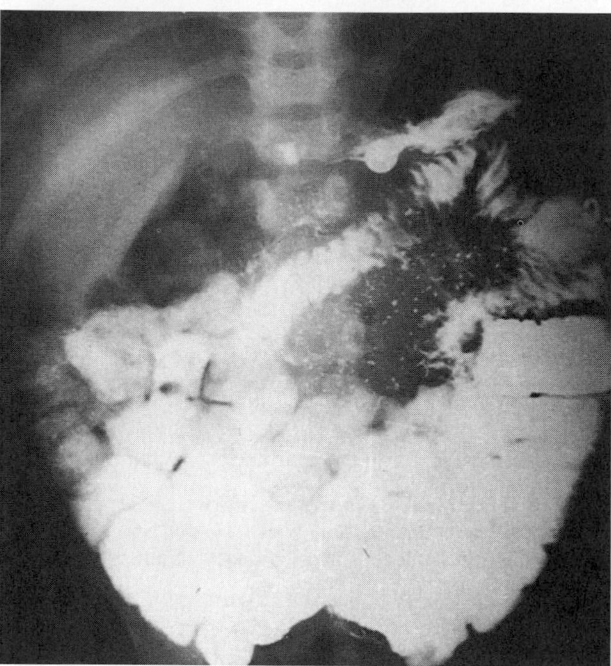

Fig. 212-4 The small bowel follow-through of this child who has growth failure shows mild dilation of loops of small bowel, some dilution of barium distally, and mild flocculation. His duodenal biopsy revealed typical celiac sprue, and he responded to a gluten-free diet.

Serological Markers in Celiac Sprue

Serological markers have emerged as a diagnostic tool and screening test for GSE.[3] These serological markers include antiendomysial, antigliadin, and antireticulin antibodies. Recently tissue transglutaminase (Ttg) has been evaluated as perhaps even more sensitive than endomysial antibody. Antiendomysial antibodies (IgA) have demonstrated the most

BOX 212-2

COMMON CAUSES OF THE FLAT VILLUS LESION

- Food sensitivity
  - GSE
  - Cow milk protein allergy
  - Soy protein allergy
  - Eosinophilic gastroenteritis
- Infections
  - Viral (rotavirus)
  - Bacterial *(Escherichia coli)*
  - Parasitic *(Giardia lamblia)*
  - Fungal *(Candida albicans)*
- Malnutrition (kwashiorkor, not marasmus)
- Tropical sprue
- Immunodeficiency disorders (most notably AIDS)
- Familial enteropathy
- Rarer causes
  - Lymphoma
  - Crohn's disease
  - Whipple's disease

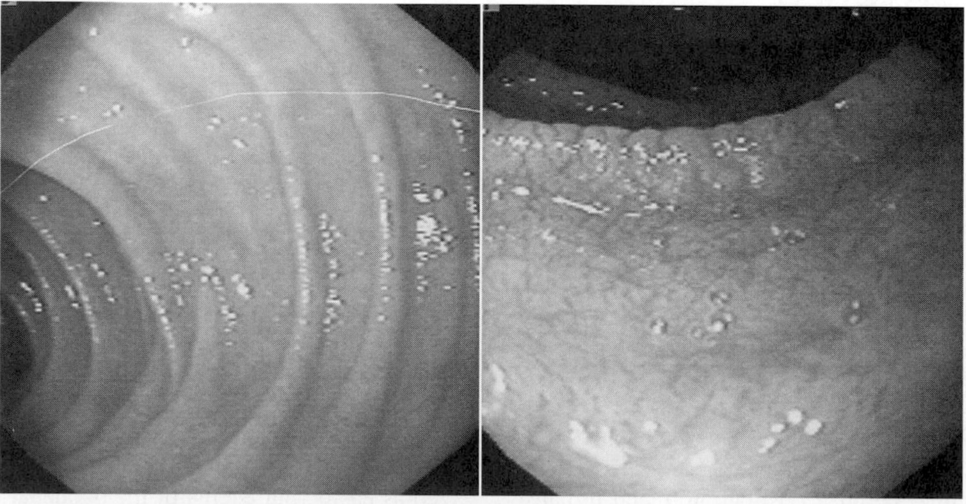

Fig. 212-5 Endoscopic study shows scalloping of the small intestinal valvulae of Kerckring, a pathognomonic finding for GSE.

sensitivity and specificity for the diagnosis of GSE compared with other antibodies at this time. This is an IgA-dependent test and, therefore, could produce a false-negative test in patients with GSE who are IgA deficient. Antigliadin antibodies appear to be less specific and less sensitive.

Serum antiendomysial antibody and serum IgA levels should be obtained together for diagnosis of GSE. If the serum IgA is low or absent then antigliadin antibodies may be obtained. A small bowel biopsy must be performed to confirm the diagnosis of GSE should serological markers be positive. About 10% to 15% of patients who have GSE may have negative markers and, therefore, a negative serological test does not exclude the diagnosis. False-positive antiendomysial antibody tests are unusual. If the subsequent small bowel biopsy is normal, the patient may need a gluten challenge and repeat small bowel biopsy.

Serological Markers in Family Screening

As has been mentioned, many patients who have celiac disease are asymptomatic. The disease is genetic; about 20% of family members may well have it without being aware of it. Parents and siblings should have serum antiendomysial antibody screening.[3] If these are positive, then small-bowel biopsies should be performed.

ASSOCIATED DISEASES

Several diseases are associated with an increased incidence of celiac disease. These include type I diabetes and Down syndrome.[4] It is appropriate to screen these patients for celiac disease with serum antiendomysial antibody.

TREATMENT

The treatment of gluten-sensitive enteropathy is complete withdrawal of gluten from the diet. Various gluten-free diets and recipes are available[7,10]; this information should be given to all patients and parents. It is important to realize that it may take a number of weeks for symptoms to disappear completely after the gluten is withdrawn. Subjective improvement, however, occurs within the first few days. In children, apathy usually is the first symptom to be alleviated, followed by progressive improvement in muscle tone, a decrease in abdominal distention, and diarrhea. Disaccharidase activity is markedly depressed in untreated cases, and a lactose-free diet is advocated during the initial 4 to 6 weeks of therapy to alleviate the diarrhea. Lactose is gradually reintroduced, provided there is no concurrent infection, severe electrolyte imbalance, dehydration, or shock (so-called celiac crisis). Replacement iron, folic acid, vitamin K, vitamin D, and calcium should be given when appropriate.

REFERENCES

1. Brocci E, et al: Endoscopic demonstration of duodenal folds in the diagnosis of celiac disease, *N Engl J Med* 319:741, 1988.
2. Caffrey C, et al: HLA-DP and celiac disease: family and population studies, *Gut* 31:663, 1990.
3. Calabuig M, et al: Serological markers and celiac disease: a new diagnostic approach? *J Pediatr Gastroenterol Nutr* 10:435, 1990.
4. Carlsson A, et al: Prevalence of IgA-antigliadin antibodies and IgA-antiendomysium antibodies related to celiac disease in children with Down syndrome, *Pediatrics* 101:272, 1998.
5. Hamilton JR, Lynch JJ, Reilly BJ: Active celiac disease in childhood, *Q J Med* 38:135, 1969.
6. Katz AJ, Falchuk ZM: Current concepts in gluten-sensitive enteropathy, *Pediatr Clin North Am* 22:767, 1975.
7. Sheedy CB, Keifeiz N: *Cooking for your celiac child,* New York, 1969, Dial Press.
8. Strober W, et al: The pathogenesis of gluten-sensitive enteropathy, *Ann Intern Med* 83:242, 1975.
9. Unsworth DJ, Brown DL: Serological screening suggests that adult coeliac disease is underdiagnosed in the UK and increases the incidence by up to 12%, *Gut* 35:61, 1994.
10. Wood MN: *Gourmet food on a wheat-free diet,* Springfield, Ill, 1967, Charles C Thomas.

SUGGESTED READINGS

Alper CA, et al: Extended major histocompatibility complex haplotypes in patients with gluten-sensitive enteropathy, *J Clin Invest* 79:251, 1987.

Misra S, Ament ME: Diagnosis of coeliac sprue in 1994, *Gastroenterol Clin North Am* 24:133, 1995.

Visakorpi JK, Maki M: Changing clinical features of coeliac disease, *Acta Paediatr Suppl* 83:10, 1994.

213 Hemolytic-Uremic Syndrome

Glenn H. Bock

Hemolytic-uremic syndrome (HUS) is defined as the triad of acute microangiopathic hemolytic anemia, thrombocytopenia, and acute renal insufficiency or failure. The syndromic nature of HUS must be emphasized. The disease manifestations undoubtedly occur as a common pathway resulting from a variety of initiating causes (Box 213-1). In North America and Western Europe, epidemic, diarrhea-associated HUS is the most common form. Atypical HUS (also known as sporadic or nondiarrhea-associated HUS) occurs less frequently in children and is classified according to the suspected underlying primary cause.

The clinical manifestations of HUS may be difficult to distinguish from those of thrombotic thrombocytopenic purpura (TTP), particularly at the time of a first episode. Classically, the kidney has been considered the primary target organ in HUS, whereas the presence of more generalized disease, particularly inclusive of the central nervous system (CNS), has been considered more characteristic of TTP. However, clinical manifestations overlap broadly.

FREQUENCY

Childhood HUS occurs worldwide, although its incidence varies among countries. Sites of epidemic outbreaks include Argentina, the United States, Western Europe, South Africa, and the Indian subcontinent. Typically the illness affects infants and young children of all races and both genders, with the majority of diarrhea-associated cases occurring in the summer months. Even in nonepidemic areas, cases commonly cluster. Although the frequency varies, typical childhood HUS is one of the most common causes of acute renal failure among pediatric patients. Atypical HUS is more common in older children and adults, although diarrhea-associated HUS is being recognized with increasing frequency in this population. The occurrence of atypical HUS tends to be sporadic without geographical or seasonal characteristics.

ETIOLOGY

There has been significant progress in our understanding of the initiating events and resultant clinical manifestations of HUS. Most forms of the syndrome appear to have in common endothelial cell injury with consequent platelet adhesion and aggregation, resulting in potentially reversible microvascular thrombosis. The diarrheal form of HUS in children is associated most commonly with colonic infection by an *Escherichia coli* (most commonly *E. coli* subtype 0157:H7) capable of producing a Shiga-like toxin (Slt). In these cases, Slt initiates the endothelial cell injury. Currently Slt (also referred to as verocytotoxin after its cytotoxic effect on the Vero cell line *in vitro*) accounts for 70% to 90% of the postdiarrheal cases of HUS in North America and Western Europe. This toxin has many characteristics in common with Shiga toxin produced by *Shigella dysenteriae,* an infectious agent known to cause HUS in underdeveloped countries. Other infectious organisms that do not produce Slt (e.g., pneumococci, clostridia, and some viruses) also have been associated with HUS. These organisms have in common the production of neuraminidase, an enzyme that can damage platelet, erythrocyte, and endothelial cell membranes. Other atypical forms of HUS may be caused by disturbances of prostacyclin regulation of platelet aggregation, by differences of host resistance to the binding of aggregate materials to endothelial cell surfaces, or from the use of certain medications (e.g., mitomycin and cyclosporine). Those patients who have inherent biochemical or endocrinological disturbances may have recurrent episodes of HUS or demonstrate familial occurrences.

HISTORY

The child who has typical HUS usually experiences a 3- to 10-day prodrome of bloody or watery diarrhea often associated with cramping abdominal pain. Nausea, vomiting, and fever are present variably but are not usually prominent features. Extreme pallor and malaise, when reported, usually occur suddenly at a time when the gastrointestinal illness has appeared to have stabilized or improved. Although the renal injury begins with the onset of the hemolytic microangiopathy, signs or symptoms attributable to acute renal failure may take several days to develop.

Extrarenal involvement in HUS often is seen (Box 213-2). In fact, with the general availability of dialysis, nonrenal disease in HUS has become the major determinant of early mortality and a significant factor in the development of long-term sequelae. Acute gastrointestinal manifestations may include abdominal distention, bleeding, intussusception, rectal prolapse, and strictures. Gangrene of the colon and intestinal perforation also have been reported. CNS abnormalities such as somnolence, irritability, seizures, or stroke, and severe chronic sequelae are observed; such symptoms now are recognized to be much more common than was appreciated when the syndrome was first described. In atypical HUS a prodrome usually is absent or consists of an upper respiratory tract infection. The manifestations at the onset of HUS

BOX 213-1

CAUSES OF HEMOLYTIC-UREMIC SYNDROME

Infection-Related
E. coli
Shigella
Neuraminidase-producing organisms
Human immunodeficiency virus

Sporadic
Familial
Pregnancy
Transplantation
Malignant hypertension
Drugs
Tumors
Collagen vascular disease

BOX 213-2

EXTRARENAL MANIFESTATIONS OF TYPICAL DIARRHEA-ASSOCIATED HUS

Common
Gastrointestinal
Central nervous system
Hepatitis
Pancreatitis

Uncommon
Pulmonary hemorrhage
Myocardial ischemia/infarction
Retinal hemorrhage
Skin necrosis
Rhabdomyolysis
Parotitis

are similar, except that gastrointestinal complaints are less common.

PHYSICAL FINDINGS

Children who have HUS usually appear acutely ill with pallor, petechiae, and/or purpura. They often are irritable or drowsy and may have hypertension. Those who have the typical childhood variety may have a distended, tympanitic abdomen with diffuse tenderness. Hepatomegaly frequently is present. The presence of congestive heart failure and pulmonary or peripheral edema results from a combination of oliguria with consequent intravascular volume overload and/or a rapidly developing anemia.

LABORATORY FINDINGS

A Coombs-negative and often-profound anemia is a typical finding. The blood smear shows the fragmented erythrocytes characteristic of the microangiopathic process as well as the thrombocytopenia. Leukocytosis often is present, and is frequently associated with more severe disease. The urinalysis usually demonstrates proteinuria, microscopic or macroscopic hematuria, cylindruria, and pyuria. Laboratory abnormalities resulting from renal dysfunction, including azotemia, hyperkalemia, hyperphosphatemia, and metabolic acidosis, are variable in their degree depending on the magnitude and duration of the renal disease and the degree of red cell hemolysis. The biochemical derangements, especially of potassium, may be life threatening and require emergent treatment to prevent potentially fatal cardiac arrhythmias. Furthermore, the child who has suspected HUS should have some form of electrocardiographic monitoring until the initial laboratory data are obtained.

DIFFERENTIAL DIAGNOSIS

The features of HUS are not specific and also may occur in disseminated intravascular coagulation (DIC), overwhelming sepsis, malignant hypertension, and some instances of vasculitis. Although the microangiopathic features of DIC and HUS are similar, coagulation pathway studies most often are normal in HUS. As mentioned, TTP, which occurs more commonly in adults, may share many of the pathophysiological features of HUS. The diagnosis of atypical (sporadic) HUS mandates an evaluation for a noninfectious underlying cause.

TREATMENT

Management of the oliguric acute renal failure, hypertension, anemia, and CNS disturbances is the most common initial therapeutic consideration in patients who have HUS. Prevention of fluid overload (which often provokes significant worsening of hypertension), correction of electrolyte imbalances, and control of uremia is achieved by careful medical management and, if necessary, dialysis. Details of the medical approach to acute renal failure are given in Chapter 295, Renal Failure.

Dialysis treatment is considered an important aspect of care in these patients, because a great deal of the morbidity of HUS in earlier reports resulted from complications of fluid overload, hypertension, and electrolyte imbalance. In addition, dialysis permits the modulation of fluid balance to allow for infusions of hyperalimentation solutions, erythrocytes, or other necessary preparations. To avoid rapid changes of intravascular volume, where possible, blood cells should be transfused in small quantities as needed to keep the hematocrit around 25%. Platelet transfusions seldom are required in patients who have HUS and should be restricted to children who have active bleeding, and those whose platelet counts are below 10,000/mm^3 to 15,000/mm^3 or who require invasive procedures. Seizures should be treated aggressively and conventionally (allowing for medication dosage adjustments for dialysis and the degree of renal failure); comatose children may require elective ventilation to protect the airway. The common symptom of irritability cannot be treated directly but resolves gradually with correction of the hemolysis and uremia.

Attempts to modify the course of HUS by treatment with corticosteroids or anticoagulants have not proved effective. Some success has been reported using several modalities, including drugs that impair platelet aggregation (aspirin, dipyridamole), plasma infusion, plasma exchange, and prostacyclin infusion. The potential benefits of these treatments seem to occur primarily in the atypical forms of HUS. However, few controlled studies assess the actual benefit of these interventions adequately. In contrast, plasma infusion has been suggested to be contraindicated in patients who have neuraminidase-associated HUS, because it may worsen the hemolysis. The complexities of acute renal failure management and the rapidly changing concepts in dialysis and treatment for HUS make early consultation with a pediatric nephrologist an important aspect of individualized patient management.

PROGNOSIS

More than 80% of children who have typical childhood HUS recover without renal or CNS sequelae. More than 10% may have some degree of persistent renal insufficiency or hypertension. Aggressive management of the renal failure and hypertension has a positive effect on survival during the acute phase of the disease. Severe CNS involvement during the early phase of the disease should raise concerns about possible long-term CNS sequelae. Children who have atypical HUS are at increased risk for permanently impaired renal function. Patients who have recurrent or familial forms of HUS also are at increased risk for progressive deterioration of renal function and often ultimately require dialysis or renal transplantation.

When to Refer

At the time of initial presentation, because rate of progression may be rapid
In the presence of rapidly progressive azotemia or hemolytic anemia
For severe or prolonged bloody diarrhea or abdominal pain
In the face of possibly evolving hyperkalemia, acidosis, or other potentially dangerous metabolic disturbances
For progressive or symptomatic hypertension
With signs of central nervous system involvement

When to Hospitalize

To provide management or comanagement with a pediatric nephrologist and other appropriate subspecialists in all but the mildest cases

SUGGESTED READINGS

Kaplan BS, et al: The pathogenesis and treatment of hemolytic uremic syndrome, *J Am Soc Nephrol* 9:1126, 1998.

Moake JL: Haemolytic-uraemic syndrome: basic science, *Lancet* 343:393, 1994.

Neild GH: Haemolytic-uraemic syndrome in practice, *Lancet* 343:398, 1994.

Neuhaus TJ: Heterogeneity of atypical haemolytic uraemic syndromes, *Arch Dis Child* 76:518, 1997.

Remuzzi G: HUS and TTP: variable expression of a single entity, *Kidney Int* 32:292, 1987.

Siegler RL: Spectrum of extrarenal involvement in postdiarrheal hemolytic-uremic syndrome, *J Pediatr* 125:511, 1994.

214 Hemophilia and Other Hereditary Bleeding Disorders

Eva G. Radel

Hemostasis requires adhesion of platelets to an injured vascular endothelium, aggregation of additional platelets with formation of a platelet plug, activation of coagulation factors resulting in the coagulation "cascade," and finally, formation of a fibrin clot that interacts with the platelet aggregate to form a stable hemostatic seal. The coagulation factors exist in the blood, mostly as precursors that become activated to become enzymes or cofactors and, in turn, activate other clotting factors. Also involved are anticoagulants, fibrinolysins, and inhibitors; all form a very complex, delicate, autoregulated system. Abnormalities of platelet function also may exist congenitally (see Chapter 161, Petechiae and Purpura).

EVALUATION TO DETECT ABNORMALITIES OF HEMOSTASIS

The most useful screening tests to study the hemostatic and coagulation mechanisms are the activated partial thromboplastin time (APTT), the prothrombin time (PT), and the bleeding time. The PT alone is not adequate for screening children for coagulation disorders, because it misses the most common congenital deficiencies. Falsely prolonged clotting tests may result from an insufficient amount of blood in the specimen tube or difficulty accessing the vein with release of tissue factor and consumption of coagulation factors. The tests are sensitive to clotting factor levels less than 30% to 40% of normal. A prolonged APTT or PT must be followed up by the performance of individual clotting factor assays. The normal activity (100%) of a clotting factor is defined arbitrarily as 1 unit/ml of plasma; the normal range of activity for different factors is from about 50% to 200%.

Factor XIII deficiency will not be detected with these tests. Prolonged PT and APTT also may be seen in the presence of lupuslike anticoagulants; these, however, are associated with thrombosis rather than with bleeding. The bleeding time can be measured with one of several commercially available disposable templates; it is prolonged in von Willebrand's disease, thrombocytopenia, and acquired and congenital abnormalities of platelet function.

HEMOPHILIA A AND B

Although factors VIII and IX are entirely different molecules that act in different ways in the coagulation cascade, their sex-linked inheritance and the clinical manifestations of their deficiencies are identical. The incidence of hemophilia is about 1 in 5000 males, 85% being hemophilia A (classic hemophilia, congenital factor VIII deficiency) and 15% hemophilia B (Christmas disease, congenital factor IX deficiency). A positive family history is present in about two thirds of cases.

Diagnosis

The diagnosis can be suspected based on the family and personal history, and laboratory tests will identify the deficiency. Severe hemophilia accounts for 80% of cases and is defined by a factor VIII or IX level of less than 1% to 2%. Levels above 5% to 10% are associated with mild disease, intermediate levels with moderate disease. Severe disease is manifested by hemarthroses and hematoma formation with minimal or no trauma. Mild disease results in bleeding only with trauma. The factor VIII and factor IX genes have both been cloned, and many different mutations have been found in both conditions.[3,8] In the majority of families, it now is possible to diagnose hemophilia prenatally by chorionic villus biopsy or amniocentesis.

Bleeding Manifestations

Hemarthrosis. Recurrent bleeding into joints is the most frequent clinical problem for patients who have severe hemophilia. The knees, ankles, and elbows are involved most often. Many patients have one particular "target" joint in which recurrent episodes occur and in which chronic changes are most likely to result. Synovial thickening and vascular friability may develop, resulting in increased susceptibility to bleeding and a vicious cycle. Synovitis accompanied by chronic effusion often develops and may progress to joint destruction (hemophilic arthropathy).[14] With prompt adequate treatment or prevention of bleeding, the incidence of these complications is much less.

Hemarthrosis must be treated as soon as pain, tingling, or limping *begins*, even if evidence of swelling is not visible. If there is marked swelling, the joint should be aspirated after factor replacement, and a few days of prednisone may be helpful (Table 214-1). Watchful waiting is *not* appropriate for the child who has hemophilia. Early synovitis should be managed by giving factor VIII or IX prophylactically for several weeks, often along with a short course of steroids. Synovectomy (open or arthroscopic) may be effective if medical management fails.[15] Intensive physical therapy also is required. Radioactive synovectomy (synoviorthesis) has been safe and effective in adults with early changes, but studies in children have been limited.[10]

Table 214-1 Products Available for Treatment of Coagulation Disorders

Product	Content	Dose/Concentration/Size of Units	Indications/Comments
Fresh-frozen plasma (FFP)	Whole plasma	5-15 ml/kg; 1 u of each of the coagulation factors/ ml; 220 or 600 ml/bag	Multiple factor deficiency; DIC; reversal of Coumadin effect; HUS or TTP; unknown coagulation defect; deficiency of factors II, V, VII, X, XI, or XIII; contains all plasma factors; not virus-inactivated
Solvent-detergent FFP	Whole plasma; does not contain high molecular weight multimers of VWF and has smaller amounts of proteins C and S	5-15 ml/kg; 1 u of each of the coagulation factors/ ml; 200 ml/bag	Same as above, but virus-inactivated*; for patients requiring multiple treatments
Cryoprecipitate	FVIII, VWF, FXIII, fibrinogen, fibronectin	1 u/kg raises FVIII 2%; 75-100 u FVIII and VWF/ bag; volume ± 20 ml; not assayed	Hemophilia A, VWD, FXIII deficiency, hypofibrinogenemia; derived from single donor units; not virus-inactivated
Factor VIII	FVIII	1 u/kg raises FVIII 2% Pre-assayed; up to 100u/ml	Hemophilia A; made by various methods, with different levels of purification; recombinant product available; virus-inactivated*
Humate P	FVIII; VWF	Pre-assayed; FVIII 20-40 u/ml; VWF 50-100 u/ml	Severe VWD; mild to moderate VWD if DDAVP ineffective or inadequate; virus-inactivated*
Factor IX	FIX	Pre-assayed; up to 100 u/ml	Hemophilia B; recombinant product available; virus-inactivated*
Prothrombin complex	FII, FVII, FIX, FX	Pre-assayed for FIX; FVII content varies among products (high and assayed in Proplex T/F-7)	Hemophilia B when purified FIX cannot be used; mild bleeding in hemophilia A with inhibitor; congenital deficiency of FII or FX; Proplex T/F-7 for FVII deficiency; Danger of thrombosis (including MI and DIC) in presence of liver disease or vascular disease, prolonged use; virus-inactivated*
Activated prothrombin complex	FII, FVII, FIX, FX; FVIII "bypassing" activity	Pre-assayed for ability to shorten PTT of plasma with high-titer FVIII inhibitor	Hemophilia A with inhibitor; cannot evaluate response by measuring FVIII activity; risk of DIC and thrombosis
Hyate:C	Porcine FVIII	Pre-assayed; 400-700 u/vial	Hemophilia A with inhibitor, which is not cross-reactive
Novoseven	Recombinant FVIIa	Pre-assayed	Hemophilia A or B with inhibitor; risk of thrombosis

DDAVP, Desmopressin; *DIC,* disseminated intravascular coagulation; *F,* factor; *HUS,* hemolytic-uremic syndrome; *MI,* myocardial infarction; *PTT,* partial thromboplastin time; *TTP,* thrombotic thrombocytopenic purpura; *VWD,* von Willebrand's disease; *VWF,* von Willebrand's factor.
*Virus attenuation processes may not inactivate parvovirus, hepatitis A, and possibly other viruses.

Soft-tissue bleeding. Superficial hematomas, unless very large, often do not require treatment. However, bleeding into muscles may result in nerve damage or muscle fibrosis and contractures; such bleeding may be difficult to diagnose because swelling often is minimal. Bleeding into the iliopsoas muscle may cause femoral nerve damage, and it must be considered whenever pain occurs in the hip or groin. Limping and flexion of the hip often are the only positive findings. Sonography or a computed tomography (CT) scan may help in making the diagnosis. Bleeding into the thigh may cause accumulation of a large amount of blood without much external change and may result in significant anemia.

Life-threatening bleeding. Intracranial bleeding can occur after trauma but also appears to occur spontaneously. All but the most minor head injury must be considered to be significant and treated promptly. A CT scan should be obtained to evaluate the extent of bleeding. Airway compromise must be considered a potential threat with any hematoma of the neck or the submental or sublingual areas, as well as the retropharyngeal or parapharyngeal regions; a severe sore throat or dysphagia also suggests bleeding and should be evaluated and treated immediately. Retroperitoneal bleeding may be quite massive before it can be detected and must be considered when abdominal or groin pain is present. In all of these situations, a CT scan or magnetic resonance imaging (MRI) may be helpful in evaluating the patient.

Mouth bleeding. The lip, tongue, and frenulum are areas of frequent trauma in young children. Factor replacement should be accompanied by the use of epsilon aminocaproic acid (EACA, Amicar) to prevent fibrinolysis of the clot, although it must be used with great caution in patients receiving prothrombin complex or any activated coagulation factors, because it can lead to thrombosis or disseminated intravascular coagulation (DIC). The dose is 50 to 100 mg/kg every 6 hours until all signs of bleeding have resolved. Tranexamic acid is used in Europe but is not available commercially in the United States.

Hematuria. Hematuria must be evaluated with noninvasive procedures, as in the normal individual. It usually resolves spontaneously with or without factor replacement. Steroid therapy is controversial. EACA should be avoided, because it can result in obstruction of the renal pelvis by clot formation.[12]

Acquired Immunodeficiency Syndrome (AIDS) and Other Viral Infections

Up to 90% of patients who had severe hemophilia in the United States in the late 1970s and early 1980s contracted HIV infection. The treatment of hemophilia with clotting factor concentrates from large donor pools in the era before the virus was identified resulted in massive exposure to HIV infection. Chronic liver disease also has been a major problem, most often caused by hepatitis C and sometimes by hepatitis B virus infection. Currently, both donor testing and several methods to inactivate viruses in the production process make the concentrates safe with regard to HIV. Hepatitis B and C also appear to have been largely eliminated. Hepatitis A and parvovirus B19 infections have been reported following treatment with some products in recent years, causing serious problems in patients who have AIDS.[17]

General Principles of Treatment

Ideal management of patients who have hemophilia is in a comprehensive center where all the needs of the patient can be met, including medical, orthopedic, physical rehabilitation, dental, and psychosocial therapies. All elective surgical procedures *must* be done in a center that has experienced personnel and immediate availability of blood clotting factor assays and a ready supply of clotting concentrates, and they should be preceded by factor inhibitor testing. Nerve blocks must be avoided. A patient who has a severe injury or life-threatening bleeding should be given an immediate dose of the appropriate clotting factor to raise its level to 100% and then be transferred to a hemophilia center.

Any significant injury must be treated promptly, even without apparent evidence of active bleeding, because bleeding often is delayed. A small superficial laceration, if not bleeding or in need of cleaning, may be managed with a simple pressure dressing, but if the dressing becomes soaked or if the laceration needs to be sutured, the appropriate clotting factor *must* be administered immediately. Casts should not be applied unless factor has been administered beforehand and is continued for several days afterward; the involved area should be watched closely for evidence of nerve compression. Treatment must be given before *all* surgical procedures, arterial punctures, and spinal taps.

Pain should be managed with acetaminophen whenever possible; however, codeine and other oral narcotics can be given if necessary. Aspirin must be avoided, but nonacetylated salicylates (choline magnesium trisalicylate) can be used, and nonsteroidal antiinflammatory agents such as ibuprofen can be given cautiously if the patient is not also on zidovudine.[13] The newer cox-2 inhibitors show promise as analgesic agents for patients who have hemophilia but have not yet been studied in this group of patients.[6]

Factor Replacement

Products available for the treatment of coagulation disorders are described in Table 214-1. Whole plasma can raise factor VIII levels to only 40% and factor IX to 20% because of the large volume and protein load that accompany its use. Early in the AIDS epidemic, it was recommended that plasma or cryoprecipitate be given when possible, rather than concentrates made from large donor pools. The safety of current concentrates makes them the preferred mode of treatment in most situations. Recombinant factors VIII and IX have become available recently and appear to be entirely free of viral contamination and effective. However, early experience indicates a higher incidence of inhibitor development with these products.[1,16]

Factor IX is available in the form of prothrombin complex, as well as in purified and recombinant forms. Mild bleeding requiring a single treatment can be managed with the complex, but if repeated doses are needed over several days or for patients who have liver disease, the more purified factor should be used because of the danger of thrombosis or DIC from activated factors in the complex. The cost of these products increases with the degree of purification.

The desired levels of factor VIII or IX for managing different clinical problems are shown in Table 214-2. Preassayed concentrates are available in vials containing varied doses. Whole vials containing the calculated, desired dose (or higher levels) should be given, because these products are too expensive to waste. Continuous infusion can be used for patients who are undergoing surgery or are bleeding extensively.[19]

Health Care Maintenance

Routine immunizations, which must include hepatitis B and hepatitis A, should be given subcutaneously if possible with a 25-gauge needle; pressure should be maintained for 5 to 10 minutes. Intramuscular injections should be minimized. Routine dental evaluation, prophylaxis, and hygiene should be begun by 3 years of age. The most difficult part of managing the child who has hemophilia is to use an adequate amount of caution but at the same time allow for the development of independence. Family education about the disease is essential, and support groups are beneficial. Psychosocial problems must be a major concern in managing patients and fam-

Table 214-2 Treatment of Bleeding Episodes in Hemophilia

Type of Bleeding	Desired Level of FVIII or FIX*	Duration of Treatment	Ancillary Treatment
Hematoma, simple	20%-40%	Usually ×1	
Hemarthrosis Mild muscle hematoma	30%-40%	×1 as soon as symptoms begin; if severe, repeat daily until better	Prednisone for severe or recurrent joint episodes (0.5-1 mg/kg/day × 3 days); aspirate joint after treatment if swelling is marked
Severe muscle hematoma	50%-100%	3-7 days	
Mouth bleeding Epistaxis Dental extractions	80%-100%	×1	Start EACA 75-100 mg/kg q6h for 3-7 days (until clot is gone)
GI bleeding	100%	3-7 days	
Hematuria	? (factor may not be needed)	3-7 days	Bed rest; hydration; ? prednisone 2 mg/kg/day; do *not* use EACA
Life-threatening CNS Airway obstruction Retroperitoneal	100%; do not allow to drop to below 50%†	7-14 days	Monitor levels
Surgery	100%; do not allow to drop to below 50%†	7-14 days	Monitor levels
Prophylaxis	25-40 u/kg	t.i.w. for FVIII b.i.w. for FIX	

*1 u/kg of FVIII increases plasma level by 2%; biological half-life = 10 to 12 hours. 1 u/kg of FIX increases level by 1%; 1 u/kg of recombinant FIX increases level by 0.8%; biological half-life = 20 to 24 hours.
Slightly lower levels of FIX than of FVIII are effective.
†Initial dose = 50 u/kg of FVIII and 80 to 100 u/kg of FIX; repeat half the FVIII dose in 8 to 12 hours, and half the FIX dose in 12 to 24 hours, or give continuous infusion of 3 to 4 u/kg/hour of either FVIII or FIX after their initial bolus dose.
EACA, Epsilon-amino caproic acid (Amicar).

ilies. Not only do they have to live with a very serious chronic illness, associated with frequent pain and limitation of normal activities, but also the impact of AIDS on this population has been devastating and in many cases has eroded trust in medical caretakers.

Home Care

If a child has reasonably easy venous access and the family dynamics allow for it, parents can be taught to administer treatment to children as young as 3 years, and 9- or 10-year-olds can be taught to self-administer factor concentrates. This allows for much earlier treatment of bleeding episodes, provides the satisfaction of self-sufficiency, and prevents some of the frustrations of having to get to a treatment center or emergency room. Indwelling venous access devices are being used with increasing frequency and have simplified home, as well as in-hospital, management.[9]

Mild Hemophilia

The patient who has mild hemophilia is more likely than the severe hemophiliac to get inadequate treatment of bleeding episodes, because neither the family nor the physicians may be aware of the need for treatment. Severe injuries require management like that of the severe hemophiliac, although smaller doses of factor concentrates may suffice to attain the desired factor levels. Desmopressin (DDAVP) is a vasopressin analog that results in release of factor VIII from the endothelial cells where it is produced. Administration of 0.3 μg/kg IV over 20 to 30 minutes usually results in a two- to fivefold increase of factor VIII in about 1 hour, which may be maintained for about 24 hours. It can be repeated in 12 to 24 hours, but its effectiveness may decrease. Overhydration must be avoided, because water retention and hyponatremia may occur with desmopressin therapy, particularly in young children. A concentrated intranasal preparation is available and has been used in children 6 years of age and older. The dose is one spray (150 μg) in children less than 50 kg and two sprays (one in each nostril) for larger individuals. A stimulation test with response assessment should be performed in each patient with both the IV and the nasal preparations before they are used therapeutically for the first time. Desmopressin is ineffective in factor IX deficiency.

Inhibitors

About 10% to 15% of patients who have hemophilia A and 3% who have hemophilia B develop antibodies that inhibit factor VIII activity, usually early in their treatment. Such patients should be managed only by experienced practitioners; the management may include the use of very large doses of factor VIII, prothrombin complex, activated prothrombin complex, porcine factor VIII, recombinant factor VIIa, induction of immune tolerance, and immunosuppression.[2]

Occasionally, patients who have hemophilia B and inhibitors develop anaphylaxis when given factor IX.[20] An inhibitor should be suspected if response to appropriate therapy is inadequate and its presence can be determined with a Bethesda inhibitor assay.[2]

Prophylaxis and Gene Therapy

Prophylactic factor concentrate treatment given three times weekly or every other day is advocated for children who have severe hemophilia to prevent hemarthrosis and joint damage and to normalize their lives.[7] Although this form of treatment is more expensive than episodic treatment for bleeding, the additional cost-saving by the prevention of future orthopedic complications and the psychological benefits also must be considered.[5,18] It is hoped that gene therapy soon will allow these conditions to be cured. Clinical trials of gene therapy for hemophilia B are already in progress.

VON WILLEBRAND'S DISEASE

Von Willebrand's disease (VWD) is the most common hereditary coagulation disorder, with estimates of an incidence as high as 1% of the population. Von Willebrand's factor (VWF) is the carrying protein for factor VIII and exists in a series of different-sized multimers of smaller subunits. Decreased VWF is associated with a corresponding decrease of factor VIII activity in most cases. The inheritance usually is autosomal dominant with variable penetrance, but autosomal recessive variants occur. The gene is on chromosome 12, it has been cloned, and several genetic defects have been identified.[11] In addition to bleeding after surgery and trauma, the major manifestation of VWD is mucosal bleeding, most frequently manifesting as epistaxis. Menorrhagia and, less commonly, gastrointestinal bleeding also may occur. Hemarthrosis and deep hematomas may be seen in very severe (Type III) VWD.

Several components of the VWF-factor VIII complex and function can be determined: factor VIII activity, VWF activity (Ristocetin cofactor), VWF antigen, and the pattern of multimers. VWF is normal in classic hemophilia. Many variants of VWD exist. The most common is type I, in which all components are similarly reduced and the multimer pattern is normal. Type II has a decrease or absence of the larger multimers; type IIB exhibits increased binding to platelets. Type III represents very severe homozygous deficiency with very low or absent levels of all components.

The bleeding time is the most sensitive but nonspecific screening test, being prolonged in most patients, and most cases are associated with decreased levels of factor VIII. However, the APTT may be normal if factor VIII is greater than 30% to 40%. All of the studies may be variable, both from patient to patient and in the same patient from time to time; if laboratory test results are normal, they should be repeated if the index of suspicion is high.

Most patients who have type I VWD will respond to DDAVP as in mild hemophilia A (see above), and this can be used for most bleeding episodes. Most patients who have type IIA and all who have type III VWD do not respond to DDAVP; its use is contraindicated in type IIB disease, because it may cause platelet aggregation and DIC. Patients who have severe bleeding or those who do not respond to DDAVP must be treated with FFP (if large volumes are not required), cryoprecipitate, or Humate P. The latter is now preferred because it is processed to inactivate viruses (see Table 214-1). Mild epistaxis often can be controlled with EACA; this agent should be used as adjunctive therapy for mucosal bleeding other than hematuria.

OTHER COAGULATION DEFECTS

The other coagulant deficiencies are inherited as autosomal recessives, with the exception of factor XI deficiency, afibrinogenemia, and dysfibrinogenemia, which are associated with bleeding in both their heterozygous and homozygous forms. Factor XIII deficiency cannot be detected with the usual screening tests; a normal screening workup in a patient who has a significant bleeding history should be followed with a clot solubility test. The contact factors prekallikrein, high molecular weight kininogen, and factor XII are necessary to initiate clotting in vitro; their absence results in a markedly prolonged APTT but is not associated with clinical bleeding.

Although all of these deficiencies can be treated with FFP, coagulation factor concentrates are preferable for treating factor VII deficiency because of its short half-life. Solvent detergent fresh frozen plasma (SD-FFP) has been treated to inactivate viruses and thus is safer than regular FFP, although it is more expensive and may not be readily available in an emergency. Factor V is labile in FFP, and studies of its availability in SD-FFP have been limited. The required doses and frequency of administration of FFP for different deficiencies vary.[4] Deficiencies of factors II, VII, and X can be treated with prothrombin complex, although the concentration of each factor in different products varies. Fibrinogen and factor XIII are concentrated in cryoprecipitate. Activated factor VII (VIIa) concentrate is available but is approved only for treatment of patients with hemophilia who have inhibitors. Activated coagulation factors may induce thrombosis, as well as DIC, and must be used with caution, particularly for patients who have liver disease. Prothrombin complex also contains activated factors. Purified concentrates of factors VII, XI, and XIII are available for compassionate use. FFP or SD-FFP can be used in an emergency for patients who are bleeding but whose deficiency has not yet been identified.

REFERENCES

1. Addiego J, et al: Frequency of inhibitor development in haemophiliacs treated with low-purity factor VIII, *Lancet* 342:462, 1993.
2. Aledort L: Inhibitors in hemophilia patients: current status and management, *Am J Hematol* 47:208, 1994.
3. Antonarakis SE, et al: Molecular etiology of factor VIII deficiency in hemophilia A, *Hum Mutat* 5:1, 1995.
4. Bauer K: Rare Hereditary coagulation factor abnormalities. In Nathan DG, Orkin S, editors: *Hematology of infancy and childhood*, ed 2, Philadelphia, 1998, WB Saunders.
5. Bohn RL, et al: Prophylactic use of factor VIII: an economic evaluation, *Thromb Haemost* 79:932, 1998.
6. Geis GS: Update on clinical developments with celecoxib, a new specific COX-2 inhibitor: what can we expect?, *J Rheumatol* 26(suppl 56): 31, 1999.
7. Liesner RJ, et al: The impact of prophylactic treatment on children with severe haemophilia, *Br J Haematol* 92:973, 1996.
8. Lillicrap D: The molecular basis of haemophilia B, *Haemophilia* 4:350, 1998.
9. Ljung R, et al: Port-A-Cath usage in children with haemophilia: experience of 53 cases, *Acta Paediatr* 87:1051, 1998.

10. Manco-Johnson M, et al: Short-term outcome of isotopic synovectomy, *Blood* 84 (suppl 1):200A, 1994.
11. Nichols WC, Ginsburg D: von Willebrand disease, *Medicine* (Baltimore) 76:1, 1997.
12. Pitts TO, et al: Acute renal failure due to high-grade obstruction following therapy with epsilon-aminocaproic acid, *Am J Kidney Dis* 8:441, 1986.
13. Ragni MV, et al: Bleeding tendency, platelet function, and pharmacokinetics of ibuprofen and zidovudine in HIV(+) hemophilic men, *Am J Hematol* 40:176, 1992.
14. Rodriguez-Merchan EC: Effects of hemophilia on articulations of children and adults, *Clin Orthop* 328:7, 1996.
15. Rodriguez-Merchan EC, et al: Hemophilic synovitis of the knee and the elbow, *Clin Orthop* 343:47, 1997.
16. Rothschild C, et al: French previously untreated patients with severe hemophilia A after exposure to recombinant factor VIII: incidence of inhibitor and evaluation of immune tolerance, *Thromb Haemost* 80:779, 1998.
17. Santagostino E, et al: Transmission of parvovirus B19 by coagulation factor concentrates exposed to 100 degrees C heat after lyophilization, *Transfusion* 37:517, 1997.
18. Smith PS, et al: Episodic versus prophylactic infusions for hemophilia A: a cost-effectiveness analysis, *J Pediatr* 129:424, 1996.
19. Varon D, Martinowitz U: Continuous infusion therapy in haemophilia, *Haemophilia* 4:431, 1998.
20. Warrier I, et al: Factor IX inhibitors and anaphylaxis in hemophilia B, *J Pediatr Hematol Oncol* 19:23, 1997.

SUGGESTED READINGS

Bussing R, Johnson SB: Psychosocial issues in hemophilia before and after the HIV crisis: a review of current research, *Gen Hosp Psychiatry* 14:387, 1992.

Cohen AJ, Kessler CM: Treatment of inherited coagulation disorders, *Am J Med* 99:675, 1995.

DiMichele D, Neufeld EJ: Hemophilia. A new approach to an old disease, *Hematol Oncol Clin North Am* 12:1315, 1998.

Werner EJ: von Willebrand disease in children and adolescents, *Pediatr Clin North Am* 43:683, 1996.

215 Henoch-Schönlein Purpura

Glenn H. Bock

Henoch-Schönlein purpura (HSP) is a diffuse necrotizing vasculitis. As a syndrome, it is distinguished most commonly from other forms of childhood vasculitis by the association of the typical rash, arthritis, gastrointestinal symptoms, and renal glomerular disease. Nonetheless, the spectrum and extent of the clinical findings may vary considerably, particularly in adults and children younger than 2 years of age. For this reason, many of the patients ultimately diagnosed with HSP are thought, initially, to have other medical or surgical conditions.

FREQUENCY

A study from northern Europe estimated the incidence of HSP to be 13.5 cases per 100,000 child population per year. This figure probably underestimates the actual incidence of HSP because it was derived from hospital admission data, thereby likely omitting patients who had milder forms of the disease. Although childhood HSP may occur at almost any age and has been reported in infants as young as 6 months, its peak incidence occurs in the 4- to 7-year age range. A slight male predominance exists, and the disease most commonly is reported in white, Native American, and Japanese children. In the Northern Hemisphere, most cases occur between November and January, although cases commonly span the fall through spring months.

ETIOLOGY

The cause of HSP is unknown, although its pathogenesis most likely involves immune-mediated processes. Recent investigations suggest that abnormalities of IgA-metabolism and/or mediation of immunological activity are important components of the disease process. However, the investigations are, as yet, incomplete and, at times, contradictory. Although many patients have upper respiratory tract infections preceding the onset of this syndrome, no consistent infectious agent has been identified. The incidence of streptococcal infections is no greater in children who have HSP than in those of the same age who do not have disease. Some cases of HSP have been associated with food allergies, certain medications, bee stings, or prior bacterial infections, but definitive proof of the relationship is lacking.

HISTORY

More than 50% of the patients will have a history of an upper respiratory tract illness 1 to 3 weeks before the onset of the HSP symptoms. A prodrome of malaise and low-grade fever also occurs frequently. The most common presenting sign of HSP is the macular/petechial rash that often coalesces and gradually becomes purpuric. Although virtually all patients who have HSP develop a rash, its appearance may not be evident at the time of initial evaluation in as many as 50% of all patients. In some patients, the rash follows other clinical manifestations of HSP; in others, it is evanescent and may escape notice. Arthritis, the second most common clinical feature, occurs in 60% to 80% of patients and may be the initial symptom in as many as 25%. Nonmigratory pain and swelling of the knee and ankle joints occur most frequently, followed by involvement of upper extremity joints (elbows, wrists, fingers); overlying erythema and tenderness to touch are uncommon findings.

Approximately 50% of the patients develop gastrointestinal problems that may include colicky abdominal pain, melena, vomiting, or bloody diarrhea. These abdominal complaints may be severe enough to suggest an acute abdominal emergency, particularly because the gastrointestinal symptoms can precede the rash and arthritis about 20% of the time. Although the need for actual surgical intervention is uncommon, intussusception is a well-recognized complication of HSP that must be considered. Presumably it results from bowel wall hemorrhage and/or edema forming a "lead point" that promotes the infolding of the bowel on itself. In two thirds of HSP patients who have intussusception, the location is ileal-ileal, with the remainder of the more typical ileal-colic variety. Thus, abdominal sonography can be a useful part of the diagnostic evaluation when this condition is suspected.

A broad spectrum of renal involvement is found in 20% to 70% of patients who have HSP. This may range from microscopic hematuria with or without mild to moderate proteinuria to fully manifested glomerulonephritis, nephrotic syndrome, or renal insufficiency. Although some patients will have recurrent episodes of hematuria, with or without proteinuria, serious renal sequelae are uncommon. However, the nephritis of HSP is an important source of long-term morbidity, because 5% of the patients will develop chronic renal-related disease or chronic renal failure. The renal manifestations usually coincide with or follow the rash; they rarely precede it. Renal involvement tends to be more severe in those patients who have recurring purpura or gastrointestinal complaints. Usually the renal abnormality manifests within 4 weeks of the onset of the joint or gastrointestinal symptoms, although nephritis has been reported to precede these manifestations in some patients and to occur as late as 2 years afterward in other patients.

Testicular swelling and pain are relatively common but under-recognized findings in HSP. Palpable tenderness and swelling of one or both testicles or the scrotum with scrotal bruising may occur. Because these findings may overshadow or precede other symptoms, careful assessment of the testicle is necessary to avoid unnecessary surgery for erroneously suspected testicular torsion. Pulmonary hemorrhage and severe central nervous system involvement are rare. Those respiratory and neurological abnormalities that uncommonly occur in patients who have HSP tend to be rather mild and of little clinical significance. The finding of severe involvement of these organ systems requires the additional consideration of other forms of systemic vasculitis.

PHYSICAL FINDINGS

The typical rash begins with symmetrical erythematous macules that usually start over the malleoli of the ankles but often spread to involve the dorsal aspect of the legs, the buttocks, and the ulnar aspects of the arms. The trunk, face, palms, and soles usually are spared. Characteristically the rash evolves rapidly to dusky red maculopapules that coalesce to form ecchymoses within 12 to 24 hours. By 2 weeks the rash becomes purple-brown and then gradually fades. Atypically the rash may not be present initially or may be more urticarial or erythematous in character, posing a diagnostic dilemma. Examination of the skin in younger patients may also disclose edema, particularly in the scalp.

The arthritis as described above usually is characterized by painful and swollen joints; erythema, warmth, and palpable tenderness usually are absent. Abdominal findings may include distention, direct or rebound tenderness, and abnormal bowel sounds. Physical signs of renal involvement usually are absent early in the illness but may develop later.

LABORATORY FINDINGS

No specific laboratory findings are diagnostic of HSP. Normal platelet counts and coagulation parameters are the rule. Neutrophilic leukocytosis may be present, and the sedimentation rate often is elevated. Serial urinalyses and monitoring of serum creatinine and albumin levels at appropriate intervals assist in the early identification of renal involvement. The presence of abnormal renal function and/or the typical biochemical abnormalities of nephrotic syndrome should alert the clinician to the possibility of a more severe or prolonged clinical illness. When measured, as many as 50% of HSP patients demonstrate transient elevations of serum IgA levels. The serum complement levels are normal in almost all cases.

DIFFERENTIAL DIAGNOSIS

HSP is a clinical diagnosis based on the characteristic rash associated with some or all of the other typical clinical findings. Similar rashes associated with renal abnormalities may occur in association with poststreptococcal glomerulonephritis and systemic lupus erythematosus. The serum complement levels usually are decreased in these conditions. Other forms of vasculitis such as polyarteritis nodosa and Wegener granulomatosis may be particularly difficult to distinguish from HSP. Although IgG-IgA nephritis (Berger disease) is thought to be the monosymptomatic variant of HSP, it is unlikely to be confused with HSP because of the absence of other organ involvement in the former. The biopsy appearances, however, are essentially indistinguishable. Purpura also may be seen in hemolytic-uremic syndrome, conditions associated with thrombocytopenia and sepsis, whereas the arthritis must be differentiated from juvenile rheumatoid arthritis and acute rheumatic fever. Other causes of an "acute abdomen" such as idiopathic intussusception, peptic ulcer disease, volvulus, and acute appendicitis must be differentiated from the gastrointestinal complaints of HSP.

TREATMENT

The general therapeutic measures for HSP mostly are supportive. Joint pain often is controlled effectively with nonsteroidal antiinflammatory agents, although these should be avoided, if possible, in the presence of significant kidney involvement. Corticosteroids and immunosuppressive medications have been used by many in attempts to modify the clinical course of more severe forms of HSP. However, there are few well-controlled data; thus, no consensus on treatment has been established.

Corticosteroids have been used most commonly in the setting of severe or prolonged gastrointestinal or renal involvement. A short course of prednisone or methylprednisolone is considered experientially, by many, to mitigate the gastrointestinal complaints, although the effect appears to shorten the duration of the symptoms rather than modify the disease. Assessing benefit from steroids in the treatment of renal disease is difficult because the majority of the patients have good long-term outcomes regardless of treatment. Nonetheless, data are accumulating, albeit largely uncontrolled, suggesting an improved prognosis using combinations of corticosteroids and immunosuppressive agents such as cyclophosphamide and azathioprine in the more severe, exudative forms of nephritis associated with HSP. Several reports also suggest a decreased incidence of renal disease in HSP patients receiving empirical courses of prednisone. A variety of other drugs have been used to treat patients who have HSP, including combinations of anticoagulant/antiaggragant/thrombolytic agents, newer immunosuppressants, and high-dose intravenous immunoglobulins. There now is insufficient convincing information to support their use.

A diagnostic and therapeutic plan for the child in whom severe renal involvement is suspected is formulated best in consultation with a pediatric nephrologist and with an accompanying renal biopsy, particularly when nephrotic or nephritic syndromes or azotemia are present.

PROGNOSIS

The rash of HSP resolves without scarring or pigmentary changes, and no permanent deformities result from even the most severe arthritis.

The most important determinant of long-term morbidity

and mortality of HSP is the degree, type, and persistence of the renal involvement. Even so, the majority of patients recover completely. In one long-term study, all of the children who had either isolated microhematuria or hematuria associated with proteinuria had normal urinalyses and renal function on follow-up 8 years later. Of those who had either nephritis or combined nephritic and nephrotic manifestations, fewer than 1% had died of renal complications, and only 2% had continued renal abnormalities. However, other studies of long-term outcome have shown that as many as 10% to 15% of HSP patients who had renal involvement have chronic sequelae, including hypertension and renal failure. These differences may be explained by the reports of worse outcomes emanating from nephrology referral institutions, in which the patient population is biased toward those who have more severe renal involvement. Clinically, patients who have both nephrotic syndrome and hematuria, especially if associated with hypertension or renal insufficiency, have the greatest likelihood of progressing to chronic renal failure. Patients having these clinical manifestations with a proliferative and crescentic glomerulonephritis on biopsy may have as great as a 50% risk of developing renal failure. Clinicopathological studies of renal biopsy findings in HSP patients also have shown histological correlates to poorer outcomes. In summary, although the vast majority of children developing HSP have uncomplicated courses with little or no long-term sequelae, increased risk for progression to renal failure has been associated with (1) the onset of HSP nephritis in the child older than 6 years of age, (2) the presence of the nephrotic syndrome, and (3) the presence of crescent formation in the glomeruli. A renal biopsy can help establish the diagnosis and improve prognostic assessment.

When to Refer

Surgical assessment of possible intestinal obstruction or intussusception

Pediatric nephrology input when there is nephritis accompanied by renal insufficiency or nephritic syndrome

General nephrology or rheumatology guidance when nature of vasculitis syndrome unclear or therapeutic intervention contemplated

When to Hospitalize

Moderate to severe gastrointestinal involvement or possible intussusception

More extensive renal involvement including nephritic syndrome and hypertension

Assessment and treatment of clinical acute vasculitis syndrome of uncertain cause, particularly with pulmonary, CNS, or cardiac manifestations

SUGGESTED READINGS

Bergstein J, et al: Response of crescentic Henoch-Schönlein purpura nephritis to corticosteroid and azathioprine therapy, *Clin Nephrol* 49:9, 1998.

Goldstein AR, et al: Long-term follow-up of childhood Henoch-Schönlein nephritis, *Lancet* 339:280, 1992.

Robson WLM, et al: Henoch-Schönlein purpura, *Adv Pediatr* 41:163, 1994.

Steward M, et al: Long-term renal prognosis of Henoch-Schönlein purpura in an unselected childhood population, *Eur J Pediatr* 147:113, 1988.

Szer IS: Henoch-Schönlein purpura: when and how to treat, *J Rheumatol* 23:1661, 1996.

216 Hepatitis

Aglaia Zellos • Kathleen B. Schwarz

Approximately 60,000 cases of viral hepatitis are reported annually to the Centers for Disease Control and Prevention. Not included in these figures are numerous unrecognized anicteric cases, especially in the pediatric population, in whom the anicteric/icteric case ratio is thought to approach 10:1. In addition, an unknown number of subclinical cases must occur, as evidenced by the presence of antibody to hepatitis A in more than 30% of the adult U.S. population and the prevalence of hepatitis B antigen-positive persons identified by bloodbank screening. Two causative agents of non-A, non-B hepatitis have been recognized: hepatitis C, which causes most transfusion-associated cases of hepatitis[25] and hepatitis E, which causes epidemic (enterically transmitted) non-A, non-B hepatitis[24] in developing countries. In addition, three new transfusion-transmitted viruses have recently been identified: hepatitis G virus (HGV)[2], GB virus-C (GBV-C), and TT-virus (TTV)[32,33]; however, whether or not these viruses cause any type of liver disease is yet to be determined. Thus, acute viral hepatitis is a major infectious disease. Although generally a self-limited illness in children, both hepatitis A (infectious hepatitis, short incubation period) and chronic hepatitis B (serum hepatitis, long incubation period) may be associated with fulminant hepatitis; superinfection with hepatitis D virus may exacerbate symptoms of hepatitis B virus infection. Chronic hepatitis C may be associated with significant lifetime morbidity and mortality. In addition, chronic hepatitis, a potential complication of acute viral hepatitis, is being recognized with increasing frequency in children.

ETIOLOGICAL AGENTS

Hepatitis A Virus[26]

Hepatitis A virus (HAV) is a 27-nm RNA virus, a member of the picornavirus group. Transmission of HAV is predominantly by the fecal-oral route, although saliva and urine are potentially important vehicles, particularly among siblings. Contaminated shellfish, polluted water, and travel to endemic areas also have been identified in the acquisition of type A infection. Viruslike particles capable of causing hepatitis A infection in primates have been demonstrated by immune electron microscopy in the stools of patients who are ill with hepatitis A. Antigen can be detected in the stool (as well as in serum and possibly in urine) as early as 2 to 3 weeks before acute illness and as much as 1 week after the onset of illness; recovery in the stool decreases as jaundice becomes evident. Aggregation of the viral particles present in stool can be achieved by adding serum containing hepatitis A antibody. This antibody is recoverable in patients' serum after antigen no longer is found in the stool. Hepatitis A antibody is present at least 10 years after infection and probably confers lifelong immunity to the virus. It now is possible to grow hepatitis A in cell culture.

Hepatitis B Virus

Hepatitis B virus (HBV) is a 42-nm hepadnavirus and consists of a surface antigen (HBsAg), a core antigen (HBcAg), an e antigen (HBeAg), and DNA with DNA polymerase.[16] Although previously thought to be transmitted only parenterally, hence the designation serum hepatitis, it now is accepted that HBV can be transmitted orally. HBsAg and HBeAg may be present in saliva and other secretions. Bloodsucking insects also have been incriminated in transmission of the virus, as has ingestion of contaminated shellfish. In hyperendemic areas (Asia, Africa, Southern Europe, Latin America), HBV infections occur in infancy and early childhood, although aggressive immunization programs in certain of these areas, such as Taiwan, have substantially lowered risks. Horizontal transmission may occur in early childhood from infectious siblings and among institutionalized patients. Improperly sterilized syringes and nosocomial transmission are means of acquisition of HBV in Eastern Europe.

Age of acquisition of the virus is an important prognostic determinant.[9] Perinatal transmission from mother to infant leads to chronic infection. Transmission is more likely if the mother is HBeAg antigen-positive but appears highly unlikely if maternal antibody to HBeAg is present. The risk of infection to the infant appears to be markedly increased (80%) if the mother has had clinical hepatitis in the third trimester of pregnancy. The route of infection may be transplacental, by the swallowing of blood at the time of delivery, or by close contact postpartum. Acquisition of HBsAg after birth is based on conversion from HBsAg negativity to positivity during the postpartum period. Infants acquiring HBsAg and HBeAg have a recognized tendency to become chronic carriers and to have features of persistent hepatitis on biopsy. However, infants of carrier mothers in whom acute fulminant hepatitis occurs during the first 6 months of life have been reported. The long-term effects of acquiring HBV in infancy include cirrhosis and hepatocellular carcinoma with an annual incidence among 6- to 14-year-old children of 0.70

per 100,000 in countries such as Taiwan, where HBV is endemic.[9]

Hepatitis C Virus[5]

Hepatitis C virus (HCV), which was recognized in 1989, is a 30- to 50-nm RNA virus present in the serum of infected individuals.[25] Multiple HCV genotypes exist because of constant mutation, and the virus fails to elicit cross neutralizing antibodies in animal models. Recent studies have shown HCV to cause the majority of cases of posttransfusion hepatitis and 50% to 60% of cases of sporadic non-A, non-B hepatitis. The prevalence of HCV in the general U.S. population is estimated at 1.8%. In children, the seroprevalence rate for those without known risk factors is 0.2% for those younger than 12 years and 0.4% for those 12 to 19 years of age. Most children are infected by parenteral exposure to contaminated blood and blood products. Increased prevalence rates are noted in children with hemophilia (60% to 90%), children with thalassemia, renal dialysis patients, cancer survivors, institutionalized children and in children who have received solid organ transplants. An outbreak in 1993-94 occurred in a group of children who had received contaminated intravenous immunoglobulin.[5,22] Currently all blood products are screened with HCV second-generation antibody tests, but the risk of HCV infection per recipient is still 0.1%. High transmission rates (up to 80% to 90%) are also noted in injection drug users and in individuals who inhale cocaine. The average rate of vertical transmission in utero from HCV-positive mothers to their infants is about 4%; rates increase in mothers coinfected with the human immunodeficiency virus and in mothers with high viral loads. Horizontal transmission from parent to child or from sibling to sibling also occurs at a rate of 4%. Sexual transmission occurs infrequently. Screening recommendations have been made by the AAP Committee on Infectious Diseases and are summarized in Box 216-1.

BOX 216-1

SCREENING RECOMMENDATIONS FOR HCV INFECTION

- Persons at high risk
- Injection drug users
- Hemodialysis patients
- Recipients of one or more units of blood or blood products before 1992
- Recipients of Gammagard intravenous immunoglobulin (Baxter Healthcare Co.) between April 1, 1993, and February 23, 1994
- Children with clinical non-A, non-B hepatitis
- Infants born to mothers infected with HCV after 12 months of age
- International adoptees born to high-risk mothers
- High-risk pregnant women

Derived from American Academy of Pediatrics, Committee on Infectious Diseases: *Pediatrics* 101:481, 1998.

Hepatitis D virus

Hepatitis D virus (HDV) replicates in the liver and is associated with a protein, the hepatitis D antigen (HDAg), which can be found in both the liver and the serum of individuals who have the disease. The virus is unique in that it is defective and requires a coat of HBsAg to replicate effectively. Acquisition of HDV is similar to that of HBV. The characteristic clinical feature of hepatitis D virus infection is that it increases the severity of hepatitis B virus infection.

Hepatitis E Virus[18,24]

Hepatitis E virus (HEV), a 27- to 34-nm single-stranded RNA virus, is the cause of epidemic, enterically transmitted hepatitis, that has occurred in India, Pakistan, Nepal, Russia, China, Algeria, central Africa, Peru, and Mexico. Only imported cases have been identified in the United States. The illness usually occurs in areas where the water supply is contaminated by feces; viruslike particles in stool specimens can be agglutinated by serum from convalescent patients. Serological identification of HesAg is diagnostic.

Hepatitis G Virus[1]

The hepatitis G virus (HGV) was identified in 1995 and is an RNA virus of the *Flaviviridae* family and a distant relative of HCV. HGV is mainly transmitted parenterally through blood and blood products and through intravenous drug use. Its prevalence was 23% in one group of patients with posttransfusion associated non-A, non-B, non-C hepatitis. The infection is self-limited but may cause a carrier state. The virus does not replicate in the liver and does not appear to alter the course and severity of those coinfected with HCV.

Hepatitis GB Virus C (HGBV-C)[41]

HGBV-C was discovered in the sera of West African individuals with high risk for hepatitis. It is a RNA virus of the *Flaviviridae* family and shares high sequence homology with HGV and may be considered a different isolate of HGV. Transmission is parenteral, and transfusion recipients are at high risk for infection. Although the prevalence of infection with HGBV-C is reported to be 5% to 13% in patients with non-A-E hepatitis and cryptogenic cirrhosis, there is little evidence that HGV causes hepatitis in humans.

TT-virus[32,33]

TT-virus (TTV) is a DNA virus discovered in 1997 in the sera of three out of five patients with biopsy-proven hepatitis and elevated serum alanine aminotransferase levels. In North America, the prevalence of TTV has been found to be 1% in blood donors, 15% in patients with cryptogenic cirrhosis, 27% in patients with idiopathic fulminant hepatic failure, 18% in patients with a history of exposure to blood products, and 4% in patients without parenteral risk factors. The role of TTV in the pathogenesis of acute and chronic liver disease is yet to be determined.

CLINICAL FEATURES

Acute Hepatitis

The clinical features of acute types A, B, and C viral hepatitis in children are reviewed in Table 216-1. HAV infection is heralded by an abrupt onset associated with fever, malaise, anorexia, nausea, vomiting, and upper abdominal discomfort. Darkening of the urine and enlargement and tenderness of the liver follow. Shortly thereafter, clinical jaundice becomes apparent. The bilirubin level increases in both direct and indirect fractions but generally does not exceed a total of 15 mg/dl. Aminotransferase elevation generally does not last more than 3 weeks. In general, the clinical and laboratory abnormalities do not persist beyond 4 weeks. The disease rarely is fulminant.

In highly endemic areas, hepatitis B is acquired either perinatally or at a very young age. In low prevalence countries, hepatitis B occurs more often in adolescents and occurs sporadically in contrast to HAV infection, which may occur in epidemics. The onset usually is insidious. Extrahepatic manifestations such as skin rash and arthralgia are common and may be prodromal. In fact, hepatitis B should be kept in mind in the differential diagnosis of serum sickness-like illness. However, younger children may be asymptomatic. The duration of illness usually is 4 to 6 weeks, generally somewhat longer than in type A. Aminotransferase elevation usually peaks approximately 1 month after the onset of illness. Although more than 90% of children recover without sequelae, fulminant hepatitis is seen more frequently than in hepatitis A.

Acute hepatitis C cannot be distinguished rigorously on clinical grounds from hepatitis B. Acute HCV infection is generally asymptomatic; however, acute liver failure has been reported in a 5-month-old who acquired HCV perinatally.

HDV infection in children presents in a more severe form than HBV infection in that there is a more marked elevation in serum transaminases and 12% to 16% of cases present with cirrhosis.

Hepatitis E is similar clinically to hepatitis A. Cholestasis may be more common than with hepatitis A, and elevation of serum aminotransferases is modest. The most unusual clinical feature of the illness is its high mortality rate in pregnant women (approximately 10%).

Fulminant Hepatitis

Fulminant hepatitis (hepatic encephalopathy within 8 weeks of onset of illness), enumerated previously, is heralded by the following laboratory aberrations[37]:

1. Prolonged prothrombin time (more than 4 seconds over control), unresponsive to large doses of vitamin K
2. Marked elevation of serum bilirubin (greater than 20 mg/dl)
3. Leukocytosis (greater than 12,500/mm^3)
4. Hypoglycemia

Fulminant disease may occur in two forms: massive hepatic necrosis or submassive hepatic necrosis. Known as acute yellow atrophy, massive hepatic necrosis rarely is asso-

Table 216-1 Clinical Features of Acute Viral Hepatitis

	HAV	HBV	HCV
Characteristics			
Age distribution	Children and young adults	All age groups	All age groups
Route of infection	Predominantly fecal-oral	Parenteral-oral	Parenteral-oral
Incubation period (days)	15-40	50-180	20-90
Onset	Acute	Insidious	Insidious
Duration of clinical illness	Weeks	Weeks to months	Weeks to months
Virus present			
Feces	Late incubation, acute	May be present	Absent
Blood	Late incubation, acute	Late incubation, acute, may persist for months	Present chronically
Signs and Symptoms			
Fever	High, common early	Moderate, less common	Moderate, less common
Nausea and vomiting	Common	Less common	Less common
Anorexia	Severe	Mild to moderate	Mild to moderate
Arthralgia or arthritis	Rare	Common	?
Rash or urticaria	Rare	Common	?
Laboratory Findings			
Aminotransferase elevation	1-3 wk	Months	Fluctuates for months
Bilirubin elevation	Weeks	May be months	Unusual
HBsAg	Absent	Present	Absent
Severity	Usually mild	Often severe	Usually mild
Progression to chronic hepatitis	Rare	More common	High rate
Immunity	Homologous, lifelong (?)	Homologous, lifelong (?)	?
Prevention	Immune serum globulin	Hyperimmune globulin; vaccine	Screen donor blood

Modified from Krugman S, Katz SL: *Infectious diseases of children*, ed 8, St Louis, 1985, Mosby; and deBelle RC, Lester R: *Pediatr Clin North Am* 22:948, 1995.

ciated with survival in the absence of liver transplantation; the patient dies within 10 days of onset of illness unless a liver transplant is performed. Submassive hepatic necrosis, often extensive, may lead to death within 3 weeks after the onset of illness or progress to chronic liver disease; a small number of patients recover completely. A characteristic form of bridging necrosis—that is, necrosis that extends from one portal area to another—has been described in patients who have submassive hepatic necrosis.

CHRONIC HEPATITIS

Continuing evidence of hepatic inflammation beyond the period generally expected for resolution of acute viral hepatitis always should suggest chronic hepatitis. However, acute hepatitis may resolve slowly over a period longer than 6 months, and alternatively, evidence of chronicity may be present earlier than 3 months. Chronic viral hepatitis can be associated with a broad spectrum of liver histology, ranging from normal to advanced cirrhosis.

In contrast to HBV, HCV, and HDV infections, hepatitis resulting from HAV or HEV do not progress to chronicity, cirrhosis, or a carrier state. Approximately 10% of patients who have acute HBV hepatitis develop chronic liver disease, many with the benign clinical pattern associated with mild nonspecific hepatitis. Host genetic factors may be relevant in the establishment of chronicity, as may characteristics of the causative agent, as suggested by the association of HBeAg with progression to chronic hepatitis.

Children with HBV infection are initially HBsAg and HBeAg positive. During this stage, which may persist for years, children are immunologically tolerant to HBV, and serum HBV-DNA levels are very high. The child is very infectious and is a source of horizontal transmission in the community. Serum aminotransferase levels fluctuate and may be in the upper limit of normal range. During childhood, conversion from HBeAg to anti-HBe may occur spontaneously with a rate of 2% to 5% per year; children born to mothers with HBsAg have a lower HBeAg clearance rate.[10] Seroconversion to anti-HBe is often preceded by a transient elevation in serum transaminases. Forty percent of children will clear HBeAg within 1 year after the transient elevation in transaminases is noted. After anti-HBe seroconversion, HBV-DNA levels remain low or undetectable, but HBV-DNA may be present by polymerase chain reaction up to 10 years after seroconversion.[7] Most children remain HBsAg positive and this chronic carrier state is generally unassociated with overt disease. The annual HBsAg clearance rate is as low as 0.56%.[19] Liver cirrhosis is encountered in 3% to 5% of children with chronic HBV. These children are at risk for developing hepatocellular carcinoma before adulthood. Serial serum alpha-fetoprotein measurements and liver ultrasound examinations should be performed on these patients.

Two characteristic clinical features of HCV infection are (1) fluctuation in the serum concentration of the aminotransferases and (2) progression to chronicity (50% to 80% of patients). The majority of patients remain asymptomatic without stigmata of chronic liver disease. Liver histology shows mild to moderate hepatitis,[23] and fibrosis increases with duration of infection. Cirrhosis has been reported in infancy. A recent study indicated that patients with chronic HCV infection who become infected with HAV are at substantial risk of fulminant hepatic failure.[44] HCV may be as common a cause of hepatocellular carcinoma as is HBV.

HGV is thought to cause a chronic carrier state but little liver damage. The potential role of HGV in cirrhosis and hepatocellular carcinoma is currently being investigated.

Other Causes of Hepatitis

Other entities are associated with chronic hepatic inflammation. These include chronic inflammation secondary to autoimmune hepatitis, drugs, metabolic liver diseases, and fatty liver secondary to obesity.

Chronic hepatitis has been associated in the pediatric population with autoimmune diseases such as ulcerative colitis, thyroiditis, and systemic lupus erythematosus. Indeed, immunological mechanisms have been invoked in its pathogenesis. For example, autoantibodies including antinuclear, antimitochondrial, anti-liver, and anti-kidney microsomal antibodies,[14] and anti-smooth muscle antibodies have been identified in chronic active hepatitis, although their presence may be an epiphenomenon. Similarly, immune complexes have been associated with the extrahepatic manifestations of both acute and chronic active hepatitis, although no definite role in the perpetuation of liver disease has been identified. Altered cell-mediated immunity to HBsAg also may play a role in pathogenesis.

Autoimmune Hepatitis

Autoimmune hepatitis (AIH) is a chronic necroinflammatory hepatitis characterized by mononuclear cell infiltration of the portal ducts, hypergammaglobulinemia and non–liver-specific autoantibodies.[31] Significant clinical, chemical, and histological findings are associated with chronic AIH.[27,30] There are two types of AIH classified according to the presence or absence of certain autoantibodies: AIH type 1 is characterized by the presence of antinuclear antibody (ANA) and anti-smooth muscle antibody (ASMA), whereas AIH type 2 is characterized by anti liver-kidney microsomal antibodies (anti-LKM).[30] The mode of presentation is highly variable; therefore, AIH should be excluded with serological testing in all children presenting with signs of liver disease. Unlike adults, in whom the onset usually is insidious, 50% or more of pediatric patients affected with both AIH types have an acute onset of disease much like that of those who have acute viral hepatitis. Fever, headache, nausea, anorexia, fatigue and jaundice are common. A small number of patients may be seriously ill, with evidence of portal hypertension or hepatocellular failure. Approximately two thirds of affected children are girls. A summary of clinical findings in 38 patients reported by Dubois and Silverman[15] revealed the following: jaundice, 87%; hepatomegaly, 79%; splenomegaly, 74%; ascites, 24%; amenorrhea, 18%; acne, 16%; clubbing, 16%; and gynecomastia, 5%. Associated extrahepatic manifestations reported included nephrotic syndrome, autoimmune thyroiditis, Behçet's disease, ulcerative colitis, insulin dependent diabetes, urticaria pigmentosa, vitiligo, hypoparathyroidism and Addison's disease.[17] Although AIH type 2 patients have higher tendency to present in acute liver failure, the overall prognosis of type 2 disease is not different from type 1 disease.[17,31]

Drug-Induced Hepatitis

Drug-induced liver disease may occur as an unexpected idiosyncratic reaction to a normally nontoxic drug or be an expected consequence to a toxic dose (acetaminophen) and may cause signs of acute hepatitis and chronic hepatitis. Up to 25% of fulminant hepatitis cases in adults are drug induced. There are some forms of drug-induced liver disease that are more common in children (e.g., valproic acid-induced liver injury). Many drugs are known to cause hepatitis, including isonicotinic acid hydrazide or isoniazid (INH), alphamethyldopa, and oxyphenisatin acetate.

Hepatitis Secondary to Metabolic Liver Disease

Metabolic liver disease may present with elevated transaminases and hyperbilirubinemia (1) in the neonatal period (e.g., galactosemia, hemochromatosis, tyrosinemia, alpha$_1$-antitrypsin deficiency, cystic fibrosis, Alagille syndrome, or defects in amino acid and organic acid synthesis and in fatty acid oxidation), (2) in infancy (progressive familial intrahepatic cholestasis [PFIC] types 1 to 4, inborn errors of bile acid synthesis, glycogen storage disease, or Niemann-Pick type C disease) and (3) later in childhood (Wilson's disease, alpha$_1$-antitrypsin deficiency, or fatty liver).

Alpha$_1$-antitrypsin (α_1AT) deficiency is the most common genetic cause of liver disease in children with an incidence of 1 in 1600 to 2000 live births. It results from the retention of the mutant α_1AT inside the endoplasmic reticulum of liver cells which may predispose certain individuals with homozygous phenotype ZZ to significant liver injury.[34]

Wilson's disease is an autosomal recessive disorder affecting 1 in 30,000 people, which results from a defect in the gene that encodes a copper-binding membrane protein regulating the transport of copper across cell membranes. Accumulation of copper in the hepatocytes and other organs results in a constellation of clinical symptoms including hepatitis, neuropsychiatric disease, and Kayser-Fleischer rings in the Descemet's membrane of the cornea.[39]

Inborn errors of metabolism including errors in bile acid synthesis, errors in amino acid and organic acid synthesis, errors in fatty acid oxidation, and peroxisomal defects may also present with hepatitis either in early infancy or childhood. Galactosemia is an autosomal recessive disorder resulting in decreased production of galactose 1-phosphate uridyl transferase that presents in the neonatal period with cholestatic jaundice and hepatitis. In newborns who have cholestasis, idiopathic giant cell hepatitis is found more frequently than is hepatitis secondary to a specific causative agent.

Tyrosinemia (hereditary tyrosinemia type 1) is an autosomal recessive disease that results in a deficiency in the enzyme fumarylacetoacetate hydrolase, the last enzyme in the tyrosine degradation pathway. This deficiency leads to an accumulation of succinylacetone, which causes hepatorenal disease characterized by progressive liver disease. Patients present in the first 2 years if life with failure to thrive, hypoproteinemia, severe coagulopathy unresponsive to vitamin K therapy, and renal Fanconi's syndrome.

Alagille syndrome, or paucity of the intrahepatic bile ducts, is the most common form of cholestatic liver disease. It is caused by mutation in the human jagged 1 gene. Patients present in the first 2 years of life with jaundice and hepatitis. Diagnostic features are discussed below. PFIC types 1 to 4 result from a variety of defects in the transport protein involved in the excretion of bile acids; patients present with pruritus and elevated transaminases. Hepatitis may be seen in the context of other systemic/metabolic diseases such as cystic fibrosis and obesity.

DIAGNOSIS

A plethora of tests are available for the diagnosis of a child with hepatitis. Referral to a pediatric gastroenterologist is recommended, because close monitoring of the child is often required. A child with acute hepatitis should be evaluated with measurement of serum alanine aminotransferase (ALT) and aspartate aminotransferase (AST), conjugated and unconjugated bilirubin, γ-glutamyl transferase (GGT), alkaline phosphatase, prothrombin time, and blood ammonia level.

The various types of viral hepatitis often can be discriminated on the basis of their clinical and epidemiological characteristics, although distinction may be difficult in sporadic cases. Sensitive radioimmunoassay techniques are available for detection of antibody to hepatitis A (anti-hepatitis A). The presence of IgM class anti-hepatitis A coinciding with clinical symptoms confirms the diagnosis of acute hepatitis A. The IgM response is followed rapidly by the development of IgG anti-hepatitis A, which persists for years.

The presence of HBsAg remains the principal means of diagnosing hepatitis B and reflects ongoing infection. This is the first marker to appear and is detected 1 to 2 weeks postexposure. HBeAg reflects increased viral replication and infectivity and appears concurrently with HBV-DNA. Both of these markers peak in parallel with symptoms. Quantitative HBV-DNA or HBV viral load testing is available and correlates with disease activity. Anti-HBs confers passive immunity and indicates resolving or past infection. Anti-HBs is seen after vaccination. Anti-HBc is the fourth serologic marker, which appears 3 to 5 weeks after HBsAg and indicates ongoing or past infection. This marker does not appear after vaccination.

A whole series of tests has been developed for the diagnosis of HCV infection. The first-generation enzyme-linked immunoassay (ELISA) for antibody to HCV (C100-3) had relatively poor sensitivity and specificity. Second generation ELISAs are highly sensitive and specific, as is the recombinant immunoblot assay (RIBA) of which the RIBA II test is thought to be best; however, neither of these tests, which now are available commercially, become positive until weeks after exposure to the virus.[2] In contrast, the highly sensitive polymerase chain reaction assay becomes positive within days after exposure to the virus. Vertically acquired infection is confirmed by the presence of HCV-RNA in serum in the first months of life or by the persistence of anti-HCV antibody beyond 18 months of age.

A fluorescence test for hepatitis E antigen in hepatocyte cytoplasm has been modified for assay of anti-HEV in the serum of affected patients. However, this assay is not available widely.[24] A test for anti-HDV is commercially available. HGV and TTV infections are diagnosed by detection of HGV-RNA and TTV-DNA by polymerase chain reaction methods.

If the history, clinical features, and serological tests leave the diagnosis in doubt, other causes, both viral and nonviral, must be ruled out. Clinical features may help discriminate among other infectious causes, for example, Epstein-Barr virus or leptospirosis. Additional infectious agents associated with inflammation of the liver include cytomegalovirus, toxoplasmosis, herpes simplex virus 6 (HSV6), echovirus, coxsackievirus, rubeola virus, adenovirus, and parvovirus B19; in children who have acquired immunodeficiency syndrome (AIDS), *Mycobacterium avium intracellulare* should be considered. Nasopharyngeal and rectal viral cultures and HIV serology should be ordered when the etiology is in doubt.

Drug-Induced Hepatitis

Noninfectious causes of hepatitis include hepatotoxic drugs and toxins. To evaluate for drug or toxin-induced hepatitis a thorough medical history should be obtained for prescribed medications, herbal teas, poisons, and ingestion of wild mushrooms. A serum acetaminophen level and a urine toxicology screen should be performed when one's index of suspicion is high.

Hepatitis Secondary to Metabolic Disease

When metabolic liver disease is suspected, the child should be evaluated with a blood ammonia level, serum glucose, blood gases with pH, blood lactate level, and urinalysis. To distinguish among different types of metabolic defects, the following tests may be ordered: serum and urine amino acids and organic acids (to evaluate for defects in the metabolism of amino acids) urine ketones, serum and urine carnitine, and dicarboxylic fatty acids (for evaluation of fatty acid oxidation defects) and serum bile acids and mass spectrometry of serum and urinary bile acids (for evaluation of inborn errors of bile acid synthesis). A very elevated GGT (800 IU/L), hypercholesterolemia, dysmorphic facies, cardiac anomalies, "butterfly" vertebra, and posterior embryotoxon on eye examination are diagnostic features of Alagille syndrome. α_1AT deficiency is diagnosed by the presence of serological phenotype ZZ or SZ, serum α_1AT less than 50 mg/dl, and by liver biopsy.

Wilson's disease is diagnosed by decreased serum ceruloplasmin (>20 mg/dl), elevated urinary copper excretion (>100 μg/24 hours), and elevated liver copper concentration (greater than 250 μg/g of dry weight). PFIC should be suspected in any child with elevated serum bile acids, low or elevated GGT, and elevated transaminases; liver biopsy may not be particularly helpful in distinguishing among the four different types. Also, in the neonatal period, urine-reducing substances and serum galactose-1-phosphate uridyl phosphatase should be measured if galactosemia is suspected; urine succinylacetone and alpha-fetoprotein should be measured for detection of tyrosinemia; and a sweat chloride test is indicated if cystic fibrosis is suspected.

In AIH, hypergammaglobulinemia is a common laboratory finding, averaging approximately twice the normal level for age. However, a normal IgG value should not exclude the diagnosis of AIH. Aminotransferases and the total bilirubin levels are elevated to a variable degree. Autoantibodies such as ANA/ASMA or anti-LKM may be present. Histologically, portal tracts are infiltrated by lymphocytes and plasma cells. Inflammatory cells often infiltrate the parenchyma, accompanied by necrosis of cells at the periphery of the hepatic lobule. Fibrosis may be seen to a variable degree, or true cirrhosis may be present.

Liver biopsy is essential for diagnosis when chronic liver disease is suspected, provided it can be performed safely. A needle biopsy is adequate, and the risks are low. An accurate diagnosis is essential because treatment is predicated, at least partially, on the degree of activity seen on biopsy. The decision to biopsy a liver should depend on the duration of illness and whether the patient conforms to the clinical course of acute viral hepatitis. If the history, clinical features, or laboratory values suggest chronicity (of 3 to 6 months duration), a biopsy should be performed. Similarly, Wilson's disease must be ruled out in any child who has hepatitis, because of the availability of therapy. Wilson's disease always must be considered in the differential diagnosis of pediatric liver disease, especially because Kayser-Fleischer rings and neurological findings may be absent and the ceruloplasmin may be normal in juveniles.[45] Thus, a liver biopsy with determination of the hepatic copper level is essential.[35] If other metabolic liver disease is suspected, the liver biopsy should also be examined with the electron microscope to determine the hepatic ultrastructure.

THERAPY AND PREVENTION

Viral Hepatitis

Hospitalization generally is unnecessary for the patient who has acute viral hepatitis. However, the infant and young child should be hospitalized and observed closely because of the rapidity with which hepatic failure can ensue in this age group. Regardless of age, if evidence of impending hepatic failure is present, the child must be hospitalized and appropriate therapy instituted. Although protein restriction coupled with high carbohydrate intake is important in hepatic failure, no benefit of a particular diet has been demonstrated with respect to course and prognosis for the child who has an uncomplicated case of acute viral hepatitis. Similarly, restriction of activity does not appear to affect the course or outcome, although the child who has hepatitis will desire increased rest.

Because recovery of HAV in the patient's stool decreases rapidly after the onset of jaundice, return to school at this point, provided the child feels well, does not appear to present an undue risk of infection to others. However, if the child appears noticeably jaundiced, his or her feelings regarding that appearance, as well as the concern of others about contact, may necessitate staying home from school until the jaundice is reduced or abated completely.

Although household contacts of the patient who has hepatitis A likely already are infected by the time of diagnosis, the physician still should stress scrupulous hand washing and the use of disposable eating utensils in the patient's home until jaundice clears. Pooled serum immune globulin (Ig) is of documented benefit in suppressing the clinical symptoms of hepatitis A. Ig for intramuscular administration when given within two weeks postexposure is 80% to 90% effective in preventing symptomatic infection. Box 216-2 shows the recent recommendations for use of Ig for postexposure prophylaxis. Household contacts should receive 0.02 to 0.04 ml/kg of body weight intramuscularly as soon as possible after exposure.

Newborn infants of infected mothers do not need special care if the mother is not jaundiced. Neither withholding of breast-feeding nor Ig administration is recommended unless the mother is jaundiced. The American Academy of Pediatrics has generated detailed recommendations for control of HAV in day care centers.[4] Children and adults with HAV infection should be excluded from the center until 1 week after onset of illness or until Ig prophylaxis has been initiated. Children traveling to endemic areas also should be immunized prophylactically.[21] Box 216-3 shows the indications for vaccination for HAV, and Table 216-2 shows the recommendations for pre-exposure immunoprophylaxis of HAV infection for travelers. There are two inactivated vaccines currently available in the United States that are approved for children 2 to 18 years old and for adults. The vaccine is given in a two- or three-dose schedule depending on the formulation. Table 216-3 shows the recommended doses for HAV vaccination. Children with underlying liver disease should receive the HAV vaccination.[29] Either pediatric formulation of Havrix induces seroconversion rates greater than 90% after the initial dose and 100% after the second dose.[40,46]

The possibility for preventing hepatitis B has been improved dramatically by introduction of safe, effective recombinant vaccines[36] and by the recommendation by the American Academy of Pediatrics that all healthy newborn infants should be immunized. Detailed recommendations regarding doses and preexposure and postexposure prophylaxis are provided in Box 216-4, Tables 216-4 and 216-5. An infant born to an HBsAg-positive mother or a mother who has had hepatitis B during pregnancy should be given 0.5 ml of hepatitis B immune globulin (HBIG) intramuscularly immediately after birth and 0.5 ml of hepatitis B vaccine intramuscularly within the first week of life and again 1 and 6 months later. A preliminary study of neonates born to mothers who were both HBsAg-positive and HBeAg-positive demonstrated that administration of recombinant hepatitis B vaccine to infants at birth, 1, and 2 months of age without concomitant immune globulin resulted in a very high protective efficacy rate against the chronic carrier state[36] and was very safe.[38] Data linking breast-feeding to the acquisition of viremia are equivocal, but HBsAg-positive mothers whose infants have received immunoprophylaxis may breast-feed without risk of transmitting HBV to the infant. The first universal vaccination program was launched in Taiwan in 1984 and included neonates, preschool children, and adults. The HBsAg carrier

BOX 216-2

PERSONS WHO SHOULD RECEIVE PROPHYLAXIS WITH IMMUNOGLOBULIN AFTER EXPOSURE TO HAV

- Household and sexual contacts of those infected with HAV
- Newborn infants whose mothers develop symptoms 2 weeks before or within 1 week after delivery
- Child care center employees
- Children and their household members who come in contact with an infected child or a child care center employee

Derived from American Academy of Pediatrics. In Peter G, editor: *1997 Red Book: Report of the Committee on Infectious Diseases*, ed 24, Elk Grove Village, Ill, 1997, American Academy of Pediatrics.

BOX 216-3

INDICATIONS FOR HAV VACCINATION

- Travelers to endemic areas
- Children more than 2 years of age living in endemic areas or areas with high rates of periodic infection (Native Americans or Alaskan Natives) if tested and have absent HAV IgM
- Patients with chronic liver disease
- Homosexual and bisexual men
- Users of injection and illicit drugs
- Those at high risk of exposure secondary to their occupation

Derived from American Academy of Pediatrics. In Peter G, editor: *1997 Red Book: Report of the Committee on Infectious Diseases*, ed 24, Elk Grove Village, Ill, 1997, American Academy of Pediatrics.

Table 216-2 Recommendations for Preexposure Immunoprophylaxis of Hepatitis A Infection for Travelers

Age (Years)	Likely Exposure (Months)	Recommended Prophylaxis
<2	<3	IG 0.02 ml/kg†
	3-5	IG 0.06 ml/kg†
	Long term	IG 0.06 ml/kg at departure and every 5 months thereafter†
≥2	<3‡	HAV vaccine*§ or IG 0.02 ml/kg†
	3-5‡	HAV vaccine*§ or IG 0.06 ml/kg†
	Long term	HAV vaccine*§

From American Academy of Pediatrics. In Pickering LK, editor: *Red Book 2000: Report of the Committee on Infectious Diseases*, ed 25, Elk Grove Village, Ill, 2000, American Academy of Pediatrics.

*To ensure protection in travelers whose departure is imminent, IG also may be given.

†IG should be administered deep into a large muscle mass. Ordinarily, no more than 5 ml should be administered in any one site in an adult or large child, and no more than 3 ml should be given to small children and infants in any one site.

‡Vaccine is preferable, but IG is an acceptable alternative.

§Dose and schedule of HAV vaccine as recommended according to age in Table 216-3.

Table 216-3 Recommended Doses and Schedules for Hepatitis A Virus (HAV) Inactivated Vaccines

Age (Years)	Vaccine*	Antigen Dose†	Volume per Dose (ml)	Number of Doses	Schedule
2 through 18	Havrix (SKB)‡	360 EL.U	0.5	3	Initial, 1 mo, and 6-12 mo later
	Havrix (SKB)	720 EL.U	0.5	2	Initial, and 6-12 mo later
	Vaqta (Merck)	25U§	0.5	2	Initial, and 6-12 mo later
19 and older	Havrix (SKB)	1440 EL.U	1.0	2	Initial, and 6-12 mo later
	Vaqta (Merck)	50 U§	1.0	2	Initial, and 6-12 mo later

From American Academy of Pediatrics. In Pickering LK, editor: *Red Book 2000: Report of the Committee on Infectious Diseases,* ed 25, Elk Grove Village, Ill, 2000, American Academy of Pediatrics.
*SKB indicates SmithKline Beecham.
†EL.U. indicates enzyme-linked immunoassay units.
‡Children receiving 360 EL.U. for the first dose should receive two additional doses of either pediatric formulation (360 EL.U. or 720 EL.U) to complete the schedule.
§Antigen units (each unit is equivalent to approximately 1 mg of viral protein).

BOX 216-4

PERSONS WHO SHOULD RECEIVE HEPATITIS B IMMUNIZATION

- All infants (infants of HBsAg-positive mothers require postexposure immunoprophylaxis with HBIG and vaccine)
- Infants and children at risk of acquisition of HBV by person-to-person (horizontal) transmission should be immunized by 6-9 mo of age
- Adolescents* (special efforts should be made to vaccinate those adolescents in the categories of high risk for hepatitis B virus [HBV] infection)
- Users of intravenous drugs
- Sexually active heterosexual persons with more than one sex partner in the previous 6 months or with a sexually transmitted disease
- Sexually active homosexual or bisexual males
- Health care workers at risk of exposure to blood or body fluids
- Residents and staff of institutions for developmentally disabled persons
- Staff of nonresidential child care and school programs for developmentally disabled persons if attended by a known HBV carrier
- Hemodialysis patients
- Patients with bleeding disorders who receive certain blood products
- Household contacts and sexual partners of HBV carriers
- Members of households with adoptees from countries where HBV infection is endemic who are HBsAg positive
- International travelers who will live for more than 6 mo in an area of high HBV endemicity and who otherwise will be at risk
- Inmates of long-term correctional facilities

Derived from American Academy of Pediatrics. In Peter G, editor: *1997 Red Book: Report of the Committee on Infectious Diseases,* ed 24, Elk Grove Village, Ill, 1997, American Academy of Pediatrics.
*Implementation can be initiated before children reach adolescence.

Table 216-4 Recommended Dosages of Hepatitis B Vaccines*

	Vaccine†‡			
	Recombivax HB§ Dose:		Energix-B‖¶ Dose:	
	μg	(ml)	μg	(ml)
Infants of HBsAg-negative mothers and children <11 yr	2.5	(0.5)#	10	(0.5)
Infants of HBsAg-positive mothers (HBIG [0.5 ml] should also be given)	5	(0.5)** (1.0)#	10	(0.5)
Children and adolescents 11-19 yr	5	(0.5)**	20	(1.0)
Adults ≥20 yr	10	(1.0)**	20	(1.0)
Dialysis patients and other immunosuppressed adults	40	(1.0)††	40	(2.0)‡‡

Modified from American Academy of Pediatrics. In Peter G, editor: *1997 Red Book: Report of the Committee on Infectious Diseases,* ed 24, Elk Grove Village, Ill, 1997, American Academy of Pediatrics.
*Vaccines should be stored at 2° to 8° C. Freezing destroys effectiveness.
†Heptavax B (available from Merck & Co.), a plasma-derived vaccine, also is licensed but no longer produced in the United States.
‡Both vaccines are administered in a three-dose schedule.
§Available from Merck & Co.
‖The Food and Drug Administration has approved this vaccine for use in an optional four-dose schedule at 0, 1, 2, and 12 months.
¶Available from SmithKline Beecham.
#Pediatric formulation.
**Adult formulation.
††Special formulation for dialysis patients.
‡‡Two 1.0-ml doses given at one site in a four-dose schedule at 0, 1, 2, and 6 to 12 months.

Table 216-5 Guide to Postexposure Immunoprophylaxis for Hepatitis B Infection

Type of Exposure	Immunoprophylaxis
Perinatal	HBIG + vaccination
Sexual—acute infection	HBIG + vaccination
Sexual—chronic carrier	Vaccination
Household contact—chronic carrier	Vaccination
Household contact—acute case with identifiable blood exposure	HBIG + vaccination
Infant (<12 mo)—acute case in primary caregiver	HBIG + vaccination
Accidental—percutaneous/permucosal	HBIG ± vaccination

Modified from American Academy of Pediatrics. In Peter G, editor: *1997 Red Book: Report of the Committee on Infectious Diseases,* ed 24, Elk Grove Village Ill, 1997, American Academy of Pediatrics.

rate decreased from 10% to less than 1% after vaccination of children more than 10 years old. Anti-HBc positivity decreased from 36% to 16% in children more than 10 years old. These findings indicate that vaccination decreased both the vertical and horizontal transmission rates. The average annual incidence of hepatocellular carcinoma dropped from 0.70 per 100,000 children between 1981 and 1986 to 0.36 between 1990 and 1994.[9,11] Hepatitis B immunization also protects against HDV infection.

Alpha-interferon is the only commercially available antiviral agent that is recommended for treatment of chronic HBV infection. Recent studies showed that 25% to 50% of children with chronic HBV treated with alpha-interferon developed seroconversion to anti-HBe. There is poor effect on HBsAg clearance, but serum transaminases and liver histology improve.[42,43] Lamivudine (or 3-TC) has been shown to increase rates of seroconversion to anti-HBe and suppress HBV-DNA in adults[12]; pediatric trials are now in progress.

Currently, no vaccine is available for the prevention of HCV infection. Natural infection does not protect from reinfection with the same or different genotypes either in patients or experimentally infected chimpanzees. The most important strategy for controlling hepatitis C is screening donor blood for anti-HCV because preliminary studies have shown that most cases of transfusion-acquired hepatitis C originate from transfusion of donor blood that was anti-HCV positive. Perinatal transmission of HCV is low in the absence of HIV infection. The American Academy of Pediatrics stated that maternal HCV-infection is not a contraindication to breastfeeding; however, mothers should be counseled that although there appears to be no increased risk of transmission, HCV-RNA has been detected in breastmilk.[5] Patients with HCV infection should be counseled to avoid hepatotoxic medications and alcohol and should receive vaccination for the prevention of HAV and HBV infections to prevent additional liver damage. Alpha-interferon was the first drug approved by the Food and Drug Administration for the treatment of adults with chronic HCV infection. The efficacy of alpha-interferon in the treatment of adults who have HCV is poor, with only approximately 10% to 15% exhibiting a sustained viral clearance once therapy is discontinued.[14] Although early studies[8] on treatment of children with chronic HCV infection with alpha interferon prompted optimism, in our experience clearance of the virus had been achieved in only 9% of patients when tested at 6 months after completion of treatment.[47] Treatment trials of HCV-positive adults using interferon and ribavirin or a long-acting interferon (pegylated interferon) have shown sustained HCV clearance rates of 35% to 40%. Similar studies have not yet been performed in children.

Prevention of hepatitis E rests on improvement of hygiene in countries where the illness is epidemic.

Autoimmune Hepatitis

Specific therapy is indicated in patients who have autoimmune hepatitis.[6,13] Prednisone alone and in combination with azathioprine helps prolong survival. Although azathioprine alone appears to be no more effective than a placebo in the treatment of autoimmune chronic active hepatitis, its use in combination with prednisone allows a smaller dosage of the steroid to be used. Some patients who are refractory to azathioprine and steroids have responded to cyclosporine.[20] Because steroids are associated with growth retardation and unpleasant side effects, the use of a small steroid dose is critical in the pediatric population.

Prednisone is begun in a dosage of 2 mg/kg/day (maximum 60 mg daily).[31] When evidence of improvement has occurred, the prednisone dosage may be tapered at weekly intervals to a dosage that achieves and maintains clinical and biochemical remission. Generally between 10 and 20 mg daily is required. Azathioprine may be added after evidence of improvement, especially if unpleasant steroid side effects are noted. Remission is defined as absence of clinical symptoms, an aminotransferase level no more than two times normal, decreasing serum gamma globulin levels, and resolution of the aggressive histological appearance on a liver biopsy specimen. Alternate-day dosages appear to be less effective in achieving remission in chronic active hepatitis but may be of value once clinical and biochemical remission has been achieved. Duration of therapy once remission is achieved is controversial. Generally, once remission is achieved, steroids may be tapered over 6 weeks.

Clinical remission generally occurs within 3 to 6 months, biochemical remission within 6 to 12 months, and histological remission within 12 to 24 months. The patient must be watched at 2- to 4-week intervals for approximately 3 months for evidence of early recurrence of disease. If a recurrence does not manifest within that time, the frequency of observation can be decreased. At least 80% of children appear to achieve initial remission. Although the adult relapse rate is 50% within 6 months, the rate of relapse tends to be lower in children.

The child with autoimmune hepatitis and fulminant hepatic failure poses a difficult therapeutic problem. Prednisone and azathioprine have been used in this situation with success[28]; however, liver transplantation may be necessary for survival.

Because of the paucity of affected children, evaluating the long-term outcome of chronic active hepatitis is difficult. However, most children are likely to have a prolonged clinical remission and perhaps a cure. Those whose disease is severe at the time of diagnosis, as indicated by prolonged prothrombin times and morphological features of extensive necrosis, frequently already have progressed or will progress to cirrhosis. Their prognosis, unfortunately, remains poor unless liver transplantation is performed.

Drug-Induced Hepatitis

Supportive care is recommended along with discontinuation of the suspected drug.

Metabolic Liver Disease

Wilson's disease is treated with the copper chelator penicillamine with an oral daily dose of $750 mg/m^2$. In case of worsening neurological disease or pregnancy, triethylene tetramine hydrochloride (trientine) has been effective in the same dose as penicillamine. Patients are counseled to avoid eating liver and shellfish, which contain high levels of copper. Drinking water should be tested, because patients with Wilson's disease cannot tolerate copper water levels higher than 0.02 ppm.[39] There is no specific therapy for α_1AT deficiency and liver transplantation should be considered for worsening liver function. Replacement of α_1AT by somatic gene therapy and hepatocyte transplantation has been discussed in the literature.[35] Dietary restriction of galactose is the treatment of choice for galactosemia. The treatment of tyrosinemia consists of dietary restriction of phenylalanine and tyrosine; however, although this improves liver transaminase levels it does not decrease the risk of developing hepatocellular carcinoma. Recently, an inhibitor of an early enzyme in the tyrosine degradation pathway, 2-(2- nitro 4-trifluoromethyl benzoyl)-1-1,3cyclohexanedione or NTBC which is thought to prevent the accumulation of toxic products in tyrosinemia has been proposed as an alternative to liver transplantation. Bile acid replacement therapy is the treatment of choice for inborn errors of bile acid synthesis. Ursodeoxycholic acid may be used in the treatment of liver disease secondary to cystic fibrosis.

Liver Transplantation

Liver transplantation has improved the outlook for children who have any of a wide variety of severe liver diseases, including disease secondary to the viruses discussed in this chapter. Evaluation of the child with hepatitis for liver transplantation should be directed toward the identification of progressive deterioration of hepatic function, portal hypertension, gastrointestinal bleeding or growth failure.[3]

For transplantation in general, 1- to 5-year survival rates in children approach 70% to 80%. Transplantation for chronic liver failure secondary to hepatitis B is complicated by almost 100% recurrence of infection; however, the use of HBIG followed by lamivudine may improve outcome. Recurrence of hepatitis C following transplantation is around 90%, but transplantation is recommended because recurrent disease usually is mild. Because successful transplantation for fulminant hepatitis has been achieved in a number of centers, the affected child must be referred to a transplant center as soon as the diagnosis of fulminant hepatitis is established. The prognosis for transplantation in the setting of viral hepatitis undoubtedly will improve with the development of new, more specific antiviral agents.

REFERENCES

1. Aikawa T, Sugai Y, et al: Hepatitis G infection in drug abusers with chronic hepatitis C, *N Engl J Med* 334:195, 1996 (letter).
2. Akader HH, Balisteri WF: Hepatitis C virus: implications to pediatric practice, *Pediatr Infect Dis J* 12:853, 1993.
3. Alonso MH, Ryckman FC: Current concepts in pediatric liver transplantation, *Semin Liv Dis* 18:295, 1998.
4. American Academy of Pediatrics: In Peter G, editor: *1997 Red Book: Report of the Committee on Infectious Diseases*, ed 24, Elk Grove Village, Ill, 1997, American Academy of Pediatrics.
5. American Academy of Pediatrics, Committee on Infectious Diseases: Hepatitis C virus infection, *Pediatrics* 101:481, 1998.
6. Arasu TS, et al: Management of chronic aggressive hepatitis in children and adolescents, *J Pediatr* 95:514, 1979.
7. Bortolotti F, et al: Long term persistence of hepatitis B virus DNA in the serum of children with chronic hepatitis B after hepatitis e antigen to antibody seroconversion, *J Pediatr Gastroenterol Nutr* 22:270, 1996.
8. Bortolotti F, et al: Recombinant interferon-alpha therapy in children with chronic hepatitis C, *Hepatology* 22:1623, 1995.
9. Chang MH: Hepatitis B: long term outcome and benefits from mass vaccination in children, *Acta Gastro-Enterologica Belgica* 61:210, 1998.
10. Chang MH, et al: Factors affecting clearance of hepatitis e antigen in hepatitis B surface antigen carrier children, *J Pediatr* 115:385, 1989.
11. Chang MH, et al: Universal hepatitis B vaccination in Taiwan and the incidence of hepatocellular carcinoma in children, *N Engl J Med* 336: 1855, 1997.
12. Conjeevaram HS: Therapy for chronic hepatitis B: nucleoside analogues in adult and pediatric patients, *Acta Gastro-Enterologica Belgica* 61: 224, 1998.
13. Czaja AJ: Current problems in the diagnosis and management of chronic active hepatitis, *Mayo Clin Proc* 56:311, 1981.
14. Davis GL, et al: Treatment of chronic hepatitis C with recombinant interferon alfa: a multicenter randomized controlled trial, *N Engl J Med* 321:101, 1989.
15. Dubois RS, Silverman A: Treatment of chronic active hepatitis in children, *Postgrad Med J* 50:386, 1974.
16. Fulginiti VA, editor: Hepatitis B virus, *Infect Dis Newsl* 1:25, 1982.
17. Gregorio G, et al: Autoimmune hepatitis in childhood: a 20-year experience, *Hepatology* 25:541, 1997.
18. Gust ID, Purcell RH: Report of a workshop: waterborne non-A, non-B hepatitis, *J Infect Dis* 156:630, 1987.
19. Hsu HY, et al: Spontaneous loss of HBsAg in children with chronic hepatitis B virus infection, *Hepatology* 15:380, 1992.
20. Hyman JS, Ballo M, Leichtner AM: Cyclosporine treatment of autoimmune chronic active hepatitis, *Gastroenterology* 93:890, 1987.
21. Immunization Practices Advisory Committee: Recommendations for protection against viral hepatitis, *MMWR* 34:313, 1985.
22. Jonas MM, et al: Clinical and virologic features of hepatitis C virus infection associated with intravenous immunoglobulin, *Pediatrics* 98: 211, 1996.
23. Kage M, et al: Pathology of chronic hepatitis C in children, *Hepatology* 26:771, 1997.
24. Krawczynski K: Hepatitis E, *Hepatology* 17:932, 1993.
25. Kuo G-L, et al: An assay for circulating antibodies to a major etiologic virus of human non-A, non-B hepatitis, *Science* 244:362, 1989.
26. Lemon SM: Type A viral hepatitis: new developments in an old disease, *N Engl J Med* 313:1059, 1985.
27. Mackay IR: Toward diagnostic criteria for autoimmune hepatitis, *Hepatology* 18:1006, 1993.
28. Maggiore G, et al: Life saving immunosuppressive treatment in severe autoimmune chronic active hepatitis, *J Pediatr Gastroenterol Nutr* 4:655, 1985.

29. Manns MP, Schuler A: Risk of hepatitis A superinfection in patients with underlying liver disease, *Acta Gastro-Enterologica Belgica* 61:206, 1998.
30. McFarlane IG: The relationship between autoimmune markers and different clinical syndromes in autoimmune hepatitis, *Gut* 42:599, 1998.
31. Mieli-Vergani G, Vergani D: Immunological liver diseases in children, *Semin Liv Dis* 18:271, 1998.
32. Nishizawa T, et al: A novel DNA virus (TTV) associated with elevated transaminase levels in posttransfusion hepatitis of unknown etiology, *Biochem Biophys Res Commun* 241:92, 1997.
33. Okamoto H, et al: Molecular cloning and characterization of a novel DNA virus (TTV) associated with posttransfusion hepatitis of unknown etiology, *Hepatol Res* 10:1, 1998.
34. Perlmutter DH: Alpha-1-antitrypsin deficiency, *Semin Liv Dis* 18:217, 1998.
35. Perman JA, et al: Laboratory measures of copper metabolism in the differentiation of chronic active hepatitis and Wilson disease in children, *J Pediatr* 94:564, 1979.
36. Poovorawan Y, et al: Protective efficacy of a recombinant DNA hepatitis B vaccine in neonates of HBe antigen-positive mothers, *JAMA* 261: 3278, 1989.
37. Ritt DJ, et al: Acute hepatic necrosis with stupor or coma: an analysis of 31 patients, *Medicine* 48:151, 1969.
38. Safety of hepatitis B vaccine confirmed, *FDA Drug Bull* 15:14, 1985.
39. Schwazenberg SJ, Sharp HL: Update on metabolic liver disease, *Pediatr Clin North Am* 43: 27, 1996.
40. Shou-Dong L, et al: Immunogenicity of inactivated hepatitis A vaccine in children, *Gastroenterology* 104:1129, 1993.
41. Simons JN, et al: Isolation of novel virus-like sequences associated with human hepatitis, *Nature Med* 1:564, 1995.
42. Sokal EM, et al: Interferon-alpha therapy for chronic hepatitis B in children: a multinational randomized controlled trial, *Gastroenterology* 114:988, 1998.
43. Vajro P, et al: Interferon: a meta-analysis of published studies in pediatric chronic hepatitis B, *Acta Gastro-Enterologica Belgica* 61:219, 1998.
44. Vento S, et al: Fulminant hepatitis associated with hepatitis A virus superinfection in patients with chronic hepatitis C, *N Engl J Med* 338: 286, 1998.
45. Werlin SL, et al: Diagnostic dilemmas of Wilson's disease: diagnosis and treatment, *Pediatrics* 62:47, 1978.
46. Werzberger A et al: A controlled trial of a formalin-inactivated hepatitis A vaccine in healthy children, *N Engl J Med* 327:453, 1992.
47. Zellos A, et al: Response to interferon alpha-2b therapy in children with hepatitis C virus (HCV) infection, *Acta Gastro-Enterologica Belgica* 61:253, 1998 (abstract).

217 Herpes Infections

Lindsey K. Grossman

Herpesvirus hominis, or herpes simplex virus (HSV), is one of the most common agents infecting humans; although 85% to 95% of primary infections may be inapparent, the disease in certain circumstances can be fatal. HSV is a deoxyribonucleic acid (DNA) virus with a protein coat. After an incubation period of 2 to 12 days, the primary infection, if apparent, usually is heralded by constitutional symptoms such as malaise, fever, anorexia, and irritability, as well as by the classic herpetic enanthem or exanthem. Lesions are painful vesicles, usually several millimeters in diameter, on an erythematous base. After healing and recovering from the initial infection, the host is not rid of the organism, rather, the organism is presumed to remain in a latent phase in the ganglion cells or nerves innervating the region of localized infection. Various stimuli, including sunlight, fever, physical or emotional trauma, or menses may induce a recurrent infection. Recurrent episodes demonstrate a similar vesicular eruption in the same general anatomical area as the primary eruption but without concomitant constitutional symptoms.

Pathologically, HSV infection is characterized by the presence of multinucleated giant cells and eosinophilic intranuclear inclusions seen in tissue scrapings taken from the base of a vesicle and stained with Giemsa (Tzanck preparation), Pap, or hematoxylin-eosin techniques. Herpes infections can be divided definitively into two immunological types that highly correlate with clinical manifestations: herpesvirus type 1 (HSV-1), which tends to be associated with disease above the waist, and herpesvirus type 2 (HSV-2), associated with disease below the waist, with sexually related transmission, or with disease acquired neonatally.

Studies have shown a sharp rise in the prevalence of antibodies to HSV-1 between 1 and 4 years of age and a slower rise of antibody acquisition between 5 and 14 years of age. From adolescence into early adulthood, coincident with the beginning of sexual activity, the presence of antibodies to HSV-2 increases markedly. Between the late 1970s and the turn of the century, the prevalence of HSV-2 infection increased by 30%, and HSV-2 antibody is now detectable in roughly one of five persons 12 years of age or older nationwide. Overall, 80% to 100% of adults in lower socioeconomic groups, where crowding probably plays an important epidemiological role, demonstrate antibodies to HSV-1; 40% or more may be positive for HSV-2. Of those of higher socioeconomic circumstances, 10% demonstrate antibodies to HSV-2, while 100% of older prostitutes have HSV-2 antibodies.

HERPESVIRUS TYPE 1

Transmission of HSV-1 is presumed to be via person-to-person respiratory spread and probably involves close contact, such as kissing an infected person. Transmission can occur whether or not the source is symptomatic with a vesicular lesion at the time. The clinical manifestation varies with site of entry, and the clinical diagnosis rarely requires laboratory confirmation.

Acute gingivostomatitis is the most common form of HSV-1 seen in children; the peak incidence is between 1 and 4 years of age. It is characterized by an abrupt onset of fever, irritability, poor feeding, and 1 to 2 days later, by very tender, red, friable mucous membranes surrounding 2- to 3-mm white ulcerations, and severe halitosis. The vesicular stage rarely is seen, but large, tender anterior cervical and submaxillary lymphadenopathy is common. The duration of the illness varies from 5 to 14 days, and the severity ranges from mild to so severe that oral intake becomes negligible and hospitalization for intravenous hydration may be required. The differential diagnosis includes coxsackievirus A herpangina, which results in lesions very similar in appearance to herpes but located in the posterior oral cavity, as contrasted with the anterior clustering of the herpetic lesions. See Chapter 268, Stomatitis, for discussion of other causes of stomatites.

Herpes labialis (or cold sores) crust and heal without scarring in 7 to 10 days. They may be found on either the upper or lower lip, and recurrence at the same site is extremely common. Traumatic herpes is the result of inoculation at the site of local trauma and includes herpetic whitlow, an extremely painful syndrome involving herpetic infection of a digit. Although it may resemble a bacterial paronychia, it should not be incised. This condition is common in thumbsuckers who have oral herpes.

Although HSV-1 infections usually are self-limited, certain syndromes are associated with ominous consequences. Ocular herpes can be extremely worrisome and is one of the most common causes of corneal blindness in the United States. The primary infection usually involves acute keratoconjunctivitis with intense swelling of the lids but without exudate. Frequently, typical herpetic vesicles are found on the skin surrounding the involved eye. Recurrent disease can be even more severe and may involve superficial or deep epithelial ulceration, stromal damage, or uveitis. Fortunately, treatment is available (see the discussion on treatment below), but these children always should be referred to an ophthalmologist for care. Indeed, the pediatrician should be aware that devastating results can occur with the use of localized steroid preparations in an unsuspected case of ocular herpes. This underlines the necessity of an ophthalmological consultation before prescribing topical corticosteroids for any use in the eye.

Certain human hosts are at more serious risk for contracting or having severe disease with HSV-1 than are others. Individuals who have deficiencies in cell-mediated immunity, those undergoing immunosuppressive therapy for cancer or transplantation, and those who are extremely malnourished may be more likely to show serious disseminated disease. The inoculation of herpes into eczematous skin can result in eczema herpeticum (Kaposi's varicelliform eruption), which can vary in severity from mild to fatal. Constitutional symptoms are the rule, and the temperatures of 39.4° to 40.6° C may last for a week or more. Wide areas of skin can become denuded, with enormous fluid, protein, and electrolyte losses, which potentially are life threatening. Secondary bacterial infection may complicate the condition. Recurrences, milder than the initial infection, occur commonly on areas of the skin affected with chronic eczema. Certain sport activities that result in close skin contact may increase the risk of HSV skin infection. Wrestlers may acquire herpes gladiatorum as a result of viral shedding from an infected opponent. Herpes rugbeiorum, or "scrum pox," may result from close skin contact between rugby players.

HSV-1 is the most common reported cause of viral encephalitis in the United States, with an estimated 250 to 500 cases per year. The disease is characterized by a rapidly progressive encephalopathy culminating in death in 1 to 2 weeks in more than 70% of untreated cases. Most often the infection localizes to a single lobe, and a definitive diagnosis often can be made by a biopsy of that area, demonstrating the typical morphological picture of herpes microscopically. Treatment now is available (see discussion below) that may improve the prognosis of this disastrous condition.

HERPESVIRUS TYPE 2

As a result of the increase in sexual activity among young adolescents in recent years, pediatricians have been faced with the challenge of diagnosing and treating all types of sexually transmitted diseases. The frequency of infection is high and underestimated by clinical history in the adolescent population.[10] The prevalence of HSV-2 infection has increased by 30% and now is detectable in roughly one in five persons 12 years of age or older. Genital HSV-2 is of increasing concern to physicians and patients alike because of its symptomatology, lack of cure, and potential for disastrous consequences to the newborn. Clinically, HSV-2 usually is manifested by typical herpetic vesicles on the penile shaft, prepuce, or glans penis in the male and on the labia minora or majora, mons, or nearby skin or within the vagina in the female. Primary infection is accompanied by significant local pain, burning, or paresthesia and constitutional symptoms of fever and malaise, dysuria, and inguinal lymphadenopathy; recurrent bouts are less severe. The 5% to 10% of cases of genital herpes associated with HSV-1 are believed to result from orogenital sex.

Viral culture is the most sensitive method of diagnosis but requires several days, depending on the size of the inoculum, for the definitive answer. When lesions are available for scraping, direct detection methods, including fluorescent antibody and immunoperoxidase assays, give a rapid answer but with lower sensitivity; therefore, a viral culture is still required for confirmation of a negative finding. Tzanck test and Pap stains are widely available and inexpensive but are not specific for HSV and also have low sensitivity. ELISA testing is available commercially but does not distinguish between HSV-1 and HSV-2. Polymerase chain reaction and Western blot are highly specific and sensitive and do discriminate between the HSV-1 and HSV-2 but are not always readily available. The application of PCR to the diagnosis of neonatal HSV disease and subsequent management issues promise to enhance the ability to treat and monitor these infants. The role of PCR in the determination of the clinical extent of disease in the skin, eye, or mouth (SEM), and especially for follow-up, in relationship to recurrences in CNS and disseminated disease awaits further investigation.[11]

NEONATAL HERPES

Although most neonatal herpes infections are caused by HSV-2, antibodies to HSV-1 are associated in 25% of cases. Transplacental transmission of HSV can occur and may induce spontaneous abortion or, in rare cases, congenital defects in newborns. More often, however, pediatricians are faced with postnatal herpetic disease contracted by the newborn during the second stage of labor while moving through an infected birth canal. The incidence is estimated to vary between 1 in 3500 to 1 in 5000 deliveries.[20] The prevalence of HSV-2 in healthy American women ranges from 10% to 60%. As many as 50% to 60% of women from lower socioeconomic groups in the United States have antibodies to HSV-2.[14] This results in an estimated 1500 to 2200 infants per year in the United States infected with HSV.[11] Postnatal transmission from a caregiver accounts for approximately 10% of cases.[5]

The greatest risk of neonatal HSV infection occurs when the mother has contracted primary herpes 2 to 4 weeks before delivery, although the disease may be transmitted to the baby in recurrent cases with or without a clinically detectable herpetic lesion. Transmission of HSV infection to the fetus most frequently is related to shedding of the virus at the time of delivery.[14] The pediatrician should note that most newborns infected with HSV at birth are delivered from women who have no history of genital herpes. Neonatal HSV disease must always be included in the differential diagnosis when a newborn or infant presents with a skin rash ranging from vesiculopapular to vesiculoulcerative.

When genital herpes occurs during pregnancy, one must worry about the risk of vertical transmission to the infant, especially at the time of delivery. HSV was isolated from 0.35% of nearly 16,000 women having no signs or symptoms, suggesting the virus was transmitted when they were admitted in early labor to a university hospital. Of those having positive HSV cultures, 35% had evidence of a recently acquired, subclinical first episode of genital HSV infection, and their infants were 10 times more likely to develop the syndrome of neonatal HSV than were those who had an asymptomatic reactivation of HSV.[3,16]

The presentation of neonatal herpes, like other infections in the neonatal period, is nonspecific, at least initially. The syndrome usually presents in the first week or so of life but uncommonly can occur as late as 3 or 4 weeks of age. The infant usually experiences poor feeding, vomiting, fussiness or lethargy, and fever or hypothermia, and often has increasing jaundice and hepatosplenomegaly. Seizures, cyanosis, and apnea also may occur. The majority of infants who have neonatal herpes eventually demonstrate a vesicular rash with either individual lesions or clumps of vesicles.

The NIAID Collaborative Antiviral Study Group[15] classifies cases of neonatal HSV infection into three categories according to clinical manifestations. Infants who have disseminated disease involving visceral organs with or without central nervous system (CNS) involvement are most likely to die (more than 80% without treatment and 54% with treatment). Babies who have HSV type 1 disseminated infection have poorer outcomes than those who have HSV type 2 infection.[17] In disseminated infection, hepatoadrenal necrosis virtually always is found, and microcephaly, hydrocephalus, mental retardation, or seizures occur in many survivors.

A second category of disease includes infants who have CNS abnormalities without involvement of viscera. In this group, mortality exceeds 50% and morbidity exceeds 90% without antiviral therapy.[18]

A third category includes infants whose skin, eyes, or mouth are involved (SEM) but not the CNS or viscera. Infants who had SEM involvement before antiviral drugs became available were not expected to die, and only 20% to 30% were left neurologically impaired; many who appeared to have SEM, however, went on to develop disseminated or CNS involvement and to suffer disastrous consequences. Classically, more than 50% of all neonatal HSV infections manifested as disseminated disease, with only a minority classified as SEM. However, apparently as a result of earlier diagnosis and treatment, 42% now manifest as SEM and 23% as disseminated disease; the remaining 35% have CNS disease, a proportion that has remained fairly stable. An NIAID study documented no deaths with appropriate therapy for SEM disease and 15% and 57% mortality in neonates who had CNS and disseminated HSV infection, respectively.[17]

Previously, stringent prenatal screening programs were recommended to attempt to prevent HSV infection in offspring of women who had recurrent genital herpes. Such programs proved costly, impractical to administer, and medically ineffective. Current guidelines for managing pregnant women who have a history of genital herpes suggest vaginal delivery if no active genital lesions are present at the time of delivery and expeditious cesarean delivery for women who have apparent genital lesions near or at term and who are in labor or have ruptured membranes. Scalp electrodes should be avoided when the mother has a history of genital HSV infection.

The American Academy of Pediatrics and the American College of Obstetricians and Gynecologists have developed joint guidelines to avoid the less likely possibility of postpartum herpes infection in the baby.[1] These guidelines specify isolation criteria to protect normal babies from their HSV-infected mothers, other infected infants, or infected staff.

TREATMENT

Although no universal cure exists for herpes infection, the prognosis for its many syndromes is improving greatly because of newly introduced therapies. One of the earliest successes was with topical idoxuridine (IDU) in the treatment of ocular herpetic infections. Unfortunately, early trials of systemic IDU and cytosine arabinoside demonstrated little value in the treatment of generalized herpes, because of high drug toxicity. Vidarabine was the first drug shown to decrease mortality and morbidity markedly without significant drug toxicity in neonatal herpes involving the CNS.[16] Although originally found to be effective in the treatment of HSV encephalitis, more recent data show acyclovir to be superior.[19]

Acyclovir clearly is the most effective weapon against HSV currently available. Topical acyclovir (Zovirax) shortens the duration of symptoms and viral shedding by several days in initial or primary genital herpes,[2,4,6] with a lessened effect in cases caused by recurrent disease.[2,12] The oral preparation is even more effective in primary infections and is of some benefit in patients who have recurrent infection, especially if administered early in the course of the recurrence. Clinical trials of chronic suppressive oral acyclovir for patients who have primary genital herpes have shown a dramatic decrease in recurrence rate.[7,13] Oral acyclovir currently is recommended for use in the treatment of initial cases of genital herpes but only for patients who have recurrent genital herpes that is very severe, frequent, or complicated. Acyclovir may be particularly useful in treating as well as preventing herpetic reactivation in immunocompromised patients.[2]

Although morbidity, mortality, and drug side effects are similar to those seen with vidarabine treatment, acyclovir usually is considered to be the treatment of choice for neonatal HSV infection on the basis of ease of administration.[16,17] Earlier diagnosis coupled with the availability of efficacious therapy has contributed to a decrease in mortality and morbidity for this potentially devastating medical problem. For specific drug doses used in the treatment of HSV infections, see Table 262-1 in Chapter 262, Sexually Transmitted Diseases.

When to Refer

- All infants who are suspected of having neonatal herpes should be considered potentially critically ill and would benefit from subspecialty involvement
- Regardless of age, patients who have known or suspected immunosuppression who contact herpes may benefit from subspecialty consultation

When to Hospitalize

- Infants who have suspected or confirmed neonatal herpes
- Patients who have severe herpes gingivostomatitis and may be unable to maintain adequate hydration status in the face of high fever and decreased oral intake; these patients may require intravenous fluid management

REFERENCES

1. American Academy of Pediatrics and American College of Obstetricians and Gynecologists: *Guidelines for prenatal care*, ed 5, Elk Grove Village, Ill, 1997, American Academy of Pediatrics.
2. American Academy of Pediatrics Committee on Infectious Disease: *1997 Red Book: Report of the committee of infectious disease*, ed 24, Elk Grove Village, Ill, 1997, American Academy of Pediatrics.
3. Brown ZA, et al: Neonatal herpes simplex virus infection in relation to asymptomatic maternal infection at the time of labor, *N Engl J Med* 324:1247, 1991.
4. Bryson YD, et al: Treatment of first episodes of genital herpes simplex virus infection with oral acyclovir, *N Engl J Med* 308:916, 1983.
5. Connelly BL, Stanberry LR: Herpes simplex virus infections in children, *Curr Opin Pediatr* 7:19, 1995.
6. Corey L, et al: A trial of topical acyclovir in genital herpes simplex virus infections, *N Engl J Med* 306:1313, 1982.
7. Douglas JM, et al: A double-blind study of oral acyclovir for suppression of recurrence of genital herpes simplex virus infections, *N Engl J Med* 310:1551, 1984.
8. Fleming DT, et al: Herpes simplex virus type 2 in the United States, 1976 to 1994, *N Engl J Med* 337:1105, 1997.
9. Hanshaw JB: Herpesvirus hominis infections in the fetus and the newborn, *Am J Dis Child* 126:546, 1973.
10. Huerta, K, et al: Epidemiology of herpes simplex virus type 2 infections in a high-risk adolescent population, *J Adolesc Health* 18:384, 1996.
11. Jacobs RF: Neonatal herpes simplex virus infections, *Semin Perinatol* 22:64, 1998.
12. Reichman RC, et al: Treatment of recurrent genital herpes simplex infections with oral acyclovir, *JAMA* 251:2103, 1984.
13. Straus SE, Takiff HE, Seidlin M: Suppression of frequently recurring genital herpes: a placebo-controlled double-blind trial of acyclovir, *N Engl J Med* 310:1545, 1984.
14. Whitley RJ: Neonatal herpes simplex virus: is there a role for immunoglobulin in disease prevention and therapy? *Pediatr Infect Dis J* 13:432, 1994.
15. Whitley RJ, et al: Changing presentation of herpes simplex virus infection in neonates, *J Infect Dis* 158:109, 1988.
16. Whitley RJ, et al: A controlled trial comparing vidarabine with acyclovir in neonatal herpes simplex virus infection, *N Engl J Med* 324:444, 1991.
17. Whitley RJ, et al: Predictors of morbidity and mortality in neonates with herpes simplex virus infections, *N Engl J Med* 324:450, 1991.
18. Whitley RJ, et al: Vidarabine therapy for mucocutaneous herpes simplex virus infection in the immunocompromised host, *J Infect Dis* 149:1, 1984.
19. Whitley RJ, et al: Vidarabine versus acyclovir therapy in herpes simplex encephalitis, *N Engl J Med* 314:144, 1986.
20. Whitley RJ, Lakeman F: Hepes simplex virus infections of the central nervous system: therapeutic and diagnostic considerations, *Clin Infect Dis* 20:414, 1995.

SUGGESTED READINGS

Carmack MA, Prober CG: Neonatal herpes: vexing dilemmas and reasons for hope, *Curr Opin Pediatr* 5:21, 1993.

Dwyer DE, Cunningham AL: Herpes simplex virus infection in pregnancy, *Baillieres Clin Obstet Gynaecol* 7:75, 1993.

Kohl S: Neonatal herpes simplex virus infection, *Clin Perinatol* 24:1, 1997.

Koutsky LA, et al: Underdiagnosis of genital herpes by current clinical and viral-isolation procedures, *N Engl J Med* 326:1533, 1992.

Nelson CT, Demmler, GJ: Superficial HSV infection: how serious is it? What should you do? *Contemp Pediatr* 13:5, 1996.

Schomogyi M, Wald A, Corey L: Herpes simplex virus-2 infection: an emerging disease? *Infect Dis Clin North Am* 12:1, 1998.

Trizna Z, Tyring SK: Antiviral treatment of diseases in pediatric dermatology, *Dermatol Clin* 16:3, 1998.

Whitley RJ: Herpes simplex virus infections of the central nervous system, *Drugs* 42:406, 1991.

218 Human Herpesvirus-6 and Human Herpesvirus-7 Infections

Jerri Ann Jenista

Human herpesvirus-6 (HHV-6) and human herpesvirus-7 (HHV-7) are two of the known causative agents of roseola,[31,38] a classic childhood exanthem also known as roseola infantum, exanthem subitum, 3-day fever, sixth disease, and pseudorubella. However, the spectrum of disease associated with these agents is now understood to be far broader than the benign illness of roseola.

ETIOLOGY

HHV-6, formerly called human B-lymphotrophic virus (HBLV), and HHV-7 are classified as herpesviruses based on physical and genetic similarities to others of the group: herpes simplex virus-1, herpes simplex virus-2, cytomegalovirus, Epstein-Barr virus, varicella-zoster virus, and the newly discovered virus associated with Kaposi sarcoma, HHV-8.[20] HHV-6 and HHV-7 can be distinguished from these other herpesviruses by DNA hybridization or by reactions with virus-specific monoclonal antibodies.

HHV-6 exists in two forms, variant A and variant B. Variant B typically is associated with childhood illnesses, such as roseola, and some adult infections. Variant A is noted most frequently in patients who have HIV infection.

Sophisticated antigen detection methods demonstrate HHV-6 and HHV-7 in many healthy persons, including those who have virus-specific antibody. HHV-6 has been isolated from saliva, plasma, and many cell lines.[20] HHV-7 is isolated most often from the saliva in healthy persons.[14]

As with other herpesviruses, latent or persistent asymptomatic viral infection occurs following the primary infection. The site of latency is not clear but may include several reservoirs, including salivary glands, peripheral blood mononuclear cells, kidneys, bronchial glands, and the cerebrospinal fluid (CSF).[5] HHV-6 infection may reactivate during primary HHV-7 infection, acute febrile illnesses, or periods of immunodeficiency. Reactivation characteristics of HHV-7 are unknown.

Both viruses interfere with the function of certain classes of T lymphocytes. Evidence is emerging that HHV-6, and perhaps HHV-7, act as cofactors in the course of human immunodeficiency virus infection. The role of these viruses in lymphoreticular malignancies, chronic fatigue syndrome, and other conditions, such as multiple sclerosis, is under investigation.

EPIDEMIOLOGY

Roseola is thought to be the manifestation of primary HHV-6, and perhaps HHV-7, infection. Roseola is so frequent an illness that fully 30% of children will suffer the clinical disease between the ages of 6 months and 2 years.[4] In Japan, the disease is even more common, noted in up to 60% of children in the first 3 years of life.[18] The diagnosis is unusual, however, in children at other ages; rare cases in adults and neonates have been reported. Most cases are sporadic, although family and institutional epidemics occasionally are noted.[25] Cases of roseola are seen year round, with an increased incidence in the late spring.

A child's first episode of roseola usually is caused by HHV-6B, occurring at an average age of 7 to 9 months.[3,11] Primary infection with HHV-7 accounts for about 10% of first and the majority of second cases of roseola. HHV-7 infection occurs somewhat later than HHV-6, at a mean age greater than 12 months.[3,6,26] Approximately 15% of episodes of roseola cannot be attributed to either HHV-6 or HHV-7.[13]

A prospective study of 2235 emergency room visits for acute childhood illness in Rochester, New York, revealed a broader role than previously recognized for HHV-6 infection.[11] Primary HHV-6 infection was documented in nearly 10% of children younger than age 3 years and in 20% of children between 6 and 12 months of age presenting with an acute febrile illness. HHV-6 infection was the cause of one third of febrile seizures in children younger than age of 2 years and resulted in hospitalization of 13% of children following emergency room presentation. Clearly, primary HHV-6 infection is a major cause of morbidity in infancy and early childhood. The contribution of HHV-7 infection to emergency room use, hospitalization, or physician visits has not been studied.

The incubation periods for HHV-6 and HHV-7 infection apparently are between 5 and 15 days; however, the modes of transmission and the period of communicability are unclear. In an extensive study of three-generation families, DNA restriction analysis of HHV-7 isolates showed similar patterns within households.[30] HHV-6 is isolated most frequently from peripheral blood mononuclear cells. HHV-6 and HHV-7 can be isolated from the saliva of 70% to 80% of healthy persons older than 1 year of age and is thought to be the most likely mode of transmission.[21,27] The rate of subclinical disease is high. Most patients have no known exposure[4], although poverty and larger family size may be risk factors for early acquisition of HHV-6. Breast-feeding may delay the acquisition of HHV-7.[19] In spite of indirect evidence of intrauterine or perinatal transmission of at least HHV-6,[1] there are no recognized sequelae attributed to such infection.

Serological surveys show that virtually all full-term infants have passively acquired maternal antibody to both HHV-6 and HHV-7 at birth. The prevalence of antibody falls, reaching a nadir by 6 months of age. By 1 year of age, nearly 90% of children have detectable antibody to HHV-6. Prevalence surveys of adults from various countries around the world show HHV-6 antibody detection rates of 88% to 90%.[21,36] The prevalence of antibody to HHV-7 also increases with age; 60% of young adolescents have detectable titers. For both viruses, these levels persist unchanged through young adulthood and then decline slightly thereafter.

DISEASE

Roseola

Recognition of roseola is based almost entirely on the observation of a classic clinical course. Interestingly, the signs and symptoms of roseola noted before the discovery of HHV-6 are essentially the same as descriptions of disease proven to be caused by HHV-6 or HHV-7[3,6,9] (Table 218-1). Typically, a fever as high as 102.2° to 105.8° F (39° to 41° C) suddenly develops in a previously well infant. Except for irritability, the child does not seem as sick as the temperature indicates. Physical findings are sparse and include only painless posterior auricular, suboccipital, or cervical lymphadenopathy accompanied by slight eyelid edema, giving the child a "sleepy-eyed" or "droopy" appearance. Nagayama spots are erythematous macules appearing on the soft palate and near the uvula and are observed regularly after a day or two of illness.[3] Rarely, mild coryza, otitis media, or a bulging fontanelle is observed.

Table 218-1 Roseola—Before and After Discovery of HHV-6 and HHV-7

Signs and Symptoms	Roseola: 1945[9]	HHV-6: 1994[3]	HHV-7: 1998[6]
Fever	100%	98%	100%
Rash	100%	98%	13%
Pruritus	1.2%	*	*
Desquamation	10%	0%	*
Pigmentation	0%	7%	*
Lymphadenopathy	97.5%	*	*
Cervical	45%	31%	*
Erythematous tympanic membranes	92.5%	*	*
Constipation	40%	*	*
Upper respiratory tract symptoms	25%	*	*
Nonspecific prodromal symptoms	*	14%	*
Diarrhea	15%	68%	38%
Meningismus	5%	*	*
Convulsions	3.7%	8%	75%
Bulging fontanelle	*	26%	*
Irritability	92.5%	*	88%
Edematous eyelids	*	30%	*
Nagayama spots†	87%	65%	*
Anorexia	80%	*	*
Abdominal pain	25%	*	*
Cough	11.2%	50%	*
Headache	5%	*	*
Earache	2.5%	*	*
Aching joints	2.5%	*	*

*Not reported using this term.
†Erythematous streaks or spots on the soft palate and uvula.

After a 2- to 5-day course, the fever resolves dramatically and a rash appears almost simultaneously. With defervescence the child seems to have recovered, despite the rash. The typical exanthem occurs as macular or maculopapular blanching patches surrounding by a lighter halo. The eruption usually begins on the neck and spreads to the trunk and extremities, sparing the face. It fades within 4 hours to 4 days and probably frequently is missed if it is faint or occurs at night.

Clinically inapparent infection occurs. Roseola also may occur in a young infant as an afebrile exanthem or as a nonspecific fever without the characteristic rash.

Seizures

HHV-6 infection is a major factor in childhood febrile seizures, associated with up to one third to one half of such incidents in children younger than the age of 2 years presenting to an emergency room.[11,15] HHV-6 can be isolated from CFS in up to 70% of children during primary infection and in 28% of children who have had past infection.[5] Seizures may be single or recurrent, prolonged, partial or focal, and may be associated with postictal paralysis or acute resolving hemiplegia.[11,16,28,32] CSF findings are normal or negative.

Even with recurrent seizures during the same illness, complete recovery is the rule.[24] The significance of HHV-6 in relation to recurrent seizures is not clear. At least one study detected no increase in the risk of recurrent seizures in the first year following a febrile seizure associated with primary HHV-6 infection versus first febrile seizures of other etiologies.

Febrile seizures also are noted in primary infection caused by HHV-7.[6,26] HHV-7 DNA has been detected in the CSF of a child who had typical roseola.[17] There is some indication that febrile seizures may be more common with primary HHV-7 than HHV-6 infection.[6]

The pathogenesis of seizures associated with HHV-6 and HHV-7 is unknown. Although there is new information that these viruses may have specific neurotropic qualities,[7,12,34] others claim that febrile seizures associated with these viruses are due to the underlying fever associated with the infection rather than actual central nervous system pathology.[15,32]

Meningoencephalitis

There are reports of severe meningoencephalitis with neurological sequelae or death in infants[2,35] and adults,[33] and fatal encephalitis attributed to HHV-6B in adult recipients of bone marrow transplants. The significance of HHV-6 in relation to recurrent seizures, chronic fatigue, multiple sclerosis, and other neurological conditions is not clear.[20]

HHV-7 infection also has been described in association with encephalopathy, hemiplegia, and atypical febrile seizures.

Mononucleosis-like Disease

HHV-6 infection in adults rarely causes a roseola-like illness. Both severe and mild infectious mononucleosis-like disease has been reported in adults who have HHV-6 infection. The disease lasts several weeks, associated with slight fatigue, headache, sore throat, cervical lymphadenopathy, and transient elevation of liver enzymes. Infectious mononucleosis-like illness associated with HHV-6 has been noted in infants.

HHV-7 was isolated from a child who had the clinical picture of chronic Epstein-Barr virus infection, characterized by pancytopenia, fever, and hepatosplenomegaly.

Hepatitis

A mild hepatitis associated with HHV-6 infection is recognized in adults and children. A few cases of fulminant and/or fatal hepatitis have been reported, usually with an associated encephalopathy.[20,22] HHV-6 infection also has been implicated in mild chronic hepatitis in childhood.[29] There has been a single case of hepatitis reported in relation to HHV-7 infection.

Infection in Immunocompromised Patients

HHV-6 infection may reactivate during periods of immunosuppression. A syndrome with fever and rash resembling graft-versus-host disease is recognized in children following bone marrow transplantation. Severe interstitial pneumonitis, disseminated infection, and encephalitis associated with HHV-6 infection have been reported in adult recipients of bone marrow transplants.[20] Some patients have recovered after treatment with foscarnet.

The role of HHV-6 in HIV infection is unclear, although there is some evidence to suggest that HHV-6 may potentiate the progression of HIV infection, especially in infants who have acquired HIV vertically. HHV-7 competes with HIV for CD-4 receptors on T cells; theoretically the virus may interfere with the progression of HIV infection.[20]

Other Diseases

HHV-6 has been isolated from patients who have many other conditions. Because HHV-6 is reactivated by many acute illnesses, it is difficult in most cases to attribute causality to the virus. Reported associations include chronic bone marrow suppression in an immunocompetent adult, idiopathic thrombocytopenic purpura, thrombocytopenia during primary HHV-6 infection,[37] hemophagocytic syndrome, fatal disseminated disease in an immunocompetent infant, lymphoproliferative disorders, and certain lymphoreticular malignancies.

The role of HHV-7 in other diseases is even less clear than its association with roseola. Several studies have purported to show evidence of reactivation of HHV-7 during relapses of adult pityriasis rosea.[10]

DIAGNOSIS

In roseola, the only helpful laboratory finding is a leukopenia that has a nadir count as low as 2000 white blood cells per cubic millimeter by the third day of fever. A relative lymphocytosis or monocytosis is typical. Results of the cerebrospinal fluid examination, urinalysis, and chest roentgenogram are normal. Because roseola is an inconsequential illness, there rarely is any need to confirm the specific diagnosis.

Neither antibody detection methods nor virus isolation techniques are standardized for HHV-6 or HHV-7. These assays are not available commercially. The presence of maternal antibody in the young infant and reactivation of herpesviruses during other infections confound interpretation of the results.[8] Except in certain situations of infection among immunocompromised hosts, there is no clinical need to confirm infection with HHV-6 or HHV-7 either serologically or virologically.

Newly developed diagnostic methods to differentiate latent versus actively replicating virus may help to shed light on both the diagnosis and pathogenesis of disease associated with HHV-6 and HHV-7.[23]

DIFFERENTIAL DIAGNOSIS

Roseola often is confused with other exanthematous diseases (see Chapter 200, Contagious Exanthematous Diseases). In rubella the rash and fever are concurrent, and enlarged lymph nodes often are tender. Coryza, respiratory symptoms, and Koplik spots distinguish rubeola. Enterovirus exanthems usually occur in epidemics, involve older as well as younger children, and are more common in the late summer and fall. Erythema infectiosum, or fifth disease, affects the school-age child and involves the face most prominently. Scarlet fever has a more confluent rash and is associated with marked pharyngitis. Drug eruptions, especially those resulting from sulfa-containing preparations, are not regularly preceded by fever and tend to be more diffuse.

TREATMENT

Management of roseola is based entirely on symptoms. Acetaminophen is quite effective in controlling the fever. Reassuring the parents that the rash is a sign of recovery often is comforting to them and may prevent unnecessary office visits.

Both HHV-6 and HHV-7 have antiviral agent profiles similar to cytomegalovirus, with limited susceptibility to acyclovir. In vitro studies show that either foscarnet or ganciclovir is somewhat effective, but there have been no clinical trials with these drugs. Because infection with either of these agents is self-limited in the immunocompetent child, antiviral therapy is reserved only for life-threatening infection.

OUTCOME

Complications are unusual in the normal child who has roseola. Febrile convulsions are noted in one third to one half of primary HHV-6 infections and in a higher percentage of HHV-7 infection.[5,11]

When to Refer

Primary HHV-6 or HHV-7 infections almost never are clinically recognized until the disease is over. Referral almost never is needed except to rule out an alternative diagnosis such as a seizure disorder or treatable encephalopathy/encephalitis. Immunocompromised patients who have severe clinical symptoms always should be managed by an infectious disease consultant.

When to Hospitalize

Primary HHV-6 or HHV-7 infections are almost never clinically recognized until the disease is over. Hospitalization usually is indicated only when an alternate disease process is suspected, such as meningitis, encephalitis, or recurrent seizures. Immunocompromised patients may have severe infection with HHV-6 or HHV-7, but they typically are hospitalized for their severe clinical presentation—that is, pneumonitis, encephalitis, suspected graft-versus-host disease, etc, rather than for suspicion of HHV-6 or HHV-7 infection.

REFERENCES

1. Adams O, et al: Congenital infections with human herpesvirus 6, *J Infect Dis* 178:544, 1998.
2. Ahtiluoto S, et al: In situ hybridization detection of human herpesvirus 6 in brain tissue from fatal encephalitis, *Pediatrics* 105:431, 2000.
3. Asano Y, et al: Clinical features of infants with primary human herpesvirus 6 infection (exanthem, subitum, roseola infantum), *Pediatrics* 93: 104, 1994.
4. Breese BB Jr: Roseola infantum (exanthem subitum), *N Y State J Med* 41:1854, 1941.
5. Caserta MT, et al: Neuroinvasion and persistence of human herpesvirus 6 in children, *J Infect Dis* 170:1586, 1994.
6. Caserta MT, et al: Primary human herpesvirus 7 infection: a comparison of human herpesvirus 7 and human herpesvirus 6 infections in children, *J Pediatr* 133:386, 1998.
7. Chan PK, et al: Presence of human herpesviruses 6, 7, and 8 DNA sequences in normal brain tissue, *J Med Virol* 59: 491, 1999.
8. Chiu SS, et al: Early diagnosis of primary human herpesvirus 6 infection in childhood: serology, polymerase chain reaction, and virus load, *J Infect Dis* 178:1250, 1998.
9. Clemens HH: Exanthem subitum (roseola infantum): report of eighty cases, *J Pediatr* 26:66, 1945.
10. Drago F, et al: Human herpesvirus 7 in pityriasis rosea, *Lancet* 349: 1367, 1997.
11. Hall CB, et al: Human herpesvirus-6 infection in children: a prospective study of complications and reactivation, *N Engl J Med* 331:432, 1994.
12. Hall CB, et al: Persistence of human herpesvirus 6 according to site and variant: possible greater neurotropism of variant A, *Clin Infect Dis* 26: 132, 1998.
13. Hidaka Y, et al: Exanthem subitum and human herpesvirus 7 infection, *Pediatr Infect Dis J* 13:1010, 1994.
14. Hidaka Y, et al: Frequent isolation of human herpesvirus 7 from saliva samples, *J Med Virol* 40:343, 1993.
15. Hukin J, et al: Case-control study of primary human herpesvirus 6 infection in children with febrile seizures, *Pediatrics* 101:e3, 1998. URL: http://www.pediatrics.org/cgi/content/full/101/2/e3
16. Jee SH, et al: Risk of recurrent seizures after a primary human herpesvirus 6-induced febrile seizure, *Pediatr Infect Dis J* 17:43, 1998.
17. Komatsu H, et al: Detection of human herpesvirus 7 DNA in the cerebrospinal fluid of a child with exanthem subitum, *Pediatr Int* 42:103, 2000.
18. Kusuhara K, et al: Attack rate of exanthem subitum in Japan, *Lancet* 340:482, 1992.
19. Lamphear BP, et al: Risk factors for the early acquisition of human herpesvirus 6 and human herpesvirus 7 infections in children, *Pediatr Infect Dis J* 17:792, 1998.
20. Levy JA: Three new human herpesviruses (HHV-6, 7 and 8), *Lancet* 349:558, 1997.
21. Levy JA, et al: Frequent isolation of HHV-6 from saliva and high seroprevalence of the virus in the population, *Lancet* 335:1047, 1990.
22. Mendel I, et al: Fulminant hepatitis in neonates with human herpesvirus 6 infection, *Pediatr Infect Dis J* 14:993, 1995.
23. Norton RA, et al: Detection of human herpesvirus 6 by reverse transcription-PCR, *J Clin Microbiol* 37:3672, 1999.
24. Ojima K, et al: Frequent convulsions in the post-eruptive stage of exanthem subitum, *No To Hattatsu* 31:310, 1999.
25. Okuno T, et al: Outbreak of exanthem subitum in an orphanage, *J Pediatr* 119:759, 1991.
26. Suga S, et al: Clinical features and virological findings in children with primary human herpesvirus 7 infection, *Pediatrics* 99:e4, 1997. URL: http://www.pediatrics.org/cgi/content/full/99/3/e4
27. Suga S, et al: Prospective study of persistence and excretion of human herpesvirus-6 in patients with exanthem subitum and their parents, *Pediatrics* 102:900, 1998.
28. Suga S, et al: Clinical characteristics of febrile convulsions during primary HHV-6 infection, *Arch Dis Child* 82:62, 2000.
29. Tajiri H, et al: Chronic hepatitis in an infant, in association with human herpesvirus-6 infection, *J Pediatr* 131:473, 1997.
30. Takahashi Y, et al: Transmission of human herpesvirus 7 through multigenerational families in the same household, *Pediatr Infect Dis J* 16: 975, 1997.
31. Tanaka K et al: Human herpesvirus 7: another causal agent for roseola (exanthem subitum), *J Pediatr* 125:1, 1994.
32. Teach SJ, et al: Human herpesvirus types 6 and 7 and febrile seizures, *Pediatr Neurol* 21:699, 1999.
33. Torre D, et al: Meningoencephalitis caused by human herpesvirus-6 in an immunocompetent adult patient: case report and review of the literature, *Infection* 26:402, 1998.
34. van den Berg JS, et al: Neuroinvasion by human herpesvirus type 7 in a case of exanthem subitum with severe neurologic manifestations, *Neurology* 52:1077, 1999.
35. Yanagihara K, et al: Human herpesvirus 6 meningoencephalitis with sequelae, *Pediatr Infect Dis J* 14:240, 1995.
36. Yoshikawa T, et al: Seroepidemiology of human herpesvirus 7 in healthy children and adults in Japan, *J Med Virol* 41:319, 1993.
37. Yoshikawa T, et al: Five cases of thrombocytopenia induced by primary human herpesvirus 6 infection, *Acta Pediatr Jpn* 40:278, 1998.
38. Yoshiyama H, et al: Role of human herpesvirus 6 infection in infants with exanthema subitum, *Pediatr Infect Dis J* 9:71, 1990.

219 Human Immunodeficiency Virus Infection and Acquired Immunodeficiency Syndrome

William Moss • Deborah Persaud

Children who have the acquired immunodeficiency syndrome (AIDS) were first identified in 1982, 1 year after the description of AIDS in adults. Approximately 7600 children younger than 13 years of age who have AIDS were reported in the United States by the end of 1996. AIDS results from progressive immune dysfunction following infection with the human immunodeficiency virus (HIV). Clinical manifestations of HIV infection range from asymptomatic infection to debilitating disease and death. In the United States, HIV infection is the ninth leading cause of death in children 5 to 14 years of age and the seventh leading cause of death in adolescents and young adults 15 to 24 years of age. Children most commonly acquire HIV infection through maternal-infant transmission, but may be infected through receipt of infected blood and blood products and through sexual intercourse. Prior to the widespread use of antiretroviral prophylaxis, an estimated 1000 to 2000 HIV-infected children were born in the United States annually.

The care of HIV-infected children is complex and requires a multidisciplinary team to address the multiple medical, psychological, social, and economic issues that confront HIV-infected children and their families. Advances in the diagnosis, treatment, and prevention of pediatric HIV infection bring hope to HIV-infected children, their families, and those who care for them; however, cure remains elusive.

TRANSMISSION OF HIV TO CHILDREN

Perinatal transmission is the most common mode of acquisition of HIV infection among children in the United States. Not all infants born to HIV-infected women acquire HIV infection; estimated perinatal transmission rates in untreated women to their infants range from 13% to 30%. Perinatal HIV transmission can occur by three mechanisms: transplacental infection in utero, intrapartum infection during labor and delivery, and postpartum infection through breast milk. Intrapartum transmission is most common. High maternal plasma HIV levels correlate with increased risk of transmission. Thus, women who have advanced HIV disease or recently acquired infection are more likely to transmit HIV to their newborns. Antiretroviral therapy administered to pregnant women during late pregnancy and delivery and to infants during the first 6 weeks of life significantly reduces the rate of perinatal HIV transmission (see below).

Routine testing of blood donors for HIV antibody began in March 1985. Children who received blood or blood products prior to this time were at risk of HIV infection. Children who had hemophilia were at particularly high risk because they received pooled factors from hundreds to thousands of donors. The risk of HIV infection from blood or blood products is now extremely small, estimated to be 1 in 38,000 to 1 in 300,000 from a single unit of blood.

HIV transmission through sexual contact occurs in children who are sexually abused or sexually active adolescents. Behaviors that place adolescents at high risk of HIV infection are initiation of sexual activity at a young age, multiple sexual partners, and unprotected sexual intercourse.

PATHOPHYSIOLOGY OF HIV INFECTION IN CHILDREN

Perinatal HIV infection occurs during the development and maturation of the immune system. This distinguishes pediatric HIV infection from adult infection and has profound effects on the clinical course, nature, and timing of opportunistic infections and immune responses to immunizations.

HIV infects several different cell types, but the primary target for HIV replication is the CD4+ T lymphocyte. In addition to the CD4 cell surface molecule, HIV requires a chemokine coreceptor to enter cells. Polymorphisms in chemokine receptors are associated with resistance to HIV infection and different rates of disease progression. Reverse transcription, in which viral DNA is synthesized from viral RNA, is carried out by the enzyme reverse transcriptase. Many antiretroviral agents inhibit HIV replication by interfering with this enzyme. Viral DNA is then transported to the nucleus and integrated into cellular DNA, persisting for the life span of the cell. A large viral polypeptide is synthesized that requires cleavage by a viral protease. Protease inhibitors interfere with this enzyme, disrupting HIV replication.

The number of copies of HIV RNA in plasma can be quantified. Plasma HIV RNA levels are useful in predicting rate of disease progression, modifying antiretroviral therapy, and understanding viral dynamics. In children who have perinatally acquired HIV infection, HIV RNA levels peak in the first few months of life and decline slowly over several years. Steady state HIV RNA levels in children are not achieved until 2 to 6 years of age. In contrast, HIV RNA levels in adults decline rapidly to steady state levels within several months after primary infection. Despite the decline in HIV RNA levels, intense viral replication continues to occur. Combination therapy with reverse transcriptase and protease inhibitors block HIV replication and can result in a dramatic decline in viral production and "undetectable" plasma HIV RNA levels. HIV persists within cellular compartments, however, and eradication is not achievable with current therapies.

Infection with HIV leads to a progressive decrease in CD4+ T lymphocytes. CD4+ T lymphocytes are helper T cells that provide stimulatory molecules to cells responsible for cellular and humoral immunity and phagocytosis. Qualitative changes in the function of CD4+ T cells occur before the decline in T lymphocyte numbers. Because CD4+ T lymphocytes are crucial to B lymphocyte function, humoral immunity can be significantly impaired in HIV-infected children, resulting in poor antibody responses to encapsulated bacteria and immunizations, despite elevated levels of total immunoglobulins.

DIAGNOSIS OF HIV INFECTION IN CHILDREN

The most important factor in identifying HIV-infected women and children is that the diagnosis be considered. Several risk factors are associated with HIV infection in women of child-bearing age, including history of multiple sexual partners, illicit drug use, and sexual contact with persons at high risk. However, the absence of identifiable risk factors does not exclude HIV infection.

Detection of HIV DNA or RNA by polymerase chain reaction (PCR) is the preferred method for diagnosing HIV infection in infants. PCR amplifies HIV DNA or RNA sequences and is extremely sensitive in detecting small amounts of virus. Almost all HIV-infected infants have a positive HIV PCR by 1 month of age, and 40% of HIV-infected infants can be identified in the first 2 days of life. False-positive results can occur because of laboratory contamination; positive results should be confirmed by PCR testing of a second blood specimen. Because early detection of HIV infection allows for the initiation of combination antiretroviral therapy at the time of primary infection, HIV-exposed infants should be tested at 48 hours of age. If negative, many experts recommend repeat PCR testing at 14 days of age. Infants negative for HIV by PCR at 48 hours and 14 days should be tested at 1 to 2 months of age. HIV infection is diagnosed by two positive HIV PCR tests performed on separate blood samples. Two negative PCR results, performed at 1 to 2 months and at 4 to 6 months of age, make the diagnosis of HIV infection extremely unlikely.

The HIV enzyme immunosorbent assay (ELISA) detects antibody to HIV and is the appropriate screening test for children older than 18 months of age. The HIV ELISA has high sensitivity but lacks specificity; thus, false positive results occur. Positive ELISA reactions for HIV are confirmed by Western blot analysis. The Western blot detects antibodies to several HIV proteins and is highly specific. False negative results may occur shortly after primary infection, because antibodies to HIV do not achieve detectable levels until 2 to 3 months after infection. Serological methods should not be used to confirm HIV infection in children younger than 18 months of age, because transplacentally derived, maternal antibodies result in a positive HIV ELISA in infants born to HIV-seropositive women. These maternal antibodies can persist for 18 months.

CLINICAL MANIFESTATIONS OF HIV INFECTION IN CHILDREN

The time from infection to onset of clinical symptoms is much shorter for children who have perinatally acquired HIV infection than for children infected through blood or blood products, and it is markedly shorter than for HIV-infected adults. Infants who have perinatal HIV infection are without symptoms in the neonatal period. Before the widespread use of *Pneumocystis carinii* pneumonia (PCP) prophylaxis and early antiretroviral therapy, a subset of HIV-infected children had rapidly progressive disease and died within the first year of life, frequently from PCP. Other children remain asymptomatic or have minimal symptoms for many years, some into adolescence. However, most children who have perinatal HIV infection develop symptoms by 2 years of age. High levels of plasma HIV levels and low CD4+ T lymphocyte cell counts are predictive of poor prognosis.

Early clinical signs and symptoms of HIV infection are nonspecific but generally indicate a systemic illness. Failure to thrive, developmental delay, persistent oral candidiasis, lymphadenopathy, hepatosplenomegaly, chronic diarrhea, recurrent bacterial infections, and recurrent herpes virus infections may be presenting conditions. Pneumonia resulting from *Pneumocystis carinii* was a frequent presenting illness in infants prior to routine prophylaxis of HIV-exposed infants. Laboratory abnormalities frequently found on presentation include anemia, thrombocytopenia, and elevated immunoglobulins.

HIV infection and secondary opportunistic infections can involve all organ systems. Pulmonary disease is common in HIV-infected children. PCP is a fulminant pulmonary infection manifested by tachypnea, cough, hypoxemia and, most commonly, diffuse alveolar infiltrates on chest radiograph. Lymphoid interstitial pneumonitis (LIP) is a chronic lung disease of HIV-infected children resulting from lymphoid hyperplasia in the lungs. Children who have LIP may be asymptomatic or have chronic cough and wheezing. Bilateral, reticulonodular densities are seen on chest radiograph, resembling miliary tuberculosis. Children who have LIP are typically older than those who have PCP and frequently have generalized lymphadenopathy and parotid enlargement.

Central nervous system disease also is common in HIV-infected children. Microcephaly, developmental delay, spasticity, abnormal reflexes, and gait abnormalities may be present. Characteristic findings on computed tomographic (CT) scan include cerebral atrophy and basal ganglia calcifications. Hematological abnormalities associated with HIV infection include leukopenia, anemia, and thrombocytopenia. Thrombocytopenia may be the presenting illness. In addition, drug-induced bone marrow suppression can follow therapy with zidovudine (ZDV), Co-trimoxazole, and ganciclovir. Hepatomegaly and elevations of hepatic transaminases are commonly seen, often in the absence of clinically apparent liver disease. HIV cardiomyopathy may lead to congestive heart failure. HIV nephropathy is a common cause of proteinuria and can progress to the nephrotic syndrome. Chronic diarrhea, resulting from several opportunistic gastrointestinal pathogens, can be debilitating.

Dermatological conditions include recurrent herpes simplex and varicella-zoster virus infections, severe molluscum contagiosum, chronic fungal infections, atopic der-

Table 219-1 Pediatric HIV Classification

	Clinical Categories			
Immunological Categories	**N: No Signs/ Symptoms**	**A: Mild Signs/ Symptoms**	**B: Moderate Signs/ Symptoms**	**C: Severe Signs/ Symptoms**
1: No evidence of suppression	N1	A1	B1	C1
2: Evidence of moderate suppression	N2	A2	B2	C2
3: Severe suppression	N3	A3	B3	C3

Immunological Categories Based on Age-Specific CD4+ T-Lymphocyte Count and Percentage of Total Lymphocytes	<12 Mo		1-5 Yr		6-12 Yr	
	μL	%	μL	%	μL	%
No evidence of suppression	≥1500	≥25	≥1000	≥25	≥500	≥25
Evidence of moderate suppression	750-1499	15-24	500-999	15-24	200-499	15-24
Severe suppression	<750	<15	<500	<15	<200	<15

Centers for Disease Control and Prevention: 1994 Revised classification system for HIV infection in children younger than 13 years of age, *MMWR* 43(No RR-12):1, 1994.

matitis, and drug-induced eruptions, particularly with Co-trimoxazole. HIV-infected children are frequently stunted in their growth, and severe wasting may be seen in advanced disease. Malignancies are not common in HIV-infected children, but lymphomas can occur.

In 1984, the Centers for Disease Control and Prevention (CDC) developed a classification system based on clinical diseases to categorize HIV infection and AIDS in children. The CDC classification was revised in 1994 to incorporate advances in the understanding of the natural history of HIV infection in children and age-specific CD4+ T lymphocyte cell counts (Table 219-1). HIV-infected children are classified into one of four clinical categories (N, A, B, or C), based on clinical signs and symptoms and into one of three immunological categories (1, 2, or 3), based on age-specific CD4+ T-lymphocyte cell counts or percentage of the total lymphocyte count. However, wide variability in clinical status exists even within a category.

COMMON CLINICAL PROBLEMS IN HIV-INFECTED CHILDREN

Most HIV-infected children who have fever and a normal clinical examination have self-limited febrile illnesses similar to those of HIV-uninfected children. However, as with other immunocompromised children, fever may indicate a serious infection. A detailed clinical history and careful physical examination, with close attention to general appearance and potential areas of focal inflammation such as skin, ears, sinuses, lungs, and gastrointestinal tract, are essential in the initial assessment of the febrile HIV-infected child. However, bacteremia with *Streptococcus pneumoniae* and salmonella can occur in the absence of physical findings. Additional diagnostic studies should be obtained based on the child's age, clinical appearance, degree of immunosuppression, and presenting signs and symptoms. Laboratory tests to be considered include a complete blood count with differential, large volume blood culture, chest radiograph, urinalysis and urine culture, and lumbar puncture. Administration of empirical antibiotic therapy is not always necessary and depends on the results of the clinical assessment and laboratory tests, as well as the likelihood of adequate monitoring and follow-up. A third-generation cephalosporin such as cefotaxime or ceftriaxone can be used as empirical antibiotic therapy to provide both gram-positive and gram-negative coverage. Increasing resistance of pneumococcal isolates to third-generation cephalosporins makes careful follow-up mandatory. Ill-appearing children should be hospitalized. Persistent fever in the HIV-infected child can be a diagnostic challenge, but identifiable causes include mycobacterial infection and drug-induced fever.

Pneumococcus is the most common bacterial cause of pneumonia in HIV-infected children. HIV-infected children are likely to develop severe disease as a result of common respiratory pathogens such as respiratory syncytial virus, parainfluenza virus, influenza virus, and adenovirus. HIV-infected children who have advanced immunosuppression are susceptible to many opportunistic pulmonary pathogens. PCP is the most common opportunistic infection in HIV-infected infants and typically presents at 3 to 6 months of age with cough, tachypnea, and hypoxemia. Early diagnosis and treatment, usually with Co-trimoxazole and corticosteroids, is critical. Physicians caring for HIV-infected children must carefully consider the diagnosis of PCP in HIV-infected children who have respiratory tract symptoms. HIV-infected children who have pulmonary disease who fail to respond to empirical antibiotic therapy, those who are severely ill, and those who are suspected of having PCP should undergo an invasive diagnostic procedure such as bronchoscopy with bronchoalveolar lavage or lung biopsy.

Persistent diarrhea can significantly compromise the quality of life and the nutritional status of HIV-infected children. Infectious causes of diarrhea in HIV-infected children include all of the pathogens of healthy children in addition to numerous opportunistic pathogens. Common parasitic pathogens causing persistent diarrhea include *Giardia lamblia*, *Entamoeba histolytica*, cryptosporidium, and Isospora. Cytomegalovirus may cause colitis in children who have advanced immunosuppression. Diagnostic studies should include stool cultures for bacterial and viral pathogens, as well as for ova and parasites. Endoscopy should be considered in refractory cases.

Bacterial and viral pathogens causing meningitis and encephalitis in HIV-infected children are similar to those in nonimmunocompromised children. Opportunistic pathogens causing meningitis and encephalitis HIV-infected children who have advanced immunosuppression include *Cryptococcus neoformans*, *Toxoplasma gondii,* and cytomegalovirus. Initial diagnostic studies include analysis of cerebrospinal fluid and brain imaging. Rarely, central nervous system lymphomas can occur.

HIV-infected children are at increased risk of disseminated varicella and recurrent zoster. HIV-infected children should receive varicella-zoster immune globulin (VZIG) promptly after exposure to varicella. Disseminated infection can occur with zoster, and oral or parenteral therapy with acyclovir is warranted.

Growth failure is common in HIV-infection in children early in the course of disease. The diagnosis of HIV infection should be considered in children who fail to thrive. Frequent measurements of weight and height are important in detecting growth disturbances early and monitoring response to interventions. Effective antiretroviral therapy with suppression of viral replication, as well as nutritional supplementation, is important to the maintenance of growth. However, supplementation with high caloric foods or formulas often results in increased body fat rather than lean body weight.

Delayed acquisition of developmental milestones or loss of previously acquired milestones also is a common manifestation of HIV-infection in children. Effective antiretroviral therapy can minimize or reverse the neurocognitive effects of HIV infection.

PREVENTION OF MATERNAL-INFANT HIV TRANSMISSION

Identification of HIV-infected women before or during pregnancy is critical in preventing perinatal HIV transmission. Prenatal HIV counseling and testing should be provided to all pregnant women. Administration of zidovudine to pregnant women during pregnancy and labor and to infants for the first 6 weeks of life reduced perinatal HIV transmission by two thirds (26% to 8%) in the Pediatric AIDS Clinical Trials Group (PACTG) 076 trial. This regimen is the standard of care for HIV-infected pregnant women and their newborns. Several clinical trials conducted in other countries have demonstrated the efficacy of shorter, less expensive regimens of zidovudine or nevirapine. Early identification of HIV-infected pregnant women also allows for appropriate care of the mother, counseling on the risks of HIV transmission through breast milk, and early institution of PCP prophylaxis for the infant at 4 to 6 weeks of age.

CARE OF THE HIV-INFECTED CHILD

Proper care of HIV-infected children requires a multidisciplinary team including pediatricians, experts in antiretroviral therapy, nutritionists, physical therapists, pharmacists, psychologists, social workers, and outreach workers. The primary care practitioner will need to rely on infectious disease specialists in the management of medication used in treatment of HIV-infected patients, which are multitudinous and change frequently as new and better regimens emerge.

Immunization of the HIV-Infected Child

Immunizations generally are safe for HIV-infected children, although the immune suppression caused by HIV results in less benefit than in non–HIV-infected children. However, the small risk of serious complications from live viral vaccines has led to special recommendations for HIV-infected children. In addition, immunization of HIV-infected children is associated with a transient increase in HIV viral load, but this increase does not appear to be clinically significant.

Toxoids, subunit vaccines, inactivated vaccines, and recombinant vaccines are not associated with increased risks of complications in HIV-infected children. Vaccines in these categories include diphtheria and tetanus toxoids, whole-cell and acellular pertussis vaccines, *Haemophilus influenzae* conjugate vaccines, and hepatitis B vaccines. These vaccines should be administered to HIV-infected children according to the routine immunization schedule. HIV-infected children may develop lower antibody titers than healthy children following immunization and are more likely to lose protective antibody earlier. The immune response to hepatitis B vaccine is particularly poor in HIV-infected children.

Because of an increased risk of invasive infection with *Streptococcus pneumoniae*, HIV-infected children should receive the pneumococcal polysaccharide vaccine at 2 years of age. Repeat pneumococcal immunization is recommended at 3 to 5 years after primary immunization. Pneumococcal conjugate vaccines should allow for immunization of HIV-infected children in infancy. Annual immunization with influenza vaccine also is recommended for HIV-infected children older than 6 months of age.

Live viral vaccines, such as oral polio vaccine and measles, mumps, and rubella vaccines, may result in infection and disease resulting from vaccine virus in immunocompromised, HIV-infected children. The risk, however, is small. Many HIV-infected children received at least one dose of oral polio vaccine (OPV) without complications before their HIV infection was known. This is a moot point, because inactivated polio vaccine (IPV) is now recommended for all children.

After the report of an HIV-infected young man who had severe immunosuppression who developed fatal infection via measles vaccine virus after immunization, advisory groups in the United States recommended withholding measles vaccine from HIV-infected children who had severe immunosuppression defined by age-specific CD4+ T-lymphocyte cell counts. However, measles immunization of children who have asymptomatic HIV infection is recommended, and consideration should be given to vaccinating symptomatic HIV-infected children who are not severely immunocompromised. As with other vaccines, the immune response to measles vaccine by HIV-infected children may be poor, and vaccinated children may remain susceptible to measles virus infection. Serious complications following mumps or rubella immunization have not been reported.

Although live varicella virus vaccine is recommended for children, experience in HIV-infected children is limited. The Advisory Committee on Immunization Practices (ACIP) recommends considering varicella vaccine for HIV-infected children who have CD4+ T-lymphocyte percentages equal to or greater than 25%.

Antimicrobial Prophylaxis

Because of the high mortality rate associated with PCP in early infancy, PCP prophylaxis should be administered to all HIV-exposed infants beginning at 4 to 6 weeks of age, even if HIV infection is not confirmed. Prophylaxis is continued until 12 months of age or until the diagnosis of HIV infection has been excluded. For children 1 to 5 years of age, PCP prophylaxis is administered if the CD4 T-lymphocyte cell count is less than 500 cells/mm^3 and for children 6 to 12 years of age if it is less than 200 cells/mm^3. Lifelong PCP prophylaxis is required for children who have a history of PCP. The recommended regimen is Co-trimoxazole taken orally 3 days a week. Alternative regimens include dapsone or pentamidine.

HIV-infected children who have recurrent oral candidiasis may benefit from antifungal prophylaxis with oral nystatin, clotrimazole, or fluconazole. Many experts recommend daily oral rifabutin for prophylaxis against *Mycobacterium avium-intracellulare* infection in children who have CD4+ T-lymphocyte cell counts of less than 100 cells/mm^3.

Monthly infusions of intravenous immunoglobulin were recommended previously to prevent recurrent bacterial infections in children who had low levels of serum IgG. However, antibiotic prophylaxis with Co-trimoxazole or penicillin is less invasive and less expensive.

Postexposure prophylaxis with immune globulin is indicated for HIV-infected children after exposure to varicella and measles, even if the child has a history of immunization. Varicella-zoster immunoglobulin (VZIG) should be given as soon as possible after varicella exposure, no later than 96 hours. Immune globulin (IG) should be given to HIV-infected children within 6 days of exposure to a person who has measles. Measles immunization should be delayed 6 months after receipt of immune globulin.

Antiretroviral Therapy

The treatment of HIV infection with antiretroviral drugs has become extremely complex. Management of antiretroviral therapy should be directed by a specialist who has knowledge of the mechanisms of action of antiretroviral agents, potential toxicity, drug interactions, and cross-resistance patterns. Often the best means of providing care to HIV-infected children, as well as determining safe and effective therapies, is to enroll HIV-infected children in clinical trials.

Because most children acquire HIV infection during or near the time of birth, antiretroviral therapy can be initiated during early primary infection. In contrast, the majority of HIV-infected adults begin therapy long after primary infection. Infants diagnosed with HIV infection in the first year of life should be treated with combination therapy consisting of three or more drugs, regardless of clinical, immunological, or virological status. For children diagnosed after 12 months of age, the decision to start treatment should be based on clinical symptoms, plasma HIV RNA levels, and CD4 T-lymphocyte cell counts. Combination therapy with reverse transcriptase and protease inhibitors is recommended. Resistance to antiretroviral drugs can develop rapidly, and as with therapy for tuberculosis, a single drug should not be used.

The choice of antiretroviral regimens for children is based on several factors, including (1) the availability of pediatric formulations; (2) the ability of the child's caregiver to administer the drug regimen; (3) potential drug interactions; and (4) the impact of the drug schedule on the child's quality of life. The last consideration includes the number and frequency of drug doses, compatibility with other medications, and compatibility with food. Because an increasing proportion of HIV-infected women receives antiretroviral therapy before or during pregnancy, exposure to these antiretroviral agents need to be considered in selecting the optimal regimen for the child. Before therapy begins, the child's clinical and nutritional status should be carefully documented, neuropsychometric testing should be performed, and baseline laboratory studies should include a complete blood count with differential, liver function tests, a CD4 T-lymphocyte cell count, and a plasma HIV RNA level.

Protease inhibitors recommended for children are nelfinavir, ritonavir, amprenavir, and saquinavir. Saquinavir is available in capsule form only. Indinavir is not yet approved for children. Commonly used combinations of nucleoside reverse transcriptase inhibitors are ZDV and ddI, ZDV and 3TC, d4T and 3TC, and d4T and ddI. Several combinations are not recommended either because of antagonism (d4T/ZDV) or because of overlapping toxicities (ddC/ddI, ddC/d4T, ddC/3TC). The non-nucleoside reverse transcriptase inhibitors nevirapine, delavirdine, and efavirenz can be used in combination with the nucleoside reverse transcriptase inhibitors.

Common side effects of nucleoside reverse transcriptase inhibitors are anemia and neutropenia with ZDV, pancreatitis with ddI, peripheral neuropathy with ddI and d4T, and a flu-like hypersensitivity reaction with abacavir. Rechallenge with abacavir can be fatal. Common side effects of the non-nucleosides reverse transcriptase inhibitors nevirapine, delavirdine, and efavirenz are rashes and hepatitis. Efavirenz can cause bad dreams, hallucinations, confusion, and impaired concentration. Gastrointestinal symptoms are the major side effects of protease inhibitors but can be minimized by slowly increasing the dose at the start of therapy.

Adherence to complex drug regimens can be difficult. Compliance is hindered by the large number or volume of medications, poor palatability, varied dosing schedules, and different effects of food on drug bioavailability. Mixing some drugs with foods, such as peanut butter or ice cream, may improve compliance in children. Behavioral therapy, begun before starting combination therapy, can be helpful in designing a routine medication schedule, teaching parents and caregivers methods to improve compliance, and teaching the child techniques for swallowing unsavory medications.

Strict adherence to the treatment regimen is essential for the prevention of drug-resistance. Because of cross-resistance, resistance to one drug can limit the effectiveness of other drugs of the same class. HIV isolates can be tested for drug resistance to guide treatment decisions. Plasma HIV-RNA levels should be measured 4 weeks after the patient has started therapy to assess response. The frequency of follow-up visits depends on many factors, including the child's clinical status and expected compliance with therapy, but should include periodic measurements of HIV RNA levels and CD4 T-lymphocyte cell counts.

Drug Interactions with Antiretroviral Therapy

HIV protease inhibitors, as well as the non-nucleoside reverse transcriptase inhibitors, are metabolized in the liver by a cytochrome P450 enzyme. Protease inhibitors have the potential to inhibit this enzyme and interfere with the metabolism of many other drugs. Protease inhibitors also can act as potent inhibitors of two other P450 enzymes active in the metabolism of analgesics, beta-blockers, and phenytoin. Ritonavir can stimulate glucuronidation, *decreasing* the concentration of drugs metabolized by this pathway, including sedatives such as lorazepam and the narcotics morphine and codeine.

Many drugs that have altered metabolism because of protease inhibitors are used in pediatric emergencies, including narcotic analgesics, anticonvulsants, antiarrhythmics, calcium-channel blockers, and corticosteroids. These drugs should be used with caution in children receiving protease inhibitors. Drugs that have narrow therapeutic margins require particularly careful monitoring for adverse effects and measurement of drug concentrations. Drugs contraindicated for use with protease inhibitors include meperidine, midazolam, astemizole, terfenadine, cisapride, and rifampin.

A number of other medications frequently prescribed for HIV-infected children are inhibitors of cytochrome P450 enzymes, including ketoconazole, itraconazole, clarithromycin, and erythromycin. Inhibition of cytochrome P450 enzymes by these medications may lead to an increase in the plasma concentration of protease inhibitors. Dosage reduction of the protease inhibitor may be required. Conversely, inducers of the cytochrome P450 enzyme system also are prescribed frequently for HIV-infected children. Antimycobacterial drugs (rifampin, rifabutin), anticonvulsants (phenobarbital, phenytoin, carbamazepine), and glucocorticoids (dexamethasone) are inducers of cytochrome P450 enzymes. Increased metabolism of protease inhibitors may result in subtherapeutic levels, with the potential emergence of drug resistance.

POSTEXPOSURE PROPHYLAXIS FOLLOWING COMMUNITY NEEDLESTICK INJURIES

Parents, caretakers, and physicians often are most concerned about transmission of HIV following accidental injury from a discarded needle. However, no consensus or recommendations are available to guide management in such circumstances. The risk of HIV transmission following occupational exposure to HIV-infected blood is 0.3%. Most experts agree that the risk following community needlestick injury is lower than the risk of occupational exposure. Factors to be considered in the use of antiretroviral agents for postexposure prophylaxis following community needlestick injuries include the potential risk of HIV transmission, toxicities, and cost of antiretroviral drugs, and the ability and willingness of the family to adhere to therapy. Regimens for occupational postexposure prophylaxis may be followed.

CHILD CARE AND SCHOOL FOR THE HIV-INFECTED CHILD

Because the risk of HIV transmission appears to be negligible, HIV-infected children should not be restricted from attending child care or school. Special consideration may be warranted for children who have unusual risk factors for transmission, such as frequent biting or scratching, severe dermatitis, or bleeding disorders. In such circumstances, the pediatrician should assess the need to protect other children.

THE HIV-INFECTED ADOLESCENT

Although the number of adolescents who have AIDS is small, an increasing number of adolescents are infected with HIV through unprotected sex. Because the onset of AIDS occurs years after sexual transmission, AIDS in young adults reflects acquisition of HIV during adolescence. Pediatricians caring for adolescents must ensure that they have knowledge of the risks of acquiring HIV and other sexually transmitted diseases through unprotected sex and be counseled on safe sexual practices.

Primary HIV infection in adolescents and adults frequently is accompanied by a mononucleosis-like illness characterized by fever, sore throat, lethargy, and lymphadenopathy. Recognition of primary HIV infection is important because it allows for early administration of antiretroviral therapy. Because HIV antibodies take several months to achieve detectable levels, PCR should be used to diagnose primary HIV infection.

THE ROLE OF THE PEDIATRICIAN IN THE CARE OF HIV-INFECTED CHILDREN

The pediatrician plays a critical role in the care of HIV-infected children and their families. As the child's primary care provider, the pediatrician can be responsible for (1) diagnosing HIV infection; (2) providing well child care, including monitoring growth and development and administering immunizations; (3) coordinating care among the multiple specialties and services, including expertise in antiretroviral therapy, developmental and psychological assessment, nutritional support, and dental care; (4) managing common medical problems; and (5) directing the family to social and financial support services.

Many parents and guardians are not willing to tell the child that he or she is infected with HIV. However, most children are made aware of their illness through frequent medical visits and medications. As the primary care provider with a close relationship with the family, the pediatrician often is in the best position to promote and assist with disclosure. Appropriate disclosure tailored to the child's cognitive level is helpful in alleviating guilt and allows for discussion between the child, caregivers, and health care professionals. Uninfected siblings of HIV-infected children also are emotionally affected by the diagnosis and should be included in support groups and counseling.

The primary care pediatrician also can play a critical role in providing advice and support as the child nears death. The pediatrician can help the family interpret the complexities of critical care and approach a decision on the appropriateness of heroic interventions. In some circumstances, the pediatrician may even be able to assist the family care for the dying child at home if critical care is deemed futile. After the death of the child, the pediatrician should continue to support the family through the grief process. Because many pediatricians invest much time and emotional energy in caring for an HIV-infected child, many take the opportunity to express their sympathy by attending the child's funeral. This can be an important gesture for both the family and the pediatrician.

RESOURCES

Information on clinical trials for HIV-infected children can be obtained by calling 800-TRIALS-A. The National Pediatric HIV Resource Center can be contacted at 800-362-0071; the telephone number for the Pediatric AIDS Foundation is 415-883-1796.

Updated information on HIV and AIDS can be obtained from the following web sites: http://www.hopkins-aids.edu and http://www.hivinsite.ucsf.edu. Updated information on potential drug interactions with protease inhibitors can be found at the Food and Drug Administration web site: http://www.fda.gov/oashi/aids/piindexl.

SUGGESTED READING

American Academy of Pediatrics: Human immunodeficiency virus infection. In Pickering LK, editor: *Red Book 2000: Report of the Committee on Infectious Diseases,* ed 25, Elk Grove Village, Ill, 2000, American Academy of Pediatrics.

220 Hydrocephalus

Dennis L. Johnson

Cerebral spinal fluid (CSF) is produced by the choroid plexus, fills the cerebral ventricles, flows out of the ventricles into the basal cisterns of the subarachnoid space, and percolates around, up, and over the surface of the brain to be absorbed into the arachnoid granulations along the sagittal sinus. If the flow in this CSF pathway is increased (e.g., by a choroid plexus papilloma) or blocked (e.g., by a medulloblastoma filling and obstructing the fourth ventricle), the rising volume of CSF dilates the ventricular system and compresses the surrounding brain.[5] Hydrocephalus is defined here as enlargement of the ventricular system associated with the accumulation of CSF under pressure. Cerebral atrophy also is associated with enlargement of the ventricular system, but in contrast to hydrocephalus, the CSF pressure is not elevated and the surrounding brain is not compressed.

Physicians throughout history have recognized hydrocephalus, and history is replete with courageous attempts to treat it. Treatment has included external CSF drainage with gold cannulas, skull binding and casting to prevent head enlargement, removal of the choroid plexus to eliminate the source of CSF, and more recently, CSF diversion through ventriculoperitoneal shunts. The history of CSF diversion is a chronicle of surgeons' courage, ingenuity, and frustration in the treatment of a condition that was hopelessly untreatable before the mid 1960s.[4] Hydrocephalus occurs in 3 to 4 of every 1000 live births; an estimated 100,000 children currently are under treatment in the United States for hydrocephalus.[2]

CLASSIFICATION

Hydrocephalus traditionally has been classified as communicating or noncommunicating. If CSF within the ventricular system does not communicate with the subarachnoid spaces at the base of the brain, the hydrocephalus is noncommunicating. Noncommunicating hydrocephalus is characterized by a relatively small fourth ventricle (which may even be distorted by tumor) on computed tomography (CT) or magnetic resonance imaging (MRI) and implies that the flow of CSF is blocked before it enters the fourth ventricle. The fourth ventricle is enlarged in communicating hydrocephalus. In the era before CT and MRI, water-soluble dye injected into the ventricles could be retrieved from the subarachnoid space by lumbar puncture (LP) in communicating hydrocephalus, but if dye could not be traced from the ventricle to the lumbar subarachnoid space, the hydrocephalus was deemed noncommunicating. Whether or not the dye appeared in the subarachnoid space had specific diagnostic and treatment implications.[11] This classification schema is still relevant in the current management of the child who has hydrocephalus.

ETIOLOGY

The further classification and cause of hydrocephalus is distinctive for each age group: infancy (birth to 12 months), childhood (1 to 12 years), and adolescence (13 to 18 years).

Infancy

The premature infant usually develops hydrocephalus following intraventricular hemorrhage associated with bleeding from the germinal matrix. The diagnosis is made and the progression of the hydrocephalus can be followed easily by weekly ultrasound examination of the head. If no fourth ventricle is visible on the scan, the block to the flow of CSF is most likely at the aqueduct of Sylvius. The hydrocephalus is noncommunicating, and LPs will not drain the ventricular system adequately. If, on the other hand, the blood has only partially obstructed the basal cisterns or the arachnoid granulations and the fourth ventricle can be identified on imaging studies, hydrocephalus is communicating, and serial LPs will drain the ventricles and avoid a shunt in the majority of cases.

Congenital hydrocephalus often is diagnosed on routine prenatal ultrasound examination and most commonly is due to aqueductal stenosis or to cytomegalic inclusion virus (CMV) or toxoplasmosis infection. Congenital hydrocephalus can be associated with Dandy-Walker malformation of the cerebellum (dilation of the fourth ventricle associated with absence of the cerebellar vermis), meningomyelocele (MM), or occipital encephalocele. Hydrocephalus may become evident only after surgical repair of MM and occipital encephalocele.

In the full-term infant, the diagnosis is suspected on the basis of macrocrania (also called macrocephaly or megalocephaly) or sequential head circumference measurements that cross percentiles on normal growth charts. The most common cause of infant macrocrania, however, is constitutional or familial megalocephaly. The differential diagnosis of progressive infant macrocrania also includes subdural hygromas, subdural hematomas, recovery from starvation, Canavan's disease, Alexander's disease, thickened skull associated with thalassemia and osteopetrosis, lead encephalopathy, and mucopolysaccharidoses. Posterior fossa tumors are not common in infancy. A rare cause of hydrocephalus in infancy is a choroid plexus papilloma or carcinoma that produces an excessive amount of CSF and enlarges the ventricles. Even after the choroid plexus tumor has been removed, hydrocephalus may persist because of postoperative distortion or stenosis of the CSF pathway. In addition, hydrocephalus can occur after meningitis and following severe head injury.

Childhood

The most common cause of hydrocephalus in a child is a posterior fossa tumor, but congenital hydrocephalus caused by aqueductal stenosis also may be discovered late. The hydrocephalus of posterior fossa tumors is associated with obstruction of the fourth ventricle and its outlets into the subarachnoid space. The most common brain tumors in childhood are medulloblastoma, cerebellar astrocytoma, and ependymoma. In a majority of cases the hydrocephalus is relieved by removing the tumor. In childhood, hydrocephalus does not manifest with macrocrania or delayed development, but rather with signs and symptoms of increased intracranial pressure—headaches, vomiting, papilledema, and ataxia.

Adolescence

In adolescence, hydrocephalus often occurs with the same constellation of signs and symptoms as in childhood; it also may manifest more subtly with a change in school performance or athletic ability. Papilledema is seen more reliably in older, more cooperative young people. In adolescence, a midbrain tumor, a pineal cyst, or a pineal region tumor is commonly the primary cause of new onset hydrocephalus. MRI is the definitive imaging study.

TREATMENT

Neonatal posthemorrhagic hydrocephalus associated with prematurity is most often communicating and can be relieved by serial LPs. However, if little or no CSF can be obtained by LP, then a presumptive diagnosis of noncommunicating hydrocephalus can be made. Because the CSF cannot pass through to the lumbar subarachnoid space, a ventricular catheter that is attached to a subgaleal reservoir is implanted. The noncommunicating hydrocephalus is relieved percutaneously until the infant has outgrown the potential morbidity of necrotizing enterocolitis (about 2 kg body weight). Then a standard ventriculoperitoneal shunt is implanted. Communicating hydrocephalus is more likely to compensate over time, and the need for a shunt may diminish. Similarly, shunt malfunction is more insidious because structures in the subarachnoid space have some capacity for absorption. The majority of shunted children remain dependent on the CSF shunt to control hydrocephalus.

In the hands of a pediatric neurosurgeon, the modern treatment of congenital hydrocephalus is straightforward, and the ventriculoperitoneal shunt is the gold standard.[13] Sufficient peritoneal tubing can be coiled in the peritoneal cavity to accommodate axial or vertical growth of the child through adulthood. Based on the experience of the past two decades, one to two revisions of a shunt can be expected in the first 10 years. Occasionally, however, especially in children who were born prematurely and who suffered posthemorrhagic hydrocephalus, shunt function is more problematic, and multiple revisions may be necessary. If the peritoneal cavity cannot be used (e.g., recent colostomy or peritonitis), a ventriculoatrial, ventriculopleural, or ventricle-to-gallbladder shunt can be substituted. Communicating hydrocephalus also can be treated with a lumboperitoneal shunt, but scoliosis and a Chiari I malformation may be acquired as a secondary effect.

Noncommunicating hydrocephalus can be treated by a variety of methods to divert the CSF around the block. The logical treatment for noncommunicating hydrocephalus is endoscopic third ventriculostomy,[3] which creates an opening from the third ventricle directly into the subarachnoid space through the lamina terminales or the floor of the third ventricle. However, third ventriculostomy will not be effective if the CSF cannot be absorbed from the subarachnoid space. Because no imaging study is available to assess CSF absorption quantitatively, the success of these alternative methods is tentative.

Children who have noncommunicating hydrocephalus, however, usually are very shunt dependent (i.e., CSF absorption is supplanted by the shunt), and shunt failure may be associated with the rapid onset of intracranial hypertension. An LP performed in a child who has noncommunicating hydrocephalus may result in life-threatening cerebral herniation. Several shunt valves and options are available to be tailored to the patient's special needs. In general, however, a low-pressure shunt is implanted in the preterm infant who has hydrocephalus associated with intraventricular hemorrhage and in the neonate who has very severe hydrocephalus (head circumference greater than 42 cm). In all other patients, a medium-pressure shunt generally is preferable. In the older child who has hydrocephalus and a very large head, an antisiphon device incorporated into the shunt (Delta valve by PS Medical) or a variable resistance valve helps to prevent collapse of the ventricular system and the development of subdural hematomas. Several devices are available to fulfill this purpose and to suit the surgeon's preference.

The medical treatment of hydrocephalus has been largely unsuccessful. Acetazolamide (Diamox) is administered to decrease the output of the choroid plexus but is not always well tolerated, and a rapid decrease in its effectiveness develops.

PROGNOSIS

An infant treated for congenital hydrocephalus shortly after birth has greater than an 85% chance of survival and 53% probability of having normal intelligence (IQ greater than 80).[10] A thin cerebral mantle and underlying abnormalities of the brain reduce the probability of a favorable outcome. A mean head circumference of 42 cm and a cerebral mantle of 1 cm thickness at birth is seen in cognitively impaired (IQ less than 65) survivors. Children who have severe hydrocephalus and no underlying abnormalities can lead normal, productive lives if the hydrocephalus is treated early.[12] With few exceptions, shunts must be maintained for the lifetime of the patient; children do not "outgrow" hydrocephalus.

MANAGEMENT AND COMPLICATIONS

Shunt Malfunction

Continuing management of the shunted hydrocephalic patient can be quite problematic. Shunt malfunction can manifest in a myriad of ways, but generally causes lethargy, vomiting, and headache, which are symptoms of many common childhood illnesses. Infants may present with a full fontanelle and irritability. In a child, shunt malfunction also can cause behavior changes and decline in school performance. Aggressive and demanding behavior is not uncommon. Parents often say the child's "eyes aren't right." Routine inspection of the shunt tract and measurement of the head circumference are important in screening for shunt complications. A slack fontanelle in an infant who is held in an upright position is reliable evidence of good shunt function. When the fontanelle closes, computed tomography (CT) scan should be done to define baseline ventricular size. Pumping the valve seldom offers useful information and may occlude the ventricular catheter by aspirating choroid plexus or debris into the tip of the catheter. With shunt malfunction, papilledema may be present, lateral eye movement may be diminished, and convergence usually disappears. The classic "sun-setting" sign (downward deviation of the eye with the iris setting on the horizon of the inferior lid margin) is not common but is a sure sign of shunt failure. Blindness occurs rarely. CT usually will show enlargement of the ventricles when compared with the baseline scan. The primary care physician must be aware, however, that a child who has severe headaches, vomiting, and increased lethargy may still have life-threatening shunt malfunction, even though a CT scan shows normal-size ventricles.[14] If the CT scan shows enlarged ventricles and obliteration of the perimesencephalic cisterns, an emergent shunt revision is in order.[8] In this author's hands, routine annual CT scans and plain radiographs of the shunt are a poor substitute for careful history and physical examination to screen for shunt malfunction.

Shunt Infection

Shunt infection complicates 5% of shunt operations. Infection commonly is associated with fever, an elevated white blood cell count, and redness along the shunt tract; however, the symptoms may be limited to low grade fever, abdominal discomfort, and anorexia. Most shunt infections occur within 3 months of shunt implantation or revision. Rarely, infection occurs many years later as focal redness and tenderness along the shunt tract. Adequate treatment dictates removal of the old shunt, placement of a temporary ventriculostomy for external CSF drainage, and administration of intravenous (IV) antibiotics.[6] *Staphylococcus epidermidis* (coagulase-negative staph) and *Staphylococcus aureus* (coagulase-positive staph) are the most common infecting organisms; vancomycin (60 mg/kg/day) is the antibiotic of choice. Intrathecal antibiotics seldom are necessary if adequate serum peak and trough levels of antibiotic are achieved. Shunts can extrude through the urethra, anus, or the vagina and must then be presumed to be infected and treated with removal of the shunt and temporary diversion by using an external drainage device. Abdominal pseudocysts or localized pockets of CSF may develop with or without infection.

If the child who has hydrocephalus develops an acute abdomen, the diagnosis may well be appendicitis. If the appendix has perforated to produce diffuse or localized peritonitis, the shunt catheter should be removed from the abdomen and connected to a drainage-collection bag until all signs of infection have disappeared. Children who have spina bifida who undergo bladder augmentation to expand the capacity of the bladder may perforate the bladder and exhibit an acute abdominal condition. Temporary externalization of the peritoneal catheter is necessary. Insufflation of the abdomen with gas during laparoscopy may obstruct absorption of CSF through the peritoneum and cause acute shunt malfunction.

Ventriculoatrial Shunts

Ventriculoatrial shunts can be complicated by septicemia, bacterial endocarditis, glomerulonephritis, pulmonary embolus, migration of the atrial catheter into the pulmonary vasculature, cardiac arrhythmias, and cor pulmonale. The complication rate is comparable to that of VP shunts, but complications are more life threatening.[9]

Seizures

Seizures occur in about 30% of shunted patients, usually because of an underlying abnormality of the brain. Recurrent seizures are an uncommon indication of shunt failure.[7]

Slit Ventricle Syndrome

Overdrainage of the ventricular system by a shunt occurs rarely and manifests as the slit ventricle syndrome.[15] Severe headaches exacerbated by activity in an upright posture are relieved at least partially by lying down. The slit ventricle syndrome is associated with nonexistent or very small slitlike ventricles. Many children have slit ventricles on CT scan but are not symptomatic. Symptoms presumably are caused by stiff, noncompliant ventricles that must first expand to push the ventricular wall away from the catheter. The treatment may be as simple as afternoon rest periods (in horizontal position) or may involve changing the valve to one that incorporates an antisiphon device or a variable resistance mechanism.

Subdural Hygromas

Subdural hygromas may occur in the child who is shunted after the fontanelle has closed and the skull has become more fixed in size and shape. Because the skull has expanded to an abnormally large size to accommodate the brain and hydrocephalus, extra space is created when the ventricles decrease in size and the brain reconstitutes itself. The accumulation of CSF in the subdural space usually resolves spontaneously. If the subdural hygroma enlarges and causes symptoms of pressure, a separate subdural-peritoneal shunt may be necessary. This complication can be avoided if an antisiphon device or variable resistance mechanism is incorporated into the valve.

Shunt Metastases

The risk of metastasis from shunting children who have primary central nervous system tumors is small and does not justify the insertion of a Millipore filter to screen tumor cells.[1] The filter often clogs and results in shunt failure.

Prophylactic Antibiotics

Prophylactic antibiotics are given during shunt implantation and revision by most pediatric neurosurgeons to prevent shunt infection. This author, however, does not recommend routine antibiotic prophylaxis for dental work on the child who has a ventriculoperitoneal shunt. Prophylactic antibiotics are recommended for children who have ventriculoatrial shunts or in children who have VP shunts who undergo abdominal procedures that involve manipulating the peritoneal catheter.

When to Refer

Unremitting headaches with or without vomiting may be sufficient reason for referring the hydrocephalic patient who has a ventriculoperitoneal shunt to his or her pediatric neurosurgeon. If the CT shows enlargement of the ventricular system compared with previous studies, then an urgent referral is indicated. However, even if no change is apparent on serial CTs, shunt malfunction still is possible. Intermittent headaches, especially those that occur in the morning and gradually subside during the day, may be associated with shunt malfunction. The classic symptom triad of shunt failure (headaches, vomiting, lethargy) is not always present and must be differentiated from common childhood illnesses.

Progressive macrocrania may be the only sign of shunt malfunction. Seizures are not a common sign of shunt malfunction. Only 4% of shunted children who are seen in an emergency room for seizures go on to have a shunt revision. Unless a seizure is associated with some other sign of shunt malfunction, the patient need not be referred or hospitalized.[7]

When to Hospitalize

The hydrocephalic patient who cannot be aroused easily should be hospitalized with the presumptive diagnosis of shunt failure. If emergent CT scan shows enlargement of the ventricles compared with previous baseline scans, an urgent revision should be done. If the basal cisterns on the CT scan are obliterated, an emergent revision will be necessary because the malfunction is life threatening.

REFERENCES

1. Berger MS, et al: The risks of metastases from shunting in children with primary central nervous system tumor, *J Neurosurg* 74:872, 1991.
2. Carey CM, Tullous MW, Walker ML: Hydrocephalus: etiology, pathologic effects, diagnosis, and natural history. In Check WR, editor: *Pediatric neurosurgery,* Philadelphia, 1994, WB Saunders.
3. Cohen AR: Endoscopic ventricular surgery, *Pediatr Neurosurg* 19:127, 1993.
4. Davidoff LM: Treatment of hydrocephalus: historical review and description of a new method, *Arch Surg* 18:1737, 1929.
5. Davson H, Welch K, Segal MB: *Physiology and pathophysiology of cerebrospinal fluid,* Edinburgh, 1987, Churchill Livingstone.
6. James HE, et al: Prospective randomized study of therapy in cerebrospinal fluid shunt infection, *Neurosurgery* 7:459, 1980.
7. Johnson DL, Conry J, O'Donnell R: Epileptic seizure as a sign of cerebrospinal fluid shunt malfunction, *Pediatr Neurosurg* 24:223, 1996.
8. Johnson DL, McCullough DC, Schwarz S: Perimesencephalic cistern obliteration: a CT sign of life-threatening shunt failure, *J Neurosurg* 64:386, 1986.
9. Johnson DL, O'Donnell R: The search for a perpetual shunt, *Concepts Pediatr Neurosurg* 9:29, 1989.
10. McCullough DM, Balzer-Martin LA: Current prognosis in overt neonatal hydrocephalus, *J Neurosurg* 57:378, 1982.
11. Milhorat TH: *Hydrocephalus and the cerebrospinal fluid,* Baltimore, 1972, Williams & Wilkins.
12. Piatt JH Jr, Carlson CV: A search for determinants of cerebrospinal fluid shunt survival: retrospective analysis of a 14-year institutional experience, *Pediatr Neurosurg* 19:233, 1993.
13. Rekate HL: Treatment of hydrocephalus. In Albright AL, Pollack IF, Adelson PD, editors: *Principles and practice of pediatric neurosurgery,* New York, 1999, Thieme.
14. Sainte-Rose C, et al: Mechanical complications in shunts, *Pediatr Neurosurg* 17:2, 1991.
15. Wisoff JH, Epstein FJ: Diagnosis and treatment of the slit ventricle syndrome, *Concepts Pediatr Neurosurg* 11:79, 1991.

221 Hyperthyroidism

Nicholas Jospe

Hyperthyroidism is the result of excessive activity of the thyroid gland. The clinical manifestation of excessive circulating thyroid hormone is called *thyrotoxicosis.*

PATHOGENESIS

With a few exceptions, thyrotoxicosis in pediatrics is the result of Graves' disease.[4] Other causes of thyrotoxicosis include the early phase of autoimmune hypothyroidism (Hashimoto's thyroiditis) before thyroid function is diminished; a hyperfunctioning thyroid nodule; pituitary resistance to thyroxine (T_4), which results in excess secretion of thyroid stimulant hormone (TSH); and factitious hyperthyroidism caused by administration of exogenous thyroid hormone. Graves' disease is most frequent in early adolescence, is rare in infancy, and is infrequent in childhood. Affected subjects frequently have a family history of thyroid disorder. The prevalence of Graves' disease is six to eight times greater in girls than in boys.

Graves' disease, like Hashimoto's thyroiditis, is an autoimmune disorder that occurs in subjects who have a genetic predisposition, which is itself linked to certain HLA haplotypes.[3] Hyperfunction of the thyroid gland in Graves' disease is caused by autoantibodies directed against the receptor for TSH.[11] These antibodies, called *thyroid receptor antibodies* (TRAb), are characterized by an overall predominant stimulatory effect on thyroid cells leading to excessive production and release of T_4. Included among TRAbs are (1) thyroid-stimulating immunoglobulins (TSI) that mimic TSH in their stimulatory action on the production of T_4, (2) TSH-binding inhibitory immunoglobulins (TBII) that prevent TSH from binding at its receptor and do not stimulate thyroid cells, and (3) TSH-blocking antibodies (TbAb). Other antibodies detected in patients who have Graves' disease include thyroid growth-stimulating antibodies, which contribute to goiter formation, and antithyroglobulin and antimicrosomal antibodies that also are found in Hashimoto's thyroiditis.[13] Graves' disease can occur in conjunction with other endocrine autoimmune diseases, such as diabetes mellitus type 1, hypoparathyroidism, and Addison's disease, or with other autoimmune diseases such as myasthenia gravis, periodic paralysis, and vitiligo.

CLINICAL FEATURES (Table 221-1)

Early nonspecific findings in Graves' disease include changes in behavior such as nervousness, sleeplessness, emotional lability, decreased school performance, or deteriorating handwriting; these largely reflect hyperactivity of the sympathetic nervous system. Graves' disease often remains undiagnosed for a long time because children can continue their normal activities without complaints overtly suggestive of hyperthyroidism. When cardiovascular signs are more prominent, these include tachycardia, a widened pulse pressure, and an overactive precordium. Neuromuscular signs and symptoms include tremor, a shortened deep tendon reflex relaxation phase, fatigability, and proximal muscle weakness. Though the child has an increased appetite, he or she loses weight more frequently than gains weight and also has frequent and loose bowel movements. Increased perspiration, warmth, heat intolerance, and smoothness of skin appear later. With long-standing disease, tall stature may accompany advanced skeletal maturation in childhood; curtailment of final height as a result of early closure of the epiphyses does not occur.

The size of the goiter when first examined is variable, and its presence frequently goes unnoticed. However, the thyroid gland usually is diffusely enlarged, is soft, and has a clearly delineated border. Examination should include palpation for the presence of a thrill and auscultation for the presence of a bruit. Measurement of the size of the lobes and of the isthmus is essential in following the course of the disease. Eye findings also are variable, although severe ophthalmopathy is far less common among children than among adults. Findings include prominence of the eyes (proptosis or exophthalmos), a conspicuous stare (caused by lid retraction and a widened palpebral fissure, as shown in Fig. 221-1), and lag of the upper lid on downward gaze. These eye findings are due to a combination of hyperactivity of the sympathetic system and of mucopolysaccharide accumulation and infiltration of the orbital fat and muscle cells. Most affected children can be treated with topical ophthalmic lubrication, but orbital fat decompression may be required in patients who have advanced conditions. In children, mucopolysaccharide accumulation in skin and subcutaneous tissue, as with pretibial myxedema, is infrequent.

LABORATORY DIAGNOSIS

The initial assessment should include measurement of serum free T_4, total T_4, and TSH concentrations. The diagnosis of Graves' disease rests on demonstrating elevated levels of T_4 and depression of TSH levels to below the lower limit of detectability. Age-appropriate normal values for T_4 must be consulted before a diagnosis of hyperthyroidism can be made.[5] Measurement of T_3 may help confirm the diagnosis, although this rarely is necessary. In thyrotoxicosis, the response of TSH to thyroid-releasing hormone (TRH) is blunted severely or is absent. The TRH stimulation test is necessary only when Graves' disease is suspected but the diagnosis is unclear. In equivocal situations, measurement of TRAbs, which are present in 95% of subjects who have Graves' disease, may help to confirm the diagnosis. In pregnant patients, high levels of TSI are predictive of neonatal Graves' disease.

The measurement of thyroid gland uptake of radioiodine (^{123}I) or technetium (^{99m}Tc) is useful only to distinguish painless thyroiditis from Graves' disease. Patients who have thyroiditis have a low uptake; patients who have Graves' disease have a high uptake. Generally, this study is not necessary.

DIFFERENTIAL DIAGNOSIS

Rarely, children who have Hashimoto's thyroiditis are thyrotoxic and have a high titer of TSI autoantibodies in addition to antithyroid antibodies. This condition has been called *Hashitoxicosis* and may be differentiated from routine Graves' disease in that the hyperthyroidism usually is a transient phase before progression to permanent hypothyroidism. Other causes of hyperthyroxinemia are rare. These include generalized resistance to thyroid hormone, found in association with attention deficit disorder,[6] factitious hyperthyroidism from excessive administration of thyroid hormone, TSH-secreting pituitary adenomas, and binding-protein changes characterized by normal free T_4 and TSH levels. Finally, hyperthyroidism caused by autonomous thyroid adenomas is rare and can be seen in association with the McCune-Albright syndrome (precocious puberty, café-au-lait pigmentation, and polyostotic fibrous dysplasia).

Table 221-1 Clinical Signs and Symptoms in Children Who Have Graves' Disease

	Prevalence (%)		
Signs and Symptoms	Saxena[10]	Mäenpää[7]	Barnes[1]
Goiter	100	100	97
Prominence of eyes	100	69	79
Exophthalmos	77		
Tachycardia	91	41	88
Nervousness	80	74	92
Increased appetite	71		67
Weight loss	67	59	50
Emotional lability	41		40
Heat intolerance	40		25
Frequent stools	16	35	13

MANAGEMENT

Antithyroid Medications

The aim of treatment is to reduce thyroid hormone production and block its effect on tissue peripherally. To this end, antithyroid medication consisting of thioamides, either methimazole (Tapazole) or propylthiouracil (PTU), usually are used first.[1,2] They are equally effective in inhibiting thyroid hormone production; however, PTU also blocks the peripheral conversion of T_4 to T_3. The half-life of PTU is 3 to 4 hours; that of methimazole is 6 to 13 hours. Both drugs cross the placenta, although PTU does so less than methimazole and therefore is the preferred drug during pregnancy. Both are present in very small quantities in breast milk, and breast-feeding may be continued. Therapy induces euthyroidism somewhat faster with methimazole than with PTU and from within weeks to a few months, depending on the size of the thyroid gland. Starting doses of PTU range from 5 to 10 mg/kg body weight, with a maximum of 300 mg/day, given in three to four divided doses; the dosage of methimazole is approximately 0.5 to 1 mg/kg, with a maximum of 30 mg/day, given in two to three divided doses. Once thyroid hormone secretion is depressed, maintenance doses may be

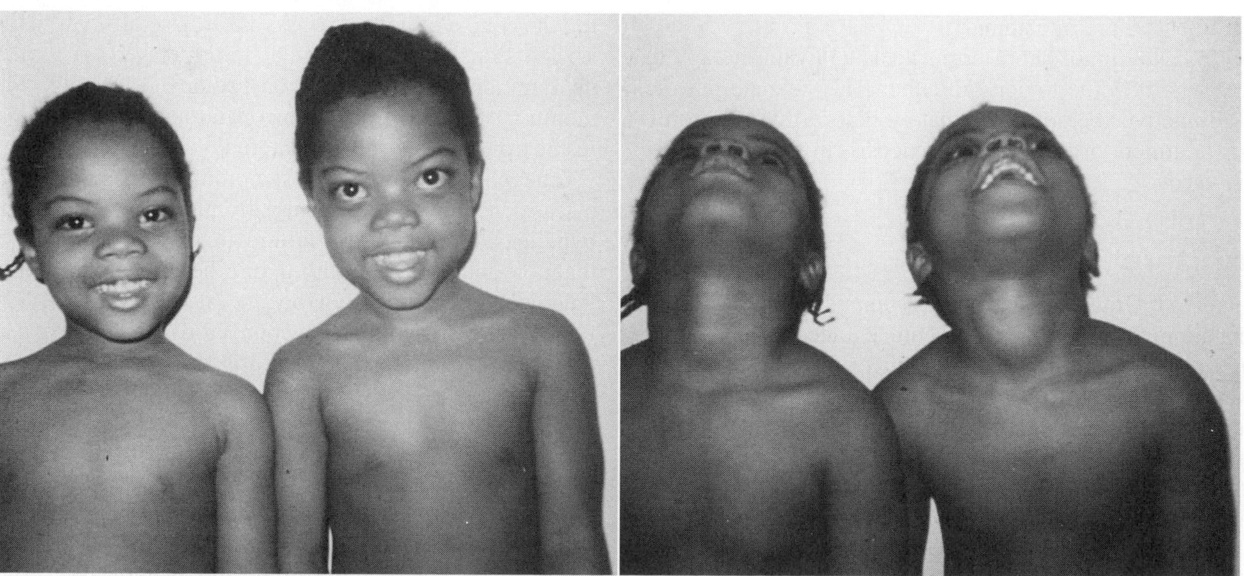

Fig. 221-1 The patient on the right exhibits a widened palpebral fissure and goiter; her twin, on the left, is unaffected at the time of this photograph, though later also developed Graves' disease.

given in two to three daily doses for PTU and one to two for methimazole.

Optimal long-term therapy for Graves' disease continues to be the subject of research and some controversy. Some physicians prefer to titrate the dose of antithyroid medication to maintain the patient in a euthyroid state. Others administer antithyroid medication until the patient becomes hypothyroid and supplement, thereafter, with thyroid hormone.

Therapy with antithyroid medication usually is maintained for a minimum of 1 year, during which time monitoring the size of the thyroid gland and following the TRAb levels can be useful, because shrinkage of the thyroid gland and falling TRAb titers predict a greater likelihood of remission after discontinuation of therapy. Thereafter, antithyroid medication can be stopped, and 20% to 40% of patients remain in remission. Continued monitoring of thyroid function tests is indicated to detect any subclinical relapse of Graves' disease.

Potential side effects of the thioamides include minor reactions that subside spontaneously. These include a purpuric, papular rash; urticaria; joint pain; stiffness; hair loss; and nausea or headaches and one serious reaction—agranulocytosis.[2] Agranulocytosis is an idiosyncratic reaction occurring in 1:500 to 1:1000 cases, usually within the first few months of therapy after either form of antithyroid medication. White blood cell count monitoring is not useful in anticipating agranulocytosis because its onset is very sudden. Patients thus need to be told about the significance of a sore throat, mouth sores, and fever as potentially heralding agranulocytosis. In addition to supportive treatment, such as antibiotic therapy, discontinuation of the thioamide is necessary. Agranulocytosis spontaneously reverses, and resumption with a different thioamide does not usually cause agranulocytosis to recur.[2] Finally, reactions such as drug fever, nephritis, hepatitis, or lupuslike reactions are rare.

In addition to antithyroid medication, adjuvant beta-adrenergic blockade may be accomplished with propranolol 0.5 to 2 mg/kg/day to control the sympathetic hyperactivity of severe Graves' disease. This form of therapy is necessary only transiently. It may be contraindicated in patients who have cardiac failure or asthma.

Iodide has a minor short-term role as adjuvant therapy in patients who develop toxicity to either PTU or methimazole or as adjunctive therapy immediately before thyroidectomy and for treatment of severe thyrotoxicosis. In practice, it seldom is used.

Definitive Therapy

If a relapse of Graves' disease occurs upon discontinuation of antithyroid medication, the therapeutic choices include either resumption of antithyroid medication or definitive therapy consisting of radioiodine or surgery. The choice depends on factors that affect the chances of success of each form of therapy, such as compliance, patient preference, and surgical expertise.

Surgery resolves the symptoms faster, but radioiodine is easy to administer, safer, and equally efficacious.[2,13] The potential for surgical complications from injury to adjacent structures (recurrent laryngeal nerve damage and hypoparathyroidism) dictates that referral be made to an experienced surgeon. Permanent hypothyroidism following surgery is frequent.[2] Radioiodine therapy is being used more extensively in the pediatric population, because fears regarding thyroid carcinoma and leukemia and radiation and genetic damage following treatment with a radioactive substance have been alleviated.[8,13] Radioactive iodine concentrates in the thyroid gland and induces cell death over time. Permanent hypothyroidism occurs within a year in 10% to 20% of patients following radioablative therapy. Pregnancy is a contraindication for radioiodine therapy because the iodine crosses the placenta and destroys the fetal thyroid.

PROGNOSIS AND COMPLICATIONS

Unfortunately, no reliable factors predict the natural course of Graves' disease in a given patient, aside possibly from goiter size and the severity of disease at onset. The clinical course ranges from progression to overt hypothyroidism on one hand to progression to thyroid storm on the other. Thyroid storm (thyrotoxic crisis) is an exceptional but severe complication.[9] This diagnosis rests on finding uncontrolled hyperthyroidism and is characterized by a constellation of findings including cardiac failure, tachycardia, hyperthermia, and central nervous system abnormalities such as confusion, apathy, or coma. Infection (even relatively minor) and trauma can be precipitating factors. Therapy must be expeditious and aggressive and should include antithyroid medication, iodide, beta-blockade, antipyresis, and medications to prevent cardiac failure.

NEONATAL THYROTOXICOSIS

Graves' disease is rare in neonates[5] and is due to the transplacental passage of thyroid-directed immunoglobulins from the mother. Transplacental passage of maternal antibodies may occur, even if the mother no longer has active autoimmune thyroid disease. In addition, stimulatory and blocking maternal thyroid antibodies may disappear at different rates, making the course of neonatal Graves' disease difficult to predict. Thus, its onset may be immediate or delayed for weeks, and its duration may be brief or prolonged, lasting up to 6 months.[12] Of note, transient neonatal hypothyroxinemia may result from the transfer of maternal TBII.

The clinical signs and symptoms of neonatal Graves' disease include microcephaly, frontal bossing, tachycardia, hypertension, irritability, failure to thrive, flushing, exophthalmos, and goiter. Vomiting, diarrhea, hepatosplenomegaly, jaundice, and thrombocytopenia also can occur. Cardiac failure and arrhythmias account for a mortality that approaches 25% when the disease is severe and treated inadequately.[5] Long-term complications are severe and include hypothyroidism, premature craniosynostosis, and intellectual deficits.

Until the disease resolves spontaneously, usually within 1 to 3 months as the maternal antibodies are degraded, adjunctive therapy may be necessary. The starting dose for methimazole is 0.5 to 1 mg/kg/day and that of PTU, 5 to 10 mg/kg/day; these doses can be increased up to 50%. Once thyroid hormone synthesis has been blocked adequately, iodide can be given as an additive. Lugol solution (5% iodide and 10% potassium iodide) is given at a dose of 1 drop every 8 hours. In severely hyperactive neonates, propranolol, 2 mg/kg/day, and digitalis, for cardiac failure, may be required. Finally, glucocorticoid therapy may be beneficial.

When to Refer

Refer all new diagnoses of hyperthyroidism to a pediatric endocrinologist, who may, in turn, use the services of nuclear medicine for radioiodine therapy or of an experienced surgeon for thyroidectomy. The endocrinologist will establish the diagnosis, initiate and then adjust treatment, review risks and benefits, and monitor the long-term course of the disease.

When to Hospitalize

Routine diagnosis and therapy of hyperthyroidism do not require hospitalization. Some of the severe complications of the disorder or of its therapy—ocular, cardiovascular, infectious—may be managed by the appropriate subspecialists and with hospitalization.

REFERENCES

1. Barnes VH, Blizzard RM: Antithyroid drug therapy for toxic diffuse goiter (Graves' disease): thirty years experience in children and adolescents, *J Pediatr* 91:313, 1977.
2. Cooper SD: Treatment of thyrotoxicosis. In Braverman LE, Utiger RD, editors: *Werner and Ingbar's the thyroid: a fundamental and clinical text,* Philadelphia, 1991, JB Lippincott.
3. Farid NR: Genetic factors in thyroid disease. In Braverman LE, Utiger RD, editors: *Werner and Ingbar's the thyroid: a fundamental and clinical text,* Philadelphia, 1991, JB Lippincott.
4. Feldmann M, et al: Mechanism of Graves thyroiditis: implications for concepts and therapy of autoimmunity, *Int Rev Immunol* 9:91, 1992.
5. Foley TP: Disorders of the thyroid in children. In Sperling MA, editor: *Pediatric endocrinology,* Philadelphia, 1996, WB Saunders.
6. Hauser P, et al: Attention deficit/hyperactivity disorder in people with generalized resistance to thyroid hormone, *N Engl J Med* 328:997, 1993.
7. Mäenpää J, Hiekkala H, Lamberg BA: Childhood hyperthyroidism, *Acta Endocrinol* 51:321, 1966.
8. Rivkees SA, Sklar C, Freemark M: Clinical review 99: the management of Graves' disease in children, with special emphasis on radioiodine treatment, *J Clin Endocrinol Metab* 83:3767, 1998 (review).
9. Roth RN, McAuliffe MJ: Hyperthyroidism and thyroid storm, *Emerg Med Clin North Am* 7:873, 1989.
10. Saxena KM, Crawford JD, Talbot NB: Childhood thyrotoxicosis: a long-term perspective, *BMJ* 2:1153, 1964.
11. Volpe R: Graves' disease. In Braverman LE, Utiger RD, editors: *Werner and Ingbar's the thyroid: a fundamental and clinical text,* Philadelphia, 1991, JB Lippincott.
12. Zakarija M, McKenzie JM, Munro DS: Immunoglobulin G inhibitor of thyroid stimulating antibody is a cause of delay in the onset of neonatal Graves' disease, *J Clin Invest* 72:1352, 1983.
13. Zimmerman D, Leif AN: Thyrotoxicosis in children, *Endocrinol Metab Clin North Am* 27:109, 1998 (review).

222 Hypospadias, Epispadias, and Cryptorchism

John P. Gearhart

The male genitalia are much more often a cause of parental preoccupation at the birth of a child than are the female. Untold variables govern this, most of them not readily apparent. The most obvious, of course, is that they are much more accessible. Less concern usually exists about the relationship of the penis to the urinary tract than to sexual function. Still, it is as a part of the urinary tract that it serves its immediate purpose at birth; it must wait until puberty to begin to realize its additional potential.

GENITAL ABNORMALITY

An external genital deformity in the newborn boy usually is obvious immediately—for example, hypospadias, epispadias, injury, swelling, and after careful palpation, undescended testes. To feel both testes is important. Although frequently of somewhat different size in a newborn, they generally are descended in a full-term infant (depending on the birth weight) and frequently undescended in the premature infant. One cause of parental distress often is not noted at birth but perhaps several weeks later as the baby gains weight: So much of a suprapubic fat pad can exist that the penis, retracted, may seem to disappear despite its being some 4 cm long. The physician, however, must not belittle the concern; the parents should be assured that the condition will correct itself in time. Only rarely does a real problem exist, namely, a micropenis, which suggests a dysmorphic abnormality. Circumcision should be delayed in infants who have micropenis and should be performed by a pediatric urologist.

Hypospadias

Among the possible penile abnormalities, hypospadias, which occurs in 8.1 : 1000 newborn boys, is the most common. In this event, the urethral meatus opens on the ventral surface of the penis, located most often on the distal half of the shaft, including the glans penis (60%), but it may be located at any proximal point along the shaft or scrotum (25%), or the perineum (15%) (Fig. 222-1). The prepuce is incompletely formed, covering only the dorsal surface of the glans penis. In approximately 10% of cases, an associated unilateral or bilateral cryptorchism is present. Any combination of hypospadias and bilateral cryptorchidism should be investigated for possible intersex anomaly.

The severity of the deformity and the position of the meatus on the undershaft of the penis will greatly influence surgical decisions. A circumcision should *not* be performed in the presence of hypospadias, however mild. None of the tissue that might be needed for repair should be sacrificed. If the hypospadias is mild and situated at or close to the corona, and if relatively little deformity is present, the repair is quite straightforward, accomplished in same-day surgery, and little more than a glorified circumcision. Occasionally a meatal stenosis is associated with hypospadias and can be corrected easily at the time of the hypospadias repair. Chordee, the downward curving of the penis as a result of abnormal ventral fibrous bands, often is present and is one of the factors that must be addressed at the time of surgical intervention. Currently, most hypospadias defects can be corrected with a single procedure. Although the frequency of an associated anomaly of the upper urinary tract is known to be low, many parents request sonography to be assured that the upper tract is normal. In any event, the pediatric urologist should be consulted as soon after birth as possible.

Even if the hypospadias defect is severe, a single-stage repair often can be performed. Multiple-stage repairs may be required when there is very severe chordee and a paucity of dorsal foreskin. The decision as to the right time for surgery and the precise approach to use must rest with the pediatric urologist but usually is performed around 1 year of age. The pediatrician, however, cannot relinquish responsibility for providing concomitant care; he or she is needed to interpret events and, in a highly charged emotional circumstance, to provide appropriate counseling to parents (and, as the child grows older, to the child). This is especially important when sexual function is threatened and sexual identity is of concern. On occasion, if the hypospadias is severe or accompanied by associated genital anomalies, a referral for endocrine evaluation is indicated. In the presence of hypospadias alone, aside from a rare defect in androgen responsiveness, little likelihood exists of significant hormonal disturbance.

Epispadias

Less frequently (1 : 112,000 live male births), the meatus is formed on the dorsum of the penis at various points along the glans and shaft and, on rare occasion, so far back as to be beneath the symphysis pubis. The more proximal deformity may be associated with complete urinary incontinence because of involvement of the bladder neck area along with distortion of the normal architecture of the pubic bones. Early consultation with the pediatric urologist is necessary; again, circumcision is to be avoided.

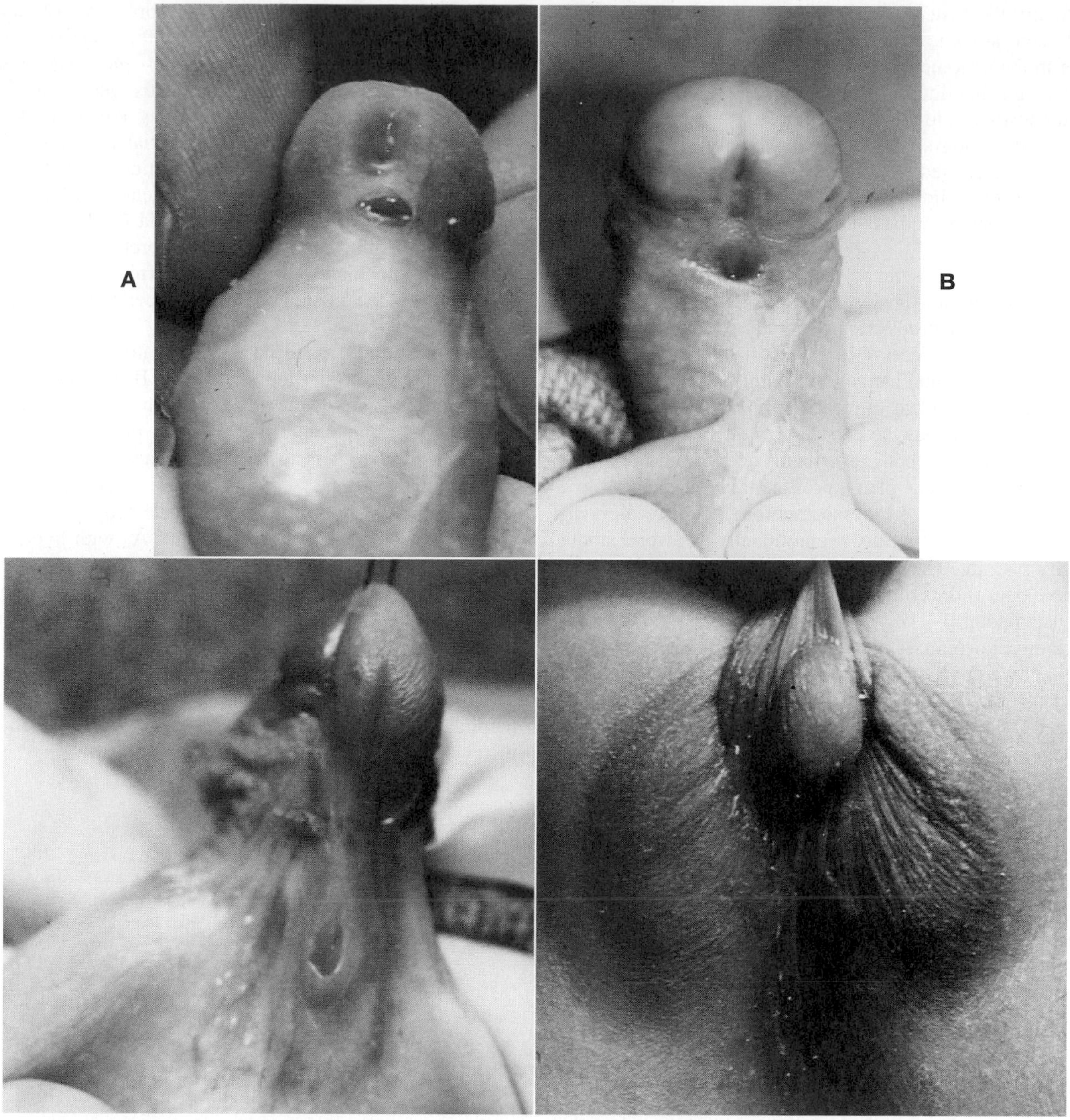

A B C D

Fig. 222-1 Varieties of hypospadias. **A,** Coronal. **B,** Distal shaft. **C,** Penoscrotal. **D,** Perineal.

CRYPTORCHISM

Given that the testes descend from within the abdomen to the scrotum usually by about week 36 of fetal life, the incidence of cryptorchism (undescended testes) is much higher in the premature infant. Any spontaneous descent of the testes after birth generally takes place well before the end of the first year; if this does not happen by the first birthday, concern is warranted. This involves the child's potential for developing testicular cancer, for reproduction capacity, and for sexual function, because with cryptorchism, testicular cellular damage is increasingly likely with each passing year, damage that probably is not reversible after the age of 4 or 5 years. On examination, one must be sure that the testis truly is undescended. Occasionally an overactive cremasteric reflex may make palpation difficult. Moving the infant or the older child into the tailor position (sitting cross-legged) or a kneeling position can help to overcome this. One must feel from above downward, "milking" the testis from the inguinal canal into the scrotum. The older patient can help this process by coughing or straining. Cold hands and abrupt palpation can invoke the cremasteric reflex. If one or the other of the testes is not palpable, one should search beyond the scrotum and the inguinal canal, to the femoral triangle and the inner thigh. Many undescended testes are associated with an inguinal hernia and possibly a hydrocele; these masses can make palpation of the testes even more difficult. If the testis is impalpable and a hernia is present, the testis usually lies just inside the internal inguinal ring.

Actually, the testes, if undescended, may have stopped their descent at some point within the inguinal canal or still may be in the abdomen. If a testis has not reached the inguinal canal, the likelihood is greater that it is abnormal; the lower the testis lies in the inguinal canal, the more likely that it is normal. Sonography has proved helpful only with the inguinal undescended testis. Computed tomography (CT) scan exposes the child to radiation, requires sedation, and has many false-positive and false-negative results. It should be avoided.

A testis that retracts simply because of an overactive cremasteric reflex obviously should not be "repaired." The truly undescended testis needs repair to improve the chance for fertility, to provide accessible examination (particularly in the event of malignant change), to diminish the possibility of testicular torsion, and to prevent the emotional trauma that frequently accompanies the condition.

Given that one or both testes truly are ectopic or "hidden," the management plan raises certain questions: How long should one wait for descent before surgical intervention? Does a "best" time exist emotionally? Is worry about infertility warranted? Can repair help in this regard? If one waits too long, is the child at greater risk for testicular malignancy as an adult?

Certainly, no one wants an unnecessary operation. Still, one cannot wait until puberty to see if natural descent occurs. If the testis is not down by 12 months of age, surgery is indicated. If the parents refuse surgery or are reticent about it, the potential for descent can be explored with a therapeutic trial of human chorionic gonadotropin (HCG), 1500 IU/m^2 body surface area intramuscularly twice a week for 4 weeks. If the testis is to descend, it generally will at this dosage level and duration. Treating with HCG over a longer period has disadvantages; it can hasten the onset of puberty and can cause testicular damage and sterility. Surgery is the desirable alternative if the testis does not descend or does, but retracts after the HCG trial. For those who respond to the administration of HCG, the outlook for full sexual maturity is excellent. If the testes lie within the abdomen and are not palpable in the inguinal canal, HCG will not bring them down into the scrotum but may bring them into the inguinal canal where they are accessible to palpation and long-term observation, thereby avoiding immediate surgery and, if the testes subsequently descend into the scrotum, avoiding surgery altogether.

The optimum time for surgical correction of cryptorchism is around 12 months of age. If, for some reason, surgical correction is delayed until adolescence (e.g., delayed diagnosis), the possibility of the testis generating viable sperm is very small. Although bringing the testis down at this time does not diminish the potential of malignancy, it increases the likelihood of early detection. Periodic examination is important. Finally, if the patient who has cryptorchism has an associated inguinal hernia (with or without a hydrocele), herniorrhaphy, along with orchiopexy, should be performed immediately. An elective herniorrhaphy is preferable to one done in the face of incarceration and possible strangulation.

Surgery may be done on an ambulatory basis when the testis is palpated in the inguinal canal. If it cannot be felt, a more extensive surgical procedure with an abdominal incision probably will be necessary unless preliminary laparoscopy reveals the testis to be absent. In specialized centers, complete laparoscopic orchiopexy now is being performed. Either way, a demonstrably abnormal testis should be removed and replaced with a prosthesis. As with hypospadias or epispadias, the role of the pediatrician in the care of the patient and his family is very important. The emotional support necessary when such a vital aspect of human function is threatened is enormous. Preparation for surgery requires full discussion about the child's and the parents' fears and concerns; these discussions should continue following surgery, particularly as the child grows older and begins to reflect on the event.

SUGGESTED READINGS

American Academy of Pediatrics: Timing of elective surgery on the genitalia of male children with particular reference to the risks, benefits, and psychological effects of surgery and anesthesia, *Pediatrics* 97:590, 1996.

Belman AB, Kass AJ: Hypospadias repair in children under one year of age, *J Urol* 128:1273, 1982.

Colodny AH: Undescended testes: is surgery necessary? *N Engl J Med* 314:510, 1986.

Docimo SG, Jordan GH: Laparoscopic surgery in children. In Marshall FF: *Textbook of operative urology,* Baltimore, 1996, WB Saunders.

Gearhart JP, Jeffs RD: Diagnostic maneuvers in cryptorchidism, *Semin Urol* VI:79, 1988.

Neely EK, Rosenfeld RG: The undescended testicle: when and how to intervene, *Contemp Pediatrics* 7:21, 1990.

Schulze KA, Pfister RR: Evaluating the undescended testis, *Am Fam Physician* 31:133, 1988.

223 Hypothyroidism

Thomas P. Foley, Jr.

Few diseases affect multiple systems so severely as hypothyroidism yet are associated with so many nonspecific symptoms and signs. Hypothyroidism can occur at any age, can occur during fetal life, and can affect the fetus as a result of maternal hypothyroidism during the first trimester of pregnancy. Its clinical manifestation during infancy differs markedly from that of childhood and adolescence; for this reason, we must distinguish between congenital and juvenile-acquired hypothyroidism.[7] The clinical distinction of hypothyroidism as a neonate and child is complicated further by reports of acquired hypothyroidism during the first year of life.[8] As a result of screening programs for the detection of congenital hypothyroidism during the preclinical stage of the disease during the first 2 weeks of life, accurate data on the incidence of congenital hypothyroidism in iodine-sufficient regions of the world indicate that approximately 1 infant is affected with congenital hypothyroidism for every 4000 live births.[5] The incidence is greater in iodine-deficient regions. The true incidence of juvenile hypothyroidism is not known. Congenital and juvenile hypothyroidism occur as familial or sporadic diseases with or without enlargement of the thyroid gland (goiter, thyromegaly) and may progress as either a permanent or a transient disorder.[7]

ETIOLOGY

In most instances the causes of hypothyroidism differ during infancy and childhood[5] (Box 223-1). An occasional patient who has a mild form of congenital hypothyroidism may be missed by newborn screening programs and not exhibit symptoms until childhood. These children usually have either familial goitrous hypothyroidism (dyshormonogenesis)[9] or thyroid dysgenesis with an ectopic thyroid gland located somewhere between the foramen cecum of the tongue and the anterior mediastinum. In most cases of permanent congenital hypothyroidism, the cause is unknown. Approximately 90% of patients have no thyroid tissue (athyreosis), an ectopic thyroid gland, or a hypoplastic thyroid gland found in the normal anterior cervical location.[7] Antibody-dependent cell-mediated cytotoxicity (ADCC) was found in 32% of infants who had permanent congenital hypothyroidism and in 24% of their mothers.[3] Several inborn errors of thyroid hormone synthesis are inherited as autosomal recessive traits and usually manifest with thyromegaly on physical examination.[9] In 2% of cases, antibodies that block the thyroid-stimulating hormone (TSH) receptor are produced by a mother who has autoimmune thyroid disease and cross the placenta and block the function of the fetal thyroid gland.[12] This form of transient hypothyroidism can persist for several weeks or months; the affected infant requires thyroxine therapy until the antibodies disappear. Other types of transient congenital hypothyroidism may occur when drugs prescribed for the mother, such as propylthiouracil, methimazole, or iodides, cross the placenta and block the fetal thyroid gland. Iodine-containing medications should not be applied to the skin or mucous membranes of neonates for more than a few days because the iodine is absorbed easily and blocks the infant's thyroid gland. Congenital primary hypothyroidism rarely is caused by mutations in the genes that code for the extracellular domain of the TSH receptor and for thyroid transcription factors;[12] rarely, congenital secondary (pituitary) hypothyroidism is caused by mutations in the genes that code for pituitary transcription factors.[12]

The most common cause of hypothyroidism in children beyond the perinatal period is goitrous or nongoitrous, autoimmune (chronic lymphocytic, Hashimoto's) thyroiditis.[13] Rarely, disease may begin as early as 6 months of age and progresses rapidly during infancy with few symptoms and signs of hypothyroidism.[8] An occasional patient who has hypothalamic or pituitary disease may be seen initially with hypothyroidism. These children usually have other clinical features to suggest an abnormality of the hypothalamus or pituitary.

HISTORY AND PHYSICAL EXAMINATION

Because hypothyroidism can affect most organ systems to varying degrees, it is very important that the clinician consider the diagnosis when the patient has many nonspecific or multisystemic complaints. Furthermore, a family history of thyroid and pituitary disease may disclose important diagnostic information. Many of the symptoms and signs of hypothyroidism are different during infancy compared with childhood.[5,10] These are summarized in Box 223-2. During the first month of life, affected infants may have no clinical symptoms or signs of hypothyroidism. Presumably, this occurs either because some transfer of thyroxine occurs in utero from mother to fetus,[16] failure of thyroid gland function (as with ectopic thyroid tissue) is incomplete, or the disease is of short duration, possibly developing during the third trimester.[5] In infants who have no functioning thyroid tissue, clinical symptoms and signs may be present at birth (rarely), develop within the first few days of life, or appear as early as the first 2 weeks of life; they are always present by 6 weeks

BOX 223-1

CAUSES OF HYPOTHYROIDISM

Congenital Hypothyroidism

A. Thyroid dysgenesis
   1. Thyroid aplasia
   2. Thyroid hypoplasia
   3. Ectopic thyroid gland
B. Familial abnormalities of thyroid hormone synthesis and metabolism (familial dyshormonogenesis)
C. Maternal disease
   1. Therapeutic doses of ^{131}I after the eleventh week of gestation
   2. Transplacental autoimmune thyroiditis
   3. Ingestion of goitrogens
D. Endemic goiter and cretinism
E. Hypothalamic-pituitary hypothyroidism
   1. Pituitary agenesis or aplasia
   2. Thyrotropin deficiency: isolated
   3. Hypothalamic hormone deficiency
      a. Isolated thyrotropin deficiency
      b. Multiple tropic hormone deficiencies
      c. Septooptic dysplasia
      d. Anencephaly
   4. Hypothalamic-pituitary lesions

Juvenile Hypothyroidism

A. Thyroiditis, autoimmune (Hashimoto's)
   1. Atrophic thyroiditis of infancy
   2. Chronic lymphocytic thyroiditis of childhood
   3. Atrophic thyroiditis of childhood and adolescence
   4. Hashimoto's thyroiditis (struma lymphomatosa)
B. Congenital thyroid dysgenesis
   1. Ectopic thyroid
   2. Hypoplastic
C. Congenital defects in thyroid hormone synthesis or metabolism
D. Iatrogenic thyroid ablation
   1. Surgical
   2. Radioactive iodine (^{131}I)
E. Ingestion of goitrogens
F. Endemic goiter
G. Hypothalamic-pituitary disease

BOX 223-2

SYMPTOMS AND SIGNS OF HYPOTHYROIDISM

Congenital Hypothyroidism

Facial edema
Large posterior fontanelle (>0.5 cm)
Rectal temperature below 95° F (35° C)
Decreased stooling (less than one stool per day)
Prolonged hyperbilirubinemia (bilirubin above 10 mg/dl after 3 days of age)
Respiratory distress in a term infant
Umbilical hernia
Birth weight above 4000 g
Macroglossia
Bradycardia (pulse below 100 beats/min)
Feeding problems and lethargy
Cutaneous mottling, vasomotor instability
Hoarse cry
Hirsute forehead

Juvenile Hypothyroidism

Growth retardation (below 4 cm/yr)
Delayed bone maturation
Delayed dental development and tooth eruption
Onset of puberty: usually delayed; rarely precocious
Myopathy and muscular hypertrophy
Menstrual disorders
Galactorrhea
Increased skin pigmentation
Physical and mental torpor
Pale, gray, cool, mottled, thickened, coarse skin
Constipation
Coarse, dry brittle hair

of age. The difficulty in diagnosing congenital hypothyroidism is evident when comparing the clinical features of three infants (Fig. 223-1). The infant on the upper left was referred at 8 months of age with clinical features very suggestive of hypothyroidism, yet her thyroid studies were normal. The infant on the upper right had documented primary hypothyroidism at 4 weeks of age. Her clinical features at this age were minimal and included only mild periorbital edema, an enlarged posterior fontanelle, decreased stooling, and abdominal distention. The 6-month-old infant pictured at bottom center, in contrast, had severe hypothyroidism.

The clinical symptoms and signs of older children who have acquired hypothyroidism may be as nonspecific and insidious in their development as those found in infants who have congenital or acquired hypothyroidism.[7] If the disease has been present for more than 6 months, growth deceleration should be evident because normal thyroid hormone secretion is essential for normal linear growth. Hence, most patients who have juvenile hypothyroidism have either thyromegaly or a deceleration of growth and usually are short in stature.[7] Deceleration of linear growth should be identified by the physician who routinely measures the height of the patient; an early diagnosis will prevent the development of long-standing hypothyroidism, cessation of linear growth, and the risk of a decrease in final adult height. The importance of this easy measurement cannot be overstressed. Frank obesity, however, is an uncommon complaint in children who have hypothyroidism because reduction in physical activity, if it occurs, usually is less than the reduction in caloric intake. On the other hand, children who have advanced hypothyroidism and myxedema usually are chubby and have periorbital edema.

Inspection and palpation of the anterior cervical area will enable the examiner to identify an enlarged thyroid gland, even in the neonate. The easiest method for examining the thyroid gland of an infant is to place the infant in the supine position with the neck hyperextended over the edge of the examining table and feel for the isthmus of the thyroid, just below the hyoid bone. After identifying the isthmus, one should palpate laterally to delineate the lobes,

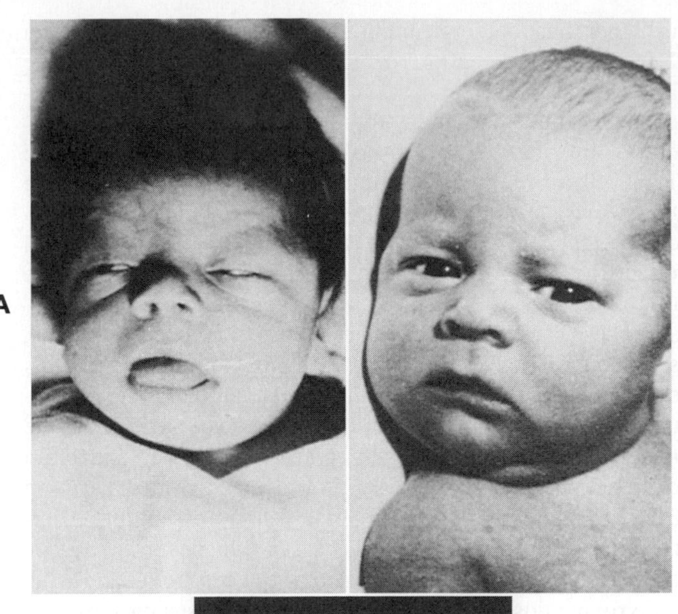

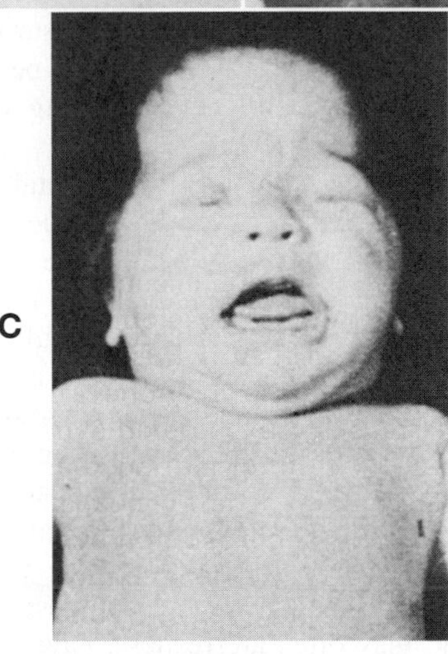

Fig. 223-1 **A,** Normal infant who has clinical signs but no clinical symptoms of congenital hypothyroidism. **B,** Affected infant who has athyreosis, age 28 days. **C,** Infant at age 6 months who has athyreosis and severe congenital hypothyroidism.

(From Foley TP Jr: Sporadic congenital hypothyroidism. In Dussault JH, Walker P, editors: *Congenital hypothyroidism,* New York, 1983, Marcel Dekker.)

which are very difficult to define in a normal infant. The thyroid examination of an older child is easier. Because the thyroid rises during swallowing, having the patient swallow water will facilitate the identification and delineation of both lobes of the thyroid gland as distinct from other adjacent tissue.

LABORATORY DATA

Although the clinical laboratory may offer a wide battery of thyroid function tests, rarely are most of these tests necessary for the diagnosis of hypothyroidism. An elevation of the serum TSH value is the single most sensitive test for primary hypothyroidism (thyroid gland failure).[7] The combination of a low serum thyroxine (T_4) value and an elevated TSH is diagnostic of primary hypothyroidism, either permanent or transient, at any age, including term and preterm infants.[10] In patients who have hypothalamic or pituitary hypothyroidism, the determination of the T_4 (low) and TSH (not elevated or suppressed, but usually normal) is not adequate for definitive diagnosis because patients who have thyroxine-binding globulin (TBG) deficiency also will have a low T_4 and normal TSH. Hence the free, or unbound, thyroxine (free T_4) and TBG values, as well as specific tests of pituitary function, usually are necessary. The free T_4 determination by direct dialysis is the most accurate method and the least likely to give false-positive or negative results from interfering drugs or other substances in serum.[7]

An occasional child or infant who has a coexisting and severe illness, such as idiopathic respiratory distress syndrome, may have the so-called euthyroid sick syndrome (or nonthyroidal illness syndrome) in which the T_4 may be low despite normal TBG levels.[7] The serum triiodothyronine (T_3) value characteristically is low; the TSH value is normal, whereas the free T_4 and reverse T_3 levels are either in the upper range of normal or are frankly elevated. This problem occurs most frequently in the preterm infant.

Tests other than the serum T_4 and TSH determinations often are not required for children in whom a diagnosis of hypothyroidism is suspected; however, thyroid antibody determinations can be very helpful in finding the cause of infantile or juvenile-acquired hypothyroidism, because the titers of the serum thyroid peroxidase (formerly known as microsomal) or thyroglobulin antibodies usually are detected in serum from children who have autoimmune thyroiditis.[1,4] Transient congenital hypothyroidism may be caused by TSH receptor-blocking antibodies (TRBAb) acquired from the mother who has autoimmune thyroid disease and primary hypothyroidism.[12] TRBAb levels diagnostically are valuable in these patients and should be measured during pregnancy in mothers receiving thyroxine therapy for primary hypothyroidism from autoimmune thyroiditis.[5] A serum T_3 determination in the infant who has congenital hypothyroidism also may be of prognostic value and often is reassuring for parents if the physician can indicate, on the evidence of a normal T_3 value, that therapy was initiated before chemical hypothyroidism developed.[10] A serum T_3 determination is not indicated, however, in the diagnostic evaluation of juvenile hypothyroidism.

Radioisotopic studies often are ordered inappropriately. Usually only a thyroid scan is needed, because the most common cause (>85%) is thyroid dysgenesis. In infants and children, the isotope iodine-131 should not be used as a diagnostic test, because other agents (iodine-123 and technetium 99m) that deliver a lower dose of radiation to the thyroid are available. A thyroid scan using either of them is important in infants who have abnormal thyroid screening tests for the following reasons:

1. It is the most rapid and definitive diagnostic test on which the initiation of therapy may be decided; the test result can be obtained 2 hours after the dose is administered.
2. The test will distinguish sporadic disease, such as thyroid dysgenesis, from familial disease (goitrous thyroid dyshormonogenesis), a distinction important for genetic counseling.[5] With dysgenesis, the scan will be consistent with agenesis and atopic thyroid tissue. In

familial dyshormonogenesis, there will be a normally sized or enlarged thyroid gland in the normal anterior cervical location of the neck.

The thyroid uptake test using only ^{123}I should be performed whenever an infant has an enlarged thyroid gland on clinical examination or when the thyroid scan demonstrates an enlarged thyroid gland.

An elevated thyroid uptake in an infant who has a goiter is very suggestive of an inborn error of thyroid hormone synthesis,[6] although it also may be seen in infants who have an iodine deficiency when living in endemic goiter regions of the world. Radioisotopic studies rarely are needed in older patients who have juvenile hypothyroidism. To exclude the possibility of thyroid carcinoma, the thyroid scan is indicated when a mass is palpated in or adjacent to the thyroid gland of a patient who has normal thyroid function and antibody tests.[4,7] Thyroid uptake studies are indicated when the patient has diffuse thyromegaly and biochemical evidence of hypothyroidism not caused by autoimmune thyroiditis or goitrogen ingestion.[4,7]

Although not essential, the assessment of skeletal maturation can provide additional data regarding the duration of hypothyroidism. A bone age determination consistent with that of a normal newborn would suggest recently acquired, mild congenital hypothyroidism, whereas notation of the absence of ossification centers at the knee in addition to the presence of only the two ossification centers in the foot indicates that the fetus was affected by hypothyroidism during the third trimester of pregnancy.

THERAPY

The treatment of choice for hypothyroidism in infancy and childhood is the daily administration of oral L-thyroxine[5,7,9,15] (Table 223-1). Other thyroid preparations are either more expensive or monitored less reliably for adequacy of dose. The initial dose in a term infant is 50 μg (0.05 mg) of L-thyroxine daily for the first 3 days to 2 weeks and should be started promptly at the initial visit when screening tests are abnormal and serum has been sent for confirmatory tests, or whenever the scan is abnormal.[9] Infants who have hypothalamic or pituitary hypothyroidism should be started on 25 μg/day because their requirements are less and their hypothyroidism mild. At the end of the first and second week, serum T_4 and TSH values should be obtained to determine that the amount of L-thyroxine is adequate but not excessive.[9] Often, after 1 or 2 weeks, those infants who were started on 50 μg/day may need to have the dose reduced to 37.5 μg/day and infrequently to 25 μg/day, (1) if clinical symptoms of hyperthyroidism develop or (2) if the serum T_4 value exceeds 16 μg/dl (the normal range for T_4 in the infant is higher than that in older children and adults) and the serum T_3 value exceeds 250 ng/dl. In athyreotic infants who have low T_4 values, it is unusual to find that 50 μg/day is inadequate. Therapy should be adjusted to maintain the serum T_4 during infancy above 8 μg/dl, preferably between 10 and 12 μg/dl, to optimize developmental outcome.[6] Within the first 4 weeks of therapy, the serum TSH value should decrease into the normal range for age, but in an occasional infant the TSH value will not return to normal even if the thyroxine dose is excessive and causes clinical thyrotoxicosis. These infants may have an abnormality in the feedback set point of TSH secretion.[13] The goal of therapy in this situation should be to maintain normal serum T_4 and T_3 values and clinical euthyroidism. Because excessive thyroxine therapy in infancy may cause cranial synostosis and brain dysfunction, monitoring of serum T_4 and TSH levels at 1- to 3-month intervals during the first year is essential.[5] Additional determinations may be necessary whenever the dose is adjusted.[5] After 2 years of age the need to change the L-thyroxine dose occurs infrequently, so measuring serum T_4 and TSH levels once or twice a year should be adequate. If linear growth and weight gain are progressing satisfactorily, no additional studies are necessary.

Table 223-1 Dose of L-Thyroxine

Age	T_4 Dose/day (μg)	T_4 Dose/kg/day (μg)
<6 mo	25-50	8-10
6-12 mo	50-75	6-8
1-5 yr	75-100	5-6
6-12 yr	100-125	4-5
>12 yr	100-200	2-3

In contrast to infants who have congenital or acquired hypothyroidism, older children who have hypothyroidism do not share the same degree of urgency in achieving the euthyroid state. Although patients who have had a recent onset of mild hypothyroidism may be started on a full replacement dose of L-thyroxine, children ages 3 years and older who have chronic hypothyroidism and clinical symptoms should be started on a low dose (25 μg/day) that gradually is increased every 2 to 4 weeks to the full replacement dose.[4,7]

The rapid correction of the hypothyroid state often can be associated with undesirable behavioral side effects. These children act as though they are thyrotoxic despite biochemical euthyroidism; they often are restless, have a short attention span, and are emotionally labile. These symptoms, in association with the expected hair loss, may lead to inappropriate discontinuance of therapy by the uninformed parent. In such cases a gradual increase in dose seems to minimize these problems in adjustment from the hypothyroid to the euthyroid state. Adequacy of L-thyroxine therapy is monitored by annual serum T_4 (or free T_4) and TSH determinations, once the patient is receiving a full replacement dose with normal values. Because patients who have acquired hypothyroidism do not have an abnormality in the feedback control of TSH secretion, an elevated TSH with or without a low T_4 value indicates either inadequate therapy or poor compliance; the latter often is characterized by variable serum T_4 and TSH values. For example, the levels may be normal on one occasion but discordant (normal or elevated T_4 with elevated TSH) on subsequent determinations, despite no change in therapy. In rare cases the medication may not contain the indicated amount of thyroxine. Studies in adults have indicated a reduced absorption of L-thyroxine when administered with meals, especially food containing fiber, and when given at the same time as iron medications[11] and possibly, calcium.[5] Hence, it is advisable, particularly in treating infants, that medication be given an hour before the next feeding.

Because an occasional infant receiving treatment merely

may have had transient congenital hypothyroidism, therapy should either be reduced to half the dose or discontinued some time after 3 years of age. Serum T_4 and TSH levels then are determined 2 to 4 weeks later and therapy restarted if the TSH is elevated. Radioisotope scan or uptake may be performed while the infant is off therapy at this age, if a definitive diagnosis was not obtained at the outset. Temporary cessation or reduction in therapy, however, is not necessary for those patients who have ectopic thyroid dysgenesis or for children who have other causes of hypothyroidism and previously had elevated TSH values after the TSH normalized during initial therapy.

PROGNOSIS

Infants who were treated adequately for congenital hypothyroidism since the first month of age have an excellent prognosis for normal intellectual function and linear growth. However, delays in diagnosis and in the institution of adequate therapy after 3 months of age usually are associated with an increased risk of mental retardation.[11] There is an increased risk for impaired intellectual function in infants who had prolonged fetal hypothyroidism because there was maternal hypothyroidism during the first trimester, or other factors blocked fetal thyroid function throughout pregnancy, such as maternal radioiodine therapy, maternal TSH receptor–blocking antibodies, and prolonged use of antithyroid drugs, including iodine. In contrast, no permanent intellectual impairment is found among patients who have juvenile hypothyroidism. Adolescents who have chronic hypothyroidism and severe growth retardation may never achieve their full growth potential. Often, their linear growth response to therapy is not accelerated, and the height percentile achieved as an adult is lower than that predicted by their growth before the development of hypothyroidism.[14]

When to Refer

1. The cause of hypothyroidism is not established on the initial evaluation.
2. Initial therapy does not normalize thyroid function tests within the normal range for age, which often is not necessarily the normal range provided by the laboratory. The physician must know the normal range of thyroid function tests for age for patient management during the first two decades of life.
3. Acquired hypothyroidism is atypical or complex: The disease occurs in infancy or early childhood, or is associated with other endocrine or nonendocrine autoimmune diseases.
4. When the diagnosis is hypothalamic or pituitary hypothyroidism based on a low free T_4 (by a method validated in infants and children) and normal or low TSH. Rarely is this form of hypothyroidism an isolated disease: It is expected to be associated with other hypothalamic-pituitary abnormalities; if it is isolated, genetic evaluation is needed to define the cause and potential for recurrence in a family.

When to Hospitalize

1. Myxedema coma
2. Parental noncompliance with treatment of the very young infant who is at increased risk for permanent impairment of CNS function if thyroid function tests are not maintained in the normal range.

REFERENCES

1. Bachrach LK, Foley TP Jr: Thyroiditis in children, *Pediatr Rev* 11:184, 1989.
2. Bogner U, et al: Cytotoxic antibodies in congenital hypothyroidism, *J Clin Endocrinol Metab* 68:671, 1989.
3. Fisher DA, et al: Screening for congenital hypothyroidism: results of screening 1 million North American infants, *J Pediatr* 94:700, 1979.
4. Foley TP Jr: Acquired hypothyroidism in infants, children and adolescents. In Braverman LE, Utiger RD, editors: *Werner and Ingbar's the thyroid,* ed 8, Philadelphia, 2000, Lippincott/Williams Wilkins.
5. Foley TP Jr. Congenital hypothyroidism. In Braverman LE, Utiger RD, editors: *Werner and Ingbar's the thyroid,* ed 8, Philadelphia, 2000, Lippincott/Williams Wilkins.
6. Foley TP Jr: Familial thyroid dyshormonogenesis. In Delange F, Fisher DA, Malvaux P, editors: *Pediatric thyroidology,* Basel, Switzerland, 1985, S Karger.
7. Foley TP Jr, Malvaux P, Blizzard RM: Thyroid disease. In Kappy MS, Blizzard RM, Migeon CJ, editors: *Wilkins the diagnosis and treatment of endocrine disorders in childhood and adolescence,* ed 4, Springfield, Ill, 1994, Charles C Thomas.
8. Foley TP Jr, et al: Acquired autoimmune mediated infantile hypothyroidism: a pathologic entity distinct from congenital hypothyroidism, *N Engl J Med* 330:466, 1994.
9. Germak JA, Foley TP Jr: Longitudinal assessment of L-thyroxine therapy in congenital hypothyroidism, *J Pediatr* 117:211, 1990.
10. Klein AH, et al: Neonatal thyroid function in congenital hypothyroidism, *J Pediatr* 89:545, 1976.
11. Klein AH, Meltzer S, Kenny FM: Improved prognosis in congenital hypothyroidism treated before age three months, *J Pediatr* 81:912, 1972.
12. Matsuura N, et al: Familial neonatal transient hypothyroidism due to maternal TSH-binding inhibitor immunoglobulins, *N Engl J Med* 303: 738, 1980.
13. Rallison M, et al: Occurrence and natural history of thyroiditis in children, *J Pediatr* 86:675, 1975.
14. Rivkees SA, Bode HH, Crawford JD: Long-term growth in juvenile acquired hypothyroidism, *N Engl J Med* 318:599, 1988.
15. Sato T, et al: Age-related change in pituitary threshold for TSH release during replacement therapy for cretinism, *J Clin Endocrinol Metab* 44: 553, 1977.
16. Vulsma T, Gons MH, de Vijlder JJM: Maternal-fetal transfer of thyroxine in congenital hypothyroidism due to a total organification defect or thyroid agenesis, *N Engl J Med* 321:13, 1989.

SUGGESTED READINGS

American Academy of Pediatrics: Newborn screening for congenital hypothyroidism: recommended guidelines, *Pediatrics* 91:1203, 1993.

Vassart G, Dumont JE, Refetoff S: Thyroid disorders. In Scriver CR, et al, editors: *The metabolic and molecular bases of inherited disease,* ed 7, vol II, New York, 1995, McGraw-Hill.

Weetman AP, McGregor AM: Autoimmune thyroid disease: further developments in our understanding, *Endocr Rev* 15:788, 1994.

224 Iatrogenic Disease

Cheston M. Berlin, Jr.

Iatrogenic (from the Greek word meaning "produced by the physician") illness is the result of therapy or diagnostic procedures used to manage the health needs of a patient. Few comprehensive studies are available to indicate its prevalence, yet a report in 1981 by Steel et al[5] found that 36% of 815 patients consecutively admitted to a general medical service had complications during their hospital stay caused by treatment or investigative procedures; 50% of these resulted from medication errors. Subsequent reports, summarized by Leape,[1] confirm that there may be significant error in treating patients.

Pediatric patients are especially vulnerable because of their size, their age, and the use of new therapies that have unknown risk for children. This is an especially significant problem in newborn medicine. Raju[3] surveyed a single pediatric journal and reported that 12.7% of articles published between 1965 and 1976 dealt with iatrogenic problems. In the pediatric intensive care unit, 8% of admissions had unanticipated complications of care; 42% of these were major. Human error was involved in 36% of cases.[4] Principi et al[2] surveyed the use of antibiotics in nine pediatric units (765 patients) and found that nearly one third of the patients received antibiotics on an "irrational" basis (no proved infection or positive laboratory test). In 75% of the patients, the antibiotic choice was not justified by the given clinical condition. This type of therapy invites iatrogenic disease.

The following is a case report of an iatrogenic illness:

Keith was referred by his family physician to an allergist at age 8 years for evaluation of continual nasal sniffing that had been present for years and was attributed to allergies, in part because of a positive family history and because decongestants were ineffective. From age 8 to 10 years he was treated with monthly injections of triamcinolone acetate by the allergist. The parents became concerned at the onset of growth failure during this period. At age 10, he was referred to an endocrinology clinic, where the evaluation revealed his height and weight to be below the 3rd percentile, with essentially no absolute gain since 8 years of age. Also noted in the history was enuresis of many years' duration. The clinic note for that visit describes the patient as "hyperactive, with constant small movements of the body and frequent repetitive sounds from the throat." He was evaluated with the following tests, all of which were normal: insulin-arginine stimulation of growth hormone release, serum thyroxine, skull roentgenograms, bone age, and buccal smear. Conclusions of the endocrine consultation were that the growth failure most likely was caused by the administration of steroids; the family was thus advised to stop the steroids. The patient was referred to a urologist for evaluation of his enuresis and to a pediatrician for evaluation of his hyperactivity.

Keith was first seen by the urologist and hospitalized. He underwent an intravenous pyelogram with voiding cystourethrogram, cystoscopy with cystometrogram, and cystourethroscopy. The results of all these studies were normal. The patient was given 25 mg imipramine at bedtime for his enuresis.

The patient was seen next in the pediatric clinic. Tourette's syndrome was diagnosed, based on multiple motor and vocal tics and coprolalia. Because of the initial delight of the patient and his family in the efficacy of imipramine in controlling the enuresis, drug therapy for controlling Tourette's syndrome was discussed but deferred. Six weeks later, with the patient's resumption of frequent enuresis while still receiving imipramine, this drug was stopped, and haloperidol, 1 mg twice daily, was started. There was prompt and considerable diminution of his tics and cessation of coprolalia within 2 days. After 1 week on this dosage, the patient experienced acute dystonic posturing of the neck and face, which was reversed by intravenous diphenhydramine, 25 mg. The dose of haloperidol was decreased to 0.5 mg twice daily; there were no further side effects.

The patient remained stable for the next 5 years on this dosage. After the initial diagnosis, Keith was placed in a special education class; subsequently, both his accomplishments and self-esteem increased. He also became a rifle marksman. The next year he returned to a regular classroom and graduated 5 years later from high school with vocational training. His height was at the 20th percentile, and his weight was at the 50th percentile. At 37 years of age, he is fully employed. After 5 years of continuous haloperidol therapy at a dose of 0.5 mg twice daily, the patient began to take the medication at the same dosage two or three times per year for 1 to 2 weeks when he was in stressful situations.

Iatrogenic illness in this patient occurred at several levels and for different reasons. First, he was misdiagnosed as being allergic because of frequent sniffing, a common symptom of Tourette's syndrome. Second, he received a potent steroid for this symptom, which stopped his growth; this led to a lengthy, expensive, and negative endocrinology evaluation. Third, he was referred to a specialist for evaluation of a common and usually benign developmental condition—enuresis. He received a lengthy, excessive evaluation that required hospitalization and the administration of an anesthetic agent. Fourth, after he was diagnosed correctly, initial drug therapy caused a severe dystonic drug reaction. And finally, failure to diagnose Tourette's syndrome early caused serious educational problems.

ETIOLOGY

Every patient contact is capable of producing iatrogenic disease. Infants younger than 1 year of age are especially vulnerable to idiosyncratic central nervous system reactions to drugs (e.g., extrapyramidal reaction to prochlorperazine).

Table 224-1 Complications That Can Arise from Diagnostic Procedures and Subsequent Therapy

	Complications
Diagnostic Procedure	
Physical examination	
Ears	Laceration of auditory canal; perforation of eardrum
Pharynx	Laceration of soft palate
Mouth or rectum (with thermometer)	Broken-glass laceration
Joints	Dislocation
Abdominal examination	Fractured spleen
Laboratory testing	
Throat culture	Gagging; vomiting; aspiration
Venipunctures	Bruising; arterial spasm
Heel sticks	Lacerated heels; infection, osteomyelitis
Roentgenographic procedures	
Position of patient	Dislocation of joints; infiltration of intravenous lines
Use of radiopaque dyes	Allergic reactions
Sedation	Central nervous system (CNS) depression; drug reaction; cardiac arrhythmias
Radiotherapy	Skin erythema; burns; sterility; alopecia
Therapy	
Drug therapy	Drug reaction; drug interaction; errors in type of drug and frequency and route of administration
Fluids and electrolytes	Overhydration or underhydration; incorrect solution; incorrect route; misplacement of intravenous line
Nutrition (including vitamins)	Deficiency states; inadequate knowledge of formula composition; hypervitaminosis
Equipment	
Infant warmers	Burns
Electric hazards	Shocks
Transillumination (fiberoptics)	Burns
Noise (especially in incubators)	Auditory damage; sleep disturbances
Constant light	CNS dysfunction (?); retinal damage (?); hormonal dysfunction (?)
Temperature control	Hypothermia or hyperthermia
Beds: mesh, rails, objects	Choking; falling out
Surgery	Wrong patient operated on; wrong part of body operated on; complication: infection, contracture, scarring, adhesions, fluid and electrolyte imbalance
Cardiopulmonary resuscitation	Fractured ribs, spleen, or liver
Instructions to patient or family	Overly restricted life at home and school; failure to appreciate impact of illness on family's and patient's life; misunderstanding of oral instructions
Immunizations	Local and systemic reactions

The risk varies from virtually zero with the insertion of a tongue depressor (the gag reflex can stimulate the vagus to produce asystole) to 100% with the use of intravenous amphotericin B. The most common but not necessarily the most serious possibilities for iatrogenic disease occur in two broad categories: diagnostic procedures and therapy (Table 224-1).

DATABASE

Recognition of iatrogenic disorders requires the physician's constant cognizance of the possibility that they may occur. The history and physical examination are most important; laboratory tests may confirm the clinical impression. Many iatrogenic disorders are obvious: ocular-gyric crisis from prochlorperazine use; sterile thigh abscesses from diphtheria-tetanus-pertussis (DTP) immunization; and a skin burn from touching an overhead warmer. Others are more subtle: rickets in the rapidly growing premature infant from failure to give sufficient vitamin D; hyponatremia from giving infants bottled "mineral" water; and thinning skin from long-term use of steroid cream for diaper rash. A careful review of systems coupled with specific questions concerning recent medications or other therapy (by nonphysicians as well as physicians) usually will uncover problem areas.

DIFFERENTIAL DIAGNOSIS

The diagnosis of the condition usually is straightforward, once considered; iatrogenic causes of disease are frequently overlooked. A list of a few iatrogenic diseases with alternative causes may be illustrative (Table 224-2).

MANAGEMENT

The management of iatrogenic disease is no different from that of any other condition, except for investigation of the iatrogenic event. The lesson usually learned is that patient-physician communication and the mechanisms of health care

Table 224-2 Differential Diagnosis of Iatrogenic Conditions

Condition (Diagnosis)	Causes
Rickets	No vitamin D supplementation Renal disease Rapid growth in a premature infant
Seizure	Seizure disorder Tap water enemas Boiled skim milk Bottled water (no electrolytes) Fever
Fever of unknown origin	Urinary tract infection Phenytoin therapy
Hearing loss	Recurrent otitis media Aminoglycoside therapy Incubator noise with concomitant aminoglycoside therapy
Short stature	Heredity Malnutrition Steroid therapy
Loose stools	Enteritis Lactose intolerance Mineral oil and senna products
Increased intracranial pressure	Meningitis Brain tumor Vitamin A intoxication
Hair loss	Emotional Thallium poisoning Vincristine therapy

delivery have broken down. Some iatrogenic events truly are unavoidable and indeed almost to be expected: limb atrophy after the application of a plaster cast and postoperative scarring in a person known to form keloids. Other iatrogenic events pinpoint serious deficiencies in medical care technology: failure to recheck the position of a decimal point in a digoxin order and inadequate postmarketing drug surveillance. The following are suggestions for preventing (or at least minimizing) iatrogenic illnesses:

1. *Careful explanation to parents and patient upon the institution of any therapy.* Preprinted handouts are helpful in anticipating and recognizing problems—for example, discussion of possible side effects of immunization. Patient information brochures on procedures and drug therapy are being developed and used more and more by practitioners and institutions.
2. *Prompt investigation of any iatrogenic event.* Comments such as "Don't worry, this happens frequently," "We see this occasionally," and "Nobody knows" hardly are reassuring to the family. Corrective measures must be instituted immediately. Iatrogenic disease frequently occurs as a systems failure. Prompt reporting of adverse events, and their immediate investigation and correction will minimize recurrence. Such investigations should not be punitive.
3. *Continuing education for all health care personnel.* It is the responsibility of the physician to investigate and report suspected links between therapy and unexpected changes in the patient's condition. Physicians should continue to educate staff on the importance of detecting, reporting, and correcting adverse events.
4. *Call for help.* This may mean additional consultative opinions from experts within and out of medicine. Social workers and teachers can assist in managing a chronically ill child whose medical regimen does not permit normal school attendance.

Iatrogenic disease may be cause for a medicolegal suit by a family. Such a malpractice risk will be considerably minimized if all the aforementioned suggestions are followed.

REFERENCES

1. Leape L: Error in medicine, *JAMA* 272:1851, 1994.
2. Principi N, et al: Control of antibiotic therapy in pediatric patients, *Dev Pharmacol Ther* 3:145, 1981.
3. Raju TNK: The injured neonate of the seventies, *J Pediatr* 91:347, 1977.
4. Stambouly JJ, et al: Complications of care in a pediatric intensive care unit: a prospective study, *Intensive Care Med* 22:1098, 1996.
5. Steel K, et al: Iatrogenic illness on a general medical service at a university hospital, *N Engl J Med* 304:638, 1981.

SUGGESTED READINGS

Fisher ES, Welsh HG: Avoiding the unintended consequences of growth in medical care, *JAMA* 281:446, 1999.

Koren G, Barzilay Z, Greenwald M: Tenfold errors in administration of drug doses: a neglected iatrogenic disease in pediatrics, *Pediatrics* 77:848, 1986.

Leape LL, et al: Promoting patient safety by preventing medical error, *JAMA* 280:1444, 1998.

Valdes-Dapena M: Iatrogenic disease in the perinatal period, *Pediatr Clin North Am* 36:67, 1989.

225 Idiopathic Thrombocytopenia

Allen E. Eskenazi • Guy Young

APPROACH TO THE THROMBOCYTOPENIC PATIENT

In evaluating the patient who has thrombocytopenia, the physician must determine (1) whether the hemostatic impairment is severe enough to warrant therapy and (2) the cause of the thrombocytopenia. Treatment undertaken without knowledge of the cause of the thrombocytopenia is arbitrary and therefore may be unsuccessful and even harmful.

The most likely cause of thrombocytopenia often may be deduced by performing a careful history and physical examination and analyzing a complete blood count (CBC), including the size of the circulating platelets. The history should focus on chronicity of the thrombocytopenia and its manifestations. The family history is helpful but is unlikely to be positive because thrombocytopenia is much more likely to be acquired than congenital. However, particular attention must be focused on the possible presence of other autoimmune diseases in family members. Petechiae are the hallmark of bleeding as a result of a low platelet count or because of platelet dysfunction. Purpura, ecchymosis, and mucosal bleeding, including epistaxis, gastrointestinal hemorrhage, and menorrhagia, commonly are seen, and bleeding from superficial cuts and abrasions usually is prolonged. In contrast, bleeding caused by plasma coagulation defects usually has a single locus (most often in deep tissues such as joints and muscles) and often occurs the day after trauma.

Thrombocytopenia is caused by accelerated destruction, impaired production, or sequestration of platelets in the spleen. Accelerated destruction of platelets is the most common cause of thrombocytopenia in childhood. For a child who appears well except for the presence of easy bleeding, this destruction likely is caused by acute idiopathic thrombocytopenic purpura (discussed below). The platelets in destructive thrombocytopenias usually are large, the hemoglobin level is normal, and the absolute neutrophil count is greater than 1500. In contrast, a febrile, ill-appearing child who has destructive thrombocytopenia is likely to have other manifestations of disseminated intravascular coagulopathy secondary to sepsis.

Thrombocytopenia caused by decreased platelet production almost always is associated with abnormalities of other cell lines, because the most common underlying disorders (e.g., malignancies, aplastic anemia, glycogen storage disorders) involve the entire bone marrow and its ability to sustain normal hematopoiesis. Many of these children are likely to be pale and appear ill, and have hepatosplenomegaly and sometimes, bone pain.

Splenic sequestration results in nonspecific removal of platelets as well as white and red blood cells from the circulation (hypersplenism). This can occur secondary to a number of diseases that result in massive splenomegaly (see Chapter 170); a normal-size or only slightly enlarged spleen precludes this diagnosis. Thus, the history, physical examination, and CBC usually can direct the clinician toward the likely cause of a patient's thrombocytopenia, resulting in a more rational diagnostic approach and therapeutic intervention.

IDIOPATHIC THROMBOCYTOPENIC PURPURA OF CHILDHOOD

Idiopathic thrombocytopenic purpura (ITP) of childhood is not truly idiopathic; it is caused by the production of autoantibodies that bind to platelets, resulting in their destruction by the reticuloendothelial system, thus leading some to label this disease *immune thrombocytopenic purpura*. The largest subset of children who have ITP also has a well-defined clinical syndrome that may be called *acute ITP of childhood* (AITPC). In other children, the ITP may be a manifestation of a more complex underlying disorder that affects the child's long-term prognosis significantly, such as a collagen-vascular disease or hypogammaglobulinemia. Still others may have chronic ITP that has no association with an underlying disorder; chronic ITP is diagnosed when the thrombocytopenia persists for longer than 6 months. Finally, 1% to 4% of children who apparently have classic AITPC suffer recurrent episodes of severe thrombocytopenia many months or years after the platelet count initially returns to normal. This disorder is called *recurrent ITP of childhood.*

The annual incidence of new cases of AITPC is roughly 4 per 100,000 children. There is no gender predilection, and the peak onset occurs between 2 and 5 years of age. Typically a previously well child suddenly develops easy bruising and petechiae 1 to 3 weeks following a viral illness. Epistaxis occurs in 20% to 30% of these children, but renal, oral, or gastrointestinal bleeding occurs in fewer than 10%. Except for the presence of bleeding, the physical examination is entirely normal. Splenomegaly rarely is seen in AITPC; the presence of splenomegaly suggests an alternative diagnosis. A very large spleen suggests hypersplenism rather than ITP. In AITPC the platelet count almost always is less than 20,000 at the time of diagnosis. Higher counts should prompt one to entertain alternative diagnoses. Thrombocytopenia is evident

BOX 225-1

CRITERIA FOR THE DIAGNOSIS OF ACUTE IDIOPATHIC THROMBOCYTOPENIA OF CHILDHOOD

- Platelet count ≤20,000/mm³
- Normal complete blood count, including the absolute neutrophil count and the examination of red blood cells, white blood cells, and platelet morphology on the blood smear
- Age 1 to 9 years
- Patient otherwise well
- Acute onset (symptomatic less than 2 weeks)
- Preceding viral illness within 1 to 3 weeks
- Normal size spleen
- No personal history or family history of other possible autoimmune disorders (e.g., hemolytic anemia, nephritis, thyroiditis, collagen-vascular disease, or frequent infections)

BOX 225-2

DIAGNOSTIC WORKUP FOR ITP

Studies to be performed when a patient who has ITP does not fit all the criteria listed in Box 225-1 or if apparent AITPC does not resolve within 6 months:
- Bone marrow examination
- Immunoglobulin levels
- Reticulocyte count
- Direct and indirect antiglobulin (Coombs) test
- Urinalysis
- Antinuclear antibody levels
- Prothrombin and partial thromboplastin times
- Bleeding time
- Human immunodeficiency virus antibody

on the peripheral blood smear, and the platelets that are present may have bizarre shapes or giant forms or be diffusely increased in size. The red and white blood cells on the smear should be normal; if they are not, other diagnoses should be considered.

The laboratory evaluation of AITPC is simple. The CBC, including an examination of the blood smear, usually is sufficient in patients who have all the characteristics listed in Box 225-1. AITPC typically presents so clearly that a routine bone marrow examination is not required. However, it is essential to examine a patient's marrow if an aregenerative thrombocytopenia is suspected or if corticosteroid treatment is contemplated. Because steroid therapy is an integral part of the treatment for acute lymphoblastic leukemia (ALL), steroid treatment of a patient who has evolving ALL but who is presumed to have AITPC not only will delay the diagnosis of ALL but also will result in the growth of leukemic cells that are resistant to steroids, which would result in a significantly poorer prognosis. Bone marrow aspiration in patients who have AITPC should reveal a normocellular marrow that has normal erythroid and myeloid maturation. Megakaryocytes are present in normal or increased numbers. Bone marrow examination will not distinguish AITPC from other forms of platelet destruction, including immune-mediated thrombocytopenic disorders other than AITPC. The bleeding time is prolonged and coagulation tests normal in patients who have AITPC, but performing these tests generally is not indicated. The measurement of platelet-associated immunoglobulin is elevated in approximately 85% of children who have ITP, including the majority who have AITPC. Platelet-associated immunoglobulin levels also are elevated in many other thrombocytopenic disorders, so the specificity of this test for AITPC is low and rarely helps to establish the diagnosis or prognosis.

Additional diagnostic tests for disorders associated with ITP should be performed in all patients who do not completely meet the criteria for the diagnosis of AITPC as outlined in Box 225-1. This diagnostic workup is summarized in Box 225-2. Bone marrow should be examined to document adequate platelet precursors. Immunoglobulin levels should be measured to rule out hypogammaglobulinemia associated with multiple autoimmune phenomena, especially autoimmune hemolytic anemia, ITP, and autoimmune neutropenia. The remaining tests search for evidence of associated autoimmune phenomena, collagen-vascular disease, or coagulopathies. The reticulocyte count is elevated during compensated hemolysis; the Coombs test is positive in most cases of autoimmune hemolytic anemia; urinalysis may reveal evidence of nephritis; the antinuclear antibody may identify patients who have systemic lupus erythematosus. Tests for infection by human immunodeficiency virus (HIV) should be performed, because isolated ITP is not an uncommon first manifestation of HIV infection.

PROGNOSIS AND MANAGEMENT

Management of ITP is based on the natural history of the disease and the desire to prevent serious intracranial or gastrointestinal bleeding. The mainstays of therapy are supportive care, corticosteroids, intravenous gammaglobulin (IVIG), anti-D immunoglobulin, and splenectomy, each of which has inherent risks and benefits. More than 90% of patients who have AITPC will have the condition resolved without therapy and without serious sequelae. However, the clinician is faced with his or her own anxiety as well as parental anxiety in attempting to restrict the activity of young children awaiting resolution of the thrombocytopenia.

The risk of serious bleeding is greatest in those patients whose platelet counts are less than 20,000/mm.[3] Therapy, therefore, is aimed at rapidly raising the platelet count above this level.[7] Many pediatric hematologists no longer recommend treatment unless the platelet count is less than 10,000/mm³ in an asymptomatic patient.[6] In a recent prospective, randomized trial, patients treated with either prednisone or IVIG had fewer days with platelet counts less than 20,000/mm³ than did patients receiving supportive care only. Patients receiving IVIG achieved a platelet count greater than 50,000/mm³ faster than either of the other two groups.[2] Adverse effects of IVIG include headache, nausea, vomiting, and fever, which are controlled easily by diphenhydramine and acetaminophen. The costs of administering the IVIG (1 g/kg/day for 2 days) are significantly greater than the costs of prednisone. Prednisone generally is administered at a dose of 2 to 4 mg/kg/day for 2 to 3 weeks. The adverse effects of corticosteroids are well known but generally are tolerable for this short duration of therapy. Long-term therapy with corticosteroids should be avoided because of their effects on growth, bone mineralization, and gastric mucosa.

Corticosteroids may have the additional benefit of stabilizing the vascular endothelium in the presence of thrombocytopenia; this may result in less clinical bleeding at a given platelet count. It again must be emphasized that all patients receiving steroids need to have their bone marrow examined carefully before therapy. Administration of IVIG will not alter the interpretation of a bone marrow examination; therefore, it may be used as empirical therapy if one chooses to avoid a bone marrow examination. Treatment with IVIG or steroids does not preclude treatment with the other modality.

Anti-D immunoglobulin is another therapeutic option for patients who have AITPC.[9] It increases the platelet count by inducing a mild immune hemolytic anemia, which saturates the splenic macrophage receptors, thereby allowing antibody-coated platelets to exit the spleen. Therefore, it is indicated only for non-splenectomized patients who are D (Rh) positive. It has been shown in randomized trials to be effective in raising the platelet count rapidly, and is given by intravenous push over 5 minutes at a dose of 50 μg/kg.[10] Recent data suggest that 75 μg/kg may be more effective.[6] Adverse effects are similar to those of IVIG; however, they occur much less frequently. In addition, a transient fall in the hemoglobin concentration by an average of 1.7 g/dl can be expected secondary to the hemolysis. Lastly, the short infusion time is more amenable to outpatient treatment than intravenous IgG and is significantly less expensive.

There is no role for routine splenectomy in the management of AITPC, but it may be useful in older children who have chronic ITP. Platelet transfusions have a very limited role in the management of AITPC. Because transfused platelets are destroyed immunologically in a fashion similar to that of the endogenous platelets, platelet transfusions will not result in a sustained increase in the patient's platelet count. Platelet transfusions may be useful and should be given to patients experiencing ongoing life-threatening hemorrhage. Defensive management also is important. Restriction of physical activity and avoidance of contact sports and playground activities are indicated. All medications that have antiplatelet activity should be avoided, including ibuprofen, aspirin, antihistamines, phenothiazines, and glycerol guaiacolate. Intramuscular injections should be avoided.

EMERGENCY MANAGEMENT OF BLEEDING

General measures should be directed at the delivery of platelets to the site of hemorrhage. Although the routine use of platelet transfusions in ITP is not indicated, platelet transfusions are useful in an emergency. A bolus infusion of 1 unit/5 kg body weight should be administered immediately because it may exert hemostatic benefit before being cleared by the reticuloendothelial system. Corticosteroids should be administered intravenously (4 mg/kg/day of prednisolone or its equivalent). IVIG also should be administered at the dose described on p. 1570. If these measures fail to control bleeding an emergency splenectomy may be indicated. Aminocaproic acid (Amicar), an inhibitor of fibrinolysis, may help to prevent serious rebleeding, especially in mucosal areas.

CHRONIC IDIOPATHIC THROMBOCYTOPENIA PURPURA

Chronic ITP is defined as a platelet count that persists below 100,000/mm^3 for more than 6 months. Approximately 20% of patients who have chronic ITP ultimately will recover spontaneously, but it is not possible to predict in which children this will occur. Chronic ITP in children is similar to ITP in adults and is caused by platelet autoantibodies that bind to specific platelet membrane glycoproteins. The female-to-male ratio for chronic ITP is 3:1. The workup for chronic ITP should include the studies outlined in Box 225-2.

Management depends on the overall impact of both platelet count and platelet function on hemostasis in the individual patient. In some patients, the antiplatelet antibody also impairs platelet function. Whereas splenectomy once was the mainstay of treating chronic ITP, other alternatives are available to prevent or postpone splenectomy. IVIG and anti-D immunoglobulin in the doses previously mentioned are effective in raising the platelet count temporarily in approximately 80% of children who have chronic ITP, although about 25% of patients eventually become refractory to their effect. In the remainder of patients, periodic doses of IVIG or anti-D immunoglobulin are effective long-term therapy and can be given as a single outpatient infusion of 1 g/kg (IVIG) or 50 μg/kg (Anti-D) every few weeks. Pulses of high doses of intravenous methylprednisolone (15 mg/kg/day for 3 days) and dexamethasone (25 mg/m^2 for 4 days every 4 weeks) also have been shown to improve the platelet count in select patients who have chronic ITP.[1,5] Thrombocytopenia in some patients also may be controlled by brief treatment with prednisone (2 mg/kg/day) or low doses of alternate-day prednisone for longer periods. This may be useful in postponing splenectomy but is not a desirable long-term option in young children because of long-term side effects. Alternative forms of immunosuppression have been used with some success, but at this point these can be recommended only for highly refractory patients and should be undertaken only after consultation at an experienced clinical center.

Splenectomy effectively raises the platelet count to levels that prevent bleeding in most children who have chronic ITP. There is no definitive test by which one can predict this response. Splenectomy itself appears to be safe in patients who have chronic ITP, and excessive bleeding during surgery is quite rare. During a splenectomy the surgeon must look carefully for an accessory spleen, because residual splenic tissue may result in the relapse of ITP after surgery. The platelet count usually starts to rise in the immediate postoperative period, and platelet counts greater than 1 million are not unusual. Because there are no reports of thrombosis at these very high levels, antiplatelet agents are not indicated.

Splenectomy should be avoided if at all possible in the younger child because the risk of postsplenectomy sepsis is highest in young children. The risk decreases dramatically with age; by 6 years of age, given proper vaccination and postsplenectomy antibiotic prophylaxis, the incidence of sepsis appears to be quite low. The increased risk of septicemia is limited to encapsulated organisms—pneumococcus, *Hemophilus influenzae* type b, and meningococcus. Rapidly overwhelming sepsis almost always is caused by pneumococcus, so penicillin prophylaxis is important and recommended for life by many pediatric hematologists. Pneumococcal and meningococcal vaccinations should be administered at least 2 weeks before splenectomy. The development of fever in children who have had a splenectomy is an indication for prompt evaluation and parenteral administration of a third-generation cephalosporin until blood cultures have been found to be negative.

IMMUNE THROMBOCYTOPENIA IN THE NEONATE

Approximately 10% of infants admitted to neonatal intensive care units have platelet counts less than 100,000/mm^3. The majority of these patients do not have immune thrombocytopenia; instead, the thrombocytopenia is secondary to sepsis, congenital infection, asphyxia, or necrotizing enterocolitis. There are, however, two immune causes of neonatal thrombocytopenia that deserve special mention, particularly given the risks associated with future pregnancies.

Maternal ITP may result in the transplacental passage of maternal autoantibodies that may destroy fetal platelets immunologically. Although these infants may become moderately thrombocytopenic (platelet count 20,000 to 50,000/mm^3), significant bleeding in the infant appears to be rare.[3] The thrombocytopenia resolves as the maternally derived antibodies are catabolized. While awaiting resolution, one can use IVIG expectantly to support the infant's platelet count.

A more serious situation exists when the mother develops antiplatelet antibodies directed against paternally derived platelet antigens that are present on the infant's platelets. This process, termed *neonatal alloimmune thrombocytopenic purpura* (NATP), is analogous to erythroblastosis fetalis (Rh disease), in which maternal anti-Rh antibodies destroy Rh-positive fetal red blood cells. NATP occurs in approximately 1 in 2000 to 1 in 5000 fetuses and results in severe neonatal thrombocytopenia. The precise incidence of intracranial hemorrhage is unknown, but estimates range between 10% and 30% of affected infants. The severity of thrombocytopenia and intracranial hemorrhage tends to increase with subsequent pregnancies. Postnatal treatment with washed, irradiated maternal platelets as well as with IVIG improve the thrombocytopenia. Identification of NATP is important because antepartum and postpartum neonatal hemorrhages may occur in future pregnancies. Antenatal treatment of the mother with IVIG and perhaps steroids are effective in raising fetal platelet counts[4] and therefore may decrease the incidence of severe injury or death from hemorrhage. A recent recommendation is to perform in utero platelet count measurements and to transfuse platelets in utero for severe thrombocytopenia.[8]

Acknowledgment

The authors acknowledge and thank Dr. Christopher N. Frantz for his prior contributions to this chapter.

When to Refer

History of fevers or bone pain
Platelet count less than 20,000/mm^3
Hepatomegaly, splenomegaly, significant lymphadenopathy
Abnormal white blood cell count

When to Hospitalize

Significant bleeding symptoms
Severe anemia
Significant concern for possible traumatic injury

REFERENCES

1. Beardsley DS: Oral dexamethasone therapy for chronic immune thrombocytopenic purpura: home run or base hit? *J Pediatr* 130:1, 1997.
2. Blanchette VS, et al: A prospective, randomized trial of high-dose intravenous immune globulin G therapy, oral prednisone therapy, and no therapy in childhood acute immune thrombocytopenic purpura, *J Pediatr* 123:989, 1993.
3. Burrows RF, Kelton JG: Fetal thrombocytopenia and its relation to maternal thrombocytopenia, *N Engl J Med* 329:1463, 1993.
4. Bussel JB, et al: Antenatal treatment of neonatal alloimmune thrombocytopenia, *N Engl J Med* 319:1374, 1988.
5. del Principe D, et al: Phase II trial of methylprednisolone pulse therapy in childhood chronic thrombocytopenia, *Acta Haematol* 77:226, 1987.
6. Freiberg A, Mauger D: Efficacy, safety and dose response of intravenous anti-D immune globulin (WinRho SDF) for the treatment of idiopathic thrombocytopenic purpura in children, *Semin Hematol* 35(suppl)1:23, 1998.
7. George JN, et al: Idiopathic thrombocytopenic purpura: a practice guideline developed by explicit methods for the American Society of Hematology, *Blood* 88:3, 1996.
8. Letsky EA, Greaves M: Guidelines in the investigation and management of thrombocytopenia in pregnancy and neonatal alloimmune thrombocytopenia, *Br J Haematol* 95:21, 1996.
9. Scaradavou A, Bussel JB: Clinical experience with Anti-D in the treatment of idiopathic thrombocytopenic purpura, *Semin Hematol* 35(suppl) 1:52, 1998.
10. Tarantino MD, Goldsmith G: Treatment of acute immune thrombocytopenic purpura, *Semin Hematol* 35(suppl)1:28, 1998.

SUGGESTED READING

Beardsley DS: Platelet abnormalities in infancy and childhood. In Nathan DG, Orkin SH, editors: *Nathan and Oski's hematology of infancy and childhood,* Philadelphia, 1998, WB Saunders.

226 Infectious Mononucleosis and Other Epstein-Barr Virus Infections

Stephen R. Barone • Leonard R. Krilov

EPIDEMIOLOGY

Infection with Epstein-Barr virus (EBV), a member of the herpesvirus group, is extremely common but often not apparent clinically. In Africa, there is a strong association between infection with EBV and development of Burkitt's lymphoma and nasopharyngeal carcinoma; this association, however, has been demonstrated less clearly in Western countries despite the demonstration of serological evidence of past infection by the great majority of children and adolescents. In the United States, interest in EBV infection centers on the typical clinical syndrome—known as *infectious mononucleosis*—that it produces and on its emerging relationship with an increasing number of tumors, noted for the most part in immunocompromised patients.

In childhood, EBV infection usually is inapparent clinically or manifested by a nonspecific, uncomplicated episode of upper respiratory tract infection or pharyngitis. Although EBV antibodies have developed in 70% to 90% of children from low socioeconomic groups by age 5 years, these antibodies occur in only 40% to 50% of those from high socioeconomic groups.[1] Primary infections that do not occur until adolescence and young adulthood are much more likely, for reasons that are unclear, to manifest as infectious mononucleosis. Thus, the annual incidence of infectious mononucleosis is highest among white high school and college students—approximately 1 in 2500 students.

CLINICAL PRESENTATION

After an incubation period of 2 to 6 weeks (normally 20 to 30 days), signs of classic infectious mononucleosis are seen: fever, sore throat, and lymphadenopathy. This constellation of signs can be preceded by vague symptoms of fatigue, malaise, and anorexia.

Because infectious mononucleosis is the result of a systemic viral infection, virtually every organ system may be involved.[5] Fig. 226-1 demonstrates the variety of clinical manifestations compatible with infectious mononucleosis.

The fever usually is not higher than 103° F (39.5° C), but the sore throat, frequently accompanied by tonsillar exudate (or in adolescents, more likely a grayish necrosis of the tonsillar surfaces) and a palatal enanthem, can be excruciating. Lymphadenopathy, perhaps the most striking feature of the illness, can be limited to the cervical nodes, but also can be so extensive as to involve virtually all lymph node groups. Posterocervical adenopathy is noted most frequently. The lymph nodes are not tender, nor do they demonstrate other signs of inflammation.

Enlargement of the spleen and possibly the liver, together with posterocervical adenopathy, are the physical signs that usually alert the clinician to the diagnosis of infectious mononucleosis. Some patients who have this illness, however, do not have any palpable splenic enlargement; massive enlargement of the spleen should suggest an alternative diagnosis. Liver enzyme levels are elevated in virtually all patients, but the frequency of jaundice is low.

The severity of illness is extremely variable, and some individuals may have relatively few signs of infection, whereas others will demonstrate virtually all the findings listed in Fig. 226-1. In general, the clinical manifestations of the illness last approximately 2 to 3 weeks, with peak involvement during the second week. Eyelid edema has been reported by some observers in about 25% of patients.

DIAGNOSIS AND SEROLOGY

Infectious mononucleosis is diagnosed by the presence of a triad of typical clinical, hematological, and serological findings. In addition to the clinical profile described in the preceding section, minimal hematological features should include a lymphocytosis of 50% or more of all leukocytes and an atypical lymphocyte count of 10% or more of all leukocytes. Other general laboratory findings usually include a decline in the number of granulocytes and platelets.

The heterophil, Paul-Bunnell antibody, an IgM antibody produced by humans during infection that reacts with horse, sheep, and beef erythrocytes, but not with guinea pig kidney cells, is the cornerstone of laboratory diagnosis. This antibody will be present in 50% or fewer of children younger than 4 years of age.[10] Among school-age children and young adults it is detectable 80% to 90% of the time during the second week of clinical illness.[5,10] Occasionally the heterophil response will be brief and minimal or will occur late in the illness and therefore may show negative results early in the course of the illness. Commercial diagnostic kits, which rely on differential adsorption to detect the heterophil antibody, are readily available and easy to use in a physician's office; they are 96% to 99% sensitive and give a result in 2 minutes.[4] False-positive results have been reported in cases of rubella, hepatitis, serum sickness, drug reactions, and systemic lupus erythematosus and through improper use of the kit or inaccurate interpretation of the agglutination reaction.

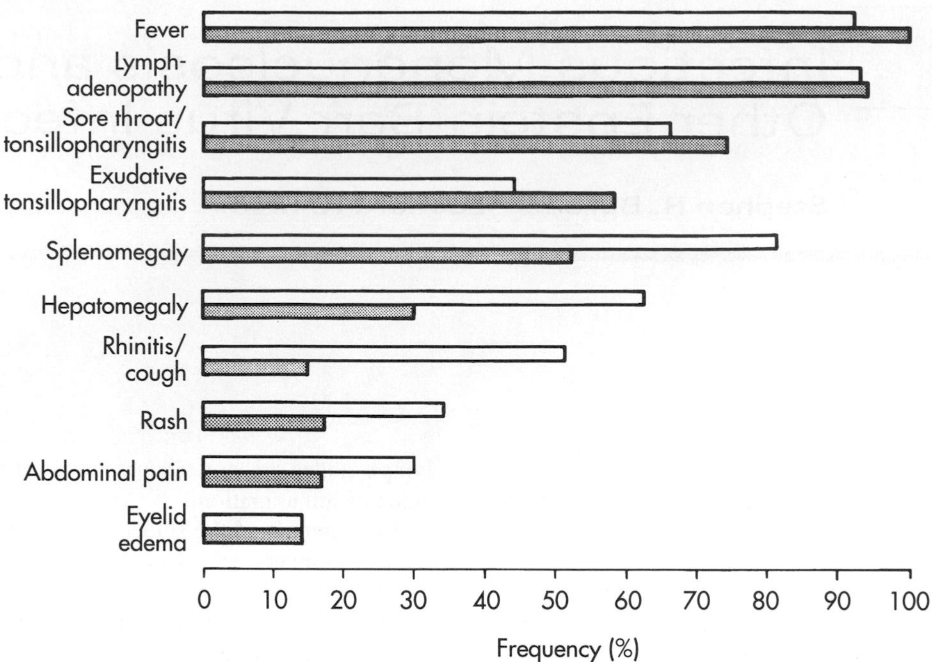

Fig. 226-1 Frequency of clinical findings in two age groups of children with documented Epstein-Barr virus infectious mononucleosis: less than 4 years old *(open bars)* and 4 to 16 years old *(shaded bars).*

(From Sumaya CV, Ench Y: *Pediatrics* 75:1005, 1985.)

The magnitude of the heterophil antibody titer does not correlate with clinical severity, and repeat testing, once a positive test result is obtained, provides no additional information regarding waxing or waning of the illness beyond that gained from clinical assessment of the patient.

If heterophil test results are negative and infection is strongly suspected, confirmation of EBV infection should be sought by other serological tests.[9] A variety of antibodies directed against various portions of EBV can be detected by numerous hospital, state health, or commercial laboratories. Patients who have negative heterophil test results will have antibodies against specific components of the virus if EBV is the cause of the clinical illness.

Four different antibodies define the EBV serological profile: IgG antibody to the viral capsid antigen (VCA-IgG), IgM antibody to viral capsid antigen (VCA-IgM), IgG antibody to early antigen (EA) and IgG antibody to Epstein-Barr nuclear antigen (EBNA). This latter antibody includes two patterns: diffuse (D) and restricted (R). These antibodies usually appear in an individual who acquires a primary EBV infection. The pattern of antibody responses, therefore, can help the practitioner to date the onset of an individual's EBV infection.

In most cases an individual develops a VCA-IgM antibody response in the acute period following an EBV infection. The same is true for the VCA-IgG antibody. Although IgG antibodies to the VCA persist for life, VCA-IgM tends to disappear in 2 to 3 months. The EA response peaks at 3 to 4 weeks into the illness and initially was thought to persist only for several months; therefore, it also was considered a good marker for an acute or recent infection. However, recent evidence suggests that the EA response may persist for years in some children and may not develop at all in others. Finally, the EBNA antibody response usually appears several weeks to months after a primary infection and, therefore, is thought to be a marker for a past or convalescent infection. However, even this antibody response has to be interpreted in light of the clinical situation, because a number of children develop this response in the acute phase of their infection; 10% to 20% of individuals never develop detectable levels of antibody to EBNA. In summary, antibodies in children who acquire an EBV infection typically develop similarly (Table 226-1); however, not all patients necessarily will follow the same pattern, and clinical judgment remains important in the interpretation of such findings. Additionally, interlaboratory variability in results of EBV antibody testing have been observed, making the reliability of these tests suspect in some cases. If both the heterophil test and specific serologies are negative, causes for a non-EBV infectious mononucleosis-like illness should be suspected.

COMPLICATIONS AND DEATHS

Most persons who have infectious mononucleosis recover uneventfully. Serious complications, however, have resulted from this illness; death occurs in approximately 1 in 3000 cases. The true complication and death rates during this illness are uncertain because many reports do not include strict diagnostic criteria for infectious mononucleosis. The relative frequencies of more common complications associated with this illness, as documented in one large study, are listed in Table 226-2.[4] A number of other complications, representing virtually every body organ, also have been reported with this disease.

Of 20 deaths clearly associated with infectious mononucleosis in one series,[7] 9 were of neurological origin, 3 were

Table 226-1 Interpretation of Epstein-Barr Virus Serology

	Heterophil Antibody	Epstein-Barr Virus Antibodies			
		VCA-IgM	VCA-IgG	EA	EBNA
No infection	–	–	–	–	–
Acute infection	+/–	+	+ (>1:320)	+/–	–
Past infection	–	–	+ (1:80-1:160)	+/–	+

Note: Other patterns may occur in an individual patient; the above profile is for a typical individual.
VCA-IgM, IgM antibody to viral capsid antigen; *VAC-IgG,* IgG antibody to viral capsid antigen; *EA,* early antigen; *EBNA,* IgG antibody to Epstein-Barr nuclear antigen.

Table 226-2 Complications Present in 113 Children with EBV Infectious Mononucleosis

Complication	No. of Children (%)
Respiratory tract	
Pneumonia	6 (5.3)
Severe airway obstruction*	4 (3.5)
Neurological	
Seizures	4 (3.5)
Meningitis/encephalitis	2 (1.8)
Peripheral facial nerve paralysis	1 (0.9)
Guillain-Barré syndrome	1 (0.9)
Hematological	
Thrombocytopenia with hemorrhages	4 (3.5)
Hemolytic anemia	1 (0.9)
Infectious	
Bacteremia	1 (0.9)
Recurrent tonsillopharyngitis	3 (2.7)
Liver	
Jaundice	2 (1.8)
Renal	
Glomerulonephritis	1 (0.9)
Genital	
Orchitis	1 (0.9)
TOTAL	31†

From Sumaya CV, Ench Y: *Pediatrics* 75:1007, 1985.
*Criteria consisted of nasal alar flaring, suprasternal retractions, or stridor.
†Because four children had more than one of these complications, this total is composed of 24 different children, or 21.2% of the study group.

caused by secondary infection, 3 by splenic rupture, 2 by hepatic failure, 1 by probable myocarditis, and 2 from an undetermined cause. Because abdominal pain is an infrequent symptom of this illness, its appearance, particularly if severe and in the left upper quadrant, should alert the clinician to the possibility of impending or actual splenic rupture. Fatal cases of Reye's syndrome associated with serological evidence of EBV infection also have been reported.

MANAGEMENT

Because most patients who have infectious mononucleosis recover uneventfully, physicians need do little except establish the diagnosis, explain the nature of the illness, and reassure the family. No specific therapy is indicated. Patients should rest to the extent that they feel necessary. As long as the patient can consume adequate amounts of fluids and calories, hospitalization is unnecessary. To minimize the danger of splenic rupture, ambulatory patients should avoid strenuous physical exercise or contact sports until the spleen no longer is palpable. Patients who have late onset of the heterophil antibody response appear to have a prolonged convalescence.

Corticosteroids are of unproved value in treating this illness.[2] They should not be used routinely merely to make the patient feel better. Most clinicians believe that their use is justified in treating severe hemolytic anemia, significant airway obstruction secondary to tonsillar hypertrophy, and thrombocytopenia. However, controlled studies documenting their efficacy for these indications are lacking. Some suggest using corticosteroids if neurological involvement is significant, but again, proof of efficacy is not available. The antiviral agent acyclovir has good activity against EBV in vitro, but it has not been shown to be beneficial in a number of clinical trials that involve patients who had infectious mononucleosis. At this time, it is not recommended for routine use. A number of antivirals (acyclovir, ganciclovir, vidarabine) and immunomodulating agents (interferon-gamma, interferon-alpha, interleukin-2) have been used in severe EBV infections, with varying degrees of success.[6] Novel therapeutic approaches under investigation for the treatment of EBV-associated lymphoproliferative disease include bone marrow transplantation, treatment with monoclonal antibodies, and infusions of donor peripheral leukocytes.

Inasmuch as the pharyngitis of infectious mononucleosis can be indistinguishable from that of streptococcal pharyngitis, culture specimens of the pharynx should be obtained, and patients who have positive culture findings should be treated accordingly.

A rash, which can be erythematous, petechial, erythema multiforme–like, urticarial, or scarlatiniform, develops in approximately 20% of children who have this illness. A rash develops in 70% to 90% of young adult patients who have this illness and who are treated with ampicillin. In some cases the ampicillin-related rash will appear after the medication has been discontinued. Although the ampicillin effect has not been well demonstrated in young children who have infectious mononucleosis, it is prudent to avoid using this drug when this infection is suspected.

Infection follows entry of the EBV into the oropharynx, and its recovery from this site can be documented up to 16 months after illness. It appears that EBV establishes latency in the epithelial cells of the oropharynx and that the virus periodically is shed from this site throughout an individual's lifetime. Transmission from one individual to another appears to occur most often through mixing of saliva (thus its description as the "kissing disease"). In the absence of such contact, transfer of infection is unlikely. In a study of families that have a childhood index case of infectious mononucleosis, seroconversion occurred in 34.6% of the susceptible siblings over a period of several months.[11] Even though the rate of transmission of the EBV infection was relatively low and slow, the development of infectious mononucleosis was quite high (55.6%) in sibling contacts who showed seroconversion.

Secondary infection in typical college settings is even lower. Consequently, strict isolation of the patient is unnecessary. Instead, separation of drinking and eating utensils (e.g., avoiding drinking from the same glass) is all that is required.

Accounts are increasing (although still rare) of infectious mononucleosis episodes that are quite severe, fatal, or result in significant long-lasting problems. Most of these patients had some form of immunological abnormality'that is, X-linked lymphoproliferative syndrome, renal or bone marrow transplant, or Chédiak-Higashi syndrome, among others. The definitive management of these patients remains unclear.

EPSTEIN-BARR VIRUS INFECTION AND CHRONIC FATIGUE SYNDROME

In the 1980's, several reports described individuals who reportedly developed a chronic EBV or mononucleosis-like syndrome following a bout of acute mononucleosis.[3,8] These patients never seemed to recover completely from their acute illnesses and complained of persistent fatigue, pharyngitis, lymphadenitis, and low-grade fevers. Subsequent studies, however, demonstrated normal immune responses to EBV and clearance of the virus in these patients. These individuals today fall under the rubric of chronic fatigue syndrome, a chronic, debilitating illness characterized by extreme fatigue, neuropsychological abnormalities, and a myriad of other problems. Although many patients who have chronic fatigue syndrome date the onset of their illness to an episode of infectious mononucleosis, virological and clinical studies have confirmed that active EBV infection is not responsible for the illness. At present there is no single infectious or other cause for chronic fatigue syndrome (see Chapter 195, Chronic Fatigue Syndrome).

EPSTEIN-BARR VIRUS–NEGATIVE INFECTIOUS MONONUCLEOSIS

Rubella, hepatitis, toxoplasmosis, cytomegalovirus (CMV), human herpesvirus-6 and adenovirus infections, systemic lupus erythematosus, and drug reactions can produce symptoms similar to those of EBV infection. Negative EBV titers and heterophil antibody responses strongly suggest one of these other agents or conditions as the cause of the illness under consideration. In hepatitis, in which the heterophil test can give a false-positive result, liver enzyme levels generally are much more elevated than those seen with infectious mononucleosis. Results of serological tests for hepatitis will be positive, as will rubella titers in rubella infection; CMV can be cultured from urine in those who have that infection as the cause of their illness. Illnesses that mimic infectious mononucleosis but lack serological confirmation of EBV infection should be classified as heterophil-negative infectious mononucleosis rather than atypical mononucleosis. The cause of most of these cases is unknown.

EPSTEIN-BARR VIRUS INFECTION AND MALIGNANCY

Lymphocytes that contain the EBV genome can be subdivided indefinitely. The virus remains dormant in human hosts for prolonged periods. These observations, together with the known association of EBV and African Burkitt's lymphoma and nasopharyngeal carcinoma, have raised speculation that EBV infection might be oncogenic in the United States as well. Some cases of leukemia occurring shortly after the onset of infectious mononucleosis have been reported, but there is no other evidence to support this speculation. Although in the United States the association between EBV and classic Burkitt's lymphoma is not as strong as in Africa, a number of lymphomas and lymphoproliferative lesions that contain EBV markers (including markers of viral replication) have been found in American patients. The EBV genome can be detected in approximately 80% of Reed-Sternberg cells found in patients with the mixed cellularity form of Hodgkin's lymphoma. However, whether EBV is an etiological agent or even a co-factor for Hodgkin's disease in unknown. Epstein-Barr virus has also been associated with a number of lymphoreticular malignancies in patients who have acquired immunodeficiency syndrome (AIDS). These include malignant B-cell lymphoma and colonic lymphoid hyperplasia. Additionally, EBV has been associated with oral hairy leukoplakia and lymphoid interstitial pneumonitis in individuals with AIDS. The precise relationship between EBV and malignancies remains unknown and is the subject of intense investigation.

REFERENCES

1. Andiman WA: The Epstein-Barr virus and EB virus infections in childhood, *J Pediatr* 95:171, 1979.
2. Collins M, et al: Role of steroids in the treatment of infectious mononucleosis in the ambulatory college student, *J Am Coll Health Assoc* 33: 101, 1984.
3. Jones JF, et al: Evidence for active Epstein-Barr virus infections in patients with persistent, unexplained illness: elevated anti-early antigen antibodies, *Ann Intern Med* 102:1, 1985.
4. Karzon DT: Infectious mononucleosis, *Adv Pediatr* 22:231, 1976.
5. Mandell GL, Douglas RG Jr, Bennett JE: *Principles and practice of infectious diseases,* vol 2, New York, 1979, John Wiley & Sons.
6. Okano M: Epstein-Barr virus infection and its role in the expanding spectrum of human disease, *Acta Paediatr* 87:11, 1998.
7. Penman HG: Fatal infectious mononucleosis: a critical review, *J Clin Pathol* 23:765, 1970.
8. Straus SE, et al: Persisting illness and fatigue in adults with evidence of Epstein-Barr virus infection, *Ann Intern Med* 102:7, 1985.
9. Sumaya CV, Ench Y: Epstein-Barr virus infectious mononucleosis in children. I. Clinical and general laboratory findings, *Pediatrics* 75:1003, 1985.
10. Sumaya CV, Ench Y: Epstein-Barr virus infectious mononucleosis in children. II. Heterophil antibody and viral-specific responses, *Pediatrics* 75:1011, 1985.
11. Sumaya CV, Ench Y: Epstein-Barr virus infections in families: the role of children with infectious mononucleosis, *J Infect Dis* 154:842, 1986.

SUGGESTED READINGS

Giffen BE, Xue S: Epstein-Barr virus infections and their association with human malignancies: some key questions, *Ann Med* 30:249, 1998.

Schuster V, Kreth HW: Epstein-Barr virus infection and associated diseases in children. I. Pathogenesis, epidemiology and clinical aspects, *Eur J Pediatr* 151:718, 1992.

Schuster V, Kreth HW: Epstein-Barr virus infection and associated diseases in children. II. Diagnostic and therapeutic strategies, *Eur J Pediatr* 151: 794, 1992.

Straus SE, et al: Epstein-Barr virus infections: biology, pathogenesis and management, *Ann Intern Med* 118:1, 1993.

227 Insect Bites and Infestations

David H. Stein • Nancy K. Barnett

INSECT BITES

Discrete, red, pruritic papules or nodules suggest the diagnosis of insect or arachnid bites. (Arachnids include mites, ticks, and spiders.) Discomfort varies from mild itch in the unsensitized child to pain caused by toxin injection or aggravating intense pruritus, especially in those with prior exposure and sensitization. Worldwide, arthropods and insects are often vectors of serious or fatal disease, including malaria, one of the most common causes of childhood deaths.

Bites are often grouped and usually found on surfaces not covered by clothing. Physical examination reveals discrete erythematous papules, nodules, and small plaques, often on several body areas. Some may have central puncta or vesicles; others are capped by a hemorrhagic or serous crust or an excoriation created by scratching. Blistering occurs with robust reactions to insect- or arachnid-associated toxins or sensitization to insect antigens. Complications include infection and eczematous changes or hypersensitivity reactions.

Papular urticaria is a common reaction to insect bites. It consists of recurrent crops of urticarial (hivelike) papules, nodules, or wheals on exposed surfaces that may be new or reactivated old bites. Papular urticaria occurs in certain sensitized individuals and can last weeks or months, plaguing the patient with profound itch, especially if repeatedly scratched or otherwise traumatized. Scratching can leave scarring or postinflammatory pigment change. Unlike the infestations discussed below, usually only one or a few family members are affected.

Insect bites can be controlled by using repellents, especially DEET (N,N-diethyl-m-toluamide) and by clothing as much of the body as possible.[3] Much controversy surrounds the use of DEET, which can cause central nervous system and systemic symptoms, in children. Many feel it is safe to use DEET intermittently and that alternate repellents may be just as toxic. Caution and attention to alternatives like clothing and bed nets is appropriate. Mosquitoes are especially attracted by carbon dioxide and lactic acid from the breath and skin, so attraction may be stronger after strenuous physical activity.[5] Topical antipruritics such as calamine are sometimes soothing, as are cold soaks or ice. Topical corticosteroid creams and oral antihistamines can relieve pruritus. Topical antihistamines should be avoided; they may cause allergic contact dermatitis and are usually ineffective. Susceptibility to mosquito bites may be decreased through avoidance of potential attractants, such as bright clothing.[5]

Flea bites tend to be vesiculo-bullous, very pruritic erythematous papules, nodules, and small plaques on the distal extremities and in places where clothes are tight. They can best be eliminated by treating the source; pets should be referred to a veterinarian for flea dipping or dusting and homes should be treated with a flea "bomb." Bedbugs reside in bedding, moldings, and floorboards and can be eradicated with insecticides.

INFESTATIONS

Pediculosis

Lice can infest the scalp as pediculosis capitis, the eyelashes as pediculosis palpebrarum, the body as pediculosis corporis, or the pubic area as pediculosis pubis. Lice are obligate human ectoparasites. They create pruritic dermatoses by puncturing the skin and injecting saliva that incites inflammation; they can also transmit diseases, including typhus.

Lice are spread by close personal contact or by fomites. Outbreaks of head lice often occur in classrooms. The grayish, crawling, six-legged louse may be seen in hair, or its eggs (nits) may be found as minute, white-gray attachments to hair shafts. Family members should be examined, especially if combs, towels, and other personal items are shared. Pruritic erythematous papules, 1 to 2 mm in diameter and presumably caused by bites of the head louse, are sometimes noted about the nape of the neck and the hairline and occasionally on other body areas.

Nits of developing lice or the insects themselves may be visible on the eyelashes or pubic hair. Transmission of pediculosis is frequent between individuals who sleep in the same bed or otherwise maintain close contact; parents, children and all close contacts should be examined for lice. Pediculosis pubis is often sexually transmitted, and affected individuals may have other sexually transmitted diseases.

Pediculosis corporis should be suspected when widespread pruritus is present. The body louse usually is not found on the body; rather, it and its nits are seen in the seams of clothing or bedding. The bites consist of erythematous macules and papules. The lesions often are obscured by the results of scratching—excoriation, impetiginization, eczematization, and pigmentation.

Treatment. The most effective treatment for body lice is the total-body application of 5% permethrin cream (Elimite) for 8 to 14 hours; other scabicides can be used but much resistance by the lice organism has been encountered to them. Simultaneously, all potentially infested clothing should be treated with wet or dry heat (or both) at a minimum of 65° C (149° F) for a minimum of 15, but preferably at least 30, minutes.[1,2,6]

Pediculosis pubis also is best treated with pyrethrins but at a concentration of only 1%; other nonprescription preparations probably are less effective and optimum lengths of application are shortest with pyrethrins.

For head lice, pyrethrins are again the drugs of choice. Older preparations, especially lindane (gamma-benzene hexachloride) are definitely more toxic and probably less effective. Pyrethrins are found in several nonprescription preparations. A fine-toothed comb or the fingernails can be used to remove nits from hair shafts after treatment. Retreatment often is necessary about 1 week after the first application to kill lice that have hatched from viable nits not killed initially. Nix cream rinse contains 1% permethrin; it and other similar products also are effective for the treatment of head lice. Malathion, another pediculicide, must be left on for 8 to 12 hours and is highly flammable. Malathion, if available, is used as a 0.5% lotion. Clothing, bedding, combs, towels, and other items used by lice-infested persons should be washed in hot water, as noted previously for body lice. Resistance of lice to usual treatments has emerged, so repeated treatments with various pediculicides such as permethrin, gamma-benzene hexachloride (GBH), and pyrethrins may be required to eradicate lice. Even the application of Elimite 5% permethrin cream to the hair may be necessary. A vinegar rinse or "Step-2" creme rinse (8% formic acid) may help to remove stubborn nits.

Pruritus may continue for 1 to 2 weeks after treatment, perhaps because of continued irritancy of dead lice or because the topical pediculicides causes irritant dermatitis. Patients should be advised that they might continue to itch so that they do not overtreat themselves through excessive repeated applications. Oral antipruritics and topical steroids can help to control pruritus.

Pediculosis palpebrarum can be treated by applying plain petrolatum to the eyelashes three to five times daily. Treatment is required for about 8 to 10 days, and a moustache comb can be used daily to remove lice and nits from the eyelashes. Other infested body areas should be treated simultaneously. If this fails, physostigmine 0.25% may be similarly applied to eyelashes and is usually curative in 3 or 4 days but may interfere with vision.[6]

The National Pediculosis Association (www.headlice.org) warns that chemical treatments for pediculosis and scabies should never be prescribed for pregnant and nursing women or for persons who have allergies, asthma, epilepsy, open wounds, or other preexisting medical conditions. These warnings include the following:

- Do not use shower caps and never leave the product on longer than directed.
- Do not use a chemical treatment on or near the eyes.
- Do not use a head lice treatment on a baby.
- Do not use lice sprays.
- Do not treat individuals who are not infested.
- Do not use treatments to prevent head lice and scabies.

Scabies

Infestation with the mite, *Sarcoptes scabiei hominis,* causes scabies, a highly pruritic dermatosis with varied and protean manifestations ranging from a few erythematous papules to diffuse scabies-laden crusts, the latter sometimes called *Norwegian scabies.*

Scabies is spread by close personal contact. Family members, sexual partners, and other close contacts of index cases should be examined and treated regardless of symptoms. Frequently the history will reveal that many people in one household are itching, in contrast to papular urticaria caused by insect bites, in which generally only the patient is affected. Fomites rarely transmit scabies to immunocompetent patients.

The burrowing of the female mite into the stratum corneum initiates scabies. Eggs are laid, and over the next 4 to 6 weeks pruritus develops gradually as the eggs hatch and the immune system reacts.[6] Reinfestation, with hypersensitivity to mite antigens, leads to more rapid development of itching.

The burrows created by female mites are helpful in establishing the diagnosis; however, they are not always obvious and often are disguised by excoriations, eczematous reactions, and superimposed infection. Signs of infestation should be looked for in the digital web spaces, the extensor surface of the elbows, and the flexor aspect of the wrists. Confirmatory ova, mites, or feces are sometimes found by light microscopy of scrapings of burrows or papules from these locations; after mineral oil is applied, the burrows or papules are scraped off with a scalpel blade and examined under low magnification.

The papules, pustules, vesicles, and hives that can occur in sarcoptic infestation justify the reputation of scabies being a great masquerader. In the face of worsening or persistent pruritus, the diagnosis of scabies must be considered, especially if close contacts also are itching. The distribution of skin changes is a clue to the diagnosis. In infants, the face, palms, and soles may also be involved, sometimes with relative sparing of the intertriginous areas, genitals, buttocks, wrists, and extensor surfaces of joints—areas usually involved in children and adults.

Treatment. The thorough application of 5% permethrin to the entire body, except the face, is the treatment of choice. An alternative treatment is lindane or a similar gamma-benzene-hexachloride (GBH) preparation. Adverse reactions from overuse of these preparations have raised concern about toxicity from percutaneous absorption. However, when used properly, lindane and other GBHs can be safe and effective but should be dispensed in limited quantity. Parents should be informed about possible neurotoxicity to deter overtreatment.

Crotamiton 10% (Eurax) is less efficacious than the GBHs. Benzyl benzoate is used widely as an inexpensive emulsion recommended by the World Health Organization. Oral ivermectin currently is being investigated for scabies treatment but should not be used until optimum dosages and schedules are established. Controlled studies of the outcomes of all of these therapies are lacking.[4]

Epidemiological studies have demonstrated a high rate of spread within families and between individuals sleeping in the same bed. Therefore, bed linens, clothing, and towels should be washed in hot water.

After successful eradication of an infestation, pruritus can persist for weeks; repeat treatment should be undertaken only when continued infestation is documented. Some individuals develop red to purple discrete nodules up to 2 cm in diameter on surfaces usually covered by clothing, particularly on the genitals or around the axillae; these may persist for months. These "nodular scabies" or "postscabetic nodules" are thought to represent a hypersensitivity reaction. The nodules usually respond to topical or intralesional injections of steroids. The same precautions regarding chemical treatments outlined previously for pediculosis apply for scabies.

REFERENCES

1. Anonymous: Drugs for parasitic infections, *Med Letter Drugs Ther* 40:1, 1998.
2. Brown S, Becher J, Brady W: Treatment of ectoparasitic infections: review of the English-language literature, 1982-1992. *Clin Infect Dis* 20(suppl 1):S104, 1995.
3. Duarte AM: Environmental hazards. In Schachner LA, Hansen RC, editors: *Pediatric dermatology,* New York, 1995, Churchill Livingstone.
4. Elgart ML: A risk-benefit assessment of agents used in the treatment of scabies, *Drug Safety* 14:386, 1996.
5. Fradin MS: Mosquitoes and mosquito repellents: a clinicians guide, *Ann Intern Med* 128:931, 1998.
6. Meinking T, Taplin D: Infestations. In Schachner LA, Hansen RC, editors: *Pediatric dermatology,* New York 1995, Churchill Livingstone.

228 Iron-Deficiency Anemia

James Palis

Iron deficiency is the most common cause of anemia in the world and affects all ages. Iron is needed not only for hemoglobin formation and tissue replacement but also for growth. Iron deficiency, as well as other nutritional deficiencies, is most common in early childhood and during adolescence, when growth rates are maximal. Iron-deficiency anemia is associated with behavioral and cognitive deficits, which may not improve despite adequate iron therapy; this makes the prevention of iron deficiency an important public health issue.

INCIDENCE

Iron deficiency is surprisingly common, even in Western societies where nutrition is generally good and the use of iron-fortified foods is widespread. Accurate estimates of iron deficiency are difficult to obtain because the incidence varies depending on the diagnostic criteria used. Several surveys of infants in various urban areas of the United States reveal a prevalence of between 17% and 44%, the highest being among infants of lower socioeconomic status. Among adolescents, females are affected more commonly than males, with a prevalence as high as 27%.[8]

IRON-CONTAINING COMPOUNDS IN THE BODY

Iron is the most abundant heavy metal in the body. The multiple iron-containing compounds found within the body can be grouped into two major categories—those serving metabolic functions and those involved with iron storage and transport.

The first category includes heme- and nonheme-containing compounds. Heme is composed of a protoporphyrin ring with noncovalently bound iron in the ferrous form (Fe^{++}). The most abundant heme-containing protein in the body is hemoglobin, which transports oxygen from the lungs to the tissues and accounts for more than 60% of total body iron. Myoglobin, which accounts for 10% of total body iron, is a heme protein that provides oxygen for use during muscle contraction. The other major heme proteins, the cytochromes, are found in the mitochondria and are necessary for the oxidative production of cellular energy. There also are several nonheme iron proteins such as the iron-sulfur complexes and flavoproteins. Many of these proteins are found in the mitochondria and also are involved in oxidative metabolism.

The second category of iron compounds is the iron transport and storage molecules. Transferrin is a beta$_1$-globulin capable of binding two atoms of iron in the ferric form (Fe^{+++}). It transports iron from the intestinal epithelium to the bone marrow where it binds to transferrin receptors on the surface of differentiating red cells. The transferrin receptor complex is then internalized and thus supplies iron for the synthesis of hemoglobin. Transferrin also plays a major role in the recycling of iron from senescent red blood cells. Ferritin, an iron storage compound found in all cells of the body, is composed of a hollow protein shell encapsulating iron molecules. Hemosiderin, which also serves to store intracellular iron, is thought to be a partially degraded form of ferritin.

ETIOLOGY AND PATHOPHYSIOLOGY

The four most important factors in the development of iron deficiency in children are (1) the iron endowment at birth, (2) the iron needs during rapid body growth, (3) exogenous iron absorption, and (4) blood loss.

During gestation the fetus is able to extract iron efficiently from the mother independently of maternal iron stores.[10] The ratio of iron content to weight in the human fetus remains constant throughout gestation. The healthy full-term infant has sufficient iron stores to last for 6 months, if sufficient small amounts of iron are ingested from the diet. The infant's iron endowment can be compromised by blood loss during the pregnancy or the perinatal period. Common causes of blood loss include third-trimester bleeding, such as abruptio placentae, placenta previa, fetomaternal hemorrhage, and twin-to-twin transfusions.

Because of their lower body weight, premature infants have a smaller absolute amount of body iron compared with full-term infants. Their increased growth requirements after birth coupled with their smaller iron endowment can lead to a rapid depletion of iron stores, resulting in iron-deficiency anemia as early as 3 months of age.[5]

Iron is needed not only for many metabolic functions and tissue replacement but also for growth. Growth rates vary with age and are maximal during infancy and adolescence, the same periods associated with the highest frequency of iron deficiency.

Because there are no mechanisms available for the active excretion of iron from the body, iron balance is maintained by regulation of iron absorption. The amount of iron absorbed depends both on the amount and the bioavailability of dietary iron, as well as on regulation of iron absorption by the intestinal mucosa. Most dietary iron occurs in the nonheme form and is much less bioavailable than that in heme proteins. The iron in hemoglobin and myoglobin is particularly bioavailable; up to 30% is directly absorbed by the gastrointestinal tract. Breast milk and cow milk contain small amounts of iron (0.5 to 1 mg/1000 ml). However, 50% of the iron in breast milk is absorbed compared with only 10% in cow milk. Full-term infants who are exclusively breast-fed for the first 6 to 9 months do not become iron deficient.[8] Nonheme iron absorption is inhibited by bran in cereals, polyphenols in many vegetables, and tannins in tea. The addition of solids to an infant's diet can impair iron absorption significantly and puts the infant at risk for developing iron deficiency. The introduced solids therefore should contain abundant amounts of iron (e.g., iron-fortified cereals).

Blood loss causes iron deficiency in children less frequently than in adults. In infancy and childhood, iron deficiency caused by blood loss most commonly is associated with the ingestion of unprocessed cow milk and with parasitic infections. Hypersensitivity to whole cow milk causes an exudative enteropathy and frequently leads to gastrointestinal blood loss. Other less common causes of blood loss in children include Meckel's diverticulum, intestinal duplication, peptic ulcer disease, hemorrhagic telangiectasia, and the chronic use of medications that prolong the bleeding time (e.g., aspirin).

CLINICAL MANIFESTATIONS

The onset and progression of iron deficiency usually is gradual, and most children will not have major symptoms. Iron deficiency in infants and children is associated with generalized weakness, irritability, easy fatigability, headaches, poor feeding, anorexia, pica, and poor weight gain.[8] The physical examination usually is unremarkable except for marked pallor of the mucous membranes and skin. Other less common physical findings associated with iron-deficiency anemia include mild hepatosplenomegaly, lymphadenopathy, glossitis, stomatitis, blue sclerae, and koilonychia (spoon-shaped nails).

Many studies have demonstrated an association between iron-deficiency anemia and lower scores on tests of mental and motor development, impaired learning, and decreased school achievement.[4,7] These findings may be related to the decreased attention span and increased irritability seen in iron-deficient children compared with nonanemic controls. To what degree iron deficiency is responsible for these clinical findings is not known because iron repletion may not completely correct the behavioral disturbances or the lower developmental, IQ, and achievement scores.[4] More studies are needed to address and clarify these issues.

STAGES OF IRON DEFICIENCY

Iron deficiency occurs when total body iron content is diminished. Iron normally is absorbed only through the gastrointestinal tract. Sites of iron loss include the skin, the gastrointestinal tract, and the urine. Iron also is lost during pregnancy and lactation. When absorption exceeds losses, the iron surplus is stored in the reticuloendothelial system, principally the liver, spleen, and bone marrow. As body iron stores increase, the gastrointestinal absorption of iron decreases so that iron balance is maintained.

Iron is removed from the reticuloendothelial storage pool to compensate for negative iron balance. The development of iron deficiency proceeds through a series of overlapping stages. The first stage of iron deficiency is storage iron depletion. During this stage, there is no deficit of iron supplied to the erythroid marrow for red cell production. If the negative iron balance continues, the second stage, iron-deficient erythropoiesis, will occur. During this stage, erythroid iron supply is diminished, but the hemoglobin concentration remains in the normal range. If the negative iron balance persists, iron-deficiency anemia finally develops. This third stage is characterized by a fall in the hemoglobin concentration and a reduction in red blood cell size and hemoglobin content.

DIAGNOSIS

Specific laboratory findings are associated with each of the three stages of iron deficiency. The hematological abnormalities and diagnostic tests characteristic of each stage are reviewed in greater depth below and are summarized in Tables 228-1 and 228-2.

Storage Iron Depletion

During this first stage of iron deficiency, the storage pool of iron in the reticuloendothelial system decreases. This can be detected by a fall in serum ferritin levels or by the absence of stainable iron on a bone marrow sample. No red blood cell changes are present at this time because there is sufficient iron to support normal erythropoiesis.

Serum ferritin. As seen in Fig. 228-1, serum ferritin levels vary with age during infancy and childhood. In healthy individuals, serum ferritin levels reflect body iron stores; levels below 12 μg/L indicate iron deficiency. Ferritin is an acute-phase reactant. Serum ferritin levels are elevated dur-

Table 228-1 Iron Status and Hematological Abnormalities in the Three Stages of Iron Deficiency

	Storage Iron Depletion	Iron Deficient Erythropoiesis	Iron Deficiency Anemia
Storage iron	↓	↓↓	↓↓↓
Erythron iron	Normal	↓	↓↓-↓↓↓
Hemoglobin concentration	Normal	Normal	↓-↓↓↓

Modified from Cecalupo AJ, Cohen HJ: Nutritional anemias. In Grand RJ, Sutphen JL, Dietz WH, editors: *Clinical nutrition: theory and practice*, Boston, 1987, Butterworth.
↓, Decreased.

ing infections and inflammatory processes as well as with liver disease. Although low serum ferritin is diagnostic of iron deficiency, an elevated ferritin level associated with inflammation or liver disease does not rule out concomitant iron deficiency (Table 228-3).

Bone marrow iron. The staining of a normal bone marrow aspirate sample with Prussian blue dye reveals the presence of iron in red blood cell precursors (normoblasts) and serves as a reliable index of body iron stores. In iron deficiency the number of iron granules in normoblasts is decreased and stainable iron in the marrow aspirate is almost completely absent.[3]

Iron-Deficient Erythropoiesis

Iron-deficient erythropoiesis characterizes the second stage of iron deficiency. The earliest hematological manifestation of iron deficiency is an elevation of the red cell distribution width.[11] The serum iron concentration decreases, and serum transferrin levels rise concomitantly. This leads to an increase in the total iron-binding capacity (TIBC), with a decrease in the percent saturation (iron/TIBC × 100). Because iron is unavailable for incorporation in the protoporphyrin ring, free erythrocyte protoporphyrin (FEP) in both red blood cells and the plasma increases during this stage of iron deficiency. The plasma loses its usual amber color and becomes clear, making inspection of the plasma on a spun hematocrit useful diagnostically.

Iron/TIBC. Serum iron levels normally fluctuate daily, with maximum levels occurring in the morning and minimal levels in the evening. The TIBC varies less than serum iron but is harder to measure accurately. The normal TIBC is 250 to 400 mg/dl, but as serum iron levels decrease, the TIBC increases to 450 mg/dl or more. Iron and TIBC measurements are useful in distinguishing iron-deficiency anemia from the anemia of chronic disease. Serum iron levels decrease with both, but the TIBC levels also decrease in chronic disease states (see Table 228-3). A useful measure of iron deficiency is the percent saturation—the serum iron divided by the TIBC and multiplied by 100. The normal ranges for serum iron and the percent saturation are shown in Table 228-4. In iron deficiency the percent saturation is reduced to less than 16%, at which point hemoglobin production becomes limited by the lack of iron. The percent saturation is a more sensitive index of iron status than are serum iron measurements alone. Because of the wide variation in serum iron and iron-binding capacity values, these should be tested in conjunction with at least one other test of iron status (e.g., ferritin, FEP) to reach a reliable diagnosis of iron deficiency.

Table 228-2 Laboratory Abnormalities in the Three Stages of Iron Deficiency

	Storage Iron Depletion	Iron-Deficient Erythropoiesis	Iron Deficiency Anemia
Bone marrow iron	Absent	Absent	Absent
Ferritin	↓	↓↓	↓↓↓
Red cell distribution width	Normal-↓	↓↓	↓↓↓
Serum iron	Normal	↓-↓↓	↓↓↓
Total iron-binding capacity	Normal	↑	↑↑-↑↑↑
Percent saturation	Normal	↓	↓↓-↓↓↓
Free erythrocyte protoporphyrin	Normal	↑	↑↑-↑↑↑
Serum transferrin receptor	Normal	↑	↑↑-↑↑↑
Red blood cell indices	Normal	Normal	↓-↓↓↓

Modified from Cecalupo AJ, Cohen HJ: Nutritional anemias. In Grand RJ, Sutphen JL, Dietz WH, editors: *Clinical nutrition: theory and practice,* Boston, 1987, Butterworth.
↑, Increased; ↓, decreased.

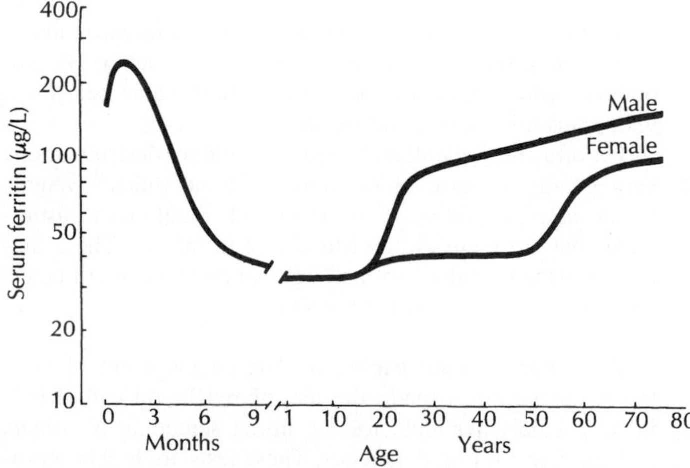

Fig. 228-1 Developmental changes in concentration of serum ferritin.

(From Dallman PR, Simes MA, Stekel A: *Am J Clin Nutrition* 33:107, 1980.)

Table 228-3 Laboratory Findings Associated with the Differential Diagnosis of Microcytic Anemias

	Iron Deficiency	Lead Poisoning	Beta-Thalassemia Trait	Chronic Disease
Ferritin	↓	Normal	Normal	↑
Serum iron	↓	Normal	Normal	↓
Total iron-binding capacity	↑	Normal	Normal	↓
Free erythrocyte protoporphyrin	↑	↑↑	Normal	↑
Red cell distribution width	↑	Normal	Normal	Normal
Serum transferrin receptor	↑	Normal	↑	Normal

↓, Decreased; ↑, increased.

Table 228-4 Means and Standard Errors of Measurement of Serum Iron and Iron Saturation Percentage by Age

Age (Years)	Serum Iron (μg/dl)	Saturation (%)
½-2	68 ± 3.6	22 ± 1.1
2-6	72 ± 3.4	25 ± 1.2
6-12	73 ± 3.4	25 ± 1.2
18+	92 ± 3.8	30 ± 1.1

Modified from Koerper MA, Dallman PR: *Pediatr Res* 11:473, 1977.

Free erythrocyte protoporphyrin. FEP accumulates in red blood cells when iron is insufficient to combine with protoporphyrin to form heme. FEP levels also are elevated in lead poisoning, infections, inflammatory diseases, and protoporphyria, but not in thalassemia trait. This makes FEP determinations helpful in distinguishing iron deficiency from alpha- or beta-thalassemia trait (see Table 228-3).

Serum transferrin receptor. The proteolytic cleavage of transferrin receptors can be measured in the serum as the serum transferrin receptor (STfR). The STfR is elevated in iron deficiency and in conditions resulting in increased production of red cells, including thalassemia and sickle cell disease.[2] However, STfR is useful in distinguishing iron deficiency from chronic inflammatory states that do not have elevated STfR (see Table 228-3). Infants have higher baseline STfR levels than do children and adults, indicating the need to establish age-specific references values.

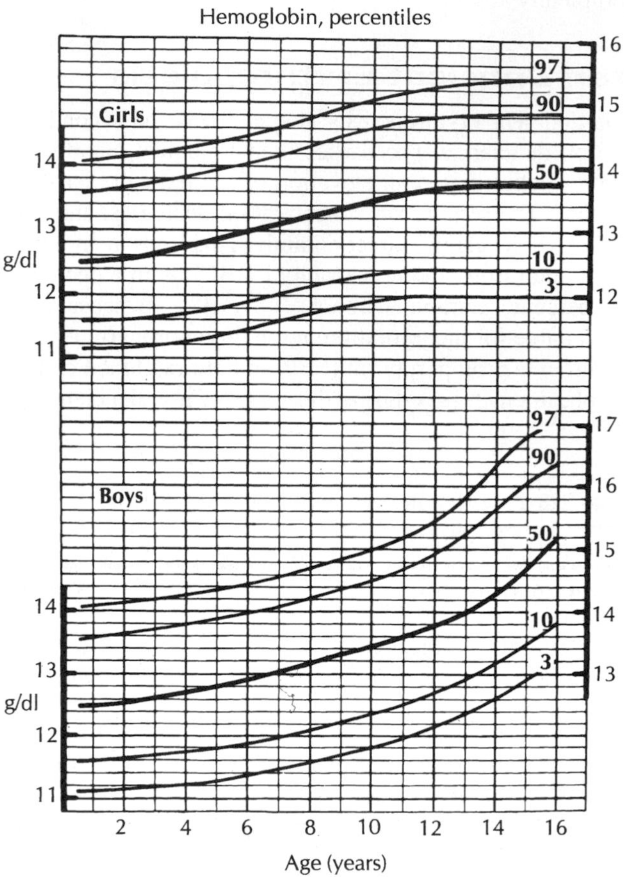

Fig. 228-2 Hemoglobin concentration in infants and children.

(Modified from Dallman PR, Simes MA: *J Pediatr* 94:28, 1979.)

Iron-Deficiency Anemia

Anemia characterizes the third stage of iron deficiency. Decreased production of red blood cells in the bone marrow leads to a decrease in hemoglobin levels and the hematocrit. The size of the red blood cells, as measured by the mean corpuscular volume (MCV), and their hemoglobin content, as measured by the mean corpuscular hemoglobin (MCH), begin to decrease as the anemia develops. Thus, persistent negative iron balance predictably leads to a microcytic, hypochromic anemia.

Hemoglobin. Percentile curves for hemoglobin values of nonindigent children living at sea level are shown in Fig. 228-2. Black children normally have a hemoglobin concentration 0.3 to 1 g/dl lower than that of white children. This difference is not explained completely by differences in socioeconomic status or prevalence of iron deficiency. By laboratory definition, anemia is a hemoglobin value below the 95th percentile for age and gender.

Unfortunately, capillary blood hemoglobin determinations vary greatly because of dilution by tissue fluids.[9] Venous blood samples produce more accurate hemoglobin measurements but are more difficult to obtain in infants. These factors limit the usefulness of hemoglobin and hematocrit determinations for screening for anemia.

Red blood cell indices. The development of electronic counters has made the use of red blood cell (RBC) indices widely available for the initial screening of infants and children for iron deficiency. These tests are highly reproducible and less subject to sampling error compared with hemoglobin determinations, because tissue fluid dilution does not affect RBC size. Because both the MCV and the MCH normally change during development, it is necessary to consult age-specific reference standards (Fig. 228-3).

Iron deficiency is the most likely diagnosis of anemia characterized by microcytosis and hypochromia. Other causes of anemia with these characteristics include alpha- and beta-thalassemia trait, hemoglobin E disease, and sometimes the anemia of infection and chronic disease. Most other anemias, however, are characterized by a normal or an elevated MCV. The laboratory findings associated with different causes of microcytic anemias are shown in Table 228-3.

The Mentzer index, defined as the MCV divided by the RBC count in millions, can help to distinguish the anemia of iron deficiency from that of beta-thalassemia trait.[6] In the former the Mentzer index often is greater than 13.5; in the latter it is less than 11.5.

Peripheral blood smear. Examination of the blood smear in iron-deficiency anemia reveals hypochromic microcytes, poikilocytes, elliptocytes, and target cells (Fig. 228-4). The presence of basophilic stippling suggests associated lead poisoning. Unfortunately, the RBC changes seen on the blood smear are not specific for iron deficiency.

The white blood cell count and morphology in iron-deficiency anemia usually are normal. Both thrombocytosis and thrombocytopenia occur with iron deficiency. The latter is more common in severe iron deficiency and resolves once iron therapy is instituted.

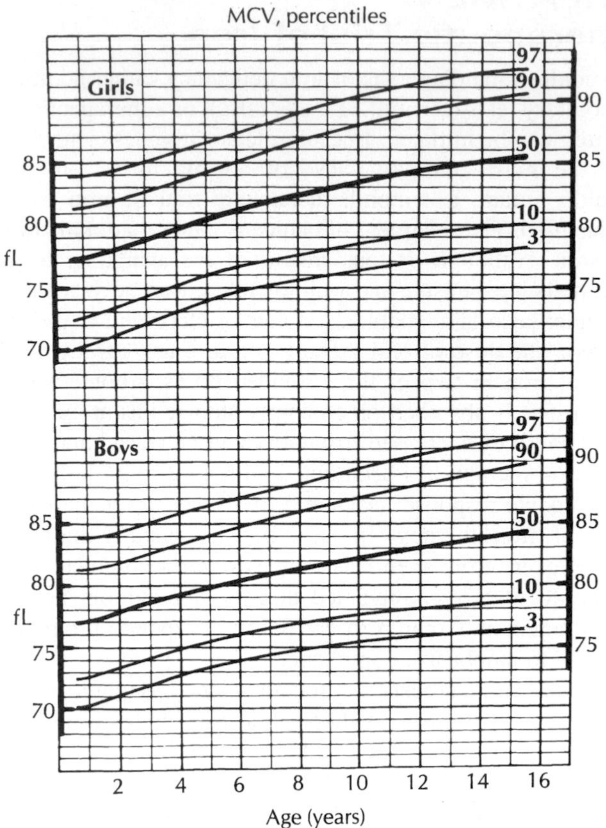

Fig. 228-3 Mean corpuscular volume (MCV) in infants and children. *fL,* Femptoliter.

(Modified from Dallman PR, Simes MA: *J Pediatr* 94:28, 1979.)

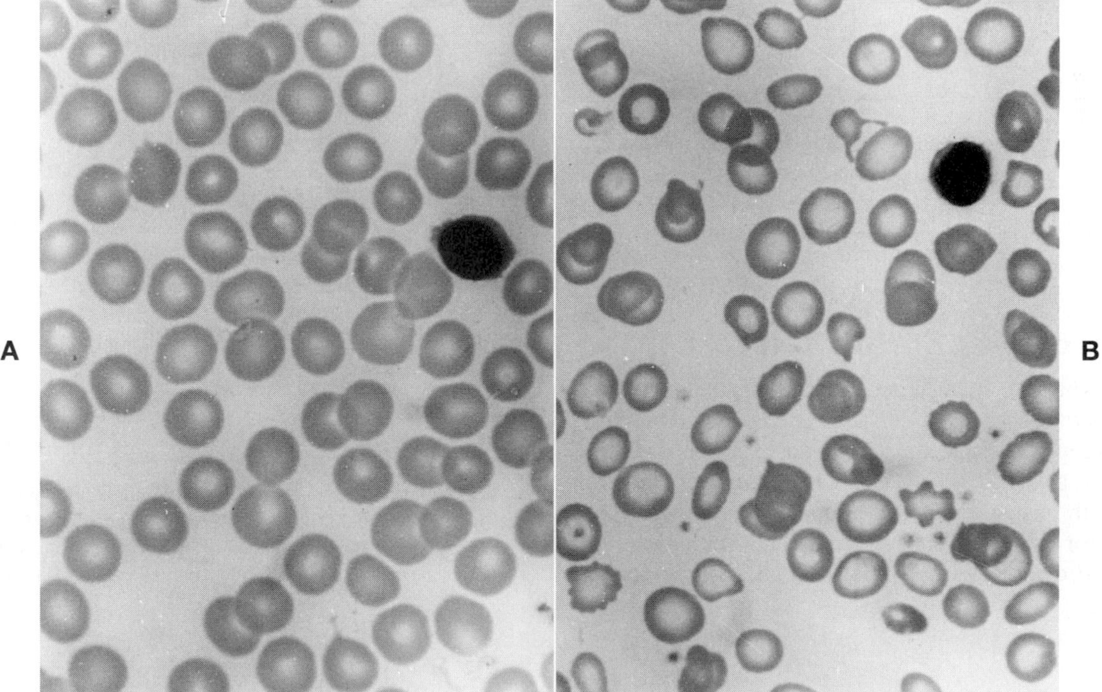

Fig. 228-4 **A,** A normal peripheral blood smear. The size of normocytic red blood cells is similar to the nucleus of a mature lymphocyte. **B,** The peripheral blood smear from an individual with iron-deficiency anemia reveals microcytosis, hypochromia, and poikilocytosis.

TREATMENT

Therapeutic Trial of Iron

To confirm the diagnosis of iron deficiency, either additional laboratory tests (ferritin, FEP, Fe/TIBC) or a therapeutic trial of iron can be initiated. Because dietary iron deficiency is by far the most common cause of anemia in an otherwise healthy infant, a 1-month therapeutic trial of iron usually is justified. The treatment of choice is the oral administration of iron. Although various iron salts are available, ferrous sulfate is inexpensive and well tolerated. Iron polysaccharide complex also is available as tablets or elixir and is well tolerated. The dose of oral therapy is 3 to 6 mg/kg/day of elemental iron in two or three divided doses. About twice as much iron is absorbed on an empty stomach as at mealtime. A response of decreased irritability and increased appetite to oral iron therapy has been noted within 12 to 24 hours. The reticulocyte response peaks at 5 to 10 days after the institution of iron therapy. In an otherwise healthy individual the recovery from anemia is about two thirds complete within 1 month. It is recommended that the hemoglobin be measured again at 1 month to check the therapeutic progress as well as to emphasize compliance.

Once the diagnosis of iron deficiency is confirmed either by a response to a therapeutic trial or by further laboratory tests, oral therapy with elemental iron at 3 to 6 mg/kg/day should be continued for 2 to 3 months after normal hemoglobin levels have been restored. This allows the repletion of body iron stores. Anemia, microcytosis, and elevated FEP levels are corrected completely with 3 to 5 months of treatment. Use of intramuscular or intravenous iron rarely is warranted. Intramuscular injections are painful, and skin discoloration is common. Anaphylactic reactions have occurred with both intramuscular and intravenous injection, and deaths have been reported. Parenteral treatment therefore should be used only when oral therapy is not possible—for example, in patients who have inflammatory bowel disease.

A blood transfusion is indicated only when severe anemia leads to congestive heart failure and cardiovascular compromise. If a blood transfusion is warranted clinically, then packed RBCs should be given slowly or a partial exchange transfusion performed. Vital signs should be monitored carefully.

Failure To Respond to Therapy

When a patient fails to respond to oral iron treatment, the following factors should be considered: (1) noncompliance with oral therapy; (2) inadequate iron dose; (3) persistent or unrecognized blood loss; (4) malabsorption of iron—for example, with primary gastrointestinal disease; (5) other diagnoses—for example, alpha- or beta-thalassemia trait and hemoglobin E disease; and (6) poor iron utilization—for example, with chronic inflammatory disease, sideroblastic anemia, lead poisoning, and congenital atransferrinemia.

PREVENTION

Although other important nutritional deficiencies of the past, such as pellagra, scurvy, and rickets, have become rare, iron deficiency remains a current public health problem.[1] Iron-deficiency anemia is associated with behavioral and cognitive deficits, some of which may not improve despite adequate iron therapy. Thus, prevention of iron deficiency is an important aspect of public health nationally. Increased iron intake in the United States over the past 30 years has resulted in a decreased incidence of iron deficiency in children.[1]

Excessive intake of cow milk during infancy leads to iron deficiency because of the low concentration and poor bioavailability of iron in cow milk. Breast-feeding or the use of milk-based infant formulas supplemented with iron should be encouraged during the first 6 months. The intake of milk thereafter should be limited to less than 1 quart per day. Because the addition of solids to an infant's diet can impair iron absorption significantly, solids should not be started before the infant is 4 months of age. The use of iron-fortified cereals should be encouraged once solids are started. Oral iron supplementation is recommended for preterm infants because they have greater iron needs than do full-term infants. In this instance 2 to 4 mg/kg/day of elemental iron in the form of ferrous sulfate drops should be started when the infant is 2 months of age.

REFERENCES

1. Centers for Disease Control and Prevention: Recommendations to prevent and control iron deficiency in the United States, *MMWR* 47(RR-3):1, 1998.
2. Cook JD, Skikne BS, Baynes RD: Serum transferrin receptor, *Annu Rev Med* 44:63, 1993.
3. Krause JR: The bone marrow in nutritional deficiencies, *Hematol Oncol Clin North Am* 2:557, 1988.
4. Lozoff B, Jimenez E, Wolf AW: Long-term developmental outcome of infants with iron deficiency, *N Engl J Med* 325:687, 1991.
5. Lundstrom U, Simes MA, Dallman PR: At what age does iron supplementation become necessary in low birth weight infants? *J Pediatr* 91:878, 1977.
6. Mentzer WG: Differentiation of iron deficiency from thalassemia trait, *Lancet* 1:882, 1973.
7. Oski FA: The non-hematologic manifestations of iron deficiency, *Am J Dis Child* 133:315, 1979.
8. Oski FA, Stockman JA: Anemia due to inadequate iron sources or poor iron utilization, *Pediatr Clin North Am* 27:237, 1980.
9. Reeves JD: Iron deficiency anemia: cost effective screening and management, *Contemp Pediatr* 1:10, 1984.
10. Rio SE, et al: Relationship of maternal and infant iron stores as assessed by determination of plasma ferritin, *Pediatrics* 55:694, 1975.
11. van Zeben D, et al: Evaluation of microcytosis using serum ferritin and red blood cell distribution width, *Eur J Haematol* 44:105, 1990.

229 Juvenile Arthritis

David M. Siegel • Harry L. Gewanter

Juvenile arthritis (JA; or juvenile rheumatoid arthritis; JRA; or juvenile chronic arthritis, JCA) is an uncommon collection of clinical syndromes that have the common feature of chronic childhood arthritis. The diagnosis is applied to any child younger than 16 years of age who has persistent arthritis of one or more joints lasting for more than 6 weeks in whom all other diseases have been excluded. JA is classified further into three subtypes (systemic-onset, pauciarticular, and polyarticular) based on the clinical course over the first 6 months of illness.[10] Many rheumatologists apply the term *juvenile rheumatoid arthritis* only to children who are seropositive for rheumatoid factor. Most recently, a new classification schema for JA has been developed in which there are seven subtypes identified, in an attempt to provide better, clinically meaningful diagnostic criteria.[12] According to this international consensus statement, juvenile arthritis would be renamed idiopathic arthritides of childhood. Despite publication some years ago, this revised categorization has yet to be widely adopted. In this chapter we use the traditional nomenclature.

Although JA is the most common of the pediatric rheumatic diseases, its true incidence and prevalence are unknown. For all subtypes taken collectively, the peak age of onset is between 2 and 4 years of age, with a smaller peak later in childhood. Overall, there is a general female predominance, but this is not the case in all subtypes. The best estimate of prevalence is about 0.5 to 1 case per 1000 children; thus, approximately 40,000 to 100,000 children in the United States have JA at any given time.[15]

ETIOLOGY

The exact cause of JA is unknown. Recent data on the frequency of certain subtypes of human leukocyte antigens (HLA) in JA (e.g., HLA-DR5 and DR8 in younger girls who have pauciarticular JA, HLA-DR4 in rheumatoid factor-positive polyarticular JA, and HLA-B27 in older boys who have pauciarticular JA)[20] have led to the concept of a genetic predisposition for the development of an inflammatory arthritis that may be triggered by any of a number of events, such as trauma, infection,[34] or emotional stress.[23]

Other areas of interesting research include investigations of immunological abnormalities involving autoantibodies,[28] cytokines, immunoregulation,[7] and the function of and communication between T and B lymphocytes and antigen-presenting cells.[20] The precise nature of these interactions and how they result in the development of JA remain to be discovered, but the recent success of specific cytokine-directed therapy (e.g., etanercept; see section on management) supports the central role of these inflammatory mediators in the clinical manifestations and course of JA.

CLINICAL PRESENTATION

The various osteochondroses and avascular necrosis syndromes, musculoskeletal trauma, chondromalacia patellae, Osgood-Schlatter disease, slipped femoral capital epiphysis, diskitis, psychogenic arthralgias, and nonspecific musculoskeletal aches and pains also can mimic JA in its early stages.

Hemophilia, sickle cell disease, inflammatory bowel disease, the collagen disorders (e.g., Ehlers-Danlos syndrome, Marfan syndrome), familial Mediterranean fever, Wegener granulomatosis, and sarcoidosis also may be associated with arthritis.

Juvenile ankylosing spondylitis and the other spondyloarthropathies can present as JA at their onset, especially in an older child who is HLA-B27 positive. Acute rheumatic fever, although in decline in the United States and other industrialized nations for many years, has undergone a bit of resurgence in the past 1 to 1½ decades. These patients can experience both arthralgia and arthritis, classically characterized as migratory.[45] Systemic lupus erythematosus has arthritis as one of its major manifestations but can be differentiated from juvenile arthritis by its other systemic features and specific laboratory test abnormalities. Although its gender distribution is equal in younger children, there is female preponderance postpubertally. Dermatomyositis is characterized more typically by inflammatory muscle involvement than by arthritis, but children can be affected with joint inflammation as well as contractures. Scleroderma occasionally is associated with arthritis but has classic dermatological and other manifestations distinguishing it from JA.

Because the diagnosis of JA is based on clinical grounds, the history and physical examination are paramount; no specific diagnostic laboratory tests yet exist. Only by considering all the data on the child's presentation and course is the physician able to diagnose JA.

The presence of arthritis or inflammation within the joint is an absolute criterion for diagnosing JA. Arthritis is defined as being present when there is (1) intraarticular swelling or effusion or (2) when two or more of the following occur: (a) joint pain or tenderness with motion, (b) limitation of joint motion, or (c) increased warmth overlying the joint.[10] Arthralgia (joint pain) is a relatively frequent pediatric symptom, but true joint inflammation, or arthritis, is much less common. Younger children rarely complain of joint pain but may instead become irritable, stop walking or using an extremity, or regress in their behavior. Other symptoms include decreased appetite, malaise, inactivity, morning stiffness, night joint pains, or failure to thrive. Features that also may present in children who have chronic arthritis (varying with the subtype as outlined below) include fever, rash, lymphadenopathy, hepatosplenomegaly, polyserositis, subcutaneous (rheumatoid) nodules, vasculitis, and growth retardation; the pattern and number of involved joints are important in classifying the disease.

SYSTEMIC-ONSET JUVENILE ARTHRITIS

Even though the hallmark of systemic-onset JA (also referred to as Still's disease) is its extraarticular manifestations, the eventual presence of arthritis is necessary to confirm the diagnosis. Affecting about 15% of all children who have JA, systemic-onset JA is slightly more common among males and usually begins at an early age, although it even has been recognized in adults (adult-onset Still's disease). The systemic features may persist for months and occur or recur independently of the arthritis.

Daily intermittent fevers characterize systemic-onset JA, with rectal temperature reaching as high as 40° C (104° F) to 41° C (106° F), most often in the afternoon, and then return to normal or subnormal levels (known as quotidian fever patterns). An evanescent, salmon-colored rash often accompanies the fevers. The lesions are small macules or papules, frequently with central clearing, and often appear in areas of increased heat (e.g., the axilla). Mild abrasion of unaffected skin can precipitate appearance of the rash (Koebner phenomenon).

Polyserositis in the form of pericarditis or pleuritis is common; enlargement of the lymph nodes, liver, and spleen may be of sufficient size to suggest the presence of a malignancy. The effusions, however, rarely are symptomatic or significant clinically. Although these children frequently complain of myalgias or arthralgias when they are febrile, they may have few symptoms when the fevers resolve. The arthritis may occur at any time following disease onset and in some patients appears only days to weeks after the presentation of systemic signs. The arthritis tends to be polyarticular, involving both large and small joints, and can be quite persistent, destructive, and severe.

Laboratory studies reveal a markedly elevated white blood cell count (WBC), with a shift to the left (predominance of band forms and polymorphonuclear leukocytes), and most patients are quite anemic. Thrombocytosis is frequent, as are significant elevations of the acute phase reactants (e.g., erythrocyte sedimentation rate [ESR] and C-reactive protein [CRP]). Rheumatoid factor (RF) and antinuclear antibody (ANA) tests rarely are positive. Serum immunoglobulin and complement levels usually are normal but may be abnormal, reflecting the degree of inflammation, and evidence of a vasculopathy and an intravascular consumption coagulopathy sometimes is found.[42]

The clinical course is extremely variable. Some children have a single systemic episode that lasts weeks to months and have few, if any, joint problems; others have multiple systemic episodes before developing the arthritis, which can be pauciarticular or polyarticular. Poor prognostic signs include the continued presence of systemic features and a platelet count greater than 600,000/mm^3 6 months after onset.[37] At least a third of these children will develop severe and crippling arthritis.

POLYARTICULAR JUVENILE ARTHRITIS

About 30% to 35% of children who have JA have the polyarticular type, which can be subdivided into IgM-rheumatoid factor (RF)-positive (about 10% of the total) and IgM-RF–negative (about 25%) forms. So-called hidden rheumatoid factors have been found in all subgroups, but their significance remains obscure.[33] It is extremely rare to find a significantly positive RF in a child younger than 7 years of age. Systemic features in polyarticular JA usually are mild and include low-grade fevers, easy fatigability, and slowing of growth. The growth problems may be local (e.g., micrognathia) or generalized and can occur regardless of whether the child receives corticosteroid treatment. Discrepancies between height and weight are seen and can be significant. For example, children who have polyarticular arthritis may be of low weight for height, whereas children who have systemic onset tend to be average in weight for height.[6] The arthritis most often is chronic and symmetrical and involves five or more joints; any joint of the body, including the temporomandibular joint and the cervical spine, can be affected. Nearly all children have wrist involvement, and small joint involvement of the hands and feet is common. Finally, these children may develop a chronic uveitis.[2]

Rheumatoid Factor-Positive Polyarticular Juvenile Arthritis

Patients who have RF-positive polyarticular JA most often are older than 8 to 10 years of age, are more likely to be girls, and are similar clinically to those patients who have adult rheumatoid arthritis. Severe, rapidly progressive, erosive, crippling arthritis, subcutaneous rheumatoid nodules, and rheumatoid vasculitis can develop, just as in adults.

Rheumatoid Factor-Negative Polyarticular Juvenile Arthritis

Children who have RF-negative polyarticular JA usually are younger and overall have a better prognosis than those who are RF-positive. However, even though children who have the RF-negative type typically respond better to therapy and have a lower frequency of severe, early, crippling arthritis than do children who have the RF-positive form, they also may develop many significant problems. Because their arthritis starts earlier, it can lead to significant deformities and problems as a result of the tendency to develop flexion contractures at the involved joints. Compared with adults, hand involvement more often affects the interphalangeal joints than the metacarpophalangeal joints. Ulnar deviation of the fingers is much less common in children compared with adults, whereas flexion contractures, boutonniere (buttonhole) deformities, and radial deviation of the fingers are seen more frequently. Ulnar deviation and subluxation at the wrist may occur. Arthritis of the apophyseal joints of the cervical spine is common and can lead to rapid and significant limitation of extension and rotation. These children are at the highest risk for developing the local and generalized growth problems mentioned above.

Pauciarticular Juvenile Arthritis

Pauciarticular JA involves four or fewer joints, most often the large joints (e.g., knee, ankle, elbow, etc.), in an asymmetrical distribution. The pattern and course of joint involvement are as important in distinguishing this form of JA from the others as are the number of joints involved. With a few exceptions, systemic features are infrequent and mild. Nearly 50% of all children who have JA fall in this subgroup, and they have the best overall prognosis.

Pauciarticular JA can be subdivided further into early and late onset.

Early-onset pauciarticular juvenile arthritis. Early-onset pauciarticular JA (5% to 10% of all patients who have JA) occurs classically in girls younger than 6 years of age and involves the large joints; these girls are at higher risk for developing chronic uveitis.[2,36] Despite the obvious arthritis, these children generally function quite well and only rarely complain of pain. Little erosive joint damage typically occurs, even though these children may have ongoing arthritis for many years. Nonetheless, these children are at risk for long-term problems, including leg-length discrepancies and muscle atrophy.[46] Perhaps paradoxically, the leg in which there is knee arthritis is the extremity that, because of prolonged hyperemia, can become longer than the contralateral leg without arthritis. Systemic signs and symptoms, except for uveitis, are few. The uveitis rarely is symptomatic until it has progressed to a severe stage and may not occur until years after the onset of the arthritis. It may even occur after the arthritis has resolved. Thus, regular ophthalmological examinations, including slit-lamp examinations, should be instituted early, performed every 4 to 6 months, and continued indefinitely. Because the risk of uveitis decreases with time, the interval between examinations can be lengthened after a number of years if no uveitis is present[2] (Table 229-1).

Except for ANA positivity, few laboratory abnormalities are noted. Although there may be mild WBC and ESR elevations or a low-grade anemia, all these tests often are normal. Most are positive for HLA-DR5 gene markers, though such investigations are not ordinarily pursued in diagnosing or managing these patients.[20]

Late-onset pauciarticular juvenile arthritis. Late-onset pauciarticular JA typically involves boys older than 8 years of age. Their arthritis more frequently is in the lower extremities, involving the knees and ankles but also occasionally the toes (resulting in a dactylitis or "sausage toe").[39] Complaints and findings of enthesopathies (i.e., inflammation of the attachment of a tendon, ligament, fascia, or capsule to bone) are extremely common in this group and may antedate the joint problems. There often is a family history of arthritis, and many of these children carry the HLA-B27 antigen. These children also seem to be at increased risk for developing spondyloarthropathies later in life, despite there being no evidence of sacroiliac disease initially. For example, some patients will progress to fulfill the criteria for ankylosing spondylitis or for Reiter's syndrome. About 10% will develop an acute iritis; in contrast to the chronic uveitis seen in early-onset pauciarticular JA, this is symptomatic, can be treated early, and usually is self-limited. As with the early-onset group, mild to moderate elevation in the ESR is expected, but other abnormal laboratory tests are found infrequently.

Table 229-1 Frequency of Ophthalmological Visits for Children Who Have Juvenile Rheumatoid Arthritis (JRA) without Known Iridocyclitis*

JRA Subtype at Onset	Age of Onset <7 yr†	Age of Onset ≥7 yr‡
Pauciarticular		
+ ANA	H§	M
− ANA	M	M
Polyarticular		
+ ANA	H§	M
− ANA	M	M
Systemic	L	L

From The American Academy of Pediatrics Section on Rheumatology's Guidelines for Ophthalmologic Examinations in Children with Juvenile Rheumatoid Arthritis, *Pediatrics* 92: 295, 1993.

*High risk (*H*) indicates ophthalmological examinations every 3 to 4 months.

Medium risk (*M*) indicates ophthalmological examinations every 6 months.

Low risk (*L*) indicates ophthalmological examinations every 12 months. *ANA* indicates antinuclear antibody test.

†All patients are considered at low risk 7 years after the onset of their arthritis and should have yearly ophthalmological examinations indefinitely.

‡All patients are considered at low risk 4 years after the onset of their arthritis and should have yearly ophthalmological examinations indefinitely.

§All high-risk patients are considered at medium risk 4 years after the onset of their arthritis.

Other subtypes of pauciarticular juvenile arthritis. At least two other subtypes of pauciarticular JA might exist. The first lies somewhere between the early-onset and the late-onset subtypes. These children seem to have the best prognosis, are ANA negative, and are at a medium risk for eye or other serious, chronic problems. About 10% to 15% of all children who have JA make up the fourth subtype. They have a pauciarticular onset but evolve into a polyarticular course (sometimes referred to as extended pauciarticular). These children more often start with three or four joints involved and/or have wrist or small finger joint arthritis.

DIFFERENTIAL DIAGNOSIS

Diseases to be considered in the differential diagnosis of JA are given in Box 229-1. The hallmark of JA is its chronicity; frequently, the best diagnostic test is "watchful waiting." Only by meeting the criterion of sustained arthritis for more than 6 weeks and excluding other possible diseases can the physician avoid mislabeling other transient entities as JA.

If the child presents with a single inflamed joint, it is critical that bacterial arthritis be considered. If there is any question as to an intraarticular septic process, arthrocentesis must be performed to establish the diagnosis. *Hemophilus influenzae* type b had been the most common organism isolated in children younger than 2 years, but its incidence has decreased with the advent of universal immunization against *H. influenza* type b. *Neisseria gonorrhoeae* is most common in adolescents, whereas various strains of staphylococci may be found at any age. Other infectious agents such as fungi, viruses (including parvovirus, rubella, and hepatitis B), and *Mycoplasma* organisms also must be considered as the cause of arthritis. Lyme disease (*Borrelia burgdorferi* infection) is a significant cause of childhood arthritis in endemic areas. Osteomyelitis, involving the bone contiguous to a joint, and reactive arthritis from a gastrointestinal (GI) bacterial infection (e.g., *Shigella, Salmonella, Campylobacter,* or *Yersinia* organisms) also may mimic some subgroups of JA. Neoplasms involving the bone, either primary or metastatic (e.g., leukemia, lymphoma, neuroblastoma), can be accompanied by musculoskeletal complaints. Although arthritis is uncommon and usually transient, complaints of pain that are out of proportion to physical findings and particularly night pain are common and potentially important clues to heed.

Children who have various immunodeficiencies can have arthritis, either from their primary problem or secondary to infections. Serum sickness and the various vasculitides, including Kawasaki disease (see Chapter 230, Kawasaki Disease) and Henoch-Schönlein purpura (see Chapter 215, Henoch-Schönlein Purpura), can produce intermittent arthritis. Finally, a number of conditions may produce significant arthralgias and myalgias and may mimic an arthropathy. The complaints and disability resulting from the hypermobility syndrome[8] and fibromyalgia (fibrositis)[40] can be sufficient to make one believe (but incorrectly) that an arthritis is present. Reflex sympathetic dystrophy deserves diagnostic consideration in children who have a hot or cold painful extremity that they refuse to move,[41] particularly when there is a premorbid history of trauma.

BOX 229-1

DIFFERENTIAL DIAGNOSIS OF JUVENILE ARTHRITIS

Rheumatic Disease of Childhood
Acute rheumatic fever
Systemic lupus erythematosus
Juvenile ankylosing spondylitis
Polymyositis and dermatomyositis
Vasculitis
Scleroderma
Psoriatic arthritis
Mixed connective tissue disease and overlap syndromes
Kawasaki disease
Behçet's syndrome
Familial Mediterranean fever
Reiter syndrome
Reflex sympathetic dystrophy
Fibromyalgia (fibrositis)

Infectious Diseases
Bacterial arthritis
Viral or postviral arthritis
Fungal arthritis
Osteomyelitis
Reactive arthritis

Neoplastic Diseases
Leukemia
Lymphoma
Neuroblastoma
Primary bone tumors

Noninflammatory Disorders
Trauma
Avascular necrosis syndromes
Osteochondroses
Slipped capital femoral epiphysis
Diskitis
Patellofemoral dysfunction (chondromalacia patellae)
Toxic synovitis of the hip
Overuse syndromes

Hematological Disorders
Sickle cell disease
Hemophilia
Inflammatory bowel disease

Miscellaneous
Growing pains
Psychogenic arthralgias (conversion reactions)
Hypermobility syndrome
Villonodular synovitis
Foreign body arthritis

MANAGEMENT

It always is necessary to individualize each patient's management in terms of the disease subtype, extent of activity, clinical course to date, and family situation. Although most physicians are accustomed to considering pharmacological therapy of primary importance, it is only one aspect of the treatment of children who have JA. A multidisciplinary team approach is the most effective means to meet the varied needs of a child who has arthritis and of his or her family. The goal of therapy is to result in the highest possible level of physical and psychological function for the child in both the present and the future.

Currently available drug therapy (Box 229-2), although not curative, can suppress the inflammatory activities in many children who have JA. Five major categories of drug

BOX 229-2

MEDICATIONS FOR JUVENILE ARTHRITIS

Nonsteroidal Antiinflammatory Drugs (NSAIDs) Currently Approved by the FDA for Use in Children
Salicylates
Indomethacin
Tolmetin sodium
Naproxen
Ibuprofen

Nonsteroidal Antiinflammatory Drugs (NSAIDs) Not Yet Approved by the FDA for Use in Children
Diclofenac sodium
Fenoprofen
Flurbiprofen
Ketoprofen
Phenylbutazone
Pirprofen
Piroxicam
Proquazone
Meclofenamate sodium
Sulindac

Slower-Acting Antirheumatic Drugs (SAARDs)
D-Penicillamine
Hydroxychloroquine
Sulfasalazine

Corticosteroids
Systemic
Intraarticular

Cytotoxic Drugs
Azathioprine
Chlorambucil
Cyclophosphamide
Methotrexate

Gold Preparations
Gold sodium aurothiomalate
Aurothioglucose
Auranofin

Other Therapies
Pheresis
Intravenous immune globulin
Cyclosporin A

therapy are available: nonsteroidal antiinflammatory drugs (NSAIDs), slower-acting antirheumatic drugs (SAARDs), corticosteroids, cytotoxic agents, and agents that possess immune and cytokine modulating effects. Significant advances in medication are taking place currently, particularly in this latter class of therapeutic agents.

Although, historically, salicylates constitute the classic NSAID, their use has declined because of concerns regarding the development of Reye's syndrome as well as the emergence of many other agents. Thus, very few pediatric rheumatologists use aspirin in treating patients who have JA. If used, aspirin should be given in divided doses sufficient to achieve a serum salicylate level between 20 and 30 mg/dl. This ordinarily is achieved by using dosages of between 80 and 100 mg/kg/day. Enteric-coated aspirin is tolerated better by children who can swallow pills, it produces less gastric upset, and it delivers adequate serum levels. If a child cannot swallow the tablets or take chewable children's aspirin, both choline salicylate and choline magnesium salicylate are available as liquid preparations. The physician always should be alert for signs of salicylism, including tinnitus, hyperpnea, GI upset, and central nervous system (CNS) alterations. Given the increased risk of Reye's syndrome in children taking salicylates,[26] it currently is recommended that these children receive varicella immunization and seasonal influenza vaccinations.

Although salicylates are no longer the initial NSAIDs of choice in treating JA, a number of other agents are available and effective, although they are more expensive than aspirin. In the past, as newer NSAIDs were introduced, they were found to be nearly equivalent in efficacy, toxicity, and mode of action to aspirin.[29] Individual responses to these agents vary widely; therefore, if a child does not improve with one of the NSAIDs after 4 to 6 weeks, it is reasonable to try others in an effort to find an efficacious drug.[30] Naproxen and ibuprofen are available as liquid preparations that can be quite useful in younger children and in those who have difficulty swallowing pills.

A new class of NSAIDs has been developed and became available for prescription in 1999; these are the cyclooxygenase (COX-II) selective inhibitors, celecoxib and rofecoxib.[13] By interfering only with COX-II, these antiinflammatory agents decrease prostaglandin production that mediates inflammation, but to a very large extent not that which is gastro-protective. Thus, the risk of gastric erosion and/or ulcer formation is reduced dramatically. These drugs remain quite expensive, and only those children who have had gastrointestinal intolerance of the more traditional (nonselective) NSAIDs are ordinarily treated with the COX-II inhibitors. It is likely that in the future as cost becomes less of a differential between selective and nonselective NSAIDs, the COX-II inhibitors will evolve to be first-line agents.

If a child continues to do poorly after 2 to 4 months of treatment with NSAIDs or has aggressive disease, the use of SAARDs should be considered.[38] These include gold, D-penicillamine, hydroxychloroquine, sulfasalazine, and methotrexate. Time of onset of clinical response to these second-line drugs varies, but patients, parents, and physicians should be prepared for at least a 1 to 2 months.

Whereas intramuscular gold (sodium aurothiomalate) was, at one time, used in the management of more severe JA, it now is rarely, if ever, employed by pediatric rheumatologists. The dosage is 0.75 to 1.0 mg/kg dose begun weekly and eventually given monthly. Careful monitoring for bone marrow, kidney, or skin toxicity is necessary with preinjection WBC and platelet counts, urinalysis, and physical examination. The presence of adverse effects, such as skin rashes, leukopenia, thrombocytopenia, eosinophilia, hematuria, or proteinuria, requires either a dosage adjustment (holding or lowering the dose) or discontinuation of the gold treatment.[9]

Auranofin was developed as an oral preparation of gold and is given as a once- or twice-daily dose of 0.1 to 0.2 mg/kg/day. In addition to the adverse effects noted above with the injectable gold preparations, it also may cause diarrhea. Although there was initial optimism for this oral alternative to injectable gold, auranofin has not proven to be of consistent benefit[16-18] and also is virtually never used in treating JA.

D-Penicillamine has been used quite extensively in Europe[4,35] and is given at a dose of 3 to 10 mg/kg/day in a single daily dose. Its adverse effects are similar to those of gold therapy, with the addition of occasional GI upset and frequent distortion of the sense of taste. The latter signs often resolve as therapy progresses and are not absolute indications for its discontinuation. Other rare adverse effects include Goodpasture's syndrome, a lupus-like syndrome, myasthenia gravis, and other autoimmune-induced effects (e.g., hemolytic anemia). Careful studies of efficacy in JA have not been plentiful, and when compared with hydroxychloroquine and placebo, it was no better.[11] Few patients who have JA currently are given D-penicillamine.

Antimalarial agents, such as hydroxychloroquine, constitute another therapeutic alternative, although consistent evidence of efficacy in JA also is lacking.[11] The dosage for hydroxychloroquine is 5 to 7 mg/kg/day given as a single dose. The primary adverse effects that require drug discontinuation are GI upset (e.g., nausea, anorexia, diarrhea), bleaching of the hair, and retinal deposits. Regular ophthalmological examinations every 6 months are necessary to detect the latter effect early; if found, therapy must be stopped. Again, this drug now is used infrequently among children who have JA.

Sulfasalazine, a drug first synthesized approximately 50 years ago as a specific antirheumatic agent, has seen a resurgence in its use in the 1990s.[3,14,24] It is given at a dosage of approximately 25 mg/kg/day, usually with food or milk. It should not be used in anyone (1) sensitive to sulfa drugs or salicylates, (2) whose renal or hepatic function is impaired, or (3) who has conditions such as glucose-6-phosphate dehydrogenase deficiency. Adverse effects caused by sulfasalazine include rashes, nausea, vomiting, dyspepsia, and a reversible decrease in sperm count. Bone marrow depression occurs in very rare cases. It may be superior to other SAARDs in patients who are HLA-B27 positive.

A significant reason for the diminished use of the above SAARDs is the advent of methotrexate in the treatment of JA. Methotrexate is a competitive inhibitor of dihydrofolate reductase and seems to exert both an antiinflammatory as well as an immunosuppressive effect on arthritis. Efficacy in treatment of JA has been established in a double-blind, placebo controlled trial,[19] and a dose-response characteristic has been documented in subsequent work.[47] There is some evidence that methotrexate may even improve carpal length (by radiological examination) in children who have JA. Methotrexate clearly has become the SAARD of first choice in treating these patients. The dose is 5 to 30 mg/m^2/week (0.15 to 1.0 mg/kg/week) given as a weekly oral dose, although at higher doses, giving the drug subcutaneously may be more effective. Potential toxicity includes hepatic, bone marrow, gastrointestinal and pulmonary; laboratory monitoring every 4 to 6 weeks is recommended.[47] Administration of folic (or folinic) acid (1 mg daily) may decrease some of the adverse effects of methotrexate, such as oral ulcers.

Other potentially more toxic forms of immunosuppression have been used to treat JA, including azathioprine, cyclosporine, chlorambucil, cyclophosphamide, and intravenous gamma globulin[43] but are not standard forms of therapy and will not be discussed here. Newly introduced (1999) and proving to be both useful and effective for children who have aggressive polyarticular JA is etanercept.[27,48] This is an agent that binds tumor necrosis factor-alpha (TNFα) and thereby interferes with its proinflammatory activity. Given at a dose of 0.4 mg/kg/dose (up to 25 mg) twice a week as a subcutaneous injection, etanercept is becoming a therapeutic consideration for patients in whom methotrexate has not been helpful and/or it has not been possible to taper corticosteroids without precipitating a flare in disease activity. Side effects have included injection-site reactions and occasional infections. The long-term impact of TNFα suppression in growing children is, of course, unknown. Other cytokine-specific preparations will undoubtedly become available in the near future for therapy of JA.

Systemic corticosteroid use in JA should follow these maxims:

1. Only use when other agents have failed or when the child is seriously ill or has progressive severe chronic anterior uveitis unresponsive to local therapy
2. Use as small a dose as possible
3. Try to taper and discontinue their use as soon as possible

Corticosteroids are effective antiinflammatory agents but do not alter the course of the disease, can be extremely difficult to discontinue in children who have JA, and their long-term use is associated with many serious adverse effects, the most important being immunosuppression, osteoporosis, and growth retardation. Alternate-day dosing regimens can be tried but often are unsatisfactory because many children develop problems on the day they do not receive the medication. Given these reservations, small (0.1 to 0.2 mg/kg) daily doses of prednisone (that eventually are tapered by 0.5 to 1 mg/day increments every 2 to 3 weeks) may be quite effective in treating pain and stiffness; higher doses (0.25 to 2.0 mg/kg/day) may be needed to manage systemic features such as pericarditis. High-dose intravenous "pulse" steroid therapy (e.g., intravenous methylprednisolone 30 mg/kg/dose to a maximum of 1 g given over 2 hours daily for 1 to 3 days) can be useful in dire situations but does not seem to be more effective when used as chronic therapy.[31]

Intraarticular steroids can be effective in controlling acute problems associated with one or several active joints but usually are used in combination with systemic, ongoing therapy. Children who have a very painful or swollen joint frequently respond to arthrocentesis and instillation of a long-acting corticosteroid preparation (e.g., triamcinolone hexacetonide).[25,44] One should be careful not to perform this procedure too frequently (more than three or four times per year) and should be sure that concomitant infectious arthritis is not the cause of the acute joint problem.

Pharmacological therapy is only one aspect of the treatment required by children who have JA. Physical therapy and occupational therapy are crucial and important adjuncts to help the child maintain strength and range of motion, to prevent contractures, and to allow the best possible quality of life. All patients should be given a home program of therapy that is reviewed and updated regularly. Heat therapy, such as taking warm baths or using a sleeping bag at night, often helps to minimize morning stiffness. Swimming is an excellent exercise; affected children should be encouraged to swim and to participate in as many other activities as possible. Normal play often is the best therapy available.

The orthopedist's contributions for those whose disease is more extensive range from the application of splints to operative tendon releases and capsulotomies. Some children may require joint resurfacing or joint replacement surgery.[21] Even though most children will not need orthopedic intervention (particularly during childhood), the orthopedist's perspective is an important part of the management.

In all its forms, JA is a chronic illness, and none of the current modes of therapy is curative. Further, JA is one of the few childhood illnesses in which pain is a primary symptom. Different expectations and attitudes, therefore, are needed when caring for the patient and family. In addition to a caring and understanding physician, a family counselor, social worker, psychologist, or similar mental health professional is of particular value in helping the family to cope with and adjust to this chronic illness. Patients, siblings, and parents will experience feelings of denial, guilt, and frustration at the time of the diagnosis and throughout the course of the disease.[5] Siblings frequently find it difficult to cope with the special and extensive treatment the affected child may receive.

Periodic depression and anger are frequent problems, especially in the early stages as the child and family realize that many changes may be necessary in their lifestyle and dreams, and again as the patient enters adolescence. Despite the frequent disruptive episodes brought on by the disease, families often are able to adapt to their child's chronic illness adequately. Poor maternal function, maternal depression, and social isolation are significant risk factors for poor psychosocial outcomes. A sense of control and mastery are important positive factors.[32]

All things being equal, most children who have JA can do well in school; thus, all efforts should be made to keep them enrolled. More recent studies of children's school and family adaptations show that children who have JA and their families develop different, albeit generally normal, styles for coping with this chronic illness.[22] Some school adjustments may be necessary, including arranging for different transportation and physical education and allowing the child extra time between classes. Having two sets of books, one for school and one for home, reduces the work of carrying the books to and from school. It may be necessary for the physician or pediatric rheumatology team to advocate on behalf of these children within the school so that they can receive all the necessary services they require.

Although it is important to concentrate on scholastic issues, one must not forget that these children will become adults. Independent living and vocational preparation must begin in childhood to reduce any potential barriers and difficulties. Anticipatory guidance about transitional issues should be provided starting in childhood and early adolescence.[49]

Although children whose disease is severe have a number of obvious problems, the child who has mild disease and a "hidden disability" also may have problems coping, adapting, and trying to accomplish the unrealistic goals set by a society that does not recognize the disability. Finally, it should be remembered that any chronic illness places a financial burden, both directly and indirectly, on the family—a burden that can add a number of further stresses. The cost per year per child who has JA is estimated to be $8670, with the average family cost being about $1524. Nationally this means that the total cost of juvenile arthritis is approximately $311 million.[1]

COURSE AND PROGNOSIS

Juvenile arthritis rarely is fatal, and in general the long-term prognosis is good, regardless of subtype. Approximately 60% to 75% of children will undergo a remission at some point, and many children will experience permanent remission. Most children who have juvenile arthritis will complete school, be gainfully employed, and raise families, just like their siblings and peers.

Several patterns of disease activity are recognized: (1) persistent active arthritis and destructive arthropathy, (2) active disease, then remission, (3) polycyclic diseases characterized by acute flares of activity followed by temporary remissions, and (4) low-grade continued activity with little if any joint destruction.

Pauciarticular JA has the best prognosis, with 40% to 50% of children undergoing a complete remission, compared with only 25% to 30% of children who have systemic-onset and polyarticular JA. Children who have IgM-RF or ANA positivity, systemic onset, and certain extraarticular manifestations (e.g., persistent fevers, thrombocytosis, subcutaneous nodules, vasculitis), as well as younger children, usually have a poorer long-term articular outcome. Younger children who have systemic-onset and polyarticular arthritis have a poorer articular prognosis; children who have pauciarticular arthritis and no chronic anterior uveitis have the best prognosis.

Children should be referred to an ophthalmologist at the time of diagnosis. Most clinical uveitis develops within the first 2 years of the diagnosis but can occur at any time. Therefore, ophthalmological examinations should be performed indefinitely. As shown in Table 229-1, The American Academy of Pediatrics recommends that children at high risk (younger children who are ANA positive and who have pauciarticular or polyarticular onset) have eye examinations every 3 to 4 months. These children are at moderate risk after 4 years, at which time they should have ophthalmological examinations every 6 months. Children who have systemic-onset JA are at low risk and should have annual eye examinations; all other children initially are at moderate risk. After 4 years, all children at moderate risk become low risk; after 7 years, all children are at low risk. If a child develops uveitis, he or she should be followed as per the ophthalmologist's recommendations; uveitis can become the child's most vexing problem.

Increasing awareness of the pediatric rheumatic diseases has resulted in earlier diagnosis and treatment. The rapid advances in understanding the diseases and their therapies are encouraging signs that the number of children disabled by these illnesses will decrease in the future.

When to Refer

- Child who has persistent oligo- or polyarticular joint inflammation
- Child who has spiking fevers and rash for whom there is no obvious infectious etiology
- Child who has persistent joint pain, limp, or asymmetrical use of an extremity for which no explanation has been found

When to Hospitalize

- Child who has systemic onset juvenile arthritis who develops severe chest pain with shortness of breath (suggesting pericarditis with hemodynamic compromise) or a change in voice quality and difficulty breathing (suggesting cricoarytenoid arthritis)
- Child who has chronic arthritis who is taking corticosteroids and develops signs of severe infection
- Child who has chronic arthritis who has been taking NSAIDs and presents with acute anemia and melanotic stools
- Child who has long-standing polyarticular arthritis complicated by multiple joint contractures and weakness who requires a period of inpatient rehabilitation (physical and occupational therapy)

REFERENCES

1. Allaire SH, et al: The economic impacts of juvenile rheumatoid arthritis, *J Rheumatol* 19:952, 1992.
2. American Academy of Pediatrics: Guidelines for ophthalmologic examinations in children with juvenile rheumatoid arthritis, *Pediatrics* 92: 295, 1993.
3. Ansell BM, et al: A multicentre pilot study of sulphasalazine in juvenile chronic arthritis, *Clin Exp Rheumatol* 9:201, 1991.
4. Ansell BW, Hall MA: Penicillamine in chronic arthritis in childhood, *J Rheumatol* 8:112, 1981.
5. Athreya BH, McCormick MC: Impact of chronic illness on families, *Rheum Dis Clin North Am* 13:123, 1987.
6. Bacon MC, et al: Nutritional status and growth in juvenile rheumatoid arthritis, *Semin Arthritis Rheum* 20:97, 1990.
7. Barron KS, et al: Abnormalities of immunoregulation in juvenile rheumatoid arthritis, *J Rheumatol* 16:940, 1989.
8. Biro F, Gewanter HL, Baum J: The hypermobility syndrome, *Pediatrics* 72:701, 1983.
9. Brewer EJ Jr, Giannini EH, Barkley E: Gold therapy in the management of juvenile rheumatoid arthritis, *Arthritis Rheum* 23:404, 1980.
10. Brewer EJ Jr, et al: Current and proposed revision of JRA criteria, *Arthritis Rheum* 20:195, 1976.

11. Brewer EJ Jr, et al: Penicillamine and hydroxychloroquine in the treatment of severe juvenile rheumatoid arthritis: results of the USA-USSR double-blind placebo controlled study, *N Engl J Med* 314:1269, 1986.
12. Fink CW: Proposal for the development of classification criteria for idiopathic arthritides of childhood. *J Rheumatol* 22:1566, 1995.
13. Fung HB, Kirschenbaum HL: Selective cyclooxygenase-2 inhibitors for the treatment of arthritis, *Clin Ther* 21:1131, 1999.
14. Gedalia A, et al.: Sulphasalazine in the treatment of pauciarticular-onset juvenile chronic arthritis, *Clin Rheumatol* 12:511, 1993.
15. Gewanter HL, Roghmann KJ, Baum J: The prevalence of juvenile arthritis, *Arthritis Rheum* 26:599, 1983.
16. Giannini EH, Brewer EJ, Person DA: Auranofin in the treatment of juvenile rheumatoid arthritis, *J Pediatr* 102:138, 1983.
17. Giannini EH, et al: Auranofin therapy for juvenile rheumatoid arthritis: results of the five-year open label extension trial, *J Rheumatol* 18:1240, 1991.
18. Giannini EH, et al: Auranofin in the treatment of juvenile rheumatoid arthritis; results of the USA-USSR double-blind, placebo controlled trial, *Arthritis Rheum* 33:466, 1989.
19. Giannini EH, et al: Methotrexate in resistant juvenile rheumatoid arthritis, *N Engl J Med* 326:1043, 1992.
20. Grom AA, Giannini EH, Glass DN: Juvenile rheumatoid arthritis and the trimolecular complex (HLA, T cell receptor, and antigen), *Arthritis Rheum* 37:601, 1994.
21. Harris CM, Baum J: Involvement of the hip in juvenile rheumatoid arthritis: a longitudinal study, *J Bone Joint Surg (Am)* 70:821, 1988.
22. Harris JA, Newcomb AF, Gewanter HL: Psychosocial effects of juvenile rheumatic disease, *Arthritis Care Res* 4:123, 1991.
23. Henoch MJ, Batson JW, Baum J: Psychosocial factors in juvenile rheumatoid arthritis, *Arthritis Rheum* 21:229, 1978.
24. Hertzberger-Ten Cate R, Cats A: Toxicity of sulfasalazine in systemic juvenile chronic arthritis, *Clin Exp Rheumatol* 9:85, 1991.
25. Huppertz H-I: Intraarticular corticosteroids for chronic arthritis in children: efficacy and effects on cartilage and growth, *J Pediatr* 127:317, 1995.
26. Hurwitz ES, et al: Public Health Service study of Reye's syndrome and medications, *JAMA* 257:1905, 1987.
27. Jarvis B, Faulds D: Etanercept: a review of its use in rheumatoid arthritis, *Drugs* 57:945, 1999.
28. Lawerence JM, et al: Autoantibody studies in juvenile rheumatoid arthritis, *Semin Arthritis Rheum* 22:265, 1993.
29. Levinson JE, et al: Comparison of tolmetin sodium and aspirin in the treatment of juvenile rheumatoid arthritis, *J Pediatr* 91:799, 1977.
30. Lovell DJ, Giannini EH, Brewer EJ Jr: Time course of response to nonsteroidal antiinflammatory drugs in juvenile rheumatoid arthritis, *Arthritis Rheum* 27:1433, 1984.
31. Miller JJ: Prolonged use of huge intravenous steroid pulses in the rheumatic disease of children, *Pediatrics* 65:989, 1980.
32. Miller JJ III: Psychosocial factors related to rheumatic diseases of childhood, *J Pediatr* 20:1, 1993.
33. Moore TL, et al: Hidden 19S IgM rheumatoid factors, *Semin Arthritis Rheum* 18:72, 1988.
34. Phillips PE: Evidence implicating infectious agents in rheumatoid arthritis and juvenile rheumatoid arthritis, *Clin Exp Rheumatol* 6:87, 1988.
35. Prieur AM, et al: Evaluation of D-penicillamine in juvenile chronic arthritis: a double-blind, multicenter study, *Arthritis Rheum* 28:376, 1985.
36. Rosenberg AM: Uveitis associated with juvenile rheumatoid arthritis, *Semin Arthritis Rheum* 16:158, 1987.
37. Schneider R, et al: Prognostic indicators of joint destruction in systemic onset juvenile rheumatoid arthritis, *J Pediatr* 120:200, 1992.
38. Siegel DM: Drug treatment of juvenile arthritis: accepted therapeutic options, *Drugs Today* 34:327, 1998.
39. Siegel DM, Baum J: HLA-B27 associated dactylitis in children, *J Rheumatol* 15:976, 1988.
40. Siegel DM, Janeway D, Baum J: Fibromyalgia syndrome in children and adolescents: clinical features at presentation and status at follow-up, *Pediatrics* 101:377, 1998.
41. Silber TJ, Majd M: Reflex sympathetic dystrophy syndrome in children and adolescents. Report of 18 cases and review of the literature, *Am J Dis Child* 142:1325, 1988.
42. Silverman ED, et al: Consumptive coagulopathy associated with systemic juvenile rheumatoid arthritis, *J Pediatr* 103:872, 1983.
43. Silverman ED, et al: Intravenous gamma globulin therapy in systemic juvenile rheumatoid arthritis, *Arthritis Rheum* 33:1015, 1990.
44. Sparling M, et al: Radiographic follow-up of joints injected with triamcinolone hexacetonide for the management of childhood arthritis, *Arthritis Rheum* 33:821, 1990.
45. Steeg CN, Walsh CA, Glickstein JS: Rheumatic fever: no cause for complacence, *Contemp Pediatr* 17:128, 2000.
46. Vostrejs M, Hollister JR: Muscle atrophy and leg length discrepancies in pauciarticular juvenile rheumatoid arthritis, *Am J Dis Child* 142:343, 1988.
47. Wallace C, Sherry D: Preliminary report of higher dose methotrexate treatment in juvenile rheumatoid arthritis, *J Rheumatol* 19:1604, 1992.
48. Weinblatt ME, et al: A trial of etanercept, a recombinant tumor necrosis factor receptor: Fc fusion protein, in patients with rheumatoid arthritis receiving methotrexate, *New Engl J Med* 340:253, 1999.
49. White PH: Educational and vocational planning: the key to success in adulthood. In Isenberg DA, Miller JJ, editors: *Adolescent rheumatology,* London, 2000, Martin Dunitz.

SUGGESTED READINGS

Ansell BM, Rudge S, Schaller JG: *Color atlas of pediatric rheumatology*, St Louis, 1992, Mosby.

Athreya BH, editor: Pediatric rheumatology, *Rheum Dis Clin North Am* 23:3, 1997.

Cassidy JT, Petty RE: *Textbook of pediatric rheumatology*, ed 3, Philadelphia, 1995, WB Saunders.

Isenberg DA, Miller JJ: *Adolescent rheumatology*, London, 1999, Martin Dunitz.

Jacobs JL: *Pediatric rheumatology for the practitioner,* ed 2, New York, 1993, Springer-Verlag.

Lovell DJ, White PH, editors: Pediatric rheumatology into the 90s, *J Rheumatol* 19:1, 1992.

Miller JJ III: Psychosocial factors related to rheumatic diseases of childhood, *J Pediatr* 20:1, 1993.

Miller ML, editor: Pediatric rheumatology, *Pediatr Clin North Am* 42:999, 1995.

Moore TL: Immunopathogenesis of juvenile rheumatoid arthritis, *Curr Opin Rheumatol* 11:377, 1999.

230 Kawasaki Disease

Michael E. Pichichero

Kawasaki disease is an acute, multisystem vasculitis of infancy and early childhood characterized by high fever, rash, conjunctivitis, inflammation of the mucous membranes, erythematous induration of the hands and feet, and cervical adenopathy. Kawasaki disease, formerly known as *mucocutaneous lymph node syndrome,* is the main cause of acquired heart disease in children.[3,12,20,40,41] It was first described in 1967 by a Japanese pediatrician, Tomisaka Kawasaki[24]; in 1974, the first cases of Kawasaki disease were reported in the United States.[6] In retrospect, illnesses that are similar to Kawasaki disease were described as early as 1871.[19] Landing and Larson compared the features of Kawasaki disease with infantile periarteritis nodosa and found that they shared many clinical signs and had indistinguishable pathological findings.[28]

EPIDEMIOLOGY

The peak age incidence of Kawasaki disease occurs during the second year of life. More than 80% of all cases occur in children under 5 years of age; the disease is quite uncommon beyond 9 years of age. Boys are more commonly affected than girls, with a male/female ratio of nearly 1.5:1. Kawasaki disease is now recognized as having a worldwide distribution. However, the greatest number of cases have been reported from Japan where more than 100,000 had been identified through 1992.[77] In Japan, three nationwide outbreaks have been documented occurring in 1979, 1982, and 1986, with the largest involving more than 15,000 cases, with an attack rate of 196/100,000 children younger than 5 years of age.[78] The Centers for Disease Control and Prevention estimates the incidence for children 8 years old or younger in the continental United States to be 2.74 cases per 100,000 in those of Asian or part Asian descent, 1.03 per 100,000 in blacks, and 0.43 per 100,000 in whites. Two nationwide surveys of children's hospitals and large general hospitals provide an alternative estimate that is perhaps more accurate relative to the incidence rate of Kawasaki disease in the United States.[68] From 1984 through 1990, just over 8,000 cases were identified, with a rising trend noted between 1986 and 1990. Extrapolation to a 100% survey response would lead to an estimate of 13,720 discharge diagnoses of Kawasaki disease for the 7-year study period, or approximately 2000 cases per year in the United States. The estimated annual attack rate for children younger than 5 years of age would therefore adjust to 9.2/100,000.[68] Outbreaks from within the United States suggest that the illness occurs more frequently in patients of middle and upper socioeconomic groups.[7,14,50] Outbreaks have tended to predominate in winter and spring.[24,35,51] Numerous temporal clusters of Kawasaki disease have been reported in the United States,[7,24,35,51,69] Japan[74,75,77,78] and worldwide.[12] This seasonality and temporal clustering of cases suggests an infectious etiology. Recurrent cases have been reported in the United States and Japan, with a rate ranging from 0.3% to 5% in Japan[75] and 1% to 2% in the United States.[16,41,53,76,77] Intravenous immunoglobulin (IVIG) therapy (discussed later in this chapter) for the first episode may increase the risk of recurrence within the following 12 months but not later.[42] Kawasaki disease occurs more commonly in siblings of patients who have had the disease than in the general population.[16,53,75] A history of Kawasaki disease among siblings ranges between 0.7% to 2.1% in epidemiological surveys in Japan[78] compared with an overall incidence of about 0.19% in the general population 0 to 4 years of age.[16] Kawasaki disease in twins is even higher than in non-twin siblings but not significantly different between monozygotic twins and dizygotic twins.[57] The interval between sibling cases is less than 10 days in 54%; sometimes the onset occurs on the same day. These findings suggest a common exposure to an infectious agent in a genetically predisposed population.[37]

ETIOLOGY

There is no established cause for Kawasaki disease.[8,53] The clinical features suggest an infectious etiology, a hypersensitivity reaction,[62] or exposure to an environmental toxin.[52] Associations have been described between Kawasaki disease and (1) rug shampooing; (2) exposure to a variant strain of *Propionibacterium acnes* infecting mites found in house dust; (3) living near stagnant water (suggesting an arthropod vector or an animal reservoir); (4) infection with Epstein-Barr virus, human herpesvirus-6, human parvovirus B19, *Streptococcus mitis*, leptospira, *Ehrlichia* species, *Staphylococcus aureus*, *Streptococcus pyogenes,* and retroviruses; and (5) exposure to mercury.*

Recently, the notion that toxin-producing staphylococcal or streptococcal bacteria are the primary etiology of Kawasaki disease has received the most attention.[29,31,32,37] These agents are attractive candidates because of the similarity of Kawasaki disease to illnesses such as staphylococcal toxic shock syndrome and streptococcal toxic shock syndrome and

*References 11, 18, 21, 22, 25, 32, 34, 37, 39, 47-49, 51, 52, 55, 59.

because of the immune response induced by the bacterial toxins released from these bacteria that act as "superantigens."[9,15] However recovery of toxin-producing bacteria has not been confirmed in all Kawasaki disease patients.[71]

PATHOGENESIS

Kawasaki disease is characterized by immunoregulatory abnormalities: a deficiency of suppressor/cytotoxic T cells, increased numbers of activated helper T cells, and increased B-cell activation reflected by high levels of spontaneous immunoglobulin synthesis.[1,2,10] These are immunological features characteristic of diseases that are caused by bacterial toxins acting as superantigens.[9,15,70] Superantigens stimulate a large fraction of the T-cell population; T-cell stimulation is mediated by the dual affinity of superantigens for the class II major histocompatibility complex on macrophages/monocytes and for the relatively invariant sequence of the variable beta region (Vβ2) of the T-cell receptor. The effectiveness of high-dose IVIG in reducing coronary vasculitis (discussed later in this chapter) might result from prevention of immune-complex deposition on blood vessel walls or from a reversal of immunoregulatory abnormalities.[30,64,65,66]

Kawasaki disease is associated with increased production of interleukin-1 beta, tumor necrosis factor-alpha, interleukin-6, interleukin-2, and interferon gamma.[33] The production of these cytokines by T cells and monocytes is thought to play an important role in the pathogenesis of vascular endothelial cell injury during acute Kawasaki disease, because these cytokines elicit proinflammatory and prothrombic responses in endothelial cells. Cytokines have been detected in tissue obtained from patients in the acute stage of Kawasaki disease.[58] More recently, increased chemokine activity has been observed in patients who have Kawasaki disease,[72] and these agents may play an important role in the pathogenesis of the vasculitis. Selectins may also contribute to localization of leukocytes to the vascular injury of Kawasaki disease.[66]

CLINICAL MANIFESTATIONS

To make the diagnosis of Kawasaki disease, five of the six major clinical characteristics associated with the condition must be present (Box 230-1), and all other illnesses having similar features must be excluded. Symptoms vary in severity, but greater than 90% of patients fulfill the first five clinical criteria. All the symptoms are not apparent simultaneously, but the timing of their appearance is remarkably constant.

The course of the disease can best be described as triphasic. The acute phase consists of fever, conjunctival hyperemia, oropharyngeal erythema, swelling of the hands and feet, a polymorphous erythematous rash, and cervical lymphadenopathy. Fever, rash, and lymphadenopathy fade after 10 to 12 days of illness, marking the beginning of the subacute phase. The subacute stage is characterized by lip cracking and fissuring, desquamation of skin overlying the tips of the fingers and toes, and the onset of arthralgias (and/or arthritis), thrombocytosis, and cardiac disease. The convalescent stage usually begins about 25 days after onset and is characterized by the absence of clinical signs of disease but the persistence of residual inflammation, marked by an elevated erythrocyte sedimentation rate (ESR).

Fever is the most prominent symptom of the acute phase of the disease. Temperatures show a high-spiking remittent pattern in the range of 38.4° C (101.1° F) to greater than 40° C (104° F). Fever persists despite the use of empirical antibiotics, corticosteroids, and standard doses of antipyretics. Fever is present on average for about 12 days, although prolonged courses of up to 5 weeks have been reported; defervescence occurs over 1 to 3 days. Discrete engorgement of the bulbar conjunctivae blood vessels (without associated discharge, exudate, keratitis, chemosis, or pseudomembrane formation) and an anterior uveitis develop shortly after the onset of fever.[60] The cornea, lens, and retina are not involved. Early oropharyngeal signs include dryness and red-

BOX 230-1

DIAGNOSTIC CRITERIA FOR KAWASAKI DISEASE

A. Principal symptoms (at least five of the following six items should be satisfied for diagnosis.)
   1. Fever of unknown cause lasting 5 days or more
   2. Bilateral congestion of ocular conjunctivae
   3. Changes of lips and oral cavity
      a. Dryness, redness, and fissuring of lips
      b. Protuberance of tongue papillae ("strawberry tongue")
      c. Diffuse reddening of oral and pharyngeal mucosa
   4. Changes of peripheral extremities
      a. Reddening of palms and soles (initial stage)
      b. Indurative edema (initial stage)
      c. Membranous desquamation from fingertips (convalescent stage)
   5. Polymorphous exanthema of body trunk without vesicles or crusts
   6. Acute nonpurulent swelling of cervical lymph nodes of 1.5 cm or more in diameter
B. Other significant symptoms or findings
   1. Carditis, especially myocarditis or pericarditis
   2. Diarrhea
   3. Arthralgia or arthritis
   4. Proteinuria and increase of leukocytes in urine sediment
   5. Changes in blood tests
      a. Leukocytosis with shift to the left
      b. Slight decrease in erythrocyte and hemoglobin levels
      c. Increased sedimentation rate
      d. Elevated C-reactive protein (CRP)
      e. Increased beta-2-globulin
      f. Thrombocytosis
      g. Negative antistreptolysin titer (ASO)
   6. Changes occasionally observed
      a. Aseptic meningitis
      b. Mild jaundice or slight increase of serum transaminase
      c. Swelling of gallbladder

dening of the lips and of the buccal and pharyngeal mucosa. The absence of aphthous ulceration or hemorrhagic bullae is noticeable. A "strawberry tongue" frequently is present. Later, as the intensity of the erythema subsides, the lips usually become cracked and fissured.

The most characteristic and unique feature of Kawasaki disease relates to changes that occur in the hands and feet. Early on, they become diffusely indurated and swollen, and the overlying skin develops a woody firmness suggestive of acute scleroderma. The palms and soles usually become erythematous or take on a purplish hue. There is fusiform swelling of the fingers, which limits the child's ability to grasp objects. The feet are painful to the touch, and many children will refuse to stand or walk. Two to 3 weeks after the onset of illness and after the early signs involving the extremities have disappeared, an unusual desquamation of the skin beginning at the subungual and periungual regions of the fingers and toes is recognizable in nearly all cases (Fig. 230-1). Progression to complete peeling of the palms and soles may occur, but exfoliation generally does not extend to the remainder of the body surface. During the convalescent phase, deep transverse grooves (Beau lines) may appear across the fingernails and toenails, presumably as a result of arrested growth during the illness.

A polymorphous, erythematous rash appears 1 to 5 days after the onset of fever; it usually begins on the extremities and spreads centripetally. The three most common patterns of rash are maculopapular (morbilliform), erythema multiforme–like with iris lesions, and scarlatiniform. The rash may be coalescent, producing large, irregular, raised plaques, and it may be pruritic. Vesicles, pustules, and bullae are not seen. The rash is not petechial or purpuric. It usually fades within a week but occasionally persists longer or recurs.

Lymphadenopathy typically involves a single cervical node measuring greater than 1.5 cm in diameter. The node usually is not tender or warm and does not become fluctuant. Generalized lymphadenopathy does not occur. The lymph node diminishes in size with defervescence of the disease. Lymphadenopathy is the one least often seen of the major criteria; it occurs in only about 60% of patients in most U.S. series, although it is more common in Japan.

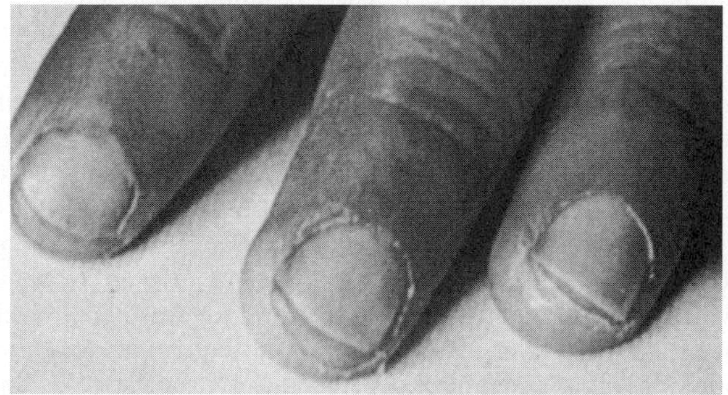

Fig. 230-1 Desquamation of the skin involving the subungual and periungual regions of the fingertips.

(From Kawasaki T, et al: A new infantile acute febrile mucocutaneous lymph node syndrome (MLNS) prevailing in Japan, *Pediatrics* 54:273, 1974. Copyright American Academy of Pediatrics, 1974.)

In addition to the six major clinical signs, other features of Kawasaki disease frequently are noted. Sterile pyuria occurs more often than lymphadenopathy in most U.S. cases; 10 to 100 white blood cells (WBCs) per high-power field may be observed on a clean-catch voided urine specimen. No WBCs will be seen on a bladder aspiration specimen, because the sterile pyuria is caused by urethral inflammation or ulceration. Occasionally a patient will demonstrate trace proteinuria or hematuria.

Irritability, mild meningismus, and lethargy are seen in nearly all of these patients, and nearly all probably have aseptic meningitis. When cerebrospinal fluid (CSF) is analyzed, it typically shows 25 to 100 WBCs/mm^3 with normal amounts of glucose and protein. Diarrhea is seen in about 50% of the patients. Passing 5 to 15 stools per day for 2 to 7 days during the acute or subacute phase is common. Stools do not contain polymorphonuclear cells and do not test positive for occult blood.

Either arthralgias, arthritis, or both occur in 30% to 40% of the children. Large joints, particularly the knees and ankles, are involved most often. Usually, no more than two or three joints will be affected. Joint symptoms occur 8 to 12 days after the onset of disease. Joint fluid, if analyzed, will reveal findings similar to those of rheumatoid arthritis.

Other findings, such as pneumonia, tympanitis, photophobia, and mild liver dysfunction, are observed somewhat less commonly. Acute hydrops of the gallbladder, jaundice, convulsions, encephalopathy, Bell's palsy, hearing loss, pancreatitis, orchitis, and pleural effusions are seen rarely, but clearly are associated complications of Kawasaki disease.[36]

The most alarming findings of Kawasaki disease are those in the cardiovascular system. Approximately 1% of children who have the disease die, usually as a result of coronary artery aneurysms. During the acute phase, tachycardia and gallop rhythms may appear; however, the most serious manifestations of cardiac involvement occur during the subacute phase. These include serious arrhythmias, congestive heart failure, pericardial effusion, mitral insufficiency, and myocardial ischemia or infarction.

Atypical Kawasaki Disease

Severe or even fatal coronary abnormalities can develop following illnesses that resemble but do not fulfill the classic diagnostic features of Kawasaki disease.* Patients who have "atypical" Kawasaki disease may display prolonged high fever, nonspecific rash, arthralgia or arthritis, fissuring of the lips, nonexudative conjunctivitis, and extreme irritability. Atypical Kawasaki disease can present occasionally with prolonged fever for 5 or more days in the absence of other clinical criteria for the illness. In other patients, unilateral cervical adenopathy refractory to antibiotic therapy is the clue that atypical Kawasaki disease may be present. Atypical Kawasaki disease is likely to present with subtle manifestations in infants less than 6 months of age; this group is at highest risk (50% or greater) for coronary artery lesions if untreated.

*References 4, 5, 8, 28, 32, 56.

LABORATORY FINDINGS

Although there are no pathognomonic laboratory findings in Kawasaki disease, certain laboratory abnormalities frequently are seen and therefore help to establish the diagnosis. In the acute phase of the disease, most patients exhibit an elevated WBC count with an associated left shift; WBC counts of 15,000 to 20,000/mm^3 are common, and may remain elevated for 1 to 3 weeks. Other laboratory abnormalities in the acute phase usually include an elevated ESR (mean = 55 mm/hr); increased C-reactive protein (CRP) and beta-2-globulin; mild normochromic, normocytic anemia; and slight elevations of the liver enzymes. As previously stated, many patients demonstrate sterile pyuria and cerebrospinal fluid (CSF) pleocytosis. In the second to third week of illness, patients characteristically develop significant thrombocytosis, with platelet counts averaging in excess of 700,000/mm^3. Importantly, a number of laboratory studies are negative. Routine cultures of blood, CSF, urine, throat, and lymph node aspirates reveal no growth or normal flora. Serological studies for bacterial and viral agents are negative, including the ASO titer. Antinuclear antibodies and the rheumatoid factor are absent, as are all other autoantibodies.

Sinus tachycardia, nonspecific ST segment and T wave changes, and evidence of mild left ventricular hypertrophy may be seen on an electrocardiogram (ECG) in the acute phase. In the subacute phase, myocardial infarction patterns on an ECG may be observed, although infrequently.

A baseline echocardiogram should be performed as soon as the diagnosis of Kawasaki disease is suspected in order to evaluate cardiac function, the presence or absence of pericardial effusion, and the anatomy of the coronary arteries. Coronary artery abnormalities generally are apparent by the third or fourth week of illness. Coronary artery disease rarely, if ever, develops after 6 to 8 weeks, although late-onset valvular disease has been reported.

DIFFERENTIAL DIAGNOSIS

The clinical picture of Kawasaki disease, after all of the major features have become manifest, is not difficult to differentiate from other mucocutaneous syndromes. In the first days of the illness, a whole spectrum of acute febrile diseases might be considered. Three to 5 days after the onset, certain clinical features may be singled out as compatible with other diagnoses—for example, strawberry tongue suggestive of streptococcal infection. Two conditions most commonly mimic Kawasaki disease; they are scarlet fever and measles.[11] However, if all the signs and symptoms are considered carefully, the diagnosis is readily apparent. The clinical features of Kawasaki disease and other mucocutaneous disorders are shown in Table 230-1. Other conditions that share some aspects of Kawasaki disease are ratbite fever, rubella, rubeola, infectious mononucleosis, toxoplasmosis, juvenile rheumatoid arthritis, systemic lupus erythematosus, Behçet's syndrome, acrodynia (mercury poisoning), and febrile drug reactions (especially those caused by anticonvulsants). The similarities between fatal Kawasaki disease and fatal infantile polyarteritis nodosa are striking; pathologically the two diseases cannot be distinguished. The exact relationship between them, however, remains undetermined. At this time one is left with the clear differentiating feature that Kawasaki disease rarely is fatal (±1% mortality), whereas infantile polyarteritis nodosa is a pathological diagnosis made at autopsy.

MANAGEMENT

IVIG with aspirin is the best available therapy for preventing coronary artery abnormalities in Kawasaki disease and should be administered to all patients diagnosed within the first 10 days of illness.[46,54] Physicians should institute treatment as soon as the diagnosis is established and as early as possible in the course of the illness. Aspirin, given in high doses (80 to 120 mg/kg/day), reduces the length and severity of Kawasaki disease during the acute phase.[27] Aspirin use early in the course of disease also may reduce coronary artery involvement. Salicylate levels should be checked to avoid toxicity. Defervescence apparently is accompanied by improvement in gastrointestinal (GI) absorption of aspirin[26,27]; therefore dosages should be reduced to 30 to 50 mg/kg/day after fever subsides and until the ESR has returned to normal. Aspirin should be continued throughout the convalescent phase because of its antithrombotic effects at 3 to 5 mg/kg/day until the platelet count has returned to normal. If coronary aneurysms are recognized, salicylates (3 to 5 mg/kg/day) should be continued until careful follow-up ECGs demonstrate aneurysm resolution.

High-dose IVIG may prevent coronary artery lesions in Kawasaki disease. A dosage of 400 mg/kg/day for 4 consecutive days was initially shown to be effective,[46] but a single dose of 2 g/kg infused over 10 to 12 hours subsequently has replaced the 4-day regimen. There appears to be no difference in efficacy among particular IVIG products currently commercially available. Patients should be monitored carefully during IVIG infusions for signs of anaphylaxis. Immune hemolysis, aseptic meningitis, serum sickness, and transmission of hepatitis C virus have been associated with IVIG therapy. Vaccination with measles, mumps, rubella, and varicella vaccine should be delayed for 9 to 12 months after administration of high-dose IVIG.[5] The efficacy of IVIG illness is not known. However, patients who remain symptomatic beyond the tenth day may still benefit from IVIG. Eighty percent to 90% of children treated with IVIG respond favorably with decreased fever and reduction in mucocutaneous findings.[37] The remainder have persistent or recurrent fever, with or without mucocutaneous signs. If ongoing fever cannot be attributed to another cause, it should be assumed that Kawasaki disease is persisting or has relapsed. Because fever may be viewed as a surrogate for continued vasculitis, retreatment with IVIG is advocated. The majority of patients retreated after a single dose of IVIG therapy has failed will respond to retreatment.[63] The decision to administer IVIG later than the tenth day of illness must be individualized.

Corticosteroids were believed to be dangerous as therapy for Kawasaki disease based on an early study in Japan in which 65% of patients treated with oral prednisolone developed coronary artery aneurysms.[23] Subsequent studies have not yielded as dramatic a detrimental effect of steroids and some have benefitted.[28,46] If IVIG therapy fails (particularly after two treatments), patients are at high risk for development of severe coronary artery complications, including death. Patients in this clinical situation may benefit from one to three pulse-doses of methyl prednisolone at 30 mg/kg/

Table 230-1 Clinical Features of Kawasaki Disease and Other Mucocutaneous Diseases

	Kawasaki Disease	Stevens-Johnson Syndrome	Streptococcal Scarlet Fever	Staphylococcal Scarlet Fever	Staphylococcal Toxic Shock Syndrome	Leptospirosis
Age (yr)	Usually <5	Usually 3-30	Usually 5-10	Usually 2-8	Usually adolescent	Usually >2
Fever	Prolonged	Prolonged	Variable	Variable	Usually <10 days	Variable
Eyes	Hyperemia of ocular conjunctivae; uveitis	Catarrhal conjunctivitis; chemosis; iritis; uveitis; panophthalmitis	No change	Hyperemia of ocular conjunctivae	Hyperemia of ocular conjunctivae	Hyperemia of ocular conjunctivae; uveitis
Lips	Red, dry, fissured	Erosions; crusted, fissured, bleeding	No change	No change	Red	No change
Oral cavity	Diffuse erythema; "strawberry tongue"	Erythema; bullae, ulcers, pseudomembrane formation	Pharyngitis; palatal petechiae; "strawberry tongue"	Pharyngitis	Erythema; pharyngitis	Pharyngitis
Peripheral extremities	Erythema of palms and soles; indurative edema; periungual, palmar, and plantar desquamation	No change	Periungual desquamation	No change	Swelling of hands and feet; dry gangrene	Gangrene of hands and feet (rare)
Exanthem	Erythematous, polymorphous	Erythematous, polymorphous; iris lesions, vesicles, bullae, crusts	Finely papular erythroderma; Pastia lines; circumoral pallor	Finely papular erythroderma; Pastia lines	Erythroderma	Erythematous, maculopapular, petechial, or purpuric
Cervical lymph nodes	Nonpurulent swelling; unilateral (frequent)	Nonpurulent swelling (occasional)	Nonpurulent or purulent swelling (frequent)	Nonpurulent or purulent swelling (occasional)	No change	Nonpurulent swelling (infrequent)
Other	Meatitis; diarrhea; arthralgia and arthritis; aseptic meningitis; rhinorrhea (uncommon): ECG changes	Malaise; cough, rhinorrhea, pneumonitis; vomiting; arthralgia; recurrent episodes	Malaise; vomiting; headache		Headache; confusion; hypotension; icteric hepatitis; diarrhea; coagulopathy; renal injury	Headache myalgia; abdominal pain; icteric hepatitis; meningitis

dose.[73] This therapy should be reserved for those patients who are clearly refractory to other more established treatments. Plasmaphoresis[71] and exchange transfusion[44] have also been reported to be of benefit in Kawasaki disease patients, but these are cumbersome and more involved treatments. Pentoxifylline at a dose of 20 mg/kg/day[17] may decrease aneurysm formation. Antibiotics are not useful.

COMPLICATIONS

The major complication of Kawasaki disease is the development of coronary artery aneurysms.[3,13,40,41,69] If IVIG is not administered, aneurysms occur in 15% to 25% of cases and usually are apparent by echocardiogram during the subacute phase of the illness. Most patients who have aneurysms are asymptomatic; in some cases, however, formation of an aneurysm, particularly a giant aneurysm (greater than 8 mm in diameter), is followed by thrombosis or rupture, resulting in a fatal myocardial infarction.[67] Limited data support the use of antiplatelet drugs such as dipyridamole and ticlopidine either alone or in combination with aspirin if there is evidence of persistent coronary artery abnormalities. Some authorities treat patients with giant aneurysms with a regimen of low-dose warfarin in combination with low-dose aspirin.[37] The indication for and timing of angiography is controversial. In children younger than 7 years of age, a radionuclide scan may help identify areas of mild cardioischemia. When echocardiography, angiography, or radionuclide scanning detect thrombi occluding a significant portion of main branches of coronary arteries, thrombolytic therapy should be instituted.[61] Percutaneous transluminal coronary angioplasty has been attempted by several groups with mixed results.[4] In the face of myocardial infarction, bypass surgery should be undertaken.

For long-term management of patients with Kawasaki disease, a risk stratification scheme may be of benefit (Table 230-2). For patients at level I risk, the primary care physician may fully assume care after the 1-year anniversary of Kawasaki disease onset. There should be no restrictions on physical activities. For patients with level II risk, a pediatric cardiologist should be consulted every 1 to 2 years; at least one stress test evaluating myocardial functioning should be done at about 10 years of age. For patients in risk level III, daily low-dose aspirin therapy and annual cardiac follow-up with echocardiography and electrocardiography may be appropriate. Periodic stress tests are recommended. For patients in risk level IV, low-dose aspirin therapy should be maintained and low-dose warfarin should be considered. Coronary angiography may be considered 6 to12 months after the acute disease has resolved to delineate coronary artery anatomy. Physical activities should be modified to minimize the risk of hemorrhage. Strenuous or competitive sports should be avoided. Patients at risk level V should receive daily low-dose aspirin, and warfarin should be considered. Patients should be evaluated for indications of bypass graft surgery. Mild to moderate recreational physical activities are permitted.

The coronary artery aneurysms seen in Kawasaki disease develop more frequently in boys than in girls; in children younger than 1 year of age; in those who have a triphasic fever pattern or fever for longer than 2 weeks, when a gallop rhythm or other arrhythmia is noted; or when the ESR exceeds 50 mm/hr[11] (Box 230-2). Cases of atypical Kawasaki disease followed by typical coronary artery involvement have led to the suggestion that an echocardiography examination be undertaken in children who have prolonged unexplained febrile illnesses associated with subsequent peripheral desquamation.[53]

A rare complication of Kawasaki disease is hydrops of the gallbladder. This occurs in approximately 3% of cases and is seen most frequently in children who are jaundiced. It becomes evident during the acute phase of the illness and is diagnosed best by ultrasound on recognition of a right upper quadrant abdominal mass. The pathogenesis is unknown.

Table 230-2 Levels of Risk for Determination of Methods for Management of Kawasaki Disease–Induced Coronary Artery Disease

Risk Level	Description
I	No coronary artery abnormalities at any stage of illness
II	Transient coronary artery ectasia followed by regression
III	Small to medium solitary coronary artery aneurysm
IV	Giant aneurysm(s) or multiple aneurysms without obstruction
V	Coronary artery obstruction (thrombosis or stenosis)

Modified from Mason WH, Takahashi M: Kawasaki syndrome, *Clin Infect Dis* 28:169, 1999.

BOX 230-2

RISK FACTORS FOR CORONARY ARTERY ANEURYSMS IN KAWASAKI DISEASE

Risk Very Increased
Fever lasts longer than 14 days
Biphasic fever pattern*†
Biphasic pattern of skin rash
Maximum WBC count ≥30,000
Maximum ESR (mm/hr) ≥101
Time until normalization of ESR or CRP ≥30 days of illness
Biphasic elevation of ESR or CRP†
Increased Q/R ratio in leads II, III, aVF >0.3
Symptoms of myocardial infarction

Risk Increased
Male sex
Age at onset under 1 year
Hemoglobin ≤10 g/dl† and RBC count ≤3.5 million
Maximum WBC count >26,000
Maximum ESR (mm/hr) >50
Cardiomegaly
Arrhythmia
Recurrence of disease

*Separated by afebrile period of 48 hours or longer.
†Causes other than Kawasaki disease must be ruled out.

Surgery is not indicated because the problem resolves spontaneously in convalescence.

PROGNOSIS

Kawasaki disease has a 0.3% mortality. Death occurs almost exclusively in children who have giant aneurysms, largely as a result of coronary artery thrombosis, massive myocardial infarction, and cardiogenic shock. Significant morbidity, in the form of coronary artery aneurysms, occurs in 15% to 25% of cases. Eighty percent of children whose aneurysms are small to moderate in size have complete resolution without apparent sequelae within 5 years.[3,20] The remaining children may experience persisting aneurysms, coronary artery stenosis or obstruction, or aortic regurgitation.[43] Emerging evidence suggests that a portion of this latter group of children may be at risk for the subsequent development of significant cardiovascular disease such as coronary arteriosclerosis or persistent aneurysms, placing some of them at risk for sudden death from aneurysm rupture or thrombosis, cardiac arrhythmias, angina, or hypertension.

PSYCHOSOCIAL ASPECTS

Kawasaki disease is almost always a self-limited illness without complications; this should be emphasized to the parents. Even if coronary artery aneurysms do develop, these resolve spontaneously in more than 50% of cases in 2 years and 80% in 5 years. Long-term risks still remain undefined, and only as we gain prospective experience with the disease over several more decades will the true incidence of cardiovascular sequelae become evident.

REFERENCES

1. Abe J, et al: Characterization of T cell repertoire changes in acute Kawasaki disease, *J Exp Med* 177:791, 1993.
2. Abe J, et al: Selective expansion of T cells expressing T-cell receptor variable regions Vβ2 and Vβ8 in Kawasaki disease, *Proc Natl Acad Sci U S A* 89:4066, 1992.
3. Akagi T, et al: Outcome of coronary artery aneurysms after Kawasaki disease, *J Pediatr* 121:689, 1992.
4. Akimoto K, et al: Percutaneous transluminal coronary angioplasty in Kawasaki disease: five case reports and literature review. In Kato H, editor: *Kawasaki disease: proceedings of the Fifth International Symposium on Kawasaki disease, Fukuoka, Japan,* Amsterdam, 1995, Elsevier Science.
5. American Academy of Pediatrics: Kawasaki disease. In Peter G, et al, editors: *1997 Red Book: report of the Committee on Infectious Diseases,* ed 24, Elk Grove Village, Ill, American Academy of Pediatrics.
6. Ammerman SD, et al: Diagnostic uncertainty in atypical Kawasaki disease, and a new finding: exudative conjunctivitis, *Pediatr Infect Dis* 4:210, 1985.
7. Bell DM, et al: Kawasaki syndrome: description of two outbreaks in the United States, *N Engl J Med* 304:1568, 1981.
8. Bierman FZ, Gersony WM: Kawasaki disease: clinical perspective, *J Pediatr* 111:789, 1987.
9. Bohach GA, et al: Staphylococcal and streptococcal pyrogenic toxins involved in toxic shock syndrome and related illnesses, *Crit Rev Microbiol* 17:251, 1990.
10. Burns JC, et al: Polymerase activity in lymphocyte culture supernatants from patients with Kawasaki disease, *Nature* 323:814, 1986.
11. Burns JC, et al: Clinical and epidemiologic characteristics of patients referred for evaluation of Kawasaki disease, *J Pediatr* 118:680, 1991.
12. Dajani AS, et al: Diagnosis and therapy of Kawasaki disease in children, *Circulation* 87:1776, 1993.
13. Daniels SR, et al: Correlates of coronary artery aneurysm formation in patients with Kawasaki disease, *Am J Dis Child* 141:205, 1987.
14. Dean AG, et al: An epidemic of Kawasaki syndrome in Hawaii, *J Pediatr* 100:552, 1982.
15. Drake CG, Kotzin BL: Superantigens: biology, immunology, and potential role in disease, *J Clin Immunol* 12:149, 1992.
16. Fujita Y, et al: Kawasaki disease in families, *Pediatrics* 84:666, 1989.
17. Furukawa S, et al: Pentoxifylline and intravenous gamma globulin combination therapy for acute Kawasaki disease, *Eur J Pediatr* 153:663, 1994.
18. Furusho K, et al: Possible role for mite antigen in Kawasaki disease, *Lancet* 2:194, 1981.
19. Gee SJ: Cases of morbid anatomy, *St. Bartholomew's Hospital Report,* 7:141, 1871.
20. Gersony WM: Long-term issues in Kawasaki disease, *J Pediatr* 121: 731, 1992.
21. Jordan SC, et al: Lack of evidence for mite-antigen-mediated pathogenesis in Kawasaki disease, *Lancet* 1:931, 1983 (letter).
22. Kato H, et al: Variant strain of *Propionibacterium acnes*: a clue to the aetiology of Kawasaki disease, *Lancet* 2:1383, 1983.
23. Kato H, Koike S, Yokoyama T: Kawasaki disease: effect of treatment on coronary involvement, *Pediatrics* 63:175, 1979.
24. Khan AS, et al: Kawasaki syndrome surveillance United States, 1991-1993. In Kato H, editor: *Kawasaki disease,* New York, 1995, Elsevier Science.
25. Kikuta H, et al: Detection of Epstein-Barr virus sequences in patients with Kawasaki disease by means of polymerase chain reaction, *Intervirology (Basel)* 33:1, 1992.
26. Koren G, MacLeod SM: Difficulty in achieving therapeutic serum concentrations of salicylate in Kawasaki disease, *J Pediatr* 105:991, 1984.
27. Kusakawa S, Tatara K: Efficacies and risks of aspirin in the treatment of Kawasaki disease, *Prog Clin Biol Res* 250:401, 1987.
28. Landing BH, Larson EJ: Are infantile periarteritis nodosa with coronary artery involvement and fatal mucocutaneous lymph node syndrome the same? Comparison of 20 patients from North America with patients from Hawaii and Japan, *Pediatrics* 59:651, 1977.
29. Lekova ES, Joffe L, Glode MP: Antigenic recognition by intravenous gamma globulin of selected bacteria isolated from throats of patients with Kawasaki syndrome, *Pediatr Infect Dis J* 9:620, 1990.
30. Leung DYM, et al: Reversal of lymphocyte activation in vivo in the Kawasaki syndrome by intravenous gamma globulin, *J Clin Invest* 79: 468, 1987.
31. Leung DYM, et al: Toxic shock syndrome toxin-secreting *Staphylococcus aureus* in Kawasaki syndrome, *Lancet* 342:1385, 1993.
32. Leung DYM, et al: Toxic shock toxin-secretory *Staphylococcus aureus* in Kawasaki syndrome, *Lancet* 342:1385, 1993.
33. Lin CY, et al: Serial changes of serum interleukin-6, interleukin-8, and tumor necrosis factor alpha among patients with Kawasaki disease, *J Pediatr* 121:924, 1992.
34. Marchette NJ, et al: Epstein-Barr virus and other herpesvirus infections in Kawasaki syndrome, *J Infect Dis* 161:680, 1990.
35. Mason WH, Schneider T, Takahashi M: The epidemiology and etiology of Kawasaki disease, *Cardiol Young* 1:196, 1991.
36. Mason WH, Takahashi M: Kawasaki syndrome, *Clin Infect Dis* 28:169, 1999.
37. Matsushita K, et al: Immunopathological activities of extracellular products of *Streptococcus mitis*, particularly a superantigenic fraction, *Infect Immunol* 63:785, 1995.
38. Melish ME, et al: Absence of significant RNA-dependent DNA polymerase activity in lymphocytes from patients with Kawasaki syndrome, *Nature* 337:288, 1989.
39. Morens DM, Anderson LJ, Huriwitz ES: National surveillance of Kawasaki disease, *Pediatrics* 65:21, 1980.
40. Nakamura Y, Yanagawa H: A case-control study of recurrent Kawasaki disease using the database of the nationwide surveys in Japan, *Eur J Pediatr* 155:303, 1996.
41. Nakamura Y, Yanagawa H, Kawasaki T: Mortality among children with Kawasaki disease in Japan, *N Engl J Med* 326:1246, 1992.

42. Nakamura Y et al: Cardiac sequelae of Kawasaki disease in Japan: statistical analysis, *Pediatrics* 88:1144, 1991.
43. Nakano H et al: High incidence of aortic regurgitation following Kawasaki disease, *J Pediatr* 107:59, 1985.
44. Netter JC, et al: Exchange transfusion for severe Kawasaki disease, *Lancet* 1:452, 1984.
45. Newberger J, et al: The treatment of Kawasaki syndrome with intravenous gamma globulin, *N Engl J Med* 315:341, 1986.
46. Nonaka Z, et al: Randomized controlled study of intravenous prednisolone and gamma globulin treatment in 100 cases of Kawasaki disease. In Kato H, editor: *Kawasaki disease: proceedings of the Fifth International Symposium on Kawasaki disease, Fukuoka, Japan,* Amsterdam, 1995, Elsevier Science.
47. Okano M, et al: Human herpesvirus 6 infection in Kawasaki disease, *J Clin Microbiol* 27:2379, 1989.
48. Orlawski JP, Mercer RD: Urine mercury levels in Kawasaki disease, *Pediatrics* 66:633, 1980.
49. Patriarca PA, et al: Kawasaki syndrome in association with the applications of rug shampoo, *Lancet* 2:578, 1982.
50. Rauch AM: Kawasaki syndrome: issues in etiology and treatment, *Adv Pediatr Infect Dis* 4:163, 1989.
51. Rauch AM: Kawasaki syndrome: review of new epidemiologic and laboratory developments, *Pediatr Infect Dis J* 6:1016, 1987.
52. Rider LG, et al: Group A streptococcal infection and Kawasaki syndrome, *Lancet* 337:1100, 1991.
53. Rowley AH, Gonzalez-Crussi F, Shulman ST: Kawasaki syndrome, *Rev Infect Dis* 10:1, 1988.
54. Rowley AH, Shulman ST: Therapy of Kawasaki disease, *Report Pediatr Infect Dis* 3:19, 1993.
55. Rowley A, et al: Failure to confirm the presence of a retrovirus in cultured lymphocytes from patients with Kawasaki syndrome, *Pediatr Res* 29:417, 1991.
56. Rowley AH, et al: Incomplete Kawasaki disease with coronary artery involvement, *J Pediatr* 110:409, 1987.
57. Sasazaki T, Harada F, Kawasaki T: Genetic analysis of Kawasaki disease, *Prog Clin Biol Res* 250:251, 1987.
58. Sato N, et al: Immunopathology and cytokine detection in the skin of patients with Kawasaki disease, *J Pediatr* 122:198, 1993.
59. Shulman ST, Rowley AH: Does Kawasaki disease have a retroviral aetiology, *Lancet* 2:545, 1986.
60. Smith LBH, Newburger JW, Burns JC: Kawasaki syndrome and the eye, *Pediatr Infect Dis J* 8:116, 1989.
61. Sonobe T, et al: Intravenous coronary thrombolysis using recombinant tissue plasminogen activator for intra-aneurysmal thrombi in Kawasaki disease. In Takahashi M, Taubert K, editors: *Proceedings of the Fourth International Symposium on Kawasaki Disease,* Dallas, Texas, 1993, American Heart Association.
62. Sugawara T, et al: Immunology of the skin lesions in Kawasaki disease, *Prog Clin Biol Res* 250:185, 1987.
63. Sundel RP, Newburger JW: Management of acute Kawasaki disease, *Prog Pediatr Cardiol* 6:203, 1997.
64. Sundel RP, et al: Gamma globulin retreatment in Kawasaki disease, *J Pediatr* 123:657, 1993.
65. Takel S, Arora YK, Walker SM: Intravenous immunoglobulin contains specific antibodies inhibitory to activation of T cells by staphylococcal toxin superantigens, *J Clin Invest* 91:602, 1993.
66. Takeshita S, et al: Circulating soluble selectins in Kawasaki disease, *Clin Exp Immunol* 108:446, 1997.
67. Tatara K, Kusakawa S: Long-term prognosis of giant coronary aneurysm in Kawasaki disease: an angiographic study, *J Pediatr* 111:705, 1987.
68. Taubert KA: Epidemiology of Kawasaki disease in the United States and world wide, *Prog Pediatr Cardiol* 6:181, 1997.
69. Taubert KA, Rowley AH, Shulman ST: Seven-year national survey of Kawasaki disease and rheumatic fever, *Pediatr Infect Dis J* 13:704, 1994.
70. Todome Y, et al: Superantigenic exotoxin production by isolates of *Staphylococcus aureus* from Kawasaki syndrome patients and age-matched control children, *J Med Microbiol* 42:91, 1995.
71. Villain E, et al: Trial of exchange or intravenous gamma globulin for the prevention of coronary artery aneurysms in Kawasaki disease, *Arch Fr Pediatr* 44:79, 1987.
72. Wong M, Silverman ED, Fish EN: Evidence for RANTES, monocyte chemotactic protein-1 and macrophage inflammatory protein-1ß expression in Kawasaki disease, *J Rheumatol* 24:1179, 1997.
73. Wright DA, et al: Treatment of immune globulin-resistant Kawasaki disease with pulsed doses of corticosteroids, *J Pediatr* 128:146, 1996.
74. Yanagawa H, Kawasaki T, Shigematsu I: Nationwide survey on Kawasaki disease in Japan, *Pediatrics* 80:58, 1987.
75. Yanagawa H, et al: A nationwide incidence survey of Kawasaki disease in 1985-1986 in Japan, *N Engl J Med* 158:1296, 1988.
76. Yanagawa H, et al: Nationwide epidemic of winter of 1985-86, *Lancet* 2:1138, 1986.
77. Yanagawa H, et al: Nationwide surveillance of Kawasaki disease in Japan, 1984 to 1993, *Pediatr Infect Dis J* 14:69, 1995.
78. Yanagawa H, et al: Results of 12 nationwide epidemiological incidence surveys of Kawasaki disease in Japan, *Arch Pediatr Adolesc Med* 149: 779, 1995.

231 Labial Adhesions

Barbara J. Howard

Adhesions of the labia minora, also called *labial fusion, synechia vulvae,* or *agglutination of the labia,* occur commonly in infants and young girls, producing considerable parental concern despite their usual lack of medical significance. What the parents see is a flap of skin formed by the adherence of the labia minora that completely covers all evidence of a vaginal opening. The fear that their daughter may have abnormal sexual anatomy may lead them to ask questions about other problems of the genital area, such as diaper rash, rather than addressing their real concern directly.

The diagnosis of labial adhesions is based entirely on the physical examination. When the labia majora are gently stretched apart, a thin, flat membrane of variable length is seen in the midline. This extends from the clitoris to the posterior fourchette in 70% of cases, the rest being cases of partial coverage.[2] There usually is a small opening near the clitoris through which the urine passes. The vaginal introitus is obscured, but one could demonstrate the space beneath the flap by inserting a small probe through the anterior opening and directing it posteriorly beneath the membrane. This, however, is not necessary once the thin line of adherence (or agglutination) between the two nonrugated, flat labia minora has been identified.

Labial adhesions rarely are present at birth, unlike congenital anomalies of the genitals such as vaginal agenesis, familial posterior labial fusion, or the ambiguous genitalia associated with the adrenogenital syndrome with which labial adhesions sometimes are confused. In adrenogenital syndrome there is no line of demarcation between the clitoral hood and the fused labia as there is with labial adhesions.[14] Imperforate hymen also differs in that it is apparent within the vaginal introitus and the labia are normal.

Occurrence of the adhesions is ascribed to a combination of bacterial inflammation and hypoestrogenization of the labia minora. Commonly the tissue is irritated (usually so mildly as to go unnoticed) through trauma (physical or chemical), infection (e.g. *Candida,* pinworms, bacteria), or poor hygiene, and the medial edges of the labia adhere to each other as they heal. Urine flow may be partially obstructed, resulting in pooling behind the fusion and further irritation, thereby continuing the cycle of inflammation, adhesion, and obstruction. Labial adhesions almost always are found in infants after 2 months of age and may occur at any time up to menarche, irrespective of race. This pattern presumably is caused by the relative immunity to inflammation of epithelium exposed to estrogen, such as that of the newborn under the influence of maternal hormones and that of postmenarchal girls. One of the rare cases found at birth was associated with infection of the infant in utero.[3] Similarly, adhesions are very rare during the reproductive years in females who have normal ovarian function, although they have been seen as a result of herpes simplex type II infection.[5] Capraro and Greenberg[3] reported the average age at diagnosis to be 2½ years, with 56% of their patients younger than 2 years of age and 94% younger than age 6 years. Leung found the peak incidence to be between 13 and 23 months, with no cases after age 5 years.[10] Earlier, Huffman reported the highest incidence to be between ages 2 and 6 years.[3] This shift to an earlier age may be the result of a greater awareness of the condition or perhaps a predisposition to inflammation from the occlusion of the plastic diapers often used today. The lack of cases after age 5 is presumed to be due to improved hygiene because there is no increase in estrogenization yet at that age.[10]

It has been estimated that 10% to 20% of girls have some period of adhesion before 1 year of age.[13] In one series of 93 girls from 3 months to 11 years of age selected for not having been sexually abused, an incidence of 38.9% was found,[4] but 19 of the 35 adhesions were less than 2 mm in length and were detected only because of examination using magnification.[11] Leung found the overall incidence in girls age 12 years and younger to be 1.8%.[9]

An association has been suggested between labial adhesions and sexual abuse, with two retrospective analyses showing that 3% of children referred for sexual abuse had had adhesions.[2] In another study, labial adhesions were the only genital abnormality in 8 of 205 sexually abused girls.[12] Although this is not an increase over the baseline prevalence, because adhesions are thought to be secondary to trauma or infection, their presence should alert clinicians at least to examine the child carefully and to ask about caretaking arrangements and elicit any concerns parents may have about inappropriate handling of the child.

Inspection of the vulvae is recommended during each health maintenance physical examination to check hygiene, monitor sexual development, and detect problems.[15] This also is important for developing a clinical baseline for normal anatomy. With the apparent increase in sexual abuse of children, in whom genital complaints may not be reported, skill in this practice becomes especially important.

Parents may be concerned that the normal self-stimulation of the genitals that starts around 10 months of age in girls and is especially prominent between 18 months and 2½ years of age is damaging to their child. It is helpful to counsel parents routinely about the normality of self-stimulation, particularly when adhesions draw attention to sexual development.[7] An effort must be made to constrain any parental overreaction. On the other hand, masturbation may be a response to genital irritation from infection or to psychological distress, especially from sexual abuse. These situations should be assessed before providing reassurance about masturbation, particularly if it is persistent or has an acute onset.

Only 20% to 38% of girls who have labial adhesions have any symptoms of dysuria, difficulty voiding, or local discomfort,[3] but urinary tract infection occurs in 14% to 57%[10]; therefore, urine culture is indicated. If there is no evidence of obstruction to voiding, repeated urinary tract infection, discomfort, or excessive parental concern, no treatment beyond explanation is needed. Because adhesions completely resolve spontaneously—50% in 6 months, 90% in 12 months, and 100% in 18 months[8]—surgical or mechanical lysis not only is unnecessary in the usual case but also is less effective in the long term; it also is potentially painful and can be psychologically traumatic and costly. Should treatment be indicated or urgently desired by the parents despite counseling, the topical application of estrogen cream (0.1% or 0.01% dienestrol) is effective.[3] Recurrence is rare after this treatment, whereas serious readhesion after mechanical lysis has been noted in 20% to 100% of cases.[1] Separation of the labia is achieved in 90% of cases after 2 weeks of twice-daily estrogen cream treatment applied with gentle pressure to the adhesion line with a swab with gentle traction of the labia laterally.[6] This should be followed by nightly application of the estrogen cream for an additional 1 to 2 weeks. Treatment is considered to have failed if separation does not occur within 8 weeks.[1] Occasionally a repeat course of treatment is needed.[6] Unresponsive cases can be managed by application of 5% xylocaine ointment and gentle teasing apart of the labia with a swab.[6] Several more weeks of application of a bland ointment (e.g., petrolatum), daily bathing, and good hygiene after separation has been established is recommended to ensure sustained labial separation.[3] This should be continued for as long as a year in the case of recurrences. The older child can be taught to apply the cream herself with supervision. Reversible vulvar pigmentation or erythema and/or breast tenderness have been reported in up to one third of children managed with topical estrogen treatment.[2] However, no serious or lasting complications of treatment have been reported.

Urine culture should be performed because 6 of 33 (18.2%) of asymptomatic girls who had labial adhesions had more than 100,000 colonies present on clean-catch urine specimens in contrast to a base rate of infection of 0.8%.[9] None of these had abnormal intravenous pyelogram or voiding cystourethrogram results. Conversely, examination for labial adhesions also is advisable in cases of urinary tract infection in girls. If a urinary tract infection is suspected as either a cause of irritation or a complication of outflow obstruction, urinalysis and culture results will dictate the necessary treatment and follow-up. Although labial adhesions are not known to be associated with congenital anomalies, Capraro and Greenberg[3] found 3 of 50 affected girls to have urinary tract anomalies (all were symptomatic). Nevertheless, further specific gynecological or renal evaluation is not needed unless urinary obstruction, persistent or recurrent urinary tract infection, or any vulvar irritation is present, or unless treatment failure is unexplained.

When to Refer

If topical treatment is ineffective and there are recurrent urinary tract infections or excessive parental concern, then referral to a gynecologist with pediatric skills could be useful. If the clinician suspects child abuse or Munchausen by proxy or is unsure if the labial findings could represent a serious condition such as lichen sclerosis or neoplasm, then prompt referral is indicated.

REFERENCES

1. Ariborg A: Topical oestrogen therapy for labial adhesions in children, *Br J Obstet Gynaecol* 82:424, 1975.
2. Berkowitz CD, Elvik SL, Logan MK: Labial fusion in prepubescent girls: a marker for sexual abuse? *Am J Obstet Gynecol* 156:16, 1987.
3. Capraro VJ, Greenberg H: Adhesions of the labia minora: a study of 50 patients, *Obstet Gynecol* 39:65, 1972.
4. Christensen EH, Oster J: Adhesions of labia minora (synechia vulvae) in childhood, *Acta Paediatr Scand* 60:709, 1971.
5. DeMarco BJ, Crandall RS, Hreshchyshyn MM: Labial agglutination secondary to a herpes simplex II infection, *Am J Obstet Gynecol* 157: 296, 1987.
6. Emans SJH, Goldstein DP: *Pediatric and adolescent gynecology,* ed 3, Boston, 1990, Little, Brown.
7. Howard BJ: One approach to anticipatory guidance of sexuality for pediatricians. In Charney E, editor: *Pediatric update,* New York, 1981, Elsevier-Dutton.
8. Jenkinson SD, MacKinnon AE: Spontaneous separation of fused labia minora in prepubertal girls, *BMJ* 289:160, 1984.
9. Leung AKC, Robson WLM: Labial fusion and asymptomatic bacteriuria, *Eur J Pediatr* 152: 250, 1993.
10. Leung AKC, Robson WLM, Tay-Uyboco J: The incidence of labial fusion in children, *J Paediatr Child Health* 29:235, 1993.
11. McCann J, et al: Genital findings in prepubertal girls selected for nonabuse: a descriptive study, *Pediatrics* 86:428, 1990.
12. Muram D: Child sexual abuse—genital tract findings in prepubertal girls. I. The unaided medical examination, *Am J Obstet Gynecol* 160: 328, 1989.
13. Parsons L, Sommers SC: *Gynecology,* ed 2, Philadelphia, 1978, WB Saunders.
14. Pokorny SF: Prepubertal vulvovaginopathies, *Obstet Gynecol Clin North Am* 1:39, 1992.
15. Williams TS, Callen JP, Owen LG: Vulvar disorders in the prepubertal female, *Pediatr Ann* 15:588, 1986.

232 Leukemias

Barbara L. Asselin

Although many primary care pediatricians only infrequently must diagnose a child as having leukemia, they play a crucial role in the treatment of these diseases. As the primary caregiver, the pediatrician is responsible for ensuring that an accurate diagnosis is made quickly, that appropriate emergency measures are initiated when necessary, and that referral to a pediatric cancer center is expedited. Once uniformly fatal diseases, the childhood leukemias now are more appropriately considered treatable and in many cases curable. However, the aggressive treatment protocols that have brought about the therapeutic successes to date also have resulted in significant acute and long-term toxicities. Pediatric subspecialists are vital members of the health care team that implements these complicated, frequently toxic, multiinstitutional clinical trials. The child's pediatrician follows up on his or her patient not only during the acute stage of treatment but also back home during periods of remission and throughout the cure. With the number of long-term survivors of childhood leukemia increasing, the pediatrician, internist, and subspecialists must be knowledgeable about the late sequelae of antileukemic therapy, alert to their emergence, and familiar with appropriate therapeutic interventions.

EPIDEMIOLOGY

Leukemia is the most common form of malignancy seen in children and the second most common cause of death in children between 5 and 14 years of age. Almost one third of cancer cases in children are a form of leukemia (Fig. 232-1). The incidence of all types of acute leukemia is 45.6 per million for white children compared with 27.8 per million for black children.[66] Each year in the United States approximately 3250 children and adolescents under 20 years of age are diagnosed with leukemia, of which 2400 are acute lymphoblastic leukemia (ALL).[66] Over the past two decades in the United States, an unexplained increase in leukemia rates among children younger than 15 years of age has occurred, with the trend primarily reflecting an increase in ALL incidence during this period. The rates of leukemias other than ALL did not appear to increase from 1977 to 1995.[30,66]

As shown in Fig. 232-2, ALL predominates, accounting for 80% of all cases of childhood leukemia. Childhood ALL has a peak incidence at approximately 4 years of age, and it is more common in boys than in girls. The observation that acute leukemia is more common in whites than in other races is based primarily on the increased peak incidence of ALL in white children between 3 and 5 years of age. In contrast to ALL, acute nonlymphoid leukemia (ANLL) in the United States shows no marked age peak.

TYPES OF LEUKEMIA

The leukemia syndromes seen in childhood can be classified as acute, chronic, congenital, and preleukemia. Acute leukemias are characterized by a predominance of immature hematopoietic precursors ("blasts") in the bone marrow (by definition, more than 25% of nucleated cells must be blasts) and a fulminant natural course, resulting in death within months unless effective treatment is instituted. In the chronic leukemias, the mature bone marrow elements hyperproliferate, resulting in an insidious onset of symptoms over months. Even without treatment patients can survive for months to years after the diagnosis of these chronic diseases. Congenital leukemia refers to conditions diagnosed in the first 4 weeks of life; they are discussed in more detail at the end of this chapter. The myeloproliferative and myelodysplastic syndromes are characterized by unexplained anemia, neutropenia, or thrombocytopenia and distorted maturation of bone marrow hematopoietic elements. These conditions, commonly referred to as *preleukemia* because of their frequent evolution into acute leukemia, are uncommon among children compared with adults.

The leukemias also are classified according to the predominant cell lines involved. This classification broadly divides the acute leukemias into lymphoblastic (ALL) and nonlymphoid forms (ANLL). Acute myelogenous leukemia (AML) is the most common subtype of childhood ANLL, followed by myelomonocytic leukemia (AMML), monocytic leukemia (AMOL), acute promyelocytic leukemia (APML), megakaryocytic leukemia, and erythrocytic leukemia. Because of recent technological advances in studies of lineage-specific immunological surface markers and gene rearrangements, very few cases are classified as undifferentiated leukemia (AUL). The chronic leukemias also can be divided into lymphocytic and myelogenous forms. Among children, chronic myelogenous leukemia (CML) is seen in 3% to 5% of patients diagnosed as having leukemia (see Fig. 232-2). Chronic lymphocytic leukemia (CLL) is extremely rare.

LEUKEMOGENESIS

Normal cell growth is controlled by a complex series of events involving growth factors that are produced by the cell itself, produced by other cells, or produced by cells in other tissues. Leukemia is a disorder of growth and proliferation in

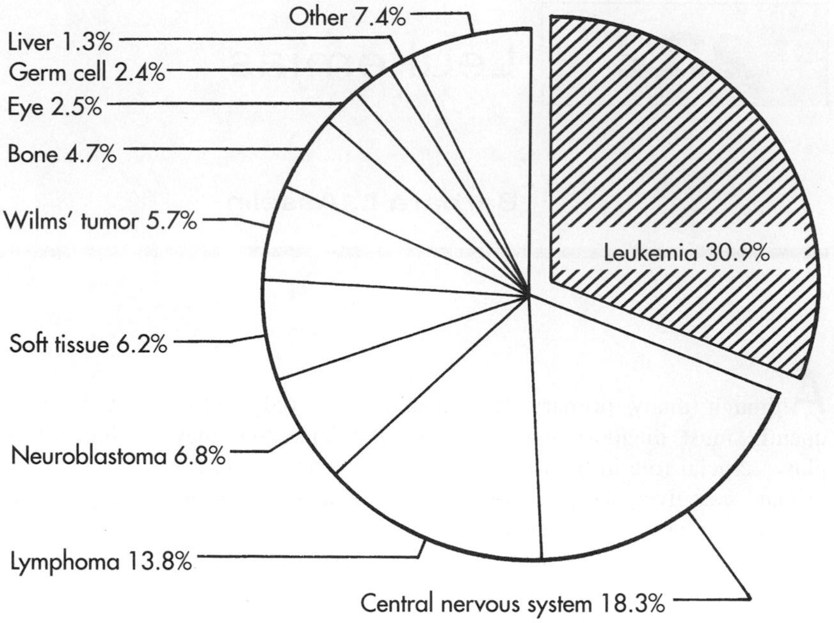

Other 7.4%
Liver 1.3%
Germ cell 2.4%
Eye 2.5%
Bone 4.7%
Wilms' tumor 5.7%
Leukemia 30.9%
Soft tissue 6.2%
Neuroblastoma 6.8%
Lymphoma 13.8%
Central nervous system 18.3%

Fig. 232-1 Major forms of cancer in American white children.

(Modified from Altman AJ, Schwartz AD: *Malignant diseases of infancy, childhood and adolescence,* ed 3, Philadelphia, 1983, WB Saunders.)

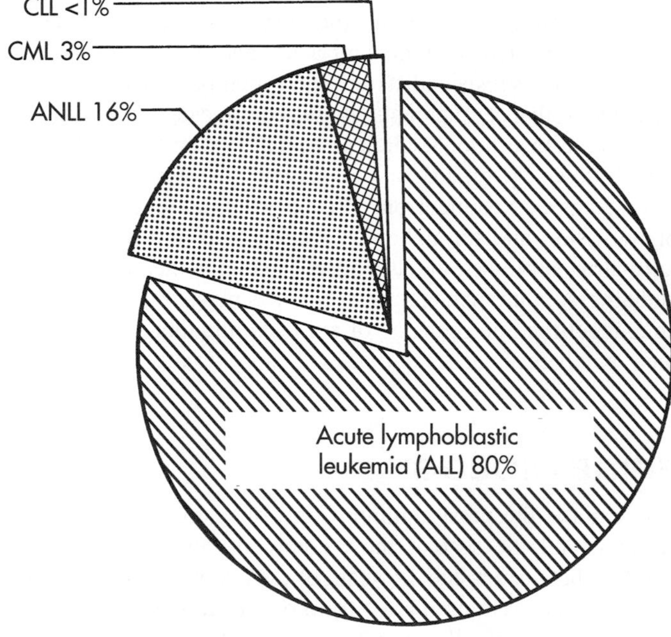

Fig. 232-2 The leukemias of childhood. *ANLL,* Acute nonlymphoid leukemia; *CML,* chronic myelogenous leukemia; *CLL,* chronic lymphocytic leukemia.

(From Nathan DG, Oski FA: *Hematology of infancy and childhood,* ed 3, Philadelphia, 1987, WB Saunders.)

which one or more of these growth-regulating events goes awry within a hematopoietic cell.[28]

The exact cause of leukemia is unknown. A number of contributing factors and possible predisposing conditions have been described, including genetic predisposition, immunodeficiency states, viruses, and environmental exposures.[16,29,63] Our current understanding of the complicated nature of normal cellular proliferation and differentiation processes suggests that the etiology of leukemia is complex, resulting from a series of multifactorial events involving "oncogenes," growth factors, and environmental conditions.

Clonal Expansion Theory

It is believed that most cases of leukemia result from a single damaged precursor cell that can self-replicate but that cannot undergo further differentiation. Because these cells do not stop dividing, the burden of leukemic cells increases. The disease apparently is a manifestation of the expansion of a single clone of cells. The clonal origin of leukemia is demonstrated best by studies involving the isoenzymes of glucose-6-phosphate dehydrogenase (G6PD) and by cytogenetics.[4,19]

Leukemic Clusters

Numerous reports of "leukemic time-space clusters" have attracted intense epidemiological study. A true leukemic cluster would suggest that a common etiological factor or horizontal transmission of an infectious agent played a role in the development of leukemia. However, the results of intense study suggest that, except for Nagasaki and Hiroshima,[6] the reports of leukemia epidemics can be explained purely by

BOX 232-1

FACTORS ASSOCIATED WITH INCREASED RISK FOR CHILDHOOD LEUKEMIA

Familial Predisposition
Twin of a patient with leukemia
Sibling of a patient with leukemia

Genetic Factors
Down syndrome
Fanconi's anemia
Bloom syndrome
Ataxia telangiectasia
Congenital hypogammaglobulinemia
Wiskott-Aldrich syndrome
Neurofibromatosis
Poland's syndrome
Klinefelter's syndrome
Schwachman syndrome

Environmental Exposure
Viral infection
Ionizing radiation (atomic bomb and nuclear accidents)
Therapeutic radiation (ankylosing spondylitis, thymic enlargement)
Prenatal diagnostic radiation exposure
Certain drugs (benzene, alkylating agents)

Modified from Neglia JP, Robinson LL: *Pediatr Clin North Am* 35:675, 1988.

chance.[1] Inherent in such epidemiological studies is the difficulty in appropriately defining the population at risk, determining the likely timing of key exposures or mutational events, and identifying all the potential confounding events that could influence the outcome.

Etiology (Box 232-1)

Familial predisposition and genetic factors. The occurrence of familial leukemia, the concordance of leukemia in monozygotic twins, and the increased incidence of leukemia in patients who have certain constitutional chromosomal abnormalities are well-documented observations suggesting that genetic factors play an important role in leukemogenesis.[32] It is hypothesized that the preexisting chromosomal defect in patients who have constitutional chromosomal abnormalities makes them more susceptible than normal to extrinsic environmental leukemogenic factors. The common finding of one or more chromosomal abnormalities in the leukemia cells of patients is further evidence of the role genetic events play in the development of leukemia.[61,73]

Molecular studies of identical twins suggest a prenatal origin for acute leukemia, both lymphoid and myeloid subtypes. Most recently, investigators have demonstrated the presence of clonotypic or patient-specific leukemia gene sequences in blood collected on Guthrie Cards at birth, thus confirming the prenatal origin of these leukemias.[25,72] It is postulated that some postnatal exposures or events are required to promote clonal expansion and progression of the fetal clone to become malignant.[22]

Patients who have congenital immune deficiency diseases (e.g., Wiskott-Aldrich syndrome, ataxia telangiectasia, and congenital hypogammaglobulinemia) all have an increased risk of developing lymphoid malignancy.[32,21] In addition, chronic therapy with immunosuppressive drugs, including long-term use of corticosteroids alone, has been associated with an increased risk of lymphoid malignancy.[50] The increased risk is thought to represent a breakdown in normal host "immune surveillance," allowing proliferation of malignant clones.

Environmental exposure. Certain viruses are known to cause leukemia in animal models, but the relationship of the leukemia that occurs in these species to human leukemia is uncertain. The role of retrovirus in human leukemogenesis was demonstrated by the association between human T-cell leukemia virus (HTLV-1) and adult T-cell leukemia.[7] Epidemiological studies have failed to show a link between exposure to cats or feline leukemia virus and the development of leukemia in humans. Epstein-Barr virus (EBV) infection, which causes infectious mononucleosis in humans, also is associated clearly with the African-type Burkitt's lymphoma. Although a link has not yet been demonstrated, EBV infection may be associated with B-cell leukemia (i.e., Burkitt's lymphoma with bone marrow involvement).

The leukemogenic potential in humans of exposure to ionizing radiation is well demonstrated by the following observations: (1) in the 1930s, radiologists had a ninefold greater incidence of leukemia than did physicians and nonradiologists[42]; (2) survivors of the 1945 atomic bomb explosions in Hiroshima and Nagasaki have a 10 to 20 times greater risk of developing leukemia[6];(3) individuals who have been treated with radiation for ankylosing spondylitis, thymic enlargement, and tinea capitis have a high incidence of leukemia[8]; and (4) children exposed to diagnostic radiation in utero have an increased risk of all childhood cancers.[31]

Controversy persists regarding the diagnostic use of radiation after birth and the development of human leukemia. Diagnostic use of ultrasonography, either before or after birth, has not been associated with an increased risk of childhood leukemia.

Investigations of adult ANLL have provided considerable information about exposure to chemical carcinogens (e.g., solvents and petroleum products) associated with an increased risk of leukemia. Partly because of the small number of cases of leukemia among children relative to adults, a link between chemical exposure and childhood leukemia has not been demonstrated. A study completed by the Children's Cancer Study Group suggests that an environmental etiological component may be involved in childhood disease similar to that found in adult cases of ANLL.[60]

A number of studies have shown a link between secondary leukemogenesis and chemotherapy, especially alkylating agents, with or without radiation treatment. For example, acute leukemia (usually AML) has been observed in patients who have Hodgkin's disease who received cyclophosphamide or nitrogen mustard as part of therapy, usually with concomitant radiation treatments,[3] or following epipodophyllotoxin treatment for leukemias and solid tumors.[52]

Other factors studied for possible association with leukemia include exposure to electromagnetic fields, herbicides and pesticides, and maternal use of alcohol, contraceptives, diethylstilbestrol (DES), or cigarettes. Definitive links between these factors and the risk of childhood leukemia have not been confirmed.[46]

CLASSIFICATION

The childhood leukemias, shown in Fig. 232-2, are actually a very heterogeneous group of disorders that can be subclassified in terms of the level of differentiation (acute versus chronic, mature versus immature) and the lineage (lymphoid versus myeloid) of the leukemogenic clone. Traditional morphological and cytochemistry techniques can help differentiate between the many subtypes of nonlymphoid leukemias but are not useful in differentiating the lymphoid subtypes. Normal hematopoietic cells undergo changes in expression of cell surface markers as they mature from stem cells into cells of a distinct lineage. The pattern of expression of these antigens, called *immunophenotype,* is lineage-specific and stage-specific. Cell surface marker expression has been helpful in differentiating AML from ALL and defining the stage of maturation of the leukemic clone and thus the subtype.[53] Newer approaches involving cytogenetic[56] and gene rearrangement[20] studies also have been used.

Immunophenotype studies of cell surface markers have defined four subsets of ALL (Table 232-1). The majority of cases of ALL are of immature B-cell lineage expressing the common ALL antigen called *CALLA* or *CD10.* These immunological subtypes of ALL are associated with specific cytogenetic findings and clinical differences (see Table 232-1). Improvements in cytogenetic and molecular technologies now make it possible to identify abnormalities in chromosome number or structure in more than 90% of cases of ALL. The most common abnormality, hyperdiploidy, is associated with a good prognosis. This is one example of how the ability to distinguish these leukemic cells, or blasts, using various cytological criteria is important therapeutically and prognostically (see the discussion of prognostic factors on p. 1611).

The French-American-British (FAB) system of classification based primarily on morphological and cytochemistry criteria defines seven subtypes of ANLL, M_1 through M_7 (see Table 232-1). The presence of myeloperoxidase in the blasts usually indicates leukemia of myelocytic origin. Nonspecific enolase-positive blasts usually indicate monocytic differentiation. Immunophenotype based on cell surface markers like in ALL are useful in establishing the specific diagnosis and degree of maturation of the leukemic clone. The identification of megakaryocyte-specific markers has been critical to the recognition of megakaryocytic leukemias as a subtype of AML in children since blast morphology and cytochemistry is indistinguishable from ALL. A number of cytogenetic abnormalities are seen in AML, but three that are pathognomonic for specific FAB subtypes are detailed in Table 232-1.

A subset of cases of leukemia have been found in which the blast cells express both lymphoid and myeloid markers or ALLs that coexpress both B- and T-cell markers.[55] The clinical significance of such "lineage infidelity" remains unclear but in most cases is treated as the higher-risk diagnosis. Rare cases of acute leukemia are biphenotypic with distinct populations of cells that exhibit characteristics of both and lymphoblasts and myeloblasts.[44]

CLINICAL MANIFESTATIONS

Presenting Signs and Symptoms

Leukemia is a process of uncontrolled proliferation of immature hematopoietic cells that results in suppression of normal hematopoiesis and infiltration of extramedullary organs. The common presenting signs and symptoms reflect the degree of bone marrow compromise, the extent and location of leukemic cell infiltration, and the general systemic effects of these processes. In most cases the presenting complaints have been present a few days, a few weeks, or, more rarely, even months. The incidence of presenting complaints among children who have ALL compared with those who have ANLL are shown in Table 232-2.

Fever is the most common feature. In most patients it is caused by the leukemia itself rather than by infection. Pallor, fatigue, petechiae, purpura, and anorexia often are present. Significant weight loss is rare. Bone pain, lymphadenopathy, hepatomegaly, and splenomegaly are more common with ALL than with ANLL. Young children who have bone pain in the lower extremities may limp or refuse to walk.

Laboratory Findings

Mild anemia and mild thrombocytopenia are common hematological abnormalities (see Table 232-2). The white blood count (WBC) may be normal, decreased, or increased. Blasts frequently, but not always, are found in the peripheral blood smear.

Other laboratory studies frequently are abnormal in children newly diagnosed with acute leukemia. In addition to hyperuricemia, serum levels of calcium, potassium, phosphate, and lactic dehydrogenase may be elevated. This constellation of abnormalities often is referred to as *tumor lysis syndrome.* The severity of these abnormalities is thought to reflect the total leukemic cell burden and the excessive production and rapid destruction of leukemia cells. These abnormalities are particularly problematical in patients who have a high initial WBC and extensive lymphadenopathy and hepatosplenomegaly. Most patients have some extramedullary disease at the time of diagnosis. An anterior mediastinal mass is present in 5% to 10% of patients newly diagnosed with ALL, making a chest roentgenogram crucial in the initial evaluation. Evidence of leukemic infiltration of the periosteum and bone often can be seen on the roentgenogram (including subperiosteal new bone formation, transverse metaphyseal radiolucent bands, osteolytic lesions, diffuse demineralization, and growth arrest lines) even in patients who have no complaints of bone pain.

Special Presentations

Central nervous system disease. The most common site of clinically apparent extramedullary leukemia is the central nervous system (CNS); this type is present in as many as 20% of patients at the time of diagnosis. Children who have CNS leukemia most often have increased intracranial pressure (causing vomiting, headache, lethargy, and

Table 232-1 Classification of Acute Leukemias

Acute Lymphoblastic Leukemia							
			Cytochemistry		Immunophenotype	Frequent Cytogenetic Abnormalities	
Common Name	**Frequency**	**Morphology**	**MP**	**TdT**	**All HLA-DR+**		**Clinical Features**
Early pre-B cell	70%	L1 or L2	(–)	+	+ CD 10, 19, 20	Hyperdiploid, t(12;21), t(11;19)	Peak incidence age 2-5 yr Infants <1 yr usually CD 10–, t(4:11), poor prognosis
Pre-B cell	15%	L1 or L2	(–)	+	+/– CD 10, 19, 20 + clg	t(1;19)	Clinically indistinguishable from early pre-B cell May carry worse prognosis
T cell	12%	L1 or L2	(–)	+	+ CD 2, 3, 7	TCR gene rearrangement t(11;14), t(7;9)	More common in boys, teens, with mediastinal mass, bulky adenopathy, organomegaly, and high WBC
Mature B cell	2%	L3	(–)	(+)	+ slg	Pathognomonic t(8;14), t(2;8) or t(8;22)	Clinically indistinguishable from Burkitt's lymphoma with marrow involvement Treated very differently than ALL

Acute Nonlymphoid Leukemia								
			Cytochemistry				Frequent Cytogenetic Abnormalities	
Common Name (Subtype)	**Frequency**	**Morphology**	**MP**	**NSE**	**Other**	**Immunophenotype**		**Clinical Features**
AML without maturation (M_1)	24%	>90% myeloblasts Auer rods	+	(–)		+ CD 15, 33, 34 + HLA-DR		
AML with maturation (M_2)	23%	30%-90% blasts Auer rods	+	(–)		+ CD 15, 33, 34 + HLA-DR	Pathognomonic t(8;21)	
Promyelocytic (M_3)	5%	Hypergranular promyelocyte Many Auer rods	+	(–)		+ CD 11, 13, 34 (–) HLA-DR	Pathognomonic t(15;17)	Often DIC at diagnosis Trans-retinoic acid part of Rx
Myelomonocytic (M_4)	27%		+	+		+ CD 11, 13, 14, 15, 33, 34		Common in children <2 yr
Monocytic (M_5)	10%	>30% myeloblasts >30% monoblasts	(–)	+		+ CD 11, 13, 14, 15, 33, 34		Common in children <2 yr ?Worse prognosis
Erythroleukemia (M_6)	2%	>80% monoblasts	(–)	(–)	Pas +	+ CD 13, 33, 34 + glycophorin		Very rare in children
Megakaryocytic (M_7)	7%	>30% megakaryoblasts, cytoplasmic blebs, myelofibrosis	(–)	(–)	Plat PO +	+ CD 13, 33, 34 + CD 41, 42, 61	t(1;22)	Most common in children with Down syndrome Rare in teens, adults

MP, Myeloperoxidase stain; *NSE,* nonspecific esterase stain; *Pas,* periodic acid-Schiff stain; *Plat,* platelet; *PO,* peroxidase.

Table 232-2 Clinical and Laboratory Features in the Diagnosis of Leukemia

Feature	Percentage of All Children with ALL*	Percentage of All Children with ANLL†
Clinical		
Fever	61	34
Pallor	55	25
Bleeding (i.e., petechiae or purpura)	48	33
Anorexia or weight loss	33	22
Fatigue, malaise	30	19
Bone or joint pain	38	18
Lymphadenopathy	50	14
Hepatosplenomegaly	68	55
Swollen gingivae	—	8
Respiratory symptoms (i.e., sore throat, cough)	—	41
Recurrent infection	—	3
Neurological symptoms	3	10
Laboratory		
Leukocyte count (mm^3)		
<10,000	53	39
10,000-49,000	30	29
>50,000	17	32
Hemoglobin (g/dl)		
<7	43	41
7-11	45	48
>11	12	11
Platelet count (mm^3)		
<20,000	28	15
20,000-99,000	47	67
>100,000	25	18
Coagulopathy	—	17

*Miller DR: *Pediatr Clin North Am* 27:269, 1980.
†Choi SR, Simone JV: *Med Pediatr Oncol* 2:119, 1976.

papilledema); occasionally, cranial nerve palsies; and, in rare cases, meningeal signs. Focal signs related to parenchymal involvement include hemiparesis, hemisensory losses, and seizure activity. Children under age 2 and those who have T-cell ALL or monoblastic subtypes of ANLL have a higher incidence of CNS leukemia. Generally, cord compression by epidural leukemic infiltrates is rare; it is more common in AML than in ALL.

Chloromas. Chloromas are solid tumor collections of immature myeloid cells that can occur in ANLL patients. These tumors frequently involve periosteal and epidural regions of the head and neck but can occur anywhere on the body. A rare chloroma has been reported to occur months or years before systemic signs of leukemia.

Testicular leukemia. Although more commonly reported in patients who have ALL, leukemic involvement of the testes in boys who have ANLL has been reported. Testicular leukemia manifests with painless enlargement of one or both testes. Although rarely reported as an initial manifestation of ALL (fewer than 5% of patients) or ANLL, it may be the first identifiable site of the recurrence of leukemia (15% of patients).

T-cell leukemia. T-cell ALL is characterized by several distinctive clinical features. It occurs more often in older boys who have a high WBC and often a mediastinal mass; these patients have a higher incidence of CNS leukemia. They also frequently have massive generalized lymphadenopathy and hepatosplenomegaly. This constellation of bulky infiltration of extramedullary sites historically has been referred to as "lymphomatous presentation" of leukemia.

Specific clinical features of ANLL subtypes. Acute promyelocytic leukemia (M_3 subtype) is associated more often with a spontaneous bleeding disorder than are the other variants of ANLL. Bleeding is the result of disseminated intravascular coagulation (DIC) and secondary fibrinolysis triggered by a substance contained within the cytoplasmic granules of the leukemic cells. Acute monoblastic leukemia (M_4 and M_5 subtypes) occurs at a younger age and is characterized by extensive extramedullary involvement at diagnosis, CNS involvement, leukemia cutis, lymphadenopathy, gingival hypertrophy, chloromas, DIC, an elevated WBC, and an elevated serum muramidase. The M_7 morphological subtype of ANLL, or acute megakaryocytic leukemia, is particularly common in children who have Down syndrome. The biopsy specimen usually shows hypocellularity with myelofibrosis.

Preleukemia. Children who have preleukemia typically have fewer than 25% blasts in the bone marrow, circulating blasts, megaloblastosis, chromosomal abnormalities, and quantitative abnormalities of at least two of the three blood cell lines. These patients may turn out to have juvenile CML, chronic myelomonocytic leukemia, or monosomy 7 syndrome, which can precede the diagnosis of ANLL.

Diagnosis and Differential Diagnosis

The challenge for the physician in diagnosing pediatric leukemias is not that the symptoms are necessarily subtle, but that subtle differences exist between the symptoms of leukemia and those of more common illnesses or infectious conditions seen in children. Box 232-2 lists the most common malignant and nonmalignant conditions that may masquerade as leukemia. Once suspicion is aroused that a patient may have leukemia, the diagnosis must be confirmed by bone marrow aspiration and the type of leukemia determined. Although leukemic cells may be identified in the peripheral blood of many patients at the time of diagnosis, morphological assessment of these cells may be misleading. Thus, examination of the bone marrow is mandatory to diagnose leukemia. Bone marrow aspirate usually provides sufficient material for diagnosis. Occasionally, however, a bone marrow biopsy may be required, particularly in patients who have pancytopenia, in which case bone marrow failure must be excluded.

Leukemias must be differentiated from a variety of infectious illnesses. Patients who have these infectious conditions may have fevers, rash, generalized lymphadenopathy, splenomegaly, peripheral blood lymphocytosis, and less frequently, thrombocytopenia or immunohemolytic anemia. Usually, these diseases can be differentiated in terms of the

BOX 232-2

DIFFERENTIAL DIAGNOSIS OF CHILDHOOD ACUTE LEUKEMIA

Nonmalignant Conditions
Juvenile rheumatoid arthritis
Systemic lupus erythematosus
Infectious mononucleosis
Idiopathic thrombocytopenic purpura
Pertussis, parapertussis
Aplastic anemia
Acute benign infectious lymphocytosis
Leukemoid reaction (more common in ANLL)
Bacterial sepsis with or without coagulopathy (more common in ANLL)
Osteomyelitis

Malignancies
Neuroblastoma
Lymphoma (especially if mediastinal mass, massive adenopathy, and organomegaly are present)
Retinoblastoma
Rhabdomyosarcoma
Ewing's sarcoma
Chronic myelogenous leukemia

Unusual Presentations
Hypereosinophilic syndrome
Cord compression or cauda equina syndrome
Eosinophilic granuloma
Parenchymal brain lesion

morphological appearance of reactive lymphocytes on the peripheral blood smear. Some conditions can be associated with a leukemoid reaction characterized by a reactive leukocytosis (WBC of 50,000 cells/mm^3 or higher), with an orderly progression of immature myeloid cells and occasional nucleated red blood cells (RBCs). Ordinarily, with idiopathic thrombocytopenic purpura, children do not have splenomegaly, anemia, or neutropenia. Juvenile rheumatoid arthritis (JRA) and systemic lupus erythematosus (SLE) may be confused with ALL because of the common complaints of fever, anemia, malaise, and painful, swollen joints. Because there is no reliable, definitive laboratory test for JRA or SLE, bone marrow aspiration may be necessary to exclude leukemia. The absence of lymphadenopathy and hepatosplenomegaly is important in diagnosing aplastic anemia. If the bone marrow aspirate is hypocellular, the marrow should be biopsied. Several pediatric malignancies may show bone marrow involvement, including neuroblastoma, lymphoma, rhabdomyosarcoma, and Ewing's sarcoma. Additional laboratory and clinical evaluation may be necessary (e.g., urinary catecholamine determination, radiological imaging) to exclude these malignancies.

Normal bone marrow contains fewer than 5% blast cells. By definition, the diagnosis of acute leukemia is confirmed when more than 25% of the nucleated cells in the marrow are blasts; typically, 90% or more of the cells in the bone marrow are blast cells. The presence of 5% to 25% blast cells in the marrow suggests several diagnostic possibilities, including non-Hodgkin's lymphoma with marrow involvement, preleukemia or myelodysplastic syndromes, chronic myelogenous leukemia, or acute monoblastic leukemia, which can manifest primarily with extramedullary disease.

As described under the discussion of classification (see p. 1608), the definitive diagnosis of specific leukemic cell type is based on review of the morphological appearance of the blast cells, use of histochemical stains (e.g., myeloperoxidase and nonspecific esterases), enzymatic analysis, immunophenotyping, and cytogenetic analysis. These sophisticated techniques are important in establishing the specific leukemic cell type. The specific immunophenotype and presence of cytogenetic abnormalities, translocations, and gene rearrangements are crucial to establish the correct diagnosis and determine appropriate therapy. It is essential, therefore, that the bone marrow aspiration or biopsy be performed in a center where cellular differentiation techniques are performed routinely.

TREATMENT

The goal of any antileukemic therapy is to eradicate the invading leukemic cells and their progenitors while preserving the expression of normal blood cell progenitors. Great strides have been made toward this goal, as evaluation, primary combination chemotherapy, bone marrow transplantation, treatment alternatives for patients who relapse, and supportive care have become more sophisticated.

Prognostic Factors

Interest in prognostic factors arose in the late 1970s as therapy became successful in most patients who had ALL. Pediatric oncologists began looking for common features among groups of patients who did well compared with patients whose disease relapsed. Through retrospective analysis of disease-free survival, certain features present at the time of diagnosis of ALL were identified that were useful in predicting which patients had a good, a fair, or a poor prognosis.

Prognostic factors are useful because they allow physicians to devise "tailored therapy," or therapy that is altered for a patient or group of patients according to the clinical features of the disease and whether it is associated with a higher or lower risk of relapse. If therapy is adequate, the bad prognostic factor no longer predicts a poor outcome but rather identifies patients who need aggressive therapy. A characteristic identified in a group of patients treated one way may not have the same significance if a different treatment is used. Thus, "good risk" patients are treated less aggressively in an attempt to minimize toxicity; "poor risk" patients get more aggressive therapy to better control the disease.

In the treatment of ALL, the initial WBC and the patient's age at diagnosis have been the two most reliable indicators of prognosis, both for the duration of remission and survival.[65] Children who are very young at diagnosis (under 2 years of age) or older (over 10 years of age) have a relatively poor prognosis compared with those in the intermediate age group.[65] The worst prognosis is for infants under 1 year of age. The presence of the Philadelphia chromosome consistently has been associated with a poor outcome among many study groups. Other clinical features that have been correlated with the prognosis include gender, race, degree of organomegaly and lymphadenopathy, presence or absence of a mediastinal mass, cytogenetic features, initial hemoglobin levels, initial platelet count, cell subtype, immunophenotype, immunoglobulin levels at diagnosis, the presence or absence of CNS leukemia at diagnosis, early bone marrow response, and human leukocyte antigen (HLA) type. Because the prognostic importance is not reproducible among different study groups, the value of these variables remains controversial.

Because only recently have more than one third of patients who have ANLL survived long term, prognostic factors in ANLL are defined less clearly than in ALL. A variety of clinical features are being examined as possibly important prognostic factors, including cytogenetic features, day-14 bone marrow response, the presence of Auer rods in affected cells, the blast cells' immune phenotype, in vitro growth characteristics, and in vitro response to chemotherapy. The factors most investigators accept as being associated with an unfavorable outcome are a WBC over 100,000 cells/mm^3, monoblastic leukemia in infants, monosomy 7 karyotype, and presentation with a preleukemia syndrome.

Death from CML usually occurs within months of the acceleration phase; therefore, the major determinant of survival is the duration of the chronic phase. One study found peripheral blood and bone marrow blast counts at presentation to be correlated with survival.[14] The juvenile form of CML is notable for an extremely poor prognosis, with a median survival of less than 9 months from the time of diagnosis.

Minimal residual disease. Traditional morphological definitions of remission are neither sensitive nor specific for leukemic progenitors. Investigations of "response to therapy" as a potential prognostic factor have resulted in development of methods for the detection of minimal residual disease.[54] Using leukemia-associated immunophenotypes,[12] fluorescence in-situ hybridization (FISH) techniques[39] or polymerase chain reaction (PCR)[9] for amplification of DNA makes it possible to identify as few as 1 leukemic cell per 104 to 106 normal cells. Development of these highly sensitive methods for the detection of rare residual cells that may be resistant to chemotherapy is of great importance to predict and eventually prevent relapse. Longitudinal studies of assays for minimal residual disease, and the significance of residual malignant cells in terms of prediction of the outcome of treatment are under way as part of the clinical trials in all forms of leukemia.

Acute Management

Initial evaluation and referral. Diagnostic evaluation of a child suspected of having leukemia has become more complex, requiring advanced laboratory techniques to perform appropriate cytogenetic, immunological, and biochemical assays. The problems and complications in a child undergoing leukemia therapy often are complex, requiring expert supportive care. A higher death rate has been reported in patients who have ALL and were treated outside of a children's cancer center without a standard protocol.[43] For these reasons and because of the intensity of current regimens, children suspected of having one of the leukemias should be referred for diagnostic testing and treatment to pediatric cancer centers that use cooperative group protocols.

The goal of initial management, often before the diagnosis has been confirmed, is to ensure that the patient does not require urgent medical intervention before transfer to another center. The major clinical problems needing to be addressed by the primary care physician and suggested emergency interventions are listed in Box 232-3. Many of these problems can be excluded as emergencies by a careful history, physical examination, and review of the complete blood count (CBC). Very few patients require specific intervention before transfer to a pediatric oncology center. For most patients, initial management involves consultation with a pediatric oncologist, referral to a pediatric oncology center, and admission to the hospital. Admission to the hospital can be helpful in facilitating the child's evaluation and the necessary diagnostic tests, stabilizing the metabolic status, starting chemotherapy, beginning patient and parent education, and building the foundation for long-term relationships between the family and health care providers. A common exception to this is the patient with CML in the chronic phase at diagnosis, who often can be treated as an outpatient if he or she is medically stable.

The primary care physician plays a vital role in ensuring a smooth transition by preparing the child and family for what may lie ahead. This includes apprising them of the facts in a positive manner early on—that is, that this may be a serious illness and that testing is important to determine the problem so that appropriate treatment can be started, emphasizing the need to enlist the help of other pediatric specialists. The primary physician can facilitate the transition by conveying information about previous displays of coping skills by the patient and family to the consulting physician. Follow-up communication between the referring physician, consulting physician, and family is essential in establishing and maintaining a strong patient-family-physician relationship.

Supportive Care

Great strides in supportive care, including transfusion therapy, better infection control, and frequent use of indwelling central venous catheters, have contributed immensely to the reduction in morbidity and mortality. The specific guidelines followed (i.e., choice of antibiotics, indwelling catheter care, isolation procedures, transfusion indications) may vary among institutions, based partly on the previous experience of the institution or investigators.

Blood product support. Myelosuppression, with resultant anemia, thrombocytopenia, and neutropenia, often is observed in these patients secondary to leukemia or chemotherapy-induced bone marrow hypoplasia or both. Irradiation of blood products has prevented graft-versus-host disease in patients who have had severe bone marrow depression and immune suppression. Administration of cytomegalovirus (CMV)-negative blood products to patients who have negative CMV antibody titers has decreased the incidence of transfusion-related CMV infection. More sophisticated techniques to test donor blood for evidence of infection such as hepatitis B, non-A, non-B hepatitis, and human immuno-

BOX 232-3

APPROACH TO ACUTE MANAGEMENT OF LEUKEMIA

A. Initial evaluation
History—Fatigue, malaise, anorexia, irritability, fever, bone pain, mouth sores
Physical examination—Pallor, petechiae, purpura, fever, lymphadenopathy, hepatosplenomegaly, respiratory distress, neurological abnormalities
Laboratory—Complete blood count with differential and platelet count, abnormal results of one or more cell lines
B. Suspicion of leukemia as a possible diagnosis and potential emergency interventions

Findings	Management
1. Temperature over 100.4° F (38° C), neutrophil count <500; symptoms of infection	Blood culture, antibiotics
2. Bleeding symptoms	Start intravenous unit for access and delivery of a fluid bolus, transfuse platelets, red cells, or plasma
3. Respiratory distress	Chest roentgenogram, oxygen
4. WBC >100,000	Blood urea nitrogen and creatinine, urate, serum potassium, serum calcium, serum phosphate, chest roentgenogram, start intravenous unit for access and delivery of a fluid bolus

C. Refer patient to a pediatric oncology center
Consult with a pediatric oncologist
Arrange for transfer of patient to the pediatric oncology center
Prepare patient and family for what to expect when they get there

deficiency virus (HIV) have reduced but not eradicated transfusion-transmitted infections.

Unless the anemia is rapid in onset (e.g., because of blood loss or hemolysis), RBC transfusion is not necessary until the hematocrit is 25 or less. Platelets generally are transfused when the platelet count falls below 20,000 cells/mm^3; use of "prophylactic" platelet transfusion when platelet counts are higher remains controversial. Indications for platelet transfusion in a patient who has thrombocytopenia, other than absolute platelet count, include fresh bleeding, fever, infection, or anticipated protracted thrombocytopenia as a result of therapy.

Granulocyte transfusions rarely are used. Their value generally is limited to treating patients who have severe neutropenia with proven gram-negative sepsis or a perirectal abscess that does not respond to appropriate antibiotics. In addition to the risk of transmission of infection, white blood cell transfusions frequently are associated with the uncomfortable side effects of fever, rigors, and allergic reactions, caused by sensitization to foreign leukocyte proteins.

Infection. Infectious complications are the most common cause of morbidity and mortality in leukemia patients, second only to relapse of leukemia. Leukemia patients who are undergoing combination chemotherapy should be considered immunocompromised hosts. Neutropenia, which can result from chemotherapy-induced bone marrow hypoplasia, contributes to an increased susceptibility to bacterial and fungal infections. In the future, strategies now being tested, including the use of growth factors and recently developed antibiotics, may reduce infectious complications significantly.

Any febrile patient whose absolute neutrophil count (ANC) is below 500 cells/mm^3 must be considered septic.*† Cultures should be obtained promptly, and the patient should be started immediately on intravenous (IV) broad-spectrum antibiotics. Because bowel, respiratory, and skin organisms commonly are identified, antibiotics that cover these gram-negative and gram-positive bacteria are used (see Chapter 31, Antimicrobial Therapy). Infections among patients who have fever and neutropenia presumably are bacterial, although specific etiological agents usually are not found. Prophylactic oral antibiotics have not proved useful. *Candida* and *Aspergillus* organisms are the major fungal pathogens reported. Prophylactic oral antifungal agents have not proved effective in preventing invasive disease. Amphotericin B is the treatment of choice for such fungal infections. Thus, patients who have neutropenia who remain febrile after 3 to 7 days of treatment with broad-spectrum antibiotics usually are treated empirically with amphotericin B, even before a definitive diagnosis of fungal disease is made.

Viral infections occur frequently in patients who have leukemia, but rarely is specific therapy indicated. Before the routine use of varicella-zoster immunoglobulin and acyclovir, chickenpox often was complicated by pneumonitis, hepatitis, encephalitis, or even death. Acyclovir particularly has contributed to a notable decline in morbidity and mortality from varicella-zoster, herpes zoster, and herpes simplex infections.

*A febrile patient is one whose oral, axillary, or tympanic membrane temperature is greater than 100.4° F (38° C); the temperature should not be taken rectally in leukemia patients.

†The ANC can be found using this formula: ANC = WBC × (% neutrophils + % bands.)

Pneumocystis carinii is another organism found to cause severe, often fatal interstitial pneumonitis in children receiving multiagent chemotherapy. Trimethoprim-sulfamethoxazole prophylaxis has been shown to reduce the incidence of *P. carinii* infections in the immunocompromised host.

Psychological aspects. The emotional impact of the diagnosis of cancer is immediate and lifelong for both patient and family; no family member is unaffected. Their lives are changed forever but, it is hoped, not irreparably. For most children, leukemia is chronic and life threatening, yet treatable. Attention to the child's and family's adaptation to the phases of diagnosis, treatment, returning to "normal," and eventual survival is essential in truly comprehensive oncological care.

The diagnosis of leukemia is a time of crisis. Feelings of anger, guilt, and loss of control are universal to patients of all ages, their parents, and their siblings. Siblings often are jealous of all the attention the patient receives, which adds to the parents' stress. In the midst of this distress, the child and parents are asked to assimilate vast amounts of information about diagnosis, prognosis, procedures, treatments, side effects, and hospital or clinical routines. Discussions should be gentle, accurate, realistic, hopeful, and, above all, honest.

Several specific techniques can help families with these early adjustments. Repeating information frequently and encouraging any and all questions (they should be written down) are important. Whenever possible, the physician should talk to the parents together to prevent misunderstandings and to avoid making one parent responsible for relaying information and answering questions for the other. Educational materials written in layperson's language are helpful supplements to verbal discussions. Information about the child's and the family's previous manner of coping with major events and previous experiences with cancer, serious illness, or death should be obtained from the primary physician and by family interview. Just as with a successful medical outcome, a positive psychosocial outcome depends on early assessment, anticipation, prevention, and intervention for complications.

Regardless of the eventual outcome—good or bad—the treatment course is full of ups and downs, discomforts, uncertainties, and both illness- and non–illness-related stress. The patient and family continue to be challenged by the pressures of day-to-day events such as jobs, school, relocation, marriage, family, finances, and other family illnesses, injury, or death, which may even precede the diagnosis of leukemia. In addition, illness-related stress factors such as separation of family members, frequent traveling, disruption of the normal routine, sleep interruptions, child care arrangements, the high cost of care, and the threat of death take an extreme emotional toll on the child and family.

During the course of therapy there are several times that can be extremely stressful and the need for increased support anticipated. Ironically, getting back to "normal," either at the time of hospital discharge, upon returning to school, or at the completion of therapy, provokes considerable anxiety. Every effort should be made to encourage the child to return to normal social, school, and physical activities as soon as possible. Early communication among family, school, and medical personnel is essential to a smooth reentry into normal routines.

Perhaps more devastating than the initial diagnosis is the news that the disease has recurred, or the realization that all treatments have failed and that the child will die. With a relapse the family must start the treatment process all over again, although with a smaller chance for a successful outcome. More than ever before, they need the support of the health care team to enable them to go on. When a cure is no longer possible, room must always be left for hope. Hope can come from changing the focus toward palliative care, with comfort as the goal. Thus, the efforts of the health care team—oncologists, psychosocial workers, family physician, and family—must be redirected toward comfort measures. Physical measures include controlling pain and bleeding without invasive diagnostic or treatment procedures. Frequent reassurance that the child and family will not be left alone are of the utmost importance in providing good, successful palliative care. At this point, perhaps more than ever before, support must be given to staff members, who, in turn, provide the most support for the child and family.

Chemotherapy

Table 232-3 lists the various chemotherapeutic agents used in treating childhood leukemias and the complications associated with their use. The specific indications for their use are described in the discussions of therapy for each type of childhood leukemia.

Bone Marrow Transplantation

The role of current bone marrow transplantation (BMT) alternatives for treating leukemia in children is shown in Fig. 232-3. BMT involves initial administration of intensive cytoreductive therapy—usually high-dose chemotherapy with or without total body irradiation—designed to eradicate 100% of the leukemia cells. This therapy is so intense that it also is lethal to normal bone marrow cells. Therefore, it must be followed by bone marrow "rescue" with intravenously infused bone marrow from a compatible donor. For an allogeneic bone marrow transplant, the donor is an HLA-matched sibling. Unfortunately, approximately only one third of patients who require transplantation are likely to have an HLA-identical sibling. For this reason, the role of bone marrow transplantation historically has been somewhat limited. With advances in transplantation technology, however, alternatives are being studied, such as autologous donation or transplantation from partially matched related donors (i.e., parents or siblings) or from matched unrelated donors.

Autologous BMT has been curative for small numbers of patients who have had ALL and ANLL. The patient undergoes bone marrow harvest during a time of remission, and the marrow is treated in an attempt to eradicate leukemic cells. The marrow cells then are cryopreserved and infused after completion of the cytoreductive therapy. Posttransplant relapse of leukemia occurs in most patients and is the major reason for failure because posttransplant mortality resulting from complications is very low. For patients who do not have

Table 232-3 Use and Complications of Chemotherapeutic Agents in Acute Leukemia

Drug	Route	Common Use	Acute Toxicity	Delayed Toxic Effects
Prednisone	PO	Induction and maintenance of ALL	Hyperglycemia, hypertension, emotional lability, increased appetite, fluid retention, weight gain, striae, cushingoid facies, peptic ulcer, diabetes mellitus	Osteoporosis, growth retardation, aseptic necrosis, cataracts, glaucoma, diabetes mellitus
Vincristine	IV	Induction and maintenance of ALL	Alopecia, constipation, paralytic ileus, peripheral neuropathy, jaw pain, SIADH,* danger with extravasation, in rare cases, myelosuppression	Peripheral neuropathy
6-Mercaptopurine	PO, IV	Maintenance of ALL	Alopecia, nausea, vomiting, diarrhea, myelosuppression, hepatic damage, cholestasis	Hepatic disease, cholestasis
Methotrexate	PO, IM, IV	Maintenance of ALL	Nausea, vomiting, mucositis, rash, myelosuppression, hepatic damage, renal toxicity	Hepatic damage, neurotoxicity
Methotrexate and/or cytosine arabinoside	Intrathecal	CNS prophylaxis of ALL and ANLL	Nausea, vomiting, headache, stiff neck, arachnoiditis, seizures	Cortical atrophy, leukoencephalopathy
L-Asparaginase	IM	Induction and consolidation of ALL	Anaphylaxis, nausea, vomiting, fever, chills, hyperglycemia, diabetes, abdominal pain, pancreatitis (increased amylase), CNS depression, coagulation defects with thrombosis or hemorrhage (i.e., stroke), hypoproteinemia, hepatic damage	Pancreatic or hepatic damage, diabetes mellitus
Doxorubicin	IV	Induction and consolidation of ALL	Myelosuppression, alopecia, nausea, vomiting, mucositis, anorexia, hepatic damage, cardiac arrhythmias, red urine, danger with extravasation	Cardiomyopathy, hepatic damage
Daunorubicin	IV	Induction and maintenance of ALL and ANLL	Myelosuppression, alopecia, nausea, vomiting, cardiac arrhythmias, hepatic damage, red urine, danger with extravasation	Cardiomyopathy
Cytosine arabinoside	IV	Induction and maintenance of ANLL Consolidation of high-risk ALL	Myelosuppression, alopecia, nausea, vomiting, diarrhea, mucositis, conjunctivitis, fever, neurotoxicity	Hepatic damage, neurotoxicity
Etoposide/tenoposide	IV	Induction and maintenance of ANLL Consolidation of high-risk ALL	Hypotension, anaphylaxis, myelosuppression, nausea, vomiting, alopecia, mucositis, danger with extravasation	Second malignancy, most commonly ANLL
6-Thioguanine	PO	Induction and maintenance of ANLL	Same as for mercaptopurine but less hepatic toxicity	
Radiation		ALL CNS prophylaxis	Alopecia, nausea, vomiting, skin hypersensitivity, mild myelosuppression	Sleeping syndrome, seizures, leukoencephalopathy, growth retardation
Trans-retinoic acid (ATRA)	PO	Induction and maintenance of APML	Myelosuppression, fever, hyperleukocytosis, fluid retention, pulmonary edema, respiratory distress, pseudotumor cerebri	None known

Data compiled from Perry MC, editor: *The chemotherapy source book,* Baltimore, 1997, Williams and Wilkins.
**SIADH,* Syndrome of inappropriate secretion of antidiuretic hormone.

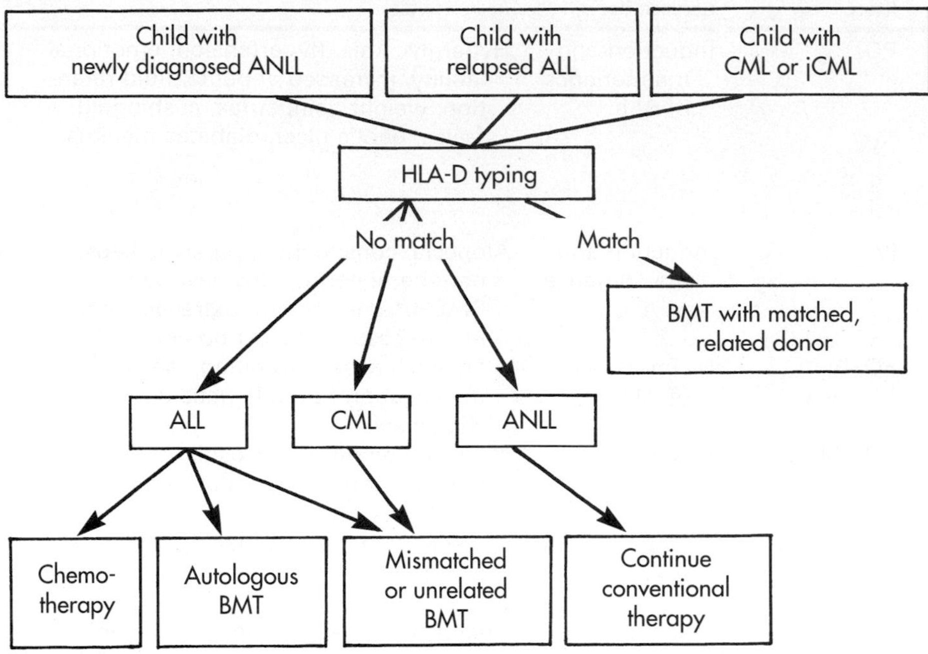

Fig. 232-3 Flow diagram of marrow transplantation for children who have leukemia. *ALL,* Acute lymphoblastic leukemia; *ANLL,* acute nonlymphoid leukemia, *BMT,* bone marrow transplantation; *CML,* chronic myelogenous leukemia; *HLA-D,* human leukocyte antigen-D; *jCML,* juvenile chronic myelogenous leukemia.

(From Trigg ME: *Pediatr Clin North Am* 35:939, 1988.)

a matched related donor available or for whom autologous transplantation is not appropriate (e.g., early relapse of ALL, patients who have any form of ANLL, or CML) transplantation is performed at some centers using matched unrelated or partially mismatched donors. To date such procedures have been associated with very poor survival rates secondary to both relapse of leukemia and treatment-related complications. The major limitations of such BMT procedures have been graft rejection and graft-versus-host disease. As progress is made in developing better prophylactic regimens and improved therapeutic strategies for overcoming these limitations, transplantation in the mismatch setting may soon be a more routine and more successful alternative. Another option being explored at some centers is the use of cord blood as a rich source of stem cells for transplantation and hematopoietic reconstitution. For these purposes, cord blood is obtained from the placenta at the time of delivery and cryopreserved. Transplantation with cord blood appears to be particularly advantageous with the mismatched or unrelated donor technique because the risk of graft-versus-host disease is reduced.

BMT can be associated with significant complications. In addition to the anticipated side effects of the cytoreductive chemotherapy (e.g., nausea, vomiting, mucositis, anorexia, and prolonged bone marrow aplasia), transplantation-related problems may occur such as graft rejection, graft-versus-host disease, and hepatic venoocclusive syndrome. As with all intensive treatment regimens, infections such as bacterial sepsis, invasive fungal disease, CMV interstitial pneumonitis, and *P. carinii pneumonia* (PCP) are significant causes of morbidity and mortality, particularly during the first 6 months after transplantation.

ACUTE LYMPHOBLASTIC LEUKEMIA

Most ALL treatment regimens divide therapy into three phases: induction of remission, CNS prophylaxis and consolidation, and maintenance treatment during remission.

Induction of Remission

The aim of the initial treatment of ALL is induction of remission. Complete remission is defined as the absence of clinical signs and symptoms of disease in the presence of a normal blood count and a normocellular bone marrow with 5% or fewer blasts. However, there is no evidence that the clinical disappearance of leukemic cells from the bone marrow indicates their total eradication.

Although the basic two-drug combination of vincristine and prednisone can induce remission in approximately 85% of children who have ALL, addition of L-asparaginase or an anthracycline improves the remission induction rate to approximately 95% and lengthens the duration of remission.[59,64]

Although a period of 4 weeks generally is required to achieve complete remission, in most cases marked regression of symptoms, organomegaly, and peripheral blasts occurs within the first week of treatment. Hospitalization during this time is common. Pancytopenia is seen routinely as a result of leukemia and chemotherapy-induced bone marrow suppression. These patients often are transfusion dependent for red cells and platelets and frequently require antibiotics for empirical treatment of fever with neutropenia.

Central Nervous System Prophylaxis

As soon as bone marrow remission has been achieved, CNS prophylaxis is instituted. The optimum and least toxic prophylaxis has not yet been determined fully. Investigators at St. Jude Children's Research Hospital showed that cranial spinal irradiation could reduce the incidence of CNS relapse to approximately 10%.[2] Because of the excessive myelosuppression and subsequent growth disturbances associated with spinal irradiation, cranial irradiation plus intrathecal methotrexate was adopted universally as the standard form of CNS preventive therapy in the 1970s. In recent years, however, concern has arisen about the apparent adverse effects of this regimen on neurological and intellectual functioning.[49] Reducing the dose of cranial irradiation may be as effective, but it is not clear whether a lower dose is associated with a lower incidence of CNS sequelae. Other approaches studied include triple intrathecal chemotherapy with methotrexate, cytosine arabinoside, and hydrocortisone; intermediate-dose systemic methotrexate, either alone or with concomitant intrathecal methotrexate; intrathecal methotrexate alone; or high-dose systemic methotrexate. For patients at standard risk, cranial irradiation does not appear to be necessary; intrathecal chemotherapy alone appears to offer adequate CNS preventive therapy.

Maintenance Therapy

The rationale for continuing to treat patients in complete continuous remission is based on historical studies in which therapy was discontinued immediately[24] or 6 months after induction of remission.[41] In both studies, relapse quickly followed discontinuation of treatment. The backbone of most maintenance regimens includes daily oral doses of 6-mercaptopurine, weekly doses of parenteral methotrexate, postinduction intravenous doses of vincristine, and oral prednisone at various intervals. These regimens often incorporate anthracyclines, L-asparaginase, and cytosine arabinoside as part of consolidation or reinduction during the first year of treatment for high-risk patients. Currently the optimum duration of therapy is unknown. Most centers continue treatment for 2½ to 3 years. For patients who successfully complete a full course of maintenance therapy, the prognosis generally is good. A study from St. Jude Children's Research Hospital demonstrated that approximately 80% of patients who complete therapy remain disease free. Of the 20% who eventually relapse, most do so in the first year off therapy.[26,54] The risk of relapse after 4 disease-free years is quite small.[23,54]

Relapse Therapy

Most patients who relapse have a grave prognosis. Several factors, such as the duration of first remission, whether relapse occurs during or after completion of therapy, and the site of relapse have been identified—factors that have some predictive value in determining the outcome of subsequent therapy. The most common site of relapse in ALL is the bone marrow. Relapse at any site must be presumed to be associated with systemic reseeding of leukemic cells. Therefore, patients who have clinically localized relapses must be treated both locally and systemically with reinduction therapy and reprophylaxis of the CNS. Most patients who have ALL can readily be induced into a second remission; however, these remissions generally last less than 1 year, and long-term remissions are uncommon.

Bone Marrow Transplantation

The current role of BMT in treating ALL is for patients who have relapsed and a select few patients during their first remission (e.g., patients who have the Philadelphia chromosome). For patients who have a bone marrow relapse and are fortunate enough to have an HLA-identical sibling, bone marrow transplantation should be strongly considered. Patients "transplanted" during remission fare better than if the procedure is attempted during relapse, and those transplanted earlier in their disease (i.e., in second remission) do better than those who receive transplantations after several previous relapses.[10,11] Autologous BMT has been curative for some patients. Its exact role in treating relapsed ALL is controversial. Data are conflicting about the benefit in terms of disease-free survival with autologous BMT compared with consolidation chemotherapy. Improved methods of purging the marrow may result in more cures in the future.

Mature B-Cell ALL

Similar to Burkitt's lymphoma, mature B-cell ALL is more common in boys, with a median age of 8 years. It frequently is associated with bulky abdominal tumor and a very high rate of cell proliferation, factors that can result in the metabolic complications associated with tumor lysis syndrome. Standard therapy includes intensive therapy with cyclophosphamide, cytarabine, high-dose systemic methotrexate, and doxorubicin administered over 6 months' time. Event-free survival is up to 70%, with relapses occurring in the first year after diagnosis[58] and being extremely refractory to treatment.

ACUTE NONLYMPHOID LEUKEMIA

Progress in the treatment of children who have ANLL has not kept pace with advances in the treatment of childhood ALL. As a result of new chemotherapeutic strategies, better supportive care, and improved transplantation technology, overall survival has increased for children who have ANLL, especially for those who have the AML and APML subtypes. In contrast to ALL, the current treatment of ANLL is very intensive for all patients. High WBCs, bleeding disorders, chloromas, and symptoms of hyperleukocytosis (see the discussion of CML on p. 1619) are much more common findings at diagnosis in ANLL than in ALL. Of importance is the recognition that APML and children with Down syndrome are conditions that require specific therapeutic interventions as discussed elsewhere on this page.

Induction of Remission

Historically, induction therapy invariably has included cytosine arabinoside (cytarabine) and anthracycline, usually daunorubicin.[67] Approximately 70% to 80% of children achieve complete remission with these two drugs. The duration of severe marrow hypoplasia with peripheral pancytopenia during a typical ANLL induction ranges from 21 to 35 days. The leukemic blasts of almost half of the 20% to 30% of patients who fail to achieve remission are refractory to the standard cytarabine and daunorubicin combination. New treatment alternatives are being studied for this group, including high-dose cytarabine or different drugs (e.g., etoposide, amsacrine, 5-azacytidine).

Central Nervous System Prophylaxis

Without some form of CNS prophylaxis, approximately 10% to 30% of children who have AML have an initial relapse in the central nervous system. Apparently effective CNS prophylaxis regimens consist of intrathecal cytarabine or methotrexate and/or cranial irradiation. High-dose intravenous cytarabine probably also has some activity against CNS leukemia.

Postinduction Continuation Therapy

The principles of treatment in ANLL remission are similar to those of ALL, but the strategy differs. Much more intensive treatment appears to be necessary. Pediatric trials have demonstrated improved outcomes with intensive postremission induction chemotherapy utilizing anthracyclines, epipodophyllotoxins, and cytarabine with 40% to 50% of patients in continuous remission at 5 years.[36,48,67] Attempts to intensify therapy by utilizing autologous bone marrow transplantation does not appear to improve outcomes significantly.[57] The consequence of such intense chemotherapy programs is severe myelosuppression and its attendant complications. The need for maintenance therapy beyond the induction-intensification phases remains a controversial issue to be addressed by future studies. There are data to support both conclusions. The answers to questions of optimum duration and drug combinations depend partly on the exact nature and intensity of the therapeutic program used for induction and intensification.

Bone Marrow Transplantation

Allogeneic BMT is the treatment of choice for patients who have ANLL in first remission, if a matched related donor is available. Five-year leukemia-free survival is reported to be 55% to 70% in children who have AML who are treated by allogeneic transplantation after chemotherapeutic induction of complete remission.[71] Both leukemia-free survival and overall survival are better than that achieved with chemotherapy alone. The price of BMT in terms of toxicity remains high, with graft-versus-host disease and infection being most problematical.

It is accepted practice to determine the HLA type of the children and family members when the initial diagnosis of ANLL is made so that therapeutic options can be established and potentially hazardous transfusions from donors or family members can be avoided. Many centers harvest bone marrow on all ANLL patients during the first remission and hold it in reserve for use in the event of relapse. As technology improves, bone marrow transplantation from unrelated or partially mismatched family members will become a more reasonable approach for ANLL patients in second remission.

Relapse Therapy

Approximately 50% of children who have ANLL who have relapsed or were refractory to initial therapy may be induced into a complete remission with one of a number of investigational treatment regimens, such as chlorodeoxyadenosine, idarubicin, etoposide, 5-azacytidine, amsacrine, and cyclocytidine. The duration of remission has been short for most of these patients. If a second remission is induced, bone marrow transplantation offers the only chance for a cure.

Special Conditions

Acute promyelocytic leukemia. In essentially all cases of APML there is a translocation, t (15;17), with the breakpoint on chromosome 17 within the gene for the retinoic acid receptor.[5] Treatment with high doses of trans-retinoic acid causes gradual cellular differentiation and cellular death, resulting in remission induction (i.e., disappearance of malignant promyelocytes from the blood and marrow) with reduced morbidity, and improved long-term outcome.[68] The standard of care for all patients with APML is to give trans-retinoic acid along with chemotherapy as part of induction and/or continuation therapy. The use of trans-retinoic acid has been associated with unique toxicities including fever, hyperleukocytosis, retention of fluid, pulmonary edema, respiratory distress (termed *retinoic acid syndrome*) and pseudotumor cerebri (see Table 232-3).

Down syndrome. Myeloproliferative disorders, which are clinically and hematologically indistinguishable from congenital AML, have been reported in newborns who have Down syndrome. These disorders are transient and typically resolve completely within weeks or months of diagnosis without specific antileukemia treatment. No test is available that can distinguish infants who have this transient disorder from those who have true congenital leukemia. Conservative therapy with close monitoring and supportive care as needed is recommended for 6 to 8 weeks to differentiate between these two disorders. Readers are referred to other sources for more detailed discussion of this fascinating phenomenon.[35]

However, children who have Down syndrome have an

increased likelihood of developing both AML and ALL.[74] These children tend to be younger and have a very high incidence of megakaryocytic leukemia. Compared with other children who have AML, children who have Down syndrome have a superior disease-free survival, but significantly higher rates of therapy-related morbidity and mortality. Thus, although children who have Down syndrome are highly responsive to current chemotherapeutic regimens, toxicity to therapy has a pronounced effect on outcome. The standard of care for all children who have Down syndrome and AML is to use moderate-intensity cytarabine and anthracycline combination chemotherapy without exposure to intensive, investigational, and potentially more toxic therapies.

CHRONIC MYELOGENOUS LEUKEMIA

Chronic myelogenous leukemia is rare in children. In childhood the disorder may appear as two distinct clinical syndromes: adult-type CML, which is virtually indistinguishable from that seen in older patients, and juvenile CML, a disease relatively restricted to very young children that has distinct clinical, laboratory, and cytogenetic features (Table 232-4).

Adult-Type CML

The adult form of CML is a clonal myeloproliferative disorder involving all of the blood progenitor lineages and at least some of the lymphoid lineages. It is characterized by expansion of the total body granulocyte pool, myeloid hyperplasia of the bone marrow, extramedullary hematopoiesis, and a specific cytogenetic marker, the Philadelphia chromosome.

The natural history of CML is divided into three phases: chronic, accelerated, and blastic. These phases represent the progressive shift in the nature of the disorder, from hyperproliferation, with production of mainly mature blood elements, to production of predominately immature blast cells.

Chronic Phase

The signs and symptoms of CML usually develop insidiously over several months. Patients usually have nonspecific complaints such as fever, night sweats, fatigue, diminished exercise tolerance, weakness, left upper quadrant pain, and early satiation of appetite. Marrow hyperplasia and marrow space expansion may result in bone pain and tenderness. The usual physical findings are pallor, low-grade fever, ecchymoses, sternal tenderness, and hepatosplenomegaly. Neurological abnormalities, visual difficulties, papilledema, retinal hemorrhages, respiratory distress with tachypnea, or priapism may complicate cases involving marked hyperleukocytosis.

Peripheral blood counts typically demonstrate a normochromic, normocytic anemia (mean hematocrit of 25%), marked leukocytosis with "a shift to the left," and thrombocytosis (mean platelet count of 500,000/mm^3). The WBC at diagnosis ranges from approximately 8000 to 800,000 cells/

Table 232-4 Differences Between Adult and Juvenile Forms of Chronic Myelogenous Leukemia

Age at Onset	Adult Form	Juvenile Form
Chromosome Studies	Philadelphia chromosome—positive Usually over age 2	Philadelphia chromosome—negative Usually under age 2
Physical Findings		
Facial rash	Absent	Present
Lymphadenopathy	Occasional	Common with tendency to suppuration
Splenomegaly	Marked	Variable
Hemorrhagic manifestations	Absent	Common
Hematological Findings		
WBC at onset	Usually >100,000/mm^3	Usually <100,000/mm^3
Monocytosis of peripheral blood and bone marrow	Absent	Usually present
Thrombocytopenia	Uncommon at onset	Common at onset
Red Blood Cell Abnormalities		
Ineffective erythropoiesis	Absent	Present
I antigen on RBC	Normal	Reduced
Fetal hemoglobin levels	Normal	15%-50%
Normoblasts in peripheral blood	Unusual	Common
Other Laboratory Findings		
Urinary and serum muramidase	Slightly elevated	Markedly elevated
Immunological abnormalities	None	Strikingly high immunoglobin levels, high incidence of antinuclear antibodies (52%) and anti-IgG antibodies (43%)
Nature of colonies produced in vitro from peripheral blood	Predominantly granulocytic	Predominantly monocytic
Response to busulfan	Uniformly good	Poor
Median survival	2½-3 yr	Less than 9 mo

Modified from Altman AJ, Schwartz AD: *Malignant diseases of infancy, childhood, and adolescence,* Philadelphia, 1983, WB Saunders.

mm^3. The peripheral blood smear is remarkable for (1) increased numbers of myeloid cells at all stages of differentiation, (2) myeloblasts and promyelocytes accounting for fewer than 15% of the total white blood cell differential count, (3) basophilia, and (4) eosinophilia. In the bone marrow, granulocytes at all stages of maturation are seen in increased numbers, although their morphological appearance is normal. The finding of the Philadelphia chromosome in approximately 90% of patients is pathognomonic for CML. The laboratory finding of a decline in leukocyte alkaline phosphatase (LAP) activity is quite helpful diagnostically. LAP activity increases in a number of conditions that can be differentiated, including infection, leukemoid reaction, hematological remission of CML, and a blast crisis of CML. Other common laboratory abnormalities include elevation of serum uric acid and lactate dehydrogenase levels.

Before any specific antileukemic therapy is initiated, the following special management problems and their treatment must be considered: hyperuricemia, hyperkalemia, hyperphosphatemia, priapism, and the neurological, retinal, or pulmonary complications of leukostasis. The goal of treatment in the chronic phase is to provide symptomatic relief by correcting the leukocytosis and organomegaly. The standard approach to hyperleukocytosis includes leukopheresis and single-agent chemotherapy, usually busulfan or hydroxyurea. Hydroxyurea is the drug of choice in children because of its increased margin of hematological safety and its reduced systemic toxicity relative to busulfan. Both drugs must be monitored carefully, and dosages must be adjusted according to the hematological response.

Conventional therapy rarely produces a true complete remission. Although the CBC may normalize and the organomegaly disappear, the bone marrow continues to show granulocyte hyperplasia and Philadelphia chromosome-positive metaphases. Attempts to ablate the Philadelphia chromosome-positive clone with aggressive multiagent chemotherapy have not succeeded.[33] Therapy does not delay acceleration to blast crisis or prolong survival. Treatment with interferon alpha can result in transient disappearance of all Philadelphia chromosome cells and may prolong the chronic phase.[37]

Acceleration Phase

Inevitably, patients develop a more malignant form of their disease. This blast crisis may be heralded by a 3- to 6-month transitional phase referred to as the *acceleration phase,* or *metamorphosis.* The clinical features observed in this period include basophilia, new-onset thrombocytosis or thrombocytopenia, leukocytosis refractory to previous therapies, anemia, and splenomegaly. Therapy should be instituted to prevent the complications of this accelerated phase of disease—renewed leukostasis, organomegaly, and hyperproliferation. No therapy short of bone marrow transplantation has been shown to prevent the inevitable development of a blastic phase and death in CML.

Blast Crisis

Acute blastic transformation occurs at a median of about 3 years and is responsible for at least 75% of deaths in CML. Leukostasis and very high WBCs are more common in the blast phase, which is quite refractory to chemotherapy regardless of whether the blastic transformation is myeloblastic or lymphoblastic. Median survival after blastic transformation is only 3 to 6 months. Long-term remissions have been reported in patients who underwent allogeneic bone marrow transplantation while in the accelerated or blastic phase, but the results generally are disappointing.

Bone Marrow Transplantation

Allogeneic BMT is the only curative approach now available for patients who have CML. The disease status at the time of transplantation is the most powerful predictor of disease-free survival. Most centers, therefore, currently recommend allogeneic BMT for any child who has the adult-type CML in the chronic phase who has an HLA-matched donor, preferably within 1 year of diagnosis. Autologous transplantation has been used as a temporizing approach, the objective being to restore the chronic phase. The bone marrow is reconstituted with Philadelphia chromosome–positive cells. Therefore, although the chronic phase may be reestablished and survival prolonged, this technique is unlikely to be curative. Advances in BMT technology have allowed successful unrelated donor transplantation and cure for small numbers of patients who have CML.[13] For the patient who has no HLA-matched sibling, this is the only alternative approach available with curative potential.

Juvenile Chronic Myelogenous Leukemia

Juvenile chronic myelogenous leukemia (JCML) is a myeloproliferative disorder seen mainly in infants and characterized by leukocytosis, splenomegaly, and decreased LAP activity.[15] Despite these clinical similarities to the adult form of CML, JCML clearly is distinguishable with respect to clinical presentation, hematological manifestations, cytogenetic analysis, response to therapy, and prognosis (see Table 232-4).

Distinctive clinical features common to JCML at diagnosis include a patient under 2 years of age, persistent respiratory infections (with tachypnea, chronic cough, wheezing), prominent lymphadenopathy, skin rash (eczema, xanthomas, and café-au-lait spots), bleeding, and failure to thrive. In addition to anemia and leukocytosis, frequent laboratory findings are thrombocytopenia, monocytosis, and nucleated RBCs in the peripheral blood. Cytogenetic analysis may be abnormal, but the Philadelphia chromosome is never found.

Most patients who have JCML die secondary to infection. Chemotherapy is of limited value. Patients who have JCML usually do not respond to busulfan or hydroxyurea. Bone marrow transplantation offers the only hope of cure at present and is the treatment of choice for the patient who has a histocompatible sibling.[17]

CONGENITAL LEUKEMIA

Congenital leukemia may be apparent at birth or may develop within the first month of life. Most patients described with this rare disorder had AML, although ALL has been reported in newborns. The etiology of congenital leukemia is unknown. Leukemia in the neonatal period has been associated with Down syndrome, Turner's syndrome, mosaic monosomy 7, and trisomy 9. No cases of congenital leukemia have been reported in infants born to women who had leukemia before or during pregnancy.

The clinical manifestations are similar to those seen with leukemia among older children except that leukemia cutis is more common. These blue-gray skin nodules represent areas of skin infiltration by leukemic cells. Petechiae, purpura, hepatosplenomegaly, and poor feeding are common findings in a newborn who has leukemia. The laboratory findings include thrombocytopenia and hyperleukocytosis.

Congenital leukemia must be differentiated from a number of conditions often found in the neonatal period, including congenital syphilis, intrauterine viral infection (CMV, rubella, toxoplasmosis), neuroblastoma, congenital thrombocytopenic purpura, leukemoid reaction in response to sepsis, hypoxemia, erythroblastosis fetalis, and the transient myeloproliferative syndrome associated with Down syndrome.

The treatment of congenital leukemia is identical to that for the older child except that cranial irradiation is omitted. The results generally have been disappointing, with many infants dying within a few days to months after diagnosis.[62] A majority of recently reported cases of congenital AML were of the monocytic (M_5) subtype. For this group of patients, treatment with etoposide or teniposide, or both, has been particularly effective.

LATE EFFECTS: THE AGONY OF SUCCESS

The advent of more successful therapy has been accompanied by a growing concern over the physical and psychological well-being of the survivors of these aggressive protocols. Studies of late effects of the childhood leukemias and their treatment, but particularly of ANLL and CML, are severely limited because of the small numbers that have been studied. The discussion of late effects pertains to studies of survivors of ALL, because there are no similar data about the survivors of ANLL or CML.

Major areas of concern identified among survivors of ALL include second malignancies, CNS damage, endocrine abnormalities with growth failure and reproductive dysfunction, cardiac toxicity, and psychological morbidity. Preliminary results of clinical research suggest that the likelihood and the type and severity of sequelae are at least partly related to (1) the patient's age at the time of diagnosis and institution of treatment, (2) the specific treatment used, and (3) the intensity of treatment. Interpretation of clinical data related to the management of long-term survivors is complicated by uncertainty as to whether a particular problem existed before the diagnosis of cancer, whether the problem is secondary to the treatment or to the life-threatening illness itself, or whether all three scenarios are involved.

Truly successful treatment of childhood cancer must incorporate care of the long-term survivor. This involves not only recognizing the delayed consequences that can emerge after cancer therapy but also actual follow-up with history, physical examination, and appropriate laboratory testing to monitor the patient's status and provide treatment for any problems identified. Unfortunately for both the patient and the physician, as yet no firm guidelines have been established as to the best method of monitoring cured patients for delayed physical or psychological sequelae. Recommendations for pertinent follow-up must be individualized according to the anticipated problems, based on the patient's disease, therapeutic history, and duration of disease-free, off-therapy survival (see Suggested Readings, Green, 1989, and Schwartz et al, 1994).

Second Malignancy

The risk of developing a second malignancy after apparently successful treatment of leukemia is estimated to be 1% to 12%.[38,47,51] Both genetics and treatment have been implicated in this increased risk, which is 20 times greater than that observed in the general population. Most second malignancies seen among survivors of childhood ALL are second leukemias or non-Hodgkin's lymphomas. Whether these represent a second carcinogenic event or a different manifestation of the primary malignant process is unknown. Brain tumors account for almost one third of secondary solid tumors, and the prognosis is poor.

In follow-up studies of a child who has had ALL, especially if cranial irradiation was used for prophylactic CNS treatment, the head and neck should be inspected carefully because most secondary carcinomas (thyroid, basal cell, parotid gland) have occurred in this region. Biopsy is recommended as soon as possible for any suspicious skin lesions, nodules, or firm, enlarged lymph nodes that do not respond completely to a trial of antibiotic therapy. If seizures, severe headaches, or symptoms of increased intracranial pressure occur in the absence of an obvious clinical explanation, computed tomography (CT) or magnetic resonance imaging (MRI) studies should be done before lumbar puncture to ensure that an intracranial mass is not present.

Central Nervous System Damage

Before the use of effective prophylaxis, the central nervous system was the most common site of first relapse in children who had ALL. Currently, CNS prophylaxis prevents isolated CNS relapse in more than 90% of patients. The functional and structural CNS changes found among long-term survivors of ALL in continuous remission after effective CNS prophylaxis are less common and less severe than among patients who relapse with CNS involvement.

The absolute incidence and natural history of long-term neurological sequelae, including memory and learning problems, among patients treated with intrathecal chemotherapy and cranial irradiation therapy are unknown. Both acute and subacute forms of neurotoxicity have been reported in patients treated with the current methods of CNS prophylaxis.[49,70] These abnormalities include structural changes, as evidenced by ventricular dilation, calcifications, focal areas of parenchymal hypodensity, and cortical atrophy visible on CT scan. Functional changes, with intellectual deficits, poor memory skills, low IQ scores, and poor school performance, also have been described. Further investigation is required to determine if a correlation exists between these structural and functional CNS changes. Severe, permanent neurological sequelae such as a seizure disorder, residual hearing loss, and hemiplegia are observed almost exclusively among children who are cured after one or more CNS relapses.

Endocrine Abnormalities

Endocrine abnormalities that involve the hypothalamic-pituitary axis probably occur secondary to cranial irradiation, whereas gonadal dysfunction probably occurs secondary to chemotherapy. Younger age appears to increase the risk for subsequent growth problems and reduce the risk for gonadal dysfunction.

Abnormally low amounts of growth hormone (GH) have been found among children who have had ALL treated with cranial irradiation. Although growth velocities after completion of therapy are not reduced significantly in these children, their final adult height is diminished.[34] Early onset of puberty and obesity is also prevalent among survivors of childhood ALL.[18,34] Studies are needed to assess the correlations between various treatments, age at diagnosis, GH secretion, pubertal development, and final height attained. The benefits of GH therapy are unknown because results from different investigators are conflicting. Follow-up studies of long-term survivors of ALL treated with cranial irradiation demonstrate approximately a 3% to 5% incidence of hypothyroidism and less than a 1% incidence of secondary thyroid malignancies. Palpation of the thyroid, review of hypothyroidism symptoms, and a low threshold for measuring serum triiodothyronine (T_3) and thyroid-stimulating hormone (TSH) should be incorporated into the routine visit of survivors.

Data on infertility and gonadal function in this group are largely unavailable. Studies in this area are complicated by the young age of most patients and the lack of an adequate way of measuring eventual reproductive capabilities. The development of secondary sex characteristics does not necessarily mean that germinal cells are present or functional. Oligospermia related to previous chemotherapy frequently improves with time. Patients who received bilateral testicular irradiation to treat testicular leukemia generally are sterile. Virtually no information is available about the reproductive capabilities of girls. Pubertal progression is more likely to be normal in girls who had leukemia and chemotherapy after onset of puberty and menarche.

Cardiac Toxicity

The anthracyclines are a vital component of the current antileukemia armamentarium for most patients. The incidence of severe cardiomyopathy has been reduced by limiting the cumulative dose to approximately 350 mg/m^2, monitoring frequently during therapy with electrocardiograms and echocardiograms, and discontinuing the anthracycline if any signs of toxicity are observed (i.e., decreased fractional shorting and arrhythmias). Unfortunately, in most patients the signs and symptoms of cardiac toxicity do not develop until months after the anthracycline treatment has been discontinued.[27,40] For many patients, congestive heart failure is reversible or at least can be controlled with medication. More sensitive diagnostic techniques, such as stress testing and electrophysiological studies, are likely to result in more frequent diagnosis of cardiac abnormalities. Comprehensive follow-up cardiac evaluation with electrocardiograms, echocardiograms, and stress testing is a crucial part of routine checkups for patients treated with anthracycline with or without chest irradiation.

Psychosocial Changes

Because only a few studies have been designed to focus on the psychosocial status of long-term survivors of ALL, information on this subject is limited. Studies of childhood cancer survivors have shown these individuals to have a significantly higher incidence of behavioral and social adjustment problems than normal, including less participation in physical activities, inadequate social relations, poor school performance, frequent somatic complaints, and behavioral maladjustment. In particular, children treated for ALL had a greater risk for school-related problems, including the number of grades repeated and special education placement.[45] Psychosocial stressors, which continue to be reported long after therapy for ALL has been completed, include anxiety about potential relapse, financial burdens, rejection for employment or insurance coverage, and rejection for military service.[69] No differences in the frequency of major depressive syndromes, suicide attempts, or hospitalizations for psychiatric reasons have been noted between these patients and their siblings and between them and the general population.

In view of the follow-up information currently available, it is clear that ongoing assessment of neurological functioning, developmental milestones, school and work performance, behavior, and overall quality of life must be an integral part of maintaining health care for the survivor of childhood leukemia.

REFERENCES

1. Alexander FE, et al: Spatial clustering of childhood leukemia: summary results from the EUROCLUS project, *Br J Cancer* 77:818, 1998.
2. Aur RJA, et al: Central nervous system therapy and combination chemotherapy of childhood lymphocytic leukemia, *Blood* 37:272, 1971.
3. Beaty O, et al: Subsequent malignancies in children and adolescents after treatment for Hodgkin's disease, *J Clin Oncol* 13:603, 1995.
4. Bhatia S, et al: Epidemiology and etiology. In Pui C-H, editor: *Childhood leukemias,* Cambridge, Mass, 1999, University Press.
5. Biondi A, et al: Retinoic acid receptor-alpha gene rearrangements as a genetic marker for diagnosis and monitoring in APML, *Blood* 77:1418, 1991.
6. Bizzozzero OJ Jr, Johnson KG, Ciocco A: Radiation-related leukemia in Hiroshima and Nagasaki, 1946-64: distribution, incidence, appearance in time, *N Engl J Med* 274:1095, 1966.
7. Blattner WA, et al: Human T-cell leukemia virus and adult T-cell leukemia, *JAMA* 250:1074, 1983.
8. Boice JD: Cancer following medical irradiation, *Cancer* 47:1081, 1981.
9. Brisco MJ, et al: Outcome prediction in childhood ALL by molecular quantification of residual disease at the end of induction, *Lancet* 343: 196, 1994.
10. Brockstein JA, et al: Allogeneic BMT after hyper-fractionated TBI and cyclophosphamide in children with acute leukemia, *N Engl J Med* 317: 1618, 1987.
11. Butturini A, et al: Which treatment for childhood acute lymphoblastic leukemia in second remission? *Lancet* 1:429, 1987.
12. Campana D, Pui C-H: Detection of minimal residual disease in acute leukemia: methodologic advances and clinical significance, *Blood* 85: 1416, 1995.

13. Casper J, et al: Unrelated bone marrow donor transplants for children with leukemia or myelodysplasia, *Blood* 85:2354, 1995.
14. Castro-Malespina H, et al: Philadelphia chromosome-positive chronic myelocytic leukemia in children: survival and prognostic factors, *Cancer* 52:721, 1983.
15. Castro-Malespina H, et al: Subacute and chronic myelomonocytic leukemia in children (juvenile CML): clinical and hematologic observations and identification of prognostic factors, *Cancer* 54:675, 1984.
16. Chow W-H, et al: Cancers in children. In Schottenfeld D, Fravmeni JF, editors: *Cancer epidemiology and prevention,* ed 2, New York, Oxford University Press, 1996.
17. Chown S, et al: Matched and mismatched unrelated donor bone marrow transplantation for juvenile chronic myeloid leukemia, *Br J Hematol* 93:674, 1996.
18. Didi M, et al: High incidence of obesity in young adults after treatment of acute lymphoblastic leukemia in childhood, *J Pediatr* 127:63, 1995.
19. Dow LW, et al: Evidence for clonal development of childhood ALL, *Blood* 66:902, 1985.
20. Felix CA, Poplack DG: Characterization of acute lymphoblastic leukemia of childhood by immunoglobulin and T-cell receptor gene patterns, *Leukemia* 5:1015, 1991.
21. Filipovich ATT, et al: Immunodeficiency in humans as a risk in development of malignancy, *Prev Med* 9:252, 1980.
22. Ford AM, et al: Fetal origins of the TEL-AML 1 fusion gene in identical twins with leukemia, *Proc Natl Acad Sci U S A* 95:4584, 1998.
23. Frei E, Sallan SE: Acute lymphoblastic leukemia: treatment, *Cancer* 42:828, 1978.
24. Freireich EJ, et al: The effect of 6-mercaptopurine on the duration of steroid-induced remission in acute leukemia: a model for evaluation of other potentially useful therapy, *Blood* 21:699, 1963.
25. Gale KB, et al: Backtracking leukemia to birth: identification of clonotypic gene fusion sequences in neonatal blood spots, *Proc Natl Acad Sci U S A* 94:3950, 1997.
26. George S, et al: A reappraisal of the results of stopping therapy in childhood leukemia, *N Engl J Med* 300:2269, 1979.
27. Giantris A, et al: Anthracycline-induced cardiotoxicity in children and young adults, *Crit Rev Oncol Hematol* 27:53, 1998.
28. Greaves M: Aetiology of acute leukemia, *Lancet* 349:344, 1997.
29. Greaves M: A natural history for pediatric leukemia, *Blood* 82:1043, 1993.
30. Gurney JG, et al: Trends in cancer incidence among children in the US, *Cancer* 78:532, 1996.
31. Harvey EB, et al: Prenatal x-ray exposure and childhood cancer in twins, *N Engl J Med* 312:541, 1985.
32. Hecht F, McCaw BK: Chromosome instability syndromes. In Mulvihill JJ, Miller, RW, Fraumeni JR, editors: *Genetics of human cancer,* New York, 1977, Raven Press.
33. Hochhaus A, et al: Quantification of residual disease in CML patients on interferon-alpha therapy by competitive polymerase chain reaction, *Blood* 87:1549, 1996.
34. Hokken-Koelega ACS, et al: Long-term effects of treatment for acute lymphoblastic leukemia with and without cranial irradiation on growth and puberty: a comparative study, *Pediatr Res* 33:577, 1993.
35. Homans AC, Verissimo AM, Vlacha VI: Transient abnormal myelopoiesis of infancy associated with trisomy 21, *Am J Pediatr Hematol Oncol* 15:392, 1993.
36. Hurwitz CA, Mounce KG, Grier HE: Treatment of patients with AML: review of clinical trials of the past decade, *J Pediatr Hematol Oncol* 17:185, 1995.
37. Kantarjian HM, et al: Chronic myelogenous leukemia: a concise update, *Blood* 82:691, 1993.
38. Kimball-Dalton VM, et al: Second malignancies in patients treated for childhood acute lymphoblastic leukemia, *J Clin Oncol* 16:2848, 1998.
39. LeBeau MM: Detecting genetic changes in human tumor cells: have scientists "gone fishing," *Blood* 81:1979, 1993.
40. Lipshultz SE, et al: Late cardiac effects of doxorubicin therapy for acute lymphoblastic leukemia in childhood, *N Engl J Med* 324:808, 1991.
41. Lonsdale D, et al: Interrupted versus continued maintenance therapy in childhood acute leukemia, *Cancer* 36:341, 1975.
42. March HC: Leukemia in radiologists, *Radiology* 43:275, 1944.
43. Meadows AT, et al: Survival in childhood acute lymphoblastic leukemia: the influence of protocol and place of treatment, *Cancer Invest* 1:49, 1983.
44. Mirro J, et al: Acute mixed lineage leukemia: clinicopathologic correlations and prognostic significance, *Blood* 66:1115, 1985.
45. Mulhern RK, et al: Social competence and behavioral adjustment of children who are long-term survivors of cancer, *Pediatrics* 83:18, 1989.
46. Neglia JP, Robison LL: Epidemiology of the childhood acute leukemias, *Pediatr Clin North Am* 35:675, 1988.
47. Neglia JP, et al: Second neoplasms after acute lymphoblastic leukemia in childhood, *N Engl J Med* 325:1330, 1991.
48. Nesbit MEJ, et al: Chemotherapy for induction of remission of childhood AML followed by marrow transplantation or multiagent chemotherapy: a report from the CCG, *J Clin Oncol* 12:127, 1994.
49. Ochs JJ: Neurotoxicity due to central nervous system therapy for childhood leukemia, *Am J Pediatr Hematol Oncol* 11:93, 1989.
50. Penn I: Second malignant neoplasms associated with immunosuppression medications, *Cancer* 37:1024, 1976.
51. Pui C-H: Childhood leukemias, *N Engl J Med* 332:1618, 1995.
52. Pui C-H, Ribeiro R, Hancock M: Acute myeloid leukemia in children treated with epipodophyllotoxins for acute lymphoblastic leukemia, *N Engl J Med* 325:1682, 1991.
53. Pui C-H, et al: Clinical and biologic relevance of immunologic marker studies in childhood acute lymphoblastic leukemia, *Blood* 82:343, 1993.
54. Pui C-H, et al: Reappraisal of the clinical and biologic significance of myeloid-associated antigen expression in childhood acute lymphoblastic leukemia, *J Clin Oncol* 16:3768, 1998.
55. Pui C-H, et al: Secondary acute myeloid leukemia in children treated for acute lymphoblastic leukemia, *N Engl J Med* 321:136, 1989.
56. Raimondi SC: Current status of cytogenetic research in childhood acute lymphoblastic leukemia, *Blood* 81:2237, 1993.
57. Ravindranath Y, et al: Autologous bone marrow transplantation vs intensive consolidation chemotherapy in childhood AML, *N Engl J Med* 13:32, 1996.
58. Reiter A, et al: Chemotherapy in 998 unselected childhood ALL patients: results and conclusions of the multicenter trial ALL-BFM 86, *Blood* 84:3122, 1994.
59. Reiter A, et al: Favorable outcome of B-cell acute lymphoblastic leukemia in childhood: a report of three consecutive studies of the BFM group, *Blood* 80:2471, 1992.
60. Robison LL, et al: Environmental exposures as risk factors for childhood ANLL, *Proc Am Assoc Cancer Res* 28:249, 1987.
61. Rubin CM, et al: Impact of chromosomal translocations on prognosis in childhood ALL, *J Clin Oncol* 9:2183, 1991.
62. Sande JE, Arceci RJ, Lampkin BC: Congenital and neonatal leukemia, *Semin Perinatol* 24:3, 1997 (review).
63. Sandler DP, Ross JA: Epidemiology of acute leukemia in children and adults, *Semin Oncol* 24:3, 1997.
64. Schorin MA, et al: Treatment of childhood acute ALL: results of DFCI-CH ALL consortium protocol 85-01, *J Clin Oncol* 12:740, 1992.
65. Smith MA, et al: Leukemia. In Ries LAG, et al, editors: *Cancer incidence and survival among children and adolescents: US SEER Program 1975-1995,* National Cancer Institute, Bethesda, MD, 1999, NIH Pub No 99-4649.
66. Smith MA, et al: Uniform approach to risk classification and treatment assignment for children with acute lymphoblastic leukemia, *J Clin Oncol* 14:18, 1996.
67. Steuver CP, Civin C, Krischer J: Comparison of induction and maintenance therapy for acute nonlymphoid leukemia in childhood: results of Pediatric Oncology Group study, *J Clin Oncol* 9:247, 1991.
68. Tallman MS: Differentiating therapy in acute myeloblastic leukemia, *Leukemia* 10:1262, 1996.
69. Teta MJ, et al: Psychosocial consequences of childhood and adolescent cancer survival, *J Chronic Dis* 39:751, 1986.
70. Waber DP, Tarbell NJ: Toxicity of CNS prophylaxis for childhood leukemia, *Oncology* 11:259, 1997.
71. Wells RJ, et al: Treatment of newly diagnosed children and adolescents with AML: a CCG study, *J Clin Oncol* 12:2367, 1994.

72. Wiemels JL, et al: Protracted and variable latency of acute lymphoblastic leukemia after TEL-AML 1 gene fusion in utero, *Blood* 94:1057, 1999.
73. Williams DL, et al: Presence of clonal abnormalities in virtually all cases of acute lymphoblastic leukemia, *N Engl J Med* 313:640, 1985.
74. Zipursky A, Poon A, Doyle A: Leukemia in Down syndrome, *Pediatr Hematol Oncol* 9:139, 1992.

SUGGESTED READINGS

Green DM: *Long-term complications of therapy for cancer in childhood and adolescence,* Baltimore, 1989, Johns Hopkins University Press.

Halperin EC, et al: *Pediatric radiation oncology,* ed 3, New York, 1999, Raven Press.

Nathan DG, Orkin SH: *Nathan and Oski's hematology of infancy and childhood,* ed 5, Philadelphia, 1998, WB Saunders.

Pizzo PA, Poplack DG: *Principles and practice of pediatric oncology,* ed 3, Philadelphia, 1997, JB Lippincott-Raven.

Pui C-H: *Childhood leukemia,* Cambridge, Mass, 1999, Cambridge University Press.

Schwartz CL, et al: *Survivors of childhood cancer: assessment and management,* St. Louis, 1994, Mosby.

233 Lyme Disease

David M. Siegel

EPIDEMIOLOGY, ETIOLOGY, AND PATHOGENESIS

Lyme borreliosis, or Lyme disease, is a spirochetal infection first described in a group of children living in and around Lyme, Connecticut, on the eastern shore of the Connecticut River. Although initially these patients mistakenly were diagnosed as having juvenile arthritis, the perceptiveness of two mothers who pinpointed the disease cluster and the follow-up epidemiological work of Steere et al[19] established the infectious etiology and vector of the disease's spread. In their landmark investigation, Steere et al found a total of 15 patients in the area of Lyme, with an overall prevalence of 4.3 cases per 1000 residents. Since then the disease has been reported on all continents except Antarctica and in 48 of the United States. The major clustering of cases in this country has occurred along the northeastern seaboard, in the northern Midwest, and in the far West. In the United States, 90% of cases have been reported from Massachusetts, Rhode Island, Connecticut, New York, New Jersey, Wisconsin, and Minnesota. Since 1982, an increasing number of Lyme disease cases have been reported to the Centers for Disease Control and Prevention (CDC), with annual totals of 12,289 in 1997 and 14,646 in 1998.[9]

Early studies revealed a tick vector as consistent with the pattern of the spread of the disease.[17,18,24] Specifically, the Lyme disease spirochete is transmitted by *Ixodes* species ticks, including *I. scapularis* (previously referred to as *I. dammini*) in the Northeastern and Midwestern United States,[18] *I. pacificus* in the western United States,[3] *I. ricinus* in Europe,[15] and *I. persulcatus* in Asia.[15] *Ixodes* ticks have a 2-year life cycle; the larval form feeds (on a blood meal) in the late summer and the following spring, and the nymph feeds in early summer. The preferred host at these times is the white-footed mouse, *Peromyscus leucopus*. These mice are able to remain infected with the spirochete without an associated inflammatory response, whereas the spirochete remains in the midgut of the larval tick and later migrates to the salivary glands of the nymph. The adult *I. scapularis* prefers the white-tailed deer as a host, although the life cycle of the spirochete does not depend on involvement of the deer.

The spirochete etiology of this multisystem disease was discovered through the integration of two pieces of information. First, the skin rash seen in most of these patients was erythema migrans (EM), described in more detail later, which had been recognized in Europe in the 1950s as an eruption of spirochetal origin. This had been established by visualization of spirochetal structures in the lesions of EM and by the subsequent response to penicillin treatment. Second, with this knowledge and with the accumulated epidemiological evidence implicating *I. dammini* (now classified as *I. scapularis*) as the vector, Burgdorfer et al[2] began a careful analysis of the digestive tract of the ticks for spirochetes. They isolated previously unrecognized spirochetes later designated *Borrelia burgdorferi*. These organisms were consistently isolated from the blood, skin lesions, and cerebrospinal fluid (CSF) of patients who had Lyme disease, confirming the causation. The infection rate of *I. scapularis* with *B. burgdorferi* in endemic areas is quite high, with spirochetes having been recovered from more than half of a sample of ticks on Shelter Island, N.Y.[1]

CLINICAL MANIFESTATIONS

Because the clinical manifestations of Lyme disease vary with the time that elapses after inoculation by the tick, the infection has been divided into early and late phases. The former is characterized by two stages. Stage 1 of early infection is seen in 60% to 80% of patients and consists of EM, sometimes accompanied by fever, minor constitutional symptoms, and regional lymphadenopathy. The EM rash begins as a red macule or papule (at the site of the tick bite), which expands to form a large annular erythematous patch with a bright red outer border and partial central clearing. In patients who have EM, the rash appears within days of the tick bite and even left untreated fades within 3 to 4 weeks. Specific serum antibody to *B. burgdorferi* usually is not present at this time. However, the spirochete is cultured more easily from the skin during stage 1 of early infection than at any other time in the illness.

Stage 2 of early infection is marked by dissemination of *B. burgdorferi,* which potentially can involve many organ systems (Table 233-1). The most commonly involved areas, however, are the skin, nervous system, and musculoskeletal system. As well, this is the stage in which patients tend to feel ill, with significant malaise and fatigue, and smaller annular skin lesions can appear at sites other than the initial EM eruption. The patient complains of a transient but severe headache and stiff neck; examination of the CSF usually is normal. Arthritis is not present early in the disease, but patients experience migratory pain in joints, bursae, tendons, muscles, and bones. At this time (3 to 4 weeks after infection) serum antibody titers to *B. burgdorferi* develop.

As stage 2 disease progresses, meningitis can develop, possibly with subtle signs of encephalitis, including somnolence, poor memory, and mood change. Unilateral or bilateral facial palsy (Bell's palsy) and/or a peripheral neuritis, which

Table 233-1 Manifestations of Lyme Disease by Stage*

System†	Early Infection: Localized (Stage 1)	Early Infection: Disseminated (Stage 2)	Late Infection: Persistent (Stage 3)
Skin	Erythema chronicum migrans	Secondary annular lesions, malar rash, diffuse erythema or urticaria, evanescent lesions, lymphocytoma	Acrodermatitis chronica atrophicans, localized scleroderma-like lesions
Musculoskeletal system		Migratory pain in joints, tendons, bursae, muscle, bone, brief arthritis attacks, myositis,‡ osteomyelitis,‡ panniculitis‡	Prolonged arthritis attacks, chronic arthritis, peripheral enthesopathy, periostitis or joint subluxations below lesions of acrodermatitis
Neurological system		Meningitis, cranial neuritis, Bell's palsy, motor or sensory radiculoneuritis, subtle encephalitis, mononeuritis multiplex, myelitis,‡ chorea,‡ cerebellar ataxia‡	Chronic encephalomyelitis, spastic parapareses, ataxic gait, subtle mental disorders, chronic axonal polyradiculopathy, dementia‡
Lymphatic system	Regional lymphadenopathy	Regional or generalized lymphadenopathy, splenomegaly	
Heart		Atrioventricular nodal block, myopericarditis, pancarditis	
Eyes		Conjunctivitis, iritis,‡ choroiditis,‡ retinal hemorrhage or detachment,‡ panophthalmitis‡	Keratitis
Liver		Mild or recurrent hepatitis	
Respiratory system		Nonexudative sore throat, nonproductive cough, adult respiratory distress syndrome‡	
Kidneys		Microscopic hematuria or proteinuria	
Genitourinary system		Orchitis‡	
Constitutional symptoms	Minor	Severe malaise and fatigue	Fatigue

From Steere AC: *N Engl J Med* 321:586, 1989.
*Classification by stages provides a guideline for the illness's manifestations, but timing and sequence call vary greatly.
†Systems are listed from the most to the least commonly affected.
‡Inclusion of this manifestation is based on one or a few cases.

usually is asymmetrical and accompanied by motor, sensory, or mixed manifestations, develops in 15% to 20% of patients in the United States. Cardiac involvement, which is seen in a smaller group (4% to 8%), is characterized most commonly by varying degrees of atrioventricular block, but it can include myopericarditis or, in rare cases, fatal pancarditis. Complete heart block usually is brief, and only temporary cardiac pacing is needed.[16] Toward the end of stage 2 (6 months after onset of the disease), patients may begin to experience brief attacks of asymmetrical, large-joint oligoarthritis, most commonly affecting the knee.

During the late phase of disease the episodes of arthritis become much more prolonged, with the possibility of chronic arthritis (a year or more of continual inflammation) developing. The arthritis remains confined to one or a few large joints, the knee being most common. While in this phase, patients also may experience neurological complications, including persistent distal paresthesia or radicular pain. Some cases have been reported in which patients who had had classic symptoms of Lyme disease in the past later showed subtle memory deficits, somnolence, or behavioral changes. These patients present a difficult dilemma, although they certainly should be treated for neurological Lyme disease if therapy was not given initially.

CONGENITAL INFECTION

The issue of congenital infection with *B. burgdorferi* is only partly understood. Transplacental transmission of the spirochete has been reported in two infants, who died during the first week of life. Spirochetes were found in the tissue of these infants, but it was not clear that they were the cause of their deaths.[12,25] In a study of 463 infants from endemic and nonendemic areas, congenital malformations were not found to be associated with the presence of *B. burgdorferi* antibody in cord blood.[26] A prospective study in which 2014

Table 233-2 Treatment Regimens for Lyme Disease

Manifestation	Regimen*
Early infection*	
Adults (except pregnant or lactating women)	Tetracycline, 250 mg orally 4× daily, 14-30 days†
	Doxycycline, 100 mg orally 2× daily, 14-30 days†
	Amoxicillin, 500 mg orally 3× daily, 14-30 days†
	Cefuroxime axetil 500 mg orally 2× daily 14-30 days
Children (≤8 yr) and pregnant or lactating women	Amoxicillin 25-50 mg/kg body weight/day in 3 divided doses, 14-30 days
	In case of penicillin allergy:
	Erythromycin, 250 mg orally 3× daily or 30 mg/kg/day in divided doses, 14-30 days
Neurological abnormalities (early or late)*	
General	Ceftriaxone, 75-100 mg/kg/day intravenously 1× daily, 14-28 days‡
	Cefotaxime, 90-180 mg/kg body weight/day intravenously 3× daily, 14-28 days
	Penicillin G, 300,000 U/kg/day intravenously, 6 divided doses daily, 14 days‡
	In case of ceftriaxone, cefotaxime, or penicillin allergy:
	Doxycycline, 100 mg orally 2× daily, 30 days
	Chloramphenicol, 250 mg intravenously 4× daily, 14 days
Facial palsy alone	Oral antibiotic regimens, as above, may be adequate
Cardiac abnormalities	
First-degree atrioventricular block (PR interval <0.3 sec)	Oral antibiotic regimens, as for early infection
High-degree atrioventricular block	Ceftriaxone, 75-100 mg/kg/day intravenously 1× daily, 14 days
	Penicillin, 300,000 U/kg/day intravenously, 6 divided doses daily, 14 days
Arthritis (intermittent or chronic)†	Doxycycline, 100 mg orally 2× daily, 30 days
	Amoxicillin and probenecid, 500 mg each orally 4× daily, 30 days
	Ceftriaxone, 75-100 mg/kg/day intravenously 1× daily, 14 days
	Penicillin, 300,000 U/kg/day intravenously, 6 divided doses daily, 14 days
Acrodermatitis	Oral antibiotic regimens for 1 mo usually are adequate

Modified from Steere AC: *N Engl J Med* 321:586, 1989; and *The Medical Letter* 39:48, 1997.
*Treatment failures have occurred with all these regimens, and retreatment may be necessary.
†The duration of therapy is based on the clinical response.
‡The appropriate duration of therapy is not yet clear for patients with late neurological abnormalities, and it may be longer than 2 weeks.

pregnant women living in a Lyme endemic area were enrolled at their first prenatal visit successfully gathered outcome data on 1929 subjects; no increase in prematurity, miscarriage, or still birth was found.[22] Steere[16] has concluded that it is unusual for *B. burgdorferi* to cause an adverse fetal outcome.

SEROLOGICAL TESTING

The major diagnostic tool in evaluating a patient for Lyme disease, other than the history of a summer exposure to a tick bite in an endemic area and development of EM, is detection of antibody to *B. burgdorferi*. Two serological tests currently are available: (1) immunofluorescence assay (IFA), now rarely used, which utilizes fluorescein-conjugated antihuman immunoglobulins to detect antibodies in patient sera, and (2) enzyme-linked immunosorbent assay (ELISA). Although IFA is relatively sensitive and specific well into stage 1 disease, it is inadequate in detecting antibody early in the illness. In one study, sera obtained from patients who had Lyme disease during the first 3 weeks of their illness showed positivity by IFA in only 38% of cases, whereas patients who had neuritis and arthritis had reactive titers 92% to 100% of the time.[11] ELISA is more sensitive and specific than IFA in diagnosing early Lyme disease, but the deficiency of both tests is their occasional false-positive result, which is caused either by the presence of other spirochetal infections in the patient (e.g., syphilis or relapsing fever) or by other confounding patient variables as yet to be defined. Another problem with both IFA and ELISA testing has been the lack of standardization and quality controls for these tests in most diagnostic laboratories, resulting in poor interlaboratory and intralaboratory agreement.[6,13] Early antibiotic therapy also can blunt antibody production. Given these limitations, most laboratories now consider a titer of 1:256 or higher in a patient who has compatible clinical symptoms as sufficient to confirm the diagnosis of Lyme borreliosis.[4] Immunoblotting (Western blot assay) should be used when the physician suspects a falsely positive ELISA. Research into improved serological testing has focused on detecting antigens by using polymerase chain reaction (PCR) techniques. The results of investigations into CSF, urine, and synovial fluid concentrations of *Borrelia* DNA suggest their potential diagnostic usefulness, especially in cases of neurological disease.[5,7,8,10] With the advent of vaccination against *B. burgdorferi*, ELISA will not be useful in screening already immunized patients for Lyme disease. In these instances, Western blotting should be performed.

DIFFERENTIAL DIAGNOSIS

In children who have what appears to be Lyme arthritis, the most likely differential diagnosis (as in the first cases of the disease) is pauciarticular juvenile arthritis. Other considerations include aseptic meningitis, Bell's palsy or a peripheral neuropathy not caused by *B. burgdorferi,* multiple sclerosis, septic arthritis, acute rheumatic fever, and fibromyalgia syndrome. Such diagnoses are ruled out easily with a history of a tick bite and EM, but many patients who have Lyme disease have no history of these events. Certainly, during the summer in an endemic area, Lyme disease should be considered when consistent symptoms are present.

MANAGEMENT

As a spirochetal infection, Lyme borreliosis can be treated successfully, depending on when in the course of the illness antibiotics are begun. With EM, oral antibiotic therapy is used; tetracycline, doxycycline, penicillin, amoxicillin, cefuroxime axetil, or erythromycin (with a penicillin allergy in a child age 8 or younger) shortens the duration of the rash and often prevents later complications. Facial palsy or peripheral neuropathy alone also can be treated with antibiotics given orally, but any other neurological abnormality, such as meningitis or general central nervous system symptoms, should be treated with parenteral ceftriaxone, cefotaxime, penicillin G, or chloramphenicol. Although first-degree atrioventricular block usually requires only oral therapy, higher-grade blocks usually are treated with parenteral therapy with ceftriaxone or penicillin G. Finally, intermittent or chronic arthritis should be treated with either parenteral or long-term oral antibiotic therapy. Specific dosages and durations are shown in Table 233-2, as recommended by both Steere[16] and others.[23]

The later antibiotic therapy is instituted, the more likely are complications and persistent problems. Thus a high level of suspicion, followed by prompt diagnosis and treatment, is rewarded with a high likelihood of a mild, short-term illness with a favorable prognosis. Should chronic arthritis persist, the usual management with antiinflammatory medications and physical therapy is required. The most recent therapeutic work in the area of Lyme disease has centered on vaccine development in which the outer surface protein A (OspA) portion of the spirochete serves as the antigenic stimulus for antibody production. In two double-blind, placebo-controlled, randomized studies involving more than 10,000 subjects (ages 15 to 70 years) in each, immunization efficacy after three doses (administered at 0, 1 and 12 months) has ranged from 76% to 92%.[14,20] One of these investigations was designed so as to determine prevention efficacy for asymptomatic Lyme disease and found this to be 100%.[20] As vaccine technology advances, those living in endemic areas or anticipating travel to such regions will have a true prevention alternative.[21] On December 22, 1998, LYMErix, manufactured by SmithKline Beecham Biologicals, was approved by the Food and Drug Administration, but only for individuals 15 years of age and older.

When to Refer

Cardiac involvement (heart block, pericarditis, myocarditis)
Neurological involvement (except isolated facial palsy in patient with definite Lyme disease diagnosis), including persistent cognitive deficits
Nonspecific clinical history, but positive or equivocal laboratory testing
Persistent arthritis

When to Hospitalize

Cardiac involvement
Meningitis or encephalopathy

REFERENCES

1. Bosler EM, et al: Prevalence of the Lyme disease spirochete in populations of white-tailed deer and white-footed mice, *Yale J Biol Med* 57:651, 1984.
2. Burgdorfer W, et al: Lyme disease: a tick-borne spirochetosis? *Science* 216:1317, 1982.
3. Burgdorfer W, et al: The Western black-legged tick, *Ixodes pacificus:* a vector of *Borrelia burgdorferi, Am J Trop Med Hyg* 34:925, 1985.
4. Eichenfield AH, Athreya BH: Lyme disease: of ticks and titers, *J Pediatr* 114:328, 1989.
5. Huppertz HI, Schmidt H, Karch H: Detection of *Borrelia burgdorferi* by nested polymerase chain reaction in cerebrospinal fluid and urine of children with neuroborreliosis, *Eur J Pediatr* 152:414, 1993.
6. Magnarelli LA: Quality of Lyme disease tests, *JAMA* 262:3464, 1989.
7. Nocton JJ, et al. Detection of *Borrelia burgdorferi* DNA by polymerase chain reaction in cerebrospinal fluid in Lyme neuroborreliosis, *J Infect Dis* 174:623, 1996.
8. Nocton JJ, et al: Detection of *Borrelia burgdorferi* DNA by polymerase chain reaction in synovial fluid from patients with Lyme arthritis, *N Engl J Med* 330:229, 1994.
9. Notifiable diseases, weekly information: United States *MMWR* 48:293, 1999.
10. Pachner AR, Delaney E: The polymerase chain reaction in the diagnosis of Lyme neuroborreliosis, *Ann Neurol* 34:544, 1993.
11. Russell H, et al: Enzyme-linked immunosorbent assay and indirect immunofluorescence assay for Lyme disease, *J Infect Dis* 149:789, 1984.
12. Schlesinger PA, et al: Maternal-fetal transmission of the Lyme disease spirochete, *Borrelia burgdorferi, Ann Intern Med* 103:67, 1985.
13. Schwartz BS, et al: Antibody testing in Lyme disease: a comparison of results in four laboratories, *JAMA* 262:3431, 1989.
14. Sigal LH, et al: A vaccine consisting of recombinant *Borrelia burgdorferi* outer surface protein A to prevent Lyme disease, *N Engl J Med* 339:216, 1998.
15. Steere AC: Lyme disease, *N Engl J Med* 308:733, 1983.
16. Steere AC: Lyme disease, *N Engl J Med* 321:586, 1989.
17. Steere AC, Broderick TF, Malawista SE: Erythema chronicum migrans and Lyme arthritis: epidemiologic evidence for a tick vector, *Am J Epidemiol* 108:312, 1978.
18. Steere AC, Malawista SE: Cases of Lyme disease in the United States: locations correlated with distribution of *Ixodes dammini, Ann Intern Med* 91:730, 1979.
19. Steere AC, et al: Lyme arthritis: an epidemic of oligoarticular arthritis in children and adults in three Connecticut communities, *Arthritis Rheum* 20:7, 1977.
20. Steere AC, et al: Vaccination against Lyme disease with recombinant *Borrelia burgdorferi* outer-surface lipoprotein A with adjuvant, *N Eng J Med* 339:209, 1998.

21. Steigbigel RT, Benach JL: Immunization against Lyme disease: an important first step, *N Engl J Med* 339:263, 1998.
22. Strobine BA, et al: Lyme disease and pregnancy outcome: a prospective study of two thousand prenatal patients, *Am J Obstet Gynecol* 169:367, 1993.
23. Treatment of Lyme disease, *The Medical Letter* 39:47, 1997.
24. Wallis RC, et al: Erythema chronicum migrans and Lyme arthritis: field study of ticks, *Am J Epidemiol* 108:322, 1978.
25. Weber K, et al: *Borrelia burgdorferi* in a newborn despite oral penicillin for Lyme borreliosis during pregnancy, *Pediatr Infect Dis J* 7:286, 1988.
26. Williams CL, et al: Lyme disease during pregnancy: a cord blood serosurvey, *Ann N Y Acad Sci* 539:504, 1988.

234 Meatal Ulceration

Mark F. Bellinger

Superficial ulceration of the male urethral meatus (urethritis orificii externi,[2] or Brennemann ulcer[1]) is a common clinical condition seen almost exclusively in circumcised boys; however, it may be seen in uncircumcised boys if the preputial opening is wide enough to expose the meatus and perimeatal portion of the glans penis. Mackenzie[7] reported meatal ulceration in 20% of boys examined within 5 weeks after neonatal circumcision but believed that the true incidence was significantly higher, based on historical data of ulcers that had healed by the time of examination.

ETIOLOGY

By approximately 16 weeks' gestation, the prepuce is completely formed, with complete fusion of the epithelium of the glans and prepuce.[5] Normal separation of the prepuce results from a gradual process of keratinization and thickening of the two layers.

Desquamation results in the formation of smegma, which mechanically separates the two layers, allowing gradual exposure of the now keratinized surfaces, which thus are more resistant to the normally harsh environment of the diaper. Preputial separation begins before birth, but in most cases continues well into infancy. Full separation and retraction of the prepuce is found in only 4% of neonates, but 90% have a retractable prepuce by the age of 3 years.[3] In contrast, forceful separation of the fused epithelial layers during neonatal circumcision exposes the raw, cherry-red translucent epithelium of the glans and meatus. Trauma to this thin epithelium from diaper contact may result in ulceration of the glans and the meatal edges.

HISTORY

Although meatal ulceration may be relatively asymptomatic, dysuria is common. Voluntary urinary retention may be the result of severe dysuria during the acute phase of ulceration, whereas involuntary retention may occur secondary to meatal crusting as the lesion heals. Acute crusting or fibrinous adhesion of the meatus may cause a deviated or split urinary stream. Recurrent cycles of ulceration and crusting may lead to scarring, gradual narrowing of the meatus, and a true stenosis with narrowing and upward direction of the urinary stream.[9]

PHYSICAL FINDINGS

Early ulcers are superficial, clean, and contiguous with the meatus, usually surrounding it. Spreading the lips of the meatus reveals normal urethral mucosa. Meatal ulceration may be seen in conjunction with diaper rash from any cause. When diaper rash is severe, inguinal adenopathy may be present. Meatal ulcers crust quickly, and a cyclical change from ulcer to crust is common as recurrent irritation disturbs the healing process. Crusting may transiently occlude the meatus with a fibrinous exudate, and urinary retention and bladder distention may result. If the crust is rubbed off, bloody spotting may be seen on the diaper. Repeated episodes of ulceration result in a healed but stenotic meatus. Visual examination of the meatus cannot adequately reveal whether significant stenosis is present, but observation of a narrowed stream with upward direction and outpouching of the meatal lips from the force of the stream indicates a urodynamically significant lesion.

DIFFERENTIAL DIAGNOSIS

Glanular trauma may result from circumcision, regardless of whether the Gomco, Plastibell, or freehand technique is used.[4] Older children may suffer glanular trauma during play, and many injuries are caused by falls during bathing. Zipper injuries to the glans are common, and adolescents may suffer trauma during intercourse. Insect bites may result in inflammation of the shaft or glans.

Balanitis (inflammation of the glans) and posthitis (inflammation of the prepuce) are most common in uncircumcised boys. Balanitis xerotica obliterans is a chronic inflammatory process of unknown etiology that may involve a whitish thickening of the glans, prepuce, and distal urethra.[8]

It is important to differentiate cutaneous lesions from urethral lesions that may protrude from the meatus. Urethral malignancies are rare in children, and most benign fibroepithiomatous polyps originate in the posterior urethra. Venereal diseases are an increasingly common source of genital lesions in adolescents. Condylomata acuminata (venereal warts) may appear on genital skin as small verrucae and may protrude from the urethral meatus as small polypoid masses. Gonorrheal or nonspecific urethritis may cause meatal edema and encrustation. Syphilitic chancre, a painless, indurated ulcer that has sharply demarcated borders, may be found on the penile shaft or glans 3 to 6 weeks after exposure. Herpes progenitalis occurs as perimeatal vesicles on an erythematous base, which may rupture to form a confluent superficial ulcer.[6] Other meatal ulcerations may result from erythema multiforme, contact dermatitis, drug eruptions, and scabies.

TREATMENT

Preventing meatal ulceration in a newly circumcised infant should not be difficult. Good hygiene, frequent diaper changes and, for babies who wear cloth diapers, proper rinsing of the diapers reduce the risk of ammoniacal dermatitis. On occasion, changing from cloth to disposable diapers or vice versa reduces irritation. Applying a protective ointment (e.g., A and D ointment) to the glans or diaper for a week or two after the circumcision reduces mechanical irritation.

When ulcers are present, local hygiene is important. Simple cleansing with soap and water and applying a protective ointment may suffice. If meatal crusting occurs, cleansing and ointment application reduce dysuria. Adherent crusts on the meatus may require mechanical debridement. Diaper rash requires appropriate topical therapy and/or acidification of the urine.

Meatal stenosis may occur after repeated episodes of meatitis.[2] The diagnosis should be made by the appearance of the voided urinary stream rather than by the appearance of the urethral meatus. A pinpoint, upward-directed stream with pouting of the meatal lips during micturition may indicate the need for meatotomy, which almost always can be performed in the office using local anesthesia. Two methods of anesthesia can be used. The first involves the injection of a small amount (less than 0.5 ml) of 1 percent lidocaine with 1:100,000 epinephrine into the ventral lip of the meatus using a 30-gauge needle. The disadvantage of this technique is that an injection is required but the advantage is that meatotomy can be performed immediately. The second technique for local anesthesia involves the application of EMLA cream to the meatus approximately 60 minutes before the procedure. Continuous contact with the skin of the glans is necessary, so that parents are instructed to apply the cream and cover the area with a piece of plastic wrap before the appointment. The technique of meatotomy is simple. A wide hemostat is clamped in the urethra, crushing the tissue of the inferior lip of the meatus for a distance of approximately 5 mm. After the hemostat has been left in place for a few seconds, it is unclamped and removed, and the crushed tissue is cut with a small scissors. The meatus then is covered with ointment. It is imperative that the patient or parent be instructed to spread the meatal lips several times a day for the next 10 to 14 days so that recurrent stenosis will be avoided.

Balanitis xerotica obliterans of the meatus may require meatotomy and topical therapy. Condylomata acuminata may be treated by topical, surgical, or laser therapy. Other genital venereal diseases require specific treatment (see Chapter 262, Sexually Transmitted Diseases).

REFERENCES

1. Brennemann J: The ulcerated meatus in the circumcised child, *Am J Dis Child* 21:38, 1921.
2. Freud P: The ulcerated urethral meatus in male children, *J Pediatr* 31: 131, 1947.
3. Gairdner D: The fate of the foreskin: a study of circumcision, *Br Med J* 2:1433, 1949.
4. Gee WF, Ansell JS: Neonatal circumcision: a 10-year overview, with comparison of the Gomco clamp and the Plastibell device, *Pediatrics* 58:824, 1976.
5. Glenister TW: A consideration of the processes involved in the development of the prepuce in man, *Br J Urol* 28:243, 1956.
6. Korting GW: *Practical dermatology of the genital region,* Philadelphia, 1980, WB Saunders.
7. Mackenzie AR: Meatal ulceration following neonatal circumcision, *Obstet Gynecol* 28:221, 1966.
8. McKay DL, Fuqua F, Weinberg AG: Balanitis xerotica obliterans in children, *J Urol* 114:773, 1975.
9. Noe HN, Dale GD: Evaluation of children with meatal stenosis, *J Urol* 114:455, 1975.

235 Meningitis

Geoffrey A. Weinberg

The meninges of the central nervous system (CNS) include three membranes that support, protect, and nourish the brain and spinal cord. The outermost layer, the dura mater, is a tough, inelastic, connective tissue layer that sheaths the brain and spinal cord and terminates caudally at the first coccygeal vertebra. The middle and innermost layers, the arachnoid and the pia mater, respectively, are similar in structure and often are referred to singly as the *leptomeninges*. The arachnoid and pia are partly separated, leaving a subarachnoid space containing cerebrospinal fluid (CSF). The CSF is formed in the choroid plexuses within the ventricles of the brain, which communicate with the subarachnoid space through the foramina of Magendie and Luschka.[8] The CSF slowly circulates around the brain and spinal cord, and is reabsorbed predominantly by the arachnoid villi of the superior sagittal sinus.[8]

Meningitis, which refers to inflammation of the meninges, most often is caused by an infectious agent, and less commonly by a chemical (medication) or malignancy. Untreated bacterial meningitis often is quickly fatal, making early diagnosis and treatment essential.

Both the incidence of bacterial meningitis and the causative organisms are related closely to age. During the first month of life the age-specific incidence is as high as 300 to 400 cases per 100,000 live births in some studies[18]; it falls to 141 per 100,000 during the second month of life, and to less than 50 per 100,000 in the second year of life. Until recent years a second peak occurred at 6 to 8 months, with an incidence of nearly 180 per 100,000 infants.[18] This second peak, which was due to *Haemophilus influenzae* type b (Hib) meningitis, has declined dramatically since 1988, when Hib conjugate vaccines were approved for use.[1,7,37,40] As illustrated in Fig. 235-1, between 1987 and 1997, the incidence of Hib meningitis fell from 40 cases per 100,000 children younger than 5 years of age to 1 case per 100,000.[11] This remarkable decline in Hib meningitis has converted bacterial meningitis to a disease predominantly of adults rather than of infants and young children, with the median age at diagnosis of 25 years in 1995 as opposed to 15 months in 1985 (Fig. 235-2).[60]

The etiology of bacterial meningitis also changes remarkably with age (Fig. 235-3). During the first month of life, more than two thirds of the cases of neonatal bacterial meningitis are caused by group B beta-hemolytic streptococci *(Streptococcus agalactiae)* or gram-negative enteric organisms, primarily *Escherichia coli, Klebsiella,* and *Enterobacter* species. In some regions the third most common isolate is *Listeria monocytogenes*. After the first month of life, *Listeria* organisms are found as the cause of meningitis only in debilitated or elderly persons.

The incidence of aseptic meningitis (predominantly caused by enteroviruses) ranges, in different years, from 1.5 to 4 cases per 100,000 population. The incidence in children actually is much higher because aseptic meningitis is still a disease of the young, with few reported cases occurring in persons over 30 years of age.

BACTERIAL MENINGITIS AFTER THE NEONATAL PERIOD

After the age of 1 month, most cases of bacterial meningitis are caused by *Neisseria meningitidis* or *Streptococcus pneumoniae* in regions where Hib conjugate vaccines are widely used (see Fig. 235-3).[60] Mortality varies with the pathogen and has been reported recently to be 21% for *S. pneumoniae,* 3% for *N. meningitidis,* and 6% for Hib.[60]

All three of these pathogens can be isolated from the throat or nasopharynx of healthy individuals. Most studies of microorganism carrier states suggest that children at highest risk for disease also are the most likely to be colonized. During an 18-month period in the pre-Hib conjugate vaccine era, 71% of the toddlers and 48% of the preschool-age children at a day care center were colonized with Hib.[38] However, no invasive Hib disease occurred. Thus, colonization with Hib, as well as that with *S. pneumoniae* and *N. meningitidis,* does not always cause meningitis; indeed, nasopharyngeal colonization may in fact be a partially immunizing event, contributing to future host defense. However, when microbial virulence factors overcome host defense, bacterial meningitis ensues.

The successful meningeal pathogen must follow several sequential steps.[44,45] Nasopharyngeal mucosal colonization is facilitated by various microbial-binding adhesins and secreted enzymes such as IgA protease, which cleaves host secretory IgA. Next, invasion across the epithelium, followed by survival of bacteria in the bloodstream (by evading the action of the alternative complement pathway) are required. Finally, the bacteria must invade the CSF by crossing the blood-brain barrier.

Meningitis occasionally may occur after head trauma, particularly with fractures of the paranasal sinuses. The pathogens most often associated with meningitis after trauma are *S. pneumoniae* (often less pathogenic capsular serotypes) and *H. influenzae* (often nontypable or encapsulated but non-type b strains). Posttraumatic meningitis can recur if CSF leakage persists. Meningitis also can occur by direct spread from a

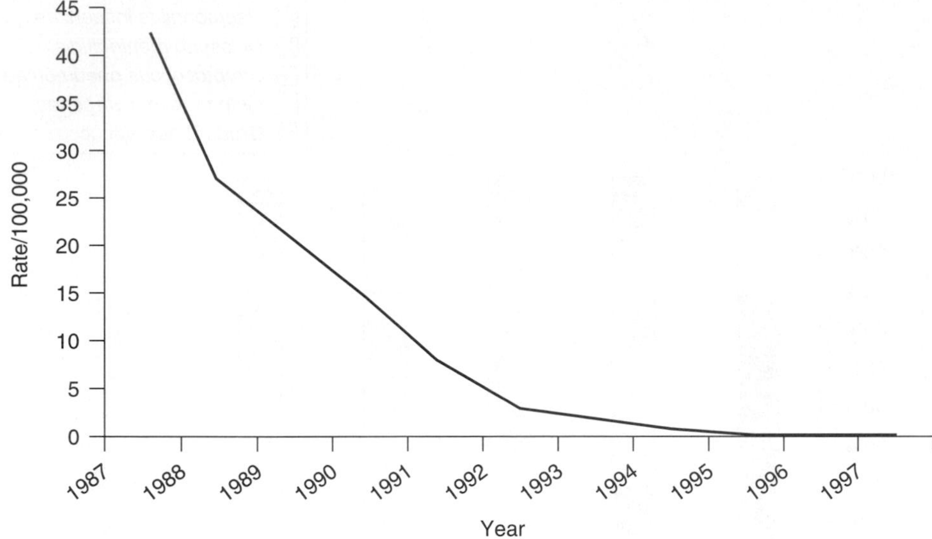

Fig. 235-1 Incidence of *Haemophilus influenzae* type b meningitis per 100,000 children younger than 5 years of age, in the United States from 1987-1997.

(Redrawn from Centers for Disease Control and Prevention: Progress toward eliminating *Haemophilus influenzae* type b disease among infants and children—United States, 1987-1997, *MMWR* 47:993: 1998.)

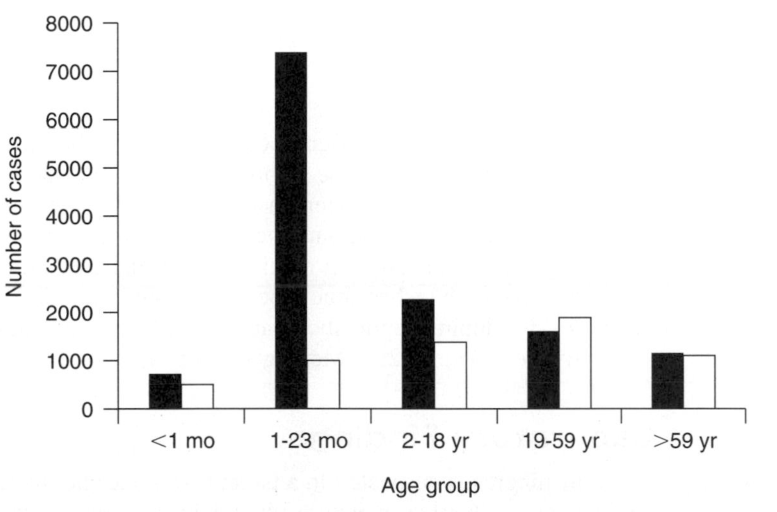

Fig. 235-2 Number of cases of bacterial meningitis caused by the five major pathogens in the United States during 1985 and 1995 according to age group.

(Redrawn from Schuchat A, et al: *N Engl J Med* 337:970, 1997.)

congenital dermal sinus that communicates with the CNS. Any time meningitis is caused by bacteria that normally reside on the skin or in the gastrointestinal tract, a diligent search of the craniospinal axis should be made. Meningitis can develop after neurosurgery and is not uncommon after procedures done to shunt ventricular fluid. Coagulase-negative staphylococci are the organisms most often associated with shunt infections.

Once bacteria establish growth in the CSF, cell wall products, such as lipopolysaccharide (endotoxin), teichoic acid, and peptidoglycans, are liberated, which in turn induce the local production and secretion of inflammatory cytokines (especially interleukin-1 [IL-1], IL-6, and tumor necrosis factor).[64] The action of these cytokines results in activation of leukocytes and vascular metabolism, which leads to leukocyte migration (diapedesis), endothelial injury, and blood-brain barrier breakdown. The injury to the cerebral microvasculature along with increasing inflammation culminate in brain edema, reduction of cerebral blood flow, thrombosis, and impairment of oxygen and glucose delivery.[18,19,44,45]

Clinical Manifestations

Children who have bacterial meningitis usually are febrile; however, the absence of fever in a child who has signs of meningeal irritation does not preclude the diagnosis.[18,19,66] Inflammation of the meninges can be manifested by irritability, anorexia, headache, nausea, vomiting, confusion, back pain, nuchal rigidity, and photophobia. The signs on physical examination described by Kernig and Brudzinski can be used to demonstrate meningeal inflammation.[68] Kernig's sign is elicited in the supine patient by extending the leg at the knee while the hip is flexed at 90 degrees. This maneuver causes extensor spasm of the knee and pain in the hamstrings of a person who has meningitis when the lower leg is extended to approximately 135 degrees. Brudzinski's sign is elicited by

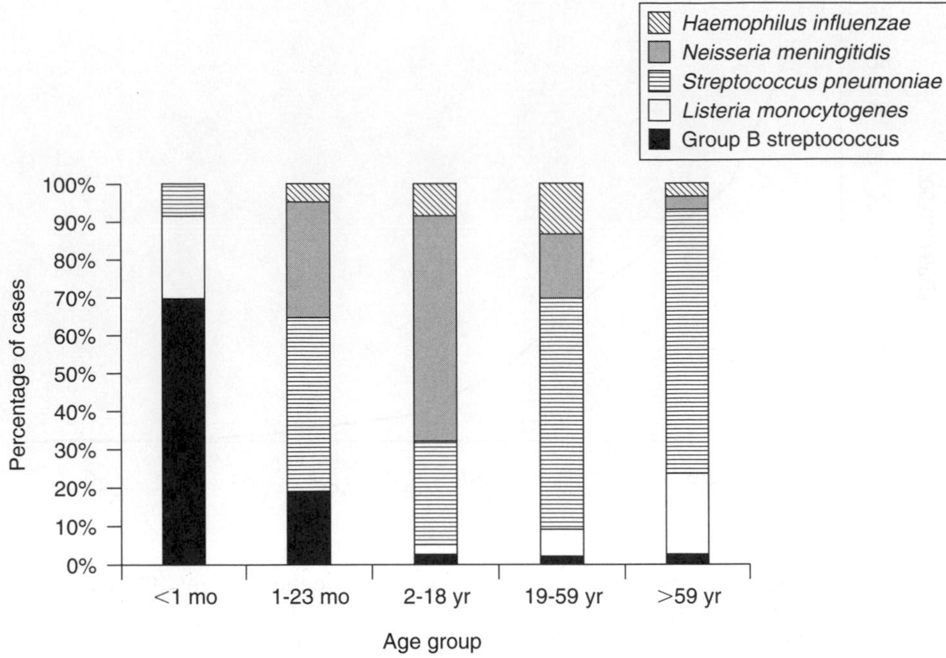

Fig. 235-3 Distribution of 248 cases of bacterial meningitis according to age group and causative organism, from an active, population-based, surveillance project performed in 22 counties across 4 states during 1995. Meningitis caused by enteric pathogens in infants younger than 1 month of age was not included in the surveillance.
(Redrawn from Schuchat A, et al: *N Engl J Med* 337:970, 1997.)

flexing the neck of a patient in the supine position and observing involuntary flexing of the hips and knees. In a young infant, signs of meningeal inflammation can be minimal or absent.[70] In infants, irritability, lethargy, poor feeding, and restlessness often are described. The patient also may have signs of increased intracranial pressure such as a headache or a bulging fontanelle. However, papilledema is uncommon with bacterial meningitis, and when it is present, other causes should be sought.

Cranial nerve involvement occurs with bacterial meningitis and, although often transient, can be permanent.[18,19] The auditory nerve often is affected, as manifested by deafness or disturbances of vestibular function. Blindness has been reported but is rare. Children also may have paralysis of extraocular or facial nerves. The degree of CNS derangement observed with bacterial meningitis ranges from irritability to coma. In a prospective series of 235 patients, Feigin and Pearlman found that about 15% of children who had bacterial meningitis were comatose or semicomatose at the time of hospitalization.[19] This occurred more often with *S. pneumoniae* or *N. meningitidis* than with Hib. Seizures occurred before or within 1 to 2 days after admission in about 30% of patients. Focal neurological signs, present in 16.5% of the patients, correlated with persistent abnormal neurological and developmental examinations 1 year after discharge.

Subdural effusions occur in about 50% of children who have bacterial meningitis but seldom are significant clinically.[18,19] Therefore, unless focal neurological signs or signs of increased intracranial pressure develop, the presence of such effusions need not be sought through the performance of subdural taps or computed tomography (CT) scans. Infection of subdural effusions is extremely rare.

Arthralgia and myalgia often occur in patients who have meningitis, particularly those who have meningococcemia.[18,19] Vasculitis can be seen in children who have any type of bacterial meningitis, but petechiae and purpura more commonly are associated with meningococcal disease. Children who have such rashes should be considered in imminent danger of developing septic shock and should be treated accordingly (see Chapter 291, Meningococcemia).

Laboratory Findings

When meningitis is suspected in a patient who does not have papilledema, a lumbar puncture should be performed, the opening pressure measured, and the CSF examined immediately. The clinical situation should influence the amount of data required before a therapeutic decision is made. If the CSF from an ill, febrile child is turbid or purulent, antimicrobial agents should be started as treatment for bacterial meningitis before further laboratory results are available. In any case, the CSF should be examined as soon as possible. If the nucleated blood cell count of the CSF is not above 6/μl the only other tests likely to be useful in diagnosing bacterial meningitis are a Gram stain and a culture of the CSF.[51] If the nucleated white blood cell count is 6/μl or above, a Gram stain, culture, and differential cell count should be done, and the CSF concentrations of total protein and glucose should be determined. If possible, the blood glucose should be measured just before the lumbar puncture so that the CSF to blood glucose ratio can be determined. (The blood glucose is best measured before the lumbar puncture because the stress of the procedure can temporarily elevate the blood glucose.) If only a small amount of CSF is obtained, the most impor-

Table 235-1 Characteristic Cerebrospinal Fluid Findings in Children with and without Meningitis

CSF Findings	Normal	Bacterial	Viral	Fungal or Tuberculous
Leukocytes/µl				
Usual	<5	>500	<500	50-750
Range	0-10	10-20,000	0-1000	10-1500
PMNs, % of Leukocytes				
Usual	2	>80	<50	<50
Range	0-20	20-100	0-100	0-80
Glucose, mg/dl				
Usual	60	<40	>40	<40
Range	45-65	0-65	30-65	5-50
Usual CSF/blood, %	≥60	<30	30-60	<40
Protein, mg/dl				
Usual	≤30	>100	<100	50-200
Range	0-40	40-500	20-200	40-1500
Other positive tests	None	Gram stain, antigen detection	PCR	Cryptococcal antigen, acid-fast stain

tant tests to perform are a Gram stain and bacterial culture. Characteristic CSF findings are shown in Table 235-1.

The CSF should be cultured on chocolate and blood agar plates and in broth. Generally, bacterial cultures will be positive within a few days if pathogens are present. The etiological agent also may be quickly identified using latex agglutination reactions or counterimmunoelectrophoresis (CIE) to detect soluble capsular antigens in CSF, and if needed, in serum or concentrated urine. Although these tests are rapid, they should *not* be viewed as essential, since their negative predictive value does not approach 100% and they appear to have little utility in patient care.[41] Rapid diagnostic tests are probably most valuable in patients in whom a significant amount of antibiotics have been given 24 hours or more before lumbar puncture.[18,41]

Blood cultures should be obtained for all children suspected of having bacterial meningitis. In one study, blood cultures were positive in 90%, 80%, and 91% of children who had not received antimicrobial agents previously and who had meningitis caused by Hib, *S. pneumoniae,* and *N. meningitidis,* respectively.[19]

Roentgenograms may help in identifying suspected bone or joint infection in selected patients. Radionuclide and CT studies have a role in complicated cases of meningitis and may be helpful for decisions on management. However, CT scans should not be obtained routinely because of prolonged or secondary fever as the results of the study are unlikely to affect management.[19,22]

A common clinical concern is how to distinguish the CSF abnormalities caused by infection from those associated with traumatic lumbar puncture. Common clinical practice is to use the ratio of red blood cells to white blood cells to "correct" the observed CSF white blood cell count, either by subtraction or by examination of the ratio of observed to "expected" cells.[8] These modifications generally are not very helpful to the clinician in deciding whether to proceed with antibiotic therapy, and bacterial or viral cultures will yield a more definitive answer within a relatively short time.

Two more common clinical concerns are when should diagnostic lumbar puncture be performed, and when may it be performed safely; a third related concern is the need to perform cranial CT scans before lumbar puncture. In general, lumbar puncture should be performed whenever the diagnosis of meningitis is known or suspected; it remains appropriate for the number of negative lumbar punctures to greatly exceed that of positive lumbar punctures if the maximum number of diagnoses of disease is to be achieved.[18] In most cases the child younger than 12 months of age (and perhaps younger than 18 months of age) with a first febrile seizure should have a lumbar puncture to exclude meningitis.[4,18]

Four reasons for delaying lumbar puncture exist: (1) clinically important cardiorespiratory compromise in a neonate; (2) signs of significantly increased intracranial pressure (e.g., retinal changes, altered pupillary responses, increased blood pressure with associated bradycardia, or focal neurological signs on exam); (3) infection in the skin, soft tissues, or epidural area through which lumbar puncture is to be performed; or (4) suspicion or history of bleeding disorders (e.g., hemophilia, severe thrombocytopenia). In these circumstances, blood cultures are obtained and antibiotics are given empirically without awaiting results of lumbar puncture. In the case of suspected increased intracranial pressure, arrangements are made for a neuroimaging study (e.g., cranial CT scan with and without contrast enhancement) during or immediately after antibiotic administration, and if the imaging study suggests that it will be safe to proceed, lumbar puncture may follow. It is not, however, necessary to perform CT scans routinely before lumbar puncture in patients with suspected meningitis, all of whom have some degree of increased intracranial pressure by virtue of the disease process; herniation of the brain on removal of a small amount of CSF is distinctly uncommon in meningitis, especially in infants with open fontanelles. Nonetheless, lumbar puncture should be performed cautiously if increased intracranial pressure is suspected, and it is reasonable to obtain CT scans before lumbar puncture in selected patients, especially in older children or adults or in those who have focal neurological signs of significantly increased intracranial pressure as noted previously.

Differential Diagnosis

Signs and symptoms suggesting meningeal inflammation or increased intracranial pressure can be seen with other infections of the CNS as well. The most common cause of meningeal inflammation is viral meningitis, which is discussed later in this chapter. Aseptic meningitis (i.e., Gram stain and routine bacterial culture are negative) can be caused by *Mycobacterium tuberculosis,* fungi, parasites, or inflammatory conditions. Meningitis or meningoencephalitis also may be present in patients who have Rocky Mountain spotted fever (RMSF), Kawasaki disease (see Chapter 230), cat-scratch disease, or toxic shock syndrome, and it often is associated with or occurs after mumps, rubeola, rubella, varicella, infectious mononucleosis, roseola, and erythema infectiosum (Table 235-2). A brain abscess, epidural abscess, primary amebic meningoencephalitis, embolic diseases (e.g., endocarditis or thrombophlebitis), venous sinus thrombosis, space-occupying lesions, reactions to medications (e.g., intravenous immunoglobulin, intravenous monoclonal antilymphocyte antibody, oral trimethoprim-sulfamethoxazole, some oral nonsteroidal antiinflammatory drugs), ingestion of toxins (e.g., lead), spider bites, pemphigus, and Behçet's syndrome can mimic bacterial meningitis. However, interpretation of the CSF findings in the context of the clinical manifestations usually differentiates bacterial meningitis from other diseases. Eosinophilic meningitis is rarely seen; the differential diagnosis includes reactions to ventriculoperitoneal shunts, unusual presentations of bacterial or *Toxoplasma* infection, or parasitic roundworms.[24,36,74] Conditions that can simulate a clinical picture of meningitis but that usually have normal CSF findings include pharyngitis, retropharyngeal abscess, cervical adenitis, cervical spine arthritis or osteomyelitis, pyelonephritis, pneumonia, torticollis, tetanus, and oculogyric crisis.[35,62]

Partially Treated Meningitis

Several studies have shown that mean values for white blood cell (WBC) counts in CSF, percentage of polymorphonuclear cells, and glucose and protein concentrations in patients who have partially treated bacterial meningitis do not differ from those values in patients not treated previously.[8,19] Even children who have received intravenous antibiotics for 44 to 68 hours have CSF findings still characteristic of bacterial meningitis.[8,19] Cultures of CSF from pretreated children with bacterial meningitis grow Hib frequently, although pneumococci and meningococci grow less often after pretreatment.[8,19] However, some patients who have partially treated bacterial meningitis will have CSF findings indistinguishable from the classic findings of aseptic meningitis. Unless there is clear evidence of a nonbacterial cause (e.g., isolation of virus from CSF or blood), antibiotics should be administered to partially treated patients for 7 to 10 days at dosages appropriate for bacterial meningitis.[8,19]

Management

General care. When initially examined, children who have meningitis may appear only mildly ill with fe-

Table 235-2 Selected Etiologies of Aseptic Meningitis*

	Common	Uncommon	Rare
Viruses	Enteroviruses Arboviruses Herpes simplex type 2 Human herpesvirus-6	HIV-1 Epstein-Barr virus Lymphocytic choriomeningitis virus Mumps	Adenovirus Varicella zoster virus Cytomegalovirus Measles Rubella Parvovirus B19 Influenza A and B
Bacteria	Pyogenic (partially treated) *Mycobacterium tuberculosis* *Borrelia burgdorferi* *Mycoplasma pneumoniae* *Leptospira* species	*Treponema pallidum* *Borrelia* species *Bartonella henselae* *Rickettsia rickettsii* *Ehrlichia canis*	*Chlamydia psittaci* *Chlamydia pneumoniae* *Rickettsia prowazekii* *Coxiella burnetii*
Fungi	*Candida* species *Cryptococcus neoformans* *Histoplasma capsulatum* *Coccidioides immitis*	*Blastomyces dermatitidis*	Various molds
Parasites		*Toxoplasma gondii* Neurocysticercosis	*Angiostrongylus cantonensis* *Baylisascaris procyonis* *Strongyloides stercoralis* Free-living amoebae
Miscellaneous	Parameningeal infections Kawasaki disease Foreign bodies (CSF shunts) CNS leukemia, tumors Acute disseminated encephalomyelitis (ADEM)	Medications (TMP-SMX, IGIV) Systemic lupus erythematosus	Sarcoidosis Behçet's syndrome Heavy-metal poisoning

**Common, uncommon,* and *rare* refer to relative frequencies within each broad category of etiological agents (e.g., viruses, bacteria). Overall, it should be noted that enteroviruses cause at least 85% of the aseptic meningitis diagnosed in children in the United States, and arboviruses approximately 5%; all other etiologies combined cause the remaining 10% or less of cases.

ver and irritability, or they may be profoundly ill with an altered state of consciousness and hypotension. The severity of illness at the time of presentation can predict morbidity and should dictate immediate management. Acute bacterial meningitis is always a medical emergency, and all infants and children who have an altered state of consciousness should be observed closely and the need for intensive care anticipated.[18,35,66]

As soon as bacterial meningitis is diagnosed, intravenous access should be secured and appropriate antimicrobial agents (and possibly antiinflammatory agents) given. The initial laboratory examination should include CSF examination and culture, blood culture, measurement of serum electrolyte and glucose concentrations, complete blood count and platelet count, and measurement of urine specific gravity. If the patient has petechiae or purpura or is in shock, the laboratory tests should include a partial thromboplastin time (PTT), prothrombin time (PT), and measurement of fibrinogen or fibrin breakdown products. Management of the child who is awake and has stable cardiorespiratory vital signs consists primarily of administering antimicrobial agents and fluids and careful monitoring for changes in level of consciousness, development of seizures, changes in vital signs, and development of the syndrome of inappropriate secretion of antidiuretic hormone (SIADH).

Other therapies should be considered in more critically ill children (see the discussion of management of septic shock in Chapter 296, Shock). Seizures should be treated with appropriate anticonvulsants, and an open airway that provides good oxygenation should be ensured. Patients who are in profound coma or whose level of consciousness deteriorates while receiving therapy should be evaluated for complications such as a cerebral abscess, obstructive hydrocephalus, or elevated intracranial pressure. A CT scan of the brain is extremely helpful in determining the diagnosis in such cases.

If significantly elevated intracranial pressure is a major clinical concern and treatment has been started or is anticipated, a neurosurgeon should be consulted and an intracranial pressure monitoring device placed (although it should be noted that all children with bacterial meningitis have some increase in intracranial pressure, and monitoring devices will not be required for the vast majority of patients). If an intraventricular catheter can be placed, increased intracranial pressure often can be treated by removing CSF. The placement of a pressure transducer affords continuous intracranial monitoring so that mannitol and hyperventilation can be used as necessary to decrease pressure and maintain cerebral perfusion. Cerebral perfusion pressure increased by 21% within 12 hours of the first dose of dexamethasone in patients who received 0.15 mg/kg per dose given every 6 hours for 4 days compared with a decline of 5% in those who received placebo.[39] Perhaps it is increased cerebral perfusion that accounts for the benefits reported by some investigators with dexamethasone therapy.[58]

Fluid management, possible antiinflammatory adjunctive treatments, and antimicrobial therapy are crucial for all patients who have bacterial meningitis. Even today, there remain controversies about mechanisms of action, utility, and choice of these interventions that would at first glance seem beyond question; these are discussed below.

Fluid therapy. Traditionally, fluids were restricted to two thirds of the total daily maintenance amount in patients who had bacterial meningitis to minimize brain edema and prevent SIADH.[18,19] Some studies found that SIADH occurred in 29% to 88% of cases of bacterial meningitis.[19] One recent study showed that plasma antidiuretic hormone (ADH) concentrations returned to normal in bacterial meningitis patients who received replacement plus maintenance fluids for 24 hours; concentrations remained elevated in patients restricted to two thirds of maintenance requirements.[43] The authors argued that maintenance fluids are necessary to perfuse, oxygenate, and deliver host defenses to the CNS, and that although SIADH occurs in bacterial meningitis, there is no evidence that fluid restriction prevents it. Others argue that these results simply confirm that dehydration produces an "appropriate" elevation of ADH, and that SIADH may still occur in nondehydrated or fluid-repleted children.[19] All authors agree that obvious fluid deficits be replaced rapidly, and that serum sodium concentrations be closely monitored several times during the first 24 hours of therapy, along with measurements of urine specific gravity. If the serum sodium concentration drops below 125 mEq/L, the test should be repeated as soon as possible. If the serum sodium is still below 125 mEq/L, fluids should be restricted to "keep the vein open" until the serum electrolyte concentrations have been corrected. Otherwise, for the usual child with bacterial meningitis, it seems appropriate to provide fluids at 75% to 80% of the maintenance rate after fluid repletion, and advance to full maintenance rates as the serum sodium increases beyond 135 mEq/L. The period of fluid restriction may only need to be one day or less.[19]

Antiinflammatory therapy. The use of glucocorticoids as adjunctive therapy in patients who have bacterial meningitis was studied by several groups in the late 1980s and the early 1990s.[33,39,69] Reviews of these studies conclude that dexamethasone most likely improves the hearing and neurological outcomes of children who have bacterial meningitis caused by Hib, [19,66,69] but that further studies are needed to confirm the utility of dexamethasone in children with bacterial meningitis caused by *S. pneumoniae* or *N. meningitidis*, or in adult patients.[45,46,66,69] Glucocorticoids and other antiinflammatory compounds produce definite salutary changes in experimental meningitis models that ought to imply better outcomes for children. However, such therapy may also cause gastrointestinal bleeding, decreased penetration of antimicrobial agents into the CSF, and obfuscation of the clinical assessment of children's response to therapy.[5,31] The American Academy of Pediatrics Committee on Infectious Diseases recommends that dexamethasone 0.6 mg/kg/day in four divided doses be given for 2 days starting at the time of the first dose of antimicrobial agents to children 6 weeks of age or older who have Hib meningitis and should be considered for use in children who have pneumococcal or meningococcal meningitis.[5] If used, dexamethasone should be administered at the time antibiotics are given or as soon as possible thereafter.

Antimicrobial therapy. Because it is not always certain which etiological agent is present at the time of diagnosis of bacterial meningitis, empirical guides to therapy are based on age (which, in turn, predicts the most likely etiology) (Table 235-3). In addition, some organism-specific points must be noted.

Until the early 1990s, all *N. meningitidis,* Hib, and most *S. pneumoniae* strains were susceptible to very low concentrations of the third-generation cephalosporins ceftriaxone and cefotaxime.[46] Since then, there have been numerous reports of infections in infants and children caused by resistant strains of pneumococci.[9,31,63] Some regions have reported that 30% of pneumococcal isolates are resistant to penicillin at some level and that many also are resistant to the third-generation cephalosporins.[10] Therefore, in areas where pneumococci are resistant to third-generation cephalosporins, infants and children suspected of having bacterial meningitis caused by pneumococci (i.e., gram-positive cocci in pairs seen on a Gram stain of the CSF) should receive vancomycin (10 to 15 mg/kg/dose given every 6 hours) in addition to either ceftriaxone (80 to 100 mg/kg/day divided in one or two daily doses) or cefotaxime (50 to 75 mg/kg/dose given every 6 hours). Because dexamethasone can decrease the CSF penetrance (and thus the activity) of vancomycin, either dexamethasone should be omitted or rifampin (10 mg/kg/dose given every 12 hours) plus vancomycin plus a third-generation cephalosporin should be used when dexamethasone is given.[5,29,46,66] As soon as the antimicrobial susceptibility of an isolate is known, vancomycin should be discontinued if the isolate is susceptible to the third-generation cephalosporins. Vancomycin must be used judiciously because it often is the last line of therapy for resistant gram-positive pathogens. If vancomycin resistance becomes prevalent, many children may die because of untreatable antibiotic-resistant bacterial infections.

Hib disease may be treated reliably with either ceftriaxone or cefotaxime; ampicillin may be used only if the isolate is known to be susceptible. Disease caused by *N. meningitidis* is treated reliably with penicillin G at high doses, or alternatively by ampicillin or a third-generation cephalosporin.

Meningitis caused by *N. meningitidis* usually is treated for 7 days, meningitis caused by Hib for 7 to 10 days, and that caused by *S. pneumoniae* for 10 to 14 days, although a 7-day course of antimicrobial therapy for uncomplicated Hib and *S. pneumoniae* meningitis has been shown to be effective.[5,26,34,46] Chloramphenicol is now rarely used for therapy in the industrialized world. Although most cases of bacterial meningitis beyond the neonatal period are caused

Table 235-3 Antimicrobial Therapy of Bacterial Meningitis

Empirical Therapy Pending Culture and Susceptibility Data		
Age	**Likely Pathogens**	**Antimicrobials**
0-1 mo	*S. agalactiae, E. coli, L. monocytogenes*	Ampicillin + cefotaxime *or* ampicillin + gentamicin
1-3 mo	*S. agalactiae, L. monocytogenes, S. pneumoniae, N. meningitidis, H. influenzae* b	Ampicillin + [cefotaxime *or* ceftriaxone] ± vancomycin
3 mo-21 yr	*S. pneumoniae, N. meningitidis H. influenzae* b if not vaccinated	[Cefotaxime or ceftriaxone] ± vancomycin

Specific Therapy			
S. agalactiae	Ampicillin or penicillin G for 14-21 days; first 3 days add gentamicin		
L. monocytogenes	Ampicillin for 14-21 days; first 3 days add gentamicin		
S. pneumoniae	MICs (μg/ml)		
	Penicillin	cefotaxime/ceftriaxone	
	<0.1	≤0.5	Penicillin G for 10-14 days
	≥0.1	≤0.5	Cefotaxime or ceftriaxone for 10-14 days
	≥0.1	1.0	[Cefotaxime or ceftriaxone] + vancomycin for 10-14 days
	≥0.1	≥2.0	[Cefotaxime or ceftriaxone] + vancomycin + rifampin for 10-14 days
N. meningitidis	Penicillin G for 7 days; alternatives: ampicillin, cefotaxime, ceftriaxone		
H. influenzae b	Cefotaxime or ceftriaxone for 7-10 days; alternative: ampicillin if isolate susceptible		

Antimicrobial Dosages			
Agent	**Dose (mg/kg/day)**		
	0-7 Days of Age	**8-28 Days of Age**	**Infants and Children**
Ampicillin	150-200 divided q8 hr	200-300 divided q6 hr	200-300 divided q6 hr
Cefotaxime	100 divided q12 hr	200 divided q8 hr	200-300 divided q6 hr
Ceftriaxone	Not recommended	80-100 divided q12-24 hr	80-100 divided q12-24 hr
Gentamicin	5 divided q12 hr	7.5 divided q8 hr	7.5 divided q8 hr
Penicillin G	100,000-150,000 units divided q12 hr	150,000-200,000 units divided q6 hr	300,000-400,000 units divided q4-6 hr
Rifampin	10 divided q12 hr	20 divided q12 hr	20 divided q12 hr
Vancomycin	20 divided q12 hr	30 divided q8 hr	40-60 divided q6 hr

by the three organisms mentioned, other bacteria can cause meningitis; in such cases, antimicrobial therapy must be individualized.

Most therapeutic failures can be related to inadequate therapy with the correct antimicrobial agent, resistant organisms, or prolonged delays in diagnosis. A repeat lumbar puncture on completion of therapy does not reflect the adequacy of therapy or predict the likelihood of recurrence and usually is not indicated. However, a delay in sterilizing the CSF beyond 24 to 36 hours has been associated with adverse outcomes; therefore, some experts recommend that another lumbar puncture be performed at that time. Repeat lumbar puncture at 24 to 48 hours of therapy also is indicated if drug-resistant *S. pneumoniae* is present, especially if dexamethasone is used.[5,29,31]

Some contacts of patients who have *N. meningitidis* or Hib meningitis are at increased risk for the disease and therefore should receive prophylaxis.[5] Prophylactic regimens for those at risk for *N. meningitidis* are described in Chapter 291, Meningococcemia. Whether all contacts of patients who have Hib disease should receive prophylaxis remains controversial. The American Academy of Pediatrics recommends that rifampin, 20 mg/kg (600 mg maximum), be given once a day for 4 days to all household contacts, including adults, in households that have at least one contact under age 4 whose immunization status against Hib is incomplete.[5] The definition of complete immunization depends on the age of the individual involved.[5] A household contact is anyone who resides with the index patient or a nonresident who has spent 4 or more hours a day with the index patient for 5 of the 7 days before the index patient was hospitalized. Prophylaxis for all household contacts, regardless of age, is given in households that have a child younger than 12 months of age. Prophylaxis for nonhousehold contacts of Hib disease does not appear to be necessary in general. The index patient also should receive rifampin either during or at the completion of treatment for Hib or meningococcal meningitis, unless ceftriaxone was used for treatment (ceftriaxone itself may clear meningococcal and likely, Hib, carriage). Many authorities still recommend that the index patient should receive rifampin either during or at the completion of treatment for Hib or meningococcal meningitis, although ceftriaxone therapy itself may clear meningococcal carriage.

Complications

Early in the course of bacterial meningitis, increased intracranial pressure, septic shock, disseminated intravascular coagulation (DIC), and even cardiorespiratory arrest may occur. Subdural effusions occasionally cause seizures or focal neurological deficits; in such cases the fluid should be removed by subdural taps. Such effusions are rarely infected directly, but subdural empyemas are occasionally reported. Inappropriate secretion of antidiuretic hormone also can complicate bacterial meningitis, as previously noted; therefore the patient should be monitored carefully for this complication, and if it occurs, fluid should be restricted severely. A brain abscess is extremely rare after bacterial meningitis except in neonates who have meningitis caused by *Citrobacter* or certain *Enterobacter* species (see p. 1641).

Sequelae

Despite the appropriate use of bactericidal antibiotics, the mortality rate for bacterial meningitis remains at 5% to 10%.[18] Approximately 15% to 25% of survivors will have long-term morbidity, including developmental delay, seizure disorder, spasticity, and hearing loss.*

It is difficult to predict long-term sequelae for an individual child at the time of discharge from the hospital. Some children who apparently are normal subsequently are found to have hearing or learning deficits or will develop a seizure disorder. Conversely, some children expected to have a dismal prognosis based on abnormal neurological examinations at discharge make remarkable gains. It therefore is important for the practitioner to be guardedly optimistic with the family while remaining sensitive to possible sequelae and observing these children closely for attainment of developmental milestones. Hearing should be tested formally before discharge from the hospital because most sensorineural hearing loss can be detected at this time. In one of the largest prospective series available,[16] the rate of persistent bilateral or unilateral sensorineural hearing loss was 31% following pneumococcal meningitis, 10.5% following meningococcal meningitis, and 6% following Hib meningitis. In young infants, brain stem-evoked response audiometry is necessary for full evaluation; in older toddlers and children, routine pure-tone audiometry may suffice. In the future, simple otoacoustic emission screening may be more useful if further study validates the technique.[49]

It is thought that much of the hearing loss in meningitis occurs soon after infection[18,19,69]; this may explain why not all studies have shown reduction of hearing loss by dexamethasone therapy. The timing of other neurological sequelae is even less certain. Some cases of bacterial meningitis present fulminantly; outcome in these cases may be poor no matter how quickly therapy is rendered.[28,30,47] In many cases, the exact onset of disease is difficult to pinpoint, and thus the length of prodromal symptoms before therapy does not correlate well with outcome.[28,30,47]

Prevention

In 1985, a purified capsular polysaccharide vaccine against Hib was licensed for use in the United States in children older than 2 years of age (in whom the risk of Hib disease was albeit substantially lower than that of the highest risk group, infants younger than 1 year).[50] Subsequently, four vaccines were made by coupling the capsular polysaccharide to a protein carrier in order to boost immunogenicity in infants.[50,71] These conjugate vaccines were also more immunogenic in older children with conditions associated with impaired responses to capsular polysaccharide vaccine.[72] Eventually, three of the four Hib conjugate vaccines were licensed for routine use in infants at 2, 4, and 6 months of age[5] (Table 235-4). Widespread use of these vaccines has resulted in the dramatic decline in the incidence of invasive Hib disease† (see Fig. 235-1). The meningococcal and pneumococcal vaccines currently available are composed of purified capsular polysaccharides and, like the prototype Hib

*References 14, 16, 18, 23, 42, 65.

†References 1, 7, 11, 37, 40, 60.

Table 235-4 *Haemophilus influenzae* Type b Conjugate Vaccines

Abbreviation	Trade Name	Manufacturer	Carrier Protein	Licensed for Use at Age (Mo)
PRP-D	ProHIBit	Aventis Pasteur	Diphtheria toxoid	12-15
HbOC	HibTITER	Wyeth Lederle Vaccines	CRM_{197} (nontoxic mutant diphtheria toxin)	2, 4, 6,12-15
PRP-OMP	PedvaxHIB	Merck & Co.	*N. meningitidis* outer membrane proteins	2, 4, 12-15
PRP-T	ActHIB OmniHIB	Aventis Pasteur SmithKline Beecham	Tetanus toxoid	2, 4, 6, 12-15
Combination Products				
HbOC + DTwP	TETRAMUNE	Wyeth Lederle Vaccines	CRM_{197} (nontoxic mutant diphtheria toxin)	2, 4, 6, 12-15
PRP-OMP + hepatitis B	COMVAX	Merck & Co.	*N. meningitidis* outer membrane proteins	2, 4, 12-15
PRP-T mixed with Aventis Pasteur DTaP (Tripedia)	TriHIBit	Aventis Pasteur	Tetanus toxoid	12-15

polysaccharide vaccine, are poor immunogens in infants under age 2 years.[5] Multivalent pneumococcal polysaccharide-protein conjugate vaccines modeled on the Hib conjugate vaccines have proved to be safe and immunogenic in children,[15] and one was licensed for use in the United States in February 2000.[5a,7a] Meningococcal polysaccharide-protein conjugate vaccines also are being developed, and although not yet licensed in the United States, are being administered in the United Kingdom.[35a]

Pneumococcal conjugate vaccine is recommended for routine universal administration to infants and children younger than 2 years of age, in a similar fashion to Hib conjugate vaccines.[5a] The pneumococcal conjugate vaccine also is suggested for high-risk children 2 to 5 years of age (including children who have sickle cell disease, functional or anatomical asplenia, immunosuppression, cancer, chronic renal disease, chronic cardiopulmonary disease, CSF leaks, and diabetes).[5a]

At present, meningococcal polysaccharide vaccine is routinely used only for children and adults at higher risk of disease, such as those with sickle cell disease, functional or anatomical asplenia, immunosuppression, and CSF leaks.[5] Meningococcal vaccine also is used as an adjunct to chemoprophylaxis in outbreak control. Recently, a controversy has developed as to whether adolescents attending college should be vaccinated routinely with meningococcal polysaccharide vaccine, in view of an apparent increase in serogroup C disease outbreaks in the United States, many of which occurred in schools and universities. Although the American College Health Association recommended such routine vaccination beginning in 1997, neither the American Academy of Pediatrics nor the Centers for Disease Control and Prevention have endorsed this recommendation fully in the absence of documented epidemics, since the actual risk of infection remains low (4.6 cases per 100,000 for freshman college students living in dormitories as opposed to 1.5 cases per 100,000 in non-college students aged 18 to 23 years).[10a] Parents and incoming college freshmen should be informed about meningococcal disease and the benefits of vaccination. Those who wish to reduce their (albeit low) risk should be vaccinated. No changes in living situations are warranted by use or non-use of meningococcal vaccine.[10a]

NEONATAL MENINGITIS

Neonatal meningitis merits separate consideration because the incidence is high, the etiological agents are unique, and it is more often fatal than is meningitis in the older child. The incidence of neonatal meningitis varies with the reporting institution, from 0.2 to 1 case per 1000 live births.[32] The age-specific incidence of bacterial meningitis in the first month of life in the United States between 1978 and 1981 was 366 per 100,000 neonates. Case fatality rates generally range from 20% to 25% in the modern era.[32,56] In general, mortality is lower for full-term infants than for infants of low birth weight (under 2500 g). Early recognition and treatment are critical because the case fatality rate falls to about 5% for neonates who survive the first 24 hours of the disease.[56]

The cause of neonatal meningitis has changed since 1970, and clinicians should be alert to the possibility of future etiological shifts.[32] During the 1960s, most cases were caused by gram-negative enteric organisms, primarily *E. coli;* gram-positive isolates were likely to be *L. monocytogenes.* During the 1970s, group B beta-hemolytic streptococci *(S. agalactiae)* became prevalent; currently this organism and *E. coli* account for 50% to 66% of cases of neonatal meningitis and *L. monocytogenes* for about 1% to 5%.[32,67] Neonatal sepsis and meningitis caused by non-group D alpha-hemolytic streptococci and coagulase-negative staphylococci also have been reported. Group B beta-hemolytic streptococci can cause sepsis and/or meningitis in the first hours of life; by definition, such infection at an age younger than 7 days is termed *early onset.* Late-onset disease—that is, group B beta-hemolytic streptococcal infection at age older than 7 days—is characteristically meningitis rather than sepsis, and tends to be associated with capsular serotype III organisms.[32,56]

The clinical signs associated with neonatal meningitis are nonspecific and therefore not very helpful. Neonates with meningitis often have apneic episodes or feed poorly, and they can be hyperthermic or hypothermic, irritable or lethar-

Table 235-5 Representative Cerebrospinal Fluid Findings in Neonates without Meningitis

CSF Findings	Full-term Neonates—Mean (Range)		Preterm Neonates—Mean (Range)	
	0-7 Days	8-28 Days	0-7 Days	8-28 Days
Leukocytes/μl	8 (1-30)	6 (0-18)	4 (1-10)	7 (0-44)
PMNs, % of leukocytes	5	3	7	9
Protein, mg/dl	81	64	150 (85-222)	148 (54-370)
Glucose, mg/dl	46	51	72 (4-96)	64 (33-217)
CSF/blood glucose, %	0.73	0.62	Not reported	Not reported

Data from Ahmed A, et al: *Pediatr Infect Dis J* 15:298, 1996; and Rodriguez AF, Kaplan SL, Mason EO Jr: *J Pediatr* 116:971, 1990.

gic, and have respiratory distress and/or diarrhea; only very infrequently do they have nuchal rigidity. They may exhibit a bulging fontanelle. The neonate has a limited repertoire of clinical responses to disease or insult; most sick neonates therefore receive a diagnostic evaluation for sepsis, including a lumbar puncture, and antimicrobial agents are started pending culture results. The cytology and chemistry of the CSF in neonates have a much broader normal range than in other age groups, especially during the first week of life (Table 235-5), and so any single test result may not appear abnormal.[2,52] However, infants who have bacterial meningitis very rarely have completely normal CSF on examination.

Antimicrobial Therapy

The principles of antimicrobial therapy for neonatal meningitis are the same as for infants and children, but because the organisms are different, the antimicrobial selection must be adjusted. Based on the most common organisms that cause neonatal meningitis, the ideal antimicrobial would be effective against *E. coli* and other enteric organisms as well as against group B beta-hemolytic streptococci and other gram-positive organisms. Two third-generation cephalosporins, cefotaxime and ceftriaxone, are extremely active against the organisms that usually cause neonatal meningitis, except for poor activity against *L. monocytogenes*. The major difference between these drugs is their pharmacokinetic profile; ceftriaxone exhibits a much longer serum half-life. In addition, because ceftriaxone is highly protein-bound and can displace unconjugated bilirubin from albumin, it generally is not used in premature infants at risk for kernicterus or in term infants who have hyperbilirubinemia. No formal comparison of these newer agents with the historical regimen of ampicillin plus an aminoglycoside such as gentamicin has taken place. However, because the third-generation cephalosporins are safe, are very active against the common pathogens, and enter the CSF relatively well, cefotaxime plus ampicillin (the latter to empirically treat *Listeria*) should be used to treat suspected neonatal meningitis (suspected disease plus abnormal CSF). Some authorities would add gentamicin as a third agent if gram-negative enteric meningitis was thought likely. Because some enteric pathogens such as *Pseudomonas aeruginosa* and *Enterobacteriaceae* readily become resistant to the third-generation cephalosporins, these antibiotics should not be used empirically for all cases of suspected sepsis in neonates (the choice of ampicillin and gentamicin remains appropriate in this situation if the CSF appears normal). Dosages and characteristics of the antimicrobials used most often to treat neonatal meningitis are listed in Table 235-3.

The role of intraventricular antimicrobial therapy remains uncertain; in one multicenter trial, infants given intraventricular therapy in addition to intravenous therapy fared worse than those receiving intravenous therapy alone did.[32] Other therapeutic considerations (e.g., fluid management and close serial monitoring) are the same for neonates as for infants and children who have bacterial meningitis, except that no data support the use of dexamethasone in infants younger than 6 weeks of age.[5] The head circumference should be measured serially to detect early signs of hydrocephalus.

Newer possible adjunctive therapies, such as intravenous immunoglobulin, do not have a defined role in neonatal bacterial meningitis. With the advent of maternal penicillin chemoprophylaxis against group B beta-hemolytic streptococci,[5] the incidence of early-onset sepsis and meningitis caused by this organism should decrease but that of late-onset meningitis will likely remain unchanged.

Prognosis

The complications of neonatal meningitis, which are similar to those seen among older infants but perhaps more common, include hydrocephalus, deafness, and blindness. The case fatality rate is 20% to 25% in general but may approach 50% in low-birth-weight babies with gram-negative enteric meningitis. Long-term follow-up studies have revealed that about 65% of survivors of coliform meningitis are normal 3 to 7 years after the illness, about 30% have mild to moderate neurological sequelae, and 5% to 10% have major sequelae.[21,56,67] About 50% of cases of group B beta-hemolytic streptococcal meningitis survivors are normal, 20% have mild to moderate sequelae, and 20% to 30% have major sequelae (i.e., hydrocephalus, seizures, or profound retardation).[21,32,56]

For unknown reasons, as many as 80% of neonates who have gram-negative enteric meningitis caused by either *Citrobacter* or certain *Enterobacter* species will develop one or more brain abscesses. This complication is distinctly unusual with meningitis caused by any other organism. Routine follow-up with cranial CT scans is indicated for neonates with *Citrobacter* species or *Enterobacter sakazakii* meningitis or sepsis. As with older infants and children, all infants recovering from meningitis should have careful audiological testing and close evaluation for attainment of developmental milestones.

ASEPTIC MENINGITIS

The syndrome of aseptic meningitis consists of a clinical picture of meningitis with CSF pleocytosis and the absence of bacteria on gram stain or culture. Although aseptic meningitis usually is a viral disease, it is important that treatable causes of this syndrome be considered in the differential diagnosis. Table 235-2 lists a wide variety of infectious and noninfectious agents and diseases that have been associated with aseptic meningitis. Nonpolio enteroviruses cause 85% of cases of aseptic meningitis in the United States, but mumps and polio should be considered in other areas of the world where they are still endemic. The CSF findings characteristic of aseptic meningitis are shown in Table 235-1. When encephalitis accompanies aseptic meningitis, the clinical course is much more severe. See Chapter 236, Meningoencephalitis.

Clinical Manifestations

Infants and children who have aseptic meningitis caused by enteroviruses often are acutely febrile, irritable, and lethargic. Their temperature usually is 38.0° to 40.5° C (100.4° to 105° F) for 4 to 5 days. Upper respiratory tract symptoms, headache, photophobia, nausea, and vomiting also are commonly present; rashes may be seen as well. In general, a child who has viral meningitis does not appear as critically ill as a child who has bacterial meningitis and is less likely to have meningeal signs.[12,18,19,70]

The diagnosis of aseptic meningitis is likely when CSF pleocytosis ranges from 10 to 500 cells that are predominantly lymphocytes, the CSF protein is mildly elevated at 50 to 150 mg/dl, and the CSF glucose concentration is normal. Early in the course of viral meningitis, polymorphonuclear neutrophils (PMNs) can predominate in the CSF. A transition from a predominance of PMNs to lymphocytes usually occurs rapidly, and a repeat lumbar puncture after 8 to 12 hours may show this transition.[6,20] Tuberculous and fungal meningitis generally have gradual onsets of illness over days to weeks.

Hypoglycorrhachia (low CSF glucose level) rarely occurs with viral meningitis caused by enteroviruses, mumps, herpes simplex, and Eastern equine encephalitis viruses. Hypoglycorrhachia caused by these viruses tends to result in CSF glucose concentrations that equal about 30% of the simultaneous blood glucose concentration, whereas bacterial meningitis usually results in CSF glucose concentrations of less than 30% of the blood glucose. The CSF glucose concentration also can be low with tuberculous and fungal meningitis.

Many physicians are reluctant to obtain specimens for viral culture because they believe that isolating viruses takes too long to affect patient management. A review of patients who had CSF specimens sent promptly on admission for viral culture showed that of 111 patients who had a discharge diagnosis of aseptic meningitis, 46 had enteroviral meningitis, 2 had herpes simplex meningoencephalitis, 1 had leukemic meningitis, and 1 had toxoplasmosis with CNS involvement.[13] It took an average of 3.7 days for CSF cultures to show a typical enterovirus cytopathic effect. The diagnosis of enteroviral meningitis frequently resulted in discontinuation of antimicrobial therapy and early discharge from the hospital. Therefore, when viral meningitis is a possibility, the CSF should be cultured for viruses, as should nasopharyngeal or throat and rectal swab specimens. Although isolation of a virus from a site other than the CSF could be misleading, if taken in the context of other clinical and laboratory findings, a presumptive diagnosis often can be made when a virus is isolated from one or more of these sites. The polymerase chain reaction (PCR) holds much promise as a rapid and sensitive method of diagnosing meningitis caused by enteroviruses, herpes viruses, and perhaps other viruses as well. PCR amplification of enteroviral RNA from CSF and serum appears to have good sensitivity, specificity, and predictive value.[3,54,59] The technique will likely continue to be studied for the diagnosis of a number of other causes of aseptic meningitis.[25,27,48]

The management of aseptic meningitis is directed mainly to supportive care. A new antienteroviral agent, pleconaril, is undergoing evaluation in both adults and children with enteroviral meningitis[57]; this or other similar drugs may be useful in the future. Meningoencephalitis caused by herpes simplex or varicella-zoster viruses should be treated with acyclovir. Aseptic meningitis caused by one of the other less common etiologies noted in Table 235-2 may also require specific therapy.

Outcome

The outcome of aseptic meningitis relates to both the causative agent and the child's age. Patients who have the most common known cause of viral meningitis, enteroviral meningitis, usually recover completely.[53,55] However, some studies [17,61,73] have reported low intelligence and delayed speech development after enteroviral meningitis in very young infants. In light of these findings, the prognosis for an infant younger than 3 months of age is somewhat guarded, and the child's development should be monitored carefully.

REFERENCES

1. Adams WG, et al: Decline of childhood *Haemophilus influenzae* type b (Hib) disease in the Hib vaccine era, *JAMA* 269:221, 1993.
2. Ahmed A, et al: Cerebrospinal fluid values in the term neonate, *Pediatr Infect Dis J* 15:298, 1996.
3. Ahmed A, et al: Clinical utility of the polymerase chain reaction for diagnosis of enteroviral meningitis in infancy, *J Pediatr* 131:393, 1997.
4. American Academy of Pediatrics: Practice parameter: the neurodiagnostic evaluation of the child with a first simple febrile seizure, *Pediatrics* 97:769, 1996.
5. American Academy of Pediatrics: Pickering L, editor: *Red Book 2000: Report of the Committee on Infectious Diseases,* ed 25, Elk Grove Village, Ill, 2000.
5a. American Academy of Pediatrics: Policy statement: recommendations for the prevention of pneumococcal infections, including the use of pneumococcal conjugate vaccine (Pravnar), pneumococcal polysaccharide vaccine, and antibiotic prophylaxis, *Pediatrics* 106: 362, 2000.
6. Amir J, et al: Shift of cerebrospinal polymorphonuclear cell percentage in the early stage of aseptic meningitis, *J Pediatr* 119:938, 1991.
7. Bisgard KM, et al: *Haemophilus influenzae* invasive disease in the United States, 1994-1995: near disappearance of a vaccine-preventable childhood disease, *Emerg Infect Dis* 4:229, 1998.
7a. Black S, et al: Efficacy, safety, and immunogenicity of heptavalent pneumococcal conjugate vaccine in children, *Pediatr Infect Dis J* 19: 187, 2000.
8. Bonadio WA: The cerebrospinal fluid: physiologic aspects and alterations associated with bacterial meningitis, *Pediatr Infect Dis J* 11:423, 1992.

9. Bradley JS, Connor JD: Ceftriaxone failure in meningitis caused by *Streptococcus pneumoniae* with reduced susceptibility to beta-lactam antibiotics, *Pediatr Infect Dis J* 10:871, 1991.
10. Butler JC, et al: The continued emergence of drug-resistant *Streptococcus pneumoniae* in the United States: an update from the Centers for Disease Control and Prevention Pneumococcal Sentinel Surveillance System, *J Infect Dis* 74:986, 1996.
10a. Centers for Disease Control and Prevention: Prevention and control of meningococcal disease and meningococcal disease and college students: recommendations of the Advisory Committee on Immunization Practices (ACIP), *MMWR* 49(RR7):1, 2000.
11. Centers for Disease Control and Prevention: Progress toward eliminating *Haemophilus influenzae* type b disease among infants and children—United States, 1987-1997, *MMWR* 47:993, 1998.
12. Cherry JD: Aseptic meningitis and viral meningitis. In Feigin RD, Cherry JD, editors: *Textbook of pediatric infectious diseases*, ed 4, Philadelphia, 1998, WB Saunders.
13. Chonmaitree T, Menegus MA, Powell KR: The clinical relevance of CSF viral culture: a 2-year experience with aseptic meningitis in Rochester, NY, *JAMA* 247:1843, 1982.
14. D'Angio CT, et al: Long-term outcome of *Haemophilus influenzae* meningitis in Navajo Indian children, *Arch Pediatr Adolesc Med* 149:1001, 1995.
15. Daum R: Pneumococcal vaccines for children: an update, *Pediatr Infect Dis J* 17:823, 1998.
16. Dodge PR, et al: Prospective evaluation of hearing impairment as a sequelae of acute bacterial meningitis, *N Engl J Med* 311:869, 1984.
17. Farmer CJ, Carpenter RL, Ray CG: A follow-up study of 15 cases of neonatal meningoencephalitis due to coxsackievirus B5, *J Pediatr* 87: 568, 1975.
18. Feigin RD, McCracken GH Jr, Klein JO: Diagnosis and management of meningitis, *Pediatr Infect Dis J* 11:785, 1992.
19. Feigin RD, Pearlman E: Bacterial meningitis beyond the neonatal period. In Feigin RD, Cherry JD, editors: *Textbook of pediatric infectious diseases*, ed 4, Philadelphia, 1998, WB Saunders.
20. Feigin RD, Shackelford PG: Value of repeat lumbar puncture in the differential diagnosis of meningitis, *N Engl J Med* 289:571, 1973.
21. Franco SM, Cornelius VE, Andrews BF: Long-term outcome of neonatal meningitis, *Am J Dis Child* 146:567, 1992.
22. Friedland IR, et al: Cranial computed tomographic scans have little impact on management of bacterial meningitis, *Am J Dis Child* 146: 1484, 1992.
23. Grimwood K, et al: Adverse outcomes of bacterial meningitis in school-age survivors, *Pediatrics* 95:646, 1995.
24. Hsu W-Y, et al: Eosinophilic meningitis caused by *Angiostrongylus cantonensis*, *Pediatr Infect Dis J* 9:443, 1990.
25. Huang C, Chatterjee NK, Grady LJ: Diagnosis of viral infections of the central nervous system, *N Engl J Med* 340:483, 1999.
26. Jadavji T, et al: Sequelae of acute bacterial meningitis in children treated for seven days, *Pediatrics* 78:21, 1986.
27. Jeffery KJM, et al: Diagnosis of viral infections of the central nervous system: clinical interpretation of PCR results, *Lancet* 349:313, 1997.
28. Kallio MJT, et al: The effect of a recent previous visit to a physician on outcome after childhood bacterial meningitis, *JAMA* 272:787, 1994.
29. Kaplan SL, Mason EO Jr: Management of infections due to antibiotic-resistant *Streptococcus pneumoniae*, *Clin Microbiol Rev* 11:628, 1998.
30. Kilpi T, et al: Length of prediagnostic history related to the course and sequelae of childhood bacterial meningitis, *Pediatr Infect Dis J* 12:184, 1993.
31. Kleiman MB, et al: Meningitis with beta-lactam-resistant *Streptococcus pneumoniae*: the need for early repeat lumbar puncture, *Pediatr Infect Dis J* 12:782, 1993.
32. Klein JO, Marcy SM: Bacterial sepsis and meningitis. In Remington JS, Klein JO, editors: *Infectious diseases of the fetus and newborn infant*, ed 4, Philadelphia, 1995, WB Saunders Co.
33. Lebel MH, et al: Dexamethasone therapy for bacterial meningitis: results of two double-blind, placebo-controlled trials, *N Engl J Med* 319: 964, 1988.
34. Lin TY, et al: Seven days of ceftriaxone therapy is as effective as 10 days' treatment for bacterial meningitis, *JAMA* 253:3559, 1985.
35. Lipton JD, Schafermeyer RW: Evolving concepts in pediatric bacterial meningitis. I. Pathophysiology and diagnosis. II. Current management and therapeutic research, *Ann Emerg Med* 22:1602, 1993.
35a. MacLennan JM, et al: Safety, immunogenicity, and induction of immunologic memory by a serogroup C meningococcal conjugate vaccine in infants: a randomized controlled trial, *JAMA* 283:2795, 2000.
36. Miron D, et al: Eosinophilic meningitis in a newborn with group B streptococcal infection, *Pediatr Infect Dis J* 12:966, 1993.
37. Murphy TV, et al: Declining incidence of *Haemophilus influenzae* type b disease since introduction of vaccination, *JAMA* 269:246, 1993.
38. Murphy TV, et al: Pharyngeal colonization with *Haemophilus influenzae* type b in children in a day care center without invasive disease, *J Pediatr* 106:712, 1985.
39. Odio CM, et al: The beneficial effects of early dexamethasone administration in infants and children with bacterial meningitis, *N Engl J Med* 324:1525, 1991.
40. Peltola H: Worldwide *Haemophilus influenzae* type b disease at the beginning of the 21st century: global analysis of the disease burden 25 years after the use of the polysaccharide vaccine and a decade after the advent of conjugates, *Clin Microbiol Rev* 12:302, 2000.
41. Perkins MD, Mirrett S, Reller LB: Rapid bacterial antigen detection is not clinically useful, *J Clin Microbiol* 33:1486, 1995.
42. Pomeroy SL, et al: Seizures and other neurologic sequelae of bacterial meningitis in children, *N Engl J Med* 323:1651, 1990.
43. Powell KR, et al: Normalization of plasma arginine vasopressin concentrations when children with meningitis are given maintenance plus replacement fluid therapy, *J Pediatr* 117:515, 1990.
44. Quagliarello V, Scheld WM: Bacterial meningitis: pathogenesis, pathophysiology, and progress, *N Engl J Med* 327:864, 1992.
45. Quagliarello V, Scheld WM: New perspectives on bacterial meningitis, *Clin Infect Dis* 17:603, 1993.
46. Quagliarello V, Scheld WM: Treatment of bacterial meningitis, *N Engl J Med* 336:708, 1997.
47. Radetsky M: Duration of symptoms and outcome in bacterial meningitis: an analysis of causation and the implications of a delay in diagnosis, *Pediatr Infect Dis J* 11:694, 1992.
48. Read SJ, Jeffery KJM, Bangham CRM: Aseptic meningitis and encephalitis: the role of PCR in the diagnostic laboratory, *J Clin Microbiol* 35:691, 1997.
49. Richardson MP, et al: Otoacoustic emissions as a screening test for hearing impairment in children recovering from acute bacterial meningitis, *Pediatrics* 102:1364, 1998.
50. Robbins JB, et al: Prevention of systemic infections, especially meningitis, caused by *Haemophilus influenzae* type b: impact on public health and implications for other polysaccharide-based vaccines, *JAMA* 276: 1181, 1996.
51. Rodewald LE, et al: Relevance of common tests of cerebrospinal fluid in screening for bacterial meningitis, *J Pediatr* 119:363, 1991.
52. Rodriguez AF, Kaplan SL, Mason EO Jr: Cerebrospinal fluid values in the very low birth weight infant, *J Pediatr* 116:971, 1990.
53. Rorabaugh ML, et al: Aseptic meningitis in infants younger than 2 years of age: acute illness and neurologic complications, *Pediatrics* 92:206, 1993.
54. Rotbart HA: Diagnosis of enteroviral meningitis with the polymerase chain reaction, *J Pediatr* 117:85, 1990.
55. Rotbart HA: Enteroviral infections of the central nervous system, *Clin Infect Dis* 20:971, 1995.
56. Sáez-Llorens X, McCracken GH Jr: Perinatal bacterial diseases. In Feigin RD, Cherry JD, editors: *Textbook of pediatric infectious diseases*, ed 4, Philadelphia, 1998, WB Saunders.
57. Sawyer MH, et al: Oral pleconaril reduces the duration and severity of enteroviral meningitis in children, *Pediatr Res* 45(Part 2):173A, 1999.
58. Schaad UB, et al: Dexamethasone therapy for bacterial meningitis in children, *Lancet* 342:457, 1993.
59. Schlesinger Y, Sawyer MH, Storch GA: Enteroviral meningitis in infancy: potential role for polymerase chain reaction in patient management, *Pediatrics* 94:157, 1994.
60. Schuchat A, et al: Bacterial meningitis in the United States in 1995, *N Engl J Med* 337:970, 1997.

61. Sells CJ, Carpenter RL, Ray CG: Sequelae of central nervous system enterovirus infections, *N Engl J Med* 293:1, 1975.
62. Stein MT, Trauner D: The child with a stiff neck, *Clin Pediatr* 21:559, 1982.
63. Tan TQ, Mason EO Jr, Kaplan SL: Systemic infections due to *Streptococcus pneumoniae* relatively resistant to penicillin in a children's hospital: clinical management and outcome, *Pediatrics* 90:928, 1992.
64. Täuber MG, Moser B: Cytokines and chemokines in meningeal inflammation: biological and clinical implications, *Clin Infect Dis* 28:1, 1999.
65. Taylor HG, et al: The sequelae of *Haemophilus influenzae* meningitis in school-age children, *N Engl J Med* 323:1657, 1990.
66. Tunkel AR, Scheld WM: Acute bacterial meningitis, *Lancet* 346:1675, 1995.
67. Unhanand M, et al: Gram-negative enteric bacillary meningitis: a twenty-one-year experience, *J Pediatr* 122:15, 1993.
68. Verghese A, Gallemore G: Kernig's and Brudzinski's signs revisited, *Rev Infect Dis* 9:1187, 1987.
69. Wald ER, et al: Dexamethasone therapy for children with bacterial meningitis, *Pediatrics* 95:21, 1995.
70. Walsh-Kelly C, et al: Clinical predictors of bacterial versus aseptic meningitis in childhood, *Ann Emerg Med* 21:910, 1992.
71. Weinberg GA, Granoff DM: Polysaccharide-protein conjugate vaccines for the prevention of *Haemophilus influenzae* type b disease, *J Pediatr* 113:621, 1988.
72. Weinberg GA, Granoff DM: Immunogenicity of *Haemophilus influenzae* type b polysaccharide-protein conjugate vaccines in children with conditions associated with impaired antibody responses to type b polysaccharide vaccine, *Pediatrics* 85:654, 1990.
73. Wilfert CM, et al: Longitudinal assessment of children with enteroviral meningitis during the first 3 months of life, *Pediatrics* 67:811, 1981.
74. Woods CR, Englund J: Congenital toxoplasmosis presenting with eosinophilic meningitis, *Pediatr Infect Dis J* 12:347, 1993.

236 Meningoencephalitis

Richard S.K. Young

Meningoencephalitis is an infection of the central nervous system (CNS) and meninges caused by a variety of agents. In children, the most common pathogens are viruses, but fungi and parasites also may cause the disorder. Depending on the extent of the infection, the patient may have signs and symptoms of meningitis, encephalitis, or myelitis. By convention, bacterial invasion of the meninges is called *bacterial meningitis* and is considered a disorder distinct from meningoencephalitis.

The actual incidence of infectious meningoencephalitis almost certainly exceeds the nearly 12,000 cases reported each year to the Centers for Disease Control and Prevention (CDC) as aseptic meningitis and encephalitis.[22] However, the difficulty in identifying the specific agent in each suspected case makes statistical accuracy impossible.

ETIOLOGY OF CHILDHOOD MENINGOENCEPHALITIS

The course of meningoencephalitis may vary from aseptic meningitis with a mild clinical presentation to a fulminant encephalitis with paresis, seizures, increased intracranial pressure, and death.[4] Although the initial signs and symptoms produced by viruses often are similar, differences in seasonal occurrence, clinical course, and outcome allow differentiation of some disorders.

Nonpolio enteroviruses, including echovirus and group B coxsackievirus, are responsible for 85% of cases of aseptic meningitis each year.[7] Enteroviral infection usually is heralded by the development of malaise and gastroenteritis, more often during the summer (see Chapter 206, Enterovirus Infections). Progression to meningoencephalitis is uncommon with most enteroviral infections. When meningoencephalitis does occur, it usually is a mild disease. Poliovirus infections have been virtually eliminated through widespread immunization and now occur primarily in immunodeficient children or among small communities of unimmunized children. Echovirus infections commonly begin with a petechial rash; coxsackie infections often start with myalgia and lesions of the palms, soles, and mouth (hand-foot-and-mouth disease). An enterovirus may infect a fetus transplacentally. Eighty-four percent of patients who develop aseptic meningitis are younger than 16 weeks of age.[20]

Herpes simplex virus commonly produces a necrotizing encephalitis, and 50% to 70% of untreated cases are fatal.[25] Herpes simplex encephalitis has a bimodal age distribution, with one third of cases occurring in childhood. Neonatal infection results from passage through an infected birth canal. Mothers of infected infants often have no symptoms of herpes infection during or before gestation, making the diagnosis of a neonatal infection more difficult. Herpes simplex in the neonate may manifest as cutaneous disease, as meningoencephalitis, or as disseminated disease. In all age groups, herpes simplex virus occasionally causes a mild, self-limited meningoencephalitis. Nervous system infection with the Epstein-Barr virus (EBV) may result in involvement of the cortex, cerebellum, or cranial nerves.[8] Neurological manifestations include combative behavior, seizures, and headache. Varicella-zoster virus is a herpes virus that causes chickenpox or herpes zoster (shingles).

Arboviral infections caused by *Bunyavirus* species and togavirus are transmitted to humans by arthropods. Arbovirus meningoencephalitis often occurs in epidemics during the summer and early fall. California virus encephalitis should be suspected in any child in a known endemic region who has signs of fever and cerebrocortical dysfunction. The course usually is mild, with a fatality rate of less than 5%. Western equine encephalitis, an arboviral disease primarily of infancy, causes a more severe syndrome. Eastern equine encephalitis has a predilection for infants and young children and usually is fatal. St. Louis encephalitis occurs most often in epidemic form and produces illness in adults more often than in children.

Other viral diseases are transmitted by vectors. The virus that causes Colorado tick fever, a reovirus transmitted by rodent arthropods, produces a denguelike illness in humans. Viral disease transmitted directly to humans from animals includes lymphocytic choriomeningitis (arenavirus), which is transmitted by infected laboratory or domestic rodents, and rabies, which is transmitted by a bite, scratch, or droplet from an infected wild animal (e.g., raccoon or bat) or an unimmunized domestic animal (e.g., cat). Recent rabies infections in children have been attributed most often to rabid raccoons, bats, and cats.[2] Rabies characteristically has a long incubation period and invariably ends in a fatal meningoencephalitis. Congenital lymphocytic choriomeningitis mimics congenital toxoplasmosis or cytomegalovirus infection with chorioretinopathy, hydrocephaly, or microcephaly.[24] Common childhood viral infections such as rubella, adenovirus, influenza, cytomegalovirus, and Epstein-Barr virus (infectious mononucleosis) occasionally can cause meningoencephalitis.[8]

Meningoencephalitis that occurs in the course of childhood exanthems (measles, mumps, rubella, varicella) may result either from the host's immunological response to the virus or from actual infection of the nervous sys-

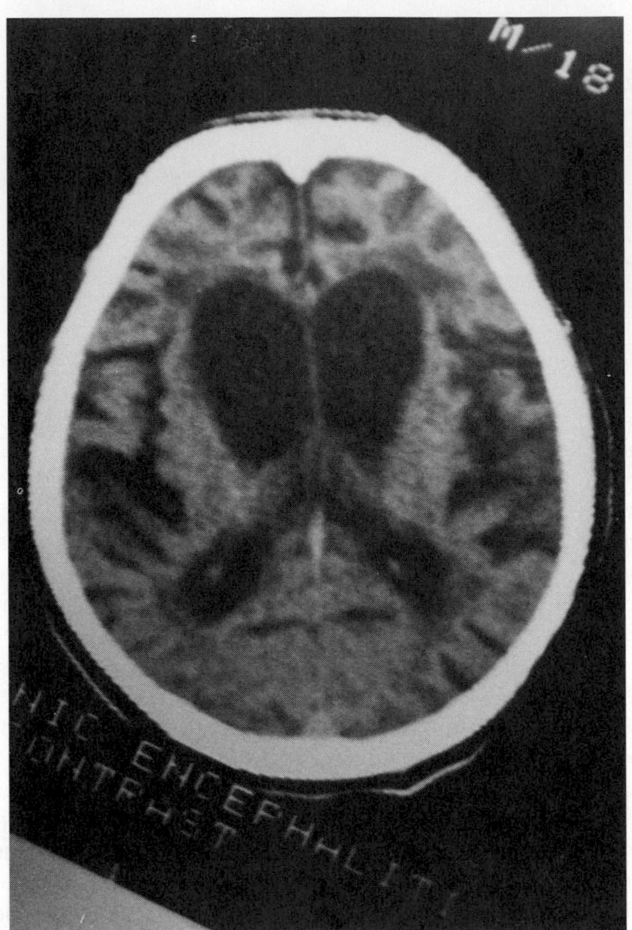

Fig. 236-1 Subacute sclerosing panencephalitis (SSPE). Marked atrophy of both the cerebral cortex and the deep gray nuclei has occurred in this child, who has long-standing SSPE.

tem. Both varicella and measles viruses cause meningoencephalitis in approximately 1 in 1000 cases and within 4 to 7 days after onset of the rash. The severity of the neurological illness (including irritability, drowsiness, and ataxia) does not appear to be related to the intensity of the systemic illness. Mortality in varicella and measles meningoencephalitis approximates 10%, and as many as half of survivors may have neurological residua. An unusual syndrome of dementia and myoclonic seizures can develop in children of school age many years after measles infection or immunization. This disorder results from a persistent measles infection known as *subacute sclerosing panencephalitis* (SSPE) (Fig. 236-1). Rubella is a less common cause of meningoencephalitis but can result in a more severe illness than can measles or varicella. In contrast, mumps meningoencephalitis is a mild illness that generally has a good prognosis. Mumps meningoencephalitis may occur without parotitis within a few weeks of exposure to the virus, or it may occur before the parotitis appears or after it has resolved.[23]

Acquired immunodeficiency syndrome (AIDS), which is caused by a retrovirus known as human immunodeficiency virus (HIV), is noteworthy for meningoencephalitides caused both by HIV and by unusual organisms such as *Toxoplasma gondii* or *Candida albicans* (Figs. 236-2 and 236-3) and Epstein-Barr virus. More than one organism, whether viral or bacterial, can be recovered in immunosuppressed patients who have AIDS.[18] Because of the immaturity of their immune responses, premature infants also are at risk for development of candidal meningitis.[14]

Nonviral causes of meningoencephalitis include infectious (fungi, spirochetes, and parasites) and postinfectious causes and noninfectious conditions associated with cerebrospinal

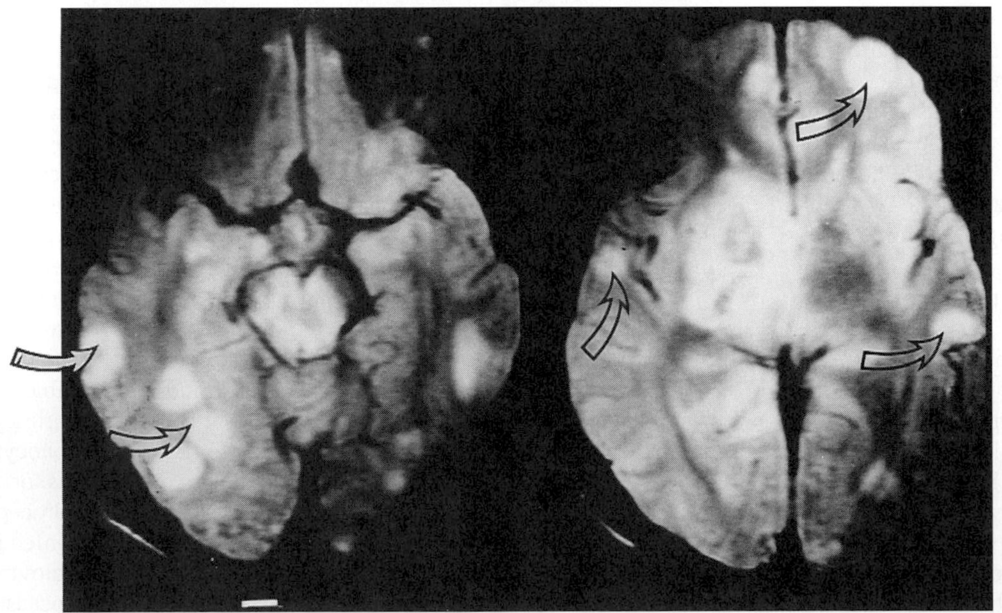

Fig. 236-2 Toxoplasmosis in acquired immunodeficiency syndrome (AIDS). Because patients who have AIDS are immunocompromised, they are at risk for opportunistic infections of the central nervous system. This T_2-weighted magnetic resonance image shows several high-intensity lesions caused by *Toxoplasma gondii* scattered throughout the frontal, temporal, and parietal lobes *(arrows)*.

(Courtesy Dr. G. Sze.)

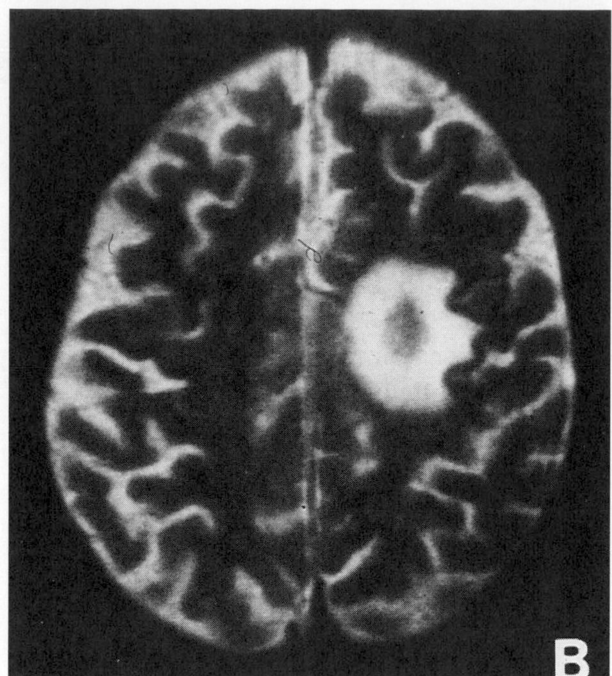

Fig. 236-3 Candidal abscess in AIDS. This T_2-weighted magnetic resonance image shows a large left parietal lesion with a mass effect. This lesion is consistent with the diagnosis of toxoplasmosis or lymphoma, but in this patient it proved to be caused by *Candida albicans.*

(Courtesy Dr. G. Sze.)

fluid pleocytosis[9] (Table 236-1). Amebic meningoencephalitis may result from swimming in infected fresh water rivers or lakes infected with *Naegleria.*[3] (See Chapter 246, Parasitic Infections.)

SIGNS AND SYMPTOMS

Depending on the extent of the viral infection, the patient may have signs and symptoms of meningitis, encephalitis, or myelitis. A patient who has meningitis characteristically complains of an intense headache, a stiff neck, and photophobia. Physical findings include meningismus, with positive Kernig's and Brudzinski's signs (see Chapter 235, Meningitis). In encephalitis, a patient who is lethargic, delirious, or hallucinating mistakenly may be diagnosed as being intoxicated or psychotic. A CNS infection should be presumed in any child with a fever who has an acute change in mental status.

Encephalitis may reveal focal neurological findings. Herpes simplex encephalitis, for example, classically is heralded by temporal lobe seizures and olfactory hallucinations. Varicella-zoster, Epstein-Barr virus, and other viruses may infect the cerebellum specifically, causing acute ataxia. With myelitis, the viral parenchymal disease causes a symmetrical limb paralysis, transverse sensory symptoms, and bowel and bladder dysfunction.

Rarely, meningoencephalitis may be occult. Ninety percent of children with facial nerve palsy caused by *Borrelia burgdorferi* had cerebrospinal fluid (CSF) pleocytosis or elevated CSF protein, although none of them had meningeal signs.[5] In contrast, other children with Lyme disease may develop pseudotumor,[13] radiculopathy, diplopia, headache, or meningismus.

LABORATORY INVESTIGATIONS

Every attempt should be made to identify and isolate the offending organism to help determine the prognosis and to document potential epidemic outbreaks. The CSF examination is crucial. Typical CSF alterations among patients who have meningoencephalitis consist of mild pleocytosis, a slight increase in protein level, and no alteration in glucose concentration (Table 236-2); however, the absence of CSF abnormalities does not rule out encephalitis. The sample of CSF should be refrigerated for later virus isolation and determination of viral antibody titers. Red cells in the CSF may indicate hemorrhagic brain necrosis, commonly seen with herpesvirus infections and Eastern equine encephalitis. A predominance of mononuclear cells in the CSF is the exception in acute bacterial meningoencephalitis but may be present with syphilis, Lyme disease,[16] listeriosis, or tuberculosis.

Computed tomography (CT) or magnetic resonance imaging (MRI) scans of the brain may demonstrate increased intracranial pressure (ventricular compression) or cerebral cortical enhancement. Temporal lobe enhancement or necrosis may be evidence of herpesvirus infection (Fig. 236-4). An electroencephalogram showing a periodic pattern in an infant who has partial motor seizures and signs of meningoencephalitis is virtually diagnostic of herpes simplex virus encephalitis.[15]

Polymerase chain reaction (PCR) is a powerful tool in the identification of enterovirus, mumps virus, cytomegalovirus, varicella zoster, and other viruses.[11] Specific identification of viruses requires isolation of the virus by tissue culture. Demonstration of a substantial convalescent antibody rise to a specific virus suggests recent viral infection. Testing the CSF and serum for other organisms may be warranted. A rapid screening test for Epstein-Barr virus (Monospot) is available at most hospitals.

Newborns who have cutaneous vesicles and who are suspected of having herpes simplex meningoencephalitis need not undergo brain biopsy for the diagnosis to be established. Rather, attempts should be made to isolate the virus from the throat, eye, or cutaneous lesions. If herpes simplex meningoencephalitis is suspected in older infants or children, a brain biopsy may be indicated for confirmation.[1] In all other nonherpetic meningoencephalitides, blood, urine, stool, and CSF samples should be obtained to facilitate later confirmation of the virus. Enteroviruses can be isolated relatively easily from throat, stool, and CSF samples. Laboratory diagnosis of mumps meningoencephalitis may be possible within the first week by demonstration of complement-fixing antibodies or by PCR.

DIFFERENTIAL DIAGNOSIS

Because laboratory tests often only suggest rather than confirm the diagnosis of meningoencephalitis, the clinician must consider the differential diagnosis carefully. Focal neurological signs often are present. Metabolic encephalopathy resulting from Reye's syndrome or from lead, alcohol, or other toxins can be ruled out by appropriate laboratory investigations. The clinical course of a brain abscess usually is slower,

Table 236-1 Causes of Meningoencephalitis

Infectious	Postinfectious or Unknown	Noninfectious Causes of Pleocytosis
Viral		
Enterovirus	Kawasaki syndrome	Intrathecal injections
Coxsackievirus	Mollaret syndrome	Leukemia
Poliovirus	Reye's syndrome	Toxins (e.g., lead)
Myxovirus		Trauma
Mumps		Lymphoma
Measles		
Influenza		
Rhabdovirus (rabies)		
Arenavirus (lymphocytic choriomeningitis)		
Bunyavirus (California encephalitis)		
Togavirus		
Eastern equine encephalitis		
Western equine encephalitis		
St. Louis encephalitis		
Rubella		
Reovirus (Colorado tick fever)		
Herpesvirus		
Epstein-Barr virus		
Varicella-zoster virus		
Cytomegalovirus		
Adenovirus		
Human immunodeficiency virus		
Nonviral		
Brain or parameningeal bacterial abscess		
Amebae (*Naegleria* and *Acanthamoeba* spp.)		
Brucellosis		
Cat-scratch disease		
Fungi (e.g., *Candida* and *Cryptococcus* spp.)		
Leptospirosis		
Lyme disease *(Borrelia burgdorferi)*		
Lymphogranuloma venereum		
Mycoplasma spp.		
Pertussis		
Rocky Mountain spotted fever		
Syphilis		
Trichinosis		
Tuberculosis		

Table 236-2 Typical Cerebrospinal Fluid Findings in Meningoencephalitis and Bacterial Meningitis

CSF Findings	Viral Meningoencephalitis	Bacterial Meningitis
Leukocytes	Initial predominance of polymorphonuclear neutrophils, followed by shift to mononuclear cells	Predominantly neutrophils
	Range: 0-2000/mm^3	Range: 0-200,000/mm^3
Glucose	>50% of serum concentration	<30% of serum concentration
Protein	Mild to moderate elevation	Marked elevation
	Range: usually <200 mg/dl	Range: usually >150 mg/dl
Gram stain	Negative	Usually reveals bacteria

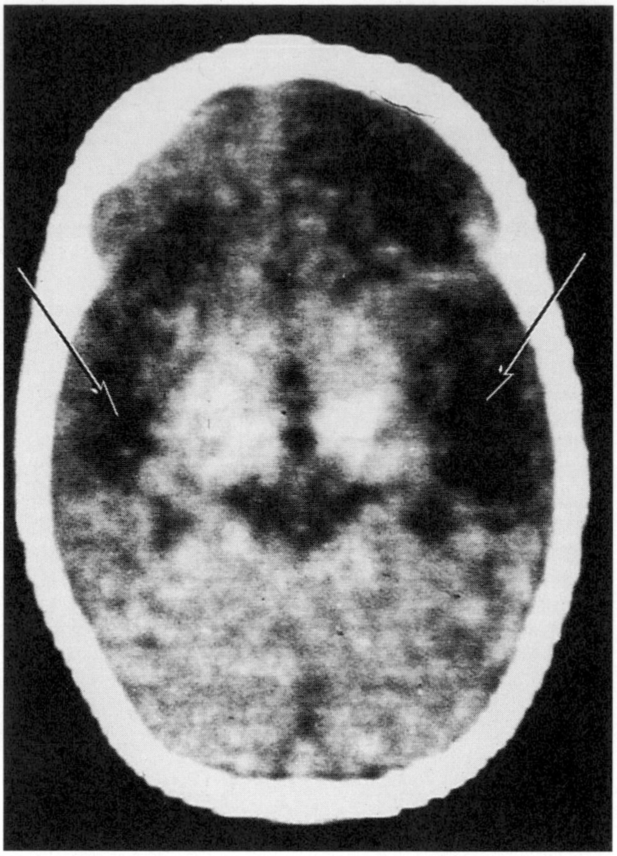

Fig. 236-4 Computed tomography (CT) brain scan of an infant who has herpes simplex encephalitis, showing complete necrosis of the frontotemporal regions *(arrows)*.

and focal findings may be present; a history of sinus infection, bronchiectasis, or congenital heart disease may be elicited. A myelitic form of viral nervous system infection may be mimicked by demyelinating disease or Guillain-Barré syndrome. MRI is superior for ruling out a spinal cord tumor, an arteriovenous malformation, or an infarction.

TREATMENT

Nonspecific treatment of a patient who has meningoencephalitis includes reducing increased intracranial pressure (see Chapter 290), respiratory support, and treating seizures. Maintaining the fluid and electrolyte balance is essential because 64% of infants who have aseptic meningitis develop inappropriate secretion of antidiuretic hormone.[20] Corticosteroids have not proved useful in treating meningoencephalitis and may blunt host defenses.

Specific treatment of acute viral infections of the nervous system is called for with herpes simplex infections. Acyclovir has proved to be superior to vidarabine (ara-A) for parenteral use in herpes infections.[1] Although it is nephrotoxic, acyclovir generally is tolerated by neonates and by children who have renal dysfunction or renal transplants. Other antiviral agents (foscarnet, S-HPMPA) are being developed. Ganciclovir, an antiviral agent similar in structure to acyclovir, has been approved for use in CMV infections.[10] The combination of zidovudine (ZDV) and didanosine (ddI) therapy is superior to monotherapy with ZDV or ddI monotherapy against CNS manifestations of human immunodeficiency virus disease.[19] Fluconazole is effective antifungal therapy even in neonates with complicated candidal infections.[12]

Another drug treatment that may be of benefit is intravenous immunoglobulin, which is known to contain viral antibodies for specific viral infections. These nonspecific immunoglobulin preparations have been used as replacement therapy or as adjuncts to treatment of meningoencephalitis in immunodeficient patients. However, immunoglobulin therapy for overwhelming viral sepsis remains controversial. Alpha-interferon has been used as prophylaxis against CMV and varicella-zoster in immunocompromised children but not as adjunct therapy in meningoencephalitis. Both active and passive postexposure prophylaxis is available for the treatment of rabies.[2]

Prevention is the most cost-effective method of reducing the morbidity and mortality caused by viral meningoencephalitis. Immunization has virtually eliminated poliomyelitis and rubella and has made mumps and measles meningoencephalitis extremely rare. Repeat measles immunizations of older children should reduce the incidence of measles encephalitis and SSPE further. The development of a varicella vaccine holds promise for lowering the morbidity from chickenpox.

PROGNOSIS

The developing nervous system may be more susceptible to viral infection and more likely to sustain serious sequelae. Eastern equine encephalitis, an infectious syndrome seen in children more commonly than in adults, often causes death within 48 hours. Those who survive frequently are severely impaired. Western equine encephalitis is associated with complete recovery in virtually all adults but causes death in 20% of children and a high prevalence of neurological residua among the survivors. Herpes simplex virus commonly produces a destructive encephalitis in neonates, infants, and children (see Fig. 236-4).[25]

Even the more "benign" meningoencephalitides of infancy, such as those caused by enteroviruses, may result in substantial reductions in head circumference, intelligence, and learning ability. California encephalitis, a relatively mild arbovirus infection, causes emotional learning disorders in 15% of affected children.[6,21] Focal epilepsy may be a sequel of a "mild" encephalitis caused by Epstein-Barr virus.

It is essential that every child who has a documented or suspected viral nervous system infection be monitored carefully for auditory, visual, and cognitive aftereffects. Carefully performed prospective, sibling-matched, controlled studies have shown that these children are at risk for cerebral cortical dysfunction.

REFERENCES

1. Arvin AA, et al: Consensus management of the patient with herpes simplex encephalitis, *Pediatr Infect Dis J* 6:2, 1987.
2. Baevsky RH, Bartfield JM: Human rabies: a review, *Am J Emerg Med* 11:279, 1993.
3. Barnett ND, et al: Primary amoebic meningoencephalitis with *Naegleria fowleri:* clinical review, *Pediatr Neurol* 15:230, 1996.

4. Bell WE, McCormick WF: *Neurologic infections in children,* ed 2, Philadelphia, 1981, WB Saunders.
5. Belman AL, et al: Cerebrospinal fluid findings in children with Lyme disease-associated facial nerve palsy, *Arch Pediatr Adolesc Med* 151: 1224, 1997.
6. Bergman I: Outcome of children with enteroviral meningitis in the first year, *J Pediatr* 110:705, 1987.
7. Centers for Disease Control: Enteroviral disease in the US, 1970-1979, *J Infect Dis* 146:103, 1982.
8. Domachowske JB, Cunningham CK, Cummings DL: Acute manifestations and neurologic sequelae of Epstein-Barr virus encephalitis in children, *Pediatr Infect Dis J* 15:871, 1996.
9. Feigin RD, Cherry JD: *Textbook of pediatric infectious diseases,* ed 2, Philadelphia, 1987, WB Saunders.
10. Ganciclovir, *Med Lett Drugs Ther* 31:79, 1989.
11. Hosoya M, et al: Application of PCR for various neurotropic viruses on the diagnosis of viral meningitis, *J Clin Virol* 11:117, 1998.
12. Huttova M, et al: Candida fungemia in neonates treated with fluconazole: report of forty cases, including eight with meningitis, *Pediatr Infect Dis J* 17:1012, 1998.
13. Kan L, Sood SK, Maytal J: Pseudotumor cerebri in Lyme disease: a case report and literature review, *Pediatr Neurol* 18:439, 1998.
14. Lee BE, et al: Comparative study of mortality and morbidity in premature infants (birth weight < 1250 g) with candidemia or candidal meningitis, *Clin Infect Dis* 27:559, 1998.
15. Mizrahi EM, Tharp BR: A characteristic EEG pattern in neonatal herpes simplex encephalitis, *Neurology* 32:1215, 1982.
16. Pachner AR, Duray P, Steere AC: CNS manifestations of Lyme disease, *Arch Neurol* 46:790, 1989.
17. Pizzo PA: Therapeutic considerations for children with HIV infection, *AIDS Update* 2:1, 1989.
18. Pizzo PA, Eddy J, Falcon J: AIDS in children, *Am J Med* 85:195, 1988.
19. Raskino C, et al: Neurologic, neurocognitive, and brain growth outcomes in human immunodeficiency virus-infected children receiving different nucleoside antiretroviral regimens. Pediatric AIDS Clinical Trials Group 152 Study Team, *Pediatrics* 104:e32, 1999.
20. Rorabaugh ML, et al: Aseptic meningitis in infants younger than 2 years of age: acute illness and neurologic complications, *Pediatrics* 92:206, 1993.
21. Sells SJ, Carpenter RL, Ray CG: Sequelae of central nervous system enterovirus infections, *N Engl J Med* 293:1, 1975.
22. Summary of notifiable diseases, US, *MMWR*, 1987.
23. Viola L, et al: Acute hydrocephalus as a consequence of mumps meningoencephalitis, *Pediatr Emerg Care* 14:212, 1998.
24. Wright R, et al: Congenital lymphocytic choriomeningitis virus syndrome: a disease that mimics congenital toxoplasmosis or cytomegalovirus infection, *Pediatrics* 100:E9, 1997.
25. Yanagihara K, et al: Human herpesvirus 6 meningoencephalitis with sequelae, *Pediatr Infect Dis J* 14:240, 1995.

237 Nephritis

William S. Varade • Edward J. Ruley

Nephritis is the general term for noninfectious inflammation of the kidney parenchyma. This inflammation may involve primarily the glomerulus (glomerulonephritis), the interstitium (interstitial nephritis), or both. Because glomerulonephritis historically has been the subject of more intense interest, when the term *nephritis* is used, many practitioners think only of glomerular lesions. Although glomerulonephritis is more common than either interstitial nephritis or combined glomerular and interstitial nephritis in children, the practitioner should have some knowledge of all three disorders.

CLASSIFICATION OF THE GLOMERULOPATHIES

Glomerulopathies previously have been classified according to a variety of schemes, such as the clinical course (e.g., acute, subacute, and chronic glomerulonephritis), the major clinical symptoms (e.g., Ellis types I and II), or some measurable serum abnormality (e.g., normocomplementemic and hypocomplementemic nephritides). All these classifications have proved to be of limited use. An ideal classification system based on cause is not possible because our understanding of the pathogenesis of many types of glomerulonephritis is incomplete. Furthermore, a great variety of renal insults manifest as only a limited number of clinical presentations. Thus, there is a great deal of overlap in the clinical signs and symptoms manifested by different disease processes. Currently the preferred method of classification is based on glomerular morphological traits.

Understanding morphological classification requires knowledge of normal renal and glomerular anatomy and of the terms *diffuse, focal, segmental,* and *global.* These terms describe the distribution of disease in the biopsy specimen (a diagram of their use is shown in Fig. 237-1). In glomerulonephritis, the terms *diffuse* and *focal* apply to the distribution of disease among the glomeruli present in the biopsy specimen; *diffuse* means that all the glomeruli are involved, and *focal* means that only some glomeruli are involved. Similarly, in interstitial nephritis the inflammation can be diffuse (i.e., general and uniform) or focal (i.e., patchy and irregular).

The terms *segmental* and *global* apply only to glomerular disease, in which they describe the extent of disease involvement in each individual glomerulus; *global* means complete glomerular involvement, and *segmental* means irregular involvement, with some loops being normal. Thus, glomerular lesions may be described as diffuse and segmental, indicating partial involvement of all the glomeruli in the biopsy specimen, or focal and global, indicating complete involvement of some of the glomeruli, and so on.

One classification scheme based on glomerular morphology is given in Box 237-1. In this scheme the category of minimal glomerular lesions includes those that have normal or minimally abnormal glomeruli. The minimal abnormalities usually consist of a mild increase in the amount of mesangium or number of cells (mild hypercellularity). The category of specific glomerular lesions includes more severe lesions characterized by morphological changes attributable to a defined cause. The largest category is that of nonspecific lesions, in which pathological patterns can be defined but may be the manifestation of more than one disease process. Finally, a category of unclassifiable glomerulopathies is included.

The following discussion deals with the common patterns of presentation of the various glomerulonephritides. It should be recognized that this is only one way of conceptualizing an approach. Furthermore, these clinical patterns are only crude categorizations, and a specific etiology may manifest in a variety of ways. Likewise, a disease may present as an acute glomerulonephritis but then run a *subacute* or *chronic* course. Examples include some cases of Henoch-Schönlein nephritis and membranoproliferative glomerulonephritis, respectively. The clinical patterns to be discussed include (1) the acute glomerulonephritides, and (2) the chronic glomerulonephritides. For each clinical pattern the classification by glomerular involvement is indicated. The indications for referral and hospitalization are listed in boxes on p. 1660. The disorders of minimal change disease, membranous glomerulopathy, and focal segmental glomerular sclerosis are discussed in Chapter 238, Nephrotic Syndrome, which is the most common pattern of presentation for these disorders.

ACUTE GLOMERULONEPHRITIS

Acute glomerulonephritis is characterized by hematuria, hypertension, and edema. The hematuria is usually grossly evident as tea-colored or cola-colored urine. In some children, however, the hematuria may be microscopic only. Red blood cell (RBC) casts and dysmorphic RBCs are present, although several urine samples may have to be examined to demonstrate them (Fig. 237-2).[3] The edema is usually periorbital and rarely severe. This clinical syndrome can be considered to present in two ways: acute nephritis with no or mild renal failure and acute nephritis with rapidly progressive renal failure.

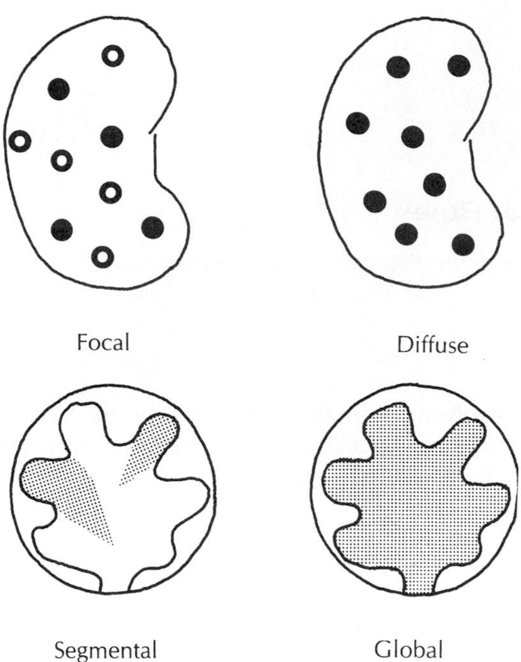

Fig. 237-1 Diagram of the use of the terms *diffuse, focal, segmental,* and *global* in describing glomerular pathological conditions.

BOX 237-1

MORPHOLOGICAL CLASSIFICATION OF GLOMERULOPATHIES

I. Minimal glomerular lesions (e.g., idiopathic nephrotic syndrome, asymptomatic proteinuria, and asymptomatic hematuria)
II. Specific glomerular lesions (e.g., malarial nephropathy, amyloidosis, diabetic glomerulosclerosis, and thrombotic microangiopathy of hemolytic-uremic syndrome)
III. Nonspecific glomerular lesions
  A. Diffuse glomerular lesions
    1. Nonproliferative (e.g., membranous nephropathy)
    2. Proliferative (e.g., mesangial proliferative glomerulonephritis, membranoproliferative glomerulonephritis, and endocapillary and extracapillary glomerulonephritis with and without crescents)
  B. Focal glomerular lesions
    1. Nonproliferative (e.g., focal glomerulosclerosis)
    2. Proliferative (e.g., focal and segmental proliferative glomerulonephritis)
IV. Unclassified glomerular lesions (e.g., Alport syndrome, focal membranoproliferative glomerulonephritis, and lesions too advanced to classify)

Modified from Habib R: Classification of glomerular nephropathies. In Rubin M, Barratt TM, editors: *Pediatric nephrology,* Baltimore, 1975, Williams & Wilkins.

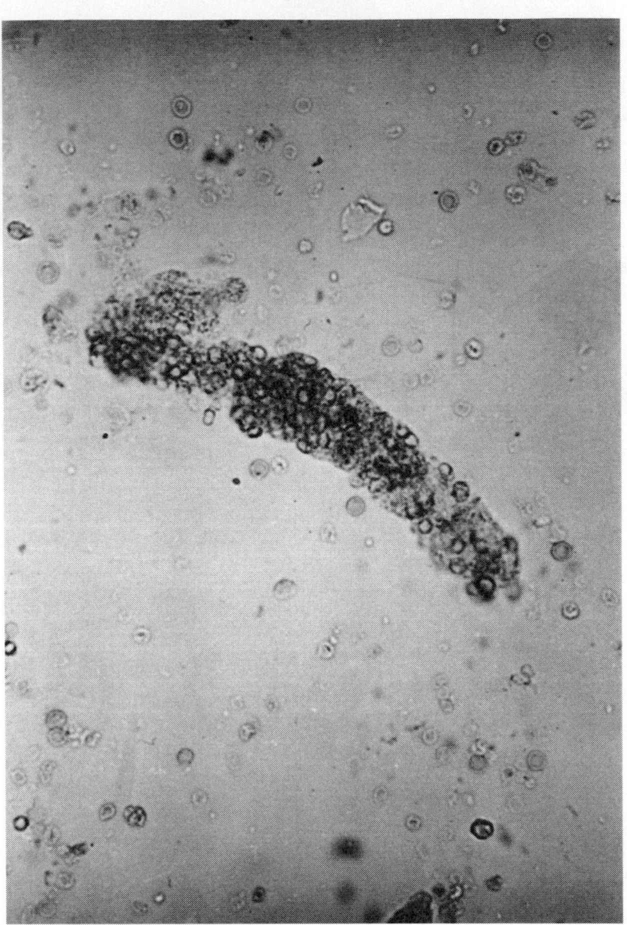

Fig. 237-2 Red blood cell cast—unstained.

Acute Glomerulonephritis with No or Mild Renal Failure

Acute nephritis is often the initial presentation of the renal diseases listed in Box 237-2.

Acute poststreptococcal glomerulonephritis. Acute poststreptococcal glomerulonephritis (APSGN) is a common form of glomerulonephritis in childhood. The true incidence is unknown, inasmuch as only a minority of patients who have this illness have symptoms. Although poststreptococcal nephritis may happen at any age, the peak incidence occurs at age 7 years, with a slight predominance among boys. It is uncommon before age 3 years and in adults.

ETIOLOGY. Poststreptococcal nephritis is the consequence of the host's immune response to a nonrenal infection with group A beta-hemolytic streptococci (GABHS). Not all GABHS strains are nephritogenic. Types 12 and 49 are the strains most commonly associated with nephritis.[23,34] How nephritogenic strains of streptococci are involved in the pathogenesis of APSGN remains uncertain. Bacterial components most recently suspected of being the nephritogenic candidates are the streptococcal preabsorbing antigen and nephritis strain-associated protein.[28,42] Both proteins generate an antibody response, can be found in the glomeruli of patients with APSGN, and can activate complement. Infection with a

BOX 237-2

DISEASES THAT USUALLY PRESENT AS ACUTE GLOMERULONEPHRITIS WITH NO OR MILD RENAL FAILURE

More Commonly
Acute poststreptococcal glomerulonephritis
Henoch-Schönlein purpura with nephritis
Postinfectious (nonstreptococcal) glomerulonephritis
Interstitial glomerulonephritis
Radiation nephritis

Less Commonly
Acute episodes in patients with chronic glomerulonephritis
Hemolytic-uremic syndrome (milder cases)
Membranoproliferative glomerulonephritis (some)
Nephritis of systemic lupus erythematosus (some)

nephritogenic strain does not guarantee an episode of nephritis, because a variety of incompletely understood factors determines the host response.

PATHOLOGY. Grossly, the kidneys are enlarged and pallid. The typical glomerular morphology is that of diffuse, uniform, cellular proliferation, although it is difficult to determine the type of cell involved. The glomerular tufts are larger than normal, and the capillary lumens are reduced. Polymorphonuclear leukocytes may be present. There is an increase in mesangial matrix, but the basement membranes are normal. By immunofluorescence microscopy, granular deposits of immunoglobulin and complement can be seen. Using electron microscopy, electron-dense "humps" (presumed to be immune deposits) can be seen on the epithelial side of the basement membrane. With healing, the increased cellularity and immune deposits become limited to the mesangial region and then gradually resolve.

CLINICAL PRESENTATION. Mild and subclinical cases are common. Renal involvement characteristically manifests 8 to 14 days after a pharyngeal infection or 14 to 21 days after a skin infection caused by the nephritogenic streptococci. Most patients who have acute poststreptococcal nephritis present as an acute glomerulonephritis, with macroscopic hematuria present in about 50% of the cases. Patients will usually have oliguria and, in rare cases, anuria. Fluid retention leads to edema that usually is periorbital and rarely, severe. Intravascular overload caused by salt and water retention can lead to signs of congestive heart failure. Approximately 60% to 70% of the patients have hypertension also related to salt and water retention. Patients who have severe hypertension may have symptoms of headache, drowsiness, vomiting, personality and visual changes, and convulsions. Although arteriolar spasm is commonly found on funduscopic examination, papilledema and hemorrhages are rare, even with severe hypertension. Anorexia and pain in the abdomen or flank are common, although palpation of the abdomen usually reveals no significant findings. Costovertebral angle tenderness often is present. Although a history of preceding skin or pharyngeal infection supports the diagnosis, such a history cannot be elicited in many cases. Patients rarely have joint symptoms or urinary outlet symptoms, such as frequency, urgency, or dysuria. In rare cases, in which convulsions or symptoms of cardiovascular dysfunction are the primary complaint, unrecognized poststreptococcal nephritis is the underlying etiology.

LABORATORY FINDINGS. The urine usually is tea colored and opaque. The specific gravity generally is increased, and hemoglobin can be detected by chemical testing. Any proteinuria that is present usually parallels the degree of hematuria and rarely reaches the nephrotic syndrome range. Microscopic examination usually reveals erythrocyturia, pyuria, and granular or cellular casts. Because identifiable erythrocyte casts and dysmorphic erythrocytes may or may not be present, serial urine specimens may need to be examined. In rare cases, a patient may have a normal urinalysis, despite having all of the other signs of acute glomerulonephritis.

Measurement of serum complement shows a reduction of C3 in 80% of the patients and, early in the course, a reduction of C4 in 50%. The erythrocyte sedimentation rate (ESR) usually is elevated. With severe oliguria, azotemia and acidosis may been seen. The plasma volume usually is expanded, causing a decline in serum protein, hemoglobin, and hematocrit levels by dilution. Hemolysis, a shortened erythrocyte half-life, and reduced erythrocyte production may contribute to these hematological changes. Salt retention with a decreased fractional excretion of sodium (FE_{Na}) often is seen even in the face of increased intravascular volume.

Evidence of a preceding streptococcal infection is important to support the diagnosis. The antistreptolysin O (ASO) titer is elevated in 80% of patients, although increases in titer are less common in patients who have skin infection and in those who receive early treatment with antibiotics. If other streptococcal antibodies (antihyaluronidase, antideoxyribonuclease B) are measured, 95% of patients will have serological evidence of preceding streptococcal infection. Cultures often are negative for GABHS by the time nephritis develops and are particularly affected by pretreatment with antibiotics.

The chest roentgenogram in patients who have hypertension usually reveals a large heart with prominent pulmonary vasculature, pulmonary edema or, in rare cases, hydrothorax.[11] Ultrasound examination usually reveals bilaterally enlarged kidneys.

COURSE. Diuresis usually ensues by one week from onset, heralding resolution of the acute illness. Creatinine should normalize by 3 to 4 weeks. Gross hematuria resolves within 1 or 2 weeks, although microscopic hematuria may persist for more than 1 year. Proteinuria should resolve by 3 months, and complement levels should normalize by 6 to 8 weeks. The presence of nephrotic-range proteinuria or extensive crescents by biopsy portends a poor prognosis. The failure of complement levels to normalize by 8 weeks suggests the presence of a form of nephritis other than ASPGN, such as membranoproliferative glomerulonephritis, the nephritis of chronic infection, or lupus nephritis.

TREATMENT. Acute poststreptococcal glomerulonephritis most often resolves spontaneously and is not affected by corticosteroids or immunosuppressive agents. Even so, the practitioner must be aggressive in treating hypertension, oliguria, and the resulting vascular overload, pulmonary edema, and encephalopathy that occur in the acute phase of the illness, because these can be fatal.

Although mild hypertension may resolve spontaneously, more severe degrees of hypertension should be controlled with antihypertensive agents that act quickly. Because increased intravascular volume is theorized to be the main determinant of hypertension in acute glomerulonephritis, diuretics are a mainstay of therapy.[11] Control of severe hypertension often will require the use of intravenous sodium nitroprusside, labetalol, nicardipine, or fenoldopam. Oral minoxidil in a dose of 0.1 to 0.2 mg/kg may be effective. Slower-acting, less potent antihypertensive drugs are not good initial choices but can be substituted once blood pressure has been acutely stabilized.

Oliguria results from decreased glomerular filtration and salt and water retention. In the absence of evidence of dehydration, administration of fluid boluses will not hasten the resolution of oliguria and excessive fluid administration will worsen hypertension. The signs of congestive heart failure usually resolve with control of the hypertension. Occasionally a patient develops acute renal failure severe enough to require dialysis.

A 10-day course of antibiotics usually is given to eradicate any remaining GABHS and, thus, prevent the spread of the organism to others. There is no evidence that such treatment affects the course of nephritis in the patient. Close contacts should be screened for streptococcal infection and treated if present.

Hospitalization for patients who have this disease needs to be determined individually (see Box 237-2). Although many children who have mild episodes do well as outpatients, the sudden development of hypertension and oliguria may produce life-threatening symptoms quite rapidly, necessitating hospitalization. After the acute phase, the child may be allowed to resume normal activities gradually. Every child should be followed up regularly until the serum complement values return to normal. To be certain of the diagnosis, a renal biopsy may be indicated for a child whose clinical or laboratory findings are atypical. Any child whose C3 value does not return to normal within 8 weeks should have a kidney biopsy.

PROGNOSIS. Studies have shown that more than 90% of children who have acute poststreptococcal glomerulonephritis recover from their illness. For most children, the critical period is early in the illness when potentially fatal hypertension or fluid overload presents a danger. Occasionally, patients who have severe involvement, as evidenced by nephrotic-range proteinuria or the presence of extensive glomerular crescents on biopsy, have some residual damage or may even progress to end-stage renal failure. In general, however, the kidneys have an outstanding recovery potential in this disease.[5] Recurrences of APSGN are rare.

Postinfectious (nonstreptococcal) glomerulonephritis. A variety of viruses are suspected of causing acute glomerulonephritis, including varicella, echovirus 10, and coxsackieviruses, as well as the viruses that cause infectious mononucleosis, measles, and mumps. However, significant renal involvement is unusual in infections caused by these viruses. Children who have such involvement have no serological evidence of recent streptococcal infection. In most cases, the acute nephritis resolves spontaneously and gradually, and renal function returns completely. There is no effective way to differentiate the nonstreptococcal postinfectious glomerulonephritides from other nephritides that progress to renal failure, except by observing the clinical course.

Henoch-Schönlein Purpura Nephritis (See also Chapter 215)

Renal involvement is the most significant complication of Henoch-Schönlein purpura. It may manifest with only isolated microscopic hematuria, as (1) an acute or subacute glomerulonephritis; (2) a rapidly progressive glomerulonephritis, leading to the nephrotic syndrome; or more rarely, (3) a chronic entity. The true incidence of renal involvement in Henoch-Schönlein purpura is difficult to ascertain and has been reported to range from 20% to 100%, depending on the definition of renal involvement used and whether the report is from a referral center or not.

Etiology. The cause of Henoch-Schönlein purpura is unknown. IgA deposition and complement activation may be involved in causing renal damage. It often appears to be triggered by an infection, although no particular infectious agent has been consistently associated with this disorder.

Pathology. The renal biopsy findings of Henoch-Schönlein purpura are indistinguishable from those of IgA nephropathy (see p. 1656). It has been suggested that these disorders may be related and represent different ends of a spectrum of disease. A necrotizing crescentic glomerulonephritis is seen in severe cases.

Clinical presentation. Renal involvement is manifested by the appearance of hematuria that may be macroscopic, proteinuria that may range from mild to nephrotic-range, and hypertension that may even occur in the face of a normal urinalysis.[1] Renal disease usually occurs within 3 months of the onset of a rash, arthritis, or gastrointestinal symptoms. The urinalysis should therefore be monitored during this time even though other symptoms may be improving. Rarely, renal disease may precede the onset of other symptoms or be delayed even years after the initial presentation. The finding of hypertension or abnormalities on the urinalysis is an indication to monitor renal function with blood urea nitrogen and creatinine determinations.

Course and prognosis. In most cases, the renal involvement of Henoch-Schönlein purpura completely resolves. However, older age at onset, the development of heavy proteinuria, renal insufficiency, hypertension, or the finding of significant numbers of glomerular crescents on kidney biopsy specimens portend a more guarded prognosis. Approximately 2% to 5% of patients with renal involvement progress to chronic renal failure. Deterioration of renal function can occur even after apparent complete resolution of urinary findings and 20 years after onset.[15] Patients should therefore be monitored with urinalyses and blood pressure monitoring over the long term.

Treatment. There is no treatment for established renal involvement in Henoch-Schönlein purpura. For severe involvement and a rapidly progressive course, pulse methylprednisolone, cyclophosphamide, or plasmapheresis have been used. The use of oral prednisone at the onset of clinical disease, but before any evidence of renal involvement, in an attempt to prevent renal disease has been suggested, although this remains a point of controversy.[26]

Other Renal Diseases That May Present as Acute Glomerulonephritis with No or Mild Renal Failure

Occasionally, patients who have undiscovered chronic renal failure suffer a sudden deterioration that may be interpreted as acute glomerulonephritis (see Box 237-2). Evaluation of these patients often reveals evidence of preexisting chronic renal failure, such as osteodystrophy or hyperphosphatemia. Hemolytic-uremic syndrome (see Chapter 213) characteristically occurs as an acute glomerulonephritis, often with significant renal failure. Systemic lupus erythematosus (SLE) may appear to be an acute glomerulonephritis but more often is discovered coincidentally during the evaluation of other complaints related to the lupus syndrome. Likewise, membranoproliferative glomerulonephritis or the nephritis of chronic infection initially may manifest acutely with low complement values. However, more often this disease appears as nephrotic syndrome or chronic glomerulonephritis. These disorders may also present at times with significant and rapidly progressing renal failure.

BOX 237-3

CLASSIFICATION OF ACUTE GLOMERULONEPHRITIS WITH RAPIDLY PROGRESSIVE RENAL FAILURE

Immune Complex
- Postinfectious reaction
  - Streptococcal infection
  - Visceral abscess
  - Other
- Collagen-vascular disease
  - Systemic lupus erythematosus
  - Henoch-Schönlein purpura
  - Mixed cryoglobulinemia
- Primary renal disease
  - IgA nephropathy
  - Membranoproliferative glomerulonephritis
  - Unknown cases (i.e., idiopathic)

No Immune Deposit
- Unknown cause
- Vasculitis
  - Polyarteritis
  - Wegener's granulomatosis
  - Hypersensitivity vasculitides

Anti-Glomerular Basement Membrane Antibody
- With lung hemorrhage (Goodpasture's syndrome)
- Without lung hemorrhage
- Complicating membranous nephropathy

Modified from Couser WG: *Am J Kidney Dis* 11:449, 1988.

Acute Glomerulonephritis with Rapidly Progressive Renal Failure

This variant of acute glomerulonephritis is characterized by symptoms of acute nephritis associated with relentless progression to renal failure over days or weeks.[20] Although acute interstitial nephritis stemming from pyelonephritis or hypersensitivity to certain drugs may occur in this way, most cases result from glomerular disease, giving rise to the term *rapidly progressive glomerulonephritis* (RPGN). As shown in Box 237-3, RPGN can be classified into three categories based on immunopathological findings as seen in kidney biopsies.[8]

The most common cause of RPGN in pediatric patients is the *postinfection reaction*, primarily poststreptococcal glomerulonephritis. The diagnosis depends on obtaining a history of a recent sore throat or skin infection and finding reduced serum complement values associated with serological evidence of a recent streptococcal infection. A large proportion of patients who have poststreptococcal RPGN recover spontaneously, provided their course is managed well during the acute phase.

RPGN may be caused by *collagen-vascular disease,* such as Henoch-Schönlein purpura, although this occurs in children considerably less often than the poststreptococcal and idiopathic (nonstreptococcal) varieties. The multisystem clinical presentation, negative streptococcal serological findings, normal serum complement values, and renal biopsy findings characterize this cause. Some reports suggest that high-dose intravenous corticosteroids, if given early in the course, promote recovery in these patients. Of the *primary renal disease group*, IgA nephropathy and membranoproliferative glomerulonephritis occur this way in rare cases.

RPGN *without immune deposits* is much less common among pediatric patients; anti-glomerular basement membrane (GBM) antibody-mediated RPGN is even more rare. Hemolytic-uremic syndrome (HUS) and disseminated intravascular coagulation (DIC) must be included in the differential diagnosis, inasmuch as hematuria and rapidly progressive renal failure are common features of their presentations. Although the characteristic clinical and laboratory features of these diseases may suggest specific etiological factors, a renal biopsy usually is indicated to make the diagnosis and to determine the extent of the disease.[20]

CHRONIC GLOMERULONEPHRITIS

The chronic glomerulonephritides may present as an acute or subacute nephritis or, more insidiously, with only an abnormal urinalysis in an asymptomatic patient. Advanced cases may present with diminished renal function associated with signs of the detrimental effects of renal failure on other organ systems. It may be discovered during investigation of nonspecific complaints such as anorexia, intermittent vomiting, and malaise that are found to result from undiagnosed chronic renal failure. The more common disorders are IgA nephropathy, Alport syndrome, the nephritis of systemic lupus erythematosus, membranoproliferative glomerulonephritis, and "chronic glomerulonephritis." Nonnephritic causes such as renal dysplasia and obstructive uropathies with significant unrecognized parenchymal damage should be considered in the differential diagnosis.

IgA Nephropathy

IgA nephropathy was first described by Berger in 1969 and has been called *IgA-IgG nephropathy,* or Berger's disease.

Etiology. The cause of IgA nephropathy is unknown. Mesangial IgA deposition and complement activation may play a role in damaging the kidneys.

Pathology. The *sine qua non* for the diagnosis of IgA nephropathy is the finding of dominant or codominant IgA staining of the glomerular mesangium by immunofluorescence microscopy. IgG and C3 generally are seen as well. The typical histological entities seen in IgA nephropathy by light microscopy include essentially normal glomeruli, mesangial hypercellularity with an increase in mesangial matrix, or a focal segmental proliferative, necrotizing, or sclerosing glomerulonephritis. By electron microscopy, immune-type deposits are seen within the mesangial matrix. IgA nephropathy is difficult to differentiate morphologically from that of Henoch-Schönlein purpura, which has led to speculation that the former is a partial clinical expression of the latter.

Clinical presentation. IgA nephropathy typically presents in the second or third decade of life but can affect all ages.[12,27] Males are affected more often than females, and it appears to occur less frequently in blacks. Characteristically, children with Berger's disease present with the sudden onset of asymptomatic gross hematuria concomitant with an infection, usually of the respiratory tract.[12] This may be associated with flank pain. The gross hematuria usually clears within a few days to a week as the infection resolves. Typically, gross hematuria may recur with subsequent infections. Microscopic hematuria may persist with or without proteinuria between episodes or the urine may clear totally. The simultaneous onset of the upper respiratory tract infection and the gross hematuria helps differentiate this disease from acute poststreptococcal glomerulonephritis, in which a delay between infection and hematuria is the rule. The absence of a rash, abdominal pain, and arthritis helps differentiate IgA nephropathy from the nephritis of Henoch-Schönlein purpura. About 10% of patients with IgA nephropathy may present with nephrotic syndrome or acute renal failure.

Laboratory findings. IgA nephropathy is characterized by a lack of abnormal laboratory findings except for the urinalysis. In particular, hypocomplementemia and serological evidence of recent streptococcal infection usually are absent. Azotemia or heavy proteinuria, when they do occur, are poor prognostic signs. A renal biopsy may be indicated in patients with renal insufficiency, nephrotic-range proteinuria, or persistent hematuria and proteinuria to confirm the diagnosis and to clarify the prognosis.

Treatment. Treatment of IgA nephropathy remains controversial. Suggested regimens for patients with poor prognostic indicators include long-term, alternate-day prednisone and fish oil.[10,17,27] Control of hypertension, as for other renal diseases, is essential.

Prognosis. Although IgA nephropathy was originally considered to be a benign disorder in children, it is now anticipated that from 10% to 30% of pediatric patients will progress to renal failure over the course of several decades. Progression has been related to the amount of proteinuria, the presence of hypertension or renal insufficiency, and the severity of the histological changes found on the kidney biopsy.[2,12,13,27]

Benign Familial Hematuria

Although not a chronic glomerulonephritis per se, benign familial hematuria is included in this section because it presents as persistent hematuria with similarly affected family members. As such, it is an important disorder in the differential diagnoses of both IgA nephropathy and Alport syndrome (see the facing page). Benign familial hematuria, as the name implies, is a benign condition inherited as an autosomal dominant trait. Undoubtedly, many of the early reports included patients who had IgA nephropathy because of the similarities of clinical presentation and because renal biopsy specimens often were not obtained. This condition has also been called *benign recurrent hematuria.*

Etiology. A mutation in the type IV collagen alpha 4 gene was found in a Dutch kindred with benign familial hematuria.[22] However, linkage to this chromosomal region was not detected in other studies, suggesting that the etiology of benign familial hematuria is heterogeneous.[29,41]

Pathology. Light and fluorescence microscopy of renal biopsy specimens are generally normal. Widespread thinning of the glomerular basement membrane is present by electron microscopy. These pathological findings may be similar to those seen early in the course of Alport syndrome. Only the family history of lack of progressive renal impairment, deafness, and eye findings distinguishes it from early Alport syndrome.

Clinical presentation. Persistent asymptomatic microscopic hematuria in the absence of hearing loss, proteinuria, or progressive renal impairment is the usual presentation.

Laboratory findings. All laboratory test results usually are normal except for the urinalysis. The presence of hematuria in family members suggests this diagnosis. The absence of notable proteinuria, deafness, ocular defects, and renal failure in older family members who have hematuria differentiates this from the hereditary nephritides.

Course. Most cases are discovered by finding microscopic hematuria on urinalysis during a routine evaluation. Benign familial hematuria may present similarly to IgA nephropathy. It was found to be the cause of isolated asymptomatic microscopic hematuria in about one third of adults while IgA nephropathy was responsible for another third of the cases.[35] The hematuria is persistent but renal failure, deafness, and eye findings do not develop, in contrast to Alport syndrome.

Treatment. No treatment is indicated for familial hematuria.

Prognosis. As indicated by the name, the course is benign and the prognosis is excellent. Neither renal failure nor deafness develop.

Alport Syndrome

Alport syndrome, or hereditary nephritis, is an inherited renal disease associated with sensorineural deafness and ocular abnormalities. Alport syndrome is inherited as an X-linked dominant trait in 80% to 85% of cases.[30] Families with Alport syndrome with autosomal recessive, or rarely, autosomal dominant inheritance, also have been described. The combination of Alport features and macrothrombocytopenia is known as *Epstein syndrome*. Rarely, X-linked Alport syndrome also can be associated with leiomyomatosis.

Etiology. X-linked Alport syndrome is due to mutation of the gene encoding the α5 chain of type IV collagen.[21] Mutations range from point mutations, leading to an amino acid substitution or a premature stop codon, to small or large deletions. The particular type of mutation may influence the severity of the clinical expression of the disease. Ten percent to 15% of cases represent new mutations.[30] X-linked Alport syndrome with leiomyomatosis appears to arise from deletions involving the contiguous genes encoding the α5 and α6 chains of type IV collagen.[21] In cases associated with platelet abnormalities, the α5 chain of type IV collagen appears to be intact, and a genetic cause has not yet been delineated. Autosomal recessive Alport syndrome has been related to mutations in the genes encoding the α3 and α4 chains of type IV collagen.[21] Autosomal dominant Alport syndrome also has been linked to the region of chromosome 2 containing the genes encoding the α3 and α4 chains of type IV collagen.[21]

Pathology. Light microscopy is nonspecific in Alport syndrome. Biopsy specimens may appear essentially normal by light microscopy early on. With progression, mesangial hypercellularity, capillary thickening, segmental sclerosis, and interstitial fibrosis develop. The usual immunofluorescent stains are negative or nonspecific. The characteristic findings are seen by electron microscopy. These include variations in the thickness of the glomerular basement membrane, with splitting and lamellation of the lamina densa of the glomerular basement membrane giving a basket weave appearance to the basement membrane. However, early on in the course of the disease the only ultrastructural abnormality may be diffuse attenuation of the glomerular basement membrane. Thus, in these cases, distinguishing patients with Alport syndrome from those with thin basement membrane nephropathy may be difficult based on biopsy findings alone. In these indeterminate cases, special stains for the individual type IV collagen chains may prove of value for making the correct diagnosis.

Clinical presentation. Renal disease is severe and progressive in males with X-linked Alport syndrome, with about 90% developing end-stage renal failure by age 40.[30] Females generally are less severely affected, with about 12% reaching end-stage renal failure by age 40 and 30% by age 60. Age at the development of renal failure tends to run true within families, although exceptions are well documented. Persistent microscopic hematuria is found early on in all affected males and in the majority of females in whom it may be intermittent. Macroscopic hematuria occurs in up to 70% of males and 33% of females, often at the time of a respiratory infection. Proteinuria develops in males with age and can reach nephrotic-range in about 30%. Sensorineural hearing loss is progressive starting with high frequencies and likewise affects males more than females. It is not, however, present in all families with Alport syndrome. Eye abnormalities are found in about 50% of patients with Alport syndrome. These include anterior lenticonus, retinal abnormalities, and corneal ulcerations.

Both males and females are equally affected in autosomal recessive Alport syndrome. The course is similar to that of males with X-linked Alport syndrome. Approximately half the carriers of the abnormal gene will also have microscopic hematuria. About two thirds of patients with the autosomal recessive form will develop hearing loss.[30]

Laboratory findings. Laboratory findings reflect the degree of renal involvement and may vary from normal early on to be indicative of advanced renal impairment as the disease progresses. Blood urea nitrogen and creatinine levels become elevated with advancing disease. Serum electrolytes may become abnormal, and hypoalbuminemia may develop in those patients who develop nephrotic syndrome. Serum complement values usually are normal. A renal biopsy may help to establish the diagnosis in some patients.

Course. The disease is progressive in males and some females with X-linked Alport syndrome and in patients of both sexes with autosomal recessive and dominant forms of Alport syndrome. Proteinuria is not present initially but usually develops later in the course of the disease. The course usually is similar for members of an affected family, although variations in the progression have been reported.

Treatment. Treatment is supportive, with medical management of hypertension and the complications of renal insufficiency. Dialysis or transplantation is instituted when medical management is no longer sufficient. Audiological screening can identify hearing impairment early and allow for the timely implementation of hearing-augmentation services.

Prognosis. As previously indicated, in affected individuals, renal disease and hearing loss are progressive. Families carrying mutations consisting of large deletions or stop codons leading to truncated proteins may be at risk for more severe disease than those with mutations leading to an amino acid substitution.[30] Dialysis and transplantation are offered when end-stage renal failure occurs. Three percent to 4 percent of patients with Alport syndrome receiving a kidney transplant develop anti-glomerular basement membrane nephritis, leading to loss of the transplanted kidney in 75% of these cases.[21]

Nephritis of Systemic Lupus Erythematosus

Systemic lupus erythematosus (SLE) is an autoimmune disease that affects multiple organ systems and is seen mainly in young women during the child-bearing years. Fifteen percent of cases, however, involve children. Blacks and Asians seem to be disproportionately affected. Up to 75% of children will have some evidence of renal involvement on presentation. However, this is rarely the presenting problem and renal disease tends to become more prominent with time in the course of SLE.[6]

Etiology. The cause of SLE is unknown. Dysregulation of the cellular and humoral branches of the immune system occurs and results in an autoimmune state, with autoantibody production and the deposition of immune complex. Female sex clearly predisposes to the development of SLE. There also appears to be a genetic predisposition to the development of SLE with increased evidence of autoimmune phenomena within these families. Some cases are related to inherited deficiencies of early components of the complement cascade.

The pathogenesis of lupus nephritis has classically been considered to be due to the deposition of immune complexes and the activation of complement. However, it is clear that other factors are involved in disease production.

Pathology. Renal histology varies greatly in patients with lupus nephritis. The World Health Organization classification of renal pathology in lupus nephritis is widely used for interpreting the renal biopsy findings in this disease. Focal proliferative (WHO class III) and diffuse proliferative (WHO class IV) lesions indicate severe disease and are found in the kidney biopsies of more than half the children with lupus nephritis.[6] Immunofluorescence microscopy demonstrates deposition of immunoglobulins and complement components in the mesangium and along the capillary loops. Dense deposits, corresponding to the immune complexes detected by immunofluorescence, are seen by electron microscopy. Cellular proliferation and basement membrane thickening also are seen.

Clinical presentation. Children with SLE usually present initially because of constitutional, cutaneous, or musculoskeletal symptoms such as fever, malaise, rash, or arthritis.[19] Initial complaints may be vague, and a high index of suspicion is warranted. Reference should be made to the criteria of the American College of Rheumatology for the classification of SLE.[32] Symptoms related to renal disease, although they may be present, rarely are the reason for initially seeking medical attention. Renal involvement usually evolves with time in most children with SLE and is an important cause of morbidity and mortality. When present, renal involvement may be manifested by isolated hematuria, hematuria with proteinuria, nephrotic syndrome, hypertension, or rapidly progressive renal failure.

Laboratory findings. Antinuclear antibodies (ANA) are positive in most children with SLE. Anti-double-stranded DNA is positive in many as well. Serum complement components frequently are decreased and tend to correlate with disease activity.

The severity and type of renal involvement (e.g., nephrotic syndrome, chronic renal failure) determine the egree of hypoproteinemia, azotemia, and other manifestations of renal failure. These changes are nonspecific. Hematological abnormalities include Coombs-positive anemia, leukopenia, and thrombocytopenia. Antiphospholipid antibodies are found in as many as 67% of children with SLE and are a risk factor for thrombotic complications.

Urinalysis findings vary greatly and range from isolated hematuria, hematuria with proteinuria, to nephrotic-range proteinuria. Pyuria is common and reflects the underlying glomerular inflammation. Red cell, white cell, and renal tubular epithelial cell casts frequently are seen.

Course. The course of SLE varies considerably. Renal manifestations can wax and wane with changes in disease activity, intercurrent illness, and type of therapy. Besides the risk for morbidity and mortality from the underlying disease, children with SLE are at risk for complications related to treatment and are at increased risk of infectious complications.

Treatment. High-dose corticosteroid therapy has been the mainstay of treatment of lupus nephritis, although accompanied by considerable morbidity. Pulse methylprednisolone is used for the treatment of rapidly progressive lupus glomerulonephritis. Oral or pulse-intravenous cyclophosphamide frequently is recommended for the treatment of WHO class III, IV, and sometimes, class V renal disease. Azathioprine and, more recently, mycophenolic acid have been used as steroid-sparing agents. Cyclosporine has been used with variable results. A renal biopsy should be performed before therapy is begun. The danger of overwhelming sepsis among these immunosuppressed patients is constant. The effectiveness of therapy can be based on changes in serological parameters, blood chemistries, and complement levels. Care of the patient who has SLE is a highly specialized endeavor that requires knowledge of current treatment modalities, the availability of highly specialized tests, and the willingness to deal with a patient who has a chronic, severe, life-threatening illness for which treatment with steroids often is disfiguring. These patients are managed best by a team trained in dealing with all aspects of this disease.

Prognosis. Overall survival of children with SLE appears to have improved over the past several decades, with many, but not all, reports citing survival rates of 70%

to 80% and higher at 15 to 20 years.[6,14,24] Reported renal survival in childhood lupus nephritis ranges form 29% to 71% at 10 years. Patients with WHO class IV diffuse proliferative glomerulonephritis have the poorest renal outcome. In addition, sclerosis on biopsy specimens, hypocomplementemia, decreased renal function, nephrotic syndrome-range proteinuria, and persistent hypertension portend a poor renal prognosis. The membranous lesion (WHO class V) also is commonly associated with nephrotic syndrome and may progress to renal failure, although progression usually is slower than with the diffuse proliferative lesion.

Membranoproliferative Glomerulonephritis

Membranoproliferative glomerulonephritis (MPGN), also referred to as *mesangiocapillary glomerulonephritis,* is a chronic inflammatory disease of the kidney with a poor prognosis.

Etiology. The etiology of membranoproliferative glomerulonephritis is unknown in most instances; some forms are associated with immune complex deposition in the glomeruli. Complement activation is prominent in all three types of MPGN, and the pattern of complement consumption suggests different mechanisms involved in each type.[36] Type 1 MPGN is thought to be mediated by immune complex formation and deposition, with activation of the classic pathway of complement as indicated by immunofluorescence and the pattern of serum complement depression. Complement consumption in MPGN types 2 and 3 is thought to be due to the presence of circulating autoantibodies called *nephritic factors* (NF) that stabilize the C3 convertases activating the alternative (NF_a) and terminal (NF_t) pathways of complement activation, respectively.[39] These can also be found in the serum of some patients with type 1 MPGN. Although thought at one time to be epiphenomena, the various nephritic factors and their resulting complement activation and consumption have more recently been considered to be of potential pathological significance.[39]

Pathology. Three types of MPGN have been described based on ultrastructural abnormalities of the glomerular basement membrane (GBM). MPGN types 1, 2, and 3 account for 44%, 20%, and 36% of cases, respectively.[38] All three types appear similar by light microscopy and have increased mesangial cellularity and matrix. By electron microscopy, type 1 shows normal-appearing GBM with subendothelial electron-dense deposits. MPGN type 2, also known as *dense-deposit disease,* appears to be a distinct disease and has thickening and increased electron density of the lamina densa of the GBM. In MPGN type 3, deposits are present on both the subepithelial and subendothelial sides of the GBM, as well as within the GBM. With special stains the GBM appears fenestrated and deposits are covered by layers of new GBM.[38] By immunofluorescence, immunoglobulin and complement components are seen along the capillary wall and in the mesangium in type 1.[9] C3 is found flanking the dense deposits in the GBM and in the mesangium in MPGN type 2. Specific immunoglobulin deposits are lacking. C3 and C5 are found along the capillary wall and in the mesangium in MPGN type 3, while immunoglobulin deposition is variable.[31]

Clinical presentation. The average age of onset of primary MPGN is about 9 years.[25] Hematuria is present in 60% to 100%, hypertension in 42% to 67%, and decreased renal function in 17% to 50% on presentation.[18,33,40] Fifty percent to 67% of patients present with nephrotic syndrome, and some of these patients may present without significant hematuria.[7,16]

Laboratory findings. The serum C3 level is depressed in 67% to 75% of patients on presentation. Blood urea nitrogen and creatinine values may be elevated and albumin may be low in severe cases. Anemia is common. Electrolyte disturbances reflect the presence of renal insufficiency. Urinalysis most commonly has both hematuria and proteinuria present. Proteinuria may reach the nephrotic range. Hematuria may be macroscopic. Cellular casts are a common finding.

Course and prognosis. Fifty percent of patients reach end-stage renal failure within approximately 11 years of diagnosis and 90% do so within 20 years.[33] Nephrotic-range proteinuria, renal insufficiency, hypertension, and sclerosis on biopsy examination are poor prognostic indicators.

Treatment. The treatment of membranoproliferative glomerulonephritis is controversial. Rigorous controlled studies are lacking. Treatment with cytotoxic agents, anticoagulants, platelet function inhibitors, and nonsteroidal antiinflammatory agents has not shown clear evidence of efficacy. The most experience reported regarding treatment of this disorder has been with high-dose, long-term, alternate-day prednisone therapy.[25,33,37,38] Cumulative renal survival of 82% at 10 years and 56% at 20 years have been reported with this therapeutic approach. Some differences in the clinical course and response to treatment may be seen according to the type of MPGN.[4]

Chronic Glomerulonephritis

Chronic glomerulonephritis is a general category for less understood, progressive renal lesions that cause renal failure. Often, patients who have severe renal lesions that have progressed so far that the initial process no longer can be recognized are grouped in this category. It is hoped that, in the future, specific disorders will be recognized and separated from this heterogeneous group.

INTERSTITIAL NEPHRITIS

Inflammation of the interstitium is much less common than glomerular inflammation. The principal manifestations of interstitial inflammation are related to the consequent tubular dysfunction: inability to reabsorb glucose, producing glucosuria despite normoglycemia; inability to reabsorb water, resulting in urine with a low fixed specific gravity; inability to reabsorb minerals, causing a "salt-losing" syndrome; and inability to reabsorb bicarbonate and secrete hydrogen ions, giving rise to renal tubular acidosis. Hypertension and fluid overload are unusual in these patients, in contrast to children who have isolated glomerulonephritis. Interstitial nephritis may be seen on renal biopsies concomitantly with severe glomerulonephritis when it is the consequence of degeneration of the tubules of the most severely affected glomeruli. This combination has a much more guarded prognosis because the combined glomerular and interstitial involvement reflects the greater severity of the renal disease. In this circumstance the interstitial inflammation tends to heal by fibrosis, thereby damaging segments of the remaining kidney. The finding of glomerulonephritis associated with tubular dysfunction should be evaluated by kidney biopsy.

When to Refer

Acute glomerulonephritis with significant complications
Acute glomerulonephritis that is not following a typical course expected of poststreptococcal glomerulonephritis
Failure of complement level to normalize within 6 to 8 weeks in suspected acute glomerulonephritis
Rapidly progressive course
Glomerulonephritis with the development of nephrotic syndrome
Persistent hematuria and proteinuria
Persistent hypertension
Elevated creatinine level for age
Family history of renal failure or deafness
Any chronic glomerulonephritis

When to Hospitalize

Severe hypertension
Renal failure with significant electrolyte disturbances
Congestive heart failure from volume overload
Oliguria/anuria
Rapidly progressive renal failure

REFERENCES

1. Alon U, Warady BA, Hellerstein S: The kidney in systemic disease. Part II. Autoimmune and vascular disorders, *Adv Pediatr* 40:325, 1993.
2. Berg UB: Long-term follow-up of renal function in IgA nephropathy, *Arch Dis Child* 66:588, 1991.
3. Birch DF, et al: Urinary erythrocyte morphology in the diagnosis of glomerular hematuria, *Clin Nephrol* 20:78, 1983.
4. Braun MC, West CD, Strife CF: Differences between membranoproliferative glomerulonephritis types I and III in long-term response to an alternate-day prednisone regimen, *Am J Kidney Dis* 34:1022, 1999.
5. Buzio C, et al: Significance of albuminuria in the follow-up of acute poststreptococcal glomerulonephritis, *Clin Nephrol* 41:259, 1994.
6. Cameron JS: Lupus and lupus nephritis in children, *Adv Nephrol* 2:59, 1993.
7. Cameron JS, et al: Idiopathic mesangiocapillary glomerulonephritis: comparison of types I and II in children and adults and long-term prognosis, *Am J Med* 74:175, 1983.
8. Couser WG: Rapidly progressive glomerulonephritis: classification, pathogenetic mechanisms, and therapy, *Am J Kidney Dis* 11:449, 1988.
9. Donadio JV, Holley KE: Membranoproliferative glomerulonephritis. *Semin Nephrol* 2:214, 1982.
10. Donadio JV, et al: A controlled trial of fish oil in IgA nephropathy, *N Engl J Med* 331:1194, 1994.
11. Fleisher DS, et al: Hemodynamic findings in acute glomerulonephritis, *J Pediatr* 69:1054, 1966.
12. Galla JH: IgA nephropathy, *Kidney Int* 47:377, 1995.
13. Gallo GR, et al: Prognostic pathologic markers in IgA nephropathy, *Am J Kidney Dis* 12:362, 1988.
14. Gloor JM: Lupus nephritis in children, *Lupus* 7:639, 1998.
15. Goldstein AR, et al: Long-term follow-up of childhood Henoch-Schönlein nephritis, *Lancet* 339:280, 1992.
16. Habib R, et al: Idiopathic membranoproliferative glomerulonephritis in children: report of 105 cases, *Clin Nephrol* 1:194, 1973.
17. Hogg RJ, Waldo B: Advances in treatment: immunoglobulin A nephropathy, *Semin Nephrol* 16:511, 1996.
18. International Study of Kidney Disease in Childhood: Nephrotic syndrome in children: prediction of histopathology from clinical and laboratory characteristics at the time of diagnosis, *Kidney Int* 13:159, 1978.
19. Iqbal S, et al: Diversity in presenting manifestations of systemic lupus erythematosus in children, *J Pediatr* 135:500, 1999.
20. Jardim H, et al: Crescentic glomerulonephritis in children, *Pediatr Nephrol* 6:231, 1992.
21. Kashtan C: Alport syndrome and thin glomerular basement membrane disease, *J Am Soc Nephrol* 9:1736, 1998.
22. Lemmink HH, et al: Benign familial hematuria due to mutation of the type IV collagen alpha 4 gene, *J Clin Invest* 98:1114, 1996.
23. Markowitz M: Changing epidemiology of group A streptococcal infections, *Pediatr Infect Dis J* 13:557, 1994.
24. McCurdy DK, et al: Lupus nephritis: prognostic factors in children, *Pediatr* 89:240, 1992.
25. McEnery PT: Membranoproliferative glomerulonephritis: the Cincinnati experience—cumulative renal survival from 1957 to 1989, *J Pediatr* 116:S109, 1990.
26. Mollica F, et al: Effectiveness of early prednisone treatment in preventing the development of nephropathy in anaphylactoid purpura, *Eur J Pediatr* 151:140, 1992.
27. Niaudet P, et al: Primary IgA nephropathies in children: prognosis and treatment, *Adv Nephrol* 2:121, 1993.
28. Peake PW, et al: Post-streptococcal glomerulonephritis: studies on the interaction between nephritis strain-associated protein (NSAP), complement and the glomerulus, *APMIS* 99:460, 1991.
29. Piccini M, et al: Evidence for genetic heterogeneity in benign familial hematuria, *Am K Nephrol* 19:464, 1999.
30. Pirson Y: Making the diagnosis of Alport's syndrome, *Kidney Int* 56: 760, 1999.
31. Strife CF, Jackson EC, McAdams AJ: Type III membranoproliferative glomerulonephritis: long-term clinical and morphological evaluation, *Clin Nephrol* 21:323, 1984.
32. Tan EM, et al: The 1982 revised criteria for the classification of systemic lupus erythematosus, *Arthritis Rheum* 25:1271, 1982.
33. Tarshish P, et al: Treatment of mesangiocapillary glomerulonephritis with alternate-day prednisone: a report of The International Study of Kidney Disease in Children, *Pediatr Nephrol* 6:123, 1992.
34. Tejani A, Ingulli E: Poststreptococcal glomerulonephritis: current clinical and pathologic concepts, *Nephron* 55:1, 1990.
35. Tiebosch A, et al: Thin-basement-membrane nephropathy in adults with persistent hematuria, *N Engl J Med* 320:14, 1989.
36. Varade WS, Forristal J, West CD: Patterns of complement activation in membranoproliferative glomerulonephritis, types I, II, and III, *Am J Kidney Dis* 16:196, 1990.

37. Warady BA, et al: Prednisone therapy of membranoproliferative glomerulonephritis in children, *J Pediatr* 107:702, 1985.
38. West CD: Idiopathic membranoproliferative glomerulonephritis in childhood, *Pediatr Nephrol* 6:96, 1992.
39. West CD, McAdams AJ: The alternative pathway C3 convertase and glomerular deposits, *Pediatr Nephrol* 13:448, 1999.
40. White RHR, Glasgow EF, Mills RJ: Clinicopathological study of nephrotic syndrome in childhood, *Lancet* 1:1353, 1970.
41. Yamazaki H, et al: No linkage to the COL4A3 gene locus in Japanese thin basement membrane disease families, *Nephrol* 1:315, 1996.
42. Yoshizawa N, et al.: Role of streptococcal antigen in the pathogenesis of acute poststreptococcal glomerulonephritis, *J Immunol* 148:3110, 1992.

238 Nephrotic Syndrome

William S. Varade

Nephrotic syndrome is defined by the clinical findings of heavy proteinuria, hypoalbuminemia, edema often to the point of frank anasarca, and hyperlipidemia. There are many causes of nephrotic syndrome, and the most likely etiology varies by age. Nephrotic syndrome may be secondary to an underlying systemic disease, or it may present as a primary idiopathic renal disorder. Examples of causes of primary and secondary nephrotic syndrome in children are listed in Box 238-1. The overall outcome of nephrotic syndrome depends on the etiology and ranges from complete remission with no long-term sequelae to inexorable progression to end-stage renal failure. Newer treatments offer alternatives for those patients with resistant forms of nephrotic syndrome or who suffer significant side effects from first-line treatments, although they carry the potential for significant side effects themselves.

PRESENTATION

Nephrotic syndrome (Fig. 238-1) typically presents with the gradual development of edema and inappropriate weight gain, although those cases associated with glomerulonephritis may have a more acute onset, with signs and symptoms of nephritis predominating. The presence of periorbital edema upon arising in the morning that resolves during the course of the day often is mistaken for allergy. Clothing may be tight and socks may leave indentations in the skin of the shins and ankles. The abdomen may be distended, and a fluid wave may be discernible on examination. Breath sounds may be decreased at the lungs bases because of accumulation of pleural fluid. Although intravascular volume is low in most children with nephrotic syndrome, in some it will be increased. These latter children may present with a gallop on auscultation of the heart, rales over the lung fields, and hepatomegaly. Boys may develop significant scrotal swelling, and girls may develop labial swelling (Fig. 238-2). The child or parents may report decreased frequency of urination and the passage of a dark, amber-colored, concentrated-appearing urine that appears to foam when voided into the toilet. Overall, 16% of children with nephrotic syndrome have diastolic hypertension on presentation.[21] The presence of significant hypertension should raise the possibility of underlying glomerulonephritis.

LABORATORY EVALUATION

Laboratory evaluation begins with a urinalysis in the child with edema. This will demonstrate significant proteinuria in cases of nephrotic syndrome. Up to about 25% of children who have primary nephrotic syndrome will also have three to five red blood cells (RBCs) per high-power field on urinalysis.[42] The presence of significant microscopic hematuria or gross hematuria should suggest that nephrotic syndrome might be secondary to an underlying nephritic process. The presence of glycosuria in untreated children with nephrotic syndrome suggests underlying tubular injury that may be seen with focal segmental glomerulosclerosis. Blood urea nitrogen and creatinine values generally are normal or only slightly elevated in primary nephrotic syndrome. Serum total protein and albumin levels are low. Mild hyponatremia may be present because of water retention. Total calcium levels are low because of the low serum albumin level, but ionized calcium levels usually are normal. The serum cholesterol level usually is elevated. The third component of complement generally is normal. A depressed level suggests membranoproliferative glomerulonephritis, poststreptococcal glomerulonephritis, or lupus nephritis. Chest radiographs usually will show a small cardiac silhouette and, in severe cases, the presence of pleural fluid. Cardiomegaly may be seen in those cases with increased intravascular volume.

Urinary protein losses can be quantified with a 24-hour urine collection or, in incontinent children, estimated with a urine protein to creatinine ratio on a random urine sample. Nephrotic-range proteinuria is defined as (1) urinary protein excretion on a timed urine collection of greater than 3.5 g/day in adults or greater than 40 mg/M^2/hr or 1 g/M^2/day in children, or (2) a urine protein to creatinine ratio (mg/mg) is greater than 1. 0 on a random urine sample. Urinary protein quantification is not critical in the management of the nephrotic child who has heavy proteinuria as demonstrated by dipstick determination and a typical clinical presentation. It is more helpful for following the response of children with resistant forms of nephrotic syndrome.

PATHOPHYSIOLOGY

The glomerular capillary wall normally possesses a net negative electrical charge and has narrow "pores" that serve as barriers, preventing the passage of proteins into the urine.[29] In nephrotic syndrome, these barriers are variably altered depending on the severity and nature of the underlying disease process. Examples of alterations in these barriers include the loss of negative charge seen in minimal change nephrotic syndrome or the altered organization of glomerular basement membrane components in Alport syndrome. The changes in the barriers allow the passage of large quantities

BOX 238-1

EXAMPLES OF PRIMARY AND SECONDARY CAUSES OF NEPHROTIC SYNDROME IN CHILDREN

Primary Nephrotic Syndrome
Minimal change nephrotic syndrome
Focal segmental glomerulosclerosis
Mesangial hypercellularity
Membranoproliferative glomerulonephritis
Membranous nephropathy

Secondary Nephrotic Syndrome
Inherited diseases (congenital nephrotic syndrome, diffuse mesangial sclerosis, Alport syndrome, nail-patella syndrome, Lowe syndrome)
Vasculitides (lupus nephritis, Henoch-Schönlein purpura nephritis, Wegener's granulomatosis, Goodpasture's syndrome)
Postinfectious (poststreptococcal, human immunodeficiency virus, hepatitis B and C, malaria, syphilis, intrauterine infections, other viruses and bacteria)
Drugs and toxins (nonsteroidal antiinflammatory drugs, gold)
Diabetes mellitus (rare in children)

of plasma proteins into the urine.[36] This, in turn, may lead to a fall in the level of proteins in the blood.

Classically, the development of edema has been explained by the massive losses of plasma proteins, in particular albumin, in the urine, with the consequent development of hypoalbuminemia.[17,19] This, in turn, leads to decreased plasma oncotic pressure and leakage of fluid from the vascular space into the interstitium. The subsequent drop in the circulating blood volume stimulates the renin-angiotensin-aldosterone system, leading to avid sodium retention, and produces a nonosmotic stimulus for vasopressin secretion and free-water reabsorption. The result of these responses is the development of massive tissue edema with the excretion of very concentrated urine in a decreased volume. This scenario, however, does not explain the edema formation in all nephrotic patients.[11,17,19,44] Studies have demonstrated that in patients going into remission diuresis often begins as the proteinuria is resolving, but before normalization of plasma albumin levels. In addition, primary sodium retention has been demonstrated with the onset of proteinuria, (but before the development of hypoproteinemia) in at least some patients having a relapse of nephrotic syndrome. This would then lead to expansion of vascular volume and the development of edema.

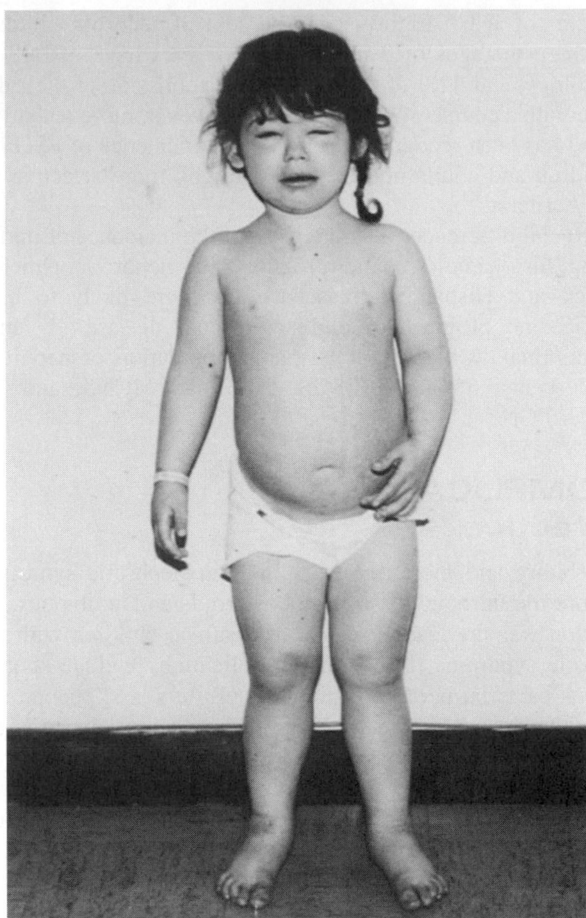

Fig. 238-1 A 2-year-old girl with nephrotic syndrome.

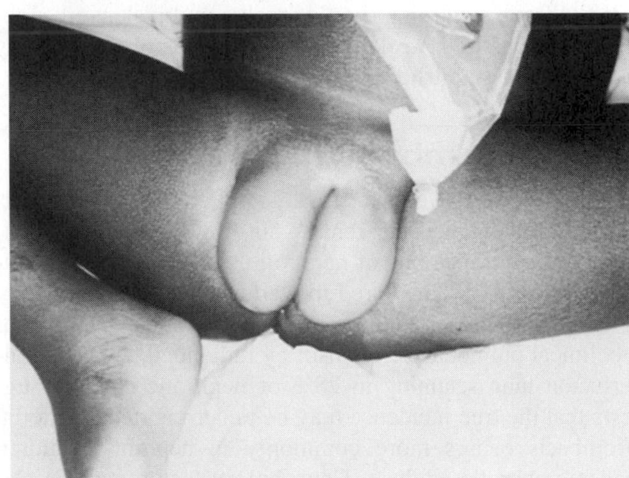

Fig. 238-2 Severe labial edema in a 3-year-old girl with nephrotic syndrome.

EPIDEMIOLOGY

The annual incidence of idiopathic nephrotic syndrome in children is estimated to be 2 to 3 cases/100,000. The incidence is tenfold lower in adults.[35] The male-to-female ratio is reported to be 2:1 for children and 1:1 in adolescents and adults. In nephrotic children 3 months to 16 years of age, 76% have minimal change nephrotic syndrome (MCNS), 7% have focal segmental glomerulosclerosis (FSGS), 2% to 5% have diffuse mesangial hypercellularity or mesangial proliferation, and 7% have membranoproliferative glomerulonephritis (MPGN) on biopsy.[8,21,46] Only 1% of nephrotic children have membranous nephropathy. This is in contrast to adults with nephrotic syndrome in whom 22% have MCNS, 12% have FSGS, 20% have membranous nephropathy, and 25% have proliferative lesions.[8] There is a peak occurrence of MCNS between 2 and

5 years of age.[46] Eighty-seven percent of nephrotic children between the ages of 3 months and 6 years have MCNS by histology, and 92% of these will have remission of their disease with a course of prednisone.[22] However, more recently a trend has been recognized for a higher incidence of FSGS in children and adults not accounted for by more selective biopsy criteria.[4,13]

Racial differences also are seen in the incidence of underlying histopathology and prognosis in nephrotic patients. Black and Hispanic adolescents are more likely to have FSGS and progress to end-stage renal disease.[20,23] In a predominantly black and Hispanic population of nephrotic adolescents, 55% had FSGS, 20% had MCNS, and 7% had MPGN.[3]

COMPLICATIONS

Infection

Morbidity and mortality were high in nephrotic syndrome before the introduction of corticosteroids and antibiotics. Infection was the leading cause of death in children with nephrotic syndrome. Infectious complications include spontaneous bacterial peritonitis, sepsis, cellulitis, and pneumonia. *Staphylococcus pneumoniae* and gram-negative bacteria are responsible for the majority of infections in nephrotic syndrome.[26] Predisposing factors for the development of bacterial infections include tissue edema that may facilitate the spread of infection, defective opsonization of invading bacteria caused by loss into the urine of small components of the alternative pathway of complement, and impaired cellular immunity. In addition, the effects of immunosuppressive therapies used in the treatment of nephrotic syndrome may increase the susceptibility to infection. Children with recurrent nephrotic syndrome should receive multivalent pneumococcal vaccination. A role for prophylactic antibiotic therapy has not been established.

Thromboembolism

Thromboembolic events such as deep-vein thrombosis, pulmonary embolism, and renal vein thrombosis are well-described complications of nephrotic syndrome in both children and adults.[15] They are reported to occur less frequently in children than in adults, although the documentation of subclinical pulmonary embolism by radionuclide ventilation-perfusion lung scanning in 28% of nephrotic children suggests that the true incidence may be underreported.[18] Arterial thrombosis occurs more commonly in nephrotic children than in nephrotic adults.[27] Contributory factors include elevated plasma levels of procoagulant factors, urinary loss of inhibitors of coagulation, and thrombocytosis.[39] The predisposition to thrombus formation may be exacerbated by decreased intravascular volume, especially in the face of vigorous forced diuresis.

Hyperlipidemia

Elevated plasma cholesterol in nephrotic syndrome results from increased hepatic lipoprotein synthesis caused by generalized increased hepatic protein synthesis in response to a lowered plasma albumin level.[34] In addition, in severe disease there may be decreased lipolysis, resulting in elevated triglycerides. The return of elevated cholesterol levels to normal upon remission of nephrotic syndrome often lags behind the normalization of serum albumin levels. In unremitting nephrotic syndrome, elevated plasma lipids may contribute to cardiovascular morbidity, and treatment of lipid abnormalities should be considered.

SPECIFIC HISTOPATHOLOGICAL ENTITIES ASSOCIATED WITH PRIMARY NEPHROTIC SYNDROME OF CHILDHOOD

Minimal Change Nephrotic Syndrome

Minimal change nephrotic syndrome (MCNS), also known as *lipoid nephrosis* and *nil* (nothing in light) *disease,* is the most common pathological diagnosis in nephrotic children and as noted previously, 92% will achieve a remission with a course of corticosteroids.[22] Hematuria is found in about 13% and hypertension in 10% to 20%.[21,46] Relapses are common, but the long-term prognosis is excellent. Relapses tend to become less frequent with age, and the disorder usually resolves around the time of puberty without permanent renal impairment. Often, the diagnosis is assumed in most children since biopsy generally is not performed in those who follow a typical course and respond to steroids. These children should more correctly be considered to have the clinical diagnosis of steroid-responsive idiopathic nephrotic syndrome of childhood, which encompasses a variety of histopathological diagnoses.

It has been proposed that MCNS may be an immune-mediated disease. Evidence suggestive for this theory includes the response of MCNS to immunosuppressive therapy, an association with allergens, an association with lymphomas, the presence of altered T-lymphocyte function, and the description of various circulating cationic proteins, immunomodulatory substances, permeability factors, and lymphokines.[36]

The histopathology of MCNS shows minimal abnormalities by light microscopy. Most pathologists allow for a small amount of mesangial hypercellularity within this classification. Immunofluorescence is negative for immunoglobulin and complement. Electron microscopy shows diffuse fusion of the glomerular epithelial cell foot processes. McAdams, Valentini, and Welch consider focal segmental scars in the presence of generalized foot process fusion to be a nonspecific finding within the category of MCNS, reflecting a more severe lesion.[23] Their subgroup of patients with MCNS and focal segmental scars was predominantly white and had a higher likelihood of being steroid resistant; they were more likely to progress to end-stage renal disease and to develop recurrence of proteinuria following renal transplantation than did those patients without scars.

Focal Segmental Glomerulosclerosis

Focal segmental glomerulosclerosis (FSGS) is found as both a primary and secondary pathological diagnosis. Secondary forms are thought to represent a final common pathway to glomerular epithelial cell injury, glomerular adaptation to significant nephron loss with glomerular hypertension or hyperfiltration, inherited abnormalities of the glomerular basement membrane, or severe glomerulonephritis.[40] Disease processes that can be associated with FSGS lesions include diabetic nephropathy, sickle cell disease, HIV nephropathy, and glomerulonephritides such as IgA nephropathy, membranoproliferative glomerulonephritis, and lupus nephritis.

Children presenting with primary FSGS tend to be older and show a disproportionately high representation of blacks.[20] Many are steroid resistant or dependent from the time of initial treatment or become steroid resistant over time. Hematuria may be found in 50% or more and hypertension in about 50%.[21,46] The prognosis of FSGS is more guarded. After an average follow-up of 11 years, 42% of children were in complete remission and none of these progressed to end-stage renal disease.[10] However, up to 50% will progress to end-stage renal disease with time and a subgroup will progress rapidly within 3 years of presentation. FSGS recurs in 20% to 50% of patients reaching end-stage renal failure who receive a renal transplant.[41,43]

Primary FSGS may actually be the manifestation of a systemic disorder. Evidence for this view includes: (1) the fact that the disease may recur in transplanted kidneys; (2) proteinuria could be induced in animals by infusion of serum from a patient with recurrent FSGS; (3) recurrent FSGS in transplanted kidneys may respond to plasmapheresis; and (4) a circulating factor capable of increasing the permeability of isolated glomeruli to albumin has been demonstrated in the serum of some patients with recurrent FSGS.[2,37,47]

The histopathology of FSGS is characterized by the presence of scars affecting portions or segments of some, but not all, glomeruli.[40] Mesangial hypercellularity, tubular atrophy, and interstitial fibrosis are seen often. Weak mesangial and segmental deposits of C3 and IgM can be seen by immunofluorescence but are thought to represent nonspecific trapping of these proteins. Electron microscopy may show widespread effacement of foot processes and separation of glomerular epithelial cells from the underlying basement membrane. Different subtypes of FSGS have been described that may reflect different stages of disease development, pathogenesis, and prognosis.[40]

In contrast to the classic view of FSGS, McAdams, Valentini, and Welch define primary FSGS as those cases in which the glomerular visceral epithelial-cell foot processes are normal in areas of the glomeruli not overlying segmental scars. Using this classification, 76% of the children in this study were black and 34% progressed to end-stage renal disease. However, there were no recurrences of nephrotic syndrome in renal transplants.[23]

Membranoproliferative Glomerulonephritis

Membranoproliferative glomerulonephritis (MPGN) is a chronic inflammatory disease of the kidney with a poor prognosis. It is discussed in more detail in Chapter 237, Nephritis. The average age of onset of primary MPGN is about 9 years.[24] Fifty percent to 67% of patients present with nephrotic syndrome, and some of these patients may present without significant hematuria.[9,25] The serum C3 level is depressed in 67% to 75% of patients on presentation.

Membranous Nephropathy

Membranous nephropathy is a chronic glomerular disease that also can be idiopathic or secondary to a systemic disorder. It can affect any age group but is rare in children and adolescents, being responsible for approximately 1% of children with nephrotic syndrome.[21] Seventy-three percent of children with membranous nephropathy present with nephrotic syndrome, 80% have microscopic hematuria, and 37% have hypertension. Six percent of children have gross hematuria at presentation while 20% will develop it sometime during the course of their illness.[7] Complement protein levels usually are normal. Spontaneous remissions are seen in the majority of patients but may not occur for several years after onset.[7,38] Approximately 13% of affected children progress to end-stage renal failure.[14] Poor prognostic factors may include persistent very heavy proteinuria (greater than 8 g/day for more than 6 months), hypertension, elevated creatinine, and significant scarring on biopsy.[16,33]

By light microscopy, membranous lesions are seen as diffuse thickening of the glomerular capillary walls.[12,14] Capillary lumens are patent, and there is little mesangial proliferation. Silver-stained biopsy specimens show "spikes" of basement membrane material projecting from the subepithelial side of the glomerular basement membrane. By electron microscopy, glomerular capillary walls are thickened by subepithelial electron-dense deposits and projections ("spikes") of the lamina densa. The extent of these projections with relation to the deposits forms the basis for classifying the stages of membranous nephropathy. Immunofluorescence studies show granular deposits of IgG along the glomerular basement membrane. C3 usually is seen in a similar distribution.

MANAGEMENT

Although a great deal of attention has been paid to the underlying pathological diagnoses in idiopathic childhood nephrotic syndrome, the clinical response to a course of corticosteroids seems to be as informative in determining long-term outcome as the underlying histopathology.[30] Eighty-five percent of nephrotic children regardless of underlying pathology will respond to a trial of prednisone. Seventy-five percent of those who will respond do so within 2 weeks of starting corticosteroids, and 94% will have responded by 4 weeks.[22] The majority of steroid-responsive patients have MCNS. However, up to 25% of steroid-resistant nephrotic children have MCNS on biopsy, whereas 5% to 10% of the steroid-responsive patients have FSGS.[22,30] Biopsy findings do not predict which children who have MCNS will be steroid resistant nor which children who have FSGS will be steroid responsive. In general, nephrotic patients who achieve a remission on steroids, whether they have MCNS or FSGS by biopsy, do not progress to renal failure if they remain steroid responsive.

Children between the ages of 1 and 6 years are most likely to have MCNS by renal biopsy and respond clinically to a trial of steroids by achieving a remission.[22] Therefore, it is now customary to treat a child in this age range (or even up to age 10) who presents with the new onset of typical, pure nephrotic syndrome with a trial of corticosteroids. Treatment consists of prednisone at 2 mg/kg/day or 60 mg/M^2/day (maximum 60 to 80 mg/day) for 4 to 6 weeks.[5,22]

This usually is given in divided doses, though some studies suggest that it can be given as a single morning dose with a similar rate of response.[45] This is followed by a single dose of 1.3 mg/kg or 40 mg/M^2 for an additional 4 to 6 weeks given in the morning on alternate days.[1,5,22] Daily prednisone was initially recommended for 4 weeks followed by 4 weeks of alternate day dosing, with the medication gradually tapered off after that.[22] More recently, studies have shown a decreased frequency of relapses in the first year and a lower total steroid dose if daily prednisone is given for 6 weeks, followed by 6 weeks of alternate-day prednisone and then tapered off over an additional 4 weeks.[5] Depending on the treatment regimen employed, from 36% to 61% of children will have a relapse of nephrotic syndrome within the first year of the initial episode.[5] A relapse is diagnosed if the urine tests 2+ or greater for protein for 3 consecutive days in the absence of edema. Relapses usually are triggered by intercurrent illnesses or allergies, and parents can be taught to use albumin test sticks or sulfosalicylic acid at home to monitor urinary protein excretion. Relapses are treated with prednisone 2 mg/kg/day or 60 mg/M^2/day until the urine is free of protein for 3 consecutive days. The prednisone dose then is changed to 40 mg/M^2 on alternate days for 4 weeks and then tapered off over an additional 4 weeks.[5]

About 25% of children with relapses will follow a frequently relapsing course, defined as 2 relapses occurring within 6 months of completing a course of steroids or 3 relapses within 1 year. Children who develop a relapse while corticosteroids are being tapered or within 2 weeks of completing a course of steroids are considered to be steroid-dependent. Both children who have frequently relapsing and steroid-dependent nephrotic syndrome are more likely to develop steroid toxicity. Secondary, tertiary, and complementary therapies for difficult cases of nephrotic syndrome are listed in Box 238-2. Consideration for treatment with these agents should be made in consultation with a pediatric nephrologist. Alkylating agents, either cyclophosphamide or chlorambucil, can induce a prolonged remission in patients with frequently relapsing and some patients with steroid-dependent nephrotic syndrome. Intravenous nitrogen mustard can be considered in noncompliant patients.[6] Levamisole has been used to decrease steroid dosage in frequently relapsing patients.[32] Nonsteroidal antiinflammatory drugs have been used to decrease proteinuria in resistant nephrotic syndrome but can lead to acute renal failure in the child who has significantly decreased intravascular volume. Cyclosporine can be used as a steroid-sparing agent in patients who do not respond to an alkylating agent.

Children who fail to respond to the initial or subsequent courses of corticosteroids have steroid-resistant nephrotic syndrome and a more guarded prognosis. Consultation with a pediatric nephrologist should be made for consideration of a renal biopsy and more aggressive treatment (see "When to Refer" on p. 1667). Likewise, children who are outside the usual age range for typical idiopathic nephrotic syndrome of childhood, who have refractory edema, or who have complicated nephrotic syndrome should be referred to a pediatric nephrologist for help with establishing the diagnosis and choosing a treatment plan. Current treatment regimens for steroid-resistant nephrotic syndrome are given in Box 238-2, which lists other therapies for nephrotic syndrome, including cytotoxic agents, high-dose, long-term intravenous methylprednisolone, cyclosporine, or tacrolimus.[28,31]

Other significant complications of therapy include the development of cushingoid features, cataract formation, glaucoma, gastritis, peptic ulcer disease, pancreatitis, hypokalemia, hypertension, increased risk of infection, behavioral changes, and growth delay if treatment is prolonged. Cytotoxic agents (e.g., cyclophosphamide, chlorambucil, nitrogen mustard, and cyclosporine) can be associated with increased risk of infection, malignancy, and sterility, but usually only with higher doses than those typically used for nephrotic syndrome or after repeated or prolonged courses. Cyclophosphamide can cause hemorrhagic cystitis. Therefore, a large fluid intake and frequent voiding should be encouraged. Chlorambucil therapy has been associated with induction of seizure activity. Nonsteroidal antiinflammatory drugs can cause salt retention and edema. There is a risk of renal failure, especially in patients with severely decreased intravascular volume. Cyclosporine and tacrolimus both have nephrotoxic potential and can cause acute and chronic renal injury. Acute renal failure can occur in severely nephrotic patients given cyclosporine who have markedly decreased intravascular volume.

Hospital admission should be considered for children during their first episode of nephrotic syndrome, especially if complications are present, and for teaching the parents home management and monitoring. Children who have severe edema compromising their ventilatory status, causing cardiovascular congestion, or interfering with ambulation should be admitted for forced diuresis. Infectious complications of nephrotic syndrome may require treatment with parenteral antibiotics. Hypertension, renal insufficiency, and electrolyte disturbances may also require hospitalization for stabilization. (See the box on p. 1667 for examples of reasons to hospitalize the nephrotic child.)

Salt intake should be restricted in edematous children given their state of avid sodium retention. Water intake usually does not need to be restricted, especially if sodium intake is adequately limited, unless significant hyponatremia develops or edema is intractable. Diuretics are used judiciously given the already reduced intravascular volume in most nephrotic patients and the attendant risk of thromboembolism. Furosemide alone or in combination with a thiazide diuretic is used for significant edema. Severe edema interfering with ambulation, compromising respiratory status, or causing tis-

BOX 238-2

SECONDARY, TERTIARY, AND COMPLEMENTARY THERAPIES FOR DIFFICULT CASES OF NEPHROTIC SYNDROME

Cyclophosphamide
Chlorambucil
Cyclosporine
Tacrolimus
Methylprednisolone infusions
Levamisole
Angiotensin-converting enzyme inhibitors
Nonsteroidal antiinflammatory drugs

sue breakdown can be treated with intravenous 25% albumin, 1 g/kg, followed by intravenous furosemide if renal function and urine output are fairly well maintained. Patients must be monitored very closely during infusion for the development of signs of intravascular overload such as rales, cardiac gallop, and hepatomegaly. This therapy can also be used in the severely edematous, steroid-resistant nephrotic patient in whom cyclosporine therapy is being considered in order to try to improve renal perfusion and prevent the precipitation of acute renal failure. Children with significant renal insufficiency may require dialysis to manage edema, electrolyte disturbances, and uremia.

Angiotensin-converting enzyme (ACE) inhibitors (e.g., captopril and enalapril) can be tried in resistant nephrotic syndrome, even in the presence of normotension, to decrease urinary protein excretion. The ACE inhibitors act by decreasing glomerular capillary pressure and can cause a reversible rise in serum creatinine and hyperkalemia that must be monitored. High doses of ACE inhibitors may decrease progressive sclerosis.

The treatment of membranous nephropathy is controversial with regard to the choice of agent and the timing of intervention. It has been suggested that therapy may be withheld in most patients given the high rate of spontaneous remission. Those who have evidence of renal insufficiency, persistent heavy proteinuria, hypertension, or sclerosis on biopsy should be considered for treatment. Agents that have been used for the treatment of membranous nephropathy include high-dose corticosteroids given orally or intravenously alone or in combination with cytotoxic agents.[7,16]

When to Refer

Complicated nephrotic syndrome
Outside the expected age range (younger than 1 year old or older than10 years old)
Accompanied by signs of glomerulonephritis (renal insufficiency, hypertension, hematuria, hypocomplementemia)
Refractory edema
Frequently relapsing nephrotic syndrome
Steroid-dependent nephrotic syndrome
Steroid-resistant nephrotic syndrome

When to Hospitalize

Initial episode for teaching of parents
Anasarca interfering with ambulation or compromising ventilation
Pleural effusions or ascites interfering with ventilation
Signs of volume overload (congestive heart failure)
Infection (e.g., severe cellulitis, peritonitis)
Significant hypertension
Significant electrolyte abnormalities
Compromised renal function

REFERENCES

1. Arbeitsgemeinschaft für Pädiatrische Nephrologie: alternate-day versus intermittent prednisone in frequently relapsing nephrotic syndrome, *Lancet* 1:401, 1979.
2. Artero ML, et al: Plasmapheresis reduces proteinuria and serum capacity to injure glomeruli in patients with recurrent focal glomerulosclerosis, *Am J Kidney Dis* 23:574, 1994.
3. Baqi N, et al: The paucity of minimal change disease in adolescents with primary nephrotic syndrome, *Pediatr Nephrol* 12:105, 1998.
4. Bonilla-Felix M, et al: Changing patterns in the histopathology of idiopathic nephrotic syndrome in children, *Kidney Int* 55:1885, 1999.
5. Brodehl J: The treatment of minimal change nephrotic syndrome: lessons learned from multicentre co-operative studies, *Eur J Pediatr* 150: 380, 1991.
6. Broyer M, et al: Nitrogen mustard therapy in idiopathic nephrotic syndrome of childhood, *Int J Pediatr Nephrol* 6:29, 1985.
7. Cameron JS: Membranous nephropathy in childhood and its treatment, *Pediatr Nephrol* 4:193, 1990.
8. Cameron JS: Nephrotic syndrome and its complications, *Am J Kidney Dis* 10:157, 1987.
9. Cameron JS, et al: Idiopathic mesangiocapillary glomerulonephritis: comparison of types I and II in children and adults and long-term prognosis, *Am J Med* 74:175, 1983.
10. Cattran DC, Rao P: Long-term outcome in children and adults with classic focal segmental glomerulosclerosis, *Am J Kidney Dis* 32:72, 1998.
11. Donkerwolcke RA, Vande Walle JG: Pathogenesis of edema formation in nephrotic syndrome, *Kidney Int* 51(suppl 58):S72, 1997.
12. Ehrenreich J, Churg J: Pathology of membranous nephropathy, *Pathol Annu* 3:145, 1968.
13. Haas M, Spargo BH, Coventry S: Increasing incidence of focal-segmental glomerulosclerosis among adult nephropathies: a 20-year renal biopsy study, *Am J Kidney Dis* 26:740, 1995.
14. Habib R, Kleinknecht C, Gubler M-C: Extramembranous glomerulonephritis in children: report of 50 cases, *J Pediatr* 82:754, 1973.
15. Harris RC, Ismail N: Extrarenal complications of nephrotic syndrome, *Am J Kidney Dis* 23:477, 1994.
16. Hebert LA: Therapy of membranous nephropathy: what to do after the after (meta) analysis, *J Am Soc Nephrol* 5:1543, 1995.
17. Hisano S, et al: Edema in childhood, *Kidney Int* 51(suppl 59):S100, 1997.
18. Hoyer PF, et al: Thromboembolic complications in children with nephrotic syndrome: risk and incidence, *Acta Paediatr Scand* 75:804, 1986.
19. Humphreys MH: Mechanisms and management of nephrotic edema, *Kidney Int* 45:266, 1994.
20. Ingulli E, Tejani A: Racial differences in the incidence and renal outcome of idiopathic focal segmental glomerulosclerosis in children, *Pediatr Nephrol* 5:393, 1991.
21. International Study of Kidney Disease in Children: Nephrotic syndrome in children: prediction of histopathology from clinical and laboratory characteristics at time of diagnosis, *Kidney Int* 13:159, 1978.
22. International Study of Kidney Disease in Children: The primary nephrotic syndrome in children: identification of patients with minimal change nephrotic syndrome from initial responders, *J Pediatr* 98:561, 1981.
23. McAdams AJ, Valentini RP, Welch TR: The nonspecificity of focal segmental glomerulosclerosis: the defining characteristics of primary focal glomerulosclerosis, mesangial proliferation, and minimal change, *Medicine* 76:42, 1997.
24. McEnery PT: Membranoproliferative glomerulonephritis: the Cincinnati experience—cumulative renal survival from 1957 to 1989, *J Pediatr* 116:S109, 1990.
25. McEnery PT, McAdams AJ, West CD: Membranoproliferative glomerulonephritis: improved survival with alternate day prednisone therapy, *Clin Nephrol* 13:117, 1980.
26. McIntyre P, Craig JC: Prevention of serious bacterial infection in children with nephrotic syndrome, *J Paediatr Child Health* 34:314, 1998.
27. Mehls O, et al: Hemostasis and thromboembolism in children with nephrotic syndrome: differences from adults, *J Pediatr* 110:862, 1987.

28. Mendoza SA, Tune BM: Treatment of childhood nephrotic syndrome, *J Am Soc Nephrol* 3:889, 1992.
29. Myers BD, Guasch A: Mechanisms of proteinuria in nephrotic humans, *Pediatr Nephrol* 8:107, 1994.
30. Niaudet P: Nephrotic syndrome in children, *Curr Opin Pediatr* 5:174, 1993.
31. Niaudet P, Gagnadoux MF, Broyer M: Treatment of childhood steroid-resistant idiopathic nephrotic syndrome, *Adv Nephrol* 28:43, 1998.
32. Niaudet P, et al: Treatment of idiopathic nephrotic syndrome with levamisole, *Acta Paeditr Scand* 73:637, 1984.
33. Pei Y, Cattran D, Greenwood C: Predicting chronic renal insufficiency in idiopathic membranous glomerulonephritis, *Kidney Int* 42:960, 1992.
34. Querfeld U: Should hyperlipidemia in children with nephrotic syndrome be treated? *Pediatr Nephrol* 13:77, 1999.
35. Ritz E: Pathogenesis of "idiopathic" nephrotic syndrome, *N Engl J Med* 330:61, 1994.
36. Savin VJ: Mechanisms of proteinuria in noninflammatory glomerular diseases, *Am J Kidney Dis* 21:347, 1993.
37. Savin VJ, et al: Circulating factor associated with increased glomerular permeability to albumin in recurrent focal segmental glomerulosclerosis, *N Engl J Med* 334:878, 1996.
38. Schieppati A, et al: Prognosis of untreated patients with idiopathic membranous nephropathy, *N Engl J Med* 329:85, 1993.
39. Schlegel N: Thromboembolic risks and complications in nephrotic children, *Semin Thrombosis Hemostasis* 23:271, 1997.
40. Schwartz MM, Korbet SM: Primary focal segmental glomerulosclerosis: pathology, histological variants, and pathogenesis, *Am J Kidney Dis* 22:874, 1993.
41. Senggutuvan P, et al: Recurrence of focal segmental glomerulosclerosis in transplanted kidneys: analysis of incidence and risk factors in 59 allografts, *Pediatr Nephrol* 4:21, 1990.
42. Strauss J, et al: Less commonly recognized features of childhood nephrotic syndrome, *Pediatr Clin North Am* 34:591, 1987.
43. Tejani A, Stablein DH: Recurrence of focal segmental glomerulosclerosis posttransplantation: a special report of the North American Pediatric Renal Transplant Cooperative Study, *J Am Soc Nephrol* 2(suppl 3):S258, 1992.
44. Vande Walle JGJ, Donkerwolcke RA, Koomans HA: Pathophysiology of edema formation in children with nephrotic syndrome not due to minimal change disease, *J Am Soc Nephrol* 10:323, 1999.
45. Warshaw BL, Hymes LC: Daily single-dose and daily reduced-dose prednisone therapy for children with nephrotic syndrome, *Pediatr* 83: 694, 1989.
46. White RHR, Glasgow EF, Mills RJ: Clinicopathological study of nephrotic syndrome in childhood, *Lancet* 1:1353, 1970.
47. Zimmerman SW: Increased urinary protein excretion in the rat produced by serum from a patient with recurrent focal glomerular sclerosis after renal transplantation, *Clin Nephrol* 22:32, 1984.

239 Obesity

Wendi G. Ehrman

Obesity is considered one of the most prevalent nutritional problems among children and adolescents in the United States. The past 20 years have seen an alarming increase in the prevalence of childhood and adolescent obesity. Obesity can lead to significant morbidity among youth and has been associated with negative social, economic, and physical outcomes in adulthood. Obesity is a complex and difficult disorder to treat. Long-term weight loss or maintenance requires family and patient commitment as well as permanent lifestyle changes.

PREVALENCE

Data from the Third National Health and Nutrition Examination Survey (NHANES III) indicate that 33% of the United States adult population is obese[40] and 11% of children and adolescents are considered overweight. An additional 14% of children and adolescents are considered "highly at risk" for becoming overweight.[72] The prevalence of being overweight has increased dramatically since the mid-1970s, with the heaviest children becoming markedly heavier than their predecessors of earlier decades and predisposing them to continuing overweight/obesity in adulthood.

ETIOLOGY

Overweight is defined as an increase in body weight in relation to height. *Obesity* is defined as the excess accumulation of body fat relative to lean body mass. Obesity results when energy intake exceeds energy expenditure and is stored as fat. However, this simplistic explanation fails to address all of the contributing social, cultural, genetic, and environmental factors that can effect accumulation of fat and weight gain.

Obesity often is viewed as a form of overnutrition since obese children tend to be taller than average, have a larger lean body mass, and have excess body fat. Despite these findings, the role of dietary intake in the development of obesity is a subject of much controversy. Earlier studies of obese children suggested that their daily intake was the same or less than their normal-weight peers.[19,35] Data in these studies came from self-reported dietary histories. Subsequent studies have shown that underreporting food intake is a common occurrence, especially among obese children and adolescents.[2,43]

In young children, diets increasingly higher in calories from fat have been associated with increasing adiposity and weight gain.[39] However, nationally the percentage of calories from fat ingested has continued to decline since the mid-1960s.[24] Caloric intake has increased for adolescents ages 16 and older, but this same increase has not been seen in younger children and adolescents. Although a positive energy balance leads to increased weight and adiposity, current nutritional data do not account for the continuing upward trend in obesity.

Recent data focus on the role of energy expenditure and lower activity levels in obese infants, children, and adults. Nonobese infants with lower total daily energy expenditures at 3 months of age went on to become overweight infants at 1 year of age.[60] Preschool children had negative correlations between physical activity and body fatness.[12] Prepubertal obese children exhibited higher energy expenditures than their nonobese peers, but these differences disappeared when energy expenditure was calculated per kilograms of weight. For these obese children, similar activities were energetically more expensive.[44] Other comparisons of obese and lean children have shown decreased activity levels, increased sedentary activities, and more time spent at rest, despite higher levels of measured energy expenditure per activity.[13] In addition, at least two studies have found a positive correlation between the amount of television viewing and the current increases seen in pediatric obesity.[15,32]

Obesity has a strong familial component that probably results from complex interactions between genetic and environmental factors. Early data from the Ten State Nutrition Survey (1968-1970) showed that children of overweight parents were more likely to be overweight and their level of "fatness" rose progressively with the level of their parents' "fatness."[28] Previous estimations showed that children of normal-weight parents had a 14% risk of obesity compared with a risk of 40% when one parent was obese and 80% if both parents were obese.[47] Adoption and twin studies also suggest a strong genetic influence on obesity. A direct relationship was seen between the body mass index (BMI) of biological parents and the weight class of adoptees.[69] In contrast, there was little or no correlation in BMIs between adoptees and their adoptive parents.Twin studies showed the BMI of monozygotic twins to be highly correlated whether or not they were reared together or apart.[71] Among overweight male twin pairs, the concordance rate for different degrees of overweight was twice as high for monozygotic than for dizygotic twins.[70] Overall, estimates of heritability for indirect measures of obesity vary greatly (10% to 80%) depending on the type of study done. Heritability estimates using direct measurements of total fat mass suggest that 25% to 40% of the variability is due to genetic factors.[4]

Current research into rodent models of obesity has identified an autosomal recessive mutation known as the *leptin*, or *lep* gene. This gene codes for an adipocyte-derived protein known as leptin that appears to play a role in energy homeostasis. Leptin has been associated with decreased food intake, increased energy expenditure, and reduced body fat when given exogenously to genetically obese leptin-deficient mice[7,33,56] and in higher doses to nonobese mice.[10] Leptin is secreted in proportion to fat mass in both animals[26] and humans.[63] Elevated leptin levels are seen early in the development of juvenile obesity and may reflect a resistance to its action.[8,41] Further animal and human research in this area may lead to specific therapies, as well as a better understanding of specific genetic abnormalities predisposing to obesity.

Childhood obesity has been associated with other factors such as geographical region, population density, season,[16] and family characteristics such as parental age,[28] marital status, family size,[58] and socioeconomic status. Results of the Ten State Nutrition Survey (1968-1970) indicated a "reversal of fatness" for black and white females.[28] White females were heavier than black females up until late adolescence at which point a reversal in weight categories was seen. This same pattern was seen when comparing low and high socioeconomic groups. Children of all ages from a higher socioeconomic group were heavier than children from lower socioeconomic groups. However, this trend was reversed for females in late adolescence and adulthood. A comprehensive review by Sobal and Stunkard showed that weight was inversely related to socioeconomic status for women but not men or children in developed countries.[68] In developing countries, socioeconomic status was positively related to weight for women, men, and children.

The substantial increase in obesity in the United States over the past decade has occurred too rapidly to attribute all to a change in genetic makeup or any other single factor. Rather, the current status of obesity is probably a reflection of a genetic predisposition modified by diets high in calorically dense foods, an overall decrease in physical activity, and other modifiable factors.

COMPLICATIONS

Obesity has a major impact on several different aspects of growth. Obese children have increased lean body mass and adipose tissue. Linear growth, bone age, and sexual maturation are often advanced.[28] Obese females tend to have earlier menarche than their nonobese peers,[20] and obese adolescent males are more likely to exhibit female-pattern adipose tissue in the mammary region, or "visible gynecomastia."[73]

Overweight adolescents are at increased risk for cardiovascular disease as adults.[52] Factors that predispose individuals to cardiovascular disease are thought to develop during early childhood. Hypertension, hyperlipidemia, and glucose intolerance are recognized cardiovascular risk factors that have been shown to occur concurrently in adults as well as obese children and adolescents.[11,67] In addition, moderately to severely obese adults have shown a significantly increased risk of mortality from all causes, including cardiovascular disease.[6]

Obese adolescents have exhibited blood pressure distributions skewed one standard deviation higher than normal. Blood pressures returned within the normal range following weight loss.[61] Cholesterol and triglycerides are related to weight in a linear fashion. Data from the National Health and Nutrition Examination Survey demonstrated that the incidence of hypercholesterolemia in a young overweight group was 2.1 times that of a nonoverweight group.[53]

Non–insulin-dependent diabetes mellitus (NIDDM) has been strongly correlated with obesity.[5] In adults, more than 80% of cases of NIDDM can be attributed to obesity. The risk for NIDDM appears to increase with the degree of obesity, duration of obesity, and central distribution of body fat.[29] Recent studies indicate a growing number of newly diagnosed cases of NIDDM among children and adolescents, paralleling recent trends of increasing pediatric obesity.[57,65] In these studies, as many as 92% to 96% of pediatric patients with NIDDM had BMIs at least as high as the 85th percentile. In addition, many of these patients also presented with hypertension and acanthosis nigricans.

Acanthosis nigricans, a skin disorder characterized by a velvety thickening and hyperpigmentation of the neck, axilla, inframammary areas, and other intertriginous body folds, is associated with obesity, hyperinsulinemia, and insulin resistance. Acanthosis nigricans often develops in puberty concurrent with the onset of obesity and may disappear following weight loss. Up to 25% of obese patients may display this skin finding.[54]

Intertrigo, a superficial inflammatory dermatitis, develops in areas of skin subject to friction and maceration. It is seen more frequently in obese children and adolescents because of the overlapping of skin folds.

Menstrual irregularities, predominately anovulatory cycles characterized by dysfunctional uterine bleeding and amenorrhea, have been associated with obesity in adolescent females. Polycystic ovary syndrome is a spectrum of clinical disorders associated with increased androgen production, abnormal gonadotropin secretion, and insulin resistance. Obesity is common in adolescents with polycystic ovary syndrome. In addition, type A HAIR-AN syndrome (a genetic disorder characterized by hyperandrogenism, insulin resistance, and acanthosis nigricans) often is associated with obesity.

Orthopedic problems may result from the stress of excess weight in obese adolescents. Slipped capital femoral epiphysis (SCFE) develops as an abrupt or gradual displacement of the femoral neck from the femoral head through the growth plate. Although numerous factors may contribute to the development of SCFE, more than 50% of the patients are classified as obese, and many are taller than the 90th percentile in height.[9,38] Blount disease, a bowing of the tibia associated with medial epiphyseal osteochondrosis, also has been associated with obesity in childhood.[17] Approximately two thirds of children and adolescents with this disorder are obese.

In adults, obesity is associated with a number of severe pulmonary complications including obesity-hypoventilation syndrome (OHS) or Pickwickian syndrome and obstructive sleep apnea (OSA). Although OHS and OSA have not been as well documented in children, recent evidence indicates that morbidly obese children and adolescents are at risk for sleep-associated breathing disorders.[45,46] These disorders have been associated with significant deficits in learning and memory.[59]

The most devastating consequences of obesity are felt to be the impact on the psychosocial functioning of the child or adolescent. Overweight children and adolescents reportedly exhibit significant depression,[75] lowered self-esteem,[64] and lower body-esteem.[49] Numerous studies have documented a pervasive "fear of fatness" among adolescent females of all weight categories. This fear can lead to inappropriate eating behaviors and attitudes among the obese and nonobese adolescent female.[50,51] In addition, a recent study showed that women who had been overweight as adolescents were less likely to be married, had completed fewer years of high school, and had lower household incomes and higher poverty levels than their nonoverweight controls. Men who had been overweight as adolescents were less likely to be married as well.[31]

Many obese children and adolescents do not suffer from impaired psychosocial functioning and demonstrate self-esteem equivalent to that of their nonobese peers.[37,74] A number of studies indicate that gender, race, parental perceptions of weight, and socioeconomic status influence self-esteem and body image of obese and nonobese children and adolescents.[14,42,55] White females of any weight category and females of higher socioeconomic status are more likely to be dissatisfied with their weight and see themselves as heavier than they actually are. Overweight blacks are less likely to see themselves as heavy and appear more satisfied with their current weight.

It is important to identify and treat obese patients with complications and counsel those at risk for obesity. However, the physical and psychological effects of obesity vary among children and adolescents. Not all obese children and adolescents will experience complications as a result of their weight. In fact, many obese children and adolescents are physically and emotionally healthy.

DIFFERENTIAL DIAGNOSIS

Obesity is a common feature of several endocrinopathies and a number of syndromes (Boxes 239-1 and 239-2). Primary obesity often is associated with average to above-average height and normal to accelerated sexual maturation. Obesity associated with a syndrome or endocrinopathy generally is associated with delayed bone age, short stature, and hypogonadism. In addition, obesity associated with syndromes such as Bardet-Biedl, Cohen, and Prader-Willi present with dysmorphic features and developmental delay.

A number of medications can cause obesity. Prolonged use of corticosteroids can lead to cushingoid obesity. Significant weight gain often is seen in asthmatic patients on chronic oral steroid treatment. Psychotropic medications including lithium, tricyclic antidepressants, and phenothiazines may also cause weight gain.

BOX 239-1

ENDOCRINE DISORDERS ASSOCIATED WITH OBESITY

Hypothyroidism
Cushing's syndrome
Polycystic ovarian syndrome
Hyperinsulinism
Growth hormone deficiency

BOX 239-2

GENETIC SYNDROMES ASSOCIATED WITH OBESITY

Syndrome	Description
1. Albright hereditary osteodystrophy (pseudoparathyroidism)	Short metacarpals, round face, developmental delays, variable hypocalcemia, hyperphosphatemia
2. Alström	Retinitis pigmentosa, deafness, insulin resistance, diabetes
3. Bardet-Biedel	Autosomal recessive, developmental delays, hypogonadism, hypotonia, small hands and feet
4. Börjeson-Forssman-Lehman	Severe cognitive delay, hypogonadism, large ears
5. Carpenter	Variable cognitive delay, acrocephaly, polydactyly and syndactyly of feet
6. Cohen	Autosomal recessive, developmental delays, hypotonia, prominent incisors
7. Prader-Willi	Developmental delays, short stature, hypogonadism, hypotonia, small hands and feet
8. Simpson-Golabi-Behmel	Prenatal and postnatal overgrowth
9. Turner (XO)	Occasional developmental delays, short female, webbed neck, low-set hair line over the nape of the neck, broad chest with wide-spaced nipples, coarctation of the aorta, gonadal dysgenesis, congenital lymphedema
10. Wilson-Turner	Developmental delays, gynecomastia, limb abnormalities

DIAGNOSIS

Obesity refers to an excess of fat or adipose tissue. Body fat can be estimated by subtracting lean body mass (or fat-free mass) from body weight. Methods for estimating lean body mass include underwater weighing to measure body density, measurement of total body water or potassium 40 levels, and measurement of total body conductivity and bioimpedance. In addition, computer tomography (CT) and magnetic resonance imaging (MRI) can define percentages of lean body mass and fat while dual-energy x-ray absorptiometry (DXA) can define percentages of lean body mass, fat, and bone. These procedures are difficult to perform technically and obviously not practical in a clinical, nonresearch setting.

Skinfold thicknesses have been used to estimate total body fat at various sites (biceps, triceps, subscapular, iliac crest) by measuring subcutaneous fat. Formulas have been developed for certain groups of children to predict body composition based on these measurements.[25,30] Although these formulas have been highly correlated with DXA, skinfold measurements are limited by interuser variability and may not reflect the body composition of pediatric subgroups.

Most methods used to estimate "obesity" do not really measure fat but rely on ratios of body weight to height. These criteria classify individuals as overweight but not obese. These methods are typically easier to perform and more precise than measurements such as skinfold thickness. In the past, measurements such as the percentage above the ideal body weight (50th percentile weight for the child's age, gender, and height) were used as an indicator of obesity. Recent recommendations from the Expert Committee on Obesity suggest the use of body mass index (BMI) as an indicator of weight status.[3] BMI is defined as weight in kilograms divided by height in meters squared. BMI has been shown to correlate highly with other measurements of obesity depending on the method used, as well as the age and sex of the subject.[18] In addition, childhood BMI values have been shown to correlate with values in adulthood.[62] However, it is important to note that BMI changes with increasing age, varies by gender, and may not be as reliable a measurement of overweight throughout childhood as it is in adulthood.

The Expert Committee on Obesity has recommended the 95th percentile BMI for age and sex as the cutoff for defining overweight children and adolescents in need of medical evaluation.[3] Children and adolescents who fall in between the 85th and 95th percentile BMI are considered "at risk" for becoming overweight and the complications of obesity. In addition, any child or adolescent with a large jump in BMI, such as 3 to 4 BMI units/year, should be considered at risk. These groups of pediatric patients should be evaluated carefully for hypertension, dyslipidemia, and current weight concerns, and considered for treatment options.

Tables are available with BMI percentiles listed by age, sex, and race.[27,34] In addition, the National Center for Health Statistics recently released revised growth charts displaying BMI percentile curves by age and sex (Figs. 239-1 and 239-2).

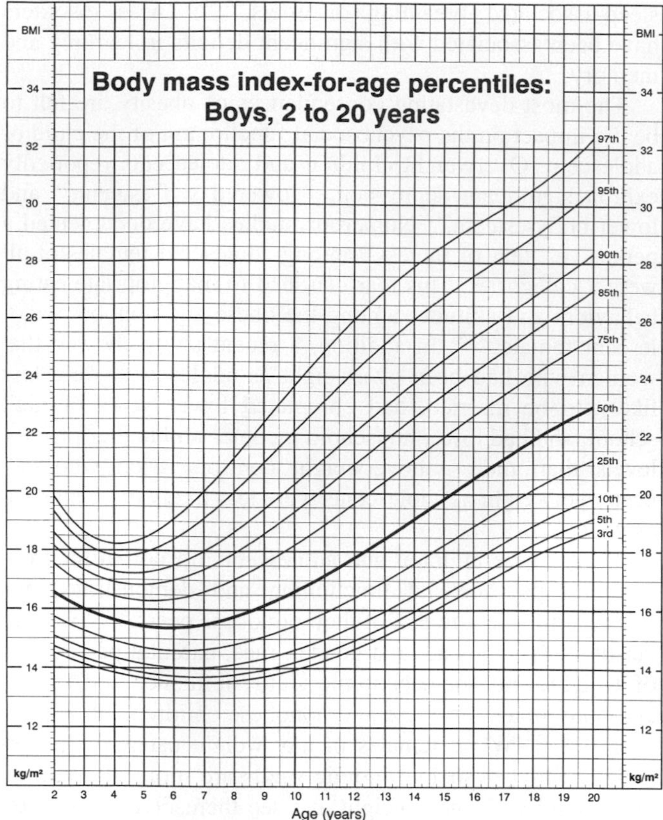

Fig. 239-1 Body mass index-for-age percentiles, boys, 2 to 20 years.

(Data from Kuczmarski RJ, et al: *CDC growth charts: United States,* No 314, US Department of Health and Human Services, Centers for Disease Control and Prevention, National Center for Health Statistics, Hyattsville, Md, 2000.)

TREATMENT

Obesity is a complex, chronic problem that provides a significant challenge to practitioners attempting to treat children, adolescents, or adults. The longer the duration of obesity, or the younger the age of onset, the poorer the outlook for permanent leanness.

Recent recommendations from the Expert Committee on Obesity stress weight maintenance, or the slowing of excessive weight gain, as the ultimate goal for healthy obese children who are: (1) ages 2 to 7 years and have a BMI in the 85th to 94th percentile or a BMI in at least the 95th percentile without complications of obesity, or (2) over age 7 years and have a BMI less than the 95th percentile with no complication of obesity.[3] Weight maintenance allows these children to grow into their height and gradually decrease their BMI. This typically is achieved through modest dietary changes and increases in activity levels.

Weight loss is recommended for obese children older than 2 years of age who have complications of obesity and a BMI higher than the 95th percentile. It also is recommended for children age who are at least 7 years of age who have a BMI in at least the 95th percentile or who have a BMI higher than the 85th percentile and a secondary health complication. For these children it is important to work with the families on first maintaining the child's weight and then working on a gradual weight loss. The primary goal with these children should be to develop healthy eating habits, with a secondary goal of achieving a BMI below the 85th percentile.

Severe weight problems in children younger than 2 years

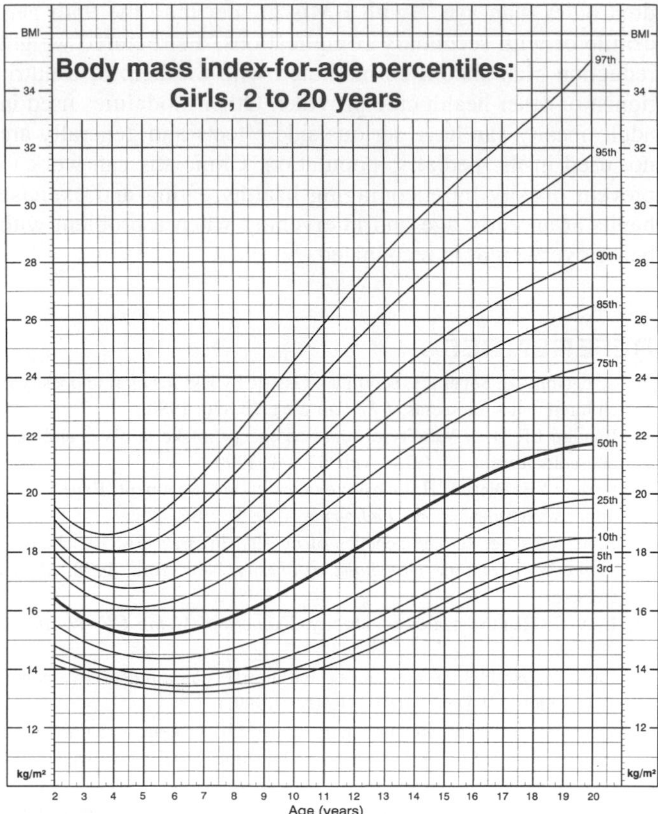

Fig. 239-2 Body mass index-for-age percentiles, girls, 2 to 20 years.

(Data from Kuczmarski RJ, et al: *CDC growth charts: United States,* No 314, US Department of Health and Human Services, Centers for Disease Control and Prevention, National Center for Health Statistics, Hyattsville, Md, 2000.)

of age are rare. However, when it does occur, the committee recommended that these children be evaluated by a pediatric obesity center.

Weight maintenance and loss is really a family health issue. Evidence has shown that maternal or family involvement with a weight loss program is associated with increased short-term weight loss and weight loss maintenance over periods of up to 10 years.[23] Before implementation of any weight control/loss plan, a family must be willing to acknowledge that their child has a weight problem and then commit to changing the child's and the family's eating habits. Failure to do so sets the child up for failure. Families that are not ready to accept their child's weight problem may benefit from counseling to improve their motivation. In addition, treatment can be deferred until the family is ready.

Weight control and loss interventions should balance healthy eating habits with increased activity levels. Families need to identify patterns of unhealthy eating behaviors, such as the consumption of high-fat or high-calorie foods, and the situations in which these eating patterns occur. A dietary calendar can be used by the parent and child to keep an accurate account of all that is eaten, when, and under what circumstances. These food diaries can be reviewed with the health care provider or nutritionist to identify areas for intervention. Once problem areas are identified, families should be encouraged to make gradually a few, small, permanent changes. Changes should be achievable and can include smaller portion sizes, substitution of lower-fat foods, less eating out, or different methods of food preparation such as baking or boiling instead of frying. High-calorie juices and sodas can be replaced with water or diet soda. Skim or 1% milk can replace whole milk. Families should be encouraged to eat regular meals together. Additional changes should only take place after the original changes are firmly in place.

Fasting and semi-starvation diets are contraindicated in growing children and adolescents because of the potential for growth arrest or retardation. In addition, these diets are difficult to maintain and do not aid in the development of healthy eating habits. Calorie-reduction diets can be instituted with the assistance of a nutritionist for those in need of substantial weight loss. The difficulty with these diets is that they can be tedious and difficult to maintain.

The Stoplight diet[21] has produced successful weight reduction in preschool and preadolescent children when part of a comprehensive treatment plan. This diet uses a structured eating plan of 900 to 1300 kcal/day that divides food into three categories. Green, or "go," foods are lower in calories and can be consumed in unlimited quantities; yellow, or "caution," foods have average nutritional value; and red, or "stop," foods are higher in fat or simple carbohydrates and should be eaten infrequently.

Commercial programs such as Shapedown are specially designed for obese/overweight adolescents. Shapedown incorporates cognitive, behavioral, and affective techniques to modify diet, exercise, relationships, lifestyle, communication, and affect. Significant short-term and long-term weight loss has been seen in some obese participants.[48] However, the cost and/or location of this type of program may limit its use among adolescents.

Parents or caretakers can aid a child's progress by encouragement and positive reinforcement. Praise should be offered for any positive behavioral change. Mistakes should not be criticized, and corrections should be directed at the behavior and not the child. Food should never be offered as a reward. Instead, increased activity time, especially with the parents or caregiver, is a preferred option. For older children, tangible rewards can be negotiated for achievement of weight or behavioral goals.

Parents or caretakers can also assist their children in other ways. Regular times should be established for meals and snacks. Parents or caretakers should determine the food being served and when, and the child should decide whether or not to eat. Snack choices should be healthy, and lower in fat and processed sugar. Older children should be encouraged to help with both the meal planning and the grocery shopping. Parents or caretakers should set their own example by purchasing, preparing, and eating healthy foods; removing temptations; and being consistent.

Regular exercise is an important component of any treatment plan. Exercise can not only improve overall fitness but also can preserve lean body mass and improve mental health. Long-term success is best achieved by changing lifestyle activities instead of incorporating rigorous exercises and programmed activities into a child or adolescent's life. This may best be achieved by a reduction in inactivity such as limitations on daily television viewing, and time spent playing video and computer games. Instead, the child or adolescent should be encouraged to increase active participation in daily routines such as walking or riding a bicycle instead of riding in a car or bus. Stairs can be used instead of elevators, and more time should be spent in active play than on the telephone. Vigorous outdoor play should be encouraged in younger children. Reduction of inactivity may be easier than vigorous aerobic exercise programs and may lead to improved long-term weight reduction.[22]

Some weight loss modalities (e.g., radical diets, drugs, surgery) are not generally recommended for children and adolescents. Anoretic drugs such as sympathomimetics, diuretics, and hormones have not shown long-term effectiveness. Stimulants have a significant risk for abuse by adolescents. Serotonin agonists such as fenfluramine and dexfenfluramine have been removed from the market because of an association with pulmonary hypertension and valvular heart disease, especially when used in combination with phentermine, a noradrenergic agent. Sibutramine (Meridia), a selective serotonin reuptake inhibitor (SSRI) has shown some effectiveness as a weight loss agent in adults but has yet to be evaluated in a pediatric population. Surgical treatments such as gastroplasty and jejunoileal bypass may lead to life-threatening side effects and should be reserved for morbidly obese adults with serious medical complications.[1,66]

PREVENTION

Prevention of obesity should start in childhood with the development of healthy eating habits and a positive feeding relationship between parent and child. Parents should pay attention to infants' hunger cues and not offer bottles or food in answer to an infant's need for attention. Feeding environments should be pleasant and supportive and allow the child to pick and choose from available food. Meals and snacks should be provided regularly and vigorous physical activity encouraged as early as 1 year of age.

Children and adolescents who may have a genetic predisposition toward obesity should be encouraged to develop or maintain healthy eating and exercise habits and develop a positive body image. Clinicians can promote these measures by incorporating dietary histories and counseling with each well-infant, child, and adolescent visit.

SUMMARY

Obesity is an increasingly common disorder of childhood and adolescence. The etiology of obesity appears to be a complex mixture of genetic, nutritional, environmental, and other social factors. In childhood and adolescence, obesity can be associated with a number of significant medical conditions that can lead to further morbidity and mortality in adulthood. A number of highly technical methods are available for measuring excess body fat, but for most clinicians body mass index is the easiest clinical measurement for estimating obesity. Body mass index can categorize children and adolescents as overweight or at risk for overweight, which can further direct treatment. Various treatment modalities are available, with the most successful involving a combination of dietary modifications, regular activity, behavior modification, and family involvement. Focus for most children and adolescents should start with weight stabilization. For children older than age 7 with BMIs greater than the 95th percentile or with secondary complications, a structured weight reduction plan should be instituted with the help of a nutritionist or other health care provider. Other modalities used in adult obesity can have serious side effects and generally are not used in the pediatric population. Clinicians can work to prevent obesity by encouraging healthy eating and exercise habits at an early age and intervening when a problem with being overweight is recognized.

REFERENCES

1. Anderson AE, Soper RT, Scott DH: Gastric bypass for morbid obesity in children and adolescents, *J Pediatr Surg* 15:876, 1980.
2. Bandini LF, et al: Validity of reported energy intake in obese and nonobese adolescents, *A J Clin Nutr* 52:421, 1990.
3. Barlow SE, Dietz WH: Obesity evaluation and treatment: Expert committee recommendations, *Pediatrics* 102:e29, 1998.
4. Bouchard C, et al: The genetics of obesity. In Bray GA, Bouchard C, James WPT, editors: *Handbook of obesity,* New York, 1998, Marcel Dekker.
5. Bray G: Health hazards of obesity, *Endocrinol Metab Clin North* 25: 907, 1996.
6. Calle EE, et al: Body-mass index and mortality in a prospective cohort of US adults, *N Engl J Med* 341:1097, 1999.
7. Campfield L, et al: Recombinant mouse OB protein: evidence for a peripheral signal linking adiposity and central neural networks, *Science* 269:546, 1995.
8. Caprio S, et al: Hyperleptinemia: an early sign of juvenile obesity. Relations to body fat depots and insulin concentrations, *Am J Physiol* 271(3 Pt 1):e626, 1996.
9. Chung S: Diseases of the developing hip joint, *Pediatr Clin North Am* 24:857, 1977.
10. Collins S, et al: Role of leptin in fat regulation, *Nature* 380:677, 1996.
11. Criqui MH, et al: Clustering of cardiovascular disease risk factors, *Prev Med* 9:525, 1980.
12. Davies PSW, White GA: Physical activity and body fatness in preschool children, *Int J Obesity* 19:6, 1995.
13. DeLany JP: Role of energy expenditure in the development of pediatric obesity, *Am J Clin Nutr* 68:950s, 1998.
14. Desmond SH, et al: Black and white adolescents' perceptions of their weight, *J School Health* 59:353, 1989.
15. Dietz WH, Gortmaker SL: Do we fatten our children at the television set? Obesity and television viewing in children and adolescents, *Pediatrics* 75:807, 1985.
16. Dietz WH, Gortmaker SL: Factors within the physical environment associated with childhood obesity, *Am J Clin Nutr* 39:619, 1984.
17. Dietz WH, Gross WL, Kirkpatrick JA Jr: Blount disease (tibia vara): another skeletal disorder associated with childhood obesity, *J Pediatr* 101:735, 1982.
18. Dietz WH, Robinson TN: Use of the body mass index as a measure of overweight in children and adolescents, *J Pediatr* 132:191, 1998.
19. Elliot DL, et al: Metabolic evaluation of obese and nonobese siblings, *J Pediatr* 114:957, 1989.
20. Ellison PT: Skeletal growth, fatness, and menarcheal age: a comparison of two hypotheses, *Hum Biol* 54:269, 1982.
21. Epstein LH, Squires S: *The stoplight diet for children,* Boston, 1988, Little, Brown.
22. Epstein LH, et al: A comparison of lifestyle, exercise, aerobic exercise and calisthenics on weight loss in obese children, *Behav Ther* 16:345, 1985.
23. Epstein LH, et al: Ten-year follow-up of behavioral, family-based treatment for obese children, *JAMA* 264:2519, 1990.
24. Federation of American Societies for Experimental Biology, Life Sciences Research Office: Prepared for the Interagency Board for Nutrition Monitoring and Related Research. *Third report on nutrition monitoring in the United States,* vol 2, Washington, DC, 1995, US Government Printing Office.

25. Forbes G, Amirhakimi GH: Skinfold thickness and body fat in children, *Hum Biol* 42:401, 1970.
26. Frederich R, et al: Leptin levels reflect body lipid content in mice: evidence for diet-induced resistance to leptin action, *Nature Med* 1:1311, 1995.
27. Frisancho AR: *Anthropometric standards for the assessment of growth and nutritional status,* Ann Arbor, 1990, University of Michigan Press.
28. Garn SM, Clark DC: Nutrition, growth, development and maturation: findings from the Ten State Nutrition Survey of 1968-70, *Pediatrics* 56:306, 1975.
29. Golay A, Felber JP: Evolution from obesity to diabetes, *Diabetes Metab* 20:3, 1994.
30. Goran MI, et al: Cross-calibration of body composition techniques against dual-energy x-ray absorptiometry in young children, *Am J Clin Nutr* 63:299, 1996.
31. Gortmaker SL, et al: Social and economic consequences of overweight in adolescence and young adulthood, *N Engl J Med* 329:1008, 1993.
32. Gortmaker SL, et al: Television viewing as a cause of obesity among children in the United States, 1986-1990, *Arch Pediatr Adolesc Med* 150:356, 1996.
33. Halaas J, et al: Weight reducing effects of the plasma protein encoded by the ob gene, *Science* 269:543, 1995.
34. Hammer LD, et al: Standardized percentile curves of body-mass index for children and adolescents, *AJDC* 145:259, 1991.
35. Hampton MC, et al: Caloric and nutrient intakes of teen-agers, *J Am Diet Assoc* 50:385, 1967.
36. Huenemann RL, et al: A longitudinal study of gross body composition and body conformation and their association with food and activity in a teen-age population: view of teen-age subjects on body conformation, food, and activity, *Am J Clin Nutr* 18:325, 1966.
37. Kaplan KM, Wadden TA: Childhood obesity and self-esteem, *J Pediatr* 109:367, 1986.
38. Kelsey JL, Acheson DM, Keggi KJ: The body build of patients with slipped capital femoral epiphysis, *AJDC* 124:276, 1972.
39. Klesges RC, et al: A longitudinal analysis of accelerated weight gain in preschool children, *Pediatrics* 95:126, 1995.
40. Kuczmarski RS, et al: Increasing prevalence of overweight among US adults: the National Health and Nutrition Examination surveys, 1960 to 1991, *JAMA* 272:205, 1994.
41. Lahlou N, et al: Circulating leptin in normal children and during the dynamic phase of juvenile obesity: relation to body fatness, energy metabolism, caloric intake, and sexual dimorphism, *Diabetes* 46:989, 1997.
42. Levinson R, Powell B, Steelman LC: Social location, significant others and body image among adolescents, *Soc Psych Q* 49:330, 1986.
43. Mafffeis C, et al: Elevated energy expenditure and reduced energy intake in obese prepubertal children: paradox of poor dietary reliability in obesity, *J Pediatr* 124:348, 1994.
44. Maffeis C, et al: Energy expenditure during walking and running in obese and nonobese prepubertal children, *J Pediatr* 123:193, 1993.
45. Mallory GB, Fiser DH, Jackson R: Sleep-associated breathing disorders in morbidly obese children and adolescents *J Pediatr* 115:892, 1989.
46. Marcus CL, et al: Evaluation of pulmonary function and polysomnography in obese children and adolescents, *Pedatr Pulmonol* 21:176, 1996.
47. Mayer J: Genetic factors in human obesity, *Ann N Y Acad Sci* 131:412, 1965.
48. Mellin LM, Slinkard LA, Irwin CE: Adolescent obesity intervention: validation of the SHAPEDOWN program, *J Am Diet Assoc* 87:333, 1987.
49. Mendelson BK, White DR: Development of self-body-esteem in overweight youngsters, *Dev Psychol* 21:90, 1985.
50. Moore DC: Body image and eating behavior in adolescent girls, *AJDC* 142:1114, 1988.
51. Moses N, Banilivy MM, Lifshitz F: Fear of obesity among adolescent girls, *Pediatrics* 83:393, 1989.
52. Must A, et al: Long-term morbidity and mortality of overweight adolescents, *N Engl J Med* 327:1350, 1992.
53. National Institutes of Health Consensus Development Panel on the Health Implications of Obesity: Health implications of obesity, *Ann Intern Med* 103:147, 1985.
54. Neptune H, Nigrin GA: Acanthosis nigricans and hyperinsulinemia: an underdiagnosed cause of obesity, *Pediatr Res* 35:104A, 1994.
55. Parnell K, et al: Black and white adolescent females: perception of ideal body size, *J Sch Health* 66:112, 1996.
56. Pellymounter M, et al: Effects of the obese gene product on body weight regulation in ob/ob mice, *Science* 269:540, 1995.
57. Pinhas-Hamiel O, et al: Increased incidence of non-insulin-dependent diabetes mellitus among adolescents, *J Pediatr* 128:608, 1996.
58. Rawelli GP, Belmont L: Obesity in nineteen-year-old men: family size and birth order associations, *Ann J Epidemiol* 109:66, 1979.
59. Rhodes SK, et al: Neurocognitive deficits in morbidly obese children with obstructive sleep apnea, *J Pediatr* 127:741, 1995.
60. Roberts SB, et al: Energy expenditure and intake in infants born to lean and overweight mothers, *N Engl J Med* 318:461, 1988.
61. Rocchini AP, et al: Blood pressure in obese adolescents: effect of weight loss, *Pediatr* 82:16, 1988.
62. Rolland-Cachera MF, Bellisle F, Sempe M: The prediction in boys and girls of the weight/height index and various skinfold measurements in adults: a two-decade follow-up study, *Inter J Obesity* 13:305, 1989.
63. Rosenbaum M, et al: Effect of gender, body composition and menopause on plasma concentrations of leptin, *J Clin Endocrinol Metab* 81:3424, 1996.
64. Sallade J: A comparison of psychological adjustment of obese vs. nonobese children, *J Psychosom Res* 17:89, 1973.
65. Scott CR, et al: Characteristics of youth-onset non-insulin-dependent diabetes mellitus and insulin-dependent diabetes mellitus at diagnosis, *Pediatrics* 100:84, 1997.
66. Silber T, Randolph J, Robbins S: Long-term morbidity and mortality in morbidly obese adolescents after jejunoileal bypass, *J Pediatr* 108:318, 1986.
67. Smoak CG, et al: Relation of obesity to clustering of cardiovascular disease risk factors in children and young adults: the Bogalusa Heart Study, *Am J Epidemiol* 125:364, 1987.
68. Sobal J, Stunkard AJ: Socioeconomic status and obesity: a review of the literature, *Psychol Bull* 105:260, 1989.
69. Stunkard AJ, Foch TT, Hrubec Z: A twin study of human obesity, *JAMA* 256:51, 1986.
70. Stunkard AJ, et al: An adoption study of human obesity, *N Engl J Med* 314:193, 1986.
71. Stunkard AJ, et al: The body-mass index of twins who have been reared apart, *N Engl J Med* 322:1483, 1990.
72. Troiano RP, Flegal KM: Overweight children and adolescents: description, epidemiology, and demographics, *Pediatrics* 101:497, 1998.
73. Voors AW, et al: Obesity and external sexual maturation: the Bogalusa Heart Study, *Prev Med* 10:50, 1981.
74. Wadden TA, et al: Dissatisfaction with weight and figure in obese girls: discontent but not depression, *Int J Obesity* 13:89, 1989.
75. Werkman SL, Greenberg ES: Personality and interest patterns in obese adolescent girls, *Psychosom Med* 29:72, 1967.

240 Obstructive Uropathy and Vesicoureteral Reflux

Melissa J. Gregory

OBSTRUCTIVE UROPATHY

Etiology

Although other causes are occasionally found, almost all cases of urinary tract obstruction in children are congenital malformations stemming from abnormal renal development[5] (Box 240-1). To understand the etiology of obstructive uropathies, some understanding of normal renal development is needed. In mammals, the final functional kidney is the *metanephros*. It develops from complex interactions between two groups of cells, the *nephrogenic blastema*, a cluster of undifferentiated mesenchymal stem cells, and the *ureteric duct*, a small epithelial bud. The metanephros is preceded by two more primitive kidneys, the *pronephros* and the *mesonephros*.[2] The pronephros is never functional in humans and regresses by the fifth week of gestation. Its remnant, the pronephric duct, becomes the mesonephric duct that eventually develops in the ureteric duct.

The mesonephroses develop between the third and fourth gestational weeks and function as interim kidneys until the metanephroses are fully developed, involuting sometime between the fifth and twelfth gestational weeks. The metanephroses begin developing as early as the fifth gestational week and are the result of reciprocal induction between the nephrogenic blastema and the ureteric duct.[8] They start to function within 4 weeks and normal fetal kidneys, with visible filling and emptying of the bladder, can be seen by ultrasound by the fifteenth week of gestation. After week 16, urine is the major contributor to amniotic fluid and has a key role in the pulmonary development.[1]

Obstruction can develop at various times and in various locations during gestation and the effect of obstruction on the fetal kidney depends on when and where it occurs.[1] For some patients, obstruction can be an almost incidental finding, as in partial ureteropelvic junction (UPJ) obstruction, whereas in others, such as the infant with severe posterior urethral valves and resultant oligohydramnios, it is a potentially fatal condition. Obstructive uropathies are the leading cause of renal failure in children under 2 years of age and account for 17% of renal transplants in children.[6] The developing kidney is more sensitive to the effects of obstruction than the adult kidney and the earlier and more complete an obstruction, the greater the damage.[4] Intuitively, it is obvious that bilateral obstruction is more problematic than unilateral obstruction, because both kidneys are affected. Obstruction of urine flow increases intrarenal pressure and changes the complex sequence of ureteric bud division and blastema induction, resulting in renal dysplasia. The pathogenesis of the renal dysplasia is controversial and may be a result of an overall abnormality in renal development or a direct consequence of obstruction. Experimental urethral ligation in animal fetuses during the first half of gestation produces a syndrome similar to that seen in human fetuses with posterior urethral valves (PUV).[6] In addition, animal models of urinary obstruction show a decreased number of nephrons in obstructed kidneys compared with unobstructed kidneys.[4] Relief of the obstruction does not lead to an increase in the number of developing nephrons, suggesting that the effect of obstruction on nephrogenesis occurs early. These studies coupled with histological analysis of fetal kidneys suggest that obstruction triggers aberrant differentiation on the interstitial mesenchyme.[6] Unilateral urinary obstruction, in addition to affecting only one kidney, enhances the growth and function of the unaffected, contralateral kidney so that, despite decreased nephrogenesis in the obstructed kidney, the absolute combined glomerular filtration rate (GFR) is minimally affected.[4]

Most congenital UPJ obstruction is secondary to an intrinsic defect in the urinary tract such as valves, polyps, abnormal musculature development, or incomplete canalization of the ureter. Extrinsic causes of UPJ obstruction, such as adhesions, ureteral kinks, or masses, also occur, although these usually develop postnatally. An exception to this is abnormal renal vasculature, which can entrap the ureter, causing obstruction. This occurs in up to 50% of cases of UPJ obstruction, often accompanying intrinsic causes of obstruction. Ureterovesical junction obstruction, more commonly called megaureter, is caused by an adynamic and/or stenotic section of the distal ureter resulting from either hypoplasia or dysplasia. Posterior urethral valves, the most common form of infravesicular obstruction, is thought to be due to abnormal migration of the terminal end of the Wolffian ducts, resulting in obliquely oriented ridges that act as a one-way valve, blocking urine flow.

Epidemiology

The onset of wide spread fetal ultrasonography has changed our understanding of the incidence of obstructive uropathies is children, because many cases are identified prior to becoming clinically evident. The incidence of prenatally diagnosed uropathies is approximately 0.5%.[4] UPJ obstruction is the most common urinary obstruction seen in children. The left kidney is affected more often than the right and there is also a slight male predominance. It is bilateral in 5% of cases. Megaureter is the second most common cause of upper tract obstruction, although its frequency is less than 5% of that of UPJ obstruction. It is also usually unilateral, occurring bilat-

BOX 240-1

CAUSES OF URINARY OBSTRUCTION IN CHILDREN

Lower Tract	Upper Tract
Posterior urethral valves*	Ureteropelvic junction obstruction*
Anterior urethral valves	***Intrinsic***
Urethral stricture	Valves
Ureterocele	Abnormal musculature
Bladder mass	Polyps
Urethral stone	Incomplete ureteral canalization
	Extrinsic
	Abnormal renal vessels
	Adhesions
	Ureteral kinks
	Masses
	Megaureter (ureterovesical obstruction)
	Ureteral valves
	Ureteral polyps
	Kidney stone

*Most common cause.

erally 10% of the time, more likely to occur on the left, and more common in boys. Lower tract obstruction is uncommon with the most common cause of infravesicular obstruction, posterior urethral valves (PUV), accounting for only 10% of neonatal hydronephrosis.[13] PUVs occur with an incidence of 1 in 5000 to 1 in 8000 males.[1]

Presentation

With the advent of prenatal ultrasounds, increasing numbers of children with both upper and lower urinary tract obstructions are being identified prenatally. The finding of unilateral hydronephrosis without hydroureter on prenatal ultrasound is suggestive of UPJ obstruction. Approximately 80% of children with prenatally diagnosed UPJ obstruction are asymptomatic at birth. Children diagnosed postnatally are most commonly found to have an abdominal mass.[1] Other presentations include intermittent nausea and vomiting, gross hematuria (because the distended ureteral mucosa is very friable), infection and, rarely, hypertension and renal failure. Older children may complain of unilateral flank pain. Megaureter can present in the same way. Lower tract obstruction such as posterior urethral valves should be suspected when prenatal ultrasound shows bilateral hydronephrosis; ureteral dilation; a thick, trabeculated bladder; and oligohydramnios.

However, PUVs can present with a wide clinical spectrum ranging from newborns found to have an abdominal mass to adults who are diagnosed when presenting with a urinary tract infection.[1] In general, the younger a child is at the time of diagnosis, the more severe the lesion. Common clinical presentations in the neonatal period include the finding of an abdominal mass, a palpable bladder, and a poor urinary stream.[1] PUVs diagnosed following the neonatal period are often present with a urinary tract infection, which in infants can be associated with nonspecific symptoms and signs such as failure to thrive, diarrhea, vomiting, feeding problems, and recurrent fevers. In addition, many of these children have polyuria resulting from a concentration defect from damage to the renal medulla, and recurrent dehydration with a relatively low urine specific gravity (less than 1.015) can be seen. Additional findings may include constipation, incontinence, gross hematuria, failure to thrive, or renal failure. Severely affected infants may present with pulmonary hypoplasia, respiratory insufficiency, and Potter's sequence.

Diagnosis

The diagnosis of urinary obstruction can be suspected on the basis of history and physical examination, but radiological evaluation is required for the diagnosis of both upper tract and lower tract obstruction. All children with suspected urinary obstruction require a triad of radiological studies: renal ultrasound, a voiding cystourethrogram (VCUG), and a functional study, either an intravenous pyelogram (IVP) or diuretic renal scintigraphy. These latter studies should not be performed until an infant is at least 2 weeks old, because the GFR of newborns is normally low and can result in false readings. The finding of hydronephrosis without hydroureter on ultrasound is suggestive of UPJ obstruction, but both a VCUG to rule out vesicoureteral reflux and studies to confirm the presence of obstruction and to provide information on renal function are needed. Megaureter can be suspected when an ultrasound shows unilateral hydroureter with a normal bladder, but again, both a VCUG and a diuretic renogram are necessary to make the diagnosis and to rule out other possible causes. A fluoroscopic VCUG is diagnostic of PUVs. In addition to showing urethral anatomy and the presence of valves, a VCUG will show if there is vesicourethral reflux (VUR), an associated finding in more than 30% of children with PUVs.[1] A VCUG also provides visualization of the bladder, which is often small and trabeculated in patients with PUVs. Renal ultrasound will provide information on the condition of the renal parenchyma, which can provide prognostic information, as well as on ureteral and bladder dilation and bladder wall thickness. Diuretic renal scintigraphy can provide information of differential function as well as confirm the absence of more proximal obstruction.

Therapy

Lower urinary tract obstruction. In patients with suspected PUVs, temporary bladder drainage can be accomplished by insertion of a sterile catheter through the urethra until the diagnosis can be confirmed and surgical correction obtained. Frequently in neonates, pulmonary issues predominate because of the association of PUVs with pulmonary hypoplasia. Acute therapy is directed toward stabilizing the patient, correcting any metabolic abnormalities, and aggressive treatment of urinary tract infection, if present. Consultation with pediatric urologists and nephrologists is required to determine the optimal surgical procedure, help with correcting metabolic abnormalities, and provide prognostic information for the parents. It is critical to bear in mind that once the obstruction is relieved, the child may develop a postobstructive diuresis with urine output reaching up to 10 to 15 ml/kg/hr and, thus, meticulous attention to fluid balance is essential.

Long-term therapy is directed toward correction of the obstruction and the accompanying metabolic abnormalities. Fulguration of the urethral valves may be all that is needed to allow adequate urine flow, although in some children vesicostomy is required. Of the children with PUVs who survive the perinatal period, 50% have or will develop renal failure, and thus, close follow-up of renal function is essential. These patients often have hyposthenuria and are unable to concentrate their urine to a specific gravity greater than 1.015. In this subpopulation, a simple gastroenteritis may be life-threatening, because the kidney cannot make adjustments for increased fluid losses and/or decreased fluid intake, and early hospitalization for parenteral hydration may be needed. In addition, many of these children have renal-salt wasting and metabolic acidosis with accompanying hyperkalemia. The use of prophylactic antibiotics to prevent urinary tract infections in those children with VURs is also important.

Recently, fetal surgery to decompress the bladder and relieve intrarenal pressure has been attempted, with mixed success. In humans, fetal survival of in utero urinary decompression does not exceed 41%.[6] Human fetal kidneys cannot be visualized by ultrasound until the fifteenth week of gestation, and much of the damage may have already been done at the time of diagnosis. The difficulty of accurately evaluating the severity and possible reversibility of renal damage is currently the main problem in predicting successful fetal surgery.

Upper urinary tract obstruction. Therapy is directed towards correcting the obstruction. In megaureter, the obstruction transmits increased pressure to the kidneys, resulting in progressive damage, and this lesion requires prompt surgical attention. In addition, even in the absence of reflux, the dilated obstructed ureter produces a stagnant collection of urine, increasing the risk of pyelonephritis. Surgical correction is performed by excising the stenotic segment of ureter and performing ureteroplasty to decrease the size of the ureter. In general, children with megaureter have no associated anomalies and, once corrected, do not require extensive reconstructive surgery.[1] The treatment of unilateral UPJ obstruction is more controversial. Individuals with severely dilated renal pelvis and obvious damage of the affected kidney, with thinning of the renal parenchyma and decreased renal function by renal scintigraphy, require prompt evaluation by a pediatric urologist with probable surgical correction of the obstruction. However, some studies suggest that neonates may have a functional obstruction that will resolve over time, leading some urologists to advocate serial radiological studies to determine persistence of the lesion before performing corrective surgery.[5]

Prognosis

Lower urinary tract obstruction. Long-term outcome of a child with valves depends on age and severity at presentation. Severe cases with associated oligohydramnios and pulmonary insufficiency may die in the newborn period as a result of respiratory complications. In those children surviving the neonatal period, 25% to 30% of boys presenting in infancy are at risk for renal insufficiency in childhood.[1] Predictors of favorable outcome in PUV is a nadir creatinine of no more than 0.8 mg/dl at 1 year of age and the presence of corticomedullary differentiation on renal ultrasound. As children with PUV become older, bladder dysfunction may become a significant factor in the progression towards renal failure, as the thickened noncompliant bladder can result in increased intrarenal pressure. Recurrent kidney infections can contribute to worsening renal function. In addition to prophylactic antibiotics, these children require strict attention to voiding habits, with some needing self-catheterization, cholinergic therapy (most commonly with oxybutynin), or surgery to increase bladder capacity. Early diagnosis is critical in improving clinical outcome and the involvement of pediatric urologists and nephrologists is required.

Upper urinary tract obstruction. Because of the predominance of unilateral disease in upper tract obstruction, with compensatory growth in the unaffected kidney, the prognosis of upper tract obstruction is superior to that of lower tract obstruction. Individual prognosis depends on the severity of the obstruction as well as the number of urinary tract infections that have occurred, making early diagnosis critical for ensuring a good outcome.

VESICOURETERAL REFLUX

Etiology

VUR is a pathological condition in which urine flows retrograde from the bladder into the ureter and, often, into the intrarenal collecting system. Under normal conditions, the ureter enters the bladder at an angle and tunnels through the smooth muscle and submucosa in a manner that allows compression of the ureteral lumen with bladder contraction, preventing the entry of urine into the ureter. VUR occurs when there is either an abnormal ureteral orifice or an abnormal submucosal ureteral tunnel that prevents this valve-like effect of the bladder smooth muscle.

VUR can be divided into primary and secondary forms. Secondary reflux is VUR associated with other renal anomalies such as PUV or multicystic dysplastic kidneys and is associated with abnormal interactions between the nephrogenic blastema and ureteric duct. This form of VUR is often associated with renal dysplasia, also due to abnormal induction of the nephrogenic blastema by the ureteric duct. It is sporadic in occurrence. Primary VUR is not associated with renal dysplasia or other forms of congenital uropathies and is the result of a primary abnormality of the anatomy of the distal ureter, which inserts lateral to its usual insertion and has a shortened intramural course. The renal pathology seen with primary VUR is renal scarring, usually acquired lesions that are the result of infection. Animal studies suggest that in primary VUR, urinary tract infection must be present in addition to reflux for renal scarring to occur, although in obstructed systems scarring can occur without infection.[7] However, some children in whom the diagnosis of VUR was made prenatally and who have never had a urinary tract infection diagnosed, have been found to have renal scarring, making the situation more confusing. Certainly the combination of VUR and infection is more likely to result in renal scarring than VUR alone.[3] Reflux nephropathy is a term that describes the coarse renal scarring of one or both kidneys associated with primary VUR and urinary tract infection.

Epidemiology

Primary VUR is often an inherited condition. Segregation analysis suggests that it is inherited via a single dominant gene and it is estimated that the gene frequency for VUR is 1 in 600.[7] This would make it the most common dominantly inherited disease in humans. The incidence of primary VUR in the general population is estimated to be 0.1% to 1.0%, with a much higher incidence occurring in children, in whom the incidence is reported to be between 12% and 50%.[7] The incidence of primary VUR is lower in boys than in girls and is significantly lower in blacks than in whites.[2] Between one half to two thirds of offspring of an affected parent will have VUR, whereas one third to one half of the siblings will have the condition.

Presentation

The majority of children with VUR are found during an evaluation for urinary tract infection. Approximately 30% of children under 5 years of age with a urinary tract infection have VUR. Less common presentations are hypertension and renal failure. Prenatal ultrasounds may also uncover VUR; 15% of prenatal hydronephrosis is due to VUR.[3]

Diagnosis

The VCUG remains the gold standard for diagnosis of VUR. Even some children with severe reflux can lack sonographic evidence of renal pelvis dilation.[14] A VCUG allows both the diagnosis of VUR and grading of its severity (Box 240-2). In most cases a VCUG is performed by instilling a contrast agent into the bladder through a urinary catheter with subsequent imaging of the bladder during filling and voiding. VCUGs can be done using one of two methods: fluoroscopy and nuclear scintigraphy. In the fluoroscopic VCUG, radiopaque contrast is instilled into the bladder and imaging is performed by fluoroscopic surveillance with interval radiographs. With nuclear scintigraphy, a radioisotope is placed in the bladder and there is continuous monitoring of the bladder and ureters via an isotope emission camera. An indirect VCUG can be done by injecting a radioisotope that is quickly and completely cleared by the kidneys and screening for reflux once the isotope has cleared the upper urinary tracts and filled the bladder. This latter method, however, relies heavily on the patient's capability for controlled voiding and is often inappropriate for children.

Both methods of VCUG have advantages and disadvantages. The fluoroscopic VCUG gives a detailed anatomical picture of bladder and urethral anatomy and, for this reason, is the method of choice for boys suspected of having PUV or for initial radiological evaluation following a urinary tract infection. Fluoroscopy also allows more precise grading of VUR. The price of enhanced anatomical details, however, is a higher gonadal radiation, with a fluoroscopic VCUG giving 100 times the radiation exposure of a radioisotope study.[2] The radioisotope study provides greater surveillance than fluoroscopy, because the isotope emission camera may run continuously without increasing the radiation exposure of the patient. Both studies, however, have a false-negative rate of up to 10%. For the initial evaluation for VUR, a fluoroscopic study is recommended to provide initial visualization of the bladder and urethra and for more precise grading of severity. Follow-up studies, however, can be by nuclear scintigraphy, to limit radiation exposure, unless circumstances arise that require reevaluation of bladder or urethral anatomy.

As reflux nephropathy is the major long-term complication of VUR, its diagnosis depends on the recognition of renal scarring in the context of past present VUR. Renal scarring is seen radiographically by the presence of focal parenchymal thinning with corresponding calyceal deformity or clubbing. The IVP has long been the gold standard for the detection of renal scars but has recently been replaced by renal scintigraphy with radioisotopes such as 99-technetium dimercaptosuccinic acid (DMSA) or glucoheptonate. Advantages of scintigraphy over IVP in the identification of renal scarring include an increased sensitivity for scar detection; the ability to perform a quantitative assessment of differential function; decreased gonadal radiation, although increased total body radiation; the absence of contrast-induced reactions; and the avoidance poor visualization of the urinary system because of bowel shadowing.

BOX 240-2

GRADING OF VESICOURETERAL REFLUX

Grade I	Retrograde flow of urine into a nondilated ureter only
Grade II	Filling of a nondilated ureter and a nondilated renal pelvis
Grade III	Filling of a dilated collecting system with sharp renal fornices
Grade IV	Filling of a dilated collecting system with blunting of renal fornices
Grade V	Filling of a massively dilated and tortuous collecting system

Therapy

VUR reflux will resolve spontaneously in most patients, so therapy is directed toward the prevention of long-term complications such as renal scarring and reflux nephropathy by the prevention of urinary tract infections. Prior to the use of antibiotic prophylaxis in reflux, children with VUR were found to have progressive renal scarring in 20% of kidneys previously identified as normal and progressive deterioration of 66% of kidneys that had been found to be damaged at the time of diagnosis. However, children with similar grades of reflux who received antibiotic prophylaxis were found to have no progression of renal scars over a 10-year follow-up period unless there were break-through infections.[2] The International Reflux Study, which evaluated more than 500 children with grades II to IV reflux who were randomly allocated to either surgical or medical treatment of their reflux, found that there were no significant differences in the incidence of recurrent UTI or in the incidence of new renal scarring between the two groups, making medical and surgical therapy of VUR equivalent in efficacy.[15]

At this time, the only reasons to advocate surgical correction of VUR are a low probability of spontaneous resolution of reflux or recurrent urinary tract infections while on appropriate antibiotic prophylaxis. Treatment should be initiated as early as possible, because significant renal damage can occur with a single episode of pyelonephritis and the younger the child, the greater the risk of incurring renal scarring. Children with abnormal prenatal ultrasounds should be maintained on antibiotic prophylaxis until proven to not have VUR by VCUG. Similarly, children under the age of 5 years who have had a single urinary tract infection should be kept on prophylactic antibiotics following the treatment of their infection until a VCUG has been performed and VUR eliminated as a cause of the UTI.

Current recommendations for antibiotic prophylaxis are, for children over 2 months of age, either co-trimazole, 2 to 4 mg/kg/day of the trimethoprim component, or nitrofurantoin, 1 to 2 mg/kg/day, not to exceed 100 mg/day. Both drugs should be given as a single daily dose. Children under 1 month of age may have difficulty metabolizing either of these drugs because of hepatic immaturity and should be given either amoxicillin (10 to 15 mg/kg/day) or cephalexin (10 to 15 mg/kg/day), again as a single daily dose. Children with recurrent infections while on appropriate antibiotic prophylaxis may require alternative drug therapy, twice-daily dosage or two-drug therapy.[2] Antibiotic suppression should be continued until VUR has resolved either spontaneously or surgically. An exception to this would be in older children (more than 8 years old) who have persistent low-grade VUR who have been without urinary tract infections for several years. In this population, a trial off of antibiotics is reasonable, although not imperative.

A careful voiding history should be obtained in children with VUR. Voiding abnormalities such as detrusor instability and voiding dyssynergy can change relatively benign, low-pressure VUR into potentially harmful, high-pressure VUR. Symptoms such as urinary urgency, dribbling, and incontinence are worrisome for voiding dysfunction. Interventions such as voiding on a timed schedule, double voiding to ensure complete bladder emptying, or treatment with anticholinergic agents such as oxybutynin may be needed. Children with these symptoms should have their bladder function evaluated by a pediatric urologist or pediatric nephrologist.

Other nonpharmacological interventions should include aggressive treatment of constipation, counseling on maintaining perineal hygiene, avoidance of chemical irritants such as bubble bath and talcum powder, and the elimination of bladder irritants from the diet: caffeinated substances, carbonated beverages, chocolate, and citrus.[14]

Prognosis

The prognosis of VUR depends on the age of the patient at the time of diagnosis and the severity of the reflux. The natural history of VUR is that 10% to 15% of cases resolve spontaneously each year, with up to 80% of low-grade (grade I-II) and 40% of high-grade VUR resolving without surgery.[2] In children over 5 years of age, however, the probability of high-grade reflux spontaneously resolving is low, and consultation with a pediatric urologist should be considered for possible surgical correction.[9] In addition, children over 1 year of age with grade V reflux or with high-grade reflux in association with other urinary abnormalities are less likely to spontaneously resolve VUR and should be referred to a pediatric urologist earlier than children with primary VUR. There is epidemiological evidence that suggests that girls with VUR are at greater risk for UTI than boys with a similar grade of VUR and, therefore, may need to be referred for consideration of surgery earlier.[9]

The major long-term complication of VUR is reflux nephropathy, which accounts for over 10% of end-stage renal failure patients.[7] Reflux nephropathy, defined as reflux-associated renal scarring, is characterized by hypertension and/or decreased renal function. It is estimated that 10% of children with renal scarring develop hypertension and the prevalence increases to 50% in adults with reflux nephropathy.[7] A study that followed 30 patients who had been diagnosed with reflux nephropathy as children showed that over the course of 27 years, 10% developed end-stage renal failure and 90% had diminished GFR.[10]

Screening for VUR

As discussed above, there is a strong familial tendency toward VUR and, subsequently, toward reflux nephropathy. Early identification of children with VUR would allow early initiation of antibiotic prophylaxis, decreasing the risk of these children developing long-term complications from VUR. A prospective study of the siblings of children with VUR has shown that 75% of siblings with VUR are asymptomatic and are less likely than the index case to have renal scarring.[12] This suggests that screening the siblings of children with VUR can help to identify at-risk children prior to the development of renal scarring. The younger the screened sibling, the more likely VUR will be present. This also is the population at greatest risk for developing renal scarring from pyelonephritis. This would suggest that screening the siblings of patients with VUR who are under the age of 5 years with a VCUG would be helpful in decreasing these children's risk of VUR-associated complications. In older siblings, who are more likely to have outgrown VUR, a renal ultrasound would be adequate to assess pelvic dilation and the renal parenchyma. If either hydronephrosis or evidence of parenchymal thinning is present, then further evaluation would be indicated. Because the incidence of VUR in the offspring of individuals with reflux is higher than in the siblings, these same guidelines should be used in this population.

FETAL HYDRONEPHROSIS

The widespread use of antenatal ultrasound has resulted in a new clinical challenge: the appropriate care of asymptomatic infants with a history of an abnormal fetal ultrasound. Hydronephrosis is a common finding on prenatal ultrasounds, occurring with a frequency of 1 in 200 to 700, whereas the incidence of prenatally diagnosed uropathy is 0.5%.[1,5,13] The significance of prenatal hydronephrosis is somewhat controversial. The reported incidence of significant urinary malformations requiring follow-up in children with a history of fetal hydronephrosis ranges from 20% to 70%.[3,4] It is clear that

BOX 240-3

FINDINGS IN FETAL HYDRONEPHROSIS ASSOCIATED WITH INCREASED RISK OF ADVERSE OUTCOME

- Sonographic findings other than hydronephrosis
  - Megacystis
  - Megaureter
  - Renal cysts
  - Increased parenchymal echogenicity
  - Oligohydramnios prior to 24 weeks gestation
- Identification of hydronephrosis before third trimester
- Bilateral disease

hydronephrosis with other associated sonographic abnormalities is more worrisome than isolated hydronephrosis (Box 240-3). Fetuses with bilateral hydronephrosis, hydroureter and oligohydramnios are suspicious for having PUV and prompt referral to a pediatric urologist familiar with fetal ultrasound is critical. Of children with isolated fetal hydronephrosis, about 60% will have UPJ obstruction and 15% to 20% have VUR.[3]

After birth, children with a history of fetal hydronephrosis should have a renal ultrasound within the first few days of life. If this ultrasound is normal, the study should be repeated after 7 to 10 days because the newborn may be relatively dehydrated, producing a falsely negative study resulting from low urine flow. If the finding of hydronephrosis is confirmed, a VCUG and diuretic renal scintigraphy, the latter done after 2 weeks of age, are needed. It is important to keep an infant with hydronephrosis on antibiotic prophylaxis until a VCUG has been done to rule out VUR as the cause of hydronephrosis. Infants with sonographic abnormalities in addition to hydronephrosis or who have persistent respiratory disturbances or feeding problems require a prompt referral to pediatric urologist or nephrologist.

REFERENCES

1. Becker N, Avner ED: Congenital nephropathies and uropathies, *Pediatr Clin North Am* 42:1319, 1995.
2. Belman AB: A perspective on vesicoureteral reflux, *Urol Clin North Am* 22:139, 1995.
3. Blachar A, et al: Clinical outcome and follow-up of prenatal hydronephrosis, *Pediatr Nephrol* 8:30, 1994.
4. Chevalier RL: Pathophysiology of obstructive nephropathy in the newborn, *Semin Nephrol* 18:585, 1998.
5. Chevalier RL, Klahr S: Therapeutic approaches in obstructive uropathy, *Semin Nephrol* 18:652, 1998.
6. Daikha-Dahmane F, et al: Development of human fetal kidney in obstructive uropathy: correlations with ultrasonography and urine biochemistry, *Kidney Int* 52:21, 1997.
7. Dillon MJ, Goonasekera CDA: Reflux nephropathy, *J Am Soc Nephrol* 9:2377, 1998.
8. Ekblom P: Embryology and prenatal development. In Holliday MA, Barratt TM, Avner ED, editors: *Pediatric nephrology*, Baltimore, 1994, Williams & Wilkins.
9. Elder JS, et al: Pediatric vesicoureteral reflux guidelines panel summary report on the management of primary vesicoureteral reflux in children, *J Urol* 157:1846, 1997.
10. Jacobson SH, et al: Long-term prognosis of post-infectious renal scarring in relation to radiological findings in childhood: a 27-year follow-up, *Pediatr Nephrol* 6:19, 1992.
11. Koff SA: Obstructive uropathy: clinical. In Barratt TM, Avner ED, Harmon WE, editors: *Pediatric nephrology*, ed 4, Baltimore, 1999, Lippincott Williams & Wilkins.
12. Noe HN: The long-term results of prospective sibling reflux screening, *J Urol* 148:1739, 1992.
13. Oliveira EA, et al: Prognostic factors in fetal hydronephrosis: a multivariate analysis, *Pediatr Nephrol* 13:859, 1999.
14. Sheldon CA, Wacksman J: Vesicoureteral reflux, *Pediatr Rev* 16:22, 1995.
15. Smellie JM, et al: Five-year study of medical or surgical treatment in children with severe reflux: radiological renal findings, *Pediatr Nephrol* 6:223, 1992.

241 Ocular Foreign Bodies

James W. McManaway III • Carl A. Frankel

Ocular foreign bodies can be classified as (1) surface, in which case they are either nonadherent or only loosely adherent to the corneal or conjunctival epithelium, (2) penetrating, in which case the foreign body goes into but not through the cornea or sclera, or (3) perforating, in which case the foreign body goes through the cornea or sclera and into the globe itself. A foreign body that goes completely through the sclera and rests in the vitreous body causes a perforating wound of the sclera and a penetrating wound of the globe. Although the terminology can be confusing, learning it allows a more accurate description of the problem. Careful examination, preferably with magnification, is necessary for all but the most superficial ocular foreign bodies, with referral to an ophthalmologist of all patients who give a history of an injury to the eye via high-velocity objects or in the setting of metal striking metal, for example, while hammering a nail.

SURFACE FOREIGN BODIES

The most likely sources of surface foreign bodies in children are small objects that can be thrown by a child (e.g., dirt, sand, and grass) and small wind-blown particles. Considering the profuse tearing associated with surface foreign bodies, it truly is the exceptional patient who requires medical care for one of these "flying" objects. In fact, even when care is sought after the acute incident, the offending agent often is absent and the cause of the ocular findings usually unknown.

When a patient consults a clinician with the complaint of a foreign body sensation—or when a nonverbal or preverbal patient seeks treatment with a history of pain, photophobia, epiphora, or rubbing of the eye(s)—the initial examination usually is accomplished more easily if a drop of topical ophthalmic anesthetic is instilled in each eye (unless a perforating wound of the cornea or sclera is suspected, in which case no medications should be used). An assessment of visual acuity should then be attempted. Once this is completed, the lids and lashes should be inspected to see if any foreign bodies can be observed and removed. Uncooperative or frightened children may need sedation to allow an adequate examination.

Attention should next be turned to the corneal and conjunctival surfaces to ascertain whether a foreign body can be identified (Fig. 241-1). At this time, magnification, either with a loupe or a slit lamp, is preferred. It may be possible to irrigate or wipe away readily observed foreign bodies with the stretched-out fibers of a cotton applicator. In a cooperative patient sitting quietly by the slit lamp, surface foreign bodies usually can be removed manually with a fine, toothless forceps. Metallic foreign bodies on the corneal surface start to oxidize within several hours; these must be removed and the "rust ring" debrided by an ophthalmologist.

After this procedure, the tarsal conjunctival surfaces should be examined. The clinician usually can pull the lower lid down by placing one finger on the middle aspect of the lid just beneath the lash line and with another, applying gentle traction inferiorly. Again, foreign bodies generally can be irrigated or brushed out and, if adherent, can be removed with a forceps. Attention then should be turned to the upper lid, which should be everted as follows: The lashes should be grasped gently between the thumb and forefinger; with the shaft of a cotton applicator placed at the superior margin of the tarsal plate, the lashes should be pulled out and up to evert the lid onto the cotton applicator (Fig. 241-2, *A*). After the lid is everted, the lashes can be pinned against the superior orbital rim and the cotton applicator removed (Fig. 241-2, *B*). Any foreign bodies that are present usually can be seen and removed readily.

After the foreign body or bodies have been removed, the eye should be checked for a corneal abrasion. This is accomplished best with a minimal amount of sterile fluorescein instilled and the eye examined with a cobalt blue light source, either at the slit lamp or via a penlight with a special filter. Corneal abrasions appear as a green line or patch; multiple fine vertical corneal abrasions that look like ice skate tracks are highly suggestive of a foreign body under the upper eyelid. If an abrasion is present, an antibiotic ointment should be instilled. If the pain was severe before instillation of the anesthetic drops, a sterile eye patch should be taped in place for 6 to 12 hours. Arrangements then should be made for follow-up the next day to ensure that the abrasion has resolved. If it has not, or if significant pain persists, the patient should be referred to an ophthalmologist to be certain that an iritis, which may require more aggressive intervention, has not developed.

PENETRATING FOREIGN BODIES

When a foreign body is imbedded in the conjunctiva, cornea, or scleral tissue (Fig. 241-3), the examiner must be concerned that it may represent a perforating wound of the cornea or sclera, allowing bacteria to gain access to the intraocular space. In these instances, visual acuity can be surprisingly normal. The examiner, therefore, must maintain a high index of suspicion and have the patient evaluated by an ophthalmologist.

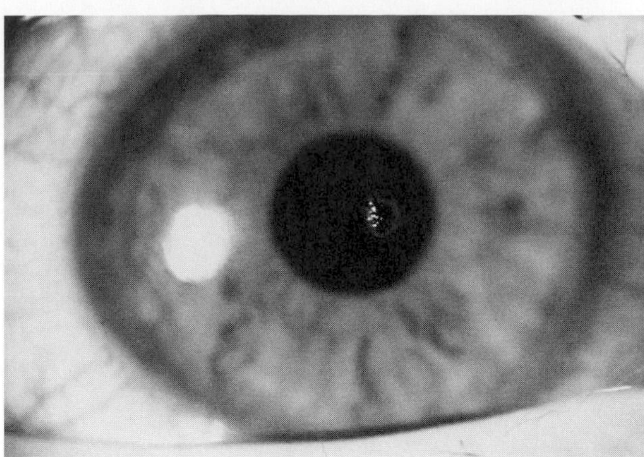

Fig. 241-1 Metallic foreign body on the surface of the cornea. Note the surrounding rust ring, which should be removed to reduce intraocular inflammation from metal breakdown.

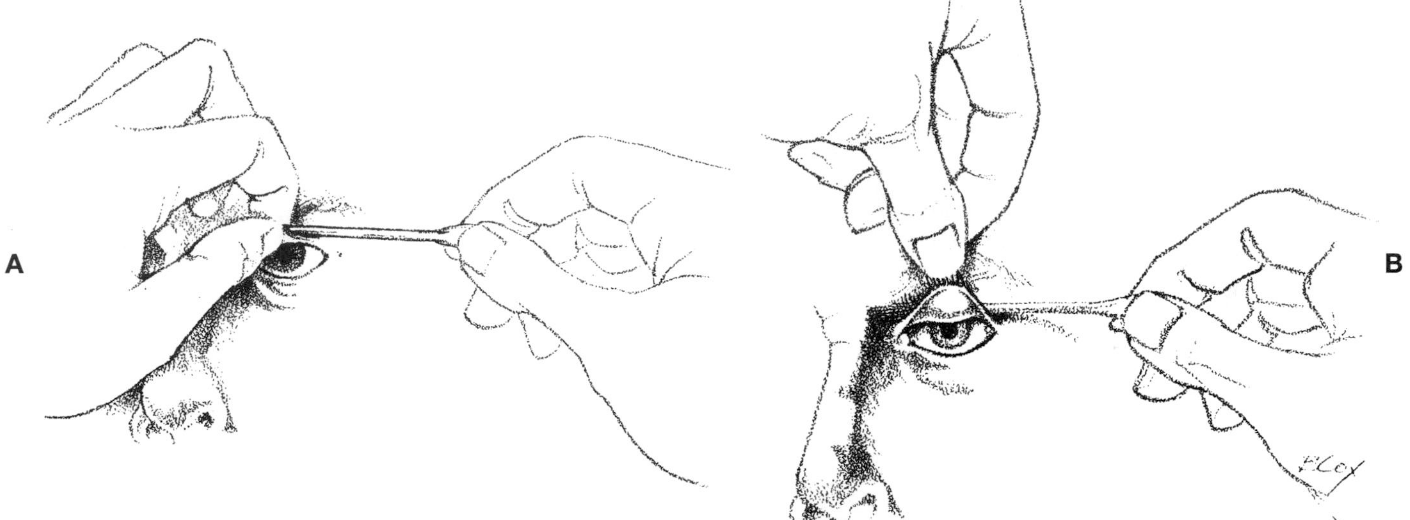

Fig. 241-2 **A,** Demonstration of an easy method for everting a patient's upper eyelid with the lashes and lid being pulled out and up from the globe. **B,** After the eyelid has been everted, the lashes are pinned against the superior orbital rim before removal of the cotton applicator. After the everted lid is examined, the lashes can be pulled inferiorly and released to reposition the lid.

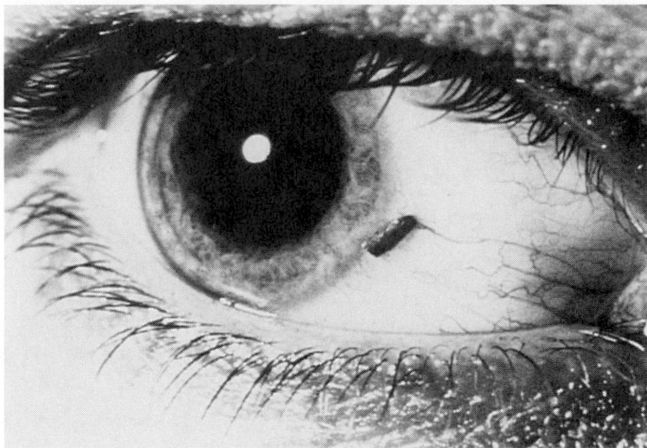

Fig. 241-3 Metallic foreign body that has penetrated the sclera. Care must be taken in determining whether this foreign body has actually perforated the sclera and entered the globe. When in doubt, an ophthalmologist should remove such foreign bodies.

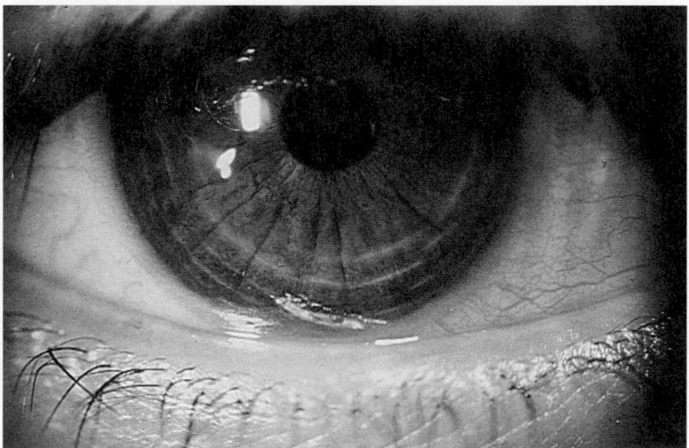

Fig. 241-4 This patient felt pain while hammering a nail. The visual acuity of this eye was 20/20. Note the metallic foreign body that has perforated the cornea and is resting on the inferior iris.

PERFORATING FOREIGN BODIES

Perforating foreign bodies go completely through the cornea or sclera. These high-velocity injuries usually are devastating to ocular integrity and frequently result in severe derangement and permanent visual loss, although initial visual acuity and cursory examination findings may be normal (Fig. 241-4). Visual loss can be minimized in some instances by prompt referral to an ophthalmologist skilled at intervention in corneal, anterior segment, and vitreoretinal trauma.

SUGGESTED READINGS

DeBustros S: Posterior segment intraocular foreign bodies. In Shingleton BJ, Hersh PS, Kenyon KR, editors: *Eye trauma*, St Louis, 1991, Mosby.

Kenyon KR, Wagoner MD: Conjunctival and corneal injuries. In Shingleton BJ, Hersh PS, Kenyon KR, editors: *Eye trauma*, St Louis, 1991, Mosby.

Smiddy WE, Stark WJ: Anterior segment intraocular foreign bodies. In Shingleton BJ, Hersh PS, Kenyon KR, editors: *Eye trauma*, St Louis, 1991, Mosby.

242 Ocular Trauma

James W. McManaway III • Carl A. Frankel

Evaluation of the patient who has ocular trauma requires a thorough knowledge of the anatomy of the eye and orbit and an understanding of the types of injuries that may result from specific types of trauma. Although it is unusual, normal or near-normal visual acuity may be achieved even after a rupture of the globe. As a result, a high index of suspicion for globe rupture must be maintained for each patient who is seen for ocular or orbital trauma. In addition, because many children who have orbital or ocular injuries are in considerable pain and have significant photophobia and fear, the very act of examining or attempting to examine the eye can create greater damage than that produced by the original injury. Uncooperative children who have signs or a history suggestive of significant ocular injury should be examined under heavy sedation or general anesthesia in the operating room by an ophthalmologist to prevent further ocular injury.

ANATOMICAL CONSIDERATIONS

The orbit is shaped roughly like a quadrilateral pyramid. The orbital roof is formed from the orbital plate of the frontal bone and the lesser wing of the sphenoid bone. The lateral orbital wall is formed by the zygoma and the greater wing of the sphenoid bone. The orbital floor is formed from the maxillary bone, the orbital plate of the zygomatic bone, and a small portion of the palatine bone. The medial orbital wall is formed by the frontal process of the maxilla, the lacrimal bone, the orbital plate of the ethmoid bone, and the body of the sphenoid bone. The orbital rim tends to absorb the impact of most large-object injuries, which may lead to fractures of the orbital bones with preservation of the integrity of the globe itself. Small-object injuries that affect the globe directly tend to cause primary injuries to the globe, with secondary injury to the thinner bones of the orbit, primarily its floor and medial wall. The contour of the object can predispose to penetrating or perforating injuries of the globe.

The globe rests in the orbit, cushioned by orbital fat, and is moved by six extraocular muscles. The lateral rectus muscle is innervated by the abducens (sixth) cranial nerve; the superior oblique muscle is innervated by the trochlear (fourth) cranial nerve. The other four extraocular muscles, the levator muscle of the upper lid, and the iris sphincter muscle are innervated by the oculomotor (third) cranial nerve. Orbital injuries can cause abnormal ocular motility as a result of cranial nerve palsies, orbital soft tissue scarring, or direct extraocular muscle injury.

The eyelids act to protect the globe from particulate debris and have an important role in maintaining the normal tear film strip over the cornea. Defects in eyelid anatomy or function can cause major problems related to corneal exposure, with subsequent infection or scarring, or both. Injuries to the eyelids can result in unsuspected injuries to the globe, especially when sharp objects lacerate or penetrate the eyelids. Eyelid lacerations that expose the orbital fat pad in the upper lid may injure the levator muscle; improper surgical repair that ignores a levator muscle injury often results in a post-traumatic ptosis. The lacrimal drainage system starts in the medial aspect of each lid and connects to the lacrimal sac via small canaliculi. Lacerations of the medial aspect of an eyelid often result in a canalicular laceration, which must be repaired carefully by an ophthalmologist skilled in this type of surgery.

Between the eyelid fissure lies the exposed surface of the globe: the bulbar conjunctiva and the cornea. These areas commonly are involved when ocular injuries occur. The bulbar conjunctiva covers the sclera from the corneal limbus to the cul-de-sac or fornix; the tarsal conjunctiva then reflects over the inner eyelid surface to the lid margin. The subconjunctival space often fills with blood after ocular injuries; a small amount of blood is spread out into a large area, giving an alarming appearance to the uninitiated. Most subconjunctival hemorrhages are benign, but they also can hide more severe ocular injuries. The clear cornea, approximately 0.5 mm thick, covers the anterior chamber, iris, and lens and provides about 66% of the refractive power of the eye. The sclera forms the wall of the eye and is thinnest (0.3 mm) under the insertions of the rectus muscles. This is a common site for the globe to rupture.

The posterior segment of the eye consists of the posterior sclera, ciliary body, choroid, retina, and vitreous body. Injuries to these areas frequently are associated with severe intraocular hemorrhage and retinal detachment, with permanent visual loss.

EVALUATION

The evaluation of the child who has ocular trauma consists of three steps: (1) recognizing life-threatening nonocular injuries and emergent ocular conditions such as ocular chemical injuries, (2) taking an adequate history to assess the potential risk of injury to the eye, to obtain significant past ocular history, and to identify medical conditions that may complicate the treatment of the injury or administration of general anesthesia, and (3) examining the eye in detail. The ocular evaluation includes visual acuity testing and examination of the external globe and eyelids, ocular motility, the pupil, the anterior segment, and the fundus.

Occasional patients initially may appear to have only ocular injuries when other severe injuries are present; one example is a patient struck in the eye with a ski-pole tip. The CT scan showed an orbital roof fracture with disruption of the frontal lobe. Ocular alkali injuries can have devastating consequences without immediate and copious ocular irrigation; any patient who has an ocular chemical injury should have irrigation first and be asked detailed questions later! In the evaluation of any child who has ocular injury, a careful history should be obtained, realizing that independent or unsupervised play (coupled with guilt and fear) may make the information obtained unreliable. As many details as possible should be obtained, specifically highlighting the source of injury, which may suggest the nature of potential injuries. Additional history taking should include the date of the last tetanus immunization, prior ocular history (such as amblyopia of either eye), medications, allergies, and when the patient last had something to eat or drink, in the event surgical intervention is necessary.

After the history has been obtained, with specific regard to symptoms, the examination should proceed in an orderly manner to ensure that nothing is omitted or overlooked. In a child who is old enough to cooperate, beginning with the nontraumatized eye usually will allay anxiety sufficiently to examine the traumatized eye next. When the traumatized eye is tested, care must be taken not to put any pressure on the globe itself.

Visual Acuity Testing

The examination should begin with testing visual acuity. Although normal visual acuity has been reported in patients who have severe injuries, the presence of significantly impaired vision is a sign that the injury is likely to be severe and the services of an ophthalmologist are needed. Children initially may display a poor visual acuity in the injured eye that improves significantly after reassurance and patience. The most objective method available should be used to establish a reliable baseline acuity measurement. The normal eye must be completely covered when the injured eye is being tested.

Preverbal children present a special challenge in measuring visual acuity, because they cannot respond to the usual visual acuity tests given to older patients. Fixation on a brightly colored toy or on the examiner's face is very useful; absence of fixation or attempts to move the head to remove the cover over the normal eye indicate poor acuity in the injured eye. Measuring the child's ability to locate small candies in the examiner's hand is well tolerated, but the child should not eat the candy if a trip to the operating room is possible.

Verbal children should have their visual acuity tested with standard picture, E-game, or letter charts. Younger children can "match" the presented picture if they cannot name it. If a child cannot identify the largest picture on the chart (usually 20/200), it should be moved closer until the figure can be identified. If the 20/200 picture is identified at 8 (not 20) feet from the chart, the acuity is recorded as 8/200. If an eye chart is not available, substitutes such as objects, faces, or facial features can be used. The examiner should record details of the objects' size and testing distance so that the data obtained can be compared with subsequent visual acuity measurements.

Patients who have significant ocular injuries still will be unable to read the eye chart even though they are very close to it. Alternative methods of measuring visual acuity under these circumstances include the ability to count fingers (recorded as "counts fingers at X feet"), distinguish the motion of a hand (recorded as "hand motion at X feet"), determine the direction of a light source (recorded as "light perception with projection"), and determine the presence of a light source (recorded as "light perception"). These methods have been listed in order of decreasing visual function.

External Examination

As with the examination of any patient, observation and inspection are important first steps. Key signs to note include edema or ecchymosis of the lids and ocular adnexal structures, asymmetry or discontinuity of the orbital and facial bones, ocular proptosis or enophthalmos, foreign bodies, subconjunctival hemorrhage, laceration(s), and the prolapse of intraocular contents (including iris, ciliary body, vitreous, and retina) through a laceration of the cornea or sclera. If the child is cooperative and no sign of a ruptured globe is present, dried blood should be removed gently to help uncover all injuries. Significant positive and negative findings should be noted; diagrams of the injuries, including details of the length and depth of lacerations, should be recorded. Photographic documentation of the injuries is very useful.

Ocular Motility

Unless a ruptured globe is suspected, ocular motility should be checked, with attention paid to both ductions (monocular eye movements) and versions (conjugate, binocular eye movements) in all gaze positions, with note made of any abnormalities. The presence of diplopia should be noted, and if possible, the examiner should obtain a description from the patient of the location of the two images with respect to each other.

Pupils

The presence of round pupils should be noted; if a pupil is not round (Fig. 242-1) (oval, teardrop, or pear shaped, for instance), a drawing of the abnormality should be made. Next, the reaction of each pupil to light should be checked, both directly and consensually. When this test is performed, the patient should be instructed to fixate on a distant point so that the accommodation reflex, with its secondary pupillary miosis, does not influence the assessment of pupillary function. The reactivity of the pupils (both direct and consensual) gives important information about both the afferent and efferent limbs of the visual pathway.

The swinging flashlight test is performed by alternately (i.e., switching eyes every 2 seconds) shining a bright light source into each eye. The normal response is for both pupils

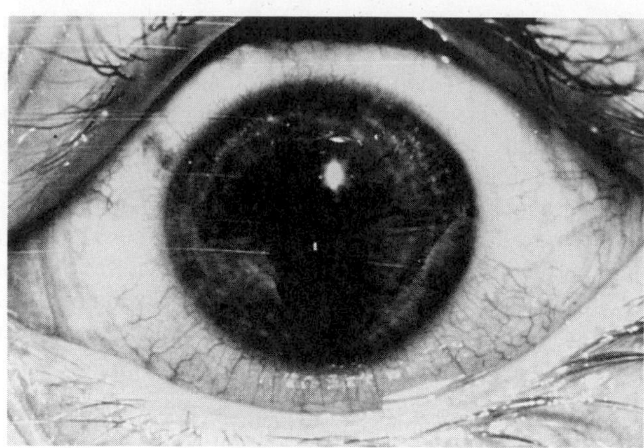

Fig. 242-1 An inverted teardrop-shaped pupil caused by an inferior corneal laceration with the iris drawn to the wound.

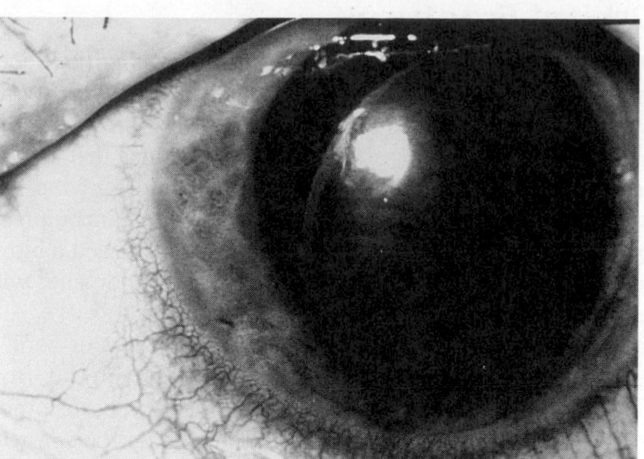

Fig. 242-2 Ocular injury from a fist, with inferior lens subluxation and minimal cataractous changes.

to stay constricted. Paradoxical dilation of a pupil when light is illuminating it indicates retinal or optic nerve dysfunction, or both. This is called a *Marcus Gunn pupil* or an *afferent pupillary defect*. The absence of an afferent pupillary defect on the swinging flashlight test is reassuring confirmation that neither significant optic nerve nor retinal damage has occurred. In the event of posttraumatic iridoplegia, both the direct and consensual reflexes would be diminished because of impairment in the terminal efferent pupillomotor organ: the iris.

Anterior Segment

If a slit lamp is available and if the patient is able, the conjunctiva, cornea, anterior chamber, iris, lens, and red reflex should be examined. Particular attention should be directed to evaluation of (1) the conjunctiva for subconjunctival hemorrhage, conjunctival lacerations, or foreign bodies (see Chapter 241); (2) the cornea for the presence of epithelial defects (abrasions), lacerations, or foreign bodies; (3) the anterior chamber for depth (shallow or deep) or the presence of red blood cells (hyphema); (4) the lens for the presence of cataracts or dislocation (Fig. 242-2); and (5) the fundus red reflex for subtle lens opacities or abnormalities that might indicate a vitreous hemorrhage or retinal detachment. If a slit lamp is unavailable, if the examiner is not familiar with its use, or if the patient cannot be brought to the slit lamp, the ophthalmoscope can be used to examine the anterior segment adequately.

Fundus

A fundus examination always should be attempted unless a ruptured globe is suspected and pressure may have to be placed on the eye to open the lids. In those circumstances, increased pressure on the globe through the eyelids may result in extrusion of intraocular contents, potentially making it impossible to restore the integrity of the visual system. In case of doubt, the examination should be delayed until the arrival of an ophthalmologist.

MANAGEMENT OF SPECIFIC INJURIES

One must keep in mind that just as the orbital relationships comprise a continuum, so too does the extent of orbital and ocular injuries. The result is that when one portion of the orbit or globe is injured, other injuries may be present.

Ecchymosis

Ecchymosis, or bruising, of the periorbital region results in the typical "black" eye. The blunt contusion injury that results in ecchymosis may be either isolated or associated with other orbital or ocular injury. An uncomplicated black eye is treated the same as a contusion anywhere else: cold compresses for the first 24 hours, followed by warm compresses until the swelling subsides, with elevation of the patient's head to help resolve the edema. The patient or parents should be advised that because of gravity, the ecchymosis and edema may appear to spread down the cheek or even to the fellow eye. Although frightening in appearance, this type of spread is not dangerous and resolves spontaneously.

Orbital Hemorrhage

When a contusion injury occurs, ecchymosis of the periorbital region may occur simultaneously with hemorrhage within the orbit itself. Because the orbit is a bony structure open on only one end, an increase in volume of the orbital contents from hemorrhage or edema increases the intraorbital pressure, which can be relieved only with anterior displacement of the globe, resulting in proptosis. If the proptosis is severe, compression of the optic nerve or acute glaucoma can permanently impair visual function. If progressive proptosis is noted, emergency lateral canthotomy and possible orbital decompression is indicated. Steroids often are used, but their effectiveness has not been demonstrated. In the absence of signs of optic nerve compromise, treatment consists of ice packs for the first 24 hours, followed by warm compresses, with elevation of the head to reduce edema.

Orbital Fractures

Direct injury to the bony orbit may result in extensive facial and orbital bone fractures and can be associated with significant intracranial and ocular injuries. When a broad concussive force is delivered to the orbit in a manner that rapidly increases the intraorbital pressure, one or more of the thin orbital walls may fracture because of the relative incompressibility of the orbital contents. This condition is called a blow-out fracture; the orbital floor is the most common site, with the medial orbital wall the next most common.

Blow-out fractures are seen more commonly in adolescents than in younger children and frequently result from motor vehicle accidents or a blow from a fist; because most people are right-handed and, thus, strike another person with the right fist, the left orbit is involved more often than the right. The patient frequently complains of diplopia and pain, with clinical signs of proptosis if orbital hemorrhage occurs or enophthalmos if the fracture is large. Movement of the affected eye is limited (typically limitation of upgaze because of inferior rectus muscle entrapment in the fracture), accompanied by eyelid edema and ecchymosis.

The evaluation of a patient who has a suspected blow-out fracture requires the use of orbital computed tomography (CT) scanning to delineate the presence and extent of the fracture accurately. Appropriate positioning of the patient to obtain 1.5 mm slices that slightly overlap is necessary for accurate imaging. Because of the nature of the orbital injury, the possibility of a coexisting injury to the globe must be considered, and an ophthalmologist should evaluate the patient before any other specialist is consulted. The concurrent presence of a ruptured globe and blow-out fracture requires delayed treatment of the fracture until the integrity of the globe is restored.

Blow-out fractures don't have to be treated immediately. Indeed, allowing time for the edema and ecchymosis to diminish may resolve the proptosis and diplopia. Frequently, diplopia is due to a muscle contusion, and the symptoms may resolve over 3 to 4 days. If surgery needs to be undertaken for entrapment of orbital contents, diplopia, or more than 2 mm of enophthalmos, it can be performed safely 5 to 7 days after the injury. Patients who have an orbital blow-out fracture should be managed by, or comanaged with, an ophthalmologist (preferably an ophthalmic plastic surgeon). Under no circumstances should an orbital blow-out fracture be repaired without prior evaluation by an ophthalmologist. When surgical intervention is indicated, the goal is to restore the anatomical location of prolapsed orbital contents and to free any restriction of ocular motility. On occasion, an artificial orbital floor needs to be created with the use of implanted material.

Eyelid Lacerations

Although eyelid lacerations and avulsion injuries may occur without significant injury to the globe, ocular injuries must be ruled out before repair of the laceration is attempted; a ruptured globe either missed altogether or not detected until after a lacerated lid has been repaired is unacceptable practice. An ophthalmologist must be consulted before eyelid repair if any question exists about the presence of ocular injuries.

Simple lid lacerations that do not involve the eyelid margin, orbicularis muscle, or other structures such as the medial or lateral canthal tendon, the levator palpebrae superioris muscle, or the lacrimal gland and drainage system can be repaired readily with local anesthesia and the use of a size 6-0 nylon suture, which usually is removed 5 to 7 days after injury. In younger children who may not be cooperative for suture removal, 6-0 mild chromic gut should be used instead. If the lid laceration involves deeper orbital structures or if the eyelid margin is involved (Fig. 242-3), an ophthalmologist should be consulted to assess the integrity of the eye and to repair the lacerations.

Conjunctival Injury

Conjunctival injury typically manifests with only mild to moderate pain because of the relative paucity of a sensory nerve supply. Most conjunctival injuries take the form of subconjunctival hemorrhages (Fig. 242-4), which can be quite frightening but actually are harmless, unless associated with more extensive ocular injuries. No treatment is neces-

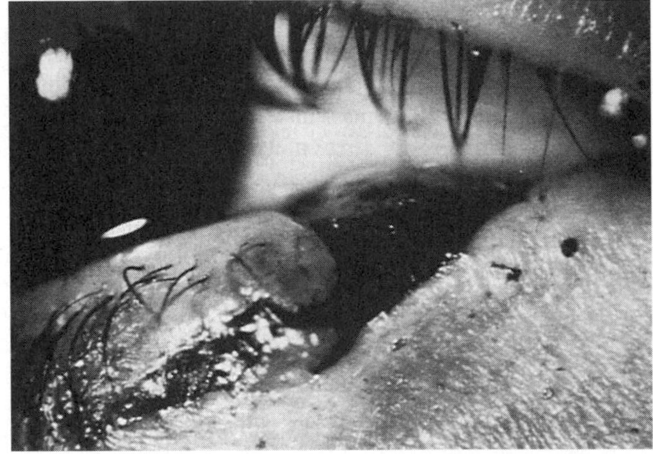

Fig. 242-3 Laceration of the lower lid that was found to involve the inferior canaliculus. Oculoplastic surgical repair was undertaken to restore the function of the inferior tear collection system.

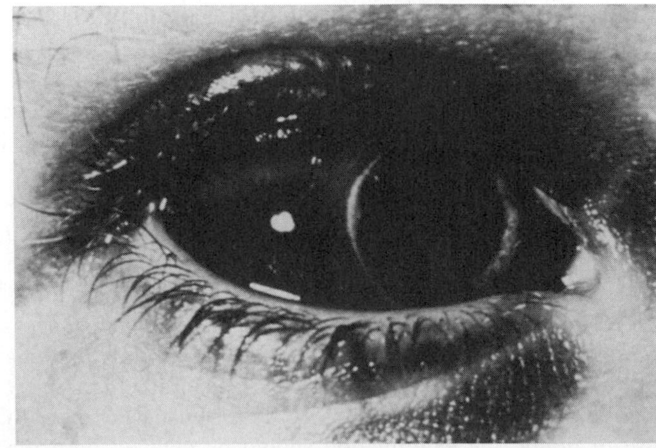

Fig. 242-4 Severe subconjunctival hemorrhage after blunt trauma.

sary for isolated subconjunctival hemorrhages, although the patient or parents should be cautioned that a brownish discoloration may result from deposition of hemosiderin. Small isolated conjunctival lacerations do not require intervention, although a thorough ophthalmic examination must be performed to rule out a laceration of the underlying sclera, choroid, or retina.

Corneal Injuries

The corneal epithelium is a multilayered structure that rests on a tough basement membrane layer called the Bowman membrane. The corneal epithelium is laced with numerous fine sensory nerve endings, resulting in extreme pain when the epithelium is disrupted. This epithelial disruption is observed easily with the use of a cobalt blue light after the instillation of sterile fluorescein (Fig. 242-5). Fortunately, most corneal abrasions heal extremely rapidly.

The initial phase of healing is characterized by migration of the remaining corneal epithelial cells over the defect, with subsequent reestablishment of the normal cell-to-cell and cell-to-basement membrane adhesions over a period of several weeks to months. In extensive corneal abrasions in which no corneal epithelium remains, conjunctival cells migrate over the corneal surface and then undergo transdifferentiation eventually to become indistinguishable from normal corneal epithelium.

During the healing phase, a tight patch after instillation of an ophthalmic antibiotic ointment may allow the patient to experience only a mild foreign-body sensation, which typically resolves after the epithelial surface of the abraded area has been restored. Typically, the eye is patched for 12 to 24 hours; in young children the occlusion may be more distressing than the injury itself. Should the abrasion not be healed substantially by 24 hours after injury, referral to an ophthalmologist should be made to rule out infection or other reasons for delayed healing.

Despite the pain that occurs from a corneal abrasion, under no circumstances should any patient be allowed to use topical anesthetic drops at home. The topical anesthetic prevents normal epithelial migration and results in a progressively larger abrasion and permanent corneal damage. These agents are to be used only in an acute setting for the diagnosis of ocular disorders or in an attempt to relieve patient discomfort for examination or for brief procedures.

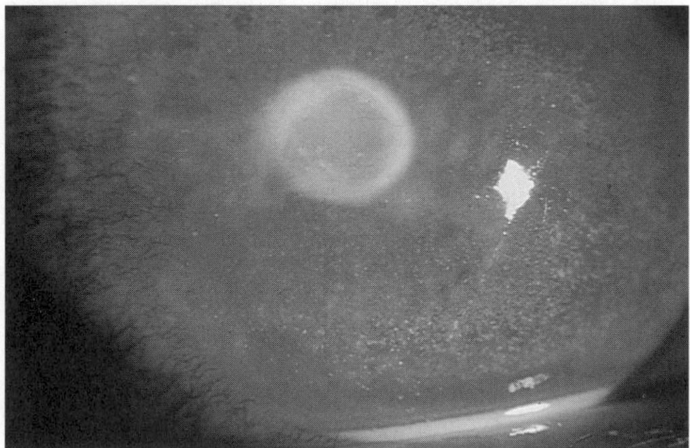

Fig. 242-5 A corneal abrasion revealed by fluorescein dye staining.

In extremely young children and infants, the plasticity of the visual system should be kept in mind so that occlusion amblyopia (poor vision in the eye under the patch because of visual deprivation) does not ensue. The susceptibility of the development of occlusion amblyopia is inversely proportional to the patient's age. In addition, as a result of impairment of the fusion mechanism, a latent deviation of an eye (typically an esophoria or exophoria—see Chapter 171, Strabismus) may convert to a manifest deviation (either an esotropia or an exotropia, respectively) because of patching of an injured eye for as short a period as 1 to 2 days. Surgical intervention occasionally may be necessary to restore normal ocular alignment.

Corneal lacerations (either full or partial thickness), no matter how well approximated, require immediate referral to an ophthalmologist. Patients who have corneal lacerations should have the eye covered with a shield to reduce the likelihood of the intraocular contents prolapsing. If a shield is unavailable, the bottom of a paper cup can be taped to the skin (Fig. 242-6) to prevent pressure on the globe.

Chemical Injuries

Chemical injuries, from either acid or alkali, are acute emergencies that require immediate, copious irrigation, followed by ocular examination by an ophthalmologist to rule out corneal or other ocular injuries. If the patient complains of pain, instillation of a topical anesthetic will reduce the discomfort from the injury and the irrigation itself. If blepharospasm during attempted irrigation is problem, a lid speculum should be used to keep the eye open; alternatively, an irrigating contact lens can be used. Overirrigation is not a problem, although the use of pH indicator paper can serve to show when the offending solution has been neutralized. Patients who have ocular alkali injuries often have permanent visual loss from corneal scarring, glaucoma, and cataract formation.

Hyphema

In blunt trauma to the globe, the forces transmitted to the intraocular structures by the noncompressible fluid contents of the globe may result in avulsion of the blood vessels at the iris root or the face of the ciliary body. When this happens, grossly visible blood enters the anterior chamber of the eye and a hyphema is formed (Fig. 242-7). When a hyphema occurs, the patient requires the care of an ophthalmologist because of potential associated complications. The purpose of this section is to provide guidelines for initial management.

Although ophthalmologists do not agree universally as to management of the patient who has a traumatic hyphema, many ophthalmologists recommend topical atropine solution, topical prednisolone acetate suspension, a clear plastic shield over the injured eye, and bed rest. The purpose of this management is to prevent rebleeding into the anterior chamber, which is associated with a worse visual prognosis. The atropine stabilizes the pupil to reduce traction on injured iris vessels and paralyzes the ciliary body to reduce discom-

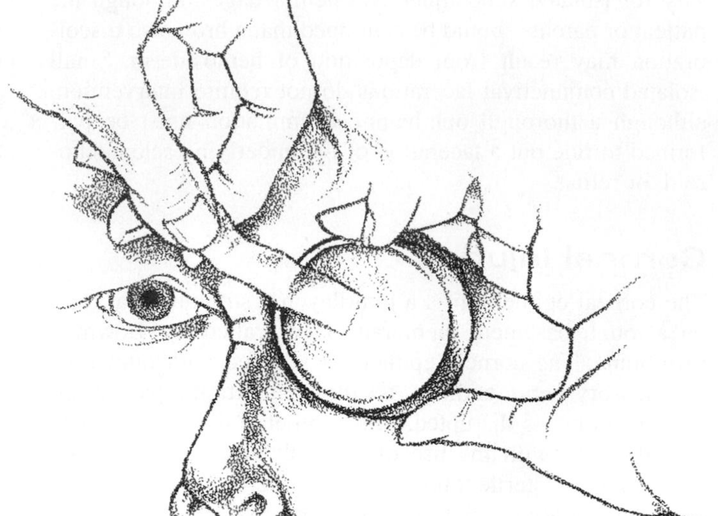

Fig. 242-6 Taping the bottom of a cup to the skin when a shield is not available to protect a suspected open globe from externally applied pressure.

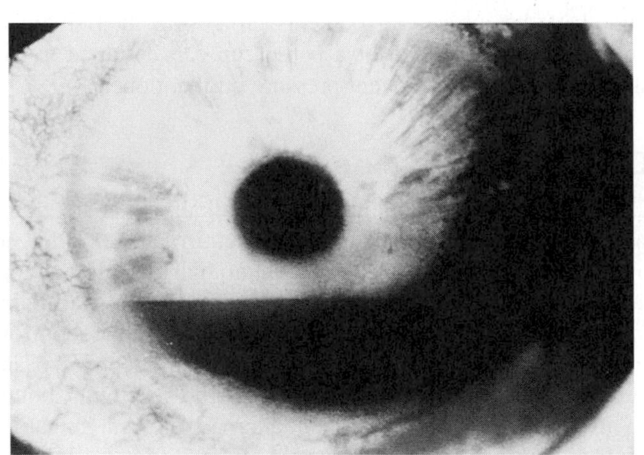

Fig. 242-7 Acute hyphema secondary to blunt ocular injury. Acute glaucoma ensued, which resolved when the hyphema cleared.

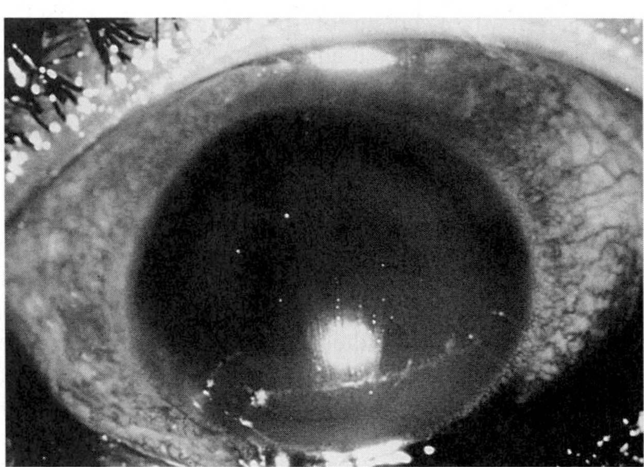

Fig. 242-8 Corneal blood staining following a hyphema in which secondary glaucoma was unable to be controlled.

fort from the associated iritis. Topical prednisolone reduces the intraocular inflammation. The shield prevents further injury to the eye, and bed rest reduces fluctuations in the venous pressure transmitted to the eye. Watching television is recommended, because the eyes are kept in nearly the same position; reading, however, is contraindicated because of the associated saccadic ocular movements. The preceding treatment can be performed at home if the patient and family are reliable and if the hyphema is small (occupying less than one third of the anterior chamber). If the hyphema is large or if the nature of the child or the social situation does not ensure adherence to this regimen, the child should be hospitalized for 5 to 6 days.

Because of the possibility of rebleeding because of clot resorption, some ophthalmologists hospitalize their patients and administer oral epsilon-aminocaproic acid (Amicar, Lederle) in an attempt to slow clot resorption, although its use is contraindicated in very large hyphemas (occupying more than 75% of the anterior chamber). If Amicar is used, it should be continued through at least the sixth postinjury day, if bleeding has not recurred. Although this agent has been shown to reduce the incidence of rebleeding significantly, hypotension and gastrointestinal side effects, including nausea and vomiting, may prompt some to restrict its use to high-risk situations in which the patient cannot be kept quiet.

Children suffering a hyphema are at risk for many ocular complications, including rebleeding, glaucoma, corneal blood staining (Fig. 242-8), and amblyopia, as well as other effects of the initial trauma, such as iris tears, angle recession, cyclodialysis (an abnormal separation between the ciliary body and sclera), cataract formation, lens subluxation, retinal tears, choroidal rupture (Fig. 242-9), and rupture of the globe. Secondary glaucoma may result from damage to the filtration angle or obstruction of the filtration angle by red blood cells; this usually resolves after the blood is absorbed totally. Glaucoma in the presence of a hyphema must be managed carefully to prevent optic nerve damage and corneal blood staining, which can cause severe amblyopia in children under 8 years of age. Glaucoma often can be controlled medically, but patients who develop uncontrolled glaucoma must have the blood surgically evacuated from the anterior chamber. Patients who have sickle cell anemia or trait are at much

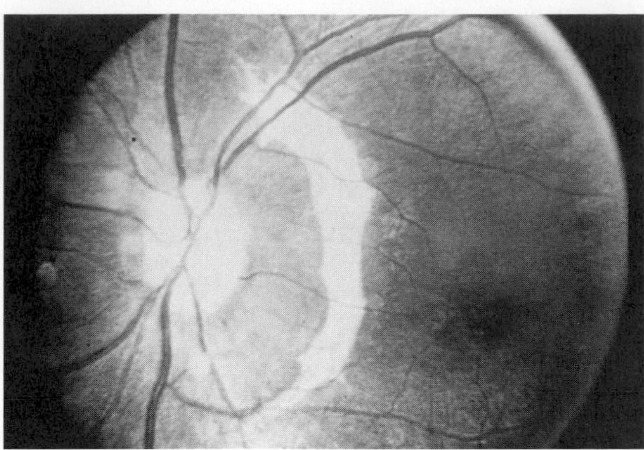

Fig. 242-9 Choroidal rupture resulting from blunt injury to the globe. The overlying retinal vessels are intact, but note the crescent-shaped area caused by absence of choroid overlying the white sclera. The typical location for choroidal and retinal ruptures is between the macula and optic nerve.

higher risk for these complications and need earlier intervention. Any patient who has a hyphema needs daily (and sometimes twice daily) intraocular pressure checks to detect the presence of glaucoma with its likelihood of causing permanent visual loss.

Ruptured Globe

Except when a perforating injury of the cornea or sclera by a small, sharp object occurs or when a posterior rupture occurs, patients who have a ruptured globe have several characteristic ocular signs. These include poor visual acuity, conjunctival edema, subconjunctival hemorrhage, compression of the anterior chamber, and hyphema. Prolapsed intraocular tissue (lens, iris, ciliary body, retina, choroid, or vitreous) may be seen if the rupture occurs at or near the limbus. If a ruptured globe is a possibility, early involvement of an ophthalmologist is essential. In the time before the ophthalmologist's arrival, the patient should be treated as follows:

1. Be kept quiet with sedation and antiemetics as needed
2. Not allowed to lie on the injured side
3. Have a shield placed over the injured eye(s) to reduce the likelihood of further injury
4. Have nothing to eat or drink in anticipation of the need for general anesthesia
5. Have no eye drops or ointments instilled until the globe is repaired
6. Receive intravenous antibiotics (gentamicin and cefazolin) in an attempt to reduce the likelihood of an endophthalmitis
7. Receive tetanus prophylaxis if it is not up to date

Nonaccidental Trauma (Child Abuse)

The manifestations of child abuse are diverse and can encompass any type of trauma; the explanation of the injury often is either inappropriate or insufficient. Unfortunately the ocular manifestations of child abuse may not be readily observable. Perhaps the most important and most often missed

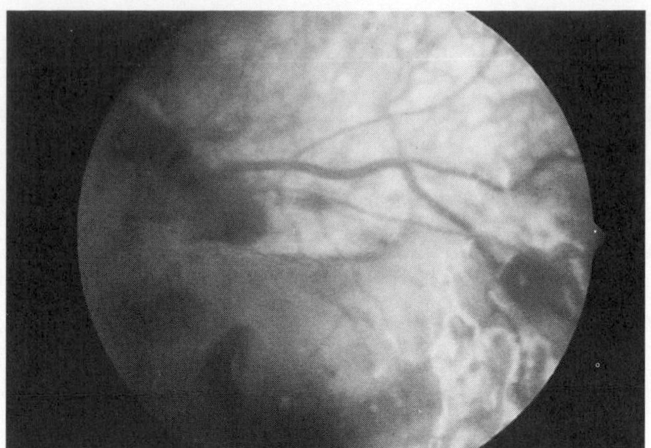

Fig. 242-10 Fundus photograph showing retinal hemorrhages in a victim of shaken-baby syndrome.

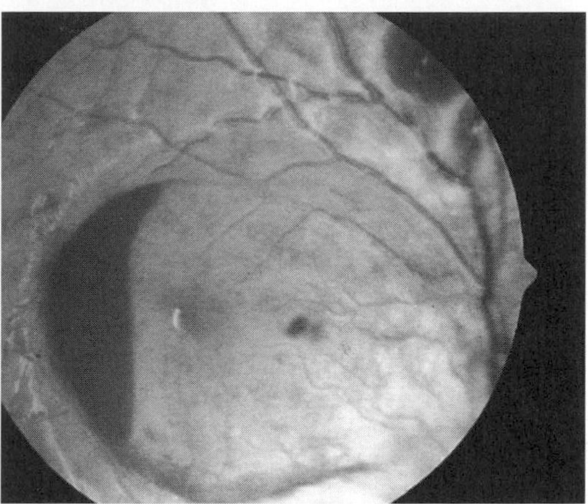

Fig. 242-11 Fundus photograph of the same patient shown in Fig. 242-10 with preretinal hemorrhage. The patient is lying on his side, hence the orientation of the pooled blood.

type of child abuse is the shaken-baby syndrome, characterized by retinal and preretinal hemorrhages (Figs. 242-10 and 242-11), subdural or subarachnoid hemorrhages, and minimal or absent signs of external trauma. A patient who has these signs needs to have a complete systemic evaluation, including evaluation by an ophthalmologist familiar with the ocular manifestations of child abuse. In any case of suspected child abuse, the ophthalmologist should be involved to document and treat any ocular injuries present. Only through the vigilance of the primary physician and the maintenance of a high index of suspicion can this form of child abuse be diagnosed.

SUMMARY

Most ocular injuries are relatively minor and easily treatable without sequelae. The circumstances surrounding some trauma, however, increase the likelihood of significant ocular or orbital injury. When such significant injury can be ruled out, involvement of the ophthalmologist may not be necessary. However, in any situation in which the primary examiner cannot determine readily the structural integrity of the globe and it contents, an ophthalmologist must be consulted.

SUGGESTED READINGS

Agapitos PJ, Noel LP, Clarke WN: Traumatic hyphema in children, *Ophthalmology* 94:1238, 1987.

Hamill MB: Clinical evaluation. In Shingleton BJ, Hersh PS, Kenyon KR, editors: *Eye trauma,* St Louis, 1991, Mosby.

Hersh PS, Shingleton BJ, Kenyon KR: Management of corneoscleral lacerations. In Shingleton BJ, Hersh PS, Kenyon KR, editors: *Eye trauma,* St Louis, 1991, Mosby.

Hoover DL, Smith LEH: Evaluation and management strategies for the pediatric eye trauma patient. In Shingleton BJ, Hersh PS, Kenyon KR, editors: *Eye trauma,* St Louis, 1991, Mosby.

Kenyon KR, Wagoner MD: Conjunctival and corneal injuries. In Shingleton BJ, Hersh PS, Kenyon KR, editors: *Eye trauma,* St Louis, 1991, Mosby.

Kylstra J: Preparation of the eye trauma patient for surgery. In Shingleton BJ, Hersh PS, Kenyon KR, editors: *Eye trauma,* St Louis, 1991, Mosby.

Shingleton BJ, Hersh PS: Traumatic hyphema. In Shingleton BJ, Hersh PS, Kenyon KR, editors: *Eye trauma,* St Louis, 1991, Mosby.

Wagoner MD, Kenyon KR: Chemical injuries. In Shingleton BJ, Hersh PS, Kenyon KR, editors: *Eye trauma,* St Louis, 1991, Mosby.

Weiss RA, McCord CD, Ellsworth RM: Orbital fractures. In Shingleton BJ, Hersh PS, Kenyon KR, editors: *Eye trauma,* St Louis, 1991, Mosby.

243 Osteochondroses

Edward M. Sills

The ossification centers of growing bones may develop irregular mineralization during childhood. Varying degrees of discomfort and dysfunction ensue associated with varying degrees of deformity. In this group of osteochondroses (Table 243-1), the disorders occur in bones preformed in cartilage and ossified from a central nucleus. The exact causal agents and mechanisms are not known. Excessive endogenous mechanical stress appears to play an important role in each of the disorders, and the degree of deformity and disability depends on the duration and degree of stress to which the softened fibrous parts are subjected. Excessive stress can lead to disordered cellular or local microvascular growth. Additional theories have pointed towards inherited tendencies to hypercoagulability as a cause of vascular thrombosis in the osteochondroses. In a study of Legg-Calvé-Perthes disease, for example, the prevalence of factor V Leiden mutation was found to be higher in patients than in controls (4.9% versus 0.7%; $p = 0.03$). Similar studies with antithrombin III, protein-C, and protein-S deficiency and activated protein C (APC) resistance have shown significant relationship to thrombotic venous occlusion in the femoral head in a few instances. The disorders that result from these alterations have been referred to as juvenile osteochondroses. Because damage to cartilage is not an instigating factor in these disorders, the root *chondro* is inaccurate. The more commonly involved areas of clinical significance and names with which they are associated include the femoral head (Legg-Calvé-Perthes), tibial tuberosity (Osgood Schlatter), tibial shaft (adolescent tibia vara or adolescent Blount), proximal tibial physis (infantile and juvenile Blount, rickets), tarsal navicular (Köhler), metatarsal heads 2, 3, or 4 (Freiberg), carpal semilunar, and lower thoracic vertebral end plates (Scheuermann).The more frequently encountered upper extremity involvement is in the distal radial epiphysis (Madelung) and in the navicular (Kienböck).

FEMORAL HEAD

Two distinctly different affections of the hip joint that occur in childhood involve damage to the femoral head. In Legg-Calvé-Perthes disease, the blood supply to the ossification center of the femoral head is interrupted, resulting in aseptic necrosis of the center. The femoral head, neck, and acetabulum become deformed and, in time, extensively reconstructed. The basis of treatment is to encourage the regaining of a spherical femoral head and to prevent irregular contour, flattening, or mushrooming of the head; shortening and broadening of the neck; and flattening of the vertical wall of the acetabulum. If these occur, osteoarthritis develops at an early age.

In the second common disorder, slipped capital femoral epiphysis, the femoral head slips gradually off the femoral neck, disrupting the epiphyseal cartilage plate. In this disorder, treatment is directed at immediately restoring normal anatomical relationships and preventing further slippage. (See Chapter 132, Extremity Pain.)

Legg-Calvé-Perthes Disease

Legg-Calvé-Perthes disease has its onset in the early school-age years and occurs in boys four times more frequently than in girls. In the vast majority of instances the disorder is unilateral. In those rare instances (less than 10%) when both hip joints are involved, the two joints are involved successively rather than simultaneously.

The earliest sign is an intermittent limp, noticed especially after exertion. This limp may be associated with hip and ipsilateral knee pain. The quadriceps muscles and adjacent thigh soft tissues atrophy, and the hip may develop adduction flexion contracture. The child experiences discomfort in the hip or knee when attempts are made to rotate the hip internally. Associated muscle spasm that anchors the hip to slight external rotation may cause distal thigh or knee tenderness. A roentgenogram taken early in the course of the disease shows widening of the hip joint and, occasionally, metaphyseal demineralization. This "acute phase" generally lasts for a week or two and is followed by the "active phase," which can last for 12 to 40 months, during which time no clinical signs or symptoms are evident; however, the process of reparative revascularization causes an increased radiodensity in the femoral head ossification center (seen on roentgenograms), which is caused by resorption of dead trabecular bone. During this remolding phase, orthopedic care should be directed to maintaining the femoral head abducted and internally rotated in relation to the acetabulum. Use of orthotic devices or surgical approaches can accomplish this goal.

Slipped Capital Femoral Epiphysis

A slipped capital femoral epiphysis causes hip and leg pain in early adolescence, at slightly younger ages in girls than in boys. The gender incidence is nearly equal, with some studies indicating a slight male preponderance. There is a greater prevalence of tall, overweight youngsters among those having this condition than among the general population of

Table 243-1 Osteochondroses

Site	Peak Age of Appearance (Years)
Upper Extremity	
Humeral head	2-8
Humeral capitulum	4-10
Lower ulna	13-20
Carpal navicular	16-24
Carpal semilunar	16-20
Bilateral entire carpus	10-14
Metacarpal heads	9-15
Basal phalanges	8-14
Lower Extremity	
Femoral epiphysis slippage	9-16*
Femoral epiphysis	3-12†
Greater trochanter	6-11
Primary patellar center	8-15
Secondary patellar center	8-10
Shaft of tibia	1.5‡ 6-12§
Tibial tubercle	10-15
Distal tibial epiphysis	4
Calcaneal epiphysis	3-18
Astragalus	2-8
Tarsal navicular	3-7
Second metatarsal	8-17
Fifth metatarsal	8-16
Spine and Pelvis	
Vertebral epiphysis	13-20
Vertebral disk	Over 16
Vertebral body	
Eosinophilic granuloma (?)	2-11
Symphysis pubis	12-18
Iliac crest	12-19
Ischial apophysis	13-18
Ischiopubic synchondrosis	12-19

*Girls are younger.
†Maximum is 6-8 years.
‡Infantile form.
§Adolescent form.

young teenagers. About 75% of cases are unilateral, and the left side is involved more often than the right.

Hip pain is the initial complaint with referral to the thigh or knee in association with a gait that is assumed to protect the hip. In the early "preslipping stage," pain often commences following a strain or minor injury. A sense of tiredness or mild pain prevails in the hip or knee, accompanied by mild limping or loss of mobility. The "preslipping stage" is succeeded by an "acute slip," with sudden acute pain, pronounced limitation of mobility, and difficulty bearing weight on the affected leg. On examination, the hip is rotated externally, with limited internal rotation and flexion. Earliest roentgenographic abnormalities are seen on a lateral view, with dorsal displacement of the capital epiphysis and widening of the zone of radiolucency between the femoral head and neck. If untreated, further posterior and medial slippage occurs. The hip must be placed in Russell traction and pinned surgically. Manipulation of the hip joint in an attempt at closed reduction may aggravate the slipping and should be avoided. The earlier the slippage is treated and the less the amount of unnecessary manipulation, the greater the likelihood that osteoarthritis can be avoided.

Tibial Tuberosity

Osgood-Schlatter disease results from avulsion of part of the patellar ligament and attached bony and cartilaginous fragments from the tuberosity. Its incidence is higher in boys, but the age of onset is earlier in girls, because ossification of the tibial tuberosity occurs earlier in females. About 25% of cases have bilateral involvement. The child's complaint is that of local pain and tenderness in the region of the knee, particularly the tuberosity. The pain is most severe at the end of active flexion or extension of the knee. If the condition has been present for several months, the tuberosity is enlarged, and one may find a bony prominence on its anterior aspect. The roentgenographic changes vary, depending on the size of the avulsed fragments, cartilage, and bone and on the duration of the condition. The best view is one with the knee rotated inward, giving a tangential view of the tibial tuberosity. One sees soft tissue swelling, an opaque patellar ligament, and a fragmented tuberosity. Treatment is directed at decreasing the stress on the tubercle until the tuberosity fuses with the tibial metaphysis. This bony fusion occurs at about 15 years of age in girls and 17 years in boys. Depending on the degree of pain, strenuous activities involving deep knee bending and jumping may have to be restricted, or casting may be required to immobilize the knee totally. The former approach usually is sufficient.

Tibial Shaft

Infants usually have some leg bowing until 18 months of age, after which time the legs straighten and then progress to a slight degree of knock-knee. Bowing of the legs that persists or progresses beyond 2 years of age should be evaluated. The differential diagnosis lies between tibia vara (Blount disease) and renal or nutritional rickets. In Blount disease, cartilage has failed to transform to bone at the medial aspect of the epiphysis. The metaphysis beneath the epiphyseal ossification center becomes demineralized, and the medial aspect of the proximal tibia fails to grow as rapidly as the lateral aspect, resulting in a bowleg deformity.

Trauma to the proximal tibial physis medially can present as unilateral tibia vara in the adolescent. Obesity appears to be a factor in adolescent-onset tibia vara, which is most common in male black teens. Dynamic gait deviations to compensate for increased thigh girth associated with obesity (fat-thigh gait) have been shown to result in increased loading of the medial compartment of the knee during the gait cycle and resultant adolescent tibia vara.

In rickets, calcification and growth of the epiphyseal cartilage of the long bones are suppressed, their metaphyses become softened, and they flare at both ends with resultant bowing. Appropriate treatment with vitamin D will produce roentgenographic evidence of healing within a few weeks and eventual straightening of the bones. Most children whose

Blount disease persists or develops beyond 6 years of age require an osteotomy to correct the bowing.

TARSAL NAVICULAR

Köhler's bone disease of the tarsal navicular bone results from an interruption of the blood supply to the developing navicular bone, causing necrosis of its ossification center. The navicular is in a crucial position in the arch of the foot; thus symptoms can be alarming. The condition is self-limited, and the ossification center becomes revascularized and completely reconstructed. The disorder is seen primarily in boys between 3 and 7 years of age, but predominantly in the younger children.

Pain is localized to the inner aspect of the midtarsal part of the foot. The foot is held in a slight varus position, and the child walks on the outer side of the foot or flat-footedly. The skin over the navicular may be warm, red, and swollen, and palpation of the bone elicits tenderness. Lateral roentgenograms of the feet show a very narrowed, waferlike, irregular navicular ossification center, with increased radiopacity and loss of trabecular markings. The process of revascularization and reconstruction takes from 1 to 3 years. Treatment primarily is directed to reassuring the child and family. Various orthotic pads can be used to absorb weight and pressure forces until the healing occurs. Surgical intervention is to be avoided.

METATARSAL HEADS

Freiberg's disease is a condition in which a part of the head of a metatarsal bone undergoes aseptic necrosis and becomes sufficiently weakened to be susceptible to functional trauma (running, jumping), which may cause compressional collapse of the metatarsal head. The second metatarsal bone most often is involved; the third metatarsal bone is the next most likely to be so. Females are affected more often than males.

Pain occurs in the region of the affected metatarsal on walking. Plantar pressure elicits tenderness, as does abrupt release of this pressure. Swelling occurs over the dorsum of the involved metatarsophalangeal joint, plantar flexion becomes limited, and the transverse arch of the involved foot becomes flattened. A callus develops on the plantar surface of the foot, overlying the involved metatarsal head. A deformed, broadened metatarsal head is seen on roentgenogram. High heels should not be worn, and long walks should be avoided until symptoms subside. Symptomatic use of nonsteroidal antiinflammatory agents is recommended.

CARPAL SEMILUNAR

Aseptic necrosis of the lunate bone (Kienböck's disease) weakens the bony structure and usually leads to a compression fracture. The lunate bone of the right hand (the usual working hand) is involved more frequently than that of the left, and males are affected more frequently than females.

Pain is experienced on movement of the wrist, and in longstanding cases the pain may be present at rest. Swelling over the dorsum of the wrist and tenderness over the affected bone often are exhibited. The roentgenogram shows a flattened fragmented lunate bone with variations in its radiodensity. The lunate, lying adjacent to the radius, is subjected to great forces and pressures; hence treatment includes wrist immobilization. On occasion, fusion of the lunate with the wrist bones of the wrist that surround it is required for stabilization and relief of pain.

LOWER THORACIC VERTEBRAE

Scheuermann's disease is a common cause of kyphosis in teenagers, occurring in about 5% of that population. The lower thoracic vertebrae are affected most often. The pathological condition involves a swelling of the intervertebral disks that exerts pressure on the cartilage plates covering the vertebral bodies; this causes the plates to thin and interferes with endochondral bone formation. The disk spaces become narrowed (more anteriorly than posteriorly), and pressure is exerted on the anterior portions of the contiguous vertebral bodies, which impedes their longitudinal growth and thus leads to kyphosis. An aching pain aggravated by physical exertion is present in the affected portion of the vertebral column. The affected area is tender to palpation. Assuming a stooping position often will cause the pain to increase. Within a year or so, the kyphosis easily is apparent as a round back deformity. In many instances the pain is so minor that the patient's complaint is that of poor posture rather than backache. Roentgenograms reveal narrowing of the anterior disk spaces and defects on the surfaces of adjacent vertebrae. In some children the condition progresses to cause severe deformity and dysfunction; in others the condition stabilizes and the deformity disappears. Treatment is aimed at preventing further deformity, occasionally with the use of casting or bracing. In those rare instances of rapid progression or of persistent, severe pain, spinal fusion is necessary. The majority of youngsters, however, require only careful observation. There have been rare instances of myopathy associated with Scheuermann's disease.

When to Refer

Whenever uncertain of diagnosis or when treatment requires orthopedic assessment or intervention

When to Hospitalize

Only for surgical intervention

SUGGESTED READINGS

Arruda VR, et al: Inherited risk factors for thrombophilia among children with Legg-Calvé-Perthes disease, *J Pediatr Orthop* 19:84, 1999.

Bowen JR, Abrams JS: Legg-Calvé-Perthes disease, *Contemp Orthop* 10: 27, 1985.

Davids JR, Huskamp M, Bagley AM: A dynamic biomechanical analysis of the etiology of adolescent tibia vara, *J Pediatr Orthop* 16:461, 1996.

Fitzsimons RB: Idiopathic scoliosis, Scheuermann's disease and myopathy: two case reports, *Clin Exp Neurol* 16:303, 1979.

Gallistl S, et al: The role of inherited thrombotic disorders in the etiology of Legg-Calvé-Perthes disease, *J Pediatr Orthop* 19:82, 1999.

Glueck CJ, et al: Thrombophilia and hypofibrinolysis: pathophysiologies of osteonecrosis, *Clin Orthop* 334:43, 1997.

Lonstein JE, et al: *Textbook of scoliosis and other spinal deformities,* ed 3, Philadelphia, 1995, WB Saunders.

Stulberg SD, Cooperman DR, Wallenstein R: The natural history of Legg-Calvé-Perthes disease, *J Bone Joint Surg (Am)* 63:1095, 1981.

Tachdjian MO: *Clinical pediatric orthopedics: the art of diagnosis and principles of management,* Stamford, Conn, 1997, Appleton & Lange.

244 Osteomyelitis

Edwards P. Schwentker

The vast majority of cases of osteomyelitis are secondary to pyogenic infection. They can result from the direct bacterial contamination of bone, which may occur with an open fracture, during operative procedures, or by direct extension from an adjacent soft-tissue infection. Most commonly, however, childhood osteomyelitis is hematogenous in origin.

Hematogenous osteomyelitis may occur at any age, but its incidence is higher in children than in adults. Unless promptly diagnosed and aggressively treated, it may lead to complications resulting in lifelong disability. Because establishing the diagnosis of osteomyelitis may at times be difficult, a high index of suspicion is required.

Pyogenic osteomyelitis initially may manifest either acutely or subacutely. In childhood these two modes of presentation are sufficiently distinct to require separate discussion. Chronic osteomyelitis is discussed with acute osteomyelitis, inasmuch as the former develops from the inadequate treatment of the latter.

ACUTE OSTEOMYELITIS

Pathogenesis

The pathogenesis and, consequently, the clinical manifestations of acute pyogenic osteomyelitis depend on the anatomy of bone, particularly its pattern of vascular supply. This anatomy is sufficiently different among infants (birth to 18 months), older children (18 months to skeletal maturity), and adults to cause a different form of acute osteomyelitis in each of the three age groups.[10] The concern here is with bone infection as it occurs during infancy and childhood.

Infancy. In anatomical studies of infants, Trueta[10] demonstrated the presence of vessels that penetrate through the growth plate to connect the metaphysis with the epiphysis. These vessels are seen most commonly before 6 months of age, but they may be present up to 18 months. Infectious spread from the metaphyseal side of the growth plate (physis) into the epiphysis is facilitated by these penetrating vessels (see Table 266-1 for the components of the growth plate). Infection thus is able to damage the growth plate and the epiphysis itself; it also is much more likely to penetrate the adjacent joint. Therefore in infancy acute osteomyelitis commonly results in an associated septic arthritis.

As in the older age group, the bone of the metaphysis and the diaphysis also can be destroyed in infancy, with subsequent formation of a sequestrum and involucrum. The richness of blood supply and the natural resilience of the infant provide an enormous capacity for repair. The development of chronic osteomyelitis is less likely in the infant than in the older child, but irreparable damage to the joint surfaces and to growth potential is far more likely.

Childhood. Hematogenous osteomyelitis in childhood (approximately 18 months to skeletal maturity) virtually always arises in the metaphyses of the long bones, gaining entrance to the bone by way of nutrient vessels. The vasculature on the metaphyseal side of the physis is characterized by loops that extend up into the layer of calcified cartilage of the physis to provide nutritional support for the formation of bone associated with growth. Bacteria within the bloodstream invade the venous side of these vascular loops. It generally is believed that a relatively sluggish blood flow within these venous sinusoids favors bacterial proliferation. Rang,[6] however, points out a relative lack of reticuloendothelial cells in the metaphyses of actively growing long bones, and he postulates that bone defenses against infection are weakest in this area.

Trauma also may play a role. The manifestation of an acute osteomyelitis frequently is associated with the history of a recent injury to the affected extremity. Morrissy and Haynes[5] have presented experimental evidence, using an immature rabbit model, to support injury to the physeal plate as a factor in the development of acute hematogenous osteomyelitis. Whatever the cause or combination of causes, the metaphysis is the predominant site of origin of hematogenous osteomyelitis in childhood.

In contrast to the situation in infancy, by 18 months of age no direct vascular connections exist between the metaphysis and the epiphysis. The physis becomes a barrier to infection, effectively preventing the spread of infection into the epiphysis.

As bacteria proliferate, local thrombosis occurs, resulting in devascularization of bone. This loss of vascularity further interferes with natural body defenses and prevents the penetration of circulating antibiotics. The result is an abscess. Untreated, infection spreads through the haversian system and Volkmann canals, eventually reaching the subperiosteal space. The periosteum then may be elevated by the infection, stripping the periosteal vascular supply from the cortex and causing further bone death.

Rupture through the periosteum at this point may result in a septic arthritis of the adjacent joint if that portion of the metaphysis happens to be intraarticular. This event is most likely in those joints in which the capsule attaches circumferentially well down on the metaphysis of the infected bone. Thus a proximal femoral osteomyelitis may result in septic arthritis of the hip. Similarly, sepsis of the elbow can result from infection of the proximal radius.

If treatment is delayed or is inadequate, the infection also may track outward to result in a spontaneously draining sinus. Devascularized bone, the sequestrum, becomes a fortress for the bacteria, against which antibiotics and natural body defenses can accomplish little more than to prevent further spread of infection. Meanwhile, the elevated hypervascular periosteum lays down a surrounding wall of new living bone known as the involucrum. An inadequately treated or untreated acute osteomyelitis thus becomes a chronic osteomyelitis.

In childhood, unlike infancy, acute osteomyelitis seldom causes growth plate or epiphyseal damage. Growth is unlikely to be retarded and may, in fact, be stimulated, possibly secondarily to the hypervascularity that attends inflammation. Damage to the epiphysis and to the physis can occur, however, when osteomyelitis is complicated by septic arthritis of the adjacent joint.

Clinical Findings

In older infants and children, osteomyelitic infection is most likely to involve a single bone. Fever and sepsis may be prominent, but systemic signs and symptoms usually are mild (or even absent), with the major signs being those localized to the affected part. This is true especially in the infant. Localized tenderness generally is present and often is exquisite. Other local signs may be associated with inflammation, including swelling, redness, and warmth. Characteristically the child is reluctant to move the adjacent joint and, when a lower extremity is involved, may refuse to bear weight. In the young infant the loss of active movement in an extremity may mimic neurological damage, a condition known as pseudoparalysis.

The diagnostic workup should include a complete blood cell count, erythrocyte sedimentation rate, C-reactive protein, blood cultures, and roentgenograms; however, findings here also may be misleading. The white blood cell count often is normal. An elevation in the sedimentation rate is more sensitive and the C-reactive protein even more so. Both are useful in monitoring clinical response to treatment.

Early in the clinical course, no bony changes are seen roentgenographically, the earliest detectable signs being those of blurred soft-tissue planes secondary to edema spreading into fatty tissues. The earliest roentgenographic changes to occur within bone itself are those of bone destruction or lysis, which generally is not apparent until at least 10 days after the onset of symptoms.

The differential diagnosis of acute osteomyelitis includes septic arthritis, acute rheumatic fever, rheumatoid arthritis, leukemia, and cellulitis. The manifestations of septic arthritis may be similar to those of acute osteomyelitis, and especially in the infant, the two entities may coexist. When septic arthritis is present, the urgency for prompt treatment is, if anything, more acute (see Chapter 261, Septic Arthritis). Rheumatoid arthritis and acute rheumatic fever generally present with less severe signs and symptoms, and tenderness, although exquisite, is not localized to the metaphysis of the involved bone as it is with osteomyelitis. Initially, leukemia may mimic or actually be an acute osteomyelitis. The presence of an anemia or a low leukocyte count may be suggestive. Distinguishing between cellulitis and osteomyelitis may be difficult. In the lower extremities a cellulitis is less likely to interfere with weight bearing. If doubt exists, management should proceed on the assumption that the infection involves the bone.

Ultrasonography can detect a subperiosteal abscess and may be helpful in guiding needle aspiration. The presence of a subperiosteal abscess is diagnostic for an acute osteomyelitis that has broken through the metaphyseal cortex. Its presence distinguishes osteomyelitis from cellulitis in an inflamed extremity, but the failure to visualize an abscess does not rule out an early osteomyelitis still contained within the bone.

Radionuclide scanning is not necessary in most cases of acute osteomyelitis, but if signs and symptoms are inconclusive, it may help in establishing the diagnosis. Scanning is far more sensitive than is radiographic examination in the early stages of the disease and is capable of differentiating most cases of soft-tissue cellulitis from infection of the bone itself. Scans are most helpful when signs of localization are poor, when multiple sites of involvement are suspected, or for the localization of sites within the axial skeleton. Technetium pyrophosphate scintigraphy is the scanning modality employed most commonly. Technetium scans provide results within 3 to 4 hours and are most helpful when performed with a three-phase protocol to evaluate blood flow, blood pool, and bone uptake.[2]

The use of gallium scans and scans with radionuclide-labeled leukocytes may be even more sensitive and specific; unfortunately these tests require 24 to 48 hours to complete, rendering them of limited usefulness in a situation in which early diagnosis is critical. Of the two techniques, indium-labeled white cell scanning may be the most useful and should be considered when needle aspiration and three-phase technetium scan both show negative results.[2]

Under no circumstances should treatment be delayed to perform a scan when clinical suspicion of osteomyelitis is high. Both false-positive and false-negative results with all scanning methods have been reported.[9]

Blood culture results are positive in 40% to 50% of cases of acute osteomyelitis. Needle aspiration of the subperiosteal space and of the metaphysis provides a positive identification of the infecting organism in most cases. In neonates the most common organisms are *Streptococcus pyogenes* (group B), *Staphylococcus aureus,* and enteric bacilli. In the older child *Staphylococcus aureus* is the predominant pathogen; *Streptococcus pneumoniae, Streptococcus pyogenes,* and *Staphylococcus epidermidis* occur less frequently. *Pseudomonas aeruginosa* is becoming more common, particularly in older children who have had penetrating trauma or who engage in parenteral drug abuse.[8]

High-risk, low-birth-weight infants present a special set of problems with respect to acute osteomyelitis. They often have multiple portals for bacterial entry into the systemic circulation, including infection of other organ systems, indwelling catheters, and heel sticks. They frequently are debilitated; as a result, osteomyelitis often develops at several sites, including the facial bones. Extension of infection from the bone into adjacent joints occurs commonly. *S. pyogenes* (group B) is a frequent offender.

The search for multiple sites of involvement in the neonate would seem to be an ideal application of radionuclide scanning. Unfortunately, false-negative results are more common in this age group. Reducing the incidence of false-negative scan results in the neonate may be possible with the use of the latest generation of cameras and the application of spot and pinhole views.[2]

Skeletal infections caused by *Candida albicans* may develop in severely debilitated infants and children who have required prolonged antibiotic therapy or hyperalimentation by central venous catheter.

Another special group is composed of patients who have sickle cell hemoglobinopathies; osteomyelitis occurring in these patients is difficult to differentiate from bony infarction. *Salmonella* spp. are the most common infecting organisms. Osteomyelitis can be differentiated from bone infarction by operative exploration and direct culture of bacteria from the involved bone or by culture of the organisms from the blood.

Because the physical signs are more difficult to interpret when osteomyelitis involves the spine or pelvis, diagnosis becomes more complex. Technetium scans are particularly helpful in making the diagnoses in such cases. Magnetic resonance imaging (MRI) is expensive and often requires patient sedation, but it too is useful in localizing infection beneath the deep tissues surrounding the spine and pelvis. This modality can identify associated epidural abscesses and can guide aspiration. MRI also can localize abscesses in the extremities that have been missed by needle aspiration.[4] MRI should be considered for patients who otherwise have inconclusive findings. Its ability to distinguish abnormal from normal bone marrow give MRI a sensitivity for diagnosing osteomyelitis that has been reported to be between 82% and 100%. Its specificity in the diagnosis of osteomyelitis is much lower, with a reported range between 53% and 94%. Conditions that may have similar MRI findings include tumors, fractures, bone infarctions, and metabolic disorders.[1]

Management

Needle aspiration is the single most helpful procedure for diagnosing infections of bones and joints. All children who have suspected osteomyelitis with localized signs should undergo aspiration of the subperiosteum with a large-bore needle; if pus is not encountered, the needle is advanced into the metaphyseal bone. The metaphysis of a long bone can be aspirated quickly without the use of general anesthesia. Aspiration confirms the diagnosis, determines the necessity for operative decompression, and provides a specimen for pathogen identification by culture, as well as material for immediate Gram stain.

Once blood cultures and needle aspiration have been performed, antibiotics should be given parenterally. In an older child who has no associated septic arthritis and in whom no risk factors for gram negative organisms exist, a penicillinase-resistant penicillin should be sufficient. Neonates should receive the same, plus an aminoglycoside. If reason exists to suspect a pseudomonal infection, the initial treatment should be a carboxypenicillin or acylureidopenicillin combined with an aminoglycoside. Children in whom a *Salmonella* infection is suspected should receive an ampicillin and aminoglycoside combination.[8]

Antibiotics should be adjusted appropriately once cultures and sensitivities are available. Antibiotics should be continued for at least 3 weeks and must be maintained at adequate concentrations in the blood. Oral antibiotics may achieve adequate bactericidal titers. Oral antibiotics, however, should be used only if the patient is responding to treatment, the parents are reliable, the antibiotic does not cause a gastrointestinal disturbance that interferes with absorption, and adequate monitored blood levels can be obtained. The erythrocyte sedimentation rate and C-reactive protein level are helpful in monitoring the clinical response and should return to normal values before therapy is discontinued.

Surgical drainage must be undertaken whenever an abscess is detected or suspected. An abscess may be assumed to be present whenever a loss of vascularity, and hence viability, has occurred in any part of the skeletal tissues. If a situation exists in which body defenses or antibiotics are ineffective, operative decompression must be used. The aspiration of frank pus is an absolute indication for surgical drainage. Similarly, lytic changes within the bone or periosteal new bone formation, as seen on initial roentgenograms in previously untreated patients, is an indication for operative drainage. On the other hand, in patients already under treatment and responding favorably both clinically and in terms of a falling sedimentation rate, the appearance of radiographic bone changes does not necessarily indicate that an abscess is present, because such changes occur in treated patients as recovery progresses.

The lack of pus on aspiration is not absolute evidence that operative decompression is not needed. The site of aspiration may have been inaccurate, or pus may be present but too thick to pass through even a large-bore needle. Persistent clinical suspicion or failure of the patient to respond to nonoperative therapy is an indication for MRI or, when localizing signs are severe, for immediate operative decompression. The risks of unnecessary surgery in the child who has an acute infection are far less than those of necessary surgery not performed.

SUBACUTE OSTEOMYELITIS

Subacute osteomyelitis in childhood is a clinical entity entirely distinct from acute osteomyelitis. The clinical course is far more benign, both systemically and with respect to the presence of localized signs and symptoms. The sites of subacute osteomyelitis are not restricted to metaphyses but may occur virtually at any site within the bony skeleton. Because of its mild clinical course, the diagnosis of subacute osteomyelitis often is delayed. This entity occurs with a variety of roentgenographic manifestations and frequently is confused with a variety of benign and malignant bone neoplasms.

Pathogenesis

Gledhill[3] has hypothesized that subacute osteomyelitis develops as the result of an altered host-pathogen relationship. As in acute osteomyelitis, bacteria appear to gain entrance to the bone through the circulation. After the infection gains a foothold, it is brought under control largely by body defenses and prevented from spreading within the bone. It may be speculated that this situation occurs when bacterial virulence is decreased, either naturally or secondary to antibiotics administered early in the infection. The acute infection also might be aborted by increased host resistance, such as is to be expected within the diaphysis or epiphysis, as compared with the metaphysis. Subacute osteomyelitis may occur in any of these three areas, whereas acute osteomyelitis arises hematogenously almost exclusively in the more susceptible metaphysis.

Whether such an "attenuated" infection occurs because of decreased virulence of the pathogen, increased natural defenses of the host, or a superimposed factor (such as the administration of suboptimal doses of antibiotics), the establishment of the subacute process is characterized by a pathological stand-off between pathogen and host, wherein the infection is contained effectively within a small area of bone. Although the bacteria cannot expand their foothold rapidly, natural body defenses are unable to eradicate the infection completely.

Clinical Findings

Subacute osteomyelitis is of insidious onset. The pain that results is mild to moderate and often intermittent. Little to no functional impairment results, and the systemic signs and symptoms of fever, malaise, anorexia, and weight loss are minimal to nonexistent. The interval between onset of symptoms and diagnosis may be measured in months, whereas the diagnosis of an acute osteomyelitis generally requires no more than a few days.

By the time medical consultation is sought, enough time generally has elapsed since onset of the infection that roentgenograms reveal positive findings. The radiographic appearance may vary considerably and may closely mimic a variety of benign and malignant neoplasms.

Roberts et al[7] have proposed an expansion of a system for radiographic classification originally proposed by Gledhill.[3] They describe seven different types of bone lesions, only one of which clearly suggests a subacute osteomyelitis. A lytic defect within the metaphysis surrounded by a dense sclerotic margin suggests the classic form of subacute osteomyelitis, often called a *Brodie abscess*. This variety is described as type IB. Type IA is similar in size and location but lacks the sclerotic rim. It most frequently is confused with an eosinophilic granuloma. Type II subacute osteomyelitis is associated with erosion of the metaphyseal cortex, and its appearance may be confused with that of an osteogenic sarcoma. A type III lesion is seen as a localized defect within the cortex of the diaphysis and resembles an osteoid osteoma. The type IV lesion is characterized by onion-skin periosteal reaction and suggests Ewing's sarcoma. The type V lesion occurs within the epiphysis and may suggest a chondroblastoma. Finally, the type VI lesion involves a vertebral body, and the roentgenographic appearance is that of erosion or destruction.

The white blood cell count and sedimentation rate in cases of subacute osteomyelitis are likely to be normal or elevated minimally. Blood cultures rarely are positive. Findings on a technetium bone scan may be positive, but if a lesion already is visible on plain roentgenograms, the scan will add little in establishing the diagnosis.

Management

Subacute osteomyelitis can be diagnosed definitively only by isolating an organism on culture of the bone or by histopathological findings consistent with infection. When the lesion involves the long bones of the extremities, curettage generally can be performed easily. Material obtained will establish the diagnosis by culture or histological findings. *S. aureus* is the most commonly isolated pathogen. Operative curettage followed by a course of antibiotic therapy, similar to that used in the treatment of acute osteomyelitis, usually is curative.

When the infection involves a vertebral body, a specimen may be obtained for biopsy with a closed-needle technique. If suspicion of infection is high, treatment may be undertaken with antibiotics and cast immobilization of the spine without resorting to biopsy or aspiration. Again, prognosis for cure is excellent.

CHRONIC OSTEOMYELITIS

Chronic osteomyelitis, characterized by sequestration and the development of fistulas draining into the surrounding soft tissues, occurs rarely among children in developed countries. Treatment consists of curettage and appropriate antibiotics administered orally over long periods until all signs of infection have disappeared.

When to Refer

To an orthopedic surgeon:
- Needle aspiration positive for abscess
- Failure to improve within 24 hours despite negative aspiration and parenteral antibiotics

When to Hospitalize

- Failure to move or use an extremity (pseudoparalysis)
- Increasing signs of localized inflammation
- Back pain with fever and an elevated erythrocyte sedimentation rate

REFERENCES

1. Boutin RD, et al: Update on imaging of orthopedic infections, *Orthop Clin North Am* 29:41, 1998.
2. Demopulos GA, Bleck EE, McDougall IR: Role of radionuclide imaging in the diagnosis of acute osteomyelitis, *J Pediatr Orthop* 8:558, 1988.
3. Gledhill RB: Subacute osteomyelitis in children, *Clin Orthop* 96:57, 1973.
4. Jaramillo D, et al: Osteomyelitis and septic arthritis in children: appropriate use of imaging to guide treatment, *Am J Radiol* 165:399, 1995.

5. Morrissy RT, Haynes DW: Acute hematogenous osteomyelitis: a model with trauma as an etiology, *J Pediatr Orthop* 9:447, 1989.
6. Rang MC: *The growth plate and its disorders,* Baltimore, 1969, Williams & Wilkins.
7. Roberts JM, et al: Subacute hematogenous osteomyelitis in children: a retrospective study, *J Pediatr Orthop* 2:249, 1982.
8. Scoles PV, Aronoff SC: Current concepts review: antimicrobial therapy of childhood skeletal infections, *J Bone Joint Surg (Am)* 66:1487, 1984.
9. Sullivan JA, Vasileff T, Leonard JC: An evaluation of nuclear scanning in orthopaedic infection, *J Pediatr Orthop* 1:73, 1981.
10. Trueta J: The three types of acute hematogenous osteomyelitis, *J Bone Joint Surg (Br)* 41:671, 1959.

245 Otitis Media and Otitis Externa

John S. Andrews

OTITIS MEDIA

Otitis media is the most common reason that children in the United States receive a prescription for an antibiotic. More than 90% of all antibiotic use in the first 2 years of life is attributable to the treatment of otitis media.[18] By the age of 7 years, between 65% and 95% of children will have been treated for at least one episode of otitis media.[13] Because it is such a prevalent condition, much attention is focused on the consequences of otitis media and its treatment. Rare suppurative complications, such as intracranial abscess, can be serious. Conductive hearing loss resulting from chronic middle ear effusions associated with otitis media may contribute to speech and language delay in some children. The use of antibiotics to treat otitis media is thought to contribute to the emergence of antibiotic-resistant bacteria.[2] Each year in the United States, more than $3.5 billion is spent on the treatment of otitis media.[20] Despite this attention, there is no consensus about the management of otitis media; it remains a source of considerable debate in the medical literature.[15]

Classification

Otitis media literally means inflammation of the middle ear. It encompasses several clinical entities. *Acute otitis media* (AOM) describes the presence of inflammatory fluid in the middle ear space accompanied by local findings such as ear pain, otorrhea, or distortion of the tympanic membrane. Systemic findings such as fever and irritability may also be present. *Otitis media with effusion* (OME), or serous otitis media, describes the presence of inflammatory fluid in the middle ear space in an asymptomatic child or in a child with mild upper respiratory tract symptoms, a common reason for examining the ears in the first place. The term *recurrent otitis media* has generally been used to refer to the occurrence of three or more episodes of AOM in 6 months or four episodes in 1 year. Recurrent otitis media should not be confused with chronic otitis media, which may be used to describe OME that lasts for greater than 3 months or a suppurative middle ear process that fails to respond to initial antibiotic therapy. Specificity in diagnosis is important because of its important implications for management.

Epidemiology

By the age of 1 year, 62% of children have experienced at least one episode of AOM.[21] Otitis media is more common in boys and in children of low socioeconomic status. Incidence rates in white and black children are similar. Several environmental factors increase the risk for developing otitis media including exposure to tobacco smoke,[6] use of a pacifier,[16] and attendance at day care centers, particularly those serving large numbers of children.[22] Exclusive breastfeeding early in life has a protective effect.[4] Children at high risk for the development of AOM include those with craniofacial anomalies, such as cleft palate, that alter the normal air and fluid dynamics of the middle ear space, those with immunodeficiencies, and those of certain ethnic groups such as Native Americans and Alaskan Natives. There appears to be a mild hereditary predisposition to develop recurrent otitis media with some of the variation in presentation and incidence explained by genetic factors; the remainder is accounted for by familial and individual environmental factors.[14]

Pathogenesis

Otitis media is an inflammatory process of the upper respiratory tract and usually results from a viral infection. As viruses infect the respiratory mucosa, edema can lead to eustachian tube dysfunction. Inflammatory fluid and pathogenic respiratory bacteria that reflux into the middle ear space do not drain normally. This process effectively leads to the formation of an abscess in the middle ear. Otitis media usually is self-limited; as the viral illness resolves, eustachian tube function is restored and the middle ear space drains normally. Although acute symptoms generally resolve spontaneously within a few days, middle ear effusions can persist for weeks following an episode of AOM. Sixty percent of middle ear effusions resolve spontaneously within 3 months, 85% within 6 months.[24] The persistence of middle ear effusions (or OME) following an episode of AOM has raised concern about the conductive hearing loss that accompanies these effusions and its impact on speech and language development, especially in younger children.

In studies of children with AOM, specimens of middle ear fluid obtained by tympanocentesis have been used to clarify the microbiology of this disease. These specimens are positive for bacteria about 70% of the time.[12] The most frequently identified pathogens are *Streptococcus pneumoniae*, *Haemophilus influenzae*, and *Moraxella catarrhalis*. Group A beta-hemolytic streptococcus is much less common. Rarely, *Mycoplasma pneumoniae* is detected but not often enough to affect the empirical selection of an antibiotic for treatment of AOM. Respiratory viruses such as respiratory syncytial virus (RSV), influenza viruses, and parainfluenza viruses also are recovered often from middle ear aspirates, either in addition to bacteria or in isolation. RSV, in particular, has a tendency to infect the mucosa of the middle ear and probably contributes substantially to the development of otitis media in children.[8]

Diagnosis

There is growing concern that overdiagnosis of otitis media and liberal use of antibiotics for its treatment has contributed to the emergence of antibiotic-resistant bacteria, particularly penicillin-resistant *Streptococcus pneumoniae*.[2] Therefore, accurate diagnosis is critical to the appropriate management of otitis media. Diagnosis is based upon recognition of the characteristic clinical context and the use of pneumatic otoscopy to document physical findings.

In the classic case of AOM, a young child with a history of a recent upper respiratory tract infection suddenly develops the acute onset of a new fever and ear discomfort. In children old enough to localize pain, the affected ear is often obvious. In younger children, discomfort may be more generalized and they may present with unexplained crying or irritability. Examination may reveal other signs of upper respiratory infection such as rhinorrhea, cough, or conjunctival injection.

The diagnosis of AOM is confirmed using pneumatic otoscopy. To perform this technique, the child must either cooperate or be restrained in a comfortable position that allows the examiner to manipulate the pinna and insert the otoscope into the external auditory canal without difficulty. Cleansing the external auditory canal must be accomplished to free it of obstructions to visualization of the tympanic membrane; cerumen or foreign bodies should be removed using a cerumen spoon or gentle irrigation with warm water. The largest speculum that will fit into the external auditory canal at a depth of ¼ inch to ½ inch should be attached to the pneumatic otoscope. This permits visualization of the largest possible area and also ensures a relatively airtight seal for effective insufflation.

Acute otitis media is present when distortion (usually bulging) of the tympanic membrane is noted on direct visualization and when restricted movement of the tympanic membrane, indicative of fluid in the middle ear, is noted with gentle insufflation and exsufflation of air using a squeeze bulb attached to the otoscope. Erythema of the tympanic membrane alone is not sufficient to make the diagnosis of AOM and may be the incidental result of fever or crying. In some cases of AOM, the tympanic membrane may be retracted rather than bulging.

Occasionally a child with AOM experiences spontaneous rupture of the tympanic membrane. This leads to marked improvement in ear pain and the presence of otorrhea on examination.

OME may be an incidental finding on physical examination and is characterized by decreased mobility of the tympanic membrane without the signs of acute inflammation seen in AOM.

Some experts advocate making a specific bacteriological diagnosis by obtaining middle ear fluid for culture and sensitivities using the technique of tympanocentesis or carbon dioxide laser-assisted myringotomy (see Appendix B, Special Procedures). These techniques are not necessary for the routine diagnosis of AOM, but are useful in specific clinical situations where identification of an organism to guide therapeutic decisions is a high priority. These situations include (1) episodes of AOM that do not respond to empirical antibiotic therapy; (2) the child who experiences frequent recurrences of AOM despite what seems to be appropriate therapy; and (3) the child who is young and particularly toxic in appearance.

Cultures of other areas of the upper respiratory tract are useful for research purposes but do not assist in the management of individual episodes of AOM. Organisms recovered from tympanocentesis or laser-assisted myringotomy specimens usually are recovered from the nasopharynx also, but the presence of an organism on a nasopharyngeal culture does not prove that it is present in the middle ear fluid.

Tympanometry is a technique for documenting tympanic membrane compliance. It can be used to document objectively the presence of fluid in the middle ear space but does not add to the information obtained on carefully performed pneumatic otoscopy. Tympanometry measurements can be useful to follow the course of an episode of OME over time.

Management

Whether an episode of AOM should be treated with antibiotics is a matter of debate. Some of the acute symptoms of AOM such as fever and ear pain may resolve more quickly with antibiotic therapy. Early empirical antibiotic therapy may also obviate the need for follow-up office visits to evaluate the patient with otitis media who is not responding to expectant management. However, most episodes of AOM resolve spontaneously, middle ear effusions may persist despite effective antibiotic therapy, and rare suppurative complications are generally easily treated with antibiotics and surgical techniques. The modest benefits of antibiotic therapy also must be weighed against the negative impact of widespread antibiotic use and its effect on producing antibiotic-resistant species of organisms such as *Streptococcus pneumoniae*.[2] In some areas of the United States, 25% to 50% of strains of this organism are resistant to penicillin.

Several guiding principles should be observed when selecting patients with AOM to be treated with antibiotics. First, the diagnosis of AOM should be clear. The presence of fever, upper respiratory symptoms, or a middle ear effusion may be consistent with AOM, but without objective findings on pneumatic otoscopy these criteria are not sufficient and should not lead to prescription of antibiotics. Second, younger patients may benefit more from empirical antibiotic therapy than older children. The positive effects of antibiotic administration have been more prevalent in children under 2 years of age. This is due, perhaps, to their more limited immune response to encapsulated organisms. Third, uniquely susceptible individuals such as those with immunodeficiencies or those with craniofacial anomalies are at greater risk of developing complications or a protracted course of illness and, therefore, warrant a lower threshold for treatment. There is growing acceptance of management that includes supportive care and observation without antibiotic treatment for the low-risk child with early AOM. If symptoms have not resolved spontaneously with 48 to 72 hours, reexamination is indicated with prescription of antibiotics if objective findings of AOM are still present.

When a decision is made to treat a child with AOM, an antibiotic with a narrow spectrum should be chosen. Many antibiotics are marketed for the treatment of this common condition including penicillins, first-, second- and third-generation cephalosporins, macrolides, and carbacephems. In the absence of specific microbiological information, the selection of empirical antibiotic therapy should be guided by knowledge of the most common bacterial pathogens identified in middle ear aspirates of children in population-based studies of children with AOM were *Streptococcus pneumoniae, Haemophilus influenzae,* and *Moraxella catarrhalis.*

Amoxicillin (40 to 50 mg/kg/day, given in 3 doses) is inexpensive, has a satisfactory spectrum of activity against these organisms, and is a good first line choice. Studies of amoxicillin treatment of AOM show cure rates of 85% to 94% based on clinical criteria, an acceptable figure given the high rate of spontaneous resolution. In the child who has had recent exposure to antibiotics, a higher dose of amoxicillin (80 to 90 mg/kg/day) may be used as a first line agent because of its greater efficacy against strains of *Streptococcus pneumoniae* with intermediate resistance to penicillin. Treatment should be administered for 10 days, although shorter courses of 5 to 7 days may be acceptable in low-risk patients, such as older children with uncomplicated histories.[17]

If fever, ear pain, and the objective findings of AOM persist despite at least 72 hours of therapy, a change of antibiotic may be warranted. Second-line agents such as second- or third-generation cephalosporins, amoxicillin plus clavulanate, or clindamycin may be used to broaden the antimicrobial spectrum to cover beta-lactamase producing strains of *Haemophilus influenzae* and *Moraxella catarrhalis,* as well as penicillin-resistant *Streptococcus pneumoniae.*

There is no proven benefit to the use of antihistamine/decongestant preparations, steroids, or nonsteroidal antiinflammatory medications in the treatment of AOM. Topical Auralgan otic solution (five drops in the external auditory canal) is somewhat effective in reducing the acute ear pain associated with AOM.[10]

Most children who respond satisfactorily to treatment of an episode of AOM do not require specific follow-up. As long as a child is asymptomatic, the main reason for follow-up is to document resolution of a middle ear effusion that may contribute to conductive hearing loss. Only 50% of middle ear effusions resolve by 6 weeks following initial presentation. Therefore, follow-up for the otherwise healthy and asymptomatic child should be scheduled no sooner than 6 weeks postdiagnosis, if at all. An effusion that is persistent at 6 weeks does not warrant specific intervention other than perhaps checking for resolution again in 6 more weeks. Further management of an effusion that persists beyond that point is described in the treatment of OME below.

OME presents a different therapeutic challenge than AOM. The goal of therapy for this disorder is to limit any potential long-term detrimental effects on speech and language development that may be due to conductive hearing loss associated with the presence of a chronic middle ear effusion. Weak associations have been found between OME and abnormal speech and language development in children younger than 4 years and problems with attention and expressive language delay in older children. However, these associations may be due to environmental influences that predispose both to OME and to developmental delays. The effects of treating OME on these outcomes are not well established.

Medical therapies for OME have produced largely unsatisfactory results. Although there is limited scientific evidence, some experts believe that empirical antibiotic therapy either early in the course of OME or later, when the effusion has persisted for 3 months or more, may hasten resolution of the effusion. There is no role for steroid medications, antihistamine/decongestant preparations, or for tonsillectomy and/or adenoidectomy in the management of OME. The most effective therapy for OME is the surgical insertion of tympanostomy tubes. Placement of tympanostomy tubes evacuates a middle ear effusion and restores near-normal hearing, but the impact of this procedure on long-term speech and language outcomes is unclear. Laser-assisted myringotomy soon may replace tympanostomy tube placement for the treatment of OME.[1]

When OME is documented in a child, follow-up at 3 months is reasonable assuming acute symptoms have not intervened. If, at 3 months, middle ear effusions are persistent and are bilateral, referral for audiological testing is indicated. If hearing is normal, further observation to allow spontaneous resolution is appropriate. If a conductive hearing loss at a threshold of 20 dB or greater is documented at the 3-month follow-up, consideration should be given to tympanostomy tube placement or laser-assisted myringotomy to drain the effusions and restore hearing. The use of these procedures for OME in otherwise healthy children with normal hearing is not recommended.

The occurrence of three or more episodes of AOM within 6 months, or of four episodes within a year satisfies many experts' definition of recurrent or chronic otitis media. The therapy of recurrent otitis media is also controversial. Studies have shown that long-term administration of prophylactic antibiotics (usually either amoxicillin or trimethoprim/sulfamethoxazole) can reduce the incidence of subsequent episodes of AOM in these children. However, the effect is modest; to improve outcome in one child, nine must be treated with daily medication, and prophylactic antibiotics contribute to the development of resistant organisms.[23] Therefore, the use of prophylactic antibiotics is not currently recommended for management of recurrent otitis media. Controlling environmental risk factors such as exposure to tobacco smoke and attendance at large day care centers is a more desirable approach to this problem.

Tympanostomy tube placement or laser-assisted myringotomy should be considered in the management of recurrent otitis media. This approach may be justified when recurrent AOM complicates OME and is accompanied by hearing loss as described above. However, frequent episodes of AOM (without OME) that respond to appropriate antibiotic therapy are not an indication for these procedures. Although AOM does tend to occur less frequently in children who have had tympanostomy tubes placed, this is a surgical procedure requiring administration of anesthesia and tubes may not remain in place for a sufficient duration to have a measurable impact on the health of an individual child.

Use of a conjugated vaccine against *Streptococcus pneumoniae*, widespread use of the influenza vaccine in healthy children, and development of an effective vaccine against

Inbox for dmontgom305@yahoo.com

Yahoo! - My Yahoo! Options - Sign Out - Help

Mail Addresses Calendar Notepad

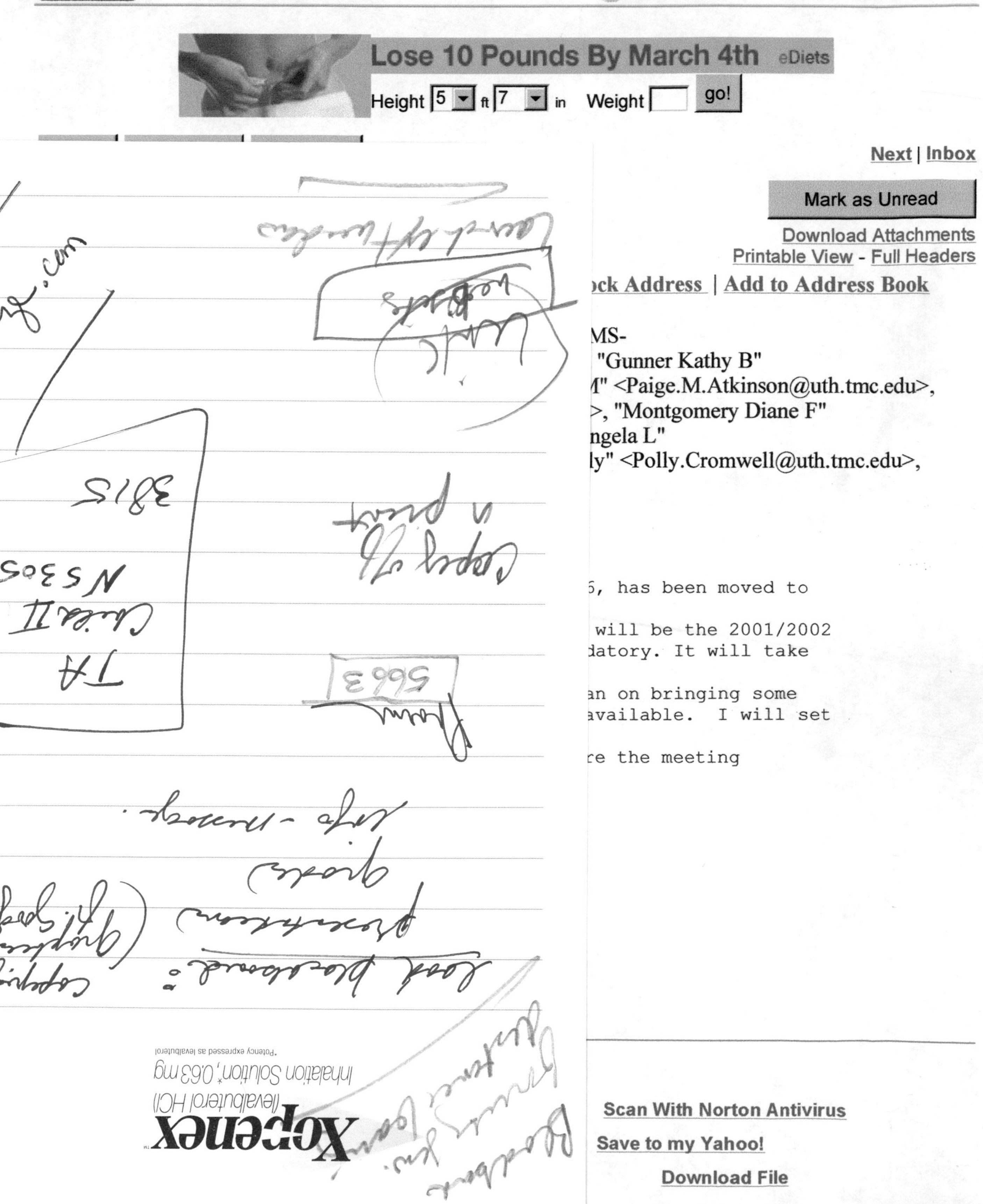

Next | Inbox

Mark as Unread

Download Attachments

Printable View - Full Headers

ock Address | Add to Address Book

MS-
"Gunner Kathy B"
M" <Paige.M.Atkinson@uth.tmc.edu>,
>, "Montgomery Diane F"
ngela L"
ly" <Polly.Cromwell@uth.tmc.edu>,

6, has been moved to

will be the 2001/2002
datory. It will take

an on bringing some
available. I will set

re the meeting

Scan With Norton Antivirus

Save to my Yahoo!

Download File

RSV are all strategies that show promise for future prevention of otitis media.

Care of the child with tympanostomy tubes. Tympanostomy tube placement is the most common surgical procedure performed in children.[11] All providers who care for children will encounter tympanostomy tubes in their practice. Examination of the child with tympanostomy tubes should show a patent tube traversing the pars flaccida. Because the tympanic membrane that contains a tympanostomy tube is not intact, its mobility is affected and pneumatic otoscopy cannot be used as a reliable indicator of the presence of AOM.

Tympanostomy tubes usually are extruded naturally sometime after insertion. Some otolaryngologists recommend actively removing tympanostomy tubes that have been in place for 2 or more years to avoid complications such as chronic perforation or tympanosclerosis. If a tympanostomy tube is visualized in the external canal and is no longer seated within the tympanic membrane, it may be removed with a cerumen spoon under direct visualization.

Occasionally a granuloma may develop at the site of tympanostomy tube insertion, which can lead to bleeding from the external auditory canal. When this occurs, these patients should be referred to an otolaryngologist for intervention.

Otorrhea is common in children with tympanostomy tubes. If otorrhea is associated with other symptoms of upper respiratory infection, it may indicate the presence of AOM and should be treated accordingly. When otorrhea occurs in isolation, it may respond to topical application of an otic solution containing neomycin, polymyxin B, and hydrocortisone. Otorrhea is no more common in children with tympanostomy tubes who swim or submerge their heads in a bathtub than it is in those who do not engage in these activities.[19] The use of topical antibiotics or earplugs does not reduce the incidence of swimming-related otorrhea. Children with tympanostomy tubes who do not dive to depths of greater than 6 feet nor swim in potentially contaminated water (such as a pond) require no special precautions in order to swim, and the use of earplugs or molds may actually increase drainage from the ears.

Complications

The possible effects of otitis media on speech and language development are discussed on p. 1704.

Suppurative complications of otitis media include mastoiditis and intracranial extension of infection. These complications are rare and occur much less frequently than in the era before routine antibiotic treatment of AOM. However, the incidence of these complications has also declined in areas of the world where routine antibiotic treatment of AOM is less common, suggesting that factors other than early antibiotic treatment have contributed to this trend.[7]

It is important to recognize the early signs and symptoms associated with suppurative complications of otitis media so that effective medical or surgical therapy can be instituted promptly. These signs and symptoms include mastoid tenderness, persistent fever associated with chronic tympanic membrane perforation, retroorbital pain on the side of the affected ear, vertigo, and nystagmus. Other focal neurological signs such as facial paralysis, meningismus, and papilledema can also signal intracranial extension of suppurative otitis media.[5]

OTITIS EXTERNA

Otitis externa (OE) is an inflammatory process that involves the structures of the outer ear, specifically the external auditory canal. The site of the inflammation is different from otitis media and the signs and symptoms associated with OE reflect this.

OE can result from trauma to the external auditory canal, the presence of a foreign body, or prolonged exposure to standing water in the canal, which occurs following swimming or bathing ("swimmer's ear"). Inflammation may be focal, at the site of trauma or an infected hair follicle, or diffuse, as is the case with swimmer's ear. When inflammation is focal and associated with infection, the organism is often *Staphylococcus aureus*, which can lead to furuncle formation at the site of the inflammation. The most common organism associated with diffuse inflammation is *Pseudomonas aeruginosa*, a hydrophilic bacterial species. Infection is often polymicrobial.[3] Enteric bacilli and fungi are less common causes of OE.

Children with OE complain of ear pain and may also report pain with chewing (because of the proximity of the temporomandibular joint to the external auditory canal) and difficulty hearing (as a result of swelling within the external auditory canal and conductive hearing loss).

Examination reveals tenderness with manipulation of the pinna or pressure on the tragus. Insertion of an otoscope into the external auditory canal can be painful and should be undertaken carefully. Within the canal, focal erythema and swelling may be seen at a site of trauma or folliculitis. If the inflammation is diffuse, swelling of the entire canal renders a boggy appearance. Edema and the presence of inflammatory debris may prevent complete visualization of the tympanic membrane. The tympanic membrane should appear normal in cases of OE unless there is coexistent otitis media.

Management

When OE is accompanied by furuncle formation, incision and drainage may be necessary. Diffuse OE usually responds to application of a topical otic solution containing neomycin, polymyxin B, and hydrocortisone four times a day. With the patient lying on the unaffected side, five drops of this solution are instilled into the affected ear. The patient should remain in this position for 5 to 10 minutes following instillation to ensure that the medication has come in contact with affected skin. Insertion of a cotton wick can prolong this contact.

OE can be prevented by keeping the external auditory canal dry and by avoiding vigorous cleaning of the canal that can lead to superficial trauma.

Malignant Otitis Externa

Malignant OE is a complicated form of OE that can develop in immunocompromised children or those with severe malnutrition. It is a necrotizing infection of the external auditory canal, usually caused by *Pseudomonas aeruginosa*, which invades the temporal bone leading to osteomyelitis of the base of the skull.[9] Treatment requires administration of intravenous antibiotics and, occasionally, surgical intervention.

REFERENCES

1. Bauer C, Waner M: Laser-assisted myringotomy, *Curr Opin Otolaryngol Head Neck Surg* 7:335, 1999.
2. Chartrand SA, Pong A: Acute otitis media in the 1990s: the impact of antibiotic resistance. *Pediatr Ann* 27:86, 1998.
3. Clark WB, et al: Microbiology of otitis externa, *Otolaryngol Head Neck Surg* 116:23, 1997.
4. Duncan B, et al: Exclusive breast-feeding for at least 4 months protects against otitis media, *Pediatrics* 91:867, 1993.
5. Elidan J, Saah D, Gomori M: Intracranial complications of otitis media, *Ann Otol Rhinol Laryngol* 106:873, 1997.
6. Ey JL, et al: Passive smoke exposure and otitis media in the first year of life, *Pediatrics* 95:670, 1995.
7. Fliss DM, Leiberman A, Dagen R: Medical sequelae and complications of acute otitis media, *Pediatr Infect Dis J* S13:34, 1994.
8. Heikkinen T, Thint M, Chonmaitree T: Prevalence of various respiratory viruses in the middle ear during acute otitis media, *N Engl J Med* 340:260, 1999.
9. Hern JD, et al: Malignant otitis externa in HIV and AIDS, *J Laryngol Otol* 11:770, 1996.
10. Hoberman A, et al: Efficacy of Auralgan for treating ear pain in children with acute otitis media, *Arch Pediatr Adolesc Med* 151:675, 1997.
11. Isaacs D: The management of otitis media with effusion: goodbye to grommets? *Curr Opin Pediatr* 6:3, 1994.
12. Klein JO: Otitis media, *Clin Infect Dis* 19:823, 1994.
13. Klein JO, et al: Epidemiology of acute otitis media in Boston children from birth to seven years of age. In Lim DJ, et al, editors: *Recent advances in otitis media with effusion,* Proceedings of the Fourth International Symposium. Toronto, Canada, 1988, BC Decker.
14. Kvaerner KJ, et al: Distribution and heritability of recurrent ear infections, *Ann Otol Rhinol Laryngol* 106:624, 1997.
15. McCaig LF, Hughes JM: Trends in antimicrobial drug prescribing among office-based physicians in the United States, *JAMA* 273:214, 1995. [Erratum, *JAMA* 279:434, 1998.]
16. Niemala M, Uhari M, Mottonen M: A pacifier increases the risk of recurrent acute otitis media in children in day care centers, *Pediatrics* 96(5 Pt 1):884, 1995.
17. Paradise JL: Short-course antimicrobial treatment for acute otitis media: not best for infants and young children, *JAMA* 278:1640, 1997.
18. Paradise JL, et al: Otitis media in 2253 Pittsburgh-area infants: prevalence and risk factors during the first two years of life, *Pediatrics* 99: 318, 1997.
19. Salata JA, Derkay CS: Water precautions in children with tympanostomy tubes, *Arch Otolaryngol Head Neck Surg* 122:276, 1996.
20. Stool SE, Field MJ: The impact of otitis media, *Pediatr Infect Dis J* 8:S11, 1997.
21. Teele DW, Klein JO, Rosner B: Epidemiology of otitis media during the first seven years of life in children in greater Boston: a prospective, cohort study, *J Infect Dis* 160:83, 1989.
22. Uhari M, Mantysaari K, Niemela M: A meta-analytic review of the risk factors for acute otitis media, *Clin Infect Dis* 22:1079, 1996.
23. Williams RL, et al: Use of antibiotics in preventing recurrent acute otitis media and in treating otitis media with effusion: a meta-analytic attempt to resolve the brouhaha, *JAMA* 270:1344, 1993.
24. Zielhaus GA, Rach GH, van den Broek P: The natural history of otitis media with effusion in preschool children, *Eur Arch Otorhinolaryngol* 247:215, 1990.

246 Parasitic Infections

Thomas Cherian • Leni G. Mathew

Parasitic infections are among the most common problems encountered in children worldwide. In 1996, the reported prevalence of malaria worldwide was 300 to 500 million clinical cases annually. Some 1.5 to 2.7 million people die of malaria each year, and approximately 1 million deaths among children under 5 years of age are attributed to malaria alone or in combination with other diseases. An additional 1 to 2 billion people are infected with helminths. Although they do not contribute significantly to mortality, helminthic infections nevertheless produce significant morbidity, especially in children. Parasites' development of resistance to antiparasitic drugs, vectors' resistance to chemicals designed to kill them, and immunosuppression caused by infection with the human immunodeficiency virus (HIV) or therapeutic agents all have expanded the prevalence and lethality of some parasitic diseases. Most of these infections occur among those living in the lesser-developed regions of the world. In the more developed countries, including the United States, infection usually is seen in travelers to endemic areas and among migrants. However, the ease of travel and increase in the number of migrants from the lesser-developed countries has resulted in an increasing number of cases of parasitic diseases being seen in the developed countries. Therefore, physicians in these countries need to be equipped with sufficient knowledge of the epidemiology, clinical manifestations, and treatment of these infections to be able to effectively deal with them.

EPIDEMIOLOGY

Most people harbor common intestinal parasites with little or no complaint of illness and with small risk of serious sequelae. It therefore is necessary to distinguish between infection and disease. *Infection* occurs when the parasite enters any part of the body, including the integument, and resides, multiplies, or develops there. Some parasites may be unable to develop after entering the human body, but their presence there still constitutes an infection. When the parasite resides on the skin or hair without penetrating the integument or any body orifice, this customarily is referred to as an *infestation. Disease* implies some associated host dysfunction that manifests itself by signs or symptoms. When an infection becomes disease, some change has taken place in the delicate balance between maintenance of the host and survival of the parasite.

Multiple host factors may influence the types, numbers, and invasiveness of parasites causing disease in a given person. These include age, sex, race, occupation, nutritional and immunological status, and the presence of concurrent infection, chronic noninfectious disease, and medications taken. For example, infection with pinworms or dwarf tapeworms is much more prevalent among children than adults, whereas amebic abscesses are more common in adults than children. Prevalence by gender often is a function of occupation or social custom, as illustrated by the increased rate of infection with *Diphyllobothrium latum* (fish tapeworm) among Jewish women because of sampling the gefilte fish before cooking it. Certain races appear to have more natural immunity against infection with a given parasite, such as the relative immunity to malaria seen in some African races. Shepherds in many parts of the world are at greater risk of contracting hydatid disease through handling of their dogs, whose feces disseminate the agent. Immunodeficiency already has been noted as a risk factor in parasitic disease.

Aside from genetic predisposition, no other host variable is as fundamental to limiting the invasiveness and duration of parasitic disease as host nutrition. Protein and iron frequently are deficient in the diets of children in tropical countries. It is in these settings that polyparasitism of children is most evident.

TRANSMISSION OF INFECTION

The spectrum of transmission modalities used by the metazoan parasites of humans is broad but can be covered largely by the following categories: direct, soil dependent, arthropod borne, foodborne, and waterborne.

Direct Transmission

The direct group includes pinworms, dwarf tapeworms, amebas, *Giardia lamblia,* and other parasites that are able to infect humans as soon as they are eliminated by an infected host. Children disseminate such parasites readily among their peers and, to a lesser extent, to adults. Parasites in the direct transmission group often are transmitted in food and water through simple contamination. Superinfections can occur with members of this group through direct reinoculation by way of the fingers—for example, from anus to mouth (i.e., autoinfection).

Soil-Dependent Transmission

Simple. Some parasites, such as *Trichuris trichiura, Ascaris lumbricoides,* and the oocyst of *Toxoplasma gondii,* require a period of development outside the body following deposition of feces onto plants or in soil before their embryos become infective for the next host. Only the embryo, still in its case or cyst, is infective. These organisms frequently reach humans on food contaminated by soil. They also may gain entry in contaminated water consumed by the host.

Complex. The embryos of other parasites (e.g., hookworms, *Strongyloides stercoralis*) molt in the soil and give rise to rhabditiform larvae. When they come into direct contact with skin, these larvae can attach themselves to and penetrate the skin. Humans who go barefoot or recline on soil contaminated by human feces containing these organisms enable the parasites to invade a new host and survive.

Arthropod-Borne Transmission

Parasites in this functional category require a period of metamorphosis in an intermediate arthropod host. Filariasis, malaria, onchocerciasis, leishmaniasis, and trypanosomiasis are examples. In all these examples except Chagas' disease (American trypanosomiasis), the parasite is introduced by the insect's bite. In Chagas' disease, the insect's feces, which contain the parasite, gain entry to the body, most commonly through the bite wound.

Foodborne Transmission

Apart from food contaminated with soil parasites, this group comprises parasites contained in the flesh of cattle, pigs, fish, snails, crustaceans, or encysted on aquatic plants. Generally, the parasite is digested free from its encysted state in the human intestine and then undergoes further metamorphosis to complete its cycle. Humans may be either the intermediate or the definitive host. In the latter case, the adult parasite with the powers of sexual reproduction are found. *Trichinella spiralis,* the tapeworms, and the endocyst of *T. gondii* are but a few examples.

Waterborne Transmission

Aside from embryos that contaminate soil and may gain entry to humans through the water they drink, members of this group gain entry because of a water-dependent life cycle. They may be free forms (e.g., schistosome cercariae, amebae, and *Giardia*), be contained in microscopic copepods (e.g., *Dracunculus medinensis*), or encysted on aquatic plants used as food (e.g., fascioliasis).

For discussions of *G. lamblia* and *Enterobius vermicularis* (pinworm) infections, see Chapters 211 and 251, respectively.

PROTOZOA

AMEBIASIS *(Entamoeba histolytica)*

Epidemiology

Entamoeba histolytica is a protozoan parasite of the human gastrointestinal tract, causing amebic dysentery and amebic liver abscess. It has been estimated that 50 million people worldwide suffer from diarrhea secondary to *E. histolytica* infection and that amebic dysentery and amebic liver abscess kill at least 50,000 individuals yearly. The disease occurs worldwide, but it is more prevalent in areas of poor hygiene and inadequate water sanitation and where human waste is used to fertilize food crops.

Two species of *Entamoeba,* a pathogenic invasive form *(E. histolytica)* and a nonpathogenic, noninvasive type *(E. dispar),* have been described. This explains why certain asymptomatic individuals excrete large number of cysts without any evidence of invasive disease.

Life Cycle and Pathogenesis

E. histolytica completes its life cycle in one host—humans. The mature quadrinuleate cysts (10 to 20 μm) are the infective forms of the parasite. The cysts, when ingested along with contaminated food or drink, enter the alimentary tract, pass through the stomach, and reach the small intestine, where excystation occurs. Ingested cysts, but not trophozoites, can survive the gastric barrier in normal humans. Each cyst liberates four metacystic trophozoites, each of which divides into two mature trophozoites measuring up to 25 μm in diameter. These continue to divide by binary fission. The actively motile trophozoites lodge in the submucous layer of the cecum and rectosigmoid, their normal habitat. After a period, trophozoites transform into precysts and then smaller true cysts, which are passed in the stool. Cysts are infective immediately. Trophozoites may be passed in the stool as well, but they are not infective.

Under certain circumstances, the trophozoites invade the bowel wall, producing flask-shaped ulcers of varying size, with sharply defined borders and a granular base. A proteolytic enzyme secreted by the trophozoites cause destruction and tissue necrosis. The organisms then gradually recede from the dead tissue toward healthy tissue. Trophozoites may also disseminate to the liver, lungs, pericardium, or brain through the blood stream.

Clinical Manifestations

The incubation period ranges from a few weeks to months. Most infected individuals are asymptomatic, but cysts are found in their feces. The most common clinical manifestations of amebiasis are due to local invasion of the intestinal epithelium and dissemination into the liver.

Intestinal amebiasis occurs within 1 to 3 weeks of infection and may manifest with acute abdominal pain, tenesmus, diarrhea, dysentery, or lower abdominal tenderness. Generalized constitutional symptoms and signs are absent in most patients. Acute amebic dysentery occurs in attacks lasting a few days to several weeks; recurrences are very common in untreated patients. Amebic colitis affects all age groups, but its incidence is strikingly high in children between the ages of 1 and 5 years. Occasionally, amebic dysentery is associated with sudden onset of fever, chills, and severe diarrhea resulting in dehydration and electrolyte imbalance. A few patients develop complications such as ameboma (a nodular, tumorlike focus of proliferative inflammation in the wall of the colon), toxic megacolon, local perforation and peritonitis, and extraintestinal extension.

Hepatic amebiasis is a serious manifestation of disseminated amebiasis occurring in less than 1% of infected individuals. It can present along with colitis, but more frequently there is no evidence or history of recent intestinal infection with *E. histolytica*. Most patients (85% to 90%) have a single abscess in the right hepatic lobe. Rarely, multiple abscesses and left hepatic lobe involvement have been documented. An abscess may develop within 2 weeks of initial symptoms or after months of intraluminal infection. Symptoms of abscess formation include pain in the right hypochondrium, fever, anorexia, and fatigue. Most patients have tender hepatomegaly. Bacterial infection occurs more often as the abscess ages. The liver abscess may extend or rupture into the lung, pleural space, peritoneum, or pericardium. Abscess formation is less common in children than adults.

Diagnosis

The diagnosis of amebiasis is based on detection of the organism in stool samples, smears obtained from ulcers by sigmoidoscopy, or tissue biopsy samples. Fresh stool samples should be examined within 30 minutes of passage for motile trophozoites containing erythrocytes. Because single stool examinations pick up only one third of infected patients, at least three stool samples should be examined before excluding the diagnosis of amebiasis.

Serological tests are useful in diagnosing invasive amebiasis and differentiating pathogenic from nonpathogenic infections. Eighty-five percent of patients with invasive intestinal amebiasis of greater than 1 week duration have serum antiamebic antibody, detected by various serological tests. Asymptomatic cyst passers infected by *E. dispar* have negative results by standard serological tests. Indirect hemagglutination antiamebic antibody titers remain higher than 1:128 for years after invasive disease. Other tests, such as counterimmunoelectrophoresis and gel diffusion precipitation, become negative after cure of invasive disease; hence, they are helpful in diagnosing active amebiasis in endemic areas. Recently, detection of serum antibodies to purified parasite antigens, such as galactose adhesin and recombinant galactose adhesin heavy subunit, has enabled specific and reproducible diagnostic methods for pathogenic *E. histolytica* infection. Direct detection of *E. histolytica* antigen in serum or feces by ELISA and epitope-specific monoclonal antibody have also been used to differentiate pathogenic from nonpathogenic infection. In addition, strain-specific DNA probes and polymerase chain reaction (PCR) have also been used to detect *E. histolytica* in feces. These antigen detection tests facilitate early diagnosis before an antibody response has occurred (<7 days) and differentiate pathogenic from nonpathogenic intestinal infection. These are also of great advantage in endemic areas where there is a high prevalence of serum antiamebic antibodies.

The diagnosis of amebic liver abscess pending serological results is based on clinical presentation, recognition of epidemiological risk factors, a lack of predisposing conditions for pyogenic liver abscess, and early use of noninvasive imaging studies. Imaging techniques available are ultrasonography, CT scan, MRI, and gallium scan. None of these are absolutely specific for establishing the diagnosis.

Treatment

Treatment depends on the anatomical location of the organism, the severity of disease, and coexisting conditions such as pregnancy, secondary bacterial infection, and drug reactions. Patients who pass cysts in their stools should be treated because of their role in transmission and the ever-present potential to develop complications such as a liver abscess. The recommended treatment for asymptomatic cyst passers is iodoquinol (30 to 40 mg/kg/day in three doses orally for 20 days) or paromomycin (25 to 35 mg/kg/day in three doses orally for 7 days). An alternative is diloxanide furoate (20 mg/kg/day in three doses orally for 10 days). For patients with intestinal amebiasis or hepatic amebiasis, the treatment of choice is metronidazole (35 to 50 mg/kg/day in three doses to a maximum of 750 mg bid, orally for 10 days). Tinidazole (50 mg/kg to a maximum of 2 g once daily orally for 3 days), a nitro-imidazole similar to metronidazole, is equally effective and better tolerated but is not available in the United States.

A suspected amebic abscess should be aspirated percutaneously when a diagnosis cannot be achieved otherwise, when the patient has not responded to treatment with appropriate therapeutic agents in 3 to 5 days, or when a large abscess, especially of the left lobe, threatens to rupture before it can be controlled with systemic amebic treatment. Surgical drainage of the abscess is seldom required. The abscess should never be drained surgically unless secondary bacterial infection is proved. When surgery is necessary, amebicidal drugs should be given before the procedure. A drainage catheter should be avoided because of the risk of amebiasis cutis.

AMEBIC MENINGOENCEPHALITIS (*Naegleria fowleri, Entamoeba histolytica,* and certain species of *Acanthamoeba, Leptomyxa, Gephyramoeba,* and *Balamuthia*)

General

Several known genera of amebae cause central nervous system (CNS) disease. *E. histolytica* may invade the brain when the agent becomes disseminated, usually when a liver abscess also is present. It causes tissue necrosis with scant, nonspecific pleocytosis and purulent exudate. Signs of meningeal irritation and hemiplegia may occur before lethargy, seizures, coma, and death. Therapy with metronidazole is indicated, but the case fatality rate with cerebral involvement is close to 100%.

Naegleria, Acanthamoeba, Leptomyxa, and *Balamuthia* are small, free-living amebas that cause meningoencephalitis in humans. Amebic meningoencephalitis has two distinct clinical presentations: an acute, fatal CNS infection occurring in previously healthy children and young adults or a chronic granulomatous meningoencephalitis occurring in immunocompromised individuals. Human infection with free-living amebae, though rare, has been reported worldwide.

Epidemiology

Naegleria has been isolated all over the world from river or lake water, domestic water supply, and polluted, heated swimming pool water. Of the six species of *Naegleria,* only *N. fowleri* and *N. australiensis* are pathogenic to humans. These are ameboflagellates that exist as cysts, trophozoites, and transient flagellate forms. Trophozoites are the only invasive form, but cysts are potentially infective since they can convert to vegetative forms.

The portals of entry for human infection are the nasal passages and olfactory neuroepithelium, which are usually exposed to the organism during swimming or bathing. Infection also can occur by inhalation of cysts from dust or soil. Once cysts are inhaled, excystation occurs and the trophozoites penetrate the nasopharyngeal mucosa, migrate to the olfactory nerves, and invade the brain through the cribriform plate. There is widespread cerebral edema and hyperemia of meninges. The olfactory bulbs usually are necrotic and hemorrhagic and are surrounded by fibrinopurulent exudate. The cerebral hemispheres, brain stem, cerebellum, and the upper portion of the spinal cord are involved. Pockets of trophozoites may be seen in the necrotic neural tissue. Cysts are not present in the CNS.

Acanthamebae are opportunistic pathogens that produce granulomatous amebic encephalitis (GAE) in immunocompromised hosts. These organisms have been isolated from soil, vegetables, and brackish and sea water as well as fresh-water sources. Unlike *Naegleria, Acanthamoeba* exists only in two forms, trophozoites and cysts. The trophozoites are slender, with spinelike acanthopodia, and the cysts are wrinkled and double walled. Of the 13 species of *Acanthamoeba,* 7 are pathogenic to humans. These are *A. castellani, A. culberstoni, A. polyphaga, A. rhisodes, A. astronyxis* and *A. palestinensis. Acanthamoeba* cause two distinct clinical syndromes, GAE and *Acanthamoeba* keratitis. The risk factors for keratitis include corneal trauma, exposure to contaminated water while wearing contact lenses, and the use of unsterile, homemade saline solution for contact lens care. The route of CNS infection is hematogenous, originating from eye, skin, or lung infections.

Clinical Manifestations

Following an incubation period of 2 to 7 days, *N. fowleri* produces a rapidly fatal disease known as *primary amebic meningoencephalitis* (PAM), which mimics acute pyogenic meningitis. It is characterized by abrupt onset of headache, fever, nausea, vomiting, pharyngitis, nasal discharge, and signs of meningitis followed by encephalitis. Rarer symptoms include abnormalities of taste and smell; cerebellar ataxia; third, fourth, and sixth cranial nerve palsies; and cardiac abnormalities. Most cases end in death within 1 week of onset of symptoms. Subclinical infections are possible in healthy people when the protozoa colonize the nose or throat.

GAE is an illness of individuals who are immunocompromised and debilitated. Underlying illnesses in these patients include acquired immunodeficiency syndrome (AIDS), neoplasms, renal transplantation, and liver disease. The incubation period ranges from weeks to months. The clinical features often are those of single or multiple space-occupying intracranial lesions. These include hemiparesis, personality changes, seizures, drowsiness, neck stiffness, headache, and fever. The disease may last from weeks to months, but the outcome has been uniformly fatal. Sinusitis; otitis media; granulomatous lesions of the skin, lungs, and genitourinary tract; and corneal ulcers all have been attributed to *Acanthamoeba* species. Dissemination to many distant body organs may occur late in the course, when blood vessel walls have been penetrated.

Diagnosis

A diagnosis of PAM should be suspected in every case of purulent meningoencephalitis in which bacteria are not found. Examination of fresh CSF is mandatory when CSF pressure is not high enough to contraindicate a lumbar puncture. The CSF appears cloudy and slightly hemorrhagic with increased numbers of erythrocytes and polymorphonuclear leukocytes. The protein content is high, and glucose is moderately low. Motile amebae may be seen on a wet mount of the CSF, but often are mistaken for lymphocytes. A cytospin instrument can be used to prepare smears, which can be fixed in Schaudinn's fixative for up to 1 hour and stained with Giemsa stain. Routine Gram stain is not useful. *N. fowleri* cysts are not likely to be seen in tissue or CSF, because infection is rapidly fatal and the patient dies before the trophozoite can encyst. It can be cultured from CSF sediment or brain biopsy samples on agar enriched with *E. coli,* on which trophozoites feed. Retrospective diagnosis can be made on tissue specimens obtained at autopsy by using immunofluorescent antibody assay or immunoperoxidase stain. Serological tests provide no help in the diagnosis of PAM.

CSF examination results in GAE resemble those of aseptic meningitis. Trophozoites are only rarely identified in the CSF. Cranial computed tomography (CT) may reveal space-occupying lesions resembling abscesses, tumors, or hemorrhagic infarction. Histology of these lesions show granulomatous encephalitis with multinucleate giant cells mainly in the posterior fossa structures, midbrain, basal ganglia, brain stem, cerebellum, and rarely, in the cervical portion of the spinal cord. Frontal lobes and olfactory bulbs usually are spared. Both trophozoites and cysts are found in the CNS lesions. Indirect immunofluorescent antibody and immunoperoxidase staining methods can be used on formalin-fixed, paraffin-embedded tissue. *Acanthamoeba,* like *Naegleria,* can be cultured on agar enriched with *Escherichia coli. Acanthamoeba* keratitis may be diagnosed by microscopy and culture of corneal scrapings.

Treatment

Treatment for PAM should be started as soon as the history and clinical picture suggest the diagnosis. Despite the dismal prognosis, treatment with amphotericin B intravenously, intrathecally, and possibly by intraventricular instillation has been recommended. There is some evidence of a synergistic effect when oral rifampin and intraspinal miconazole are administered along with amphotericin B. Survival has been the exception, even with combined therapy.

Effective treatment for acanthamebic encephalitis has

not been established. In vitro research with strains taken from fatal cases has shown the organisms are susceptible to paromomycin, 5-fluorocytosine, pentamidine, ketoconazole, polymyxin B, hydroxystilbamidine, amphotericin B, and sulfa drugs. Treatment with sulfadiazine has been successful in experimental animal infection but only partially effective in human infection.

Combinations of topical propamidine, neomycin, polyhexamethylene biguanide, various azoles, and topical corticosteroids have been used successfully in the treatment of *Acanthamoeba* keratitis.

Surgery has been tried for amebic foci in the brain and elsewhere as a means of halting this highly fatal disease; however, its use must be weighed carefully because of the intrinsic danger of brain surgery where infection is involved and the uncertainty about both the portal and the limiting boundaries of the infection.

All cases of CNS infection from amebae should be treated in a medical setting where neurological, neurosurgical, and infectious disease expertise can be brought to bear on management. Life support systems are essential. Consultation with the Centers for Disease Control and Prevention (CDC) is advisable to make a single repository of experience available to all.

Prevention

Diving or just swimming in contaminated water, especially heated pools, picking one's nose, or aspirating water into the nose all may be ways of acquiring *N. fowleri,* if not other amebic species. Although the route of transmission for Acanthamoeba and other GAE-producing strains is known, it has been suggested that individuals who have a chronic disability or immunodeficiency are at increased risk. This has not been confirmed in all cases. Maintaining a level of 1 part per million (ppm) free chlorine in swimming pools and sterilizing filters frequently is advisable. Waters known to be high in fecal organisms, warm, or stagnant should be avoided for swimming and bathing. Persons using contact lenses must make sure that only fresh, sterile fluids are used to clean lenses and that soiled fingers are not used to handle them.

BABESIOSIS (*Babesia microti, B. divergens, B. bovis,* and other species)

Babesiosis is a malaria-like illness caused by the intraerythrocytic parasite, *Babesia.* It is a tickborne protozoan parasite that infects a broad variety of vertebrate hosts. At least 99 species of *Babesia* infect mammals. Human infections are caused by *B. bovis* and *B. divergens* in Europe (cattle species); by *B. microti* (rodent species) and a recently identified species, *WA 1,* in the Northeastern United States; and by *B. canis* in Mexico. This zoonotic infection is transmitted from wild or domestic animal reservoirs to humans by ixodid ticks, the same vector that transmits *Borrelia burgdorferi,* the causative agent of Lyme disease (see Chapter 233). Rarely, babesiosis may be acquired through blood transfusion or by mother-to-infant transmission.

Epidemiology

Human babesiosis has been reported almost exclusively from the United States and Europe. Most human infections with *B. microti* occur from June through August, when human outdoor activities are at their peak. For efficient transmission of *Babesia,* the tick must be attached to human skin for more than 24 hours. Because of the small size of the tick and painless nature of the bite, the tick may remain attached for a long time without being discovered. Hence, only 10% to 20% of infected persons recall a tick bite. Typically, babesiosis is a mild disease in healthy people; however, in immunocompromised and asplenic individuals the disease can be overwhelming.

Pathogenesis and Life Cycle

With few exceptions, the life cycle of *Babesia* resembles that of malaria. Sporozoites introduced following a tick bite rapidly invade the host red cells, replicate, and eventually rupture the erythrocytes. The intracellular parasite is pleomorphic and exists in tetrads or pairs. The daughter forms, or merozoites, liberated from the erythrocytes then infect other red blood cells (RBCs) and the cycle continues.

Intraerythrocytic multiplication of organisms leads to massive hemolysis and acute renal failure. The mechanism of hemolysis is not known, but parasite-induced damage or autoimmune reactions to the RBC membrane have been implicated. The spleen plays an important role in limiting the intensity of parasitemia by trapping and phagocytosing parasitized erythrocytes. Asplenic patients have a higher level of parasitemia and hence a more severe disease. Both humoral and cell-mediated immunity (CMI) have been demonstrated in babesiosis. However, CMI plays the major role in control of infection.

Clinical Manifestations

The incubation period ranges from 1 to 4 weeks. Symptoms include the insidious onset of malaise, anorexia, and fatigue, followed by high-grade fever with shaking chills, sweating, myalgia, headache, and dark urine. Physical examination may reveal jaundice, pallor, and mild hepatosplenomegaly. Laboratory features include mild to moderate hemolytic anemia, reticulocytosis, thrombocytopenia, and a near normal leukocyte count. In addition, hyperbilirubinemia and elevated transaminases, alkaline phosphatase, and lactic dehydrogenase are observed. An elevated sedimentation rate, a positive direct Coombs' test, hemoglobinuria, and low serum haptoglobin also occur frequently. The proportion of erythrocytes parasitized ranges from 3% to 20% in patients with normal splenic function, but it can be as high as 85% in asplenic patients.

The clinical manifestations of babesiosis differ markedly between European and North American cases. Most of the cases from Europe are caused by *B. bovis* and *B. divergens;* the fatality rate is high in splenectomized patients. In contrast, the North American cases are caused by *B. microti,* and the majority of infections are subclinical or mild. Coinfection with Lyme disease is well known. Patients with both Lyme disease and babesiosis have more severe symptoms and a longer duration of illness than those with either infection alone. Because babesiosis can be transmitted through blood transfusion, it should be considered in the differential diagnosis of a febrile hemolytic disorder following blood transfusion in an endemic area.

Diagnosis

Diagnosis is based on identification of intraerythrocytic parasites on Gram- or Wright-stained, thick or thin peripheral blood smears. Diagnostic criteria include the presence of mild parasitemia, 1% to 10% erythrocytes with multiple ring forms, the presence of extracellular merozoites, and the absence of the malarial pigment, hemozoin. Demonstration of tetrad forms of merozoites is pathognomonic, but these are rare. Absence of hemozoin, schizonts, and gametocytes distinguishes *Babesia* from *Plasmodium falciparum*. Serological tests, including indirect immunofluorescence assays for IgG and IgM antibody, also are diagnostic. In acute infection the titer may be 1:1024 or more, but a titer of 1:64 is considered positive. Antibody titers rise 2 to 4 weeks after the onset of disease and then gradually decline over 6 to 12 months.

Treatment

B. microti infection in individuals with normal splenic function generally is self-limited. Severe symptomatic infection is treated with a combination of quinine (25 mg/kg/day orally in three divided doses) and clindamycin (20 to 40 mg/kg/day intravenously in two doses) for at least 7 days. Clindamycin can be administered orally also. In fulminant cases with a high degree of parasitemia and hemolysis, exchange transfusion is useful. Inadequate response and relapses following treatment with quinine and clindamycin have been reported in patients with HIV infection. Recently, a combination of azithromycin and quinine has been shown to reduce parasitemia and prolong survival in hamsters.

In Europe, babesiosis usually runs a fulminant course, with rapidly increasing parasitemia and massive intravascular hemolysis. Several patients have been treated successfully with quinine and clindamycin. A combination of pentamidine with trimethoprim-sulfamethoxazole was successfully used in a splenectomized patient with mild infection with *B. divergens*.

Prevention

Wearing long sleeves and trousers tucked in at the boot and waist level and using diethyltoluamide (Deet) or permethrin repellent are helpful, as is avoiding known areas of high tick infestation during tick season. However, *Ixodes* ticks are found in urban areas as well as in woods and fields. It is important to inspect the body after outings and to remove promptly any ticks found crawling on the clothing. Hard ticks remain on the body for up to a week or more. A tick should be removed by grasping it with a thin forceps as close to the skin as possible and applying steady, gentle pressure until the tick releases its pincer grasp. It is essential to examine both the tick and the skin site under magnification to ensure that mouth parts were removed. Applying an antiseptic (isopropyl alcohol) and leaving the wound to air dry is adequate treatment if no secondary infection is obvious.

MALARIA *(Plasmodium falciparum, P. vivax, P. ovale, P. malariae)*

Epidemiology

Despite heroic efforts to eradicate malaria after World War II, the problem has worsened since 1965 because of the ban on the use of DDT as an insecticide, the expanding population in endemic areas, growing resistance to antimalarial drugs, vector resistance to other insecticides, and erratic control efforts on the part of governments faced with competing economic needs. The annual incidence of malaria globally is estimated to be 300 to 500 million cases. Approximately 1.5 to 2.7 million people die of malaria each year; approximately 1 million deaths in children under 5 years of age are attributed to malaria alone or in combination with other diseases. The great majority of deaths and 90% of total malaria cases occur in countries in tropical Africa.

Malaria is transmitted from person to person by the bite of the female *Anopheles* mosquito. Four species of plasmodia infect humans: *P. falciparum, P. vivax, P. malariae,* and *P. ovale*. *P. falciparum,* which is the most dangerous, is the predominant malarial parasite in tropical Africa, Southeast Asia, and Oceania; *P. vivax* is the most widely distributed; *P. malariae* is the least common and tends to occur in the cooler climates; and *P. ovale* is uncommon and found largely in Africa.

Life Cycle

When a female *Anopheles* mosquito feeds on a human who has circulating gametocytes (the sexual stage of malaria), the male microgametes fertilize the female macrogametocytes in the mosquito, and the sporogony phase begins. In 1 to 3 weeks, the infective-stage sporozoites are found in the mosquito's saliva and can enter the bloodstream of a human when he or she is bitten by the infected mosquito. Each sporozoite released into the human circulation travels to and enters a liver parenchymal cell (extraerythrocytic stage), where it divides into as many as 40,000 tiny merozoites. When the cell finally ruptures, these merozoites attach to and enter erythrocytes (erythrocytic stage) by a complex process that causes abnormalities on the RBC surface. In the erythrocytes, the parasites mature successively into the ring trophozoite and schizont stages. After maturation, the schizont stage lyses the host erythrocyte, releasing the next generation of merozoites, which invade previously uninfected erythrocytes.

Pathogenesis

The paroxysms of fever in malaria occur when the schizonts rupture from the host erythrocytes to release merozoites. This accounts for the typical pattern of fever seen when synchronous maturation of the parasite occurs in partially immune hosts. This phenomenon has been ascribed to the release of a malarial toxin when the schizont ruptures; however, the nature of this toxin has remained elusive. Recent evidence suggests that tumor necrosis factor (TNF), which is released in response to erythrocyte rupture, is the mediator of the fever. Although a number of substances manufactured by the parasite, including hemozoin, can induce TNF release, it appears that a major toxin, which may be a complex of malarial surface proteins, is responsible for all or most of the response. It also is likely that TNF, which also is a critical mediator for endotoxic shock, is responsible for algid malaria, a form of falciparum malaria involving the gastrointestinal tract that presents with vomiting and/or bloody diarrhea.

The pathogenesis of cerebral malaria still is not well understood. The more persuasive explanations for its causation include the so-called mechanical and toxin-cytokine hypothesis. Parasitization of the erythrocytes by *P. falciparum* results in the expression of a family of proteins, known as the *P. falciparum erythrocyte membrane protein-1* (PfEMP-1), on the surface of the erythrocytes. These proteins are concentrated under electron-dense knobs and cause the adherence of the erythrocytes to a number of endothelial receptors and to one another. The cytoadherence results in mechanical obstruction of the cerebral and other vascular beds. Another suggestion is that a malarial toxin, which may be a complex of malarial surface proteins, may stimulate the release of TNF and other cytokines, which contribute to the severity and neurological sequelae of cerebral malaria.

Clinical Manifestations

The incubation period of malaria varies from 9 to 30 days, depending on the infecting species of plasmodium (*P. falciparum* has a shorter incubation period, whereas *P. malariae* tends to have a longer incubation period) and the acquired immunity produced by the patient. *P. vivax* and *P. ovale* have exoerythrocytic cycles, which are not eradicated with treatment with chloroquine and may result in relapses years after the original infection.

Mild malaria, caused by all species of plasmodium, is characterized by irregular fever. The classic periodicity (tertian, quartan, and quotidian fever) only appears if the disease is protracted without treatment. It rarely is seen in cases of imported malaria. Other features include anorexia, irritability, cough, vomiting, and diarrhea. Anemia and hepatosplenomegaly may be detected on physical examination.

Severe malaria is caused exclusively by *P. falciparum*. In endemic areas, children 1 to 5 years of age are at highest risk; travelers from nonendemic areas are at risk at any age. Severe malaria may present with multiorgan failure, which often is indistinguishable from severe bacterial sepsis. In fact, malaria is a great mimic and must be suspected in any severely ill patient who has traveled to a malaria-endemic area.

Manifestations of severe malaria and complications of falciparum malaria include: (1) cerebral malaria, (2) severe normocytic anemia, (3) renal failure, (4) pulmonary edema or acute respiratory distress syndrome (ARDS), (5) hypoglycemia, (6) circulatory collapse or shock (algid malaria), (7) disseminated intravascular coagulation (DIC), (8) repeated generalized convulsions, and (9) jaundice. Cerebral malaria is the most dreaded form of malaria and is seen more often in children in endemic areas and in nonimmune adults. It is characterized by the presence of unrousable coma (no localizing response to pain), presence of asexual forms of *P. falciparum* in the blood, exclusion of other causes of encephalopathy, and characteristic cerebral histopathological appearances in fatal cases. If the patient has had a seizure, coma must have persisted for more than 6 hours to qualify diagnostically. Generalized convulsions are reported in up to 80% of children with cerebral malaria. Other manifestations include symmetrical upper motor neuron signs, abnormal extensor or flexor posturing, dysconjugate gaze, and retinal hemorrhages. Hypoglycemia is a common complication. The case fatality of strictly defined cerebral malaria is 15% to 20%. Most children who have cerebral malaria have full neurological recovery, but sequelae have been reported in up to 12% of survivors. The common sequelae are hemiplegia, cortical blindness, aphasia, and ataxia. Factors predisposing to sequelae include prolonged coma, protracted convulsions, severe anemia, and a biphasic course characterized by recovery followed by recurrent convulsions and coma.

Congenital malaria may occur in babies born to mothers who have malaria. The infants present in the first few weeks of life with fever, severe anemia, jaundice, and hepatosplenomegaly.

Diagnosis

Examination of a stained peripheral blood smear is still the most reliable method of confirming the diagnosis. A thick blood smear is used to detect the malarial parasite, although species may be identified only by a thin smear. A trained microscopist can detect as few as 10 to 20 parasites per milliliter of blood. Blood smears may be falsely negative because of observer error, prior treatment or prophylaxis, or sequestration of *P. falciparum* in the deep-tissue capillaries. Hence, repeated blood smears must be performed if malaria is suspected.

The quantitative buffy coat (QBC) analysis using acridine orange stain is a rapid screening test. However, it requires the use of a fluorescent microscope and special QBC tubes. Also, the diagnosis has to be confirmed by peripheral smear. Serology is not useful in the diagnosis of acute disease but may be used in epidemiological surveys. Newer tests include the use of DNA and RNA probes, antigen detection using radioimmunoassay and dot ELISA, and PCR.

The search for malaria should not hamper the search for other pathogens since gram-negative sepsis may be a complication in patients with severe malaria. Also, patients residing in endemic areas may have parasitemia without ill effects and may require workup for other suspected pathogens.

Treatment

Chemotherapy. The single most important aspect of managing malaria is early recognition and treatment of *P. falciparum* infection to prevent cerebral malaria and death. Only *P. vivax* and *P. ovale* have the potential for recurrent attacks after the initial circulating disease is treated, because these two species continue to release new "crops" of merozoites from infected liver cells. When a diagnosis of malaria is entertained but the species is unknown, the patient should be treated for *P. falciparum* infection immediately and the

Table 246-1 Chemotherapy of Malaria

Drug	Dosage
All *Plasmodium* Species Except Chloroquine-Resistant Species	
Oral drug of choice:	
Chloroquine phosphate	10 mg/kg base (max: 600 mg) initial dose followed by 5 mg/kg base (max: 300 mg) 6, 24 and 48 hours later
Parenteral drug of choice:	
Quinidine gluconate *or*	10 mg/kg (max: 600 mg) loading dose in saline, IV over 1-2 hr, then 0.02 mg/kg/min continuous infusion until oral therapy can be started.
Quinine dihydrochloride	30 mg/kg/day. Give one third of daily dose IV in 5% dextrose over 2-4 hr every 8 hr until oral therapy can be started (max: 1800 mg/day)
P. falciparum **Acquired in Areas of Known Chloroquine Resistance**	
Oral regimen of choice:	
Quinine sulfate *and*	25 mg/kg/day in three divided doses for 3-7 days
Tetracycline	5 mg/kg (max: 250 mg) four times a day for 7 days
Alternative regimen:	
Oral: Quinine sulfate	25 mg/kg/day in three divided doses for 3 days
Parenteral: Quinidine gluconate or	Same dose as above
Quinine dihydrochloride *and*	Same dose as above
Pyrimethamine-sulfadoxine (Fansidar)	Single dose Age <1 yr: ¼ tablet* 1-3 yr: ½ tablet 4-8 yr: 1 tablet 9-14 yr: 2 tablets >14 yr: 3 tablets
or Mefloquine	15-25 mg/kg PO followed by 10 mg/kg PO 8-12 hr later; maximum total dose, 1250 mg
Prevention of relapses: *P. vivax* and *P. ovale* only	
Primaquine phosphate	0.3 mg base/kg/day (max: 26.3 mg base) for 14 days

Modified in part from Pickering LK, editor: *Red Book 2000: Report of the Committee on Infectious Diseases,* ed 25, Elk Grove Village, Ill, American Academy of Pediatrics.
*25 mg pyrimethamine and 500 mg sulfadoxine.

diagnostic workup continued while the success of treatment is monitored with repeated blood smears. Recurrence of the malaria without continued or repeated exposure can mean drug resistance or the presence of *P. vivax* or *P. ovale*. The standard drug treatment of malaria is summarized in Table 246-1. Quinidine must be substituted for quinine when intravenous (IV) treatment is indicated because IV quinine no longer is available in the United States. Both of these drugs may cause hypoglycemia, even if the patient is given IV glucose. Close attention must be paid to contraindications and warnings supplied by the manufacturer. Consultation with the CDC is advisable when questions of resistance or adverse reactions arise.*

Artemisinin (quinghaosu) derivatives such as artemether and artesunate are replacing quinine in some areas, particularly in China and Southeast Asia. These compounds have been shown to be as effective as quinine in reducing case fatality in severe malaria and have an additional advantage in that some of the derivatives can be administered orally or as rectal suppositories. However, neurotoxicity, in the form of prolonged duration of coma and excess convulsions, in artemether-treated cases compared with those treated with quinine has been a cause for concern. Another concern is the high rate of recrudescence of parasitemia after initial clinical cure. The recrudescence rate after use of artesunate suppositories for 3 days was 40% to 50%. Hence, this drug should be used only when quinine resistance is suspected. It should be administered for a minimum period of 3 days and followed up with an effective dose of mefloquine or any other long-acting effective drug in order to achieve a cure rate of greater than 90%.

Early studies with atovaquone, a new antimalarial drug, showed good initial control but high rates of recrudescence. Combining of atovaquone with proguanil has been shown to have synergistic action, both in vitro and in clinical studies. A fixed combination of atovaquone (25 mg) and proguanil hydrochloride (100 mg) is now available for the treatment of acute, uncomplicated falciparum malaria and results in cure rates of more than 98%. In randomized trials, the combination has been shown to be more effective than mefloquine, chloroquine, or chloroquine plus pyrimethamine/sulfadoxine.

*The CDC's Drug Service telephone number in Atlanta, Georgia, is 1-404-639-3356. The CDC's Parasitic Disease telephone number is 1-770-488-7760.

Table 246-2 Chemoprophylaxis for Malaria*

Drug	Dosage
Areas with Chloroquine-Sensitive Plasmodia	
Chloroquine phosphate	5 mg/kg base (max: 300 mg base) once a week
Areas with Chloroquine-Resistant Plasmodia	
Mefloquine	<15 kg: 5 mg/kg 15-19 kg: ¼ tablet† per week 20-30 kg: ½ tablet per week 31-45 kg: ¾ tablet per week >45 kg: 1 tablet per week
Alternatives	
Doxycycline	2 mg/kg/day (max: 100 mg) orally in children 8 years of age or older
or	
Chloroquine phosphate	Same dose as above
with or without	
Proguanil	<2 yr: 50 mg daily 2-6 yr: 100 mg daily 7-10 yr: 150 mg daily >10 yr: 200 mg daily
and	
Pyrimethamine-sulfadoxine (Fansidar)	Carry a singe dose for presumptive treatment of febrile illnesses. Dosage as under treatment in Table 246-1

Modified in part from Pickering LK, editor: *Red Book 2000: Report of the Committee on Infectious Diseases,* ed 25, Elk Grove Village, Ill, American Academy of Pediatrics.
*Chemoprophylaxis should begin 1 week before entry into an endemic area and continued weekly until 4 weeks after return to a nonendemic area.
†250 mg.

Parasites isolated during recrudescence following treatment with this combination have not been resistant to atovaquone in vitro.

Supportive treatment. Convulsions may be treated with phenobarbital or diazepam. Close attention must be paid to fluid and electrolyte balance. Hypoglycemia is a common complication of severe malaria and should be looked for and corrected, if present. Anemia should be corrected with packed RBC transfusions. Although there are no controlled trials evaluating the use of exchange transfusion, this procedure has the potential to rapidly reduce parasitemia and remove harmful metabolites while replacing the erythrocytes, platelets, and clotting factors. The procedure often is used in nonimmune patients when peripheral parasitemia exceeds 5% to 10%. Gram-negative sepsis must be suspected in patients who present with shock and appropriate antibiotics started after obtaining blood for culture. Corticosteroids, dextran, heparin, and osmotic diuretics have not been shown to be beneficial.

Prevention

The methods used for prevention of malaria include reduction in the population of anopheles mosquitoes, prevention of contact with mosquitoes, chemoprophylaxis, and chemotherapy of infected individuals.

For travelers from nonendemic areas to endemic areas, chemoprophylaxis is the preventive method of choice, though measures to prevent contact with mosquitoes may be taken in addition. The recommended regimes for chemoprophylaxis in travelers are summarized in Table 246-2. Chemoprophylaxis should begin 1 week before entry into an endemic area and continued for 4 weeks after return to a nonendemic area. In endemic areas, chemoprophylaxis may be used in select high-risk populations such as young children and pregnant women.

In endemic areas, measures to control malaria have mainly consisted of chemotherapy of infected individuals, control of the mosquito population, and prevention of contact with mosquitoes.

Most anopheles, which have picked up an infecting dose of gametocytes, die of natural causes before they can transmit infection. Increasing the mosquito mortality by the use of residual insecticides reduces the number of infective mosquitoes to almost zero. DDT was a cheap and effective insecticide. However, mosquitoes are increasingly resistant to DDT. Currently, pyrethroids are the insecticides of choice, because they kill mosquitoes more quickly than DDT and do not accumulate in mammalian tissues. Where the breeding sites of anopheles are limited and can be found easily, the use of larvicides can substantially reduce the density of the adult mosquito population. The organophosphorus compound temefos is the standard insecticide for this purpose and is safe in drinking water.

Measures to prevent contact with mosquitoes have included the use of pyrethroid-treated bed nets, house screening to prevent entry of mosquitoes, use of electrically heated vaporizing mats containing volatile pyrethroids, and the use of repellents such as DEET (*N*-diethyl-meta-toluamide). Pyrethroid-treated bed nets have been used extensively in China and Vietnam, with significant impact on malaria transmission and morbidity. Studies in Africa have shown that these bed nets can reduce the incidence of clinical attacks of malaria by 50% and reduce overall childhood mortality by 20% to 50%.

The malaria peptide vaccine SPF66 has undergone field trials in South America and Africa. In South America the vaccine was associated with significant protective efficacy. However, a study in Gambian infants showed no protective effect. A study in Tanzanian children aged 1 to 4 years demonstrated 30% protective efficacy. Several other malaria vaccines currently are undergoing field trials while new generations of vaccines, including DNA vaccines, are under development.

CHAGAS' DISEASE (American Trypanosomiasis)

Epidemiology and Life Cycle

Chagas' disease is limited to the Western hemisphere and is widely prevalent in Central and South America. It is estimated that as many as 16 to 18 million people are infected with *Trypanosoma cruzi,* the agent that causes American trypanosomiasis, and about 100 million are at risk of infection. It has been estimated that as many as 100,000 immigrants in the United States are carrying the trypanosome. However, a 68% reduction in the rate of infection in the age group 0 to 14 years has occurred since 1985 in a program in Argentina, Brazil, Chile, Paraguay, and Uruguay for control of Chagas' disease.

The human disease is incurred most commonly when feces of the reduviid bug containing the metacyclic trypomastigote of Chagas' disease are rubbed into the bug's bite wound; these insects defecate while sucking blood. The bite wound frequently occurs at the lateral canthus of the eye, the mucocutaneous border of the lip, or other exposed sites on the face or upper limbs. Transmission may also occur transplacentally, by transfusion, or by ingestion or inhalation of reduviid feces.

Once the metacyclic trypomastigote gains access through broken skin, mucous membrane, or conjunctiva, it is engulfed by a macrophage, where it changes into a leishmanial form. This form, the amastigote (without flagellum), divides every 12 hours. Some transform into the blood trypomastigote form before the cell ruptures, while the remaining amastigotes disintegrate after cell rupture. When trypomastigotes enter the bug during a vertebrate blood meal, they change into the epimastigote form in the midgut of the bug and multiply actively in this form without apparent harm to the bug. The epimastigotes undergo another metamorphosis to the infective metacyclic trypomastigote before being passed in the bug's feces.

The wild cycle occurs away from human habitats and involves an unknown number of vertebrate species as definitive hosts and reduviid bugs as intermediate hosts. Fowl and amphibians seem to be immune to infection. The paradomestic and domestic cycles involve wild vertebrates that frequent the yards and barns of humans (e.g., opossums, armadillos, rats, bats) or domestic pets and farm animals.

Clinical Manifestations

Acute phase. The course of Chagas' disease is divided clinically into acute, latent, and chronic phases. The acute phase usually lasts several weeks to several months. The bloodstream largely is cleared of its high-grade parasitemia at this point, but low-grade parasitemia and tissue damage continues for 10 to 20 years or longer. The damage may be due to direct cell infection or autoimmune or toxic inflammation from the continuous disintegration of cells and release of parasitic antigens.

The usual incubation period is 4 days to 2 weeks after percutaneous infection and 20 to 40 days after transmission by transfusion. At the time the patient presents to the physician, the disease may be expressed systemically, but this often is preceded by a localized "chagoma," which consists of an erythematous swelling that may be tender and warm to the touch, at the site of original inoculation. When a chagoma occurs at the lateral canthus of the eye (Romaña's sign), it appears as unilateral, bipalpebral edema associated with enlargement of the lacrimal gland and conjunctival injection. Regional lymphadenopathy usually is present. With the Romaña's sign, the preauricular node is palpable.

With dissemination of the parasite in the bloodstream, the patient experiences fever, often high fever (100.4° to 104° F [38° to 40° C]), which may be intermittent or recurring. Evening peaks or two daily peaks have been described. A transient rash, usually morbilliform, is not uncommon. Edema, which is gelatinous, may be localized to the face or other region of initial infection and to the lower extremities. It can become generalized, especially in fatal cases. Nausea, vomiting, and a persistent diarrhea may be present.

Some degree of myocarditis probably is present in all cases of symptomatic acute Chagas' disease. It usually is mild and may be overshadowed by other aspects of the disease, but it can become severe and is responsible for most deaths occurring in the acute phase. Although organisms occasionally may be found in the CSF, meningoencephalitis is a rare cause of death.

Latent phase. Individuals who survive the acute phase may enter a latent or indeterminate phase during which they are asymptomatic. Low levels of parasitemia persist during this phase and may be demonstrated by xenodiagnosis, which is a method involving laboratory-reared insect vectors. This phase can persist for 10 to 40 years, even for the life of the patient, before chronic manifestations of the disease ensue. Although not much is known about this phase, it is likely that tissue destruction is occurring because the chronic phase is heralded by loss of reserve function.

Chronic phase. The chronic phase manifests most commonly as chagasic heart disease. Chronic heart failure is the most common cardiac presentation. Because the failure is biventricular, it usually is not accompanied by pulmonary congestion. The heart may become grossly enlarged. Tricuspid and mitral valves may manifest regurgitation. A pathognomonic "apex aneurysm," typically of the left ventricle, is present in many cases. However, rupture of this or other aneurysms is extremely rare. All chambers become enlarged, but the right auricle is notable as the source of pulmonary emboli. Loss of cardiac parasympathetic control, with resultant tachycardia, often is blamed for chronic stress on the heart. Most patients show some electrocardiographic (ECG) changes. PR and QT intervals may be prolonged, and partial or complete atrioventricular (AV) blocks and premature ventricular contractions (PVCs) are common. More than half of all cases develop a right bundle branch block, with an anteriorly directed QRS axis. The QRS complexes often show low voltage. Arrhythmias are a common clinical feature of the chronic phase. Complete heart block with Stokes-Adams attacks, high-grade ventricular ectopy, and atrial fibrillation may cause sudden death.

Another common but less life-threatening problem is that created by loss of autonomic control and/or damage to smooth muscle in the hollow viscera. This type of clinical pattern may reflect strain differences in *T. cruzi* or an unexplained host factor. It is most prevalent in central Brazil but has been described elsewhere. Megacolon is slightly more common than megaesophagus. Extreme enlargement of the gallbladder, urinary bladder, ureters, and even the trachea and bronchi have been reported. Symptoms can be remarkably few with megacolon. Some patients go 4 or 5 months without having a bowel movement. The viscous walls are greatly hypertrophied and the lumens grossly enlarged. Fecaloma, volvulus, and rupture of the bowel accompanied by peritonitis are encountered. In megaesophagus, dysphagia, regurgitation, aspiration, and pneumonia occur. Emaciation, anemia, and general disability are common in advanced cases. Esophageal cancer reportedly is more common in Chagas' disease with megaesophagus.

Diagnosis

In the acute phase, the parasite may be detected in blood either by a Giemsa-stained smear or a direct wet mount preparation. In chronic infections, which are associated with low levels of parasitemia, identification of the organism by culture or by xenodiagnosis is required. A number of serological tests, including complement fixation, indirect hemagglutination, indirect immunofluorescence, and enzyme-linked immunosorbent assays (ELISA), are available. The ELISA tests using recombinant antigens are highly sensitive and specific and are currently used for screening blood donors in endemic areas.

Treatment

Two drugs have shown considerable promise in treating acute-phase Chagas' disease. A nitrofuran derivative, nifurtimox, is available from the CDC in the United States (see the footnote on p. 1714). For children 1 to 10 years old, the dosage is 15 to 20 mg/kg/day, administered orally and divided into four doses and given for 90 days. For children 11 to 16 years old, the dosage is 12.5 to 15 mg/kg/day orally, divided into four doses and given for 90 days. For those over age 16, the dosage is 8 to 10 mg/kg/day orally, divided into four doses and given for 120 days. The alternative drug, benzimidazole (Radinil), is available from Roche Laboratories (telephone: 1-800-526-6367), is given at a dosage of 5 to 7 mg/kg/day orally in two divided doses for 30 to 120 days. The addition of gamma interferon to nifurtimox for the first 20 days of treatment has been shown to shorten the acute phase of disease in a limited number of patients and in experimental animals. These drugs are not effective against the forms of the parasite seen in chronic forms of the disease.

Traditional therapy for heart failure is less successful than expected in Chagas' disease, probably because of the reduction in cardiac reserve already present when the patient is first seen and the absolute loss of autonomic neural control that cannot be adequately compensated. Surgery is indicated in the megasyndromes, largely for the complications, previously described.

Prevention

Homes of patients should be examined for vectors. If these are found, the homes should be disinfected with insecticides, the rodent population on which the vectors feed controlled, and habitats for the vectors eliminated. Windows and doors should be screened to prevent further entry of vectors. For campers and hunters, using mosquito netting on an overhead frame and tucked under the bedding, as well as insect repellents (e.g., permethrin) may be useful. Use of new, rapid serological tests to screen blood donors is essential. Six South American countries already require routine blood bank testing for *T. cruzi* antigen. With the many Latin American immigrants already in the United States and Canada, it seems prudent to perform periodic serosurveys of the blood and organs of donors living in areas that have significant populations of immigrants from endemic regions.

LEISHMANIASIS/KALA-AZAR *(Leishmania donovani, L. tropica, L. mexicana, L. braziliensis, L. major, L. aethiopica, L. infantum, L. chagasi)*

Leishmaniasis is a disease of the skin, mucous membranes, and/or the reticuloendothelial (RE) system, depending on which species of this protozoan parasite has infected the host. In recent years, leishmaniasis has acquired significance for several reasons. These include (1) the occurrence of major epidemics of visceral leishmaniasis in India, Bangladesh, and Sudan; (2) the acquisition of infection by American soldiers during the Persian Gulf war; (3) the inclusion of visceral leishmaniasis as a complication of AIDS; and (4) the interest of immunologists in this organism, which survives solely within phagolysosomes.

The World Health Organization (WHO) estimates that leishmaniasis currently affects 12 million people in 88 countries, all but 16 of which are in the developing world. Currently, the global annual incidence is estimated at 1 to 1.5 million cases of cutaneous leishmaniasis and 500,000 cases of visceral leishmaniasis.

Pathogenesis and Life Cycle

The flagellated promastigote of leishmaniasis (15 to 26 μm by 2 to 5 μm) divides by binary fission in the midgut of the phlebotomine fly and escapes through the proboscis, which the fly sticks into the human host's skin to suck blood. These promastigotes are rapidly engulfed by macrophages, but until cellular immunity develops some weeks or months later, the macrophages are unable to kill all the parasites. The promastigote transforms into the oval, nonflagellated amastigote form (2 to 3 μm), which divides in the macrophages by binary fission. Upon cell rupture, the amastigotes are taken up by other macrophages and monocytes, and the cycle continues. These collections of parasitized cells evoke a chronic granulomatous response from the host involving lymphocytes, plasma cells, multinucleated giant cells, and histiocytes. The course of the disease appears to be governed by the interplay of factors that promote spread of the disease (interleukins 4 and 10) and those that inhibit it (gamma-interferon).

Epidemiology

Visceral leishmaniasis typically is caused by *L. donovani* in India and Africa; by *L. infantum* in southern Europe, the Middle East, and North Africa; and by *L. chagasi* in Latin America. Occasionally, species of *Leishmania* that are commonly associated with cutaneous disease, such as *L. mexicana* and *L. major,* have been associated with visceral disease. A small group of American troops who were infected with *L. tropica* during the Persian Gulf War developed a disseminated viscerotropic disease. Classically, the disease occurs sporadically in endemic areas but major epidemics associated with famines, mass migration, and civil disturbance have been reported.

Cutaneous leishmaniasis typically is a sporadic disease in endemic areas. Most cases in the Mediterranean basin, the Middle East, Southern Asia, and Africa are caused by three species—*L. major,* which is endemic in rural desert areas in central Asia, the Middle East and North Africa; *L. tropica,* which is endemic in urban areas in the Middle East, the Mediterranean basin, India, Pakistan, and Central Asia; and *L. aethiopica,* which is endemic in the Ethiopian highlands. In Central and South America, cutaneous leishmaniasis is caused by *L. mexicana* and *L. braziliensis*. The latter, which is endemic in Central America, produces mucosal leishmaniasis in a subset of infected persons.

Clinical Manifestations

Three main clinical presentations of leishmaniasis are described—visceral, cutaneous, and mucosal.

Visceral disease. Most persons infected with *L. donovani, L. chagasi,* or *L. infantum* are asymptomatic or have a mild, self-limiting disease that may not be recognized as leishmaniasis. Only a minority of cases progress to classic visceral leishmaniasis, which presents with insidious onset of fever, malaise, and weight loss. Occasionally the onset may be abrupt. The fever usually is intermittent or remittent, with twice-daily spikes. Physical findings typically include hepatomegaly and splenomegaly; the spleen often is massively enlarged. Peripheral lymphadenopathy has been described in Chinese and Sudanese patients with visceral leishmaniasis. Patients in India often develop hyperpigmentation, which gives this syndrome the name *kala-azar,* or black fever. Less common manifestations include jaundice, bacteremia, and Guillain-Barré syndrome. Laboratory investigations characteristically reveal anemia, neutropenia, thrombocytopenia, and hypergammaglobulinemia. The latter abnormality may be striking, with globulin levels in the range of 9 to 10 g/dl.

Patients with visceral leishmaniasis may develop post-kala-azar dermal leishmaniasis after treatment. This presents with hyperpigmented macules and frank nodules, which may persist over the trunk and extremities for months or years.

Coinfection of HIV and leishmania has been described and occurs most frequently in the Mediterranean basin. Visceral leishmaniasis is the most frequent clinical form, though in HIV-infected populations, involvement of the gastrointestinal and respiratory tracts occurs more frequently.

Viscerotropic leishmaniasis caused by *L. tropica* was described in American troops who served in Saudi Arabia during Operation Desert Storm. These patients presented with chronic low-grade fever, malaise, fatigue, and diarrhea. Massive splenomegaly, wasting, or progressive deterioration associated with classic visceral disease was not encountered, though leishmania were isolated from bone marrow specimens.

Cutaneous disease. Cutaneous forms of leishmaniasis produce a spectrum of disease ranging from a single chronic ulcer (oriental sore) to disseminated, nonulcerative nodular lesions (diffuse cutaneous leishmaniasis). The lesions usually begin with a small, erythematous papule at the site of inoculation of the promastigote. This progresses to form a nodule that then ulcerates, leading to an open sore with raised, firm, reddened borders and either a crusted or weeping granular center. The ulcer widens in most cases, sometimes reaching 5 cm in diameter. When not infected secondarily, the ulcer is painless. It heals slowly from its center, eventually leaving a depressed and hypopigmented scar. In chronic cutaneous cases, the process continues for years, with continuous lesions in an active state.

Patients with anergy may develop disseminated cutaneous nodules that do not ulcerate, developing multiple cutaneous nodules over the face and extremities that progress slowly and persist for decades.

Mucosal leishmaniasis (espundia). Mucosal lesions involving the nose, mouth, pharynx, or larynx may occur in a few patients infected with *L. braziliensis* months to years after the cutaneous lesions have healed. The disease typically begins with nasal congestion followed by ulceration of the nasal mucosa and perforation of the nasal septum. In rare instances the cheeks, soft palate, pharynx, or larynx are involved. Although mortality is low, the disease may produce considerable morbidity and disfigurement.

Diagnosis

Smears of aspirates or scrapings and biopsy material, when stained with Giemsa, may demonstrate the amastigotes in macrophages. The highest yield is from splenic aspirates, though the organism may often be demonstrated on a bone marrow aspirate. Flagellated forms are found in positive tissue cultures on NNN (Novy, Nicolle, and McNeal) medium. The Montenegro (leishmanin) skin test does not yield a positive result until the ulcerative phase and is of little value in diagnosis. It has been useful as a survey tool to establish endemic zones. A number of serological tests and molecular diagnostic tests, using PCR, have been described but there have been concerns about their specificity. Conventional methods using microscopy and culture remain the mainstay of diagnosis.

Treatment

Pentavalent antimonials and amphotericin B have been used as therapy for decades, but a high rate of toxicity has encouraged the development and testing of a number of other potentially curative agents. Stibogluconate sodium, a pentavalent antimonial drug, is the standard drug of choice and is given in a dose of 20 mg/kg/day intravenously or intramuscularly for 20 to 28 days. Chemical pancreatitis is seen in the majority of patients treated with stibogluconate, but this does not always necessitate discontinuation of therapy.

Amphotericin B is effective in cases of kala-azar that are clinically resistant to antimony and pentamidine. It has been used at a dose of 0.25 to 1 mg/kg by slow IV infusion on a daily or every-other-day basis for periods up to 8 weeks. Amphotericin in a dose of 0.5 mg/kg every other day for 14 days (total dose 7 mg/kg) has been shown to be as effective as higher doses. Liposomal or lipid-associated amphotericin B at a dose of 3 mg/kg daily or every other day for 5 or 6 doses has also shown high efficacy.

Pentamidine (diamidinophenoxypentane) has been used as a second-line drug. Ketoconazole and allopurinol, local heat, and cryotherapy also have been credited with some success.

Aminosidine, produced by *Streptomyces rimosus* (and virtually identical to paromomycin) has been used with considerable success and has been well tolerated. However, ototoxicity occurs and must be considered a risk, especially if serum titers of aminosidine exceed the recommended dosage.

Combinations of the above agents have been used in clinically resistant cases.

Intralesional stibogluconate and topical paromomycin-containing formulations have been successfully used for the treatment of cutaneous leishmaniasis.

Prevention

Because of the wild parasitical life cycles that perpetuate the disease, which cannot be eradicated, and because of the absence of safe, inexpensive drugs that can attack the intracellular parasite, vaccines are the most viable long-term hope for reducing the human burden of leishmaniasis. Screening domiciles effectively, using insect repellents, and limiting exposure to phlebotomine fly bites from dusk to dawn are important. Early presentation and appropriate treatment can reduce complications.

Several candidate vaccines against leishmaniasis are in different stages of development and testing. The approaches to vaccine development that have been used include killed *Leishmania* organisms in combination with BCG; live, attenuated organisms (e.g., the DHFR/TS-strain); subunit vaccines; crude fractions of the organism; and recombinant viruses and bacteria expressing leishmanial antigens. Although several antigens have been shown to induce protective immunity in animal models, it is unlikely that any one molecule alone will be sufficient to protect against the complex group of parasites that cause leishmaniasis. A combination of well-defined antigens is more likely to overcome the strain/species specificity that is likely to be observed when one molecule alone is used.

TOXOPLASMOSIS *(Toxoplasma gondii)*

Toxoplasma gondii is an obligate intracellular protozoan parasite of the class Sporozoa that can infect most vertebrate animals, including avians and some reptiles. It was first described by Nicolle and Manceaux in 1908. Members of the cat family are the definitive hosts of the organism. Humans and other vertebrates become intermediate hosts when they ingest the oocysts shed in the feces of cats. *T. gondii* exists in three forms: an oocyst that produces sporozoites; a proliferative and invasive form known as *tachyzoite;* and the tissue cyst, which has an intracystic form termed *bradyzoites*. The tachyzoites and tissue cysts occur in the extraintestinal tissues of cats and are the only form of parasite in other mammalian and avian hosts. The oocyst is formed only during the enteroepithelial stage of infection in members of the cat family. *T gondii* infection is acquired when bradyzoites within tissue cysts or sporozoites within oocysts are ingested.

Epidemiology

T. gondii infection is ubiquitous and is one of the most common latent infections of humans throughout the world. The prevalence of infection varies considerably with geographical location—colder regions and hot, dry places have a lower incidence than warmer, humid areas. Higher rates of seropositivity have been noticed in areas where there is more frequent ingestion of under-cooked meat or environmental contact with cat excrement. Congenital infection results from acquisition of primary infection in seronegative mothers during pregnancy. It is least frequent but most severe when the mother acquires and transfers infection in the first trimester and most frequent but with fewer clinical signs at birth when the infection is acquired in the third trimester.

Pathogenesis and Life Cycle

The asexual cycle in humans begins with ingestion of oocysts from the environment or the ingestion of tissue cysts in uncooked or inadequately cooked meat. The trophozoites are liberated in the gastrointestinal (GI) tract and immediately invade the epithelial cells, where the parasite-bearing vacuole protects the parasite from lysis by methods not fully clarified. Trophozoites divide repeatedly by endodyogeny until the cell ruptures and releases more trophozoites. The trophozoites are oval or curved, approximately 3 to 7 μm long, and infective; they may be disseminated via the circulatory and lymphatic vessels. They typically attack the cells of the skeletal muscles, brain, cardiac muscle, lymph nodes, eye, and lung but may infect other organs. A mild initial mononuclear cell response (with some polynuclear cells) is typical, and edema usually is present. In immunocompetent individuals, the dissemination of trophozoites soon diminishes, and both humoral and cellular immunity components become measurable. Oocysts are not shed in the feces of animals other than the cat family. However, not all *Toxoplasma* organisms are killed, even in an immunocompetent host. Some trophozoites develop into a tissue cyst that may remain dormant and viable for life or may rupture in response to a change in the host's immune status. Necrosis may occur in the initial infection but usually is limited in an immunocompetent host. Necrosis that occurs secondary to release of trophozoites after a fully active immune response has developed may cause significant impairment, especially in the eye and brain. The inflammatory response in these later lesions involves a granulomatous picture with plasma cells, monocytes, lymphocytes, and sometimes, the organisms. Edema and endarteritis are reported.

The cycle of infection in cats begins with ingestion of infected cat "kills" (rats, mice, birds) or inadequately cooked kitchen scraps. Licking its own dirt-contaminated fur might also cause infection. The trophozoites released from ingested oocysts or tissue cysts invade the GI epithelial cells and multiply, as in humans, but the sexual stage of trophozoite differentiation into gametocytes occurs in the second generation of multiplication. Their union leads to the oocyst (10 to 12 μm), that is passed in the cat's feces. After an incubation period that varies in length (days to several weeks) and systemic infection, a cat having its first infection passes millions of oocysts in its feces daily for as long as 3 weeks, sometimes longer.

Clinical Manifestations

Congenital disease. The risk for the fetus depends on when the mother has her first infection with *T. gondii*. The risk of acquiring the infection is less for the first trimester (15% to 20%) and greatest for the last trimester (60% to 65%). However, when infection does occur earlier in gestation, the risk of a serious outcome is much greater because of the expansion of the impact of a few cells destroyed in early development. Some infections in fetuses remain undetected after birth, but such infants can show significant impairment later. Others are born with hepatosplenomegaly, hydrocephalus or microcephaly, seizures, neurological deficits, jaundice, rash, chorioretinitis, and anemia. Symptoms and signs of meningoencephalitis may be present. Roentgenograms may show bilateral, scattered punctate calcifications (infection with cytomegalovirus [CMV], conversely, has a pattern of paraventricular calcifications). Obstruction of the aqueduct of Sylvius can result in ventricular enlargement and hydrocephalus. Cerebromalacia can lead to microcephaly and microphthalmia. The CSF may show xanthochromia, increased protein (as high as 2 g/dl in the ventricular fluid), and increased numbers of RBCs and WBCs. The latter predominantly are mononuclear. At autopsy, widespread vasculitis and parenchymal cell necrosis is found, including myocarditis, encephalitis, pneumonitis, and polymyositis. Stillbirths occur, and mortality in the first few months of life is high in live births that demonstrate the classic picture. A third type of congenital clinical picture is the infant who appears normal at birth but proves to have had slowly progressive lesions of the brain or eye that are detected much later. Most survivors develop sequelae, usually serious, involving the brain or eye. *T. gondii* infection in more than one child of a given mother is possible in cases of maternal HIV infection.

Acquired disease. Primary infection in an immunocompetent child could be asymptomatic or self limiting, with nonspecific symptoms and signs. Cervical lymphadenopathy with or without fever, myalgia, fatigue, and neck stiffness are the common clinical features. Lymphadenopathy is sometimes generalized and tender but without suppuration. Rarely, acute infection can cause myocarditis, pericarditis, encephalitis, meningitis, or hepatitis and can be fatal. Primary infection not involving the vital organs always resolves without treatment.

Disease in immunodeficient patients. Infection in immunocompromised patients may be primary or reactivation of latent infection. The infection is widespread and often fatal. The CNS, lungs, and eyes frequently are involved. Rarely, multiorgan involvement presenting with respiratory failure and hemodynamic abnormalities similar to septic shock occurs. *Toxoplasma* infection of the brain in patients who have AIDS may be localized or disseminated. Typical symptoms and signs include fever, headache, altered mental status, psychosis, seizures, and focal neurological deficits. Because serological tests are likely to be negative and culture of the organism requires time, a high index of suspicion is warranted for early recognition and treatment. For this reason, some advise therapy if infection is suspected at all.

Ocular disease. *Toxoplasma* infection is an important cause of chorioretinitis in the United States and Western Europe. In the majority of patients, it is congenitally acquired and is bilateral. Approximately 35% to 40% of acquired chorioretinitis is due to *Toxoplasma* infection. Acute chorioretinitis presents with blurred vision, photophobia, epiphora, and loss of central vision caused by involvement of the macula. On funduscopic examination, the characteristic lesions appear to be yellowish, creamy, and raised, with distinct margins and satellite lesions. On healing, the lesions become pale and atrophic, with black pigment along the border giving a rosette appearance. Rarely, panuveitis may occur. Papillitis usually is associated with overt CNS disease. Acquired infections are characteristically unilateral. Relapses are frequent but rarely are associated with systemic symptoms or signs. Other ophthalmic manifestations in congenital infections include strabismus, nystagmus, microphthalmia, phthisis, microcornea, cataract, retinal detachment, and optic atrophy.

Diagnosis

The diagnosis of *Toxoplasma* infection can be made either by demonstration of the organism in various specimens or by serological tests.

Organisms are isolated by inoculating body fluids, leukocytes, or tissue specimens into mice or tissue culture. Body fluids should be processed and inoculated immediately. Six to 10 days after inoculation, or earlier if the mouse dies, tachyzoites can be demonstrated in the peritoneal fluid. At 6 weeks, tissue cysts can be seen in the mouse brain. Tissue culture specimens demonstrate areas of necrosis with numerous extracellular tachyzoites. Tachyzoites can be stained with Giemsa or Wright stain but are best demonstrated with immunoperoxidase stain or immunofluorescent antibody technique. Tissue cysts are diagnostic of infection but do not differentiate between acute or chronic infection; however, the presence of numerous cysts suggests acute infection. The tissue cysts stain well with Periodic acid Schiff and silver stain, as well as with immunoperoxidase.

Various serological tests are used to confirm the diagnosis of *Toxoplasma* infection. The Sabin Feldman dye test, measuring IgG antibody, is sensitive and specific. It is based on the observation that parasites obtained from peritoneal exudates of mice, when incubated with normal serum for 1 hour at 37° C, appear swollen and stain deep blue when alkaline methylene blue is added. The results are expressed as IU/ml. IgG or IgM florescent antibody tests, IgM, IgA or IgE ELISA, IgM or IgE immunosorbent assay (ISAGA), enzyme linked immunofiltration assay, indirect hemagglutination tests, PCR, and lymphocyte blastogenesis to *Toxoplasma* antigen are various other tests available for the diagnosis of Toxoplasma infection.

Ideally, a woman's serological status should be known before she conceives. If seropositive, no further tests are needed unless she is immunocompromised. When this information is not available, it is useful to determine the serological status of pregnant women at the initial visit. If the test is positive, serum should be tested for IgM antibody or for a rise in titer of IgG antibody after 3 weeks. If these suggest a recent infection and she is in the first or second trimester, therapeutic abortion may be considered. In immunocompromised mothers, the fetus is at risk for congenital *Toxoplasma* infection even if the mother was seropositive before pregnancy. Fetal blood sampling, fetal ultrasound examination, and analysis of amniotic fluid are used in prenatal diagnosis of congenital toxoplasmosis. Isolation of *T. gondii* from fetal white blood cells or from amniotic fluid, PCR testing of the amniotic fluid, or detection of *Toxoplasma*-specific IgM antibody in the fetal blood are diagnostic of congenital infection. When congenital infection is suspected after birth, the following studies should be performed: general, neurological, and ophthalmic examination; CT scan of the brain; isolation of the organism from the placenta or from umbilical cord WBCs; and measurement of *Toxoplasma*-specific IgG, IgM, IgA, or IgE antibodies, as well as total serum IgG and IgM. CSF should be analyzed for cells, glucose, protein, and *Toxoplasma*-specific antibodies.

In immunocompetent patients, the presence of *Toxoplasma*-specific IgM antibody or a fourfold rise in *Toxoplasma*-specific IgG titer in sera obtained 3 weeks apart and tested in parallel is diagnostic. Recent seroconversion is suggestive of infection, provided the patient has not acquired antibodies from a blood transfusion. Demonstration of classic histopathological changes or isolation of organisms from various tissues are definitive indications of infection. In immunocompromised patients, IgG antibody titers may be low and *Toxoplasma*-specific IgM is often negative. Demonstration of *Toxoplasma* antigen or DNA in serum, blood, or CSF signifies disseminated infection. A CT scan or MRI showing a space-occupying lesion in the brain or resolution of a radiological lesion following a therapeutic trial of pyrimethamine and sulfadiazine also are suggestive of infection. Rarely, a brain biopsy is indicated to establish the diagnosis of *Toxoplasma* encephalitis. The diagnosis of ocular infection is based on characteristic fundal changes and abnormal serology.

Treatment

Treatment of acquired toxoplasmosis in an immunocompetent host rarely is necessary. Treatment should be considered when HIV infection or other immunosuppression is a factor, when visual problems are present and progressive, when signs and symptoms become chronic, or when known accidental inoculation occurs in a seronegative host. Currently, combined therapy with pyrimethamine and sulfadiazine is believed to prevent replication of the organism, but it does not inactivate tissue cysts or kill trophozoites. The pediatric dose of pyrimethamine is 2 mg/kg/day for 3 days, then 1 mg/kg/day to a maximum daily dose of 25 mg given for 4 weeks. Sulfadiazine is given in a dose of 85 to 100 mg/kg/day in four divided doses for 3 to 6 weeks. Adequate hydration should be maintained, and folinic acid, in a daily dose of 5 mg, is given with the pyrimethamine to counteract its inhibition of folate synthesis. The patient should be monitored by means of complete blood and platelet counts twice weekly to detect bone marrow suppression. The decision whether to treat a pregnant woman involves balancing the risk of teratogenic effects on the fetus from pyrimethamine with those from untreated congenital toxoplasmosis; expert consultation is advised. For adult patients with HIV who have *T. gondii* encephalitis, a multicenter study found the following regimen to be effective: sulfadiazine (1 to 2 g four times daily), pyrimethamine (25 to 50 mg/day), and leucovorin calcium (5 to 10 mg/day) for up to 180 days. Toxicity (especially bone marrow depression) necessitated treatment cessation in a large percentage of cases, most often between days 14 and 28 of therapy. This regimen was followed by daily therapy for life using pyrimethamine/sulfadiazine. Azithromycin, clindamycin, clarithromycin, and spiramycin have been tried both alone and in combination with pyrimethamine, with mixed results. The author recommends consultation with a pediatric AIDS treatment group or the CDC (see the footnote on p. 1714), since most trials reported involve adults. Some experts recommend the use of corticosteroids for active ocular disease in conjunction with the therapy described above. Sulfadiazine is available through the CDC (telephone: 1-404-639-3356) and spiramycin through the U.S. Food and Drug Administration (telephone: 1-301-594-1012).

Prevention

The ubiquitous nature of *T. gondii* and the ease of its transmission make prevention difficult, especially in children. Those who would benefit most from prevention are women of childbearing age and immunodeficient individuals. Avoiding contact with cats, cat litter, and yard or farm dirt (e.g., no gardening, at least without gloves, and very thorough washing and nail cleaning afterward) is important, as is cooking meat adequately, especially pork and mutton. Holding meat below –4° F (–20° C) until ice crystals form on the outside may reduce or destroy infectivity. Cooking the center of meat to at least 151° F (66° C) kills the infective cysts. An oven thermometer should be used. All fruit and vegetables should be washed thoroughly, and raw meat and unwashed fruit and vegetables should be handled with impermeable gloves.

CRYPTOSPORIDIOSIS *(Cryptosporidium parvum)*

Cryptosporidium parvum is a coccidian protozoan parasite that belongs to the same family as *Isospora* and *Toxoplasma*. Although it was discovered in 1907, its importance as a human pathogen has been recognized only since 1982. In recent years it has been recognized as a cause of diarrhea in previously healthy individuals and severe, life-threatening diarrhea in patients with AIDS. The organism is 2 to 6 μm in diameter and infects the epithelial cells lining the digestive tract of fish, birds, reptiles, and mammals, including humans.

Epidemiology

Cryptosporidium is an ubiquitous parasite. It is associated with diarrheal illness worldwide, especially in developing countries. Reported rates of *Cryptosporidium* infection in patients who have diarrhea are 2.1% and 6.1% in industrialized and developing countries, respectively. About 3.5% of children with AIDS reported to the CDC have cryptosporidiosis. Reviews of HIV-infected persons with diarrhea showed cryptosporidium infection in 14% to 24%. Seroepidemiological studies have shown that 17% to 32% of healthy individuals in the United States have evidence of infection by young adulthood. In contrast, more than half of children under the age of 5 in rural China and 90% of infants in an impoverished area in Brazil have been reported to have serological evidence of infection. Several well-documented outbreaks of cryptosporidiosis have occurred, including a large waterborne outbreak in Milwaukee in 1993, which affected an estimated 403,000 people. Although contamination of the water supply was responsible for this outbreak, outbreaks involving swimming pools and wading pools and ingestion of contaminated pressed apple cider have also been reported. Person-to-person spread of *Cryptosporidium* in households and institutions such as day care centers and hospitals also is well documented.

Pathogenesis and Life Cycle

Infection is acquired by ingestion of thick-walled oocysts. The oocysts are not destroyed by chlorination or removed by routine filtration, accounting for the outbreaks involving public water supplies and swimming pools. In the upper small bowel, the action of proteolytic enzymes and bile salts enhances excystation and release of four infectious sporozoites, which enter the brush border of the surface epithelium. Here the trophozoites develop into merozoites. After release the merozoites may enter adjacent cells and continue asexual reproduction or enter the sexual form of reproduction, resulting in the formation of microgametocytes and macrogametocytes. The sexual stages combine to form oocysts; the thin-walled oocysts sporulate and cause infection in the same person, whereas the thick-walled oocysts are excreted. Infection generally is limited to the superficial surface of the intestinal epithelium, but in immunocompromised individuals, infection may spread to involve the biliary tree and pancreas. Extraintestinal infection has been reported rarely, most commonly in the respiratory tract.

The precise mechanism by which *Cryptosporidium* causes diarrhea is not known. Studies in animal models have demonstrated the loss of vacuolated villous tip epithelium accompanied by an approximate 50% reduction in glucose-coupled sodium cotransport. Based on further studies in animal models, researchers have proposed a prostaglandin-dependent secretory effect that occurs through a bumetanide-inhibitable chloride secretory pathway and by the inhibition of neutral sodium chloride absorption through the amiloride-sensitive sodium hydrogen exchanger, predominantly in the junctional or transitional epithelium.

Clinical Manifestations

Acute infection is characterized by watery diarrhea, abdominal cramps, fatigue, weight loss, myalgia, fever, and vomiting. The incubation period is 2 to 14 days. The mean duration of diarrhea among those affected in the Milwaukee outbreak was 12 days (range 1 to 55 days). The mean maximum number of stools was 19 per day (range 1 to 90 per day), and the median weight loss was 10 lb (range 1 to 40 lb). Thirty-nine percent of those affected during this outbreak had a recurrence of diarrhea after a 2-day, symptom-free period. Recurrence was thought to be due to reinfection through exposure to their own oocyst-laden feces, to the presence of a specific stage of the organism, or to the expression of a specific pathogenic factor.

Among patients with HIV infection, those with preserved immunological function are able to clear infection whereas those with CD4 counts less than 180 cells/mm^3 tend to have chronic diarrhea of waxing and waning nature and significant weight loss. About 10% to 15% of HIV-infected persons with cryptosporidiosis have involvement of the biliary tree, leading to sclerosing or acalculous cholangitis. This presents with fever, right upper quadrant pain, jaundice, and nausea and vomiting, with or without diarrhea. Investigations reveal elevated alkaline phosphatase and gamma glutamyl transpeptidase. Sonograms may reveal a dilated, thick-walled gall bladder. If there is stenosis of the common bile duct, the extrahepatic ducts usually are dilated. Rarely, pancreatitis may occur as a result of infection of the pancreatic duct. *Cryptosporidium* oocysts have been detected in the respiratory tract of patients presenting with cough, dyspnea, wheezing, croup, and hoarseness. However, not all symptoms can be attributed to *Cryptosporidium,* since other pathogens often are present conjointly.

Diagnosis

The diagnosis is made by demonstration of oocysts in the stool by acid-fast or immunofluorescence staining. Appropriate concentration methods and testing multiple stool specimens will enhance detection. Several ELISA methods are available for detection of cryptosporidial antigen in stool specimens, though these methods may have low sensitivity in formed stool specimens. Endoscopic biopsy specimens reveal *Cryptosporidium* in less than 10% of patients in whom stool specimens are negative. PCR may help in detection of *Cryptosporidium* in water supplies or in asymptomatic carriers.

Treatment

In immunocompetent patients, cryptosporidiosis is a self-limiting disease and no therapy, except maintenance of hydration, is required. In those who have severe infection, including immunocompromised patients, several antimicrobial agents have been used but with no consistent success. Paromomycin, a nonabsorbable aminoglycoside, has been shown to improve symptoms in approximately 50% of patients, though complete resolution with eradication of the parasite occurs in only 10%. Other agents that have been tried with varying success include the macrolide antibiotics spiramycin and azithromycin.

Immune-based therapies such as hyperimmune bovine colostrum and bovine transfer factor have shown some benefit, though trials have been limited because of cumbersome production techniques and difficulty in standardizing batches of the products.

Cryptosporidial diarrhea is voluminous, and utmost attention must be paid to correction of dehydration and electrolyte abnormalities. Nutritional support is required, especially for those with chronic symptoms. Nutritional supplements containing medium-chain triglycerides may be better absorbed in patients with small intestinal abnormalities. Milk and dairy products should be avoided because lactose intolerance is common. Antimotility drugs such as loperamide and diphenoxylate/atropine (Lomotil) may be used for symptomatic relief. New approaches to speeding repair of the disrupted intestinal barrier using glutamine and its derivatives currently are being evaluated.

Prevention

Resistance to chlorination and ineffectiveness of conventional methods of filtration are responsible for some waterborne and swimming pool outbreaks. Immunocompromised individuals who want to take independent precautions may reduce risk by boiling water intended for drinking for 1 minute. Alternatively, microstraining filters or high-quality bottled water may be used. Filters that are considered effective in removing cryptosporidial oocysts include those that filter water by reverse osmosis, those that have "absolute" 1-µm filters and those that meet National Sanitation Foundation (NSF) standard (No. 53) for cyst removal. Strict contact precautions must be observed for hospitalized patients, especially those who are incontinent or diapered.

CESTODES

TAPEWORM/CYSTICERCOSIS *(Taenia saginata, T. solium)*

Human infestations may be caused either by the adult tapeworms residing in the intestinal lumen or by the larval forms, which infect the tissues. Humans are the definitive hosts for the intestinal forms, which are acquired by ingestion of the larval forms in infected meat or fish. In case of tissue infection with the larval forms, humans are accidental intermediate hosts.

Humans acquire *Taenia solium* (pork tapeworm) and *T. saginata* (beef tapeworm) when they consume inadequately cooked meat containing the larval form of one of these cestodes. As a definitive host, humans harbor the adult tapeworm in the small intestine. If a human happens to ingest eggs of the pork tapeworm, as by contamination of food or drink with feces from a person harboring the worm, the eggs release larvae that form cysts in the victim's tissues. Both parasites have a worldwide distribution, the actual prevalence varying greatly depending on the number of animals, meat-eating habits, and the amount of human fecal contamination of rangeland. Tapeworm disease caused by *Taenia* species can be prevented by cooking all meat adequately—that is, to at least 150° F (65.5° C) measured at the center of the meat with a meat thermometer.

With the increasing availability of neuroimaging studies and serosurveys using the enzyme-linked immunotransfer blot (EITB) assay, it has become clear that cysticercosis is more widely prevalent than previously appreciated. It has been estimated that about 50 million people are infected with the cyst stage worldwide. The areas with highest prevalence are Mexico, Central and South America, India, and sub-Saharan Africa. Studies in Mexico showed the presence of at least one CNS cysticercus in 0.4% to 3.5% of unselected autopsies. Studies in India have shown that up to half of all patients with afebrile seizures have serological evidence of cysticercosis. With the recent influx of immigrants from Latin America and Asia, cysticercosis is being increasingly recognized in the United States.

Pathogenesis and Life Cycle

The adult worms (strobilae) are segmented and consist of a head (four suckers and a rostellum armed with 22 to 32 hooklets in *T. solium* but no hooklets in *T. saginata*), a neck, and proglottids. Proglottids may be immature, mature, or gravid and contain both male and female reproductive organs and large numbers of eggs. These proglottids eventually drop off, or strings of them may break off the worm, and are carried or migrate out of the anus. *T. saginata* proglottids are more muscular, but those of either species may actually crawl after exiting the body. The eggs may leave the proglottid before or after it detaches from the rest of the strobila. Eggs are infective for weeks to months under favorable conditions. They continue their cycle when ingested from plant or soil by an appropriate intermediate host animal. The larvae released from the eggs penetrate the intestinal mucosa, reach the lymphatic or blood vessels, and are carried to all parts of the body, especially muscles and connective tissues. In 2 months or more, they become encysted scolices and remain viable in the muscle for years. The scolex matures fully to a tapeworm when meat containing a live scolex is eaten. Both *T. solium* and *T. saginata* gain maturity in the human bowel in about 12 weeks, eventually reaching lengths of 2 to 7 meters and 5 to 15 meters, respectively. The eggs of the two species cannot be distinguished microscopically. When a human ingests the pork tapeworm eggs (or possibly when these move in a retrograde direction in the bowel after release from a proglottid), the larvae are digested free from the eggs and enter the circulation. The larvae may attach and encyst anywhere in the body. An increase in size of the cysticercus may produce a significant pathological condition, especially when it is present in the intracranial space.

Clinical Manifestations

A single tapeworm of either pork or beef origin is likely to be "silent" in an otherwise healthy host. Either can cause abdominal pain or epigastric hunger pains, an increased appetite, weight loss, weakness, and general malaise. Findings elicited less commonly are diarrhea, upper abdominal distention, postprandial vomiting, and in rare cases, intestinal obstruction. Tapeworms have been known to live up to 25 years.

Cysticercus infections produce few general symptoms unless large numbers of larvae develop simultaneously. Localized findings are largely a result of the expanding mass and the functions with which it interferes. The brain is the most common site for cysticercosis and also the site of infections that most often causes symptomatic disease. Seizures are the most common clinical manifestation and occur in 70% to 90% of recognized cases. Less common manifestations include headache, visual problems, altered mental status (including psychosis), ataxia, focal deficits, and hydrocephalus.

Diagnosis

Eggs in the stool reveal only the presence of taeniasis. Study of a gravid proglottid for its number of main lateral uterine branches has been used as a means to identify the species of *Taenia,* but this has been questioned recently. *T. solium* is believed to have 7 to 13 main lateral uterine branches; *T. saginata* is said to have 15 to 20 on each side. Cysticercosis is identified by finding calcified "rice grains" on roentgenograms of any part of the body. A negative series of films does not rule out infection, however, because the calcification usually occurs 5 or more years after initial invasion of larvae. Excision of a cyst provides the opportunity to examine the evaginated scolex (head) of the larva and to look for the typical rostellum and hooklets of *T. solium.* The indirect hemagglutination (IHA) test has been valuable in the serological diagnosis of difficult cases. Some laboratories also use indirect fluorescent and counterimmunoelectrophoresis tests. The CDC has begun to use an immunoblot test that uses a semipurified extract of *T. solium* cysticerci, which has given a sensitivity of 98% and a specificity of 100%. Although previous serological assays were only positive in patients with multiple cysts, with the newer immunoblot test diagnosis is possible without multiple cysts being present in the patient.

Treatment

Because of the potential for cysticerci to develop with *T. solium,* this species of tapeworm always should be treated. Praziquantel in a single dose of 5 to 10 mg/kg is the treatment of choice. It should be taken with a fatty meal to enhance absorption. The alternative drug is niclosamide, which is administered in a single dose of 1 g for those weighing 11 to 34 kg and 1.5 g for those weighing more than 34 kg; the adult dose is 2 g.* The tablets must be chewed thoroughly before swallowing or should be crushed and administered mixed in liquids or pureed foods.

Treatment of neurocysticercosis depends on the location of the cyst(s), their viability, and the degree of inflammatory response. There is no role for antiparasitic drugs in the treatment of inactive disease—that is, patients who have seizures and only calcified lesions on neuroimaging. Such patients should be treated with anticonvulsants alone. Praziquantel in a dose of 50 to 60 mg/kg/day in three daily doses for 15 days or albendazole in a dose of 15 mg/kg/day in two or three daily doses for 8 to 30 days are equally effective in hastening the resolution of the cysts, although some patients may develop worsening inflammation with resultant headaches, vomiting, and seizures. Therefore, the routine use of corticosteroids is recommended to prevent this complication. Although antiparasitic drugs cause resolution of cysts and seizures, the results are not obviously different from the natural history of the disease. Hence, there is no consensus about the use of these drugs in neurocysticercosis. Antiparasitic drugs may be reserved for patients with multiple parenchymal cysts or those with solitary cysts that have not resolved after 6 to 12 months of follow-up. Because of the risk of worsening symptoms, hospitalization or close monitoring is advisable if antiparasitic drugs are administered. Antiparasitic drugs, in conjunction with shunting procedures, also are recommended for patients with hydrocephalus and ependymitis.

HYDATID DISEASE *(Echinococcus granulosus, E. multilocularis, E. oligarthrus, and E. vogeli)*

Epidemiology

Echinococcosis is caused by the larval (metacestode) stage of various cestode species. *Echinococcus granulosus* is the cause of cystic echinococcosis and is the most common form in humans. *E. multilocularis,* the etiological agent of alveolar echinococcosis, is less common. *E. vogeli,* the cause of polycystic echinococcosis is very rare. *E. oligarthrus* infection is limited to sylvatic animals in Central and South America, and no human cases have been reported.

E. granulosus infection occurs worldwide. Areas of high endemicity are China, India, Africa, Iraq, the Mediterranean basin, Uruguay, Argentina, and Chile. Disease occasionally occurs in Great Britain, the United States, southern and eastern Europe, Australia, and New Zealand. *E. multilocularis* infection is limited to the northern hemisphere's subarctic regions of Alaska, Canada, and northern Europe.

Pathogenesis and Life Cycle

Humans become infected through accidental ingestion of eggs or gravid proglottids passed in the feces of infected dogs. The embryo emerges from the ova in the human duodenum, penetrates a small blood vessel, and is filtered out in the liver (60%), in the lung (20%), or by the capillaries of other tissues (20%). The bladderlike cyst (larva) expands at about 1 mm/month until body defenses overwhelm it or its size causes its discovery and treatment. It may manifest as an expanding mass (intracranial) or an inflammatory mass (pulmonary), or it may cause anaphylactic shock if it begins leaking fluid in a hypersensitive person. Secondary bacterial infection has been the cause of leakage or rupture of the cysts. The cyst is filled with fluid but has a germinal layer and a multilayered acellular membrane surrounding the fluid. The germinal layer produces brood capsules that in time collectively contain thousands of tiny protoscolices (embryos). These eventually break loose and float in the cyst fluid as "hydatid sand." Each protoscolex can develop into either another hydatid cyst or a tapeworm, depending on whether it escapes from the original cyst into the intermediate host's body or is ingested by the definitive host, respectively. In

*Praziquantel and niclosamide are available from Miles, Inc., West Haven, Conn., (203) 937-2000. Praziquantel also is available from SmithKline Beecham, Philadelphia, Pa., (215) 751-4000.

cases of *E. multilocularis,* the boundary of the cyst is poorly demarcated. It rarely produces brood capsules or mature protoscolices. It most commonly is found in the liver and extends its growth to other organs.

Clinical Manifestations

Echinococcosis can mimic a variety of conditions, depending on the location of the cysts. The course of the disease is variable. Infection may occur in childhood, but because of the slow growth of the cysts it may not produce symptoms until middle age. *E. granulosus* cysts are most often found in the liver (65%) and lungs (25%). On the other hand, *E. multilocularis* cysts occur almost exclusively in the liver (98%), but metastatic lesions can form in the lungs, brain, and other organs.

Hydatid cysts may be asymptomatic and accidentally discovered on routine chest roentgenogram or abdominal ultrasound. When they do cause symptoms, they usually are related to compression of the surrounding structures. Liver cysts give rise to right upper quadrant and epigastric pain, hepatomegaly, jaundice, and portal hypertension. Lung cysts may present with hemoptysis, pleural effusion, and atelectasis. Cysts in the brain produce signs and symptoms of a cerebral tumor while those in the kidney produce hematuria and may resemble a hypernephroma. Cysts in the bone may present as spontaneous fractures of the long bones or compression fractures of the vertebrae. Cysts may rupture spontaneously, resulting in fever, urticaria, and signs of anaphylaxis. Seeding of protoscolices may result in secondary cysts at other sites. Fatalities are rare but may occur as a result of cyst rupture, compression of vital structures, or septicemia from infected cysts.

Alveolar cysts tend to grow rapidly and metastasize and therefore result in symptoms early in the course of disease. They are associated with high mortality if not diagnosed and treated early.

Diagnosis

Hydatid cyst must be suspected in any patient from an endemic area who presents with signs and symptoms of a space-occupying lesion. Radiographic studies such as chest roentgenograms, ultrasound, CT scan, and MRI will reveal the presence of the typical fluid-filled cysts, sometimes with enclosed daughter cysts and brood capsules.

A number of serological tests using hydatid cyst fluid or antigen 5 are available. These tests have a sensitivity of 80% to 100% and specificity of 88% to 96% for diagnosing liver cysts; sensitivity is lower for pulmonary cysts (50% to 56%) and cysts in other sites (25% to 56%). At present, imaging remains more sensitive than serodiagnosis, and a positive scan would suggest echinococcosis even though serological tests are negative.

Treatment

Surgery is recommended for single unilocular *E. granulosus* cysts. Because infection may spread if the cyst ruptures, the recommended procedure is to inject the cyst with a scolicidal agent such as hypertonic (30%) saline, 95% ethanol, or iodophor before attempting excision.

Albendazole* is effective against echinococcal cysts and may be used as an adjunct to surgery, when surgery is not possible or would be associated with significant morbidity; its use in itself is associated with significant morbidity when cysts in the brain or bone or multiple cysts are present. Albendazole administration results in improvement in about 75% of cysts in the liver, lung, or peritoneum and in cure in 30% to 50%. Cure rates are lower for bone cysts (25%), with improvement in about half the patients. The recommended treatment schedule with albendazole is 10 to 15 mg/kg/day in two to three divided doses given as three 28-day cycles with 14 days between cycles. Preoperative use of albendazole for 28 days renders the cysts nonviable and reduces the risk of recurrence. Two 28-day cycles of albendazole may be used postoperatively to reduce the risk of recurrences.

For alveolar cysts, wide surgical resection is recommended to ensure total removal of the cyst. Albendazole may be used as an adjuvant to surgery, either to reduce the size of the cyst preoperatively or to prevent intraoperative spread.

DWARF TAPEWORM *(Hymenolepsis nana)*

Epidemiology

Hymenolepsis nana is a tapeworm of rats and mice. However, it is well adapted to humans and completes its entire life cycle in them, making autoinoculation a problem. Transmission occurs directly from child to child or through contamination of food and drink with human or rodent feces. The parasite is found worldwide, and the prevalence is much higher among children than adults. Children at special risk are those under age 3 years, those on a protein-deficient diet, immunodepressed children, or those living in a crowded, unhygienic environment infested with rodents. The decreasing prevalence with age reflects a decrease in exposure, but serological studies suggest that previous exposure evokes a measure of resistance against recurrent infestation. The current world prevalence is estimated to be about 50 million cases.

Pathogenesis and Life Cycle

H. nana is the smallest tapeworm that infests humans. The adult worm measures only 5 to 45 mm in length and has a scolex with four suckers and a short rostellum with 20 to 30 hooks. Infection generally is acquired by ingestion of *H. nana* eggs from the feces of infected individuals. The eggs hatch in the stomach or small intestine. The liberated oncospheres penetrate the villi of the upper small intestine. The larvae mature into the cysticercoid stage in the villi and then migrate back into the lumen where the scolices evaginate and attach themselves to the mucosa. The adult worm matures within a few weeks.

Clinical Manifestations

Most patients are asymptomatic. However, a variety of symptoms, including anorexia or increased appetite, abdominal pain, nausea, vomiting, diarrhea, irritability, dizziness, and

*Albendazole is available from SmithKline Beecham, Philadelphia, Pa., (215) 751-4000.

headache have been described, especially in those with heavy worm burden. Seizures have been described in patients in the former Soviet Union. Autoinfestation, in which the eggs hatch in the intestine and complete the life cycle within the same host, may result in heavy infestation in immunocompromised patients.

Diagnosis

Diagnosis is established by the demonstration of eggs in the feces; proglottids are rarely expelled. A moderate eosinophilia is present with heavy infections. Serological tests are of no real value in the diagnosis of *H. nana*.

Treatment

Praziquantel in a single dose of 25 mg/kg is the treatment of choice (see the footnote on p. 1724). A repeat dose may be necessary. Stools should be checked for eggs every 2 weeks for 3 months. Timing repeat drug therapy for 2 weeks after initial treatment carries the best chance of ridding the patient of the parasite. Close contacts (e.g., family and other closed populations) should be treated simultaneously.

FISH TAPEWORM *(Diphyllobothrium latum)*

Epidemiology

D. latum, or "fish tapeworm," belongs to the pseudophyllidean cestode group. This group has a scolex with two "bothria" (sucking organs) rather than the typical four seen in the *Taenia* group. Fish tapeworms consist of 3000 to 4000 proglottids and measure up to 25 m in length. The proglottids have a characteristic rosette-shaped uterus. An individual may be infected with more than one worm at a time. Infestation is mainly seen in the lake and delta areas in Siberia, Scandinavia, the Baltic regions, and adjacent areas of the former Soviet Union, and in the northern United States, Canada, and South America. Infestation may be maintained by fish-eating mammals in the absence of humans.

Life Cycle

Infestation is acquired by ingestion of raw, poorly cooked or pickled freshwater fish. The worm matures in 3 to 6 weeks after ingestion of eggs, after which both eggs and proglottids are passed in the stool. The eggs develop in fresh water and hatch to release ciliated coracidium larvae, which are ingested by the first intermediate host, the copepod. The copepods containing the second-stage larvae (procercoids) are ingested by fish and develop into more advanced stages in the muscles of the fish. Smaller fish may be ingested by larger fish, resulting in parasitization of the muscles of the larger fish. The cycle is completed when humans or other fish-eating mammals ingest infected fish.

Clinical Manifestations

Infestation may be asymptomatic, although patients may notice the passage of proglottids in the stool. Infestation with multiple worms may lead to abdominal discomfort and, occasionally, intestinal obstruction. Chronic infestation may be associated with vitamin B_{12} deficiency and megaloblastic anemia. The vitamin B_{12} deficiency is partly the result of parasite-mediated vitamin B_{12}-intrinsic factor dissociation leading to decreased absorption, and partly caused by high uptake of the vitamin by the parasite itself. Megaloblastic anemia is seen much more commonly in Finland and adjacent areas than in North America. Increased uptake of vitamin B_{12} by strains of the parasite in Finland and a genetic predisposition to megaloblastic anemia are the postulated reasons for this phenomenon.

Diagnosis

Diagnosis is made by recovery of the characteristic eggs or proglottids in the feces.

Treatment

Praziquantel (5 to 10 mg/kg as a single dose) is the treatment of choice (see the footnote on p. 1724). Severe vitamin B_{12} deficiency should be treated with parenteral vitamin injections.

NEMATODES

INTESTINAL NEMATODES

ASCARIASIS/LARGE ROUNDWORM *(Ascaris lumbricoides)*

Epidemiology

Ascaris lumbricoides is the largest roundworm that infests humans. Globally, it is believed to be the most common nematode parasite of humans. The number of infested persons worldwide is estimated to be 1 billion; three-quarters live in developing countries. It probably is second only to pinworms in prevalence in the United States; an estimated 4 million people, mainly in the Southeast, are infected. The adult worm measures 15 to 30 cm in length and resides in the lumen of the jejunum and the ileum.

Pathogenesis and Life Cycle

Infestation occurs by ingestion of embryonated eggs via contaminated fingers or food or by geophagy. The adult female worm produces an average of 200,000 eggs per day, which are passed in the feces and develop in the soil in about 2 to 3 weeks. Once swallowed, the fertile egg hatches in the small intestine. The larvae then penetrate the intestinal wall, enter the venous circulation, and travel to the lungs. A local hypersensitivity reaction (Splendore-Hoeppli's phenomenon) may occur at the site of entry of the larvae into the lung tissue. After further development in the lungs, the larvae ascend to the trachea, are coughed up and then swallowed, and develop into adults in the small bowel.

Clinical Manifestations

Most cases of ascariasis are asymptomatic or so mild that medical attention is not sought. The most common clinical manifestations are nonspecific, colicky abdominal pain and distention. These symptoms are caused by metabolic products of the worms that irritate the sensory receptors in the intestine, with resultant interference with normal peristalsis, leading to spasmodic contraction and sometimes, ischemia of the bowel wall. Heavy infestation with ascaris can result in small-bowel obstruction. Migration of worms can cause obstruction of biliary and pancreatic ducts. In regions where it is endemic, ascaris is a common cause of acute abdominal emergencies and biliary and pancreatic disease. Migration of larvae through the lungs may result in Loeffler's syndrome presenting as fever, productive cough, wheezing, eosinophilia, and pulmonary infiltrates.

Chronic ascariasis is known to precipitate malnutrition in undernourished children, probably as a result of malabsorption of vitamin A, fat, and protein, and of lactose intolerance.

Diagnosis

Diagnosis is made by the demonstration of the distinctive golden-coated embryonated and unembryonated eggs in the feces. Adult worms may sometimes be passed via the rectum or, less commonly, coughed up through the mouth or nose. Eosinophilia is seen during the pulmonary migration phase of the larvae but may not be seen in uncomplicated intestinal infestation.

Treatment

The recommended treatment for symptomatic or asymptomatic infestation is pyrantel pamoate 11 mg/kg but not exceeding 1 g, as a single dose or mebendazole in a fixed dose of 100 mg twice daily for 3 days. Albendazole in a single dose of 400 mg is equally effective (see the footnote on p. 1725). Experience with these drugs is limited in children younger than 2 years; nevertheless these drugs do not seem to act differently at this age compared with older age groups.

In cases where intestinal or biliary obstruction is suspected, piperazine citrate solution, 75 mg/kg/day not exceeding 3.5 g, may be given through a nasogastric tube. Piperazine paralyzes the worms, allowing them to be passed by peristalsis without migrating into other sites. Piperazine is antagonistic to pyrantel pamoate, so the two should not be used together. If pharmacological treatment has not been successful after 48 hours, surgery is recommended. With a laparotomy, small-bowel obstructions usually can be "milked" down into the cecum without opening the bowel itself. The patient then can be treated with drugs postoperatively for final removal of the parasites. Entering the bowel should be a last resort.

Prevention

Sanitary disposal of human excreta, reasonable personal hygiene, and avoiding food or water potentially contaminated with human feces constitute the first line of defense against ascariasis. Single oral doses of albendazole (400 mg) or mebendazole (500 mg) administered every 6 months have been shown to be effective in reducing the worm burden and alleviating morbidity, as well as reducing transmission. Because schoolchildren have the most intense infestation, which adversely affects their growth and school performance, they should be the targets for disease control. In areas in which more than 25% of children are mild to moderately underweight and parasites are known to be widespread, the children may be targeted for regular deworming programs. In highly endemic areas in which more than 50% of the population are infested, mass treatment of the entire community is justified.

HOOKWORM DISEASE/ ANCYLOSTOMIASIS *(Ancylostoma duodenale, A. ceylonicum, Necator americanus)*

An estimated 900 million people worldwide are infested with two species of hookworm, *Ancylostoma duodenale* and *Necator americanus*. The near-universal use of modern plumbing and the reduction in barefoot children in the United States has reduced the burden of hookworm infestation significantly in this country. Currently, most cases are imported. In developing countries, hookworm infection is a common cause of iron-deficiency anemia and hypoproteinemia.

Pathogenesis and Life Cycle

Adult hookworms are cylindrical, grayish-white, and approximately 1 cm in length. They reside in the upper small intestine. The adult female worm may produce 9000 to 30,000 eggs daily, which are passed in the feces. Under suitable soil conditions of temperature and humidity, the eggs hatch into larvae, molt once, and become infective. Infective larvae penetrate exposed skin that comes into contact with contaminated soil, enter the venous circulation, and are carried to the lungs. In the lungs the larvae penetrate the alveoli, travel up the trachea, and are coughed up and swallowed. In the gastrointestinal tract the larvae mature into adult worms, which attach themselves to the jejunal mucosa, sucking minute quantities of blood. The worms move location every 4 to 8 hours, producing small mucosal ulcerations. The daily blood loss from a single adult worm is 0.16 to 0.34 ml for *Ancylostoma duodenale* and 0.03 to 0.05 ml for *Necator americanus*. Thus, moderate (100 to 500 worms) and severe (500 to 1000 worms) infection can cause significant blood loss daily.

Clinical Features

An intense pruritus, erythema, and vesicular rash (ground itch) may develop at the site of the entry of the infective larvae. Passage through the lungs may cause a Loeffler-like syndrome, with cough, pulmonary infiltrates, and eosinophilia.

The intestinal phase of the infection may cause epigastric pain, abdominal tenderness, and diarrhea. However, the major clinical manifestations of infection in children are anemia and hypoproteinemia as a result of chronic blood loss. Iron deficiency may lead to geophagia in young children, which in endemic areas may result in other nematode infections.

Diagnosis

The diagnosis is made by finding the characteristic ovoid eggs in the feces. With egg counts of more than 1200/ml of feces, direct examination of the feces is sufficient. Concentration techniques may be required for light infection.

Treatment

Mebendazole (100 mg twice daily for 3 days) is the drug of choice. Albendazole (see the footnote on p. 1725) (400 mg as a single dose) or pyrantel pamoate (11 mg/kg, not exceeding 1 g) also are effective. A stool examination, using a concentration technique, should be repeated 2 weeks after treatment. If it is positive, treatment should be repeated. Supplemental iron should be given for at least 3 months after the hemoglobin concentration reaches the level of 12 g/dl.

Prevention

Sanitary disposal of feces prevents contamination of the soil but may be difficult to achieve in many poor countries. Screening of high-risk populations and treatment of those who have known infection reduces transmission. The use of footwear may also reduce the risk of infection.

TRICHURIASIS/WHIPWORM *(Trichuris trichiura)*

Trichuriasis is among the common helminthic infections, with an estimated 500 million cases worldwide. Infection is commonest in warm, humid regions. In the United States, trichuriasis is limited to the Southeastern states and to migrants from the tropics. The adult worm has a cylindrical body (mean length of 40 mm), with a thin, whiplike anterior end that anchors to the intestinal mucosa and a coiled, thicker posterior end exposed to the lumen. It normally inhabits the cecum and the ascending colon.

Life Cycle

The adult female worm produces approximately 13,000 eggs per day that are passed in the feces. In warm, moist, shaded soil, the eggs mature over a period of 3 weeks and become infective. Infection is acquired by the ingestion of the embryonated eggs, which release the larvae in the upper small intestine. Unlike other nematodes, *Trichuris* does not have the tissue migratory phase. The complete development of the larvae to mature adult worms takes place during passage through the intestine.

Clinical Features

Most infections are asymptomatic. However, heavy infection (more than 1000 worms) may cause severe colitis and proctitis presenting with abdominal pain, bloody diarrhea, and rectal prolapse. The clinical presentation may mimic Crohn's disease. The worms also are known to suck minute quantities of blood (0.005 ml/worm/day), so heavy infections may result in mild anemia.

Diagnosis

The diagnosis is established by demonstration of the characteristic lemon-shaped eggs in the stool. Because of the relatively high egg counts in the feces, concentration techniques generally are not required.

Treatment

The drug of choice for the treatment of trichuriasis is mebendazole (100 mg twice daily for 3 days, regardless of age). A single 400-mg dose of albendazole (see the footnote on p. 1725) may be used for light and moderate infections; a 3-day course is recommended for heavy infection.

STRONGYLOIDIASIS *(Strongyloides stercoralis)*

Strongyloides stercoralis is less common than other nematode infections but has the potential to cause overwhelming infection, particularly in immunosuppressed individuals. It is widely distributed throughout the world, particularly in the tropics. In the United States, it is prevalent in the Southeastern states. The adult female worm is colorless and measures about 2.2 mm in length. The male worm is shorter, measuring 0.7 mm. They inhabit the upper small intestine.

Life Cycle

S. stercoralis has a more complex life cycle than that of other nematodes. The mature females lay eggs, which embryonate within the intestine, develop into rhabditiform larvae, and are deposited on the soil along with feces. In the soil, the larvae may either develop into free-living adult males or females, which continue their existence in the soil, or into infective filariform larvae. The infective larvae penetrate the skin to enter the venous circulation, pass to the lungs, and finally to the intestine, where they develop into adult worms. The *Strongyloides* rhabditiform larvae may also develop into infective larvae while still in the intestine. These penetrate the intestinal wall or the skin of the perianal region and are carried through the circulation to the lungs and then to the intestine. This "autoinfection" may result in hyperinfection in immunocompromised hosts.

Clinical Features

The clinical manifestations of strongyloidiasis correspond to the various stages of infection. Penetration of the skin and migration through the lungs may produce a pruritic skin rash (larva currens) and a Loeffler-like syndrome, respectively. The intestinal phase of infection often is asymptomatic but may produce epigastric pain, vomiting, and diarrhea. In heavy infection, chronic malabsorption and weight loss may be seen. In immunocompromised individuals, including those infected with HIV, hyperinfection strongyloidiasis may be seen, with invasion of all tissues, including the CNS. In such patients, penetration of the intestinal wall by filariform larvae may result in translocation of intestinal flora into the blood stream, leading to sepsis.

Diagnosis

Diagnosis of *Strongyloides* is made by demonstration of larvae in the feces or in the duodenal fluid. Sampling of duodenal contents is achieved by the use of the string test (Enterotest). Diagnosis of uncomplicated infection may be difficult, and repeated examinations may be necessary. Serodiagnosis for *Strongyloides* is available in a few reference laboratories, but false-positive tests are known to occur. Eosinophilia is common, and in disseminated infections, the larvae may be found in the sputum.

Treatment

Thiabendazole is the drug of choice. It is administered orally in a dose of 50 mg/kg/day in two doses on 2 consecutive days. In disseminated infection, the drug must be continued for 5 days. Albendazole, 400 mg daily for 3 consecutive days, is better tolerated and may eradicate 80% of infections. Ivermectin (200 mg/kg/day for 1 to 2 days) also is effective but is not approved for use in the United States except as an investigational drug.

ABERRANT INFECTION WITH INTESTINAL NEMATODES

TOXOCARIASIS/VISCERAL LARVA MIGRANS *(Toxocara canis, T. cati, others)*

Most nematodes have only one host in whom their life cycle can be completed. Infection of an unnatural host results in failure to complete the cycle, and no disease occurs. Occasionally, infection of an unnatural host results in aberrant migration of the larvae, which may cause more symptoms than natural infection. Infections with *T. canis* or *T. catis* are examples of this phenomenon. These nematodes infect dogs or cats and have a life cycle similar to that of *Ascaris lumbricoides*. A sizable percentage of domestic pets are infected and routinely contaminate school grounds, yards, and sandboxes used by children. Small children, especially those in the 1- to 4-year-old age group, are prone to eating dirt and putting soiled hands or toys into their mouths, thus increasing their risk of infection. Higher rates of infection are found in the southern United States and are associated with rural living, increasing age of children, number of persons living in the home, lower income, less education, and fewer rooms in the house. The presence of a litter of puppies in the home or the habit of pica in a child also have been correlated with the presence of toxocariasis. It has been estimated that 20% of dogs and 98% of puppies in the United States are infected.

Life Cycle and Pathogenesis

When ingested by humans, the eggs hatch in the intestine, releasing larvae that penetrate the intestinal mucosa to enter the circulation. Because they cannot mature further in humans, they tend to migrate for a prolonged period, passing through several organs and tissues of the body, before they are overwhelmed by the host immune response. During tissue migration, the larvae form granulomas and induce a significant peripheral eosinophilia and IgE response. The tissue identified most often as the site of infection is the liver, but involvement of the lungs, kidneys, brain, heart, skeletal muscle, eyes, and other tissues have been reported.

Clinical Manifestations

The severity of the illness in visceral larva migrans (VLM) is determined in part by the number of fertile viable eggs ingested, the organ system or systems involved, and the host's immunological status. Several larvae could be encysted in the liver and produce minimal or no symptoms, whereas even a single larva in the eye or brain can be devastating. Toxocariasis can manifest in a number of ways, and a high index of suspicion is essential in making the diagnosis.

Asymptomatic type. Mild constitutional symptoms may be present but apparently do not prompt the person to seek medical attention. Incidental findings of eosinophilia, an enlarged liver, or hypergammaglobulinemia may prompt a search for the diagnosis.

Hepatopulmonary type. This form primarily involves the liver and lungs but should be distinguished from the migration phase of other nematodes. The child may be mildly to severely ill. Typical findings include episodic fever to 104° F (40° C) with night sweats, hepatomegaly, and pulmonary findings (e.g., wheezing, dyspnea, cough, and patchy pneumonitis or pneumonia). Transient GI disturbances that may recur are anorexia, nausea, vomiting, abdominal pain, and distention. A variety of rashes have been described, but urticaria is the most common. Other common findings include marked leukocytosis with fluctuating eosinophilia (20% to 90%), hypergammaglobulinemia, elevated isohemagglutinins, anemia, a positive test result for blood in the stool, and eosinophils in the sputum. Chest roentgenograms demonstrate pulmonary infiltrates. No form of the parasite is found in the sputum or stool.

Generalized type. When larvae migrate directly from the intestine or reach the left ventricle, they may enter virtually any organ system, with subsequent development of corresponding clinical signs and symptoms. These include myalgia, arthralgia, subcutaneous nodules, loss of weight or failure to gain weight, myocarditis, neuritis, and neurological dysfunction, including grand mal or petit mal seizures.

Ocular type. This form is found most commonly among individuals older than age 4 and is not associated with concomitant systemic manifestations or eosinophilia. This form manifests as insidious or sudden impairment of vision in one eye. Ophthalmoscopic examination reveals a raised, rounded, or umbilicated granuloma, frequently near the macula. If the larva protrudes into the vitreous, there may be serious inflammation farther anteriorly, carrying with it a high likelihood for impaired vision. This lesion usually is painless and must be distinguished from retinoblastoma.

Diagnosis

Infection produces a high degree of eosinophilia (up to 80%) and hypergammaglobulinemia associated with elevated titers of isohemagglutinins to A and B blood group antigens. These, along with a characteristic clinical presentation, would suggest the diagnosis. Because of the high degree of eosinophilia, hepatomegaly (with or without associated splenomegaly), and lymphadenopathy, eosinophilic leukemia may have to be ruled out by bone marrow examination. The larvae may occasionally be demonstrated in the affected tissues by histological examination. Serodiagnosis using an ELISA test often is helpful in diagnosing visceral larva migrans but may be negative in ocular larva migrans.

Treatment

Most patients recover without specific treatment. Treatment should be reserved for symptomatic infection. Diethylcarbamazine, in a dose of 6 mg/kg/day in three divided doses for 7 to 10 days, is the drug of choice. Alternatives include albendazole 400 mg twice daily for 3 to 5 days or mebendazole 100 to 200 mg twice daily for 5 days.

CUTANEOUS LARVA MIGRANS (*Ancylostoma caninum, A. braziliense,* others)

Epidemiology

Cutaneous larva migrans, or "creeping eruption," commonly is caused by nonhuman hookworm filariform larvae such as *Ancylostoma braziliense, Ancylostoma caninum,* and other species. Because these species only rarely are able to penetrate the full thickness of the skin and reach the GI tract of humans, they wander aimlessly in the skin, producing raised, erythematous, pruritic tracks. They are acquired when a human's exposed skin comes into contact with soil or sand contaminated with animal feces containing nonhuman hookworm eggs. The parasite is most prevalent where warm, moist, sandy soil with a high humus content is used by dogs and cats to defecate, and subsequently for gardening, a children's playground, or sports field. Beaches also have been the sites of transmission. In the United States, the Southeast has the highest incidence.

Life Cycle and Pathogenesis

Although ground itch caused by human hookworm and *Strongyloides* larvae is a form of cutaneous larva migrans, it differs from the condition caused by nonhuman species in that the latter cannot complete their cycle. The tunneling migrations of these nonhuman hookworms evoke an intense neutrophilic and eosinophilic infiltrate and produce edema and vascular congestion.

Clinical Manifestations

The serpiginous track through the skin is visualized easily. It is pruritic, often highly so, and has been described as painful by a minority of patients. Localized swelling and rash also may occur. The lesions often are found on the feet, thighs, or buttocks. In some reported series, secondary bacterial infection is present, perhaps enhanced by scratching.

Diagnosis

The diagnosis of creeping eruption is made clinically, although the species of larva responsible may remain unknown. Biopsy generally is unwarranted and may often be negative for larval forms.

Treatment

Topical use of 15% thiabendazole cream applied two or three times a day or given orally in a dose of 50 mg/kg/day in two divided doses for 2 to 5 days is adequate for cure. Albendazole (see the footnote on p. 1725) 200 mg twice daily for 3 days is an alternative. Oral ivermectin (150 to 200 mg/kg once) has proved very successful and had no side effects in at least one series of patients.

TISSUE NEMATODES

FILARIASIS (*Wuchereria bancrofti, Brugia malayi*)

Epidemiology

Bancroftian and brugian filariasis are clinically similar conditions caused by *Wuchereria bancrofti* and *Brugia malayi,* respectively. The estimated prevalence of cases (infection and chronic disease) caused by *W. bancrofti* worldwide is 106 million. More than 80% of these occur in sub-Saharan Africa and India. An estimated 13 million cases caused by *B. malayi* are reported worldwide annually, mainly in Southeast Asia and the Pacific islands. Infection is most common in the age group of 15 to 44 years. However, a significant proportion of cases occur in children younger than 15 years of age.

Life Cycle

Infection is acquired through the bite of an infected anopheline mosquito. The infective larvae pass into the lymphatic system where they mature into threadlike adult worms. The male and female worms measure 40 mm and 100 mm in length, respectively. The fertilized females liberate microfilariae that enter the blood stream, usually in a surge during the night, and are ingested by mosquitoes in which they mature into infective larvae, completing the cycle.

Clinical Manifestations

In endemic areas, a sizable proportion of the population may have microfilaremia without having any symptoms. Symptoms usually are caused by acute inflammation resulting in lymphangitis, which presents as painful, cordlike swellings with reddish streaks on the overlying skin, and as lymphadenitis. Other manifestations include acute epididymitis, orchitis, funiculitis, or lymphatic obstruction with lymphedema or hydrocele. In elephantiasis, the skin overlying the area of lymphedema becomes thick and warty. Rupture of distended lymphatics into the peritoneal cavity or into the urinary tract results in chylous ascites and chyluria, respectively.

Diagnosis

Diagnosis is established by the demonstration of microfilaria in stained smears of blood, urine (in chyluria), or hydrocele fluid. Concentration techniques may be necessary when low microfilarial densities are suspected. A number of serological tests have been described, but these do not differentiate between recent and past infection. Serological assays may be positive in the presence of microfilaremia but not in other forms of the disease. Antigen detection assays are available but are not very sensitive in detecting nonmicrofilaremic infection.

Treatment

Diethylcarbamazine is the drug of choice for the treatment of filariasis in children. It is administered orally in a dose of 6 mg/kg/day in two to three divided doses for 12 to 14 days (for *W. bancrofti*) or 3 to 6 mg/kg/day in divided doses for 6 to 12 days (for *B. malayi*). Because reactions induced by disintegrating microfilaria may occur in patients with heavy infection, initiation of treatment with lower doses during the first 4 to 5 days is recommended. Ivermectin in a single oral dose of 200 mg/kg has been shown to have equal efficacy and tolerability.

Control

The two methods used for filariasis control include vector control and systematic individual or community chemotherapy. Vector control may be achieved by indoor spraying of houses with insecticides, use of mosquito nets impregnated with pyrethroids, and larval control of mosquito breeding sites. These are difficult to achieve in most endemic areas. The other option is to use mass treatment of entire communities with diethylcarbamazine. In Polynesia, a single dose of 6 mg/kg administered once a year has been reported to reduce the prevalence of microfilaremia and clinical manifestations of filariasis. In India and China, similar results have been achieved by the addition of diethylcarbamazine to table salt in a concentration of 0.1% to 0.3%.

ONCHOCERCIASIS/RIVER BLINDNESS *(Onchocerca volvulus)*

Epidemiology

Onchocerca volvulus is a long nematode (females are 300 to 400 mm long and males, 20 to 40 mm). Worms of both sexes live curled up in an encapsulated nodule, in the subcutaneous tissues of humans. Onchocerciasis is endemic to West and Central Africa, Central and South America, and Yemen. An estimated 17 million people in Africa and 100,000 in Central and South America are infected.

Life Cycle

Infection is transmitted by the bite of female black flies (*Simulium* species), which breed along rivers and streams, hence the name "river blindness." Infective larvae may take 12 months to develop into adult worms. The fertilized females produce unsheathed microfilariae, which migrate to the skin, where they remain till they are ingested by biting black flies.

Clinical Manifestations

Microfilariae in the skin produces a pruritic, erythematous, papular rash. Severe infection is associated with lymphedema and depigmentation of the skin (leopard skin). Adult worms in the subcutaneous tissue produce firm, mobile, nontender nodules located mainly over bony prominences. With chronic infection, the skin may lose its elasticity, which, with chronic lymphadenopathy, gives rise to pedunculus sacs, particularly in the inguinal region (hanging groin). Hernia, hydrocele, and elephantiasis are reported. Leonine facies is seen, especially in patients in the Americas.

Microfilariae in the eyes may give rise to iridocyclitis, chorioretinitis, optic atrophy, and ultimately, corneal fibrosis and blindness.

Diagnosis

Diagnosis is established by demonstration of microfilariae in skin snips or in the eye by slit lamp examination. Adult worms can be identified in excised nodules. When the diagnosis is strongly suspected but the parasite cannot be demonstrated, if a single oral dose of diethylcarbamazine results in exacerbation of the rash within a few hours (Mazzotti reaction), infection is likely.

Treatment

The current drug of choice is ivermectin. This drug kills microfilariae but not the adult worm. However, a dose of 150 μg/kg repeated every 3 months will suppress the disease to a degree that will avoid complications. Surgical excision of nodules on the head, especially in children, may reduce the risk of blindness. Diethylcarbamazine is no longer the drug of choice for onchocerciasis because of the frequency with which it causes severe host (Mazzotti) reactions.

Control

Control is mainly by reduction of the vector population at the breeding sites by spraying insecticides and by teaching communities at risk how to avoid contact with black flies. More recently, mass treatment with the microfilaricide ivermectin has been used. The major obstructions to prevention now are ineffective host education and unreliable distribution and consumption of ivermectin.

TRICHINOSIS *(Trichinella spiralis)*

Of five recognized species of *Trichinella, Trichinella spiralis* is responsible for most human infection. Adult worms are small, with the female measuring 2 to 4 mm in length and the males 1.0 to 1.5 mm. *Trichinella* is ubiquitous in its distribution and infects a wide variety of domestic and wild animals. The United States and Europe are the major endemic zones of transmission. Domestic pork is the most common source in these countries, but wild bear, walrus, and boar meats have been the source of infection for humans in North America and Africa. The incidence of trichinosis in the United States has shown a marked decline, presumably as a result of laws governing the feeding of swine, mandatory slaughterhouse surveillance, food service sanitation, and general public awareness of the cause. Because the parasite is killed by being frozen at 5° F (–15° C) for 21 days, the use of home freezers to store meat also has played an important role in reducing the incidence. Heating meat to 171° F (77° C) provides a safe margin against trichinosis.

Life Cycle

Trichinosis is acquired by ingestion of animal muscle containing the encysted larvae. In the intestine, larvae are liberated from the cysts and enter the columnar epithelium of the intestine where they mature into adults. The fertilized female adult worm produces larvae at the rate of approximately 50 per day for a few weeks, after which it dies. The larvae enter the blood stream and are disseminated throughout the body. On reaching the striated muscle, they enter individual muscle cells, which transform into nurse cells. In a few weeks the larvae become infective and the nurse cells become thick-walled capsules (cysts).

Clinical Manifestations

Symptoms may be related to the intestinal, muscle invasion, and convalescent stages of infection. The intestinal phase of the infection starts 1 to 7 days after ingestion of infected meat and consists of abdominal pain, nausea, vomiting, and malaise. The muscle invasion phase occurs in the second week and may last 1 to 5 weeks or longer. It is characterized by eyelid edema, myalgia, weakness, fever, and eosinophilia. Less commonly encountered symptoms include headache, facial flushing, urticaria, profuse sweating, conjunctivitis, splinter hemorrhages, hoarseness, dyspnea, and dysphagia.

In rare instances, involvement of the cardiac muscle may result in arrhythmias or myocardial failure, whereas CNS involvement may result in a meningitis-like illness or focal neurological deficits.

Diagnosis

The triad of myalgia, eosinophilia (20% to 90%), and periorbital edema, in the presence of fever and a history of eating inadequately cooked meat about 2 to 3 weeks earlier, is presumptive of the diagnosis of trichinosis. If others who shared the food are ill with similar symptoms, the diagnosis is strengthened. Available serological tests from state laboratories and the CDC may establish the diagnosis, but only when the disease has reached the muscle stage. Muscle biopsy may test positive after the larvae reach muscle (second week postingestion), but negative test results do not rule out trichinosis. Fresh specimens of muscle are crushed between two microscope slides and inspected for the encysted larvae. If any meat from the suspect meal has been saved, it may be examined for the cysts.

Treatment

All cases of confirmed or suspected trichinosis should be treated to prevent the continued production of larvae. Mebendazole 200 to 400 mg thrice daily for 3 days followed by 400 to 500 mg thrice daily for 10 days is the recommended treatment. Concomitant administration of prednisolone may be required to reduce the allergic and inflammatory symptoms.

Control

Control is achieved by inspection of carcasses and thorough cooking of pork and game. Freezing at –30° C (–22° F) for 24 hours also kills the larvae.

SCHISTOSOMIASIS *(Schistosoma mansoni, S. japonicum, S. hematobium, S. mekongi,* and *S. intercalatum)*

Schistosomiasis is an infection caused by a trematode, *Schistosoma,* that requires two generations, one asexual and one sexual, to complete its life cycle. It affects more than 200 million people worldwide, primarily children and young adults. About 120 million of these are symptomatic, 20 million severely. The mortality associated with schistosomiasis is estimated to be 20,000 per year. Five Schistosoma species infect humans. These are *S. mansoni, S. japonicum, S. hematobium, S. mekongi,* and *S. intercalatum.* The life cycle involves a sexual phase of multiplication in humans, the definitive host, and asexual multiplication in freshwater snails, the intermediate hosts. The adult males range from 6 to 20 mm in length by 0.5 to 1 mm in width. The female parasite measures 7 to 25 mm by 0.3 mm. The females are held within a gynecophoral canal in the ventral surface of the male parasite. Adult schistosomes usually live for 5 to 10 years, but survival up to 30 years has been reported. Human infections can result in significant pathology in the gastrointestinal tract, liver, urinary bladder, and kidneys.

Epidemiology

Each of the five species of schistosomes that infect humans has a specific geographical distribution. *S mansoni* is prevalent in Arabia, Africa, South America, and the Caribbean; *S. japonicum* in Japan, China, and the Philippines; *S. hematobium* in Africa and the Middle East; *S. mekongi* in southeast Asia; and *S. intercalatum* in West and Central Africa. The prevalence of schistosomiasis has declined considerably because of the success of control programs. *S. japonicum* and *S. hematobium,* which were the main cause of infection 50 years ago, have now declined considerably, and *S. mansoni* has become the most prevalent and widespread of the three species. *S. japonicum,* which was the most prevalent of the three species and the most difficult to control, is now endemic in only three countries, namely China, Indonesia, and the Philippines. The major factors responsible for endemicity of schistosomiasis in these areas are the presence of specific snails as intermediate hosts and the method of disposal of human excreta.

Life Cycle and Pathogenesis

Humans are infected through contact with water contaminated with cercariae, the free-living infective stage of the parasite. These motile, forked-tailed organisms emerge from infected snails and are capable of penetrating intact human skin. In the subcutaneous tissue, cercariae change into the next stage of development, schistosomula, and migrate to the lungs and finally to the liver. As they reach sexual maturity, adult worms migrate to specific anatomical sites, characteristic of the species. *S. hematobium* reside in the perivesical and periurethral venous plexus, *S. mansoni* in the inferior mesenteric veins, *S. japonicum* in the superior mesenteric veins, and *S. intercalatum* and *S. mekongi* in the mesenteric veins. Upon fertilization, the female worms begin oviposition in the small venous tributaries. The eggs of the three main species have characteristic morphological features; *S. hematobium* has a terminal spine, *S. mansoni* has a lateral spine, and *S. japonicum* is smaller in size, with a short curved spine. Eggs reach the lumen of the urinary tract or intestine and are carried to the outside environment where they hatch if deposited in fresh water. Motile miracidia emerge and infect specific freshwater snails, the intermediate hosts, and multiply asexually. In 4 to 6 weeks, infective cercariae are released in the water.

Diseases can occur at each of the major steps of the parasite's life cycle: cercarial invasion, schistosomula migration and maturation, and finally, egg retention in the tissues. The earliest manifestation of schistosomiasis is an immunologically mediated dermatitis. Acute schistosomiasis, a febrile illness, is an immune-complex disease associated with early infection and oviposition. The major pathology of infection is chronic granulomatous injury secondary to retention of eggs in the host tissues. The live embryo within each egg secretes antigenic material through ultramicroscopic pores in the shell. These antigens are continually released for about 2 to 4 weeks, and they induce host sensitization and granulomatous response. When the embryos within the eggs die, antigenic secretion stops and granulomas undergo healing, with deposition of fibrous tissue. Granulomas in the urinary bladder wall or the ureterovesical junction lead to hematuria, dysuria, and obstructive uropathy. Intestinal lesions can lead to ulceration and fibrosis of the intestinal wall, where hepatic lesions lead to hepatosplenomegaly and portal hypertension. Patients who have a higher lymphocyte proliferation response to egg antigen have a more severe form of chronic schistosomiasis.

Clinical Features

Most infected individuals are asymptomatic; symptoms occur mainly in those who are heavily infected. Cercarial penetration of human skin may result in a papular pruritic rash, known as *swimmer's itch.* Acute schistosomiasis or Katayama fever occurs 4 to 8 weeks after exposure in those who are heavily infected. It is a serum sickness-like illness characterized by acute onset of fever, chills, sweating, lymphadenopathy, hepatosplenomegaly, and eosinophilia. Acute schistosomiasis usually occurs in patients who experience primary infection at an older age. Chronic infection with *S. hematobium* presents with dysuria, hematuria, or urinary frequency. Microscopic examination of urine may reveal red blood cells, leukocytes and parasite eggs. More than 50% of infected children in endemic areas develop moderate to severe lesions in the urinary tract. These can lead to chronic renal failure or carcinoma of the bladder. The other four species of schistosomiasis produce intestinal symptoms, namely colicky abdominal pain, bloody diarrhea, hepatosplenomegaly, portal hypertension, and ascites. Rarely, *Schistosoma* eggs may escape into the lungs, causing pulmonary hypertension and cor pulmonale. *S. japonicum* may migrate to the brain and may produce localized lesions and focal seizures. Transverse myelitis is a rare complication of chronic infection by *S. hematobium* or *S. mansoni*.

Diagnosis

Demonstration of eggs of *S. mansoni, S. japonicum,* and *S. mekongi* in stool or eggs of *S. hematobium* in urine is diagnostic of infection. A Kato thick smear using 25 to 50 mg of stool sample gives a better yield than a direct stool smear obtained from 1 to 2 mg of stool. The sensitivity of urine examination can be increased by obtaining a mid-day sample or a sample after light exercise when excretion of eggs is the maximum. Serological tests are not useful in endemic areas.

Treatment

The drug of choice for any species of schistosomiasis is Praziquantel (see the footnote on p. 1724). It is administered orally in a dose of 40 mg/kg in two divided doses for 1 day for *S. hematobium* and *S. mansoni* and 50 mg/kg in three divided doses for 1 day for *S. japonicum.* For *S. mekongi,* praziquantel may be administered in a dose of 60 mg/kg in three divided doses for 1 day. An alternative for treatment for *S. mansoni* is oxamniquine 20 mg/kg in a single dose.

Prevention

Improved sanitation and control of vector snails through environmental engineering or the use of molluscocides are the primary means of prevention. Individuals traveling to endemic areas should be warned about the hazard associated with swimming or wading in fresh water. Chemoprophylaxis or vaccines are not currently available.

When to Refer

Amebiasis

Severe colitis

Liver abscess with impending rupture

Pericardial, pleural, cerebral, or pleuropulmonary abscess

All patients who have amebic meningoencephalitis

When to Hospitalize

Amebiasis
Amebic liver abscess
Severe colitis
Pericardial, pleural, cerebral, or pleuropulmonary abscess
Patients who require treatment with dehydroemetine
All patients who have amebic meningoencephalitis

When to Refer

Babesiosis
Splenectomized or immunocompromised individuals
Patients who have a parasitic index greater than 10%
Failure of conservative treatment

When to Hospitalize

Babesiosis
Severe hemolytic anemia
Jaundice
Respiratory distress
Patients who require exchange transfusion

When to Refer

Malaria
If an experienced microscopist is not available to establish the diagnosis
If more than 5% of RBCs are parasitized
If facilities for intensive care of patients who have severe malaria are not available

When to Hospitalize

Malaria
If more than 5% of RBCs are parasitized
Signs of CNS or other end-organ involvement
Acidosis
Hypoglycemia
Severe anemia
Patients who require exchange transfusions

When to Refer

Chagas' Disease
If appropriate diagnostic facilities are not available
If drugs for treatment are not available
All patients who have the chronic phase of the disease

When to Hospitalize

Chagas' Disease
All patients who have the chronic phase of the disease

When to Refer

Leishmaniasis
If appropriate diagnostic facilities are not available
Patient has HIV or other immunocompromising conditions

When to Hospitalize

Leishmaniasis
All patients who have visceral leishmaniasis
All patients who have diffuse cutaneous leishmaniasis
All patients who have mucosal leishmaniasis

When to Refer or Hospitalize

Toxoplasmosis
Acute toxoplasmosis in an immunocompromised patient
Toxoplasma encephalitis
Pneumonia presenting as acute respiratory failure
Severe disease presenting with multiorgan failure

When to Refer

Cryptosporidiosis
If appropriate diagnostic facilities are not available
Patients who have HIV or immunocompromising conditions

When to Hospitalize

Cryptosporidiosis

Patients who have voluminous diarrhea, requiring intravenous rehydration

Patients who have involvement of the biliary tree or pancreas

Immunocompromised patients with wasting syndrome

When to Refer

Tapeworm Disease

All patients with neurocysticercosis who are difficult to diagnose based on radiology alone or who have altered mental status, focal deficits, or hydrocephalus

All patients who have hydatid cyst

When to Hospitalize

Tapeworm Disease

Patients who have neurocysticercosis when antiparasitic therapy is planned

Patients who have neurocysticercosis with altered mental status, focal deficits, or hydrocephalus

All patients who have hydatid cyst requiring excision

When to Refer or Hospitalize

Ascariasis

Patients who have suspected small-bowel obstruction, perforation, or ischemia

Patients who have involvement of the biliary tract or pancreas

When to Refer or Hospitalize

Hookworm Disease

Patients who have severe anemia (<5 g/dl)

When to Refer or Hospitalize

Trichuriasis

Patients who have severe infestation manifesting with colitis, proctitis, or rectal prolapse

When to Refer

Strongyloidiasis

All patients who have immunocompromising conditions, including HIV

Suspected hyperinfection

When to Hospitalize

Strongyloidiasis

Patients who have evidence of disseminated disease

Patients who have suspected sepsis

When to Refer

Visceral Larval Migrans

All cases of suspected ocular involvement

If diagnosis is suspected but difficult to establish

When to Refer

Filariasis

Patients who have acute lymphangitis when diagnosis is suspected but cannot be confirmed

Patients who have elephantiasis

Patients with chylothorax, chylous ascites, hydrocele or diarrhea, or chyluria

When to Hospitalize

Filariasis

All patients who require surgical treatment for complications

When to Refer

Onchocerca volvulus

All patients who have suspected ocular involvement

When to Refer or Hospitalize

Trichinosis

Patients who have CNS manifestations

Patients who have ECG abnormalities or evidence of myocardial failure

SUGGESTED READINGS

General

Abramowicz M: Drugs for parasitic infections, *Med Lett Drugs Ther* 35:111, 1993.

American Academy of Pediatrics: *Red Book 2000: Report of the Committee on Infectious Diseases,* ed 25, Elk Grove Village, Ill, 2000, American Academy of Pediatrics.

Benenson AS, editor: *Control of communicable diseases manual,* ed 16, Washington, DC, 1995, American Public Health Association.

Connolly KJ, Kvalsvig JD: Infection, nutrition, and cognitive performance, *Parasitology* 107:S187, 1993.

deSilva N, Guyatt H, Bundy D: Anthelminthics: a comparative review of their clinical pharmacology, *Drugs* 53:769, 1997.

Feigin RD, Cherry JD, editors: *Textbook of pediatric infectious diseases,* ed 3, Philadelphia, 1992, WB Saunders.

Liu LX, Weller PF: Antiparasitic drugs, *N Engl J Med* 334:1178, 1996.

Maddison SE: Serodiagnosis of parasitic diseases, *Clin Microbiol Rev* 4:457, 1991.

Shulman IA, Appleman MD: Transmission of parasitic and bacterial infections through blood transfusion within the US, *Crit Rev Clin Lab Sci* 28:447, 1991.

Warren KS, Mahmoud AAF: *Tropical and geographic medicine,* ed 2, New York, 1990, McGraw-Hill.

Amebiasis

Barnett ND, et al: Primary amebic meningoencephalitis with *Naegleria fowleri:* clinical review, *Pediatr Neurol* 15:230, 1996.

Bruckner DA: Amebiasis, *Clin Microbiol Rev* 5:356, 1992.

Clark CG: Amebic disease: *Entameba dispar,* an organism reborn, *Trans R Soc Trop Med Hyg* 92:361, 1998.

Ma P, et al: *Naegleria* and *Acanthamoeba* infections: review, *Rev Infect Dis* 12:490, 1990.

Sison JP, et al: Disseminated acanthamoeba infection in patients with AIDS: a case report and review, *Clin Infect Dis* 20:1207, 1995.

Stanley SL, Jr: Progress towards development of a vaccine for amebiasis, *Clin Microbiol Rev* 10:637, 1997.

Babesiosis

Dobroszycki J, et al: A cluster of transfusion-associated babesiosis cases traced to a single asymptomatic donor, *JAMA* 28:927, 1999.

Garnham PCC: Human babesiosis: European aspects, *Trans R Soc Trop Med Hyg* 74:153, 1980.

Gombert ME, et al: Human babesiosis: clinical and therapeutic considerations, *JAMA* 248:3005, 1982.

Krause PJ, et al: Concurrent Lyme disease and babesiosis: evidence for increased severity and duration of illness, *JAMA* 275:1657, 1996.

Quick RE, et al: Babesiosis in Washington State: a new species of *Babesia? Ann Intern Med* 119:284, 1993.

Cestodes

Botero D, et al: Taeniasis and cysticercosis, *Infect Dis Clin North Am* 7:683, 1993.

Clinton White, A Jr: Neurocysticercosis: a major cause of neurological disease worldwide, *Clin Infect Dis* 24:101, 1997.

Davis A, Pawlowski ZS, Dixon H: Multicentre clinical trials of benzimidazole carbamates in human echinococcosis, *Bull World Health Organ* 64:383, 1986.

Kammerer WS, Schantz PM. Echinococcal disease, *Infect Dis Clin North Am* 7:605, 1993.

Morris DL: Pre-operative albendazole therapy for hydatid cyst, *Br J Surg* 74:805, 1987.

Morris DL, Taylor DH: Optimal timing of post-operative albendazole prophylaxis in *E. granulosus, Ann Trop Med Parasitol* 82:65, 1988.

Rajshekhar V, et al: Differentiating solitary small cysticercus granuloma and tuberculoma in patients with epilepsy, *J Neurosurg* 78:402, 1993.

Schaefer JW, Khan MY: Echinococcosis (hydatid disease): lessons from experience with 59 patients, *Rev Infect Dis* 13:243, 1990.

Chagas' Disease

Cimo PL, Luper WE, Scouros MA: Transfusion-associated Chagas' disease in Texas: report of a case, *J Texas Med* 89:48, 1993.

Krieger MA, et al: Use of recombinant antigens for the accurate immunodiagnosis of Chagas' disease, *Am J Trop Med Hyg* 46:427, 1992.

Marsden PD: South American trypanosomiasis (Chagas' disease), *Int Rev Trop Med* 4:97, 1971.

Moncayo A: Chagas' disease. *Tropical Disease Research Progress 1991-1992 Report,* 1993.

Cryptosporidiosis

Guerrant RL: Cryptosporidiosis: an emerging, highly infectious threat, *Emerg Infect Dis* 3:51, 1997.

Juranek DD: Cryptosporidiosis: sources of infection and guidelines for prevention, *Clin Infect Dis* 21:S57, 1995.

MacKenzie WR, et al: A massive outbreak in Milwaukee of *Cryptosporidium* infection transmitted through the public water supply, *N Engl J Med* 331:161, 1994.

MacKenzie WR, et al: Massive outbreak of waterborne *Cryptosporidium* infection in Milwaukee, Wisconsin: recurrence of illness and risk of secondary transmission, *Clin Infect Dis* 21:57, 1995.

Ramratnam B, Flanigan TP: Cryptosporidiosis in persons with HIV infection, *Postgrad Med J* 73:713, 1997.

Leishmaniasis

Alvar J, et al: Leishmania and human immunodeficiency virus coinfection: the first 10 years, *Clin Microbiol Rev* 10:298, 1997.

Berman JD: Human leishmaniasis: clinical, diagnostic and chemotherapeutic developments in the last 10 years, *Clin Infect Dis* 24:684, 1997.

Pearson RD, Sousa A deQ: Clinical spectrum of leishmaniasis, *Clin Infect Dis* 22:1, 1996.

Malaria

Gera R, Khalil A: Artemisinine and its derivatives, *Indian Pediatr* 34:813, 1997.

Greenwood BM: What's new in malaria control, *Ann Trop Med Parasitol* 91:523, 1997.

Kain KC, Keystone JS: Malaria in travelers: epidemiology, disease and prevention, *Infect Dis Clin North Am* 12:267, 1998.

Kondrachine AV, Trigg PI: Global overview of malaria, *Indian J Med Res* 106:39, 1997.

Kwiatkowski D, Marsh K: Development of malaria vaccines, *Lancet* 350: 1696, 1997.

Kwiatkowski D, et al: The malarial fever response: pathogenesis, polymorphism and prospects for intervention, *Ann Trop Med Parasitol* 91:533, 1997.

Lee LH, Caserta MT: Malaria: update on treatment, *Pediatr Infect Dis J* 17:342, 1998.

Looareesuwan S, Chulay JD, Canfield CJ: Malarone (atovaquone and proguanil hydrochloride): a review of its clinical development for the treatment of malaria. Malarone Clinical Trials Study Group, *Am J Trop Med Hyg* 60:533, 1999.

Makler MT, Palmer CJ, Ager AL: A review of practical techniques for the diagnosis of malaria, *Ann Trop Med Parasitol* 92:419, 1998.

Snow RW, Marsh K: New insights into the epidemiology of malaria relevant for disease control, *Br Med Bull* 54:293, 1998.

Warrell DA: Cerebral malaria: clinical features, pathophysiology and treatment, *Ann Trop Med Parasitol* 91:875, 1997.

Nematodes

Anderson RM: The population dynamics and epidemiology of intestinal nematode infections, *Trans R Soc Trop Med Hyg* 80:686, 1986.

Bundy DAP: The global burden of intestinal nematode disease, *Trans R Soc Trop Med Hyg* 88:259, 1994.

Dolin R, editors: *Principles and practice of infectious diseases,* ed 4, New York, 1995, Churchill Livingston.

Gelhand H: Diethylcarbamazine salt in the control of lymphatic filariasis, *Am J Trop Med Hyg* 50:655, 1994.

Genta RM: Diarrhea in helminthic infections, *Clin Infect Dis* 16(suppl 2): S122, 1993.

Grove DI: Tissue nematodes (trichinosis, dracunculiasis, filariasis). In Mandell GL, et al, editors: Re-assessing the global prevalence and distribution of lymphatic filariasis, *Parasitology* 112:409, 1996.

Hlaing T: Ascariasis and childhood malnutrition. *Parasitology* 107(suppl): S125, 1993.

Igra-Siegman Y, et al: Syndrome of hyperinfection with *Strongyloides stercoralis, Rev Infect Dis* 3:397, 1981.

Khuroo MS: Ascariasis, *Gastroenterol Clin North Am* 25:553, 1996.

Koontz F, Weinstock JV: The approach to stool examination for parasites, *Gastroenterol Clin North Am* 25:435, 1996.

McCarthy JS, Nutman TB: Perspective: prospects for development of vaccines against helminths infection, *J Infect Dis* 174:1384, 1996.

Michael E, Bundy DAP, Grenfell BT: Re-assessing the global prevalence and distribution of lymphatic filariasis, *Parasitology* 112:409, 1996.

Michael E, Meyerowitsch DW, Simonsen PE: Cost and cost-effectiveness of mass diethyl carbamazine chemotherapy for the control of bancroftian filariasis: comparison of four strategies in Tanzania, *Trop Med Int Health* 1:414, 1996.

Ottensen EA: Filarial infections, *Infect Dis Clin North Am* 7:619, 1993.

Pritchard DI, et al: Hookworm *(Necator americanus)* infection and storage iron depletion, *Trans R Soc Trop Med Hyg* 85:235, 1991.

Stephenson LS, et al: Treatment with a single dose of albendazole improves growth of Kenyan school children with hookworm, *Trichuris trichiura,* and *Ascaris lumbricoides* infection, *Am J Trop Med* 41:78, 1989.

Schistosomiasis

Cook JA, Mecaskey JW: A look ahead in research and control of schistosomiasis, *R I Med* 75:217, 1992.

De Cock KM: Hepatosplenic schistosomiasis: a clinical review, *Gut* 27:734, 1986.

El-Garem AA: Schistosomiasis. *Digestion* 59: 589, 1998.

el Kouni, MH: Chemotherapy of schistosomiasis, *R I Med* 75:212, 1992.

Jarallah JS, et al: Role of primary health care in the control of schistosomiasis, *Trop Geogr Med* 45:297, 1993.

Lucey DR, Maguire JH: Schistosomiasis, *Infect Dis Clin North Am* 7:635, 1993.

Morris W, Knauer CM: Cardiopulmonary manifestations of schistosomiasis. *Semin Respir Infect* 12:159, 1997.

Pittella JE: Neuroschistosomiasis. *Brain Pathol* 7:649, 1997.

Strickland TG, et al: Clinical characteristics and response to therapy in Egyptian children heavily infected with *Schistosoma mansoni, J Infect Dis* 146:20, 1982.

Wiest PM, Olds GR: Clinical schistosomiasis, *R I Med* 75:170, 1992.

Toxoplasmosis

Guerrina NG, et al: Neonatal serologic screening and early treatment for congenital *Toxoplasma gondii* infection, *N Engl J Med* 330:1858, 1994.

Nussenblatt RB, Belfort R: Ocular toxoplasmosis, *JAMA* 271:304, 1994.

247 Pectus Excavatum and Pectus Carinatum

J. Alex Haller, Jr.

Significant chest wall deformities in children may cause physiological, structural, and cosmetic problems that often require surgical correction. If 100 children who have chest wall deformities are referred for surgical evaluation, the most common abnormality is pectus excavatum (funnel chest) (90%); many fewer (about 6%) have pectus carinatum (pigeon or chicken chest) (Figs. 247-1 and 247-2). The remaining conditions in which various chest wall deformities occur include Poland's syndrome,[7] Cantrell's syndrome,[4] Noonan's syndrome, and Jeune's syndrome.[5,11,12] Although not thought to be genetic, the exact cause of these chest deformities is unclear. The primary defect in pectus excavatum and pectus carinatum is due to an overgrowth of the length of the anterior costal cartilages. This cartilaginous tissue, for some reason, appears to grow excessively and distorts the entire chest wall, either by holding the sternum posteriorly (pectus excavatum) or by thrusting it anteriorly (pectus carinatum). For pectus excavatum the overgrowth of the ribs occurs in utero; therefore, a sunken chest usually is noted at birth or shortly thereafter. Overgrowth in pectus carinatum usually occurs during the pubertal growth spurts; therefore, this diagnosis is made most frequently in early adolescence. The cartilage in both conditions appears to be histologically normal. Patients with Marfan syndrome may have pectus excavatum or pectus carinatum.

The surgical repair of both these abnormalities involves removal of the overgrown rib cartilage, which allows the sternum to be repositioned.[8-11,16] The cartilage then regenerates from the remaining perichondrium. The chest wall is healed solidly and is fully stable after 6 to 8 weeks. Only then can children safely be released to full activity, including contact sports.

A major difficulty in assessing chest wall deformities in children is deciding which of them requires surgical correction. Unfortunately, no absolute criteria prevail. The physician should evaluate each child frequently so as to monitor chest wall growth and development. Sequential evaluations include (1) measurement, with calipers, of the anteroposterior diameter of the chest and (2) determination of any limitation of central thoracic expansion, of abnormalities in posture, and of structural changes in the upper portion of the abdomen.

PECTUS EXCAVATUM

The vast majority of chest wall deformities seen by primary care physicians are some variation of pectus excavatum. If the deformity is severe, it should be repaired in early childhood for three important reasons: (1) chest wall growth and development will be abnormal if correction is not effected; (2) pulmonary and cardiac function will be affected adversely during adolescence, even though this may not be apparent during childhood; and (3) the cosmetic abnormality will be of increasing concern to the patient. A cosmetic concern is not the primary indication for repairing a pectus excavatum deformity because the structural deformity must be significant enough in and of itself to require intervention.

With pectus excavatum a significant structural problem is considered to be present if the depression is greater than 2 cm. Such measurements, however, often are not absolute. By the time a child reaches 5 to 6 years of age, deformities severe enough to cause difficulties usually are obvious. Fortunately, this is early enough to alleviate secondary cosmetic concerns, and the condition can be repaired before any significant psychological problems associated with the deformity occur.

Physiological derangement in breathing and cardiac function can be documented in teenagers and young adults who have severe deformities,[1,2] but such derangements are more difficult to demonstrate in children because of the invasiveness of the evaluative procedures.[3,13] In severe forms of pectus excavatum, the heart is shifted laterally in the left hemithorax, and thoracic compliance is compromised; these changes are reversible if the repair is effected before adolescence. The pectus excavatum deformity should be repaired before the teenage growth spurt if normal growth and development of the chest wall are to be achieved. Thereafter, the deformity can be corrected cosmetically, and the basic abnormal chest wall configuration and posture will be improved. The surgeon can employ some plastic surgical procedures to fill the defect with prosthetic material and provide cosmetic correction, but this is not the procedure of choice since these methods do not correct the physiological and structural aberrations.

Waiting until a child reaches 5 to 6 years of age before performing elective repair of pectus excavatum is important so that the child is more mature emotionally and thus may have a better hospital experience and, to some extent, may participate in the decision for surgical repair of the deformity. Even for young children, alterations in the configuration of the body may affect their perceptions of their body image significantly in later years. Postoperative management of 5- to 6-year-olds is far easier than that of 2- to 3-year-olds, and earlier repair has no technical surgical advantage. More-

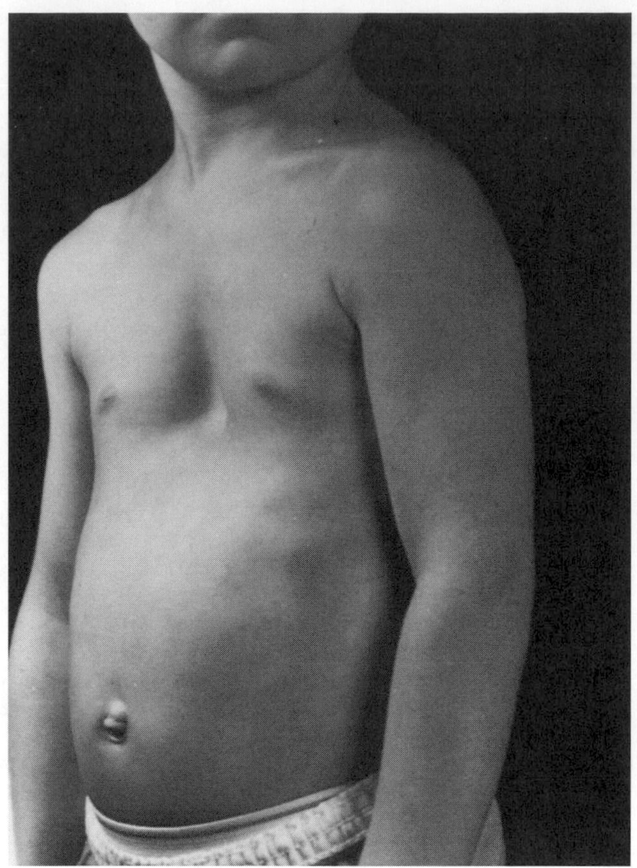

Fig. 247-1 Pectus excavatum.

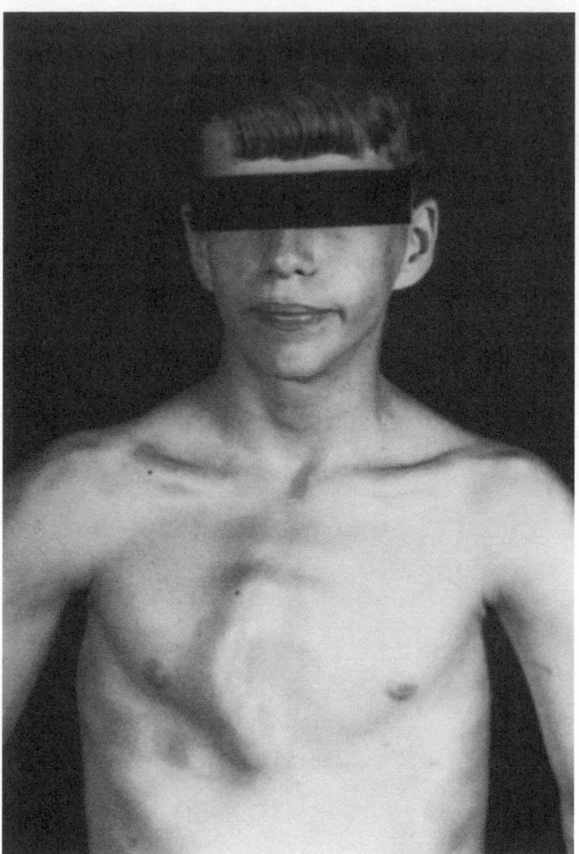

Fig. 247-2 Pectus carinatum.

over, a 5- to 6-year-old can avoid trauma and rough-house activities better in the postoperative healing period of 6 to 8 weeks than can a young child.

The minimally invasive endoscopic surgical correction has become standardized in most children's centers.[9,14] A minimally invasive operative procedure has been introduced in recent years[6,13,14] that employs a curved metal rod inserted intrathoracically at the fourth or fifth intercostal space via small incisions at the anterior axillary line bilaterally. The rod is advanced through one incision transpleurally and transmediastinally, with its convex surface facing posteriorly behind the sternum to exit through the other incision; it is then rotated 180 degrees to elevate the sternum. The bar is sutured on each side to a rib to support it, and left in place for 2 years. No cartilage is removed, and usually no injury to the heart or other mediastinal structures, or to the lungs occurs. Correction occurs immediately but long-term results are not yet available to determine if the correction persists with the teenage growth spurt. This technique is still in controlled experimental trials. The standard operation of removing the abnormal cartilages is essentially bloodless when electrocoagulation is used, and blood transfusions are not needed. The operation, nevertheless, is major because it requires 3 hours of anesthesia followed by considerable discomfort, requiring intravenous sedation and analgesia. Children recover within 48 hours and usually are discharged by the fourth day after surgery.

Traditional, standard surgery yields excellent results in more than 95% of patients. Long-term results remain good, with a low 1% to 2% recurrence rate during adolescence.[6] Complications are extremely uncommon; they include (1) collection of serosanguineous fluid in the substernal and subcutaneous spaces (which is avoided by placement of plastic drains connected to suction), (2) infection (which is avoided by careful sterile technique and prophylactic antibiotics for 48 hours postoperatively), and (3) bleeding (which is controlled with electrocoagulation). None of these is life threatening. The only postoperative precaution necessary is avoidance of vigorous activities, including contact sports, for 6 to 8 weeks until the cartilages have all regenerated. A postoperative patient may be swimming and jogging in 2 weeks. Postoperative cardiopulmonary exercise studies have shown improved cardiac output, especially in competitive athletes.[15] Recent studies from Poland have shown that correcting the sunken sternum takes pressure off the right ventricle of the heart. This may explain the increase in cardiac output with strenuous exercise after correction because there is better filling of the right side of the heart. If these echocardiographic studies during exercise can be duplicated, we may finally have a physiological explanation for the symptomatic improvement that so many postoperative pectus excavatum patients have reported for years!

PECTUS CARINATUM

Pectus carinatum is much less common than is pectus excavatum, occurring in only 6% of all children who have chest wall deformities. It also appears to result from overgrowth of the involved costal cartilages, which push the sternum into an exaggerated anterior position. Unlike pectus excavatum, which usually is noted in infancy, carinatum deformities occur during rapid pubertal growth. This abnormality is purely cosmetic and does not appear to be associated with any physiological abnormality. Unlike pectus excavatum deformities, recurrence of pectus carinatum is likely after repair in early childhood because of subsequent chest wall growth in which the regenerated cartilage replicates the initial abnormal growth pattern. Therefore, surgery should be delayed until the patient is 15 or 16 years old, when maximal growth generally has occurred and the deformity can be corrected with little chance of recurrence. The surgical procedure for the correction of pectus carinatum consists of removing the abnormal costal cartilages and repositioning the sternum posteriorly by means of a transverse osteotomy.[11] Healing occurs within 6 to 8 weeks; the patient then can participate in active contact sports.

REFERENCES

1. Beiser GD, et al: Impairment of cardiac function in patients with pectus excavatum, with improvement after operative correction, *N Engl J Med* 287:267, 1972.
2. Bevegard S: Postural circulatory changes at rest and during exercise in patients with funnel chest, with special reference to factors affecting the stroke volume, *Acta Med Scand* 171:695, 1962.
3. Cahill JL, Lees GM, Robertson HT: A summary of preoperative and postoperative cardiorespiratory performance in patients undergoing pectus excavatus and carinatum repair, *J Pediatr Surg* 19:430, 1984.
4. Cantrell JR, Haller JA Jr, Ravitch MM: A syndrome of congenital defects involving the abdominal wall, sternum, diaphragm, pericardium, and heart, *Surg Gynecol Obstet* 107:602, 1958.
5. Finegold MJ, et al: Lung structure in thoracic dystrophy: case reports, *Am J Dis Child* 122:153, 1971.
6. Haller JA Jr, et al: Correction of pectus excavatus without prostheses or splints: objective measurement of severity and management of asymmetrical deformities, *Ann Thorac Surg* 26:78, 1978.
7. Haller JA Jr, et al: Early reconstruction of Poland's syndrome using autologous rib grafts combined with a latissimus muscle flap, *J Pediatr Surg* 19:423, 1984.
8. Haller JA, et al: Evolving management of pectus excavatum based on a single institutional experience of 664 patients, *Ann Surg* 209:578, 1989.
9. Haller JA, et al: Operative correction of pectus excavatum: an evolving perspective, *Ann Surg* 184:554, 1976.
10. Haller JA, et al: Pectus carinatum: results of surgical therapy, *J Pediatr Surg* 14:228, 1979.
11. Hull D, Barnes ND: Children with small chests, *Arch Dis Child* 47:12, 1972.
12. Jeune M, Beraud C, Carron R: Dystrophic thoracique asphysiante de caractere familial, *Arch Fr Pediatr* 12:886, 1955.
13. Nuss D, Kelly RE, Croitory DP, Swoveland: Repair of pectus excavatum, *Pediatr Endosc Innovative Tech* 2:34, 1998.
14. Nuss D, et al: Review of minimally invasive techniques for the correction of pectus excavatum, *J Pediatr Surg* 33:545, 1998.
15. Peterson RJ, Young WG, Goodwin JD: Noninvasive assessment of exercise cardiac function before and after pectus excavatus repair, *J Thorac Cardiovasc Surg* 90:215, 1985.
16. Ravitch MM: *Congenital deformities of the chest wall and their operative correction,* Philadelphia, 1977, WB Saunders.

248 Pertussis (Whooping Cough)

Fred J. Heldrich

Few illnesses have a clinical picture as characteristic as pertussis. At the height of the illness, the harsh, persistent cough occurring in paroxysms and ending with an inspiratory whoop and vomiting certainly suggests pertussis as the most probable diagnosis. Although undoubtedly a disease of antiquity, pertussis was first described in 1906 by Bordet and Gengou, who associated it with the *Bordetella pertussis* microorganism. Although pertussis is one of the communicable diseases of childhood that can be prevented with proper immunization, it nonetheless still occurs, usually in preschool-age children. The reported incidence and the severity of the disease remain highest in patients under 1 year of age. Adolescents and adults who have waning immunity may develop a clinical illness that is not recognized and continue to serve as a reservoir for infecting nonimmunized or partially immunized infants and children.

A well-documented decline in levels of pertussis immunization led to an increased incidence in pertussis in several countries, including the United States,[1,2,11] where the annual incidence rose from 0.82 per 100,000 population in 1982 to 1.74 per 100,000 in 1986.[4] In 1991, the incidence was 1.1 per 100,000, perhaps reflecting an improvement in pertussis immunization efforts; however, by 1997 the incidence was more than 2 per 100,000.[9] There has been a shift in age among pediatric cases. Although 41% of recent cases were children younger than 1 year of age, 28% were older than 10 years.[2] This may reflect a reservoir of infection in older patients whose immunity has waned and in whom the illness has been attenuated. Nonetheless, they represent a source of infection capable of infecting unimmunized infants. Unless immunization policies continue to be implemented, outbreaks of pertussis will continue.

ETIOLOGY

B. pertussis, a motile, gram-negative rod, is the etiological agent in most cases. A special medium (Bordet-Gengou) and special care in obtaining the specimen are required to obtain a positive culture with this fastidious organism. Either coughing directly onto the culture medium or inoculating the medium directly from a nasopharyngeal swab gives the best results. Of the two methods, the nasopharyngeal culture is preferred, especially for younger patients. The direct fluorescent antibody (DFA) test is a more sensitive and rapid diagnostic procedure than culture. It increases the possibility of laboratory confirmation.[8,11,12]

PATHOLOGY

The tissue most involved is the respiratory epithelium, extending from the upper respiratory tract to the trachea, bronchi, and bronchioles. Histologically, the organisms are lodged in the cilia of the epithelial cells, with underlying epithelial cell changes consisting of edema and necrosis; also, inflammatory cells infiltrate the interstitial tissues. A mucopurulent exudate, which may cover the respiratory epithelium, can lead to airflow obstruction. Alveolar exudate is thought to be caused by secondary bacterial invasion. The ability of pertussis to elaborate an endotoxin may be responsible for lymphocytic predominance in the peripheral blood count, local tissue damage, and hypoglycemia.

CLINICAL PRESENTATION

Typically, the child who has pertussis progresses through three stages, characterized by varying symptoms and clinical severity: the catarrhal stage, the acute stage, and the stage of convalescence. Each stage lasts approximately 2 weeks. The illness may extend longer than the usual 6 weeks, especially with prolongation of the acute stage. In such instances, other causes of persistent cough should be seriously considered.

The incubation period is from 7 to 14 days, with an average of 10. The illness is ushered in with symptoms of a "cold"—sneezing, rhinitis, lacrimation, and cough. The cough soon becomes more pronounced than is customary with the usual cold and becomes a dominant feature by the end of the first week. Fever, if present, usually is low grade. Systemic, nonspecific symptoms of malaise and anorexia also are seen.

In infants younger than 2 months of age, apnea, bradycardia, cyanosis, and seizures are symptoms that frequently are seen in early stages of the disease and should not be considered as complications only. Classic symptoms usually follow in infants who present in this fashion.

Unless exposure to pertussis is known, the diagnosis may not be seriously considered until the second week of illness or until the cough has become more persistent and annoying. The cough occurs in bursts or paroxysms and has been described as harsh, dry, irritating, and rapid. It accompanies the expiratory phase of respiration and may be especially prominent at night, disturbing the child's (and the parents') sleep. When these bursts of explosive coughing increase in frequency and are followed by an exaggerated inspiratory effort or "whoop," the acute, or paroxysmal, stage has begun.

When coughing is of this magnitude, the patient also shows signs of respiratory distress. The face becomes suffused and red or cyanotic. Neck veins become more prominent, and the child becomes alarmed and anxious. The face appears swollen, the eyes prominent. The tongue may protrude, and perspiration may be profuse. The child vomits thick, tenacious material and may appear to be "strangling." Facial petechiae, conjunctival hemorrhage, and epistaxis may occur because of the severe coughing episodes. Paroxysms may last 10 to 15 seconds; after these episodes the child frequently is exhausted and obtunded. The frequency of these paroxysmal outbursts may range from several per day to several per hour and may be precipitated by eating or drinking. External stimuli such as smoke, examination of the pharynx, or pressure on the trachea also may precipitate the attack. In younger patients the inspiratory whoops may be absent; however, these patients are at risk for respiratory arrest and may require resuscitation.

After approximately 2 weeks of severe distress (by the fourth week of illness), symptoms begin to abate; the vomiting and whoop clear first. By the sixth week the cough usually has diminished markedly and, barring complications, the patient is well on the way to recovery. After recovery the patient may experience bouts of paroxysmal coughing, with further episodes of respiratory tract infection for the next few months or longer.[7]

Partial immunity provided by inadequate primary immunization, or a prolonged interval since immunization leading to a deficiency in immunological protection, may produce an atypical or attenuated form of illness characterized primarily by persistent cough. These patients become a reservoir for *B. pertussis,* which may result in disease in the unimmunized or incompletely immunized infant.

The physical examination in patients whose pertussis is uncomplicated may reveal, in addition to signs of upper respiratory tract infection, a low-grade fever and, on auscultation of the lungs, rhonchi.

LABORATORY FINDINGS

Success in culturing *B. pertussis* from the nasopharynx is greatest in the prodromal stage of the illness. A cotton swab wrapped on an aluminum wire allows easy access to the nasopharynx. Growth of the organism on a Bordet-Gengou plate should occur in 3 days; it can be identified by the use of specific antiserums to produce agglutination. Pertussis may be diagnosed rapidly by the direct fluorescent antibody test (DFA) or by the enzyme-linked immunosorbent assay (ELISA).[8] Polymerase chain reaction (PCR) diagnosis may soon emerge as a reliable test leading to early diagnosis.[10] The most distinctive, though nonspecific, laboratory finding is a marked leukocytosis, with more than 50% of the cells being lymphocytes. When associated with a cough, a total white blood cell (WBC) count greater than 20,000/mm^3 strongly suggests pertussis. The total WBC may rise as high as 100,000/mm^3, with as many as 90% lymphocytes.

Acute and convalescent sera may be compared if there is doubt about the diagnosis and should demonstrate a rise in pertussis antibody titers; this test, however, is most useful for a retrospective assessment of the illness and most often is not necessary. Ten to 14 days should elapse between the collection of specimens.

COMPLICATIONS

Death from pertussis, although extremely rare today, is most likely to occur in infants. Permanent damage to the lung may lead to bronchiectasis. Bronchopneumonia, usually resulting from secondary invaders, is the most common complication. Although petechiae or purpura, subconjunctival hemorrhage, or epistaxis may occur secondary to the increase in venous pressure associated with the paroxysmal cough, intracranial hemorrhage is a more ominous complication. Another central nervous system complication, encephalopathy, may occur. Although its exact cause is unknown, some have suggested that it may result from hypoxemia or hypoglycemia. Inguinal hernias and rectal prolapse secondary to severe coughing also have been reported.

DIFFERENTIAL DIAGNOSIS

Conditions to be considered and ruled out by history, physical examination, and appropriate laboratory studies are chlamydial pneumonia, a pertussis-like syndrome caused by other infectious agents (especially parapertussis organisms); foreign body aspiration; paratracheal lymph node enlargement; and allergic cough. A functional cause also must be considered. Although not an extensive list, these conditions share a common feature—a persistent, irritating cough.

Chlamydial Pneumonia

Frequently found in infants, chlamydial pneumonia is characterized by a dry, staccato-like cough and a chest roentgenogram that reveals pneumonic infiltrates. Patients usually are afebrile. The past history may indicate a chlamydia conjunctivitis perhaps not treated with systemic antibiotics. Eosinophilia may be noted on the peripheral blood smear. Chlamydiae can be grown on tissue culture from respiratory tract secretions. Serological blood study reveals an elevated antibody titer.

Other Infectious Agents

The adenovirus has been associated with a clinical syndrome indistinguishable from pertussis. Other organisms that may produce an illness similar to pertussis include *Mycoplasma pneumoniae, Bordetella parapertussis,* and *Bordetella bronchiseptica.* Marked lymphocytosis usually is not found with these infections.

Foreign Body Aspiration

Although the act of aspiration may not be observed, a definite choking episode usually ushers in this condition. Localized changes may appear on the chest roentgenogram secondary to obstruction, or the foreign body may be radiopaque and easily visualized.

Paratracheal Lymph Nodes

If paratracheal lymph nodes are enlarged, diseases such as tuberculosis, histoplasmosis, infectious mononucleosis, or malignancies of the reticuloendothelial system must be considered.

Allergic Cough

In the allergic individual, a persistent, irritating cough may be the earliest manifestation of bronchospasm. A family history of allergy or a history of allergic manifestations in the patient should strengthen the diagnostic suspicion. Upper respiratory tract symptoms, such as clear nasal discharge, sneezing, conjunctivitis, or "allergic shiners," also may be suggestive. Frequently, the serum IgE level will be elevated. A therapeutic trial with a bronchodilator will relieve symptoms and thus confirm the diagnosis.

Factitious

On rare occasions a patient with a functional cough may present with a cough so significant that pertussis is considered. Organic pathology must be carefully excluded by a careful history and physical examination; chest roentgenogram, including inspiratory and expiratory phases; and a complete blood count. Finding the patient to be asymptomatic when not observed or sleeping is helpful.

TREATMENT

Supportive care is the mainstay of therapy for the acute phase of pertussis. The patient should be disturbed as little as possible. The paroxysms of coughing, especially in younger patients, may necessitate the removal of secretions via aspiration. Hypoxia, as manifested by cyanosis, may indicate a need for oxygen and hospitalization. Optimum hydration and adequate nutrition usually can be maintained by frequent but small feedings. In infants, intravenous fluid therapy may be required.

Erythromycin, the antibiotic of choice, has been shown to reduce the frequency and severity of coughing and also has been shown to reduce the period during which *B. pertussis* can be recovered from the respiratory tract. Seven days of therapy has been shown to be as effective as 14.[5] In very young infants, periods of apnea may require intubation and assisted ventilation.

Routine immunization procedures call for pertussis vaccination—usually combined with diphtheria and tetanus (DPT)—at 2 months, 4 months, and 6 months of age. In the event of a community outbreak, immunization may be started at 2 weeks of age. An acellular pertussis vaccine now is available and recommended for all doses of the DPT series for children younger than 7 years of age. This vaccine reduces side effects and produces effective immunity.[3]

Graduates of intensive care nurseries who have chronic pulmonary disease are at great risk of significant morbidity or mortality should they develop pertussis. Pertussis immunization should be initiated at 2 months of age, even if the infant has yet to be discharged from the hospital.[6]

Complications of whooping cough require specific therapy. Antibiotics should be prescribed for secondary bacterial infections such as pneumonia or otitis media. Bronchial aspiration may be required to relieve segmental atelectasis. Pneumothorax secondary to obstructive emphysema caused by tenacious secretions in the bronchial tree may necessitate the use of closed-tube drainage. Ventilatory assistance may be required for infants who experience prolonged intervals of apnea and hypoxia. Patients may develop seizures because of tetany precipitated by alkalosis, caused by severe vomiting. Correction of blood pH abnormalities is indicated. Direct damage to the central nervous system by anoxia or hemorrhage may occur and may require anticonvulsant medication.

Although the prognosis for most patients who acquire whooping cough is good, the proper management is prevention. This can be accomplished by adhering to recommended immunization schedules.

REFERENCES

1. Broome CV, Fraser DW: Pertussis in the United States, 1979: a look at vaccine efficacy, *J Infect Dis* 144:187, 1981.
2. Centers for Disease Control: Pertussis surveillance: United States, January 1992-June 1995, *MMWR* 44:525, 1995.
3. Committee on Infectious Diseases, AAP: Recommended childhood immunization schedule—United States, January-December 1999, *Pediatrics* 103:182, 1999.
4. Fulginiti VA: The current state of pertussis and pertussis vaccines, *Am J Dis Child* 143:532, 1989.
5. Halpern SA, et al: Seven days of erythromycin estolate is as effective as fourteen days for the treatment of *Bordetella pertussis* infection, *Pediatrics* 100:65, 1997.
6. Koblen BA, et al: Response of preterm infants to diphtheria-tetanus-pertussis vaccine, *Pediatr Infect Dis J* 7:704, 1988.
7. Krugman S, Katz SL, editors: Pertussis (whooping cough). In *Infectious diseases of children,* ed 8, St Louis, 1985, Mosby.
8. Mertsola J, et al: Serologic diagnosis of pertussis: comparison of enzyme linked immunosorbent assay and bacterial agglutination, *J Infect Dis* 147:252, 1983.
9. Pertussis by year—United States, 1967-1997, *MMWR* 46 (No 54):47, 1997.
10. Pertussis. In Pickering LK, editor: *Red Book 2000, report of the Committee on Infectious Diseases,* ed 25, Evanston, Ill, 2000, American Academy of Pediatrics.
11. Robinson RJ: The whooping cough immunization controversy, *Arch Dis Child* 56:577, 1981.
12. Strebel PM, et al: Pertussis in Missouri: evaluation of nasopharyngeal (NP) culture, direct fluorescent antibody (DFA) testing and clinical case definitions in the diagnosis of pertussis, *Clin Infect Dis* 16:276, 1993.

249 Pharyngitis and Tonsillitis

Philip E. Thuma

Acute pharyngitis is one of the diagnoses made most frequently by pediatricians, exceeded only by otitis media and generalized upper respiratory tract infections. The term *pharyngitis* means an infection or inflammation of the throat; when the tonsils are affected the most, the term *tonsillitis* is more appropriate. Pharyngitis may be associated with other inflammatory conditions of the mucous membranes or may be the sole finding in an illness. Generally, a clinical complaint of sore throat indicates some degree of pharyngitis, even though this may not be the main focus of the illness.

ETIOLOGY

Although pharyngitis most commonly is due to viral infection, a major concern is to establish whether group A beta-hemolytic streptococcus (GABHS) is the cause, because of the possible sequela, acute rheumatic fever. In younger children, especially those below the age of 2 years, GABHS is uncommon, and viruses predominate. In children older than 2 years, it has been estimated that 15% to 20% of pharyngitis episodes are caused by GABHS. The cause of pharyngitis varies somewhat depending on the geographical location and season of the year; GABHS, respiratory viruses, or other organisms, such as *Mycoplasma,* may predominate. In addition to these, many other infectious agents have been associated with pharyngitis. (Box 249-1)

Viruses

Although many practitioners associate pharyngitis and tonsillitis with a bacterial infection, viruses play a major role in the cause of these illnesses. In fact, whenever pharyngitis is associated with symptoms of nasal congestion and rhinorrhea, viral infection is the most likely cause.

Adenoviruses. At least 12 different types of adenoviruses have been found to cause pharyngitis in children and adolescents, accounting for up to 23% of cases in some reports.[13] These viruses cause both a nasopharyngitis and a tonsillitis that can be exudative. Outbreaks of a pharyngoconjunctival fever caused by adenovirus type 3 also have been reported and often are accompanied by a high fever, cough, and myalgias, in addition to pharyngitis and conjunctivitis.

Enteroviruses. Two prominent members of the enterovirus class of viruses—coxsackie A and echovirus—have been shown to cause pharyngitis, often accompanied by respiratory symptoms, commonly in the late summer or early fall. Herpangina is a specific entity caused by coxsackie A, typified by pharyngitis associated with small, shallow, ulcerated areas on the soft palate and peritonsillar area.

Epstein-Barr virus. This etiological agent of infectious mononucleosis characteristically causes a rather severe exudative pharyngitis and tonsillitis. In older children, this is accompanied by fever, adenopathy, and malaise, as well as splenomegaly in some cases.

Herpes simplex. Although traditionally believed to cause only "cold sores," this virus can cause a gingivostomatitis and pharyngitis with initial infection in infants. Studies in a college-age population also have documented that it accounts for 5.7% of pharyngitis cases.[11]

Other viruses. Many other viruses cause a pharyngitis, although pharyngitis usually is not the primary manifestation of the illness. These include influenza, parainfluenza, respiratory syncytial virus (RSV), measles, coronavirus, and rhinoviruses.[16]

Bacteria

One of the main considerations in evaluating a child who has pharyngitis and tonsillitis is to determine whether the cause is bacterial, thus requiring specific antibiotic therapy. Group A beta-hemolytic streptococcal infections are the major bacterial cause, but other organisms should be considered and sought in certain situations.

Streptococcus pyogenes. *Streptococcus pyogenes* causes complete hemolysis when grown on blood agar and hence has been called *beta-hemolytic streptococcus*. In addition, it has been subdivided into groups based on the C-substance in the cell wall, and it has been found that most human pathological disease is caused by the A group. Group A beta-hemolytic streptococcus (GABHS) was not fully recognized as a frequent cause of pharyngitis with the possibility of subsequent rheumatic fever until the 1940s. Whereas other groups of streptococcus (B, C, F, and G) have been associated at times with pharyngitis,[2] GABHS is by far the most frequent bacterial cause. GABHS can be divided into M and T serotypes, and certain of these have been associated with both the rash of scarlet fever (T4)[14] and the development of rheumatic fever (M3 and M18).[6]

The pharyngitis caused by GABHS characteristically be-

BOX 249-1

CAUSES OF PHARYNGITIS

Bacteria	Viruses
Streptococcus pyogenes	Epstein-Barr
Corynebacterium diphtheriae	Adenovirus
Arcanobacterium haemolyticum	Enteroviruses
Neisseria gonorrhoeae	Herpes simplex
Group C streptococci	Influenza
Group G streptococci	Parainfluenza
Chlamydia pneumoniae	Rhinoviruses
Chlamydia trachomatis	Coronavirus
Mycoplasma pneumoniae	Respiratory syncytial
Yersinia enterocolitica	
Francisella tularensis	
Coxiella burnetii	

From Tanz RT, Shulman ST: Pharyngitis. In Long SS, Pickering LK, Prober CG, editors: *Principles and practice of pediatric infectious diseases,* New York, 1997, Churchill Livingstone.

gins after a 2- to 5-day incubation period, usually following exposure to another individual who has the infection. Spread is thought to be by way of respiratory secretions, although fomites, such as shared silverware or household pets, have been shown to be vectors. The ingestion of GABHS-contaminated food also has led to outbreaks of pharyngitis. The illness is heralded by sudden onset of fever, sore throat, and dysphagia, often associated with headache and abdominal pain. Examination of the throat reveals an erythematous pharynx and tonsillar area, often with exudate present. Small petechiae (enanthem) sometimes are seen on the uvula and soft palate. Cervical lymph nodes usually are enlarged and tender. These symptoms can last for 4 days and gradually subside, even if no antibiotic therapy is instituted.

Neisseria gonorrhoeae. Pharyngitis in sexually active adolescents or sexually abused children can be caused by gonorrhea acquired from oral sex, and the organism should be looked for where appropriate.

Hemophilus influenza type b (Hib). The possible involvement of the Hib organism in pharyngitis and tonsillitis has been controversial, but recent evidence suggests that it may contribute to infection in some children, especially those with recurrent tonsillitis. Fine-needle aspiration of tonsils during acute tonsillitis and pathological specimens from tonsillectomy have documented that as many as 20% of sampled tonsils have Hib infection.[4,15] However, with Hib immunization of most infants in the United States in recent years, this organism may be less likely to play a role in the pathogenesis of acute tonsillitis and pharyngitis.

Other bacteria. A century ago, *Corynebacterium diphtheria* was a frequent and deadly cause of pharyngitis, with a characteristic gray pseudomembranous exudate over the posterior pharynx and tonsils. Fortunately, this now is rare in North America, although it still is seen in some developing countries. Various reports have been published of other bacteria causing pharyngitis and tonsillitis, including *Actinomyces, Arcanobacterium haemolyticum,*[8] *Chlamydia trachomatis* and *pneumoniae, Yersinia enterocolitica, Coxiella burnetii, and Francisella tularensis,* the organism that causes tularemia.

Other Causes

Mycoplasma. Two types of mycoplasma have been shown to cause pharyngitis, namely *M. pneumonia* and *M. hominis.* In children, the former causes a mild pharyngitis, often associated with a laryngotracheitis or progressing to bronchitis or pneumonia. In school-age children, as much as 5% of pharyngitis may be caused by this organism.

Fungi. *Candida* is an uncommon cause of pharyngitis but certainly can be so in immunocompromised patients or those taking steroids.

Parasites. *Toxoplasma gondii* is a rare cause of pharyngitis, but its exact incidence is unclear.

Kawasaki disease. Of unknown cause, Kawasaki disease manifests mostly in preschool children who have pharyngitis associated with erythema and fissuring of the lips, as well as palmar and pedal edema and erythema. An association with staphylococcal toxin has been postulated,[9] as have other etiologies (see Chapter 230, Kawasaki Disease).

Exposure to cigarette smoke. Although smoke itself has not been reported to cause pharyngitis or tonsillitis, it has been shown that there is a highly significant association between the incidence of tonsillectomy in children and parental smoking.[5] Children of smokers also had a much higher frequency of attacks of acute tonsillitis compared with children in a smoke-free environment. Whether this association will be confirmed in other studies remains to be seen, but among children seeking treatment for frequent tonsillitis, a history of parental smoking should be sought. If such a history exists, it would be prudent to recommend measures to reduce the child's exposure to cigarette smoke.

DIFFERENTIAL DIAGNOSIS

Sore throats are common in pediatric practice. The astute clinician wishes to determine which are caused by GABHS so that he or she may administer antibiotic therapy. Unfortunately, multiple studies have shown that "strep throats" cannot be distinguished purely on clinical grounds. Streptococcal infections should be considered in children over the age of 2 years who have pharyngitis, even if no exudate is present. However, pharyngitis associated with nasal, chest, or "cold" symptoms is much more likely to be a viral illness.

When a pharyngitis is atypical, either in its duration or its severity, the clinician should suspect infectious mononucleosis or one of the rarer bacterial causes, including those that are sexually transmitted. A peritonsillar abscess or cellulitis also may manifest as a sore throat, but careful examination will reveal swelling extending into the soft palate, with deviation of the uvula and a change in the tonal quality of the voice. Allergies may lead to chronic inflammation of the mucous membranes, which could include the pharynx, but pharyngitis would be infrequent as a sole manifestation. Postnasal drip from a viral respiratory tract infection or allergies has been thought to irritate the posterior pharynx, but this is not well documented.

The one entity in the differential diagnosis not to be missed is epiglottitis, which can be life threatening. Generally, the child who has epiglottitis has severe throat pain, rapidly becomes ill, appears to have a toxic condition, and experiences respiratory distress accompanied by stridor or a croupy cough. (See Chapter 284, Epiglottitis.)

MANAGEMENT

Laboratory Procedures

Rapid streptococcal test and cultures. The traditional method for determining whether a pharyngitis or tonsillitis was caused by a virus or by GABHS was to take a throat swab and do a culture. Many pediatricians' offices had a candle jar incubator in which culture plates containing bacitracin disks were placed daily and read the following morning. Fortunately, with the availability of "rapid strep" tests, this process was made simpler, allowing a result to be obtained in minutes, rather than waiting 1 to 2 days. Unfortunately, with the advent of strict federal guidelines for office laboratories, even the use of these rapid tests requires certification. Despite such encumbrances, most clinicians now perform a rapid strep diagnostic test on all patients whose pharyngitis is suggestive of GABHS.

The various rapid strep tests claim differing levels of specificity and sensitivity. They appear to be very specific (95% to 98%), but their sensitivity can be as low as 70% to 85%, so some cases of GABHS are not detected. For this reason, a positive rapid strep screen is sufficient indication to treat the patient; however, if the test is negative, a culture should be sent. The physician also needs to be aware that some individuals are strep carriers, and they may well be found to be "strep positive" during a viral illness. Because doing pre- and post-illness titers on every child who presumably has GABHS pharyngitis is impractical, all those who are positive are treated.

Serological tests. In cases in which Epstein-Barr virus (EBV) infection is suspected, a heterophile antibody or specific EBV test can be ordered. One needs to ascertain with the reference laboratory whether an IgG or IgM test is done because a positive heterophile test may confirm only that the child was exposed sometime in his or her life to EBV. Specific IgG and IgM levels of antibody to various components of EBV are available but usually are rather expensive and may take some time to get results, making it a less than ideal test to determine the cause of an acute pharyngitis. See Chapter 226, Infectious Mononucleosis and Other Epstein-Barr Virus Infections.

Although serological tests exist to determine recent streptococcal infections, they rarely are helpful in evaluating an acute pharyngitis. An antistreptolysin-O titer is used more commonly in diagnosing rheumatic fever, by documenting a recent exposure to streptolysin with production of antibody.

White blood cell count. The only real value in performing a white blood cell count is if infectious mononucleosis is suspected. Patients who have an acute EBV infection tend to have a relative lymphocytosis, with 10% to 20% atypical lymphocytes. Thus, a blood count may be a helpful diagnostic study, together with a heterophile or specific EBV antibody test in a child who has a severe pharyngitis and is culture-negative for GABHS.

Treatment

Pharyngitis caused by viruses generally is treated symptomatically with saline gargles, throat lozenges, and analgesics such as acetaminophen. When GABHS has been documented, either by a positive rapid strep test or by culture, antibiotics are indicated primarily to prevent the subsequent development of rheumatic fever. Various antibiotic regimens have been used for GABHS pharyngitis or tonsillitis, but the standard therapy has been a 10-day oral course of potassium penicillin V given three or four times a day. Alternatively, intramuscular benzathine penicillin G may be given as a single injection, although these injections often are painful not only initially but for a few days afterward. Patients allergic to penicillin may be given erythromycin or a cephalosporin, again for a full 10 days. Although shorter courses of newer antibiotics have been studied and shown to be effective in eradicating GABHS from the pharynx,[12,17] their efficacy in preventing rheumatic fever is not clear, although presumed. A recent study comparing 10-day regimens of amoxicillin once daily to penicillin three times daily showed equivalency.[3] If confirmed by larger studies, once-a-day amoxicillin may become an alternative treatment for GABHS pharyngitis.

Controversy exists over whether to begin antibiotics for presumptive GABHS pharyngitis while waiting for culture results. Because rheumatic fever can be prevented even if treatment is started as late as the ninth day of symptoms, the decision to begin therapy immediately rests with the individual physician who knows the circumstances of his or her patients. Although some practitioners believe that early antibiotic treatment will shorten the duration and severity of symptoms, this has not been well documented. What has been shown in a number of studies is that *communicability essentially is eliminated after 24 hours of antibiotic therapy.* Thus, it generally is recommended that children not return to school or day care until they have been taking antibiotics for a full 24 hours.

In cases of gonococcal pharyngitis, one intramuscular injection of ceftriaxone is recommended. In young children who have this diagnosis, sexual abuse must be investigated. Other possible bacterial causes of pharyngitis are treated with appropriate antibiotics, once the causative organism has been determined.

The question of tonsillectomy often is raised by parents after a child has more than one episode of pharyngitis or tonsillitis. Except in cases of documented recurrent, frequent streptococcal infection or the development of a peritonsillar abscess, tonsillectomy is not indicated in children who have recurrent pharyngitis. See Chapter 270, Tonsillectomy and Adenoidectomy.

Although the administration of steroids to decrease pain in acute exudative pharyngitis has been studied in adults and found to provide some benefit,[10] their use in children is not recommended except in rare situations such as infectious mononucleosis infection with imminent airway obstruction.[1]

COMPLICATIONS

Most cases of pharyngitis present no unusual complications because so many of them are viral and resolve with or without therapy. However, the physician must be aware of the possibility of a peritonsillar or retropharyngeal abscess or cellulitis developing and should reexamine the throat of any patient who is not improving. Other suppurative complications also can develop, such as cervical adenitis, otitis media, sinusitis, and pneumonia. In addition, hematogenous spread of a bacterial organism is possible and can result in bacteremia, joint, bone, or meningeal infection.

Rheumatic fever (see Chapter 257) is the one complication of streptococcal pharyngitis that can be life threatening, although it occurs some time after the acute throat infection. Although the incidence of rheumatic fever is low in North America, it still occurs and has been seen in increasing numbers at some centers.[7] Although acute glomerulonephritis is possible after streptococcal throat infections, it is much more likely after streptococcal skin infections.

REFERENCES

1. Boglioli LR, Taff ML: Sudden asphyxial death complicating infectious mononucleosis, *Am J Forensic Med Pathol* 19:174, 1998.
2. Dudley JP, Sercarz J: Pharyngeal and tonsil infections caused by non-group A streptococcus, *Am J Otol* 12:292, 1991.
3. Feder et al: Once-daily therapy for streptococcal pharyngitis with amoxicillin, *Pediatrics* 103:47, 1999.
4. Gaffney RJ, Cafferkey MT: Bacteriology of normal and diseased tonsils assessed by fine-needle aspiration: *Haemophilus influenzae* and the pathogenesis of recurrent acute tonsillitis, *Clin Otolaryngol* 23:181, 1998.
5. Hinton AE, et al: Parental cigarette smoking and tonsillectomy in children, *Clin Otolaryngol* 18:178, 1993.
6. Johnson DR, Stevens DL, Kaplan EL: Epidemiologic analysis of group A streptococcal serotypes associated with severe systemic infections, rheumatic fever, or uncomplicated pharyngitis, *J Infect Dis* 166:374, 1992.
7. Kaplan EL: Return of rheumatic fever: consequences, implications, and needs, *J Pediatr* 111:244, 1987.
8. Karpathios T, et al: *Arcanobacterium haemolyticum* in children with presumed streptococcal pharyngotonsillitis or scarlet fever, *J Pediatr* 121:735, 1992.
9. Leung DYM, et al: Toxic shock syndrome toxin-secreting *Staphylococcus aureus* in Kawasaki syndrome, *Lancet* 342:1385, 1993.
10. Marvez-Valls EG, et al: The role of betamethasone in the treatment of acute exudative pharyngitis, *Acad Emerg Med* 5:567, 1998.
11. McMillan JA, et al: Pharyngitis associated with herpes simplex virus in college students, *Pediatr Infect Dis J* 12:280, 1993.
12. Mehra S, et al: Short course therapy with cefuroxime axetil for group A streptococcal tonsillopharyngitis in children, *Pediatr Infect Dis J* 17: 452, 1998.
13. Moffet HL, Seigel AC, Doyle HK: Non-streptococcal pharyngitis, *J Pediatr* 73:51, 1985.
14. Ohga S, et al: Outbreaks of group A beta-hemolytic streptococcal pharyngitis in children: correlation of serotype T4 with scarlet fever, *Scand J Infect Dis* 24:599, 1992.
15. Stjernquist-Desatnik A, Preller K, Schalen C: High recovery of *Haemophilus influenzae* and group A streptococci in recurrent tonsillar infection or hypertrophy as compared with normal tonsils, *J Laryngol Otol* 105:439, 1991.
16. Tanz RR, Shulman ST: Pharyngitis. In Long SS, Pickering LK, Prober CG, editors: *Principles and practice of pediatric infectious diseases*, New York, 1997, Churchill Livingstone.
17. Venuta A, et al: Azithromycin compared with clarithromycin for the treatment of streptococcal pharyngitis in children, *Int Med Res* 26:152, 1998.

250 Phimosis

Dennis M. Super

Phimosis (derived from the Greek word for muzzling) occurs when the tip of the foreskin becomes scarred (Fig. 250-1). The scarred foreskin loses its suppleness and no longer can be retracted over the glans penis. The incidence of phimosis in uncircumcised males ranges from 2% to 10%. The signs and symptoms of a child who has a scarred, unretractable foreskin are dysuria, hematuria, poor urinary stream, and tenderness of the foreskin. If the tip of the foreskin is severely scarred and if the opening of the foreskin is stenotic, the child's foreskin will "balloon" during urination. If the stenosis progresses, the child develops hydronephrosis and renal failure from the atretic opening of the foreskin.

The actual cause of a scarred, unretractable foreskin is unknown. Some of the proposed theories for the etiology of phimosis are trauma from forcible retraction of the foreskin, irritation from soiled diapers, improperly performed circumcision, congenital anomalies, and recurrent infection of the foreskin.

Most young children who have an unretractable foreskin do not have phimosis. Almost 96% of male neonates have foreskins that cannot be retracted over the glans. These infants do not have phimosis because their foreskins are still supple. The difficulty in retracting the foreskin is caused by remnants of the tissue plane that normally bridges the area between the foreskin and the glans. In 90% of these cases the tissue plane will be resorbed sufficiently by age 3 years to allow retraction of the foreskin. If this tissue plane is torn prematurely, the foreskin may become scarred and phimotic.

DIFFERENTIAL DIAGNOSIS

Balanoposthitis

Balanoposthitis is an inflammation of the glans (balano) and the foreskin (posthe). This inflammation can occur from trauma (acute injury: caught in a zipper fastener; chronic injury: masturbation), irritants (diaper dermatitis, allergy to laundry products), poor penile hygiene, and infection. With poor penile hygiene, a few drops of urine coupled with smegma, which is a "cheesy" substance composed of desquamated epithelial cells and the secretions of sebaceous glands, becomes trapped between the foreskin and glans. In this intertriginous area the trapped urine and smegma begin to macerate the delicate surfaces of the glans and foreskin. The moist, macerated skin may then become infected. The foreskin and the glans may be tender, warm, erythematous, edematous, and suppurative. The child may suffer from dysuria and urinary frequency, and he may be febrile. Some of the organisms that can cause this secondary infection are *Staphylococcus aureus*, groups A and D streptococci, coliforms, *Pseudomonas aeruginosa*, *Candida albicans*, and *Trichomonas vaginalis*.

Children who have recurrent balanoposthitis or who have phimosis secondary to balanoposthitis may have diabetes mellitus. The glucose in a diabetic child's urine enhances the chance for secondary infections in this intertriginous space. In their retrospective review, Cates, Finestone, and Bogash[2] reported that their adult patients who had recent onset of phimosis secondary to balanoposthitis had a tenfold increase in the prevalence of diabetes mellitus over the general population. Almost 20% of these patients previously were undiagnosed diabetics.

Another type of balanoposthitis that may lead to phimosis is balanitis xerotica obliterans. This type of balanoposthitis is a chronic inflammation of the foreskin and glans. It begins as an erythematous lesion and eventually forms a thickened white plaque that may erode into the urethral meatus. These lesions histologically resemble lichen sclerosus et atrophicus, and there is some evidence linking balanitis xerotica obliterans with squamous cell carcinoma of the penis. Balanitis xerotica obliterans is present in about 9% of all children undergoing a circumcision between 2 and 15 years, with a rate of 19% in those presenting with phimosis or balanitis.[1]

Paraphimosis

Paraphimosis is a condition in which a snugly fitting foreskin or a foreskin that has a partially scarred tip is retracted over the glans and becomes trapped behind it. This incarcerated foreskin begins to obstruct venous return from the tip of the penis, which results in further edema and ischemia. Paraphimosis is a medical emergency because with each passing minute, the amount of edema and the degree of ischemia increases. If the incarcerated foreskin is not released quickly, paraphimosis can lead to necrosis of the glans penis.

MANAGEMENT

For mild to moderate phimosis, initial management is directed toward preserving the foreskin. Treatment involves topical steroids, lysis of adhesions after inducing anesthesia with an eutectic mixture of lidocaine and prilocaine (EMLA technique), and stretching of the prepuce, with lysis

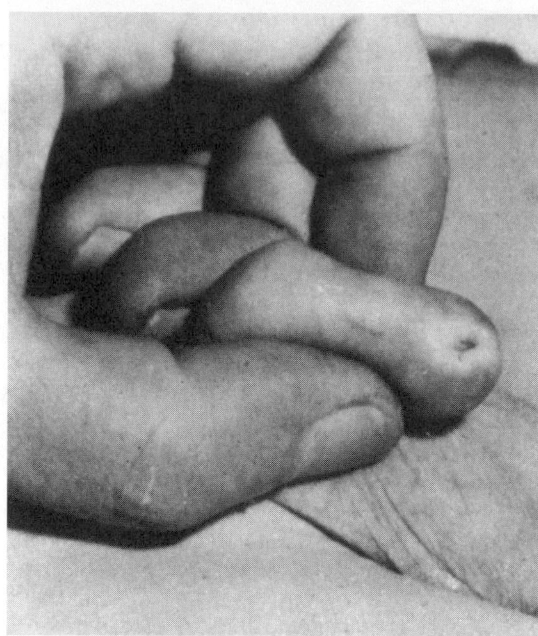

Fig. 250-1 In phimosis, the tip of the foreskin is whitish, scarred, and stenotic.

(From Rickwood AMK, et al: *Br J Urol* 52:147, 1980.)

of adhesions using general anesthesia. In one study of boys who had a nonretractable foreskin and ballooning of the foreskin with micturition, the two conditions resolved in 84 of 111 cases (76%) after a 1- to 2-month course of betamethasone valerate (0.5%), which was applied to the tip of the foreskin three times a day.[9] In this study, more than half the children who failed topical steroids and who were later circumcised had balanitis xerotica obliterans. In the study by Lafferty, MacGregor, and Scobie, lysis of adhesions with EMLA produced a retractable foreskin in 85% of the cases, and stretching of the prepuce was successful in 73% of the cases.[4]

If the aforementioned regimens fail to produce a retractable foreskin, the child should be circumcised. Circumcision also is the preferred treatment if the phimosis occurs secondary to balanitis xerotica obliterans or if significant renal impairment develops secondary to the phimosis.

In balanoposthitis, a wet mount preparation, a potassium hydroxide (KOH) preparation, a rapid antigen study for group A beta hemolytic streptococcus, and a Gram stain of the exudate may help determine which organism is causing the infection. If the history or physical examination (urethral exudate with stripping of the urethra) is suggestive of sexual abuse, the evaluation includes appropriate studies for sexually transmitted diseases.[7] Because of the association between balanoposthitis and diabetes mellitus, children who have balanoposthitis also should be tested for diabetes mellitus by either a urinalysis or a glucose tolerance test.

The treatment for balanoposthitis consists of reducing edema by elevating the penis and improving penile hygiene by Sitz baths, warm soaks to the glans, and proper care of the foreskin.[5] Depending on the cause of the inflammation, the child may also need antimicrobial therapy and/or topical steroids. Broad-spectrum systemic antibiotics may be needed if the infection is severe. If the KOH preparation contains yeast forms, the treatment also should include topical nystatin for *C. albicans*. The patient should be treated with metronidazole (Flagyl) if the wet mount preparation or urinalysis contains *T. vaginalis*.

Untreated balanoposthitis can cause severe edema, resulting in an ischemic glans penis. A dorsal slit of the foreskin will reduce this strangulation of the glans. After the edema and the ischemia have resolved, the slitted foreskin can be removed by circumcision. Circumcision also can prevent recurrent episodes of balanoposthitis in children who cannot maintain proper penile hygiene.

The treatment for balanitis xerotica obliterans is circumcision, especially if the patient has phimosis. Penile lesions are removed surgically. If removal of the lesion is impractical, topical or intralesional corticosteroids are used.[6]

The treatment of paraphimosis is a medical emergency because of possible ischemia of the glans. In the outpatient setting, the clinician may try to release the trapped foreskin by gently applying outward traction on the foreskin while pushing the glans inward. If this fails, the outpatient treatment options are the iced-glove technique and the multiple puncture method.[3,8] In the iced-glove technique, the foreskin is lubricated and anesthetized by applying a lidocaine jelly to it for 2 minutes. The foreskin then is retracted, and the glans and shaft are inserted into the thumb of a sealed glove filled with ice water. The entire glove is pushed down the shaft of the penis until it rests on the symphysis pubis. The glove is held in place for about 5 minutes or until the edema is reduced. Finally, the iced glove is removed and the constricting foreskin is slipped over the glans.[3] In the multiple-puncture method, the foreskin can be anesthetized with a local anesthetic, using a penile ring block; 20 to 30 punctures can be made in the foreskin with a 20- to 25-gauge needle. Usually, this results in the seepage of enough transudate to allow reduction of the foreskin.[8] If these methods fail to reduce the paraphimosis or if, at any time, the blood supply to the glans is severely compromised, the patient should receive a general anesthetic and undergo either a manual reduction or a dorsal slit of the foreskin. Following reduction of the paraphimosis, the child should be circumcised to prevent recurrence.

When to Refer

Phimosis
Obstructive uropathy
Failure of topical steroids
Parents desire a circumcision

Paraphimosis
Failure of manual reduction in the outpatient setting
Prevention of future episodes by elective circumcision

Balanoposthitis
Recurrent episodes
Balanitis xerotica obliterans
Vascular comprise of the glans

When to Hospitalize

Phimosis
Renal failure
Unable to urinate or severe dysuria

Paraphimosis
Failure of manual reduction in the outpatient setting
Vascular compromise to the glans
Unable to urinate or severe dysuria

Balanoposthitis
Severe systemic infection (sepsis, cellulitis)
Vascular compromise of the glans
Unable to urinate or severe dysuria

REFERENCES

1. Bale PM, et al: Balanitis xerotica obliterans in children, *Pediatr Pathol* 7:617, 1987.
2. Cates JL, Finestone A, Bogash M: Phimosis and diabetes mellitus, *J Urol* 110:406, 1973.
3. Houghton GR: The "iced-glove" method of treatment of paraphimosis, *Br J Surg* 60:876, 1973.
4. Lafferty PM, MacGregor FB, Scobie WG: Management of foreskin problems, *Arch Dis Child* 66:696, 1991.
5. Osborn LM, Metcalf TJ, Mariani EM: Hygienic care in uncircumcised infants, *Pediatrics* 67:365, 1981.
6. Rickwood AMK, et al: Phimosis in boys, *Br J Urol* 52:147, 1980.
7. Schwartz RH, Rushton HG: Acute balanoposthitis in young boys, *Pediatr Infect Dis J* 15:176, 1996.
8. Walters TC, Sripathi V: Reduction of paraphimosis, *Br J Urol* 66:660, 1990.
9. Wright JE: The treatment of childhood phimosis with topical steroid, *Aust N Z J Surg* 64:327, 1994.

251 Pinworm Infestations

Craig M. Wilson

ETIOLOGY

Pinworm *(Enterobius vermicularis)* infestation is exceptionally common. When looked for carefully, the parasite can be found in at least 30% of children worldwide, and infestation rates may approach 100% in boarding schools and institutions. Good sanitation and advanced socioeconomic status are feeble deterrents to pinworms. Adults often are infested (in one study, 31% of Army recruits were found to be infested), and it is not uncommon to find pinworms in all members of a family. The discovery of *Enterobius* eggs in human coprolites from the Hogup and Danger caves in Utah (10,000 BC) proves that the parasite was no stranger to our ancestors.

E. vermicularis is a white, threadlike worm that lives primarily in the cecum and adjacent bowel. The gravid female, which is 1 cm long, migrates to the perianal area to deposit up to 10,000 eggs and dies shortly thereafter. Thus. the infestation would be self-limited were it not for reinfestation. Unfortunately, the eggs, which are 50 × 30 μg, oval, flat on one side, and thin shelled, become infective in about 6 hours. Autoinfestation occurs readily through ingestion of eggs if the host scratches the perianal area or does not wash the hands thoroughly after defecating. Moreover, *Enterobius* eggs are rather hardy and may survive for weeks in dirt, house dust, clothing, and bed sheets. Survival is enhanced by lower temperature and if inhaled and swallowed. Pets may carry eggs in their fur. Once ingested, the eggs hatch in the upper small intestine and the worms mature while migrating to the lower ileum and ascending colon. The cycle from ingestion to deposition of eggs is approximately 4 to 6 weeks. The worm burden within an individual may reach the hundreds, but within an infested population most individuals would be harboring few parasites.

CLINICAL MANIFESTATIONS

Localized perianal pruritus is the most commonly reported symptom but most infestations are asymptomatic. Restlessness and fitful sleep are common complaints, as well as secondary excoriation and dermatitis. Multiple clinical entities have been anecdotally linked to pinworm infestation, including masturbation, enuresis, vaginitis, urinary tract infections, nausea and vomiting, diarrhea, and vague abdominal pain, but it seldom is clear that the pinworm is the cause of these problems.

In rare cases, pinworms invade tissue and cause a granulomatous reaction and granulomas containing worms have been an incidental finding in the fallopian tubes, peritoneum, and bladder. Inflammation associated with the parasite has been found in cases of appendicitis, but in such patients it is difficult to be certain whether the acute attack actually was caused by *E. vermicularis.*

LABORATORY EVALUATION

Diagnosis is dependent on identifying either the adult worms or eggs. Occasionally, adult pinworms may be noted near the anus, particularly in the morning. Eggs seldom are found in the patient's feces even if concentration techniques are used. The best way to make a diagnosis is to use the cellophane tape technique. When the child awakens in the morning, the adhesive side of a 2-inch strip of clear cellophane tape should be pressed against the perianal skin; this is most easily done using a tongue depressor. The tape then should be placed on a microscope slide with the adhesive side down and scanned for eggs. Placing a drop of toluene on the slide beneath the tape will make the preparation easier to read. A single test should detect at least 50% of infestations, three tests will detect 90%, and five tests will detect virtually 100%.

PREVENTION AND THERAPY

Zealous physicians who try to eliminate pinworm from their patients are doomed to frustration and failure. The ubiquity and infectivity of the parasite and its persistence in the environment make eradication extremely difficult. Moreover, vigorous pursuit of a permanent cure may provoke needless turmoil and anxiety in the family. When the diagnosis is confirmed in a patient who has symptoms, the following approach seems reasonable.

The entire family should be treated with one of several drug regimens. A single dose of either mebendazole (100 mg for all ages) or albendazole (400 mg for all ages) is extremely effective and has virtually no side effects. Pyrantel pamoate, administered as a single does of 11 mg/kg (maximum 1 g), also is effective; a transient headache and abdominal complaints have been reported with this therapy. All of these treatments are effective against the adult worms only. Therapy usually is repeated in 2 weeks to eradicate any emerging parasites.

Other simple, prudent measures can be followed, such as clipping the fingernails (a favorite repository for eggs), washing the hands frequently, and showering daily in the morning. Wearing tight-fitting cotton underpants and applying a bland ointment (e.g., petroleum jelly) to the perianal region may limit dispersal of the eggs. The floors in sleeping areas should be cleaned thoroughly, particularly in cases of recurrence. Clothing and bedding should be washed at the time of treatment. The most important aspects of treatment, however, are humility on the part of the physician and reassurance of the family.

SUGGESTED READINGS

Cook GC: *Enterobius vermicularis* infection, *Gut* 35:1159, 1994.

Drugs for parasitic infections, *Med Lett Drugs Ther* 40:1, 1998.

Pearson RD, Schwartzman JD: Enterobiasis. In Strickland GT, editor: *Hunter's tropical medicine,* Philadelphia, 1991, WB Saunders.

Russell LJ: The pinworm, *Enterobius vermicularis, Primary Care* 18:13, 1991.

252 Pneumonia

Christopher E. Harris • Thomas A. Hazinski

Pneumonia in infants and children is a common cause for families to seek medical attention throughout the world. However, infections of the lower respiratory tract have varying morbidity and mortality when comparing illness in developed and developing countries. The combined effects of malnutrition and inadequate immunization may cause much more severe respiratory disease for children living in developing countries who also may not have the benefits of advanced therapy to treat the underlying infection and subsequent complications. This, then, leads to many more deaths resulting from pneumonia in the developing world. However, the general concepts regarding pneumonia are the same and will be reviewed here.

EPIDEMIOLOGY

The incidence of acute pneumonia varies throughout the pediatric age range. Infants and toddlers are more commonly infected by respiratory pathogens. Children in the first 5 years of life have an incidence of 30 to 45 episodes of acute lower respiratory illness per 1000 children per year. This figure drops to about 16 to 20 cases in the 5- to 9-year-old age group. In older children and adolescents, the incidence of pneumonia is estimated to be 6 to 12 cases per 1000 patients. Multiple factors have been investigated that may alter the risk for developing pneumonia. Importantly, exposure to environmental tobacco smoke and airway pollutants have been shown to be associated with more than 190,000 cases of pneumonia per year in the United States among those in the youngest age groups.[2] Other factors that may increase the risk of pneumonia include malnutrition, immune deficiency, or severe developmental delay. Infants who have a history of prematurity and chronic lung disease may also be higher at risk for acute lower respiratory infection.

ETIOLOGY

The etiology of pneumonia in infants and children depends on the age of the patient. However, research into etiologies has often used indirect evidence to prove causation. Some investigators have evaluated acute and convalescent serology, while others have used antigen tests of nasopharyngeal secretions or urine to indirectly determine pathogens in the lower respiratory tract. Also, blood cultures have often been obtained to provide etiological information but are infrequently positive (i.e., 3% to 30% of cases), depending on the organism.

In the neonatal period, acute pneumonia is caused by bacteria that may cause sepsis and meningitis. Most importantly, group B streptococci (GBS) cause a severe lower respiratory tract infection with major morbidity and mortality. Infections caused by GBS have been found in infants up to 8 months of age, but in a recent series, 75% presented by 2 months of age.[1] Other organisms that cause pneumonia in the first few months of life include *Escherichia coli*, *Klebsiella pneumoniae,* and other enteric gram-negative bacteria. *Listeria monocytogenes* must also be considered as a cause of pneumonia in newborns. Less frequently, nontypeable *Hemophilus influenzae*, other strains of streptococci, and enterococci may be implicated in episodes of lower pulmonary infections. Rarely, anaerobic bacteria may be found infecting the respiratory tract of neonates. Infants may also be infected with *Chlamydia trachomatis,* leading to pneumonia with significant auscultatory findings. Frequently, conjunctivitis may precede or accompany the respiratory infection in these infants. It is felt that colonization occurs during vaginal delivery.

With regard to bacterial causes of acute lower respiratory tract illness in all children beyond the neonatal period, *Streptococcus pneumoniae* is the most important pathogen both in terms of the numbers of cases and potential for complications. Various studies have shown that the pneumococcus may be the etiological agent in 25% to 38% of pneumonia cases. Patients may be gravely ill, and complications such as sepsis and meningitis may be seen. The significant overuse of antibiotics in treating young children who have upper respiratory tract infections has led to the development of antibiotic-resistant pneumococci. Resistance may be to both penicillins and advanced-generation cephalosporins. Resistance to other antibiotics may also occur in these bacteria because resistance genes are frequently plasmid borne and may be transferred from one bacteria to another.

Other bacterial pathogens associated with acute lower respiratory infections in toddlers and young children include *Hemophilus influenzae* type B and other nontypeable strains of *H. influenzae*, *C. trachomatis*, *Mycoplasma pneumoniae*, and *Moraxella catarrhalis*. Recently, cases of severe group A beta-hemolytic streptococcal pneumonia have been reported, often with marked co-morbidity (pleural effusion, empyema, and shock).

Among school-age children and adolescents, *M. pneumoniae* is the major treatable cause of pneumonia. *Chlamydia pneumoniae* also may cause pneumonia in this age group. As with younger children, *Streptococcus pneumoniae* may be the cause of significant lower respiratory tract infections. *Legionella pneumophila* is a rare cause of lower respiratory tract infection in older children and adolescents.

Children younger than 5 years of age also are significantly at risk for viral pneumonias. Respiratory syncytial virus (RSV) infects almost all toddlers by the age of 3, with 1% being sufficiently ill to require hospitalization (see Chapter 192, Bronchiolitis). Other viral etiologies that may be seen in the first years of life include parainfluenza virus, influenza virus, and adenovirus. Influenza virus may cause significant respiratory illness within all pediatric age groups, and infants are particularly at risk during yearly influenza outbreaks. It is important to remember that multiple pathogens may be found in the same patient. Also, viral infections, with consequent epithelial loss and inflammation, may lead to secondary bacterial infections. Many studies confirm this concept, with 16% to 50% of patients who have pneumonia harboring more than one pathogen.[3,5]

PRESENTATION

During the neonatal period, signs and symptoms may be nonspecific; infants may present with fever, irritability, altered feeding patterns, cough, and either tachypnea or apnea. Findings on examination may include retractions, nasal flaring, and grunting. Auscultation may reveal crackles, decreased breath sounds, and occasionally, wheezing, especially if RSV is the causative agent.

Among older children, tachypnea, cough, fever, crackles, and respiratory distress also correlate with pneumonia. Complaints of pleuritic chest pain may accompany pneumonia and will help localize attention to the chest. It is important to remember that abdominal pain may be associated with acute lower respiratory tract infections. Milder cases of pneumonia may be associated with findings in the upper respiratory tract, usually pharyngitis and hoarseness. This is especially true for illnesses caused by *Mycoplasma* and *Chlamydia*.

DIAGNOSIS

Diagnosis involves careful assessment of respiratory signs, attention to details of the history, and a complete physical examination. Signs that suggest a pneumonic process include fever, increased respiratory rate, cough, nasal flaring, grunting, retractions, and the use of accessory muscles of respiration. The cough may be dry or productive of purulent sputum. Features noted on physical examination that particularly correlate with acute lower respiratory tract infection include abnormal findings on palpation, percussion, or auscultation.

If pneumonia is suspected, roentgenograms of the chest are indicated. Radiographic patterns may be helpful in suggesting whether a pneumonia is bacterial or viral, but often such characterization is not possible. Lobar involvement, pleural effusions, pneumatoceles, and pulmonary abscess often point to a bacterial process, while bilateral perihilar infiltrates and increased interstitial markings suggest a viral etiology. Focal or interstitial infiltrates often accompany mycoplasmal infection. This also aids in decision making about the need for antimicrobial therapy. Repeat chest roentgenograms are important for documenting resolution of the pneumonic process and should be obtained within 3 to 6 weeks after diagnosis. Lack of radiological resolution may suggest the presence of a congenital lung malformation, a foreign body, or a neoplastic process.[4]

To assist in determining viral etiologies, direct antigen testing is currently available for influenza A virus and RSV. Because of the availability of effective therapies against influenza, consideration should be given to obtaining nasal or respiratory secretions for testing.

Sputum culture is extremely valuable in determining the cause of pneumonia in adult patients. However, it is infrequent that patients in the pediatric age group can reliably produce a quality sputum sample. In patients with significant respiratory distress and a clinical picture that fails to fall into a readily recognized category, bronchoalveolar lavage may yield important diagnostic information that may help define therapeutic choices. It may also allow the discontinuation of certain antimicrobials, thereby alleviating risks of adverse reactions associated with these agents. Bronchoscopy with lavage is particularly valuable in patients with immune defects. This procedure may be done quickly with minimal morbidity in almost any pediatric patient. It often is desirable to consider this important diagnostic test early in the illness before multiple antibiotics have been started so as to increase the yield of the test. Unfortunately, bronchoscopy may not be available to every practitioner.

TREATMENT

In devising a treatment plan for the patient with pneumonia, a primary consideration must be the need for hospitalization (see "When to Hospitalize" on the facing page). Overall clinical assessment is most important in making this decision. Attention must be paid to hydration status, degree of respiratory distress, hypoxemia, and the presence of other medical conditions. The ability of the family to assess the patient for clinical deterioration or to bring the child back for further care also influences whether a child is discharged home. If a clinician feels that a patient requires admission to the hospital, parenteral antibiotics should be given. For patients who have less severe illness, oral antibiotics may be prescribed.

For young infants with bacterial pneumonia, hospitalization usually is necessary. Here, ampicillin along with either an aminoglycoside or third-generation cephalosporin is recommended. This combination provides good coverage for those organisms frequently seen in the neonatal period—group B streptococci, gram-negative enteric bacteria, and *Listeria*. Older infants and toddlers requiring hospitalization may be treated with intravenous cefuroxime or high doses of ampicillin. Many of these illnesses will be caused by pneumococci, which are increasingly resistant to beta-lactam antibiotics, as previously mentioned. Therefore, if patients worsen significantly on either of the above choices of antibiotics, consideration should be given to the institution of therapy with vancomycin. Fortunately, treatment failures are rather uncommon because of penicillin-nonsusceptible strains of *S. pneumoniae*. For children who have severe illness, additional antibiotic coverage with erythromycin or a newer macrolide should be considered. These antibiotics may also be chosen as agents of first choice in the treatment of pneumonia for school-age children and adolescents, thereby covering *M. pneumoniae* and *C. pneumoniae*.[6]

Patients who have less severe illness may be treated orally with those antibiotics mentioned above that can be given orally, again providing adequate coverage for the organisms mentioned.

SUMMARY

Many infants and children will present with episodes of respiratory distress caused by infection with a common bacterium or virus. Clinical assessment and radiographs are necessary in establishing a diagnosis of pneumonia. Careful consideration must be given to the general assessment of the illness and to the need for antimicrobials. Clinicians should ensure that patients recover fully from acute lower respiratory tract infections.

When to Hospitalize

If the child is younger than 3 months of age
If the child has significant respiratory distress (presence of grunting, nasal flaring, or retractions)
If the child is hypoxic
If the child appears toxic
If the family cannot adequately assess and care for the child
If the child cannot maintain adequate hydration
If the child cannot be brought back for reassessment after out-patient therapy is instituted
If the child has other medical conditions that might influence the response to treatment adversely
If this is a recurrent episode of pneumonia

REFERENCES

1. Bonadio WA, et al: Systemic infection due to group B beta-hemolytic streptococcus in children, *Clin Pediatr* 31:230, 1992.
2. DiFranza JR, Lew RA: Morbidity and mortality in children associated with the use of tobacco products by other people, *Pediatrics* 97:560, 1996.
3. Korppi M, et al: Aetiology of community-acquired pneumonia in children treated in hospital, *Eur J Pediatr* 152:24, 1993.
4. Oermann CM, Moore RH: Foolers: things that look like pneumonia in children, *Semin Respir Infect* 11:204, 1996.
5. Ruuskanen O, et al: Pneumonia in childhood: etiology and response to antimicrobial therapy, *Eur J Clin Microbiol Infect Dis* 11:217, 1992.
6. Schutze GE, Jacobs RF: Management of community-acquired bacterial pneumonia in hospitalized children, *Pediatr Infect Dis J* 11:160, 1992.

253 Postoperative Management of the Pediatric Outpatient: Surgical and Anesthetic Aspects

Myron Yaster • Charles N. Paidas • Lynne G. Maxwell

Over the past 20 years, outpatient or "ambulatory" anesthesia and surgery have revolutionized the way surgery and anesthesia are practiced in the North America.[49] Safe, reliable, inexpensive, and convenient, outpatient surgery is an attractive option for parents, children, their health care providers, and, perhaps most importantly, their insurers. Surgical procedures that routinely required 1 or 2 days of preadmission hospitalization and 1 to 7 days of postoperative recuperation now are commonly performed without any inpatient hospitalization at all. The cost savings are substantial; the average cost of 1 day in an American hospital is more than $1000. Government and private health care insurers are demanding the increasing use of ambulatory surgery services and will pay for fewer and fewer inpatient procedures. Besides cost savings, there are additional advantages. Ambulatory anesthesia and surgery reduces the psychological trauma of hospitalization and family separation, produces fewer nosocomial infections, and hastens recovery.[49] In children, examples of surgical procedures that now are routinely performed on an outpatient are listed in Box 253-1.

Although the incidence of serious postoperative complications in healthy children undergoing ambulatory surgery is relatively low (<1%), some minor postoperative problems occur commonly.[12,49] These common anesthetic and surgical postoperative problems can be classified into early and late, depending on their time of onset. Often, it will be the primary health care provider rather than the surgeon or anesthesiologist who will be called upon by the family to diagnose and treat these problems.

SELECTION OF PATIENTS

Guidelines to select appropriate procedures and patients for outpatient surgery and anesthesia are continually evolving and are discussed in greater detail in Chapter 9, Preoperative Assessment.[6,22,51] In general, the procedure itself should not involve excessive bleeding or open entry into a major body cavity. Additionally, the patient should not require any special postoperative nursing care and must have a responsible adult at home who will be available to provide care until recovery is complete. The patient's physical condition and health also play a role.[6,22,51] Anesthesiologists and surgeons often use a shorthand description of a patient's physical status to decide on the suitability of outpatient surgery. This shorthand code, developed by the American Society of Anesthesiologists (ASA) is listed in Table 253-1. In general, patients undergoing outpatient surgery usually are healthy (ASA Class 1, 2) or have a well-controlled systemic illness (ASA Class 3). The ex-premature infant poses a unique problem, because these patients are at an increased risk to develop apnea and bradycardia following general anesthesia.[3,20,43] It is our practice to either defer surgery until the ex-premature infant is no longer at risk (institutionally defined; we use 60 postconceptual [gestational and postnatal] weeks of age; others use 44, 48, or 52 postconceptual weeks of age) or admit these children to the hospital for 12 to 24 hours of cardiorespiratory monitoring following surgery and anesthesia.[3,21]

POSTOPERATIVE ANESTHETIC PROBLEMS—EARLY

The most frequent complications or "side effects" of general anesthesia are postoperative nausea, retching, and vomiting.[29,39] Indeed, this is the most common cause of delayed discharge from the post anesthesia care unit (PACU, formerly called the recovery room), and the most common cause of unanticipated hospitalization following outpatient surgery.[29] The etiology of this side effect is multifactorial. Important factors include predisposition (previous history of perioperative vomiting), the anesthetic drugs or techniques used, the procedure being performed, the skill of the anesthesiologist providing the anesthetic, and motion. Certain surgical procedures, such as strabismus surgery, middle ear surgery, orchiopexy, and umbilical hernia repair are associated with a greater than 50% incidence of postoperative vomiting. Similarly, the perioperative use of *any* opioid is associated with a very high incidence of postoperative nausea and vomiting even when less nauseating general anesthetic drugs such as propofol are used.[23,42]

The complex act of vomiting involves coordination of the respiratory, gastrointestinal, and abdominal musculature and is controlled by the emetic center. Stimuli from several areas within the central nervous system (CNS) can affect the emetic center. These include afferents from the pharynx, gastrointestinal tract, and mediastinum, as well as afferents from the higher cortical centers (including the visual center and the vestibular portion of the eighth nerve) and the chemoreceptor trigger zone in the area postrema of the ventral lateral nucleus. The area postrema of the brain is rich in dopamine, opioid, and serotonin receptors.[39] Indeed, blockade of these receptors is an important mechanism of action of the most commonly used antiemetics currently used in practice (Fig. 253-1 and Table 253-2). There are several techniques to treat, or prevent, postoperative nausea and vomiting. These include altering the anesthetic technique (e.g., avoiding the perioperative use of opioids), using antiemetics perioperatively (e.g., droperidol, phenothiazines, ondansetron, or antihistamines, Tables 253-2 and 253-3), and limiting oral intake postoperatively.[2,32,35,39]

Certain anesthetic agents and techniques produce more vomiting than others. The effects of the general anesthetic inhalational agents halothane, enflurane, and nitrous oxide on vomiting are controversial.[5,25] Some studies report significantly more vomiting when these anesthetics are used while others do not. A new intravenous general anesthetic agent, propofol, produces significantly less vomiting and nausea than others, if opioids are not given concomitantly.[40] Indeed, the "culprit" that has been consistently shown to cause nausea and vomiting in virtually every study to date are the opioids.[24] All of the commonly used opioids, whether morphine, meperidine, fentanyl, codeine, oxycodone, or hydromorphone, produce nausea and vomiting.[46] Individual patients may find one drug more nauseating than another and sometimes changing from one drug to another may decrease the amount of nausea and vomiting. Finally, regional anesthetic techniques that use local anesthetics produce less vomiting than general anesthetic techniques.[47]

Avoiding opioids perioperatively may solve only part of the puzzle. Obviously, pain control is essential in children who undergo surgery and opioids are the most commonly used analgesic drugs for this purpose (see Chapter 26, Management of Acute Pain in Children). An alternative may be the use of ketorolac, a powerful nonsteroidal antiinflammatory drug (NSAID), which is almost as potent as morphine as an analgesic but does not produce nausea, vomiting, or respiratory depression.[8,10,45] Because NSAIDs affect platelet aggregation and adhesiveness, their use is limited in many postoperative patients, particularly in children who have undergone tonsillectomy.[8,30]

Insisting that children drink or ambulate when they are experiencing nausea is as good a recipe for vomiting as any one can think of. Many anesthesiologists prefer to keep patients NPO until they are ready and willing to drink and eat, even if this means that the child leaves the hospital while still fasting.[32,34] In essence the child must say that he or she is thirsty, or, better still, hungry, and must specifically ask for something to drink or eat before any food or liquid is offered. Even in the youngest of patients there is little, if any risk, of dehydration, particularly if intravenous fluid management was appropriately administered perioperatively. In current anesthetic practice, virtually all pediatric patients undergoing surgery and anesthesia receive salt and sugar containing intravenous fluids in the operating room and PACU. If sufficient fluids to supply maintenance and replacement requirements were given in this period, a postoperative fast will be readily tolerated. Nausea and vomiting that persists beyond 12 to 24 hours is extraordinarily unusual and requires investigation to rule out an alternative pathology. Thus, just as anesthesiologists are abandoning stringent, prolonged preoperative fasts, they are increasingly appreciating its benefits postoperatively.[32,36] Unfortunately, many institutions continue to require that patients drink and ambulate before they can be discharged from the hospital or same-day-care unit.

BOX 253-1

COMMON OUTPATIENT SURGICAL PROCEDURES BY SPECIALTY

General Surgery
Femoral, inguinal, and umbilical herniorrhaphies
Lymph node and other diagnostic biopsies
Central line insertion
Fistulotomy

Genitourinary Surgery
Orchiopexy, hydrocele
Circumcision
Hypospadias repair

Otorhinolaryngeal Surgery
Myringotomy and tube placement
Adenoidectomy
Tonsillectomy
Bronchoscopy

Ophthalmological Surgery
Strabismus
Examination under anesthesia

Orthopedic Surgery
Tendon lengthening
Spica changes
Fracture reductions

Table 253-1 American Society of Anesthesiologists (ASA) Physical Status Categories

Physical Status	Description
1	Healthy patient who has no organic, physiological, biochemical, or psychiatric disturbance
2	Mild to moderate systemic disturbance caused either by the condition to be treated surgically or by other pathophysiological processes; examples include hypertension, extreme obesity, mild asthma or diabetes, or extremes of age (neonates)
3	Severe systemic disturbance or disease from whatever cause, even though it may not be possible to define the degree of disability with finality; examples include severe diabetes, congenital heart disease, pulmonary insufficiency (BPD)
4	Severe systemic disease that is life threatening, not always correctable by operation; examples include severely limiting congenital heart disease with evidence of cardiac insufficiency, advanced pulmonary, renal, or hepatic insufficiency
5	A moribund patient who has little chance of survival but is submitted to surgery in desperation; examples include major cerebral trauma with rapidly increasing intracranial pressure, necrotizing enterocolitis with profound shock, and presumptive dead bowel

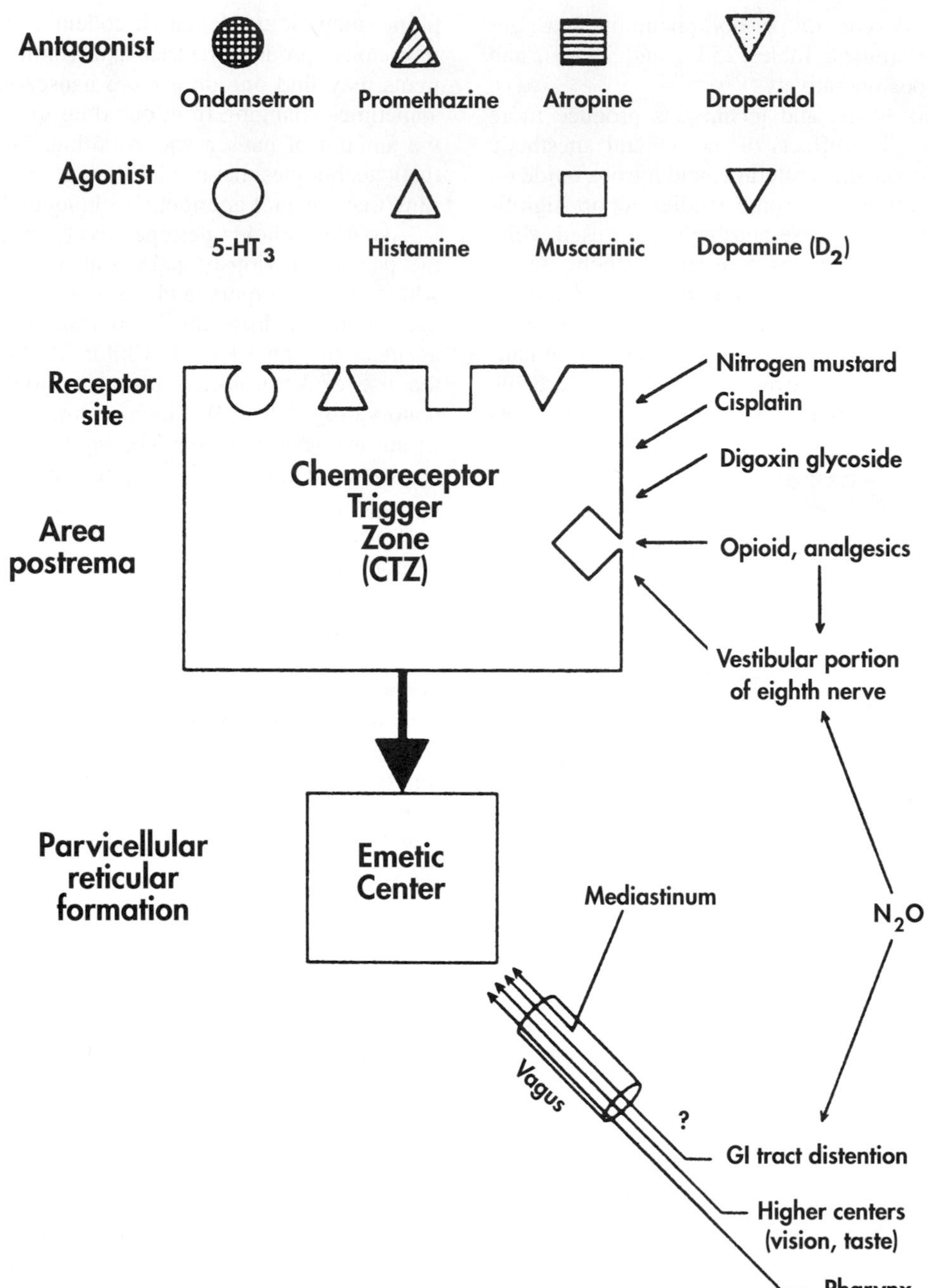

Fig. 253-1 The chemoreceptor trigger zone and the emetic center with the agonist and antagonist sites of action of various anesthetic-related agents and stimuli.

(Reprinted with permission from Watcha MF, White PF: *Anesthesiology* 77:162, 1992.)

This almost certainly contributes to the high incidence of unanticipated admission to the hospital following outpatient surgery because of vomiting.

The treatment of nausea and vomiting is the same as for viral gastroenteritis. A "cooling off" period of 2 to 4 hours is followed by sips of clear sugar and salt containing fluids (e.g., oral rehydration solution, Gatorade [see Chapter 278, Dehydration]). Each sip is separated by several minutes. Giving fluids or solids prematurely only aggravates the problem. Very rarely, excessive air swallowing in the postoperative period may lead to acute gastric dilation in young children. Recognition of the characteristic distended abdomen and gastric splash, if present, should be followed by nasogastric decompression. Finally, antiemetics can be used either prophylactically or to treat the problem once it develops. The most common antiemetics are those that block receptors within the vomiting center. Four major neurotransmitter systems play a role in mediating the emetic response: dopaminergic, histaminic, cholinergic, and serotonergic. Antiemetic drugs may act at more than one receptor, but they tend to have a more prominent action at one or two receptors.[39] The most commonly used antiemetics include

Table 253-2 Receptor Site Affinity of Antiemetic Drugs

Pharmacological Group Drug	Dopamine	Muscarinic Cholinergic	Histamine	Serotonin
Phenothiazines				
Chlorpromazine	++++	++	++++	+
Prochlorperazine	++++			
Butyrophenones				
Droperidol	++++	—	+	+
Haloperidol	++++	—	+	—
Antihistamines				
Promethazine	++	++	++++	—
Diphenhydramine	+	++	++++	—
Benzamides				
Metoclopramide	+++	—	+	++
Anticholinergics				
Scopolamine	+	++++	+	—
Antiserotonin				
Ondansetron	—	—	—	++++

From Watcha MF, White PF: *Anesthesiology* 77:162, 1992.

Table 253-3 Dosage Guidelines for Commonly Used Antiemetics

Pharmacological Group (Generic)	Brand Name	Dosage (mg/kg)	Comments
Phenothiazines			Adverse effects include drowsiness, hypotension, arrhythmias, extrapyramidal symptoms; potentiates effects of opioids, sedatives
Chlorpromazine	Thorazine	IV, PO: 0.5-1 q6-8 hr	
Prochlorperazine	Compazine	PO, PR: 0.1 q6-8 hr (maximum dose 10 mg)	
Butyrophenones			Adverse effects include drowsiness, hypotension, arrhythmias, extrapyramidal symptoms; lowers seizure threshold; potentiates effects of opioids, sedatives
Droperidol	Inapsine	IV: 0.01-0.03 q6-8 hr	
Haloperidol	Haldol	IV: 0.01 q8-12 hr	
Antihistamines			Adverse effects include drowsiness, hypotension, arrhythmias; contraindicated in patients taking MAO inhibitors
Promethazine	Phenergan	IV: 0.25-0.5 q6 hr	
Diphenhydramine	Benadryl	0.5-1.0 q4-6 hr (maximum dose 50 mg)	
Benzamides			Adverse effects include extrapyramidal symptoms
Metoclopramide	Reglan	IV, PO: 0.05-0.1 q6 hr	
Anticholinergics			Adverse effects include dry mouth, blurred vision, fever, tachycardia, constipation, urinary retention, drowsiness, amnesia
Scopolamine	Hyoscine, transdermal scopolamine	IV, PO: 0.005 q4-6 hr apply behind ear 4 hr before needed; lasts 72 hr	
Antiserotonin			Adverse effects include bronchospasm, tachycardia, headaches, lightheadedness
Ondansetron	Zofran	IV, PO: 0.15 q8hr, (maximum dose 4 mg)	

phenothiazines (chlorpromazine and phenergan), butyrophenones (droperidol, haloperidol), antihistamines (hydroxyzine, diphenhydramine), anticholinergics (scopolamine, atropine), benzamides (metoclopramide), and serotonin antagonists (ondansetron).[39,41] Unfortunately, virtually all of these antiemetics produce sedation, which can interfere with rapid return to baseline function. Site of action, dosage, and route of administration of the most commonly used antiemetics are listed in Tables 253-2 and 253-3. The dose and cost of serotonin antagonists can be reduced by the co-administration of dexamethasone (Decadron).[37]

Finally, postoperative vomiting may interfere with the resumption of chronic oral medication regimens. With few exceptions (monoamine oxidase [MAO] inhibitors, oral hypoglycemics, and diuretics), all chronically administered oral medications should be taken on the morning of surgery.[22] Indeed, the question of whether patients should take oral medications on the morning of surgery has become moot because of the liberalization of preoperative fasting guidelines. This ability of patients to take their medications preoperatively has greatly reduced the stress associated with deciding when oral medications can be restarted postoperatively. Most chronically administered drugs, such as anticonvulsants, bronchodilators, and digitalis, have half-lives of elimination that are long (>12 hours). This means that missing a dose of these drugs for one or two half-lives (12 to 24 hours) will have minimal, if any, effect on blood levels. Of course, this assumes that therapeutic blood levels existed before surgery began. If vomiting persists beyond 24 hours, parenteral drug administration may be required.

POSTOPERATIVE PAIN MANAGEMENT

The treatment and alleviation of pain is fundamental to medical care.[31,48] The physician's obligation to manage pain and relieve patient suffering is a crucial element of our professional commitment to patient care. This is not merely a lofty ideal; effective pain management produces a myriad of patient benefits, including reduced morbidity and mortality, early mobilization, and more rapid recovery and return to work, school, and play. A detailed discussion of pain management can be found in Chapter 26, Management of Acute Pain in Children.

EMERGENCE PHENOMENA FOLLOWING GENERAL ANESTHESIA

Emergence from general anesthesia in healthy patients is often accompanied by transient symmetrical neurological changes that usually are considered pathological reflexes. These otherwise pathological reflexes include sustained and nonsustained ankle clonus, bilateral hyperreflexia, the Babinski reflex, and decerebrate posturing. These reflexes can often be detected within minutes of discontinuing a general anesthetic and may persist for hours. It is unknown why this happens. However, the discovery of focal neurological deficits in a postoperative patient is never normal and should point to a possible central or peripheral nervous system injury.

Children are prone to disorientation, hallucinations, and at times, uncontrollable physical activity during emergence from general anesthesia. This hyperexcitable, hyperactive state is sometimes referred to as *emergence delirium* and most commonly occurs if a patient awakens in pain after receiving a potent vapor anesthetic (e.g., halothane, sevoflurane, isoflurane, and desflurane).[4] Other causes include sensory deprivation (eye bandages, eye lubricant); residual anesthetic; awakening in a foreign, "unfriendly" environment (PACU); and the perioperative use of ketamine.[44] Regardless of etiology, before discharge from the PACU, the majority of the disorientation, hyperactivity, excitability, and hallucinatory visual disturbances should be completely resolved.

Occasionally, some lingering evidence of it may persist for 12 to 24 hours. Thus, some children who have undergone general anesthesia and surgery may experience sleep disturbances, nightmares (terrors), separation anxiety, aggression toward authority, and even loss of nighttime bladder control on the night following surgery. Indeed, children who are extremely anxious during the induction of anesthesia are more at risk of developing postoperative negative behavioral changes compared with children who appear calm during the induction process.[13] These children clearly benefit from premedication with a benzodiazepine (midazolam) before the induction of anesthesia. In fact, Kain et al have clearly demonstrated that oral premedication with midazolam is more effective than either parental presence or extensive behavioral preoperative programs at reducing preoperative anxiety and postoperative, delayed emergence phenomenon.[14,15] Ketamine in particular is associated with sleep disturbances following its administration.[44] Although the incidence of nightmares following ketamine administration is less in children than adults, it has been reported to occur in 5% to 10% of patients who receive it. Fortunately, regardless of the cause, sleep disturbance is time limited and rarely persists beyond 48 hours following surgery and general anesthesia. If sleep disturbances become overwhelming, they can be treated with oral diazepam (0.02 mg/kg). Usually, one dose given at bedtime "cures" the problem completely.

INTUBATION-RELATED COMPLICATIONS

Upon awakening from a general anesthetic, many children who have been endotracheally intubated or who have experienced either airway manipulation or instrumentation (laryngeal mask airway, cuffed oral pharyngeal airway) will complain of a sore throat.[11] This discomfort can be alleviated with fruit-flavored ice pops, ice chips, or common throat lozenges once cough, gag, and swallowing reflexes have returned to baseline. Analgesics are rarely required, but if they are, acetaminophen usually will suffice.

POSTINTUBATION CROUP

Postintubation croup, or postextubation subglottic edema, has been a well-recognized entity since airways were first secured by intubation. Children are more prone to develop croup following intubation than are adults because of differences in their airway anatomy. Children have narrower laryngeal and tracheal lumens that are more readily obstructed by mucosal edema. Additionally, the narrowest portion of the child's airway is at the level of cricoid cartilage and not at the level of the larynx. This invites internal tracheal injury since an endotracheal tube can easily pass through the vocal cords and become wedged in the subglottic area. Other contributing factors to the development of croup are traumatic or repeated intubations, coughing ("bucking") on the tube, changing the patient's position after intubation, and providing general anesthesia to children who have a current or recent upper respiratory tract infection.[18,33]

The incidence of postintubation croup has been lowered from 6% to 1% of all endotracheally intubated children.[18] This reduction has occurred through the use of sterile, implant-tested endotracheal tubes and the routine intraoperative use of heated, humidified gases, and in children younger than 5 years of age, by using appropriately sized (air leak pressure of less than 30 cm water), noncuffed endotracheal tubes.[17] Children who have Down syndrome appear to be particularly prone to develop this problem.

The treatment of postintubation croup is the same as

for viral laryngotracheitis. Humidification is effective in most cases. Rarely is nebulized racemic epinephrine therapy necessary. If it is, these patients should not be discharged from the PACU to their homes. Rather, they must be admitted to the hospital for overnight observation because of the potential for rebound edema formation. The efficacy of corticosteroids in treating postintubation croup has been controversial, although most studies have shown it to be effective.[1,16] Most anesthesiologists will prescribe dexamethasone, 0.3 to 0.4 mg/kg, for this problem, even though there are no controlled, prospective trials to validate its use for this purpose. Doses as low as 0.15 mg/kg have been shown to be effective also.[9]

SUCCINYLCHOLINE-INDUCED MYALGIA

Succinylcholine, a short-acting, depolarizing muscle relaxant, was once very commonly used by many anesthesiologists to facilitate intubation of the trachea. Because of the risk of fatal hyperkalemia in children with undiagnosed Duchenne's muscular dystrophy, it no longer is.[38] Succinylcholine administration in all children normally will result in damage to the muscle cell. In fact, myalgia and increased blood levels of creatinine phosphokinase (CPK) and myoglobin are expected "complications" of succinylcholine administration.[19,23] To some degree, much of this can be avoided by pretreating the patient with small doses of a nondepolarizing muscle relaxant or of calcium. The myalgia is intense and is as debilitating as the myalgia produced by an influenza infection. Treatment is supportive, and the pain usually resolves over several days.

POSTOPERATIVE ANESTHETIC PROBLEMS—LATE

Jaundice

The development of hepatic dysfunction (jaundice, abnormal liver enzymes and function) several days to weeks following general anesthesia and surgery has many etiologies, and arriving at a specific diagnosis may be very difficult. Postoperative hepatic dysfunction may be caused by the surgical procedure, the stress of surgery, ischemia, infection, preexisting but unsuspected liver disease, or drugs. One of the more sensationalized and feared is halothane-induced hepatitis. Halothane, a potent vapor general anesthetic, can induce hepatotoxicity in adults and animals by direct drug injury, allergy, or tissue hypoxia.[26-28] In adults, 25% of patients exposed to halothane will develop a mild postoperative increase in serum aminotransferase concentrations that may last for 2 weeks. What, if any, connection this increase in liver enzymes has to do with fulminant halothane-induced hepatitis is unknown. In adults, severe, fulminant halothane-induced hepatitis develops 6 to 11 days after exposure to halothane and has an incidence of between 1:35,000 to 1:200,000 halothane administrations. In the pediatric age group, however, there is no substantiated evidence that halothane hepatitis occurs. Thus, if liver dysfunction occurs in a child following surgery, other causes should be sought. Nevertheless, the fear of producing halothane hepatitis has resulted in the virtual elimination of this drug from the anesthesiologist's armamentarium.

POSTOPERATIVE SURGICAL PROBLEMS—EARLY

Fever

Pyrexia (rectal temperature greater than 101.2° F [38.5° C]) within 24 hours of operation and general anesthesia is very common and usually is caused by atelectasis (Table 253-4).[50] There are many causes of postoperative atelectasis. Endotracheal intubation, inhalational general anesthetics, and the use of nonhumidified gases all depress ciliary motion within the tracheal-bronchial tree and thereby interfere with normal pulmonary toilet. When these factors are combined with small tidal volume breathing, somnolence, splinting secondary to pain, and cough suppression caused by pain or opioid analgesics, the result is atelectasis. Early ambulation, deep breathing, and coughing can be extremely helpful in alleviating or preventing atelectasis and postoperative fever. Indeed, this may be one of the important medical advantages of ambulatory surgery since patients are more likely to be up and about when they are at home rather than in the hospital.

Other causes of postoperative pyrexia are rare. Yeung, Buck, and Filler, in a retrospective analysis of the postoperative course of 256 febrile children at the Hospital for Sick Children in Toronto found that only 4 had infections that required treatment.[50] Interestingly, all four of these children had significant and obvious accompanying signs of infection (local tenderness, crepitance, or erythema at the incision site, tachypnea, cough, dysuria, headache, and so on). Thus, most patients with low-grade postoperative fevers require nothing more than a physical examination to differentiate between a septic and nonseptic process. Extensive (and expensive) diagnostic workups rarely are indicated. Indeed, in the majority of patients, fever in the early postoperative period is so common that it can actually be regarded as a normal response to operative trauma and general anesthesia. Other unusual causes of postoperative fever include urinary tract infections, dehydration, infected intravenous access sites, thyroid storm, pheochromocytoma, and malignant hyperthermia. Urinary tract infections do not usually produce symptoms in the immediate postoperative period. Rather, they are a cause of late postoperative fever, usually occurring 3 to 5 days after operation. These children generally are symptomatic and complain of dysuria, or in infants, may have hematuria.

Wound infection as a cause of fever is rare.[50] The postoperative day on which a given wound infection becomes apparent and the local signs of sepsis produced by the infection vary according to the organism and the concomitant use of antibiotics (Table 253-5). As a general rule, the earlier the onset of wound sepsis the more destructive and life-threatening the infection is. The majority of wound infections do not usually become apparent until the fifth to tenth postoperative day. Two rare exceptions are beta-streptococcal, *Clostridium difficile,* and *C. perfringens (welchii).* These organisms produce wound infections that can become apparent within 24 to 48 hours of surgery. *Clostridium* and streptococ-

Table 253-4 Common Causes of Postoperative Fever

Site	Etiology	Time	Incidence	Sign Symptoms	Diagnosis	Therapy
Wind (lungs)	Atelectasis	24-48 hr	Very common	Cough, shortness of breath, retractions	Examination, CXR	Cough, deep breathing, incentive spirometer
Wound (operative site)	Infection	<24 hr-7 days	Rare	Pain, erythema, induration	Examination, wound cultures	Antibiotics, open wound
Water (urinary tract)	Urinary tract infection	3-5 days	Very rare	Dysuria, hematuria	Examination, urinalysis, culture	Remove indwelling catheter, ± antibiotics
Walker (legs)	Deep-vein thrombosis	>3 days	Extremely rare	Swelling, heaviness of lower extremities, superficial venous congestion, palpable cord	Examination, duplex Doppler, venogram	Bed rest, elevation, heparin/coumadin, thrombolytics

Table 253-5 Postoperative Wound Infections

Onset (PO Day)	Usual Pathogens	Wound Appearance	Other Signs
1-3	*Clostridium welchii*	Brawny, hemorrhagic, cool Occasional gaseous crepitance Putrid "dishwasher" exudate Intense local pain	High standard fever (39°-40° C) Irrational behavior Leukocytosis >15,000/mm^3 Occasional jaundice
2-3	Streptococcus	Erythematous, warm, tender Occasionally, hemorrhagic with blebs Serous exudate	High, spiking fever (39°-40° C) Irrational at times Leukocytosis >15,000 mm^3 Rare jaundice
3-5	Staphylococcus	Erythematous, warm, tender Purulent exudate	High, spiking fever (38°-40° C) Irrational behavior at times Leukocytosis 12,000-20,000/mm^3
>5	Gram-negative rods	Erythematous, warm, tender Purulent exudate	Sustained low-grade to moderate fever (38°-40° C) Rational behavior Leukocytosis 10,000-16,000/mm^3
>5	Symbiotic (usually anaerobes plus gram-negative rods)	Erythematous, warm, tender Focal necrosis Purulent, putrid exudate	Moderate to high fever (38°-40° C) Leukocytosis >15,000/mm^3 Occasional jaundice Mentation variable

cal wound infections are life threatening, and children with these infections appear acutely toxic. Usually, they develop high, spiking fevers (102.2° to 105.8° F [39° to 41° C]), become irrational, and may even develop jaundice. The surgical incision site is red, warm, and intensely painful on palpation. Additionally, vesicle formation, wound crepitance, and an exudate may be present. Obviously, patients who develop this type of wound infection require immediate hospitalization and treatment (see p. 1764).

Drainage

A small amount of serosanguinous drainage in the postoperative dressing is normal and should not be a cause for alarm. This is easier said than done; most parents and children are not at all sanguine about the presence of blood in a dressing. It is only persistent bleeding that requires immediate surgical attention. Persistent bleeding is defined as bleeding and bloody ooze that continues for more than 6 to 8 hours after the operation, or a need to change a blood-soaked wound dressing more than twice in the first 6 to 8 hours after surgery. It almost always indicates inadequate hemostasis and usually is due to a superficial skin arterial bleeding site. Until the bleeding site is investigated and controlled by the operating surgeon or his or her designee, direct digital pressure applied to the wound will slow or stop the flow of blood.

Serosanguinous discharge from the operative site 2 to 3 days after the operation may be due to a superficial hematoma just below the incision site. A hematoma can be recognized by its characteristic ecchymoses and fluctuance. Small hematomas directly below a wound, umbilicus, or scrotum usually spontaneously drain or resorb. If the hematoma progressively expands, it may require operative exploration to evacuate the clot and control any ongoing bleeding. In general, a nonexpanding hematoma usually will resolve within 4 to 6 weeks following surgery. If the wound hematoma is associated with pain, the child should be examined by the operating surgeon.

Serous drainage from a wound may be caused by creation of a large dead space during the operative procedure or by liquefaction of adipose tissue. In general, seromas caused by dead space usually drain 4 to 7 days after surgery, whereas liquefaction of adipose tissue, characterized by yellow drainage, occurs 2 to 3 weeks after surgery.

Regardless of size, both hematomas and seromas are excellent culture media for bacteria, and increase the likelihood of wound infection.[50] Both of these postoperative problems should be closely watched for and usually are characterized by the triad of pain, wound dehiscence, and persistent drainage.

Urinary Retention

In contrast to adults, urinary retention is rare in the pediatric surgical outpatient. Indeed, Fisher et al recently reported that 92% (85/92) of all children who underwent surgery through the inguinal canal voided within 8 hours of the operation, regardless of their intraoperative anesthetic technique or their postoperative analgesic regimen.[7] The latter included parenteral and enteral opioids, regional anesthesia (caudal epidural blockade or ilioinguinal-iliohypogastric nerve blocks) or both. This is a significant finding because theoretically opioids and regional anesthetics, particularly caudal epidural blockade, may interfere with the neural mechanisms responsible for evacuation of the bladder. In fact, many who argued against the routine use of caudal anesthesia and/or opioids for the treatment of postoperative surgical pain based their opinions on the theoretical risk of urinary retention. Fortunately, Fisher's data should put these hypothetical concerns to rest.[7]

Fisher et al's data also have important clinical implications in terms of discharge criteria from ambulatory care centers. Many surgeons, anesthesiologists, and ambulatory care administrators have insisted that children void before discharge following outpatient procedures requiring anesthesia. Many patients simply cannot void on command, particularly in the very strange setting of a PACU or hospital. In Fisher et al's study, only 8.5% of patients (7/92) required more than 8 hours to void. All of these patients voided at home without the need for any medical intervention.[7] The knowledge that all patients void within 24 hours of operation and virtually all spontaneously void within 10 hours of a procedure strongly suggests that voiding before discharge is unnecessary.

To minimize bladder distention, the child or adolescent should be encouraged to urinate immediately before coming to the operating room and as soon as possible postoperatively. In our practice, we do not routinely require patients to void before postoperative discharge from the PACU. Exceptions to this rule include patients who complain of lower abdominal distention and discomfort. These patients are initially treated with ambulation, in the case of the older child or adolescent, or palpation of the lower abdomen in infants. If these measures do not lead to voiding and amelioration of symptoms, bladder catheterization ("straight cath") should be performed. Patients requiring bladder catheterization should then be observed for their ability to voluntarily urinate. If bladder function does not return, the patient should be admitted to the hospital, a specimen of urine should be sent for urinalysis and culture, and a decision should be made by the patient's surgeon about reinsertion of a bladder catheter. Nevertheless, the need for bladder catheterization is very rare. In our experience, urination following outpatient surgery requires a "less is more" attitude—that is, the more attention one pays to this issue, the more problems one creates.

Scrotal Swelling

Scrotal swelling and concomitant discoloration of the scrotum commonly occur following inguinal herniorrhaphy and/or hydrocelectomy. Initially, this process can manifest as swelling alone, and may progress to bluish discoloration as bleeding and clot lysis occur. In general, the problem usually is the result of bleeding from the cut edge of the peritoneal sac derived from either a hernia or hydrocele. The swelling and color change should resolve in 4 to 6 weeks. However, if there is fever, erythema, tenderness, and progressive enlargement of the hemiscrotum, an urgent consultation with the patient's surgeon is needed. Oftentimes, this requires reexploration and operative evacuation of the hematoma via a suprainguinal or trans-scrotal approach.

POSTOPERATIVE SURGICAL PROBLEMS—LATE

Infection

Pyrexia (rectal temperature greater than 101.2° F [38.5° C]) 48 hours or more after outpatient surgery is unusual and may indicate a serious wound infection (Tables 253-5 and 253-6).[50] It requires evaluation and examination by the patient's pediatrician or surgeon. The wound is examined for signs of inflammation, such as heat, pain, redness, and swelling. If any of these signs or symptoms are present, the operating surgeon should be informed. If the wound appears to be the source of the fever and infection, the wound can be probed with a sterile swab (Q-tip) and a Gram stain and culture obtained. If pus is present, the wound should be opened, copiously irrigated, and debrided. Regardless of the presence of pus, a culture swab should always be sent for Gram stain and culture.

Gram-positive infections are the most common causes of wound infection. Wound infections caused by *Staphylococcus aureus* or *S. epidermidis* usually are characterized by a milky white, purulent drainage and usually occur 3 to 5 days after surgery (Table 253-6). Staphylococcal infections usually present with high, spiking fevers (102.2° to 104° F [39° to 40° C]) and leukocytosis (>12,000 white blood cells/mm^3). Following Gram stain and culture, the patient is treated with a penicillinase-resistant antibiotic such as oxacillin. Enteric, encapsulated, gram-negative organisms such as *Escherichia coli* usually are associated with significant erythema, tenderness, and possibly, purulent discharge and usually occur more than 5 days after surgery (see Table 253-6). Enteric organisms such as *E. coli* are sensitive to penicillin, cephalosporins, and aminoglycosides.

Finally, in patients who develop fevers more than 5 days after an operational procedure, one should suspect an anaerobic infection or a mixed (symbiotic) infection of anaerobic and gram-negative rods. The skin surrounding the wound should be examined closely for the presence of crepitus and vesicle formation, purulent and putrid discharge, and focal necrosis. All of these indicate the development of gas gangrene or necrotizing fasciitis. These anaerobic types of infections can be caused by the gram-positive cocci, *Clostridium perfringens* or the gram-negative rods of the *Bacteroides* species (usually *Bacteroides fragilis*). *C. perfringens* causes exquisite pain, brown discoloration, and a wound that is crepitant to palpation. Gas may be seen in the subcutaneous tissues on a plain roentgenogram. Wound infections caused by *Bacteroides* usually are purulent and malodorous. Both of these anaerobic infections are life threatening and require immediate hospitalization, resuscitation, and operational evaluation and intervention.

The treatment of a serious wound infection is straightforward and consists of inpatient hospitalization, opening the wound along its entire length, drainage, wide debridement of necrotic tissue, high-dose intravenous antibiotics (penicillin, clindamycin, metronidazole, cefotetan) and, if available, hyperbaric oxygen therapy. These wounds are not closed. Rather, they are allowed to close spontaneously by contracture. If only cellulitis is detected, the wound should not be opened, but the patient should be started on intravenous antibiotic therapy. Lymphangitis, manifested by its characteristic red streaks and tender regional adenopathy, should also be treated with intravenous antibiotics in the hospital.

If the surgical incision site does not appear to be responsible for the development of fever, a thorough history and physical examination should be performed. Particular attention should be devoted to the lungs and intravenous administration sites. As stated previously, atelectasis often follows general anesthesia and surgery. Infected IV insertion sites, phlebitis, or thrombophlebitis, especially in the adolescent female taking birth control pills, also can occur. Additionally, "routine" causes of pyrexia in children can occur in the postoperative patient and include upper respiratory tract infections, gastroenteritis, and otitis media.

PRACTICAL ASPECTS OF THE POSTSURGICAL WOUND

Wound healing represents a highly dynamic, integrated series of cellular physiological and biochemical events. The morphological events that make up the healing of closed wounds include the following: inflammation, epithelialization, cellular influx, and fibroplasia. The inflammatory phase begins immediately. During its early stages, white blood cells migrate into the wound and engulf and remove cellular debris and tissue fragments. This phase sets the stage for subsequent events in the healing process.

After dead material is removed, the epidermis and dermis immediately adjacent to the wound edges begin to thicken within 24 hours after injury. Within 48 hours, the entire wound surface is reepithelialized. This is the critical period during which the wound should be kept dressed and dry. Thus, wound dressings are not required after 48 hours. Wound contamination with stool and urine should be cleansed with water or saline and the overlying dressing should be replaced. Detergent soaps and peroxide should be avoided.

Between days 2 and 3, deep to the epithelium there is an influx of fibroblasts into the wound. By the fourth or fifth day the fibroblasts begin to lay down collagen fibers. This continues for several months. However, remodeling of collagen takes place for more than 1 year. Practically speaking, by postoperative day 4 the wound may be washed with warm water and a bland soap (e.g., Ivory, Dove, Neutrogena).

From the surgeon's point of view, all of the morphological events of wound healing lead to a single important conclusion: wounds become stronger with time. Closing the wound with suture material only serves to hasten the process. Normally, a simple wound will attain 50% of the strength of surrounding uninjured tissue by 28 days. Most wounds are closed using absorbable suture material, which maintains tensile strength for 60 to 90 days, supplies an appreciable amount of wound strength to allow for the normal healing process to take place, and does not require suture removal. This allows the child to return to activity at an earlier time. For instance, adolescents with uncomplicated inguinal hernia repair may return to nonstrenuous activity 7 to 10 days postoperatively. They may return to full activity by 4 to 6 weeks. Whenever possible, toddlers are kept off tricycles and bicycles for 7 to 10 days. As for infants, we advise the family to treat the baby as if no operation was performed (i.e., full bath by the fourth postoperative day and no restrictions for carrying the baby).

SCAR FORMATION

Blacks and whites of Mediterranean descent are predisposed to hypertrophic scars and keloid formation. Keloids are tumors characterized by massive formation of scar tissue in and beneath the skin after any trauma, including surgery. The keloid grows well beyond the borders of the incision, and this is what differentiates it from hypertrophic scar formation. Furthermore, a hypertrophic scar tends to resolve with time and as a rule is not associated with prolonged itchiness. Keloids tend to recur after excision. Children have a greater tendency to form and re-form keloids than adults do. A careful family history may be a predictor of this pathological process. An abnormal scar should be observed for a minimum of 6 months postoperatively. If it does not resolve, a trial excision should be attempted, staying within the confines of the lesion to see what response is obtained. If it recurs, it should be reexcised and a mixture of triamcinolone/ Kenalog 1% injected beneath the scar. This mixture will produce some keloid resolution. A hypertrophic scar, on the other hand, should be treated with pressure. Overall, the management of the abnormal scar should be determined by the anatomical position of the wound, the age of the patient, and any underlying associated diseases.

Finally, all skin wounds and surgical skin incision sites will scar regardless of the expertise of the surgeon or the use of "plastic surgical techniques" in closing the skin. Indeed, it is a myth that plastic surgery is "scarless." Further, the scar tissue will permanently pigment (usually it will become red to dark brown-black) when exposed to intense sunlight during the first 6 months of its formation. Thus, patients and their families should be advised that when going outdoors and exposing the surgical incision site to the sun, the incision site should be completely covered or be protected with zinc oxide or a sunblock with an SPF number higher than 30 for 6 months following surgery.

REFERENCES

1. Ausejo M, et al: The effectiveness of glucocorticoids in treating croup: meta-analysis, *BMJ* 319:595, 1999.
2. Christensen S, Farrow-Gillespie A, Lerman J: Incidence of emesis and postanesthetic recovery after strabismus surgery in children: a comparison of droperidol and lidocaine, *Anesthesiology* 70:251, 1989.
3. Cote CJ, et al: Postoperative apnea in former preterm infants after inguinal herniorrhaphy: a combined analysis, *Anesthesiology* 82:809, 1995.
4. Davis PJ, et al: Recovery characteristics of sevoflurane and halothane in preschool-aged children undergoing bilateral myringotomy and pressure equalization tube insertion, *Anesth Analg* 88:34, 1999.
5. Divatia JV, et al: Omission of nitrous oxide during anesthesia reduces the incidence of postoperative nausea and vomiting: a meta-analysis, *Anesthesiology* 85:1055, 1996.
6. Fisher QA, Feldman MA, Wilson MD: Pediatric responsibilities for preoperative evaluation, *J Pediatr* 125:675, 1994.
7. Fisher QA, et al: Postoperative voiding interval and duration of analgesia following peripheral or caudal nerve blocks in children, *Anesth Analg* 76:173, 1993.
8. Forrest JB, Heitlinger EL, Revell S: Ketorolac for postoperative pain management in children, *Drug Saf* 16:309, 1997.
9. Geelhoed GC, Macdonald WB: Oral dexamethasone in the treatment of croup: 0.15 mg/kg versus 0.3 mg/kg versus 0.6 mg/kg, *Pediatr Pulmonol* 20:362, 1995.
10. Gillis JC, Brogden RN: Ketorolac: a reappraisal of its pharmacodynamic and pharmacokinetic properties and therapeutic use in pain management, *Drugs* 53:139, 1997.
11. Greenberg RS, et al: A randomized controlled trial comparing the cuffed oropharyngeal airway and the laryngeal mask airway in spontaneously breathing anesthetized adults, *Anesthesiology* 88:970, 1998.
12. Hannallah RS: Pediatric outpatient anesthesia, *Urol Clin North Am* 14: 51, 1987.
13. Kain ZN, et al: Distress during the induction of anesthesia and postoperative behavioral outcomes, *Anesth Analg* 88:1042, 1999.
14. Kain ZN, et al: Parental presence during induction of anesthesia versus sedative premedication: which intervention is more effective? *Anesthesiology* 89:1147, 1998.
15. Kain ZN, et al: Preoperative preparation programs in children: a comparative examination, *Anesth Analg* 87:1249, 1999.
16. Kairys SW, Olmstead EM, O'Connor GT: Steroid treatment of laryngotracheitis: a meta-analysis of the evidence from randomized trials, *Pediatrics* 83:683, 1989.
17. Khine HH, et al: Comparison of cuffed and uncuffed endotracheal tubes in young children during general anesthesia, *Anesthesiology* 86:627, 1997.
18. Koka BV, et al: Postintubation croup in children, *Anesth Analg* 56:501, 1997.
19. Laurence AS: Serum myoglobin release following suxamethonium administration to children, *Eur J Anaesthesiol* 5:31, 1988.
20. Liu LM, et al: Life-threatening apnea in infants recovering from anesthesia, *Anesthesiology* 59:506, 1983.
21. Malviya S, Swartz J, Lerman J: Are all preterm infants younger than 60 weeks postconceptual age at risk for postanesthetic apnea? *Anesthesiology* 78:1076, 1993.
22. Maxwell LG, Deshpande JK, Wetzel RC: Preoperative evaluation of children, *Pediatr Clin North Am* 125:675, 1994.
23. McLoughlin C, Leslie K, Caldwell JE: Influence of dose on suxamethonium-induced muscle damage, *Br J Anaesth* 73:194, 1994.
24. Mendel HG, et al: The effects of ketorolac and fentanyl on postoperative vomiting and analgesic requirements in children undergoing strabismus surgery, *Anesth Analg* 80:1129, 1995.
25. Muir JJ, et al: Role of nitrous oxide and other factors in postoperative nausea and vomiting: a randomized and blinded prospective study, *Anesthesiology* 66:513, 1987.
26. Njoku DB: Effects of halogenated agents on the liver and kidney. In Yaster M, editor: *Current issues in pediatric anesthesia,* Philadelphia, 1998, Lippincott Williams and Wilkins.
27. Njoku D, et al: Biotransformation of halothane, enflurane, isoflurane, and desflurane to trifluoroacetylated liver proteins: association between protein acylation and hepatic injury, *Anesth Analg* 84:173, 1997.
28. Nomura F, et al: Halothane hepatotoxicity and reductive metabolism of halothane in acute experimental liver injury in rats, *Anesth Analg* 67: 448, 1988.
29. Patel RI, Hannallah RS: Anesthetic complications following pediatric ambulatory surgery: a 3-year study, *Anesthesiology* 69:1009, 1988.
30. Rusy LM, et al: A double-blind evaluation of ketorolac tromethamine versus acetaminophen in pediatric tonsillectomy: analgesia and bleeding, *Anesth Analg* 80:226, 1995.
31. Schechter NL, Berde CB, Yaster M: *Pain in infants, children, and adolescents,* Baltimore, 1993, Williams and Wilkins.
32. Schreiner MS: Preoperative and postoperative fasting in children, *Pediatr Clin North Am* 41:111, 1994.
33. Schreiner MS, et al: Do children who experience laryngospasm have an increased risk of upper respiratory tract infection? *Anesthesiology* 85: 475, 1996.
34. Schreiner MS, et al: Should children drink before discharge from day surgery? *Anesthesiology* 76:528, 1992.
35. Schreiner MS, Nicolson SC: Pediatric ambulatory anesthesia: NPO—before or after surgery? *J Clin Anesth* 7:589, 1995.
36. Schreiner MS, Triebwasser A, Keon TP: Ingestion of liquids compared with preoperative fasting in pediatric outpatients, *Anesthesiology* 72: 593, 1990.
37. Splinter WM, Rhine EJ: Low-dose ondansetron with dexamethasone more effectively decreases vomiting after strabismus surgery in children than does high-dose ondansetron, *Anesthesiology* 88:72, 1998.
38. Sullivan M, Thompson WK, Hill GD: Succinylcholine-induced cardiac arrest in children with undiagnosed myopathy, *Can J Anaesth* 41:497, 1994.
39. Watcha MF, White PF: Postoperative nausea and vomiting: its etiology, treatment, and prevention, *Anesthesiology* 77:162, 1992.
40. Watcha MF, et al: Effect of propofol on the incidence of postoperative vomiting after strabismus surgery in pediatric outpatients, *Anesthesiology* 75:204, 1991.
41. Watcha MF, et al: The dose-response relationship of ondansetron in preventing postoperative emesis in pediatric patients undergoing ambulatory surgery, *Anesthesiology* 82:47, 1995.
42. Weir PM, et al: Propofol infusion and the incidence of emesis in pediatric outpatient strabismus surgery, *Anesth Analg* 76:760, 1993.

43. Welborn LG, Greenspun JC: Anesthesia and apnea: perioperative considerations in the former preterm infant, *Pediatr Clin North Am* 41:181, 1994.
44. White PF, Way WL, Trevor AJ: Ketamine: its pharmacology and therapeutic uses, *Anesthesiology* 56:119, 1982.
45. Yaster M: Non-steroidal antiinflammatory drugs. In Yaster M, et al, editors: *Pediatric pain management and sedation handbook,* St Louis, 1997, Mosby Year Book.
46. Yaster M, Deshpande JK, Maxwell LG: The pharmacologic management of pain in children, *Compr Ther* 15:14, 1989.
47. Yaster M, Maxwell LG: Pediatric regional anesthesia, *Anesthesiology* 70:324, 1989.
48. Yaster M, et al: *Pediatric pain management and sedation handbook,* St. Louis, 1997, Mosby Year Book.
49. Yaster M, et al: The night after surgery: postoperative management of the pediatric outpatient: surgical and anesthetic aspects, *Pediatr Clin North Am* 41:199, 1994.
50. Yeung RS, Buck JR, Filler RM: The significance of fever following operations in children, *J Pediatr Surg* 17:347, 1982.
51. Zuckerberg AL: Perioperative approach to children, *Pediatr Clin North Am* 14:15, 1987.

254 Preseptal and Orbital Cellulitis

James W. McManaway III • Carl A. Frankel

Periorbital infections in children can lead to serious complications, including permanent loss of vision, bacterial meningitis, and death. Although noninfectious disorders can cause eyelid edema and proptosis and can limit ocular motility, bacterial cellulitis always must be ruled out. Noninfectious causes of eyelid edema include trauma, allergic dermatitis (Fig. 254-1), insect stings, sunburn, and systemic diseases, including nephrotic syndrome and congestive heart failure. The differential diagnosis of proptosis in children is outlined in Box 254-1.

PRESEPTAL CELLULITIS

A sagittal section through the eyelids reveals an extension of the periorbita (periosteum of the orbit) known as the *orbital septum.* The orbital septum extends from the orbital rim to the lid margins and provides a natural resistance to the spread of bacteria from the eyelids into the orbit. As defined by the orbital septum, preseptal cellulitis is limited to the eyelids, although in reality there is a continuum between the preseptal and orbital processes.

Preseptal cellulitis (Fig. 254-2) typically occurs with a 12- to 24-hour history of increasing swelling, ptosis, erythema, and edema localized to the eyelids. Occasionally an insect bite, puncture wound, or area of impetigo may be found to be the origin of this localized infection but usually no proximate cause is found. The area is warm to the touch and usually nontender. Early on, the patient may be uncomfortable but rarely shows toxicity. These children should have normal visual acuity, normal ocular motility, and no sign of proptosis. Without treatment, preseptal cellulitis progresses rapidly to orbital cellulitis, with possible meningitis, cavernous sinus thrombosis, and death.

The management of patients who have preseptal cellulitis consists of ruling out signs of orbital cellulitis, obtaining appropriate cultures, deciding if hospitalization is necessary, starting appropriate oral or intravenous antibiotics, and monitoring for worsening clinical signs. Any patient who has diminished visual acuity, limitation of ocular motility, or evidence of proptosis must have a computed tomography (CT) scan of the orbits to rule out orbital cellulitis. Conjunctival and skin cultures may yield the causative agent; blood cultures should be obtained from children who show signs of toxicity. Because toxicity develops so quickly in children under age 3, hospitalization should be considered in this age group, using intravenous antibiotics for treatment. Older patients who develop toxicity or any patient suspected of having *Haemophilus influenzae* preseptal cellulitis should be hospitalized.

The most likely causative organism in preseptal cellulitis depends on the clinical situation.[4] *Staphylococcus aureus* and *Streptococcus pyogenes* are associated with a preexisting skin wound or area of impetigo. These patients should be treated initially with intravenous nafcillin (inpatient) or oral cloxacillin (outpatient).[1] *H. influenzae* type b and *Pneumococcus* species are associated with a preexisting upper respiratory tract infection. Patients who have purple discoloration of the eyelid often have *H. influenzae* preseptal cellulitis and should be watched especially for worsening clinical signs and for evidence of other sites of *H. influenzae* infection, albeit *H. influenzae* infections are rare since the introduction of the Hib vaccine. These patients should be treated initially with intravenous ceftriaxone and later can be converted to oral amoxicillin-clavulanate if this treatment is supported by culture and sensitivity results.[1] Antibiotics should be used for a minimum of 10 days. All patients who have preseptal cellulitis need daily follow-up examinations until significant improvement is noted to ensure that orbital cellulitis is not developing. No clinical sequelae are anticipated when preseptal cellulitis is treated appropriately.

ORBITAL CELLULITIS

Orbital cellulitis usually is a disease of children older than 5 years of age and nearly always is due to spread from adjacent sinuses, usually the ethmoid. Rare causes of orbital cellulitis include orbital trauma, complications of retinal detachment, orbital or strabismus surgery, dental infections, or necrosis of an orbital tumor. Children who have orbital cellulitis typically have moderate to severe eyelid edema, ptosis, and proptosis (Fig. 254-3, *A*). When the lid is elevated, the eye shows conjunctival hyperemia and chemosis and typically is deviated compared with the fellow eye (Fig. 254-3, *B*). While the patient's lid is elevated, he or she may report diplopia, pain on attempted eye movement, or inability to move the globe; visual acuity may be reduced significantly. When visual acuity is reduced, especially in the presence of an afferent pupillary defect detected by the swinging flashlight test, optic neuritis or optic nerve compression is present, and aggressive management is necessary to prevent permanent visual loss. These patients usually appear acutely ill and almost always have fever and a leukocytosis with a left shift.

The management of patients who have orbital cellulitis

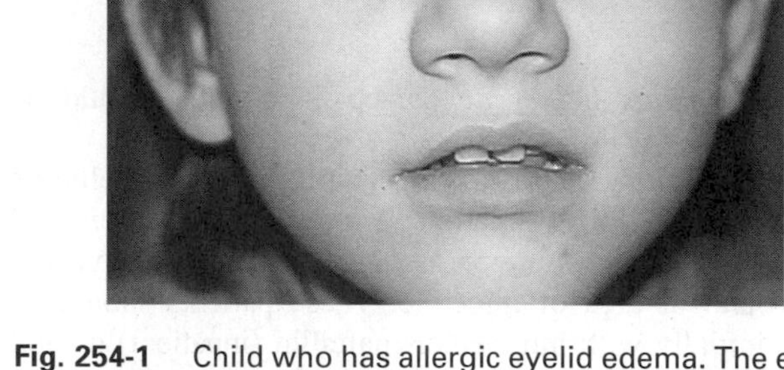

Fig. 254-1 Child who has allergic eyelid edema. The eye beneath the swollen eyelid was quiet and had normal visual acuity and motility. Proptosis was absent.

BOX 254-1

DIFFERENTIAL DIAGNOSIS OF PROPTOSIS IN CHILDREN

Capillary hemangioma
Craniosynostosis
Dermoid cyst
Glaucoma (secondary buphthalmos)
Histiocytosis X
Hyperthyroidism
Idiopathic inflammatory pseudotumor
Leukemia
Lymphangioma
Meningoencephalocele
Neuroblastoma
Neurofibroma
Orbital cellulitis
Optic nerve glioma
Rhabdomyosarcoma
Trauma

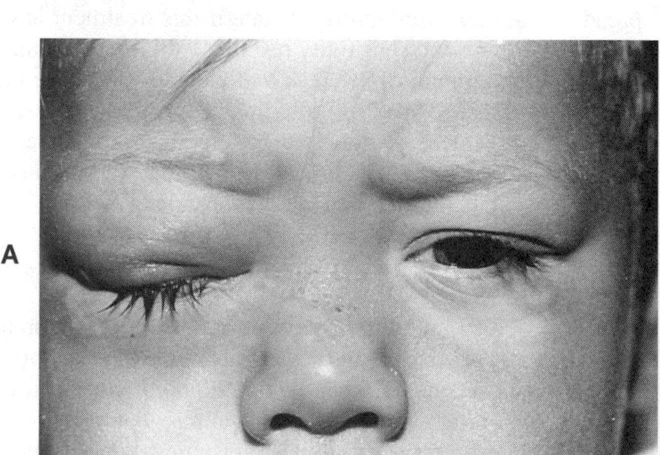

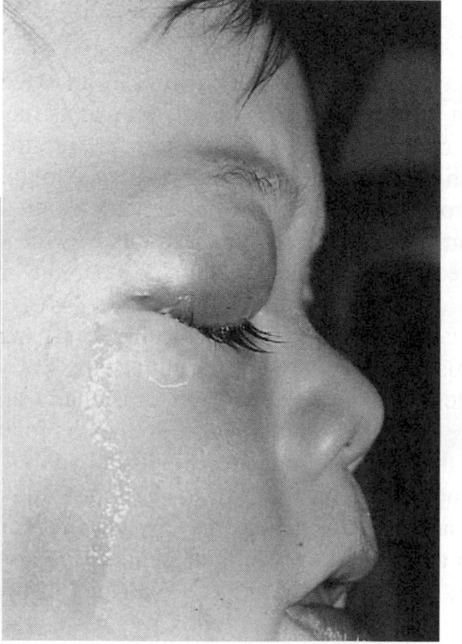

Fig. 254-2 **A,** Frontal view of a patient who has bacterial preseptal cellulitis. When the eyelid was elevated, the eye showed no restriction of motility and produced no pain with movement. Systemic antibiotics readily resolved the condition. **B,** Lateral view of the same patient. Lid edema is significant; however, when the lid was elevated, no evidence of proptosis was noted.

includes hospitalization, a CT scan of the head and orbits, blood and conjunctival cultures, appropriate intravenous antibiotics, and ophthalmological and otolaryngological consultation. The purpose of the CT scan is to distinguish exogenous infections (trauma, orbital surgery) from endogenous infections (bacterial sinusitis) and to rule out an orbital abscess, which must be drained surgically. If CT scanning reveals an orbital subperiosteal abscess, a trial of intravenous antibiotics should be given, as reliable correlation has not been shown between orbital subperiosteal abscesses as suspected by CT scanning and the actual findings at the time of surgical drainage.[2,3] A subperiosteal abscess should be drained if the patient's condition worsens despite appropriate antibiotic therapy.

Children who have typical bacterial orbital cellulitis that occurs secondary to sinusitis in which *S. pneumoniae,* group A beta-hemolytic streptococci, *H. influenzae,* and *S. aureus* are the most likely offending organisms should be given

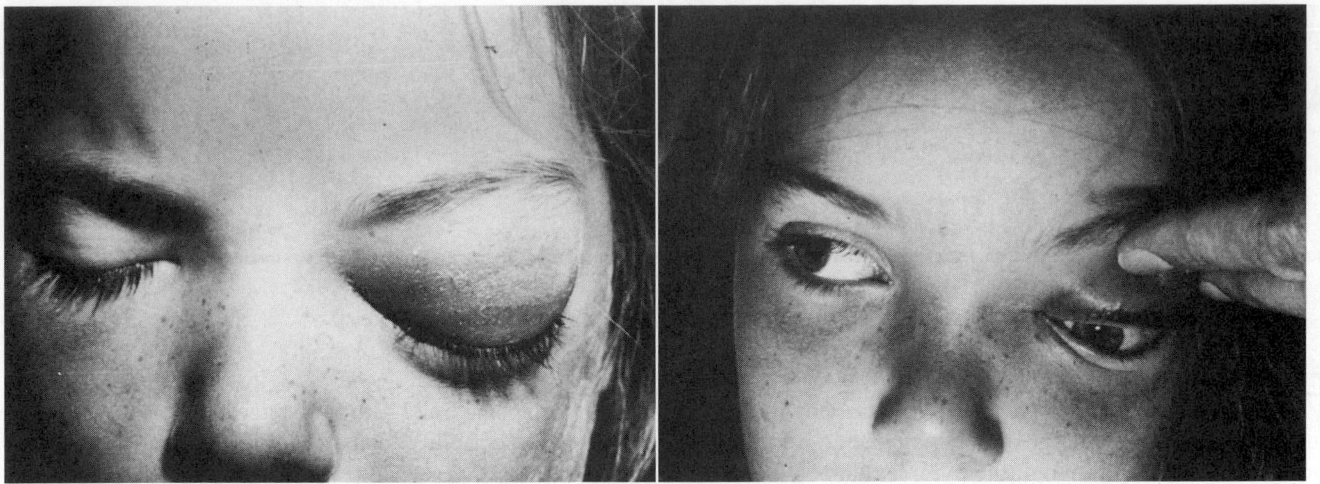

Fig. 254-3 **A,** A girl who has severe periorbital inflammatory edema and a suggestion of inferior displacement of the globe. **B,** The same patient; on elevation of the eyelid, proptosis and limited movement of the eye were noted. Patients who have this condition also may complain of pain when they attempt to move the affected eye, and their vision may be reduced as a consequence of inflammatory or infectious optic neuritis.

intravenous ceftriaxone (100 mg/kg/day in two divided doses—maximum of 4 g/day) and intravenous vancomycin (40 mg/kg/day in two to three divided doses).[1] Patients who have orbital cellulitis that occurs secondary to orbital trauma or surgery in which *S. aureus* and streptococcal species are the most likely infecting organisms should be treated with intravenous nafcillin or tobramycin or both, depending on the Gram stain result of the wound drainage. An ophthalmologist should be consulted to detect and manage potential ophthalmological complications such as corneal exposure, secondary glaucoma, septic retinitis, exudative retinal detachment, central retinal artery occlusion, optic neuritis, and cavernous sinus thrombosis. Otolaryngological consultation may be obtained to manage sinus disease and to assist in orbital abscess drainage if it becomes necessary. The condition of patients who have orbital cellulitis may worsen for the first 24 hours; thereafter they usually improve dramatically. Intravenous antibiotics should be continued until the patient is afebrile for 24 hours; oral antibiotics then should be substituted. If the patient remains free of fever for 24 hours on an oral antibiotic regimen, discharge from the hospital is reasonable, with oral antibiotics continued so that the patient receives antibiotics for 2 weeks.

CAVERNOUS SINUS THROMBOSIS

Cavernous sinus thrombosis is a dreaded complication of orbital cellulitis. Because the orbital venous system has no valves, bacteria can leave the orbit via the ophthalmic veins and gain access to the cavernous sinus, leading to thrombosis. Patients who have cavernous sinus thrombosis have the typical signs of orbital cellulitis but are more toxic. Proptosis is marked owing to poor orbital venous drainage; cranial nerves III, IV, V, and VI often are involved. The thrombosis can spread to the contralateral cavernous sinus, causing abnormal ocular motility of the uninvolved eye. The condition should be managed by a neurosurgeon; treatment involves high-dose intravenous antibiotics, anticoagulants and, possibly, systemic steroids.

REFERENCES

1. Rhee DJ, Pyfer MF: Orbital cellulitis. In Rhee DJ, Pyfer MF, editors: *The Wills eye manual—office and emergency room diagnosis and treatment of eye disease,* ed 3, Philadelphia, 1999, Lippincott Williams & Wilkins.
2. Rubin SE, et al: Medical management of orbital subperiosteal abscess in children, *J Pediatr Ophthalmol Strabismus* 26:21, 1989.
3. Tannenbaum M, et al: Medical management of orbital abscess, *Surv Ophthalmol* 30:211, 1985.
4. Weiss A, et al: Bacterial periorbital and orbital cellulitis in childhood, *Ophthalmology* 90:195, 1983.

SUGGESTED READINGS

Catalano RA, Smoot CN: Subperiosteal orbital masses in children with orbital cellulitis: time for a reevaluation? *J Pediatr Ophthalmol Strabismus* 27:141, 1990.

Eustis HS, et al: Staging of orbital cellulitis in children: computerized tomography characteristics and treatment guidelines, *J Pediatr Ophthalmol Strabismus* 23:246, 1986.

Lessner A, Stern GA: Preseptal and orbital cellulitis, *Infect Dis Clin North Am* 6:933, 1992.

Noel LP, Clarke WN, MacDonald N: Clinical management of orbital cellulitis in children, *Can J Ophthalmol* 25:11, 1990.

Powell KR: Orbital and periorbital cellulitis, *Pediatr Rev* 16:163, 1995.

255 Pyloric Stenosis

Jeff C. Hoehner

Pyloric stenosis (PS) is an acquired hypertrophy of the circumferential muscle of the pyloric sphincter, resulting in elongation and obliteration of the pyloric channel. The resultant gastric outlet obstruction, with compensatory hyperperistalsis and dilation of the stomach, causes progressively worsening nonbilious vomiting and consequent dehydration. The mainstays of treatment are hydration and surgical pyloromyotomy.

INCIDENCE AND ETIOLOGY

The incidence of PS ranges between 0.1% and 1% in the general population. Studies conducted in the 1950s reported rates of 1 in 300 to 1 in 900. More recent population-based studies from the United Kingdom and the United States confirm a rise in incidence from approximately 0.1% to near 0.8%,[16,29]; however, contradictory reports also exist.[3] PS appears to be an acquired disorder. A longitudinal study of 1400 randomly selected preterm neonates confirmed an ultrasonographically normal pylorus at birth in all 9 infants who thereafter developed PS.[34] There is a significant male predominance of about 4:1, although the belief that PS primarily afflicts first-born males has not been confirmed. The incidence in whites exceeds that of black, Indian, and Asian infants. The development of PS involves the variable transmission of an inheritable trait through generations. Maternal transmission is more frequent than paternal; PS develops in 19% of boys and 7% of girls whose mothers had PS and in 5% of boys and 2.5% of girls whose fathers were afflicted.[7]

The etiology and pathophysiology of PS is unclear, although various theories have been entertained. One proposal is that dyscoordinated gastric peristalsis and pyloric relaxation results in gastric contraction against a closed pylorus. This could potentially cause work hypertrophy of the pyloric muscle and initiate a cycle of increasing pyloric obstruction. Other theories incriminate alterations in gastrin levels,[33] changes in breast-feeding practices,[17] and variations in infant milk formulas,[46] among others. Myectomy specimens from patients with PS show a reduction in smooth muscle vasoactive amines,[25] neurons and nerve fibers,[20] as well as the interstitial "pacemaker" cells of Cajal,[44] suggesting that impaired neuronal function may be involved. Other recent observations suggest that local decreases in nitric oxide, a ubiquitous mediator of smooth muscle relaxation, is involved. Nitric oxide synthase (NOS), which is identified throughout the smooth muscle layers and myenteric plexus of normal controls, is selectively depleted in the circular muscle of PS patients.[18,43] Investigations of neuronal NOS gene polymorphisms in 27 families suggested that the gene represents a susceptibility locus for PS.[9]

CLINICAL PRESENTATION

The typical clinical presentation is a term male infant between 3 and 6 weeks of age who has progressively worsening, nonbilious, projectile vomiting. The age of onset may vary somewhat, with PS documented both in the newborn period and as late as the fourth month of age. Prematurity does not appear to alter the age of onset, rather it is the postnatal age that is important. In the typical case, an infant begins to regurgitate a small amount of formula immediately following a feed, although he or she continues to gain weight at first. Later the vomiting becomes more frequent and more forceful (i.e., projectile) and eventually occurs after every feed. The baby continues to be hungry and active, lethargy does not ensue until significant dehydration has occurred. The vomitus does not contain bile, but if vomiting has occurred for a considerable period, it may become brownish as a result of hemorrhagic gastritis. Weight loss, dehydration, and a hypochloremic, hypokalemic contraction metabolic alkalosis (with paradoxical aciduria when severe) result if the vomiting is prolonged. Hypoglycemia may be present and cause seizures. Unconjugated hyperbilirubinemia is common, correlates with a decrease in hepatic glucuronosyltransferase activity, and resolves following treatment.

Although the majority of infants with PS are otherwise healthy and genetically normal, PS has been reported with increased frequency in infants with hiatal and inguinal hernias.[15] Associations with malrotation, junctional epidermolysis bullosa, Hirschsprung's disease, ovarian cysts, ichthyosis, and deletions of the long arm of chromosome 11 also have been reported in the literature.[27,30,39]

DIAGNOSIS

The diagnosis is best confirmed by palpating the firm, mobile, ovoid-shaped, enlarged pylorus, the so-called olive. This can be accomplished in approximately 80% to 90% of cases, if the infant can be made calm and relaxed. Two or three fingertips are gently placed in the right upper abdomen and gently advanced into the deeper tissues below the liver edge. They are then slowly swept caudally toward the umbilicus. The olive can be felt to roll under the fingertips during this sweeping motion, likened to palpating a pistachio inside a pillow. The feet with the knees flexed should be elevated with the examiner's nonpalpating hand to aid in relaxing the

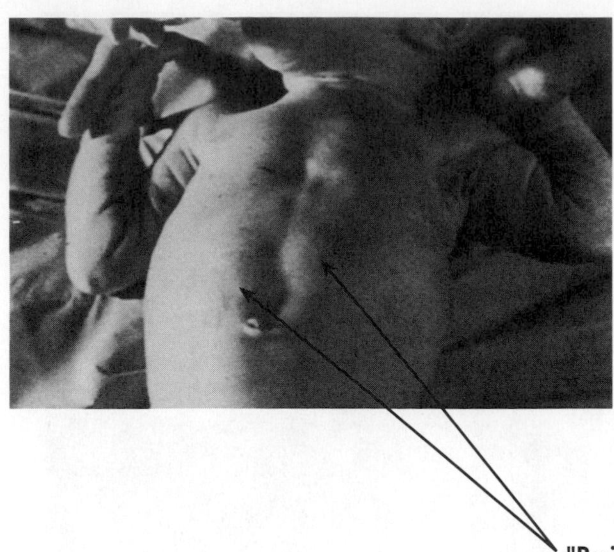

Fig. 255-1 Peristaltic waves seen in the upper abdomen (moving from left to right) in a baby who has pyloric stenosis.

(From Hoekelman RA: The physical examination of infants and children. In Bickley LS, editor: *Bates' A guide to physical examination and history taking,* ed 7, Philadelphia, 1999, JB Lippincott.)

muscles of the abdominal wall. The art of detecting the olive lies in performing the examination under conditions conducive to deep abdominal palpation in a quiet, cooperative infant; sometimes 10 to 20 minutes of preparation may be required. The olive can almost never be identified in an agitated, crying infant with a contracted abdominal wall. Gastric contractions may be seen moving across the upper abdomen from left to right (Fig. 255-1). This is best viewed standing at the foot of the examining table with a bright light at table height, directed across the abdomen from the patient's side. Emptying the stomach with a nasogastric tube and feeding the baby a small amount of dextrose water allows the examiner to palpate the abdomen while it is fully relaxed. The best time to palpate for the pyloric tumor is immediately after projectile vomiting occurs because the pylorus is fully contracted and at its firmest consistency. If the olive is unequivocally felt, the diagnosis is established, and no further diagnostic maneuvers are necessary. If the olive is not felt with the baby supine, palpation while the baby is lying prone may be more successful.

If the pylorus is not detected and the clinical presentation is sufficient to warrant further evaluation, radiological studies can be definitive. Teele and Smith observed the hypertrophied pylorus to have a characteristic appearance on B-mode ultrasound.[41] Subsequent measurement of various pyloric dimensions, including overall diameter, pyloric wall thickness, and pyloric channel length, accurately establishes the diagnosis of PS. A pyloric muscle wall thickness of 3.7 mm or greater, and a channel length of 17 mm or greater have been shown to have a greater than 90% positive predictive value. In infants up to 30 days of age, diagnostic criteria for wall thickness may be reduced to 3 mm.[19,37] Additionally, an upper GI contrast study can be diagnostic in cases in which ultrasound is equivocal by demonstrating an elongated and narrowed pyloric channel (string sign), the shoulders of the hypertrophied pylorus characteristically bulging into the intestinal lumen. Additional observations, including the volume of fluid aspirated from the stomach of a fasting infant, may prove helpful.[26]

Although an accurate diagnosis based on physical examination alone should be possible in most cases, and should be attempted in all, it is evident that an increasing reliance on radiological tests will continue to erode the skills of examiners. In a recent study, even when a pyloric mass was palpable in 85% of cases, 80% still underwent some unnecessary diagnostic imaging procedure.[6] A review comparing diagnostic accuracy between two eras in a single pediatric institution found that the sensitivity of physical examination declined by half during a period of increasing reliance on ultrasound,[23] a finding confirmed by others.[32] It is likely that ultrasound, a noninvasive, highly accurate, and relatively inexpensive technology, will experience even greater popularity in the future.[8]

When a diagnosis of PS cannot be established in a baby who vomits persistently and who has a normal ultrasound examination and GI series, the possibilities of sepsis, a poor feeding regimen, gastroesophageal reflux, intracranial disease, renal failure, or adrenal insufficiency should be entertained. In these cases it may be crucial to make a prompt diagnosis. Infants who have congenital adrenal hyperplasia who are "salt losers" may require immediate therapy. Clues to the latter diagnosis include an infant who is more ill than expected, possesses abnormal genitalia, and presents with hyponatremia and hyperkalemia. Otherwise, the infant should be reevaluated in a week or 10 days when the pyloric mass may become palpable or the ultrasound examination or GI series may become diagnostic.[13]

TREATMENT

Preoperative Management

The fluid and electrolyte disturbance in PS is similar to that seen in a patient who has an obstructing duodenal ulcer. Gastric losses result in a deficit of sodium, potassium, chloride, and water. Because gastric secretions contain more chloride than sodium, a hypochloremic, hypokalemic metabolic alkalosis develops. Potassium shifts out of the cell and sodium into the cell; much of the potassium is lost in the urine and a lesser amount in the vomitus. Although metabolic alkalosis has been regarded as the classic electrolyte derangement, recent studies suggests that a spectrum of electrolyte abnormalities may be seen, and variations from the expected pattern are not unusual.[42] Fortunately, infants of the current era rarely present with the overwhelming malnutrition and electrolyte abnormalities seen in past decades.[31] The cardinal point to be emphasized in the management of a depleted, alkalotic baby with PS is that anatomical correction is not a surgical emergency. Even though PS is a form of intestinal obstruction, gangrene and intestinal perforation do not occur. No infant should be operated for PS until the fluid and electrolyte deficits have been corrected. If infants come to surgery with uncorrected alkalosis, the profound effect that surgical stress has on the urinary excretion of sodium may intensify the electrolyte abnormalities.

Patients who present with mild to moderate dehydration usually can be hydrated within 24 hours, using intravenous saline solutions. Although numerous protocols have and can be used for replacement, the author prefers a continuous maintenance infusion of 5% dextrose in 0.45N NaCl, adding 20 mEq/L KCl once urine output is established. In addition, repeated boluses of isotonic NaCl at 20 ml/kg should be given until a serum chloride of 100 mEq/L is achieved. The volume replaced depends on the extent of dehydration, determined by the history in conjunction with physical and laboratory examinations. A severely depleted, lethargic infant may require more vigorous therapy. Fresh frozen plasma in volumes of 5 ml/kg and/or small-volume blood transfusions may be necessary in rare instances.

Nasogastric decompression is recommended during fluid and electrolyte resuscitation. This ensures the necessary gastric decompression required both at the time of technical repair, as well as during the induction of anesthesia.

Surgical Management

The mainstay of current treatment for PS is surgical pyloromyotomy. The classic open procedure is performed through a transverse right upper quadrant, right subcostal, or periumbilical incision. As the peritoneal cavity is entered, the pylorus can be delivered from the wound holding traction on the stomach. The hypertrophic pylorus has a pale white appearance, rubbery texture, and a palpably thickened muscular wall. After the overlying pyloric serosa is incised, the pyloric muscle is split or "cracked" by blunt means (Fig. 255-2). A myotomy of 2 cm in length is generally adequate. Bleeding from the circular muscle will cease after the pylorus is returned to the peritoneal cavity, as local venous hypertension resolves. Particular care must be taken at the most distal extent of the myotomy, near the pyloric vein, to avoid entrance into the duodenal lumen. Deliberate attention to the possibility of a mucosal tear is important because the morbidity associated with a recognized injury is minimal, while nonrecognition may be lethal. The abdominal wound is closed in layers. Success is enjoyed in nearly all patients, with low morbidity and mortality. Reoperation is required rarely.

More recently, pyloromyotomy has been achieved through laparoscopic means.[1] Although often successful, initial reports indicate the frequency of mucosal injuries to be greater than with the open technique.[2,12,38] The laparoscopic procedure also adds the real dangers associated with establishing a pneumoperitoneum.[14,36] The cosmetic result, length of hospitalization, and cost may or may not be improved. More rigorous evaluation and experience with the technique is required before it can be considered standard therapy.[11]

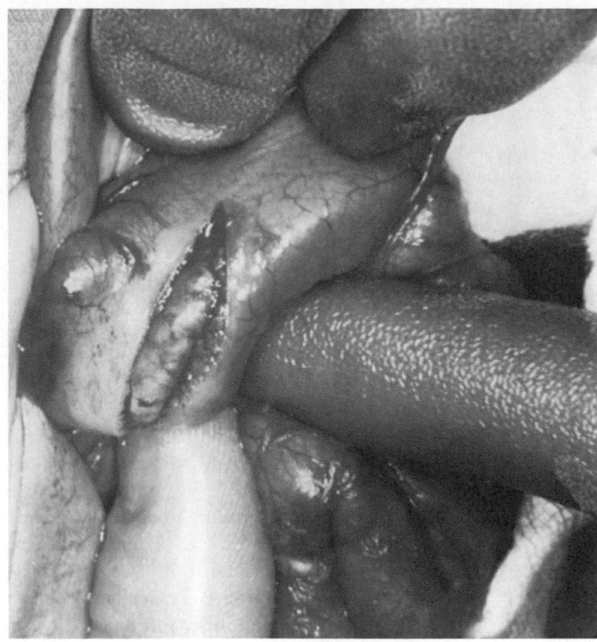

Fig. 255-2 The operative appearance following pyloromyotomy. The submucosa is seen to bulge out from the margins of the split, hypertrophic pyloric muscle.

Medical Management

Because of the reliability and relative safety of surgical myotomy, medical therapy alone has been largely discarded over the past several decades. Nonetheless, medical management may deserve another look. Indeed, hydration, observation, and transpyloric nasoduodenal feeding alone was successful therapy in 45 of 50 infants.[47] Although truly unsuccessful in only 3 infants, the downside was that the mean duration of hospitalization was 39 days. Medical therapies, including the anticholinergic, atropine sulfate, have been used. Nagita et al, employing an atropine sulfate regimen of 0.04 mg/kg/day IV, increased by 0.01 mg/kg/day until vomiting ceased, followed by 2 weeks of oral atropine sulfate at twice the effective IV dose, experienced success in 21 of 23 infants.[28] The remaining two were not considered medical failures. Pyloric hypertrophy resolved ultrasonographically in all infants by 4 to 12 months, not dissimilar from results following surgical myotomy. Later studies comparing two groups receiving either a predominantly oral atropine sulfate regimen or surgical myotomy reported similar successes (12 of 14 versus 20 of 20 respectively).[48] Medical therapy might be most beneficial in the occasional infant who remains hospitalized for other reasons and incidentally develops concomitant PS. Controlled prospective trials comparing outcomes and cost of medical versus surgical therapy are necessary before the former can be recommended.

Postoperative Management

Most infants will continue to vomit postoperatively; however, this usually will cease by the second to fifth feed. It is important to explain this to parents before an operation is undertaken. Tradition directs infants to be fed 12 to 24 hours following operative repair, with small amounts of dextrose water, and later to be advanced to dilute and finally full-strength formula. The author prefers to begin full-strength formula feeds, or breast feeds, every 3 to 4 hours, 6 hours following operation. If the baby vomits during a feed, the current feed only is held, and regular feeding is resumed at the next scheduled interval. This schedule works and is simple to understand for the physicians, nurses, and parents involved. Discharge from the hospital usually takes place 24 to 48 hours postoperatively. It is important that both the parents and health care providers alike are satisfied that the infant is feeding reliably at discharge.

Complications

Postoperative obstruction. In the rare instance in which vomiting persists beyond several days, radiographic examinations should be obtained. Although distal intestinal obstruction is uncommon in infants with PS, it must be excluded. Gastroesophageal reflux may also contribute to prolonged and persistent vomiting. An upper GI contrast series may be helpful but also difficult to interpret. Narrowing and elongation of the pyloric channel usually persists weeks to months following a successful operation, even in babies who have minimal or no postoperative vomiting.[35,48]

A second operation for gastric outlet obstruction following pyloromyotomy should not be undertaken hastily; the physician should wait 10 to 14 days before making this decision, unless the infant's condition deteriorates. If persistent pyloric obstruction is the culprit, an inadequate pyloromyotomy is the most likely cause; this typically is on the proximal stomach end, not the duodenal. Reoperation may be indicated in these circumstances.

Hypoglycemia. Reactive hypoglycemia has been recorded in depleted infants who have a wide variety of medical and surgical conditions. This may cause unexpected respiratory arrest and unexplained death. Increases in insulin secretion, a result of constant dextrose infusion, can result in severe hypoglycemia if the infusion is suddenly terminated before oral alimentation is adequate. This is particularly likely if liver glycogen stores have been depleted, as has been shown in babies with PS. Fatalities from postoperative hypoglycemia in babies with PS have been reported.

Apnea. Anesthesia in infants with PS may prove difficult. After completion of the operation and anesthetic, apnea may develop in the immediate postoperative period. When the painful stimulus of the surgical procedure is no longer present, the level of anesthesia may deepen. Hypoventilation then may proceed to respiratory arrest. Careful attention to respiratory efforts as the baby enters the recovery room is necessary, and stimulation or assisted breathing may be necessary during the postoperative period. Administration of naloxone may be helpful.[5]

Death. The mortality in infants with PS has fallen to well under 1%.[49] Although this is encouraging, the goal is to prevent deaths altogether. Modern anesthetic management has contributed to these improved results.[24] On review of 754 consecutive patients with PS, 8 causes of death could be identified: (1) delayed diagnosis, (2) inadequate preoperative rehydration, (3) pulmonary aspiration, (4) unrecognized perforation, (5) hypoglycemia, (6) persistent obstruction, (7) hemorrhage, and (8) the presence of other associated congenital anomalies.[10] Almost all such deaths are avoidable.

Long-term outcome. The long-term outcome for patients treated for PS is excellent. Although at least one study revealed increased gastric emptying and duodenogastric reflux in some patients who had undergone pyloromyotomy for PS 5 to 7 years earlier,[40] other studies with longer follow-up have shown no differences between previous PS patients and controls.[4,21,22,45]

REFERENCES

1. Alain JL, et al: Extramucosal pyloromyotomy by laparoscopy, *Eur J Pediatr Surg* 6:10, 1996.
2. Alain JL, et al: Extramucosal pyloromyotomy by laparoscopy, *J Laparoendosc Surg* 6(suppl 1):S41, 1996.
3. Applegate MS, Druschel CM: The epidemiology of infantile hypertrophic pyloric stenosis in New York State, 1983 to 1990, *Arch Pediatr Adolesc Med* 149:1123, 1995.
4. Asai A, et al: Ultrasonographic evaluation of gastric emptying in normal children and children after pyloromyotomy, *Pediatr Surg Int* 12:344, 1997.
5. Beilin B, et al: Naloxone reversal of postoperative apnea in a premature infant with pyloric stenosis, *Anesthesiology* 63:317, 1985.
6. Breaux CW, et al: Changing patterns in the diagnosis of hypertrophic pyloric stenosis, *Pediatrics* 81:213, 1988.
7. Carter CO, Evans DA: Inheritance of congenital pyloric stenosis, *J Med Genet* 6:233, 1969.
8. Chen EA, et al: Pyloric stenosis in the age of ultrasonography: fading skills, better patients? *J Pediatr Surg* 31:829, 1996.
9. Chung E, et al: Genetic evidence for the neuronal nitric oxide synthase gene (NOS1) as a susceptibility locus for infantile pyloric stenosis, *Am J Hun Genet* 58:363, 1996.
10. Colodny AH: Pyloric stenosis. In Hoekelman RA, et al, editors: *Primary pediatric care,* ed 3, St Louis, 1997, Mosby.
11. Ford WD, et al: The learning curve for laparoscopic pyloromyotomy, *J Pediatr Surg* 32:552, 1997.
12. Fujimoto T, et al: Laparoscopic extramucosal pyloromyotomy versus open pyloromyotomy for infantile hypertrophic pyloric stenosis: which is better? *J Pediatr Surg* 34:370, 1999.
13. Geer LL, et al: Evolution of pyloric stenosis in the first week of life, *Pediatr Radiol* 15:205, 1985.
14. Holland AJ, Ford WD: The influence of laparoscopic surgery on perioperative heat loss in infants, *Pediatr Surg Int* 13:350, 1998.
15. Iijima T, et al: Hypertrophic pyloric stenosis associated with hiatal hernia, *J Pediatr Surg* 31:277, 1996.
16. Jedd MB, et al: Trends in infantile hypertrophic pyloric stenosis in Olmsted County, Minnesota, 1950-1984, *Paediatr Perinat Epidemiol* 64:138, 1988.
17. Knox EG, et al: Changing incidence of pyloric stenosis, *Arch Dis Child* 58:582, 1983.
18. Kusafuka T, Puri P: Altered messenger RNA expression of the neuronal nitric oxide synthase gene in infantile hypertrophic pyloric stenosis, *Pediatr Surg Int* 12:576, 1997.
19. Lamki N, et al: Hypertrophic pyloric stenosis in the neonate: diagnostic criteria revisited, *Can Assoc Radiol J* 44:21, 1993.
20. Langer JC, et al: Hypertrophic pyloric stenosis: ultrastructural abnormalities of enteric nerves and the interstitial cells of Cajal, *J Pediatr Surg* 30:1535, 1995.
21. Ludtke FE, et al: Gastric emptying 16 to 26 years after treatment of infantile hypertrophic pyloric stenosis, *J Pediatr Surg* 29:523, 1994.

22. Ludtke FE, et al: Long-term analysis of ultrasonic features of the antro-pyloric region 17-27 years after treatment of infantile hypertrophic pyloric stenosis, *J Clin Ultrasound* 22:299, 1994.
23. Macdessi J, Oates RK: Clinical diagnosis of pyloric stenosis, a declining, *Br Med J* 306:553, 1993.
24. MacDonald NJ, et al: Anaesthesia for congenital hypertrophic pyloric stenosis, *Br J Anaesth* 59:672, 1987.
25. Malmfors G, Sundler F: Peptidergic innervation in infantile hypertrophic pyloric stenosis, *J Pediar Surg* 21:303, 1986.
26. Mandell GA, et al: Cost-effective imaging approach to the nonbilious vomiting infant, *Pediatrics* 103(6 Pt 1):1198, 1999.
27. Muller H, et al: Herlitz syndrome and pyloric obstruction, *Helvetica Paediatrica Acta* 43:457, 1989.
28. Nagita A, et al: Management and ultrasonographic appearance of infantile hypertrophic pyloric stenosis with intravenous atropine sulfate, *J Pediatr Gastroenterol Nutr* 23:172, 1996.
29. O'Donoghue JM, et al: The increasing incidence of infantile hypertrophic pyloric stenosis, *Ir J Med Sci* 162:175, 1993.
30. O'Hare AE, et al: Deletion of the long arm of chromosome 11, *Clin Genet* 25:273, 1984.
31. Papadakis K, et al: The changing presentation of pyloric stenosis, *Am J Emerg Med* 17:67, 1999.
32. Poon TS, et al: Changing patterns of diagnosis and treatment of infantile hypertrophic pyloric stenosis: a clinical audit of 303 patients, *J Pediatr Surg* 31:1611, 1996.
33. Rogers JM: Plasma gastrin in congenital hypertonic pyloric stenosis, *Arch Dis Child* 50:467, 1975.
34. Rollins MD, et al: Pyloric stenosis: congenital or acquired? *Arch Dis Child* 64:138, 1989.
35. Sauerbrei EE, Paloschi GG: The ultrasonic features of hypertrophic pyloric stenosis with emphasis on the postoperative appearance, *Radiology* 147:503, 1983.
36. See WA, et al: Predictors of laparoscopic complications after formal training in laparoscopic surgery, *JAMA* 270:2689, 1993.
37. Shkolnik A: Applications of ultrasound in the neonate, *Radiol Clin North Am* 23:141, 1985.
38. Sitsen E, et al: Is laparoscopic pyloromyotomy superior to open surgery? *Surg Endosc* 12:813, 1998.
39. Stoll C, et al: Hypertrophic pyloric stenosis associated with X-linked ichthyosis in two brothers, *Clin Exp Dermatol* 8:61, 1983.
40. Tam PK, et al: Pyloric function 5 to 7 years after Ramstedt's pyloromyotomy, *J Pediatr Surg* 20:236, 1985.
41. Teele RL, Smith EH: Ultrasound in the diagnosis of congenital hypertrophic pyloric stenosis, *N Engl J Med* 296:1149, 1977.
42. Touloukian RJ, Higgins E: The spectrum of serum electrolytes in hypertrophic pyloric stenosis, *J Pediatr Surg* 18:394, 1983.
43. Vanderwinden JM, et al: Nitric oxide synthase activity in infantile hypertrophic pyloric stenosis, *N Engl J Med* 327:511, 1992.
44. Vanderwinden JM, et al: The pathology f infantile hypertrophic pyloric stenosis after healing, *J Pediatr Surg* 31:1530, 1996.
45. Vilmann P, et al: A long-term gastrointestinal follow-up in patients operated on for congenital hypertrophic pyloric stenosis, *Acta Paediatr Scand* 75:156, 1986.
46. Webb AR, et al: Infantile hypertrophic pyloric stenosis: effects of changes in feeding practices, *Arch Dis Child* 58:586, 1983.
47. Yamashiro Y, et al: Conservative management of infantile pyloric stenosis by nasoduodenal feeding, *Eur J Pediatr* 136:187, 1981.
48. Yamataka A, et al: Pyloromyotomy versus atropine sulfate for infantile hypertrophic pyloric stenosis, *J Pediar Surg* 35:338, 2000.
49. Zeiden B, et al: Recent results of treatment of infantile hypertrophic pyloric stenosis, *Arch Dis Child* 63:1060, 1988.

256 Reye's Syndrome

Rebecca Ribovich Matsakis

Reye's syndrome, as a distinct clinical and pathological entity, was first reported in 1963 from Australia by Reye, Morgan, and Baral[11] in 1963 when they described a syndrome of encephalopathy and fatty degeneration of the liver. Since then, cases of this syndrome have been reported from all over the world.

The number of Reye's syndrome cases in the United States has decreased markedly since the reported peak of more than 500 in 1980.[3] About 100 cases a year were reported in 1985 and 1986. From 1994 through 1997, no more than two cases were reported annually.[3] Temporal and geographical associations of Reye's syndrome with cases of varicella, influenza B, and influenza A have been observed. Reye's syndrome has occurred in infants and children of all age groups, and cases have been reported in adults. The highest incidence is in the 5- to 14-year-old age group. There is no gender predilection; 90% of the cases have occurred in whites and 8% in blacks. There have been case reports of recurrent Reye's syndrome, familial Reye's syndrome, and Reye's syndrome following live virus vaccination.

DEFINITION

The case definition for Reye's syndrome as established by the Centers for Disease Control and Prevention[4] in 1980 is as follows:

1. Acute noninflammatory encephalopathy with one of the following:
   a. Microvesicular fatty metamorphosis of the liver confirmed by biopsy or autopsy
   b. A serum aspartate aminotransferase (AST), a serum alanine aminotransferase (ALT), or a serum ammonia (NH_3) that is greater than three times normal
2. Cerebrospinal fluid, if obtained, with fewer than eight leukocytes/mm^3
3. No other more reasonable explanation for the neurological or hepatic abnormalities

PATHOLOGY

In Reye's syndrome, pathological changes have been described in the liver, brain, kidney, heart, pancreas, and skeletal muscle. The liver has a diffuse yellowish appearance caused by lipid accumulation within the cytoplasm of the hepatocytes. Glycogen stains show diffuse depletion of glycogen. There is no necrosis, nor are there inflammatory infiltrates. The mitochondria of the hepatocytes are swollen, and their outer cellular membranes are deformed.

On gross examination, the brain is swollen, with flattening of the gyri. Microscopic examination shows cerebral edema. The ultrastructural abnormalities include focal areas of swelling in myelin sheaths and accumulation of edema fluid in glial cells. The brain mitochondria show variable changes, including matrix distortion and swelling.

Lipid accumulation also has been described in the kidney, heart, and skeletal muscle. Evidence of mitochondrial injury also has been reported in cardiac and skeletal muscle. Focal necrosis, hemorrhage, and inflammatory changes have been described in the pancreas.

BIOCHEMICAL ABNORMALITIES

Since the original report of Reye's syndrome in which elevated serum aminotransferases and hypoglycemia were described, numerous other metabolic abnormalities have been documented. The serum ammonia level is elevated in almost all patients who have Reye's syndrome, but this is transient, with levels returning to normal in 24 to 48 hours. Levels greater than 350 μg/dl usually are associated with a less favorable prognosis for survival.

There are various explanations for the hyperammonemia. Reductions in the hepatic activities of ornithine transcarbamoylase and carbamyl phosphate synthetase, which are mitochondrial enzymes of the urea cycle, may explain the hyperammonemia. Also, because of the anorexia and vomiting that occur, the patient is in a catabolic state, which results in increased release of amino acids from muscle; this too may lead to the hyperammonemia.

The serum aminotransferase levels always are elevated, but the bilirubin is normal or elevated only minimally. Hypoglycemia occurs in about 40% of patients, is seen primarily in children under 4 years of age, and is thought to result from deficient hepatic gluconeogenesis.

Elevated serum lactic acid concentrations frequently are found and may be related to impaired oxidative metabolism of glucose or to accelerated production by extrahepatic tissues such as muscle. Total serum free fatty acids, particularly short-chain fatty acids, are elevated in patients who have Reye's syndrome. In some studies, clinical improvement has been associated with the clearance of these short-chain fatty acids. Possible explanations for the fatty acidemia include an increased release from adipose tissue secondary to the anorexia and vomiting or a lipolytic response to a virus.

Coincident with the increased free fatty acid concentrations, dicarboxylic acids appear in urine and serum. This finding suggests that mitochondrial beta-oxidation of fatty acids is compromised or overwhelmed by a massive influx of fatty acids. Alternative routes of oxidation then are used.

Other reported abnormalities include elevations in serum amino acids, creatinine phosphokinase, uric acid, blood urea nitrogen (BUN), amylase, and serum osmolality. Transient acute renal failure has been described on occasion.

The prothrombin time is prolonged, but the platelet count usually is normal in patients who have Reye's syndrome. Fibrin split products usually are absent from the circulation. Decreased coagulation factors (except for factor VIII) have been observed. Disseminated intravascular coagulation has been described only rarely.

Respiratory alkalosis is present as a result of primary stimulation of the respiratory centers in the brainstem. A mixed metabolic acidosis often is found in addition to the respiratory alkalosis. The hyperthermia that is present early in the disease may be the result of hypothalamic dysfunction.

ETIOLOGY AND PATHOGENESIS

The etiology of Reye's syndrome remains unclear, but available evidence suggests a multifactorial cause. Contributing factors may include genetic susceptibility and an exogenous toxin, whether a medication or an environmental agent, which modifies the reaction to a viral infection.

An increased incidence of Reye's syndrome has been reported during outbreaks of varicella, influenza B, and influenza A. Both influenza A and B infections have been demonstrated serologically in many patients who have Reye's syndrome. Adenovirus, coxsackieviruses A and B, echovirus, Epstein-Barr virus, parainfluenza virus, reovirus, rubella virus, rubeola virus, type I poliomyelitis virus, and herpes simplex viruses also have been linked to Reye's syndrome.

Much attention has been given to the role of salicylates in the origin of Reye's syndrome. Epidemiological studies,[5,7,15,20] including a Public Health Service study,[8] have found a higher rate of salicylate ingestion (by history) in patients who have Reye's syndrome compared with control children who have similar antecedent illnesses. These epidemiological studies suggest a strong association between salicylate use and Reye's syndrome and have resulted in the recommendation that the use of salicylates be avoided for children who have varicella infections and during influenza outbreaks. Since the publicity about the association between Reye's syndrome and aspirin began in late 1980, much of the decline in its reported incidence has been attributed to the reported decrease in the use of salicylates in treating children who have viral illnesses.[1,2] It has been suggested that salicylates, in conjunction with certain viral infections, may inhibit mitochondrial enzymes in susceptible individuals.[9] The precise role of salicylates in the pathogenesis of Reye's syndrome remains unclear.

Environmental toxins such as aflatoxins and insecticides have been implicated in the etiology of Reye's syndrome, but there is little evidence that these toxins play a major role.

The pathogenesis of the encephalopathy in Reye's syndrome remains unclear. Some etiological factors that have been suggested are hyperammonemia, lactic acidemia, short-chain fatty acidemia, and direct brain cell mitochondrial damage paralleling that seen in the liver cells.

It also has been suggested that generalized mitochondrial insult and dysfunction are the bases of the metabolic abnormalities found. As noted, there is strong evidence for insult to hepatic mitochondria in terms of both morphological and enzymatic abnormalities. The evidence for a similar primary mitochondrial dysfunction in brain cells is less substantial.

CLINICAL FEATURES

Patients who have Reye's syndrome have a viral prodromal illness usually consisting of an upper respiratory tract infection, gastroenteritis, or varicella. The child appears to be recovering from that illness, but then develops repetitive vomiting. Within 24 to 48 hours the child becomes agitated, combative, disoriented, and behaves irrationally. Periods of lethargy may alternate with the combative behavior. Hyperventilation also may be prominent. Approximately 85% of patients have hepatomegaly, but jaundice is absent. Pancreatitis is found in up to 22% of autopsied cases. The pancreatic involvement can be so severe as to produce hemorrhagic necrosis and death. Seizures can occur at any time during the encephalopathic stages.

The child may begin to recover spontaneously or may deteriorate further into full obtundation. Central nervous system dysfunction progresses from stupor to coma with intact brainstem function, to decorticate or decerebrate posturing, and finally to a flaccid and areflexic state.

Various systems have been devised to stage the severity of the illness in Reye's syndrome. The National Institutes of Health Consensus Development Conference on the Diagnosis and Treatment of Reye's syndrome held in 1981 generated the revised staging system shown in Table 256-1. This was

Table 256-1 Staging of Reye's Syndrome

	I	II	III	IV	V
Level of consciousness	Lethargy; follows verbal commands	Combative/stupor; verbalizes inappropriately	Coma	Coma	Coma
Posture	Normal	Normal	Decorticate	Decerebrate	Flaccid
Response to pain	Purposeful	Purposeful/nonpurposeful	Decorticate	Decerebrate	None
Pupillary reaction	Brisk	Sluggish	Sluggish	Sluggish	None
Oculocephalic reflex (doll's eyes)	Normal	Conjugate deviation	Conjugate deviation	Inconsistent or absent	None

From National Institutes of Health Consensus Development Conference: *JAMA* 246:2442, 1981.

done in an attempt to introduce a uniform staging system for use by all treatment centers.

The clinical presentation of Reye's syndrome in infants is somewhat different from that previously outlined, so early recognition is more difficult. Following the prodromal illness, vomiting may be minimal or absent. Diarrhea, however, is a frequent occurrence. Seizures also are frequently present, can occur early in the course of the illness, and may be the presenting sign. Respiratory disturbances, such as hyperventilation and apnea, are prominent and also may occur early in the course of the illness.

DIAGNOSIS

The diagnosis of Reye's syndrome should be considered when a history of an antecedent viral illness is followed by vomiting, progressive lethargy, agitation, and obtundation. Early diagnosis is important because prompt treatment may provide a better chance for complete recovery.

Laboratory Tests

Laboratory tests that should be obtained to help establish the diagnosis include serum ammonia, serum aminotransferases, bilirubin, prothrombin time, blood glucose, and urine and blood toxicology screens. A lumbar puncture should not be performed routinely if Reye's syndrome is suspected, because of the associated cerebral edema and increased intracranial pressure. If meningitis is suspected, a lumbar puncture should be performed using a small-gauge needle, with removal of as little cerebrospinal fluid as possible to minimize the likelihood of cerebral herniation. A cerebrospinal fluid specimen containing fewer than eight leukocytes/mm^3 and normal protein and glucose concentrations, except when there is concomitant hypoglycemia, is consistent with Reye's syndrome.

Special Studies and Computed Tomography

A liver biopsy is not essential to diagnose most cases of Reye's syndrome because the clinical and laboratory features are typical. However, a liver biopsy to establish the diagnosis firmly should be considered in patients under 1 year of age, in children who have recurrent episodes, in familial cases, in atypical cases that have no antecedent viral infection or vomiting, and when new and potentially dangerous therapeutic regimens are planned.

Computed tomographic (CT) brain scanning is not needed for diagnosing Reye's syndrome. A CT scan performed early in the course of the illness will either be normal or show evidence of diffuse brain edema. The electroencephalogram also will be nonspecific and will not help to establish the diagnosis, alter treatment regimens, or determine prognosis.

DIFFERENTIAL DIAGNOSIS

The conditions that should be considered in the differential diagnosis of Reye's syndrome are as follows[18]:

1. Infections: meningitis, varicella, hepatitis, encephalitis
2. Toxins: salicylates, methyl bromide, hypoglycin, isopropyl alcohol, aflatoxin, lead, valproic acid
3. Anoxic encephalopathy
4. Inborn metabolic defects: disorders of fat oxidation, hyperammonemia syndromes, and organic acid disorders.

Meningitis may follow an upper respiratory tract infection and can produce vomiting and lethargy. Aminotransferase elevations may occur in children who have varicella without concomitant Reye's syndrome and in hypoxia resulting from a wide variety of causes. Excessive salicylate ingestion can cause vomiting, seizures, obtundation, hyperventilation, hypoglycemia, and abnormal liver function. A serum salicylate level of 25 mg/dl or more suggests salicylism rather than Reye's syndrome. Other toxins, such as methyl bromide, hypoglycin, isopropyl alcohol, aflatoxin, lead, and valproic acid may produce disturbances of consciousness and elevation of serum aminotransferase levels.

An increasing number of metabolic disorders have been described that may mimic Reye's syndrome, especially in infants and younger children.[6,12,13] These disorders also are associated with vomiting and altered consciousness. The inborn errors of ureagenesis that may mimic Reye's syndrome include partial ornithine transcarbamoylase deficiency and partial carbamoyl-phosphate synthase deficiency. Defects of fatty acid metabolism, such as systemic carnitine deficiency and various acetyl-CoA dehydrogenase deficiencies, also can resemble Reye's syndrome in presentation. Clinical features that suggest an underlying metabolic disorder include an atypical prodrome with rapid onset, patient age under 2 years, and familial or recurrent episodes of Reye's syndrome–like illness.

It has been observed that, as the incidence of Reye's syndrome declines, an increasing proportion of patients who seem to have its "typical" features may have one of the metabolic disorders that mimic this syndrome.[13] Therefore, it has been recommended that investigations to exclude metabolic disorders be considered seriously in all patients suspected of having Reye's syndrome.

TREATMENT

Once the diagnosis of Reye's syndrome is suspected, the severity of the patient's illness should be staged, using a staging system such as the one shown in Table 256-1. All patients, regardless of their stage of disease, should be hospitalized for careful observation because neurological deterioration can progress rapidly. The primary care physician should arrange for the patient to be transferred to a regional pediatric intensive care unit (PICU) as soon as possible, using a transport team prepared to provide support for all vital functions. Supportive care for patients in stages I and II includes frequent evaluations of neurological status. A 10% dextrose solution containing balanced electrolytes should be administered intravenously at the rate needed to deliver daily maintenance fluid requirements. The use of a high-glucose concentration is designed to decrease lipolysis. Any abnormalities in the serum electrolytes and fluid balance should be corrected.

Children at later stages of the disease require intensive

monitoring and aggressive therapy directed toward correction of metabolic abnormalities and reduction of increased intracranial pressure.

Some authorities recommend that fluids be given at two-thirds maintenance; others recommend full maintenance fluid volumes, with adjustments according to electrolyte levels and urinary output. A nasogastric tube should be placed to decompress the stomach and prevent vomiting and aspiration, and a Foley catheter should be inserted so that accurate urinary output can be determined. An arterial catheter, which permits continuous blood pressure measurement and arterial blood gas sampling, should be placed. Temperature should be maintained at normal levels via a cooling blanket. The head of the patient's bed should be elevated 30 degrees. Endotracheal intubation should be performed and assisted ventilation instituted in comatose patients. Seizures may be treated with lorazepam and, at the same time, the patient should be loaded with intravenous phenytoin or phenobarbital.[10]

Vitamin K (5 mg, given intramuscularly) can be administered in an attempt to correct the clotting abnormalities. If a significant amount of bleeding occurs, the administration of fresh-frozen plasma (10 ml/kg) may be helpful.

Arterial blood gases, serum osmolality, glucose, electrolytes, BUN, and hematocrit should be monitored closely. Once the patient is admitted to a PICU, more definitive therapeutic measures can be undertaken. A central venous catheter should be placed to monitor blood volume and cardiac function. In addition, it is recommended that patients receive hypertonic glucose solutions of 15% dextrose; a central line is required for administration of such hypertonic solutions. A pulmonary artery catheter may be required to monitor the pulmonary artery pressure and cardiac output of seriously ill children.

Peritoneal dialysis has been used to clear the hyperammonemia. Other ammonia-reducing strategies, including exchange transfusion, charcoal hemoperfusion, and heart-lung bypass total body washout, have not been found to be effective.[17] However, double-volume exchange transfusion with fresh blood has been used to replenish coagulation factor deficiencies.

Management of the cerebral edema associated with Reye's syndrome is the major factor that affects the outcome. The most significant adjunct to management has been the development of techniques to monitor intracranial pressure. Most centers recommend that children beyond stage II have an intracranial pressure monitor inserted. Monitoring provides a mechanism to titrate management of the patient and is designed to maintain the intracranial pressure within normal ranges until the illness resolves. The monitoring device can be either an intraventricular cannula or a subarachnoid bolt, and it should be placed after the prothrombin time is brought to normal levels. Controlling intracranial pressure requires maintenance of adequate cerebral perfusion while preventing herniation. Intracranial pressure greater than 20 mm Hg should be treated. The cerebral perfusion pressure should be maintained above 50 mm Hg to prevent cerebral ischemia. Cerebral perfusion pressure is equal to the mean arterial pressure minus the intracranial pressure.

The following measures can be undertaken to treat elevated intracranial pressure:

1. Mannitol, 0.25 g/kg/dose, should be administered intravenously. Hyperosmolality is a complication of osmotherapy. Fluid should be replaced to keep the serum osmolality below 320 mOsm, thereby preventing any compromise of renal function. The addition of the diuretic furosemide, 0.5 to 1 mg/kg IV, also can help to decrease the intracranial pressure.[10] The use of mannitol requires careful monitoring of the patient's fluid balance.
2. Hyperventilation should be controlled by a mechanical respirator to maintain a PCO_2 of 25 to 35 mm Hg.[10] A PCO_2 above this leads to increased pressure from vasodilation, and values below this range can be correlated with inadequate cerebral blood flow.
3. Sedation can be achieved through the use of a sedative/hypnotic agent, such as midazolam. If intracranial pressure control remains a problem, a paralytic agent such as pancuronium can be added.[10]
4. If an intraventricular catheter is used, small amounts of cerebrospinal fluid can be released through the catheter for immediate control of intracranial pressure elevations.

Corticosteroids have not been shown to be effective in controlling the intracranial pressure.

If the aforementioned measures are unsuccessful, high-dose barbiturate therapy may be indicated, although its use remains controversial.[14,19] Varying success rates have been reported with this therapy. Barbiturates are thought to decrease cerebral metabolic demands and cerebral blood flow and thereby control intracranial pressure. This therapy involves the administration of intravenous pentobarbital to maintain a blood level of 30 to 50 μg/dl and is carried out until the intracranial pressure returns to normal. Because possible complications of this therapy include a drop in arterial blood pressure, a change in cardiac output, or unexplained hypoxia, monitoring devices are necessary to measure these indices accurately.

Some centers have used hypothermia when the aforementioned therapeutic measures have failed to control the elevated intracranial pressure.[16] Surface body cooling to a target body temperature of 89.6° F (32° C) is achieved with hypothermia blankets. However, this therapy increases the risk of infection because the immune system does not function as well during hypothermia.

A final mode of therapy that has been used for patients who have increased intracranial pressure refractory to all other measures is decompressive craniectomy. Because infection and bleeding are potential risks with this therapy, it should be reserved for the most difficult cases.

PROGNOSIS

Early reports indicated that the mortality from Reye's syndrome was 80%, with the usual cause of death being herniation secondary to cerebral edema; this rate has decreased to less than 30%. Some of this decrease may be the result of increased recognition of the illness, especially of mild cases, in addition to greater use of intensive medical support.

Recent studies have attempted to evaluate neurological sequelae in survivors of Reye's syndrome. It is estimated that 10% of survivors have incurred severe brain damage. Several studies suggest that those children who have the most severe illness (as evidenced by the degree and duration of increased intracranial pressure) and those who are younger than 2 years of age when affected are most likely to suffer sequelae. However, the vast majority of children older than 2 years of age who survive Reye's syndrome appear to recover completely.

Neuropsychological testing has shown that some children who have recovered from Reye's syndrome have difficulty achieving in school and with visual motor integration, sequencing, tactile problem solving, and concept formation. These more subtle deficits may persist for many months or years. In general, extensive psychological and educational testing of Reye's syndrome survivors appears to be unnecessary.

Overprotectiveness of the child by the family should be avoided because this can contribute to behavioral or school problems; family guidance and counseling are essential in this regard.

When to Refer

When Reye's syndrome is suspected, the patient should be referred to an emergency department.

When to Hospitalize

When Reye's syndrome is suspected, the patient should be hospitalized.

REFERENCES

1. Arrowsmith JB, et al: National patterns of aspirin use and Reye syndrome reporting—United States, 1980 to 1985, *Pediatrics* 79:858, 1987.
2. Barrett MJ, et al: Changing epidemiology of Reye syndrome in the United States, *Pediatrics* 77:598, 1986.
3. Belay ED, et al: Reye's syndrome in the United States from 1981 through 1997, *N Engl J Med* 340:1377, 1999.
4. Centers for Disease Control: Follow-up on Reye syndrome—United States, *MMWR* 29:321, 1980.
5. Forsyth BE, et al: New epidemiologic evidence confirming that bias does not explain the aspirin/Reye's syndrome association, *JAMA* 261:2517, 1989.
6. Greene CL, Blitzer MG, Shapira E: Inborn errors of metabolism and Reye syndrome: differential diagnosis, *J Pediatr* 113:156, 1988.
7. Halpin TJ, et al: Reye's syndrome and medication use, *JAMA* 248:687, 1982.
8. Hurwitz ES, et al: Public Health Service study of Reye's syndrome and medications: report of the main study, *JAMA* 257:1905, 1987.
9. Pinsky PF, et al: Reye's syndrome and aspirin: evidence for a dose-response effect, *JAMA* 260:657, 1988.
10. Poss WB, et al: Pathophysiology and management of the intracranial vault. In Rogers MC, editor: *Textbook of pediatric intensive care,* Baltimore, 1996, Williams and Wilkins.
11. Reye RDK, Morgan G, Baral J: Encephalopathy and fatty degeneration of the viscera: a disease entity in childhood, *Lancet* 2:749, 1963.
12. Robinson RO: Differential diagnosis of Reye's syndrome, *Dev Med Child Neurol* 29:110, 1987.
13. Rowe PC, Valle D, Brusilow SW: Inborn errors of metabolism in children referred with Reye's syndrome, *JAMA* 260:3167, 1988.
14. Shaywitz BA, Lister G, Duncan CC: What is the best treatment for Reye's syndrome? *Arch Neurol* 43:730, 1986.
15. Starko KM, et al: Reye's syndrome and salicylate use, *Pediatrics* 66:859, 1980.
16. Swedlow DB, Schreiner MS: Management of Reye's syndrome, *Crit Care Clin* 1:285, 1985.
17. Tasker RC, Poss WB, Dean JM: Reye syndrome and metabolic encephalopathies. In Rogers MC, editor: *Textbook of pediatric intensive care,* Baltimore, 1996, Williams and Wilkins.
18. Trauner DA: Reye's syndrome, *Curr Probl Pediatr* 12:1, 1982.
19. Trauner DA: What is the best treatment for Reye's syndrome? *Arch Neurol* 43:729, 1986.
20. Waldman RJ, et al: Aspirin as a risk factor in Reye's syndrome, *JAMA* 247:3089, 1982.

SUGGESTED READINGS

DeLong GR, Glick TH: Encephalopathy of Reye's syndrome: a review of pathogenetic hypotheses, *Pediatrics* 69:53, 1982.

Heubi JE, et al: Reye's syndrome: current concepts, *Hepatology* 7:155, 1987.

Hurwitz ES: Reye's syndrome, *Epidemiol Rev* 11:249, 1989.

Huttenlocker PR, Trauner DA: Reye's syndrome in infancy, *Pediatrics* 62:84, 1978.

National Institutes of Health Consensus Development Conference: Diagnosis and treatment of Reye's syndrome, *JAMA* 246:2441, 1981.

257 Rheumatic Fever

Welton M. Gersony • Thomas J. Starc

Acute rheumatic fever is a systemic connective tissue disorder that is clinically manifested by polyarthritis, carditis, and chorea, either singly or in combination. The major long-term consequence is the potential for inflammatory cardiac valvar involvement leading to chronic heart disease. The other manifestations are self limiting with no late sequelae; arthritis clears without joint dysfunction or deformity; chorea leaves no neuromuscular impediment. Therefore, the most important concern is the prevention of recurrent attacks, which carry the risk of recrudescent heart involvement and further cardiac damage.

Because it has been established that an immunological reaction to group A beta-hemolytic streptococci is the cause of rheumatic fever, it has been shown that the incidence of the first attack of rheumatic fever can be reduced by adequate penicillin treatment of all cases of streptococcal pharyngitis. The incidence of rheumatic fever observed in epidemics of streptococcal pharyngitis is approximately 2% to 3%, whereas the attack rate following sporadic streptococcal upper respiratory tract infection is only about 0.2% to 0.3%. In those who have already had one or more attacks of rheumatic fever, however, the recurrence rate of carditis rises to about 15% following subsequent streptococcal infection.[11]

Numerous community primary prevention programs have demonstrated the efficacy of identifying streptococcal infection by performing throat cultures on susceptible children and treating them early. Furthermore, the widespread application of secondary prevention in the form of antistreptococcal prophylaxis programs for patients after their first attack has significantly reduced the recurrence rate and the additive effects of repeated bouts of carditis.

The incidence of acute rheumatic fever has declined in the past four decades in the United States and Europe. However, in underdeveloped countries, rheumatic fever remains a common illness in childhood. Continued immigration from the Caribbean Islands, South America, and Southeast Asia also is a factor in the prevalence of the disease in the United States. An apparent resurgence of acute rheumatic fever in certain areas of the United States, both urban and suburban, was reported between 1984 and 1988,[3,6,8,14] but there is no evidence that this trend has continued. Although the disease persists, the annual incidence may be so low, even at large teaching medical centers, that during 3 years of pediatric training, a resident physician may not see more than one or two children who have acute rheumatic fever.

DIAGNOSIS

Because there are neither pathognomonic clinical findings nor specific laboratory tests to confirm the diagnosis of rheumatic fever, the diagnosis must be somewhat arbitrary and empirical. A list of "major" and "minor" criteria to offer guidelines for the evaluation and diagnosis of rheumatic fever and rheumatic heart disease was published more than 50 years ago by Dr. T. Duckett Jones.[7] These have been accepted as diagnostic criteria throughout the world. The guidelines have been "modified" (1955) and "revised" (1984) by specifically appointed committees of the American Heart Association. The most recent review of the Jones criteria was designated as a "1992 Update."[2] These are shown in Table 257-1. The five major manifestations in order of decreasing frequency are polyarthritis, carditis, chorea, erythema marginatum, and subcutaneous nodules. The two major manifestations involving the skin, especially the nodules that were most often seen only after multiple attacks of rheumatic fever, have been extremely uncommon during the late 1900s in the United States.

The category of minor manifestations includes two laboratory findings: (1) elevated acute phase reactants (erythrocyte sedimentation rate and C-reactive protein) and (2) electrocardiographic (ECG) evidence of prolongation of the PR interval. The clinical observation of fever, usually a temperature under 102° F (38.8° C), may be present early in the course of polyarthritis or carditis. Arthralgia, another minor manifestation, is nonspecific and may affect any joint without objective signs of inflammation; it should not be considered to be a minor manifestation if arthritis is counted as a major manifestation.

Under current guidelines, laboratory confirmation of recent streptococcal infection should be part of the diagnostic evaluation. The absence of evidence of streptococcal infection should make one suspicious of the diagnosis except in cases in which indolent carditis or chorea are the major manifestations. The tendency to label as rheumatic fever any low-grade febrile illness with arthralgia for which no obvious cause can be found should be avoided.

The Jones criteria should be viewed as a guide to the probability of rheumatic fever, but the final diagnosis must remain a clinical judgment. The institution of prophylactic regimens requires prolonged administration of antistreptococcal agents, and this places an important responsibility on the physician who diagnoses rheumatic fever. It often is advisable to hospitalize a youngster who has arthritis and/or

Table 257-1 1992 Jones Criteria for the Diagnosis of an Initial Episode of Rheumatic Fever

Major Manifestations
Carditis
Polyarthritis
Chorea
Erythema marginatum
Subcutaneous nodules
Minor Manifestations
Clinical findings
Arthralgia
Fever
Laboratory findings
Elevated acute phase reactants
Erythrocyte sedimentation rate
C-reactive protein
Prolonged PR interval
Supporting Evidence of Antecedent Group A Streptococcal Infections
Positive throat culture or rapid streptococcal antigen test
Elevated or rising streptococcal antibody titer
Evidence of antecedent group A streptococcal infections, two major manifestations, or one major and two minor manifestations indicates a high probability of acute rheumatic fever as the diagnosis.

Data from the American Heart Association Committee on Rheumatic Fever, Endocarditis and Kawasaki Disease of the Council of Cardiovascular Disease in the Young, *JAMA* 268: 2069, 1992.

carditis for observation and appropriate documentation of a poststreptococcal illness, and initiation of treatment. This also emphasizes to the family the seriousness of the disease and the importance of prophylaxis to prevent recurrence. Because of the specific association of Sydenham's chorea with rheumatic fever, hospitalizing a child who has this manifestation should not be mandatory if abnormal neuromuscular activity is mild and unlikely to cause self-inflicted injury.

Age

Rheumatic fever is predominantly a disease of school-age children, with most first attacks occurring between 5 and 15 years of age. It is uncommon under 5 years of age and extremely rare before 3 years. When occurring in infancy, acute rheumatic fever usually is associated with severe carditis and congestive heart failure. Polyarthritis caused by rheumatic fever is unusual in the preschool-age group; rheumatoid arthritis and other inflammatory diseases of the joint are more likely diagnoses. Chorea also is uncommon in early childhood; most of the cases occur in patients older than 8 years of age.

Host Susceptibility

Rheumatic fever has often been referred to as a "social status disease," and the majority of studies have noted its strong association with poverty. The major social risk factors that predispose to rheumatic fever appear to be crowding and lack of medical attention. Crowding increases the likelihood of transmission of the group A beta-hemolytic streptococcus from person to person, and lack of medical care precludes timely treatment of "strep" throats and leads to late attention to signs and symptoms of acute rheumatic fever.[9]

The tendency for rheumatic fever to occur in more than one member of a family has long been recognized. The observation is noted even when family members are not concurrently living in the same household, indicating that environmental influences are probably not solely responsible for the disease. No genetic factors have been clearly established.[13]

There is no gender predisposition in the incidence of arthritis or carditis in childhood, although chorea has been noted to be more common in girls. However, there are gender differences in the type of valvular lesions that develop with carditis; boys having a higher incidence of aortic regurgitation. In young adults, mitral stenosis is more common in women.

STREPTOCOCCAL INFECTION AND LATENT PERIODS

Streptococcal pharyngitis presumptively precedes an attack of rheumatic fever, even though some patients fail to report such a history. Scarlet fever occasionally will be followed by signs of polyarthritis or carditis, but suppurative streptococcal disease, such as skin infection, is not a precursor of rheumatic fever. Throat cultures may be misleading in the evaluation of patients suspected of having rheumatic fever because the streptococcal infection antedates the common manifestations of polyarthritis and carditis by periods varying from 3 to 8 weeks; only 50% or fewer of patients who have rheumatic fever continue to harbor streptococci during the course of their illness.[11]

The most reliable evidence of a preceding streptococcal infection is obtained by demonstration of an antibody response to one or more of the streptococcal antigens. The most common of these, the antistreptolysin O (ASLO) titer, reaches maximal levels 3 to 5 weeks after infection and gradually declines to preinfection levels 6 to 12 months later. The ASLO titer is elevated in about 85% of patients who have rheumatic fever; titers are never extremely low. Serological evidence of an antecedent streptococcal infection rises to 95% if other streptococcal antibody tests (e.g., antihyaluronidase, antideoxyribonuclease B, and antistreptokinase) are performed.

The temporal relationship between the onset of the common manifestations of rheumatic fever and the antecedent streptococcal infection is illustrated in Fig. 257-1. As shown, polyarthritis and carditis usually occur 3 to 5 weeks after infection. The streptococcal antibody titer (ASLO) peaks before the onset of the clinical symptoms and then declines gradually. Occasionally, children complain of abdominal pain after a streptococcal infection for which medical or surgical evaluation is sought, and occasionally this symptom may precede signs of joint or cardiac involvement.

The sequence of the manifestations of rheumatic fever is noteworthy: polyarthritis, when it occurs, usually is present before the onset of carditis. Although carditis may be present without preceding joint symptoms, most often the apical sys-

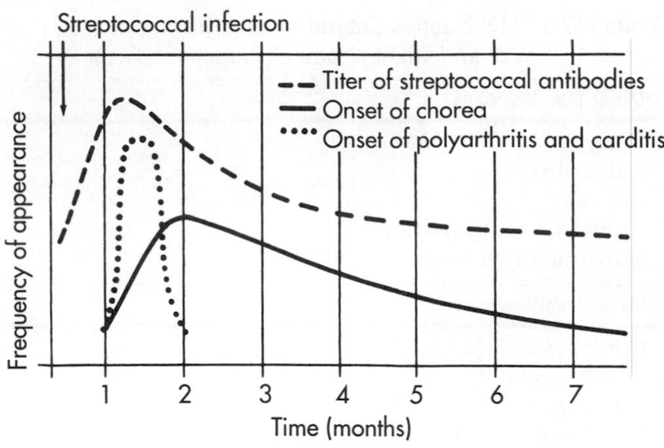

Fig. 257-1 Onset of rheumatic manifestations in relationship to antecedent streptococcal infection and ASLO titer.
(Modified from Stollerman GH: *Rheumatic fever and streptococcal infection,* New York, 1975, Grune & Stratton.)

tolic murmur of mitral valvulitis occurs within 2 weeks of the onset of arthritis. The diastolic murmur of isolated aortic valvulitis takes longer to appear and may not be heard for 6 to 8 weeks after the joint signs and symptoms appear. Chorea may develop during the convalescent phase of carditis, although there usually is a longer latent period. Classically, chorea appears as an independent manifestation of rheumatic fever long after the initial streptococcal infection. The majority of cases begin 2 months following streptococcal infection, with episodes still occurring up to 6 months afterward. Although chorea and carditis may coexist, chorea and polyarthritis rarely appear concurrently, presumably because of the difference in the latent periods.

MAJOR CLINICAL MANIFESTATIONS

Polyarthritis

Polyarthritis is the most common single manifestation of rheumatic fever at the onset, and usually involves the large joints of the lower extremities, particularly ankles or knees. This may result in the complaint of joint pain while walking; this often is initially considered to be secondary to trauma. Other large joints—for example, wrists or elbows—become involved in a migratory fashion. An affected joint characteristically is warm and reddened, but minimally swollen. Involved joints are exquisitely sensitive to touch, as well as painful on motion. Arthralgias, or aching in the joints without objective signs of inflammation, are suggestive, but are not specific for rheumatic fever. Fever almost always is present but usually below 102° F (38.8° C).

Carditis

Inflammation of cardiac tissue is characteristically expressed as endocarditis (valvulitis), but pancarditis involving the myocardium and pericardium may be present in severe cases. The murmurs audible in rheumatic carditis are the result of mitral and/or aortic valvulitis, with mitral involvement by far the most common. The auscultatory diagnosis of valvulitis often includes the presence of an apical mid-diastolic murmur. Pericarditis typically is silent, but a friction rub and distant heart sounds may occasionally be noted. However, isolated pericarditis without associated auscultatory findings of mitral and/or aortic involvement is not consistent with the diagnosis of acute rheumatic fever. Although viral inflammation of the heart by coxsackie B virus or Kawasaki disease may be associated with myocarditis and pericarditis, these entities do not cause valvulitis.

Carditis, clinically diagnosed by the presence of valvulitis with characteristic murmurs, arbitrarily may be designated as *mild, moderate,* or *severe.* Such a categorization is useful in the approach to management and to establishing a prognosis for developing rheumatic heart disease. Auscultation of the heart and evaluation of murmurs are influenced by fever and tachycardia; therefore, the patient should be reexamined frequently following the diagnosis of acute rheumatic fever and after the temperature has normalized with aspirin therapy. It is important to note that a "changing" functional murmur in an anxious and/or febrile child does not indicate the presence of carditis.

Mild carditis characteristically is defined by the presence of a prominent, high-pitched, apical systolic murmur typical of mitral insufficiency. This usually is of grade 2 to 3 (on a scale of 1 to 6) intensity and occupies all or most of systole. A mid-diastolic rumble at the apex is not present. Heart size on chest roentgenogram usually is normal.

Moderate carditis designates patients who have (1) both long systolic and prominent mid-diastolic apical murmurs, reflecting greater severity of mitral valvulitis; (2) a basilar diastolic murmur of aortic valvulitis; or (3) a combination of mitral and aortic valvulitis. An aortic diastolic murmur, which is high pitched and decrescendo in character, usually is heard best during end expiration with the diaphragm of the stethoscope firmly held at the third left intercostal space. A chest roentgenogram may show mild cardiac enlargement.

Severe carditis is defined by the presence of either pericarditis or congestive heart failure in addition to mitral and/or aortic valvulitis. The quality of the heart sounds may be poor, either because of pericardial effusion or low cardiac output. Murmurs may become more intense as cardiac compensation improves. The chest roentgenogram will show obvious cardiomegaly and may reveal pulmonary vascular congestion compatible with left-sided heart failure and pulmonary edema, an appearance also may be consistent with what is referred to as "rheumatic pneumonia."

Two-dimensional echocardiography is invaluable for the documentation and quantification of pericardial effusion.

However, the interpretation of valvular regurgitation by Doppler ultrasound should not constitute the basis of a diagnosis of carditis without auscultatory evidence of significant mitral or aortic involvement. Doppler studies in normal subjects frequently show a small degree of regurgitation across the mitral valve; trivial aortic valve regurgitation also occasionally may be noted.[10]

Chorea

The clinical picture of Sydenham's chorea includes that of poor neuromuscular coordination, sometimes first detected by a change or sloppiness in handwriting. A wide variety of jerky, involuntary movements may occur during the period of 6 to 8 weeks during which most cases of chorea are active. Neurological examination may give evidence of specific deficiencies particularly in trunk and upper extremity control of movements. A protective environment is recommended while the process is active. Occasionally, mild sedation is indicated, and there may be a role for agents such as clonazepam (Clonopin) or haloperidol (Haldol) for more severe movement disorders.

When chorea occurs as an isolated manifestation, the patient usually is afebrile, and the sedimentation rate is normal. Because of the long interval following the initiating streptococcal infection, the ASLO titer typically is normal or only mildly elevated. The murmur of mild mitral insufficiency may be noted.

Erythema marginatum. Erythema marginatum is a transient pink rash that has irregular, deeper-colored serpiginous borders that may be seen on the smooth, hairless surfaces of the inner aspect of the upper arms and thighs or trunk. This manifestation, although a specific finding for acute rheumatic fever, has been encountered infrequently in recent decades.

Subcutaneous nodules. Subcutaneous nodules characteristically are pea-sized and usually are located on extensor surfaces of fingers and toes, elbows and other joints, and less often on the occiput. They usually reflect a long-standing or smoldering illness following severe carditis; nodules may persist for weeks or months. Subcutaneous nodules rarely are found in children with rheumatic fever in the present era.

MINOR CLINICAL MANIFESTATIONS

Fever, although almost always present, is nonspecific, as is arthralgia without objective signs of joint inflammation. An elevated acute-phase reactant, such as the erythrocyte sedimentation rate, is an invaluable though nonspecific laboratory sign of inflammation in acute rheumatic fever. Initial values usually range between 60 and 120 mm/hr. It should be noted, however, that in chorea the sedimentation rate is normal because of the long interval beyond the antecedent streptococcal infection. Elevated C-reactive protein, although very helpful in diagnosing cases with borderline findings, also is elevated in a variety of other diseases.

Prolongation of the PR interval (first-degree heart block) on the electrocardiogram (ECG) is considered to be vagal and supports the diagnosis of rheumatic fever. It most commonly is noted while polyarthritis is apparent and is not necessarily associated with carditis. The ECG is almost always otherwise normal regardless of cardiac involvement. Although PR interval prolongation is the common manifestation, occasionally, second- or third-degree heart block occurs, indicating further heightening of vagal tone, perhaps more pronounced in the rheumatic state than in other acute illnesses. First- or second-degree heart block is not a major criterion for carditis, a harbinger of potential rheumatic heart disease, a threat to progress to complete heart block, or a cause of symptoms.

MANAGEMENT

Therapeutic management of acute rheumatic fever includes the use of antistreptococcal antibiotics and antiinflammatory agents.

Antistreptococcal Therapy

Eradication of group A beta-hemolytic streptococcal infection (even in the absence of a positive throat culture) by antibiotic treatment is the foremost principle in management of acute rheumatic fever. Antibiotic treatment always must be immediately followed by institution of a prophylactic program to prevent reinfection (see the discussion of rheumatic fever prophylaxis on p. 1784). Penicillin is the drug of choice prescribed initially in dosage and duration to maintain therapeutic blood levels for 10 days. Several treatment schedules, which periodically are revised, are outlined by the American Heart Association.[4] The intramuscular administration of the long-acting repository benzathine penicillin G (Bicillin) is the preferred treatment method, because it ensures therapeutic levels for a sufficient length of time. A single injection of 1.2 million units for children 5 to 15 years of age is recommended, to be followed by prophylactic injections of 1.2 million units every 3 to 4 weeks. An alternative method is (1) oral penicillin, 200,000 or 250,000 units (penicillin G or V), given three or four times a day for a full 10 days, followed by the same dose twice daily thereafter, or (2) a combination of oral and intramuscular penicillin (see the discussion of rheumatic fever prophylaxis on p. 1784).

For patients sensitive to penicillin, erythromycin may be used for antistreptococcal therapy. The sulfonamide drugs, which are bacteriostatic rather than bactericidal, are not effective for streptococcal eradication, although they can be used in rheumatic prophylaxis programs to prevent reinfection.

Antiinflammatory Agents

Salicylates are indicated in the presence of acute, painful arthritis during the febrile phase of acute rheumatic fever. The duration of salicylate therapy in polyarthritis or carditis in childhood usually ranges from 4 to 8 weeks; the average initial amount prescribed should be approximately 50 to 75 mg/kg/day, given in four divided doses.[12] Extremely high doses are not required; aspirin is used for symptomatic relief only. Aspirin administration usually is associated with a rapid and dramatic improvement in objective arthritis signs and symptoms, and with almost immediate defervescence of fever. Specific blood levels do not need to be reached or maintained if clinical signs have disappeared. There is no evidence that salicylate administration affects the clinical course or later manifestations of cardiac involvement. The administration of steroid hormones, most commonly prednisone (1 to 2 mg/kg/day), is indicated for severe cardiac involvement manifested by pancarditis with congestive heart failure. When myocarditis appears to be fulminant, steroid therapy has been shown to significantly improve survival; but, as with salicylates, there is no evidence of long-term palliative effects on chronic rheumatic valvular disease.[1] The duration of steroid treatment may be extended to 1 to 3 months in severe cases, with varying schedules of tapering the dosage and possibly adding salicylate therapy.

Additional, specific therapeutic measures to control congestive heart failure may be useful (i.e., diuretics and digitalis). Furosemide (Lasix) is used for the management of pulmonary congestion with left ventricular failure. Digitalis (digoxin) should be administered cautiously; the threshold for toxicity may be lower in the presence of inflammatory myocarditis. It may be prudent to withhold digitalis for 1 or 2 days until steroid therapy has begun to suppress the myocarditis. Serum potassium levels should be monitored, because steroids and furosemide both decrease body potassium, predisposing to digitalis intoxication. Aldactone is a potassium-sparing diuretic agent that can be added to the medical regimen.

Limitation of Activity

The role of bed rest in the treatment of rheumatic fever has been deemphasized in recent years. For children with arthritis, ambulation can be permitted when the pain and joint tenderness improve. Patients who have stable mild cardiac involvement can be allowed to ambulate when they feel well enough. For those who have more severe carditis, the length of restricted activity is individualized according to the severity of cardiac involvement.

EVOLUTION OF RHEUMATIC HEART DISEASE

In the months and years that follow an attack of rheumatic fever, the auscultatory findings frequently change from those heard during the acute episode. Apical systolic murmurs heard initially may diminish or even completely disappear. This is in contrast to the aortic diastolic murmur, which will almost always persist during the follow-up period. An initial diagnosis of "carditis" does not necessarily imply progression to permanent heart damage. When a child is labeled with "history of acute rheumatic fever," the additional appellation of "rheumatic heart disease" must be reevaluated continually. Even patients with severe carditis in the acute phase will show remarkable improvement in the weeks and months after the recuperative period; more than half of murmurs of mild/moderate mitral insufficiency will disappear completely. Nevertheless, the ultimate development of rheumatic heart disease following a first attack of rheumatic fever can be correlated with the severity of the acute carditis. It has been shown in the 10-year follow-up study of treatments begun in 1951 that approximately 30% of those who had mild carditis and 50% of those who had moderate carditis develop chronic rheumatic heart disease (mitral insufficiency/stenosis and/or aortic regurgitation). With severe carditis, nearly 75% of the patients will have residual heart disease.

The majority of children who develop rheumatic heart disease after a single attack of rheumatic fever have mitral regurgitation. The others either have both mitral and aortic regurgitation or aortic regurgitation alone. Mitral stenosis evolves slowly, usually after repeated attacks of acute rheumatic fever, but at times unexpectedly, many years after initial mild mitral valvitis, perhaps previously undiagnosed. Isolated mitral stenosis is unusual before early adulthood and has become a rare finding in developed nations.

An issue that arises in the follow-up of children who have rheumatic heart disease is the amount of physical activity permitted. In general, those who have mild mitral regurgitation with normal heart size should be allowed to engage in all athletic activities, except perhaps for the most strenuous, competitive sports. Those who have more severe mitral regurgitation and/or aortic insufficiency with cardiomegaly should have some restriction of their activities, and a continuing appropriate regimen. If symptoms of fatigue or of exercise intolerance persist despite medical management, a full diagnostic evaluation should be carried out; if appropriate, surgical intervention with valvuloplasty or valve replacement should be considered.

RHEUMATIC FEVER PROPHYLAXIS

The rationale for antibiotic prophylaxis in a known rheumatic patient is protection against recurrence of rheumatic fever through prevention of group A streptococcal infection. The most effective method for reducing streptococcal infections and rheumatic fever recurrence is by intramuscular injections of long-acting penicillin (benzathine penicillin G, 1.2 million units).[4] This preventive regimen is most effective when given every 3 to 4 weeks; with residual cardiac involvement, this approach is recommended for at least a 1- or 2-year period, before initiating oral prophylaxis. An every-3-week regimen is recommended for the first 6 to 12 months. Parenteral therapy is the most effective method of prophylaxis, since strict adherence to a program of daily oral medication is especially difficult for children and adolescents. Some transient discomfort at the injection site (anterior thigh or buttock) may be relieved by a hot bath and aspirin on the evening of injection.

Alternative methods of prophylaxis include the oral administration of penicillin G (200,000 or 250,000 units, twice a day) or sulfisoxazole (Gantrisin, 0.5 g twice a day). For the exceptional patient who may be sensitive to both penicillin and sulfa, daily prophylaxis with another agent may be considered. Successful oral prophylaxis is hard to maintain, and if employed, its value and need for compliance should be reinforced constantly by the pediatrician. Because rheumatic fever recurrence is less likely after 2 to 5 years, for patients with chronic rheumatic heart disease, an oral regimen can be substituted for intramuscular penicillin. Oral prophylaxis can be instituted immediately for patients who did not have carditis during the acute attack, because under these circumstances recurrences with carditis are extremely rare.

RECURRENCE OF RHEUMATIC FEVER

One of the most striking characteristics of rheumatic fever is its tendency to recur. Before the introduction of preventive measures, the great majority of patients who had an initial attack of rheumatic fever had one or more recurrences. The recurrence rate is highest during the first 3 years following an initial attack; it diminishes with time after the original episode, and recurrence is rare in adulthood.

Continuous antimicrobial prophylaxis should be carried out in all children who have a history of rheumatic fever, including those who present with chorea. If by the time of high school graduation or at 18 years of age there is no auscultatory evidence of heart disease in patients who initially had cardiac involvement, prophylaxis may be discontinued. If, however, there is chronic mitral or aortic valvular disease, prophylaxis should be maintained into adulthood. In children who had no cardiac involvement during the initial attack, prophylaxis can be discontinued after 5 years.

Bacterial Endocarditis

Individuals who have a history of rheumatic fever without evidence of significant murmurs on follow-up examination are not susceptible to bacterial endocarditis, because they do not have damaged heart valves. However, those who do have rheumatic heart disease should have specific antimicrobial coverage before dental manipulation or extraction in addition to their regular rheumatic fever prophylaxis. With dental work or oropharyngeal surgery, including tonsillectomy and adenoidectomy, antibiotics should be administered to protect the patient from *Streptococcus viridans* bacteremia. The latest recommendation of the American Heart Association is to administer amoxicillin 2 g orally 1 hour before the procedure.[5] For amoxicillin/penicillin-allergic patients, clindamycin, cephalexin, or azithromycin are prescribed. For genitourinary procedures, appropriate antibiotic coverage should be directed against enterococci and gram-negative organisms.

CONTRACEPTION AND PREGNANCY

Patients who have severe rheumatic heart disease are at high risk during pregnancy and delivery. Mitral stenosis has an especially high-risk profile. However, mild rheumatic heart disease is well tolerated during pregnancy.

The adolescent girl who has rheumatic heart disease should be counseled in regard to contraceptive methods. Oral medication with a low level of estrogen can be prescribed and instructions given on the use of a diaphragm. An intrauterine device, however, should be avoided because of the risk of bacteremia.

Because of the added cardiovascular burden during pregnancy, careful obstetrical care should be provided from the first trimester through delivery. Prophylaxis against streptococcal infection should be continued. Psychosocial support may be needed, especially for the pregnant teenager with significant rheumatic heart disease who may face medical complications during pregnancy. If early termination of a pregnancy is sought, therapeutic abortion should be carried out in the hospital; intravenous antibiotic prophylaxis against bacterial endocarditis should be administered.

REFERENCES

1. Albert DA, Harel L, Karrison T: The treatment of rheumatic carditis: a review and meta-analysis., *Medicine* 74:1, 1995.
2. American Heart Association Committee on Rheumatic Fever, Endocarditis and Kawasaki Disease of the Council of Cardiovascular Disease in the Young: Guidelines for the diagnosis of rheumatic fever: Jones criteria, 1992 update, *JAMA* 268:2069, 1992.
3. Centers for Disease Control: Acute rheumatic fever at a navy training center—San Diego, California, *Morbidity and Mortality Weekly Report* 37:101, 1988.
4. Dajani A, et al: Treatment of acute streptococcal pharyngitis and prevention of rheumatic fever: a statement for health professionals, *Pediatrics* 96:758, 1995.
5. Dajani AS, et al: Prevention of bacterial endocarditis: recommendations by the American Heart Association, *JAMA* 277:1794, 1997.
6. Griffiths SP, Gersony WM: Acute rheumatic fever in New York City (1969 to 1998): a comparative study of two decades, *J Pediatr* 116:882, 1990.
7. Jones TD: Diagnosis of rheumatic fever, *JAMA* 126:481, 1944.
8. Kaplan EL, Hill HR: Return of rheumatic fever: consequences, implications and needs, *J Pediatr* 111:244, 1987.
9. Massell BF: *Rheumatic fever and streptococcal infection,* Boston, 1997, Harvard University Press.
10. Stollerman GH: Rheumatic fever, *Lancet* 349:935, 1997.
11. Stollerman GH: *Rheumatic fever and streptococcal infection,* New York, 1975, Grune & Stratton.
12. Taranta A, Markowitz M: *Rheumatic fever,* Boston, 1989, Kluwer Academic Publishers.
13. Veasy LG, Hill HR: Immunologic and clinical correlations in rheumatic fever and rheumatic heart disease, *Pediatr Infect Dis J* 16:400, 1997.
14. Veasy LG, et al: Resurgence of acute rheumatic fever in the intermountain area of the United States, *N Engl J Med* 316:421, 1987.

258 Rocky Mountain Spotted Fever

Fred J. Heldrich

Rocky Mountain spotted fever (RMSF), an acute infectious disease caused by *Rickettsia rickettsii*, is characterized by fever, headache, myalgia, and a distinctive exanthem. The major pathological lesion, vasculitis, makes RMSF a multisystem disease. Most important, it is a disease that requires clinical diagnosis and treatment before laboratory confirmation.

The disease was first reported in patients from the Rocky Mountain region. Today, however, the incidence of the disease is greatest east of the Mississippi River, with most cases being reported from the southeastern and south central United States. Although the disease occurs predominantly in the United States, it has been reported from other areas in the Western Hemisphere, specifically Canada, Central America, and South America. The reported frequency of the disease in the United States has decreased slightly over the past several years.

EPIDEMIOLOGY

Ticks serve as a vector for the infectious agent *R. rickettsii*. Transmission to humans occurs when the tick takes a blood meal or when the abraded skin is contaminated by tick feces or a crushed tick, which may occur when ticks are removed. Two specific ticks serve as major carriers: the wood tick, *Dermacentor andersoni,* is the more important vector in the West; the dog tick, *Dermacentor variabilis,* is the usual vector in the East. Ticks, in turn, acquire the rickettsiae by feeding on infected wild mammals. Infection of laboratory workers has been reported independent of exposure to ticks. The seasonal incidence of RMSF—primarily occurring in spring, summer, and fall—is in accordance with the activity of ticks.[6] Dog ticks infected with *R. rickettsii* have been found in urban areas, which suggests this tick's ubiquitous nature and places individuals at risk without travel to endemic areas.[8] In adults, occupational or recreational exposure to ticks increases the risk of infection; however, children are affected with greatest frequency, and boys more often than girls.

Exposure to a tick is not elicited in every case, although a history of removing a tick before the onset of illness is not unusual. The tick bite is painless and leaves no local lesion or regional lymphadenopathy; it is important, therefore, to question specifically about prior tick removal activities that increase the risk of exposure (e.g., removal of a tick from a pet dog and camping or picnicking in a high-risk area).

PATHOLOGY

RMSF is an infectious disease that produces a vasculitis, giving rise to symptoms in multiple organ systems including skeletal muscle, brain, lungs, kidneys, testes, adrenal glands, liver, and heart. Rickettsiae multiply in endothelial cells and may produce cellular injury by various mechanisms. These include cell wall penetration, disturbance of intracellular metabolism, production of toxic metabolites, and utilization of metabolites required by the host cell. Necrosis of endothelial cell walls, an increase in vascular permeability, fibrin extravasation, and thrombosis of small blood vessels ensue. Resulting cell damage in multiple locations is responsible for the clinical picture.[3]

CLINICAL FEATURES

After inoculation with the rickettsiae, the incubation period ranges from 3 to 12 days; the usual period is 5 to 7 days. In general, shorter incubation periods are associated with most serious disease.

In the typical case,[5] there is a short prodromal period of 2 to 3 days, with low-grade fever, chills, and muscle aches predominating. Headache also is an early symptom. Younger patients indicate muscle pain and headache by crying. Malaise, anorexia, vomiting, and photophobia also frequently are present. The prodrome is followed by accentuation of symptoms, especially of the fever, which remains elevated, often as high as 104° F (40° C) or more. The lowest temperatures, although still elevated, are recorded in the mornings. Lethargy and mental obtundation become prominent. Although the symptoms seen at this stage are not diagnostic, the triad of fever, headache, and myalgia, combined with a history of tick bite or removal within the previous 2 weeks, mandates treatment for RMSF until the diagnosis can be excluded.

Of RMSF symptoms and signs, it is the rash that is most distinctive. It usually appears on the fourth day of fever and begins peripherally on the wrists, ankles, hands, and feet. Initially, the lesions are macular, discrete, and erythematous and blanch on pressure. The rash rapidly spreads centrally, involving the arms, legs, axillae, buttocks, trunk, neck, and face. The lesions deepen in color, becoming dusky red, maculopapular and petechial. Petechial lesions may coalesce and form large ecchymotic areas. Even before the frank appearance of petechiae, a tourniquet applied for phlebotomy may produce petechial lesions distal to the tourniquet. In severe cases and when treatment is delayed, these ecchymotic areas may ulcerate, and distal regions (e.g., fingers and toes) may become gangrenous. Nonpitting edema, especially notable around the eyes, face, hands, and feet, also occurs frequently.

Tachycardia and an elevated pulse rate are noted early and are proportional to the degree of hyperpyrexia. A sudden increase in pulse rate or fall in blood pressure is ominous and may indicate peripheral circulatory collapse, severe bleeding, or myocardial failure. Photophobia is associated with conjunctival ecchymosis involving both bulbar and palpebral conjunctivae. Retinal hemorrhages also may be seen.

Abdominal pain and vomiting, with generalized abdominal tenderness, may occur,[2] as may hepatomegaly and splenomegaly. Jaundice usually is not seen, except in the most critically ill patients. Fever, poor fluid intake, and vomiting all contribute to a diminished urinary output. Mild azotemia should respond to rehydration. In addition to the lethargy and obtunded state of consciousness, the patient may exhibit nuchal rigidity. Disorientation and confusion, as well as seizures, may occur. Vasculitis, hemorrhage, or secondary metabolic changes are responsible for these neurological manifestations.[1] When these symptoms occur early in the course of RMSF, they may mask its diagnosis.

DIFFERENTIAL DIAGNOSIS

Illnesses to be considered and differentiated from RMSF, especially after the rash appears, include rubeola, atypical measles, meningococcemia, Henoch-Schönlein purpura, Kawasaki disease, idiopathic thrombocytopenic purpura, leukemia, typhus, ehrlichiosis, and infectious mononucleosis. Of these, meningococcemia and ehrlichiosis, because of their severe consequences, require immediate differentiation from RMSF.

The petechial rash of meningococcemia differs from that of RMSF in its distribution, rapid extension, and coalescence of lesions into larger hemorrhagic, purpuric areas. Prostration develops rapidly if the patient remains untreated and often is present on admission. Absence of myalgia and an extremely abrupt onset are helpful points in differentiating meningococcemia from RMSF. Although the white blood cell count may be elevated in meningococcemia, the sickest patients frequently are leukopenic. Meningitis with pleocytosis, low glucose levels, and organisms in the cerebrospinal fluid (CSF) also may be present.

Ehrlichiosis is a rickettsial disease with clinical similarity to RMSF. Although a rash occurs with less frequency, it has been noted in more than 60% of pediatric patients and, while variable in location and appearance, it may be petechial. Early diagnosis and treatment of patients with ehrlichiosis with either tetracycline or doxycycline reduces morbidity.

Rubeola (measles) is characterized by a macular rash (infrequently becoming hemorrhagic), which always begins on the face and neck and is preceded by an enanthem—Koplik spots on the buccal mucosa. The coryza and cough in the prodromal stage of illness are not consistent with RMSF. A history of adequate immunization with rubeola vaccine greatly diminishes this possibility.

Atypical measles has a prodromal period similar in duration to RMSF but differs in that upper respiratory tract symptoms usually are prominent. From 1963 to 1968, killed measles vaccine was used for immunization against rubeola. Atypical measles occurs in patients previously immunized with killed vaccine who are subsequently exposed to natural measles. An Arthus reaction may be noted at the site of prior inoculation. Additionally, joint pain is common in atypical measles but is not found in RMSF.

Henoch-Schönlein purpura may produce a petechial or purpuric rash, which frequently is concentrated on the lower extremities and buttocks. These cutaneous lesions may be multiform and occur on other parts of the body. Frequently, there is an arthralgia with periarticular swelling and accompanying signs and symptoms of upper respiratory tract inflammation, gastroenteritis, or nephritis.

Kawasaki disease shares many of the features of RMSF: fever, puffy hands and feet, rash, and conjunctival injection. Usually, Kawasaki disease is not considered strongly until 5 days of fever, and an enlarged cervical node, pharyngeal hyperemia, dry cracked lips, strawberry tongue, and marked irritability tend to set it apart. Although patients who have Kawasaki disease do have a rash, it typically does not begin peripherally and spread centrally or become petechial in 1 to 2 days. Leukocyte and erythrocyte sedimentation rates usually are elevated significantly. An elevated platelet count begins during the second week of illness. See Chapter 230 for a more detailed discussion of Kawasaki disease.

Other illnesses that produce petechiae must also be mentioned, even though they lack the distinctive distribution of the rash. Idiopathic thrombocytopenic purpura is seen as a petechial rash in an otherwise healthy patient. Leukemic patients who have fever and petechiae at initial presentation would be expected to be anemic and have lymphadenopathy or hepatosplenomegaly. Patients who have infectious mononucleosis, if they have a petechial eruption, usually have lymphadenopathy, hepatosplenomegaly, and a more gradual onset. Typhus is a rickettsial infection to be excluded. Murine typhus produces a milder disease, with a rash that is macular and not petechial. Epidemic typhus may produce a petechial rash that typically begins proximally and extends peripherally, but usually does not involve the palms or soles; history of a tick bite also is absent.

LABORATORY EVALUATION

The diagnosis of RMSF is made clinically, and treatment should be started before laboratory diagnosis is confirmed. Immunofluorescent staining of the skin biopsy may identify *R. rickettsii* and may provide early proof of RMSF, but this study is not readily available to most clinicians.[4] Appropriate antibiotic therapy started 3 days before biopsy has resulted in negative immunofluorescence. Therefore, when appropriate treatment has been initiated before biopsy, clinical criteria justify a full course of antibiotic therapy. Polymerase chain reaction (PCR) testing, if available, provides a specific diagnostic tool for early diagnosis.[3]

Complement fixation and immunofluorescent antibody studies will identify patients who have RMSF, but these do not become positive until the second week of illness or later if antibiotic therapy has begun early. The Weil-Felix reaction, agglutination of *Proteus vulgaris* by the patient's serum, is at best a nonspecific test for RMSF. Again, acute and convalescent serums must be compared, although *Proteus* agglutinins may appear by the end of the first week of illness. Availability of the more specific and sensitive tests make this test obsolete.

Rickettsiae can be isolated from body fluid or tissue specimens when grown in laboratory animals or chick embryos. However, the high rate of disease transmission to laboratory technicians makes such techniques feasible only in laboratories engaged in rickettsia-related research in which all workers are immunized; thus, culture identification of rickettsiae is not available in most clinical settings.

Blood leukocyte counts and differential counts usually are within normal limits. Thrombocytopenia is a complication seen in the later stages of the disease. In seriously ill patients, metabolic derangements such as hyponatremia and hypochloremia may occur but are nonspecific findings. Only with the complication of intravascular coagulation will such tests as prothrombin time, partial thromboplastin time, fibrinogen, and fibrin split products become abnormal.

In patients who have neurological symptoms, the CSF pressure, white and red blood cell counts, and protein level all may be elevated.

COURSE

Experience with RMSF before effective therapy was discovered indicated that the illness persisted for 2 to 3 weeks and that the overall mortality was 20%. RMSF now has a mortality of approximately 5% in recognized cases, but RMSF patients have been identified by serological evidence who escaped clinical detection, suggesting that the disease may occur in a mild or even subclinical form.[7] The importance of abdominal pain mimicking an acute abdominal condition and dominating as an early symptom before the development of a rash must be emphasized. Rocky Mountain spotless fever also has been described.[9] Of great concern is a report suggesting that patients who have "spotless or almost spotless" fever have a significantly higher mortality.[9,10]

It is appropriate to consider RMSF a potentially lethal illness, even though younger patients are likely to be less severely affected. Early diagnosis and prompt therapy lessen disease severity. Under such circumstances, death would be extremely unusual; in the majority of patients, early clinical diagnosis and adequate therapy shorten the duration of illness appreciably. Normal temperatures within the first 3 to 4 days may be expected, and patients recover rapidly from other signs of illness (e.g., headache, myalgia, and lethargy). Extension of the rash ceases.[5] Recovery from the illness is accompanied by permanent immunity.

COMPLICATIONS

Vascular necrosis and thrombosis may result in local gangrene and loss of tissue. Although uncommon, disseminated intravascular coagulation (DIC) may develop. This is an ominous sign, and patients with this complication have the greatest risk of dying. Myocardial failure may result from myocarditis and arrhythmias. Edema may be generalized as a result of an increase in capillary permeability secondary to the vasculitis, of heart failure, and/or of iatrogenic fluid overload.

Neurological complications, in addition to the lethargy, have already been discussed. Hematuria and anemia also may occur.

TREATMENT

Specific therapy with either chloramphenicol (100 mg/kg/24 hr; maximum 4 g/24 hr), tetracycline (20 mg/kg/24 hr; maximum 2 g/24 hr), or doxycycline (5 mg/kg/24 hr, maximum 200 mg/24 hr) may be used. Although studies in children are few, those reported indicate a good response to doxycycline. Because of the potential for dental injury, the effectiveness of tetracycline has not been studied. Some may prefer doxycycline, because of a diminished risk of tooth staining, although a course of tetracycline sufficient to treat RMSF is unlikely to result in dental injury. If therapy is started before a definitive diagnosis of RMSF has been made, it may be prudent not to use chloramphenicol because it has not been proved to be as effective for ehrlichiosis. The intravenous route is indicated for patients moderately or severely ill or for those who are vomiting. Oral medication should be reserved for the mildly ill.

Hospitalization is desirable initially for all patients, both to confirm the diagnosis and to observe the effect of therapy. Therapy should be continued until the patient has improved and has been afebrile for 48 hours.

Supportive therapy includes maintenance of hydration and nutrition with appropriate intravenous fluids and oral feedings (if tolerated), or both. Management of DIC remains unsatisfactory, but therapeutic maneuvers such as giving fresh-frozen plasma, transfusing fresh platelets and packed red blood cells, and administering vitamin K may be helpful. The use of corticosteroids is believed to be warranted in the most severely ill and toxic patients. Seizures may require the use of anticonvulsant medications.

PREVENTION

The use of vaccine is not indicated except in those individuals at highest risk for exposure. Even then, the availability of effective therapy reduces the need for vaccination. When exposure is likely, ticks should be searched for daily, and for those in tick-infested areas, twice daily. Careful inspection at bath time is an excellent way to discover the presence of ticks. They may be removed by gentle traction with forceps or tweezers, but care must be taken not to crush them.

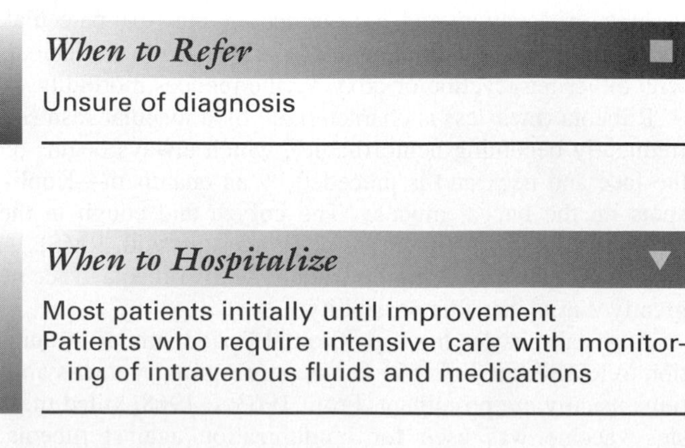

When to Refer

Unsure of diagnosis

When to Hospitalize

Most patients initially until improvement

Patients who require intensive care with monitoring of intravenous fluids and medications

REFERENCES

1. Bell WE, Lacari AD: Rocky Mountain spotted fever: neurologic symptoms in the acute phase, *Neurology* 20:841, 1970.
2. Davis AE, Bradford WD: Abdominal pain resembling acute appendicitis in Rocky Mountain spotted fever, *JAMA* 247:2811, 1982.
3. Edwards MS, Feigen RD: Rickettsial disease. In Feigen RD, Cherry JD, editors: *Textbook of pediatric infectious diseases,* ed 4, Philadelphia, 1998, WB Saunders.
4. Fleisher G, Lennette ET, Honig P: Diagnosis of Rocky Mountain spotted fever by immunofluorescent identification of *Rickettsia rickettsii* in skin biopsy tissue, *J Pediatr* 95:63, 1979.
5. Haynes RE, Sanders DY, Cramblett HG: Rocky Mountain spotted fever in children, *J Pediatr* 76:685, 1970.
6. Lange JV, Walker DH, Wester TB: Documented Rocky Mountain spotted fever in wintertime, *JAMA* 247:2403, 1982.
7. Marx RS, et al: Rocky Mountain spotted fever: serological evidence of previous subclinical infection in children, *Am J Dis Child* 136:16, 1982.
8. Salgo MP, et al: A focus of Rocky Mountain fever within New York City, *N Engl J Med* 318:1345, 1988.
9. Sexton DJ, Corey GR: Rocky mountain "spotless" and "almost spotless" fever: a wolf in sheep's clothing, *Clin Infect Dis* 15:439, 1992.
10. Westerman EL: Rocky Mountain spotless fever: a dilemma for the clinician, *Arch Intern Med* 142:1106, 1982.

259 Seborrheic Dermatitis

Ana M. Duarte • Lawrence A. Schachner

Seborrheic dermatitis (SD) is a common, usually asymptomatic dermatosis of unknown etiology that is seen primarily in infants, but also in adolescents and adults. It presents in 50% of affected infants before 5 weeks of age.[1] There is an incidence of 2% to 5% in the general population.[1] Although SD occasionally is seen in infants who are infected with the human immunodeficiency virus (HIV), a true increased incidence has not been documented.[4] No evidence suggests a genetic predisposition. Studies have indicated that infants who present with seborrheic dermatitis may be at an increased risk of developing atopic dermatitis and, less often, psoriasis.[3]

CLINICAL FEATURES

Seborrheic dermatitis may present most commonly as a greasy, scaly dermatitis, less often as psoriasiform seborrheic dermatitis, and rarely as erythrodermic seborrheic dermatitis.

Seborrheic dermatitis presents in infancy with diffuse, red, crusted, and yellow scaling plaques on the vertex of the scalp (cradle cap). Similar lesions also may be found in the retroauricular creases, the eyebrows, and the nasolabial folds, as well as in the axillary and inguinal folds, the neck, and the diaper area. The lesions usually are asymptomatic and distributed symmetrically.

The presentation is similar in adolescents. Patients may note a greasy, scaling, pruritic eruption on the scalp. Except for lack of inguinal area involvement, the distribution of the lesions is the same as for infants.

HIV-positive children aged 2 to 5 years may manifest SD with lesions similar to those seen in adolescents and adults. This is distinctly unusual in immunocompetent children and appears to be a manifestation of HIV infection.[4]

Psoriasiform seborrheic dermatitis, also known as *sebopsoriasis* or *seborrhiasis,* presents with features of both SD and psoriasis and may represent a bridge between the two conditions. Psoriasiform plaques—that is, annular, red-brown plaques having a silvery scale—may be present among the classic greasy, yellow, scaling lesions of SD. Patients may or may not have "pitted" nails, which are seen with classic psoriasis.

Erythrodermic seborrheic dermatitis is rare and presents with widespread exfoliative erythroderma. Diffuse desquamation usually begins in the flexures and then spreads. The patient may exhibit signs and symptoms of systemic involvement—that is, fever, chills, lymphadenopathy, peripheral edema, and dehydration. This also may be the presentation of Leiner's disease (see the discussion of differential diagnosis on the facing page).

PATHOGENESIS

The etiology of seborrheic dermatitis remains unknown; several different pathogenic mechanisms are proposed. Based on the distribution of the lesions that involve areas of highest sebaceous gland concentration, an abnormality in the sebaceous gland or an increased sensitivity to circulating maternal or endogenous hormones has been suggested. However, these patients have normal sebaceous secretion and hormonal levels. Recent studies have found that altered essential fatty acids may be important in the pathogenesis of this disorder.[5] In addition, *Pityrosporum ovale* may play a role in the evolution of SD in infant and adult patients.[2]

DIFFERENTIAL DIAGNOSIS

The differential diagnosis of seborrheic dermatitis includes atopic dermatitis, psoriasis, dermatophyte infection, diaper dermatitis, histiocytosis X, and Leiner's disease.

Atopic dermatitis usually is distinguished by the presence of extreme pruritus, extensoral distribution in infancy and flexural distribution in older children (tending to spare the scalp and to involve the hands and feet), as well as a family history in 70% of those affected. Seborrheic dermatitis also may occur concomitantly with atopic dermatitis (see Chapter 189).

Psoriasis is a common inherited papulosquamous skin disorder characterized by well-demarcated, annular, thick, red-brown, scaling plaques usually present on the trunk, the extensor areas on the arms, the knees, the elbows, the diaper area, and the scalp, as well as by nail pitting. It usually lacks the specific distribution and the greasy component of SD. However, some cases of SD may overlap with psoriasis. Extensive cases of SD become persistent; when there is a positive family history of psoriasis, patients should be referred to a dermatologist for biopsy and, potentially, long-term follow-up.

Dermatophyte infection of the scalp (tinea capitis) may present with scaling, pruritus, and redness of the scalp. It usually results in alopecia, a distinguishing feature. Tinea corporis may be distinguished by its annular configuration. In addition, a potassium hydroxide preparation of the scalp hair roots or scales from body lesions will demonstrate septate hyphae.

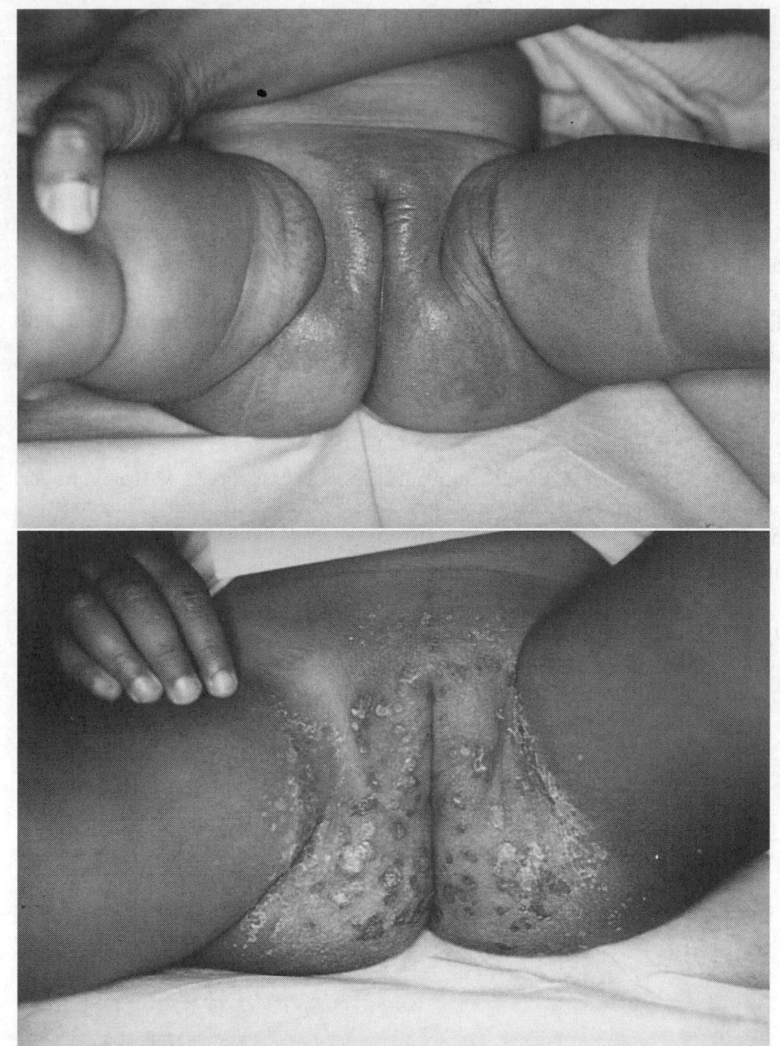

Fig. 259-1 A, Irritant diaper dermatitis. B, Candidal diaper dermatitis.

Diaper dermatitis, or irritant diaper rash (ammoniacal diaper dermatitis), is characterized by involvement primarily of the convex surfaces by red, scaling plaques; the inguinal folds are spared (Fig. 259-1, *A*). In candidal diaper dermatitis, similar red, scaling plaques involve the skin folds, but there also are satellite pustules in areas not covered by the diaper (Fig. 259-1, *B*). Seborrheic dermatitis in the diaper area involves the skin folds; however, there are no satellite lesions.

Histiocytosis X refers to a group of Langerhans' cell histiocytoses: Letterer-Siwe disease (diffuse disseminated histiocytosis), Hand-Schüller-Christian disease, and eosinophilic granuloma (chronic multifocal or focal histiocytosis). Letterer-Siwe disease may be confused with seborrheic dermatitis because its pattern of distribution is similar. However, Letterer-Siwe disease also is characterized by axillary, inguinal, and oral mucosal erosions, purpura and petechiae, and hepatosplenomegaly. A skin biopsy specimen will distinguish the two disorders easily and is recommended in cases of seborrheic dermatitis that are unresponsive to treatment.

Leiner's disease, sometimes referred to as *erythrodermic seborrheic dermatitis,* is an inherited immunological disorder characterized by generalized seborrheic dermatitis, persistent diarrhea, failure to thrive, and recurrent gram-negative infections. The diagnosis is made by demonstrating deficient yeast opsonic activity in the patient's serum.

MANAGEMENT

Therapy for seborrheic dermatitis (infantile cradle cap) includes the application to the scalp of a 1% to 2% salicylic acid in liquid or petrolatum form, followed by a keratolytic shampoo (e.g., Sebulex) and a topical low-potency corticosteroid (Synalar solution or Derma-Smoothe). The salicylic acid solution or petrolatum should be applied only for 10 minutes and then shampooed out carefully, avoiding the face and particularly the eyes because severe contact irritation may occur. The corticosteroid solution should be applied sparingly and left on for several hours. This regimen may be repeated up to twice daily as needed and then tapered. Dramatic improvement occurs usually within a week. Lesions occurring on the face, intertriginous areas, and the diaper area may be treated with a low-potency topical corticosteroid cream (1% hydrocortisone cream) twice a day. A mid-potency corticosteroid such as 0.1% Kenalog cream may be used on the body twice a day. A mid-potency or strong halogenated corticosteroid should not be used on the face, intertriginous areas, and diaper area. Topical ketoconazole (Nizoral), which has been used to treat adult SD, has been found to be beneficial in treating infantile SD. Lesions in the diaper and intertriginous areas may become superinfected with *Candida* species and require topical Mycostatin cream twice a day in addition to a topical corticosteroid.

Therapy for adolescent seborrheic dermatitis consists of topical corticosteroids and keratolytic shampoos applied to the scalp similar to those described for infants. In addition, topical Nizoral cream and oral ketoconazole may be used in severe cases.

Psoriasiform seborrheic dermatitis of the scalp is treated as described for cradle cap. Psoriasiform lesions on the face and truck respond to treatment with topical corticosteroid ointments and emollients. If lesions persist into childhood, a modified Goeckerman regimen consisting of application of a tar preparation followed by outdoor exposure to sunlight and topical corticosteroids[1] is therapeutic.

Generalized erythrodermic seborrheic dermatitis may require systemic corticosteroids and antibiotics to control superinfection in addition to the antiseborrheic therapies already mentioned. Hospitalization for intravenous antibiotic administration may be required.

PROGNOSIS

The prognosis for infantile seborrheic dermatitis usually is good. Most cases resolve within the first 6 months of life. Adolescent-onset and HIV-related seborrheic dermatitis may be more persistent; however, it usually responds readily to topical therapy. Infants who have seborrheic dermatitis are at an increased risk of developing atopic dermatitis or psoriasis later.

REFERENCES

1. Caputo R: Papulo-squamous disease. In Schachner LA, Hansen R, editors: *Pediatric dermatology,* New York, 1988, Churchill Livingstone.
2. Maldonado RR, et al: *Pityrosporum ovale* in infantile seborrheic dermatitis, *Pediatr Dermatol* 6:16, 1989.
3. Menni SM, et al: Infantile seborrheic dermatitis: seven-year follow-up and some prognostic criteria, *Pediatr Dermatol* 6:13, 1989.
4. Prose N: HIV infection in children, *J Am Acad Dermatol* 22:1223, 1990.
5. Tollesson A, et al: Essential fatty acids in infantile seborrheic dermatitis, *J Am Acad Dermatol* 28:957, 1993.

260 Seizure Disorders

Sarah M. Roddy • Margaret C. McBride

Seizures are caused by abnormal discharges of neurons and may have a wide variety of clinical manifestations. A seizure should be considered a symptom of systemic or central nervous system (CNS) dysfunction. Management consists not only of controlling seizures but also of diagnosing any potentially treatable underlying condition. Acute conditions associated with seizures include metabolic disturbances, fever, meningitis, encephalitis, and toxic encephalopathy. The terms *seizure disorder* and *epilepsy* are synonymous and are applied to the condition in which there is a tendency for recurrent, unprovoked seizures. Care of patients who have epilepsy includes managing the psychosocial impact of epilepsy on the child and family.

CLASSIFICATION

Classification of seizures has provided a means to study seizures that have similar pathophysiology and to determine which medications are effective for which seizure types. Electroencephalographic (EEG) monitoring has aided in the current classification,[10] which is based on characterization of seizure onset and progression. Seizures are either partial or generalized. *Generalized* seizures result from involvement of both cerebral hemispheres simultaneously from the onset of the seizure. Types of generalized seizures include absence, myoclonic, atonic, tonic, clonic, and tonic-clonic. *Partial* seizures are caused by seizure discharges that begin in one hemisphere. Partial seizures are divided further into *simple partial seizures,* in which consciousness is preserved, and *complex partial seizures,* in which consciousness is impaired. Partial seizures of either type may progress to become secondarily generalized.

Epilepsy syndromes also have been defined in terms of a cluster of signs and symptoms, including age of onset, severity, diurnal or nocturnal occurrence, clinical course, associated neurological dysfunction, inheritance, and EEG findings.[9] Generalized epilepsy syndromes include juvenile myoclonic epilepsy, Lennox-Gastaut syndrome, infantile spasms (West's syndrome), and childhood absence epilepsy. A common partial epilepsy syndrome is benign partial epilepsy of childhood. Neonatal seizures can be generalized or focal and therefore are considered separately, as are febrile seizures. Box 260-1 outlines the classification of the various seizure types and epilepsy syndromes.

Generalized Seizures

Absence seizures. Absence seizures are generalized, nonconvulsive seizures characterized by interruption of activity, staring, and unresponsiveness; they usually last between 5 and 15 seconds. The episode starts abruptly, without warning, and ends abruptly with resumption of the child's preictal activity. The child may be unaware that the episode occurred. At times, unresponsiveness is accompanied by eyelid fluttering and upward rotation of the eyes and occasionally by mild clonic movements or automatisms such as lip smacking, grimacing, or swallowing. Seizures may occur more than 100 times per day and may interfere with the child's learning ability. The age of onset generally is between 4 and 8 years of age; rarely does it occur before 3 years or after 15 years. Girls are affected more commonly than boys. The influence of genetic factors in the etiology of absence seizures is suggested by 15% to 44% of first-degree relatives having a history of absence seizures, paroxysmal EEG abnormalities, or both.[1]

The classic finding on the EEG in patients who have absence seizures is bilaterally synchronous 3-Hz spike-and-wave discharges. Hyperventilation may be used to precipitate the electrical discharge as well as a clinical seizure. Photic stimulation during the EEG also induces the seizure discharge in some patients. Generalized tonic-clonic seizures may occur in some children, especially those who have an onset of absence seizures after 8 years of age. The prognosis for remission is good for children in whom absence is the sole seizure type but less favorable for those who have associated tonic-clonic seizures.

Monotherapy with ethosuximide or valproate usually controls absence seizures effectively. Valproate is the drug of choice if there are associated tonic-clonic seizures. Lamotrigine has been shown to be effective as an add-on medication when absence seizures are not completely controlled with valproate.[17] Benzodiazepines also are effective in controlling absence seizures, but their adverse effects on behavior make them second-line therapeutic agents. Phenytoin, phenobarbital, and carbamazepine usually are ineffective for treatment of absence seizures and may exacerbate them.

Myoclonic seizures. Myoclonic jerks are characterized by brief, sudden muscle contractions that may involve only part of the body or may be generalized. They may occur in clusters, especially during the period of falling asleep or shortly after awakening. There may be no alteration in consciousness associated with the jerks.

Atonic seizures. Atonic, or astatic, seizures also have been termed *drop attacks.* They are characterized by a sudden decrease in muscle tone, which may result in head nodding or mild flexing of the legs. More significant decreases in

BOX 260-1

CLASSIFICATION OF SEIZURES AND EPILEPSY SYNDROMES

Primary Generalized
Seizure types
Absence
Myoclonic
Atonic/astatic
Tonic-clonic

Epilepsy syndromes
Infantile spasms (West's syndrome)
Lennox-Gastaut syndrome
Childhood absence epilepsy
Juvenile myoclonic epilepsy

Partial
Seizure types
Simple partial
Complex partial
Partial seizures with secondary generalization

Epilepsy syndromes
Benign partial epilepsy of childhood
Epilepsia partialis continua

Unclassified
Neonatal seizures
Febrile seizures
Pseudoseizures

Data from Commission of Classification and Terminology of the International League Against Epilepsy: *Epilepsia* 26: 268, 1985.

muscle tone may cause the patient to slump to the floor. There usually is no detectable alteration in consciousness with these seizures.

Generalized tonic-clonic seizures. Generalized tonic-clonic seizures also are known as *grand mal seizures* and consist of motor manifestations and loss of consciousness. The tonic phase is characterized by a sustained contraction of muscles; as a result the patient falls to the ground, usually in opisthotonus. There usually is extensor posturing with tonic contraction of the diaphragm and intercostal muscles. This halts respirations, which, in turn, produces cyanosis. The tonic phase lasts less than 1 minute and is followed by the clonic phase, which consists of bilateral and rhythmic jerking. The jerks may be accompanied by expiratory grunts produced by diaphragmatic contractions against a closed glottis. The frequency of the clonic jerks decreases as the seizure progresses, although the intensity actually may increase. The tongue may be bitten, and bowel and bladder incontinence may occur. The clonic activity usually stops after several minutes. The seizure may be followed by vomiting, confusion, and lethargy, with gradual recovery of consciousness over a period of minutes to hours.

Generalized tonic-clonic seizures may be primary generalized or secondary generalized. Primary generalized seizures usually are idiopathic or genetic in origin and are associated with bilaterally synchronous electrical discharges on EEG. Secondary generalized seizures begin as partial seizures but may generalize so rapidly that any suggestion of focal origin is lacking. The EEG may demonstrate a focal discharge that may spread to both hemispheres or may show only bilateral synchronous discharges. The history that is helpful in determining that a seizure is secondary generalized is the presence of an aura, head or eye deviation, or focal clonic movement at the onset of the seizure. Neurological examination may reveal subtle focal signs such as a mild hemiparesis or visual field defect. Complete seizure control is less likely in secondary generalized epilepsy than in primary generalized epilepsy.[1] Effective antiepileptic medications for the treatment of generalized tonic-clonic seizures include phenobarbital, phenytoin, primidone, and carbamazepine. Valproate also is an effective anticonvulsant for generalized tonic-clonic seizures with or without focal features.

Infantile spasms (West's syndrome). Infantile spasms are a unique form of epilepsy, with onset during the first year of life. The seizures are characterized by a sudden contraction of neck, trunk, and extremity muscles. The spasms may be flexor, extensor, or mixed flexor-extensor and last only a few seconds each, but they often occur in clusters of up to 100 individual spasms. A typical episode is characterized by dropping of the head with abduction of the shoulders and flexion of the lower extremities. The infant may cry during or following the spasm. Pallor, flushing, grimacing, laughter, and nystagmus are observed during some episodes. Episodes are common on awakening from sleep, during drowsiness, and with feedings but are rare during sleep. The peak age of infantile spasm onset is between 3 and 7 months,[1] with an estimated incidence of 0.24 to 0.60 per 1000 infants.[22] Males are more likely to be affected than females.

Infantile spasms usually are divided into symptomatic and cryptogenic groups based on the presence of a predisposing etiological factor. Included among symptomatic infantile spasms are infants who have abnormal neurological development before the onset of spasms. Causes include structural abnormalities of the brain, hypoxic-ischemic insults, CNS infections or hemorrhages, and inborn errors of metabolism. Children who have tuberous sclerosis account for up to 25% of patients who have infantile spasms.[1] The cryptogenic group includes those patients in whom no etiological factor can be found. Infants in this group tend to be older at the onset of infantile spasms compared with infants in the symptomatic group.

The EEG pattern associated with infantile spasms is known as *hypsarrhythmia* and is characterized by high-voltage slow waves with irregularly interspersed multifocal spike and sharp waves. Hypsarrhythmia may precede the onset of clinical manifestations, or it may occur later or not at all. Over time, the hypsarrhythmia usually evolves into other focal or generalized abnormalities; in some cases the EEG may normalize.

Infantile spasms are resistant to treatment with most anticonvulsants. The treatment used most commonly is adrenocorticotropic hormone (ACTH). ACTH in a long-acting form is administered as a single daily intramuscular dose of 20 to 40 IU. Adverse effects of ACTH and steroids are significant and include Cushing's syndrome, hypertension, susceptibility to infections, hyperglycemia, gastrointestinal bleeding, and electrolyte disturbance. The benzodiazepines also are effective in controlling infantile spasms. Nitrazepam seems to be more effective than clonazepam or diazepam. Both valproic acid and topiramate are effective therapy for infantile spasms in some infants.[19]

The prognosis for infants who have infantile spasms remains grave. The average mortality is approximately 20%, with aspiration pneumonia being a common cause of death.[1] Approximately 80% of survivors are mentally retarded. The spasms usually remit by a few years of age, but 55% to 60% of patients subsequently develop other forms of seizures.[1] The prognosis is more favorable for those infants whose neurological development had been normal before the onset of the spasms.

Lennox-Gastaut syndrome. Lennox-Gastaut syndrome is a severe epileptic encephalopathy characterized by a variety of primary generalized seizures. Tonic seizures cause sudden, sustained contraction of the muscle groups, at times causing the patient to fall. Atypical absence seizures consist of a brief period of staring and immobility. The onset and recovery of atypical absence seizures are less abrupt than those of typical absence seizures. The episodes may be associated with mild tonic motor manifestations, automatisms, or loss of postural tone. Atonic seizures occur and may be preceded by myoclonic jerks. Tonic-clonic seizures and partial seizures also may occur in patients who have Lennox-Gastaut syndrome.

The majority of these patients begin to have seizures between 3 and 5 years of age[18]; boys are affected slightly more frequently than girls. Many patients have neurological deficits before the onset of Lennox-Gastaut syndrome, including mental retardation and cerebral palsy, which may be related to hypoxic encephalopathy or other insults to the brain. Patients may have a history of infantile spasms. The EEG typically shows an irregular, high-voltage, slow (2.5 Hz or slower) spike-wave pattern. The discharges are bilaterally synchronous.

The treatment of the seizures associated with Lennox-Gastaut syndrome is disappointing. Valproic acid has been the most successful in treatment of the different seizure types and is the drug of choice. Both felbamate and topiramate as add-on drugs have been shown to reduce the frequency of atonic and generalized tonic-clonic seizures significantly.[16,20] The benzodiazepines also have been successful in controlling atonic, myoclonic, and atypical absence seizures. Unfortunately, with increasing doses the frequency of adverse side effects also increases. The development of tolerance also is a problem associated with their use. Ethosuximide can help control the atypical absence episodes, and phenytoin can be used for tonic seizures. A ketogenic diet also has been beneficial in seizure control, but because of the nature of the diet, compliance is poor. Generally the goal of treatment is to achieve reasonable seizure control with as few medications as possible so as to minimize adverse effects. Sometimes the seizures typical of Lennox-Gastaut syndrome occur in otherwise normal preschool-age children, associated with normal background and fast polyspike-and-wave changes on EEG. These children have a much better prognosis for seizure control and cognitive development.

Juvenile myoclonic epilepsy. Juvenile myoclonic epilepsy is a primary generalized epilepsy with an age of onset of 12 to 18 years. It represents 7% of all epilepsy and is characterized by myoclonic jerks that affect mainly the upper extremities and less commonly the lower extremities. The jerks usually occur shortly after awakening, and patients may complain of clumsiness or difficulty holding objects early in the morning. Approximately 80% of patients have generalized tonic-clonic seizures, and 25% have absence seizures in addition to myoclonic seizures.[23] Myoclonic jerks almost always precede the onset of generalized tonic-clonic seizures by months to years. A teenager who has generalized tonic-clonic seizures should be questioned carefully regarding myoclonic jerks. Both the myoclonic jerks and the tonic-clonic seizures may be precipitated by sleep deprivation, stress, alcohol, and hormonal changes. Patients remain neurologically normal. Juvenile myoclonic epilepsy is genetic; a locus on the short arm of chromosome 6 has been identified.[12] The ictal EEG typically shows generalized, symmetrical polyspike and waves at 4 to 6 Hz. Photic stimulation precipitates the electrical discharges in some patients. The recommended treatment for juvenile myoclonic epilepsy is valproate. Valproate will control the myoclonic jerks, absence seizures, and generalized tonic-clonic seizures in more than 80% of patients. Other anticonvulsants may control certain seizure components of the syndrome, but valproate controls all the seizure components. There is a high rate of seizure recurrence among patients who discontinue valproate. Juvenile myoclonic epilepsy therefore is considered a lifelong condition that requires continuous treatment.

Partial Seizures

Simple partial seizures. Simple partial seizures are characterized by seizure activity restricted to one side of the body, with preserved consciousness. The symptoms may be motor, sensory, or cognitive, depending on the location of the neuronal discharge. Motor seizures may be restricted to part of the body, such as the face or a limb, or they may spread to involve the entire side. If the seizure discharge spreads to structures involved in consciousness, the seizure will become a complex partial seizure. The seizure activity also may spread to the opposite side of the brain, causing a generalized seizure. A partial seizure may be followed by Todd's paralysis, a weakness of the limbs involved in the seizure. Partial sensory seizures most often are manifested by paresthesias lasting less than 1 to 2 minutes. Seizure discharges from one occipital lobe may cause visual symptoms such as scintillating colored spots or scotomata in the visual field contralateral to the discharge. Seizures with more complex visual hallucinations often progress to complex partial seizures with diminished consciousness. Auditory seizures are manifested by hearing noises and less commonly by having elaborate but usually nonverbal auditory hallucinations such as hearing music.

Although simple partial seizures are caused by focal epileptiform discharges, a focal structural lesion may not be found in 30% to 50% of patients. Causes associated with these seizures include prenatal and perinatal insults, CNS malformations, and metabolic disturbances such as hypocalcemia, hypoglycemia, and inborn errors of metabolism. Carbamazepine, phenytoin, and valproic acid are effective drugs in the treatment of simple focal seizures.

Complex partial seizures. Complex partial seizures are seizures that originate in a limited area of one cerebral hemisphere and result in impaired consciousness. A complex partial seizure may begin as a simple partial seizure that progresses to impairment of consciousness. The initial portion of a seizure that occurs before consciousness is lost is referred to as the *aura.* The aura may consist of any of a wide variety of symptoms, depending on the location of cortical discharges. There may be auditory, olfactory, or visual illusions or hallucinations. Affective symptoms such as fear or other unpleasant feelings can occur. Anger or rage are extremely rare as a seizure manifestation but may occur during postictal confusion if the patient is restrained.

Déjà vu, the feeling that an experience has occurred before, and jamais vu, the feeling that a previously experienced sensation is unfamiliar and strange, have been described. Young children have difficulty describing déjà vu and may say only that there was a "funny feeling" that occurred in the head or stomach. Staring and automatisms, which are involuntary coordinated motor activity, occur when there is clouding of consciousness. Automatisms include simple phenomena such as chewing, lip smacking, swallowing, and hissing and more complicated activities such as picking at clothes, searching, or ambulating. Automatisms usually are followed by postictal amnesia. The child may become tired and go to sleep.

Complex partial seizures must be distinguished from absence seizures, which also are characterized by staring and unresponsiveness. Episodes of absence seizures have an abrupt onset and termination, compared with complex partial seizures, which have a more gradual onset and termination. Absence seizures last less than 30 seconds and are not associated with postictal confusion. Automatisms can occur if absence episodes are prolonged, but they often are just a continuation of motor activity present before the onset of the seizure.

The most frequent EEG finding in complex partial seizures is an anterior temporal lobe spike discharge, although some patients will have spike discharges from other areas. Interictal EEGs often are normal. Repeating the EEG increases the likelihood of demonstrating the abnormal discharge. Nasopharyngeal or sphenoidal electrodes rarely add information that is not obtained by scalp recordings that include special temporal placements.

Causes of complex partial seizures include perinatal insults, head trauma, encephalitis, and possibly, status epilepticus, all of which may be associated with scarring of the temporal lobe. Indolent tumors such as hamartomas and low-grade gliomas also can cause complex partial seizures and are found in approximately 20% of persons who have intractable partial seizures. Genetic factors play a secondary role in the etiology of complex seizures.[1]

Anticonvulsant drugs used in the treatment of complex partial seizures include carbamazepine, phenytoin, phenobarbital, primidone, and valproate. Carbamazepine is the drug of choice in children because of its efficacy and relatively mild adverse effects. If seizures are not controlled with carbamazepine, the addition of acetazolamide may result in improved seizure control.[37] Patients who have medically intractable partial seizures should be evaluated at a comprehensive epilepsy center to determine their candidacy for surgical intervention, which results in complete seizure control in up to 90% of patients.[14]

Benign partial epilepsy of childhood. Benign partial epilepsy of childhood also is known as *rolandic epilepsy, sylvian seizures,* and *centrotemporal epilepsy.* This epilepsy syndrome is a common type of partial motor epilepsy in childhood. The onset usually is between 5 and 8 years of age. Males more often are affected than females. Genetic factors play a role in the etiology. The seizures typically occur during sleep, although patients occasionally may have an episode during wakefulness. Episodes are characterized by the child awakening with one side of the face twitching. The oropharyngeal muscles often also are involved, causing the child to make unintelligible gurgling sounds. The ipsilateral upper extremity may be involved, but only rarely is the lower extremity involved. In rare cases a seizure episode will become generalized. Consciousness often is retained during the seizure, although the child may not be able to speak. Most seizure episodes last less than 2 minutes. The frequency of seizures is low, with 25% of patients having a single seizure episode and 50% having fewer than five episodes.[1] The typical EEG findings are midtemporal or centrotemporal spike discharges that usually are unilateral, often very frequent, and present in light sleep. Neuroradiological studies show no abnormalities to correlate with the EEG focus. If a child has infrequent episodes, no treatment may be needed. If the episodes frighten the child and a decision is made to initiate treatment, carbamazepine is the drug of choice. Other effective drugs include phenytoin and valproate. The seizure episodes remit when the child is around 9 to 12 years of age, but no later than 17 years. Remission is long lasting, and no developmental or neurological impairment is associated with these seizures.

Epilepsia partialis continua. Epilepsia partialis continua is a rare type of seizure in which twitching is continuous and limited to one side of the body. The twitching frequently involves only a few muscles and occurs most often in the hand or foot. Consciousness is preserved, but the seizure activity might weaken the extremity involved. Seizure activity may persist for hours to months. Focal encephalitis and tumor have been associated with this type of seizure. Medical treatment of epilepsia partialis continua generally is unsuccessful, although carbamazepine, phenytoin, and benzodiazepines have been used with varying degrees of success.

Unclassified Seizures

Neonatal seizures. Seizures are the most common manifestation of neonatal neurological disease and occur in approximately 0.5% of all newborns.[30] For a long time, seizures have been identified only clinically but as EEG has become more available to intensive care nurseries, it has been recognized that acute injury of the neonatal brain results in frequent subclinical electrographic seizures that can only be recognized with an EEG running. In fact, particularly after the initiation of antiseizure medication, only 10% or fewer of electrographic seizures in the neonate may be recognized clinically. Additionally, the antiseizure medications that are available for newborns in parenteral forms (phenobarbital, phenytoin, and lorazepam) are not very effective in stopping these electrographic seizures, which tend to run a course of several days after the injury. Genuine debate exists about whether seizures in the neonate can further the brain damage that caused them.[21] Hence, there is no uniformity of opinion about how aggressive to be about identifying and treating neonatal seizures, particularly the larger portion of neonatal seizures that are not recognized clinically.[26]

The combination of clinical manifestations of neonatal seizures and their likelihood to be associated with simultaneous electrographic seizures has led to revised classifications of seizures in the neonate. The clinical manifestations are classified as follows:

1. Subtle seizures occur in both full-term and premature infants and often are overlooked. These seizures consist of eye deviation, blinking, sucking, swimming movements of the arms, pedaling movements of the legs, and apnea. EEG recordings do not always show correlation of electrical seizure discharges with the clinical seizure activity. This has raised the possibility that in some instances the abnormal movements arise from regions of the brain from which abnormal electrical activity cannot be detected with surface electrodes, or that they may not be seizures. Subtle seizures usually occur in infants who have severe CNS insults.
2. Clonic seizures are either focal or multifocal. Focal clonic seizures are characterized by clonic jerking that remains localized and is almost always associated with electrographic seizure discharges from the central part of the opposite hemisphere. Although focal clonic seizures can result from focal CNS lesions such as cerebral infarction, they also can occur with metabolic disturbances. Multifocal clonic seizures are characterized by clonic activity in one extremity that migrates randomly and often rapidly from side to side and place to place within the body. The EEG shows multifocal independent areas of electrical discharge.

   Clonic seizures should be differentiated from benign neonatal sleep myoclonus, which consists of small-amplitude clonic activity that may wax and wane in various parts of the body. These occur only in sleep in healthy neonates and infants and are accompanied by a normal EEG throughout the jerking period. Benign neonatal sleep myoclonus is self limited and is not associated with later epilepsy.
3. Tonic seizures are focal or generalized. Focal tonic seizures are characterized by sustained posturing of a limb or asymmetrical posturing of the neck and trunk. There may be accompanying subtle seizure activity such as eye deviation. Generalized tonic seizures are characterized by tonic extension of the limbs. Less commonly, the upper extremities are flexed and the lower extremities are extended. They often have no electrographic correlate and may not be seizures but are possibly some kind of brainstem phenomenon. They usually are associated with severe EEG background abnormalities. In premature infants they may occur at the onset of severe intraventricular bleeding.
4. Myoclonic seizures are flexion jerks of the upper or lower extremities. They may occur singly or in a series of repetitive jerks, and they sometimes are associated with tonic spasms and multifocal seizures. Myoclonic seizures may persist into infancy and become or be followed by infantile spasms. The EEGs in infants with myoclonic seizures usually are very abnormal. They may show a burst suppression pattern although the EEG may not change during the myoclonic event. Infants with myoclonic seizures tend to have severely abnormal dysgenetic brains, or metabolic defects. Occasionally the seizures are cryptogenic. Infants with these seizures may later develop infantile spasms. These myoclonic seizures should be differentiated from benign myoclonic jerks that occur during sleep in neonates and are accompanied by a normal EEG.

Jitteriness is a movement in neonates that may be confused with seizure activity. The movement is a tremor that is stimulus sensitive and can be stopped by passively flexing the affected limb. There is no associated eye deviation or other abnormal eye movements. Some investigators advocate identification of neonatal seizures by EEG recording, maintaining that only electrical seizures are true seizures and require treatment. However, this remains controversial because identical clinical seizures in the same infant may at times not be associated with electrical seizures.[48] It is clear, however, that electrical seizures may not have clinical correlates; hence, EEG recording should be done for all infants at risk for seizures so as to identify these silent electrical seizures.

ETIOLOGY. There are multiple etiologies of neonatal seizures; however, only a few causes account for most cases. Determining the etiology of neonatal seizures is important because specific treatment may be indicated. The etiology of the seizures also is an important factor influencing prognosis. Some of the most common causes of seizure are described as follows:

1. Hypoxia-ischemia is the most common cause of seizure in both premature and full-term infants.[47] These seizures usually begin within the first 24 hours of life and may be very difficult to control for several days. Metabolic disturbances in the infant also may complicate seizure control.
2. Intracranial hemorrhage is another cause of seizures in both premature and full-term infants. Intraventricular hemorrhage is seen mainly in premature infants within the first 3 days of life. Generalized tonic seizures may be associated with severe hemorrhage involving the brain parenchyma. Infants who have a primary subarachnoid hemorrhage may not have any clinical symptoms or may develop seizures on the second day of life. These infants often are full-term infants who are normal neurologically except for the seizure. Subdural hemorrhage is associated with trauma and may result in focal seizure activity.
3. Metabolic disturbances, especially hypoglycemia and

hypocalcemia, also are associated with seizures in neonates. Infants who are small for gestational age and infants of diabetic mothers are at risk for hypoglycemia, and the blood glucose level should be monitored closely. Low-birth-weight infants and infants of diabetic mothers are at risk for hypocalcemic seizures, which occur when calcium levels drop below 7 mg/dl during the first 2 to 3 days of life. Often, infants who have hypocalcemia also have a history of hypoxia, which contributes to the risk of seizure. Hypocalcemic seizures that occur later usually are related to a low calcium and high phosphate intake. Late hypocalcemic seizures are now rare as a result of the development of formula that has an appropriate ratio of calcium and phosphorus supplementation. Other metabolic disturbances less frequently associated with seizures in neonates include hyponatremia, hypernatremia, local anesthetic intoxication, pyridoxine dependence, and a variety of inborn errors of metabolism.

4. Infection, including bacterial and viral intracranial infections, is an important cause of neonatal seizures. The most common bacterial causes are group B streptococci and *Escherichia coli.* Onset of seizures with meningitis usually is after the first 3 to 4 days of life. Prenatal nonbacterial infections causing neonatal seizures include toxoplasmosis, rubella, herpes simplex virus, coxsackie B virus, and cytomegalovirus.
5. Malformations of the brain can cause seizures at any time during the newborn period. The malformations associated most commonly with seizures are those that have cortical dysgenesis such as lissencephaly, pachygyria, and polymicrogyria.[47]

MANAGEMENT. Treatment of neonatal seizures is urgent if they interfere with vital functions such as maintaining good arterial oxygen saturation. When neonatal seizures are suspected clinically, it is important to pursue rapidly the treatable causes such as hypoglycemia, electrolyte imbalance, and infection and also to pursue EEG confirmation of seizure activity to help avoid the pitfall of treating coarse jitteriness or other transient abnormal movements with antiseizure medication.[45] The following is an approach to the treatment of seizures:

1. Ensure adequate ventilation and perfusion.
2. Obtain blood for glucose, calcium, magnesium, and electrolyte studies. Check a Dextrostix for an immediate determination of glucose.
3. Correct any associated metabolic abnormality.
   A. Hypoglycemia: If glucose is low as shown by Dextrostix (<40 mg/dl), immediately give 10% dextrose intravenously in a dose of 2 ml/kg. Maintain blood glucose levels above 40 mg/dl by continuous intravenous infusion and monitor the levels in both full-term and premature infants.
   B. Hypocalcemia: Correct by administering 5% calcium gluconate solution, 4 ml/kg intravenously at a rate of 1 ml/min to maintain serum calcium levels above 7 mg/dl, while monitoring cardiac rate and rhythm.
   C. Hypomagnesemia: Correct serum magnesium levels to 1 mmol/L with 50% magnesium sulfate solution, 0.2 ml/kg intramuscularly.
4. Continued seizure activity requires administration of anticonvulsants.
   A. Phenobarbital is given in a loading dose of 20 mg/kg intravenously over 10 minutes. Additional doses of 5 or 10 mg/kg can be given, up to a total of 40 mg/kg.
   B. Phenytoin or fosphenytoin is given in a loading dose of 20 mg/kg intravenously while monitoring cardiac rhythm.
   C. Lorazepam can be given in doses of 0.1 mg/kg intravenously for persistent seizures.[28] Respiratory status should be monitored.

After seizures are controlled via loading doses of anticonvulsants, electrographic seizures may continue and if frequent or prolonged may merit further anticonvulsant therapy. In general, seizures related to acute injuries such as asphyxia, stroke, or acute CNS infections other than herpes are self limited and stop after several days though they may recur months or years later. There is no evidence that continuing treatment past the neonatal period will change the chance of recurrence later. Therefore, seizures caused by acute injuries usually are treated short-term and in many nurseries, infants are not sent home on anticonvulsants, or if they are, anticonvulsants are continued for just a few weeks. Because phenobarbital has a long half-life, especially in asphyxiated infants, it will remain at good levels after a full loading dose for several days and no maintenance therapy may be needed. Seizures related to brain malformations or inborn errors of metabolism may be much more persistent, and the duration of treatment will depend on the infant's clinical course.

PROGNOSIS. The prognosis of neonatal seizures relates mainly to the underlying diseases that caused them. Mental retardation and cerebral palsy are more common sequelae than are seizures. Infants who have seizures related to hypoxic-ischemic encephalopathy, hypoglycemia, or bacterial meningitis have a 50% chance of developing normally; those whose seizures result from late-onset hypocalcemia and primary subarachnoid hemorrhage have a greater than 90% chance of developing normally.[47] The interictal EEG is helpful in determining the prognosis. A normal background EEG pattern usually is associated with a good neurological outcome; a markedly abnormal background pattern such as burst-suppression or marked suppression of voltage is associated with a high risk of neurological sequelae.

Febrile seizures. Febrile seizures are seizures that occur in young children who have fever but no evidence of intracranial infection or acute neurological illness. Simple febrile seizures are generalized tonic-clonic convulsions that last less than 15 minutes and do not recur within 24 hours. Complex febrile seizures are less common and are focal or prolonged beyond 15 minutes or recur within 24 hours. Febrile seizures occur in children between 3 months and 5 years of age; the median age of occurrence is 18 to 22 months. Approximately 2% to 5% of children will experience a febrile convulsion; boys are more susceptible than girls. Familial clustering of febrile seizures suggests that genetic factors play a role in the etiology.[1]

A febrile seizure may be the first sign that a child is ill. It is not known whether the seizure activity is triggered by the rapid rise of fever or the actual height of the temperature.

Febrile seizures can be triggered by any illness that causes fever, most frequently by otitis media and upper respiratory tract infections. There is a high rate of febrile seizures with shigellosis, salmonellosis, and roseola, possibly related to a direct effect the causative organism has on the CNS or to a neurotoxin they produce.

One third of children who have a febrile seizure will have another one with another febrile illness. The younger the child at the time of the first episode, the greater the risk of recurrence. Approximately 50% of the recurrences occur within 6 months of the initial seizure; 75% occur within 1 year.

Usually, seizure activity has stopped by the time the child is evaluated. However, if the seizure continues, lorazepam or diazepam should be administered (see Chapter 298, Status Epilepticus). The temperature should be brought down by using rectal antipyretics, removing blankets and clothing, and sponging. Once seizure activity is controlled, evaluation is directed toward finding the cause of the fever. If the child is under 1 year of age or if the child has not rapidly returned to normal, a lumbar puncture should be strongly considered to evaluate for meningitis.

The EEG generally is not helpful in the evaluation of children who have febrile seizures. EEG tracings recorded within 1 week of the seizure often show posterior slowing. Paroxysmal activity is seen in the EEGs of 35% to 45% of patients who are followed up for several years.[1] These EEG abnormalities do not predict recurrence of febrile seizures or the development of epilepsy.

Treatment of febrile seizures includes family education that addresses the benign nature of the seizures, the use of antipyretics, and first aid for seizures. Administration of oral diazepam (0.33 mg/kg body weight administered every 8 hours during febrile illness) reduces the risk of recurrent febrile seizures.[38] Administration of phenobarbital, however, at the onset of a febrile illness does not prevent seizure activity because therapeutic blood levels are not achieved soon enough. Prophylactic treatment with anticonvulsant agents should be considered if neurological development is abnormal, it is a complex febrile seizure, or the child is under 1 year of age. Administration of phenobarbital in doses that achieve blood levels of 15 μg/ml reduces the recurrence of febrile seizures. Valproate also appears to be effective in prophylaxis; phenytoin and carbamazepine do not prevent recurrences. The adverse effects of anticonvulsant therapy must be weighed against the possible benefits. There is no evidence that prophylactic treatment reduces the risk of subsequent epilepsy.

The risk of subsequent epilepsy in children who have febrile seizures is less than 5%. Factors associated with subsequent development of afebrile [sic] partial seizures include focal seizures, prolonged seizures, and repeated episodes of seizures with the same febrile illness. Factors associated with development of afebrile [sic], generalized seizures include more than three febrile seizures, a family history of afebrile seizures, and age over 3 years at the time of the first febrile seizure.[2]

Pseudoseizures. Pseudoseizures are uncommon but must be recognized if inappropriate treatment is to be prevented. They differ from true epileptic seizures in several respects. The movements usually are not clonic but may be quivering or random thrashing movements. Usually, no incontinence, injury, or tongue biting is associated with pseudoseizures. Episodes may be dramatic, with screaming and shouting. Episodes also may vary greatly in the same patient. Usually, there is no postictal period. Pseudoseizures can occur in early childhood but are more frequent in adolescence, especially in females.[1] Pseudoseizures are most likely to occur in children who have true epileptic seizures. A detailed history and observation of an episode often is all that is needed to diagnose pseudoseizures; EEG monitoring can be used in patients in whom the distinction cannot be made clinically. Once the diagnosis is established, treatment is directed toward the psychosocial issues involved.

APPROACH TO THE MANAGEMENT OF AN INITIAL SEIZURE

The first step in treating the child who has an initial seizure is making the correct diagnosis. The risk of seizure recurrence is important when deciding whether to initiate antiepileptic therapy. Some types of seizures, such as absence, myoclonic, akinetic, and infantile spasms, have a recurrence rate of virtually 100% and usually have recurred by the time the child is seen by the physician. These types of seizures require treatment. However, children who have a generalized tonic-clonic or partial seizure have a recurrence risk of about 40%.[4,41] Factors that increase the risk of recurrence include a partial complex seizure, an abnormal neurological examination, and focal epileptiform abnormalities on the EEG. The best prognosis is in those children who have a generalized seizure, a normal neurological examination, and a nonepileptiform EEG. Many patients who have a single seizure should be observed for recurrence but should not be started on antiepileptic medication. More than 50% of the recurrences occur within 6 months, up to 90% within 1 year. If a second seizure occurs, initiation of antiepileptic medication should be considered because approximately 80% of children who have a second seizure will have more seizures.[8]

Diagnostic Procedures

Laboratory tests. Laboratory tests usually performed at the time of the initial seizure include measurement of serum electrolytes, calcium, magnesium, and blood glucose. In some cases the history or examination may indicate that a more extensive laboratory evaluation is required.

Electroencephalography. The EEG, which measures the physiological function of the brain, changes throughout childhood, reflecting brain maturation. The EEG is important in the evaluation of a child who has seizures because it helps to define the seizure type. An epileptiform EEG may support the diagnosis of epilepsy, but a normal tracing does not exclude the diagnosis. Other abnormalities, such as slowing and background disorganization, are much less specific. Repeat tracings increase the likelihood of detecting epileptiform discharges in patients who have seizures. Procedures such as hyperventilation, photic stimulation, and sleep should be used when obtaining EEG recordings. Nasopharyngeal and sphenoidal electrodes may be used to detect mesial temporal discharges, but they rarely add information to that obtainable by special scalp electrode placements. Video EEG monitoring is useful in correlating clinical symptoms with electrical seizure activity and may be useful when clinical manifestations are atypical. Although the EEG provides electrophysiological evidence to support the diagnosis of epilepsy, EEG abnormalities must be interpreted in view of the clinical symptomatology. Some individuals have epileptiform discharges and other EEG abnormalities without ever having a clinical seizure; treatment is not indicated for such individuals.

Neuroimaging studies. Plain skull roentgenograms can detect calcifications that may be seen in some syndromes, but they rarely help in the evaluation of children who have epilepsy. Computed tomography (CT) and magnetic resonance imaging (MRI) have replaced skull roentgenograms in the evaluation of seizures. CT and MRI scanning detect structural abnormalities; MRI is more sensitive than CT in the detection of low-grade tumors, changes in myelination, and heterotopic gray matter. Neuroimaging studies are not warranted in every child who has epilepsy; however, MRI or CT should be performed in children who have focal neurological abnormalities on examination or have intractable epilepsy. Positron emission tomography (PET) is useful in evaluating metabolic alterations with seizure activity, but the clinical relevance of PET in individual patients is not clear, and its availability is limited.

Lumbar puncture. The cerebrospinal fluid should be examined in patients in whom meningitis or encephalitis is suspected. In other patients the lumbar puncture rarely is helpful and is not indicated routinely.

TREATMENT WITH ANTIEPILEPTIC MEDICATION

Once the child has had recurrent seizures and antiepileptic medication is indicated, the physician is faced with the decision of which medication to prescribe. Diagnosing seizure type correctly is the critical first step in treatment because some seizure disorders respond to certain medications. In choosing among potentially effective antiepileptic agents, the drug that has the least adverse effects should be selected. The medication is started at a dose that will result in a low therapeutic blood level. The dose should be increased until seizures are controlled or adverse effects become intolerable. If the initial medication is not fully effective, a second medication may be added. Consideration should be given to discontinuing the first medication if seizures are fully controlled with the second medication. It is important to use monotherapy if possible, since polytherapy often does not improve seizure control but may increase toxicity dramatically.

To devise an optimum dosing regimen it is important to consider the pharmacokinetics of the various antiepileptic medications. The dosing frequency is determined by the *half-life,* defined as the time in which the serum level falls to 50% of the initial value. The dosing interval should be no longer than the half-life of the medication, which means that most antiepileptic agents may be administered twice a day and some only once daily. The efficacy of an antiepileptic medication should be evaluated only after five half-lives have elapsed, since this is the period required for the medication to reach a steady state. In antiepileptic medications that induce hepatic enzymes (e.g., carbamazepine), the half-life decreases over the first weeks of treatment. If breakthrough seizures occur at times of low (trough) serum drug levels or if toxicity occurs at times of peak serum drug levels, the frequency of dosing should be increased.

Patients requiring higher antiepileptic medication levels usually need more frequent dosing to avoid toxicity.

Serum drug levels can guide the adjusting of doses of antiepileptic medications. A baseline level should be obtained when the patient has been taking an appropriate dose long enough to have stable levels. Other indications for obtaining levels include verification of compliance, breakthrough seizures, and toxic effects. Levels also may be checked when other medications have been added or deleted from the patient's regimen. The timing of the sample in relation to the last dose is important in the interpretation of the levels, especially in drugs with short half-lives.

SPECIFIC ANTIEPILEPTIC MEDICATIONS

Table 260-1 outlines commonly used antiepileptic medications and their properties.

Phenobarbital

Phenobarbital is one of the oldest antiepileptic agents still in use. Because of its long half-life, it has the advantage of requiring dosing only once or twice a day. The recommended dose per kilogram decreases as the weight increases. Failure to decrease the per-kilogram dose levels in older children will result in toxic levels. Because phenobarbital is a relatively safe medication in terms of serious toxic effects, monitoring of parameters other than serum levels usually is not necessary. The major disadvantage of phenobarbital is its effect on behavior and cognitive function, including hyperactivity, irritability, and attention deficits. Maintaining serum levels at the minimum level for seizure control may help decrease these adverse effects. Phenobarbital administration will lower the serum levels of carbamazepine and valproate. Administration of valproate will increase phenobarbital levels; therefore, phenobarbital doses should be decreased by 25% to 50% to prevent toxicity when prescribed concomitantly with valproate.

Phenytoin

Phenytoin also is among the older antiepileptic medications and has been used widely. Because of its pharmacokinetics, blood levels vary dramatically with small changes in dosage. Therefore, changes in dosage should be monitored via serum levels, and only very small dose changes should be made when serum levels are close to or within the therapeutic range. Phenytoin commonly is used for treatment of status epilepticus because intravenous administration results in rapid penetration into the CNS. Fosphenytoin is a water-soluble prodrug of phenytoin with a more neutral pH and less tissue irritation. It can be administered intravenously or intramuscularly.[34] Although phenytoin is an effective antiepilep-

Table 260-1 Common Antiepileptic Medications

Drug	Indications	Half-life (hours)	Usual Dose (mg/kg/day)	Therapeutic Levels (μg/ml)	Adverse Effects
Carbamazepine	Partial, secondary generalized	3-23 (18-55 initially)	5-25 5-10 (monotherapy)	4-12	Allergic rashes, nausea, diplopia, blurry vision, dizziness, hypersensitivity hepatitis, aplastic anemia
Phenytoin	Partial, secondary generalized, primary generalized	7-42 (nonlinear kinetics)	5-7	10-20 (occasionally lower)	Rashes, hirsutism, gingival hyperplasia, coarse features, psychomotor slowing, neuropathy, folate deficiency, myelosuppression, drug-induced lupus
Valproic acid	Primary generalized, absence, myoclonic, akinetic, febrile, infantile spasms, some partial	6-16	10-30 20-50 (infants and in polytherapy)	50-100 (150 if tolerated)	Nausea, tremor, weight gain, hair loss, thrombocytopenia, hepatic failure, pancreatitis
Phenobarbital	Neonatal, febrile, partial, secondary generalized, primary generalized, akinetic	36-120	3-5 (<25 kg) 2-3 (25-50 kg) 1-2 (>50 kg)	10-40	Sedation, inattention, hyperactivity, irritability, cognitive impairment, rare hypersensitivity reactions
Ethosuximide	Absence, myoclonic, akinetic	15-68	15-40	40-100	Nausea, abdominal discomfort, hiccups, drowsiness, behavioral problems, dystonias, myelosuppression, drug-induced lupus
Primidone	Partial, secondary generalized, primary generalized	3-20	5-10 (1-2 initially)	5-12	Sedation, irritability, psychomotor slowing, rare hematological and hypersensitivity reactions
Clonazepam	Absence, primary generalized, infantile spasms	20-36	0.01-0.2	0.01-0.07	Sedation, hyperactivity, inattention, aggressiveness, tolerance, ataxia, withdrawal seizures
Acetazolamide	Absence, myoclonic, akinetic, partial	10-12	10-20	10-14	Diuresis, paresthesias, sedation, CO_2 retention, rashes
Felbamate	Partial (in patients >12 years), Lennox-Gastaut syndrome	20 (in monotherapy)	15-45 (maximum of 3600 mg)	—	Anorexia, weight loss, nausea, insomnia, headache, fatigue, aplastic anemia
Gabapentin	Partial, with or without secondary generalized seizures in patients >12 years	5-7	Total daily dose 900-1800 mg	—	Somnolence, dizziness, ataxia, fatigue
Lamotrigine	Partial, primary generalized, absence, atypical absence, atonic, and myoclonic	7 to 45	5-15 without valproic acid, 1-5 with valproic acid	—	Somnolence, rash, vomiting
Topiramate	Partial, primary generalized, tonic, atonic, atypical absence	20-30	1-9	—	Somnolence, anorexia, fatigue, difficulty with concentration, nervousness
Tigabine	Partial	3-9	0.25-1.5 (maximum of 56 mg)		Dizziness, somnolence, headache, depression

tic agent in generalized tonic-clonic and partial seizures, its adverse effects limit its use. Cosmetic adverse effects include gingival hypertrophy, hirsutism, and coarsening of the facial features. Also of concern are its effects on mood and cognitive function, which include depressed mood, slowed psychomotor functioning, and, in a few, depressed IQ scores.[43] Other adverse effects include folate-deficiency anemia, cerebellar degeneration, and allergic dermatitis. Valproic acid may lower total serum phenytoin, but the free phenytoin level transiently increases and then returns to its original level; thus, no adjustment in dosage is necessary. Phenytoin may decrease carbamazepine levels and increase phenobarbital levels.

Carbamazepine

Carbamazepine is widely used because it has relatively few effects on cognitive function. It may also affect behavior positively.[43] The most serious adverse effect associated with carbamazepine has been aplastic anemia. This is extremely rare, occurring at a rate of less than 1 case per 200,000 treatment years.[25] A complete blood count should be obtained before carbamazepine therapy is initiated and should be repeated after 2 to 3 weeks. It is not clear whether further blood counts are useful when the initial counts are normal, but they should be obtained more readily when the child is ill and often are repeated biannually or annually. Neutropenia as low as $3000/mm^3$ may occur but does not predict more serious myelosuppression. The dose of carbamazepine may need to be changed during the course of treatment because the drug tends to induce its own metabolic breakdown. Phenobarbital, phenytoin, primidone, and clonazepam decrease carbamazepine serum levels.

Valproic Acid

Valproic acid has a broad spectrum of efficacy and also has the advantage of minimal cognitive adverse effects. Tremor may occur with high serum levels. Other adverse effects include increased appetite, weight gain, transient hair loss, nausea, and vomiting. Fatal hepatotoxicity also has been associated with valproic acid. Most cases occur during the first 3 months of treatment. Those patients at greatest risk for hepatotoxicity are children younger than 2 years of age who receive valproic acid as part of antiepileptic polytherapy.[11] Successful treatment of valproic acid-associated hepatotoxicity via *N*-acetylcysteine has been reported.[15] Valproic acid should be administered extremely cautiously to patients who have preexisting hepatic dysfunction. Liver function should be monitored in patients taking valproic acid, especially those in the high-risk group. Valproic acid raises the level of phenobarbital; therefore, the dose of phenobarbital must be decreased by 25% to 50% if valproic acid is added. Carbamazepine, phenobarbital, and phenytoin decrease valproic acid serum levels.

Ethosuximide

Ethosuximide has a limited spectrum of efficacy; it is used mainly for treating absence seizures and some forms of myoclonic seizures. Behavioral disturbances can occur in some children taking ethosuximide, and pancytopenia has been associated with chronic administration. Periodic blood counts therefore may be necessary. Ethosuximide does not interact significantly with other antiepileptic medications.

Primidone

Primidone is not a commonly used antiepileptic agent because it has no specific advantage over other agents. Primidone is metabolized to phenobarbital and phenylethylmalonamide and has many of the same characteristics of phenobarbital, including behavioral and cognitive adverse effects. It may be more sedating than phenobarbital. Because one third of primidone is metabolized to phenobarbital, phenobarbital levels should be monitored. Phenobarbital levels may be 1.3 to 2 times higher than primidone levels. Valproate increases primidone serum levels; phenytoin and carbamazepine increase the phenobarbital-to-primidone ratio.

Clonazepam

Clonazepam, a benzodiazepine, is not a first-line antiepileptic medication because of its adverse effects. It causes significant behavioral changes, including hyperactivity, decreased attention span, aggressiveness, and restlessness. Because withdrawal of the drug may cause irritability, myoclonus, and increased seizures, it should be withdrawn slowly. Treatment with clonazepam usually is reserved for absence and myoclonic seizures that are refractory to ethosuximide and valproic acid.

Acetazolamide

Acetazolamide is an inhibitor of the enzyme carbonic anhydrase. It is an effective adjunctive therapy for treatment of several types of seizures, although its antiepileptic properties are not well understood. Acetazolamide can be used in combination with valproic acid for treatment of absence, myoclonic, and akinetic seizures. Adding acetazolamide to carbamazepine may improve control of partial seizures.[37] Acetazolamide metabolism is not affected significantly by other medications.

Felbamate

Felbamate was approved by the U.S. Federal Drug Administration (FDA) in 1993 for treatment of partial seizures in adults and for adjunctive therapy in children who have Lennox-Gastaut syndrome. A placebo-controlled trial of add-on felbamate in patients who have Lennox-Gastaut syndrome demonstrated that felbamate significantly reduced the frequency of atonic and generalized tonic-clonic seizures.[16] The most common side effects of felbamate are anorexia, weight loss, nausea, insomnia, headache, and fatigue. No serious cardiac effects have been reported. However, more than 20 cases of aplastic anemia among persons taking felbamate have been reported. The true incidence and severity of this problem has not yet been determined. Cases of hepatic toxicity have also been reported. It currently is recommended that felbamate be used only in patients whose epilepsy is so severe that the benefits from its use outweigh the risk of aplastic anemia. Dosage of felbamate is based on weight, with a current maximum recommended total daily dose of 3600 mg. It is not necessary to follow felbamate levels. Felbamate interacts with phenytoin, carbamazepine, and valproate; therefore, doses of these medications must be reduced by 25% to 50% when felbamate is added. Felbamate levels are lowered by medications that induce liver enzymes; consequently, felbamate doses may need to be increased.

Gabapentin

Gabapentin was approved in 1994 by the FDA for treatment of partial seizures with and without secondary generalization in adults who have epilepsy. Safety and effectiveness in children below the age of 12 years have not been established in the United States.

In a multicenter, placebo-controlled, double-blind study among patients refractory to conventional anticonvulsants, gabapentin treatment resulted in a significant reduction in seizure frequency.[7] Gabapentin does not interact with other drugs; consequently, doses of other antiepileptic medications do not have to be adjusted when gabapentin is added. In add-on trials the most common side effects were somnolence, dizziness, ataxia, and fatigue. The effective dose of gabapentin is 900 to 1800 mg/day although higher doses may result in better seizure control. Because of its relatively short half-life of 5 to 7 hours, it has to be administered three to four times a day. It is not necessary to monitor levels.

Lamotrigine

Lamotrigine was approved for treatment of partial seizures in patients older than 16 years of age. Studies in children who have epilepsy reveal that lamotrigine reduces the frequency of both partial and generalized seizures.[5,29,39] It was particularly effective in patients with absence, atypical absence, and atonic seizures.[5] The most common side effects of lamotrigine are somnolence, rash, and vomiting. The rash usually is maculopapular or morbilliform, but a few cases of Stevens-Johnson syndrome have occurred. Comedication with valproic acid increases the incidence of rash. Starting a low dose of lamotrigine in patients who already are being treated with valproic acid and slowly increasing the dose of lamotrigine helps to minimize the risk of rash. Lamotrigine administration has no effect on the metabolism of other antiepileptic drugs; however, phenobarbital, phenytoin, and carbamazepine decrease the half-life of lamotrigine. Valproic acid increases the half-life of lamotrigine by two- or threefold; therefore, doses of lamotrigine should be lower when given in combination with valproic acid. Therapeutic plasma concentration has not been established for lamotrigine.

Topiramate

Topiramate is a new antiepileptic drug that has received FDA approval for treatment of partial seizures in adults. Studies in children show that topiramate is effective as an add-on therapy for partial seizures and Lennox-Gastaut syndrome.[13,20] Topiramate has also been effective for treatment of infantile spasms in some patients.[19] The most common side effects of topiramate are somnolence, anorexia, fatigue, difficulty with concentration, and nervousness. Topiramate administration has minimal effects on the metabolism of other antiepileptic drugs. However, concomitant therapy with phenytoin or carbamazepine will lower topiramate levels. Therapeutic plasma concentrations have not been established for topiramate.

Tiagabine

Tiagabine is a recently approved antiepileptic medication for adjunctive therapy of partial seizures in adults. Studies show that tiagabine is effective as adjunctive or monotherapy for partial seizures in some children.[6,44] Its efficacy in generalized seizures is unclear. Side effects include dizziness, somnolence, and headache. Tiagabine does not alter the concentrations of other antiepileptic drugs except for a slight decrease in valproate levels. Enzyme inducers such as carbamazepine, phenytoin, and phenobarbital lower tiagabine levels. Therapeutic plasma concentrations for tiagabine have not been established.

OTHER TREATMENT FOR SEIZURES

Ketogenic Diet

In some cases, seizures may not be controlled by medication and the ketogenic diet has proved to be an effective alternative treatment. The benefits of fasting as a treatment for seizures were reported years ago, but the diet was not consistently used. During the past decade there has been renewed interest in the diet. A recent multicenter prospective study of the efficacy of the ketogenic diet in children with intractable epilepsy found that 10% of treated patients were seizure-free at 1 year. A greater than 50% decrease in seizure frequency occurred in an additional 50% of the patients. Seizure type, patient age, and EEG abnormalities were not related to outcome.[46]

The exact mechanism by which the diet controls seizures is unknown although ketone body formation is critical for the diet to be effective. To achieve ketosis the patient is given a calorie-restricted, high-fat, low-protein, and low-carbohydrate diet. The patient must be admitted to the hospital for initiation of the diet. This allows for monitoring for hypoglycemia and other complications. During the hospitalization the dietitian teaches the parents about the diet, giving them sample menus and explaining how to measure foods. Strict adherence to the diet is needed for it to be successful. Complications of the diet include constipation, renal stones, fatigue, and metabolic acidosis.

Vagal Nerve Stimulation

A treatment for intractable epilepsy that emerged during the late 1980s and the 1990s is vagal nerve stimulation. The first vagal nerve stimulation device was implanted into a human in 1988.[35] More recently there have been reports of the use of vagal nerve stimulation in children. Patients selected for the treatment had seizures that were intractable to medical treatment. Some patients were continuing to have seizures despite having had epilepsy surgery. After 2 years of treatment with vagal nerve stimulation, approximately 40% of children had a greater than 50% reduction in seizure frequency, with a few patients becoming seizure-free.[27,32]

The vagal nerve stimulation device is surgically implanted subcutaneously in the anterior chest wall and stimulates the left vagus nerve. The mechanism for the antiepileptic effect of vagal nerve stimulation is not known, but changes in cerebrospinal fluid amino acids and activation of the noradrenergic system in the locus ceruleus occur with the stimulation.[3,24,31] Side effects associated with vagal nerve stimulation include infection, hoarseness, and neck pain.

PSYCHOSOCIAL ISSUES

Treatment of the child with a seizure disorder also must address psychosocial issues. Parents and patients may have many fears and need reassurance. The terms *epilepsy* and *seizure disorder* must be explained, and parents need to understand that the diagnosis of epilepsy does not mean that their child has mental retardation or a psychiatric disorder. Guidelines should be given on what to do when a child has a seizure, including positioning on the side and putting nothing in the mouth. Witnessing a seizure can be very frightening. Parents may be afraid that the child is going to die and should be told that death from a seizure is very rare.

Activities of patients with seizures should be restricted as little as possible. A child with a seizure disorder should not swim alone or go bike riding without a helmet. However, these rules apply to all children, whether or not they have epilepsy. Contact sports are permissible when epilepsy is controlled. The decision about climbing up to certain heights should be based on how well the child's seizures are controlled. Older children, who are not supervised when bathing, should be encouraged to take showers rather than baths to minimize the risk of drowning if a seizure occurs. Parents need encouragement to treat the child normally and not be overprotective. The National Epilepsy Foundation and its local chapters can be a valuable resource for families by providing free literature and many other helpful services.

DISCONTINUATION OF ANTIEPILEPTIC MEDICATIONS

After seizures have been controlled for a period of 2 years, consideration should be given to discontinuing antiepileptic medications. Studies have shown that approximately 75% of children who were seizure free for more than 2 years remained seizure free after antiepileptic medications were discontinued.[36] The EEG can be helpful when considering discontinuing antiepileptic medications. In children who have idiopathic epilepsy and a normal EEG, the prognosis for remaining seizure free after discontinuation of medications is good except in juvenile myoclonic epilepsy (discussed on p. 1795). However, if the EEG demonstrates slowing, there is a higher risk of seizure recurrence.[40] The risk of recurrence is not increased if medication is tapered over a period as short as 6 weeks.[42] Long-term follow-up of children after withdrawal of medication has shown that 50% of the recurrences occur within 6 months and 60% to 80% within 2 years.[40]

INTRACTABLE SEIZURES

When seizures continue despite anticonvulsant therapy, it is important to consider three possibilities before deciding that the child's seizures are intractable to anticonvulsant therapy:

1. Seizures may be occurring at times that the child has lower blood levels of medication because of incomplete compliance or because dosing intervals are too long.
2. The medication may not be appropriate to the child's type of seizures. Primary generalized seizures often will not respond and may even worsen if treated with medications that are indicated for partial or secondary generalized seizures (e.g., carbamazepine).
3. The child's repeated events may represent one of the nonepileptiform paroxysmal disorders rather than an electrical seizure. Pseudoseizures can be especially difficult to differentiate from seizures because they tend to occur in persons who have epilepsy.

If a child is having electrographic seizures and the seizures continue despite appropriate amounts of the correct medications, the child has intractable seizures. About 15% of children who have epilepsy have intractable seizures, and about 50% of these may be appropriate candidates for epilepsy surgery. Therefore, children who have intractable seizures should be referred to a center that has a multidisciplinary team of professionals including epileptologists, specialized neurosurgeons, neurophysiologists, neuropsychologists, neuroradiologists, psychologists, and family therapists. These professionals can best determine the location of the epileptic zone within the child's brain and the potential morbidity from loss of function in that area or adjacent tissue, can perform the surgery, and can treat the secondary effects of the surgery on the child and his or her family. Although epilepsy surgery can be done at any age, if it is done soon after intractability of seizures has been established, some of the secondary physiological and psychosocial effects of growing up with epilepsy may be prevented, and the child is more likely to be able to live up to his or her potential in adult life.

Epilepsy surgery consists either of resecting the epileptic focus, such as a temporal lobectomy or a cortical resection, or of disconnecting the pathways that may facilitate the spread of epileptic activity within the brain, such as a corpus callosotomy.

The outcome from temporal lobectomies in appropriately chosen children is as good as in adults—at least 65% become seizure free and another 15% are significantly improved; morbidity is minimal.[14,49] Hemispherectomies in children who have a congenital hemiparesis and resistant seizures originating in the damaged hemisphere result in control of seizures in 75% of cases and often result in improvement of function because the normal, opposite hemisphere is no longer being interrupted by seizure discharges.[33] A few cases of intractable infantile spasms also may benefit from partial or complete hemispherectomies.[45] The corpus callosotomy is a palliative procedure for individuals who do not qualify for a local resection. It can be quite effective in controlling "drop" attacks and the resultant injuries in children who have multiple seizure types. Results are best in higher-functioning individuals who have localized CNS dysfunction as opposed to diffuse CNS dysfunction.

When to Refer

Type of seizure is unclear
Seizures refractory to medication

When to Hospitalize

Uncontrolled or prolonged seizures
Video EEG monitoring needed
Need to rapidly change anticonvulsant medication
Initiation of the ketogenic diet

REFERENCES

1. Aicardi J: *Epilepsy in children,* New York, 1986, Raven Press.
2. Annegers JF, et al: Factors prognostic of unprovoked seizures after febrile convulsions, *N Engl J Med* 316:493, 1987.
3. Ben-Menachem E, et al: Effects of vagus nerve stimulation on amino acids and other metabolites in the CSF of patients with partial seizures, *Epilepsy Res* 20:221, 1995.
4. Berg AT, Shinnar S: The risk of seizure recurrence following a first unprovoked seizure: a meta-analysis, *Neurology* 41:965, 1991.
5. Besag FMC, et al: Lamotrigine for the treatment of epilepsy in childhood, *J Pediatr* 127:991, 1995.
6. Boellner SW, Deaton R, Sommerville KW: Long-term treatment of partial seizures with tiagabine in children, *Epilepsia* 38(suppl 8):208, 1997.
7. Bruni J, et al: Efficacy and safety of gabapentin (Neurontin): a multicenter, placebo-controlled, double-blind study, *Neurology* 41(suppl 1):330, 1991.
8. Camfield PR, Camfield C: Pediatric epilepsy: an overview. In Swaiman K, Ashwal S, editors: *Pediatric neurology principles and practice,* St Louis, 1999, Mosby.
9. Commission on Classification and Terminology of the International League Against Epilepsy: Proposal for classification of epilepsies and epileptic syndromes, *Epilepsia* 26:268, 1985.
10. Commission on Classification and Terminology of the International League Against Epilepsy: Proposal for revised clinical and electroencephalographic classification of epileptic seizures, *Epilepsia* 22:489, 1981.
11. Dreifuss FE, et al: Valproic acid hepatic fatalities: a retrospective review, *Neurology* 37:379, 1987.
12. Durner M, et al: Localization of idiopathic generalized epilepsy on chromosome 6p in families of juvenile myoclonic epilepsy patients, *Neurology* 41:1651, 1991.
13. Elterman RD, et al: A trial of topiramate as adjunctive therapy for partial onset seizures in children, *Neurology* 52:1338, 1999.
14. Engel J Jr, editor: *Surgical treatment of the epilepsies,* ed 2, New York, 1993, Raven Press.
15. Farrell K, et al: Successful treatment of valproate hepatotoxicity with *N*-acetylcysteine, *Epilepsia* 30:700, 1989.
16. The Felbamate Study Group in Lennox-Gastaut Syndrome: Efficacy of felbamate in childhood encephalopathy Lennox-Gastaut syndrome, *N Engl J Med* 328:29, 1993.
17. Ferrie CD, et al: Lamotrigine as an add-on drug in typical absence seizures, *Acta Neurol Scand* 91:200, 1995.
18. Genton P, Dravet C: Lennox-Gastaut syndrome and other childhood epileptic encephalopathies. In Engel J, Pedley TA, editors: *Epilepsy: a comprehensive textbook,* Philadelphia, 1997, Lippincott-Raven.
19. Glauser TA, Clark PO, Strawsburg R: A pilot study of topiramate in the treatment of infantile spasms, *Epilepsia* 39:1324, 1998.
20. Glauser TA, et al: Topiramate in Lennox-Gastaut syndrome: a double blind trial, *Neurology* 48:1729, 1997.
21. Holmes GL: Do seizures cause brain damage? *Epilepsia* 32(suppl 5): S14, 1991.
22. Holmes GL, Vigevano F: Infantile spasms. In Engel J, Pedley TA, editors: *Epilepsy: a comprehensive textbook,* Philadelphia, 1997, Lippincott-Raven.
23. Janz D: Juvenile myoclonic epilepsy with typical absences. In Duncan JS, Panayiotopoulos CP, editors: *Typical absences and related syndromes,* London, 1994, Churchill.
24. Krahl SE, et al: Possible mechanism of the seizure attenuating effects of vagus nerve stimulation, *Soc Neurosci Abst* 20:1453, 1994.
25. Kriel RL, Birnbaum AK, Cloyd JC: Antiepileptic drug therapy in children. In Swaiman K, Ashwal S, editors: *Pediatric neurology principles and practice,* St Louis, 1999, Mosby.
26. Lombroso CT: Neonatal seizures: historic note and present controversies. *Epilepsia* 37(suppl 3):5, 1996.
27. Lundgren J, et al: Vagal nerve stimulation in 16 children with refractory epilepsy, *Epilepsia* 39:809, 1998.
28. Maytal J, et al: Lorazepam in the treatment of refractory neonatal seizures, *J Child Neurol* 6:319, 1991.
29. Mims J, et al: Treatment with high doses of lamotrigine in children and adolescents with refractory seizures, *J Child Neurol* 12:64, 1997.
30. Mizrahi EM, Kellaway P: *Diagnosis and management of neonatal seizures,* Philadelphia, 1998, Lippincott-Raven.
31. Naritoku DK, Wendy JT, Helfert RH: Regional induction of fos immunoreactivity in the brain by anticonvulsant stimulation of the vagus nerve, *Epilepsy Res* 22:53, 1995.
32. Parker APJ, et al: Vagal nerve stimulation in epileptic encephalopathies, *Pediatrics* 103:778, 1999.
33. Peacock WJ: The role of hemispherectomy in the treatment of intractable seizures in childhood, *Int Pediatr* 7:291, 1992.
34. Pellock JM: Fosphenytoin use in children, *Neurology* 46:S14, 1996.
35. Penry JK, Dean JC: Prevention of intractable partial seizures by intermittent vagal stimulation in humans: preliminary results, *Epilepsia* 31: S40, 1990.
36. Quality Standards Subcommittee of the American Academy of Neurology: Practice parameter: a guideline for discontinuing antiepileptic drugs in seizure-free patients—summary statement, *Neurology* 47:600, 1996.
37. Ramsey RE, De Toledo J: Acetazolamide. In Engel J, Pedley TA, editors: *Epilepsy: a comprehensive textbook,* Philadelphia, 1997, Lippincott-Raven.
38. Rosman NP, et al: A controlled trial of diazepam administered during febrile illness to prevent recurrence of febrile seizure, *N Engl J Med* 329:72, 1993.
39. Schlumberger E, et al: Lamotrigine in treatment of 120 children with epilepsy, *Epilepsia* 35:359, 1994.
40. Shinnar S, et al: Discontinuing antiepileptic drugs in children with epilepsy: a prospective study, *Ann Neurol* 35:534, 1994.
41. Shinnar S, et al: The risk of seizure recurrence after a first unprovoked afebrile seizure in childhood: an extended follow-up, *Pediatrics* 98:216, 1996.
42. Tennison MB, et al: Rate of taper of antiepileptic drugs and the risk of seizure recurrence in children, *N Engl J Med* 330:1407, 1994.
43. Trimble MR, Cull CA: Antiepileptic drugs, cognitive function, and behavior in children, *Cleve Clin J Med* 56(suppl 1):140, 1989.
44. Uldall P, et al: Single-blind study of safety, tolerability, and preliminary efficacy of tiagabine as adjunctive treatment of children with epilepsy, *Epilepsia* 36(suppl 3):S147, 1995.
45. Uthman BM, et al: Outcome for West syndrome following surgical treatment, *Epilepsia* 32:668, 1991.
46. Vining EPG, at al: Multi-center study of the efficacy of the ketogenic diet, *Ann Neurol* 40:300, 1996.
47. Volpe JJ: *Neurology of the newborn,* ed 3, Philadelphia, 1995, WB Saunders.
48. Weiner SP, Scher MS, Painter MJ: Neonatal seizures: electroclinical disassociation, *Epilepsia* 30:691, 1989.
49. Wyllie E, et al: Seizure outcome after epilepsy surgery in children and adolescents, *Ann Neurol* 44:740, 1998.

261 Septic Arthritis

Edwards P. Schwentker

Septic arthritis most commonly involves lower extremity joints and characteristically affects young children and infants. Septic arthritis constitutes a true clinical emergency because its complications may include dissolution of articular cartilage, necrosis of the underlying epiphysis, destruction of the adjacent growth plate, and dislocation of the joint itself. Complications can be minimized only by a high index of clinical suspicion, prompt diagnosis, and aggressive treatment.

PATHOGENESIS

Bacteria may reach a joint by any of three routes. Direct introduction may occur through percutaneous puncture, with the needle being either introduced purposely into the joint for diagnostic or therapeutic purposes, or wandering from adjacent structures such as from blood vessels during an attempted venipuncture or arterial puncture. Second, hematogenous bacterial seeding may occur directly to the membrana synovialis. Finally, septic arthritis may develop from a contiguous metaphyseal osteomyelitis that decompresses into the joint capsule. In young infants, bone infection may extend from the metaphysis into the epiphysis via transepiphyseal vessels and then from the epiphysis directly into the joint. (For a more complete discussion of osteomyelitis, see Chapter 244, Osteomyelitis.)

With few exceptions, the organisms most commonly responsible for septic arthritis are the same as those causing acute osteomyelitis; thus the leading offender is *Staphylococcus aureus*. Particularly in very young children, streptococci of various types are seen. *Haemophilus influenzae* type b was a common pathogen in young children in the past, but the advent of vaccination against this organism significantly reduced the incidence of such infections.[6] Gonococcal arthritis is fairly rare; when it occurs, however, it often involves several joints. Meningococcal arthritis also can occur and may develop without meningitis or meningococcemia.[4]

The consequences of an established septic arthritis can be severe. Enzymes destructive to both cartilage matrix and collagen are released by leukocytes and synovial cells as part of the inflammatory process. With infections caused by *S. aureus* and some of the gram-negative bacteria, the potential for destruction of joint surfaces is increased because these organisms also produce proteolytic enzymes. By raising intraarticular pressure, intracapsular infection may obstruct blood flow, leading to necrosis of the epiphysis and the underlying growth plate. Finally, an untreated joint infection can result in joint instability through destruction of the ligamentous fibers of the capsule. Dislocation of the hip and shoulder particularly is likely.

Considering the possible consequences and, particularly in the young child, the potential for permanent deformity and disability, the need for accurate diagnosis and expeditious treatment of a septic arthritis cannot be exaggerated.

CLINICAL FINDINGS

The source of a hematogenous septic arthritis may be a preexisting infection elsewhere in the body, but frequently none is recognized. As the septic arthritis develops, it generally is accompanied by an acute onset of fever and malaise and marked localized signs and symptoms.[2,5] Swelling, erythema, and tenderness often are prominent but may be hard to detect in a deep joint such as the hip. The most characteristic finding is pain with joint motion. When a lower extremity joint is involved, the patient usually refuses to bear weight.

The joint will be held immobile by muscle spasm in a position that maximizes capsular volume, thus minimizing the intraarticular pressure. For the hip, the preferred position is a combination of moderate flexion, abduction, and external rotation; for the knee, gentle flexion; and for the shoulder, adduction against the trunk. It is not at all unusual for a child to appear entirely well and in no distress so long as the affected joint is allowed to remain undisturbed.

The pediatrician should rely most on the physical examination. The only absolutely reliable laboratory tests are Gram stain and culture of aspirated joint fluid. White blood cell (WBC) counts may be within normal limits or only mildly elevated. The erythrocyte sedimentation rate is elevated more consistently, but even this test may be unremarkable in the newborn. C-reactive protein level elevation is even more sensitive than the sedimentation rate. Blood cultures should be drawn when septic arthritis is suspected because they frequently are positive for the offending organism.

Early in the course of septic arthritis, radiographs are negative for any bone change but frequently demonstrate soft tissue changes, including swelling and edematous infiltration into fatty tissue planes. Radionuclide scanning is not necessary if localizing signs are clear-cut. Scans are contraindicated if they delay appropriate treatment in any way. Scanning may help find or rule out other sites of involvement, particularly in very sick or very young children.

Ultrasonography has proven useful in detecting the capsular distention that accompanies septic arthritis of the hip.[8] In the hands of an experienced radiologist, this noninvasive test can exclude the presence of a joint effusion or, if one is present, assist the operator in accurate needle placement during diagnostic aspiration.

Joint aspiration with a large-bore needle is the most important diagnostic maneuver. This generally can be performed in most joints without the use of an anesthetic. An orthopedist should be consulted to aspirate suspected joints, unless the primary care physician is skilled in this procedure. Fluoroscopy or, possibly, ultrasonography should be used to confirm entrance into the relatively inaccessible hip and shoulder joints. A diagnostic aspiration yields fluid with a WBC count exceeding 50,000 and a percentage of polymorphonuclear leukocytes greater than 90. Lower counts can be found early in the course of a septic arthritis. An effusion with a low WBC count also may be associated with acute osteomyelitis of an adjacent metaphysis, the effusion being sympathetic. In most instances of septic arthritis, the aspiration yields frank pus. In any case, aspirated fluid should be cultured and Gram stained.

In septic arthritis, as in osteomyelitis, the neonate presents a unique challenge.[2] Systemic signs may be absent, and laboratory findings may be within normal limits. Nonetheless, localized signs almost always are prominent, particularly pain with motion of the involved joint.

The failure of an infant to move an infected joint is a condition known as pseudoparalysis and may be seen in a child who otherwise appears completely normal. The clinician may be misled into seeking a neurological deficit as the primary disorder, on the assumption that the lack of motion is caused by true muscle paralysis. In fact, it is possible for a septic arthritis of the shoulder to cause a brachial plexus neuropathy and septic arthritis of the hip to cause neuropathies of the femoral and sciatic nerves.[1] Such occurrences are rare, however, and even in such cases, the primary disorder is a joint infection, which must be promptly diagnosed and definitively treated. When a septic arthritis is present, passive movement of the affected extremity almost invariably elicits severe pain, a finding not characteristic of an isolated neuropathy. To make the diagnosis of septic arthritis, the pediatrician must suspect infection; in any infant, failure to move an extremity spontaneously must be considered a result of septic arthritis until proved otherwise.

MANAGEMENT

Following an expeditious clinical, roentgenographic, and laboratory evaluation, the suspected joint should be aspirated with a large-bore needle using local anesthesia and sedation. Blood cultures should be obtained. If pus is obtained from the joint, the material should be Gram stained and cultured, and parenteral antibiotics should be initiated immediately based on the Gram stain findings. If bacteria are not seen, antibiotic therapy should be instituted empirically while culture results are pending. Neonates should be treated with a penicillinase-resistant penicillin and an aminoglycoside. A penicillinase-resistant penicillin given alone is appropriate therapy for a child more than 5 years of age. For younger children who have not been vaccinated against *Haemophilus influenzae* type b, coverage for ampicillin-resistant strains of *H. influenzae* should be added. Immunocompromised patients and older patients suspected of parenteral drug abuse should have coverage against enteric gram-negative bacilli and *Pseudomonas*. These patients should receive a broad-spectrum penicillin and an aminoglycoside.[7]

Aspiration of a distal extremity joint together with administration of appropriate antibiotics may be sufficient treatment for selected patients.[3] Such patients should have an uncomplicated acute hematogenous septic arthritis of less than 6 days' duration and have no evidence of clinical osteomyelitis, immune deficiency, or other chronic illness. If aspiration and antibiotics fail to provide a prompt clinical response, the involved joint must be drained operatively under general or spinal anesthesia depending on the joint that is involved. Because the hip joint is relatively inaccessible and the capital femoral epiphysis is susceptible to avascular necrosis secondary to increased intraarticular pressure, an infected hip joint should be drained operatively and not treated with aspiration and antibiotics alone.

Operative drainage unquestionably is more effective than percutaneous aspiration. The findings at the time of arthrotomy often indicate the futility of attempting to eradicate an abscess by needle aspiration, because heavy fibrin deposits frequently are encountered. Such deposits cannot be debrided by needle aspiration. The pediatrician should be quicker to call a surgical colleague when the offending organism is *S. aureus* or a gram-negative bacterium that can produce cartilage-damaging enzymes.

Failure to obtain pus from a joint that is otherwise suspected of harboring sepsis must be viewed with skepticism. Fibrin debris or thick pus may prevent aspiration. Exquisite pain with passive joint motion, discretely localized soft tissue swelling and tenderness, and evidence of joint effusion should overrule the negative aspiration and prompt operative exploration. The risks of an unnecessary exploration are minimal compared with the certainty of joint damage that attends a neglected septic arthritis.

Parenteral antibiotics should be continued and adequate blood levels maintained following operative drainage. The choice of antibiotics should be adjusted after the results of cultures are obtained. If methods are available for determining bactericidal activity, substitution of oral medications for parenteral antibiotics may be possible. Oral antibiotics, however, should be used only if the patient is responding to treatment, the parents are reliable, the antibiotic does not cause a gastrointestinal disturbance that interferes with absorption, and blood levels can be monitored adequately. Antibiotic therapy should continue for a minimum of 3 weeks, but treatment should not be discontinued until the clinical response indicates that the condition has been corrected and the C-reactive protein level and erythrocyte sedimentation rate have returned to normal.[4]

Immobilization is the final principle of treating septic arthritis.[5] Splinting should be provided for comfort and rest of the affected distal joints of the upper and lower extremities after drainage, but it need be continued only while swelling, tenderness, and pain with motion persist. Neglected infection of a shoulder or hip may lead to subluxation or frank dislocation; thus, these joints should be immobilized long enough for the capsule to restabilize. If diagnosis and treatment are accomplished soon after the onset of the disease, 1 or 2 weeks of immobilization may be adequate. A prolonged infection, particularly of the hip, may require immobilization for 2 to 3 months. The shoulder can be protected adequately with a simple sling and swathe. The hip may be immobilized in a spica cast, or once pain has subsided, protection may be provided by a simple Pavlik harness or any similar device that maintains reduction by centering the hip deeply within the acetabulum. The need for immobilizing a joint should be determined according to the individual's condition, to maximize joint stability while avoiding unnecessary stiffness.

When to Refer

- Failure to move or use an extremity (pseudoparalysis)
- Severe pain with passive movement of a joint

When to Hospitalize

To an orthopedic surgeon:
- Joint aspiration positive for pus
- Primary care physician not experienced in aspiration of suspected joint

REFERENCES

1. Gabriel SR, Thometz, JG, Jaradeh S: Septic arthritis associated with brachial plexus neuropathy. A case report, *J Bone Joint Surg (Am)* 78:103, 1996.
2. Griffin PP, Green WT Sr: Hip joint infections in infants and children, *Orthop Clin North Am* 9:123, 1978.
3. Herndon WA, et al: Management of septic arthritis in children, *J Pediatr Orthop* 6:576, 1986.
4. Jackson MA, Nelson JD: Etiology and medical management of acute suppurative bone and joint infections in pediatric patients, *J Pediatr Orthop* 2:313, 1982.
5. Paterson DC: Acute suppurative arthritis in infancy and childhood, *J Bone Joint Surg (Br)* 52:474, 1970.
6. Peltola H, Kallio MJT, Unkila-Kallio L: Reduced incidence of septic arthritis in children by *Haemophilus influenzae* type-b vaccination, *J Bone Joint Surg (Br)* 80:471, 1998.
7. Scoles PV, Aronoff SC: Current concepts review: antimicrobial therapy of childhood skeletal infections, *J Bone Joint Surg (Am)* 66:1487, 1984.
8. Wingstrand H, et al: Sonography in septic arthritis of the hip in the child: report of four cases, *J Pediatr Orthop* 7:206, 1987.

262 Sexually Transmitted Diseases

Alain Joffe

For a variety of reasons, teenagers are at high risk for acquiring sexually transmitted diseases (STDs) (Box 262-1). Although rates of sexual activity among adolescents have decreased modestly since the early 1990s, they increased dramatically in the prior three decades, especially among white adolescents. Hence, many teenagers now are exposed to these infectious agents. Furthermore, by virtue of their cognitive developmental level, adolescents often feel invulnerable and minimize their potential for becoming infected. They may ignore symptoms or believe that as long as they are symptom free, they are neither infected nor infectious.

A large body of evidence indicates that condoms provide substantial protection against many STDs. Although use of condoms by teenagers has increased over the last decade, most teenagers do not use them consistently and some use them not at all. Oral contraceptives, still a popular method of contraception, do not protect against acquisition of STDs, although they may protect against the development of symptomatic pelvic inflammatory disease (PID) among infected teenagers. Depot medroxyprogesterone acetate injections, an increasingly popular method of contraception among teens, also do not provide protection against STDs.

Adolescents often have difficulty discussing sexual matters with partners or with parents and may be reluctant to reveal that they are infected or have been treated. They may postpone a visit to a physician because they are embarrassed, fear a lecture, are concerned about the physician maintaining confidentiality, or lack the money or social skills to get to a source of health care. Some physicians hesitate to provide confidential services to an adolescent with an STD because they are uncertain about the adolescent's capacity to consent to treatment without parental involvement. Currently, all 50 states have laws that permit a physician to treat most minors seeking treatment for STDs without parental consent or notification.

There may be a physiological basis for adolescent girls being particularly susceptible to STDs on exposure. The transformation zone of the cervix, which is relatively large among pubertal girls, is particularly vulnerable to infection with *Chlamydia trachomatis* and human papillomavirus (Fig. 262-1). Not surprisingly, therefore, current data indicate that adolescent and young adult females have higher infection rates because of these agents than any other age group in the United States. The most recent age-specific infection rates from the Centers for Disease Control and Prevention (CDC) for *Chlamydia trachomatis* and *Neisseria gonorrhoeae* are shown in Fig. 262-2. Rates of infection among 10- to 19-year-olds may actually be higher than indicated, because the pool of truly susceptible individuals (those sexually active) is smaller in this age group than in the older ones. For example, only 50% of 15- to 19-year-olds, compared to close to 100% of those over 19, are sexually active. Both sexually active males and females in the 15- to 19-year age group are likely to have the highest rates of infection caused by those two organisms of any age group in the United States.

The list of infectious agents that can be transmitted sexually is extensive. Box 262-2 lists the most common of these. Gonorrhea, chlamydia, herpes, human papillomavirus, and syphilis are discussed in detail in this chapter. (See Chapter 217, Herpes Infections, and Chapter 219, Human Immunodeficiency Virus Infection and Acquired Immunodeficiency Syndrome for discussion of these topics. Chapter 178, Vaginal Discharge, provides an overview of agents causing vaginal discharge. Information about other STDs should be sought through the index.)

An alternative way of conceptualizing the spectrum of problems attributable to STDs is to focus on symptoms or diseases rather than on specific agents. More than one organism can produce various signs, symptoms, or syndromes, and many teenagers deny or are reluctant to discuss sexual activity for the reasons outlined above. Hence, when an adolescent has a symptom or sign that may be caused by STDs, the physician must proceed with appropriate diagnostic tests or therapy, even though the history may appear to exclude such an etiology. Most sexually active teenagers, however, will be truthful when questioned respectfully without a parent or guardian present and when given appropriate guarantees about confidentiality. Box 262-3 lists a variety of symptoms and clinical entities that frequently are caused by sexually transmitted organisms.

Pediatricians generally concern themselves with the short-term morbidity associated with STDs, but the complications may extend into adulthood. Cervical cancer, infertility, ectopic pregnancy, and chronic pelvic pain are all long-term sequelae of infections acquired during adolescence and young adulthood. In addition, there is now ample evidence that STDs increase one's risk for acquiring HIV infection. Also, HIV-positive individuals who contract STDs shed increased amounts of HIV in genital body fluids and, therefore, are more likely to transmit HIV to an uninfected partner.[4] In Africa, aggressive control of STDs was accompanied by a reduction in the incidence of cases of HIV infection.

This perspective underscores the importance of preventing, diagnosing and treating STDs among adolescents. Hence, the FDA approval and commercial availability of DNA amplification tests for the diagnosis of *Chlamydia trachomatis* and *Neisseria gonorrhoeae* infections represents a major advance in achieving this goal. These tests are more sensitive than both culture and previous generations of nonculture tests, do not require the recovery of viable organisms, and can be performed on urine specimens.[18] By eliminating or reducing the need for invasive testing, use of these tests has the potential to greatly expand the number of at-risk youth who are screened.[5] Similarly, self-collection of specimens and elimination of the pelvic exam for diagnosing vaginal infections may also enhance detection efforts.[1,14]

SPECIFIC AGENTS

Chlamydia trachomatis

The obligate intracellular chlamydia microorganism causes a wide spectrum of disease and is the most common sexually transmitted *bacterial* agent in the United States. Of greatest importance is its causative role in urethritis and epididymitis in males and cervicitis and pelvic inflammatory disease in females.

Chlamydia appears to cause 30% to 40% of symptomatic nongonococcal urethritis among males; use of DNA amplification tests (see below) may reveal a higher prevalence. The organism can also be recovered from 15% to 25% of men with urethral gonorrhea. Approximately 5% to 10% of asymptomatic adolescent males will test positive for chlamydia, depending on the population studied. Symptoms generally develop 1 to 3 weeks after infection. Adolescents may complain only of mild dysuria or itching at the terminal urethra, or they may have a scanty, mucoid discharge that is easily ignored and will disappear without treatment. The optimal time to examine a male with a suggestive history, but no discharge, is the first thing in the morning, without his having voided overnight. Alternatively, having him strip his urethra may produce some discharge. A profuse, purulent discharge should raise the possibilities of *Neisseria gonorrhoeae* coinfection or of its being the single causative agent. Males also may complain of testicular or scrotal pain or both, suggesting that urethral infection has spread to the epididymis.

Because the organism can infect the urethra as well as the cervix, a female may complain of dysuria as the primary manifestation of infection. Hence, *Chlamydia trachomatis* infection should be considered in any adolescent female suspected of having a urinary tract infection. She may complain of spotting between periods as a result of cervicitis or, if the infection has spread to the upper genital tract, of low abdominal pain or right upper quadrant pain (Fitz-Hugh-Curtis syndrome). The latter is caused by organisms tracking up the abdominal cavity and causing inflammation of the liver capsule along with adhesions to the diaphragm. Unless a careful history is obtained, the combination of dysuria and right upper quadrant or right flank pain could lead a clinician to the erroneous diagnosis of pyelonephritis. Lower abdominal pain suggests the possibility of pelvic inflammatory disease. Vaginal discharge is more likely to indicate the presence of another infection (see Chapter 178, Vaginal Discharge), although chlamydia may be found incidentally. Chlamydia also may infect Bartholin's ducts, resulting in an exudative vaginal discharge or an abscess.

As with males, infections in females are often asymptomatic. Rates of infection vary according to region of the country and other factors. Among 16- to 24-year-old females entering the United States Job Corps program, infection rates varied from 4% to 6% in Maine and in the Northwest to 16% to 17% in Indiana and the Southeast. On pelvic examination, clues to infection are the presence of mucopurulent discharge

BOX 262-1

WHY ADOLESCENTS ARE AT RISK FOR STDS

- Increased prevalence of sexual activity at earlier ages
- Sense of invulnerability ("It can't happen to me.")
- Lack of information ("If I don't feel sick, I can't be sick.")
- Infrequent use of barrier methods of contraception
- Poor communication skills with partners and physicians
- Barriers to care (legal obstacles, concerns about confidentiality)
- Poor compliance
- Physiological changes associated with puberty

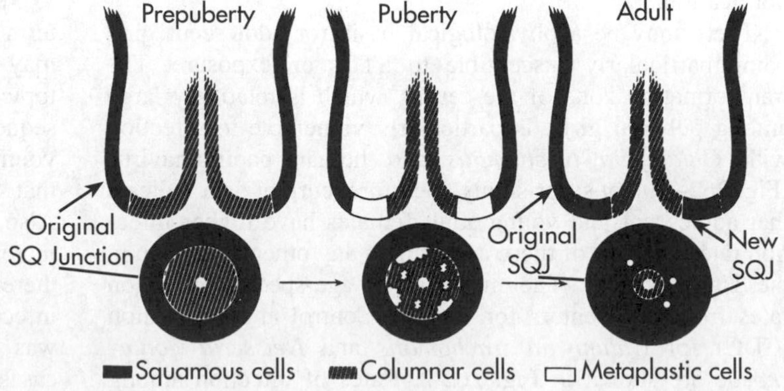

Fig. 262-1 Cervical development. In most prepubertal females, the original squamocolumnar junction is located well onto the ectocervix. During puberty, uncommitted germ cells of the columnar epithelium differentiate into squamous cells during a process called squamous metaplasia. This process begins at the original squamocolumnar junction at various areas and continues caudally. Thus the pubertal cervix is in a transitional state. By adulthood the transformation results in a new squamocolumnar junction, now found near or in the ectocervix.

(From Moscicki B, Shafer MB: *J Adolesc Health Care* 7:505, 1986.)

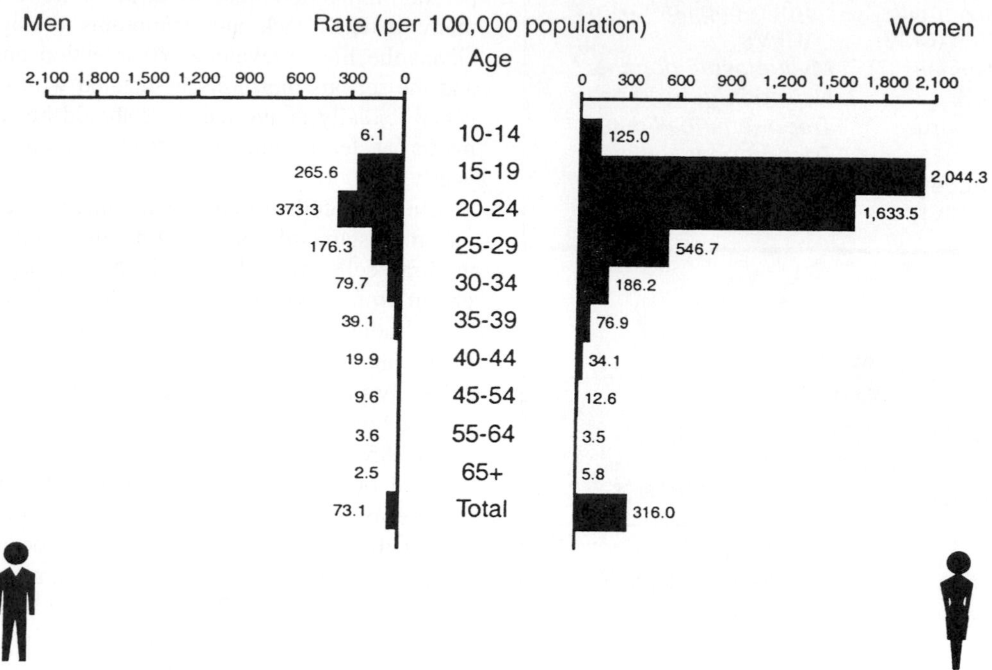

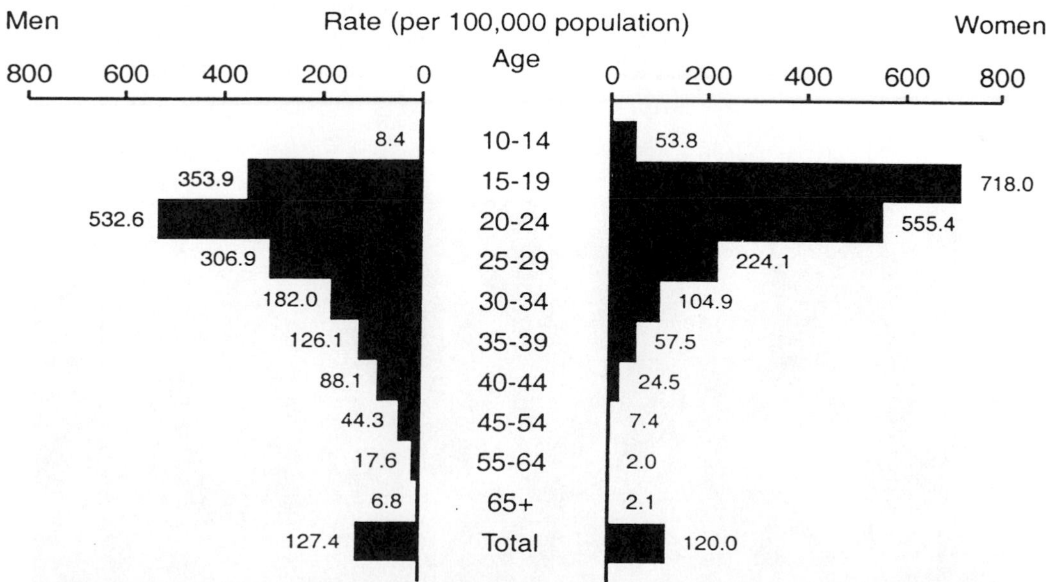

Fig. 262-2 Rates of infection of *Chlamydia trachomatis* and *Neisseria gonorrhoeae* in the United States, by age and gender, 1997 data.

(Data from Division of STD Prevention, STD Surveillance, 1997, US Department of Health and Human Services, Public Health Service, Atlanta, September, 1998, Centers for Disease Control and Prevention.)

BOX 262-2

SEXUALLY TRANSMITTED INFECTIOUS AGENTS

Chlamydia trachomatis	Human papillomavirus (HPV)
Cytomegalovirus (CMV)	*Mycoplasma hominis*
Gardnerella vaginalis (?)	*Neisseria gonorrhoeae*
Hepatitis B	*Treponema pallidum*
Herpes simplex virus (HSV)	*Trichomonas vaginalis*
Human immunodeficiency virus (HIV)	*Ureaplasma urealyticum*

BOX 262-3

SIGNS, SYMPTOMS, AND CLINICAL ENTITIES SUGGESTING SEXUALLY TRANSMITTED DISEASE IN ADOLESCENTS

Males
- Dysuria, urethritis
- Epididymitis (scrotal pain, swelling)

Female
- Mucopurulent cervicitis
- Vaginitis
- Dysuria
- Right upper quadrant pain
- Pelvic inflammatory disease (low abdominal pain)

Both
- Genital ulcers
- Genital warts
- Hepatitis B infection
- HIV infection
- Proctitis
- Septic arthritis

from the cervical os ("mucopus," Fig. 262-3), cervical erythema, and friability. A cervical Gram stain will reveal the presence of 30 or more polymorphonuclear white blood cells per oil immersion field in three or more fields. However, many patients lack any symptoms or signs of infection. Given the high prevalence of infection among adolescents and the serious morbidity associated with untreated disease, every sexually active teenager should be screened for chlamydia at least annually; some recommend testing twice yearly.[2]

Culturing cells for chlamydial infection at present remains the gold standard for detecting infection. Endocervical or urethral cells must be obtained; the organism cannot be grown from vaginal discharge alone. However, recent data from studies that use multiple tests to detect the presence of *C. trachomatis* indicate that DNA amplification tests are considerably more sensitive than other methods.[11] For example, among females, the sensitivity of cultures is 70% to 85% versus 85% to 96% using ligase chain-reaction testing of cervical or urine specimens. Such tests currently are more expensive than other methods but have a distinct advantage in that they are noninvasive (that is, specimens can be obtained without performing a pelvic examination or swabbing the urethral orifice). Older nonculture tests, such as DNA probes or enzyme-linked immunoabsorbent assays, are only 54% to 84% sensitive. Because detection of infection is critical to preventing serious morbidity, the clinician should use the most sensitive diagnostic test available.[15] Screening programs for chlamydia have been shown to reduce the incidence of pelvic inflammatory disease among enrollees in a health maintenance organization.[17]

Uncomplicated cervical or urethral chlamydial infection should be treated orally with azithromycin (1 g as a single

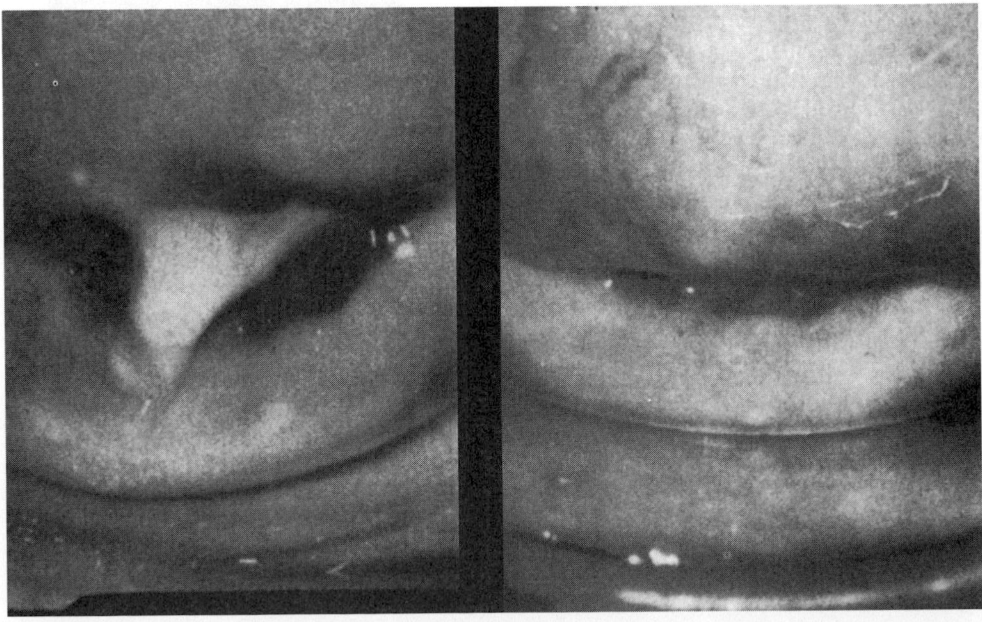

Fig. 262-3 Colpophotograph showing mucopurulent cervicitis before and 2 weeks after treatment with 500 mg of tetracycline four times daily for 7 days. Note disappearance of endocervical exudate after therapy.
(From Brunham RC, et al: *N Engl J Med* 311:2, 1984.)

BOX 262-4

1998 GUIDELINES FOR TREATMENT OF SEXUALLY TRANSMITTED DISEASES

Chlamydial Infection in Adolescents and Adults

Treatment

Treatment of infected patients prevents transmission to sex partners; and, for infected pregnant women, treatment might prevent transmission of *C. trachomatis* to infants during birth. Treatment of sex partners helps to prevent reinfection of the index patient and infection of other partners.

Coinfection with *C. trachomatis* often occurs among patients who have gonococcal infection; therefore, presumptive treatment of such patients for chlamydia is appropriate (see Gonococcal Infection, Dual Therapy for Gonococcal and Chlamydial Infections). The following recommended treatment regimens and the alternative regimens cure infection and usually relieve symptoms.

RECOMMENDED REGIMENS

Azithromycin 1 g orally in a single dose, OR

Doxycycline 100 mg orally twice a day for 7 days

ALTERNATIVE REGIMENS

Erythromycin base 500 mg orally four times a day for 7 days, OR

Erythromycin ethylsuccinate 800 mg orally four times a day for 7 days, OR

Ofloxacin 300 mg orally twice a day for 7 days

The results of clinical trials indicate that azithromycin and doxycycline are equally efficacious. These investigations were conducted primarily in populations in which follow-up was encouraged and adherence to a 7-day regimen was good. Azithromycin should always be available to health care providers to treat at least those patients for whom compliance is in question.

In populations with erratic health-care–seeking behavior, poor compliance with treatment, or minimal follow-up, azithromycin may be more cost-effective because it provides single-dose, directly observed therapy. Doxycycline costs less than azithromycin, and it has been used extensively for a longer period. Erythromycin is less efficacious than either azithromycin and doxycycline, and gastrointestinal side effects frequently discourage patients from complying with this regimen. Ofloxacin is similar in efficacy to doxycycline and azithromycin, but it is more expensive to use and offers no advantage with regard to the dosage regimen. Other quinolones either are not reliably effective against chlamydial infection or have not been adequately evaluated.

To maximize compliance with recommended therapies, medications for chlamydial infections should be dispensed on site, and the first dose should be directly observed. To minimize further transmission of infection, patients treated for chlamydia should be instructed to abstain from sexual intercourse for 7 days after single-dose therapy or until completion of a 7-day regimen. Patients also should be instructed to abstain from sexual intercourse until all of their sex partners are cured to minimize the risk for reinfection.

Follow-up

Patients do not need to be retested for chlamydia after completing treatment with doxycycline or azithromycin unless symptoms persist or reinfection is suspected, because these therapies are highly efficacious. A test of cure may be considered 3 weeks after completion of treatment with erythromycin. The validity of chlamydial culture testing at less than 3 weeks after completion of therapy to identify patients who did not respond to therapy has not been established. False-negative results can occur because of small numbers of chlamydial organisms. In addition, nonculture tests conducted at less than 3 weeks after completion of therapy for patients who were treated successfully could be false-positive because of continued excretion of dead organisms.

Some studies have demonstrated high rates of infection among women retested several months after treatment, presumably because of reinfection. In some populations (e.g., adolescents), rescreening women several months after treatment might be effective for detecting further morbidity.

Modified from the Centers for Disease Control and Prevention: 1998 guidelines for treatment of sexually transmitted diseases, *MMWR* 47:RR1, 1998.

Continued

dose) or doxycycline (100 mg bid for 7 days).[3] Azithromycin is more expensive but has the advantage of being a single dose and, if the clinician wishes, of directly observable therapy. Alternative regimens include erythromycin and ofloxacin (Box 262-4).

As with treatment for any STD, the patient's abstinence from intercourse is imperative until therapy is complete and his or her partner is notified and treated. Short-term complications of chlamydial infection include epididymitis and pelvic inflammatory disease; long-term complications include Reiter's syndrome and the sequelae of pelvic inflammatory disease. Although clearly not an independent risk factor for the development of cervical dysplasia, chlamydia infection may play some role. An untreated, infected woman can pass the infection to her infant through colonization during birth.

Neisseria gonorrhoeae

Infection with the gonococcus produces a constellation of symptoms very similar to that produced by chlamydia. Approximately 45% of males who have urethral discharge have gonococcal infection. In general, patients who are symptomatic with gonococcal infection tend to have more pronounced symptoms (more severe dysuria and a greater amount of and more purulent discharge) and usually seek health care within a shorter period of time than those infected with chlamydia. However, many patients have no symptoms

Text continued on p. 1822

BOX 262-4

1998 GUIDELINES FOR TREATMENT OF SEXUALLY TRANSMITTED DISEASES—cont'd

Gonococcal Infection in Adolescents and Adults

Dual therapy for gonococcal and chlamydial infections

Patients infected with *N. gonorrhoeae* often are coinfected with *C. trachomatis;* this finding led to the recommendation that patients treated for gonococcal infection also be treated routinely with a regimen effective against uncomplicated genital *C. trachomatis* infection. Routine dual therapy without testing for chlamydia can be cost-effective for populations in which chlamydial infection accompanies 20% to 40% of gonococcal infections, because the cost of therapy for chlamydia (e.g., $0.50 to $1.50 for doxycycline) is less than the cost of testing. Some experts believe that the routine use of dual therapy has resulted in substantial decreases in the prevalence of chlamydial infection. Because most gonococci in the United States are susceptible to doxycycline and azithromycin, routine cotreatment might hinder the development of antimicrobial-resistant *N. gonorrhoeae.*

Since the introduction of dual therapy, the prevalence of chlamydial infection has decreased in some populations, and simultaneous testing for chlamydial infection has become quicker, more sensitive, and more widely available. In geographic areas in which the rates of coinfection are low, some clinicians might prefer to test for chlamydia rather than treat presumptively. However, presumptive treatment is indicated for patients who may not return for test results.

Uncomplicated gonococcal infections of the cervix, urethra, and rectum

RECOMMENDED REGIMENS

Cefixime 400 mg orally in a single dose, OR
Ceftriaxone 125 mg IM in a single dose, OR
Ciprofloxacin 500 mg orally in a single dose, OR
Ofloxacin 400 mg orally in a single dose, PLUS
Azithromycin 1 g orally in a single dose, OR
Doxycycline 100 mg orally twice a day for 7 days

Cefixime has an antimicrobial spectrum similar to that of ceftriaxone, but the 400-mg oral dose does not provide as high nor as sustained a bactericidal level as that provided by the 125-mg dose of ceftriaxone. In published clinical trials, the 400-mg dose cured 97.1% of uncomplicated urogenital and anorectal gonococcal infections. The advantage of cefixime is that it can be administered orally.

Ceftriaxone in a single injection of 125 mg provides sustained, high bactericidal levels in the blood. Extensive clinical experience indicates that ceftriaxone is safe and effective for the treatment of uncomplicated gonorrhea at all sites, curing 99.1% of uncomplicated urogenital and anorectal infections in published clinical trials.

Ciprofloxacin is effective against most strains of *N. gonorrhoeae.* At a dose of 500 mg, ciprofloxacin provides sustained bactericidal levels in the blood; in published clinical trials, it has cured 99.8% of uncomplicated urogenital and anorectal infections. Ciprofloxacin is safe, relatively inexpensive, and can be administered orally.

Ofloxacin also is effective against most strains of *N. gonorrhoeae,* and it has favorable pharmacokinetics. The 400-mg oral dose has been effective for treatment of uncomplicated urogenital and anorectal infections, curing 98.4% of infections in published clinical trials.

ALTERNATIVE REGIMENS

Spectinomycin 2 g IM in a single dose. Spectinomycin is expensive and must be injected; however, it has been effective in published clinical trials, curing 98.2% of uncomplicated urogenital and anorectal gonococcal infections. Spectinomycin is useful for treatment of patients who cannot tolerate cephalosporins and quinolones.

Single-dose cephalosporin regimens other than ceftriaxone 125 mg IM and cefixime 400 mg orally that are safe and highly effective against uncomplicated urogenital and anorectal gonococcal infections include

(a) ceftizoxime 500 mg IM, (b) cefotaxime 500 mg IM, (c) cefotetan 1 g IM, and (d) cefoxitin 2 g IM with probenecid 1 g orally. None of these injectable cephalosporins offers any advantage in comparison with ceftriaxone, and clinical experience with these regimens for treatment of uncomplicated gonorrhea is limited.

Single-dose quinolone regimens include enoxacin 400 mg orally, lomefloxacin 400 mg orally, and norfloxacin 800 mg orally. These regimens appear to be safe and effective for the treatment of uncomplicated gonorrhea, but data regarding their use are limited. None of the regimens appears to offer any advantage over ciprofloxacin at a dose of 500 mg or ofloxacin at 400 mg.

Many other antimicrobials are active against *N. gonorrhoeae;* however, these guidelines are not intended to be a comprehensive list of all effective treatment regimens. Azithromycin 2 g orally is effective against uncomplicated gonococcal infection, but it is expensive and causes gastrointestinal distress too often to be recommended for treatment of gonorrhea. At an oral dose of 1 g, azithromycin is insufficiently effective, curing only 93% of patients in published studies.

Uncomplicated gonococcal infection of the pharynx

Gonococcal infections of the pharynx are more difficult to eradicate than infections at urogenital and anorectal sites. Few antigonococcal regimens can reliably cure such infections more than 90% of the time.

Although chlamydial coinfection of the pharynx is unusual, coinfection at genital sites sometimes occurs. Therefore, treatment for both gonorrhea and chlamydia is suggested.

Modified from the Centers for Disease Control and Prevention: 1998 guidelines for treatment of sexually transmitted diseases, *MMWR* 47:RR1, 1998.

BOX 262-4

1998 GUIDELINES FOR TREATMENT OF SEXUALLY TRANSMITTED DISEASES—cont'd

Gonococcal Infection in Adolescents and Adults—cont'd

Uncomplicated gonococcal infection of the pharynx–cont'd

RECOMMENDED REGIMENS

Ceftriaxone 125 mg IM in a single dose, OR
Ciprofloxacin 500 mg orally in a single dose, OR
Ofloxacin 400 mg orally in a single dose, PLUS
Azithromycin 1 g orally in a single dose, OR
Doxycycline 100 mg orally twice a day for 7 days

Disseminated Gonococcal Infection (DGI)

DGI results from gonococcal bacteremia. DGI often results in petechial or pustular acral skin lesions, asymmetrical arthralgia, tenosynovitis, or septic arthritis. The infection is complicated occasionally by perihepatitis, and rarely by endocarditis or meningitis. Strains of *N. gonorrhoeae* that cause DGI tend to cause minimal genital inflammation. In the United States, these strains have occurred infrequently during the past decade.

No studies of the treatment of DGI among persons in North America have been published recently. The following recommendations reflect the opinions of experts. No treatment failures have been reported.

Treatment

Hospitalization is recommended for initial therapy, especially for patients who cannot be relied on to comply with treatment, for those in whom the diagnosis is uncertain, and for those who have purulent synovial effusions or other complications. Patients should be examined for clinical evidence of endocarditis and meningitis. Patients treated for DGI should be treated presumptively for concurrent *C. trachomatis* infection unless appropriate testing excludes this infection.

RECOMMENDED INITIAL REGIMEN

Ceftriaxone 1 g IM or IV every 24 hours

ALTERNATIVE INITIAL REGIMENS

Cefotaxime 1 g IV every 8 hours, OR
Ceftizoxime 1 g IV every 8 hours, OR
For persons allergic to β-lactam drugs:
Ciprofloxacin 500 mg IV every 12 hours, OR
Ofloxacin 400 mg IV every 12 hours, OR
Spectinomycin 2 mg IV every 12 hours

All regimens should be continued for 24-48 hours after improvement begins, at which time therapy may be switched to one of the following regimens to complete a full week of antimicrobial therapy:

Cefixime 400 mg orally twice a day, OR
Ciprofloxacin 500 mg orally twice a day, OR
Ofloxacin 400 mg orally twice a day

Human Papillomavirus Infection

Genital warts

TREATMENT

The primary goal of treating visible genital warts is the removal of symptomatic warts. Treatment can induce wart-free periods in most patients. Genital warts often are asymptomatic. No evidence indicates that currently available treatments eradicate or affect the natural history of HPV infection. The removal of warts may or may not decrease infectivity. If left untreated, visible genital warts may resolve on their own, remain unchanged, or increase in size or number. No evidence indicates that treatment of visible warts affects the development of cervical cancer.

REGIMENS

Treatment of genital warts should be guided by the preference of the patient, the available resources, and the experience of the health care provider. None of the available treatments is superior to other treatments, and no single treatment is ideal for all patients or all warts.

The available treatments for visible genital warts are patient-applied therapies (i.e., podofilox and imiquimod) and provider-administered therapies (i.e., cryotherapy, podophyllin resin, trichloroacetic acid [TCA], bichloroacetic acid [BCA], interferon, and surgery). Most patients have from 1 to 10 genital warts, with a total wart area of 0.5 to 1.0 cm^2, that are responsive to most treatment modalities. Factors that might influence selection of treatment include wart size, wart number, anatomical site of wart, wart morphology, patient preference, cost of treatment, convenience, adverse effects, and provider experience. Having a treatment plan or protocol is important, because many patients will require a course of therapy rather than a single treatment. In general, warts located on moist surfaces and/or in intertriginous areas respond better to topical treatment (e.g., TCA, podophyllin, podofilox, and imiquimod) than do warts on drier surfaces.

The treatment modality should be changed if a patient has not improved substantially after three provider-administered treatments or if warts have not completely cleared after six treatments. The risk-benefit ratio of treatment should be evaluated throughout the course of therapy to avoid overtreatment. Providers should be knowledgeable about, and have available to them, at least one patient-applied and one provider-administered treatment.

Complications rarely occur if treatments for warts are employed properly. Patients should be warned that scarring in the form of persistent hypopigmentation or hyperpigmentation is common with ablative modalities. Depressed or hypertrophic scars are rare but can occur, especially if the patient has had insufficient time to heal between treatments. Treatment can result rarely in disabling chronic pain syndromes (e.g., vulvodynia or hyperesthesia of the treatment site).

External genital warts, recommended treatments

Patient-applied:

Podofilox 0.5% solution or gel. Patients may apply podofilox solution with a cotton swab, or podofilox gel with a finger, to visible genital warts

Continued

BOX 262-4

1998 GUIDELINES FOR TREATMENT OF SEXUALLY TRANSMITTED DISEASES—cont'd

Human Papillomavirus Infection—cont'd

Genital warts—cont'd

REGIMENS—CONT'D

External genital warts, recommended treatments—cont'd

twice a day for 3 days, followed by 4 days of no therapy. This cycle may be repeated as necssary for a total of four cycles. The total wart area treated should not exceed 10 cm^2, and a total volume of podofilox should not exceed 0.5 mL per day. If possible, the health care provider should apply the initial treatment to demonstrate the proper application technique and identify which warts should be treated. *The safety of podofilox during pregnancy has not been established.*

OR

Imiquimod 5% cream. Patients should apply imiquimod cream with a finger at bedtime, three times a week for as long as 16 weeks. The treatment area should be washed with mild soap and water 6 to 10 hours after the application. Many patients may be clear of warts by 8 to 10 weeks or sooner. *The safety of imiquimod during pregnancy has not been established.*

Provider-administered:

Cryotherapy with liquid nitrogen or cryoprobe. Repeat applications every 1 to 2 weeks.

OR

Podophyllin resin 10% to 25% in compound tincture of benzoin. A small amount should be applied to each wart and allowed to air dry. To avoid the possibility of complications associated with systemic absorption and toxicity, some experts recommend that application be limited to no more than 0.5 mL of podophyllin or no more than 10 cm^2 of warts per session. Some experts suggest that the preparation should be thoroughly washed off 1 to 4 hours after application to reduce local irritation. Repeat weekly if necessary. *The safety of podophyllin during pregnancy has not been established.*

OR

TCA or BCA 80% to 90%. Apply a small amount only to warts and allow to dry, at which time a white "frosting" develops; powder with talc or sodium bicarbonate (i.e., baking soda) to remove unreacted acid if an excess amount is applied. Repeat weekly if necessary.

OR

Surgical removal either by tangential scissor excision, tangential shave excision, curettage, or electrosurgery.

External genital warts, alternative treatments

Intralesional interferon OR

laser surgery

For patient-applied treatments, patients must be able to identify and reach warts to be treated. Podofilox 0.5% solution or gel is relatively inexpensive, easy to use, safe, and self-applied by patients. Podofilox is an antimitotic drug that results in destruction of warts. Most patients experience mild/moderate pain or local irritation after treatment. Imiquimod is a topically active immune enhancer that stimulates production of interferon and other cytokines. Before wart resolution, local inflammatory reactions are common; these reactions usually are mild to moderate.

Cryotherapy, which requires the use of basic equipment, destroys warts by thermal-induced cytolysis. Its major drawback is that proper use requires substantial training, without which warts are frequently overtreated or undertreated, resulting in poor efficacy or increased likelihood of complications. Pain after application of the liquid nitrogen, followed by necrosis and sometimes blistering, are not unusual. Although local anesthesia (topical or injected) is not used routinely, its use facilitates treatment if there are many warts or if the area of warts is large.

Podophyllin resin contains a number of compounds, including the podophyllin lignans that are antimitotic. The resin is most frequently compounded at 10% to 25% in tincture of benzoin. However, podophyllin resin preparations differ in the concentration of active components and contaminants. The shelf life and stability of podophyllin preparations are unknown. It is important to apply a thin layer of podophyllin resin to the warts and allow it to air dry before the treated area comes into contact with clothing. Overapplication or failure to air dry can result in local irritation caused by spread of the compound to adjacent areas.

Both TCA and BCA are caustic agents that destroy warts by chemical coagulation of the proteins. Although these preparations are widely used, they have not been investigated thoroughly. TCA solutions have a low viscosity comparable to water and can spread rapidly if applied excessively, thus damaging adjacent normal tissue. Both TCA and BCA should be applied sparingly and allowed to dry before the patient sits or stands. If pain is intense, the acid can be neutralized with soap or sodium bicarbonate (i.e., baking soda).

Surgical removal of warts has an advantage over other treatment modalities in that it renders the patient wart-free, usually with a single vsit. However, substantial clinical training, additional equipment, and a longer office visit are required. Once local anesthesia is achieved, the visible genital warts can be physically destroyed by electrosurgery, in which case no additional hemostasis is required. Alternatively, the warts can be removed either by tangential excision with a pair of fine scissors or a scalpel or by curettage. Because most warts are exophytic, this can be accomplished with a resulting wound that only extends into the upper dermis. Hemostasis can be achieved with an electrosurgical unit or a chemical styptic (e.g., an aluminum chloride solution). Suturing

Modified from the Centers for Disease Control and Prevention: 1998 guidelines for treatment of sexually transmitted diseases, *MMWR* 47:RR1, 1998.

BOX 262-4

1998 GUIDELINES FOR TREATMENT OF SEXUALLY TRANSMITTED DISEASES—cont'd

Human Papillomavirus Infection—cont'd

Genital warts—cont'd

REGIMENS—CONT'D

External genital warts, alternative treatments—cont'd

is neither required nor indicated in most cases when surgical removal is done properly. Surgery is most beneficial for patients who have a large number or area of genital warts. Carbon dioxide laser and surgery may be useful in the management of extensive warts or intraurethral warts, particularly for those patients who have not responded to other treatments.

Interferons, either natural or recombinant, used for the treatment of genital warts have been administered systemically (i.e., subcutaneously at a distant site or IM) and intralesionally (i.e., injected into the warts). Systemic interferon is not effective. The efficacy and recurrence rates of intralesional interferon are comparable to other treatment modalities. Interferon is believed to be effective because of antiviral and/or immunostimulating effects. However, interferon therapy is not recommended for routine use because of inconvenient routes of administration, frequent office visits, and the association between its use and a high frequency of systemic adverse effects.

Because of the shortcomings of available treatments, some clinics employ combinaion therapy (i.e., the simultaneous use of two or more modalities on the same wart at the same time). Most experts believe that combining modalities does not increase efficacy but may increase complications.

Cervical warts

For women who have exophytic cervical warts, high-grade squamous intraepithelial lesions (SIL) must be excluded before treatment is begun. Management of exophytic cervical warts should include consultation with an expert.

Vaginal warts

Cryotherapy with liquid nitrogen. The use of a cryoprobe in the vagina is not recommended because of the risk for vaginal perforation and fistula formation.

OR

TCA or BCA 80% to 90% applied only to warts. Apply a small amount only to warts and allow to dry, at which time a white "frosting" develops; powder with talc or sodium bicarbonate (i.e., baking soda) to remove unreacted acid if an excess amount is applied. Repeat weekly if necessary.

OR

Podophyllin 10% to 25% in compound tincture of benzoin applied to a treated area that must be dry before the speculum is removed. Treat no more than 2 cm^2 per session. Repeat application at weekly intervals. Because of concern about potential systemic absorption, some experts caution against vaginal application of podophyllin. *The safety of podophyllin during pregnancy has not been established.*

Urethral meatus warts

Cryotherapy with liquid nitrogen,

OR

Podophyllin 10% to 25% in compound tincture of benzoin. The treatment area must be dry before contact with normal mucosa. Podophyllin must be applied weekly if necessary. The safety of podophyllin during pregnancy has not been established.

Anal warts

Cryotherapy with liquid nitrogen

OR

TCA or BCA 80% to 90% applied to warts. Apply a small amount only to warts and allow to dry, at which time a white "frosting" develops; powder with talc or sodium bicarbonate (i.e., baking soda) to remove unreacted acid if an excess amount is applied. Repeat weekly if necessary.

OR

Surgical removal

NOTE: Management of warts on rectal mucosa should be referred to an expert.

Oral warts

Cryotherapy with liquid nitrogen OR

Surgical removal

FOLLOW-UP

After visible genital warts have cleared, a follow-up evaluation is not mandatory. Patients should be cautioned to watch for recurrences, which occur most frequently during the first 3 months. Because the sensitivity and specificity of self-diagnosis of genital warts is unknown, patients concerned about recurrences should be offered a follow-up evaluation 3 months after treatment. Earlier follow-up visits also may be useful a) to document a wart-free state, b) to monitor for or treat complications of therapy, and c) to provide the opportunity for patient education and counseling. Women should be counseled regarding the need for regular cytologic screening as recommended for women without genital warts. The presence of genital warts is not an indication for cervical colposcopy.

Management of sex partners

Examination of sex partners is not necessary for the management of genital warts because the role of reinfection is probably minimal and, in the absence of curative therapy, treatment to reduce transmission is not realistic. However, because self- or partner-examination has not been evaluated as a diagnostic method for genital warts, sex partners of patients who have genital warts may benefit from examination to assess the presence of genital warts and other STDs. Sex partners also might benefit from counseling about the implications of having a partner who has genital warts. Because treatment of genital warts probably does not eliminate the HPV infection, patients and sex partners should be cautioned that the patient might remain infectious even though the

Continued

BOX 262-4

1998 GUIDELINES FOR TREATMENT OF SEXUALLY TRANSMITTED DISEASES—cont'd

Human Papillomavirus Infection—cont'd

Management of sex partners—cont'd

warts are gone. The use of condoms may reduce, but does not eliminate, the risk for transmission to uninfected partners. Female sex partners of patients who have genital warts should be reminded that cytological screening for cervical cancer is recommended for all sexually active women.

Genital Herpes Simplex Virus (HSV) Infection

First clinical episode of genital herpes

Management of patients with first clinical episode of genital herpes includes antiviral therapy and counseling regarding the natural history of genital herpes, sexual and perinatal transmission, and methods to reduce such transmission. Five percent to 30% of first-episode cases of genital herpes are caused by HSV-1, but clinical recurrences are much less frequent for HSV-1 than HSV-2 genital infection. Therefore, identification of the type of the infecting strain has prognostic importance and may be useful for counseling purposes.

RECOMMENDED REGIMENS

Acyclovir 400 mg orally three times a day for 7 to 10 days, OR

Acyclovir 200 mg orally five times a day for 7 to 10 days, OR

Famciclovir 250 mg orally three times a day for 7 to 10 days, OR

Valacyclovir 1 g orally twice a day for 7 to 10 days.

NOTE: Treatment may be extended if healing is incomplete after 10 days of therapy.

Higher dosages of acyclovir (i.e., 400 mg orally five times a day) were used in treatment studies of first-episode herpes proctitis and first-episode oral infection, including stomatitis or pharyngitis. It is unclear whether these forms of mucosal infection require higher doses of acyclovir than used for genital herpes. Valacyclovir and famciclovir probably are also effective for acute HSV proctitis or oral infection, but clinical experience is lacking.

Counseling is an important aspect of managing patients who have genital herpes. Although initial counseling can be provided at the first visit, many patients benefit from learning about the chronic aspects of the disease after the acute illness subsides. Counseling of these patients should include the following:

- Patients who have genital herpes should be told about the natural history of the disease, with emphasis on the potential for recurrent episodes, asymptomatic viral shedding, and sexual transmission.
- Patients should be advised to abstain from sexual activity when lesions or prodromal symptoms are present and encouraged to inform their sex partners that they have genital herpes. The use of condoms during all sexual exposures with new or uninfected sex partners should be encouraged.
- Sexual transmission of HSV can occur during asymptomatic periods. Asymptomatic viral shedding occurs more frequently in patients who have genital HSV-2 infection than HSV-1 infection and in patients who have had genital herpes for less than 12 months. Such patients should be counseled to prevent spread of the infection.
- The risk for neonatal infection should be explained to all patients, including men. Women of childbearing age who have genital herpes should be advised to inform health-care providers who care for them during pregnancy about the HSV infection.
- Patients having a first episode of genital herpes should be advised that a) episodic antiviral therapy during recurrent episodes might shorten the duration of lesions and b) suppressive antiviral therapy can ameliorate or prevent recurrent outbreaks.

Recurrent episodes of HSV disease

Most patients with first-episode genital HSV-2 infection will have recurrent episodes of genital lesions. Episodic or suppressive antiviral therapy might shorten the duration of lesions or ameliorate recurrences. Because many patients benefit from antiviral therapy, options for treatment should be discussed with all patients.

When treatment is started during the prodrome or within 1 day after onset of lesions, many patients who have recurrent disease benefit from episodic therapy. If episodic treatment of recurrences is chosen, the patient should be provided with antiviral therapy, or a prescription for the medication, so that treatment can be initiated at the first sign of prodrome or genital lesions.

Daily suppressive therapy reduces the frequency of genital herpes recurrences by at least 75% among patients who have frequent recurrences (i.e., six or more recurrences per year). Safety and efficacy have been documented among patients receiving daily therapy with acyclovir for as long as 6 years, and with valacyclovir and famciclovir for 1 year. Suppressive therapy has not been associated with emergence of clinically significant acyclovir resistance among immunocompetent patients. After 1 year of continuous suppressive therapy, discontinuation of therapy should be discussed with the patient to assess the patient's psychological adjustment to genital herpes and rate of recurrent episodes, as the frequency of recurrences decreases over time in many patients. Insufficient experience with famciclovir and valacyclovir prevents recommendation of these drugs for more than 1 year.

Suppressive treatment with acyclovir reduces but does not eliminate asymptomatic viral shedding. Therefore, the extent to which suppressive therapy may prevent HSV transmission is unknown.

Modified from the Centers for Disease Control and Prevention: 1998 guidelines for treatment of sexually transmitted diseases, *MMWR* 47:RR1, 1998.

BOX 262-4

1998 GUIDELINES FOR TREATMENT OF SEXUALLY TRANSMITTED DISEASES—cont'd

Genital Herpes Simplex Virus (HSV) Infection—cont'd

Recurrent episodes of HSV disease—cont'd

RECOMMENDED REGIMENS FOR EPISODIC RECURRENT INFECTION

Acyclovir 400 mg orally three times a day for 5 days, OR

Acyclovir 200 mg orally five times a day for 5 days, OR

Acyclovir 800 mg orally twice a day for 5 days, OR

Famciclovir 125 mg orally twice a day for 5 days, OR

Valacyclovir 500 mg orally twice a day for 5 days

RECOMMENDED REGIMENS FOR DAILY SUPPRESSIVE THERAPY

Acyclovir 400 mg orally twice a day, OR

Famciclovir 250 mg orally twice a day, OR

Valacyclovir 500 mg orally once a day, OR

Valacyclovir 1,000 mg orally once a day

Valacyclovir 500 mg once a day appears less effective than other valacyclovir dosing regimens in patients who have very frequent recurrences (i.e., at least 10 episodes per year). Few comparative studies of valacyclovir and famciclovir with acyclovir have been conducted. The results of these studies suggest that valacyclovir and famciclovir are comparable to acyclovir in clinical outcome. However, valacyclovir and famciclovir may provide increased ease in administration, which is an important consideration for prolonged treatment.

Primary and Secondary Syphilis

Treatment

Parenteral penicillin G has been used effectively for four decades to achieve a local cure (i.e., healing of lesions and prevention of sexual transmission) and to prevent late sequelae. However, no adequately conducted comparative trials have been performed to guide the selection of an optimal penicillin regimen (i.e., the dose, duration, and preparation). Substantially fewer data are available concerning nonpenicillin regimens.

RECOMMENDED REGIMEN FOR ADULTS

Patients who have primary or secondary syphilis should be treated with the following regimen:

Benzathine penicillin G 2.4 million units IM in a single dose

RECOMMENDED REGIMEN FOR CHILDREN

After the newborn period, children in whom syphilis is diagnosed should have a CSF examination to detect asymptomatic neurosyphilis, and birth and maternal medical records should be reviewed to assess whether the child has congenital or acquired syphilis. Children with acquired primary or secondary syphilis should be evaluated (including consultation with child-protection services) and treated by using the following pediatric regimen.

Benzathine penicillin G 50,000 units/kg IM, up to the adult dose of 2.4 million units in a single dose

Other management considerations

All patients who have syphilis should be tested for HIV infection. In geographical areas in which the prevalence of HIV is high, patients who have primary syphilis should be retested for HIV after 3 months if the first HIV test result was negative. This recommendation will become particularly important if it can be demonstrated that intensive antiviral therapy administered soon after HIV seroconversion is beneficial.

Patients who have syphilis and who also have symptoms or signs suggesting neurological disease (e.g., meningitis) or ophthalmic disease (e.g., uveitis) should be evaluated fully for neurosyphilis and syphilitic eye disease; this evaluation should include CSF analysis and ocular slit-lamp examination. Such patients should be treated appropriately according to the results of this evaluation.

Invasion of CSF by *T. pallidum* accompanied by CSF abnormalities is common among adults who have primary or secondary syphilis. However, neurosyphilis develops in only a few patients after treatment with the regimens described in this report. Therefore, unless clinical signs or symptoms of neurological or ophthalmic involvement are present, lumbar puncture is not recommended for routine evaluation of patients who have primary or secondary syphilis.

Follow-up

Treatment failures can occur with any regimen. However, assessing response to treatment often is difficult, and no definitive criteria for cure or failure have been established. Serological test titers may decline more slowly for patients who previously had syphilis. Patients should be reexamined clinically and serologically at both 6 months and 12 months; more frequent evaluation may be prudent if follow-up is uncertain.

Patients who have signs or symptoms that persist or recur or who have a sustained fourfold increase in nontreponemal test titer (i.e., in comparison with either the baseline titer or a subsequent result) probably failed treatment or were reinfected. These patients should be retreated after reevaluation for HIV infection. Unless reinfection with *T. pallidum* is certain, a lumbar puncture also should be performed.

Failure of nontreponemal test titers to decline fourfold within 6 months after therapy for primary or secondary syphilis identifies persons at risk for treatment failure. Such persons should be reevaluated for HIV infection. Optimal management of such patients is unclear. At a minimum, these patients should have additional clinical and serologic follow-up. HIV-infected patients should be evaluated more frequently (i.e., at 3-month intervals instead of 6-month intervals). If additional follow-up cannot be ensured, retreatment is recommended. Some experts recommend CSF examination in such situations.

Continued

BOX 262-4

1998 GUIDELINES FOR TREATMENT OF SEXUALLY TRANSMITTED DISEASES—cont'd

Primary and Secondary Syphilis—cont'd

Follow-up—cont'd

When patients are retreated, most experts recommend retreatment with three weekly injections of benzathine penicillin G 2.4 million units IM, unless CSF examination indicates that neurosyphilis is present.

Latent Syphilis

Latent syphilis is defined as those periods after infection with *T. pallidum* when patients are seroreactive but demonstrate no other evidence of disease. Patients who have latent syphilis and who acquired syphilis within the preceding year are classified as having early latent syphilis. Patients can be demonstrated as having early latent syphilis if, within the year preceding the evaluation, they had a) a documented seroconversion, b) unequivocal symptoms of primary or secondary syphilis, or c) a sex partner who had primary, secondary, or early latent syphilis. Almost all other patients have latent syphilis of unknown duration and should be managed as if they had late latent syphilis. Nontreponemal serological titers usually are higher during early latent syphilis than late latent syphilis. However, early latent syphilis cannot be reliably distinguished from late latent syphilis solely on the basis of nontreponemal titers. Regardless of the level of the nontreponemal titers, patients in whom the illness does not meet the definition of early latent syphilis should be treated as if they have late latent infection. All sexually active women with reactive nontreponemal serological tests should have a pelvic examination before syphilis staging is completed to evaluate for internal mucosal lesions. All patients who have syphilis should be tested for HIV infection.

Treatment

Treatment of latent syphilis is intended to prevent occurrence or progression of late complications. Although clinical experience supports the effectiveness of penicillin in achieving these goals, limited evidence is available for guidance in choosing specific regimens. There is minimal evidence to support the use of nonpenicillin regimens.

RECOMMENDED REGIMENS FOR ADULTS

The following regimens are recommended for nonallergic patients who have normal CSF examination (if performed):

Early latent syphilis:

Benzathine penicillin G 2.4 million units IM in a single dose

Late latent syphilis or latent syphilis of unknown duration:

Benzathine penicillin G 7.2 million units total, administered as three doses of 2.4 million units IM each at 1-week intervals

Follow-up

Quantitative nontreponemal serologic tests should be repeated at 6, 12, and 24 months. Limited data are available to guide evaluation of the treatment response for patients who have latent syphilis. Patients should be evaluated for neurosyphilis and retreated appropriately if a) titers increase fourfold, b) an initially high titer (at least 1:32) fails to decline at least fourfold (i.e., two dilutions) within 12 to 24 months, or c) signs or symptoms attributable to syphilis develop in the patient.

Pelvic Inflammatory Disease (PID)

PID comprises a spectrum of inflammatory disorders of the upper female genital tract, including any combination of endometritis, salpingitis, tubo-ovarian abscess, and pelvic peritonitis. Sexually transmitted organisms, especially *N. gonorrhoeae* and *C. trachomatis,* are implicated in most cases; however, microorganisms that can be part of the vaginal flora (e.g., anaerobes, *Gardnerella vaginalis, Haemophilus influenzae,* enteric gram-negative rods, and *Streptococcus agalactiae*) also can cause PID. In addition, *M. hominis* and *U. urealyticum* might be etiological agents of PID.

Treatment

PID treatment regimens must provide empiric, broad-spectrum coverage of likely pathogens. Antimicrobial coverage should include *N. gonorrhoeae, C. trachomatis,* anaerobes, Gram-negative facultative bacteria, and streptococci. Although several antimicrobial regimens have been effective in achieving a clinical and microbiologic cure in randomized clinical trials with short-term follow-up, few investigations have a) assessed and compared these regimens with regard to elimination of infection in the endometrium and fallopian tubes or b) determined the incidence of long-term complications (e.g., tubal infertility and ectopic pregnancy).

All regimens should be effective against *N. gonorrhoeae* and *C. trachomatis,* because negative endocervical screening does not preclude upper-reproductive tract infection. Although the need to eradicate anaerobes from women who have PID has not been determined definitively, the evidence suggests that this may be important. Anaerobic bacteria have been isolated from the upper-reproductive tract of women who have PID, and data from in vitro studies have revealed that anaerobes such as *Bacteroides fragilis* can cause tubal and epithelial destruction. In addition, bacterial vaginosis also is diagnosed in many women who have PID. Until treatment regimens that do not adequately cover these microbes have been shown to prevent sequelae as well as the regimens that are effective against these microbes, the recommended regimens should have anaerobic coverage. Treatment should be initiated as soon as the presumptive diagnosis has been made, because prevention of long-term sequelae has been linked directly with immediate administration of appropriate antibiotics. When selecting a treatment regimen, health care providers should consider availability, cost, patient acceptance, and antimicrobial susceptibility.

Modified from the Centers for Disease Control and Prevention: 1998 guidelines for treatment of sexually transmitted diseases, *MMWR* 47:RR1, 1998.

BOX 262-4

1998 GUIDELINES FOR TREATMENT OF SEXUALLY TRANSMITTED DISEASES—cont'd

Pelvic Inflammatory Disease (PID)—cont'd

Treatment—cont'd

There are no efficacy data comparing parenteral with oral regimens. Experts have extensive experience with both of the following regimens. Also, there are multiple randomized trials demonstrating the efficacy of each regimen. Although most trials have used parenteral treatment for at least 48 hours after the patient demonstrates substantial clinical improvement, this is an arbitrary designation. Clinical experience should guide decisions regarding transition to oral therapy, which may be accomplished within 24 hours of clinical improvement.

PARENTERAL REGIMEN A

Cefotetan 2 g IV every 12 hours, OR

Cefoxitin 2 g IV every 6 hours, PLUS

Doxycycline 100 mg IV or orally every 12 hours

NOTE: Because of pain associated with infusion, doxycycline should be administered orally when possible, even when the patient is hospitalized. Both oral and IV administration of doxycycline provide similar bioavailability. In the event that IV administration is necessary, use of lidocaine or other short-acting local anesthetic, heparin, or steroids with a steel needle or extension of the infusion time may reduce infusion complications. Parenteral therapy may be discontinued 24 hours after a patient improves clinically, and oral therapy with doxycycline (100 mg twice a day) should continue for a total of 14 days. When tuboovarian abscess is present, many health-care providers use clindamycin or metronidazole with doxycycline for continued therapy rather than doxycycline alone, because they provide more effective anaerobic coverage.

Clinical data are limited regarding the use of other second- or third-generation cephalosporins (e.g., ceftizoxime, cefotaxime, and ceftriaxone), which also might be effective therapy for PID and might replace cefotetan or cefoxitin. However, they are less active than cefotetan or cefoxitin against anaerobic bacteria.

PARENTERAL REGIMEN B

Clindamycin 900 mg IV every 8 hours, PLUS

Gentamicin loading dose IV or IM (2 mg/kg of body weight), followed by a maintenance dose (1.5 mg/kg) every 8 hours. Single daily dosing may be substituted

NOTE: Although use of a single daily dose of gentamicin has not been evaluated for the treatment of PID, it is efficacious in other analogous situations. Parenteral therapy may be discontinued 24 hours after a patient improves clinically, and continuing oral therapy should consist of doxycycline 100 mg orally twice a day or clindamycin 450 mg orally four times a day to complete a total of 14 days of therapy. When tuboovarian abscess is present, many health-care providers use clindamycin for continued therapy rather than doxycycline, because clindamycin provides more effective anaerobic coverage.

Oral treatment

As with parenteral regimens, clinical trials of outpatient regimens have provided minimal information, regarding intermediate and long-term outcome. The following regimens provide coverage against the frequent etiological agents of PID, but evidence from clinical trials supporting their use is limited. Patients who do not respond to oral therapy within 72 hours should be reevaluated to confirm the diagnosis and be administered parenteral therapy on either an outpatient or inpatient basis.

REGIMEN A

Ofloxacin 400 mg orally twice a day for 14 days, PLUS

Metronidazole 500 mg orally twice a day for 14 days

Oral ofloxacin has been investigated as a single agent in two well-designed clinical trials, and it is effective against both *N. gonorrhoeae* and *C. trachomatis.* Despite the results of these trials, ofloxacin's lack of anaerobic coverage is a concern; the addition of metronidazole provides this coverage.

REGIMEN B

Ceftriazone 250 mg IM once, OR

Cefoxitin 2 g IM plus Probenecid 1 g orally in a single dose concurrently once, OR

Other parenteral third-generation cephalosporin (e.g., ceftizoxime or cefotaxime), PLUS

Doxycycline 100 mg orally twice a day for 14 days (Include this regimen with one of the above regimens.)

The optimal choice of a cephalosporin for Regimen B is unclear; although cefoxitin has better anaerobic coverage, ceftriaxone has better coverage against *N. gonorrhoeae.* Clinical trials have demonstrated that a single dose of cefoxitin is effective in obtaining short-term clinical response in women who have PID; however, the theoretical limitations in its coverage of anaerobes may require the addition of metronidazole (see Regimen A). The metronidazole also will effectively treat bacterial vaginosis, which is frequently associated with PID. No data have been published regarding the use of oral cephalosporins for the treatment of PID.

Proctitis, Proctocolitis, and Enteritis

Sexually transmitted gastrointestinal syndromes include proctitis, proctocolitis, and enteritis. Proctitis occurs predominantly among persons who participate in anal intercourse, and enteritis occurs among those whose sexual practices include oral-fecal contact. Proctocolitis can be acquired by either route, depending on the pathogen. Evaluation should include appropriate diagnostic procedures (e.g., anoscopy or sigmoidoscopy, stool examination, and culture).

Proctitis is an inflammation limited to the rectum (the distal 10 to 12 cm) that is associated with anorectal pain, tenesmus, and rectal discharge. *N. gonorrhoeae, C. trachomatis, T. pallidum,* and HSV usually

Continued

BOX 262-4

1998 GUIDELINES FOR TREATMENT OF SEXUALLY TRANSMITTED DISEASES—cont'd

Proctitis, Proctocolitis, and Enteritis—cont'd

are the sexually transmitted pathogens involved. In patients coinfected with HIV, herpes proctitis may be especially severe.

Proctocolitis is associated with symptoms of proctitis plus diarrhea and/or abdominal cramps and inflammation of the colonic musoca extending to 12 cm. Fecal leukocytes may be detected on stool examination depending on the pathogen. Pathogenic organisms include *Campylobacter* sp., *Shigella* sp., *Entamoeba histolytica,* and, rarely, *C. trachomatis.* CMV or other opportunistic agents may be involved in immunosuppressed HIV-infected patients.

Enteritis usually results in diarrhea and abdominal cramping without signs of proctitis or proctocolitis. In otherwise healthy patients, *Giardia lamblia* is most frequently implicated. Among HIV-infected patients, other infections that usually are not sexually transmitted may occur, including those caused by CMV, *Mycobacterium avium-intracellulare, Salmonella* sp., *Cryptosporidium, Microsporidium,* and *Isospora.* Multiple stool examinations may be necessary to detect *Giardia,* and special stool preparations are required to diagnose cryptosporidiosis and microsporidiosis. Additionally, enteritis may be a primary effect of HIV infection.

When laboratory diagnostic capabilities are available, treatment should be based on the specific diagnosis. Diagnostic and treatment recommendations for all enteric infections are beyond the scope of these guidelines.

Treatment

Acute proctitis of recent onset among persons who have recently practiced receptive anal intercourse is most often sexually transmitted. Such patients should be examined by anoscopy and should be evaluated for infection with HSV, *N. gonorrhoeae, C. trachomatis,* and *T. pallidum.* If anorectal pus is found on examination, or if polymorphonuclear leukocytes are found on a Gram-stained smear of anorectal secretions, the following therapy may be prescribed pending results of additional laboratory tests.

RECOMMENDED REGIMEN

Ceftriaxone 125 mg IM (or another agent effective against anal and genital gonorrhea), PLUS

Doxycycline 100 mg orally twice a day for 7 days

Modified from the Centers for Disease Control and Prevention: 1998 guidelines for treatment of sexually transmitted diseases, *MMWR* 47:RR1, 1998.

at all. In large-scale studies, approximately 2% of sexually active males have been shown to be infected with gonorrhea; 70% of these were asymptomatic. The proportion of women with infection who are asymptomatic is unclear; estimates range from 25% to 80%. The gonococcus can cause pharyngitis and proctitis; females may harbor the organism in the rectum, even though they do not engage in anal intercourse.

The gonococcus can be grown from urethral or cervical discharge; from swabs of the vagina, cervix, urethra, pharynx, or rectum; and in many instances from urine sediment. Historically, the diagnosis of gonococcal infection rested on culture or on the classic findings of white blood cells and gram-negative intracellular diplococci in Gram stains of discharge or material obtained from a urethral swab. Even under ideal conditions, the organism can be difficult to grow, and each physician should be familiar with the yield from the laboratory he or she uses. In the male, a typical Gram stain from a urethral discharge is diagnostic (Fig. 262-4). For samples taken from females, sorting out gram-negative organisms that truly are intracellular versus those that may be overlying or near the cells is more difficult. However, when at least eight pairs of such diplococci are seen in at least two polymorphonuclear leukocytes, the culture will be positive 96% of the time.

As is the case with chlamydia, diagnosis of *N. gonorrhoeae* infections is now possible by amplified DNA testing. These tests are at least as sensitive as culture results but have the added advantage of eliminating the need for pelvic examination or swabbing the urethral meatus to obtain specimens; instead, a urine specimen can be used.[18]

Uncomplicated gonococcal infections can be treated with any of the following single-dose regimens: 400 mg cefixime orally, 125 mg ceftriaxone intramuscularly, 500 mg ciprofloxacin orally, or 400 mg ofloxacin orally (see Box 262-4). Because of the high likelihood that coinfection with chlamydia is present, any treatment for gonorrhea must include an effective regimen for *Chlamydia trachomatis* as well (azithromycin or doxycycline). Pharyngeal infection is more difficult to treat than infection at other sites; only the doses of ceftriaxone, ciprofloxacin or ofloxacin listed above are indicated for treatment. Again, because of the possibility of coinfection with chlamydia, azithromycin or doxycycline also should be administered.

Gonorrhea also may produce epididymitis and pelvic inflammatory disease. In addition and in contrast to chlamydia, the gonococcal organism has the capacity to become bloodborne and can lead to what has been called the arthritis-dermatitis syndrome, or disseminated gonococcal infection (DGI). About 1% to 3% of untreated patients develop DGI; women, especially pregnant women, are more likely to develop DGI, as are adolescents with pharyngeal infection. Strains of *N. gonorrhoeae* that lead to DGI characteristically tend to cause little in the way of genital symptoms. Typically, the patient develops fever (although not always) and may have anorexia or malaise or both. Skin lesions then appear, generally distributed on the extremities (arms more often than legs). These lesions typically are erythematous macules less than 5 mm in diameter; they become pustular and occasionally hemorrhagic or necrotic. They most often are noticed near the small joints of the hands and feet. Such lesions last several days, during which time, blood cultures are positive in 25% of cases. Accompanying the dermatitis is a teno-

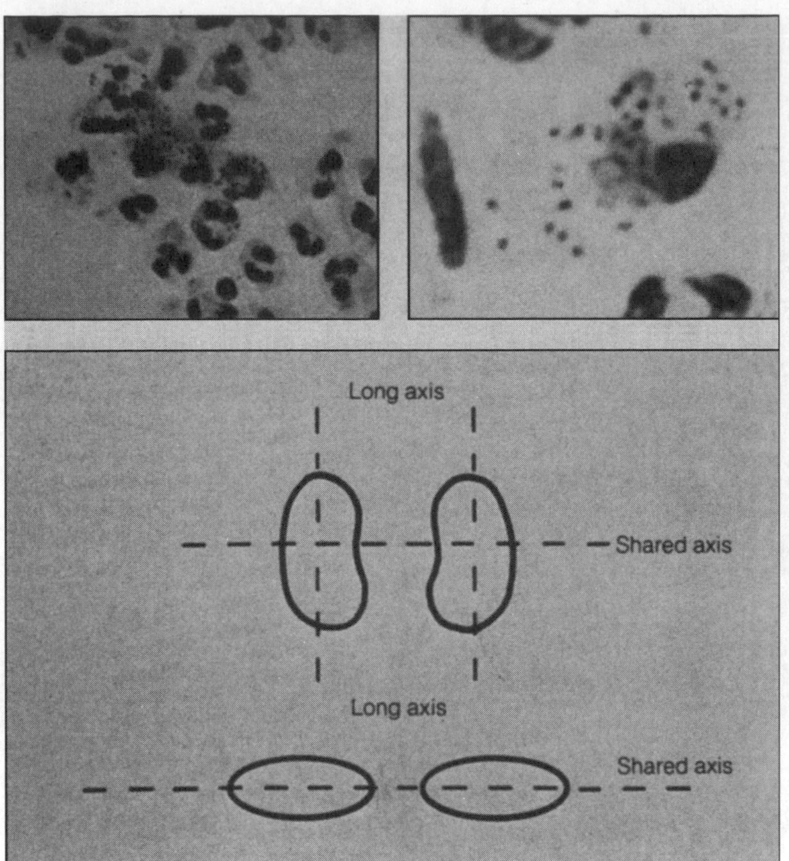

Fig. 262-4 *Neisseria gonorrhoeae* on Gram stain of male urethral smears (×1500 and ×4000) appear as tiny gram-negative diplococci within polymorphonuclear leukocytes pink-stained nuclei). *Neisseria* organisms are kidney bean-shaped, and their long axes are perpendicular to the shared axis, as shown in the diagram.

(From Gilchrist MJR, Rauch JL: *Contemp Pediatr* 4:54, 1987.)

synovitis that tends to occur over the extensor and flexor tendons of the hands and feet.

In general, once the tenosynovitis and dermatitis clear, the patient develops polyarthralgias but usually seeks care only at the point that an oligoarthritis develops. The knee is the joint most commonly infected, followed by the elbow, ankle, and small joints of the hands and feet. Hence, among adolescents, DGI should be considered in the differential diagnosis of septic arthritis. Aspirates of joint fluid reveal the typical changes of septic arthritis, but joint fluid cultures usually are negative. Meningitis or endocarditis may also be present. Patients with DGI, especially those with arthritis, should be hospitalized for treatment (see Box 262-4).

Genital Warts (Human Papillomavirus)

Infections with human papillomavirus (HPV) are the most prevalent STD in the United States. Such infections have always drawn attention because they cause unsightly warts (condylomata acuminatum), and, among adolescent girls, HPV infection represents the most common cause of abnormal Pap smears. Recent concerns about HPV focus on its role in the development of cervical neoplasia.[10]

More than 70 different types of HPV have been identified: "benign" genital warts usually are caused by types 6 and 11; types 16,18, 31, 33, 35, 45, 51, 52 and 56 are associated most commonly with squamous intraepithelial neoplasia (SIL) changes on Pap smear. These types have the oncogenic potential to transform normal cells into malignant ones. An individual can be infected with more than one type. HPV infection has been associated with more than 90% of cervical dysplasia worldwide.

As with other STDs, infection rates among adolescents and young adults are quite high—up to 40% in some studies. Detection of infection is not always easy. Although 50% to 60% of women who have external genital warts have cervical infection, only 3% to 6% of those who have cervical disease have external genital warts. Hence, offering Pap smears to all sexually active females is extremely important in screening for infection, even among those who have no visible signs of external genital infection.

Males constitute a significant reservoir of undetected HPV infection. In one study, only 21 of 156 male partners of HPV positive women had clinical evidence of warts. However, with use of magnification and acetic acid "soaks" to produce the "acetowhite" changes seen in HPV-infected skin, 77% of male partners were shown to be infected (Fig. 262-5). Almost all data regarding HPV among males is drawn from samples aged 18 and over; very few data exist on younger adolescent males.

Overt warts develop in roughly two thirds of persons having intercourse with an infected individual. Visible warts usually develop in 6 weeks to 8 months, but the length of the incubation period may be even longer. The typical pedunculated wart with a keratotic and irregular surface is easy to recognize, but warts also may be flat and more difficult to detect. The use of a handheld magnifying glass or even a colposcope is extremely helpful. Among males, warts usually are seen on the penile shaft, prepuce, frenulum, corona, and glans but also may be present on the skin of the scrotum and the anus (Fig. 262-6). The presence of anal warts often is

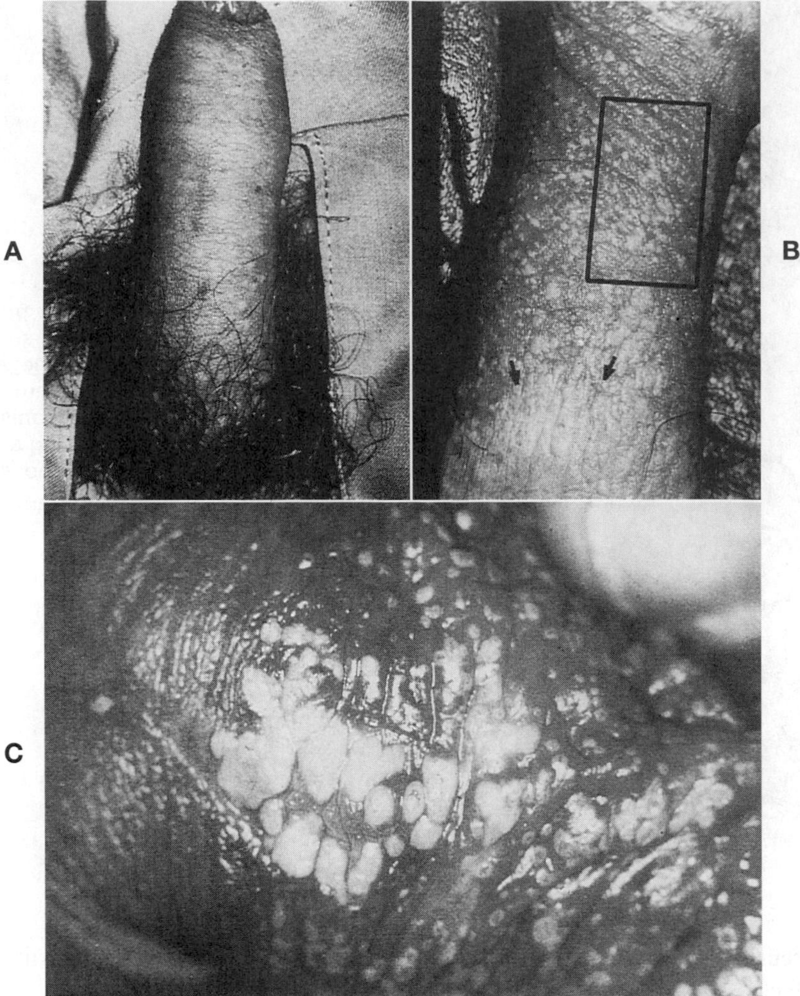

Fig. 262-5 Demonstration of subclinical lesions. **A,** Appearance of penis before acetic acid application. **B,** Penis after 5-minute application of gauze soaked in 5% acetic acid. Note coalescing sheets *(arrows)* and discrete dots of acetowhite staining *(inset).* **C,** Magnified view of apparent subclinical human papillomavirus infection shown in **B.**

(From Ketelaris PM, et al: *J Urol* 140:302, 1988.)

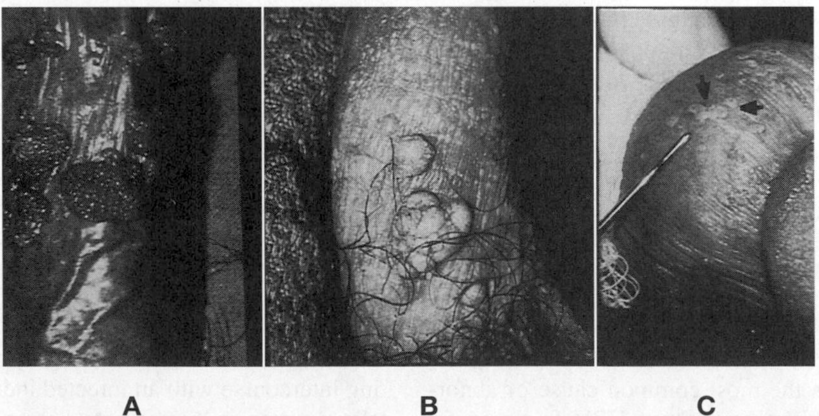

Fig. 262-6 Morphology of macroscopic warts. **A,** Condylomata demonstrated by preputial retraction. **B,** Verrucous wart at penoscrotal junction. **C,** Small, flat warts *(arrows)* on distal third of penis.

(From Ketelaris PM, et al: *J Urol* 140:302, 1988.)

associated with anal receptive intercourse, but warts in this location have been described in males who deny this type of behavior. Occasionally, warts are seen at the urethral opening.

The posterior vaginal introitus, labia minora, and vestibule represent the most common sites of infection among females (Fig. 262-7); again, however, warts can be seen anywhere on the external or internal genitalia. Subclinical disease is most likely to occur on the cervix; the relatively large transformation zone of the maturing adolescent cervix affords a hospitable site of infection for the virus. Extensive disease in males or females should raise the possibility of underlying HIV disease.

Evidence continues to accumulate linking the presence of HPV with the development of dysplastic and malignant changes in the cervix.[13] Hence, the role of the routine Pap smear in the care of sexually active teenagers has assumed increased importance. Depending on the clinical situation, some females who have (1) atypical squamous cells of undetermined significance (ASCUS), (2) low-grade squamous intraepithelial lesions (LGSIL), representing the previous diagnostic category of carcinoma in situ type 1 (CIN1), or (3) high-grade squamous intraepithelial lesions (HGSIL, previously referred to as CIN2 or CIN3) may need immediate referral for colposcopy.

Guidelines for management of abnormal Pap smears have been developed by Kurman.[12] Better management of women with abnormal Pap smears requires a clearer understanding of the natural history of HPV infection and risk factors for persistence of infection. Recent data indicate that the median duration of new infections was 8 months and that 70% of women had HPV regression by 24 months. Risk factors for persistent infection included infection with multiple types of HPV and infection with a high-risk type such as 16 or 18. However, 88% of women with persistently positive HPV tests for high risk types did not develop HGSIL during the course of the study.[8,11]

A variety of treatments for genital warts exist, including those applied by the patient (see Box 262-4); treatment is primarily directed towards symptomatic warts. There is no

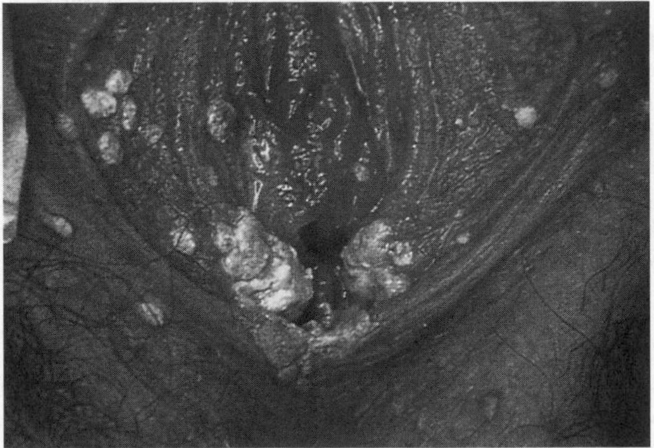

Fig. 262-7 Condyloma acuminatum of the vulva appears as a polypoid mass with a keratotic fissured and irregular surface.

(From Moscicki B: *Contemp Pediatr* 6:24, 1989.)

evidence that the natural history of infection or of dysplasia is altered by treatment or that treatment reduces an individual's infectivity. Each physician who chooses to treat genital warts should determine which technique is most suitable to his or her practice and become familiar with that technique. Regardless of which approach is chosen, careful follow-up (initially at weekly intervals) is essential to monitor the results and prevent regrowth between too widely spaced treatment intervals. The benefit of treating subclinical HPV infection in the absence of cervical dysplasia is unclear. Examination and treatment of sex partners is of uncertain benefit.

Because HPV infection is so prevalent and treatment does not alter the natural course of the infection, current approaches to the prevention and eradication of HPV infection and the treatment of abnormal PAP smears are focusing on HPV vaccines. Preliminary evidence indicates that these vaccines may be useful in preventing or eradicating infection and in causing regression of abnormal PAP smears and precancerous lesions.[9,16]

Herpes Genitalis

Herpes simplex viral infections of the male and female genital tract are particularly distressing to patients because of the high likelihood of recurrence after an initial episode. Both herpes simplex type 1 (HSV-1) and type 2 (HSV-2) can cause genital tract disease, although type 2 infections still tend to predominate. Infection rates have increased in the 1980s and the 1990s. Although genital herpes infections were believed at one time to be associated with the development of cervical cancer, current evidence indicates that HSV more likely acts as a cofactor.

Infections with the virus can be classified as primary or nonprimary. Primary infection refers to infection with HSV-1 or HSV-2 in an individual without prior antibody to either virus. Nonprimary infection occurs in those with existing antibody to either type 1 or type 2 who become infected with the other strain. This type of infection, almost always occurring in individuals who have existing antibody to type 1 who then become infected with type 2, tends to be less symptomatic.

In primary infection, symptoms usually occur within 2 to 20 days after sexual exposure. The patient experiences burning or itching at the site of inoculation, followed by erythema and the development of discrete vesicles. Initially the vesicles contain clear fluid, but they rapidly form pustules with an erythematous base. Typically, a patient may have 15 to 30 vesicles, each full of infectious viral particles. Lesions are located on the vulva, cervix, clitoris, or perineum. In males they may occur on the penile shaft, glans, or prepuce. Infection also can involve the urethra, leading to dysuria or urinary retention. Vesicles can be seen on the thighs, buttocks, groin, or perianal region as a result of autoinoculation or anal receptive intercourse.

Because primary infection represents the first episode of infection with the particular virus type, systemic symptoms such as fever, malaise, and headache are common. About 50% of patients have tender inguinal lymphadenopathy.

After 2 to 4 days, the pustules break open and coalesce to form wet ulcers. This is usually the time at which patients are seen by physicians. New lesions still may be developing at this point (with a peak at 7 to 11 days), but within 20 days all the lesions have crusted over, and the pain and other symptoms have disappeared. Herpetic lesions generally heal without scarring.

The diagnosis of herpes genitalis is made most often on clinical grounds. Cultures of intact vesicles generally are positive, as are cultures of the cervix. A Tzanck preparation or a Wright-Giemsa stain of a scraping from an ulcer demonstrates the presence of multinucleated giant cells.

Following resolution of the infection, the virus remains latent in the sacral ganglia and may reactivate at any time. This reactivation is referred to as recurrent disease. Recurrences may occur in association with stress, local trauma, fever, or menstruation and tend to be shorter, less symptomatic, and lacking in systemic symptoms. Vesicles usually occur near the initial infection site but tend to be fewer in number. Just before the recurrence, the patient may experience burning or itching at the site of infection. Healing takes place within 1 to 2 weeks.

Females whose only site of recurrence involves the cervix may be unaware of it, although they are shedding the virus. About one third of males also may have inapparent recurrences but still are infectious. Asymptomatic reactivation is most likely to happen within 6 months after the initial infection. Hence, unless sex partners reveal their history of infection, many exposures can occur without an individual being aware that he or she has come into contact with the virus. Recent prospective studies indicate that many HSV seropositive patients who deny a history of genital herpes actually have lesions that they fail to recognize as herpetic. Nevertheless, they are capable of infecting their sex partners.

The risk of recurrence depends on a number of factors. Males are somewhat more likely to have recurrent disease, as are those individuals whose infection was caused by HSV-2. In one study, 86% of patients who had HSV-1 infection *did not* have recurrences, compared with 40% of those who had HSV-2. Once a second episode occurs, the patient is likely to have multiple recurrences.

Development of antiviral drugs such as acyclovir, famciclovir, or valacyclovir has altered the nature of herpes therapy dramatically. These agents significantly reduce the symptoms associated with primary episodes of genital herpes and decrease both the duration of viral shedding and the time to resolution of lesions (see Box 262-4). Some patients who have recurrent disease may derive benefit from therapy if the medication can be started during the prodrome or within 1 day after onset of lesions. Those who have six or more recurrences per year have a 75% reduction in recurrences with daily suppressive therapy (see Box 262-4). Two recent randomized controlled trials of a glycoprotein vaccine for prevention of HSV-2 infection showed a protective effect at 5 months but not at 1 year for those receiving the vaccine.[6]

Syphilis

In 1990, an epidemic of syphilis occurred in the United States; since then syphilis rates have declined. On the other hand, given that more than 16,000 cases occurred in 1995 and that genital ulcer disease increases one's risk for acquiring HIV infection, clinicians must remain knowledgeable about this infection.

The typical chancre of syphilis develops at the site of intimate sexual contact approximately 2 to 3 weeks after exposure to an infected individual (range 10 to 90 days). This lesion, varying from a few millimeters to a few centimeters, is clean-based, painless, and has sharply demarcated, indurated borders. Multiple ulcers may be present. Lymphadenopathy is usually present, often bilaterally. Because the ulcer is painless, its appearance in the vagina or rectum or even in the mouth is likely to go unnoticed. While the ulcer is present, the exudate overlying it is highly infectious. Untreated, the chancre disappears in 3 to 6 weeks.

The rash of secondary syphilis appears 4 to 10 weeks after the chancre appears in the untreated patient. Hence, the rash and the chancre may coexist. Because the spirochetes spread hematogenously from the site of initial infection, constitutional symptoms such as fever, malaise, sore throat, and generalized lymphadenopathy may be present.

The rash typically is papulosquamous but can be macular or pustular. Initially, it involves the trunk and flexor surfaces of the arms but then spreads to the entire body, including the palms and soles, and mucous membranes. Hence, any sexually active adolescent with a generalized eruption (such as that seen with pityriasis rosea) should be screened for syphilis. Annular papules can appear on the face, and the rash can resemble impetigo or eczema. Sometimes moist, fissured papules or elevated, thickened papules (condyloma lata) are seen; both are highly infectious. Finally, loss of scalp or eyebrow hair can be associated with secondary syphilis. The rash disappears spontaneously 3 to 12 weeks after its appearance; at this point, the patient is classified as having latent syphilis.

At the time the chancre is present, a darkfield examination of the nonbloody exudate should be performed by someone expert in darkfield microscopy. If performed on 3 successive days, the likelihood of obtaining a positive result from an infected individual is extremely high. If the results of all three examinations are negative, the diagnosis of primary syphilis should be reconsidered.

If the darkfield examination is unavailable, a serological test for syphilis should be obtained. A variety of tests for detecting syphilis are available; their relative sensitivities and specificities are outlined in Table 262-1. If the examiner is relatively certain that the chancre is one of primary syphilis, he or she should request the fluorescent treponemal antibody-absorption (FTA-ABS) test, since the sensitivity of the Venereal Disease Research Laboratory (VDRL) flocculation test, the rapid plasma reagin (RPR) test and the microhemagglutination assay for antibody to *T. pallidium* (MHA-TP) at this point in the disease process are relatively low. Alternatively, a second specimen can be obtained 2 to 4 weeks later.

In one study of 59 urban adolescents diagnosed with syphilis, only a minority (15%) presented with a chancre, 24% presented with a rash, and 20% had adenopathy. The majority (46%) were identified only through routine serological screening, underscoring the importance of testing at-risk youth.

The recommended CDC treatment guidelines for primary and secondary syphilis are outlined in Box 262-4. Follow-up with repeat serological tests should occur at 6-month intervals until the RPR reverts to negative. The FTA-ABS test

Table 262-1 Comparison of Diagnostic Tests for Syphilis

	Sensitivity and Specificity of Serological Tests for Syphilis* at Different Stages							
	Percent Sensitivity (Sens.) and Specificity (Spec.)							
	VDRL		RPR		FTA-ABS		MHA-TP	
Stage of Syphilis	**Sens.**	**Spec.**	**Sens.**	**Spec.**	**Sens.**	**Spec.**	**Sens.**	**Spec.**
Primary	80 (59-87)	98 (80-99)	86 (81-100)	98 (80-99)	98 (93-100)	98 (84-99)	82 (64-90)	99 (98-100)
Secondary	100 (99-100)	98	100 (99-100)	98	100 (99-100)	98	100 (96-100)	99
Latent	96 (73-100)	98	99	98	100 (96-100)	98	100 (96-100)	99
Late	71	98	73	98	96	98	94	99

From Dans PE: Syphilis. In Barker LR, Burton JR, Zieve PD, editors: *Principles of ambulatory medicine,* ed 2, Baltimore, 1986, Williams & Wilkins.

*The consensus figures for the sensitivity and specificity are for tests done in the Centers for Disease Control Reference Laboratory on samples derived from a well-run STD clinic. The figures in parentheses demonstrate the variability in published reports. Responsible factors include (*a*) study of populations with different prevalences of syphilis and other confounding illnesses, (*b*) variable performance by the laboratory, and (*c*) different clinical criteria for the diagnosis of syphilis.

always remains positive. Criteria for reevaluation or retreatment include persistence or recurrence of clinical signs and symptoms, a sustained fourfold or greater rise in titers, or the persistence of a higher than 1:8 titer for more than 1 year after adequate treatment. All patients with syphilis should be screened for HIV infection. Patients who are seroreactive but do not have any physical findings of infection are classified as having latent syphilis. Patients who are known to have seroconverted within the previous 12 months are classified as early latent syphilis; those for whom the chronology of seroconversion cannot be clearly determined are treated as if they have late latent syphilis. Patients with latent syphilis should be managed according to the guidelines in Box 262-4.

Congenital Syphilis

In 1998, 801 cases of congenital syphilis were reported in the United States; of these, 80% occurred because the mother either failed to receive penicillin therapy or received substandard care before or during her pregnancy. The clinical manifestations of this entirely preventable disease are protean.[7] Infected infants may be identified early in life via routine serological screening or on the basis of various symptoms (early congenital syphilis). Alternatively, some may escape detection and appear after 2 years of age with the sequelae of untreated infection (late congenital syphilis).

Most infected liveborn infants (congenital syphilis is a major cause of stillbirths) are asymptomatic. Common signs of infection include hepatomegaly (with or without splenomegaly or jaundice), nephrotic syndrome (limb edema and proteinuria), eye abnormalities (chorioretinitis, glaucoma, uveitis), generalized nontender lymphadenopathy (especially involving the epitrochlear nodes), anemia or thrombocytopenia or both, persistent rhinitis (snuffles), which can be clear, blood tinged, or purulent, and intrauterine growth retardation. Involvement of the central nervous system can mimic bacterial meningitis, although the cerebrospinal fluid (CSF) generally shows a monocytosis with an elevated protein and a normal glucose level.

Skin manifestations also are extremely important. Congenital syphilis always should be suspected when an infant has a persistent diaper rash or an exanthem involving the palms and soles. Mucocutaneous fissuring of the mouth and lips (rhagades) may be present. About 30% to 60% of infected infants have skin lesions, the most common being a large, round, pink macule that turns coppery and fades in 1 to 3 months without treatment. The lesions tend to spare the anterior trunk. A fine scale may cover the involved areas. The rash also can be vesiculobullous or, lacking bullae, can manifest as desquamation. Eczematoid, often impetiginized lesions have a predilection for the perineum, for the intertriginous areas, and for the middle third of the face (including the tongue and palate). Darkfield examination or direct fluorescent antibody staining of material obtained by scraping skin lesions provides a straightforward confirmation for the diagnosis of congenital syphilis.

Some two thirds of infants also have bony involvement, although in many cases this can be detected only by radiological means. The epiphyses involved most commonly are those of the radius, femur, humerus, tibia (saber shins) and fibula, with infection generally in multiple, symmetrical sites. Bony tenderness can lead to decreased movement of the affected limb and thus a false diagnosis of paralysis secondary to birth trauma (pseudoparalysis of Parrot). Frontal bone prominence and nasal bridge depression (saddle nose) also may be present.

Dorfman and Glaser reported on seven infants who had congenital syphilis diagnosed between 3 and 14 weeks of age, six of whom were RPR negative at birth.[8] In four cases, the mothers had a negative serological test at delivery; the other three were not tested because of a negative test before delivery. All the infants had hepatomegaly and elevated serum transaminase levels, but other physical findings were inconstant. To ensure complete identification of all infected children, testing of *both* maternal and infant sera is essential. The Centers for Disease Control and Prevention recommend testing infant serum rather than cord blood because of lower false-positive and -negative rates with this approach. A cerebrospinal fluid VDRL (not RPR) should be performed on all infants suspected of having congenital syphilis.

Box 262-5 lists the CDC criteria for surveillance case definition for congenital syphilis. The diagnosis is more difficult in an asymptomatic infant whose treponemal test for syphilis is positive and whose mother also has a positive test. In this case, consultation with an infectious disease specialist may be warranted to differentiate active infection from passive transfer of maternal antibody.

Infants younger than 4 weeks of age classified as confirmed or presumptive cases of congenital syphilis according to the CDC criteria should be treated for 10 to 14 days with aqueous crystalline penicillin G (100,000 to 150,000 U/kg/day intravenously every 8 to 12 hours). If the infant's mother has not been treated adequately, if it cannot be determined whether the treatment was adequate, or if the infant's mother is HIV antibody positive, a similar regimen should be used. If the mother has been treated adequately, the decision to treat the infant depends on assurances regarding careful follow up and a normal CSF examination. Under optimum circumstances, no treatment is needed at birth, but serial antibody titers should be obtained at 1, 2, 4, 6 and 12 months. Infants who cannot reliably be followed up but who have normal CSF should receive a single dose of benzathine penicillin (50,000 U/kg intramuscularly). Infants older than 4 weeks should be treated with aqueous crystalline penicillin, 200,000 to 300,000 U/kg per day intravenously every 6 hours for 10 to 14 days. Nontreponemal tests should be repeated at 3, 6, and 12 months after treatment or until titers return to zero.

BOX 262-5

SURVEILLANCE CASE DEFINITION FOR CONGENITAL SYPHILIS

For reporting purposes, congenital syphilis includes cases of congenitally acquired syphilis in infants and children, as well as syphilitic stillbirths.

A CONFIRMED CASE of congenital syphilis is an infant in whom *Treponema pallidum* is identified by darkfield microscopy, fluorescent antibody, or other specific stains in specimens from lesions, placenta, umbilical cord, or autopsy material.

A PRESUMPTIVE CASE of congenital syphilis is either of the following:

A. Any infant whose mother had untreated or inadequately treated syphilis at delivery, regardless of findings in the infant

OR

B. Any infant or child who has a reactive treponemal test for syphilis and any one of the following:
   1. Any evidence of congenital syphilis on physical examination or
   2. Any evidence of congenital syphilis on long-bone radiograph or
   3. Reactive cerebrospinal fluid VDRL or
   4. Elevated CSF cell count or protein (without other cause) or
   5. Quantitative nontreponemal serological titers that are fourfold higher than the mother's (both drawn at birth) or
   6. Reactive test for FTA-ABS-19S-IgM antibody

A SYPHILITIC STILLBIRTH is defined as a fetal death in which the mother had untreated or inadequately treated syphilis at delivery of a fetus after a 20-week gestation or of a fetus weighing more than 500 g.

From Congenital syphilis—New York City, 1986-1988, *MMWR* 38:825, 1989.

SYNDROMES ASSOCIATED WITH SEXUALLY TRANSMITTED DISEASES

Pelvic Inflammatory Disease

Pelvic inflammatory disease (PID) refers to infection involving the upper genital tract (uterus, fallopian tubes, ovaries, and pelvis) occurring as a result of undetected or inadequately treated STDs of the lower genital tract (endocervix). In the short term, PID can lead to such problems as a ruptured tuboovarian abscess. In the long run, infertility, chronic pelvic pain, and increased risk for ectopic pregnancy are attributable to this condition, even when the acute episode has been managed appropriately. Among all sexually active females, teenagers under 19 years of age are at greatest risk for contracting this disease; the risk is 1:8 for sexually active 15-year-olds, 1:16 for 16-year-olds but only 1:80 for 24-year-olds.[19] Because a major risk factor for developing PID is a prior episode, adolescent girls who experience this illness early in their reproductive life cycle are at great risk for having further significant problems.

Even though the condition is common, the diagnosis of PID is imprecise. Signs and symptoms can be nonspecific, and the only sure method for diagnosis, laparoscopy, is not routinely performed for diagnostic purposes in this country. Hence pediatricians must maintain a high index of suspicion, obtain a thorough history, and perform a careful physical examination to avoid the pitfalls of misdiagnosis.

When eliciting a history from a patient who has lower abdominal pain, the physician should keep in mind those factors that place an individual at risk for infection. Hence, failure to use barrier methods of contraception, douching, the presence of an intrauterine device (IUD), multiple partners, a recent change in partner, or history of other STDs or PID should raise concern. The presence of a new vaginal discharge (or a change in odor, color, or amount), abnormal menstrual bleeding (increased or prolonged or occurring at the wrong time in the cycle), or dyspareunia all suggest PID. Oral contraceptive pills appear to protect against the development of PID due to chlamydia but not gonorrhea. Whether the newer formulations of oral contraceptive pills also are protective is unknown.

Other symptoms include dysuria, dysmenorrhea (usually more severe than normal), nausea, vomiting, diarrhea, fever, and malaise. Except for dysmenorrhea, these symptoms also can be seen in patients who have diseases of the urinary tract (e.g., pyelonephritis) or gastrointestinal tract (e.g., appendicitis).

Depending on the extent of upper genital tract involvement, physical signs may include pain on cervical movement and endometrial or adnexal tenderness or both. Fever is present in fewer than 50% of patients who have documented PID. If the infection has "tracked" up to involve the capsule of the liver, right upper quadrant tenderness also may be elicited. With extensive infection, signs of peritonitis, particularly rebound tenderness, are present. The palpation of an adnexal mass raises the concern of a coexisting tuboovarian abscess. Mucopus visible in the cervical os strongly suggests the presence of infection, but its absence does not rule out the diagnosis. Acute-phase reactants lack the necessary sensitivity and specificity to be routinely helpful in establishing the diagnosis of PID. Although 60% to 80% of patients have an elevated white blood cell count, sedimentation rate, or C-reactive protein, so do 20% to 50% of patients with abdominal pain who do not have PID. Conversely, it is estimated that up to 60% of cases of PID are subclinical.

In an attempt to guide clinicians and minimize the potential for diagnostic confusion, several investigators have suggested diagnostic criteria for infections localized to the female pelvic organs. The criteria for diagnosing PID are indicated in Box 262-6. Despite use of these diagnostic criteria, several studies have indicated substantial false positive and false negative rates in the diagnosis of PID. The physician should take particular note that certain surgical emergency conditions can mimic PID in their manifestation. Hence one should keep in mind the differential diagnosis, as outlined in Box 262-7. Because many teenagers at risk for PID are similarly at risk for pregnancy and because ectopic pregnancy can mimic PID, a urine or serum pregnancy test should be obtained routinely at the time of evaluation. If an

BOX 262-6

PELVIC INFLAMMATORY DISEASE: DIAGNOSTIC CONSIDERATIONS

Acute PID is difficult to diagnose because of the wide variation in the symptoms and signs. Many women with PID have subtle or mild symptoms that do not readily indicate PID. Consequently, delay in diagnosis and effective treatment probably contributes to inflammatory sequelae in the upper reproductive tract. Laparoscopy can be used to obtain a more accurate diagnosis of salpingitis and a more complete bacteriological diagnosis. However, this diagnostic tool often is not readily available for acute cases, and its use is not easy to justify when symptoms are mild or vague. Moreover, laparoscopy will not detect endometritis and may not detect subtle inflammation of the fallopian tubes. Consequently, a diagnosis of PID usually is based on clinical findings.

The clinical diagnosis of acute PID also is imprecise. Data indicate that a clinical diagnosis of symptomatic PID has a positive predictive value (PPV) of 65% to 90% for salpingitis in comparison with laparoscopy. The PPV of a clinical diagnosis of acute PID differs depending on epidemiological characteristics and the clinical setting, with higher PPV among sexually active young (especially teenaged) women and among patients attending STD clinics or from settings in which rates of gonorrhea or chlamydia are high. In all settings, however, no single historical, physical, or laboratory finding is both sensitive and specific for the diagnosis of acute PID (i.e., can be used both to detect all cases of PID and to exclude all women without PID). Combinations of diagnostic findings that improve either sensitivity (i.e., detect more women who have PID) or specificity (i.e., exclude more women who do not have PID) do so only at the expense of the other. For example, requiring two or more findings excludes more women who do not have PID but also reduces the number of women with PID who are identified.

Many episodes of PID go unrecognized. Although some cases are asymptomatic, others are undiagnosed because the patient or the health care provider fails to recognize the implications of mild or nonspecific symptoms or signs (e.g., abnormal bleeding, dyspareunia, or vaginal discharge [atypical PID]). Because of the difficulty of diagnosis and the potential for damage to the reproductive health of women even by apparently mild or atypical PID, health care providers should maintain a low threshold for the diagnosis of PID. Even so, the long-term outcome of early treatment of women with asymptomatic or atypical PID is unknown. The following recommendations for diagnosing PID are intended to help health care providers recognize when PID should be suspected and when they need to obtain additional information to increase diagnostic certainty. These recommendations are based partially on the fact that diagnosis and management of other common causes of lower abdominal pain (e.g., ectopic pregnancy, acute appendicitis, and functional pain) are unlikely to be impaired by initiating empiric antimicrobial therapy for PID.

Empirical treatment of PID should be initiated in sexually active young women and others at risk for STDs if all the following minimum criteria are present and no other cause(s) for the illness can be identified:

- Lower abdominal tenderness
- Adnexal tenderness
- Cervical motion tenderness

More elaborate diagnostic evaluation often is needed, because incorrect diagnosis and management might cause unnecessary morbidity. These additional criteria may be used to enhance the specificity of the minimum criteria listed previously. Additional criteria that support a diagnosis of PID include the following:

- Oral temperature >101° F (>38.3° C)
- Abnormal cervical or vaginal discharge
- Elevated erythrocyte sedimentation rate
- Elevated C-reactive protein
- Laboratory documentation of cervical infection with *N. gonorrhoeae* or *C. trachomatis*

From the Centers for Disease Control and Prevention: 1998 guidelines for treatment of sexually transmitted diseases, *MMWR* 47:RR1, 1998.

BOX 262-7

DIFFERENTIAL DIAGNOSIS OF ACUTE LOWER ABDOMINAL PAIN IN THE ADOLESCENT FEMALE BY ORGAN SYSTEM

URINARY
Cystitis
Pyelonephritis
Urethritis
Other

GASTROINTESTINAL
Appendicitis
Constipation
Diverticulitis
Gastroenteritis
Inflammatory bowel disease
Irritable bowel syndrome
Other

REPRODUCTIVE
Acute PID
Cervicitis (?)
Dysmenorrhea (primary/secondary)
Ectopic pregnancy
Endometriosis
Endometritis
Mittelschmerz
Ovarian cyst (torsion/rupture)
Pregnancy (intrauterine, ectopic)
Ruptured follicle
Septic abortion
Threatened abortion
Torsion of adnexa
Tuboovarian abscess

From Shafer M, Sweet RL: *Pediatr Clin North Am* 36:513, 1989.

adnexal mass is palpated or suspected, an ultrasound should be obtained to determine if a tuboovarian abscess is present. Cultures for *C. trachomatis* and *N. gonorrhoeae* should be obtained routinely.

The hospital admission of any teenager who has PID is recommended by many authorities in an attempt to minimize future sequelae and because teenagers often comply poorly with the lengthy regimens needed for successful treatment. Others argue that if careful follow-up can be ensured, outpatient management can be attempted. The other indications for admission are shown in Box 262-8.

Treatment is directed toward eradicating the organism responsible for the infection. Unfortunately, the exact nature of the infection is established with great difficulty. Cultures obtained from the cervix do not necessarily reflect the nature of the tubal infection. Many organisms believed to play a role in PID are difficult to grow; thus studies that did not use state-of-the-art culture techniques may not have identified all relevant organisms. Those studies that have been performed carefully point to the polymicrobial nature of the infection. *N. gonorrhoeae* and/or *C. trachomatis* are recovered from approximately 25% to 75% of adolescents and young adults with PID. Facultative and anaerobic bacteria as well as organisms associated with bacterial vaginosis have been recovered from various points in the upper genital tract of women who have PID.

As a result of the uncertainty concerning the nature of the infecting organisms and the lack of controlled treatment and outcome studies, the CDC treatment regimens outlined in Box 262-4 reflect empirical therapy based on the assumption that the infection is polymicrobial. The recommendation for doxycycline as part of therapy, with its potential to stain developing teeth, underscores the need for obtaining a pregnancy test before treatment. If outpatient therapy is to be attempted, careful follow-up at 48 hours must be ensured, and a mechanism for hospitalizing the patient before that time if symptoms worsen must be in place. Otherwise, admission should occur at the time of diagnosis.

BOX 262-8

INDICATIONS FOR HOSPITALIZATION OF PATIENTS WHO HAVE PELVIC INFLAMMATORY DISEASE

In the past, many experts recommended that all patients who had PID be hospitalized so that bed rest and supervised treatment with parenteral antibiotics could be initiated. However, hospitalization is no longer synonymous with parenteral therapy. No currently available data compare the efficacy of parenteral with oral therapy or inpatient with outpatient treatment settings. Until the results from ongoing trials comparing parenteral inpatient therapy with oral outpatient therapy for women who have mild PID are available, such decisions must be based on observational data and consensus opinion. The decision of whether hospitalization is necessary should be based on the discretion of the health care provider.

The following criteria for HOSPITALIZATION are based on observational data and theoretical concerns:

- Surgical emergencies such as appendicitis cannot be excluded
- The patient is pregnant
- The patient does not respond clinically to oral antimicrobial therapy
- The patient is unable to follow or tolerate an outpatient oral regimen
- The patient has severe illness, nausea and vomiting, or high fever
- The patient has a tubo-ovarian abscess or
- The patient is immunodeficient (i.e., has HIV infection with low CD4 counts, is taking immunosuppressive therapy, or has another disease)

Most clinicians favor at least 24 hours of direct inpatient observation for patients who have tubo-ovarian abscesses, after which time home parenteral therapy should be adequate.

From the Centers for Disease Control and Prevention: 1998 guidelines for treatment of sexually transmitted diseases, *MMWR* 47:RR1, 1998.

Once therapy is initiated, the patient should improve within 48 hours. Failure to see improvement should raise concerns about the accuracy of the diagnosis or the presence of complications. The pelvic examination should be repeated to look for a tuboovarian abscess if one has not already been detected.

Approximately 10% to 20% of patients who have PID develop a tuboovarian abscess; 3% to 15% of these abscesses rupture. If an abscess is detected or if the patient fails to improve, the physician should seek gynecological consultation (or surgical consultation if appendicitis is suspected).

The patient may be discharged from the hospital 24 to 48 hours after she demonstrates substantial clinical improvement. Treatment must include a total of 14 days of doxycycline (or other suitable oral regimens), and follow-up at completion of treatment is essential. The patient should be instructed not to have intercourse until her therapy is completed and her partner is notified and treated. Because an episode of PID is a major risk factor for development of a second episode, the use of barrier methods of contraception must be stressed to the patient.

Even with optimum diagnosis and treatment, the long-term morbidity from a single episode of PID can be significant. Long-term complications include tubal factor infertility, increased risk for ectopic pregnancy and chronic pelvic pain. Risk for infertility and ectopic pregnancy increases with the number of episodes of PID and with the severity of infection; women younger than 25 years of age at time of diagnosis are less likely to develop either complication.

Perihepatitis (Fitz-Hugh-Curtis Syndrome)

Perihepatitis associated with gonococcal salpingitis was described in 1920. Subsequently, Fitz-Hugh described a patient who had "violin string" adhesions between the liver and anterior abdominal wall, and Curtis described localized peritonitis of the liver's anterior surface in a woman who had upper abdominal pain and tenderness who was undergoing laparotomy for suspected gallbladder disease. Since then, it has been well documented that *C. trachomatis* infections can cause a similar picture.

Onset of upper abdominal pain usually follows the onset of lower abdominal pain, but it can precede it. The pain generally occurs on the patient's right side and can radiate to the shoulder. Fewer than 50% of patients have mildly elevated liver enzymes. Treatment for pelvic inflammatory disease also eliminates the perihepatitis.

Enteric Infections

The syndromes of proctitis, proctocolitis, and enteritis are limited mostly to adolescent males who practice anal receptive intercourse. Symptoms include anorectal pain, tenesmus, constipation, and anal discharge. Those who have proctocolitis or enteritis will have diarrhea. Patients who have proctitis should be examined with anoscopy and evaluated for *C. trachomatis, N. gonorrhoeae,* and *Treponema pallidum* infection. Treatment should be with standard doses of cefixime and doxycycline.

Those who have symptoms suggesting proctocolitis or enteritis should receive more extensive evaluation. Organisms such as *Campylobacter jejuni, Shigella* spp., and *Giardia lamblia* can be sexually transmitted.

Vaginitis

As discussed in Chapter 178, Vaginal Discharge, *Trichomonas vaginalis*, an important cause of vaginitis among sexually active adolescents, is a sexually transmitted infectious agent. Some evidence suggests that bacterial vaginosis, associated with the overgrowth of *Gardnerella vaginalis,* also is sexually transmitted. Male sex partners of women who have bacterial vaginosis more often have *G. vaginalis* recovered from the urethra than do controls. However, this same organism can be recovered from approximately 15% of females who have never been active sexually. Treatment of male partners does not appear to influence recurrence risks for females who are treated for bacterial vaginosis.

Vaginitis, in and of itself, can be distressing enough to females. However, current concerns about bacterial vaginosis center on its possible role in the pathogenesis of pelvic inflammatory disease. Nongonococcal, nonchlamydial pathogens associated with PID are recovered more often from the endometrium of women who have bacterial vaginosis than from those who do not. Bacterial vaginosis has been related causally to postpartum endometritis. Hence, treatment of symptomatic women who have bacterial vaginosis is warranted.

REFERENCES

1. Blake DR, et al: Evaluation of vaginal infections in adolescents: can it be done without a speculum? *Pediatrics* 102:939, 1998.
2. Burstein GR, et al: Incident *Chlamydia trachomatis* infections among inner-city adolescent females, *JAMA* 280:521,1998.
3. Centers for Disease Control and Prevention: 1998 Guidelines for treatment of sexually transmitted diseases, *MMWR* 47:RR1, 1998.
4. Centers for Disease Control and Prevention: HIV prevention through early detection and treatment of other sexually transmitted diseases—United States, *MMWR* 47:RR-12, 1998.
5. Cohen DA, et al: A school-based chlamydia control program using DNA amplification technology, *Pediatrics* 101:E1, 1998.
6. Corey L, et al: Recombinant glycoprotein vaccine for prevention of genital HSV-2 infection: two randomized controlled trials, *JAMA* 282: 331, 1999.
7. Darville T: Syphilis, *Pediatr Rev* 20:160, 1999.
8. Dorfman DH, Glaser JH: Congenital syphilis presenting in infants after the newborn period, *N Engl J Med* 323:1299, 1990.
9. Galloway DA: Is vaccination against human papillomavirus a possibility? *Lancet* 351(suppl):22, 1998.
10. Ho GYF, et al: Natural history of cervicovaginal papillomavirus infection in young women, *N Engl J Med* 338:423, 1998.
11. Howell MR, et al: Screening women for *Chlamydia trachomatis* in family planning clinics, *Sex Transm Dis* 25:108, 1998.
12. Kurman RJ, et al: Interim guidelines for the management of abnormal cervical cytology, *JAMA* 271:1866, 1994.
13. Moscicki A-B, et al: The natural history of human papillomavirus infection as measured by repeat DNA testing in adolescents and young women, *J Pediatr* 132:277, 1998.
14. Polaneczky M, et al: Use of self-collected vaginal specimens for detection of *Chlamydia trachomatis* infection, *Obstet Gynecol* 91:375, 1998.
15. Rome ES: Sexually transmitted diseases: testing and treating, *Adolesc Med* 10:231, 1999.
16. Rowen D, Lacey C: Towards a human papillomavirus vaccine, *Dermatol Clin* 16:835, 1998.
17. Scholes D, et al: Prevention of pelvic inflammatory disease by screening for cervical chlamydial infection, *N Engl J Med* 334:1362, 1996.
18. Smith KR, et al: Evaluation of ligase chain reaction for use with urine for identification of *Neisseria gonorrhoeae* in females attending a sexually transmitted disease clinic, *J Clin Microbiol* 33:455, 1995.
19. Westrom L, Eschenbach O: Pelvic inflammatory disease. In Holmes KK, et al, editors: *Sexually transmitted diseases*, ed 3, New York, 1999, McGraw Hill.

263 Sinusitis

John S. Andrews

Infection of the paranasal sinuses in children occurs frequently. It is estimated that 5% to 10% of viral upper respiratory tract infections in children are complicated by acute bacterial sinusitis.[11] On average, children develop 5 to 10 upper respiratory tract infections yearly. The distinction between viral infections and acute bacterial sinusitis is based on the persistence and severity of upper respiratory symptoms.

PATHOPHYSIOLOGY

The paranasal sinuses arise during fetal development as outpouchings beneath the turbinates in the nasopharynx. Only the maxillary and ethmoid sinuses are present at the time of birth. The sinuses continue to develop and grow until adulthood (Table 263-1). Growth may be asymmetrical, and some individuals lack one or more sinuses altogether. Various functions have been ascribed to the sinuses, but none have been proved. These functions include warming and humidifying inspired air, reducing the weight of the skull, providing thermal insulation to the central nervous system and sensory organs, affecting facial form, and serving as vocal resonators. Recently, it has been suggested that the sinuses serve as reservoirs for production and absorption of antigens, tolerating infections until effective specific immunity develops.[1]

The lining of the mucosa of the sinuses is similar to that of the nasopharynx, with pseudostratified, ciliated, columnar epithelium interspersed with goblet cells and submucosal glands. Cilia beat toward the ostium of the sinus to expel mucus and particulate matter into the nasopharynx.[7] The ostia of the maxillary sinuses are located in the upper part of the chamber where cilia must battle gravity to clear secretions. This probably contributes to the high frequency of infection in these sinuses.[10] Occlusion of the ostia, impairment of ciliary motility, and alterations in the consistency of mucus secretions alone or in combination can predispose the sinuses to infection.

Sinusitis occurs most frequently after a viral upper respiratory tract infection or as the result of nasal allergy. Inflammation and edema of the respiratory mucosa lead to obstruction of the ostium. Pressure changes in the sinus that result from occlusion or from blowing and sniffing through the nose allow bacteria to invade the normally sterile sinus cavity. Other disorders associated with sinusitis in children are listed in Box 263-1.

Respiratory viruses such as adenoviruses, influenza viruses, parainfluenza viruses, and rhinoviruses contribute to the development of sinusitis. The most common bacterial pathogens associated with acute sinusitis are *Streptococcus pneumoniae, Haemophilus influenzae,* and *Moraxella catarrhalis. Staphylococcus aureus* and anaerobes are prevalent in chronic sinusitis.[2,10]

CLINICAL PRESENTATION AND DIAGNOSIS

Differentiating upper respiratory tract infections or allergic rhinitis from acute sinusitis can be difficult in children. Most uncomplicated upper respiratory tract infections improve after 5 to 7 days. Symptoms that persist without improvement for more than 10 but fewer than 30 days suggest bacterial superinfection, and a diagnosis of acute sinusitis can be made.[12] Cough and nasal discharge are the most common clinical manifestations of acute sinusitis. The cough occurs during the day and frequently is worse at night or when the child is lying supine. Nasal discharge may be clear or purulent. Parents of young children may report fetid breath. Headache and facial pain are manifestations of acute sinusitis that are uncommon in children. Painless swelling of periorbital tissues, usually in the morning, is an occasional manifestation of sinusitis that may be confused with periorbital cellulitis in its early stage.

A less common presentation of acute sinusitis is as an unusually severe upper respiratory tract infection. In most cases of viral upper respiratory infection, fever precedes the onset of watery nasal discharge and is associated with constitutional symptoms. Thickening of nasal secretions occurs later in the course, prior to resolution. When high fever and purulent discharge coexist for several days, this suggests the diagnosis of acute sinusitis.

Cough and nasal discharge persisting for more than 30 days occurs with subacute or chronic sinusitis.[12]

On physical examination, the nasal mucosa usually is erythematous and swollen but may be pale and boggy.[11] Mucopurulent material sometimes can be seen in the nose or draining into the nasopharynx. The presence of a foreign body in the nose must be ruled out. Palpation or percussion of the sinuses may elicit tenderness.

Sinus roentgenograms can help confirm the diagnosis of sinusitis.[4] When clinical signs and symptoms suggest acute sinusitis and maxillary sinus roentgenograms show air-fluid levels, complete opacification, or mucosal thickening of at least 4 to 5 mm, bacteria are present in a sinus aspirate 75% of the time.[11] Routine use of roentgenograms to confirm the diagnosis of uncomplicated sinusitis is not recommended in young children. Sinus roentgenograms are more specific and therefore more helpful in children older than

Table 263-1 Sinus Development

Sinus	First Appearance	Size (ml) Birth	3 Years	10 Years	14 Years	Age of Clinical Importance
Maxillary	3 wk of fetal life	0.13	2.5	10.4	11.6	Birth
Ethmoid	6 mo of fetal life	0.06	0.16	2.4	4.8	Birth
Sphenoid	3 mo of fetal life	0.02	0.68	1.8	2.1	5 yr
Frontal	1 yr of life	—	0.08	1.0	3.6	10-12 yr

Modified from Schaeffer JP: *The embryology, development and anatomy of the nose, paranasal sinuses, nasolacrimal passageways and olfactory organ in man,* Philadelphia, 1920, Blakiston.

BOX 263-1

DISORDERS ASSOCIATED WITH PARANASAL SINUSITIS

1. Anatomical
   a. Nasal malformations
   b. Nasal trauma
   c. Tumors and polyps
   d. Cleft palate
   e. Foreign bodies
   f. Dental infection
   g. Cyanotic congenital heart disease
2. Physiological—barotrauma
3. Abnormalities of local defense mechanisms
   a. Allergy
   b. Cystic fibrosis
   c. Immotile-cilia syndrome and Kartagener syndrome
4. Abnormalities of systemic defense mechanisms—immunodeficiency, primary or secondary

From Shurin PA: *Ann Otol Rhinol Laryngol* 90(suppl 84):72, 1981.

6 years of age. Cysts and polyps may also be seen on sinus roentgenograms.

Computed tomography (CT) imaging of the sinuses should be reserved for patients who have frequent recurrences, those who have complicated sinusitis accompanied by orbital or intracranial complications, and those for whom sinus surgery is being contemplated.[10,13]

Transnasal aspiration of the maxillary sinuses can be performed by an otolaryngologist for diagnostic purposes in specific situations. Nasopharyngeal culture results correlate poorly with sinus culture results. Sinus aspiration and lavage are indicated only in children who fail to respond to conventional antibiotic therapy, in immunosuppressed patients, and in those whose illness is severe or life threatening.

COMPLICATIONS

Complications of sinusitis most often are due to local extension of the disease. Orbital cellulitis is the most common serious complication of sinusitis. The ethmoid sinus is separated from the orbit by the thin lamina papyracea. Erosion of this bone leads to invasion of the orbit by bacterial pathogens. Staging of orbital cellulitis is described in Table 263-2. The eyelids appear intensely red and swollen on physical examination. Fever, malaise, and an increased white blood cell count are present. Orbital pain, proptosis, and limitation of eye movement (ophthalmoplegia) help distinguish this condition from preseptal (periorbital) cellulitis, although CT scanning may be needed to differentiate the two. Treatment of orbital cellulitis involves parenteral antibiotics; an ophthalmologist and an otolaryngologist should be consulted to determine whether surgical drainage is indicated.[12]

Intracranial infection, most commonly subdural empyema, is the second most common complication of sinusitis. This can occur by direct extension through necrotic bone or by bacterial spread through the venous system. Because the frontal sinuses are involved most often, the peak age of incidence of this complication is between 10 and 20 years, although it can develop in younger children. Patients have a low-grade fever, malaise, and a frontal headache. Vomiting and a decreased level of consciousness appear as the disease progresses.

If a patient is suspected of having an intracranial abscess, a head CT should be obtained. Lumbar puncture should be avoided until intracranial mass effect has been ruled out. Treatment with high-dose parenteral antibiotics and neurosurgery to drain the abscess and to debride necrotic bone are required. Steroids and hypertonic agents such as mannitol or glycerol may be necessary to control intracranial hypertension.

Other less common complications of sinusitis in children include meningitis, osteomyelitis ("Pott's puffy tumor"), and cavernous sinus thrombosis.

TREATMENT

Treatment of sinusitis in children involves antibiotic therapy, symptomatic relief measures, and drainage, if necessary.[9] Amoxicillin (40 to 60 mg/kg/day divided twice a day) is an appropriate choice for the treatment of uncomplicated sinusitis in geographical areas where the prevalence of beta-lactamase–producing strains of *H. influenzae* and *M. catarrhalis* is low.[8] Broader coverage with amoxicillin plus clavulanate, a carbacephem, a macrolide, or a third-generation cephalosporin should be considered for children who are allergic or fail to respond to amoxicillin. These alternatives should also be considered for the child who has recently been treated with amoxicillin, has frontal or sphenoid sinusitis, has complicated ethmoid sinusitis, or has very protracted symptoms.[10] Clinical improvement should be expected within 48

Table 263-2 Classification of Orbital Cellulitis

Stage	Description
I Inflammatory edema	Inflammatory edema beginning in medial or lateral upper eyelid; usually nontender with only minimal skin changes. No induration, visual impairment, or limitation of extraocular movements
II Orbital cellulitis	Edema of orbital contents with varying degrees of proptosis, chemosis, limitation of extraocular movement, and visual loss
III Subperiosteal abscess	Proptosis down and out with signs of orbital cellulitis (usually severe). Abscess beneath the periosteum of the ethmoid, frontal, or maxillary bone (in that order of frequency)
IV Orbital abscess	Abscess within the fat or muscle cone in the posterior orbit. Severe chemosis and proptosis; complete ophthalmoplegia and moderate to severe visual loss present (globe displaced forward or down and out)
V Cavernous sinus thrombosis	Proptosis, globe fixation, severe loss of visual acuity, prostration, signs of meningitis; progresses to proptosis, chemosis, and visual loss in contralateral eye

From Wald ER, et al: *Pediatr Clin North Am* 28:787, 1981; modified from Chandler JR, Langenbrunner DJ, Stevens ER: *Laryngoscope* 80:1414, 1970.

hours, and 10 days of antibiotic therapy usually is adequate. If a patient's symptoms fail to resolve completely within 10 days, he or she should be treated for 7 days beyond the resolution of symptoms.[12]

Decongestants, antihistamines, and saline nose drops have been recommended to help drain the sinuses, but no proof of the efficacy of these agents exists.[3] Intranasal steroids may provide some benefit, particularly in the second week of therapy, but further research is necessary to define their role in management.[10]

In unusually severe cases, parenteral antibiotics may be required and otolaryngological consultation is indicated. Some experts have recommended antibiotic prophylaxis for the child who has recurrent sinusitis and no underlying disorder, although no scientific studies support this practice.[12] Surgery may be required in cases of medically recalcitrant severe chronic sinusitis in children.[5,6]

Acknowledgment

The author acknowledges the contributions of Rickey L. Williams, M.D., to the preparation of this manuscript in the previous editions.

REFERENCES

1. Altemeier WA, Ward C: Why do we have paranasal sinuses? *Pediatr Ann* 27:784, 1998.
2. Brook I: Bacteriologic features of chronic sinusitis in children, *JAMA* 246:967, 1981.
3. Giebink GS: Childhood sinusitis: pathophysiology, diagnosis and treatment, *Pediatr Infect Dis J* 13(suppl):55, 1994.
4. Kovatch AL, et al: Maxillary sinus radiographs in children with nonrespiratory complaints, *Pediatrics* 73:306, 1984.
5. Lund VJ: Bacterial sinusitis: etiology and management, *Pediatr Infect Dis J* 13(suppl):58, 1994.
6. Parsons DS, Phillips SE: Functional endoscopic surgery in children: a retrospective analysis of results, *Laryngoscope* 103:899, 1993.
7. Rachelefsky GS, Katz RM, Siegel SC: Diseases of paranasal sinuses in children, *Curr Probl Pediatr* 12:1, 1982.
8. Siegel JD: Diagnosis and management of acute sinusitis in children, *Pediatr Infect Dis J* 6:95, 1987.
9. Wald ER: Management of sinusitis in infants and children, *Pediatr Infect Dis J* 7:449, 1988.
10. Wald ER: Sinusitis, *Pediatr Ann* 27:811, 1998.
11. Wald ER: Sinusitis, *Pediatr Rev* 14:345, 1993.
12. Wald ER: Sinusitis in children, *N Engl J Med* 326:319, 1992.
13. Yousem DM: Imaging of sinonasal inflammatory disease, *Radiology* 188:303, 1993.

264 Spina Bifida

Gregory S. Liptak

Meningomyelocele (myelomeningocele) is a serious and complex congenital malformation, occurring at a rate of 0.4 to 0.8 case per 1000 live births in the United States.[12,19] The incidence is higher among females, among those of lower socioeconomic status, and among families of English, Irish, or Welsh extraction. The incidence of meningomyelocele (and other neural tube defects) has been declining for the past several decades. The establishment of prenatal diagnosis with elective termination has significantly decreased the birth prevalence in the United States.[14,44]

ETIOLOGY

Meningomyelocele belongs to the family of neural tube defects that includes abnormalities of the head (anencephaly, cranial meningocele, encephalocele) and of the spine (spina bifida occulta, meningocele, and meningomyelocele). In spina bifida occulta (occult spinal dysraphism), the spinal cord and soft tissues are normal, but the vertebral arches are incomplete. In meningocele, the spinal cord is normal, but the meninges protrude through abnormal vertebral arches and soft tissue. On rare occasions, the meningocele may appear as an anterior mass in the pelvis, abdomen, or thorax. In meningomyelocele, the malformed spinal cord and nerve roots protrude through abnormal vertebral arches and soft tissue. Lipomas or dermoid cysts may accompany meningomyelocele or occult spinal dysraphism.

The cause of neural tube defects is unknown, although faulty closure of the neural groove by day 28 of gestation seems to be the primary mechanism. The most recent etiological hypothesis is that neural tube defects result from the interaction of many genes (polygenic expression) that can be modified by factors in the fetal (maternal) environment. Abnormalities in the gene that regulates methylenetetrahydrofolate reductase (MTHFR), an enzyme associated with folate metabolism, have been associated with neural tube defects.[39] Assuming an overall incidence of 1 per 1000, the risk for a second affected child from the same parent is 2 or 3 per 100; for a third, it is 10 per 100. An adult who has meningomyelocele has a 2% to 3% chance of having a child who has a neural tube defect—the same risk that exists for the sibling of an affected child.

Environmental factors such as potato blight, organic solvents, maternal hyperthermia, aminopterin, valproic acid, and ethanol have been implicated in the origin of neural tube defects.[36] The incidence of neural tube defects is greater in mothers who are obese; however, maternal malnutrition, especially folic acid deficiency, appears to be the most important variable.[2,35] Meningomyelocele may be seen with certain syndromes, including trisomy 13, trisomy 18, maternal thalidomide and valproate ingestion, and cri du chat syndrome. It also may be associated with cryptorchism, imperforate anus, ventricular septal defect, cleft palate, inguinal hernias, tracheoesophageal fistula, renal anomalies, and diaphragmatic hernia. Most cases, however, are isolated occurrences.

PATHOLOGY

As shown in Figs. 264-1 and 264-2, four major malformations account for the findings of meningomyelocele: soft-tissue malformation, brain malformation, vertebral body malformation, and spinal cord malformation.

Soft-Tissue Malformation

The failure of skin and other soft tissues to close leaves the spinal cord open to infection. The lipomas that occasionally accompany the defect may grow larger, compressing the spinal cord, and may cause progressive neurological symptoms as the child grows. The surgery to cover the cord may itself result in loss of neurological function or may lead to scar tissue that tethers the cord and results in further neurological deterioration as the child grows.

Brain Malformation

Malformations of the brain include the Chiari type II deformity, in which the pons and medulla are distorted and elongated and the cerebellar vermis is displaced inferiorly into the spinal canal.[32] This abnormality often is associated with progressive hydrocephalus. Brainstem malformations also may lead to laryngeal nerve palsy and difficulty in swallowing, as well as hypoventilation,[17] apnea, and sudden death. Subtle abnormalities of cranial nerve nuclei may occur in many affected children. Brain malformations and ventricular shunts also result in the 15% to 20% occurrence of grand mal seizures experienced by children and adolescents who have spina bifida.[6,42]

About 25% of children who have meningomyelocele are born having evidence of hydrocephalus, with an additional 25% to 60% developing such signs within the first year of life.[23] The higher (i.e., the more cephalad) the spinal lesion, the greater the likelihood of hydrocephalus developing. In

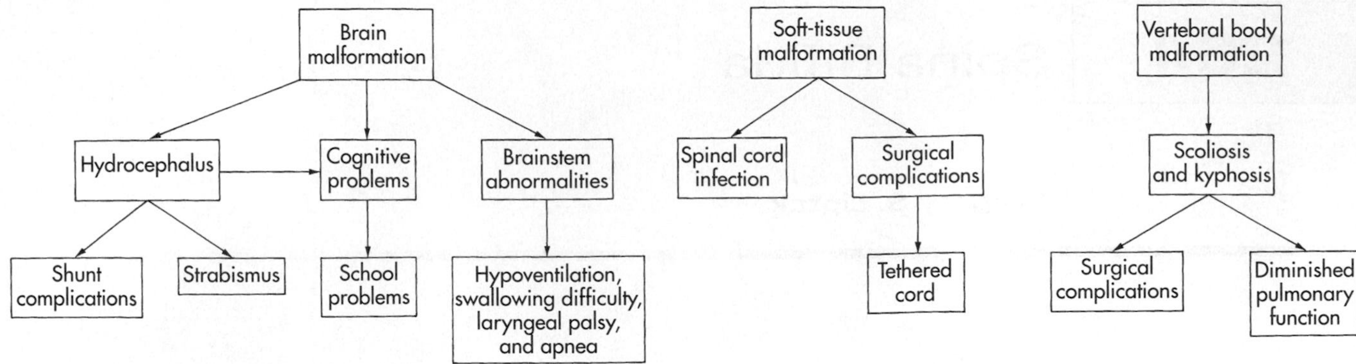

Fig. 264-1 Problems related to meningomyelocele with brain, soft-tissue, and vertebral body malformations.

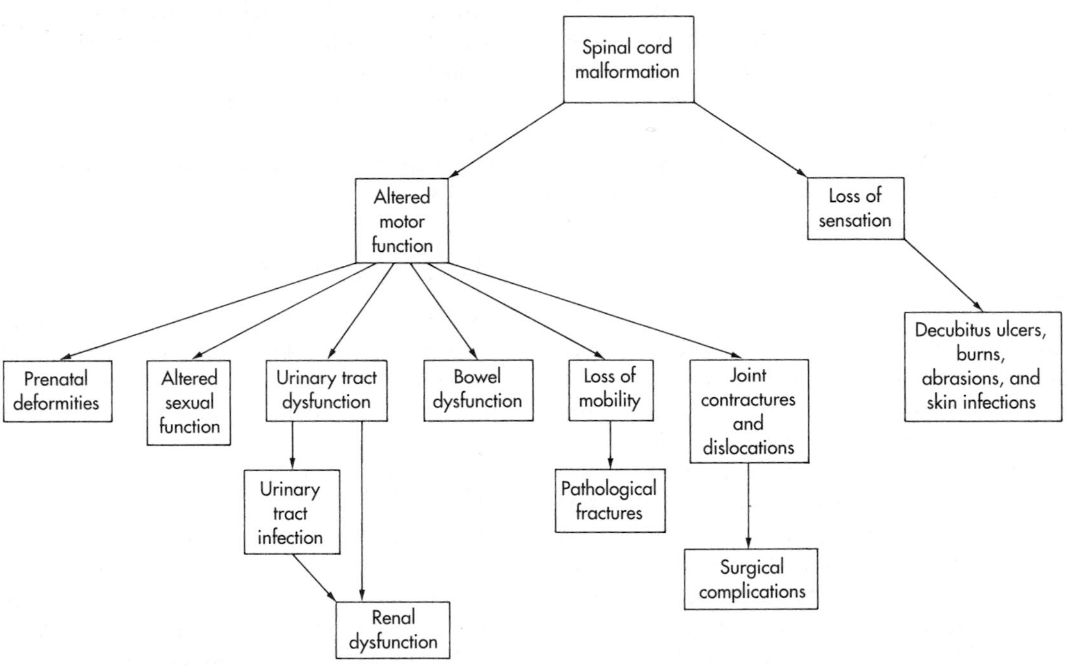

Fig. 264-2 Problems associated with meningomyelocele with spinal cord malformation.

addition to the usual manifestations of hydrocephalus and complications of shunt placement, strabismus secondary to anomalies of the centers that control conjugate gaze occurs in about 50% of children who have hydrocephalus and meningomyelocele. In addition, central precocious puberty develops in many children who have hydrocephalus.

Sudden shunt malfunction in children shunted for hydrocephalus may produce life-threatening elevations of intracranial pressure requiring emergency intervention. Signs and symptoms of acute shunt malfunction include headache, lethargy, irritability, paralysis of upward gaze, sixth cranial nerve palsy, a bulging fontanelle (in infants), and vomiting. Progression to loss of consciousness, abnormal pupillary reflexes, papilledema, deterioration of vital signs, and death may occur rapidly.

Most children who have meningomyelocele have normal overall intelligence quotient (IQ) scores. Yet most of these youngsters have selective cognitive disabilities and score better on verbal than on performance scales. Even those children who have very low performance scores may have surprising verbal fluency, a trait sometimes referred to as the "cocktail party syndrome." Specific cognitive testing often reveals deficiencies of selective visual attention, visual-spatial perception, tactile perception, auditory concentration, and higher-order functioning (such as organizational skills). Children who have hydrocephalus and higher spinal lesions are more likely to have these deficits. Manifestations seen in school include short attention span, distractibility, perseveration (the constant repetition of a meaningless word or phrase), poor comprehension, poor handwriting, disorganization, poor memory, faulty problem solving and decision making, diminished motivation and initiative, reduced social skills, emotional instability, impulsivity, irritability, tearfulness, inappropriate laughter, and difficulty with subjects requiring visual-motor integration, such as arithmetic.

Vertebral Malformation

Vertebral malformations caused by abnormal segmentation or formation include absent vertebrae, fused vertebrae, hemivertebrae, and butterfly vertebrae. Occasionally, bony or ligamentous spurs lead to diastematomyelia. Of children who

Table 264-1 Correlation Between Function and Level of Motor Involvement

Functional Area —Level of Lesion	Bowel and Bladder Function	Toe Intrinsics	Foot: Dorsiflexion—Inversion	Foot: Plantar Flexion—Eversion
S2-3	±*	±	+*	±
S1-2	–*	–	+	±
L5-S1	–	–	+	–
L4-5	–	–	±	–
L3-4	–	–	–	–
L2-3	–	–	–	–
L1-2	–	–	–	–

Functional Area —Level of Lesion	Knee: Extension	Knee: Flexion	Hip: Flexion	Hip: Adduction	Hip: Abduction	Hip: Extension
S2-3	+	+	+	+	+	+
S1-2	+	+	+	+	+	±
L5-S1	+	±	+	+	+	–
L4-5	+	–	+	+	–	–
L3-4	+	–	+	+	–	–
L2-3	±	–	±	±	–	–
L1-2	–	–	–	–	–	–

*±, May be present; +, present; –, absent.

have thoracic lesions, 10% are born with kyphosis; by adolescence this rate increases to 33%. Children who have lumbar lesions have a 5% occurrence of kyphosis by adolescence. In addition to cosmetic deformity, severe kyphosis can lead to back pain, pulmonary dysfunction, and recurrent skin ulceration; it also interferes with walking.[8]

The occurrence of scoliosis is related to the level of the lesion, with curves of 30 degrees or more appearing in 81% of adolescents who have thoracic lesions and 23% of those who have lower lumbar lesions. The consequences of scoliosis are similar to those of kyphosis. Lordosis also occurs but is much less common.

Spinal Cord Malformation

Spinal cord malformation results in both loss of sensation and loss of motor function. Loss of sensation leaves these children vulnerable to burns and abrasions. Decubitus ulcers also occur, especially among adolescents and adults who spend large amounts of time in wheelchairs. All three skin lesions are susceptible to infection and may lead to osteomyelitis.

Loss of motor function leads to decreased movement in utero, which may lead to deformities seen at birth, such as clubfoot (talipes equinovarus) and dislocated hip.

Loss of efferent nerve stimuli to the urinary bladder and sphincter results in neurogenic voiding dysfunction in virtually all children who have meningomyelocele. Voiding dysfunction may be classified as (1) failure to store urine or (2) inability to void completely. Failure to store urine may result from a hypotonic urinary outlet or a spastic, hypertonic bladder or both. Inability to void completely may result from spastic urinary sphincter or hypotonic bladder or both. The combination of spastic outlet and hypertonic bladder is especially serious because of the reflux and hydronephrosis that occur frequently with this combination. In addition to incontinence and hydronephrosis, these children have frequent urinary tract infections.[31, 37] These infections lead to fibrosis of the bladder and to chronic renal damage, which remains a significant source of morbidity and mortality.[24]

Altered sexual function also occurs, especially in males. Approximately 25% of males who have meningomyelocele are unable to have erections, and of those who can, most have retrograde ejaculation with decreased fertility. Although females have decreased sensation, most can experience orgasm and have normal fertility.

Children who have meningomyelocele usually have fecal incontinence as a result of diminished function of the external rectal sphincter and the levator ani muscles. Most children have intact internal rectal sphincter function, and many have intact rectal sensation. Abnormal migration of neural cells in utero can lead to bowel immotility similar to that seen in Hirschsprung's disease.[27] Abnormal rectal function, immobility, and the use of a low-fiber diet because of fear of incontinence may lead to constipation or obstipation with overflow soiling.[21]

Loss of motor function in the lower extremities leads to loss of mobility. The degree of mobility is related closely to the level of the lesion; thus, children who have intact quadriceps (L2-4) are much more likely to be ambulatory through adolescence than are those who lack such function.[40] As Table 264-1 illustrates, muscle function around the joints is related directly to the level of the lesion. Contractures and dislocations are more likely to develop in children who have an imbalance of forces around a joint than in those who have either full function or no function. For example, children who have a lesion at the L4-5 level are more likely to develop foot and ankle contractures than are those who have L1-3 or S2-3 lesions. Loss of mobility and innervation also increases the risk for pathological fractures in the lower extremities.

HISTORY

Because meningomyelocele is inherited polygenically, affected newborns may have a family history of neural tube defects or spontaneous abortions (miscarriages). Other historical facts worth noting in the newborn period include length of gestation, type of delivery, complications with and length of labor, maternal nutrition and environmental exposures, current family functioning (including social support and stress), and parental expectations and understanding of the problem. For the older child, information about current and past therapies for neurosurgical, orthopedic, urological, dermatological, and gastrointestinal problems should be obtained. Educational and social functioning at school, relations with peers and with family members, and sexual function and understanding of sexuality should be ascertained. The child's growth, development, mobility, and activities of daily living (personal hygiene, ability to feed oneself, self-help skills) also should be assessed. The onset of new neurological symptoms, such as weakness, changes in bowel and bladder function, tripping, and clumsiness, should be sought because these usually indicate treatable conditions such as tethered spinal cord, diastematomyelia, syringomyelia, or ventricular shunt malfunction. Up to 50% of children who have meningomyelocele may have allergies to latex.[30,41] A history of reactions to products made of latex, such as balloons, bandages, and balls, should be sought. Contact to latex-containing products should be restricted from the first day of life in these children. All operative procedures should be performed in a latex-free environment.

PHYSICAL EXAMINATION

The backs of all children should be examined for pigmented spots, hairy patches, and sinuses that extend into the spine, because these may be signs of occult spinal dysmorphism.[1,15] These children are at high risk for meningitis and for neurological deterioration secondary to diastematomyelia, lipoma, and tethering of the spinal cord.[4]

Children who have meningomyelocele should have a complete physical examination that emphasizes neurological, orthopedic, and developmental aspects. The neurological examination should include motor function (see Table 264-1) and sensory level. A rectal examination and assessment of an anal wink can assist in the evaluation of lesions at S2-4. Upper extremity strength, including grip, should be assessed because deterioration may indicate syringomyelia or malfunction of the ventricular shunt. Palpation of the anterior fontanelle, ophthalmoscopic visualization of the eyegrounds, assessment of the cranial nerves (especially of extraocular movements), and palpation of the shunt valve and tubing help to evaluate shunt functioning.

The orthopedic examination should include an assessment of posture (scoliosis, lordosis, kyphosis) as well as of joint mobility and stability. Erythema and swelling of a joint or bone in an area that lacks sensation represent a fracture until proved otherwise.[8] The skin should be examined for evidence of sores and ulcers in insensate areas.

Formal and informal developmental assessments should be part of the routine examination of these children and should include visual-spatial functioning and verbal, performance, and educational measures, as well as the more standard areas—fine motor, gross motor, language, and social-adaptive skills. These are especially important to perform before school entry to enable the school to provide interventions that will optimize the child's learning.

LABORATORY DATA

Laboratory assessments of the newborn should include measurement of length, weight, and head circumference—the latter, daily. Ultrasound or computed tomography (CT) scan or both of the head, radiograms of the spine and hips, and a urine culture also should be performed. The kidneys should be examined by ultrasound; serum BUN and creatinine levels should be obtained as a baseline assessment of renal function. As the child grows, urinalysis and urine cultures should be performed routinely, and head circumference, height, and weight should be monitored. Some clinicians recommend substituting arm span for height because growth below the waist is disproportionately slow.[5] A CT scan of the head should be performed routinely to detect asymptomatic ventricular enlargement. The condition of the spine and joints should be monitored by radiograms. The kidneys should be screened by using routine renal ultrasound, voiding cystourethrograms, renal scans, and urodynamics.

Special studies that may be indicated include (1) grip strength measurement to monitor for syringomyelia, (2) skinfold thickness measurements to evaluate nutritional status, (3) magnetic resonance imaging (MRI)[34] of the spine and hind brain (posterior fossa), and (4) injection of radiopaque dye into the shunt and measurement of pressure to evaluate its function. A child who has signs and symptoms suggestive of ventricular shunt malfunction should have a head CT scan and a shunt series (to evaluate the integrity of the tubing) performed.

PSYCHOSOCIAL CONSIDERATIONS

The birth of a child who has meningomyelocele is potentially devastating.[25] Most parents are shocked and begin a journey through a series of phases characteristic of people undergoing a loss (in this case a loss of the expected normal child). These stages include shock, denial, sadness, anger, guilt, and ultimately, acceptance and equilibrium.[16] In addition to grieving, parents must share in difficult medical decisions. For these reasons, parents require support from medical professionals and others. An evaluation of their current levels of social support and the presence of other stressors is critical in helping them through this time. Because most children who have meningomyelocele have multiple medical problems, they require the expenditure of much money,[3] time, patience, and understanding. Such demands stress parents and can lead to isolation of one from the other. This isolation may be reinforced by a medical system that sees patients during working hours and that is content to deal exclusively with mothers.[26] The stresses also may affect siblings, who may have an increased occurrence of behavioral problems.

Parents may begin mourning but never reach equilibrium, and the clinician may notice manifestations of denial, guilt, or anger. In addition, one spouse may be able to reach equilibrium but be emotionally unavailable to the spouse still struggling with the earlier stages.[16]

Children who have meningomyelocele may have difficulty at home with parents unable to provide affection or set consistent limits. They may have difficulty with peers who see them as "cripples" rather than as children who have disabilities. They may have difficulty performing academically and may lose interest in school because of frequent negative reinforcement. They may have no adult role models. Finally, they may lose self-esteem from frequent visits to clinicians—visits that often are characterized by the identification of new problems without any positive reinforcement of their successes.

MANAGEMENT[23]

The two goals in the management of these patients are (1) to prevent dysfunctions (e.g., neurological defects) from becoming disabilities (e.g., "can't walk") and (2) to prevent the disabilities from becoming handicaps (the social disadvantages experienced from the disabilities, e.g., "can't get a job"). Achieving these goals requires comprehensive, coordinated care,[26] as well as routine care such as immunizations and anticipatory guidance.[33]

The newborn and family should be evaluated by a team, usually consisting of a pediatrician, nurse, social worker, neurosurgeon, orthopedist, physical therapist, and urologist. Once the neonate has been examined and given supportive care, central nervous system infection must be prevented. For infants who have an open lesion, parenteral antibiotics that provide coverage against gram-negative bacilli and *Staphylococcus aureus* organisms should be given as soon as possible. Surgery to close the open defect may occur within the first 72 hours of life.

Daily measurement of the head circumference and frequent ultrasound or CT scans of the head should be used as guides for ventriculoperitoneal shunt placement to reduce hydrocephalus. No universally accepted criteria exist to determine the need for or the timing of shunt placement. Furosemide (Lasix) and acetazolamide (Diamox) may be administered to delay the insertion of the shunt if the child cannot tolerate surgery immediately.[20]

Deformities such as clubfeet or dislocated hips should be managed with range-of-motion exercises, splinting, and casting. The urological system should be evaluated by urine culture and renal ultrasound. Baseline radiograms of the spine and hips should be taken. Genetic counseling and social support should be provided to the family, and assistance with finances should be a priority. As the child grows, the primary care physician should coordinate the child's care and be his or her advocate. Enhancing environmental stimulation for the maximization of cognitive development should be another goal in the care of these children. In most instances, children may benefit from formal early-intervention programs, which are mandated under the Individuals with Disabilities Education Act (IDEA). Opportunities for interactions with people and objects (toys) should be provided. Similarly, the child should be encouraged to develop the best social interaction and self-help skills possible, including the development of independence in hygiene and eating.

According to Bronfenbrenner,[7] learning and development are facilitated by the participation of the developing person in progressively more complex patterns of reciprocal activity with someone with whom that person has developed a strong and enduring emotional attachment and when the balance of power gradually shifts in favor of the developing person. A child who has a disability has the same psychosocial needs as healthy children, and the clinician should help the family achieve this shifting of power.

Orthopedic management may include surgery for joint contractures, scoliosis, or kyphosis. To prevent contractures and dislocations, regular passive range-of-motion exercises, splints, body jackets, and casts may be used.[8]

Various exercises and orthoses (braces) may be used to enhance locomotion. The parapodium—a standing brace that allows the child to be in an upright position with hands unencumbered—and reciprocal gait orthosis can be started between 18 and 24 months of age.[22,40] Crutches or walkers that have more standard bracing may be used, and early use of wheeled mobility is encouraged, especially for those children who have quadriceps paralysis. Adaptive equipment such as carts and hand-pedaled tricycles also can enhance the function and self-esteem of these children.

Goals of urological management include prevention of renal damage and attainment of continence.[38] In the past, urinary diversion via ileal loops was performed in most children who had meningomyelocele to achieve these goals. Clean intermittent catheterization, introduced in 1972, is safer, is more acceptable, and results in better renal function than does urinary diversion. Vesicostomy may be indicated in the infant who has vesicoureteral reflux or hydronephrosis or both. Most families are able to perform clean intermittent catheterization when the child is 4 to 5 years of age, and many children, even those this young, are able to perform the procedure themselves. Clean intermittent catheterization also has been used in children younger than 3 years of age and can be helpful in the management of vesicoureteral reflux with or without hydronephrosis or in those who have frequent urinary tract infections.[45] The addition of drugs that relax the detrusor muscle or increase sphincter tone, such as imipramine hydrochloride, oxybutynin chloride, or pseudoephedrine, can enhance continence. For older children in whom catheterization does not provide continence, the use of a surgical procedure such as bladder augmentation plus the creation of a continent stoma with clean intermittent catheterization may provide continence.[11]

Obtaining regular urine cultures to detect urinary tract infection and administering prophylactic antibiotics in those children who have frequent infections may prevent renal damage. Trimethoprim-sulfamethoxazole, sulfisoxazole, nitrofurantoin, and cephalexin given in less than the therapeutic dosage have been used for prophylaxis.

Bowel continence after 4 years of age and avoidance of severe constipation often is difficult to achieve. However, a high-fiber diet, stool softeners, regular toileting, regular stimulants, and biofeedback in those children who have rectal sensation may be used singly or in combination to attain these goals. Regular enemas, using 20 ml/kg of normal saline, have been shown to be effective in some children.[21] Several surgical procedures have been developed to help the child achieve fecal continence. One surgical procedure removes the appendix, opens its distal end, and uses it to create a "fistula" between the colon and the abdominal wall.[13] In a related procedure, an opening is made in the cecum, either surgically or in the radiology suite, and a gastrostomy button is placed into the cecum.[10] Both procedures allow forward-flowing irrigation of the colon on a regular basis and show promise for a select group of children and adolescents in whom more conventional constipation-relieving techniques have failed.

Impotence in the male may be managed surgically via penile implants, vacuum pumps, and the injection or insertion of prostaglandin, or possibly with sildenafil (Viagra). Pregnant women who have meningomyelocele may need to have their babies delivered by cesarean section because of hip contractures. Their intervertebral disks also may become herniated, with neurological sequelae; therefore, they should have frequent neurological evaluations throughout pregnancy.

Because 50% or more of children who have meningomyelocele may have allergies to latex,[30] including anaphylaxis during surgery, contact with products made from latex should be avoided. For example, all surgical procedures should occur in latex-free settings. Catheterization should be performed with nonlatex catheters; gloves used during care should be of nonlatex material; toys that contain significant amounts of latex should be avoided, as should products that contact the skin, such as adhesive or Ace bandages.

Even though the execution of all these interventions requires tremendous resources and effort, they still may be inadequate in the absence of social changes. To prevent disabilities from becoming handicaps, society's attitudes and practices must be altered. The clinician can advocate for these children by helping remove architectural barriers in the community, which will allow people who have disabilities access to places such as banks, public buildings, transportation, and recreation areas. Altering the attitudes of people who have no disabilities may be more difficult, but the clinician can help to enable the child and adult who have disabilities to serve as role models in the community—for instance, by encouraging the hiring of workers who have disabilities. Performing all the aforementioned tasks requires constant effort and can be achieved only with a multidisciplinary team that is willing to collaborate with the family.

PREVENTION

Periconceptual supplementation of the diets of mothers of children who have neural tube defects has been shown to decrease the recurrence of these defects and decreases the primary occurrence of such defects as well.[28,29] The American Academy of Pediatrics and Centers for Disease Control recommend that all women of child-bearing age receive 0.4 mg of folic acid daily. Women who have a first-degree relative who has a neural tube defect should receive 4.0 mg of folic acid daily.

Open neural tube defects may be diagnosed prenatally by the measurement of alpha-fetoprotein levels in maternal serum between 14 and 16 weeks of gestation, coupled with confirmation of the diagnosis via high-resolution ultrasound. Amniocentesis is recommended for those who have elevated serum alpha-fetoprotein levels to confirm the diagnosis. The prenatal detection of a neural tube defect allows the family to plan rationally, whether or not they elect to continue the pregnancy. If they elect to deliver, the fetus should be monitored for the development of hydrocephalus, which may necessitate delivery before term. Prenatal endoscopic surgery to cover the open lesion on the back during the second trimester has been shown to decrease neurological involvement after delivery[9] and diminish the severity of the Chiari malformation.[43] Whether this procedure will become the standard of treatment or another disappointing prenatal surgical intervention, like previous attempts to treat hydrocephalus in utero, remains to be seen. The infant may benefit from delivery by cesarean section to avoid trauma to the head and back.[18] Social support should be provided to these families, whatever their decision.

When to Refer

Infants born with meningomyelocele should be referred to a tertiary medical center that specializes in the care of these children. They all should be followed during childhood by a multidisciplinary team that includes experts in child development, neurosurgery, orthopedics, urology, orthotics, social work, nursing, physical and occupational therapies, and plastic surgery. Referral to a psychologist and educational specialist should be accomplished early on.

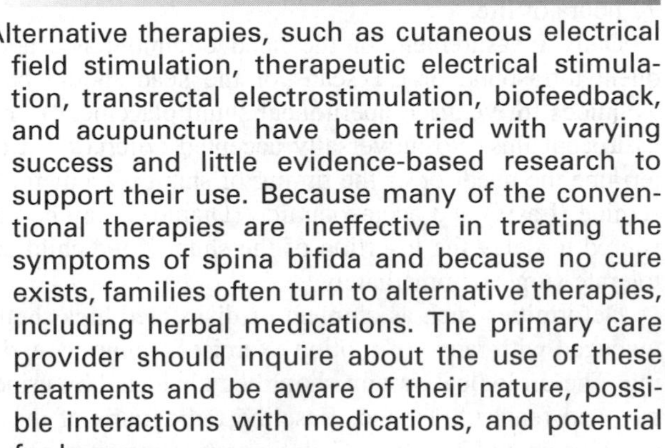

Use of Alternative Medicine

Alternative therapies, such as cutaneous electrical field stimulation, therapeutic electrical stimulation, transrectal electrostimulation, biofeedback, and acupuncture have been tried with varying success and little evidence-based research to support their use. Because many of the conventional therapies are ineffective in treating the symptoms of spina bifida and because no cure exists, families often turn to alternative therapies, including herbal medications. The primary care provider should inquire about the use of these treatments and be aware of their nature, possible interactions with medications, and potential for harm.

When to Hospitalize

When the child is acutely ill and cannot be managed at home, and when he or she requires surgical intervention.

REFERENCES

1. Albright AL, Gartner JC, Wiener ES: Lumbar cutaneous hemangiomas as indicators of tethered spinal cords, *Pediatrics* 83:977, 1989.
2. American Academy of Pediatrics Committee on Genetics: Folic acid for the prevention of neural tube defects, *Pediatrics* 92:493, 1993.
3. Anonymous: Economic burden of spina bifida: United States, 1980-1990, *MMWR* 38:264, 1989.
4. Bartonek A, et al: Ambulation in patients with myelomeningocele: a 12-year follow-up, *J Pediatr Orthop* 19:202, 1999.

5. Bartoshesky LE, et al: Seizures in children with meningomyelocele, *Am J Dis Child* 139:400, 1985.
6. Belt-Niedbala BJ, et al: Linear growth measurement: a comparison of single arm-lengths and arm-span, *Dev Med Child Neurol* 28:319, 1986.
7. Bronfenbrenner U: *The ecology of human development,* Cambridge, Mass, 1979, Harvard University Press.
8. Broughton NS, Menelaus MB, editors: *Menelaus' orthopaedic management of spina bifida cystica,* New York, 1998, WB Saunders.
9. Bruner JP, et al: Endoscopic coverage of fetal myelomeningocele in utero, *Am J Obstet Gynecol* 180:153, 1999.
10. Chait PG, et al: Fecal incontinence in children: treatment with percutaneous cecostomy tube placement: a prospective study, *Radiology* 203: 621, 1997.
11. Cher ML, Allen TD: Continence in the myelodysplastic patient following enterocystoplasty, *J Urol* 149:1103, 1993.
12. Cragan JD, et al: Surveillance for anencephaly and spina bifida and the impact of prenatal diagnosis—United States, 1985-1994, *MMWR CDC Surveill Summ* 25:1, 1995.
13. Curry JI, Osborne A, Malone PS: The MACE procedure: experience in the United Kingdom, *J Pediatr Surg* 34:338, 1999.
14. Forrester MB, Merz RD, Yoon PW: Impact of prenatal diagnosis and elective termination on the prevalence of selected birth defects in Hawaii, *Am J Epidemiol* 148:1206, 1998.
15. Gibson PJ, et al: Lumbosacral skin markers and identification of occult spinal dysraphism in neonates, *Acta Paediatr* 84:208, 1995.
16. Irvin NA, Kennell JH, Klaus MH: Caring for the parents of an infant with a congenital malformation. In Klaus MH, Kennell JH, editors: *Parent-infant bonding,* ed 2, St Louis, 1982, Mosby.
17. Kirk VG, Morielli A, Brouillette RT: Sleep-disordered breathing in patients with myelomeningocele: the missed diagnosis, *Dev Med Child Neurol* 41:40, 1999.
18. Kuller JA, et al: Cesarean delivery for fetal malformations, *Obstet Gynecol Surv* 51:371, 1996.
19. Lary JM, Edmonds LD: Prevalence of spina bifida at birth—United States, 1983-1990: a comparison of two surveillance systems, *MMWR CDC Surveill Summ* 19:15, 1996.
20. Libenson MH, et al: Acetazolamide and furosemide for posthemorrhagic hydrocephalus of the newborn, *Pediatr Neurol* 20:185, 1999.
21. Liptak GS, Revell GM: Management of bowel dysfunction in children with spinal cord disease or injury using the enema continence catheter, *J Pediatr* 120:190, 1992.
22. Liptak GS, et al: Mobility aids in children with high-level meningomyelocele: parapodium versus wheelchair, *Dev Med Child Neurol* 34:787, 1992.
23. Liptak GS, et al: The management of children with spinal dysraphism, *J Child Neurol* 3:3, 1988.
24. Little DM, et al: Renal transplantation in patients with spina bifida, *Urology* 44:319, 1994.
25. McCormick MC, Charney EB, Stemmler MM: Assessing the impact of a child with spina bifida on the family, *Dev Med Child Neurol* 28:53, 1986.
26. McInerny TK: The general pediatrician as care coordinator for children with chronic illness, *Pediatrician* 15:102, 1988.
27. Merkles RG, Solish SB, Scherzer AL: Meningomyelocele and Hirschsprung disease: theoretical and clinical significance, *Pediatrics* 76:299, 1985.
28. Milunsky A: Prenatal detection of neural tube defects. VI. Experience with 20,000 pregnancies, *JAMA* 244:2731, 1980.
29. Milunsky A, et al: Multivitamin/folic acid supplementation in early pregnancy reduces the prevalence of neural tube defects, *JAMA* 262: 2847, 1989.
30. Niggemann B, et al: Latex provocation tests in patients with spina bifida: who is at risk of becoming symptomatic? *J Allergy Clin Immunol* 102:665, 1998.
31. Ottolini MC, et al: Relationship of asymptomatic bacteriuria and renal scarring in children with neuropathic bladders who are practicing clean intermittent catheterization, *J Pediatr* 127:368, 1995.
32. Pollack IF, Kinnunen D, Albright AL: The effect of early craniocervical decompression on functional outcome in neonates and young infants with myelodysplasia and symptomatic Chiari II malformations: results from a prospective series, *Neurosurgery* 38:703, 1996.
33. Raddish M, et al: The immunization status of children with spina bifida, *Am J Dis Child* 147:849, 1993.
34. Rindahl MA, et al: Magnetic resonance imaging of pediatric dysraphism, *Magn Reson Imaging* 7:217, 1989.
35. Rush D: Periconceptional folate and neural tube defects, *Am J Clin Nutr* 59(suppl 2):511, 1994.
36. Sandford MK, Kissling GE, Joubert PE: Neural tube defect etiology: new evidence concerning maternal hyperthermia, health and diet, *Dev Med Child Neurol* 34:661, 1992.
37. Schlager TA, et al: Nitrofurantoin prophylaxis for bacteriuria and urinary tract infection in children with neurogenic bladder on intermittent catheterization, *J Pediatr* 132:704, 1998.
38. Selzman AA, Elder JS, Mapstone TB: Urologic consequences of myelodysplasia and other congenital abnormalities of the spinal cord. *Urol Clin North Am* 20:485, 1993.
39. Shaw GM, et al: Maternal vitamin use, genetic variation of infant methylenetetrahydrofolate reductase, and risk for spina bifida, *Am J Epidemiol* 148:30, 1998.
40. Shurtleff DB: Mobility. In Shurtleff DB, editor: *Myelodysplasia and exstrophies: significance, prevention, and treatment,* New York, 1986, Grune & Stratton.
41. Szepfalusi Z, et al: Latex sensitization in spina bifida appears disease-associated, *J Pediatr* 134:344, 1999.
42. Talwar D, Baldwin MA, Horbatt CI: Epilepsy in children with meningomyelocele, *Pediatr Neurol* 13:29, 1995.
43. Tulipan N, Hernanz-Schulman M, Bruner JP: Reduced hindbrain herniation after intrauterine myelomeningocele repair: a report of four cases, *Pediatr Neurosurg* 29:274, 1998.
44. Velie EM, Shaw GM: Impact of prenatal diagnosis and elective termination on prevalence and risk estimates of neural tube defects in California, 1989-1991, *Am J Epidemiol* 144:473, 1996.
45. Wu HY, Baskin LS, Kogan BA: Neurogenic bladder dysfunction due to myelomeningocele: neonatal versus childhood treatment, *J Urol* 157: 2295, 1997.

265 Spinal Deformities

Edward M. Sills

Back pain in children usually is a sign of an underlying disorder. Postural abnormalities may or may not indicate an underlying disorder, and the challenge to the physician is to determine whether the child's posture is caused by an underlying skeletal deformity or merely is a habit that exaggerates, increases, or decreases in the normal spinal curves. Abnormal curvatures and protrusions merit careful investigation. The thoracic spine normally has some kyphosis, and the lumbar spine normally has slight lordosis. If either condition is excessive, progressive, or painful, concern is appropriate. Scoliosis, a side-to-side curve, always is abnormal (a classification of spinal deformities is provided in Box 265-1).

CONGENITAL MALFORMATIONS

The newborn is relaxed when placed prone in the examiner's palm. The infant's back falls into slight flexion, allowing detection of meningomyelocele, congenital scoliosis, kyphosis, or dorsolumbar hyperflexion. Lumbar spinal deformity may be indicated by a hair tuft, dimple, discoloration, or a palpable spina bifida lamina defect (see Chapter 264, Spina Bifida).

Congenital scoliosis is the result of asymmetrical growth. It is characterized by a lateral curvature of the spine caused by an asymmetrical structural vertebral deformity. The curve is fixed and inflexible. When located near the middle of the spine, the segments of the spine above and below compensate for it by curving in opposite directions. The result is a balanced spine and a straight back. Treatment is unnecessary. When, however, the asymmetrical vertebra is at the base of the spine, the compensatory curve that develops above is insufficient, and a curvature progresses as the patient grows. This condition requires surgical correction before adolescence. When the deformity occurs in the cervical spine, a "wryneck" deformity results, and thoracolumbar compensatory curvature severely distorts posture. Unilateral surgical fusions are required to minimize deformity.

Congenital kyphosis is caused by lack of segmentation of vertebral bodies anteriorly or by lack of formation of a vertebral body. Surgical fusion is required to prevent paraplegia.

Other congenital malformations of the spine include Klippel-Feil syndrome, which is characterized by a short neck, limitation of head motion, and a low posterior hairline. Spina bifida often is present in the cervical spine; it is caused by failure of the two lateral halves of the vertebral arch to fuse. Exercises to maintain the neck's functional range of motion are indicated, but surgery is contraindicated because of the danger of injuring the cervical spinal cord.

Spina bifida can be mild and of no clinical significance (occulta), or it can be severe (vera), with meningeal and neural elements protruding posteriorly. When the protrusion includes bony elements, it may transfix the spinal cord. This transfixing spur is called *diastematomyelia*. Severe forms of spina bifida require prompt neurosurgical correction.

Congenital vertebral anomalies also are seen in several syndromes in which other anomalies may be present. These include the following:

1. Larsen's syndrome—vertebral, joint, facial, and palate
2. Waardenburg's syndrome—spine and ribs
3. Goldenhar's syndrome—oculoauriculovertebral dysplasia
4. Morquio's syndrome (mucopolysaccharidosis, type IV)—odontoid dysplasia with atlantoaxial subluxation
5. VATER association—*v*ertebral anomalies, *a*nal atresia, *t*racheo*e*sophageal fistula, and *r*adial dysplasia. Sometimes, VATER association includes congenital heart disease and renal dysplasia.

ACQUIRED ABNORMALITIES

Scoliosis

Scoliosis can be nonstructural (corrects with side bending) or structural (no improvement with position change). Nonstructural scoliosis results from posture habit, splinting because of pain, muscle spasm, or hysteria. Of the structural forms of scoliosis, the congenital (e.g., absent or fused spinal segments), metabolic (e.g., juvenile osteoporosis), or neuromuscular (e.g., poliomyelitis or cerebral palsy) types are less common than idiopathic scoliosis, which accounts for 75% of all cases. Although most cases are idiopathic, an increased familial risk exists for scoliosis. Idiopathic scoliosis can appear clinically at any age, although the majority of cases begin in adolescence and most are girls who usually exhibit a right thoracic or right thoracolumbar pattern. The infantile form begins before age 3 years, is predominant in boys, and usually resolves without treatment because of vertebral compensations above and below the area of curve. The juvenile form occurs between ages 6 and 10 years, has no gender predilection, and usually consists of a right thoracic curve. Although some of the mild curves do not progress, the juvenile and adolescent curves tend to progress rapidly during growth spurts.

Scoliosis usually is painless and is discovered on routine physical examinations or at school scoliosis screening programs. When the patient bends forward, prominence of one scapula, of one side of the rib cage, or of the lumbar para-

BOX 265-1

CLASSIFICATION OF SPINAL DEFORMITY

A. Idiopathic
   1. Infantile
   2. Juvenile
   3. Adolescent
B. Neuromuscular
   1. Neuropathic
      a. Upper motor neuron lesion
         (1) Cerebral palsy
         (2) Spinocerebellar degenerations
         (3) Syringomyelia
         (4) Spinal cord tumor
         (5) Spinal cord trauma
      b. Lower motor neuron lesion
         (1) Poliomyelitis
         (2) Other viral myelitis
         (3) Trauma
         (4) Spinal muscular atrophy
         (5) Meningomyelocele (paralytic)
      c. Dysautonomia (Riley-Day)
   2. Myopathic
      a. Arthrogryposis
      b. Muscular dystrophy
      c. Fiber-type disproportion
      d. Congenital hypotonia
      e. Myotonia dystrophica
C. Congenital
   1. Congenital scoliosis
      a. Failure of formation
         (1) Wedge
         (2) Hemivertebra
      b. Failure of segmentation
         (1) Unilateral bar
         (2) Bilateral bar
   2. Congenital kyphosis
      a. Failure of formation
      b. Failure of segmentation
      c. Mixed

C. Congenital—*cont'd*
   3. Congenital lordosis
   4. Associated with neural tissue defect
      a. Meningomyelocele
      b. Meningocele
      c. Spinal dysraphism (diastematomyelia)
D. Neurofibromatosis
E. Mesenchymal
   1. Marfan syndrome
   2. Ehlers-Danlos syndrome
F. Traumatic
   1. Fracture or dislocation
   2. After irradiation
   3. After laminectomy
G. Soft-tissue contractures
   1. After thoracoplasty
   2. Burns
H. Osteochondrodystrophies
   1. Achondroplasia
   2. Spondyloepiphyseal dysplasia
   3. Diastrophic dwarfism
   4. Mucopolysaccharidosis
I. Scheuermann disease
J. Infection
K. Tumor
L. Rheumatoid disease
M. Metabolic
   1. Rickets
   2. Juvenile osteoporosis
   3. Osteogenesis imperfecta
N. Lumbosacral anomalies
O. Hysterical
P. Functional
   1. Postural
   2. Secondary to short limb
   3. Secondary to pain

Modified from Scoliosis Research Society.

spinous muscles can indicate the site and direction of the scoliosis. An erect anteroposterior spinal roentgenogram determines the degree of curvature and the structure of the vertebrae.

Treatment is undertaken because pulmonary restriction, significant back pain, and cosmetic deformity are the sequelae of untreated severe scoliosis. Exercises are of no benefit in retarding or reversing the progress of scoliosis. A curvature in excess of 40 degrees requires surgical fusion regardless of the patient's age. Curves between 20 and 40 degrees should not require treatment if skeletal maturation is complete, but bracing often is recommended in the growing child. A curve milder than 20 degrees should be observed for possible progression but does not require treatment.

Kyphosis

An acquired dorsal hump can be secondary to a spinal tumor, radiation, infection, or surgery. The most common cause of acquired kyphosis is an osteochondrosis known as Scheuermann's disease (see Chapter 243, Osteochondroses), which occurs in 5% of the population. Alternatively, glucocorticoid-induced osteoporosis, caused either by supraphysiological levels of endogenous (Cushing's disease) or exogenously administered glucocorticoids, can provoke kyphosis. Excess glucocorticoids often act to suppress bone formation and increase bone resorption, leading to trabecular bone loss, vertebral body collapse, and pathological fractures causing an increased propensity toward kyphotic spinal malalignment. The most common site is in the lower thoracic vertebrae, but this condition can occur in any site in the vertebral column. The initial event is a bulging of the intervertebral disks in the direction of contiguous vertebral bodies, which exerts pressure against the cartilage plates covering the bodies, causing thinning of the plates. This interferes with endochondral bone formation on the growth surface of the plates, causing gaps that are the basis for the herniation of the disk into the bodies, isolating the apophyseal ossification center from the vertebral body. The disk space narrows, more so anteriorly, causing increased pressure on the anterior portions of contiguous vertebral bodies and impeding their longitudinal growth anteriorly, resulting in attendant kyphosis.

An aching pain aggravated by physical exertion is present in the affected part of the vertebral column. The affected area is tender to palpation. Having the patient assume a stooping position often causes the pain to increase. Once the backache has been present for a year or so, the kyphosis easily is apparent as a round-back deformity. In many instances the pain is so minor that the patient first complains to the physician about pain caused by "poor posture," and then the kyphosis is noted. Roentgenograms reveal a narrowing of the anterior disk space and defects on the surfaces of adjacent vertebrae at sites where the disk tissue has penetrated the bodies. The prolapsed disk tissue, in time, becomes walled off by osseous tissue, forming a bulbous mass of extruded tissue appearing as an area of lucency in the affected body (Schmorl nodule). In some children the condition can progress to cause severe deformity and dysfunction; in others, it stabilizes and the deformity may disappear. Treatment is aimed at preventing further deformity by casting or bracing. In those rare instances of rapid progression or very severe pain, spinal fusion is necessary. The majority of youngsters, however, require careful observation with intervention only if there is progression of the deformity.

BACK PAIN

Although scoliosis and kyphosis can be painful, usually they are painless postural deformities. The pediatrician should be aware of several painful disorders related to spinal deformity (see also Chapter 118, Back Pain).

Spondylolysis and Spondylolisthesis

Spondylolysis, a defect in the continuity of the pars interarticularis of the posterior portion of L4 or L5, may lead to forward slippage of the vertebral body, known as *spondylolisthesis*. The horizontal slippage usually involves the fifth lumbar vertebral body moving anteriorly in relationship to S1. This deformity, however, can occur anywhere in the vertebral column. Spondylolysis often causes back pain before the spondylolisthesis develops. Because spondylolysis is fairly common in young athletes with low back pain, primary care physicians need to have a high index of suspicion with this group of patients. Trauma, causing disruption of the pars interarticularis, is believed to be the cause of spondylolysis in a genetically susceptible host. The propensity for spondylolysis to become spondylolisthesis with forward slippage is increased during growth spurts. Single photon emission computed tomography (SPECT) scans are important aids in diagnosis.

A flattening of the normal lumbar lordosis with posterior tilting of the pelvis is noted in spondylolysis. An oblique roentgenogram reveals the pars interventricularis defect; a standing lateral roentgenogram demonstrates spondylolisthesis. Activities that hyperextend the lumbar spine should be avoided, and exercises to reduce lumbar lordosis relieve the pain of spondylolysis. Once slippage occurs, surgical spinal fusion is necessary.

Infections

Infections involving the spinal structures are exceedingly rare. Acute pyogenic osteomyelitis and tuberculosis (Pott's disease) cause bone destruction, initially in the anterior portion of the vertebrae, leading to collapse. Vigorous antibiotic therapy and immobilization are indicated.

Disk space inflammation, or diskitis, can appear as a fever of unknown origin accompanied by a limp, low back pain, or refusal to walk. Narrowing of the disk space is the usual roentgenographic finding. In all cases, blood cultures are indicated. The majority of younger patients do not evidence bacterial infection and require only immobilization. Children older than age 8 years occasionally are found to have staphylococcal infections. The indications for using antibiotics include positive blood culture results, recurrences of back pain accompanied by systemic signs such as fever, leukocytosis with a "left shift" in the differential white blood cell count, erythrocyte sedimentation rate elevation, bone erosion, or clinical advancement of disease despite immobilization.

Tumors

Bone tumors occur most commonly in adolescence and usually appear at the end of growth peaks. Of the malignant bone tumors, none primarily involve the spine, although chondrosarcomas and the marrow tumors (leukemias, lymphomas, Ewing's tumor, and histiocytic lymphoma) often invade the pelvis early and can cause low back pain in adolescents.

Roentgenograms display bony lesions surrounded by a soft-tissue mass. Calcification of periosteum lifted away from bone causes a characteristic sunburst appearance.

Of the nonmalignant tumors, the osteogenic group often involves the spine. Both osteoid osteoma and osteoblastoma are reparative rather than infiltrative. Osteoid osteoma occurs in long bones and in the posterior portion of the vertebrae; osteoblastoma occurs in the neural arches of the vertebral column. Pain, usually occurring at night, is the common complaint and is relieved quickly by aspirin. On roentgenogram, the examiner sees a hyperostotic lesion surrounding a nidus of sclerotic bone separated by a radiolucent zone. Surgical excision is curative.

When to Refer

Whenever uncertain as to diagnosis or treatment

Use of Alternative Medicine

Nonsurgical physical therapies have been recommended to correct alignment deficits, but none have been subjected to clinical trial.

When to Hospitalize

Whenever surgery or intensive intravenous therapy is indicated

SUGGESTED READINGS

Burgos-Vargas R, Petty RE: Juvenile ankylosing spondylitis, *Rheum Dis Clin North Am* 18:123, 1992.

Congeni J, McCulloch J, Swanson K: Lumbar spondylolysis: a study of natural progression in athletes, *Am J Sports Med* 25:248, 1997.

Freehill AK, Lenke LG: Severe kyphosis secondary to glucocorticoid-induced osteoporosis in a young adult with Cushing's disease: case report and literature review, *Spine* 24:189, 1999.

Gary JP, McShane J: Lumbar scoliosis in adolescent athletes, *J Fam Pract* 47:145, 1998.

Harvey CJ, et al: The radiological investigation of lumbar spondylolysis, *Clin Radiol* 53:723, 1998.

Hensinger RN: Current concept review: spondylolysis and spondylolisthesis in children and adolescents, *J Bone Joint Surg (Am)* 71:1098, 1989.

King HA: Evaluating the child with back pain, *Pediatr Clin North Am* 33:1489, 1986.

Letts M, et al: Fractures of the pars interarticularis in adolescent athletes: a clinical-biomedical analysis, *J Pediatr Orthop* 6:40, 1986.

Mitcheli LJ, Wood R: Back pain in young athletes: significant difference from adults in causes and patterns, *Arch Pediatr Adolesc Med* 149:15, 1995.

Oestreich AE, Young LW, Poussaint TY: Scoliosis circa 2000: radiologic imaging perspective. I. Diagnosis and pretreatment, *Skeletal Radiol* 12: 591, 1998.

Oestreich AE, Young LW, Poussaint TY: Scoliosis circa 2000: radiologic imaging perspective. II. Treatment and follow-up, *Skeletal Radiol* 12:651, 1998.

Papanicolaou N, et al: Bone scintigraphy and radiography in young athletes with low back pain, *Am J Roentgenol* 145:1039, 1985.

Portenoy RK, et al: Back pain in the cancer patient: an algorithm for evaluation and management, *Neurology* 37:134, 1987.

Riseborough E, Herndon JH: *Scoliosis and other deformities: deformities of the axial skeleton,* Boston, 1975, Little, Brown.

Rittler M, Paz JE, Castilla EE: VACTERL association, epidemiologic definition and delineation, *Am J Med Genet* 63:529, 1996.

Schmorl G: *The human spine in health and disease,* New York, 1959, Grune & Stratton.

Sills EM: What's causing the back pain? *Contemp Pediatr* 5:85, 1988.

Sward L, et al: Back pain and radiologic changes in the thoracolumbar spine of athletes, *Spine* 15:124, 1990.

Tachdjian M: *Pediatric orthopedics,* Philadelphia, 1979, WB Saunders.

Theiss SM, Smith MD, Winter RB: The long-term follow-up of patients with Klippel-Feil syndrome and congenital scoliosis, *Spine* 22:1219, 1997.

Williams HJ: Vertebral epiphysitis, *Am J Roentgenol* 90:1236, 1963.

266 Sports Injuries

Michael T. Busch • David E. Hall

Increasing numbers of young athletes are involved in organized sports. Many athletes now train in sports year-round and frequently several sports at a time. Organized sports count for only about one third of sports injuries, with the remainder occurring in physical education classes and in recreational sports. Wrestling and football have the highest significant injury rates per participant in high school, followed by softball, gymnastics, track and field, and soccer. Tennis and swimming produce the fewest injuries. Other sports fall somewhere in between. Frequency of injury, however, is not always the best measure of a sport's risk. The trampoline, for example, accounts for a disproportionately large number of injures that cause paralysis. Although intuitively it seems that younger athletes would be at greater risk for injury, statistics from soccer and American football demonstrate just the opposite. The risk of injury is much greater among senior high school students than among junior high and younger participants.

Although many sports injuries are random events, it is estimated that nearly two thirds of all injuries could be reduced by improvements in conditioning, equipment, compliance with rules, coaching and supervision, rehabilitation of existing injuries, and efforts to prevent reinjury. Many schools now use certified athletic trainers for the prevention and rehabilitation of sports injuries. These programs should be encouraged and supported. Inexperienced coaches with high expectations of young athletes and a poor understanding of training may contribute to injury.

Competition often is emphasized, but the greatest value of sports participation may lie in fostering lifelong habits of exercise and recreation. Especially for younger children, programs should emphasize participation by all children, not just the physically gifted.

This chapter will discuss some of the medical issues regarding sports participation such as heat stroke and drug use, overuse syndromes, and acute trauma. It also discusses the common problem of anterior knee pain in young athletes.

Sports medicine is a discipline in itself. This chapter can serve as only an introduction to some of the more common problems. The reader is referred to references on sports medicine for information on treatment and exercises for rehabilitation.[2,5,25] Sports medicine centers, located in many urban areas, provide consultation and continuing education for interested physicians.

HEAT INJURY

Heat injury is commonly divided into three syndromes: heat cramps, heat exhaustion, and heat stroke.

Heat is lost in five ways[2]:

1. Convection: when heat from the body is transferred to cooler air moving across its surface
2. Conduction: heat transfer to another object by direct contact, as occurs when the skin comes in direct contact with a cooler object, such as a wet towel or shirt
3. Radiation: when heat from the body radiates into a cooler environment. This is not very effective when the ambient temperature is greater than the typical skin temperature, which is about 87° F
4. Respiration: when heat is lost during exhalation and cooler air is inspired
5. Evaporation: typically of sweat

When the environmental temperature is warmer than the body temperature, the primary method of heat loss is evaporation of sweat, and heat loss methods 1 through 4 become less effective. Blood vessels close to the surface of the skin dilate to increase blood flow and heat dissipation. As the humidity increases, evaporation is less effective in producing loss of heat. Interestingly, some acclimatization to high humidity occurs with training and exposure to warmer temperatures.

Heat exposure syndromes include heat cramps, heat exhaustion, and heat stroke. All appear to be more common in athletes who do not take adequate fluids, are not acclimatized to local heat and humidity, and are poorly conditioned. Most authorities recommend that adult-size athletes take ½ liter of fluids per hour during persistent activity. Water usually is adequate. Thirst is not a reliable indicator of fluid requirements during vigorous exercise. Salt tablets are not recommended, since most athletes receive abundant salt in their diet.

Heat cramps usually involve the arms, abdomen, or legs. Affected individuals usually have been sweating profusely. Treatment consists of rest in a cool environment, stretching, and fluids. Many fail to recognize that these cramps are a symptom of dehydration and heat stress, rather than a muscle problem.

Heat exhaustion is a more severe syndrome probably caused by ineffective cardiovascular and autonomic responses to heat. Patients feel weak, faint, dizzy, and nauseous. They may vomit and look pale. Syncope sometimes occurs. They may sweat profusely, or if severely dehydrated, the skin may feel warm and dry. Surprisingly, body temperature often is normal. Treatment consists of cool fluids and placement in a cool environment. Cool compresses and fanning also will help. If the affected athlete is unable to tolerate oral fluids, administering intravenous fluids should be considered.

Heat stroke is a medical emergency in which mechanisms for cooling are overwhelmed. The rectal temperature is markedly elevated. The skin is hot and dry. Patients show signs of central nervous system dysfunction, such as irritability, combativeness, and disorientation, that may progress to obtundation. Tachycardia and hypotension often are present. Heat stroke is most often seen in long-distance runners and is the second most common cause of fatality in football players (head and neck injuries are the first).[2] To treat heat stroke, ice-water-soaked towels or wet sheets with fans (if ice is not available) should be applied. The patient should be taken to an emergency room immediately. Heat stroke is most common when the temperature is greater than 95° F and the humidity is higher than 50%.

DRUG USE IN ATHLETES

Athletes frequently use drugs and nutritional supplements they believe will give them a competitive advantage or will improve their strength or appearance. The American Academy of Pediatrics and the American College of Sports Medicine have issued policy statements condemning the use of these supplements.[1] Despite this, their use is exceedingly common. Anabolic steroid use, for example, has been reported to be as high as 5% to 11% among high school males and 2.5% among high school females.[3,11,26]

Anabolic steroid use is most common among football players and track participants. Clues to excessive use include jaundice, increased acne, behavioral changes (aggressiveness, irritability, marked mood swings), gynecomastia, and testicular atrophy. Hirsutism and deepening of the voice may occur in women. Liver function tests may be elevated. Anabolic steroid withdrawal also may cause side effects such as mood changes, irritability, hot flashes, nausea, myalgia, malaise, tachycardia, and hypertension.[1] Although controversy exists, anabolic steroids do appear to increase muscle mass and decrease catabolism of muscle in some situations.[12] Anabolic steroids adversely affect lipid profiles. Unfortunately, physicians may have overestimated and overstated short-term side effects, causing them to lose credibility with athletes, who see their peers taking these drugs without obvious problems.[12,23] Little information is available on long-term effects.

The Anabolic Steroids Control Act of 1990 made most anabolic steroids schedule III controlled substances. Illicit distribution is a felony. However, androstenedione, often mentioned in the media as a drug used by major league baseball player and home-run king Mark McGwire, is still available without a prescription.

Creatine supplements, often advertised in body building magazines and sold at many gyms and health food stores, also are popular with adolescents. Unlike most androgen supplements, they can be obtained legally. In fact, some colleges provide them free of charge to athletes. They are not banned in professional sports or in the Olympic games.

Creatine is converted to phosphocreatine in muscle with the help of the enzyme creatine kinase. Phosphocreatine is believed to serve as a reservoir for the high-energy phosphate bonds of ATP, which are the sources of energy for muscle contraction. The idea behind the supplements is that excess phosphocreatine will lead to a higher rate of ATP resynthesis during exertion and delay the fatigue that results from ATP depletion.[20]

Some studies do show some benefit from creatine for activities requiring short bursts of high-intensity muscle contraction.[6,13] There is little evidence that creatine is helpful in endurance sports. Some athletes argue that it helps them train more vigorously by reducing the time to recover from exertion.

Creatine supplements appear to elevate serum creatinine levels. This is not an indication of any renal dysfunction, but just a reflection of an increased load of creatinine. Long-term effects are unknown, and most sports medicine experts do not recommend its use.

Over-the-counter supplements are not under government control, and it is difficult to be sure that these medications contain what is printed on their the labels. In addition, some supplements have been found to contain small doses of stimulants that cause athletes to test positive for banned substances.[15]

INJURIES TO BONE AND SOFT TISSUES

Injuries related to sports participation fall into the general categories of overuse syndromes that develop over time and acute traumatic injuries.

Overuse Syndromes

Overuse injuries are characterized by injury to bone, cartilage, or soft tissue caused by repetitive submaximal physical stress. In contrast to an acute fracture or soft-tissue injury, the tissue breakdown in overuse injuries occurs gradually. This phenomenon of hard- and soft-tissue breakdown is a normal, daily occurrence. The body continually remodels these tissues, so that they recuperate fully.

Athletic training is a process of repetitively stimulating the musculoskeletal system and relying on remodeling and ultimately hypertrophy and strengthening to occur. Training not only strengthens the muscles but also strengthens bones and connective tissues.

When an imbalance occurs between the rate of breakdown of the connective tissues and the body's ability to remodel them, stress injuries occur. In young athletes, the frequency with which these problems occur has grown tremendously over the past several decades Box 266-1 lists factors that contribute to overuse injuries in young athletes.

More and more young athletes are training harder and longer as competition grows. A larger proportion of youths also are becoming involved in competitive sports. Many athletes now train year-round for participation in one sport, while others participate in multiple sports each year and frequently several sports at a time. Frequently, time off is not considered a priority. Inexperienced coaches may have unrealistic expectations of young athletes. All of these factors contribute to the growing number of training errors that often underlie these conditions.

Prevention of overuse syndromes involves the education of young athletes, their parents, their coaches, and the entire health care team from trainers to physicians. Understanding these principles is crucial to successfully returning an athlete to sports after sustaining one of these overuse conditions. Failure to change the underlying problem often simply results in reinjury.

Overuse syndromes of bone. Stress fracture of bone is conceptually the simplest overuse syndrome of the musculoskeletal system. Repetitive loading of this relatively rigid tissue leads to work hardening. Unless remodeling occurs, the bone becomes brittle and eventually breaks. Along the way, the athlete begins to experience progressive discomfort with activities. This most commonly occurs with long-distance running.

METAPHYSEAL/DIAPHYSEAL STRESS INJURIES. The athlete may experience gradual onset of symptoms. Eventually, pain may preclude running. In some circumstances, the weakened bone may fail completely and result in a complete and/or displaced fracture.

Although the majority of these occur in later adolescence (ages 16 to 19 years) some do occur at younger ages. Typically, there is an equal distribution of male and female patients.

Only about 10% of radiographs are abnormal at the onset of symptoms. A bone scan is much more sensitive for detecting an early stress fracture of the metaphysis or diaphysis (Table 266-1). The bone scan findings, however, must be correlated to the clinical symptoms. As many as 50% of adolescents with stress fractures will show on bone scan multiple areas of stress response, many of which do not correlate to areas of symptoms. Currently, magnetic resonance imaging (MRI) probably is the most sensitive study for stress fractures.

BOX 266-1

FACTORS CONTRIBUTING TO OVERUSE INJURIES IN YOUNG ATHLETES

Training errors
Increased recreational time
Increased intensity and duration of competition
Increasing standards in competition
Inadequate preseasoning conditioning
Suboptimal facilities and equipment
Overly enthusiastic coaches and parents
Participation in multiple sports
Endless seasons

Metaphyseal and diaphyseal stress fractures in young athletes most commonly involve the fibula, metatarsals, tibia, femur, and ulna; but virtually any bone can be affected. Fortunately, stress fractures of the metatarsals (typically the second or third) and the distal fibula rarely have complications other than pain and temporary disability. Fractures of the tibia, humerus, and forearm rarely displace but have the potential to do so. Stress fractures of the hip are rare but have the highest potential for morbidity; displaced femoral neck fractures can disrupt the blood supply to the femoral head and lead to avascular necrosis and arthritis.

Most diaphyseal and metaphyseal stress fractures are managed by rest. Crutches often are necessary. Occasionally, casts and immobilization are needed. Healing time ranges from 4 to 12 weeks. A well-designed plan of alternative training, gradual resumption of participation in sports, and monitoring for recurrent symptoms is necessary.

Occasionally, stress fractures require surgical intervention. A suspected stress fracture of the proximal femur is probably best managed by an orthopedic surgeon. A slipped capital femoral epiphysis must be considered. Screw stabilization for either the slipped epiphysis or stress fracture may be needed. Stress fractures of the fifth metatarsal tend to be recurrent and often are best managed with an intramedullary screw.

APOPHYSEAL CONDITIONS

Osgood-Schlatter disease. In 1903, Osgood and Schlatter separately described a disorder of the proximal tibial apophysis that commonly affects young athletes but may bother other active youngsters who are not involved in formal, organized sports.[14] See Chapter 243, Osteochondroses. The tubercle of the proximal tibia is the insertion site of the patellar tendon. The quadriceps is the strongest muscle group in the body, and the tensions it generates through the patellar tendon are enormous. Stresses applied at the interface between the tendon and the apophysis create a disruption of the normal transition from the ossified and unossified tubercle into the tendon.[21] Although mechanics undoubtedly play a key role, some individuals appear to be predisposed to this condition.

Patients typically are 10 to 15 years of age at the onset of this disorder. Boys are more commonly affected than girls; however, female gymnasts are particularly prone to this problem. Approximately 15% of teenage boys and 10% of teenage girls have complained of pain at their tibial tubercle at some point. Bilaterality is high, although its reported incidence varies considerably. The average youngster with symptomatic Osgood-Schlatter disease has significant pain, ten-

Table 266-1 Parts of the Growth Plate of a Long Bone

Name	Root Origin	Definition
Physis		Specialized area of growth cartilage occurring at both ends of major long bones or at one end of the smaller tubular bones, such as metatarsals and phalanges
Epiphysis	Epi- (on)	Secondary ossification center interposed between the physis and joint articulation
Metaphysis	Meta- (next to)	Flared transition from the primary spongiosa of the physis to the dense tubular bone of the diaphysis
Diaphysis	Dia- (in between)	Dense cortical and tubular bone comprising the shaft
Apophysis	Apo- (arising from)	Specialized growth cartilage area to accommodate insertion of a major tendon

derness, and swelling of the tubercle on the presenting side and usually has some degree of findings on the contralateral side as well.

Many of these patients have a prior history of heel pain compatible with Sever's disease (calcaneal apophysitis—see below). As many as 20% to 30% have siblings who also have had apophysitis.

The pain in Osgood-Schlatter disease usually is well localized to the tibial tubercle; it typically increases with activity. Signs or symptoms of intraarticular problems of the knee joint itself are absent. A lateral radiograph of the knee can help to confirm the diagnosis by showing irregularity of the tibial tubercle and rule out a tumor or infection, which can mimic Osgood-Schlatter disease.

In the vast majority of patients, Osgood-Schlatter disease will simply run its course with time. Symptoms can last for 1 to 4 years. In approximately 3% of patients, a persistent ossicle will form that can remain symptomatic and ultimately require surgical excision.

Fracture of the tibial tubercle has been reported in patients with Osgood-Schlatter disease; its incidence is not known, but it appears to be very low. As such, it is not an absolute contraindication to remaining active in sports.

The symptoms are often relieved with:

1. Topical application of an ice pack to the area
2. Intermittent use of oral, nonsteroidal antiinflammatory drugs (NSAIDs)
3. Application of a compressive band over the area
4. Activity modifications as indicated by the symptoms
5. Hamstring stretching

Casts are not used routinely because immobilization may weaken ligament insertions. However, brief periods of rigid immobilization may be necessary for acute exacerbations.

Sinding-Larsen-Johansson disease. Sinding-Larsen-Johansson (SLJ) disease affects the inferior pole of the patella as a result of the same stresses that create the problem of Osgood-Schlatter disease.[17] Although an apophysis is not present at the inferior pole of the patella, there is a transition of the patellar ligament fibers as they join the bone. In response to chronic repetitive stresses, the patellar periosteum can create a bony reaction that is classic of SLJ.

Affected youngsters typically are 10 to 13 years of age. They complain of very well localized pain at the inferior pole of the patella. Like those with Osgood-Schlatter disease, they have no signs or symptoms of internal derangement of the knee joint itself. On physical examination, they exhibit point tenderness at the inferior edge of the patella and typically have no other abnormal findings.

A lateral radiograph of the knee may demonstrate irregular ossification at the inferior pole of the patella. Some clinicians mistake this for a fracture.

Pain in the same area without radiographic change often is due to patellar tendonitis or "jumper's knee." This is an early stage of SLJ disease. With advanced skeletal maturity, the periosteal reaction usually is not seen.

This entity is self-limited and typically lasts 3 to 12 months. Like Osgood-Schlatter disease, ice, NSAIDs, and activity modification may be helpful. Immobilization rarely is necessary, as is surgery. Rupture of the patellar tendon or a "sleeve fracture" (avulsion of the inferior pole of the patella with attached cartilage) is not a well-recognized complication of this disorder. In general, athletes may participate in sports as tolerated.

Calcaneal apophysitis. Calcaneal apophysitis, or Sever's disease, occurs at the apophyseal insertion of the Achilles tendon into the calcaneus.[19] The patient typically is 9 to 14 years of age, with a substantial peak at 10 and 11 years of age. Most (60% to 80%) of cases are bilateral.

Patients may present with complaints of heel, ankle, or foot pain. On physical examination, however, the discomfort typically is well localized at the region of the calcaneal apophysis. It typically is medial or posterior, though occasionally the tenderness may be on the lateral side. It is rare for the tenderness to be distal near the origin of the plantar fascia. There should be no swelling, warmth, or limitation of motion. Occasionally, because of a concurrent tendonitis, there is some tenderness along the course of the Achilles tendon itself. There is no classic radiographic change of calcaneal apophysitis. Significant irregularity of the ossifying calcaneal apophysis is a normal finding at this age and should not be confused as evidence of a fracture.

Radiographs of the heels can be obtained to rule out other osseous processes, such as tumor or infection. In bilateral cases, radiographs are only necessary if there is some atypical component of the history and physical examination that raises concern about some other diagnosis.

Treatment focuses primarily on symptom management. This condition almost always resolves with time, and complications are extremely rare.

Shoe inserts that provide padding beneath the heel can be very helpful. The material must be resilient enough so that it does not collapse. Typically, a ⅜-inch silicone or felt pad works best. Ice, NSAIDs, and activity modification are dictated by symptoms. Casts or Cam walkers occasionally are necessary for severe cases. Surgery is not indicated.

REPETITIVE PHYSEAL INJURIES

Little League shoulder. "Little League shoulder," or physiolysis of the proximal humerus, is a widening of the proximal humeral physeal plate.[24] It occurs almost exclusively in Little League baseball players. It typically affects pitchers, but occasionally, individuals who do a lot of throwing from other positions can develop it as well.

Usually, the patient is a 12- to 15-year-old male who complains of pain in the shoulder related to overhead throwing. The key consideration in the differential diagnosis is rotator cuff tendonitis. Many of the signs and symptoms are the same. The patient with Little League shoulder typically has more pain in the deltoid region as opposed to the subacromial region.

Another differential diagnostic consideration is impending pathological fracture from a simple bone cyst in the upper humerus. Radiographic widening of the proximal humeral physis on the affected side confirms the diagnosis of Little League shoulder.

The essence of treatment is rest. Complications are uncommon. If the symptoms are minimal, the young baseball player can often be allowed to bat and play in infield position that involves minimal throwing. Clinical and radiographic resolution can take up to 6 months. A carefully planned resumption of pitching can then begin, but monitoring for recurrence of symptoms is necessary.

Physeal widening of the distal radius. Physeal stress injury of the distal radius occurs almost exclusively in young female gymnasts. These injuries usually present with progressive pain in the wrists. Most often the pain is bilateral but may be more prominent on one side. On physical examination, point tenderness often is present and a prominence may be noted on the dorsum of the distal radial physis.

Differential diagnoses include carpal laxity with dorsal wrist capsular impingement, posterior interosseous neuroma, and avascular necrosis of the lunate.

Anteroposterior and lateral radiographs should demonstrate the physeal widening. Comparison films of the other side almost always are obtained, though both sides may be involved. Typically, there is some asymmetry.

Premature closure of the distal radial physis has been described, resulting in relative overgrowth of the ulna at the wrist. This causes asymmetrical loading of the carpal bones that can lead to chronic wrist disability. The goal of treatment is resolution of symptoms and normalization of the radiographs. This usually takes 3 months or longer. Once the athlete returns to gymnastics, clinical and radiographic monitoring are required.

EPIPHYSEAL OVERUSE CONDITIONS. Perhaps the best example of a repetitive stress-related injury of the epiphyses occurs at the capitellum (the lateral condyle of the distal humerus where it articulates with the radius). These injuries are typically classified as "osteochondroses" rather than "stress fractures." In osteochondroses, a segment of epiphyseal bone and overlying articular cartilage becomes loose.

Panner disease. Panner described a lesion of a young boy's capitellum that he compared with Legg-Calvé-Perthes disease. In patients younger than 10 years of age who develop irregularity of the capitellum, the course usually is benign. There appears to be an avascular segment in the center of the capitellum. With time it will revascularize. There is a substantial cartilaginous cap around this area, and loose bodies typically do not form. Sequelae are rare, and treatment simply involves rest.

Osteochondritis dissecans of the capitellum. Although the term *osteochondritis dissecans* implies that an inflammatory process is present, histological studies have failed to confirm this. This is clearly a repetitive stress phenomenon and most commonly occurs in baseball pitchers. As the ball is released during the pitching motion, a valgus movement occurs at the elbow. Tension occurs on the medial side of the elbow, and compressive forces are created across the radial capitellar articulation. The capitellum has an end-arterial blood supply, which may be partially responsible for its susceptibility to developing avascular necrosis from these chronic repetitive compression forces.

Any pitching style that releases the ball lateral to the body's midsagittal plane accentuates the valgus moment at the elbow. Therefore, side arm pitches, many curve ball techniques, and others can increase the compression loads across the lateral side of the elbow.

Patients typically complain of aching pain in the lateral side of the elbow. With time, they can lose range of motion. Osteochondral fragments can displace acutely, resulting in a loose body sensation, a locked elbow, and/or significant synovitis and pain.

Plain radiographs often will demonstrate a lesion of the capitellum. Either a sclerotic region or simply radiolucency may be present. Tangential views may be necessary to see this. Occasionally, computed tomography (CT) scanning and/or magnetic resonance imaging (MRI) are helpful.

Unlike most overuse syndromes in young athletes, the sequelae of this condition are not always benign. Osteochondritis of the capitellum can result in permanent arthrosis of the elbow joint.

The most important lesson about this condition is the opportunity for prevention. Junior baseball programs typically have rules limiting the frequency and duration youngsters can pitch. Typically, this is three innings per game and up to six innings per week. Young athletes, parents, and coaches need to be educated about this condition so that excessive pitching does not occur at other times.

Cases of osteochondritis dissecans of the capitellum occasionally heal with prolonged rest. However, surgery often is necessary to remove an unstable or displaced bone fragment.

Overuse syndrome of soft tissues

TENDONOSES. Overuse injuries of tendons can occur in younger patients. In adults, tendonitis is divided into three stages based on the progression of the disease from inflammation of the paratenon (the fatty or synovial tissue between a tendon and its sheath) through inflammation of the tendon itself, and finally into degenerative change of the tendon that ultimately results in rupture. Typically in young athletes, only the earliest inflammatory stage is seen.

The most common tendonitis in young athletes is that of the Achilles tendon. The etiology is not clear. Symptoms typically are located 2 to 6 cm above the insertion of the Achilles tendon into the calcaneus. Some lack of flexibility in the gastrocnemius muscle group may be found on physical examination.

The diagnosis typically is made clinically. Radiographs and MRIs rarely are indicated. The treatment in young athletes is entirely nonoperative. If analysis of lower extremity mechanics during gait suggest a hyperpronation pattern, custom foot orthoses to control this can be very helpful. Ice, stretching, and NSAIDs also are used. Training modifications and heel lifts can be helpful as well. Immobilization rarely is necessary.

Occasionally a physical therapist may aid in a carefully planned program of muscle strengthening, and gradual reintroduction of sporting activities is achieved.

Rotator cuff tendonitis. The rotator cuff is a convergence of the tendons of the subscapularis, supraspinatus, infraspinatus, and teres minor muscles. These extend laterally from the scapula over the humeral head. Together, they function to help stabilize the humeral head in the glenoid fossa of the scapula. A particularly important function of the rotator cuff is preventing the upper humerus from rubbing beneath the arch of the acromion. The supraspinatus muscle is the most important for this function.

Many factors contribute to rotator cuff tendonitis.[7] In young athletes, inherent laxity of the glenohumeral capsule (ligament complex) is likely to be a significant factor. Sporting activities that stress the shoulder joint with the arm extended overhead are particularly prone to precipitate symptoms. Some typical activities include overhead throwing in baseball, swimming, tennis serves, and gymnastics. Once a shoulder becomes irritated, a reflex arc inhibits the firing of the rotator cuff muscles. This precipitates further dysfunction of the shoulder muscle and leads to impingement of the humeral head beneath the acromion. With time, a well-established bursitis and tendonitis develop.

Typically, the patient complains of pain with overhead activities. Often, the athlete will complain of the arm becoming heavy, tired, or "dead."

A thorough examination of the neck and shoulder should be conducted, looking for range-of-motion limitation, muscle atrophy, and focal tenderness in the subacromion region, both anteriorly and laterally. There may be tenderness along the course of the biceps tendon as well. Bringing the shoulder fully overhead may produce pain; this finding is referred to as a *positive "impingement" test*. The supraspinatus strength should be tested and glenohumeral laxity should be assessed as well.

Plain radiographs are not diagnostic of rotator cuff tendonitis but often are obtained to rule out other bony abnormalities. An MRI can be diagnostic for rotator cuff tendonitis but often is not necessary. The diagnosis usually can be made clinically. Full-thickness rotator cuff tears are almost never seen below 18 years of age.

Acute Trauma

Acute injuries include sprains, muscle tears, and fractures. Sprains are injuries to ligaments, and they typically are graded from mild to severe (Table 266-2).

The fundamental principles of treatment for many musculoskeletal injuries go by the acronym RICE (*r*est, *i*ce, *c*ompression, and *e*levation). Rest is especially important for the first 24 to 72 hours after a significant injury. For lower extremity injuries, crutches should be used to avoid weight bearing. Randomized studies have demonstrated that athletes can return to full activity faster if cryotherapy is begun immediately after the injury.[8] Ice may be applied for 20 minutes every 2 to 4 waking hours. A wet cloth can be used between the ice and skin to decrease the chance of cold injury. Many trainers advise continuing the use of ice until the swelling disappears completely. Compression may be applied with an elastic bandage. The goal of elevation is to place the injured extremity above the level of the heart to aid in reducing edema.

Ankle sprains. Ankle sprains are the most common musculoskeletal injury in sports.[22] Approximately 97% involve the lateral ankle ligaments. The typical mechanism of injury involves inversion and external rotation of the foot. This results in a sequential tearing of the anterior talofibular ligament, calcaneal fibular ligament, and finally the posterior talofibular ligament. Occasionally the anterior talofibular ligament and the syndesmosis complex are involved. These are much more severe injuries. The deltoid ligament also may be injured.

The presence of bony tenderness should be determined, particularly over the distal fibula, the anterolateral tibia, the medial malleolus, the base of the fifth metatarsal, or the proximal fibula. In the skeletally immature athlete, the bone usually is weaker than the ligaments, so lateral ankle injuries often result in physeal fractures of the distal fibula. Sometimes, separating focal tenderness over the physis from diffuse tenderness of the lateral ankle ligaments can be difficult initially. Percussing with the tip of the examiner's finger can often separate tenderness at the proximal physis from tenderness around the ligaments.

The decision to obtain radiographs is based on a myriad of factors including the patient's age, history of injury, physical findings, ability to bear weight, and progress since injury. One should keep in mind that the typical fracture of the distal fibular physis has a Salter I fracture pattern without displacement, which results in a normal radiograph of the bone, showing only soft-tissue swelling. The diagnosis, therefore, is made clinically. The radiograph simply excludes displacement of the fracture or other fractures being present.

As simple as the injury may sound, the treatment options for ankle sprains are complicated. Treatment modalities vary widely and are chosen based on the severity of the injury (see Table 266-2), the demands of the athlete, and the experience of the treating health care team.

If the injury does not appear severe, the RICE principles can be applied and the ankle reevaluated periodically. Some injuries respond remarkably quickly. At reevaluation, if the pain is minimal, then the ankle should be tested for stability. The athlete then should be observed in functional tasks such as running, cutting, and twisting. If these tasks are performed well without significant pain, then he or she may return to competition. Ideally, the ankle should be taped or splinted to lessen the risk of reinjury, and a preventive physical therapy program considered.

For ankle sprains of moderate grade, numerous other options come into play. For the less serious athlete, an expectant approach can be used, including crutches, Ace wrap, and gradual progression of weight bearing, with return to sports only after resolution of symptoms. Occasionally a cast or Cam walker (removable rigid walking splint) is helpful.

Table 266-2 Severity Grading of Sprains

Grade	Description	Clinical Presentation	Typical Recuperation
I (mild)	Stretching of the ligament with minimal microscopic injury	Mild swelling, limp	0-2 wk
II (minor)	Partial disruption of the ligament	Modest swelling, diffuse tenderness, difficulty weight bearing	1-4 wk
III (severe)	Complete disruption of the ligament	Extensive swelling and bleeding, instability, and disability	4-12 wk

For the more serious athlete with moderate-grade sprains, referral to a physical therapist often is helpful. A variety of physical therapy modalities can help to reduce the swelling. Range of motion is begun early, and strengthening is emphasized. As the ankle becomes comfortable, a proprioception training phase of rehabilitation begins. A variety of lace-up and Velcro ankle supports are available. For some athletes, taping may be an option. In all cases, functional criteria for return to sports, prevention of reinjury, and reassessment of progress are key components.

Severe-grade sprains should be managed by someone with more advanced musculoskeletal skills. This might be an experienced primary care physician or an orthopedic surgeon. Often, a period of immobilization to reduce bleeding and swelling is helpful. A myriad of rehabilitation protocols can be used successfully. Assessment for chronic laxity and tarsal coalitions should be made.

Persistent anterolateral ankle pain can occur even after mild ankle sprains. Often, this is due to an area of fibrosis or synovial hypertrophy in the anterior lateral corner of the joint. The differential diagnosis should include chondral and osteochondral injuries at the dome of the talus, chronic laxity of the ankle and/or subtalar joints, and tarsal coalition. Initial treatment includes NSAIDs, ankle supports, and physical therapy modalities. Occasionally, steroid injection is helpful. If symptoms persist, referral to an orthopedist or sports medicine specialist is indicated.

Collateral ligament injuries of the knee. Although classically, the physis is "the weak link in the chain," injuries to the ligaments do occur in skeletally immature individuals. The collateral ligaments of the knee originate from the epiphyses of the femur and insert into the epiphyses of the tibia and fibula with one exception. The distal portion of the superficial medial collateral ligament inserts over a broad area of the proximal tibial metaphysis. Like the lateral ankle, physeal injuries should always be suspected in those with open growth plates. Plain radiographs may not be diagnostic. Stress radiographs or an MRI occasionally are needed to make this diagnosis. Concurrent injury to the cruciate ligaments, menisci, and articular surfaces need to be considered as well.

Most medial collateral ligament injuries heal satisfactorily.[9] Initially, the principles of RICE are employed. Depending on the severity, the knee is mobilized as the swelling and tenderness diminish. As range of motion returns, strength should be assessed. A physical therapist or athletic trainer can be very helpful in designing an adequate rehabilitation program. For moderate- and severe-grade sprains, consideration should be given to using a dual, upright, hinged, functional knee orthosis.

Lateral knee and ligament injuries are much less common in young athletes. This diagnosis should raise suspicion that there is another explanation for the patient's signs and symptoms, and referral is wise. For true lateral collateral ligament injuries, the principles of treatment are similar to those for medial collateral ligament injuries.

Anterior cruciate ligament injuries. As adolescents become skeletally mature, the incidence of anterior cruciate ligament (ACL) injuries rises rapidly. The incidence of injuries to young female athletes, particularly in soccer, basketball, and gymnastics, is rising rapidly. For boys, American football, soccer, and basketball are very common sources of these injuries.

The ACL is a key stabilizer of the knee joint, particularly to rotational movements. As such, it is frequently injured in sports that involve cutting and twisting. Alternatively, the knee may be struck from the lateral side, first injuring the medial collateral ligament and then the ACL.

Classically, athletes describe an acute "pop and pain" in the knee. They often fall to the ground and have moderate to severe pain. The knee may not swell immediately, but typically it does swell within the first few hours because of the development of a hemarthrosis.

Occasionally the tenderness is not marked, and athletes will attempt to return to their sporting competition only to discover that the knee is not stable; this may result in a significant exacerbation of the injury. One should maintain a high index of suspicion for anterior cruciate ligament injury, and make certain it is ruled out before the young athlete who has a knee injury returns to practice or competition.

The physical examination will vary considerably depending on the severity, the other structures involved, the time that has elapsed, and whether the injury is truly acute or actually an exacerbation of a chronic instability.

The most sensitive physical examination component is the Lachman examination. This is performed with the patient lying supine; the knee is gently flexed to about 30 degrees. The patient must be able to relax the quadriceps and hamstrings enough to allow the examiner to attempt to slide the proximal tibia anteriorly. Although the amount of movement of the tibia has some importance, the key factor is the end point. If the test is negative (i.e., the ligament is intact), then a very distinct end point or cessation of forward movement should be felt. This end point should feel like holding the two ends of a short piece of rope in your hands and pulling the ends apart rapidly until the movement suddenly stops.

Comparison with the uninjured knee can be helpful. Performing this examination competently requires experience. The size of the patient's leg, the ability of the patient to relax, and the size of the examiner's hands all are factors that contribute to successful performance of the test. If there is doubt, the knee should be reevaluated later on or the patient referred to an orthopedist. Occasionally an MRI is indicated, but in most cases a properly performed Lachman physical examination is diagnostic.

In contrast to the collateral ligaments of the knee, the healing potential of the anterior cruciate ligament is very limited because of its susceptible vascular supply. As a result, most injuries to the anterior cruciate ligament do not heal well, and primary surgical repairs (as opposed to reconstructive surgery) are not effective.

Left without the stability of the ACL, most knees in young, active patients eventually will become symptomatically unstable and sustain reinjury.[16] In older and less active individuals, there is a role for nonoperative management of these injuries; however, most ACL injuries in young athletes should be reconstructed. Leaving the knee unstable makes it vulnerable to injury to the other ligaments, the joint capsule, and the menisci.

Most reconstructive techniques currently in use involve

drilling holes through the proximal tibia and distal femur to insert grafts along the anatomical course of the ACL. For the skeletally immature individual, this raises some concerns about potential injury to the physis.

Numerous factors go into the decision to reconstruct the ACL. During the last year that the physes are open, there is very little growth of the distal femur and proximal tibia so any disturbance to them should result in minimal problems. Most studies have not demonstrated any complications of ACL reconstruction in skeletally immature individuals, although little data exist about youngsters younger than 10 years of age. The risk of further damaging the knee ligaments and the menisci by not repairing the ACL must be weighed against the risk of surgical injury to the physis, which is unusual and largely correctable. For the very young patient, a brace, physical therapy, and significant activity modifications probably are the more advisable approach to managing ACL injuries.

Meniscal tears. The meniscal cartilages have several important functions within the knee joint. These include providing mechanical shock absorption between the weight-bearing articular cartilages of the femur and tibia, enhancing the distribution of synovial fluid, which provides nourishment to the superficial portion of the articular cartilage, and enhancing the stability of the articulation between the tibia and femur.

Loss of the meniscal cartilages has little detectable effect on the knee joint initially. However, over the ensuing decades, particularly after 20 years, the rate of degenerative joint disease rises significantly. As a result, all reasonable efforts should be made to protect, preserve, and repair menisci of younger patients.[4]

For many years, it was felt that the menisci, relatively avascular structures, had virtually no ability to heal. Microangiographic studies have shown, however, that even the adult meniscus is vascular in its capsular one-third. Very early in life, the vascular proportion is even greater. Clearly, a significant number of meniscal tears, particularly in younger patients, have the potential to heal.

In youths 10 years of age and younger, the majority of meniscal tears are related to discoid menisci. These are congenitally abnormal menisci that are almost always on the lateral side of the joint. When viewed from the top down, the discoid meniscus does not have the usual C shape but rather has a variable degree of excessive tissue covering the tibial plateau. The complete discoid meniscus covers the plateau entirely. Discoid menisci are smaller than normal menisci, less mobile, and much more prone to tear. A discoid variant, the Wrisberg type, has thick margins and usually is not attached to the capsule posteriorly. These patients present with a classic finding of a "snapping knee." As the knee actively extends, it suddenly shifts and pops as the thick, mobile discoid meniscus shifts between the weight-bearing surfaces of the tibia and femur.

Often, the diagnosis of a discoid lateral meniscus can be made clinically by the sound and shift of the cartilage itself, but MRI confirmation often is sought. Symptomatic discoid lateral menisci require surgical intervention. The principles of treatment are to preserve as much of a normal functioning rim of meniscal cartilage as possible while alleviating the mechanical snapping that ultimately leads to degenerative changes of the articular surfaces.

For patients older than 10 years of age, the incidence of tearing of normal menisci rises. Most commonly, this occurs in association with significant ligament injury, such as a tear of the ACL. Rarely do normal menisci in teenagers tear without a substantial injury. As a result, meniscal tears typically are not at the top of the differential diagnosis of a young person with gradual onset of nonspecific knee pain.

If a meniscal tear is suspected, referral or MRI is appropriate. Arthrograms are now performed much less commonly. If a normal meniscus is torn, the general principles of surgical treatment are preservation of meniscal tissue and reconstruction of the unstable joint. The pattern and location of the tear determine whether the meniscus may heal on its own, or will require arthroscopic partial removal or repair.

Quadriceps contusion. Minor contusions of the quadriceps muscle are common events in contact sports such as American football, soccer, and lacrosse. However, significant hematomas can develop within the quadriceps. These can be quite disabling.[10] More extensive hematomas have a propensity to rebleed. Myositis ossificans traumatica (heterotopic ossification of the muscle) may develop, which can be disabling.

The key finding for separating minor hematomas from major ones is limitation of knee flexion. Minor hematomas should not limit knee motion, whereas large ones can. Occasionally, it becomes challenging to differentiate a large quadriceps hematoma from a malignant tumor of the thigh, such as Ewing's sarcoma and osteosarcoma, both of which have a propensity to occur in teenagers, and, themselves, may bleed internally.

Initial treatment of quadriceps hematoma involves RICE and crutches. As pain and swelling diminish, active knee flexion exercises are begun. Full return of motion is the minimal requirement for return to contact sports, at which time a padded guard should be used. Monitoring for reinjury is essential.

Avulsion fractures of the pelvis. Six major apophyses are present on each side of the pelvis. These include the iliac crest, the anterior/superior iliac spine, the anterior/inferior iliac spine, the lesser trochanter, the greater trochanter, and the ischial apophysis. Each of these is prone to develop an apophysitis and, except for the greater trochanter, avulsion fractures also are fairly common.[18]

An avulsion fracture typically presents with acute onset of pain during a sudden athletic motion. Examples include an explosive start for a sprint, an extreme pike maneuver (hips flexed and knees extended) in gymnastics, or a combination twisting movement and direct blow to the iliac crest. Careful history sometimes will reveal mild antecedent symptoms consistent with a preexisting apophysitis.

Findings include focal tenderness to palpation over the affected apophysis and pain with resisted strength testing of the corresponding muscle insertion or origin. Often, the diagnosis can be confirmed with plain radiography. Special oblique views and occasionally a CT scan or an MRI are helpful.

Most of these avulsions do not displace significantly. Almost all heal with time and rest. Typically, crutches and rest are recommended for the first few weeks. Stretching may inhibit healing and should be avoided until the site is pain-free. Complete healing typically takes 6 weeks to several months. The athlete should be gradually returned to activity and monitored for recurrence of symptoms.

Muscle strains. Injuries to muscle tendon units almost always occur at the musculotendinous junction. Like sprains, they vary in severity from mild through severe. Mild injuries heal fairly rapidly, whereas severe strains can lead to large areas of scar tissue that are prone to reinjury.

The diagnosis of muscle strain has several pitfalls. Muscle strains are not as common in young athletes as in older ones. Too often, the diagnosis of "strain" is applied to a musculoskeletal malady for which the true diagnosis is not obvious to the examiner. Particularly around the hip and thigh area, one should be careful not to miss a slipped capital femoral epiphysis, an avulsion fracture, an infection, or a tumor as causes of pain.

Slipped capital femoral epiphysis is the most common disorder of the hip in adolescents (see Chapter 132, Extremity Pain, and Chapter 243, Osteochondroses). Although classically presenting with hip pain, discomfort may be referred to the thigh or knee joint. Delay in diagnosis and treatment is a common problem and can result in the severe complication of avascular necrosis of the femoral head.

The most common muscle strain in teenage athletes is of the hamstring. Hamstring strain presents with pain at the musculotendinous junction, which is at the junction of the middle and distal thirds of the posterior thigh. More proximal hamstring tenderness should raise suspicion of an occult injury to the ischial apophysis.

The treatment principles for hamstring strain initially involve RICE and crutches. Reduction of tenderness can take days to weeks, depending on initial severity. Once comfortable, a gradual stretching and strengthening program is initiated. The athlete is returned to activities as tolerated and monitored for recurrent symptoms. Reinjury is a problem with hamstring strains.

Dislocations. The most common dislocations of young athletes include patella, shoulder (glenohumeral joint), elbow, and digits of the hand. With severe trauma, dislocations and fracture dislocations can occur in virtually any joint, and musculoskeletal specialists generally manage these injuries.

PATELLAR DISLOCATION. The most common musculoskeletal dislocation in young athletes involves the patella. Patellar dislocation should not be referred to as "knee dislocation," which denotes displacement of the articulation between the tibia and femur. The latter is a high-energy injury and has a high associated morbidity including, occasionally, loss of limb.

By contrast, patellar dislocation often is the result of a trivial injury. Many individuals are predisposed to dislocation of the patella by virtue of genetic variability in their knee extensor mechanism. Variations leading to easy dislocation include a shallow sulcus in the distal femur, lateral translation of the insertion of the patellar tendon into the tibia, relative underdevelopment of the vastus medialis muscle, and tightness of the lateral retinaculum.

Almost all patellae dislocate to the lateral side. Occasionally the patient will report having seen a medial prominence, but this typically is due to the medial femoral condyle being exposed by the displaced patella.

The history of injury can vary from a minor twisting episode to a significant direct blow to the knee. The patella may spontaneously reduce or remain displaced and require manipulation.

Manipulative reduction often can be achieved relatively easily. Ideally, the patient is placed in a prone position, which facilitates hip extension and thereby starts to relax the hamstrings. The knee then is gently extended, and as it extends, the patella should reduce without forced manipulation.

Unless the patellar dislocation or subluxation is a trivial event that incites very little pain in the joint, radiographs should be obtained to look for osteochondral fragments. These loose pieces typically arise from the lateral femoral condyle or the patella.

Following a significant patellar dislocation, the knee is immobilized and the principles of RICE are used. As the pain and swelling subside, a rehabilitation program is initiated emphasizing strengthening of the quadriceps muscles, particularly the vastus medialis. The hamstrings are stretched, and a lower extremity rehabilitation program is undertaken. A patellar stabilizing knee sleeve is used during the initial phases of return to activity.

Most patellar dislocations can be successfully managed with a single therapeutic program. Recurrent patellar instability, particularly in those with a familial history, may require reconstruction.

SHOULDER DISLOCATION. Much like patellar dislocation, dislocations of the glenohumeral joint can occur from relatively minor trauma in predisposed individuals or as a result of major trauma in the average person. Reduction can occur spontaneously; however, fixed dislocations can be difficult to reduce. These may require transportation to an emergency care facility. Reduction may require expertise, local anesthesia, sedation, and occasionally, general anesthesia. Unless the episode is minor, radiographs generally are obtained to confirm reduction and rule out an associated fracture. Remember to think of pathological collagen disorders, such as Marfan syndrome, in these patients. Physical findings consistent with Marfan syndrome include tall, thin body habitus; arachnodactyly; pectus excavation; heart murmur; dislocated lens; and myopia.

Traditionally, shoulder dislocations have been treated with 3 weeks of immobilization, followed by a rigorous physical therapy program. The therapy should be directed at strengthening the rotator cuff muscles. The principle is to strengthen these dynamic stabilizers of the joint to help compensate for laxity of the shoulder joint capsule (ligaments). The patient's program is advanced, and an experienced therapist monitors progress.

Recurrent instability despite a therapy program generally is an indication for surgical stabilization. Support is growing for earlier surgical intervention, particularly with the less invasive arthroscopic techniques that are evolving. The exact indications and preferred techniques currently are in a significant state of evolution.

ANTERIOR KNEE PAIN IN YOUNG ATHLETES

The most common knee complaint of adolescents is that of anterior knee pain. This ubiquitous symptom can arise from a wide variety of disorders. In many cases, a specific diagnosis such as Osgood-Schlatter disease, Sinding-Larsen-Johansson syndrome, patellar tendonitis, or patellar instability can be made. Careful history, physical examination, and diagnostic studies can help to reach these diagnoses.

Unfortunately, a specific diagnosis cannot always be made. In some instances, there is a degree of psychological overlay to the symptoms, and this can make management challenging.

For patients who have anterior knee pain, diagnostic imaging, including MRI, often does not reveal its source. Occasionally, these studies are indicated to rule out other definable abnormalities. In general, consultation from a physician with appropriate expertise should be obtained before embarking on diagnostic studies beyond plain radiographs.

Some of the more common causes of anterior knee pain are discussed above and two additional entities, chondromalacia patella and patellofemoral pain syndrome, are discussed below. A wide variety of less common disorders not discussed herein can cause anterior knee pain. These include quadriceps tendonitis, bipartite patella, osteochondritis dissecans of the femur or patella, iliotibial band tendonitis, popliteus tendonitis, inflamed plica, prepatellar bursitis, and synovial flat pin impingement syndrome. Osteomyelitis, septic arthritis, inflammatory arthritis, and tumors should always be kept in mind.

Chondromalacia Patella

The term *chondromalacia patella* refers to softening of the articular surface of the patella, which can occur in mild to severe grades, ranging from edema of the cartilage to complete ulceration of the articular surface. This term had previously been misapplied to virtually any case of anterior knee pain. The diagnosis should be reserved for specific instances of symptomatic articular change of the surface of the patella.

Particularly in more mild cases, the pain from chondromalacia patella will abate with intermittent use of NSAIDs, a quadriceps-strengthening program, and judicious activity modifications. A therapy program can be helpful, but the patient must have a clear understanding that the goal is to reduce symptoms. It may not be possible to completely eliminate symptoms. Occasionally, surgical intervention to alter the patella's articular surface becomes indicated.

Patellofemoral Pain Syndrome

Many adolescents complain of a symptom complex that shares many similar features. Although seen in males, the typical patient is a teenage girl older than 12 years of age who complains of a diffuse pain over the anterior surface of her knee.[27]

The typical onset is insidious without a specific history of trauma. Usually, there is no history of erythema, warmth, induration, or true effusion. Occasionally, patients describe the knee having become slightly "puffy." Typically, there are no mechanical complaints of catching or locking. Popping may be present, because this is a fairly ubiquitous symptom, but the popping usually is not painful.

On physical examination, tenderness often is present along the medial and lateral sides of the patellofemoral articulation. There may be mild discomfort over the anterior portion of the joint line, but typically no tenderness over the middle or posterior portion of the tibial femoral articulation. The joint has full range of motion with no crepitation. The knee is stable. Predisposing biomechanical factors, including femoral anteversion, external tibial torsion, pronating gait, and increased valgus alignment at the knees, may be present. Plain radiographs usually are negative. Further diagnostic evaluation is not indicated.

The etiology of this problem is not clear. It is commonly thought that an abnormality of the tracking of the patella is responsible. Abnormal stresses in the patellofemoral articulation or the surrounding soft tissues are probably responsible. To date, better clarification is not available. Typically, the long-term natural history of this presentation is benign, although the symptoms can be troublesome.

The most important role of the physician is to rule out other more serious or more specifically treatable disorders. From there, education, reassurance, and symptom management are the cornerstones of treatment. Psychological concerns need to be considered as well.

In some cases, the syndrome may result from training errors. Sudden increase in mileage, running on hard surfaces, poor preseason conditioning, and inadequate footwear may be contributing factors. For patients with significant flexible flatfeet, foot orthoses (arch supports) may reduce pronation at the foot and thereby diminish torsional stresses applied at the knee.

Stretching and strengthening of the quadriceps muscles often reduces anterior knee pain. The principles are to strengthen the vastus medialis and improve patellar tracking. Occasionally, taping or supportive knee sleeves will provide relief. The intermittent and judicious use of NSAIDs may help as well. In some cases, adjustment of expectations and activities are necessary.

In refractory cases, referral to a musculoskeletal specialist may become appropriate. Surgery occasionally is performed, although the exact indications and preferred techniques are controversial.

REFERENCES

1. American Academy of Pediatrics: Adolescents and anabolic steroids: a subject review, *Pediatrics* 99:904, 1997.
2. *Athletic training and sports medicine:* Rosemont, Ill, 1984, American Academy of Orthopedic Surgeons.
3. Buckley WE, et al: Estimated prevalence of anabolic steroid use among male high school seniors, *JAMA* 260:3441, 1988.
4. Busch MT: Meniscal injuries in children and adolescents, *Clin Sports Med* 9:661, 1990.
5. Busch MT: Sports medicine. In Morrissy RT, Weinstein SL, editors: *Lovell & Winter's pediatric orthopedics,* ed 4, Philadelphia, 1996, Lippincott-Raven.
6. Grindstaff PD: Effects of creatine supplements on repetitive sprint performance and body composition in competitive swimmers, *Int J Sport Nutr* 7:330, 1997.
7. Hawkins RJ, Kennedy JC: Impingement syndrome in athletes, *Am J Sports Med* 8:151, 1980.

8. Hocutt JE, et al: Cryotherapy in ankle sprains, *Am J Sports Med* 10:316, 1982.
9. Indelicato PA: Non-operative treatment of complete tears of the medial collateral ligament of the knee, *J Bone Joint Surg* 65A:323, 1983.
10. Jackson DW, Feagin JA: Quadriceps contusions in young athletes, *J Bone Joint Surg* 55A:95, 1973.
11. Johnson MD, et al: Anabolic steroid use by male adolescents, *Pediatrics* 83:921, 1989.
12. Knopp WD, Wang TW, Bach BR: Primary care of the injured athlete. Part 1. Ergogenic drugs in sports, *Clin Sports Med* 16:375, 1997.
13. Kreider RB: Effects of creatine supplementation on body composition, strength, and sprint performance, *Med Sci Sports Exerc* 30:73, 1998.
14. Kujala UM, Kvist M, Heinonen O: Osgood-Schlatter's disease in adolescent athletes, *Am J Sports Med* 13:236, 1985.
15. Leach RE: Supplements. *Am J Sports Med* 27:275, 1999.
16. McCarroll JR, Rettig AC, Shelbourne KD: Anterior cruciate ligament injuries in the young athlete with open physes, *Am J Sports Med* 16:44, 1988.
17. Medlar RC, Lyne ED: Sinding-Larsen-Johansson disease: its etiology and natural history, *J Bone Joint Surg* 60A:1113, 1978.
18. Metzmaker JN, Pappas AM: Avulsion fractures of the pelvis, *Am J Sports Med* 13:349, 1985.
19. Micheli LJ, Ireland ML: Prevention and management of calcaneal apophysitis in children: an overuse syndrome, *J Pediatr Orthop* 7:34, 1987.
20. Mujika I: Creatine supplementation as an ergogenic acid for sports performance in highly trained athletes: a critical review, *Int J Sports Med* 18:491, 1997.
21. Ogden JA, Southwick WO: Osgood-Schlatter's disease and tibial tuberosity development, *Clin Orthop Related Res* 116:180, 1976.
22. Smith RW, Reischl SF: Treatment of ankle sprains in young athletes, *Am J Sports Med* 14:465, 1986.
23. Sturmi JE, Diorio JD: Sports pharmacology: anabolic agents, *Clin Sports Med* 17:261, 1998.
24. Torg JS, Pollack H, Sweterlitsch P: The effect of competitive pitching on the shoulders and elbows of preadolescent baseball players, *Pediatrics* 49:267, 1972.
25. Torg JS, Welsh RP, Shepherd RJ: *Current therapy in sports medicine,* ed 2, Philadelphia, 1990, BC Decker.
26. Windsor RE, Dumitru D: Prevalence of anabolic steroid use by male and female adolescents, *Med Sci Sports Exerc* 21:494, 1989.
27. Yates C, Grana WA: Patellofemoral pain: a prospective study, *Orthopedics* 9:663, 1986.

267 Staphylococcal Toxic Shock Syndrome

Michael E. Pichichero

Staphylococcal toxic shock syndrome (TSS) is a distinct clinical entity characterized by fever; diffuse, nonexudative mucous membrane inflammation; vomiting and profuse diarrhea; generalized myalgia; scarlatiniform erythroderma; hypotension; and shock associated with multiple organ failure—renal, myocardial, pulmonary, hepatic, hematological, and central nervous system (CNS).*

Staphylococcal TSS is an important consideration in the evaluation of toxic exanthematous diseases in children. It must be distinguished from other serious or potentially life-threatening disease, including streptococcal toxic shock syndrome, staphylococcal scalded skin syndrome, Stevens-Johnson syndrome, Kawasaki disease, streptococcal scarlet fever, measles, leptospirosis, and drug-related toxic epidermal necrolysis.

Although first described in association with menstruation and tampon use,† public health information resulted in a shift to predominantly nonmenstrual cases. Currently, the incidence of nonmenstrual TSS exceeds that of menstrual TSS.[5,6,23,26,38] Staphylococcal TSS may occur whenever a patient becomes colonized or infected with a strain of *Staphylococcus aureus,* which produces a toxin, and the patient lacks protective antibody to that toxin. Clinical associations of staphylococcal TSS are shown in Table 267-1. TSS is probably under recognized in children because of a persistent misconception that a foreign body is required for development of illness.[23] The overall annual incidence of staphylococcal TSS is 0.53 cases per 100,000 population, although wide variations exist in different geographical regions; both genital and nongenital cases occur more often in whites than in nonwhites.[13]

CLINICAL PRESENTATION

Strict criteria for case definition have been established by the Centers for Disease Control and Prevention (Box 267-1). The time sequence of the clinical manifestations of staphylococcal TSS is outlined in Fig. 267-1. Patients usually are healthy before the onset of symptoms. Occasionally a prodrome consisting of low-grade fever, malaise, myalgia, or vomiting occurs in the week preceding the beginning of the acute illness. The patient abruptly develops a spiking fever of 102.2° to 105.8° F (39° to 41° C), chills, and severe gastrointestinal symptoms consisting of abdominal cramps, nausea, vomiting, and profuse, watery, nonbloody diarrhea. Many patients also complain of headache, myalgia, and a sore throat. At this stage of the illness a diagnosis of acute viral gastroenteritis may well be entertained incorrectly and the youngster treated symptomatically. However, over the next 24 to 72 hours additional clinical signs develop suggestive of the diagnosis of staphylococcal TSS. A diffuse, blanching, macular erythroderma (sunburnlike) or scarlatiniform rash appears. The rash may be faint or evanescent and therefore sometimes is missed or attributed to high fever. The rash is not pruritic but occasionally is petechial. Patients demonstrate bilateral conjunctival hyperemia without discharge and may complain of photophobia. Oropharyngeal inflammation, sometimes with an associated strawberry tongue or buccal ulcerations, also occurs, as does vaginal erythema with minimal clear watery discharge in cases associated with menstruation.

Within 24 to 72 hours of onset, most patients experience orthostatic dizziness or syncope or both because of orthostatic hypotension. These symptoms can manifest abruptly and may precede the development of hypovolemic shock. The peak of illness occurs on the second or third day and involves multiple organ systems. CNS dysfunction may appear as headache, confusion, disorientation, hallucinations, and complaints of paresthesias of the hands and feet. Some patients have a stiff, tender neck. If a lumbar puncture is performed, normal values for cerebrospinal fluid (CSF) glucose and protein are found, although patients may have up to 100 white blood cells/mm^3, 50% of which may be polymorphonuclear cells. Abdominal musculature tenderness, absent or hypoactive bowel sounds, and radiological evidence of a nonobstructive ileus are common. Azotemia and a diminished creatinine clearance occur as evidence of renal involvement. Oliguria is typical; complete renal shutdown occurs rarely. The musculoskeletal system nearly always is affected. Exquisite muscle tenderness and severe myalgias are common. Arthralgias and joint effusions may be seen. Nonpitting edema over the wrists and ankles and synovitis of the small joints of the hands and feet have been reported to occur. Patients may experience shock lung or adult-type respiratory distress syndrome. Hematological involvement includes a progressive normochromic normocytic anemia, thrombocytopenia, and leukocytosis. Arrhythmias or prolonged shock may lead to eventual myocardial failure.

LABORATORY FINDINGS

No laboratory test is available for confirming the diagnosis of staphylococcal TSS. Initial laboratory findings often include

*References 6, 12, 18, 21, 23, 26, 38, 39.

†References 8, 13, 18, 25, 27, 35, 39.

Table 267-1 Summary of Clinical and Laboratory Data Associated with Staphylococcal TSS

Condition	Relative Frequency of Occurrence (%)	Condition	Relative Frequency of Occurrence (%)
Clinical		Prolonged prothrombin time	70
Fever	100	Decreased fibrinogen	68
Temperature >40° C (>104° F)	70	Thrombocytopenia	64
Rash	100	Prolonged partial thromboplastin time	60
Diffuse erythema	87	***Metabolic***	
Desquamation	90	Hypoproteinemia	95
Myalgia	99	Hypoalbuminemia	85
Hypotension (orthostatic hypotension or syncope)	95	Hypocalcemia	83
Disorientation, irritability, or lethargy	89	Hypokalemia	75
Diarrhea	83	Hypophosphatemia	62
Vomiting	82	Hyponatremia	47
Sore throat	80	***Hepatic***	
Strawberry tongue	80	Elevated hepatic enzymes	67
Headache	78	Hyperbilirubinemia	63
Abdominal pain and tenderness	70	***Renal***	
Vaginal hyperemia	67	Pyuria	100
Conjunctivitis	65	Increased creatinine	82
Vaginal discharge	42	Increased BUN	75
Stiff neck	36	Proteinuria	70
Arthralgia	15	Microscopic hematuria	50
Joint effusion	12	***Musculoskeletal***	
Adult respiratory distress syndrome	10	Increased creatinine phosphokinase	75
Laboratory		Metabolic acidosis	75
Hematological		Myoglobinuria	66
Increased fibrinolytic split products	100		
Immature neutrophils	95		
Anemia	82		
Leukocytosis	76		

BOX 267-1

CASE DEFINITION OF STAPHYLOCOCCAL TOXIC SHOCK SYNDROME

Fever: temperature >38.9° C

Rash: diffuse macular erythroderma; desquamation of palms and soles 1 to 2 weeks after onset of illness

Hypotension: systolic blood pressure 90 mm Hg for adults or below 5th percentile by age for children under 16 years of age; orthostatic drop in diastolic blood pressure 15 mm Hg from lying to sitting, or orthostatic syncope

Multisystem involvement—three or more of the following:

- Gastrointestinal: vomiting or diarrhea at onset of illness
- Muscular: severe myalgia or creatinine phosphokinase level at least twice the upper limit of normal for laboratory
- Mucous membrane: vaginal, oropharyngeal, or conjunctival hyperemia
- Renal: blood urea nitrogen (BUN) or creatinine at least twice the upper limit of normal for laboratory or urinary sediment with pyuria (>5 white cells per high-power field) in the absence of urinary tract infection
- Hepatic: total bilirubin, serum glutamic-oxalo-acetic transaminase (SGOT), or serum glutamic-pyruvate transaminase (SGPT) at least twice the upper limit of normal for laboratory
- Hematological: platelets <100,000/mm^3
- CNS: disorientation or alterations in consciousness without focal neurological signs when fever and hypotension are absent

Negative results on the following tests, if obtained:

- Blood, throat, cerebrospinal fluid (CSF) cultures
- Rise in antibody titer: Rocky Mountain spotted fever, leptospirosis, and rubeola

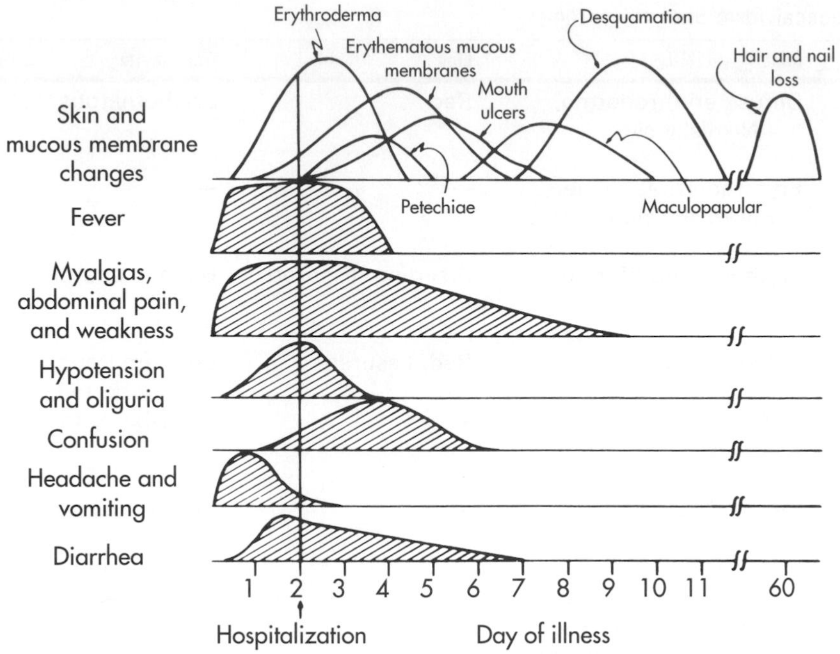

Erythroderma
Erythematous mucous membranes
Mouth ulcers
Desquamation
Hair and nail loss
Skin and mucous membrane changes
Petechiae
Maculopapular
Fever
Myalgias, abdominal pain, and weakness
Hypotension and oliguria
Confusion
Headache and vomiting
Diarrhea
1 2 3 4 5 6 7 8 9 10 11 60
Hospitalization
Day of illness

Fig. 267-1 Major systemic, skin, and mucous membrane manifestations of toxic shock syndrome.

(From Chesney PJ, et al: *JAMA* 246:743, 1981.)

leukocytosis, with a striking increase in the percentage of immature neutrophils, progressive anemia, and thrombocytopenia. These hematological abnormalities are self-correcting during the convalescent stage. Thrombocytopenia may be accompanied by prolongation of prothrombin time and partial thromboplastin time and the appearance of increased fibrin split products. However, neither serious bleeding during the acute phase of illness nor thrombosis resulting from rebound thrombocytosis during recovery has been a significant clinical problem. A majority of patients have hypoproteinemia and hypoalbuminemia, probably as a consequence of increased capillary permeability caused by exotoxin-mediated vascular cell membrane change (see the following section on etiology and pathogenesis). A number of patients also experience metabolic acidosis from inadequate tissue perfusion, and this may be complicated by hyponatremia and hypokalemia as a result of accompanying persistent vomiting and diarrhea. Serum concentrations of calcium may appear dangerously low; however, tetany rarely is seen. The BUN and creatinine usually are elevated early in the illness. Peak abnormal values occur after 5 to 7 days and then return rapidly to normal. However, some patients have required acute hemodialysis or peritoneal dialysis to correct these and other metabolic imbalances. Despite abnormal renal function, hypophosphatemia typically is present in the first days of illness. The creatinine phosphokinase level often is elevated, and occasionally, patients experience myoglobinemia. These findings normalize with resolution of the myalgias, usually between the fifth and tenth day of disease. Hepatic enzyme and bilirubin levels typically are elevated initially but tend to revert to normal in convalescence. The relative frequency of these abnormal laboratory findings is presented in Table 267-1.

ETIOLOGY AND PATHOGENESIS

Patients who develop staphylococcal TSS are colonized or infected with specific strains of *S. aureus*. A specific staphylococcal exotoxin known as *TSS toxin 1* (TSST-1) has been identified as the most common cause, or a mediator of, the pathophysiological events associated with almost all cases of genital (menstrual) staphylococcal TSS.* Sixty percent to 80% of nongenital (nonmenstrual) cases of TSS also are caused by TSST-1,† whereas the remainder are produced by staphylococcal enterotoxins B and C.‡ Approximately 20%

BOX 267-2

MANAGEMENT OF STAPHYLOCOCCAL TOXIC SHOCK SYNDROME

1. Consider other possible diagnoses
2. Remove potentially infected foreign bodies (e.g., tampons)
3. Obtain cultures of blood, throat, vagina, nares, rectum, and other appropriate sites
4. Drain and irrigate infected sites
5. Give an intravenous antistaphylococcal beta-lactamase–resistant antimicrobial agent at maximum dosage for weight and age
6. Consider methylprednisolone for severe cases
7. Treat aggressively and monitor for the following:
   - Hypovolemia and inadequate tissue perfusion
   - Adult respiratory distress syndrome
   - Myocardial dysfunction
   - Acute renal failure
   - Cerebral edema
   - Hypocalcemia/hypophosphatemia
   - Metabolic acidosis
   - Disseminated intravascular coagulation
   - Fluid and electrolyte abnormalities

*References 2, 10, 15, 21, 29, 31, 33.
†References 2, 9, 15, 19, 21, 23, 29-31.
‡References 2, 4, 19, 21, 23, 29, 30, 34.

Table 267-2 Differential Diagnosis of Staphylococcal Toxic Shock Syndrome

Disease	Hypotension	Rash	Lips	Oral Cavity
Staphylococcal toxic shock syndrome	Yes	Diffuse erythroderma, – Nikolsky sign	Red	Erythematous
Staphylococcal scalded-skin syndrome	No	Erythroderma, bullae, ± Nikolsky sign	—	—
Stevens-Johnson syndrome	No	Erythema multiforme	Bleeding, fissured	Bullous enanthem
Kawasaki disease	No	Polymorphous	Red, fissured	Erythematous, strawberry tongue
Scarlet fever	No	Diffuse erythroderma, circumoral pallor, Pastia lines	—	Strawberry tongue
Measles	No	Morbilliform	—	Koplik spots
Leptospirosis	Sometimes	Erythematous, macular, petechial, purpuric	—	± Pharyngitis
Toxic epidermal necrolysis (drug related)	Sometimes	Painful erythroderma, bullae, + Nikolsky sign	—	—
Streptococcal toxic shock syndrome	Yes	Diffuse erythroderma, maculopapular	Cracked	Erythematous

of all clinical isolates of *S. aureus* produce TSST-1, which is regulated by a gene known as *agr.*[16] All strains possessing the agr gene produce TSST-1, but the amount of toxin produced varies by strain. Physical and chemical factors are known to influence production of TSST-1. These include pH (toxin production increases between pH 6 to 8), oxygen concentration (toxin production increases at lower PO_2 levels), concentration of CO_2 (toxin production increases with rising CO_2 levels), and concentration of divalent cations (especially magnesium).[15] TSST-1 production is associated with massive release of tumor necrosis factor alpha and interleukin 1.[24] These cytokines produce the fever, rash, hypotension, tissue injury, and shock associated with the syndrome.[14] The absence of antibody to TSST-1 is a major risk factor for acquisition of TSS, and failure to generate anti-TSST-1 antibody after an episode of TSS predisposes patients to recurrent episodes.[3,20,29] Staphylococcal enterotoxins also are potent mediators of cytokine production and release. They behave in a similar fashion to TSST-1 in producing clinically similar TSS disease.

MANAGEMENT

The initial steps in management of staphylococcal TSS are outlined in Box 267-2. Nearly all patients should be hospitalized, although a few who have a very mild form of the illness may be managed cautiously as outpatients. The first and major resuscitative goal is to administer large volumes of crystalloid (lactated Ringer's) or colloid (fresh-frozen plasma or albumin) solutions to restore normal intravascular volume and correct hypotension, since shock is the initial threat to intact survival. Patients may require enormous volumes of fluid (two to four times normal daily maintenance) to maintain tissue perfusion. Adequate treatment of hypotension also may require vasopressor therapy such as dopamine or dobutamine. Much of the administered fluid is sequestered outside the intravascular space, and many patients become markedly edematous. Therefore, it is advisable to have a central venous pressure line or a Swan-Ganz catheter in place to monitor left ventricular end-diastolic pressure to prevent the development of congestive heart failure caused by overvigorous fluid resuscitation. If significant hypotension exists, multiple organ system failure likely is imminent. The management outlined in Box 267-2 should be pursued while transport to a tertiary care medical facility is arranged. There, continued management largely will be supportive and dictated by the degree of organ dysfunction.

A multidisciplinary approach usually is required to manage the patient who has staphylococcal TSS. Patients who develop adult-type respiratory distress syndrome or shock lung require endotracheal intubation and ventilatory assistance with positive end-expiratory pressure and high oxygen flow rates. Renal failure, severe electrolyte and acid-base abnormalities, ventricular ectopy, refractory ventricular arrhythmias, and disseminated intravascular coagulation (DIC) all can occur.

Because staphylococcal TSS appears to be an exotoxin-mediated disease, the importance of antibiotics could be questioned. However, administration of an anti-streptococcal antibiotic is important in nongenital (nonmenstrual) TSS to arrest staphylococcal growth and thereby toxin production. Empirical therapy with a beta-lactamase-resistant penicillin (nafcillin) or a cephalosporin (cefazolin) is appropriate.[41] Clinical reports and laboratory studies suggest that clindamycin may be a more effective alternative because it interferes with staphylococcal division at the ribosome level, as op-

Eyes	Hands and Feet	Desquamation	Other Findings	Diagnosis
Nonpurulent conjunctivitis	Erythematous, edematous	Hands and feet—can be generalized	Diarrhea, renal, hepatic, CNS, hematological abnormalities	Clinical, culture of *S. aureus* from nasopharynx, vagina, or wound
± Purulent conjunctivitis	Relatively spared or grossly involved	Gross	—	Clinical, culture of *S. aureus* from nasopharynx or wound, skin biopsy
Purulent conjunctivitis	Involved	Involves only individual lesions	Respiratory and GI tract involvement	Clinical, skin biopsy
Nonpurulent conjunctivitis	Erythematous, edematous	Fingertips	Coronary aneurysms, generalized vasculitis	Clinical, no diagnostic test
—	Relatively spared	Fine, flaky	Rheumatic fever, glomerulonephritis	Clinical, culture of group A streptococci from pharynx, serology
Conjunctivitis	Involved	Fine	Respiratory tract involvement	Clinical, serology
Conjunctivitis	Relatively spared	—	CNS, renal, hepatic involvement	Clinical, serology
± Conjunctivitis	± Involved	Gross	—	Clinical, serology
Injected	—	—	Confusion, abdominal pain and vomiting, hyperesthesia	Clinical, culture of group A streptococci

posed to interfering with cell wall synthesis.[32,37] The combination of an aminoglycoside, such as gentamicin, with nafcillin or cefazolin may be appropriate.[11]

High levels of antibody to TSST-1 have been found in intravenous immunoglobulin (IVIG) preparations; animal model studies and small case series suggest that its administration early in the course of disease can reduce the morbidity and mortality of staphylococcal TSS.[1] The usual dose of IVIG is 400 mg/kg over a period of 4 to 8 hours as a single dose.[1,17,22] Use of high-dose corticosteroids has sometimes been advocated to be of possible benefit in the treatment of shock syndromes. However, such therapy should not be administered routinely to patients with TSS. Such therapy may result in a shorter time to defervescence and clinical stability while making no difference in overall risk of mortality.[40] Nonsteroidal antiinflammatory agents are contraindicated because they actually may increase the progression to TSS by enhancing production of tumor necrosis factor.[36]

DIFFERENTIAL DIAGNOSIS

In some aspects, staphylococcal TSS might be confused with staphylococcal scalded-skin syndrome, staphylococcal scarlet fever, Stevens-Johnson syndrome, Kawasaki disease, streptococcal scarlet fever, streptococcal TSS, measles, leptospirosis, or toxic epidermal necrolysis. The differentiating features among these diagnoses are presented in Table 267-2. The strict case definition presented in Box 267-1 particularly is useful for epidemiological purposes and serves to exclude patients who have other diseases. However, recent experience suggests that this strict definition also may exclude patients who have milder forms of staphylococcal TSS, and this should be kept in mind when confronted with a patient who demonstrates some but not all of the clinical findings of staphylococcal TSS.

PROGNOSIS AND CONVALESCENCE

The majority of patients who have staphylococcal TSS recover within 7 to 10 days. The case fatality rate is 2% to 5%. Although most patients with TSS do not experience pulmonary compromise, mortality is increased significantly if early or prolonged adult respiratory distress syndrome becomes manifest.[11] Nongenital TSS seems to carry a worse prognosis than genital disease, probably because of delayed diagnosis and the more serious nature of the primary infection.[23] Refractory hypotension is associated with mortality rates of up to 50%. Convalescence is characterized by a desquamation of the palms and soles within 1 to 2 weeks after the onset of illness. Some patients also experience hair and nail loss. Fatigue and weakness for as long as 3 months may occur in the recovery phase.

The incidence of recurrent staphylococcal TSS may be as high as 28% if antistaphylococcal antibiotics are not employed and if antibody to toxin is not produced. The criteria for recurrent disease are less stringent than those required for defining an initial episode. Recurrent nongenital TSS occurs but much less frequently than genital disease. Persistent neuropsychological symptoms, such as fatigue, depression, and memory loss, have been described in up to 50% of patients who recover from nongenital TSS.[7,28]

REFERENCES

1. Barry W, et al: Intravenous immunoglobulin therapy for toxic shock syndrome, *JAMA* 267:3315, 1992.

2. Bohach GA, et al: Staphylococcal and streptococcal pyrogenic toxins involved in toxic shock syndrome and related illnesses, *Crit Rev Microbiol* 17:251, 1989.
3. Bonventre PF, et al: Antibody responses to toxic-shock syndrome (TSS) toxin by patients with TSS and by healthy staphylococcal carriers, *J Infect Dis* 150:662, 1984.
4. Bonventre PF, et al: Production of staphylococcal enterotoxin F and pyrogenic enterotoxin C by *Staphylococcus aureus* isolates from toxic shock syndrome-associated sources, *Infect Immun* 40:1023, 1983.
5. Centers for Disease Control: Reduced incidence of menstrual toxic-shock syndrome—United States: 1980-1990, *MMWR* 39:421, 1990.
6. Chesney PJ: Clinical aspects and spectrum of illness of toxic shock syndrome: overview, *Rev Infect Dis* 11(suppl):S1, 1989.
7. Chesney PJ, et al: Toxic-shock syndrome: management of long-term sequelae, *Ann Intern Med* 96:847, 1982.
8. Chow AW, et al: Toxic shock syndrome: clinical and laboratory findings in 30 patients, *Can Med Assoc J* 130:425, 1984.
9. Crass BA, Bergdoll MS: Involvement of staphylococcal enterotoxin in nonmenstrual toxic shock syndrome, *J Clin Microbiol* 23:1138, 1986.
10. Crass BA, Bergdoll MS: Toxin involvement in toxic shock syndrome, *J Infect Dis* 153:918, 1986.
11. Davis D, Gash-Ki TL, Heffernan EJ: Toxic shock syndrome: case report of a postpartum female and a literature review, *J Emerg Med* 16:607, 1998.
12. Davis JP, et al, and the Investigation and Laboratory Team: Toxic-shock syndrome: epidemiologic features, recurrence, risk factors, and prevention, *N Engl J Med* 303:1429, 1980.
13. Gaventa S, et al: Active surveillance for toxic shock syndrome in the United States: 1986, *Rev Infect Dis* 11(suppl 1):S28, 1989.
14. Ikejima T, et al: Induction by toxic-shock-syndrome toxin-1 of a circulating tumor necrosis factor-like substance in rabbits and of immunoreactive tumor necrosis factor and interleukin-1 from human mononuclear cells, *J Infect Dis* 158:1017, 1998.
15. Kass EJ, Parsonnet J: On the pathogenesis of toxic shock syndrome, *Rev Infect Dis* 9:482, 1987.
16. Kreiswirth BN: Genetics and expression of toxic shock syndrome toxin 1: overview, *Rev Infect Dis* 11(suppl 1):S97, 1989.
17. Lamothe F, et al: Clinical usefulness of intravenous human immunoglobulins in invasive group A streptococcal infections: case report and review, *Clin Infect Dis* 21:1469, 1995.
18. Larkin SM, et al: Toxic shock syndrome: clinical, laboratory, and pathologic findings in nine fatal cases, *Ann Intern Med* 96:858, 1982.
19. Lee VY, Chang AH, Chow AW: Detection of staphylococcal enterotoxin B among toxic shock syndrome (TSS) and non-TSS-associated *Staphylococcus aureus* isolates, *J Infect Dis* 166:911, 1992.
20. Leung DYM, Travers JB, Norris DA: The role of superantigens in skin disease, *J Invest Dermatol* 105(suppl):37s, 1995.
21. Manders SM: Toxin-mediated streptococcal and staphylococcal disease, *J Am Acad Dermatol* 39:383, 1998.
22. Melish ME, et al: Use of IVIG for therapy in the rabbit model of TSS, *Clin Res* 35:220, 1987.
23. Parsonnet J: Nonmenstrual toxic shock syndrome: new insights into diagnosis, pathogenesis, and treatment, *Curr Clin Top Infect Dis* 16:1, 1996.
24. Parsonnet J, et al: Induction of human interleukin-1 by toxic-shock-syndrome toxin-1, *J Infect Dis* 151:514, 1985.
25. Reingold AL, et al: Risk factors for menstrual toxic shock syndrome: results of a multistate case-control study, *Rev Infect Dis* 11(suppl 1): S35: 1989.
26. Reingold AL, et al: Toxic-shock syndrome not associated with menstruation, *Lancet* 1:1, 1982.
27. Reingold AL, et al: Toxic shock syndrome surveillance in the United States, 1980 to 1981, *Ann Intern Med* 96(Part 2):875, 1982.
28. Rosene KA, et al: Persistent neuropsychological sequelae of toxic shock syndrome, *Ann Intern Med* 96:865, 1982.
29. Rosten PM, Bartlett KH, Chow AW: Serologic responses to toxic shock syndrome (TSS) toxin-1 in menstrual and nonmenstrual TSS, *Clin Invest Med* 11:187, 1988.
30. Schlievert PM: Staphylococcal enterotoxin B and toxic-shock syndrome toxin-1 are significantly associated with non-menstrual TSS, *Lancet* 1:1149, 1986.
31. Schlievert PM: TSST-1: structure, function, purification, and detection—role of toxic shock syndrome toxin 1 in toxic shock syndrome: overview, *Rev Infect Dis* 11:107, 1989.
32. Schlievert PM, Kelly JA: Clindamycin-induced suppression of toxic-shock syndrome-associated exotoxin production, *J Infect Dis* 143:509, 1981.
33. Schlievert PM, et al: Identification and characterization of an exotoxin from *Staphylococcus aureus* associated with toxic-shock syndrome, *J Infect Dis* 143:509, 1981.
34. Schlievert PM, et al: Molecular structure of staphylococcus and streptococcus superantigens, *J Clin Immunol* 15(suppl):4s, 1995.
35. Shands KN, et al: Toxic-shock syndrome in menstruating women: association with tampon use and *Staphylococcus aureus* and clinical features in 52 cases, *N Engl J Med* 303:1436, 1980.
36. Stevens DL: Could nonsteroidal antiinflammatory drugs (NSAIDS) enhance the progression of bacterial infections to toxic shock syndrome, *Clin Infect Dis* 21:977, 1995.
37. Stevens DL, Yan S, Bryant AE: Penicillin-binding protein expression at different growth stages determines penicillin efficacy in vitro and in vivo: an explanation for the inoculum effect, *J Infect Dis* 167:1401, 1993.
38. Strausbaugh LJ: Toxic shock syndrome: are you recognizing its changing presentations, *Postgrad Med* 94:107, 1993.
39. Todd J, Fishaut M: Toxic shock syndrome associated with phage-group-I staphylococci, *Lancet* 2:1116, 1978.
40. Todd JK, et al: Corticosteroid therapy for patients with toxic shock syndrome, *JAMA* 252:3399, 1984.
41. Van Langervelde P, et al: Combinations of flucloxacillin and gentamycin inhibits toxic shock syndrome toxin 1 production by *Staphylococcus aureus* in both logarithmic and stationary phases of growth, *Antimicrob Agents Chemother* 41:1682, 1997.

SUGGESTED READINGS

Allen ST, et al: Toxic shock syndrome associated with use of latex nasal packing, *Arch Intern Med* 150:2587, 1990.

Bartlett P, et al: Toxic shock syndrome associated with surgical wound infections, *JAMA* 247:1448, 1982.

Bracero L, Bowe E: Postpartum toxic shock syndrome, *Am J Obstet Gynecol* 143:478, 1982.

Britto J, et al: Systemic complications associated with bacterial tracheitis, *Arch Dis Child* 74:249, 1996.

Dann EJ, et al: Bacterial laryngotracheitis associated with toxic shock syndrome in an adult, *Clin Infect Dis* 18:437, 1994.

Dorman KJ, et al: Toxic shock syndrome in the postoperative patient, *Surg Gynecol Obstet* 154:65, 1982.

Faich G, et al: Toxic shock syndrome and the vaginal contraceptive sponge, *JAMA* 255:216, 1986.

Ferguson MA, Todd JK: Toxic shock syndrome associated with *Staphylococcus aureus* sinusitis in children, *J Infect Dis* 161:953, 1990.

Finkelstein S, Hyland RH: Toxic shock syndrome as the AIDS-defining diagnosis, *Chest* 104:950, 1993.

Graham DR, et al: Postoperative toxic shock syndrome, *Clin Infect Dis* 20:895, 1995.

Griffith JA, Perkin RM: Toxic shock syndrome and sinusitis: a hidden site of infection, *West J Med* 148:580, 1988.

Hirsch B, et al: Toxic shock syndrome from staphylococcal pharyngitis, *Ear Nose Throat J* 63:494, 1984.

Hull HR, et al: Toxic shock syndrome related to nasal packing, *Arch Otolaryngol* 109:624, 1983.

Jacobson JA, Kaswork EM: Toxic shock syndrome after nasal surgery: case reports and analysis of risk factors, *Arch Otolaryngol Head Neck Surg* 112:329, 1986.

Kain KC, Schulzer M, Chow AW: Clinical spectrum of nonmenstrual toxic shock syndrome (TSS): comparison with menstrual TSS by multivariate discriminant analyses, *Clin Infect Dis* 16:100, 1993.

MacDonald KL, et al: Toxic shock syndrome: a newly recognized complication of influenza and influenza-like illness, *JAMA* 257:1053, 1987.

Nahass RG, Cocke DJ: Toxic shock syndrome associated with use of a nasal tampon, *Am J Med* 8:4629, 1988.

Reingold AL, et al: Nonmenstrual toxic shock syndrome: a review of 130 cases, *Ann Intern Med* 96:875, 1982.

Reiser RF, et al: Staphylococcal enterotoxin antibodies in pediatric patients from Utah, *J Infect Dis* 158:1105, 1988.

Schwartz G, et al: Nonmenstrual toxic shock syndrome associated with barrier contraceptives: report of a case-control study, *Rev Infect Dis* 11(suppl 1):S43, 1989.

Shah A, et al: Nonmenstrual toxic shock syndrome in a young child with human immunodeficiency virus infection, *Pediatr Infect Dis J* 15:639, 1996.

Solomon R, Truman T, Murray DL: Toxic shock syndrome as a complication of bacterial tracheitis, *Pediatr Infect Dis* 4:298, 1985.

Sparano J, Ferranti E: The acquired immunodeficiency syndrome and nonmenstrual toxic shock syndrome, *Ann Intern Med* 105:300, 1986.

Sperber SJ, Francis JB: Toxic shock syndrome during an influenza outbreak, *JAMA* 257:1086, 1987.

Surh L, Read SE: Staphylococcal tracheitis and toxic shock syndrome in a young child, *J Pediatr* 105:585, 1984.

Thomas SW, Baird IM, Frazier RD: Toxic shock syndrome following submucous resection and rhinoplasty, *JAMA* 247:2402, 1982.

Tolan RW Jr: Toxic shock syndrome complicating influenza A in a child: case report and review, *Clin Infect Dis* 17:43, 1993.

Van Lierde S, et al: Toxic shock syndrome without rash in a young child: link with syndrome of hemorrhagic shock and encephalopathy, *J Pediatr* 131:130, 1997.

Whitfield JW, Valenti WM, Magnussen CR: Toxic shock syndrome in puerperium, *JAMA* 246:1806, 1981.

Wilkins EG, et al: Probable toxic shock syndrome with primary staphylococcal pneumonia, *J Infect Dis* 11:231, 1985.

Wolfe MW, Bennett JT: Pyomyositis with toxic shock syndrome presenting as back pain and fever: a case report and literature review, *Am J Orthoped* 26:135, 1997.

Wood SD, et al: Maxillary sinusitis: the focus of toxic shock syndrome in a male patient, *West J Med* 147:467, 1987.

Woods SL, Jackson B: The human immunodeficiency virus and nonmenstrual toxic shock syndrome: a female case presentation, *Nurse Pract* 19:68, 1994.

268 Stomatitis

Julius G. Goepp

Stomatitis (ulceration and inflammation of the mucosa of the oral cavity) is a common problem in children at all ages beyond the neonatal period, with incidence as high as 50% in some populations.[2] Although most cases of stomatitis are mild and self-limited, several types may cause more severe or recurrent disease. Specific treatments exist for only a few types of stomatitis, and management usually consists of measures to support comfort and hydration.

ETIOLOGY

Stomatitis in children has numerous causes, including infections (generally viral), trauma, and the effects of cancer chemotherapy. Stomatitis may also occasionally be found in association with systemic disease, and rarely occurs as the presenting sign. Aphthous stomatitis, which accounts for the largest proportion of cases in otherwise healthy children, has no clear-cut cause.

Infectious Causes

Viral causes. Several viral classes are capable of causing stomatitis of distinct clinical appearance, whereas others are suspected as causes, although not proved.

Herpes simplex virus. Herpes simplex virus, type 1 (HSV1), causes acute primary herpetic gingivostomatitis (APHGS) in previously uninfected children. Less commonly, HSV2 may be the cause. Most pediatric cases occur in children between 10 months and 3 years. The virus usually is acquired from an individual who has a mouth sore caused by HSV1 or who has a herpetic whitlow of a finger or a toe. Illness begins 5 to 10 days after exposure and is heralded by fever, chills, and a nonspecific "viral syndrome," with subsequent development of a sore throat and cervical adenopathy. Older children may complain of a burning sensation in the mouth. Vesicles develop anywhere on the oral mucosa but primarily in the anterior oropharynx and on the lips, tongue, and buccal mucosa. They may spread to the perioral skin.[2] Vesicles rupture within 1 to 2 days. The resulting small ulcers may coalesce, while new lesions will continue to appear for 3 to 5 days after the initial outbreak. Anorexia resulting from pain is common and may produce dehydration severe enough to warrant hospitalization. Some children, especially in the younger age groups, may autoinoculate fingers, eyes, or genitals, resulting in spread of the lesions.

Recovery from APHGS is spontaneous in 7 to 10 days. About 50% of patients develop at least one episode of "cold sores" subsequently, but APHGS does not recur in immunocompetent children.

Enteroviruses. Milder forms of stomatitis are caused by the enteroviruses, especially coxsackieviruses.[2] Herpangina is caused most commonly by coxsackie A4. The lesions usually are extremely painful, small vesicles that may enlarge slowly over several days. Lesions develop a red "halo" that may ultimately reach 1 cm in size. The lesions typically are found in the posterior portion of the oropharynx, posterior to the anterior tonsillar pillars. Fever in the moderate to high range, as high as 105.8° F (41° C) is common, as are generalized myalgias and malaise, with diminished oral intake. Dehydration is unusual, but the combination of high fever, irritability, and decreased oral intake may lead to the suspicion of sepsis, particularly in the younger child. Careful and thorough examination of the posterior pharynx and soft palate may reveal the characteristic lesions, thereby sparing a child the extended sepsis evaluation. Herpangina is seasonal in the United States, being especially prominent in the summer. Herpangina usually resolves spontaneously in 3 to 5 days.

Coxsackie A16 (and other enterovirus) infections may produce hand, foot, and mouth disease (HFMD). In this condition, 4- to 8-mm vesicles appearing in the posterior oropharynx may erode to produce small, painful ulcers. A characteristic rash, which may be vesicular or appear only as blanching red spots, appears on the palms and soles. The cutaneous lesions may also develop red surrounding halos, and may be mildly tender to palpation. Fever, malaise, and decreased oral intake are common. HFMD usually resolves in about 1 week.

Enteroviral stomatitis may be differentiated from APHGS by the location of the lesions (more posterior in enteroviral illness) and the lack of exudate and coalescence. Generally, APHGS is a more severe stomatitis than that seen with enteroviral infections.

Bacterial causes. Acute necrotizing ulcerative gingivitis (ANUG, trench mouth) is caused by fusiform bacilli and spirochetes, which may be part of normal oral flora. The condition is characterized by a rapid progression from gingival redness and pain to ulceration and spontaneous bleeding. Necrotic material accumulates as a pseudomembrane over the gums and is the cause of a characteristic foul breath odor. Children who have ANUG may have fever and malaise and generally do not eat well.

Other bacterial pathogens generally do not cause stomatitis but may play a significant role in superinfection of existing oral ulcers. Oral flora poses a real threat to the immunocompromised patient who may acquire serious systemic bacterial infection when the oral mucosa breaks down.

Noninfectious Causes

Trauma. Minor oral trauma such as cheek-biting or vigorous toothbrushing can cause local oral ulcers that are not recurrent and that resolve spontaneously. Trauma can be significant in the immunocompromised patient and as a precipitant for recurrent aphthous stomatitis (discussed after the section on chemotherapy below).

Chemotherapy. Children undergoing cancer chemotherapy are at high risk of developing stomatitis.[3] Its severity depends on the type and duration of chemotherapy, as well as on the state of the oral cavity at the onset of treatment.

Chemotherapeutic drugs are toxic to tissues such as oral mucosa, which normally have high rates of cell turnover. Within 5 days of beginning anticancer treatment, patients may experience thinning of the oral mucosa accompanied by inflammation and pain. Ulceration may follow by day 7, with potential for local and systemic bacterial infection. Routine intraoral trauma may cause or exacerbate local lesions, as can the presence of orthodontic devices.

Aphthous Stomatitis

Aphthous stomatitis (AS) is the most common ulcerative oral disease in children.[2,9] The condition often is recurrent. Terminology in this condition is confusing, in part because the term *aphthae* has been used to describe any undefined oral ulcers. Aphthous stomatitis can occur in isolation or as part of multiorgan disease.[9]

Three categories of AS have been defined based on the size, duration, and tendency of lesions to produce scarring.[2] "Minor" AS lesions are less than 1 cm in diameter, are round or oval, and appear in groups of one to five. They are yellow-gray in the center and have a red "halo"; they occur mainly on the labial and buccal mucosa and tongue. The recurrence interval is variable and occasionally cyclical. Healing without scarring occurs in 7 to 14 days. About 80% of AS are the "minor" form. "Major" AS is found in about 10% of cases. Lesions exceed 1 cm in diameter and may occur on any part of the oral mucosa, especially the lips, soft palate, and tonsillar pillars. Lesions may take up to 6 weeks to heal, and submucosal scarring may occur. "Herpetiform" AS also accounts for about 10% of disease. Despite the name, "herpetiform" AS does not resemble herpetic stomatitis. Up to 100 1- to 2-mm yellow vesicles appear, which may coalesce and produce ulcers. The lesions, which may scar, heal in 7 to 10 days. The anterior mouth, tongue, and floor of the mouth are affected most commonly.

The pathogenesis of AS is unclear for any of the categories. No convincing evidence has been produced for bacterial or viral causes. Strong genetic predisposition appears to exist,[4,6] but specific genetic factors remain unidentified. Minor local trauma is a precipitant[10] but not a cause. Stress and anxiety also are recognized as precipitating factors in susceptible individuals.[7]

Accumulated evidence points to an immunopathological mechanism for AS,[2] but the specific process remains unclear. No good direct evidence exists for an autoimmune process in response to specific antigens.

Stomatitis with an aphthous appearance may occur as part of a number of systemic conditions that should be considered in evaluation. These conditions include various nutritional deficiency states (iron, folate, B_{12}, zinc), as well as blood dyscrasias and inflammatory bowel disease. Cyclic neutropenia is associated with oral ulcers, which recur periodically during neutropenia nadirs. Its cause is unknown. In Behçet's disease, aphthouslike ulcers occur in the mouth in conjunction with urethral ulcers and eye findings such as conjunctivitis and uveitis.

Other Causes of Stomatitis

Several systemic disease entities are associated periodically with stomatitis and should be considered in children whose pattern of outbreak and nature of lesions are not readily explained by one of the more common conditions already described. Recently, a syndrome known as PFAPA (periodic fever, aphthous stomatitis, pharyngitis, and cervical adenitis) has been described and characterized.[8] PFAPA is first manifested before the age of 5 years, in otherwise well children. Diagnosis is made in the context of a child under age 5 years with regularly recurring fevers (fevers lasting for about 5 days and recurring roughly every month) who does not have upper respiratory tract symptoms. Children with PFAPA have at least one of the following: aphthous stomatitis, cervical adenitis, or pharyngitis. Markers of acute inflammation (elevated white blood cell count and erythrocyte sedimentation rate) are present during the febrile episodes. Children are completely well between febrile episodes and exhibit normal growth and development. Bacterial and viral cultures obtained during the episodes are negative. The differential diagnosis for PFAPA includes cyclic neutropenia, familial Mediterranean fever (FMF), hyperimmunoglobulinemia D syndrome, and Behçet's syndrome. PFAPA is not accompanied by neutropenia and is characterized by negative cultures, unlike cyclic neutropenia. The serositis and arthralgias that are typical of FMF are absent in PFAPA. Immunoglobulin levels are normal, and the characteristic genital lesions and uveitis found in Behçet's syndrome are absent in PFAPA.

Pyostomatitis vegetans is an oral ulcerative condition associated with inflammatory bowel disease in adults. Although rare in children, it has recently been described in siblings aged 5 and 7 years. This unusual condition consists of characteristic gingival pustules and erosions that may fuse to form "snail track" ulcers. Its significance lies in its strong association with inflammatory bowel disease. A hereditary predisposition has been suggested.[1]

DATABASE

History

When mouth sores are the chief complaint, the history should include the duration, site, and initial appearance of the lesions. Any prior history of stomatitis and pattern of recurrence should be noted. A relationship to oral trauma or to anxiety or stress may be identified. A family history of recurrent stomatitis is helpful in diagnosing aphthous stomatitis. The presence of fever may point to one of the viral causes of stomatitis or to PFAPA. Finally, a general medical history and review of systems may help to identify associated systemic conditions.

The possibility of stomatitis should also be entertained in the young child who presents during the summer and early fall with complaints of fever, malaise or fussiness, and decreased oral intake. Because the lesions of herpangina and hand, foot, and mouth disease are small and posterior, they may have escaped the parents' notice.

Physical Examination

Physical examination, noting the size and especially the location (anterior or posterior) of lesions and any accompanying signs such as fever, adenopathy, and lethargy, often leads to a specific diagnosis. Table 268-1 shows the various features of the most common types of stomatitis. Because lesions in the oral cavity tend to break down rapidly and become ulcerated, a search for new lesions may be the best way to detect any characteristic appearances.

Laboratory Tests

Laboratory findings usually are not helpful in determining the cause of stomatitis. In rare cases, determination of viral titers may be desirable. In recurrent aphthous stomatitis, hematological screening is recommended[1] to exclude iron or folate deficiency. The initial screen should include a complete blood count with red cell indices and hemoglobin. Ferritin, B_{12} level, and serum and red cell folate levels may be needed for further evaluation when anemia is detected. In a child with regularly recurring fevers, a complete blood count obtained both during the febrile episode and during a well interval may reveal a diagnosis of cyclic neutropenia, while elevated white blood cell counts in such children may suggest the diagnosis of PFAPA in the presence of other criteria.

DIFFERENTIAL DIAGNOSIS

The differential diagnosis of stomatitis in children consists of the entities discussed previously and listed in Table 268-1. Generally, a specific diagnosis is not critical, unless symptoms are exceptionally severe or protracted or unless serious systemic disease is suspected.

PSYCHOSOCIAL CONSIDERATIONS

Severe stomatitis resulting in diminished or absent oral intake can be stressful for families. Parents may experience a sense of loss of control and attendant anxiety. Fears of dehydration, while appropriate, may be exaggerated. If a child is reasonably well hydrated, the physician can reassure the parents by pointing out how well they are managing the child's illness.

Pain, particularly with APHGS, may be a significant concern. Adequate analgesia is important, and occasionally, hospitalization is indicated for pain control and hydration. The physician should remember that a fussy or irritable child who is refusing to drink is at increased risk for physical abuse when parents become stressed and exhausted.

In APHGS, parents frequently are concerned that the herpetic condition was acquired through venereal contact. Such transmission is rare, and parents should be counseled about the innocent fashion in which the disease usually is transmitted, unless a high index of suspicion exists. In addition, parents should be counseled about the likelihood of recurrence but that the recurrence consists of isolated cold sores, not full-blown stomatitis.

The role of stress in precipitating recurrent AS is well established and should be discussed with parents and older patients.

MANAGEMENT

Primary concerns in management of the child who has any type of stomatitis are comfort and hydration. Supportive therapy alone is sufficient in hand, foot, and mouth disease; herpangina; and mild AS. Pain can be managed with acetaminophen or ibuprofen. Topical relief may be obtained with application, every 4 hours, of occlusive gels such as Orajel or Anbesol, of a 1:1 mixture of diphenhydramine and Kaopectate, or in more severe cases, of 2% viscous lidocaine. Systemic toxicity has occurred with the latter, so the dose should be restricted to less than 2 ml, the dosing interval strictly limited, and the parent cautioned to keep the bottle away from children.

In addition, APHGS usually can be managed supportively; occasionally, however, pain may be severe enough to warrant parenteral medication. Hydration via intravenous fluids may become necessary. Acyclovir may be helpful if started early enough in the course.

Therapy for trench mouth (ANUG) consists of topical chlorhexidine 0.2% rinses and curettage, which usually are curative. Oral penicillin may be added when systemic signs, such as fever, are present.[5]

Recurrent AS has responded well to treatment via daily oral washes with triamcinolone acetate 0.1% or 0.2% aqueous solution.[9]

PFAPA may respond to short (5-day) courses of prednisone 1 to 2 mg/kg/day, and may resolve entirely following tonsillectomy and adenoidectomy.

COMPLICATIONS

Complications are unusual in most forms of stomatitis. Scarring is unusual in APHGS and minor AS, but submucosal scarring may occur in major AS and herpetiform AS. In the immunocompromised patient, stomatitis or mucositis may be the site of bacterial invasion, with resulting systemic infection.

PROGNOSIS

Hand, foot, and mouth disease and herpangina rarely recur, although second infections with different viral strains are possible. APHGS does not recur, but up to 50% of patients experience one or more episodes of cold sores. Aphthous stomatitis commonly recurs, exacerbated by trauma and stress, and occasionally occurs cyclically. PFAPA generally

Table 268-1 Features of Stomatitis by Category

Type	Organism	Location in Mouth	Appearance of Lesion	Time to Healing	Associated Features	Recurrence
Acute primary herpetic gingivostomatitis	HSV1	Anywhere, especially anterior mucosa	Vesicles on red base	7-10 days	Fever, pain, cervical adenopathy, anorexia, dehydration	As cold sores
Herpangina	Enteroviruses, especially coxsackie A4	Posterior, especially soft palate	Small, gray-white vesicles	3-5 days	Mild pain, fever	None
Hand, foot, and mouth disease	Enteroviruses, especially coxsackie A16	Posterior	Small vesicles erode to small ulcers	7 days	Ulcers painful, papular or vesicular rash on palms and soles, fever common	None
Acute necrotizing ulcerative gingivitis (trench mouth)	Oral spirochetes and fusiform bacilli	Gingiva	Red swelling of gums progressing to ulcers with necrotic, gray pseudomembrane	Variable, depends on treatment	Fever, malaise, foul breath	Possible
Aphthous stomatitis						
Minor	Unknown or none	Tongue, labial, and buccal mucosa	Ulcers <1 cm diameter, round or oral, yellow-gray with red halo	7-14 days	Groups of one to five lesions	Common
Major	Unknown or none	Any part of mucosa, especially lips, soft palate, tonsillar pillars	Ulcers >1 cm diameter, deeper than minor	Up to 6 weeks	Submucosal scarring	Common
Herpetiform	Unknown or none	Any part, especially anterior mouth and tongue	Multiple (up to 100) vesicles 1-2 mm diameter	7-10 days	Vesicles may coalesce to small ulcers	Common

resolves completely following the fifth birthday, without long-term sequelae.

When to Refer

Failure of lesions to resolve with 7 to 10 days
Development of extraoral manifestations (rash, conjunctivitis)
There is suspicion of nutritional deficiency

When to Hospitalize

Inability to maintain hydration orally
Severe pain not adequately managed with oral medication
Occasionally, exhausted parents may benefit from an overnight hospitalization of the child for respite purposes.

REFERENCES

1. Al-Rimawi HS, et al: Pyostomatitis vegetans in childhood, *Eur J Pediatr* 157:402, 1998.
2. Field EA, Brookes V, Tyldesley WR: Recurrent aphthous ulceration in children: a review, *Int J Paediatr Dentistry* 2:1, 1992.
3. Hebert AA, Berg JH: Oral mucous membrane diseases of childhood. I. Mucositis and xerostomia. II. Recurrent aphthous stomatitis. III. Herpetic stomatitis, *Semin Dermatol* 11:80, 1992.
4. Miller MF, Ship II, Ram C: Inheritance patterns in recurrent aphthous ulcers, *Oral Surg Oral Med Oral Pathol* 43:886, 1977.
5. Piecuch JF, Topazian RG: Infections of the oral cavity. In Feigin RD, Cherry JD, editors: *Textbook of pediatric infectious diseases,* Philadelphia, 1987, WB Saunders.
6. Ship II: Epidemiologic aspects of recurrent aphthous ulcerations, *Oral Surg Oral Med Oral Pathol* 33:400, 1972.
7. Ship II, et al: Recurrent ulcerations and recurrent herpes labialis in a professional student population, *Oral Surg Oral Med Oral Pathol* 13: 1191, 1960.
8. Thomas KT, Edwards KM: Periodic fever syndrome, *Pediatr Infect Dis J* 18:68, 1999.
9. Vincent SD, Lily GE: Clinical, historic, and therapeutic features of aphthous stomatitis, *Oral Surg Oral Med Oral Pathol* 74:79, 1992.
10. Wray D, Graykowski EA, Notkins AL: Role of mucosal injury in initiating recurrent aphthous stomatitis, *BMJ* 283:1569, 1981.

269 Sudden Infant Death Syndrome

John G. Brooks • Robert A. Darnall

Sudden infant death syndrome (SIDS) remains the leading cause of death in the United States for children between 1 month and 1 year of age, despite reductions in the SIDS rate over the past few years in many countries, including the United States. Although numerous hypotheses have been advanced and extensive research has been done over the past several decades, the cause of SIDS remains unknown. The loss of a baby to SIDS is devastating for the family, as well as for the health care providers, and it is the pediatrician's responsibility to see that the family receives appropriate support, accurate information about SIDS, and the results of their infant's autopsy.

DEFINITION AND DIAGNOSIS

SIDS is defined as "the sudden death of an infant under 1 year of age that remains unexplained after a thorough case investigation, including performance of a complete autopsy, examination of the death scene, and review of the clinical history."[7] For clinical purposes, the diagnosis of SIDS should not be excluded because of the absence of a death scene investigation, if all other findings point to SIDS. This diagnosis usually is restricted to deaths during the first year of life, although rare deaths that have the same clinical picture have occurred in the second year. Throughout most of this country there are no mandatory autopsy laws for unexpected infant deaths, so pediatricians should do their best to see that an autopsy is performed on any suspected SIDS cases. Because SIDS is mostly a diagnosis of exclusion, the autopsy is essential to rule out the 10% to 20% of sudden, unexpected infant deaths that are due to other causes such as intracranial hemorrhage, myocarditis, meningitis, and sometimes, trauma, which may not be easily distinguished from SIDS without an autopsy. The autopsy results also are very important for counseling of the bereaved family so that they can be reassured that they had not missed the signs of some potentially treatable disease.

The autopsy characteristic essential for the diagnosis of SIDS is the absence of any finding that would constitute an "adequate cause of death," such as myocarditis, significant pneumonia, or intracranial hemorrhage. The most subjective aspect of the diagnosis of SIDS is the determination of what pathological findings constitute an "adequate cause of death." Small amounts of inflammation, in the trachea, for example, or small, isolated foci of pneumonia certainly would not be thought to cause death and therefore are compatible with the diagnosis of SIDS. Some infants who have chronic, stable, underlying diseases such as bronchopulmonary dysplasia (BPD) may die suddenly and unexpectedly, and although their autopsy findings are not normal, no abnormality explains the death. These infants' deaths also can be classified as SIDS. From the perspective of public health and the clinician, it is more important to understand which infants are at risk of sudden and unexpected death than to determine which autopsy findings constitute an "adequate cause of death." Clinicians should assume that sudden unexpected infant deaths are SIDS until proved otherwise so that family support and counseling can be implemented promptly. Investigating the scene of death and speaking directly with the individuals who found the dead infant are essential aspects of diagnosing SIDS accurately. It is of utmost importance that this search for evidence of environmental risk to, or maltreatment of, the infant is carried out with extraordinary sensitivity to the feelings of the bereaved family. Individuals who conduct death scene investigations of possible SIDS cases must be sensitive and knowledgeable about SIDS, bereavement processes, and child abuse. They must be aware of any of their own biases toward or against any socioeconomic or ethnic groups or child care practices so that such personal biases do not influence the sensitivity, thoroughness, or conclusions of the death scene investigation.

INCIDENCE

The current incidence of SIDS in the United States has decreased dramatically since 1992 and as of 1997 averages about 0.8 per 1000 live births (Fig. 269-1). Black and Native American infants probably have a twofold to threefold greater incidence than white infants. In both the United States and England, Asian populations have a lower incidence of SIDS than is found in the general population, and the incidence is lowest among Asians who have immigrated most recently. Nationally, the incidence of SIDS among non-Hispanic white infants is similar to that among Hispanic infants, despite the significant difference in mean socioeconomic status. There also is a wide variation in the incidence of SIDS in populations outside the United States. SIDS occurs relatively infrequently (less than 1 per 1000 live births) in most Scandinavian countries, Japan, Hong Kong, and Israel. Until recently the SIDS rate in New Zealand and Australia was 3 to 4 per 1000 live births, but this diminished significantly over the past few years at the same time that public education campaigns to prevent SIDS were implemented in those two countries. Although some of this variability between populations may be due to differences in reporting procedures and diagnostic criteria, the differences

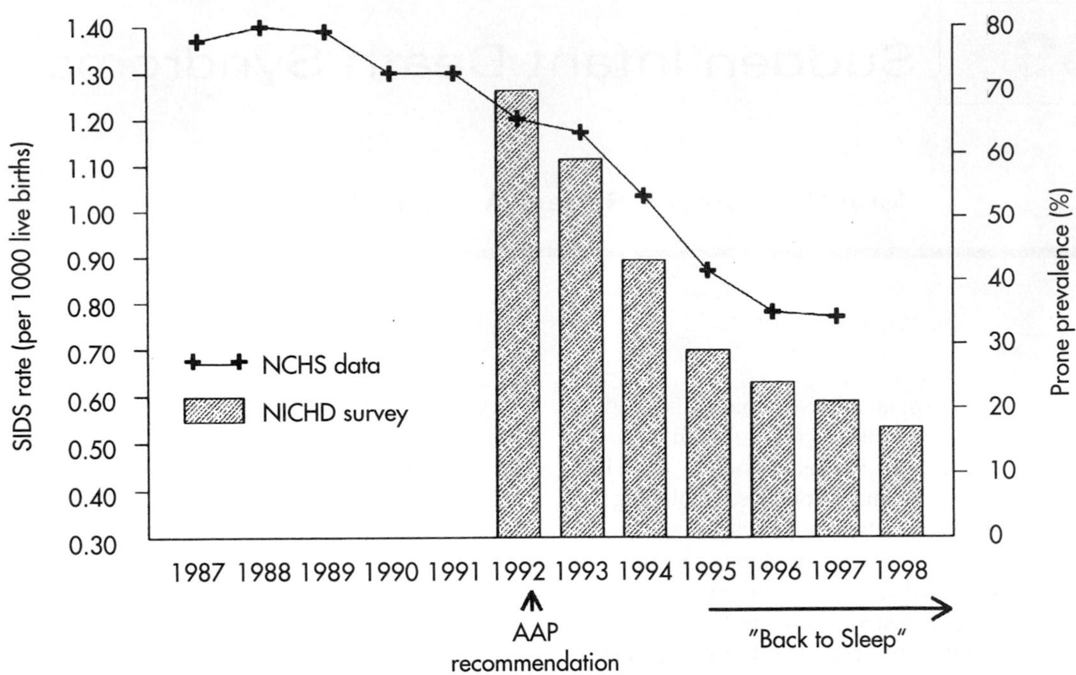

Fig. 269-1 Sudden infant death syndrome rate in the United States (line) from National Center for Health Statistics data and prone positioning rate from National Institute for Child Health and Human Development surveys (bars). The American Academy of Pediatrics recommendation was made at the April 1992 spring meeting and was published in June 1992. The "Back to Sleep" campaign was begun in mid 1994.

probably are due mostly to other, possibly cultural, diversities. In most countries where accurate SIDS incidence data are available, the incidence has been declining for the past 3 to 7 years. In the United States, the incidence of SIDS has fallen by almost 50%, from about 1.2 per 1000 live births in 1992 to approximately 0.8 per 1000 live births in 1997 (see Fig. 269-1). More recent data are not available since there is a 2-year lag in the availability of accurate national data in this country.

There is a characteristic frequency distribution of age at death of SIDS victims, although the 2- to 4-month peak is significantly less prominent in some recently reported data from Australia and England after their SIDS prevention campaigns. In this country, about 5% of SIDS cases occur in the first month of life, 60% by 3 months of age, 85% by 6 months, and more than 99% in the first year of life. SIDS has been reported to be rare in the first week of life, but this is at least partly because most incidence studies have excluded deaths in the first week of life. In up to 10% of neonatal autopsies, the cause of death remains unexplained, and these may represent SIDS cases. Countries that have low SIDS rates also have low total infant mortality.

POSTMORTEM STUDIES OF SIDS VICTIMS

The diagnosis of SIDS cannot be established without an autopsy. Many states still lack legislation requiring an autopsy and death scene investigation for unexpected infant deaths. Autopsies of such infants should follow standardized, comprehensive protocols. Although nonspecific findings such as vascular congestion, mild pulmonary edema, mild pulmonary inflammation, and an increased number of minor congenital anomalies are common, no diagnostic findings are seen on routine autopsy. The most characteristic finding is the presence of intrathoracic petechiae, which are found on the visceral surfaces of the heart, lungs, and thymus in approximately 80% of SIDS victims. Although intrathoracic petechiae are not unique to SIDS, their localization to the thoracic cavity has led to an unproved hypothesis that they may result from inspiratory efforts against an occluded upper airway.

For the past several decades, studies that have used specialized techniques on tissues obtained from SIDS victims and control infants who died suddenly from an explained cause have indicated that group mean differences exist for some autopsy findings between the SIDS babies and their controls. However, these group differences lack sufficient sensitivity or specificity for SIDS to be of any use in establishing the diagnosis. Although there still is some controversy about which "SIDS tissue markers" have been clearly established, those that are most generally accepted include extramedullary hematopoiesis, delayed postnatal resorption of periadrenal brown fat, abnormal pulmonary surfactant, and brainstem gliosis. It is not known whether any of these are related causally to SIDS. Some of these "tissue markers" are consistent with the hypothesis that SIDS deaths are preceded by in utero or postnatal hypoxic insults or both, but this hypothesis remains unproved. In addition, numerous microbiological studies have failed to identify any specific viral or bacterial infection associated with SIDS. Because of methodological shortcomings and conflicting data, it is unclear whether either viral or bacterial infections are more common in SIDS victims than in appropriate controls matched for age and time of year.

EPIDEMIOLOGY

Of the diverse methodologies, disciplines, and approaches to SIDS research, epidemiology has provided the most important and conclusive contributions to an understanding of the disorder. Several clinical, demographic, and environmental characteristics of mothers and infants have been shown to be associated with an increased risk for SIDS. It is important that only those studies that meet minimal criteria for methodological acceptability be considered. The minimal criteria for an acceptable, epidemiological SIDS study are (1) the study must be population based; (2) the SIDS definition must be clearly stated, acceptable, and consistently adhered to; (3) all SIDS cases must be confirmed by autopsy; and (4) control infants must be appropriately selected. Identification of risk factors for SIDS is important for two reasons: first, true risk factors (in contrast to confounding variables or effect modifiers) should provide clues to the etiology of SIDS; second, these data will serve as the basis for developing a focus for efforts to prevent SIDS.

Maternal risk factors for SIDS that have been reported most consistently include maternal smoking, maternal age under 20, poor prenatal care, and social deprivation. In unadjusted analyses, each of these generally confers a threefold to fourfold increased risk compared with mothers who do not have the particular risk factor. Each of these risk factors is still significantly associated with SIDS after socioeconomic status and race have been controlled for. Maternal smoking is one of the strongest and most consistently reported risk factors for SIDS. Both prenatal and postnatal maternal smoking increase the risk for SIDS. Recent emphasis has been placed on the dangers of smoke in the infant environment, and a few studies have identified this as a separate risk factor.[46,58] However, it is difficult to sort the effects of "second-hand" smoke from those of maternal smoking, per se. The complexity of the relationship between risk factors and SIDS is well illustrated by the synergistic effect of maternal smoking and maternal anemia on SIDS risk.[8] Anemia is not a risk factor for SIDS in nonsmoking mothers; in smoking mothers, however, a maternal hematocrit below 30% is associated with an increased risk of SIDS. There have been several reports of a dose-response effect of maternal smoking, with the risk of SIDS being proportional to the number of cigarettes smoked per day. Interestingly, the effect of maternal smoking on SIDS risk appears to be stronger for infants who die in the first 3 months of life than for older SIDS infants. This is in contrast to most of the other risk factors that are more highly associated with the risk of SIDS in older infants. To date, no intervention studies have reported a relationship between a decrease in the incidence of maternal smoking and a decrease in the SIDS rate.

The seasonal occurrence of SIDS has been a consistent factor. Wintertime is a major environmental risk factor for SIDS, with approximately 65% to 75% of SIDS cases in this country occurring during the 6 winter months. A peak SIDS incidence in the colder months is reported in both the Northern and Southern hemispheres. The winter risk factor will need to be closely evaluated, however, since it appears that in both Australia and England the seasonal differences in the incidence of SIDS have diminished since the implementation of SIDS prevention campaigns.

Characteristics of infants that confer an increased risk of SIDS include low birth weight, prematurity, small for gestational age, multiple births, male gender, prone sleeping position, and soft sleep surfaces and loose bedding.* Both prematurity and multiple births remain significantly associated with SIDS after adjustment for birth weight and race. The association of SIDS with low birth weight remains significant after adjusting for smoking, race, and gestational age. Approximately 60% of SIDS infants are boys.

It now is recognized that prone positioning during sleep is a major risk factor for SIDS.† A causal relationship between prone positioning and SIDS is strongly supported by the dramatic reductions in the SIDS rates in countries, including the United States, in which programs have been instituted to change the prevalence of prone sleeping. In this country, the incidence of SIDS has declined almost 50% since the American Academy of Pediatrics Task Force on Infant Positioning Statement in 1992[25] and the U.S. "Back to Sleep" program was instituted in 1994. Several epidemiological studies have also identified soft surfaces such as pillows and comforters in the infant's environment as additional risk factors.‡ Pillows filled with polystyrene beads were found to be associated with increased risk to young infants,[29] and these items have been removed from the marketplace in the United States. Loose bedding, particularly when it can easily cover the infant's head, has also been found to be associated with an increased risk for SIDS.§ Overheating may be a separate risk factor for SIDS,[15,19,52,53,68] although it is more likely that relative overheating represents an "effect modifier" of the risk associated with prone sleeping and the time of year. This is suggested by studies showing that the risk associated with overheating is more evident when the infant is in the prone position.[52]

Under certain circumstances, bed sharing can be a risk factor for SIDS. Sofa sharing with an adult or bed sharing with multiple family members may be particularly dangerous.[61] Some reports have indicated that the risk related to bed sharing is particularly high when the co-sleepers have been using alcohol, mind-altering drugs, or are smokers.[32,40,60,61] Although there is a definite relationship between race and the risk of SIDS in this country, this finding most likely is due to confounding effects of other variables, so race probably is not a true risk factor for SIDS. Of all the well-established SIDS risk factors, sleeping prone clearly is the one that can be avoided most simply. This is well supported by the success of campaigns to reduce prone sleeping in many countries. On the other hand, there are several well-documented reports in which the prevalence of risk factors such as low birth weight and having a teenage mother declined, but

*References 6, 30, 41, 43, 51, 52, 57.
†References 12, 40, 42, 50, 52, 67.
‡References 6, 30, 41, 43, 51, 57.
§References 4, 6, 14, 35, 40, 51.

the SIDS incidence did not change. Despite anecdotal reports to the contrary, SIDS is not associated with diphtheria-pertussis-tetanus (DPT) immunizations. Minor clinical symptoms may be more common in SIDS victims in the 2 weeks before death compared with appropriate controls, but this observation has no clinical role in identifying infants at high risk for SIDS because of the high prevalence of minor clinical symptoms and the low occurrence of SIDS.

A few activities have been shown to have a potential protective effect against SIDS. For example, breast-feeding often is cited as being protective against SIDS.[16,23] Unfortunately, the studies demonstrating this effect have been retrospective and their results have not been confirmed in prospective cohort studies.[18,22,33,45,54] Most recently, the use of pacifiers has been reported to be related to lower incidence of SIDS compared to non-use.[3,35,40,44] There has been some speculation as to the possible mechanisms but there are no data linking any of these potential mechanisms to SIDS.

PHYSIOLOGY

Despite major efforts to define physiological characteristics that could prospectively identify infants at high risk for SIDS and delineate the mechanism of SIDS death, no clinically useful physiological characteristics have been identified to date. The only data that can illuminate the physiology of the SIDS infant are those collected on SIDS infants before death. Because SIDS is relatively rare, the study of large numbers of normal infants is necessary, and such studies rarely have been carried out. Those who subsequently die of SIDS have in some cases demonstrated more tachycardia, variability in heart rate, and fewer respiratory pauses than those who do not die of SIDS, but these differences are not sufficiently specific or sensitive to be of any clinical usefulness. There is no evidence that increased respiratory pauses or increased periodic breathing is predictive of SIDS in the general population. In addition, there is no evidence that any abnormalities of cardiac rhythm predict the infant at high risk for SIDS. Reports of recordings obtained from home monitors while infants were dying of SIDS have demonstrated variability in heart rate and, in some cases, bradycardia before the final cardiac arrest, but it is not clear in some cases whether periods of hypoxia or any respiratory difficulty preceded the bradycardia.

PROSPECTIVE IDENTIFICATION OF INFANTS AT HIGH RISK FOR SIDS

Efforts to identify infants at high risk for SIDS prospectively generally have focused on three different approaches. First is the unwarranted evaluation of 12- to 24-hour recordings of cardiorespiratory activity (pneumogram), based on the assumption that increased amounts of respiratory irregularity (pauses, periodicity) identify infants at high risk for SIDS. A second approach, although not appropriate for clinical use, is at least based on a more defensible rationale—the development of scoring systems based on various clinical or demographic characteristics of the infant or the infant's mother.[7] The scoring systems were derived from epidemiological data, but because of high false-positive and false-negative rates when they were tested prospectively, the scoring systems are not useful clinically. If "high risk" is defined by a score that would identify 20% of the general population as being at high risk, only 50% of the population of SIDS cases would be in the high-risk group. Because there is no proven successful intervention, use of the scoring systems is not clinically indicated at this time.

Finally, the incidence of SIDS among certain clinically identifiable groups has been noted to be greater than among the general population; this has been the most clinically useful and most widely used method for identifying infants at high risk for SIDS. The two clinical groups for which an increased risk has been established most clearly are infants who have experienced apparent life-threatening events (ALTE) and prematurely born infants. The subgroup of ALTE infants who are perceived to have required cardiopulmonary resuscitation for episodes occurring during sleep may have a subsequent mortality of 8% to 10%, and those who have more than one such severe spell (a very small subgroup) may have a risk as high as 28% of subsequently dying.[48] Those who develop a seizure disorder around the time of their ALTE episodes also have a very high risk of dying subsequently. Premature infants have an increased risk for SIDS, and this is not explained by the high incidence of apnea of prematurity in this group while still in the hospital.[52] It remains unclear whether the increased incidence of chronic lung disease contributes to the increased risk for SIDS in premature infants.[20] Although some of these clinical subgroups have a high risk of SIDS, as shown in Fig. 269-2, they do not account for most SIDS cases. Only about 5% of SIDS victims have been noted to have experienced apparent life-threatening events, and about 18% of babies who die of SIDS were born prematurely.

The notion that subsequent siblings of SIDS victims are at increased risk for SIDS has always been difficult to prove, and the true risk remains unknown. Although some studies have shown a threefold to fivefold increase in the risk for SIDS in subsequent siblings,[21,52] others have not shown a relationship.[24] Most recently, this idea has been challenged by reports of covert videos of mothers trying to harm their infants and that in some cases where multiple infants in a

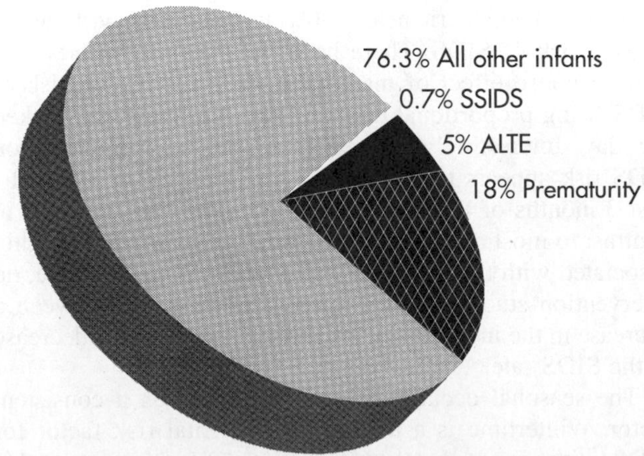

Fig. 269-2 Sources of SIDS cases as a percentage of all SIDS cases. *SSIDS,* Sibling of a SIDS victim; *ALTE,* prior acute life-threatening event.

family died of "SIDS," infanticide was ultimately found to be the cause of death.[13,65,66] Published estimates of the incidence of infanticide among deaths attributed to SIDS has ranged from less than 1% to 10%.[1,2,34,55,65] This is an important example of why a thorough investigation of the death scene and the case is critical in every case of suspected SIDS. A high index of suspicion should accompany the investigation of any case in which two infants in the same family have died of SIDS. It should be emphasized, however, that infanticide is rare, and it is of utmost importance that any search for evidence of maltreatment of the infant is carried out with extraordinary sensitivity to the feelings of the bereaved family.

It is likely that infants of mothers who use cocaine are at an increased risk for dying of SIDS, but it is difficult to prove that the cocaine is the important risk factor because of the clustering of other adverse characteristics in this same population.

ETIOLOGY OF SIDS

Neither the cause of SIDS nor the mechanism of death have been clearly established, and SIDS most likely results from a variety of causes. Studies that provide clues to hypotheses that are consistent with epidemiological data are more likely to contribute to our knowledge about the causes of SIDS and the mechanisms of death. One important hypothesis that may explain a subset of SIDS cases is that SIDS is related to abnormalities, maldevelopment, or delayed maturation of regions of the brain responsible for cardiorespiratory control and/or arousal. Anatomical and histochemical examinations of the brain stems of infants dying of SIDS have revealed hypoplasia and/or decreased neurotransmitter binding of regions on or near the surface of the ventral brain stem thought to be involved in the control of breathing, heart rate, and blood pressure. Homologous areas in animal models have been found to play major roles in chemosensitivity and control of sympathetic tone.[31,49] The hypothesis is that abnormalities or delayed development in these regions of the brain stem, called the "arcuate nucleus," result in an impaired ability to mount an adequate protective physiological response to normal stresses such as hypercapnia, hypoxia, or upper airway reflex apnea. These protective responses include arousal, an increase in the rate and depth of breathing, and termination of apnea. This hypothesis is closely associated with another theory that SIDS may be related to rebreathing of expired air, resulting in progressive hypercapnia and hypoxia. This might occur in an infant sleeping prone on soft bedding where a pocket develops around the infant's face, possibly in association with some rebreathing into the soft bedding, or possibly in combination with some component of upper airway obstruction.*

Some evidence exists that all infants are particularly at increased risk of sudden and unexplained death between 2 and 4 months of age, possibly because of interrelations of developing control systems for arousal and cardiac and respiratory rhythms. Hyperthermia has also been hypothesized, perhaps in combination with asphyxia, to be responsible. Importantly, both prone positioning and soft bedding could increase the probability of rebreathing and/or hyperthermia. There is little support for a primary cardiac arrhythmia, although neurally mediated bradycardia as a contributing factor is a possibility. A recent report identified a prolonged QT interval in SIDS victims in Italy.[59] However, serious concerns about this report have been raised by many SIDS investigators.[38] Currently, there are little data to support electrocardiographic screening to identify potential SIDS victims. Rarely, cases of SIDS may be due to botulism or rare metabolic disorders.

SIDS PREVENTION

Over the past two decades, three different approaches to preventing SIDS have been promoted. Electronic home cardiorespiratory monitors, usually using thoracic impedance technology, have been used as a preventive intervention with infants from clinically identifiable groups at high risk for SIDS, such as those who have experienced ALTE. There is no convincing evidence that home monitoring programs have lowered the incidence of SIDS. There is also no evidence that infants with an increased risk for SIDS can be identified by in-hospital cardiorespiratory monitoring.[39] It is clear that some monitored infants have succumbed despite prompt initiation of effective resuscitation, both at home and in the hospital. In a large proportion of the reported cases when infants have died despite the prescription of home monitors, the monitor was not being used properly or the resuscitative efforts were not initiated properly. There is no new information that would lead to a major modification of the 1985 American Academy of Pediatrics statement on infantile apnea[2] or the 1986 National Institutes of Health Consensus Development Conference report.[47]

A second SIDS prevention approach, most widely used in England, has involved increased numbers of home visits by health visitors (community health nurses) to assess the infant and to advise the caregiver about appropriate care practices and available support services and other resources. This intervention has not been evaluated adequately in terms of its ability to lower the incidence of SIDS.

In Australia, New Zealand, England, and some Scandinavian countries, national public education campaigns to prevent SIDS were implemented. These efforts to educate the general public and health professionals by using a variety of media and teaching tools have focused on some combination of encouraging breast-feeding and discouraging maternal smoking and prone positioning for infants, avoidance of overwrapping or otherwise overheating infants, and discouraging soft bedding for infants. These campaigns have been associated with dramatic decreases in the prevalence of prone sleeping among infants, a slight reduction in the prevalence of other targeted risk factors, and a dramatic drop of approximately 50% in the incidence of SIDS. Some countries have almost completely eliminated prone sleeping.[11,40,56] The success of the campaign to reduce the incidence of prone sleeping in the United States has confirmed the wisdom of this approach. Since the American Academy of Pediatrics recommended that infants be placed to sleep on their backs and institution of the National "Back to Sleep" program, the frequency of prone sleeping has decreased from 70% to approx-

*References 9-11, 15, 17, 27-30, 37, 52, 62, 64.

imately 20%, and the SIDS rate has fallen 50%, similar to the experience in other countries. In the United States, strategies to reduce the incidence of prone sleeping have included providing information to hospital nurseries and physicians, focusing on childcare education programs, and initiating public media campaigns.[26] Despite the dramatic reduction in the SIDS rate in the United States, infants in the age range at highest risk for SIDS still sleep prone about 20% of the time.[69] Also, it has been recently reported that some caregivers revert back to putting infants asleep prone.[5,36] There is also some evidence that infants who normally sleep supine may be at a higher risk for SIDS when allowed to sleep prone.[35,36,63]

For the future, it seems reasonable to continue strategies that have been successful and to work on changing those elements that have been the most clearly shown to be risk factors. Besides prone positioning, maternal smoking is a risk factor that is potentially changeable, notwithstanding the difficulties in changing smoking habits. The American Academy of Pediatrics has made the following recommendations: Infants should clearly be placed on their backs for sleep. Side positioning has been recommended in the past as an alternative to supine positioning, but many side-sleeping infants roll to the prone position. A safe sleeping environment should be provided, including a crib that conforms to current safety standards. A plain mattress with a tight-fitting sheet and sleep clothing without blankets or other coverings is best. Infants should not be put to sleep on waterbeds, sofas, soft mattresses, or other soft surfaces. Soft materials such as pillows, comforters, stuffed toys, loose bedding, and other potentially gas-trapping objects should not be in the sleeping environment. Bed-sharing is dangerous and should be discouraged. Alternatives might include putting the infant's crib near the parent's bed to provide convenience for breast-feeding and parent contact. Overheating should be avoided. Although devices have been developed to help maintain sleep position, there are no data as to their efficacy or safety. Electronic cardiorespiratory monitors may be of value for infants who have experienced abortive SIDS episodes. The 1986 NIH Consensus Development Conference Report is the most current guideline for home monitor use at the time of this writing. There is no evidence that home monitoring prevents SIDS or that monitoring in the hospital before discharge is of any value.[26]

MANAGEMENT AND SUPPORT

The loss of an infant to SIDS is devastating to the family and health care providers. The important role for the physician is to remain informed about SIDS; to ensure that an autopsy is performed in all cases of sudden, unexpected infant death; to see that the family is given accurate, appropriate information about SIDS and the results of the autopsy on their child as soon as possible; and that opportunities for ongoing support and counseling are readily available and are offered to the family. The family should be provided support for age-appropriate discussions with surviving siblings. The common bereavement reactions of shock, denial, anger, and sadness should be discussed with the family, and it should be directed to local counseling and support groups. Current information about SIDS and local counseling and support groups can be obtained through the National SIDS Alliance (1-800-221-SIDS).

REFERENCES

1. American Academy of Pediatrics Committee on Child Abuse and Neglect: Distinguishing sudden infant death syndrome from child abuse fatalities, *Pediatrics* 94:124, 1994.
2. American Academy of Pediatrics. Task Force on Prolonged Infantile Apnea: Prolonged infantile apnea: 1985, *Pediatrics* 76:127, 1985.
3. Arnestad M, Andersen M, Rognum TO: Is the use of a dummy or carry-cot of importance for sudden infant death? *Eur J Pediatr* 156:968, 1997.
4. Beal SM, Byard RW: Accidental death or sudden infant death syndrome? *J Paediatr Child Health* 31:269, 1994.
5. Brenner RA, et al: Prevalence and predictors of the prone sleep position among inner-city infants, *JAMA* 280:341, 1998.
6. Brooke H, et al: Case-control study of sudden infant death syndrome in Scotland 1992-95, *BMJ* 314:1516, 1997.
7. Brooks JG: Evaluation of the Oxford and Sheffield SIDS risk prediction scores, *Pediatr Pulmonol* 14:171, 1992.
8. Bulterys MG: Chronic fetal hypoxia and sudden infant death syndrome: interaction between maternal smoking and low hematocrit during pregnancy, *Pediatrics* 86:535, 1990.
9. Campbell AJ, Taylor BJ, Bolton DPG: Comparison of two methods of determining asphyxial potential of infant bedding, *J Pediatr* 130:245, 1997.
10. Chiodini BA, Thach BT: Impaired ventilation in infants sleeping face-down: potential significance for sudden infant death syndrome, *J Pediatr* 123:686, 1993.
11. Dwyer T, et al: The contribution of changers in prevalence of prone sleeping position to the decline in sudden infant death syndrome in Tasmania, *JAMA* 273:783, 1995.
12. Dwyer T, et al: Prospective cohort study of prone sleeping position and sudden infant death syndrome, *Lancet* 337:1244, 1991.
13. Firstman R, Talan J: *The death of innocents: a true story of murder, medicine, and high stakes science,* New York, 1997, Bantam.
14. Fleming PJ, et al: Environment of infants during sleep and risk of the sudden infant death syndrome: results of 1993-95 case-control study for confidential inquiry into stillbirths and deaths in infancy, *BMJ* 313:191, 1996.
15. Fleming PJ, et al: Interaction between bedding and sleeping position in the sudden infant death syndrome: a population-based case-control study, *BMJ* 301:85, 1990.
16. Ford RP, Taylor BJ, Mitchell EA: Breastfeeding and the risk of sudden infant death syndrome, *Int J Epidemiol* 22:366, 1993.
17. Galland, BC: The micro-environment of the sleeping newborn piglet covered by bed clothes: gas exchange and temperature, *J Paediatr Child Health* 30:144, 1994.
18. Gilbert R, et al: Bottle feeding and the sudden infant death syndrome, *BMJ* 311:123, 1995 (reply).
19. Gilbert R, et al: Combined effect of infection and heavy wrapping on the risk of sudden unexpected infant death, *Arch Dis Child* 67:171, 1992.
20. Gray PH, Rogers Y: Are infants with bronchopulmonary dysplasia at risk for sudden infant death syndrome? *Pediatrics* 93:774, 1994.
21. Guntheroth WG: Risk of sudden infant death syndrome in subsequent siblings, *J Pediatr* 116:520, 1990.
22. Henderson-Smart D, Ponsonby A-L, Murphy E: Reducing the risk of sudden infant death syndrome: a review of the scientific literature, *J Paediatr Child Health* 34:213, 1998.
23. Hoffman HJ, et al: Risk factors for SIDS: results of the National Institute of Child Health and Human Development SIDS Cooperative Epidemiological Study, *Ann N Y Acad Sci* 533:13, 1988.
24. Irgens LM, Skjaerven R, Peterson, DR: Prospective assessment of recurrence risk in sudden infant death syndrome siblings, *J Pediatr* 104:349, 1993.
25. Kattwinkel J, Brooks JG, Myerberg D: Positioning and SIDS: AAP Task Force on Infant Positioning and SIDS, *Pediatrics* 89:1120, 1992.

26. Kattwinkel J, et al: Changing concepts of sudden infant death syndrome: implications for infant sleeping environment and sleep position: AAP Task Force on Infant Sleep Position and SIDS, *Pediatrics* 105:650, 2000.
27. Kemp JS, Thach BT: A sleep position-dependent mechanism for infant death on sheepskins, *Am J Dis Child* 147:642, 1993.
28. Kemp JS, Thach BT: Quantifying the potential of infant bedding to limit CO_2 dispersal and factors affecting rebreathing in bedding, *J Appl Physiol* 78:740, 1995.
29. Kemp JS, Thach BT: Sudden death in infants sleeping on polystyrene-filled cushions, *N Engl J Med* 324:1858, 1991.
30. Kemp JS, et al: Unintentional suffocation by rebreathing: a death scene and physiologic investigation of a possible cause of sudden infant death, *J Pediatr* 122: 874, 1993.
31. Kinney HC, et al: Decreased muscarinic receptor binding in the arcuate nucleus in sudden infant death syndrome, *Science* 269:1446, 1995.
32. Klonoff-Cohen H, Edelstein SL: Bed sharing and the sudden infant death syndrome, *BMJ* 311:1269, 1995.
33. Kraus JF, Greenland S, Bulterys M: Risk factors for sudden infant death syndrome in US collaborative perinatal project, *Int J Epidemiol* 18:113, 1989.
34. Kukull WA, Peterson DR: Sudden infant death and infanticide, *Am J Epidemiol* 106:485, 1977.
35. l'Hoir M, Engleberts AC, vanWell GTJ: Risk and preventive factors for cot death in the Netherlands, a low incidence country, *Eur J Pediatr* 157:681, 1998.
36. Lesko SM, et al: Changes in sleep position during infancy: a prospective longitudinal assessment, *JAMA* 280:336, 1998.
37. Lijowska AS, et al: Sequential arousal and airway-defensive behavior of infants in asphyxial sleep environments, *J Appl Physiol* 83:219, 1997.
38. Lucey JF: Comments on a sudden infant death article in another journal, *Pediatrics* 103:812, 1999.
39. Malloy MH, Hoffman HJ: Home apnea monitoring and sudden infant death syndrome, *Prev Med* 25:645, 1996.
40. Markestad TB, et al: Sleeping position and sudden infant death syndrome (SIDS): effect of an intervention programme to avoid prone sleeping, *Acta Paediatr* 84:375, 1995.
41. Mitchell EA, Scragg L, Clements M: Soft cot mattresses and the sudden infant death syndrome, *N Z Med J* 109:206, 1996.
42. Mitchell EA, Scragg R, Stewart AW: Results from the first year of the New Zealand cot death study, *N Z Med J* 104:71, 1991.
43. Mitchell EA, Thompson JM, Ford RP: Sheepskin bedding and the sudden infant death syndrome, *J Pediatr* 133:701, 1998.
44. Mitchell EA, et al: Dummies and the sudden infant death syndrome, *Arch Dis Child* 68:501, 1993.
45. Mitchell EA, et al: Risk factors for sudden infant death syndrome following the prevention campaign in New Zealand: a prospective study, *Pediatrics* 100:835, 1997.
46. Mitchell EA, et al: Smoking and the sudden infant death syndrome, *Pediatrics* 91:893, 1993.
47. National Institutes of Health Consensus Development Conference Statement: Infantile apnea and home monitoring, *Pediatrics* 79:292, 1987.
48. Oren J, Kelly D, Shannon DC: Identification of a high-risk group for sudden infant death syndrome among infants who were resuscitated for sleep apnea, *Pediatrics* 77:495, 1986.
49. Panigrahy A, et al: Decreased kainate binding in the arcuate nucleus of the sudden infant death syndrome, *J Neuropathol Exp Neurol* 56:1253, 1999.
50. Platt MJ, Pharoah POD: Child health statistical review—1996, *Arch Dis Child* 75:527, 1996.
51. Ponsonby AL, et al: Association between use of a quilt and sudden infant death syndrome: case-control study, *BMJ* 316:195, 1998.
52. Ponsonby A, et al: Factors potentiating the risk of sudden infant death syndrome associated with the prone position, *N Engl J Med* 329:377, 1993.
53. Ponsonby AL, et al: Thermal environment and sudden infant death syndrome: case-control study, *BMJ* 304:277, 1992.
54. Ponsonby AL, et al: The Tasmanian SIDS case-control study: univariable and multivariable risk factor analysis, *Paediatr Perinatol Epidemiol* 9:256, 1995.
55. Reece RM: Fatal child abuse and sudden infant death syndrome: a critical diagnostic decision, *Pediatrics* 91:423, 1993.
56. Report of the Chief Medical Officer's Expert Group on the Sleeping Position Cot Death—1993, London, Her Majesty's Stationery Office (HMSO).
57. Scheers NJ, Dayton CM, Kemp JS: Sudden infant death with external airways covered: case-comparison study of 206 deaths in the United States, *Arch Pediatr Adolesc Med* 152:540, 1998.
58. Schoendorf KC, Kiely JL: Relationship of sudden infant death syndrome to maternal smoking during and after pregnancy, *Pediatrics* 90: 905, 1992.
59. Schwartz PJ, Stramba-Badiale M, Segantini A: Prolongation of the QT interval and the sudden infant death syndrome, *N Engl J Med* 338:1709, 1998.
60. Scragg RK, Mitchell EA: Side sleeping position and bed sharing in the sudden infant death syndrome, *Ann Med* 30:345, 1998.
61. Scragg R, Mitchell EA, Taylor BJ: Bed sharing, smoking, and alcohol in the sudden infant death syndrome, *BMJ* 307:1312, 1993.
62. Skadberg BT, Markestad T: Consequences of getting the head covered during sleep in infancy, *Pediatrics* 100:E6, 1997.
63. Skadberg BT, Morild I, Markestad T: Abandoning prone sleeping: effect on the risk of sudden infant death syndrome, *J Pediatr* 132:340, 1998 (comments).
64. Skadberg BT, et al: CO_2 rebreathing: a possible contributory factor to some cases of sudden infant death? *Acta Paediatr* 84:988, 1995.
65. Southall DP, et al: Covert video recordings of life-threatening child abuse: lessons for child protection, *Pediatrics* 100:735, 1997.
66. Steinschneider A: Prolonged apnea and the sudden infant death syndrome: clinical and laboratory observations, *Pediatrics* 50:646, 1972.
67. Taylor JA, Drieger JW, Reay DT: Prone sleep position and the sudden infant death syndrome in King County, Washington: a case-control study, *J Pediatr* 128:626, 1996.
68. Williams SM, Taylor BJ, Mitchell EA: Sudden infant death syndrome: insulation from bedding and clothing and its effect modifiers, *Int J Epidemiol* 25:366, 1996.
69. Willinger M, et al: Factors associated with the transition to nonprone sleep positions of infants in the United States: the National Infant Sleep Position Study, *JAMA* 280:329, 1998 (comments).

SUGGESTED READINGS

Guntheroth WG: *Crib death: the sudden infant death syndrome,* ed 2, Mt Kisco, New York, 1990, Futura Publishing.

Harper RM, et al: *Sudden infant death syndrome: risk factors and basic mechanisms,* New York, 1988, PMA Publishing.

Henderson-Smart D, Ponsonby AL, Murphy E: Reducing the risk of sudden infant death syndrome: a review of the scientific literature, *J Paediatr Child Health* 34:213, 1998.

Hunt CE, editor: Apnea and SIDS, *Clin Perinatol* 19:701, 1992.

Kiely M: *Reproductive and perinatal epidemiology,* Boston, 1990, CRC Press.

Valdes-Dapena M, et al: *Histopathology of the sudden infant death syndrome,* Washington, DC, 1993, Armed Forces Institute of Pathology.

270 Tonsillectomy and Adenoidectomy

Robert A. Hoekelman

During the twentieth century the most frequently performed operation on children in the United States that required general anesthesia was the removal of the tonsils, the adenoids, or both.

The decline in the frequency of these operations beginning in the early 1970s was the result of the gradual resolution of the controversy that had raged within the medical community for several decades regarding the indications for performing the procedures.[3] This was so because the function of tonsils and adenoids, which constitute the major elements of the Waldeyer ring within the nasopharynx, is not well understood, and evaluative studies of the worth of tonsillectomy and adenoidectomy (T&A) were inconclusive until the 1980s. Consequently, each practitioner had to rely on "clinical judgment and individual experience" in recommending that a given child be subjected to one of these surgical procedures. Naturally, these approaches varied considerably and formed the basis for much of the controversy.[6]

INDICATIONS AND RISKS

The indications for T&A that have been advanced by practitioners (and parents) include both those that are generally accepted and those that are more suspect or even capricious (Box 270-1). There can be little argument about the absolute indications listed at the top of the box; however, all those listed below (in relative order of validity) have been controversial.

Of particular note is the development of a method to measure the severity of obstructive sleep apnea (OSA)[5] quantitatively and to relate that score to abnormalities in right ventricular function, even before clinical signs of cor pulmonale are present.[13] OSA scores higher than 3.5 are highly predictive of the need for T&A (see Box 270-1).

Ultimately, the worth of T&A must be measured by weighing the benefits it may provide to the patient against the risks involved. In general, the morbidity and mortality from T&A are poorly documented. The mortality has been estimated in the past to be as high as 1 in every 1000 operations[4] and as low as 1 in 27,000 operations.[3] However, in the current climate of modern anesthetic techniques, high technology, and professional competence in monitoring and managing postoperative complications of hemorrhage, shock, and airway obstruction, mortality and severe morbidity following T&A surgery are extremely rare.

The true morbidity rate from T&A, however, is unknown, because no nationwide reporting mechanism is available. Predictors of complications following T&A include cerebral palsy, seizures, age younger than three years, obstructive sleep apnea, bleeding disorders, congenital heart disease, and prematurity. Patients who have one or more of these risk factors should be considered for inpatient, postoperative management.[2,14] Preoperative screening with chest radiographs and electrocardiograms is of little predictive value for postoperative cardiorespiratory complications. Preoperative screening for bleeding disorders, using prothrombin and partial thromboplastin times need be done only when there is a family history of a bleeding disorder[2,7]; nevertheless, most surgeons require that these two tests be performed preoperatively.

Otitis media has been reported to be a frequent sequel of adenoidectomy, but the incidence of otitis media in children who have similar indications for adenoidectomy but who did not have surgery has not been assessed over the same interval. The incidence and severity of psychological complications are unknown, but asocial and aggressive behavior, excessive dependency, night terrors, and enuresis have been attributed to emotional trauma surrounding hospitalization, separation from parents, anesthesia, and the discomfort associated with T&A.

The benefits that can be attributed to tonsillectomy, adenoidectomy, or both, although attested to by many parents and physicians, were not demonstrated in an adequate, prospective, randomized, controlled study until the late 1970s and early 1980s, in a study conducted at the Children's Hospital of Pittsburgh.[8] In this study, 95 children severely affected with recurrent throat infections were subjected to tonsillectomy or tonsillectomy with adenoidectomy, whereas 92 children who had similar histories and "matched" with the "tonsillectomized" children (through both randomized and nonrandomized techniques) were not subjected to surgery. During the subsequent 2 years, the surgical group had a significantly lower incidence of throat infection than did the nonsurgical group. On the other hand, many of the children in the nonsurgical group had fewer throat infections during the two-year follow-up period than previously, and most of these episodes were mild. During the third year of follow-up, the surgical group had fewer throat infections, but these differences overall were not statistically significant. The criterion for tonsillectomy in the Pittsburgh study was recurrent throat infection (tonsillitis, pharyngitis, or tonsillopharyngitis) characterized by the following:

1. At least three episodes in each of 3 years, or five episodes in each of 2 years, or seven episodes in 1 year

BOX 270-1

INDICATIONS THAT HAVE BEEN ADVANCED FOR TONSILLECTOMY, ADENOIDECTOMY, OR BOTH

Absolute Indications

Alveolar hypoventilation (obstructive sleep apnea) or cor pulmonale, secondary to airway obstruction
Dysphagia
Malignancy
Uncontrollable hemorrhage from tonsillar blood vessels
Nasal obstruction causing discomfort in breathing and severe distortion of speech

Controversial Indications

Recurrent peritonsillar abscess
Chronic or recurrent tonsillitis
Chronic or recurrent otitis media
Chronic cervical lymphadenitis
Hyponasality, "hot potato" voice, or both
Sensorineural or conductive hearing loss
Chronic mastoiditis
Cholesteatoma
Chronic sinusitis or nasopharyngitis
Diphtheria or streptococcal carrier state
Chronic bronchitis or pneumonia
Mouth breathing, snoring, or both (without obstructive sleep apnea)
Rheumatic fever, when compliance with anti-streptococcal prophylaxis cannot be assured
Parental anxiety
Frequent colds with loss of time from school
Adenoidal facies
Allergic respiratory diseases
Chronic cough
Failure to thrive
Poor appetite
Focus of infection
Scarred or cryptic tonsils
Halitosis

2. Each episode having been characterized by one or more of the following:
   a. Oral temperature 100.9° F (38.3° C) or higher
   b. Enlarged (more than 2 cm) or tender anterior cervical lymph nodes
   c. Tonsillar or pharyngeal exudate
   d. Positive culture for group A beta-hemolytic streptococci
3. Apparently adequate antibiotic therapy having been administered for proven or suspected streptococcal episodes
4. Each episode having been confirmed by examination and its qualifying features described in a clinical record at the time of occurrence

Those who received concurrent adenoidectomy met one of the following criteria:

1. Recurrent suppurative or serious otitis media, if myringotomy and insertion of tympanostomy tubes had been performed at least once previously
2. Persistent nasal obstruction
   a. Manifested by stertorous breathing or mouth breathing with or without episodes of obstructive sleep apnea, and by hyponasal speech
   b. Accompanied by both clinical and roentgenographic evidence of adenoid hypertrophy
   c. Apparently not caused by allergy
3. Chronic sinusitis or nasopharyngitis
   a. Accompanied by both clinical and roentgenographic evidence of adenoid hypertrophy
   b. Apparently not caused by allergy
   c. Persisting despite appropriate antimicrobial and other medical therapy

Although the Pittsburgh study provided evidence of the efficacy of tonsillectomy (with or without adenoidectomy) in reducing the number of throat infections by using these criteria, T&A performed for less stringent criteria (those used at that time for most T&A surgery in the United States) did not prove to reduce the frequency of pharyngitis in a similar Pittsburgh-based study.[11] A nationwide collaborative study on a larger sample representative of all socioeconomic and geographical childhood populations would be needed to determine a set of absolute criteria for performing T&As to reduce the frequency of throat infections that would be acceptable to all, but the difficulties in mounting and conducting such a study reliably have been too formidable to date and probably will never be overcome.

Thus, it is likely that the controversy over indications for T&A will continue. Data from the National Center for Health Statistics National Hospital Discharge Surveys (NHDS) indicate that some overall restraint and discrimination have been exercised in the removal of tonsils and adenoids in recent years. In 1971, 1.019 million tonsillectomies, adenoidectomies, or T&As were performed on inpatients of all ages discharged from hospitals in the United States. This number fell to 584,000 in 1979, to 259,000 in 1987, and to 76,000 in 1992. However, these figures are misleading because in the mid-1980s, changes in reimbursement for these procedures resulted in more being done on ambulatory surgical patients (not included in NHDS) than on hospitalized patients. One study reported that between 1985 and 1988, 60% of these operations occurred in ambulatory surgical centers (ASCs).[12] Since then, almost all adenoidectomies and T&As have been performed in ASCs. In 1994, 140,000 adenoidectomies and 286,000 T&As were performed on children younger than 15 years of age.[7]

The probability of a child receiving T&A surgery may be determined more by parental and physician opinion regarding the worth of T&A than on the basis of the child's health status. Because at least 25% of all visits to pediatricians' offices are for upper respiratory tract infections, including tonsillitis and otitis media, it is not surprising that parental and physician attention frequently is focused on decisions concerning the removal of tonsils and adenoids. The decision to recommend removal of the tonsils or adenoids should be an individual matter, taking into consideration not only the frequency with which they become infected but also possible relationships to (1) mechanisms of speech, hearing, and swallowing; (2) airway obstruction; and (3) cardiorespiratory function. Many of these relationships, it must be emphasized, are at best hypothetical. Because the worth of T&A, using less stringent criteria than those used in the first Pittsburgh study,[9] has not been demonstrated,[11] conservatism in recommending such surgery in this latter group is indicated. Under certain circumstances, reasonable alternatives such as antibiotic prophylaxis or placement of tympanostomy tubes should be considered.

Although it is not the purpose here to recommend specific indications for T&A, it seems that tonsillectomy and/or adenoidectomy should not be performed on any child whose criteria for surgery do not approximate those used in the Pittsburgh studies. In addition, certain indications are considered "absolute," whereas others are considered "reasonable" but in need of verification.

The absolute indications are so considered because (as in cor pulmonale) surgical intervention is of established value for a serious or life-threatening condition or because surgery, although of uncertain benefit, may help prevent worsening of the impairment. Absolute indicators are as follows:

1. Alveolar hypoventilation (obstructive sleep apnea) with or without cor pulmonale and secondary to severe chronic upper airway obstruction (Box 270-2). Depending on the respective size and anatomical relationships of the tonsils and adenoids, this condition may call for either tonsillectomy or adenoidectomy or both.
2. Tonsillar enlargement sufficient to cause significant difficulty swallowing (tonsillectomy only)
3. Uncontrollable tonsillar bleeding (tonsillectomy only)
4. Tonsillar malignancy (tonsillectomy only)
5. Nasal obstruction caused by hypertrophied adenoids and resulting in manifest discomfort in breathing and severe distortion of speech (adenoidectomy only)

Any one of the following is sufficient as a reasonable indication:

1. Recurrent peritonsillar abscess
2. Chronic or recurrent tonsillitis, using the Pittsburgh criteria[9]
3. Chronic or recurrent otitis media, using the Pittsburgh criteria[10]
4. Muffled, "hot potato" voice if the child is at least 6 years old
5. Chronic (minimum 6 months) enlargement (more than 2 cm) or tenderness of anterior cervical lymph nodes, persisting despite appropriate antibiotic therapy

BOX 270-2

OBSTRUCTIVE SLEEP APNEA SCORE

OSA Score = 1.42D + 1.41A + 0.71S − 3.83
D = Difficulty of breathing during sleep (O = never, 1 = occasionally, 2 = frequently, and 3 = always)
A = Apnea observed during sleep (0 = No and 1 = yes)
S = Snoring (0 = never, 1 = occasionally, 2 = frequently, and 3 = always)
Scores of >3.5 are highly predictive of the need for T&A
Scores of <−1 rule out OSA
Scores of −1 to 3.4 require polysomography to determine whether OSA requiring T&A exists

CONTRAINDICATIONS

Removal of the adenoids is contraindicated in children who have hypernasality resulting from velopharyngeal insufficiency. The most common cause of this is complete or incomplete cleft palate. Removal of the adenoids in this circumstance may result in a marked increase in hypernasality. Children who have a cleft palate, repaired or unrepaired, should not be subjected to adenoidectomy without specialists being consulted in the management of cleft palate. All children scheduled for adenoidectomy should be examined carefully to rule out a submucous cleft, which involves the palatal muscles but not the overlying mucous membrane. The presence of a bifid uvula, a shortened and widened median raphe of the soft palate, and a palpable V-shaped midline notch (rather than a smooth, rounded curve) at the junction of the hard and soft palate is indicative of a submucous cleft (see Fig. 8-26). When hypernasality resulting from velopharyngeal insufficiency is suspected, irrespective of the physical findings, consultation with a speech pathologist for palatal function studies should be sought.

Local infection is considered a contraindication to T&A because of the patient's increased risk for anesthetic complications, systemic spread of infection, and hemorrhage during and after surgery. Ordinarily, surgery should be delayed for at least 3 weeks following an acute local infection except in cases in which prolonged antibiotic therapy has been ineffective and when the upper airway is severely obstructed.

Respiratory allergy is considered by some physicians to be a contraindication for T&A for fear that the surgery may precipitate bronchial asthma. Although such a relationship has not been proven clinically, these physicians advocate at least six months of antiallergic treatment for the patient's symptoms before T&A is performed.[1]

ROLE OF THE PRIMARY CARE PHYSICIAN

The pediatrician's responsibility does not end once a decision has been made in favor of T&A. The risks of ASC or hospital admission, anesthesia, and the surgery itself must be minimized. The pediatrician must assume responsibilities in this regard by choosing a surgeon, anesthesiologist, and hospital that will provide the best expertise and facilities available in the technical performance of the surgery and administration of the anesthesia, and by working closely with them in providing preoperative and postoperative care for the child and the parents.[1] The role of each physician and that of supporting professionals in preparing the child for surgery and caring for the patient during and afterward should be discussed and agreed on beforehand so that a coordinated team approach to care can be effected, misunderstanding among the involved professionals and between the professionals and the parents can be avoided, and the experience for the patient and parents can be as pleasant as possible.

Parents and the child should be well informed of the circumstances of the surgery beforehand through preadmission visits to the hospital and age-appropriate literature (see Chapter 24, The Ill Child). The parents' presence throughout is extremely important in minimizing the potential for psychological trauma. It is particularly important, in both inpatient and ambulatory settings, to have one or both parents present immediately before the child's anesthesia induction and when the child first awakens after surgery. Assessment of the patient for surgery, anesthesia, and risk for complications should be shared by the team of physicians. Under ordinary circumstances, this requires only a careful history and physical examination. Children who have underlying cardiac anomalies, and who therefore are at risk for bacterial endocarditis, should receive antibiotic prophylaxis.

Tonsillectomy and adenoidectomy carry the potential of grave risks for each child subjected to the procedures. The physician must consider the risks and weigh them against the potential benefits to be gained from the operation in reaching a decision to recommend that tonsillectomy and/or adenoidectomy be performed. If this evaluation is done carefully and conservatively, the benefits of surgery relative to its costs will be maximized.

REFERENCES

1. Avery AD, Harris LJ: Tonsillectomy, adenoidectomy, and tonsillectomy with adenoidectomy: assessing the quality of care using short-term outcome measures. In *Quality of medical care assessment using outcome measures: eight disease-specific applications,* Santa Monica, Calif, 1976, Rand.
2. Biavati MJ, Manning SC, Phillips DL: Predictive factors for respiratory complications after tonsillectomy and adenoidectomy in children, *Arch Otolaryngol Head Neck Surg* 123:517, 1997.
3. Bluestone DC, et al: Workshop on tonsillectomy and adenoidectomy, *Ann Otol Rhinol Laryngol* 84(suppl 19):1, 1975.
4. Bolger WE, Parsons DB, Potempa L: Preoperative hemostatic assessment of the adenotonsillectomy patient, *Otolaryngol Head Neck Surg* 103:396, 1990.
5. Browlette R, et al: A diagnostic approach to suspected OSA, *J Pediatr* 105:10, 1984.
6. Giebink GS, Thell TE: Tonsillectomy and adenoidectomy practice patterns in Minnesota: a retrospective, multi-hospital audit, *Minn Med* 63: 421, 1980.
7. Hall MJ, et al: National survey of ambulatory surgery, *Stat Bull Metrop Insur Co* 78:18, 1997.
8. Howells RC II, Wax MK, Ramadon HH: Values of preoperative prothrombin time/partial thromboplastic time as a predictor of postoperative hemorrhage in pediatric patients undergoing tonsillectomy, *Otolaryngol Head Neck Surg* 117:628, 1997.
9. Paradise JL, et al: Efficacy of tonsillectomy for recurrent throat infection in severely affected children: results of parallel randomized and nonrandomized clinical trials, *N Engl J Med* 310:674, 1984.
10. Paradise JL, et al: Efficacy of adenoidectomy for recurrent otitis media in children previously treated with tympanostomy tube placement: results of parallel randomized and nonrandomized clinical trials, *JAMA* 263:2066, 1990.
11. Paradise JL, et al: Comparative efficacy of tonsillectomy for recurrent throat infection in more vs. less severely affected children, *Pediatr Res* 31(part 2):126A, 1992.
12. Paradise JL, et al: Adenoidectomy and adenotonsillectomy (T&A) for recurrent otitis media in children not previously subjected to tympanostomy tube placement. Paper presented at the Sixth International Congress of Pediatric Otolaryngology, Rotterdam, The Netherlands, May 30, 1994.
13. Reiner SA, et al: Safety of outpatient tonsillectomy and adenoidectomy, *Otolaryngol Head Neck Surg* 102:161, 1990.
14. Tal A, et al: Ventricular dysfunction in children with obstructive sleep apnea (OSA), *Pediatr Pulmonol* 4:139, 1998.

SUGGESTED READINGS

Deutsch ES: Tonsillectomy and adenoidectomy: changing indications, *Pediatr Clin North Am* 43:1219, 1996.

Paradise JL: Tonsillectomy and adenoidectomy. In Bluestone CD, Stoll SE, Sheetz MD, editors: *Pediatric otolaryngology,* ed 2, Philadelphia, 1990, WB Saunders.

271 Tuberculosis

Cynthia Christy • Jeffrey R. Starke

Tuberculosis is one of the most important infectious diseases of humans. One third of the world's population is infected with *Mycobacterium tuberculosis*. The World Health Organization (WHO) estimates that 8 million cases of tuberculosis disease and 3 million deaths resulting from tuberculosis occur annually; 1.3 million cases and 450,000 deaths occur annually in children.[8,11] In the United States, an estimated 15 million people are infected with *M. tuberculosis*, 10% of whom will develop clinical tuberculosis if not properly treated. The tuberculin skin test is the only clinical test available to identify infected individuals. However, the accuracy of this test changes dramatically, depending on the population in which it is used. Although most children in developed countries are at low risk of contracting tuberculosis infection and should not routinely undergo the skin test, some groups in the United States have a high risk of acquiring tuberculosis infection and therefore should be tested.

Tuberculosis occurs in three basic stages: exposure, infection, and disease. Because each of these stages requires different therapy, it is imperative to classify each patient properly. Exposure occurs when a child comes in contact with an adult or adolescent who has been confirmed as having or is suspected of having infectious pulmonary tuberculosis. The infectious case (called a *source case*) typically is a member of the patient's household, although a contagious adult in a school or child care center can be a source of significant exposure. Children who have pulmonary tuberculosis almost never are infectious. The exposed individual has a negative Mantoux skin test reaction (under 5 mm), a normal chest roentgenogram, and no signs or symptoms of tuberculosis disease. If infectious droplet nuclei have been deposited in the lungs of the exposed individual, it may take up to 3 months for a delayed-type hypersensitivity reaction to tuberculin (positive tuberculin skin test result) to develop. Because of the short incubation period of tuberculosis in children age 5 or younger, some of these infected children (as many as 15% in one study[9]) develop severe tuberculosis disease in less than 3 months if left untreated. For this reason, children younger than 5 years old who have possible or confirmed exposure should receive chemotherapy for possible infection until 3 months after contact with the source case is broken by physical means, or by instituting antituberculosis chemotherapy for the source case. A second tuberculin skin test then should be done; if the result is negative, the chemotherapy can be discontinued. If the result is positive (5 mm or larger), tuberculosis infection is present and 6 to 9 months of chemotherapy should be given.

An individual has tuberculosis infection if he or she is harboring *M. tuberculosis* but does not have systemic or local manifestations of tuberculosis disease. The chest roentgenogram usually is normal, but it may show small calcifications and still not be considered indicative of tuberculous disease. In this stage, the Mantoux skin test usually yields a positive result. Approximately 5% to 10% of adults who have untreated tuberculosis infection develop tuberculosis disease during their lifetime, with half of these cases occurring in the 2 years after the initial infection. This risk is increased markedly to 7% to 10% per year among those coinfected with HIV. Among children, the likelihood of an untreated infection developing into tuberculosis depends on the age at the time of the primary infection, with rates as high as 40% for those younger than 2 years of age, 15% to 25% for children 2 to 5 years of age, and 5% to 15% among older children and adolescents. All children with *M. tuberculosis* infection should receive chemotherapy to prevent disease from developing.

If an infected individual develops clinical manifestations or has an abnormal chest roentgenogram, including hilar or mediastinal adenopathy, he or she has tuberculosis disease, commonly referred to as "tuberculosis" (TB). The Mantoux skin test result usually is positive. However, among adults and children who are not infected with the human immunodeficiency virus (HIV), 10% may have a negative result on the Mantoux test[15,16]; among HIV-infected individuals, as many as 50% may have a negative result. Tuberculosis in adults and some adolescents usually occurs when previously dormant *M. tuberculosis* reactivates years or even decades after the initial infection. In contrast, within 1 year of exposure, children and most adolescents develop tuberculosis disease as a complication of the initial infection rather than as a reactivation of a previous infection.

EPIDEMIOLOGY

M. tuberculosis is transmitted to children almost exclusively through inhalation of infected aerosol droplets into the alveoli of the lungs. Individuals most likely to be infectious are adults or adolescents who (1) have cavitary pulmonary tuberculosis, (2) cough frequently, and (3) have a positive result with acid-fast staining of sputum. Most children under age 12 who have pulmonary tuberculosis are unable to cough forcefully, rarely produce sputum, have a comparatively low burden of organisms, and therefore rarely are contagious. Because transmission of *M. tuberculosis* usually requires repeated or prolonged (not casual) contact, understanding tuberculosis infection and disease among children necessitates an understanding of contagious pulmonary tuberculosis among adults.

The incidence of tuberculosis in the United States increased by 20% (from 22,201 cases to 26,673 cases) from 1985 to 1992.[2] In the past, tuberculosis disease was diagnosed predominantly in older adults. From 1985 to 1992, however, the median age of those who had tuberculosis disease in the United States dropped, especially among young Hispanic and nonwhite adults and children. During the same period, the incidence of tuberculosis disease increased 27% (from 7592 cases to 9623 cases annually) among blacks and 75% (from 3092 cases to 5397 cases annually) among Hispanics. Although data are fairly complete for tuberculosis disease because it is reportable in all states, tuberculosis infection in children is reportable only in Indiana, Kentucky, Missouri, and Texas, making true epidemiological patterns of infection among adults and children difficult to determine.

Tuberculosis has received much attention in the United States over the past decade because of its increased incidence from 1985 to 1992, the increase in certain groups of patients, and the development of multidrug-resistant tuberculosis strains caused mainly by poor adherence to treatment. The good news is that the total number of TB cases reported in 1998 is 31% lower than that reported in 1992. The largest decrease occurred among children younger than 15 years of age and in adults 25 to 44 years of age. Five states—California, Florida, Illinois, New York, and Texas—reported the highest number of cases in 1998, representing 54% of all reported TB cases. From 1992 to 1998, the number of cases in U.S.-born persons decreased 44% and the number of cases in foreign-born persons increased 4%. The proportion of TB cases among foreign-born persons increased steadily from 27% in 1992 to 42% in 1998. The TB rate in foreign-born persons remained four to six times higher than for U.S.-born persons. Among foreign-born persons with TB, the most frequent countries of birth were Mexico, the Philippines, and Vietnam.[10]

Although the risk of acquiring tuberculosis infection depends mostly on environmental factors—that is, the chance that a child has significant contact with an adult who has contagious pulmonary tuberculosis—the risk of developing tuberculosis disease depends mostly on host-related factors (Box 271-1). One of the most important risk factors for infection is contact with an HIV-infected adult. These adults are at far greater risk than the general population of developing pulmonary tuberculosis, and they are significantly more likely to harbor a multidrug-resistant organism.[3] Contact with foreign-born adults, especially those who have immigrated recently, is another risk factor. In 1993, 29.6% of tuberculosis cases in the United States occurred among foreign-born individuals. Adults of Hispanic, Asian, or Pacific Island descent who have immigrated in the past 5 years have a particularly high risk of developing pulmonary tuberculosis and becoming source cases. Certain congregate facilities (e.g., prisons, homeless shelters, nursing homes, and other chronic-care facilities) are high-risk settings for *M. tuberculosis* infection and transmission. Finally, the incidence of tuberculosis disease is higher in metropolitan areas; 40% of U.S. children age 4 or younger who were diagnosed with tuberculosis disease in 1991 lived in cities that had populations greater then 250,000. In general, however, the vast majority of people in the United States and other industrialized countries are at low risk for tuberculosis infection.

BOX 271-1

CHILDREN AT HIGH RISK FOR TUBERCULOSIS IN THE UNITED STATES

- Children who were born or resided in countries that have a high prevalence of tuberculosis
- Children from families that have a recent history of tuberculosis
- Foster children
- Children who have present or past contact with adults who are or were:
  - Residents of high-prevalence countries
  - Residents of correctional institutions or long-term care facilities
  - Homeless
  - Users of intravenous or other drugs of abuse
  - Infected with the human immunodeficiency virus

Host-related factors help to determine which infected individuals develop tuberculosis. Most cases of childhood tuberculosis occur in children under age 5, and these young patients are more likely to develop severe or life-threatening forms of disease. School-age children (5 to 12 years of age) have been called the "favored age" because most of them who are infected do not develop primary tuberculosis disease (although they are more likely to develop reactivation tuberculosis disease as adults than are children who are infected at a younger age). Children who have chronic immunosuppressive medical problems (e.g., malignancy) or who receive medications such as corticosteroids or antineoplastic chemotherapy also are at increased risk of developing tuberculosis disease if infected with *M. tuberculosis*. Infection with HIV appears to be a strong risk factor for the development of tuberculosis disease in children infected with *M. tuberculosis*.[4]

THE TUBERCULIN SKIN TEST

The tuberculin purified protein derivative (PPD) skin test, derived from supernatant extracts of cultures of *M. tuberculosis*, has been in use since 1939. Although more than six decades have passed since the first batch was prepared in Philadelphia, PPD skin testing remains the only clinical test for diagnosing tuberculosis infection.

There are two ways to administer PPD or another antigen, called old Tuberculin: multiple-puncture devices (MPDs), which typically have metal or plastic prongs coated with dried or liquid antigen, and the Mantoux 5 tuberculin unit intradermal injection, which is considered the gold standard skin test. MPDs should no longer be used because of their inherent inaccuracies and limitations.[14]

A Mantoux skin test is best administered by anchoring the side of the hand that is holding the syringe against the side of the child's arm and injecting solution containing five tuberculin units of PPD (0.1 ml) intradermally in a transverse direc-

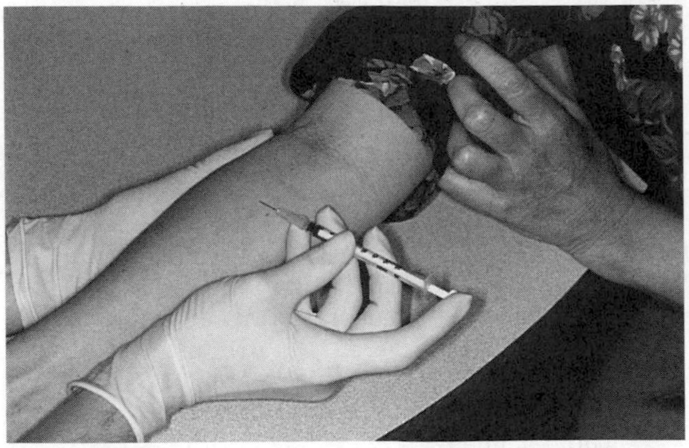

Fig. 271-1 Tuberculin skin test placement.

tion on the volar surface of the forearm (Fig. 271-1). The fluid should make a palpable wheal of 5 to 8 mm in diameter that is reabsorbed over the next hour. The reaction size is measured no sooner than 48 hours and preferably at 72 hours. If further induration occurs after 72 hours, regardless of its initial size, the reaction should be considered positive. Erythema, although common, is not considered a positive reaction; only the diameter of the induration, even mild, is palpated, measured, and recorded in millimeters (never as "positive" or "negative"). A positive reaction depends on the risk factors that are present; these are detailed in Box 271-1. The test should be interpreted only by a trained health professional; parents never should be allowed to interpret the test because many studies have shown that they cannot do so with adequate accuracy.

Neither tuberculosis infection nor disease can be ruled out in a child who has a negative result on a Mantoux tuberculin skin test. A number of factors may reduce responsiveness to tuberculin (Box 271-2). Overwhelming tuberculosis disease itself may lower tuberculin reactivity in children. Approximately 10% of immunocompetent children who have culture-proven tuberculosis disease have a negative result on the initial Mantoux tuberculin skin test; most of these children develop positive skin test results several months after chemotherapy is started.

Previous immunization with BCG (which is administered routinely in all countries except the United States and the Netherlands) may cause confusion when a Mantoux skin test is interpreted. The BCG vaccines are produced from *M. bovis* organisms that have been passed in serial culture to diminish their virulence. Currently, four principal strains of BCG vaccine, which have widely varying characteristics, are in common use, and immunization schedules vary among countries in the number of immunizations given, the method of administration, and the age at which initial or booster doses are administered.[11] Because of these variations, it is difficult to make standard recommendations for interpreting Mantoux skin reactions after BCG immunization. However, it generally has been demonstrated that only 50% of infants who receive a BCG vaccine shortly after birth have a positive result on a tuberculin skin test at 6 to 12 months of age, and virtually all immunized children have a negative result by age 5. Patients who receive a BCG vaccine as an older child or an adult are more likely to develop and retain a reaction to a tuberculin skin test than those who are immunized as infants, but by 10 years postvaccination, 80% to 90% of these individuals have little or no reaction to a skin test.[6,7] It is presumed that most recipients of a BCG vaccine will have a PPD reaction below 10 mm after a few months to years. Skin test reactions should be interpreted in the same manner for individuals who have or have not received BCG. Prior BCG immunization is never a contraindication for tuberculin testing.

Although the Mantoux skin test is considered the gold standard, the accuracy of the test depends on proper placement, correct assessment of the reaction's size, and the population being tested. Because *M. tuberculosis* infection in the United States is concentrated mostly in discrete subset populations, most children in the United States are at low risk for tuberculosis infection and disease. Under the best conditions, the sensitivity and specificity of the Mantoux skin test are about 90% (which is very low for a diagnostic test), yielding a high positive predictive value in high-risk populations.[12] However, the predictive value of a positive test result drops dramatically in populations that have a low rate of infection. In other words, most positive Mantoux skin test results in high-risk children are true positives, whereas the vast major-

BOX 271-2

FACTORS THAT DIMINISH TUBERCULIN REACTIONS

Host-Related Factors

Infections
- Viral (rubella, rubeola, varicella, influenza)
- Bacterial (typhoid fever, brucellosis, leprosy, pertussis, overwhelming tuberculosis)
- Fungal (blastomycosis)

Vaccines (live viral)
Chronic renal failure
Malnutrition
Diseases affecting lymphoid organs (leukemia, lymphoma, HIV infection)
Certain drugs (corticosteroids, antineoplastic agents)
Age (newborns and the elderly)
Stress (surgery, burns, mental illness)

Tuberculin-Related Factors

Improper storage (exposure to light or heat)
Improper dilutions
Chemical denaturation
Contamination
Adsorption to glass or plastic

Administration-Related Factors

Injection of too little antigen
Delay in administration after antigen is drawn into the syringe
Insufficient interval between injections

Reading-Related Factors

Inexperienced reader
Conscious or unconscious bias
Error in recording

Table 271-1 Cut-off Size of the Induration Area for a Positive Mantoux Tuberculin Reaction in Children Who Have Various Risk Factors for Having Tuberculosis

≥5 mm	≥10 mm	≥15 mm
Contacts of infectious tuberculosis cases Children suspected of having tuberculous disease based on clinical findings and a chest roentgenogram consistent with the diagnosis HIV-infected and other immunosuppressed patients	Children born in or who have lived in countries that have a high prevalence rate for tuberculosis Residents of prisons, nursing homes, and other institutions in which many persons are housed Users of intravenous street drugs Medical risk factors—e.g., Hodgkin's disease, lymphoma, diabetes mellitus, chronic renal failure, and malnutrition Locally identified high-risk populations Children in close contact with high-risk adults Children younger than 4 yr of age	Children 4 yr of age or older who have no risk factors

ity (more than 80%) of "positive" Mantoux skin test reactions in low-risk populations are false positives. Therefore, populations at low risk for tuberculosis infection should not undergo routine testing with the Mantoux skin test.

In 1994, the American Academy of Pediatrics (AAP) with the American Thoracic Society and the Centers for Disease Control and Prevention (CDC) developed guidelines for interpreting Mantoux skin test results based on the patient's clinical, social, and medical history (Table 271-1).[1] This set of guidelines is scientifically valid, but it may be difficult to classify an individual into the proper risk category because of an inability to elicit an accurate medical and social history. A further difficulty is that the risk factors for children depend largely on the risk factors of the adults who care for them. For instance, a child may live with an uncle who recently has been released from a jail that has a population with a high rate of tuberculosis. A careful history is crucial to classify the child properly. It also may be socially stigmatizing to place into different risk categories students in the same classroom who have identical reactions, since this may create the appearance of cultural, economic, or racial bias. However, if children who have no risk factors for tuberculosis are not tested, the scheme for interpretation is much simplified, and the number of skin tests done and interpreted will be diminished greatly in most pediatric practices or clinics.

DETECTION OF TUBERCULOSIS IN CHILDREN

Infected children are discovered as a result of routine screening, when they develop tuberculosis disease and become symptomatic, or as a result of a health department contact investigation. Routine, periodic screening should be conducted only among children who have risk factors for infection (see Box 271-1).

Children most commonly are discovered to have tuberculosis infection or disease through contact investigation of an adult source case. Contact investigations not only have a high yield, but they also find the more recently infected children who are at higher risk of developing primary tuberculosis disease. When a case of suspected contagious pulmonary tuberculosis is reported to the health department, a contact investigation is initiated, ideally within several days of the report. The health department performs a Mantoux skin test on all significant contacts of the index case, beginning with those at highest risk (usually those in the household or immunosuppressed individuals). Individuals who have a Mantoux skin test reaction of 5 mm or larger receive a chest roentgenogram and physical examination to determine if disease is present, and then all are placed on proper chemotherapy regardless of the findings. On average, 30% to 50% of household contacts of an infectious adult have a positive Mantoux skin test result, and 1% to 2% already have the disease.[5] About half of childhood tuberculosis cases in the United States are discovered through contact investigation; most of these children are asymptomatic, but significant signs of disease can be seen on the chest roentgenogram.

Any ill child who has signs or symptoms consistent with tuberculosis disease, even in the absence of any identifiable risk factors, should receive a full medical evaluation, including tuberculin skin testing. Specifically, most children who have pneumonia, cervical adenopathy or lymphadenitis, osteomyelitis or chronic arthritis, or meningitis should receive a tuberculin skin test, and their history should be reviewed for tuberculosis exposure if another cause of disease is not readily apparent.

HIV-infected children may benefit from annual Mantoux skin testing. HIV-infected children are more likely to be in contact with HIV-infected adults and have other significant risk factors for tuberculosis infection. Many HIV-infected children have anergy to tuberculin and other antigens, so a negative skin test result should not dissuade the clinician from pursuing a diagnosis of tuberculosis infection or disease in a child who has a significant exposure or signs and symptoms of disease. A difficult situation arises when an anergic, HIV-infected child has significant contact with an adult who has contagious pulmonary tuberculosis. The child should have a careful evaluation for tuberculosis disease. If no disease is found, most experts would treat the child for tuberculosis infection even though its presence cannot be proved.

MANAGEMENT OF CHILDREN WHO HAVE A REACTIVE MANTOUX SKIN TEST

Once a child is found to have a positive tuberculin skin test result, clinical evaluation determines if the child has tuberculosis infection or disease. About 50% of children who have pulmonary tuberculosis are asymptomatic. Infants are much more likely to develop severe respiratory symptoms and extrapulmonary or disseminated disease; older children, particularly adolescents, frequently have fewer clinical manifestations.

The first step in evaluating a child who has a positive result on the Mantoux tuberculin skin test, whether placed for screening or because of a contact investigation, is to obtain a complete history. Specific and nonjudgmental questions must be asked because many families may feel stigmatized by the infection and may be reluctant to disclose possibly embarrassing information about themselves or other family members and friends. It is important to ask every question of every family, regardless of ethnic or social background. The patient or parents should be asked about the immediate family first; then the scope of questions should be widened to include friends, child care, school, or work, and finally social contacts, such as those in a church or other large congregations. Questions must be asked about contacts known to have or to have had tuberculosis infection or disease, whether previously treated or currently receiving therapy; contacts who showed weight loss or were coughing or sick; contacts in nursing homes, prisons, or homeless shelters; and contacts who had immigrated during the past 5 years. The patient's travel history also should be explored. Any history of contacts diagnosed with or treated for tuberculosis disease should be confirmed by the local health department's division of tuberculosis control to determine the extent of the previous contact investigation and treatment. Questions also must be asked about the past and present health of a child who has a positive result on the tuberculin skin test.

After the history is taken, a careful physical examination of the child should be performed because 25% to 35% of tuberculosis disease in children is extrapulmonary. The most common sites are cervical lymph nodes, meninges, pleura, bones, joints, and skin. Often, no abnormalities will be discovered. The child should be checked for adenopathy, central nervous system (CNS) abnormalities, lung involvement, and liver enlargement. All patients also should have high-quality posteroanterior and lateral roentgenographic views of the chest taken to detect any pulmonary involvement. The need for additional testing is determined by the demonstration of any abnormality on the chest roentgenogram or physical examination and by the history.

PULMONARY AND INTRATHORACIC TUBERCULOSIS

The most common sites for tuberculosis disease are the lung and perihilar lymph nodes. The spectrum of pulmonary involvement can range from none in an asymptomatic infection to progressive pulmonary tuberculosis. Small, calcified densities in the lung parenchyma or lymph nodes indicate areas of a healed primary complex and are not considered evidence of active disease in the absence of other abnormalities. Perihilar lymph node involvement (Fig. 271-2) may be seen as an enlarged silhouette but also may be seen to encircle and compress a mainstem bronchus or to impinge unilaterally on the trachea or mainstem bronchus, causing deviation. Pulmonary disease commonly is manifested as atelectasis, a discrete pulmonary infiltrate (Fig. 271-3), pleural effusion, a miliary pattern (more common in infants) (Fig. 271-4) or, in rare cases, cavitary disease in older children and adolescents.

At the beginning of the tuberculosis infection, the child typically is asymptomatic. Occasionally the child may present with nonspecific symptoms such as low-grade fever, malaise, and cough. Primary infection leads to lymphangitis and regional lymphadenitis, enhanced by the development of tuberculin hypersensitivity. The child usually remains asymptomatic and the radiograph remains normal more commonly among school-age children (80% to 90%) than among infants less than 1 year old (40% to 50%). In some children, hilar lymph node enlargement can cause bronchial compression, leading to air trapping and secondary bacterial pneumonia. Partial bronchial obstruction can occur when the infected node erodes into a bronchus, leading to endobronchial tuberculosis. As the obstruction progresses, atelectasis and infiltrates can occur. Despite extensive pulmonary disease, many children are asymptomatic at the time of diagnosis. Infants are more likely to be symptomatic, presenting with cough (79%), fever (64%), loss of appetite (43%), or localized rales or wheezing (38%).[18] In a study of 47 infants younger than 1 year of age in Houston, intrathoracic disease alone was present in 70% of cases and 21% had meningitis. Ten infants

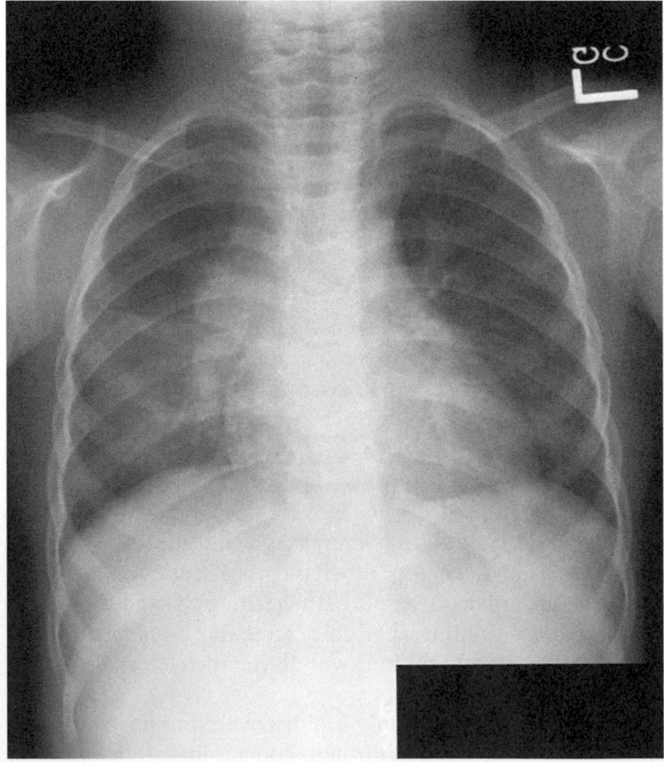

Fig. 271-2 A posteroanterior chest roentgenogram from a 3-year-old child who has cough, fever, and a positive Mantoux skin test shows enlarged hilar lymph nodes and atelectasis on the right side, suggestive of TB disease.

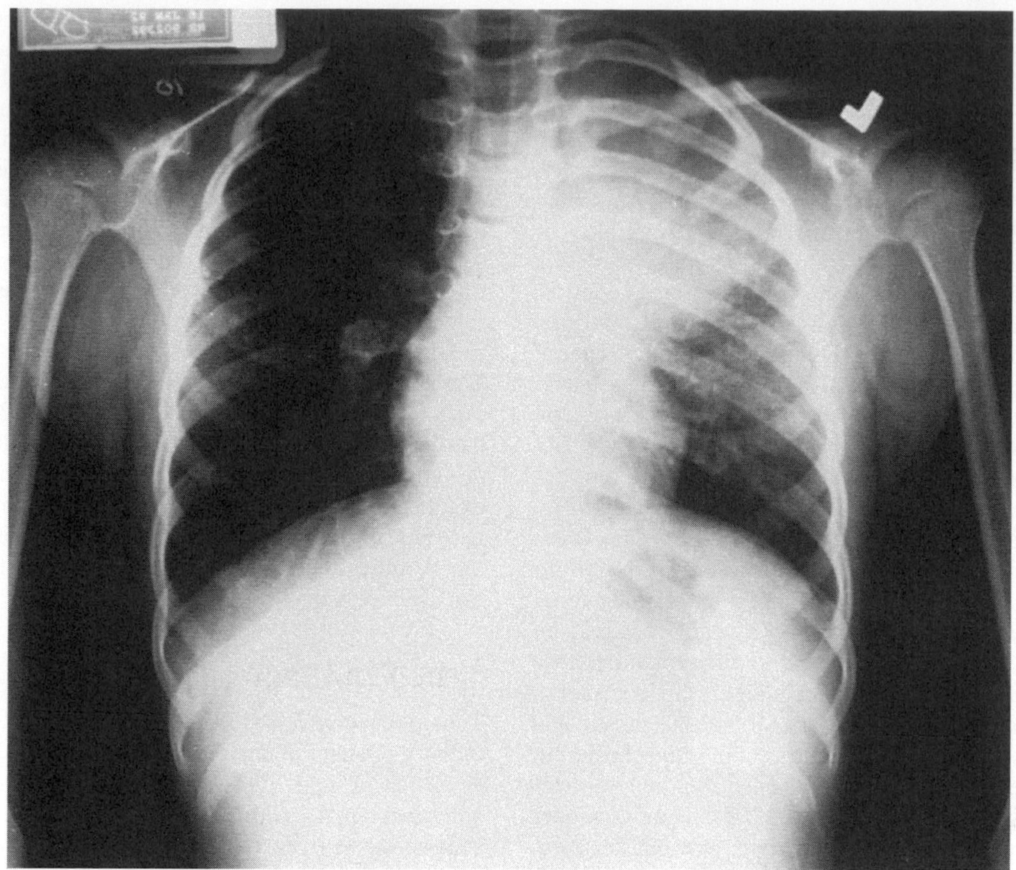

Fig. 271-3 A posteroanterior chest roentgenogram from a 6-year-old black boy with left upper lobe pneumonia. The tuberculin skin test was 12 mm.

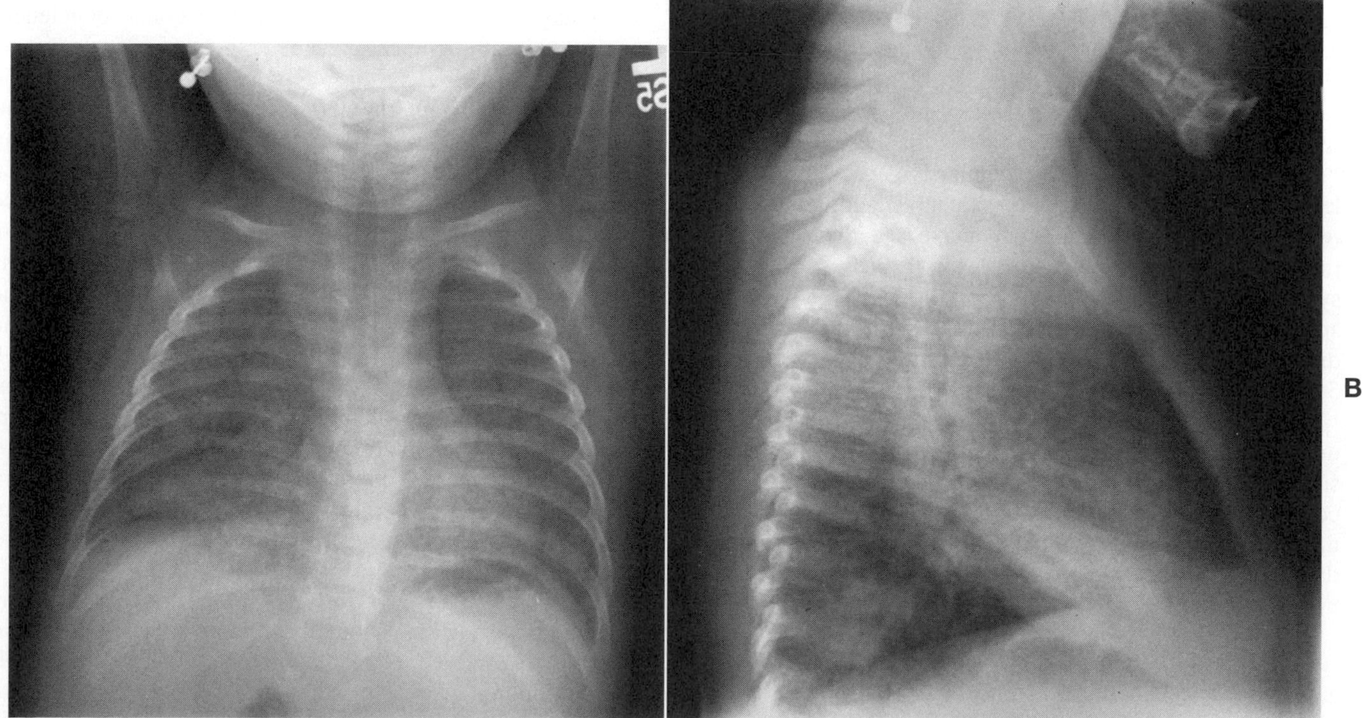

Fig. 271-4 Miliary tuberculosis in an infant. The numerous tubercles can be seen on both the posteroanterior **(A)** and lateral **(B)** views.

(22%) had no reaction to their Mantoux skin test when their disease was diagnosed. Seventy-two percent of the patients had cultures yielding *M. tuberculosis*.

EXTRATHORACIC DISEASE

Extrapulmonary sites are involved less commonly but may be associated with significant morbidity or mortality if treated inadequately. The most common extrapulmonary site of involvement is the cervical lymph nodes; surgery rarely is required for treatment, and this disease usually is managed effectively by antituberculosis chemotherapy. Mycobacterial lymphadenitis occurs most often in the neck, usually causing an indolent, nontender enlargement of one or several nodes, without systemic signs or symptoms. Of the mycobacteria isolated from children younger than 12 years old, approximately 10% are *M. tuberculosis*, with 90% caused by atypical mycobacteria (65% to 80% *Mycobacterium avium-intracellulare* complex, 10% to 20% *Mycobacterium scrofulaceum*). More than 90% of culture-proved mycobacterial lymphadenitis in children older than 12 years is caused by *M. tuberculosis*. Because it is difficult to differentiate disease caused by *M. tuberculosis* and nontuberculous mycobacteria, surgical excision usually is necessary for both diagnostic and therapeutic reasons (i.e., for nontuberculous mycobacteria).

CNS involvement is the second most common form of extrapulmonary disease and is always fatal without proper treatment. Many patients have symptoms of malaise, irritability, and fever for many days or weeks before manifesting cranial nerve abnormalities, hydrocephalus, and basilar meningitis. Up to 3% of children infected but not treated before the age of 2 years develop this form of tuberculosis. This frequency decreases to 1% or less in later life. Meningitis occurs within 3 to 6 months of the initial infection. Typical cerebrospinal fluid (CSF) findings include a lymphocystic pleocytosis, a low glucose level, and an elevated protein concentration. Hyponatremia is a common complication. Most children with tuberculosis meningitis have abnormal chest radiographs. The tuberculin skin test, however, can be negative in 40% of children at the time of diagnosis.

Miliary or disseminated tuberculosis is caused by the release of organisms into the bloodstream, leading to disease in two or more organs. Children, and especially infants, are more prone to develop miliary disease than adults. Signs and symptoms may include fever, weight loss, hepatomegaly, splenomegaly, generalized lymphadenopathy, and respiratory distress. Meningitis accompanies miliary disease in 30% to 50% of children at diagnosis.

Bone and/or joint tuberculosis complicates 1% to 6% of untreated infections with *M. tuberculosis* in children, and spinal involvement is seen in 50% to 60% of cases. Less common sites of infection with skeletal tuberculosis include the femur, tibia, and fibula. Skeletal tuberculosis may be undiagnosed for months to years because of its indolent presentation.

Other extrapulmonary sites of involvement (e.g., pleura, skin, pericardium, kidney, and gastrointestinal tract) are less common.

An attempt should be made to determine the drug susceptibility pattern of the organism in all cases of suspected or proved tuberculosis infection or disease. If the drug susceptibility results are known for the isolate from the adult source case, it may be presumed that the child's isolate has the same pattern. However, if the source case has not been found for a child who has tuberculosis disease, isolating the organism from the child should be attempted. Children should be evaluated by acid-fast stain and mycobacterial culture of either expectorated sputum (from an adolescent), if it is available, or of early-morning aspiration of gastric contents on 3 successive days (from infants and children). Collection of gastric aspirates requires hospitalization because the desired sample is the pooled overnight secretions that have been swallowed and remain in the stomach before the child arises. The culture yield of three consecutive morning gastric aspirates for *M. tuberculosis* in children is only 30% to 50%, but the yield from infants can be up to 70%. Decisions about the need for further cultures (urine, CSF) or histopathological examination of biopsied tissue are dictated by the extent and anatomical location of suspected disease. The culture yield of other body fluids in children with extrapulmonary disease usually is less than 50%.

TREATMENT

Tuberculosis infection and disease are treated with chemotherapy. Commonly used antituberculosis drugs and doses are listed in Table 271-2. Unlike adults, children who take antituberculosis medication experience few side effects. Transient gastrointestinal (GI) distress sometimes is encountered, resulting in vomiting during the first few days of administration. Although rare, the most common serious problem is hepatotoxicity, principally induced by isoniazid (INH) but occasionally associated with rifampin (RIF) or pyrazinamide (PZA). Peripheral neuritis or convulsions caused by inhibition of pyridoxine metabolism in children receiving INH are very rare, and pyridoxine supplementation is not necessary unless the patient has nutritional deficiencies (meat- and milk-deficient diet), is pregnant, or is a breast-fed infant. Discolored secretions are common with RIF administration and may stain contact lenses permanently. Oral contraceptives may be rendered ineffective by RIF, so an alternative form of birth control should be used while RIF is taken. Reversible optic neuritis is a serious but rare side effect caused by ethambutol (EMB); therefore, visual acuity and color discrimination should be monitored monthly in patients receiving this drug. Streptomycin (STM) administration may be associated with ototoxicity and hearing loss. The drug should be avoided as a long-term agent, and hearing should be tested before, during, and after STM therapy. Because hepatotoxicity is rare in children, many tuberculosis experts do not monitor blood chemistries routinely for evidence of abnormalities but rely instead on early identification of clinical manifestations. Allergic reactions associated with antituberculosis medications, manifested primarily by skin rashes and pruritus, also are rare.

Children who have a positive Mantoux skin test result and no other abnormalities have tuberculosis infection, and treatment with INH for 6 to 9 months is considered optimal.[12] Children who have been coinfected by HIV and *M. tuberculosis* should be treated for 12 months. For patients who cannot tolerate INH or who are infected with INH-resistant organisms, RIF for 9 months is a satisfactory alternative. If

Table 271-2 Drugs Used Commonly for the Treatment of Tuberculosis Among Infants, Children, and Adolescents

Drugs	Dosage Form	Daily Dose (mg/kg/day)	Twice Weekly Dose (mg/kg/dose)	Maximum Dose	Adverse Reactions
Ethambutol	Tablets 100 mg, 400 mg	15-25	50	2.5 g	Optic neuritis (reversible), diminished visual acuity, reduced red-green color discrimination, GI disturbance
Isoniazid*	Scored tablets: 100 mg, 300 mg Syrup: 10 mg/ml	10-15	20-30	Daily: 300 mg; twice weekly: 900 mg	Mild hepatic enzyme elevation, hepatitis, peripheral neuritis, hypersensitivity
Pyrazinamide*	Scored tablets: 500 mg	20-40	50	2 g	Hepatotoxicity, hyperuricemia
Rifampin*	Capsules: 150 mg, 300 mg Syrup formulated from capsules	10-20	10-20	Daily: 600 mg; twice weekly: 900 mg	Orange discoloration of secretions/urine, staining of contact lenses, hepatitis, flu-like reaction, thrombocytopenia; may render birth control pills ineffective
Streptomycin (intramuscular administration)	Vials: 1 g, 4 g	20-40	20-40	1 g	Ototoxicity, nephrotoxicity, skin rash

*Rifamate is a combination drug capsule containing 150 mg of isoniazid and 300 mg of rifampin. Rifater is a combination drug tablet containing 50 mg of isoniazid, 120 mg of rifampin, and 300 mg of pyrazinamide. Each of these combination drug preparations can be used when combined therapy is indicated to reduce the number of capsules and tablets that need to be administered to pediatric patients.

the adult source case is known to have a multiple drug-resistant isolate of *M. tuberculosis* (INH and RIF resistant), at least two drug therapies based on the susceptibility pattern should be instituted, if possible. It is imperative to search for the adult source case and the drug susceptibility pattern of his or her isolate to be sure the correct drugs are given to the child.

Children who have drug-susceptible pulmonary tuberculosis (including hilar or mediastinal adenopathy) may be treated adequately with 6 months of INH and RIF, with the addition of PZA for the first 2 months.[14] If drug resistance is suspected (especially if the adult source case was treated previously for tuberculosis, came from a country or region that has high rates of drug-resistant tuberculosis, or is HIV infected), a fourth drug, usually EMB or STM, should be added to the initial regimen. Extrapulmonary tuberculosis disease may be treated adequately with INH, RIF, and PZA, but longer courses of 9 to 12 months and the initial addition of EMB or STM (to guard against unknown drug resistance) are indicated for complicated, severe, or CNS disease. As with tuberculosis infection, if the adult source case is known to have a multiple drug-resistant *M. tuberculosis* isolate and/or a resistant organism is cultured from a child who has tuberculosis disease, at least a four-drug therapy should be instituted, based on the susceptibility pattern. Consultation with an infectious-disease specialist or other appropriate specialist is recommended for any case of drug-resistant tuberculosis infection or disease.

The greatest challenge in treating tuberculosis is patient failure to fulfill treatment requirements; this leads to relapse, development of secondary drug resistance, and possible transmission of organisms to others. All patients being treated for tuberculosis disease should have their therapy administered and monitored by a health care worker, usually a member of the health department. This directly observed therapy (DOT) is necessary to monitor for drug side effects and to ensure compliance in taking medications, which essentially eliminates the emergence of secondary drug resistance. Antituberculosis drugs may be given twice weekly under DOT for drug-susceptible tuberculosis infection and for pulmonary and uncomplicated extrapulmonary tuberculosis disease. For these forms of tuberculosis, twice-weekly DOT is as effective as daily therapy, has the same or fewer adverse reactions, and is more effective in preventing the emergence of drug resistance.[17]

All household and close contacts under age 5 years of a patient with suspected contagious pulmonary tuberculosis (even if the Mantoux skin test result was nonreactive) should be given INH to prevent disease from occurring rapidly. Some young children, if infected, develop disseminated disease before a tuberculin skin test result becomes apparent. The Mantoux test should be repeated 3 months after contact with the source case has ended. If the second reaction is positive, infection has occurred and the patient should remain on INH and be evaluated for possible tuberculosis disease. If the Mantoux skin test remains nonreactive, the patient should discontinue INH, provided the source case is undergoing adequate, monitored antituberculosis therapy and his or her sputum tests negative for acid-fast organisms on a smear.

Congenital tuberculosis disease is extremely rare. The more common situation is the newborn in whose family an adult (sometimes the mother) is suspected of having contagious pulmonary tuberculosis. The infant should remain separated from a mother who has a newly recognized reactive tuberculin skin test result until she has had a chest roentgenogram. If the mother has no evidence of pulmonary disease, the infant may safely stay with her. If the mother or any member of the household is suspected of having pulmonary disease but there is no evidence or suspicion of INH-resistant *M. tuberculosis*, the infant should be treated with INH (given daily by the mother or a public health nurse) and a Mantoux skin test should be done 3 months after the mother (or other family member) is no longer contagious. If a member of the household is undergoing treatment for tuberculosis disease, that individual should not have contact with the infant, if possible, unless his or her sputum smear tests negative on acid-fast staining. If the infant and infected family member cannot be separated, the family member must be followed up carefully to ensure compliance with treatment; the infant should be given INH for 3 months, and a Mantoux skin test should be done before therapy is discontinued. If the second tuberculin skin test reaction is positive, infection has occurred, and the infant should continue receiving INH for 9 months and be evaluated for possible tuberculosis disease.

OUTCOME

Children infected with tuberculosis who are treated adequately are nearly universally free of tuberculosis disease on completion of treatment, and most patients who have uncomplicated pulmonary and extrapulmonary disease have complete resolution of the disease. Patients who have the least favorable prognosis are infants who have severe disseminated disease, children who have tuberculosis meningitis, patients who have multiple drug-resistant tuberculosis disease, and patients who have underlying problems such as immunosuppression (especially HIV infection) or debilitating chronic disorders. Patients should be examined every 4 to 6 weeks during therapy so that their adherence to therapy and any medication side effects may be monitored. Roentgenographic abnormalities should show improvement but may take many months or years to resolve completely. Most children's roentgenograms still show abnormalities after 6 months of therapy, but this does not indicate treatment failure. Patients who have completed medical therapy should be examined within 3 to 6 months to ensure that there is no evidence of recurrent disease.

CONCLUSION

The clinician must be aware of who is at increased risk for tuberculosis and administer and interpret Mantoux skin tests accordingly. Reporting suspected and confirmed cases of tuberculosis disease in adolescents and adults to the health department is essential to prevent source cases from continuing to infect children and other adults. Most important, the physician must institute directly observed therapy whenever possible to ensure complete eradication of infection or disease in the patient. When the patient, the clinician, and the health department interact effectively, nearly all patients with TB recover fully.

When to Refer

All cases of tuberculosis infection and disease should be referred to the local and state health department.

Cases of tuberculosis disease should be managed collaboratively with an infectious disease or pulmonary specialist.

When to Hospitalize

Any child or infant suspected of having pulmonary TB for initial evaluation and gastric aspirate culture collection

Any child when the clinical condition justifies admission based on symptoms (e.g., disseminated disease, respiratory distress, meningitis)

REFERENCES

1. American Academy of Pediatrics: Tuberculosis. In Pickering LK, editor: *Red Book 2000: Report of the Committee on Infectious Diseases,* ed 25, Elk Grove Village, Ill, 2000, American Academy of Pediatrics.
2. Cantwell MF, et al: Epidemiology of tuberculosis in the United States, 1985 through 1992, *JAMA* 272:535, 1994.
3. Frieden TR, et al: The emergence of drug-resistant tuberculosis in New York City, *N Engl J Med* 328:521, 1993.
4. Gutman LT, et al: Tuberculosis in human immunodeficiency virus-exposed or -infected United States children, *Pediatr Infect Dis J* 13:963, 1994.
5. Hsu KHK: Contact investigation: a practical approach to tuberculosis eradication, *Am J Public Health* 53:1761, 1963.
6. Karalliede S, Katughan LP, Uragoda CG: The tuberculin response of Sri Lankan children after BCG vaccination at birth, *Tubercle* 68:33, 1987.
7. Lifschitz M: The value of the tuberculin skin test as a screening test for tuberculosis among BCG-vaccinated children, *Pediatrics* 36:624, 1965.
8. Miller FSN, Seale RME, Taylor MD: *Tuberculosis in children,* Boston, 1963, Little, Brown.
9. Nolan RC Jr: Childhood tuberculosis in North Carolina: a study of the opportunities for intervention in the transmission of tuberculosis to children, *Am J Public Health* 76:26, 1986.
10. Progress toward the elimination of tuberculosis—United States, 1998, *MMWR* 48:732, 1999.
11. Raviglione MC, Snider DE Jr, Kochi A: Global epidemiology of tuberculosis: morbidity and mortality of a worldwide epidemic, *JAMA* 273: 220, 1994.
12. Snider DE Jr: The tuberculin skin test, *Am Rev Respir Dis* 125(suppl): 108, 1982.
13. Starke JR, Connelly KK: Bacille Calmette-Guérin vaccine. In Plotkin SA, Mortimer EA Jr, editors: *Vaccines,* ed 2, Philadelphia, 1994, WB Saunders.
14. Starke JR, Jacobs RF, Jereb J: Resurgence of tuberculosis in children, *J Pediatr* 120:839, 1992.
15. Starke JR, Taylor-Watts KT: Tuberculosis in the pediatric population of Houston, Texas, *Pediatrics* 84:28, 1989.
16. Steiner P, et al: Persistently negative tuberculin reactions: their presence among children who culture positive for *Mycobacterium tuberculosis, Am J Dis Child* 134:747, 1990.
17. Weis SE, et al: The effect of directly observed therapy on the rates of drug resistance and relapse in tuberculosis, *N Engl J Med* 330:1179, 1994.
18. Vallejo JG, Ong LT, Starke JR: Clinical features, diagnosis and treatment of tuberculosis in infants, *Pediatrics* 94:1, 1994.

272 Umbilical Anomalies

Robert W. Marion

"It [the umbilicus] is all that remains of the stem that bound us to the parental stalk. It is a reminder that we have been plucked and must sooner or later die. It might be said that when the stem is severed, we cease to live in any true sense. We may be ornamental like roses or useful like cabbages but only for a little while. Our dissolution has begun."[5]

Despite its essential role in the survival of the fetus during prenatal life, the umbilicus, the external vestige of the umbilical cord, frequently is ignored or overlooked by the pediatric primary care provider. However, aberrations in either the formation or the position of this structure can offer helpful clues to underlying pathology in the young child. Major congenital anomalies of the ventral abdominal wall, such as omphalocele, gastroschisis, and exstrophies of the bladder and cloaca, are described in detail elsewhere (see Chapter 49, Critical Neonatal Illnesses). This chapter will deal with minor anomalies in configuration, placement, and formation of the umbilicus. In addition to the conditions described here, the umbilicus can be the site of both tumors (either vascular or teratomatous neoplasms) and infections (omphalitis).[3]

To understand the etiology and significance of anomalies of the umbilicus, it is necessary to review some basic fundamentals of the embryological development of the umbilical cord.

Embryological Development of the Umbilical Cord

Appearing within the first 6 weeks of gestation, the umbilical cord is derived from the fusion of three separate embryonic structures: (1) the primitive or primary yolk sac, which contains the allantois and a portion of the vitelline duct, transient structures that ultimately form the central portion of the embryonic gut, the urinary bladder, the urachus, and the umbilical blood vessels (usually two arteries and one vein); (2) the secondary yolk sac, composed of the remainder of the vitelline duct; and (3) the mesenchyme of the connecting body stalk of the embryo, the tissue which produces Wharton's jelly, the packing substance that holds the cord together. After fusion is complete, these unified structures become covered by the amnion and ultimately are surrounded by amniotic fluid.[2]

Many of these embryonic structures that form the umbilical cord are transitory, present for only brief periods during embryogenesis. Following the seventh week of gestation, the vitelline duct regresses and ultimately becomes completely resorbed. Similarly the allantois, which is contiguous with the urinary bladder, degenerates, forming a fibrous cord called the *urachus,* which connects the apex of the bladder with the umbilicus. Anomalies may result when these structures fail to undergo normal regression, causing them to persist into postnatal life.

ANOMALIES

Abnormalities of Position and Morphology

Anatomically, the level of the umbilicus usually is at the top of the iliac crest ventral to the third or fourth lumbar vertebra.[6] Variations in the position of the umbilicus can result from abnormalities in the way in which the abdominal wall itself has formed and, as such, may be a clue to the diagnosis of specific dysmorphic syndromes. For example, as described in Table 272-1, the umbilicus has been noted to be low-set in entities such as achondroplasia (in which disproportionate growth of the trunk accounts for the aberration in position), bladder and cloacal exstrophy,[8] and in association with various anomalies of the urinary tract.[1] Higher-than-normal placement of the umbilicus occurs in Robinow syndrome, a condition also known as *fetal face syndrome* because of the striking ocular hypertelorism and macrocephaly that occurs in affected individuals.[8]

Not only abnormal location but also variations in the appearance of the umbilicus can suggest the presence of a syndrome. In Aarskog syndrome, a disorder that combines abnormalities of the face (ocular hypertelorism, small nose with anteversion of the nares, minor anomalies of the ears), digits (mild soft-tissue webbing with blinobrachydactyly of the fifth fingers), and genitalia ("shawl" scrotum, cryptorchidism), the umbilicus is prominent and appears pouting and protuberant. In Robinow syndrome, previously described, the umbilical scar is broad and poorly epithelized.[8] Hypoplasia of the umbilicus occurs in Cornelia de Lange syndrome, a disorder combining growth and developmental retardation with a characteristic facial appearance and multiple congenital anomalies. Finally, in Rieger syndrome, which combines iris dysplasia and other ophthalmological malformations with hypodontia (absence of the upper incisors), there is failure of involution of the periumbilical skin, leading to a protruding umbilicus.[9]

Embryonic Umbilical Remnants

As previously noted, the umbilical cord is formed of the vitelline duct, which connects the yolk sac to the midgut, the allantois, which ultimately degenerates into the urachus, a structure that forms a connection between the apex of the urinary bladder and the umbilicus, and the umbilical blood vessels. Persistence of these structures can lead to the presence of anomalies within the newborn.

Failure of the closure and total regression of the vitelline duct by the seventh week of gestation may lead to the presence of Meckel's diverticulum (an outpouching of the gut without attachment to the anterior abdominal wall), a vitelline cyst or enterocystoma (a connection between the midgut and umbilicus without communication with either structure), an enteric or vitelline fistula (formed from a communicating connection between the midgut and the umbilicus), or a urachal sinus, cyst, or fistula (resulting from a connection between the bladder and the urachus)[2] (Fig. 272-1). In the child, the presence of these anomalies may be signaled by the presence of signs of infection and of a lower midline abdominal mass (caused by infection of a vitelline cyst); the discharge of feces and urine, which can lead to an erosive dermatitis (from enteric and urachal fistulas); and urinary tract infections (also resulting from urachal fistulas). Further, the persistence of a fibrous band of tissue attached to the gut, the result of incomplete involution, may serve as the lead point for a volvulus or the cause of intestinal obstruction.

Of all these anomalies, Meckel's diverticula clearly are the most common. Present in 2.5% of American newborns,[2] they are a well-known cause of clandestine lower intestinal bleeding in children and adults. The bleeding results from the presence of ectopic gastric mucosa within the diverticulum, which is prone to ulceration and hemorrhage. Also, since these diverticula (which can occur anywhere from the ileocecal valve to a point 3 feet or more proximal to the valve) resemble a supernumerary vermiform appendix, their presence may be signaled by symptoms and signs of acute appendicitis.

Table 272-1 Conditions Associated with Abnormalities in Position or Morphology of the Umbilicus

Disorder	Abnormality in Position	Abnormality in Morphology
Aarskog syndrome	—	Prominent, protruding, pouting
Achondroplasia	Low placement	—
Bladder exstrophy	Low placement	—
Cloacal exstrophy	Low placement	—
Cornelia de Lange syndrome	—	Hypoplasia
Rieger syndrome	—	Prominent, broad, redundant periumbilical skin
Robinow syndrome	High placement	Broad, scar is poorly epithelialized

From Curry CJR, Honore L, Boyd E: The ventral wall of the trunk. In Stevenson RE, Hall JG, Goodman RM, editors: *Human malformations and related anomalies,* vol 2, New York, 1993, Oxford University Press.

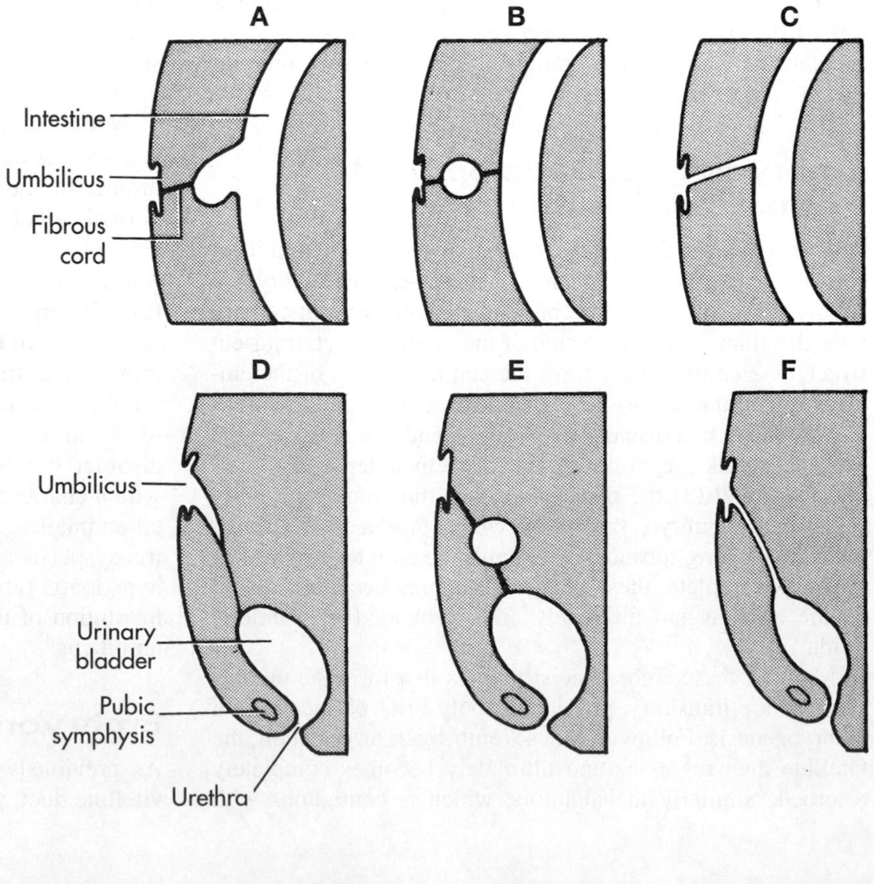

A B C
Intestine
Umbilicus
Fibrous cord
D E F
Umbilicus
Urinary bladder
Pubic symphysis
Urethra

Fig. 272-1 Embryonic umbilical remnants. **A,** Meckel's diverticulum. **B,** Enterocystoma. **C,** Enteric (vitelline) fistula. **D,** Urachal sinus. **E,** Urachal cyst. **F,** Urachal fistula.

Embryonic umbilical remnants that are lined with gastric mucosa can be detected by gastrointestinal radionuclide scans using ^{99m}Tc pertechnetate. Sonography or computed tomography (CT) is helpful in delineating vitelline cysts that, following infection, present as abdominal masses. The presence of a urachal fistula can best be documented by noting the presence of methylene blue dye in the urine after it has been instilled at the umbilicus. The treatment of all internal umbilical cord remnants that are symptomatic is surgical excision and repair.

Vascular Abnormalities of the Umbilical Cord

Derived from the primitive or primary yolk sac, the blood vessels are the most important structures present in the umbilical cord. Although usually consisting of two arteries and one vein, variations on this pattern are well known, occurring in 0.7% of all births.[2] By far, the most common variation is the presence of only two vessels in the cord, consisting of one vein and one artery. In 25% to 50% of cases, this arrangement is associated with various additional anomalies, including malformations of the central nervous system (CNS), the genitourinary tract, the spine and the extremities.

The pattern of anomalies seen in infants with aberrant cord vessels often depends on which vessels are present and which are missing. Blackburn and Cooley describe three separate patterns.[2] In the first, the single umbilical artery is of allantoic origin; this pattern is associated with growth retardation, anomalies of the CNS such as anencephaly and spina bifida, and abnormalities of the lower genitourinary tract. In the second pattern, the single artery is of vitelline origin; associated anomalies include sirenomelia, sacral agenesis, reduction defects of the lower extremities, anal atresia (features of the VACTERL association), and trisomy 18. Infants with the third pattern have cords that have three vessels, including a single umbilical artery (of either allantoic or vitelline origin), a left umbilical vein, and a persistent and aberrant right umbilical vein; such a pattern has been described in some children with Noonan's syndrome and 47,XXY karyotype.

Umbilical Hernia

The predisposition to develop an umbilical hernia occurs during the second trimester, after the midgut, which has until then been developing extraabdominally, returns to the abdominal cavity. Failure to form the normal fascial reinforcements that keep the midgut in place leads to a weakness in the abdominal wall.[6]

Umbilical hernias are so common that they should be thought of as a variation of normal. The incidence varies with race and age. Evans found that at 6 weeks of age, 32% of black infants had umbilical hernias, whereas only 4% of white babies did. At 1 year, the prevalence decreased to 12% and 2%, respectively.[7] Low-birth-weight babies also are at markedly increased risk.[7] There is, however, no gender predilection; boys and girls are equally affected.

In the vast majority of affected individuals, umbilical hernias are associated with no medical sequelae. One study revealed that incarceration, strangulation, rupture, or skin breakdown occurred in less than 5% of 590 children.[7] Other studies have revealed even lower rates of complication. Further, in most cases, the hernia will close spontaneously without any medical intervention.[10] Thus, the major indication for surgical treatment of the condition is cosmetic. As such, surgery should only be considered in carefully selected individuals.

Although most umbilical hernias occur as isolated findings in otherwise healthy children, they also can be associated with a variety of known conditions, many of which are associated with increased abdominal girth or hypotonia. As shown in Table 272-2, these conditions include the common autosomal trisomies, the mucopolysaccharidoses and other inborn errors of metabolism that are associated with organomegaly, and various dysmorphic syndromes, such as Beckwith-Wiedemann syndrome.

Umbilical Granulomas

At birth, the normal umbilical cord contains only the umbilical vessels surrounded by the protective Wharton's jelly. Within the first 2 weeks after birth, the umbilical stump normally dries and separates from the abdomen; the region is completely covered by skin in 3 to 4 weeks. Delayed healing with the accumulation of excessive amounts of granulation tissue produces an umbilical granuloma, a small, reddened mass. The lesion may be associated with infection at its base or with a foreign body such as talcum, but it recedes rapidly after repeated topical applications of silver nitrate. Persistence of a granulomatous-appearing lesion after treatment, the presence of erosive dermatitis at the site, or the egression of gas, feces, or urine from it should suggest the persistence

Table 272-2 Some Conditions Associated with Umbilical Hernias

Chromosomal Anomalies	Metabolic Disorders	Dysmorphic Syndromes
Trisomy 21	Hypothyroidism	Aarskog syndrome
Trisomy 18	Mucolipidosis III (Pseudo-Hurler syndrome)	Beckwith-Wiedemann syndrome
Trisomy 21	Mucopolysaccharidoses	Fetal hydantoin syndrome
Deletion 9p	Type 1 (Hurler syndrome)	Marfan syndrome
Duplication 3q	Type 2 (Hunter syndrome)	Opitz syndrome
	Type 4 (Morquio syndrome)	Weaver syndrome
	Type 6 (Maroteaux-Lamy syndrome)	

From Curry CJR, Honore L, Boyd E: The ventral wall of the trunk. In Stevenson RE, Hall JG, Goodman RM, editors: *Human malformations and related anomalies,* vol 2, New York, 1993, Oxford University Press.

of one of the embryonic remnants described in more detail beginning on p. 1889.[4]

Umbilical Polyps

Although they may superficially resemble umbilical granulomas, polyps at the umbilicus actually represent external remnants of the umbilical cord. They may be sinuses of the vitelline duct or the urachus. Often larger in size than granulomas, they are bright red and do not respond to treatment with silver nitrate. Diagnosis depends on histological examination, and treatment is surgical excision.

REFERENCES

1. Aase JM: Caudal displacement of the umbilicus: implications for diagnosis of genitourinary anomalies, *Proc Greenwood Genet Center* 10: 120, 1991.
2. Blackburn W, Cooley NR: The umbilical cord. In Stevenson RE, Hall JG, Goodman RM, editors: *Human malformations and related anomalies,* vol 2, New York, 1993, Oxford University Press.
3. Campbell J, et al: Clinical diagnosis of umbilical swellings and discharges in children, *Med J Aust* 145:450, 1986.
4. Cresson SL, Pilling GP: Lesions about the umbilicus in infants and children, *Pediatr Clin North Am* 6:1085, 1959.
5. Cullen TS: *Embryology anatomy and disease of the umbilicus together with disease of the urachus,* Philadelphia, 1916, WB Saunders.
6. Curry CJR, Honore L, Boyd E: The ventral wall of the trunk. In Stevenson RE, Hall JG, Goodman RM, editors: *Human malformations and related anomalies,* vol 2, New York, 1993, Oxford University Press.
7. Evans AG: Comparative incidence of umbilical hernias in colored and white infants, *J Natl Med Assoc* 33:158, 1944.
8. Friedman JM: Umbilical dysmorphology, *Clin Genet* 28:343, 1985.
9. Jones KL: *Smith's recognizable patterns of human behavior,* ed 5, Philadelphia, 1997, WB Saunders.
10. Walker SH: The natural history of umbilical hernia, *Clin Pediatr* 6:29, 1967.

SUGGESTED READINGS

Blackburn W, Cooley NR: The umbilical cord. In Stevenson RE, Hall JG, Goodman RM: *Human malformations and related anomalies,* New York, 1993, Oxford University Press.

Curry CJR, Honore L, Boyd E: The ventral wall of the trunk. In Stevenson RE, Hall JG, Goodman RM: *Human malformations and related anomalies,* New York, 1993, Oxford University Press.

273 Urinary Tract Infections

Glenn H. Bock

INCIDENCE

Infection is the most common disease of the kidneys and urinary tract encountered in pediatric practice. In newborns, the incidence of urinary tract infections (UTI) has been estimated to be as high as 5 per 1000 live births; boys are affected more than five times as often as girls. Among infants who develop first-time symptomatic UTI during the first year, most cases occur during the first 3 months, and boys account for as many as 75% of cases. Thereafter, and throughout childhood and adolescence, the overwhelming majority of first cases of UTI occur in girls, affecting 5% or more during this period. The prevalence of covert (asymptomatic) bacteriuria in preschool girls is 0.8%; in school-age girls it is nearly 2%. After infancy, covert bacteriuria is extremely uncommon in boys.

Numerous clinical guidelines for diagnostic and therapeutic management of childhood UTI have been proposed. It seems clear, however, that the extent of diagnostic evaluation and the form of therapeutic intervention merit substantial individualization in many cases. In addition to the actual bacteriological diagnosis, the presence of coexisting risk factors and a realistic assessment of the likelihood of UTI-associated morbidity must be considered as a care plan is formulated.

ETIOLOGY

Both infection-related (bacterial) and patient-related (host) factors contribute to the overall risk of UTI. Among the bacteria causing urinary tract infections, *Escherichia coli* accounts for 75% to 80% of cases. Bacterial virulence appears to be an important determinant in many of these infections. Recent data suggest that binding sites (pili, or P-fimbriae) are present on the surface of certain uropathogenic *E. coli* organisms, enabling them to combine with receptors on uroepithelial cells; this process is thought to enhance bacterial virulence. Insights into the nature of these and other virulence factors may give rise to new therapeutic approaches to preventing and treating UTI in the future. Less common among the enteric uropathogens are *Enterobacter aerogenes, Enterobacter cloacae,* and the *Klebsiella* and *Proteus* species. Of the nonenteric gram-negative pathogens, *Pseudomonas aeruginosa* is the most common. In a sexually active adolescent, gram-positive *Staphylococcus saprophyticus* is the most common pathogen after *E. coli.* Infection with *Neisseria gonorrhoeae* should be suspected in boys who have a urethral discharge or purulent balanitis. Urinary voiding symptoms may result from gonococcal vulvovaginitis in girls. Although the presence of gram-negative intracellular diplococci in a stain of the discharge strongly suggests gonococcal infection, a culture is necessary to confirm the diagnosis. Other causes of urethritis syndrome include such sexually transmitted organisms as *Chlamydia trachomatis* and *Ureaplasma urealyticum.*

Viral uropathogens are relatively unimportant except for the adenovirus in acute hemorrhagic cystitis. Fungal infections rarely are significant except in immunocompromised or diabetic patients. Fungal overgrowth, however, may complicate antibiotic treatment of immunologically normal children with abnormal urinary tract emptying or those with indwelling urinary catheters. Although protozoan infections of the urinary tract are important in many parts of the world, they remain uncommon in the United States. Urinary infections with *Mycobacterium tuberculosis* occur rarely in secondary tuberculosis but should be considered when sterile pyuria is found in a suspect clinical setting, particularly since the prevalence of tuberculosis currently is increasing.

A number of host characteristics appear to be important contributing risk factors for UTI. Among newborns, the higher incidence of congenital urinary anomalies in males undoubtedly affects the risk of neonatal UTI in infant boys. However, many infant boys who have UTI have anatomically normal urinary tracts. Insofar as the ratio of sepsis in boys compared with girls is similar to the ratio of UTI, the hematogenous route of urinary infection might also contribute to the gender difference. The incidence of UTI in newborns also appears to be inversely related to gestational age, being greatest in low-birth-weight and premature infants. This has led to speculation that an immature kidney more readily allows the bacteria to pass the renal filtration barrier than does a mature kidney.

In older infants and children, most UTIs are "ascending." The high incidence in girls has been attributed to anatomical features of the lower urinary tract, including the comparatively short urethra, its proximity to the anus, and its exit within the folds of the vulva. Sexually active females are rendered susceptible to infection when, during coitus, bacteria are introduced into the urethra, which often becomes inflamed and swollen as a result of coital friction. In all patients, conditions that result in incomplete urinary drainage and/or stasis in the urinary system increase susceptibility to primary and recurring UTI. Frequent, complete bladder emptying is an essential element in host resistance to infections. Incomplete voiding may result from either structural or functional disturbances of voiding, and these may be congenital or acquired (Box 273-1).

BOX 273-1

CONDITIONS ASSOCIATED WITH ABNORMAL URINARY DRAINAGE

Congenital
- Urethral valves (males)
- Ureteropelvic junction obstruction
- Ureterovesical junction obstruction
- Vesicoureteral reflux
- Neurogenic bladder
- Nonobstructive dilation (e.g., megacystis, megaureter conditions)

Acquired
- Urolithiasis
- Urethral stricture
- Bladder dysfunction (as result of prior obstruction, acquired neurogenic lesion, voiding dysfunction syndromes, etc.)
- Behavioral or psychiatric conditions with urine holding
- Foreign body
- Retroperitoneal fibrosis
- Neoplasms (causing urinary obstruction)

Vesicoureteral reflux deserves particular emphasis given its importance in urinary tract infections and renal scarring. The prevalence of pyelonephritis is high among patients who have reflux and UTI, and there appears to be a substantial risk of renal parenchymal scarring in those who have pyelonephritis and reflux. It must be remembered, however, that the majority of infants and young children who have pyelonephritis do *not* have urinary reflux. (Obstructive urinary lesions and vesicoureteral reflux are discussed in Chapter 240, Obstructive Uropathy and Vesicoureteral Reflux.)

Circumcision may also be considered a structural issue with respect to UTI risk. The overwhelming majority of male infants who develop UTI are uncircumcised, and the relative risk of UTI among uncircumcised males is higher than in their circumcised counterparts at all ages. Nonetheless, routine circumcision of infant males cannot be justified based on the reduction of UTI incidence alone since the actual number of serious long-term sequelae prevented would be rather small.

The contributory role of functional disturbances of micturition to UTI risk cannot be overemphasized. Most children with dysfunctional voiding have persistence of an unstable urinary bladder, and children with unstable bladders are at increased risk for UTI. The diagnosis of voiding dysfunction may be delayed because the daytime incontinence and/or symptoms of urgency and uninhibited bladder contractions characteristic of the unstable bladder syndrome are easily attributed to a UTI, itself. As a result, many children are treated for recurring UTIs without identification of the underlying condition. Behavioral factors also contribute to the risk of urinary tract infections, particularly in females. These factors include voluntary deferral of micturition and failure to void promptly after coitus. Chronic constipation also is associated commonly with both voiding dysfunction and UTI. Chemical irritation of the urethra from soaps and detergents, masturbation, the presence of foreign bodies in the introitus, and infestation of the bowel with *Enterobius* organisms (pinworms) all have been suggested to increase the frequency of UTIs in girls. Although certain aspects of hygiene, such as "wiping forward" after bowel movements, have been purported to contribute to the risk of UTI in females, there is little objective data to support such notions.

Nonobstructive renal malformations in which there is an increased incidence of UTI include renal hypoplasia/dysplasia, ectopia, and both autosomal dominant and recessive polycystic kidney diseases. The reason for the increased incidence of infection in these conditions is unknown. A number of metabolic disorders also are associated with increased risk of urinary tract infection. Although severe malnutrition is of considerable importance as a contributing factor in UTI worldwide, other disorders associated with an increased incidence of urinary tract infections are hypokalemia, nephrocalcinosis, vitamin A deficiency, diabetes mellitus, and uremia.

CLINICAL FINDINGS

History

Urinary tract infections may occur without symptoms, with symptoms that direct attention to the urinary system, or with symptoms that divert the attention to other organ systems. Thus, the clinician must maintain a high index of suspicion for UTI, particularly in infants and young children with vague or nonspecific infectious symptoms. This concept cannot be overemphasized since, by the time a "first" UTI is diagnosed in a child, preexisting renal scars may already be present, indicating antecedent, previously undetected infection. Nonspecific or extraurinary symptoms occurring commonly in infants include malaise, anorexia, feeding problems, unexplained jaundice, failure to thrive, and fever of unknown origin. In addition, newborns and infants with UTI also may display signs and symptoms referable to the gastrointestinal (GI) system such as diarrhea or vomiting (sometimes so severe as to mimic hypertrophic pyloric stenosis), as well as neurological symptoms, such as irritability, lethargy, or hypertonicity. If present, specific urinary tract symptoms in this age group are often subtle and, therefore, easily overlooked. They include changes of the caliber and force of the urinary stream, dribbling of urine, or diapers that seem constantly wet. In older children, specific urinary tract symptoms are more frequently identified. They include dysuria; urinary frequency or urgency; burning on urination; foul-smelling urine; pain in the abdomen, back, or flank; or development of nocturnal or diurnal enuresis. Nonetheless, the symptoms of UTI, even in older children, may be quite subtle and the infection is discovered only by urine culture.

Many children with covert bacteriuria have recurrent UTIs, renal scars, or symptoms of a dysfunctional bladder. It also has been noted in untreated patients with UTI that fever and urinary symptoms may resolve after several weeks, even though cultures remain positive. Investigators have reported that spontaneous cures in such circumstances are uncommon despite resolution of the symptoms.

The importance of recognizing the role of dysfunctional voiding syndromes in children who have recurrent UTI has already been stated. The history is invaluable in identifying those children at risk. A detailed interview must seek the presence of often subtle (or frequently denied) signs and symptoms, including urinary urgency, squirming, recurring "pain" in the suprapubic area, and primary or secondary daytime enuresis (often with small amounts of urine). Too often, the symptoms pointing to significant bladder dysfunction are attributed to normal child behavior (e.g., "... waits until the last minute ...", "... too busy playing to go...").

Physical Findings

Findings in infants who have a UTI may be normal except for fever and irritability. Older children may report direct tenderness on palpation of the abdomen, suprapubic area, or costovertebral angle (CVA). Patients who have urinary tract obstruction may have palpable abdominal masses, whereas girls with sexually transmitted infections often have a concomitant vulvovaginitis. Examination of the external genitalia should include inspection for vaginal discharge, inflammation of the urethral meatus, and the state of penile and foreskin hygiene. As dictated by clinical circumstances, children who have UTI also may need assessment of their state of hydration, possible sexual abuse, psychiatric or behavioral disorders, and central or peripheral nervous system dysfunction.

Localization of Infection

Sites of infection within the urinary system have been described with "classic" clinical presentations. However, there is a surprising degree of symptom overlap when groups of children who have upper and lower UTI are evaluated. Discussions of the most common ones follow.

The *urethritis* syndrome (with or without fever) may be sudden or insidious in onset but usually varies somewhat in intensity from day to day. The complaints primarily are related to urinary outlet irritation. The patients, usually girls, void small volumes of urine. Prominent symptoms are frequency, urgency, and dysuria. Although microscopic hematuria is common, gross hematuria is unusual, and urinary casts are never seen. Fever is uncommon. Such symptoms usually are attributable to irritation of the vulva. Potential causes of this irritation include bacterial infection (often with repeated low colony counts of single organisms), poor hygiene, vulvitis, vaginitis, chemical irritation (from soaps or bubble bath), foreign bodies, masturbation, urethral trauma (bicycle seat hematuria), and *Enterobius* infestations. In these circumstances, the child has burning on urination because of the urethral or vaginal irritation. This pain causes the child to stop and start the urinary stream, leading to frequent small voidings, hesitancy, and urgency. In boys, such stop-and-start voiding may lead to dilation of the urethra and subsequent microhematuria. Urinalysis may reveal pyuria and bacteriuria as a result of local infection and denudation, although urine cultures still are necessary to identify a bacterial infection.

In the *cystitis* syndrome, the outlet symptoms are more severe, and back and suprapubic pain, as well as fever, may occur. Gross hematuria (without casts) is a common finding. Bacterial infection, particularly with *E. coli,* is the most common cause of this syndrome in girls whereas in boys, adenovirus infection occurs frequently and produces intense dysuria, urinary frequency, and gross or microscopic hematuria. The urine culture will reveal the offending organisms in the former instance and will be sterile in the latter.

In the classic *pyelonephritis* syndrome, the patient has generalized symptoms that may include a toxic appearance, high fever, chills, vomiting, diarrhea, and abdominal pain in addition to the urinary outlet symptoms. However, it is clear that in a significant proportion of patients, neither high fever nor CVA tenderness discriminates uncomplicated cystitis from pyelonephritis. The urinalysis usually reveals typical pyuria and bacteria, and often, white blood cell (WBC) casts are observed. There may be relatively impaired renal concentrating capacity that can persist for 8 to 12 weeks after infection because of medullary dysfunction caused by an ascending infection. Urographic evidence of the loss of renal parenchyma noted in a patient during or shortly after an episode of pyelonephritis indicates *previous* kidney infection or congenital structural maldevelopment, inasmuch as such scars take time to form. Blood cultures should be obtained from ill-appearing patients suspected of having pyelonephritis because bacteremia is common.

LABORATORY AND IMAGING STUDIES

Recent data indicate that, by conventional testing, neither pyuria nor bacteriuria alone have sufficient levels of specificities or positive predictive values to be accurate predictors of the presence or absence of UTI. However, when the urine dipstick is negative for both leukocyte esterase and nitrite, the negative predictive value for UTI may be as high as 98% to 99% in infants and children. Thus, the urinalysis can be useful as a screening test in children undergoing evaluation for infectious illnesses. However, the urinalysis is insufficient documentation alone, and urine cultures are mandatory for the diagnosis of UTI in children.

Urine Culture

Although patient comfort and office efficiency favor collection of urine for culture by the simplest and least painful method, this is difficult to accomplish accurately in very young patients and those who do not yet have voluntary control of urination. In these patients, the use of sterile plastic bags attached to a washed perineum is an unsatisfactory method for obtaining urine for culture because the bags are contaminated easily by skin or fecal bacteria and the time of voiding usually is unknown. Thus, the urine-filled bag may remain attached to the child in a warm environment for a prolonged period. Even in cohorts with a high prior probability of UTI, a single "bagged" urine culture has a positive predictive value of under 20%! The only setting in which such a specimen may be useful is as a screening culture (that turns out to be negative) in a sick infant or young child with a normal urinalysis in whom empirical antibiotic therapy is not prescribed.

BOX 273-2

FACTORS THAT CAN CAUSE LOW COLONY COUNTS DESPITE SIGNIFICANT URINARY INFECTION

High-volume urine flow	Bacteriostatic agents in the urine
Recent antimicrobial therapy	Complete obstruction of a ureter
Fastidious organisms	Chronic or indolent infection
Low urine pH (<5.0) and specific gravity (<1.003)	Use of inappropriate culture techniques

Suprapubic needle aspiration of the bladder and bladder catheterization are far more accurate methods for obtaining urine (1) from very young and not-yet-continent patients, (2) when a urine specimen is urgently needed because of the severity of the illness, and (3) to confirm suspected infection in a child who has had several cultures with equivocal colony counts. Direct bladder aspiration of urine through puncture of aseptically prepared suprapubic skin is safe and reliable (see Appendix B, Special Procedures, for details of this procedure). Any bacterial growth from urine obtained by this method is significant.

Many clinicians find bladder catheterization a preferable alternative to suprapubic aspiration in most clinical circumstances. It is less invasive and better accepted by patients and parents. The smallest bladder catheter or feeding tube possible can be used. Although there is an increased theoretical risk of contamination from skin or distal urethral bacterial flora, in practice this is uncommon when the procedure is done by an experienced individual and the urine specimen is handled appropriately. Catheterization may also be considered more useful than bladder aspiration because it will more likely result in a specimen for culture; if no urine is present upon introduction of the catheter into the bladder, the catheter may be closed with a sterile cap and left in place for a brief time during which further hydration can be provided to generate urine, if necessary.

In children with urinary control, a midstream, clean-catch urine specimen usually suffices. Proper collection of a clean-caught specimen from a girl requires that the sample be obtained after the vaginal vestibule, vulva, and perineum have been cleansed thoroughly with a nonirritating antiseptic solution. The cleaned area should be rinsed with sterile water or saline and gently wiped dry with a sterile towel before voiding. Care should be taken not to get the cleaning solution into the urine culture. Inadvertent contamination by vulvar flora can be further decreased by having the girl sit "backward" on the seat. This often will provide for better labial separation and less contact of urine with external structures. In boys, a midstream urine sample should be obtained after the glans penis has been cleaned with an antiseptic solution, with care taken to retract the foreskin in an uncircumcised individual.

Contamination of the urine collection by bacteria from the external genitalia is the most confounding problem in evaluating a positive urine culture result. An important aspect of obtaining accurate culture results is the handling of the urine after it has been obtained and once it passes from the clinicians to the transport and laboratory personnel. Cultures should be promptly transported on ice to the laboratory and "plated out" as soon as possible. Cultured specimens may be accurate with minimal contaminant growth even after storage for up to 24 hours before plating if kept at 39.2° F (4° C).

Bacterial colony counting has been used as a technique to improve the accuracy of cultures. The diagnosis of bacterial urinary tract infection traditionally is based on a colony count of more than 100,000/ml grown from a clean-caught, midstream urine specimen, or 50,000 colonies/ml from catheterized specimens. Colony counts of this magnitude rely on the premise that bacteria thrive in urine at body temperature and multiply significantly in the bladder before voiding occurs. Certain conditions that may produce low colony counts despite significant infection are given in Box 273-2. Counts below 50,000 colonies/ml from voided specimens most commonly are due to contaminants although consideration of the identity of the isolated organisms also is important. Certain organisms such as enterococci and *S. saprophyticus* grow slowly and thus may be pathogenic when the colony counts are less than the usual values. Single ("pure") isolates are seen more commonly in actual infections, particularly of the acute variety, whereas multiple species found on culture usually indicate contamination. Multiple isolates, however, are more common in recurrent infections or in cultures taken from sites of urinary diversions.

Imaging

Several radiographic studies have been advocated as essential parts of the evaluation of UTI, both for localizing the infection and identifying co-existing urinary tract anomalies. Currently, the three imaging studies most commonly obtained are sonography of the kidneys and bladder, nuclear or contrast (voiding) cystography, and renal scintography using ^{99m}Tc dimercaptosuccinic acid (DMSA), ^{99m}Tc diethylene triamine pentaacetic acid (DTPA), or mercaptoacetyl triglycine (MAG-3). These studies, taken together, provide a good deal of information regarding the structural and infectious state of the urinary system. However, from the clinical decision-making viewpoint, the actual usefulness of performing *all* of these studies in *all* younger children who have UTI is being challenged with increasing frequency. For example, with the common use of prenatal fetal sonography in the United States, it has been proposed that routine sonography in children who have UTI rarely identifies previously undiagnosed significant urinary tract anomalies. This remains controversial and at least for now, sonographic imaging of the kidneys and urinary system, particularly in younger children and those who have recurring UTI, remains advisable. Many clinicians no longer are obtaining routine DMSA renal scans at the time of an acute, febrile UTI. Rather, in the at-risk child, information regarding the development of renal scars can be obtained by performing this study at least 4 to 6 months after the episode of clinical pyelonephritis. It gener-

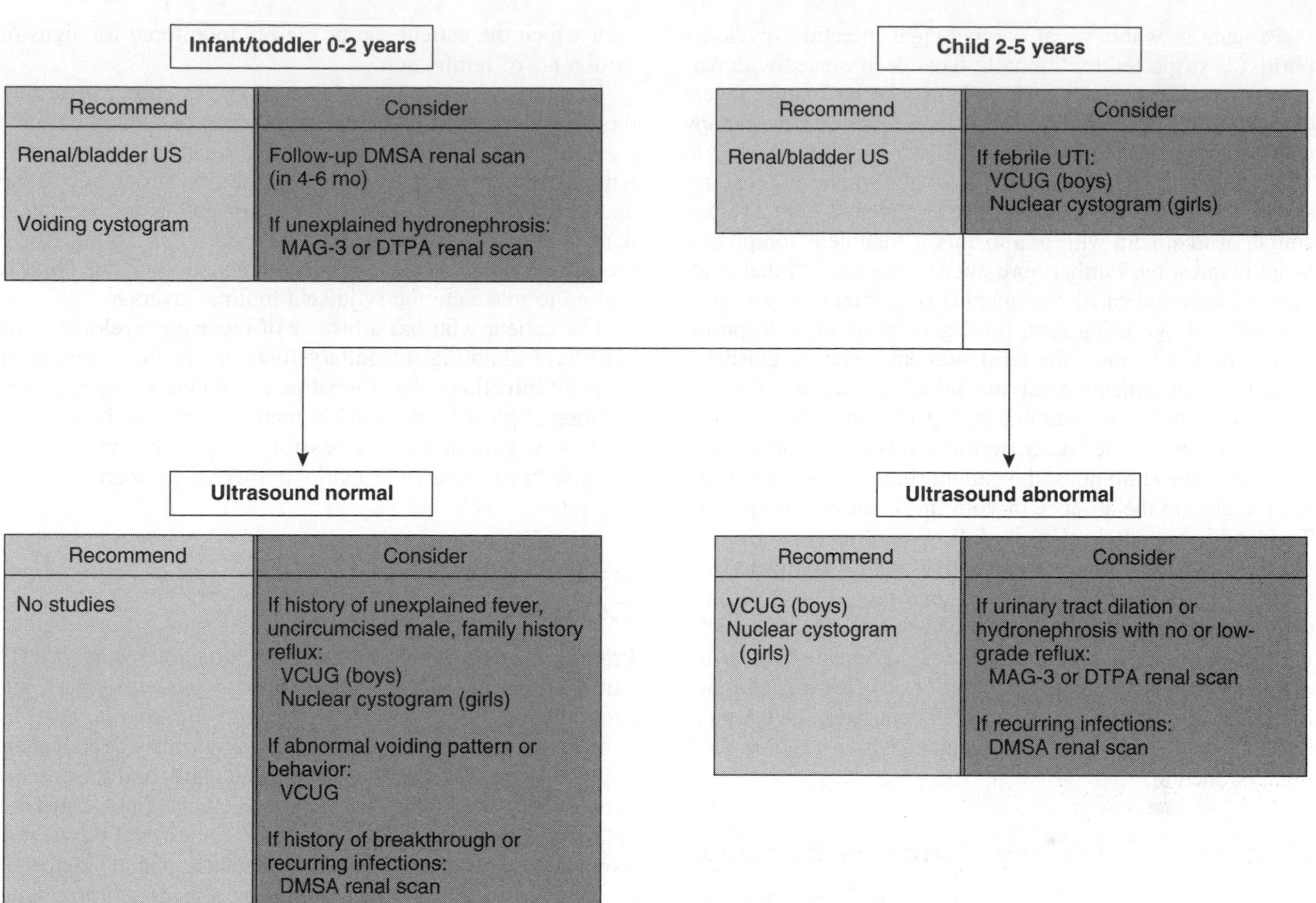

Fig. 273-1 General guidelines for imaging studies for patients who have UTI.

ally is agreed that there is an increased risk of upper urinary tract infection among patients with vesicoureteral reflux. However, young infants who have normal bladder and upper tract anatomy by sonography frequently are treated empirically with antimicrobial prophylaxis for 6 to 12 months following an episode of pyelonephritis given the suspected risk of UTI recurrence. In addition, although reflux is a risk factor for pyelonephritis, acutely abnormal DMSA renal scans have been demonstrated in similar proportions of infected children who do or do not have reflux. Therefore, the discovery of low-grade reflux would not alter the initial medical management. Thus, it could be concluded that in such patients the cystogram could be deferred until the time a decision is made as to continuing or not continuing prophylaxis.

Considering the aforementioned reasons, as well as the differences of the clinical course and co-existing risk factors in individual patients, specific algorithms for imaging studies are difficult to develop. The diagram in Fig. 273-1 does provide some general guidelines for infants and young children. Prepubescent children over the age of 5 to 7 years with first infections should undergo renal/bladder sonography screening. Further investigations are based on sonogram findings and the presence or absence of co-existing risk factors. For children who require a cystogram, if delayed only 1 week, the timing of the study with regard to the infection does not appear to affect the results.

TREATMENT

The goals of treatment are to eradicate the infection in a timely manner, address and treat any significant anatomical or functional abnormalities, and prevent recurrences. Achieving these goals requires the cooperation of the parents and the patient in diagnostic evaluation and treatment.

In cases of symptomatic acute UTI, treatment may begin before culture data are available. Oral treatment with trimethoprim-sulfamethoxazole or third-generation cephalosporins are reasonable choices for most children who have uncomplicated lower UTI, because most first bacterial UTIs are caused by *E. coli*. Ampicillin monotherapy must be used with caution because some surveys show that nearly half of the *E. coli* cultured in UTI are ampicillin resistant. The antibiotic sensitivities of the initial urine culture are useful in deciding whether to change the initial drug choice. If the patient does not improve clinically, a repeat urine culture should be done 48 to 72 hours after beginning therapy. If the initial culture is sterile, antibiotics should be discontinued and causes other than a bacterial infection considered. Most uncomplicated initial UTIs are effectively treated with a 7- to 10-day antibiotic course. Although acceptance of shorter courses of therapy in children remains controversial, increasing numbers of studies are demonstrating comparative efficacy of 3-day courses to the longer initial treatment regimens.

Patients in whom renal parenchymal infection (pyelonephritis) is suspected traditionally have been treated with parenteral antibiotics. Except for patients who have more severe clinical illness, the duration rather than route of drug therapy appears to be more important. Most patients older than 2 to 3 months of age who have a good 48-hour clinical response to parenteral antibiotics can complete a 12- to 14-day course of treatment with oral agents if treatment compliance is not in question. Furthermore, recent data suggest that treatment of uncomplicated pyelonephritis in infants as young as 2 months of age using oral, third-generation cephalosporins results in short- and long-term outcomes indistinguishable from those in patients receiving initial intravenous therapy. Nitrofurantoin is not a suitable therapeutic agent for pyelonephritis because tissue bacteriostatic levels are suboptimal. In addition to the antibiotics, the patient should have a good oral fluid intake (in the absence of vomiting) and void frequently. To identify potential relapses, follow-up cultures should be obtained within 1 to 2 weeks after treatment is completed and several repeat screening urine cultures should be performed over the subsequent several months to identify patients who have covert bacteriuria. In this case, the sensitivities of the organism are useful in the selection of an effective antibiotic if clinical reinfection occurs. Also, patients who have asymptomatic bacteriuria should be evaluated for co-existing voiding dysfunction.

Recurrent Urinary Tract Infections

Recurrent UTIs are most common in girls. Most often, their symptoms are associated with fever, but as already mentioned, they can develop insidiously. When UTIs recur, approximately 50% do so within the first year and another 25% during the second year. The risk of recurrence within 2 years of the first infection is 80% in white girls and 60% in black girls. The reason for this racial difference is unclear.

As previously mentioned, infections may recur, particularly in the absence of structural urinary tract abnormalities, in children who have asymptomatic bacteriuria and/or dysfunctional voiding syndromes. Many of these children will have little improvement of their UTI recurrences from antibiotic treatment regimens until the treatment focuses on management of the functional disturbance as well. Depending on the clinical characteristics of the voiding dysfunction, therapy often requires the addition of voiding behavior modification/bladder "rehabilitation" measures and/or an agent, such as oxybutynin, to attenuate uninhibited bladder contractions.

In a child with a history of recurring UTI, the frequency of infections may be reduced substantially by using long-term antibiotic prophylactic therapy. The drugs of choice for patients older than 2 months of age are trimethoprim-sulfamethoxazole (2 mg/kg/day given once at bedtime) or nitrofurantoin (1 to 2 mg/kg/day given once at bedtime). These drugs have excellent antibacterial spectra for the more common urinary pathogens, are rapidly absorbed and excreted in the urine and, in low doses, are not generally associated with alterations of GI bacterial resistance. In the absence of urinary reflux, other underlying risk factors, and renal scars, prophylaxis can be continued for 6 to 12 months after which the patient can be closely monitored for signs or symptoms of reinfection.

Recently, a resurgence of interest has occurred regarding the possible benefit of cranberry juice in patients who have recurring UTI, based on a proposed mechanism whereby certain constituents in the juice attenuate bacterial adherence and hence virulence of *E. coli* urinary pathogens. Although data thus far are insufficient to support this notion, there seems to be little to deter this recommendation if the child is willing to make cranberry juice a routine beverage.

The patient who has a history of recurring pyelonephritis may have abnormal medullary function. In more severe or frequent infection-related renal parenchymal damage, abnormalities of glucose and sodium reabsorption may be present, as well as permanent and possibly progressive impairment of renal function as reflected by a lowered glomerular filtration rate.

PSYCHOSOCIAL CONSIDERATIONS

Prompt diagnosis and treatment of serious or recurring UTI can decrease the risk of UTI-associated sequelae. Thus, appropriate ongoing monitoring and treatment program compliance is essential for the short- and long-term success of therapy. The patient (if old enough to understand) and the parents should be advised of the treatment plan (including the follow-up cultures) and have some understanding of the overall goals of management so that a maximal degree of cooperation may be elicited. This should be done frankly but in a way that does not create undue anxiety. The need to complete the full course of antibiotics and the reasons for the long follow-up with cultures should be stressed. Patients and parents should agree that urine cultures will be obtained when fevers that have no apparent origin occur.

REFERRAL

Patients who have complex clinical conditions, recurring infections, or suboptimal treatment response often benefit from consultation with, or ongoing collaborative management by an experienced pediatric nephrologist or pediatric urologist. Although some urological abnormalities require surgical correction, the primary care physician should be aware that many childhood urinary structural disorders are equally well managed by nonsurgical means. Under most circum-

When to Refer

Patients who have the following conditions can benefit from consultation with a pediatric nephrologist or a pediatric urologist (depending on local expertise):

- The occurrence of complex or recurring upper or lower UTI
- Those who have suspected voiding dysfunction complicating UTI
- Evaluation and recommendations regarding structural urinary tract abnormalities identified on initial radiographic evaluation

When to Hospitalize

Treatment of suspected pyelonephritis in an infant younger than 3 months of age or patients who have clinical urosepsis
Patients who have clinical pyelonephritis whose symptoms worsen despite 24 hours of appropriate antibiotics or those not significantly improved within 48 to 72 hours
For initiation of parenteral therapy if home treatment compliance is in question

stances, the primary care physician can implement and monitor the treatment plan developed in conjunction with the consultant. Thus, the frequency of required return visits to the consultant can be kept to a minimum while maximizing patient convenience and quality of care.

SUGGESTED READINGS

American Academy of Pediatrics, Committee on Quality Improvement, Subcommittee on Urinary Tract Infection: Practice parameter: the diagnosis, treatment, and evaluation of the initial urinary tract infection in febrile infants and young children, *Pediatrics* 103:843, 1999.

Hellerstein S: Urinary tract infections in children: why they occur and how to prevent them, *Am Fam Physician* 57:2440, 1998.

Hoberman A, et al: Oral vs initial intravenous therapy for urinary tract infections in young febrile children, *Pediatrics* 104:79, 1999.

Hoberman A, et al: Prevalence of urinary tract infection in febrile infants, *J Pediatr* 123:17, 1993.

Majd M, et al: Relationship among vesicoureteral reflux, P-fimbriated *Escherichia coli,* and acute pyelonephritis in children with febrile urinary tract infection, *J Pediatr* 119:578, 1991.

Shapiro E, et al: The office management of recurrent urinary tract infections and vesicoureteral reflux in children, *Urol Clin North Am* 25:725, 1998.

Sharief N, et al: Use of rapid dipstick tests to exclude urinary tract infection in children, *Br J Biomed Sci* 55:242, 1998.

Zhanel GG, et al: Asymptomatic bacteriuria: which patients should be treated? *Arch Intern Med* 150:1389, 1990.

274 Verrucae (Warts)

Judith V. Williams • Donald P. Lookingbill

ETIOLOGY

Warts are virus-induced tumors of the skin.[2,6,7] The wart virus is a human papillomavirus[2,7] (HPV) that infects epidermal cells and causes focal epidermal proliferation, expressed clinically as a verrucous papule.

In recent years, deoxyribonucleic acid (DNA) hybridization analysis has been used to identify different types of human papillomaviruses. To date, more than 60 types have been characterized, and the number continues to grow. Specific DNA types have been associated with specific warts. For example, HPV type 1 (HPV-1) is found in plantar warts, HPV-2 and HPV-4 in common warts, HPV-3 and HPV-10 in flat warts, HPV-6 and HPV-11 in "benign" genital warts and laryngeal papillomas, and HPV-16 and HPV-18 in genital warts that have malignant potential (e.g., cervical carcinoma). Thus, HPV typing holds promise in helping to identify premalignant warts as well as sources of the transmission of warts.[7,12]

EPIDEMIOLOGY

The wart virus presumably is inoculated into the skin from some external source, but neither the source nor the event of inoculation usually is elicitable. Frogs and toads have been unfairly incriminated as carriers.[15] It is reasonable, however, to ask about and search for warts on other areas of the body; for example, patients who have warts on their lips often have them on their fingers. Because warts are transmissible, other family members also may have them.

In young infants, warts (including those in laryngeal and genital locations) are assumed to have been acquired from the mother's vaginal tract during delivery. Genital warts in children raise the possibility of sexual abuse.[4,14] However, several recent studies of anogenital warts in children found no evidence of sexual abuse in most of the subjects under the age of 3 years.[8,12] Based on HPV typing, anogenital HPV infection in most infants appears to be acquired either by nonsexual transmission or perinatally through an infected birth canal.[8,12] The latter process also may result in the acquisition of laryngeal papillomas. A careful social history and physical examination may be helpful in determining the need for further evaluation for possible sexual abuse.

Patients who have systemic defects in self-mediated immunity are more susceptible to warts, which often are recalcitrant to treatment.[1] Also, because cellular immune responses in the skin are impaired with atopic dermatitis, these patients, too, have more difficulty with warts and other viral infections of the skin.

PHYSICAL FINDINGS

The clinical appearance of warts varies, depending on the type and the location on the skin. The common wart, or verruca vulgaris, is easily recognized as a superficial, light-colored papule that has a coarse, roughened surface. Warts often are studded with black specks, which many patients call "seeds" but which actually are small, superficial dermal capillaries. Warts sometimes are found in linear array, presumably as a result of autoinoculation through scratching. Not all warts appear as verrucous papules. Variants include flat (planar) warts, plantar warts, periungual warts, and anogenital warts.

LABORATORY FINDINGS

Warts almost always are diagnosed clinically. If there is doubt, a skin biopsy can provide histological confirmation.

DIFFERENTIAL DIAGNOSIS

The distinctive clinical appearance of the common wart usually presents no problem in diagnosis. Epidermal nevi, which are hamartomas, may be confused with warts, but they usually are softer, more pigmented, more persistent, and much less common. Flat (planar) warts appear as small, flesh-colored papules (Fig. 274-1). When located on the face, they often are confused with the closed comedones (whiteheads) seen in acne. On very close inspection, however, flat warts are seen to have sharp borders and a finely verrucous surface, whereas closed comedones are smooth, dome-shaped lesions.

Plantar warts are so named because they appear on the plantar surface of the foot (Fig. 274-2). They often are confused with calluses and corns, although corns are much less common in children than are warts. Large plantar warts often are composed of confluent smaller ones, which form a mosaic wart around which satellite lesions often occur. Additionally, plantar warts differ from corns by having a verrucous surface that interrupts the skin markings and often is punctuated with black specks. Sometimes the two entities can be distinguished only by paring down the surface; wart

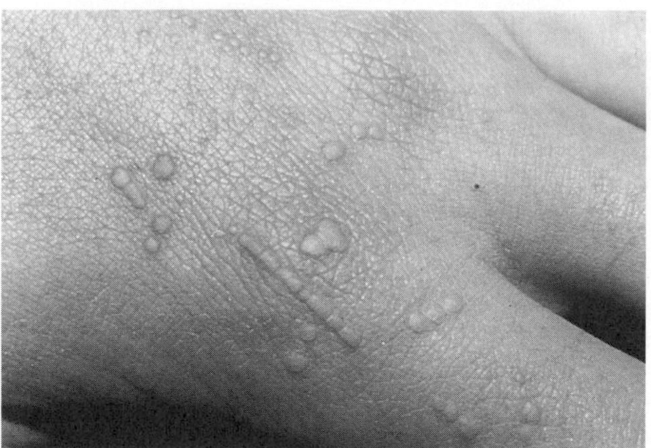

Fig. 274-1 Flat warts. The streaks of warts are due to autoinoculation from scratching. When smaller and located on the face, flat warts may be confused with comedones.

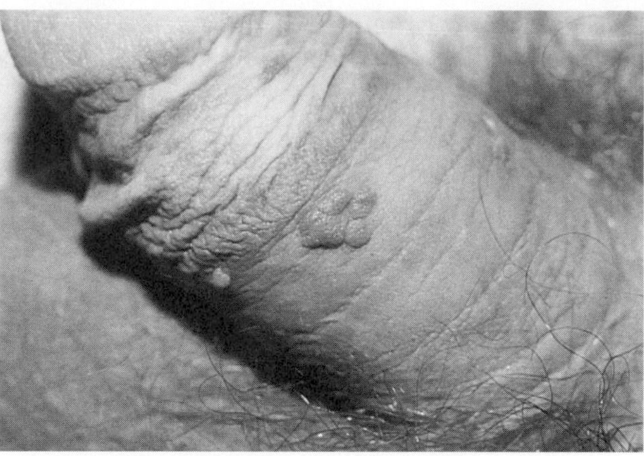

Fig. 274-3 Condylomata acuminata, shown here as verrucous papules on the penis.

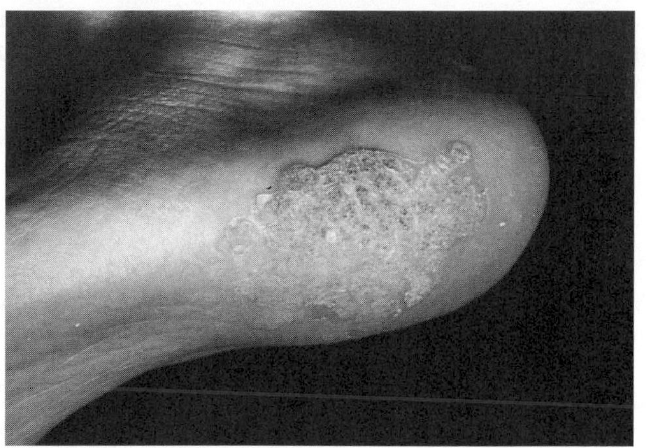

Fig. 274-2 A mosaic plantar wart with a roughened surface punctuated with black specks.

tissue still has a roughened texture, whereas a corn is smooth. A corn also becomes smaller in diameter as it is pared; a wart does not.

Periungual warts that occur around the nail fold should not pose diagnostic difficulty. Warts under the free edge of the nail, however, can cause the nail plate to separate from the nail bed and may be confused with a fungal infection. On close inspection, the verrucous nature of the wart usually can be appreciated.

Anogenital warts (condylomata acuminata) sometimes, but not always, are acquired by sexual contact.[8,12,14] They usually can be identified easily as verrucous papules (Fig. 274-3), but sometimes they are small and/or flat and therefore more difficult to see. In this situation the acetowhitening technique can aid in the diagnosis. A compress of 5% acetic acid is applied for several minutes to the suspected area, which then is reexamined, ideally under magnification. With this technique, warty tissue turns white and, thus, is visualized more easily.

Genital warts may be confused with the less common condylomata lata, which are skin lesions found in secondary syphilis. In general, condylomata acuminata are drier and usually more verrucous than condylomata lata, which are flat and moist. If there is doubt, a serological test for syphilis should settle the issue.

PSYCHOSOCIAL CONSIDERATIONS

Among schoolchildren, warts often are a focus for teasing and insensitive remarks. Consequently, when children ask that their warts be treated, they usually do so because of social pressure. Successful therapy gives patients the opportunity to feel better about themselves and their appearance.

MANAGEMENT

Over the years a wide variety of treatments have been recommended, including some interesting unscientific approaches (such as applying banana peels or slices of raw potato), which probably "worked" because most warts eventually regress spontaneously. One recent prospective study of untreated common warts in children showed that two thirds of the warts underwent spontaneous regression within 2 years.[7] This must be kept in mind when physicians credit their treatment for a successful result. Nonetheless, when a patient requests treatment of a wart, practitioners usually are inclined to oblige. However, because a specific antiviral medication for warts has not yet been developed, nonspecific destructive techniques still are relied on as therapy; the following are the most commonly used techniques.

Cryotherapy

Tissue is frozen by applying liquid nitrogen (−195° C) to the wart either with a swab or by means of a cannister delivery system. The freezing should extend beyond the wart to include a 1- to 2-mm rim of normal skin. To destroy tissue better, the wart may be refrozen after the initial thaw. The patient must be advised that the frozen area will be sore for several days, that a blister may form, and that it usually takes several weeks for the wart to turn dark and "drop off." This is a favorite office therapy for common warts. For small warts, a single treatment often is successful, but large warts frequently need to be refrozen at about 3-week intervals. Scars may result but are uncommon. The skin also may become hypopigmented. In freezing warts on the fingers, care must be taken not to freeze too deeply, because underlying structures such as digital nerves can be damaged.

Electrodesiccation and Laser Therapy

Electrodesiccation of a wart can be preceded or followed by curettage. One advantage of this technique is that the patient leaves the office without visible evidence of the wart, although the cure rate probably is no higher than with cryotherapy. The disadvantages are that the procedure must be preceded by injection of a local anesthetic, and scarring is more likely. The carbon dioxide laser can be used to destroy large or refractory warts, but the risk of scarring is significant. The pulsed dye laser, which destroys the vascular component of the wart, may prove to be another alternative, with less risk of scarring. It is used for some recalcitrant warts, particularly in palmar/plantar and periungual locations.[10]

Acid Therapy

Acid therapy is slower and involves more patient participation, but it is less immediately painful and is least likely to cause scarring. A variety of acids are available for treating warts. A convenient outpatient medication incorporates 17% salicylic acid in a polyacrylic or flexible collodion vehicle (Occlusal-HP and Duofilm). The vehicle dries rapidly to prevent spread of the acid onto surrounding skin. The patient is instructed to put the medication on the wart at bedtime and to cover the area with a bandage. At the end of each week, superficial necrotic tissue should be pared. This usually can be done at home either with a pumice stone or an emery board. Because of its minimal discomfort, this approach is useful with multiple warts and those on very young children. Plantar warts often require a stronger acid, such as a 40% salicylic acid plaster. These can be bought over the counter (Mediplast and Duofilm patch), but the patient needs instruction in application. A piece of plaster the size of the wart is cut, and the adhesive, medicated side is applied to the wart and held in place with tape. The plaster is changed every 24 hours and the macerated wart pared weekly, as already described.

Flat warts often are treated successfully with vitamin A acid (Retin A), which probably acts as a "peeling" agent in this situation. Retin A gel or liquid is applied nightly to the entire affected area. Painful irritation may occur, necessitating less frequent use.

These home acid therapies usually require a minimum of a month of continuous use to be effective. If no progress has been made after several months, other treatments should be considered. For deeply seeded warts, paring, followed by a combination of acid and cryotherapy, usually provides successful treatment. Caustic acids such as trichloroacetic acid at concentrations of 30% to 100% are reserved for office treatment of palmar or plantar warts. They must be carefully applied, because they can cause destruction of normal tissue as well. Cantharidin is a vesiculating agent derived from the blister beetle and can be used for almost all nongenital warts.[10] Repeat application may be required at 1- to 3-week intervals. It has the advantage of being painless when initially applied, and causes little risk of scarring. Occasionally a "ring wart" will develop at the edge of the treated site.

The efficacy of oral cimetidine in the treatment of warts is still controversial.[3,9,11,13,18] It may be useful in the treatment of flat warts at a dose of about 40 mg/kg/day for up to 2 months.[11] Its use in other types of warts is under investigation.

All these treatments are nonspecific, and none is foolproof. Sometimes, different modalities are used in sequence. Although warts commonly regress spontaneously, the time required for this varies considerably. In some patients, therapy may only serve to appease the patient while nature takes its course; in others, perhaps the destructive techniques initiate an inflammatory reaction, exposing the wart viral antigen to the body's immune system, which finally rejects the wart. This may explain the phenomenon observed by some, wherein by "treating the mother wart, the baby goes away." In any event, whenever warts are treated, the physician must guard against doing harm by being overzealous. Accordingly, surgical excision usually should be discouraged, and radiotherapy is contraindicated.

TREATMENT OF GENITAL WARTS

Although condylomata in children usually are asymptomatic, they may be treated to curtail their spread and to allay parental concerns. None of the accepted therapeutic options has been systematically studied in children, nor has been approved by the Food and Drug Administration (FDA) for use in pediatric patients.[16] Several forms of therapy may be painful, and recurrence rates may be as high as 50%. It is wise to weigh the risks versus the benefits before treating genital warts in children.

Podophyllin is derived from the May apple plant and is available in 10% to 25% solutions in alcohol or benzoin. It is exclusively for office use. It is painless when applied but can be toxic if used over large areas. It must be washed off within 4 to 6 hours of application. Purified 0.5% podophyllotoxin solution or gel (Condylox) is FDA approved for the treatment of condylomata in adults. It is available for home use but can be very irritating for some patients. Imiquimod is an immune-response modifier that induces a variety of cytokines.[5] It is available in a 5% cream that is effective in some patients who have genital warts. Other options for treatment of condylomata include cryotherapy, lasers, caustic acids, and cimetidine.

COMPLICATIONS

The major complications of warts are those caused by overzealous therapy, resulting in short-term discomfort or scarring. The annoyance of the presence of a wart, which usually is temporary, must be balanced against a scar, which usually is lifelong, may be unsightly, and sometimes is tender, particularly if present on a pressure-bearing surface such as the sole of the foot.

PROGNOSIS

As already mentioned, most warts eventually involute spontaneously, probably through immunological rejection.[1] Because the time required for this varies greatly, it is impossible to predict for an individual patient when this might occur. The goal of therapy, then, is to shorten the time it takes for the wart to disappear. The therapies outlined in this chapter result in clearing in most cases, but patients who have resistant, persistent warts will continue to be plagued by them. It is especially for these patients that more specific therapy is needed.

When to Refer

If child older than 3 years of age has genital warts
Unresponsive/persistent or extensive warts of any type

REFERENCES

1. Adler A, Safai B: Immunity in wart resolution, *J Am Acad Dermatol* 1:305, 1979.
2. Androphy EJ: Human papillomavirus: current concepts, *Arch Dermatol* 125:683, 1989.
3. Bauman C, et al: Cimetidine therapy for multiple viral warts in children, *J Am Acad Dermatol* 35:271, 1996.
4. Bender ME: New concepts of condylomata acuminata in children, *Arch Dermatol* 122:1121, 1986.
5. Beutner KR, et al: Treatment of genital warts with an immune-response modifier (imiquimod), *J Am Acad Dermatol* 38:230, 1998.
6. Birkett DA: Warts and their management, *Practitioner* 226:1251, 1982.
7. Cobb MW: Human papillomavirus infection, *J Am Acad Dermatol* 22: 547, 1990.
8. Cohen BA, Honig P, Androphy E: Anogenital warts in children: clinical and virologic evaluation for sexual abuse, *Arch Dermatol* 126:1575, 1990.
9. Glass AT, Solomon BA: Cimetidine therapy for recalcitrant warts in adults, *Arch Dermatol* 132:680, 1996.
10. Goldfarb MT, et al: Office therapy for human papillomavirus infection in nongenital sites, *Dermatol Clin* 9:287, 1991.
11. Karablut AA, Sahin S, Eksioglu M: Is cimetidine effective for nongenital warts? A double-blind, placebo-controlled study, *Arch Dermatol* 133: 533, 1997.
12. Obalek S, et al: Condylomata acuminata in children: frequent association with human papillomaviruses responsible for cutaneous warts, *J Am Acad Dermatol* 23:205, 1990.
13. Orlow SJ, PallerA: Cimetidine therapy for multiple viral warts in children, *J Am Acad Dermatol* 28:794, 1993.
14. Rock B, et al: Genital tract papillomavirus infection in children, *Arch Dermatol* 122:1129, 1986.
15. Ross MS: Warts in the medical folklore of Europe, *Int J Dermatol* 18:505, 1979.
16. Siegfried EC, Frasier LD: Anogenital warts in children, *Adv Dermatol* 12:141, 1997.
17. Webster GF, et al: Treatment of recalcitrant warts using the pulsed dye laser, *Cutis* 56:230, 1995.
18. Yilmaz E, Alpsoy E, Bajaran E: Cimetidine therapy for warts: a placebo-controlled, double-blind study, *J Am Acad Dermatol* 34:1005, 1996.

part nine

Critical Situations

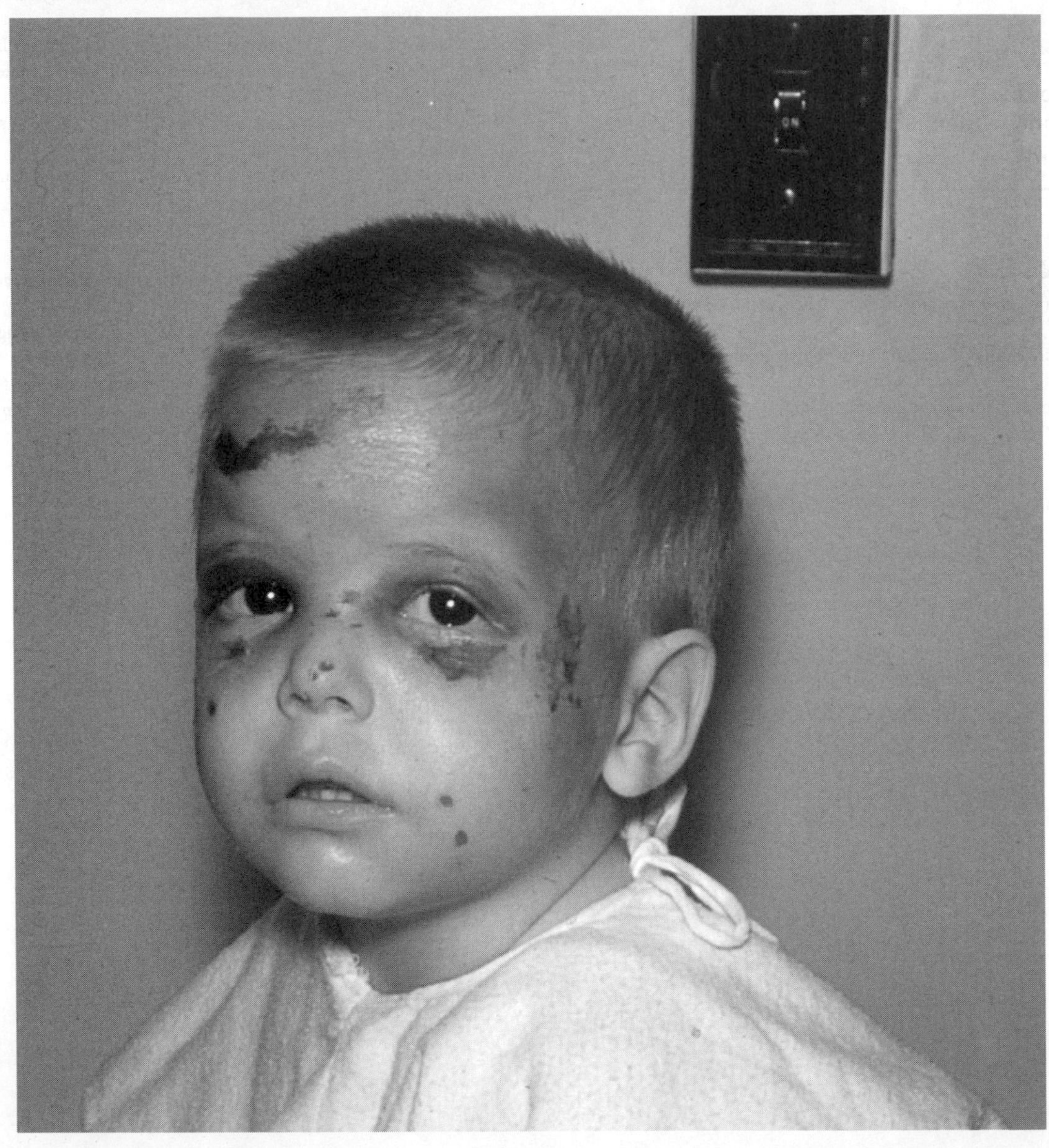

275 Airway Obstruction

Steven E. Lucking

Acute upper airway obstruction presents an immediate threat to life. Because of the fourth-power relationship between airway diameter and airway resistance, the same amount of airway encroachment or edema in millimeters causes a far greater physiological obstruction in a child than in an adult.[13] Inspiratory stridor (a high-pitched sound) is the hallmark of upper airway obstruction. This is not to say, however, that upper airway obstruction cannot occur in the absence of stridor, because profound degrees of obstruction may manifest silently if airflow is nearly absent. When confronted with a child who has acute upper airway obstruction, the practitioner must assess the degree of obstruction quickly and accurately. The possibility of progression to complete airway obstruction with hypoxemia and cardiac arrest must be appreciated.[5] Delaying intervention in a child whose airway is unstable may be costly, but unnecessary instrumentation in a child who has stable upper airway obstruction may precipitate a crisis.

The cause of death in patients who have airway obstruction is progressive hypoxemia and cardiac arrest causing brain damage. Thus, the immediate concern when first assessing the child is to provide oxygen and assess the degree of oxygen saturation. A previously healthy infant or child can tolerate significant degrees of hypercapnia without end-organ damage. In addition, the degree of hypercapnia can vary over a matter of minutes as a result of factors such as the child's level of agitation, the degree of airway obstruction, the response to palliative therapies, and the onset of fatigue. For these reasons, arterial blood gas (ABG) measurement, which provides an assessment of only one moment in time, generally is not considered sufficiently worthwhile to warrant the amount of distress it causes the child.

HISTORY AND PHYSICAL EXAMINATION

The clinician first should assess the child's level of distress from a distance so as not to agitate the child. One useful approach is to obtain a brief history from the parents or caretaker while merely observing the child. The parents also can be asked to remove the child's clothes to facilitate a quicker assessment of the patient's general appearance. The physician should attempt to obtain as complete an assessment as possible in the least threatening manner because agitation and crying worsen the relative degree of airway obstruction and the attendant work of breathing. After noting all physical signs that do not require direct physical contact with the patient, the examiner should gently approach the child to auscultate the chest and assess the circulation.

The child's appearance gives important clues to the degree of respiratory compromise. The degree of the child's anxiety can be an important clue to the severity of the airway obstruction. Many children who have croup appear quite calm and contented sitting in their parent's arms when not being "threatened" by an examiner. Although these children may have significant stridor, their level of comfort indicates that they are not significantly hypoxic or hypercarbic. Conversely, a child who remains persistently anxious or who has become somnolent to the point of no longer interacting with those around him may be significantly hypoxic or hypercarbic.

Use of accessory muscles indicates the degree of inspiratory effort. Stridor needs to be assessed in the context of the inspiratory breath sounds. Generally, stridor becomes less loud as airway obstruction lessens. However, in extreme cases, stridor may become barely audible as inspiratory flow almost ceases. It is the quality of the inspiratory breath sounds that differentiates improvement (breath sounds clearly heard) from rapid deterioration (breath sounds barely audible) as the reason for diminishing stridor. Respiratory rate has been reasonably well correlated with hypoxemia, but little correlation has been established with hypercapnia.[10] Currently, the degree of hypoxemia is easily assessed by pulse oximetry monitoring, which most children tolerate well. In the differential diagnosis of acute infectious upper airway obstruction, the presence of fever, drooling, or cough,[8] a forward-leaning posture, or the appearance of toxicity is useful in leading toward a specific diagnosis and approach to therapy (see Chapters 277, Croup [Acute Laryngotracheobronchitis], and 284, Epiglottitis).

Various scoring systems have been proposed to aid in assessing the degree of upper airway obstruction. Such systems help focus observation and provide a guide to the effects of therapy (Table 275-1).

DIFFERENTIAL DIAGNOSIS OF AIRWAY OBSTRUCTION

Upper airway obstruction in children can be categorized according to certain features of the presentation and history (Box 275-1).

Early Infancy

Abnormalities of the airway may manifest with airway obstruction and stridor starting early in infancy and occasion-

Table 275-1 Scoring System for Assessing the Severity of Upper Airway Obstruction

Sign	Score*
Stridor	
None	0
Inspiratory	1
Inspiratory and expiratory	2
Cough	
None	0
Hoarse cry	1
Bark	2
Retractions and nasal flaring	
None	0
Flaring and suprasternal retractions	1
Flaring plus suprasternal, subcostal, and intercostal retractions	2
Cyanosis	
None	0
In room air	1
In 40% oxygen	2
Inspiratory breath sounds	
Normal	0
Harsh, with wheezing or ronchi	1
Delayed	2

From Downes JJ, Goldberg AI: Airway management, mechanical ventilation, and cardiopulmonary resuscitation. In Scarpelli EM, Auld PAM, Goldman HS, editors: *Pulmonary disease of the fetus, newborn, and child,* Philadelphia, 1978, Lea & Febiger.

*A score of 4 or higher indicates significant airway obstruction.

BOX 275-1

CAUSES OF AIRWAY OBSTRUCTION

Congenital Causes
Craniofacial dysmorphism
Hemangioma
Laryngeal cleft/web
Laryngoceles, cysts
Laryngomalacia
Macroglossia
Tracheal stenosis
Vascular ring
Vocal cord paralysis

Acquired Infectious Causes
Acute laryngotracheobronchitis
Bacterial tracheitis
Diphtheria
Epiglottitis
Laryngeal papillomatosis
Mononucleosis
Retropharyngeal abscess
Spasmodic croup

Acquired Noninfectious Causes
Anaphylaxis
Angioneurotic edema
Foreign-body aspiration
Supraglottic hypotonia
Thermal/chemical burn
Trauma
Vocal cord paralysis

ally in the immediate newborn period. Laryngomalacia is the single most common cause of stridor that begins in early infancy.[11] Most patients have a history of stridor that is audible whenever the child is excited, agitated, or crying, beginning from the first days of life. This is a developmental disorder in that the "floppy" larynx becomes more rigid and less obstructing with time. Endoscopically, the epiglottis is seen to fold over the larynx on inspiration. Another finding is varying degrees of prolapse of the arytenoid cartilages into the center of the larynx on inspiration. These infants typically may have feeding problems, and the stridor often worsens with minor respiratory tract infections. Through continuous noninvasive monitoring, it has been demonstrated that infants who have laryngomalacia are more likely than age-matched controls to have transient episodes of hypoxemia and hypercapnia, although none of the episodes was life threatening.[9] Because the disorder improves over time, these infants rarely require an artificial airway.

Unilateral or bilateral vocal cord paralysis may occur in otherwise healthy newborns and has been associated with birth trauma. However, vocal cord paralysis also may be associated with other neurological diseases and increased intracranial pressure.[11] In an otherwise healthy child whose vocal cord paralysis is thought to be due to birth trauma, improvement over time is the rule.

Craniofacial dysmorphism (as in Pierre Robin and Treacher Collins syndromes) causes stridor as a result of micrognathia with posterior displacement of the tongue. Macroglossia (as in Beckwith-Wiedemann syndrome, congenital hypothyroidism, glycogen storage diseases, Down syndrome, and other conditions) also may cause stridor in the newborn period.

Congenital laryngeal webs and subglottic stenosis may cause critical airway obstruction in the immediate newborn period. Some of these children may not be diagnosed correctly at presentation because endotracheal intubation in the newborn period not only provides a lifesaving airway but also temporarily corrects the abnormality. With subsequent scarring, the child may manifest the condition again later in infancy during an upper respiratory tract infection.

Vascular rings and slings may cause some degree of airway obstruction in infancy.[11] An infant who has a vascular ring may have persistent wheezing if the obstruction is in the lower trachea near the carina. Conversely, the major symptom may be stridor if the obstruction is higher up in the extrathoracic trachea.

Laryngeal clefts are uncommon and may manifest with either stridor or symptoms of recurrent aspiration. Congenital cysts and laryngoceles also are uncommon causes of stridor in early infancy. Congenital tracheal stenosis, a rare disorder, has an extreme form in which the entire trachea may have circumferential cartilaginous rings much like lobar and segmental bronchi.

Hemangiomas may develop at any level of the airway in

infancy, and these may be associated with cutaneous hemangiomas. Corticosteroids (systemic or intralesional) may promote shrinkage, although the hemangiomas generally regress spontaneously after the infant is 1 year old.

Acquired Infectious Causes of Airway Obstruction

The most common cause of acute infectious airway obstruction is viral laryngotracheobronchitis (croup). The typical patient is between 3 months and 4 years of age, has had a preceding upper respiratory tract infection, and has a barking cough and loud inspiratory stridor (see Chapter 277, Croup [Acute Laryngotracheobronchitis]). Bacterial tracheitis, also called *membranous laryngotracheobronchitis,* is becoming the most common cause of acute infectious upper airway obstruction, culminating in respiratory failure and requiring referral to a tertiary care pediatric intensive care unit. The consensus is that this condition represents a bacterial superinfection of viral croup.[4] The most common offending agents are *Staphylococcus aureus* and *Moraxella catarrhalis,* although *Streptococcus* and *Haemophilus* organisms have been implicated. The patient initially has a crouplike illness that progresses in severity, with rising fever and increasing toxicity, culminating in respiratory failure, with thick, purulent secretions noted upon intubation. This disorder usually is diagnosed at the time of intubation when the child's condition progresses to respiratory failure. Contrary to initial reports, tracheostomy generally is not necessary for treatment, and mortality should be very uncommon in children who have not suffered cardiac arrest before admission to an appropriate intensive care setting. Acute spasmodic croup manifests with recurrent nighttime onset of inspiratory stridor and croupy cough. Patients generally are afebrile, and episodes are short-lived.

Retropharyngeal abscess is a relatively rare infectious cause of stridor in children. It usually involves high fever and difficulty swallowing, with airway obstruction to a lesser degree.

Acute epiglottitis has been seen far less frequently in the past 10 years, most probably the result of the development of effective vaccines. It most commonly is due to infection with *Haemophilus influenzae* type b and may occur at any age, including in adulthood (see Chapter 284, Epiglottitis).

Acute infectious mononucleosis may cause significant upper airway obstruction as a result of tonsillar hypertrophy. This condition rarely leads to respiratory failure, and the airway obstruction generally responds promptly to a short course of corticosteroids. Laryngeal papillomatosis may cause persistent stridor in children and adults at any age. Rarely, it may present as recurrent wheezing mimicking asthma.[14] Multiple, recurrent, rough-surfaced laryngeal tumors are caused by infection with the human papillomavirus (HPV). Repeated surgical excision generally is required to maintain a patent airway. Most recently, immunological therapy with interferon-alpha has proved beneficial.[7] The condition tends to improve with time, presumably as the child develops immunity to the virus.

Diphtheria is an extremely rare infection in the United States, but it still may occur in unimmunized children.

Other Acquired Causes of Airway Obstruction

Foreign body aspiration may manifest with airway obstruction at almost any level of the pediatric airway.[5] Stridor may be one of the presenting symptoms when a foreign body lodged in the upper esophagus has caused progressive airway obstruction secondary to localized edema that develops over days to weeks. Foreign bodies lodged in the upper airway itself often cause sudden death. Foreign bodies aspirated into the lower airway generally manifest with a combination of wheezing, cough, and infection. Clinical suspicion can be confirmed by appropriate roentgenographic studies. The definitive therapy is removal of the foreign body using rigid bronchoscopy techniques in an operating room, thereby permitting tracheostomy or thoracotomy if the foreign body cannot be removed by bronchoscopy.

Thermal or chemical trauma of the airway may cause sufficient swelling to precipitate respiratory failure. Flash burns of the face from injudicious use of volatile liquids to start fires commonly causes oropharyngeal and laryngeal edema that may seriously compromise the airway. Empirical use of parenteral corticosteroids is not beneficial for an inhalational injury.[6] Ingestion of corrosive substances likewise may cause sufficient burns of the oropharynx and larynx to require placement of an artificial airway.

External trauma to the head and neck may cause upper airway obstruction by dislocating the laryngeal cartilages or by causing a hematoma or edema.[15] This type of injury is rare in the spectrum of pediatric traumatic injury.

Vocal cord paralysis may occur as a consequence of a variety of serious intracranial injuries. Typical patients have required a tracheostomy, although vocal cord function may improve over ensuing months, allowing decannulation.[2] Children who have suffered brain injuries may have upper airway obstruction secondary to poor supraglottic motor control and hypotonia. The tongue may obstruct the airway, or the pharynx may collapse on inspiration. This can occur as the result of long-standing severe psychomotor retardation or may be acquired as a result of hypoxic, infectious, or traumatic brain injury.

Upper airway swelling can develop suddenly after ingestion of an allergen (e.g., milk, shellfish), an insect sting, or an environmental exposure (e.g., heat, sulfur dioxide, chlorine, ammonia). This may occur with highly allergic individuals (anaphylaxis) or with hereditary angioneurotic edema, an extremely rare condition. If an airway can be secured in time, the prognosis is good.

DIAGNOSTIC EVALUATION

With acute, infectious upper airway obstruction, diagnostic assessment of the cause of obstruction is urgent because, depending on the cause, the child's condition may change dramatically in a very short time. Diagnosis is relatively easy when a young child has the classic symptoms of viral croup (upper respiratory tract infection prodrome with subsequent development of stridor, a barking cough, and a mildly elevated temperature).[8] Likewise, an older child who has the classic presenting features of epiglottitis (acute onset of a sore throat; a high fever; a muffled voice; unwillingness to swallow; a toxic, distressed appearance; and rapidly progressive respiratory distress) also presents no special diagnostic dilemma. In practice, however, many children have varying combinations of these features. Indeed, the emergence of bacterial tracheitis has complicated the diagnosis because this disorder's clinical findings seem to evolve over time from those of more typical croup to those suggestive of epiglottitis.

Considerable controversy still exists over whether roentgenographic neck examinations should be done in a moderately ill child of any age who has acute upper airway obstruction. Although roentgenographic confirmation of the diagnosis of croup may be comforting in some situations, this type of evaluation can be counterproductive. In an uncooperative child who has classic croup, it is not uncommon for a lateral neck roentgenogram (usually an oblique view) to be of such poor quality that it is misinterpreted as showing a swollen epiglottis when evaluated by someone other than an experienced pediatric radiologist. This usually results in an unnecessarily high level of anxiety and referral to a tertiary care pediatric center. The more important scenario, however, is the child who has epiglottitis who develops acute upper airway obstruction and respiratory arrest while being positioned for roentgenographic evaluation, necessitating emergency resuscitation in a suboptimal environment. Finally, membranous laryngotracheobronchitis has no specific roentgenographic features. Because of these considerations, many pediatric institutions forgo routine roentgenographic evaluation of the upper airway if epiglottitis is suspected. Rather, the airway is visualized in the operating room by a pediatric anesthesiologist who has surgical backup and provisions for emergency tracheostomy, if necessary. This approach affords maximal safety for children who have the most dangerous disease—epiglottitis; it also affords an opportunity for early diagnosis and intervention in cases of bacterial tracheitis. Some institutions that have not abandoned the use of lateral neck films in cases of suspected epiglottitis now require that an anesthesiologist experienced in managing the pediatric airway accompany the child to the radiology department.

In the case of a neonate who has chronic stable or intermittent stridor and no significant respiratory embarrassment, a number of diagnostic approaches can be taken. A barium swallow or fluoroscopic evaluation of the airway can be helpful in demonstrating a number of congenital lesions. In addition, flexible laryngoscopy and bronchoscopy allow direct diagnostic evaluation and videotaping of airway dynamics. With experienced personnel and appropriate monitoring, this procedure can be done at the bedside.

Blood sampling is a low priority in a child who has an obstructed airway because the crying elicited by this painful procedure increases both the metabolic rate and the inspiratory work of breathing through the obstructed airway. Children who have croup or epiglottitis may have mild hypoxemia in room air, which may be due to atelectasis or early secondary pneumonia. Noninvasive pulse oximetry is a more appropriate way to monitor hypoxemia than intermittent sampling of blood gases. Cultures of blood, purulent tracheal secretions, or the surface of the epiglottis can be obtained, if desired, with the child anesthetized for examination and possible nasotracheal intubation.

MANAGEMENT

Triage

A child who has significant airway obstruction from any cause, as well as any child suspected of having foreign-body aspiration or an acute airway injury, should be hospitalized immediately. These children should be placed in a pediatric intensive care unit or in a continuously monitored area in an institution that contains a pediatric intensive care unit to which the child can be transferred immediately should deterioration occur. A child who has mild croup without stridor during quiet breathing need not be hospitalized. A child who has croup with stridor at rest, but who responds well to specific therapies, need not be transferred to a pediatric tertiary care center.

A child who has significant airway obstruction should be transported by ambulance and receive oxygen continuously. The child must be accompanied at all times during transport by personnel skilled in airway management. Children suspected of having epiglottitis should not be transported before endotracheal intubation because the medical literature contains numerous reports of cardiorespiratory arrests during transport when the airway has not been secured beforehand. It is a rare circumstance when a community hospital cannot assemble a team for controlled endoscopic examination and nasotracheal intubation in the operating room before transport.

Initial Stabilization

Any child who has significant airway obstruction should be monitored by pulse oximetry and receive supplemental oxygen. Allowing the child or parent to hold the oxygen mask may make this unfamiliar equipment less frightening. The child should be allowed to maintain the position that is most comfortable. Most children who have an obstructed airway prefer to sit up if they are developmentally capable of doing so. If airway obstruction is severe or if controlled examination in the operating room is contemplated, the child should be given nothing by mouth.

When acute laryngotracheobronchitis is the most likely diagnosis, aerosolized racemic epinephrine (2.25%, 0.5 ml in 2.5 ml of saline) or L-epinephrine (1%, 0.5 ml in 2.5 ml of saline) in oxygen via face mask generally provides prompt temporary improvement in airflow. Most practitioners hospitalize any child given nebulized epinephrine treatment in an emergency department, regardless of the degree of improvement. However, more recently, some are advocating a prolonged observation period and discharge home if significant airway obstruction does not recur over a number of hours. The most significant toxicity of aerosolized epinephrine in a healthy child is tachycardia, which is well tolerated. Indeed, sometimes the heart rate declines after administration of epinephrine aerosol, coincident with the improvement in airflow. Aerosol treatments may be repeated every 15 to 30 minutes, as necessary, for palliation of upper airway obstruction in croup, provided no signs of toxicity develop.

Most children who have tracheobronchial foreign bodies are not in respiratory distress on arrival because the foreign bodies usually are not located in the proximal airway. In the very rare instance in which the patient is moribund, back blows, chest thrusts, or Heimlich abdominal thrusts may be performed (as appropriate for age) if foreign-body aspiration is deemed likely. If these procedures are unsuccessful, direct examination of the airway with a laryngoscope is warranted. If a foreign body is seen to be wedged in the larynx or subglottic space, an emergency cricothyroidotomy may be necessary. If no foreign body is seen, endotracheal intubation should be performed because a foreign body may have migrated to the distal trachea. The only recourse in such circumstances is to push the foreign body forcibly into the right mainstem bronchus and ventilate the left lung. This situation is exceedingly rare.

Definitive Therapy

The definitive therapies for the three most common causes of upper airway obstruction—viral croup, epiglottitis, and bacterial tracheitis—are very different. Most patients who have croup respond to supportive medical treatment, which includes humidified oxygen, inhalation of epinephrine aerosol, and systemic or inhaled corticosteroids.[1,12] It is the unusual patient who has laryngotracheobronchitis who requires an artificial airway. A diminishing response to epinephrine or the development of hyperpyrexia and toxicity may be evidence of bacterial superinfection, heralding the onset of bacterial tracheitis.

Helium has been used to replace nitrogen as the carrier gas for oxygen (Heliox) to reduce the work of breathing in patients who have critical narrowing of the upper or lower airway.[3] Helium concentrations of 60% or greater (i.e., oxygen concentration of 40% or lower) lower the density of inspired gas significantly and reduce airway resistance. Although Heliox temporarily may relieve and palliate airflow obstruction, it is not a specific therapy in itself and cannot be used effectively in children requiring oxygen concentrations above 40%. Heliox should not be used in cases of acute epiglottitis.

Optimal treatment in all cases of acute epiglottitis is securing the child's airway, preferably by nasotracheal intubation. Tracheostomy for treatment of acute epiglottitis is unusual. Inspection and intubation are carried out in the operating room, with the patient undergoing general anesthesia and a pediatric anesthesiologist managing the airway. A surgeon must be present to perform either rigid bronchoscopy or tracheostomy if intubation is not possible. Intubation for epiglottitis generally lasts 18 to 36 hours, until parenteral antibiotics effective against *H. influenzae* have controlled the infection. A second- or third-generation cephalosporin generally is used because of the current emergence of ampicillin-resistant strains. Repeated visualization of the epiglottis is not necessary for determining the timing of elective extubation.

Most cases of bacterial tracheitis reported to date have required endotracheal intubation to secure an adequate airway. Consequently, most diagnoses are made at the time of intubation. Milder forms of the disease can be treated with appropriate antibiotics and other conservative measures. The usual antibiotic regimen consists of an antistaphylococcal penicillin paired with a second- or third-generation cephalosporin active against *Moraxella* and *Haemophilus* organisms. Generally, extubation is attempted only after thick, purulent secretions have diminished markedly and an air leak is heard on inspiration around the endotracheal tube. The requirement for an air leak is arbitrary because some children have a successful trial of extubation after 5 to 7 days of intubation even without an air leak.

Another scenario encountered in the emergency department involves a child with long-standing, mild upper airway obstruction who has a sudden exacerbation of obstruction. This may be an infant who has mild to moderate laryngomalacia who has increasing difficulty with oropharyngeal secretions arising secondary to a viral infection. Or it may be a child who has poor supraglottic muscle tone as a result of severe psychomotor retardation who has an increase in upper airway obstruction caused by a further decrease in mental status secondary to seizures or the effects of medications.

The clinician is guided in responding to the needs of all of these children by remembering the "ABCs" of basic life support—airway, breathing, and circulation.[3] Initial assessment of the child's upper airway function focuses on the degree of airway obstruction and the efficiency of ventilation. The clinician must determine whether the airway is stable and patent (which requires no intervention), or maintainable (the airway is compromised but can be maintained with basic interventions of oxygen, suctioning, and positioning). The third possibility is that the airway is judged to be unstable; this requires immediate placement of an artificial airway to maintain patency. Nasopharyngeal and endotracheal airways are the adjuncts of choice to maintain patency of an unstable airway.

Further Care

After a critically impaired airway has been diagnosed and appropriate therapy has been started, the issue of where the child will be cared for must be addressed. A child whose life depends on the patency and stability of an endotracheal tube, nasotracheal tube, or newly created tracheostomy requires the constant attention of nurses, therapists, and physicians experienced in pediatric intensive care. No amount of monitoring equipment can substitute for experienced personnel. Hence, it is only in dire circumstances that a child should be cared for in an intensive care unit that deals primarily with adults. The focus of care in a pediatric intensive care unit revolves around vigilant provision of adequate sedation (and paralysis if necessary) to prevent additional trauma to the airway, or even its inadvertent loss. Airways can be kept patent by suctioning and chest physiotherapy. Providing adequate ventilation and lung expansion will prevent parenchymal complications. Attention to other organ system derangements, as well as to the routine needs of a critically ill child, also is essential. When it becomes appropriate to do so, extubation is performed only by personnel experienced in the care of the pediatric airway.

REFERENCES

1. Ausejo M, et al: The effectiveness of glucocorticoids in treating croup: meta-analysis, *BMJ* 319:595, 1999.
2. Chaten FC, et al: Stridor: intracranial pathology causing postextubation vocal cord paralysis, *Pediatrics* 87:39, 1991.

3. Curtis JL, et al: Helium-oxygen gas therapy: use and availability for the emergency treatment of inoperable airway obstruction, *Chest* 90:455, 1986.
4. Donnelly BW, McMillan JA, Weiner LB: Bacterial tracheitis: report of eight new cases and review, *Rev Infect Dis* 12:729, 1990.
5. Downes JJ, Goldberg AI: Airway management, mechanical ventilation, and cardiopulmonary resuscitation. In Scarpelli EM, Auld PAM, Goldman HS, editors: *Pulmonary disease of the fetus, newborn, and child,* Philadelphia, 1978, Lea & Febiger.
6. Herndon DN, et al: Treatment of burns in children, *Pediatr Clin North Am* 32:1311, 1985.
7. Leventhal BG, et al: Long-term response of recurrent respiratory papillomatosis to treatment with lymphoblastoid interferon-alpha-1, *N Engl J Med* 325:613, 1991.
8. Mauro RD, Poole SR, Lockhart CH: Differentiation of epiglottitis from laryngotracheitis in the child with stridor, *Am J Dis Child* 142:679, 1988.
9. McCray PB, et al: Hypoxia and hypercapnia in infants with mild laryngomalacia, *Am J Dis Child* 142:896, 1988.
10. Newth CJ, Levision H, Bryan AC: The respiratory status of children with croup, *J Pediatr* 81:1068, 1972.
11. Quinn-Bogard AL, Potsic WP: Stridor in the first year of life: the clinical evaluation of the persistent or intermittent noisy breather, *Clin Pediatr* 16:913, 1977.
12. Super DM, et al: A prospective, randomized, double-blind study to evaluate the effect of dexamethasone in acute laryngotracheitis, *J Pediatr* 115:323, 1989.
13. *Textbook of pediatric advanced life support,* Elk Grove Village, Ill, 1988, the American Heart Association and the American Academy of Pediatrics.
14. Wilson NW, Millman E, Hogan MB: Laryngeal papilloma presenting as steroid-dependent asthma in a 3-year-old child without recurrent stridor, *Allergy Asthma Proc* 19:11, 1998.
15. Yarington CT: Trauma involving the air and food passages, *Otolaryngol Clin North Am* 12:321, 1979.

276 Coma

Allen R. Walker

Coma, strictly defined as "a state of unarousable psychologic unresponsiveness in which the subjects lie with eyes closed . . . ,"[3] is relatively rare in children and most commonly is caused by blunt trauma to the head. However, the more general syndrome of altered mental status, which includes coma as the most extreme manifestation, is vastly more common and has a more extensive list of possible etiologies.

Alterations in mental status include "clouding of consciousness,"[3] reflecting a primary problem of attentiveness, in which patients seem to be less awake or aware than normal. Delirious patients are out of touch with their environment and may have visual hallucinations. The delirium may be intermittent, alternating with periods of full orientation. Stuporous patients typically seem comatose but can be aroused from their unresponsiveness with strong stimuli, particularly painful ones.

Few studies document the incidence of coma or other alterations of mental status in children[4]; however, it occurs often enough that every primary care physician must have an approach in mind, ready to be called into play quickly. The early management of comatose children can influence the outcome, particularly when the cause is recognized quickly.

ETIOLOGY

Coma and other changes in mental status typically result from processes that involve either both cerebral hemispheres or the brainstem's reticular activating system. Coma may be caused by direct destruction of brain cells and tissues (trauma, tumor), impairment of function or cell death as a result of insufficient supply of substrate (shock, infarction, hemorrhage, increased intracranial pressure), or impairment of function by endogenous (e.g., carbon dioxide) or exogenous (e.g., barbiturates) toxins. Trauma is the most common cause of coma among children; traumatic brain injury caused by child abuse is prominent among infants and young children.[1] The most common nontraumatic cause of coma is intracranial infection, followed by hypoxic-ischemic injury, metabolic abnormalities, and seizures.[4] The list of possible causes of coma is extensive, requiring a logical plan for establishing a diagnosis as therapy is initiated.

Plum and Posner[3] have suggested categorizing coma as being due to (1) supratentorial lesions, (2) subtentorial lesions, or (3) diffuse, multifocal, or metabolic causes. Such a classification is useful because it can lead directly to diagnostic and therapeutic considerations early in the management of coma. Box 276-1 lists some of the general causes of coma according to this categorization scheme. Boxes 276-2, 276-3, and 276-4 provides some examples of causes of coma by age group.

Immediate Assessment of Threat to Intact Survival

The "ABC" (airway, breathing, circulation) approach to initial management of emergencies, with the addition of "D" and "E" (disability and exposure), is particularly relevant to coma. Meticulous airway management is the first step in coma therapy, with respect for the possibility of a cervical spine injury. Not only is appropriate management of the airway a critical step in dealing with threats to intact survival but also under some circumstances it may offer a means of treating increased intracranial pressure by hyperventilation, with resultant hypocapnia and diminished cerebral blood flow. If there is any suspicion of head trauma, careful in-line immobilization of the cervical spine during airway maneuvers is crucial for protecting the spinal cord.

Comatose children may need help with breathing, either because they are not breathing on their own or because hyperventilation to produce a modest hypocapnia (PCO_2 of 25 to 35 mm Hg) may be used in managing their increased intracranial pressure. Provision of extra oxygen during resuscitation and initial stabilization has not been shown to be deleterious and may be helpful; ventilation with 100% oxygen should be the rule during the early phases of management.

The goal of maintaining circulation is to provide oxygen and other substrates to the central nervous system (CNS). Clearly, shock must be treated aggressively. Perfusion of the brain to supply oxygen, glucose, and other substrates depends on the difference between mean systemic arterial blood pressure and intracranial pressure; if the systemic arterial pressure is low, cerebral blood flow will be reduced or absent. Fluid restriction has no place in the management of a child in shock, even with a head injury. Restoring circulating intravascular volume, and red blood cell (RBC) mass if necessary, is the critical first step to ensuring adequate perfusion of the CNS. Once normal intravascular volume and adequate perfusion have been achieved, fluid administration can be modestly restricted when good evidence of increased intracranial pressure is present.

Arrhythmias rarely are a concern in the management of children in coma, except for bradycardia resulting from increased intracranial pressure and ventricular tachyarrhyth-

BOX 276-1

DIFFERENTIAL DIAGNOSIS OF COMA: GENERAL CAUSES*

Supratentorial Causes
- Closed head trauma
  - Concussion
  - Hemorrhage
- Hemorrhage/infarction secondary to vascular disease
- Neoplasms
  - Herniation, obstruction of cerebrospinal fluid, invasion of activating structures
- Subdural empyema

Subtentorial Causes
- Arteriovenous malformation
- Basilar migraine
- Cerebellar abscess
- Cerebrovascular disease
- Rupture of vertebrobasilar artery aneurysm
- Trauma
  - Posterior fossa subdural hematoma

Diffuse, Multifocal, and Metabolic Causes
- Acid-base disorders
- Altered temperature regulation
- Central nervous system (CNS) infection or inflammation
- Dysfunction of non-CNS organs
  - Endocrine
  - Nonendocrine
  - Sepsis
- Electrolyte disorders
- Failure to provide substrate
  - Hypoglycemia
  - Hypoxia
  - Ischemia
- Poisoning

*These causes apply to all pediatric age groups.

BOX 276-3

DIFFERENTIAL DIAGNOSIS OF COMA: CHILDREN

Supratentorial Causes
- Arteriovenous malformation
- Hydrocephalus
  - Malfunction of ventricular shunt
- Trauma
- Tumor

Subtentorial Causes
- Arteriovenous malformation
- Basilar migraine
- Cerebellar abscess
- Trauma

Diffuse, Multifocal, and Metabolic Causes
- Acidosis
- Altered temperature regulation
- Encephalitis
- Hepatic failure
- Hypertension
  - Encephalopathy
- Hypoglycemia
- Hyponatremia
- Hypoxia
- Meningitis
- Poisoning
- Pulmonary disease
  - Hypoxia
  - Hypercapnia
- Renal failure
- Seizures/postictal state
- Sepsis
- Shock
- Suicide attempt

BOX 276-2

DIFFERENTIAL DIAGNOSIS OF COMA: INFANTS

Supratentorial Causes
- Hydrocephalus
- Intraventricular hemorrhage
- Subdural empyema
- Trauma
  - Closed head trauma
  - Shaken-baby syndrome
  - Subdural hematoma

Subtentorial Causes
- Arteriovenous malformation
- Subdural hemorrhage

Diffuse, Multifocal, and Metabolic Causes
- Asphyxiation (child abuse)
- Encephalitis
- Epilepsy/postictal state
- Hypoglycemia
- Hyponatremia
- Hypothermia
- Hypoxia
- Inborn errors of metabolism
  - Carbohydrate metabolism
  - Amino acid metabolism
- Intentional poisoning (child abuse)
- Intussusception
- Meningitis
- Sepsis
- Shock

BOX 276-4

DIFFERENTIAL DIAGNOSIS OF COMA: ADOLESCENTS

Supratentorial Causes
- Arteriovenous malformation
- Hemorrhage
- Hydrocephalus
  - Malfunction of ventricular shunt
- Trauma
- Tumor

Subtentorial Causes
- Arteriovenous malformation
- Basilar artery migraine

Diffuse, Multifocal and Metabolic Causes
- Asphyxiation
  - Autoerotic
- Drug overdose
- Encephalitis
- Hepatic failure
- Hypertension
  - Encephalopathy
- Hyperthermia
  - Heat stroke
- Hypoglycemia
- Hypothermia
- Hypothyroidism
- Hypoxia
- Meningitis
- Occupational exposure to toxins
- Poisoning
- Pulmonary disease
  - Hypoxia
  - Hypercapnia
- Renal failure
- Seizures/postictal state
- Sepsis
- Shock
- Suicide attempt
- Vasculitis
  - Lupus erythematosus
  - Epstein-Barr virus

mias arising as manifestations of intoxicants (especially tricyclic antidepressants) that can cause coma.[2,5]

Assessment of disability is part of the initial management of coma. A brief and focused neurological examination, with attention paid particularly to pupillary size and degree of constriction, level of responsiveness (if any), and position and function of the extremities, will give some information. Assessment of disability also is done by using a coma scale, the best known of which is the Glasgow Coma Scale (GCS). Coma scales offer a reproducible method for assessing neurological disability in a way that can be communicated easily and is useful both for immediate management and for determining the prognosis. A number of coma scales have been developed especially for children[6] because some of the items on the GCS are inappropriate; however, none has the widespread acceptability and familiarity of the GCS, modified for pediatric patients (see Table 286-1).

Exposure of the comatose child's whole body permits a search for evidence of trauma, particularly among infants, because even trauma not directed at the head may cause brain injury, subdural hematomas, and coma (shaken-baby syndrome[1]). During full-body examination, evidence should be sought for other life-threatening diagnoses, such as petechiae/purpura, suggesting sepsis or meningococcemia, or an abdominal mass and rectal bleeding, suggesting intussusception.

Diagnosis and treatment must proceed hand-in-hand in the successful management of a child in coma. The initial resuscitation priorities start with a major therapeutic maneuver, that of assuming control of the airway and hyperventilating the child when evidence of increased intracranial pressure is present.

Referral for Care

Many of the conditions that cause coma are within the knowledge and management skills of the general pediatrician. For example, treating diabetic ketoacidosis or meningitis resolves the coma as the underlying disease process improves. Just as clearly, though, some causes of coma require knowledge, skills, and equipment not often within the province of the general pediatrician. Direct measurement of intracranial pressure is one such skill that has assumed increasing importance in the management of traumatic brain injury. Decisions about referral are best made early in the course of management to allow the receiving physician and institution to apply their knowledge and skills to the fullest.

Recognition of local capabilities is crucial to decisions about referral. If 24-hour ventilatory management and one-to-one nursing care are not available, local management of a child in frank coma is not advisable if feasible, safe alternatives are available. The advice of a tertiary care expert should be sought as to the necessity for and timing of transfer so that the potential for destabilization during transport is minimized and the child arrives at the most appropriate site—one that is prepared to assume care immediately.

Appropriate transport of a comatose child requires personnel who have the highest level of advanced life-support training, as well as careful decisions about mode of transport (air or ground, fixed wing or helicopter, normal speed or flashing lights and sirens). Most crucial is maximal stabilization before transport. The more stable the child is before transport, the fewer problems will have to be dealt with under difficult conditions aboard a helicopter or an advanced life-support ambulance. The receiving institution may be able to send a transport team to assist with stabilization and transport.

Common Pitfalls

A number of pitfalls can complicate the management of a child in coma. The most fundamental is underestimating the severity of the symptom. Coma, or any variant of altered mental status, is a medical emergency, whether it results from head injury, ethanol overdose, status epilepticus, or other serious cause. Management of the comatose child must include plans to deal with worsening of the condition (e.g., brainstem herniation in the case of trauma, aspiration in the case of a drug overdose, or continued seizures requiring long-term phenobarbital therapy) should that occur.

Concern about increased intracranial pressure may lead to undertreatment of fluid deficits, including frank shock, with disastrous results.

Secondary Needs for General Homeostatic Support

During a short period of coma, most homeostatic needs are met easily by providing intravenous fluids and a neutral thermal environment, in which caloric expenditure for maintaining body temperature is minimal. After 24 to 48 hours, however, nutritional support becomes a major issue, necessitating full parenteral nutrition or enteral nutrition by nasogastric tube or gastrostomy tube.

BRAIN HERNIATION

A critical step in managing coma in children is assessing the risk of herniation of the brain through a bony foramen or its encroachment against a membranous barrier (the falx cerebri or tentorium). There are a number of specific syndromes of herniation, which have been well outlined in classic references.[6] Quick observations should be made repeatedly during management to detect signs of impending herniation. Respiratory pattern and rate, pupillary size, response of the eyes to the doll's head maneuver, and the motor system's function at rest and with stimulation all give clues to suggest impending herniation. These signs follow predictable patterns as herniation progresses, with initial changes reflecting reversible lesions and later changes reflecting irreversible lesions resulting from ischemia or hemorrhage (see Chapter 286, Head Injuries).

Respiratory patterns during the early, reversible stages of herniation may appear normal, but more typical are yawns and deep sighs or classic Cheyne-Stokes respirations, with periodic crescendo-decrescendo tachypnea followed by short periods of apnea. As herniation progresses, the respiratory pattern may change to (1) sustained hyperventilation, (2) a pattern indistinguishable from normal breathing, or (3) a slow, irregular pattern.

Coincident with changes in respiratory pattern are changes in pupillary responsiveness. Unilateral pupillary changes are typical of "uncal" herniation, in which midbrain structures are displaced laterally. In "central" (symmetrical) herniation, pupillary changes are bilateral. The earliest pupillary change may be a decrease in the size of the pupils, with limited additional constriction in bright light. As herniation continues, becoming progressively irreversible, the pupils become midposition in size, lose their responsiveness to light, and may become unequal. An early sign of uncal herniation is the development of a unilaterally dilated pupil that initially may be somewhat responsive to light but is progressively less so as the herniation continues.

The doll's head maneuver is accomplished by turning the patient's head to one side and then the other (clearly, one must be sure that there is no cervical spine injury before performing this test). In a conscious patient, the eyes normally turn with the head in the direction of the turning. In a comatose patient whose brainstem function is intact, the eyes typically deviate conjugately in the direction opposite that in which the head is turned (doll's eyes are present). Once brainstem function begins to fail, movement of the eyes becomes dysconjugate or totally absent. Should uncal herniation occur, dysconjugate eye movements may be apparent quite early in the herniation sequence.

Motor responses to herniation are assessed both at rest and with stimulation. Early in the course, motor responses may be symmetrical and appropriate, although there may be extensor plantar responses. As central herniation progresses, the child may be motionless at rest and respond to stimulation with stiffened legs and flexed arms (referred to as *decorticate rigidity*),[3] then with extension of both arms and legs *(decerebrate rigidity),* and ultimately *flaccidity.* Motor deterioration during uncal herniation typically is more rapid, often manifesting with decerebrate posturing.

Clearly, herniation is a life-threatening event; impending herniation must be dealt with aggressively. Immediate intubation and hyperventilation to achieve a PCO_2 in the range of 25 to 30 mm Hg is the initial treatment of choice. Mannitol, an osmotic diuretic, given in a dose of 0.5 to 1 g/kg intravenously, may be helpful. Recently, the use of hypertonic (3%) saline has been explored, and such use may soon become standard. Routine administration of dexamethasone is controversial, but this drug does appear to be useful in the management of increased intracranial pressure resulting from brain tumors. It generally is given intravenously in a dose of 1 to 2 mg/kg.

Definitive management of herniation depends on the results of diagnostic studies. Possible etiologies include subdural hematomas in infants, brain tumors in children and adolescents, strokes in children who have underlying vascular anomalies or sickle cell disease, and malfunctioning ventricular shunts in children who have hydrocephalus. Emergency brain imaging, usually by computed tomography (CT) scanning, ordinarily is required after consultation with radiological and neurosurgical specialists to confirm the diagnosis.

INFECTION

If life-threatening herniation syndromes and trauma have been ruled out, intracranial infection is the next most likely cause of the coma.[4] Empirical antibiotic and antiviral treatment may need to be initiated before the infectious etiology is defined clearly. In the presence of signs of increased intracranial pressure or cardiorespiratory instability, lumbar puncture should be deferred.

Treatment of presumed infection (meningitis) should be directed at the most likely etiologies (see Chapter 235, Meningitis). In young infants, particularly those under 2 months of age, broad-spectrum antibacterial coverage, including an antibiotic active against *Listeria monocytogenes* and an antiviral agent directed against herpes simplex virus, are indicated. In older children, broad-spectrum coverage includes drugs with particular effectiveness against *Streptococcus pneumoniae* and *Neisseria meningitidis. Haemophilus influenzae* type b, now rare, is a consideration in children with deficient or absent immunizations. Antibiotic therapy should never be delayed because of fear that the results of the lumbar puncture may be affected; eliminating infection is, after all, the point of treatment. If an infectious agent is never recovered but other evidence points to infection, treatment for the most likely organisms should be completed if the child survives the immediate crisis.

ANOXIA/ISCHEMIA

Seshia, Seshia, and Sachdeva[4] found that survivors of cardiopulmonary arrest constituted 24% of their series of children with nontraumatic coma. Management of hypoxic-ischemic encephalopathy requires the same knowledge and skills as the management of coma and increased intracranial pressure in general, keeping in mind the overall goal of preventing any further injury to CNS cells that may have the potential to recover after the initial injury. Critical to successful management of children who have suffered hypoxic and/or ischemic brain damage are (1) paying meticulous attention to delivery of oxygen and other nutrients to the CNS, and (2) not overlooking other, potentially treatable causes of coma, particularly metabolic or toxic causes.

SEIZURES

The identification and treatment of seizures that are obvious clinically are discussed in detail in Chapter 260, Seizure Disorders. When stupor or coma is unexplained, the possibility of nonconvulsive seizures should be kept in mind. An electroencephalogram (EEG) may lead to a diagnosis and appropriate therapy.

METABOLIC CAUSES OF COMA

The few metabolic causes of coma are relatively common and vary by age group. Rarer causes are listed in Boxes 276-2 to 276-4. In neonates and infants, inborn errors of metabolism must be considered, and measurement of the pH, blood ammonia, lactic acid, and organic and amino acids may be diagnostic. Managing metabolic coma may require avoiding or adding specific substances, and consultation with a metabolic specialist is advised.

In infants, particularly those who are bottle-fed water during the summer, water intoxication with resultant hyponatremia and seizures is not uncommon. Measuring electrolyte levels confirms the diagnosis, and treatment with isotonic or occasionally, hypertonic saline resolves the problem.

BOX 276-5

POISONS ASSOCIATED WITH COMA

Alcohol	Iron
Anesthetics	Lead
Antihistamines	Lithium
Barbiturates	Meprobamate
Benzodiazepines	Monoamine oxidase (MAO) inhibitors
Bromide	Narcotics
Butyrophenone	Organophosphates
Carbamates	Phenothiazines
Carbon monoxide	Salicylates
Clonidine	Sedative-hypnotics
Cyanide	Strychnine
Hydrocarbons	Theophylline
Hypoglycemics (oral and injectable)	Tricyclic antidepressants

From Mandl KD, Lovejoy FH: *Pediatr Rev* 15:151, 1994; and Woolf AD: *Pediatr Rev* 14:411, 1993.

Abnormalities of blood sugar, both low and high, are relatively common causes of metabolic coma. Both may be due directly to diabetes and either too much or not enough insulin, respectively. Hypoglycemia also may complicate ethanol ingestion or may be seen as the distinct entity, ketotic hypoglycemia, particularly in toddlers.

Poisonings, intentional (child abuse or suicide) or unintentional, must be considered in the differential diagnosis of coma early in the course.[2,5] Box 276-5 lists some of the common ingestants that can cause coma as part of an overall symptom complex picture; further details on poisoning can be found in Chapter 293, Poisoning.

Differential Diagnosis

Boxes 276-2, 276-3, and 276-4 offer a number of specific illnesses and conditions that may cause coma in infants, children, and adolescents, respectively. These lists are not exhaustive but rather represent common and some of the uncommon etiologies to be considered in the differential diagnosis.

Plum and Posner's classification of coma etiologies into supratentorial, subtentorial, and diffuse, multifocal and metabolic is helpful not only in predicting who is likely to be at acute risk of herniation but also in ensuring consideration of the full range of etiologies. Clearly, a child with impending herniation caused by brain injury does not require consideration of the diffuse, multifocal, and metabolic causes of coma; however, the child with undifferentiated coma, particularly an infant, requires consideration of both structural and nonstructural etiologies.

The early steps of differential diagnosis proceed in concert with the early steps of management. Initial observations allow early classification of trauma victims, children who have impending herniation, children who have the petechiae and purpura of meningococcemia, and the like. Early provision of oxygen, along with aggressive fluid resuscitation of those in shock, provides substrate for the brain deprived by poor perfusion. A therapeutic trial of glucose allows identification of some hypoglycemic children. Naloxone reverses the CNS depression of opiates. Flumazenil may help to reverse the CNS depression caused by benzodiazepines, although its use must be carefully considered because it is not a pure antagonist like naloxone; its use may precipitate seizures in some children. In many instances, brain imaging can provide crucial information to guide the neurosurgeon and the intensive care physician.

Coordination of Multidisciplinary Care

When coma persists over an extended period, the pediatrician plays a central role in the management of the child, either as a direct provider or coordinator of care. Comatose children often are seen by several subspecialty consultants. The general pediatrician can assume the role of advocate for the child, coordinating the efforts of the subspecialists, interpreting their opinions in light of the child's overall condition, and regularly talking with the family. Involving rehabilitation medicine specialists early in the child's course helps ensure the most favorable outcome possible. The pediatrician must know the rehabilitation plans and be sure that acute care interventions in the rehabilitation phase do not interfere with other treatment strategies.

Potential for Organ Donation

Children in coma who ultimately are declared brain dead may be potential organ donors. A responsible organ procurement agency can provide the pediatrician with personnel skilled in discussing donation with families who may, in turn, see organ donation as allowing some good to come from their loss.

SUMMARY

The primary care pediatrician is crucial to the management of comatose children. Preventing coma by counseling children and parents on injury and poisoning prevention during well-child visits is a daily duty. Evaluating sick and injured children in the office and the emergency department, identifying comatose children early, and rapidly initiating a logical plan for management and diagnosis is a role all primary care pediatricians should be able to assume. Some general pediatricians choose to maintain skills and involvement in the critical care of the comatose child. All can serve as advocates for their comatose patients during the most critical, intensive phases of their care, as well as during rehabilitation.

When to Refer

- If the need for subspecialty expertise is not available locally
- If the need for 24-hour-per-day ventilatory management and one-to-one nursing care is not available locally
- If the need for invasive treatment of increased intracranial pressure is not available locally

When to Hospitalize

When the etiology of altered mental status is unclear (may get worse)
Always for a child in coma
Virtually always for a child with significant alteration in mental status, unless the problem can be definitively diagnosed and managed in the emergency department

REFERENCES

1. Committee on Child Abuse and Neglect: Shaken baby syndrome: inflicted cerebral trauma, *Pediatrics* 92:872, 1993.
2. Mandl KD, Lovejoy FH: Common poisonings, *Pediatr Rev* 15:151, 1994.
3. Plum F, Posner JB: *The diagnosis of stupor and coma,* ed 3, Philadelphia, 1980, FA Davis.
4. Seshia SS, Seshia MMK, Sachdeva RK: Coma in childhood, *Dev Med Child Neurol* 19:614, 1977.
5. Woolf AD: Poisoning in children and adolescents, *Pediatr Rev* 14:411, 1993.
6. Yager JY, Johnston B, Seshia SS: Coma scales in pediatric practice, *Am J Dis Child* 144:1088, 1990.

SUGGESTED READINGS

Dietrich AM, et al: Head trauma in children with congenital coagulation disorders, *J Pediatr Surg* 29:28, 1994.

Duhaime AC, et al: Head injury in very young children: mechanisms, injury types, and ophthalmologic findings in 100 hospitalized patients younger than 2 years of age, *Pediatrics* 90:179, 1992.

Goetting MG, Tiznado-Garcia E, Bakdash TF: Intussusception encephalopathy: an underrecognized cause of coma in children, *Pediatr Neurol* 6:419, 1990.

Levi L, et al: Diffuse axonal injury: analysis of 100 patients with radiological signs, *Neurosurgery* 27:429, 1990.

Levin HS, et al: Severe head injury in children: experience of the Traumatic Coma Data Bank, *Neurosurgery* 31:435, 1992.

Plum F, Posner JB: *The diagnosis of stupor and coma,* ed 3, Philadelphia, 1980, FA Davis.

Simpson DA, et al: Head injuries in infants and young children: the value of the Pediatric Coma Scale: review of literature and report on a study, *Childs Nerv Syst* 7:183, 1990.

277 Croup (Acute Laryngotracheobronchitis)

Caroline Breese Hall • William J. Hall

DEFINITION

Viral croup, or acute laryngotracheobronchitis, is an age-specific syndrome caused by various viral agents. It is characterized by subglottic swelling, respiratory distress, and inspiratory stridor. This syndrome, recognized and respected by physicians for centuries, inherited its name, croup, from the Anglo-Saxon word *kropan*,[4] or from an old Scottish word *roup,* which meant to cry out in a hoarse voice. *Spasmodic croup* is a term sometimes used to denote recurrent episodes of croup that affect some children. Airway hyperreactivity resulting from allergens may play a role in predisposing these children to repetitive bouts of croup.

Important advances in our understanding of the etiology, pathophysiology, and treatment of croup have led to better management and outcome for these distressed children. An understanding of the physiological abnormalities underlying the child's distress is basic to proper management.

ETIOLOGY

As shown in Table 277-1, a variety of agents may be associated with croup. However, the parainfluenza viruses are the agents identified most frequently as causing this disease, and parainfluenza virus type 1 is the major single agent.[7,11,15,28] In an 11-year study of croup in a private practice in Chapel Hill, North Carolina, the parainfluenza viruses constituted 75% of all the viral isolates obtained from children who had croup; 65% of the parainfluenza viral isolates were parainfluenza virus type 1.[7] Respiratory syncytial virus (RSV), influenza viruses A and B, and *Mycoplasma pneumoniae* were the only other agents isolated with appreciable frequency in this study. Measles (once a major cause of croup) again became a significant cause of severe croup in several large cities most affected by the resurgence of measles cases during the 1989-91 upswing in the United States.[10,40]

EPIDEMIOLOGY

Croup occurs primarily in children between 3 months and 3 years of age, with the peak incidence being in the second year of life. Studies of both hospitalized and ambulatory patients have shown that boys tend to be affected more often than girls.[7,11,15] The incidence of croup varies not only according to age but also by geographical location and season. A prospective study by Hoekelman[19] found that during the first year of life, 1.2% of infants in pediatric practice developed croup. In a prepaid group practice in Seattle, the annual incidence of croup was 7 per 1000 children under age 6 years.[11] However, between 1 and 2 years of age, this incidence approximately doubled. In the Chapel Hill practice, the attack rate during the second year of life was 4.7 per 100 children per year, and the yearly incidence per 100 children for all ages was 1.82 for boys and 1.27 for girls.[7]

The seasonal flourishes of croup depend on the epidemiological personality of the viral agents (see Table 277-1, Fig. 277-1). Parainfluenza virus type 1, the most common cause of croup (Fig. 277-2), has the distinctive pattern of producing epidemics of croup and other associated respiratory illnesses every other year in the autumn.[28] In a continuing surveillance program done in Monroe County, New York, from 1976 to 1992, the parainfluenza viruses overall constituted about 17% of all the viral isolates obtained from outpatients in private practices and for 67% of the isolates from children who had croup.[28] Smaller peaks of croup are associated with outbreaks of influenza, RSV, and parainfluenza virus types 2 and 3.[7,15,28] Although the proportion of RSV infections that are manifest as croup is relatively small (about 5%), RSV is associated with up to 11% of croup cases. Cases of croup that occur in the fall are most likely related to the parainfluenza viruses, especially type 1, and to a lesser extent type 2. Winter cases are associated most frequently with influenza and RSV. In the warmer months of spring and summer, parainfluenza type 3 is the agent isolated most often.

Croup in children 5 years of age or older has been associated with the influenza viruses or *Mycoplasma pneumoniae*.[7] RSV tends to cause croup in younger children (in the first year of life) and results more often in prolonged symptoms and hospitalization. The parainfluenza viruses predominately cause croup in toddlers, but they may infect younger and sometimes school-age children.

PATHOPHYSIOLOGY

Infection with one of these viruses usually occurs through close person-to-person contact and occasionally through contact with infected secretions. The upper respiratory tract serves as the route of inoculation. The respiratory epithelium offers fertile fields for most of these agents, and viral multiplication occurs easily. Subsequently, the infection spreads farther down the respiratory tract. Involvement of the subglottic tissue appears particularly pronounced. Nevertheless, the infection may extend from the large airways to the alveoli. However, the characteristic diagnostic features of croup, stridor, hoarseness, and cough are engendered primarily by inflammation in the larynx and trachea. Inflammation at the subglottic area is especially apt to obstruct airflow seriously

Table 277-1 Causes of Croup

Agent	Epidemiology
Most Frequent	
Parainfluenza type 1	Epidemic, fall
Less Frequent	
Influenza A	Epidemic, winter
Influenza B	Epidemic, winter
Respiratory syncytial virus	Epidemic, winter-spring
Mycoplasma pneumoniae	Endemic
Parainfluenza type 2	Occasionally epidemic, fall
Parainfluenza type 3	Spring to summer
Uncommon	
Adenoviruses	Endemic
Rhinoviruses	Endemic, fall, spring-summer
Reoviruses	Endemic
Coronaviruses	Epidemic, winter
Herpesvirus hominis	Endemic

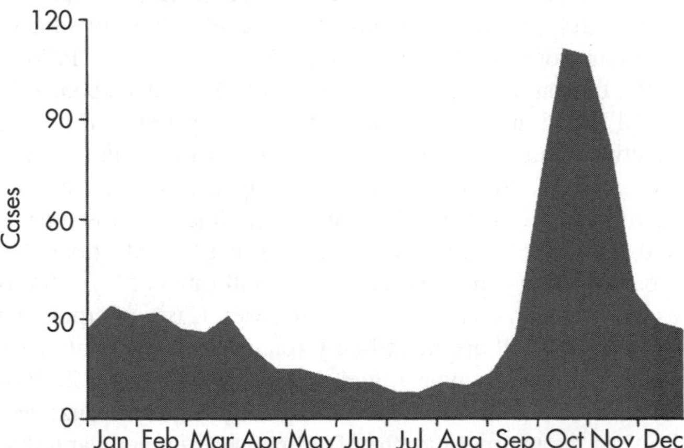

Fig. 277-1 Seasonal occurrence of croup from 1975 to 1998 in patients in pediatric practices participating in an ongoing community surveillance program in Monroe County, New York. Most cases observed in the fall resulted from outbreaks for parainfluenza virus type 1 occurring during odd-numbered years.

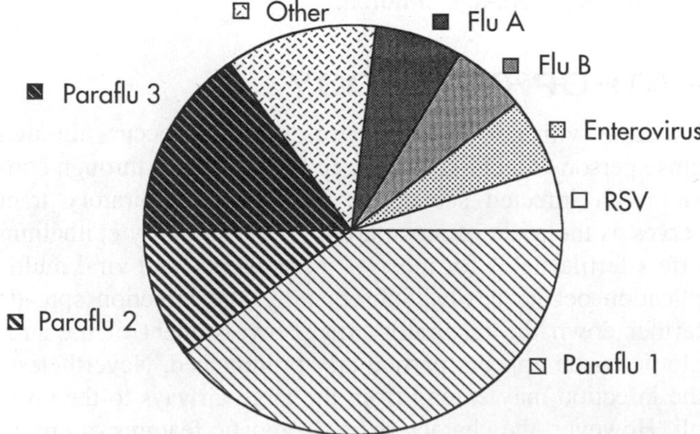

Fig. 277-2 Viral etiology of croup in patients in pediatric practices participating in a community surveillance program in Monroe County, New York.

because the anatomy of the cricoid and thyroid cartilage make this area both the narrowest and the least distensible part of the larynx. Inflammation, however, commonly affects the conducting airways at all levels. Necrosis of the epithelium is prominent, and the inflammatory exudate and secretions may add to the obstruction.

The age predilection of viral croup can be partly explained by the anatomy of the airway. Smaller airways are prone to greater degrees of obstruction from any inflammation of the lining membranes as illustrated by the fact that resistance to airflow is inversely related to the fourth power of the radius of the airway. The subglottic trachea of a young child is relatively smaller and also more pliable than that of an older individual. The narrowing that occurs with inspiratory effort, therefore, may be exaggerated in a young child with croup. In addition, obstruction above the subglottic area, such as may occur with nasal congestion, increases the collapsing force, and an increased respiratory rate associated with crying or anxiety may compromise the child's ventilation further.

Other host factors (e.g., genetic and immunological mechanisms), as yet poorly defined, are likely to contribute to the development and severity of croup. Atopy or hyperreactivity of the airways has been suggested as playing a role in spasmodic or recurrent croup by the higher incidence of a family history of allergy and positive skin tests for allergens in such children.[18,30,33,52] Serum IgA levels also have been noted to be lower in these predisposed patients.[53] Abnormalities in the immune response to parainfluenza viral antigens have been observed in children who developed croup compared with those who had other upper respiratory tract illnesses associated with parainfluenza virus infection.[49]

CLINICAL FEATURES

Symptoms of an upper respiratory tract infection usually precede the laryngotracheobronchitis. As the infection progresses, the characteristic cough develops. The cough may be spasmodic, with a deep "brassy" or "barking" tone. This classic sign thus has aptly earned the name "seal's bark" and is likened to the notes of a "brass bell" and even to a "crowing cock" or "braying ass." Laryngitis with a raspy-sounding voice may also develop. Fever commonly is present, particularly with influenza and parainfluenza viral infections.

These signs herald the usually abrupt onset of the inspiratory stridor. The child may awaken at night with a spasmodic cough and respiratory distress. Although airflow is impeded during both inspiration and expiration, the impediment is most marked on inspiration. Because the subglottic region is outside the pleural cavity, the negative pressures generated on inspiration tend to narrow the passage further, much like sucking on a plugged straw. The child's distress is marked audibly by each stridulous note of inspiration and is accentuated visibly by the retractions of the accessory muscles of the chest wall. The suprasternal, supraclavicular, and substernal retractions particularly are characteristic of the inspiratory obstruction. Further distress may be marked by asynchronous movements of the chest wall and abdomen.

The respiratory rate is increased but usually not more than 50 breaths/min. This is in contrast to bronchiolitis, in which the picture of respiratory distress may be accompanied by respirations of 80 to 90 breaths/min. Auscultation of the chest reveals a prolonged inspiration, often accompanied by coarse rales. Wheezes and rhonchi may be heard on expiration. With more severe obstruction, the breath sounds may be diminished. Cyanosis may occasionally be noted, particularly about the lips and nail beds.

The varying intensity of the respiratory distress is characteristic of croup. The child may appear severely compromised and an hour later appear improved, only to worsen over the next hour. Often, for unknown reasons, the symptoms appear to abate on waking in the morning but may worsen again as the day progresses. For most children, the signs of croup extend over 3 or 4 days, but the upper respiratory tract signs and cough may last longer.

In a few children, the respiratory distress may be unremitting or associated with significant pneumonitis and hypoxemia.[37] As the child tires, his or her respirations may become more rapid but also shallow, indicating the need for ventilatory assistance.

DIFFERENTIAL DIAGNOSIS

Viral croup must be differentiated from the two bacterial causes of stridor, bacterial tracheitis and epiglottitis, that without immediate therapy may be fatal. Since the conjugated *Haemophilus influenzae* type b (Hib) vaccines were licensed and incorporated into the routine immunization schedule of young children, epiglottitis has become rare in the United States. The differentiating features of epiglottitis are described in Chapter 284. The rapidly progressive and unrelenting course, the drooling, and the toxicity of epiglottitis tend to distinguish it from croup.

Bacterial tracheitis is the second emergent entity that needs to be differentiated from viral croup.[8,9,32,34] Bacterial tracheitis is an uncommon infection that may affect children of any age, resulting in the acute onset of respiratory stridor, high fever, and often copious, purulent secretions. As with epiglottitis, the child may appear toxic, and because the respiratory obstruction rapidly progresses, tracheal intubation is necessary. The pathogens most often involved are *Staphylococcus aureus,* and group A beta-hemolytic streptococci. The diagnosis may be confirmed by direct laryngoscopy, which shows the purulent secretions and inflammation in the subglottic area, and sometimes by a lateral neck roentgenogram, which may reveal an area of subglottic narrowing with a shaggy, purulent membrane.

Fortunately, other infectious agents that may mimic croup are now rare.[21] Diphtheria may be excluded by a history of adequate immunizations and by the absence of the characteristic gray pharyngeal or laryngeal diphtheritic membrane. However, a number of noninfectious entities cause stridor, most of which (e.g., congenital malformations and trauma) can be differentiated by obtaining a good history.[36,45] An aspirated foreign body may produce stridor. Abrupt onset of the stridor, respiratory distress, and the lack of preceding respiratory symptoms and fever should suggest this diagnosis. Laryngeal edema caused by an allergic reaction may cause abrupt and severe respiratory distress, occasionally with stridor. The history of the circumstances of the abrupt onset, the lack of previous respiratory signs, and manifestations of an allergic reaction elsewhere should help to differentiate laryngeal edema from other causes of croup.

DIAGNOSIS

Croup usually is diagnosed based on the characteristic clinical findings and a compatible history.[21,36,45] In cases that are atypical or apt to be confused with other syndromes characterized by stridor, the diagnosis of croup may be aided by a lateral inspiratory and expiratory roentgenogram or by a posteroanterior (PA) roentgenogram of the neck.[6,39,50] The air shadow of the larynx will be seen to narrow like an hourglass or a steeple in the subglottic region, as a result of the characteristic inflammation in this area (Fig. 277-3).[39] However, the sensitivity and specificity of diagnosing viral croup by use of the neck roentgenogram has been variable.[20,39,42,44] Sometimes the roentgenogram is not interpretable or the classic signs may not be evident.

The diagnosis of spasmodic croup has been applied by some to children who have recurrent episodes of croup in which an allergic diathesis is believed to play a role.[52] However, the illness in almost all instances is still triggered by a viral infection, and spasmodic croup cannot be differentiated clinically from the usual cases of croup.

Laboratory findings are not specific for the diagnosis of acute laryngotracheobronchitis. They may be more helpful in

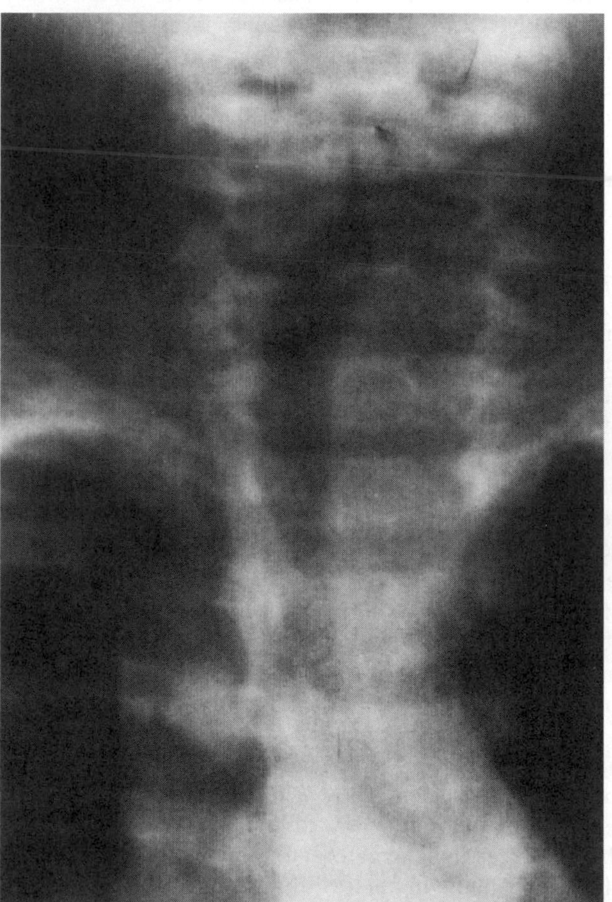

Fig. 277-3 Roentgenogram of the posteroanterior neck of a child with viral croup, showing narrowing in the subglottic area.

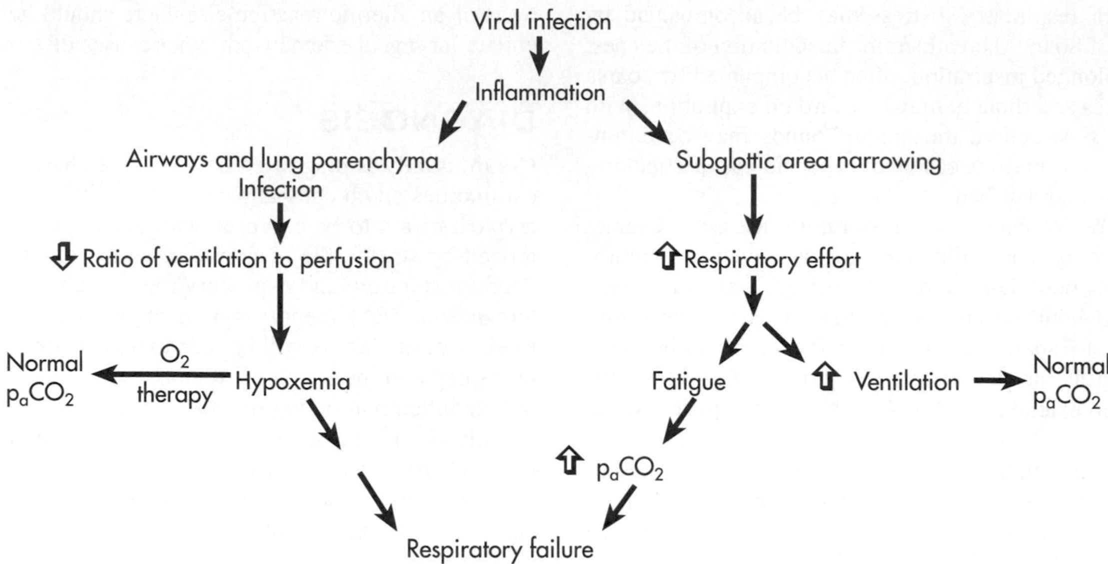

Fig. 277-4 Physiological abnormalities in viral croup. Viral infection of the subglottic area produces inflammation and obstruction, resulting in an initial decrease in the child's tidal volume. To maintain an adequate alveolar ventilation, the child increases the respiratory rate. With greater degrees of obstruction, however, the work of breathing may increase such that the child can no longer compensate by the increased respiratory effort. The ensuing decrease in tidal volume and respiratory rate may then result in hypercapnia and secondary hypoxemia.

the management than in diagnosis. The total white blood cell count (WBC) and differential counts in children who have croup may be normal or shifted slightly to the left in the more distressed child. Children with hypoxemia may have an increased proportion of bands in their peripheral count. Most hospitalized children with acute laryngotracheobronchitis have some degree of hypoxemia.[37] Hypercapnia is unusual except in the severely distressed child (Fig. 277-4).

MANAGEMENT

An understanding of the physiological changes that occur during acute laryngotracheobronchitis is basic to the management of these patients.[1,17,23,31] As depicted in Fig. 277-4, the infecting virus causes inflammation in the subglottic area and lower in the respiratory tract, resulting in two different types of physiological abnormalities. Obstruction at the subglottic area forces the child to increase his respiratory effort, causing the respiratory rate to rise. This increased ventilation compensates for the impeded flow of air and results in a normal arterial PCO_2. A few children will become fatigued from the increased effort of breathing. As their respirations become shallow, the carbon dioxide no longer can be eliminated adequately, and the arterial PCO_2 rises.

The inflammation of the airways and lung parenchyma causes concurrent physiological abnormalities that often are not appreciated adequately.[37] Infection of the parenchyma results in an abnormally low ratio of ventilation to perfusion. This produces hypoxemia, seen in more than 80% of hospitalized patients.[37] In contrast to the abnormalities associated with obstruction at the subglottic area, a child who has lower respiratory tract inflammation has little means of compensating. Raising the arterial oxygen saturation requires therapeutic intervention—the administration of supplemental oxygen. In the severely distressed child, the hypoxemia contributes to the fatigue. The resulting hypercapnia aggravates the hypoxemia, and respiratory failure may ensue.

The first phase of management is to evaluate which children may be managed at home and which require hospitalization. Severity often is difficult to determine in this fluctuating disease, and no clinical signs are reliably prognostic of a complicated course or of hypoxemia. The severity of the stridor and retractions is better correlated with the degree of subglottic obstruction and the respiratory effort than with hypoxemia. Toxicity, dehydration, and fatigue are indications for hospitalization.

Children who are to be managed at home should be made comfortable to avoid unnecessary anxiety and fatigue. Crying and anxiety tend to make the young child take rapid, short breaths, which aggravate the narrowing of the airway and the metabolic need for gas exchange. Fluids should be encouraged, and antipyretics should be given for fever. Despite a cornucopia of cures passed down from generation to generation, few other home therapies have proved beneficial. Because of croup's fluctuating nature, a number of unverified therapeutic modalities may appear to work. Vaporizers and home-devised mist tents, from showers to teakettles, commonly have been tried. The water particles produced by these devices, nevertheless, are too large to reach the lower respiratory tract and can humidify only the anterior nares and oropharynx. Furthermore, devices that use hot water and steam pose the potential hazard of accidental burns. A cool mist may help to cool the airway and may be beneficial in some children who have croup. This may also explain the improvement some children experience when taken out in the cold night air. Cold-dry, cold-mist, and warm-dry air all tend to cool the airway and, therefore, may be beneficial in croup as suggested by animal studies.[41,51]

In the hospital, the child may be evaluated by the objective criteria of measurements of arterial oxygen saturation. Oximetry provides a simple, noninvasive method for such measurements. Occasionally the PCO_2 may need to be assessed in managing the more severely ill child. Laboratory evaluation, however, should be kept to a minimum to avoid upsetting the child further.

Humidification in the hospital may be achieved by use of an ultrasonic nebulizer fitted to either a mask or an oxygen tent. This device can produce water particles of a size small enough to reach the bronchioles, although the value of such therapy has not been proved. Two small studies that have evaluated the use of humidification could show no benefit.[3,31]

Nebulized racemic epinephrine has appeared beneficial in children hospitalized with croup.[2,29,43,46] Clinical improvement occurs in most cases by reducing the degree of stridor and retractions, probably as a result of local vasoconstriction and diminished subglottic swelling from the alpha-adrenergic effect. Such an agent, therefore, may prevent fatigue in the distressed child, but it should be used only with the understanding that (1) amelioration of the clinical signs is transient, and the child may worsen within a couple of hours with rebound mucosal vasodilation and respiratory distress, and (2) the arterial oxygen saturation is not affected.[47] L-epinephrine, which contains only the active isomer, has been shown to be similarly beneficial and has the advantage of fewer side effects.[24,48]

Use of corticosteroid therapy had been controversial.[2,22,43,47] Many controlled studies using steroids have been published[2,22,43,47] that, when subjected to meta-analysis, indicated that for hospitalized children, corticosteroid administration provided significant clinical improvement when used at higher dosages—0.3 mg/kg to 0.6 mg/kg of dexamethasone (or its equivalent), given as single dose or up to four doses at 6-hour intervals.[22,43] Most recent studies have confirmed the clinical benefit of the administration of corticosteroids to both inpatients and outpatients with croup.[5,12-14,24-27] Furthermore, such trials have shown the efficacy of corticosteroids administered by multiple routes, including intramuscular, oral, and by nebulization. The beneficial clinical effect of corticosteroids may be noted within a few hours of administration but generally is not appreciated for about 6 hours.[13,29] Nevertheless, their use has allowed effective management of children with severe, as well as mild, croup and has resulted in a diminished need for hospitalization.

Because croup is of viral etiology, antibiotics usually are not indicated. Secondary bacterial infection is unusual, and antibiotics should be reserved for such documented episodes.[38,43]

With these supportive measures, few children require assisted ventilation. General guidelines for determining when the child requires assisted ventilation are (1) progressive carbon dioxide retention, (2) hypoxemia unresponsive to supplemental oxygen administration, and (3) copious secretions not mobilized by coughing.

PROGNOSIS

The severity of croup is related in part to the type of infecting virus and in part to unknown host factors. In most children, croup is a self-limited disease that resolves within a few days. However, several studies have suggested that children who have had croup have a high incidence of bronchial reactivity in subsequent years.[16,33,35,52]

REFERENCES

1. Barker GA: Current management of croup and epiglottitis, *Pediatr Clin North Am* 26:565, 1979.
2. Bass JW, Bruhn FW, Merritt WT: Corticosteroids and racemic epinephrine with IPPB in the treatment of croup, *J Pediatr* 96:173, 1980.
3. Bourchier D, Dawson KP, Fergusson DM: Humidification in viral croup: a controlled trial, *Aust Paediatr J* 20:289, 1984.
4. Cherry JD: Croup. In Kiple KF, editor: *Cambridge History and Geography of Human Disease Project,* Bowling Green, Ohio, 1990, University of Cambridge Press.
5. Cruz MN, et al: Use of dexamethasone in the outpatient management of acute laryngotracheitis, *Pediatrics* 96:220, 1995.
6. Currarino G, Williams B: Lateral inspiration and expiration radiographs of the neck in children with laryngotracheitis (croup), *Radiology* 145: 365, 1982.
7. Denny FW, et al: Croup: an 11-year study in a pediatric practice, *Pediatrics* 71:871, 1983.
8. Donnelly BW, McMillan JA, Weiner LB: Bacterial tracheitis: report of eight new cases and review, *Rev Infect Dis* 12:729, 1990.
9. Dudin AA, Thalji A, Rambaud-Cousson A: Bacterial tracheitis among children hospitalized for severe obstructive dyspnea, *Pediatr Infect Dis J* 9:293, 1990.
10. Fortenberry JD, et al: Severe laryngotracheobronchitis complicating measles, *Am J Dis Child* 146:1040, 1992.
11. Foy HM, et al: Incidence and etiology of pneumonia, croup and bronchiolitis in preschool children belonging to a prepaid medical care group over a four-year period, *Am J Epidemiol* 97:80, 1973.
12. Geelhoed GC: Croup, *Pediatr Pulmonol* 23:370, 1997.
13. Geelhoed GC, MacDonald WBG: Oral and inhaled steroids in croup: a randomized, placebo-controlled trial, *Pediatr Pulmonol* 20:355, 1995.
14. Geelhoed GC, MacDonald WBG: Oral dexamethasone in the treatment of croup: 0.15 mg/kg versus 0.6 mg/kg, *Pediatr Pulmonol* 20:362, 1995.
15. Glezen WP, Denny FW: Epidemiology of acute lower respiratory disease in children, *N Engl J Med* 228:498, 1973.
16. Gurwitz D, Corey M, Levison H: Pulmonary function and bronchial reactivity in children after croup, *Am Rev Respir Dis* 122:95, 1980.
17. Hen J Jr: Current management of upper airway obstruction, *Pediatr Ann* 15:274, 1986.
18. Hide DW, Guyer BM: Recurrent croup, *Arch Dis Child* 60:585, 1985.
19. Hoekelman RA: Infectious illness during the first year of life, *Pediatrics* 59:119, 1977.
20. Jones JL, et al: False positives in lateral neck radiographs used to diagnose epiglottitis, *Ann Emerg Med* 12:797, 1983 (letter).
21. Kaditis AG, Wald EG: Viral croup: current diagnosis and treatment, *Pediatr Infect Dis J* 17:827, 1998.
22. Kairys SW, Olmstead EM, O'Connor GT: Steroid treatment of laryngotracheitis: a meta-analysis of the evidence from randomized trials, *Pediatrics* 83:683, 1989.
23. Kilham H, Gills J, Benjamin B: Severe upper airway obstruction, *Pediatr Clin North Am* 34:1, 1987.
24. Klassen TP: Managing croup: racemic epinephrine versus L-epinephrine, *J Respir Dis* 16:245, 1995.
25. Klassen TP, et al: Nebulized budesonide and oral dexamethasone for treatment of croup, *J Am Med Assoc* 279:1629, 1998.
26. Klassen TP, et al: Nebulized budesonide for children with mild-to-moderate croup, *N Engl J Med* 331:285, 1994.
27. Klassen TP, et al: The efficacy of nebulized budesonide in dexamethasone-treated outpatients with croup, *Pediatrics* 97:463, 1996.
28. Knott A, et al: Parainfluenza viral infections in pediatric outpatients: seasonal patterns and clinical characteristics, *Pediatr Infect Dis J* 13: 269, 1994.

29. Kuusela AL, Vesikari T: A randomized double-blind, placebo-controlled trial of dexamethasone and racemic epinephrine in the treatment of croup, *Acta Paediatr Scand* 77:99, 1988.
30. Laufer P: The relationship of respiratory allergies to croup, *J Asthma* 23:9, 1986.
31. Lenney W, Milner AD: Treatment of viral croup, *Arch Dis Child* 53:704, 1978.
32. Liston SL, et al: Bacterial tracheitis, *Am J Dis Child* 137:764, 1983.
33. Litmanovitch M, et al: Relationship between recurrent croup and airway hyperreactivity, *Ann Allergy* 65:239, 1990.
34. Long SS: Bacterial tracheitis, *Rep Pediatr Infect Dis* 2:29, 1992.
35. Loughlin G, Taussig LM: Pulmonary function in children with a history of laryngotracheobronchitis, *J Pediatr* 94:365, 1979.
36. McBride JT: Stridor in childhood, *J Fam Practice* 19:782, 1984.
37. Newth CJL, Levison H, Bryan AC: Respiratory status of children with croup, *J Pediatr* 81:1068, 1972.
38. Pianosi P, et al: Inappropriate use of antibiotics in croup at three types of hospitals, *Can Med Assoc J* 134:357, 1986.
39. Rapkin RH: The diagnosis of epiglottitis: simplicity and reliability of radiographs of the neck in the differential of the croup syndrome, *J Pediatr* 80:96, 1972.
40. Ross LA, et al: Laryngotracheobronchitis as a complication of measles during an urban epidemic, *J Pediatr* 121:511, 1992.
41. Sasaki CT, Suzuki M: The respiratory mechanism of aerosol inhalation in the treatment of partial airway obstruction, *Pediatrics* 59:689, 1977.
42. Shackelford GD, et al: Subglottic edema in acute epiglottitis in children, *Am J Roentgenol* 131:603, 1978.
43. Skolnik NS: Treatment of croup, *Am J Dis Child* 143:1045, 1989.
44. Stankiewicz JA, Bowes AK: Croup and epiglottitis: a radiologic study, *Laryngoscope* 95:1159, 1985.
45. Tan HKK, Holinger LD: Tachypnea is often the first sign of respiratory distress: how to evaluate and manage stridor in children, *J Respir Dis* 15:245, 1994.
46. Taussig LM, et al: Treatment of laryngotracheobronchitis (croup): use of intermittent positive-pressure breathing and racemic epinephrine, *Am J Dis Child* 129:790, 1975.
47. Tunnessen WW, Reinstein AR: The steroid-croup controversy: an analytic review of methodologic problems, *J Pediatr* 96:751, 1980.
48. Waisman Y, et al: Prospective randomized double-blind study comparing L-epinephrine and racemic epinephrine aerosols in the treatment of laryngotracheitis (croup), *Pediatrics* 89:302, 1992.
49. Welliver RC, Sun M, Rinaldo D: Defective regulation of immune responses in croup due to parainfluenza virus, *Pediatr Res* 19:716, 1985.
50. Wildin SR, Chonmaitree T, Swischuk LE: Roentgenographic features of common pediatric viral respiratory tract infections, *Am J Dis Child* 142:43, 1988.
51. Wolfsdorf J, Swift DL: An animal model simulating acute infective upper airway obstruction of childhood and its use in the investigation of croup therapy, *Pediatr Res* 12:1062, 1978.
52. Zach M, Erban A, Olinsky A: Croup, recurrent croup, allergy, and airways hyperreactivity, *Arch Dis Child* 56:336, 1981.
53. Zach M, Messner H: Serum IgA in recurrent croup, *Am J Dis Child* 137:184, 1983.

278 Dehydration

Julius G. Goepp

Dehydration resulting from diarrheal illness remains the primary cause of infant and child mortality in the world, accounting for roughly 4 million deaths annually.[8] Although not a leading cause of death in the United States, gastroenteritis and related disorders result in a substantial amount of morbidity and generate significant health care costs. In a recent review, Glass[2] estimated that 16.5 million children younger than 5 years of age have at least one episode of diarrhea annually in the United States: 3 million episodes result in a physician visit, and 220,000 hospitalizations occur each year, accounting for about 10% of all pediatric hospitalizations. There are still between 300 and 500 pediatric deaths annually in the United States resulting from dehydration, mainly in the southern states and primarily among Hispanic and black children.

ETIOLOGY

Dehydration in infants and children overwhelmingly is the result of infectious processes. Of these, viral agents are of primary importance in the industrialized countries. Rotavirus and the Norwalk agent account for most cases of viral gastroenteritis in the pediatric population.

Bacterial pathogens also cause significant disease, with the commonest agents being *Salmonella* species, *Shigella sonnei, Campylobacter* species, and *Yersinia enterocolitica.* In addition, enterotoxigenic strains of *Escherichia coli* are increasingly prevalent as etiological agents producing significant morbidity, both from dehydrating diarrhea and from associated conditions such as hemolytic-uremic syndrome.

Noninfectious causes of dehydration in children include agents that produce osmotic diarrhea, such as laxatives or cathartics containing high concentrations of sugars; obstructive processes in the gastrointestinal tract; and occasionally, vomiting as a sign of elevated intracranial pressure. Although each of these conditions occurs only rarely, they should be borne in mind in the evaluation of the child who is dehydrated and has a history that is not typical for infectious gastroenteritis.

PATHOPHYSIOLOGY OF DEHYDRATION IN GASTROENTERITIS

To make the best-informed decisions about appropriate treatment of dehydration, practitioners should understand the basic principles underlying dehydrating diarrhea and the mechanisms by which rehydration occurs. In this section, the mechanisms of diarrheal dehydration and the principles of coupled co-transport on which therapy is based are discussed.

Regardless of which pathogen is involved, diarrhea and fluid loss ultimately result when intestinal fluid secretion exceeds the rate of absorption. In the case of viral agents and cytopathic bacteria such as *Shigella, Salmonella, Campylobacter,* and enteropathogenic strains of *E. coli,* fluid absorption is diminished because absorptive cells at the intestinal villus tip are destroyed, whereas secretory processes that occur at the level of intestinal crypt cells remain unimpaired. On the other hand, toxin-producing bacterial pathogens such as *Vibrio cholerae*, toxigenic *E. coli*, and some strains of *Shigella* cause dramatic increases in fluid secretion from crypt cells by deranging modulation of ion channels in the crypt cell membranes. Intestinal absorptive function is normal in such cases but does not keep pace with secretion, and diarrhea results.

Substantial fluid loss from the intestines depletes intravascular volume, resulting in end-organ hypoperfusion and poor nutrient and oxygen delivery; ultimately, tissue acidosis develops. Elevated aldosterone levels resulting from hypovolemia lead to renal potassium loss. Eventually, circulatory collapse and shock are manifest; irreversible organ damage and death may follow. The chain of events can be interrupted by very rapid repletion of fluids to restore circulating volume, reverse acidosis, and improve perfusion and end-organ function.[3] Traditionally in the United States, volume has been restored directly by administering intravenous (IV) fluids, and deficits have been replaced rather slowly, over a 24-hour period. There is now growing recognition that even moderate to severe intravascular fluid deficits may be replaced by the enteral (usually oral) route and that better results are obtained with rapid repletion.[3] The balance of this discussion will be devoted primarily to the use of oral rehydration therapy (ORT).

ORAL REHYDRATION

Fluid absorption can be promoted by the enteral administration of properly designed fluids, even in the face of ongoing losses. Oral rehydration exploits a normal cellular process known as *co-transport,* in which absorption of a molecule of an organic substrate promotes the absorption of an ion of sodium from the small intestine. With enhanced absorption of sodium, water, in turn, is absorbed rapidly into the circulation. Intravascular fluid volume can be restored in this fashion rapidly and reliably.[5]

Fluids designed to promote water and electrolyte absorption through the co-transport system in the gut are referred to as *oral rehydration solutions* (ORS). Physiologically appropriate ORS contains 70 to 90 mEq/L sodium and not more than 25 g/L glucose. In addition, ORS typically contains 20 mEq/L potassium and 30 mEq/L base in the form of citrate. It should be noted that almost all juices, soft drinks, and punches contain much higher concentrations of sugars, and almost no sodium, making them inappropriate for use as ORS. In fact, the higher sugar concentrations in these fluids may exacerbate diarrhea by presenting a large osmotic load within the intestinal lumen.

DATABASE

In evaluating an infant or child at risk for dehydration, the pathophysiology of the condition should be kept in mind. The interviewer should elicit the duration of symptoms, the frequency and quality of stool (characterized as watery, loose, pasty, or formed), the frequency and approximate volume of emesis, the frequency and volume of urination, and the overall level of activity and appetite displayed by the child. The child who remains active and playful is much less likely to be significantly dehydrated than the child who is listless or irritable at home. It is important to bear in mind that infants and younger children may become dehydrated much more rapidly than older children.

The examiner's attention should be directed first to the overall appearance of the child. An alert, interactive, and engageable child is reassuring, whereas irritability and lethargy are of concern. Specific physical findings in dehydration reflect the degree of intravascular volume depletion. Findings suggesting dehydration include a depressed anterior fontanelle, sunken eyes, loss of moisture of the oral mucosa (not dry lips, which may result from mouth-breathing), diminished skin turgor, and delayed capillary refill. To check for the latter, the skin of the thenar eminence is pressed firmly for 1 second and then released. Capillary refill time is the time elapsing before the blanched tissue returns to its normal color. A time longer than 3 seconds is considered indicative of some degree of diminished intravascular volume. Cool extremities and absence of tears do not necessarily denote significant dehydration. Table 278-1 shows a scheme for the assessment of the degree of dehydration as a proportion of total body weight by using physical findings, as well as initial treatment recommendations.

A variety of laboratory studies has been recommended in the past as indicators of the degree of dehydration present in a child. In practice, few such studies are truly necessary in the assessment of the child who has uncomplicated dehydration from gastrointestinal fluid losses. An accurate sense of the severity of dehydration may be formed from the physical examination and history. Therapy of dehydration is straightforward and rarely needs to be guided by laboratory studies, which should be reserved for unusual or refractory cases. In such cases, measurement of serum sodium, potassium, and bicarbonate levels may be useful, as may determination of the blood urea nitrogen (BUN). It should be noted that ORS can be used to restore both fluid and electrolyte balance in children who have a wide range of initial serum sodium values. By the end of the rehydration period, both hypernatremia and hyponatremia generally have resolved.

Stool diagnostic studies should similarly be used sparingly. Bacterial cultures should certainly be obtained in ill-appearing children, those with significant fever, those who have bloody or mucoid stools, or those in whom a travel or exposure history is suggestive of enteric pathogens. Most children will not meet these criteria, and routine stool cultures should be discouraged. Similarly, little additional diagnostic or therapeutic guidance is provided by detection of rotavirus antigen in stool, and such studies should rarely be obtained.

Table 278-1 Fluid Therapy for Dehydration

Degree of Dehydration*	Signs†	Rehydration Phase‡ (First 4 Hours; Repeat Until No Signs of Dehydration Remain)	Maintenance Phase (Until Illness Resolves)
Mild (3%-5%)	Slightly dry mucous membranes, increased thirst	ORS 60 ml/kg	Breast-feeding, undiluted lactose-free formula, ½-strength cow milk or lactose-containing formula
Moderate (6%-9%)	Sunken eyes, sunken fontanelle, loss of skin turgor, dry mucous membranes, decreased urine output	ORS 80 ml/kg	Same as above
Severe (>10%)	Signs of moderate dehydration plus one or more of the following: rapid thready pulse, hypotension, cyanosis, rapid breathing, delayed capillary refill, markedly reduced or absent urine output, lethargy, coma	IV or IO isotonic fluids (0.9% saline or lactated Ringer's), 20 ml/kg over 1 hr; repeat until pulse and state of consciousness return to normal, then 50-100 ml/kg of ORS based on remaining degree of dehydration§	Same as above

*Percent of total body weight lost.
†If no signs of dehydration are present, the rehydration phase may be omitted. Proceed with maintenance therapy and replacement of ongoing losses.
‡In addition to the rehydration amounts shown, replace ongoing stool losses and vomitus with ORS, 10 ml/kg for each diarrheal stool and 5 ml/kg for each episode of vomitus.
§While parenteral access is being sought, nasogastric infusion of ORS may be begun at 30 ml/kg/hr, provided airway protective reflexes remain intact.

MANAGEMENT

The overwhelming majority of dehydrated children can be rehydrated successfully without resorting to parenteral (intravenous or intraosseous) therapy. The combined use of ORS and an appropriate regimen of refeeding is referred to as *oral rehydration therapy* (ORT).

The first step in ORT is assessment of the degree of dehydration as a proportion of total body weight. Children who have mild dehydration, with thirst as the only presenting sign, are considered to have lost 5% or less of their total body weight. Losses of 6% to 9% of body weight are characterized as moderate dehydration and heralded by sunken eyes, dry mucous membranes, diminished skin turgor, delayed capillary refill time (CRT), and diminution in urine output. Fluid loss of 10% or more of body weight results in severe dehydration and generally produces signs of shock. Severe dehydration is characterized by marked changes in sensorium (lethargy or irritability), markedly delayed CRT, markedly reduced or absent urine output, tachycardia, and in extreme cases, hypotension. As can be seen from the overlap in descriptors, classifying dehydration is somewhat arbitrary. Therefore, fluid replacement calculations are considered to be approximate rather than rigidly accurate. It should be emphasized that in U.S. populations, dehydration of greater than mild severity is unusual, when objective signs are considered. Many children with only minimal dehydration are subjected to unnecessary intravenous rehydration as a result of inaccurate estimations of fluid deficit.

Intravenous Rehydration

Patients who present with severe dehydration (shock) should receive initial rehydration fluids parenterally, either intravenously or, when line placement proves difficult, via the intraosseous route. Patients treated parenterally should be given rapid boluses of 0.9% sodium chloride in initial volumes of 20 ml/kg over not more than 20 minutes. Fluid boluses should be repeated until signs of shock begin to disappear. In especially severe cases, it is not unusual for patients to require 60 to 100 ml/kg before the restoration of circulating volume is apparent. Even in such cases, however, enteral fluid therapy may begin immediately either by mouth or by nasogastric tube, provided the patient is conscious and that airway protective reflexes are intact.

Oral Rehydration

In the conscious child who has mild or moderate dehydration, fluid replacement always should be initiated orally. Successful ORT depends on proper fluid selection and skilled administration.[3] Simply instructing parents to purchase and feed a child ORS is unlikely to result in success and satisfaction.[4]

Types of ORS. Oral rehydration solutions are most widely available commercially in the industrialized world as premixed liquids. These solutions contain sodium levels varying from 50 to 70 mEq/L. For the mildly dehydrated child, any of these solutions is appropriate. For more significantly dehydrated infants and children, a solution containing 70 to 90 mEq/L of sodium should be chosen. Packets of oral rehydration salts for preparation of a solution containing 90 mEq/L of sodium are available for mixing with 1 liter of water to provide an inexpensive and reliable alternative. These packets always should be distributed with a 1-liter bottle to promote proper mixing. It should again be noted that juices, punches, and other soft drinks are inappropriate solutions for children who have diarrhea because of the high osmotic load they present to the intestines. Table 278-2 lists the most commonly available solutions and their compositions. Information on juices and soft drinks is provided for comparison.

Although homemade sugar-salt solutions can be prepared to produce appropriate ORS, the risk of incorrect mixing is high. Such homemade solutions are not recommended when commercial solutions are available.

Administration of ORT. In general, ORT can be started in the office or emergency department immediately after assessment excludes acute abdominal processes (such as appendicitis, volvulus, intussusception, and pyloric stenosis) and extraintestinal causes of fluid losses (such as intracranial hypertension caused by tumor, meningitis, or hydrocephalus, all of which may induce volume loss as a result of vomiting). Ideally the goal is to replace the entire fluid deficit in the first 4 to 6 hours. A child who is mildly dehydrated is given 60 ml/kg, and one who is moderately dehydrated is given 80 ml/kg; severe losses are replaced with 100 ml/kg (including any fluids given parenterally). In addition, 10 ml/kg of ORS for each diarrheal stool and 5 ml/kg for each episode of vomiting should be given.

Table 278-2 Solutions Commonly Used in Children Who Have Diarrhea

Solution	Glucose/CHO (g/L)	Sodium (mEq/L)	Base (mEq/L; Citrate or HCO_3)	Potassium (mEq/L)	Osmolality (mmol/L)
Physiologically Appropriate Solutions					
Pedialyte	25	45	30	20	270
Ricelyte	30*	50	30	25	200
Rehydralyte	25	75	30	20	310
WHO/UNICEF ORS	20	90	30	20	310
Physiologically Inappropriate Solutions					
Cola	700	2	13	0.1	750
Apple juice	690	3	0	32	730
Gatorade	255	20	3	3	330

*Rice syrup solids.

Fluids are best administered initially by a parent, who is instructed to place into the child's mouth (via a needleless syringe) 1 teaspoon (5 ml)/minute for infants, 10 ml/minute for toddlers, and 15 ml/minute for older children. This steady rate of administration provides 300, 600, and 900 ml/hour, respectively, which generally replaces the calculated deficit within a 4- to 6-hour period. Frequent reassessment of the child and encouragement of the parent is crucial during this period, referred to as the *rehydration phase*. The rehydration phase should be completed in the office, clinic, or emergency department before the child is sent home.

In general, vomiting is not a contraindication to ORT. Even when vomiting occurs, steady fluid replacement is continued orally. Children usually do not discharge their entire stomach contents when they vomit. As dehydration and tissue acidosis are corrected, the frequency and severity of vomiting generally are reduced. It should be borne in mind, however, that children who present with vomiting only (without diarrhea) warrant especially careful evaluation for conditions other than gastroenteritis (such as appendicitis, intussusception, volvulus, or pyloric stenosis, depending on age).

At the end of 4 hours, the state of hydration should be reassessed by using the original clinical criteria. If detectable dehydration remains, the rehydration phase should be repeated based on the remaining calculated volume deficit. If rehydration has been completed, the "maintenance phase" is begun. In this phase, the parent is instructed to continue to administer ORS in ad libitum quantities, but to alternate this fluid intake with breast milk, formula, or other appropriate feedings. Regular feedings should not be withheld once rehydration is complete. Strong evidence suggests that both the volume and duration of diarrhea are reduced when children are fed immediately following rehydration.[6,7]

It is becoming apparent that the subpopulation of children who present to emergency departments may represent a somewhat distinct group of patients. These children have often seen a primary care physician earlier in the illness, and may have had attempts made at oral rehydration. Although use of ORT in the emergency room should be strongly encouraged, and always should be attempted in the mild and moderately dehydrated child, one should also consider the possibility that these children are one step closer to a decision that ORT has failed, and that they might require intravenous treatment. This is especially the case in the older (school-aged) child in whom vomiting is the most prominent feature. Such children not infrequently are simply too exhausted to continue with efforts to drink. A brief trial of ORT, followed, if necessary, by a brief course of intravenous fluids and subsequent reintroduction of liquids and solids, is a reasonable approach in such children.[1] See also Chapter 29, Fluid Therapy, and Chapter 124, Diarrhea and Steatorrhea.

COMPLICATIONS

Complications of inadequately treated dehydration may be severe, ultimately including full-blown shock and multiorgan dysfunction syndrome, with end-organ damage to the kidneys, liver, and brain, culminating in death. In practice, such extreme consequences may be avoided readily by early and aggressive fluid therapy, using the oral or occasionally the intravenous or intraosseous routes. As a rule, it is far better to risk overhydration than to be exceptionally cautious with fluid administration. On rare occasions, aggressive oral hydration has resulted in mild overhydration, with some transient periorbital puffiness and a 2% to 3% weight gain.[4] These findings generally are self-limited and of no clinical consequence.

Hypokalemia, which results from the losses of total body potassium as a consequence of the increased aldosterone activity in the kidney, is a common occurrence in severe dehydration. As sodium is avidly retained, potassium is lost in urine. Hypokalemia can result in ileus, which may impair fluid and electrolyte absorption from the intestines. ORS generally contains 20 mEq/L of potassium chloride; such solutions are capable of restoring potassium balance.

PROGNOSIS

Although diarrheal dehydration is the leading cause of death among children globally, when appropriately treated it carries an excellent prognosis. Rapid restoration of circulating volume coupled with proper dietary management results in maintenance of hydration and earlier resolution of diarrheal symptoms. Parents should be warned, however, that even with ideal therapy, typical episodes of gastroenteritis last 3 to 7 days. Parents and providers should be reassured about the child's state of good hydration. The physician should reinforce the idea that the diarrheal illness itself is of little consequence so long as hydration is maintained and feeding reintroduced in a timely fashion.

SUMMARY

Dehydration resulting from gastroenteritis is a common condition generally managed by ORT on an outpatient basis. Little laboratory evaluation is necessary. Parenteral therapy is reserved for severe or unusual cases. Regardless of route of delivery, fluid should be administered rapidly, with the intent to restore the entire fluid deficit in 4 to 6 hours. Proper dietary management is essential to minimize the severity and duration of symptoms.

When to Refer

Most children in the industrialized world come to medical attention before gastroenteritis results in significant dehydration. Such children almost always can be managed directly from the office or clinic. Children who have moderate or severe dehydration, however, require rehydration under observation, which is not possible in some sites. Such children may be referred to a hospital emergency department for ORT. Emergency department staffs should be trained to initiate and administer ORT and to instruct parents in its use. Children who cannot be fully rehydrated within 6 hours, or those with persistently abnormal mental status, persistently abnormal electrolytes, or chronic diarrhea (more than 14 days' duration) should be referred to an emergency department at which pediatric gastroenterologists are available.

When to Hospitalize

In the industrialized world, otherwise healthy children treated with proper ORT for gastroenteritis and dehydration rarely need to be hospitalized. Most can be rehydrated in the office, clinic, or emergency department and discharged to home for the maintenance phase. Hospitalization should be reserved for the child who has other medical problems (e.g., short-gut and inflammatory bowel disease) or for children whose hydration status cannot be restored or maintained after a 6-hour outpatient treatment period. The expense and occasional adverse consequences of inpatient intravenous therapy warrant keeping dehydrated children who have no complications out of the hospital.

REFERENCES

1. Conners GP, Goepp JGK: Emergency department oral rehydration of children: the best solution? *Clin Pediatr Emerg Med* 1:27, 1999.
2. Glass RI, et al: Estimates of morbidity and mortality rates for diarrheal diseases in American children, *J Pediatr* 118:27, 1991.
3. Goepp J: Oral rehydration. In Henretig FJ, King C, editors: *Textbook of pediatric emergency procedures,* Baltimore, 1994, Williams & Wilkins.
4. Goepp J, Katz S: Oral rehydration therapy: a practice-oriented approach, *Am Fam Physician* 47:843, 1993.
5. Hirschhorn N: The treatment of acute diarrhea in children: an historical and physiological perspective, *Am J Clin Nutr* 33:637, 1980.
6. Santosham M, et al: Role of soy-based, lactose-free formula during treatment of acute diarrhea, *Pediatrics* 76:292, 1985.
7. Santosham M, et al: Role of a soy-based, lactose-free formula in the outpatient management of diarrhea in infants, *Pediatrics* 87:619, 1991.
8. Snyder JD, Marson MH: The magnitude of the global problem of acute diarrhoeal disease: a review of active surveillance data, *Bull WHO* 60: 605, 1982.

279 Diabetic Ketoacidosis

Robert E. Greenberg

Ketoacidosis may be the initial event leading to the diagnosis of diabetes of diabetes mellitus. Coexistence of coma is a much less common occurrence because of improvement in the early clinical recognition of the diabetic state. Yet, intercurrent episodes of ketoacidosis remain a frequent occurrence, especially among those diabetic children whose psychosocial and biological factors impose barriers to effective diabetic management or impede the metabolic response to insulin. Although mortality is low, even from coma, meticulous management of diabetic ketoacidosis is required to prevent death.

DEFINITION

Diabetic ketoacidosis occurs when the rate of endogenous glucose production continues unrestrained, despite the presence of markedly curtailed peripheral glucose utilization. The resultant increase in the breakdown of fat leads to the accumulation of nonesterified fatty acids and, because of the subsequent hepatic conversion of fatty acids to ketone bodies, to the release of hydrogen ion. The combined effects of osmotic diuresis and increased generation of protons lead to both dehydration and acidosis. If these events are prolonged or severe, stupor, drowsiness, and coma may occur.

ETIOLOGY

Glucose Metabolism

The concentration of glucose in blood is remarkably constant in a normal child, even during periods of fasting. Fasting involves the physiological suppression of insulin secretion, with consequent reduction of peripheral glucose utilization and mobilization of substrate (free or nonesterified fatty acids) from triglyceride stores. The reduction in insulin secretion leads to a marked curtailment of glucose utilization by insulin-sensitive tissues. Glucose utilization is compromised further during fasting by the direct inhibitory effects of both free fatty acids and ketone bodies (Fig. 279-1); it may be impeded still further during severe metabolic acidosis, when the binding of insulin to membrane receptors is impaired.

The reduction in glucose utilization that normally occurs during fasting is necessary to conserve body protein as effectively as possible. Were ongoing glucose utilization not curtailed, increased rates of new glucose formation *(gluconeogenesis)* would be mandatory to replace missing exogenous carbohydrate during fasting. However, gluconeogenesis requires precursor amino acids, so the duration of a prolonged fast would be markedly restricted were body protein stores not guarded most zealously.

Gluconeogenesis is not finely modulated in diabetic ketoacidosis but rather persists at a physiologically uncontrolled rate. This lack of control is the complex result of reduced insulin availability, impaired insulin action, increased substrate flow from muscle and adipose tissue, and an increase in counterregulatory hormones (which accelerate glucose production). Thus, at the very time when glucose utilization is compromised, glucose production is paradoxically increased, with resultant hyperglycemia and consequent osmotic diuresis and dehydration.

Alternate Energy Sources

When the availability of glucose as a substrate for intracellular energy metabolism is reduced, alternate energy sources must be made available. Hence triglyceride (neutral fat) is broken down into glycerol and fatty acids; the fatty acids release hydrogen ion during their subsequent hepatic conversion to ketone bodies (Fig. 279-2). Ketone bodies accumulate in blood as a consequence of both increased production and reduced peripheral utilization, as documented by prolonged turnover rates for ketone bodies in diabetic ketoacidosis (Figs. 279-2 and 279-3).

Role of Counterregulatory Hormones

The action of insulin in diabetic ketoacidosis is resisted for reasons other than the direct effects of acidosis. One such reason is the increased secretion of counterregulatory hormones, a clear example of which is seen in the control of triglyceride breakdown (Fig. 279-4). Insulin inhibits lipolysis, an aspect of its action that is partially independent of its effects on glucose transport. However, catecholamines, cortisol, growth hormone, glucagon, and thyroid hormones all exert—either directly or indirectly—an opposite effect on fat breakdown as to enhance lipolytic rates, even in the presence of adequate insulin. Activation of counterregulatory hormone secretion, in response to either biological or emotional stimuli, leads to accelerated rates of lipolysis, which in persons who have diabetes impairs metabolic regulation further. Increased secretion of counterregulatory hormones in the presence of relative insulin insufficiency thus compounds the decreased utilization and increased production of glucose and ketone bodies.

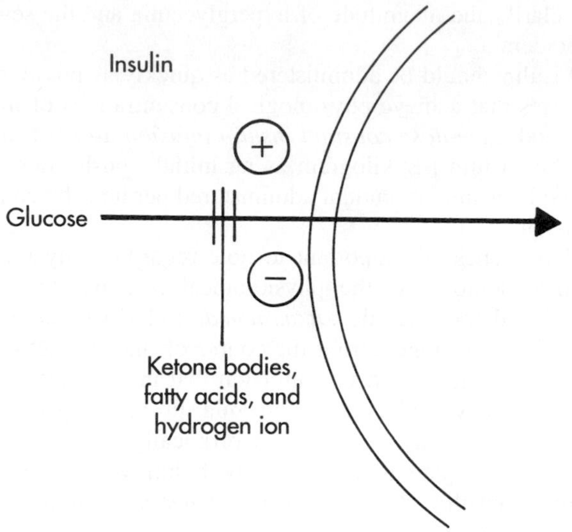

Fig. 279-1 Factors affecting glucose transport across cell membranes. +, Increase; –, decrease.

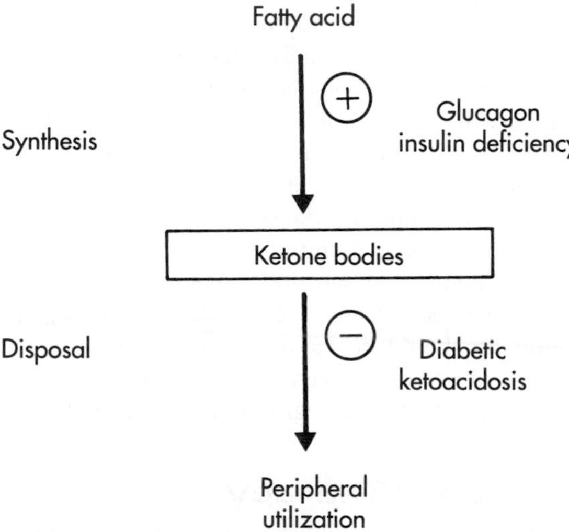

Fig. 279-2 Control of ketone body synthesis and disposal. +, Increase; –decrease.

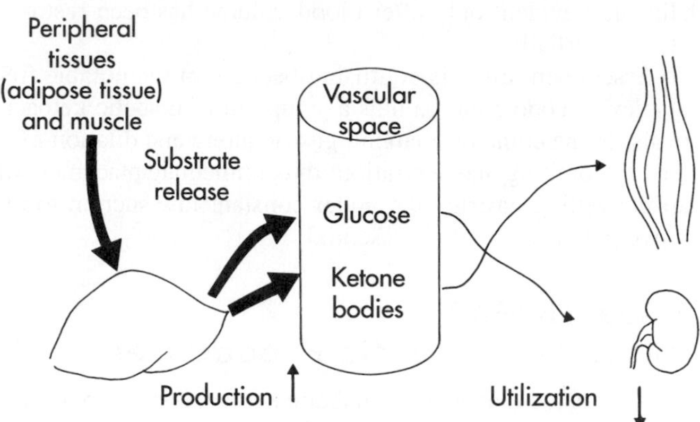

Fig. 279-3 Substrate production and utilization in diabetic ketoacidosis.

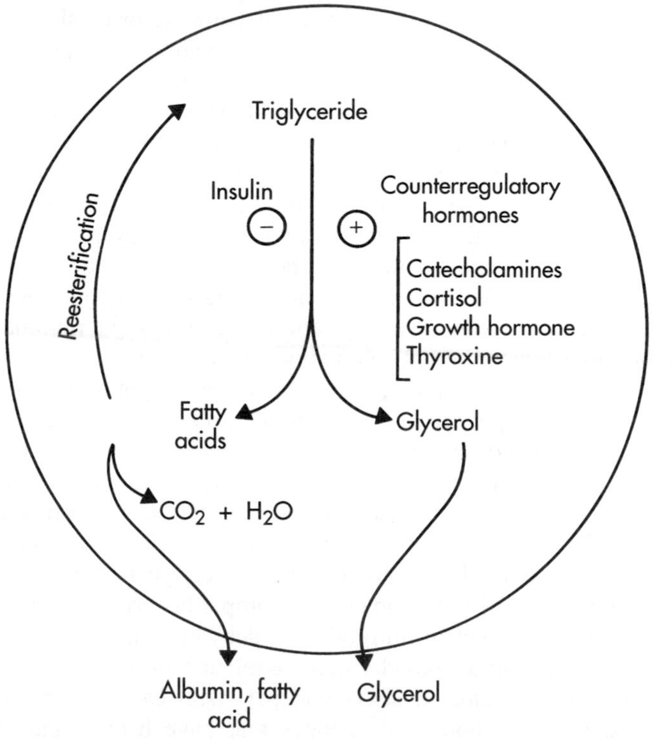

Fig. 279-4 Control of triglyceride breakdown. +, Increase; –, decrease.

INITIAL ASSESSMENT

The severity of acidemia in diabetic ketoacidosis is the summation of increased hydrogen ion generation and reduced hydrogen ion excretion, the latter as a consequence of dehydration. Reversal of this process requires the biological actions of exogenously supplied insulin and replacement of water and electrolytes. The diagnosis of diabetic ketoacidosis usually is not difficult, except when a previously undiagnosed patient is admitted in coma. The antecedent symptoms of nausea and vomiting, thirst and polyuria, weakness, weight loss, and visual disturbances most often lead to a rapid clinical diagnosis.

In the initial assessment, two urgent issues are (1) the evaluation of effective blood volume and (2) the differential diagnosis of coma. Tachycardia, hypotension, and hypothermia all should suggest reduced circulating blood volume; its rapid increase with isotonic saline or colloid is essential. The precise cause of stupor, drowsiness, and coma in a diabetic child may be difficult to discern and hence to treat accurately and might well involve hypoglycemia, ketoacidosis, lactic acidosis, or hyperglycemic-hyperosmolar nonketotic coma. Where there is doubt as to the cause of coma, *immediate intravenous administration of glucose (2 to 3 ml/kg of a 50% dextrose solution) may prevent significant neurological damage;* if hypoglycemia is not present, the amount of glucose given under such a policy is insignificant compared with the total pool of available glucose.

When blood volume is depleted markedly or when ketoacidosis is especially severe, respiratory compensation for metabolic acidosis may not be clinically apparent; that is, the classic Kussmaul respirations of ketoacidosis may become clinically evident only after blood volume has been restored at least partially.

Assessment often is confusing because of the notable frequency of abdominal pain as a symptom of diabetic ketoacidosis. In the comatose patient, gastric atony and dilation may lead to vomiting and aspiration; thus immediate placement of an indwelling gastric tube under constant low suction to remove gastric contents is essential.

TREATMENT

Initial Therapeutic Procedures

The suspected diagnosis of diabetic ketoacidosis is confirmed rapidly by use of methods available in any emergency room that demonstrate elevated glucose and ketone body concentrations in both blood and urine. Blood glucose can be measured accurately using glucometers; similarly the severity of ketonemia can be estimated by noting the dilution of serum that still gives a positive test result with use of crushed or powdered Acetest tablets. Although there are exceptions, it is possible to derive semiquantitative estimates of blood ketone body concentration by multiplying by 0.1 mM the highest dilution still giving a positive test result; this yields a rough estimate of acetoacetate concentration. Because the normal ratio of beta-hydroxybutyrate to acetoacetate is 3:1, multiplying the estimated concentration of acetoacetate by 4 provides the final estimate for total ketone body concentration. The patient who is dehydrated, has an altered state of consciousness, and has Kussmaul respirations, yet has only a minimal rise in estimated serum ketone body concentration, is the one in whom alternate proton donors must be sought, especially lactic acid. A difficult clinical problem may be presented by the dehydrated, acidemic child who has been given parenteral glucose–containing solutions before blood glucose has been measured; in this setting reduced peripheral perfusion may be associated with impaired glucose utilization to produce "artifactual" (i.e., nondiabetic) hyperglycemia. The correct diagnosis depends on eliciting proper historical evidence to reveal the mechanism producing dehydration.

The severity of blood volume depletion in the child who has diabetic ketoacidosis (blood pH <7.2) can be appreciated from the hormonal changes that have been found in such patients: serum concentrations of arginine vasopressin, plasma renin activity, aldosterone, and norepinephrine are increased threefold to twentyfold, and the concentration of atrial natriuretic peptide is reduced markedly.

After establishing the diagnosis of diabetic ketoacidosis, the physician should center attention quickly on (1) *restoring blood volume* and (2) *initiating a physiological response to insulin*. The overall management can be stated simply to be *hurry up* to replace reduced blood volume and start insulin replacement, then *slow down* in terms of subsequent fluid and electrolyte replacement. In the presence of significant hyperosmolality (i.e. hyperglycemia) the rapid administration of hypotonic fluids may cause cerebral edema; accordingly, initial intravenous fluids should be isotonic and rapidly administered (10 to 20 ml/kg/hr), even in the absence of evident blood volume depletion, until the results of laboratory tests can clarify the magnitude of hyperglycemia and the severity of acidemia.

Insulin should be administered as quickly as possible and in doses that achieve physiological concentrations of insulin in blood. *Low-dose constant insulin infusion* uses 0.1 unit of regular insulin per kilogram as an initial "push" dose, followed by a similar amount administered per hour by constant infusion.

Two issues are important to note regarding any form of insulin therapy: (1) the physiological response to insulin must be demonstrated, *not assumed*, and (2) sensitivity to insulin may change during the course of diabetic ketoacidosis so that a rate of insulin infusion that initially effects stabilization may produce hypoglycemia subsequently. Subcutaneous insulin may be absorbed erratically or poorly by a hypovolemic patient, compared with intravenous infusion, although insulin administered subcutaneously remains an effective form of therapy.

Demonstrating that insulin is exerting a biological effect may not be easy during the first hours of therapy. Blood glucose concentration sharply falls as a result of blood volume repletion alone (leading to a marked increase in glucose excretion). Bedside estimation of ketone body concentration often does not reflect accurately total ketone bodies in serum because of interconversions between acetoacetate and beta-hydroxybutyrate as acidosis is corrected. Demonstrating an improving state of metabolic acidosis provides indirect evidence supporting the effectiveness of infused insulin.

If clinical evaluation indicates that the blood volume is beginning to be restored and appropriate amounts of insulin are being provided, the question of patient transfer, if necessary, can be decided. A flow sheet should be started, on which the following should be recorded and monitored carefully: the nature and rate of intravenous fluids administered, insulin dosage, urine output, vital signs, and laboratory data.

Subsequent Therapy

During the 6 to 12 hours after initial stabilization, therapeutic concerns should center on the following series of definable problems:

Prevention of cerebral edema. The occurrence of cerebral edema appears to be common as a subclinical finding during therapy for diabetic ketoacidosis; clinically evident cerebral edema represents the primary cause of death in diabetic ketoacidosis. Patients at risk for development of cerebral edema include those whose condition has been in prolonged poor control, those who have severe acidemia (blood pH <7.2), those who have normal serum sodium concentrations in the presence of hyperglycemia, those whose serum sodium concentration falls to low levels during blood volume repletion, and those who have early signs of increased intracranial pressure. Although blood volume depletion initially must be addressed vigorously, the rate of subsequent infusion of hypotonic fluids should not be excessive and must be monitored carefully. A maximum of 4500 ml fluids/M^2/24 hr should guide therapy.

Management of acidemia. The definitive approach to the management of ketoacidosis is to reduce the generation of increased hydrogen ion (by insulin administration) and to improve the capacity to excrete an acid load (by blood volume expansion). In the presence of severe acidemia (pH <7.0), the irritability of cardiac muscle increases with resultant increased likelihood of cardiac arrhythmias. Because of negative inotropic effects on the heart, cardiac output may fall. When the pH is reduced markedly, the ability of insulin to bind to its membrane receptors is impaired, reducing still further the physiological response to insulin.

Correction of severe acidosis with bicarbonate may thus be necessary before insulin can be effective and, certainly, is necessary in instances of aberrant cardiac function. However, use of bicarbonate is not without significant hazard; when it is administered in large amounts, serum bicarbonate rises, raising blood pH values and reducing the stimulus for respiratory compensation so that carbon dioxide accumulates. Because carbon dioxide equilibrates across the blood-brain barrier much more rapidly than does bicarbonate, the intracerebral space may become more acidotic, even as extracellular pH values climb. Further, severe hypokalemia may be precipitated by bicarbonate administration, requiring frequent monitoring and potassium supplementation.

Prevention of hypoglycemia. The occurrence of significant and even dangerous hypoglycemia during management of diabetic ketoacidosis can be a severe complication. It occurs primarily when glucose is not being provided in the intravenous fluids, excessive amounts of insulin are administered, or the patient's changing sensitivity to insulin is not recognized. Early administration of exogenous glucose and use of the low-dose constant insulin infusion technique minimize the risk of hypoglycemia.

Hyperosmolar nonketotic diabetic coma in childhood is a rare condition; when it does occur, however, the mortality is much higher than in diabetic ketoacidosis. Hyperosmolar nonketotic hyperglycemic coma is defined as a marked increase in blood glucose concentration (usually >800 mg/dl), the absence of ketoacidosis, an altered state of consciousness, and significant dehydration. Thus the initial laboratory studies demonstrating severe hyperglycemia without significant ketonemia in a child who has an altered state of consciousness should alert the physician to the presence of this syndrome. A hyperosmolar state also can develop during treatment and is detected by demonstrating marked hyperglycemia and by often noting an excessive rate of diuresis in relation to the observed clinical state of hydration and rate of intravenous fluid administration. Because of the rarity of hyperosmolar coma relative to the frequency of therapy-induced hypoglycemia, glucose should be incorporated into intravenous fluids just as soon as it is clear that the blood glucose concentration either is not markedly elevated or is falling during insulin infusion and blood volume expansion.

Replacement of water and electrolyte deficits. The child who has severe diabetic ketoacidosis has marked deficits of water and electrolytes. However, in contrast to other conditions in which dehydration secondary to gastrointestinal losses is the presenting problem, ongoing renal fluid and electrolyte losses in diabetic ketoacidosis may be excessive, as a consequence of osmotic diuresis. When blood glucose values are brought below 200 mg/dl, urinary losses diminish markedly; in that situation excessive urine formation usually is secondary to excessive fluid administration. Because cerebral edema and hypokalemia are the primary reasons for fatality in diabetic ketoacidosis, therapy should be directed primarily toward preventing those complications. Accordingly, full correction of dehydration and resolution of ketoacidosis need not be accomplished during the initial 24 hours after therapy is initiated, as long as clinical assessment indicates normalization of circulating blood volume and no clinical or laboratory evidence of hypokalemia.

Osmotic diuresis produces water losses in excess of electrolyte losses. Thus, as soon as blood volume has been expanded and the danger of hyperosmolality assessed, the introduction of hypotonic fluids becomes appropriate. The usual fluid contains the following approximate contents: Na^+, 30 to 40 mEq/L; K^+, 30 to 40 mEq/L; HCO_3^-, 10 to 20 mEq/L; and Cl^-, 40 to 50 mEq/L; and PO_4^-, 20 to 30 mEq/L. Because prolonged use of chloride ion as the only anion is itself acidifying, the administration of bicarbonate in amounts found in extracellular fluid represents physiological replacement in this case, rather than the use of bicarbonate to combat established acidosis.

Prevention of hypokalemia. Total body potassium losses may well be excessive in diabetic ketoacidosis and may continue during ongoing osmotic diuresis. Further, the reincorporation of available extracellular potassium into the intracellular space may lead to profound hypokalemia. Adequate amounts of potassium used early in the intravenous fluid program and careful monitoring of both serum potassium and electrocardiographic tracings minimize the hazard of hypokalemia, the danger of which is greatest during the first 12 hours after the initiation of corrective therapy.

Detection of lactic acidosis. Lactic acidosis may occur in several situations in diabetes: (1) lactic acid may accumulate, to some degree, as part of ketoacidosis, (2) it may accumulate during therapy as a complication of tissue hypoxia accompanying severe *hypophosphatemia*, and (3) lactic acidemia may be a presenting problem in the absence of significant ketonemia. This latter occurrence is much more common in adults, especially in the elderly, than in children.

Serum phosphate predictably falls during the management of diabetic ketoacidosis. With significant hypophosphatemia, levels of red blood cell 2,3-diphosphoglycerate also fall, thus reducing the ability of hemoglobin to release oxygen. The resultant tissue hypoxia leads to lactic acidosis, which is corrected with phosphate infusions. The presence of lactic acidosis should be suspected whenever the clinical appearance of the child (e.g., Kussmaul respirations) or the measurement of blood pH indicates a degree of acidemia unexplained by the measured or estimated concentration of serum ketone bodies.

The Acetest tablet reflects only acetoacetate and does not detect beta-hydroxybutyrate. On initial examination the patient's degree of ketonemia may be underestimated because the beta-hydroxybutyrate/acetoacetate ratio is increased in diabetic ketoacidosis. Upon correction, the degree of ketonemia may be overestimated inasmuch as the aforementioned ratio decreases, so a greater proportion of the total ketone bodies are present as measurable (by Acetest) acetoacetate. Thus the occurrence of a significant anion gap and acidemia in the absence of detectable ketone bodies is an important clue to the presence of other causes for persistent metabolic acidosis.

Treatment of precipitating conditions. Diabetic ketoacidosis may be precipitated by other events, including infection. Presence of an underlying infection may be difficult to document because leukocytosis with increased release of nonsegmented leukocytes can occur in diabetic ketoacidosis without infection. Careful observation and repeated physical examination usually clarify coexistent disease and delineate the significance of concurrent abdominal pain.

IATROGENIC DANGERS

The main predisposing factor in iatrogenic complications is the physician's failure to monitor the child as his or her physiological state changes under therapy. Attention to the physiology of the primary problems to be ameliorated and careful observation of the child during the first 6 to 12 hours of treatment should minimize the danger of complications. The most important consideration in evaluating the need to transfer a patient is the availability of competent professionals; interactions with physicians experienced in the management of diabetic ketoacidosis in person or by phone may provide valuable guidance.

CONVALESCENT CARE

Subcutaneous insulin can be initiated after oral intake of fluids and nutrition becomes adequate. The principal task then must be to focus on exploring reasons for the occurrence of diabetic ketoacidosis. If the onset of ketoacidosis heralded the initial diagnosis of diabetes mellitus, primary attention must be focused on patient and family education and on helping the family adapt to the new diagnosis of a chronic (and incurable) disease. Where the ketoacidosis represents a recurrent problem in a known diabetic child, primary attention must be focused on determining and resolving the biological and psychosocial factors that lead to aberrant metabolic control.

When to Refer

- Newly diagnosed type I diabetes
- No physicians experienced in management of diabetic ketoacidosis are present
- Uncertain precipitating events
- Child/youth who has recurrent episodes of diabetic ketoacidosis

When to Hospitalize

- When oral fluids are not tolerated
- When blood pH is less than 7.2
- When there is no prior experience with the child or family

SUGGESTED READINGS

Brink SJ: Diabetic ketoacidosis, *Acta Paediatr Suppl* 427:14, 1999.

Cahill GF Jr, et al: Hormone-fuel interrelationships during fasting, *J Clin Invest* 45:1751, 1966.

DeFronzo RA, Matsuda M, Barrett EJ: Diabetic ketoacidosis: a combined metabolic-nephrologic approach to therapy, *Diabetic Rev* 2:209, 1994.

Finberg L: Fluid management of diabetic ketoacidosis, *Pediatr Rev* 17:46, 1996.

Finberg L: Why do patients with diabetic ketoacidosis have cerebral swelling and why does treatment sometimes make it worse? *Arch Pediatr Adolesc Med* 150:785, 1996.

Glaser NS, et al: Variation in the management of pediatric diabetic ketoacidosis by specialty training, *Arch Pediatr Adolesc Med* 151:1125, 1997.

Hale PM, et al: Factors predicting cerebral edema in young children with diabetic ketoacidosis and new onset type I diabetes, *Acta Paediatr* 86:626, 1997.

Mel JM, Werther GA: Incidence and outcome of diabetic cerebral oedema in childhood: are there predictors? *J Paediatr Child Health* 31:17, 1995.

Rosenbloom AL: Intracerebral crises during treatment of diabetic ketoacidosis, *Diabetes Care* 13:22, 1990.

Silink M: Practical management of diabetic ketoacidosis in childhood and adolescence, *Acta Paediatr Suppl* 425:673, 1998.

Tulassay T, et al: Atrial natriuretic peptide and other vasoactive hormones during treatment of severe diabetic ketoacidosis in children, *J Pediatr* 111:329, 1987.

280 Disseminated Intravascular Coagulation

John T. Horan • David N. Korones

Disseminated intravascular coagulation (DIC) is not a distinct disease, but rather a process stimulated by a variety of underlying clinical disorders. DIC is marked by widespread microvascular thrombosis and fibrinolysis, which lead to the depletion of hemostatic factors and platelets. Severe DIC frequently results in life-threatening hemorrhage and end-organ damage resulting from microvascular thrombosis.

INCIDENCE AND ETIOLOGY

Few published data exist regarding the incidence of DIC in children or adults. In a recent analysis of the experience of one pediatric tertiary care center, a diagnosis of DIC was made in 0.4% of all inpatient admissions.[15] DIC has been associated with numerous diseases, but illness specific rates are lacking; in pediatrics, infections and traumatic injury are among the more frequent causes. A list of common triggers is presented in Box 280-1. In infants and children, DIC typically is an acute and often fulminant disorder. It can also present in a more chronic and indolent manner, often with few clues from the history, physical examination, and laboratory tests. The latter form is seen much more frequently in adults, and thus something pediatricians are unlikely to encounter. The discussion in this chapter is limited to acute DIC.

PATHOPHYSIOLOGY

Physiological coagulation is initiated by tissue factor, a transmembrane glycoprotein that is synthesized on cells in the vascular media and adventitia, as well as on cells in the extravascular connective tissue. Normally, coagulation is limited to sites of vascular injury. Following such injury, platelets adhere to the exposed extracellular matrix, leading to primary hemostatic plug formation. Simultaneously, as tissue factor is produced, it binds factor VIIa. This complex then combines with factor X, factor IX, and Ca^{++} on a negatively charged phospholipid cell membrane to form the extrinsic tenase complex. Formation of this complex sets off a cascade of reactions that leads to thrombin formation on the platelet surface. Once thrombin is generated, it converts fibrinogen to fibrin, which enmeshes the platelet plug, forming a secondary hemostatic plug. This process is kept in check by circulating anticoagulants such as protein C, protein S, antithrombin III, the fibrinolytic system, and the normally antithrombotic endothelium.

In DIC, there appears to be an acceleration of thrombin formation through the normal tissue-factor pathway of coagulation, which overwhelms natural regulatory mechanisms. In animal models of gram negative sepsis-associated DIC, it has been demonstrated convincingly that this uncontrolled thrombin formation is initiated by endotoxin-stimulated increases in tissue factor.[23,24] Plasma tissue factor antigen is increased in patients with DIC in association with various underlying diseases, providing indirect proof that this surface bound glycoprotein is also an important trigger in clinical DIC.[8,12] The source of tissue factor is likely to vary depending on the associated underlying disease. Cytokines and endotoxin can stimulate white blood cell and endothelial cell tissue factor production[1,5,6,19]; this is likely to be important in sepsis. Alternatively, in obstetrical accidents or traumatic brain injury, exposure to tissues normally rich in tissue factor, such as the placenta or brain, may be sufficient. Hemostatic abnormalities other than excessive tissue factor can also lead to the up-regulation of the tissue factor pathway in DIC. For instance, severe congenital or acquired deficiencies of proteins C or S, which are anticoagulants, can cause DIC.[13,14,16]

The tissue factor coagulation pathway is activated in both normal clotting and in DIC, and in this respect the difference between DIC and normal clotting is a matter of degree. However, two important qualitative differences exist: first, in DIC the clotting occurs intravascularly; second, although platelets are activated and consumed in DIC, they do not directly participate in clot formation.[1]

Bleeding in DIC is likely caused by platelet and procoagulant factor consumption, inhibition of platelets and fibrin formation by fibrin degradation products and secondary fibrinolysis. A less common but important and often unrecognized complication is injury to the liver, kidneys, lungs and other organs from the widespread microvascular thromboses.

With recent advances in our understanding of vascular biology, it has become apparent that some illness-related coagulopathies, thought to be forms of DIC, are in fact pathophysiologically distinct. For example, the coagulopathy associated with acute promyelocytic leukemia is in many ways clinically indistinguishable from DIC, appears to be primarily a fibrinolytic disorder.[17] In the future, many other illness-related coagulopathies, now thought to be forms of DIC, may also be found to be distinct entities.

DIAGNOSIS

DIC is usually diagnosed in the context of a critical illness. Moderate-to-severe cases are often accompanied by oozing from venipuncture sites, mucosal bleeding, and petechiae. Purpura fulminans can sometimes complicate DIC and is

BOX 280-1

CAUSES OF DIC IN PEDIATRIC PATIENTS

Infection
Bacteria (e.g., *Neisseria meningitides, Escherichia coli, Streptococcus pneumoniae, Staphylococcus aureus)*
Viruses
Fungi
Protozoa

Trauma
Burns, brain injury

Cancer
Acute leukemia

Hematological
Transfusion reactions
Congenital or acquired severe protein C or S deficiency

Obstetrical Complications
Placental abruption, retained dead fetus, amniotic fluid embolism

Liver Disease
Fulminant hepatitis
Advanced cirrhosis

Miscellaneous
Collagen vascular diseases
Antiphospholipid syndrome

marked by large ecchymotic lesions, often with central bullae and gangrene of the digits. This entity is most often seen in meningococcemia,[9] pneumococcal sepsis,[10] and severe protein C or protein S deficiencies.[13,14,16]

Laboratory testing is essential. The associated physical examination findings are frequently absent and when present are nonspecific and often observed in other illnesses. Laboratory testing helps detect DIC when physical examination findings are lacking and should be considered for any patient with an illness that is highly associated with this disorder (e.g., sepsis, brain trauma, acute leukemia). Likewise, laboratory assays can be used to rule out coagulopathies with otherwise similar clinical manifestations. A complete blood count with peripheral blood film and differential, prothrombin time, activated partial thromboplastin time, fibrinogen level, and either a fibrin degradation products (FDP) or D-Dimer assay should be obtained. The classic laboratory findings of DIC include thrombocytopenia, fragmented red blood cells on the peripheral smear, hypofibrinogenemia, and prolongation of the prothrombin time and the activated partial thromboplastin time. All of these are relatively insensitive and nonspecific laboratory markers, which are more useful for guiding management. Some or all of these abnormalities may be absent in less severe cases, and they are frequently found alone or in combination in other coagulopathies.

Elevation of either FDPs or D-Dimer, each a measure of fibrin degradation by plasmin, is crucial for the diagnosis of DIC. In small clinical studies, they both displayed good sensitivity, specificity and predictive value, and there is no apparent clinically relevant difference in accuracy between the two assays.[3,4] These two markers virtually always will be elevated above the normal range in severe DIC and within the normal range in vitamin K deficiency, hemolytic-uremic syndrome and most other disorders considered in the differential diagnosis of DIC. Coagulopathy from liver disease however, is often quite difficult to differentiate from DIC, because it can produce all of the laboratory abnormalities seen with DIC, including elevated FDP/D-Dimer (because of decreased clearance). In many critically ill patients, both processes are present.

Recent advances in the study of thrombosis have led to the development of specific laboratory markers of procoagulant activation (e.g., prothrombin fragment 1.2), fibrinolytic activity (e.g., plasmin-antiplasmin complexes), and anticoagulant activity (e.g., anti-thrombin III) and many of these assays are now commercially available. Quantitative abnormalities in all of these markers are likely in DIC, and diagnostic criteria incorporating these assays have been formulated. However, there remain few data regarding the accuracy and reliability of these tests.

CLINICAL COURSE AND THERAPY

Most children with DIC require admission to an intensive care unit, because of the multiple complications stemming from the underlying disorder. Effective therapies for DIC have yet to be identified, so its resolution is contingent upon effective treatment of the underlying disorder. It is unclear whether DIC has any independent impact on patient mortality. It can however, cause significant morbidity. Bleeding is the most frequent complication and can often be severe. Gastrointestinal, urinary tract, and intracranial bleeding can all be seen with DIC.[22] Microvascular thrombosis can lead to renal cortical necrosis and to the gangrene of the digits seen with purpura fulminans.[20,21] Patients with purpura fulminans often require amputation of the affected digits.

Unfortunately, most currently available practice guidelines for the specific treatment of DIC are not evidence-based. The conventional therapeutic approach to this disorder relies on hemostatic replacement therapy and is not derived from clinical trials in DIC, but rather from experience with consumptive coagulopathies (e.g. massive hemorrhage). Typically, PT/PTTs, fibrinogens and platelet counts are obtained every 8 to 12 hours depending on the severity of the DIC. Fresh frozen plasma is administered to replace coagulation factors, anticoagulants, and fibrinolytic factors. Cryoprecipitate is given for hypofibrinogenemia, and platelet transfusions are administered for thrombocytopenia. Accepted guidelines are given in Box 280-2.

The safety and efficacy of replacement therapy in DIC remains largely untested, and there are theoretical concerns with this approach. As previously mentioned, elevated plasma FDPs, which are not directly affected by replacement therapy, may contribute significantly to the bleeding diathesis in DIC by interfering with fibrin polymerization and platelet function. Some investigators have expressed the concern that replacement therapy "fuels the fire," potentiating ongoing microvascular thrombosis and the resulting end-organ dysfunction.[2]

Novel approaches have been developed and are largely

BOX 280-2

MANAGEMENT OF ACUTE DIC

Laboratory Monitoring

PT, APTT, Fibrinogen, platelet count every 8 to 12 hours

CBC, D-Dimer or FDP every 24 hours

Therapy

Platelets, 1 unit/5 kg (maximum of 6 units) for platelet count less than 50,000; cryoprecipitate, 1 bag/5 kg (maximum of 10 bags) for fibrinogen less than 100 mg/dl; fresh-frozen plasma, 10 ml/kg for APTT or PT greater than 1.5 normal control.

aimed at inhibiting intravascular thrombosis. These include heparin therapy, and anticoagulant replacement therapy with either antithrombin III concentrate or protein C concentrate.[7,11,18] Unfortunately, there have been no large clinical studies of any of these agents in DIC, and no recommendations can be made regarding their use at this time.

CONCLUSION

Advances have been made in the understanding of the biology of disseminated intravascular coagulation. This knowledge has been translated into new potential diagnostic markers and treatment modalities. Because of the lack of clinical research in this area, these technological advances have had little impact on patient outcomes.

REFERENCES

1. Bevilacqua MP, et al: Recombinant tumor necrosis factor induces procoagulant activity in cultured human vascular endothelium: characterization and comparison with the actions of interleukin 1, *Proc Natl Acad Sci U S A* 83:4533, 1986.
2. Bick RL: Disseminated intravascular coagulation: objective criteria for diagnosis and management, *Med Clin North Am* 78:511, 1994.
3. Bick RL, Baker WF: Diagnostic efficacy of the D-dimer assay in disseminated intravascular coagulation (DIC), *Thromb Res* 65:785, 1992.
4. Carr JM, McKinney M, McDonagh J: Diagnosis of disseminated intravascular coagulation: role of D-dimer, *Am J Clin Pathol* 91:280, 1989.
5. Colucci M, et al: Cultured human endothelial cells generate tissue factor in response to endotoxin, *J Clin Invest* 71:1893, 1983.
6. Conkling PR, Greenberg CS, Weinberg JB: Tumor necrosis factor induces tissue factor-like activity in human leukemia cell line U937 and peripheral blood monocytes, *Blood* 72:128, 1988.
7. Feinstein DI: Diagnosis and management of disseminated intravascular coagulation: the role of heparin therapy, *Blood* 60:284, 1982.
8. Gando S, et al: Significant correlations between tissue factor and thrombin markers in trauma and septic patients with disseminated intravascular coagulation, *Thromb Haemost* 79:1111, 1998.
9. Giraud T, et al: Adult overwhelming meningococcal purpura: a study of 35 cases, 1977-1989, *Arch Intern Med* 151:310, 1991.
10. Hautekeete ML, et al: Purpura fulminans in pneumococcal sepsis, *Arch Intern Med* 146:497, 1986.
11. Inthorn D, et al: Antithrombin III supplementation in severe sepsis: beneficial effects on organ dysfunction, *Shock* 8:328, 1997.
12. Koyama T, et al: Determination of plasma tissue factor antigen and its clinical significance, *Br J Haematol* 87:343, 1994.
13. Levin M, et al: Postinfectious purpura fulminans caused by an autoantibody directed against protein S, *J Pediatr* 127:355, 1995.
14. Mahasandana C, et al: Neonatal purpura fulminans associated with homozygous protein S deficiency, *Lancet* 335:61, 1990 (letter).
15. Manco-Johnson MJ: Disseminated intravascular coagulation. In Hoekelman RA, et al, editors: *Primary pediatric care,* ed 3, St Louis, 1997, Mosby.
16. Marciniak E, Wilson HD, Marlar RA: Neonatal purpura fulminans: a genetic disorder related to the absence of protein C in blood, *Blood* 65:15, 1985.
17. Menell JS, et al: Annexin II and bleeding in acute promyelocytic leukemia, *N Engl J Med* 340:994, 1999.
18. Rivard GE, et al: Treatment of purpura fulminans in meningococcemia with protein C concentrate, *J Pediatr* 126:646, 1995.
19. Rivers RP, Hathaway WE, Weston WL: The endotoxin-induced coagulant activity of human monocytes, *Br J Haematol* 30:311, 1975.
20. Robboy SJ, et al: Pathology of disseminated intravascular coagulation (DIC): analysis of 26 cases, *Hum Pathol* 3:327, 1972.
21. Robboy SJ, et al: The skin in disseminated intravascular coagulation: prospective analysis of thirty-six cases, *Br J Dermatol* 88:221, 1973.
22. Spero JA, Lewis JH, Hasiba U: Disseminated intravascular coagulation: findings in 346 patients, *Thromb Haemost* 43:28, 1980.
23. Thomas LGR: Studies on the generalized shwartzman reaction. I. General observations concerning the phenomenon, *J Exp Med* 96:605, 1952.
24. Warr TA, Rao LV, Rapaport SI: Disseminated intravascular coagulation in rabbits induced by administration of endotoxin or tissue factor: effect of anti-tissue factor antibodies and measurement of plasma extrinsic pathway inhibitor activity, *Blood* 75:1481, 1990.

281 Drowning and Near-Drowning

Steven E. Lucking

Drowning is the second leading cause of accidental death among children and adolescents.[11] Motor vehicle injuries remain the leading cause of accidental death in this age group, although rates have declined in the decade ending in 1988. Deaths caused by drowning and other accidents also have shown a decline, whereas the death rates from suicide and homicide have increased.[5] In 1997, 1237 deaths from drowning were reported in children 19 years of age and younger, with the highest rate—2.9 per 100,000—in the 1- to 4-year age group.[11] It also has been estimated that for each drowning fatality in childhood, there are three to four hospital admissions for nonfatal near-drownings.[29] In addition it has been estimated that for each hospital admission, four children are seen in an emergency department for a water-related accident and are released.

The circumstances by which drownings and near-drownings occur vary by age. Bathtub drownings generally occur in children less than 1 year of age who are left in the care of an older sibling and without adult supervision. A strong correlation exists between the incidence of drowning in toddlers and the presence of family swimming pools. Drownings among older children and adolescents may occur as a result of diving accidents. Adolescent and adult drowning incidents often are associated with the use of alcohol.

Community education and mandated barriers around private pools may help to decrease the incidence of this clearly preventable source of morbidity and mortality. However, in the late 1990s children still suffered significant morbidity from near-drowning, even in supervised public pools that have lifeguards on duty.

The oldest and most common definition of drowning is "death from suffocation from submersion in liquid." Additional definitions have been developed over time to reflect certain specific pathophysiological events that may occur. Near-drowning most typically defines survival of at least 24 hours after suffocation from submersion in liquid. The term *secondary drowning* usually refers to the development of cardiorespiratory compromise after a variable latent period. The term *dry drowning* is commonly used to reflect that suffocation from submersion in liquid can occur without fluid aspiration into the lung. This phenomenon also is referred to as *drowning* or *near-drowning without aspiration*. Finally, some have defined immersion syndrome as indicating the sudden development of asystole and death upon immersion in cold water; this event probably is mediated vagally.

PATHOPHYSIOLOGY OF DROWNING

The physiological response to submersion is variable.[18] The classic description of the initial response to submersion includes a period of panic, characterized by vigorous struggling, breath-holding, and automatic swimming. A number of eyewitness reports, however, describe the victim's response as being much more subdued or placid. Children, for instance, are reported to stop playing suddenly and become motionless as if subdued by panic, although it is unknown what actually occurs at this moment. Some children will ingest a large amount of water early in the sequence of events. With progressive loss of consciousness, they may vomit then aspirate the vomitus with the onset of gasping respirations. As loss of consciousness progresses, airway reflexes eventually are lost and fluid may enter the lungs passively. Conversely, 10% to 20% of autopsy cases of drowning show no fluid aspirated into the lungs. These dry drownings are believed to be caused by laryngospasm occurring early in the sequence of events, preventing aspiration.

Fluid and Electrolyte Shifts

Early interest in the study of drowning in the 1960s focused on fluid and electrolyte abnormalities. Salt water has an osmolarity approximately 3½ to 4 times that of plasma. When aspirated into the lung in sufficient quantities, this hypertonic fluid draws additional fluid into the alveolar space. Intravascular hypovolemia and hemoconcentration result, and the serum concentration of major electrolytes increases. Conversely, fresh water is hypotonic with respect to plasma. Aspiration of sufficient quantities of fresh water will result in intravascular hypervolemia with dilutional hyponatremia as water is absorbed from the lung. Hemodilution and hemolysis may occur in severe cases, presumably as a result of regional osmolar changes. This may lead to hemoglobinuria, acute renal failure, and hyperkalemia. The electrolytic phenomena, which are reported in humans and are easily reproducible in the laboratory, actually are quite uncommon in the clinical setting. In laboratory animals one must instill at least 22 ml/kg into the lung to produce electrolyte changes.[20] It is unusual for nearly drowned humans to aspirate more than 4 ml/kg, and in one study, less than 15% of near-drowning victims aspirated more than 22 ml/kg.[19] Thus, significant electrolyte abnormalities are uncommon in patients who survive to reach a medical facility.

Pulmonary Injury

The most important aspect of the fluid aspiration itself is the pulmonary injury that ensues. It has been demonstrated in laboratory animals that fresh water inactivates pulmonary surfactant on contact, whereas salt water will cause surfactant wash-out.[10] Thus, the aspiration of sufficient quantities of either fresh or salt water causes loss of functional surfactant, with resultant poor lung compliance. This in turn leads to increased work of breathing, atelectasis, and hypoxemia.

Any child who has a submersion injury may vomit and aspirate during the event. Regardless of the type of liquid in which the submersion occurred, pulmonary aspiration of acid gastric contents may be associated. This can lead to tracheobronchial inflammation with bronchospasm and the development of alveolar capillary injury. Finally, if the patient has suffered a cardiac arrest and has some degree of cardiogenic shock in the aftermath, a secondary pulmonary capillary injury may occur with resultant capillary leak, diffuse pulmonary edema, and hypoxemia (acute lung injury, adult respiratory distress syndrome [ARDS]).

Neurological Injury

The single most important determinant of morbidity and mortality in near-drowning is the extent of brain injury. Prolonged submersion under water leads to hypoxia and hypercapnia. It is primarily the hypoxemia that leads to myocardial depression and eventual cardiac arrest. During cardiac arrest the entire body is subject to global ischemia and anoxia. Although all organs are affected by global ischemia, the brain tends to be the least forgiving of this insult.

Beginning in the 1980s a considerable amount of interest has focused on the issue of anoxic brain injury and on attempts to improve neurological outcome after global anoxia: an approach called cerebral resuscitation.[15]

Within 2 minutes of the onset of anoxia there is loss of substrate for energy production within the body's cells. This is accompanied by potassium efflux from cells, coupled with the influx of calcium and sodium.[27,28] Following anoxia, as much as a 90% reduction in ionic calcium concentration in brain interstitial fluid with toxic accumulation of calcium within neuronal mitochondria has been noted. The enzyme phospholipase A2 is activated by elevated intracellular calcium, resulting in rapid liberation of free fatty acids (predominantly arachidonic acid) from the plasma membrane. Arachidonic acid becomes the substrate for the enzymes cyclooxygenase and lipoxygenase, triggering production of prostaglandins, thromboxanes, leukotrienes, and endoperoxides.[15,27,28] All these mediators may contribute to neuronal damage through vasoconstriction, by local accumulation of platelets and neutrophils after reperfusion, or by other mechanisms as yet undefined.

In looking at the circulatory status of the brain as a whole, numerous investigators have described and reproduced the phenomenon of postischemic cerebral hypoperfusion. With reperfusion following global cerebral anoxia, there is a period of transient vasodilation during which blood flow to the brain is as much as two times the baseline level before the anoxic injury. This phase of hyperemia usually lasts 20 to 30 minutes. What follows then is a prolonged period of oligemia with markedly reduced blood flow.[28] In its extreme form, this pathophysiological event is referred to as the no reflow phenomenon.[1] In these circumstances, one can often demonstrate the absence of cerebral blood flow by contrast angiography or radionuclide flow scan and the patient almost always is clinically brain dead.

In recent years, research in cerebral resuscitation has focused on ameliorating reperfusion injury by using one or more compounds designed to block some of the pathways in the pathophysiological sequence of events as we understand them.[15,27,28] Drugs such as corticosteroids, barbiturates, and calcium channel blockers show efficacy in certain animal models but have not proved effective in treating humans who have hypoxic brain injury. Presently, the use of drugs to block the action of xanthine oxidase (allopurinol),[13] cyclooxygenase or lipoxygenase, and free radical scavengers is being investigated. Although these approaches have been successful in specific animal models, their ability to treat reperfusion injury in humans, when administered sometime after reperfusion has occurred, is questionable.

INITIAL STABILIZATION AT THE SCENE

The factor most crucial to survival after near-drowning is the prompt restoration of ventilation and circulation. In addition to the effects of submersion, the rescuer also must keep in mind that any preexisting condition that can lead to cardiac arrest under ordinary circumstances can also do so in the water. All victims of diving-related or unwitnessed submersions must be considered to have suffered a head or cervical spine injury as the cause of their failure to resurface. Beyond these considerations, the initial efforts at rescue should follow the procedures of pediatric basic life support, the approach based on the "ABCs" of airway, breathing, and circulation (see Appendix A, Pediatric Basic and Advanced Life Support). Abdominal thrust (Heimlich maneuver) should not be used routinely in submersion victims because of the risk of vomiting and pulmonary aspiration of gastric contents.[26] Oxygen should be administered to all spontaneously breathing patients regardless of their level of consciousness. Thereafter, immediate transport to the nearest medical facility is crucial.

TREATMENT IN THE HOSPITAL

The management of the nearly drowned child in the hospital must be tailored to the patient's clinical condition. The condition on presentation can vary from the child who, by history, had a serious submersion but who looks essentially well, to the child who presents in cardiorespiratory arrest. One can define reasonably the minimal criteria for a significant submersion to be the presence of cyanosis or the requirement of any form of assisted breathing before spontaneous respirations occur.

Children who have suffered a significant submersion should be monitored for some time, regardless of how well they look in the emergency department, because lung injury may not be apparent immediately. Numerous reports have demonstrated that the initial chest radiograph may be normal in children who later develop the "secondary drowning" syndrome. Arterial blood gases may be abnormal, even in the presence of a normal chest radiograph, and appear to be a more sensitive indicator of early pulmonary injury. Most would recommend an observation period of 12 to 24 hours for these children, with documentation of a normal respiratory rate and oxygen saturation in room air before discharge.[17]

Guidelines for managing childhood victims of near-drowning who present as being more severely ill are given below, according to an organ systems approach. This discussion presupposes that basic cardiopulmonary resuscitation has been successful and that spontaneous circulation has been restored, although the child may not be breathing spontaneously.

Central Nervous System

Unfortunately, no specific cerebral resuscitation therapies to date have been shown to be effective in the treatment of hypoxic encephalopathy. Intracranial pressure (ICP) monitoring was practiced widely in the early to mid-1980s in the treatment of comatose children following near-drowning episodes.[8] It was learned that ICP usually is not elevated within the first 72 hours, even in the most severely brain-injured children. Its elevation beyond 72 hours has been shown to be a marker of the most severe cortical injuries; specific treatment of the increased ICP had no effect on outcome.[24] At present, routine ICP monitoring cannot be recommended in comatose children following near-drowning, because it has no therapeutic value for the child and because there are numerous other prognosticators that are noninvasive.

Similarly, we have learned that corticosteroids, barbiturates, and hypothermia have not improved the neurological outcome after near-drowning.[12,21,25] On the contrary, high-dose barbiturates probably increase the likelihood of cardiopulmonary death, whereas hypothermia actually increases the risk of septicemia.[4] Similarly, the routine use of hyperventilation is of no benefit in the treatment of hypoxic encephalopathy. Because intracranial pressure generally is not elevated in the first 72 hours and cerebral blood flow already is reduced, hyperventilation probably does little more than decrease cardiac output.[24]

The most important therapy for the treatment of hypoxic encephalopathy is an approach that seeks to minimize the possibility of additional neuronal injury following the hypoxic event. The goal therefore is to achieve adequate arterial oxygenation and a systemic blood pressure that is at least within the normal range, if not slightly elevated. Seizures should be treated as they would be with any other neurological condition. Hyperthermia should be treated when it occurs to minimize the metabolic demands placed on the brain and the other organs.

Pulmonary Injury

All children who are breathing spontaneously after a near-drowning initially should receive supplemental oxygen. A common situation facing the clinician in the emergency room is that of a child who required some resuscitation at the scene, usually poolside, and who is now lethargic but is making good respiratory efforts. If his or her oxygen saturation by pulse oximeter is in the high 90s while receiving supplemental oxygen, the child does not need to be intubated immediately. The initial blood gas often will show a mixed metabolic and respiratory acidosis. This also is not an indication for immediate intubation because most of these children will continue to improve. So long as oxygenation and mental status do not deteriorate, the child should continue to be given supplemental oxygen and observed closely because subsequent blood gas levels usually will improve. If one does choose to manage such a patient without intubation, the appropriate setting is the pediatric intensive care unit, where intervention can be undertaken immediately should pulmonary injury worsen. Children in this condition usually are not hypotensive and therefore should not require aggressive fluid infusions. Conversely, if at all possible, the early institution of diuretic therapy will improve their pulmonary condition.

The child who has more severe pulmonary injury is treated as one would treat any other child who has diffuse pulmonary injury and hypoxemic respiratory failure (acute lung injury, ARDS). The same strategies for enhancing oxygenation should be used that are applied to other forms of acute lung injury in children.[23]

The pathophysiology of lung injury caused by near-drowning includes the possibility of significant pulmonary capillary injury. In this situation crystalloid or colloid infusions to increase intravascular volume invariably will increase pulmonary capillary pressure and thus increase the rate of pulmonary edema formation.[30] Early attempts at diuresis should be considered. The pulmonary injury in near-drowning, however, is rarely the determinant of overall morbidity and mortality. It is the rare child who has a good neurological prognosis but dies of the pulmonary injury caused by near-drowning.

Cardiovascular Injury

Some degree of circulatory impairment will be present in the victims of a near-drowning episode affected most seriously. The same pathophysiological events that occur during anoxia and reperfusion in the brain also will occur within the myocardium and may lead to impaired ventricular function after resuscitation. There is no particular reason to believe that children who suffer near-drowning are hypovolemic intravascularly, but invasive monitoring of children following global anoxic injury has demonstrated a vasoconstricted state.[16] Hence it is appropriate that the initial intervention in the hypotensive child be a bolus administration of 20 ml/kg of isotonic crystalloid or colloid solution. If the hemodynamic response to the initial fluid bolus is not impressive, one then should consider the use of inotropic support early in the course, particularly if there is evidence of pulmonary injury. The response to moderate doses of dobutamine is often so impressive that diuresis can be accomplished early.

Any child who requires mechanical ventilation for significant cardiopulmonary derangements following a near-drowning should have a multilumen central venous catheter placed. Focus on this procedure, however, should not distract the clinician from attention to the initial priorities of stabilization. The purpose of the catheter is to provide multiple stable sites of vascular access so that vasoactive drug infusion and other therapies may proceed uninterrupted. Central venous pressure monitoring is not itself particularly useful, because it does not necessarily reflect events of the left heart and because there is no single optimal range for central venous pressure in the treatment of hypoxemic respiratory failure.

A small subset of nearly drowned children will develop progressive cardiovascular instability with hypotensive shock and metabolic acidosis. This almost invariably occurs in those children who have the most profound global anoxic brain injuries. These events often are heralded by the development of hyperthermia and neutropenia, which may signify the onset of systemic bacterial sepsis.[4] Additional cardiovascular support with fluids, dopamine, or epinephrine may be undertaken, but the prognosis is grim.

Another cardiovascular phenomenon, occasionally displayed in the pediatric patient who has a profound cerebral anoxic injury, is the development within the first 48 hours of marked hypertension and tachycardia. Infants may have blood pressures as high as 180/130 with heart rates greater than 260/min. The rhythm almost invariably is sinus, and the cause is believed to be the unchecked sympathetic outflow from the brainstem cardiovascular center. The phenomenon generally lasts a matter of hours, can be treated with short-acting beta blockers, resolves spontaneously, and almost always indicates a profound neurological injury.

Infection

The infectious complications of near-drowning episodes range from bronchopneumonia to aspiration pneumonia to septicemia. The child who has fever and pulmonary infiltrates should receive antibiotics. Intubated children following near-drownings may develop fever with purulent tracheal secretions. Under these circumstances, regardless of whether there are well-defined parenchymal infiltrates, antibiotic coverage is warranted. The offending organisms include airway flora, gram negative rods, and occasionally *Staphylococcus aureus*.

In the children most severely asphyxiated, the scenario of high fever and progressive neutropenia develops. These findings may or may not initially be associated with cardiovascular instability, but often herald the onset of systemic bacterial sepsis. It is not clear whether the neutropenia is entirely caused by the severe global anoxia with migration of neutrophils to anoxic tissue during reperfusion or whether the bacterial invasion produces the neutropenia. These patients may develop a rapidly fulminant cardiopulmonary deterioration. The infecting organisms are the same as those listed above for tracheobronchial infection. The use of induced hypothermia appears to increase the risk of neutropenia with sepsis in nearly drowned children.[4] Anoxic injury seems to diminish in some way the normal barriers to systemic infection, and induced hypothermia only increases the risk.

PROGNOSIS

Numerous attempts have been made to predict outcome after near-drowning. Certain aspects of the history and initial physical examination have been shown to have reasonably good predictive value for outcome. If the child arrives awake or blunted (confused, combative, responsive to voice or pain), chances for a good outcome are quite high. In one study all children who had a Glasgow Coma Scale score greater than 5 had a normal or near-normal outcome[9] (see Table 286-1). For children who arrive comatose with a Glasgow Coma Scale of 3 or 4, the outcome is mixed. In such patients the presence of spontaneous respirations in the emergency department indicates the potential for a good outcome, whereas the presence of flaccidity with apnea after resuscitation suggests a very poor neurological outcome.[14]

The neurological outcome of children suffering a near-drowning is related to the severity of brain anoxia occurring at the time of submersion. The prognostic information helps the clinician to prepare the parents for the likely outcome because most parents desire some estimate of prognosis at the time of admission.

A child who drowns in cold water may represent an exception to outcome predictions. Cold water (water temperature less than 68° F [20° C]) rapidly cools the victim, decreasing metabolic rate. Children may cool more rapidly than adults because of a greater relative body surface area. Loss of vasomotor tone occurs in water less than 53.6° F (12° C), further increasing the rate of cooling. The "diving reflex" also may be more prominent in children. This reflex slows heart rate and produces profound redistribution of blood flow so that the heart and brain receive preferential circulation at the expense of the skin, muscle, and gut. Thus rapid cooling with hypothermia and the diving reflex may act to preserve brain function, particularly in small children immersed in very cold water.[17] Intact survival has been reported with up to 40 minutes of submersion in icy water.

A recent review of 55 pediatric near-drowning victims examined the variables of core temperature and presence or absence of vital signs upon arrival at an emergency department.[3] All patients who arrived with a detectable pulse, regardless of temperature, survived without neurological sequelae. All patients who had absent vital signs and a temperature greater than 91.4° F (33° C) either died or survived in a persistent vegetative state. For the patients who arrived with absent vital signs and hypothermia (temperature less than 91.4° F [33° C]), the outcome was mixed. Four of fourteen such patients had intact survival; all four had been submerged under ice or in very cold water. Thus, it appears that pediatric near-drowning victims, who present in cardiac arrest but who are profoundly hypothermic, may warrant cardiopulmonary resuscitation throughout the warming phase, provided their hypothermia was secondary to submersion in very cold water. Conversely, presentation of one who is in cardiorespiratory arrest and who has not been rapidly cooled in very cold water at the time of submersion is strongly predictive of poor neurological outcome.[12,25]

ORGAN DONATION

Organs have varying tolerances to hypoxic injury. It is possible for a pediatric victim of near-drowning who has satisfied criteria for brain death to become a donor for kidneys, heart, liver, corneas, and other tissues. The suitability for organ donation should be explored in every child who meets brain death criteria because the criteria for organ donation continue to be liberalized. When organ donation is possible, the parents or legal guardians should be approached to determine their willingness to make such a gift, once brain death is diagnosed. The making of such a gift can be a comfort to parents in their remembrance of an otherwise terrible sequence of events.

PREVENTION

As a form of accidental injury, drowning and near-drowning ultimately are preventable. Statements from the American Academy of Pediatrics and the Centers for Disease Control have addressed approaches to drowning prevention.[6,7] On the local level it is up to pediatricians, as child safety advocates, both by educating the public and by lobbying public officials, to help to prevent accidental death or disability from submersion injuries in children. However, a recent survey of members of the American Academy of Pediatrics has demonstrated that the majority of pediatricians do not routinely provide written materials or give anticipatory guidance about drowning, and only 4% of pediatricians are involved in community or legislative efforts aimed at drowning prevention.[22]

REFERENCES

1. Ames A, et al: Cerebral ischemia. II. The no-reflow-phenomenon, *Am J Pathol* 52:437, 1968.
2. Babbs CF: Reperfusion injury of postischemic tissues, *Ann Emerg Med* 17:1148, 1988.
3. Biggart M, Bohn D: Effect of hypothermia and cardiac arrest on outcome of near-drowning accidents in children, *J Pediatr* 117:179, 1990.
4. Bohn D, et al: Influence of hypothermia, barbiturate therapy, and intracranial pressure monitoring on morbidity and mortality after near-drowning, *Crit Care Med* 14:529, 1986.
5. Centers for Disease Control: Mortality trends and leading causes of death among adolescents and young adults—United States, 1979-1988, *MMWR* 42:459, 1993.
6. Centers for Disease Control: Setting the national agenda for injury control in the 1990s: home and leisure injury prevention, *MMWR* 41:9, 1992.
7. Committee on Injury and Poison Prevention: Drowning in infants, children and adolescents, American Academy of Pediatrics Committee on Injury and Poison Prevention, *Pediatrics* 92:292, 1993.
8. Conn AW, et al: Cerebral salvage in near-drowning following neurological classification by triage, *Can Anaesth Soc J* 27:201, 1980.
9. Dean JM, Kaufman ND: Prognostic indicators in pediatric near-drowning: the Glasgow Coma Scale, *Crit Care Med* 9:536, 1981.
10. Giammona ST, Modell JH: Drowning by total immersion: effects on pulmonary surfactant of distilled water, isotonic saline and sea water, *Am J Dis Child* 114:612, 1967.
11. Guyer B, et al: Annual summary of vital statistics—1997, *Pediatrics* 102:1333, 1998.
12. Habib DM, et al: Prediction of childhood drowning and near-drowning morbidity and mortality, *Pediatr Emerg Care* 12:255, 1996.
13. Itoh T, et al: Effect of allopurinol on ischemia and reperfusion-induced cerebral injury in spontaneously hypertensive rats, *Stroke* 17:1284, 1986.
14. Jacobsen W, et al: Correlation of spontaneous respiration and neurologic damage in near-drowning, *Crit Care Med* 11:487, 1983.
15. Kirsch JR, et al: Current concepts in brain resuscitation, *Arch Intern Med* 146:1413, 1986.
16. Lucking SE, Pollack MM, Fields AI: Shock following generalized hypoxic-ischemic injury in previously healthy infants and children, *J Pediatr* 108:359, 1986.
17. Martin TG: Near-drowning and cold water immersion, *Ann Emerg Med* 13:263, 1984.
18. Modell J: Drowning, *Curr Concepts* 328:253, 1993.
19. Modell JH, Davis JH: Electrolyte changes in human drowning victims, *Anaesthesia* 30:414, 1969.
20. Modell JH, Moya F: Effects of volume of aspirated fluid during chlorinated fresh water drowning, *Anaesthesia* 27:662, 1966.
21. Nussbaum E, Maggi C: Pentobarbital therapy does not improve neurologic outcome in nearly drowned, flaccid-comatose children, *Pediatrics* 81:630, 1988.
22. O'Flaherty JE, Pirie PL: Prevention of pediatric drowning and near-drowning: a survey of members of the American Academy of Pediatrics, *Pediatrics* 99:169, 1997.
23. Royall J, Levin D: Adult respiratory distress syndrome in pediatric patients, *J Pediatr* 112:169, 1988.
24. Sarnaik A, et al: Intracranial pressure and cerebral perfusion pressure in near-drowning, *Crit Care Med* 13:224, 1985.
25. Spack L, et al: Failure of aggressive therapy to alter outcome in pediatric near-drowning, *Pediatr Emerg Care* 13:98, 1997.
26. Standards and guidelines for cardiopulmonary resuscitation (CPR) and emergency cardiac care (ECC), *JAMA* 255:2905, 1986.
27. Vannucci RC: Experimental biology of cerebral hypoxia-ischemia: relation to perinatal brain damage, *Pediatr Res* 27:317, 1990.
28. White BC, et al: Possible role of calcium blockers in cerebral resuscitation: a review of the literature and synthesis for future studies, *Crit Care Med* 11:202, 1983.
29. Wintemute GJ: Childhood drowning and near-drowning in the United States, *Am J Dis Child* 144:663, 1990.
30. Wood L, Prewitt R: Cardiovascular management in acute hypoxemic respiratory failure, *Am J Cardiol* 47:963, 1981.

282 Drug Overdose

Cheston M. Berlin, Jr.

Drug overdose, whether from accidental ingestion, a therapeutic mistake, or a suicide attempt, is a major problem in pediatric practice. In 1997, 2,192,088 case reports of exposure to potentially toxic substances were tabulated by the American Association of Poison Control Centers, Toxic Exposure Surveillance System.[3] The participating Poison Control Centers serve a population of 250.1 million; thus, the data reported involve approximately 93.5% of the U.S. population. Children under 6 years of age accounted for 52.5% of case reports, and 39.3% occurred in children 2 years of age or younger. Annually, 1.3 million children age 12 years or younger are exposed to drugs that are potentially able to cause toxicity; 36% of the total exposures in 1997 resulted in clinical symptoms and 29 in deaths.

DEFINITION

Drug overdose or toxicity occurs when a child accidentally ingests or is given an amount of a substance that exceeds the recommended dosage or that causes an idiosyncratic reaction within the recommended dosage.

EPIDEMIOLOGY AND ETIOLOGY

The epidemiology of drug overdose is related to the patient's age, as shown in Table 282-1, which lists the number of exposures and deaths from drugs and other compounds according to patient age. The bimodal frequency of deaths peaks at 5 years or below and again at 15 to 19 years. The former reflects accidental ingestions, the latter, usually suicidal events. For some compounds, acetaminophen being a prime example, therapeutic mistakes may play a significant role. Many acetaminophen poisonings are drug overdosages caused by errors in one of the following: calculating the dose, errors in measurement, use of the wrong preparation (e.g., drops instead of elixir), or the use of nonprescription cough and cold preparations that may also contain acetaminophen.[1,2,6] Preventive measures, such as child-resistant bottle tops, are effective in eliminating acute, single-dose accidental exposures. Substances causing deaths are carbon monoxide, pesticides, antidepressants, acetaminophen, hydrocarbons, iron, and alcohol. Chapter 293, Poisoning, provides detailed information on the management of the most common drug ingestions that occur in pediatric practice.

IMMEDIATE ASSESSMENT

An optimum therapeutic response will be achieved if the following steps are taken immediately on encountering the overdosed patient: Detain the person(s) who brought the child to the hospital or office. If initial contact is by telephone, obtain the caller's name and telephone number and then instruct the caller to proceed immediately with the child to the hospital. Be sure to obtain the precise description of the drug thought to have been ingested: name, dose, pharmacy of origin, and prescription number. Instruct the parents to bring the actual container when they come with the patient. Try to determine the amount of drug ingested. This frequently is impossible, and such information, even if obtained, occasionally is misleading. Assume maximal exposure unless a precise tablet or liquid count is available.

Initial Procedures for Stabilization and Life Support

The vital signs (temperature, pulse, respirations, blood pressure) should be determined and pulse oximetry and continuous electrocardiography instituted. The sensorium should be monitored frequently—that is, every 15 minutes until the patient's condition is stable. Changes in frequency and duration of monitoring will depend on the drug, dose, and clinical course.

The adequacy of the airway requires close assessment. Most drug overdoses will not affect the upper airway (larynx, trachea) but will interfere with air exchange by either depressing the central nervous system (CNS) or paralyzing neuromuscular transmission. An intravenous line should be established. If danger of respiratory depression or ingestion of drugs that alter cardiovascular status exists, placing an arterial line should be considered. Some toxic substances, such as insecticides, have significant dermal absorption, especially if the skin is inflamed or abraded, and in such instances, the skin needs to be cleansed.

Decontamination of the patient after oral ingestion has undergone recent changes. The use of ipecac has decreased from 13% of childhood ingestions under 6 years of age in 1983 to 1.5% in 1997.[3] Syrup of ipecac may be used within 30 minutes of ingestion in the alert patient with no sensorium changes and no history of ingestion of hydrocarbons, acids, lye, or other corrosive substances.[7] This may be important

Table 282-1 Substances Causing Toxic Exposure (by Patient Age)

Substance	Age (yr) <6	6-19
Pharmaceutical agents	504,725	168,053
Nonpharmaceutical agents (chemicals, plants, gases)	725,941	188,002

	<6 yrs	6-12 yrs	13-19 yrs
Deaths	25	4	48

Data modified from Litovitz TL, et al: *Am J Emerg Med* 11:494, 1993.

when the patient can be seen immediately in a hospital setting. Studies have been disappointing as emesis appears not to improve patient outcome compared with administration of activated charcoal.[4] Gastric lavage is reserved for patients who have ingested a near lethal or lethal amount of a toxic agent within the prior 1 to 2 hours. Activated charcoal is now considered the best method of gastrointestinal decontamination.[5] It is given at a dose of 1 g/kg usually via nasogastric tube; most children refuse to drink the slurry. Use of a cathartic remains controversial, with no firm evidence supporting its use.[5,6] Only a very small number of compounds appear not to be absorbed to the charcoal (acids, alkali, iron salts). For substances poorly absorbed to charcoal, the use of whole-bowel irrigation (with a polyethylene glycol/electrolyte solution [Colyte or Golytely]) at a dose of 25 to 40 ml/kg/hr may be used. This technique may be especially helpful for the increasing numbers of delayed-release drugs.[7] Gastrointestinal fluid obtained by any of the aforementioned methods should be saved for drug analysis.

DIFFERENTIAL DIAGNOSIS

Considerations of other conditions that can mimic the signs and symptoms of drug overdose will depend on the drug ingested. For patients who have alterations in sensorium, head trauma is of prime consideration. Adolescents who have head trauma may have ingested ethanol. Near-drowning victims also may have ingested ethanol. Spontaneous intracranial hemorrhages in the pediatric age group are rare; they usually produce focal neurological signs rather than global depression of consciousness.

Metabolic conditions such as diabetes mellitus, hypoglycemia, and Addisonian crisis may cause clinical states that resemble drug ingestion. Awareness of these possibilities will help narrow the diagnostic considerations. Head injury with drug overdose in the child may indicate child abuse.

The most difficult situation of all is presented by the patient who has a psychiatric illness, who may develop tremors, hallucinations, or hysterical paralysis. In these patients, precise and rapid laboratory analyses are most important in ruling out drug ingestion. If the patient has been receiving psychoactive medications and is having an untoward reaction, management is identical to that presented above, with special attention directed to the emotional needs of the patient.

MANAGEMENT

The two factors to consider in deciding location and personnel for management of the patient are (1) expertise of the physician in the management of drug overdose and (2) available hospital support facilities. The latter is of most concern because even the best-trained physician cannot provide care properly in an institution that is inadequately equipped with support staff, equipment, and laboratory facilities. The well-trained pediatrician will not always be able to predict the clinical course of a patient who has "overdosed." Will the patient require charcoal perfusion, renal or peritoneal dialysis, or an exchange transfusion? Is the hospital able to offer pediatric intensive care unit monitoring? Can the hospital provide prolonged ventilation and airway management? Can the nursing staff monitor intracranial and/or intraarterial pressure properly? It is best to decide very early in the clinical course whether special facilities will be needed. It is preferable to transfer a stable patient early than a critically ill child requiring mobile life support later. It is important to maintain frequent and smooth communication with the patient's family. Regardless of the cause of their child's poisoning, these families are in constant need of counseling, especially with regard to any guilt feelings they may be experiencing.

Need for General Homeostatic Support

Thermal monitoring is an important aspect of management in drug overdose. Centrally and peripherally induced hypothermia is a common problem—for example, the hypothermia that occurs with phenothiazine ingestion. Hyperthermia can occur with salicylate and atropine poisoning.

Monitoring fluid balance and electrolyte homeostasis is important. Deficits must be replaced, and the amount of maintenance fluids needed will depend on changes in the vital and physical signs. For example, hyperventilation and increased body temperature require increases beyond normal in the amount of maintenance fluids administered. Continuing losses through vomiting and diarrhea should be replaced as they occur.

Monitoring central venous pressure and arterial pressure to assess vascular volume and tone is important. Respiratory function and oxygenation (with pulse oximetry) also require monitoring. Intracranial pressure may need to be assessed to determine the need for treatment of cerebral edema. The need for peritoneal dialysis, hemodialysis, charcoal perfusion, or exchange transfusion to remove the ingested drug must be considered.

Nutritional considerations frequently are neglected in patients who require prolonged intensive care. Feeding via a nasogastric tube or with parenteral alimentation should be considered, especially if coma exceeds 3 days.

Diagnostic Procedures

Assays of blood, urine, and gastric contents for barbiturates, antidepressants, phenytoin, iron, digoxin, salicylate, acetaminophen, narcotics, alcohol, cocaine, and propoxyphene must be available. Rapid drug screens should be available; quantitative analyses should follow as quickly as possible.

Table 282-2 Common Antidotes

Drug	Diagnostic Findings Requiring Treatment	Antidote	Dosage
Acetaminophen	History of ingestion and toxic serum level	*N*-acetylcysteine	140 mg/kg/dose PO, then 70 mg/kg/dose q 4 hr PO × 17
Anticholinergics Antihistamines Atropine Phenothiazines Tricyclic antidepressants	Supraventricular tachycardia (hemodynamic compromise) Unresponsive ventricular dysrhythmia, seizures, pronounced hallucinations or agitation	Physostigmine	Child: 0.5 mg IV slowly (over 3 min) q 10 min prn (maximum: 2 mg) Adult: 1-2 mg IV slowly q 10 min prn (maximum: 4 mg in 30 min)
Cholinergics	Cholinergic crisis: salivation, lacrimation, urination, defecation, convulsions, fasciculations	Atropine sulfate Physostigmine Insecticides	0.05 mg/kg/dose (usual dose 1-5 mg; test dose for child 0.01 mg/kg) q 4-6 hr IV or more frequently prn
Carbon monoxide	Headache, seizure, coma, dysrhythmias	Oxygen, hyperbaric oxygen	100% oxygen (half-life 40 min); consider hyperbaric chamber
Cyanide	Cyanosis, seizures, cardiopulmonary arrest, coma	Amyl nitrite	Inhale pearl q 60-120 sec
		Sodium nitrite (3%)	0.27 ml (8.7 mg)/kg (adult: 10 ml [300 mg]) IV slowly (Hb ≥10 g/dl)
		Sodium thiosulfate (25%) Also consider hyperbaric oxygen	1.35 mL (325 mg)/kg (adult: 12.5 g) IV slowly (Hb ≥10 g/dl)
Ethylene glycol	Metabolic acidosis, urine Ca^{++} oxalate crystals	Ethanol (100% absolute, 1 ml-790 mg)	1 ml/kg in D_5W IV over 15 min, then 0.16 ml (125 mg)/kg/hr IV; maintain ethanol level of 100 mg/dl
Iron	Hypotension, shock, coma, serum iron >350 mg/dl (or greater than iron-binding capacity)	Deferoxamine	Shock or coma: 15 mg/kg/hr IV for 8 hr; if no shock or coma 90 mg/kg/dose IM q 8 hr
Phenothiazines Chlorpromazine Thioridazine	Extrapyramidal dyskinesis, oculogyric crisis	Diphenhydramine (Benadryl)	1-2 mg/kg/dose (maximum: 50 mg/dose) q 6 hr IV, PO
Methanol	Metabolic acidosis, blurred vision; level >20 mg/dl	Ethanol (100% absolute)	1 ml/kg in D_5W over 15 min, then 0.16 ml (125 mg)/kg/hr IV
Methemoglobin Nitrate Nitrites Sulfonamide	Cyanosis, methemoglobin level >30%, dyspnea	Methylene blue (1% solution)	1-2 mg (0.1-0.2 ml)/kg/dose IV; repeat in 4 hr if necessary
Narcotics Heroin Codeine Propoxyphene	Respiratory depression, hypotension, coma	Naloxone (Narcan)	0.1 mg/kg up to 0.8 mg initially IV, if no response give 2 mg IV
Organophosphates Malathion Parathion	Cholinergic crisis: salivation, lacrimation, urination, defecation, convulsions, fasciculations	Atropine sulfate	0.05 mg/kg/dose (usual dose 1-5 mg; test dose for child 0.01 mg/kg) q 4-6 hr IV or more frequently prn
		Pralidoxime	After atropine, 20-50 mg/kg/dose (maximum: 2000 mg) IV slowly (<50 mg/min) q 8 hr IV prn × 3

From Barkin RM: *Pediatr Ann* 19:632, 1990.

A flat plate of the abdomen may be required to identify radiopaque tablets (e.g., iron) or foreign bodies. A computed tomography (CT) scan of the head should be performed if intracranial hemorrhage is suspected following amphetamine or cocaine ingestion. A chest roentgenogram is needed if narcotic-induced pulmonary edema or aspiration is suspected.

It is important to remember that trauma may have occurred in any poisoned patient, especially in adolescents. Half of adolescent drownings are associated with alcohol use. Because near-drownings often follow diving, in which the head and neck may be injured, immobilization of the cervical spine should be accomplished immediately on site.

Definitive Therapy

Specific antidotes exist for some drugs but unfortunately not for most. Thus, definitive therapy consists of intensive supportive care and treatment of signs and symptoms as they develop (e.g., hypotension and hypertension, thermal instability, cardiac arrhythmias). The following steps should be taken in treating drug overdosage:

1. Stabilize the patient.
2. Identify the drug ingested and determine the amount ingested.
3. Contact the local poison control center for toxicology data and information regarding the signs and symptoms and clinical course. "POISINDEX" (Micromedex, Englewood, Colorado) is an excellent comprehensive reference and is updated quarterly.
4. Use gastrointestinal decontamination as discussed on p. 1943.
5. If a specific antidote exists, administer it. It is most helpful to have a table prepared of specific antidotes and their location in the hospital (Table 282-2); the best location is the emergency department. All staff members must know the precise location.
6. Provide supportive care in an intensive or intermediate care unit as appropriate.
7. Meet social service needs as indicated (e.g., drug ingestion by a toddler as a symptom of chaotic family structure or by an adolescent as a symptom of depression or as a suicidal gesture).
8. Provide counseling concerning the institution of poison control measures in the home.

Complications

Possible complications of drug overdose are many and varied. Therapy itself can have side effects, such as too rigorous treatment of seizures causing apnea and the need for mechanical ventilation. Many poisoned patients require ventilator therapy. Such therapy, especially if prolonged, may lead to complications such as pneumothorax, oxygen toxicity, and airway infections. Nosocomial infections are not uncommon, especially hypostatic pneumonia, urinary tract infection (secondary to catheter placement), or septicemia from vascular catheters. Thrombotic and embolic episodes also can result from vascular catheters.

Permanent CNS damage sometimes follows periods of hypoxia or hypoglycemia—usually before therapy is instituted. Topical skin, mucous membrane, and deeper-tissue injuries often result from acids, lyes, or corrosives. Specific compounds can cause permanent organ damage (e.g., to the lungs from hydrocarbons, the kidneys from ethylene glycol, the liver from acetaminophen, and the retina from methanol).

Hazards of treatment for drug overdosage include overtreatment, the wrong treatment, an insufficient period of observation, and failure to appreciate drug ingestion as an indication of child neglect or abuse. Especially suspect is the child under age 12 months who is admitted with "accidental ingestion" or the child who has a history of repeated drug ingestions. Overtreatment occurs when errors are made in assessing the amount of drug ingested. A nontoxic ingestion may be vigorously but inappropriately treated with potentially toxic antidotes—for example, using sodium nitrate-sodium thiosulfate for the treatment of cyanide ingestion.

The wrong treatment can occur when a mistake is made in identifying the drug ingested—for example, from a mislabeled prescription vial. An insufficient period of observation can worsen the situation. For example, hepatic necrosis may not occur until day 3 after acetaminophen ingestion, and renal disease may not occur until day 7 to 10.

When to Refer

Ingestion of any substance unfamiliar to the primary care physician

Any patient who potentially may require a therapy unfamiliar to the primary care physician

When to Hospitalize

Any patient strongly suspected of ingesting a toxic or lethal dose of any substance

An unstable patient

Any patient requiring gastrointestinal decontamination, intravenous therapy, hemoperfusion, or charcoal perfusion, even if clinically well

A patient in an environment suggesting child abuse

REFERENCES

1. Heubi J, Barbacci M, Zimmerman H: Therapeutic misadventures with acetaminophen: hepatotoxicity after multiple doses in children, *J Pediatrics* 132:22, 1998.
2. Kearns G, Leeder J, Wasserman G: Acetaminophen overdose with therapeutic intent, *J Pediatr* 132:5, 1998.
3. Litovitz TK, et al: 1997 annual report of the American Association of Poison Control Centers Toxic Exposure Surveillance System, *Am J Emerg Med* 16:444, 1998.
4. Neuvonen P, Vartiainen M, Tokola O: Comparison of activated charcoal and ipecac syrup in prevention of drug absorption, *Eur J Clin Pharmacol* 24:557, 1983.
5. Perry H, Shannon M: Emergency department gastrointestinal decontamination, *Pediatr Ann* 25:19, 1996.
6. Rivera-Penera T, et al: Outcome of acetaminophen overdose in pediatric patients and factors contributing to hepatotoxicity, *J Pediatr* 130:300, 1997.
7. Snodgrass WR: Clinical toxicity. In Klaasen CD, editor: *Casarett and Doull's toxicology,* ed 5, New York, 1996, McGraw-Hill.

283 Envenomations

Steven D. Salhanick

An *envenomation* is the injection of venom via bite or sting of venomous creatures. Bites refer to the injection via structures associated with the mouth and are primarily evolved for handling prey, whereas stings are delivered via a posterior structure (sting) and are primarily defensive.[74] Envenomations are common presenting complaints to primary care and emergency medicine physicians; concerns regarding serious allergic reactions result in referrals to allergy and immunology specialists. Although most cases are minor in nature, serious local and systemic injury can result. Consequently, the primary care clinician must be aware of local venomous species and be able to recognize and treat the injuries caused by them. In North America the predominant vectors for envenomations include arthropods, specifically Hymenoptera (bees, wasps, ants), arachnids (spiders, scorpions), and snakes.

HYMENOPTERA

In the United States, social Hymenoptera are responsible for most insect stings; family Apidae (honeybees), family Bombidae (bumblebees), superfamily Vespoidae (paper wasps, white-faced hornets, yellow hornets, and yellowjackets), and superfamily Formicidae (harvester ants and native and imported fire ants).[38,83] All possess a sting located posteriorly.

Hymenoptera stings can cause local or systemic reactions. Reactions may be a direct effect of the venom, or they may occur through IgE-mediated allergic reaction. Systemic reactions occur in less than 5% of patients.[45]Anaphylactic reactions are uncommon. Their prevalence in the general population ranges from 0.15% to 3.9%.[16] Large local cutaneous reactions to stings occur in approximately 2.3% to 18.6% of the general population.[33,57] Biphasic anaphylactic reactions, characterized by return of symptoms 6 to 10 hours after initial symptom resolution, may occur in up to 20% of patients.[43]

Winged Hymenoptera

Characteristics and distribution. Winged Hymenoptera are found in most areas of the United States. Honeybees usually nest in hollow trees and crevices, whereas bumblebees prefer nesting underground. Wasp nests often can be found under roofs and eaves, hornets prefer to nest in the branches of trees, and yellowjackets tend to build their nests in the ground.

The majority of social bees and wasps sting primarily in the defense of the nest. Yellowjacket wasps are common near exposed food and garbage, resulting in stings not associated with nest protection. Yellowjackets have also been implicated in frequent stings in late summer associated with "yellowjacket delirium," a poorly understood seasonal behavior characterized by aggressiveness towards objects that are not threatening or provocative.[10]

Honeybees differ from other Hymenoptera in that they possess a barbed stinger that anchors into the skin. Because of this, bees die from evisceration after they sting. Wasps also have barbed stingers, but they usually are able to withdraw them from the skin and can sting multiple times.[83]

A great deal of attention has been paid recently to the presence of Africanized honey bees, commonly referred to as killer bees, which now are found in southern Texas, Arizona, and California.[60] The original colonies of these bees were imported to South America to breed with European varieties in an attempt to increase honey production. Unfortunately, ensuing generations of these bees retained the ferocity of the African bees. The bees are not more individually dangerous than the European bees. Their venom is similarly potent and similar amounts are delivered on a per-sting basis. Their aggressive nature, however, results in massive envenomations secondary to the number of stings delivered in an attack.[43]

Winged Hymenoptera venoms contain many protein components that account for the various observed reactions. Phospholipase A_2, hyaluronidase, histamine, apamin, mellitin, mast cell-degranulating peptide, acid phosphatase, norepinephrine, dopamine, and allergen C are the main constituents of honeybee venom. Bumblebee venom contains acid phosphatase, triptic amadase, and melittin. The major vespid allergens are antigen 5 and hyaluronidase, but they also contain histamine, kinins, serotonin, phospholipase A_1 and B, and mastoparans.[38,83] Cross-reactivity between the apid and vespid venoms is limited, but a significant cross-reactivity exists between the different vespid venoms.[33,51]

The most common areas to be stung are the head, neck, feet, and hands. Stinging is most common during the summer months, and children often are affected.[83] Most patients cannot reliably identify the insect that stung them.

Physical examination

LOCAL. Types of local reactions to stings are nonallergic and allergic. The nonallergic reaction is a direct result of envenomation via mast cell degranulation and the production of a wheal-and-flare response. This produces erythema, swelling, pain, and itching. These signs and symptoms usually subside in a few hours.

Allergic local reactions occur in about 17% of people stung by winged hymenoptera. They consist of erythema and local edema of greater than 10 cm in diameter, they often persist for 48 to 72 hours, and may become indurated for a period of up to 5 days.[57,83] Some patients may experience headache, nausea, or malaise with these reactions.

As mentioned previously, a stinger sometimes may be found at the sting site. This usually indicates a honeybee or, in some cases, a yellowjacket sting.

SYSTEMIC. The more common systemic manifestations of an allergic reaction to hymenoptera stings include urticaria, angioedema, wheezing, shortness of breath, stridor, nausea, vomiting, diarrhea, abdominal pain, malaise, dizziness, and anaphylaxis. Dysphagia, dysarthria, hoarseness, weakness, and confusion also have been described. Respiratory and cardiovascular complications are seen in adults more frequently than in children.[57] Fatal anaphylaxis is rare, especially in children.[33,60] However, the sheer number of exposures makes hymenoptera the second leading cause of anaphylactic reactions after penicillin exposure with upwards of 40 deaths per year documented in the United States.[72]

The risk of developing a systemic reaction appears to be greater with a history of multiple stings or within a few weeks after a previous sting. The risk is higher in patients who have a previous history of anaphylaxis. Their risk of anaphylaxis with subsequent stings is 35% to 60%.[51,57] However, the pattern of reaction is difficult to predict.[33] Atopic patients do not appear to be at greater risk of developing systemic complications, but the severity of their symptoms may be greater than in nonatopic individuals.[57] A history of a large local reaction does not reliably predict progression to systemic complications. The risk of subsequent anaphylaxis after a large local reaction is about 5% to 10%.[33,85]

Systemic reactions may also be caused by direct action of bee venom. In rare cases, serum sickness, vasculitis, encephalopathy, neuritis, and renal disease are seen.[53] The presence of Africanized bees may result in high doses of venom, resulting in hemolysis, thrombocytopenia, rhabdomyolysis (skeletal and myocardial), and characteristically acute tubular necrosis.[6,28,54,65]

Differential diagnosis. Differential diagnosis of the local reaction include other arthropod envenomations, puncture wounds with reactive erythema or cellulites, or simple cellulites.[85] Differential diagnosis of systemic reactions include any other cause of allergic reaction, reactive airway disease, or infectious processes. Other causes of stridor, wheezing, and allergic reaction should be considered if a sting site cannot be identified.

Laboratory studies. No specific laboratory test is useful in the acute management of hymenoptera stings.

Management. Insect sting sites should be inspected for the presence of a stinger. Honeybee stingers remain present and will further imbed and continue to pump venom after separation from the bee, and the venom sack is emptied within 2 minutes of entering the skin.[64,74] Consequently, rapid removal of the stinger is imperative.[8,67,75] Traditional teaching advocates removal of the stinger by scraping with a hard-edged object, such as a credit card, to prevent pressure on the venom sack. Such pressure would theoretically result in an increase in envenomation.[45] Recent experimental data shows that removal of the stinger with fingers does not increase envenomation,[75] and suggests that rapid removal of the stinger by any means is most effective in minimizing envenomation.

Nonallergic local reactions require symptomatic treatment including ice, elevation, and local wound care. No further evaluation is necessary. If local itching is significant, an oral H_1 antihistamine such as diphenhydramine may be useful.

Local allergic reactions require similar care as nonallergic reactions. For very large cutaneous reactions, prednisone (0.5 to 2 mg/kg/day given in 1 to 4 doses for 3 to 5 days) may be useful.[45,60]

Mild systemic allergic reactions may be treated with diphenhydramine or another H_1 antihistamine, supportive care, and observation. Epinephrine is the mainstay of therapy for severe systemic allergic reactions* along with H_1 antagonists, corticosteroids, and intensive supportive care.[43] Severe systemic reactions from direct toxic effects of massive envenomation require intensive supportive care, therapy similar to that for anaphylactic reactions as exposure to large numbers of stings can stimulate the production of IgE antibodies, and careful monitoring for rhabdomyolysis, thrombocytopenia, cardiac arrhythmias and renal failure. Dialysis may be required.[43,54,65]

Patients with systemic reactions who respond completely to therapy in the emergency department should be observed for 6 to 8 hours after the sting because of the possibility of a delayed anaphylactic episode. The mechanism of this delayed complication is poorly understood.[51] Patient who presented with severe symptoms including airway, cardiovascular or pulmonary compromise, or persistent symptoms should receive a short course of corticosteriods.[45]

At the time of discharge following a systemic reaction, all patients should be given a prescription for a self-administered epinephrine kit. The patient or caretaker should be instructed in the proper use of this kit before discharge from the emergency department. They also should be encouraged to wear a MedicAlert bracelet identifying them as being allergic to insect stings. Patients should be told how to avoid further stings (Box 283-1).

Children who sustain extracutaneous systemic reactions should be referred to an allergist for risk analysis and possible venom immunotherapy.[52,73,83] Various immunotherapy regimens exist, consequently susceptible patients may be effectively protected within hours to days, although typical regimens take weeks to months.[56] Immediate access to aqueous epinephrine and a thorough understanding of its administration remain important aspects of care for children undergoing immunotherapy until maintenance doses are reached.[52,73]

---

*A 0.01 ml/kg dose of 1:1000 aqueous epinephrine solution is injected subcutaneously. The original dose should not exceed 0.3 ml, but it may be repeated in 15 minutes. Alternatively, Sus-Phrine (0.005 ml/kg) can be used. It is highly recommended that susceptible individuals carry epinephrine self-administered kits when outdoors. After such a kit is used, medical help should be sought because the drug's duration of action is brief.

BOX 283-1

HOW TO AVOID INSECT STINGS

Do not disturb nests or hives—have someone else remove them.
Do not wear perfume, cologne, scented sunscreens, or hairspray when outdoors.
Use footwear when outside.
Avoid picnic areas, garbage sites, orchards, fields of clover, and flowerbeds.
Be extra careful when gardening and cover your hands and body.
Avoid trips outdoors if medical help is not readily available or until maintenance immunotherapy is established.
Do not wear brightly colored clothes or jewelry.
Install screens on windows and doors to prevent insects from entering the home.

Fire Ants

Characteristics. There are approximately 20 species of ants of the genus *Solenopsis* (commonly known as fire ants) in the United States. Of these, two imported species have the most clinical importance: *Solenopsis invicta* and *Solenopsis richteri*. Three common species of native fire ant, *Solenopsis xyloni, Solenopsis geminata,* and *Solenopsis aurea* are less aggressive, have limited geographical range and have largely been displaced by the imported species.[39]

S. invicta is red, 3 to 4 mm in length, and native to northern Argentina, Paraguay, and western Brazil. It arrived in Mobile, Alabama, in the late 1930s and has spread aggressively throughout the Southeast from Texas to Virginia, as well as into California. *S. invicta* is expected to spread north along the west coast and may reach the Canadian boarder by the end of the next decade, displacing native species as it spreads.[70] In infested areas, imported fire ants can make up 90% of the ant population.[61]

S. richteri is black, slightly larger than *S. invicta*, and is native to Argentina and Uruguay. *S. richteri*'s importation to southern Alabama preceded *S. invicta* by approximately 20 years and has been largely displaced by it.[70] Currently, *S. richteri* is found only in northeastern Mississippi and northwestern Alabama. Significant changes in the characteristics of imported fire ants have occurred in this country. *S. invicta* and *S. richteri* have formed hybrid species with a greater tolerance to cold, which will likely increase their geographical distribution.[37] Spread of fire ants is largely passive, commonly via soil or plant matter.[37]

Imported fire ants are extremely aggressive, resulting in a high frequency of envenomation among humans in endemic areas. The preponderance of the literature supports a 20% to 30% annual attack rate in endemic areas, although rates as high as 58% have been reported.[25,37] Children are especially vulnerable. Adams and Lofgren[3,4] have noted the highest sting rate (close to 50%) in persons younger than 20 years of age. Trespassing into the fire ants' territory or disturbing a nest will incite aggressive, swarming behavior, often resulting in multiple stings. Cases of ants attacking victims indoors are not uncommon.[26,27,36] Heavy rains appear to increase this occurrence, although increasingly the ants are noted to nest in manmade structures.[25]

Fire ants bite the skin of their victims with their mandibles, then arch their bodies to inject venom through a lancet-shaped stinger located at the distal end of their abdomen. If undisturbed they will continue to sting the victim repeatedly in a circular pattern using their mandibles as a pivot; venom is injected with each sting.[19,29,31,69]

Fire ant venom is mostly composed of alkaloid piperidine compounds and contains very little protein. However, it is this protein moiety that is responsible for the IgE-mediated allergic reactions sometimes encountered with fire ant stings. The alkaloid portion is believed to be responsible for the more common local dermal reactions, as well as having some neurotoxicity.[3,19,31,36,38]

Physical Examination: Signs and Symptoms

Local. Stings from imported fire ants frequently occur on children's ankles and feet in the summer. Stings tend to be multiple and cause immediate local burning and itching. Soon after, the area becomes erythematous and raised. This reaction usually subsides after 30 to 60 minutes. The classic, pathognomonic finding of small, sterile pustules develops between 4 and 24 hours of the sting and is more common with imported fire ant stings.[37,45] Pustules may occur in rings or lines consistent with fire and stinging behavior. Pustules usually resolve over a period of 3 to 10 days. Some patients develop a large local reaction similar to the of other hymenoptera stings. An initial wheal and flare reaction evolves into an erythematous, pruritic, warm, indurated area around the sting site. Large local reactions may progress for 48 hours and may not subside for 7 days. The pathophysiology of large local reactions is not clear, and they may be confused with cellulites.

Secondary bacterial infections are not uncommon after stings. These are usually minor and localized. However, sepsis may result from superinfected lesions.[27]

Systemic. Systemic allergic reactions occur in up to 16% of patients treated for fire ant stings, with serious reactions, including anaphylaxis, occurring in up to 2%.[37,70] Systemic allergic reactions are similar to those associated with other insects and include bronchospasm, angioedema, urticaria pruritus, and anaphylaxis. The venoms of native and imported fire ants are highly cross reactive, and phospholipase components of fire ant venom have been shown to be cross reactive with vespid venom phospholipases.[38,39] Direct systemic toxic effects of fire ant venom are not well understood. Currently, no deaths have been attributed to fire ant venom toxicity. Most systemic toxic effects reported have been neurological including seizures, neuropathy, and Guillain-Barré syndrome.[37,70]

Laboratory studies. The diagnosis of fire ant sting is a clinical one; there is no confirmatory laboratory test.

Management. Mild local reactions are treated conservatively with ice, analgesia, and wound care. Large local reactions may require systemic antihistamines and prednisone.[43,70] Large local reactions must be carefully examined to differentiate them from cellulitis. The absence of lymphadenopathy and lymphangitis supports the diagnosis of large localized reaction.[43] Systemic allergic reactions are treated similarly to those from any cause. Epinephrine is the mainstay of therapy, coupled with H_1 blockers, systemic steroids, and vigorous supportive care as appropriate.[43,70] Patients who have had severe allergic reactions to stings should be referred to an allergist for immunotherapy assessment.[30,60]

Harvester Ants

Harvester ants (genus *Pogonomyrmex*) belong to the Hymenoptera order, subfamily Myrmicinae, which includes the genus *Solenopsis* (fire ants). More than 20 native species inhabit the United States, but only three have been associated with anaphylaxis: *Pogonomyrmex barbatus, Pogonomyrmex rugosus,* and *Pogonomyrmex maricopa.*[69] Harvester ants occupy a wide geographical area and are found in the southern and western United States and in Mexico.

Like fire ants, harvester ants attach to the skin with their mandibles and envenomate their victim through a sting. Their venom differs from fire ant venom in that it contains a much larger fraction of protein constituents; hence it is more like other Hymenoptera venoms.

Unlike imported fire ants, harvester ants do not leave characteristic skin lesions. Their sting resembles that of other insects and may be associated with allergic reactions. Treatment of *Pogonomyrmex* stings is the same as that for other hymenoptera.

ARACHNIDS

Arachnids belong to the phylum Arthropoda, which includes the orders Araneae (spiders) and Scorpionidae (scorpions). Although both of these can inflict envenomations with significant morbidity, fatalities are rare.

Spiders

Most of the 30,000 species of spiders in the world are harmless to humans, but approximately 50 species are of medical importance. In North America, *Loxosceles* (which includes the brown recluse spider), *Latrodectus* (black widow spider), and tarantulas are the species most commonly implicated.

Prevention. Eradicating *Loxosceles* and black widow spiders is difficult or impossible. Prevention, therefore, is focused chiefly on caution in areas inhabited by these spiders.

Loxosceles

Characteristics. There are two species of *Loxosceles* spiders in the United States commonly implicated in envenomations: *Loxosceles reclusa* and *Loxosceles deserta. L. reclusa* is found in most of the continental United States but is most common in the South and Midwest.[84] They commonly are called violin, or fiddleback, spiders. They are hearty and live in dry areas such as wood piles, rodent burrows, vacant buildings, attics, or closets. They are reclusive and nonaggressive unless disturbed. Their web is irregular and common in appearance.

Loxosceles' body is oval (10 to 15 mm long, 4 mm wide) and light fawn to dark chocolate in color. The leg span is about 25 mm. The most distinguishing feature is the violin-shaped marking on the dorsal aspect of the cephalothorax, with the neck pointing toward the abdomen. Another distinguishing feature is the presence of three pairs of eyes instead of the four pairs usually seen in other species.

Bites usually are a result of accidental contact, such as looking through boxes or wood piles, or contact with linens or clothing in which the spider has become trapped.

Distribution. *Loxosceles* spiders are found throughout the world. Many species are found in the United States, mostly in the south and central areas. Only six of these are known to cause necrotic skin lesions: *Loxosceles reclusa, Loxosceles laeta, Loxosceles rufescens, Loxosceles unicolor, Loxosceles arizonica,* and *Loxosceles devia.*[6,82]

Physical examination: signs and symptoms

LOCAL MANIFESTATIONS. The bite itself does not cause much discomfort and may go unnoticed. Sometimes a minor stinging or burning sensation may be felt at the site. Erythema, pruritus, pain, and edema typically develop within 2 to 8 hours. These may be followed in the next 24 to 48 hours by the appearance of a blue-gray halo surrounding the erythematous center. Vesicles or bullae containing serous or hemorrhagic fluid soon follow.

Local ischemia and necrosis result in the formation of a black eschar within 7 to 10 days of the bite. This necrotic area may expand slowly in diameter for weeks, especially in fatty areas that have delicate blood supplies such as the abdomen, buttocks, and thighs.[77] The eschar is shed after 2 to 5 weeks and an ulcer remains; the latter may take weeks to months to heal.

SYSTEMIC MANIFESTATIONS. Systemic manifestations of loxoscelism are less common than cutaneous ones. The most common symptoms are fever, chills, and malaise. Symptoms usually occur within 24 hours of the bite and also may include nausea, vomiting, diarrhea, arthralgia, urticaria or maculopapular rash, hemolytic anemia, disseminated intravascular coagulation, jaundice, renal failure, transverse myelitis, seizures, and shock.[5,41]

Differential diagnosis. In the absence of a definitive history of spider bites, other diagnostic possibilities must be considered, such as emboli, thrombi, focal vasculitis, envenomation by other insects or reptiles, fat herniation with infarction, pressure sore, pyoderma gangrenosum, poison oak or ivy, cutaneous manifestation of gonorrhea or herpes simplex, diabetic ulcer, purpura fulminans, erythema nodosum, or abusive or self-inflicted trauma.

Other species of spiders have been implicated in the cause of necrotic skin lesions similar to loxosceles. These are *Argiope* (orbweaver spider), *Chiracanthium* (sac spider), *Lycosa* (wolf spider), *Phidippus* (jumping spider), and *Tegenaria agrestis.*[5,79]

Laboratory studies. No laboratory study can confirm the presence of necrotic arachnidism. Complete blood counts, coagulation profiles, electrolytes, and renal function should be monitored in systemic illness.

Management. Management is controversial because the unpredictable natural course of the wounds make prospective trials difficult. Serial observations, cleansing, cool compresses, splinting of the affected extremity, and tetanus prophylaxis commonly are recommended wound care measures. Symptomatic relief with antipruritics and analgesics may be useful in some cases.

Different therapies have been proposed, including systemic steroids, antibiotics, antihistamines, dapsone, colchicine, surgical excision, hyperbaric oxygen, and observation. The most suitable therapy in the pediatric population is unclear, but there is general agreement on delaying any surgical repair of skin defects until the necrotic demarcation is discrete and there is no further spread; this takes about 8 weeks.

Black Widow Spider *(Latrodectus)*

Characteristics. Although both male and female black widow spiders have venom, only the female has fangs that are powerful enough to bite through skin and envenomate humans. Black widow spiders are among the largest spiders in the world, with a leg span of 40 mm and a body of 1.5 cm. The mature female is black, with a red or orange hourglass-shaped marking on the ventral surface. The immature female may be red, brown, or cream in color, and the hourglass marking may be cream colored or even incomplete.[5]

The web, usually built close to the ground in dimly lit, moist areas, is distinguishable by its irregular pattern. It may be found in barns, outhouses, lumber piles, and sheds where insects are plentiful. Bites usually are a result of the spider being disturbed and acting in self-defense.

Distribution. *Latrodectus* spiders are found in both temperate and tropical climates throughout the world. Five species are found in the United States; Alaska is the only state that does not have this genus. The most common spiders implicated in latrodectism are *Latrodectus mactans, Latrodectus variolus,* and *Latrodectus hesperus.*[17] Envenomations by any of these results in the same clinical syndrome.

Physical examination: signs and symptoms

LOCAL. A bite may go unnoticed or may be experienced as a pinprick or burning sensation. Two small punctate lesions may be visible. Within half an hour, pain at the site and in the regional lymph nodes develops. Central pallor at the bite site with surrounding erythema also has been described.[3,12,33] Unlike the bite of loxosceles (violin or fiddleback spiders), the black widow bite usually does not induce an impressive inflammatory response.

SYSTEMIC. The onset of systemic symptoms frequently is sudden, with crampy, skeletal muscle pains in the legs, abdomen, back, and chest and associated autonomic dysfunction. A review of 163 cases by Clark et al[17] showed the most frequent systemic signs and symptoms to be generalized abdominal pain or back pain (56%), local or extremity pain (38%), hypertension (29%), diaphoresis (22%), and isolated abdominal (18%) or chest (17%) pains. Nausea and vomiting and tachycardia were present in 11% of patients. Restlessness, salivation, bronchorrhea, priapism, urinary retention, periorbital edema, tremor, and convulsions also may be seen.[5,59] Abdominal rigidity may mimic peritoneal irritation. Respiratory paralysis and heart failure also have been reported.

Patients who do not receive antivenom may have protracted symptoms that last for weeks to months. Symptoms can include fatigue, weakness, paresthesias, generalized aches, diaphoresis, headache, sleeplessness, excessive sweating, impotence, mental status changes, and transient hemiparesis.[55]

Laboratory studies. No specific laboratory test helps to establish this diagnosis. Leukocytosis and hyperglycemia are common. Creatine phosphokinase may be elevated because of increased muscle activity. Serum calcium is normal.

Differential diagnosis. The causes of acute abdominal pain should be part of the differential diagnosis. Of interest is the close resemblance of the autonomic hyperactivity seen after black widow spider bites and that seen in organophosphate poisoning.

Management. The vast majority of black widow spider bites require only cool compresses, elevation of the affected extremity, tetanus status update (if needed), and analgesics. In more severe cases oxygen, cardiac monitoring, and intravenous access are recommended.

Muscle cramps may be relieved with opiates and muscle relaxants. Diazepam, methocarbamol, and calcium gluconate have been used with varying results. Recently the efficacy of 10% calcium gluconate has been questioned by Clark et al[17] in their retrospective study. Patients who do not receive antivenom gradually will improve over the next 12 to 48 hours. As previously mentioned, some individuals may have protracted symptoms.

Latrodectus antivenom of equine origin is available and neutralizes venom from all related species.[5] Patients should be tested for horse serum hypersensitivity before it is administered. It should be considered in severe envenomations that have evidence of respiratory distress, significant hypertension, and cardiovascular compromise, as well as for pregnant women and for protracted symptoms unresponsive to analgesics and muscle relaxants. Prompt response within an hour of infusion is mandated. The administration of antivenom may decrease length of stay in hospital and prevent lingering neurological complications.[5,55]

Tarantulas (Mygalomorphs)

Characteristics. Tarantulas, more appropriately called mygalomorphs, are considered primitive forms of true spiders. In the United States the species spends most of the daytime hours in burrows and hunts at night.[82] They are docile, and bites are unusual. Body size varies and can reach up to 10 cm. These spiders possess large vertically oriented fangs that require them to lean back on their hind legs to bite; this is a characteristic defensive posture. More than 30 species of tarantulas are found in the tropical and subtropical desert areas of the southwestern United States. Some North American and foreign species are kept as pets.

Physical examination: signs and symptoms. Most bites are no more severe than a bee sting and occasionally result in local erythema, swelling, and pain. Nausea and vomiting may occur from the bite. Some genera (*Lasiodora, Grammostola, Acanthoscurria,* and *Brachypelma*) are capable of releasing urticaria-producing hairs from their abdomen by rubbing their hind legs on the area. This can result in local histamine release with mild pruritus. However, the itching can last for weeks.[5,82] The hairs may become itching in eyes or airways causing considerable discomfort.[74]

Management. Local wound care and tetanus update as required are all that is needed in most cases; antihistamines and oral analgesics may be helpful. Adhesive tape may be useful to remove the urticaria-producing hairs from the skin. Saline solution irrigation may also be used for the removal of hairs.

Scorpions

Characteristics. *Centruroides exilicauda,* formerly *Centruroides sculpturatus,* or bark scorpion, is the only medically relevant species in the United States. It measures 1.3 to 7.5 cm in length and envenomates its victim with a stinger located at the distal end of the tail. The venom is a potent neurotoxin that activates neuronal sodium channels and results in excessive firing of the affected neurons, including both adrenergic and parasympathetic systems.[9,62] Patients may present with both adrenergic and cholinergic symptoms.

Stings usually result from accidental contact with a scorpion trapped in linen or clothing or during play outdoors. Fortunately, not all stings result in clinical evidence of envenomation. Although most stings take place in scorpion-endemic areas, scorpions can be accidentally transported to other areas by travelers. Scorpions are found in Arizona and parts of southern California, Nevada, New Mexico, and Texas. *C. exilicauda,* considered a climbing scorpion, can be sighted on trees, fence posts, and rocks and in cracks and rubbish piles.

Physical examination: signs and symptoms

LOCAL. Pain at the sting site with or without paresthesias is common, especially with species other than *C. centruroides*. In mild envenomations this may be the only symptom. Infants may manifest this symptom as unexplained crying.[9] Local erythema and swelling may surround a small puncture wound, but the sting site more often is unidentifiable.

SYSTEMIC. Systemic manifestations of scorpion envenomation can be dramatic and usually develop within 60 minutes of the sting. They tend to be more common in children less than 10 years of age.[62] Cardiovascular findings include tachycardia or bradycardia.[35,46] Severe hypertension is common. Severe cases may show a terminal hypotension unresponsive to fluids or pressors.[42] Echocardiographic, scintigraphic, and hemodynamic evaluations reveal hypodynamic ventricular[35,42] motion with decreased systolic performance. Pulmonary edema is a common feature and is likely due to decreased ventricular performance in the setting of increased venous return, arterial hypertension, kinin-induced increased permeability of the pulmonary vasculature and impaired left ventricular filling caused by tachycardia.[1,35,42,44] Electrocardiographic changes are common and include nonspecific ST-T changes or ST elevation or depression consistent with myocardial infarction.[35,42]

Pathological cardiac specimens show evidence of ischemia as well as direct toxicity.[35,42] The primary mechanism of cardiovascular toxicity is thought due to excessive stimulation of the autonomic nervous system with the sympathetic influence being generally greater than the parasympathetic. Cardiac effects may also be mediated by electrolyte changes, in particular a relative hyperkalemia.[42]

Neurological toxicity includes excessive cholinergic stimulation resulting in salivation, sweating and vomiting.[35] Skeletal muscle findings include twitching or jerking of the extremities, which in some cases may be severe enough to be mistaken for seizure activity; rhabdomyolysis may result from this.[9] Seizures and agitation may occur as well.

Differential diagnosis. Two factors make it difficult to establish the correct diagnosis. The first is that the sting site may not be identifiable; the second is that the child may not be able to communicate the history of a sting clearly. Seizure disorders, intraabdominal catastrophes, phenothiazine or cholinergic poisoning, and allergic reactions are some of the differential diagnostic possibilities. Some children have been misdiagnosed as having asthma in the presence of wheezing and respiratory distress.[62]

Progression of symptoms is not predictable. A review of cases from Arizona's Regional Poison Management Center revealed that progression to serious symptoms always occurred in less than 5 hours if at all. Numbness, tingling, and pain may persist for 2 weeks.[21] Rimsza, Zimmerman, and Bergeson[62] found the duration of symptoms to be related inversely to the age of the patient.

Laboratory studies. Scorpion envenomation is a clinical determination; there is no confirmatory laboratory test. Leukocytosis, CSF pleocytosis, and elevated creatine phosphokinase have been reported.[9,35]

Management. The treatment of scorpion envenomation primarily is supportive, with the use of cold compresses and analgesics.

Severe cases require aggressive supportive therapy. Various therapies have been tried and there is no clear standard therapy.[1,35,42] Antihypertensives including calcium channel blockers, hydralazine, prazosin, and captopril have all been used. At present afterload reducers such as ACE inhibitors, calcium channel blockers or prazosin are front-line therapeutic agents for hypertension.[35,42] Concern about reflex tachycardia has led some authors to favor prazosin and captopril.[35,42] The use of diuretics for pulmonary edema is controversial.[35,42] Atropine may be used with caution if cholinergic symptoms become severe.[35,42] Therapy should be strongly influenced by thorough hemodynamic investigation.

Benzodiazepines are generally recommended for the treatment of seizures and agitation.[42] Steroids have been shown to be of no benefit.[2]

The use of scorpion antivenom is controversial.[11,34,42,68] Antivenom therapy may decrease the need for hospitalization, the length of stay, and the number of intensive care procedures the child has to undergo.[9,11] Goat serum-derived antivenom to *C. centruroides* is available from the Antivenom Production Laboratory of Arizona State University. It is not approved by the FDA. As with other xenobiotic sera, there is a risk of immediate anaphylaxis with its administration and a possibility of delayed serum sickness. In the United States, to *C. centruroides* antivenom is available only in the state of Arizona, where it is distributed on an "absolutely must have to survive" basis. Use of antivenom should only be considered with severe envenomations and in consultation with a toxicologist via one of the regional poison centers.

SNAKES

The venomous snakes of North America can be divided into two families: Crotalidae and Elapidae. The Crotalidae includes genera *Crotalus* (rattlesnakes) *Agkistrodan,* (water moccasins or cottonmouths, and copperheads), and *Sistrurus* (pygmy rattlesnakes and massasaugas). As a group these snakes are known as pit vipers because of a heat-sensitive pit found behind and below their nostrils used to locate the victim of a strike. The Elapidae family includes coral snakes as well as the nonindigenous cobras and mambas.

Epidemiology

Type of snake. Envenomations by snakes in North America are overwhelmingly caused by indigenous crotalids, whereas Elapidae constitute less than 1% of envenomations.[40] Nonindigenous snakes in North American zoos, or kept as exotic pets are responsible for a small percentage of envenomations as well.[32] All sea snakes are venomous, but fortunately none inhabits the coastal waters of North America.[71]

Host factors. Usually, the person bitten is a young adult white male. Approximately 40% of bites occur while handling or playing with a snake; 40% of those bitten have a blood alcohol level greater than 0.1%.[80] In one study of rattlesnake bites, only 43% occurred before an encounter with a snake was recognized or while the person was attempting to move away from the snake.[17] The 1975-1980 incidence of snake venom poisoning by state is illustrated in Fig. 283-1.[63] More recent data are not available.

Body area. Most bites are sustained on the upper extremity. A review of inpatient and outpatient cases of snake

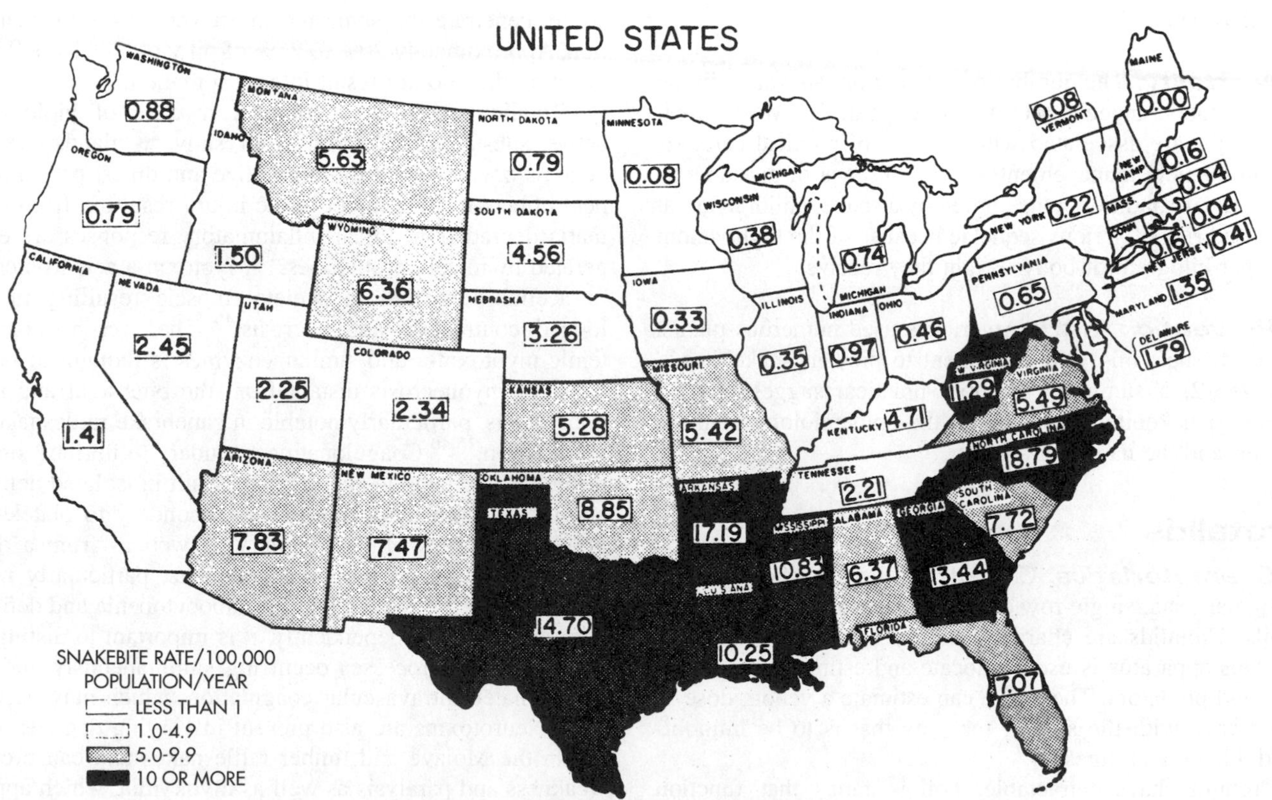

Fig. 283-1 Incidence of snake venom poisoning by state.
(From Russell FE: *Snake venom poisoning*, New York, 1983, Scholium International.)

BOX 283-2

SNAKEBITE PREVENTION

1. It is impossible to differentiate poisonous from nonpoisonous snakes without years of experience. Therefore, children should not approach, disturb, play with, capture, or kill *any* snake. These practices are dangerous for both the human and the snake.
2. Children should not put their hands or feet in places they cannot see. Children should not put their hands or feet anywhere without first looking.
3. Snakes frequently can be found under rocks, boulders, fallen trees, fences, rubbish piles, and boats that have been left on shore for several hours; in tall grass and heavy underbrush; or sunning themselves on logs, boulders, trees, walls, or cliffs. Extra caution should be used in these areas.
4. The striking distance of a snake is roughly half its length. Children should be taught to keep a good distance from snakes.
5. The striking reflex remains intact for up to an hour after the snake is dead. Therefore, even if one is sure that the snake is dead, it must be examined or transported at the opposite end of a long stick.
6. Rattlesnakes are nocturnal feeders and therefore are active after dark. Never gather firewood after dark. Camp should be set up on open ground; never near wood, rubbish piles, swampy areas, or the entrance of a cave.
7. Children should wear boots when walking in endemic areas.
8. Children should not be allowed to walk alone in an endemic area.
9. Children should not be allowed to swim in waters known to be infested with snakes.
10. Once bitten, everyone present should get away from the snake as quickly as possible. The benefit of identifying the snake is small in comparison to the risk of additional bites.

bite in California reported the following site distribution: 70% finger, 15% hand, 2% arm, 12% leg or foot, and 1% torso.[81] Given the high percentage of bites sustained while the snake was being handled intentionally, these statistics are less surprising than reports of snakebites to the tongue[23] and the glans penis.[20]

Mortality. The number of deaths from snakebite in the United States ranged from 0 to 14 per year.[40,63] Most snakebite deaths are associated with absence of medical care, errors in medical management, or the presence of an underlying medical condition. Once bitten by a snake, children are at increased risk of serious sequelae because of the high venom dose per kilogram of body weight they receive.

Prevention. Native Americans used numerous plants, animal tissues, oils, and excrement to prevent snakebites.[63] Box 283-2, a summary of more practical suggestions for avoiding snakebites, is based on the epidemiology of these injuries and the nature of snakes.

Crotalids

Characteristics. Crotalids can be identified by their triangular head, single row of subcaudal scales, and elliptical pupils. Crotalids are characterized by a heat-sensing facial pit. This apparatus is used to locate and estimate the size of prey and predators. The snake can estimate a venom dose in accordance with the size of the prey that is to be immobilized, killed, and digested.[7]

Crotalids have retractable, hollow fangs that function much like a hypodermic needle. Usually, they penetrate to subcutaneous tissue, but large snakes can reach a depth of 8 to 19 mm.[80] Consequently, larger snakes may penetrate dermal or subcutaneous structures and deposit venom intramuscularly. Venom is generally absorbed via the lymphatic system, although there are rare cases of intraarterial and intravenous deposition of venom. For an envenomation to take place, the pit viper must be venomous at the time of the strike, penetrate the skin, and inject venom during penetration. Approximately 20% to 25% of pit viper bites are "dry," meaning they do not result in envenomation.[48]

Crotalid venom is a complex mixture of biologically active substances. Derived from salivary glands, crotalid venoms have evolved to immobilize and digest prey. Prominent effects include direct tissue injury resulting from enzymatic degradation. Local inflammatory responses are exaggerated by metalloprotienases.[40] Myotoxin-a acts to increase intracellular calcium in skeletal muscle resulting in prolonged contraction and necrosis.[40] The presence of systemic myotoxin-a and similar enzymes is thought to be the cause of myonecrosis distant from the bite sight and rhabdomyolysis, particularly notable in canebrake rattlesnake envenomation.[15,40] Coagulopathy secondary to fibrinolysin and thrombin-like peptide actions may result in isolated defibrination.[40] Thrombocytopenia occurs secondary to platelet aggregation at sites of tissue injury as well as from a direct effect of venom on individual platelets, particularly rattlesnake venom.[12,40] Given that thrombocytopenia and defibrination both occur independently, it is important to distinguish between these processes occurring simultaneously and true disseminated intravascular coagulation, which may occur as well. Neurotoxins are also present in varying degrees, notably in the Mojave and timber rattlesnakes and can produce weakness and paralysis as well as myokymia, which appears as involuntary wormlike muscle movements under the skin.[18] The cause of crotalid induced neurotoxicity remains under study.[18,40]

BOX 283-3

INDIGENOUS LOCATIONS FOR NORTH AMERICAN PIT VIPERS

Southeast
- Cottonmouths and copperheads*
- Eastern diamondback *(Crotalus adamanteus)*
- Timber *(Crotalus horridus horridus)*
- Southeastern pygmy rattlesnakes *(Sistrurus miliarius barbouri)*

Midwest
- Cottonmouths and copperheads*
- Eastern diamondback *(Crotalus adamanteus)*
- Timber *(Crotalus horridus horridus)*
- Prairie *(Crotalus viridis viridis)*

Northeast
- Cottonmouths and copperheads*
- Eastern diamondback *(Crotalus adamanteus)*
- Timber *(Crotalus horridus horridus)*
- Eastern Massasauga rattlesnakes *(Sistrurus catenadus catenatus)*

Northwest
- Great Basin *(Crotalus viridis lutosus)*
- Northern Pacific *(Crotalus viridis oreganus)*

Southwest
- Western diamondback *(Crotalus atrox)*
- Sidewinder *(Crotalus cerastes)*
- Rock *(Crotalus lepidus)*
- Speckled *(Crotalus mitchelli)*
- Black-tailed *(Crotalus molossus)*
- Twin-spotted *(Crotalus pricei pricei)*
- Red diamond *(Crotalus ruber)*
- Mojave *(Crotalus scutulatus)*
- Tiger *(Crotalus tigris)*
- Prairie *(Crotalus viridis viridis)*
- Grand Canyon *(Crotalus viridis abyssus)*
- Southern Pacific *(Crotalus viridis helleri)*
- Great Basin *(Crotalus viridis lutosus)*
- Ridge-nosed *(Crotalus willardi)*

From Banner W: *Curr Probl Pediatr* 18:1, 1988.
**Agkistrodrodon* species.

Distribution. Box 283-3 lists the indigenous locations for North American pit vipers.[7]

First aid. Commonly accepted guidelines for snakebite first aid are summarized in Box 283-4.[7,81] Other forms of first aid are controversial and are discussed here because the physician may see patients less damaged by the snake than by the field treatment of well-meaning but untrained (and possibly inebriated) attendants.

Identification. The utility of identifying the type of snake is controversial. No time should be lost in getting the victim to medical attention, nor should the rescue party expose themselves to risk while trying to find and identify the snake.

Cryotherapy. This form of snakebite treatment is used to constrict blood flow and thus diminish systemic venom absorption. Unfortunately the consequent ischemia is limb threatening. Thus, cryotherapy is contraindicated.

BOX 283-4

FIRST AID FOR SNAKEBITES

1. Observe the approximate size and characteristics of the snake if this can be done without danger of remaining within the snake's striking range.
2. Move the patient as little as possible.
3. Mark the victim's skin with a pen denoting the area of swelling and the time. Repeat this every 15 minutes.
4. Remove all rings from the victim's fingers.
5. Immobilize the affected limb by splinting as if for a fracture and keep the limb below the level of the heart.
6. Regardless of early symptoms, transport the victim to the nearest medical facility at a safe speed.
7. Avoid the use of ice (tissue damage), aspirin (anticoagulation), alcohol or sedative drugs (vasodilation), or stimulants such as caffeine (acceleration of venom absorption).
8. As soon as possible start basic life support, including volume expansion and Trendelenburg position for hypotensive patients.

Incision and suction. Incision at the bite sight and suction has shown mixed results in clinical and laboratory trials.[13,40,49] Complications of incision and suction include damage to underlying neurovascular structures, increased rate of wound infection and further tissue damage.[40,49] Given that no clear benefit has been demonstrated, incision and suction is not recommended.

Constricting bands. Constricting bands that impede blood flow are contraindicated. Only loose-fitting bands placed in an effort to reduce lymphatic flow have been advocated but have not been shown to be of clear benefit.[40,49] Consequently, constricting bands of either type are not currently recommended.[40,49]

Immobilization. Splinting of the affected extremity should be performed if this can be done without significant delay in transfer.

Inhospital care

HISTORY-TAKING. Information elicited in the medical history of known envenomations include the size and species of the snake, the circumstances of the bite (e.g., through clothing, alcohol related), the number of bites and body area affected, first aid methods used, time of bite and transport time, previous snakebite episodes and exposure to horse serum, allergies (e.g., horse serum, antibiotics), and tetanus immunization status.[81]

PHYSICAL EXAMINATION: SIGNS AND SYMPTOMS

Local. Local signs and symptoms usually include the presence of fang marks as well as pain, edema, ecchymosis, and erythema from 15 minutes to 4 hours after the bite. Fang marks typically have ragged edges but may be obscured by secondary trauma sustained in the flight from the snake or the first aid attempts. Because of the hematoxic effects of pit viper venom, blood may ooze from the puncture sites and hemorrhagic bullae may develop. Muscle necrosis also may become apparent.

Systemic. Hemolysis, coagulopathy, thrombocytopenia and generalized hemorrhage frequently are present in serious envenomations. The physical examination also should be directed to detecting signs of ARDS, respiratory depression, circulatory collapse, and renal failure. Symptoms may include malaise, weakness, lightheadedness, diaphoresis, visual disturbances, nausea, vomiting, syncope, myokymia, paraesthesias, and a metallic taste.[14]

LABORATORY STUDIES. Laboratory studies have been found to be of "minor assistance in assessing the severity of (rattlesnake) envenomation."[81] However, they may be useful in determining if envenomation has occurred early in the course of treatment.[40] Studies should include a complete blood count with differential, red blood cells morphology (to evaluate for spherocytosis), prothrombin time, plasma thromboplastin time, fibrinogen levels, fibrin-split products, and platelet count. If the just-mentioned studies demonstrate any abnormality or if the patient has clinical symptoms, envenomation must be assumed and electrolytes, blood urea nitrogen, blood type and cross-match and urinalysis should be done. Ill patients may require further testing as the clinical situation dictates.

Therapy

LOCAL. Local wound care includes gentle cleansing, nonconstrictive immobilization, elevation of the bitten extremity and close observation. Intercompartmental pressures should be measured as compartment syndrome may occur or may be closely mimicked by the effects of the venom. Fasciotomy has not been shown to be of benefit.[40,49] No solid evidence exists for the use of excisional therapy.[40,49] Digital dermotomy may be indicated on clinical grounds.[40]

SHOCK. Patients may have marked decrease in intravascular volume as a result of hemorrhage, third spacing of fluids, vomiting, and diaphoresis. Crystalloid replacement should begin immediately in envenomated patients.

FLUID AND ELECTROLYTE ABNORMALITIES. Extensive third-space losses may cause fluid and electrolyte imbalances. Electrolyte and urine output monitoring with fluid and electrolyte replacement becomes essential under these conditions.

HEMATOLOGICAL COMPLICATIONS. Treatment of thrombocytopenia and anemia (caused by hemolysis) may require multiple transfusions. Transfusions of fresh frozen plasma and cryoprecipitate may be required in severely envenomated patients. Therapy with blood products is rarely effective, however, in the absence of antivenom therapy. Thrombocytopenia often corrects with antivenom alone, and clotting factor levels rarely improve when blood products are given without antivenom.[40] Disseminated intravascular coagulopathy caused by snakebite does not respond to heparin; antivenom is the treatment of choice.

USE OF ANTIVENOM. The antivenom currently available in the United States is polyvalent, and is produced by injecting horses with venom from *Crotalus adamanteus, Crotalus atrox, Crotalus durissus terifficus,* and *Bothrops atrox.* There is a high incidence of serum sickness and serious allergic reaction associated with its use. Skin testing is necessary before administration of antivenom. Instructions are included with the antivenom kit. Patients with positive skin tests, those with known horse serum allergy, or those with previous horse serum therapy should be assumed allergic.

Indications for antivenom therapy include rapid progression of swelling, significant coagulopathy, defibrination, thrombocytopenia, neurological toxicity, and shock. Some reserve its use for large rattlesnake, water moccasin, or unidentified snake bites.[76] Recent studies support the treatment of copperhead envenomations without antivenom, because copperhead envenomations tend to be less severe than those of other crotalids.[50,78]

Antivenom use should proceed simultaneously with supportive therapy, as shown in Box 283-5. The starting dose should be 10 to 20 vials.[40] Pediatric dosing is the same as adult dosing.[40] Antivenom therapy (even when the skin test is negative) should be instituted only in an environment with full resuscitation capabilities, given the risk of anaphylaxis. Epinephrine, corticosteroids, antihistamines and airway maintenance equipment should be at the bedside. Volume depletion should be aggressively treated prior to initiating antivenom therapy because of the risk of rapid vasodilatation and third space fluid loss associated with anaphylaxis. Administration of the initial vial should be over 5 to 10 minutes, observing for untoward effects, then administration should be as rapidly as is clinically allowable, watching for anaphylactoid reactions that may be associated with overly rapid administration.[40] Therapy should be continued until the patient's clinical and hematological profile has improved. Anaphylaxis associated with antivenom therapy should be treated in the standard fashion.[40]

Crotalid F(ab) antivenom is currently under investigation in the United States. Preliminary reports indicate that it is effective in the treatment of thrombocytopenia, neurotoxicity and tissue injury with no evidence of immune mediated complications, even though repeat dosing may be required.[18,24,66]

PREVENTION AND TREATMENT OF SERUM SICKNESS. Up to 80% of patients develop serum sickness sometime within 4 weeks after being treated with antivenom, but only 3% require hospitalization for this complication. Oral corticosteroids should be prescribed at the first signs (usually urticaria and pruritus) and should be continued for 24 hours after all symptoms have subsided. The steroid then should be tapered over 72 hours. If necessary, diphenhydramine may be added to control pruritus.

ADDITIONAL THERAPEUTIC MEASURES

Pain control. Analgesics should not be overlooked in the management of snakebites. Adequate pain control allows rehabilitation to begin as early as possible to prevent contractures.

Infection control. Although snakes have been found to carry a wide variety of bacteria in their mouths (histotoxic

BOX 283-5

STEPS IN USING ANTIVENOM

1. *Prepare to manage anaphylaxis.* Because development of an anaphylactic reaction is unpredictable,[37] all patients receiving antivenom should be monitored and have two intravenous catheters—one for the antivenom and one for emergency drugs and fluids. Intravenous epinephrine, diphenhydramine, and plasma expanders, as well as respiratory support, must be readily available.
2. *Test for sensitivity to horse serum.* Skin testing, detailed on the package insert* of the antivenom, is not reliable.[26] Therefore, a negative skin test should not lull one into a sense of false security. However, some physicians have used the antivenom in very serious cases despite a positive skin test. To decrease the risk of an allergic reaction in these cases, give the saline-diluted antivenom slowly with diphenhydramine premedication and a simultaneous infusion of epinephrine.[37]
3. *Start the infusion.* In the child who weighs more than 45 kg, the initial dose should be estimated based on the clinical grading system (Table 283-1). Children under this weight usually require *50% more* than this dose. The intravenous antivenom solution infusion should begin at 1 ml/hour and be increased over 30 minutes to a maximum of 150 ml/hour. "One to two vials per hour is appropriate to avoid the risks associated with higher infusion rates."[6]
4. *Repeat infusion.* If, after the initial infusion, the local signs progress or the systemic signs persist, the initial antivenom dose (usually five vials in children) should be repeated. Although the incidence of serum sickness is proportional to the person's sensitivity and the volume of antivenom received, morbidity and mortality after serious envenomations are related to giving too little hyperimmune serum or giving it too late. Large doses of antivenom may be associated with metabolic acidosis, because each vial contains 0.25% formalin.[5]

*Antivenom polyvalent is hyperimmunized horse serum active against the venom of all species of pit vipers. It is available from Wyeth-Ayerst Laboratories, Box 8299, Philadelphia, PA 19101.

Table 283-1 Extent of Envenomation and Dosage of Antivenom

Grade	Signs and Symptoms	Initial Treatment
No envenomation	Fang marks present; no local or systemic reactions	No antivenom; local care. Tetanus prophylaxis when indicated. Observation in emergency department for at least 4 hours
Mild envenomation	Fang marks present; local swelling but no systemic reaction. Pain may be present or absent	Three to five vials of antivenom
Moderate envenomation	Swelling that progresses beyond the site of the bite with systemic reaction or laboratory changes (e.g., fall in hematocrit and fibrinogen levels or platelets or hematuria)	Six to 10 vials of antivenom
Severe envenomation	Marked local and systemic reaction. Bleeding diathesis, DIC, shock, or ARDS with marked laboratory changes	15+ vials of antivenom

clostridia, *Bacteroides,* many gram positive and gram negative aerobes), infection is unlikely in the absence of severe necrosis, and good wound care is believed to be sufficient to prevent secondary infection. Systemic and local changes produced by envenomation and the subsequent vascular damage may be difficult to differentiate from infection. If infection is suspected, antibiotic therapy should be instituted. Antibiotic prophylaxis is not currently recommended.[40,46]

TETANUS PROPHYLAXIS. *Clostridium tetani* are not part of the mouth flora of snakes. Updating the patient's tetanus immunization status is the only necessary intervention.

Coral Snakes

Coral snakes are the members of the Elapidae family that are indigenous to North America. Although their venom can cause a life-threatening paralysis, coral snakes tend to be small, secretive, and mild-mannered unless provoked. Few bites are reported, and mortality is rare.

Characteristics. The Eastern coral snake often is mistaken for the nonvenomous scarlet king snake because of similar colorful bands encircling the body. The mnemonic "red to yellow, kill a fellow; red to black, venom lack; head of black, step back, Jack!" refers to the color patterns of these snakes. The poisonous black-snouted snake has broad red and black bands separated by narrow yellow ones; the nonpoisonous variety's snout is red, and its broad red bands are separated by narrow yellow ones bounded on each side by black. Despite these distinctions, a large proportion of people bitten by coral snakes thought they were handling a scarlet king snake.[47]

Unlike pit vipers, coral snakes lack facial pits, are diurnal, and have fixed fangs and nearly round pupils. Their bites may produce superficial scratches or definite fang marks. Their retroverted teeth gnaw or chew on their prey and make coral snakes difficult to shake off. Because they must stay attached long enough for their venom to be deposited around their teeth, 50% of coral snake bites are dry. Elapidae venom is primarily neurotoxic; systemic neurological symptoms are the rule and local tissue injury is uncommon. Elapidae venom causes paresthesias and paralysis by inhibiting acetylcholine receptors at the neuronal synapse.

Distribution. Three types of coral snakes are found in the United States: the Eastern coral snake, the Texas coral snake, and the Arizona or Sonoran coral snake. Their distribution is shown in Fig. 283-2. The bite of the Sonoran coral snake produces no more than local pain and a small amount of nausea.

First aid. Cryotherapy, incision and suction (including the Sawyer extractor), and constricting bands have no proven value in coral snakebites. However, Russell[63] recommends the following: "No food or drink should be given. if the victim is more than 1 hour's distance from a medical facility, a tourniquet might be placed immediately proximal to the bite area. It should be released for 1 minute every 10 minutes, and it should be left in place until 3 minutes after intravenous antivenom has been started."

Physical examination: signs and symptoms

LOCAL. Erythema and local pain from a coral snake bite are transient or absent. Although 85% of patients have evident fang marks, envenomations have been reported that were not associated with apparent fang marks on close examination.[58]

SYSTEMIC. Systemic manifestations may be delayed for 12 hours and may appear precipitously. They may include bulbar paralysis with ptosis, dysphagia, dysarthria, excessive salivation, paresthesias, euphoria or apprehension, drowsiness, dizziness, weakness, confusion, nausea, vomiting, diaphoresis, muscle tenderness or fasciculations, and ophthalmoplegias causing visual disturbances. These may be followed by seizures, respiratory paralysis, and pulmonary hemorrhage. It often is unclear which findings are primary and which are secondary to hypoxia.

Laboratory studies. Coral snake bites do not mandate routine laboratory screening.

Supportive therapy. Elective intubation before impending respiratory paralysis tends to prevent aspiration

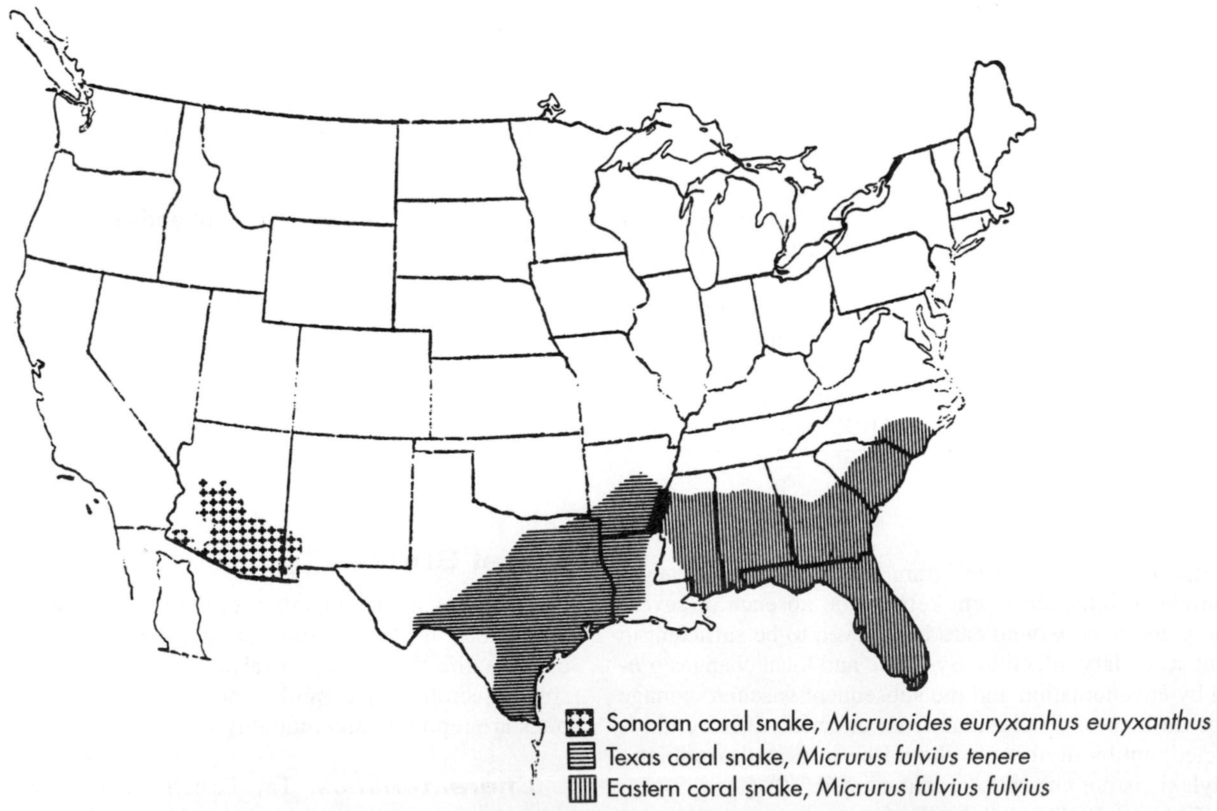

Fig. 283-2 Distribution of coral snakes by type in the United States.
(From Russell FE: *Snake venom poisoning,* New York, 1983, Scholium International)

pneumonia. Elective intubation is recommended if any signs of bulbar paralysis develop.[47]

USE OF ANTIVENOM. Russell[63] recommends the use of antivenom effective against Eastern and Texas snake venom (*Micrurus fulvius*; produced by WyethAyerst) if a patient definitely has been bitten (five vials) or if any signs[63] or symptoms develop (three vials).[63] These guidelines are based on the judgment that the risks of intravenous hyperimmune horse serum are offset by the potential prevention of respiratory paralysis, which may ensue if therapy is not given early in the disease.

As with pit viper antivenom, skin testing yields many false negatives and the same precautions must be taken as outlined above. Three to five vials of antivenom are mixed in 250 to 500 ml of normal saline, and 1 to 2 ml are given intravenously over 3 to 5 minutes. If the patient does not exhibit any signs of an allergic reaction, the remainder of the solution is infused slowly as tolerated. A second three to five vials of antivenom-saline mixture may need to be infused if the patient's signs and symptoms do not abate or worsen.

ADDITIONAL THERAPEUTIC MEASURES. Recommendations for infection and tetanus prophylaxis are the same as for pit viper bites. Additional measures may become necessary if aspiration pneumonia develops. Patients should be aware that muscular weakness may persist for 3 to 6 weeks.

Nonindigenous Snakes

The variety of imported snakes is too great to detail in this text. If an exotic species is suspected, the recommended approach includes local wound care, supportive care, and consultation with experts at a regional poison control center.[7]

When to Refer

Hymenoptera
Systemic reactions should be evaluated for immunotherapy

Arachnids
Loxosceles
Surgical intervention necessary for wound care
Latrodectus
Prior to use of antivenom therapy
Tarantulas
Hairs in eyes that are not easily removed
Scorpions
Considered use of antivenom

Snakes
Pit vipers
Considered use of antivenom
Surgical intervention necessary for wound care
Coral snakes
Anticipated need for airway control or intensive care unit monitoring

When to Hospitalize

Hymenoptera
Severe systemic allergic reactions or severe systemic reactions secondary to massive envenomation

Arachnids
Loxosceles
Secondary infection requiring intravenous antibiotics
Inability to provide adequate wound care at home
Severe systemic symptoms
Latrodectus
Severe systemic symptoms
Following use of antivenom
Tarantulas
Significant comorbidity
Inability to tolerate oral fluids
Scorpions
Cardiac or neurological toxicity
Severe systemic signs or symptoms

Snakes
Pit vipers
Any signs or symptoms more severe than mild local reaction
Coral snakes
Significant chance of envenomation

REFERENCES

1. Abroug F, et al: Assessment of left ventricular function in severe scorpion envenomation: combined hemodynamic and echo-Doppler study, *Intens Care Med* 21:629, 1995.
2. Abroug F, et al: High-dose hydrocortisone hemisuccinate in scorpion envenomation, *Ann Emerg Med* 30:23, 1997.
3. Adams CT, Lofgren CS: Red imported fire ants (Hymenoptera: formicidae): frequency of sting attacks on residents of Sumter County, Georgia, *J Med Entomol* 18:378, 1981.
4. Adams CT, Lofgren CS: Incidence of stings or bites of the red imported fire ant (Hymenoptera:Formicidae) and other arthropods among patients at Ft. Stewart, Georgia, USA, *J Med Entomol* 19:366, 1982.
5. Allen C: Arachnid envenomations, *Emerg Med Clin North Am* 20:269, 1992.
6. Ariue B: Multiple Africanized bee stings in a child, *Pediatrics* 94:115, 1994.
7. Banner W: Bites and stings in the pediatric patient, *Curr Probl Pediatr* 18:1, 1988.
8. Bansal AS: Bee stings, *Lancet* 348:900, 1996.
9. Berg RA, Tarantino MD: Envenomation by the scorpion Centruroides exilicauda *(C. sculpturatus)*: severe and unusual manifestations, *Pediatrics* 87:930, 1991.
10. Bischof RO: Seasonal incidence of insect stings: autumn "yellow jacket delirium," *J Fam Pract* 43:271, 1996.
11. Bond GR: Antivenin administration for Centruroides scorpion sting: risks and benefits, *Ann Emerg Med* 21:778, 1992.
12. Bond GR, Burkhart KK: Thrombocytopenia following timber rattlesnake envenomation, *Ann Emerg Med* 30:40, 1997.
13. Bronstein AC, et al: Negative pressure suction in suction in field treatment of rattlesnake bite, *Vet Hum Toxicol* 27:297, 1985.
14. Burch JM, et al: The treatment of crotalid envenomation without antivenin, *J Trauma* 28:35, 1988.

15. Carroll RR, Hall EL, Kitchens CS: Canebrake rattlesnake envenomations, *Ann Emerg* Med 30:45, 1997.
16. Charpin D, et al: Prevalence of allergy to Hymenoptera stings in different samples of the general population, *J Allerg Clin Immunol* 90:331, 1992.
17. Clark RF, et al: Clinical presentation and treatment of black widow spider envenomation: a review of 163 cases, *Ann Emerg Med* 21:782, 1992.
18. Clark RF, et al: Successful treatment of crotalid-induced neurotoxicity with a new polyspecific crotalid fab antivenom, *Ann Emerg Med* 30:54, 1997.
19. Cohen PR: Imported fire ant stings: clinical manifestations and treatment, *Pediatr Dermatol* 9:44, 1992.
20. Crane DB, Irwin JS: Rattlesnake bite of glans penis, *Urology* 26:50, 1985.
21. Curry SC, et al: Envenomation by the scorpion *Centruroides sculpturatus, J Toxicol Clin* Toxicol 21:417, 1983.
22. Curry SC, et al: The legitimacy of snakebites in central Arizona, *Ann Emerg Med* 18:658, 1989.
23. Danzl DF, Carter GL: "Kiss and yell": a rattlesnake bite to the tongue, *Ann Emerg Med* 17:549, 1988 (letter).
24. Dart RC, et al: Affinity-purified, mixed monospecific crotalid antivenom ovine fab for the treatment of crotalid venom poisoning, *Ann Emerg Med* 30:33, 1997.
25. deShazo RD: The continuing saga of imported fire ants: evolution before our eyes, *Ann Allergy, Asthma, Immunol* 77:85, 1996.
26. deShazo RD, Banks WA: Medical consequences of multiple fire ant stings occurring indoors, *J Allergy Clin Immunol* 93:847, 1994.
27. deShazo RD, Butcher BT, Banks WA: Reactions to the stings of the imported fire ant, *N Engl J Med* 323:462, 1990.
28. dosReis MA, et al: Acute renal failure in experimental envenomation with Africanized bee venom, *Renal Failure* 20:39, 1998.
29. Fox RW, Lockey RF, Bukantz SC: Neurologic sequelae following the imported fire ant sting, *J Allerg Clin Immunol* 70:120, 1982.
30. Freeman TM, et al: Imported fire ant immunotherapy: effectiveness of whole body extracts, *J Allerg Clin Immunol* 90:210, 1992.
31. Ginsburg CM: Fire ant envenomation in children, *Pediatrics* 73:689, 1984.
32. Gold BS: Neostigmine for the treatment of neurotoxicity following envenomation by the Asiatic cobra, *Ann Emerg Med* 28:87, 1996.
33. Golden DBK: Diagnosis and prevalence of stinging insect allergy, *Clin Rev Allergy* 5:119, 1987.
34. Gueron M, et al: The management of scorpion envenomation, *Toxicom* 31:1071, 1993.
35. Gueron M, Ilia R, Sofer S: The cardiovascular system after scorpion envenomation: a review, *Clin Toxicol* 30:245, 1992.
36. Hardwick WE, et al: Near-fatal fire ant envenomation of a newborn, *Pediatrics* 90:622, 1992.
37. Hoffman DR: Fire ant venom allergy, *Allergy* 50:525, 1995.
38. Hoffman DR: Hymenoptera venom proteins, *Natural Toxins* 10:169, 1996.
39. Hoffman DR: Reactions to less common species of fire ants, *J Allergy Clin Immunol* 100:679, 1997.
40. Holstege CP, et al: Crotalid Snake Envenomation, *Med Toxicol* 13:889, 1997.
41. Ingber A, et al: Morbidity of brown recluse spider bites: clinical picture, treatment and prognosis, *Acta Dermatol Venereol* 71:337, 1991.
42. Ismail M: The scorpion envenoming syndrome, *Toxicon* 11:825, 1995 (review).
43. Jerrard DA: ED Management of insect stings, *Am J Emerg Med* 14:429, 1996.
44. Karnad DR: Haemodynamic patterns in patients with scorpion envenomation, *Heart* 79:485, 1998.
45. Kemp ED: Bites and stings of the arthropod kind, *Postgrad Med* 103:88, 1998.
46. Kerrigan KR, et al: Antibiotic prophylaxis for pit viper envenomation: prospective, controlled trial, *World J Surg* 21:369, 1997.
47. Kitchens CS, Van Mierop LHS: Envenomation by the Eastern coral snake *(Micrurus fulvius), JAMA* 258:1615, 1987.
48. Kunkel DB, et al: Reptile envenomations, *J Toxicol Clin Toxicol* 21:503, 1983-1984.
49. Lawrence WT, et al: Pit viper bites: rational management in locales in which copperheads and cottonmouths predominate, *Ann Plast Surg* 36: 276, 1996.
50. Lawrence WT, Giannopoulos A, Hansen A: Pitviper bites: comments, *Ann Plast Surg* 38:302, 1997.
51. Li JTC, Yunginger JW: Management of insect sting hypersensitivity, *Mayo Clin Proc* 67:188, 1992.
52. Lockey RF: Immunotherapy for allergy to insect stings, *N Engl J Med* 323:1627, 1990.
53. Maguire JF, Geha RS: Bee, wasp, and hornet stings, *Pediatr Rev* 8:5, 1986.
54. Mejia G, et al: Acute renal failure due to multiple stings by Africanized bees, *Ann Intern Med* 104:210, 1986.
55. Miller TA: Latrodectism: bite of the black widow spider, *Am Fam Phys* 45:181, 1992.
56. Mosbech H: Hymenoptera immunotherapy, *Allergy* 52:1, 1997.
57. Muller UR: Epidemiology of insect sting allergy: epidemiology of clinical allergy, *Monogr Allergy* 31:131, 1993.
58. Norris RL, Dart RC: Apparent coral snake envenomation in a patient without visible fang marks, *Am J Emerg Med* 7:402, 1989.
59. Rauber A: Black widow spider bites, *J Toxicol Clin Toxicol* 21:473, 1983-1984.
60. Reisman RE: Insect Stings, *N Engl J Med* 331:523, 1994.
61. Rhoades RB, Stafford CT, James FK: Survey of fatal anaphylactic reactions to imported fire ant stings, *J Allerg Clin Immunol* 84:159, 1989.
62. Rimsza ME, Zimmerman DR, Bergeson PS: Scorpion envenomation, *Pediatrics* 66:298, 1980.
63. Russell FEL: *Snake venom poisoning*, Philadelphia, 1980, JB Lippincott.
64. Schumacher MJ, Tveten MS, Egen NB: Rate and quantity of delivery of venom from honeybee stings, *J Allergy Clin Immunol* 93:831, 1994.
65. Schumacher MJ, Egen NB: Significance of Africanized bees for public health, *Arch Intern Med* 155:2038, 1995.
66. Seifert SA, et al: Relationship of venom effects on venom antigen and antivenom serum concentrations in a patient with *Crotalus atrox* envenomation treaded with a fab antivenom, *Ann Emerg Med* 30:49, 1997.
67. Simini B: Bee stings, *Lancet* 348:900, 1996.
68. Sofer S, Shahak E, Gueron M: Scorpion envenomation and antivenom therapy, *J Pediatr* 124:973, 1994.
69. Stablein JJ, Lockey RF: Adverse reactions to ant stings, *Clin Rev Allergy* 5:161, 1987.
70. Stafford CT: Hypersensitivity to fire ant venom, *Ann Allergy Asthma Immunol* 77:87, 1996.
71. Tu AT: Biotoxicology of sea snake venoms, *Ann Emerg Med* 16:1923, 1987.
72. Valentine M: Insect sting anaphylaxis, *Ann Intern Med* 118:225, 1993.
73. Valentine MD, et al: The value of immunotherapy with venom in children with allergy to insect stings, *N Engl J Med* 323:1601, 1990.
74. Vetter RS, Visscher PK: Bites and stings of medically important venomous arthropods, *Int J Derm* 37:481, 1998.
75. Visscher PK, Vetter RS, Camazine S: Removing bee stings, *Lancet* 348: 301, 1996.
76. Wagner CW, Colladay ES: Crotalid envenomation in children: selective conservative management, *J Pediatr Surg* 24:128, 1989.
77. Wasserman GS, Anderson PC: Loxoscelism and necrotic arachnidism, *J Toxicol Clin Toxicol* 21:451, 1983-1984.
78. Whitley RE: Conservative treatment of copperhead snakebites without antivenin, *J Trauma Injury Infect Crit Care* 41:219, 1996.
79. Willis GA: Loxoscelism in Canada, *CMAJ* July 1988.
80. Wingert WA: Poisoning by animal venoms, *Top Emerg Med* 2:89, 1980.
81. Wingert WA, Chan L: Rattlesnake bites in southern California and rationale for recommended treatment, *West J Med* 148:37, 1988.

82. Wong RC, Hughes SE, Voorhees JJ: Spider bites, *Arch Dermatol* 123: 98, 1987.
83. Wright DN, Lockey RF: Local reactions to stinging insects (Hymenoptera), *Allerg Proc* 11:23, 1990.
84. Wright SW, et al: Clinical presentation and outcome of brown recluse spider bite, *Ann Emerg Med* 30:28, 1997.
85. Zuckerberg AL, Schweich PJ: An arm red and hot: infection or not? *Pediatr Emerg Care* 6:275, 1990.

SUGGESTED READINGS

Ismail M: The scorpion envenoming syndrome, *Toxicon* 11:825, 1995 (review).

Jerrard DA: ED Management of insect stings, *Am J Emerg Med* 14:429, 1996.

Reisman RE: Insect stings, *N Eng J Med* 331:523, 1994.

Vetter RS, Visscher PK: Bites and stings of medically important venomous arthropods, *Int J Derm* 37:481, 1998.

284 Epiglottitis

Caroline Breese Hall • William J. Hall

Epiglottitis, or supraglottitis, is an acute infection manifested by progressive, severe respiratory obstruction. Licensure of the conjugated *Haemophilus influenzae* type b vaccines has resulted in a dramatic reduction in epiglottitis cases and changes in the primary ages affected and causative organisms.* Nevertheless, epiglottitis remains the same clinically, a potentially fatal disease that requires prompt recognition and treatment.

ETIOLOGY

Before the widespread use of the conjugated *H. influenzae* type b (Hib) vaccines, epiglottitis was caused almost exclusively by *H. influenzae* type b. *H. influenzae* organisms were first discovered by Pfeiffer during the pandemic of influenza in 1890. Believing these to be the cause of influenza, he titled the organism the "influenza bacillus." These gram-negative, aerobic bacilli were later designated *H. influenzae*. In clinical specimens, these organisms appear pleomorphic, often coccobacillary. Epiglottitis is caused only by the type b organisms, which are distinguished by their capsular polysaccharide. The organisms may be seen to be encapsulated in clinical specimens by stained smears or by the swelling reaction, which produces capsular swelling with type-specific antiserum. On laboratory growth media and broth, the capsules can be demonstrated easily during the first few hours of growth, but with age, the morphological traits change.

The effectiveness of the conjugated Hib vaccines has resulted in a significant drop in the proportion of cases caused by *H. influenzae* type b and in a relative increase in organisms previously considered rare.† In Philadelphia from 1979 through 1983, *H. influenzae* type b caused 82% of the cases of epiglottitis and in 1984 through 1989, 75% of cases[12] (Fig. 284-1). However, from 1990 through 1992, only 25% of cases were identified as being caused by *H. influenzae* type b. Group A beta-hemolytic streptococcus (GABHS) was the only other organism isolated in the Philadelphia study, constituting 4.2% of the total group (six patients); 50% of these cases occurred from 1990 to 1992. In 20% of patients, no organism was identified. Other bacteria have been identified occasionally as causing epiglottitis, including pneumococci, group B and C streptococci, and *Haemophilus parainfluenzae*.[2,4,8,18] Epiglottitis may occur secondary to asymptomatic colonization by these organisms in the upper respiratory tract or, particularly with pneumococci and streptococci, may be secondary to spread from a nearby focus of infection.

INCIDENCE

The dramatic decline in the incidence of epiglottitis cases and *H. influenzae* type b infections closely chronicles the history of the Hib vaccines.[5,7,32] Introduction and use in 1988 of the Hib conjugate vaccines for children age 18 months produced the initial decline in *H. influenzae* disease, reported at 41 cases per 100,000 in 1987 to less than 30 cases per 100,000 reported in 1988.[7] Licensure of the *H. influenzae* type b conjugate vaccines for infants 2 months of age and older in 1990 resulted in a decline to 2 cases per 100,000 in 1993. Of note, however, is that cases of *H. influenzae* type b in patients 5 years of age and older, who would not have received the vaccine, remained essentially stable from 1987 through 1993. The annual incidence of epiglottitis cases over the 14 years reviewed in Philadelphia was 8.9 cases per 10,000 hospital admissions. Before 1990, the yearly incidence was 10.9 per 10,000 admissions and was 1.8 per 10,000 from 1990 through 1992, thus declining by 84%.[14] In the first 9 months of 1998, only 39 cases of invasive *H. influenzae* type b infections have been reported to the Centers for Disease Control.[6]

Epiglottitis when caused by *H. influenzae* type b, and previous to the current vaccine era, was primarily a disease of children 3 to 7 years of age.* In contrast, other serious disease caused by *H. influenzae* type b, such as meningitis, occurred primarily in infants, whereas viral croup primarily affects children in the second year of life.[28,31] Because other organisms, particularly GABHS, currently make up a greater proportion of the epiglottitis cases, a change in the age distribution may be expected. In Philadelphia, the median age range of cases of epiglottitis increased from 35.5 months before 1990 to 80.5 months from 1990 through 1992.[14] This reflected the older median age for patients who had GABHS epiglottitis (117.5 months) compared with that for patients who had *H. influenzae* type b epiglottitis (35 months). Epiglottitis also may occasionally occur during adulthood.[24] Currently in institutions treating both children and adults, the majority of cases of epiglottitis are in adults.[12]

Epiglottitis has had no distinctive seasonal predilection. However, cases caused by GABHS would be expected to be

*References 7, 10, 14, 19, 23, 29, 30.

†References 9, 16, 19, 23, 34, 35.

*References 1,2, 8, 25, 28, 31.

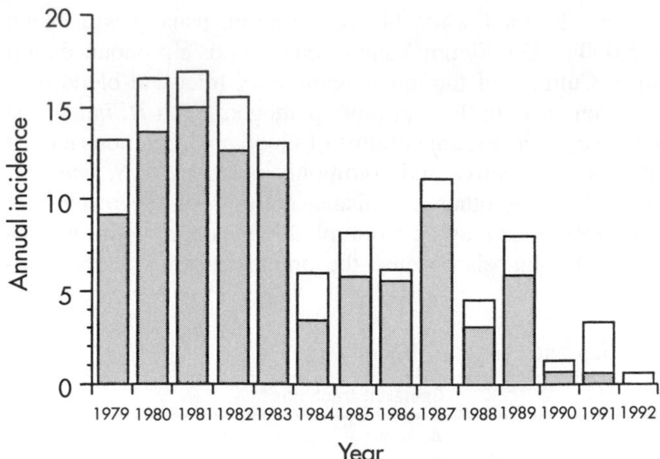

Fig. 284-1 Incidence of epiglottitis. Bars show cases per 10,000 hospital admissions. Solid portion represents cases known to be caused by *Haemophilus influenzae* type B. (From Gorelick MH, Baker D: *Arch Pediatr Adolesc Med* 148:47, 1994.)

more likely to occur during the seasons when GABHS infections are more prevalent, which in temperate climates is in the winter, usually peaking in February and March.

PATHOGENESIS

The organisms causing epiglottitis commonly reside asymptomatically in the upper respiratory tract or cause other forms of respiratory disease, usually much less severe than epiglottitis. Why certain children should develop epiglottitis is not understood. One hypothesis is that invasion by these organisms colonizing the upper respiratory tract may occur secondary to stress, trauma, or concurrent viral respiratory tract infection. Whether or not the causative organism initially is responsible for clinical signs, such as nasopharyngitis, infection commonly spreads from the upper respiratory tract to involve the epiglottis, producing marked inflammation and edema. The inflammation is not limited to the epiglottis, however, but involves the surrounding area, the arytenoids, the arytenoepiglottic folds, the vocal cords, and to some extent the subglottic region. The characteristically rapid and pronounced inflammatory response of these structures mechanically obstructs the flow of air. Inspiratory obstruction is particularly pronounced because of the narrowing force generated by the negative intrathoracic pressure. The edematous epiglottis, like a ball valve, is pulled down into the larynx during inspiration and may obstruct the airway completely. In addition, secretions and exudate are formed by the inflammation, which may include the lower tracheobronchial tree as well. The secretions and edema compound the obstruction to the flow of air. The work of breathing increases, and hypoxemia and carbon dioxide retention may result. Thus, even without total occlusion of the airway by the epiglottis, assisted ventilation commonly is required in children.[21,27]

CLINICAL FEATURES

Although the demographics of epiglottitis and the causative organisms have changed recently because of vaccine use, the classic clinical features of epiglottitis in children remain unchanged.[14] Hence, the clinical manifestations appear related to common pathophysiological processes of the inflamed epiglottis and surrounding structures, whatever the differences in the organisms that initiate the inflammatory response.

Children who have epiglottitis usually have been well previously, although up to 25% may have had some prior upper respiratory tract symptoms that may or may not be related. Since the advent of the conjugated Hib vaccines, the proportion of children with a concurrent or previous condition who develop epiglottis has appeared to increase. The hallmarks of epiglottitis are the abrupt onset of severe sore throat, fever, and toxicity in a formerly healthy child.[1,2,4,31] With fulminant progression, the other classic symptoms and signs occur: dysphagia, drooling, and respiratory distress. Stridor eventually develops, but toxicity and respiratory distress may be present initially without overt stridor. Retractions of the chest wall become evident, particularly in the supraclavicular and suprasternal areas, and indicate high airway obstruction. Cough usually is not a prominent part of the picture but may develop as the child tries to clear the increasing secretions. As noted in Table 284-1, the preceding spasmodic, brassy cough and laryngitis are more characteristic of viral croup. With progression of the epiglottitis, voice changes do occur, however. These may be described more correctly as dysphonia rather than the "scratchy" or "rasping" hoarseness associated with viral laryngotracheobronchitis.

The general appearance of the child who has epiglottitis should suggest the diagnosis although bacterial tracheitis may have a very similar presentation. The child who has epiglottitis often appears to have a toxic condition and classically is in a sitting position, leaning forward with the mouth open, tongue protruding, and drooling. The drooling is a particularly characteristic and helpful clinical sign.

Examination of the child reveals a markedly inflamed, "beefy red" pharynx, bathed by copious secretions. Although the "cherry red" epiglottis often may be seen by examination of the pharynx with a tongue depressor, this generally should not be attempted. Fatal occlusion of the airway may result. Inspiratory stridor and expiratory rhonchi may be heard on auscultation, and with progressive obstruction the breath sounds may become diminished.

Bacteremia may occur with development of secondary sites of infection or the epiglottitis may be secondary to bacteremia with a focus of infection elsewhere.[9,25,35] Most frequent of these are pneumonia, otitis media, and cervical lymphadenitis.

DIAGNOSIS

Because of the gravity of epiglottitis, the tentative diagnosis must be made based on the history and clinical manifestation.[2,27] If epiglottitis is suspected, the child should be sent to the hospital immediately, where the diagnosis may be confirmed and trained personnel and equipment are available for establishing an artificial airway.[13,22] Only with these precautions may visualization of the epiglottis be attempted to confirm the diagnosis.

Roentgenograms of the lateral neck can confirm the diagnosis, but these usually are unnecessary and unwise for the distressed child who has epiglottitis.[26,27] When a roentgenogram is taken, the child should be accompanied at all times by personnel equipped to handle an airway occlusion. As shown in Fig. 284-2, the characteristic swelling of the epiglottis may be seen as an enlarged, rounded shadow that resembles an adult thumb. This has been called the "thumb sign" by Podgore and Bass[26] and may be compared with the "little finger sign" of the normal epiglottis (Fig. 284-3). The normal epiglottis appears narrower, with the configuration of an adult little finger viewed from the side, as seen in the figure. The total white blood cell count usually is elevated (15,000 to 25,000/mm^3) and often contains a pronounced left shift. Cultures of the upper respiratory tract and blood usually demonstrate the causative pathogen. With *H. influenzae* type b epiglottitis, the cultures of blood and secretions almost always are positive and commonly positive for *S. pneumoniae* also. For other organisms, cultures of the respiratory tract secretions may be an unreliable means of definitive etiological diagnosis because the organisms are isolated com-

Table 284-1 Characteristic Signs of Epiglottitis Compared with Viral Croup and Bacterial Tracheitis

	Epiglottitis	Viral croup	Bacterial tracheitis
Peak age	3-7 yr	3 mo-3 yr	Any age (mostly ≤12 yr)
History	Previously well	Preceding upper respiratory tract infection common; may have had croup previously	Preceding upper respiratory tract infection common; sometimes viral croup; occasionally, previous trauma or manipulation of trachea and upper respiratory tract
Onset	Acute (hours)	Less acute (days)	Acute (hours)
Appearance	Toxic; drooling, dysphagia; sitting forward, mouth open	Less toxic; no drooling	Toxic; respiratory distress and stridor; drooling and sitting forward not characteristic
Cough	Unusual	Very characteristic, spasmodic, "seal's bark"	May be absent or may be present from preceding viral upper respiratory tract infection
Temperature	High (usually ≥39° C)	Lower (usually <39° C, sometimes none)	High (usually >39° C)
Pharynx	"Beefy" erythema	Normal or slight erythema	Normal or minimal inflammation
White blood cell count and differential	High; left shift	Normal or slight increase; normal or slight left shift	High; left shift
Roentgenogram of neck	"Thumb" sign on lateral view (edematous epiglottis)	Subglottic narrowing on posteroanterior view	Normal epiglottis; subglottic narrowing with membranous tracheal exudate occasionally visible on lateral view

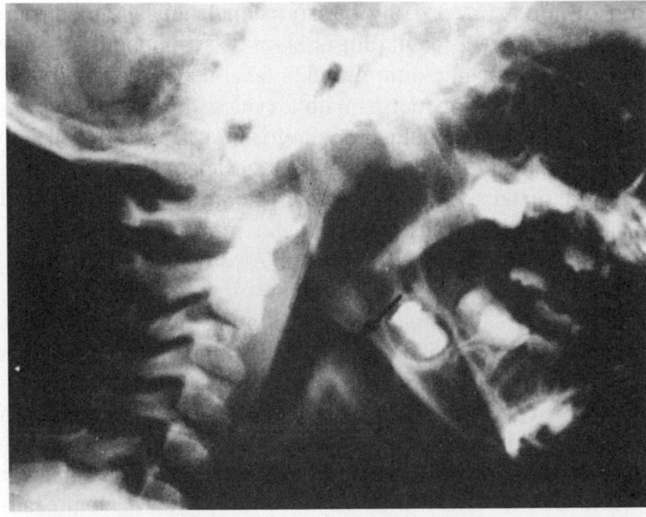

Fig. 284-2 Roentgenogram of lateral neck of a child who has epiglottitis. The arrow points to the shadow of the epiglottis, which is enlarged and resembles the anteroposterior view of a thumb.
(From Hall CB, Hall WJ: *Update* 2:655, 1975.)

Fig. 284-3 Roentgenogram of lateral neck of a normal child. In contrast to Fig. 284-2, the epiglottis is not enlarged and resembles an adult's fifth finger, viewed laterally.
(From Hall CB, Hall WJ: *Update* 2:655, 1975.)

monly from the upper respiratory tract without associated disease. Nevertheless, the causative organism is likely to be recovered, along with other organisms, from the respiratory secretions. Such cultures, as a means of diagnosis, therefore, usually are sensitive but not specific.[9,25,35]

MANAGEMENT

Few illnesses in pediatrics require more swift and careful management.[1] As has been stressed previously, suspicion of the diagnosis of epiglottitis is indication enough to rush the child to the hospital. Once the diagnosis is established, an adequate airway must be maintained. In some intensive care settings, with highly trained personnel in continuous attendance, some children who have early disease have been managed without an artificial airway. In most centers, however, immediate airway intervention is chosen.[2,3,33] With experienced personnel available, nasotracheal intubation is the procedure of choice. Fewer complications occur with this method, and in most patients extubation is possible within 1 to 3 days.

Intravenous antibiotic therapy also should be started immediately. Previously, antibiotic therapy has been directed almost exclusively at *H. influenzae* type b. Currently, the choice of therapy must be broadened to include not only sensitive and resistant *H. influenzae* type b organisms but also gram-positive organisms, such as *Streptococcus pyogenes* and *S. pneumoniae*. In special circumstances, such as nosocomially acquired infection and in patients with recent courses of antibiotic therapy, antibiotic coverage for *Staphylococcus aureus*, gram-negative bacilli, and resistant pneumococci should be considered.[9] In most cases, a cephalosporin that is stable against the beta-lactamases, such as several third-generation cephalosporins, should be adequate until initial culture results are available. In areas in which pneumococci resistant to both penicillins and cephalosporins have been identified, vancomycin may be added pending the results of antibiotic sensitivity tests.

Supportive care in epiglottitis is of the utmost importance. Direct humidification of the airway and removal of the secretions should be maintained. As with any mechanical airway, its position and patency should be monitored carefully. A short course of corticosteroids may be used to help reduce the postintubation edema. Antipyretics may be given during the initial period of high fever. Intravenous fluid should be monitored carefully. The acute onset of the disease means that most of these children are not dehydrated and only maintenance fluids are necessary.

PROGNOSIS

The outcome for these children often depends on the primary care physician. The clinical acumen of the physician and a high index of suspicion of the diagnosis, even over the telephone, will allow the child to reach the hospital rapidly and will prevent an unexpected calamity. The prognosis of epiglottitis is related directly to the speed with which therapy and the precautions against fatal asphyxia are initiated. Once an airway has been established and appropriate antibiotic therapy has been begun, the clinical response usually is rapid in children, but less so in adults.[12] Progression of the infection usually is controlled in less than 24 hours, and the nasotracheal tube usually may be removed within the next few days.

PREVENTION

Immunization of all children starting at 2 months of age with the conjugated Hib vaccines has been the most effective means of prevention for *H. influenzae* type b epiglottitis.[14,15] For epiglottitis caused by other organisms, no vaccine or means of prevention is available currently. Conjugated pneumococcal vaccines are being developed for use in young children. Whether such vaccines could affect the occurrence and epidemiological status of epiglottitis remains to be determined.

DIFFERENTIAL DIAGNOSIS

The major entities to be distinguished from epiglottitis are viral croup and bacterial tracheitis. The distinguishing features of these diseases are listed in Table 284-1. Bacterial tracheitis, in particular, may mimic epiglottitis in its severity and rapid progression and requires equally prompt treatment.[10,11] This unusual entity may affect children of any age. The onset is similar in its acuteness, fever, and toxic condition but is characterized by respiratory stridor, more severe than that usually observed with viral croup, and the production of copious, purulent sputum. The diagnosis may be made by direct laryngoscopy, which shows the purulent secretions and an exudate localized to the inflamed subglottic area. The epiglottic and supraglottic structures usually are involved minimally. Roentgenograms of the lateral neck can demonstrate the subglottic narrowing and occasionally even a fibrinous exudate obstructing the airway.[11] The organisms most commonly causing this syndrome are *S. aureus* and GABHS, both of which usually can be recovered in almost pure culture from the secretions obtained on laryngoscopy.[10,17]

Diphtheria with pharyngolaryngeal involvement may be confused with epiglottitis. However, the slower onset, other signs of diphtheria, and a pharyngeal grayish membrane may help to differentiate the two. Most helpful in the differentiation is the history of inadequate immunizations. Specific diagnosis of diphtheria may be obtained by Gram-stained smear and culture of the diphtheritic membrane.

Aspiration of a foreign body should be suspected in a child, usually a toddler, who has a history of acute onset of choking and respiratory distress. Fever is not present early in the course, and the pharynx does not show the "beefy" erythema characteristic of acute bacterial infection. Roentgenograms of the lateral neck will not show the "thumb" sign. Further roentgenographic examination may show the foreign body, if opaque, or endoscopy may be required. In rare cases, thermal injury to the epiglottis has been reported in young children drinking hot beverages, resulting in a clinical picture markedly similar to that of epiglottitis.[20]

REFERENCES

1. Ashcraft CK, Steele RW: Epiglottitis: a pediatric emergency, *J Respir Dis* 9:48, 1988.
2. Bass JW, Steele RW, Weide RA: Acute epiglottitis: a surgical emergency, *JAMA* 229:671, 1974.

3. Battaglia JD, Lockhart CH: Management of acute epiglottitis by nasotracheal intubation, *Am J Dis Child* 129:334, 1975.
4. Berenberg W, Kevy S: Acute epiglottitis in childhood, *N Engl J Med* 258:870, 1958.
5. Black SB, et al: Immunization with oligosaccharide conjugate *Haemophilus influenzae* type b (HbOC) vaccine on a large health maintenance organization population: extended follow-up and impact on *Haemophilus influenzae* disease epidemiology, *Pediatr Infect Dis J* 11: 610, 1992.
6. Centers for Disease Control: *MMWR Morb Mortal Wkly Rep* 47:844, 1998.
7. Centers for Disease Control: Progress toward elimination of *Haemophilus influenzae* type b disease among infants and children—United States, 1987-1993, *MMWR Morb Mortal Wkly Rep* 43:144, 1994.
8. Dajani AS, Asmar BI, Thirumoorthi MC: Systemic *Haemophilus influenzae* disease: an overview, *J Pediatr* 94:355, 1979.
9. Daum RS, et al: Nosocomial epiglottitis associated with penicillin- and cephalosporin-resistant *Streptococcus pneumoniae* bacteria, *J Clin Microbiol* 32:246, 1994.
10. Davidson S, Yahav BJ, Rubinstein E: Bacterial tracheitis: a true entity? *J Laryngol Otol* 96:173, 1982.
11. Denneny JC, Handler SD: Membranous laryngotracheobronchitis, *Pediatrics* 70:705, 1982.
12. Freeman L, Wolford R: Acute epiglottitis caused by methicillin-resistant *Staphylococcus aureus* in adults, *Clin Infect Dis* 26:1240, 1998.
13. Fulginiti VA: Acute supraglottitis (epiglottitis): to look or not? *Am J Dis Child* 142:597, 1988.
14. Gorelick MH, Baker D: Epiglottitis in children, 1979 through 1992: effects of *Haemophilus influenzae* type b immunization, *Arch Pediatr Adolesc Med* 148:47, 1994.
15. Hoekelman RA: A pediatrician's view: Hib vaccination now! *Pediatr Ann* 19:683, 1990.
16. Hussain SM, et al: Invasive group B streptococcal disease in children beyond infancy, *Pediatr Infect Dis J* 14:278, 1995.
17. Jones R, Santos JI, Overall JC Jr: Bacterial tracheitis, *JAMA* 242:721, 1979.
18. Jones RN, Slepack J, Bigelow J: Ampicillin-resistant *Hemophilus paraphrophelus* laryngoepiglottitis, *J Clin Microbiol* 4:405, 1976.
19. Kucera CM, et al: Epiglottitis in adults and children in Olmstead County, Minnesota, 1976 through 1990, *Mayo Clin Proc* 71:1155, 1996.
20. Kulick RM, et al: Thermal epiglottitis after swallowing hot beverages, *Pediatrics* 81:441, 1988.
21. Margolis CZ, Ingram DL, Meyer JH: Routine tracheotomy in *Haemophilus influenzae* type b epiglottitis, *J Pediatr* 81:1150, 1972.
22. Mauro RD, Poole SR, Lockhart CH: Differentiation of epiglottitis from laryngotracheitis in the child with stridor, *Am J Dis Child* 142:679, 1988.
23. Mayo-Smith MF, et al: Acute epiglottitis: an 18-year experience in Rhode Island, *Chest* 108:1640, 1995.
24. Mayo-Smith MF, et al: Acute epiglottitis in adults, *N Engl J Med* 314: 1133, 1986.
25. Molteni RA: Epiglottitis: incidence of extraepiglottic infection: report on 72 cases and review of the literature, *Pediatrics* 58:526, 1976.
26. Podgore JK, Bass JW: The "thumb sign" and "little finger sign" in acute epiglottitis, *J Pediatr* 88:154, 1976.
27. Rapkin RH: Acute epiglottitis: pitfalls in diagnosis and management, *Clin Pediatr* 10:312, 1971.
28. Robbins JB: *Haemophilus influenzae* type b: disease and immunity in humans, *Ann Intern Med* 78:259, 1973.
29. Schoendorf KC, et al: National trends in *Haemophilus influenzae* meningitis mortality and hospitalization among children, 1980 through 1991, *Pediatrics* 93:663, 1994.
30. Senior BA, et al: Changing patterns of pediatric supraglottitis: a multi-institutional review 1980-1992, *Laryngoscope* 104:1314, 1994.
31. Todd JK, Bruhn FW: Severe *Haemophilus influenzae* infections, *Am J Dis Child* 129:607, 1975.
32. Vadheim CM, et al: Eradication of *Haemophilus influenzae* type b in southern California, *Arch Pediatr Adolesc Med* 148:51, 1994.
33. Weber ML, et al: Acute epiglottitis in children: treatment with nasotracheal intubation: report of 14 consecutive cases, *Pediatrics* 57:152, 1976.
34. Wenger JK: Supraglottitis and group A S*treptococcus, Pediatr Infect Dis J* 16:1005, 1997.
35. Young N, Finn A, Powell C: Group B streptococcal epiglottitis, *Pediatr Infect Dis J* 15:95, 1996.

285 Esophageal Caustic Injury

Walter Pegoli, Jr. • George T. Drugas

Caustic injury of the esophagus, a disease of industrialization, is a major pediatric health concern. Corrosive esophageal injuries continue to occur despite federal legislation mandating preventive packaging and labeling, injury prevention programs designed for children and parents, and laws restricting the potency and availability of caustic substances. Nearly 5000 caustic burns of the esophagus occur annually in the United States. Most ingestions afflict children younger than 3 years of age, and they are entirely preventable. Sixty percent of esophageal caustic injuries occur in boys. During adolescence, when intentional suicide attempts are more prevalent, girls are more likely to be afflicted.[5] Twenty percent of caustic ingestions result in some form of esophageal injury. Although death from caustic ingestion is rare, morbidity can be devastating. Early management strategies after caustic ingestion are now well accepted, yet controversy persists with regard to the prevention and management of caustic esophageal strictures.

PATHOPHYSIOLOGY

The extent of injury after a caustic ingestion is dependent on the type of agent, whether the substance was liquid or solid, the concentration, the volume ingested, and the duration of contact the agent has had with the esophageal mucosa. Ingestion of liquid laundry detergents and dishwasher solutions found in the home usually results in mild esophageal injury that heals without complication. Household bleaches rarely have been associated with severe esophageal injury because of their low concentration of sodium hypochlorite. Ingestion of strong acids and alkalis are particularly deleterious, with acute and chronic implications. Strong alkalis are destructive because they cause liquefaction necrosis, which allows penetration of the corrosive agent transmurally through the esophagus and potentially into adjacent mediastinal tissues. The ensuing inflammatory reaction can result in gangrene, perforation, mediastinitis, fibrosis, or severe contracture of the esophagus. Liquid lye ingestion is the most common cause of esophageal caustic injury, and it is associated with the greatest number of deaths. Lye is odorless, tasteless, and viscous. These properties allow lye to be easily ingested by children and in massive volumes by suicidal teens and adults. Lye's high viscosity retards transit through the esophagus, making it particularly injurious. Lesions caused by lye injury occur in three phases. The acute *necrotic* phase usually lasts 24 to 96 hours after ingestion. An intense inflammatory reaction surrounds nonviable tissue. During the second *ulceration and granulation* phase 3 to 5 days after injury, superficial necrotic tissue sloughs, and it is replaced by an ulcerated, inflamed granulation bed. This phase lasts 10 to 12 days, and it is during this period that the esophagus is most vulnerable to perforation. The third phase of *scarring and cicatrization* begins during the third week after injury. In this period, contracture of the wound may lead to stricture formation. In contrast, solid alkalis, like Clinitest tablets and batteries, tend to lodge during transit, which results in focal burns and perforations at their point of impaction.

Strong acids, unlike alkalis, have an offensive odor and bitter taste that usually results in rapid expectoration after accidental ingestion. Acids exhibit rapid esophageal transit; they are more likely to damage the stomach or intestine. Esophageal injury is less common after acid ingestion because of rapid transit time and the presumed intrinsic resistance of the esophageal mucosa to acid. Acids cause coagulation necrosis, which results in superficial eschar formation that, in turn, prevents penetration into deeper tissues. Acids and alkalis can induce pylorospasm that results in pooling of the caustic agent in the gastric antrum.

DIAGNOSIS AND INITIAL MANAGEMENT

After caustic ingestion, symptoms can consist of searing or burning pain of the mouth and lips, drooling or hypersalivation, and burning pain and difficulty with swallowing. Epiglottic or vocal cord edema may result in stridor, dysphonia, or aphonia. Substernal or back pain usually results from esophageal disruption and mediastinitis. Acute epigastric pain may indicate gastric perforation. The presence of fever is strongly correlated with significant esophageal injury. It is imperative to recognize that the absence of oral burns does not exclude an esophageal burn injury and that 20% to 45% of patients with such burns have no evidence of oral burns.[6] Bleeding can occur and results from mucosal sloughing with persistent ooze from the exposed submucosa or muscularis. Life-threatening hematemesis from the development of an aortoesophageal fistula is, however, a rare event.

Every attempt should be made to identify the agent ingested. In the case of young children, parents usually are aware of the offending agent and often bring the container to the emergency department. With suicidal ingestion, the caustic agent may be unknown. Stridor or aphonia from laryngoepiglottic injury should be monitored carefully and may require urgent orotracheal intubation. Occasionally, severe laryngeal destruction necessitates emergency cricothyroidotomy or tracheostomy. Adequate vascular access should

BOX 285-1

GRADING OF CAUSTIC ESOPHAGEAL BURNS

Grade I	Mucosal hyperemia and edema
Grade II	Mucosal hemorrhage, exudate, ulceration, sloughing, and pseudomembrane formation
Grade III	Deep ulceration, massive hemorrhage, obliteration of the lumen, charring, and perforation

be obtained to correct hypovolemia or hypotension. A chest roentgenogram may identify concomitant aspiration, subcutaneous cervical emphysema, or pneumomediastinum suggestive of perforation. Emetics should be avoided because of the risk of reexposing the esophagus to the ingested corrosive agent and because of the threat of aspiration. Placement of a nasogastric tube should be deferred because of the risk of esophageal perforation. Any attempt to neutralize an ingested caustic agent poses an additional danger because the resultant exothermic reaction frequently exacerbates the burn injury. Gastric lavage is not necessary because the caustic agent frequently is regurgitated immediately and lavage may result in propagation of injury beyond the level of the pylorus.

When the patient is stabilized, early endoscopic examination should be performed to establish the extent of injury even in the absence of oral pharyngeal burns.[3] Flexible rather than rigid esophagoscopy is preferred to minimize the risk of iatrogenic perforation. The extent to which the endoscopist continues the examination is controversial. Most endoscopists fearing perforation will advance the scope only to the level at which maximal injury is encountered. Others advocate full examination of the stomach and, if possible, the duodenum. The degree of injury can be graded similarly to that of thermal skin burns (Box 285-1).[10] Contrast radiographic examination is unreliable in the presence of early esophageal injury, but it is important in later follow-up to identify strictures.

TREATMENT

Therapy for a caustic injury to the esophagus depends on the grade of injury assigned at endoscopy. Children with no injury or grade I injuries usually are admitted and observed for 24 to 48 hours. Any intentional ingestion mandates inpatient psychiatric evaluation regardless of the extent of esophageal injury. Strictures after grade I injury are rare, and follow-up contrast esophagography is unnecessary. Patients with grade II or grade III injury are begun empirically on broad-spectrum parenteral antibiotics. Although no controlled trials supporting the use of antimicrobials have been performed, empirical therapy is reasonable. After disruption of the mucosal barrier by caustic ingestion, bacterial translocation and secondary bacterial invasion are likely events. Parenteral nutrition is instituted, and oral feedings are withheld until the dysphagia of the initial phase has regressed and there has been no further evidence of clinical or radiographic deterioration. A barium esophagogram for the early detection of stricture development is performed 2 to 4 weeks after discharge. It is preferable to detect a stricture before the development of symptoms when stricture dilation may prove more challenging. The use of steroids to limit fibrosis after caustic injury has debatable efficacy in humans although they have been shown to be effective in experimental animals. Most studies demonstrate a lack of proven benefit, and the potential side effects of steroids argue against their routine use.[1] Various methods have been proposed for prophylaxis against stricture formation.[2,4] Esophageal bougienage to prevent adhesion formation in the injured segment, intraluminal stenting, and prolonged esophageal rest (by keeping the patient NPO) have demonstrated no proven benefit.

SURGICAL INTERVENTIONS

Surgical indications after caustic ingestion include uncontrollable hemorrhage, pneumomediastinum or pneumoperitoneum, mediastinitis, or overt peritonitis. The constellation of unrelenting substernal pain, abdominal pain, and refractory metabolic acidosis can substantiate the need for exploratory laparotomy. The operative field extends from the xiphoid to the pubis. Inspection of the stomach wall for black discoloration indicative of transmural necrosis will determine the extent of gastric resection. If there is a question of tissue viability, a second-look operation may be necessary in 24 to 36 hours. When a total gastrectomy is needed, the injury to the esophagus usually will be severe. Transhiatal thoracic esophagectomy is performed along with cervical esophagostomy, and a feeding jejunostomy is placed. Morbidity after full-thickness necrosis of the esophagus is nearly 100%, with a 20% mortality rate.

When strictures develop, esophageal dilation is the first treatment modality. Dilation therapy usually is started 4 to 6 weeks after injury to reduce the risk of perforation. Prograde or retrograde dilation via a gastrostomy site may be helpful. In either circumstance, dilation should be repeated every other week until the stricture softens. The length of time a surgeon should persist with dilation before consideration of esophageal substitution is problematic. An adequate lumen usually should be attained within 6 months to 1 year, with progressively longer intervals between dilations. Beyond that time, operative intervention for esophageal replacement should be considered.

Esophageal substitution is reserved for multiple diffuse strictures, complete stenosis with failure to establish lumen, recalcitrant strictures over a year of dilation therapy, or complications of dilation such as perforation, fistula formation, or mediastinitis. Skin tube esophagoplasties are mainly of historical interest. The colon, stomach, and jejunum are currently used as esophageal substitutes in children. Colonic interposition, gastric advancement, gastric tube esophagoplasty, and jejunal interposition are accepted procedures to replace the injured esophagus.[9] Esophagoplasty with a colonic patch over less extensive but persistent strictures also has been advocated.[7] Whatever technique is selected, these procedures may result in serious or even fatal complications because of minor errors of judgment or deviations in technique.

The management of the bypassed, damaged esophagus after injury also is problematic. The residual esophagus, if left in place, is predisposed to ulceration from gastroesophageal reflux and the development of cancer. The extensive dissection necessary to remove the damaged esophagus can result in significant morbidity. Retention of the esophagus may preserve vagal function to the distal bowel, but the retained damaged esophagus can result in multiple blind pouches and the subsequent development of mediastinal abscesses years later. Most surgeons advocate removal of the esophagus unless the operative risk is prohibitive.[9]

DELAYED COMPLICATIONS

The long-term outcome after caustic injury to the esophagus correlates with grade of injury. Strictures are exceedingly rare after grade I burns, but they develop in 20% to 30% of patients who have grade II burns and almost 90% of patients who have grade III injuries. The risk for postcorrosive esophageal carcinoma is estimated to be 500- to 1000-fold higher than the incidence for esophageal cancer in the general population. These carcinomas usually arise in the mid-esophagus and usually are of the squamous cell type. Local dissemination seems to occur less frequently; the potential for curative resection is, therefore, slightly improved. The interval between burn injury and the development of carcinoma ranges from 10 to 70 years, with a mean of 50 years.[8] Long-term follow-up of children who have grade II and III burns is warranted, regardless of their symptoms. Esophagography or surveillance esophagoscopy should be performed annually or biannually.

REFERENCES

1. Anderson KD, Rouse TM, Randolph JG: A controlled trial of corticosteroids in children with corrosive injury of the esophagus, *N Engl J Med* 323:637, 1990.
2. Berkovits RN, et al: Caustic injury of the esophagus: sixteen years experience, and introduction of a new model of esophageal stent, *J Larnygol Otol* 110:1041, 1996.
3. Ferguson MK, et al: Early evaluation and therapy for caustic esophageal injury, *Am J Surg* 157:116, 1989.
4. Lahoti D, et al: Corrosive esophageal strictures: predictors of response to endoscopic dilation, *Gastrointest Endosc* 41:196, 1995.
5. Litovitz TL, et al: 1997 Annual Report of the American Association of Poison Control Centers Toxic Exposure Surveillance System, *Am J Emerg Med* 16:443, 1998.
6. Lovejoy FH, Woolf AD: Corrosive ingestions, *Pediatr Rev* 16:473, 1995.
7. Ochersen HB Jr, et al: Save the child's esophagus. Part II. Colic patch repair, *J Pediatr Surg* 32:328, 1997.
8. Ribeiro U, et al: Risk factors for squamous cell carcinoma of the esophagus, *Br J Surg* 83:1174, 1996 (review).
9. Watson TJ, et al: Esophageal replacement for end-stage benign esophageal disease, *J Thorac Cardiovasc Surg* 115:1241, 1998.
10. Zargar SA, et al: The role of fiberoptic endoscopy in the management of corrosive ingestion and modified endoscopic classification of burns, *Gastrointest Endosc* 37:165, 1991.

286 Head Injuries

David E. Hall • Edward M. Goldstein

Head injuries are exceedingly common and a cause for great concern to parents. About 50% of patients hospitalized with head injury are younger than 20 years of age.[11] Boys are injured at least twice as often as are girls. More than 75% of trauma deaths in children are due to brain injury.[22]

The causes of severe head injury vary with age. In infants, falls and child abuse predominate; in preschool and school-age children, vehicular accidents are most common; and during the adolescent years, sports injuries and assault are seen most frequently. For all ages combined, falls are the most common cause of head trauma, but vehicular accidents are the leading cause of serious injury. In most vehicular accidents, the child is a pedestrian. As many as 70% of children hit by a vehicle are not supervised by an adult at the time of the accident.[15] Education regarding prevention of head injury is an essential role for the pediatrician. Anticipatory guidance regarding appropriate supervision of children, high-risk activities, and recommendations regarding protective equipment such as car seats for infants and bicycle helmets for older children, can dramatically reduce morbidity and mortality resulting from head injury.[17,29]

Physicians should be familiar with the initial management of the child who has a severe head injury. However, the most common problem faced by the practitioner is distinguishing those patients who require treatment from those who do not. Because these two aspects of care are so different, they are dealt with separately.

INITIAL CARE OF THE SEVERELY INJURED PATIENT

The improved prognosis for survival and neurological recovery of the child after a severe head injury compared with an adult,[3,20] plus the potential for organ donation in those patients who are brain dead, dictate that the physician providing emergency care make every effort to resuscitate the child who has a severe head injury. The basic ABC's of resuscitation (airway, breathing, and circulation) should be addressed first. As Haldane stated in 1919, "Anoxia not only stops the machine but wrecks the machinery."[18] In addition, ischemia, increased intracranial pressure, and uncontrolled seizures may cause further brain injury. The correction of anoxia and poor cerebral perfusion is more important than detection of an intracranial hematoma.

In patients with severe head injury, a coexisting cervical spine injury should be assumed until proved otherwise. The neck should not be moved until cervical spine films are performed to rule out a fracture or dislocation, which may result in spine trauma if movement occurs. The preferred initial radiographs are cross-table lateral, anteroposterior, and odontoid views. In the severely injured patient, the airway requires intubation to ensure adequate ventilation to reduce the chance of developing increased intracranial pressure. When possible, an anesthesiologist should perform the intubation. This usually is accomplished with a combination of a sedative to induce anesthesia, atropine to reduce secretions and prevent vagal reflexes, and a neuromuscular-blocking agent to produce paralysis. Close attention to blood pressure is necessary because sedatives may cause hypotension. Cricoid pressure may be applied to reduce the risk of aspiration. At one time, prolonged hyperventilation was recommended in patients with acute severe head injury. This no longer is the case.[1] Although hyperventilation constricts intracranial blood vessels and lowers intracranial pressure, there are concerns that hyperventilation may decrease cerebral perfusion.[7] Meticulous attention to $PaCO_2$ is required, to avoid hypercapnia at all costs. The optimal level of $PaCO_2$ is unknown and may vary from patient to patient. Acute hyperventilation may be useful, however, in an emergency situation in which the patient deteriorates acutely because of increased intracranial pressure.

Vital signs should be assessed frequently to ensure adequacy of circulation. Shock leads to further brain injury despite adequate airway management and oxygenation. Vigorous fluid therapy to restore adequate circulating blood volume and sufficient cerebral perfusion is essential. Isotonic solutions or blood products should be used, because hypotonic solutions may promote movement of free water into damaged brain tissue, increasing the potential for cerebral edema. Some have even argued for the use of hypertonic solutions in acute severe brain trauma,[28] although this has not achieved widespread use. If shock exists, a source of bleeding should be sought. Patients rarely sequester sufficient blood volume in the head to produce shock (notable exceptions include the infant with an expansible skull, and in the presence of a large subgaleal hematoma). Additional measures directed at reducing secondary brain injury include elevating the patient's head 30 degrees and keeping it in a midline position to maximize venous outflow from the cranial vault.

Cushing's response (hypertension and bradycardia) is an ominous sign that implies elevated intracranial pressure. This and unilateral pupillary dilation (a sign of impending catastrophic temporal lobe herniation) should prompt the admin-

Table 286-1 Glasgow Coma Scale*

Eye-Opening Response		
Score	**>1 Year**	**<1 Year**
4	Spontaneous	Spontaneous
3	To verbal command	To shout
2	To pain	To pain
1	None	None

Motor Response		
Score	**>1 Year**	**<1 Year**
6	Obeys commands	Spontaneous response
5	Localizes pain	Localizes pain
4	Withdraws from pain	Withdraws from pain
3	Displays abnormal flexion to pain (decorticate rigidity)	Displays abnormal flexion to pain (decorticate rigidity)
2	Displays abnormal extension to pain (decerebrate rigidity)	Displays abnormal extension to pain (decerebrate rigidity)
1	None	None

Verbal Response			
Score	**>5 Years**	**2 to 5 Years**	**0-23 Months**
5	Is oriented and converses	Uses appropriate words and phrases	Babbles, coos appropriately
4	Conversation is confused	Use inappropriate words	Cries, but is consolable
3	Words are inappropriate	Cries or screams persistently to pain	Cries or screams persistently to pain
2	Sounds are incomprehensible	Grunts or moans to pain	Grunts or moans to pain
1	None	None	None

Modified from Simon J: Accidental injury and emergency medical services for children. In Behrman RE, editor: *Nelson textbook of pediatrics.* Philadelphia, 1992, WB Saunders.

*Glasgow coma score = sum of best eye opening, motor, and verbal responses. Range = 3 to 15. Usual definitions of severity of head injury: Severe = score of <9; Moderate = score of 9 to 12; Mild = score of 13 to 15.

istration of mannitol at doses of 0.25 g/kg of body weight. Steroids do not improve outcome when used in the acute phase management of traumatic brain injury.[1,13]

Antipyretics should be given if fever exists. Hyperthermia may increase cerebral metabolic demands, further taxing delivery of nutrients to the injured brain. Similarly, seizures greatly increase the metabolic demands of the brain and should be treated promptly with intravenous diazepam or lorazepam, followed by 20 mg/kg of intravenous phenytoin. The latter should be given if the patient is pharmacologically paralyzed and, thus, seizure activity cannot be detected. This also is advisable before transfer to another medical center.

A more detailed neurological evaluation should be performed only when adequacy of the airway, breathing, and circulation are ensured. The Glasgow Coma Scale (Table 286-1) can be used to assess mental status and is valuable in assessing prognosis and in following the patient's progress. The scale is based on the patient's response in three areas: motor response, verbal response, and eye-opening response. Severe head injury may be defined as that resulting in a Glasgow Coma Score (GCS) of less than 9, whereas moderate head injury is associated with a GCS of 9 to 12. A GCS of 13 to 15 is consistent with mild head injury. Motor response is evaluated by noting symmetry of tone, movement, and reflexes. Cranial nerve examination may reveal signs of focal injury to the brainstem. Pupil size, symmetry, and reactivity should be noted carefully, and the fundus examined for signs of papilledema. Retinal hemorrhages suggest child abuse from shaken-baby syndrome. Pontine and midbrain function may be assessed by examination of oculovestibular reflexes. In the unconscious patient, the head should be rotated briskly from side to side after making certain the cervical spine has not been injured. Normally, when the head moves to the right, the eyes move to the left, and vice versa. Loss of these reflex eye movements in a comatose patient suggests an injury to the midbrain or pons. Alternatively, if the tympanic membranes are intact, ice water caloric responses should be elicited. With the patient's head elevated to 30 degrees, 120 ml of ice water is infused alternately into each ear canal. The eyes should turn toward the irrigated ear. If they do not, a brainstem injury is likely. To assess pontine function further, the quality and symmetry of the grimace evoked by painful stimulation of the face should be observed. In patients who do not respond to this stimulation, or do so minimally, the corneal reflex should be tested. Failure to react by blinking is consistent with pontine injury or deep coma. Medullary function is evaluated by assessing the patient's gag reflex and tongue movement. Examination of the patient's craniospinal axis should be done in concert with the neurological assessment, looking for signs of trauma. Swelling and bony depression of the skull suggest an underlying fracture. Ecchymoses behind the ear (Battle's sign) or around the orbits (raccoon sign), cerebrospinal fluid rhinorrhea, otorrhea, or hemotympanum suggest a basilar skull fracture. Basilar fractures or scalp lacerations overlying fractures are important to detect, because they serve as portals of entry for bacteria into the subarachnoid space and may cause meningitis. This neurological evaluation forms the baseline for serial assessments of neurological function while obtaining neuroimaging studies, and transferring the patient to the care of pediatric neurosurgeons and intensivists.

Neuroimaging studies for the severely injured patient typically consist of cervical spine films to rule out fracture or subluxation, and a noncontrast computed tomography (CT) scan of the brain with bone windows. The bone windows identify skull fractures and obviate the need for a skull roentgenogram. CT scan is the imaging study of choice in acute trauma. It is easier to obtain than a magnetic resonance image (MRI) and may not require sedation. It identifies the relationship between bone fragments and intracranial contents, and reveals extraaxial fluid collections such as epidural and subdural hematomas, as well as injury to brain parenchyma. The MRI may be useful later on, because it is more sensitive at detecting intrinsic brain injuries.[21]

CARE OF THE LESS SEVERELY INJURED PATIENT

Most physicians have little trouble identifying those patients who require intensive care at a regional medical center. More difficult is deciding whether to admit the less severely injured child to the hospital for observation. Information from published studies concerning the indications for such action is scant because most head trauma studies have focused just on hospitalized patients.[4] Decisions regarding the hospitalization of less severely injured patients must be made individually.

When taking the history, the possibility of abuse must be kept in mind. Children rarely sustain a serious injury when they fall out of bed, so such a history when given as the cause of severe injury is suspect. Loss of consciousness, seizures, amnesia for the circumstances surrounding the injury, and focal neurological deficits are indicators of more severe head trauma. Vomiting and headache are common symptoms after head trauma and their presence, if not persistent or severe, is not particularly ominous or suggestive of any specific pathological finding.[8] Persistent clouding of consciousness is the most reliable sign of a significant brain injury. In addition, the duration of posttraumatic amnesia, defined as an inability to generate new memories after head injury, correlates positively with the severity of injury.[27]

Examination of the patient should begin with assessment of mental status and assignment of a GCS. Neurological examination should proceed with assessment of the cranial nerves. Particular care needs to be given to pupillary responses and symmetry, funduscopic examination (to rule out papilledema or hemorrhage), eye movements (looking for dysconjugate gaze), asymmetries of facial sensation or movement, tongue movement, and gag reflex. As a sensory screening examination, symmetrical responses to pain in all four limbs should be determined. Symmetry of muscle tone and movement and of the deep-tendon reflexes and plantar responses needs to be determined, as should the alert, cooperative child's ability to manipulate small objects. The child's gait and station also need to be assessed.

The general physical examination should focus on the presence of injury to other body systems, and on seeking evidence of physical neglect or abuse.

The decision to perform neuroimaging studies is difficult and must be individualized. As a general rule, if the clinician is sufficiently worried about a child's clinical status to desire radiographic studies, a noncontrast CT with bone windows is the preferred imaging study and has supplanted the use of skull roentgenograms.[12] As already mentioned, the CT scan is highly sensitive in the detection of fractures and extraaxial fluid collections. In addition, it often detects parenchymal brain injury.

Like the performance of neuroimaging studies, the decision to admit a child with mild to moderate head trauma must be individualized. It seems prudent to obtain a CT scan when the patient has (1) a history of loss of consciousness exceeding several minutes in duration, (2) residual depression of mental state, (3) focal neurological deficits, (4) posttraumatic seizures (5) headache of increasing severity, (6) persistent vomiting, (7) serious facial injury, (8) an unreliable history of injury suggesting child abuse, and (9) signs of a basilar skull fracture or possible skull penetration. CT scans usually are not ordered when the patient has no history of loss of consciousness, a GCS of 15, and a normal neurological examination.[11] Many physicians have lower thresholds for obtaining CT scans in children younger than 2 years old.[12] Normal CT scans are extremely reassuring but do not totally eliminate the possibility of intraparenchymal injury.[8] Whenever a head injury occurs, there is always the question of a coexisting cervical spine injury. Most emergency department physicians do not obtain cervical spine radiographs if mental status and neurological examinations are normal, there is no tenderness of the spine, and the child moves his or her head around without difficulty, especially if the child is older than 5 years. The younger the child, the lower the threshold for obtaining cervical spine films.[14]

Electroencephalograms and lumbar punctures are not indicated in the acute phase management of pediatric head injury.

Patients with mild head injury who sustain prompt recovery of neurological function, are not suspected of being abused, and who have reliable caregivers can be discharged home with appropriate instructions. Children with normal neurological examinations and negative CT scans rarely have neurological deterioration after discharge from the emergency department.[9,26] Parents often are instructed to observe the child carefully for at least 24 hours, awakening him or her periodically during periods of sleep. Caregivers should return immediately to the emergency department if their child (1) cannot be awakened, (2) demonstrates decreasing mental status while awake, or (3) develops seizures, focal weakness, increasing headache, progressive instability, or vomiting to the point of dehydration. Linear skull fractures do not mandate admission to the hospital if the child is asymptomatic, but they do require close observation because the force required to fracture a child's skull is significant. A reliable observer at home is required.

Following hospital or emergency room discharge, office follow-up is recommended at 2 weeks. The child's recovery can be reviewed and further anticipatory guidance provided to the family regarding relevant neurological sequelae of the

BOX 286-1

CLASSIFICATION OF CONCUSSION

Grade 1
1. Transient confusion
2. No loss of consciousness
3. Concussion symptoms* or mental status abnormalities on examination resolve in less than 15 minutes

Grade 2
1. Transient confusion
2. No loss of consciousness
3. Concussion symptoms* or mental status abnormalities on examination lasting more than 15 minutes

Grade 3
1. Any loss of consciousness, either brief (seconds) or prolonged (minutes)

Modified from McQueen JK, et al: *J Neurol Neurosurg Psychiatry* 46:899, 1983.
*Concussion symptoms: *Early* (minutes and hours)—headache, dizziness or vertigo, lack of awareness of surroundings, nausea or vomiting. *Late* (days to weeks)—persistent low-grade headache; light-headedness; poor attention and concentration; memory dysfunction; easy fatigability; irritability and low frustration tolerance; intolerance of bright lights or difficulty focusing vision; intolerance of loud noises, sometimes ringing in the ears; anxiety or depressed mood; sleep disturbance.

child's head injury. Children younger than 2 years of age who have diastatic fractures (fractures that involve normal suture lines) should be evaluated again in 6 to 8 weeks, to check for a "growing fracture" secondary to leptomeningeal cyst formation. These enlarging fractures frequently require neurosurgical closure.

A special situation occurs in the child who sustains a concussion after a sports injury. Physicians often are asked to make recommendations regarding return to sports participation. The Colorado Medical Society and the American Academy of Neurology have published guidelines to assist in making these decisions.[24] Proper care is especially important because the effects of head injuries are cumulative and repeated minor injuries closely spaced in time may cause permanent harm. Box 286-1 presents criteria with which to classify concussions into three grades, and Box 286-2 defines when a child may return to play after sustaining each grade of concussion. Patients with grade 1 concussions may return to the sports event if all symptoms resolve at rest and exertion within 15 minutes. A second grade 1 concussion in the same contest eliminates the player from competition that day, and he or she may only return after 1 week if asymptomatic. Patients with grade 2 concussions may return to sports participation after 1 week if there are no symptoms at rest or on exertion. Patients with grade 3 concussion may not return to participation for 1 week if the symptoms lasted only seconds, but if loss of consciousness greater than a minute occurred, the athlete may not play for at least 2 weeks after he or she has been asymptomatic at rest and with exercise.

BOX 286-2

WHEN TO RETURN TO PLAY AFTER REMOVAL FROM SPORTS CONTEST FOR CONCUSSION*

Grade 1: May return to play if all symptoms resolve within 15 minutes
Multiple grade 1: 1 week
Grade 2: 1 week
Multiple grade 2: 2 weeks
Grade 3 (brief loss of consciousness [seconds]): 1 week
Grade 3 (prolonged loss of consciousness [minutes]): 2 weeks
Multiple grade 3 concussions: 1 month or longer

Modified from McQueen JK, et al: *J Neurol Neurosurg Psychiatry* 46:899, 1983.
*Patients must be asymptomatic, with normal neurological assessment at rest and with exercise.

PROGNOSIS

Children who have mild head trauma (GCS 13 to 15) are indistinguishable from their peers at 1 year following their injuries.[16] Despite this, significant neurological dysfunction may be seen in the period immediately after the child's injury, and may persist for as long as 8 weeks. Symptoms include irritability, sleep disturbance, clinging behavior, hyperactivity, and headache.[7,10] It is important to provide anticipatory guidance to parents regarding the transient nature of these symptoms in mild head injuries.

Children who have moderate head injury (GCS 9 to 12) and severe head injury (GCS 3 to 8) may suffer from multiple physical, cognitive, and psychological disabilities. However, prognosis generally is more favorable for head-injured children than adults.[2] For example, children with an initial GCS of 6 or more have an 80% chance of achieving functional independence.[3] Intellectual recovery continues for as long as 2 years following head injury in children,[6] so long-term rehabilitative services are needed. Formal psychological assessment for staging school reentry, and for ongoing adjustment of the child's academic curriculum should be obtained.[5,19]

Five percent of patients will have seizures within the first week following their head injury. The occurrence of these "early-onset" seizures does not accurately predict the development of later posttraumatic epilepsy.[16] The risk of subsequently developing epilepsy is significantly increased if seizures are present beyond the first week after head injury, particularly when severe head trauma, intraparenchymal hematoma, or depressed skull fracture occurs. With these risk factors, approximately one third of patients will develop posttraumatic epilepsy.[16] Electroencephalographic studies do not accurately predict its subsequent development,[15,25] and the use of prophylactic anticonvulsant medications does not appear to reduce the risk of its occurrence. These medications generally are not used in mild brain injury.[23,30,31] They are indicated for children who have had severe brain injury to prevent increased intracranial pressure caused by the seizures per se.

When to Refer

Deteriorating mental status
Coma or persistent alteration in mental status
GCS <9
Subdural, epidural, or intraparenchymal hematoma
Focal abnormalities on neurological examination
Seizures after the first week or recurrent seizures
Shock
Signs of Cushing's response (bradycardia and hypertension)
Suspicion of child abuse (refer to appropriate local governmental agency)
Cervical spine injury
Basilar skull fracture
Depressed skull fracture
Increasingly severe headaches
Facial laceration or suspicion of significant trauma at other locations

When to Hospitalize

Persistent alteration in mental state
Focal neurological deficits
Seizures
Persistent vomiting that precludes adequate hydration
Severe headache
Suspicion of abuse
Unreliable caregivers or observers at home
Any injury requiring neurosurgical intervention
CT scan indicating intracranial bleeding or brain injury

REFERENCES

1. Allen E, et al: Head and spinal cord injury. In Rogers MC, Helfaer M, editors: *Handbook of pediatric intensive care,* Baltimore, 1999, Williams and Wilkins.
2. Bacco E, et al: Early outcome prediction in severe head injury: comparison between children and adults, *Child Nerv Syst* 2:67, 1986.
3. Bruce DA: Outcome: does it work? In Harris BH, editor: *Progress in pediatric trauma,* Boston, 1985, Nobb Hill Press.
4. Casey R, Ludwig S, McCormick MC: Morbidity following minor head trauma in children, *Pediatrics* 78:497, 1986.
5. Chadwick O, Rutter M: Intellectual performance and reading skills after localized head injury in childhood, *J Child Psychol Psychiatry* 22:117, 1981.
6. Chadwick O, et al: A prospective study of children with head injuries. II. Cognitive sequelae, *Psychol Med* 11:49, 1981.
7. Chesnut R: Hyperventilation in traumatic brain injury: friend or foe? *Crit Care Med* 25:1275, 1997.
8. Cheung D, Kharasch M: Evaluation of the patient with closed head trauma: an evidence based approach, *Emerg Med Clin North Am* 17:9, 1999.
9. Davis RL, et al: The use of cranial CT scans in the triage of pediatric patients with mild head injury, *Pediatrics* 95:345, 1995.
10. Farmer MY, et al: Neurobehavioral sequelae of minor head injuries in children, *Pediatr Neurosci* 13:304, 1987.
11. Field JH: *Epidemiology of head injuries in England and Wales,* London, 1976, Her Majesty's Stationery Office.
12. Frush D, O'Hara, SM, Kliewer M: Pediatric imaging perspective: acute head trauma—is skull radiography useful? *J Pediatr* 132:553, 1998.
13. Gudeman SK, Miller JD, Becker DP: Failure of high-dose steroid therapy to influence intracranial pressure in patients with severe head injury, *J Neurosurg* 51:301, 1979.
14. Hall D, Boydston W: Pediatric neck injuries, *Pediatr Rev* 20:13, 1999.
15. Jennett B: *Epilepsy after non-missile head injuries,* ed 2, London, 1975, William Heinermann.
16. Jennett WB, Lewin W: Traumatic epilepsy after closed head injuries, *J Neurol Neurosurg Psychiatry* 23:295, 1960.
17. Johnston C, et al: Children in car crashes: analysis of data for injury and use of restraints, *Pediatrics* 2:960, 1994.
18. Kalbag RM: Management of head injuries. In Cartilidge NEF, Shaw DA, editors: *Head injury,* London, 1981, WB Saunders.
19. Levine HS, Bento AL, Grossman RG: *Neurobehavioral consequences of closed head injury,* New York, 1982, Oxford University Press.
20. Luersson T, Klauber M, Marshall L: Outcome from head injury related to patient's age: a longitudinal prospective study of adult and pediatric head injury, *J Neurosurg* 68:409, 1988.
21. Mansfield RT: Common issues in pediatric and adult clinical care, *Crit Care Clin* 13:611, 1997.
22. Mayer T, et al: Causes of morbidity and mortality in severe pediatric trauma, *JAMA* 245:719, 1981.
23. McQueen JK, et al: Low risk of late posttraumatic seizures following severe head injury: implications for clinical trials of prophylaxis, *J Neurol Neurosurg Psychiatry* 46:899, 1983.
24. Quality Standards Subcommittee, American Academy of Neurology: Practice parameter: the management of concussion in sports (summary statement) report of the Quality Standards Committee, *Neurology* 48: 581, 1997.
25. Raimondi AJ, Hirschauer J: Head injury in the infant and toddler, *Childs Brain* 11:12, 1984.
26. Roddy S, Cohn S, Moller B, et al: Minimal head trauma in children revisited: is routine hospitalization required? *Pediatrics* 101:575, 1998.
27. Rutter M, et al: A prospective study of children with head injuries, *Psychol Med* 10:633, 1980.
28. Simma B: A prospective, randomized, and controlled study of fluid management in children with severe head injury: lactated Ringer's solution versus hypertonic saline, *Crit Care Med* 26:1265, 1998.
29. Thompson RS, et al: A case-control study of the effectiveness of bicycle safety helmets, *New Engl J Med* 320:1361, 1989.
30. Yablon S: Posttraumatic seizures, *Arch Phys Med Rehabil* 74:983, 1993.
31. Young B, et al: Failure of prophylactically administered phenytoin to prevent late posttraumatic seizures, *J Neurosurg* 58:236, 1983.

287 Heart Failure

Steven E. Lipshultz

Congestive heart failure means in the broadest sense an inability to adequately perfuse the body tissues. Congestive heart failure can occur in infants or children of any age, but up to 90% of cases occur during the first year of life, and most of these occur during the neonatal period.[17] In this chapter, four aspects of congestive heart failure will be discussed. First, the pathophysiology of congestive heart failure will be reviewed, especially as it relates to differences in age at presentation. The therapy of congestive heart failure in children then will be presented. The third section covers signs and symptoms of congestive heart failure. The fourth section reviews the specific etiologies and associated findings in children presenting with congestive heart failure at different ages, an important topic because in many children, congestive heart failure takes a chronic, smoldering course and may not be recognized early. Understanding the causes and associations for pediatric congestive heart failure, as well as its presenting signs and symptoms, will help with early identification, which may, in turn, reduce morbidity and mortality.

PATHOPHYSIOLOGY

Left ventricular force generation differs at different developmental stages.[1] The inotropic forces of myocardial contractions are higher in neonatal animals than in fetal animals, and higher in adult animals than in neonatal animals. Thus, for a particular left ventricular preload, cardiac output or stroke volume rises as animals progress from fetal to neonatal to adult stages of life. Although the mechanisms are not entirely clear, differences in the properties of contractile proteins are expressed at different developmental stages, as well as in the properties of ion channels and cell surface receptors. All of these affect contractility of the left ventricular myocardium at different developmental stages. Animal studies also suggest that neonatal animals operate closer to their maximal inotropic potential than adults do and may have less reserve to handle excess ventricular preload, making them more likely to have episodes of congestive heart failure. Several human clinical examples suggest this as well. For example, during the third trimester of pregnancy, intravascular volume in pregnant women is approximately 50% greater than baseline. Yet, only one in 4000 pregnant women develops peripartum cardiomyopathy. In contrast, in a normal 3-kg neonate, intravascular volume may be 240 ml, and a 50% increase of 120 ml would likely result in congestive heart failure. Although this simplified scenario does not take into account the difference between acute and longer-lasting increases in intravascular volume, it indirectly suggests that animal study data may be applicable to human situations.

PHARMACOTHERAPY FOR CONGESTIVE HEART FAILURE IN CHILDREN

Four classes of pharmacotherapy are used most frequently in the management of congestive heart failure in children: diuretics, inotropes, agents to reduce afterload, and beta-adrenergic antagonists.[2,5] Each addresses a different aspect of the pathophysiology of congestive heart failure, and they often are used in combination. The treatment of congestive heart failure in children should be directed by a pediatric cardiologist.

In children, symptomatic left ventricular dysfunction or congestive heart failure can result from many mechanisms. One of them is preload excess. In this situation, even though the left ventricular myocytes are healthy and have normal contractility, the overall systolic performance of the ventricle is reduced.[13] Frequently, preload reduction with diuretic therapy is of therapeutic benefit.[14]

Congestive heart failure may also follow from depressed contractility of unhealthy left ventricular myocytes. In this case, inotropic support frequently brings early symptomatic relief.[10] Digoxin, an inotrope that can be administered orally or intravenously, will raise a child to a somewhat higher inotropic state, and in the process, lead to some reduction in preload. Frequently, digoxin is used in combination with a diuretic. Some studies suggest a synergy between digoxin and diuretics, which potentiates both an improved inotropic state and a reduction in preload,[8] more so than either agent would accomplish if not coupled therapeutically with the other.[14] Combination therapy frequently will reduce the chance of individual agent toxicity.

The third major class of pharmacotherapy for the management of heart failure consists of agents that reduce afterload. Reducing left ventricular afterload in a child with symptomatic left ventricular dysfunction will improve that function and reduce symptoms. Several types of afterload reducers are available. One commonly used is the angiotensin-converting enzyme (ACE) inhibitors.[6] Two examples are captopril and enalapril. Like hydralazine and nifedipine, these agents are vasodilators, but in addition, they affect neurohormonal mechanisms. In adults with asymptomatic left ventricular dysfunction or congestive heart failure, the use of ACE inhibitors has been associated with slowing the progression from asymptomatic left ventricular dysfunction to congestive heart failure, as well as reducing mortality from heart failure. It is thought that these beneficial effects are due to the combination of vasodilatory and neurohormonal activation. The vasodilatory effects of ACE inhibitors often will move a child to a more favorable preload state as well as reducing afterload, slightly improving left ventricular contractility.

A fourth class of therapy for left ventricular dysfunction in children is the beta-adrenergic antagonists.[16] Beta-adrenergic antagonists appear to reverse adrenergically mediated intrinsic myocardial dysfunction and remodeling. In adults who have congestive heart failure, beta antagonists improve symptoms, ventricular function, and survival. Some reports suggest that beta antagonists may improve ventricular function in some children who have congestive heart failure, but these agents have not been used extensively in children.

No large, controlled clinical trials have been conducted on the indications, dosages, and optimal use of existing therapy for congestive heart failure in children. The basis for using these agents, therefore, is extrapolation from adults, and they generally are used usually for the palliative relief of symptoms. Treatments directed at prevention or cure of congestive heart failure in children have also not been evaluated.

SIGNS AND SYMPTOMS OF CONGESTIVE HEART FAILURE

Congestive heart failure occurs most often in very young children. In a 6-week-old infant who develops congestive heart failure secondary to a ventricular septal defect (used here as an example), the history often is helpful, as it is in all cases of congestive heart failure.

Feeding

A feeding history helps quantify nutritional intake and allows it to be compared with weight gain. The average 6-week-old child may be expected to take roughly 3 to 4 ounces of formula per feeding and to nutritively suck no longer than 20 minutes per feed. Much lower intake or much longer feeding times may be a basis for concern. Most healthy, full-term, 6-week-old infants gain 10 to 30 g/day and consume more than 90 kcal/kg/day. Children who have congestive heart failure frequently have greater nutritional needs because of increased metabolic demands and often require 150 kcal/kg/day or more to gain adequate weight. Frequently, children who have congestive heart failure are not vigorous in their feeding and may feed only in short, interrupted periods. It is not uncommon to obtain a history that suggests that the child is feeding all day long. However, such a child may have a nutritional intake of only 65 kcal/kg/day or less, and may gain little or no weight. Typically, the longer a child is in congestive heart failure, the more wasting occurs. Weight usually is the initial anthropometric measurement to be affected, followed by height and ultimately head circumference.

Activity Level

Infants who have congestive heart failure usually change their activity level. In some cases they become less active, and in others they become more irritable.

Tachycardia

At this age, a sleeping child is expected to have a resting heart rate less than 160 beats/min. Children who have congestive heart failure may have persistent sinus tachycardia with heart rates higher than 160 beats/min.

Tachypnea

Healthy full-term children at this age typically have sleeping respiratory rates of less than 60 breaths/min. Higher rates frequently are found in children who have congestive heart failure.

Rales

Clinically evident pulmonary distress symptoms are less likely to be found in infants and young children who have congestive heart failure than in older patients. In a young child, rales may suggest active pulmonary disease.

Jugular Venous Distention

Although found in many older patients who have heart failure, jugular venous distention is less likely to be found in infants, largely because it is difficult to observe their jugular veins.

Hepatomegaly

The liver frequently is enlarged in infants and children who have congestive heart failure. Measuring the total liver span by percussion may be more useful than determining how far the liver edge extends below the right costal margin. The left lobe of the liver also is frequently enlarged in infants and young children who have congestive heart failure, and therefore a palpable liver edge that crosses the midline is notable.

S_3 Gallop

An S_3 gallop frequently is observed in children of all ages who have congestive heart failure. However, during the neonatal period, an S_3 gallop may not indicate congestive heart failure. For example, a child with a patent ductus arteriosus with a left-to-right shunt will experience increased left ventricular preload, often resulting in an S_3 gallop.

Pulses and Perfusion

By definition, congestive heart failure is an inability to perfuse the tissues adequately. It therefore is not uncommon to note decreased pulses and perfusion. Palpating the upper and lower extremity pulses simultaneously may reveal differences in intensity or timing of the pulses, indicating a coarctation of the aorta, an interrupted aortic arch, or another lesion interfering with arterial blood flow.

LEADING CAUSES OF CONGESTIVE HEART FAILURE AT DIFFERENT AGES

Prenatal Period

Fetuses can develop congestive heart failure from a variety of causes. Infections such as those caused by parvovirus can lead to congestive heart failure with or without myocarditis. Abnormalities of heart rhythm can lead to congestive heart failure as well. Prolonged supraventricular tachycardia is poorly tolerated by fetuses, and frequently the mother must be treated with antiarrhythmic medications to control the condition in the fetus. The more chronic or severe the congestive heart failure in a fetus, the more likely is hydrops fetalis and ultimately, fetal death.

The First Day of Life

The leading cause of congestive heart failure in the first day of life is persistent fetal circulation or persistent pulmonary hypertension of the newborn. Often, meconium aspiration and neonatal acidosis are present. Newborns who have persistent pulmonary hypertension often have congestive heart failure that may not be clinically apparent. Many of the therapies for these patients are specifically directed to congestive heart failure. When the condition is recognized early, careful use of fluids, inotropes, and oxygen can be beneficial.

Another leading cause of congestive heart failure in the first day of life is neonatal sepsis. Prolonged rupture of membranes, maternal infection, and associated findings are suggestive. In these cases, the congestive heart failure usually is accompanied by the classic signs or symptoms. Treating the sepsis with antibiotics and judicious use of fluids in conjunction with anticongestive therapy often is effective.

Congestive heart failure on the first day of life may have hematological or metabolic causes. Children who have hematocrits that are too high or too low are at risk for heart failure. Polycythemia resulting in sludging and hyperviscosity can lead to congestive heart failure, more commonly in infants of diabetic mothers. A partial exchange transfusion often will lead to a rapid improvement in signs of heart failure.

Severe anemia in the first day of life can also cause congestive heart failure. It is important to determine whether the reduced red blood cell numbers have an acute or a chronic cause. An acute blood loss such as occurs from abruptio placentae can be managed with blood transfusion and by otherwise increasing intravascular fluid volume. On the other hand, a chronic anemia such as that caused by Rh sensitization may also present with a low red blood cell count and a low hematocrit. However, in these cases, the intravascular volume may actually be high, so transfusion may worsen the heart failure. Such patients may benefit from double-volume exchange transfusion.

Metabolic causes of cardiomyopathy in the first day of life include hypoglycemia. The neonatal myocardium uses glucose for energy metabolism by which fat reserves are diminished. A newborn who has low blood sugar and signs or symptoms of congestive heart failure often will improve significantly when blood sugar levels are normalized. Another metabolic cause of congestive heart failure in the first day of life is hypocalcemia. Normalization of calcium, a potent inotrope, may reduce signs or symptoms of congestive heart failure. Hypoglycemia and hypocalcemia often are seen together in infants of diabetic mothers.

Rare congenital heart defects such as absent pulmonary valve syndrome, free tricuspid orifice, or severe anomaly of the tricuspid valve associated with severe pulmonary stenosis may cause congestive heart failure in the first day of life.

Heart rate abnormalities may also lead to congestive heart failure in the first day of life. A newborn can tolerate supraventricular tachycardia of 250 to 300 beats/min for only 12 to 36 hours before developing signs and symptoms of congestive heart failure. Sinus rhythm should be established immediately in symptomatic neonates who have supraventricular tachycardia and congestive heart failure. If vagal maneuvers or intravenous administration of adenosine do not convert the child to normal sinus rhythm, and if a pacemaker is unavailable, then cardioversion should be attempted, followed by pharmacological management. Heart rates that are too slow may also lead to congestive heart failure in a newborn. Heart rates less than 60 beats/min have also resulted in symptomatic congestive heart failure in newborns—for example, those with congenital complete heart block. The heart rate should be raised pharmacologically with a chronotropic agent such as isoproterenol, and ultimately a pacemaker may be indicated. When congenital complete heart block is diagnosed in a child, the mother should be screened for rheumatologic and connective tissue disorders.

Day 1 to 2

Between 1 and 2 days of age, congestive heart failure may develop in an infant who has persistent or progressive tachypnea and hypoxia, whose chest radiographs show a "snowman" or "snowball" pattern with vessels radiating from a small cardiac silhouette. This scenario is typical for a child who has obstructed total anomalous pulmonary venous return. This condition should be identified early because it must be corrected with surgery. Echocardiography can confirm the diagnosis.

Day 2 to 3

The leading cause of congestive heart failure at this point in life is ductus arteriosus dependent lesions. These include (1) right-sided obstructive lesions such as pulmonary atresia, maximal tetralogy of Fallot, or tricuspid atresia; (2) transposition of the great arteries (the most common type of cyanotic heart disease); and (3) left-sided obstructive lesions such as hypoplastic left heart, critical aortic stenosis, or complex coarctation of the aorta. Congestive heart failure is less likely when any of these conditions is accompanied by a patent ductus arteriosus but may develop at 2 to 3 days of age after the ductus arteriosus has closed, especially in cases of left-sided obstructive lesions. If diagnosed in time, these patients can often be stabilized by infusions of prostaglandin E_1, which maintains patency of the ductus arteriosus.

Days 3 to 7

Later in the first week of life, congestive heart failure can follow from endocrine disorders, including congenital adrenal hypoplasia or hyperthyroidism, or renal disorders, including renal vein thrombus, renal artery stenosis, and hypertension or oliguria of any cause.

Week 1 to 2

Between 1 and 2 weeks of age, a leading cause of congestive heart failure is complex coarctation of the aorta. Other similar lesions such as an interrupted aortic arch also may present at this age. These conditions present at 1 to 2 weeks of age when the ductus arteriosus, which was open, closes. The ductus arteriosus usually closes by 3 days of life in children who do not have these conditions. A child who has coarctation of the aorta presenting with congestive heart failure at 1 to 2 weeks of age may have no pulse differential if cardiac output is very low, so any suspected complex coarctation or interrupted aortic arch should be investigated by echocardiography. When diagnosed early, the child can often be stabilized quickly, with anticongestive therapy and prostaglandin E_1.

1 to 2 Months

Left-to-right shunt lesions are most common at 1 to 2 months of age. A typical example is a child who has a ventricular septal defect in whom pulmonary artery resistance has fallen over the first few postnatal weeks, resulting in increased left-to-right shunting. Other examples include atrial level shunts (such as an atrial septal defect), common atria, ventricular-level left-to-right shunts (such as complete atrioventricular canal defects, ventricular septal defects, and single ventricle), and great vessel-level shunts such as patent ductus arteriosus. The timing of presentation often suggests that a left-to-right shunt is present. It is unclear whether congestive failure in this circumstance is easily treated. Inotropes, diuretics, and afterload reduction agents are commonly used alone or in combination in this situation. Hypertransfusion therapy to reduce shunting has been found to be beneficial historically but is not commonly used at this time.

6 to 12 Months

This period is characterized by causes of congestive heart failure that include metabolic and genetic cardiomyopathies and infectious and inflammatory cardiomyopathies.[15] The typical scenario of a child who has a metabolic genetic cardiomyopathy would be an unremarkable first 6 months of life according to the family, and upon contracting a viral illness, the child presents with congestive heart failure. The child also may have growth failure and associated findings such as hypotonia. An example would be a child who has glycogen storage disease. Infectious and inflammatory diseases can cause myocarditis at this age. These include, among others, HIV and enterovirus infections and Kawasaki disease.[3,11]

1 to 18 Years

These years are characterized by congestive heart failure occurring most commonly in children who have severe or chronic illnesses. For example, the child treated for cancer may be at risk for congestive heart failure while[9] being treated with anthracycline chemotherapy[12] or receiving radiation[4] to the cardiovascular system or for many years thereafter. Nevertheless, during childhood, beyond the first year of life, it is unusual to see congestive heart failure. Children who have congenital heart disease, other than those who have had corrective surgery, rarely develop congestive heart failure. In fact, the leading indications for pediatric heart transplantations (indicative of a failure of the medical management of congestive heart failure) are congenital heart disease during the first year of life and cardiomyopathies thereafter.[7]

SUMMARY

Congestive heart failure can occur at any age in infants and children. It is most common in the neonatal period and the first year of life. Although it can be acute and fulminant, most often it is a chronic, smoldering process and is associated with significant morbidity and mortality. It is important that signs and symptoms of congestive heart failure in infants and children be recognized as soon as possible since therapeutic options exist that can reduce morbidity and improve the quality of life. Some may even affect mortality. The causes of congestive heart failure vary with the age of the infant or child. Prenatally, infectious and heart rate abnormalities are most common. In the first day of life, persistent fetal circulation and neonatal sepsis are common as well as metabolic and hematological causes. Day 2 and 3 of life are associated with ductus arteriosus-dependent cardiovascular lesions. One to 2 weeks of age is associated with complex coarctation and other aortic obstructions. One to 2 months of age finds congestive heart failure onset most commonly associated with left-to-right cardiovascular shunts. The second half of the first year of life is most commonly associated with metabolic genetic cardiomyopathy as well as infectious and inflammatory conditions. Later on, the onset of congestive heart failure is most commonly associated with chronic illnesses, including toxic exposures and infectious and inflammatory conditions. The early recognition and effective management of infants and children who have mild congestive heart failure may significantly improve their outcome. The goal should be to strive for early diagnosis and the institution of effective etiology-specific treatment under the direction of a pediatric cardiologist.

REFERENCES

1. Auslender M: Pathophysiology of heart failure, *Prog Pediatr Cardiol* 2000 (in press).
2. Auslender M, Artman M: Overview of the management of heart failure, *Prog Pediatr Cardiol* 2000, (in press).
3. Bowles NE, et al: The detection of viral genomes by polymerase chain reaction in the myocardium of pediatric patients with advanced HIV disease, *J Am Coll Cardiol* 34:857, 1999.
4. Cameron EH, et al: Cardiovascular disease in long-term survivors of pediatric Hodgkin's disease, *Prog Pediatr Cardiol* 8:139, 1998.
5. Giantris A, Lipshultz SE: Cardiac therapeutics in HIV-infected patients. In Lipshultz SE, editor: *Cardiology in AIDS,* New York, 1998, Chapman and Hall.

6. Grenier MA, et al: Angiotensin converting enzyme inhibitor therapy for ventricular dysfunction in infants, children, and adolescents, *Prog Pediatr Cardiol* 2000 (in press).
7. Grenier MA, et al: Design and implementation of a North American pediatric cardiomyopathy registry, *Am Heart J* 139(2 pt 3):S86, 2000.
8. Hougen TJ: Digitalis use in children: an uncertain future, *Progr Pediatr Cardiol* 2000 (in press).
9. Krischer JP, et al: Clinical cardiotoxicity following anthracycline treatment for childhood cancer: the pediatric oncology group experience, *J Clin Oncol* 15:1544, 1997.
10. Latifi S, Lidsky K, Blumer JL: Pharmacology of inotropic agents in infants and children, *Prog Pediatr Cardiol* 2000 (in press).
11. Lipshultz SE, et al, for the Pediatric Pulmonary and Cardiovascular Complications of Vertically Transmitted HIV Infection Study Group: Cardiac structure and function in children infected with human immunodeficiency virus: the prospective P2C2 HIV multicenter study, *Circulation* 97:1246, 1998.
12. Lipshultz SE, et al: Female sex and higher drug dose as risk factors for late cardiotoxic effects of doxorubicin therapy for childhood cancer, *N Engl J Med* 332:1738, 1995.
13. Lipshultz SE, et al: Limitations of fractional shortening as an index of contractility in HIV-infected children, *J Pediatr* 125:563, 1995.
14. Lowrie L: Diuretic therapy of heart failure in infants and children, *Prog Pediatr Cardiol* 2000 (in press).
15. Schwartz ML, et al: Clinical approach to genetic cardiomyopathy in children, *Circulation* 94:2021, 1996.
16. Shaddy RE, et al: Beta-blocker treatment of dilated cardiomyopathy with congestive heart failure in children: a multiinstitutional experience, *J Heart Lung Transplant* 18:269, 1999.
17. Towbin JA, Lipshultz SE: Genetics of neonatal cardiomyopathy, *Curr Opin Cardiol* 14:250, 1999.

SUGGESTED READINGS

Auslender M, Artman M, Lipshultz SE: Therapeutics for pediatric ventricular dysfunction, *Prog Pediatr Cardiol* 2000 (in press).

Auslender M, Lipshultz SE, Artman M: Pathophysiology of pediatric ventricular dysfunction, *Prog Pediatr Cardiol* 2000 (in press).

288 Hypertensive Emergencies

Glenn H. Bock

Acute hypertensive emergencies are relatively infrequent in the pediatric population. However, their full clinical manifestations represent potential life-threatening events demanding prompt identification and carefully implemented therapeutic intervention. The increasing array of potent oral and parenteral antihypertensive agents, as well as the widespread availability of dialysis, has resulted in significant reductions of morbidity and mortality associated with hypertensive crises. The term *malignant hypertension* describes those conditions in which there is significant end-organ injury, most particularly involving the brain, heart, or kidneys. Vascular endothelial damage with resultant microangiopathic hemolysis also may occur. Clinically, among patients who have acute or progressive end-organ dysfunction, it is useful to differentiate between those who have hypertensive emergencies and those who have hypertensive urgencies. Emergencies refer to those conditions that are life threatening or in which there is an imminent risk of serious long-term morbidity. Those conditions occurring most frequently in children include acute heart failure with or without pulmonary edema, symptoms of hypertensive encephalopathy, and acute intracranial or retinal hemorrhages. Hypertensive urgencies include otherwise uncomplicated malignant hypertension, acute renal failure, postoperative hypertension, and compensated states of left ventricular dysfunction. Emergent conditions mandate immediate reduction of blood pressure; in urgent conditions, less aggressive blood pressure reduction is necessary. Because acute blood pressure reduction may, itself, result in end-organ ischemia or infarction, aggressive, immediate treatment should be reserved for those in whom the risks of less aggressive treatment are considerable.

ETIOLOGY

In most reports, malignant hypertension in children and adolescents almost always is the result of an identifiable secondary cause rather than of an acute exacerbation of primary (essential) hypertension. The probability of secondary hypertension in the pediatric population increases with younger age and the magnitude of the blood pressure elevation. Box 288-1 lists some of the more common secondary causes that may be associated with acute hypertension in pediatric-age patients. Although the list is not all-inclusive, renal parenchymal diseases, renovascular abnormalities, and coarctation of the aorta account for more than 90% of the cases. Initial consideration of these three conditions allows the practitioner to focus on the hypertensive workup, thereby limiting unnecessary invasive and often time-consuming tests. For the majority of the remaining diagnoses, the history and physical findings frequently point to a specific condition. Box 288-1 lists some useful initial screening information that can be obtained rapidly during the initial assessment of the acutely hypertensive patient. The more uncommon causes of acute hypertension should be sought only if the initial history and physical examination strongly suggest their presence or after the three most common causes have been ruled out.

HISTORY AND PHYSICAL EXAMINATION FINDINGS

As part of the initial physical assessment, all pediatric patients evaluated for hypertension must have their blood pressure measured in both upper extremities and in at least one lower extremity.

The magnitude of blood pressure elevation at which malignant hypertension becomes clinically manifest varies considerably. This is the result of both the rapidity of the rise of blood pressure as well as the actual level that occurs. Also, the presence of chronic underlying hypertension offers some protection against the development of a hypertensive emergency. Regardless, the clinical manifestations of malignant hypertension usually result from some combination of neurological, cardiovascular, or visual system perturbations. The neurological abnormalities result from failure of arteriolar blood pressure autoregulation in the brain with consequent hypertensive encephalopathy. Signs and symptoms of hypertensive encephalopathy include headache, anxiety, restlessness, dizziness, blurred vision, diplopia, nausea, and vomiting. Later, mental confusion, changing levels of consciousness, cranial nerve palsies, and convulsions can occur. Hypertension should be considered in any patient who has unexplained convulsions. Papilledema and vascular changes in the ocular fundus are much less common in hypertensive children than in adults.

Congestive heart failure can be the predominant manifestation in some patients, particularly neonates and children who have underlying heart disease. Cardiac dysfunction is the result of a number of factors, including increased peripheral vascular resistance and reduced left ventricular function. Underlying chronic hypertension may contribute to ventricular dysfunction as the result of chronic myocardial hypertrophy. Consideration of the diagnosis of acute hypertension is particularly difficult in neonates and infants in whom the clinical signs tend to be vague and nonspecific. In these groups, severe hypertension may manifest only as irritability, poor feeding, poor sleeping, restlessness, or vomiting. The

BOX 288-1

SCREENING ELEMENTS OF THE HISTORY AND PHYSICAL EXAMINATION IN THE ASSESSMENT OF SEVERE HYPERTENSION IN CHILDREN

Present or Past Medical History of:	**Suggests**
• Headache, visual disturbance, irritability, abdominal pain (in young child)	Malignant or accelerated hypertension
• Drug use	Drug-induced hypertension
• Umbilical artery catheter	Renovascular hypertension
• Sore throat	Glomerulonephritis
• Recurrent cough, shortness of breath	Preexisting congestive heart failure, pulmonary edema
• Weight loss or gain	Hyperthyroidism, pheochromocytoma, Cushing's syndrome, congestive heart failure, renal failure, nephrosis
• Palpitations, flushing, diarrhea	Hyperthyroidism, pheochromocytoma
• Bloody diarrhea	Hemolytic-uremic syndrome
• Purpuric-petechial rash	Vasculitis syndrome
Physical Findings of	
• Thin general appearance	Hyperthyroidism, pheochromocytoma
• Obese general appearance (truncal)	Cushing's syndrome
• Blood pressure normal or much lower in lower extremity than upper extremity	Aortic coarctation
• Edema	Congestive heart failure, renal failure, nephrosis
• Skin	
Ash-leaf spots	Tuberous sclerosis
Café-au-lait spots	Neurofibromatosis
Rash	Vasculitis
Pyoderma	Glomerulonephritis
• HEENT	
Rounded (moon) facies	Cushing's syndrome
Proptosis, goiter	Hyperthyroidism
Papilledema	Intracranial mass or hemorrhage
• Heart	
Cardiomegaly	Congestive heart failure or long-standing hypertension
Murmur	Aortic coarctation
• Abdomen	
Mass involving flank(s)	Tumor (Wilms' neuroblastoma) obstructive uropathy, polycystic kidney disease
Bruit	Renal artery stenosis
• Ambiguous genitalia	Virilizing adrenal hyperplasia

diagnosis in these age groups is complicated further by the technical difficulties inherent in accurate blood pressure measurement. A greater awareness by the practitioner is necessary to prevent overlooking this diagnostic possibility. Other clinical findings attributable to possible underlying diagnoses are listed in Box 288-1.

LABORATORY FINDINGS

As mentioned previously, hypertensive emergencies mandate immediate treatment, although some basic laboratory studies can be readily obtained for later interpretation. The initial laboratory tests should include a urinalysis (including a carefully performed microscopic examination of the centrifuged urinary sediment) and measurements of blood urea nitrogen, serum creatinine, and plasma renin and aldosterone. In patients in whom pheochromocytoma is suspected, a plasma or urine catecholamine quantitation or both should be done. If an acquired glomerulonephritis is suspected, serum complement and streptococcal antibody titers should be obtained. Adolescents who have acute hypertension should have urine tests for illicit drug use. Performing thyroid, adrenal, or other endocrine tests is unnecessary unless the patient has multisystem complaints to suggest such diagnoses.

Radiographic imaging studies are useful in the assessment of possible renal causes of acute hypertension. Renal radionuclide scans (MAG-3 or DTPA) and ultrasound allow noninvasive assessment of kidney number, size, location, relative blood flow, and function. High-quality nuclear and sonographic pediatric studies usually are readily available at most tertiary medical institutions. The kidneys of patients who have acute forms of glomerulonephritis may be swollen and frequently have abnormal echogenicity. In renal artery stenosis the involved kidney often is smaller and has a delay in the blood flow and excretory phases compared with the uninvolved kidney. Obtaining a second radionuclide renal scan after a brief course of an angiotensin II-converting enzyme inhibitor often increases the sensitivity of the study for detecting renal artery stenosis. In this circumstance, the scan done after the converting enzyme inhibitor is administered

Table 288-1 Antihypertensive Drugs for Parenteral or Sublingual Administration in Hypertensive Emergencies in Pediatric Patients

Drug	Route	Dosage	Onset	Peak
Sodium nitroprusside*	IV infusion	0.5 μg/kg/min titrated to a maximum of 10 μg/kg/min	Within 30 sec	—
Diazoxide*	IV bolus injection	1-3 mg/kg repeated q5-15 min until BP controlled (minibolus)	1-5 min	1-5 min
Hydralazine	30 min IV infusion or IM	0.15-0.2 mg/kg q6hr	10-20 min	10-90 min
Nifedipine	Sublingual	0.25 mg/kg/dose q4-6hr	10-15 min	60-90 min
Labetalol*	IV infusion	0.5 mg/kg over 2 min. For nonresponse, double dose and repeat q 10 min to a maximum cumulative dose of 5 mg/kg	2-5 min	5-15 min
Phentolamine	IV bolus injection	0.05-0.1 mg/kg	Within 30 sec	2 min

*Manufacturer's warning: safety in children not established.
†Vasodilation symptoms include sweating, flushing, feelings of warmth, orthostatic hypotension, tachycardia, palpitations, nausea, and vomiting.
‡Neurological symptoms include headache, blurred vision, dizziness, and light-headedness.
sx, Symptoms; *BP,* blood pressure; *D/C,* discontinue.

often shows poorer function on the involved side compared with the function of the same kidney scan done before the converting enzyme inhibitor is administered. When these screening tests are abnormal or if the plasma renin value is elevated significantly in the absence of dehydration, obvious renal parenchymal disease, or any medication that could raise renin directly, a renal angiogram and renal vein renin measurement should be performed. As mentioned in Chapter 240, Obstructive Uropathy and Vesicoureteral Reflux, imaging studies are important in differentiating the various obstructive conditions of the kidney, many of which can produce hypertension. They also are important in the investigation of renal tumors. Physical findings that suggest a coarctation of the aorta should be evaluated by echocardiography, cardiac catheterization, or both.

TREATMENT

Immediate control of blood pressure in a child who has accelerated or malignant hypertension should take precedence over determination of the precise cause. Complicated diagnostic tests, which often require transportation to various departments in the hospital, should be delayed until the practitioner believes that the blood pressure is controlled. Intravenous access should be established immediately in these patients. In hypertensive emergencies in which the airway is compromised or there are seizures, conventional treatment approaches usually are adequate initial measures. It must be reemphasized that in the context of hypertensive emergencies or urgencies, blood pressure control should not be equated to blood pressure normalization. A child who has had chronically elevated blood pressure with uncomplicated malignant hypertension may experience further end-organ injury with excessive blood pressure reduction. In contrast, the child who has a true acute blood pressure elevation would be expected to have little risk from rapid blood pressure normalization. Often in an emergency, however, whether the blood pressure elevation is acute or more chronic is unclear. Therefore, the rapid reduction of blood pressure to normal levels generally should be avoided until a better understanding of the patient's overall condition can be achieved. It generally is considered that, initially, a 15% to 25% reduction of blood pressure ameliorates the symptoms and is well tolerated regardless of the underlying condition. Despite the admonition about diagnostic testing interfering with acute therapeutic intervention, some etiological possibilities should be considered because certain medications should be avoided in certain conditions (such as beta-adrenergic blockade in a patient who has possible pheochromocytoma). Also, several basic drug properties should be considered when selecting an initial antihypertensive agent. Drugs such as diazoxide, hydralazine, minoxidil, and calcium channel blockers (e.g., nifedipine) cause reflex sympathetic activity, thereby potentially augmenting myocardial or cerebral ischemia. Sodium nitroprusside must be used with caution in patients who have abnormal renal function or if used for prolonged periods in high doses. In these settings, serum thiocyanate and cyanide levels must be monitored.

Duration	Adverse Effects	Relative Contraindications	Comments
Length of infusion	Nausea, vomiting; vasodilation sx†; neurological sx‡; apprehension, restlessness	Hepatic insufficiency	Solution good for 24 hr; photosensitive (wrap in foil); monitor blood thiocyanate if used longer than 72 hr (D/C for thiocyanate level greater than 10 mg/dl); tachyphylaxis and metabolic acidosis—early cyanide poisoning
Variable; usually <12 hr	Arrhythmias; hyperglycemia; sodium and water retention; vasodilation sx†; neurological sx‡	Thiazide sensitivity; severe tachycardia; diabetes; coarctation	Ineffective in pheochromocytoma; give diuretics to decrease sodium; may displace highly protein-bound substances
3-6 hr	Headache; nausea, vomiting; tachycardia, palpitation	Hypersensitivity to hydralazine ("hyperdynamic syndrome")	Undergoes color change in most infusion fluids, which does not indicate loss of potency
Variable; usually 2-3 hr	Headache; palpitations; flushing	Concomitant use of beta-blocking drugs; cimetidine	Dose can be drawn from the 10-mg capsule via a 1-ml syringe and then squirted sublingually
Variable; usually 2-4 hr	Neurological sx‡; bronchospasm; tingling scalp	Jaundice or hepatic dysfunction; pheochromocytoma; asthma; diabetes	Keep supine for 3 hr after administration; ambulate gradually
15-30 min	Tachycardia; arrhythmias; marked hypotension	None	Specific for pheochromocytoma

In hypertensive emergencies the initial use of parenteral, rapidly acting agents allows blood pressure control to be achieved quickly and predictably. This process requires establishing the means to measure the blood pressure response closely on a continuous basis. Often, this initially requires intra-arterial blood pressure monitoring. Sodium nitroprusside is the drug of choice in most hypertensive emergencies; intermittent or continuous infusion of labetalol also is effective in most settings. For hypertensive urgencies, less aggressive means such as oral medications (if tolerated) may be used to achieve the targeted level of blood pressure control over the course of several hours. Some of the more effective medications for acute blood pressure control are given in Table 288-1. Oral medications should be substituted for parenteral agents as soon as practical. With the determination of cause, the medication that is most specific for the altered pathophysiological condition producing hypertension is preferred. In renovascular hypertension, revision or bypass of the renovascular lesion is preferred to long-term medical therapy or nephrectomy. Consultation with a pediatric nephrologist, cardiologist, or vascular surgeon is important in defining a therapeutic plan to serve best the patient's long-term interests.

PROGNOSIS

The immediate prognosis of the child who has symptoms resulting from a hypertensive emergency depends on the rapidity of recognition of the problem and, thereafter, achievement of appropriate blood pressure reduction. Although the initial neurological and visual disturbances may improve or resolve with time, risks remain for residual abnormalities such as seizure disorders, cranial nerve palsies, hemiplegia, and blindness. Renal function often deteriorates acutely in patients who have chronic renal diseases following a hypertensive emergency or urgency. With sustained blood pressure control, renal function may improve over a period of weeks or longer. The long-term prognosis also depends, to some extent, on the underlying cause as well as the success in managing the malignant hypertension. Some causes, such as acute poststreptococcal glomerulonephritis, may resolve spontaneously. Others, such as isolated vascular abnormalities, are amenable to correction. In other settings, such as hypertension associated with chronic glomerulonephritis, the condition may be controlled by continued antihypertensive therapy, although periodic medication noncompliance is a continual threat. Regardless, the longevity of the patient and the subsequent development of end-organ damage (e.g., hypertensive cardiomyopathy and stroke) are directly related to the adequacy of long-term blood pressure control.

When to Refer

- Consultation with a pediatric nephrologist for diagnostic evaluation of hypertension etiology, or for short- and long-term management recommendations
- Consultation with a pediatric cardiologist or pediatric neurologist if assessment of end-organ cardiac or CNS injury is suspected or if there is a question of the relationship between end-organ dysfunction and hypertension

When to Hospitalize

For treatment of all hypertensive emergencies and most cases of hypertensive urgencies

SUGGESTED READINGS

Dillon MJ: Investigation and management of hypertension in children, *Pediatr Nephrol* 1:59, 1987.

Guignard JP, et al: Arterial hypertension in the newborn infant, *Biol Neonate* 55:77, 1989.

Kitiyakara C, et al: Malignant hypertension and hypertensive emergencies, *J Am Soc Nephrol* 9:133, 1998.

Wright RR, et al: Hypertensive encephalopathy in childhood, *J Child Neurol* 11:193, 1996.

289 Hypoglycemia

Craig C. Orlowski

Diagnosing hypoglycemia promptly is essential because low blood glucose levels that persist or recur may have catastrophic effects on the brain, particularly in infants. Accordingly, the primary care physician must recognize the clinical symptoms associated with hypoglycemia, document the low blood glucose level, and treat appropriately with glucose. Delineating the cause of the hypoglycemia is necessary so that effective continuing treatment can be initiated.

DEFINITION

A child who has a serum or plasma glucose concentration less than 40 mg/dl or a whole blood glucose concentration less than 35 mg/dl should be investigated and treated for hypoglycemia[13]; those who have plasma glucose concentrations between 40 and 50 mg/dl should be followed up on carefully.[13] If hypoglycemia is suspected, the blood glucose level may be approximated quickly at the bedside using a visual test strip or glucometer and later confirmed by an appropriate chemical laboratory test. Although these thresholds have been commonly quoted and used, the level of plasma glucose that is safe is uncertain and some advocate a therapeutic goal of maintaining a plasma glucose level above 60 mg/dl in both neonates and older children to prevent permanent brain damage.[28]

CLINICAL MANIFESTATIONS

The clinical findings in hypoglycemia are those caused mainly by cerebral dysfunction and adrenergic discharge. Incoordination of eye movements, strabismus, excessive irritability, motor incoordination, and convulsions may occur after 1 month of age. In the older child, pallor, tachycardia, sweating, limpness, inattention, staring, listlessness, hunger, abdominal pain, ataxia, stupor, coma, and convulsions are frequent findings. It should be noted that episodes of hypoglycemia may be present at any age without obvious clinical manifestations.

IMMEDIATE MANAGEMENT

At the time hypoglycemia is suspected in a child, a diagnostic blood sample for glucose, insulin, growth hormone (GH), cortisol, ketone bodies, lactic acid, and amino acids must be obtained, generally before the low blood glucose has been corrected.[1,6] These measurements provide important information concerning cause. Unnecessary blood sampling can be minimized by using a bedside glucometer to decide if the patient is truly hypoglycemic during a symptomatic episode. If available blood volume is a limiting factor, judgment must be used in ranking the importance of these tests with measurement of the blood glucose and insulin levels receiving priority. Urinary ketones, as well as specific tests for urinary glucose and nonglucose-reducing substances, should also be determined. If ketones are present, the urine should be tested further for presence of amino acids and organic acids. For diagnostic purposes, the administration of glucagon can be useful; a robust glycemic response to glucagon strongly suggests hyperinsulinism.[6]

Once these essential diagnostic blood samples are obtained, the child should immediately receive an intravenously administered bolus of 2 to 4 ml/kg body weight of 10% to 25% glucose to alleviate acute symptoms. Intravenous fluids containing appropriate electrolytes and glucose should then be given at a rate sufficient to maintain plasma or serum glucose levels above 50 to 60 mg/dl. A common mistake is to consider the hypoglycemia resolved after the initial bolus and fail to follow up with sufficiently frequent blood glucose monitoring to determine the adequacy of the continuous glucose infusion. The blood glucose level should be monitored initially every 30 to 60 minutes at the bedside until stable then every 2 to 4 hours, and the rate of glucose administered should be adjusted accordingly. Overcorrection with subsequent hyperglycemia may complicate fluid management by causing an osmotic diuresis.

Significant hypoglycemia should be evaluated as an inpatient to allow for close monitoring. During transport to the hospital, personnel experienced in intravenous techniques and rapid bedside blood glucose determinations must ensure that adequate amounts of glucose are infused continuously. The previously obtained diagnostic blood samples should be sent with the patient to the hospital, preferably on ice. The patient who has hypoglycemia should be under the combined care of a pediatric specialist and the child's primary physician.

ETIOLOGY

The blood glucose level is the final balance between the sum of hepatic glucose production and dietary intake minus peripheral glucose use. An adequate fasting blood glucose concentration depends on sufficient amounts of endogenous nonglucose precursors (e.g., alanine, lactate, and glycerol), effective hepatic enzyme pathways for gluconeogenesis and glycogenolysis, and normal hormonal activities (insulin, GH, cortisol, glucagon, and epinephrine) for the mobilization of substrates and the regulation of these processes.

Many healthy infants and young children, in contrast to adults, cannot maintain normoglycemia during a 24-hour fast.[4] The glycogen stores of healthy infants are sufficient only to meet glucose requirements for 8 to 12 hours in the absence of caloric intake,[24] so after 24 to 36 hours of fasting the young child depends totally on gluconeogenesis for glucose production.[19] Because of relatively lower protein and fat stores, fasted infants and young children may not be able to supply sufficient substrates for adequate glucose production. Hence, the physician caring for a child requiring surgery or other procedures accompanied by fasting must prevent hypoglycemia by ensuring that extended fasting is avoided, by administering parenteral glucose before and after surgery, and by monitoring the patient's blood glucose level.

CLINICAL APPROACH

Hypoglycemia reflects the failure of one or more factors that regulate the concentration of glucose in the blood. These may be classified as in Box 289-1. Clinical clues enable the physician to plan a logical approach to the diagnostic evaluation of a patient who has hypoglycemia. The age at onset of hypoglycemia is important. The inborn errors of carbohydrate, amino acid, organic acid metabolism, and hormonal deficiencies become apparent during the first 2 years of life.[7] Hyperinsulinism has two peak times of onset: during the first year

BOX 289-1

CAUSES OF HYPOGLYCEMIA IN CHILDHOOD

Hyperinsulinism
Islet cell dysplasia (functional beta-cell secretory disorder)
Islet cell adenoma
Adenomatosis
Beckwith-Wiedemann syndrome

Hereditary Defects in Carbohydrate Metabolism
Glycogen storage diseases
Glucose-6-phosphatase deficiency, types Ia, Ib
Amylo-1,6-glucosidase deficiency, type III
Defects of liver phosphorylase enzyme system

Enzyme Deficiencies of Gluconeogenesis
Fructose-1,6-diphosphatase (FDPase)
Phosphoenolpyruvate carboxykinase
Pyruvate carboxylase

Other Enzyme Defects
Galactose-1-phosphate uridyltransferase (galactosemia)
Fructose-1-phosphate aldolase (hereditary fructose intolerance)
Glycogen synthetase

Hereditary Defects in Amino Acid and Organic Acid Metabolism
Maple syrup urine disease
Propionic acidemia
Methylmalonic aciduria
Tyrosinosis
3-Hydroxy-3-methylglutaric aciduria
Glutaric aciduria, type II

Hereditary Defects in Fat Metabolism
Systemic carnitine deficiency
Carnitine palmitoyl transferase deficiency
Long- and medium-chain acyl-CoA dehydrogenase deficiencies

Hormone Deficiencies
Congenital hypopituitarism or hypothalamic abnormality
Growth hormone
Cortisol
Adrenocorticotropic hormone (ACTH)
ACTH unresponsiveness
Glucagon
Thyroid hormone
Catecholamine

Ketotic Hypoglycemia

Nonpancreatic Tumors
Mesenchymal tumors
Epithelial tumors
Hepatoma
Adrenocortical carcinoma
Wilms' tumor
Neuroblastoma

Poisoning or Toxins
Salicylate
Alcohol
Propranolol
Oral hypoglycemic agents (e.g., sulfonylureas)
Insulin
Unripe ackees (hypoglycin) (Jamaican vomiting sickness)
Pentamidine

Liver Disease
Hepatitis, cirrhosis
Reye's syndrome

Other Causes
Malnutrition
Malabsorption
Chronic diarrhea
Cyanotic congenital heart disease
Postsurgery

Data from Cornblath MD, Schwartz R: *Disorders of carbohydrate metabolism in infancy,* ed 2, Philadelphia, 1976, WB Saunders. From Kogut MD: Hypoglycemia: pathogenesis, diagnosis, and treatment. In Gluck L, et al, editors: *Current problems in pediatrics,* Chicago, 1974, Mosby; and Kogut MD: Neonatal hypoglycemia: a new look. In Moss AJ, editor: *Pediatrics update: review for physicians,* New York, 1980, Elsevier.

of life and after age 3 years.[7,15] Ketotic hypoglycemia is the most likely cause of hypoglycemia with onset after 1 year of age.[7] In toddlers, hypoglycemia may result from ingestion of alcohol, aspirin, and other drugs (see Box 289-1). Hypoglycemia is rare after age 5 years.[6]

A history of other affected family members or the occurrence of unexplained infant deaths among close relatives suggests the possibility of one of the inherited metabolic disorders. Some disorders associated with hormonal deficiencies[18] and hyperinsulinism[29] also may be familial. The physician should inquire carefully about the frequency of hypoglycemic episodes, the possibility of drug ingestion, and the malicious administration of drugs.[1,6] The temporal relation of symptoms to food intake is important in assessing hypoglycemia. In hereditary defects of amino acid and organic acid metabolism, hypoglycemic symptoms may occur shortly after the ingestion of protein.[15] Symptoms that occur after the ingestion of lactose suggest galactosemia; those that occur after sucrose ingestion suggest hereditary fructose intolerance (HFI).[15] In contrast, fasting hypoglycemia is characteristic of ketotic hypoglycemia, hormonal deficiencies, hyperinsulinism, glycogen storage diseases (GSD), and fructose-1,6-diphosphatase (FDPase) deficiency[17] (Table 289-1).

Metabolic acidosis, ketonemia, or hepatomegaly in association with hypoglycemia strongly suggests the presence of an inborn error of metabolism of carbohydrate, amino acid, or organic acid[15] (see Chapter 20 [Three], Recognition of Genetic-Metabolic Diseases by Clinical Diagnosis and Screening). Hypotonia and hyperammonemia may also be present in infants who have defects in organic acid and amino acid metabolism. The presence of nonglucose-reducing substances in the urine may indicate galactosemia or HFI. Nonketotic hypoglycemia in patients who have hepatomegaly, with or without metabolic acidosis, suggests 3-hydroxy-3-methylglutaric aciduria,[23] glutaric aciduria type II,[9] systemic carnitine deficiency,[30] carnitine palmityl transferase deficiency,[2] or long- and medium-chain acyl-CoA dehydrogenase (MCAD) deficiencies.[13] In contrast, hepatomegaly, ketonuria, and metabolic acidosis are usually absent in patients with hypoglycemia accompanied by hyperinsulinism.[16] The findings of ketonuria and hypoglycemia without hepatomegaly among small and underweight males older than 1 year of age suggest ketotic hypoglycemia,[7,15] although ketosis may be present in some hypoglycemic patients who have hypopituitarism[20] and adrenocorticotropic hormone (ACTH) unresponsiveness.[14]

Because children who have an inborn error of metabolism may manifest a Reye's syndrome–like illness, the physician must be alert to the possibility of an underlying metabolic defect, particularly in young children or in a child who has a recurrence of Reye's syndrome–like symptoms.[11,13]

DIFFERENTIAL DIAGNOSIS AND MANAGEMENT OF HYPOGLYCEMIA

Hyperinsulinism

Hyperinsulinism may be caused by any of several abnormalities of the beta cell (see Box 289-1) and is the most common cause of persistent or recurrent hypoglycemia in the first year of life.[27] In Beckwith-Wiedemann syndrome (omphalocele,

Table 289-1 Hypoglycemia in Infancy and Childhood

	Inborn Metabolic Errors of Carbohydrate and Amino Acids	Hormone Deficiency	Hyperinsulinism
Family history	+	Variable	Variable
Hypoglycemia			
Fasting	GSD, fructose-1,6-diphosphatase deficiency	+	+
After lactose	Galactosemia	–	–
After sucrose	Hereditary fructose intolerance	–	–
After protein	Amino acids, organic acids	–	Variable
Hepatomegaly	+	Variable	–
Ketosis	+	Variable	–
Acidosis	+	–	–
Tests	Glucose, glucagon, galactose, fructose tolerance tests; amino acids, gas chromatography	Blood growth hormone, cortisol; stimulation tests	Random blood glucose and immunoreactive insulin; leucine tolerance test
Liver biopsy (enzymes)	Diagnostic for carbohydrate errors (not for galactosemia; use red blood cells)	Not indicated	Not indicated
White blood cells, fibroblasts (enzymes)	Amino acids, organic acids		
Treatment	Specific	Specific	Diazoxide; somatostatin analog; partial excision of the pancreas

Data from Cornblath MD, Schwartz R: *Disorders of carbohydrate metabolism in infancy,* ed 2, Philadelphia, 1976, WB Saunders. From Kogut MD: Hypoglycemia: pathogenesis, diagnosis and treatment. In Gluck L, et al, editors: *Current problems in pediatrics,* Chicago, 1974, Mosby; and Kogut MD: Neonatal hypoglycemia: a new look. In Moss AJ, editor: *Pediatrics update: review for physicians,* New York, 1980, Elsevier.

+, Present; –, absent; *GSD,* glycogen storage diseases, types I, III, and defects of liver phosphorylase enzyme system.

macroglossia, and gigantism), hypoglycemia occurs in many of the affected infants and resolves at several months of age.[25] Some of these infants also have hemihypertrophy. An increased incidence of adrenal, liver, and kidney (Wilms') tumors occurs in these patients. More commonly, hyperinsulinism is transient and associated with infants of diabetic mothers.[28]

Most children who have hypoglycemia caused by persistent hyperinsulinism (previously called *nesidioblastosis, islet cell dysplasia*,[13] or, more recently, *congenital hyperinsulinism*,[29]) have symptoms beginning during the first year of life. The understanding of the genetic basis of this condition has advanced enormously in the last several years. Pancreatic β-cell insulin secretion is regulated through a multistep signaling pathway. Glucose, amino acids, and other fuels are metabolized in the β-cells raising the ATP : ADP ratio. This in turn activates a plasma protein, the sulfonylurea receptor (SUR), to close a potassium channel (K_{ATP}), depolarizing the membrane and leading to an influx of calcium and release of insulin. The rate-limiting step in glucose metabolism is the enzyme glucokinase. The most severe form of congenital hyperinsulinism has been found to be caused by a recessive mutation in the potassium channel. Other forms of congenital hyperinsulinism are caused by mutations in the SUR, potassium pore, glucokinase, and other steps of the signaling path. Congenital hyperinsulinism appears to occur associated with either focal or diffuse abnormalities of the β-cells.

Pancreatic islet cell adenomas are uncommon in children. Although hypoglycemia caused by varying histological types of insulinoma may have its onset in the newborn period, symptoms begin after age 4 years in 85% of patients.[7]

Laboratory investigation. Hyperinsulinism in infants and older children usually is characterized by fasting hypoglycemia, even if of only a few hours' duration,[26] and low fasting plasma levels of beta-hydroxybutyrate (β-OHB) and free fatty acids (FFAs).[26] Frequent random simultaneous measurements of blood glucose and insulin levels, particularly before feeding and as hypoglycemia occurs, help identify patients who have hyperinsulinism (see Table 289-1). The diagnosis depends on detecting inappropriate insulin secretion by demonstrating insulin levels disproportionately high relative to blood glucose values, particularly during hypoglycemia. A high rate of glucose infusion (greater than 12 mg/kg/min) is often necessary to maintain euglycemia. Leucine or tolbutamide challenges are not helpful in delineating the specific cause of hyperinsulinism.[15,27]

In any child who has intermittent attacks of nonketotic hypoglycemia, the physician should always investigate the possibility of malicious or self-administration of insulin or oral sulfonylurea drugs.[8,18,22] Measurement of C-peptide, insulin, and insulin antibodies in blood may identify the patient who has an exogenous source of insulin. In contrast to patients who have endogenous hyperinsulinism, C-peptide levels are suppressed; insulin antibodies may be present in patients to whom insulin has been administered.[18,22] In children who have received oral hypoglycemic agents, plasma insulin and C-peptide levels may be misleading; however, the drug may be detected in the child's blood or urine.[22]

Management. Acute hypoglycemic episodes must be treated promptly and adequately with intravenously administered glucose. The rate of glucose administration required to maintain normal blood glucose levels among hyperinsulinemic infants often can exceed 12 to 14 mg/kg/min.

Further management of the patient depends on the age at onset of disease. An infant's response to diazoxide is of great diagnostic and therapeutic value. Diazoxide raises blood glucose levels primarily by suppressing pancreatic insulin secretion.[21] In patients in whom diazoxide results in restoration of normal glucose levels, the drug is continued and the patients are assessed periodically until approximately 5 to 7 years of age. Some patients remain euglycemic without medication by this age.[21] The knowledge that many of these patients harbor genetic defects supports the concept that although clinical improvement may occur with increasing age, abnormalities of glucose regulation remain. Because hyperglycemia, ketosis, and hyperosmolar nonketotic coma can occur with diazoxide therapy, the parents should be instructed to monitor urinary glucose and ketones.[15]

Diazoxide acts by inhibiting the β-cell SUR. Although it is effective in many children, hyperinsulinism caused by SUR mutations may not respond to this drug. If hypoglycemia associated with hyperinsulinism persists or recurs despite diazoxide therapy, octreotide, a long-acting analog of somatostatin, may be used. Tachyphylaxis has prevented its long-term use in all but a small number of severely effected children.[25]

Surgery is needed if medical therapy fails. Although the traditional recommendation has favored controlling hyperinsulinism with removal of 95% of the pancreas, resulting in a significant risk of subsequent diabetes, new insights may change this approach. Preoperative catheterization and intraoperative histological studies may allow partial pancreatectomy in about 40% of infants with focal abnormalities, thus reducing the postoperative incidence of diabetes.[17]

Inborn Errors of Metabolism

Carbohydrate enzyme defects. Several enzymatic defects of carbohydrate metabolism result in deficiencies of hepatic glucose formation and release.[15] Glucose-6-phosphatase deficiency is the most common deficiency, and the symptoms are more severe than in other GSD types (see Box 289-1).[15] Patients who have GSD types Ia and Ib have growth retardation, cherubic facies, a protuberant abdomen, a large smooth liver, enlarged kidneys, normal intelligence, fasting hypoglycemia of only a few hours' duration, ketosis, lacticacidemia, hyperlipidemia, hyperuricemia, and bleeding diathesis. In type Ib the patients also have neutropenia and an increased frequency of infections. Among infants and young children, poor food intake during an illness may result in severe lactic acidosis and hypoglycemia. Death may result if hypoglycemia and hyperlacticacidemia are not treated adequately and promptly with intravenous glucose and sodium bicarbonate.[15] A dramatic advance in treatment has been the introduction of continuous nocturnal glucose-containing gastric feedings.[12] To maintain normal blood glucose levels during the day, frequent feedings, at least every 3 to 4 hours, are essential. Foods rich in fructose and galactose should be avoided. The daily oral administration of an uncooked cornstarch suspension has been beneficial in older children but not as effective in infants in maintaining normoglycemia and attaining adequate metabolic control.[5]

Table 289-2 Differential Diagnosis of Hepatic Enzyme Defects

Blood Values	GSD—I	GSD—III	GSD, Phosphorylase Enzyme System	FDPase	HFI
Fasting					
Glucose	↓	↓ or nl	↓ or nl	↓	nl
Lactic acid	↑	nl	nl	↑	nl
After glucose*					
Glucose	↑	↑	↑	↑	↑
Lactic acid	↓	↑	↑	↓	↔
After glucagon*					
Glucose	↔	↑†	↑ or ↔	↑ or ↔‡	↑§
Lactic acid	↑	↔	↔	↓ or ↑	↔
After galactose*					
Glucose	↔	↑	↑	↑	↑
Lactic acid	↑	↑	↑	↔	↔
After fructose*					
Glucose	↔	↑	↑	↓	↓
Lactic acid	↑	↑	↑	↑	↑

*Tolerance tests done after variable fasting period.
†Two hours after feeding.
‡Variable, dependent on duration of fast.
§No increase in glucose at time of fructose-induced hypoglycemia.
GSD, Glycogen storage diseases; *FDPase,* fructose-1,6-diphosphatase; *HFI,* hereditary fructose intolerance; ↑, increased; ↓, decreased; ↔, no change; *nl,* normal.

Galactosemia in a lactose-fed infant is characterized by failure to thrive, jaundice, vomiting, susceptibility to infection, hepatomegaly, edema, ascites, a tendency to bleed, cataracts, proteinuria, aminoaciduria, and galactosuria.[15] Mental retardation, progressive liver failure, and death may occur unless galactose-containing feedings are eliminated. Symptomatic hypoglycemia is not a common finding and is reversed quickly by intravenous glucose. When the diagnosis of galactosemia is suspected, the patient should be given a galactose-free diet immediately. This diet should be maintained carefully while the physician awaits the results of erythrocyte enzyme studies and should be continued if the diagnosis is confirmed. Clinical manifestations of HFI develop only after fructose ingestion and include vomiting, profound hypoglycemia, and convulsions.[15] Continued ingestion of fructose is associated with failure to thrive, prolonged vomiting, jaundice, hepatosplenomegaly, hemorrhage, abnormal liver function, fructosuria, defects in proximal renal tubular function (including proteinuria, glucosuria, and aminoaciduria), and, in some, hepatic failure and death. The acute episodes of hypoglycemia are reversed promptly by the intravenous administration of glucose. Long-term treatment consists of strict elimination of dietary fructose and of fructose in cough syrups and other drugs.

Patients who have FDPase deficiency may have episodic hyperventilation, fasting hypoglycemia, lactic acidosis, ketosis, hyperuricemia, and hepatomegaly.[15] Refusal to eat and vomiting, often associated with febrile illness, precipitates the attacks. The disorder is life threatening in the neonate and in young children. In contrast to those who have HFI, these patients do not vomit after fructose intake and do not develop an aversion to sweets. Treatment of the acute attack consists of correcting the hypoglycemia and acidosis by intravenous infusion of glucose and sodium bicarbonate. Long-term management should emphasize the avoidance of fasting and the provision of a fructose-free, high-carbohydrate diet.

Laboratory investigation. A suggested outline for the investigation of hypoglycemia caused by inborn errors of carbohydrate metabolism has been included in Tables 289-1 and 289-2. These studies should be done in a pediatric metabolic center but only when the child's condition is stable and the blood glucose level is normal. Judgment must be exercised in choosing the proper diagnostic test to delineate the underlying abnormality. The presence of specific hepatic enzyme deficiencies may be determined by the use of other tolerance tests (see Table 289-2). The tolerance tests are done after a variable period of fasting and only with a physician in attendance who must be prepared to interrupt the test by administering intravenous glucose should symptoms and signs of hypoglycemia occur or should a low blood glucose level be detected. Definitive diagnosis of any of the inherited disorders of carbohydrate metabolism (see Box 298-1) except galactosemia depends on assay of specific hepatic enzyme activities (see Table 289-2). Galactosemia, on the other hand, may be detected by the absence of galactose-1-phosphate uridyltransferase activity in red blood cells, so liver biopsy is unnecessary for its definitive diagnosis.

Amino acid and organic acid metabolic defects. Hypoglycemia has been noted in a variety of inborn errors of amino acid and organic acid metabolism (see Box 289-1).[15] Although symptoms usually begin in the neonatal period, they may occur later. The infants tend to improve when protein feedings are discontinued and 10% glucose is administered intravenously. Occasionally peritoneal dialysis or exchange transfusion may be lifesaving. Amino acid analysis and gas chromatography of blood and urine often are helpful in detecting these inborn errors (see Table 289-1). Diagnosis and treatment of a specific disorder depend on detection of its characteristic metabolites in blood and urine and on assays of specific enzyme activities in skin fibroblasts or white blood cells.

MCAD deficiency is the most common defect of fatty

acid oxidation. This condition may present with nonketotic hypoglycemia (similar to Reye's syndrome), an acute life-threatening event, or even sudden death. In fact, an association has been made between infants with known MCAD deficiency and a history of a sibling dying of sudden infant death syndrome. Initial screening for defects of fatty acid oxidation is best done with analysis of urine organic acids, plasma acylcarnitine profile, and measurement of serum carnitine.[3]

Hormonal Deficiencies

GH deficiency, cortisol deficiency, or combined hormonal deficiencies may cause hypoglycemia.

Hypopituitarism. Congenital hypopituitarism, caused either by a hypothalamic abnormality or by aplasia of the anterior pituitary gland, is associated with severe hypoglycemia during the first few days of life.[1,7,16] Occasionally, however, hypoglycemia may appear first later in infancy or childhood. A few patients may have midline deformities, including hypotelorism, abnormality of the frontonasal process, and cleft lip or palate. Septooptic dysplasia (optic nerve hypoplasia and absence of the septum pellucidum) is present in some patients and may be accompanied by nystagmus. Some patients who have congenital hypopituitarism may have a small penis (microphallus). Measurement of height and weight is essential for the evaluation of a child in whom GH deficiency is suspected because these children have significant growth retardation, which may begin within the first 1 to 2 years of life. These children also tend to be pudgy, and affected boys may have small genitalia.

Cortisol deficiency. Deficient cortisol production may be secondary to Addison's disease, congenital adrenal hyperplasia, ACTH deficiency, or ACTH unresponsiveness.[1,7,14,16] Patients who have ACTH unresponsiveness and Addison's disease may have abnormal pigmentation.

Laboratory investigation and treatment. Laboratory studies should include determination of GH and cortisol in the blood, particularly when the child has hypoglycemia (see Table 289-1). Hypoglycemia is an excellent stimulus for GH and cortisol secretions, so low values of either hormone in the presence of hypoglycemia raise suspicion of deficiencies of those hormones and the need for further studies. In patients who have suspected hypopituitarism or GH deficiency, magnetic resonance imaging and computed tomography of the brain may be of diagnostic help. Correction of hypoglycemia by intravenous administration of glucose makes up the treatment of acute episodes. Specific treatment depends on identifying the underlying hormonal deficiency. However, if GH or cortisol deficiency is suspected on clinical grounds, empiric replacement therapy should be started while awaiting test results. Patients should be encouraged to avoid prolonged fasting.

Ketotic Hypoglycemia

Although the pathogenesis of hypoglycemia in ketotic hypoglycemia has not been defined, the evidence suggests that it represents an exaggeration of the starvation state.[7] During hypoglycemia, blood insulin levels are appropriately low; blood alanine levels also may be low; GH, glucagon, cortisol, β-OHB, and FFA levels in the blood are elevated; urinary ketones are present; and blood glucose levels fail to rise after the administration of glucagon.

Ketotic hypoglycemia is the most common cause of hypoglycemia after 1 year of age.[7,15] Symptoms mimicking those noted in ketotic hypoglycemia have occurred in children who have GH deficiency, ACTH unresponsiveness, FDPase deficiency, glycogen synthetase deficiency, and Reye's syndrome. Before a child is classified as having ketotic hypoglycemia, therefore, careful laboratory investigation to consider these and other diseases must be accomplished.

The combination of ketonuria, hypoglycemia, and central nervous system symptoms, which may vary from unresponsiveness, pallor, and vomiting to coma and convulsions, and which often occur in the early morning hours in association with an upper respiratory tract infection or prolonged fast, is typical of ketotic hypoglycemia for which no cause is known.[15] The onset is between 9 months and 5½ years of age, with a peak incidence at 2 years. Hypoglycemic episodes occur at intervals of from a few months to a year or more; they then decrease in frequency and tend to disappear, usually by 7 to 8 years of age.

The physician should document hypoglycemic blood glucose levels at the time of symptoms by obtaining a diagnostic blood sample. After the child has had several days to recover from the acute episode and is eating well, the administration of a provocative low-calorie, high-fat ketogenic diet has been useful in establishing the diagnosis if an acute blood sample is unobtainable.[7,15] The child must be observed carefully for hypoglycemia during the test period.

The acute hypoglycemic attacks are reversed by the intravenous administration of glucose; glucagon usually has no effect. Because the attacks occur infrequently, long-term drug therapy is not indicated. A liberal carbohydrate diet, including a bedtime snack, is recommended. Prolonged overnight fasting, particularly during weekends or holidays and periods of illness, should be avoided. The parents should be encouraged to test their child's urine for ketones during illness or periods of fasting. Carbohydrate-containing foods, given promptly when acetonuria develops, usually are successful in aborting attacks.

REFERENCES

1. Aynsley-Green A: Hypoglycemia in infants and children, *Clin Endocrinol Metab* 2:159, 1982.
2. Bougneres PF, et al: Fasting hypoglycemia resulting from hepatic carnitine palmitoyl transferase deficiency, *J Pediatr* 98:742, 1981.
3. Burton BK: Inborn errors of metabolism in infancy: a guide to diagnosis, *Pediatr* 102:E69, 1998.
4. Chaussain JL: Glycemic response to 24 hour fast in normal children and children with ketotic hypoglycemia, *J Pediatr* 82:438, 1973.
5. Chen YT, Cornblath M, Sidbury JB: Cornstarch therapy in type I glycogen-storage disease, *N Engl J Med* 310:171, 1984.
6. Cornblath M: Hypoglycemia in infancy and childhood, *Pediatr Ann* 10:356, 1981.
7. Cornblath M, Schwartz R: *Disorders of carbohydrate metabolism in infancy,* ed 2, Philadelphia, 1976, WB Saunders.

8. Dershewitz R, et al: Transient hepatomegaly and hypoglycemia: a consequence of malicious insulin administration, *Am J Dis Child* 130:998, 1976.
9. Dusheiko G, et al: Recurrent hypoglycemia associated with glutaric aciduria type II in an adult, *N Engl J Med* 301:1405, 1979.
10. Glaser B, Hirsch HJ, Landau H: Persistent hyperinsulinemic hypoglycemia of infancy: long-term octreotide treatment without pancreatectomy, *J Pediatr* 123:644, 1993.
11. Greene CL, Blitzer MG, Shapira E: Inborn errors of metabolism and Reye syndrome: differential diagnoses, *J Pediatr* 113:156, 1988.
12. Greene HL, et al: Type I glycogen storage disease: five years of management with nocturnal intragastric feeding, *J Pediatr* 96:590, 1980.
13. Haymond MW: Hypoglycemia in infants and children, *Endocrinol Metab Clin North Am* 18:211, 1989.
14. Kershnar AK, Roe TF, Kogut MD: Adrenocorticotropic hormone unresponsiveness: report of a girl with excessive growth and review of 16 reported cases, *J Pediatr* 80:610, 1972.
15. Kogut MD: Hypoglycemia: pathogenesis, diagnosis and treatment. In Gluck L, et al, editors: *Current problems in pediatrics,* vol 4, Chicago, 1974, Mosby.
16. Kogut MD: Neonatal hypoglycemia: a new look. In Moss AJ, editor: *Pediatrics update: review for physicians,* New York, 1980, Elsevier.
17. Lonlay-Debeney P, et al: Clinical features of 52 neonate with hyperinsulinism, *N Engl J Med* 340:1169, 1999.
18. Mayefsky JH, Sarnaik AP, Postellon DC: Factitious hypoglycemia, *Pediatrics* 69:804, 1982.
19. Pagliara AS, et al: Hypoglycemia in infancy and childhood, part 1, *J Pediatr* 82:365, 1973.
20. Roe TF, Kogut MD: Hypopituitarism and ketotic hypoglycemia, *Am J Dis Child* 121:296, 1971.
21. Roe TF, Kogut MD: Idiopathic leucine-sensitive hypoglycemia syndrome: insulin and glucagon responses and effects of diazoxide, *Pediatr Res* 16:1, 1982.
22. Scarlett JA, et al: Factitious hypoglycemia: diagnosis by measurement of serum C-peptide immunoreactivity and insulin-binding antibodies, *N Engl J Med* 297:1029, 1977.
23. Schutgens RBH, et al: Lethal hypoglycemia in a child with a deficiency of 3-hydroxy-3-methylglutaryl coenzyme A lyase, *J Pediatr* 94:89, 1979.
24. Shelly HJ, Neligan GA: Neonatal hypoglycemia, *Br Med Bull* 22:34, 1966.
25. Stanley CA: Hyperinsulinism is infants and children, *Pediatr Clin North Am* 44:363, 1997.
26. Stanley CA, Baker L: Hyperinsulinism in infancy: diagnosis by demonstration of abnormal response to fasting hypoglycemia, *Pediatrics* 57: 702, 1976.
27. Stanley CA, Baker L: Hyperinsulinism in infants and children: diagnosis and therapy, *Adv Pediatr* 23:315, 1976.
28. Stanley CA, Baker L: The causes of neonatal hypoglycemia, *N Engl J Med* 340:1200, 1999.
29. Thornton PS, et al: Familial and sporadic hyperinsulinism: histopathologic findings and segregation analysis support a single autosomal recessive disorder, *J Pediatr* 119:721, 1991.
30. Ware AJ, et al: Systemic carnitine deficiency: report of a fatal case with multisystemic manifestations, *J Pediatr* 93:959, 1978.

290 Increased Intracranial Pressure

Todd F. Barron • Peter L. Himber • Maher Saqqur

Increased intracranial pressure (ICP) is a potentially life-threatening problem that can be a neurological or neurosurgical emergency if it occurs acutely. Rapid identification of the cause and expedient management can prevent serious morbidity and possible mortality. Increased ICP has many causes, and symptoms can be acute, subacute, or chronic.

PATHOPHYSIOLOGY

In older children and adults the skull is a closed, rigid space. This container is filled with three compartments—the brain accounting for 80% to 90% of the volume, the circulating cerebrospinal fluid (CSF) accounting for 5% to 10%, and the circulating blood accounting for the remainder.[1,14] In that the relative volume is fixed, small increases in any one of these compartments result in a compensatory decrease in the other two. If the increase exceeds normal compensatory mechanisms, ICP rises. Also affecting this is the compliance (stiffness) of the brain, which is altered in various disease states. Because the brain accounts for most of the intracranial volume, changes in brain compliance dampen compensatory mechanisms.[14]

The normal ICP in older children and adults usually is 15 mm Hg in the recumbent position; in young children it is less.[17] ICP is pulsatile and varies around a baseline; variation is a result of cardiac and respiratory activity.[10,14] Transient increases up to 50 mm Hg or higher occur normally with actions that increase intrathoracic pressure or that impede venous return such as coughing, sneezing, and straining. However, with discontinuation of these maneuvers, ICP returns rapidly to baseline.

Under normal conditions, blood flow to the brain is autoregulated, maintaining a constant level of perfusion over a range of blood pressures.[10,14] Any disruption in this makes blood flow pressure passive, which in turn can lead to significant changes in cerebral perfusion with any change in blood pressure. The cerebral perfusion pressure (CPP) is defined as the mean arterial pressure minus the ICP.[14] With increasing ICP, the CPP falls, leading to further cerebral compromise ischemia, swelling, and further increases in ICP. This cycle, if untreated, persists and ultimately causes death.

ETIOLOGY

The causes of increased ICP in children are numerous and can be classified as shown in Box 290-1. Depending on the cause, intracranial hypertension can be chronic (as with pseudotumor cerebri) or acute (as with head trauma with resultant cerebral edema or intracerebral hemorrhage). Common causes of increased ICP in children include head trauma, infection, hydrocephalus, and mass lesions.

SIGNS AND SYMPTOMS

Signs and symptoms of both acute and chronic increased ICP are presented in Box 290-2. Many of these are the same, demonstrating their somewhat nonspecific nature. The temporal pace of development differs between the two. Acute signs of rapidly increasing ICP are the result of displacement of neuronal tissue through the several dural openings with subsequent compression and ischemic changes to the cerebral structures. For example, with uncal herniation in association with supratentorial masses, the uncus is displaced through the tentorial opening, leading to compression of the ipsilateral third nerve and displacement of the peduncles and brainstem laterally[11] (Fig. 290-1). Clinically, the patient is in a comatose state and has an ipsilateral pupillary dilation (third nerve palsy) and ipsilateral hemiparesis, which suggests a lesion in the contralateral hemisphere that is falsely localizing. The pupil reliably localizes the side of the lesion. Downward herniation of the cerebellar tonsils through the foramen magnum leads to compression and vascular compromise of the lower brainstem structures (medulla) (see Fig. 290-1). Patients are comatose and exhibit decorticate or decerebrate rigidity and autonomic (respiratory and circulatory) changes. Classically, the symptoms of a widened pulse pressure, bradycardia, and deep, slow respiration are referred to as "Cushing's triad." Clinically, this triad rarely is seen.[11]

DIAGNOSIS

Key to the management of increased ICP is the rapid recognition of the patient who has intracranial hypertension. As with any individual who has neurological complaints, the history and physical AND neurological examinations are the most important aspects of the initial diagnostic evaluation. These provide the physician information on the pace of illness and therefore allow him or her to discern the need for urgent versus emergent management. If a rapidly evolving process (e.g., impending herniation) is evident, stabilizing the patient is essential before proceeding to definitive diagnosis and therapy.

Performing a lumbar puncture (LP) provides an opportunity to evaluate the ICP by inserting a spinal needle into the thecal sac, attaching a manometer, and measuring the height of the column of CSF while the patient is in the lateral decu-

BOX 290-1

CAUSES OF INCREASED ICP IN CHILDREN

Head Trauma
Cerebral edema
Intracerebral hemorrhage
Extracerebral hemorrhage (subdural, epidural)

Vascular Causes
Arterial/venous infarctions
Intracerebral hemorrhage
Dural sinus thrombosis
Subarachnoid hemorrhage
Vascular anomalies (vein of Galen malformation, arteriovenous malformations)

Neoplastic Causes
Primary brain tumors
Metastatic (intracerebral, meningeal infiltration)

Hydrocephalus
Congenital or acquired
Communicating or noncommunicating

Pseudotumor Cerebrii (Benign Intracranial Hypertension)

CNS Infections
Meningitis (bacterial, fungal, mycobacterial)
Encephalitis (focal or diffuse)
Abscess

Metabolic Causes
Inborn errors of metabolism (hyperammonemia)
Hepatic encephalopathy
Diabetic ketoacidosis
Renal failure
Reye syndrome
Hypoxic-ischemic encephalopathy
Fluid-electrolyte abnormalities (hyponatremia, hypernatremia)

Structural Causes
Craniosynostosis

Status Epilepticus

Modified from Pickard JD, Czosnyka M: *J Neurol Neurosurg Psychiatry* 56:845, 1993.

BOX 290-2

SYMPTOMS AND SIGNS OF ACUTE AND CHRONIC INCREASED INTRACRANIAL PRESSURE IN CHILDREN

Infants
Acute
Irritability
Poor feeding/emesis
Split sutures (especially lambdoidal)
Bulging fontanelle
Altered mental status
Seizures
Parinaud sign (upgaze paresis)

Chronic
Irritability
Poor feeding/emesis
Increased head circumference
Bulging fontanelle
Split sutures (especially lambdoidal)
Apparent developmental arrest or regression
Parinaud sign (upgaze paresis)

Children
Acute
Severe, acute headache
Seizures
Emesis
Rapidly deteriorating mental status
Decerebrate/decorticate posture
Focal neurological deficits
+/– Papilledema
Pupillary abnormalities
Autonomic dysfunction (Cushing's triad)

Chronic
Chronic, progressive headache
Seizures
Early morning emesis
Change in school performance
Altered mental status
Cranial neuropathy (e.g., sixth cranial nerve palsy)
Focal neurological deficits
Papilledema
Visual changes

bitus position with the legs extended. Between 12 and 18 cm is normal. However, if a mass lesion is suspected, the withdrawal of CSF may precipitate a herniation syndrome; therefore neuroimaging generally is recommended before an LP. The one exception is in children who are suspected of having meningitis, in which case, in general, neuroimaging before performance of an LP is unnecessary.[6] If meningitis is a serious consideration and a computed tomography (CT) scan is still desired, institution of antibiotic therapy should not be delayed pending completion of the CT scan and, in turn, the LP. A spinal fluid analysis always should include measurement of glucose and protein and a differential cell count.

Depending on the clinical situation, other studies can be obtained, including microbial cultures (bacterial, fungal, viral, mycobacterial), special stains, and cytology.

Neuroimaging

CT or magnetic resonance imaging (MRI) can provide essential information in the diagnosis and management of patients who have increased ICP. Although MRI provides better anatomical differentiation, it is frequently unavailable in the emergency setting; therefore, CT is performed most often. If a mass lesion is suspected, neuroimaging, regardless of modality, should include contrast enhancement. Both the modalities are effective in evaluating the cause of intracranial hypertension and are done primarily to determine the presence of a mass lesion. The one exception is in the patient suspected of having a subarachnoid hemorrhage, when CT followed by LP remain the mainstays of initial diagnosis. And finally, in infants suspected of having aqueductal stenosis, ultrasonography is a reasonable alternative to CT or MRI

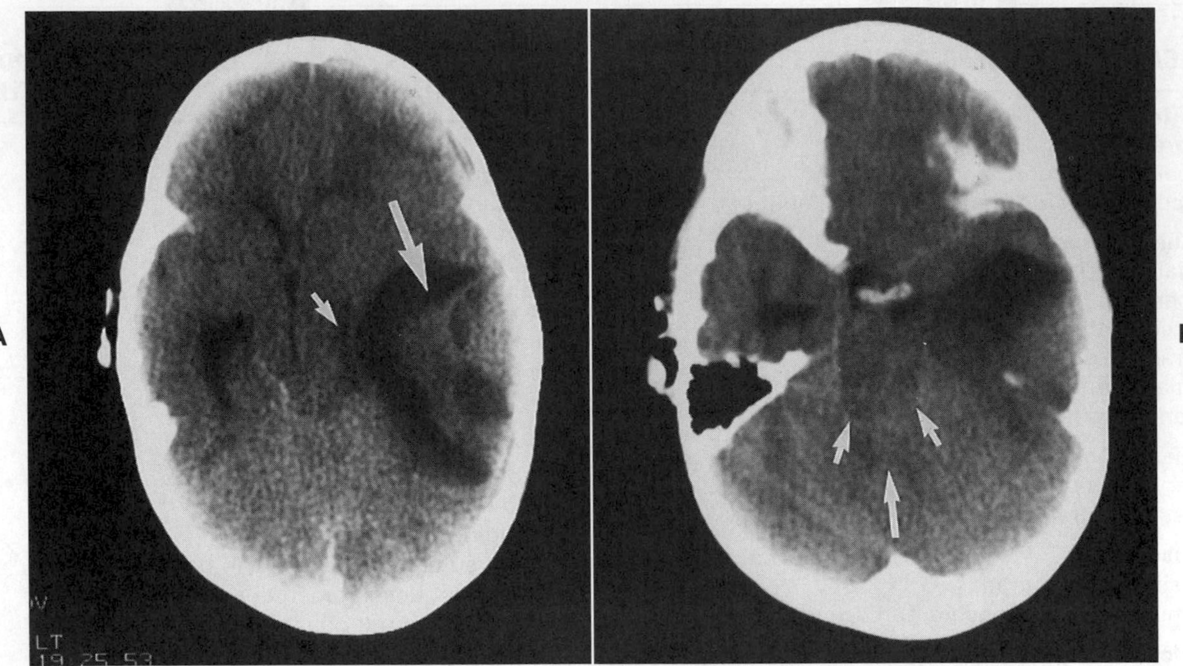

Fig. 290-1 Two sections from a computed tomography scan of a 5-year-old girl who is comatose and has increased intracranial pressure. **A,** Large, cystic left temporal lobe mass *(large arrow)* causing left uncal herniation *(small arrow)* with loss of perimesencephalic cistern and midline shift. **B,** A lower cut demonstrating loss of the fourth ventricle (large arrow) and a quadrigeminal cistern (small arrows), suggesting downward (tonsillar) herniation.

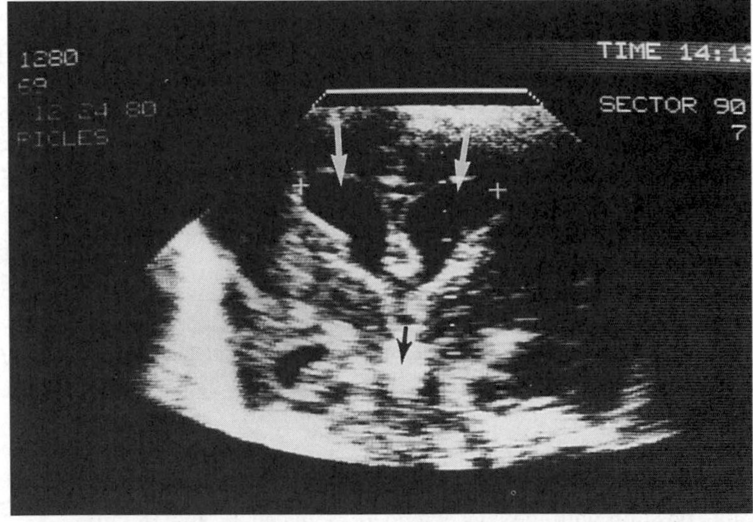

Fig. 290-2 A coronal head ultrasound of a baby born at 30 weeks' gestation with a history of an intraventricular hemorrhage now with increasing head circumference. Prominent dilated lateral ventricles *(white arrows)* and a clot-filled third ventricle *(black arrow)* are demonstrated.

(Fig. 290-2). Other neuroimaging studies, such as angiography, rarely play a role in the initial diagnostic management of intracranial hypertension.

MANAGEMENT

Rapid recognition and stabilization of the patient suspected of having acutely increased ICP is essential in preventing greater morbidity and mortality. The goal of early management is to lower ICP without compromising cerebral perfusion and to identify the cause so that more definitive therapy can be provided, be it medical or neurosurgical. In patients who have evidence of chronically elevated ICP, management usually is directed toward definitive therapy.

As in any emergency situation, the first step in management is to assess the airway, breathing, and circulation (the ABCs). It also is useful to obtain a urine Dextrostick and, in the case of the trauma patient, to expose the patient completely so that injuries can be identified. When acute increased ICP is suspected, the following initial steps should be taken:

1. Stabilize the airway. In most instances this requires rapid, controlled intubation, taking care to minimize any patient Valsalva maneuvers, which increase ICP further, albeit transiently.
2. Obtain IV access. Use only isotonic solutions, minimizing fluids initially unless circulatory compromise is evident.

3. Measure the vital signs and assess the neurological state rapidly and frequently.
4. Position the head at 30 degrees and maintain a midline position in the event that there might be an injury to the cervical spine.
5. Maintain adequate intravascular volume and blood pressure.
6. Maintain adequate oxygenation.

After these maneuvers, the interventions detailed in the following sections should be attempted depending on the patient's clinical situation. The goal of therapy is to keep the ICP ≤20 and to keep the CPP ≥70 without sacrificing cerebral perfusion or oxygenation.

Hyperventilation

Cerebral blood flow is exquisitely sensitive to CO_2 levels. Low CO_2 levels lead to cerebral vasoconstriction, whereas elevated levels lead to dilation. Early hyperventilation (HV) of the patient who has increased ICP leads to a decrease in cerebral blood volume and, therefore, a decrease in the ICP. This provides the most rapid, effective method of lowering ICP acutely. This effect is transient; therefore other methods must be employed to maintain normal or near-normal ICP. In general, CO_2 should be lowered to the low thirties (mm Hg). Further decreases can lead to a significant decrease in cerebral blood flow, producing ischemia and increasing ICP further. Failure to respond to HV often is a poor prognostic sign.[15] Evidence suggests that the alkalizing effect of HV and, therefore, lowered ICP can be minimized through the use of intravenous buffers such as tris hydroxymethyl aminomethane (THAM).[15]

HV, although long a mainstay in the treatment of increased ICP, has recently been called into question as possibly causing more harm than good.[1,16,19] HV induces a more pronounced change in cerebral blood flow than in cerebral blood volume. This can lead to a reduction in PO_2 despite the beneficial effect on CPP and ICP.[2] One study found that of patients with early, severe head trauma those who had early, aggressive HV had worse outcomes than those who were normocapnic.[9] Although HV is the most rapid method to lower ICP acutely, it is probably not beneficial for the chronic treatment of increased ICP.[1] HV should be used judiciously with monitoring of cerebral oxygenation if at all possible.

Osmotic Agents and Diuretics

Intravenous osmotic agents (mannitol and glycerol) are unable to permeate the blood-brain barrier and therefore draw fluid from the intracellular brain compartment to the vascular space, thereby reducing ICP and allowing increased cerebral perfusion.[3] Traditionally, mannitol has been favored over glycerol. However, one study found that although mannitol decreased ICP, it did not improve cerebral PO_2.[5] Mannitol is given rapidly in an initial IV bolus of 0.75 to 1 g/kg. Following this, additional boluses ranging from 0.25 to 0.5 g/kg should be given every 3 to 5 hours, depending on the status of the patient. Response to IV mannitol is rapid and occurs usually within 10 to 20 minutes. Serum osmolarity should be maintained in the 295 to 320 mOsm/L range. Because mannitol is excreted renally, it cannot be given in the face of renal failure because this can provoke potentially life-threatening pulmonary edema.[13]

Glycerol acts in a similar fashion to mannitol.[3] The advantages include that it is a physiologic agent that has caloric value, which can be beneficial for nutritional support. It has less diuretic effects so that unlike mannitol, it does not depend solely on renal function and can be given in patients with renal insufficiency. The main side effect is intravascular hemolysis that can be avoided by giving a low concentration (<20%) at a slow rate of infusion (>1 hour). Glycerol is most effective via enteroduodenal administration. Direct oral intake or gastric tube administration is less effective. As opposed to mannitol, which is most effective if given as intermittent boluses, glycerol is usually given as a continuous drip. In summary, mannitol and glycerol are probably equally effective and may be complementary because of their different properties.

Loop diuretics such as furosemide act to reduce ICP by provoking a diuresis of water and electrolytes, thereby establishing a gradient between the intravascular compartment and the brain. Diuretics must be used cautiously in traumatic brain injury and subarachnoid hemorrhage because volume depletion can worsen outcome. They frequently are used in combination with osmotic diuretics but are used alone infrequently. In using any of the aforementioned agents, care must be given to maintain intravascular volume and adequate blood pressure. Electrolytes must be monitored carefully.

Hypertonic Saline

A more recent treatment of increased ICP is the intravenous administration of 3% to 23.4% hypertonic saline.[12,13,18] Intravenous boluses can reduce ICP and augment CPP for several hours.[11,14] It creates an osmotic gradient and draws water from the intracellular and extracellular spaces into the intravascular compartment.[10,11] Hypertonic saline can be given quickly and requires lower volumes of fluid than do osmotic agents. There is no immediate concern for volume depletion as can occur with mannitol. The potential side effects include hyperosmolar central pontine myelosis, congestive heart failure, subdural hematomas, and rarely, coagulopathy. Studies are under way to determine the most effective osmolarity.[12] The volume given depends on the osmolarity volume status of the patient and the patient's age.

Neuromuscular Blockade

Use of agents such as pancuronium and vecuronium can be effective in decreasing ICP by preventing maneuvers that increase intrathoracic pressure such as coughing, straining, or "bucking" the ventilator. The physician must remember that these agents do not provide analgesia or sedation; therefore, they should be used in conjunction with analgesic agents and short-acting sedatives.

Temperature Control

Hyperthermia leads to greater cerebral metabolism; therefore measures should be taken to avoid body temperature elevation. This generally includes judicious use of antipyretics, cooling blankets, and antibiotics if infection is suspected. Conversely, hypothermia decreases cerebral metabolism and may be advantageous in the management of elevated ICP as long as shivering is prevented and efforts are made to maintain full cardiorespiratory function. Body temperature should be maintained between 96.8° and 98.6° F (36° and 37° C).[10,17]

Seizure Control

Seizure activity, whether clinical or subclinical, places an excessive metabolic demand on already compromised brain tissue. Treatment with antiepileptic drugs is necessary for any patient who is having or is suspected of having seizures, especially if neuromuscular blocking agents are to be used. In general, diazepam (0.1 mg/kg/dose IV) or lorazepam (0.05 to 0.1 mg/kg/dose IV) is the drug to be used in treating acute seizures. For more prolonged therapy, either phenytoin, fosphenytoin (a water-soluble prodrug of phenytoin), or phenobarbital can be used. Phenytoin and fosphenytoin have the distinct advantage of not depressing mental status. Phenytoin needs to be given slowly (50 mg/mm). Although fosphenytoin can be given more rapidly (150 mg/min), it is water soluble so it can also be given intramuscularly. If possible, the cause of seizure activity (e.g., fever, drug toxicity, hypoglycemia, and electrolyte abnormalities) should be identified and treated.

Corticosteroids

The use of corticosteroids remains controversial in the management of acutely elevated ICP associated with head trauma, intracerebral hemorrhage, and ischemic stroke.[15] Several controlled studies involving the use of glucocorticoids in head injury did not find any change in outcome or benefit for the control of increased ICP.[4] Thus steroids rarely have a role in the treatment of increased ICP in head injury patients. However, they do have clear utility in the management of edema associated with brain tumors and in the management of refractory pseudotumor cerebri. Their mechanism of action is unknown, but hypotheses include stabilization of the blood-brain barrier, enhancement of brain energy supplies, decrease in tumor growth, reduction of CSF production, and stabilization of cellular membranes.[10,17] In general, dexamethasone is used.

Glycemic Control

Hyperglycemia after head injury is associated with a poorer outcome than that for patients who were normoglycemic.[4] Many centers now remove glucose from intravenous fluids and aggressively treat hyperglycemia.

High-Dose Barbiturates

In situations of refractory increased ICP, treatment with high doses of barbiturates can sometimes be effective. These agents act to decrease cerebral blood flow and metabolism. Pentobarbital is the agent of choice for prolonged therapy; in general, a loading dose of 3 to 10 mg/kg IV is given followed by a maintenance infusion of 1 to 2 mg/kg/hr. The dose should be titrated on the electroencephalogram, with a goal of obtaining a burst-suppression pattern. This therapy should be maintained for 24 hours or more and then tapered. Side effects are frequent and include myocardial suppression and hypotension, often requiring the use of pressors. Which groups of refractory increased ICP patients benefit from this therapy has not yet been determined.[10,15] It should be used only when all other medical and surgical therapies have failed.

Intracranial Pressure Monitoring and Removal of Cerebrospinal Fluid

Numerous invasive devices are available for assessing ICP. These include intraventricular catheters that have the advantage of allowing drainage of CSF and, therefore, reducing ICP. The disadvantage of this device is the higher risk of infection, seizures, and hemorrhage compared with the other devices available. Fluid-filled catheter and fiberoptic monitoring systems can be placed both extradurally and intradurally, allowing relatively accurate assessment of ICP with fewer complications. Measuring cerebral venous oxygenation via a jugular bulb-indwelling catheter and noninvasively by transcutaneous, transcranial near infrared spectroscopy can assess ICP and cerebral perfusion indirectly.[8,10,15]

Surgical Decompression

Obviously, in children who have large intracranial masses causing acutely increased ICP, surgical removal of the mass can be life saving. Surgery also may play a role in decreasing ICP in those patients who have large intracerebral hemorrhages by removing the clot and in trauma patients who have massive edema and contusion or in patients who have a large cerebral infarction through either craniectomy or decompression of the edematous mass. In the latter two instances, surgery is performed only after all other measures have failed and increased ICP has become refractory.[1,10] Its effectiveness remains anecdotal.[15]

Future Trends

In the future, cerebral protectants such as free radical scavengers, excitotoxic amino acid antagonists, lazeroids, and *N*-methyl-D-aspartate (NMDA) receptor antagonists may be part of the "cocktail" in the initial emergent management of acutely increased ICP.[10,15]

With respect to patients who exhibit evidence of chronically increased ICP who are neurologically stable, management is directed toward definitive therapy—that is, evacuation of the chronic subdural hematoma, appropriate tumor management (surgery or radiation and chemotherapy or both), and treatment with acetazolamide, loop diuretics, steroids, or a lumbar drain in patients who have more benign causes of intracranial hypertension.

OUTCOME

In at least 50% of children who have severe head injuries and in children who are comatose from other cerebral insults (hypoxia, infections, metabolic disorders), increased ICP is a major complication that affects morbidity and, possibly, ultimate outcome.[2,7,19] Which of the variables—ICP, CPP, or initial Glasgow Coma Scale score (see Table 286-1)—are helpful in predicting prognosis remains uncertain.[2,7] In any regard, significant morbidity remains for children who have increased ICP. Clearly, in those children who have mass lesions or treatable metabolic disorders, early identification and treatment before a catastrophic increase in ICP occurs will improve outcome.

When to Refer

Macrocephaly/accelerating head growth ("crossing percentiles")
Chronic unremitting headache or new onset of severe headache
Mild papilledema
Visual abnormalities (field cuts, diplopia)
Developmental arrest/regression

When to Hospitalize

Bulging fontanel
Altered mental status
Prolonged seizures
New focal neurological deficits
Moderate to severe papilledema
Cushing's triad (widened pulse pressure, bradycardia, and deep, slow respirations)

REFERENCES

1. Allen CH, Ward JD: An evidence based approach to management of increased intracranial pressure, *Crit Care Clin* 14:485, 1998.
2. Barzilay Z, et al: Variables affecting outcome from severe brain injury in children, *Intensive Care Med* 14:417, 1988.
3. Biestro A, et al: Osmotherapy for increased intracranial pressure: comparison between mannitol and glycerol, *Acta Neurochir (Wein)* 139:725, 1997.
4. Giannotta SL, et al: High dose glucocorticoids in the management of severe head injury, *Neurosurgery* 15:497, 1984.
5. Härtl R, et al: Mannitol decreases ICP but does not improve brain-tissue pO_2 in severely head-injured patients with intracranial hypertension, *Acta Neurochir (Wein)* 70(suppl):40, 1997.
6. Haslam RHA: Role of computed tomography in the early management of bacterial meningitis, *J Pediatr* 119:157, 1991.
7. Lieh-Lai MW, et al: Limitations of the Glasgow Coma Scale in predicting outcome in children with traumatic brain injury, *J Pediatr* 120:193, 1992.
8. McKinley BA, Parmley CL, Tonneson AS: Standardized management of intracranial pressure: a preliminary clinical trial, *J Trauma* 46:271, 1999.
9. Muizelaar JP, et al: Adverse effects of prolonged hyperventilation in patients with severe head injury: a randomized clinical trial, *J Neurosurg* 75:731, 1991.
10. Pickard JD, Czosnyka M: Management of raised intracranial pressure, *J Neurol Neurosurg Psychiatry* 56:845, 1993.
11. Plum F, Posner JB: *The diagnosis of stupor and coma,* ed 3, Philadelphia, 1982, FA Davis.
12. Prough DS, Zornow MH: Hypertonic maintenance fluids for patients with cerebral edema: does the evidence support a "phase II" trial? *Crit Care Med* 26:421, 1998.
13. Prough DS, Zornow MH, Mannitol: an old friend on the skids, *Crit Care Med* 26:997, 1998.
14. Ropper AH, Rockoff MA: Physiology and clinical aspects of raised intracranial pressure. In Ropper AH, editor: *Neurological and neurosurgical intensive care,* ed 2, New York, 1993, Raven Press.
15. Ropper AH: Treatment of intracranial hypertension. In Ropper AH, editor: *Neurological and neurosurgical intensive care,* ed 2, New York, 1993, Raven Press.
16. Schneider GH, et al: Influence of hyperventilation on brain tissue-PO_2, pCO_2, and pH in patients with intracranial hypertension, *Acta Neurochir* 71(suppl):62, 1998.
17. Shapiro K, Morris WJ, Teo C: Intracranial hypertension: mechanisms and management. In Cheek WR, editor: *Pediatric neurosurgery,* ed 3, Philadelphia, 1994, WB Saunders.
18. Suarez JI, et al: Treatment of refractory intracranial hypertension with 23.4% saline, *Crit Care Med* 26:1118, 1998.
19. Young A: Controversies in management of acute brain trauma, *Lancet* 352:165, 1998.

291 Meningococcemia

Mary T. Caserta

Meningococcemia is a classic example of fulminant bacterial sepsis and is the most dreaded consequence of infection with *Neisseria meningitidis*. Although occult or chronic meningococcemia occasionally is detected, children who have the severe form of the disease can progress from a state of good health to death in hours, regardless of whether meningitis is present.

EPIDEMIOLOGY

N. meningitidis is a gram-negative coccus that appears typically in pairs (diplococci) with the adjacent sides flattened. The organism is enclosed by a cell envelope containing outer membrane proteins and a lipopolysaccharide (LPS or endotoxin) and by a polysaccharide capsule. Nine serogroups have been identified based on the antigenic structure of the capsular polysaccharide.

N. meningitidis is found only in the human nasopharynx and is spread from person to person via respiratory droplets or direct contact with secretions. Invasive meningococcal disease is a relatively uncommon event, with most individuals colonized only intermittently with the organism. Approximately 5% to 20% of adults in nonepidemic conditions are colonized. Subgroups, such as military recruits, can have rates as high as 80%, and carriage rates are even higher in household contacts of patients who have infection or in noninfected carriers.[5] Colonization with both pathogenic and nonpathogenic *Neisseria,* in addition to other gram-negative organisms that have similar capsular polysaccharides, induces the development of natural immunity to *N. meningitidis*. Nonetheless, *N. meningitidis* causes both epidemic and endemic disease worldwide. Since the introduction of an effective vaccine against *Haemophilus influenzae* type B, the meningococcus is the leading cause of meningitis and sepsis in children and young adults in the United States (approximately 3308 cases in 1997). Data from the Centers for Disease Control and Prevention show that in 1997 the overall incidence of meningococcal disease was 1.24 cases per 100,000 people.[7] The highest incidence of disease consistently is found in infants, with a peak attack rate of 26.4 cases per 100,000 population. From 25% to 33% of all cases of meningococcal disease occur in children younger than 1 year of age. Almost 50% of all cases of meningococcemia occur in children younger than age 2 years, when passively acquired maternal antibody concentrations have reached their nadir and substantial numbers of children have not yet acquired protective antibodies following colonization. By age 5 years the incidence reaches adult levels (Fig. 291-1).

Historically, the majority of cases of invasive meningococcal disease in the United States have been caused by serogroup B meningococcus. In the early 1990s, however, organisms of serogroup B and C were each identified in approximately 45% of cases of meningococcal disease. Despite this relative equality, 69% of disease caused by group C occurred in persons older than 2 years of age, whereas only 37% of disease caused by group B occurred in those children, making group B meningococcus more of a threat to the younger age groups. During the past several years the number of cases of meningococcal disease caused by group Y has increased. In 1997, 29% of all cases were due to group Y, with group B and C each causing approximately 33% of cases. Data are not yet available to determine whether this change is due to disease in specific age groups. The occurrence of meningococcal infection also varies with the seasons. Winter and spring constitute the peak time of disease in the United States. Several studies have shown an association between meningococcal disease and influenza and other viral respiratory infections, although the exact nature of the interaction is not clear.[6]

Sixty percent of cases of invasive meningococcal disease are associated with meningitis; approximately 40% are classified as sepsis without central nervous system involvement. The overall mortality for meningococcal disease is 10% to 15%. Subgroups of patients, such as those who have fulminant meningococcemia, can have fatality rates as high as 50% to 80% despite aggressive intensive care therapy.

DIAGNOSIS AND DIFFERENTIAL DIAGNOSIS

The early recognition of meningococcemia is an important determinant of survival. In a study of 100 children who had meningococcal infections reported by Wong, Hitchcock, and Mason,[29] the predominant findings on examination were fever and rash, each noted in 71% of patients. Other important symptoms and signs included irritability or lethargy in just over 50% of the patients; vomiting occurred in approximately 35% of children, and shock was noted in 42%. Less common symptoms include delirium, headache, coryza, diarrhea, myalgia, and hypothermia. In almost all cases of invasive meningococcal disease the patient appears very ill.

The type and duration of the rash provide important information about the course and prognosis of the disease. Early in the infection a tender, pink, maculopapular rash similar to that seen in rubella, secondary syphilis, or disseminated gonorrhea can appear on any part of the skin. The rash often

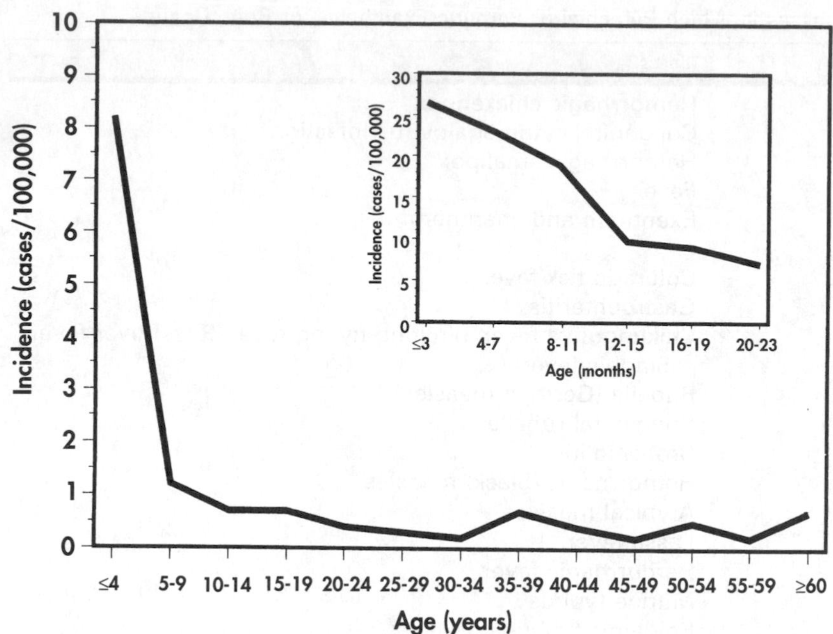

Fig. 291-1 Incidence of meningococcal disease, by age group, in selected areas in the United States, 1989-1991.
(From Jackson LA, Wenger JD: *MMWR* 42:25, 1993.)

fades rapidly with treatment, and patients who have this type of manifestation are less likely to have a fulminant course. A generalized petechial rash most prominent on the distal extremities, including the palms and soles, usually is associated with meningococcal disease. Initially the lesions are discrete, 1 to 2 mm in diameter, and found in clusters where clothing puts pressure on the skin.[2] This rash must be differentiated from that seen with Rocky Mountain spotted fever, bacterial endocarditis, and enterovirus infections. Scrapings of petechial lesions reveal the organism approximately 70% of the time.

The most ominous manifestation of meningococcal disease is an ecchymotic or purpuric rash with a centrifugal distribution usually present in cases of fulminant meningococcemia. The differential diagnosis includes Rocky Mountain spotted fever, plague, rubeola, septicemia with other bacteria (Table 291-1), and Henoch-Schönlein purpura. Meningococcemia is the most common cause of purpura. In the classic series by Toews and Bass,[26] of 151 patients who had meningococcal infections, 7 of the 16 patients who had ecchymotic or purpuric lesions died; only 4 of the 135 patients who had either maculopapular or petechial lesions, or no rash at all, died. A 1991 report also noted an association between the presence and type of rash with outcome.[23] The authors demonstrated that mortality in children who had invasive meningococcal disease and a petechial or purpuric rash was 19%, compared with no deaths in those children who had no rash. Similarly, in the aforementioned review of 100 children, patients who had purpura fulminans had a 50% mortality. The case fatality rate also is significantly higher in patients who have petechiae for 12 hours or less. Therefore, a febrile child who has purpura or petechiae that have been present for fewer than 12 hours should be managed as a medical emergency.

MANAGEMENT

An infant or child who has an acute onset of fever and a purpuric or petechial rash requires aggressive monitoring and treatment as soon as possible. If the patient must be transported to a pediatric intensive care unit, blood should be drawn, antibiotics given, and intravenous access secured beforehand. The patient should be attended during transport by a physician prepared to treat shock and respiratory failure because the disease may worsen when endotoxin is liberated after antibiotic therapy. Initial laboratory tests should include a blood culture, a complete blood count and differential, a partial thromboplastin time (PTT), a prothrombin time (PT), measurement of fibrin breakdown products, and serum chemistries. If the patient is stable when first evaluated, a lumbar puncture should also be performed to determine if meningitis is present in order to examine the CSF for organisms, obtain cultures, and assess the prognosis more accurately. If the patient is unstable on initial assessment, the lumbar puncture should be deferred until a later time.

The recommended antibiotic regimen for treatment of meningococcemia is aqueous penicillin G 250,000 to 400,000 units/kg/day in four to six divided doses. No resistance of the meningococcus to penicillin is reported in the United States. However, strains that have decreased susceptibility to penicillin have been reported from several other countries in Europe and Africa. Ceftriaxone, cefotaxime, and chloramphenicol are alternative antibiotics recommended for penicillin-allergic patients or in the rare instance in which resistance might be present. Antibiotic therapy generally is continued for 5 afebrile days or 7 days total. Rifampin (10 mg/kg per dose given twice a day for 2 days) is added at the end of the course of penicillin to eliminate carriage of the organism from the nasopharynx.[1] Rifampin is not necessary if the patient has been treated with a third-generation cephalosporin because these agents are effective in eliminating carriage.

In addition to antibiotic therapy, children who have meningococcemia often require aggressive supportive therapy in a pediatric intensive care setting with invasive monitoring of hemodynamic, neurological, and respiratory function. Mechanical ventilation often is necessary to treat respiratory failure. Maintenance of optimal plasma expansion with intra-

Table 291-1 Infectious Agents Associated with Illnesses in Which Petechial or Purpuric Exanthems, or Both, Occur

Infectious Agent	Illness
Varicella-zoster virus	Hemorrhagic chickenpox
Cytomegalovirus	Congenital cytomegalovirus infection
Variola virus	Hemorrhagic smallpox
Coxsackieviruses A4, A9	Fever
Coxsackieviruses B2 to B4	Exanthem and enanthem
Echoviruses 4, 7, 9	
Colorado tick fever virus	Colorado tick fever
Rotavirus	Gastroenteritis
Alphaviruses	Chikungunya fever, o'nyong-nyong fever, Ross River fever, Sindbis fever
Rubella virus	Rubella (German measles) Congenital rubella
Respiratory syncytial virus	Bronchiolitis
Measles virus	Hemorrhagic (black) measles Atypical measles
Lassa virus	Lassa fever
Marburg virus	Hemorrhagic fever
Rickettsia typhi	Murine typhus
Rickettsia prowazekii	Epidemic typhus
Rickettsia rickettsii and other tickborne rickettsiae	Rocky Mountain spotted fever
Ehrlichia canis	Ehrlichiosis
Mycoplasma pneumoniae	Atypical pneumonia
Streptococcus pyogenes	Scarlet fever; septicemia
Streptococcus pneumoniae	Pneumococcal septicemia
Enterococcal and viridans group streptococci	Endocarditis
Neisseria gonorrhoeae	Gonococcemia
Neisseria meningitidis	Meningococcemia
Moraxella catarrhalis	Sinusitis, otitis media, sepsis
Haemophilus influenzae	*H. influenzae* septicemia
Pseudomonas aeruginosa	Ecthyma gangrenosa
Streptobacillus moniliformis	Rat-bite fever
Yersinia pestis	Septicemic plague (Black Death)
Bartonella henselae	Cat-scratch fever
Treponema pallidum	Congenital syphilis
Borrelia spp.	Relapsing fever
Toxoplasma gondii	Congenital toxoplasmosis
Trichinella spiralis	Trichinosis

Modified from Cherry JD: Cutaneous manifestations of systemic infections. In Feigen RD, Cherry JD, editors: *Textbook of pediatric infectious diseases,* Philadelphia, 1992, WB Saunders.

venous fluids is the first step in stabilizing the circulatory system. Large amounts of fluid may be needed because of the capillary leak associated with endotoxic shock. In addition, multiple transfusions with platelets and fresh-frozen plasma may be necessary to correct the coagulopathy associated with meningococcemia. Several studies have demonstrated that myocardial dysfunction precedes shock in adult and pediatric patients who have meningococcal sepsis.[18] This phenomenon is believed to be secondary to endotoxemia. The use of inotropic agents aimed at reversing myocardial depression and improving tissue perfusion is recommended based on these observations.

Supportive measures for severe purpura include treatments aimed at relieving the ischemic complications associated with vasculitis. Case reports have demonstrated the successful use of continuous epidural anesthesia in improving perfusion of the lower extremities and preventing gangrenous necrosis.[25] The mechanism of action is thought to be vasodilation of partially occluded vessels via sympathetic blockade. If no evidence exists of coagulopathy, an anesthesiologist can perform this type of regional block with an indwelling catheter in the caudal space without an appreciable effect on overall cardiovascular status. Systemic thrombolytic therapy with tissue plasminogen activator (r-TPA) has been used in a limited number of patients in an attempt to dissolve microthrombi and restore organ perfusion.[30] The topical administration of nitroglycerin also has been reported to be useful in restoring blood flow to limited areas of skin and superficial tissues without notable adverse effects.[15]

Other ancillary treatments evaluated experimentally are aimed at interrupting the disease process pathophysiology via interference with secondary mediators of inflammation induced by the release of endotoxin. These treatments include plasmapheresis, whole blood exchange, extracorporeal membrane oxygenation, continuous veno-venous hemodiafiltration, or the administration of monoclonal antibodies directed against endotoxin or specific mediators such as tumor necrosis factor.[3,14] Several studies have shown a correlation between plasma levels of endotoxin or tumor necrosis factor and multiorgan failure or disease severity, making these strategies theoretically attractive.[4,28] Recombinant human bactericidal/permeability-increasing protein ($rBPI_{21}$) is the N-terminal fragment of a human protein naturally found in the azurophilic granules of polymorphonuclear leukocytes. This compound binds to bacteria and endotoxin and inhibits the inflammatory response caused by these substances. In a preliminary trial of $rBPI_{21}$ in children who had severe meningococcemia, mortality was reduced compared with historical controls, prompting a larger randomized efficacy trial of this substance.[13] Heparin therapy was advocated in the past to treat disseminated intravascular coagulation caused by sepsis, but it has not been found to alter the disease course or the mortality in human or animal studies. Recent reports have associated purpura fulminans induced by sepsis with acquired deficiencies of the natural anticoagulation factor proteins C and S.[29] Several small case series have reported positive results from treating adult and pediatric patients who had purpura fulminans with concentrates of antithrombin III or activated protein C.[12,19,20] These results support future large-scale trials of this type of therapy among patients who have meningococcal sepsis and purpura fulminans. In patients who have meningitis, adjunctive treatment with dexamethasone (0.15 mg/kg per dose every 6 hours for 4 days) to prevent neurological sequelae is supported by limited studies involving small numbers of patients who have meningococcal disease. The use of high-dose steroids in the treatment of adults who have sepsis and shock, caused primarily by gram-negative bacteria, has not proved to be of benefit in decreasing either morbidity or mortality. The use of high-dose steroids in children who have meningococcal disease remains controversial.

Numerous investigators have attempted to predict the outcome for individual patients who have meningococcal disease, based on various laboratory and clinical data. In 1966, Stiehm and Damrosch[22] developed a prognostic score whereby patients who had three or more of these findings—the presence of petechiae for fewer than 12 hours before admission, shock, the absence of meningitis, normal or low white blood cell counts, or normal or low erythrocyte sedimentation rates—had fatality rates of 85% or greater when the score was validated. The Glasgow Meningococcal Septicemia Prognostic Score was developed in 1987 (Box 291-1) and is designed for rapid bedside assessment without the need for multiple laboratory tests.[24] Points are assigned for shock, a skin-to-rectal temperature differential of greater than 3° C, a pediatric-modified coma scale score of less than 8, absence of meningismus, an extending purpuric rash, deterioration in the hour before scoring, and a base deficit greater than 8. The scale was tested retrospectively on a group of 123 children who had meningococcemia in an effort to predict mortality reliably. A score of 10 or greater had a positive predictive value of 87.5% and a negative predictive value of 100%. In a recently reported combined prospective and retrospective study comparing eight different prognostic scores in children, the Glasgow Meningococcal Septicemia Prognostic Score performed significantly better than the others and accurately identified a large number of survivors (see Box 291-1).[10] In general, these scoring systems are used to determine which patients might benefit from more aggressive or experimental therapies and to help evaluate the usefulness of newer treatments.

BOX 291-1

GLASGOW MENINGOCOCCAL SEPTICEMIA PROGNOSTIC SCORE

	Points
BP <75 mm Hg systolic, age <4 yr <85 mm Hg systolic, age >4 yr	3
Skin/rectal temperature difference >3° C	3
Modified Glasgow Coma Scale score less than 8* or deterioration of at least 3 points in 1 hour	3
Clinical deterioration in hour before scoring	2
Absence of meningitis	2
Extending purpuric rash or widespread ecchymoses	1
Base deficit (capillary or arterial) >8.0	1
Maximum score	15

From Thomson AJ, Sills JA, Hart A: Validation of the Glasgow Meningococcal Septicemia Prognostic Score: a 10-year retrospective survey, *Crit Care Med* 19:26, 1991.
A score of at least 9 has a sensitivity of 100%, a specificity of 95%, a positive predictive value of 73.7%, and a negative predictive value of 100% in predicting mortality.
*See Table 286-1.

COMPLICATIONS

The majority of children who survive meningococcal disease recover completely; 15% to 40% of patients, however, develop a complication of infection that may be categorized broadly as suppurative, neurological, ischemic, or allergic. The suppurative complications include subdural effusions, subdural empyema, and acute suppurative arthritis. In a retrospective review by Edwards and Baker,[11] suppurative complications were detected in approximately 9% of children. Deafness is the most common neurological sequelae and was noted in 6% of children by Edwards and Baker. Most other series report deafness in 2% to 3% of patients. The percentage of survivors who have ischemic complications such as gangrenous necrosis of the skin or extremities requiring skin grafting or amputation varies from 3% to 20%, depending on the series.[16] Arthritis and pericarditis are the most common sequelae of meningococcal infection and are reported in 8% to 24% of cases. Both of these complications are thought to be secondary to an allergic phenomenon with immune complex deposition rather than a direct invasion of the heart or joints by the organism. Allergic arthritis and pericarditis are late in onset and more common in adults than in children. The symptoms usually are self limited. Specific therapy generally is not required; however, drainage of pericardial or joint fluid occasionally is necessary.

Although not a true complication, complement deficiency can be detected in 8% of adults and children who have meningococcal disease. These patients are at high risk for recurrent episodes of invasive infection. Mayatepek et al[17] detected a terminal complement component abnormality in 26.6% of patients who had meningococcal disease caused by the uncommon serotypes Y and W135. Similarly, the rate of deafness in patients infected with uncommon serotypes is increased significantly compared with those who had disease caused by the group B meningococcus (26.6% versus 3.3%). Based on this information, screening for complement deficiencies with a total hemolytic complement assay should be considered in any pediatric patient who has meningococcal disease.

DISEASE CONTROL AND PREVENTION

Antimicrobial chemoprophylaxis is an integral component in the control of meningococcal disease. Several studies have demonstrated that household, child care, and preschool contacts of patients who have invasive disease have a rate of infection approximately 100 to 800 times that in the general population.[9] In addition, 50% of secondary cases occur within 5 days of the index case and 70% within 1 week. Rifampin is 90% effective in eliminating carriage of the meningococcus from the nasopharynx. In addition, the recent Centers for Disease Control and Prevention surveillance study did not detect any resistance to rifampin in isolates from disease cases. Based on these data, the American Academy of Pediatrics and the Canadian Paediatric Society recommend that all household, child care, or preschool contacts or anyone directly exposed to a patient's secretions be given rifampin within 24 hours of recognition of the primary case.[8] The dosage is 10 mg/kg per dose (maximum adult dose is 600 mg) every 12 hours for 2 days for children older than 1 month of age and 5 mg/kg per dose every 12 hours for 2 days for infants younger than 1 month of age.

Newer agents being evaluated for use in chemoprophylactic regimens include ceftriaxone and ciprofloxacin. Schwartz et al[21] demonstrated that a single 250-mg dose of intramuscular ceftriaxone was 97% effective at eliminating nasopharyngeal carriage of group A meningococcus. Although ceftriaxone is not recommended for widespread chemoprophylactic use, this regimen has the advantage of being safe for pregnant women. Several studies also have shown that use of ciprofloxacin results in a greater than 90% meningococcal carrier reduction.[27] Although not approved for children or pregnant women, ciprofloxacin can be used in older adolescents and young adults and has the advantage of being administered as a single oral 500-mg dose.

Another important aspect of disease control and prevention is vaccination. A quadrivalent meningococcal vaccine, composed of purified capsular polysaccharide of meningococcal groups A, C, Y, and W135, is licensed for use in the United States. The dose for adults and children is 0.5 ml administered as a single dose subcutaneously. The American Academy of Pediatrics and the Advisory Committee on Immunization Practices of the Centers for Disease Control and Prevention recommend routine vaccination only for those individuals at high risk of contracting meningococcal disease either through travel to highly endemic areas such as sub-Saharan Africa or via altered host defenses such as individuals who have asplenia or complement deficiencies. In 1997, the American College Health Association recommended consideration of meningococcal vaccination for all college students as a result of outbreaks of serogroup C meningococcal disease on college campuses. Vaccination is a key component of outbreak control and has been used in selected areas in the United States and Canada for this purpose. The immunity induced by vaccination is serogroup specific; therefore, no cross-reactive antibody to other serogroups is produced by this vaccine. In general, protective antibody levels are achieved 10 to 14 days after administration, and the vaccine can be given concurrently with other immunizations if necessary. Adverse reactions are mild and infrequent, and usually are limited to local reactions.

The group A polysaccharide vaccine is safe, immunogenic, and efficacious in protecting against epidemic disease among adults and children as young as 3 months. Although not a major cause of disease in the United States, serogroup A is responsible for the majority of epidemic disease worldwide and for most cases of disease in the meningitis belt of Africa. Group C vaccine is neither immunogenic nor efficacious in children younger than 2 years of age. Efficacy is 90% or more in adults, and this vaccine has been very useful in controlling outbreaks in the military. Group Y and W135 vaccines are safe and immunogenic in adults and children older than age 2 years. Unfortunately, no vaccine is available for protection from group B meningococcal disease. The group B capsule is not immunogenic in humans and has been found to share cross-reacting antigens with human neural tissue. Attempts to create vaccine by using outer membrane proteins are being investigated.

REFERENCES

1. Alvez F, et al: Effect of chemoprophylaxis on the meningococcal carrier state after systemic infection, *Pediatr Infect Dis J* 10:700, 1991.
2. Baxter P, Priestley B: Meningococcal rash, *Lancet* 1:1166, 1988.
3. Best C, et al: Early haemo-diafiltration in meningococcal septicaemia, *Lancet* 347:202, 1996.
4. Brandtzaeg P, et al: Plasma endotoxin as a predictor of multiple organ failure and death in systemic meningococcal disease, *J Infect Dis* 159: 195, 1989.
5. Cartwright KAV, Stuart JM, Robinson PM: Meningococcal carriage in close contacts of cases, *Epidemiol Infect* 106:133, 1991.
6. Cartwright KAV, et al: Influenza A and meningococcal disease, *Lancet* 338:554, 1991.
7. Centers for Disease Control and Prevention: Summary of notifiable diseases, US 1997, *MMWR* 46:1, 1998.
8. Committee on Infectious Diseases, American Academy of Pediatrics; Infectious Diseases and Immunization Committee, Canadian Paediatric Society: Meningococcal disease prevention and control strategies for practice-based physicians, *Pediatrics* 97:404, 1996.
9. De Wals P, et al: Meningococcal disease in Belgium: secondary attack rate among household, day-care nursery and pre-elementary school contacts, *J Infect* 3:53, 1981.
10. Derkx HHF, et al: Meningococcal disease: a comparison of eight severity scores in 125 children, *Intensive Care Med* 22:1433, 1996.
11. Edwards MS, Baker CJ: Complications and sequelae of meningococcal infections in children, *J Pediatr* 99:540, 1981.
12. Fourrier F, et al: Meningococcemia and purpura fulminans in adults: acute deficiencies of proteins C and S and early treatment with antithrombin III concentrates, *Intensive Care Med* 16:121, 1990.
13. Giroir BP, et al: Preliminary evaluation of recombinant amino-terminal fragment of human bactericidal/permeability-increasing protein in children with severe meningococcal sepsis, *Lancet* 350:1439, 1997.
14. Goldman AP, et al: Extracorporeal support for intractable cardiorespiratory failure due to meningococcal disease, *Lancet* 349:466, 1997.
15. Irazuzta J, McManus ML: Use of topically applied nitroglycerin in the treatment of purpura fulminans, *J Pediatr* 117:993, 1990.

16. Kirsch EA, et al: Pathophysiology, treatment and outcome of meningococcemia: a review and recent experience, *Pediatr Infect Dis J* 15:967, 1996.
17. Mayatepek E, et al: Deafness, complement deficiencies and immunoglobulin status in patients with meningococcal diseases due to uncommon serogroups, *Pediatr Infect Dis J* 12:808, 1993.
18. Monsalve F, et al: Myocardial depression in septic shock caused by meningococcal infection, *Crit Care Med* 12:1021, 1984.
19. Powars DR, et al: Purpura fulminans in meningococcemia: association with acquired deficiencies of proteins C and S, *N Engl J Med* 317:571, 1987.
20. Rivard GE, et al: Treatment of purpura fulminans in meningococcemia with protein C concentrate, *J Pediatr* 126:646, 1995.
21. Schwartz B, et al: Comparative efficacy of ceftriaxone and rifampicin in eradicating pharyngeal carriage of group A *Neisseria meningitidis, Lancet* 1:1239, 1988.
22. Stiehm ER, Damrosch DS: Factors in the prognosis of meningococcal infection: review of 63 cases with emphasis on recognition and management of the severely ill patient, *J Pediatr* 68:457, 1966.
23. Tesoro LJ, Selbst SM: Factors affecting outcome in meningococcal infections, *Am J Dis Child* 145:218, 1991.
24. Thomson APJ, Sills JA, Hart CA: Validation of the Glasgow meningococcal septicemia prognostic score: a 10-year retrospective survey, *Crit Care Med* 19:26, 1991.
25. Tobias JD, et al: Use of continuous caudal block to relieve lower-extremity ischemia caused by vasculitis in a child with meningococcemia, *J Pediatr* 115:1019, 1989.
26. Toews WH, Bass JW: Skin manifestations of meningococcal infection: an immediate indicator of prognosis, *Am J Dis Child* 127:173, 1974.
27. Visakorpi R: Ciprofloxacin in meningococcal carriers, *Scand J Infect Dis Suppl* 60:108, 1989.
28. Waage A, Halstensen A, Espevik T: Association between tumour necrosis factor in serum and fatal outcome in patients with meningococcal disease, *Lancet* 1:355, 1987.
29. Wong VK, Hitchcock W, Mason WH: Meningococcal infections in children: a review of 100 cases, *Pediatr Infect Dis J* 8:224, 1989.
30. Zenz W, et al: Treatment of fulminant meningococcemia with recombinant tissue plasminogen activator, *Thromb Haemost* 74:802, 1995.

292 Pneumothorax and Pneumomediastinum

David I. Bromberg • Michael Milobsky

Pneumothorax and pneumomediastinum are defined as the presence of air in the potential pleural or mediastinal spaces, respectively. These conditions are relatively rare in pediatric patients, having their greatest incidence in the neonatal period. However, in several clinical situations, pneumothorax is a serious complication, and failure to recognize its presence could result in serious morbidity. Pneumothorax may play a prominent role (1) in the neonatal period; (2) as a complication of specific respiratory diseases, especially asthma and cystic fibrosis; (3) as a complication of mechanical ventilation; (4) as a result of trauma; and (5) when it occurs spontaneously.

The classic studies of Macklin and Macklin[1] have helped elucidate the mechanism of pneumothorax and pneumomediastinum. When a pressure gradient exists between the alveolus and interstitial tissue (usually as a result of high inspiratory pressures), alveolar rupture may result, with escape of air into the perivascular interstitium. This accumulation of air travels along the vascular ray (seen clinically as pulmonary interstitial emphysema) to the surface of the lung or to the mediastinum and eventually may result in a pneumothorax or pneumomediastinum. The entities, then, of pulmonary interstitial emphysema, pneumothorax, and pneumomediastinum all are expressions of a single pathological process.

The clinical manifestation varies with the extent of disease. Pain almost universally is present. As the size of the pneumothorax increases, tachypnea, dyspnea, and cyanosis may occur. Physical findings also vary from a normal examination to the presence of hyperresonance to percussion, the absence of breath sounds, and a mediastinal shift to the opposite side of the thorax.

When air enters the pleural space through a ball valve mechanism, a tension pneumothorax is produced. The pneumothorax increases in size, with each inspiration greatly reducing lung volume. Clinical findings in addition to severe and progressive tachypnea, dyspnea, and cyanosis may include shock. This constitutes an emergency in which thoracentesis can be lifesaving.

Pneumothorax has been demonstrated by radiological studies to occur in between 1% and 2% of all newborns. Some of these, undoubtedly, are related to overaggressive resuscitation, but others have been shown to occur spontaneously. Fewer than 50% of the total number are symptomatic. The incidence of pneumothorax is much greater in neonates who have pulmonary disease, especially hyaline membrane disease, meconium aspiration, and pulmonary hypoplasia. An increased incidence of renal anomalies in association with neonatal pneumothorax and pneumomediastinum has been noted.

Pneumothorax in older children, rather than occurring spontaneously, is seen as a complication of an underlying pulmonary disease or as a result of trauma or mechanical ventilation. Although rare, it has been reported in conjunction with asthma, cystic fibrosis, pneumonia (especially staphylococcal), and tuberculosis. Any entity that pathologically includes interstitial emphysema may progress to include pneumothorax or pneumomediastinum as well. In a study of patients hospitalized with asthma, more than 5% were found to have pneumomediastinum, with the incidence increasing to greater than 15% among patients older than 10 years of age. The therapeutic significance of this is clear, contraindicating the use of positive-pressure breathing in these patients. In thoracic trauma cases, many patients have pneumothorax, which usually is apparent. These patients may have tension or "sucking" pneumothoraces and require immediate attention.

In late adolescence and young adulthood, in addition to the causes listed above, spontaneous pneumothorax becomes a significant entity, occurring predominantly in otherwise healthy males who have no known underlying respiratory disease. These individuals are believed to have a pulmonary or pleural site of structural weakness or abnormality, but this seldom is proved. Activity levels appear to have little correlation with the onset of symptoms, which may begin while the patient is at rest. Fewer than 20% have a recurrence; those who do frequently have the ipsilateral side involved within a year of the initial attack.

The diagnosis of pneumothorax and pneumomediastinum should be entertained seriously in patients who fall into the clinical categories discussed and who manifest sudden onset of sharp chest pain. Confirmation is made by obtaining posteroanterior and lateral chest roentgenograms and demonstrating the presence of free pleural or mediastinal air. Quantification of the pneumothorax also should be attempted. In the neonatal nursery, fiberoptic transillumination has proved a valuable adjunctive tool for the rapid bedside diagnosis of pneumomediastinum and pneumothorax.

Iatrogenic causes of pneumothorax also must be considered. Pneumothorax can occur as a complication of tracheostomy, internal jugular puncture, subclavian vein line insertion, and mechanical ventilation. When a patient is given pressurized oxygen, care must be taken to ensure that the system is vented, or a tension pneumothorax could result.

Therapy depends on the size of the lesion, the cause, and the clinical status of the patient. In neonates, most pneumothoraces are managed with the insertion of a thoracostomy tube attached to a water seal. In symptomatic patients who have underlying pulmonary disease, needle aspiration of the pneumothorax is attempted while continuing to direct therapy toward the primary disease. If air reaccumulates in the pleural space, insertion of a thoracostomy tube connected to a water seal is indicated. The therapeutic approach to spontaneous pneumothorax usually is conservative. In the patient who is asymptomatic but has a minor pneumothorax, observation alone is sufficient. In the case of larger lesions, the physician should perform thoracentesis, removing as much air as possible. In cases of spontaneous pneumothorax without an identifiable cause, the patient and family should be reassured that the initial therapy is curative and that the majority of patients will not have recurrences.

After resolution, no activity reduction is indicated. Pneumomediastinum rarely produces symptoms. When this lesion becomes large enough to produce respiratory or circulatory distress, aspiration under fluoroscopic control is indicated. General supportive care is of the utmost importance in managing both lesions and should include adequate pain control and cough suppression when necessary.

REFERENCE

1. Macklin MI, Macklin CC: Malignant interstitial emphysema of the lungs and mediastinum as an important occult complication in many respiratory diseases and other conditions: an interpretation of the clinical literature in the light of laboratory experiment, *Medicine* 23:281, 1944.

SUGGESTED READINGS

DeVries WC, Wolfe WG: The management of spontaneous pneumothorax and bullous emphysema, *Surg Clin North Am* 60:851, 1980.

Melton LJ, Hepper NGG, Offord KP: Influence of height on the risk of spontaneous pneumothorax, *Mayo Clin Proc* 56:678, 1981.

Peters JI: When to suspect—and how to treat—a pneumothorax, *J Respir Dis* 7:17, 1986.

Pollack MM, Fields AI, Holbrook PR: Pneumothorax and pneumomediastinum during pediatric mechanical ventilation, *Crit Care Med* 7:536, 1979.

293 Poisoning

Teresa M. Herbert • Michael L. Weitzman

EPIDEMIOLOGY

Ingestion of potentially toxic substances is a common pediatric problem. Of the 2.2 million reports of ingestion received in 1997 by the American Association of Poison Control Centers (AAPCC), 1.5 million (67%) of exposures occurred in children. Fifty-two percent of the children were younger than 6 years of age, with 39% less than three years old. In younger children, ingestion usually is accidental, resulting from the natural curiosity, increasing mobility, and indiscriminate oral gratification displayed by this age group. The morbidity and mortality in this high-incidence age group is small; only 23% of reported ingestions among children younger than 6 years of age resulted in any symptoms and there were 25 deaths.[10] In the adolescent and the adult, the ingestion of a potentially toxic substance generally is the result of a willful act (i.e., attempted murder or suicide), although the resulting toxicity may be unintentional (e.g., adverse experience with an illicit drug). More than 60% of adolescent ingestions are symptomatic, and poisoning deaths in adolescents and adults are not unusual.

Significant morbidity and mortality occur in both age groups as a result of therapeutic misuse of medications. This may be accidental, as in the administration of multiple doses to a child by the two parents, each unaware of the actions of the other, or intentional, excessive dosage administration to achieve an enhanced therapeutic effect (e.g., fever reduction with aspirin or acetaminophen, antienuretic effect with imipramine).

Categories of agents most frequently involved in childhood poisonings are medications (32%), caustics and cleaning agents (11%), cosmetics (13%), plants (7%), insecticides or pesticides (4%), and hydrocarbons (3%). A significant incidence of exposure does not imply resultant toxicity; most ingested cosmetics and plants, for example, are harmless. The major categories of agents responsible for fatal poisoning among children younger than 6 years of age reported by the AAPCC from 1988 through 1992 are medications (53%), carbon monoxide inhalation (14%), hydrocarbons (11%), insecticides or pesticides (7%), and caustics or cleaning agents (7%). Iron-containing medications, psychotropic agents (including tricyclic antidepressants), and analgesics (salicylates and acetaminophen) in rank order account for almost 70% of the fatal medication ingestions among children younger than 6 years of age.

Over the past 30 years, mortality from accidental poisoning and the agents involved in poisoning episodes have changed significantly. Currently, mortality in the preschool-age child is about 10% of the rate during the mid-1960s. The causes for this decline generally are believed to include child-resistant closures (although the declining death rate clearly antedated implementation of the Poison Prevention Packaging Act of 1970), increased public awareness, improved diagnosis and management of the poisoned child, and a decreased need for certain highly toxic substances (e.g., kerosene, lye) in the home. Aspirin used to be the substance ingested most frequently by children, but the prevalence of aspirin ingestion has declined both absolutely and as a percentage of total ingestions. Fatalities from salicylates have declined more than tenfold, with the downward trend accelerating since the early 1980s when the link between aspirin and Reye's syndrome resulted in a rapid decline in aspirin use in children. Childhood ingestions of iron-containing medications and psychotropic agents each account for more than three times as many fatalities as does aspirin.

Males predominate slightly in early-childhood ingestions, whereas females predominate in adolescent ingestions. Family stress, social isolation, poor parenting skills, and maternal depression are among the family variables that predispose to accidental early childhood poisonings. They tend to occur at times of family disorganization, with deviations from normal routines (e.g., household moving, spring cleaning, vacation, or holidays), and during times of family stress (e.g., sickness, death, or divorce). Recidivism is high, with estimates ranging from 10% to 40%.

The majority of early-childhood ingestions occur in the child's home. The homes of grandparents who have medications of significant toxicity (e.g., cardiovascular medications and psychotropic agents) and a potential lower level of vigilance and "child proofing" also is a common site of ingestions. Ingestions occur most frequently in the kitchen, where cleansing products, polishing fluids, and other toxic household products are stored beneath the sink or on easily accessible lower cabinet shelves. The bathroom also is a common site for an accidental ingestion; agents involved most frequently are medications and cosmetics. Improper storage of solvents and cleaning agents in drinking glasses, cups, or beverage bottles also are contributing factors.

PREVENTION

Every child is at risk for toxic ingestions, so effective prevention is directed toward the environment of all children and in most instances requires parental compliance. The only preventive measure of proved efficacy is societal intervention through the legislated requirement of child-resistant closures for toxic household products and drugs.

Appropriate selection of products to be stored in a household that has young children, selection of reasonable sites of storage, and prompt, proper disposal of unnecessary toxic materials are facets of the protective parental obligation. The environment may be rendered safer by the use of locked cabinets or boxes for all drugs and toxic household products. All drugs and household products should be kept in their original containers. Materials no longer required should be discarded in a manner that precludes access by the child, such as flushing them down the toilet. Certain compounds can be fatal to an average size toddler when 1 to 2 teaspoons or capsules are ingested. Highly toxic medications; camphor, chloroquine, desipramine, hydroxychloroquine, imipramine, methyl salicylate, and quinine require special safeguarding. Other highly toxic substances commonly found around the home include acetonitrile (artificial finger-nail remover), ammonium fluoride (wheel-cleaner, derusting agent), selenious acid (gun bluing compound), and brodifacoum ("superwarfarin").[4]

Advising parents and caretakers of children about safe storage and disposal and alerting parents to the dangers of failing to supervise children during periods of family stress are recommended anticipatory guidance practices. In addition, the physician should provide educational materials in the office, participate in community education programs, limit prescribed drugs to necessary quantities, and instruct parents to use the entire prescribed quantities.

PRINCIPLES OF MANAGEMENT

General Considerations

The pediatrician should be able to deal effectively with the vast majority of acute ingestions. To facilitate this care, specific textbooks on poisonings should be readily available in the office library. Two excellent books are *Clinical Toxicology of Commercial Products* by Gosselin et al[6] and *Clinical Management of Poisoning and Drug Overdose* by Haddad and Winchester.[8] The POISINDEX system,[13] a poison information software package, is widely available in emergency treatment facilities. The POISINDEX system can be accessed by most office computers.

Prompt removal of the offending agent can obviate the need for future treatment and may ameliorate subsequent developing symptoms. Cleansing from the skin any toxins that can produce a local effect or that can be absorbed cutaneously is accomplished easily in the home or office. Prompt gastric evacuation with syrup of ipecac to induce emesis and administration of an adsorbent, such as activated charcoal, or of a demulcent, such as evaporated milk or milk of magnesia, can be accomplished in the home or office. Further definitive treatment of seriously poisoned children is accomplished more easily in the hospital or emergency facility.

The physician should be familiar with and have ready access to community resources that may provide information or practical help with acute poisonings. A hospital emergency room or treatment facility should be readily available for the transfer of patients who are in need of care beyond that available in the office. Poison control centers are an excellent source of information on management of ingestions. From 1953 to 1970, local poison control centers were established throughout the United States; improved data retrieval and communication technologies during the 1970s led to regionalization and by 1997 about 93% of the U.S. population was served by poison control centers of the AAPCC. These regional centers offer comprehensive information 24 hours a day, toll-free telephone access, and access to a regional treatment facility for patient referral. Protocols for giving advice are used for the initial management of consumer calls.

Poison control centers can help in the identification of an unknown ingestion. Pharmacists can also provide information about medications when the name of the medication or the amount dispensed does not appear on the label. Similarly, manufacturers may need to be called to determine the ingredients in a household product. A list of many manufacturers with their addresses and telephone numbers can be found in *Clinical Toxicology of Commercial Products*.[6]

Telephone Calls

Most poisoning episodes are handled over the telephone. The person answering the telephone needs to be calm and firmly directive. Initially, the practitioner needs to determine the agent, the quantity ingested, the weight of the child, and the presence or absence of symptoms. From this information, the risk of toxicity can be determined. This depends on the relative toxicity of the agent involved and the amount of the agent ingested. Alternatively, the presence of symptoms may suggest that toxicity is a risk, despite neither the agent nor the amount ingested seeming to be toxic.

If no toxic risk is present, the appropriate response is reassurance. If, however, a toxic risk exists, further data must be collected before advice can be given. The resources available to the caller need to be identified, such as the presence of first-aid drugs in the home (e.g., syrup of ipecac) or the proximity to a pharmacy or to a hospital and whether transportation is readily available. Using this information, the practitioner can recommend appropriate management.

Poisoning and injury prevention should be discussed with the parents within a few days of such a call; experience has shown that addressing prevention at the time of the initial call is less effective than doing so later. A recent accidental ingestion focuses the minds of the parents, providing a valuable opportunity to impart advice on poison prevention.

Approach to the Symptomatic Patient

Diagnosing poisoning in patients who are symptomatic can be difficult when an ingestion has not been observed. Although some poisons produce characteristic signs and symptoms, most do not; they may simulate many acute illnesses seen in pediatrics. The physician always should consider the possibility of poisoning when faced with a puzzling situation in which the diagnosis is not clear. The rapid onset of central nervous system (CNS), gastrointestinal, or respiratory symptoms should alert the physician to ask about medications or toxins within the home. Unexplained signs of CNS stimulation, such as delirium or convulsions, or of CNS depression, such as stupor or coma, should be considered to result from poisoning until proved otherwise. The presence of hyperpnea in a child or a young infant who has a febrile illness may be caused by the overzealous use of salicylates by the parents. A characteristic odor of specific poisons on the breath or in the vomitus sometimes can be discerned.

Therapeutic Modalities

The important principles of management of acute poisonings are (1) elimination of the poison from the body, (2) adsorption and inactivation of the poison, (3) administration of specific antidotes, and (4) provision of supportive measures. A calm and reasoned approach is far more effective than overtreatment with stimulants, depressants, or antidotes. Heroic measures are not needed with most poisoning episodes.

Syrup of ipecac has long been recommended to induce vomiting when an ingestion has occurred. Its main advantage is that it is readily available in most homes, so it may be administered within a short time of an ingestion. Although ipecac induces vomiting in the majority of patients, experimental studies have shown a highly variable response in the recovery of ingested material (from 17.5% to 62%) when administered within the first hour after ingestion. Ipecac should not be administered for caustic ingestions, most hydrocarbon ingestions, and antiemetic ingestions. It should not be given when the patient manifests neurological symptoms (depressed level of consciousness, seizures) or has a rapidly deteriorating clinical picture. Infants younger than 6 months of age have a poorly developed gag reflex and should not receive syrup of ipecac. Close medical observation is required when syrup of ipecac is administered to infants 6 to 9 months of age. Ipecac may delay the administration or reduce the effectiveness of activated charcoal. While ipecac-induced emesis has the temporal advantage of immediate home administration, there are insufficient data to support or exclude ipecac administration soon after poison ingestion. The American Academy of Pediatrics currently is reviewing its recommendations on the use of ipecac in the management of ingestions.

Gastric lavage should be considered if a patient has ingested a potentially life-threatening amount of a poison and the procedure can be performed within 60 minutes of ingestion. In the conscious, alert patient, it has the advantage of being a controlled means of gastric evacuation. Unless a patient is intubated, gastric lavage is contraindicated if airway protective reflexes are lost. It is contraindicated in caustic and most hydrocarbon ingestions. A large-bore plastic catheter should be passed into the stomach, and the stomach should be irrigated with 50 to 200 ml aliquots of isotonic saline until the returns are clear. Tap water should not be used in children because of the danger of producing water intoxication. Before the catheter is withdrawn, activated charcoal may be instilled. On withdrawal, the tube should be either pinched off or the suction maintained to prevent aspiration of material into the lungs.

Activated charcoal is an effective adsorbent for most drugs, including acetaminophen, aspirin, sedative hypnotics, tricyclic antidepressants, stimulants (amphetamines and cocaine), and phenothiazines. It is ineffective in alcohol, cyanide, iron, and other heavy-metal poisonings. Given as a water slurry (20 to 50 g in children, 50 to 100 g in adolescents), it is effective immediately after ingestion and can be given safely by nonprofessionals. In general, charcoal should be administered as soon as possible, preferably within the first hour after the ingestion. Repeated administration of activated charcoal every 3 to 4 hours effectively can "trap" a toxin in the intestinal lumen. Cathartics (sorbitol) may be required because activated charcoal can be constipating. Activated charcoal is contraindicated in caustic ingestions because it is ineffective and will obscure later endoscopic findings; it also should not be used simultaneously with syrup of ipecac because charcoal adsorbs the ipecac, rendering it ineffective. It should be administered after emesis has been induced or lavage completed successfully.

Relatively few effective specific antidotes exist. Oxygen is the specific effective antidote for carbon monoxide poisoning. Naloxone hydrochloride (Narcan) safely and effectively antagonizes the pharmacological effects of natural and synthetic narcotics. Flumazenil improves consciousness in ingestions of benzodiazepine. Specific antibody fragments can reverse the arrhythmias associated with ingestions of digitalis. Ethanol infusion or the new antidote fomepizole[1] effectively blocks the alcohol dehydrogenase conversion of ethylene glycol or methanol to more toxic metabolites. Pyridoxine reduces isoniazid-induced seizure activity. For the treatment of organophosphate poisoning, pralidoxime (2-PAM) is highly effective if used in conjunction with atropine. *N*-acetylcysteine is effective when administered early in severe acetaminophen poisoning. Of the chelating agents used to treat heavy-metal poisonings, deferoxamine mesylate (Desferal) is specific for iron poisoning; dimercaprol (BAL) combines with arsenic, bismuth, lead, and mercury; and calcium EDTA chelates cadmium, copper, iron, and lead. Methylene blue may be lifesaving in drug-induced methemoglobinemia; sodium thiosulfate and inhalation of amyl nitrate combined with intravenous sodium nitrite (both of which may cause methemoglobinemia) may be lifesaving in cyanide poisoning. Fresh-frozen plasma and repeated doses of vitamin K may be required to counteract the anticoagulant properties brodifacoum. Vitamin K rarely is required when coumarin or warfarin is ingested, because repeated ingestions over a period of days are necessary to produce toxicity.

When an ionizable drug has been ingested, intracellular and CNS drug levels may be reduced and renal excretion increased by therapy directed toward achieving "ion trapping." Ionizable drugs, such as amphetamine, phencyclidine, salicylate, and phenobarbital, cross lipid membranes (the cell wall or blood-brain barrier) only in the nonionized state. Gradients in pH across the membrane "trap" the ionized drug in the milieu, favoring dissociation. A more alkaline pH favors dissociation (and hence, ion trapping) of weakly acidic drugs (e.g., phenobarbital, salicylate); a relatively acidic milieu favors higher concentrations of weakly basic drugs (e.g., amphetamines, phencyclidine). Occasionally in acute salicylism, and almost invariably in chronic salicylism, potassium depletion (with or without hypokalemia) precludes the excretion of an alkaline urine. Drugs with a small volume of distribution, such as salicylates, theophylline derivatives, and amphetamines can be "cleansed" from the body by hemodialysis, charcoal hemoperfusion, exchange transfusion, or peritoneal dialysis. Drugs that have high degrees of tissue binding and a high degree of distribution, such as digoxin and phenothiazines, are removed poorly by those techniques.

Supportive therapy is the mainstay of treatment in most intoxications. This consists of protecting the airway, supporting respiration, administering intravenous fluids, and treating symptoms such as shock, convulsions, temperature instability, cardiac arrhythmias, hypotension, and cerebral edema.

SALICYLATE POISONING

Salicylism is seen in all age groups, including congenital salicylism caused by maternal ingestion of toxic quantities, accidental ingestion in early childhood, and attempted suicide in adolescence and adulthood. Poisoning also can occur following excessive topical application of oil of wintergreen to denuded skin. More than 50% of hospitalized cases of salicylism result from chronic ingestion associated with therapeutic misuse; 25% of patients who have salicylism have an associated intercurrent infection. Oil of wintergreen (1400 mg methyl salicylate/ml) was the cause of the majority of fatal acute salicylate ingestions in children younger than 6 years of age reported from 1989 to 1997.

Laboratory Findings

Diagnosis depends on either eliciting a history of ingestion or recognition of the characteristic clinical findings. A high index of suspicion is necessary in adolescent ingestions. In many cases of deliberate self-harm the patient frequently is unclear or evasive about the agents he or she ingested. A positive urine ferric chloride reaction can confirm salicylate ingestion but not toxic exposure because the test is sensitive to ordinary therapeutic doses. The anion gap usually is elevated. The serum salicylate level confirms the diagnosis. Single acute ingestions of greater than 150 mg/kg generally result in clinical symptoms; acute ingestions greater than 500 mg/kg are potentially fatal. The nomogram introduced by Done[5] (Fig. 293-1) correlates the serum salicylate level with the time since ingestion and is essential to assessment of clinical severity following ingestion of a single dose. The serum salicylate level is of limited value in assessing clinical severity when the drug has been administered repeatedly or ingested chronically. The clinical picture of salicylism is characterized by tinnitus, vomiting, hyperpnea, and dehydration. Salicylism should be considered in the diagnosis of cryptogenic metabolic acidosis, particularly in the 18-month to 4-year age group.

Clinical Findings

The major toxic effects of salicylate are (1) local gastrointestinal irritation, (2) direct stimulation of the CNS respiratory center, (3) increased metabolic rate, (4) interference with carbohydrate metabolism through the inhibition of several Krebs cycle enzymes and the uncoupling of oxidative phosphorylation, and (5) interference with normal blood coagulation mechanisms.

The net disturbance in hydrogen ion concentration in salicylism is the product of two simultaneously occurring challenges to acid-base homeostasis. CNS-mediated inappropriate hyperpnea may lead to respiratory alkalosis. Deranged

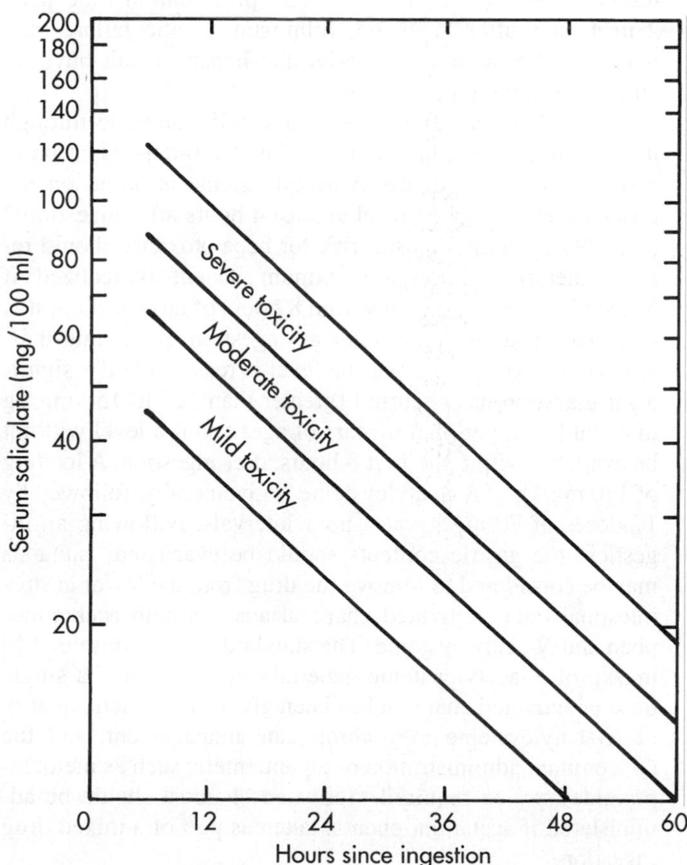

Fig. 293-1 Done nomogram for estimating the severity of poisoning after a single acute salicylate ingestion. (Modified from Done AK: *Pediatrics* 26:800, 1960.)

carbohydrate metabolism and dehydration are potent stimuli for metabolic acidosis. In children younger than 4 years of age, metabolic acidosis generally predominates clinically; in older children and adults, however, the patient frequently has respiratory alkalosis. Profound acidemia among older children and adults heralds a poor prognosis. Hyperthermia, resulting from the increased and dysregulated metabolic state, is common.

The clinical findings of hyperglycemia, hyperpnea, polyuria, glucosuria, and ketonuria early in the course of intoxication simulate diabetic ketoacidosis closely. In salicylism, however, blood glucose exceeding 200 mg/dl is unusual. Hypoglycemia may supervene as glycogen stores are depleted. Dehydration causing decreased renal blood flow often results in oliguria later in the course. Hypokalemia is common, and total body stores of potassium often are depleted.

Therapy

Therapy has three objectives: (1) prevention of further salicylate absorption, (2) correction of existent solute and fluid deficits, and (3) reduction of tissue salicylate levels. Further salicylate absorption is prevented by removing salicylate from the gastrointestinal tract through lavage or induced emesis and by binding the medication within the gastrointestinal lumen through the repeated administration of activated charcoal.

The initial consideration in fluid therapy is the establishment of an adequate circulating fluid volume. In the presence of shock or impending shock, an isotonic solution should be administered at a rate of 20 ml/kg/hr. This may be continued safely a second hour in the absence of improved tissue perfusion. Blood pressure, pulse, capillary filling, and in extreme circumstances, central venous pressure are effective monitors of adequate volume expansion.

The correction of existent solute and water deficits may require total fluid volumes from 115 ml/kg/24 hr to 250 ml/kg/24 hr. A solution containing 40 to 50 mEq/L of sodium should be used. A urine volume of 2000 ml/m^2/day and a specific gravity less than 1.010 (300 mmol/liter) are reasonable goals.

Both hypokalemia and hypoglycemia can present life-threatening situations. A minimum of 25 mEq/L of potassium should be included once adequate renal function has been established; all intravenous fluids should include a minimum of 5 g/dl of glucose; with hypoglycemia or neurological symptomatology, the use of 10 g/dl of glucose should be considered. Correction of acidemia and hypokalemia is essential to the lowering of tissue salicylate levels; the establishment of an alkaline urine dramatically increases urine salicylate excretion. Sufficient bicarbonate should be administered intravenously to raise the urine pH to 8. Although a forced alkaline diuresis is ideal, diuresis in the absence of alkalinization is not effective in eliminating salicylates, and alkalinization of the urine may be difficult to achieve during a rapid diuresis.

Peritoneal dialysis and hemodialysis are effective therapies for serum salicylate values in excess of 100 mg/dl, coma, renal insufficiency, refractory acidosis, or failure of response to conservative therapy.

ACETAMINOPHEN

Ingestion of acetaminophen is a common cause of death among adults and adolescents who have suicidal intent. A widespread lack of appreciation of the toxicity of acetaminophen and the frequent delay in onset of symptoms increase the potential for fatal outcomes in adolescent suicide gestures. Although nearly 60% of the acetaminophen ingestions reported by the AAPCC in 1996 and 1997 occurred in children younger than 6 years of age, less than 1% of the fatalities reported were in that age range. Fatal ingestions in young children are the result of therapeutic misuse.

More than 90% of an ingested acetaminophen load is inactivated in the liver through conjugation with sulfate or glucuronide. A third hepatic metabolic pathway dependent on cytochrome P-450 detoxifies acetaminophen through conjugation with glutathione. This pathway produces a variety of hepatotoxic metabolites from acetaminophen if the hepatic glutathione reserves are depleted. A diminished toxic state occurs in children younger than 6 years of age as a result of relatively increased glutathione stores or lessened metabolic detoxification by the P-450 pathway. Comparable toxic doses are five to ten times more likely to be hepatotoxic in the child older than 6 years of age.

Clinical Findings and Therapy

During the first 24 hours after ingestion, the child who has toxic plasma levels of acetaminophen may have anorexia, nausea, and vomiting. A latent period follows during which gastrointestinal symptoms resolve concurrent with evolving liver function abnormalities in the untreated individual. The transaminases, bilirubin levels, and prothrombin time peak 2 to 4 days after ingestion; fulminant hepatic failure may intervene. Children who survive the hepatic insult have no clinical or pathological sequelae.

N-acetylcysteine functions as a specific antidote through its substitution for glutathione in the P-450-dependent pathway. The decision to use *N*-acetylcysteine is based on the plasma acetaminophen level at least 4 hours after ingestion[14] (Fig. 293-2). Individuals at risk for hepatotoxicity should receive therapy. Although maximum benefit is realized if *N*-acetylcysteine is begun within 8 hours of an ingestion, it is indicated up to 24 hours after an ingestion. Beginning therapy without knowing a plasma level is reasonable if a significant ingestion has occurred (greater than 125 to 150 mg/kg in a child younger than 6 years of age) and if a level will not be available within the first 8 hours after ingestion. A loading of 140 mg/kg of *N*-acetylcysteine is given orally, followed by 17 doses of 70 mg/kg at 4-hour intervals. Following an ingestion, the gastric contents should be evacuated; catharsis may be considered to remove the drug from the lower gastrointestinal tract. Activated charcoal adsorbs both acetaminophen and *N*-acetylcysteine. The standard loading dose of 140 mg/kg of *N*-acetylcysteine generally is sufficient if a single dose of activated charcoal has been given. The emetic quality of *N*-acetylcysteine may complicate management, and the concomitant administration of an antiemetic such as metoclopramide may be required. Activated charcoal should be administered if acetaminophen is taken as part of a mixed drug ingestion.

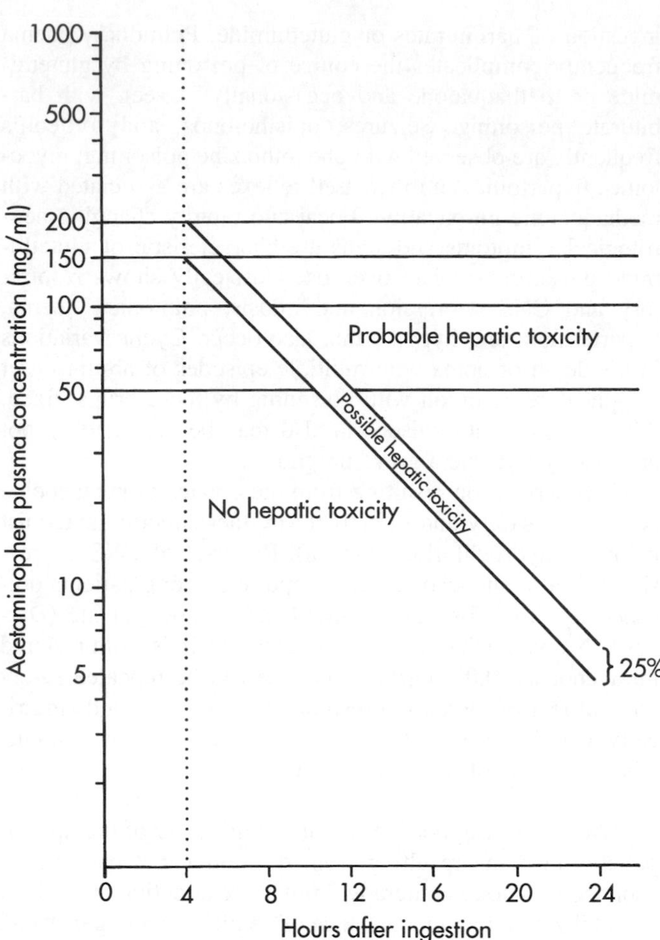

Fig. 293-2 Rumack-Matthew nomogram for estimating the probability of hepatic toxicity after a single acute acetaminophen ingestion. The lower solid diagonal line is placed 25% below the upper solid diagonal line, which divides the "no hepatic toxicity" area. This allows for potential errors in estimating the time after ingestion of the acetaminophen and potential errors in the measurement of acetaminophen plasma levels.

(Modified from Rumack BH, Matthew H: *Pediatrics* 55:871, 1975.)

ORGANOPHOSPHATES

Pesticides continue to be a source of serious poisoning among children in both rural and urban settings. The particular substance or the particular chemical group into which it falls must be identified. Standard references are invaluable in this regard.[6]

Organophosphates account for most reported pesticide exposures and most deaths from such exposures. These insecticides, with few exceptions, are highly toxic to humans. Because organophosphates are readily absorbed from the skin, lungs, and gastrointestinal tract, they need not be ingested to cause symptoms of toxicity. Contaminated clothing can lead to symptoms.

Organophosphate insecticides and their metabolic byproducts inhibit acetylcholinesterase. The result is the accumulation of unhydrolyzed acetylcholine. This causes excessive and continued stimulation and then depression of the parasympathetic nervous system, the somatic motor nerves, and the CNS.

Clinical Findings

The clinical manifestations of organophosphate poisoning are protean. Stimulation of the autonomic nervous system leads to increased sweating, salivation, and miosis. Bradycardia may develop. Bronchial secretions and bronchial constriction are increased, with resultant cough, dyspnea, and cyanosis. Pulmonary edema may occur. Gastrointestinal symptoms include vomiting, abdominal cramps, and intestinal hypermotility. Effects on striated muscle are evidenced by incoordination, tremors, and weakness, then muscle fasciculations followed by paralysis, particularly of the respiratory muscles. CNS manifestations are headache, confusion, anxiety, emotional lability, ataxia, convulsions, coma, and eventual depression of the respiratory and circulatory centers. Hypotension or hypertension may be seen.

Children who are poisoned commonly exhibit pinpoint pupils, excessive respiratory tract secretions, CNS excitement or depression, and respiratory arrest. The onset of symptoms may be extremely rapid, and death generally occurs within 24 hours. After sublethal doses, with reversal of inhibition of cholinesterase, the symptoms disappear; the rate of recovery varies with different compounds, from a few hours to several weeks.

Proximal limb paralysis and respiratory muscle compromise can occur in occasional patients after the resolution of cholinergic symptoms, the "intermediate syndrome." These patients require appropriate supportive measures. Organophosphates may cause a delayed (1 to 4 weeks after exposure) polyneuropathy accompanied by ataxia and spasticity.

Diagnosis

Once thought of, the diagnosis of organophosphate poisoning is not difficult to make. The diagnosis should be made based on (1) a history of exposure or a reasonable possibility of exposure, (2) the onset of symptoms within 12 hours of exposure, and (3) a clinical picture consistent with this diagnosis. In addition, these insecticides have a disagreeable garliclike odor, and children who have been poisoned may have a garliclike odor on their clothes or breath. This diagnosis can be confirmed by determining depression of serum and red blood cell cholinesterase levels at presentation. Although serum concentrations (pseudocholinesterase) are measured in most hospitals, many hospitals are not prepared to do the more specific erythrocyte (true cholinesterase) determination. Treatment should be initiated without waiting for laboratory results.

Therapy

Treatment of organophosphate poisoning involves both general measures and specific antidotes. If the skin has been exposed, all clothing should be removed and the skin washed with copious amounts of soap and water. If intoxication has resulted from ingestion, the gastric contents should be emptied. Health care providers should avoid contact with the contaminated clothing, vomitus, or lavage fluid. Activated charcoal adsorbs many of the organophosphates. The upper airway should be cleared of secretions and an airway inserted. Endotracheal intubation and mechanical ventilation may be required to treat respiratory depression. Atropine 0.05 to 0.10 mg/kg should be administered every 10 to 30 minutes until complete atropinization (clearing of excessive oral and pulmonary secretions) and the reversal of cholinergic signs has been achieved. Very large quantities of atropine may be required initially. Atropinization should be maintained intermittently for 24 to 48 hours. Atropine blocks the action of acetylcholine without restoring the action of cholinesterase. After atropinization, in moderate to severe intoxication, pralidoxime (Protopam or 2-PAM), a cholinesterase reactivator, 25 to 50 mg/kg (up to 0.5 to 1 g) should be given intravenously in saline solution over 15 to 30 minutes. The dose may be repeated in 1 to 2 hours if muscular weakness does not resolve and every 6 to 8 hours thereafter if symptoms warrant. Pralidoxime does not cross the blood-brain barrier; reversal of CNS symptoms depends on atropine therapy. Pralidoxime is of minimal benefit if given more than 36 to 48 hours after exposure.

Atropine should be tapered slowly under close observation and reinstituted if symptoms recur. Observation for a minimum of 24 hours is necessary after the cessation of atropine and pralidoxime therapy. Diazepam can help control the agitation and muscle fasciculations.

PSYCHOACTIVE DRUGS

Sedatives, Hypnotics, and Opiates

Clinical findings. CNS depression (e.g., somnolence, stupor, coma) may constitute the presenting signs for patients whose toxicity results from the ingestion of sedatives, hypnotics, anxiolytics, or opiates. There frequently are no distinguishing clinical features. Occasionally a constellation of findings may suggest a specific drug class. Hypotension and respiratory depression are seen frequently following ingestion of toxic quantities of barbiturates or glutethimide; they are observed occasionally with phenothiazine or methaqualone poisoning. Hypothermia usually is associated with the ingestion of barbiturates or glutethimide. Pulmonary edema frequently complicates the course of poisoning by glutethimide or methaqualone and occasionally is seen with barbiturate poisoning. Seizures, opisthotonos, and torticollis frequently are observed with phenothiazine poisoning; myoclonus, hypertonia, and increased reflexes are associated with methaqualone intoxication. Focal and rapidly changing neurological symptoms and signs are characteristic of glutethimide poisoning. Opiate overdose classically shows respiratory and CNS depression and miosis; pulmonary edema, hypertension, and hypothermia also occur. Cyclic variations in the depth of coma with multiple episodes of abrupt onset of apnea are common with poisoning by these drugs; fixed, dilated pupils with anisocoria also may be seen and do not necessarily indicate a grave prognosis.

CNS depression resulting from the opiates or pentazocine is reversed safely and effectively by the narcotic antagonist naloxone hydrochloride (Narcan). Reversal of CNS depression by naloxone also has been reported among patients poisoned by diphenoxylate (Lomotil) and propoxyphene (Darvon). Naloxone has no agonist activity. It is administered intravenously, 0.01 mg/kg; this dose can be repeated safely without fear of increasing respiratory depression and empirically can be used safely and effectively among patients whose coma is of unknown origin.

Therapy. Supportive care is the mainstay of therapy for patients in coma resulting from poisoning that has not responded to naloxone therapy. Immediate attention is directed to stabilization and maintenance of ventilation and perfusion. Patients in coma require intubation. Atelectasis and aspiration pneumonia frequently are complications of coma from poisoning. Gastric lavage late in the course of ingestion-induced coma is hazardous and of questionable efficacy; it should be undertaken only after a protected airway has been carefully secured. Hypotension resulting from barbiturate ingestion generally is caused by decreased peripheral vascular resistance and hypovolemia and usually responds to plasma volume expansion. The frequency of pulmonary edema as a complication of methaqualone or glutethimide poisoning precludes rapid fluid administration in these poisonings in the absence of careful central venous pressure monitoring. In the profoundly ill, comatose, poisoned patient, a central venous pressure monitor is essential. Analeptic drugs are not indicated in the management of poison-induced coma. Forced diuresis, with alkalinization of the urine to achieve ion trapping, is effective in facilitating clearance of phenobarbital but is of no value in treating poisoning from the short-acting barbiturates and is contraindicated in the management of methaqualone poisoning.

Phencyclidine, Amphetamine, and Cocaine

Poisoning by phencyclidine (PCP) is characterized by aggressive, even assaultive, behavior, which may seriously impede evaluation and therapy of the gravely ill patient. Symptoms and signs may include confusion, irritability, hallucinations, tremor, chest pain, palpitations, hypertension, tachycardia, auditory hyperesthesia, sweating, excessive salivation, anxiety, panic, hyperpyrexia, hyperreflexia, and rhabdomyolysis. Coma and convulsions occur with severe poisoning. Psychotic states (which may persist), nystagmus (horizontal or vertical), increased muscle tone (which may be associated with opisthotonos), and fixed staring are prominent features of PCP intoxication.

Amphetamines and cocaine, although structurally different, are powerful CNS stimulants. Abuse of cocaine, particularly the free-base form, "crack," which can be smoked, has reached epidemic proportions. Cocaine deaths reported to the AAPCC more than doubled since the mid-1980s. Severe morbidity or death may occur from high-dose chronic or "binge" use or may occur after a single exposure. Intoxication results in a sense of enhanced energy, which may progress to violent and bizarre behavior, delirium, seizures, paranoia, agitation, and death. Adverse effects include systemic hypertension, tachycardia and other cardiac arrhythmias, hyperthermia, and respiratory depression. Myocardial infarction, stroke, aortic rupture, and rhabdomyolysis have been reported.

Therapy. Immediate therapy includes careful limitation of sensory stimuli and supportive care. Seizures may be difficult to control. Diazepam is the preferred anticonvulsant. Diazoxide or hydralazine is preferred for the management of hypertension. Additional alpha-adrenergic blocking drugs (phentolamine) may be required. Chlorpromazine, highly useful in the treatment of amphetamine poisoning, is contraindicated in PCP intoxication. Amphetamine and PCP levels in the CNS can be reduced and excretion in the urine increased by acidification to achieve ion trapping. Careful monitoring of serum pH, potassium, and ammonia levels is required. In addition, the physician should interrupt the gastroenteric recirculation of PCP by initiating repeated doses of activated charcoal every 3 to 4 hours (independent of the PCP's route of administration).

Date-Rape Drugs: Flunitrazepam, Clonazepam, Gamma Hydroxybutyrate

Designer drugs wax and wane in popularity so the primary care pediatrician needs to be cognizant of current trends, but all produce altered mental status, often with associated amnesia and dissociation. The primary intent of their use may be to get "high;" however, the trend increasingly is to use these substances to assist in sexual assaults. Although flunitrazepam (rohypnol, or "roofies") is not manufactured or sold in the United States, it has been available through black market channels since the early 1990s. Flunitrazepam, a benzodiazepine, enhances the high from low-quality heroin and eases the crack user down from a crack binge. When used with alcohol it produces disinhibition and amnesia.[15] Gamma hydroxybutyrate, a food supplement, is a GABA analogue.

Tricyclic Antidepressants

The widespread use, accessibility, and toxicity of the tricyclic antidepressants imipramine, amitriptyline, nortriptyline, desipramine, amoxapine, maprotiline, protriptyline, and doxepin make these medications the most common cause of fatal ingestion with prescription drugs in individuals younger than 17 years old. The newer tricyclics are used for depression in adults and adolescents; several are used to treat enuresis and hyperkinesis in children. Accidental ingestion and therapeutic misuse predominate in the younger population.

Clinical findings. Patients have anticholinergic effects, such as dry mouth and skin, mydriasis, urinary retention, delayed gastric emptying and intestinal ileus, and hyperthermia. Tricyclic poisoning should be suspected when hypotension and cardiac arrhythmias or coma are present. Evidence of CNS toxicity may include initial excitement that progresses to coma; myoclonus or choreoathetosis, central respiratory depression, and seizures also occur. The primary cause of death in tricyclic overdose is cardiac malfunction; arrhythmias and myocardial depression are common.

Therapy. Initial treatment of tricyclic ingestion is aimed at removing the gastric contents. Lavage rather than emesis is the preferred means of gastric decontamination because of the potential for coma and seizures. The decreased gastric motility secondary to the anticholinergic effects of the ingestion makes gastric decontamination beneficial up to 18 hours after the ingestion. Repeated administration of activated charcoal should follow gastric emptying. All patients should be hospitalized for continuous electrocardiogram (ECG) monitoring, preferably in an intensive care unit. The pharmacokinetics of tricyclic ingestion are complex. Drug levels should not be used as the sole criterion for therapeutic intervention; initial management should be based on the patient's clinical status. A QRS complex of greater than 100 milliseconds is the most reliable indicator of tricyclic toxicity (occurring in patients who have tricyclic levels greater than 1000 ng/ml) and is correlated strongly with the risk of serious arrhythmias, most commonly ventricular tachycardia degenerating into ventricular fibrillation. Life-threatening arrhythmias usually occur within 24 hours of ingestion but can occur as long as 5 days after ingestion. ECG monitoring should continue for at least 24 hours after the resolution of signs of cardiac toxicity (QRS interval less than 100 milliseconds).

Treatment of intoxication is symptomatic and supportive. The mainstay of treatment is alkalinization to a pH of 7.45 to 7.55 with intravenous sodium bicarbonate, which decreases the risk of arrhythmias that are potentiated by acidosis. Ventricular tachycardia or fibrillation should be treated with a 1 to 2 mEq/kg sodium bicarbonate bolus and appropriate resuscitative measures. Direct ventricular pacing may be necessary. Excessive alkalinization (pH > 7.6) is unnecessary and is associated with increased mortality.

Hypotension should be treated with volume expansion. Excessive fluids can result in pulmonary edema because of decreased myocardial contractility. Norepinephrine, dopamine, or dobutamine are recommended as pressor agents if volume therapy is insufficient. Seizures may be difficult to control; they respond best to diazepam followed by phenytoin.

HOUSEHOLD CLEANING AGENTS AND CAUSTICS

Household disinfectants and cleaning agents (e.g., ammonia and bleach, laundry detergent, automatic dishwater detergent, and oven, drain, and toilet cleaners) contain variable amounts of acidic or alkaline caustics. The severity of damage to the oropharynx, esophagus, and stomach upon ingestion depends on the volume and concentration of the caustic and its duration of contact with the mucosal surfaces. The concentration of the caustic must be determined through history, examination of the container, or consultation with a regional poison control center.

Household bleach (sodium hypochlorite), weak ammonia solutions, and phosphate-based laundry detergents usually do not damage tissue but may irritate the mucosa. Industrial-strength ammonia, bleaches, and detergents brought to the home from the work place constitute a significant hazard. Children on farms who have access to industrial-strength liquid alkaline cleaners are a high-risk group. Ecologically sound "low phosphate" detergents containing carbonates and other alkaline agents, such as trisodium phosphate, and dishwater detergents have a high pH and may destroy tissue. Most caustic injuries are caused by ingestion of liquid or particulate alkaline drain or oven cleaners. Recent reductions in the alkali concentration of liquid cleaners to the 8% to 10% range have reduced, but not eliminated, morbidity. Adolescents and adults who ingest caustics with suicidal intent are more likely to have severe burns than are children who have unintentional exposures.

Clinical Findings

Alkali ingestions generally result in greater tissue destruction than do acid ingestions. The bitter taste and instantaneous burning sensation associated with strong acids limit the volume of the ingestion and prompt immediate expectoration. A greater volume of the relatively tasteless liquid alkaline preparation may be swallowed before the child experiences significant distress. Acid mucosal injury results in a coagulation necrosis, with the formation of a dense eschar that tends to limit tissue penetration. The liquefaction necrosis characteristic of an alkali injury permits deep penetration of the alkali through the mucosa, submucosa, and muscular layers of the upper gastrointestinal tract. Acidic agents generally cause greater damage to the gastric mucosa, particularly the lesser curvature and the prepyloric area; alkaline ingestions result in greater damage to the esophagus. Liquid ingestions often produce circumferential burns; particulate ingestion causes spotty or streaklike burns. The intense inflammatory response may cause acute or subacute viscus perforation or stricture formation 14 to 28 days after the ingestion.

The patient may be in severe distress, with drooling, inability or refusal to swallow, abdominal pain, and violent retching. Air hunger and stridor may result from burns and subsequent edema of the glottic structures. Circumferential or patchy burns or ulcerations of the oral mucosa may be present, with edema of the oral and pharyngeal tissues. Significant ingestions may show minimal symptomatology. Esophageal damage with the potential for stricture formation may occur in the complete absence of oral lesions.

Therapy

Management is supportive and expectant. Induction of emesis is contraindicated. The child should be kept upright to minimize vomiting and reflux. If the child is able to swallow, several ounces of water or milk may be given to dilute the poison. Attempts to neutralize an alkali ingestion with a mild acid such as vinegar are contraindicated because the resulting exothermal reaction will result in further tissue damage. Although serious burns are more likely in symptomatic patients, the initial presenting symptoms are not reliably predictive of esophageal injury; endoscopy should be considered in all patients who have a credible history of caustic ingestion. The efficacy of steroids (prednisolone 2 mg/kg/day) to reduce the inflammatory response and subsequent potential for stricture formation is based on anecdotal and retrospective data; controlled prospective studies have shown no benefit. H_2-blockers may be used to suppress gastric acid production and secondary gastric or esophageal acid injury. Parenteral fluid therapy and antibiotics are used as clinically indicated. Bougienage may be used to prevent or dilate strictures. Long-term morbidity results from esophageal or pyloric strictures and the attempts to maintain patency through chronic dilation or surgical reconstruction.

HYDROCARBONS

Hydrocarbon ingestion is a leading cause of death from poisoning with household products. Hydrocarbons include petroleum distillates such as gasoline, kerosene, mineral seal oil, lighter fluids, paint thinners, and pine oil derivatives such as turpentine. Deaths from hydrocarbon poisoning are the result of pulmonary involvement.

Pulmonary Complications

The pulmonary complications of hydrocarbon ingestions are the result of aspiration into the tracheobronchial tree. With significant ingestions, symptoms usually begin within 30 minutes and often are associated with choking, gagging, and vomiting. Signs of pulmonary involvement include grunting respirations; a persistent, nonproductive cough; intercostal retractions; cyanosis; tachypnea; tachycardia; and fever. Rales, rhonchi, or diminished breath sounds may be heard. Frequently, the sensorium is depressed, and the odor of the ingested hydrocarbon can be smelled on the breath. A depressed sensorium signifies hypoxemia. Signs and symptoms of respiratory involvement usually peak in the first 24 hours and then regress over the next 2 to 5 days.

Radiographic Findings

The risk of aspiration depends on the chemical and physical properties of the hydrocarbons ingested. Low surface tension allows a hydrocarbon to spread rapidly over the mucosal surfaces, and low viscosity enables deeper penetration of the fluids into the distal airways. Highly volatile hydrocarbons cause acute chemical pneumonitis. Highly viscous, nonvolatile petroleum distillates such as mineral oil, motor oil, most baby oils, and liquid petrolatum are not aspirated as easily and do not cause chemical pneumonitis unless large amounts are aspirated.

Chest roentgenographic changes can be seen as early as 30 minutes after ingestion. Initially, multiple, small, mottled densities are seen in the perihilar area and may extend into the midlung field. The mottled densities may become confluent and give a picture of consolidation. Lower airway obstruction with air trapping often is evident. Pleural effusions may develop. Occasionally, pneumatoceles form. Correlation between the chest roentgenographic findings and the clinical symptoms is poor. Whereas approximately 75% of patients who have ingested hydrocarbons exhibit roentgenographic evidence of lung involvement, only 25% to 50% of these have respiratory symptoms.

Therapy

Management of hydrocarbon ingestion is nonspecific, symptomatic, and supportive. Because aspiration is the principal hazard, vomiting should not be induced. Gastric lavage is not recommended. (Hydrocarbons that act as carriers for heavy metals or insecticides, as well as certain halogenated or aromatic hydrocarbons that have systemic toxicity such as carbon tetrachloride or benzene, should be evacuated from the stomach.) Patients who are asymptomatic should be observed for up to 6 hours after ingestion. Patients who have respiratory symptoms warrant hospitalization. Oxygen administration, humidification of inspired air, and intravenous fluids should be instituted. The severely symptomatic patient may require mechanical ventilation with positive end-expiratory pressure. Adrenocorticosteroids have not been effective in preventing or ameliorating pulmonary complications and are not recommended. Leukocytosis and fever are common findings in hydrocarbon aspiration without infection. The use of antimicrobial therapy is not warranted initially. Damage to the pulmonary clearance mechanisms and aspiration of oral flora may cause a secondary bacterial pneumonia requiring antimicrobial therapy.

PLANTS

Because definitive identification of the ingested plant usually is not available, most practitioners find the management of plant ingestions confusing and frustrating. Most plants produce minimal symptoms in the quantities usually ingested. Fatalities are rare. In doubtful situations, most physicians prefer to empty the stomach. Activated charcoal adsorbs many plant toxins.

The ingestions reported most commonly involve members of the arum family (dieffenbachia, philodendron, caladium, colocasia). These plants contain needlelike calcium oxalate crystals, which produce intense mucosal irritation. Although treatment at home with a demulcent usually suffices, upper airway obstruction and esophageal erosions occur in rare cases and can be life threatening. Corneal damage may result from contact with the crystals. Oleander and lily of the valley contain cardiac glycosides similar to foxglove's digitalis. Digitalis toxicity has occurred following ingestions of these plants, particularly if they are used in the brewing of "herbal" tea. Digoxin-specific antibody fragments have been used to treat plant-ingestion digitalis toxicity.

Jimsonweed (locoweed, angel trumpets) contains belladonna alkaloids that produce anticholinergic symptoms. Therapy with physostigmine may be required but should not be used for mild symptomatology. Mistletoe berries, Jerusalem cherries, and holly berries represent seasonal hazards and may poison when consumed in quantity; lavage or induced emesis then is indicated. The ingestion of poinsettias usually does not result in symptoms but occasionally is followed by oral or anal irritation or mild gastrointestinal symptoms. Improperly prepared pokeweed (pokeweed salad) produces severe gastrointestinal symptoms and occasionally, neurotoxicity. Dangerously poisonous plants, occasionally ingested, include castor bean, jequirity bean, rosary pea, and lantana berry. Ingestion of water hemlock, a highly toxic plant toxin, may result in the rapid onset of seizures and death.

Most toadstools that grow in the yard are not poisonous. Mushroom poisoning is most common with mycetophiles and their families. Because wild mushrooms are difficult to identify accurately, all such ingestions must be considered potentially toxic. Ingestion of *Amanita* species may cause irreversible hepatic failure. Appropriate supportive management should follow gastric decontamination, catharsis, and the administration of activated charcoal.

VITAMINS

The accidental ingestion of modest amounts of the routinely used pediatric multiple vitamins with or without fluoride (not containing iron) does not present a toxic risk. Ingestions of elemental fluoride of 4 to 8 mg/kg of body weight has been associated with nausea, vomiting, diarrhea, and abdominal pain. Fluoride ingestions in excess of 8 mg/kg can cause electrolyte disturbances, particularly hypocalcemia with resultant convulsions, cardiac arrhythmias, and coma. Fatalities have been reported following the ingestion of sodium fluoride insecticides, sodium fluoride tablets, and 4% stannous fluoride solution. The standard toothpaste preparations present minimal risk of acute toxicity.

Toxicity may result from the chronic ingestion of excess quantities of both vitamin A and vitamin D. Excess intake of vitamin D may result in renal damage secondary to nephrocalcinosis, as well as hypercalcemia, bone pain, nausea, and vomiting. Chronic ingestion of excessive vitamin A may result in skin changes, hair loss, cortical thickening of tubular bones, and anorexia.

Acute intoxication with vitamin A results in the abrupt onset of increased intracranial pressure (pseudotumor cerebri). Symptoms include drowsiness, irritability, severe headache, and vomiting. A bulging fontanel may be present in infants. Desquamation, usually beginning around the mouth, may follow over the next few days. Induced emesis or gastric lavage should be considered in patients who have ingested 100,000 units or more of vitamin A.

Toxicity from excessive ingestion of water-soluble vitamins has been reported, usually in association with fad diets or megavitamin "ortho molecular" therapy. Dosages of pyridoxine and vitamin B_6 in excess of 2 g per day, cause peripheral nerve degeneration. Excessive dosages of vitamin C may result in chronic diarrhea and kidney stone formation.

IRON

Ingestion of iron-containing medications, particularly the commonly prescribed maternal prenatal 325-mg ferrous sulfate (65-mg elemental iron) tablets, is a major cause of death among accidental ingestions by toddlers. Lack of widespread public appreciation of the toxicity of iron and the close resemblance of prenatal ferrous sulfate to M & M brand candies contribute to the incidence of this common ingestion. Iron has a direct corrosive effect on the small bowel and gastric mucosa. The lesion is pathologically similar to the coagulation necrosis caused by acid ingestions. Significant ingestions cause severe abdominal pain, diarrhea, vomiting, and gastrointestinal hemorrhage. Shock may ensue as a result of the hemorrhage and attendant coagulopathy; significant hypovolemia can occur secondary to "third spacing" of fluid in the injured bowel in the absence of hemorrhage. Free iron in the circulation causes dysregulation of the coagulation cascade. Inhibition of cellular oxidative metabolism and the conversion of ferrous ions to ferric ions in the circulation may intensify the metabolic acidosis. Acute hepatic failure may complicate the course of acute iron poisoning. Scarring and stricture formation, usually at the pylorus, may occur as late as 4 weeks after the ingestion. The asymptomatic or quiescent period traditionally described as occurring after the gastrointestinal symptoms have subsided and before the onset of shock may represent a failure to recognize early signs of hypovolemia.

Therapy

The minimal toxic dose is 20 to 60 mg of elemental iron/kg of body weight. Ingestions in this range or greater should be managed with gastric emptying by induced emesis or gastric lavage. A plain roentgenogram of the abdomen is helpful in detecting residual iron tablets. Large concentrations of iron tablets in the stomach or small bowel should be removed by whole-bowel irrigation with a polyethylene glycol electrolyte solution (250 to 500 ml/hr via nasogastric tube). Endoscopic or surgical removal of iron tablet bezoars may be necessary.

Serum iron concentrations in excess of 500 μg/dl, measured 4 to 6 hours postingestion, are associated with a significant risk of shock; levels less than 300 μg/dl often are tolerated. Ingested doses exceeding 60 mg/kg of body weight usually are associated with toxic levels. Symptomatic individuals who have levels greater than 300 μg/dl and all individuals with levels greater than 500 μg/dl should receive chelation therapy. An elevated serum total iron-binding capacity is not protective and does not diminish the need for chelation therapy in the iron-intoxicated child.

The slow, continuous intravenous infusion of deferoxamine at 15 mg/kg/hr may cause the color of the urine to change to "vin rose" in the intoxicated individual. Lack of a urine color change in severely poisoned children (levels greater than 500 μg/dl), particularly in those in early shock or whose urine output is decreased, is not unusual. Because the vin rose color change is unreliable, the duration of chelation therapy is based on the child's clinical status and generally should continue until the serum iron level is below 300 μg/dl. Supportive care with early intensive management of shock through volume therapy is essential.

LEAD

Lead poisoning (plumbism) in the young child most often is a chronic disease. The ingestion of lead-based paint chips and paint-soaked plaster and putty remains the most significant source of high-dose lead exposure for young children. Household dust from crumbling wall fixtures and dirt contaminated by automobile emissions before the deleading of gasoline in the 1970s and by deteriorating exterior paint constitute "intermediate dose" sources of lead for the toddler through repetitive hand-to-mouth contamination. Studies conducted over the past decade clearly indicate that lead-contaminated household dust is the most common source of exposure for most children with elevated lead levels.

Toxicity also can result from a variety of less common exposures. Water and food contamination can result from lead-soldered plumbing systems or containers. Acidic foods and beverages can be contaminated through storage in improperly lead-glazed ceramic ware. Smelter dust, the contaminated work clothing of lead-acid storage battery factory workers, and the burning of discarded battery casings are a hazard. Slow absorption from ingested lead weights, sinkers, and retained bullets or shotgun pellets may result in poisoning. Certain Mexican-American and Asian Indian folk remedies may contain up to 86% lead by weight (e.g., azarcon and greta).

Physiological Effects

Blood lead levels reflect the equilibrium among absorption, excretion, and soft tissue and bone pools. A variable percentage of ingested lead, 5% to 10% in adults and up to 50% in younger children, is absorbed. Iron, zinc, and calcium deficiency and the excessive dietary intake of fat are believed to potentiate gastrointestinal lead absorption. Respiratory absorption of lead depends on particle size. Lead is excreted at a relatively limited rate in the urine, bile, and sweat. Ingestion of greater than 5 mg/kg of body weight per day generally results in retention, which results in increased tissue levels and toxic effects on bone marrow, kidneys, and nervous system and deposition of lead in bone (Fig. 293-3).

Lead in soft tissues has serious but reversible effects on hemoglobin production, renal function, and vitamin D metabolism. Lead interferes with the biosynthesis of heme, leading to decreased activity of delta-aminolevuline acid dehydratase, increased erythrocyte protoporphyrin levels, and increased excretion of coproporphyrin in urine. Globin synthesis also is impaired. The effect on the bone marrow is confounded by the frequent coexistence of iron-deficiency anemia. A reversible Fanconi's syndrome (hypophosphatemia with hyperphosphaturia, glycosuria, and generalized aminoaciduria), caused by proximal renal tubular damage, rarely may be seen in acute poisoning.

The most important aspect of lead's toxicity is that it has irreversible effects on the CNS. Severe intoxication causes cerebral edema with resultant acute encephalopathy. Capillary permeability is increased, with transudation of protein-containing fluid into the brain. Necrosis of vessel walls is present and may be accompanied by petechial hemorrhages. Neurons are damaged irreversibly. Lower-level intoxications result in mild neurological disabilities. High-level intoxication causes peripheral nervous system injury with a motor neuropathy; lower-level exposure results in an asymptomatic decrease in motor nerve conduction velocity.

Diagnosis and Clinical Findings

The blood lead level reflects the risk of symptomatic lead intoxication and acute encephalopathy as well as the potential for subtle but serious neurocognitive impairments at

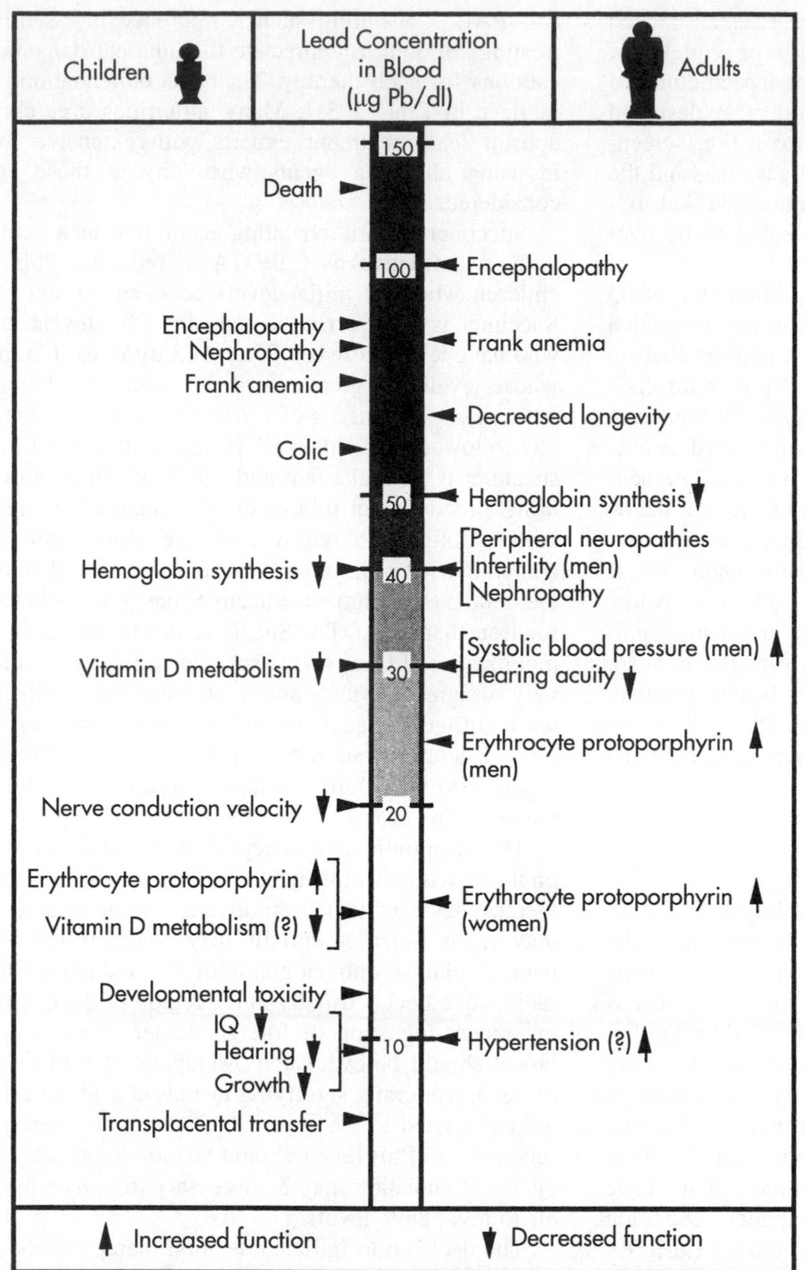

Fig. 293-3 Effects of inorganic lead on children and adults—lowest observable adverse-effect levels.

(From Agency for Toxic Substances and Disease Registry, US Department of Health and Human Services.)

lower levels. The Centers for Disease Control and Prevention (CDC) revised its guidelines for lead toxicity in 1991[2] and again in 1998[3] to reflect the fact that blood lead levels (PbB) as low as 10 µg/dl result in neurological toxicity (see Chapter 20 [Six], Screening for Lead Poisoning, for further discussion of this topic). Erythrocyte protoporphyrin, as an index of the metabolic effect of lead poisoning, often is elevated in association with lead levels greater than 25 µg/dl. The frequent coexistence of iron deficiency in high-risk populations may account for some of the hematological effects traditionally ascribed to lead intoxication.

The symptomatology of chronic lead poisoning is protean, nonspecific, and may wax and wane. Initial symptoms may include anorexia, constipation, and bouts of abdominal pain, nausea, and vomiting. Apathy, lethargy, and irritability may be mistaken for a primary behavioral disturbance. Incoordination, ataxia, and loss of recently acquired developmental milestones may occur. The process may abate or may progress to the gross ataxia, persistent vomiting, lethargy, coma, and intractable convulsions characteristic of acute encephalopathy. Absence of papilledema and vital sign changes does not exclude the possibility of cerebral edema in acute encephalopathy. A child may suffer recurrent symptomatic episodes without developing obvious acute encephalopathy. These nonspecific complaints may seem to be explained adequately by a minor intercurrent illness. A lumbar puncture generally is contraindicated because of the risks associated with increased intracranial pressure. Long-term sequelae of encephalopathy include seizure disorders, nonspecific mental retardation, and hyperkinetic behavior disorders. Widespread public recognition of the dangers of lead intoxication, screening programs, the decreased use of leaded gasoline, and the reduction of lead content in household paints have led to a dramatic reduction in the incidence of encephalopathy over the past 30 years.

Neuropsychiatric deficits, distractibility, diminution of IQ scores, and decreased academic achievement are associated with lead levels as low as 10 μg/dl, and it appears that on average there is a decrease of IQ of 2 to 3 points for each 10 μg/dl increase in blood lead above 10 μg/dl.[11] Intrauterine exposure to maternal PbB levels greater than 10 μg/dl results in quantifiable and persistent developmental delay. The neurotoxicity of low-level lead exposure (PbB levels below 25 μg/dl) has been adequately documented despite the coexistence of confounding variables such as socioeconomic class in exposed populations. The threshold lead level below which adverse biological effects in general, and neurocognitive deficits in particular, do not occur has yet to be defined.

For further discussion of the public health problem presented by PbB levels between 10 and 25 μg/dl in the general population, see Chapter 20 (Six), Screening for Lead Poisoning.

Therapy

Chelation therapy is adjunctive to the most imperative intervention in lead poisoning: separation of the child from the source of lead. Acute encephalopathy is a medical emergency. In addition, because the course of encephalopathy is fulminant and its onset unpredictable, any child who has an elevated PbB, particularly 45 μg/dl or higher, who has symptoms potentially referable to lead should be treated as an emergency. CaEDTA, dimercaptopropanol (BAL), and meso-2, 3-dimercaptosuccinic acid (Succimer) are the three chelating agents used to treat plumbism. Piomelli et al[12] have extensively described the protocols for inpatient chelation therapy of children who have lead poisoning using CaEDTA and BAL. Consulting such a reference is essential before treating children to appreciate the inherent dangers and precautions for such therapy. Their recommendations are summarized in Table 293-1. Many authorities urge clinicians to consult lead treatment experts with extensive experience in using chelating agents when any of these agents are considered.

Succimer, an oral chelating agent, has been demonstrated to be as effective as CaEDTA in reducing PbB levels in children who had initial levels between 50 and 69 μg/dl.[7] Succimer is as effective in reducing PbB levels in children who have levels between 25 and 45 μg/dl as it is in children whose levels are greater than 45 μg/dl.[9] Chelation therapy with succimer consists of 5 days of 10 mg/kg three times a day followed by 14 days of 10 mg/kg twice a day. Because succimer is an oral agent and can be given on an outpatient basis, this does not relieve the physician of his or her paramount obligation: removal of the child from the lead-contaminated environment and removal of lead sources from the child's environment. Succimer has a much lower affinity for iron than CaEDTA. Succimer penetrates and effectively mobilizes lead from soft tissues, including the brain. It has a very disagreeable taste and odor. Adherence with its use often is difficult to achieve, and within several weeks of stopping its administration the child's blood lead level tends to rebound to two thirds to three fourths of the level before receiving the drug.

The symptomatic or encephalopathic child should be hospitalized without oral intake. After cautious parenteral fluid therapy has established an adequate urine output, chelation may begin. Seizures initially may be controlled with diazepam. If plain roentgenograms of the abdomen demonstrate radiopaque flecks, usually in the region of the colon, signifying recent ingestion of foreign matter containing lead, the bowel should be evacuated. Metaphyseal lead lines present on roentgenogram, signifying increased lead storage in bone, are not related to the severity of symptoms. Renal and liver function and PbB levels should be monitored daily. Repeated cycles of chelation may be necessary to reduce the PbB levels to acceptable levels.

The decision to initiate chelation therapy in the clinically

Table 293-1 Chelation Therapy of Lead Poisoning

Status	Therapy	Comments
Encephalopathy	BAL* 75 mg/m^2 IM every 4 hr for 5 days CaEDTA† 1500 mg/m^2/day IV over 6 hr for 5 days	Give BAL 4 hr before CaEDTA infusion. Treat 5 additional days (after 2-day break) if PbB remains high. Additional cycles may be necessary depending on PbB rebound.
PbB of 70 μg/dl or higher or nonencephalopathic symptomatology	BAL 50 mg/m^2 IM every 4 hr for 3-5 days CaEDTA 1000 mg/m^2/day IV over 6 hr for 5 days	Give BAL 4 hr before CaEDTA infusion. BAL may be stopped after 3 days if the PbB falls below 50 μg/dl. Additional cycles may be necessary depending on PbB rebound.
PbB of 45 to 69 μg/dl PbB of 25 to 44 μg/dl	CaEDTA 1000 mg/m^2/day IV over 6 hr for 5 days	Additional cycles may be necessary depending on PbB rebound.

Modified from Piomelli S, et al: *J Pediatr* 105:527, 1984.
*Medicinal iron should not be given concurrently with BAL therapy.
†Adequate diuresis is essential (IV or oral fluid) to minimize renal toxicity.

asymptomatic child who has an increased lead burden depends on the lead level. Although chelation therapy has never been definitively demonstrated to benefit the asymptomatic child or reverse subtle neurotoxicity, the general consensus is that asymptomatic children who have PbB levels greater than 45 μg/dl should be chelated. The increasing appreciation of the toxic effects of lower lead levels and the availability of an effective oral chelating agent has led many physicians to chelate children whose PbB levels are between 25 and 45 μg/dl. Use of the CaEDTA provocation test (lead mobilization test) to determine which asymptomatic children who have PbB levels below 45 μg/dl should be chelated has been tempered by the potentially undesirable shifts of lead into the soft tissues (brain) during the test. At this time there is no evidence to support the use of chelating agents for children who have blood lead levels below 25 μg/dl. Children who have low-level lead elevations (i.e., blood lead levels between 10 and 24 μg/dl) require careful monitoring of blood lead levels, identification and removal of sources of ongoing lead exposure, and for those with blood lead levels of 20 or more μg/dl, or sustained elevations above 15 μg/dl, thorough medical, nutritional, and environmental evaluation.

Children receiving chelation therapy should not be released from the hospital until lead hazards in their environment are controlled or suitable alternative housing has been arranged. Exposure to aerosolized leaded dust during the deleading of a home containing lead-based paint is particularly hazardous, with the potential for precipitating encephalopathy in the lead-intoxicated child. Children must be excluded from the dwelling until the procedure is complete. Following chelation therapy, children still are at high risk and should have follow-up blood lead determinations at 1- to 2-week intervals until these levels stabilize or show a decline continually for at least 6 months. Thereafter, they should be followed up at 1- to 3-month intervals until 6 years of age or longer. Neurological and psychological conditions should be assessed at the time of diagnosis and in the following years.

The systematic screening of high-risk toddlers to detect lead deposits in soft tissue before symptoms occur is essential. Therapy does not prevent neurological sequelae after elevated blood lead levels. The cornerstone of treatment involves effective removal of lead from children's environments, case management, and the sustained cooperation of health department personnel, the medical social worker, visiting nurse, and pediatrician.

Acknowledgment

The authors gratefully acknowledge the contributions of the previous author, Dr. Robert Nolan.

REFERENCES

1. Brent J, et al: Fomepizole for the treatment of ethylene glycol poisoning, *N Engl J Med* 340:833, 1999.
2. The Centers for Disease Control: *Preventing lead poisoning in young children: a statement by the Centers for Disease Control,* Atlanta, 1991, US Department of Health and Human Services.
3. The Centers for Disease Control: *Screening young children for lead poisoning: guidance for state and local public health officials,* The Centers for Disease Control, Atlanta, 1997, US Department of Health and Human Services.
4. Chua JD, Friedenberg WR: Superwarfarin poisoning, *Arch Intern Med* 158:1929, 1998.
5. Done AK: Salicylate intoxication: significance of measurements of salicylate in blood in cases of acute ingestion, *Pediatrics* 26:800, 1960.
6. Gosselin RE, et al: *Clinical toxicology of commercial products,* ed 5, Baltimore, 1984, Williams & Wilkins.
7. Graziano JH, et al: Controlled study of meso-2,3-dimercaptosuccinic acid for the management of childhood lead intoxication, *J Pediatr* 120:133, 1992.
8. Haddad LM, Winchester JF: *Clinical management of poisoning and drug overdose,* ed 2, Philadelphia, 1998, WB Saunders.
9. Liebelt EL, Shannon M, Graef JW: Efficacy of oral meso-2,3-dimercaptosuccinic acid therapy for low-level childhood plumbism, *J Pediatr* 124:313, 1994.
10. Litovitz TL, et al: 1996 annual report of the American Association of Poison Control Centers Toxic Exposure Surveillance System, *Am J Emerg Med* 11:494, 1996.
11. National Research Council: *Measuring lead exposure in infants, children, and other sensitive populations,* Washington, DC, 1993, National Academy Press.
12. Piomelli S, et al: Management of childhood lead poisoning, *J Pediatr* 105:527, 1984.
13. Rumack BH: *POISINDEX information system,* ed 84, Denver, 1994, Micromedex.
14. Rumack BH, Matthew H: Acetaminophen poisoning and toxicity, *Pediatrics* 55:871, 1975.
15. Waltzman ML: Flunitrazepam: a review of "roofies," *Pediatr Emerg Care* 15:59, 1999.

SUGGESTED READINGS

Anderson KD, Rouse TM, Randolph JG: A controlled trial of corticosteroids in children with corrosive injury of the esophagus, *N Engl J Med* 323:637, 1990.

Bellinger DC, Stiles KM, Needleman HL: Low-level lead exposure, intelligence and academic achievement: a long-term follow-up study, *Pediatrics* 90:855, 1992.

Clark M, Royal J, Seeler R: Interaction of iron deficiency and lead and the hematologic findings in children with severe lead poisoning, *Pediatrics* 81:247, 1988.

Fine JS, Goldfrank LR: Update in medical toxicology, *Pediatr Clin North Am* 39:1031, 1992.

Gawin FH, Ellinwood EH: Cocaine and other stimulants: actions, abuse, and treatment, *N Engl J Med* 318:1173, 1988.

Gilman AG, Goodman LS, Gilman A: *Goodman and Gilman's the pharmacological basis of therapeutics,* ed 8, New York, 1990, Pergamon Press.

Gorman RL, et al: Initial symptoms as predictors of esophageal injury in alkaline corrosive ingestions, *Am J Emerg Med* 10:189, 1992.

Haddad LM: Managing tricyclic antidepressant overdose, *Am Fam Physician* 46:153, 1992.

Lampe KF, McCann MA: *AMA handbook of poisonous and injurious plants,* Chicago, 1985, American Medical Association.

Mortenson ML: Management of acute childhood poisonings caused by selected insecticides and herbicides, *Pediatr Clin North Am* 33:421, 1986.

Peterson RG, Peterson LN: Cleansing the blood: hemodialysis, exchange transfusion, charcoal hemoperfusion, forced diuresis, *Pediatr Clin North Am* 33:675, 1986.

Smilkstein MJ, et al: Efficacy of oral *N*-acetylcysteine in the treatment of acetaminophen overdose: analysis of the national multicenter study (1976-1985), *N Engl J Med* 319:1557, 1988.

Spiller HA, et al: A prospective evaluation of the effect of activated charcoal before oral *N*-acetylcysteine in acetaminophen overdose, *Ann Emerg Med* 23:519, 1994.

294 Rape

Margarete I. Parrish • Kathleen Lord Feroli • Marianne E. Felice

Because rape is a legal definition, not a medical diagnosis, every state has its own statutory definitions of sexual assault and rape. Clinicians should therefore be familiar with the statutes in their local jurisdictions. An accurate definition of rape includes three elements: (1) the absence of, or the impossibility of, obtaining consent from the victim; (2) the use of physical force, coercion, threats, punishments, or rewards; and (3) acts of sexual intimacy involving penetration.[11] This definition includes both statutory rape (consensual relations between a legal minor and an adult) and date or acquaintance rape (the victim and the perpetrator know each other socially or professionally). In general, *rape* refers to sexual intercourse with force or the threat of force or without a person's consent. Rape entails an assault acted out sexually, rather than a sexual act per se. Not only is rape an unchosen act for the victim but also it causes health risks unchosen by the victim.

INCIDENCE

Exact statistics on the incidence and prevalence of rape vary because many victims never report the crime. Estimates of unreported rape range from 40% to 90%.[20] Between 40% to 60% of all rape victims are younger than 18 years of age, and most are adolescents.[2,22] Worldwide, it is estimated that between one third and two thirds of rape victims are age 15 years and younger.[17] Although most rape victims are female, 5% to 10% are male.[2,23] Ninety percent of adolescent rape victims are assaulted by someone they know, and more than 50% of these cases occur on a date.[15] Survivors of prior sexual abuse are at particular risk of revictimization.[25] Adolescents who engage in high-risk behaviors, such as running away and the use of drugs and alcohol, are at an increased risk for rape.[19] About half of all reported rapes in the United States eventually lead to arrests; about two thirds of those arrested are prosecuted, and about half of those prosecuted are found guilty. In other words, for every 100 reported rapes, there are 16 convictions.[20] On behalf of pediatric rape victims seeking justice, providers of care need to be mindful of such prospects.

TYPES OF RAPES

Types of rape vary considerably, based on the relationship of the victim to the assailant. The various types of rapes raise different issues that are crucial to consider when providing care for the pediatric survivor. Psychosocial sequelae of rape often vary according to the type of rape involved.

Known Assailant

In most reported pediatric rape cases the victim knows the assailant, who may be a parent, a stepparent, an adult relative or friend of the family, a neighbor, an acquaintance, or a classmate. The victim-assailant relationship may cause conflicting family or social loyalties. In these cases, victims are less likely to report the rape, thereby contributing to the high estimates of underreporting. Rape victims who know their assailants also are prone to self-doubt and self-blame, and when they do report the rape, their reports may be received with skepticism and disbelief, even by the professionals to whom they turn for help. The "wish to forget" is a consistent factor in the delay of and resistance to reporting rape.[21]

Stranger Rape

An estimated 15% to 55% of reported rapes are committed by individuals who are not known by the victim.[1] Stranger rape is more likely to entail threats or use of violence and fear of immediate danger, and it is associated with a higher incidence of reporting the rape and of subsequent conviction of the assailant. Stranger rape is most likely to occur in areas of poverty and in high-crime districts, in which walking and playing also pose risks of danger.

Date Rape

Estimates of the incidence of date rape are unclear. However, in one survey of middle and high school students, nearly 20% of the females and more than 10% of the males reported a history of unwanted sexual activity on dates.[12] Surveys of college students indicate that about 25% of female students and 6% of male students report a history of sexual assault that meets the definition of rape while on a date.[12,23] Almost none of the college students in those surveys reported the sexual assault to authorities. Particularly in cases of young adolescent females (ages 10 to 15) and older males, questions of statutory rape arise, along with questions of consent, refusal skills, and exploitation.[10] Given the current incidence of sexually transmitted diseases among females under age 20, and the likelihood of their having been contracted from an older partner, health care providers are encouraged to consider the implications of age and power differentials between sexual partners.

Of the various types of rape, date rape is the least likely to be reported. It is of particular concern to adolescents that the incidence of date rape appears highly correlated with one or both parties having been drinking or using other drugs before the rape. As would be expected, date rapes are more likely to occur on weekends between 10 PM and 1 AM, in automobiles or at the home of the assailant.[1]

Youthful date rape victims frequently are new to an environment (e.g., a newcomer to school or town, or a college freshman). She may lack a strong social support system and may lack refusal skills; she may not be particularly assertive in establishing limits and boundaries with others and may have been intoxicated at the time of the incident. The date rape perpetrator typically is more sexually active than others his age and has a history of aggressive and/or antisocial behavior toward women. He typically perceives a victim's passivity as permission and denies the element of coercion. He, too, is likely to be intoxicated.[1] Manipulative verbal threats and physically trapping the victim are tactics used commonly by the date rapist.

Long-term issues of trust, self-blame, and vulnerability are important issues for victims of date rape, as in any other form of rape. The date rape victim may not trust her judgment concerning men, and she may blame herself for the rape, erroneously believing that she did not resist clearly or did not resist convincingly enough. She may be ashamed that she ended up in a situation that resulted in rape. It is easy to understand why victims have reservations about reporting date rape. Unfortunately, such secrecy also applies to discussing the incident in general, making catharsis, as well as verbal and emotional support from others, difficult to obtain.

Gang Rape

Gang rape typically involves a group of young males raping a solitary female victim. This type of rape may be associated with ritualistic behavior as well as displaced rage on the part of the assailants. Issues of sexualized rites of passage apply both to stereotypical adolescent gangs as well as to college fraternities. Victims of college campus gang rapes are more likely to drop out of college following the rape than to pursue legal recourse,[1] thus perpetuating the dynamics of avoiding confrontation with the perpetrators at the long-term expense of the victim.

Male Rape

In this discussion, *male rape* refers to same-sex rape. Although there are sporadic reports of male rape by females, the law is very unclear in this area, and data are limited.[21] The area of male rape remains understudied and is far less understood than female rape.

Specific subgroups of young men are at particular risk for sexual abuse: those in institutionalized settings (such as the criminal justice system), street youth (who may engage in prostitution), young male homosexuals (who may be runaways), and youth who have a parental history of physical or sexual abuse (parents who were abused themselves may become abusers as adults).[16] The occurrence of male rape in institutionalized settings often is attributed to displaced heterosexual behavior or undifferentiated sexual orientation, along with aggressive dominance of a weaker partner.[5,18] Male rape outside institutions often occurs through coercion by an individual perceived as an authority figure to the victim.[20]

Although male rape victims are more likely than their female counterparts to sustain physical trauma, the treatment of male victims should parallel that described for females. Issues of loss of control are particularly relevant for the male rape victim, along with subsequent symptoms of depression, anxiety, sleep disturbances, and suicidal ideation. Conflicted sexual identity is common among all male rape victims, whether or not they are homosexual. Male rape victims nearly always perceive the rape as a life-threatening event; this may result in long-term psychological problems.[18] Because of the pervasive reluctance of males to report rape, the preclusion of social support and intervention is a particularly challenging issue in this population.

LEGAL ISSUES

All states have laws that require physicians to report cases involving violent assault, including rape. This is particularly true of minors because rape obviously is a form of physical abuse. Some states require parental notification of a minor's sexual assault, and in those states, this statute overrides issues of confidentiality; most states permit a minor to receive treatment for sexual assault without parental consent. It is essential that all clinicians be familiar with local statutes.

Giving consent for treatment of rape is different than giving consent for collection of evidence. In most states, patients may limit their consent to a confidential report that includes only the patient's name, address, type of crime, and extent of injuries, rather than a full evidentiary examination. The physician must ask the patient for permission to complete a full evidentiary examination and to release the evidence to the police. Many victims are reluctant to give permission because they fear social isolation and possible retribution by the perpetrator. Furthermore, the evidentiary examination may be viewed as another form of assault by the victim.

From a medical-legal perspective the physician must realize that his or her responsibility is limited to the documentation of evidence. It is not the physician's role to determine whether a rape really occurred; that is a court decision. The physician will be of most help to the victim and the authorities by presuming that the victim is telling the truth, being thorough in the evaluation, and keeping accurate medical records.

MEDICAL EVALUATION

Rape is a serious medical and psychological emergency for both the victim and family. The purpose of the initial evaluation is fourfold: treatment of injury and infection; prevention of pregnancy, collection of evidence, and psychological assessment with referral for follow-up counseling.

General Concepts

Many metropolitan areas have treatment centers with trained interdisciplinary teams available for adolescent and child victims of rape; these treatment centers are ideal sites for an initial evaluation.[3] For various reasons, most pediatric rape victims do not use such specialized facilities.[8] To minimize the physical and psychological trauma of the evaluation, eliminate the need for repeat evaluations, and maximize the probability of collecting forensic evidence of good quality, the initial evaluation should be performed by the most skilled professional available. The gender of the examiner is less important than the individual's comfort with adolescents and children, skill at conducting the examination, and compassion.

The rape evaluation can be long and tedious, but it should never be rushed. While the youngster is coping with his or her personal outrage and physical and psychological pain, he or she is expected to tolerate and cooperate with uncomfortable procedures that may appear to be similar to the acts of intrusion and aggression experienced previously. Hence it is crucial that the approach to the evaluation be calm, gentle, and private. Rape protocols, if available, are helpful and will serve to minimize the chance for error or omission in the evidence collection process. Most jurisdictions have printed standardized forms for the evidence procurement process[17]; prior to examining a victim, the clinician should become familiar with these forms.

It is important that the clinician avoid making inappropriate assumptions about the victim based on his or her psychological state. Many victims are in a state of shock or denial immediately after the event. How a patient responds in the emergency room varies and depends on numerous factors, including developmental maturity. It is not uncommon for a 13-year-old child to look older physically but function cognitively at the level of a preadolescent. The physician should assume that the patient is uncomfortable with the assault and the ongoing rape assessment and attempt to minimize the victim's sense of personal guilt, shame, and anxiety by offering reassurance immediately. Taking a few minutes to empathize with the patient and acknowledge her feelings before proceeding with the evaluation helps both the patient and the physician. Particularly in cases in which acute trauma may compromise a pediatric patient's existing coping skills, the establishment of the patient's safety is crucial. Do not leave him/her alone if at all possible.

It always is prudent to take whatever time is necessary at the beginning of the evaluation to explain the process of the examination and allow for questions. This is particularly true for those rape victims who never had previous sexual relationships or a prior gynecological examination, but it also is helpful for more experienced patients who understandably still may be anxious and fearful of anticipated pain and discomfort. Whenever possible, allow the patient some control over the proceedings; let the patient set the pace of the examination. Be careful to inform the patient in advance of what tasks must be accomplished. Let them signal when to begin the procedure. If the victim becomes visibly agitated with the proceedings, stop and allow her to regain composure before continuing with the examination. At no point should a physician continue to examine a child or adolescent against his or her will.

Whenever it is applicable, making reference to prior experience with other similar-aged rape survivors may help establish that he/she is not the only child or adolescent to whom this has happened. It also establishes that you are not shocked at such circumstances, and have some practical knowledge with which to anticipate their concerns. Examples such as, "Sometimes when someone your age has been attacked, they ask me about . . . "

After obtaining consent from the patient, the physician should obtain a detailed and relevant history, followed by a thorough general physical examination and a gentle but complete pelvic examination. It is essential to have a female nurse or assistant present during this process, and for small children or very young adolescents it usually is helpful to have a parent present during the examination if the parent is reassuring, rather than openly distraught during the procedure. Some aspects of the evaluation will change depending on the temporal proximity of the evaluation to the alleged event. The following guidelines are recommended for evaluations conducted within 72 hours of the assault. Modifications are necessary if the evaluation is conducted after this time. In some centers the interdisciplinary team obtains the history simultaneously and together so that the victim does not have to repeat his or her story unnecessarily.

History

History-taking necessarily entails asking some very personal and potentially awkward questions. Thus, the patient needs to be assured of privacy and respectful compassion. The history should include the time, date, and location of both the event and the examination. Recalling the event may be emotionally traumatic for the patient, so it sometimes is useful to begin with a relevant, but relatively neutral medical history. Such information as a thorough menstrual history, including the age of menarche, the date of the last menstrual period, the frequency of menses, sexual activity if relevant, previous pregnancies, miscarriages, and abortions, and the use of contraceptives and feminine hygiene products, is very important.

Next, the event itself should be focused upon. Questions should be asked calmly and with sensitivity and patience. Some of the questions asked may seem invasive and, when taken out of context, inappropriate, but it is important to obtain all relevant information the first time the interview is conducted. Studies show that repeated attempts at obtaining a history are emotionally traumatic, often confusing to the victim, and actually may discredit the victim's testimony. The victim's own words should be recorded whenever possible. The medical chart is a legal document and will be subjected to the same scrutiny as any other form of evidence. Only the historical facts, without embellishment or interpretation, should be recorded.

The patient should be asked about the use of intoxicating substances before or during the event, as well as whether there was any loss of consciousness. One needs to ask whether weapons or restraints were used during the assault. The patient should be asked to describe in detail the location of the event, the appearance of the perpetrator, the type of sexual contact and the positions used, the utilization of force (by both the perpetrator and the victim), the removal of clothing and the manner in which it was removed, and what measures, if any, the patient took to cleanse or relieve himself or herself (e.g., bathing, douching, changing clothes, urinating, or defecating). It should be determined whether the assailant used a condom or any other means of contraception. Finally, the physician should ask about the presence of clinical symptoms in the musculoskeletal, gastrointestinal, and genitourinary system.

Physical Examination

A complete physical examination from "head to toe" is warranted. Although no visible physical injuries occur in 40% to 60% of sexual assaults, an inspection of the entire body may provide the corroborative evidence necessary to convict the perpetrator.

The patient's physical appearance and emotional state, and the condition of his or her clothing should be noted. If the patient presents in the same clothing worn at the time of the event, its condition should be noted and each piece saved in a separate, labeled bag. Applying a Wood light to the clothing may illuminate the presence of dried semen. These specimens should be marked for later analysis for the presence of seminal vesicle-specific antigen. Next, a topical survey of the body, documenting any evidence of recent trauma or bruising, should be done. The use of photographs may be useful during subsequent litigation. Use of a diagram to indicate locations of visible injuries can be very helpful.

Particular attention should be given to the examination of the head and neck. Compression injuries of the neck are fairly common if force is used. This may lead to obstruction of venous return from the head, causing the development of neck bruising and/or petechial hemorrhages in the eyelids and conjunctiva. The inner surface of the lips may have tiny abrasions resulting from forced pressure applied to the mouth by the perpetrator to prevent the victim from screaming. If the patient reports biting the assailant in self-defense, an imprint of the bite plate and a saliva sample should be taken for later comparison. Two common injuries to the mouth include torn frenulum of the lip and tears beneath the tongue.

The breasts may show bite marks or bruises. Tanner staging to determine the victim's level of sexual maturation (breasts and pubic hair in females; genitalia and pubic hair in males) should be done also. It is not improbable that by the time a case comes to trial, a child may progress from a Tanner stage 2 to a stage 3 or 4. This significant physical change may bias an uneducated jury inappropriately.

Genital Examination

The female patient. After the initial physical examination, the patient can be draped and placed in the lithotomy position. If the patient seems too anxious and a speculum examination is not required to investigate for a source of undiagnosed internal bleeding, the knee-chest position may be a suitable alternative, particularly for younger adolescents or children. In some cases it may be necessary to perform the pelvic examination with the patient under sedation or, on rare occasions, under general anesthesia.

The pelvic examination should begin with inspection of the thighs and perineum for evidence of trauma, bruising, semen, or blood. Appropriate forensic evidence should be taken at this time (Box 294-1). The inguinal lymph nodes should be palpated for evidence of ongoing or previous genital infection. Erythema and engorgement of the clitoris is common after intense local stimulation. The effect usually wears off in 1 to 2 hours.

In myths and legends, an intact hymen is synonymous with virginity. Hence the patient, and often her parents, may want to know about the structural integrity of the hymen. It is next to impossible, however, to ascertain from a visual inspection of the hymen whether rape has taken place. The presence of hymenal tears is not proof of rape because such tears may be old and the result of nonrape trauma (e.g., forceful use of a tampon). Nevertheless, because of the emphasis placed on this area of the anatomy, careful inspection and documentation of the hymen's condition is essential. A saline-moistened cotton swab rolled around the edges of the hymen, the use of an otoscope, or the application of toluidine blue to the hymenal margin may help to locate and identify fresh tears. Many experts use colposcopy for this purpose, but because standards for this procedure have not been defined clearly and because many emergency facilities do not have a colposcope available, its use still is considered investigational. Measurements of the width of the hymenal opening should be recorded.[11]

BOX 294-1

RECOMMENDED PROCEDURES FOR THE COLLECTION OF FORENSIC DATA

Combed and plucked pubic hair
Wet mount of secretions from the vaginal vault
Wet mount and fixed smear for the detection of both motile and dead sperm
Vaginal aspirate for acid phosphatase
Vaginal aspirate for p30 and MH-5 testing
Cervical cultures for both chlamydia and gonorrhea
Rectal cultures for gonorrhea even if sodomy has not occurred
Oral culture for gonorrhea if fellatio occurred
Dried secretions from skin, pubic hair, or clothing for analysis
Blood tests: ABO typing, syphilis, pregnancy test, and HIV test (if patient requests it)

Most female adolescents should be able to undergo a speculum examination of the internal genitals, which will allow a clear view of the vaginal walls, fornices, and cervix. Appropriate specimens for culture and forensics should be obtained (see Box 294-1).

After the speculum examination is completed, a vaginal bimanual and rectovaginal examination should be conducted to rule out the presence of trauma. A history of sodomy in both male and female victims indicates the need to conduct a careful anal inspection and digital examination. In addition to looking for evidence of rectal bleeding (hemorrhoids, erythema, engorgement, and, if the offense is chronic, constipation), particular attention should be paid to the quality of anal sphincter tone.

The male patient. A detailed history and physical examination, as well as specimens for forensic and laboratory evaluation, should be obtained in the male rape victim. Particular focus should be placed on the evaluation of the oral cavity, the genitals, and the anus. One should look for evidence of infection in the mouth and pharynx. The testes, epididymis, vas deferens, penile shaft, foreskin, and glans penis should be examined thoroughly for the presence of infection or trauma. Inguinal lymphadenopathy may indicate the presence of an infectious process. The physician should check for the presence of external hemorrhoids, rectal fissures, or fistulas. A digital evaluation of sphincter tone, the internal anal canal, and prostate should be performed. The use of an anoscope or a large-bore otoscope may be helpful to inspect the internal anal canal.

Summarizing the Examination

When the physical examination is completed, the patient should be given ample time to dress and regain his or her composure before discussing any findings. Most patients will benefit from knowing that their genital anatomy is normal. It also is important to discuss physical findings, treatment options, and plans for follow up.

Forensic and Laboratory Information

The recovery of laboratory and forensic data is probably the most controversial aspect of the evaluation.[26] This is especially true when it comes to the recovery of semen and sperm, yet the finding of male ejaculate is neither predictive nor essential for criminal conviction. In one study, physical evidence of rape was found in only 23% of all of the cases that resulted in felony convictions.[9] The newest developments in forensic science have occurred in the laboratory analysis of semen and include the demonstration of quantifiable levels of acid phosphatase and a positive monoclonal antibody test, MH-5 ELISA (specific for seminal vesicle antigen) in vaginal fluids.

Sexually Transmitted Disease

Most patients are concerned about the risk of acquiring a sexually transmitted disease (STD) as a result of the rape. This risk is related directly to the health status of the assailant and the victim, the site of the assault, and the infectivity of the disease in question. Overall, the risk of contracting an STD from a single encounter is small. Repeat assaults or assaults by more than one assailant increase the risk of infection. Many adolescent victims of rape, however, also engage in high-risk behaviors that put them at increased risk of having a preexisting sexually transmitted disease. Additionally, as many as 50% of sexual assault survivors do not return for follow-up appointments. The Centers for Disease Control and Prevention recommends the use of prophylactic antibiotics for treatment of potential sexually acquired infections (see Chapter 262, Sexually Transmitted Diseases).[6,7] A prophylactic hepatitis B vaccination against possible exposure is recommended.

Regardless of the antibiotics given, it must be emphasized to the patient that the incubation period for STDs varies, and it is highly possible that an infection may not be detected or may be missed or treated inadequately at the time of the evaluation examination. Therefore, while baseline studies should be obtained at the initial evaluation, medical follow-up, no matter how discomforting a thought to the patient, is absolutely crucial. After 2 weeks the patient should be reexamined for the presence of an STD. Serological tests for syphilis and HIV infection should be performed 12 weeks after the assault in most cases.

Pregnancy

The occurrence of pregnancy after unprotected exposure is strongly influenced by whether or not a female is in the fertile interval of her menstrual cycle, as well as the possible sexual dysfunction of the assailant (e.g., failure to maintain an erection or to ejaculate).[16,22,24] Many adolescents, however, have irregular menstrual cycles; therefore, the occurrence of ovulation for any particular cycle may be in question. If the assault occurred within 48 to 72 hours of the evaluation, a form of postcoital contraception (see the discussion of postcoital "morning after" contraception in Chapter 41, Contraception and Abortion) should be offered to the patient after a negative pregnancy test has ruled out the presence of an already existing pregnancy[14] (see Chapter 41, Contraception and Abortion). With pregnancy prophylactics, antiemetics should be offered because of the frequent side effects of nausea and vomiting. The occurrence of pregnancy following unprotected exposure should be strongly suspected when menses does not occur within 4 weeks of the rape, at which point the patient should return for a repeat evaluation.

PSYCHOLOGICAL ASSESSMENT

The psychosocial and emotional implications of rape in children and adolescents are complex. Three distinct areas must be considered nonconsensual: a sexual act or acts that may be the victim's initial sexual experience, the threat of physical danger or violence, and the victim's feelings of loss of control. These three factors are tempered further by the young person's stage of development and the family's response to the rape. For example, a young adolescent who is just beginning to grapple with his or her own sexuality may feel that he or she deserved to be raped because of having begun to experience sexual urges. A child who sees her mother respond with tearful distress to the news that her child was raped may feel guilt not just because of the rape but because of the emotional trauma inflicted on the mother.

How the youngster copes with the rape also is related to how society responds to victims of rape. Unlike most crimes, the crime of rape often is blamed on the victim rather than on the perpetrator, particularly in adolescents. Following no other crime is the victim's prior reputation, appearance, and behavior as subject to scrutiny as in rape. Prior behaviors such as running away, sexual activity, and even hitchhiking are used as justification for the rape, placing further blame on an already troubled young victim. Providers of care must avoid compounding such punitive dynamics.

Role of Interdisciplinary Care

The evaluation of a rape victim is best conducted by an interdisciplinary care team, usually consisting of a physician, nurse, and social worker. An interdisciplinary approach is beneficial for several reasons, including the ability to provide support to the child and family simultaneously and to serve as a resource for future services. Ideally, a supportive health professional should be available to the child or adolescent upon presentation and, if possible, should stay with the young rape victim throughout the evaluation process. This individual is in a position to establish trust and continuity for the successful provision of future needed services at a time when the rape victim may be afraid to trust anyone.

Ideally, the child should be able to relate the account of the rape just once to all the professionals involved. For legal reasons, the parents should not be present during this narrative in the event that any aspect of the assault involves the family. Also, this enables the child to give his or her version of the events without parental interruption or coaching. However, the family's needs should not be ignored, and another supportive health professional can address the many questions that concerned parents or friends may have.

Immediate Response to Rape by the Victim

Immediate responses to rape vary considerably, ranging from distraught histrionics to near-mute withdrawal. Most victims have intense levels of fear and anxiety. This postrape acute phase also is characterized by varying levels of cognitive disorganization, "shock," and disbelief.[4] As occurs in any crisis, many children and adolescents regress to previous stages of development. An adolescent rape victim who previously was self-assured and appropriately independent may become clinging and dependent on the parent or health professional.

The potential for confusion and further trauma on the part of the victim also should be considered. For example, the natural reaction to embrace or try to comfort a rape victim in fact may be unwelcome, if not traumatic, following rape. Many victims, including children and adolescents, may not want to be touched by any stranger after the rape, including caring health professionals. Following the trauma of rape, some victims experience psychological symptoms that are both foreign and frightening. For example, a previously articulate individual may have difficulties describing the rape and simply may not be able to speak about the event. Obviously, a minor's level of cognitive development may contribute to this difficulty.

Immediate Response by the Family

Unlike other crime victims, the victim of rape rarely contacts the police immediately. Typically, there is an intermediary (a friend or family member) whom the victim contacts first. That individual's response is crucial in the ensuing medical and legal processes, but most family and friends need guidance to know how best to be supportive to the victim. The disclosure of rape usually is traumatic for the family as well as the victim. Parents may blame themselves inappropriately for the rape. In other instances, parental activities (e.g., neglect) may have contributed to the rape. In either scenario, the issues are highly sensitive and need to be addressed with skill and compassion.

Familial responses to a child's rape range from denial and disbelief to shame and outrage. There is no guarantee that a family is prepared to respond appropriately to a raped child's needs at this time. In some cases, a victim's mother's financial dependence on a perpetrator may confound reactions. During the initial evaluation session, health care professionals, therefore, must spend some time with the family members and/or friends of the victim to determine their own psychological response and their ability to be supportive of the victim.

Follow-up Care

After the initial evaluation is completed, arrangements should be made for follow-up care not only for the medical issues discussed previously but also to assess the victim's ability to cope with the rape and to accept counseling concerning the rape. All rape victims and their families should be seen as soon as possible after the rape by a mental health professional who is trained to work with children or adolescents and who is knowledgeable about the emotional sequelae to rape.

Rape Trauma Syndrome

The term *rape trauma syndrome* is used to group the constellation of emotional and behavioral symptoms that follow rape. This term encompasses both short- and long-term considerations and addresses both mental and physical reactions. It was introduced by Burgess and Holstrom[4] to describe the responses of adult women to rape, but it also has been applied to younger rape victims. It is still used as a variation of posttraumatic stress disorder (PTSD), and to distinguish among the three phases of response following rape—the acute trauma period, followed by an adaptive period, and then a long-term reorganizational period. In the acute phase (days to weeks following the rape), symptoms associated with an acute stress disorder frequently are noted—increased startle response, diminished concentration, and sleep disturbances including nightmares, mood swings, and flashbacks. Such symptoms usually are short-lived, but they have been reported to persist in some patients from 1 to 3 years after the rape.[5] During the adaptive phase, the child is faced with readjustment to a normal lifestyle. Normal eating and sleeping patterns usually resume (although nightmares may continue), and the rape victim usually grapples with fear, anxiety, and issues of self-worth. Finally, during the reorganization phase, survivors face the disruption caused by the rape. They usually question why they were victims and others were not, and they search for explanations to help them understand why the rape occurred.

Short- and Long-Term Psychological Sequelae

Multiple factors will determine how a child or adolescent responds to the rape, such as level of social support, coping styles and strengths, and developmental variables and cognitive functions. Hence, one cannot predict how any given individual will respond to rape. However, it does appear that children and adolescents who have been rape victims consistently have lower levels of self-esteem following rape than the general population.[17] In addition, sexually traumatized children have been noted to have higher levels of precocious sexualization than nontraumatized children.[2,13] There may be confusion about what is normal adult sexual behavior, sometimes leading to inappropriate sexual, "acting out" behaviors. Some children experience developmental arrests at the time of the trauma; such arrests are not necessarily readily apparent. Although child and adolescent studies are still too scarce to be considered definitive, it appears that the earlier and more traumatic the rape, the greater chance of developmental and functional impairment.[5]

Behavioral concerns frequently associated with childhood and adolescent rape sequelae include school phobias, generalized fearfulness and withdrawal, and especially in adolescents, the onset of truancy. Suicidal ideations are not uncommon, with increased lifetime risks of major depression and suicide attempts being associated with women in the aftermath of rape.[5] For male rape victims the existing research is less clear, but it appears that male sexual trauma in childhood may be associated with sexually abusive behavior toward other boys during adolescence.[16,18] Obviously, not all children and adolescents who have been raped will have psychiatric sequelae, but all of those who have been raped should be assessed and monitored for serious sequelae. Particularly in cases in which sexual "acting out" follows a rape, careful clinical attention to issues such as PTSD and depression is required. Self-medication with various substances is an ongoing clinical hazard following rape and deserves consideration as a "red flag" for care providers working with at-risk patients.

MALE PERPETRATORS

Just as adolescent females constitute a large proportion of reported rape victims, adolescent males make up a large proportion of convicted rape assailants; 40% of convicted rapists are 16 to 20 years of age, and another 25% are between 20 and 24 years of age.[20]

Perpetrators tend to fall into one of three clusters: those for whom anger is the primary dynamic; those for whom power or conquest is the central issue; and the sadistic, for whom anger and control are in and of themselves erotic.[4] For the anger-driven rapist, the act tends to be impulsive, with the intent of hurting, humiliating, and degrading the victim. Physical brutality is common. Rape functions as the outlet for anger, essentially by using sex as a weapon. The power-oriented rapist is more likely to engage in premeditated, obsessive, and/or stalking behavior, in which the rape essentially compensates for social and sexual incompetence or inadequacy. Aggression for the power-oriented rapist is less likely to be violent than a means of dominating his prey. Both anger- and power-driven rapists have serious deficits in social skills and the inability to interpret and respond to social cues from others. For the sadistic rapist, eroticism and violence are enmeshed; victims typically are subjected to premeditated, deliberate acts of cruelty and dehumanization. The sadistic perpetrator finds gratification in his victim's pain and powerlessness.

Although some rapists are dysfunctional sexually at the time of the rape,[22] most rapists are sexually active with available, consensual partners outside the rape.[4] Perpetrators usually appear ordinary by most standards; most do not have symptoms of major psychiatric illnesses such as psychoses, nor is there a preponderance of mental retardation. However, other conditions such as antisocial, schizoid, paranoid, and narcissistic personality disorders are noted more commonly among convicted rapists than in the general population.[16,22]

Alcohol and drug use have been associated with the occurrence of rape. Ironically, alcohol intoxication sometimes seems to have the effect of both diminishing a perpetrator's sense of responsibility and increasing a victim's culpability. Specifically, victim intoxication consistently is linked with the process of "unfounding," or disproving, rape charges. For date rape victims, having been seen drinking with the perpetrator before the attack has serious implications in relation to public, social, and legal responses to the charges.

SUMMARY

Rape is an act of violence that involves a disparity of power between the perpetrator and the victim. Because of its sexual context, rape is easily misinterpreted as erotic or sexual behavior, which it is not.

Children and adolescents who have been raped should have sensitive, careful, and thorough evaluations and follow-up assessments. From the time of initial disclosure through eventual legal outcome, many developmental, familial, and social variables can shape the experience for young survivors and their families. Long-term adjustment following rape varies considerably, with both developmental and familial factors having considerable impact.

REFERENCES

1. Allison J, Wrightsman LS: *Rape: the misunderstood crime,* Newbury Park, Calif, 1993, Sage.
2. American Academy of Pediatrics, Committee on Adolescence: Sexual assault and the adolescent, *Pediatrics* 94:761, 1994.
3. American Academy of Pediatrics, Task Force on Adolescent Assault Victim Needs: Adolescent assault victim needs: a review of issues and a model protocol, *Pediatrics* 98:991, 1996.
4. Burgess A, Holstrom L: *Rape: crisis and recovery,* Bowie, Md, 1979, Prentice-Hall.
5. Calhoun K, Atkeson B: *Treatment of rape victims: facilitating psychosocial adjustment,* New York, 1991, Pergamon.
6. Centers for Disease Control (CDC): 1998 Guidelines for treatment of sexually transmitted diseases, *MMWR* 47:1, 1998.
7. Centers for Disease Control: Sexual assault and STDs, *MMWR* 42:97, 1993.
8. Crowell NA, Burgess AW: Understanding violence against women, Washington, DC, 1996, National Academy Press.
9. De Jong AR, Rose M: Legal proof of child sexual abuse in the absence of physical evidence, *Pediatrics* 88:506, 1991.
10. Elstein S, Davis N: *Sexual relationships between adult males and young teen girls: exploring the legal and social responses,* Chicago, 1997, American Bar Association.
11. Emans SJH, Woods ER, Allen EN: Hymenal findings in adolescent women: impact of tampon use and consensual sexual activity, *J Pediatrics* 125:153, 1994.
12. Erickson PI, Rapkin AJ: Unwanted sexual experiences among middle and high school youth, *J Adolesc Health* 12:319, 1991.
13. Friedrich W: Behavior problems in sexually abused children. In Wyatt GE, Powell GJ, editors: *Lasting effects of child sexual abuse,* Newbury Park, Calif, 1988, Sage.
14. Hatcher R, et al: Emergency contraception. In Hatcher R, et al, editors: *Contraceptive technology,* ed 17, New York, 1998, Ardent Media.
15. Heger A, et al: *Evaluation of the sexually abused child: a medical textbook and photographic atlas,* New York, 1992, Oxford University Press.

16. Knight R, Rosenberg R, Schneider B: Classification of sex offenders: perspectives, methods, and validation. In Burgess AW, editor: *Rape and sexual assault: a research handbook,* New York, 1985, Garland Press.
17. Koss MP, Heise L, Russo NF: The global health burden of rape, *Psychol Women Qtrly* 18:509, 1994.
18. Lacey HB, Roberts R: Sexual assault of men, *Int J STD AIDS* 2:258, 1991.
19. Nagy S, Adcock AG, Nagy MC: A comparison of risky health behaviors of sexually active, sexually abused, and abstaining adolescents, *Pediatrics* 93:570, 1994.
20. Neinstein LS, editor: *Adolescent health care: a practical guide,* ed 3, Baltimore, 1996, Urban & Schwarzenberg.
21. Petrak JA: Current trends in the psychological assessment and treatment of victims of sexual violence, *Sexual Marital Therapy* 11:37, 1996.
22. Raine A: *The psychopathology of crime,* San Diego, 1993, Academic Press.
23. US Department of Justice: *Sex offenses and offenders: an analysis of data on rape and sexual assault,* Bureau of Justice Statistics, NCJ-163392, Washington, DC, 1997.
24. Wilcox AJ, Weinberg CR, Baird DD: Timing of sexual intercourse in relation to ovulation, *N Engl J Med* 333:1517, 1995.
25. Wyatt GE, Guthrie D, Notgrass C: Differential effects of women's child sexual abuse and subsequent sexual revictimization, *J Consult Clin Psychol* 60:167, 1992.
26. Young WW, et al: Sexual assault: review of a national model protocol for forensic and medical evaluation, *Obstet Gynecol* 80:878, 1992.

295 Renal Failure

Glenn H. Bock

Acute renal failure (ARF) is a syndrome of sudden diminution or cessation of renal function that may arise in a broad spectrum of clinical settings. Data over the past three decades show substantially increased morbidity and mortality in most ARF subgroups, despite improvements in renal replacement therapies. Although this has been attributed largely to the tendency for "sicker" patients to be disproportionately represented in ARF cohorts, some recent data suggest that perturbed renal function in itself is a significant risk factor. Clinical symptoms and signs in patients who have ARF result from both the inciting disease process and the altered homeostasis produced by the reduction of renal function. Acute renal failure may occur at any age, but although less common in children and adolescents than in adults, its exact incidence is unknown because self-limited episodes may go undetected. This especially is true for the nonoliguric form of ARF.

ETIOLOGY

Factors leading to diminished renal function often are grouped according to prerenal, renal (parenchymal), and postrenal causes or a combination thereof. Prerenal causes are those that diminish renal perfusion without producing actual parenchymal injury. In the pediatric age group, hypovolemia is the most common clinical situation in which this occurs. In children, the hypovolemia usually results from dehydration associated with acute gastrointestinal losses, although it also may occur in shock as the result of hemorrhage, burns, sepsis, and trauma. Less common causes of prerenal azotemia are those that diminish renal blood flow in the absence of hypovolemia, such as congestive heart failure, renal vascular obstruction from thrombosis or embolism, and increased renal vascular resistance as is seen occasionally following anesthesia or surgery. Although oliguria and/or azotemia occur in the prerenal syndrome, normal compensatory renal tubular function usually persists, manifesting as high urinary osmolality and low urinary sodium concentrations as the result of renal water and sodium conservation.

Acute renal failure from intrinsic renal parenchymal injury may result from glomerular, renal tubular, or interstitial disorders. Acute renal failure from glomerular injury results most commonly from any of the glomerulonephritides or the microangiopathy of the hemolytic-uremic syndrome. Processes primarily causing tubular injury frequently are the result of prolonged, unrecognized, or inadequate renal perfusion, as may be seen in hypotensive episodes, severe dehydration, sudden hemorrhage, or sepsis. Tubular toxins (e.g., hemoglobin and myoglobin) and various chemicals (e.g., carbon tetrachloride, diethylene glycol, and heavy metals) may cause acute parenchymal renal failure. Drugs can produce renal failure because of either direct toxic effects or hypersensitivity reactions. Diffuse pyelonephritis also may result in ARF, particularly in infants. Renal cortical necrosis associated with infection, hemorrhage, or dehydration can produce significant injury to both glomeruli and tubules.

Postrenal causes of acute renal failure refer to processes that impair urinary drainage. These are discussed in Chapter 186, Anuria/Oliguria.

History

The process(es) contributing to renal functional impairment frequently can be identified from the patient's history. It is important to note that the volume of urine production is not included in the definition of ARF because renal failure occurs not only in anuric states but also in those with oliguric (urine volume less than 240 ml/m^2/day), or nonoliguric (normal or increased urinary output) states. Some renal insults, such as various glomerulonephritides and hemolytic-uremic syndrome, frequently are associated with oligoanuric ARF; others, such as aminoglycoside toxicity, more often will cause nonoliguric renal failure. Determination of the type of insult provides the clinician with insights into the possible manifestations of renal failure, the probable duration of renal insufficiency, and the overall prognosis. The history often helps to distinguish between an episode of ARF in an otherwise healthy child and the acute deterioration of renal function in a child who has preexisting, undiagnosed, chronic renal disease. A preceding history of urinary abnormalities, fatigue, pallor, slowed linear growth, poor school performance, and anorexia extending over a period would lead the practitioner to suspect the latter.

Physical Findings

Obviously, the child who has oligoanuric acute renal failure will have markedly diminished urine output. Complete anuria is unusual and leads to consideration of a catastrophic renovascular event or urinary obstruction. In the child who has anuria or oliguria, fluid retention can produce edema, water intoxication, vascular overload with congestive heart failure, pulmonary edema, and/or hypertension. Often, the fluid overload is iatrogenic, resulting from attempts to increase urinary output by increasing fluid intake. Early detection of fluid retention is determined best by short-term weight gain on serial measurements and carefully recorded intakes and outputs, with appropriate allowances for insensible fluid losses. In contrast, acute nonoliguric renal failure may be clinically covert; it usually is suspected only after the laboratory tests reveal azotemia.

Laboratory Findings

The biochemical disturbances that contribute to clinical findings in acute renal failure are complex and interrelated. Inherent to the diagnosis of acute renal failure is the accumulation of nitrogenous waste products, manifested by a rise in blood urea nitrogen and creatinine. If hypotonic fluids have been used in excess to hydrate the patient, dilutional hyponatremia and anemia may affect central nervous system (CNS) and cardiac function adversely, respectively.

Hyperkalemia often is the result of injudicious potassium administration or inadequate renal potassium excretion. It is a potentially life-threatening complication of ARF and can be especially severe in disease states associated with cellular damage and the consequent release of intracellular potassium. These states include hemolysis, burns, trauma, and infections. Hyperkalemia produces a state of increased neuromuscular excitability, including a vulnerability to cardiac arrhythmias. Unfortunately, there are no consistent physical signs of hyperkalemia; diagnosis depends on the measurement of serum potassium and, if indicated, assessment of the electrocardiogram (ECG) for evidence of altered cardiac electrical activity. In ARF, metabolic acidosis develops as the result of the kidney's failure to excrete hydrogen ions and reabsorb bicarbonate. Furthermore, any state associated with increased catabolism, such as shock, fever, poor caloric intake, or extensive tissue damage, may accentuate the degree of acidosis as a result of increased production of organic and inorganic acid radicals. The acidosis promotes further hyperkalemia resulting from movement of intracellular potassium into the extracellular space as the body attempts to accommodate the higher hydrogen ion concentration. Respiratory compensation for an underlying metabolic acidosis may manifest as tachypnea or Kussmaul breathing.

Failure of phosphate excretion can lead to hyperphosphatemia. The hypocalcemia associated with hyperphosphatemia may manifest clinically as tremors, tetany, or seizures. Other causes of seizures in acute renal failure include hypertensive encephalopathy, uremia, and water intoxication. It is not unusual for a child to present first with the sudden onset of seizures and other signs of CNS dysfunction, only to be found to have acute renal failure.

In children who have the nonoliguric form of ARF, severe fluid and electrolyte problems are less common, unless attention given to the appropriate fluid, salt, and mineral replacements mandated by the excessive urinary losses that occur frequently is inadequate.

DIFFERENTIAL DIAGNOSIS

The sine qua non of acute renal failure is the detection of retained nitrogenous waste products in the blood. A recommended clinical approach to the child who has anuria and oliguria is discussed in Chapter 186, Anuria/Oliguria. and is portrayed in Fig. 186-1. All children who have ARF in whom the cause is unclear should undergo renal and bladder ultrasonography.

In considering prerenal and parenchymal renal failure, it first is important to correct any preexisting hypovolemia before evaluating the state of renal function. Various tests often are useful in differentiating prerenal (functional) from intrinsic (parenchymal) renal failure (Table 295-1). Rates of urine sodium and water excretion usually are low in prerenal azotemia, reflecting maximal sodium and water reabsorption by the kidney in order to expand the circulating fluid volume. Normally, urinary sodium concentration varies according to the amount of sodium in the diet. Despite enhanced sodium conservation in hypovolemic states, the variability of measured urine sodium concentrations often limits the usefulness of this measurement alone in discriminating between these two conditions. Calculation of the fractional excretion of sodium (Table 295-1) improves the discriminant value of urine sodium excretion. In general, tests of renal sodium conservation are not interpretable if the child has received large amounts of sodium intravenously, has been given diuretics, or has a nonoliguric form of ARF. The state of renal water conservation is assessed by the urine osmolality or the ratio of urine osmolality to plasma osmolality. Although the latter is a more useful index, it should be interpreted with caution in children who have received hypotonic intravenous rehydration solutions, in those who have nonoliguric acute renal failure, and in those who are malnourished.

Finally, the renal response to mannitol or furosemide after

Table 295-1 Clinical Tests to Differentiate Functional from Parenchymal Oliguric Acute Renal Failure (ARF)

Test	Functional ARF	Parenchymal ARF	Discrimination
Sodium conservation			
Urine sodium concentration (UNa)*	<20 mEq/L	>40 mEq/L	Poor
Fractional excretion of sodium (FENa)	<1	>1	Good
$FENa = \frac{UNa/SNa}{UCr/SCr^*} \times 100$			
Water conservation			
Urine osmolality (Uosm)	>500 mosm/L	>350 mosm/L	Poor
Urine-serum osmolality ratio (Uosm/Sosm)	>2	<1.1	Fair
Response to diagnostic challenge with IV mannitol and furosemide (see text)	Urine flow increase	No change	Good

* *U*, Urine; *Na*, sodium; *Cr*, creatinine; *S*, serum.

a fluid challenge also has been used to differentiate prerenal conditions from intrinsic renal disease. Although mannitol (0.5 g/kg intravenously) and furosemide (1 mg/kg intravenously) were evaluated initially as separate challenges, many clinicians combine these agents to decrease the incidence of false-negative responses. A good provocative response is the formation of 6 to 10 ml of urine per kilogram over the 1 to 3 hours subsequent to the infusion. To evaluate the response accurately, the patient often requires urinary catheterization. Repetitive doses of mannitol and furosemide in instances of nonresponse generally should be avoided because fluid shifts and convulsions as the result of the former and potential ototoxicity from the latter may occur.

Prompt differentiation of prerenal ARF from the oliguria of renal parenchymal injury is extremely important in view of the nature of subsequent fluid management. If prerenal oliguria is unrecognized, adequate fluids may not be given, leading to the development of intrinsic renal damage as a result of prolonged hypoperfusion. In contrast, if intrinsic renal oliguria already is present but unrecognized, vigorous fluid administration to induce diuresis may lead to clinically significant fluid overload.

PREVENTION

Numerous reports have proposed that infusion of "low-dose" dopamine (3 to 5 μg/kg/min), with or without concomitant furosemide early in the course of the ARF may attenuate the severity of the ARF or convert oligoanuric to nonoliguric forms of the injury. These clinical observations are in contrast to several recent studies in a variety of ARF situations that failed to demonstrate a significant clinical role for dopamine in the prevention of ARF. The aforementioned independent association of ARF with increased morbidity and mortality risks and the potential limitations placed on other essential therapies are important clinical considerations. Thus, the single most effective means of ARF management is its prevention through prompt recognition and aggressive elimination of contributory factors wherever possible.

TREATMENT

Management of oliguric parenchymal renal failure requires attention to many details. Hyperkalemia is a particular immediate risk to the patient and must be treated immediately when present. The electrocardiographic changes of hyperkalemia often reflect the state of potassium balance more accurately than does the serum potassium measurement. Peaking of T waves on the ECG is one of the earliest signs of potassium-induced disturbances of myoelectrical activity in the heart. The emergence of hyperkalemia-associated T wave changes must be addressed promptly, since there is considerable variability of the time that PR interval prolongation, QRS complex widening, and tachyarrhythmias appear, with the more serious conduction abnormalities often ensuing rapidly. Various means to lower serum potassium are outlined in Table 295-2. The administration of calcium salts, sodium bicarbonate, and insulin in combination with dextrose are immediate measures whose effects, although of short duration, may be lifesaving. The action of these treatments is by either decreasing the sensitivity of the myocardium to the elevated levels of serum potassium or transiently displacing potassium from the extracellular space. These treatments do not reduce the increased body burden of potassium. Actual net potassium may be removed effectively, but slowly, through the use of enteral potassium-exchange resins (see Table 295-2). Often, it becomes necessary to make an anticipatory decision in the child who has potentially life-threatening hyperkalemia to initiate emergency dialysis to reduce the serum potassium concentration to a safe level quickly when time is of the essence.

Table 295-2 Treatment of Hyperkalemia in Pediatric Patients

Agent	Dose	Effect	Remarks
Calcium gluconate (10%)	0.5 ml/kg IV over 2-4 min	Rapid but transient	Monitor ECG for bradycardia during injection; may be repeated but *not likely* to be effective
Sodium bicarbonate (7.5%)	2.5 mEq/kg (approximately 3 ml/kg) IV by slow push	Rapid but transient	Repetition *not* recommended
Glucose (50%)	1 ml/kg IV by slow push	Within 1-2 hr	Attempt to increase blood glucose to 250 mg/dl; may be maintained by infusion of 30% glucose at rate equal to insensible fluid loss
Insulin (regular)	0.1 U/kg IV	Rapid	Give *only* with hypertonic glucose infusion (30%)
Sodium polystyrene sulfonate (Kayexalate)	1 g/kg PO or PR	3-6 hr	Side effects: gastric irritation (nausea and vomiting), diarrhea, *or* fecal impaction; PO more effective than PR; enemas should be retained >60 min—removed by cleansing enema; may cause *hypokalemia:* use cautiously in patients who tolerate sodium loads poorly; also chelates Ca^{++} and Mg^{++}

Strict attention must be given to fluid, electrolyte, and caloric intake in these patients to minimize other potentially dangerous homeostatic disturbances and to avoid the development of uremia-enhancing catabolism. If acute renal failure persists, the patient may be given intravenous alimentation, which should include essential amino acids, to provide calories, promote healing, and minimize uremia.

The management of children who have nonoliguric acute renal failure generally is less complex compared with those who have the oliguric form, to a great extent because strict fluid restrictions are not necessary. In addition, the volume of fluid these children require gives the clinician a means of providing calories, alkalinizing agents, calcium, and other therapies that are needed to manage the biochemical abnormalities of the ARF and any underlying conditions.

The patient who has any type of acute renal failure is managed best in collaboration with a pediatric nephrologist. With vigorous attention to details of management, dialysis may be unnecessary. However, peritoneal dialysis often is useful to treat those disturbances resistant to more conservative measures, regardless of the age of the patient. Hemofiltration, hemofiltration-dialysis, and hemodialysis may be indicated in situations in which peritoneal dialysis is inadequate or not feasible. The first two forms of invasive therapy are more suited for use in neonates and smaller infants than is hemodialysis. All these procedures should be performed in collaboration with a pediatric nephrologist who has experience with their use.

COMPLICATIONS

The most common complications of acute renal failure in children, beyond the immediate biochemical and fluid problems already mentioned, are infection and gastrointestinal hemorrhage. Infection is more common in patients who have had trauma or surgery and is a factor in as many as two thirds of the deaths occurring in patients who have ARF. As previously mentioned, part of the increased risk of serious bacterial infection in ARF appears to be independent of underlying conditions. The urinary system is the most common site of infection, followed by the bloodstream (septicemia) and the respiratory tract. Although urinary catheterization may be required in the initial evaluation of the oliguric child, prolonged urinary catheterization predisposes the child to infection. Antibiotics given prophylactically to catheterized patients who have ARF also increase the risk of serious urinary infection. Therefore, neither prolonged urinary catheterization for monitoring of urine output nor prophylactic antibiotics are recommended as part of routine management of these patients. Meticulous care should be given to all intravenous catheters to decrease the risk of septicemia.

PROGNOSIS

The short-term outcome of ARF depends on the physician's ability to recognize it and to construct an individualized treatment plan that will minimize the biochemical abnormalities as well as complications. The long-term prognosis depends most on the nature of the underlying condition that produced the renal failure. For example, a patient who has ARF following cardiac surgery has a poor prognosis if the cardiac function remains inadequate; a patient who has renal failure following hemolytic-uremic syndrome generally has a good prognosis.

When to Refer

Consultation from a pediatric nephrologist for the following:
- Guidance on diagnostic evaluation
- Management of complex fluid, mineral, electrolyte, and blood pressure abnormalities
- Evaluation of dialysis options, preparation for and implementation of dialysis or hemofiltration treatment
- Disease-specific management

When to Hospitalize

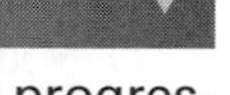

- When renal failure is unexplained, rapidly progressive, or oligoanuric
- In the presence of severe or potentially dangerous fluid or metabolic abnormalities (e.g., hyperkalemia, hypocalcemia, acidosis, clinical fluid overload, or dehydration)
- For renal biopsy

SUGGESTED READINGS

Bock GH: Acute renal failure. In Kher KK, Makker SP, editors: *Clinical pediatric nephrology*, New York, 1992, McGraw-Hill.

Dixon BS, Anderson RJ: Nonoliguric acute renal failure, *Am J Kidney Dis* 6:71, 1985.

Ellis EN, et al: Use of urinary indices in renal failure in the newborn, *Am J Dis Child* 136:615, 1982.

Levy EM, et al: The effect of acute renal failure on mortality: a cohort study, *JAMA* 275:1489, 1996.

Schaffer SE, et al: Renal function and renal failure in the newborn, *Clin Perinatol* 16:199, 1989.

Weiss L, et al: Continuous arteriovenous hemofiltration in the treatment of 100 critically ill patients with acute renal failure: report on clinical outcome and nutritional aspects, *Clin Nephrol* 31:184, 1989.

296 Shock

Joseph R. Custer

The traditional method of writing about and teaching the diagnosis and treatment of shock can be bewildering to a primary care practitioner who rarely encounters such critically ill children.[34] However, the practitioner should bear in mind that the cause of the shock state rarely affects its treatment, especially in its early stages. Prompt recognition and management of shock minimizes mortality and morbidity, even if transfer to a tertiary care facility is required.[8]

The clinician should recognize that simple principles of fluid and pressor therapy are effective in the management of shock regardless of its etiology. When treating shock the clinician should be confident in treating the hemodynamic abnormalities first and establishing the etiology later.

Several guidelines are axiomatic:

1. Vascular access must be established immediately.
2. Volume restoration is always the correct first step.
3. Children who require more than two 20 ml/kg fluid boluses usually require tertiary ICU care.
4. Dopamine is almost uniformly the vasopressor of first choice in pediatric age groups.
5. Sequelae are minimized if hypoxemia is avoided; therefore, adequate ventilation and oxygenation must be assured.
6. Children in septic and cardiogenic shock require referral for definitive care after primary care stabilization.

These few axioms are supported by consideration of pitfalls encountered in the initial management of children referred to a tertiary unit for definitive care (Box 296-1). All of these issues can be addressed easily by the primary care provider.

CLASSIFICATIONS OF SHOCK

Etiology

Shock is classified by mechanism: hypovolemic, distributive, and cardiogenic. The diagnosis, treatment, and therapy of shock has fascinated investigators; a textbook chapter published recently cites 320 references![37] Shoemaker has commented on the complex literature surrounding the etiology and mechanism of shock and the seemingly paradoxical simplistic approach to treatment:

> "The traditional approach is simple, clear, logical, straightforward, readily understandable, and generally accepted by most textbooks and educators. The only problem with this conceptualization is that it is wrong. Real life is not that simple. *Irrespective of the initiating event, the interacting circulatory alterations of flow, volume, and oxygen transport produce characteristic patterns that lead to survival or to circulatory failure, shock, and death.*"[34]

The clinician who initially encounters a child in shock must resist the temptation to perform elaborate, complex diagnostic tests before the patient is stabilized. Securing the airway, establishing vascular access, administering fluids, and providing 100% oxygen are urgent priorities. Once the patient is stabilized, diagnostic tests and evaluation of response to therapy lead to an appropriate comprehensive differential diagnosis.

Underscoring the need to treat first and establish etiology later is the observation of common physiological and hemodynamic patterns in studies that compare children who have either septic or cardiogenic shock. No significant differences in the early or later stages of disease could be found when patients in cardiogenic shock were compared with those in septic shock in terms of cardiac index and oxygen consumption or delivery.[9]

Shock traditionally has been classified as follows:

Hypovolemic
- Dehydration
- Gastrointestinal losses
- Blood loss
- Excess urine output
  - Diabetes mellitus
  - Diabetes insipidus
- High-output renal failure
- "Third space" fluid losses
  - Peritonitis
  - Burns
  - Hypoalbuminemia
- Mannitol administration
- Diuretic agent administration

Distributive
- Septic shock
- Hypoadrenal states
- Anaphylaxis
- Drug overdose

Cardiogenic
- Pump or inotropic
  - Myocarditis
  - Myocardiopathy
  - Decreased contractility acquired in sepsis syndromes
  - Hypoplastic left heart syndrome
  - Arrhythmia
- Obstructive
  - Coarctation of the aorta
  - Pericardial tamponade

BOX 296-1

COMMON PITFALLS NOTED IN A POPULATION OF CHILDREN WHO HAVE SHOCK PRESENTING FOR TERTIARY INTENSIVE CARE

Failure to obtain or delay in obtaining adequate intravenous or intraosseous access
Failure to infuse adequate fluid volume
Failure to document vital signs
Failure to protect the airway
Failure to determine or treat hypoglycemia
Failure to recognize hypoxemia
Failure to recognize occult blood loss
Failure to diagnose an acute abdomen as a source of sepsis

HYPOVOLEMIC SHOCK

Hypovolemic shock is by far the most common form of shock encountered among children. Etiologies include trauma, loss of plasma volume subsequent to burns, gastrointestinal losses, or third space fluid losses.[36]

Shock is defined by hypoperfusion rather than by hypotension. Shock may be present in a child who maintains a near-normal blood pressure but has tachycardia, poor capillary refill, oliguria, and mental status changes. The child will not demonstrate hypotension until all homeostatic mechanisms are exhausted.

The rate at which an infant loses vascular volume and the age of the patient alter the presentation. For example, an acute blood or fluid loss of 15% of body weight precipitates all the classic signs of shock—pallor, tachycardia, poor perfusion, and coma. However, compared with adults, an infant has a much larger extravascular fluid compartment. Thus, slow fluid losses over days are compensated for modestly, so clinical signs of shock are blunted.[14]

Blood Loss

Blood loss resulting from trauma is the most common cause of shock in children. Gastrointestinal bleeding, which occasionally can be rapid and severe, may be seen with esophageal variceal ulcers, Meckel's diverticulum, intussusception, volvulus, or inflammatory bowel disease. Hemolytic-uremic syndrome may present with bloody diarrhea, azotemia, and a coagulopathy.

Plasma Loss

Plasma loss occurs with severe burns; the degree of loss is related to the extent and depth of the burn. Peritonitis produces a significant loss of plasma through the peritoneal surface; this loss, being hidden in a "third space," frequently is underestimated.

Electrolyte Loss

Electrolyte loss and imbalance are seen most commonly in pediatric conditions associated with vomiting and diarrhea. Significant electrolyte loss also occurs in paralytic ileus and intestinal obstruction; large volumes of fluid can fill dilated loops of bowel, and continuous suctioning of gastric content can remove significant amounts of fluid and electrolytes. Excessive diuresis from mannitol or furosemide also may produce significant iatrogenic fluid and electrolyte loss. Hyperosmolar agents, as used in radiological diagnostic procedures, can produce an osmotic diuresis.

The advanced trauma life support classification of shock (Box 296-2) emphasizes the relationship of volume loss to physical signs.[37]

BOX 296-2

ADVANCED TRAUMA LIFE SUPPORT CLASSIFICATION OF SHOCK

Class I
15% or less loss of acute blood volume
Blood pressure normal
Age-related pulse increased 10% to 20%
No change in capillary refill

Class II
20% to 25% loss of blood volume
Tachycardia >150 beats/min
Tachypnea 35 to 40 breaths/min
Capillary refill prolonged >3 sec
Systolic blood pressure decreased
Pulse pressure decreased
Orthostatic hypotension
Urine output >1 ml/kg/hr

Class III
30% to 35% blood volume loss
All of the above signs
Urine output <1 ml/kg/hr
Lethargic, clammy skin, and vomiting

Class IV
40% to 50% blood volume loss
Nonpalpable pulses
Obtunded

DISTRIBUTIVE SHOCK

The many causes of distributive shock produce vasodilation and decreased blood flow to some organs but spare others. As in the other "classes" of shock, early rapid restoration of fluid volume and stabilization of the airway are the foundations of successful therapy.

Causes of distributive shock include sepsis, drug overdose, some poisonings, and anaphylaxis. The hallmark of the clinical presentation is peripheral vasodilation, with warm, red skin in the presence of tachycardia, and altered mental status and oliguria, a constellation often referred to as *hyperdynamic shock*.[24] Septic shock may be more common than historical reports would suggest.[17,25]

The bacterial etiology of septic shock has been altered by vaccination against *Haemophilus influenzae* type B, beginning in 1988. If sepsis in the (increasingly common) immunocompromised patient is excluded, meningococci and streptococci are the bacterial causes of sepsis encountered most frequently. In a retrospective analysis of 2110 admissions to a pediatric intensive care unit before 1989, 564 patients had septic shock; 48% (268) required inotropic support. In the patients who had positive blood cultures, causes were *H. influenzae* type b in 41%, *Neisseria meningitidis* in 18%, and *Streptococcus pneumoniae* in 11%.[17]

Studies of children who have meningococcemia highlight important issues in the care of children in septic shock (see Chapter 291, Meningococcemia).[6,33] Mortality remains high, despite modern advances in critical care.[34] Clinicians who encounter these clinical stigmata in primary care settings should recognize the importance of early stabilization, the need for referral for definitive therapy, and the high mortality despite aggressive intervention.

The development of multisystem organ failure in a group of 100 children who had meningococcemia was predictive of death. Patients in shock, who had a white blood count less than 10,000 cells/mm^3 and coagulopathy, had extremely high mortality.[2] Multisystem organ failure among patients in septic shock correlates with the development of cardiac depression. The hallmark of this presentation is persistent tachycardia despite restoration of blood volume.[24] When cardiac failure can be controlled with catecholamines and judicious fluid management aided by Swan-Ganz catheters, survival is possible. If aggressive volume replacement and catechol therapy do not correct the plasma volume and cardiac failure occurs, death is likely.[18,30]

Toxic shock syndrome is caused by local infection with toxin-producing strains of bacteria, often *Staphylococci* or *Streptococci*. The condition may affect children of any age and of either gender. Cases have been associated with the use of tampons by menstruating women. Closed-space infections, such as retropharyngeal abscess, and infections involving elaboration of large amounts of toxin may be associated with the syndrome. Clinicians should know that only 50% of cases occur in menstruating females. Any focal staphylococcal infection can produce the syndrome (see Chapter 267, Staphylococcal Toxic Shock Syndrome). The patients present with a remarkably rapid downhill course. Fever, accompanied by vomiting, diarrhea, headache, and myalgia, proceeds abruptly to cardiovascular collapse. A scarlatiniform exanthem with flexor surface accentuation and palmar-plantar erythema are common cutaneous manifestations. The differential diagnosis includes Kawasaki disease (Chapter 230), Rocky Mountain spotted fever (Chapter 258), rubeola, and erythema multiforme.[31]

CARDIOGENIC SHOCK

The heart may fail because of primary muscle failure, secondary functional depression, or an obstruction to blood flow. Causes of primary or secondary cardiac pump failure include myocarditis, overwhelming sepsis (bacterial and viral), hypoxemia, myocardial ischemia from inadequate coronary perfusion associated with hypovolemia and hypoxemia, and pericardial tamponade from blood, other fluid, or air.[3]

Decreased preload is the term used to describe inadequate return of blood to the heart. Preload is measured clinically by determining central venous pressure (CVP).[13] Fig. 296-1 demonstrates the interaction of adequate volume status (preload, or CVP) and contractility (cardiac output). In uncomplicated shock, restoration of blood volume alone increases preload and thus restores cardiac output. Acidosis, hypoglycemia, and hypocalcemia decrease cardiac output.

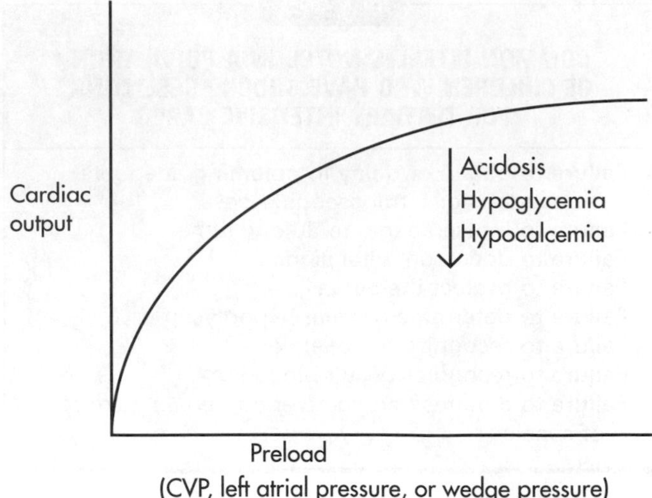

Fig. 296-1 Relationship of stroke volume to preload, determining myocardial contractility (Starling curve). A depressed response may be caused by hypoxemia, acidosis, hypocalcemia, sepsis, or drug toxicity.

Cardiac failure is a rare cause of shock in children. The possibility of a cardiac etiology for shock should not delay venous access, and it is safe to administer a fluid bolus of 10 to 20 ml/kg. If the patient develops symptoms of congestive heart failure—pulmonary edema, an enlarged heart, and hepatomegaly—and exhibits clinical signs of poor perfusion, a cardiac etiology should be suspected. An electrocardiogram, echocardiogram, and chest radiograph should be obtained.

Management of cardiogenic shock is complex and requires sophisticated monitoring devices, cardiac catheterization, and technically complex treatment. Consultation with an intensivist or cardiologist is needed, and transport to a tertiary pediatric intensive care facility usually is necessary.[15]

OTHER COMMON TYPES OF SHOCK

Hypoxic-Ischemic Shock

The primary cause of cardiac arrest in children is hypoxemia.[20] The type of shock following hypoxemic-ischemic insults, a common occurrence in the pediatric age group, is unique. Cardiac output is reduced, oxygen delivery inadequate, and systemic vascular resistance elevated. The poor perfusion and cool, "clamped-down" appearance of the child may be misinterpreted as hypovolemia. In this circumstance aggressive volume infusion can produce symptoms of congestive heart failure. Dopamine, in doses greater than 10 µg/kg/minute, may intensify vasoconstriction and produce tachyarrhythmia. Epinephrine is the agent of choice in this situation.[38]

Hypoadrenal Shock

Many pediatric patients with increasingly complex chronic disease are cared for in primary-care settings. Many of these children are treated with steroids; these include patients who have asthma, rheumatic disease, or renal disease and post–organ transplant patients. Patients who may have secondary depression of the adrenal response should be treated with steroids, usually hydrocortisone (Solu-Cortef), in stress doses of 150 mg/m^2.[10]

SEQUELAE OF SHOCK

The molecular biology of shock, especially septic shock, is complex; detailed reviews are available.[37] When oxygen transport to the tissues is reduced and cellular hypoxemia and anaerobic glycolysis occur, the resultant production of lactic acid causes a fall in blood pH and bicarbonate levels. Inflammatory mediators, such as tumor necrosis factor and interleukins, are released. In turn, a cycle of complement activation and endothelial interaction with leukocytes, macrophages, and platelets is initiated, resulting in tissue ischemia and cell death. General metabolic changes during shock include increased glucagon production, decreased insulin response to glucose, and marked protein catabolism. Metabolism of the cell is disrupted, and less adenosine triphosphate (ATP) is available. Cellular changes include the passage of sodium into and potassium out of the cell, as well as intracellular calcium accumulation. Lysozymes are broken down, and the cell finally is destroyed. However, restoration of adequate tissue perfusion may reverse some of these cellular changes.

Several organ systems may be affected by shock. A common form of hypoxemic respiratory failure known as adult respiratory distress syndrome (ARDS) occurs 24 to 48 hours after initial presentation. The child becomes dyspneic and has significant hypoxemia (PaO_2/FiO_2 ratio <150). Physical examination reveals rales and tachypnea; a chest roentgenogram reveals "diffuse infiltrates." These changes may be delayed and may appear for the first time 12 to 24 hours after the onset of the dyspnea. The interstitial edema that develops appears to be caused by a capillary leak syndrome. This complication is life threatening, and the patient should be referred to a pediatric ICU. Mechanical ventilation and positive end–expiratory pressure, right heart catheters, high-frequency oscillatory ventilation, or extracorporeal membrane support may be required.[5]

Inadequate perfusion and the presence of inflammatory mediators of the heart affect contractility and may lead to a decrease in cardiac output. Myocardial depression is encountered commonly in septic shock.[24]

Renal failure, especially acute tubular necrosis, is common. Renal failure is suspected when the urine output is less than 0.5 ml/kg/hr, despite adequate restoration of blood volume as evidenced by a central venous pressure greater than 5 cm H_2O. An increase in the blood urea nitrogen and creatinine levels supports this diagnosis. Aggressive use of dialysis and hemofiltration has minimized the morbidity resulting from this complication. Unrecognized renal failure increases the mortality resulting from shock. Serum levels of drugs in the blood become uncertain. Doses of antibiotics, sedatives, and analgesics must be monitored carefully, following blood levels in serum whenever possible. Fluid therapy must be titrated carefully to insensible fluid loss replacement; otherwise congestive heart failure results. Anuria complicating shock requires referral or consultation with a nephrologist or intensivist.[19]

BOX 296-3

CAUSES OF SHOCK IN THE YOUNG INFANT

Cardiac
Hypoplastic left heart syndrome
Coarctation of the aorta
Myocarditis
Arrhythmia

Infectious
Bacterial meningitis
Urinary tract sepsis
Herpes (meningitis and sepsis)
Streptococcal sepsis

Metabolic
Hypoglycemia
Inborn errors of metabolism

Traumatic
Child abuse
Occult CNS hemorrhage

Surgical
Bowel obstruction
Occult blood loss

The central nervous system is most susceptible to hypoxemia and ischemia. A child may suffer significant neurological impairment while other organs are spared. Early central nervous system signs of shock include delirium, irritability, confusion, and coma. Signs of increased intracranial pressure usually are delayed 24 to 72 hours after a hypoxemic-ischemic insult. The presence of increased intracranial pressure accompanying the acute presentation of shock implies a traumatic or metabolic etiology.[37]

Liver function may become impaired as a result of inadequate perfusion. Bilirubin and transaminase levels are elevated, and clotting factors may be diminished. In septic shock, liver perfusion may be adequate, but bacteria or toxins may damage hepatic cells. Liver failure is usually transient.

Adrenal failure is uncommon but may occur in septicemia. Meningococcemia may result in the lethal complication of Waterhouse-Friderichsen syndrome. The common use of steroid therapy in asthma, other allergic states, and immune suppression therapy has produced a population of patients in whom "stress doses" of steroids need to be administered should such patients show symptoms in shock. Such a child exhibits hypotension that is refractory to intravascular volume infusion and pressor therapy.[10]

DIAGNOSIS OF SHOCK

History

Appreciation of the effects of age and circumstance helps the examiner to arrive at a more precise differential diagnosis, minimize time and expense of extraneous laboratory tests, and determine appropriate consultation.

Age

Newborns less than 6 weeks of age who are in shock merit special attention, and a broader differential diagnosis should be considered compared with older children. Early discharge of well babies shortly after birth requires attention to both acquired and congenital or inherited conditions. Algorithmic diagnostic and treatment flow sheets designed for older children have proved too general in the evaluation of this age group. Box 296-3 lists the most common diagnoses to consider when approaching infants who are in shock.[28,29]

Shock in toddlers usually has a determinable, apparent cause. The clinician should recognize the propensities unique to this age group, especially poisonings, ingestions of medications, inhalation and swallowing of foreign bodies, exposure to day care compatriots, and trauma resulting from falls, playground and household accidents, and child abuse.

The adolescent may not be forthright in volunteering an accurate history. The risk-taking behavior of the teen years should be considered when a differential diagnosis is generated in this age group. Ingestion and poisoning after attempted suicide may not be reported by those available to give a history. Experiments with drugs and alcohol can have catastrophic consequences.

In all age groups, history of travel may lead to further etiological clues. Rocky Mountain spotted fever and Lyme disease rarely present with cardiovascular collapse. In a child with recent exposure to pets and who has diarrhea, the possibility of *Salmonella* infection must be considered. Recent ingestion of possibly contaminated meat as well as bloody diarrhea with early onset of central nervous system symptoms imply hemolytic uremic syndrome. Exposure to organophosphates should be sought if weakness is part of the presentation.[26]

Physical Diagnosis of Shock

Hypotension and tachycardia are the hallmarks of shock (Box 296-4). In uncomplicated shock, restoration of blood pressure and reduction of heart rate are indicators of therapeutic success. Normal vital signs are seen in Table 296-1.[24,30]

The signs and symptoms of shock are a result of inadequate perfusion, which is a clinical representation of the combined effects of cardiac output and peripheral resistance. Cardiac output is the product of heart rate and stroke volume expressed in liters of blood flow per minute. In older children and adults, hypotension (loss of peripheral vascular tone) is sensed by baroreceptors, which act to increase the heart rate and stroke volume. Infants cannot increase stroke volume as readily and increase cardiac rate as a compensatory mechanism.

BOX 296-4

SYMPTOMS AND SIGNS ASSOCIATED WITH SHOCK

- Tachycardia
- Hypotension
- Oliguria
- Capillary refill >3 seconds
- Tachypnea
- Dry mucous membranes
- Altered mental status

From Crone RK: *Pediatr Clin North Am* 27:525, 1980.

Table 296-1 Normal Vital Signs

	Heart Rate	Blood Pressure (S/D)
Neonate	140±40	65±10/40
<1 year	120±30	80±20/50
1-2 years	110±20	90±20/55
2-5 years	90±20	90±20/60
>5 years	80±10	100±20/60

Heart rate is a valuable clinical sign in shock. Infants are not able to increase stroke volume as well as adults can; therefore cardiac output in the very young is affected by increasing the heart rate.[13] Thus, an infant in shock whose heart rate is 2 standard deviations above normal is attempting to increase cardiac output. The improvement of the infant correlates with the heart rate decreasing to the normal range. Thus, pulse rate is a valuable predictor of success.[3,9,24]

Mental status is a remarkably sensitive and important indicator of degree of illness and response to therapy. Presence of coma or neurological compromise implies significant brain hypoperfusion. Restoration of neurological well-being is the goal of therapy. Shock must be ruled out in children who demonstrate changes in mental status, such as agitation, lethargy, confusion, and coma.[37]

Urine output is usually an accurate indicator of blood volume and perfusion. However, several caveats are important. Many children have multiple caretakers during a typical day, so the frequency and volume of urination may not be accurately recounted. Patients who have high output renal failure or hyperglycemia from diabetes mellitus, patients on diuretics, and children who have received mannitol have high obligatory urine losses.

Capillary refill within 3 seconds is not helpful as a single clinical sign, but when interpreted in constellation with heart rate, blood pressure, and mental status, it does help to determine the degree of illness.[4]

TREATMENT

Early volume resuscitation and vasopressor therapy always are indicated in the treatment of shock. One should be conservative in using these treatments only if patients demonstrate pulmonary edema, congestive heart failure, or renal failure. In these cases judicious use of fluid and evaluation of response to therapy by measurement of the central venous pressure lead astute clinicians to a diagnosis of shock due to cardiac or renal causes. Rather than fearing fluid overload and thus undertreating the vast majority of patients, the clinician should use the patient's response to fluid administration as a diagnostic test.[27] A simple algorithm is displayed in Fig. 296-1.

Treatment of shock, especially in primary care settings, is based on simple principles of restoring adequate circulating blood volume, thereby achieving adequate delivery of glucose and oxygen to all tissues. Timely documentation of response to each intervention is essential.

Clinicians not involved customarily with critically ill children often worry about which type of fluid and vasopressor is most effective.[36,39] This concern is unwarranted. The type of resuscitation fluid has not been demonstrated to improve outcome. The most important therapy, often overlooked or delayed, is the immediate establishment of an intraosseous or large-bore intravenous device; standards of care require this to be placed within minutes of presentation.[23] The second most important priority is giving adequate fluid volume and restoring the circulation. This can be accomplished with commonly available fluids, such as normal saline or lactated Ringer's solution with glucose added to maintain adequate blood glucose levels. A reasonable volume is 20 ml/kg with a range of 10 to 30 ml/kg.[36]

The next urgent priority in all shock patients is to ensure that the airway is patent. All patients in shock should immediately be given 100% oxygen; oxygenation should be monitored continuously with a pulse oximeter and the values documented in the patient's record. Because a normal oxygen saturation does not reflect adequate oxygen content, the hemoglobin (the carrying vehicle for oxygen) must be at a normal level. Clinicians need to appreciate that a normal oxygen saturation does not imply adequate tissue delivery.[32]

Acidosis is a common sequela of shock. The salutary effects of restoring the pH to greater than 7.25 are crucial: myocardial contractility is enhanced, sensitivity to catecholamines is improved, and potassium is returned to the intracellular space.

Sodium bicarbonate may be required to improve blood pH to greater than 7.25 and serum bicarbonate levels to greater than 15 mEq/dl.[18] See Chapter 29, Fluid Therapy.

Hypocalcemia may accompany shock. Total calcium measurements do not correlate with measurements of the biologically more important ionized calcium.[21] Restoring ionized calcium to normal levels can be an important component of later stages of therapy.

Clinicians must appreciate the crucial role of hemoglobin, especially when low cardiac output is combined with hypoxemia. Clinicians should also realize that a normal oxygen saturation and "adequate" arterial PO_2 are not accurate reflections of adequate tissue oxygen delivery.[1,22,32]

Blood transfusions are an essential component in blood loss and anemic states. If the circulation is compromised and cardiac output falls, oxygen delivery to tissues will be compromised. Oxygen delivery is merely the product of the blood's oxygen content and cardiac output. Blood oxygen content = 1.36 × % saturation × hemoglobin (in grams) and is expressed as milliliters of O_2/100 ml blood. Cardiac output is the product of heart rate and stroke volume expressed as liters of flow per minute (L/min).

In shock states, tissue oxygen consumption needs may increase simultaneously with inadequate cardiac output, leading to inadequate tissue oxygenation. If lung disease is present or hypoventilation occurs, hemoglobin is less than 100% saturated and oxygen delivery is compromised further.[9,26] Transfusion is indicated if anemia is present. For the patient in shock, a hemoglobin of at least 12 g must be maintained.

Preservation of coagulation balance is in the second tier of therapies. In general, unless bleeding is evident, platelet counts of 20,000 to 50,000/mm^3 are tolerated well. Prothrombin time and partial thromboplastin time should be maintained at 1.3 times the normal values. Fresh-frozen plasma, administered at 10 ml/kg, is a reasonable method both of repairing volume deficit and replenishing coagulation factors.[11,35]

Glucose replacement is crucial, especially in the very young. Glucose should be maintained at greater than 60 mg/dl in infants and at least at 80 mg/dl in adolescents. Clinicians who use normal saline or lactated Ringer as a volume expander need to remember to provide 10% glucose to these fluids in infants and 5% in other age groups. Rapid serum glucose determinations are available. These values should be monitored and recorded as a "vital sign" whenever blood pressures are measured. Persistent hypoglycemia is an ominous sign in sepsis and may indicate the presence of an inherited metabolic disorder in infants.

VASOPRESSOR DRUGS

The clinician should not be misled or seduced by unneeded complexities when choosing an appropriate vasopressor[39] In the vast majority of situations that a primary care physician encounters, knowledge of the effects of dopamine carries the day. A very basic knowledge of vasopressor physiology is required (Table 296-2).[38]

Catecholamine drugs commonly used in shock include dopamine, epinephrine, and dobutamine. Catecholamines are classified by their relative effects on the alpha or beta receptor. The alpha receptor produces vasoconstriction, which accounts for its salutary effect in raising blood pressure. Alpha agonists are not delivered with peripheral intravenous devices because skin and muscle necrosis can result. Intense alpha stimulation can decrease renal and splanchnic blood flow, but this can be offset by the dopaminergic effect of low-dose dopamine.[37]

Beta-agonists have type 1 and 2 receptors. Beta 1 recep-

Table 296-2 Specific Vasopressor Agents Used to Treat Shock

Agent	Site of Action (Receptor)	Dose* (μg/kg/min)	Effect
Dopamine	δ	1-3	"Dopaminergic"; renal vasodilation; inotropic
	$\alpha > \beta$	5-20	Peripheral vasoconstriction; increased systemic vascular resistance; dysrhythmias
Dobutamine	β_1, β_2	1-20	Inotropic, chronotropic; vasodilation (β_2); lowers systemic vascular resistance; lowers pulmonary vascular resistance; tachycardia and arrhythmia (β_1)
Epinephrine	$\alpha > \beta$	0.05-1.0	Inotropic Tachycardia; arrhythmia; decreased renal flow from α effect; increase in myocardial oxygen consumption; intense vasoconstriction
Norepinephrine	$\alpha > \beta$	0.005-1.0	Profound vasoconstriction; inotropic; dramatic increase in myocardial oxygen consumption and systemic vascular resistance

*The doses listed are suggested starting ranges. The drugs can be titrated to the desired effect depending on the patient's response.

tors stimulate heart rate and cardiac muscle contractility; thus, toxicity is reflected in cardiac tachyarrhythmias and ischemia. Beta-2 agonists occur in bronchial and arteriole smooth muscle; thus, these muscles relax when stimulated. At low doses (1 to 4 μg/kg/min) dopamine acts at a unique dopaminergic receptor that can enhance or preserve renal blood flow.

A vasoactive drug should be infused continuously with a calibrated infusion pump; continuous heart rate and blood pressure monitoring is required, preferably with an intraarterial catheter and transducer. Vasoactive agents should be infused into a central venous catheter. Norepinephrine, epinephrine, and dopamine increase blood pressure by vasoconstriction, which can decrease renal blood flow. These drugs are only adjuncts to volume replacement in hypovolemic shock; blood and fluid replacement is the cardinal therapeutic modality.[12,39]

Dopamine is used frequently to increase cardiac output and augment renal perfusion in the critically ill child. The effects are dose dependent, with renal (dopaminergic, δ) effects seen at the low-dose range (1 to 4 μg/kg/min). At higher doses (>10 μg/kg/min) alpha-adrenergic effects predominate with vasoconstriction and reduced peripheral perfusion.

Dobutamine differs from dopamine because of its enhanced inotropic effect with less chronotropic effect than dopamine; also, it has less effect on systemic vascular resistance. In some circumstances, especially shock induced by hypoxemia-ischemia, epinephrine or dobutamine may be preferred because dopamine may precipitate tachyarrhythmias and increase myocardial oxygen consumption.[18]

Epinephrine is a valuable agent when dopamine proves futile, which may occur in severe septic shock. It is the preferred second-line drug when dopamine fails. It is primarily indicated for the shock that occurs following a hypoxic-ischemic event.[38]

Steroids are not indicated in shock therapy except when adrenal suppression occurs after corticosteroid treatment. In large prospective human trials, steroids used to treat septic shock have increased mortality and the incidence of secondary infection.[7] Therefore, steroids are indicated only in patients suspected of having secondary adrenal suppression from prior steroid use.[10]

In selected situations and in tertiary settings only, the use of vasodilator drugs (nitroprusside, milrinone, nitroglycerin) may be beneficial in reducing afterload when increased afterload is detrimental to myocardial performance. This therapy optimizes myocardial contractility and improves cardiac output but requires sophisticated monitoring, including pulmonary arterial oximetry, cardiac output measurement, and pulmonary vascular pressure catheters.[27,37]

Trials of several new therapies have been unsuccessful and have not affected outcomes for pediatric patients. Extracorporeal membrane oxygenation has not been explored adequately and should be performed only at the few centers capable of supporting this technology.[5] A randomized trial of methylprednisolone demonstrated more complications and no reduction in mortality.[7] Trials of ibuprofen, antibody to endotoxin, and antibody to tumor necrosis factor alpha have not met expectations for improving survival in cases of septic shock.[33]

EVALUATION

Response to therapy is important, simple to assess, and of diagnostic value. Documentation of serial interventions and responses is a standard of care. Pulse, respiratory rate, O_2 saturation, blood pressure, capillary refill, urine output, mental status, and glucose level should be recorded every 15 minutes while the patient remains unstable.

Several laboratory tests help to determine further therapy or appropriate consultation. A persistent anion-gap metabolic acidosis (HCO_3 <15 mEq) may support the diagnosis of renal failure, ketoacidosis, lactic acidemia from sepsis, or poisoning from a salicylate, ethanol, or methanol.

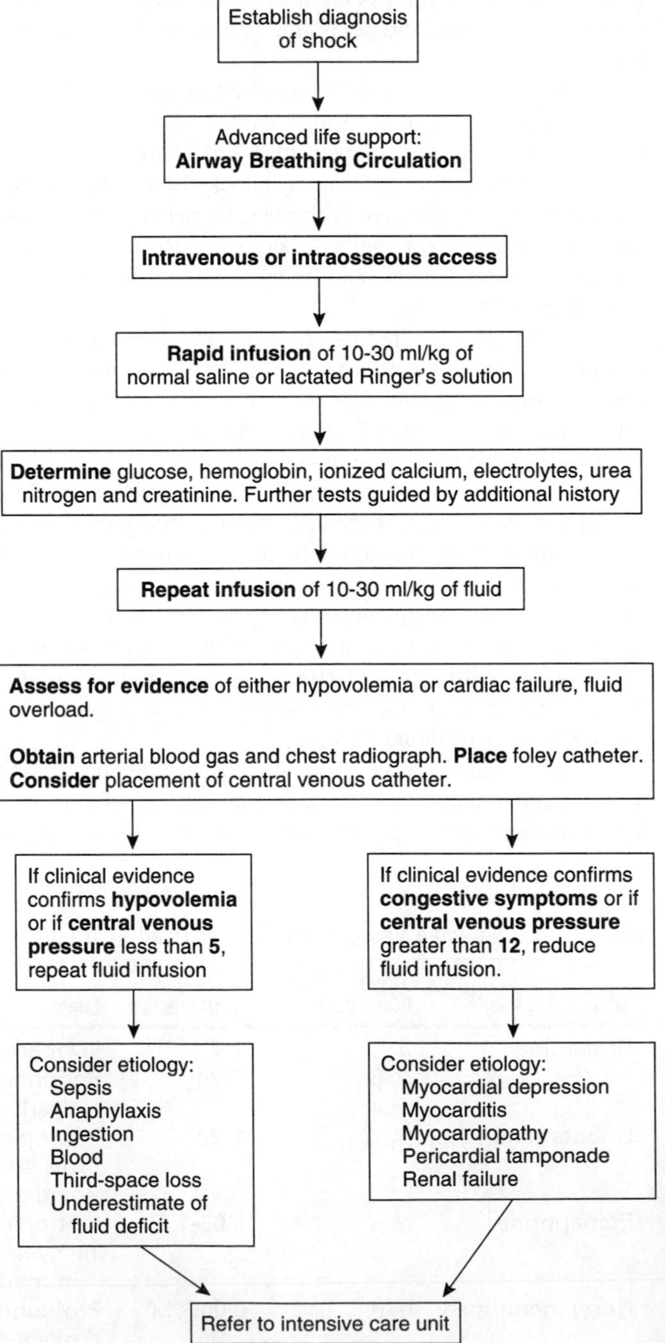

Fig. 296-2 Algorithm for the treatment of shock.

Patients who remain in coma or have a depressed sensorium despite evidence of adequate volume repletion are at high risk for neurological sequelae. An inherited metabolic disorder, hypoglycemia, hepatic failure, azotemia, trauma, and poison ingestion must be considered if normalization of blood pressure does not improve mental status.

If two bolus infusions do not result in an improvement, determination of central venous pressure (CVP) is invaluable. If the CVP is less than 5 cm H_2O, another bolus infusion (10 to 30 ml/kg) and additional pressor therapy should be administered (Fig. 296-2).

If the CVP is greater than 12 cm H_2O and congestive failure, pulmonary edema, and poor perfusion are present, a cardiac etiology should be suspected and the fluid infusion rate reduced. An ECG, echocardiogram, and chest radiograph are indicated, and consultation with a pediatric cardiologist should be obtained.

REFERENCES

1. Akingbola OA, et al: Management of severe anemia without transfusion in a pediatric Jehovah's Witness: case report and literature review, *Crit Care Med* 22:524, 1994.
2. Algren JT, et al: Predictors of outcome in acute meningococcal infection in children, *Crit Care Med* 21:447, 1993.
3. Bangur AR, Meliones JN: Cardiogenic shock, *New Horiz* 6:139, 1998.
4. Barraff LJ: Capillary refill: is it a useful clinical sign? *Pediatrics* 92:723, 1993.
5. Beca J, Butt W: Extracorporeal membrane oxygenation for refractory septic shock in children, *Pediatrics* 93:726, 1994.
6. Bone RC: Let's agree on terminology: definitions of sepsis, *Crit Care Med* 19:973, 1991.
7. Bone RC, Fisher CJ Jr, Clemmer TP: A controlled clinical trial of high-dose methylprednisolone in the treatment of severe sepsis and septic shock, *N Engl J Med* 317:653, 1987.
8. Carcillo JA, Davis AL, Zaritsky A: Role of early fluid resuscitation in pediatric septic shock, *JAMA* 266:1242, 1991.
9. Carcillo JA, Pollack MM, Ruttimann UE: Sequential physiologic interactions in pediatric cardiogenic and septic shock, *Crit Care Med* 17:12, 1989.
10. Chamberlin P, Meyer WJ III: Management of pituitary-adrenal suppression secondary to corticosteroid therapy, *Pediatrics* 67:245, 1981.
11. Colman RW, Robboy SJ, Minna JD: Disseminated intravascular coagulation: a reappraisal, *Annu Rev Med* 30:359, 1979.
12. Fisher DG, Schwartz PH, Davis AL: Pharmacokinetics of exogenous epinephrine in critically ill children, *Crit Care Med* 21:111, 1993.
13. Friedman WF, George BL: Treatment of congestive heart failure by altering loading conditions of the heart, *J Pediatr* 106:697, 1985.
14. Friis-Hansen B: Body water compartments in children, *Pediatrics* 28: 169, 1961.
15. Girour BP, Perkin RM, Levin DL: Shock. In Levin DL, Morriss FC, editors: *Essentials of pediatric intensive care,* London, 1997, Churchill Livingstone.
16. Hesselvick JF, Bradin B: Low-dose norepinephrine in patients with septic shock and oliguria: effects on afterload, urine flow, and oxygen transport, *Crit Care Med* 17:179, 1989.
17. Jacobs RF, et al: Septic shock in children: bacterial etiologies and temporal relationships, *Pediatr Infect Dis J* 9:196, 1990.
18. Kirsch EA, Barton P, Kitchen L: Pathophysiology, treatment, and outcome of meningococcemia: a review and recent experience, *Pediatr Infect Dis J* 15:967, 1996.
19. Lucas CE: The renal response to acute injury and sepsis, *Surg Clin North Am* 56:953, 1976.
20. Lucking SE, Pollack MM, Fields AI: Shock following generalized hypoxic-ischemic injury in previously healthy infants and children, *J Pediatr* 108:359, 1986.
21. Meliones JM, Moler FW, Custer JR: Hemodynamic instability after the initiation of extracorporeal membrane oxygenation: role of ionized calcium, *Crit Care Med* 19:1247, 1991.
22. Mink RB, Pollack M: Effect of blood transfusion on oxygen consumption in pediatric septic shock, *Crit Care Med* 18:1087, 1987.
23. Orlowski JP: Comparison study of intraosseous central intravenous and peripheral intravenous infusions of emergency drugs, *Am J Dis Child* 144:112, 1990.
24. Parker MM, et al: Serial cardiovascular variables in survivors and nonsurvivors of human septic shock: heart rate as an early predictor of prognosis, *Crit Care Med* 15:923, 1987.
25. Parrillo JE, et al: Septic shock in humans, *Ann Intern Med* 113:227, 1990.
26. Perkin RM: Shock states. In Fuhrman BH, Zimmerman JR, editors: *Pediatric critical care,* St Louis, 1992, Mosby.
27. Perkin RM, Anas NG: Cardiovascular evaluation and support in the critically ill child, *Pediatr Ann* 15:30, 1986.
28. Perkin RM, Levin DL: Shock in the pediatric patient. I. Therapy, *J Pediatr* 101:319, 1982.
29. Perkin RM, Levin DL: Shock in the pediatric patient. II. Therapy, *J Pediatr* 101:613, 1982.
30. Pollack MM, Fields AI, Ruttiman UE: Distributions of cardiopulmonary variables in pediatric survivors and nonsurvivors of septic shock, *Crit Care Med* 13:454, 1985.
31. Resnsick SD: Toxic shock syndrome: recent developments in pathogenesis, *J Pediatr* 116:321, 1990.
32. Rodriguez LR, et al: A study of pediatric house staff's knowledge of pulse oximetry, *Pediatrics* 93:810, 1994.
33. Saez-Llorens X, McCracken GH Jr: Sepsis syndrome and septic shock in pediatrics: current concepts of terminology, pathophysiology, and management, *J Pediatr* 123:497, 1994.
34. Shoemaker WC: Circulatory mechanisms of shock and their mediators, *Crit Care Med* 15:787, 1987.
35. Sinclair JF: The management of fulminant meningococcal septicaemia in children, *Intensive Care World* 5:89, 1988.
36. Thomas NJ, Carcillo JA: Hypovolemic shock in pediatric patients, *New Horiz* 6:120, 1998.
37. Tobin JR, Wetzel RC: Shock. In Rogers M, editor: *Textbook of pediatric intensive care,* ed 3, Baltimore, 1996, Williams & Wilkins.
38. Zaritsky A: Recent advances in pediatric cardiopulmonary resuscitation and advanced life support, *New Horiz* 6:201, 1998.
39. Zaritsky A, Miles M: Too much pharmacokinetics? *Crit Care Med* 21: 1620, 1993.

297 Status Asthmaticus

Nienke P. Dosa • Robert K. Kanter

Asthma is the most common chronic illness of childhood (see Chapter 188), affecting 4% to 7% of American children.[8,33] Status asthmaticus, defined as airway obstruction refractory to conventional treatment and necessitating hospital admission, is the acute exacerbation of a chronic disease for which the cornerstone of management is preventive therapy. Both the prevalence and the severity of asthma are increasing. Between 1982 and 1991, asthma diagnoses among Americans increased approximately 40%, and the number of deaths from asthma jumped by 68%.[8,53] Approximately 0.5% of hospitalized asthmatic patients require intubation or cardiopulmonary resuscitation.[14] Mortality due to status asthmaticus has been related to inadequate or delayed treatment and the use of inappropriate medications, such as over-reliance on beta-adrenergic agonists and avoidance of corticosteroids.[29,48,50] Psychological problems, recurrent emergency room or hospital admissions, diurnal variation in pulmonary function, use of more than two canisters of short-acting beta-2 agonists per month, current use or recent withdrawal from oral steroids, race, and socioeconomic status have been associated with an increased mortality risk.[15,22,35,41,49] The two risk factors most closely correlated with fatal asthma are a prior near-fatal attack and hospitalization within the previous year.[47] Overall, approximately 5000 people die of asthma in the United States each year, with increasing mortality noted among adolescents and young adults.[2,12,52] Morbidity represents an even greater burden. Asthma is now the most common discharge diagnosis for patients admitted to pediatric hospitals.[5,14] Asthmatic children miss more than 10 million schooldays per year, and loss in productivity by working parents caring for these children is estimated to approach $1 billion per year.[4]

As defined by National Institutes of Health (NIH) guidelines, asthma is a chronic inflammatory disorder of the airways caused by the triad of bronchial wall inflammation, smooth muscle hyperreactivity (bronchospasm), and excessive intraluminal mucus. Status asthmaticus is an acute episode of airway obstruction that is resistant to bronchodilator therapy. Most children have a history of gradual deterioration. However, a subset of patients who may have a blunted perception of their symptoms[24] have "sudden asphyctic asthma" or "hyperacute asthma," defined as status asthmaticus necessitating intubation within the first 3 hours of medical attention. In addition, asthma exacerbations triggered by an allergen can occur in two phases. The immediate phase is caused by mast cell degranulation and results in abrupt bronchoconstriction. The late phase, which occurs 8 or more hours later, is caused by progressive airway inflammation and is often associated with mucus plugging that can be difficult to treat. Significant individual variation can exist in the presentation of status asthmaticus.

The diagnosis of asthma is based on the clinical symptoms of recurrent episodes of wheezing and coughing. Other symptoms and signs include dyspnea, chest tightness, use of accessory muscles of respiration, and cyanosis. For children older 5 years of age, spirometry is used to establish the degree of airflow obstruction. Alternative diagnoses such as vocal cord dysfunction, vascular rings, and foreign bodies need to be excluded in patients with atypical asthma. Imaging studies are indicated in this setting. During the winter, bronchiolitis needs to be considered, and response to beta-2 agonist therapy carefully monitored, since evidence for its efficacy for this disease remains inconclusive.[13] If allergy or gastroesophageal reflux disease are suspected, nasal examination, allergy testing, or a pH probe study may be indicated. Finally, medically complex children may require a more extensive evaluation to establish whether respiratory symptoms are pulmonary in origin. For example, children with heart disease may have increased bronchoreactivity because of high pulmonic blood flow or beta-blocker therapy. The child with spina bifida and Chiari II malformation may have wheezing episodes because of palatopharyngeal dysfunction or latex allergy. For children who require a long-term tracheostomy, improperly humidified oxygen tubing may cause bronchospasm. These children may also develop granulomatous lesions that can cause wheezing. Polypharmacy may contribute to bronchospasm in the medically complex population as well.

Once asthma is diagnosed, the goal is preventive care and patient education. The four key components for long-term control of asthma are assessment and monitoring, pharmacological therapy, control of factors contributing to asthma severity, and patient education. A stepwise approach to the management of asthma is outlined by the National Institutes of Health Expert Panel Guidelines.[32] In addition, programs specifically directed to patients with life-threatening asthma may prevent asthma deaths. Such programs include daily pulmonary function testing and a community-based emergency communication and response network.[47] Cost-saving algorithms for children hospitalized for status asthmaticus have been developed in recent years,[27] but care should be taken to recognize that significant individual variation exists in clinical presentation and that some children may have idiosyncratic responses to therapies. Treatment should be based on assessment of a child's response to therapy and a careful history of previous presentations. Avoiding repeat exacerbations and treating acute episodes require an understanding of the pathophysiology of asthma so that effective treatments, both medical and educational, can be designed for the child and the family.

PATHOPHYSIOLOGY

During severe exacerbations of asthma, the central event is irregular airway narrowing secondary to bronchospasm, mucosal edema, epithelial sloughing, and the formation of mucus plugs. The relative contribution of each of these processes to airway obstruction varies according to the age of the child, the size of the airway, and the duration and severity of asthma. Obstruction of airways is the final common pathway for acute asthma, whether the stimulus is nonimmunological (viruses, smoke, cold air, exercise) or an immunological antigen. Initially, the resultant hyperinflation compensates for intraluminal airflow obstruction by causing airway distention. Altered pulmonary mechanics increase the work of breathing, however, and cause the sensation of breathlessness. As hyperinflation increases, tidal volume approaches the volume of pulmonary dead space and alveolar hypoventilation develops. Large amounts of negative pleural pressure during the inspiratory phase of respiration increases the afterload imposed on the left ventricle. In addition, hypoxia causes pulmonary vasoconstriction, which increases right ventricle afterload. This causes the intraventricular septum to shift to the left, further impeding left ventricular filling. These factors combine to diminish cardiac output and oxygen delivery to tissue beds.[28]

Furthermore, children acutely affected by asthma often have poor oral intake and increased insensible fluid loss because of increased ventilatory drive and fever, resulting in the development of a fluid deficit. This fluid deficit increases the viscosity of secretions and contributes to hypoperfusion and hypoxemia. Dehydration, work of breathing, and hypoxia all contribute to an escalating metabolic acidosis. Alveolar hypoventilation due to narrowed airways leads to ventilation-perfusion ($\dot{V}/\dot{Q}$) mismatch. Hypoxemia is common in early status asthmaticus, even in mildly symptomatic children. Whether or not the patient is hypoxic, an effective central response to the mechanical load of breathing results in hyperventilation and a drop in $PaCO_2$. As the obstruction becomes more severe, fatigue develops and CO_2 retention occurs. The additive effect of late acute respiratory acidosis to the preexistent metabolic acidosis can produce a sharp decline in intravascular pH. Acidosis may impair cardiac contractility and increases pulmonary vascular resistance. These factors contribute to the rapid progression of respiratory failure by depressing oxygen delivery to the tissues further, impairing adenosine triphosphate (ATP) synthesis, and leading to muscle fatigue and cardiorespiratory collapse.[1,20,42,54]

An understanding of the cell and molecular biology of asthma is key to the future management of the disease. At present, asthma is a disease that is preventable but not curable. There is evidence that long-term undertreatment of this inflammatory disease may result in airway remodeling of musculature and connective tissue. Histologically, smooth muscle cell hyperplasia and hypertrophy occur, as well as increased collagen deposition in the basement membrane. In addition, mucosal edema and increased mucus production result from damage to the airway at the cellular level by eosinophilic cytokine products and mast cell proteases. Research in immunology and signal transduction pathways may yield more specific and effective asthma therapy in the future.[34]

MANAGEMENT

Assessment of Severity

Subjective and objective signs of the magnitude of airflow limitation and respiratory fatigue should be evaluated initially upon patient presentation and frequently during therapy. The respiratory rate and pattern correlate with the severity of the asthmatic attack; tachypnea, tachycardia, expiratory grunting, and accessory muscle use are ominous signs. The use of sternocleidomastoid muscles for movement of the chest wall correlates with peak expiratory flow rates of less than 50%.[56] Dyspnea can be assessed by determining the degree of breathlessness, that is, the inability of the verbal patient to speak without appearing short of breath. Fatigue and lethargy may be signs of hypercapnia; confusion, or combativeness are signs of hypoxia. Some signs, however, may be insensitive. For instance, wheezing may not be heard if airway obstruction is severe, as in sudden asphyctic asthma, and cyanosis may be absent in the anemic patient despite severe hypoxia.

Peak expiratory flow rates (PEFR) provide a useful objective measure of airway obstruction. Ideally, home peak flow measurements are obtained when a child is well, providing a peak flow meter diary and establishing a "personal best." Trends away from this baseline then can be identified promptly and preventive therapy initiated. This may be particularly important to the management of the subset of children who have impaired perception of their symptoms. A drop of 20% from personal best may predict an exacerbation within 12 to 24 hours. A drop of 50% signifies a severe exacerbation.[32] In the acute setting serial measurements of PEFR are used to quantify the severity of acute airway obstruction and its response to therapy. Forced expiration may exacerbate severe bronchospasm and should be avoided among patients with severe respiratory distress.

Pulse oximetry (SpO_2) is a good noninvasive monitor of oxygenation and response to therapy. Continuous oximetry should be performed on all patients in status asthmaticus. Blood gas analysis reflects early mild impairment of oxygenation and hypocapnia, or late severe hypoxia and combined metabolic and respiratory acidosis. Decisions regarding intubation and assisted ventilation often must be made urgently based on clinical appearance, without awaiting results of blood gas measurements. In the severely distressed patient, arterial puncture may increase the child's anxiety and work of breathing and should be avoided. Because improvement in response to therapy or progression of respiratory failure may be rapid, blood gas measurements are of limited value in guiding therapy unless available within minutes.

Chest radiographs should be reserved for first-time wheezers and children who exhibit clinical signs of pneumothorax, pneumonia, or atelectasis.

Therapy

Successful management of status asthmaticus requires the reversal of hypoxia and treatment of the two pathological components of asthma: bronchospasm and inflammation (Table 297-1). Standard initial treatment in the medical setting consists of oxygen, beta-2 agonists, and corticosteroids.

Oxygen. Humidified oxygen is the first line of treatment in any child who is in respiratory distress. Benefits of oxygen therapy include correction of hypoxia caused by $\dot{V}/\dot{Q}$ mismatching and a reduction of pulmonary hypertension. Pulse oximetry should be used to assess oxygenation; oxygen saturation should be kept greater than 90%. NIH guidelines recommend that infants, children with coexistent heart disease, and pregnant women maintain oxygen saturation greater than 95%.

BRONCHODILATORS. The most effective therapies for status asthmaticus are the bronchodilators. These include beta-2 agonists and anticholinergics. Methylxanthines are not indicated in rescue treatment of status asthmaticus.[7,31,32,51] Short-acting inhaled beta-2 agonists such as albuterol or ter-

Table 297-1 NIH-Recommended Dosages of Drugs for Rescue Treatment of Status Asthmaticus

	Dosages		
Medication	**Adults**	**Children**	**Comments**
Inhaled Short-Acting Beta$_2$-Agonists			
Albuterol Nebulizer solution (5 mg/ml)	2.5 to 5 mg every 20 min for 3 doses, then 2.5 to 10 mg every 1 to 4 hr as needed, or 10 to 15 mg/hr continuously	0.15 mg/kg (minimum dose 2.5 mg) every 20 min for 3 doses, then 0.15 to 0.3 mg/kg up to 10 mg every 1 to 4 hr as needed, or 0.5 mg/kg/hr by continuous nebulization	Only selective beta$_2$-agonists are recommended. For optimal delivery, dilute aerosols to minimum of 4 ml at gas flow of 6 to 8 L/min
Metered-dose inhaler (90 µg/puff)	4 to 8 puffs every 20 min up to 4 hr, then every 1 to 4 hr as needed	4 to 8 puffs every 20 min for 3 doses, then every 1 to 4 hr as needed	As effective as nebulized therapy if patient is able to coordinate inhalation maneuver. Use spacer/holding chamber
Bitolterol and pirbuterol			Have not been studied in severe asthma exacerbations
Systemic (Injected) Beta$_2$-Agonists			
Epinephrine 1:1000 (1 mg/ml)	0.3 to 0.5 mg every 20 min for 3 doses SQ	0.01 mg/kg up to 0.3 to 0.5 mg every 20 min for 3 doses SQ	No proven advantage of systemic therapy over aerosol
Terbutaline (1 mg/ml)	0.25 mg every 20 min for 3 doses SQ	0.01 mg/kg every 20 min for 3 doses then every 2 to 6 hr as needed SQ	No proven advantage of systemic therapy over aerosol
Anticholinergics			
Ipratropium bromide Nebulizer solution (0.25 mg/ml)	0.5 mg every 30 min for 3 doses then every 2 to 4 hr as needed	0.25 mg every 20 min for 3 doses, then every 2 to 4 hr	May mix in same nebulizer with albuterol. Should not be used as first-line therapy; should be added to beta$_2$-agonist therapy
Metered-dose inhaler (18 µg/puff)	4 to 8 puffs as needed	4 to 8 puffs as needed	Dose delivered from MDI is low and has not been studied in asthma exacerbations
Steroids			
Prednisone Methylprednisolone Prednisolone	120-180 mg/day in 3 or 4 divided doses for 48 hr, then 60 to 80 mg/day until the peak expiratory flow rate (PEFR) reaches 70% of predicted personal best	1 mg/kg every 6 hr for 48 hr, then 1 to 2 mg/kg/day (maximum = 60 mg/day) in 2 divided doses until the peak expiratory flow rate (PEFR) reaches 70% of predicted or personal best	Adult "burst" at discharge: 40 to 60 mg in single or 2 divided doses for 3 to 10 days Child "burst" at discharge: 1 to 2 mg/kg/day, maximum 60 mg/day for 3 to 10 days

From National Asthma Education and Prevention Program: Expert Panel Report II: *Guidelines for the diagnosis and management of asthma,* Pub No 97-4051, Bethesda, Md, 1997, US Department of Health and Human Services.

butaline should be administered every 20 to 30 minutes for three treatments, with close monitoring for response. The onset of action is in about 5 minutes, and peak effect occurs in about 20 minutes. Equivalent bronchodilation can be achieved if the same dose of the beta-2 agonist is given by a metered dose inhaler (MDI) with a spacer or by nebulizer therapy.[10,21] Continuous administration with a nebulizer may be more effective in young children and severely obstructed asthmatics[23,25,44] and has been shown to result in a more rapid improvement in pulmonary function as compared with intermittent therapy.[36] Subcutaneous beta-2 agonists provide no benefit over inhaled medication. However, some patients benefit from an initial subcutaneous injection of epinephrine or terbutaline to improve air movement and delivery of aerosolized drugs.

Agents such as albuterol and terbutaline dilate smooth muscle by stimulating beta 2–adrenergic receptors. Side effects of beta-2 agonists are dose related and include cardiac arrhythmias, tremors, headaches, hyperglycemia, hypokalemia, and nausea. Patients needing nebulizations more frequent than every 3 hours require a cardiorespiratory monitor. Overuse of beta-2 agonists can result in the development of tachyphylaxis because of down-regulation of beta receptors.[6] Other studies have suggested that repeated use of beta-2 agonists may result in increased airway hyperresponsiveness from exercise- or allergen-induced bronchospasm[34,38] Some studies have linked overreliance on beta-2 agonists with increasing asthma mortality.[48] Subsequent studies have refuted this conclusion and implied that the increased mortality is caused by the underuse of antiinflammatory agents as well as various socioeconomic factors.[9,30] Deaths have also been reported in patients who mistakenly use the long acting salmeterol inhalers in the acute setting.[26] Studies to further evaluate the safety of beta-2 agonists are ongoing. At present, short-acting beta-2 agonists remain the first-line treatment for acute asthma exacerbations. Anticholinergic agents, such as ipratropium bromide, produce bronchodilation by blocking the activity of acetylcholine on airway smooth muscle receptors. The effect on airway obstruction is modest; studies have shown approximately one tenth the efficacy of albuterol, when measured in terms of improvement in FEV_1.[40,46] The onset of action is slow (20 minutes), and peak effect occurs at 60 minutes.[16] It should not be used as a first-line therapy, but clinical trials have found ipratropium bromide to have an additive effect when coadministered with beta-2 agonists.[19,37,57]

ANTIINFLAMMATORY AGENTS. Until more specific antiinflammatory agents are developed, corticosteroids remain the most effective drugs for treating airway obstruction caused by inflammation. They are known to improve beta-receptor regulation in the airway, inhibit the activation and influx of inflammatory cells, and interfere with the metabolism of arachidonic acid to prostaglandins and leukotrienes.[32] Oral or parenteral administration appears to be equally potent.[18,39] In the acutely dyspneic child, parenteral administration is preferred to ensure adequate delivery of the medication. Steroids should be administered to patients with moderate to severe exacerbations, to patients who fail to respond promptly to inhaled beta-2 agonists, and to patients admitted to the hospital. Onset of action is approximately 4 hours.[11,43,45] A 3- to 10-day course speeds recovery and reduces the likelihood of recurrence. For patients who take oral steroids long term, supplemental doses are indicated, even if the exacerbation is mild. Inhaled corticosteroids are the most effective long-term treatment for moderate to severe asthma, and should be reinstituted before discontinuation of oral therapy, since withdrawal of the latter is usually accompanied by a rapid return to airway hyperresponsiveness.[17,55] Studies are under way to evaluate the role of inhaled steroids in acute situations and among intubated patients.

Other antiinflammatory agents, including mast-cell stabilizers and medications that inhibit lipoxygenase products, offer benefits for the long-term management of asthma but do not play a role in the acute management of status asthmaticus.

Alternative forms of therapy for refractory cases of status asthmaticus are reserved for use in pediatric intensive care units. These therapies include intravenous magnesium sulfate, theophylline, inhalational anesthetics, calcium channel blockers, extracorporeal membranous oxygenation, and heliox (helium with oxygen). No randomized studies evaluating these modalities in pediatric patients have been published yet, but sporadic case reports have offered hope for severe cases of asthma.

Supportive care. Dehydration caused by increased insensible fluid loss, poor oral intake, and vomiting is corrected by an initial intravenous bolus of 5 to 10 ml/kg of normal saline. Thereafter, intravenous hydration to meet maintenance requirements and replace remaining deficits helps to improve tissue perfusion and decreases viscosity of respiratory secretions.

Chest physiotherapy (CPT) and postural drainage may be indicated in patients who have significant mechanical obstruction because of mucus plugging, but the therapeutic effect of routine CPT for status asthmaticus is not well documented.[3]

Bacterial and viral infections are known triggers of airway responsiveness, but routine use of antibiotics should be withheld, except for those patients exhibiting signs of bacterial infection.

Most patients presenting in status asthmaticus exhibit signs of irritability and agitation because of high levels of endogenous and exogenous catecholamines, hypoxia, and sleep deprivation. The use of sedation in these patients may be of benefit in a controlled setting where endotracheal intubation and mechanical ventilation can be accomplished without delay, but they are contraindicated otherwise.[32]

Criteria for Discharge, Admission to Hospital, and Transfer to Intensive Care Unit

NIH guidelines state that patients may be discharged to home after 60 to 90 minutes of standard therapy if symptoms have resolved and peak flow or FEV_1 is more than 70% of the patient's "personal best." Before discharge, patients should be provided sufficient medications to complete the course of therapy, written and verbal instructions on when to increase medications or return for care if symptoms worsen, training on how to monitor peak flow, training on necessary environmental control measures, and referral to a follow-up appointment within 3 to 5 days. Communication with the primary physician assures continuity of care for this chronic disease. Patients whose symptoms have improved but who have peak flow readings between 50% and 70% of their "personal best" are assessed for discharge on an individual basis.[32] Conservative management is recommended for those who have significant risk factors as ascertained by a careful history. Patients who remain symptomatic are admitted to the hospital for continued treatment with aerosolized bronchodilators, systemic steroids, oxygen, and frequent assessments.

Indications for transfer to an intensive care setting include any patient in severe distress or moderate distress unrelieved by initial therapy. In addition, any patient who has signs of respiratory fatigue, such as somnolence or diminishing respiratory effort, hypoxemia with modest levels of supplemental oxygen (SaO_2 <90 in 60% FiO_2), extreme tachycardia, or symptomatic air leak (pneumothorax, pneumomediastinum, or pneumoperitoneum) should be transferred to a PICU for escalation of therapy. The first-line treatment for these children usually is IV steroids and continuous beta-2 agonist nebulizations. With worsening respiratory or neurological status, mechanical ventilation may be required.

Status asthmaticus remains a complex problem among pediatric patients. It requires prompt intervention, frequent patient observation, and titration of therapies, including transfer of appropriate patients to a pediatric intensive care setting. Aggressive preventive management of all patients, including broad use of both antiinflammatory and bronchodilatory agents, remains the cornerstone of therapy for this chronic disease.

REFERENCES

1. Anderson MN, Borden JR, Mouritzen CV: Acidosis, catecholamines and cardiovascular dynamics: when does acidosis require correction? *Ann Surg* 166:344, 1967.
2. Arrighi HM: US asthma mortality: 1941-1989, *Ann Allergy Asthma Immunol* 74:321, 1995.
3. Asher MI, et al: Effects of chest physical therapy on lung function in children recovering from acute severe asthma, *Pediatr Pulmonol* 9:146, 1990.
4. *Asthma: a concern for minority populations,* National Institute of Allergy and Infectious Diseases, January, 1997.
5. Asthma mortality and hospitalization among children and young adults—United States, 1986-1996, *MMWR Morb Mortal Wkly Rep* 45: 350, 1996.
6. Bhagat R, et al: Rapid onset of tolerance to the bronchoprotective effect of salmeterol, *Chest* 108:5, 1995.
7. Carter E, et al: Efficacy of intravenously administered theophylline in children hospitalized with severe asthma, *J Pediatr* 122:470, 1993.
8. Centers for Disease Control and Prevention: Surveillance for asthma: United States, 1960-1995, *MMWR Morb Mortal Wkly Rep* 47(SS-1):1, 1998.
9. Chang CC, et al: Asthma mortality: another opinion: is it a matter of life and . . . bread? *J Asthma* 30:93-103, 1993.
10. Colacone A, et al: A comparison of albuterol administered by metered-dose inhaler (and holding chamber) or wet nebulizer in acute asthma, *Chest* 104:835, 1993.
11. Connett GJ, et al: Prednisolone and salbutamol in the hospital treatment of acute asthma, *Arch Dis Child* 70:170, 1994.
12. Evans R III, et al: National trends in the morbidity and mortality of asthma in the US: prevalence, hospitalization, and mortality of asthma over two decades: 1965-1984, *Chest* 91:65s, 1987.
13. Flores G, Horwitz RI: Efficacy of beta 2-agonists in bronchiolitis: a reappraisal and meta-analysis, *Pediatrics* 100:233, 1997.
14. Gergen PJ, Weiss KB: Changing patterns of hospitalizations among children: 1979-1987, *JAMA* 264:1689, 1990.
15. Greenberger PA, Miller TP, Lifschultz B: Circumstances surrounding deaths from asthma in Cook County (Chicago), Illinois, *Allergy Proc* 14:321, 1993.
16. Gross NJ: Ipratropium bromide, *N Engl J Med* 319:486, 1988.
17. Haahtela T, et al: Effects of reducing or discontinuing inhaled budesonide in patients with mild asthma, *N Engl J Med* 331:700, 1994.
18. Harrison BD, et al: Need for intravenous hydrocortisone in addition to oral prednisolone in patients admitted to hospital with severe asthma without ventilatory failure, *Lancet* 1:181, 1986.
19. Higgins RM, Stradling JR, Lane DJ: Should ipratropium bromide be added to beta-agonists in treatment of acute severe asthma? *Chest* 94: 718, 1988.
20. Howarth PH, Redington AE, Montefort S: Pathophysiology of asthma, *Allergy* 48(suppl 17):50, 1993.
21. Idris AH, et al: Emergency department treatment of severe asthma: metered-dose inhaler plus holding chamber is equivalent in effectiveness to nebulizer, *Chest* 103:665, 1993.
22. Kallenbach JM, et al: Determinants of near fatality in acute severe asthma, *Am J Med* 95:265, 1993.
23. Kelly HW, Murphy S: Beta-adrenergic agonists for acute severe asthma, *Ann Pharmacother* 26:81, 1992.
24. Kikuchi Y, et al: Chemosensitivity and perception of dyspnea in patients with a history of near fatal asthma, *N Engl J Med* 330:1329, 1994.
25. Lin RY, et al: Continuous versus intermittent albuterol nebulization in the treatment of acute asthma, *Ann Emerg Med* 22:1847, 1993.
26. Mann RD: Results of prescription event monitoring study of salmeterol, *BMJ* 309:1018, 1994.
27. McDowell KM, et al: A cost-saving algorithm for children hospitalized for status asthmaticus, *Arch Pediatr Adolesc Med* 152:977, 1998.
28. McFadden ER, Gilbert IA: Asthma, *N Engl J Med* 327:1928, 1992.
29. Molfino NA, et al: Respiratory arrest in near-fatal asthma, *N Engl J Med* 324:285, 1991.
30. Mullen M, Mullen B, Carey M: The association between beta-agonist use and death from asthma: a meta-analytic integration of case-control studies, *JAMA* 270:1842, 1993.
31. Murphy DG, et al: Aminophylline in the treatment of acute asthma when beta 2-adrenergics and steroids are provided, *Arch Intern Med* 153:178, 1993.
32. National Asthma Education and Prevention Program: Expert Panel Report II: *Guidelines for the diagnosis and management of asthma*, Pub No 97-4051, Bethesda, Md, 1997, US Department of Health and Human Services.
33. Newacheck PW, Taylor WR: Childhood chronic illness: prevalence, severity, and impact, *Am J Public Health* 82:364, 1992.
34. O'Connor BJ, et al: Selective airway responsiveness in asthma, *Trends Pharmacol Sci* 20:9, 1999.
35. O'Hollaren MT, et al: Exposure to an aeroallergen as a possible precipitating factor in respiratory arrest in young patients with asthma, *N Engl J Med* 324:359,1990.
36. Papo MC, Frank J, Thompson AE: A prospective, randomized study of continuous versus intermittent nebulized albuterol for severe status asthmaticus in children, *Crit Care Med* 21:1479, 1993.
37. Qureshi F, et al: Effect of nebulized ipratropium on the hospitalization rates of children with asthma, *N Engl J Med* 339:1030, 1998.
38. Ramage L, et al: Reduced protection against exercise induced bronchoconstriction after chronic dosing with salmeterol, *Respir Med* 88:363, 1994.
39. Ratto D, et al: Are intravenous corticosteroids required in status asthmaticus? *JAMA* 260:527, 1988.
40. Reisman J, et al: Frequent administration by inhalation of salbutamol and ipratropium bromide in the initial management of severe acute asthma in children, *J Allergy Clin Immunol* 81:16, 1988.
41. Rodrigo C, Rodrigo G: Assessment of the patient with acute asthma in the emergency department: a factor analytic study, *Chest* 104:1325, 1993.

42. Roos A, Boron WF: Intracellular pH, *Physiol Rev* 61:296, 1981.
43. Rowe BH, Keller JL, Oxman AD: Effectiveness of steroid therapy in acute exacerbations of asthma: a meta-analysis, *Am J Emerg Med* 10:301, 1992.
44. Rudnitsky GS, et al: Comparison of intermittent and continuously nebulized albuterol for treatment of asthma in an urban emergency department, *Ann Emerg Med* 22:1842, 1993.
45. Scarfone RJ, et al: Controlled trial of oral prednisone in the emergency department treatment of children with acute asthma, *Pediatrics* 2:513, 1993.
46. Schuh S, et al: Efficacy of frequent nebulized ipratropium bromide added to frequent high-dose albuterol therapy in severe childhood asthma, *J Pediatr* 126:639, 1995.
47. Sherman JM, Capen CL: The red alert program for life-threatening asthma, *Pediatrics* 100:187, 1997.
48. Spitzer WO, et al: The use of beta-agonists and the risk of death and near death from asthma, *N Engl J Med* 326:501, 1992.
49. Suissa S, et al: A cohort analysis of excess mortality in asthma and the use of inhaled beta-agonists, *Am J Respir Crit Care Med* 149(3 Pt 1) 604, 1994.
50. Targonski PV, et al: Trends in asthma mortality among African Americans and whites in Chicago, 1968-1991, *Am J Public Health* 84:1830, 1994.
51. Weinberger M, Hendeles L: Theophylline in asthma, *N Engl J Med* 334:1380, 1996.
52. Weiss KB, Wagener DK: Changing patterns of asthma mortality: identifying target populations at high risk, *JAMA* 264:1683, 1990.
53. Weitzman M, et al: Recent trends in the prevalence and severity of childhood asthma, *JAMA* 268:2673, 1992.
54. Wildenthal K, et al: Effects of acute lactic acidosis on left ventricular performance, *Am J Physiol* 214:1352, 1968.
55. Woolcock A, et al: Comparison of addition of salmeterol to inhaled steroids with doubling of the dose of inhaled steroids, *Am J Respir Crit Care Med* 153:1481, 1996.
56. Wright BM, McKerrow CB: Wright peak flow meter, *BMJ* 2:1041, 1959.
57. Zorc JJ, et al: Ipratropium bromide added to asthma treatment in pediatric emergency department, *Pediatrics* 103:748, 1999.

298 Status Epilepticus

Sarah M. Roddy • Margaret C. McBride

Status epilepticus is defined by the World Health Organization as "a condition characterized by an epileptic seizure that is sufficiently prolonged or repeated at sufficiently brief intervals as to produce an unvarying and enduring epileptic condition."[1] There has been much variability in the interpretation of what constitutes an "unvarying and enduring epileptic condition." The most widely accepted criterion for diagnosis of status epilepticus is any seizure that continues for 30 minutes, or intermittent seizures lasting for 30 minutes or longer in which the person does not regain consciousness between the episodes.

Status epilepticus can be classified in terms of the type of seizure. Generalized convulsive status epilepticus is the most common and easily recognized type in children. The seizure activity usually is tonic-clonic or clonic and less often is tonic or myoclonic. In simple partial status epilepticus or epilepsia partialis continua, focal seizure activity is prolonged and restricted to one side of the body without loss of consciousness. Nonconvulsive status epilepticus manifests as a confused, drowsy state in which the patient moves in slow motion. This condition results from continuing or repetitive absence seizures or partial complex seizures (see Chapter 260, Seizure Disorders).

The incidence of status epilepticus in patients who have epilepsy ranges from 4% to 16%.[3] Its frequency is highest in the younger age groups.[4,7] Infants and children also are much more likely than adults to have status epilepticus as the manifestation of their first seizure.[7] Up to 70% of children with epilepsy beginning before the age of 1 year experience status epilepticus.[3]

In approximately 25% of cases, status epilepticus is idiopathic. In another 20% to 25% it is provoked solely by fever.[9] Acute symptomatic status epilepticus accounts for another 25% of cases and is an expression of an acute encephalopathy or brain injury. Causes in this group include meningitis, electrolyte disturbance, drug ingestion, and poor compliance with antiepileptic medication. Remote symptomatic status epilepticus occurs in patients with a prior history of central nervous system insult known to be associated with increased risk of seizure. This group accounts for another 20% of the cases of status epilepticus in children, with the majority having cerebral palsy or mental retardation. The etiology of status epilepticus in a small percentage of cases is a progressive encephalopathy. This category includes neurodegenerative diseases and neurocutaneous syndromes (phakomatoses).

Nonconvulsive status epilepticus and epilepsia partialis continua require prompt treatment, but there is less urgency because these seizures do not alter the body's homeostatic mechanisms to the degree that convulsive status epilepticus does. Convulsive status epilepticus is considered a medical emergency because it is life threatening and sometimes is followed by severe neurological sequelae. The longer convulsive status epilepticus continues, the more resistant it is to therapy and the greater the incidence of mortality and morbidity. Experimental studies have shown that continued seizure activity for more than 60 minutes results in permanent cell damage, even in ventilated animals whose metabolic parameters are kept in the normal range. Neurological sequelae from status epilepticus include intellectual impairment and motor dysfunction. Over the past 20 years, morbidity and mortality from status epilepticus have declined, probably because of better access to medical care, more aggressive treatment, and the availability of benzodiazepines. In children with idiopathic or febrile status epilepticus, less than 5% develop new neurological dysfunction.[2] Mortality in children attributable to status epilepticus currently does not exceed 6%,[6] with most deaths caused by the illness that precipitated the seizure.[2]

The objectives of treating convulsive status epilepticus are to maintain vital functions, identify and correct any precipitating factors, and control seizure activity. A plan for management is outlined in Box 298-1. A history should be obtained from an accompanying family member and should include any history of previous seizures, chronic and recent medication use, intercurrent illness, head trauma, and details of the onset of status epilepticus. On physical examination, fever, any evidence of head trauma, increased intracranial pressure, or infection should be noted. A urine toxicology screen is helpful in determining if the seizures were precipitated by drug ingestion. Computed tomography (CT) scanning may be required to rule out an intracranial lesion if the etiology of status epilepticus remains obscure. If the history or physical examination suggests a central nervous system infection, antibiotics should be administered immediately and a lumbar puncture performed as soon as seizure activity has been controlled. Because neurological sequelae of status epilepticus can result from precipitating factors such as hypoxia, hypotension, and acidosis, attention should be given immediately to the respiratory and cardiovascular status of the child. If the patient is febrile, reducing body temperature is extremely urgent because

BOX 298-1

TREATMENT OF STATUS EPILEPTICUS

A. Assess cardiovascular function by making sure the airway is clear, the patient is breathing, and circulation is adequate. Provide oxygen or respiratory support and cardiac stimulation (CPR) as necessary.
B. Establish an intravenous line and obtain blood samples for electrolytes, blood urea nitrogen, calcium, a complete blood count, and anticonvulsant medication levels. A blood Dextrostix test should be performed immediately, and if the glucose is under 60 mg%, 1 to 2 ml/kg of $D_{25}W$ should be administered.
C. One member of the emergency team should obtain a history while another does a brief physical examination.
D. Administer anticonvulsant drugs in the following order until seizure activity is controlled:
   1. Initial therapy
      a. Lorazepam should be the initial anticonvulsant administered intravenously at a dose of 0.1 mg/kg (maximum 4 mg) over 2 minutes; a dose of 0.05 to 0.1 mg/kg may be repeated every 5 minutes if necessary up to a maximum of 0.5 mg/kg, but not over 10 mg in toto.
      b. If lorazepam is not available, diazepam should be administered intravenously at a dose of 0.1 to 0.2 mg/kg (maximum 10 mg) by "pushing" half the dose over 1 minute and the remainder at 1 mg/min. A dose of 0.1 mg/kg may be repeated in 5 minutes if necessary. Because of diazepam's short duration of anticonvulsant effect, another anticonvulsant such as phenytoin must be administered immediately.
      c. If the patient is known to be receiving phenytoin on a chronic basis, it should be administered as the initial anticonvulsant (see D.2.).
   2. If status epilepticus continues, administer phenytoin or fosphenytoin, which is a water-soluble prodrug of phenytoin with a more neutral pH value. The dose for both drugs is 15 to 20 mg/kg up to a total dose of 1000 mg. Phenytoin must be given intravenously, but fosphenytoin can be given intramuscularly if IV access is not available. A quarter of the dose may be administered during the first 2 minutes and then at a rate of 1 to 2 mg/kg/min (maximum rate of 50 mg/min) for phenytoin and 3 mg/kg/min (maximum rate of 150 mg/min) for fosphenytoin. If the patient is known to be receiving phenytoin chronically, 5 to 8 mg/kg of phenytoin may be administered as the initial anticonvulsant. Monitor the heart rate, and slow the rate of phenytoin infusion if bradycardia occurs. If seizure activity continues despite a full loading dose of phenytoin, correction of underlying acidosis with sodium bicarbonate (0.25 to 0.5 mEq/kg) is indicated.
   3. If status epilepticus continues, administer phenobarbital 15 to 20 mg/kg intravenously up to a total dose of 800 mg. Administer this amount over 15 minutes, monitoring respirations and blood pressure, especially if the patient has been given a benzodiazepine.
E. If seizure activity still persists, consult a neurologist to determine the need for other anticonvulsants, general anesthesia, or induction of pentobarbital, diazepam, or midazolam coma.

of the synergism of fever and status epilepticus in producing brain damage.[5,10] Fortunately, most episodes of status epilepticus are controlled by one or more of the drugs listed in Box 298-1.

Once seizure activity is controlled, management should be directed toward preventing recurrence of seizures, including maintenance anticonvulsant therapy. The appropriate duration of therapy following an initial episode of idiopathic status epilepticus is not clear. Recurrence of seizures in this situation may be as low as 25%,[6] and recurrence of status epilepticus only 4%.[8]

When to Refer

The need for pediatric neurology expertise cannot be met locally
Seizure activity cannot controlled

When to Hospitalize

Always for a child who has sustained status epilepticus
Virtually always for a child who is unresponsive following status epilepticus

REFERENCES

1. Gastaut H, editor: *Dictionary of epilepsy,* I. Definitions, Geneva, 1973, World Health Organization.
2. Gross-Tsur V, Shinnar S: Convulsive status epilepticus in children, *Epilepsia* 34(suppl 1):S12, 1993.
3. Hauser WA: Status epilepticus: epidemiologic considerations, *Neurology* 40(suppl 2):9, 1990.
4. Hesdorffer DC, et al: Incidence of status epilepticus in Rochester, Minnesota, 1965-1984, *Neurology* 50:735, 1998.
5. Lundgren J, et al: Hyperthermia aggravates and hypothermia ameliorates epileptic brain damage, *Exp Brain Res* 99:43, 1994.

6. Maytal J, et al: Low morbidity and mortality of status epilepticus in children, *Pediatrics* 83:323, 1989.
7. Shinnar S, et al: In whom does status epilepticus occur: age-related differences in children, *Epilepsia* 38:907, 1997.
8. Shinnar S, et al: Recurrent status epilepticus in children, *Ann Neurol* 31:598, 1992.
9. Shinnar S, et al: The risk of seizure recurrence after a first unprovoked afebrile seizure in childhood: an extended follow-up, *Pediatrics* 98:216, 1996.
10. van Esch A, et al: Outcome after febrile status epilepticus, *Dev Med Child Neurol* 38:19, 1996.

299 Thermal Injuries

L.R. Scherer III

The leading cause of death among children between 1 and 15 years of age is traumatic injury. Thermal injuries affect an estimated 1 million children in the United States annually; 100,000, require hospitalization.[1] Of these, 3000 die as a result of their injuries, making thermal injuries the third leading cause of traumatic death in children, after motor vehicle accidents and drowning. Permanent disability remains a major complication in pediatric patients.

ETIOLOGY

Most childhood thermal injuries occur in the child's home. Approximately 80% to 90% of these injuries are potentially preventable.[1] The pattern of injury is related to the child's age and gender. During the first 2 years of life, 60% of the injuries are caused by scald burns from hot liquids; they involve boys twice as often as girls,[4] which may be due to the seemingly more active and inquisitive nature of males in this age group. Most scald burns occur when a young child accidentally pulls a pan or pot of hot liquid off the stove or table onto the head, chest, and arms. Occasionally a small child may manage to turn on the hot water in the bathtub, or a parent may carelessly or deliberately place a child in a bathtub of scalding water, causing burns, most often to the arms, buttocks, legs, and feet. Although scald burns more commonly involve only partial-thickness injury, infants and toddlers have skin that is quite thin, and scald burns may result in full-thickness loss.

Because toddlers insist on exploration, the next most common childhood burn results from contact with hot surfaces in the home. These injuries usually involve only the "exploring" surfaces of the hands.

Flame burn injuries are more common in children over 3 years of age. There is no gender predilection in this age group.[1] Causes include the careless use of matches, space heaters, outdoor fires, and stoves. Governmental restrictions on the manufacture of children's sleepwear have decreased the risk of flame injury in young children, but flammable products still are involved in most flame burn injuries. Because of the intense thermal energy of flame burns, large body surface area full-thickness injury is more common, and the associated inhalation injury increases the morbidity and mortality in this age group.

PATHOPHYSIOLOGY

During the assessment of the burn patient it is necessary to determine the depth and extent of injury so that a treatment plan can be developed. Classically, the depth of a burn has been categorized as first, second, or third degree. A first-degree burn is a superficial burn that involves only the epidermis. They are erythematous and painful and do not produce blisters. The most common first-degree burn occurs after overexposure to the sun. Occasionally, first-degree burns are seen as a result of flashburns from an explosion. First-degree burns should not be included in the estimation of the total extent of a burn wound injury. A second-degree burn, more commonly regarded as a partial-thickness skin loss, is usually erythematous or appears mottled red. The epidermal and dermal injury is evident with blistering, is moist to the touch, and is extremely painful to touch and exposure. A deep, partial-thickness, second-degree burn appears mottled and waxy because of complete injury to the entire epidermis and dermis; therefore, it may look like a full-thickness injury. A full-thickness, third-degree burn injury involves the epidermis, dermis, and subcutaneous tissue. These injuries appear dry or waxlike. There are no blisters, and the skin may be white or black. The texture of the skin is hard, dry, and leathery with no elasticity, and coagulated veins are noticeable. These injuries are painless to touch because of complete injury to the nerve supply to the skin.

Injury from partial-thickness and full-thickness burns results in increased capillary permeability and sequestration of large quantities of fluids within the extravascular space. Because of the larger surface area/volume ratio of infants and children, as well as their thinner skin and subcutaneous tissue, young burn victims tend to lose more fluid and body heat than do adolescents and adults. These greater evaporative water and body heat losses necessitate the use of larger quantities of fluid for resuscitation and external temperature regulation.

Significant morbidity and mortality occur as a result of inhalation thermal injuries. The manifestations of these injuries may not be apparent for the first 24 hours. Major injuries to the respiratory tract result from inhaling products of incomplete combustion and toxic fumes or from direct thermal injury to the upper or lower respiratory tract.

Inhaling products of incomplete combustion or toxic fumes may lead to chemical tracheobronchitis and pneumonia. Carbon monoxide (CO) exposure should always be assumed in children who sustain burns in an enclosed space. CO causes a direct hypoxic injury to the mucosa or an ischemia-reperfusion injury to the lung resulting in acute respiratory distress syndrome.[16] Because of the high affinity of CO for hemoglobin (240 times that of oxygen), CO displaces oxygen from the hemoglobin molecule and shifts the dissociation curve to the left. Carbon monoxide dissociates from hemoglobin very slowly; when breathing room air, 50% of the patient's CO dissociates within 250 minutes, whereas it takes only 40 minutes for this to happen when the patient breathes 100% oxygen. Therefore the patient who has suspected smoke inhalation should be treated with 100% oxygen.

Inhaling heated gases causes direct thermal injury; it rarely causes injury below the vocal cords except when volatile gases or steam is inhaled. Airway injury produces edema and obstruction, mucosal sloughing, bronchorrhea, and pulmonary edema. Early management of inhalation injuries includes endotracheal intubation and administration of 100% oxygen.

Children with significant airway injury because of inhalation require critical care management. Treatment strategies include mechanical ventilation, aerosolized heparin, and *N*-acetylcystine,[3] positive end-expiratory pressure, inverse ratio ventilation, high-frequency oscillating ventilation, nitric oxide administration,[13] and extracorporeal life support.[7]

HISTORY

A detailed clinical history is extremely important in the evaluation of a burned pediatric patient. This should include when, where, and how the burn occurred and the nature of the burning agent. If the injury occurred within an enclosed environment, a smoke inhalation injury should be suspected and aggressive airway management initiated. Evaluation should include the child's general health, any preexisting medical problems, allergies, and most important, tetanus immunization status. Recent infection should be noted, especially the possibility of a streptococcal organism. A careful clinical history helps to determine the depth of the wound, potential associated trauma, particulate or thermal airway injury, and CO poisoning.

The diagnosis of child abuse can be obtained from detailed information of the history of the injury. The physician obtaining a history that includes the following should suspect child abuse: (1) an accident that occurs when the child is alone, (2) an injury incurred by a sibling, (3) an unclear or inconsistent history, (4) a previous history of accidental injury, (5) an injury incompatible with the description of the event, (6) a delay in seeking medical attention, and (7) an unstable social environment.[5]

CLINICAL FINDINGS

On initial evaluation all clothing should be removed from the child to stop the burning process and to allow complete assessment of all potential injuries. Airway assessment is particularly important in flame injuries and injuries encountered in an enclosed environment. The child should be assessed for facial burns, singed eyebrows and nasal hairs, carbon deposits in the oropharynx, and carbonaceous sputum, all of which indicate significant airway injury. Early airway management includes endotracheal intubation; delayed intubation may compromise airway management critically because of upper airway edema. Early and rapid assessment for associated injuries is necessary when the child has neurological impairment, a history of trauma, an electrical injury, or evidence of abuse. Unrecognized visceral or long bone injuries result in significant morbidity and mortality in the burned child.

At this point a careful, thorough inspection of the burn wounds is necessary. The child should be disrobed completely and all wounds covered with sterile dry linens or towels. Mask, gown, and gloves are worn to inspect the depth and extent of the burn. The burned surface area in children is estimated by using the Lund and Browder chart (Fig. 299-1), because in younger children the surface area of the head is relatively large and the surface area of the lower extremities is small. Estimation of the surface area is required for the management of fluid therapy and for wound care and prognosis. Pitfalls in estimation occur in chemical and electrical injuries, in which extensive tissue damage may manifest few signs of injury to the skin.

OUTPATIENT MANAGEMENT

As stated earlier, approximately 90% of childhood burns can be treated outside the hospital. Minor burns may be classified as partial-thickness burns involving no more than 10% of the body surface or full-thickness burns involving no more than 2% of the body surface (Box 299-1).

Generally the aforementioned patients can be treated with oral fluids and burn wound care in the emergency department or the pediatrician's office. The wounds should be cleansed with water or saline and a mild antibacterial solution. Blisters should be left intact, since this provides greater comfort and ease of care; however, open blisters should be debrided. Silver sulfadiazine cream is applied to the wound twice daily after cleansing, and dry, sterile, occlusive dressing is applied to the wound. Close observation is required in the initial management of burns, and the child should be seen at least every 48 hours for evaluation of the depth of the burn and potential complications. Once intact blisters begin to leak or are no longer tense, the blisters should be debrided. Over the past 30 years, laboratory and clinical research has found that the maintenance of a moist wound environment facilitates wound healing. The beneficial effects include prevention of tissue dehydration and cell death, accelerated angiogenesis, increased breakdown of dead tissue and fibrin, and accelerated interaction of tissue growth factors and target cells.[8]

As an alternative to the conventional antimicrobial gauze dressing, the burn wound may be covered with an occlusive moisture-retentive dressing such as the semipermeable membrane film or the hydrocolloid occlusive dressing. Clinical research documents a healing rate that is 3 to 4 days faster and involves less pain during and between dressing changes.[8] Recent technology is introducing nylon mesh dressings coated with silicone or cultured fibroblasts.[2,10] Initial results report earlier wound healing and improved epithelial covering of burn wounds. In the overall care of a minor injury, the child should be managed with oral hydration; pain should be alleviated with acetaminophen or codeine. Most important, the child's tetanus immunization status must be documented and updated, if necessary. Facial burns may be treated with open dressings, applying an antibacterial ointment such as bacitracin, Neosporin, or polymyxin B to the partial-thickness burn wound areas three times daily. Partial-thickness burns should regenerate epithelium within 14 to 21 days. Follow-up care calls for monitoring wound healing and

Burn Estimate Age versus Area

Area	Birth-1 yr	1-4 yr	5-9 yr	10-14 yr	15 yr	2°	3°	Total
Head	19	17	13	11	9			
Neck	2	2	2	2	2			
Ant. Trunk	13	13	13	13	13			
Post. Trunk	13	13	13	13	13			
R. Buttock	2 1/2	2 1/2	2 1/2	2 1/2	2 1/2			
L. Buttock	2 1/2	2 1/2	2 1/2	2 1/2	2 1/2			
Genitalia	1	1	1	1	1			
R.U. Arm	4	4	4	4	4			
L.U. Arm	4	4	4	4	4			
R.L. Arm	3	3	3	3	3			
L.L. Arm	3	3	3	3	3			
R. Hand	2 1/2	2 1/2	2 1/2	2 1/2	2 1/2			
L. Hand	2 1/2	2 1/2	2 1/2	2 1/2	2 1/2			
R. Thigh	5 1/2	6 1/2	8	8 1/2	9			
L. Thigh	5 1/2	6 1/2	8	8 1/2	9			
R. Leg	5	5	5 1/2	6	6 1/2			
L. Leg	5	5	5 1/2	6	6 1/2			
R. Foot	3 1/2	3 1/2	3 1/2	3 1/2	3 1/2			
L. Foot	3 1/2	3 1/2	3 1/2	3 1/2	3 1/2			
					Total			

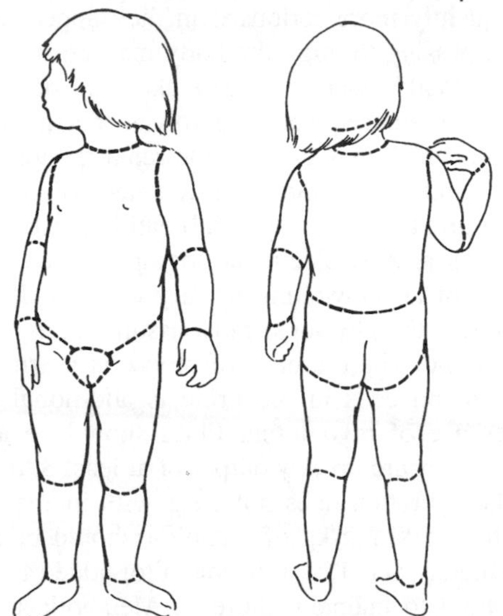

Fig. 299-1 Burn chart for estimating extent of injury. Numbers equal percentage of total body surface.

BOX 299-1

TRIAGE CRITERIA FOR THERMAL INJURIES

Outpatient Management

Partial-thickness burn <10% body surface area (BSA)
Full-thickness burn <2% BSA

Inpatient Management

Primary care hospital

Partial-thickness burn 10% to 20% BSA
Full-thickness burn 2% to 10% BSA
Partial-thickness burn to face, perineum, hands, or feet
Questionable burn wound depth or extent
Inadequate family support
Suspected abuse

Burn center

Partial-thickness burn >20% BSA
Full-thickness burn >10% BSA
Full-thickness burn to face, perineum, hands, or feet
Respiratory tract injury
Associated major trauma
Significant coexisting illness
Chemical or electrical burns

patient compliance with the healing regimen, comfort, and early rehabilitation.

PRIMARY CARE HOSPITAL MANAGEMENT

More extensive burns necessitate hospitalization for wound care and intravenous fluid therapy (see Box 299-1). Hospital treatment is required in cases of partial-thickness burns involving 10% to 20% of the body surface. The following factors necessitate initial inpatient evaluation and management: full-thickness burns involving 2% to 10% of the body surface; partial-thickness injury to the face, hands, feet, and perineum; questionable burn wound depth and extent; minor chemical burns; inadequate family support; and suspected abuse. In the emergency department the assessment of a child who has a thermal injury involves evaluation of the airway and associated injuries and estimation of the burned area and depth of injury. Intravenous fluid resuscitation is required for severe injuries, and one or two peripheral intravenous lines are required for intravenous fluid therapy. In the approach to fluid management, and in burns involving more than 15% of the body surface, the practitioner should administer a formula using 3 to 4 ml of lactated Ringer's solution per kilogram per percent burn, in addition to the child's regular maintenance fluid, during the first 24 hours after the burn occurs. Half of the fluid is given over the first 8 hours after injury, and the remaining half is delivered over the following 16 hours. The adequacy of fluid therapy is determined by urinary output, which should be maintained at 1 to 2 ml/kg/hr (measuring output may require the use of a Foley catheter). With extensive burns a central venous pressure line may be required in the management of fluid therapy. Children who have a burn covering 15% or more of the body surface often develop a paralytic ileus, and therefore nasogastric tube decompression often is required. All medications, including antibiotics, analgesics, or sedatives should be given intravenously because gastrointestinal absorption and parenchymal perfusion is unpredictable. Initial management of the wound is similar to that of minor wounds except for the extent and potential depth of the wound. Therefore, early involvement by the surgical team is required for the overall assessment and management of the burned child.

BURN CENTER MANAGEMENT

Thermal injuries of greatest magnitude, that is, partial-thickness burns involving more than 20% of body surface area; full-thickness burns involving more than 10% of body surface area; full-thickness burns of the face, hands, feet, or perineum; a respiratory tract injury; an associated major injury; or major chemical or electrical burns necessitate the special facilities and personnel of a regional burn center (see Box 299-1). A burn center offers specialists involved in the long-term physical, psychological, and social needs of these infants and children.[6,9,14] These centers have produced remarkable improvements in the morbidity and mortality of those who have major burns. The injured child needs to be carefully evaluated and adequately resuscitated before he or she is transferred to a burn center. Initial evaluation and resuscitation include early airway stabilization, adequate intravenous access, fluid resuscitation with lactated Ringer's solution, tetanus immunization, and covering the burn wounds with sterile, dry linens or towels. To initiate the transfer, early telephone communication between the referring physician and the coordinator of the burn center is important. All pertinent information regarding vital signs, laboratory evaluation, fluids administered, and urinary output should be recorded and a flowchart sent with the patient. Any other information deemed important by either the referring physician or the burn center physician should be sent with the child. At the time of transport, the child must be well prepared and have a secure airway, an established and secure intravenous line, burn dressings, adequate pain relief, and a nasogastric tube and Foley catheter in place.

SPECIAL BURN REQUIREMENTS: ELECTRICAL BURNS

Electrical burns result when a source of electrical power makes contact with a person's body.[12,15] Electrical burns are frequently more serious than they appear externally. A current passing through the body may destroy muscles, nerves, and blood vessels but spare skin and bone because of their high resistance. Rhabdomyolysis results in myoglobin release, which may cause acute renal failure. As with any serious injury, immediate management of the patient includes attention to the airway and breathing, establishment of intravenous access, electrocardiographic monitoring, and placement of an indwelling urinary catheter. If the urine is cola colored, the physician must assume myoglobin is present in the urine. The presence of blood on a urine dipstick and no red blood cells in the urine is additional evidence for the presence of myoglobin. Fluid should be administered at a rate to ensure urinary output of at least 3 to 5 ml/kg/hr. If the cola coloration does not clear with increased fluid administration, 500 mg/kg of mannitol should be administered immediately and 12.5 g of mannitol added to subsequent liters of fluid to maintain diuresis. Metabolic acidosis should be corrected by maintaining adequate perfusion, and sodium bicarbonate should be used to alkalinize the urine and increase the solubility of myoglobin.

The most common electrical burn in children is sustained by the toddler, when the corner of the mouth is injured by chewing on an electrical cord. Initial management of these injuries involves standard wound care and topical application of an antibiotic ointment. These wounds should be allowed to demarcate, and a plastic surgeon should be involved in their early assessment and management.

COMPLICATIONS

A number of complications may occur in the early management of thermal injuries in children[5]; the most catastrophic occurs when an inhalation injury is not recognized or not adequately treated. The second most common complication arises from underestimating the size and depth of a burn, which often occurs in scald burns of young children. Early and repeated methodical examination using a burn chart (see Fig. 299-1) helps in estimating the size of the injury. A common unrecognized complication is failure to suspect child abuse. Burns frequently are encountered as part of a spectrum of injuries inflicted on children.

Later complications in the management of children who have moderate to severe burns requiring hospitalization include pneumonia, septic thrombophlebitis, burn wound sepsis, peptic ulcer disease, and behavior disorders. The use of appropriate antibiotic therapy, vigorous pulmonary toilet, and intensive ventilatory support are the mainstays of preventing pulmonary complications in a burn patient.

Potentially lethal infections include suppurative skin lesions or thrombophlebitis when both peripheral and central venous catheters are used. The usual organisms involved are *Staphylococcus aureus, Staphylococcus epidermidis,* or a variety of gram-negative bacterial organisms. Burn wound sepsis remains a complication with significant morbidity and mortality; thus prevention is essential. Early aggressive debridement and excision of the wound, use of surveillance quantitative culture, and institution of appropriate topical and systemic antibiotic therapy are the cornerstones of prevention and management of burn wound sepsis. One of the lethal complications in a child who has a burn injury is a gastroduodenal ulcer (curling ulcer). Mortality is higher than 60% for children who suffer more than 60% of blood loss over a 24-hour period from peptic ulcer disease as a result of burns.[11] The prevalence, morbidity, and mortality have diminished with the use of antacids, histamine-antagonist therapy, and early enteral feeding of burn patients. Because of the severe and chronic nature of burns, psychological changes often occur in children: characteristically they regress to earlier stages of development. Behavior changes include hostility and self-destructiveness. Treatment may necessitate sedation, but usually the members of the burn team need to provide a great deal of understanding and support for the patient and the family. A cheerful environment, an experienced staff of child-life personnel, and a humane approach to the numerous painful procedures are most beneficial.

PROGNOSIS

The morbidity and mortality of thermal injuries have declined in the past 20 years because of advances in fluid therapy, management of pulmonary complications, control of wound infections by topical antibiotic agents, and advances in surgical wound management, nutrition, and regionalization of care.[6,14]

The most remarkable areas of improvement involve burn care. The use of topical antibacterial therapy has changed the 50% mortality level expected from 35% of body surface area (BSA) burns to 65% of BSA burns.[1,6,14] Since the development of early excision and grafting of large BSA burns, several authors have reported 50% mortality for greater than 90% of BSA burns.[1,6,14] Aggressive fluid resuscitation, early excision and grafting, and the overall improved management of the burned child have improved the survival rate and the quality of survival.

The early determinants of unnecessary mortality include inadequate volume resuscitation and inappropriate assessment of inhalation injury.[6] Later predictors of mortality include secondary development of renal, cardiovascular, and pulmonary organ failure.

Since the evolution of these new therapies, the child who has a burn under 70% BSA has an excellent prognosis, but the morbidity remains high because these children may develop hypertrophic scarring and contractures. Physical and occupational therapy and the use of long-term compressive garments have diminished the morbidity of these wound complications, but further investigation of the prevention of these scars and contractures is required. Ninety percent of children suffering from burns can be treated as outpatients, with the expectation of epithelial regeneration within 5 to 14 days. Further investigation and development of therapies for the 10% who require long-term hospitalization, physical therapy, and rehabilitation of their burn wounds is required to decrease the morbidity of their long-term care, which may require 4 to 6 months of hospitalization.

REFERENCES

1. Brigham PA, McLoughlin E: Burn incidence and medical care used in the United States: estimates, trends, and data sources, *J Burn Care Rehabil* 17:2, 1996.
2. Bugmann P, et al: A silicone-coated nylon dressing reduces healing time in burned paediatric patients in comparison with standard sulfadiazine treatment: a prospective randomized trial, *Burns*, 24:609, 1998.
3. Desai MH, et al: Reduction in mortality in pediatric patients with inhalation injury with aerosolized heparin/*N*-acetylcysteine therapy, *J Burn Care Rehabil* 19:210, 1998.
4. Feldman KW, et al: Tap water scald burns in children, 1997, *Inj Prev* 4:238, 1998.
5. Harmel RP, Vane DW, King DR: Burn care in children: special consideration, *Clin Plast Surg* 13:95, 1986.
6. Herndon DN, et al: Determinants of mortality in pediatric patients with greater than 70% full-thickness total body surface area thermal injury treated by early total excision and grafting, *J Trauma* 27:208, 1987.
7. Kane TD, et al: Pediatric burn patients with respiratory failure: predictors of outcome with the use of extracorporeal life support, *J Burn Care Rehabil* 20:145, 1999.
8. Kerstein MD: A symposium: wound infection and occlusion—separating fact from fiction, *Am J Surg* 167:1A, 1994.
9. Moore P, et al: Psychologic adjustment after childhood burn injuries as predicted by personality traits, *J Burn Care Rehabil* 14:80, 1993.
10. Noordenbos J, Dore C, Hansbrough JF: Safety and efficacy of TransCyte for the treatment of partial-thickness burns, *J Burn Care Rehabil* 20:275, 1999.
11. Prasad JK, Thomson PD, Feller I: Gastrointestinal hemorrhage in burn patients, *Burns* 13:194, 1987.
12. Remensnyder JP: Acute electrical injuries. In Martyn JA, editor: *Acute management of the burned patient,* Philadelphia, 1990, WB Saunders.
13. Sheridan RL, et al: Low-dose inhaled nitric oxide in acutely burned children with profound respiratory failure, *Surgery* 126:856, 1999.
14. Tompkins RG, et al: Significant reductions in mortality for children with burn injuries through the use of prompt eschar excision, *Ann Surg* 208: 577, 1988.
15. Volinksy J, Hansen J, Lustig J: Lightning burns, *Arch Pediatr Adolesc Med* 148:529, 1994.

appendixes

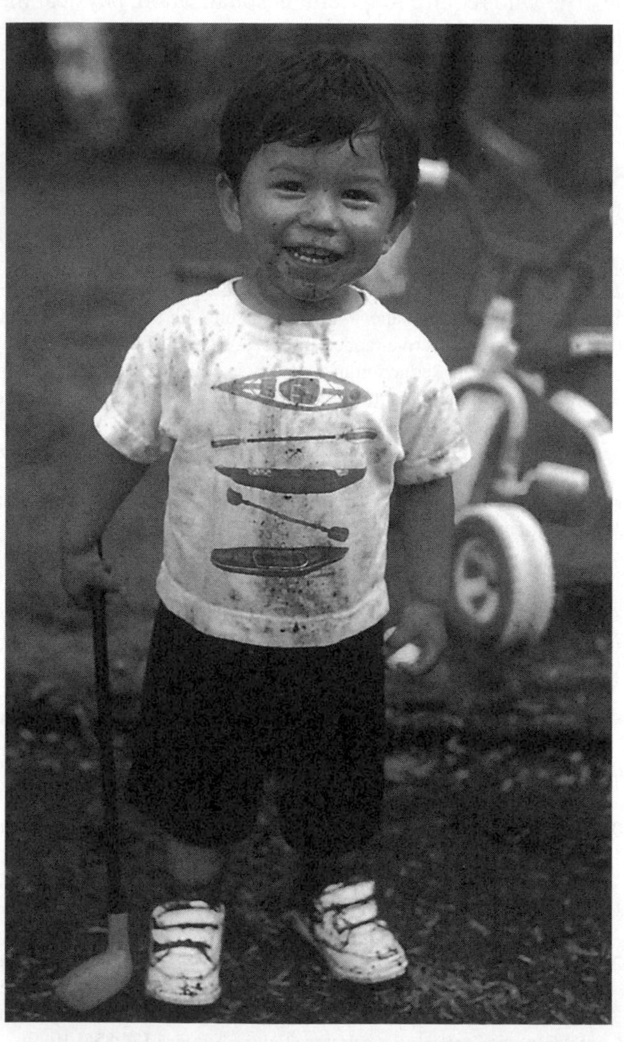

- **A** Pediatric Basic and Advanced Life Support
- **B** Special Procedures
- **C** Miscellaneous Values
- **D** Common Psychological and Educational Tests

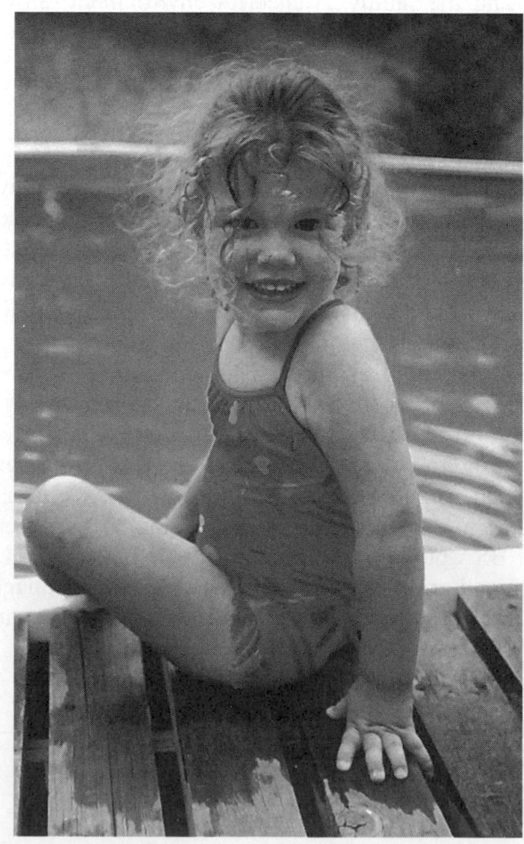

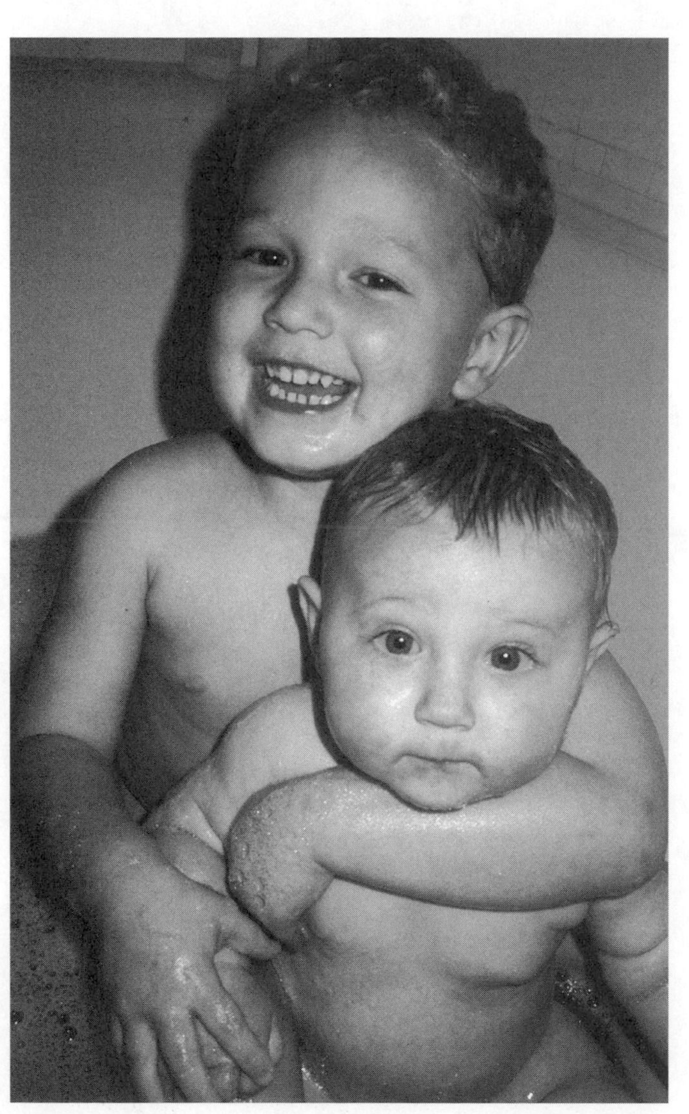

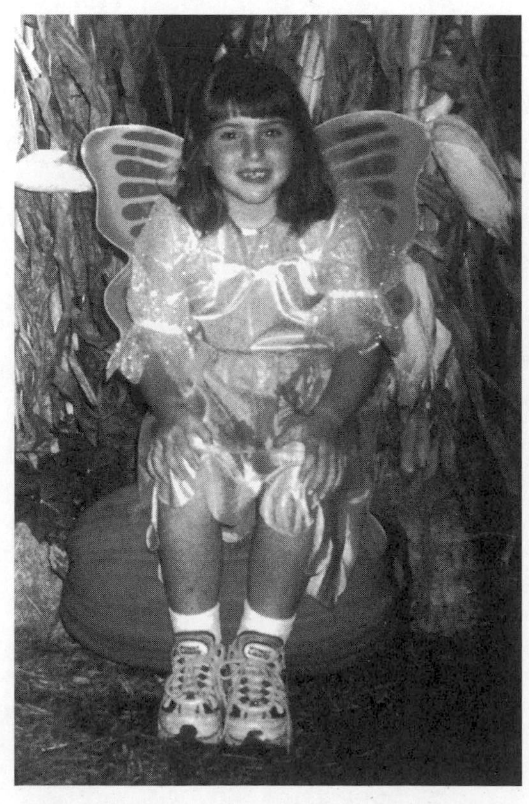

A Pediatric Basic and Advanced Life Support

Joseph Greensher • Pramod Narula

An estimated 40,000 infants younger than 1 year of age and 16,000 children between 1 and 14 years of age die each year in the United States from various causes (see Chapter 3, Morbidity and Mortality Among the Young). Most deaths in infants under 1 year of age occur before the child is 4 months old.[2]

Pediatric cardiopulmonary arrest (CPA) occurs biphasically, with the incidence peaking in infants under 1 year of age and in teenagers. During infancy, when most CPAs occur, the most common causes of death are sudden infant death syndrome (SIDS), respiratory diseases, airway obstruction, submersion, sepsis, and neurological diseases. After 1 year of age, injuries are the most common cause of death. The mortality of children under 15 months of age who suffer cardiac arrest outside a hospital is almost 100%.[32] Even in-patient cardiac arrests carry a mortality above 90%, and half of the survivors have major neurological damage.[10]

However, the survival rate approaches 50% after prompt resuscitation in children who have respiratory arrest alone.[34] The amount of time that elapses between arrest and initiation of life-support measures appears to be critical in determining the effectiveness of those measures. This appendix reviews and updates the guidelines for pediatric basic cardiopulmonary resuscitation (CPR) and advanced life support (ALS). It is not intended as a substitute for participation in the basic and ALS courses given by the American Heart Association and the American Academy of Pediatrics. Ideally, basic life support should be integrated into a community effort on education in injury prevention and easy access to emergency medical services (EMS).

Primary care practitioners, fortunately, do not encounter CPA often, but when they do, they must be skilled in administrating basic life support and resuscitation measures. When these are not successful, ALS measures must be used. It is clear that most primary care practitioners do not have all of the knowledge and skills needed to conduct the complicated process of ALS described in this appendix. However, help is available from Emergency Medical Technicians, local hospital emergency room physicians, and regional medical center pediatric intensivists, who deal with CPA all too frequently. Because of their lack of expertise in this area, primary care practitioners should familiarize themselves with the processes involved in resuscitating children with CPA by reading this appendix carefully. If the primary care practitioner practices in a community in which he or she is the only source of pediatric care, the physician should become proficient in the management of this devastating event through continuing education courses that address CPR and ALS.

In the discussion that follows, an infant is defined as 1 year of age or younger, a child as 1 to 8 years of age, and an older child as older than 8 years. CPA is the failure of both effective ventilation and circulation. *Respiratory arrest* is the lack of effective ventilation, as evidenced by absence of breath sounds or air movement or of thoracoabdominal movement. *Cardiac arrest* is the loss of effective circulation, as evidenced by the absence of pulsation in a major artery.

Basic life support is designed to generate perfusion of the vital organs with some oxygenated blood during cardiac arrest. To be successful, it must be coupled with ALS measures. It is important that EMS personnel are optimally trained and equipped to care for pediatric emergencies and that hospital emergency departments receiving acutely ill or injured children have transfer agreements with a pediatric tertiary care facility, where advanced pediatric postresuscitative care can be rendered if necessary.

In 1992, the Fifth National Conference on Cardiopulmonary Resuscitation and Emergency Cardiac Care revised the national guidelines for pediatric basic life support, ALS, and neonatal resuscitation. These changes were published in *The Journal of the American Medical Association* (JAMA) October 28, 1992.[7,26] The conference based changes in therapeutic interventions on supporting scientific evidence, and each recommendation was assigned to one of the following classes:

Class I: "A therapeutic option that is usually indicated, always acceptable, and is considered useful and effective." Examples are oxygen, endotracheal (ET) intubation, and defibrillation.

Class II: "A therapeutic option that is acceptable but of uncertain efficacy and may be controversial."

- *Class IIa:* "A therapeutic option for which the weight of evidence is in favor of its usefulness and efficacy." An example is a standard dose of epinephrine in ventricular fibrillation (VF).
- *Class IIb:* "A therapeutic option that is not well established by scientific evidence but may be helpful and probably not harmful." An example is using high-dose epinephrine in adults.

Class III: "A therapeutic option that is inappropriate, is without supporting data, and may be harmful." An ex-

The authors of this chapter owe a huge debt of gratitude to Howard C. Mofenson, M.D., for the major contribution of material reproduced from his chapter in the previous edition.

ample is using sodium bicarbonate in hypoxic lactic acidosis.

The new recommendations also emphasize the importance of following guidelines established by the Occupational Safety and Health Administration (OSHA) to avoid transmitting disease from the victim to the rescuer, and they advocate use of gloves and mechanical ventilation equipment, including resuscitative masks, that divert expired air away from the rescuer.

1992 BASIC LIFE SUPPORT CHANGES

1. Children should receive 1 minute of CPR before EMS is summoned because respiratory arrest is the most common cause of cardiac arrest in children and VF is rare. In adults it is recommended that a lone rescuer summon EMS immediately, before starting CPR.
2. To manage an obstructed airway in infants, a series of five back blows and chest thrusts is recommended (this number makes it easier to remember because it is the same as for cardiac compressions). (The 1986 recommendations specified four back blows and chest thrusts to manage the obstructed airway.)
3. In rescue breathing for adults it is recommended that the duration of inspiratory filling of the lungs be increased to 1½ to 2 seconds to prevent gastric distention. However, the inspiratory filling time for children is unchanged (1 to 1½ seconds) because children have smaller tidal volumes and higher ventilatory rates.

1992 ADVANCED LIFE SUPPORT CHANGES

1. Epinephrine is to be administered endotracheally in a dose of 0.1 mg/kg (1 : 1000 solution) except in neonates. (The 1986 recommendation for epinephrine administered endotracheally was 0.01 mg/kg [1 : 10,000 solution]) (a class IIb recommendation).[14]
2. Other drugs administered endotracheally are administered in doses two to three times that of the intravenous (IV) route. (The 1986 recommendations for the doses of atropine, lidocaine, and naloxone were the same as for the IV doses.)
3. In asystolic pulseless arrest, the second and subsequent doses of IV and intraosseous epinephrine for unresponsive and pulseless arrest are higher than the initial dose of 0.01 mg/kg (1 : 10,000) and are administered as 0.1 mg/kg (1 : 1000) except in neonates. This is a class IIa recommendation in children because of scientific evidence of better neurological outcome.[23] (The 1986 recommendations were for an initial dose of 0.01 mg/kg [1 : 10,000] of epinephrine, and subsequent doses were the same.)
4. The management of paroxysmal supraventricular tachycardia (SVT), the most common dysrhythmia to cause circulatory instability in infants, includes a rapid bolus (1 to 3 seconds) of adenosine (0.1 mg/kg) initially in a stable patient and continuous cardiac monitoring. If the initial dose is ineffective, the dose can be doubled. The maximum single dose is 12 mg. In an unstable child, adenosine can be given before 0.5 J/kg cardioversion if an IV line is already in place. This is a class I recommendation. (The 1986 recommendations did not include adenosine.)
5. The management of bradycardia no longer includes atropine or isoproterenol. (The 1986 recommendations included atropine in the management of bradycardia.)
6. The management of asystole does not include atropine.
7. Intracardiac administration of emergency drugs is no longer included.
8. It is recommended that pulse oximetry be used in respiratory compromise during stabilization and transport.
9. Use of the Broselow Pediatric Emergency Tape to determine a child's approximate weight by measuring the recumbent length has been validated and can help in calculating drug doses in emergencies. It is suggested that manufacturers print recommended doses on prefilled syringes.
10. The 1992 recommendations advocate a simple protocol for establishing intravascular access quickly. In a child younger than age 6, an intraosseous line should be established if reliable venous access cannot be achieved within 90 seconds or in three attempts. This technique is not reliable in children older than age 6 because the red marrow has been replaced by fat in the long bones. If the intraosseous line cannot be established in 3 to 5 minutes, medications should be given via the ET tube—the least preferred route. An infusion pump is recommended for rapid administration of viscous fluids and large amounts of fluid to overcome the resistance of the emissary veins encountered with intraosseous infusions.

DIFFERENCES BETWEEN CARDIOPULMONARY ARREST IN CHILDREN AND ADULTS

Adults

The cause of CPA in adults commonly is an acute cardiac insult, such as myocardial infarction, which leads to a disturbance in cardiac rhythm. It usually occurs in patients whose hearts are damaged already. Ventricular fibrillation (VF) is common, and unmonitored defibrillation may be attempted to restore normal cardiac rhythm.

Children

The cause of CPA in children usually is severe hypoxia and acidosis or circulatory collapse, or both. Management focuses on preventing these events with prearrest assessment and anticipatory intervention through respiratory ventilation. Establishing airway patency and adequate ventilation often makes further resuscitative measures unnecessary if the child is not yet in CPA and is experiencing only respiratory arrest or compromise. Because asystole occurs in 90% of pediatric patients who have cardiac arrest, unmonitored defibrillation is not recommended.[2]

Table A-1 summarizes the distinguishing features of CPA in adults and children.

Children need oxygen more than drugs to correct rhythm disturbances; however, they do require medications for some arrhythmias, such as epinephrine and bicarbonate for asystole, digoxin for SVT, and lidocaine for ventricular arrhyth-

Table A-1 Differences Between Adults and Children in Cardiopulmonary Arrest

Feature	Adults	Children
Cause	Myocardial infarction	Hypoxia and acidosis
Cardiac status	Damaged heart	Healthy heart
Arrhythmia	Ventricular fibrillation	Asystole
Defibrillation	Unmonitored	Only monitored
Predominant therapy	Defibrillation	Oxygen

mias. The anatomical and physiological differences of children, compared with adults, present special problems. For example, in pediatric patients major differences exist in the anatomy of the airways, the airway diameter, the methods used for vascular access, and the choice of medication. A special cart with age-labeled equipment and precalculated drug doses should be available.

CPA in children usually does not occur suddenly. It often can be prevented if respiratory failure and shock are recognized early and treatment is begun promptly.[2,27] Respiratory failure and shock can be recognized within 30 seconds by assessing the ABCs of CPR—*a*irway, *b*reathing, and *c*irculation.

RESPIRATORY FAILURE

Respiratory failure occurs when ventilation and oxygenation become inadequate. Its clinical definition is based on the inability of pulmonary gas exchange to satisfy the body's metabolic demands for transporting oxygen and eliminating carbon dioxide. Its presence is confirmed by abnormal levels for blood gas (the arterial oxygen [PO_2] and carbon dioxide [PCO_2] pressures), and pH, not by physical signs, except for apnea. The presence of respiratory failure or impending respiratory failure is detected by evaluating airway patency and the quality of breathing and by checking for signs of hypoxia and hypercarbia (cyanosis, central nervous system [CNS] depression, and bradycardia).

Airway Patency

The airway is determined clinically to be (1) patent, requiring no intervention, (2) maintainable with noninvasive procedures (e.g., positioning, suctioning, or a bag-valve-mask system), or (3) nonmaintainable, requiring invasive procedures (e.g., use of airway adjuncts, ET intubation, cricothyroidotomy, or removal of a foreign body).

Breathing

The effectiveness of breathing and oxygenation is evaluated clinically by analyzing the respiratory rate, air entry, respiratory effort, skin and mucosal color, and level of consciousness.

The respiratory rate is classified as apnea, bradypnea, or tachypnea. The rate varies and is nonspecific for age. Tachypnea without respiratory distress may result from attempts to compensate for metabolic acidosis (quiet tachypnea). Bradypnea is ominous and may be caused by fatigue or CNS depression. Any respiratory rate over 60 breaths/min or under 10 breaths/min is abnormal at any age.

The adequacy of tidal volume (5 to 7 ml/kg) is best assessed by auscultating for breath sounds and air entry at the periphery of the lung fields, over the apices and laterally, and by observing excursions of the chest wall. The minute volume equals the tidal volume times the respiratory rate. Minute volume may be low because of breaths that are too shallow or a respiratory rate that is too slow.

Increased respiratory effort indicates respiratory distress and represents compensation for inadequate gas exchange. The signs of increased respiratory effort are head bobbing, nasal flaring, grunting, stridor, use of the accessory muscles, retractions, seesaw movement of the chest and abdomen, and prolonged expiration. These findings mandate measurement of arterial blood gases (ABGs).

The skin color reflects the level of tissue oxygenation and perfusion. Diminished oxygenation produces an ashen gray or cyanotic color of the skin and mucosa. It is a late sign of hypoxia.

The level of consciousness reflects oxygenation and perfusion of the brain. Patients are classified according to their responsiveness (i.e., alertness, verbal response, pain response, or unconscious). In infants over 2 months of age, an early sign of diminished cerebral oxygenation and perfusion is failure to recognize his or her parents.

SHOCK (CIRCULATORY FAILURE)

Shock (see also Chapter 296) is a clinical state characterized by failure of the cardiovascular system to perfuse vital organs adequately, resulting in inadequate oxygen and substrate delivery to meet the needs of the tissues and to remove their metabolites. This results in anaerobic metabolism and accumulation of acids. Shock may occur with normal, increased, or decreased cardiac output and blood pressure. In compensated shock the cardiac output is low and the blood pressure is normal. In decompensated shock the blood pressure and cardiac output are low.

Shock is classified as either hypovolemic or cardiogenic. Hypovolemic shock, or distributive shock, the most common type in pediatric patients, is caused by a loss of vascular space volume as a result of dehydration or blood loss or a loss of vascular tone, such as occurs in sepsis, anaphylaxis, and an acute CNS pathological condition. Cardiogenic shock caused by heart failure or arrhythmias is relatively rare among children except in postcardiac arrest patients in whom it is the primary cause of shock.

Cardiovascular performance can be evaluated by assessing the peripheral pulses, skin perfusion, level of consciousness and heart rate, and, later, the blood pressure and urinary output.

Pulse

Palpating the peripheral pulse (a reflection of peripheral perfusion) allows the examiner to estimate the stroke volume and heart rate. The stroke volume is the volume of blood pumped by each heartbeat. The cardiac output is the volume of blood pumped by the heart every minute (heart rate ×

stroke volume). Organ perfusion is determined by the cardiac output and the peripheral vascular resistance.

Skin Perfusion

The skin is a relatively nonessential organ and loses its perfusion first. This is assessed by capillary refill time, or the time it takes for normal skin color to return after blanching pressure is applied; this should be less than 2 seconds, or less than the time it takes to say "capillary refill." When testing for capillary refill, the extremity used should be elevated above the level of the heart. Poor perfusion also can be identified by mottled skin color, cool hands and feet, and a line of demarcation that separates the warm skin from the cool skin of an extremity.

Level of Consciousness

Evidence of diminished brain oxygenation and perfusion was discussed previously in the section on respiratory failure.

Heart Rate

Changes in the heart rate reflect changes in cardiac output but, unfortunately, are nonspecific. Tachycardia is defined as a heart rate above 180 beats/min in patients younger than age 5 years; above 160 beats/min in patients between 5 and 10 years of age; and above 100 beats/min in patients older than age 10 years. If tachycardia is present, the examiner must distinguish between benign and serious causes. When tachycardia fails to compensate adequately for tissue oxygen needs, hypoxia, hypercapnia, acidosis, and bradycardia develop. Bradycardia in a distressed child is an ominous sign of impending cardiac arrest.

Blood Pressure

The blood pressure is the product of cardiac output times the peripheral vascular resistance. Hypotension is a late and ominous finding in patients who are in shock. The systolic blood pressure should be above 60 mm Hg from birth to 1 month of age and above 70 mm Hg in infants 1 month to 1 year of age. A formula for determining the lower limit for systolic blood pressure in children over 1 year of age is as follows:

$$70 + (2 \times \text{Age in years})$$

This represents a level that is greater than two standard deviations below the mean.

Urinary Output

The normal urinary output is 1 to 2 ml/kg/hr. Although this measure is unavailable to help in the initial evaluation, it is a valuable indicator of kidney perfusion later on. The bladder urine obtained initially by catheterization should not be used for calculating urinary output.

In respiratory failure the blood is delivered adequately to the body tissues, but the blood delivered is deficient in oxygen. In shock the blood contains adequate oxygen, but it is delivered poorly. Both conditions can lead to hypoxia, hypercapnia, anaerobic metabolism, acidosis, and CPA. Table A-2 summarizes the ABCs of cardiorespiratory assessment.

Table A-2 Summary of Cardiorespiratory Assessment

Respiratory Assessment	Cardiovascular Assessment
A. Airway patency	C. Circulation
Able to maintain independently	Heart rate
Requires adjuncts/assistance to maintain	Blood pressure
B. Breathing	Volume/strength of central pulses
Rate	Peripheral pulses
Mechanics	Present/absent
Retractions	Volume/strength
Grunting	Skin perfusion
Accessory muscles	Capillary refill time (consider ambient temperature)
Nasal flaring	Temperature
Air entry	Color
Chest expansion	Mottling
Breath sounds	Central nervous system perfusion
Stridor	Responsiveness
Wheezing	Awake
Paradoxical chest movement	Responds to voice
Color	Responds to pain
	Unresponsive
	Recognizes parents
	Muscle tone
	Pupil size
	Posturing

Modified from Chameides L, Hazinski FN, editors: *Pediatric advanced life support,* The American Academy of Pediatrics and the American Heart Association, Dallas, 1997, The Association.

PEDIATRIC BASIC LIFE SUPPORT

In applying pediatric basic life support measures, the priorities of management should be based on clinical assessment. Questionable cases, as well as patients successfully resuscitated in CPA, require frequent reassessment by means of arterial blood gas (ABG) determinations and chest roentgenograms.

The patient's condition should be classified as one of the following:

1. *Stable:* requires no intervention but does require continued reassessment
2. *Questionable:* requires very frequent reassessment
3. *Definite respiratory failure or shock:* requires immediate intervention
4. *Cardiopulmonary failure:* requires basic life support and ALS

General Priorities of Management

1. With upper airway obstruction the child should be allowed to stay with the parents and remain in the selected position of comfort. Feedings are withheld, the normal body temperature is maintained, and the maximum amount of oxygen tolerated is delivered.

Table A-3 Methods of Chest Compression

Age	Site	Applicator	Depth	Pressure	Rate/min
Infant (<1 yr)	1 fb below internipple line	Middle and ring fingers	½-1 in (1.3-2.5 cm)	Hand	At least 100
Child (1-8 yr)	2 fb above xiphoid	Heel of the hand	1-1½ in (2.5-3.8 cm)	Arm	80-100
Child (>8 yr)	2 fb above xiphoid	Both hands clasped	1½-2 in (3.8-5 cm)	Body	80-100

fb, Fingerbreadth.

2. Respiratory failure requires securing an airway, establishing adequate ventilation, administering maximum supplemental oxygen, instituting cardiorespiratory monitoring and pulse oximetry, and obtaining frequent ABG values and chest roentgenograms.
3. Shock requires delivering maximum supplemental oxygen, establishing vascular access, expanding blood volume, administering appropriate vasopressors (if necessary), obtaining an electrocardiogram (ECG), and instituting cardiorespiratory monitoring and pulse oximetry.
4. Cardiopulmonary failure requires instituting ventilation and oxygenation, establishing cardiorespiratory monitoring and pulse oximetry, gaining vascular access to expand blood volume, and obtaining frequent ABG values and chest roentgenograms.

Basic Airway, Breathing, and Circulation of Cardiopulmonary Resuscitation[1,7,27]

If unconscious, the patient should be placed supine, turned as a unit with firm support to the head and the neck to prevent spinal injury, and placed on a firm, flat surface. The airway should be maintained by using the head-tilt/chin-lift maneuver or, if a neck injury is suspected, by using the jaw-thrust maneuver. If the patient is not breathing, CPR should be performed for 1 minute before help is sought. If the patient is conscious and in respiratory distress, the child's position of comfort should be respected and transport in a properly equipped ambulance should be accomplished without disturbing him or her.

Airway. The *head-tilt* maneuver consists of placing a hand on the forehead and tilting the head backward into a "sniffing," or neutral, position. The *chin-tilt* maneuver consists of placing the fingers under the chin and lifting it upward. The neck should not be overextended. The *jaw-thrust* maneuver is accomplished by placing two or three fingers on each side of the lower jaw at its angle and lifting upward with both elbows resting on the surface on which the victim is lying. If the airway is not maintainable with these maneuvers, an oropharyngeal airway or an ET tube should be placed.

Breathing. The patency of the airway must be maintained. The examiner should place his or her ear close to the patient's mouth and nose to listen for breath sounds. The chest should be felt for air movement, and the chest and abdomen observed for movement.

If the patient is not breathing, mouth-to-mouth resuscitation must be instituted. With an infant, this involves tilting the head and sealing the mouth and nose; with a toddler or older patient, the rescuer pinches the nose and seals the patient's mouth with his or her own. The rescuer delivers slow puffs of air (1 to 1½ seconds' duration), breaking the mouth seal after each puff to allow the patient to exhale. The force and volume of the puff should be sufficient to cause the chest to rise. Using this volume of air and the slow puffs prevents gastric distention in the patient. If air enters the lungs freely and the chest rises, the airway is patent. The most common cause of airway obstruction is improper head positioning; it should be readjusted and mouth-to-mouth breathing repeated. If the chest still does not rise, a foreign body lodged in the upper airway should be suspected and the methods for removing it (given below) should be instituted. The patient should receive ventilation with a bag (with reservoir) and mask attached to oxygen as soon as possible.

Gastric distention with vomiting and aspiration can be minimized in unconscious patients by applying cricoid pressure (using one fingertip in infants and the thumb and index finger in children) to occlude the proximal esophagus. The pressure is released once ET intubation is accomplished.

Circulation. Inefficient cardiovascular performance is recognized by the absence of the pulse in a large artery or by bradycardia that does not respond to ventilation and oxygenation. For patients older than 1 year of age, the carotid artery should be palpated; for patients younger than age 1, the brachial artery is palpated. If the pulse is present but respirations are absent, the head-tilt maneuver and mouth-to-mouth breathing should be maintained.

Chest compression. Compression of the chest is performed to effect cardiac compression. Table A-3 summarizes the methods used for chest compression for pediatric patients of varying ages.

The indications for chest compression are asystole (as evidenced by absent pulses) or bradycardia below 60 beats/min in a child or 80 beats/min in a neonate unresponsive to ventilation and oxygenation.

The patient should be horizontal and supine on a firm surface. With small infants, the palm of the rescuer's hand should support the back.

The site at which compression is applied varies with the patient's age.[9,18,21]

In infants, compressions should be applied one fingerbreadth (fb) below the intersection of the internipple line with the sternum; compression should not be applied over the xiphoid. The middle and ring fingers should be used to compress the chest to a depth of ½ to 1 inch (1.3 or 2.5 cm) at a rate above 100/minute. The pressure is released without lifting the fingers off the sternum but allowing it to return to its normal position. Equal time is allotted for each phase (compression and decompression). In applying compressions for a neonate or a small infant, the hands should encircle the thorax, and the thumbs should be placed side by side just below the internipple line over the lower third of the sternum. Chest compressions should then be applied with the thumbs to the same depth and at the same rate as for an older infant.

In children older than 1 year of age, the resuscitator places the heel of one hand 2 fb above the sternal notch (where the lower margin of the rib cage and sternum meet) and uses the pressure generated by his or her arm to compress the sternum 1 to 1½ inches (2.5 to 3.8 cm) at a rate of 80 to 100/minute, taking care to keep the fingers off the ribs. Again, the compression and decompression phases are equal. The compression rate for children older than age 8 is also 80 to 100/minute, but the depth of compression is increased to 1½ to 2 inches (3.8 to 5 cm), with the resuscitator using the pressure generated by his or her whole body applied through clasped hands just above the sternal notch.

The adequacy of the compressions is determined by palpating the pulse during compression. External cardiac compressions must be accompanied by head tilt and ventilations. At the end of every fifth compression, a pause of 1 to 1½ seconds should be made to allow for mouth-to-mouth or bag-and-mask ventilation (5:1 compression to ventilation ratio). The victim should be assessed after 10 cycles of compressions and ventilations (approximately 1 minute). With a single rescuer, the head-tilt maneuver must be performed with each ventilation. ECG monitoring should be instituted as soon as possible and blood specimens obtained for glucose, serum electrolyte, and gas analysis.

Relieving airway obstruction.[2,6,27] The sequence for managing an obstructed airway is as follows:

- I. Conscious patient
  - A. Breathing and coughing→No intervention
  - B. Ineffective cough and increasing stridor with a witnessed or suspected foreign body aspiration
    1. Infant→Back blows and chest thrusts
    2. Child→Heimlich maneuver (abdominal thrusts)
- II. Unconscious, nonbreathing patient
  - A. Nonspontaneous breathing→Head tilt, chin lift, and assisted ventilation
  - B. Assisted ventilation—No chest rise
    1. Reposition head and repeat assisted ventilation
    2. Attempt to relieve obstruction
       - a. Infant: Up to five back blows and chest thrusts
       - b. Child: Up to five Heimlich maneuver abdominal thrusts
    3. Perform tongue-jaw lift, and manually remove a foreign body if one is seen

Infant back blows and chest thrusts. With the infant straddled over the rescuer's forearm, the head positioned lower than the trunk, and the jaw held open by the rescuer's fingers, up to five back blows are delivered with the heel of the hand between the shoulder blades. If this does not remove the foreign body, the infant should be turned over so that the head, neck, and back are well supported on the rescuer's forearm. If this too is unsuccessful, up to five chest thrusts similar to cardiac compressions, but deeper, should be administered.

The Heimlich Maneuver (Abdominal Thrusts)

1. *Standing patient.* From behind, the thumb of one fisted hand is placed in the midline above the navel and well below the xiphoid. The fist is grasped by the other hand and a quick upward thrust is administered. Each thrust is separate. Up to five thrusts should be completed in an attempt to dislodge and expel the foreign body.
2. *Supine, unconscious patient.* With the child lying supine, the rescuer should kneel at his or her feet. The heel of one hand is placed on the child's abdomen above the navel and well below the xiphoid. The other hand is placed on top of the first and pressed into the abdomen with a quick upward thrust in the *midline*. A series of five thrusts are performed or fewer if the foreign body is expelled.
3. *The tongue maneuver.* This maneuver is used if back blows, chest thrusts, and subdiaphragmatic thrusts fail. The child's mouth is opened, and the tongue and lower jaw are grasped between the rescuer's thumb and index finger and are lifted. This maneuver may relieve airway obstruction even with a foreign body still in place. If a foreign body is seen, it should be removed with the thumb and forefinger of the other hand, or if available, a hemostat. Blind sweeps of the throat with the examiner's index finger are contraindicated because they may force a foreign body farther down the airway.

Table A-4 summarizes the basic life support measures used in infants and children.

PEDIATRIC ADVANCED LIFE SUPPORT

When pediatric basic life support measures such as CPR are ineffective in resuscitating and stabilizing affected infants and children, ALS measures must be taken immediately. These measures include airway access and management, administration of oxygen, vascular access, administration of fluids and electrolytes, and drug therapy. To implement these measures the physician must be familiar with the ranges of body surface area, weight, and vital signs for pediatric patients (Table A-5) and the guidelines for use of resuscitation equipment of various sizes, according to the patient's age and weight (Table A-6). Resuscitation of newborns is presented in Chapter 45 (One), Peripartum Considerations.

Airway Access and Management

Ventilation can be assisted without the placement of an endotracheal (ET) tube. The purpose of CPR is to get oxygen into the airway. Oxygen delivery systems include an oropharyngeal airway, a nasal cannula, oxygen hoods and tents, and face shields and masks; however, these methods do not reliably provide oxygen concentrations over 40%. The most effective, noninvasive, assisted ventilation method is the self-inflating bag and mask with a reservoir connected to an oxygen source. Airway patency must be maintained and as-

Table A-4 Summary of Basic Life Support Maneuvers in Infants and Children

Maneuver	Infant (<1 yr)	Child (1 to 8 yr)
Airway	Head tilt—chin lift (if trauma is present, use jaw thrust)	Head tilt—chin lift (if trauma is present, use jaw thrust)
Breathing		
Initial	Two breaths at 1 to 1½ s/breath	Two breaths at 1 to 1½ s/breath
Subsequent	20 breaths/min (approximate)	20 breaths/min (approximate)
Circulation		
Pulse check	Brachial/femoral	Carotid
Compression area	Lower half of sternum	Lower half of sternum
Compression with	Two or three fingers	Heel of one hand
Depth	Approximately one third to half the depth of the chest	Approximately one third to half the depth of the chest
Rate	At least 100/min	100/min
Compression-ventilation ratio	5:1 (pause for ventilation)	5:1 (pause for ventilation)
Foreign-body airway obstruction	Back blows/chest thrusts	Heimlich maneuver

Modified from Chameides L, Hazinski FN, editors: *Pediatric advanced life support,* The American Academy of Pediatrics and the American Heart Association, Dallas, 1997, The Association.

Table A-5 Ranges of Body Surface Area, Weight, and Vital Signs for Infants, Children, and Adults

Age	Body Surface Area (m^2)	Weight (kg)	Pulse*/Min	Systolic Blood Pressure† (mm Hg)	Respiratory Rate‡/Min
Newborn	0.19	3.5	90-200	60	30-60
1 mo	0.30	4.0	90-180	65	30-60
6 mo	0.38	7.0	90-180	70	24-30
1-2 yr	0.50-0.55	10-12	70-140	72-74	20-24
3-5 yr	0.54-0.68	15-20	60-120	76-80	16-22
6-9 yr	0.68-0.85	20-28	60-120	82-88	14-20
10-12 yr	1.00-1.07	30-38	60-110	90	12-20
12-14 yr	1.07-1.22	38-48	50-100	90	12-20
15-16 yr	1.30-1.60	53-58	50-100	90	12-18
Adult	1.40-1.70	60-70	50-100	90	12-18

*Pulse range includes sound sleep and vigorous crying.
†Systolic blood pressure less than fifth percentile.
‡Respiratory rate >60 or <10/min is abnormal at any age.

sessed frequently by observing for adequate symmetrical chest movements, adequate breath sounds, and good color.

Oropharyngeal and nasopharyngeal airways. The oropharyngeal airway can be used in an unconscious patient to support the tongue. It is not used in conscious patients because it may stimulate vomiting. To estimate the proper size, the flange should be placed at the level of the central incisors and the tip of the appropriate-size airway should reach the angle of the jaw. The tongue should be depressed with a tongue depressor, and the airway should be inserted into the oropharynx in the position of function and rotated into proper position as it approaches the back of the oropharynx. Proper head extension must be maintained.

Conscious patients tolerate a nasopharyngeal airway better than an oropharyngeal airway; however, the nasopharyngeal type may injure enlarged adenoidal tissue and cause bleeding in children younger than age 10.

Suctioning should not last longer than 5 seconds and should be preceded and followed by ventilation with 100% oxygen. The heart rate should be monitored for bradycardia during suctioning.

Endotracheal airway. Placement of an ET tube should be considered early in the care of an unconscious patient because it prevents aspiration, permits suctioning of the trachea and main bronchi, is a route for administering resuscitative medications,[11,12,30] allows for hyperventilation, and permits application of positive end-expiratory pressure (PEEP) when 100% oxygen does not improve oxygenation sufficiently. Hyperventilation may help reduce increased intracranial pressure and can compensate for metabolic acidosis. PEEP may increase the functional residual capacity of the lungs and improve ventilation and perfusion. If prolonged ventilation is anticipated or if bag-mask and other airway adjuncts cannot accomplish adequate ventilation, an ET tube should be inserted. See Appendix B, Special Procedures, for methodology of ET intubation.

The ET tube should be translucent, of uniform diameter (not tapering), and equipped with a standard 15-mm adapter; preferably the tube should have distance markers and an opening on its side wall as well as at its end. Cuffed ET tubes should be used only in children older than age 8. An air leak with an uncuffed ET tube should be present when a breath is given at 20 cm H_2O pressure; if it is not, the tube is too large

Table A-6 Pediatric Resuscitation Equipment Guidelines[1]

Age	Weight (kg)	ET Tube (mm Internal Diameter*)	Laryngoscope Blade (No.)	Suction Catheter (Fr)	Distance from Midtrachea to Teeth (cm)	Chest Tube (Fr)	Venous Catheter (Gauge)	Foley Catheter and Nasogastric Tube (Fr)
Newborn, premature	<1	2.5	0	5 or 6	8	10-14	22-24	5 fdt
Newborn, full term	3	3.0	1	6	10	12-18	22-24	6 fdt
6 mo	7	3.5	1	8	12	14-20	22-24	8
1 yr	10	4.0	1	8	12	14-24	20-22	10
18 mo	11	4.0	1	8	14	14-24	20-22	10
3 yr	14	4.5	2	8	16	18-26	20-22	10
5 yr	18	5.0	2-3	10	16	20-32	20-22	10-12
8 yr	25	6.0 cuff	3	10	18	28-34	20-22	12
10 yr	34	6.5 cuff	3	10	18	30-38	18-20	12
12 yr	38	6.5-7 cuff	3	10	20	34-38	18-20	12-14
16 yr	55	7.5-8 cuff	3	12	22	34-38	18-20	12-14
Adult		8-8.5 cuff	3	12	22	34-38	18-20	12-14

Cuff, Cuffed endotracheal tube; *ET,* endotracheal; *Fdt,* feeding tube.

*Internal diameter of the ET tube = $\frac{\text{Child's age} + 16}{4}$

and should be replaced with a smaller one. The internal diameter of the ET tube should equal approximately 16 plus the patient's age in years, divided by 4; after 1 year of age the external diameter of the ET tube used should equal the size of the patient's external nasal orifice or the width of the patient's fifth finger.

Straight-blade laryngoscopes are preferred in children. Before laryngoscopy is begun, the examiner should check the equipment and the light source. Attempts at ET intubation should not exceed 30 seconds, and the heart rate and oxygenation should be monitored during the procedure. Bradycardia below 80 beats/min in a neonate or 60 beats/min in a child mandates interruption of the procedure and administration of 100% oxygen by face mask and bag. The ET tube should be passed into the trachea to a length that places the distance marker at the level of the vocal chords.

Once intubation has been established, the ET tube should be held securely in position and its position confirmed by (1) observing symmetrical movements of the chest, (2) auscultating the lungs to detect bilateral breath sounds, (3) auscultating over the stomach to ensure that air entry sounds are absent, and (4) looking for condensation in the ET tube during exhalation. An end-tidal carbon dioxide detector allows verification of ET tube placement or displacement during stabilization and transport.

Asymmetrical right-sided breath sounds usually indicate intubation of the right main bronchus. When this occurs, the tube should be withdrawn until breath sounds are heard in both lungs; the ET tube should then be withdrawn another 1 to 2 cm to ensure a midtracheal position. The final position of the ET tube must be confirmed by chest roentgenogram.

A properly placed tube but inadequate lung expansion indicates that (1) the tube is too small, (2) a large laryngeal air leak is present (detected by auscultating the neck), (3) the "pop-off" valve on the ventilator bag is not depressed, (4) the bag-valve device leaks, or (5) an insufficiently strong air bag puff was administered.

The tube's position should be verified by noting the distance marked on the tube at the lips; it should be secured to the patient's face with benzoin and tape (see Fig. B-22). Its position should be assessed frequently by observing chest wall expansion, listening for bilateral breath sounds, and noting improvement of color and perfusion, obtaining blood gas values, and checking pulse oximeter readings.

Drugs can be administered through the ET tube while vascular access is sought. These drugs are *a*tropine, *n*aloxone, *e*pinephrine, and *l*idocaine (ANEL). Two to three times the usual IV dose (diluted in 1 to 2 ml of 0.9% saline) is administered through a catheter that has been passed beyond the ET tube as deeply as possible into the tracheobronchial tree. The dose of epinephrine, however, should be 10 times the IV dose (0.1 mg/kg of a 1:1000 solution), except in neonates.[14] After the drug has been instilled, several positive pressure puffs should be given.[3,11,12,30]

Cricothyrotomy. In patients younger than age 8, airway obstruction may occur at the cricoid ring, the narrowest portion of the larynx in this age group. Because the ring is located below the thyrocricoid membrane, cricothyrotomy may not be effective in establishing an airway. In general, this route is not recommended in infants and small children.[15]

Airway emergencies with endotracheal tubes. When emergencies occur, the gas delivery system should be disconnected and the patient should receive manual ventilation by means of a resuscitation bag and use of 100% oxygen. Auscultation should be used to determine the tube's position and patency. Problems that may be encountered include (1) loss of oxygen supply to the tube, (2) occlusion or kinking of the tube, or (3) displacement of the tube. If obstruction or displacement is the problem, poor breath sounds, a lack of chest movements, and increased resistance to inflation should be observed. Decreased resistance to inflation occurs when the ET tube has been misplaced into the esophagus. If the ET tube is obstructed, it should be irrigated with 1 ml of saline and suctioned for 3 to 4 seconds. After suctioning, the breath sounds, airway resistance, and adequacy of chest movements should be evaluated. If proper positioning and adequate manual ventilation of the ET tube are ensured, the problem should be assumed to lie with the gas delivery systems, which should be disconnected and manual ventilation instituted. If it is unclear whether the ET tube has been dislodged, its placement can be determined by direct laryngoscopy or by using a capnometer (an end-tidal carbon dioxide detector). Sometimes the tube has to be removed and reinserted.

Oxygen Administration

The rational for administering oxygen is that establishing an adequate airway alone cannot reverse the pathophysiology of hypoxemia. Mouth-to-mouth breathing delivers only 16% fractional inspiratory oxygen (FiO_2) and results in an oxygen tension (PaO_2) of only 80 mm Hg. Normally, when one breathes room air, the PaO_2 is 104 mm Hg. Chest compression generates only 25% to 30% of the normal circulation in adults. Oxygen is indicated in any situation in which hypoxia is suspected. Oxygen should be administered even if the PaO_2 is high because a low cardiac output may not deliver sufficient oxygen to the tissues. The oxygen concentration should be 100% (preferably humidified and warmed) to achieve an adequate PaO_2 and tissue saturation. Once the airway has been established, if the respiration is not adequate, oxygen should be administered through an appropriate-size face mask connected to a self-inflating bag with an attached reservoir that delivers oxygen at a rate of 10 to 15 L/min. When a self-inflating bag is used, the "pop-off" valve should be occluded because the pressures needed to ventilate the lungs may exceed the valve's limit. Administering oxygen through a nasal cannula, a face mask, or a face shield does not provide oxygen concentrations above 40% with sufficient reliability.[2,7,27]

Vascular Access

In children younger than age 6, if venous access cannot be established in 90 seconds or after three attempts, the intraosseous fluid access route should be used. For patients older than age 6, the lesser saphenous vein or a femoral vein should be accessed.[2]

Infusion pumps or minidrip chambers should be used for infusion therapy. Head and neck vessels should not be used because this interferes with resuscitative measures. Cannulation of central veins should be supervised by experienced operators.

The intraosseous space is a plexus of noncollapsible veins through which any fluid or medication may be infused.[16,24,28,29] Interosseous infusion is recommended for children younger than age 6 if vascular access cannot be established in 90 seconds or after three percutaneous attempts.[2,27] It is an easily learned and quickly accomplished technique. An 18-gauge short spinal needle with a stylet or a large-bore marrow needle may be used. The favorite site is 2 cm below the tibial tuberosity on the edial surface of the tibia. Intraosseous infusions are equivalent to those given intravenously and are preferable to the ET route for administering drugs. Appendix B, Special Procedures, describes in detail the methods used in intraosseous infusions.

Resuscitative and Postresuscitative Fluids and Drugs

The purposes of the pharmacological agents used during cardiac arrest and the postresuscitation period are (1) to expand intravascular volume and increase perfusion; (2) to stimulate spontaneous, forceful myocardial contractions; (3) to accelerate the cardiac rate; (4) to correct metabolic acidosis; and (5) to suppress ventricular conduction ectopy. The pharmacological agents used, their indications and doses, and the precautions to apply in using them are discussed below and are presented in Table A-7.

Volume expansion. The types of fluids available for volume expansion include the following:

1. Crystalloids—lactated Ringer's or 0.9% saline. Lactated Ringer's is preferred because it contains less chloride and does not aggravate acidosis. Because only one fourth of crystalloids remain in the vascular space, four times the deficit is required to restore plasma volume.
2. Colloids and blood products—albumin, fresh frozen plasma, human plasma protein fraction (Plasmanate), whole blood or packed red blood cells (RBCs). In general, the patient requires that these products constitute half the amount of the crystalloids given to restore plasma volume.
3. Glucose[2,4,7,25,27]—Glucose is not administered in the initial resuscitative fluids unless hypoglycemia exists. In response to stress, the endogenous catecholamines cause glycogenolysis and increase the blood glucose. Excess glucose may be metabolized to lactate and cause an osmotic diuresis.

Small infants and chronically ill children have limited glycogen stores, and hypoxemia-like hypoglycemia may develop. Glucose is a major metabolic substrate for the neonatal myocardium. A rapid blood glucose test should be obtained, and if hypoglycemia exists, glucose should be administered. In children a $D_{25}W$ solution should be used (dilution of $D_{50}W$ 1:1 with sterile water), and in infants a $D_{10}W$ solution (dilution of $D_{50}W$ 1:4 with sterile water) should be used. Sufficient amounts should be given to keep the blood glucose level above 100 mg/dl. Repeated hyperosmolar doses have been associated with intracranial hemorrhage in premature infants.

The principle in fluid resuscitation is to administer a bolus of fluid over a period of 10 to 15 minutes and then reevaluate the patient's hydration status. In hypovolemic shock a 20-ml/kg dose of crystalloid is administered as soon as vascular access is established. A child who is in hypovolemic shock often requires 40 to 60 ml/kg of fluid in the first hour of resuscitation and, occasionally, up to 100 to 200 ml/kg in the first few hours. A three-way stopcock attached to a 20-ml or 50-ml syringe may be useful in "pushing" fluids with the aid of the syringe. Subsequently, volume expanders may be needed (e.g., colloid or blood); a 20-ml/kg dose of 5% albumin, a 1-g/kg dose of 25% albumin, or a 20-ml/kg dose of fresh frozen plasma may be used. Whole blood (20 ml/kg) is administered if hemorrhage has occurred, and packed RBCs (10 ml/kg) are given to a patient who has had chronic blood loss.

Fluid resuscitation should be monitored by reassessing perfusion frequently. Fluid overload is detected by auscultating the chest for signs of pulmonary edema and by noting the size of the heart on a chest roentgenogram. In hypovolemia the heart is normal or small in size; in cardiogenic shock or fluid overload, it usually is enlarged.

Resuscitation medications.* The resuscitative medications described here are listed in Table A-7 along with their recommended doses and means of administration. The normal values for arterial blood pH, gases, oxygen saturation, and bicarbonate for newborns, infants, and children are shown in Table A-8.

The vagus nerve, through its neurotransmitter acetylcholine, inhibits conduction at the sinoauricular and atrioventricular (AV) nodes. The sympathetic nervous system, through its alpha-adrenergic receptors, enhances perfusion by causing vasoconstriction and increased peripheral vascular resistance. Its beta-1 adrenergic receptors increase heart rate, cardiac conductivity, and myocardial contractility, resulting in increased cardiac output. The sympathetic nervous system's beta-2 adrenergic receptors cause vasodilation of skeletal muscle blood vessels and bronchodilation; they do not play a role in CPR.

Epinephrine. Epinephrine is an endogenous catecholamine that has alpha- and beta-adrenergic receptor properties. In doses used for CPR, it has alpha, beta-1, and beta-2 effects. Its mechanism of action relates to its alpha effect, which increases systemic vascular resistance, leading to increased coronary artery perfusion pressure and increased oxygen delivery to the myocardium. It is indicated in asystole, unstable bradyrhythmias, which constitute 90% of rhythm disturbances in pediatric patients, and VF, which occurs in only 10% of children who have rhythm disturbances. Epinephrine renders VF more susceptible to conversion by countershock.

Sodium bicarbonate. Respiratory acidosis is corrected by establishing effective ventilation. By inducing hyperventilation (and thereby reducing the $PaCO_2$), respiratory alkalosis results and compensates for any metabolic acidosis that may be present because of poor oxygen delivery. The

*References 2, 4, 9, 15, 16, 23, 25, 30.

Table A-7 Drugs Used in Pediatric Advanced Life Support

Drug	Dose	Comments
Adenosine	0.1-0.2 mg/kg (max: 12 mg in a single dose)	Rapid IV bolus
Atropine sulfate	0.02 mg/kg/dose Minimum dose: 0.1 mg Maximum single dose: *Child:* 0.5 mg *Adolescent:* 1 mg	
Bretylium	5 mg/kg; may be increased to 10 mg/kg	Rapid IV bolus
Calcium chloride 10% (100 mg/ml)	20 mg/kg/dose	Administer slowly Not for cardiac arrest Use for hypocalcemia, hypermagnesemia, and channel blocker overdose
Dobutamine HCl	2-20 μg/kg/min	Titrate to desired effect
Dopamine HCl	2-20 μg/kg/min	Titrate to desired effect
Epinephrine		
For bradycardia	*IV/IO:* 0.01 mg/kg (0.1 ml/kg) 1:10,000 *ET:* 0.1 mg/kg (0.1 ml/kg) 1:1000	Be aware of preservative administered when large doses are used
For asystole or pulseless arrest	**First dose:** *IV/IO:* 0.01 mg/kg 1:10,000 *ET:* 0.1 mg/kg 1:1000 Doses as high as 0.2 mg/kg may be effective **Subsequent doses:** *IV/IO/ET:* 0.1 mg/kg 1:1000 Doses as high as 0.2 mg/kg may be effective	Be aware of preservative administered when large doses are used
Epinephrine infusion	*Initial:* 0.1 μg/kg/min Use higher infusion dose with asystole: 20 μg/kg/min	Titrate to desired effect 0.1-1 μg/kg/min Lower dose with effective pulses
Lidocaine	1 mg/kg/dose	
Lidocaine infusion	20-50 μg/kg/min	
Sodium bicarbonate	1 mEq/kg/dose or 0.3 × kg × base deficit Subsequent doses are based on blood gas analysis every 10 min of arrest	Infuse slowly and only if ventilation is adequate Not for cardiac arrest Use for metabolic acidosis

Modified from Chameides L, Hazinski FN, editors: *Pediatric advanced life support,* The American Academy of Pediatrics and the American Heart Association, Dallas, 1997, The Association.
ET, Endotracheal; *IO,* intraosseous; *IV,* intravenous.

Table A-8 Normal Values for Arterial Blood (pH, Gases, Oxygen Saturation, Bicarbonate)

		Infants and Children			
Parameter	Unit	Mixed Venous	Capillary	Arterial	Newborn
pH	units	7.31-7.41	7.35-7.40	7.40-7.45	7.11-7.30
Pco_2	torr	35-40	40-45	35-40	27-40
Po_2	torr	41-51	45-50	80-100	33-75
Sao_2	%	60-80	>70	>90	40-90
HCO_3^-	mEq/L	22-25	22-26	22-26	14-22

Modified from Gordon IB: Reference ranges for laboratory tests. In Behrman RE, Vaughan VC, editors: *Nelson's textbook of pediatrics,* ed 12, Philadelphia, 1983, WB Saunders.
HCO_3^-, Bicarbonate; *Pco_2,* carbon dioxide pressure; *Po_2,* oxygen pressure; *Sao_2,* oxygen saturation.

resultant pH is less acidotic. If acidemia persists despite respiratory compensation and the pH is persistently below 7.20 to 7.25, sodium bicarbonate should be administered to correct the residual metabolic acidosis. Bicarbonate should not be used with inadequate ventilation. The interpretation of blood pH, gases, oxygen saturation, and bicarbonate determinations is complex and can be simplified in terms of determining the acid-base balance and its origins by applying the following "golden rules"[2]:

Rule 1: An acute change in $PaCO_2$ of a 10 torr increase or decrease is associated with an increase or decrease of 0.08 units in the pH.

To assess the respiratory component of acidosis, determine the amount of the measured partial pressure of carbon dioxide in arterial blood ($PaCO_2$) that falls below or above 40 torr. Calculate the pH using rule 1. Compare the measured pH with the calculated pH; if they are reasonably close, all acidotic changes are respiratory in origin.

Rule 2: A pH change of 0.15 units is equivalent to (or the result of) a change in bicarbonate (HCO_3^-) of 10 mEq/L from its 20-mEq/L baseline.

To assess the metabolic component, determine the calculated pH using rule 1 and compare with the measured pH value. If they are not reasonably close, determine the following:

1. If the measured pH is less than the calculated pH (a negative number), the acidosis is metabolic in origin; subtract the measured pH from the calculated pH to determine the base deficit or fixed acid.
2. If the measured pH is greater than calculated (a positive number), metabolic alkalosis is present; subtract the calculated pH from the measured pH to determine the base excess (or negative base excess).

Rule 3: The dose of bicarbonate (mEq) required to correct the metabolic acidosis fully is the base deficit (mEq/L × patient's weight [kg] × 0.3). Usually only half this amount is administered and then the acid-base status is reassessed, which ordinarily indicates that 1 mEq/kg sodium bicarbonate is needed.

If the arrest is observed and brief, bicarbonate usually is unnecessary and, in children, may worsen existing respiratory acidosis. Bicarbonate may be required in prolonged arrest (longer than 10 minutes) after initial ventilation and perfusion are established and when the arterial pH remains below 7.2.

Excessive administration of bicarbonate can have adverse effects because it (1) shifts the oxygen dissociation curve to the left and reduces the delivery of oxygen to the tissues, (2) shifts the potassium intracellularly, lowering the serum potassium level, (3) reduces plasma-ionized calcium, (4) lowers the fibrillation threshold, (5) increases the risk of hypernatremia and water overload, (6) increases the risk of hyperosmolality, and (7) may produce paradoxical cerebrospinal fluid and intracellular acidosis.[17]

Atropine. Atropine is a parasympatholytic drug by virtue of its competitive antagonism of acetylcholine. It accelerates sinus and atrial pacemaker discharge and AV conduction. In low doses (less than 0.1 mg) a paradoxical CNS vagal nuclei stimulation may produce AV node slowing. Higher doses are used in asystole to shorten the response time.

Atropine is indicated to treat hemodynamically unstable bradycardia accompanied by poor perfusion or hypotension and asystole. Bradycardia most often results from hypoxia, and initial treatment should be directed at improving ventilation, oxygenation, and perfusion.

The vagolytic dose is 0.02 mg/kg with a minimum dose of 0.1 mg. The duration of action is 2 to 4 hours; the pupils remain dilated for 6 hours or longer after injection and thus cannot provide a basis for neurological evaluation of the patient. Repeat doses during asystole can be given every 15 minutes up to a total dose of 1 mg in a child and 2 mg in an adolescent.

Calcium chloride. Calcium has a positive inotropic effect on the heart, but calcium entry into cell cytoplasm is the final common pathway in cell death. Its use is no longer recommended in cardiac arrest protocols. The indications for calcium are documented hypocalcemia (total serum calcium below 8.1 mg/dl or ionized calcium below 2.4 mg/dl), hyperkalemia, hypermagnesemia, and calcium channel blocker overdose. Calcium chloride is used in emergency hypocalcemia because it delivers the ionized calcium directly. Calcium always should be injected slowly, concurrently with ECG and blood pressure monitoring. The injection should be discontinued if bradycardia or hypotension occurs.

Lidocaine. Lidocaine in usual doses has no effect on myocardial contractility, blood pressure, or cardiac conduction. Its action suppresses ectopic foci, reduces automaticity, raises the fibrillation threshold, and inhibits the formation of reentry circuits that lead to ventricular tachycardia (VT) and VF. VF occurs in fewer than 10% of pediatric patients in cardiac arrest. If VF is present, a metabolic cause (abnormalities of calcium, potassium, and glucose), hypothermia, and drug intoxication (especially tricyclic antidepressants) should be considered.

The indications for lidocaine administration are (1) VT, (2) VF, and (3) frequent (more than six per minute) or potentially serious premature ventricular contractions (couplets, multifocal), particularly if associated with hemodynamic instability. Lidocaine infusion is recommended after successful conversion of VT or VF.

To ensure adequate plasma concentrations, a bolus of 1 mg/kg should be given when the IV infusion is placed. If the patient is in shock or has liver disease, beginning doses of 1 ml/kg/hr (20 µg/kg/min) should be used to prevent toxicity from impaired lidocaine clearance. The dose for an adolescent is a 50- to 100-mg bolus followed by infusion of 1 to 4 mg/min. The antiarrhythmic effect occurs at a serum concentration of 1 to 5 µg/ml. Concentrations above 6 µg/ml may cause seizures, and those above 10 µg/ml may cause myocardial depression. The practitioner should be prepared to treat bradycardia and hypotension. Lidocaine is contraindicated in severe heart block. Widening of the QRS complex by more than 0.02 seconds or significant ventricular slowing suggests cardiac toxicity. It is important to monitor ECG activity and plasma lidocaine concentrations because of the erratic pharmacokinetics of lidocaine in patients who have CPA.

Bretylium. Bretylium is a quaternary ammonium compound with postganglionic adrenergic properties and antiarrhythmic activity. It has a biphasic effect. Initially, through

Table A-9 Effects of the Infusion Rate of Dopamine on the Cardiovascular System

Infusion Rate	Cardiac Output	Inotropic Effect	Vascular Resistance	Renal Blood Flow
2-5 μg/kg/min	0	0	0	+
6-20 μg/kg/min	+	+	+/–	+
>20 μg/kg/min	+	+	+	0

Table A-10 Effects of the Rate of Epinephrine Infusion on the Cardiovascular System

Dose (μg/kg/min)	Chronotropic (Heart Rate) Effect	Inotropic (Cardiac Contractibility) Effect	Vasodilation	Vasoconstriction
0.05-0.3	+	+	+	0
0.3-1.5	+	+	0	+

norepinephrine release, it increases the blood pressure and heart rate; this is followed by adrenergic blockade of norepinephrine and epinephrine, but cardiac output remains unchanged. Bretylium may raise the fibrillation threshold and prevent reentry. It is a second-line drug after lidocaine and is indicated in refractory VT or VF. Bretylium improves the susceptibility of a refractory heart to defibrillation, cardioversion, and lidocaine in adults. It is important to continue CPR for 2 minutes after administering bretylium to allow for its circulation before attempting defibrillation. The drug's adverse effects are nausea, vomiting, hypotension, and transient hypertension; it may worsen arrhythmias in digitalized patients.

Postresuscitative medications.* Postresuscitative medications should be administered if the blood pressure or peripheral perfusion remains unstable.

The current teaching is that the following drugs are important in a post-CPA patient:

With hypotension: epinephrine and norepinephrine
With normotension but poor cardiac output: dobutamine and epinephrine
With septic shock accompanied by hypotension: epinephrine and norepinephrine
With septic shock accompanied by normotension and poor cardiac output: dopamine and dobutamine

Dopamine. Dopamine is an endogenous catecholamine that is an immediate precursor of norepinephrine. At low doses (2 to 5 μg/kg/min) it binds to dopamine receptors in splanchnic, coronary, and renal vascular beds, causing vasodilation and increased contractility without affecting the heart rate and blood pressure. At higher doses (6 to 20 μg/kg/min) beta-1 adrenergic effects (inotropic and chronotropic) and alpha-adrenergic effects (vasoconstriction) predominate, causing blood pressure to rise as a result of general vasoconstriction and increased cardiac output. At doses above 20 μg/kg/min, dopamine produces predominantly vasoconstrictive effects. The indications for its use are hypotension or poor peripheral perfusion in the presence of a stable rhythm and with adequate vascular volume.

A reasonable starting dose of dopamine for a patient in shock is 5 to 10 μg/kg/min. It is not recommended that infusion rates rise above 20 μg/kg/min; if a further inotropic effect is needed, epinephrine and dobutamine should be used. Dopamine may cause tachycardia (which increases myocardial oxygen demands), hypertension, arrhythmias, and extremity ischemia. It should be given in a central vein, if possible. ECG activity should be monitored and the skin observed for ischemia; the blood pressure and urinary output also should be monitored closely. Extravasation of dopamine causes tissue necrosis. Table A-9 summarizes the effects of dopamine infusions at various rates.

Dobutamine. Dobutamine is a synthetic catecholamine prepared by manipulation of isoproterenol. It is a direct-acting catecholamine with selective beta-1 adrenergic action and a mild peripheral beta-2 effect (vasodilation), resulting in increased cardiac contractility and heart rate and decreased afterload (systemic resistance); all of this increases the cardiac output. It is less effective in septic shock and in infants younger than 12 months of age. Its major indication is the treatment of cardiogenic shock. It may cause tachyrhythmias, nausea, vomiting, hypotension, and hypertension.[20]

Epinephrine infusion. Epinephrine is indicated in the treatment of shock with diminished systemic perfusion from any cause. An epinephrine infusion is the treatment of choice and is preferable to dopamine in patients with marked circulatory instability. The initial dose is 0.1 μg/kg/min; it can be increased up to 1 μg/kg/min, with the dose titrated to reach the desired effect. Higher infusion rates may be used in asystole. It should be administered through a well-secured peripheral line or, preferably, a central line. The adverse effects of epinephrine infusion are arrhythmias and, at doses exceeding 0.5 μg/kg/min, profound vasoconstriction that compromises skin and extremity blood flow (Table A-10). Epinephrine vasoconstriction reduces renal blood flow but improves renal function through increased cardiac output and tissue perfusion. Extravasation causes tissue necrosis.[33]

EMERGENCY PEDIATRIC CARDIAC RHYTHM DISTURBANCES[4]

Emergency pediatric cardiac rhythm disturbances usually result from hypoxemia and acidosis and rarely cause cardiac arrest thus ventilation and oxygenation are important in their management. The principle of therapy is to initiate treatment only if the rhythm disturbance compromises the cardiac output or can potentially deteriorate into a lethal

*References 2, 7, 10, 17, 20, 25, 27, 33.

Table A-11 Normal Ranges of ECG Parameters

Age (yr)	Heart Rate (beats/min)	PR Interval (sec)	QRS Complex (sec)
<1	90-180	0.07-0.16	0.03-0.08
1-3	70-140	0.08-0.16	0.04-0.08
4-10	60-120	0.09-0.17	0.04-0.07
>10	55-110	0.09-0.20	0.04-0.08

Modified from Garson A: *Electrocardiogram in infants and children: a systematic approach,* Philadelphia, 1983, Lea & Febiger.

rhythm. Electrical therapy includes (1) defibrillation, an untimed depolarization of the myocardium to allow for a spontaneous organized beat, and (2) cardioversion, a timed polarization designed to avoid the vulnerable period in the cardiac cycle.

Table A-11 shows the normal ranges for heart rates, PR intervals, and QRS complexes at various ages; these values are important in interpreting ECGs as part of the assessment and management of cardiac rhythm disturbances.

In children younger than age 10, a PR interval longer than 0.18 second and a QRS complex longer than 0.10 second are abnormal. The P wave almost always is upright in lead II; if it is not, or if it is absent, a normal sinus rhythm is not present. An inverted P wave in lead II most commonly is a result of incorrect placement of one of the ECG leads. A wide QRS complex may be ventricular in origin or a result of an aberrantly conducted supraventricular beat. However, a wide QRS complex should always be considered as VT because of its serious implications and the relative rarity of aberrant SVT in children.[2,19]

A useful clinical classification of emergency arrhythmias in pediatrics would be (1) rhythms that are too fast (tachyrhythmias) or too slow (bradyrhythmias) associated with hemodynamic instability and reduced cardiac output, (2) rhythms that are disorganized (VF), or (3) rhythms that are absent altogether (asystole). Other arrhythmias may need evaluation and treatment but usually do not constitute an emergency.[2]

Tachyrhythmias

In infants, supraventricular tachycardia (SVT) usually is associated with a heart rate above 230 beats/min; P waves are difficult to find, and the QRS complex is narrow in 98% of cases. If the patient is hemodynamically stable, vagal maneuvers can be tried (e.g., inverting the infant quickly or applying an ice bag to the face). Adenosine, administered intravenously, is the drug of choice for converting the rhythm to normal. Adenosine is an endogenous nucleoside that causes a temporary block through the AV node; it is very effective, and side effects are minimal because its half-life is only 10 seconds. Adenosine is given by rapid IV bolus (see Table A-7). If hemodynamic instability and reduced cardiac output are present, synchronized cardioversion (0.5 J/kg) should be attempted immediately if no IV access is available. If SVT persists, the cardioversion dose should be increased to 2 J/kg. If it still persists, the diagnosis may be incorrect. Verapamil should not be used to treat SVT in infants or children because cardiovascular collapse has been reported following its use.[2,7,8,22]

VT usually has wide QRS complexes, absent P waves, and T waves that are the opposite in polarity to the QRS complex. VT may degenerate into VF.

If the patient is hemodynamically unstable and cardiac output is reduced, synchronized cardioversion (0.5 to 1 J/kg) should be attempted immediately. If a lidocaine bolus can be given without delaying cardioversion, the success of conversion will be greater. If VT recurs, an infusion of lidocaine given after cardioversion will help maintain the converted rhythm. If this is unsuccessful, cardioversion at a higher voltage (2 J/kg) should be used. If success still is not achieved, bretylium should be given initially instead of lidocaine, but there are no published data on its usefulness; this is a class IIb recommendation.[7]

Bradycardia

Bradycardia (a heart rate below 80 beats/min) requires resuscitation if accompanied by poor perfusion, even if the blood pressure is normal. Epinephrine is the drug of choice. The neonatal dose remains the same (0.01 to 0.03 mg/kg given IV or by ET tube).[7] Atropine is now a class IIb drug if epinephrine is ineffective or bradycardia is caused by AV block. Atropine is administered in doses of 0.02 mg/kg, or paradoxical bradycardia may result. Because bradycardia may be caused by hypoxia, atropine should be administered only after adequate oxygenation and ventilation have been established. Isoproterenol is no longer recommended to treat bradycardia (Fig. A-1).

Absent or Disorganized Rhythms

Asystole and pulseless cardiac arrest. In making the diagnosis of asystole it is important to be sure that the clinical picture (no pulse and absent spontaneous respirations) correlates with the ECG activity that has been monitored. Ventilation, oxygenation, and volume repletion are the standards of treatment. Ventricular arrhythmias rarely occur in children who do not have congenital heart disease; however, the new guidelines endorse prompt defibrillation of pulseless VT. If an initial dose of 2 J/kg fails, the dose is doubled and administered twice. If this fails, epinephrine is given followed by lidocaine and then a rapid infusion of bretylium (5 mg/kg given as the first dose, followed by 10 mg/kg as the second dose). The treatment for asystole and electromechanical dissociation (EMD) is epinephrine. Atropine is no longer recommended (Fig. A-2).

VF is characterized by a disorganized series of depolarizations seen on the ECG with no detectable pulse and reduced cardiac output. The ECG pattern is classified as coarse or fine on the basis of the height of the electrical waves.

CPR measures should be continued until defibrillation can be applied, using an initial dose of 2 J/kg. If this is unsuccessful, the dose should be doubled and repeated twice. If this also is unsuccessful, ventilation and correction of any metabolic disturbance (hypoxia, hypoglycemia, and severe metabolic acidosis) should be accomplished followed by a bolus of epinephrine and another attempt at defibrillation. If this, too, fails, a bolus of lidocaine and further defibrillation should be attempted. Finally, if that fails, bretylium should be given initially at a dose of 5 mg/kg and subsequently at doses

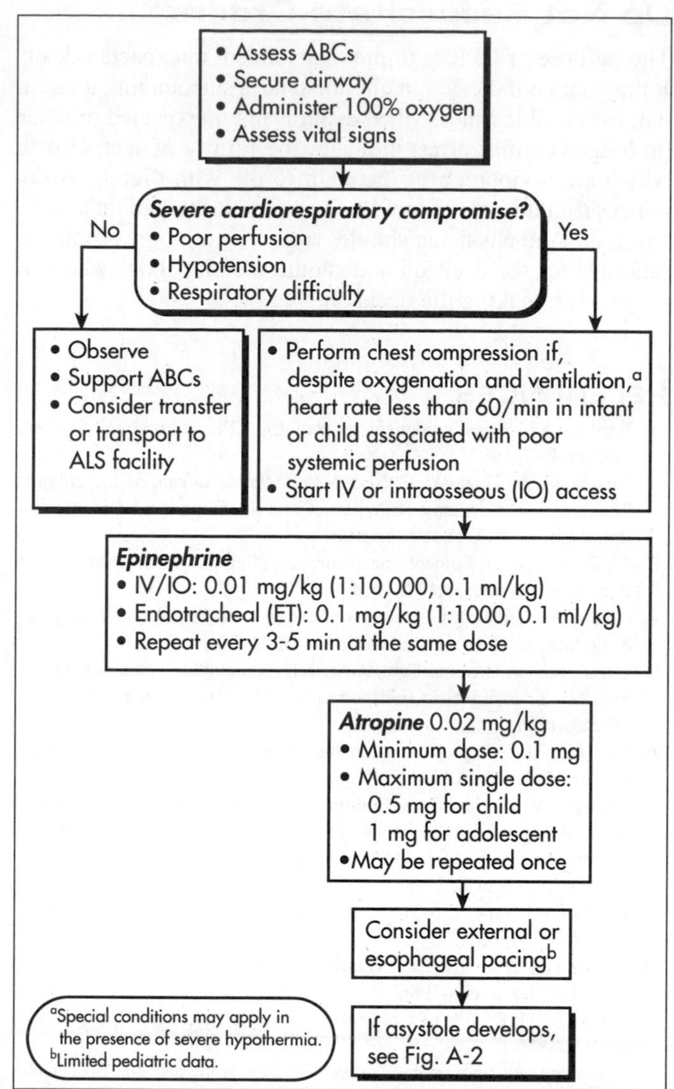

Fig. A-1 Bradycardia algorithm. *ABC,* Airway, breathing, and circulation; *ALS,* advanced life support; *IO,* intraosseous; *IV,* intravenous.

From Chameides L, Hazinski FN, editors: *Pediatric advanced life support,* The American Academy of Pediatrics and the American Heart Association, Dallas, 1997, The Association.

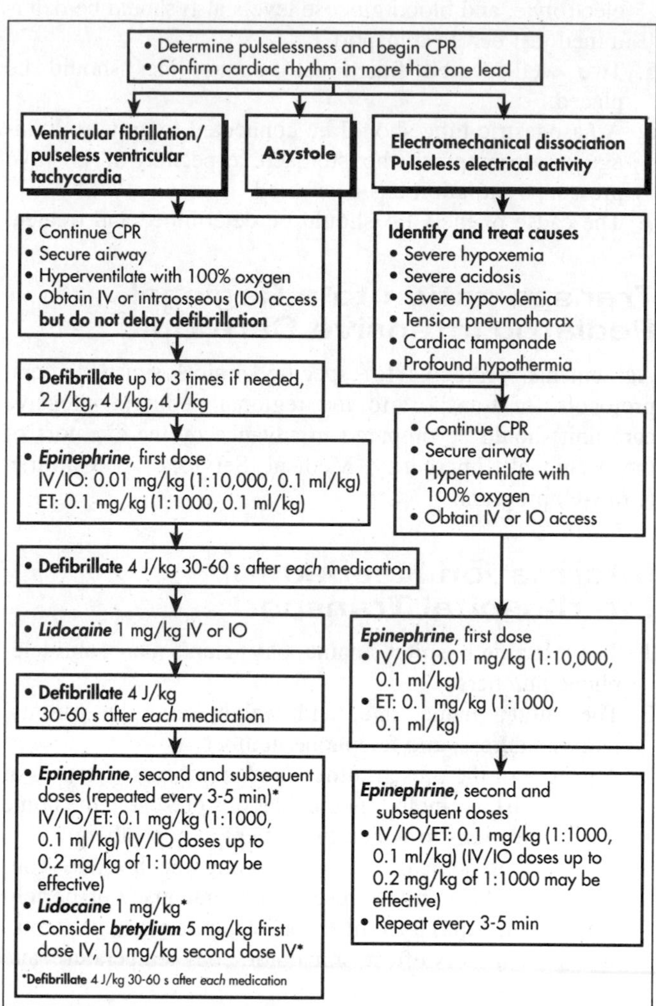

Fig. A-2 Algorithm for asystole and pulseless arrest. *CPR,* Cardiopulmonary resuscitation; *ET,* endotracheal; *IO,* intraosseous; *IV,* intravenous.

From Chameides L, Hazinski FN, editors: *Pediatric advanced life support,* The American Academy of Pediatrics and the American Heart Association, Dallas, 1997, The Association.

of 10 mg/kg in place of lidocaine before defibrillation is attempted. Some have recommended lidocaine infusion after cardioversion (see Fig. A-2).

EMD is characterized by the presence of organized electrical activity with ineffective myocardial contractions, as evidenced by the absence of a pulse. Causes include hypoxia, acidosis, volume depletion, tension pneumothorax, and cardiac tamponade. Treatment consists of ventilation, oxygenation, volume repletion, administration of an epinephrine bolus (see Fig. A-2), and relief of pneumothorax and pericardial effusion.

POSTRESUSCITATIVE CARE OF INFANTS AND CHILDREN[2]

Postresuscitative care involves stabilization, frequent assessment, and care during transport to a tertiary care facility, as well as the care rendered in that facility's intensive care unit. Any infant or child who has suffered respiratory or cardiac arrest should be admitted to a pediatric intensive care unit.

Elements of Postresuscitative Care

1. Cardiovascular function should be assessed by determining tissue perfusion clinically and by monitoring urinary output, blood pressure, and continuous ECG recordings.
2. Ventilation should be evaluated clinically and by interpretation of ABG levels and pulse oximeter or transcutaneous PO_2 readings.
3. Serial neurological examinations should be performed, with attention given to the level of consciousness and evidence of increased intracranial pressure and seizures.
4. Humidified, warm oxygen at the highest attainable concentration should be administered until ABG levels are available. These levels should be measured after a venti-

lation system has been in use for at least 15 minutes and before the patient is transported. The hematocrit, serum electrolyte, and blood glucose levels also should be determined just before transport.
5. Two well-secured functional venous lines should be placed.
6. A nasogastric tube should be connected to gravity drainage to decompress the stomach, especially if positive pressure ventilation has been used.
7. The cause of the CPA should be determined and treated.

Transportation to a Regional Pediatric Intensive Care Unit[5]

Agreements, protocols for specific clinical situations, and protocols for transport to the regional pediatric intensive care unit should be prepared in advance by the directors of the Regional Emergency Medical Services for Children (EMS-C) program.

Information Needed for Interhospital Transport

1. The referring hospital's name, physician's name, and telephone numbers
2. The child's name, age, and weight, and the parents' names, address, and telephone number
3. A history of the present illness and significant elements of the past history, including medications present in the home and medications to which the patient may be allergic
4. The current clinical status, including the level of consciousness, heart rate, presence and adequacy of peripheral pulses, capillary refill time, respiratory rate, air entry status, respiratory effort, skin color, body temperature, and blood pressure
5. Laboratory test data, including all roentgenograms and ECG tracings
6. All medications administered, including dosages and times given
7. The number of IV lines and fluids administered, including their infusion rates
8. The ventilator settings if the patient is receiving assisted ventilation
9. The availability of parents or their designates for providing consent for treatment

Brain Death[13]

Brain death, the ultimate criterion for removing life support mechanisms, is defined as (1) irreversible cessation of circulation and respiratory function or (2) irreversible cessation of all brain functions, including those of the brainstem. Caution should be used in reaching the determination of brain death if the patient (1) is younger than age 5, (2) has hypothermia, (3) nearly drowned, and (4) ingested neuromuscular blocking agents or barbiturates because early in these circumstances electroencephalographic recordings may be unreliable.*

*The determination of brain death is very difficult and must be done precisely. Guidelines for the determination of brain death in children have been drawn up by the Task Force for the Determination of Brain Death in Children, *Arch Neurol* 44:587, 1987.

Do Not Resuscitate Orders[31]

The purpose of CPR is to prevent sudden, unexpected death. It may not be indicated in circumstances surrounding a terminal, irreversible illness when death is not unexpected or when prolonged cardiac arrest indicates the futility of such efforts, which are a violation of the right to die with dignity. A do-not-resuscitate order should be written on the patient's order sheet, and the physician should explain in a progress note the rationale for the decision and should identify those who participated in making the decision.

REFERENCES

1. Bardossi K: Newest guidelines on pediatric CPR and first aid, *Contemp Pediatr* 4:47, 1987.
2. Chameides L, Hazinski FN, editors: *Pediatric advanced life support*, The American Academy of Pediatrics and the American Heart Association, Dallas, 1997, The Association.
3. Chernow R, et al: Epinephrine absorption after endotracheal administration, *Anesth Analg* 63:629, 1984.
4. Committee on Drugs, American Academy of Pediatrics: Emergency drug doses in children, *Pediatrics* 81:462, 1988.
5. Committee on Hospital Care, American Academy of Pediatrics: Guidelines for air and ground transportation of pediatric patients, *Pediatrics* 78:943, 1986.
6. Day RL: Differing opinions on the emergency treatment of choking, *Pediatrics* 71:975, 1983.
7. Emergency Cardiac Care Committee and Subcommittees, American Heart Association: Guidelines for cardiopulmonary resuscitation and emergency cardiac care, *JAMA* 268:2171, 1992.
8. Epstein ML, Kiel EA, Victoria BE: Cardiac decompensation following verapamil therapy in infants with supraventricular tachycardia, *Pediatrics* 75:737, 1985.
9. Finholt DA, et al: The heart is under the lower third of the sternum, *Am J Dis Child* 646:649, 1986.
10. Gillis J, et al: Results of inpatient pediatric resuscitation, *Crit Care Med* 14:469, 1986.
11. Greenberg MI: Endotracheal drugs: the state of the art, *Ann Emerg Med* 13:789, 1984.
12. Greenberg MI, Roberts RJ: Drugs for the heart by way of the lungs, *Emerg Med* 12:209, 1980.
13. Guidelines for the determination of death: Medical Consultants on the Diagnosis of Death to the President's Commission for the Study of Ethical Problems in Medicine and Biomedical and Behavioral Research Report, *JAMA* 246:2184, 1981.
14. Johnston C: Endotracheal drug delivery, *Pediatr Emerg Care* 8:94, 1992.
15. Mace SE: Cricothyrotomy, *J Emerg Med* 6:309, 1988.
16. Mofenson HC, Caraccio TR: Guidelines for intraosseous infusion, *J Emerg Med* 6:143, 1988.
17. Nieman JT, Rosborough JP: Effects of acidemia and sodium bicarbonate therapy in advanced life support, *Ann Emerg Med* 13:781, 1984.
18. Orlowski J: Optimum position for external cardiac compression in infants and young children, *Ann Emerg Med* 15:667, 1986.
19. Park MK, Guntheroth WG: *How to read pediatric ECGs*, Chicago, 1982, Mosby.
20. Perkin RM, et al: Dobutamine: a hemodynamic evaluation in children in shock, *J Pediatr* 100:977, 1982.
21. Phillips GWL, Zideman DA: Relationship of infant heart to sternum: its significance in cardiopulmonary resuscitation, *Lancet* 1:1024, 1986.
22. Radford D: Side effects of verapamil in infants, *Arch Dis Child* 58:465, 1983.
23. Rose JS, Koenig KL: Code blue: what's new? *J Emerg Med* 12:187, 1994.
24. Rosetti VA, et al: Intraosseous infusion: an alternate route of pediatric intravascular access, *Ann Emerg Med* 14:885, 1985.
25. Schuman AJ: Pediatric advanced life support: an update and review, *Contemp Pediatr* 6:26, 1989.

26. Schuman AJ: The latest guidelines on pediatric life support, *Contemp Pediatr* 10:25, 1993.
27. Seidel JS, Burkett DL, editors: *Instructor's manual for pediatric advanced life support,* Dallas, 1988, American Heart Association.
28. Seigler RS, Tecklenburg FW, Shealy R: Prehospital intraosseous infusion by emergency medical services personnel: a prospective study, *Pediatrics* 84:173, 1989.
29. Spivey WH: Intraosseous infusions, *J Pediatr* 111:639, 1987.
30. Stewart RD, Lacovery DC: Administration of endotracheal medication, *Ann Emerg Med* 14:136, 1985.
31. Tomlinson T, Brody H: Ethics and communications in do-not-resuscitate orders, *N Engl J Med* 316:43, 1988.
32. Tsai A, Kallsen G: Epidemiology of pediatric prehospital care, *Ann Emerg Med* 16:284, 1987.
33. Zaritsky A, Chernow B: Use of catecholamines in pediatrics, *J Pediatr* 105:341, 1984.
34. Zaritsky A, et al: CPR in children, *Ann Emerg Med* 16:1107, 1987.

B Special Procedures

Joseph R. Custer

The information presented here details the methods by which samples of normal and abnormal body fluids are obtained to enhance diagnosis and treatment of pediatric patients, how therapeutic fluids are introduced parenterally, and how endotracheal intubation can be accomplished in children with respiratory difficulties.

PATIENT PREPARATION

General Approach

The first step in performing any pediatric procedure is to establish an understanding among physician, parents, and child of what is to be done. Failure to do this compromises the physician-patient-parent relationship. The physician who dismisses the parents' and patient's concerns or fears of an impending procedure loses their confidence. Procedures that the physician may consider routine and ordinary have great significance to parents and patients. They have a right to know what will be done and why it will be done.

The information to be gained from the simplest procedure must be explained. The parents and the patient should be informed about the indications for each test and procedure. Parents should be given a reason for their child's inconvenience and discomfort. Reassurance that the physician understands the child and the child's perceptions must be conveyed to the parents.[5]

The spectrum of ages and stages of development of pediatric patients dictates that an adaptive approach be taken by the practitioner. Appreciation of the child's fears and the parents' reservations requires a calm, empathic, reassuring posture. The newborn, toddler, and older child all present different problems. If one forgets the newborn's individuality in the frustration of repeated attempts at venipuncture, normal protective emotions in the parents may be aroused and the physician-parent relationship may suffer.

The toddler, just beginning to develop a new vocabulary and new emotions, may react to painful procedures submissively or obstinately. The toddler's fear of pain, of being handled by strangers, and of separation from the parents must be respected. A calm, authoritative approach conveys to the child that the adults present are in control.

In older children it is important to appreciate their perception of what will happen. Here the expression "blood test" may conjure up all sorts of mysterious images in the child's mind. A more explicit explanation of what is to be done helps to dispel those mysteries. The older child also responds to contracts of cooperation, such as, "You may cry, but hold your arm still, and we will finish the test quickly," or "You can help by holding very still." One must not violate this contract by denying the child's feelings of pain or discomfort. If the operator sees that the child is terribly upset by a procedure, a few minutes given to reassurance will not be wasted.

Before any procedure is done, a decision as to whether the parents should be in attendance during the procedure should be considered. This depends on the relative comfort of both the physician and the parents. If their presence causes anxiety for the physician, the success of the procedure may be hampered; on the other hand, children's cooperation may be enhanced by the reassuring presence of their parents. The presence of a parent will not totally allay all of a child's apprehension, and a sedative agent will still be needed.[16] The adolescent at times may feel the presence of parents to be embarrassing.[4] Although tradition has kept parents from the bedside and treatment rooms when procedures are performed on their child, this determination should be made on an individual basis.

An "open-door" policy that allows parents to be present when procedures are performed must never represent a demand for demonstration of parenting behavior. Therefore, the wishes of those parents who do not want to be present should be respected. Parents should never be involved in restraining their child or in assisting in the performance of a painful procedure.

Restraint and Immobilization

It may be necessary to immobilize infants and some children to complete quickly and safely most of the procedures described here. An assistant is required to help hold the child and to reassure and comfort the child. In general, parents should not be asked to serve in this role.

For infants and younger children, the "papoose" board can be used effectively for immobilization. Children up to about age 5 can be immobilized by wrapping, as demonstrated in Fig. B-1. The assistant stands at the side or foot of the wrapped child, leans lightly on the trunk, stabilizing the patient's thorax with the elbows, and with the hands fixes the patient's head or free arm for the procedure.

Monitoring During a Procedure

Children are particularly susceptible to hypoxia and ischemia. Safe, efficient performance of a procedure requires se-

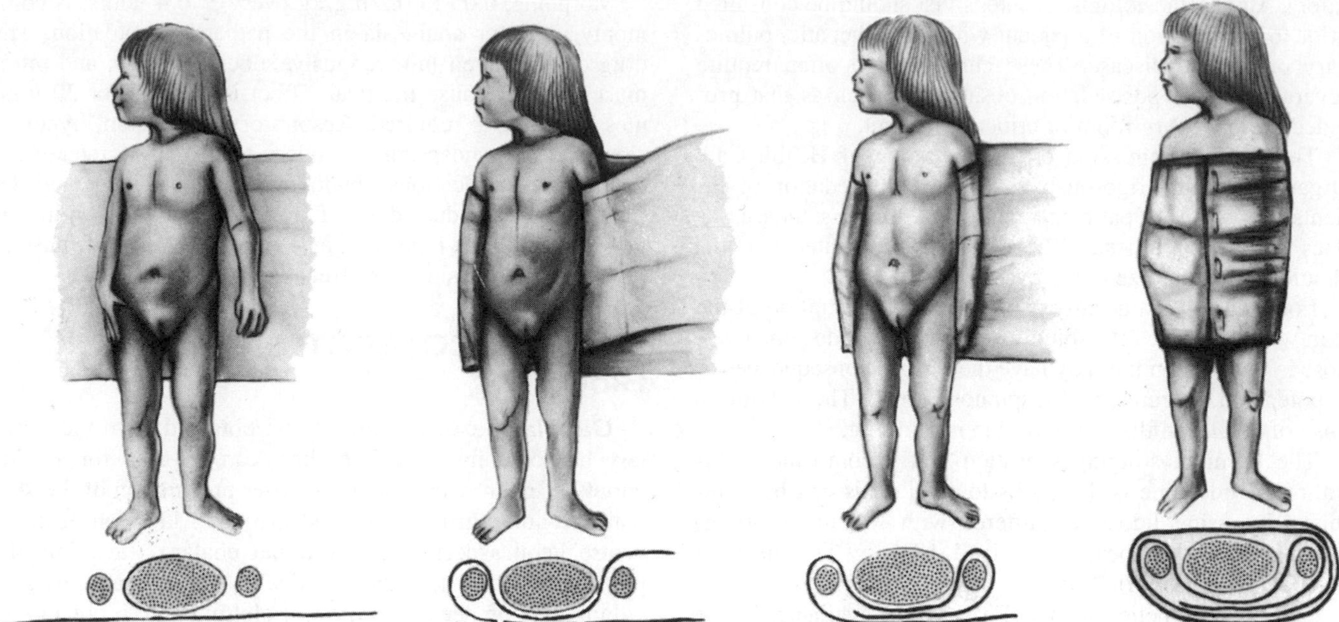

Fig. B-1 Method of mummy-wrapping an infant or child to restrain the upper extremities. The four steps are illustrated with frontal and cross-sectional views. A wider sheet or blanket may be used to restrain the lower extremities.

dation. Monitoring of oxygenation, heart rate, and respiratory rate is mandatory. Patients who receive systemic sedatives and analgesics should be treated as if they were undergoing general anesthesia.

The child's recovery from the procedure also should be supervised. Sedation has inherent risks that can be anticipated. The Academy of Pediatrics has developed clearly stated standards of care for the monitoring and management of patients before, during, and after procedures.[1]

The patient's record must show documentation of assessment of risk, doses and timing of drugs administered, vital signs, the intravenous (IV) fluids administered, and the child's recovery from the procedure.

Assessment of Risk

If systemic analgesia or sedation is required, the risks of hypoxemia, hypotension, and hypoventilation must be assessed.

The patient's medical history should be reviewed for allergies. The major complication of sedation is loss of respiratory drive and the ability to protect the airway. The patient may require intubation or bag mask ventilation. The adequacy of a patient's airway can be estimated.[2,22] An anesthesiologist or intensivist should be consulted if the patient has a potential risk for a difficult airway. The possibility of renal or hepatic disease, which will alter drug pharmacology, should be considered. Pulmonary disease that requires chronic oxygen use places a patient at higher risk for hypoxemia. Patients with cardiac disease require careful monitoring, reduced drug doses, and in some circumstances precautions against bacterial endocarditis. Anemia increases the risk of dysoxia (adequate oxygen saturation but diminished tissue delivery) or the attainment of analgesia when given conventional drug doses. The stomach should be empty.

Monitoring devices and equipment for highly invasive procedures should include the following:

Pulse oximeter
Blood pressure cuff
Cardiotachometer
Respiratory rate monitor
Resuscitation equipment
Intubation equipment
Airway suction equipment
Flowsheet
Oxygen delivery equipment
Antidotes (Flumazenil, Narcan)
IV access and fluid

The ability to monitor the child's respiratory rate and effort and airway patency continuously is paramount. A common error is to cover the patient's chest and airway with sterile drapes and towels; this deprives the clinician of the most reliable monitor—direct observation. An assistant who is free to circulate during the procedure is invaluable for documenting vital signs, helping to ensure sterility, observing the patient's chest excursion, and monitoring the patency of the airway.

Anesthesia

In general, if the procedure involves only a needle puncture, local anesthesia may be dispensed with, inasmuch as it itself necessitates a needle puncture.[15]

Sedation and Analgesia

The primary care clinician can safely administer and monitor sedation in most pediatric patients. Patients who have a chronic disease, especially those who have neuromuscular, pulmonary, cardiac, or renal disease, are difficult to sedate safely. An anesthesiologist or intensivist should be consulted prior to the sedation of a patient with renal, hepatic, pulmonary or cardiac disease. These children also often require several hours of postsedation observation such as that provided in a recovery room or critical care unit.

The Joint Commission on Accreditation of Health Care Organizations has rigorously scrutinized the sedation of patients. Sedation of patients requires the same standards as does general anesthesia. The care for all sedated patients should be standardized wherever it occurs.[10]

Local anesthesia usually is produced by infiltration of the skin with lidocaine (1% solution, 10 mg/ml). Lidocaine overdose is uncommon but may have the serious consequences of hypotension, seizures, and respiratory arrest. The maximum dose of locally infiltrated lidocaine is 5 mg/kg.

The burning, stinging sensation that accompanies infiltration of lidocaine is due to its low pH. This can be minimized by using lidocaine buffered with sodium bicarbonate ($NaHCO_3$). Lidocaine is mixed 10:1 by volume with $NaHCO_3$ (1 mEq/ml).[34]

Topical anesthetic creams (EMLA) are available. These are applied to the venipuncture site and covered with a patch. However, 20 to 30 minutes of exposure is required. Cost and time should be considered when using these agents. In some extremely anxious children, this technique is helpful when repeated blood sampling is required.[14]

Deep sedation for invasive procedures may be required. The risks of sedation include respiratory and central nervous system (CNS) depression, hypotension, and emesis. Therefore, patients who are sedated require monitoring of their vital signs, as well as pulse oximetry. Judgment is required in the choice of sedative dose. The clinician should be familiar with the pharmacology of the agent used.[3] Patients who have cardiorespiratory embarrassment need a reduced dose. The best practice is to titrate the dose to the desired effect while carefully monitoring the patient.[21]

When one desires cooperation with relatively pain-free procedures, such as immobilization for an echocardiogram or a computed tomographic (CT) scan in infants and toddlers, chloral hydrate is the drug of choice.[23] This drug may be given orally or by rectum in doses of 25 to 75 mg/kg. Commonly perceived as harmless, the drug has its risks.[31] Side effects include movement disorders, respiratory depression, and vomiting. An alternative is oral fentanyl in a candy base, Fentanyl Oralet. The dose is 10 to 15 micrograms per kilogram. The time of onset is 20 minutes and the duration of sedation is several hours.[4]

Midazolam is a water-soluble imidazobenzodiazepine with a rapid onset of 1 to 5 minutes and short duration of action. The drug produces good anxiolytic effect and retrograde amnesia. The usual initial dose of 0.05 to 0.1 mg/kg is given by slow push IV, followed by 0.005 to 0.01 mg/kg every 2 minutes for 1 to 3 doses. Respiratory depression is the drug's most serious side effect.[3] Flumazenil partially reverses respiratory depression. The initial dose is 0.005 to 0.01 mg/kg IV. If no effect is observed in 60 seconds, an additional dose of 0.005 to 0.01 mg/kg/hour should be given by continuous infusion to a total cumulative dose of 1 mg. Flumazenil is contraindicated in children who have seizures treated with a benzodiazepine and in cases of tricyclic overdose.[4]

Morphine, 0.05 to 0.2 mg/kg every 3 to 4 hours, is commonly used for analgesia in the pediatric population. The drug can be given intravenously, subcutaneously, and intramuscularly. Because the peak effect is delayed for 30 minutes, patience is required. Respiratory depression, hypotension, and bronchospasm secondary to histamine release are common complications. Naloxone, 0.1 mg/kg given IV (maximum individual dose of 2 mg) every 3 to 5 minutes, will reverse the hypotension and apnea; however, it must be given repeatedly, since its effect is transient.

SAMPLE COLLECTION

Blood

Capillary puncture. Blood obtained from the capillary bed of a finger, toe, or heel can be used for a wide variety of microdeterminations. After preparation of the skin with alcohol, a firm stab wound is made with a lancet in the ventrolateral aspect of the terminal phalanx, (avoiding the pad and joint) or the posterior edge of the heel pad. Frequent wiping may be needed to prevent clotting and to obtain free flow without squeezing. Local pressure applied with a dry sponge will stop the bleeding after the sample has been obtained. The procedure is painful and osteomyelitis can result from deep penetration.

Venipuncture. Fig. B-2 illustrates the location of superficial veins commonly used to obtain blood samples. The largest superficial veins are those of the cervical and femoral areas, although these should be avoided for routine blood sampling.

For venipuncture of the arms, legs, hands, and feet, the child is immobilized and the skin is prepared with alcohol. A tourniquet is applied to the extremity above the point of planned venous puncture tightly enough to produce venous stasis and vein distention, yet loosely enough to allow arterial perfusion. This can be demonstrated, if there is capillary refilling after blanching created by direct pressure on the extremity distal to the tourniquet. A 20- or 22-gauge needle or "butterfly" infusion needle attached to a syringe may be used. The vein is stabilized by traction on the overlying skin along the longitudinal axis of the vein. The skin is pierced with the needle bevel up. The needle tip is then advanced subcutaneously, and the vein is entered with a short jab to prevent its rolling away. Negative pressure in the syringe is used to withdraw the amount of blood needed. After the blood is obtained, the tourniquet is released, the needle removed, a dry sponge applied with pressure to the site, and the extremity elevated for a minute or two to prevent bleeding at the puncture site.

For external jugular venipuncture, the child is positioned on a table with the head rotated to one side and extended over the edge of the table 45 degrees toward the floor. The assistant, leaning over the mummy-wrapped child, holds the head firmly in this position. After preparation of the skin with alcohol, a butterfly needle is attached to a syringe and used to penetrate the skin in a caudal direction where the vein crosses the sternocleidomastoid muscle. The vein is then entered with a separate thrust, and negative pressure is created within the syringe. If a hematoma appears, the procedure should be discontinued at that site. After the sample has been

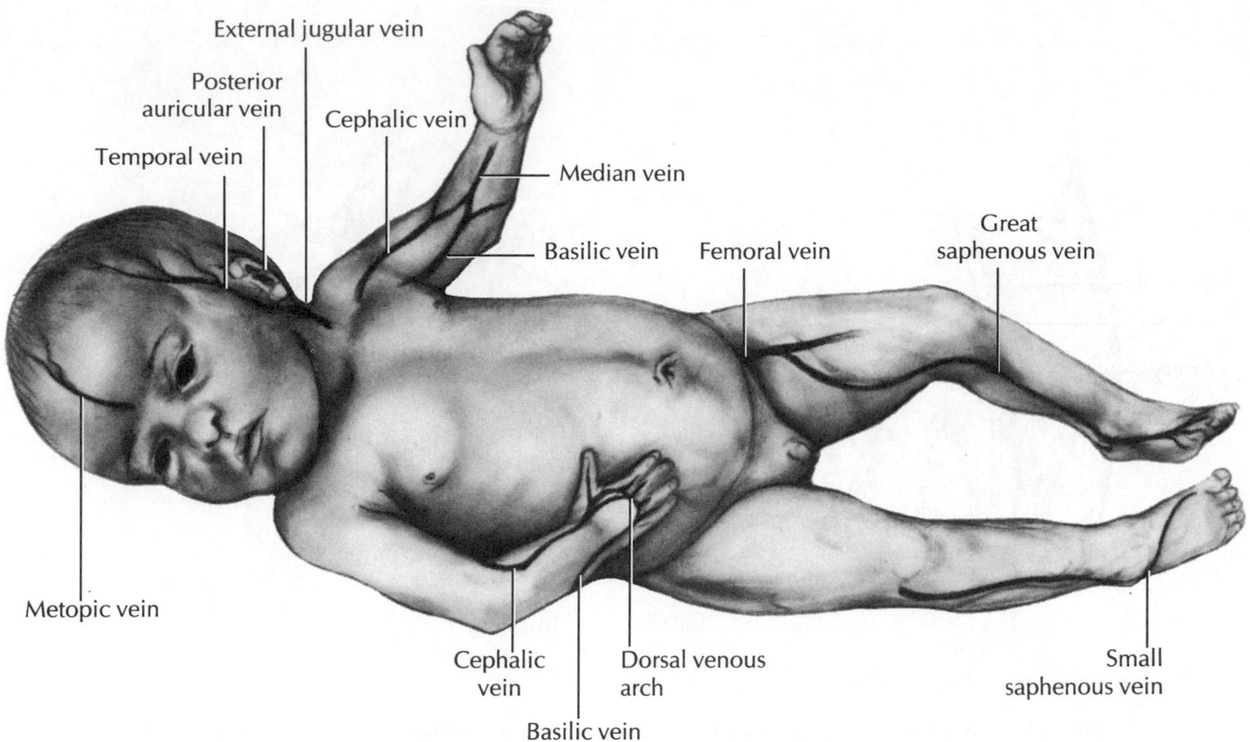

Fig. B-2 Accessible veins for blood sampling and administration of intravenous infusions.

obtained, firm pressure is applied over the venipuncture site for 3 to 5 minutes with the child sitting upright.

For puncture of the femoral vein, the child is placed in the supine position with the leg slightly flexed at the knee and externally rotated. The assistant holds this position while leaning over the child's trunk from one side. The femoral artery is identified by palpation just distal to the inguinal (Poupart) ligament and medial to the midpoint of the ligament. The femoral vein lies medial and parallel to the artery here (Fig. B-3). The skin is prepared with alcohol, and while the artery is being palpated, the skin is entered 1 to 2 cm distal to the flexion crease of the groin. The needle should be directed medial to the arterial pulsations and cephalad, at a 30-degree angle, while negative pressure is applied to the syringe during insertion and withdrawal. Blood will enter the syringe as soon as the vein is entered. Complications of the procedure, which are caused by faulty needle placement, include septic arthritis of the hip, osteomyelitis of the femur, and femoral arteriospasm.

Arterial puncture. Arterial puncture has become a necessary technical skill for physicians who care for critically ill children. Assessment of arterial blood gases is essential in monitoring and diagnosing a variety of cardiopulmonary diseases.

The right radial artery is the preferred site for arterial puncture. It is in a consistent anatomical position and is well fixed by surrounding connective tissue. In the newborn, the site has the added advantage of providing preductal arterial blood samples. Other available sites are the brachial and femoral arteries.

Arterial punctures may be hazardous because arterial laceration, spasm, or insufficiency secondary to hematoma may occur.[7] The adequacy of collateral circulation for the radial artery is good, but it may be less so for the femoral and brachial arteries. Septic arthritis of the hip is an infrequent complication of femoral artery puncture. The data from blood gases may be erroneous if venous blood is sampled, if the sample is exposed to air, if the equipment used for analysis is improperly standardized, or if the oxygen concentration to which the patient is exposed during the sampling is not considered or is reported inaccurately.

The wrist is supported in a position of supination and slight dorsiflexion. The artery may be located at the wrist by feeling for the point of maximal pulsation. In newborns it usually is found along the first flexor crease one sixth of the width of the wrist measured from its radial edge (Fig. B-4).

Specially designed blood gas syringes containing dry or liquid lithium heparin are preferred. The type of syringe will influence laboratory results.[19] If liquid heparin is used the syringe needs only to be rinsed with heparin; then all the heparin is ejected. The trace amount of heparin remaining coating the walls is adequate for anticoagulation. If heparin solution is left in the syringe, a dilutional artifact will result.

The size of the needle used varies with the patient's age (25 gauge for newborns and infants to 22 gauge for older children and adolescents). Care must be taken to avoid compressing the artery during restraint. The syringe is held as one would hold a pencil or a dart, and the needle is introduced into the artery at approximately a 45-degree angle. A "flash" of blood spurting into the syringe indicates a successful puncture. Gentle aspiration is required when plastic, dispos-

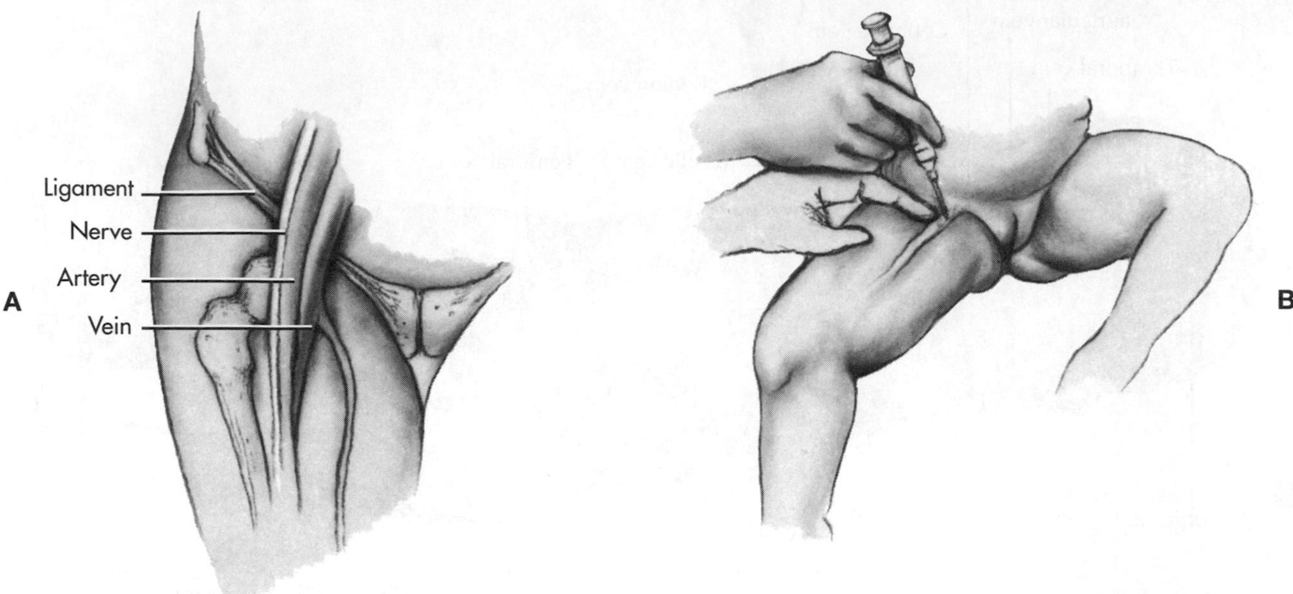

Fig. B-3 Femoral vein or artery puncture. **A,** Anatomical structures. **B,** Position of the patient, with needle poised for piercing the skin, subcutaneous tissue, and femoral vein. The procedure for femoral artery puncture is identical except that the needle is aimed more laterally, directly into the pulsating femoral artery.

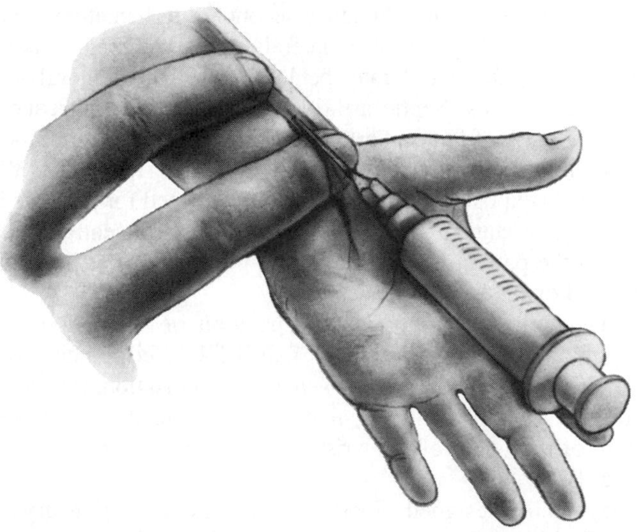

Fig. B-4 Radial artery puncture. The position of the radial artery is determined by palpation; it is fixed with the index and middle fingers while the needle is inserted at a 45-degree angle.

able syringes are used. A butterfly needle may also be used. The butterfly needle, without the syringe attached, is introduced into the artery as described above. A pulsatile flow of blood into the tubing ensures that arterial puncture has been accomplished. The syringe then is connected to the butterfly tubing, and the sample is collected. The sample should be sealed, placed in ice, and sent to the laboratory for analysis. Direct pressure on the puncture site for a minimum of 5 minutes prevents bleeding and hematoma formation.

The brachial artery in the antecubital fossa is a less desirable choice for sampling because collateral circulation is not always adequate and because a vein may be sampled mistakenly. The artery is located by palpation. Either a 22- or 25-gauge needle and syringe or, for infants, a 23- or 25-gauge butterfly needle may be used. The needle should be held at a 45-degree angle and the skin punctured at the point of maximal pulsation. Pressure must be applied to the site of puncture for 5 to 10 minutes after the needle is withdrawn.

The femoral artery is the least desirable choice for sampling because the hip joint can be inadvertently entered and contaminated. This area is more apt to be contaminated than are other arterial puncture sites; therefore extra attention to skin preparation is required. The puncture site may be found at the point of maximal pulsation, just inferior to the inguinal ligaments (see Fig. B-3). The femoral nerve is lateral, and the femoral vein medial, to the artery. The artery should be punctured at approximately a 60-degree angle. Gentle aspiration as the needle penetrates the soft tissue aids in detecting a successful puncture. Once the sample has been obtained, careful pressure on the puncture site is necessary for at least 10 minutes.

Cerebrospinal Fluid

The need to perform a lumbar puncture to rule out meningitis and other CNS infections must be weighed against the dangers inherent in performing a lumbar puncture in the presence of a supratentorial space-occupying lesion. Increased intracranial pressure is a contraindication to lumbar puncture. Its presence dictates immediate neurosurgical consultation if collection of cerebrospinal fluid (CSF) is judged clinically necessary. If meningitis is suspected, however, antibiotic therapy must not be delayed.

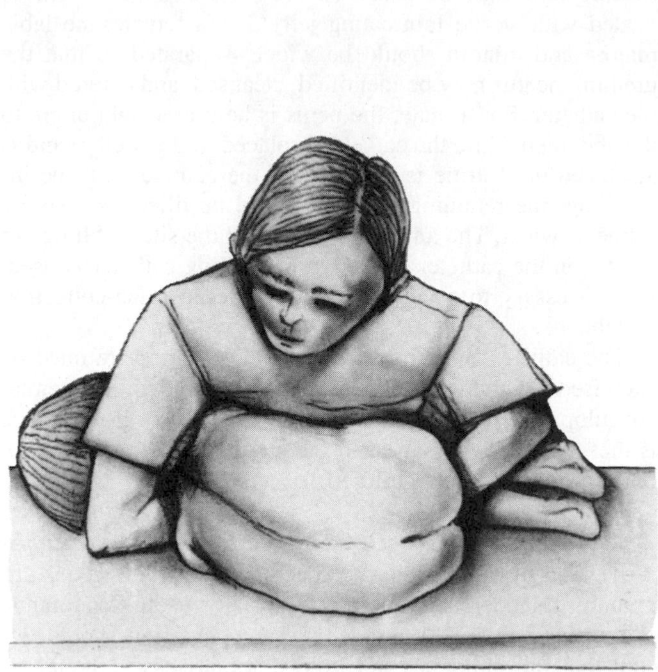

Fig. B-5 Restraining a child during lumbar puncture. The patient's nuchal and popliteal surfaces are in contact with the assistant's antecubital fossae.

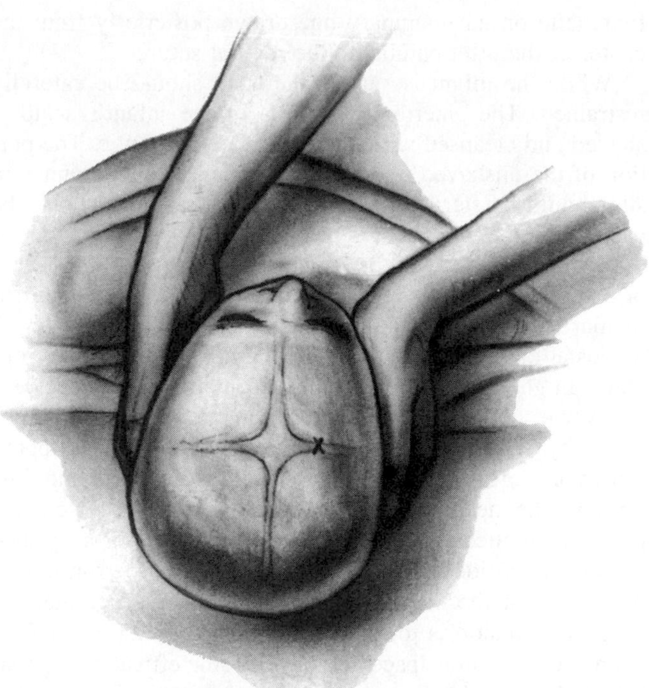

Fig. B-6 Subdural tap. Position of the child for a subdural tap. The subdural needle should be inserted into the coronal suture 1 to 2 cm lateral to the edge of the anterior fontanelle.

A relative contraindication to lumbar puncture is the presence of a coagulopathy or thrombocytopenia. Again, if bacterial meningitis is suspected, antimicrobial therapy must not be delayed.

The position of the patient during lumbar puncture should be dictated by the mutual comfort of the patient, the assistant, and the operator. Some prefer infants to be held upright; others prefer the lateral recumbent position (Fig. B-5). Use of a local anesthetic is not necessary for infants. Reassurance, an explanation of what is to occur, and a tranquil atmosphere may be as important as a local anesthetic for an older child (see Chapter 27, Self-Regulation Therapies: Hypnosis and Biofeedback).

The preferred site is the L3-L4 interspace. It is located by determining the site at which an imaginary line drawn between the superior edge of the right and left posterior iliac crests crosses the spine. The interspace above and below also may be used. The skin is prepared thoroughly with appropriate antiseptic, the site is draped, and sterile gloves are worn.

Care must be taken that the needle enters the intervertebral space in the sagittal plane. This requires several different perspectives of the proposed line of entry with the needle "aimed" toward the umbilicus.

Once the skin is penetrated, the needle is advanced slowly in the sagittal plane. Although a distinct "pop," or give, may be felt in the older patient when the dura is pierced, this is not the case in the infant. When the physician suspects that the spinal canal has been entered, the stylet is removed and the needle gently rotated to maximize the flow of cerebrospinal fluid through the needle. If no flow is obtained, the stylet is reinserted and the needle is advanced further or withdrawn and redirected. Care must be taken to avoid a "bloody tap," or traumatic tap, caused by pushing the needle into the venous plexus along the anterior wall of the spinal canal. A syringe should never be used to enhance the aspiration of cerebrospinal fluid, because this creates undue negative pressure and might produce herniation of the brainstem through the foramen magnum.

A stopcock and manometer are attached to the spinal needle to measure the opening and closing pressure of cerebrospinal fluid. These measures may be useless with the struggling child. One milliliter of fluid is collected in each of three sterile test tubes to be used for bacteriological, chemical, and cytological determinations. In the case of a traumatic tap, the red cells in both the first and the third tubes should be counted. A traumatic tap usually gives fewer red cells in the third tube than in the first. Blood from a central nervous system hemorrhage will have the same number of red cells in both samples. Once the fluid is removed, the stylet is replaced and the needle is withdrawn. Direct pressure is applied to the puncture site briefly. No dressing is required.

Subdural Fluid

The purpose of a subdural tap is to detect a posttraumatic subdural hematoma or postinfectious subdural effusion. With closed sutures and ossified fontanelles, neurosurgical assistance should be sought.

The incidence of postinfectious subdural effusions has declined markedly with the advent of vaccination against *Haemophilus influenzae*, type b. However, the clinician should remain vigilant for this complication. Persistent fever, an increasing head circumference, and transillumination provide clues to the diagnosis.

Fig. B-6 illustrates the preferred site of puncture. This is a point in the coronal suture 1 to 2 cm lateral to the anterior fontanelle on an imaginary line drawn posteriorly from the center of the orbit parallel to the sagittal suture.

While the infant is supine, the head should be carefully restrained. The anterior two thirds of the infant's scalp is shaved and cleansed with an appropriate antiseptic. The portion of the unshaved scalp posterior to the planned puncture site should be sterilely draped, and sterile gloves should be used while the procedure is performed.

A short, beveled 19- or 20-gauge lumbar puncture needle or a subdural tap needle is inserted through the skin perpendicular to the scalp and slowly is advanced 2.5 to 5 mm. A hemostat clamped to the shaft of the needle will aid the operator in gauging the depth of insertion and prevent accidental overpenetration. Perforation of the dura usually is recognized by a sudden decrease in resistance and a popping sensation. A few drops of fluid normally are present and flow through the needle when the stylet is removed. Negative pressure applied to the needle with the aid of a syringe should be avoided. The procedure usually is performed on both sides of the head. Current practice in the treatment of subdural effusion is to remove no more than 25 ml of fluid from each subdural space per day. Chronic effusions necessitate daily taps. After removal of the subdural specimen, the needle is withdrawn and a sterile cotton and collodion dressing is applied.

Urine

Urethral catheterization. To collect a sterile specimen of urine from a child who cannot produce a midstream, clean-catch, voided specimen, or to monitor the urine output continuously, a catheter is inserted into the bladder through the urethra. The child is placed in a supine frog-leg position and prepared with sterile technique, including drapes, gloves, and skin cleansing. A small (8 Fr) straight or indwelling catheter should be used for a child; for an infant, a No. 5 feeding tube may be used. The catheter or tube should be coated with sterile lubricating jelly. For a female, the labia majora and minora should be widely separated so that the urethral meatus may be identified, cleansed, and entered with the catheter. For a male, the penis is held at a right angle to the abdomen while the catheter is placed in the urethra and is advanced until urine is obtained. If the catheter is to be indwelling, the retaining balloon should be filled with sterile saline or water. The amount of fluid and the site of filling are shown on the catheter. When an indwelling catheter is used, it is necessary to establish a closed, sterile urine-collection system.

The catheter should not be forced. Extreme care must be exercised in children who have an acquired or congenital coagulopathy. It is possible to force the catheter if resistance is met during its passage and thereby damage the urethra in both male and female children.

Percutaneous suprapubic bladder aspiration. To obtain sterile urine specimens, a percutaneous suprapubic bladder aspiration is especially useful in infants. Before attempting this procedure, the physician should ensure that the child has not voided for at least 1 hour. An assistant should hold the child in the supine frog-leg position while the operator percusses the bladder above the symphysis pubis and prepares the skin with alcohol. To prevent urination during the procedure, the urethra should be compressed by pressure through the rectum of the female or by direct pressure to the penis of the male. The abdominal wall is entered in the midline 1 to 2 cm above the symphysis pubis with a 22-gauge, 1-inch needle attached to a syringe (Fig. B-7). The needle should be directed slightly cephalad, and negative pressure maintained in the syringe as it is advanced. Urine entering the barrel of the syringe signals a successful bladder tap.[4]

The procedure may be repeated once if no urine is ob-

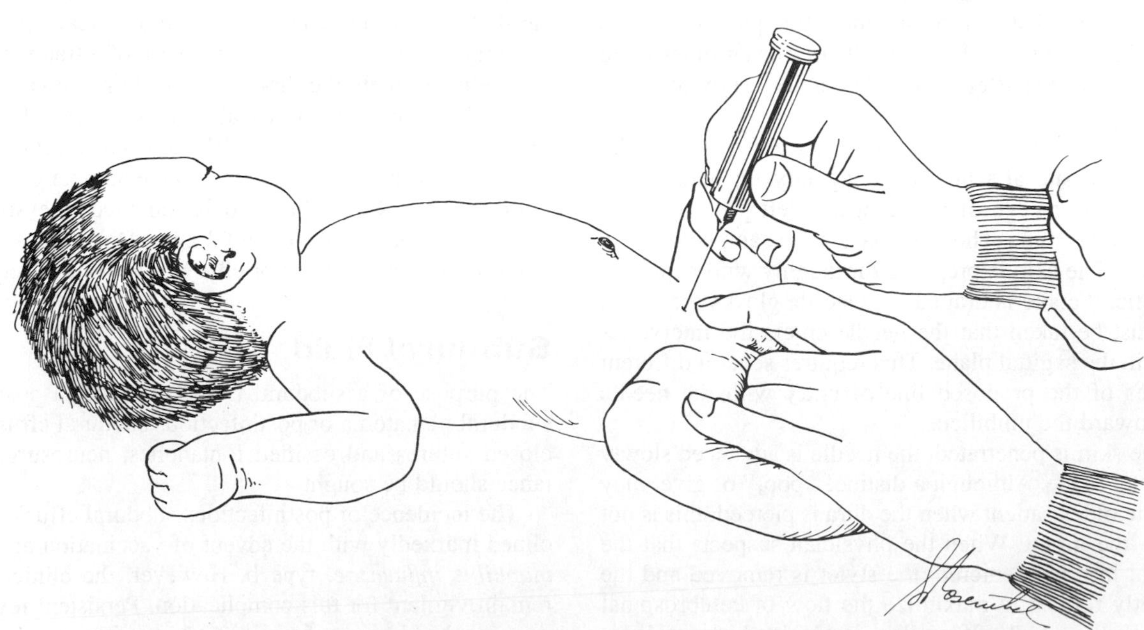

Fig. B-7 Position of an infant before aspiration of urine by suprapubic aspiration. A right-handed physician's left index finger is placed on the symphysis pubis.

tained with the first attempt. If the repeat attempt is unsuccessful, an hour should be allowed to elapse before another attempt is made. When urine is obtained, the needle is withdrawn, and the entry site is covered with a dry dressing. Complications include transient hematuria and, rarely, perforation of the bowel.

Other Body Cavities

Tympanocentesis. Tympanocentesis may be required for bacteriological diagnosis of otitis media in infants and compromised hosts in whom identification of gram negative and other organisms is particularly important. This maneuver also may be therapeutic because it reduces middle-ear pressure and removes infected fluid. The procedure is contraindicated if the patient has a bleeding disorder.

The child is mummy-wrapped and restrained by the assistant, who should hold the child's head absolutely immobile. The otic canal is cleansed with cotton swabs and alcohol or benzalkonium chloride. After cleansing and before the puncture, specimens should be taken from the ear canal and cultured to identify contaminating organisms.

The tympanic membrane is visualized through the open-ended otoscope. A 3½-inch, 20- or 22-gauge spinal puncture needle with a double bend (Z shape) allows clear visualization of the tip along its axis (Fig. B-8). The needle is connected directly to a tuberculin syringe. The plunger of the syringe is removed, and one end of a length of tubing is

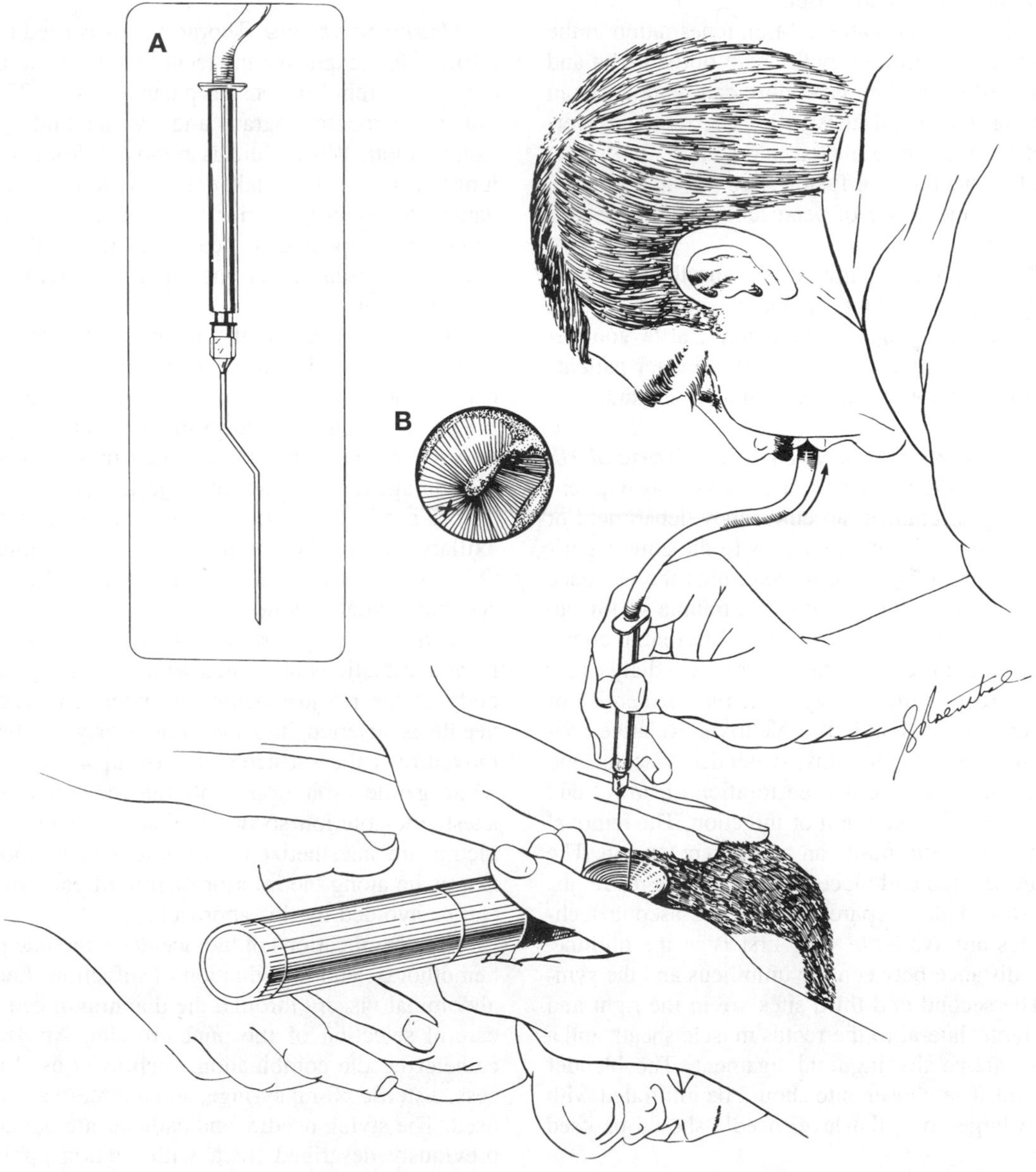

Fig. B-8 Tympanostomy. **A,** A 3-inch, 22-gauge spinal needle that has been shaped to allow direct visualization of the tympanic membrane through the operating otoscope. A tuberculin syringe barrel is attached to the needle, and tubing is attached to the syringe barrel. **B,** The preferred site on the right tympanic membrane for puncture and aspiration of the middle ear. Once the middle ear has been entered, the physician applies negative pressure through the end of the tubing placed in his or her mouth, as illustrated.

placed over the proximal end of the syringe's barrel. The other end of the tubing is placed in the physician's mouth so that controlled negative pressure can be created within the needle-syringe-tubing apparatus. The needle is used to pierce the posteroinferior quadrant of the tympanic membrane, and gentle negative pressure is applied to withdraw middle-ear fluid. A drop should be Gram stained and the remainder cultured appropriately. If there is no visible fluid, the needle should be flushed with 2 to 3 ml of blood culture medium, which may then be Gram stained and cultured.

Laser-assisted myringotomy. A novel approach to myringotomy utilizes a carbon dioxide laser (OtoLAM, ESC Sharplan Medical Systems; Tel Aviv, Isreal; SurgiTouch Sharplan Laser, Inc., Allendale NJ). The device includes a handpiece attached with an articulated arm to a conventional continuous wave carbon dioxide laser.[9]

In this method the laser creates a 2 mm fenestration in the tympanic membrane of children with acute otitis media and otitis media with effusion. The procedure can be done in an ambulatory setting with local anesthetic. The reported average duration of ventilation achieved is 24 days. Early data reports 60% of patients as effusion free at the 3-month follow-up visit. The incidence of persistent perforations at 3 months is less than 1%.[6]

The patient's tympanic membrane is anesthetized with 16% tetracaine solution 1 hour before the procedure. The laser makes an audible "pop," which may startle younger children. Because the patient must be still, younger patients may require additional conscious sedation and restraint.

Abdominal paracentesis and peritoneal dialysis catheter placement. The physician who encounters a critically ill child in an emergency department or an inpatient unit can easily obtain access to the child's peritoneal cavity. This might be done to determine the presence of and to remove extravasated blood in a trauma victim; to obtain specimens for a white blood cell or differential count, or a Gram stain and culture; to institute peritoneal dialysis for the treatment of renal failure, hyperkalemia, azotemia, or fluid overload; or to remove a dialyzable toxin. Relative contraindications include coagulopathy, distended viscera, and local skin infection. Risks include perforation of bowel and bladder, bleeding, and introduction of infection. The removal of large amounts of ascitic fluid can cause hypotension. The patient should be sedated and placed in appropriate restraints. The abdomen should be prepared with strict aseptic technique. Three sites are available. The first is in the midline, one third of the distance between the umbilicus and the symphysis pubis. The second and third sites are in the right and left lower quadrants, lateral to the rectus muscle sheath and a few centimeters above the inguinal ligament. The bladder should be emptied. The chosen site should be infiltrated with 1% lidocaine. A large-bore, flat-level needle should be used for entry.

For paracentesis, lavage, and dialysis, guide wire-placed peritoneal dialysis catheters are used.* They are available in diameters of 9 French (Fr) and 11 Fr, and have multifenestrated tips. The catheter is made with the last few centimeters set at approximately a 30-degree angle, which aids placement.

The technique for guide wire-aided placement of a dialysis catheter for lavage or dialysis is simple. The paracentesis needle is supplied with the manufacturer's prepackaged "kit." Immediately after the peritoneum is entered, a guide wire of appropriate size is placed through the needle and advanced. The dialysis catheter is advanced over the wire until resistance is encountered. The wire and needle are removed, and the catheter is attached to a syringe or intravenous tubing. Care must be taken to ensure that all the catheter's side holes are inside the abdominal cavity. A purse-string suture placed around the introduction site helps to prevent leakage. One then can proceed with removal of fluid or blood, lavage, or dialysis.

Thoracentesis. Thoracentesis is used to remove pleural fluid for diagnosis; the technique also can be used for the emergency relief of tension pneumothorax. The site is determined by roentgenogram and by the findings on physical examination. When fluid is removed from the bases of the lungs, care must be taken that abdominal viscera are not damaged. Anteroposterior, supine, and lateral radiographs should be inspected to determine if the fluid is loculated. Ultrasound examination may help to determine the location of an effusion.

The positioning of the patient depends on whether the anterior or posterior aspect of the chest is to be entered. The patient should be sitting and leaning forward, either against the back of a chair while sitting, or against a bed stand when in bed. An infant or a small toddler may be held in a hugging fashion against an assistant's chest.

The needle is inserted in the anterior, middle, or posterior axillary line in the fourth, fifth, or sixth intercostal space. Other sites may be elected as dictated by the location of specific loculated collections of fluid.

A wide area is prepared with an appropriate antiseptic, and local anesthetic is infiltrated with a 25-gauge needle over the body of the rib just below the intended puncture site. The needle is inserted into the skin overlying the rib and then moved over the surface of the rib upward to the interspace, while gentle aspiration is alternated with infiltration of the anesthetic solution so that the subcutaneous tissues and the pleura are anesthetized. The intercostal blood vessels and nerves lie along the inferior margin of each rib and therefore can be avoided by this approach.

The complications of thoracentesis include pneumothorax, hemothorax, and introduction of infection. Laceration of the abdominal viscera through the diaphragm can be avoided by careful selection of the puncture site. An 18- to 22-gauge catheter needle combination, such as is used for venous access, a sterile 50-ml syringe, and a three-way stopcock can be used. The stylet, needle, and catheter are advanced along the previously described tract, with suction applied to the syringe. When the pleura is entered, the plastic cannula is threaded over the needle-stylet and advanced. The three-way stopcock is attached to the syringe and cannula, and fluid is aspirated and placed in appropriate containers for fungal, viral, and bacteriological cultures and Gram staining. Pleural fluid also may be examined for its white blood cell and dif-

*Cook, Inc., Bloomington, Ind.

ferential counts, its protein, glucose, and lactate dehydrogenase (LDH) levels, and its cytological characteristics.[26]

An alternative to tube thoracostomy for long-term drainage of effusions is placement of a pigtail catheter by use of a modified Seldinger technique.[20] An 8.5 Fr, 15 cm polyurethane tube is placed over a 0.035-inch guide wire.* A kit is supplied that contains the pigtail catheter, an 8 Fr dilator, a needle, a guide wire, and a "Christmas tree" adapter that Luer locks to the catheter and can be firmly attached to large-bore rubber tubing for continuous suction.

The tube is inserted by advancing the needle over the superior margin of a rib, usually T4 to T6, in the midline or anterior axillary line, into the pleural space. A guide wire is advanced through the needle into the pleural cavity. A small stab wound, 2 to 4 mm in diameter, is made at the site where the guide wire enters the skin. An 8 Fr, hard, polyurethane dilator is advanced over the wire. This enlarges the tract to facilitate passage of the catheter. With the wire position fixed, the dilator is withdrawn. The pigtail catheter then is threaded over the wire and advanced into the pleural space; then the wire is withdrawn. The pigtail catheter finally is attached to large-bore rubber tubing with the Christmas tree adapter placed on the appropriate suction device. The pressure in the suction device should be set at 15 to 20 cm H_2O. A chest roentgenogram should be taken to document the catheter's position. The pigtail catheter can be secured to the chest with a small adhesive dressing and/or simply sutured and tied in place. This technique is quick, simple, complication free, and easy to learn; it also is especially valuable to transport and emergency room teams for treatment of pneumothorax.

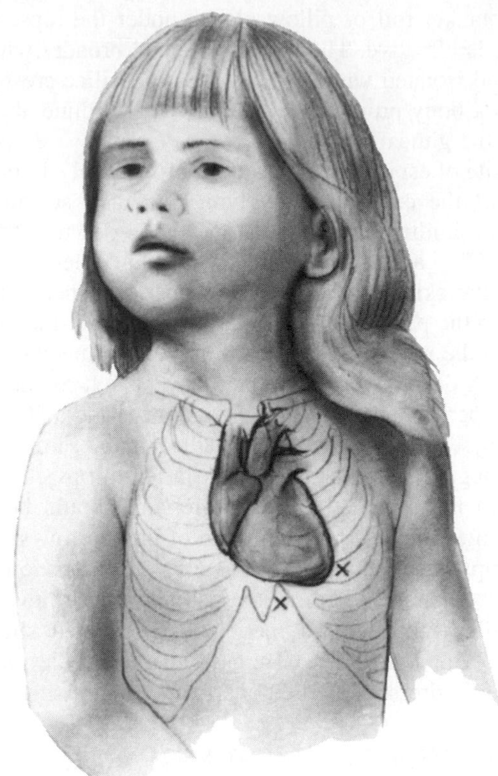

Fig. B-9 Pericardiocentesis. Two sites for aspiration of the pericardial sac are shown. These vary with the extent of the effusion, as determined by examination, contrast study, and/or echocardiography.

Pericardiocentesis. Pericardiocentesis is a high-risk procedure. Its dangers must be weighed against the urgency of diagnosing a pericardial effusion or an unchecked cardiac tamponade.

Myocardial injury, laceration of a coronary artery, cardiac arrhythmia, and infection are possible complications of pericardiocentesis. The internal mammary arteries are within 2.5 cm of the sternal border, and they also may be damaged.

The alternate points of entry into the chest are illustrated in Fig. B-9. The best site is at the left chondroxiphoid angle. The others are in the left fourth, fifth, and sixth intercostal spaces, 1 to 2 cm medial to the border of percussible cardiac dullness. A roentgenogram, fluoroscopy, and ultrasound examination also may aid in determining the border of the pericardium.

The patient, who may require sedation, should be supine at approximately a 30-degree angle and carefully restrained. A wide area of the precordium is prepared with an appropriate antiseptic. The chosen site is infiltrated with lidocaine. A 50-ml syringe then is connected to a three-way stopcock and an 18-gauge needle. An electrocardiogram V lead, with an alligator clip, is attached to the needle to detect an injury current should the myocardium or coronary artery be entered.

The needle is directed inward and medially when the intercostal approach is used. When the chondroxiphoid approach is used, the needle is aimed upward and posteriorly.

Gentle negative pressure should be applied to the syringe as the needle is advanced. The ECG should be monitored constantly and the needle withdrawn if an injury current is detected. The fluid should be aspirated slowly. The needle then is withdrawn, and a simple sterile dressing is applied over the puncture site.[18]

Bone marrow aspiration. Bone marrow samples aid in the diagnosis of leukemia, thrombocytopenia, some forms of anemia, suspected metastatic disease, and several of the "storage" diseases, such as the lipidoses. Culture of the bone marrow occasionally is indicated in cases of suspected sepsis. Bone marrow aspiration has few risks; infection is the greatest. It usually is performed safely in those who have thrombocytopenia.

The preferred site is the posterior iliac crest because it is easy to locate, the patient can be easily restrained for its performance, and the site contains active marrow in patients of all ages. Other sites include the tibia, femur, sternum, spinous vertebral process, and anterior iliac crest. The tibia is most useful in children under 18 months of age. The femur also is a useful site in this age group, but overlying muscle tissue makes the procedure more difficult. The sternum is the least safe site for children. The spinous vertebral process requires exceptional restraint of the patient and in general is a technically difficult site to use.

The needle used is a commercially available bone marrow needle and stylet.

The technique for using the posterior iliac crest is described here. The child is restrained in the prone position

*Cook, Inc., Bloomington, Ind.

with a blanket roll or pillow placed under the hips. Use of sedation is effective. The site is scrubbed broadly with antiseptic and isolated with sterile drapes. The iliac crest is palpable as a bony prominence lateral to the midline above the level of the gluteal cleft.

The site of aspiration is located approximately 1 cm below the lip of the crest. The overlying skin and subcutaneous tissues are infiltrated with local anesthetic down to the periosteum. The aspiration needle with its stylet is pushed through the skin, angled toward the patient's head, and advanced to the periosteum. A steady, screwdriver-like rotation of the needle with applied pressure forces the needle into the marrow. A decrease in resistance may be felt as the bone's cortex is perforated. The stylet is removed, and a 20-ml sterile syringe is attached to the needle's hub. Firm, quickly applied negative pressure will cause a few drops of blood to spurt into the syringe. Negative pressure should be terminated immediately to avoid dilution of the marrow specimen with peripheral blood. Approximately 1 ml of bone marrow should be aspirated. The syringe is carefully removed from the needle, and 6 to 10 meticulously cleaned slides are smeared. The stylet then is reinserted, the needle removed, and a sterile dressing applied over the puncture site.

EMERGENCY THERAPEUTIC PROCEDURES

Emergency Intravenous Access Protocol

Significant delay can be encountered in the establishment of intravenous access in the critically ill child.[25] The small size of the pediatric patient, the stress of the situation, and venous collapse make insertion of a peripheral intravenous device difficult. An algorithmic, protocol approach to the problem of establishing venous access has been suggested.[17] In one series of pediatric resuscitations, more than 10 minutes was required to establish venous access, and in 6% of the subjects no access could be established. In an algorithm suggested for use in cardiopulmonary resuscitation, attempts at peripheral vein insertion would be made for only 1½ minutes.[24]

Physicians who might encounter critically ill children should consider the development of such venous access protocols and algorithms. These should be tailored to the needs of the institution or site and to those of the practitioner.

Standard of care guidelines demand early use of the intraosseous needle. All clinicians who might encounter children in cardiovascular collapse should familiarize themselves with this quick, simple, and easy-to-learn technique.

When caring for a child in cardiovascular or respiratory collapse, undue time must not be spent on attempts at placing peripheral or central venous lines. Placement of a central venous catheter should not be attempted by those inexperienced in the technique. Central venous access is not required for cardiopulmonary resuscitation or in the early, important stages of shock treatment. If venous access cannot be achieved in 90 seconds, an intraosseous device should be placed.

Likewise, even if the practitioner is skilled in the saphenous vein cutdown procedure, it should not be attempted for venous access in an arrest or shock resuscitation because of the length of time required for placement.[14] Cutdown may be indicated for chronic venous access after successful resuscitation.

Intraosseous Infusions

Intraosseous infusion is a procedure that should be familiar to all who provide care to children.[29] This easily learned technique can be used for any critically ill child under 6 years of age whenever a delay in establishing venous access might compromise the patient. In many situations, obtaining venous access is time consuming. A surgeon, intensivist, or anesthesiologist must be brought in to establish a central venous catheter by guide wire or to perform a cutdown. These actions can cause needless delay in treatment. The ability to place an intraosseous needle allows even a technically inexperienced person to gain immediate access to the intramedullary venous system, which is continuous with the venous circulation (Fig. B-10). Crystalloid and colloid for fluid resuscitation, blood, plasma, catecholamines (e.g., epinephrine and dopamine), glucose, calcium, and sodium bicarbonate all can be administered by the intraosseous route.[23] Although a standard 18- or 20-gauge spinal needle with stylet and bone marrow biopsy needles are useful in extreme situations, intraosseous needles, manufactured specifically for this purpose, are available and preferable. The proximal and distal tibias are the sites of choice. The iliac crest, sternum, and femur are alternate sites. The anterior medial surface of the proximal tibia or the medial surface of the distal tibia proximal to the medial malleolus are preferred sites (Figs. B-11 and B-12). The epiphysis must be avoided when the proximal tibia is used. The cortex in the midshaft of the tibia is difficult to penetrate, although this sometimes is used in emergencies.

In a child older than age 6, the thick cortex at the proximal and distal tibia prevents easy use of these sites, although one might be successful with the latter site in some children older than 6 years of age. The site is aseptically prepared. Then the needle is advanced perpendicular to the bone, with firm pres-

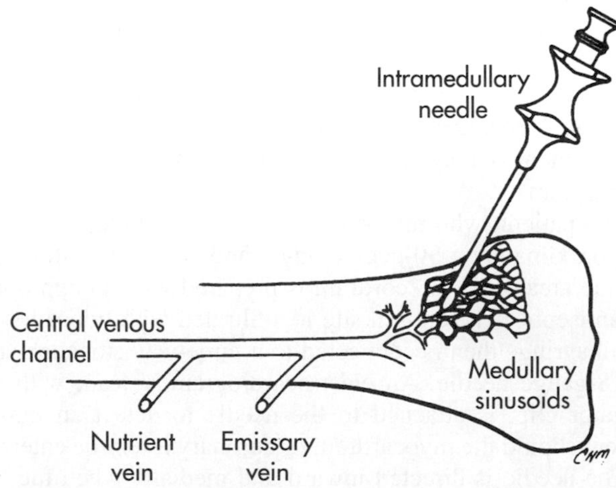

Fig. B-10 The intramedullary venous system demonstrates the position of an intraosseous needle in the medullary sinusoids. Blood may be aspirated from the sinusoids to confirm the position of the needle.

(From Spivey WH: *J Pediatr* 5:111, 1987.)

sure and a rotary motion. Entry to the marrow cavity is detected by decreasing resistance. Aspiration with a syringe should produce blood and marrow. To clear the needle, it should be flushed with 3 to 5 ml of sterile saline in a sterile syringe. The device then is connected to standard intravenous tubing. Although the flow rate is slower than that observed in a standard device, it should be steady, with no evidence of extravasation at the site. If the needle dislodges or fluid extravasates, the opposite leg should be used. If large volumes are required, two devices should be placed. A second device should not be placed on the same leg after removal of the first device, because leakage will occur. Resuscitative drugs should be "flushed" in after 3 to 5 ml of saline have been injected. Compartment syndrome has been described when fluid extravasates. This complication can be limited by changing the site if there is evidence of edema or vascular compromise.[33]

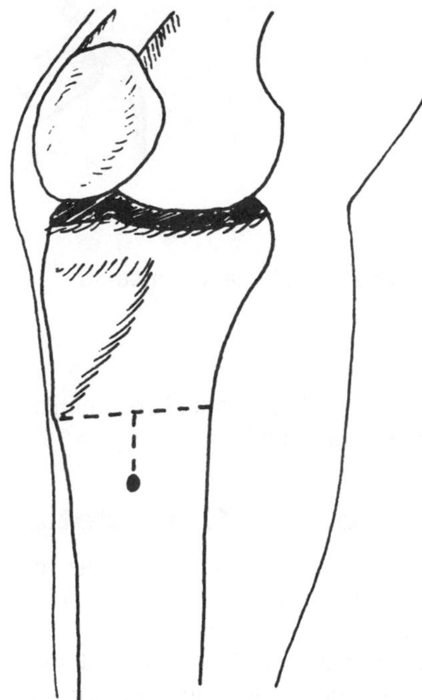

Fig. B-11 Insertion site in the proximal tibia. The tibial tuberosity and medial border of the tibia are palpated. The needle is inserted halfway between these points and 1 or 2 cm distally, pointing away from the joint space and in a caudal direction.

(From Spivey WH: *J Pediatr* 5:111, 1987.)

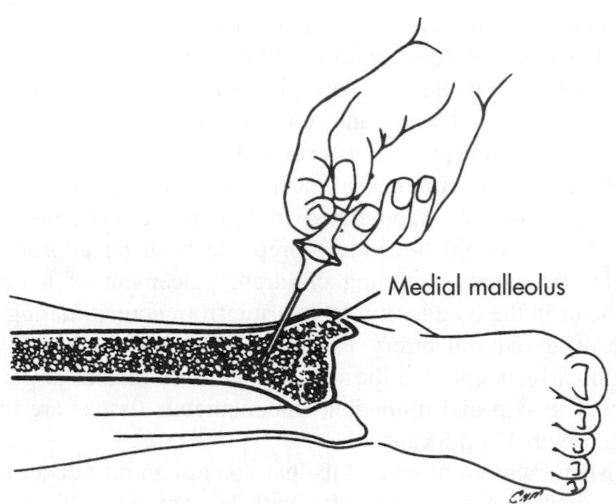

Fig. B-12 The position of an intraosseous needle in the distal tibia. The needle is inserted into the medial surface of the distal tibia at the junction of the malleolus and shaft of the tibia. It is inserted away from the joint space in a cephalad direction.

(From Spivey WH: *J Pediatr* 5:111, 1987.)

INFUSIONS

Percutaneous Intravenous Infusion

Fig. B-2 depicts the location of accessible superficial veins suitable for percutaneous intravenous infusions. The veins of the extremities and scalp are commonly used; the latter have no valves and can be punctured in either direction. Skin preparation should be especially meticulous when scalp veins are used because they communicate by means of emissary veins with the dural sinuses.

The child is positioned and immobilized, and the extremity is immobilized further by being taped firmly to a padded board or sandbag. A tourniquet is applied above the vein to be infused, and the skin is cleansed with alcohol. A butterfly 22- or 25-gauge needle or a 20- or 22-gauge intravenous catheter/needle is filled with saline and attached to the intravenous tubing and solution bottle and is used to enter the vein in the direction of venous flow. When the vein is entered, the tourniquet is removed and the blood flow is tested by opening the intravenous tubing to allow the solution to be infused to flow. Alternatively, saline can be injected through the needle with a syringe.

If the flow is adequate and there is no extravasation of fluid, a piece of tape is placed over the entry site and the wings of the butterfly needle are taped to the skin. A pad may be used under the hub of the needle to maintain the angle that best allows free flow of fluid. A protective cover is taped over the needle, and the adequacy of the restraints is checked (Fig. B-13). If percutaneous needle catheterization is performed, the vein is entered as described above. When blood is seen in the hub of the needle, it is stabilized and the catheter sleeve is advanced up the vein. The catheter then is stabilized, the needle removed, and the blood flow checked before the catheter hub is taped in position and the intravenous tubing attached.

Cutdown Intravenous Infusion

A cutdown intravenous infusion may be required if a vein cannot be entered percutaneously. Generally, these children are chronically ill, and conventional percutaneous catheter placement sites have been exhausted. The useful "life" of a cutdown is less than 5 days. Thus, if chronic access will be a continuing requirement, a long-term indwelling Silastic catheter placed by a surgeon is more appropriate.[14]

The great saphenous vein is preferred because its position is constant, anterior to the medial malleolus running cephalad, so it may be found even when not visible through the

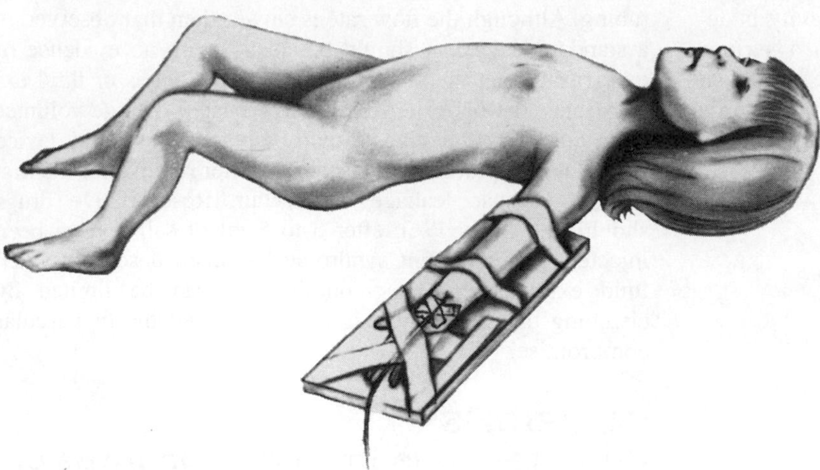

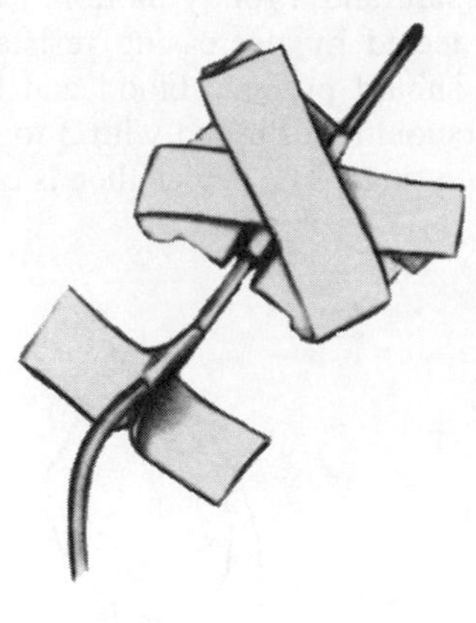

Fig. B-13 Immobilization of the upper extremity for intravenous infusion and a method of securing the needle and tubing with tape.

skin. The child is positioned and the limb restrained on a padded board, as for a percutaneous infusion. A tourniquet is applied in the midcalf region, and surgical aseptic technique is observed. Local anesthesia is produced by infiltration of the skin over the site of the incision with 1% lidocaine. A 2- to 3-cm transverse incision should be made 1 cm superior and anterior to the medial malleolus, and the skin and superficial fascia should be widely spread. Blunt dissection is used to identify and isolate the vein (Fig. B-14). A curved hemostat is used to scoop the vein off the periosteum and up into the wound. The vein should be freed from connective tissue for 1 to 2 cm along its length by blunt dissection and two No. 000 silk ligatures passed under it. The distal ligature is used to tie off the lower portion of vein and to provide caudal traction on the vein.

An intravenous catheter needle may be used to enter the vein, as described in the section on percutaneous intravenous infusion, or a small nick may be made in the vein and an intravenous cannula threaded cephalad for 2 to 5 cm. The proximal ligature is then firmly tied around the vein and cannula. The wound is closed with fine silk sutures, one of which should be tied around the catheter to anchor it. The wound is dressed with a gauze bandage and cleansed daily.

Heparin Lock

An intravenous catheter needle or a plastic indwelling catheter may be converted to heparin lock for intermittent administration of medications or drawing of blood samples. The great saphenous vein at the ankle is the preferred site, but one of the anterior cubital veins will suffice.

Heparin in normal saline solution is used to flush and fill the needle and tubing or the catheter. A concentration of 10 units of heparin per milliliter avoids heparinization of the patient but still prevents clotting within the needle or catheter; a stopcock is attached to the hub of the indwelling needle or catheter. Prolonged use of any indwelling device carries the risk of local and disseminated infection. Care must be taken to sterilize the ports with iodophor solution before each use. When the device is used, 1 to 2 ml of blood should be aspirated before sampling to avoid contamination with heparin and the indwelling fluid.

Femoral Venous Cannulation

The femoral vein is a safe, easily accessible vessel for cannulation with a single- or multiple-lumen catheter. With reasonable care it can be used for relatively long-term access as well. Several investigators have reported successful use of femoral venous catheters with minimal infectious complications. In fact, femoral venous catheters compare favorably over other sites in complications from infection.[28] The consistent anatomy of the area and proximity to the femoral arterial pulse allow the vessel to be easily located, because it lies 1 to 2 cm medial to the artery and 2 to 4 cm below the inguinal ligament. A transcutaneous Doppler device with a hand-held probe and earphones can help locate the artery when the pulse is difficult to palpate.* When the femoral arterial pulse cannot be located because of obesity or hypotension, as is the case in cardiac arrest, the femoral artery easily can be confused with the vein and inadvertently catheterized. In severe cardiorespiratory embarrassment, the color of aspirated blood and blood gas tensions may confuse the operator and prevent discrimination of artery from vein.

Placement is simple and easily learned (Fig. B-15). The patient should be supine and in four-point restraints. The groin area should be widely prepared with an appropriate antiseptic agent. In young children, placement of a Foley catheter in the bladder prevents urine from contaminating the site. The femoral artery is palpated 2 to 4 cm below the inguinal ligament, and the vein is 1 to 2 cm medial to the artery. The skin and immediate subcutaneous tissues are infiltrated with 1% lidocaine.

Manufacturer-supplied kits that contain an introducer needle, dilator, guide wire, and catheter are available.† The appropriate-size catheter has an outer diameter of 3 to 4 Fr for patients under 1 year of age, 5 to 6 Fr to age 7, and 7 Fr

*Parks Electronics Laboratory, Beaverton, Ore.

†Cook, Inc., Bloomington, Ind.; Arrow International, Inc., Reading, Pa.

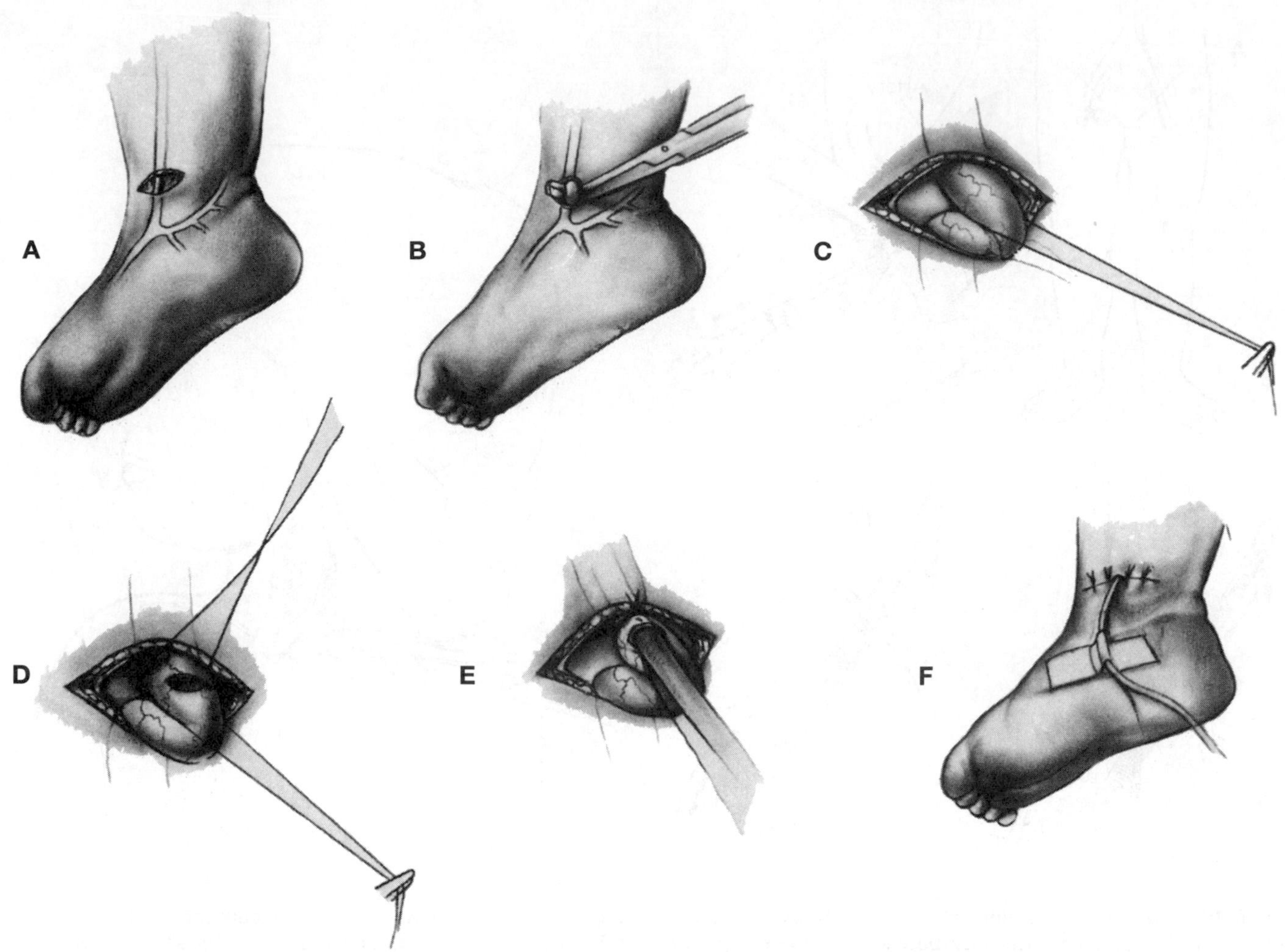

Fig. B-14 Procedure for cutdown of the great saphenous vein. **A,** Site of incision anterior to the medial malleolus. **B,** Elevation of the vein into the wound with a curved clamp. **C,** Application of distal ligature for traction. **D,** Loosely placed proximal ligature and venostomy incision. **E,** Venous catheter tied in place. **F,** Wound sutured and catheter secured.

for children 8 years or older. A syringe that contains 2 to 3 ml of heparinized saline is attached to the introducer needle. The needle is introduced at a 30- to 45-degree angle from horizontal and aimed at the umbilicus. Care should be taken to avoid advancing the needle beyond the inguinal ligament because the peritoneum, bowel, and bladder can be perforated. With continuous, gentle aspiration the needle is advanced into the vein. When good blood return is documented, the syringe is removed. The guide wire then is advanced into the vein. There should be minimal resistance to the passage of the wire. If resistance is encountered, the needle and wire must be removed simultaneously to avoid shearing the wire off in the patient's vein. The needle is then withdrawn, leaving the wire in place. An incision, 2 to 4 mm, is made with a scalpel where the guide wire enters the skin. A dilator is threaded over the wire and passed through skin and subcutaneous tissue into the vessel, then withdrawn, again leaving the wire in place. The catheter is threaded over the wire. Care must be taken to ensure that at least 1 to 2 cm of the guide wire extends from the proximal end of the catheter before it is threaded into the vein. Otherwise, the wire can be "lost" in the vessel. Being careful not to change the position of the wire, the practitioner slowly advances the catheter over the wire to the desired distance, then removes the wire. For central venous pressure measurement, the catheter tip should be placed just above the diaphragm. The position should be verified by roentgenogram. The catheter then is sutured in place.

Complications include bleeding, infection, inadequate venous drainage, thrombus formation, and inadvertent penetration of viscera or a vessel wall. These must be weighed against the benefits of obtaining secure, large-bore venous access and the need to determine the central venous pressure.[11]

Subclavian Vein Catheter Placement

The subclavian vein is a readily accessible site that provides a secure central conduit for (1) fluid administration (including hypertonic or irritating solutions that cannot be infused into peripheral veins), (2) maintenance of cardiac output by direct infusions of pressor drugs, and (3) central venous pressure monitoring.[32]

Risks include pneumothorax or accidental penetration of the subclavian artery, with hematoma formation, hemorrhage, or thrombosis. The risk of this procedure must be

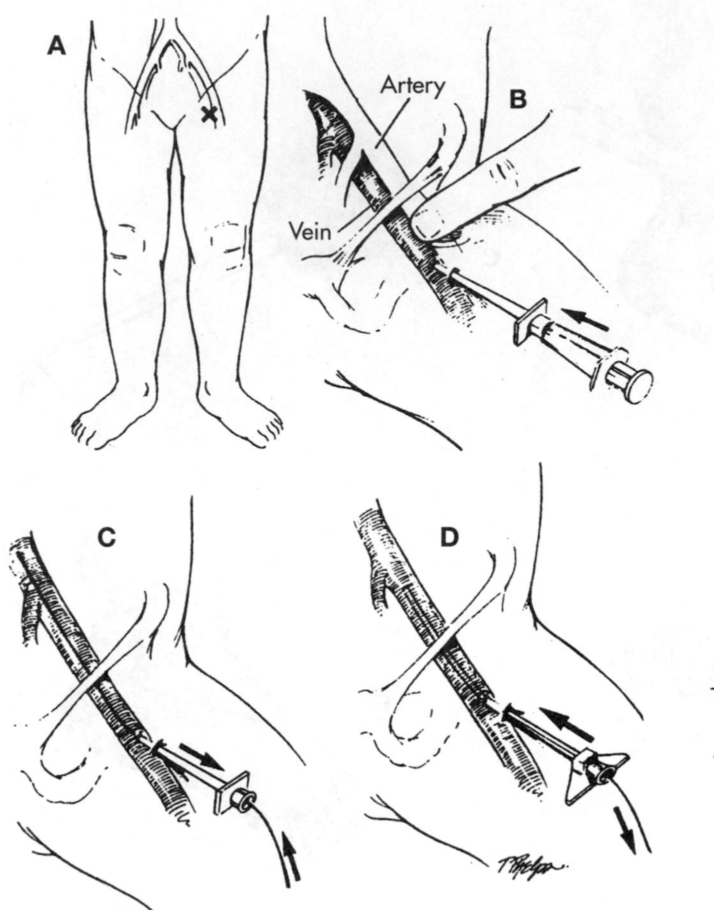

Fig. B-15 Femoral vein line placement (Seldinger technique). **A,** Femoral vein midway between anterior superior iliac crest and symphysis pubis. **B,** Insertion of needle into femoral vein just medial to femoral arterial pulse. **C,** Insertion of guide wire through needle in the vein. Needle removed once guide wire in place. **D,** Infusion catheter advanced over guide wire into vein. Guide wire removed after catheter in place.

(From Nichols DG, Yaster M, Lappe DG, Haller JA: *Golden hour: the handbook of advanced pediatric life support,* ed 2, Mosby, St Louis, 1996.)

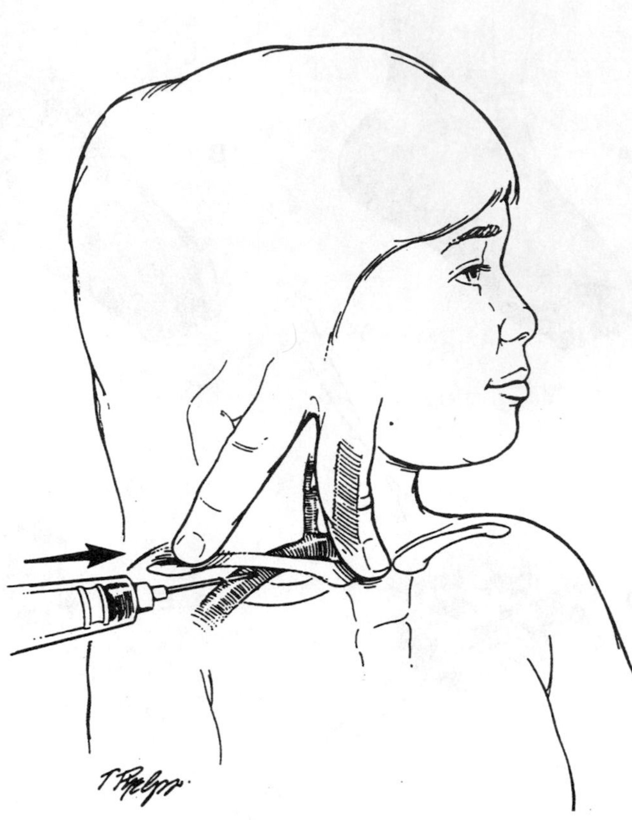

Fig. B-16 Subclavian vein line placement. Landmarks identified by placing operator's thumb in the sternal notch and index finger at the junction of the clavicle and first rib. Needle puncture 1 cm medial and 1 cm inferior to clavicle-rib junction aiming for the sternal notch. Then use Seldinger technique (see Fig. B-15) for line placement.

(From Nichols DG, Yaster M, Lappe DG, Haller JA: *Golden hour: the handbook of advanced pediatric life support,* ed 2, Mosby, St Louis, 1996.)

balanced with the skill of the physician and the benefit to the patient.[8] The operator first should be familiar with the use of the Seldinger technique for percutaneous placement of a catheter over a guide wire placed through an introducer needle.

Catheterization kits* provide a guide wire, catheters, and an introducer needle. The following sizes of catheters are used: 3 Fr in infants, 4 Fr in toddlers, 5 Fr in children 4 to 12 years of age, and 7 Fr for adolescents. The right subclavian vein is preferred over the left because of its more direct entry to the superior vena cava and because there is less risk of pneumothorax (the right lung lies lower in the thorax than the left) and injury to the thoracic duct, which lies in the left hemithorax. Fig. B-16 illustrates this technique.

The patient is placed in the Trendelenburg position and is restrained. The child's face is turned 90 degrees away from the intended puncture site. A 3-inch thick towel roll is placed along the long axis of the thoracic spine between the shoulder blades.

The area overlying the puncture site is cleansed widely, and drapes are used to provide an aseptic field. Masks, gloves, and gowns are used.

The subclavian vein is cannulated by the infraclavicular approach. The vein lies approximately parallel to the proximal third of the clavicle and is accessed in a triangle bounded by the medial third of the clavicle, the anterior scalene muscle, and the upper surface of the first rib. The subclavian artery runs posterior to the vein behind the anterior scalene muscle. Using a 1½-inch, 22-gauge needle, the skin overlying the puncture site and intended insertion tract is infiltrated with 1% lidocaine.

The introducer needle is placed just medial to the midclavicular line 2 to 3 cm below the inferior border of the clavicle. The needle is aimed toward the midsternal notch and is advanced to the inferior border of the medial portion

*Cook, Inc., Bloomington, Ind.

of the clavicle. A syringe containing a few milliliters of heparinized saline is attached to the introducer needle, and with negative pressure applied to the barrel of the syringe, the needle is advanced deep to the clavicle on a course nearly parallel to its medial portion. Small cephalad adjustments of the target point (approximately 0.25-cm increments) can be made if the vein is not entered immediately.

When the vein has been entered, as evidenced by blood entering the syringe, the hub of the introducer needle should be held securely in place, and the syringe removed.

Caution must be exercised, because air may be introduced into the vein as the patient increases the negative pleural pressure when initiating a breath. Therefore, the patient must be instructed to hold his or her breath, or, with infants, the proximal orifice of the needle must be occluded temporarily. The flexible, spring loaded end of the catheter's guide wire is inserted into the introducer needle and advanced through the bore of the needle into the subclavian vein and beyond into the superior vena cava. A minimum of 3 cm of wire is passed beyond the estimated tip of the needle. A cardiac arrhythmia may signal that the guide wire has been passed too far into the right ventricle, in which case it should be drawn back a bit. The proximal end of the wire should be held securely as the introducer needle is removed.

The catheter is flushed with heparin solution and advanced over the guide wire to the desired position in the superior vena cava; care should be taken not to advance the wire simultaneously. The guide wire then is removed, and the proximal end of the catheter is attached to the desired intravenous fluid-administration system or the central venous pressure-monitoring system.

The position of the catheter should be verified roentgenographically. The catheter must be placed so that the distal tip is in the distal third of the superior vena cava, above its junction with the right atrium.

Umbilical Vein Catheterization

Catheterization of the umbilical vein is useful in newborns for emergency correction of acidosis, hypoglycemia, and hypotension, in the performance of exchange transfusions, and for the measurement of central venous pressure. The complications of umbilical vein catheterization include sepsis and microembolization from catheter-induced thrombosis. An umbilical venous catheter easily can be misplaced into a branch of the portal venous system, and the injection of hyperosmolar solutions containing substances such as glucose and sodium bicarbonate can lead to portal vein thrombosis and hepatic necrosis. Umbilical vein catheters also have been implicated in cases of necrotizing enterocolitis and spontaneous perforation of the large bowel.[13]

A radiopaque catheter must be used in umbilical vein catheterization to allow verification of its position by roentgenogram. The small premature infant is susceptible to chilling during the catheterization procedure, and use of a radiant warmer is necessary. The equipment found on a cutdown tray, with the addition of fine-toothed pickup forceps, is adequate. The catheter size is selected on the basis of the weight of the baby: a 3.5 Fr catheter should be used for infants weighing less than 1500 g and a 5 Fr catheter for those weighing more. Special attention to aseptic techniques, including surgical scrubbing of the operator's hands, antiseptic preparation of the baby's abdomen and umbilical cord, and maintenance of a sterile field, is essential. The physician should be gloved, masked, and gowned as for any surgical procedure.

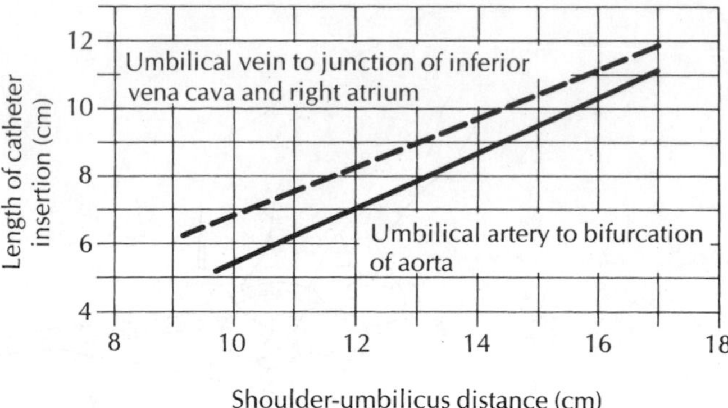

Fig. B-17 Method of determining the optimal length for umbilical catheter insertion.

The length that the catheter is to be inserted should be determined by measuring the distance from the infant's shoulder to the umbilicus by the conversion method shown in Fig. B-17. This length ideally places the catheter at the junction of the inferior vena cava and the right atrium. Care must be taken not to cover the infant's chest in such a manner that apnea or malfunction of the heat probes or monitor leads will go undetected. An assistant provides gentle traction to the cord stump while the physician transects the cord with a scalpel 1 to 1.5 cm above the skin. Gauze sponges should be available for tamponade to control oozing of blood from the umbilical vein; the amount of oozing usually is insignificant. The cord stump is inspected to locate the thin-walled umbilical vein and the two thick-walled umbilical arteries. The catheter is attached to a three-way stopcock and a syringe containing heparinized saline solution (1 unit of heparin per milliliter of saline), and the catheter is filled. Minimal traction on the superior edge of the cord stump may be helpful in locating the orifice of the umbilical vein; this is dilated gently with pickup forceps or a small probe, and the catheter is introduced the predetermined distance (Fig. B-18). Resistance occasionally is met at the level of the abdominal wall or at the level of the ductus venosus. Very gentle pressure and partial withdrawal and rotation of the catheter usually overcomes this resistance; force should not be used. The position of the catheter should be verified by roentgenogram except under emergency circumstances.

Care must be taken to avoid iatrogenic blood loss through accidental dislodgment of the catheter. A purse-string suture around the umbilical stump and careful taping of the catheter to the abdominal wall help to avoid this. Antibiotic ointment and a dressing that will show any significant blood loss from the stump should be applied lightly over the umbilicus after successful catheterization. Current practice discourages keeping umbilical vein catheters in place for long periods; however, if neonatal transport requires fixation of the catheter, this can be accomplished with a purse-string suture, a bridge of adhesive tape (see Fig. B-18), or umbilical cord tape. Fortunately, these rarely are needed for hemostasis. Application of an antibiotic ointment and daily inspection of the

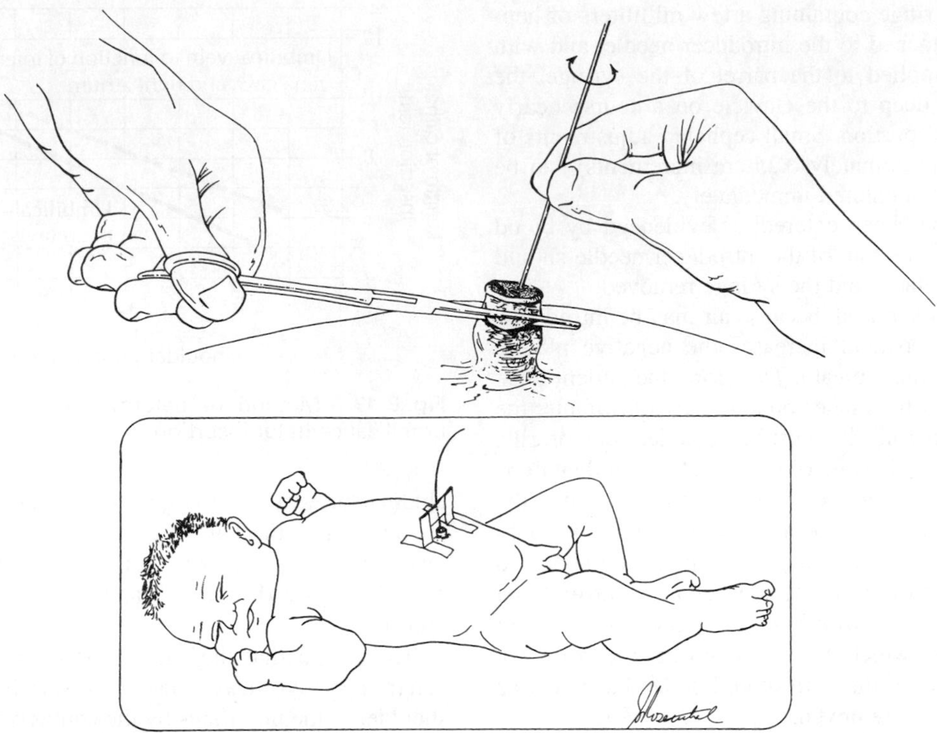

Fig. B-18 Umbilical vessel cannulation. The hemostat is used to grasp the edge of the cord stump, which then is rolled toward the physician to allow visualization and provide stability. A probe is shown in the physician's right hand. Gentle pressure and a rolling motion are used to dilate the orifice of the vessel. The lower portion of the illustration shows a method of taping that fixes the catheter's position, preventing it from penetrating deeper or becoming dislodged. A light dressing can be placed over the umbilicus to guard against local infection.

umbilical vein and stump for signs of local infection should follow removal of the catheter.

Umbilical Artery Catheterization

Catheterization of the umbilical artery is accomplished in a manner similar to catheterization of the umbilical vein, and the equipment used is the same. Its purpose is to provide access to the arterial circulation for monitoring blood pressure and blood gases and for infusion of selected solutions. Even in skilled hands, the procedure carries risks of embolization, sepsis, extravasation of blood, and distal arterial insufficiency. These complications must be considered in any determination of the risk/benefit ratio before performance of the procedure. Samples from the radial and temporal arteries are of preductal arterial blood and for single-measurement purposes are safer and more precise than is umbilical artery catheterization. Catheter placement at the point of bifurcation of the aorta is desirable to avoid damage to the renal arteries. The shoulder-umbilical length is measured, and the distance to the bifurcation of the aorta is determined by the conversion method shown in Fig. B-17.

Attention to aseptic techniques is essential. The heavy-walled artery may be dilated gently. A rim of vessel wall is picked up gently with fine-toothed forceps. The catheter, filled with heparinized saline and attached to a closed three-way stopcock, then is introduced into the artery. Advancement of the catheter may be hindered by vasospasm; this can be overcome by applying slow, gentle pressure. Forceful probing should be avoided. If the catheter cannot be advanced, the other umbilical artery should be used. If resistance again is encountered and gentle pressure fails to advance the catheter, 0.1 to 0.2 ml of 1% or 2% lidocaine, without epinephrine, is instilled into the lumen of the artery. After 2 or 3 minutes the catheter usually can be advanced more easily.

The position of the catheter at the bifurcation of the aorta should be verified by roentgenogram. The catheter must be fixed carefully to the cord stump with a purse-string suture and to the abdomen with adhesive tape. An antibiotic ointment and a sterile dressing should be applied lightly, so as not to obscure blood loss, and the dressing should be changed daily.

The danger of iatrogenic accidents must be emphasized. Dislodgment of the catheters, stopcock leakage, and inadequate tamponade on removal of the catheter may result in significant blood loss. Failure to record and replace blood removed from the catheter may result in anemia and a deficit of fluid. Catheter removal is indicated when signs of ischemia of the lower extremities are present.

Exchange Transfusion

Prepackaged exchange transfusion sets with appropriate four-way stopcocks are available commercially for treatment of erythroblastosis fetalis and other conditions requiring exchange transfusion. The physician must take time to become familiar with the function of the stopcock. If two standard stopcocks are used rather than the four-way stopcock, extra care must be taken to prevent directional-flow accidents.[12]

Needed are materials for an umbilical catheterization, a source of heat (preferably an overhead radiant warmer), sterile surgical drapes, gown and gloves, a cap and mask, monitors for pulse and respiration, blood matched to infant and mother, resuscitation equipment, and 5 to 10 ml of 10% calcium gluconate solution. The blood should be warmed with a blood warmer.

Acid-citrate-dextrose blood, citrate-phosphate-dextrose blood, or heparinized preserved blood may be used. The first is adequate and usually available. A two-volume exchange should be performed. The amount of blood required is 170 ml/kg body weight, up to 500 ml. If possible, the blood bank should adjust the hematocrit of the donor blood to 55%. The hydropic infant, however, may require a very slow, careful exchange with packed red blood cells, while an assistant monitors central venous pressure and observes the patient for signs of congestive heart failure.

The infant should be restrained and the stomach emptied. The umbilicus should be prepared and draped and the venous catheter inserted. Plastic tubing connects the stopcock to the waste bag, the donor blood, and the umbilical vein catheter. The central venous pressure, blood pressure, pulse, and respirations should be recorded throughout the procedure.

Initially, blood is withdrawn from the baby and sent to the laboratory for determination of hematocrit, bilirubin, glucose, total protein, and serum electrolytes (sodium, chloride, carbon dioxide, calcium, potassium, and blood urea nitrogen).

Aliquots of 5 to 20 ml may be withdrawn and replaced, depending on the infant's age and cardiovascular stability. A rate of 3 to 5 ml/kg/min, or 1 to 1½ minutes per aliquot withdrawn and replaced, is desirable.

An assistant is required to record the vital signs, each volume exchanged, and a running exchange total. A person skilled at resuscitation and appropriate equipment to accomplish this should be available.

If acid-citrate-dextrose blood is used, 1 ml of 10% calcium gluconate should be given for every 100 ml exchanged. Irritability, tachycardia, and prolongation of the QT interval on the ECG are signs of hypocalcemia. If heparinized blood is used, 0.5 mg of protamine is given intramuscularly after the procedure.

Box B-1 lists the potential complications of exchange transfusions.

The final aliquot of blood removed is sent to the laboratory for typing and cross-matching and for hematocrit and electrolyte determinations. The catheter then is withdrawn, and a sterile dressing is applied to the umbilicus. The infant is monitored intensively over the next 4 hours for cardiovascular stability. During this time, the infant should receive nothing by mouth and have intravenous hydration. From 4 to 6 hours after the procedure, determinations of hematocrit, bilirubin, and calcium should be made.

BOX B-1

COMPLICATIONS OF EXCHANGE TRANSFUSIONS

Vascular
- Embolization with air or clots
- Thrombosis

Cardiac
- Arrhythmias
- Volume overload
- Arrest

Electrolyte
- Hyperkalemia
- Hypernatremia
- Hypocalcemia
- Acidosis

Hematological
- Overheparinization
- Thrombocytopenia

Infectious
- Bacteremia
- Serum hepatitis

Miscellaneous
- Mechanical injury to donor cells
- Hypothermia
- Hypoglycemia

Tube Thoracostomy

Pneumothorax is a common complication in the emergency care of infants, children, and adolescents. Placement of a thoracostomy tube (for drainage of air and fluid that has accumulated in the pleural cavity) by blunt dissection of a tract in the intercostal space with a hemostat is more tedious but safer than using a trocar unless the operator is experienced in the latter technique. A 12 Fr catheter should be used for infants and children up to age 3, a 16 Fr catheter for children up to age 10, and a 20 Fr catheter for older children and adolescents.

The fourth or fifth intercostal space in the anterior axillary line is the appropriate site. The pectoralis muscle, the nipple, and the intercostal arteries (at the inferior aspect of each rib) are to be avoided. The infant or child is placed in the supine position with the arm restrained above the head. The site is prepared and draped aseptically. Local anesthetic is infiltrated into the skin overlying the fifth or sixth rib by using a 22-gauge, 1½-inch needle. While the needle is advanced subcutaneously within the fourth or fifth intercostal space, the anesthetic is infiltrated within the soft tissues down to the level of and including the pleura.

A 2-cm skin incision over the intercostal space is made, and with blunt dissection a hemostat is introduced through the previously anesthetized tissues into the pleural cavity, as illustrated in Fig. B-19. The chest tube then is clamped in the curved jaws of the hemostat and advanced through the dissected intercostal space tract to the pleural cavity. The tube ideally should lie anterior to the lung at its apex. The lateral orifices of the catheter must be well within the pleural cavity. The tube is secured with skin sutures, one on either side of the incision, wrapped around the tube, and tied tightly enough to crimp the tube slightly. A minimal dressing is applied so that malpositioning may be detected. Bulky dressings are not warranted. The dissected tract heals rapidly.

Common errors in the placement of thoracostomy tubes are subcutaneous placement, resulting from incomplete blunt dissection, and dislodgement caused by inadequate securement. Bleeding and infection rarely are encountered.

An alternative technique for immediate placement of a catheter in the chest for drainage involves using a guide wire and a pigtail catheter and is useful in emergencies and transport.

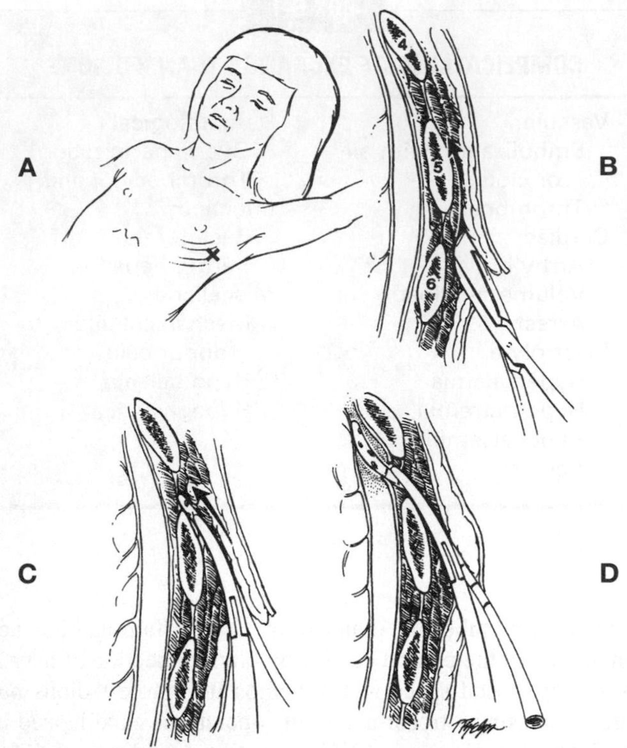

Fig. B-19 Steps in chest tube placement. **A,** Sterile prep and local anesthesia to the fifth intercostal space between the anterior and midaxillary line. **B,** Horizontal skin incision of 2 cm followed by blunt dissection with a hemostat just above the rib. **C,** Chest tube is clamped between the teeth of the hemostat and **D,** advanced into the pleural space. The incision then is closed and a dressing applied to stabilize the tube.

(From Nichols DG, et al, editors: *Golden hour: the handbook of advanced pediatric life support,* ed 2, St Louis, 1996, Mosby.)

Endotracheal Intubation

It is essential for every physician who cares for children to master endotracheal intubation. Several hazards commonly accompany this process; they are listed in Box B-2.

The key to success in intubation is approaching the procedure in a calm, deliberate way with a much-practiced technique and with equipment that is readily available and properly prepared. The equipment required for intubation is listed in Box B-3. A well-organized emergency tray, which is checked daily, is one of the most important items needed to perform this emergency procedure.

Preparation of the patient. Protection of the airway and adequate oxygenation guarantee safe and successful intubation. Medications undoubtedly will improve patient safety.[27] Intubation always should be accompanied by administration of atropine (0.01 to 0.02 mg/kg, with a maximum dose of 1 mg). Use of a muscle relaxant to reduce respiratory effort may be indicated. When used, it should be accompanied by sedation. Succinylcholine (1 to 2 mg/kg given intravenously) is preferred as a muscle relaxant because it is metabolized rapidly. Succinylcholine is contraindicated in patients with hyperkalemia, in patients with burn injuries, and patients with muscular diseases. Atracurium, 0.4 to 0.5 mg/kg is an alternative.

Methohexital (Brevital) may be given as a light anesthetic during intubation (1 to 2 mg/kg intravenously), but it should be used with caution in a patient whose cardiovascular system is compromised secondary to shock or cyanotic congenital heart disease.

Midazolam, 0.1 mg/kg., is a useful, quick-acting induction agent.

Emesis and subsequent aspiration are hazards encountered in emergency intubation. When the urgency of the situation does not allow for an anesthetist to be called, reasonable precautions can prevent complications.

Before any airway manipulation, a source of suction and a supply of suction catheters should be readily available. Downward pressure exerted on the cricoid cartilage effectively closes the esophagus and can prevent passive regurgitation and aspiration of oral or gastric material. This maneuver is crucial and is easily learned (Fig. B-20).

When possible, preoxygenation of the patient (3 minutes of breathing 100% oxygen) reduces complications. A pulse

BOX B-2

HAZARDS OF INTUBATION

- Hyperextension or hyperflexion of the neck
- Failure to clear the oropharynx of secretions
- Failure to ventilate the patient manually with mask oxygen before and after unsuccessful attempts
- Prolonged attempts, lasting longer than 30 seconds
- Intubation of the esophagus
- Intubation of the right main stem bronchus
- Faulty or unavailable equipment
- Haste

BOX B-3

EQUIPMENT REQUIRED FOR INTUBATION

- Laryngoscope handle: extra bulbs, batteries
- Blades: Miller, sizes 00, 0, 1, and 2
- Suction catheters: 5, 8, 10, 12, and 14 Fr
- Source of suction
- Endotracheal tubes: one size larger than deemed appropriate by age, one of adequate size, and one size smaller than deemed appropriate by age
- Sterile lubricant
- Oxygen supply
- Ventilator bag with 15-mm universal female adapter (Hope, Ambu, Ohio)
- Mask for ventilator bag: infant, child, and adult sizes
- Tape
- Tincture of benzoin
- Nasogastric tubes

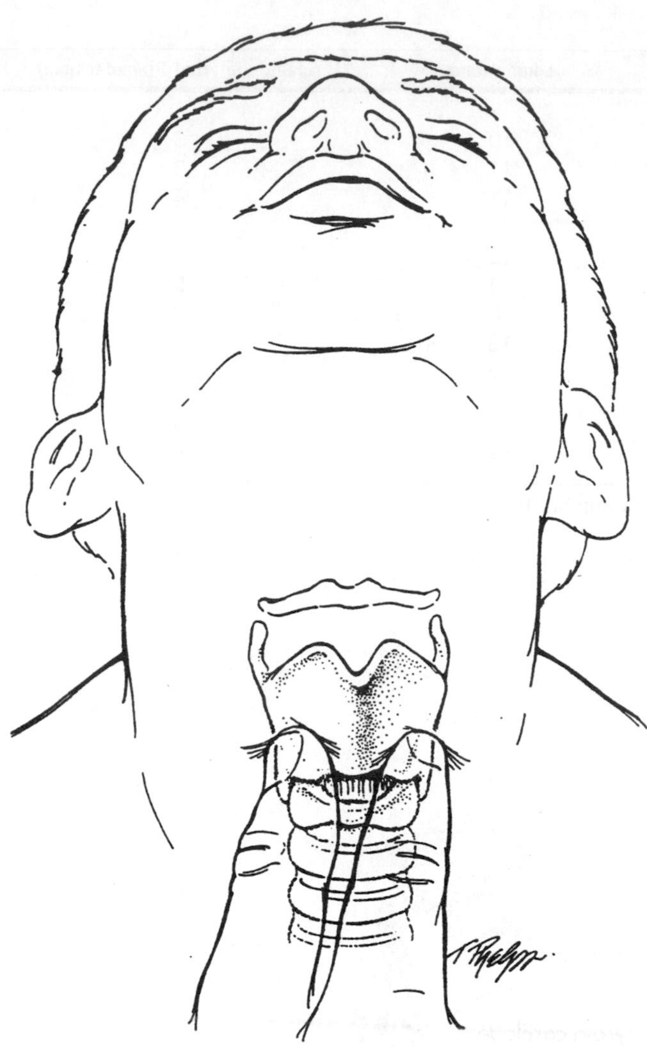

Fig. B-20 Cricoid pressure prior to intubation should be used to avoid passive regurgitation during sedation and intubation.

(From Nichols DG, Yaster M, Lappe DG, Haller JA: *Golden hour: the handbook of advanced pediatric life support,* ed 2, Mosby, St Louis, 1996.)

oximeter, ECG leads, and a blood pressure monitor should be placed if time allows.

Technique of intubation. During intubation, care must be taken to avoid damaging the teeth with the laryngoscope blade. Loose teeth should be removed. A straight laryngoscope blade may be easier to use for most pediatric practitioners; Portex or Murphy endotracheal tubes are recommended because they are uniform in diameter and biologically nonreactive. A slight air leak is to be expected with a tube of appropriate size. The recommended sizes, according to the patient's weight and age, are shown in Table B-1.

Fig. B-21 illustrates the relationship of the laryngoscope blade to the epiglottis and vocal cords. The endotracheal tube ideally should be positioned midway between the vocal cords and the carina. The patient should be placed on a firm surface with the head and neck extended. The neck is extended only slightly and the jaw pulled forward only slightly. The nose and mouth are suctioned gently, and the patient is given oxygen by bag and mask for no more than 1 minute. The laryngoscope is held in the left hand. The blade is introduced into the mouth to the right of the tongue so that the tongue will be deflected to the left. The tip of the blade is inserted to the vallecula. The handle of the laryngoscope is tilted slightly backward and upward toward the operator. Care must be taken not to use the teeth or alveolar ridge as a fulcrum. The vocal cords should be in view. The endotracheal tube can be advanced along the right side of the patient's mouth, inserted between the cords into the trachea, and advanced further to a position below the level of the vocal cords. Immediate auscultation of the lungs for symmetry of air movement is essential. If the right main stem bronchus is cannulated accidentally, the tube can be withdrawn to a safe position above the carina and checked again by auscultation. A chest roentgenogram should be obtained to ensure appropriate placement. The size, position of the tip of the tube in the trachea, and distance inserted from the patient's lip must be documented in the patient's record.[30]

Stabilizing the tube. Stabilizing the tube is subject to many variations. Fig. B-22 illustrates one method. Some common problems encountered include the following:

1. Increased extension or flexion of the neck causes the tube to move up and down the trachea; therefore, care must be taken to stabilize the position of the neck when handling the patient. The rule of thumb is that the tip of the endotracheal tube follows the chin up or down.
2. Using too much tape may prevent adequate nasal and oral suctioning, and inspection for leaks and kinks in the tube may be hampered.
3. Tincture of benzoin may spill into the eyes.

Postintubation care. The intubated infant or child requires exacting nursing care. The patient needs monitoring of vital signs and frequent physical examinations to ascertain the adequacy of ventilation. Pneumothorax, tube obstruction, and dislodgement of the tube must be anticipated in the care of these children.

Suctioning reduces tidal volume and available oxygen. It predisposes the patient to apnea and bradycardia. The physician and nurse should decide jointly how often suctioning should be done. Once an hour is a reasonable initial schedule. Suctioning of the tube is a nursing task primarily, but the physician should be aware of certain potential problems. The following is a safe method:

1. The endotracheal tube is disconnected from the ventilator.
2. Normal saline (0.25 to 0.5 ml) is instilled into the tube.
3. The infant receives ventilation for 60 seconds.
4. The head is turned to one side.
5. A sterile, end-hole catheter is passed a premeasured 1 to 2 cm beyond the tracheal tube's distal orifice.
6. Suction is applied after the catheter has been pulled back 1 cm.
7. Suction is applied as the catheter is withdrawn, over a 5-second interval.
8. The endotracheal tube is reconnected to the ventilator.
9. The head is turned to the opposite side, and the procedure is repeated.

Table B-1 Recommended Sizes of Endotracheal Tubes*

Patient's Age	No. (Fr)	Internal Diameter (mm)	Length (cm)	Adapter, Internal Diameter (mm)
Newborn				
<1 kg	11-12	2.5	10	3
>1 kg	13-14	3.0	11	3
1-6 mo	15-16	3.5	11	4
7-12 mo	17-18	4.0	12	4
13-18 mo	19-20	4.5	13	5
19-36 mo	21-22	5.0	14	5
3-4 yr	23-24	5.5	16	6
5 yr	25	6.0	18	6
6-7 yr	26	6.5	18	7
8-9 yr	27-28	7.0	20	7
10-11 yr	29-30	7.5	22	8
12-14 yr	32-34	8.0	24	8

*Tube should be of material labeled "I.T.-Z79" to satisfy standard tissue implant tests.

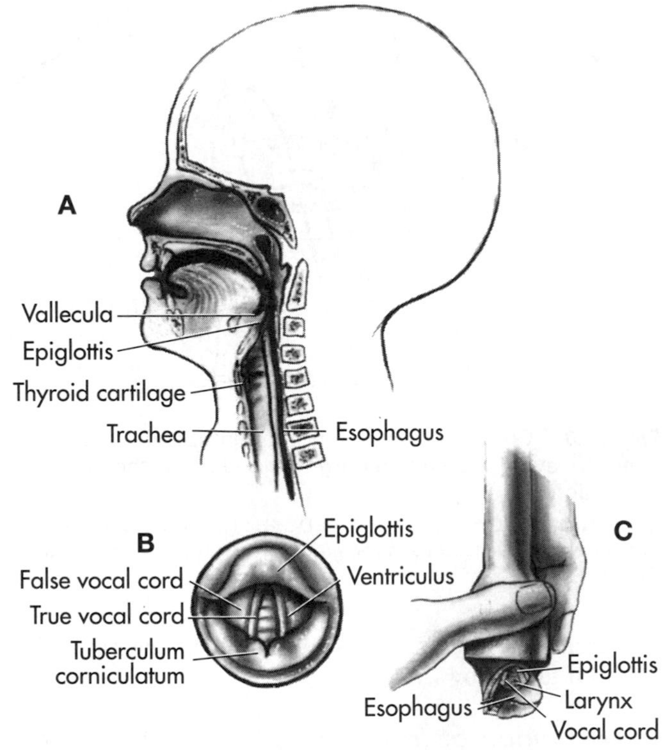

Fig. B-21 Endotracheal intubation. Relationship of the vallecula, the epiglottis, and the base of the tongue; note the cephalad position of the larynx in the infant, **A**; an older child's larynx is positioned more caudally. **B,** The laryngeal structures as viewed from above. **C,** The small size and relative position of the vocal cords, the epiglottis, and the larynx as viewed through the laryngoscope.

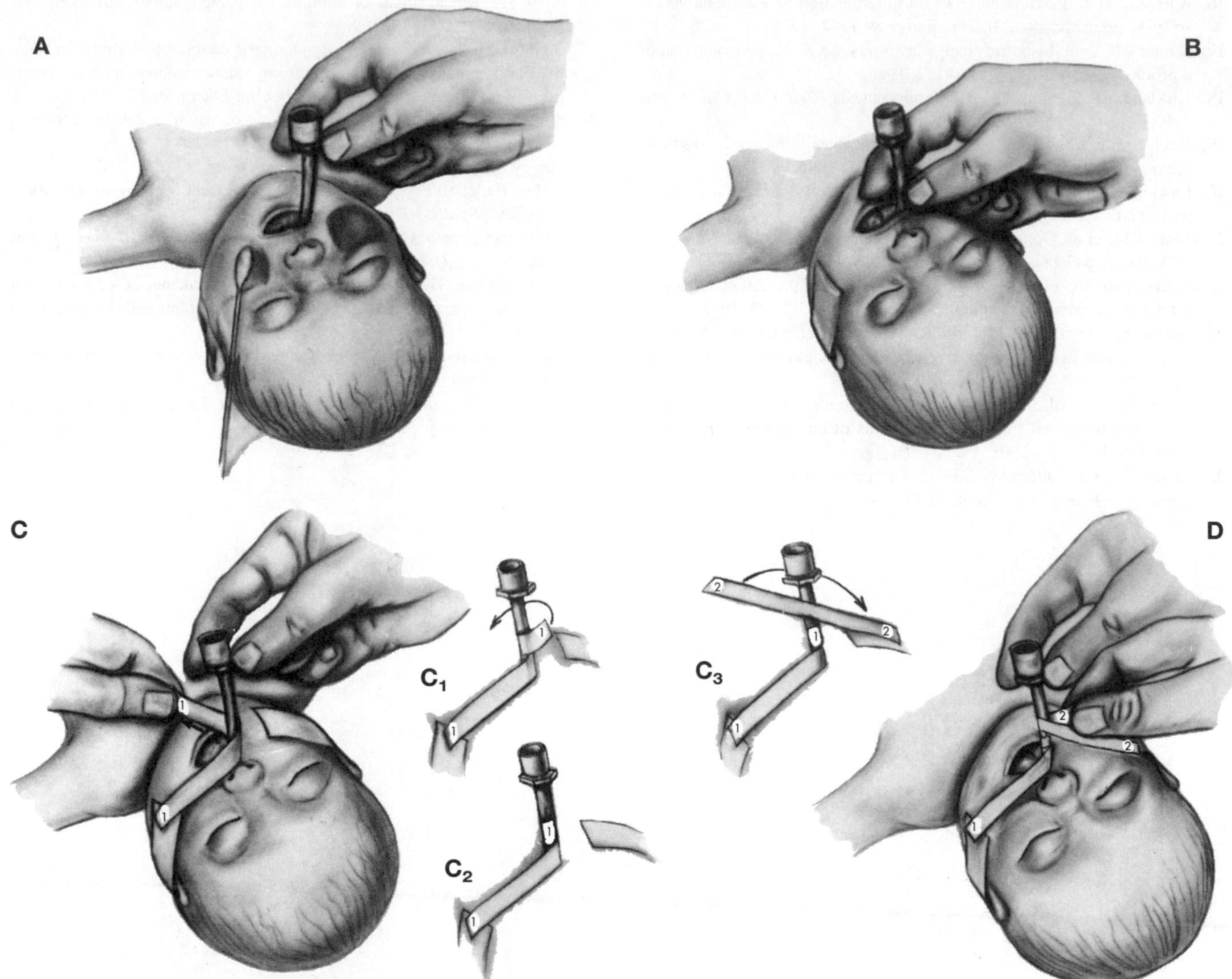

Fig. B-22 Securing an endotracheal tube. **A,** The cheeks and sides of the face are painted with tincture of benzoin (some neonatal intensive care units do not use benzoin because of its absorption and potential toxic effects). **B,** Wide pieces of elastic tape (Elastikon, Johnson & Johnson, New Brunswick, NJ) are placed over the sides of the face and pinnae. **C** to **C_2,** With the tube pulled to the right side of the mouth, a thin piece of tape *(1)* secures the tube on the left side of the face. **C_3** and **D,** Another piece of tape *(2)* then secures the tube on the right side of the face in a similar fashion.

REFERENCES

1. American Academy of Pediatrics, Committee on Drugs: Guidelines for monitoring and management of pediatric patients during and after sedation for diagnostic and therapeutic procedures, *Pediatrics* 89:1110, 1992.
2. American Society of Anesthesiology Report of Task Force on Management of the Difficult Airway, *Anesthesiology* 78:597, 1993.
3. Arnold JH, Truog RD: Sedation in neonatal and pediatric intensive care, *J Intensive Care Med* 7:244, 1992.
4. Barrone MA: Analgesia. In *The Harriet Lane Handbook*, ed 15, St Louis, 2000, Mosby.
5. Bauchner H: Procedures, pain, and parents: commentaries, *Pediatrics* 87:563, 1991.
6. Bauer C, Waner M: Laser-assisted myringotomy, *Curr Opin Otolaryngol Head Neck Surg* 7:335, 1999.
7. Butt W: Complications resulting from use of arterial catheters: retrograde flow and rapid elevation in blood pressure, *Pediatrics* 76:250, 1985.
8. Casado-Flores J, et al: Subclavian vein catheterization in critically ill children: analysis of 322 cannulations, *Int Care Med* 17:250, 1991.
9. Cohen D: Middle ear laser office ventilation (LOV) with a carbon dioxide laser flash scanner, *Med Surg* 16:107, 1998.
10. Coté CJ: Sedation protocols: why so many variations, *Pediatrics* 94: 281, 1994 (editorial).
11. Durbec O, et al: A prospective evaluation of the use of femoral venous catheters in critically ill adults, *Crit Care Med* 25:1986, 1997.
12. Hansen AR, Simmons CF: Management of the sick newborn. In Graef JW, editor: *Manual of pediatric therapeutics*, ed 6, Philadelphia, New York, 1977, Lippincott-Raven.
13. Hijazi OM, et al: Venous access and catheters. In Levin DL, Moriss FC, editors: *Essentials of pediatric intensive care*, ed 2, Edinburgh, 1997, Churchill-Livingston.
14. Iserson KV, Criss EA: Pediatric venous cutdowns: utility in emergency situations, *Pediatr Emerg Care* 2:231, 1986.
15. Joyce TH III: Topical anesthesia and pain management before venipuncture, *J Pediatr* 122:S24, 1993.

16. Kain ZN, et al: Parental presence during induction of anesthesia versus sedative premedication, *Anesthesiology* 89:1147, 1998.
17. Kanter RK, et al: Pediatric emergency intravenous access: evaluation of a protocol, *Am J Dis Child* 140:132, 1986.
18. Kirkland LL, Taylor RW: Pericardiocentesis, *Crit Care Clin* 8:699, 1992.
19. Koch SM, et al: Arterial blood sampling devices influence ionized calcium measurements, *Crit Care Med* 23:1825, 1995.
20. Lawless S, et al: New pigtail catheter for pleural drainage in pediatric patients, *Crit Care Med* 17:173,1989.
21. Marx CM, et al: Optimal sedation of mechanically ventilated pediatric critical care patients, *Crit Care Med* 22:163, 1994.
22. Mellampati SR, et al: A clinical sign to predict the difficult tracheal intubation: a prospective study, *Can Anesth Soc J* 32:429, 1985.
23. Napoli KL, Ingall CG, Martin GR: Safety and efficacy of chloral hydrate sedation in children undergoing echocardiography, *J Pediatr* 129: 287, 1996.
24. Orlowski JP, et al: Comparison study of intraosseous, central intravenous, and peripheral intravenous infusions of emergency drugs, *Am J Dis Child* 144:112, 1990.
25. Rosetti V, et al: Difficulty and delay in intravenous access in pediatric arrest, *Ann Emerg Med* 13:406, 1984.
26. Sahn SA: Management of complicated parapneumonic effusions, *Am Rev Resp Dis* 148:813, 1993.
27. Sivilotti MLA, Ducharme J: Randomized double-blind study on sedatives and hemodynamics during rapid-sequence intubation in the emergency department: the SHRED study, *Ann Emerg Med* 31:313, 1998.
28. Smith-Wright DL, et al: Complications of vascular catheterization in critically ill children, *Crit Care Med* 12:1015, 1984.
29. Spivey WH: Intraosseous infusions, *J Pediatr* 111:639, 1987.
30. Todres ID, et al: Endotracheal tube displacement in the newborn infant, *J Pediatr* 89:126, 1976.
31. US Pharmacopeia: Chloral hydrate overdoses result in children's deaths, *Drug Produce Quality Rev* 33, 1993.
32. Venkataraman ST, Orr RA, Thompson AE: Percutaneous infraclavicular subclavian vein catheterization in critically ill infants and children, *J Pediatr* 113:480, 1988.
33. Vidal R, Kissoon N, Gayle M: Compartment syndrome following intraosseous infusion, *Pediatrics* 91:1201, 1993.
34. Yaster M: The management of acute pain in children with a local anesthetic: a primer for the nonanesthesiologist, *Compr Ther* 15:14, 1989.

C Miscellaneous Values

Kathleen A. Woodin

BONE AGE

Sontag Method

The Sontag method is used to evaluate the skeletal development of children from 1 to 60 months of age:

1. Roentgenograms are taken of all epiphyseal centers on the left side of the body: shoulder, elbow, wrist and hand, hip, knee (anteroposterior [AP] views before 24 months of age, lateral views after 24 months), and ankle and foot (AP views before 48 months of age, lateral views after 48 months).
2. All ossification centers in the left half of the body are counted. A center is counted as soon as it casts any shadow on the roentgenogram.
3. The number of ossification centers is compared with normal values for the patient's age (Table C-1).

Gruelich and Pyle Method

The Gruelich and Pyle method is used to evaluate the skeletal development of girls from 5 to 18 years of age and for boys from 5 to 19 years:

1. A roentgenogram is taken of the left hand and wrist.
2. Calculation of the skeletal development is based on the order of appearance and maturation of the epiphyseal centers. (For normal values, see Gruelich and Pyle's *Radiographic Atlas of Skeletal Development of the Hand and Wrist.*[1])

DETERMINATION OF BODY SURFACE AREA

Based on the nomogram shown in Fig. C-1, a straight line joining the patient's height and weight will intersect the center column at the calculated body surface area (BSA).

CONVERSION FORMULAS

Height (Length)

1 millimeter (mm) = 0.04 inch
1 centimeter = 0.4 inch
2.54 centimeters = 1 inch
1 meter (m) = 39.37 inches

Weight

60 milligrams (mg) = 1 grain
28.35 grams (g) = 1 ounce
454 grams = 1 pound
1000 grams (1 kilogram [kg]) = 2.2 pounds

Table C-1 Mean Total Number of Centers on the Left Side of Body Ossified at Given Age Levels

	Boys		Girls	
Age (mo)	Mean	SD*	Mean	SD
1	4.11	1.41	4.58	1.76
3	6.63	1.86	7.78	2.16
6	9.61	1.95	11.44	2.53
9	11.88	2.66	15.36	4.92
12	13.96	3.96	22.40	6.93
18	19.27	6.61	34.10	8.44
24	29.21	8.10	43.44	6.65
30	37.59	7.40	48.91	6.50
36	43.42	5.34	52.73	5.48
42	47.06	5.26	56.61	3.98
48	51.24	4.59	57.94	3.91
54	53.94	4.35	59.89	3.36
60	56.24	4.07	61.52	2.69

From Sontag LW, Snell D, Anderson M: *Am J Dis Child* 58:949, 1939.
**SD,* Standard deviation.

Milligram-Milliequivalent Conversions

mEq/L = mg/L × Valence/Atomic weight
mg/L = mEq/L × Atomic weight/Valence
Equivalent weight = Atomic weight/Valence

Milliosmols

The milliequivalent (mEq) is roughly equivalent to the milliosmol (mOsm), the unit of measure of osmolarity or tonicity.

Prefixes for Decimal Factors

Prefix	Symbol	Factor
mega	m	10^6
kilo	k	10^3
hecto	h	10^2
deka	da	10^1
deci	d	10^{-1}
centi	c	10^{-2}
milli	m	10^{-3}
micro	μ	10^{-6}
nano	n	10^{-9}
pico	p	10^{-12}
femto	f	10^{-15}

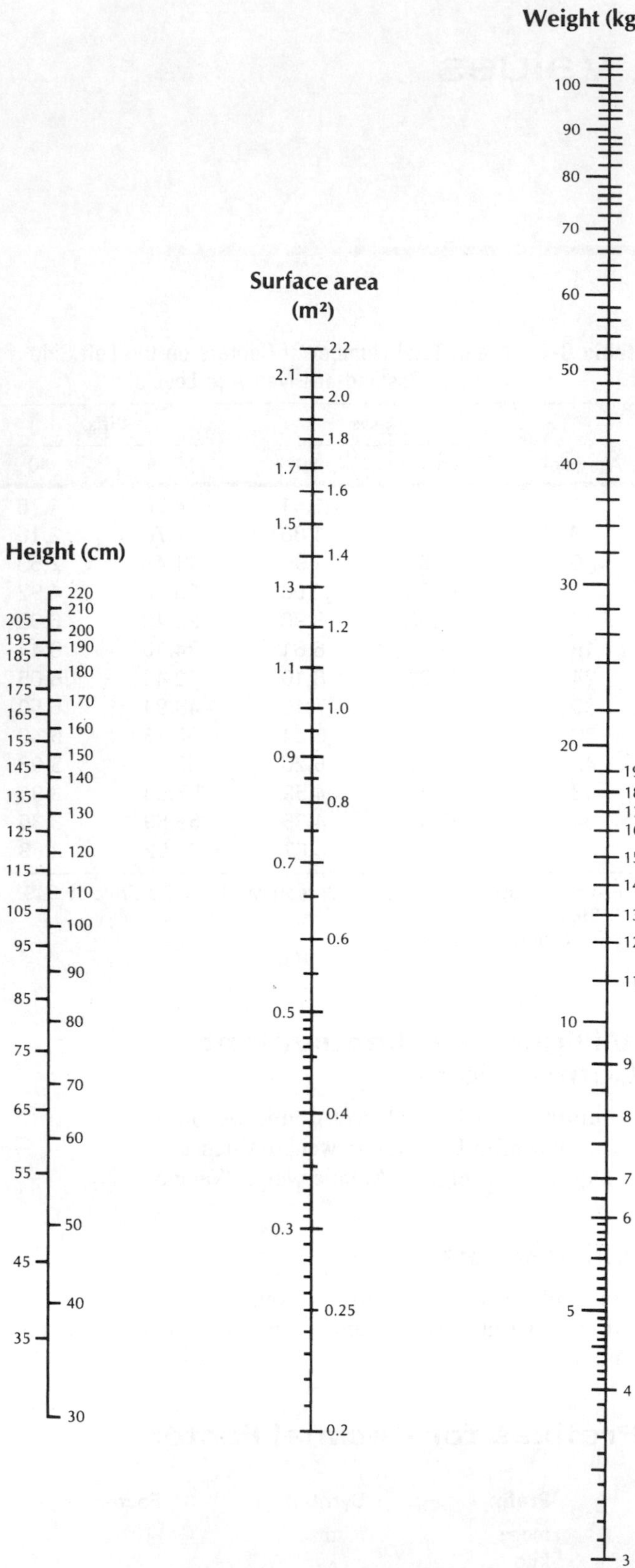

Fig. C-1 Nomogram to determine body surface area.

(Redrawn from Cole CH, editor: *The Harriet Lane handbook,* ed 10, Chicago, 1984, Mosby. Based on data from Gelian EA, George SL: *Cancer Chemother Rep* 54:225, 1970.)

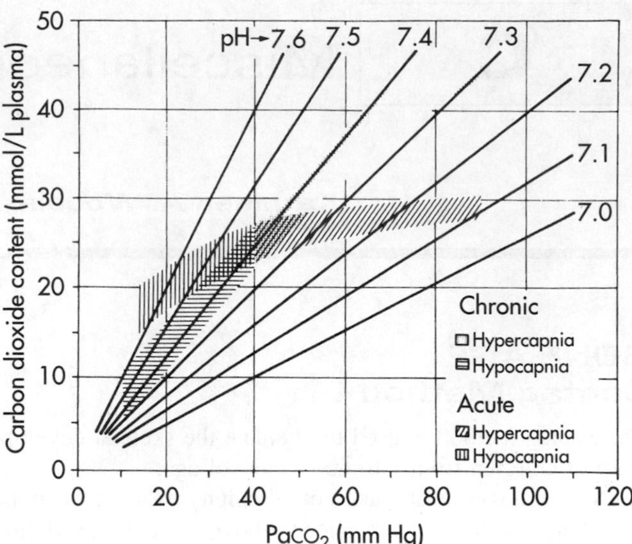

Fig. C-2 Acid-base response in respiratory acidosis and alkalosis.

(Modified from Arbus GS: *Can Med Assoc J* 109:291, 1973.)

ACID-BASE RESPONSE IN RESPIRATORY ACIDOSIS AND ALKALOSIS

The nomogram in Fig. C-2 shows confidence bands for the normal adjustment in carbon dioxide content and pH made to accommodate acute and chronic changes in arterial PCO_2.

1. The pH is determined on the nomogram from the plotted $PaCO_2$ and carbon dioxide content obtained from blood gas measurements.
2. If the pH value is not within confidence bands, the change in carbon dioxide content and pH is different from that expected from a pure respiratory condition; thus a metabolic abnormality also is present.
3. To estimate the effect of acute and chronic changes in PCO_2 on pH, the following formulas are used:
   Acute change in PCO_2: $(\Delta\ PCO_2)\ (0.008) = \Delta$ pH
   Chronic change in PCO_2: $(\Delta D\ PCO_2)\ (0.003) = \Delta$ pH

REFERENCE

1. Gruelich WW, Pyle SI: *Radiographic atlas of skeletal development of the hand and wrist,* San Francisco, 1974, Stanford University Press.

SUGGESTED READINGS

Normal laboratory values (case records of the Massachusetts General Hospital), *N Engl J Med* 314:39, 1986.

Queen PM, Wilson SE: Growth and nutrient requirements of infants. In Grand RJ, Sutphen JL, Dietz WH, editors: *Pediatric nutrition: theory and practice,* Boston, 1987, Butterworth.

Tietz NW, editor: *Clinical guide to laboratory tests,* Philadelphia, 1983, WB Saunders.

Young SD: Normal laboratory values in SI units, *N Engl J Med* 292:795, 1975.

Table C-2 Cerebrospinal Fluid

	Mean	Range	Polymorphonuclear Cells
Cell Count*			
Preterm newborn	9.0	0-29	57%
Term newborn	8.2	0-32	61%
Child (>1 mo)		0-6	
Glucose			
Preterm newborn	50 mg/dl	24-63 mg/dl	
Term newborn	52 mg/dl	34-119 mg/dl	
Child		40-80 mg/dl	
Pressure, Opening			
Newborn	<110 mm H_2O		
Child	<200 mm H_2O		
Protein			
Preterm newborn	115 mg/dl	65-150 mg/dl	
Term newborn	90 mg/dl	20-170 mg/dl	
Child		5-40 mg/dl	
Volume			
Child	60-100 ml		
Adult	100-160 ml		

Data from Klein JO, Feigin RD, McCracken GH: *Pediatrics* 78(suppl):959, 1986; Portnoy JM, Olson LC: *Pediatrics* 75:484, 1985; Sarff LD, Platt LH, McCracken GH: *J Pediatr* 88:473, 1976.
*Traumatic lumbar punctures (>1000 red blood cells/mm^3) are uninterpretable because correction formulas may underestimate the true white blood cell count.

Table C-3 Synovial Fluid Analysis

	Cells Per Microliter (µl)	Polymorphonuclear Leukocytes (PMNL)	Glucose (mg/dl)	Mucin Clot	Protein (mg/dl)
Normal	50-200	<5%	>80	Good	1.8
Inflammatory*					
Bacterial	>10,000	>90%	<50	Poor	>4
Nonseptic	<10,000	<90%	50-80	Poor	2-4

Modified from Rudy P, DuPont HL: Infectious arthritis. In Pickering LK, DuPont HL, editors: *Infectious diseases of children and adults,* Menlo Park, Calif, 1986, Addison-Wesley.
*Fluid should be evaluated for the presence of urate crystals that occur in gout and pseudogout.

Table C-4 Clinical Chemistry

Determination	Standard Units	Factor	SI Units
Alanine aminotransferase (ALT or SGPT)			
Infant	5-54 U/L	NA*	NA
Child	3-37 U/L	NA	NA
Adult	8-45 U/L	NA	NA
Aldolase			
Newborn	5.2-32.8 U/L	1.00	5.2-32.8 U/L
Child	2.6-16.4 U/L	1.00	2.6-16.4 U/L
Adult	1.3-8.2 U/L	1.00	1.3-8.2 U/L
Alkaline phosphatase			
Newborn	35-213 U/L	1.00	35-213 U/L
Child	71-142 U/L	1.00	71-142 U/L
Adolescent	106-213 U/L	1.00	106-213 U/L
Adult	32-92 U/L	1.00	32-92 U/L
Ammonia	15-49 μg/dl	0.7333	11-35 μmol/L
Amylase			
Serum	60-160 U/dl	NA	NA
Urine	17-200 U/dl	NA	NA
Aspartate aminotransferase (AST or SGOT)			
Newborn	25-75 U/L	NA	NA
Infant	15-60 U/L	NA	NA
Child	20-50 U/L	NA	NA
Adult	8-40 U/L	NA	NA
Bicarbonate	18-25 mEq/L	1.00	8-25 mmol/L
Bilirubin (>1 mo)			
Total	<0.2-1.0 mg/dl	17.10	<3.4 μmol/L
Direct	<0.2 mg/dl	17.10	<3.4-17.1 μmol/L
Calcium			
Total	8.8-10.8 mg/dl	0.2495	2.20-2.70 mmol/L
Ionized	4.48-4.92 mg/dl	0.2495	1.12-1.23 mmol/L
Carotene			
Infant	20-70 μg/dl	0.0186	0.37-1.30 μmol/L
Adult	40-130 μg/dl	0.0186	0.74-2.42 μmol/L
Child	60-200 μg/dl	0.0186	1.12-3.72 μmol/L
Chloride	98-106 mEq/L	1.00	98-106 mmol/L
Cholesterol, fasting			
Newborn	53-135 mg/dl	0.0259	1.37-3.50 mmol/L
Infant	70-175 mg/dl	0.0259	1.81-4.53 mmol/L
Child	120-200 mg/dl	0.0259	3.11-5.18 mmol/L
Adolescent	120-210 mg/dl	0.0259	3.11-5.44 mmol/L
Adult	140-250 mg/dl	0.0259	3.63-6.48 mmol/L
Copper			
Infant	20-70 μg/dl	0.1574	3.14-10.99 μmol/L
Child	90-190 μg/dl	0.1574	14.13-29.83 μmol/L
Adolescent	80-160 μg/dl	0.1574	12.56-25.12 μmol/L
Adult	70-155 μg/dl	0.1574	10.99-24.34 μmol/L
Creatinine			
Newborn	0.8-1.4 mg/dl	88.4	70.7-123.8 μmol/L
Infant	0.7-1.7 mg/dl	88.4	61.9-150.3 μmol/L
Adult	0.6-1.5 mg/dl	88.4	53-133 μmol/L
Creatinine kinase			
Female	10-55 U/L	1.00	10-55 U/L
Male	12-80 U/L	1.00	12-80 U/L
Glucose	55-100 mg/dl	0.05551	3.055-5.55 mmol/L

**NA,* Not available or not applicable.

Table C-4 Clinical Chemistry—cont'd

Determination	Standard Units	Factor	SI Units
Haptoglobin	40-336 mg/dl	0.01	0.4-3.36 g/L
Iron, serum			
Newborn	100-250 μg/dl	0.1791	17.90-44.75 μmol/L
Infant	40-100 μg/dl	0.1791	7.16-17.90 μmol/L
Child	50-120 μg/dl	0.1791	8.95-21.48 μmol/L
Adult	40-160 μg/dl	0.1791	7.16-28.64 μmol/L
Iron-binding capacity, total (TIBC)			
Infant	100-400 μg/dl	0.1791	17.90-71.60 μmol/L
Child	250-400 μg/dl	0.1791	44.75-71.60 μmol/L
Adult	250-400 μg/dl	0.1791	44.75-71.60 μmol/L
Lactate	0.6-1.8 mEq/L	1.00	0.6-1.8 mmol/L
Lactic dehydrogenase			
Newborn	160-450 U/L	NA	NA
Infant	100-250 U/L	NA	NA
Child	60-170 U/L	NA	NA
Adult	45-90 U/L	NA	NA
Lead (child)	<10 μg/dl	0.0483	<0.48 μmol/L
Lipids			
Phospholipids	180-295 mg/dl	0.01	1.8-2.95 g/L
Triglycerides	40-150 mg/dl	0.01	0.4-1.5 g/L
Lipoprotein, HDL	150-330 mg/dl	0.01	1.5-3.3 g/L
Lipoprotein, LDL	28%-53% total		
Magnesium			
Newborn	1.0-1.8 mEq/L	0.5	0.5-0.9 mmol/L
Child	1.5-2.0 mEq/L	0.5	0.8-1.0 mmol/L
Osmolarity	275-295 mOsm/kg	1.00	275-295 mmol/kg
pH (arterial)	7.35-7.45	1.00	7.35-7.45
PCO_2	35-45 mm Hg	0.1333	4.7-6.0 kPa
PO_2	83-108 mm Hg	0.1333	11.04-14.36 kPa
Phosphorus, inorganic			
Newborn	5.5-9.5 mg/dl	0.3229	1.78-3.07 mmol/L
Infant	4.5-6.5 mg/dl	0.3229	1.45-2.10 mmol/L
Child	4.5-5.5 mg/dl	0.3229	1.45-1.78 mmol/L
Adult	2.7-4.5 mg/dl	0.3229	0.87-1.45 mmol/L
Potassium	3.5-5.1 mEq/L	1.00	3.5-5.1 mmol/L
Proteins (NOTE: Globulin = Total protein – Albumin)			
Albumin/total protein			
Newborn	2.4-4.8/4.6-7.0 g/dl	10.0	24-48/46-70 g/L
Infant	3.0-4.5/5.1-7.3 g/dl	10.0	30-45/51-73 g/L
Child	3.8-5.6/6.0-8.0 g/dl	10.0	38-56/60-80 g/L
Adult	3.5-5.5/6.4-8.3 g/dl	10.0	35-55/64-83 g/L
Sodium	136-145 mEq/L	1.00	136-145 mmol/L
Urea nitrogen			
Newborn	4-12 mg/dl	0.3569	1.4-4.3 mmol/L
Child/adult	5-18 mg/dl	0.3569	1.8-6.4 mmol/L
Uric acid	3.0-7.0 mg/dl	0.0595	0.18-0.42 mmol/L
Vitamin A	30-80 μg/dl	0.0349	1.05-2.79 μmol/L
Vitamin E (tocopherol)	0.5-2.0 mg/dl	23.22	11.6-46.4 μmol/L

Table C-5 Newborn Clinical Chemistry

Determination*	Cord Sample†	Capillary Samples† 1-12 hr	12-24 hr	24-48 hr	48-72 hr
Sodium (mmol/L)	147 (126-166)	143 (124-156)	145 (132-159)	148 (134-160)	149 (139-162)
Potassium (mmol/L)	7.8 (5.6-12)	6.4 (5.3-7.3)	6.3 (5.3-8.9)	6.0 (5.2-7.3)	5.9 (5.0-7.7)
Chloride (mmol/L)	103 (98-110)	100.7 (90-111)	103 (87-114)	102 (92-114)	103 (93-112)
Calcium (mg/dl)	9.3 (8.2-11.1)	8.4 (7.3-9.2)	7.8 (6.9-9.4)	8.0 (6.1-9.9)	7.9 (5.9-9.7)
Phosphorus (mg/dl)	5.6 (3.7-8.1)	6.1 (3.5-8.6)	5.7 (2.9-8.1)	5.9 (3.0-8.7)	5.8 (2.8-7.6)
Blood urea (mg/dl)	29 (21-40)	27 (8-34)	33 (9-63)	32 (13-77)	31 (13-68)
Total protein (g/dl)	6.1 (4.8-7.3)	6.6 (5.6-8.5)	6.6 (5.8-8.2)	6.9 (5.9-8.2)	7.2 (6.0-8.5)
Glucose (mg/dl)	73 (45-96)	63 (40-97)	63 (42-104)	56 (30-91)	59 (40-90)
Lactic acid (mg/dl)	19.5 (11-30)	14.6 (11-24)	14 (10-23)	14.3 (9-22)	13.5 (7-21)
Lactate (mmol/L)‡	2.0-3.0	2.0			

Modified from Avery GB: *Neonatology, pathophysiology and management in the newborn,* ed 3, Philadelphia, 1987, JB Lippincott.
*Acharya PT, Payne WW: *Arch Dis Child* 40:430, 1965.
†Numbers in parentheses indicate a normal range.
‡Daniel SS, Adamsons K Jr, James LS: *Pediatrics* 37:942, 1966.

Table C-6 Hematology

Age	Hemoglobin (grams %): Mean (−2 SD)	Hematocrit (%) Mean (−2 SD)	Mean Cell Volume (Fluid) Mean (−2 SD)	Mean Corpuscular Hemoglobin Concentration (grams/% RBC) Mean (−2 SD)	Reticulocytes (%)	WBC/mm^3 × 100 Mean (−2 SD)	Platelets (10^3 mm^3) Mean ±2 SD)
26-30 wk gestation*	13.4 (11)	41.5 (34.9)	118.2 (106.7)	37.9 (30.6)	—	4.4 (2.7)	254 (180-327)
28 wk	14.5	45	120	31	(5-10)	—	275
32 wk	15.0	47	118	32	(3-10)	—	290
Term† (cord)	16.5 (13.5)	51 (42)	108 (98)	33 (30)	(3-7)	18.1 (9-30)‡	290
1-3 days	18.5 (14.5)	56 (45)	108 (95)	33 (29)	(1.8-4.6)	18.9 (9.4-34)	192
2 wk	16.6 (13.4)	53 (41)	105 (88)	31.4 (28.1)		11.4 (5-20)	252
1 mo	13.9 (10.7)	44 (33)	101 (91)	31.8 (28.1)	(0.1-1.7)	10.8 (4-19.5)	
2 mo	11.2 (9.4)	35 (28)	95 (84)	31.8 (28.3)			
6 mo	12.6 (11.1)	36 (31)	76 (68)	35 (32.7)	(0.7-2.3)	11.9 (6-17.5)	
6 mo-2 yr	12.0 (10.5)	36 (33)	78 (70)	33 (30)		10.6 (6-17)	(150-350)
2-6 yr	12.5 (11.5)	37 (34)	81 (75)	34 (31)	(0.5-1.0)	8.5 (5-15.5)	(150-350)
6-12 yr	13.5 (11.5)	40 (35)	86 (77)	34 (31)	(0.5-1.0)	8.1 (4.5-13.5)	(150-350)
12-18 yr							
Male	14.5 (13)	43 (36)	88 (78)	34 (31)	(0.5-1.0)	7.8 (4.5-13.5)	(150-350)
Female	14.0 (12)	41 (37)	90 (78)	34 (31)	(0.5-1.0)	7.8 (4.5-13.5)	(150-350)
Adult							
Male	15.5 (13.5)	47 (41)	90 (80)	34 (31)	(0.8-2.5)	7.4 (4.5-11)	(150-350)
Female	14.0 (12)	41 (36)	90 (80)	34 (31)	(0.8-4.1)	7.4 (4.5-11)	(150-350)

Modified from Siberry GK, Iannone R, editors: *The Harriet Lane handbook*, ed 15, St Louis, 2000, Mosby.
*Values are from fetal samplings.
†Under 1 mo of age, capillary hemoglobin exceeds venous hemoglobin: age 1 hr—by 3.6 g; age 5 days—by 2.2 g; age 3 wk—by 1.1 g.
‡Mean (95% confidence limits.)

Table C-7 Conversion of Centimeters to Inches

cm	in	cm	in	cm	in	cm	in
1	0.39	51	20.08	101	39.76	151	59.45
2	0.79	52	20.47	102	40.16	152	59.84
3	1.18	53	20.87	103	40.55	153	60.24
4	1.57	54	21.26	104	40.94	154	60.63
5	1.97	55	21.65	105	41.34	155	61.02
6	2.36	56	22.05	106	41.73	156	61.42
7	2.76	57	22.44	107	42.13	157	61.81
8	3.15	58	22.83	108	42.52	158	62.20
9	3.54	59	23.23	109	42.91	159	62.60
10	3.94	60	23.62	110	43.31	160	62.99
11	4.33	61	24.02	111	43.70	161	63.39
12	4.72	62	24.41	112	44.09	162	63.78
13	5.12	63	24.80	113	44.49	163	64.17
14	5.51	64	25.20	114	44.88	164	64.57
15	5.91	65	25.59	115	45.28	165	64.96
16	6.30	66	25.98	116	45.67	166	65.35
17	6.69	67	26.38	117	46.06	167	65.75
18	7.09	68	26.78	118	46.46	168	66.14
19	7.48	69	27.17	119	46.85	169	66.54
20	7.87	70	27.56	120	47.24	170	66.93
21	8.27	71	27.95	121	47.64	171	67.32
22	8.66	72	28.35	122	48.03	172	67.72
23	9.06	73	28.74	123	48.43	173	68.11
24	9.45	74	29.13	124	48.82	174	68.50
25	9.84	75	29.53	125	49.21	175	68.90
26	10.24	76	29.92	126	49.61	176	69.29
27	10.63	77	30.31	127	50.00	177	69.68
28	11.02	78	30.71	128	50.39	178	70.08
29	11.42	79	31.10	129	50.79	179	70.47
30	11.81	80	31.50	130	51.18	180	70.87
31	12.20	81	31.89	131	51.57	181	71.26
32	12.60	82	32.28	132	51.97	182	71.65
33	13.00	83	32.68	133	52.36	183	72.05
34	13.39	84	33.07	134	52.76	184	72.44
35	13.78	85	33.46	135	53.15	185	72.83
36	14.17	86	33.86	136	53.54	186	73.23
37	14.57	87	34.25	137	53.94	187	73.62
38	14.96	88	34.65	138	54.33	188	74.02
39	15.35	89	35.04	139	54.72	189	74.41
40	15.75	90	35.43	140	55.12	190	74.80
41	16.14	91	35.83	141	55.51	191	75.20
42	16.54	92	36.22	142	55.91	192	75.59
43	16.93	93	36.61	143	56.30	193	75.98
44	17.32	94	37.01	144	56.69	194	76.38
45	17.72	95	37.40	145	57.09	195	76.77
46	18.11	96	37.80	146	57.48	196	77.17
47	18.50	97	38.19	147	57.87	197	77.56
48	18.90	98	38.58	148	58.27	198	77.95
49	19.29	99	38.98	149	58.66	199	78.35
50	19.69	100	39.37	150	59.06	200	78.74

Table C-8 Conversion of Pounds to Grams

	1 lb	2 lb	3 lb	4 lb	5 lb	6 lb	7 lb	8 lb
Ounces	**Grams**							
0	454	907	1361	1814	2268	2722	3175	3629
1	482	936	1389	1843	2296	2750	3204	3657
2	510	964	1418	1871	2325	2778	3232	3686
3	539	992	1446	1899	2353	2807	3260	3714
4	567	1021	1474	1928	2381	2835	3289	3742
5	595	1049	1503	1956	2410	2863	3317	3771
6	624	1077	1531	1985	2438	2892	3345	3799
7	652	1106	1559	2013	2466	2920	3374	3827
8	680	1134	1588	2041	2495	2948	3402	3856
9	709	1162	1616	2070	2523	2977	3430	3884
10	737	1191	1644	2098	2552	3005	3459	3912
11	765	1219	1673	2126	2580	3033	3487	3941
12	794	1247	1701	2155	2608	3062	3515	3969
13	822	1276	1729	2183	2637	3090	3544	3997
14	851	1304	1758	2211	2665	3119	3572	4026
15	879	1332	1786	2240	2693	3147	3600	4054

Table C-9 Temperature Equivalents

Celsius*	Fahrenheit†	Celsius*	Fahrenheit†
34.0	93.2	38.6	101.4
34.2	93.6	38.8	101.8
34.4	93.9	39.0	102.2
34.6	94.3	39.2	102.5
34.8	94.6	39.4	102.9
35.0	95.0	39.6	103.2
35.2	95.4	39.8	103.6
35.4	95.7	40.0	104.0
35.6	96.1	40.2	104.3
35.8	96.4	40.4	104.7
36.0	96.8	40.6	105.1
36.2	97.1	40.8	105.4
36.4	97.5	41.0	105.8
36.6	97.8	41.2	106.1
36.8	98.2	41.4	106.5
37.0	98.6	41.6	106.8
37.2	98.9	41.8	107.2
37.4	99.3	42.0	107.6
37.6	99.6	42.2	108.0
37.8	100.0	42.4	108.3
38.0	100.4	42.6	108.7
38.2	100.7	42.8	109.0
38.4	101.1	43.0	109.4

*To convert Celsius to Fahrenheit: $\frac{9}{5}$ × (Temperature) + 32).
†To convert Fahrenheit to Celsius: $\frac{5}{9}$ × (Temperature) − 32).

Table C-10 Laboratory Parameters of Acid-Base Disturbances*

	pH	Arterial Carbon Dioxide Pressure ($Paco_2$)	Bicarbonate (HCO_3^-) (mEq/L)	Carbon Dioxide (CO_2) Content (mEq/L)
Normal values	7.35-7.45	35-45	24-26	25-28
Disturbances				
Metabolic acidosis	↓	↓	↓	↓
Acute respiratory acidosis	↓	↑	↔	Slight ↑
Compensated respiratory acidosis	↔ or slight ↓	↑	↑	↑
Metabolic alkalosis	↑	Slight ↑	↑	↑
Acute respiratory alkalosis	↑	↓	↔	Slight ↓
Compensated respiratory alkalosis	↔ or slight ↑	↓	↓	↓

*Values obtained by arteriolized capillary blood or direct arterial puncture.

Table C-11 Carbohydrate Content of Formulas

	Lactose	Sucrose and Glucose Polymers	Glucose Polymers	Minimal Carbohydrate
Common ingredient names		See glucose polymers	Glucose polymers Maltodextrins Corn syrup solids Modified tapioca starch	
Comments	Requires lactase enzyme for digestion Contraindicated in galactosemia	Requires sucrase enzyme for digestion (see also glucose polymers)	Easily digested For individuals with lactose malabsorption	For severe carbohydrate intolerance
Infants	Enfamil Enfamil 22* Enfamil AR Enfamil Premature Carnation Follow-up Carnation Good Start Neosure* Similac Similac PM 60/40 Similac Special Care	Alimentum Alsoy Isomil Isomil DF (Fiber) Portagen	Isomil SF Lactofree Neocate Nutramigen Pregestimil ProSobee Similac Lactose Free	MJ3232A RCF
Toddlers and young children	Next Step*	Compleat Pediatric† Kindercal (Fiber) Neocate One Plus Next Step Soy Nutren Junior PediaSure (also w/Fiber) Peptamen Junior ProPeptide for Kids Resource Just for Kids	Vivonex Pediatric L-Emental Pediatric	
Older children and adolescents	Carnation Instant Breakfast Scandishake	All other formulas in Table C-17	Criticare HN Deliver 2.0 Glucerna Isocal Jevity (fiber) L-Emental L-Emental Plus Peptamen PropPeptide Tolerex Vivonex TEN Vivonex Plus	

*Also contains glucose polymers.
†Also contains fruit and vegetable purees.
From Siberry GK, Iannone R, editors: *The Harriet Lane handbook,* ed 15, St Louis, 2000, Mosby.

Table C-12 Protein Content of Formulas

	Cow's Milk	Soy	Hydrolysate	Free Amino Acids
Common ingredient names	Cow's milk protein Nonfat milk Demineralized whey Reduced mineral whey Sodium, calcium, magnesium caseinate Casein	Soy protein Soy protein isolate	Casein hydrolysate Hydrolyzed whey, meat, and soy	—
Comments	Requires normal protein digestion and absorption	Requires normal protein digestion and absorption Not recommended for premature infants or those with cystic fibrosis	For individuals with protein allergy and/or malabsorption	For individuals with severe protein allergy and/or severe protein malabsorption
Infants	Enfamil Enfamil 22 Enfamil AR Follow-up Lactofree Neosure Portagen Enfamil Premature Similac Similac PM 60/40 Similac Special Care Similac Lactose Free	Alsoy Follow-up Soy Isomil Isomil DF ProSobee RCF	Alimentum Good Start Nutramigen Pregestimil MJ3232A	Neocate
Toddlers and young children	Compleat Pediatric* Resource Just for Kids Kindercal Next Step Nutren Junior PediaSure	Next Step Soy	Peptamen Junior Pro-Peptide for Kids	Vivonex Pediatric Neocate One Plus EleCare L-Emental Pediatric
Older children and adolescents	All other formulas in Table C-17	Ensure† Ensure with Fiber† Isocal† Osmolite† Promote† Sustacal† Boost High-Protein† Boost with Fiber†	Criticare HN Peptamen Vital HN ProPeptide	Tolerex Vivonex TEN Vivonex Plus L-Emental L-Emental Plus

*Blenderized protein diet of meat, vegetables, and fruit.
†Also contains cow's milk.
From Siberry GK, Iannone R, editors: *The Harriet Lane handbook,* ed 15, St Louis, 2000, Mosby.

Table C-13 Fat Content of Formulas

	Long-Chain Triglycerides		Medium-Chain and Long-Chain Triglycerides	
Common ingredient names	Safflower oil Soy oil Palm olein Coconut oil	Sunflower oil Corn oil Canola oil Butterfat	Medium-chain triglycerides (MCT oil) Fractioned coconut oil	
Comments	Requires normal fat digestion and absorption		For individuals with fat malabsorption Bile digestion not required Absorbed directly into portal circulation	
Infants	Alsoy Enfamil Enfamil AR Carnation Follow-up Carnation Follow-up Soy Carnation Good Start	Isomil (all) Lactofree Neocate Nutramigen ProSobee RCF Similac Similac PM 60/40 Similac Lactose Free	Alimentum Enfamil Premature Enfamil 22 Pregestimil Portagen Neosure Similac Special Care	
Toddlers and young children	Next Step Compleat Pediatric Toddler's Best		Resource Just For Kids Kindercal Neocate One Plus Nutren Junior PediaSure L-Emental Pediatric Peptamen Junior Vivonex Pediatric	
Older children and adolescents	Carnation Instant Breakfast Ensure Ensure with Fiber Ensure Plus Glucerna	Nepro Pulmocare Scandishake Suplena Boost Plus Boost High-Protein Boost with Fiber	Deliver 2.0 Isocal Jevity Lipisorb Nutren 2.0 Nutrivent	Osmolite Promote Respalor Traumacal Ultracal

From Siberry GK, Iannone R, editors: *The Harriet Lane handbook,* ed 15, St Louis, 2000, Mosby.

Table C-14 Analysis of Human Milk and Fortifiers (Per Liter)

Formula	kcal/mL (kcal/oz)	Protein g (% kcal)	Carbohydrate g (% kcal)	Fat g (% kcal)	Na (mEq)	K (mEq)	Ca (mg)	P (mg)	Fe (mg)	Osmolality (mOsm/kg water)	Suggested Uses
Human milk (mature)	0.69 (20)	9 (5) Human milk protein	73 (42) Lactose	42 (54) Human milk fat	8	13	280	147	0.4	286	Infants
Preterm human milk*	0.67 (20)	14 (8) Human milk protein	66 (40) Lactose	39 (52) Human milk fat	11	15	248	128	1.2	290	Preterm infants
Enfamil Human Milk Fortifier (per packet) (Mead Johnson)	3.5 (–)	0.15 (20) Whey protein concentrate Na caseinate	0.68 (76) Corn syrup solids	0.02 (3.9) From caseinate Lactose	0.08	0.1	23	11	0	—	Fortifier for preterm human milk
Similac Natural Care Human Milk Fortifier (Ross)	0.8 (24)	22 (11) Nonfat milk Whey protein concentrate	86 (42) Corn syrup solids Lactose	44 (47) MCT oil Soy oil Coconut oil	15	26.6	1694	935	3	280	Fortifier for preterm human milk
Preterm Human Milk + Similac Natural Care 75:25 ratio	0.7 (21)	16 (9) Human milk protein Nonfat milk Whey protein concentrate	71 (40) Lactose Corn syrup solids	40 (51) Human milk fat MCT oil Soy oil Coconut oil	12	18	610	330	1.65	288	Preterm infants
Preterm Human Milk + Similac Natural Care 50:50 ratio	0.74 (22)	18 (10) Human milk protein Nonfat milk Whey protein concentrate	71 (40) Lactose Corn syrup solids	41 (50) Human milk fat MCT oil Soy oil Coconut oil	13	21	971	531	2.1	285	Preterm infants
Preterm Human Milk + Similac Natural Care 25:75 ratio	0.77 (23)	19.9 (10) Nonfat milk Whey protein concentrate Human milk protein	81 (42) Lactose Corn syrup solids	43 (50) MCT oil Soy oil Coconut oil Human milk fat	14	24	1332	734	2.5	282	Preterm infants
Preterm Human Milk + Enfamil Human Milk Fortifier (1 pkt/50 mL)	0.73 (22)	17.3 (9) Human milk protein Whey protein concentrate Na caseinate	79 (43) Lactose Corn syrup solids	39 (48) Human milk fat	12	16	688	348	1.2	350	Preterm infants
Preterm Human Milk + Enfamil Human Milk Fortifier (1 pkt/25 mL)	0.78 (24)	20.5 (10) Human milk protein Whey protein concentrate Na caseinate	91 (46) Lactose Corn syrup solids	39 (44) Human milk fat	13	17	1166	561	1.2	410	Preterm infants

From Ross Products Division, Abbott Laboratories, Inc.[7]
*Composition of human milk varies with maternal diet, stage of lactation, within feedings, diurnally, and among mothers.
From Siberry GK, Iannone R, editors: *The Harriet Lane handbook,* ed 15, St Louis, 2000, Mosby.

Table C-15 Analysis of Infant Formulas (Per Liter)

Formula	kcal/mL (kcal/oz)	Protein g (% kcal)	Carbohydrate g (% kcal)	Fat g (% kcal)	Na (mEq)	K (mEq)	Ca (mg)	P (mg)	Fe (mg)	Osmolality (mOsm/kg water)	Suggested Uses
Alimentum (Ross)	0.67 (20)	19 (11) Casein hydrolysate Cystine, Tyr, Trp Methionine	69 (41) Sucrose 67% Modified tapioca starch	38 (48) MCT oil (50%) Safflower oil (40%) Soy oil (10%)	13	20	709	507	12	370	Infants with food allergies, protein or fat malabsorption
Alsoy (Carnation)	0.67 (20)	19 (11) Soy Isolate Methionine	75 (44) Sucrose Maltodextrin	36 (45) Soy oil	10	20	709	412	12	200	Infants with allergy to cow's milk, lactose malabsorption, galactosemia
Enfamil [w/Fe] (Mead Johnson)	0.67 (20)	14 (9) Nonfat milk Demineralized whey	73 (43) Lactose	36 (48) Palm olein (45%) Soy oil (20%) Coconut oil (20%) HO Sun oil (15%)	8	19	530	360	5 [12.5]	300	Infants with normal GI tract
Enfamil AR (Mead Johnson)	0.67 (20)	16.7 (10) Nonfat milk Demineralized whey	73 (44) Lactose (57%) Rice starch (30%) Maltodextrins (13%)	34 (46) Palm olein (45%) Soy oil (20%) Coconut oil (20%) HO sun oil (15%)	11	18	520	353	12	230	When a thickened feeding is desired
Enfamil 24 [w/Fe] (Mead Johnson)	0.8 (20)	17 (9) Nonfat milk Whey	88 (43) Lactose	43 (48) Palm olein (45%) Soy oil (20%) HO Sun oil (15%)	10	22	630	430	6 [15]	360	Infants with normal GI tract requiring additional calories
Enfamil Premature Formula 20 [w/Fe] (Mead Johnson)	0.67 (20)	20 (12) Demineralized whey Nonfat milk	75 (44) Corn syrup solids Lactose	35 (44) MCT oil (40%) Soy oil Coconut oil	11	18	1120	560	1.7 [12]	260	Preterm infants
Enfamil Premature Formula 24 [w/Fe] (Mead Johnson)	0.8 (24)	24 (12) Demineralized whey Nonfat milk	9 (44) Corn syrup solids Lactose	41 (44) MCT oil (40%) Soy oil Coconut oil	14	21	1340	670	2 [15]	310	Preterm infants
Enfamil 22 with iron (Mead Johnson)	0.73 (22)	20.6 (11) Nonfat milk Demineralized whey	79 (43) Corn syrup solids Lactose	39 (48) HO sun oil Soy oil MCT oil Coconut oil	11	20	890	490	13	—	Preterm infants after hospital discharge until goal catch-up growth

milk formula*	[illegible] (21)	[illegible] Cow's milk	[illegible] Lactose Corn syrup	[illegible] Butterfat	[illegible]	[illegible]	[illegible]	[illegible]	[illegible]	—	Infants with normal GI tract; need vitamin C and iron supplement
Follow-up (Carnation)	0.67 (20)	18 (10) Nonfat milk	89 (53) Corn syrup (43%) Lactose (37%)	28 (37) Palm olein (47%) Soy oil (26%) Coconut oil (21%) HO saff oil (6%)	11	23	912	608	13	328	Infants 4-12 months with normal GI tract
Follow-up Soy (Carnation)	0.67 (20)	21 (12) Soy isolate Methionine	81 (48) Maltodextrin Sucrose	29 (40) Palm olein (47%) Soy oil (26%) Coconut oil (21%) HO saff oil (6%)	12	20	912	608	12	200	Infants 4-12 months with allergy to cow's milk, lactose malabsorption, galactosemia
Good Start (Carnation)	0.67 (20)	16 (10) Hydrolyzed whey	74 (44) Lactose Maltodextrins	3.5 (46) Palm olein (47%) Soy oil (26%) Coconut oil (21%) HO saff oil (6%)	7	17	432	243	10	265	Infants with normal GI tract
Isomil (Ross)	0.67 (20)	17 (10) Soy isolate Methionine	70 (41) Corn syrup Sucrose	37 (49) Soy oil Coconut oil	13	19	709	507	12	230	Infants with allergy to cow's milk, lactose malabsorption, galactosemia
Isomil DF (Ross)	0.67 (20)	18 (11) Soy isolate Methionine	68 (40) Corn syrup Sucrose Soy fiber	37 (49) Soy oil Coconut oil	13	19	709	507	12	240	Short-term management of diarrhea; contains fiber
Lactofree (Mead Johnson)	0.67 (20)	14 (9) Milk protein isolate	7 (43) Corn syrup solids	36 (48) Palm olein (45%) Soy oil (20%) Coconut oil (20%) HO Sun oil (15%)	9	19	550	370	12	200	Infants with lactose malabsorption

*13 ounces evaporated whole milk, 119 ounces water, 12 tbsp corn syrup.
From Siberry GK, Iannone R, editors: *The Harriet Lane handbook,* ed 15, St Louis, 2000, Mosby.

Continued

Table C-15 Analysis of Infant Formulas (Per Liter)—cont'd

Formula	kcal/mL (kcal/oz)	Protein g (% kcal)	Carbohydrate g (% kcal)	Fat g (% kcal)	Na (mEq)	K (mEq)	Ca (mg)	P (mg)	Fe (mg)	Osmolality (mOsm/kg water)	Suggested Uses
MJ3232A (Mead Johnson)	0.42 (12.6)	19 (17) Casein hydrolysate Cystine, Tyr, Trp	28 (25) Tapioca starch CHO selected by physician	28 (57) MCT oil (85%) Corn oil (15%)	13	19	630	420	13	250	Infants with severe CHO intolerance (CHO must be added)
Neocate (Scientific Hospital Supply)	0.69 (21)	20 (12) Free amino acids	78 (47) Corn syrup solids	32 (41) Safflower oil Coconut oil Soy oil	8	16	826	620	10	342	Infants with severe food allergies
Nutramigen (Mead Johnson)	0.67 (20)	19 (11) Casein hydrolysate Cystine, Tyr, Trp	74 (44) Corn syrup solids Modified cornstarch	34 (45) Palm olein (45%) Soy oil (20%) Coconut oil (20%) HO Sun oil (15%)	14	19	640	430	13	320	Infants with food allergies
Portagen (Mead Johnson)	0.67 (20)	24 (14) Na caseinate	78 (46) Corn syrup solids Sucrose	32 (40) MCT oil (85%) Corn oil (15%)	16	22	640	470	13	230	Infants with fat malabsorption
Pregestimil (Mead Johnson)	0.67 (20)	19 (11) Casein hydrolysate Cystine, Tyr, Trp	69 (41) Corn syrup solids (60%) Modified corn-starch (20%) Dextrose (20%)	38 (48) MCT oil (55%) Corn oil (20%) Soy oil (12.5%) HO Saff oil (12.5%)	11	19	640	430	13	320	Infants with food allergies, protein or fat malabsorption
ProSobee (Mead Johnson)	0.67 (20)	20 (12) Soy isolate Methionine	73 (42) Corn syrup solids	37 (48) Palm olein (45%) Soy oil (20%) Coconut oil (20%) HO Sun oil (15%)	10	21	710	560	12	200	Infants with allergy to cow's milk, lactose malabsorption, galactosemia
RCF† (Ross) [w/Fe]	0.4 (12)	20 (20) Soy isolate	— Selected by physician	36 (80) Soy oil Coconut oil	13	19	709	507	12	—	Infants with severe CHO intolerance (CHO must be added) Modified for ketogenic diet

(Ross)	(20)	Nonfat milk Whey protein	Lactose	Soy oil Coconut oil HO saff oil	7	18	327	284	15 [12]	300	Infants with normal GI tract
Similac 24 [w/Fe] (Ross)	0.8 (24)	22 (11) Nonfat milk	85 (42) Lactose	43 (47) Soy oil Coconut oil	12	27	726	565	1.8 [15]	380	Infants with normal GI tract requiring additional calories
Similac Lactose Free (Ross)	0.67 (20)	14.5 (9) Milk isolate	72.3 (43) Corn syrup solids Sucrose	36.5 (49) Soy oil Coconut oil	9	18.5	568	378	12	230	Infants with lactose malabsorption
Similac Neosure (Ross)	0.75 (22)	19 (10) Nonfat milk Whey	77 (41) Corn syrup solids (50%) Lactose (50%)	41 (49) MCT oil Soy oil Coconut oil HO saff oil	11	27	784	463	13	250	Preterm infants, after hospital discharge, until goal catch-up growth
Similac PM 60/40 (Ross)	0.67 (20)	15 (9) Whey Na caseinate	69 (41) Lactose	38 (50) Soy oil Coconut oil Corn oil	7	15	378	189	1.5	280	Infants who require lowered calcium and phosphorus levels
Similac Special Care 20 [w/Fe] (Ross)	0.67 (20)	18 (11) Nonfat milk Whey	72 (42) Corn syrup solids Lactose	37 (49) MCT oil Soy oil Coconut oil	13	22	1216	676	2.5 [12]	235	Preterm infants
Similac Special Care 24 [w/Fe] (Ross)	0.8 (24)	22 (11) Nonfat milk Whey	86 (42) Corn syrup solids Lactose	44 (49) MCT oil Soy oil Coconut oil	15	27	1452	806	3 [15]	280	Preterm infants

†Available as concentrated liquid. Nutrient values vary depending on amount of added carbohydrate (CHO) and water. A total of 12 fl oz of concentrated liquid with 15 g CHO and 12 fl oz water yields 20 kcal/fl oz formula with 68 g CHO/L.

From Siberry GK, Iannone R, editors: *The Harriet Lane handbook,* ed 15, St Louis, 2000, Mosby.

Table C-16 Analysis of Toddler and Young Child Formulas (Per Liter)

Formula	kcal/mL (kcal/oz)	Protein g (% kcal)	Carbohydrate g (% kcal)	Fat g (% kcal)	Na (mEq)	K (mEq)	Ca (mg)	P (mg)	Fe (mg)	Osmolality (mOsm/kg water)	Suggested Uses
Compleat Pediatric (Novartis)	1 (30)	38 (15) Meats Vegetables Na caseinate Ca caseinate	125 (50) Vegetables Fruit Hydrolyzed cornstarch	39 (35) HO sun oil Soy oil MCT oil	30	38	1000	1000	13	380	For those who desire a blenderized tube feeding
Cow's milk, whole	0.63 (19)	Cow's milk 34 (22)	Lactose 48 (31)	34 (49) Butterfat	22	40	1226	956	0.5	285	Children >1 year of age with normal GI tract
EleCare (Ross)	1 (30)	30 (15) Free L-amino acids	110 (44) Corn syrup solids	47.6 (42) HO saff oil MCT oil Soy oil	19.6	38.4	1082	808	17	596	Children with malabsorption, protein allergy
Kindercal (contains fiber) (Mead Johnson)	1.06 (32)	34 (13) Na caseinate	135 (50) Maltodextrins (83%) Sucrose (17%)	44 (37) Canola oil (50%) HO sun oil (15%) Corn oil (15%) MCT oil (20%)	16	34	850	850	11	310	Tube feeding and oral supplement for children with normal GI tract
L-Emental Pediatric (GalaGen/ Nutrition, Medical)	0.8 (24)	24 (12) Free L-amino acids	130 (63) Maltodextrins Modified starch	24 (25) Soy oil MCT oil (68%)	17	31	970	800	10	360	Children with malabsorption, protein allergy
Neocate One Plus (Scientific Hospital Supply)	1 (30)	25 (10) Free amino acids	146 (58) Maltodextrins Sucrose	35 (32) MCT oil (35%) Safflower oil Canola oil	9	24	620	620	8	835	Children with malabsorption, protein allergy
Next Step (Mead Johnson)	0.67 (20)	17 (10) Nonfat milk	74 (45) Lactose Corn syrup solids	34 (45) Palm olein (45%) Soy oil (20%) Coconut oil (20%) HO [illegible] oil (15%)	12	22	800	560	12	270	Toddlers with normal GI tract

[illegible] (Mead Johnson)	[illegible] (20)	[illegible] Soy protein	[illegible] Corn syrup solids Sucrose	[illegible] Palm olein (45%) Soy oil (20%) Coconut oil (20%) HO sun oil (15%)	13	26	767	600	12	260	Toddlers with cow's milk allergy, galactosemia
Nutren Junior (also with fiber) (Clintec)	1 (30)	30 (12) Casein Whey	128 (51) Maltodextrins Sucrose Soy polysaccharides	42 (37) Soy oil Canola oil MCT oil	20	34	1000	800	14	350	Tube feeding and oral supplement for children with normal GI tract
PediaSure (also with fiber) (Ross)	1 (30)	30 (12) Na caseinate Whey protein	110 (44) Hydrolyzed corn-starch (70%) Sucrose (30%) (Soy fiber)	50 (44) HO saff oil (50%) Soy oil (30%) MCT oil (20%)	16.5	33.5	970	800	14	310	Tube feeding and oral supplement for children with normal GI tract
Peptamen Junior (Clintec)	1 (30)	30 (12) Hydrolyzed whey	138 (55) Maltodextrin Sucrose (flavored) Cornstarch	38.5 (33) MCT oil (60%) Soy oil Canola oil Lecithin	20	34	1000	800	14	260 (unflavored) 365 (flavored)	Children with malabsorption
ProPeptide for Kids (GalaGen/ Nutrition, Medical)	1 (30)	30 (12) Enzymatically hydrolyzed whey protein	137.5 (55) Maltodextrin Sucrose Cornstarch	38.5 (33) Medium-chain triglycerides (18.5%) Soy oil (22%) Canola oil (60%)	20	34	1000	800	14	360	Children with malabsorption
Resource Just for Kids (Novartis)	1 (30)	30 (12) Na caseinate Ca caseinate Whey protein concentrates	110 (44) Hydrolyzed cornstarch Sucrose	50 (44) HO Sun oil Soy oil MCT oil	17	33	1140	800	14	390	Tube feeding and oral supplement for children with normal GI tract
Vivonex Pediatric (Novartis)	0.8 (24)	24 (12) Free amino acids	130 (63) Maltodextrins Modified starch	24 (25) MCT oil (68%) Soy oil (32%)	17	31	970	800	10	360	Children with malabsorption, protein allergy

From Siberry GK, Iannone R, editors: *The Harriet Lane handbook,* ed 15, St Louis, 2000, Mosby.

Table C-17 Analysis of Older Child and Adult Formulas (Per Liter)

Formula	kcal/mL (kcal/oz)	Protein g (% kcal)	Carbohydrate g (% kcal)	Fat g (% kcal)	Na (mEq)	K (mEq)	Ca (mg)	P (mg)	Fe (mg)	Osmolality (mOsm/kg water)	Suggested Uses
Carnation Instant Breakfast w/whole milk (Clintec)	1.2 (36)	53 (18) Cow's milk	161 (54) Lactose Maltodextrin Sucrose	34 (26) Butterfat	42	67	1632	1400	17	590	High-calorie supplement for patients with normal GI tract
Criticare HN (Mead Johnson)	1.06 (32)	38 (14) Hydrolyzed casein Amino acids	220 (81.5) Maltodextrin Modified cornstarch	53 (4.5) Safflower oil	27	34	530	530	9.5	650	Patients with malabsorption
Deliver 2.0 (Mead Johnson)	2 (60)	75 (15) Ca caseinate Na caseinate	200 (40) Corn syrup	102 (45) Soy oil (70%) MCT oil (30%)	35	43	1000	1000	18	640	Oral supplement or tube feeding for patients with fluid restriction or increased calorie needs
Ensure (Ross)	1.06 (32)	37 (14) Na caseinate Ca caseinate Soy protein	145 (55) Corn syrup (70%) Sucrose (30%)	37 (32) Corn oil	36	40	530	530	9.6	470	Oral supplement or tube feeding for patients with normal GI tract
Ensure Plus (Ross)	1.5 (45)	55 (15) Na caseinate Ca caseinate Soy protein	200 (53) Corn syrup Sucrose	53 (32) Corn oil	46	50	705	705	13	690	Oral supplement or tube feeding for patients with higher calorie needs, normal GI tract
Ensure with Fiber (Ross)	1.1 (33)	40 (15) Na caseinate Ca caseinate Soy protein	162 (55) Hydrolyzed cornstarch (58%) Sucrose (32%) Soy polysaccharide (10%)	37 (31) Corn oil	37	43	719	719	13	480	Oral supplement or tube feeding with fiber, normal GI tract
Glucerna (Ross)	1 (30)	42 (17) Na caseinate Ca caseinate	94 (33) Glucose polymers (53%) Soy polysaccharide (25%) [illegible] (21%)	56 (50) HO saff oil (85%) Soy oil (15%)	40	40	704	704	13	375	Patients with impaired glucose tolerance, also contains fiber

Isocal (Mead Johnson)	1.06 (32)	34 (13) Na caseinate Ca caseinate Soy protein	135 (50) Maltodextrin	44 (37) MCT oil (20%) Soy oil (80%)	23	34	630	530	10	270	Tube feeding for patients with normal GI tract
Jevity (Ross)	1.06 (32)	44 (17) Na caseinate Ca caseinate	152 (53) Hydrolyzed cornstarch Soy polysaccharide	36 (30) HO saff oil (50%) Canola oil (30%) MCT oil (20%)	40	40	909	758	14	300	Tube feeding with fiber, normal GI tract
L-Emental (GalaGen/ Nutrition, Medical)	1 (30)	38 (15) Free L-amino acids	205 (82) Maltodextrins	2.85 (2.5) Safflower oil	20	20	500	500	9	630	Patients with malabsorption, protein allergy
L-Emental Plus (Nutrition, Medical)	1 (30)	45 (18) Free L-amino acids	190 (76) Maltodextrins	6.7 (6) Soy oil	26	27	556	556	10	650	Patients with malabsorption, protein allergy
Lipisorb (Mead Johnson)	1.35 (40)	57 (17) Na caseinate Ca caseinate	161 (48) Maltodextrin Sucrose	57 (35) MCT oil (85%) Soy oil (15%)	59	43	850	850	15	630	Patients with fat malabsorption
Nepro (Ross)	2 (60)	70 (14) Ca caseinate Mg caseinate Na caseinate	215 (43) Hydrolyzed cornstarch (88%) Sucrose (12%)	96 (43) HO saff oil (90%) Soy oil (10%)	36	27	1373	686	19	635	Patients with renal failure undergoing dialysis
Nutren 2.0 (Clintec)	2 (60)	80 (16) K caseinate Ca caseinate	196 (39) Sucrose Corn syrup solids Maltodextrin	106 (45) MCT oil (75%) Canola oil Corn oil Soy oil Lecithin	57	49	1340	1340	24	720	Oral supplement or tube feedings for patients with fluid restriction or increased calorie needs
Nutrivent (Clintec)	1.5 (45)	68 (18) Ca caseinate K caseinate	100 (27) Maltodextrin Sucrose	95 (55) MCT oil (40%) Canola oil (43%) Corn oil (13%) Lecithin (4%)	50	42	1200	1200	18	330	Patients requiring higher percentage of calories from fat
Osmolite (Ross)	1.06 (32)	37 (14) Na caseinate Ca caseinate Soy protein	145 (55) Hydrolyzed cornstarch	38 (31) HO saff oil (50%) Canola oil (30%) MCT oil (20%)	28	26	530	530	9.5	300	Tube feeding for patients with normal GI tract

From Siberry GK, Iannone R, editors: *The Harriet Lane handbook,* ed 15, St Louis, 2000, Mosby.

Continued

Table C-17 Analysis of Older Child and Adult Formulas (Per Liter)—cont'd

Formula	kcal/mL (kcal/oz)	Protein g (% kcal)	Carbohydrate g (% kcal)	Fat g (% kcal)	Na (mEq)	K (mEq)	Ca (mg)	P (mg)	Fe (mg)	Osmolality (mOsm/kg water)	Suggested Uses
Peptamen (Clintec)	1 (30)	40 (16) Hydrolyzed whey	127 (51) Maltodextrin (88%) Hydrolyzed corn-starch (12%)	39 (33) MCT oil (67%) Sunflower oil (18%) Lecithin (6%) Milk fat (9%)	22	32	800	700	120	270	Patients with malabsorption
Promote (Ross)	1 (30)	63 (25) Na caseinate Ca caseinate Soy protein	130 (52) Hydrolyzed corn-starch (91%) Sucrose (9%)	26 (23) HO saff oil (50%) Canola oil (30%) MCT oil (20%)	40	51	960	960	14	330	Oral supplement or tube feeding for patients with increased protein needs
ProPeptide (unflavored) (GalaGen/ Nutrition, Medical)	1 (30)	40 (16) Hydrolyzed whey	127 (51) Maltodextrins Starch	39 (33) Sunflower oil (30%) MCT oil (70%)	22	32	800	700	14	270	Patients with malabsorption
Pulmocare (Ross)	1.5 (45)	63 (17) Na caseinate Ca caseinate	106 (28) Hydrolyzed corn-starch (46%) Sucrose (54%)	92 (55) Corn oil	57	44	1056	1056	19	465	Patient's requiring higher percentage of calories from fat
Respalor (Mead Johnson)	1.5 (45)	76 (20) Ca caseinate Na caseinate	148 (39) Corn syrup Sucrose	71 (41) Canola oil (70%) MCT oil (30%)	55	38	710	710	13	580	Patients requiring higher percentage of calories from fat
Scandishake w/ whole milk (Scandi-pharm)	2.5 (75)	50 (8) Cow's milk	292 (47) Lactose Maltodextrin Soy oil	125 (45) Coconut oil Safflower oil Palm oil	240	103	391	478	trace	1094	High-calorie supple-ment and for fat malabsorption
Suplena (Ross)	2 (60)	30 (6) Na caseinate Ca caseinate	255 (51) Hydrolyzed corn-starch (90%) Sucrose (10%)	96 (43) HO saff oil (90%) Soy oil (10%)	34	29	1385	728	19	600	Patients with renal failure not under-going dialysis
Boost High Protein (Mead Johnson)	1 (30)	61 (24) Na caseinate Ca caseinate Soy protein	140 (55) Corn syrup Sucrose	23 (21) Partially hydrogenated soy oil	40	54	1010	930	17	650	Oral supplement or tube feeding for patients with increased protein needs

Boost Plus (Mead Johnson)	1.5 (45)	61 (16) Na caseinate Ca caseinate	190 (50) Corn syrup solids Sucrose	57 (34) Corn oil	37	38	850	850	15	670	Oral supplement or tube feeding for patients with high calorie needs, normal GI tract
Boost with Fiber (Mead Johnson)	1.06 (30)	46 (17) Na caseinate Ca caseinate Soy protein	140 (53) Maltodextrin Sucrose	35 (30) Corn oil	31	36	850	710	13	480	Oral supplement or tube feeding with fiber, normal GI tract
Tolerex (Novartis)	1 (30)	21 (8) Free amino acids	230 (91) Maltodextrin	1.5 (1) Safflower oil	20	31	560	560	10	550	Patients with malabsorption or severe food allergy
Traumacal (Mead Johnson)	1.5 (45)	82 (22) Na caseinate Ca caseinate	142 (38) Corn syrup Sucrose	68 (40) Soy oil (70%) MCT oil (30%)	51	36	750	750	9	560	Patients with increased protein and calorie needs
Ultracal (Mead Johnson)	1.06 (30)	44 (17) Na caseinate Ca caseinate	123 (46) Maltodextrin Soy fiber Oat fiber	45 (37) MCT oil (40%) Canola oil (60%)	40	41	850	850	15	310	Oral supplement or tube feeding with fiber, normal GI tract
Vital HN (Ross)	1 (30)	42 (17) Hydrolyzed whey, meat, and soy (87%) Free amino acids (13%)	185 (74) Hydrolyzed cornstarch (83%) Sucrose (17%) Lactose (<0.5%)	11 (9) Safflower oil (55%) MCT oil (45%)	25	36	667	667	12	500	Patients with malabsorption
Vivonex Plus (Novartis)	1 (30)	45 (18) Free amino acids	190 (76) Maltodextrin	6.7 (6) Soybean oil	27	28	560	560	10	650	Patients with malabsorption or severe food allergy
Vivonex TEN (Novartis)	1 (30)	38 (15) Free amino acids	210 (82) Maltodextrin	2.8 (3) Safflower oil	20	20	500	500	9	630	Patients with malabsorption or severe food allergy

From Siberry GK, Iannone R, editors: *The Harriet Lane handbook,* ed 15, St Louis, 2000, Mosby.

D Common Psychological and Educational Tests

Philip W. Davidson • Kyle D. Houser • Olle Jane Z. Sahler

During the 1980s and 1990s, the number of preschool and school-age children seeing allied health professionals for psychological and educational assessment rose dramatically. At the same time, the assessment armamentarium of the psychoeducational specialist has expanded to the point that many of the materials commonly used are unfamiliar to the pediatrician. The physician frequently receives reports from psychologists and educational specialists, speech and language pathologists, and pediatric occupational therapists—reports that must be interpreted or explained to the parents. Because these materials must be described succinctly to simplify the physician's assignment, summaries are provided in Box D-1 (which groups tests by the function they measure) and Table D-1 (which lists tests alphabetically and gives some of the tests' characteristics).

Table D-1 provides a quick reference to a wide range of psychoeducational screening and diagnostic tools commonly used by school health teams, special-child educators, clinical psychologists, and other allied health professionals. Only individually administered tests are included, inasmuch as they are less familiar to both parents and physicians than are the group-administered standardized tests used by schools.

The information provided for each procedure is useful in identifying the general nature of each, the usual professional training of the person administering the test, and whether it is "normed." For some procedures, special features or characteristics also are noted.

The list of tests is not all-inclusive, but most procedures that are likely to be described in a typical consultant's report are included. Screening procedures are presented because more and more states are requiring preschool and kindergarten readiness screening for all children. These screening tools often trigger more extensive evaluations for children who do not pass, a decision in which the pediatrician should participate. The diagnostic procedures given include many standard methods, as well as a variety of nonstandard methods designed for children who have disabilities that may interfere with routine testing procedures. Finally, some "parent report" procedures also are included because many preschool assessments may depend on such tools.

Clearly, interpreting the results of a screening or a complete diagnostic assessment cannot be accomplished fully by referring only to Table D. Communicating directly with the evaluator is the only reliable means of clarifying results. Such contact often must be initiated by the pediatrician because personnel from many schools and mental health facilities may not communicate routinely with the primary health care provider.

REFERRAL BY THE PEDIATRICIAN FOR PSYCHOLOGICAL OR EDUCATIONAL TESTING

Often the primary care pediatrician is in the best position to identify a child's developmental or behavioral difficulties, such as developmental delay in the infant or preschool child, learning difficulty or school failure in the school-age child, or adjustment difficulty in the latency-age child or adolescent. In these and similar situations the pediatrician quite appropriately might consider initiating a referral for psychological or educational testing, or both.

Several types of resources are available to accept referrals. The local county health department or the school district in which the child resides are generally good contacts with which to begin, since both are statutorily obliged by the Individuals with Disabilities Education Act (IDEA, 1990) and its predecessors the Education for All Handicapped Children Act (PL 94-142 and reauthorized under PL 99-457). Under this "landmark legislation," each state must guarantee a meaningful, individually appropriate, publicly supported education suited to the needs of the child regardless of the type of degree of his or her mental, physical or emotional disability or impairment (IDEA, 1990). This process begins with an evaluation of the child's strengths and weaknesses and culminates in a contextually appropriate Individual Education Plan (IEP) for any child needing such educational and other supports. This IEP process for each child is guaranteed under law, reviewed at least annually and modified as appropriate. Federal law is implemented differently for preschool children ages birth through 2 years 11 months, and for school-age children ages 3 to 21 years, but services must be provided at public expense and without cost to the family. Preschoolers may be evaluated by any community resource certified as qualified by the state agency administering Part H of the law pertaining to preschoolers. Such resources must be interdisciplinary and must include a medical examination, a developmental assessment, and a family assessment. The results are incorporated in an Individualized Family Service Plan (IFSP) to be carried out by the school district or other local entity as designated by the state.

Evaluations for school age children must be provided by the local school district and usually are performed by school

Text continued on p. 2130

BOX D-1

CLASSIFICATION OF COMMON PSYCHOLOGICAL AND EDUCATIONAL TESTS BY FUNCTION

Developmental Scales
Battelle Developmental Inventory (BDI)
Bayley Scales of Infant Development-II (BSID-II)
Callier-Azusa Scale
Cattell Infant Intelligence Scale
Clinical Adaptive Test/Clinical Linguistic Auditory Milestone Scale (CAT/CLAMS)
Denver Developmental Screening Test (DDST)
Gesell Developmental Schedules
Infant Mullen Scales of Early Learning (Infant-MSEL)
Infant Psychological Development Scale
Kaufman Developmental Scale (KDS)
Kaufman Infant and Preschool Scale (KIPS)
Minnesota Child Development Inventory
Neonatal Behavioral Assessment Scale (Brazelton)
Ordinal Scales of Psychological Development
Prescreening Developmental Questionnaire (PDQ)
School Readiness Survey

Temperament Measures
Infant Temperament Questionnaire (ITQ) (Carey-McDevitt)
Temperament Assessment Battery for Children (TABC)
Temperament Scales

Sensory/Perceptual/Motor/Auditory/Visual Scales
Auditory Discrimination Test
Bender Visual Motor Gestalt Test
Bruininks-Oseretsky Test of Motor Proficiency
Developmental Test of Visual Motor Integration (DTVMI)
Frostig Developmental Test of Visual Perception
Goldman-Fristoe-Woodcock Auditory Skills Test Battery
Motor Free Test of Visual Perception (MFTVP)
Peabody Developmental Motor Scales and Activity Cards
Sequenced Inventory of Communication Development–Revised Edition
Southern California Sensory Integration Test

Intelligence/Cognitive/Neuropsychological Tests
Brown Attention Deficit Disorder Scales
Columbia Mental Maturity Scale
Draw-A-Man
Goodenough-Harris Drawing Test
Halstead Reitan Neuropsychological Test Battery for Older Children
Kaufman Assessment Battery for Children (K-ABC)
Luria-Nebraska Neuropsychological Battery: Children's Revision (LNNB-C)
McCarthy Scales of Children's Abilities
Merrill-Palmer Scale
Raven's Progressive Matrices (RPM)
Reitan-Indiana Neuropsychological Test Battery for Children
Slosson Intelligence Test–Revised (SIT-R)
Stanford-Binet Intelligence Test–Fourth Edition (SBFE)
Wechsler Intelligence Scale for Children-III (WISC-III)

Intelligence/Cognitive/Neuropsychological Tests—cont'd
Wechsler Memory Scale–Revised (WMS-R)
Wechsler Preschool and Primary Scales of Intelligence-Revised (WPPSI-R)
Wisconsin Card Sorting Test (WCST)

Nonverbal/Nonsighted/Nonhearing
Blind Learning Aptitude Test (BLAT)
French Pictorial Intelligence Test
Hiskey-Nebraska Test of Learning Aptitude
Leiter International Performance Scale (LIPS)
Perkins-Binet Test of Intelligence for the Blind
Test of Nonverbal Intelligence–Revised (TONI-2)

Adaptive Behavior Scales
AAMR Adaptive Behavior Scale (ABS)
Adaptive Behavior Inventory for Children (ABIC)
California Adaptive Behavior Scale
Vineland Adaptive Behavior Scale (VABS)

Behavior/Personality/Problem Scales and Checklists
Childhood Autism Rating Scale (CARS)
Child Behavior Checklist (CBC) and Revised Child Behavior Profile
Children's Apperception Test (CAT)
Connors Parent and Teacher Rating Scales
Devereux Child Behavior Rating Scale (DCB)
Functional Analysis Interview Form (FAIF)
House-Tree-Person (H-T-P) Projective Technique
Kinetic Drawing System for Family and Schools (KFD and KSD)
Motivation Assessment Scale (MAS)
Personality Inventory for Children–Revised Format (PIC-R)
Preschool Behavior Questionnaire
Reiss Scales for Children's Dual Diagnosis
Rorschach Psychodiagnostic Test
Sentence Completion Test
Thematic Apperception Test (TAT)
Wisconsin Behavior Rating Scale (WBRS)

Achievement/Aptitude/Other Educational Tests
ADD-H Comprehensive Teacher's Rating Scale (ACTeRS)
Assessing Prelinguistic and Early Linguistic Behaviors
Attention Deficit Disorders Behavior Rating Scales (ADDBRS)
Autism Screening Instrument for Educational Planning (ASIEP)
Detroit Test of Learning Aptitude-3 (DTLA-3)
Illinois Test of Psycholinguistic Abilities-2 (ITPA-2)
Kaufman Test of Educational Achievement (K-TEA)
KeyMath Revised: a Diagnostic Inventory of Essential Mathematics
Peabody Individual Achievement Test–Revised (PIAT-R)
Peabody Picture Vocabulary Test–Revised (PPVT-R)
Physician Developmental Quick Screen for Speech Disorders
Piers-Harris Children's Self Concept Scale (PHCSCS)

Continued

BOX D-1

CLASSIFICATION OF COMMON PSYCHOLOGICAL AND EDUCATIONAL TESTS BY FUNCTION—cont'd

Achievement/Aptitude/Other Educational Tests—cont'd

Preschool Language Scale (PLS)
Receptive-Expressive Emergent Language Scale (REEL)
Silvaroli Reading Inventory
Stanford Measurement Series
Sucher-Allred Reading Placement Inventory
Test of Language Development-2 (TOLD-2)

Achievement/Aptitude/Other Educational Tests—cont'd

Test of Written Language-2 (TOWL-2)
Test of Written Spelling-2 (TWS-2)
Wide Range Achievement Test-3 (WRAT-3)
Woodcock Reading Mastery Test–Revised (WRMT-R)
Woodcock-Johnson Psychoeducational Battery-Revised (WJ-R)

Table D-1 Common Psychological and Educational Tests

Test Name	Age Range	Purpose and Description
AAMR Adaptive Behavior Scales (ABS) Residential and Community (ABS-RC:2) School (ABS-S:23)	3 yr-adult	The third and latest revision (1992) of this widely used scale; assesses social, daily living, domestic, and other skills of children whose behavior indicates possible mental retardation, emotional disturbance, or other handicaps; used for screening and instructional planning as well as for documenting progress; generally administered by a psychologist or educational specialist.
Adaptive Behavior Inventory for Children (ABIC)	5-11 yr	Interview inventory to assess child's social role performance in family, peer group, and community; section two includes age-graded questions.
ADD-H Comprehensive Teacher's Rating Scale (ACTeRS)	Grade K-5	Also widely known as the ACTeRS; aids in assessing behavior in the classroom that may be relevant to a diagnosis of attention deficit disorder; four subscales include hyperactivity, social skills, oppositional, and attention; ACTeRS Profile for either boys or girls is generated; psychologist administers and interprets.
Assessing Prelinguistic and Early Linguistic Behaviors	9-24 mo	A "normed" measure containing five scales assessing prelinguistic and linguistic development, including cognitive antecedents to word meaning, play, communicative interaction, language comprehension, and language production; speech pathologist administers.
Attention Deficit Disorder Behavior Rating Scales (ADDBRS)	6-16 yr	A screening device used by a teacher or parent and evaluated by an examiner; results aid in the differential diagnosis of attention deficit with and without hyperactivity.
Auditory Discrimination Test (ADT)	4-8 yr 11 mo	Gross screening measure of auditory discrimination for preschool and early elementary school-age children; designed to measure a child's ability to hear spoken language accurately; administered by an educational specialist, psychologist, or speech pathologist.
Autism Screening Instrument for Educational Planning (ASIEP)	18 mo-adult	Battery of five tests useful in assessing children, adolescents, and adults who have autism; assesses interactional, vocal, and functional skills and provides a prognosis for learning rate; includes Autism Behavior Checklist (ABC); used to establish IEPs; administered by a psychologist or educational specialist.
Battelle Developmental Inventory (BDI)	Birth-8 yr	Developmental inventory encompassing five domains: personal-social, adaptive, motor, communication, and cognitive; uses a mixture of test item, interview, and observational data: results heavily dependent on an informant's ability to provide accurate information; administered by a psychologist or educational specialist.
Bayley Scales of Infant Development-II	1-42 mo	One of the most widely used tools for assessing developmental status; newly revised second edition has an extended age range that measures cognitive, perceptual, and motor behavior; scale yields normed developmental indices useful in comparing a child with age peers; generally administered by a psychologist.
Bender Visual Motor Gestalt Test	3 yr-adult	Widely known and used screening test of visual-motor integration, usually administered by a psychologist; two normed scoring forms: Koppitz for children ages 4-12 yr; Hutt for adolescents and adults; test also yields indicators of neurological and emotional status.

Table D-1 Common Psychological and Educational Tests—cont'd

Test Name	Age Range	Purpose and Description
Blind Learning Aptitude Test (BLAT)	6-16 yr	Nonverbal cognitive test for use with blind children that assesses general reasoning and abstraction; test seems to work best with children ages 6-12 yr; should be used in conjunction with a verbal test; usually administered by a psychologist or other trained professional.
Brown Attention Deficit Disorder Scales (Brown ADD Scales)	12 yr-adult	Reliable, clinician administered instrument that elicits cognitive and affective indications of ADD in adolescents and adults; the "Ready Score" form indicates overall impairment from a broad range of symptoms and is used as an efficient screening instrument; the "Diagnostic Form" aids in conducting a more comprehensive evaluation based on *DSM-IV* criteria. Also screens for comorbid disorders.
Bruininks-Oseretsky Test of Motor Proficiency	4½-14½ yr	A normed performance scale that assesses motor proficiency and neurological development; yields a gross and fine motor composite as well as a battery composite; age equivalents available; generally administered by an occupational or physical therapist.
California Adaptive Behavior Scale	Birth-18 yr	Measures overall adaptive behavior in the areas of self-help, socialization, language and gross motor, perceptual motor, vocational, independent living, and academic skills; also assesses school and vocational readiness; psychologist or educational specialist administers and interprets.
Callier-Azusa Scale-H	Severely and profoundly mentally retarded individuals	Developmental scale designed to assess communicative abilities of the deaf-blind and severely and profoundly handicapped; scale should be administered by individuals who are familiar with the child's behavior.
Cattell Infant Intelligence Scale	3-30 mo	Diagnostic test of developmental status in infancy that measures cognitive and perceptual adaptive behaviors; a well-established tool, but the norms are dated; has been displaced by the Bayley Scales; usually administered by a qualified developmental specialist (e.g., a pediatric psychologist).
Child Behavior Checklist and Revised Child Behavior Profile	2-16 yr	Commonly known as the CBC and CBCL and developed by Achenbach; assesses behavioral problems and competencies of children and adolescents; four versions available, including Parent, Teacher, Youth Self-Report, and Direct Observation; a version for evaluating the mentally retarded is available from the author.
Childhood Autism Rating Scale (CARS)	Child, adolescent	Useful in the diagnosis of children functioning on the autistic spectrum and for distinguishing them from developmentally delayed children and others who are not autistic; used in psychological, medical, and educational assessment.
Children's Apperception Test (CAT)	2-10 yr	Diagnostic test of personality and social development in children and adolescents that usually is administered by a psychologist; used to help characterize the child's interpersonal relationships; test has three forms: one based on picture stories of humans (CAT-H), another on picture stories of animals, (CAT-A) and a supplemental form based on animal figures in family situations (CAT-S).
Clinical Adaptive Test/ Clinical Linguistic Auditory Milestone Scale (CAT/CLAMS)	1-36 mo	A parental report (CLAMS) and direct assessment (CAT) measure developed for pediatricians to assess early development; normed developmental quotients (DQ) provided for nonlanguage, visual, motor, and language abilities as well as a composite score; brief and easy to administer; reported to discriminate children who have mental retardation from those who have communication disorders; preliminary data suggest that individual and composite DQs correlate with Bayley Scales of Infant Development (BSID).
Columbia Mental Maturity Scale	3½-10 yr	Diagnostic test of cognitive ability used to evaluate children who have sensory or motor defects or difficulty speaking or writing; developmental index is derived from norms; usually administered by a psychologist.

Continued

Table D-1 Common Psychological and Educational Tests—cont'd

Test Name	Age Range	Purpose and Description
Connors Parent and Teacher Rating Scale	School age	Screening test of personality and social development completed by teachers to evaluate possible hyperactivity and other patterns of behavior in students; used widely in research settings.
Denver Developmental Screening Test (DDST)	Birth-6 yr	Office screening test of developmental status that evaluates performance in four developmental areas: gross motor, fine motor, language, and personal and social skills; can be administered by a physician, nurse, or other trained worker; requires multiple data points, and up to 10% of all results are either abnormal, questionable, or unobtainable; shorter form (DDST-R) available for preliminary screening (see Chapter 20 [Thirteen]).
Detroit Test of Learning Aptitude-3	6-18 yr	Diagnostic test of learning potential that was revised in 1988; useful as a test of general intellectual ability; standard scores used for each of 11 subtests; usually administered by a trained psychologist or special educator.
Developmental Test of Visual Motor Integration (DTVMI or VMI)	4-13 yr	Sometimes known as the Beery, Beery-Buktenica, or simply the VMI; perceptual motor ability test that aids in identifying children who have visual perception, hand control, and eye-hand coordination problems; also used with developmentally delayed adults; usually administered by a psychologist, educational specialist, or occupational or physical therapist.
Devereux Child Behavior Rating Scale (DBC)	6-12 yr	Diagnostic and screening procedure used to assess overt behavior patterns in children; examiner evaluates ratings made by parent or caregiver on 17 subscales; also used with mentally retarded and emotionally disturbed children.
Draw-a-Man	3-16 yr	See Goodenough-Harris Drawing Test.
French Pictorial Intelligence Test	3-8 yr	Diagnostic test of cognitive development independent of verbal expression—requires "pointing" responses to visual stimuli; most often used with speech-, language-, or hearing-impaired children; yields a developmental quotient based on norms; administered by a trained psychologist.
Frostig Developmental Test of Visual Perception	Infancy-8 yr	Drawing and copying test of perceptual motor ability that measures five areas of visual perception, including eye-hand coordination, figure-ground perception, form constancy, position in space, and spatial relationships; usually administered by a psychologist or specially trained teacher.
Functional Analysis Interview Form (FAIF)	Any age	Semiinstructed, interview-based, functional analysis protocol used to define both biomedical and environmental antecedents and conditions that may contribute to or set the occasion for problem behavior; aids in developing a "behavior support plan" (BSP) based on the teaching of "replacement behaviors" that meet the same function as the problem behavior; contributes to a descriptive, structural, and functional behavior assessment.
Gesell Developmental Schedules	4 wk-5 yr	Assesses physical and mental abilities in the adaptive, gross motor, fine motor, language, and personal-social areas; infant performance usually observed by a psychologist; norms yield an age-equivalent score.
Goldman-Fristoe-Woodcock Auditory Skills Test Battery	3 yr-adult	A normed scale that assesses ability to hear clearly under difficult conditions; subtests measure auditory attention, discrimination, memory, and sound symbol skills; administered by an educational specialist or other qualified professional.
Goodenough-Harris Drawing Test	3-16 yr	Also informally known as Draw-A-Man Test; brief, nonverbal test of intelligence and mental maturity that requires child to draw a person; points are given for various body parts; Harris revision includes an extensive objective scoring system as well as Draw-A-Woman and Self-Drawing tests; assesses perception, abstraction, generalization, and concept formation; male and female norms; administered by a psychologist or skilled examiner.

Table D-1 Common Psychological and Educational Tests—cont'd

Test Name	Age Range	Purpose and Description
Halstead-Reitan Neuropsychological Test Battery for Older Children	9-14 yr	Neuropsychological test battery that falls between the Reitan-Indiana Battery and the adult version of the Halstead-Reitan in age applicability; multihour battery of cognitive and perceptual measures that includes a version of the Wechsler Intelligence Scale for Children (WISC) and various sensory-perceptual, academic, and achievement measures; as with other neuropsychological batteries, it is administered by a psychologist or specialist trained in neuropsychological assessment; used to evaluate children suspected of brain damage and cognitive dysfunction; short screening battery available.
House-Tree-Person (H-T-P) Projective Technique	3 yr-adult	Diagnostic test of personality and cognitive status usually administered by a trained psychologist as a projective device to evaluate self-image and other ego functions.
Hiskey-Nebraska Test of Learning Aptitude	3-18 yr	Nonverbal diagnostic test of cognitive ability usually used for deaf and hearing-impaired children; separate norms available for deaf and for hearing children; usually administered by a trained psychologist.
Illinois Test of Psycholinguistic Abilities–Revised (ITPA-R)	2-10 yr	Normed diagnostic test of cognitive ability designed specifically to evaluate verbal abilities and auditory-verbal and visual-motor processing; can be administered by a psychologist, speech pathologist, or educator; both the norms and the test's usefulness in a psychoeducational battery have been questioned.
Infant Mullen Scales of Early Learning (Infant MSEL)	Birth-36 mo	Comprehensive scale of mental and motor ability; measures specific learning abilities and patterns in gross motor, visual, and language areas; yields strengths and weaknesses and generates an IEP predicated on child's receptive-expressive learning style; administered by a psychologist or educational specialist.
Infant Psychological Development Scale	2 wk–2 yr	Developed by Uzgiris and Hunt based on Piagetian theory; measures cognitive processes associated with natural stages of development; subscales measure development of a specific ability and consist of a number of ordinal steps; can be useful in planning sequenced curriculum; has both clinical and educational use; administered by a psychologist or educational specialist.
Infant Temperament Questionnaire (ITQ)	4-8 mo	Helps to determine infant temperament; questions relate to the nine categories of behavior described by Thomas, Chess, and Birch (see Temperament Scales described later in this table); takes approximately 30 minutes; this questionnaire, which is completed by parents, can be used to supplement information about parent-child interaction derived from the clinical interview.
Kaufman Assessment Battery for Children (K-ABC)	2½-12½ yr	Diagnostic test that should be administered by a qualified professional; intended for use in schools and clinical settings to provide a measure of intelligence and achievement; does not include measures of verbal cognitive processes in the composite score.
Kaufman Developmental Scale (KDS)	Up to 9 yr	Evaluates school readiness and developmental deficiencies among children through age 9; yields a developmental age and developmental quotient, as well as individual age scores in several areas; also useful in evaluating mental retardation; administered by a psychologist.
Kaufman Infant and Preschool Scale (KIPS)	1 mo-4 yr	Screening test for early cognitive processes; indicates possible need for intervention in normal children and in mentally retarded individuals who have mental ages of 4 years or less; administered by a psychologist, physician, or special education teacher.
Kaufman Test of Educational Achievement (K-TEA)	6-18 yr	Screening measure of achievement in the areas of reading, mathematics, spelling, decoding, and comprehension; used for educational planning by a psychologist or educational specialist.
Key Math Test	Kindergarten-grade 8	Normed diagnostic test of arithmetic achievement that can be administered by a teacher or psychologist; evaluates 14 areas of mathematics content, including operations and applications; weak in the area of computation.

Continued

Table D-1 Common Psychological and Educational Tests—cont'd

Test Name	Age Range	Purpose and Description
Kinetic Family Drawing	5 yr-adolescence	Diagnostic test of personality and social development that measures, in particular, family interactions; special features include identification of trends or characteristics commonly seen in various subgroups (e.g., learning disabled, developmentally disabled, or perceptual-motor–handicapped children); usually administered by a psychologist or trained clinician.
Leiter International Performance Scale	2 yr-adult	Normed diagnostic test of cognitive development usually administered by a psychologist and particularly appropriate for evaluating speech- and hearing-impaired individuals.
Luria-Nebraska Neuropsychological Battery: Children's Revision (LNNB-C)	8-12 yr	Considered the downward extension of the Adolescent-Adult Luria-Nebraska Battery; a verbal observational adaption designed to assess cognitive strengths and weaknesses and aid in selection and assessment of rehabilitation programs; administered by a psychologist or specialist trained in neuropsychological evaluation.
McCarthy Scales of Children's Abilities	2½-8½ yr	Relatively new diagnostic test of cognitive and perceptual ability that yields IQ-like indices of verbal, memory, perceptual, quantitative, and motor function; the General Cognitive Index (GCI), an overall estimate of cognitive function, is also derived; must be administered by a trained professional; particularly useful for diagnosing learning disabilities.
Merrill-Palmer Intelligence Test	18 mo-4 yr	Diagnostic test of cognitive and adaptive skills usually performed by a psychologist; because the test contains many "timed" items, it is highly demanding of the child being examined; yields a normal cognitive level score; extended version also available.
Minnesota Child Development Inventory	12 mo-6 yr	Parent questionnaire inventory that assesses general development and fine motor, gross motor, expressive language, comprehension-cognition, self-help, and personal-social skills.
Motivation Assessment Scale (MAS)	Any age	A 16-item, informant-rated scaled protocol used to generate hypotheses regarding the function or purpose of an individual's problem behavior(s) within a particular environmental setting; should be completed separately by different informants in different settings to assess for possible differences in maintaining variables across settings; contributes to a descriptive, structural, and functional behavior assessment.
Motor Free Test of Visual Perception (MFTVP)	4-9 yr	Diagnostic test of cognitive ability that measures the same five areas of visual perception evaluated by the Frostig Test, except that the child is not required to give motor responses requiring eye-hand coordination; useful in differentiating perceptual-motor problems from purely visual-perceptual difficulties; can be administered by a psychologist or teacher.
Neonatal Behavioral Assessment Scale	Birth-1 mo	Diagnostic test of developmental status in infancy that evaluates early social behaviors; results give a profile of infant behavior rather than an overall score; subscale ratings for different item types (e.g., neurological development) can be obtained; administered by an examiner who must be certified in its administration and interpretation
Peabody Developmental Motor Scales and Activity Cards	Birth-7 yr	Normed task performance test consisting of a sequence of gross and fine motor skills; identifies children whose gross or fine motor skills are delayed; activity cards include 170 gross motor and 112 fine motor items; activities referenced to items on the test can be used to set developmental-instructional objectives; administered by an educational specialist, physical therapist, or occupational therapist.
Peabody Individual Achievement Test–Revised (PIAT-R)	5-18 yr	Achievement test usually administered by an educational specialist or psychologist; provides wide-range screening in six areas—general information, reading recognition, reading comprehension, mathematics, spelling, and written expression; useful in diagnosing an individual's general level of achievement but does not provide in-depth assessment of specific areas of skill.

Table D-1 Common Psychological and Educational Tests—cont'd

Test Name	Age Range	Purpose and Description
Peabody Picture Vocabulary Test–Revised (PPVT-R)	2½ yr-adult	Screening test of receptive vocabulary administered by a speech and language specialist, teacher, or psychologist; correlates highly with IQ tests but cannot be used in place of a more intensive test of cognitive ability.
Perkins-Binet Tests of Intelligence for the Blind	3 yr-adult	Test of general intelligence with two forms—one for children who have usable vision and one for children who have no usable vision; yields IQ score based on the same method as that used in the Stanford-Binet intelligence tests.
Personality Inventory for Children–Revised (PIC-R)	3-16 yr	Screening test of personality and social development completed by parents; areas evaluated are achievement, intellectual screening, somatic concerns, depression, family dysfunction, withdrawal, anxiety, psychosis, hyperactivity, and social skills.
Physician Developmental Quick Screen for Speech Disorders (PDQ)	6 mo-6 yr	Office screening test performed by a physician, nurse, or other trained individual; measures various aspects of language, rhythm of speech, articulation, speaking mechanisms, and voice.
Piers-Harris Children's Self-Concept Scale	4-12 yr	Screening test for personality and social development that evaluates six facets of self-concept, including physical, social, family, and school precepts; the face validity of this test appears to be quite good; usually administered by a psychologist or teacher.
Preschool Behavior Questionnaire	3-6 yr	Observational screening scale for behavior problems in preschool children; measures hostile-aggressive, anxious, and distractible behaviors; administered by a teacher or psychologist.
Preschool Language Scale (PLS)	1-7 yr	Diagnostic test measuring expressive and receptive language skills that yield normed age-equivalent score for each skill; usually administered by a teacher, psychologist, or speech and language pathologist; revised in 1993.
Prescreening Developmental Questionnaire (PDQ)	3 mo–6 yr	Parent questionnaire used to determine whether DDST screening is necessary; addresses motor, language, social, and cognitive items; either office staff members or parents can complete items.
Raven Progressive Matrices	5½ yr–adult	Normal diagnostic test of cognitive ability that relies heavily on visual-spatial abstract reasoning; claimed to be culture free; usually administered by a psychologist; Coloured Progressive Metrics (CPM) used for younger children and special populations.
Receptive-Expressive Emergent Language Scale (REEL)	Birth-36 mo	Sometimes prefaced by authors' names (Bzoch and League); 132-item scale assesses emerging factors of receptive and expressive language as being present or absent; identifies those needing further evaluation; items are answered by a parent or reliable correspondent and evaluated by an educational specialist or speech pathologist.
Reiss Scales for Children's Dual Diagnosis	4-21 yr	Informant-rated, standardized assessment instrument with empirically derived scales. Its primary purpose is to aid in identifying a child or adolescent with mental retardation who also may have psychopathology, hence the term "dual diagnosis." Best results are obtained on the 60-item, 20-scale protocol when average scores from two or more informants are used.
Reitan-Indiana Neuropsychological Test Battery for Children	5-8 yr	Related to the Halstead-Reitan Neuropsychological Test Battery, which is used with older children and adults; a 4- to 6-hour battery of cognitive and perceptual tests that includes a version of the Wechsler Intelligence Scale for Children (WISC), a modified Reitan, an Aphasia Screening Test, and other sensory-perceptual measures; used to evaluate children suspected of brain damage and cognitive dysfunction; administered by a psychologist or specialist trained in neuropsychological assessment.
Rorschach Psychodiagnostic Test	3 yr-adult	Projective test of personality and social development specifically designed to evaluate personality structure; administered by a trained psychologist; extensive scoring criteria required to interpret results.

Continued

Table D-1 Common Psychological and Educational Tests—cont'd

Test Name	Age Range	Purpose and Description
School Readiness Survey	4-6 yr	Screening test of learning ability in children that can be administered by a teacher, psychologist, or parent; identifies areas in which a child may be ready for school or deficient with regard to entrance into kindergarten.
Sentence Completion Tests	All ages	Projective tests of personality and social development usually administered by a psychologist; responses differentiating between adjustment and maladjustment can be identified; a number of different versions of the technique are in use, some of which have been validated and others in which scoring usually is achieved by clinical interpretation.
Sequenced Inventory of Communication Development–Revised Edition	4 mo-4 yr	Normed 210-item inventory assessing language disorders in young children; behaviorally based receptive and expressive sections result in an overall Communication Profile; used in developing remedial programs for language-disordered, mentally retarded, hearing-impaired, and visually impaired children; can also be used with autistic and other difficult-to-test children; administered by a psychologist, educational specialist, or speech pathologist.
Silvaroli Reading Inventory	Preschool-grade 8	Screening test of achievement usually administered by an educational specialist; assesses word recognition, passage comprehension, and spelling; scores for children in kindergarten to grade 6 appear to be somewhat inflated; reliability appears to be better at higher grade levels.
Slosson Intelligence Test–Revised (SIT-R)	Birth-27 yr	Diagnostic test of cognitive ability usually administered by a teacher or psychologist; designed to be a quick assessment, it is widely used in schools and is less well normed than the more intensive individual intelligence tests.
Southern California Sensory Integration Test	4-8 yr	Test usually administered by a certified occupational therapist; 18 subtests evaluate sensory integration; findings are not widely accepted by many psychologists or educators, although a sizable literature suggests substantial construct validity.
Stanford-Binet Intelligence Test, fourth edition	2 yr-adult	Well-known diagnostic test of cognitive ability administered by a psychologist; yields 15 subtest scores organized into four areas, including verbal reasoning, quantitative reasoning, and short-term memory; full battery requires more than 2 hours to administer, making it perhaps the longest standardized test of general intelligence; an option to shorten the scales for briefer administration is available, but validity has not yet been established for shortened version; may not be as effective as the WISC-R for diagnosing educational difficulties and for language handicaps; because of uneven range of standard scores, profile analysis should be used with caution.
Stanford Measurement Series	School age	Not to be confused with the Stanford-Binet Intelligence Test; a series of tests that measures mathematics, reading, and overall achievement; may be used for diagnosing specific student needs; administered by an educational specialist.
Sucher-Allred Reading Placement Inventory	Kindergarten-grade 9	Diagnostic test of reading ability containing a word recognition test and an oral reading test; provides an informal measure of a child's reading ability, not an in-depth assessment of reading difficulties; usually administered by an educational specialist or a classroom teacher to screen students for placement in reading.
Temperament Assessment Battery for Children (TABC)	3-7 yr	Multiple-item measure assessing six temperamental variables: activity, adaptability, approach-withdrawal, intensity, distractibility, and persistence; each is rated on a 7-point scale; parent, teacher, and clinical forms available; administered by a psychologist or educational specialist.
Temperament Scales	Infancy	Uses nine scales (activity level, rhythmicity, response to new stimuli, adaptability, intensity, threshold of responsiveness, mood, distractibility, attention span) to assess infant temperament; evaluation usually performed by a trained clinician.

Table D-1 Common Psychological and Educational Tests—cont'd

Test Name	Age Range	Purpose and Description
Test of Language Development-Primary (TOLD)	4 yr 8 mo-11 yr	Diagnostic test of language development in children usually administered by a speech and language pathologist but also can be administered by a teacher, psychologist, or other professional; measures spoken language, listening, semantics, and syntax; age scores and language quotients result from norms. Intermediate version available.
Test of Non-Verbal Intelligence (TONI-2)	5-86 yr	Language-free measure of intelligence that may be used for hearing-, language-, and motor-impaired persons; has been suggested that the TONI should be used only as a supplemental test (as part of a battery) and that it should not be used with children under age 7.
Test of Written Language (TOWL-2)	7-17 yr	Diagnostic test usually administered by an educational specialist; helps to determine a student's general writing proficiency and to recognize a student's strengths and weaknesses.
Test of Written Spelling-2 (TWS-2)	6½-18½ yr	Uses a dictated work format to measure student's ability to spell words with readily predictable and with less predictable sound-letter patterns; can provide diagnostic information relative to specific spelling strategies; an excellent instrument for assessing written spelling ability; can be administered by a teacher, psychologist, or other professional.
Thematic Apperception Test (TAT)	School age-adult	Projective test of personality and social development measuring interpersonal relationships and usually administered by a trained psychologist; useful in identifying emotional disorders; extensive scoring criteria are applied to interpret results.
Vineland Adaptive Behavior Scale (VABS)	Birth-19 yr	Assesses social competence of handicapped and nonhandicapped individuals; usually administered by a trained interviewer; has three versions: survey form, expanded form, and classroom edition; each version measures adaptive behavior in four domains: communication, daily living skills, socialization, and motor skills; survey and expanded forms include a maladaptive behavior domain; respondent is a caregiver, parent, or teacher; also used with mentally retarded and low-function adults.
Wechsler Intelligence Scale for Children–3	6 yr–16 yr 11 mo	Intelligence test used most commonly for school-age child and adolescent; third edition published in 1991; gives separate verbal and performance quotients as well as Full Scale IQ scores. Subscale profiles can be used to evaluate learning ability and special learning disabilities; also used as part of Halstead-Reitan and Reitan-Indiana neuropsychological test batteries; usually administered by a psychologist or school psychologist.
Wechsler Memory Scale–Revised (WMS-R)	16-74 yr	Used primarily in neuropsychological testing to assess memory functioning; also used to evaluate aphasic, brain-impaired, and elderly individuals; has subtests for verbal and nonverbal memory functioning; three new subtests and more explicit scoring guidelines are improvements over Wechsler's original memory scale; administered by a psychologist or skilled examiner.
Wechsler Preschool and Primary Scales of Intelligence–Revised (WPPSI-R)	3-7 yr	Wechsler test designed to be used with preschool children and designed similarly to the WISC-III.
Wide Range Achievement Test-3	5-74 yr	A commonly used and recently revised brief screening test of achievement; evaluates reading, spelling, and arithmetic; usually administered by an educational specialist.
Wisconsin Behavior Rating Scale (WBRS)	Birth-3 yr	An adaptive behavior rating scale designed for persons who function developmentally at or below the 3-year-old level; assesses basic survival skills, using items that are developmentally arranged and sequenced under several subcategories of adaptive behavior: gross motor, fine motor, expressive communication, play skills, socialization, domestic activities, eating, toileting, dressing, and grooming; usually administered by a trained interviewer.

Continued

Table D-1 Common Psychological and Educational Tests—cont'd

Test Name	Age Range	Purpose and Description
Wisconsin Card Sorting Test Test (WCST)	16 yr-adult	Used primarily in neuropsychological testing to assess abstract thinking and perseveration; a nonverbal test that has an individual match card in two response decks to one of four stimulus cards based on color, form, or number; helps identify frontal lobe dysfunction; administered by a psychologist or skilled examiner.
Woodcock-Johnson Psychoeducational Battery–Revised (WJ-R)	All ages	Diagnostic test of achievement usually administered by an educational specialist; measures cognitive ability, achievement, and interest; more reliable at the elementary than the secondary educational level.
Woodcock Reading Mastery Test–Revised (WRMT-R)	5 yr or older	Tests specifically for reading skills; usually administered by an educational specialist; measures word and letter identification, word attack, and passage and word comprehension; norms available.

psychologists, who typically specialize in standard educational testing and are less intensively trained in dealing with complex psychoeducational and emotional problems. According to Reschly (1999) approximately 21,000 to 23,000 school psychologists exist. The national ratio of students to school psychologist is approximately 1800:1 (Lund et al, 1998). Unfortunately, the referral may not be acted upon promptly because of the large caseloads carried by school psychologists, who usually serve many schools within a district. The benefit of a school psychologist referral is that results, once available, may be acted on more expeditiously because the psychologist is a member of the Committee on Special Education (CSE), the school district–based, decision-making body required by law to address the needs of children who have educational challenges.

Other referral resources include an appropriately trained and licensed psychologist or an educational specialist. Such resources may be useful in obtaining an independent second opinion following a school district evaluation, especially if results are in question by involved parties or the parents. Parental preference for a particular evaluator should be considered in making the decision to obtain a second opinion.

Licensed psychologists are the best resources for determining both cognitive and emotional status by means of psychological evaluations. In most states, psychologists who are eligible for third-party reimbursement must be licensed. In general, licensed psychologists must hold a doctoral degree in psychology and have postdoctoral training. The postdoctoral subspecialization areas of most interest to pediatricians include clinical child psychology, pediatric psychology, counseling psychology, neuropsychology, and educational psychology. In some instances referral to specialists would be appropriate. For example, a child who has experienced a brain injury with suspected or actual neurological impairment should be evaluated by a clinical neuropsychologist.

A child's age may determine which specialist should be consulted. For instance, almost all child neuropsychological tests are not suitable for children under age 6 or 7. Despite the new requirement for evaluation and intervention for preschoolers, relatively few school psychologists have extensive training in preschool evaluation. Although this situation is being corrected by school psychology graduate curriculum reform, some time will pass before local districts develop sufficient expertise. Thus preschool children might be referred better to a clinical child psychologist or pediatric psychologist.

Some psychologists may perform psychoeducational assessments—evaluations of the child's learning styles and determination of the best teaching approaches. Alternative resources for these services include special educators and educational consultants. No licensure is required to practice in this specialty, nor are many of the services provided by educational consultants eligible for third-party reimbursement. Nevertheless, the pediatrician may decide that children who have certain complex problems require special education studies to clarify appropriate interventions and consider referral to such consultants as the most appropriate option.

Recent evaluation approaches to young children and adolescents who exhibit problem behavior increasingly involve behavior assessment. This is especially true for children who have learning and emotional difficulties, mental retardation, or autism, and for those who have suffered traumatic brain injury. In fact, under the new revisions to IDEA, functional behavior assessments and positive behavioral interventions are specifically targeted. A behavioral assessment should be requested when the child's behavior is disruptive to his or her own learning process or that of others. Behavior assessment involving a functional analysis of why the problem behavior is occurring is generally the purview of a behavior consultant or specialist who typically has at least a Master's degree in behavioral psychology. Usually, licensure is not required for these professionals.

CHARACTERISTICS OF A GOOD PSYCHOEDUCATIONAL OR PSYCHOLOGICAL REPORT

A written report that clearly and concisely summarizes the findings leading to concrete recommendations should be provided concerning the child being assessed. A good assessment should include identifying information, background and history, behavioral observations, results of psychometric and other scales, and a valid indication of the abilities and performance of the child within the context of the assessment process on that given day. Identification of assets, limitations, and undeveloped strengths of the child is also important. The assessment should include quantitative and qualitative aspects of the child's performance, and test scores should be supplemented with concrete recommendations for interventions. Ideally, a good assessment answers a referral question or set of questions from the referral source and is complete only after it has been discussed with the referral source. If any of these elements are missing from the report, the pediatrician should request their inclusion from the professional.

Usually, the psychologist shares the report with the child's parents. In cases in which this practice has not been followed, the pediatrician should ask the psychologist the reasons for withholding the data. It may be that the child refused to allow release of some part of the report to his or her parents, or the psychologist may believe that the release of some parts of the report is not in the child's or the family's best interest. Knowing this, the pediatrician is in a better position to preserve requested confidentiality and thus can be discrete in developing an effective management strategy that is acceptable to the child and the family.

SUGGESTED READINGS

Education for All Handicapped Children Act, Pub L No 94-142, 20 USC §1400 (1975).

Education for the Handicapped Act Advancement, Pub L No 99-457, 20 USC §1400 (1986).

Fewell RR: Trends in the assessment of infants and toddlers with disabilities, *Except Child* 58:166, 1991.

Gilbride KE: Developmental testing, *Pediatr Rev* 16:338, 1995.

Goldstein G, Hersen M: *Handbook of psychological assessment,* ed 2, New York, 1990, Pergamon Press.

Hebbeler KM, Smith BJ, Black TL: Federal early childhood special education policy: a model for the improvement of services for children with disabilities, *Except Child* 58:104, 1991.

Hoon AH Jr, et al: Clinical Adaptive Test/Clinical Linguistic Auditory Milestone Scale in early cognitive assessment, *J Pediatr* 123:S1, 1993.

Individuals With Disabilities Education Act, Pub L No 102-119, 20 USC §1400 (1990).

Keyser DJ, Sweetland RC: *Test critiques,* vol 1-9, Kansas City, Kan, 1984, Test Corp of America.

Kramer JJ, Conoley JC: *The eleventh mental measure yearbook,* Lincoln, Neb, 1992, University of Nebraska Press.

Lund AR, Reschly DJ, Martin LM: School psychology personnel needs: correlates of current patterns and historical trends, *Sch Psychol Rev* 27: 106, 1998.

Mitchell JV Jr: *Tests in print III,* Lincoln, Neb, 1983, University of Nebraska Press.

Reschly DJ: Assessing educational disabilities. In Hess AK, Weiner IB, editors: *Handbook of forensic psychology,* ed 2, New York, 1999, John Wiley & Sons.

Sweetland RC, Keyser DJ: *Tests: a comprehensive reference for assessments in psychology, education, and business,* ed 3, Austin, Texas, 1991, Pro-Ed.

Woodrich DL: *Children's psychological testing: a guide for nonpsychologists,* ed 3, Baltimore, 1997, Paul H Brooks.

Index

*Page numbers followed by *t*, *f*, or *b* indicate text in tables, figures, or boxes, respectively. Numbers followed by *n* indicate text in footnotes.

D

E

F

J

O

W